15 Nursing Care Highlight charts emphasize important aspects of "hands on" nursing care.

16 Education Guide charts provide instructions for nurses to provide to clients and their families.

17 The Continuing Care subsection includes information on case management, health teaching, home care, and other aspects of care across the health care continuum.

18 Case Study boxes present brief clinical scenarios and pose pertinent questions designed to stimulate critical thinking abilities.

19 Selected Bibliography and Suggested Readings guide students to other sources of pertinent information.

10 The Analysis subsection identifies pertinent nursing diagnoses and collaborative problems that may apply to a client problem.

11 In Planning and Implementation, expected outcomes and interventions are discussed for common nursing diagnoses and collaborative problems.

12 Nursing Focus on the Elderly charts highlight normal age-related changes that affect care and specify individualized care that elderly clients need.

13 Expected outcomes are identified in the Evaluation: Outcomes subsection.

14 Research Applications for Nursing boxes provide synopses of recent nursing research articles and other scientific articles applicable to nursing.

The following are reproductions of sample textbook pages shown on this guide page.

816 UNIT 7 ▪ Problems of Cardiac Output and Tissue Perfusion: Management of Clients with Problems of the Cardiovascular System

are elevated in left-sided heart failure because volumes and pressures are increased in the left ventricle. (See Chapter 35 for a more detailed description of the pulmonary artery catheter.)

▶ Analysis

▶ Common Nursing Diagnoses and Collaborative Problems

The most common nursing diagnoses pertinent to the client with heart failure are

1. Impaired Gas Exchange related to altered oxygen supply
2. Decreased Cardiac Output related to a reduction in stroke volume as a result of mechanical malfunctions
3. Activity Intolerance related to an imbalance between oxygen supply and demand, fatigue, or an electrolyte imbalance

The primary collaborative problem is Potential for Pulmonary Edema.

▶ Additional Nursing Diagnoses and Collaborative Problems

Some clients have one or more of the following:
- Ineffective Management of Therapeutic Regime related to failed social support systems, inadequate follow-up, inadequate discharge planning, or knowledge deficit
- Ineffective Individual Coping related to physical inactivity, major changes in lifestyle, loss of control over body function, or fear of death
- Altered Thought Processes related to impaired gas exchange or fear of the unknown
- Impaired Physical Mobility related to fatigue and activity intolerance

Some clients are also at risk for the following collaborative problems:
- Potential for Pneumonia
- Potential for Dysrhythmias

▶ Planning and Implementation

▶ Impaired Gas Exchange

Planning: Expected Outcomes. The client is expected to have a normal rate, rhythm, and depth of respiration and to have an O_2 saturation greater then 92%.

Interventions. The nurse or assistive nursing personnel monitors the client's respiratory rate, rhythm, and character every 1 to 4 hours and auscultates breath sounds. If clients are experiencing pulmonary congestion, the oxygen content of their blood is often markedly reduced. The nurse may titrate the amount of supplemental oxygen delivered to the client within a range prescribed by the health care provider to maintain the client's oxygen saturation at 92% or greater.

If the client experiences respiratory difficulty, the nurse or assistive nursing personnel places the client in a high

Fowler's position with pillows under each arm to maximize chest expansion and improve oxygenation. Repositioning the client and having the client perform coughing and deep breathing exercises every 2 hours helps to improve oxygenation and to prevent atelectasis.

▶ Decreased Cardiac Output

Planning: Expected Outcomes. The primary outcome is that the client is expected to resume and maintain an adequate cardiac output.

Interventions. Interventions are aimed at improving cardiac output. A critical pathway for congestive heart failure that reflects an interdisciplinary approach to client care is included in this chapter. Therapy may be directed toward optimizing the two major components of cardiac output: stroke volume (determined by preload, afterload, and contractility) and heart rate.

Interventions to optimize stroke volume include reducing afterload, reducing preload, and improving cardiac muscle contractility.

Reducing Afterload. By relaxing arterioles, arterial vasodilators can reduce impedance to left ventricular ejection (afterload) and improve cardiac output. In the strictest sense, these drugs do not act as vasodilators but reverse some of the inappropriate or excessive vasoconstriction that is common in heart failure.

Clients with even mild heart failure due to left ventricular dysfunction should be given a trial of angiotensin-converting enzyme (ACE) inhibitors. ACE inhibitors, a group of arterial vasodilators such as enalapril (Vasotec), moexipril (Univasc), and captopril (Capoten), generally prolong and improve the quality of life of clients in heart failure (see Chart 37–3). Studies have shown that these

Chart 37–4

Nursing Focus on the Elderly: Heart Failure

- Assess older clients with confusion for indications of heart failure. People older than 80 years often present with restlessness or confusion as the initial manifestation of heart failure.
- Auscultate the lungs carefully, recognizing that dependent crackles may not be an indication of heart failure in the older adult.
- Do not expect crackles to clear rapidly after treatment. Crackles may persist in the lung bases of older adults for an extended period after pulmonary congestion has decreased.
- Be especially alert for the signs of digitalis toxicity in the elderly client because it occurs frequently.
- If loop diuretics are used for diuresis, monitor the client closely for signs of excessive diuresis, dehydration, and hypokalemia.
- In older clients receiving drug therapy for heart failure, monitor for orthostatic hypotension. Cardiovascular changes associated with aging make this likely to develop.

---

820 UNIT 7 ▪ Problems of Cardiac Output and Tissue Perfusion: Management of Clients with Problems of the Cardiovascular System

1. After the recipient is placed on cardiopulmonary bypass, the heart is removed.
2. The posterior walls of the recipient's left and right atria are left intact.
3. The left atrium of the donor heart is anastomosed to the recipient's residual posterior atrial walls, and the other atrial walls, the atrial septum, and the great vessels are joined.

POSTOPERATIVE RESULT

Figure 37–6. Heart transplantation.

For equipment needs, such as home oxygen therapy or a hospital bed, medical supply companies provide set-up and maintenance services. A detailed description of home oxygen therapy is found in Chapter 30.

▶ Evaluation: Outcomes

On the basis of the identified nursing diagnoses and collaborative problems, the nurse evaluates the care of the client with heart failure. Outcomes include that the client will

- Have a normal rate, rhythm, and depth of respiration

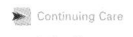

▶ **Research Applications for Nursing**

Mortensson, J., Karlsson, J. E., & Fridlund, B. (1997). Male patients with congestive heart failure and their conception of the life situation. Journal of Advanced Nursing, 25, 579–586.

This qualitative study examined the experiences of 12 male Swedish clients with heart failure. Clients ranged from 2 months to 2 years following diagnosis. Clients ranged from NYHA Classification II (5) to IV (2), and most were married.

Six categories emerged that described how clients with heart failure perceived of their situation. Six men described feeling a belief in the future. These more hopeful men were more engaged in daily activities, possibly ignoring certain aspects of their illness. Eight men mentioned gaining aware-

---

CHAPTER 37 ▪ Interventions for the Client with Cardiac Problems **821**

ing heart also increases its oxygen requirement. The nurse should be alert for the possibility that the client may experience angina (chest pain) in response to digoxin. Intravenous medications that increase contractility are described in Chapter 40.

▶ Activity Intolerance

Planning: Expected Outcomes. The client is expected to perform activities of daily living and walk at least two blocks without dyspnea or excessive fatigue.

Interventions. Initially, the client in severe heart failure requires physical and emotional rest. On the first day of hospitalization, clients may sit up in a chair for meals and do basic leg exercises while up. Nursing care should

▶ Potential for Pulmonary Edema

Planning: Expected Outcomes. The client is expected to be free of pulmonary edema.

Interventions. The nurse monitors clients for acute pulmonary edema, a life-threatening event that can result from severe heart failure. In pulmonary edema, the left ventricle fails to eject sufficient blood, and pressure increases in the lungs because of the accumulated blood. The increased pressure causes fluid to leak across the pulmonary capillaries and into the pulmonary interstitium.

Clients often respond dramatically and quickly to these interventions, but their condition can also deteriorate rapidly because of pulmonary congestion and severe hypoxemia. Clients occasionally require Bipap or intubation and ventilation to survive the acute episode. A skilled nurse is needed to assist with intubation. (Management of the client who is critically ill with heart failure is detailed in Chapter 40.)

Chart 37–6

Education Guide: Digoxin Therapy

- Noon is the best time of day to take this medication if you can remember to take it then.
- Continue administration of this medication unless you are told to stop it by your health care provider.
- Do not take digoxin at the same time as antacids or cathartics (laxatives).
- Take your pulse rate before taking each dose of digoxin. Notify your health care provider of a change in pulse rate (60–100 beats per minute is normal) or rhythm as well as increasing fatigue, muscle weakness, confusion, or loss of appetite (signs of digitalis toxicity).
- If you forget to take a dose, it may be delayed a few hours. However, if you do not remember it until the next day, you should take only your usual daily dose.
- Report for scheduled laboratory test (such as potassium and digoxin levels).
- If potassium supplements are prescribed, continue the dose until told to stop by your health care provider.

▶ **Continuing Care**

▶ Case Management

Clients who have not been adequately prepared for discharge or who do not have good community support and follow-up are at high risk for recurrent hospital admissions for heart failure (Dracup et al., 1995). In a case management system, the case manager or care coordinator assesses the client's needs for health care resources and facilitates appropriate placement. It is imperative that the case manager assess the available social supports because inability to obtain help in such activities as food shopping and obtaining medications is a major contributor to hospital readmission (Dracup et al., 1995). If home support is available, the client may be discharged home in the care of a family member or other caregiver. Home care nurses may direct the care, while aides may provide assistance with ADLs.

If the client has multiple health problems or has been severely compromised by heart disease, he or she may require admission to a subacute unit or traditional nursing home for either transitional or long-term care. Home care services cost about $125 per nursing visit compared with $150 to $300 per day in a traditional nursing home and up to $1,000 per day for hospital care.

▶ Health Teaching

Activity Schedule. Medicare usually provides reimbursement for client assessment and teaching, so that a home care nurse can continue teaching and assessment when the client returns home. The nurse encourages clients with heart failure to stay as active as possible and to develop a regular exercise regimen. Clients who are more active appear to have better outcomes (Dracup

Chart 37–5

Nursing Care Highlight: Care of the Client with Pulmonary Edema

- Identify the client's chief complaint.
- If the client's blood pressure is adequate, place the client in a high-Fowler's position.
- Auscultate the client's lungs briefly (posterior assessment).
- Ensure that vascular access is present and check for patency.
- Provide oxygen as ordered.
- Provide IV diuretic (usually furosemide) as prescribed.
- Anticipate urinary output in 5–15 min after diuretic administration; catheterize if ordered.
- Monitor blood pressure, respiratory rate, pulse oximetry, pulse, and cardiac rhythm, and the client's subjective feelings of ability to breathe.
- Provide additional medications as prescribed (usually morphine sulfate or nitroglycerin).
- Provide comfort measures and reassurance.
- Notify the physician if the client does not have a rapid

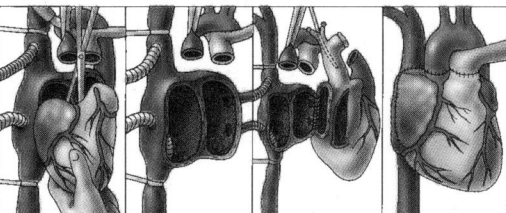

CHAPTER 37 ▪ Interventions for the Client with Cardiac Problems **835**

aged to participate in a regular exercise program but cautioned to allow at least 10 minutes of warm up and cool down for the denervated heart to adjust to changes in activity level.

CASE STUDY for the Client with Heart Failure

▪ An 85-year-old woman is one of your nursing home residents. She has a long history of heart failure, myocardial infarction, pulmonary emphysema, hypertension, and degenerative joint disease. Her medications include Lasix 20 mg qd, Vasotec 5 mg qd, digoxin 0.125 mg qd, KCI 40 mEq qd, and Motrin 200 mg qd.

Today the resident complains that she "just doesn't feel right." The nursing assistant reports that her pulse is weak and irregular at 116 bpm, and her skin feels cooler than usual. You go to her room for further assessment.

QUESTIONS:

1. When taking a history from this client, what important questions would you ask?
2. What physical assessments techniques would you perform?
3. During the assessment, you find that she is dyspneic at rest, has a respiratory rate of 32, a blood pressure of 180/95, is very anxious, and has crackles in the bases of her lungs. What should you do first?

SELECTED BIBLIOGRAPHY

Abelmann, W. H. (Ed.). (1995). Atlas of heart diseases: Volume II. Cardiomyopathies, myocarditis, and pericardial disease. Philadelphia: Current Medicine.
American Heart Association. (1996). Heart and stroke facts. Dallas: American Heart Association.
Baker, D. W., Konstam, M. A., Bottorff, M., & Bertram, B. (1994). Management of heart failure: 1. Pharmacologic treatment. JAMA, 272(17), 1361–1365.
Boehrer, M. F., & Ignatavicius, D. D. (1996). Infusion therapy: Techniques and medications. Philadelphia: W. B. Saunders.
Bove, L. A., et al. (1996). Nursing care of patients undergoing dynamic cardiomyoplasty. Critical Care Nurse, 15(3), 96–104.
*Braunwald, E. (1997). Heart disease: A textbook of cardiovascular medicine (5th ed.). Philadelphia: W. B. Saunders.
Byars, J. F., & Goshorn, J. (1995). How to manage diuretic therapy. AJN, 95(2), 38–43.
Cash, A. (1996). Heart failure from diastolic dysfunction. Dimensions of Critical Care Nursing, 15(4), 171–177.
Dec, G. W., & Fuster, V. (1994). Idiopathic dilated cardiomyopathy New England Journal of Medicine, 331(23), 1564–1573.
Dracup, K., et al. (1994). Management of heart failure: II. Counseling

care nursing: Body-mind-spirit (3rd ed. p. 523). Philadelphia: J. B. Lippincott.
Hawthorne, M. H., & Hixon, M. E. (1994). Functional status, quality of life and mood disturbance in patients with heart failure. Progress in Cardiovascular Nursing, 9(1), 22–32.
Jaarsma, T., Dracup, K., Walden, J., et al. (1996). Sexual function in patients with advanced heart failure. Heart and Lung, 25(4), 262–270.
Jensen, G. A., & Miller, D. S. (1995). The heart of aging: Special challenges of cardiac ischemic disease and failure in the elderly. AACN Clinical Issues, 6(3), 471–481.
Kayser, S. R. (1994). Management of chronic congestive heart failure: Part II—Selection of treatment. Progress in cardiovascular nursing, 9(2), 30–37.
Martens, K. H., & Mellor, S. D. (1997). A study of the relationship between home care services and hospital readmission of patients with congestive heart failure. Home Healthcare Nurse, 15(2), 123–129.
Matthews, D. (1994). The prevention and diagnosis of infective endocarditis. Nurse Practitioner, 19(8), 53–59.
McGrath, D. (1997). Clinical snapshot: Mitral valve prolapse. AJN, 97(5), 40–41.
Miner, P. D. (1994). Infective endocarditis. Nursing Clinics of North America, 29(2), 269–283.
Moser, D. K. (1996). Maximizing therapy in the advanced heart failure patient. Journal of Cardiovascular Nursing, 10(2), 29–46.
Newkirk, T., & Leeper, B. (1994). Congestive heart failure: Mapping the way to quality outcomes. AJN: Critical Care Issues Supplement, 96(5), 25–28.
Pratt, N. G. (1995). Pathophysiology of heart failure: Neuroendocrine response. Critical Care Nursing Quarterly, 18(1), 22–31.
Recker, D. (1994). Patient perception of preoperative cardiac surgical teaching—Done pre- and postadmission. Critical Care Nurse, 14(1), 52–58.
Redfield, M. (1996). Evaluation of congestive heart failure. In E. Giuliani (Ed.). Mayo Clinic practice of cardiology (3rd ed., p. 569). St. Louis: C. V. Mosby.
Schwabauer, N. J. (1996). Retarding progression of heart failure: Nursing actions. Dimensions of Critical Care Nursing, 15(6), 307–317.
Shine, L., & Howland-Gradman, J. (1996). Aortic stenosis in elderly Valvuloplasty versus surgery. AJN: Critical Care Issues Supplement. May, pp. 7–11.
Sullivan, M. J. (1994). New trends in cardiac rehabilitation in patients with chronic heart failure. Progress in Cardiovascular Nursing, 9(1), 13–21.
Swearingen, P. L., & Keen, J. H. (Eds.). (1995). Manual of critical care (3rd ed.). St. Louis: Mosby–Year Book.
UNOS. (1998). Donation and transplantation. Nursing source.richmond. UNOS
U.S. Department of Health and Human Services. Agency for Health Care Policy and Research. (1994). Heart failure. Evaluation and care of patients with left-ventricular systolic dysfunction. Rockville, MD: U.S. Department of Health and Human Services.

SUGGESTED READINGS

Cash, A. (1996). Heart failure from diastolic dysfunction. Dimensions of Critical Care Nursing, 15(4), 171–177.
This article presents a detailed explanation of the pathophysiology of diastolic heart failure. It describes tests to differentiate diastolic from systolic heart failure and describes possible management strategies for diastolic heart failure.
Konick-McMahon, J. (1997). Discharged with dobutamine. RN, 60(4),

To Stephanie and Charles, who continue through the years to tolerate my unending hours of travel, computers, and phone calls—I love you both so very much for your support; and to Lee Henderson, whose mentoring helped me grow and develop as a writer—thank you for your patience and guidance.

DDI

To my father, Homer D. Workman, the gentle giant who was my first, best, and most inspiring teacher; and to the other men in my life, my husband John and sons David and Gregory, for their love, patience, and humor.

MLW

To Laura Vogel, my daughter, a sophomore at Boston University School of Communication, and to Aaron Vogel, my son, a sophomore at Ithaca College School of Music; you have made my life more interesting and fulfilling than you can possibly imagine—love you always!

MAM

About the Authors

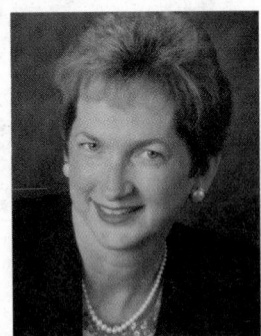

Donna D. Ignatavicius received her diploma in nursing from the Peninsula General Hospital School of Nursing in Salisbury, Maryland, in 1969. After working as a staff and charge nurse in medical-surgical nursing, she became Instructor in Staff Development at the University of Maryland Medical Center. In 1976 she received her BSN from the University of Maryland School of Nursing. For 5 years she taught in several schools of nursing while working toward her MS in nursing, which she received in 1981. Ms. Ignatavicius then taught in the baccalaureate program at the University of Maryland School of Nursing for 6 years, after which she pursued her interest in gerontology by becoming Director of Nursing at a skilled nursing facility. She has been a certified gerontological nurse since 1989 and was certified in nursing case management in 1998. Through her consulting and seminar business, Ms. Ignatavicius has gained national recognition in case management, including an appointment as the national Education Chair for the Case Management Society of America. She is currently employed as a clinical nurse specialist in medical-surgical/gerontological nursing at the Calvert Memorial Hospital in Prince Frederick, Maryland.

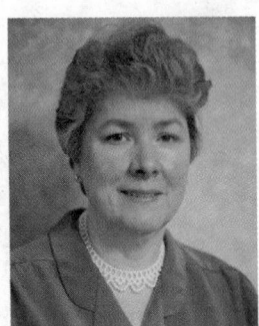

M. Linda Workman received her BSN from the University of Cincinnati College of Nursing and Health. After serving in the U.S. Army Nurse Corps and working as an Assistant Head Nurse and Head Nurse in civilian hospitals, Dr. Workman, a native of Canada, earned her MSN from the University of Cincinnati College of Nursing and Health and a PhD in developmental biology from the University of Cincinnati College of Arts and Sciences. Dr. Workman's 18 years of academic experience include teaching at the diploma, associate degree, baccalaureate, and master's levels. Her areas of teaching expertise include physiology, pathophysiology, genetics, oncology, and immunology. She is a former American Cancer Society Professor of Oncology Nursing and currently is an Associate Professor of Nursing at the Frances Payne Bolton School of Nursing at Case Western Reserve University, Cleveland.

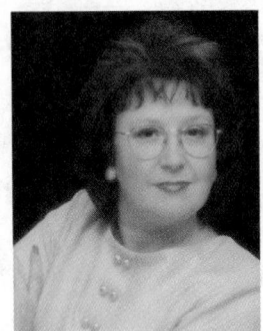

Mary A. Mishler has practiced medical-surgical nursing throughout her entire nursing career. She has worked as a staff nurse, staff development coordinator, clinical nurse specialist, nursing supervisor, and assistant director of nursing as well as a consultant. She has also served as senior-level course coordinator at a school of nursing. A 1971 graduate of Temple University Hospital School of Nursing in Philadelphia, Ms. Mishler received her BSN in 1973 and her MSN in 1977 from the University of Pennsylvania. A member of Sigma Theta Tau, Ms. Mishler is a faculty member at the Helene Fuld School of Nursing in Camden County and at Gloucester County College, both in New Jersey. She is certified both as a Clinical Specialist in Medical-Surgical Nursing and as a Nephrology Nurse. In 1993 she received a Certificate for Excellence in Nursing from the New Jersey State Department of Health. She has served as a member of the Standard Setting Panel for the NCLEX-RN examination and on the Editorial/Advisory Board of *Nursing Spectrum*. She also teaches continuing education seminars throughout the United States.

About the Authors

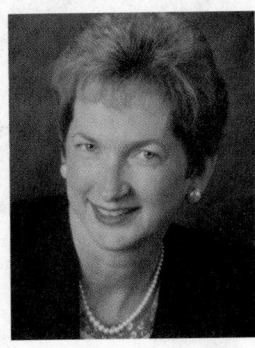

Donna D. Ignatavicius received her diploma in nursing from the Peninsula General Hospital School of Nursing in Salisbury, Maryland, in 1969. After working as a staff and charge nurse in medical-surgical nursing, she became Instructor in Staff Development at the University of Maryland Medical Center. In 1976 she received her BSN from the University of Maryland School of Nursing. For 5 years she taught in several schools of nursing while working toward her MS in nursing, which she received in 1981. Ms. Ignatavicius then taught in the baccalaureate program at the University of Maryland School of Nursing for 6 years, after which she pursued her interest in gerontology by becoming Director of Nursing at a skilled nursing facility. She has been a certified gerontological nurse since 1989 and was certified in nursing case management in 1998. Through her consulting and seminar business, Ms. Ignatavicius has gained national recognition in case management, including an appointment as the national Education Chair for the Case Management Society of America. She is currently employed as a clinical nurse specialist in medical-surgical/gerontological nursing at the Calvert Memorial Hospital in Prince Frederick, Maryland.

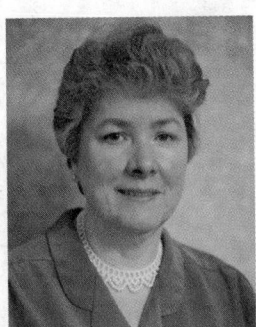

M. Linda Workman received her BSN from the University of Cincinnati College of Nursing and Health. After serving in the U.S. Army Nurse Corps and working as an Assistant Head Nurse and Head Nurse in civilian hospitals, Dr. Workman, a native of Canada, earned her MSN from the University of Cincinnati College of Nursing and Health and a PhD in developmental biology from the University of Cincinnati College of Arts and Sciences. Dr. Workman's 18 years of academic experience include teaching at the diploma, associate degree, baccalaureate, and master's levels. Her areas of teaching expertise include physiology, pathophysiology, genetics, oncology, and immunology. She is a former American Cancer Society Professor of Oncology Nursing and currently is an Associate Professor of Nursing at the Frances Payne Bolton School of Nursing at Case Western Reserve University, Cleveland.

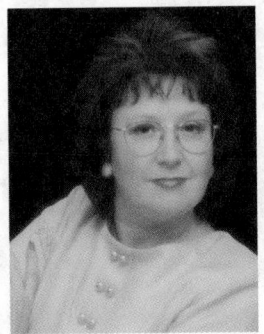

Mary A. Mishler has practiced medical-surgical nursing throughout her entire nursing career. She has worked as a staff nurse, staff development coordinator, clinical nurse specialist, nursing supervisor, and assistant director of nursing as well as a consultant. She has also served as senior-level course coordinator at a school of nursing. A 1971 graduate of Temple University Hospital School of Nursing in Philadelphia, Ms. Mishler received her BSN in 1973 and her MSN in 1977 from the University of Pennsylvania. A member of Sigma Theta Tau, Ms. Mishler is a faculty member at the Helene Fuld School of Nursing in Camden County and at Gloucester County College, both in New Jersey. She is certified both as a Clinical Specialist in Medical-Surgical Nursing and as a Nephrology Nurse. In 1993 she received a Certificate for Excellence in Nursing from the New Jersey State Department of Health. She has served as a member of the Standard Setting Panel for the NCLEX-RN examination and on the Editorial/Advisory Board of *Nursing Spectrum*. She also teaches continuing education seminars throughout the United States.

To Stephanie and Charles, who continue through the years to tolerate my unending hours of travel, computers, and phone calls—I love you both so very much for your support; and to Lee Henderson, whose mentoring helped me grow and develop as a writer—thank you for your patience and guidance.

DDI

To my father, Homer D. Workman, the gentle giant who was my first, best, and most inspiring teacher; and to the other men in my life, my husband John and sons David and Gregory, for their love, patience, and humor.

MLW

To Laura Vogel, my daughter, a sophomore at Boston University School of Communication, and to Aaron Vogel, my son, a sophomore at Ithaca College School of Music; you have made my life more interesting and fulfilling than you can possibly imagine—love you always!

MAM

Contributors

Barbara Diebold Ahlheit, MSN, RN, CS; Adjunct Faculty, Vanderbilt School of Nursing, Nashville, Tennessee; Family Nurse Practitioner, Veterans Administration Medical Center, Nashville, Tennessee

Suzanne Cushman Beyea, PhD; Co-Director, Perioperative Nursing Research, Association of Operating Room Nurses, Denver, Colorado

Marilyn Booker, RN, MS, CRNI; Infusion Consultant, Sunnybrook Services; Case Manager, Diversified Health Services, Inc., Baltimore, Maryland

Marcia Sue DeWolf Bosek, DNSc, RN; Associate Professor, Department of Adult Health Nursing, College of Nursing, Rush University, Chicago, Illinois

Janice Cuzzell, MA, RN; Vice-President of Service Development/Business Models, Clinical Service Consultant, Island Health Care, Inc., Savannah, Georgia

Lucille Sanzer Eller, PhD, RN; Assistant Professor, College of Nursing, Rutgers University, Newark, New Jersey

Kathleen Ellstrom, MS, RN, CS; Pulmonary Clinical Nurse Specialist, Pulmonary and Critical Care Division, UCLA Medical Center, Los Angeles, California

Cynthia Gerrett, MSN, RNC; Women's Health Clinical Nurse Specialist, University of North Carolina Hospital, Chapel Nill, North Carolina

Kathy Hausman, PhD, RNC; Instructor, University of Maryland, Baltimore County, Baltimore, Maryland; Director of Education Services, Harbor and Franklin Square Hospitals, Baltimore, Maryland

Donna D. Ignatavicius, MS, RNC, CM; Clinical Nurse Specialist, Calvert Memorial Hospital, Prince Frederick, Maryland; Former Professor, Charles County Community College, La Plata, Maryland

Ann Putnam Johnson, EdD, MSN, BSN; Associate Dean, College of Applied Sciences, Associate Professor, Department of Nursing, Western Carolina University, Cullowhee, North Carolina

Kathleen J. Jones, MS, RN, ANP; Adult Nurse Practitioner, Hematology/Oncology Clinic, Walter Reed Army Medical Center, Washington, D.C.

Mary K. Kazanowski, PhD, RN, CS, OCS, CRNH; Associater Professor, Department of Nursing, Saint Anselm College, Manchester, New Hampshire; Hospice Nurse, Optima VNA Hospice, Manchester, New Hampshire

Anne Keane, MSN, EdD, FAAN; Associate Director, Program Direction, Acute/Tertiary Nurse Practitioner Program, University of Pennsylvania School of Nursing, Philadelphia, Pennsylvania

Deitra Leonard Lowdermilk, PhD, RNC, FAAN; Clinical Professor, Department of Community, Family, Mental, and Women's Health, School of Nursing, University of North Carolina, Chapel Hill, North Carolina

Judy Malkiewicz, PhD, RN; Professor, School of Nursing, University of Northern Colorado, Greeley, Colorado

Tina M. Marrelli; MA, MSN, RNC; Editor, Home Care Nurse News; President, Marelli and Associates, Inc., Boca Grande, Florida

Jan Hoot Martin, PhD, RN, GNP; Associate Professor, School of Nursing, University of Northern Colorado, Greeley, Colorado

Margaret Elaine McLeod, MSN, RNCS, CDE; Clinical Nurse Specialist/Diabetes Educator, VA Medical Center, Nashville, Tennessee

Mary A. Mishler, MSN, RNCS, CNN; Adjunct Faculty, Helene Fuld School of Nursing, Camden County, Blackwood, New Jersey; Adjunct Faculty, Gloucester County College, Sewell, New Jersey; Faculty, American Health Care Institute, Silver Spring, Maryland

Phyllis Naumann, MA, MSN, CRNP; Coordinator, Undergraduate Program; Assistant Professor, The Johns Hopkins University School of Nursing, Baltimore, Maryland

Kathleen Ouimet Perrin, MS; Associate Professor, Nursing, Saint Anselm College, Manchester, New Hampshire

Carmen J. Petrin, RN; Cardiac Services Educator, Catholic Medical Center, Manchester, New Hampshire

Charon A. Pierson, RN, PhD, GNP, CS; Instructor, Advanced Practice Nursing, University of Hawaii School of Nursing, Honolulu, Hawaii; Geriatric Nurse Practitioner/Clinical Nurse Specialist, Kaiser Permanente Long-Term Care Team, Honolulu, Hawaii

Rosemary Polomano, MSN, PhD, FAAN; Pain Clinical Nurse Specialist, Department of Surgical Nursing, University of Pennsylvania Medical Center, Philadelphia, Pennsylvania

Lynn Rew, EdD, RNC, FAAN; Associate Professor, and Graduate Advisor, School of Nursing, The University of Texas, Austin, Texas

Denise A. Sadowski, RN, MSN; Independent Burn and Wound Care Nurse Consultant and Educator, Cincinnati, Ohio

Theresa A. Savage, PhD, RN; Adjunct Assistant Professor, Maternal–Child Nursing; Postdoctoral Research Fellow in Primary Health Care/Social Ethics, College of Nursing, University of Illinois, Chicago, Illinois

Susan M. Schneider, PhD, CS, OCN; Assistant Professor, Frances Payne Bolton School of Nursing, Case Western Reserve University, Cleveland, Ohio; Pediatric Oncology Nurse, Ireland Cancer Center, University Hospitals of Cleveland, Cleveland, Ohio

Susan N. Shelton, RD, LD, MA; Consultant Dietitian, Arnold, Maryland

Deborah Shpritz, PhD, RN, CCRN; Assistant Professor, Department of Adult Health, School of Nursing, University of Maryland, Baltimore, Maryland

Ann E. Furiel Sievers, MA, RN, CORLN; Clinical Associate, Department of Physiological Nursing, School of Nursing, University of California, San Francisco, San Francisco, California; Otolaryngology Clinical Nurse Specialist, University of California, Davis Health System, Sacramento, California

Karen M. Stanley, MS, RN, CS; Psychiatric Consultation Liaison Nurse, Medical University of South Carolina, Charleston, South Carolina

Georgeanne V. Stilley, RN, MSN, OCN; Clinical Nurse Specialist, Pain Management/Oncology, Our Lady of Lourdes Medical Center, Camden, New Jersey

Judith Sturgis, RN, BSN, CIC; Director of Infection Control, Calvert Memorial Hospital, Prince Frederick, Maryland

Debera Jane Thomas, DNS, ANP; Associate Professor, Florida Atlantic University College of Nursing, Boca Raton, Florida

Connie Visovsky, RN, MS, ACNP; University Hospitals of Cleveland, Cleveland, Ohio

M. Linda Workman, PhD, RN, FAAN; Associate Professor of Nursing, Frances Payne Bolton School of Nursing, Case Western Reserve University, Cleveland, Ohio

Reviewer List

Marianne Adam, RN, MSN; St. Luke's Hospital, Bethlehem, Pennsylvania

Jeanette Adams, ADCN, APN, DrPH; University of Texas–Houston, Houston, Texas

Janice Allen, RN, MS, CNOR; University of Arizona College of Nursing, Tucson, Arizona

Lisa K. Anderson-Shaw, RNC, MSN, MA; University of Illinois at Chicago, Chicago, Illinois

Linda Craig Baker, RNC, MSN, FNP; Scottsdale Community College, Phoenix Children's Hospital, Phoenix, Arizona

Sharon Beasley, RN, MSN; Rend Lake College, Ina, Illinois

Barbara J. Benz, RN, MS; Roswell Park Cancer Institute, Buffalo, New York

Madalyn A. Biggs, RN, BSN; Johns Hopkins Hospital, Baltimore, Maryland

Phyllis Ann Bonham, RN, MSN, CCRN; University of North Carolina; North Carolina Jaycee Burn Center, Chapel Hill, North Carolina

Kennith Culp, PhD, RN, CS; University of Iowa, College of Nursing, Iowa City, Iowa

Maria Piccolo-Cvach, RN, MS, CCRN, ACLS; Johns Hopkins Hospital, Baltimore, Maryland

Sharon L. Daut, RN, MS; Erie Community College–North, Williamsville, New York

Karen Keady Davis, RN, MS, CCRN; Johns Hopkins Hospital, Baltimore, Maryland

Carrie Dowdy, MSN, RNC; Piedmont Virginia Community College, Charlottesville, Virginia

Julie Doyon, BScN, MScN; University of Ottawa, Ottawa, Ontario, Canada

Cathy Eddy, MSN, RN, CCRN; University of South Dakota; Rapid City Outreach, Rapid City, South Dakota

Barbara Fitzsimmons, RN, MS, CNRN; Johns Hopkins Hospital, Baltimore, Maryland

Nancy Nightingale Gillespie, PhD, PHN II, RN; Saint Francis College, Fort Wayne, Indiana

Mary Ann Goetz, MS, BSN, RN, CANP; Ohio University, Zanesville, Ohio

Margaret J. Greene, EdD, RN; Fairleigh Dickinson University, Teaneck, New Jersey

Elisabeth Greenfield, RN, MSN, CCRN; U.S. Army Institute of Surgical Research, Fort Sam Houston, Texas

Susan J. Hart, MSN, RN, CS, CCRN; Seton Hall University College of Nursing, South Orange, New Jersey

Janie Heath, MS, RN, CS, CCRN, ANP, ACNP; Veterans Administration Medical Center; Medical College of Georgia School of Nursing, Augusta, Georgia

Gale Hess, RN, MS; Mayo Medical Center, Rochester, Minnesota

Robin R. Higley, RN, MS, CNA; Fairview Hospital, Cleveland, Ohio

Sr. Esther Holzbauer, BS, MSN, RN, ANAC; Mount Marty College, Yankton, South Dakota

Renée S. Hyde, RN, MSN, CNRN; Carolinas College of Health Sciences, Charlotte, North Carolina

Mary Jane Jones, RN, BSN, MN; Henderson Community College, Henderson, Kentucky

David R. Johnson, DNSc, RN, CS; Saint Francis College, Fort Wayne, Indiana

Lorene M. Kimzey, RNC, MEd; National Institutes of Health, Bethesda, Maryland

Donna Lee Kistler, RN, MS; University of California–Davis Medical Center, Sacramento, California

Pamela Sue Laughlin, RN, AD; W.S. Major Hospital, Shelbyville, Indiana

Jean Marie Lucas, RN, BSN, CEN; Johns Hopkins Hospital, Baltimore, Maryland

Suzanne K. Marnocha, RN, MSN, CCRN; University of Wisconsin, Oshkosh, College of Nursing, Oshkosh, Wisconsin

Michel S. Martin, RN; Mayo Medical Center, Rochester, Minnesota

Lisa J. Massarweh, RN, MSN, CCRN; Kent State University, Ashtabula, Ohio

Preface

The first edition of this text, titled *Medical-Surgical Nursing: A Nursing Process Approach,* found widespread acclaim as the medical-surgical nursing text of the 1990s. The second edition built on that achievement and further solidified the text's position. Now, with the publication of the third edition, a title change signals the text's focus on the changing nature of nursing and health care as we prepare to enter the 21st century.

The title *Medical-Surgical Nursing Across the Health Care Continuum* was carefully chosen to reflect an emphasis on collaborative care and continuing care that extend beyond the hospital setting into the community and home. Our goal has been to ensure that the book you hold today is as current and as accessible as possible to help nursing students provide state-of-the-art health care in today's—and tomorrow's—rapidly evolving health care system.

Medical-Surgical Nursing Across the Health Care Continuum embraces collaborative, interdisciplinary client care in a variety of health care settings. This revision provides expanded coverage of women's health issues, transcultural care, and special needs of the elderly. Case management and managed care concepts are interwoven throughout to help the reader understand these new emerging roles and variables. Simple, but effective, complementary therapies that nurses can use to relieve pain and manage chronic illness are also discussed. Finally, critical thinking is promoted through case studies with questions provided at the end of most chapters.

Clinical Currency and Comprehensiveness

To ensure the text's currency, accuracy, and comprehensiveness, we listened to the readers of the first two editions—their impressions of and experiences with the text. We also listened to experts' opinions on the current state of nursing and the health care system and trends that are driving change. Based on this input, we formulated our revision plan. We assembled a team of clinical experts to revise, rewrite, and in some cases draft entirely new chapters. We then commissioned in-depth reviews of each chapter by clinicians and instructors from across the United States and Canada, using their reviews to guide us in revising the chapters into their final form.

The results are reflected in the third edition's strong, consistent focus on pathophysiology, collaborative care, and continuing care; foundation of relevant nursing research; and emphasis on the critical "need to know" information that nurses must master to provide safe, effective care.

Ease of Access

To make the text as easy to use as possible, we maintained the second edition's approach of smaller chapters of more uniform length. The third edition now has 80 chapters, including new chapters on complementary therapies, continuing care, managed care and case management, and infusion therapy. We also maintained the second edition's unit structure, with vital body systems (cardiovascular, respiratory, and neurologic) appearing earlier in the book. In these three units, we also maintained the approach of providing critical care content in separate chapters on managing critically ill clients with coronary artery disease, respiratory problems, and neurologic problems. Within each chapter, we carefully edited to ensure maximum readability for all levels of students. To help break up long blocks of text and also highlight key information, we included numerous headings, bulleted lists, tables, charts, and in-text highlights. We end each chapter with Selected Bibliography (with classic sources noted by an asterisk*) and Suggested Readings lists.

One of the most obvious changes in the third edition is the new full-color design. Color is used not only in the photographs and drawings, enhancing their usefulness as learning tools, but also in the design of the text itself to help distinguish key features and clarify chapter organization.

A Collaborative Approach

As in the previous two editions, we take a collaborative approach to client care. We believe that in the real world of health care, nurses, clients, physicians, and other health care providers share responsibility for the management of client problems. Thus, we present client care in a *collaborative management* framework. In this framework, we make no artificial distinctions between medical treatment and nursing care—instead, we cover the entire range of approaches that health care providers of all disciplines take in dealing with client problems.

Nonetheless, because this text is first and foremost a *nursing* text, we organize discussion of client problems and their management using a *nursing process* approach. Discussions of key disorders follow the full nursing process format, with the following structure:

DISORDER

Overview
   Pathophysiology
   Etiology
   Incidence/Prevalence

Collaborative Management

 Assessment

 Analysis
   Common Nursing Diagnoses/Collaborative
      Problems
   Additional Nursing Diagnoses/Collaborative
      Problems

 Planning and Implementation
   Nursing Diagnoses/Collaborative Problems
   Planning: Expected Outcomes
   Interventions

 Continuing Care
   Health Teaching
   Home Care Management
   Health Care Resources

 Evaluation

Discussions of other disorders, while not given this complete subhead structure, nonetheless follow the same basic format: a discussion of the disorder itself, including pertinent pathophysiology, etiology, and incidence information, followed by a section on collaborative management of clients with the disorder.

Integral to this collaborative management approach is a clear delineation of just who is responsible for what. When a responsibility is primarily the nurse's, the text says so. When a decision must be made jointly by the client, nurse, physician, and therapist, this is clearly stated. When different health care providers in different care settings might be involved in the client's care, this is stated, too.

Multinational, Multicultural, Multigenerational Focus

Reflecting the increasing diversity of our society in general and the health care system in particular, *Medical-Surgical Nursing Across the Health Care Continuum* includes a number of special features.

To address the needs of American and Canadian readers, we have included examples of trade names of drugs available in the United States and drugs available in Canada. A maple leaf icon identifies the Canadian trade names.

To help nurses provide quality care for clients whose race, culture, or ethnic background differs from their own, numerous *Transcultural Considerations* throughout the text highlight important aspects of culturally competent care.

Increased life expectancy means a steadily increasing elderly population. To help nurses prepare for this trend, the third edition features expanded coverage of the care of elderly clients. This edition includes a greater number of *Nursing Focus on the Elderly* charts and highlights laboratory values and drug dosages typical for elderly clients. Charts specifying normal physiologic changes to expect in the elderly are included in each assessment chapter. In addition, highlighted *Elderly Considerations* presented throughout the text emphasize key points to consider when caring for these clients.

Also appearing throughout the text, *Women's Health Considerations* address topics of concern to female clients and their health care providers. Specifically, this feature highlights gender-related differences in assessment parameters and in the incidence, severity, treatment, or expected client responses to health problems.

Organization

The 80 chapters of *Medical-Surgical Nursing Across the Health Care Continuum* are grouped into 16 distinct units. Unit 1, Health Promotion and Illness, lays the groundwork for the health care concepts incorporated throughout the text. It includes new chapters on integration of care across the health care continuum (Chapter 2), case management and managed care (Chapter 3), and complementary, holistic therapies (Chapter 4). Unit 2 covers specific biopsychosocial concepts, including pain, stress, and sexuality. Unit 3 comprises six chapters on the management of clients with fluid, electrolyte, and acid-base imbalances. This unit includes a new chapter on infusion therapy (Chapter 17).

Unit 4 presents the perioperative nursing content that medical-surgical nurses need to know. This content provides a solid foundation to help the student better understand the coverage of specific surgeries throughout the remainder of the text. Unit 5 provides core content on health problems related to immune system function. This content includes normal inflammation and the immune response, altered cell development and growth, and interventions for clients with connective tissue disease, AIDS, and other immunologic disorders, cancers, and infections.

The remaining 11 units cover medical-surgical content by body system. Each of these units begins with a chapter on assessment and then continues with one or more chapters on interventions for clients with specific health problems related to the subject body system.

Pedagogical Features

The third edition includes various features to help the student quickly identify and retain key information and to serve as study aids:

- At the beginning of each chapter, a list of *Chapter Highlights* provides a guide to the chapter's contents and organization.
- *Nursing Care Highlight* charts emphasize important "hands-on" nursing care.
- *Nursing Focus on the Elderly* charts highlight normal age-related changes that affect nursing care and specify the individualized care that nurses need to provide to elderly clients with specific conditions or undergoing specific procedures.
- Written in "client-friendly" language, *Education Guide* charts provide the kind of instructions that nurses must learn to provide to clients and their families to help them cope with life changes caused by illness.
- *Health Promotion Guide* charts, also written in client-oriented language, give examples of instructions that nurses can provide to help clients and their families prevent illness and maintain optimum health.
- *Laboratory Profile* charts summarize important information on laboratory tests commonly ordered to evaluate health problems. Information typically includes normal ranges of laboratory values (including differences for elderly clients, when appropriate) and the possible significance of abnormal findings.
- *Drug Therapy* charts summarize important information about commonly used drugs. These charts include U.S. and Canadian trade names, usual dosages (including dosages for elderly clients, as appropriate), and nursing interventions with rationales.
- *Key Features* charts highlight the clinical manifestations of important disorders.
- *Research Applications for Nursing* boxes, provided in nearly every chapter, give synopses of recent nursing research articles and other scientific articles applicable to nursing. Each box provides a summary of the article, a brief critique, and a summary of possible implications for nursing practice. The goal of this feature is to help the student identify the strengths and weaknesses of the research and see how research can help guide nursing practice.
- A selection of representative *Client Care Plans* provides detailed plans of nursing care for specific client problems.
- Various *Clinical Pathways* provide examples of how hospitals are implementing a collaborative approach to client care.
- Included at the end of most chapters, a *Case Study* presents a brief clinical scenario and poses pertinent questions designed to stimulate critical thinking.
- To further guide students in locating important information, a list of *Resources*—including Internet resources—is included in an appendix.

Complete Teaching and Learning Package

A full complement of companion, or ancillary, publications accompany *Medical-Surgical Nursing Across the Health Care Continuum,* providing a complete teaching and learning package for both instructors and students.

Every effort has been made to correlate content among these ancillary publications and to focus the content on a set of core concepts developed specifically for this purpose. An editor of this text has been involved in writing each of the ancillaries to ensure consistency and cohesion with the text itself.

Resources for instructors include an *Instructor's Manual, Test Manual, ExaMaster,* and *LectureView.* The *Instructor's Manual,* written by Elaine Kennedy, an expert in cooperative learning, and Donna Ignatavicius, is a truly groundbreaking educational ancillary. It provides content on how to promote collaborative or cooperative learning with features never before presented in any comparable instructor's manual, including critical learning outcomes, suggested learning activities, and a list of supplemental resources arranged in a unique three-column format. Learning activities that involve group work are included, as are time frames for learning and strategies for promoting active learning, including aspects of teaching/learning via distance education. Supplemental resources, which foster independent exploration, include transparency masters, Internet resources, and materials from community organizations. Numerous graphic organizers are provided, including concept maps, algorithms, team concept maps, and sequence chains to assist students in making connections among isolated pieces of information and to encourage them to assemble the puzzle of today's complex health care system. The focus of content is on the Core Concepts Grids, which are provided for each unit and serve as the basis for material presented therein. Also provided are answer guidelines for the questions posed in the case studies that appear in the text.

A printed *Test Manual* and a computerized *ExaMaster* provide instructors with more than 1,500 completely new test questions coded for correct answer, rationale, and cognitive level. These questions, prepared by M. Linda Workman, have been written in response to feedback from the market to be both more challenging and reflective of the scope of questions on the NCLEX examination. Most are application-based questions, and only about 10 percent are knowledge-level or comprehension-level questions. Questions were written focusing on the Core Concepts Grids presented in the *Instructor's Manual* and the *Critical Thinking Study Guide.* The *ExaMaster,* now on CD-ROM, allows the instructor to generate comprehensive tests by selecting questions based on instructor-chosen criteria.

Representing a quantum leap from the former acetate transparencies, *LectureView,* a new CD-ROM presentation program, includes 500 full-color images from the text with slide copy for projection in the classroom. This PowerPoint-compatible ancillary allows the instructor to provide lecture material and key illustrations, using powerful new classroom presentation software.

For students, the *Critical Thinking Study Guide* provides material to enhance learning in various formats to promote mastery of the text. Echoing one of the text's themes, the study guide emphasizes questions aimed at enhancing critical thinking skills. The guide was written by Elaine Kennedy and Donna Ignatavicius in conjunction with the *Instructor's Manual* to ensure consistency. Its focus is also on the Core Concepts Grids in the *Instructor's Manual,* which are also included here for student review.

The *Pocket Companion for Medical-Surgical Nursing,* authored by Donna Ignatavicius and Kathy Hausman, retains the alphabetical format that proved so popular in the first two editions. It also includes extensive cross-referencing to help the student access vital information quickly.

In summary, we feel that *Medical-Surgical Nursing Across the Health Care Continuum* and its teaching-learning package provide all of the resources needed by students preparing to meet the challenge of practicing nursing in the 21st century.

Donna D. Ignatavicius
M. Linda Workman
Mary A. Mishler

Acknowledgments

Publishing a textbook of this depth and breadth would not be possible without the combined efforts of many people. Our contributors provided consistently excellent manuscripts in a timely fashion. Our reviewers, expert clinicians and instructors from around the United States and Canada, provided invaluable suggestions and encouragement throughout the book's development.

The staff of the W.B. Saunders Company once again provided us with crucial guidance and support throughout the planning, writing, revision, and production of the third edition. In particular, two Senior Editors—first Barbara Nelson Cullen, followed by Robin Carter—kept us on schedule and encouraged us every step of the way. Senior Developmental Editor Kevin Law—with the invaluable assistance of Senior Developmental Editor Lee Henderson; Assistant Developmental Editors Rachel Hubbs and Marie Pelcin; Editorial Assistants Beth Dean, Ross Landy, and Amelia Cullinan; and freelance developmental editors Neal Fandek, Marian Sandmaier, and Debra Osnowitz—helped us translate our conceptual vision into a consistently formatted and pedagogically sound reality.

W.B. Saunders Copy Editors Blair Davis and Scott Filderman, aided by freelance copy editors Mary McCoy and Debra Adleman, assumed the monumental task of checking all of the text's editorial details and ensuring consistency throughout. They did an outstanding job. Other W.B. Saunders staff deserving special thanks include Production Managers Laurie Sanders and Peter Faber, Illustration Coordinator Lisa Lambert, Marketing Manager Jean Rodenberger, and Marketing Assistant Linda Lee.

Creating a new, full-color design and art program for a major textbook is a enormous undertaking. Our thanks go to W.B. Saunders Designer Gene Harris for the text's clean yet visually arresting design; Academy Artworks for the hundreds of wonderful line drawings; and Rick Williams and John Workman for the clear, instructive color photographs.

Contents

Guide to Special Features

TRANSCULTURAL CONSIDERATIONS

Obesity (Chapter 64)
Osteoarthritis (Chapter 24)
Osteoporosis (Chapter 53)
Paget's Disease (Chapter 53)
Pain (Chapter 9)
Peripheral Arterial Disease (Chapter 38)
Pneumococcal and Influenza Vaccine (Chapter 33)
Prolapsed Uterus (Chapter 78)
Pulmonary Fibrosis (Chapter 32)
Renal Disease, End-Stage (Chapter 72)
Renal/Urinary System (Chapter 72)

Respiratory Disorders (Chapter 29)
Rheumatoid Arthritis (Chapter 24)
Sarcoidosis (Chapter 32)
Sexuality (Chapter 11)
Sexuality and Reproduction (Chapter 76)
Sexually Transmitted Diseases and Pelvic Inflammatory Disease (Chapter 80)
Sickle Cell Disease (Chapter 42)
Stroke (Chapter 47)
Tuberculosis (Chapter 33)
Ulcerative Colitis (Chapter 60)

WOMEN'S HEALTH CONSIDERATIONS

Alzheimer's Disease (Chapter 44)
Angina (Chapter 40)
Cardiovascular Disease and Obesity (Chapter 35)
Chronic Back Pain (Chapter 45)
Chronic Obstructive Pulmonary Disease and Chronic Airflow Limitation (Chapter 32)
Colles' Fracture (Chapter 54)
Colorectal Cancer (Chapters 55 and 59)
Coronary Artery Disease and Atherosclerosis (Chapter 38)
Eating Disorders (Chapter 63)
Fluid and Electrolyte Balance (Chapter 14)
Fractures (Chapter 54)
Gallbladder Disease (Chapter 62)
Genitourinary Tract Infection (Chapter 28)
Health Promotion (Chapter 1)
Hematologic, Blood Cell Counts (Chapter 41)
HIV Infection and AIDS (Chapter 25)
Hypertension (Chapter 38)

Hypocalcemia (Chapter 16)
Hyponatremia (Chapter 16)
Malnutrition (Chapter 64)
Mitral Stenosis (Chapter 37)
Musculoskeletal Disorders (Chapter 52)
Myocardial Infarction (Chapter 40)
Myocardial Infarction and Chest Pain (Chapter 40)
Obesity (Chapter 64)
Peripheral Vascular Disease (Chapter 38)
Pregnancy and Burns (Chapter 71)
Pregnancy and Gallstones (Chapter 62)
Pregnancy and Leukemia (Chapter 42)
Respiratory Disorders (Chapter 29)
Rheumatoid Arthritis (Chapter 24)
Sexually Transmitted Diseases (Chapter 80)
Sickle Cell Disease (Chapter 42)
Stroke (Chapter 47)

NURSING FOCUS ON THE ELDERLY CHARTS

Chart 1–2	Teaching the Older Adult
Chart 1–3	Interviewing
Chart 5–2	Effects of Aging on Body Systems
Chart 6–5	Social Services Provided by the Older Americans Act of 1965
Chart 7–1	Myths and Ethical Issues Related to Care of the Elderly
Chart 8–2	Reducing Stress
Chart 9–1	The Elderly Client Experiencing Pain
Chart 11–1	Changes Affecting Sexuality
Chart 14–1	Impact of Age-Related Changes on Fluid and Electrolyte Balance
Chart 14–2	Normal Plasma Electrolyte Values for People Older Than 60 Years
Chart 17–4	Special Considerations for the Elderly Client Receiving Peripheral Intravenous Therapy
Chart 18–2	Age-Related Risk Factors for Acid-Base Disturbances
Chart 19–1	The Elderly Client Experiencing Acid-Base Imbalance
Chart 20–1	Changes of Aging as Surgical Risk Factors
Chart 20–2	Specific Considerations When Planning Care for the Elderly Preoperative Client

Chart 21–3	Intraoperative Nursing Interventions
Chart 22–2	Postoperative Skin Care
Chart 23–1	Changes in Immune Function Related to Aging
Chart 24–2	Total Hip Replacement
Chart 26–1	Cancer Assessment Considerations
Chart 28–3	Infection
Chart 29–1	Changes in the Respiratory System Related to Aging
Chart 32–1	Respiratory Disorders
Chart 35–1	Changes in the Cardiovascular System Related to Aging
Chart 36–7	Dysrhythmias
Chart 37–4	Heart Failure
Chart 38–4	Hypertension
Chart 40–6	Coronary Artery Disease
Chart 40–7	Coronary Artery Bypass Graft Surgery
Chart 41–1	Hematologic Assessment
Chart 42–13	Transfusion Therapy
Chart 43–1	Changes in the Nervous System Related to Aging
Chart 45–2	Factors Contributing to Low Back Pain
Chart 47–5	Head Injury
Chart 48–1	Changes in the Eye Related to Aging

FOCUSED ASSESSMENT CHARTS

LABORATORY PROFILE CHARTS

HEALTH PROMOTION GUIDE CHARTS

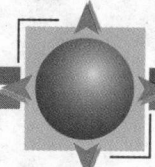

Health Promotion

and Illness

Chapter 1

MEDICAL-SURGICAL NURSING AND THE ROLE OF THE MEDICAL-SURGICAL NURSE

Medical-surgical nursing is a quickly changing specialty practice that is influenced by increasing knowledge about disease etiology, rapid advances in technology, reform of the health care system, and trends in health promotion and protection. A major focus of medical-surgical nursing is to promote well-being and prevent complications of illness and disease.

HEALTH

Beliefs about health and illness are a major feature of every known culture. How one views himself or herself as a person and as a part of the environment affects how health is defined. Health is often viewed as a continuum on which optimal wellness, at one end, is the highest level of function, and illness, at the other end, results in death (Fig. 1–1). Every person is somewhere on the continuum. As one's health state changes, the location on the continuum changes.

Although the term *health* is used every day, no universally accepted definition has been established. Over time, the focus and expression of health have varied, depending on knowledge, theories, and beliefs. Some people have

viewed health and disease as reward or punishment for their actions. Others have considered health as a soundness or wholeness of the body.

Definitions of Health

A typical dictionary may define health in terms of a person's ability to function in society. Some definitions also describe health as a disease-free state or condition. Definitions such as these do not make clear what constitutes health and illness and seem to present an "either/or" situation—that is, a person is either healthy or ill.

World Health Organization Definition of Health

As science has progressed, the definition of health has evolved. One of the most frequently quoted definitions is the one presented in 1947 by the World Health Organization (WHO). WHO stated that health is "a state of complete physical, mental, and social well-being and not merely the absence of disease or infirmity" (WHO, 1947, p. 1). Thus, according to WHO, to be healthy a person

3

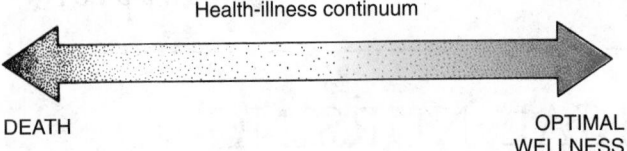

Health-illness continuum

DEATH   OPTIMAL
                         WELLNESS

Figure 1–1. Common concept of health as a continuum ranging from optimal wellness at one end to illness culminating in death at the other end.

must be in a state of well-being physically, mentally, and socially. Health professionals have found this concept problematic because achieving a state of "health" seems to be an unrealistic goal. This definition does not allow for degrees of health or illness, and it fails to reflect the dynamic, ever-changing nature of health.

A concept related to health is *homeostasis,* or internal equilibrium or balance. When a person experiences a disturbance in homeostasis, he or she is considered to be "unhealthy." Like the WHO definition of health, this concept is losing popularity because "stasis" implies an unchanging state, and most theorists today believe that health is always changing.

Sociologic Definitions of Health

Sociologists view health as a condition that allows for the pursuit and enjoyment of desired cultural values. Studies that have polled laypeople for their definitions of health concur that health is the absence of symptoms and a feeling of well-being. "Good health" includes the ability to carry out "normal," daily activities, such as going to work and performing household chores.

Holistic Health

A term frequently used when health and wellness are discussed is *holistic health.* The holistic view considers the body, mind, and spirit as interrelated parts of a person's being. The concept of high-level wellness, which consid-

ers the needs of the whole person, has led to the growth of holistic health care. Holistic health focuses on promoting health and preventing illness, with emphasis on the person's responsibility to achieve high-level wellness. There is also concern with bringing the person's mind, body, and spirit into harmony with the environment. Various complementary therapies, sometimes referred to as alternative medicine practices, have been used for many years to promote mind-body-spirit harmony. Chapter 4 describes some commonly used therapies and how they can be incorporated into medical-surgical nursing practice.

Definition of Health Used in This Book

In this text, health is defined as a person's level of wellness. This level of wellness is a process in which a person is striving to attain his or her full potential. Health reflects one's biological, psychological, and sociologic state (Fig. 1–2). The *biological* (physical) state refers to the structure of body tissues and organs as well as to the biochemical interactions and functions within the body. The *psychological* state includes a person's mood, emotions, and personality. The *sociologic* (social) state involves the interaction between a person and the environment. *Spiritual health* is sometimes considered as part of sociologic health but may be described as a separate aspect of one's overall health state.

Factors that affect a person's biological, psychological, or social well-being require additional energy and thus alter the level of wellness. Therefore, a high level of wellness is achieved when one's biopsychosocial needs are met.

One of nursing's primary functions is to assist clients in reaching a high level of wellness. Understanding the concept of health and high-level wellness is therefore essential. As nurses assess clients, they must be aware of factors that affect a person's health state and must use nursing interventions to promote and maintain an optimal level of wellness (Fig. 1–3).

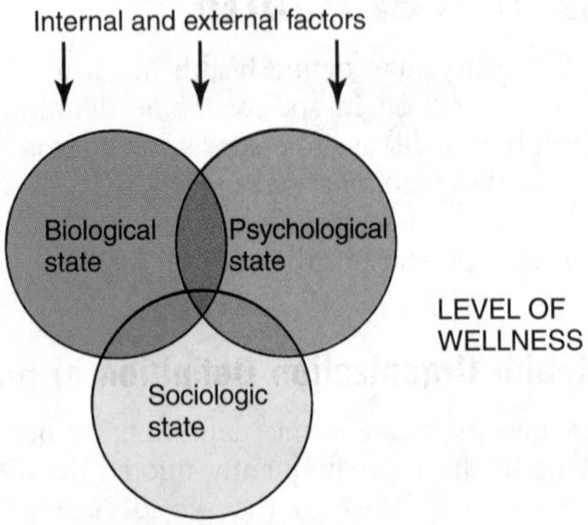

Internal and external factors

Biological state   Psychological state

Sociologic state

LEVEL OF WELLNESS

Figure 1–2. Textbook definition of health—one's biological, psychological, and sociologic state. Internal and external factors affect a person's level of wellness.

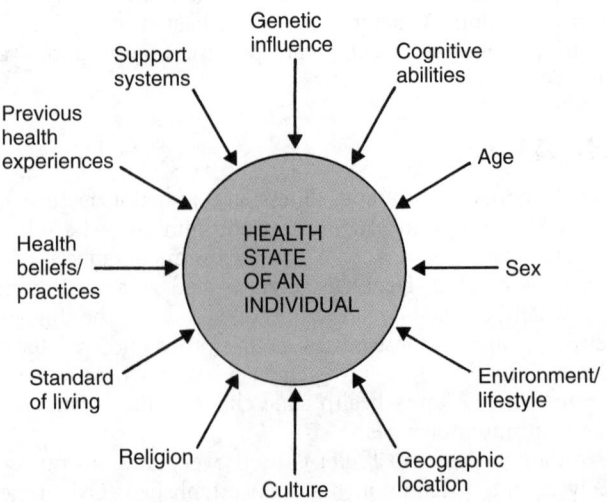

Figure 1–3. Multiple variables influence health and illness.

HEALTH PROMOTION

Health promotion refers to activities that are directed toward developing a person's resources to maintain or enhance well-being as a protection against illness. Reversing the emphasis from curing a disease to promoting health provides a more positive orientation for health care. Illness no longer needs to be the primary focus of health care. In addition, illness care is much more expensive than promoting health.

The U.S. Department of Health and Human Services (1990) joined the world mission to promote health in its "Healthy People 2000" campaign. The expectation was that by the year 2000 people would be healthier and practicing healthier lifestyles. In particular, the agenda calls for health care access for everyone, a longer life expectancy, and equal life expectancy for people of all cultures. At present, some ethnic groups in the United States (especially Hispanics, African/Americans, and Asian Americans and Pacific Islanders) have shorter life expectancies than others.

TRANSCULTURAL CONSIDERATIONS

The demographic profile of the U.S. population is rapidly changing. Whereas the African-American population is currently the largest nonwhite ethnic group in the country, by the year 2010 the Hispanic population will outnumber African-Americans. The Census Bureau projects that by the year 2000, 11% of the population will be Hispanic, for a total of 31 million people. People of Mexican origin make up the largest subgroup. Access to health care, lifestyle, and environmental factors affect the health of Hispanics. Among adults, heart disease, diabetes mellitus, cancer, and liver disease are much higher in Hispanics than in non-Hispanic whites (Castillo & Torres, 1995). Many Hispanics use "folk healing" remedies because they are more available, affordable, and user friendly. Chapter 4 describes some of these nontraditional health practices.

Nearly a third of African-Americans live in poverty, compared with 11% of Caucasians. Cancer, heart disease, and acquired immune deficiency syndrome (AIDS) lead to higher mortality rates among African-Americans compared with Caucasians. This is partly because many African-Americans lack access to health care and have a reluctance to seek health promotion care, especially primary prevention and early detection (Douglas, 1995).

Asian-Americans and Pacific Islanders (AAPIs) presently represent between 3% and 4% of the U.S. population, but that number is expected to jump to 11% by the year 2050 (Louie, 1995). Chen and Hawks (1995) reported that the mortality rates for AAPIs with lung cancer and cardiovascular disease will probably exceed those of other ethnic groups in 20 years. In addition, the prevalence of hepatitis B and tuberculosis is higher among AAPIs than among any other ethnic group. Like Hispanics, many AAPIs lack access to health care and have lifestyle and environmental factors that influence their health status. Beliefs about health and illness for AAPIs are strongly guided by religion (Louie, 1995).

WOMEN'S HEALTH CONSIDERATIONS

Historically, women's health issues have not been studied, especially for women of color (non-Caucasian). Recent interest in women's health has shown that many women in the United States do not receive necessary health care; have many undetected, treatable problems; and experience long-lasting effects of abuse. Women of color are more likely to be poor and uninsured when compared with Caucasian women. All women are at serious risk of heart disease, lung cancer, and osteoporosis, and they lack the knowledge about how to prevent these health problems (Allen & Phillips, 1997).

Today, the National Institutes of Health strongly support research on women's health. Throughout this book, women's health considerations are highlighted, as appropriate, and research on women's health issues is included when possible.

Several nursing theorists have developed nursing health promotion models. One of the best-known models is that advocated by Pender. In her model, Pender (1987) makes a distinction between health promotion and illness prevention: Health promotion is not "health problem–specific," but prevention (sometimes called health protection) is. In addition, Pender believes that health promotion is a positive activity, whereas illness prevention is an avoidance activity.

Although this text integrates illness prevention with health promotion, it recognizes that the two concepts are somewhat different. The goal of both types of activities, explained later, is to improve or maintain the client's health. Throughout this text, Health Promotion Guide charts help the nurse in teaching clients about health promotion activities.

Part of the health promotion movement in nursing is reflected in the use of the term *client* rather than *patient*. Whereas the word *patient* is associated with a dependent position in a hospital, the word *client* suggests an active partnership in the process of health care delivery and maintenance in any setting. *Client* is therefore the term used for the health care consumer in this text.

Practices to Promote Health

Researchers have found certain health practices to have a positive correlation with health promotion in adults. Some of these general health practices include

- Eating well-balanced meals that incorporate foods from the food pyramid, as recommended (see Fig. 64–1)
- Moderate eating to maintain ideal weight and prevent obesity
- Moderate exercising on a routine schedule
- Sleeping regularly, about 7 to 8 hours each day
- Limiting consumption of alcohol to a moderate amount
- Not smoking
- Keeping exposure to the sun to a minimum

These practices have been associated with high-level wellness regardless of sex, age, or economic status. The greater the number of these practices followed in a consistent, routine manner, the better the health state.

Practices to Prevent Illness

Illness prevention is related to health promotion and maintenance. In an effort to decrease the occurrence of illness, prevention is essential. Preventive health behavior is described as voluntary action taken by a person or group to decrease the potential or actual threat of illness and its harmful consequences. As mentioned earlier, some ethnic groups are not focused on health promotion activities, especially prevention and early detection. Throughout this text, where appropriate, these transcultural considerations are discussed.

People must be motivated and educated to make health-related changes. Three levels of illness prevention are summarized in Table 1–1: primary, secondary, and tertiary.

Primary Prevention

Primary prevention is used to avoid or delay the actual occurrence of a specific disease. Strategies for health maintenance raise the general level of health and well-being of a person, family, or community. Smoking cessation clinics, immunizations, use of seat belts, and use of helmets by motorcyclists are examples of primary prevention strategies.

Secondary Prevention

The purpose of secondary prevention is early detection of a disease or condition, sometimes before the signs and symptoms are evident. Emphasis is on early diagnosis and treatment as well as on intervention to prevent or limit permanent disability or death. Screening procedures such as the Papanicolaou (Pap) smear for cervical cancer and the purified protein derivative (PPD) skin test for tuberculosis are examples.

Tertiary Prevention

Tertiary prevention involves rehabilitation and begins when the disease or condition has stabilized and no further healing is expected, such as cardiac rehabilitation after a myocardial infarction. The goal is to return the person to the highest level of function and to prevent severe disabilities.

Consumer Education and Awareness

Consumer education and awareness have been the major focus in an attempt to influence people and promote wellness. Information about nutrition, exercise, stress management, and routine health examinations is available at schools, work sites, and community centers and in the media. This abundance of information and materials is a major resource for increasing public awareness of the need for health promotion. The Internet also provides access to a vast amount of public health information. (See Appendix for a list of commonly used web sites.)

ROLE OF THE MEDICAL-SURGICAL NURSE

Medical-surgical nursing is one of the many specialties in nursing, yet its scope is much broader than other specialties such as cardiovascular or orthopedic nursing. In 1991, the Academy of Medical-Surgical Nurses (AMSN) was formed as the first specialty organization for this group of nurses. AMSN has published standards for medical-surgical nursing and a core curriculum. The official journal of the AMSN is *MEDSURG Nursing*.

The focus of medical-surgical nursing is on the adult client with acute or chronic illness in any health care setting. Nurses who specialize in medical-surgical nursing need a broad knowledge of the biological, psychological, and social sciences because of the range of clients for whom they care. The overall outcome of care is similar to that for any other specialty—the achievement of an optimal level of wellness and prevention of illness, as discussed earlier in this chapter.

Medical-surgical clients range in age from 18 years to more than 100 years, and their health problems are usually complex. Because the typical client is usually older than 65 years, medical-surgical nurses need a strong background in *gerontology*, or care of the elderly. In this text, charts entitled Nursing Focus on the Elderly highlight the special nursing interventions that this group of clients requires.

As medical-surgical nursing meets changing health care needs, the expectations for providing client care have expanded and increased. Medical-surgical nurses assume various roles and functions within a number of health

TABLE 1–1

Examples of Health Behaviors for the Three Levels of Illness Prevention	
Level	**Examples of Behaviors**
Primary prevention	• Wearing seat belts, helmets • Eating well-balanced meals • Not smoking • Consuming no or minimal alcohol • Being immunized • Maintaining ideal body weight
Secondary prevention	• Having yearly Papanicolaou (Pap) smear tests • Doing monthly breast or testicular self-examination • Having mammograms as recommended • Getting skin tests for tuberculosis screening • Having routine tonometry tests to detect glaucoma
Tertiary prevention	• Following a cardiac rehabilitation program • Pursuing rehabilitation programs for stroke, head injury, or arthritis

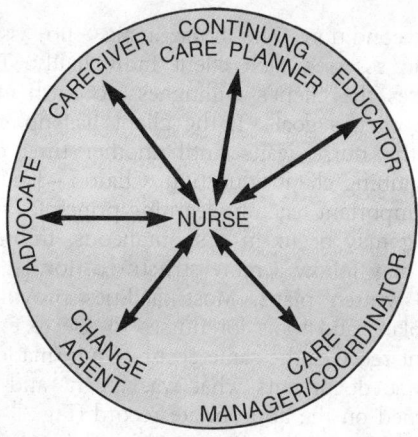

Figure 1–4. Major roles of the medical-surgical nurse.

care settings (Fig. 1–4). Although each role is associated with specific responsibilities, some aspects of each role are interrelated and are common to all nursing positions and specialties.

Care Manager or Coordinator

As a result of health care reform during the 1990s, *managed care* has become the predominant health care delivery system in the United States and other countries. Simply defined, managed care is a system to contain health care costs through a case management process.

Case management targets high-risk, high-cost, complex-problem clients and aims to improve their care by meeting cost-effective clinical outcomes. Most case managers are nurses. Although nurses are not typically taught how to become case managers in their basic education programs, they should learn how to manage and coordinate care. As a *care manager*, the medical-surgical nurse coordinates client care through collaboration with the health care team: The nurse does not provide all of the direct care. Chapter 3 discusses case management, care management, and managed care in more detail.

Caregiver

Another role commonly associated with the medical-surgical nurse is *caregiver*. In this role, nurses assess clients, analyze collected information to determine clients' needs, develop nursing diagnoses and collaborative problems, plan care and carry out the plan with the health team, and evaluate the care given. This process, referred to as the *nursing process* and discussed later, is used throughout this text as an organizational and practice framework.

As a caregiver, the nurse provides physical care through skills such as administering medications and performing comprehensive assessments. Some nursing tasks and activities may be delegated to unlicensed assistive personnel. Throughout this textbook, activities that the nurse may delegate are indicated. The nurse also implements psychosocial interventions, such as encouraging the client to discuss concerns or offering measures to reduce the client's anxiety.

The activities performed by the nurse caregiver are often categorized as *collaborative* (interdependent) or *independent*. *Collaborative* functions include

- Those mutually determined by the nurse and the physician or other health care team member, such as setting activity limitations or providing a special diet
- Those directed or prescribed by the health care provider (physician, nurse practitioner, or physician's assistant) but requiring nursing judgment to perform, such as giving medications

Independent nursing functions are those initiated and carried out by the nurse without direction from the health care provider. Examples include

- Weighing a client
- Listening to bowel sounds
- Testing blood glucose with a fingerstick

This text discusses both types of functions—collaborative and independent—in an interrelated framework under the heading *Collaborative Management*. Charts entitled Nursing Care Highlights identify the most important nursing care for clients with selected health problems.

Continuing Care Planner

Because health care continues to emphasize early discharge from the hospital, nursing home, and home care, the role of the medical-surgical nurse as continuing care planner has become increasingly important. This process involves an assessment of the client's health needs across the health care continuum. A large part of this process is health teaching and assessment of the home or other setting to which the client is discharged for available resources, support systems, and equipment, if needed.

Continuing care planning may be coordinated by a designated discharge planner employed by the agency in collaboration with the staff nurse, or by a case manager. The discharge planner or case manager is usually a nurse or social worker. If the agency does not employ designated discharge planners, the staff nurse caring for the client is typically responsible for the continuing care planning process. Throughout this text, a section entitled Continuing Care is included to facilitate planning.

Educator

Client education is a major component of medical-surgical nursing care. In collaboration with the interdisciplinary health team, the nurse tries to improve health by providing information on health promotion, disease and illness, and specific treatment. As educators, nurses work with individual clients as well as with family members or other caregivers. The role of education has become increasingly important because clients are discharged "quicker and sicker" from the hospital, subacute unit, or nursing home to their homes. Nurses often become frustrated when they feel that they do not have as much time as they need to teach in these fast-paced settings.

Chart 1–1

Nursing Care Highlight: Principles of the Adult Teaching-Learning Process

- Assess the client's goals and willingness to learn.
- Before beginning teaching, assess how the client is feeling (e.g., a client in acute pain is unlikely to learn)
- Include family and significant others in teaching as appropriate
- Assess factors that may influence the client's ability or motivation to learn, such as educational level, socioeconomic status, and cultural background
- Provide pictures or other types of visual aids to reinforce learning
- Break complex information or skills into small parts until the client learns them
- Provide the client with "hands-on" experience for psychomotor skills, and request a return demonstration by the client (e.g., insulin administration, dressing change, colostomy care)
- Provide the client with a health resource contact for follow-up questions or concerns

---

The Teaching-Learning Process

Before educating clients, the nurse, in collaboration with members of the health care team, assesses the client's learning needs. A client with a disease of 20 years' duration may need as much teaching as one who has a newly diagnosed condition. The nurse makes no assumptions but instead assesses each client individually. The nurse also assesses the client's willingness to learn and determines the client's goals. If the client has no interest in learning, the nurse waits until another time or setting before beginning client education. Chart 1–1 summarizes the most important teaching-learning principles for adults.

Teaching may occur in a spontaneous, informal manner, or it may follow a more structured, formal approach based on written plans. Most facilities provide written teaching plans and tools for nurses to use to ensure that every client receives the same accurate information.

The nurse documents what was taught and what the client learned on the appropriate record (Fig. 1–5). Some health care agencies use a lay version of the clinical pathway (discussed later in this chapter), which outlines care in a sequential manner for the client. A summary of the teaching-learning process for each client generally becomes a part of the client's medical record. A copy is also given to the client or family member or significant other at the time of discharge. Each Continuing Care section within this text includes a section entitled Health Teaching. Education Guides for teaching clients are also included as appropriate throughout the text.

Factors Affecting the Teaching-Learning Process

As interdisciplinary team members assess the teaching-learning needs of each client, they evaluate many factors.

Teaching-Learning Record for Insulin Self-Administration			
Client Steps	**Taught/Demonstrated (Initial)**	**Date**	**Return Demonstration (Initial)**
1. Selects correct insulin type.			
2. Selects correct syringe.			
3. Cleans top of vial.			
4. Draws up correct insulin amount(s).			
5. Selects appropriate site for injection.			
6. Cleans skin with alcohol swipe.			
7. Uses 90-degree angle when injecting insulin.			

Figure 1–5. A sample teaching-learning record for self-administration of insulin.

Some of the most important factors include the client's educational level, socioeconomic level, support system, age, and transcultural considerations.

Educational Level

The client's educational level directly affects the nurse's plans for teaching. In the United States, it is estimated that more than a third of adults do not have a high school diploma. Consequently, illiteracy in the United States is quite widespread. Information written for the public should therefore not be above the eighth-grade reading level and often needs to be lower. Albright et al. (1996) found that most health education materials are typically written at a level between the 8th and 13th grades (see the Research Applications for Nursing box).

For illiterate clients and those with limited reading skills, the nurse uses other types of visual aids, such as pictures and symbols. When possible, the nurse explains and interprets information for clients rather than merely offering them a booklet or instruction sheet.

▷ Research Applications for Nursing

Reading Level of Education Materials Too High for Most Clients

Albright, J., de Guzman, C., Acebo, P., et al. (1996). Readability of patient education materials: Implications for clinical practice. Applied Nursing Research, 9, 139–143.

The purpose of this nursing study was to examine the readability of education materials at one medical center across four units as well as hospital-wide. A government study reported that 47% of people in the United States lack basic reading skills. Other studies have shown that reported grade completion level is higher than actual reading level.

The results showed that mean readability scores (grade level) ranged from 8.62 for diabetes education materials to 11.37 for surgery education materials. Many of the materials were commercially prepared by manufacturers. Recommendations for the hospital where this study was conducted include

- Provide verbal explanation as well as written materials
- Begin to write new education materials at a sixth-grade reading level
- Inform manufacturers of the high readability levels
- Build a bank of education materials for use in a variety of areas
- Assess the reading level of clients who receive health care at the hospital

Critique. The researchers reviewed a wide variety of educational materials from various suppliers of educational tools. Although they limited their study to one setting, many health care agencies use these same materials and can benefit from the study findings.

Possible nursing implications. Nurses must augment the written client education materials with verbal teaching and provide answers to client questions. For nurses involved in writing educational materials, a fifth- or sixth-grade reading level is most appropriate.

Socioeconomic Level

When teaching clients how to care for themselves at home, the nurse must consider their financial resources. For example, if the client needs to perform muscle-strengthening exercises using small weights, the nurse cannot always expect the client to purchase expensive commercial weights. Instead, the nurse suggests the use of 1- or 2-pound coffee cans or bags, bags of sugar or flour, or similar available household items.

Another concern for the nurse is the cost of required medication, equipment, or supplies. For instance, clients who do not qualify for medical assistance but work for an employer that does not provide group health insurance may not be able to afford the necessary medical items or follow-up care. As part of continuing care planning, the nurse attempts to locate resources, such as community health organizations like the American Cancer Society, that can provide the necessary resources. In addition, clinics that specialize in providing care for working uninsured clients are available in some parts of the United States. Some of these clinics are nurse-managed community centers.

Support Systems

The nurse assesses the client's support systems and should include part or all of these systems in client education. Examples of support systems include families, significant others, churches, and social community clubs and organizations. In general, people tend to be more compliant with their health regimen if they have the encouragement of others. Support is particularly important if the client must follow many lifestyle restrictions. For instance, a farmer who may be accustomed to eating fried foods and red meat may find it difficult to change to a low-fat, low-sodium diet. If the farmer's wife has always been the cook in the home, the nurse includes her in the teaching process to help to ensure compliance with the new dietary restrictions.

Age

Age affects the teaching-learning process as well. An elderly client may take longer than a younger person to process information or may have visual or hearing deficits (Chart 1–2). The nurse provides small amounts of information at one time and checks with the client before proceeding to make sure that he or she has understood. Too much information is difficult to comprehend and absorb and usually results in the client's frustration and noncompliance.

TRANSCULTURAL CONSIDERATIONS

The nurse considers the client's cultural background before teaching. If the client does not clearly understand the nurse's language, the nurse locates resources that can help with the teaching process. For example, many people who emigrated to the United States in the 1940s have attempted to retain their language and culture and not become too "Americanized." As a result, when

---

Chart 1–2

Nursing Focus on the Elderly: Teaching the Older Adult

- Ensure that the client wears glasses or hearing aids if needed
- Be sure that the area for teaching has ample lighting and minimal distraction
- Provide most of the teaching in the morning (after breakfast), before the client becomes too fatigued
- Speak slowly, and provide small amounts of new information at a time
- Ask the client to repeat the information to make sure that he or she has learned it
- Provide written information so that the client can refer to it later if needed

---

they interact with health care professionals, they often cannot understand and need someone to interpret for them.

Another factor to consider during health teaching is the health practices of various cultures. For example, Mexican-Americans, particularly those living near the Mexican border, often use *curandismo,* or folk medicine, because they cannot afford Westernized health care or prefer their own medical traditions. Another reason that these clients avoid the health care system is that they may have limitations in speaking, reading, or writing English or Spanish. The nurse needs to know this information so that she or he can incorporate cultural beliefs and practices into the teaching-learning process.

The nurse also considers spiritual and religious differences. A client whose spiritual beliefs forbid taking medication is not likely to comply with instructions about drug therapy.

Advocate

As a client advocate, the medical-surgical nurse assists the client and family in interpreting information from other health care team members. The nurse offers additional information that the client needs to make decisions about health care. This assistance may include explanations about the implications of the client's decisions about health and ensuring that the client receives appropriate care. For example, a client scheduled for a total knee replacement may not understand that the knee joint will be removed and replaced with a prosthesis. If the nurse determines that the client does not fully understand the operative procedure, he or she notifies the surgeon of the need for additional preoperative education. The nurse reinforces the information even if another health team member has provided it.

Client advocacy is closely associated with the field of ethics. Chapter 7 discusses ethics in detail and illustrates examples of ethical dilemmas that medical-surgical nurses encounter in their practice.

Change Agent

The medical-surgical nurse serves as a change agent within the work setting and within the profession. The role of change agent involves planning and implementing a system to change the client's health-related behaviors. In the work setting, the nurse assesses health behaviors of the client and family to identify those that need altering. The most important factor in this process is to assess the client's readiness to change. If the client is not ready, he or she will not comply with the change and the nurse will be ineffective in this role.

Within the community, medical-surgical nurses serve as role models and assist consumers in bringing about changes to improve the environment, work conditions, or other factors that affect health. Nurses also work together to bring about change through legislation. For example, nurses provide and support bills for legislation that can affect a person's health status, such as those mandating increased hospital stays for clients having mastectomies.

PRACTICE SETTINGS FOR MEDICAL-SURGICAL NURSES

Medical-surgical nurses have opportunities to provide health care in a variety of settings, including hospitals, long-term care facilities, and community-based settings. The hospital setting is described in this chapter. Chapter 2 discusses community-based settings.

Hospitals, or acute care facilities, are the largest employers of nurses; approximately 57% of all nurses work within hospitals. However, this number is declining.

In the United States, the cost of hospital care is usually paid for by third-party payers, or insurers. Medicare Part A (in-hospital coverage), a federal program, pays for most of the care given to people older than 65 years and to any client who is disabled. Private insurers and managed care organizations pay for most or part of the care provided to clients with insurance. State medical assistance programs pay for some of the health care provided for clients of any age who are indigent.

In Canada, all people are entitled to free comprehensive health care for life. In the 1960s, the Canadian government started this system with the belief that health care should be accessible to all Canadian citizens.

There are three general types of inpatient units in most hospital settings:

- Critical care units
- Intermediate care units
- Long-term care units (including subacute units)

Critical Care Units

Critical care units are areas for the intense care of critically ill clients. Examples are surgical or medical intensive care units, shock trauma and "step-down" units, and neurosurgical intensive care units. Emergency and operating departments are also considered critical care areas because of the acute and intense nature of the care provided in these parts of the hospital. Critical care areas require nurses who thrive in crisis situations and work effectively under high stress. Nurses must be highly skilled in making accurate observations of clients' conditions and interpreting findings quickly and correctly. The nurse-to-client ratio in critical care units is typically 1:2.

Intermediate Care Units

Intermediate care units have changed dramatically over the past decade. The clients on these units today are much sicker than those in the past. Examples of intermediate care areas are neuroscience (neurology) units, urology units, and orthopedic units. In hospitals that are too small to separate clients by specialty, intermediate care units provide treatment for a combination of medical and surgical health problems.

Nurses in intermediate care areas must be able to adapt to caring for various types of illness and must be interested in health teaching and discharge planning. As in critical care areas, nurses must also be highly skilled in making accurate assessments and performing technical procedures.

Long-Term Care Units

Long-term care (LTC) units are areas within or adjacent to the hospital in which clients have chronic illnesses or health problems requiring constant care and rehabilitation. Examples are rehabilitation and chronic disease units. Some hospitals also offer a skilled nursing facility (SNF) or subacute unit as part of the in-hospital system. Chapter 2 describes long-term care in detail.

Overview of the Nursing Process

The nursing process is an organized, systematic approach used by medical-surgical nurses to meet the individualized health care needs of their clients, families, and communities. The term *nursing process* emerged in the mid-1960s. As nursing became more recognized and respected as a profession, there was a growing need to define more clearly what nurses do.

Comparison of the Nursing Process with the Scientific Method

The nursing process is a decision-making approach that promotes critical thinking. Critical thinking exercises are found in this text at the end of the body system interventions chapters and in the accompanying *Student Study Guide.*

Many books compare the nursing process with the scientific method of solving problems. The steps are similar in the two approaches as they proceed from identification of the problem to evaluation of the solution. However, one difference is that the scientist identifies the problem first and then collects the data. In contrast, the nurse collects the data first and then determines the problem.

Intuitive Judgment in Nursing Practice

Over the past 20 years, research has shown that nurses sometimes use (and should use) intuitive judgment in clinical practice (Benner & Tanner, 1987). *Intuition* is the ability to understand immediately without using formal analysis and is based on experience and knowledge. Intuition helps the nurse act quickly if necessary, particularly in critical care settings or emergency situations in which he or she must assess the client and intervene at once.

The authors of this book use the nursing process as the organizing framework for its content. We do not believe that the nursing process is merely a technical skill with rules that apply in all situations but rather that nurses need to use intuition as well as a scientific basis for nursing care.

Steps of the Nursing Process

Most literature citations list five steps of the nursing process: assessment, analysis (nursing diagnosis), planning, implementation, and evaluation.

The steps initially are followed in sequence, from assessment to evaluation. However, once the nursing process begins, it is continuous or cyclic (Fig. 1–6). For example, if the client's outcomes are not met on the basis of the initial evaluation, the nurse may need to reassess the client or implement new actions to help the client achieve the desired outcomes. To understand the nursing process as a whole, it is first necessary to briefly review each step and its associated activities. A more detailed discussion of the nursing process may be found in basic nursing textbooks.

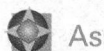 **Assessment**

Assessment, the first step of the nursing process, is a systematic method of collecting data about the client, family, or community for the purpose of identifying actual and potential health problems. The data base is the organization of assessment data and frequently refers to the tool or chart form used to record the data.

Types of Data Bases. Jarvis (1996) names four kinds of data bases: complete; episodic, or problem-centered; follow-up; and emergency.

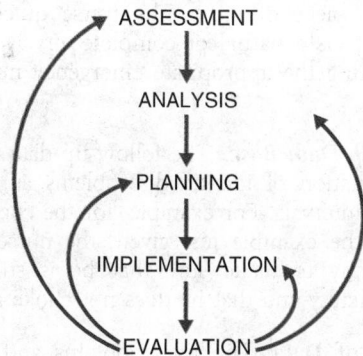

Figure 1–6. The nursing process cycle.

Complete Data Base. The complete, or total, data base includes a thorough health history and physical assessment. In the acute care setting, the data base is usually completed during the first 8 hours after a client's admission to the hospital. In the home, the nurse completes the data base during the first visit. In the nursing home, the nursing assessment is documented within the first 24 hours; the federally mandated interdisciplinary Minimum Data Set (MDS) requires completion within 14 days of admission. For Medicare A residents, the MDS must be completed and electronically transmitted to the Health Care Finance Administration (HCFA) within 7 days of admission. A copy of the MDS is located in the Appendix.

The information collected by the nurse is *not* a repetition of the medical history that the health care provider records. Rather, the nurse collects additional data regarding the client's response to health problems, functional ability, ability to perform activities of daily living, usual health behaviors, coping patterns, health goals, and support systems.

Episodic, or Problem-Centered, Data Base. An episodic data base is collected for a limited or short-term problem. It focuses on one problem, and data collected are associated with the problem. For example, an elderly hospitalized woman falls when trying to get out of bed and complains of hip pain. The nurse's history focuses on how the fall occurred, which parts of the client's body made contact with the floor, and what position she assumed after she fell. The physical assessment is centered on the neurologic and musculoskeletal systems, especially the head, hip, and knee. These data are usually not recorded on a data base form as such, but the information is documented according to agency policy.

In other situations, the nurse documents assessment findings frequently during the day on a flow sheet. For example, the client who is receiving patient-controlled analgesia (PCA) for pain control must be monitored carefully to determine whether the intervention is successful. The Daily Pain/PCA Flow Sheet shown in Figure 1–7 is an episodic data base that requires the nurse to assess and document the client's level of pain and sedation.

Emergency Data Base. The emergency data base is similar to the episodic data base in that the nurse focuses on the immediate problem. However, the assessment must be more rapid to prevent life-threatening consequences. For example, a hospitalized client begins to choke on a piece of meat. The nurse quickly assesses whether there is a partial or complete airway obstruction before selecting the appropriate emergency nursing intervention.

Follow-Up Data Base. The follow-up data base is simply an evaluation of identified problems at regular and appropriate intervals. For example, for the client who was choking in the example just given, the nurse checks on him frequently to make sure that he is still breathing without difficulty and that he does not choke again.

Sources of Data. The nurse obtains and documents data from several sources in the client's medical record according to the policies of the health care agency.

Client. The client is the primary source of data. This information is direct and firsthand and is collected by interview. Interviewing is a communication skill by which a nurse can explore the thoughts, feelings, and perceptions of the client. As in the teaching-learning process, the interview process is affected by many variables, including timing, environment, and demographic factors such as age. Chart 1–3 provides tips for interviewing an elderly person.

A medical history differs from a nursing history. A *medical* history is taken by the health care provider to determine the presence of a pathologic condition and to provide a basis for planning medical care. A *nursing* history is obtained by the nurse and focuses on the meaning of the illness and/or hospitalization to the client and family. It is used as a basis for planning nursing care.

Family and Significant Others. The client's family members or significant others are secondary sources of data. They can often supplement or verify information provided by the client. They may also be able to offer information about the client before the illness, provide family history related to health and illness, and describe the client's home environment.

Records. Previous medical histories, laboratory records, vital signs, and diagnostic reports provide pertinent data.

Chart 1–3

Nursing Focus on the Elderly: Interviewing

- Review old records and the medical history, if available, before interviewing the client
- Provide privacy as much as possible
- Ask the client whether family or significant others should be present during the interview
- Refer to the client by his or her last name (e.g., Mrs. Brown) unless the client prefers another name
- Make sure that eyeglasses, contact lenses, and hearing aids are available and working properly, if the client wears these devices
- Conduct the interview when the client is not experiencing pain and after basic comfort needs have been met
- Before conducting the interview, allow the client to adjust to a new environment
- Sit at the client's eye level during the interview
- Speak clearly, slowly, and in a low-pitched voice; do not shout
- Be aware that the client may not be able to distinguish soft consonant blends, like "sh" or "ch"
- Interview in the morning, after breakfast, or in the early afternoon, after the client has rested
- Use open-ended questions, when possible, to gather more information; avoid questions that can be answered "yes" or "no"
- Consider the client's education, culture, and age when phrasing questions, especially about sensitive or controversial issues
- Observe the client's nonverbal behavior as well as what he or she says

MEMORIAL HOSPITAL AT EASTON, MD. INC.

<u>DAILY PAIN / PCA FLOW SHEET</u>

Initial Assessment & Plan

1. Has MD told pt. about PCA?

　_____ YES _____ NO

2. Does patient verbalize understanding?

　_____ YES _____ NO

3. BP: _____ PULSE: _____

　NOTE:　Actual settings in Blue/Black ink.

Nurse Initials & Signature

Init.	Signature	Init.	Signature

ASSESSMENT INFORMATION

DATE/TIME	DRUG NAME & CONC.	PCA DOSE (ML)	LOCKOUT INTERVAL (MIN.)	4 HR LIMIT (ML)	PAIN LEVEL 0-5	SEDATION LEVEL 1-5	RESPIRATORY RATE	INITIALS	I.E. AMOUNT WASTED, WITNESS, ETC. INJECTOR VIAL CHANGED COMMENTS

<u>LEVEL OF PAIN</u>　　　　<u>SEDATION LEVEL</u>

0 - ASLEEP AT TIME OF CHARTING
1 - COMFORTABLE
2 - MILD DISCOMFORT
3 - IN PAIN
4 - IN BAD PAIN
5 - IN VERY BAD PAIN

1 - ALERT AND AWARE
2 - DROWSY
3 - DOZING INTERMITTENTLY
4 - MOSTLY SLEEPING
5 - DIFFICULT TO AROUSE

REVISED 1/90

FORM# 140265

Figure 1-7. An example of an episodic data base: a Daily Pain/PCA Flow Sheet. (Courtesy of Memorial Hospital at Easton, Easton, MD.)

These data validate information identified in the current history and physical examination or serve as a comparison to indicate changes in the client's health condition. Records from previous admissions to the hospital also supply additional pieces of information. The client's health care provider usually requests the old records from the agency's medical records department or other health care facility where the client has sought health care.

Collaboration. A nurse may gather client information in collaboration with other health care team members. The physician or nurse practitioner is a key source of information. A social worker or home care nurse who has worked with the client can also contribute valuable information.

When a client is admitted to the hospital from another health care facility, such as a nursing home, the hospital nurse should contact the nurse who cared for the client in the facility for specific client information. Most nursing homes supply a nursing transfer form that accompanies the client to the hospital or other facility. The transfer form describes the client's abilities and limitations, drug therapy, diet therapy, and past and current health state. This information is particularly helpful when the client cannot communicate and if no family is available.

 Analysis

The second step of the nursing process is the analysis of data. In this phase, the nurse summarizes and analyzes the data and draws conclusions to determine what health problems the client may have or is at risk for. Client data are compared with "normal" findings and behaviors for the client's age, education, and cultural background. Abnormal data are reviewed to determine patterns of altered functioning. Client health problems are identified and categorized as potential problems requiring prevention or actual problems being managed or requiring interventions.

In a classic book, Aspinall and Tanner (1981) state that nurses make two types of judgments or conclusions about the health state of a client: (1) those health problems that nurses, "by virtue of their education and experience, are licensed and able to treat" (p. 4) (nursing diagnoses) and (2) those problems that are diagnosed and treated by other members of the health team but require continued nursing assessment and implementation of therapeutic interventions (collaborative problems).

This textbook uses nursing diagnoses and collaborative problems that incorporate both types of client health problems.

Nursing Diagnoses. The nursing profession's acknowledgment and endorsement of the term *nursing diagnosis* began in 1973, when the American Nurses' Association (ANA) published its first *Standards of Nursing Practice.* Since then, other countries have also adopted nursing diagnoses as a way to describe client health problems.

In the early 1980s, the North American Nursing Diagnosis Association (NANDA) was formed to serve as the official organization for the development and dissemination of nursing diagnoses. Nurses from all over the world belong to this organization, although most are from countries within North America. The official journal of

NANDA is *Nursing Diagnosis,* which is published quarterly. Other countries or continents such as Europe have formalized nursing diagnosis associations.

Although many definitions of nursing diagnosis have been proposed by various nursing leaders, the authors of this book recognize the official definition approved by NANDA at its Ninth Conference in 1990: "A nursing diagnosis is a clinical judgment about an individual, family, or community response to actual or potential health problems/life processes which provides the basis for definitive therapy toward achievement of outcomes for which the nurse is accountable" (Carpenito, 1995, p. 65).

Unlike medical diagnoses, which identify illness, nursing diagnoses identify the *responses* to health problems and life processes, such as aging or death. A medical diagnosis is the basis for medical interventions; a nursing diagnosis is the basis for nursing interventions. Nursing diagnoses are not diagnostic tests, medical treatments, or problems experienced by the nurse while caring for the client. Table 1–2 differentiates medical and nursing diagnoses. The current nursing diagnosis list is located on the inside back cover of this text.

Collaborative Problems. Collaborative problems, as identified in this text, are potential health problems for which the nurse monitors. The nurse then reports on these problems, if they occur, to the health care provider. Measures that help prevent the problem are implemented. Through keen assessment skills, the nurse detects the health problem as early as possible if it occurs. Then, in collaboration with members of the interdisciplinary care team, he or she carries out interventions to resolve the problem. An example of a collaborative problem is Potential for Hemorrhage following a vaginal hysterectomy.

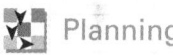 Planning

The planning step follows the analysis step of the nursing process. Throughout the planning process, the nurse performs several important functions: setting priorities and expected outcomes, selecting nursing interventions, and determining resources.

TABLE 1–2

Differentiation Between Medical and Nursing Diagnoses	
Medical Diagnosis	**Nursing Diagnosis**
Identifies the pathologic basis for an illness	Identifies a response to illness
Focuses on the physical condition of the client	Focuses on the physical, psychosocial, and spiritual needs of the client
Addresses actual, existing problems	Addresses actual and potential problems
Is not validated with the client	Is validated with the client if possible
Uses standardized goals and treatments	Uses individualized outcomes and intervention
May not be resolvable	Is usually resolvable

Setting Priorities and Outcomes. After analyzing the needs of the client to identify client health problems, the nurse decides on the urgency of the problems. This step is vital because some problems are more critical than others. Problems of higher priority require more immediate intervention than problems of lower priority. Setting priorities helps the nurse organize and plan care that solves the most urgent problems first.

Establishing Priorities. In determining the priority of the problems, the nurse must consider the impact on the client. Several classic theorists have presented hierarchies that are still used today to assist in determining priorities.

Bower (1972) offers a three-level approach, in descending order of priority:

- First priority—problems that threaten life, dignity, and integrity of the client
- Second priority—problems that destructively change the client
- Third priority—problems that affect normal growth and development

Maslow's hierarchy of needs can also serve as a useful guide for establishing priorities. These needs form five levels. The client progresses up the hierarchy when attempting to satisfy needs. As shown in Figure 1–8, physiologic needs are of greatest priority and must be met first. Once they are met, the client is more willing and able to seek fulfillment of higher-level needs.

Priorities may fluctuate as the client's level of wellness changes. The nurse should consider both actual and high-risk problems when establishing priorities. Actual problems are usually more important than high-risk problems; at times, however, high-risk problems may be more important. For example, in a client who is asthmatic, the high-risk problem of Ineffective Airway Clearance is more life-threatening than an actual problem of constipation.

The establishment of priorities reflects an agreement between the client and nurse when possible. In addition to the guidelines for priorities that theorists have offered, the nurse must be aware of factors such as the client's health goals, the availability of resources, and the client's knowledge of the problem. The priorities of the client are often more important to the client than the priorities outlined by theoretical guidelines.

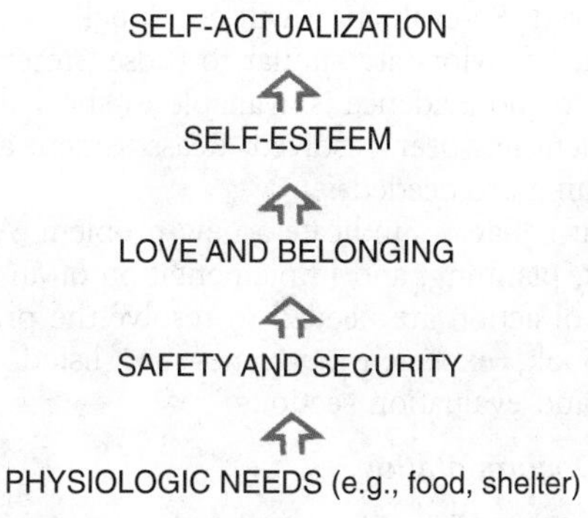

SELF-ACTUALIZATION

⇑

SELF-ESTEEM

⇑

LOVE AND BELONGING

⇑

SAFETY AND SECURITY

⇑

PHYSIOLOGIC NEEDS (e.g., food, shelter)

Figure 1–8. Maslow's hierarchy of needs. Needs must be met in ascending order. For example, safety and security must be achieved before love and belonging.

Establishing Outcomes. After establishing priorities, the client and nurse mutually try to decide on expected outcomes on the basis of identified nursing diagnoses and collaborative problems. Outcomes serve as guides in selecting nursing interventions and in determining criteria for evaluating nursing interventions. The purpose of writing expected outcomes is to assist in the evaluation of the client's progress and to determine resolution, if possible, of the client's problem.

Expected outcomes should be
- Client-centered
- Realistic in terms of the client's potential for achievement and the nurse's ability to help the client achieve them
- Specific and measurable to the extent possible

When writing outcomes, the nurse should state them in a clear, concise manner that can be understood and measured by all health care team members. Any health care professional caring for the client should be able to determine whether the outcomes have been achieved. For example, "The client will state that pain is reduced within 45 minutes after interdisciplinary intervention" is a specific outcome for one client that can be measured easily. If after 45 minutes the client states that pain is reduced, the outcome has been met.

Selecting Nursing Interventions. After determining the outcomes, the nurse develops strategies to accomplish them. Nursing interventions, also known as nursing actions or measures, are designed to assist the client in achieving goals. They are based on the client's health problems and define activities required to promote, maintain, or restore the client's health.

Bulachek and McCloskey (1989) define nursing interventions as "any direct care treatment that a nurse performs on behalf of a client. These treatments included nurse-initiated treatments resulting from nursing diagnoses, physician-initiated treatments resulting from medical diagnoses, and performance of the daily essential functions for the client who cannot do these" (p. 25).

Although the definition of nursing interventions proposed by these experts seems to imply that a nurse performs only treatments or technical skills, these authors have broadened their definition. In a more recent book, Bulechek and McCloskey (1992) discuss interventions that range from physical interventions (positioning, feeding) to psychosocial interventions (therapeutic touch, reminiscence therapy). In 1992 they also published the results of the first phase of the Iowa Intervention Project. This research produced a Nursing Interventions Classification (NIC) system of 336 standardized nursing interventions. Like the development of nursing diagnoses, NIC is intended to help nurses standardize their terminology and practice. Most recently, the authors have developed a Nursing Outcomes Classification (NOC).

Nurse-initiated interventions, also called nurse-prescribed interventions or *nursing orders,* are independent activities that address nursing diagnoses. In the North American Nursing Diagnosis Association (NANDA) definition of nursing diagnosis, "definitive therapy" refers to nurse-initiated interventions. For example, the nurse teaches relaxation techniques for a client experiencing the nursing diagnosis of Ineffective Coping.

For some of the currently approved nursing diagnoses, the nurse may implement health care provider–initiated interventions. For example, the nurse gives analgesic medication to relieve pain. The health care provider prescribes the medication, but the nurse uses clinical judgment about when and how to administer the medication. The nurse may also use non-drug interventions, like imagery or massage, to help reduce the client's pain. Thus, the nurse and health care provider *collaborate* in an effort to resolve the client's problem of pain.

Developing the Collaborative Plan of Care. The collaborative plan of care (POC) is an interdisciplinary document that outlines the essential aspects of client care, often across a time sequence. The format commonly used is a clinical pathway, which is also called a critical path, care map, or coordinated POC.

The clinical pathway delineates what care must be provided, who will provide the care, and when the care will be provided. It is a guideline for care that can be individualized if needed. Most pathways also list expected outcomes for the client, which may be hourly, daily, or weekly, depending on the nature of the health care setting. This textbook provides samples of clinical pathways. When possible, one pathway may view care across the health care continuum.

This text also includes Client Care Plans. Although these plans of care are not interdisciplinary, they are necessary for beginning students to help them follow the steps of the nursing process and to identify the rationale for selected nursing interventions. In most clinical practice settings, this format is no longer used because the accrediting agency for hospitals and other health care facilities, the Joint Commission on the Accreditation of Healthcare Organizations (JCAHO), does not require the use of columnar care plans. Instead, JCAHO requires evidence that nurses plan and implement care based on identified client health problems in collaboration with the interdisciplinary team.

To save time and duplication, a number of computer programs and books have been developed to create standardized plans of care or clinical pathways that can be individualized as needed. As technology advances, these programs should be more widely available to nurses in all health care settings.

Determining Resources. While planning the nursing interventions, the nurse determines which resources are necessary to implement them. The client is a valuable source of information about health care resources that were successful in the past. For example, the client with an irritated stoma may mention that an enterostomal therapist was helpful with previous problems with an ileostomy. Including the client and family in planning care often promotes their cooperation during the implementation phase.

Other nurses and health care team members are valuable resources. An interdisciplinary conference or "walking rounds" during which health care team members

identify problems and resources to solve them may be very helpful, especially for continuing care planning.

When the financial feasibility of the plan is explored, the nurse takes into account the availability of other resources for the client, such as equipment, time, personnel, and money. The client's value system is also considered. For instance, if the client requires dialysis in the home, the type of system implemented depends on the home water supply, electrical capability, space, available money, spiritual beliefs, and personal support system.

 Implementation

Implementation involves the actual carrying out of a specific, individualized POC. This step of the nursing process is the action phase, in which the nurse assumes the responsibility for implementing the POC based on the nursing diagnosis and collaborative problems. Interventions are based on scientific principles and, at times, intuitive judgment.

Because planning and implementation are closely related, this book discusses them under one heading: Planning and Implementation. However, expected outcomes and interventions are clearly labeled.

 Evaluation

Evaluation, the fifth step of the nursing process, is a cognitive activity that completes the nursing process by indicating the degree to which the client's goals have been met.

Although evaluation is given as the final step of the nursing process, it is an ongoing and integral part of each step of the process (see Fig. 1–6). The nurse reviews the data to determine whether sufficient information was collected and whether the behaviors identified were appropriate. Client health problems are evaluated for their accuracy and completeness. The nurse examines the expected outcomes and interventions to determine whether they were realistic, achievable, and effective.

The outcome of evaluation may be one or a combination of the following:

- The client responded as expected and the problem is resolved. No additional nursing actions are needed.
- Client behaviors indicate that the client's problem has not been resolved. Outcomes have been accomplished, but the overall long-term goal has not been achieved. Re-evaluation will continue.
- Client behaviors are similar to those present initially. Little or no evidence is available to show that the problem has been resolved. Reassessment and re-planning are needed.
- Client behaviors indicate a new problem. Assessment, planning, and implementation of an additional plan of action are needed to resolve the problem.

In this book, expected outcomes are listed under the planning and evaluation sections.

Documentation

Documentation of each phase of the nursing process is essential and is accomplished by various means. Two gen-

Date/Time	Focus/Problem	Notes
4/18/98 2:15 P.M.	Fever	D: T = 102.2° (R); face flushed; diaphoretic A: Give Tylenol 2 tab as ordered. Recheck temp. in 1 hr. *R. Jones, RN*
4/18/98 3:15 P.M.	Fever	R: T = 100.2° (R); face not flushed; not diaphoretic *D. Ignas, LPN*
4/19/98 3:30 A.M.	Impaired skin	D: 2-cm reddened area over coccyx; blanches A: Positioned on (L) side *N. Smith, RNC*

Figure 1–9. A sample of focus charting.

eral, traditional methods of documentation are still used in many health care settings: (1) source-oriented charting, which usually includes narrative notes that organize varied data that are entered into the medical record by health care professionals (e.g., nurses' notes, physicians' progress notes, dietary notes) and (2) the problem-oriented record (POR), in which a master health problem list is developed. Each problem is numbered, and all chart entries refer to one of the problems identified on the list.

The notes may be recorded in a SOAP, SOAPIER, or PIE format (or one of its many variations) on the same progress note form in the chart by all health profession-als. The initials represent **S**ubjective data, **O**bjective data, **A**nalysis, **P**lan of action, **I**nterventions, **E**valuation, and **R**evision of the plan. This technique of documentation is systematic and limits data to only pertinent information related to the identified problem. Although this system assists the nurse in addressing each step of the nursing process, it is very time-consuming and promotes duplication of record-keeping. Many physicians, social workers, and dietitians still use the SOAP format, but new systems for nursing documentation have been and are being developed.

Documentation Systems

Focus Charting. A commonly used format in documentation is focus charting. Focus charting is not limited to specific client health problems but, rather, encourages nurses to document any significant changes in the client's condition, any client concern, or any significant client event. As seen in Figure 1–9, the record has three columns. The actual notes are divided into **D**ata, **A**ction, and **R**esponse information. An **E** may be added for documenting client **E**ducation. This technique helps locate desired information but still uses the familiar narrative approach to recording pertinent data.

Charting by Exception. Another system is charting by exception (CBE). CBE was started at St. Luke's Hospital in Milwaukee, Wisconsin, in an attempt to save nursing time. It incorporates three basic components (Burke and Murphy, 1988):

- Comprehensive flow sheets that list normal findings and require the nurse to initial them if they are present. If the findings are not present, the nurse writes an entry into the notes.
- Reference to pre-established nursing standards. The nurse initials the appropriate space when they are completed.

Chart 1–4

Nursing Care Highlight: Legal Tips for Nursing Documentation

- Write clearly and legibly
- Do not erase or "white-out" any part of the client's record
- To correct an error, use one line to cross out the incorrect entry, then initial the change
- Use only standard and facility-approved abbreviations and symbols
- Document significant information as close as possible to the time it is collected instead of waiting until the end of a shift
- Transcribe physicians' orders carefully and correctly
- If using nurses' notes or progress notes, do not leave blank spaces between entries
- Time and date each entry on the client's record
- Use only blue or black ink (it visualizes best for copies or microfilm)
- Document like a reporter: State facts objectively and avoid judgment or criticism
- Do not state that "an incident report has been completed" or refer to any unusual occurrence or special event as an "incident"
- Follow all facility policies for documentation
- To add one or two words, use a caret (^) and insert the words, then initial the change; if agency policy does not allow this practice, write a late entry
- To make a late entry, begin by stating that it is a "Late entry for (date and time);" if the entry is more than a day late, state the reason for the late entry (e.g., "on vacation for 3 days")
- If an order is discontinued on the record as indicated by a highlighter, be sure that the original can still be read, especially on copies

		2300-0300	0300-0700	0700-1100	1100-1500	1500-1900	1900-2300
MENTAL	ALERT - ORIENTED X 3						
	COOPERATIVE						
	EMOTIONAL SUPPORT						
CARDIOVASCULAR	RADIAL PULSE REGULAR						
	MONITOR						
	(CIRCLE) COMPRESSION STOCKINGS / TEDS						
	CIRCULATION CHECKS Q HRS TO						
	A.V. GRAFT THRILL & BRUIT						
RESPIRATORY	RESPIRATIONS EASY AND REGULAR						
	BREATH SOUNDS CLEAR						
	FREQUENT BREATH SOUNDS Q						
	DYSPNEA ON EXERTION						
	O_2 L/MIN VIA						
	O_2 VIA % VENTI-MASK						
	POST-OP COUGH & DEEP BREATH						
	SUCTIONED VIA						
	TRACH CARE						
	COUGH						
	HUMIDIFIER						
	ORAL / NASAL AIRWAY UTILIZED						
IV THERAPY	IV SITE PATENT WITHOUT SIGNS OF INFECTION/ INFILTRATION						
	SOLUTION AND RATE CHECKED						
	IVAC						
	(CIRCLE) HEP LOCK / CENTRAL LINE PATENT W/O SIGNS OF INFECTION/ INFILTRATION						
	PCA						
	BLOOD						
TREATMENT	FINGERSTICK BLOOD SUGAR						
	HYPO/HYPER THERMIA MACHINE						
	ISOLATION						
	PAIN MANAGEMENT						
MUSCULOSKEL	CIRCULATION CHECKS						
	CPM						
	TRACTION						
	IMMOBILIZATION DEVICE						
	(CIRCLE) CAST / SPLINT LOCATION						
	TEMP PUMP						
DIRECTIVES	PLAN OF CARE WRITTEN						
	(CIRCLE) PLAN OF CARE REVIEWED / REVISED						
	ATTENDING PHYSICIAN IN						
	CONSULTING PHYSICIAN IN						
	PATIENT TEACHING						
MISC							

Figure 1–10. A portion of a daily flow sheet used for charting by exception. (Courtesy of Dorchester General Hospital, Cambridge, MD.)

■ Bedside accessibility of forms. All flow sheets are kept at the bedside, which prevents wasting the nursing time in looking for a client's chart. Bedside charting also prevents transcription of data from one form to another, which can lead to errors as well as wasted time. The information is available for any health care professional to read.

Like all charting systems, variations of the concept are being implemented. A portion of a flow sheet used in a CBE system is found in Figure 1–10.

Computerized Nursing Information Systems. A major advantage of documentation systems, such as CBE, is the ability to transfer the concept to computerization. Bedside computer charting, also known as point-of-care charting and online documentation, is beginning to appear in hospitals, nursing homes, home care agencies, and ambulatory care settings.

The literature suggests that the major advantages of point-of-care documentation are accuracy and time savings. Electronic charting at the bedside also increases the time that the nurse spends in the client's room. Kirk (1995) noted that in addition to improving the quality of care, handheld documentation devices decreased costly nursing overtime. The goal of any system should be to streamline or diminish paperwork and save valuable nursing time, giving nurses more time for direct client care.

The Methodist Hospital in Arcadia, California, established criteria for point-of-care technology, including the following (Gianni, Beasley, & Linson, 1996):

- It must take the same time as or less time than manual charting.
- Radio frequency must be reliable, with no lost data.
- Charting cannot be redundant.
- Hardware must be standardized on all units.
- Assistance is readily available.

Legal Aspects of Documentation. Regardless of the type of documentation system used, the nurse remembers that the client's chart is a legal document. Chart 1–4 lists basic charting guidelines that all nurses should follow.

SELECTED BIBLIOGRAPHY

Albright, J., de Guzman, C., Acebo, P., et al. (1996). Readability of patient education materials: Implications for clinical practice. *Applied Nursing Research, 9,* 139–143.

Allen, K. M., & Phillips, J. M. (1997). *Women's health across the lifespan: A comprehensive perspective.* Philadelphia: Lippincott-Raven.

*Aspinall, M. J., & Tanner, C. (1981). *Decision-making for patient care.* Norwalk, CT: Appleton & Lange.

Barry, R., & Burggraf, V. (1996). Healthy people: Objective look at the elderly. *Journal of Gerontological Nursing, 22*(10), 9–11.

*Benner, P., & Tanner, C. (1987). How expert nurses use intuition. *American Journal of Nursing, 87,* 23–31.

*Bower, F. (1972). *The process of planning nursing care.* St. Louis: C. V. Mosby.

*Bulechek, G., & McCloskey, J. (1989). Nursing interventions: Treatments for potential nursing diagnoses. In R. M. Carroll-Johnson (Ed.), *Classification of nursing diagnoses: Proceedings of the eighth conference* (pp. 23–30). Philadelphia: J. B. Lippincott.

*Bulechek, G. M., & McCloskey, J. C. (1992). *Nursing interventions: Essential nursing treatments* (2nd ed.). Philadelphia: W. B. Saunders.

*Burke, L. J., & Murphy, J. (1988). *Charting by exception: A cost-effective, quality approach.* New York: John Wiley.

Bush, A. M. P., & Ebel, C. A. (1996). Testing an electronic documentation system. *Nursing Management, 27*(7), 40–42.

Carpenito, L. J. (1995). *Nursing care plans and documentation: Nursing diagnoses and collaborative problems.* Philadelphia: J. B. Lippincott.

Castillo, H., & Torres, S. (1995). Cultural considerations: Providing quality nursing care to Hispanics. *Imprint, 42*(5), 52–55.

Chen, M. S., & Hawks, B. L. (1995). A debunking of the myth of the healthy Asian Americans and Pacific Islanders. *American Journal of Health Promotion, 8,* 261–268.

Clay, J. C., Wyatt, L. K., & Norris, G. M. (1996). Patient and family education: An interdisciplinary process. *MEDSURG Nursing, 5*(5), 333–338, 354.

Cordell, B. (1994). Streamlined charting for patient education. *Nursing94, 24*(1), 57–59.

Douglas, C. Y. (1995). Cultural considerations for the African-American population. *Imprint, 42*(5), 57–59.

*Dunn, H. L. (1980). *High level wellness.* Thorofare, NJ: Charles B. Slack.

Eggland, E. T. (1995). Charting smarter—Using mechanisms to organize your paperwork. *Nursing95, 25*(9), 35–41.

Gianni, N., Beasley, E., & Linson, D. (1996). Online documentation: Making it work with POC technology. *Health Management Technology, April,* 46–50.

Gruber, M. (1995). Documentation is communication. *Gastroenterology Nursing, 18*(3), 107–108.

Ignatavicius, D. D., & Hausman, K. (1995). *Clinical pathways for collaborative practice.* Philadelphia: W. B. Saunders.

Jarvis, C. (1996). *Physical examination and health assessment* (2nd ed.). Philadelphia: W. B. Saunders.

Johnson, D., & Martin, K. (1996). Preparing for electronic documentation. *Nursing Management, 27*(7), 43–44.

Jones, M., & Nies, M. A. (1996). The relationship of perceived benefits of and barriers to reported exercise in older African American woman. *Public Health Nursing, 13,* 151–158.

King, C., & Macmillan, M. (1994). Documentation and discharge planning for elderly patients. *Nursing Times, 90*(20), 31–33.

Kirk, T. (1995). On the front lines of patient care. *Healthcare Informatics, June,* 50, 54.

Krause, C. R., Westdorp, J. M., Coonen, D. A., & Jenks, D. L. (1996). Forming an integrated documentation system. *Nursing Management, 27*(8), 25–26.

Leddy, S. K. (1996). Development and psychometric testing of the Leddy Healthiness Scale. *Research in Nursing and Health, 19,* 431–440.

Louie, K. B. (1995). Cultural considerations: Asian-Americans and Pacific Islanders. *Imprint, 42*(5), 41–46.

*Maslow, A. (1970). *Motivation and personality.* New York: Harper & Row.

Maidwell, A. (1996). The role of the surgical nurse as a health promoter. *British Journal of Nursing, 5*(15), 898–904.

*McCloskey, J. C., & Bulechek, G. M. (1992). *Nursing interventions classification (NIC).* St. Louis: Mosby-Year Book.

Northam, S. (1996). Access to health promotion, protection, and disease prevention among impoverished individuals. *Public Health Nursing, 13,* 353–364.

*Pender, N. J. (1987). *Health promotion in nursing practice* (2nd ed.). Norwalk, CT: Appleton & Lange.

Rasmussen, N., & Gengler, T. (1994). Clinical pathways of care: The route to better communication. *Nursing94, 24*(2), 47–49.

Schielke, C. (1997). Patient advocacy: The shield that empowers. *Continuing Care, 16*(3), 22–26.

*U.S. Department of Health and Human Services, Public Health Service. (1990). *Healthy people 2000: National health promotion and disease prevention objectives.* Washington, D. C.: U.S. Government Printing Office.

Weiler, K. (1994). Legal aspects of nursing documentation for the Alzheimer's patient. *Journal of Gerontological Nursing, 20*(4), 31–40.

*World Health Organization. (1947). *Constitution of the World Health Organization: Chronicle of the World Health Organization.* Geneva: Author.

Zander, K., & McGill, R. (1994). Critical and anticipated recovery paths: Only the beginning. *Nursing Management, 25*(8), 34–40.

Zink, M. R. (1994). Nursing diagnosis in home care: Audit tool development. *Journal of Community Health Nursing, 11*(1), 51–58.

SUGGESTED READINGS

Castillo, H., & Torres, S. (1995). Cultural considerations: Providing quality nursing care to Hispanics. *Imprint, 42*(5), 52–55.

This article begins with a thorough description of the demographic characteristics of the Hispanic population in the United States. The authors then discuss health care beliefs and health status of Hispanics. Finally, they make suggestions regarding how to use the nursing process with this growing subgroup of the population.

Clay, J. C., Wyatt, L. K., & Norris, G. M. (1996). Patient and family education: An interdisciplinary process. *MEDSURG Nursing, 5*(5), 333–338, 354.

This article describes an interdisciplinary education and discharge plan developed in a 404-bed teaching hospital. The Learner Assessment, Education Plan, and Discharge Plan forms are included in the article to demonstrate the necessary documentation.

Louie, K. B. (1995). Cultural considerations: Asian-Americans and Pacific Islanders. *Imprint, 42*(5), 41–46.

The author points out that there are 23 subgroups of Asian-Americans and a number of subgroups of Pacific Islanders living in the United States. The article disputes a 1985 report that concluded that the AAPI population is at a lower risk of early death than the Caucasian population. Newer findings show that this fast-growing minority group has higher mortality rates when compared with other groups, especially for lung cancer and cardiovascular disease. The remainder of the article describes specific characteristics of some of the Asian-American subgroups.

CONTINUING CARE

Continuing care for medical-surgical clients can be provided in a number of settings. Continuing care may be needed after a hospital or nursing home stay or as an alternative to inpatient hospital care. Although the majority of health care currently occurs in the hospital, the trend is rapidly moving toward care in alternative settings, such as ambulatory care, home care, and long-term care in rehabilitation centers, nursing homes, and chronic care facilities. This chapter provides a brief description of each of these settings.

This textbook covers care for clients in all settings in which medical-surgical nurses practice. Continuing Care sections after discussions of major health problems highlight the most important aspects of care in nonhospital environments.

AMBULATORY CARE

Ambulatory health care is a general term for client care provided in myriad community settings, such as physician offices, hospital or freestanding outpatient clinics, freestanding surgicenters, and health maintenance organizations, a type of managed-care organization (see Chap. 3). The purpose of ambulatory care is health promotion, health protection (illness prevention), short-term treatment, and follow-up for existing health problems.

Client visits to ambulatory care settings are episodic and based on need. For example, clients may visit their health care provider for annual physical examinations (health promotion). Alternatively, they may seek out providers for acute health care problems or selected surgeries, such as cataract removal or laparoscopic cholecystectomy (removal of the gallbladder). Still others are monitored periodically for chronic health conditions, such as diabetes mellitus and hypertension.

Clients discharged from the hospital are frequently followed in one or more ambulatory care settings. The cost of ambulatory care is typically far less than that provided by a nursing home or home care agency.

Role of the Nurse in Ambulatory Care

One of the major roles of the nurse working in an ambulatory care setting is health promotion activities, including client education, health screening, and comprehensive assessment. In a surgicenter, for example, the nurse provides preoperative teaching to prepare clients for the surgical procedure and postoperative expectations. Clients' vital signs and general condition are assessed to ensure that clients are ready to have the surgery.

Some physician offices employ nurses to assist in their practice. These nurses often triage clients who call; that is, the nurse decides which clients need priority care and intervenes accordingly. In some parts of the country, large physician practices employ nurse case managers who monitor high-risk, high-cost, problem-prone clients throughout the continuum of health care in all settings. Case management is discussed in Chapter 3.

Nursing Community Centers

Nursing community centers are ambulatory care settings operated by nurses. Although the organizational structure and services provided vary among centers, most centers are affiliated with large university schools of nursing. The primary health care providers are typically nurse practitioners, nurse midwives, clinical nurse specialists, and students preparing to become one of these advanced-practice specialists. Funding for nursing community centers also varies. Some monies come from city, state, and federal governments, whereas others come from grants obtained by university faculty.

HOME CARE

Home care in the United States is a diverse and rapidly growing industry. For many clients, the home is the lowest-cost health care setting.

History of Home Care Nursing

Modern home care nursing has its roots in public health nursing and community health nursing models. In the mid-1880s, visiting nurse associations evolved in Philadelphia, Boston, and Buffalo, New York. The traditions of Lillian Wald, regarded as the founder of public health nursing, began with the Henry Street Settlement in New York City in 1893.

Home care, however, was a small entity until the passage of the Medicare Law in 1965. At that time, Medicare required agencies to provide a minimum of nursing services plus one additional service, such as physical or occupational therapy, speech-language pathology, medical social services, or home health aide services. The advent of Medicare began the trend toward and basis for reimbursement of home care services. In 1963, 3 years before Medicare became law, it has been estimated that there were only 1100 home care programs. Today, more than 16,000 home care organizations provide some kind of

service or product to clients in their homes. About one half of these are Medicare certified and provide skilled nursing services.

Many factors have contributed to the growth and acceptance of home care, including the following:

- The continued shift from inpatient-based care to community-based and home care
- The increasing need for health care for the elderly
- Technology, such as mobile x-ray machines, apnea monitors, electrocardiography (ECG) machines, and others that help clients remain at home
- The increased general acceptance of home care as a care site
- The generally lower cost of home care (compared with inpatient care)
- The hospitals' continuing incentives to reduce lengths of stays in a managed-care environment
- The growth of hospital-based home health agencies

Types of Home Care

The term *home care* can be confusing and can refer to different kinds of products or services. There are different specialty areas within the home care industry, and nurses may work in any of these segments (Fig. 2–1). In addition, some companies may provide all or just one of these home care segments. There are generally four markets or segments of the home health care industry.

1. The home medical equipment (HME) market, which can also include durable medical equipment (DME) (such as hospital beds and wheelchairs). HME companies provide products to clients such as walkers, beds, wheelchairs, oxygen equipment, and other equipment. Medicare and other insurers pay for products that are "covered" (reimbursed) based on the insurance programs rules.
2. The home infusion or intravenous (IV) company. These companies deliver and administer infusion therapies in the client's home. Home infusion includes antibiotic therapies, hyperalimentation, blood and blood products, and other infusion therapies. Nursing services may be covered under Medicare or

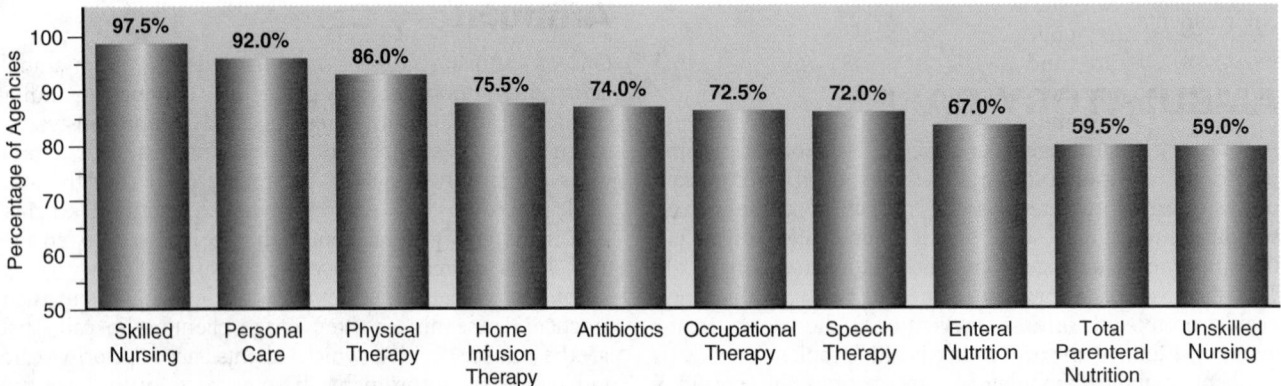

Figure 2–1. Ten most commonly offered home care services. (Courtesy of Marion Merrell Dow, Inc., Managed Care Digest Series, *Institutional Digest*, 1995, and SMG Marketing Group, Inc.)

other insurers for such services as IV site care and observation and assessment. The medications may or may not be reimbursed based on the insurance or managed-care company's rules.

3. Personal care or private duty services. These agencies may provide "shifts" of nurses or home health aides or private duty nurses to clients in their homes. They may provide other services such as respite for caregivers, homemakers, and meal preparation, among others. Usually these services are paid for privately by the client or family. Some insurance programs may pay for limited services related to health care based on medical necessity.

4. Skilled home care services (the largest type). These agencies employ most of the home care nurses as well as other health professionals to provide care as needed. Skilled home care services are provided by home care organizations that are usually Medicare certified and provide the six services of nursing, physical and occupational therapy, speech-language pathology services, medical social services, and home health aides. They may also provide dietitian services and have specialists such as enterostomal therapist nurses or others based on the program's mission. The interdisciplinary aspects of home care make it truly client centered.

Role of the Nurse in Home Care

Home health nursing is a synthesis of community health nursing and selected skills from other specialty nursing practices. In 1986 the American Nurses' Association (ANA) published its *Standards of Home Health Nursing Practice*, identifying home care nursing as a component of community health nursing that incorporates public health principles and practice. The standards include both health promotion and care of the sick and are targeted toward communities, families, and individuals. Activities necessary to achieve goals may warrant preventive, maintenance, and restorative emphasis to avoid potential deficits from developing (ANA, 1986).

Home care has come to mean a variety of specialized and generalized nursing care provided to clients whose primary health care site is their home. Adult health (medical-surgical) care, child care, perinatal care, elder care, mental health care, and many other specialties are practiced routinely in the community setting by home care nurses. Effective home care nursing incorporates aspects of comprehensive assessment skills of community health with technology and "hi-touch" care of skilled, caring nursing intervention, planning, and evaluation (Table 2–1).

Home care nursing incorporates the client care plan with effective care coordination and ongoing communication, also called *case management*. In addition, in home care, collaborative communication among team members, along with active and ongoing client participation, ensures that clients are truly equal partners in their health care.

TABLE 2–1

Major Differences Between Nursing Care in the Home and Inpatient Settings

Home Setting	Inpatient Setting
Nurse is more autonomous.	Nurse relies heavily on physician directives.
Environment is controlled by the client.	Environment is controlled by the facility and its staff.
Nurse must be knowledgeable about care of all types and ages of clients.	Nurse is typically knowledgeable about care of specific types of clients, often based on diagnosis.
Nurse must know reimbursement for home care and document care accordingly.	Financial officer and accounting department usually handle reimbursement.
For elderly clients, only selected skilled services are reimbursed by Medicare.	For elderly clients, hospital care is largely reimbursed by Medicare.
There is limited direct supervision of assistive staff, such as home health aides.	There is continuous direct supervision of assistive staff. Nurse and staff work on a single unit.

Home Visits

Home care is usually provided in "visits," not shifts or hours as in the inpatient area. A visit is usually composed of preparation time for the client's visit, such as telephone calls to the physician for clarification of orders for the client's care, obtaining and organizing needed supplies (e.g., wound dressings, catheters, venipuncture supplies), and equipment or insurance authorization of care. There is also travel time, such as driving to clients' homes, and the actual visit time spent in the home for the provision of ordered care. In addition, there is the time for completion of assessment findings, analysis, and care planning and the completion of required, often lengthy documentation.

The usual number of visits per day can vary from four to seven. Clearly, the range is based on the geographic location of the clients and the distance between them, the unique needs of the clients (examples of long visits would be the admitting visit or those involving very ill or terminally ill clients), as well as other factors. The actual client assignments are usually based on the diagnosis and the nurse's expertise as well as physical location.

Client Plan of Care

Like other care settings, a physician's order is needed for care interventions and care plan changes. Because home care nursing practice is more autonomous than in many traditional inpatient settings, it is imperative that orders are obtained from physicians for care and care changes. Sometimes physicians do not see the home care client for months and rely on the home care nurse's judgments and reports. Therefore, verbal or telephone orders are a large

Department of Health and Human Services
Health Care Financing Administration

Form Approved
OMB No. 0938-0357

HOME HEALTH CERTIFICATION AND PLAN OF CARE

1. Patient's HI Claim No.	2. Start Of Care Date	3. Certification Period		4. Medical Record No.	5. Provider No.
		From:	To:		

6. Patient's Name and Address

7. Provider's Name, Address and Telephone Number

8. Date of Birth	9. Sex ☐ M ☐ F

10. Medications: Dose/Frequency/Route (N)ew (C)hanged

11. ICD-9-CM	Principal Diagnosis	Date

12. ICD-9-CM	Surgical Procedure	Date

13. ICD-9-CM	Other Pertinent Diagnoses	Date

14. DME and Supplies

15. Safety Measures:

16. Nutritional Req.

17. Allergies:

18.A. Functional Limitations
1 ☐ Amputation   5 ☐ Paralysis   9 ☐ Legally Blind
2 ☐ Bowel/Bladder (Incontinence)   6 ☐ Endurance   A ☐ Dyspnea With Minimal Exertion
3 ☐ Contracture   7 ☐ Ambulation   B ☐ Other (Specify)
4 ☐ Hearing   8 ☐ Speech

18.B. Activities Permitted
1 ☐ Complete Bedrest   6 ☐ Partial Weight Bearing   A ☐ Wheelchair
2 ☐ Bedrest BRP   7 ☐ Independent At Home   B ☐ Walker
3 ☐ Up As Tolerated   8 ☐ Crutches   C ☐ No Restrictions
4 ☐ Transfer Bed/Chair   9 ☐ Cane   D ☐ Other (Specify)
5 ☐ Exercises Prescribed

19. Mental Status: 1 ☐ Oriented   3 ☐ Forgetful   5 ☐ Disoriented   7 ☐ Agitated
2 ☐ Comatose   4 ☐ Depressed   6 ☐ Lethargic   8 ☐ Other

20. Prognosis: 1 ☐ Poor   2 ☐ Guarded   3 ☐ Fair   4 ☐ Good   5 ☐ Excellent

21. Orders for Discipline and Treatments (Specify Amount/Frequency/Duration)

22. Goals/Rehabilitation Potential/Discharge Plans

23. Nurse's Signature and Date of Verbal SOC Where Applicable:	25. Date HHA Received Signed POT

24. Physician's Name and Address	26. I certify/recertify that this patient is confined to his/her home and needs intermittent skilled nursing care, physical therapy and/or speech therapy or continues to need occupational therapy. The patient is under my care, and I have authorized the services on this plan of care and will periodically review the plan.
27. Attending Physician's Signature and Date Signed	28. Anyone who misrepresents, falsifies, or conceals essential information required for payment of Federal funds may be subject to fine, imprisonment, or civil penalty under applicable Federal laws.

Form HCFA-485 (U-4) (02-94)

Figure 2–2. Health Care Financing Administration Form 485.

part of home care practice and communication with physicians. For Medicare clients, physicians must sign HCFA Form 485, which is the client's home health certification and plan of care (Fig. 2–2).

Medicare pays for 15 skills that are attributable to nursing knowledge and licensure. Medicare coverage is predicated on the client meeting defined eligibility criteria (e.g., the client is a Medicare beneficiary, Medicare is the correct payer, the client is homebound [see Homebound Consideration]), and other rules. These 15 skills are

1. Observation and assessment of the client's condition when only the specialized skills of a medical professional can determine a client's status
2. Management and evaluation of a client care plan
3. Teaching and training activities
4. Administration of medications
5. Tube feedings
6. Nasopharyngeal and tracheostomy suctioning
7. Catheters
8. Wound care
9. Ostomy care
10. Heat treatments
11. Gas administration, such as oxygen
12. Rehabilitation nursing
13. Venipuncture
14. Nursing visits
15. Psychiatric evaluation and therapy

Documentation Systems

Reimbursement for home health care relies heavily on the documentation of care. In many home care and other community-based settings, the Omaha Problem Classification System is used instead of the nursing diagnoses from the North American Nursing Diagnosis Association (see Chap. 1). The Omaha system delineates four general areas that represent community and home health practice and provide organizational groupings for client problems: environmental, psychosocial, physiologic, and health-related behaviors. More than 40 nursing diagnoses with modifiers, such as potential deficit, deficit, and health promotion, are then listed within their appropriate domains (Martin & Scheet, 1992). The Omaha Problem Classification System may be found in the Appendix.

NURSING HOME CARE

Long-term care (LTC) has become synonymous in clinical practice with nursing home or chronic care. However, LTC for adult clients with medical-surgical problems occurs in either the home or in facilities such as nursing homes, subacute units, or rehabilitation centers. In general, LTC implies that clients receive care for a prolonged period of time, usually weeks or months. A small percentage of clients may remain in a facility indefinitely, perhaps a lifetime.

Nursing homes in the United States provide care for clients with physical and cognitive impairments as well as those with chronic illness. Clients admitted to a nursing home are called *residents* because the facility is considered their home. The majority of residents are female and older than 65. However, nursing homes are experiencing an increase in the number of younger residents as people live longer with debilitating chronic illnesses, such as multiple sclerosis and muscular dystrophy.

Nursing homes are undergoing another major change. If Medicare certified, most facilities increasingly admit short-term (1–3 weeks) residents for rehabilitation or recovery from an illness or injury. Many of these clients are discharged from hospitals "quicker and sicker," and these individuals often require complex care.

Types of Nursing Homes

Nursing homes can be divided into residential care homes, nursing facilities, and skilled nursing facilities. Some nursing homes are part of retirement communities, and others have specialty units, such as dementia, ventilator, or subacute units.

Residential facilities include domiciliary homes, care homes, rest homes, assisted-living facilities, and group homes. Most of these facilities are small and much like boarding homes before the advent of Medicare (Ignatavicius, 1998). The typical resident in a residential facility is fairly independent and able to perform most or all self-care activities.

Formerly called intermediate care facilities, *nursing facilities* (NFs) provide an intermediate level of care. Certified, licensed NFs receive Medicaid funding for the care of residents who cannot independently perform activities of daily living. Each state has specific guidelines for reimbursement.

Skilled nursing facilities (SNFs, pronounced "snifs") provide care that requires licensed health care professionals, such as nurses and therapists. Only a small portion of most nursing home residents are categorized as skilled and are, therefore, eligible for Medicare reimbursement. Examples of skilled care include tube feedings, daily rehabilitation for postoperative fractured hips, and care of stage 3 and 4 wounds.

Role of the Nurse in Nursing Home Care

Nurses employed by nursing homes are generally more autonomous than those working in hospitals. Physicians are usually not present in the LTC facility on a continuous basis, because residents are considered to be more medically "stable" than those in acute care. However, with early discharge, nursing home nurses are caring for sicker residents than in the past.

Most nurses are placed "in charge" of a unit or shift, because there are more unlicensed personnel (geriatric nursing assistants) than professional nurses. Therefore, the nursing home or LTC nurse needs leadership, management, and clinical competencies to function in this interdisciplinary care environment. One nurse may be the only nurse on that unit in charge of 30 to 35 residents.

SUBACUTE CARE

Subacute care (SAC), one of the newest concepts in health care, is designed for clients who are too ill to be discharged from the hospital to a traditional nursing

TABLE 2–2

Categories of Subacute Care

Definition of Category	Examples of Services
Transitional Subacute Care	
A substitute or alternative for continued hospital stays	Deep wound management Stroke rehabilitation Vascular or cardiac surgery Oncology surgery with chemotherapy Medically complex care Complicated orthopedic surgery
Medical-Surgical Subacute Care	
A setting for stable residents who require moderate level of care	Uncomplicated orthopedic surgery Individuals with human immunodeficiency virus Intravenous therapy Uncomplicated tracheostomy care Stroke rehabilitation
Chronic Subacute Care	
A setting for residents with little or no hope of recovery	Long-term comatose residents Ventilator-dependent residents Progressive neurologic diseases
Long-Term Transitional Subacute Care	
A setting for medically complex conditions with residents	Acute ventilator support Medically complex residents requiring an extended stay

Data from Stahl, D. A. (1994). Subacute care: The future of health care. *Nursing Management, 25*(10), 34–40. Used with permission from Ignatavicius, D. D. (1998). *Introduction to long term care nursing: Principles and practice.* Philadelphia: F. A. Davis.

home or the client's own home. SAC "fills the gap" between the hospital and LTC. Most SAC units are located in freestanding nursing home settings; a smaller percentage are located in hospital settings.

The American Health Care Association (AHCA), which represents the long-term care industry, defines subacute care as a "comprehensive inpatient program designed for the individual who has an acute event as a result of an illness, injury or exacerbation (flare-up) of a disease process; has a determined course of treatment; and does not require intensive diagnostic and/or invasive procedures" (AHCA, 1994). About one third of health care provided by SA units are rehabilitation services; the remainder are medical-surgical services (Stahl, 1994).

Types of Subacute Care

Most SAC units are part of traditional nursing homes. Some units are diagnostic specific, whereas others admit clients with a variety of health problems. Health problems for SAC can be divided into four broad categories: transitional, general medical-surgical, chronic, and long-term

transitional SAC (Stahl, 1994). Table 2–2 lists examples of services provided by each type.

Role of the Nurse in Subacute Care

Little has been published about the role of the nurse in SAC. Nurses who work in SAC must be knowledgeable about LTC and have medical-surgical, critical care, or rehabilitation skills, depending on the type of unit in which they work.

Few nurses have a background that encompasses all of the necessary SAC skills. Nursing homes and hospitals employing nurses for their units are responsible for educating them to ensure that clients' needs are met.

REHABILITATIVE CARE

Rehabilitation is designed for clients who have experienced an acute injury or illness or for those coping with chronic conditions. Rehabilitation services may be provided in the home setting, nursing home, or rehabilitation unit or center. Chapter 13 discusses rehabilitation of individuals with chronic or disabling health problems in detail.

SELECTED BIBLIOGRAPHY

American Health Care Association. (1994). *Blueprint for the future vision.* Washington, DC: Author.
American Nurses' Association. (1986). *Standards of home health nursing practice.* Washington, DC: Author.
Anderson, A. (1996). Nursing clinics in urban settings. *Home Healthcare Nurse, 14,* 542–546.
Bradley, P. J., & Alpers, R. (1996). Home healthcare nurses should regain their family focus. *Home Healthcare Nurse, 14,* 281–288.
Brown-Goebler, S. (1994). Subacute care: Nursing for the next century. *MedSurg Nursing, 3,* 497–499.
Erickson, G. P. (1996). Clinical pearls for home health nursing: Recollections from an oral history. *Home Healthcare Nurse, 14,* 907–913.
Hyatt, L. (1995). *Subacute care: Redefining healthcare.* Burr Ridge, IL: Irmin Professional.
Ignatavicius, D. D. (1998). *Introduction to long term care nursing: Principles and practice.* Philadelphia: F. A. Davis.
Jones, A. M., & Foster, N. (1997). Transitional care: Bridging the gap. *MedSurg Nursing, 6*(1), 32–38.
Marrelli, T. (1994). *Handbook of home health standards and documentation guidelines for reimbursement.* St. Louis: C. V. Mosby.
Marrelli, T., & Hilliard, L. S. (1996). *Home care and clinical paths.* St. Louis: C. V. Mosby.
Marrelli, T., & Whittier, S. (1996). *Home health aide: Guidelines for care.* Westerville, OH: Marrelli.
Martin, K. S., & Scheet, N. J. (1992). *The Omaha system: Applications for community health nursing.* Philadelphia: W. B. Saunders.
Stahl, D. A. (1994). Subacute care: The future of health care. *Nursing Management, 25*(10), 34–40.
Walsh, G. G. (1995). How subacute care fills the gap. *Nursing95, 25*(3), 51.

SUGGESTED READINGS

Anderson, A. (1996). Nursing clinics in urban settings. *Home Healthcare Nurse, 14,* 542–546.
This article examines the roots of nurse-managed clinics and describes the experience of the Regis College School of Nursing as they developed and implemented two nursing clinics in elderly housing establishments in Boston. The school collaborated with a large medical center in creating the clinics to provide care as well as excellent practice for both students and faculty.

Brown-Goebler, S. (1994). Subacute care: Nursing for the next century. *MedSurg Nursing, 3,* 497–499.

This article emphasizes the growth of subacute care and the corresponding opportunities in the 21st century. It describes the purpose and components of subacute care as well as the roles and skills of nurses working in subacute units.

Ignatavicius, D. D. (1998). *Introduction to long term care nursing: Principles and practice.* Philadelphia: F. A. Davis.

This concise reference focuses on care in the nursing home, the largest component of the long-term care industry. The first half of the book explores clinical issues, such as common health problems, comprehensive assessment, and medication use. The second half discusses the role of nurses as leaders in the nursing home (e.g., the charge nurse, the survey process, and total quality management).

Chapter 3

INTRODUCTION TO MANAGED CARE AND CASE MANAGEMENT

CHAPTER HIGHLIGHTS

Until the 1980s, health care costs in the United States escalated at a much greater rate than the general inflation rate. Duplication and fragmentation of health care services, as well as advanced technology, have contributed to rising costs.

Since the late 1980s, managed care has grown to be the largest provider system for health care in the United States. Managed health care is a system that "seeks to control the cost of health care by using a select group of providers, who have agreed to a predetermined payment, with the clinical intervention being managed via utilization and/or a case management process" (Owens, p. 1). In other words, the managed care concept integrates providing health care with paying for health care in an attempt to control costs while ensuring the quality of care.

MANAGED CARE

The managed care system is very different from the traditional way of paying for health care. Prior to the managed care movement, hospitals, physicians, and other health care providers were paid by health insurance companies on the basis of what the providers billed for their services. Under this *fee-for-service* arrangement, two physi-

cians could perform identical services but could bill at their own rates. For example, one physician might bill $3000 for a surgical procedure, and another might bill $1800 for the same service. Therefore, under the fee-for-service system, the "risk" was largely taken by the insurance companies.

Purpose of Managed Care

Managed care organizations (MCOs) seek to standardize costs and keep them reasonable. Under the managed care payment system, health care providers receive a uniform amount of money for each client; this is referred to as a *capitated reimbursement system* (Table 3–1).

Balancing costs with quality is an important concept for managed care. Health care providers have been concerned that some MCOs may be too focused on saving money rather than providing high-quality client care (Powell, 1996). The National Committee for Quality Assurance (NCQA) reviews and accredits MCOs that demonstrate high-quality care.

As discussed in Chapter 1, an important role for the nurse is to advocate for clients to ensure that they receive necessary and appropriate care. As a client advocate, care manager, and consumer, nurses need to know about

TABLE 3–1

Glossary of Terms Related to Managed Care	
Authorization	The process used by managed health care organizations to grant authorization of services for a specified period for reimbursement of specific services
Capitation	A managed care reimbursement arrangement that prepays the physician or other health care provider a set dollar amount on a per-member–per-month basis for the delivery of services to a specified group of members
Deductible	The amount of money that an insured person must pay toward health care costs before the insurance company begins reimbursement for health care
Fee-for-service	A reimbursement arrangement in which health care services are paid for as billed by the provider
Indemnity	An arrangement in which benefits are paid in a predetermined amount in the event of a covered loss
Integrated delivery system (IDS)	A system created to manage or provide health care services ranging from primary to tertiary inpatient care and all other settings for care
Risk sharing	A mechanism that provides incentives to physicians and other health care providers to deliver cost-effective and efficient services

managed care and the need for collaborative management of client care.

Role of Nurse Practitioners

Nurse practitioners (NPs) have become more predominant health care providers in the managed care environment because they can deliver more cost-effective health care. In addition, NPs work from a wellness model, with a focus on empowering clients to stay well and care for themselves. Several studies are underway to compare the outcomes from care provided by nurse practitioners with that provided by physicians.

As a result of the increased demand for this advanced practice role, many schools of nursing now offer graduate programs to prepare nurses to become NPs.

Types of Managed Care Organizations

Health care costs have become a national concern to consumers, employers, and health care providers in the United States. Many employers have contracted with a variety of MCOs to reduce health benefit costs. Govern-

ment reimbursement systems have also entered into managed care arrangements to control escalating costs. For example, Medicare, a federal program for the elderly and qualified disabled, is expected to become a managed care system by the year 2000. Many states' Medicaid programs, which pay for health services for the poor, have entered managed care agreements as well.

The oldest and most common type of MCO is the health maintenance organization (HMO), sometimes referred to as a membership organization. Many models for HMOs are used, but all either employ health care professionals to serve subscribing members (enrollees) in an ambulatory setting or contract with physicians and other providers to treat clients in their private offices. The enrollee usually pays a small copayment, typically $5 or $10, for each physician visit.

Another popular type of MCO is the preferred provider organization (PPO). PPOs provide contractual arrangements with physicians, hospitals, and other providers who meet their criteria. In other words, they are the "preferred" providers who render care to a group of subscribers in the health plan.

A point of service (POS) plan is actually an HMO that lets enrollees receive care outside of its network but at a higher copayment or deductible.

COLLABORATIVE MANAGEMENT

As the United States has been moving forward with the managed care system, health care professionals have realized that they must work together as an interdisciplinary team to provide comprehensive care. Although this idea is not new in certain settings, such as rehabilitation, home care, and long-term care, health care professionals in hospitals have not always worked as well as a team. One of the constraints in acute care is the short-term stay. However, the Joint Commission on Accreditation of Healthcare Organizations (JCAHO) mandates that *all* JCAHO-accredited agencies must provide collaborative, interdisciplinary care for their clients.

This text has advocated collaborative management of care since its first edition was published in 1991. This edition continues to discuss client care under "Collaborative Management" headings. Nurses often take the lead role in the interdisciplinary team because they tend to be with the clients for longer periods as they coordinate comprehensive, holistic care.

Focus on Outcomes

The primary focus of collaborative management is on the outcomes of care. The interdisciplinary team identifies expected outcomes for the client and provides interventions to help the client meet those outcomes. Both clinical and cost outcomes are established. This text identifies common clinical outcomes for clients with a number of diseases and illnesses. However, each client is an individual with unique problems and circumstances that may require modification of the commonly identified expected outcomes.

From Collaborative Care Management to Case Management

Whereas all clients need to have their care managed in a collaborative manner, not all clients need to be case managed. *Case management* is not a new concept. Since the turn of the 20th century, social workers, psychologists, and others have "carried a case load" of clients in the community for a variety of purposes. For instance, social workers have worked with at-risk elderly to keep them at home rather than admitted to a nursing home.

In the mid-1980s, Karen Zander and her colleagues at New England Medical Center introduced a nursing case management (NCM) model. The case managers followed up on high-risk, high-cost clients during their hospital stay to coordinate resources and ensure quality outcomes. Physician-nurse collaboration was a primary focus in this model.

The Carondolet integrated health system in Arizona expanded on the NCM model by using case managers across the health care continuum. Sometimes referred to as "beyond the walls" case management, this model incorporated the ethnic values and culture of the community.

Process of Case Management

Case management is "a collaborative process which assesses, plans, implements, coordinates, monitors, and evaluates services and options to meet an individual's health needs through communications and available resources to promote quality, cost-effective outcomes" (Case Management Society of America [CMSA], 1995, p. 8). Sometimes case managers may meet the health needs of a population, rather than a single individual (e.g., all diabetic clients in a given community).

The case management process is reserved for clients who have complex health problems (high risk) and incur a high cost to the health care system. An example of a client who could benefit from case management is an elderly woman with pulmonary emphysema and congestive heart failure who has had repeated admissions to the hospital for pneumonia and lives alone at home. The *Study Guide* and *Instructor's Guide* that accompany this text provide clinical scenarios to show how the case management process is used.

Part of the definition of case management endorsed by CMSA is similar to the steps of the nursing process (Chart 3–1). The individual who practices case management is called a *case manager*. In some agencies, the case manager is referred to as the care coordinator or care manager. Most case managers are nurses, although some are social workers or mental health workers. A few case managers have little or no clinical health background.

In general, case managers can be considered as internal or external. *Internal* case managers are employed by a health care agency and are usually nurses or social workers. Although these individuals manage resources, the primary focus of internal case managers is clinical care. *External* case managers are either employed by an MCO or traditional insurance company or are self-employed and

---

Chart 3–1

Nursing Care Highlight

The Process of Case Management

Needs Assessment

- Assesses/collects data
- Conducts case screening
- Identifies client's support systems and care providers
- Reviews history and determines current health care needs
- Obtains approvals for contracts

Plan Development

- Identifies services and funding options
- Reviews plan for consensus
- Advocates for client as needed
- Develops plan, including life care needs, if indicated

Implementation and Coordination

- Communicates regularly with clients and support systems
- Coordinates treatment plan
- Promotes coordinated and efficient care
- Identifies needs for additional services

Outcomes Monitoring and Evaluation

- Assesses benefit value to cost and value to quality of life
- Reviews plan for continuity of care
- Evaluates client satisfaction and compliance with treatment plan

Documentation

- Records services and outcomes
- Submits reports and other documentation as needed

---

contract with the MCO or traditional insurance company. The primary focus of external case managers is the utilization of resources for insurance companies.

Standards for Case Management Practice

As the largest professional case management organization, CMSA published standards that specify the recommended preparation for a case manager (Table 3–2). As listed in these criteria, the recommended educational preparation is a baccalaureate degree in a health or human service. Although most case managers today are approximately 40 years of age and are nurses prepared at the associate degree level, it is likely that new case managers in the 21st century will be at least baccalaureate prepared. A number of graduate nursing programs offer masters' preparation as a case manager. The developers of these programs believe that case management is an advanced practice role for nurses.

According to CMSA, the criteria for preparation as a case manager also includes working toward obtaining a certified case manager degree (CCM). This certification process requires that the experienced case manager (with at least 2 years experience) successfully complete a na-

TABLE 3–2

Recommended Preparation for a Case Manager

- Maintain current professional licensure or national certification in a health and human services profession or both
- Have a baccalaureate or higher degree for health and human services personnel
- Complete training and experience with the health needs of the population served
- Have knowledge of health, social service, and funding sources
- Maintain continuing education appropriate to case management and professional licensure
- Work toward and maintain case management certification

Adapted from the Case Management Society of America. (1995). *Standards of Practice for case management*. Little Rock, AR: Author.

tional standardized examination. The CCM designation is a valued credential in the field of case management for any discipline. A new certification is available for nurses who want to be credentialed by their professional organization as a nursing case manager. In October 1997, the first nursing case management examination was given by the American Nurses Credentialing Center (ANCC).

Other certifications may also be acquired by case managers, such as the CRRN for case managers in rehabilitation nursing. Resources in the book's appendices list the names and addresses of certifying organizations.

Roles of Case Managers

Although models for case management vary, all case managers assume a common set of roles and functions. The CMSA *Standards of Practice* outlines the major case manager roles, including assessment, planning, facilitation, and advocacy. For nurses, many of the skills needed to fulfill these roles can be learned as part of basic nursing education.

Case management is being used in a number of countries around the world, including Australia and Singapore. Nursing educators are revising curricula to better prepare their graduates for functioning in a managed care environment.

From Case Management to Disease State Management

Some parts of the United States are practicing disease state management, sometimes called disease management. Put simply, disease state management is a focus on care of clients with chronic disease or illness, such as asthma, diabetes, or congestive heart failure. The purpose of this care approach is to keep clients with chronic conditions as well as possible in the community. If successful, health management would be the goal and health care professionals would be reimbursed for wellness care rather than illness care.

The Role of Clinical Pathways

As mentioned in Chapter 1, the clinical pathway (CP) is a commonly used format for delineating the client's plan of care. It is an interdisciplinary guideline for care that optimally sequences interventions and expected outcomes for a client. Other names for the pathway include the collaborative plan of care (POC), multidisciplinary action plan (MAP), critical pathway, and care path.

The CP is developed by clinical experts for diagnoses, treatments, procedures, or symptoms that are costly, complex, and variable. The health team follows the pathway in managing the client's care. If expected outcomes are not met, the nurse or other health professional records variances, or deviations, on a data collection tool. These variances are then analyzed to identify actual or potential problems needing improvement. An action plan is then implemented and followed up to determine if the infection rate decreases. This entire sequence of data collection, problem identification, action plan, and follow-up is part of the continuous quality improvement (CQI) process that every health care agency uses to monitor and improve the care that it provides.

This textbook provides a number of examples of CPs with varying formats. Traditional client care plans are also included in the book to help students see the difference between a nursing focused care plan and an interdisciplinary plan of care, the CP.

SELECTED BIBLIOGRAPHY

Case Management Society of America. (1995). *Standards of practice for case management*. Little Rock, AR: Author.

Cohen, E. L. (1996). *Nurse case management in the 21st century*. St. Louis: Mosby-Year Book.

Hogan, T. D. (1997). Case management in a wound care program. *Nursing Case Management, 2*(1), 2–15.

Howe, R. S. (1996). *Clinical pathways for ambulatory care case management*. Gaithersburg, MD: Aspen.

Ignatavicius, D. D., & Hausman, K. (1995). *Clinical pathways for collaborative practice*. Philadelphia: W. B. Saunders.

Lee, S. S. (1996). Hospital-home care critical pathways in disease management: Improving case management and patient outcomes in postoperative cardiothoracic surgical patients. *The Journal of Care Management, 2*(3), 42–54.

Marrelli, T. M., & Hilliard, L. S. (1996). *Home care and clinical paths: Effective care planning across the continuum*. St. Louis: Mosby-Year Book.

Mullahy, C. M. (1995). *The case manager's handbook*. Gaithersburg, MD: Aspen.

Owens, M. (1997). Hi, I'm your case manager. *Home Care Provider, 2*(6), 307–310.

Pacala, J. T., & Boult, C. (1996). Factors influencing effectiveness of case management in managed care organizations: A qualitative analysis. *The Journal of Care Management, 2*(3), 29–35.

Powell, S. K. (1996). *Nursing care management: A practical guide to success in managed care*. Philadelphia: Lippincott-Raven.

Romaine, D. S. (1995). Case management challenges: Present and future. *Continuing Care, 14*(1), 24–31.

Siefker, J. M., Garrett, M. B., Van Genderen, A., & Weis, M. J. (1998). *Fundamentals of case management: Guidelines for practicing case managers*. St. Louis: Mosby-Year Book.

SUGGESTED READINGS

Hogan, T. D. (1997). Case management in a wound care program. *Nursing Case Management, 2*(1), 2–15.
This article uses a case study approach to show how case managers make a difference in care of clients with various types of wounds

being cared for at home. A complete plan of care with expected outcomes is also included in the article. A quiz at the end of the article can be completed for continuing education credit or practice.

Lee, S. S. (1996). Hospital-home care critical pathways in disease management: Improving case management and patient outcomes in post-operative cardiothoracic surgical patients. *The Journal of Care Management, 2*(3), 42–54.

This article is from the official journal of the Case Management Society of America. The author describes the development and implementation of a pathway for a cardiothoracic client across the health care continuum, from the hospital through home care.

Chapter 4

COMPLEMENTARY THERAPIES

CHAPTER HIGHLIGHTS

Health problems can no longer be separated into solely "physical" or "mental" categories. Research has clearly demonstrated that healing is successful when the mind, body, and spirit are integrated (Dossey et al., 1995). Complementary therapies, sometimes called complementary modalities or alternative medicine, allow clients to integrate the mind, body, and spirit, and make them active participants in their health care and healing.

Despite the increasing use of complementary therapies in the United States, the concept of "alternative" medicine remains controversial. Physicians have shown a growing openness to the possibility that these therapies can be effective. Younger physicians tend to be more receptive than older ones (American Health Consultants, 1997). Nurses have contributed a great deal to the acceptance and use of therapies that help promote healing.

HOLISTIC NURSING

Holistic nursing practice is a rapidly growing specialty field. According to the American Holistic Nurses' Association, the goal of holistic nursing is about healing the whole person (Dossey, 1997). Therefore, the role of the holistic nurse is to incorporate mind-oriented modalities to treat the physiologic as well as the psychological and spiritual results of illness. Holistic nurses specialize in supplementing traditional medical therapies with mind therapies to augment (not replace) the effects of drugs, surgery, and technology.

All nurses can use aspects of holistic care to enhance healing. Medical-surgical nurses in a variety of settings care for clients who are physically ill, but have psychological and spiritual effects associated with their conditions as well.

Traditional medical therapies, sometimes referred to as the allopathic approach, focus on the body to treat illness. Complementary therapies, many of which have been used for thousands of years, focus on the mind-body-spirit connection. Examples of complements to conventional medical therapies include relaxation, imagery, biofeedback, prayer, humor, music therapy, and touch. Table 4–1 lists and defines some of the most common complementary therapies. Resources from which more information can be obtained are listed in the Appendix.

OFFICE OF ALTERNATIVE MEDICINE

In their classic study, Eisenberg and his colleagues (1993) found that one third of all adults in the United States used some type of alternative health care in their lifetime. This finding translates into 425 million visits to practitioners of alternative medicine, such as acupuncturists and chiropractors, at a cost of almost $14 billion. The authors divided alternative therapies into high-risk and low-risk groups. Examples of high-risk therapies are certain herbal preparations and some types of spinal manipulation (usually performed by chiropractors). Examples of low-risk therapies are relaxation, imagery, massage, and hypnosis. Not surprisingly, most of the money spent on

TABLE 4–1

Definitions of Common Complementary Therapies

Acupressure	Use of pressure from the fingers and hands to stimulate the energy points in the body, thereby removing energy blocks that are believed to produce health problems
Acupuncture	Use of needles to stimulate certain points on the surface of the body to treat pain, diseases, or dysfunctions of the body; the World Health Organization currently lists a number of medical conditions that may be effectively treated, including migraine, asthma, and arthritis (practitioners are usually licensed by the state)
Aromatherapy	Use of medicinal properties of essential oils extracted from plants and herbs; may be administered via inhalation, topically, or through ingestion
Biofeedback	Use of an electrical device to help the client become aware of certain body functions, such as heart rate, blood pressure, and muscle activity
Chiropractic medicine	Use of adjustments to realign the spine and nervous system so that the body can heal (practitioners are usually licensed by the state)
Imagery	Use of a technique in which a client experiences memories, dreams, and fantasies to relieve stress, decrease pain, and promote healing
Hypnotherapy	Use of hypnosis, posthypnotic suggestion, or any similar process in which the client is susceptible to suggestion or direction
Massage therapy	Manipulation of skeletal muscle to relieve stress or muscle tension; includes stroking, kneading, or stretching on muscles
Naturopathy	A system of prevention, diagnosis, and management of health problems using natural medicines and therapies to stimulate the client's healing process
Osteopathy	Use of body mechanics and manipulative techniques to detect faulty body structure and function

complementary therapies was not reimbursed by health insurance companies. Eisenberg et al. also found that consumers of alternative medicine tended to be educated, upper-income Caucasians in the 25- to 49-year age group.

TRANSCULTURAL CONSIDERATIONS

More recent studies have shown that ethnicity and culture may play a part in determining who seeks complementary therapies. For example, Arcury at al. (1996) found that rural clients in North Carolina used a variety of conventional and alternative remedies for arthritis. Prayer was the most common modality used (92% of the sample used it). African-Americans used alternative methods more often than Caucasians.

Another transcultural study revealed that 44% of Mexican-Americans in the Texas Rio Grande Valley visited an alternative practitioner one or more times during the study year (Keegan, 1996). The most commonly sought therapies were herbal medicine, spiritual healing and prayer, relaxation, and massage.

Paramore (1997) attempted to update national estimates of the use of complementary therapies using the 1994 Robert Wood Johnson Foundation National Access to Care Survey (N = 3450). The results showed that 10% of the U.S. population, or almost 25 million people, saw a professional in 1994 for at least one of the following therapies: chiropractic, relaxation, therapeutic massage, or acupuncture. The researcher concluded that alternative, or complementary, therapies could have a larger role in the health care system of the future.

Recognizing the growing trend toward complementary modalities, the National Institutes of Health created the Office of Alternative Medicine (OAM) in 1992 to evaluate therapies that hold the most promise in treating illness and disease. The ultimate goal of the OAM is to integrate validated complementary therapies into current conventional medical practice. At this time, a number of studies are being conducted around the country by physicians, nurses, and others interested in holistic health practice to determine which therapies are the most effective for which conditions. Many of the studies are focusing on mind-body control therapies, such as biofeedback and imagery; structural and energetic therapies, such as acupressure and therapeutic touch; and ethnomedicine, such as homeopathic medicine and herbal medicine. The safety, efficacy, mechanism of action, and cost effectiveness of individual therapies are being examined.

In 1996, the OAM cosponsored the first conference on medical and nursing education in complementary therapies. Schools of medicine and nursing were encouraged to continue to include content on complementary modalities in their curricula.

MANAGED CARE AND THE HOLISTIC APPROACH

As discussed in Chapter 3, the health care system in the United States has become managed care. Whereas traditional health insurance companies have not typically paid for complementary care, health maintenance organizations (HMOs) around the country are adding alternative medicine practitioners to their list of preferred providers. A study of HMOs in 13 states showed that subscribers are requesting alternative care therapies as part of the health plan. Many HMOs reported that they will offer a blend of conventional and alternative therapies, especially for clients with chronic illness (American Health Consultants, 1997; Eisenberg, 1997).

COMMONLY USED COMPLEMENTARY THERAPIES

It is beyond the scope of this chapter to describe all of the many therapies used by consumers and health care professionals. Some of the most common, low-risk therapies are briefly discussed here. In addition to this chapter's description, complementary therapies are found throughout the text as part of discussions related to management of health problems, such as pain (Chap. 9), fibromyalgia (Chap. 24), acquired immunodeficiency syndrome (Chap. 25), cancer (Chap. 27), and burns (Chap. 71). Many of these interventions can be independently used by nurses in medical-surgical nursing practice settings.

Prayer

Spirituality and religion are not the same. Spirituality gives meaning to a person; that is, it is an aspect of humanity that simply exists. Religion, on the other hand, is not essential for existence and is chosen by an individual. Religion refers to a belief system and practices of worship that are related to that system (Dossey, 1997).

Prayer is an activity related to religion. It has many forms and expressions, but can be generally defined as "a representation of one's longing for communion or communication with God or the Absolute" (Dossey, 1997, p. 45).

Research has demonstrated that faith and prayer can positively affect healing. For example, a qualitative study of adults undergoing coronary artery bypass grafting showed that spiritual-religious issues become very important when a person is faced with a crisis or potentially life-threatening event (Camp, 1996) (see Research Applications for Nursing).

Because religion and prayer take many forms, the medical-surgical nurse explores the way that clients express these beliefs. For instance, the nurse can help clients reflect on the meaning of prayer in their lives as well as other expressions of spirituality and religion, including inspirational readings and music. Questions that a nurse might ask clients to help them find meaning in spiritual or religious activities are listed in Chart 4–1.

Relaxation

Relaxation is one of the simplest and easiest complementary therapies to use. The purpose of relaxation techniques is to reduce physical, mental, and emotional tension, resulting in changes opposite to those of the fight-or-flight mechanism (Dossey, 1997). The physiologic effects of relaxation involve the autonomic, immune, and endocrine systems as summarized in Table 4–2. Com-

monly used relaxation techniques include progressive muscle relaxation (PMR), hypnosis, and biofeedback.

Progressive Muscle Relaxation

Progressive muscle relaxation is based on the tenet that stress increases skeletal muscle tension. Intentional tensing and releasing of successive muscle groups promotes relaxation and decreases anxiety. PMR has been used successfully for clients with hypertension, asthma, and panic attacks.

▷ Research Applications for Nursing

Meeting the Spiritual Needs of Clients

Camp, P. E. (1996). Having faith: Experiencing coronary artery bypass grafting. Journal of Cardiovascular Nursing, 10(3), 55–64.

Clients perceive coronary artery bypass grafting (CABG) as a potentially life-threatening event. The purpose of this qualitative study was to explore the spiritual needs of 17 clients (ages 34–83 years) who recently had CABG surgery (4–7 days postoperatively). The major findings from the client interviews were that spiritual needs centered around faith in their decision making, faith in the hospital staff (especially the nurses), and an overwhelming faith in God.

Critique. Although the sample size in this study was limited, the information obtained by a qualitative research methodology provides insight into the spiritual needs and resources of clients who are stressed by potential life-threatening events or illnesses. Few studies investigating spirituality have been conducted.

Possible Nursing Implications. Because nurses are with clients on a consistent basis, they are in the unique position of assessing and identifying spiritual needs of their clients. Nurses should be educated about how to assess these needs and provide the necessary spiritual resources for clients.

Chart 4–1

Nursing Care Highlight

Questions That Can Be Used as Part of a Spiritual Assessment

- What gives your life meaning?
- What brings you joy and peace in your life?
- What helps you cope when you are troubled or worried?
- How do you feel about yourself?
- Who are significant people in your life?
- Are worship and religion important to you?
- Do you believe in God or a higher power?
- Do you pray?
- Is faith important in your life?
- What is the most important or powerful thing in your life?

TABLE 4–2

Physiologic Effects of Relaxation
Increased peripheral blood flow
Decreased respiratory rate and volume
Decreased heart rate
Decreased blood pressure
Decreased epinephrine level
Decreased gastric acidity and motility
Increased activity of killer cells
Decreased oxygen consumption
Decreased sweat gland activity

Hypnosis

Hypnosis also relaxes skeletal muscles and enhances the clients' ability to use images through suggestions made when the clients are in an altered state of consciousness. In many cases, hypnosis has been successful for smoking cessation.

Biofeedback

Biofeedback is a technique in which clients learn to become aware of certain body functions, such as heart rate, blood pressure, and muscle activity. It involves instrumentation that allows clients to alter these functions using various relaxation techniques.

Biofeedback can also be used for muscular or neuromuscular retraining. For example, Jackson at al. (1996) successfully used biofeedback to help clients achieve continence after radical prostatectomy by increasing their ability to contract pelvic floor muscles. Twenty of 27 clients studied improved: 13 had complete success and 7 had significant improvement. The researcher also found that client motivation is an important factor for success.

The medical-surgical nurse can easily use PMR without special training. Hypnosis and biofeedback are more advanced relaxation techniques that require special training.

When caring for a client who is tense or anxious, the nurse assesses the client's (1) perception of the need for relaxation, (2) readiness and motivation to learn relaxation strategies, and (3) past experience, if any, with relaxation techniques. The nurse also determines whether the client can remain still for a short period of time and assesses his or her ability to see and hear.

To begin PMR, with eyes closed, the client takes several deep breaths, in through the nose and out through the mouth. Then the client tenses and releases each muscle group for several seconds, starting with the head and progressing to the toes. The entire procedure can be completed in a few minutes. The nurse evaluates the success of relaxation strategies by asking the client how he or she feels before and after the intervention.

ELDERLY CONSIDERATIONS

 Muscle relaxation can also help promote sleep. Richards (1996) found that caring interventions that focus on the body-mind connection, such as muscle relaxation, back rubs, music, and imagery, promote sleep in the hospitalized elderly.

Imagery

Imagery is a technique in which a person experiences memories, dreams, and visions as a bridge for making the body-mind-spirit connection. Images can occur spontaneously or be induced deliberately. All senses may be involved, but most images are visual; that is, people see positive "mental pictures," such as a beautiful sunset or magnificent ocean. Herbs and aromas, sometimes referred to as aromatherapy, can enhance the formation of images.

Imagery produces physiologic effects that affect healing. Images and thoughts are transmitted through the hypothalamus and limbic system of the brain by neurotransmitters, especially norepinephrine and acetylcholine. These substances affect both the peripheral and autonomic nervous systems to promote relaxation. Clients with cancer or severe pain often use imagery as a complementary therapy.

The nurse assesses the client's history of using imagery and his or her readiness to participate actively in the imagery session. Each session should begin with a relaxation exercise, described in the last section. Sessions may last from 10 to 60 minutes depending on the desired outcomes. Scripts can be used to facilitate the process. Table 4–3 describes several types of imagery that can be employed. The nurse facilitates imagery sessions until the client feels comfortable with the technique and can induce images without assistance.

TABLE 4–3

Commonly Used Types of Imagery	
Interactive guided imagery	Uses a client's own images, both positive and negative; is facilitated by a practitioner
Receptive imagery	Occurs spontaneously when daydreaming and immediately on wakening
Active imagery	Occurs when a client intentionally focuses on forming an image
End-state imagery	Occurs when the client rehearses about being in a healed state
Packaged imagery	Uses tapes, such as relaxation or hypnosis tapes, to create images
Symbolic imagery	Occurs when a client creates images of people, objects, or events to achieve a desired result (e.g., cancer cells are mentally destroyed by a bomb)

Music

Soothing music produces a hypometabolic response in which the autonomic, immune, and endocrine systems are affected. Music also establishes a means of communication between the right and left sides of the brain. Because music is nonverbal, it appeals to the right side of the brain; traditional verbalization appeals to the left side of the brain.

Music can complement conventional medical therapy by reducing pain, anxiety, isolation, and stress. For example, music has been used for surgical clients in both the preoperative and postoperative phases of care. After listening to music of their choice, preoperative clients have reported less anxiety than those who did not. Music can also lower heart rates, blood pressures, and respiratory rates of preoperative clients (Augustin & Hains, 1996). Another nursing study showed that music in the immediate postoperative period helped clients relax and functioned as a distractor (Heiser et al., 1997).

Music can also reduce anxiety in clients receiving chemotherapy. Sabo and Michael (1996) found that music significantly reduced anxiety associated with chemotherapy treatment for cancer.

Like prayer, relaxation, and imagery, music therapy can be used in any health care setting or in the client's home. The nurse assesses the types of music that the client prefers and how it makes him or her feel. Recorded tapes can be played for several daily sessions, each lasting between 20 and 30 minutes. The nurse then evaluates the client's response to the therapy, including vital signs and the client's description of the experience (if possible) and its effects, such as decreased insomnia, pain relief, or decreased agitation.

ELDERLY CONSIDERATIONS

For elderly clients who are confused and restless, the calming effect of music may improve behavioral manifestations, such as agitation and combativeness (Ragneskog et al., 1996). Music causes a variety of experiences for the client, including imagery, sensory stimulation, and relaxation.

Touch

The use of touch for healing was documented more than 5000 years ago. All cultures have developed some form of touch therapy. The Oriental world view is founded on energy. Examples of touch therapies based on energy are acupressure and reflexology (see Table 4–1). The Western world view is based on reduction of matter; examples are massage and therapeutic touch.

Research has demonstrated that touch slows heart rate, decreases diastolic blood pressure, and reduces anxiety. Yet most nurses do not frequently use touch as a comfort or healing measure.

Many types of touch therapies are available, including therapeutic massage, therapeutic touch, acupressure, reflexology, and healing touch. Nurses have been administering back rubs for most of the 20th century, but time constraints have limited this intervention in most settings.

Yet back rubs are a type of therapeutic massage. Back rubs and massage of other parts of the body can promote relaxation and sleep and provide a distraction for clients with anxiety or pain.

Therapeutic touch is more involved. It is a healing modality that involves touching with the intent to help or heal. Therapeutic touch decreases anxiety, facilitates healing, and relieves pain. This modality works by mobilizing areas in the client's energy field that are not flowing and directing one's excess body energies to assist the client to repattern his or her own energies (Dossey et al., 1995).

Acupressure is based on the Oriental energy system of meridian lines and points. The application of the healer's finger and/or thumb to one or more of 657 energy points that run along 12 pathways, or meridian lines, releases congestion and promotes energy flow.

In the early 1900s, Dr. William Fitzgerald noted that pressure applied to certain parts of the hands caused anesthesia in other parts of the body. His work was used by others to explore the field of reflexology, based on the theory that there are 10 equal, longitudinal zones running the length of the body. Like acupressure, applying pressure to certain points releases congestion and promotes energy flow. The other major goal of this therapy is relaxation. Figure 4–1 shows a foot reflexology chart and the location of some of the pressure points.

Healing touch is an advanced group of touch therapies. It is a collection of noninvasive energy-based techniques to make energy available to the client and requires specialized training.

Like the previously described complementary therapies, the nurse can use touch in any health care setting or in the client's home. Massage or simple touching are most commonly used by medical-surgical nurses. Before using touch, however, the nurse assesses the client's feeling about touching, including cultural and age considerations. The nurse also evaluates the client's response to touch.

ELDERLY CONSIDERATIONS

Older clients are likely to receive the least amount of touch; these clients need touch as much as or more than any other age group. Elderly clients often have no family members or significant others. In addition, some elderly cannot communicate and need touch as an effective communication tool (Dossey et al., 1995).

Severely agitated elderly clients may not want to be touched; indeed, touch can cause an increase in aggressive behaviors. The severely cognitively impaired elderly may view touch as an invasion of their personal space.

Laughter and Humor

Laughter and humor have been shown to have physiologic effects on the body by strengthening the immune system, increasing circulation, and stimulating the cortex of the brain. Laughter decreases serum cortisol levels (which increases during stress), increases the numbers of helper T cells and natural killer cells (to destroy tumor cells), and increases salivary immunoglobulin A (to protect against upper respiratory and oral infections) (Berk & Tan, 1993). The physical activity of laughter dilates pe-

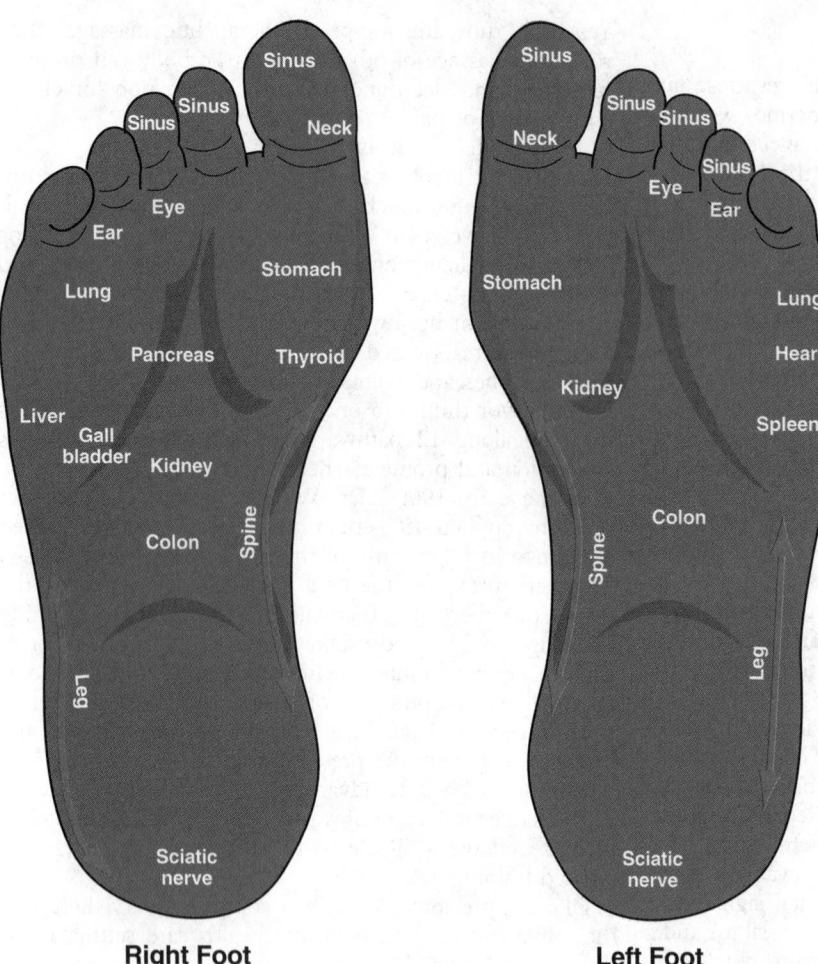

Right Foot **Left Foot**

Figure 4–1. Reflexology chart of the foot. (From Dossey, B. M. [1995]. Using imagery to help your patient heal. *American Journal of Nursing, 95*[6], 41–46. Used with permission.)

ripheral blood vessels, increasing blood flow to extremities (Dossey, 1997).

Humor is a cognitive skill that involves both the logical left brain and the creative right brain. For example, the left side of the brain is active during joke telling, but the right side perceives the humor.

Laughter and humor also have psychological effects, resulting in relaxation, stress reduction, and distraction. Individuals who have a strong sense of humor generally deal better with stress than those who do not.

Nurses often use laughter and humor when caring for clients. Before using this therapy with clients, the nurse assesses the client's sense of humor as well as his or her own level of comfort with humor therapy. Humor can be very therapeutic for both the client and the nurse.

Some health care agencies use therapeutic, mobile comedy carts, humor rooms, or clown visitation programs. All of these techniques help distract the client, relieve pain, and promote stress reduction.

Nutrition

It has long been established that nutrition plays a major part in the healing process. The importance of trace elements, such as zinc, has been shown to impact healing, especially of skin lesions. Chapter 64 discusses the role of nutrition as well as nutritional assessment and interventions that the nurse can use.

IMPLICATIONS FOR HEALTH CARE PROVIDERS

Physicians, nurses, and other health care professionals need to learn more about complementary therapies as research becomes available. As discussed earlier in the chapter, healing requires a body-mind-spirit approach.

Eisenberg (1997) suggested that physicians should incorporate the use of complementary therapies into their practices. He recommended that physicians discuss safety and efficacy issues with their clients and help them identify suitable licensed providers of alternative medicine. He further suggested that a follow-up visit after treatment by a practitioner of alternative therapies be made to review response to treatment.

Medical and nursing education programs should incorporate low-risk therapies into their basic curricula. Practicing health care providers need continuing education to keep up with the public's demand for alternative care. Continued nursing research is needed to better delineate the nurse's role in the use of complementary therapies.

SELECTED BIBLIOGRAPHY

American Health Consultants. (1997). HMOs moving more toward alternative care coverage. *Case Management Advisor, 8*(1), 18–19.

Arcury, T. A., Bernard, S. L., Jordan, J. M., & Cook, H. L. (1996). Gender and ethnic differences in alternative and conventional arthritis remedy use among community-dwelling rural adults with arthritis. *Arthritis Care Research, 9,* 384–390.

Augustin, P., & Hains, A. A. (1996). Effect of music on ambulatory surgery patients' preoperative anxiety. *AORN Journal, 63,* 750, 753–758.

*Berk, L. S., & Tan, S. A. (1993). Eustress of humor associated laughter modulates specific immune system components. *Annals of Behavioral Medicine, 15,* S111.

Bryant, J. P. (1996). Therapeutic touch in home healthcare: One nurse's experience. *Home Healthcare Nurse, 14,* 580–586.

Camp, P. E. (1996). Having faith: Experiencing coronary artery bypass grafting. *Journal of Cardiovascular Nursing, 10*(3), 55–64.

Collins, J. A., & Rice, V. H. (1997). Effects of relaxation intervention in phase II cardiac rehabilitation: Replication and extension. *Heart and Lung, 26,* 31–44.

Corley, M. C., Ferriter, J., Zeh, J., & Gifford, C. (1995). Physiologic and psychologic effects of back rubs. *Applied Nursing Research, 8*(1), 39–42.

Dossey, B. M. (1995). Using imagery to help your patient heal. *American Journal of Nursing, 95*(6), 41–46.

Dossey, B. M. (1997). *Core curriculum for holistic nursing.* Gaithersburg, MD: Aspen.

Dossey, B. M., Keegan, L., Guzzetta, C. E., & Kolkmeier, L. G. (1995). *Holistic nursing: A handbook for practice.* Gaithersburg, MD: Aspen.

Eisenberg, D. M. (1997). Advising patients who seek alternative medical therapies. *Annals of Internal Medicine, 127,* 61–69.

*Eisenberg, D. M., Kessler, R. C., Foster, C., et al. (1993). Unconventional medicine in the United States—Prevalence, costs, and patterns of use. *New England Journal of Medicine, 328,* 246–252.

Fascione, J. (1995). Healing power of touch. *Elder Care, 7*(1), 19–21.

Fawcett, J., Sidney, J. S., Riley-Lawless, K., & Hanson, M. J. (1996). An exploratory study of the relationship between alternative therapies, functional status, and symptom severity among people with multiple sclerosis. *Journal of Holistic Nursing, 14,* 115–129.

Ferrara-Love, R., Sekeres, L., & Bircher, N. G. (1996). Nonpharmacologic treatment of postoperative nursing. *Journal of Perianesthesiology Nursing, 11,* 378–383.

Heiser, R. M., Chiles, K., Fudge, M., & Gray, S. E. (1997). The use of music during the immediate postoperative recovery period. *AORN Journal, 65,* 777–778, 781–785.

Jackson, J., Emerson, L., Johnston, B., et al. (1996). Biofeedback: A noninvasive treatment of incontinence after radical prostatectomy. *Urology Nurse, 16*(2), 50–54.

Keegan, L. (1996). Use of alternative therapies among Mexican Americans in the Texas Rio Grande Valley. *Journal of Holistic Nursing, 14,* 277–294.

Mackey, R. B. (1995). Discover the healing power of therapeutic touch. *American Journal of Nursing, 95*(4), 26–33.

Maxwell, J. (1997). The gentle power of acupressure. *RN, 60*(4), 53–56.

McCain, N. L., Zeller, J. M., Cella, D. F., et al. (1996). The influence of stress management training in HIV disease. *Nursing Research, 45,* 246–253.

Paramore, L. C. (1997). Use of alternative therapies: Estimates from the 1994 Robert Wood Johnson Foundation National Access to Care Survey. *Journal of Pain and Symptom Management, 13*(2), 83–89.

Ragneskog, H., Kihlgren, M., Karlsson, I., & Norberg, A. (1996). Dinner music for demented patients: Analysis of video-recorded observations. *Clinical Nursing Research, 5*(3), 262–277.

Richards, K. C. (1996). Sleep promotion. *Critical Care Clinics of North America, 8*(1), 39–52.

Rimmer, L. (1998). The clinical use of aromatherapy in the reduction of stress. *Home Healthcare Nurse, 16*(2), 123–126.

Sabo, C. E., & Michael, S. R. (1996). The influence of personal message with music on anxiety and side effects associated with chemotherapy. *Cancer Nursing, 19,* 283–289.

Skinner, S. (1996). How homeopathy works. *RN, 59*(12), 53–56.

Turkosis, B., & Lance, B. (1996). The use of guided imagery with anticipatory grief. *Home Healthcare Nurse, 14,* 878–888.

Wallace, K. G. (1997). Analysis of recent literature concerning relaxation and imagery interventions for cancer pain. *Cancer Nursing, 20*(2), 79–87.

SUGGESTED READINGS

Bryant, J. P. (1996). Therapeutic touch in home healthcare: One nurse's experience. *Home Healthcare Nurse, 14,* 580–586.

This article describes how one nurse used therapeutic touch with 27 home health clients. It describes the technique she used and the positive results she obtained. The author believes that the clients recovered quicker than they would have without this important intervention.

Corley, M. C., Ferriter, J., Zeh, J., & Gifford, C. (1995). Physiological and psychological effects of back rubs. *Applied Nursing Research, 8*(1), 39–42.

This nursing study examined the benefits of back rubs on elderly residents living in nursing homes. The significant physiologic effects were increased skin temperature and relaxation of the trapezius muscle. However, change in mood (improved) was the most significant finding of the study.

Dossey, B. M. (1995). Using imagery to help your patient heal. *American Journal of Nursing, 95*(6), 41–46.

The author describes types of imagery that can be used with a variety of clients. She discusses how the nurse should conduct an imagery session, including client assessment and evaluation. At the end of the article, a continuing education quiz is available for contact hours.

ADULT DEVELOPMENT

The medical-surgical nurse needs an understanding of each stage of adult development because it affects the client's response to illness and other stressors. However, nurses must also remember that each person is unique and, therefore, may not follow all expected patterns of the developmental stage.

THEORIES OF ADULT DEVELOPMENT

The developmental stage of adolescence seems to fade gradually into adulthood. Adulthood is commonly described as having its onset at some point after a person achieves physical maturity. In contrast to earlier periods of the life cycle, adulthood has no established landmarks that precisely characterize its onset or its stages.

People share certain traits with respect to age and the rate of maturation. Age in years may indicate that several social milestones have passed. Designating arbitrary ages for the onset of maturity, middle age, and old age, however, may promote a stereotypic view of the stages of adulthood. The nurse should remember that there are many individual differences that result from factors such as heredity, gender, health history, and life experience.

A single theory explaining changes during adulthood has been difficult to construct. Thus, many theories have

been developed, each representing a different view. Theories of adult development can be divided into two broad areas: developmental theories and theories of aging.

Developmental Theories

Developmental theories imply that certain psychosocial growth mechanisms can be assigned to various ages. The classic theories expressed by Erikson, Peck, and Havighurst are the most commonly cited. However, these theories were constructed more than 30 years ago and may not reflect the developmental patterns of all adults in the 21st century.

Erikson's Eight "Stages of Man"

Erikson (1968) proposed that personalities continue to evolve throughout adult life in a gradual, continuous manner. The first five stages of Erikson's theory largely expand on Freud's stages of childhood development. The last three stages provide a useful model for understanding some general issues of adult developmental changes during the adult years. Table 5–1 explains these adult stages and related nursing assessment.

For example, the task of the older adult is ego integrity versus despair. If older adults cannot adjust to the physical, psychological, and sociologic changes that may occur

TABLE 5–1

Erikson's Adult Developmental Tasks		
Developmental Stage	**Developmental Task**	**Nursing Assessment**
Young adulthood	• Intimacy versus isolation	• Assess whether the client has meaningful, intimate relationships. • If the client has no intimate relationships, ask whether he or she has had one or more in the past. • Assess other support systems that the client may have.
Middlescence	• Generativity versus stagnation	• Assess whether the client is employed. • Ask the client what he or she does for leisure or recreation. • If the client is not employed or has no regular leisure activity, ask the client what he or she does during a 24-hour day. • Assess for signs of depression, such as excessive sleeping and decreased appetite.
Older adulthood	• Ego integrity versus despair	• Assess what the client does each day. • Ask about the client's family and other relationships. • Ask the client if he or she feels lonely; if so, assess for signs of depression.

as they age, they are at risk for despair. The result may be depression. The nurse assesses the older adult to determine whether this task has been accomplished successfully or whether the person is at a high risk for depression or is already depressed.

Peck's Developmental Tasks of Adulthood

The last two of Erikson's stages encompass all the middle adult and late years of the life cycle. This view of adulthood may be too simplistic and general. Using Erikson's model as a foundation, many developmental psychologists have expanded his theory to more realistically represent adulthood. Peck (1968) identified seven crucial developmental tasks for the last two periods of the life cycle: middlescence (middle adulthood) and late adulthood (Table 5–2). Peck believed that there are four major tasks in middlescence and three tasks in late adulthood that must be confronted for healthy adjustment. If these tasks

are not accomplished, a person's state of health may decline.

For example, in the period of "old age," one task is body transcendence versus body preoccupation. Peck included this task because he observed many older adults beginning to focus on the declines in their physical functioning, resulting in a preoccupation with their body. Peck said that to age successfully, older adults need to accept these body changes and adapt to them as well as possible. When caring for an older adult, the nurse assesses the person's view of body changes and how he or she has coped with them.

Havighurst's Theory of Adult Developmental Tasks

Havighurst's (1972) ideas have also contributed to the understanding of adult development. His theory has a

TABLE 5–2

Peck's Developmental Tasks of Adulthood		
Period of Life Cycle	**Developmental Task**	**Clinical Applications**
Middlescence	• Valuing wisdom vs physical powers • Socializing vs sexualizing in human relationships • Cathectic flexibility vs cathectic impoverishment • Mental flexibility vs mental rigidity	• The client is likely to have strong relationships with family or significant others. • The client is likely to be more flexible in his or her lifestyle if necessary. • The client is able to make and adapt to changes as needed.
Old age	• Ego differentiation vs work role preoccupation • Body transcendence vs body preoccupation • Ego transcendence vs ego preoccupation	• The client is able to have a meaningful life after retirement from work. • The client accepts and adapts to changes in body structure and function without difficulty. • The client accepts the inevitability of death and approaches it in a positive manner, feeling that he or she has lived a "good" life.

TABLE 5-3

Havighurst's Developmental Tasks of the Adult	
Stage	**Developmental Task**
Early adulthood	• Selecting a mate • Learning to live with a marriage partner • Starting a family • Rearing children • Managing a home • Getting started in an occupation • Assuming civic responsibility • Finding a congenial social group
Middle age	• Achieving adult civic and social responsibility • Establishing and maintaining an economic standard of living • Assisting teenage children to become responsibile and happy adults • Developing leisure activities • Accepting and adjusting to the physiologic changes of middle age • Adjusting to the aging of parents
Later maturity	• Adjusting to decreasing physical strength and health • Adjusting to the death of a spouse • Adjusting to retirement and reduced income • Establishing an explicit affiliation with one's age group • Meeting social and civic obligations • Establishing satisfactory physical living arrangements

broad definition of successful aging that addresses social competency and adaptation to new roles. He viewed developmental tasks as a continual discovery of new and meaningful roles. This positive view of aging helps people "successfully age." He divided the life cycle into six age periods, each containing 6–10 developmental tasks. The tasks for the adult periods are summarized in Table 5–3.

A major criticism of Havighurst's ideas is his stereotypic presentation of the tasks in each age period (which were perhaps appropriate for the 1960s and 1970s). For example, he stated that people typically marry and start a family in young adulthood. Today, it is increasingly common for young adults to postpone marriage or not marry at all. Many couples choose to have children later in life or not at all. In addition, Havighurst did not acknowledge same-sex relationships.

Theories of Aging

In addition to theories of adult development, numerous theories are associated with the aging process. These include biological (physiologic), sociologic, and psychological theories. Several of the most commonly cited theories are briefly presented here.

Biological Theories of Aging

Biologists exploring the aging process concluded that aging can be viewed as a progression through a continuum of events that occur from birth to death. From this perspective, the aging process has been defined as the sum total of all changes that occur in a person over the life span. On the basis of this broad definition, it has been proposed that aging can best be understood by studying physiologic development. Over the years, many biological, or physiologic, theories have emerged, including exhaustion theories, genetic theories, single-organ theories, the free radical theory, and the immunity theory.

A number of very large studies are being conducted across the country to follow people as they age and learn more about the normal aging process.

Exhaustion Theories

Early theorists on aging proposed that there is a fixed store of energy available to the body. As time passes, the energy available is depleted, and, because it cannot be restored, the person dies.

Later, other related theories emerged. The *wear and tear theory* stated that the body is like a machine that wears out its parts with repeated use and comes to a grinding halt. Today, the concept of wear and tear is not widely accepted as an explanation for the aging process. However, this theory may explain the development of certain diseases, such as degenerative joint disease, in which the joint cartilage degenerates with prolonged use.

A more popular theory is the *stress theory,* which focuses on the physical and psychological wear and tear from sudden and unexpected stressors over which a person has no control. This theory maintains that a person copes with stressors through a three-stage process of alarm, resistance, and exhaustion (see Chap. 8). This process eventually leaves the person weakened because of the accumulation of successive stressful events over the life span. Stress theory suggests that as people age they are no longer capable of fighting off the various stressors as a result of the accumulation of wear and tear.

Genetic Theories

A major breakthrough to help explain biological development was the identification of deoxyribonucleic acid (DNA) molecules as the information center of the cell. This discovery led to the theory that cellular death results from DNA damage. The possibility that biological aging results when the wrong information is provided for normal cell function has been considered and is called *error theory.*

Several theories suggest that aging changes may occur as a result of an alteration in cellular genetic information. For example, the *cross-link theory* proposes that a chemical reaction occurs that produces irreparable damage to DNA and consequent cell death (Matteson et al., 1997).

In clinical practice, it is interesting to note the trend for similar life expectancies in families. It is not unusual for a person of advanced age to state that he or she had parents who also lived to be very old.

Single-Organ Theories

Other physiologic theories of aging have attempted to explain aging and the life span on the basis of changes in a single organ or in terms of impairments in control mechanisms. One theory suggests that aging results primarily from lowered oxygen supply delivered to crucial body tissue, such as brain tissue. Other theories suggest that thyroid gland function might be responsible for the slowing of metabolic processes at the cellular level (because cellular metabolism is regulated by the thyroid gland). The slowing of metabolic processes would then promote aging.

Free Radical Theory

Free radicals are highly reactive cellular components that replace genetic information at the cellular level. Lipofuscin is a material that is associated with free radicals and is rich in lipids and protein. This abnormal substance has been found in large quantities in body organs as they age. Some researchers suggest that the accumulation of lipofuscin interferes with cellular metabolism and may play an important role in the aging process (Matteson et al., 1997).

Immunity Theory

According to the immunity theory, as people age, mutations occur in some cells, resulting in the formation of proteins that the body does not recognize. The immune system then produces antibodies against these new proteins and attempts to destroy them, causing an autoimmune response (Matteson et al., 1997). With increasing age, there would then be a reduction in the function of the immune system. The antibodies fail to recognize abnormal cells, allowing them to divide and multiply. Immune system failure might then promote such late-life diseases as cancer, diabetes, and emphysema.

Sociologic Theories of Aging

The concept of socialization during adulthood refers to the process by which people, over the course of their adult lives, acquire ways to perform new roles. Several theories are relevant to how adults learn which roles bring rewards and which roles are considered undesirable and how they adjust to changing roles and role losses in society. These include Rosow's role theory and the activity theory.

Rosow's Role Theory

Rosow (1974) maintained that socialization for roles is a continuous and cumulative process that corresponds to the developmental stages of the life cycle. Socialization for roles begins in infancy and extends through adolescence. However, the actual learning of specific role demands begins and continues as a person moves through the stages of adulthood.

The concept of role continuity suggests that role demands of the previous stage prepare the person for the responsibilities associated with the next status or position

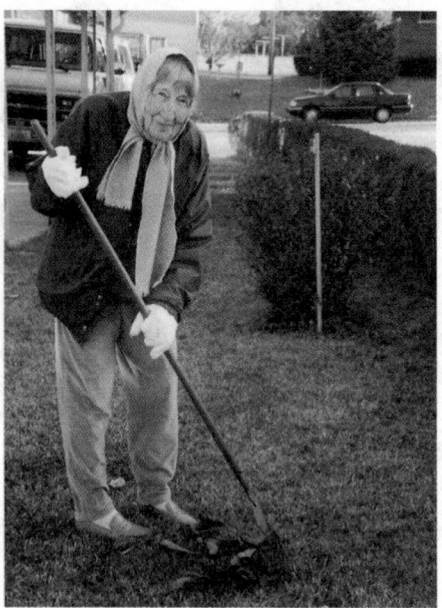

Figure 5–1. An active elderly woman.

that the adult assumes. Thus, role transitions through the life span progress in a smooth manner from one age level to the next.

Activity Theory

The activity theory holds that the maintenance of activities is important to most people as a basis for obtaining satisfaction, self-esteem, and health. Most research has shown the importance of activity as the basis for the promotion of vigor and satisfactory adjustment in the elderly (Fig. 5–1). People who restrict their activities as they age may tend to experience a reduction in overall life satisfaction. The significance of this theory to nurses is that they should encourage older adults to remain active to the extent they are able. Continued activity includes both physical actions and cognitive stimulation.

Psychological Theories of Aging

Psychological theories of aging are often the extension of sociologic and developmental theories. Personality theories usually consider the human needs and forces that motivate thought and behavior within a physical and social environment. The problem with studying personality changes throughout adulthood is that, as people pass through life, they become increasingly different rather than more similar. Theorists who have addressed adult personality development have primarily focused on one central issue: whether adult personality is characterized by continuity or by change.

Jung (1928/1971) was one of the first psychologists to consider that the latter half of life has a purpose of its own, quite apart from that of survival: namely, the development of self-awareness through reflective activity. He strongly believed in the importance of the latter half of life. This phase is characterized by inner discovery, as opposed to the first half of life, which is oriented toward biological and social goals. Jung's work regarding the life review process clearly defined the growth potential for aged adults. A review of past events, or reminiscence, helps with personal growth and evolving identity.

STAGES OF ADULTHOOD

Adulthood can be divided into three broad categories: young adulthood, middle adulthood, and older adulthood. In general, experts in adult development do not agree on the age span for each category. Therefore, differences in the professional and popular literature are common.

The medical-surgical nurse should know about normal adult development as a basis for physical and psychosocial assessment. A review of normal development and associated health issues follows.

Young Adulthood

Young adulthood is generally designated as the period between the 18th and 35th year. Many young adults are able today to postpone the tasks of adulthood, to experiment, and to prolong their own transition from childhood by exploring the many choices available to them. This period offers the time needed for the person to grow and make the necessary and complex linkages with adult society.

Physiologic Changes
Musculoskeletal Changes

Even though growth essentially ceases at adolescence, minimal growth can continue. Fusion of the epiphyses of long bones occurs approximately at age 18 to 25 years. Muscular efficiency is at its peak level between ages 20 and 30 years. Thereafter, muscular strength declines. Regular exercise is important to maintain a healthy body. People often become more sedentary in the postadolescent years as a result of the lack of a regular exercise plan, changes in work and leisure activities, and alterations in eating patterns.

Cardiopulmonary Changes

Physical development of the heart, blood vessels, and lungs stops in adolescence. Maintaining cardiopulmonary functioning and preventing pathologic changes during the second half of life largely depend on the young adult's lifestyle practices that are carried into middle age and late life.

Although arteriosclerotic disease becomes clinically evident in middle adulthood, it represents the result of progressive changes in the arterial walls that began in childhood. Studies are currently under way to examine the lifestyles of children and to find ways to improve health during childhood to prevent later problems.

TRANSCULTURAL CONSIDERATIONS

Although heart disease is not usually associated with the young adult age group, heart-related mortality for young Native Americans is about twice that for all other young adults living in the United States (Jarvis, 1996).

Integumentary Changes

The abundance of skin care and hair-coloring products attests to the aging changes that begin in young adulthood. These changes are often traumatic if a young adult has accepted the youth-oriented value system in Western countries like the United States and Canada.

Wrinkling of the skin occurs with aging and is markedly increased by exposure to the sun. Facial wrinkling becomes obvious in most adults in their 20s and tends to be progressive thereafter. Early wrinkling is usually related to habitual facial expressions, such as frowning and smiling. The skin loses its moisture and gradually dries. In later years, the atrophy of fat accelerates and increases the appearance of wrinkles.

The onset of graying hair and baldness often begins in young adulthood as well. Graying of hair results from the inability of melanocytes to provide hair with pigment granules over time. Hair loss with aging results from a number of factors. Although it is more common in men, it also occurs in women. Early balding is a result of genetic factors and is related to the amount of androgens, such as testosterone, that are produced (Fig. 5–2).

Dental Changes

The third molars, or wisdom teeth, normally erupt in an adult's early 20s. There are four third molars, although in some adults all four may not develop fully. Wisdom teeth frequently present problems and require dental care.

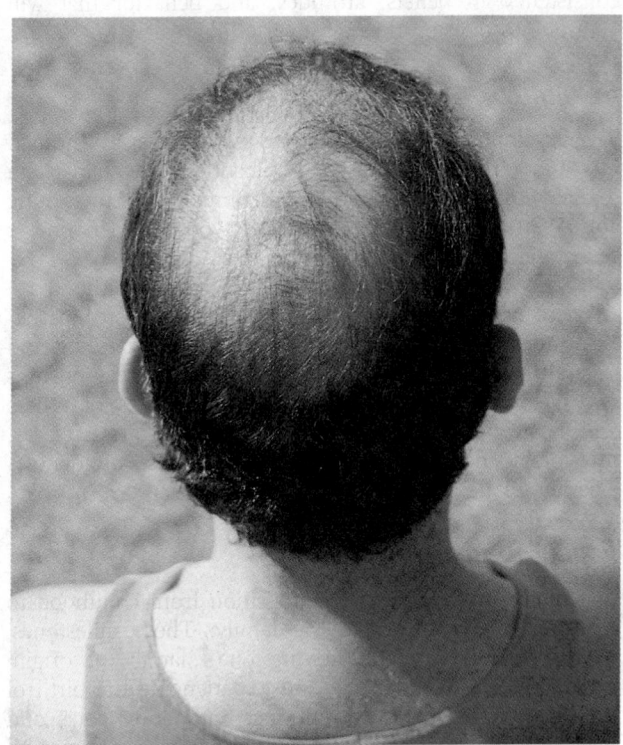

Figure 5–2. Early balding. This man is in his early 30s.

Their eruptions are unpredictable, and it is not uncommon for them to be malaligned or to remain impacted in the gums.

Psychosocial Development

The central issues of psychosocial development in young adulthood are related to the final resolution of the identity crises begun in adolescence. People work through these issues rather slowly. By the time the adolescent reaches young adulthood, some of these issues are nearing resolution.

The young adult struggles with expanding a sense of self in determining who he or she is within various social roles. In this stage of identity development, the prime concern is the relationship between the person and the social system. Young adults seek to resolve several psychosocial issues in their quest for maturity.

Self-Identity

In young adulthood, the sense of self usually becomes sharper and clearer, more consistent, and less influenced by others. This identification is quite different from that in the adolescent, who is self-conscious and concerned with seeing the self from the viewpoint of others.

Young adults become increasingly more comfortable with making decisions when faced with unexpected life events. In the mature young adult, coping with the unexpected does not easily disrupt the sense of continuity and integration.

As young adults participate in adult roles, they select lifestyle patterns and role combinations that endure through later life. These decisions solidify their self-identity and enable the young adult to develop a sense of consistency in beliefs, attitudes, and behavior that will continue to develop through their adult years.

Sexuality

The development of contraceptive pills, the fear of human immunodeficiency viral (HIV) infection, and changes in sexual mores have resulted in a dilemma for many young adults. Much conflict and confusion occur when one is questioning values related to sexuality.

Change in the sexual aspects of young adulthood relates to more than just sexual behavior. Relationships become increasingly more responsive to understanding and accepting others as they are. Interpersonal relationships depend more on appreciating the uniqueness of others and less on a projection of one's adolescent fantasies, physiologic needs, and a search for a sense of identity. Chapter 11 describes sexuality in detail.

Family Structure

The major milestones of the transition from childhood to adulthood largely involve the family. These milestones, which typically include leaving one's family of origin, selecting a mate, marrying, and experiencing the birth of the first child, mark the entrance into adult roles and functions (Fig. 5–3). Not all young adults experience all of these milestones. Not everyone marries or has children.

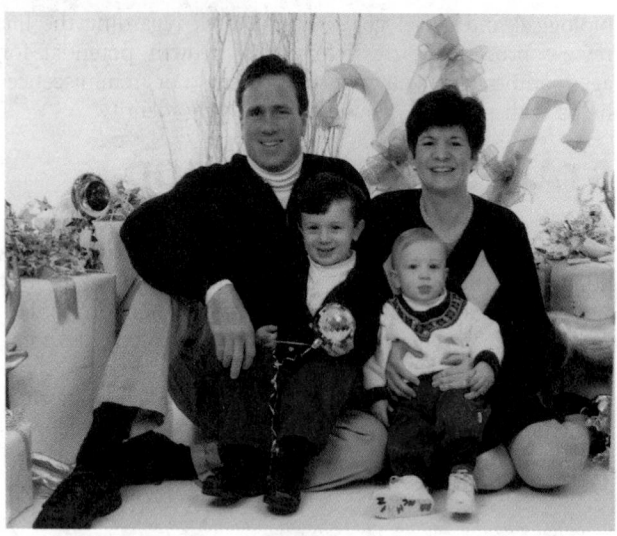

Figure 5–3. A young family.

Some adults select homosexual rather than heterosexual relationships.

In the United States, two general types of family structures exist: patriarchal (headed by men) and matriarchal (headed by women).

TRANSCULTURAL CONSIDERATIONS

About half of all African-American families are matriarchal, in contrast to one fourth of Hispanic families and one sixth of Caucasian families (Giger & Davidhizar, 1995).

Patriarchal Family Structure

If the young adult marries and has children, the event of marriage and the establishment of the family bring about many changes and crisis points. The birth of a child requires a major shift from a primarily spousal role to the demands and responsibilities of a parental role. This resocialization requires not only the learning of a new role but also the ability to combine this new role into a set pattern with other roles. The addition of a dependent, demanding third person may disrupt the established couple relationship as well as one's routine patterns of living.

Matriarchal Family Structure

In the United States, one of every two marriages ends in divorce. More often than not, children of divorced parents live with their mother, which can place a physical, financial, and emotional burden on the single parent. Some single mothers have never been married or may not have ongoing contact with the father of their children. Financial or child care support may not be available, and the mother is left with the total responsibility of childrearing. The single mother often ignores personal needs to balance child care, work, and home responsibilities. This family structure, rather than the traditional patriarchal structure described by Havighurst (1972), is becoming increasingly more common in the late 1990s and into the 21st century.

Work

Entrance into the work world for the young adult involves a twofold process. The first aspect is the choice of an occupation, followed by socialization into the role demands of the job. The process of selecting and maintaining an occupation is characterized by more flexibility than in years past. The traditional factors of social class, culture, intelligence, gender, aptitudes, role models, and experiences that once operated to limit the range of choices have lost much, but not all, of their impact.

Both partners in a relationship may work outside the home. Not infrequently, one person may need to work at two jobs. Over the past decade, unemployment in the United States has dramatically increased as a result of restructuring and re-engineering of most major businesses. Finding jobs has become more difficult and has greatly increased stress for many adults. Homelessness has increased, and an increasing number of people have no health insurance or are underinsured.

Many young adults see prolonged or continuous education as the means to obtain desired standards of living. This often means postponing intimate relationships or combining the roles of student, temporary worker, partner, and parent. Balancing these responsibilities at a time when young adults are still acquiring basic knowledge and skills needed to resolve their developmental tasks can create considerable stress.

Leisure

Leisure in adulthood is often a difficult concept to define. Most adults consider their work to be the most meaningful activity in their lives. Work provides the necessities of life. It is also the major aspect of one's identity and status. Therefore, to many people, leisure is a negative concept rather than a potentially positive, healthful experience in its own right.

Health Issues

The young adulthood years are usually the healthiest years in the life cycle. Most young adults are not seriously ill or incapacitated. As a result, young adults often feel a sense of immunity to illness and neglect health promotion and maintenance activities. The greatest potential for improving health is in what people do and do not do for themselves. Young adults' decisions about diet, exercise, smoking, and drug use are of critical importance to their health status in middle age and later life.

Health Promotion

For young adults to maintain optimal health, the nurse should encourage them to have regular physical examinations, with more frequent visits if there are particular problems. For early detection of cancer, young women should have routine Papanicolaou (Pap) tests and perform breast self-examination (BSE) once a month. The nurse teaches BSE to women and teaches testicular self-examination (TSE) to young men. Young adults should schedule annual dental examinations to avoid dental and periodontal disorders. In addition, young adults should have

---

Chart 5–1

Health Promotion Guide: Activities to Promote Health and Prevent Illness

- Have regular (yearly) physical examinations.
- For women, have regular Pap tests and perform breast self-examination monthly.
- For men, perform testicular self-examination on a regular basis.
- Have annual dental examinations and prophylaxis.
- Have regular eye examinations (every 1–2 years).
- Exercise regularly at least three times a week for 30 minutes.
- Do not smoke; avoid second-hand (passive) smoke.
- Avoid alcohol and so-called recreational drugs.
- Decrease fat and increase fiber in the diet.

---

regular eye examinations every 1 to 2 years (Chart 5–1). Despite a general state of good health, young adults are susceptible to a few major health concerns.

Accidents

In the United States, accidents are the most frequent cause of death among young adults. Injuries occur as a result of work-related incidents, thrill-seeking pleasures, violent crimes, automobile accidents, and war. Men are consistently more frequently involved in accidents throughout the life cycle than women. Between the ages of 15 and 34 years, the death rate among males is more than three times that among females, largely because of the high rate of accidental deaths.

The everyday lives of young adults present stressful experiences, such as driving in city traffic and caring for small children, that contribute to accidents. Excessive fatigue occurs in young adults who attempt to balance too many roles. Stress overload combined with excessive fatigue can lead to accidents as well as psychosomatic illnesses.

Young adults should be especially aware of maintaining good health care practices, such as well-balanced diets, regular exercise, and adequate sleep. Because accidents and their consequences present major threats to their health, young adults should take care when engaging in potentially hazardous activities. This care includes using seat belts, avoiding drinking when driving, following speed limits, and observing caution around machinery. In many states in this country, nurses have advocated for legislation that mandates the use of seat belts and motorcycle helmets to help prevent serious injuries from accidents.

Homicide and Suicide

After accidents, the leading causes of death in young adults are homicide and suicide. The highest incidence of homicide is associated with young African-Americans living in urban areas (Giger & Davidhizar, 1995). Some of the deaths are related to substance abuse, such as drugs and alcohol, and the formation of gangs.

Drug and Alcohol Use and Misuse

Few issues have received as much recent attention as drug and alcohol abuse. Use of alcohol and other illicit drugs has increased significantly in the last two decades. Even though the use of tobacco has declined, the use of potentially addictive agents in young adulthood has not decreased, despite the numerous efforts to control this problem. Many law enforcement agencies have united in an effort to identify and prosecute drug dealers, buyers, and users. Clinics and programs have also been established to help people wean themselves from drugs. National prevention and awareness programs like DARE (Drug Awareness Resistance Education) have been conducted in elementary and middle schools across the United States for a number of years.

Regardless of the health care setting, the role of the nurse is affected by the growing problem of substance abuse. In the medical-surgical setting, the nurse often provides care for the client who is or has been a substance abuser. As a result, the planning of nursing interventions is typically more difficult and complicated. For example, the client in pain from a fractured tibia may want pain medication by injection on a regular basis. If the nurse's assessment does not validate that the client is in severe pain, the nurse is faced with an ethical dilemma as well as a care management decision.

Even though alcohol and drug problems are often associated with young adults, this age group is not the only one affected by these addictive agents. Middle-aged and older adults often use addictive agents, but the nurse may have more difficulty in assessing this problem in these groups.

Middle Adulthood

The time between 35 and 64 years of age is generally considered the period of middle age. This period has been described as the "best years" in the life cycle. During this span of time, adults refer to being in the "prime of life." If healthy development has occurred, the struggles of young adulthood are past and have been resolved, and middle-aged adults should be able to enjoy the results of their labor as established, mature, social, and personally valued people. Yet this time is fraught with its own difficulties.

Middlescence (middle age) is recognized as the midpoint in the life cycle. Most people reflect on and evaluate their lives during this period. Evaluation is not an unusual experience, but it takes on special meaning at this time. The accomplishments of young adulthood shape the life of the middlescent. At this point, people may suddenly realize that this transitional period is the last chance to change life's direction. Many middlescents begin to examine the results of their life work against what they want to do with the rest of their lives. Most of the young adulthood years were spent in working toward achieving goals set in youth. Middlescents reassess their choices and wonder if their chosen directions will progress toward realizing their life goals or desires. This examination may result in massive lifestyle changes for some. This often unsettling time of life, which entails the transition to old age, is often referred to as the midlife crisis.

Physiologic Changes

From young adulthood through the middle years, physiologic changes occur gradually.

Sensory Changes

Visual Changes

All people eventually experience a change in visual acuity. The decreased ability of the eyes to accommodate for close and detailed work (presbyopia) becomes evident at about age 35 and continues throughout the rest of one's life. Pupil size becomes smaller, which decreases the amount of light that reaches the retina. This change limits the ability of the pupil to constrict and dilate and affects the ability to adapt one's vision in dim light and darkness.

Toward the end of middlescence, the eyes are less able to detect the blues, violets, and greens of the color spectrum and more easily adapt to reds, yellows, and oranges. This change in color perception is linked to the yellowing of the lens with advancing age, but it is not actually a color vision impairment (Matteson et al., 1997).

People in their 50s need about twice as much light to see things as they did when they were in their 20s. There is a need for more light for all visual perception with advancing age. The nurse teaches middle-aged and older adults to use extra lighting at home to prevent falls. In the health care setting, the nurse provides adequate lighting, especially at night.

Hearing Changes

Hearing loss typically begins in late middlescense. Changes in the efficiency of the cochlea and the hair cells of the organ of Corti are responsible for the impaired transmission of sound waves along the nerve pathways of the brain. These changes are considered to be the most common cause of presbycusis, which is progressive hearing loss associated with aging (Ney, 1993). Presbycusis primarily affects the ability to hear high-pitched sounds and soft consonants or consonant blends. For example, the "s," "sh," and "ch" sounds are difficult for people with presbycusis to differentiate in conversations. Vowels that have a low pitch are more easily heard. Background noise interferes with conversation, so that it is difficult to hear what is being said.

The abilities to see and to hear are major contributors to communication. Age-related changes in these abilities are not only frustrating but also threatening to security and self-esteem. Yet many middlescents are reluctant to wear eyeglasses or hearing aids, even when vision or hearing problems significantly affect functioning. Many seem to want to deny the problem rather than to admit to age-related changes. The nurse teaches middle and older adults the importance of wearing assistive devices if needed to help prevent falls or other accidents.

Neuromuscular Changes

For many middlescents, sedentary or slower paced lifestyles result in loss of muscle strength and mass. This loss of muscle tone is noticed as the waistline thickens, the abdomen protrudes, and facial tissue sags.

There is a gradual decline in motor and sensory functioning from its peak during a person's 20s to lower levels in the middle years. Reflexes that entail responses to sudden changes in the environment may be slowed, but for the most part the alterations in function occur gradually and go unnoticed.

Middle-aged adults view neuromuscular changes as relatively insignificant because their progress is so gradual that most people have learned to compensate for them. For example, driving ability is considered to be *better* in middle-aged adults than in younger people, despite declines in coordination, increased reaction time, and sensitivity to glare. It seems that the improvements in judgment and caution compensate for the physical declines. The same is true for manual workers. Middle-aged people usually have fewer disabling injuries and are more conscientious and careful than their younger counterparts.

Cardiopulmonary Changes

Coronary and pulmonary diseases are among the leading causes of morbidity and mortality in middlescence. These problems are more probably related to lifestyle and genetic factors than to aging per se.

Heart function, rate, and rhythm usually remain unchanged in middlescence. However, when lifestyles become sedentary, anatomic and physiologic changes may occur. Lack of regular exercise over time causes the heart muscle to lose its tone, and changes in rate and rhythm result. Among the most significant factors implicated in atherosclerosis and heart disease are poor nutrition, lack of physical exercise, smoking, and stress.

Pulmonary changes in middlescence are largely related to whether the person is or has been a smoker. Smoking decreases respiratory efficiency and increases the risk of lung disease. Smoking and chronic lung disease largely account for the loss of functioning in lung tissues seen in middlescence. These risk factors, coupled with environmental or occupational pollution, inactivity, and altered cardiac status, can result in decreased breathing capacity. The nurse assesses for risk factors and provides health teaching, such as smoking cessation and regular exercise, to reduce them.

Dental Changes

Dental problems tend to be a major concern throughout middlescence. Many people older than 55 years have lost some of their teeth. This problem is related to lack of dental care throughout the earlier years rather than to the aging process. The nurse teaches the importance of proper dental health care to prevent further problems.

Endocrine Changes

Throughout the adult life span, there is a progressive decrease in a person's ability to metabolize glucose efficiently. In fact, this deterioration in performance is so great that nearly all older adults are thought to have increased glucose levels.

The levels of male and female sex hormones decrease in middlescence. Reduced hormone levels result in atrophy of the ovaries, uterus, and vaginal tissues in women. Women lose their ability to have children, but men can father children well into their 70s.

Women are also highly predisposed to osteoporosis, which can lead to painful fractures and heart disease. The decrease in estrogen production after menopause is associated with these health problems. In men, a tendency for benign prostatic hypertrophy occurs during the middle years.

Psychosocial Development

Middlescence (middle age) is an often unsettling time of questioning former goals, determining what a person wants for the future, and making decisions or changes that will influence the second half of life. It is the time when most people acknowledge that they have begun to grow older. Although middle-aged adults recognize that they are in their prime of life, they also realize that time is limited, and many accept that they cannot achieve all that they had once hoped. For many people, middlescence is the last chance to identify and pursue new goals and interests. For others, it is merely a plateau into old age.

Self-Concept

If the maturing years of young adulthood have been handled successfully, middlescents usually have the wisdom and skills to see themselves and their world more realistically. Awareness of their future assists them to see middlescence as a point in the life cycle when they must make changes, if changes are to be made at all. Typically, middle-aged adults are assessing what they have achieved in the second half of life regarding their careers, marriages or other intimate relationships, families, lifestyles, social roles, and friendships. For some, this reassessment can result in drastic changes in any or all of these aspects. Others may elect to continue with their established patterns for the remainder of their lives.

Sexuality

Biologically, the most significant milestone in middlescence is the so-called change of life. This change is signaled by the *climacteric* in both women and men, but it is far less dramatic in men. Climacteric in women, or *menopause,* refers to the process during which menses (menstrual periods) cease, ovaries stop producing ova and female sex hormones, and the genitals atrophy. Other possible signs are sweats, hot flashes, palpitations, dizziness, and emotional changes, such as irritability and depression.

Climacteric for men involves a decrease in the levels of the male sex hormones. This decline is so gradual that most men can produce sperm until well into old age. The male climacteric is not as abrupt or intense as menopause.

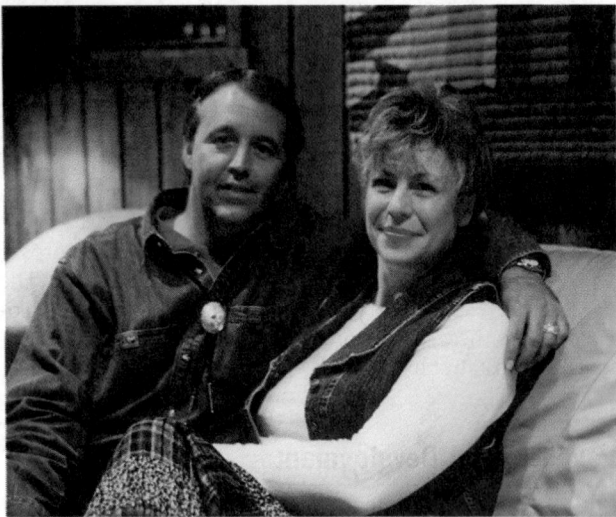

Figure 5–4. A middle-aged couple whose relationship is stronger after active parenting.

Family Structure

Changes within family relationships, such as children leaving home, separation and divorce, aging of parents, and death of a spouse or partner, are often experienced in the middle years. Coping adequately with these changes is a major task of middlescense. Ideally, people should deal with these considerable changes in a manner that helps them grow toward emotional maturity and feel secure and independent rather than depressed, ill, or dependent.

Child Launching

The child-launching phase begins when the first child leaves the parental home and ends when the parents face each other again as a couple. Because of their usually greater emotional and time investments in childrearing, readjustment tends to be more critical and profound for women than for men. The arrival of this change often coincides with menopause, and for family-oriented women the combination of these events may be very stressful. Some women seem unable, for a time, to develop an alternative workable identity, find new ways of nurturing, or find new interests and goals to fill empty time.

Reactions to child launching depend on individual differences and life situations. Women who have combined the work role with motherhood may find it a time of freedom from family responsibilities and financial pressures. Other women may continue to find satisfaction through the roles of wife, partner, or grandmother or through work or other activities. Other women may find their lives lonely, frustrating, and generally unsatisfying. To cope effectively, a strong sense of self-identity and an ability to shift roles are crucial.

Change in Intimate Relationships

The stage after active parenting in the family life cycle also greatly influences the marital or intimate relationship.

The couple must learn to divert the energy and feelings that flowed to their children back to each other. For many couples, the happiest years of the relationship are those before the children are born and after the children are on their own. In these latter years, the couple often experiences a sense of freedom and privacy they have not had for years. This freedom provides an opportunity to get to know each other as people. Divorce or dissolution of an intimate relationship may occur during this time if the relationship has been shaky over the childrearing years. If the relationship has been good, however, it is likely to improve at this time (Fig. 5–4).

If divorce has occurred, a middle-aged adult may remarry and begin a second family. It is not unusual for a middlescent to have several adult children and preschool children from a second or third marriage.

Caring for Aging Parents

During middlescence, a drastic change seems to occur in the relationship between middle-aged children and their parents. Parents suddenly seem old. Aged parents begin to seek their children's help in making decisions and may become dependent for physical and financial support. Middlescents may have to make tough decisions about their parents' living arrangements. Strain is often placed on married middlescents as they weigh their responsibilities toward their parents against those toward their spouse and children. When parents move in with their children, conflict can occur. There may be competition for existing family roles, financial strains, space constraints, or anger over increased responsibilities if the aged person is ill. If the decision to institutionalize the elder is made, the adult child often experiences guilt about the perceived abandonment of the parent. The middle-aged adult who has to care for an older parent while continuing to rear children is sometimes referred to as belonging to the "sandwich generation" (Fig. 5–5).

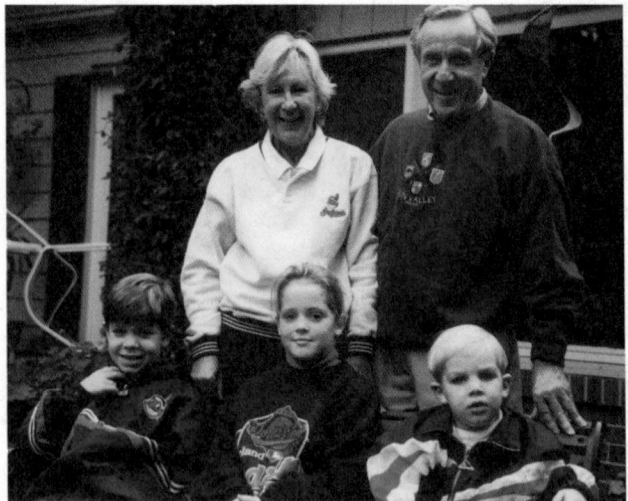

Figure 5–5. Grandparenting roles vary, but everyone involved may benefit from the relationships regardless of the roles.

TRANSCULTURAL CONSIDERATIONS

The overall institutionalization rate for elderly African-Americans is less than that for Caucasians. A greater number of African-Americans and other minorities choose to care for their elders themselves as a result of a greater sense of responsibility to their older family members and strong religious beliefs (Ignatavicius, 1998).

The medical-surgical nurse needs to be aware that families often are or will be the caregivers after a hospitalized older adult is discharged. The caregivers are usually wives or daughters. Chapter 8 discusses the caregiver stress experienced by these family members.

Work

For almost all adults, the work role provides a major source of esteem, satisfaction, happiness, and identity. It is a frequently observed phenomenon that career-oriented men and women become increasingly preoccupied with their work as they grow older. This preoccupation with work is a common phenomenon, tending to exclude leisure activities and other roles.

Most adults peak in their careers during middlescence and continue in their chosen fields until retirement. However, there is a new tendency toward changing occupational directions in the middle years. Seeking a second career is an emerging trend within some groups. One such group comprises people who are forced to find new directions because of technological or economic factors, such as unemployment. Another group includes women who, after devoting their adulthood years to marriage and children, seek a career as an avenue of financial gain and personal growth and satisfaction. Similarly, many people who joined the work force in early adulthood and are eligible for early retirement seek a second career rather than face retirement, which they perceive as boring, idle, and wasteful. Yet another group includes those who made career choices in young adulthood that did not provide them with a sense of satisfaction.

Leisure

During the later middle adult years, most people find themselves with more time on their hands than their experience or interests can accommodate. Settling into careers, launching children, and retiring result in much unstructured time. Adjustment to this free time is largely related to the person's attitudes toward these events. If the person perceives these losses negatively, fears the loss of accustomed roles or friends, or is uncertain about the future, adjustment may be difficult.

People seek to enhance a positive self-concept through numerous pursuits and interests beyond those of the work and family roles. These alternatives can make the pending loss of roles a means for greater involvement in challenges that are equally important. It is vital for all middlescents to sustain feelings of self-worth by having several alternative life pursuits as the means for achieving a continuing sense of personal growth.

Health Issues

Although there are inevitable physical changes and an increasing incidence of chronic conditions as one passes through the middle years, most of the changes from young adulthood are minor ones. Few middlescents are affected by conditions or diseases that necessitate a change in lifestyle or that have a substantial effect on their future. The most common causes of death during the middle years are heart disease, cancer, strokes, and respiratory tract disease. People who smoke, drink alcohol, are obese, have high cholesterol levels, and are inactive are at high risk for these health problems.

General health during middlescence is better than most people expect. Yet it is important for middlescents to engage in preventive and health promotion practices to retain optimal health. The nurse encourages middle-aged adults to schedule annual physical and eye examinations and semiannual dental examinations to detect and treat any significant changes. Because of the relationship of smoking and cardiopulmonary diseases, the nurse encourages smokers to limit or stop their habit. The nurse may refer clients to a smoking cessation program, if available. A regular exercise program and sound nutritional practices, such as reducing the intake of cholesterol and saturated fats, are also effective preventive health measures.

Marital state appears to influence health maintenance as well; married people often live longer than single or widowed people. When roles are lost in middlescence, it is important for one's mental health to move into another lifestyle that will be satisfying. Prolonged psychological stress throughout these transition periods can cause injury, illness, and physical and emotional threats.

Late Adulthood

Over the past century, the elderly population (those 65 years of age and older) has increased at rates far higher than those for other segments. The proportion of elderly people in the United States is expected to increase. In 1990, there were 30.1 million older adults, making up 13.3% of the U.S. population. By the year 2030, that proportion is expected to double. Advances in health care and improved health maintenance habits have resulted in a healthier aged population, with greater numbers of elderly living longer.

The aged person has unique attributes that can be either used or allowed to remain dormant. Many societies neglect or fail to activate the potential of these people because of stereotypic beliefs about older people. Gerontological research has indicated that there is a systematic stereotyping of and discrimination against people who are old. This is also called *ageism*. It is clear that an accurate understanding of the aged is often lacking.

Physiologic Changes

As in every other age cycle, there is no arbitrary dividing line to mark when middle age ends and old age begins. The most popular dividing point is 65 years of age, but some theorists use 55 or 60 years as a division point.

Chart 5-2

Nursing Focus on the Elderly: Effects of Aging on Body Systems

System/Function	Normal Changes	Abnormal Changes and Diseases
Cardiovascular	• Increase in the size of the heart • Increase in collagen • Increase in the thickness of valves and blood vessels • Decrease in cardiac output • Decrease in cardiac reserve • Decrease in blood flow to organs	• Hypertension • Coronary artery disease • Congestive heart failure • Peripheral vascular disease • Varicose veins
Endocrine		
Pancreas	• Decreased ability to metabolize glucose • Reduced insulin secretion • Delayed insulin response	• Diabetes mellitus
Gonads	• Decreased hormone levels • Atrophy of the ovaries, uterus, and vagina • Development of firmer testes • Benign prostatic hypertrophy	• Cancer of the uterus, ovaries, or vagina • Cancer of the prostate gland
Integumentary	• Thinning of epithelial cells and subcutaneous fat layers • Lines and wrinkles in the skin • Age spots • Roughness or dryness of the skin • Thinning and loss of color of the hair • Thickening and brittleness of the nails	• Infections: viral, bacterial, fungal • Abnormal cell growth • Tumors: benign and malignant • Skin ulcerations
Musculoskeletal	• Loss of flexibility in the joints • Cartilage degeneration • Bony growths at the edges of joints • Decreased muscle mass	• Osteoporosis • Rheumatoid arthritis • Fracture • Loss of height as a result of spinal column changes
Neurologic	• General slowing of reaction time • Slow responses to heat and cold • Changing sleep patterns • Decreased cerebral blood flow	• Cerebrovascular disease • Parkinson's disease • Senile dementia and Alzheimer's disease

Physical changes take place at different rates in different people. However, all the body systems are affected somewhat by the aging process. Although some changes become apparent in earlier stages, old age seems to be the time in the life cycle when the progressive changes become more readily apparent and degenerative changes occur more rapidly (Chart 5-2).

In each body system assessment chapter in this text, Nursing Focus on the Elderly charts list major physiologic changes in older people and the nursing implications associated with each change. In addition, normal laboratory values that differ in the elderly are included in Lab Profile charts when appropriate.

Integumentary Changes

Of all body tissue, the fatty tissue layer fluctuates the most throughout life and with aging is subject to the greatest change. Peripheral body parts display the most striking examples of this alteration. For example, veins and bones of the hand become prominent under a parchment-like, thin layer of skin, and deep hollows appear in the clavicular and axillary areas of the body. The elderly person is susceptible to skin tears, which heal slowly as a result of decreased blood flow to the skin and soft tissues. Breasts sag and become pendulous, and the eyes seem to sink, because of the disappearance of the fat layer around the orbit and decreased skin elasticity.

Subcutaneous tissue has a significant role in the body's adjustment to temperature change. The natural insulation that subcutaneous fat provides is lost. It is not uncommon to hear elderly people say that they are cold, nor is it uncommon to see them wearing a sweater or sitting with a lap blanket when environmental temperatures are comfortable for younger people.

Although subcutaneous tissue does not affect the aged person's tolerance of heat, problems with heat tolerance do exist. Changes in the sweat glands, which diminish in size, number, and activity, cause a decline in the efficiency of the body's cooling mechanism. The elderly do not perspire freely, leaving them at high risk for heat exhaustion. They need to be aware of these changes and learn how to compensate. The nurse teaches them to avoid extreme heat conditions. Sudden changes in room temperature or exposure to overly heated bath water causes the blood vessels in the skin and muscles to dilate.

Chart 5–2		

Nursing Focus on the Elderly: Effects of Aging on Body Systems *Continued*

System/Function	Normal Changes	Abnormal Changes and Diseases
Pulmonary	• Increase in the diameter of the chest • Decrease in coughing ability • Decrease in vital capacity and tidal volume • Increase in the production of mucus • Progressive kyphosis • Calcification of the cartilage connecting the ribs to the spinal column and sternum • Decreased strength of the expiratory muscles • Thickening of the alveolar walls, decreased recoil	• Asthma • Bronchitis • Emphysema • Pneumonia • Tuberculosis
Sensory Sight	• Presbyopia • Lowered acuity • Altered accommodation to light and dark • Difficulty in color discrimination • Decreased lens clarity	• Cataracts • Glaucoma • Senile ocular degeneration
Hearing	• Decreased discrimination of pitch and acuity • Decreased sensitivity to higher frequency sounds • Excessive cerumen	• Deafness
Touch	• Decreased receptors • Lowered ability to distinguish temperature and feel pain	• Total loss of feeling
Taste	• Decreased number of taste buds • Diminished ability to distinguish specific tastes	• Total loss of taste
Smell	• Decreased olfactory function • Diminished sensation to distinguish specific odors	• Total loss of smell
Urinary	• Diminished kidney function • Decreased glomerular filtration rate • Decreased number of nephrons • Decreased muscle tone to bladder • Decreased bladder capacity • Decreased sphincter control	• Urinary retention • Urinary tract infection

This can result in temporary slowing of blood to the brain, leading to a temporary changes in mental status or to dizziness.

Sleep Changes

The aged take longer to move through the relaxation stages of non–rapid eye movement (non-REM) sleep. The number of awakenings and their duration increase. When asked about the quality of sleep, the aged often respond that they hardly slept all night. Typically, their sleep is more fragmented than that of the young. These interruptions are often caused by nocturia (urination at night), leg cramps, and mental stimulation through worry, bereavement, or extraneous noises (Johnson, 1991). It was thought at one time that the elderly needed more sleep, but this is not usually true. The aged seem to sleep less. If one sleeps more, it is usually because of boredom, depression, sedation, or symptoms of disease.

The aged who are not aware that these changes are normal may worry, and the more they worry, the less they sleep. Noisy environments, unresolved fears, worries, and concerns also disrupt sleep quality and patterns. Health care providers often attempt to address the problem by prescribing sleep medications. However, few hypnotic drugs have been found to promote the entire sleep cycle. Instead, these drugs depress REM sleep, or deep sleep, which is necessary for intellectual functioning and for the relief of tension and anxiety. When medications are discontinued, normal sleep patterns usually return but not until fully re-established dreaming patterns emerge.

Neurologic and Sensory Changes

With aging, the central nervous system loses neurons, has a decreased blood supply, and undergoes a decrease in electrical activity. Short-term memory may be affected, but long-term memory is usually intact. For the older adult, these changes may cause altered sensory perception and decreases in reaction time and movement time. It often takes the elder a longer time to respond and initiate action in a given situation.

Visual and hearing changes that started in a person's 30s become much more pronounced in old age. Vestibular (inner ear) functioning decreases, causing dizziness and poor balance. As a result, the elderly person is more prone to falls and accidents.

According to Ney (1993), 25% to 40% of all adults older than 65 are hearing impaired. Ninety percent of people in their 80s have a hearing handicap. Several anatomic changes contribute to hearing loss in the elderly. The cartilage of the auditory canal loses its elasticity and may become narrowed or collapse. In men, stiff coarse hairs in the auditory canal can block the outward flow of cerumen (Ney, 1993). Cerumen impaction sometimes results and can cause hearing impairment.

Cardiopulmonary Changes

All of the body systems and organs change with age, but the most serious changes affect the heart and lungs. The output of the heart is decreased, and the volume of oxygen-carrying blood to all parts of the body is reduced. The continuation of the arteriosclerotic process in the blood vessels ("hardening of the arteries") accentuates this problem.

Respiratory movements of the chest decrease as a result of reduced chest wall muscle activity and deterioration of the alveoli, which alters inspiratory and expiratory volumes. Less oxygen is consumed, and lower respiratory tract infections occur more frequently in older adults. The activity of the cilia diminishes, which allows pathogens and other foreign matter to enter the respiratory tract more easily. The cough reflex, another protective mechanism, is also diminished.

Musculoskeletal Changes

Musculoskeletal problems are very common in old age. The most frequent conditions are

- Degenerative joint changes
- Osteoporosis resulting from increased bone resorption
- Extra-articular pathologic changes of obscure origin, including fibrositis and bursitis
- Fractures caused by trauma and osteoporosis (bone loss)

In addition to these changes, posture and gait changes put the older person at risk for falls. The nurse teaches the older person how to prevent falls at home (e.g., by removing scatter rugs, wearing supportive shoes, and using ambulatory devices if needed).

A complete discussion of osteoporosis can be found in Chapter 53.

Urologic and Renal Changes

As a person ages, bladder capacity and muscle tone decrease, sometimes causing urinary retention and frequency. As a result, the older adult is prone to urinary tract infections and calculi. The older person typically has to wake in the middle of the night to void (nocturia).

Urinary incontinence is not a normal change associated with aging. However, many elderly people are incontinent. Because the urinary sphincter tone also decreases with age, stress incontinence, particularly in women, is fairly common. Stress incontinence, or urine leakage, occurs when the woman coughs, sneezes, or laughs. Although this can be very embarrassing, many lightweight protective products are available. If the condition worsens, treatment with exercises, medication, or surgery may be necessary.

Older men often experience benign prostatic hypertrophy, which causes overflow incontinence. Overflow incontinence is the constant dribbling of urine that results from an overly distended bladder. The enlarged prostate gland causes urine to be retained in the bladder.

The kidneys are also affected by the aging process. Renal nephrons decrease in number, resulting in a decreased ability to concentrate urine. Blood urea nitrogen (BUN) also increases as a result of a decreasing glomerular filtration rate.

Gastrointestinal Changes

In older people, the entire gastrointestinal tract undergoes atrophic changes that may interfere with the efficiency of its function. The capacity of the stomach may decrease, and gastric secretions may diminish. The nurse encourages the older adult to eat small, frequent meals. Digestion and absorption of nutrients from the small intestine are also slower. Constipation is a common complaint, usually caused by decreased peristalsis, decreased appetite, inadequate fluid consumption, and lack of exercise. Chronic laxative abuse over the years worsens the problem.

Nutritional Changes

As a result of a lack of proper dental care in earlier years, loss of teeth, gum disease, and bone degeneration may make eating more difficult for the elderly person. Chewing may become more difficult. Poor muscle tone, loss of digestive juices, and impaired circulation often create problems with digestion and elimination. Atrophy of the taste buds, coupled with problems related to dentition and digestion, diminishes the pleasure of eating for many older adults.

Changes in eating patterns often lead to anemia, malnutrition, and increased susceptibility to infections. The medical-surgical nurse should be aware that these problems can lead to serious complications when the client is ill or has had surgery.

Psychosocial Development

The last years of a person's life cycle constitute the final stage of development in which adults can grow and change. It is the phase in which the person has the opportunity to make final revisions. How well adults adapt to old age depends in part on how well they have resolved the tasks of the previous stages. People who enter old age with many unresolved crises from prior years experience a difficult time. For others, old age is a time to pass on the wisdom of one's experiences, continue fulfilling productive roles, and enjoy a sense of fulfillment for a life well lived.

Self-Concept

The way people regard themselves determines their life satisfaction. Self-concept is developed by a continuous interaction between a person and the environment. Loss of a significant other and loss of roles such as parent, spouse, and worker often affect the elder's sense of self and psychological well-being. The need to be creative and productive is particularly important in old age to gain attention and approval from others.

Other people may attempt to maintain a positive self-concept in several ways. These include such reactions as denial of illness, regression, or retreat into fantasy. Reminiscence may also be used as a defense against present threats to self-esteem. These reactions, although adaptive to conditions or events outside the control of the older person, do not help people to develop their personal potentials. Good health, adequate income, a useful role, opportunities for social interactions, and lively interests are the main determinants of a happy old age. An estimated 10% to 15% of the elderly population in the United States are in poor health and do not have adequate financial support to meet basic needs. (See Research Applications for Nursing.)

Sexuality

Studies of sexual behaviors and interest in these behaviors among the elderly have been limited and inconsistent in their findings. Many studies suggest that elders retain an interest in sexual function and are sexually active. Other studies conclude that there is a decline of sexual interest and behavior among the aged. Reported declines are largely the result of social, cultural, and psychological factors rather than biological and physical factors. Factors that determine sexual activity include present health status, past and present life satisfaction, and the status of marital or intimate relationship. For example, many older women are widowed or divorced and lack available sexual partners, which probably accounts for their decline in sexual interest.

Physiologic changes associated with the aging process occur in both men and women. In women, vaginal secretions diminish and the vagina atrophies. In men, the time required to attain an erection increases. With age, men are also able to maintain an erection for an extended period of time without ejaculation. After ejaculation, the older man often cannot have a subsequent erection for 12 to 24 hours. Despite these physiologic changes, both elderly men and women are capable of sexual activity, including intercourse.

▶ Research Applications for Nursing

Culture Influences Functional Health Status of Older Women

Gale, B. J., & Templeton, L. A. (1995). Functional health status of older women. Journal of the American Academy of Nurse Practitioners, 7, 323–327.

Two groups of elderly women were studied to determine differences in functional health status. Participants in the first group were 98% Caucasian and well educated, and reflected the profile of middle-class older women. The second group consisted of multiethnic women with lower socioeconomic indicators, including low income and less than high school preparation. As assessed by the Sickness Impact Profile tool, measuring physical, independent, and psychosocial health, the second study group had a poorer functional health status than the first group.

Critique. Most of the volunteers in the sample came from churches and volunteer community agencies. However, even though the study used a convenience sample, there was a total of 211 participants.

Possible Implications for Nursing. There has been a growing concern for the health of older women, who comprise most of the elderly population. All older women, especially non-Caucasians, need to be educated more about health promotion activities. The prescription of drugs that decrease functional ability should be discouraged among health care providers.

Family Structure

Three principal factors affect family structure and function in late life:

- Health status and expected life span
- Social changes, such as industrialization and urbanization
- Normal aging processes

Many married couples see their last child leave home when the couple are in their 40s or 50s and can expect to live another 30 or more years. This long period that follows active parenting responsibilities presents a variety of problems that elders have not had to deal with in previous generations, such as widowhood.

Widowhood

Although most elderly men are married, two thirds of all elderly women are widowed. Even when men have been widowed, their chances for remarriage are twice those of women (Matteson et al., 1997).

The elderly widowed person may confront the prospect of becoming socially isolated. The ability to prevent social isolation may be related to advanced level of education, residence in a small town or a rural area, or, most important, the presence of friends and neighbors with whom one can relate. Older widowed people may adjust better to bereavement because of anticipatory grieving and the tendency to view death as one of the developmental tasks of old age.

Factors other than choice frequently operate to isolate the widowed person. Those who lack skills, money, health, and transportation for engaging in society encounter more difficulties in adjusting to a change in role status. The isolated status of widows may be related to the socialization of women in past generations as dependent on men. Like any other life crisis, the loss of a spouse affects people in various ways. Adjustment is related to the person's previous lifestyle and coping patterns.

Family Support

The relationship between adult children and their elderly parents depends on a variety of factors, such as distance, economics, health, and emotional health. Relationships are often taxed by a complex mixture of conflicts. Pulls between love and resentment, duty to parents and obligations for others, and wanting to do what is right and not wanting to change one's lifestyle are not unusual in families. Yet, from the literature available, most families seem able to resolve problems in a way that provides the elder with a sense of support, belonging, and love.

Most older people live within an hour's traveling distance of their children and manage to see them often. There are, however, some differences according to social class. Upper- and middle-class adults are likely to live greater distances from their parents than are lower-class adults. This difference is more a result of professional career patterns than a desire to be separated. Although patterns of aid and contact vary among the socioeconomic classes, there is no difference in caring. Greater distance results in fewer visits, but the quality of the visits and frequent long-distance communication may compensate for periods of absence. Distance between family members also alters the type of support exchanged. Families living close to one another tend to exchange services, such as shopping and household maintenance tasks, whereas family members who live some distance apart tend to confine their assistance to monetary support.

Fewer than one third of the elderly live with their children. Many elders want their privacy, independence, and freedom rather than having to adjust to their children's lifestyle.

There is a growing proportion of frail, dependent elders. For this group, several options are available. They can live in a retirement community or other group setting or can remain in the community, sustained by families and friends. Most elders prefer to reside in their own communities, but there are problems that make realization of this preference difficult. Families generally attempt to help but may be limited in their ability. Most adult couples are active members of the work force and still have dependent children at home or in school.

Grandparenting

Grandparenting is often the most important role in the life of the elderly, providing them with a sense of purpose, value, and esteem. A relationship with grandparents often brings a sense of stability and perspective to the

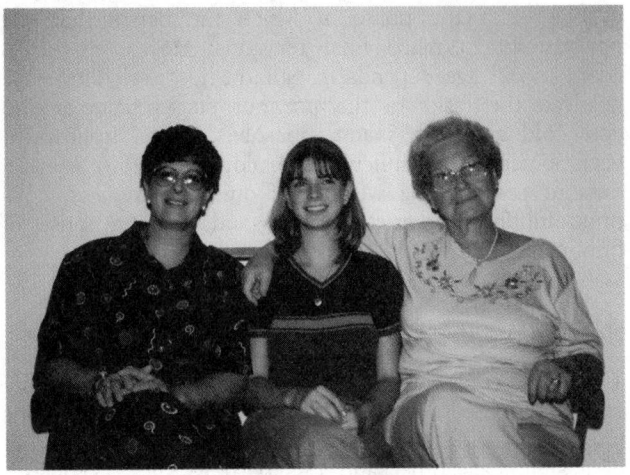

Figure 5–6. The woman on the left is in the "sandwich generation."

children and grandchildren (Fig. 5–6). Grandparents provide the young with advice, affirmation, and a sense of roots and continuity. In addition, grandparents may relieve some of their children's parenting burden by assuming actual caretaking responsibilities, especially when both parents are working.

Regardless of the type of role assumed, grandparenting benefits the older adult, the adult child, and the grandchild. Through the role of grandparent, the elder can maintain ego integrity (Erikson) and approach death with a sense of fulfillment and a feeling of extension of his or her influence into future generations. Many schools and senior citizen centers have joined forces to help children appreciate the pleasure of relationships with older adults other than their grandparents. This intergenerational visiting has also helped the elderly feel wanted and useful (MacPhail, 1993).

Work and Retirement

In 1900, every two out of three older men were employed. In recent years, retirement has become less a matter of choice, with only one of six older men employed. Because women were less likely to be working outside the home earlier in the century, the numbers of older female workers were less and have remained stable. This picture may change as the increased numbers of younger women who have entered the labor force become older. Adjustment to retirement remains a significant crisis for a working person. One survey of retirees revealed that one third of all retirees would prefer to work (Ferraro, 1990).

To most elderly people, it comes as a grim surprise that their income may be less than adequate. For those who depend solely on Social Security benefits, their incomes may fall below the poverty levels established by the U.S. government. For some people, therefore, one of the most serious problems retirement creates is inadequate financial resources.

Some older people prefer to work rather than retire. Some need to work to supplement income from other

HEALTH CARE OF OLDER ADULTS

Nurses have frequent contact with the elderly in both their professional and personal lives. Because much of their professional contact is through health care settings such as hospitals, nursing homes, and community health agencies, nurses sometimes have a tendency to stereotype the typical older adult as a confused, dependent person.

This chapter describes major health issues associated with late adulthood. The care of older adults with specific health problems, such as diseases and the need for surgical procedures, is discussed throughout this text under each body system as appropriate. In addition, Nursing Focus on the Elderly charts and Implications for the Elderly headings highlight the most important information related to care of the elderly client with a selected health problem.

SUBGROUPS OF LATE ADULTHOOD

Late adulthood, consisting of people older than 65 years, can be divided into four subgroups:

- Age 65–74 years: the young old
- Age 75–84 years: the middle old
- Age 85–99 years: the old old
- Age 100 years or more: the elite old

The fastest growing subgroup is the old old, sometimes referred to as the advanced elderly population. Their needs and problems are generally different from those of adults between 65 and 74 years old. The incidence of chronic disease increases markedly when a person is older than 80. At any age, the older adult has specific needs and problems.

DISTRIBUTION OF OLDER ADULTS IN THE HEALTH CARE SYSTEM

About 80% to 85% of older adults are relatively healthy and living in the community at home, in assisted-living facilities, or in retirement complexes. Five percent are in long-term care facilities (nursing homes), and another 10% to 15% are ill but are being cared for at home (Matteson et al., 1997). The elderly from any setting usually experience one or more hospitalizations in their lifetime. Seventy percent to 90% of clients on most medical-surgical units in hospitals are older than 65.

ADMISSION OF THE OLDER ADULT TO A HOSPITAL OR NURSING HOME

Being admitted to a hospital or nursing home is often a traumatic experience for anyone, especially for the older adult. Many elders suffer from *relocation stress,* also known as relocation trauma or relocation syndrome. Most of the early studies on this syndrome examined the increased mortality rate associated with moving elderly people from their own homes to a nursing home or hospital

---

Chart 6-1

Nursing Care Highlight: Minimizing the Effects of Relocation Stress in the Elderly

- Provide opportunities for the client to assist in decision making.
- Carefully explain all procedures and routines to the client before they occur.
- Ask the family or significant others to provide familiar or special keepsakes to keep at the client's bedside (e.g., family picture, a favorite hairbrush).
- Reorient the client frequently to where he or she is.
- Ask the client what his or her expectations are during hospitalization or nursing home placement.
- Encourage the client's family and friends to visit often.
- Establish a trusting relationship with the client as early as possible.
- Assess the client's usual lifestyle and daily activities, including food likes and dislikes and preferred time for bathing.
- Avoid unnecessary room changes.
- If possible, have a family member, significant other, staff member, or volunteer accompany the client when leaving the unit for special procedures or therapies.

(Coffman, 1981). Other studies have investigated other effects of relocation on behavior and health. Few studies have examined the negative impact of relocation on health status and function, although physical and mental changes have been noted (Matteson et al., 1997).

In some cases, the elderly person who is admitted to the hospital or nursing home from the community can become disoriented, confused, agitated, or abusive. Risk factors thought to contribute to relocation syndrome are the lack of choice or preparation time and the major environmental change. Men older than age 75 who are physically and mentally impaired are at a very high risk for relocation syndrome. Chart 6-1 lists interventions that may help minimize the effects of relocation for the elderly client.

HEALTH ISSUES

This book presents many discussions of health problems that are experienced by the elderly, particularly in the institutional health care setting. Most of this chapter focuses on health issues and problems that may not warrant hospital or nursing home admission.

Health Promotion

Health is a major concern of most elderly people. Elderly clients' health status can affect their ability to perform basic activities of daily living and to participate in social roles. Failure in the performance of these activities may increase their dependence on others and may have a negative effect on morale and life satisfaction.

The health problems most frequently observed among older clients tend to be chronic and degenerative rather than acute. Further, the health problems of the aged are frequently the result of multiple causes, including physical, psychological, and social components, in a complex mixture.

For both middle-aged and older adults, heart disease and cancer are the most frequent causes of death. Most fatalities among older adults are due to disorders resulting from diminished physiologic defenses, such as a severe infection related to cancer or cancer treatment.

Like younger adults, older adults need to practice health promotion and prevention of illness to maintain or achieve a high level of wellness (Chart 6-2). The nurse working with the elderly in any setting needs to teach them the importance of promoting wellness and strategies for accomplishing this goal.

Health is related to a person's level of functioning. In assessing older people's level of functioning, the nurse considers self-responsibility and self-management, nutritional awareness, physical fitness and mobility, stress management, and environmental factors.

Self-Responsibility and Self-Management

The elderly's ability to maintain a positive self-concept and self-control may be hampered by the loss of re-

---

Chart 6-2

Health Promotion Guide: Lifestyles and Practices to Promote Wellness

Health-Protecting Behaviors

- Have yearly influenza vaccinations.
- Obtain pneumococcal vaccinations.
- Wear seat belts when you are in an automobile.
- Use alcohol in moderation or not at all.
- Avoid smoking.
- If you smoke at home, do not smoke in bed.
- Install and maintain working smoke detectors.
- Create a hazard-free environment to prevent falls; eliminate hazards such as scatter rugs and waxed floors.
- Use medications according to your physician's orders.
- Avoid over-the-counter medications unless your physician directs you to use them.

Health-Enhancing Behaviors

- Have a yearly physical examination; see your physician more often if health problems occur.
- Reduce dietary fat to not more than 30% of calories; saturated fat should provide less than 10% of your calories.
- Increase your dietary intake of complex carbohydrate- and fiber-containing food to five or more servings of fruits and vegetables and six or more servings of grain products daily.
- Allow at least 10 to 15 minutes of sun exposure two to three times weekly for vitamin D intake.
- Exercise regularly three to five times a week for 30 minutes per session.
- Manage stress through coping mechanisms that you have used successfully in the past.
- Get together with people in different settings.
- Reminisce about your life.

sources in the late years of life. The elderly may also experience a number of losses that can affect their sense of control over their lives: the death of a spouse and significant others, the loss of social and work roles, and a decrease in physical mobility. The nurse can support older clients' self-esteem and feelings of competency by encouraging them to maintain as much control as possible over their lives, participate in decision making, and perform as many tasks as possible.

Regardless of the situation, it is important that elderly clients direct their lifestyle in a manner that encourages them to feel capable and valued. The elderly need to find opportunities to be productive and take care of themselves as well as others.

The nurse in the community health setting often has the opportunity to assess older adults' self-care or self-management ability. A number of assessment tools are available for this, but most are too long and complex to be used in a hospital setting. When elderly clients are admitted, the nurse also needs to assess their self-management capabilities for discharge planning.

Nutritional Awareness
Nutrition Needs in the Community

A person's need for adequate nutrition remains constant throughout the life span, yet many elderly people eat an inadequate diet. Inflation, reduced income, and the lack of transportation are factors that may contribute to inadequate nutrition among older adults. Elderly people whose diets consist of inappropriate or unbalanced foods (e.g., an excess of carbohydrates) may also be poorly nourished. Some elders reduce their intake of food to near-starvation levels, even with the availability of assistive programs, such as food stamps, free food, and Meals on Wheels. The lack of transportation, the necessity of traveling to obtain such services, and the inability to carry large quantities of groceries prohibit some elders from taking advantage of food programs.

Poor nutrition among the elderly may also be related to loneliness. Elders may respond to loneliness, depression, and boredom by not eating, which can lead to malnutrition. Many elderly who live alone have lost the incentive to prepare or eat balanced diets. Still others respond to stress by overeating, which leads to obesity.

Nutritional Requirements

The human body's minimal nutritional requirements from youth through old age remain consistent, with a few exceptions. Older adults need increased dietary intake of calcium, vitamin C, and vitamin A because alterations with age disrupt the ability to store, use, and absorb these substances. Sedentary lifestyles and reduced metabolic rate require a reduction in total caloric intake to maintain ideal body weight.

Physical Changes Affecting Nutrition

Other physical aging changes influence the older adult's nutritional status or ability to consume needed nutrients. Diminished senses of taste and smell often result in a loss of appeal of food. Elderly people experience a greater decline in the ability to taste sweet and salt than in the discrimination of bitter and sour. This phenomenon often results in the elder's overuse of table sugar and salt to compensate. The nurse teaches the elderly client to use herbs and spices to season food or to vary the textures of food substances to achieve satisfaction from food rather than increase the intake of sugar and salt.

The loss of teeth and poorly fitting dentures from inadequate dental care can also cause the elderly to avoid important foodstuffs. The extensive use of prescribed and over-the-counter drugs may affect one's appetite, food tolerances, and food absorption and utilization. Older people with dentition problems frequently resort to eating soft, high-calorie foods, like ice cream and mashed potatoes, which lack roughage and fiber. Unless the person carefully chooses more nutritious soft foods, vitamin deficiencies, constipation, and other disorders can result.

The aged person sometimes responds to problems associated with mobility, prescribed diuretics, and limited bladder capacity by limiting fluid intake, especially in the evening. The nurse teaches older adults that fluid restrictions make them prone to dehydration and electrolyte imbalances that can cause serious illness or death.

Nutrition Needs in the Hospital and Nursing Home

In addition to the nutritional needs that have been described for older adults living in the community, those who are in the hospital or nursing home have special needs related to their illness and general health state. For example, an elderly client with a pressure ulcer needs additional protein, vitamin C, and zinc to heal the open skin lesion. The health care provider, nurse, and dietitian collaborate to determine the best sources of these nutrients. The health care provider may prescribe a multivitamin tablet with zinc to be given every day. The dietitian may recommend a high-calorie, high-protein supplement like Ensure Plus to be given several times a day. The nurse encourages the client to select and eat high-protein foods to promote healing. (See Chapter 64 for further discussion of nutrition in the elderly.)

Physical Fitness and Mobility

Exercise and activity are important to older adults as a means of promoting and maintaining health (Fig. 6–1). Physical activity can help keep the body in shape and maintain an optimal level of functioning. In addition, regular, moderate exercise typically results in feelings of well-being. Numerous studies have shown a lower incidence of coronary artery disease in individuals who engage in regular physical activity compared with those who do not. Karper and Boschen (1993) found that moderate exercise in the elderly also helped to strengthen the immune system and, therefore, prevent the high incidence of acute respiratory infections that are common in this age group.

Without exercise, muscles, organs, and tissues tend to atrophy, and motor, sensory, and cognitive functions can become impaired. It is estimated that 50% of the physical

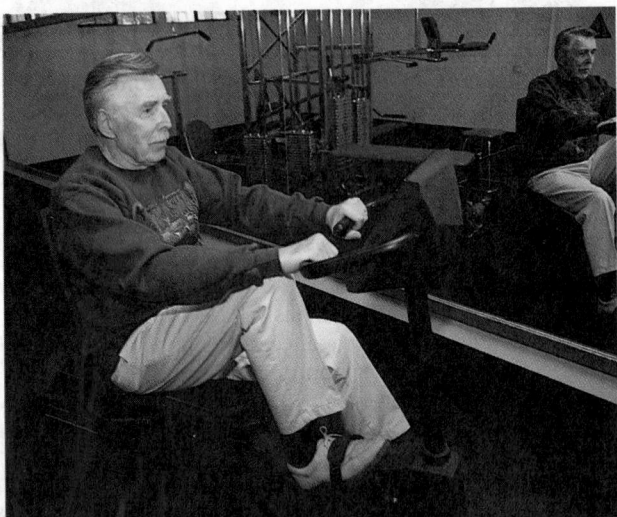

Figure 6–1. Exercise is important to the elderly for health promotion and maintenance.

decline of the elderly is caused by disuse rather than by the aging process or illness. A study by Mills (1994) showed the beneficial effects of low-intensity aerobic exercise on flexibility and balance (see Research Applications for Nursing).

The benefits and purposes of regular exercise are to improve circulation, improve blood pressure, improve respiratory function, maintain muscle tone throughout the body, reduce muscle tension, reduce muscle pain, and promote relaxation. One of the best exercises for older adults is to walk three to five times a week for at least 30 minutes each session (Karper & Boschen, 1993). Swimming is also recommended but does not offer the weight-bearing advantage of walking. Elders who have been sedentary should start their exercise programs slowly and gradually increase the frequency and duration of activity over time.

When older adults are hospitalized, the opportunity for continuing a program of physical fitness is interrupted, at least temporarily. During severe or prolonged illness, older adults are at high risk for complications of decreased physical mobility, such as pneumonia, skin impairment, contractures, muscle atrophy, constipation, and renal calculi. These problems are addressed elsewhere in this text.

Stress Management
Factors Contributing to Stress in the Elderly

According to many physiologic and psychological theories of aging, stress and disease play significant roles. Stress can speed up the aging process over time, or it can lead to diseases that increase the rate of degeneration (see Chap. 8). Stress can impair the reserve capacity of the elderly and lessen their ability to respond and adapt to changes in their environment.

Although no period of the life cycle is free from stress, the later years can be a time of especially high risk. Frequently observed sources of stress for the older popu-

lation include rapid environmental changes that require immediate reaction, changes in lifestyle resulting from retirement or physical incapacity, acute or chronic illness, loss of significant others, financial hardships, and relocation. How people react to these stresses depends on their personal coping skills and support networks. The loss of roles experienced by the elderly often limits the availability of external support networks. For instance, for a number of elderly, successive role losses have left them without friends to whom they can turn for support and help. As a result, many elderly have to rely solely on their personal resources to maintain their mental health. When poor physical health is combined with social problems, older people are susceptible to stress overload, which can result in illness and premature death.

Coping with Stress

The ways in which people adapt to old age largely depend on the personality traits and coping strategies that have characterized them throughout their lives. Establishing and maintaining relationships with others throughout life are especially important to the elderly's happiness. Even more important than having friends at all is the nature of the friendships. People who have close, intimate, stable relationships with others in whom they confide are more likely to maintain integrity in times of crises.

Environmental Factors

Most older adults live in and own their own homes. Physical incapacity or economic problems may force some to relocate (Matteson et al., 1997). If an older person

---

▷ Research Applications for Nursing

Does Exercise Help to Increase the Mobility of Sedentary Elders?

Mills, E. M. (1994). The effect of low-intensity aerobic exercises on muscle strength, flexibility, and balance among sedentary elderly persons. Nursing Research, 43(4), 207–211.

In this small experimental study, 20 sedentary elders were monitored for 8 weeks during a program of stretching and strengthening chair exercises. The control group consisted of 27 older adults who performed their usual activity level. At the end of the 8 weeks, there was a significant difference in flexibility but not in muscle strength or balance. However, balance among the experimental group was 22% better than among the control group at the end of the study period.

Critique. This was a very small study, but it used an experimental research design. The study needs to be replicated using a larger sample size and a random sample. It is an attempt, however, to show the importance of health promotion among the elderly population.

Possible Nursing Implications. Nurses need to teach the importance of exercise to their elderly clients as part of a comprehensive wellness program. Exercise does improve mobility in this population.

must move to a retirement center or a long-term care facility, family members and facility staff need to be aware that the older person needs personal space in the new surroundings. Older people need to participate in deciding how the space will be arranged and what they can keep in the new environment. Such participation helps to offset the feelings of powerlessness and depersonalization that often accompany relocation to a group setting. The nurse suggests that the client or family bring in personal items, such as pictures of relatives and friends, favorite clothing, and valued knickknacks to assist in making the new setting seem more familiar and comfortable. The same intervention can be carried out in a hospital setting.

Changes in vision, touch, and motor ability can create difficulties for the elderly in functioning in any environment. For example, decreased vision in old age, especially the poor perception of distance, may make walking more difficult; the person is less aware of where each step is. The reduced sense of touch gives the older person a decreased awareness of body orientation (e.g., whether the foot is squarely on the step). Decreased reaction time that commonly results from age-related changes in the neurologic system may also impair the older adult's ability to recognize or move from a dangerous setting.

Accidents

Accidents in the Community

The nurse teaches older adults about the need to be aware of safety precautions that should be taken to prevent accidents. The prevention of injury to muscles, bones, and other body parts that have grown fragile with age not only is critically important but also is probably the area in which aging people can do the most to preserve their fitness. Incapacitating accidents are a primary cause of restricted physical fitness and decreased mobility in old age.

Safeguards such as installing and holding onto hand rails when using steps and getting into and out of the shower or bathtub, securing rugs with slip-proof underpads, and making sure treacherous places are well lighted are essential. To minimize sensory overload in the elderly, the nurse advises the older person to concentrate on one activity at a time. If needed, the nurse encourages the use of visual, hearing, or ambulatory assistive devices. High costs and fear of appearing old sometimes prevent the elderly from obtaining or using hearing aids, eyeglasses, walkers, or canes.

Accidents in the Hospital and Nursing Home

The most common accident among elderly clients in a hospital or nursing home setting is falling. Many falls result in serious injuries such as fractures and head trauma. The nurse should be aware that these injuries are potentially life threatening and should take action to prevent them.

Risk Assessment for Falls

The nurse assesses the client for risk for falls. Many risk assessment tools have been developed to help the nurse

---

Chart 6–3

Nursing Care Highlight: Risk Factors and Measures for Preventing Falls in the Elderly

Assess for the presence of these risk factors:

- History of falls
- Advanced age (>80 years)
- Multiple illnesses
- Generalized weakness or decreased mobility
- Disorientation or confusion
- Use of drugs that can cause increased confusion, mobility limitations, or orthostatic hypotension
- Urinary incontinence
- Communication impairments
- Major visual impairments or visual impairment without correction
- Substance abuse
- Location of client's room away from the nurses' station (in the hospital or nursing home)
- Change of shift or mealtime (in the hospital or nursing home)

Implement these nursing interventions:

- Monitor the client's activities and behavior as often as possible, preferably every 30 to 60 minutes.
- Remind the client to call for help before getting out of bed or a chair.
- Help the client to get out of bed or a chair.
- Provide, or remind the client to use, a walker or cane for ambulating.
- Remind the client to wear eyeglasses or a hearing aid if needed.
- Toilet the incontinent client every 1 to 2 hours.
- Clean up spills immediately.
- Arrange the furniture in the client's room or hallway to eliminate clutter or obstacles that could contribute to a fall.
- Provide adequate lighting at all times, especially at night.
- Observe for side effects and toxic effects of drug therapy.

---

focus on factors that increase an older person's risk of falling. Chart 6–3 lists some of the common risk factors that the nurse should assess and measure to help prevent falls.

Once an elderly client has been identified as being at a high risk for falls, the nurse chooses interventions that help to prevent falls and possible serious injury. One of the most controversial issues in fall prevention is the use of side rails on the bed, and physical and chemical restraints, especially in the hospital setting.

Nursing Interventions to Prevent Falls

As a result of being in an unfamiliar environment and because of increased nocturia (urination at night), the elderly client commonly gets out of bed at night to go to the bathroom. In the darkness and disorientation of the room, the client may forget to ask for assistance to the bathroom and subsequently fall. In some cases, the client may crawl over the bed rail, which can make the results of a fall more serious. Because of this, side rails are used less often in both hospitals and nursing homes.

Similar considerations are being given to the use of physical and chemical restraints. A restraint is any device or medication that prevents the client from moving freely. The federal government enforced a law in 1990 that gives residents in nursing homes the right to be restraint-free. In a nursing home, bedside rails are classified as restraints. Although the majority of hospitals have not adopted this policy, most have policies that limit the use of restraints and require careful nursing assessment. The Joint Commission on Accreditation of Healthcare Organizations (JCAHO) has specific standards that limit the use of restraints in hospitals.

Physical Restraints

Experts agree that elderly clients should not be placed in a Posey vest or be sedated just because they are elderly. However, if all other interventions, such as reminding clients to call for assistance when needed or asking a family member to stay with the clients, are ineffective in fall prevention, the nurse may need to use a physical restraint for a specified period of time. Applying a restraint is a serious intervention and should be analyzed for its risk versus benefit (Wilson, 1996). The nurse checks the client in a restraint every 30 to 60 minutes and releases the restraint every 2 hours for turning, repositioning, and toileting. Physical restraints like cloth vests have caused serious injury and even death. If restraint is needed, the least restrictive device should be used.

Chemical Restraints

Chemical restraints, or psychoactive drugs, are often overused in hospital settings. Clients who are noisy, agitated, abusive, or combative may have an "as needed" order for a psychoactive drug. Such medications include

- Antipsychotic drugs, such as haloperidol (Haldol, Peridol✱)
- Antianxiety drugs, such as alprazolam (Xanax)
- Antidepressant drugs, such as nortriptyline (Pamelor)
- Sedative-hypnotic drugs, such as chloral hydrate

These drugs produce serious side and toxic effects and should, therefore, be reserved for clients who cannot be managed in any other way. Clients receiving these medications must be closely monitored for therapeutic and adverse effects.

The most potent group of psychoactive drugs is the antipsychotics. These drugs may be appropriate for the control of certain behavioral symptoms, such as hallucinations, delusions, and violent episodes. However, fewer than half of clients respond to these drugs.

If a psychoactive drug is used as a last resort, a low dose should be given. Table 6–1 lists some of the drugs commonly used as chemical restraints.

TABLE 6–1

Drugs Commonly Used as Chemical Restraints
Low Potency (High Sedation, High Anticholinergic Effects)
Chlorpromazine (Thorazine)
Thioridazine (Mellaril)
Chlorprothixene (Taractan)
Mesoridazine (Serentil)
Medium Potency (Medium Sedation, Medium Anticholinergic Effects)
Triflupromazine (Vesprin)
Acetophenazine (Tindal)
Loxapine (Loxitane)
Molindone (Moban)
High Potency (Low Sedation, Low Anticholinergic Effects)
Trifluoperazine (Stelazine)
Thiothixene (Navane)
Fluphenazine (Prolixin)
Haloperidol (Haldol)
Pimozide (Orap)

From Ignatavicius, D. D. (1998). *Introduction to long term care: Principles and practice.* Philadelphia: F. A. Davis. Used with permission.

Drug Use and Misuse

Drug therapy for the elderly population in general is another major health issue. Because of the multiple chronic and acute illnesses that occur in this age group, drugs for elderly people account for about a third of all prescription drug costs.

Older adults also frequently use nonprescription drugs, such as analgesics, antacids, cold and cough preparations, laxatives, and vitamins, often without consulting a physician. The occurrence of adverse drug reactions is directly related to the number and frequency of drug exposures. Elders are, therefore, at high risk for adverse drug reactions or interactions and are often admitted to the hospital for these problems.

Physiologic Changes Affecting Drug Use

It has been recognized only recently that older adults may not tolerate the standard dosage of medications traditionally prescribed for younger adults. The physiologic changes related to aging make drug therapy more complex and challenging. These changes affect the absorption, distribution, metabolism, and excretion of drugs from the body.

Age-related changes that can potentially affect drug absorption from an oral route include an increase in gastric pH, a decrease in gastric blood flow, and a decrease in gastrointestinal motility. Despite these changes, most elderly do not have difficulty with absorption because of age-related changes alone. Age-related changes that affect the distribution of a drug include smaller amounts of total body water, an increased ratio of adipose tissue to lean body mass, a decreased albumin level, and a decreased cardiac output. Increased adipose tissue in proportion to lean body mass can cause increased storage of lipid-soluble drugs. This leads to a decreased concentration of the drug in plasma but an increased concentration in tissue.

Drug metabolism most often occurs in the liver. Age-related changes affecting metabolism include a decrease in liver size, a decrease in liver blood flow, and a decrease in liver enzyme activity. These changes can result in increased plasma concentrations of a drug. Changes in the kidneys can also result in high plasma concentrations of drugs. Excretion of drugs most often involves the renal system. Age-related changes of the renal system include a decrease in renal blood flow and reduced glomerular filtration rate. These changes result in a decreased creatinine clearance and thus a slower excretion time for medications (Matteson et al., 1997)

Effects of Drugs in the Elderly

Because of age-related physiologic changes, older adults are at a high risk for side and toxic effects from drugs. In 1991, the Geriatric Drug Therapy Research Institute was established to study and make recommendations for drug therapy in the elderly. Currently, the institute is developing tools that physicians and other health care professionals can use when caring for the older adult.

When chronic disease is added to the physiologic changes of aging, drug reactions have a more dramatic effect and take a longer time to correct. This is because elders have less reserve capacity in most organ systems. Often a lower dose of medication is necessary to prevent adverse effects. The policy of "start low, go slow" is appropriate when health care providers prescribe drugs for the elderly. However, the physiologic changes of aging are highly individual. Thus, alterations in drug therapy should always be individualized according to the actual physiologic changes present and the occurrence and severity of chronic disease.

Common adverse drug reactions in elders include edema, nausea, vomiting, anorexia, dry mouth, fatigue, weakness, dizziness, urinary retention, diarrhea, constipation, and confusion. Many of these signs and symptoms can be mistakenly attributed to a concurrent illness clients might be experiencing or may be assumed to be part of the aging process. The nurse assesses all elderly clients with such symptoms for possible adverse reactions to medications.

Self-Administration of Medication

Most people older than 65 years live at home and are responsible for taking their own medications. Because the risk of drug toxicity is considerably increased in the elderly population, the nurse should assist elderly clients in assuming this task responsibly. The nurse helps prevent problems by educating clients and their caregivers, providing clear and concise directions, and developing ways to assist elders in overcoming self-administration handicaps or difficulties.

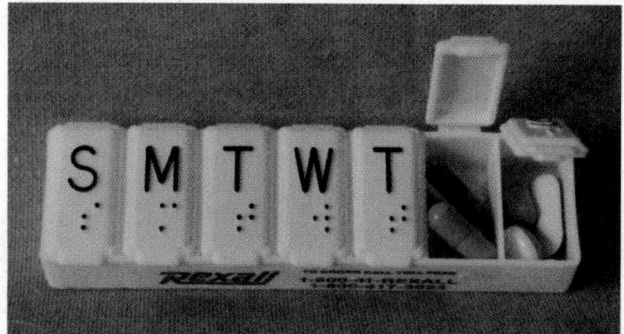

Figure 6–2. A medication system for safe self-administration.

Older adults make errors in self-administration for several reasons. First, they may simply forget. In the rush of daily activities, they may not take the drug at all or may take it too often because of an inability to remember when or whether medications have been taken. It can be helpful if clients associate pill taking with daily events, such as meals, or keep a simple chart or calendar. Pill boxes have been devised so that a daily, weekly, or monthly supply of medicine can be placed in appropriate compartments (Fig. 6–2). Large print on the drug label assists those clients with poor visual acuity. Writing the drug regimen on the top of the bottle with large letters and numbers is also helpful.

A second reason that elderly people frequently commit errors in taking medications is poor communication with health care professionals. These difficulties stem from such sources as inadequate explanations to elderly clients or explanations they cannot understand because of educational limitations or language barriers. Health care professionals frequently presume that if they tell the elder about the drugs, the elder has acquired the knowledge. The nurse or other health care provider needs to help older adults plan their medication schedules.

A third reason for medication errors is one's attitude and long-ingrained feelings about taking medicine. Some people are chronic pill takers; they think no physician can help them unless he or she is the one who prescribed the medication. These people often add to their drug regimen by taking over-the-counter drugs that can interact with prescription drugs and cause serious problems. For example, a client receiving warfarin (Coumadin, Warfilone✱) for anticoagulation may take aspirin (Ancasal✱) regularly for arthritis. Aspirin is also an anticoagulant, which can cause overt or occult bleeding.

Conversely, other elderly people avoid taking medication whenever they can. The fear of drug dependency or the cost of the drugs may cause many to discontinue medications too soon. In addition, the action or side effects of some drugs may not be desirable. For example, diuretics may cause incontinence when clients cannot get to the bathroom quickly enough. Others think that two pills will be twice as effective as one; some elders take medication that is left over from a previous illness or a drug that has been prescribed for someone else.

Health care providers can influence the attitudes of

elders toward their medication and their health problems. Laypersons of the same socioeconomic or cultural background as that of the elder can be effective instructors. A method that is being tried in some hospitals and nursing homes is supervised drug self-administration. Clients are allowed to take their own medications under supervision. In this way, the nurse can be sure of a client's understanding and ability to self-administer medications at home or in another health care setting.

Mental Health

A few changes in cognition have been identified as age-related. These changes are linked to specific functions of cognition as opposed to intellectual capacity. They include a decreased reaction time to stimuli and an impairment of memory of recent events. It is certain, however, that gross cognitive impairment, depression, hallucinations, and delusions are not part of the normal aging process. Most elders are mentally sound.

Losses in income and physical health, lack of comprehensive health care and social services, loss of social roles, and death of significant others may affect a person's emotional stability. It is not surprising that mental illness occurs among the aged population. Elders are often unaware of early symptoms of emotional or mental impairments. Symptoms may go unnoticed by family and friends and thus are allowed to progress until crisis results. The three most common cognitive problems among the elderly are depression, dementia, and delirium.

Depression

Depression, as a response to multiple life stresses, a single situation (situational depression), or a problem associated with dementia, is one of the major disturbances in cognitive functioning in elders. It is often underdiagnosed by physicians and, therefore, undertreated. Without treatment, depression can result in suicide.

Elderly people with the early clinical manifestations of depression may experience early morning insomnia, excessive daytime sleeping, poor appetite, a lack of energy, and an unwillingness to participate in social and recreational activities. The treatment for depression usually includes drug therapy and psychotherapy. Electroconvulsive therapy (ECT) may also be used, either as a last resort or when drugs are not effective. Table 6–2 lists commonly used drugs for depression. Most of these drugs take 2 to 3 weeks to become effective. More information on this disorder is available in mental health nursing textbooks.

Transcultural Considerations

Caucasian males older than 70 years are at the highest risk for suicide during older adulthood. Older adults contemplating suicide usually do not talk about their plans and choose a method, such as gunshot, that will ensure death.

Dementia

Dementia is a broad term used for a syndrome that is characterized by a disturbance in cognition in elders. For-

TABLE 6–2

Medications Commonly Used for Depression in the Elderly and Their Adverse Effects

Medication	Adverse Effects
***Tricyclic Antidepressants**	
Amitriptyline (Elavil, Endep) Clomipramine (Anafranil) Desipramine (Norpramin) Doxepin (Sinequan, Adapin) Imipramine (Tofranil) Nortriptyline (Pamelor) Protriptyline (Vivactil) Trimipramine (Surmontil)	Cardiac dysrhythmias, orthostatic hypotension, weight gain, drowsiness, anticholinergic effects (dry mouth, constipation, urinary retention, visual disturbances) (amitriptytine has the most anticholinergic effects of any in this group)
†Heterocyclic Antidepressants	
Amoxapine (Asendin) Bupropion (Wellbutrin) Maprotiline (Ludiomil) Trazodone (Desyrel)	Drowsiness (maprotiline has the longest half-life in this group)
†Selective Serotonin Reuptake Inhibitors (SSRIs)	
Fluoxetine (Prozac) Paroxetine (Paxil) Sertraline (Zoloft)	Insomnia, agitation, gastrointestinal distress, weight loss (fluoxetine has the longest half-life in this group)
Monoamine Oxidase Inhibitors	
Isocarboxazid (Marplan) Phenelzine (Nardil) Tranylcypromine (Parnate)	Weight gain, insomnia, agitation Hypertensive crisis (avoid foods containing tyramine)

*Do not give with antidysrhythmics or monoamine oxidase inhibitors.
†Do not give with monoamine oxidase inhibitors.
Data compiled from *Depression in Primary Care: Volume 2. Treatment of major depression. Clinical Practice Guideline. Number 5.*
From Ignatavicius, D. D. (1998). *Introduction to long-term care: Principles and practice.* Philadelphia: F. A. Davis. Used with permission.

merly called organic brain syndrome (OBS) and chronic brain syndrome (CBS), dementia represents global impairment of intellectual function and is generally chronic and progressive. There are many types of dementia; the most common is Alzheimer's disease (senile dementia, Alzheimer type). Multi-infarct dementia, the second most common dementia, is a vascular disorder and accounts for 20% to 25% of all dementias. Chapter 44 discusses dementias in detail, with a focus on Alzheimer's disease.

Delirium

Whereas dementia is a chronic, progressive disorder, delirium is an acute state of confusion. Delirium is also different from dementia in that it is usually short-term and reversible. Delirium is often seen in the hospital setting or in a setting with which the client is unfamiliar. The client may try to climb out of bed, pull out invasive

TABLE 6–3

Differences in the Characteristics of Delirium and Dementia

Variable	Dementia	Delirium
Description	• A chronic, progressive cognitive decline	• An acute confusional state
Onset	• Slow	• Fast
Duration	• Continuous	• Usually 1 month or less
Cause	• Unknown, possibly familial, chemical	• Multiple, such as surgery, infection, drugs
Reversibility	• None	• Usually
Treatment	• Treat signs and symptoms	• Remove or treat the cause
Nursing interventions	• Reorientation not effective in the late stages; use validation therapy (acknowledge the client's feelings and don't argue); provide a safe environment; observe for associated behaviors, such as delusions and hallucinations	• Reorient the client to reality; provide a safe environment

catheters (e.g., oxygen or intravenous cannulas), or become quite agitated and combative.

The nurse should use a calm voice in reorienting the client and try to divert attention away from devices or tubes. A number of innovative nursing interventions have been used with some success. For example, playing tapes of soothing music in the client's room may have a calming effect. Giving the client a doll or stuffed animal to "fidget" with may prevent the client from removing important medical instrumentation. Some nurses believe that providing dolls and stuffed animals is treating the adult like a child, but, when used for therapeutic purposes, this intervention can be very effective with some clients. If the client already has a favorite item, such as an afghan or picture, the nurse asks the client's family or significant others to provide it for the same purpose.

There are multiple causes of delirium, including

- Medication (especially anticholinergic drugs)
- Metabolic disturbances
- Infections
- Surgical operations
- Circulatory, renal, and pulmonary disorders
- Nutritional deficiencies
- Major loss

Table 6–3 briefly differentiates delirium and dementia and the major nursing considerations for each. The most difficult challenge is caring for a client with both problems at the same time.

Elder Neglect and Abuse

Another problem that is sometimes encountered by the elderly is neglect and abuse, both verbal and physical. Some elders are very vulnerable to this problem, especially widowed women, who may have difficulty being assertive. Studies have shown that older persons who are neglected or abused are often physically dependent. The abuser may be a family member who becomes frustrated or distraught over the burden of caring for the elder (Greenberg, 1996; Lynch, 1997).

Role theorists propose that prolonged caregiving by a family member is a new, unexpected role for adult children, most often women. This new role may result in role fatigue and role conflict. Caregiver Role Strain and High Risk for Caregiver Role Strain have been added to the list of North American Nursing Diagnosis Association (NANDA)–approved nursing diagnoses (NANDA, 1992). From their research, McCloskey and Bulechek (1992) identified Caregiver Support as a major nursing intervention (Chart 6–4). Chapter 8 discusses caregiver stress in more detail.

The nurse carefully assesses the elderly client for signs of abuse. If the older adult is too weak or has no other resources or support system, the client may not acknowledge that the abuse is occurring. If physical abuse is suspected, the nurse notifies the physician and social

---

Chart 6–4

Nursing Care Highlight: Interventions for Family Caregiver Support

- Determine the caregiver's preparation and acceptance of his or her new role.
- Assess the caregiver's level of knowledge about the role and the client's health status.
- Teach stress management techniques to the caregiver (see Chap. 8).
- Monitor for signs of caregiver stress.
- Help the caregiver identify sources of respite care.
- Teach the caregiver health promotion practices for his or her own health.
- Help the caregiver identify caregiver support groups, and encourage participation in them.
- Teach the caregiver about the grieving process.
- Help the caregiver identify financial and other health care resources.
- Encourage the caregiver to share responsibilities with other members of the family or significant others.

worker to investigate the situation. Many states in the United States and some Western countries have laws requiring health care professionals to report suspected elder abuse.

ECONOMIC ISSUES
Income

Most adults hope that throughout their life cycle they can provide for their own needs. One of the greatest fears many adults have related to aging is becoming dependent on family, friends, or society. In many cases, older adults have not achieved economic self-sufficiency. One fifth of the total population of the United States is poor, and one fifth of the poor are older than 65 (Brock, 1992).

Most people expect financial resources to decline in their retirement years compared with their working years. However, they also expect that the level of their expenses will decline as well, and this may not occur. In the United States, for example, the inflation that began in the 1970s reduced the value of financial assets. The elderly were especially hard hit because most rely on Social Security benefits or pension funds for the bulk of their income. These assets are usually fixed and cannot be altered by the person. Therefore, many elders are unable to adjust their income to changing economic circumstances and hence are powerless to combat declining real income. Health care purchases are paid for in substantial part by private insurance and federal health and social programs. Yet the rising cost of these programs contributes substantially to rising government costs and may result in more out-of-pocket costs for the aged health care consumer.

Housing

The popular belief that the elderly are frail, dependent, senile people living out their last years in an institution has no factual basis. Only about 5% of the aged population reside in institutions providing long-term care (Ignatavicius, 1998). Many elders live in their own homes and have paid off their mortgages. Yet living arrangements are a major problem for some people as they age. The nurse needs to be aware of this issue because it can increase the client's stress level and have an impact on health care planning.

Rising energy and housing costs in many countries have joined the high costs of food and health care as factors that contribute to the economic hardship of aging people. In addition to financial difficulties, housing for the aged may be a problem because environmental supports that would help them to remain residing and participating in the community are lacking.

Deterioration of property, escalation of property taxes, and maintenance service costs create many problems for elder homeowners wishing to keep their homes. In some areas, elderly renters are extremely vulnerable to high rent fees, real estate speculation, and loss of living quarters because of removal of substandard, low-rent apartment or hotel buildings. Physical impairments and a lack of available, affordable support services, such as household help, transportation, home health care, and assistance with meals, prevent some aged people from being able to manage adequately in their own homes.

The need for special housing for the aged has long been recognized. Numbers of government and privately funded experiments in alternative housing for the aged have been tested. These projects incorporate such variables as personal care services, special health and safety remedies, and recreation and leisure plans. Although most of these projects provide security, improve life satisfaction, and prove cost effective, in many countries there is no overall plan for alternative living arrangements for the elderly.

RESOURCES FOR THE ELDERLY

In the United States, Canada, and other countries, a broad range of government benefits and services is available to assist older people with problems related to income, health insurance, housing, and social services. The nurse informs older adults and their families about the types of services available to help them achieve a higher quality of life.

Government Resources
Income

In the United States, the major portion of federal funds supporting programs for the elderly is devoted to the Social Security programs. The Social Security Act was passed in 1935, after the Depression, when many elderly were economically impoverished. Since that time, there has been a gradual shift from a program that was intended to provide a minimal supplement to retirees' sources of income to one that is the primary source of retirement income for many people. Other provisions of this act that are significant for people younger than 65 years are the disability and survivors' insurance provisions.

Health Insurance

Medicare was enacted as part of the amendments to the Social Security Act of 1965. This program was created to help older people meet the cost of health care. Despite its deficiencies, Medicare has provided a means for elders to obtain needed health care in times of escalating costs without decimating their total personal savings.

Medicare provides health insurance to people 65 years of age and older and to qualified disabled people of any age. Medicare A primarily pays for most of in-hospital care and is paid for by the federal government. It covers only a very small portion of care required in long-term care and minimal home health services. Currently, traditional Medicare requires a 3-day qualifying hospital stay before admission to a nursing home. Medicare B is an optional insurance and requires payment of a monthly premium. Medicare B pays most of the outpatient costs associated with physicians' visits, medication, and home health services. This traditional Medicare program is changing to managed care. It is predicted that all of

Medicare will be managed care shortly after the turn of the century. (See Chapter 3 for information on managed care.)

Medicaid (medical assistance) is a program designed to provide payment for medical services for the poor, including the poor elderly. For eligible people who are age 65 or older, it supplements the Medicare insurance program. Eligibility is related to determination of poverty level, and each state program determines its own criteria for eligibility. A number of states have completed the transition to managed care for their Medicaid recipients.

Housing Programs

In the United States, Congress has passed a number of legislative acts designed to alleviate housing problems for older citizens. Among these programs is rental assistance for lower-income families, the elderly, and the disabled. Direct low-interest loans are available to individuals to construct special rental housing facilities for the handicapped and the elderly. The federal government supports construction and rehabilitation of nursing homes. It subsidizes rental facilities, which can be rented by the aged at rates below the existing market price. For information related to these housing programs, nurses can contact the local public housing authority or the Housing and Urban Development area office in most communities.

Social Services

The Older Americans Act of 1965 provided social services to the aged. Under this legislation, each state created an office to provide leadership in the coordination and development of services for the elderly (Office on Aging). Some of the more significant programs and services carried out under this legislation are described in Chart 6–5.

Chart 6–5

Nursing Focus on the Elderly: Social Services Provided by the Older Americans Act of 1965

- Senior centers to meet the need for a central place for older people to congregate, develop new interests, and socialize.
- Nutrition programs to provide nutritious meals in a centralized setting as well as to the homebound elderly. Recreation, education, and health activities are incorporated in many sites as a regular part of the program.
- Transportation services to accommodate the elderly via special fares on existing public transportation systems and the operation of specially equipped vehicles for the frail and the handicapped elderly.
- Information and referral services to direct the elderly to the appropriate agency that provides needed services.
- In-home services, such as household help, telephone reassurance, chore maintenance, and visitation by home health aides, to enable the impaired elderly to remain living in the community.

Research Agencies

The National Institute on Aging was established in 1974. Its purpose is to conduct research on the biological, population-related, and sociologic aspects of aging at its Gerontology Research Center in Baltimore. It also supports research by others at universities and laboratories across the United States.

Within the National Institute for Mental Health, one division is devoted exclusively to problems of the aged: the Center for Studies of the Mental Health of the Aging. Its major role is to stimulate, coordinate, and support research training and to offer technical assistance relating to aging and mental health. Although it provides no monies for programs of service delivery to older people, it significantly affects the training of those working with elderly clients in community mental health centers and other service settings.

Community Resources

Over the years, it has become evident that government programs cannot provide all services needed by the aged. In many areas, private efforts can supply the same services at lower costs and without the red tape that some government programs involve. Transportation is an area in which the private sector and local, state, and federal governments all have roles.

In many urban areas, governments have provided Dial-A-Ride or similar services that provide free transportation. The federal government has subsidized the development and operation of transit systems, but its aid has been focused mainly on high-use systems and routes. For occasional travel, particularly in rural areas, the best solution may be for the elder to rely on a friend or a neighbor. Churches and community groups often help organize this approach by using sign-up sheets and recruiting volunteers to drive 1 day a week.

Education, recreation, and cultural activities help maintain a person's physical condition, mental alertness, and social contact. Education helps older people keep up with a rapidly changing world. Although advances in cable and satellite television systems, as well as the Internet, provide a broad range of new educational experiences at home, the value of person-to-person discussion and the need to focus some educational activities on local issues means that community discussion groups and other informal education will remain important.

Recreation and cultural activities are best managed on a local, nongovernment basis because personal preference plays such a large role in determining individual participation. A variety of activities run by different organizations or informal groups is more likely to please more people than a large program run by a government agency. For example, in the Midwest, elders have formed square dance groups and gourmet groups that meet frequently for socialization and compete with similar local, regional, and state groups.

Churches and other religious institutions serve the elderly in many ways. In addition to their primary role of providing organized worship, they sponsor many activities that bring the elderly together with their peers as well as with younger people. Clergypersons and other spiritual leaders are often excellent counselors, and other members of the congregation or religious group are sometimes willing to help older members in time of trouble.

Many communities have access to community resource books (e.g., those published by the United Way). Area agencies on aging are excellent referral centers. Some of these agencies publish directories of services that are specifically geared to the elderly. The nurse can help to inform elderly clients about community resources that they may need, depending on their specific life situation.

THE FUTURE OF GERONTOLOGICAL NURSING

Nurses in most adult health care settings encounter the challenges of caring for both well and ill older adults. In view of the rapidly increasing elderly population, especially the over-85 group, nurses in many settings are specializing in gerontological nursing or geriatric case management. Nurses can practice these specialties in acute care, long-term care, and community-based settings. Just as nurses can achieve certification in medical-surgical nursing, they can become certified in gerontological nursing or case management. The American Nurses Credentialing Center (ANCC) provides three gerontology examinations for certification for those who qualify: gerontological nurse, gerontological clinical specialist, and gerontological nurse practitioner. The ANCC also offers a nursing case management examination, which is broad-based and not specific for geriatric case management. Other professional organizations also certify case managers, including geriatric case managers (see Chap. 3).

SELECTED BIBLIOGRAPHY

All, A. C. (1994). A literature review: Assessment and interventions in elder abuse. *Journal of Gerontological Nursing, 20*(7), 25–32.

Baldwin, R. L., Craven, R. F., & Dimond, M. (1996). Falls: Are rural elders at greater risk? *Journal of Gerontological Nursing, 22*(8), 14–21.

Bradley, L., Siddique, C. M., & Dufton, B. (1995). Reducing the use of physical restraints in long-term care facilities. *Journal of Gerontological Nursing, 21*(9), 21–34.

*Brock, A. M. (1992). Economics and the aged. In E. Baines (Ed.), *Perspectives on gerontology nursing*. Boston: Sage.

Broussard, M. C., & Pitre, S. (1996). Medication problems in the elderly: A home healthcare nurse's perspective. *Home Healthcare Nurse, 14*(6), 441–443.

Burke, M. M., & Walsh, M. B. (1997). *Gerontologic nursing: Wholistic care of the older adult* (2nd ed.). St. Louis: C. V. Mosby.

*Coffman, T. L. (1981). Relocation and survival of institutionalized aged: A re-examination of the evidence. *Gerontologist, 21,* 483–500.

Commodore, D. I. (1995). Falls in the elderly population: A look at incidence, risks, healthcare costs, and prevalence strategies. *Rehabilitation Nursing, 20*(2), 84–89.

*Department of Health and Human Services. (1990). *Healthy people 2000*. Rockville, MD: Author.

Dunning, S. (1994). Elder abuse is our fight, too. *RN, 57*(8), 76.

Frost, M. H., & Willette, K. (1994). Risk for abuse/neglect: Documentation of assessment data and diagnoses. *Journal of Gerontological Nursing, 20*(8), 37–45.

Greenberg, E. M. (1996). Violence and the older adult: The role of the acute care nurse practitioner. *Critical Care Nursing Quarterly, 19*(2), 76–84.

Ignatavicius, D. D. (1998). *Introduction to long-term care: Principles and practice.* Philadelphia: F. A. Davis.

*Karper, W. B., & Boschen, M. B. (1993). Effects of exercise on acute respiratory tract infections and related symptoms. *Geriatric Nursing, 14*(1), 15–18.

Kuehn, A. F., & Sendelwick, S. (1995). Acute health status and its relationship to falls in the nursing home. *Journal of Gerontological Nursing, 21*(7), 41–49.

Lange, M. (1996). The challenge of fall prevention in home care: A review of the literature. *Home Healthcare Nurse, 14*(3), 198–206.

Lay, T. (1994). The flourishing problem of elder abuse in our society. *AACN Clinical Issues in Critical Care Nursing, 5*(4), 507–515.

Loughran, S. (1996). Medication use in the elderly: A population at risk. *MedSurg Nursing, 5*(2), 121–124.

Lynch, S. H. (1997). Elder abuse: What to look for, how to intervene. *American Journal of Nursing, 97*(1), 26–32.

Matteson, M. A., McConnell, E. S., & Linton, A. D. (1997). *Gerontological nursing: Concepts and practice* (2nd ed.). Philadelphia: W. B. Saunders.

*McCloskey, J. C., & Bulechek, G. M. (1992). *Nursing interventions classification (NIC)*. St. Louis: Mosby-Year Book.

Mills, E. M. (1994). The effect of low-intensity aerobic exercises on muscle strength, flexibility, and balance among sedentary elderly persons. *Nursing Research, 43*(4), 207–211.

*North American Nursing Diagnosis Association. (1992). *Definitions and classification 1992.* St. Louis: Author.

Rosen, S. L. (1994). Managing delirious older adults in the hospital. *MedSurg Nursing, 3*(3), 181–189.

Wilson, E. B. (1996). Physical restraint of elderly patients in critical care: Historical perspectives and new directions. *Critical Care Nursing Clinics of North America, 8*(1), 61–70.

SUGGESTED READINGS

Bradley, L., Siddique, C. M., & Dufton, B. (1995). Reducing the use of physical restraints in long-term care facilities. *Journal of Gerontological Nursing, 21*(9), 21–34.

This article presents the findings of a longitudinal study that documented the positive outcomes of a structured restraint education program in reducing the use of physical restraints and promoting nonrestrictive alternatives. The researchers showed that restraint-free elder care can be attained in a cost-effective manner and without an increase in resident falls and injuries.

Lange, M. (1996). The challenge of fall prevention in home care: A review of the literature. *Home Healthcare Nurse, 14*(3), 198–206.

This article provides an extensive review of the literature regarding falls and outlines successful clinical nursing strategies that can be used to prevent falls in the home. These interventions address primary, secondary, and tertiary activities.

Lynch, S. H. (1997). Elder abuse: What to look for, how to intervene. *American Journal of Nursing, 97*(1), 26–32.

This comprehensive article examines the four types of elder abuse: physical, psychological, and financial abuse and neglect by self or others. The author describes detection and interventions for abuse as well as strategies to prevent abuse in long-term care settings. Resources are also presented in a chart. A continuing education quiz is available at the end of the article.

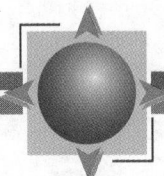

Biopsychosocial Concepts

Related to Health Care

ETHICS

Medical-surgical nurses in all settings experience a variety of ethical issues every day. These ethical issues vary in intensity from seemingly minor issues, such as whether a nurse should tell a client a "white lie," to extremely emotional issues about euthanasia or how to allocate scarce health care resources. Frequently, nurses realize that they are in the midst of an ethical dilemma when two or more equally unfavorable options exist (Curtin & Flaherty, 1982). At other times, however, the nurse may not recognize that an ethical issue has occurred until after the situation is over.

WHAT IS ETHICS?
Definition

Ethics is the study of what is right or what people ought to do in a specific situation. The nurse decides "what is right" by consulting a variety of resources, including

- Ethical theories and principles
- Legal statutes
- Decision-making models
- The values of the persons involved
- Professional codes
- Policies
- Nursing and ethics consultants

Thus, a nurse cannot learn the one correct answer for resolving any specific ethical issue because each clinical ethical issue is unique.

Ethical Theories

Ethical theories are a way of approaching ethical problems and determining what is the right action to implement. The two most common ethical theories are utilitarianism and deontology.

Utilitarianism

The guiding rule in utilitarianism is the greatest happiness principle, in which decisions are based on whatever action would bring about the greatest happiness for the greatest number of people. Recently, this principle has been expanded beyond happiness to include other intrinsic values, such as close relationships, success, personal freedom, good health, and beauty (Beauchamp & Childress, 1994). The consequences of the possible options are evaluated regarding their ability to promote group happiness or good rather than individual happiness. Utilitarians believe that rules such as "never lie" can be broken if the consequence of lying will bring about the most happiness. For example, if an unstable myocardial infarction client voices concern that his spouse has not visited, a utilitarian would justify not telling the client his spouse had been killed in an automobile accident if telling would cause a setback in recovery (Beauchamp & Childress,

1994; Beauchamp & Walters, 1982; Curtin & Flaherty, 1982; DeWolf, 1989b).

Deontology

In contrast, deontologists believe that actions are right or wrong despite their consequences and that a person's intentions to do good should be praised. Deontology emphasizes the importance of the individual person, not the group. Rules are rarely broken. In addition, a deontologist would agree that answers for an ethical issue can be identified and generalized to similar ethical issues (Beauchamp & Childress, 1994; Beauchamp & Walters, 1982; Curtin & Flaherty, 1982; DeWolf, 1989b). To return to the example given for utilitarianism, a deontologist would tell the unstable myocardial infarction client that his spouse had been killed because truth-telling is always the right action. However, rarely are people purely utilitarian or purely deontological in their approach to ethical decision-making. Generally, ethical decisions reflect a combination of theoretical approaches and ethical principles.

Ethical Principles

Ethical principles can also help the nurse determine what a correct action is for resolving an ethical issue. Four major ethical principles are nonmaleficence, beneficence, justice, and autonomy. However, one difficulty with using ethical principles is that no criteria exist for choosing between competing or conflicting principles (Beauchamp & Childress, 1994).

Nonmaleficence

The principle of nonmaleficence requires that no matter what other outcomes are achieved during an ethical issue, the nurse must prevent harm. "Do no harm" is the minimal standard of behavior for health care professionals. The principle of nonmaleficence is supported when a nurse follows the "five rights" of medication administration or helps a postoperative client to turn, cough, and deep breathe.

Beneficence

Beneficence builds on the principle of nonmaleficence. Besides doing no harm, the nurse must benefit the client by promoting good. Thus, the principle of beneficence requires the nurse to perform an action. For example, a nurse is acting beneficently when he or she relaxes visitation rules in a hospital to allow a family member to spend the night with a confused elderly client.

Justice

The principle of justice is concerned with how resources are divided among individual people and/or groups in the society. Typically, justice is concerned only with resources that are in short supply, such as financing for specialized health care services like organs for transplantation. How-ever, little agreement exists whether resources should be allocated by a person's effort, need, merit, or social contribution or by free market exchange. Nurses make decisions based on justice when they decide how to allocate their time among clients.

Autonomy

The principle of autonomy requires that a person be involved in decisions that affect his or her life. Making a decision for a person when he or she could have made the decision is paternalistic and negates the person's autonomy. A nurse promotes client autonomy by advising the client of options in care, ensuring that the client has adequate information to make a decision, and supporting the client's decision.

Ethical Versus Legal Actions

Actions determined to be ethical for a given situation may not be considered legal actions. For example, it may be ethically justifiable to facilitate a client's death based on the principle of beneficence and utilitarian theory. However, assisted suicide is not a legal option in most countries. Typically, legal statutes reflect the ethical mindset held by society 10 to 15 years ago. Thus, new technology can create conflicts between current ethical reasoning and the law.

Because of conflicts between ethical and legal opinions, people may bring suit in the hopes of overturning current law and establishing a new legal precedent. For example, *Cruzan v. Director, Missouri Department of Health* (1990) addressed the right of a family to have a client's treatment—in this case, gastrostomy tube feedings—removed.

Values

A value is a way of looking at life that ultimately directs the person's behavior and gives life meaning. Values are beliefs that have been freely chosen, communicated to others, and acted on repeatedly throughout life. The development of values is influenced by one's family, religion, culture, interpersonal relationships, and activities. Despite being of long standing, values do change and are never stagnant (Steele & Harmon, 1983). Examples of personal values include a comfortable life, world peace, happiness, salvation, and love.

A nurse's personal values serve as the foundation for the development of professional values. Thus, nurses sometimes have difficulty in balancing their personal and professional values. Examples of professional values include promoting health, being truthful with clients, providing client advocacy, and having a nonjudgmental attitude.

Values serve as rationale for determining whether an action is right or wrong. The nurse may experience an ethical quandary when personal and professional values conflict. For example, when a client requires a valve replacement because of endocarditis caused by intravenous

TABLE 7-1

An Exercise for Clarifying Personal and Professional Values

- Step 1. Choosing freely
  - a. Am I sure I've thought about this value and have chosen to believe it for myself?
  - b. Who first taught me this value?
  - c. How do I know I'm "right"?
- Step 2. Choosing from among alternatives
  - a. What other alternatives are possible?
  - b. Which alternative has the most appeal for me and why?
  - c. Have I thought much about this value alternative?
- Step 3. Choosing after considering the consequences
  - a. What consequences do I think might occur as a result of my holding this value?
  - b. What price will I pay for my position?
  - c. Is this value worth the price I might pay?
- Step 4. Complement to other values
  - a. Does this value "fit" with other values, and is it consistent with them?
  - b. Am I sure this value doesn't conflict with other values I deem important?
- Step 5. Pride and esteem
  - a. Am I proud of my position and value? Is this something I feel good about?
  - b. How important is this value to me?
  - c. If this were not my value, how different would my life be?
- Step 6. Public affirmation
  - a. Am I willing to speak out for this value?
- Steps 7 and 8. Action
  - a. Am I willing to put this value into action?
  - b. Do I act on this value? When? How consistently?
  - c. Is this a value that can guide me in other situations?
  - d. Would I want others who are important to me to follow this value?
  - e. Do I think I'll always believe this? How committed to this value am I?
  - f. Am I willing to do anything about this value?
  - g. How do I know this value is "right"? How do I know? Are my values ethical?

Reprinted with permission from Fowler, M. D. M., & Levine-Ariff, J. (1987). *Ethics at the bedside: A source for the critical care nurse.* Philadelphia: J. B. Lippincott (pp. 160–161).

drug abuse, the nurse may experience conflict between professionally believing everyone deserves high-quality health care and personally believing that a person who uses illegal intravenous drugs does not deserve aggressive treatment.

Values clarification is a process of analyzing alternatives and exploring the associated feelings and beliefs (Table 7–1). The process serves to identify the conscious and unconscious values that guide behavior. When clarifying values, people ask themselves, "What is important to me?" or "What are my beliefs?" Values clarification can facilitate the nurse's understanding of competing values displayed by other health care professionals and clients.

ETHICAL DECISION-MAKING
Variables Influencing Ethical Decision-Making

Many variables can influence a nurse's ethical decision-making in any medical-surgical setting. The nurse's ethical decision-making can become more complex, depending on the variety and number of variables involved. These variables can be described as nurse, task, or environmental (Simon, 1978).

Nurse Variables

Variables that can influence ethical decision-making processes include those inherent within the nurse, such as values and beliefs, gender, age and maturity, assumptions, and self-image. A nurse's knowledge, education, moral reasoning, and communication skills and previous experiences can also influence how the nurse perceives an ethical issue (DeWolf, 1989a).

Task Variables

Task variables influence the process used to resolve ethical issues. Ethical decision-making is influenced by the amount of time available to make a decision. The complexity of the decision to be made also influences the decision-making task. Often nurses attempt to use a "rule of thumb," such as "Never give pain medication early," to simplify the decision task. Another variable influencing a decision task is the perceived costs and benefits associated with a possible option (DeWolf, 1989a).

Environmental Variables

Environmental variables can be classified as either institutional (health care agency) characteristics or community variables.

INSTITUTIONAL CHARACTERISTICS. Institutional characteristics identified by hospital-based nurses during a study by Crisham (1981) include

- Hospital policies
- Time limitations created by work shifts
- Conflicting loyalties between client, profession, and institution
- Difficulties applying knowledge in the clinical setting
- Diversity of expectations of clients, supervisors, and other health care professionals
- Limited awareness by nurses regarding their responsibilities and authority during clinical ethical decision-making

Other institutional characteristics that influence ethical decision-making are philosophy, tolerance for ethical questions, staffing patterns, client acuity, available technology or equipment, economic stability of the health care agency, the nurse's job description and associated responsibilities, overall quality of working relationships between nurses and other health care professionals, and accessibility of ethics resources (DeWolf, 1989a). Additional variables may enter into the decision-making process depending on the setting (e.g., home, clinic, nursing home, or ambulatory surgical center).

COMMUNITY VARIABLES. The ethical decision-making environment is also influenced by changing community variables. For example, the lay public is becoming more informed about health care issues, and community groups are involved in health care reform. Health care decisions are influenced by laws, public beliefs about how resources should be allocated, and current events in the media. Because communities are generally heterogeneous, each community reflects a specific mix of ethnic, religious, and cultural perspectives. Thus, these factors may influence how an ethical issue is resolved.

Normative Ethical Decision-Making Models

A variety of ethical decision-making models have been created to assist the nurse with clinical ethical decision-making. In each model, a specific concept is emphasized, such as rights (Curtin & Flaherty, 1982), biblical principles (Shelly, 1980), or the application of bioethical stan-

dards (Husted & Husted, 1994). Each model requires the decision-maker to

- Identify the ethical problem
- Identify and consider alternatives
- Implement a choice
- Evaluate the decision-making process and its outcome

Thus, normative decision-making models parallel the nursing process even though some models may require extra steps, such as values clarification or application of ethical principles. Frequently, nurses do not perceive these normative decision-making models as helpful. Nurses have difficulty considering a variety of options and their associated consequences during urgent, time-limited situations. Therefore, these normative models are more useful for retrospective or hypothetical case analysis. The more often nurses use a normative model for retrospective or hypothetical case review, the more apt they will be to use a logical decision-making process to resolve real clinical ethical situations.

Descriptive Ethical Decision-Making Models

The process nurses use to resolve clinical ethical situations in an acute medical-surgical setting has been investi-

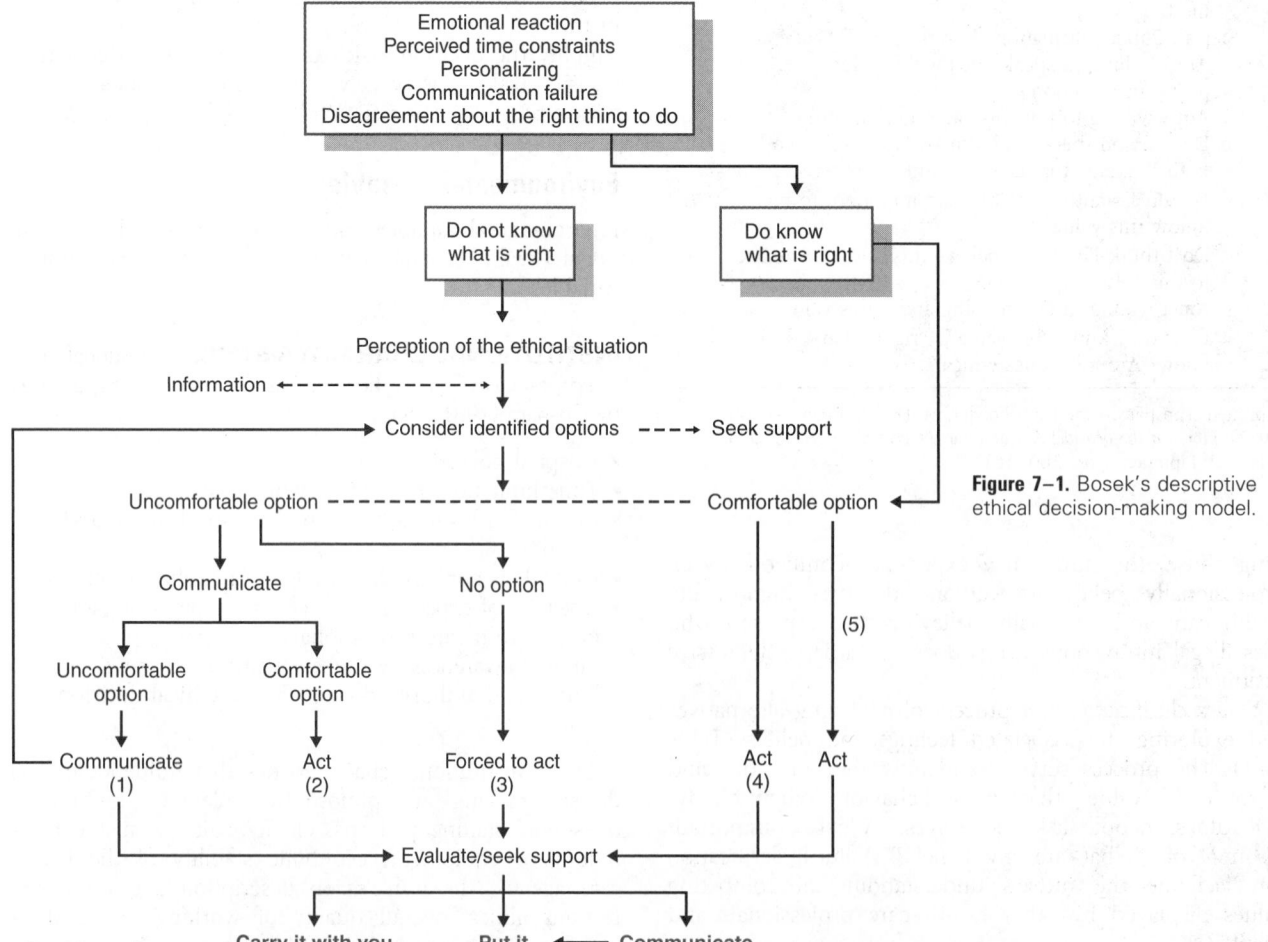

Figure 7–1. Bosek's descriptive ethical decision-making model.

gated and is described in the Descriptive Ethical Decision-Making Model (Fig. 7–1). From this model, several difficulties with the nurses' ethical decision-making process have been identified (DeWolf, 1989a).

First, the nurses did not perceive that an ethical situation was occurring until after they

- Experienced an emotional reaction
- Perceived a limited amount of time available to make a decision
- Considered what they would want done if they were the client
- Experienced a communication failure
- Did not know what was the right thing to do to resolve the ethical situation

Second, the nurses did not identify possible options; instead, they considered options identified by others. The nurses evaluated all possible options on a comfortable-uncomfortable continuum. Comfort was defined as the nurse's personal psychological comfort and the amount of physical comfort the client would experience as a result of implementing the option. If nurses were forced to choose between their own psychological comfort and the client's physical comfort, they always favored their own psychological comfort (DeWolf, 1989a).

Third, nurses often had difficulty putting the ethical issue behind them. Some nurses described their need to keep discussing the ethical issue and the fact that they continued to experience the same emotional reactions years after the issue occurred. Thus, for some nurses, the ethical issue was never resolved.

ETHICAL RESOURCES

Various ethical resources exist that may facilitate a nurse's ethical decision-making in a medical-surgical setting. These resources may vary among health care agencies. Nurses need to learn what resources are available in their practice setting. These resources may include professional codes, policies and procedures, nursing administrators, and institutional ethics committees or consultants.

Ethical Codes for Nurses

In Canada and the United States, major nursing associations have codes of ethics. The *Code for Nurses,* developed by the American Nurses' Association (1976; 1985) (Table 7–2) is undergoing revision. One of the requirements for a profession is the existence and adherence to an ethical code to regulate professional conduct. Each code signifies the profession's acknowledgment of the responsibility and faith entrusted by society to the nursing profession. Nurses are expected to follow the code in their daily practice.

Policies and Procedures

Ethical codes represent standards for ideal behavior. However, the codes do not tell nurses the exact actions to take in specific ethical situations. One way that health care agencies have addressed this lack of specificity is

TABLE 7–2

The American Nurses' Association Code for Nurses

1. The nurse provides services with respect for human dignity and the uniqueness of the client, unrestricted by considerations of social or economic status, personal attributes, or the nature of health problems.
2. The nurse safeguards the client's right to privacy by judiciously protecting information of a confidential nature.
3. The nurse acts to safeguard the client and the public when health care and safety are affected by the incompetent, unethical, or illegal practice of any person.
4. The nurse assumes responsibility and accountability for individual nursing judgments and actions.
5. The nurse maintains competence in nursing.
6. The nurse exercises informed judgment and uses individual competence and qualifications as criteria in seeking consultation, accepting responsibilities, and delegating nursing activities to others.
7. The nurse participates in activities that contribute to the ongoing development of the profession's body of knowledge.
8. The nurse participates in the profession's efforts to implement and improve standards of nursing.
9. The nurse participates in the profession's efforts to establish and maintain conditions of employment conducive to high-quality nursing care.
10. The nurse participates in the profession's efforts to protect the public from misinformation and misrepresentation and to maintain the integrity of nursing.
11. The nurse collaborates with members of the health professions and other citizens in promoting community and national efforts to meet the health needs of the public.

Reprinted with permission. American Nurses' Association. (1976; 1985). *Code for nurses with interpretive statements.* Kansas City, MO: Author.

through the development of policies and procedures that reflect the intents found in the codes.

Nurses have a responsibility to participate in the development and ongoing review of policies and procedures that facilitate ethical practice in their agency. For example, a preoperative policy requires that consent for surgery be obtained before the client receives preoperative sedation. This policy reflects the need to respect the client's autonomy and legal right to informed consent. At times, a nurse may experience intense pressure from others to "keep on schedule" and send the client to the operating suite although consent has not yet been obtained. In this situation, the policy provides legal and ethical support for a nurse's refusal to send the client to surgery before informed consent is obtained.

Nursing Administrators

Nursing administrators, including unit nurse managers, can be valuable resources when ethical issues arise. Most administrators have had experience as staff nurses and are also familiar with available agency resources and applicable policies and procedures that may assist in resolving an ethical issue. Nurses sometimes hesitate to consult a nursing administrator because of fears that they will be perceived as incompetent. However, the opposite is usually true. Nurses should keep nursing administrators informed of any potential or actual ethical situations and should seek an administrator's advice, because administrators have the authority to mobilize resources, redistribute responsibilities, and use discipline, if necessary, in resolving an ethical situation.

Institutional Ethics Committees

Ethical issues arise when a nurse does not know what is a correct course to follow. The Joint Commission on Accreditation of Healthcare Organizations (JCAHO) (1997–1998, 1998, 1998–1999a, b) requires all agencies to have a mechanism for dealing with ethical issues. Health care agencies may provide specific ethics resources through institutional ethics committees (IECs), ethics consultants, or a combination of both.

Most health care agencies have an interdisciplinary ethics committee that serves as an advisory group for ethical deliberation. In long-term care agencies, this committee is called the patient care advisory committee (PCAC). This committee has three functions:

- Providing agency and community education about ethical issues and ethical analysis
- Developing policies relevant to ethical decisions, such as resuscitation, refusal of treatment, or informed consent
- Deliberating on cases

Depending on agency policy, referral of an ethical issue to an ethics committee may be optional or mandatory. In addition, whether a health care professional must follow the recommendations of the IEC may be considered optional or mandatory.

Ethics committees may be composed of administrators, physicians, nurses, occupational therapists, physical therapists, dietitians, social workers, lay people, and someone with an extensive background in ethics (e.g., a philosopher, theologian, and/or clinician with advanced education in bioethics). The group process of analyzing a problem reflects the opinions and advice that many minds can contribute on a case. However, ethics committees can be bureaucratic and unwieldy with outspoken members who intimidate quieter members (Savage, 1994).

The following is an example of a home health case referred to an agency's ethics committee: A 78-year-old man with gangrenous feet was refusing amputation. He was legally competent, but the home health team was uncomfortable with his refusal. They referred his case to the committee. After considering relevant data, the committee concluded that if the client is determined to be competent, his wishes must be respected and the health care team should not amputate his feet. If he is determined to be incompetent, then a legal guardian should be appointed to decide what treatment is in the client's best interest. The committee also found that the client's refusal for amputation was consistent with earlier expressions of

valuing his independence. The home health team considered the committee's conclusions and recommendations. After the home health team followed the protocol to determine the client's competency, they believed that the client was competent to refuse amputation. Although the home health team regretted the client's decision, the committee's recommendation fortified their resolve to respect the client's right to make this difficult decision.

Ethics Consultants

An ethics consultant may be a health care professional, such as a physician, nurse, chaplain, or philosopher. This consultant gathers and reviews data and offers an ethical analysis. An ethics consultant model overcomes the bureaucratic problem of coordinating an agency ethics committee meeting, but the interdisciplinary perspectives of a committee are lacking. Nurses should be aware of the various ethics resources in their practice settings.

SELECTED ETHICAL ISSUES
Futility

One of the major ethical issues to be faced in the future is the concept of futility. Technology can extend human life beyond the point when a person cares to live, has consciousness, or has the possibility of recovery. The determination of futile treatment is made by analyzing the cost of treatment (financial, physical, emotional) and the likely outcome (cure, recovery, prolongation of life, death). The value of the costs and outcomes should be determined by the client or, if the client is unable, by the family and friends closest to the client. This is a gross oversimplification, however. Even if a client requests futile treatment (e.g., resuscitation in terminal disease), such requests are not automatically honored. The determination of futility also relies on the clinical judgment of health care professionals. Although treatment is thought to be futile, it may be continued because the health care agency may fear a lawsuit. However, discussion and education must occur to learn the client's values, goals, fears, and motives. A request for futile treatment may represent a client's fear of dying.

Do Not Resuscitate Orders

Cardiopulmonary resuscitation (CPR) was originally designed to treat witnessed cardiac arrests. Based on the principle of beneficence, the use of CPR has expanded. However, initiating CPR for persons with terminal illnesses, such as acquired immunodeficiency syndrome or cancer, or the severely ill or aged elderly may be perceived as causing harm. Discussions about the client's wishes and the benefits and burdens of CPR should occur periodically during any acute, chronic, or terminal illness. However, the presence of a written advance directive does not translate into an automatic do not resuscitate (DNR) order.

The agency DNR policy should be available in a prominent place so that health care professionals are familiar with the policy. The policy should stipulate how the DNR

TABLE 7–3

Components in a Do Not Resuscitate Order

Specify	Examples
Resuscitative measures	Cardiopulmonary arrest Pulmonary arrest Hypotensive event Life-threatening cardiac event Dysrhythmia
Measures to be withheld	External cardiac massage Endotracheal intubation Cardiotonic medications Vasopressors Cardioversion Ventilator or changes in ventilator settings
Measures to be continued	All current therapies Pain medications Oxygen Comfort medications (e.g., antibiotics, diuretics, steroids, chemotherapy)
Measures to be initiated	Artificial ventilation with a mask Cardiotonic drug trial Increased ventilator rate setting Increase oxygen to 100%
Who to notify in case of cardiac arrest	Attending physician House officer Nurse practitioner Consultant

order must be written (Table 7–3), how frequently the order must be reviewed, and under what conditions it is suspended. For example, DNR orders are frequently suspended when a client needs surgery requiring ventilator support, based on the principle of beneficence at the risk of violating client autonomy (Clarke et al., 1994; Langslow, 1995; Rhodes, 1994; Rosner et al., 1994).

Quality of Life

Quality of life (QOL) remains an elusive concept; no single definition exists. According to studies by Ferrans and Powers (1985), QOL is determined by the client's judgment about the importance of certain elements in his or her life and satisfaction with those elements. A client who is confined to a wheelchair, for example, may believe that mobility is very important. Although being in a wheelchair is not as good as walking, using a wheelchair may be better than being immobilized, according to this client. However, other people who believe that walking is crucial for happiness may perceive the client's QOL as being poor. If clients are unable to communicate, whether they never had this ability or have irreversibly lost this ability, it is impossible to know how they view their QOL.

Utilitarian Versus Deontological Approach

From a utilitarian standpoint (for the good of *all*), two perspectives can be taken when evaluating QOL. First, a person warrants resources on the basis of real or potential productivity that that person offers society. Second, humanity is served by protecting vulnerable individuals in society because one never knows when one may be in the vulnerable group. This perspective does not offer guidance in determining the quantity resources one should expend.

The deontological approach to QOL is based on respect for an *individual* person's life. Deontologists maintain that human life has intrinsic value and should be preserved at all costs.

When conflict exists in a specific case of whether to continue treatment for someone lacking decisional capacity and the client's wishes are unknown, the health care system turns to the legal system.

Legal Perspective

Through the legal system, society has grappled with how best to preserve the autonomy of incompetent clients, as in the cases of Nancy Cruzan and Karen Ann Quinlan (Weir, 1989), who were in irreversible comas. In these cases, the central issue was the incompetent person's right to refuse treatment and how this right is exercised. If the person's wishes are unknown, the law presumes that a person, even an incompetent person, prefers to live. While the state has an interest in preserving life, society is not in agreement on whether the financial burden of preserving life at all costs is justifiable.

The current health care system in the United States forces allocation based on accessibility to services and ability to pay. The uninsured and underinsured forego treatment except in emergency care, and then they may receive services only after a lengthy wait. Similarly, some people often must wait for appointments or referrals to specialists when they are in health maintenance organizations (HMOs). In Canada, however, clients are not limited by ability to pay, but they may have to wait for certain procedures or surgeries or they may not have access to some procedures available in the United States. Many groups, especially nursing associations, have worked tirelessly for universal access to health care and believe the health care system should be revamped to focus on preventive care and health maintenance rather than acute inpatient care.

The state of Oregon proposed an allocation of health care dollars based on a quality-of-life-year (QOLY) and probability of medical benefit. A prioritized list of more than 700 treatments was compiled as a method of determining what treatments would be supported and what treatments would not be funded with state dollars (Hadorn, 1991). The Bush administration (1989–1993) opposed this plan, arguing that it potentially discriminated against disabled clients. Thus, by 1993, the Oregon Health Plan was still not fully implemented. After making changes mandated by the federal government, Oregon was $83.6 million short of funding the plan, was losing

DECLARATION UNDER ILLINOIS LIVING WILL ACT

This declaration is made this _____ day of _____ 19___.
I, _____, being of sound mind, willfully and voluntarily make known my desires that my moment of death shall not be artificially postponed.

If at any time I should have an incurable and irreversible injury, disease, or illness judged to be a terminal condition by my attending physician who has personally examined me, and has determined that my death is imminent except for death delaying procedures, I direct that such procedures which would only prolong the dying process be withheld or withdrawn, and that I be permitted to die naturally with only the administration of medication, sustenance, or the performance of any medical procedure deemed necessary by my attending physician to provide me with comfort care.

In the absence of my ability to give directions regarding the use of such death delaying procedures, it is my intention that this declaration shall be honored by my family and physician as the final expression of my legal right to refuse medical or surgical treatment and accept the consequences from such refusal.

Signed _____

City, County and State of Residence   _____

_____

_____

The declarant is personally known to me and I believe the declarant to be of sound mind. I did not sign the declarant's signature about, for or at the direction of the declarant. At the date of this instrument, I am not entitled to any portion of the estate of the declarant according to the laws of intestate succession or, to the best of my knowledge and belief, under any will of declarant or other instrument taking effect at declarant's death, or directly financially responsible for the declarant's medical care.

Witness _____

Witness _____

Figure 7–2. An example of a living will.

support of the business community, and faced cutting the education budget to fund health care (Campbell, 1993).

Palliative Versus Curative Care

There may come a point in the course of a disease when a cure may not be possible. For example, clients with cardiomyopathy, neoplastic diseases, or degenerative diseases may no longer respond to treatment; thus, they might perceive continued treatment with poor probability of cure unbearable. These clients may opt for treatment that provides symptom management but does not cure the condition. Palliative care—aimed toward comfort, not cure—may involve radiation, chemotherapy, or surgery to reduce tumor mass; administration of analgesics in high and frequent doses; and/or variation in nutrition routes.

Nurses often have an opportunity to practice the art as well as the science of nursing in palliative care. During palliative care, nurses make a commitment to provide relief for the client until death. A client's comfort is often related to the tenacity of the nurse in advocating and providing client care.

Intentionality

The doctrine of the "double effect" (Garcia, 1995) is moral reasoning presented by some Catholic theologians in defending the use of analgesics in terminal illness. The double effect doctrine holds that it is morally permissible to medicate a client to relieve pain even if there is a risk that the medication may suppress respirations and cause the client to stop breathing. If the *intent* is to relieve pain, the action is permissible. If the *intent* is to kill the person, it is not permissible. For example, a nurse gives morphine sulfate to a client dying of lung cancer. The nurse realizes that morphine can depress respirations, which are already compromised by the cancer. Nevertheless, the nurse intends to provide pain relief and is aware that an untoward side effect may be death due to apnea. The nurse is ethically justified in giving the morphine because the intent is to relieve pain, not to cause death.

Competency

Two forms of competency exist: legal and clinical competency. A person is considered to be *legally* competent if he or she is

- 18 years of age or older
- Pregnant or a married minor
- A legally emancipated minor who is self-supporting
- Not declared incompetent by a court of law

If a court determines that a person is legally incompetent, a guardian is appointed to make health care and/or financial decisions.

A person is considered to be *clinically* competent if he or she is legally competent and possesses decisional capacity. Decisional capacity is determined by the person who is the most knowledgeable about the issue. Decisional capacity is determined by assessing the client's ability to

- Identify the problem
- Recognize options and their potential consequences
- Make a decision
- Provide rationale supporting the chosen option

Thus, a surgeon would determine a client's decisional capacity related to surgery, an internist would assess capacity related to medical treatment, and a nurse would determine the client's ability to make decisions about nursing activities (Bosek, 1993).

Written Advance Directives

Written advance directives are "legal documents which provide a mechanism for individuals to indicate their decisions about future medical care" (Bosek & Fitzpatrick, 1992, p. 33). The U.S. Patient Self Determination Act of 1990 requires health care professionals to inform each client who is admitted to a hospital or nursing home about the availability of advance directives. If the client has a written advance directive on admission, a copy is placed with the medical record so that the directive will be available if needed.

There are two common types of written advance directives: living wills and durable power of attorney for health care.

Living Wills

Living wills, sometimes referred to as "death with dignity" documents, allow persons to document their wishes regarding life-sustaining treatment in case they are ever unable to speak for themselves and are imminently dying of a terminal illness (Fig. 7–2). Some states in the United States and provinces in Canada do not recognize living wills as legal documents. Nurses must investigate whether living wills are legally recognized in their state or prov-

ince. This information can be obtained from an ethicist or their agency's legal consultant or department. In most states, "imminent death" refers to when death is expected within a few hours or days according to best medical estimates (Kilner, 1990). In some states, imminent death may be defined as death that is expected to occur within a few months.

Durable Power of Attorney for Health Care

A durable power of attorney for health care (DPOA), sometimes called a durable medical power of attorney, is a legal document in the United States. This document allows people to

- Identify someone to make decisions for them if unable to speak for themselves
- Identify how aggressive treatment should be if they should ever be in a coma or a persistent vegetative state (PVS)
- List any medical treatments they would never want performed (Fig. 7–3)

Each state in the United States has legislation that describes the scope and execution of a DPOA.

The following example illustrates the use of advance directives: A client who sustained head trauma in an accident is now in a PVS and requires ventilator support. The spouse presents a copy of the client's living will and DPOA to the hospital staff and requests that the ventilator be discontinued. The living will does not apply in this situation because the client is not considered terminally ill. The DPOA, however, does apply and identifies the spouse as the agent to make the health care decisions. In addition, the client has documented the desire to forego artificial life support in the event of irreversible coma. The health care team respects the client's autonomy, as exercised by the spouse and the written advance directive, and discontinues the ventilator. Nurses should become familiar with applicable laws on advance directives in their state or province as well as remember that written advance directives are not to be implemented until the person has lost decisional capacity.

Verbal Advance Directives

Occasionally, family members, friends, or health care professionals are able to remember conversations with the client when specific comments were made about life-sustaining treatments. These comments may be considered verbal advance directives when the client has no written directives and is unable to communicate his or her wishes. A common myth is that the physician is obligated to follow the next-of-kin consent when the client cannot participate in decision-making. In most cases, next-of-kin do not have legal authority to consent or refuse treatment for an adult relative without becoming declared the legal guardian or the agent in a DPOA. Traditionally, however, health care professionals have obtained next-of-kin approval to minimize the chance of being sued.

If a client tells a nurse or other health care professional about his or her wishes regarding health care and life-sustaining treatment, the professional should encourage

DURABLE POWER OF ATTORNEY FOR HEALTH CARE

Power of Attorney made this _____ day of _____ , 19____

   1. I, the undersigned hereby appoint (insert name and address of agent)

_____

as agent to act for me and in my name to make any and all decisions for me concerning my personal care, medical treatment, hospitalization and health care and to require, withhold or withdraw any type of medical treatment or procedure, even though my death may ensue. My agent shall have the same access to my medical records that I have, including the right to disclose the contents to others. My agent shall also have full power to make a disposition of any part or all of my body for medical purposes, authorize an autopsy and direct the disposition of my remains. (Neither the attending physician nor any other health care provider may act as your agent.)

   2. The powers granted above shall be subject to the following rules or limitations (if none, leave blank):

_____

(The subject of life-sustaining treatment is of particular importance. For your convenience in dealing with that subject some general statements concerning the withholding or removal of life-sustaining treatment are set forth below. If you agree with one of these statements, you may initial that statement; but do not initial more than one.)

   (I do not want my life to be prolonged nor do I want life-sustaining treatment
   (to be provided or continued if my agent believes the burdens of the treatment
   (outweigh the expected benefits. I want my agent to consider the relief of
   (suffering the expense involved and the quality as well as the possible extension
_____(of my life in making decisions concerning life-sustaining treatment.

   (I want my life to be prolonged and I want life-sustaining treatment to be
   (provided or continued unless I am in a coma which my attending physician
   (believes to be irreversible, in accordance with reasonable medical standards at
   (the time of reference. If and when I have suffered irreversible coma, I want
_____(life-sustaining treatment to be withheld or discontinued.

   (I want my life to be prolonged to the greatest extent possible without regard to
_____(my condition, the chances I have for recovery or the cost of the procedures.

   3. This power of attorney shall become effective on _____

Figure 7–3. An example of a durable power of attorney for health care.

the client to specifically elaborate on vague phrases, like "do everything" or "when my time comes, let me go." The health care professional helps the client to document these directives in written form when possible. In addition, the nurse should document the conversation in the medical record (Fig. 7–4). All health care professionals should refer to agency policies and procedures about the use of verbal advance directives for guiding clinical ethical decision-making.

Euthanasia

Euthanasia means "good death" (Bandman & Bandman, 1995, p. 308). Although this concept is an ethical issue,

in the United States it is dealt with more from a legal perspective. Chapter 12 includes a complete discussion on euthanasia.

Placebo Administration

A placebo is an inert substance or benign action intentionally administered as a treatment, usually as a modality for pain relief. For instance, a client may receive a normal saline injection for a complaint of pain. When prescribing a placebo, the physician is intentionally attempting to deceive the client and thus is limiting the client's autonomy. When clients are deceived, they are unable to make

4. This power of attorney shall terminate on _____

_____

5. If any agent named by me shall die, become legally disabled, resign, refuse to act or be unavailable, I name the following (each to act alone and successively, in the order named) as successors to such agent:

_____

_____

6. If a guardian of my person is to be appointed, I nominate the following to serve as such guardian (if same as agent, leave blank):

_____

7. I am fully informed as to all the contents of this form and understand the full import of this grant of power to my agent.

Signed _____

Principal

The principal has had an opportunity to read the above form and has signed the form or acknowledged his or her signature or mark on the form in my presence.

_____ Residing at _____

Witness

(You may, but are not required to, request your agent and successor agents to provide specimen signature below. If you include specimen signature in this Power of Attorney, you must complete the certification opposite the signatures of the agents.)

Specimen signatures of agent   I certify that the signature of my agent
(and successors)   (and successors) are correct.

_____   _____
(agent)   (principal)

_____   _____
(successor agent)   (principal)

_____   _____
(successor agent)   (principal)

Figure 7–3. *Continued*

informed decisions. In addition, the use of placebos denies that the client is experiencing pain and jeopardizes client trust in both the physician's and nurse's motives. When clients seek health care assistance, they are assuming that health care professionals will act in their best interest; thus, the use of a placebo threatens this assumption (Elander, 1991).

When a nurse cannot ethically implement a placebo order, he or she is obligated to explain this position to the physician. If the physician continues the placebo order after this discussion, the nurse is obligated to work toward a resolution of this ethical issue by seeking ethics consultation. When a nurse cannot follow a physician's

order, the nurse must follow the health care agency's policy and lines of nursing authority precisely while documenting each communication. Fox (1994) described the arduous but satisfying task of getting the policy on use of placebos changed in one health care agency.

Many nurses have no moral opposition to using placebos if a client expresses pain relief after receiving the placebo. Often, clients do experience increased comfort because of personal attention and associated nursing interventions, such as repositioning or relaxation techniques, provided with the placebo (Beauchamp & Childress, 1994; Elander, 1991).

When administering a placebo, the nurse has a basic

Nursing Focus Note

5/1/97   12 noon   Focus: HIV with lymphadenopathy

D: C/O cheek and neck swelling. R=20 and easy. Denies dysphagia.

A: Initiated discussion regarding use of emergency treatment for respiratory distress or arrest. Instructed on purpose and use of advance directives. Dr. Jones notified of swelling.

R: Stated: "I won't live much longer...I want all the usual emergency treatments...I wouldn't want a machine continued if there was no hope that I'd get better. I'm not sure if my Mom could actually carry out this request. I'll talk to her this afternoon."

A: Client discussed wishes with mother.

R: Durable Power for Attorney completed with mother as agent.

A: Dr. Jones notified of DPOA. Is a full code. *Marcia Bosek, RN*

Nursing Narrative Note

8 am	C/O neck swelling. Left cheek and entire neck obviously swollen. No C/O dysphagia. R = 20 and easy. Lungs clear bilaterally. *Marcia Bosek, RN*
8:30 am	Dr. Jones notified of cheek and neck swelling. *Marcia Bosek, RN*
10 am	Informed of O$_2$ saturation tests q shift, instructed to notify nurse of respiratory distress. Discussion initiated by RN regarding wishes about emergency treatment for respiratory arrest. Stated: "I won't live much longer. I want all the usual emergency treatments. I wouldn't want a machine continued if there was no hope that I'd get better. I'm not sure if my Mom could actually carry out this request. I'll talk to her this afternoon. "Provided with copy of DPOA and instructed on use. Verbalized understanding of process. *Marcia Bosek, RN*

Figure 7–4. Sample documentation of verbal directives.

obligation to prevent harm. The nurse needs to conduct a thorough client assessment before and after administering a placebo. When a client does not experience pain relief, the nurse must notify the physician and request other treatment options. With the patient's permission, alternating pain medication with a placebo as a trial to determine the extent of genuine pain is ethically acceptable.

Restraints

Restraints are interventions that limit a person's freedom to move. Restraints can be physical (e.g., vest, limb, or geri-chair with lap table in place) or chemical (e.g., haloperidol [Haldol, Periodol✦]). Because restraints limit movement, they also limit autonomy. Before deciding whether to restrain a client, the nurse needs to identify the desired outcome and consider the related risks and benefits of all possible options.

When planning client care, the nurse may desire a variety of outcomes, such as preventing harm to the client and to the other clients, and/or maintaining the client's autonomy. However, balancing these two outcomes may be difficult when a client's autonomy is compromised by an illness such as Alzheimer's disease. A client with Alzheimer's disease may be free from harm if he or she has a steady gait, yet wandering may cause harm to other clients. Therefore, on the basis of nonmaleficence (preventing harm to others), the nurse in a case such as this would be justified in limiting the client's autonomy by preventing the wandering (Reigle, 1994).

When using a restraint, nurses must always consider both the risks and benefits (Table 7–4) and use the least restrictive method possible (Robbins, 1986). For instance, a waist restraint is less restrictive than a vest restraint, and a vest restraint is less restrictive than limb restraints. Chemical restraints (drugs) are the most restrictive be-

TABLE 7–4

Potential Benefits and Risks of Physical Restraints

Potential benefits
- Prevention of falls, which might result in injury
- Protection from other accidents or injuries
- Allowing medical treatment to proceed without client interference
- Protection of other clients or staff from disturbances or physical harm
- Increased client feelings of safety and security

Potential risks
- Injury from falls
- Accidental death by strangulation
- Functional decline
- Skin abrasions or skin breakdown
- Biochemical, physiologic, and psychological sequelae of prolonged immobilization
- Cardiac arrest
- Reduced appetite and dehydration
- Disorganized behavior
- Emotional desolation
- Possible increased mortality

Reprinted with permission from Evans, L. K., & Strumpf, N. E. (1989). Tying down the elderly: A review of the literature on physical restraint. *Journal of the American Geriatrics Society, 37,* 65–74.

cause they affect the client's physical and mental abilities.

As always, a nurse follows both state statutes and the health care agency's policies and procedure when using restraints. A client's mental and physical condition is routinely re-evaluated and documented along with justification for continued use of restraints (also see Chapter 6). Restraints should be discontinued as soon as possible or when an alternate intervention has been implemented (Bosek, 1993). Miles and Meyers (1994) suggest a restraint reduction program that includes "reviewing medications, allowing for naps to prevent fatigue, social stimulation, using nonrestraining postural supports, treating pain or Parkinson's disease or other debilitating conditions, physical therapy, and providing a safe and enclosed area for ambulating or wandering" (p. 522).

Personal Rights

A right is a justifiable claim that all persons can make (Curtin & Flaherty, 1982). In the past, health care was acquired through bartering. However, in the late 20th century, health care has evolved into a business industry. When health care is a right, every citizen will be able to access health care services and society will have an obligation to provide health care.

In Canada and several other countries, health care is recognized as a right. National health care programs have been implemented to guarantee that every citizen has equal access to health care; however, not all treatments and procedures are available.

In the United States, many people believe that health care is a right, but no universal health care system exists at this time. At present, health care is available to those who can afford to pay, have insurance, or qualify for Medicare and Medicaid. Emergency care is available to the uninsured, but access to other forms of health care is limited. A growing segment of the U.S. population is uninsurable or unemployed or does not have access to insurance through an employer. There has been much debate about how to deal with this access issue. Many advocate a two-tiered system that would provide basic health care to all while allowing each person to purchase additional "high-tech" medical treatment. Others propose a universal, single-payer system emphasizing health promotion and disease prevention.

Obligation

If a person has a specific right to health care, that person also has an obligation to maintain and protect his or her health. Rights and their associated responsibilities are inherently in conflict with autonomy. Life insurance companies often compensate for high correlations between voluntary behavior and disease by charging higher premium rates to people who smoke, drink alcoholic beverages, or engage in high-risk activities, such as auto racing.

Confidentiality

Confidentiality is a major ethical issue. Confidentiality requires that a person can expect that personal information will be kept in confidence and not shared without consent (Winslade, 1995). Some information may be perceived as sensitive and thus should be shared only on a "need-to-know" basis. For example, release of genetic test results could have long-reaching consequences for job and insurance discrimination. Thus, nurses must be ever vigilant to protect client information from any person without expressed permission from the client (McLure, 1995).

The nursing codes of the American Nurses' Association and the Canadian Nurses Association require nurses to maintain client confidentiality. Too often, nurses and other health care professionals discuss client cases in elevators, cafeterias, and other public places. Although they do not intend to breach a client's confidentiality, others may overhear the conversations.

Cultural and Spiritual Practices

Values are critical in ethical issues and are shaped by many influences—family, experiences, culture, and spirituality. Health care decisions involve clarification of values and interpreting the meaning that a client places on illness (see Table 7–4). Clients often interpret the meaning of their illness through the tenets of their faith. For example, they may view illness as a punishment for wrongdoings or lack of faith and may refuse pain medication because of the belief that suffering leads to redemption.

How clients cope with illness is also affected by their faith. When addressing ethical issues, the nurse assesses the client's spirituality. Often clients are asked to list their religious preference when admitted to a health care agency, but religion is only a part of the broader concept of spirituality. A nurse discusses the client's spiritual needs to learn how the client relies on spirituality during major life changes. Often clients share thoughts and feelings with the nurse, who can help them clarify questions and fears to discuss with family, physician, or others.

At times, a conflict can occur between the medical treatment plan and a client's spiritual beliefs. For example, consider a client who is a Jehovah's Witness and has multiple trauma injuries that necessitate blood transfusions. This is an ethical issue because the client requires blood but his religion prohibits accepting a blood transfusion. Facing this conflict can be emotionally taxing for the client and health care team. Strategies for dealing with similar issues can be developed to prepare for future challenging clients. Nurses and health care providers may also need to consult the hospital chaplain or other religious leaders to understand spiritual practices. These resources may also help health care professionals to deal with the dissonance created when they must implement acts contrary to their own personal beliefs.

Tube Feeding

Certain conditions prevent clients from taking food and fluids orally. For example, a client may have had extensive treatment for cancer of the head and neck or may have a neurologic disorder, such as PVS or permanent unconsciousness. For clients who hope to recover and take oral feedings again, tube feedings are a temporary intervention to ensure adequate nutrition and hydration. The ethical issue occurs when recovery is unlikely and tube feeding becomes death-delaying instead of life-prolonging treatment. Controversy exists over whether tube feeding (nasogastric, gastrostomy, or jejunostomy) is considered a medical treatment or a basic need that must be met. The American Academy of Neurology views artificial nutrition and hydration as medical therapy that competent patients or surrogate decision makers may refuse (Bernat et al., 1996).

Ethical Debate

Some ethicists (Weir, 1989) argue that feeding, whether oral or tube, is a basic need, like oxygen, that must be met regardless of prognosis. One is obligated to feed the client if the client would die of starvation and dehydration rather than of the underlying disease or disorder. The exception is if the client's condition would actually worsen if feedings were given, as with pulmonary edema, aspiration pneumonia, or renal failure. Other ethicists believe that tube feedings are a medical procedure that can be withheld or withdrawn if no medical benefit (improvement or recovery) is foreseen. For clients in a PVS who will not regain consciousness, tube feedings maintain but do not alter their condition.

If the client has expressed wishes in the form of an advance directive stating that tube feedings should not be initiated if there is no hope of recovery, then tube feedings should not be started or they should be discontinued

on presentation of this advance directive. However, if a client has no advance directive, the decision to initiate and continue tube feedings becomes more difficult, as in the Cruzan case (*Cruzan v. Director, Missouri Department of Health,* 1990). Tube feedings may have been started before the prognosis was certain (a diagnosis of a PVS is usually made 1 to 6 months after an initial injury). Hodges and Tolle (1994) defend the use of quality of life (QOL), medical goals, and patient preferences as criteria to consider when making decisions regarding tube feedings in the elderly.

Nursing Dilemma

Nurses often express ethical discomfort in caring for clients in a PVS who are receiving tube feedings. Nurses may respect the right to life of such clients but also may question what purpose is being served by expending resources for those who probably will not benefit. Alternatively, nurses may believe that all clients deserve basic comfort measures—food, warmth, protection from harm—and may resist withdrawing feedings. Deeper issues of respect for life, spirituality, QOL, and allocation of resources are involved in the question of whether to use tube feedings (see the Research Applications for Nursing box).

Nurses must first examine their feelings and beliefs about tube feedings and then participate in a team conference that explores the benefits and burdens of this treatment for a particular client. Decisions on whether to tube feed rest with the client (by advance directive) or family and the physician with input from other health care professionals who know the client and family. Legal requirements may necessitate obtaining a court order to withdraw feedings. In some states, the living will statute specifically mandates that nutrition, hydration, and medication must be provided, although all other treatments may be discontinued.

In some states of the United States, laws exist that allow a family and health care team to make the decision to withhold or withdraw feedings without obtaining a court order, provided that specific steps are taken and documented in the medical record. When the nurse does not personally agree with the decision that is made, two courses can be pursued: (1) even if the nurse would not make the same decision, he or she should respect the client's autonomy and the process that produced this decision and believe that the best decision was made under these circumstances; or (2) if the nurse morally objects to this decision, he or she can state the objection and rationale to the nursing supervisor and request to be reassigned to another client if necessary.

Unethical Professional Conduct

In the American Nurses' Association Code for Nurses (1976; 1985), the third plank addresses the responsibility of nurses to uphold the highest standards and protect clients from health care professionals who engage in illegal, unethical, or incompetent practice. The *Code of Ethics for Nursing* by the Canadian Nurses Association (1991)

▷ Research Applications for Nursing

Level of Moral Certainty Influences View of Artificial Nutrition

Wurbach, M. W. (1996). Long-term care nurses' ethical convictions about tube feeding. Western Journal of Nursing Research, 18(1), 63–76.

Using a descriptive exploratory design, Wurbach interviewed 25 long-term care nurses about their experiences when artificial nutrition was withheld or withdrawn from elderly patients at the end of life. The interview data were analyzed, and five categories of moral conviction were identified from the interview data.

Moral conviction is the "willingness to act on strong beliefs, sometimes assuming risk to oneself personally or professionally" (p. 68). The nurses described experiencing absolute moral conviction (20%), strong moral conviction (16%), moderate moral conviction (48%), moral uncertainty with conviction (12%), and moral uncertainty (4%). Those nurses experiencing moral certainty described significant positive and negative experiences with artificial nutrition; however, the nurses experiencing moral uncertainty had little or no direct experiences with providing artificial nutrition. Morally certain nurses had a negative opinion regarding the use of artificial nutrition and took actions, such as education, to stop or prevent the use of artificial nutrition for elders in the last stage of life. In contrast, nurses with moral uncertainty rarely acted. Despite the level of moral certainty experienced, each nurse subject described making decisions on "gut feeling" rather than by a problem-solving approach.

Critique. The researcher investigated a frequently occurring yet little researched phenomenon. Actions were taken to ensure the trustworthiness of the data analysis, such as evaluation of the findings by subjects and process trail auditing by a second person. The convenience sampling method may have resulted in a skewed proportion of nurses with moral certainty participating because morally uncertain nurses may have been reluctant to discuss their uncertainty.

Possible Nursing Implications. The findings from this study appear to support Benner's (1984) theory described in *From Novice to Expert.* Nurses with practical experience with artificial nutrition described higher levels of moral certainty. Thus, nursing administrators and educators need to establish decision-making resources to facilitate the novice nurse's decision-making abilities regarding the withdrawing or withholding of artificial nutrition. Safeguards must also be in place to prevent nurses with high levels of moral certainty from using their beliefs to coerce clients or family members to refuse artificial nutrition. Further research is needed to describe whether the nurse's level of moral certainty changes when a written advance directive is present.

lists "Value VIII: Protecting Clients from Incompetence. Value: The nurse takes steps to ensure that the client receives competent and ethical care" (p. 15). In the health care system, however, it is not very easy to report another's unethical conduct ("whistleblowing") without suffering unpleasant and sometimes devastating consequences.

The nurse who observes or discovers an act that jeopardizes a client's safety (e.g., seeing a medication error or witnessing another health care professional verbally or physically abusing a client) has an obligation to take steps to protect the client. This includes notifying the physician if a medication error was made, verifying information as thoroughly as possible, and documenting each incident according to agency policy. Next, the nurse follows the lines of authority for reporting the incident. Some nurses may wish to discuss the incident with other professionals involved, advising them that an incident was discovered and giving them an opportunity to take corrective action or clarify their behavior. In the spirit of collegiality and peer review, nurses can assist each other in keeping the standards of practice of nursing at the highest level.

Some nurses, however, have found themselves in situations in which they are made a party to unethical practices and have been threatened with loss of their job or license and even bodily harm when they followed channels of communication (Witt, 1983). Nurses must realistically evaluate the consequences of their actions in whistleblowing. The American Nurses' Association published guidelines on reporting incompetent, unethical, or illegal practices (1994). To maintain the public's trust and to self-regulate, nurses must continue to monitor their practices and the practices of others.

Chart 7–1

Nursing Focus on the Elderly

Myths and Ethical Issues Related to Care of the Elderly

Myths

- The older the client, the less likely he or she is to be competent.
- Adult children have the right to know their parent's medical status or to make health care decisions for their parents.
- The elderly are more likely to have articulated their beliefs about death and life-sustaining treatment than are younger clients.
- When a client can no longer control his or her bodily functions, he or she is also unable to make informed decisions about health care.

Ethical Issues

- How should health care resources be allocated for the frail and terminally ill elderly?
- Should health care services be rationed by age?
- Should elderly clients be able to choose the time to die?
- Does society have an obligation to provide for the elderly?
- Should health care treatment decisions be influenced by the elderly client's ability to pay? by the type of payment (private insurance/Medicare/Medicaid)?
- What is "the best interest" standard for the elderly?
- What constitutes elder abuse?
- Do the elderly have clearly defined values because of life experiences?
- When is it appropriate to provide comfort care for the elderly, versus using all available technology?

OTHER ETHICAL ISSUES THAT MEDICAL-SURGICAL NURSES FACE

Some of the ethical issues that nurses in medical-surgical settings face have been described in this chapter, but many others also exist, especially in the care of the elderly (Chart 7–1). Other ethical issues that occur include

- Use of fetal tissue for Parkinson's disease treatment
- Allocation of organs for transplantation
- Mandatory direct observed therapy for tuberculosis or drug abuse treatment
- Health care professional whose judgment is impaired by alcohol, drugs, or lack of knowledge
- Confidentiality of computerized records
- Disclosure of the health care professional's human immunodeficiency virus (HIV) status to clients
- Mandatory genetic screening for insurance or employment
- Maintaining quality of care during downsizing
- Conflict between client advocacy and financial responsibility in managed care

Many of these issues are presented and discussed elsewhere in this text.

SELECTED BIBLIOGRAPHY

* American Nurses' Association. (1976, 1985). *The Code for Nurses with Interpretive Statements.* Kansas City, MO: Author.

American Nurses' Association. (1994). *Guidelines on reporting incompetent, unethical, or illegal practices.* Washington D. C.: American Nurses Publishing.

Bandman, E. L., & Bandman, B. (1995). *Nursing ethics through the life span* (3rd ed.). Norwalk, CT: Appleton-Lange.

* Beauchamp, T. L., & Childress, J. F. (1994). *Principles of biomedical ethics* (4th ed.). New York: Oxford University Press.

* Beauchamp, T. L., & Walters, L. (1982). *Contemporary issues in bioethics* (2nd ed.). Belmont, CA: Wadsworth.

* Benner, P. (1984). *From novice to expert: Excellence and power in clinical nursing practice.* Menlo Park, CA: Addison-Wesley.

Bernat, J. L., Goldstein, M. L., & Viste, K. M. (1996). The neurologist and the dying patient. *Neurology, 46,* 598–599.

* Bosek, M. S. D. (1993). Ethical issues with the use of restraints. *MEDSURG Nursing, 2*(2), 154–156.

* Bosek, M. S. D., & Fitzpatrick, J. (1992). A nursing perspective on advance directives. *MEDSURG Nursing, 1*(1), 33–38.

* Campbell, C. S. (1993). Gridlock on the Oregon Trail. *Hastings Center Report, 23*(4), 6–7.

*Canadian Nurses Association. (1991). *Code of ethics for nursing.* Ottawa: Author.

Clarke, D. E., Goldstein, M. K., & Raffin, T. A. (1994). Ethical dilemmas in the critically ill elderly. *Clinics in Geriatric Medicine, 10*(1), 91–101.

* Corley, M. C., & Selig, P. M. (1992). Nurse moral reasoning using the Nursing Dilemma Test. *Western Journal of Nursing Research, 14,* 380–388.

* Crisham, P. (1981). Decision analysis: A step by step guide for making clinical decisions. *Nursing & Health Care, 7,* 148–154.

* *Cruzan v. Director, Missouri Department of Health.* 110 S. Ct. 2841 (1990).

* Curtin, L., & Flaherty, M. J. (1982). *Nursing ethics: Theory and pragmatics.* Bowie, MD: Robert J. Brady.

* DeWolf, M. S. (1989a). *Clinical ethical decision-making: A grounded theory method.* Chicago: Rush University.

* DeWolf, M. S. (1989b). Ethical decision making. *Seminars in Oncology Nursing, 5*(2), 77–81.

* Elander, G. (1991). Ethical conflicts in placebo treatment. *Journal of Advanced Nursing, 16,* 947–951.

* Evans, L. K., & Strumpf, N. E. (1989). Tying down the elderly: A review of the literature on physical restraint. *Journal of the American Geriatric Society, 36,* 65–74.

* Ferrans, C. E., & Powers, M. J., (1985). Quality of life index: Development and psychometric properties. *Advances in Nursing Science, 8,* 15–24.

* Fowler, M. D. M., & Levine-Ariff, J. (1987). *Ethics at the bedside: A source book for the critical care nurse.* Philadelphia: J. B. Lippincott.

Fox, A. E. (1994). Confronting the use of placebos for pain. *American Journal of Nursing, 94*(9), 42–46.

* Fromer, M. J. (1981). *Ethical issues in health care.* St. Louis: C. V. Mosby.

Garcia, J. L. A. (1995). Double effect. In W. T. Reich (Ed.), *Encyclopedia of bioethics* (Rev. ed., Vol. 2, pp. 636–641). New York: Simon & Schuster Macmillan.

* Hadorn, D. C. (1991). The Oregon priority-setting exercise: Quality of life and public policy. *Hastings Center Report, 21*(3, Suppl), 11–16.

Hodges, M. O., & Tolle, S. W. (1994). Tube-feeding decisions in the elderly. *Clinics in Geriatric Medicine, 10*(3), 475–488.

Husted, G. L., & Husted, J. H. (1994). *Ethical decision making in nursing* (2nd ed). St. Louis: Mosby-Year Book.

Joint Commission on Accreditation of Healthcare Organizations. (1997–1998). *Comprehensive accreditation manual for home care.* Oakbrook Terrace, IL: Author.

Joint Commission on Accreditation of Healthcare Organizations. (1998). *Comprehensive accreditation manual for hospitals.* Oakbrook Terrace, IL: Author.

Joint Commission on Accreditation of Healthcare Organizations. (1998–1999a). *Comprehensive accreditation manual for ambulatory health care.* Oakbrook Terrace, IL: Author.

Joint Commission on Accreditation of Healthcare Organizations. (1998–1999b). *Comprehensive accreditation manual for long term care.* Oakbrook Terrace, IL: Author.

* Kilner, J. F. (1990). *Who lives? Who dies? Ethical criteria in patient selection.* New Haven: Yale University Press.

Langslow, A. (1995). "Not for CPR" orders: Current developments. *Australian Nursing Journal, 2*(10), 36–38.

McLure, H. (1995). The insurance industry's use of genetic information: Legal and ethical concerns. *Journal of Health and Hospital Law, 28*(4), 231–242.

Miles, S. H., & Meyers, R. (1994). Untying the elderly: 1989 to 1993 update. *Clinics in Geriatric Medicine, 10*(3), 513–525.

* Newell, A., & Simon, H. A. (1972). *Human problem solving.* Englewood Cliffs, NJ: Prentice-Hall.

Parkman, C. A., & Carfee, B. E. (1997). Advance directives: Honoring your patient's end-of-life wishes. *Nursing '97, 27*(4), 48–53.

Pinch, W. J. E. (1996). Feminism and bioethics. *MEDSURG Nursing, 5*(1), 53–56.

* Ratzan, R. M. (1987). The use of physical force. *Postgraduate Medicine, 81*(1), 125, 128.

Reigle, J. (1994). HealthCare Ethics Forum '94: Ethical challenges in the critically ill: Use of restraints. *AACN Clinical Issues, 5*(3), 329–332.

Rhodes, R. (1994). An alternate opinion: Do-not-resuscitate orders in the operating room. *Mount Sinai Journal of Medicine, 61*(6), 498–499.

* Robbins, L. J. (1986). Restraining the elderly patient. *Clinics in Geriatric Medicine, 2*(3), 591–597.

Rosner, F., Bennett, A. J., & Sechzer, P. H. (1994). Do-not-resuscitate orders in the operating room. *Mount Sinai Journal of Medicine, 61*(6), 493–496.

*Rushton, C. H., & Lynch, M. E. (1992, June). Dealing with advance directives for critically ill adolescents. *Critical Care Nurses,* 31–37.

Savage, T. (1994). The nurse's role on ethics committees and as an ethics consultant. *Seminars for Nurse Managers, 2*(1), 41–47.

*Shelly, J. A. (1980). *Dilemma.* Downers Grove, IL: InterVarsity Press.

*Simon, H. A. (1978). Information-processing theory of human problem solving. In W. K. Estes (Ed.). *Handbook of learning and cognitive processes* (Vol. 5, pp. 271–295). Hillsdale, NJ: Lawrence Erlbaum Associates.

*Steele, S. M., & Harmon, V. M. (1983). *Values clarification in nursing* (2nd ed.). Norwalk, CT: Appleton-Century-Crofts.

*Thompson, J., & Thompson, H. O. (1985). *Bioethical decision-making for nurses.* Norwalk, CT: Appleton-Century-Crofts.

*Veatch, R. M. (1980). Voluntary risks to health. *Journal of the American Medical Association, 243*(1), 50–55.

*Weir, R. F. (1989). *Abating Treatment with Critically Ill Patients: Medical* *and Legal Limits to the Medical Prolongation.* New York: Oxford University Press.

*Wicclair, M. R. (1991). Differentiating ethical decisions from clinical standards. *Dimensions of critical care nursing, 10*(5), 280–288.

Winslade, W. (1995). Confidentiality. In W. T. Reich (Ed.) *Encyclopedia of bioethics* (Rev. ed., Vol. 1, pp. 451–459). New York: Simon & Shuster MacMillan.

*Witt, P. (1983). Notes of a whistleblower. *American Journal of Nursing, 83,* 1649–1651.

Wurbach, M. E. (1996). Long-term care nurses' ethical convictions about tube feedings. *Western Journal of Nursing Research, 18*(1), 63–76.

SUGGESTED READINGS

Bandman, E. L., & Bandman, B. (1995). *Nursing ethics through the life span* (3rd ed.). Norwalk, CT: Appleton-Lange.

Individual chapters are devoted to the various stages in the life span. In each of these chapters, the authors present selected cases with related ethical principles and identify nursing judgments and actions. Traditional and contemporary theories of ethical decision-making and the pitfalls that can occur in moral reasoning are also discussed.

Keffer, M. J. (1996). Nurse advocate: Advocate for whom? *MEDSURG Nursing, 5*(2), 125–126.

Nurses are taught to be patient advocates; however, this advocacy role can be undermined by agency policy or politics. Three categories of influence (persuasion, manipulation, and coercion) are described. Policies should be evaluated to identify potential situations in which the nurse may be coerced to place agency issues before the patient's best interests. Nurses need to be involved in creating and revising policies that keep the patient's interests as top priority.

STRESS, COPING, AND ADAPTATION

When laypeople speak of stress, they may say that it is an actual feeling of being overwhelmed. To others, stress is the cause of this feeling. In the social sciences, including nursing, the concept of stress has evolved to include both the feeling and the event.

OVERVIEW
Definitions
Stress

Stress is a relationship between a person and the environment that the person perceives as taxing or dangerous (Lazarus & Folkman, 1984). The cognitive evaluation, or thought process, through which a person determines that an event is stressful is called an "appraisal" of stress. A *stressor* is the taxing or dangerous physical, psychological, social, or environmental event that leads to the appraisal of stress. Following are some examples of stressors:

- *Physiologic:* Injuries; infectious, viral, or fungal agents; radiation; drugs; and alcohol
- *Psychological:* Frustrations, loss of control, and anger
- *Social:* Losses of social support, problems in living arrangements, and the difficulties associated with low economic status
- *Environmental:* Pollution, the hazards of the workplace, and extremes of temperature

Coping

To deal with stress effectively, people try to cope by using specific strategies. Coping strategies are the ways by which people try to control the causative problem or stress-related feelings. Some examples of coping strategies are denial, use of social supports, confrontation of the problem, and consideration of the positive aspects of the situation. These strategies are described later in this chapter.

Adaptation

Adaptation occurs when a person has mastered, changed, or accepted the stressful event. Adaptation implies that a sense of equilibrium is restored to the person disordered by stress. Adaptation is reflected in one or more changes in a person's psychological, social, or physical health.

THE IMPORTANCE OF STRESS IN MEDICAL-SURGICAL NURSING PRACTICE

Stress is particularly important in the practice of medical-surgical nursing for adults because its presence may cause, prolong, or aggravate a client's illness. Stress can interfere with other aspects of clients' lives because it may contribute to family, spiritual, and social crises.

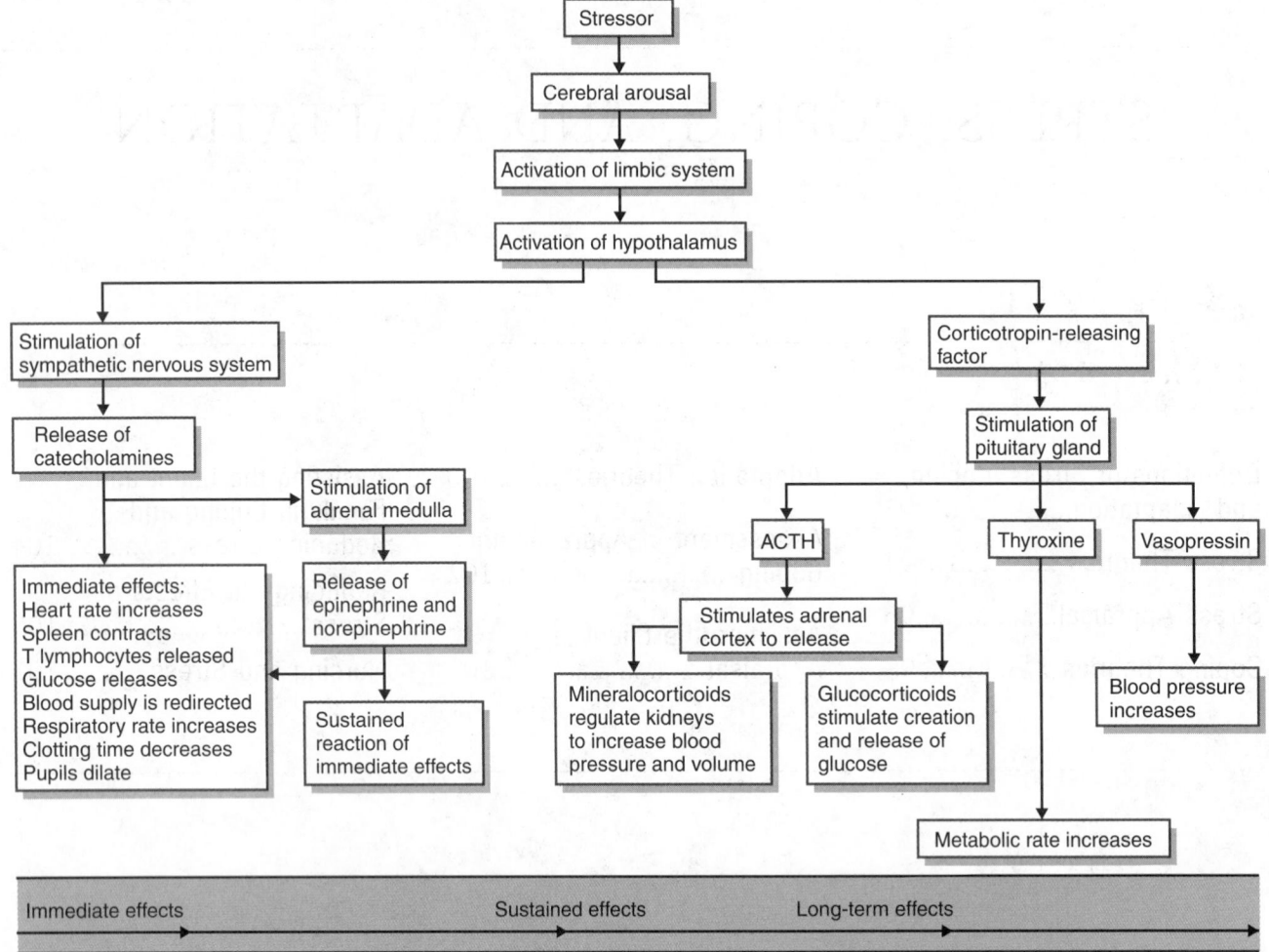

Figure 8–1. The general adaptation syndrome.

Clients use a variety of strategies to deal with stress. Nurses are commonly in positions in which they can aid the clients' coping, either through assisting the clients' self-initiated efforts or by suggesting alternatives. Successful coping and adaptation are the goals of both the client and the nurse. All clients want stress to be reduced to manageable levels or eliminated.

Theories About Stress

Stress has been studied from three major viewpoints. First, researchers have viewed stress as the body's physical response to threat. Second, stress has been considered to be a stimulus, or outside force, that causes a reaction. Third, stress has been examined as a transaction between the person and the event.

Stress as a Response

The biological and medical sciences have traditionally viewed stress as the body's response to an event; that is, stress is the physiologic response or change that occurs within the body. The idea of stress as a response gained prominence through the classic work of Hans Selye, who defined stress as "the nonspecific response of the body to any demand made upon it to adapt, whether that demand produces pain or pleasure" (1946, p. 230).

From Selye's definition, three phenomena are immediately apparent. First, Selye thought that the body's response to stress is nonspecific: The body reacts as a whole organism. Second, stress is considered a physiologic response, not a psychological one. Third, Selye believed that it is not just the "bad" things in life that cause stress but the "good" things as well. From Selye's viewpoint, a wedding can cause the same physiologic response as a funeral. Selye called the body's generalized response to a stressor the *general adaptation syndrome* (GAS) (Fig. 8–1). This syndrome has three distinct stages:

1. The alarm stage
2. The stage of resistance
3. The stage of exhaustion

In addition to recognizing the body's *generalized* response, Selye noted a *localized* response. He labeled the body's limited, localized response as the *localized adaptation syndrome* (LAS). Inflammation at a surgical site is an example of the LAS.

THE ALARM STAGE. The physiologic response to a stressor begins with the alarm stage, in which the body prepares itself for survival. Cannon (1931) called this initial physiologic response the "fight-or-flight response." As outlined by Cannon, this response process prepares all animals, including humans, for survival. When faced with danger, the body prepares to either fight the danger or flee from it. Either reaction is thought to cause the same changes in the body.

The stress-related changes are coordinated by the central nervous system (CNS). Within the CNS, the limbic system is the emotional response center that triggers the fight-or-flight response. The limbic system then activates the hypothalamus. The hypothalamus in turn initiates the stress response and directs the activities of the autonomic nervous system (ANS), composed of the sympathetic and parasympathetic systems. The ANS controls the body's involuntary responses, such as hormone secretions, metabolism, and fluid regulation.

The sympathetic system of the ANS is responsible for dynamic change, and the parasympathetic system is responsible for restoring the body to its normal resting state. In response to stress, the sympathetic nervous system stimulates the adrenal medulla, which in turn secretes the catecholamines norepinephrine and epinephrine. The adrenal cortex is also stimulated by the pituitary gland's release of adrenocorticotropic hormone (ACTH). The circulating ACTH causes the adrenal cortex to release glucocorticoids (cortisol, corticosterone, and cortisone) and mineralocorticoids (aldosterone and deoxycorticosterone). As a result of the CNS and adrenal activity, seven major changes occur within the body:

- *Increase in heart rate,* to ensure that adequate oxygen and nutrients are available to the muscles and organs
- *Contraction of the spleen,* to reduce the amount of blood lost from the spleen in case of injury and to release T lymphocytes into the bloodstream for defense
- *Release of glucose,* to fuel the body for response to danger
- *Redirection of blood supply,* to ensure blood flow to the vital organs, such as the brain
- *Changes in the respiratory system* (increased respiratory rate and depth), to provide for effective oxygen–carbon dioxide exchange
- *Decrease in blood clotting time,* to decrease blood loss in case of body injury
- *Dilation of pupils,* to enhance vision

These major changes, plus minor changes, such as increased perspiration and piloerection (hairs standing on end), appear to occur whenever a person is threatened. Selye called these collective processes the alarm stage in the body's preparation for survival. Although these preparations may have been useful to human beings in the past, they have limited utility in most of today's threat situations. It is unfortunate that these reactions persist, because they result in tremendous wear and tear on the body. If these reactions occur frequently or are sustained, a person may experience damage to the body's systems or illness, such as heart disease and diabetes mellitus.

THE STAGE OF RESISTANCE. The second stage in the GAS is called the stage of resistance. When the body recognizes continued threat, physiologic forces are mobilized to maintain an increased resistance to stressors. This resistance begins with a decrease in the production of ACTH. The body concentrates its activities on those organs or organ systems that are most involved in the specific stress response. Successful adaptation implies positive growth toward a return to or improvement in physical health. The efforts of the body to resist stress may be ineffectual, leading to a state of maladaptation in which deterioration occurs in levels of physical functioning. Chronic resistance eventually causes damage to the involved systems.

THE STAGE OF EXHAUSTION. The body enters the stage of exhaustion when organs or organ systems show evidence of deterioration. Selye determined that the overwhelmed body exhibits a triad of symptoms: hypertrophy of the adrenal glands, ulcerations in the gastrointestinal tract, and atrophy of the thymus gland. In this final stage, all energy for adaptation has been used, ACTH secretion increases, and a more generalized response is seen once again. This third stage can also result in what health care professionals call the diseases of adaptation, or stress-related diseases, and even death. Conditions and diseases in Table 8–1 represent examples thought to be related to or worsened by stress.

Stress as a Stimulus

Realizing that people do not react to all stressors as threats, theorists and researchers began to explore the stress associated with a stimulus. In the stimulus theory,

TABLE 8–1

Conditions and Diseases Thought to Be Stress-Related
• Cancer
• Hypertension
• Myocardial infarction
• Cerebrovascular accident
• Peripheral vascular disease
• Asthma
• Tuberculosis
• Emphysema
• Gastrointestinal ulcers
• Irritable bowel syndrome
• Sexual dysfunctions
• Obesity
• Anorexia nervosa
• Bulimia nervosa
• Connective tissue disease
• Ulcerative colitis
• Crohn's disease
• Infections
• Allergic and hypersensitivity diseases

stress is seen as the event itself, or the stressor, not as the response to the event.

With the advent of the stimulus concept of stress, research efforts were directed toward determining which life events were stressful and how stressful they were. Scales were developed by researchers, such as Holmes and Rahe (1967), to quantify the stress associated with different life events. These stress scales listed events such as death, divorce, and monetary and health concerns. Each event was assigned a score that reflected its relative stressfulness. The idea behind the scales was that the accumulation of a certain number of "stress points" would result in a reaction, such as illness. Despite the popularity of these scales in both the scientific and the lay literature, they have not proved to be valid as predictors of stress, especially in relation to illness. No research has been able to show more than a limited predictive relation between stressful life events and illness, hospitalization, and mortality.

Although the usefulness of stress scales has not proved valid, common sense indicates that certain events can and do provoke physiologic manifestations and feelings of stress. It seems, however, that the events that provoke stress symptoms may not always be life's major events but, rather, the minor annoyances of everyday life. These daily stresses, or "hassles," have shown more relation to illness than have the major life events (DeLongis et al., 1982). Within the hospital setting, there are many potential hassles that can increase stress. Table 8–2 presents examples of environmental and psychological hassles common to hospitalization and illness.

Stress as a Transaction Between a Person and the Environment

Gradually, nurse researchers and others have come to realize that all events have different meanings for different

TABLE 8–2

Potential Stressors Common to Hospitalization and Illness

- Eating different foods at different times
- Having a stranger for a roommate
- Sleeping in a different bed
- Using a different pillow
- Being awakened at odd hours
- Feeling too hot or too cold
- Smelling hospital odors
- Hearing strange hospital noises
- Having movement restricted
- Being unable to obtain desired objects
- Having too many, no, or few visitors
- Worrying about bills, job, or family concerns
- Being uncertain of one's diagnosis
- Not understanding medical language
- Being dependent on others for bathing or toileting
- Being embarrassed about revealing body parts or intimate details
- Having to deal with large numbers of health care workers

people. The perception of stress appears to be related to the person and event within a certain environment. The view of stress as a relation between the person and the environmental event is called the *transactional model of stress* (Lazarus & Folkman, 1984).

In this model, people are more than passive recipients of stress and are not merely unthinking reactors to the events around them. The person's interpretation of the event is important to consider, and the meaning given to the event by the person determines the perception of stress. Stress occurs only when a person appraises a situation as stressful.

In the transactional model of stress, there are few universal stressors because of the differences in individual appraisal. *Appraisal* is the cognitive evaluation of events (primary appraisal) and available coping resources (secondary appraisal). No event can be considered inherently stressful—not even tornadoes, hurricanes, and other disasters that are generally thought of as stressful. The transactional model states that there is no way of predicting how a person will respond to events. Although some people experience a stress reaction to these major events, many others do not. These differences are a result of individual appraisal.

Several factors contribute to a person's perception that an event is stressful. These include factors specific to the person, the environment, or the event itself. Effective nursing care must include an understanding of the many factors that enter into a client's decision that an event is stressful.

Appraisal Factors Related to the Person
Depth of Feeling

One important factor in an appraisal of stress is the depth of feeling that the event arouses in a person. Events about which people feel strongly are more likely to produce stress than events that arouse little or no feeling. For example, if hospitalization interferes with an important life event, such as marriage, the client's appraisal of hospitalization may result in a perception of stress.

Beliefs

Along with commitments, beliefs also influence the appraisal of stress. For example, a person with a strongly held religious belief that God can influence the course of life's events may appraise events differently from someone with other spiritual beliefs.

Control

Control is also important to the stress-coping response. Many researchers have reported that most people want to maintain a sense of control over their world. For that reason, not having control can be appraised as a stressor. The key to understanding control is the recognition that control means different things to different people and in different situations. Although it is obvious that ill or hospitalized clients cannot control situations such as the course of illness, research has identified a list of areas in which most people seek control even when they are sick (Moos & Tsu, 1977). These areas include

- Avoidance of pain and incapacitation
- The immediate hospital environment
- Treatments and procedures
- Relationships with hospital personnel
- Emotional balance
- A satisfactory self-image
- Relationships with family and friends
- Preparing for an uncertain future

This list is important for three reasons. First, it alerts nurses to the fact that people may seek control over most aspects of their lives, whether they are ill or not. Second, the loss of a sense of control, which is stressful to many people, can occur because of the nature of the hospital environment. Third, some people do not want active control. People who do not desire control may experience stress when they are given control. Nurses should ascertain how much control clients want before insisting or recommending that they take control.

Environmental Event Factors Related to Stress Appraisal

Differences in the appraisal of environmental event factors influence whether a person perceives an event as stressful.

Unpredictability of Events

One factor that can make a difference in the appraisal of events is their unpredictability. People generally believe that a predictable event is less stressful than a similar unpredictable event. This is partly because with time, people can prepare. Being able to prepare for events appears to be related to a reduction in stress. Without the necessary time or information needed for preparation, events may appear more stressful than they need to be. If possible, the nurse should give a client sufficient information and time to comprehend a potentially stressful event, such as an uncomfortable procedure, before he or she experiences it.

Uncertainty of Events

The client's uncertainty about an event can also increase its potential stressfulness. It appears that most people like to know what to expect. Although this is true of life events in general, people especially like to know the odds about health-related events. The key to understanding much of the stress experienced by clients with chronic disease may lie in their uncertainty about the disease course. Not knowing how a disease will evolve or the chances of recovery can be very stressful. For example, clients with cancer often experience such uncertainty. Despite such treatments as extensive surgery, chemotherapy, and radiation, many clients with cancer can never be

completely sure of a cure. Thus, the uncertainty of the event enhances its appraisal as stressful.

Timing of Events

The timing of events also has an impact on the level of stress. Events that are considered to be in the distant future are usually perceived as less stressful than events that are closer in time. The time that elapses between the client's hearing about an event and its occurrence can also influence appraisal. Although the stress may be manageable for a period of time, the longer a person is kept waiting, the harder it is to control the thoughts about what is to come. Thus, the appraisal of threat can build up when too much time elapses. People need sufficient time to prepare for events. However, too long a period of anticipation can have a negative effect. Unfortunately, there are no set guidelines as to timing for nurses who prepare clients for tests and procedures.

The timing of an event in relation to one's stage of life is also important. Having a heart attack at age 25 may be more stressful than at age 80. Any life event that occurs at an unexpected time can be more stressful than one occurring at a time of life when it is expected.

Duration of Events

Another factor related to timing is the duration of events. Chronic, long-term events can sometimes wear down a person's ability to cope. As in Selye's stage of exhaustion, constant demands over a long time can have massive psychological as well as physical effects. However, people can also become accustomed to long-term events. The difference between the two reactions may lie in a person's appraisal or in the coping strategies used.

Ambiguity of Events

Knowing what will happen, when it will happen, and how long it will last is important in the appraisal of stress. Yet, even with this information, unknown elements of an event always are present and contribute to the ambiguity, or vagueness, of the experience. Ambiguity is important to appraisal. Generally, the more vague a situation, the more stressful. Ambiguity can also influence what coping strategies are used. People usually choose their coping strategies on the basis of the information that they have. If information is missing, however, the planning of specific and appropriate coping strategies is not possible.

According to Lazarus and Folkman's theory (1984), the effectiveness of coping mechanisms depends on the accuracy of the appraisal of a stressful situation. Because people may not correctly appraise a situation and because no one can predict the future, misappraisals cannot be avoided—they are part of life. It is the degree of difference between the appraisal of what will happen and the reality of what occurs that makes a difference in coping effectiveness. Because situations are constantly changing, coping effectiveness also depends on the person's ability to reappraise and change strategies as necessary (Fig. 8–2).

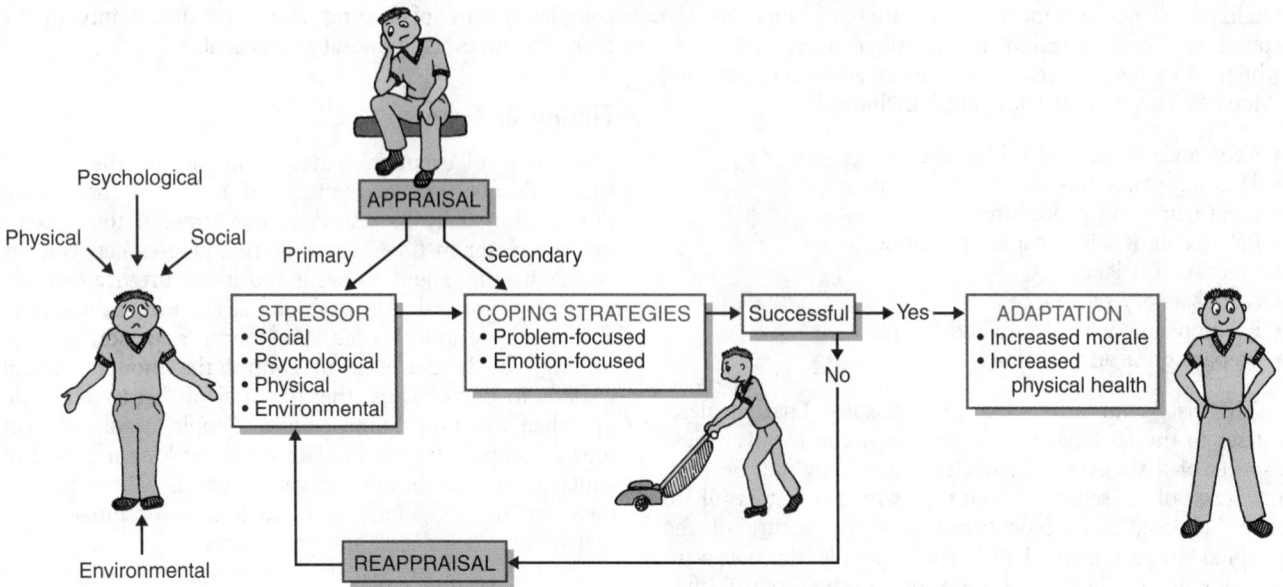

Figure 8–2. Appraisal and coping mechanisms.

THEORIES ABOUT COPING

Coping is any behavioral or cognitive activity that is used to deal with stress. If an event is perceived as taxing or dangerous, coping should occur. The concept of coping implies that most people do not remain passive and allow events to happen; rather, they react. The reactions to a stress-provoking event can be either to use the problem-solving approach to change the event (problem-focused coping) or to change emotional reactions to the event (emotion-focused coping). Coping strategies vary from person to person and event to event. It is thought that people generally use coping strategies that they have found successful in the past. If a strategy is not successful in the current situation, others may be considered.

Problem-Focused Coping
Problem-Solving

In many cases, the best way to deal with a causative stressor is to try to change or eliminate the problem. A major coping strategy is problem-solving.

Problem-solving as a coping strategy involves the same skills that are used in the nursing process. In problem-solving coping, a person defines the problem, lists alternatives, chooses the best alternative, and applies it to the problem. When asked about problem-solving coping, people may state that they try to find out more about the problem at hand, analyze the problem, make a plan, and follow it.

Some problem-solving activity is also directed inward. In this case, the coping activity is directed at how the problem is faced. Inward-focused problem-solving solutions might include learning new skills, changing aspirations, or finding other avenues of personal reward.

When people use problem-solving, they need accurate information and accurate appraisal so that their plans to deal with the stressor are based on reality. Nurses can ask clients if they have made any plans, on what the plans are based, and what is involved in these plans. When plans are unrealistic, the nurse helps the client by sharing his or her expertise and information.

Confrontive Coping

Many people cope by confronting the problem that is causing the stress. Confrontive coping is often used successfully in dealing with life's problems, such as those in the workplace. In addition, confrontive coping may be used when less forceful coping strategies have failed to alleviate the perception of stress. Clients in health care situations may use confrontive coping by aggressively seeking information, refusing treatments, and expressing their anger. Many times anger is the primary indicator that the client feels stressed and is attempting to cope. However, not all confrontive-type coping activities reflect aggression; sometimes the expressions of anger in confrontive coping reflect feelings of anxiety and powerlessness in the client.

Although these two problem-focused coping strategies are commonly used, they are not the only ways to cope. Nurses who are interested in supporting the client should find out how the client has coped in the past, how he or she plans to cope with the new stresses, and how other clients with the same problem have coped.

Emotion-Focused Coping

Some people are more skilled at problem-solving than others, and some problems are easier to resolve than others. When problem-focused strategies are not appropriate or are not sufficient, emotion-focused strategies are used. In some cases, a person may use both problem-focused and emotion-focused coping. Emotion-focused strategies reduce the emotional manifestations of stress, such as anxiety and anger.

Distancing Strategies

A vast array of distancing strategies are frequently used for coping in health-related situations. Some people deny a problem or blame others, and some people accept responsibility for their contribution to the occurrence of stress—they appear to be seeking a sense of control over life events. The refusal of a person who has had a motor vehicle accident while drinking alcohol to accept some blame is an example of distancing.

Drawing Strength from Adversity

A related coping strategy is drawing strength from adversity by growing as a person, finding new faith, and rediscovering what is important in life. At other times, strategies that emphasize the positive aspects of an event can be effective. Trying to have a positive outlook, looking on the bright side, and telling oneself that things could be worse are examples of this form of coping.

Tension Reduction

Coping strategies aimed at tension reduction can also be used to deal with stress. Some healthy means of reducing tension may include meditation, yoga exercises, biofeedback, and physical exercise. Other ways of coping, although not healthy, are to reduce tension through the use of alcohol or other so-called recreational drugs. Eating modifications, such as overeating or undereating, can also be used as inappropriate attempts to cope.

Hostility Versus Humor

Hostility, reflected through anger, irritability, childish reactions, or demonstration of temper, may reflect coping activity in some clients. A more positive expression of feelings that can reflect coping is humor. Humor is a commonly used coping activity (Weinberger, 1991). Many clients tell jokes or make light of serious situations when they are under stress.

Fatalism

Even fatalism can be used as a coping strategy. When using fatalism, clients say they will take a wait-and-see attitude, leave it in God's hands, or accept what has happened to them. Fatalism is usually accompanied by a sense that there is nothing that can be done about the problem.

Social Support

Social support by family, friends, and the community often can be a powerful aid in coping and can be extremely important to those in need of health care. By seeking support from others, people can gain information, physical help, and other forms of assistance. Both the type of help and the number of people willing to help can make a difference in the client's coping success.

Hospital rules and regulations often interfere with a client's ability to obtain the social support he or she needs. The interference with support can be especially acute within ethnic groups with large, close, and supportive families, such as in the Hispanic culture. Loss of social support can result when hospitalization occurs at a physical distance from the client's family, when elderly clients have outlived friends and relatives, or when the client has a socially stigmatizing illness, such as acquired immunodeficiency syndrome (AIDS). The inability to use a coping strategy on which one had previously depended, such as social support, can result in further stress.

Faith

Faith in God, a deity, or an ultimate meaning of life can be an effective aid to coping. For people who have a strong faith, the attitude of relinquishing control to God or believing in transcendence can be beneficial. Prayer, increased religious activity, and even a calm acceptance of God's will or an ultimate purpose are all forms of coping when they help reduce the perception of stress.

Event Rehearsal

If time allows, coping often begins before the stress event occurs, through event rehearsal. Event rehearsal involves mental or physical preparation in anticipation of an event or the practice of coping strategies before the event occurs. For example, clients who are to undergo elective surgery begin to plan their coping strategies before the actual surgery occurs. If time allows before a potentially stressful event, clients may mentally envision how they will react or handle the situation. Some authors have called this preparatory coping the "work of worrying" (Janis, 1985). However, that phrase implies that clients are concerned with only the negative aspects of an upcoming experience and ignores the fact that clients may focus on the positive aspects as well.

Event Review

After a stressful event, many people cope by reviewing the event. This review can be mental, verbal, or both. Event review probably helps people to cope by giving them the opportunity to understand what has happened to them. Often, there is no time during a stress event to process the incoming information. Review after an event occurs when there is time and energy available for processing. Nurses aid coping through review by encouraging clients to think or talk about their experiences.

People cope with the same problem in a variety of ways. Most nurses agree that coping in the hospital setting can be successfully accomplished through any one of a number of avenues. Common coping strategies are presented in Table 8–3.

TABLE 8–3

Common Coping Strategies	
Coping Strategy	**Examples**
Event rehearsal	• Mental and verbal preparation • Practice of coping strategies
Confrontation	• Aggressive information-seeking • Anger • Refusal of treatments
Distancing or denial	• Unwillingness or inability to talk about events • Going on as if nothing has happened
Self-control	• Stoicism • Showing no feelings
Social support	• Seeking out family, friends, or others in similar situations
Accepting responsibility	• Verbally placing responsibility for a situation on oneself
Faith	• Praying • Reading religious material • Seeking out clergy or religious guidance
Problem-solving	• Making plans • Verbally outlining what to do next
Positive reappraisal	• Speaking of how the situation has fostered growth
Event review	• Discussing situations or coping that has occurred

THEORIES ABOUT ADAPTATION

If a client has coped effectively, the stress or the emotional reaction to stress is eliminated or managed and a sense of equilibrium is restored. Restored equilibrium that results from coping is called adaptation. Some nurse theorists, such as Roy and Roberts (1981), have incorporated the concept of adaptation into their theory or model of nursing practice.

Adaptation is dependent on accurate appraisal of a stressful situation and effective coping. Adaptation can have many outcomes. The two results with the most significance to nursing are psychological and physical well-being.

Psychological Adaptation: Morale

People who cope adequately, it is hoped, will be satisfied with how they coped and the outcome reached. If a client believes that the correct decision was made with regard to health care issues, such as agreeing to hospitalization, choosing medical professionals, or handling pain or discomfort, the challenge of the stress has been met and coping is viewed as effective. The ability to see stress as a challenge to be overcome is important to the long-term maintenance of morale.

Morale is related to emotional equilibrium and the sense of well-being. In the past, many researchers considered well-being as the absence of depression or other signs of poor psychological health. More recently, the approach has changed: well-being is assessed through positive indicators, such as happiness and contentment. Healthy psychological adaptation is reflected in the client's sense of well-being.

Physical Adaptation: Somatic Health

Stress is consistently blamed for causing all illness and unhappiness. Diseases in which it can be determined that the mind influences the body's processes are called *psychophysiologic* (previously called psychosomatic). Stress is thought to be a major factor in psychophysiologic disease. Interestingly, the link between stress and illness is far from clear. Some evidence indicates that stress may suppress the effectiveness of the immune system and thus predispose a person to infection, cancer, and other diseases thought to be related to the immune system (see Table 8–1). Stress may also weaken the body so that any pathogens or toxic agents are more damaging than they would otherwise be. Other evidence indicates that stress may precipitate damage so that it occurs at a faster rate than normal, such as in cardiovascular disease.

At one time, it was hoped that a direct link could be found either between the stress event and illness or between personality type and illness. At that time, it was not uncommon to hear professionals speak of a colitis, ulcer, or arthritis personality. However, none of these theories has held up under study. No research has been able to show a strong relationship among incidence of illness, personality type, and stress.

The Concept of Hardiness

Research into the relationship between illness and personality characteristics is currently focused on hardiness, which is the ability to resist the effects of stress. The attribute of hardiness may be one reason why some people are negatively affected by exposure to stress and others are not. Hardiness is related to three personality characteristics:

■ Hardy people have a sense of *commitment* to work, a way of life, or ideals that provides them with a sense of satisfaction, motivation, and possibly achievement.
■ Hardy people look at life's occurrences as *challenges,* not threats. These people welcome change for the growth it promotes. They are optimistic and curious about life.
■ Hardy people have a sense of *control* over their lives. They do not feel helpless in the face of what happens to them. On the other hand, people who are low in measures of hardiness usually appear bored, are hopeless, and lack enthusiasm.

Commitment, challenge, and control may be three rea-

TABLE 8-4

Techniques for Increasing Hardiness

Personality Characteristic	Techniques
Commitment	• Capitalize on skills and interests to develop hobbies • Reduce time spent watching television • Develop a list outlining why one's work is important to the community • Recognize and acknowledge self-worth • Join a volunteer organization that provides services to help others • Join political, social, or religious organizations
Challenge	• Take a controlled physical risk, e.g., become involved in Outward Bound, take a glider flight or parachute jump, or undertake a new sport • Take a vacation that involves little or no planning • Take a course or attend a talk on a topic that questions one's own values • Vary daily activities and change routines
Control	• Set aside a period of time each week to do exactly what one wants • Volunteer for leadership positions in clubs and organizations • Become active in the political process; vote • Seek work situations in which control is increased • Recognize the enormous amount of control one can exercise over his or her own life

sons why differences exist in the ability to adapt to stress. Hardiness may actually help buffer the effects of stress. People who are hardy may be more resilient, or "tougher," in the face of life's ups and downs.

Because hardiness may be a personality characteristic, experts are unsure as to whether people can be taught to be hardy. However, attempts to increase hardiness may be beneficial. Table 8–4 shows a few examples of ways in which clients may increase commitment, challenge, and control in everyday life.

COLLABORATIVE MANAGEMENT

 Assessment

The first step in helping clients to deal with stress is to obtain an accurate assessment of the stress situation. The problem may be in the client's appraisal of the situation, in how the client is coping, or in the inherent stressfulness of the situation, which cannot be controlled or changed. The nurse should assess all aspects of the stress response before determining which nursing interventions are appropriate.

➤ Assessment of Stress

The nurse assesses for physiologic signs that identify that the client is experiencing stress (Chart 8–1).

Physical Assessment: Clinical Manifestations

One of the most obvious physiologic indicators is increased heart rate. Although increased heart rate is a stress-related response, heart rate by itself has not proved to be a reliable indicator of the presence of stress. Among the reasons for this unpredictability is that heart rate

Chart 8-1

Nursing Care Highlight: Assessing for Common Signs of Stress

Physical Signs
• Sleep problems
• Headaches
• Shaking
• Inability to sit still
• Muscle tension
• Rapid speech, stuttering, or stammering
• Fatigue
• Increased heart rate
• Digestive troubles
• Increased perspiration
• Light-headedness
• Cold chills
• Hot flashes
• Palpitations
• Dry mouth
• Frequent urination
• Menstrual cycle changes
• Crying

Psychosocial Signs
• Resentment toward health care workers
• Anger, loss of temper
• Feelings of helplessness
• Resistance to treatments or tests
• Overuse of drugs, including prescription and over-the-counter drugs
• Withdrawal from friends and family
• Overuse of alcohol
• Excessive excitement
• Confusion and forgetfulness
• Nervousness
• Irritability
• Complaints of anxiety

varies with almost any stimulus, from movement to illness. Thus, heart rate is not specific enough to be a valid sign of stress. The correlation of stress and blood pressure has demonstrated the same problem.

A variety of physical complaints may also reflect stress in the client. Examples of stress-related complaints are headaches, neckaches, stomachaches, muscular cramping, and other signs of muscular tension. Some people perspire, some get pale, and others become flushed under stress. Many people experience alterations in their patterns of elimination, both bowel and urinary. Eating patterns may also reflect change, with some people eating more than usual and others eating less. Sleep patterns may be disrupted, with some clients experiencing insomnia and others wanting to sleep more than usual. The patterns of these changes are as different as the people involved.

Psychosocial Assessment

Nurses use many obvious psychosocial signs to assess stress behavior (see Chart 8–1). Many of the signs used to assess stress actually reflect coping activity. The more common signs attributed to stress include emotional excesses, such as agitation, anxiety, anger, and apathy. Other signs may include inappropriate or ineffectual coping behaviors, such as denial and blaming. Stress in people may be signaled by expressions of hopelessness, powerlessness, or loss of control; alterations in normal communication patterns, such as a change from extreme talkativeness to silence; and changes in thought processes. Even signs that are considered pathologic, such as manipulative behavior, depression, and withdrawal, may only reflect a person's reaction to tremendous stress.

Laboratory Assessment

Levels of epinephrine and norepinephrine are somewhat more predictive of stress than other laboratory values. Unlike steroid products, epinephrine and norepinephrine are released almost instantly in response to stress. Initial research has focused on athletes, astronauts, and others exposed to intense but transient stress-provoking episodes. Norepinephrine levels almost always rise when a person is subjected to a stressor, but epinephrine levels tend to stabilize after a brief period of elevation. Although these results are promising, they are only preliminary findings. In addition, it is not always possible to obtain blood for laboratory analysis, and this procedure is invasive.

➤ Assessment of Appraisal and Coping

The study of coping, including individual appraisal, is a new area of research, and many questions remain unanswered. Until further studies are available, nurses are best guided by the client in the perception of what is stressful and the best coping strategies to be used.

Assessment of Appraisal

The nurse first tries to determine what the client perceives as stressful. The nurse asks specific questions about which aspects of hospitalization or illness are stressful.

The assessment relates specifically to the appraisal process, with the nurse considering such factors as perceived ambiguity, predictability, and uncertainty of events. The nurse also asks specific questions about how much the client knows about diagnosis, diagnostic testing, and expected length of hospitalization.

The nurse next attempts to learn how stressful these items are perceived to be by the client. Stress is an individual matter, so it is the client's perception, or appraisal, that is important. One way of determining the level of stress is to ask the client to name the most stressful event possible and then compare the new stressor with that event.

After determining the client's appraisal of the event and the coping methods used, the nurse learns the successful coping strategies that the client has used in the past for similar problems.

Figure 8–3 depicts a guide for interviewing clients about stress and coping.

Assessment of Specific Coping Strategies

Nurses should remember that different individuals cope with the same problem in a variety of ways. If the chosen coping strategy is working, the nurse should support the client in that effort. If the coping strategy is not effective, the nurse works with the client to develop alternatives.

The nurse may note that clients are using event rehearsal if they discuss or talk about the upcoming event or if, when asked, say they have been thinking about the situation. If the event rehearsal is to be effective, clients need information about the stressor. Nurses may also make an assessment that clients are using event rehearsal when clients seek information. Many clients actively solicit information from health care providers, friends, or relatives.

Calling friends and family on the telephone, encouraging visitors, and socializing with others who are in the hospital may reflect the client's use of social support as a coping strategy. Talking with others about what has occurred may reflect the use of event review.

Developing a plan to eliminate or reduce the effect of the stressor can be another form of coping that is reflected in information-seeking behavior. When clients use planned problem-solving, they need accurate information so that the plans they make are based on reality.

If clients purposefully appear to keep their emotions or behaviors in check, they may be using self-control to aid their coping. Stoicism can reflect a personality type or even a culturally approved coping strategy. Other, more expressive clients may not keep their emotions and feelings in check and may be using confrontive coping strategies. The nurse may also assess anger, hostility, and argumentative behavior in the client as coping strategies.

Nurses may make an assessment of denial or distancing in clients who exhibit avoidance behavior, such as refusing to look at surgical scars or not learning self-care. Clients who do not talk about their conditions, do not prepare for upcoming events, or appear to go on as if nothing had happened to them may also be using denial. Some clients may even exhibit withdrawal behavior by

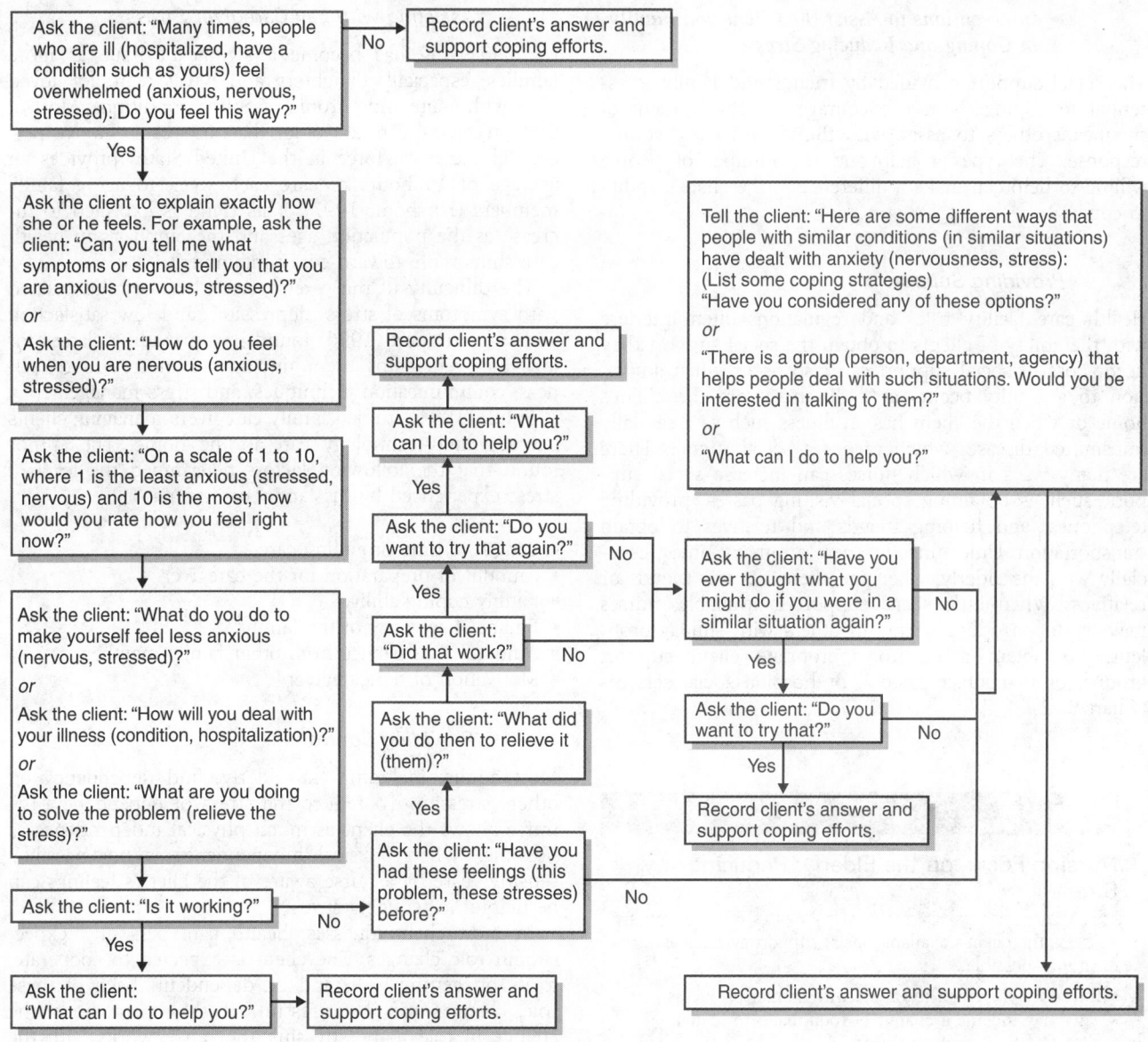

Figure 8–3. A guide for interviewing clients for stress and coping.

refusing to communicate or by communicating only minimally.

Clients who blame themselves for their illness or hospitalization may be using the coping strategy of self-blame. Clients who use faith as a coping strategy may request clergy visits, use religious articles, and engage in prayer, which are signs that the nurse can observe.

Interventions

After the nurse has assessed that there is a problem in the client's ability to appraise or to cope, many interventions are available. Because of the personal nature of stress, appraisal, and coping, the nurse must remember that there are no universal, standard nursing interventions.

➤ Interventions to Assist the Client in Appraisal

Nurses can help clients make more accurate appraisals through client education. Nurses assist clients to recognize and correct faulty appraisal, and they provide positive reinforcement of correct appraisal. Appraisal depends on accurate information. For example, nurses aid clients in appraisal by supplying information about the scheduling and the duration of events in an attempt to avoid ambiguity, confusion, and fear of the unknown.

Another important step in assisting clients with appraisal is exploring perceptions of stress and stressors to determine whether appraisals are accurate. The nurse encourages the client to verbalize perceptions and to help the nurse identify and correct faulty appraisal. If appraisals are inaccurate, the nurse intervenes to supply correct information and aids clients in changing their perception.

➤ *Interventions to Assist the Client and Family in Coping and Reducing Stress*

The social support provided by friends and family is essential to coping. Nurses encourage the involvement of significant others to assist with the client's stress-coping response. The type of help and the number of people willing to help can make a difference in the client's ability to cope.

Providing Support

Health care facility rules and regulations often interfere with the ability of clients to obtain the social support they need. Loss of social support can also occur when admission to a facility occurs at a distance from the client's home or when the client has an illness such as a sexually transmitted disease, which carries a social stigma. There are many ways in which nurses can increase social support, such as obtaining special visiting passes, providing telephones, and helping friends and relatives to obtain transportation. Unfortunately, there are many times, especially with the elderly, when the client has few friends or relatives. When little social support is available, nurses may try to introduce clients to others with similar problems, to obtain access to appropriate client support groups, or to contact pastoral or hospital social services (Chart 8–2).

Chart 8–2

Nursing Focus on the Elderly: Reducing Stress

- Assess the client's available social support systems as early as possible.
- Introduce the client to others with similar problems. This may include a change of roommates to match clients to help meet this need.
- Request spiritual support by contacting clergy, requesting religious articles, or saying a prayer, depending on the client's preference. Consider the client's cultural background.
- Take time to listen to the client's concerns.
- Collaborate with the social services department in identifying support systems for the client.
- Allow the client to be as independent as possible, even if it takes more time for a task, such as feeding, to be completed.
- To the extent possible, give the client an opportunity to make decisions about activities of daily living, hospital activities, and nursing interventions.
- Teach information about surgery, procedures, tests, and so forth at a slower pace than for a younger adult.
- Teach the importance of proper rest, sleep, exercise, and nutrition.
- Teach progressive muscle relaxation and guided imagery, if appropriate.

Assisting with Lay Caregiver Stress

Lay caregiving has become a significant issue as more families, especially daughters and wives, care for loved ones with acute and chronic disabling conditions. Most of those receiving care are older than 65 years. Twelve percent of the work force in the United States provides an average of 15 hours of care each week to aging family members (Hirshom, 1997). This trend is expected to increase as the population ages and the emphasis in health care shifts more toward cost containment.

The difficulty of the caregiver role has been associated with symptoms of stress, depression, and low satisfaction with life. Ruppert (1996) found that providing classes for lay caregivers helps them understand more about wellness, communication techniques, and stress management.

Smith (1994) studied family caregivers managing clients needing high-technology care in the home. The author found that the following factors determined the level of stress experienced by the family caregivers:

- Length of time providing care
- Amount of preparation for the caregiver
- Family coping ability
- Financial solvency of the family
- Amount of assistance from other family members
- Motivation of the caregiver

Providing Control

Most adults, including the elderly, find dependency on others stressful. To reduce the stress of dependency, the nurse allows the client as much physical independence as possible. When physical independence is not possible, sensitive care by a nurse aware of the client's feelings can be helpful in reducing stress.

In most client illnesses, health care personnel expect certain role changes. The client is expected to cooperate, focus on getting well, and be dependent. Each of these role changes can be stressful. If the client finds the change in role to be stressful, the nurse works with the client to develop a plan of care that incorporates maintenance of important role behaviors. Whenever possible, nurses should allow clients who desire it to have control over other activities of daily living, hospital activities, and nursing interventions. Control over such things as times of bathing, food choices, awake and sleep times, and scheduling of therapies and procedures can be very helpful in reducing stress and in maintaining self-esteem.

Providing Information

Adequate knowledge may also help clients gain control. Nursing research has shown the importance of client preparation for diagnostic tests and procedures (Johnson & Lauver, 1989). Among the content that should be included in client education is knowledge of the duration of events, expected behaviors, sensations involved, and sequencing of activities. Nurses should remember that even everyday experiences in the hospital or nursing home, such as the administration of intravenous therapy, can be extremely stressful to the client and the family.

Research Applications for Nursing

Communicating with Families Can Reduce Stress and Anxiety

Johnson, M. J., & Frank, D. I. (1995). Effectiveness of a telephone intervention in reducing anxiety of families of patients in an intensive care unit. Applied Nursing Research, 8, 42–43.

This study evaluated the results of a program designed to keep family members apprised of their loved one's status while in the intensive care unit. A total of 24 telephone calls were made to family members of the experimental group over a 48-hour period. The calls were brief, lasting less than 5 minutes. An additional 10 verbal contacts were made with this group. The anxiety scores of the experimental group decreased significantly more than those of the control group who did not receive the calls.

Critique. Although the sample was fairly small (20 families in each group), the study showed how a simple nursing intervention can help relieve the stress and anxiety of family members who are critically ill. This study supports the findings of other researchers who also had success with telephone programs.

Possible Nursing Implications. This study suggests that nurses need to take the time to communicate with families to minimize their anxiety. Some of the nurses who made calls in the study were reluctant to do so because they thought they were too time-consuming or not part of their role. Nurses in all health care settings should incorporate the family and significant others in their client care.

Not all clients and their families want to know about *all* aspects of care and hospitalization. For clients who want to know, it is vital that they receive detailed information about those areas in which lack of knowledge is perceived as stressful.

Families also experience anxiety and stress when they are not informed or an unpredictable event occurs. A study by Johnson and Frank (1995) showed that a telephone intervention helped reduce anxiety of families of clients in an intensive care unit (see the Research Applications for Nursing box).

A client's coping strategy of event rehearsal also depends on adequate and correct information about events. Many clients actively seek information from health care providers, friends, relatives, and even comparative strangers who have undergone similar experiences.

After a stress-provoking event, nurses can aid clients' coping through event review by encouraging clients to think or talk about their experiences. Nurses should allow clients to verbally review as much as they need to, even when the account is repetitive. The repetition of thoughts about a threatening event can facilitate coping.

Recognizing Client Feelings

When experiencing or responding to stress, clients can have a number of feelings. For example, if the client becomes hostile, nurses should not react personally. In-

stead, acknowledging the client's feelings of anger and aggression is often helpful. For example, the nurse might say, "I can understand why you're angry. I would be angry too, if that had happened to me." After anger is acknowledged, it often decreases or disappears. If the anger does not diminish, the nurse allows the client to explore his or her anger no matter how irrational it may seem. After the anger has been reduced, the nurse can explore the more logical reasons why the feelings arose.

Occasionally, people become so angry that they become a danger to themselves or others around them. If the client loses control over his or her emotions, the nurse should follow institutional guidelines governing such situations.

The nurse can often best facilitate coping by supporting the client's own coping strategies. For example, when clients use self-controlling mechanisms, they should be supported in those efforts rather than forced to share their feelings or to demonstrate their emotions if they are not comfortable in doing so.

➤ Interventions to Aid Family Coping

Families also experience many of the same stressors that the ill or hospitalized client does. Families under stress also use coping strategies, such as seeking social support, reviewing events, and venting hostility. Nurses can aid the family and significant others in appraisal of stress and coping just as they do for the client. The nurse can also refer them to social service agencies and other support services.

➤ Interventions to Reduce the Effects of Stress

When clients are facing illness, surgery, and other health-related events, they may experience a high level of stress that is not immediately reducible. The introduction of further stress can inhibit coping effectiveness. Nursing action that eliminates or reduces additional stress allows the client to concentrate his or her coping activities on the major stressor and not divert his or her energies to coping with annoyances.

Although many stressful aspects of illness or hospitalization can be reduced or eliminated, there are still many other aspects with which clients either cannot or will not cope. Some stressors cannot be eliminated or avoided. In such cases, effective nursing care may involve teaching the client techniques that may reduce the physical impact of stress on the body as well as provide a means of physical or emotional control to the client. Examples are biofeedback, progressive muscle relaxation (PMR), meditation, and guided imagery. These interventions are also considered complementary therapies (see Chapter 4). If these techniques are not effective, psychotherapy and/or medication, such as antianxiety drugs, may help.

Biofeedback

Biofeedback can be an effective treatment when obvious signs of stress, such as headaches, high blood pressure, muscle tension, and heart palpitations, occur frequently, are debilitating, or may be dangerous. Biofeedback works

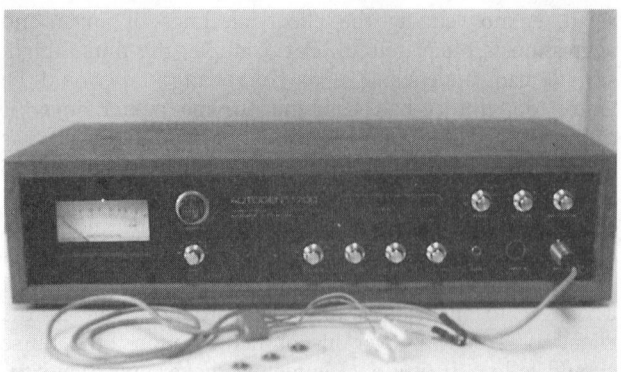

Figure 8–4. An example of a biofeedback system used to reduce stress. (Courtesy of Autogenic Systems, Inc., Newton, MA.)

by training the client to reverse the subtle changes that lead to a somatic, or physical, response. For instance, if a headache is the result of muscle tension in the forehead, the client can be trained to relax that tension before a headache results.

Biofeedback involves using electronic instrumentation to signal the user about selected somatic changes. The machinery is sensitive to minute changes within a body system. For example, if the biofeedback is directed toward sampling muscle activity, the machine detects small changes in the electrical activity of the muscles. If brain wave activity is the variable considered, the machine signals the type of brain waves that are occurring at a given moment. Cardiovascular and skin surface activity can also be monitored. After the physical clues are learned, the client can use them to gain control over and to reduce the undesired activity (Fig. 8–4).

Many hospitals and clinics have biofeedback equipment and trained personnel available. If not, referrals can usually be made to a local practitioner.

Progressive Muscle Relaxation

Stress commonly causes muscle tension, which results in many of the nagging physical symptoms of stress, such as headaches and neckaches. Control of muscle tension appears to help reduce the physical effects of such tension as well. PMR is one method used to reduce muscular tension.

PMR involves the tensing and then the relaxing of all the major muscle groups, usually in sequential steps. In PMR, the nurse guides the client through relaxation of each major body part, having the client first tighten and then relax each part. The following is a suggested sequence: feet, thighs, buttocks, stomach, chest, hands, forearms, shoulders, neck, and head. The nurse instructs the client in PMR until he or she can comfortably perform it alone without prompting. If time is a problem, the client can use a tape recorder and prerecorded PMR tape after completing the initial instruction (Chart 8–3). PMR is useful in nursing practice because it is easy to teach and can be used for a wide spectrum of clients. It is also inexpensive, unlike methods that use machinery, such as biofeedback.

Meditation

Meditation is a learned process through which a person attempts to quiet the mind. The methods used to quiet the mind involve consciously removing disturbing thoughts or filling the mind with only one thought, such as a *mantra* or prayer. By removing other thoughts, it is believed that stress can be reduced. Meditation is probably best learned through a mentor, although books and other audiovisual aids are available. If clients are inter-

---

Chart 8–3

Education Guide: Progressive Muscle Relaxation

- Take a minute and feel your body's different parts. Think about what portions of your body feel tense and which parts feel relaxed.

- We are going to do an exercise that will help you to relax and remove the tension from your body. I am going to talk you through this exercise, so just relax and follow my directions.

- I am going to ask you to tense one body part at a time. When you tense the body part, try to make the muscle as tight as possible. If you feel pain or a cramp when you tighten, reduce the tightness. This tightening is called tension.

- After you hold that muscle tightness for 5 to 10 seconds, I am going to ask you to let all the tightness out of that body part—to let it go limp. This is called relaxation.

- First, point your feet and curl your toes. Feel the tension in your feet. Hold that feeling until I tell you to relax.

- Relax—let your feet go limp. Feel the difference in going from tension to relaxation. Take a few moments to feel the relaxation.

- Now tighten the muscles in your lower legs. Feel the tension in your calves. Feel the tightness of your muscles. Hold that feeling until I say relax.

- Now relax your lower legs. Let them go limp. Feel the tightness leave and the feeling of relaxation take over.

- Now tighten the muscles of your neck by clenching your lower jaw. Feel the tightness of your muscles. Feel the tenseness as you clench your jaw.

- Relax your neck and jaw. Let the tightness go—feel the relaxation take over. Feel the difference between tension and relaxation.

- Close your eyes tightly and try to tighten all the other muscles in your face. Feel how tight your face feels.

- Now relax your face and let the tenseness flow out.

- Finally, I want you to let your whole body go limp—let it all relax. Remember those feelings of relaxation and let those feelings take over. Release any feelings of tension.

- Now, it is time to end this exercise. I want you to take your time as you slowly begin to move. When you are ready, you may resume your normal activities.

ested in learning meditative techniques, they should be referred to an appropriate source.

Guided Imagery

Similar to meditation, imagery also attempts to control the mind's thoughts. Guided imagery seeks to fill the mind with positive and pleasant mental pictures. Usually, imagery involves thinking about a peaceful scene or one in which there is total relaxation. Thinking processes are directed toward the promotion of relaxation rather than stress.

NURSING AND STRESS

Nurses as well as clients experience stress. Many nurses are affected by stress that exceeds their ability to cope. Nurses are exposed to tremendous numbers of stressors in their work each day, from exposure to death to sometimes unrealistic expectations of the work environment.

The effect of managed care in the 1990s and into the 21st century has been especially stressful for nurses in all health care settings, particularly hospitals. The decreasing census of many hospitals has led to layoffs of nurses and, in some cases, replacements of nurses with unlicensed assistive personnel. All health care agencies are attempting to contain costs in a number of ways. Nurses are very concerned that quality of care may be sacrificed in this cost containment era.

Many programs are available to aid the nurse in reducing stress, and there are also a variety of strategies that the nurse may use. In addition to the strategies outlined for clients, the following stress management techniques may be effective (Schultes, 1997):

- Learn assertiveness techniques to present feelings and thoughts in an honest, direct, and acceptable manner. Remember that hostile expression of anger and aggression usually inflame, rather than reduce, stress feelings.
- Acknowledge the positive aspects of work and do not dwell on the negatives. Happier people have been found to be less "realistic" in their assessments of situations, in that they focus on the funny and the positive aspects of life.
- Develop alternative plans for situations known to cause stress. For example, if transportation is a problem, arrange for a friend or coworker to serve as a back-up when trouble develops.
- Follow the same health care practices that nurses recommend to others. Get adequate sleep, eat a healthy diet, reduce caffeine consumption, get regular exercise, stop smoking, and use alcohol only in moderation, if at all.
- Use humor to cope with stress as well as to help clients cope and heal.

SELECTED BIBLIOGRAPHY

*Cannon, W. B. (1931). *The wisdom of the body.* New York: W. W. Norton.
Corley, M. C., Ferriter, J., Zeh, J., & Gifford, C. (1995). Physiological and psychological effects of back rubs. *Applied Nursing Research, 8,* 39–42.
*DeLongis, A., Coyne, J. C., Dakof, G., Folkman, S., & Lazarus, R. S. (1982). Relationship of daily hassles, uplifts and major life events to health status. *Health Psychology, 1,* 119–136.
Gio-Fitman, J. (1996). The role of psychological stress in rheumatoid arthritis. *MedSurg Nursing, 5*(6), 422–426.
Hirshom, E. (1997). Case study: Meeting the challenges of dementia management. *Continuing Care, 16*(2), 19–21.
*Holmes, T. H., & Rahe, R. H. (1967). The social readjustment rating scale. *Journal of Psychosomatic Research, 11,* 213–218.
Hunt, R. & Zurek, E. L. (1997). *Introduction to community based nursing.* Philadelphia: J. B. Lippincott.
*Janis, I. L. (1985). Coping patterns among patients with life-threatening diseases. *Issues in Mental Health Nursing, 7,* 461–476.
*Johnson, J. E., & Lauver, D. R. (1989). Alternative explanations of coping with stressful experiences associated with physical illness. *Advances in Nursing Science, 11,* 39–52.
Johnson, M. J., & Frank, D. I. (1995). Effectiveness of a telephone intervention in reducing anxiety of families of patients in an intensive care unit. *Applied Nursing Research, 8,* 42–43.
*Kobasa, S. C. (1979). Stressful life events, personality, and health: An inquiry into hardiness. *Journal of Personality and Social Psychology, 37,* 1–10.
*Lazarus, R. S., & Folkman, S. (1984). *Stress, appraisal and coping.* New York: Springer.
*Moos, R. H., & Tsu, V. D. (1977). The crisis of physical illness. In R. H. Moos (Ed.), *Coping with physical illness.* New York: Plenum.
*Pollock, S. E. (1989). The hardiness characteristic: A motivating factor in adaptation. *Advances in Nursing Science, 11,* 53–62.
*Pollock, S. E., Christian, B. J., & Sands, D. (1990). Response to chronic illness: Analysis of psychological and physiological adaptation. *Nursing Research, 39,* 300–304.
*Pollock, S. E., & Duffy, M. E. (1990). The health-related hardiness scale: Development and psychometric analysis. *Nursing Research, 39,* 218–222.
*Robinson, L. (1990). Stress and anxiety. *Nursing Clinics of North America, 25,* 935–943.
*Roy, C., & Roberts, S. (1981). *Theory construction in nursing: An adaptation model.* Englewood Cliffs, NJ: Prentice-Hall.
Ruppert, R. A. (1996). Caring for the lay caregiver. *American Journal of Nursing, 96*(3), 40–45.
Sarna, L., van Servellen, G., & Padilla, G. (1996). Comparison of emotional distress in men with acquired immunodeficiency syndrome and in men with cancer. *Applied Nursing Research, 9,* 209–212.
Schultes, L. S. (1997). Humor with hospice clients: You're putting me on. *Home Healthcare Nurse, 15*(8), 561–566.
*Selye, H. (1946). General adaptation syndrome and diseases of adaptation. *Journal of Clinical Endocrinology, 6,* 117–230.
Smith, C. (1994). A model of caregiving effectiveness for technologically dependent adults residing at home. *Advances in Nursing Science, 17*(2), 27–40.
*Weinberger, R. (1991). Teaching the elderly stress reduction. *Journal of Gerontological Nursing, 17*(10), 23–27.

SUGGESTED READINGS

Corley, M. C., Ferriter, J., Zeh, J., & Gifford, C. (1995). Physiological and psychological effects of back rubs. *Applied Nursing Research, 8,* 39–43.
This nursing pilot study examined the physiologic and psychological effects of a back rub on elderly residents in a nursing home. Mood ratings improved in both the experimental group (those receiving back rubs) and the control group (those who rested), but the mood was significantly better in the experimental group. The study has implications for nursing practice because back rubs are often not provided for residents in long-term care.
Ruppert, R. A. (1996). Caring for the lay caregiver. *American Journal of Nursing, 96*(3), 40–45.
This article discusses the effects of prolonged caregiving by family members in the home. The author shares her experience providing classes for caregivers to help them prepare for their caregiving experience as well as alert them to the need to take care of themselves.

PAIN

Pain is a protective mechanism for the body in that it occurs when tissues are being damaged (Guyton, 1996). The person in pain usually takes action to remove the pain or its cause, if possible. Indeed, pain is the number one symptom or complaint that causes people to seek health care. It alters or compromises the quality of life more than any other single health-related problem.

OVERVIEW

Everyone experiences pain at some time in life, but although this is likely a universal experience, it is also a complex and private one. Because it is such a personal experience, it is very difficult to describe or explain to others. Many factors make hard to understand and assess, including psychosocial, cultural, and developmental factors and the influence of gender, the environment, and the subjectivity of pain itself. The interpretation of pain, based solely on the person's actions or behaviors can be misleading, because the amount of pain and responses to it vary from person to person.

Definitions of Pain

Several attempts have been made to define pain in descriptive or measurable terms; however, no one definition is more accepted than another. Among the most popular definitions of pain are those of Sternbach (1968), Mc-

Caffery (1979), and the International Association on Pain (1979). Sternbach (p. 8) asserted that pain is "an abstract concept which refers to:

- A personal, private sensation of hurt
- A harmful stimulus which signals current or impending tissue damage
- A pattern of responses to protect the organism from harm"

This comprehensive definition serves to explain pain through a physiologic, psychological, and social approach.

McCaffery (1979) offered a more personal explanation of pain when she stated that pain "is whatever the experiencing person says it is and exists whenever he says it does" (p. 11). This understanding of pain requires that the client be seen as the authority on the pain and the only one who can define the experience.

Finally, the International Association on Pain (1979) described pain as an unpleasant sensory and emotional experience associated with actual or potential tissue damage.

Regardless of the definition, most people agree that pain has both sensory and behavioral components and is strongly influenced by various physiologic, psychological, and sociologic factors. A comprehensive understanding of pain requires a knowledge of the descriptive definitions, theories, and physiology of pain. The nurse can use this knowledge as a basis to develop an appreciation of the variety of clinical pain situations and skill in pain intervention. This understanding can also help the nurse develop a personal philosophy of pain management.

Theoretical Bases for Pain

Several theories have been proposed to explain the complex phenomenon of pain. Early theories emphasized the recognition of specific pathways of pain transmission. Later theories attempted to uncover the complexity of central processing of pain in specific areas of the brain. More recently, the concept of a pain-modulating network was introduced. This concept describes the various links and connections in the spinal cord and brain, specifically the medulla and the midbrain. The identification of chemical mediators involved in the pain response has helped in an understanding of pain transmission and perception.

Early Theories of Pain

The specificity theory was first proposed in the early 1800s and was accepted for almost 100 years as the most popular theoretical explanation for pain. This theory emphasized the highly specific structures and pathways responsible for pain transmission. Its premise was based on the existence of free nerve endings in the periphery of the body that were capable of accepting sensory input and transmitting it along highly specific nerve fibers. Although this theory set the stage for further research, its major biological orientation was not sufficient to account for the complexity of pain.

Later, in the early 1900s, an opposing pattern theory was developed. Goldscheider (cited in Melzack, 1973), the originator of this theory, identified two major pain fibers: a rapidly conducting fiber and a slowly conducting fiber. Both fibers synapse in the spinal cord and relay information to the brain. The concept of central summation was introduced: As pain fibers converge at the level of the spinal cord, the summation of impulses from these fibers ascends to various levels of the brain. The amount, intensity, and type of sensory input permit the brain to interpret the sensation.

Both the pattern theory and the specificity theory failed to explain the influences of psychological variables, such as anxiety and depression, on pain. Also, neither theory provided a reasonable explanation for failure of pain to resolve after pain pathways and spinal nerves were interrupted.

Gate Control Theory

The gate control theory was proposed to explain the observed relationship between pain and emotion. Melzack and Wall (1982), who first introduced this theory, concluded that pain is not just a physiologic response, but that psychological variables, such as behavioral and emotional responses, also influence the perception of pain.

According to the gate control theory, a gating mechanism occurs in the spinal cord. Pain impulses are transmitted from the periphery of the body by nerve fibers (A delta and C fibers). The impulses travel to the dorsal horns of the spinal cord, specifically to the area of the cord called the *substantia gelatinosa*. The cells of the substantia gelatinosa can inhibit or facilitate pain impulses that are transmitted to the trigger cells (T cells). When T-cell activity is inhibited, the gate is closed and impulses are less likely to be transmitted to the brain. When the gate is opened, pain impulses ascend to the brain (Fig. 9–1).

Similar gating mechanisms exist in the descending nerve fibers from the thalamus and cerebral cortex. These areas of the brain regulate a person's thoughts and emotions, including beliefs and values. When pain occurs, a person's thoughts and emotions can modify perceptual phenomena as they reach the level of conscious awareness.

The gate control theory has helped nurses and other

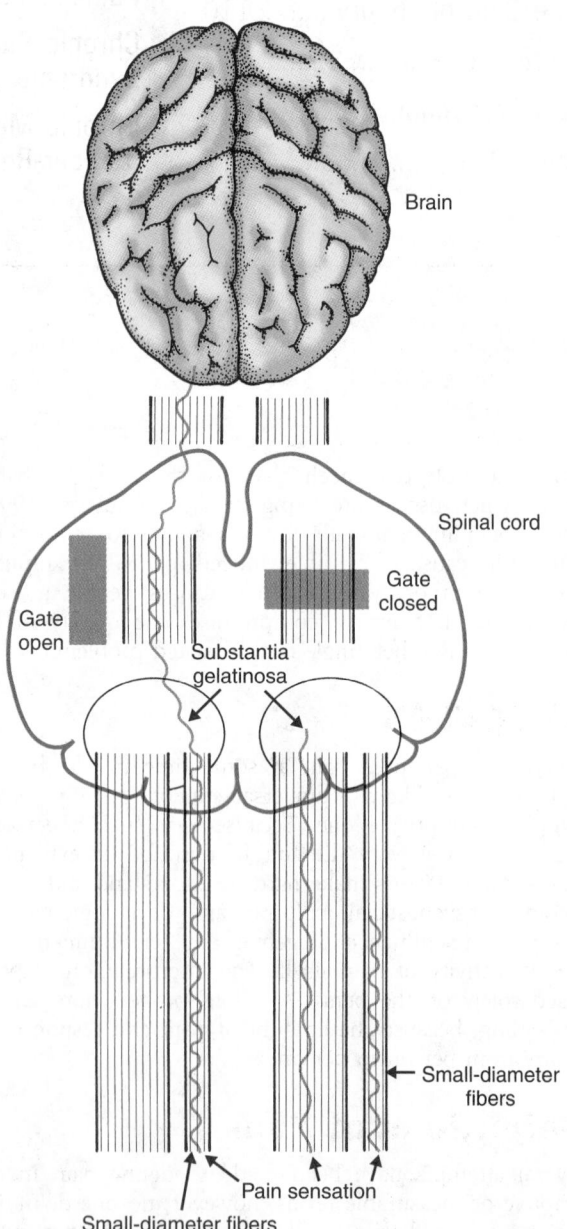

Figure 9–1. The gate control theory of pain.

health care professionals recognize the *holistic* nature of pain. As a result, many interventions, such as imagery and distraction (discussed later), are used to help relieve a client's pain.

Anatomic and Physiologic Bases for Pain

Pain Stimuli

Various types of noxious pain stimuli account for the perception of pain. A wide range of sensory input is capable of producing pain. In addition, tissue ischemia and muscle spasm cause pain. Free nerve endings, or receptors capable of responding to painful stimuli, are often referred to as nociceptors. Nociceptors are located in various body tissues and are activated by thermal, mechanical, and chemical stimuli. In addition to nociceptors, other receptors in the body respond to almost any type of intense stimulation, sometimes resulting in pain.

In most circumstances, painful stimuli cause actual tissue damage, which leads to the release of certain chemical substances, such as histamine, bradykinin, serotonin, norepinephrine, and certain acids that sensitize the nociceptors, including leukotrienes, prostaglandins, and substance P. These chemicals are believed to activate pain receptors. For example, the accumulation of lactic acids leads to the pain associated with ischemic tissue damage (Guyton, 1996). Muscle contraction or spasm can also produce ischemic-type pain. The muscle's oxygen demands are increased, but the blood supply is limited because of compressed blood vessels.

Pain Fibers and Pathways

Usually, painful stimuli originate in the periphery of the body. For the painful stimuli to be perceived, however, they must first be transmitted to the spinal cord and then to the central areas of the brain, as described by the gate control theory of pain (Fig. 9–1). In the periphery, two specific fibers can transmit stimuli: A delta fibers, which are found primarily in the skin and muscle, and C fibers, which are distributed in muscle, periosteum, and viscera. Both of these nerve fibers comprise the first-order neurons capable of accepting nociceptive stimuli.

A delta fibers are myelinated fibers that carry rapid, sharp, pricking, or piercing sensations. A person feeling these sensations can generally localize them readily to a fairly well-defined area. Because these fibers respond predominantly to mechanical stimuli, rather than to chemical or thermal stimuli, they are called mechanical nociceptors.

C fibers are unmyelinated or poorly myelinated fibers that conduct thermal, chemical, and strong mechanical impulses. Pain conduction from C fibers is more diffuse and dull, burning, or achy—quite different from the sensations of A delta fibers. In contrast to the intermittent nature of A delta sensations, C fibers usually produce constant pain.

Second-order neurons or pain pathways of the ascending pain tracts are found in the dorsal horn of the spinal cord and terminate in the thalamus. The spinothalamic tract is divided into two spinal tracts known as the lateral or neospinothalamic tract and the medial or paleospinothalamic tract. The neospinothalamic tract is responsible for sensory pain discrimination, as it transmits painful stimuli more directly to the sensory cortex where pain is eventually perceived and interpreted. The paleospinothalamic tract synapses in other parts of the brain, such as the limbic system (or emotional center) and the reticular formation (or sleep-wake center), subjecting the painful stimuli to emotional and behavioral influences.

Central Nervous System Processing

The central processing of pain occurs at three different levels of the brain: the thalamus, midbrain, and cortex. These areas of the brain cooperate to raise the awareness of pain, interpret the painful stimuli, and produce a response to the pain. The thalamus acts as the relay station for sensory input from the spinothalamic tract of the spinal cord. The midbrain signals the cortex to increase the awareness of the stimuli. The cortex seems to be involved in the discrimination of well-localized pain as well as in the interpretation of the pain experience.

Inhibitory and Facilitatory Mechanisms

Sensory input to the spinal cord may be influenced by chemical substances known as *neuroregulators*. These are classified as neurotransmitters or neuromodulators.

Neurotransmitters

Neurotransmitters are chemicals that exert inhibitory or excitatory activity at postsynaptic nerve cell membranes. Acetylcholine, norepinephrine, epinephrine, and dopamine are documented neurotransmitters.

Neuromodulators

Neuromodulators, also called endogenous opiates, are protein hormones found in the brain. They have been implicated in the modification of pain. These substances are composed of large amino acid peptides called *alpha-* and *beta-endorphins* and *enkephalins*. The speculation that these natural opiate-like substances were responsible for pain relief was confirmed when induced analgesic effects were reversed with naloxone (Narcan), an opioid antagonist.

Endorphins and enkephalins are similar to morphine-like substances, only more potent. They are believed to play a major role in the biological response to pain. The larger peptides (endorphins) exert more prolonged analgesic effects than do the enkephalins. Endorphins are produced by the anterior pituitary gland and the hypothalamus. The smaller peptides (enkephalins) tend to be more widespread throughout the brain and the dorsal horn of the spinal cord. Several types of endorphins and enkephalins have been identified. Each acts on highly specific opiate receptors in the central nervous system.

Opioid receptors are binding sites for not only endogenous opiates but also opioid analgesics that are taken to relieve pain also bind to these receptors. There are several types of opioid receptors: mu, kappa, delta, epsilon, and sigma. The mu receptors are found throughout the central nervous system, especially in the periaqueductal gray matter in the brain stem, the limbic system, and the dorsal horn. Morphine and morphine agonists bind to the mu receptors. Specific subtypes of the mu receptor are responsible for analgesia, bradycardia and sedation, and opioid agonist binding, which is associated with respiratory depression, euphoria, and physical dependence.

Various factors influence the production of neuromodulators. The activity of endorphins and enkephalins may be enhanced by prolonged strenuous activity (Fig. 9–2), transcutaneous electrical nerve stimulators (see later discussions about interventions for pain and chronic pain), and antidepressant therapy, which often increases serotonin levels in the body. Adequate amounts of serotonin, a neurotransmitter, have been shown to enhance analgesia through the activity of endorphins and enkephalins. Similarly, pain and stress are strong activators of the endogenous opiate system.

Sources of Pain

There are three major categories of pain sources: somatic, visceral, and neuropathic. Another arbitrary classification for the physiological sources of pain is based on pain that involves the activation of nociceptors and nonnociceptive pain or neuropathic pain. For a complete characterization of the physiological sources of pain, consult Table 9–1.

Somatic Pain

Somatic structures are the first source of pain. These structures are further classified as cutaneous and deep.

Cutaneous structures make up the superficial parts of the body, such as the skin and subcutaneous tissue. The cutaneous structures are well supplied with nerves; therefore, painful stimuli are well defined and localized.

Deep somatic structures include nerve receptors originating in bone, blood vessels, nerves, muscles, and other supporting tissues. Because these structures are poorly supplied with nerves, this pain is usually dull and poorly localized. Deep pain may produce an autonomic nervous system response, including nausea, pulse and blood pressure changes, and sweating.

Visceral Pain

The second source of pain is visceral and is defined as pain arising from body organs. The scarcity of nerve receptors in these structures produces poorly localized and diffuse pain. Visceral receptors are sensitive to stretching, inflammation, and ischemia, but they are not sensitive to cuts and extremes of temperature.

Visceral pain is well known for its ability to produce referred pain, which is a type of pain that a person perceives in an area other than the site of the stimuli. Referred pain occurs because visceral fibers synapse at the level of the spinal cord, close to fibers supplying certain subcutaneous tissue areas of the body. A common example of referred pain is pain in the right posterior shoulder that is related to gallbladder disease. The referred pain occurs because the subcutaneous tissue fibers of the scapula are close to the fibers of the gallbladder that are transmitting the painful stimuli. Other referred pain sites are illustrated in Figure 9–2.

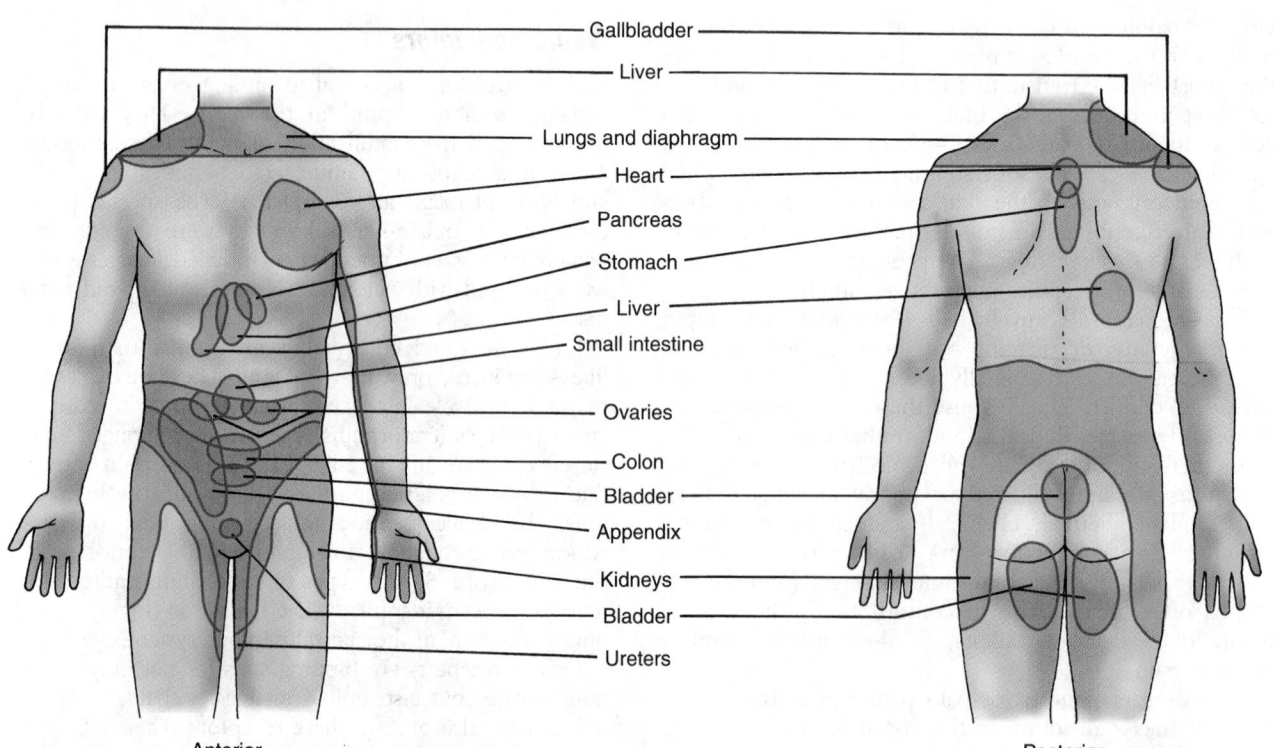

Figure 9–2. Anterior and posterior referred pain sites.

TABLE 9–1

Physiologic Sources of Pain					
Type of Pain	**Physiologic Structures**	**Mechanism of Pain**	**Characteristics of Pain**	**Sources of Acute Postoperative Pain**	**Sources of Chronic Pain Syndromes**
Somatic pain	Cutaneous: skin and subcutaneous tissues Deep somatic: bone, muscle, blood vessels, connective tissues	Activation of nociceptors	Well localized Constant and achy	Incisional pain, pain at insertion sites of tubes and drains, wound complications, orthopaedic procedures, skeletal muscle spasms	Bony metastases, osteo- and rheumatoid arthritis, low back pain, peripheral vascular disease
Visceral pain	Organs and the linings of the body cavities	Activation of nociceptors	Poorly localized Diffuse, deep, cramping or splitting	Chest tubes, abdominal tubes and drains, bladder distention or spasms, intestinal distention	Pancreatitis, liver metastases, colitis
Neuropathic pain	Nerve fibers, spinal cord, and central nervous system	Nonnociceptive Injury to the nervous system structures	Poorly localized Shooting, burning, fiery, shock-like, sharp, and painful numbness	Phantom limb pain, postmastectomy pain, and pain from nerve compression	Diabetic, human immunodeficiency virus, chemotherapy-induced neuropathies, postherpetic neuralgia, cancer-related nerve injury

Neuropathic Pain

The third major source of pain is neuropathic. Neuropathic pain is that caused by injury or destruction to peripheral nerves, pathways in the spinal cord, and neurons located in the brain. This injury results in disruptions in the transmission of afferent and efferent impulses in the periphery, spinal cord, and brain. Interruptions in the processing of painful stimuli give rise to peripheral and/or central perceptual phenomena, alterations in sensory modalities (touch, pressure, and temperature), and sometimes motor dysfunction. Central pain may be evident when the brain senses painful stimuli even though there may be no obvious or documented physiologic cause for the pain. Phantom limb pain, which may occur after the removal of an extremity or body part or severe damage to a major nerve plexus that innervates a particular extremity is one example of neuropathic pain.

Neuropathic pain represents a variety of complex painful mechanisms. This category of pain is receiving increased attention in the literature because it may not be as easily relieved by opioid analgesics as is somatic or visceral pain. Successful treatment of neuropathic pain usually requires a combination of pharmacologic approaches and sometimes pain-relieving procedures.

Pain Perception

The subjectivity of the pain experience limits our understanding of the perception and response to pain. This situation is further complicated by the knowledge that even when pain pathways are surgically interrupted, the perception of pain may persist. However, even though the perception of pain is difficult to measure, it can be characterized as the actual awareness of the painful feeling or sensation.

The pain threshold is the amount or degree of noxious stimuli that leads a person to first interpret a sensation as painful. More specifically, this term refers to the point at which a person feels pain and reports it as such.

Even though all pain is real, it sometimes persists without any detectable physical cause. Such pain may be highly influenced by emotional and social factors. In these situations, the lack of a physiologic or organic cause may lead health professionals, families, and clients to doubt the validity of the pain.

Pain tolerance refers to the ability of a person to endure the intensity of pain. Pain tolerance is usually characterized by an overt expression of behavior. Unlike pain perception and pain threshold, the ability to tolerate pain is more a function of psychological and social variables than of biological characteristics.

The nurse should be aware that many variables affect a person's perception of and response to pain. Demographic factors, such as age, gender, and sociocultural background, personality characteristics, and cognition, may influence the client's ability to process pain sensations and react to them.

Age

ELDERLY CONSIDERATIONS

Researchers agree that there are some variations in threshold associated with the chronologic age of the nervous system, but there are no clear trends (Zatzick & Dimsdale, 1990). Some researchers believe that the perceptual acuity of pain diminishes as a result of aging, although this finding has not been validated (Acute Pain Management Guideline Panel, 1992; Neeley, 1993). The perception of cutaneous pain may diminish because of age-related skin changes, but the perception of visceral pain may increase in older adults (Egbert, 1991).

Little attention has been paid to assessing pain in elderly people who are cognitively impaired and hospitalized, those residing at home, or residents of long-term care facilities (Harkins, 1996; Miller et al., 1996). Miller et al. (1996) examined various ways of assessing pain in elderly clients who were acutely confused.

Older adults generally receive less analgesia and tend to report pain less often than do younger adults (Neeley, 1993). These findings may be related to beliefs and concerns that the elderly have about pain and the reporting of pain. Many elderly people hold the following beliefs and concern about pain (Neeley, 1993):

- Pain is something that they must live with.
- Expressing pain is unacceptable or is a sign of weakness.
- Complaining of pain will label them as "bad" clients.
- Nurses are too busy to listen to complaints of pain.
- Pain signifies a serious illness or impending death.

Nurses should be aware of the beliefs that elderly clients hold to manage their pain. Nurses and other caregivers frequently undermedicate elderly clients and are sometimes reluctant to administer prescribed analgesics. Unfounded concerns about overmedication, addiction, and decreases in pain perception may contribute to undermedication (Champlin, 1992; Ferrell et al., 1992b; Greipp, 1992; Haviley et al., 1992).

Gender

Gender differences in types of pain and responses to it have been described by several researchers (Faucett, 1994; Vallerand, 1995). Physiologic, hormonal, and anatomic influences on pain are unclear, but it is apparent that some painful conditions are more common in either men or women (Ruda, 1993). Women suffer more frequently from migraine headaches, arthritis, and facial pain, whereas cluster headaches, back pain, and chest pain are more common among men (Faucett, 1994; Vallerand, 1995).

Gender effects on pain in clinical situations have been identified in some studies but not in others. Such studies must be interpreted with caution, as gender-oriented pain research is based largely on male responses. Women may be more likely to discuss their pain and distress and therefore are mistakenly labeled as less likely to deal effectively with their pain. Some investigators have demonstrated that men tolerate pain better than women do, whereas others have found no gender differences. It is widely believed that men exhibit greater stoicism than do women (Zatzick & Dimsdale, 1990). Research has shown that nurses expect men to be stoic but accept more emotional responses from women in pain (Walding, 1991).

Whatever gender differences do exist in the perception of and response to pain, nurses must acknowledge the effects of gender bias. Studies investigating the attitudes of caregivers toward the client in pain suggest that women are treated less aggressively, and their complaints are viewed with suspicion (Vallerand, 1995). In a recent study of physicians' pain management practices for clients with cancer, being female was an important predictor of inadequate analgesia (Cleeland et al., 1994).

TRANSCULTURAL CONSIDERATIONS

The American Nurses' Association emphasizes the need for nurses to appreciate the cultural diversity of their clients in all aspects of nursing practice. Weber (1996) contends that cultural sensitivity is critical to the understanding of factors that influence pain and expressions of pain. More importantly, the evolving integration of traditional ethnic heritage and modern American socialization gives rise to unique and highly individualized cultural expressions of pain. Yet, sociocultural groups are still sometimes categorized according to their ability to tolerate pain. This leads to unfair stereotypes and expectations of certain ethnic groups; for example, "Italian-Americans are very dramatic when they are in pain" or "Mexican-Americans have a low pain tolerance" (Calvillo & Flaskerud, 1991). A recent investigation of ethnic pain styles in clients experiencing myocardial infarction found few ethnographic correlates of pain dimensions (Neill, 1993), although higher mean pain scores and lower socioeconomic status were related. The dominant social class in the United States may still value less expressive responses to pain.

Many studies have shown a relationship between pain and a person's culture, but the study methods and results have not been consistent (Zatzick & Dimsdale, 1990). Descriptions of the study sample must be carefully evaluated for similar and dissimilar characteristics compared with patients in clinical practice. Findings from ethnic groups studied in other countries may not apply to culturally diverse populations living in America and socialized in the American culture. Also, studies that lack evidence of acceptable psychometric or measurement properties for the pain instruments must be interpreted cautiously. Finally, cross-cultural comparisons performed on pain measurement data substantially improve the ability to identify similarities and differences in the perceptions of and responses to pain across cultures.

Few nursing studies have examined the transcultural aspects of pain, yet nurses assess pain and make decisions regarding pain management for individuals in various ethnic groups. For example, many Mexican-American clients, especially women, moan or cry when they are uncomfortable. As a result, they are often identified by nurses as complainers who cannot tolerate pain (Calvillo & Flaskerud, 1991). Nurses who value the stoic model or "norm" for pain response interpret behaviors such as moaning and crying as an inability to tolerate pain and a request for intervention. In the Mexican culture, however, these behaviors might help the client relieve pain rather than communicate a need for intervention (Calvillo & Flaskerud, 1991).

Nurses must also consider language when dealing with people from various cultures. If English is not the person's first language within an English-speaking culture, the ability of the person to express pain may be limited, or expressions of pain may be misinterpreted. The nurse may need to rely on nonverbal communication, which can also be misinterpreted. Gaston-Johansson and colleagues (1990) examined the similarities in pain descriptions from four different cultural groups and found that people with diverse cultural and educational backgrounds may use similar words to describe the terms pain, hurt, and ache. Fortunately, some researchers have provided evidenced-based data to support the use of several standardized pain measures in clinical practice among culturally diverse groups diagnosed with cancer. Research on 536 persons with cancer of different ethnic backgrounds showed that evaluations of sensory pain using the McGill Pain Questionnaire were congruent across ethnic populations; however, descriptions of pain using affective terminology varied significantly (Greenwald, 1991). The multidimensional structure of the Brief Pain Inventory (BPI) has consistently demonstrated a high degree of reliability and validity when administered to samples from other countries (Cleeland & Ryan, 1994; Cleeland et al., 1996).

Personality Traits

According to the gate control theory of pain, a person's perception of pain and pain tolerance can be influenced by personality and other psychosocial factors. For example, people who are outgoing, or extroverts, may be more likely to express their pain than those who are quiet and shy.

Another personality factor that can influence pain perception and tolerance is anxiety. Many researchers have linked the presence of anxiety with pain. Other associated characteristics are feelings of powerlessness and the inability to cope with anxiety and pain. Nursing interventions to reduce anxiety and increase the ability to cope have also helped to relieve pain (Walding, 1991). However, the way in which pain is interpreted or appraised influences the coping strategies or methods selected by clients to deal with their pain (Arathuzik, 1991).

In addition to personality and other factors that cannot be changed, such as age and gender, other factors that are present at a given time may influence a person's experience of pain. Factors that tend to *decrease* the threshold for and tolerance of pain include discomfort, insomnia, fatigue, anxiety, fear, anger, sadness, depression, mental isolation, introversion, and past experience. Factors that tend to *increase* the threshold for and tolerance of pain include relief of symptoms, sleep, rest, sympathy, understanding, diversion, elevation of mood, analgesics, anxiolytic agents, and antidepressants. Because many of these factors can be altered, nursing interventions for pain often include minimizing factors that lower the pain threshold and tolerance and increasing or maximizing factors that increase the pain threshold and tolerance.

Research on Pain

Nurse-researchers have been concerned with the concept of pain, most often in relation to measuring the effects of nonpharmacologic interventions aimed at relieving pain. It is important for nurses to recognize the value of non-drug measures in alleviating pain and the associated distress. However, these techniques, when used for surgical pain and cancer-related pain, should compliment and not replace analgesic therapy.

In a classic study by Wells (1982), the effects of postoperative relaxation training were evaluated in a small sample of clients who had undergone cholecystectomy. Relaxation training reduced the psychological discomforts related to pain but demonstrated no measurable changes on any physiologic measures, such as blood pressure or pulse rate.

The overall effectiveness of relaxation techniques, including exercise, imagery, rhythmic breathing, and medication, has been evaluated by several investigators (Hyman et al., 1989). The result of their meta-analysis of published clinical studies indicated that relaxation techniques positively affect some clinical symptoms. Headaches were found to be consistently relieved through these techniques, whereas effects for chronic pain and anxiety were low to moderate and for acute pain were quite low.

In another evaluation of the effects of nursing intervention, Keller and Bzdek (1986) investigated the effects of therapeutic touch on tension headache pain. In this study, the McGill-Melzack Pain Questionnaire (Fig. 9–3) was used to demonstrate an average 70% pain reduction in the group who received touch intervention compared with the group who did not. Ferrel-Torry and Glick (1993) successfully used therapeutic massage as a nursing intervention to modify anxiety and the perception of cancer pain. Mulloney and Wells-Federman (1996) documented the powerful healing potential for therapeutic touch, including relief of pain, for selected clients. More recently, the benefits of progressive muscle relaxation and of therapeutic touch on pain and distress associated with degenerative arthritis were compared in older persons. Although both were effective, the greatest benefits for pain and distress were found with progressive muscle relaxation (Eckes Peck, 1997).

Music therapy as an intervention for pain has been shown to reduce postoperative pain and promote restorative sleep (Zimmerman et al., 1996). Benefits of music therapy have also been noted for clients experiencing cancer-related pain.

Pain Attitudes and Practices

Negative and mistaken beliefs about pain and its treatment currently prevail in the health care system. When such beliefs are perpetuated in clinical settings, it is difficult for health professionals to accept research-based information over traditional practices that are shaped by myths and misconceptions. Numerous studies have been conducted to help health professionals be more insightful and sensitive to these misconceptions that continue to obstruct views of pain and efforts to management it.

Attitudes of Nurses

Nurses' attitudes toward pain easily influence the way they perceive clients in pain and interact with them. Studies have suggested that practicing nurses perceive nu-

McGill-Melzack
PAIN QUESTIONNAIRE

Patient's name _____ Age _____
File No. _____ Date _____
Clinical category (e.g., cardiac, neurologic)
Diagnosis: _____
_____
_____

Analgesic (if already administered):

1. Type _____
2. Dosage _____
3. Time given in relation to this test _____

Patient's intelligence: circle number that represents best estimate.

1 (low)   2   3   4   5 (high)

****

This questionnaire has been designed to tell us more about your pain. Four major questions we ask are

1. Where is your pain?
2. What does it feel like?
3. How does it change with time?
4. How strong is it?

It is important that you tell us how your pain feels now. Please follow the instructions at the beginning of each part.

_____
© R. Melzack, Oct. 1970

Part 1. Where Is Your Pain?

Please mark, on the drawings below, the areas where you feel pain. Put E if external, or I if internal, near the areas you mark. Put EI if both external and internal.

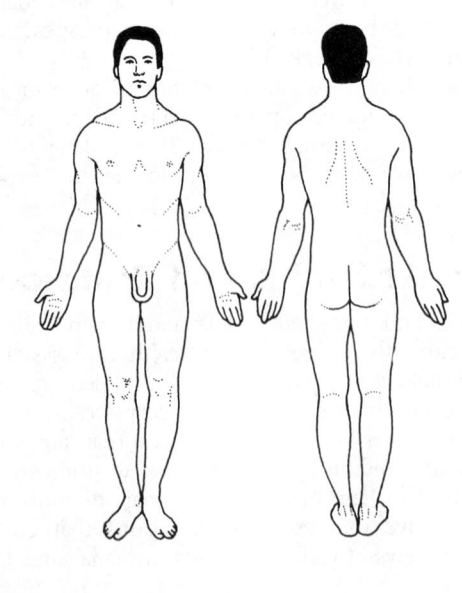

Part 2. What Does Your Pain Feel Like?

Some of the words below describe your *present* pain. Circle *ONLY* those words that best describe it. Leave out any category that is not suitable. Use only a single word in each appropriate category — the one that applies best.

1	6	11	16
Flickering	Tugging	Tiring	Annoying
Quivering	Pulling	Exhausting	Troublesome
Pulsing	Wrenching	**12**	Miserable
Throbbing	**7**	Sickening	Intense
Beating	Hot	Suffocat-	Unbearable
Pounding	Burning	ing	**17**
2	Scalding	**13**	Spreading
Jumping	Searing	Fearful	Radiating
Flashing	**8**	Frightful	Penetrating
Shooting	Tingling	Terrifying	Piercing
3	Itchy	**14**	**18**
Pricking	Smarting	Punishing	Tight
Boring	Stinging	Grueling	Numb
Drilling	**9**	Cruel	Drawing
Stabbing	Dull	Vicious	Squeezing
Lancinating	Sore	Killing	Tearing
4	Hurting	**15**	**19**
Sharp	Aching	Wretched	Cool
Cutting	Heavy	Blinding	Cold
Lacerating	**10**		Freezing
5	Tender		**20**
Pinching	Taut		Nagging
Pressing	Rasping		Nauseating
Gnawing	Splitting		Agonizing
Cramping			Dreadful
Crushing			Torturing

Part 3. How Does Your Pain Change With Time?

1. Which word or words would you use to describe the *pattern* of your pain?

1	2	3
Continuous	Rhythmic	Brief
Steady	Periodic	Momentary
Constant	Intermittent	Transient

2. What kind of things *relieve* your pain?

3. What kind of things *increase* your pain?

Part 4. How Strong Is Your Pain?

People agree that the following 5 words represent pain of increasing intensity. They are:

1	2	3	4	5
Mild	Discomforting	Distressing	Horrible	Excruciating

To answer each question below, write the number of the most appropriate word in the space beside the question.

1. Which word describes your pain right now? ____
2. Which word describes it at its worst? ____
3. Which word describes it when it is least? ____
4. Which word describes the worst toothache you ever had? ____
5. Which word describes the worst headache you ever had? ____
6. Which word describes the worst stomach ache you ever had? ____

Figure 9–3. The McGill-Melzack Pain Questionnaire. (From Melzack, R. [1975]. The McGill Pain Questionnaire: Major properties and scoring methods. *Pain, 1,* 272–281.)

merous barriers to effective pain management outcomes (Ferrell et al., 1992a; Fife et al., 1993; Wallace et al., 1995). Without an adequate knowledge of pain and principles of analgesic therapy, nurses may not be able to understand their clients' pain and confidently participate with physicians and other professionals in its treatment. Similarly, surveys of nursing faculty have shown that they too are ill prepared to care for clients in pain (Deikmann & Wassem, 1991; Ferrell et al., 1993)

Nurses who may have little personal experience with pain may not appreciate the magnitude of painful conditions associated with diseases and medical and surgical interventions. Nurses may expect that clients with chronic pain will react similarly to those with acute pain. They may assume that reactions to pain, including complaints about pain, will fall within a certain norm on the basis of their own cultural values. The more the response of a person with pain varies from these expected norms, the more likely it is that the attitude of the nurse toward the client will be biased, either positively or negatively.

Attitudes of Clients

Many client are reluctant to report pain, and when they do, they may underestimate its severity (Von Roenn et al., 1993). Clients may not complain of pain because they want to be a "good" client or they may not want to bother or distract their caregivers from other issues in their care. In clients with a history of cancer, pain can be an unwanted reminder of the disease and its progression.

Clients may also be reluctant to take pain medication, especially opioid analgesics, because of fear that they will become addicted or used to the medication (Ward & Gatwood, 1994). Compliance with medications can be affected by the complexity of the medication schedule or experience with untoward side effects, such as sedation or constipation.

Attitudes of Physicians

Undertreatment of pain, especially cancer pain, is a serious problem in the United States and elsewhere in the world. In 1983, the World Health Organization estimated that on any given day, 3.5 million people in the world experience cancer pain that could be relieved (Haviley et al., 1992).

Despite increased education about pain, many physicians underprescribe medication for clients in pain, especially opioids such as morphine. Some investigators have assessed several factors that account for this practice (Von Roenn et al., 1993).

First, cultural and societal attitudes exist about opioid use, especially in the United States. In some states, clients who use these drugs have to register with state regulatory agencies in a manner similar to that required of people enrolled in methadone programs. Requiring this procedure equates the client with a drug abuser. Some state regulations make it mandatory that triplicate prescriptions are used for schedule II controlled substances, which can deter physicians from prescribing some opioid analgesics.

Second, government regulatory agencies do not set practical guidelines for drug use in people with severe or chronic pain. A physician may be reprimanded by the medical board for prescribing what the board considers an inappropriate amount or type of pain medication.

Third, there is still a lack of knowledge about the effects of analgesics. Most of the studies on a person's response to drug therapy have been done with people who were not in pain. In many of these studies, subjects were volunteers who were former drug addicts imprisoned for drug abuse. The fear of respiratory depression that some physicians have is unnecessary because pain prevents or diminishes the respiratory effect of opioids (Haviley et al., 1992; Hill, 1990).

Types of Pain

There are several ways to classify types of pain. In 1986, the National Institutes of Health Consensus Conference on Pain categorized pain according to its cause. The participants at the conference identified three types of pain: acute, chronic malignant, and chronic nonmalignant. Acute pain results from acute injury, disease, or surgery. Chronic nonmalignant pain is associated with tissue injury that is not progressive or that has healed. Pain that is associated with cancer or another progressive disease is called chronic malignant pain. The nurse is usually concerned with two basic types of pain in practice: acute pain and chronic pain.

Acute Pain
Characteristics of Acute Pain

Acute pain is experienced by almost everyone at some time. Certain characteristics distinguish this type of pain from the more chronic, or long-term pain that is often associated with chronic illness. A major distinction between acute and chronic pain is the effect of pain on biological responses. Acute pain serves a biological purpose. It acts as a warning signal because it can activate the sympathetic nervous system. This stimulation causes the release of catecholamine neurotransmitters, such as epinephrine, which give rise to various physiologic responses. As a result, clients experiencing acute pain exhibit physiologic responses similar to those found in "fight-or-flight" reactions (see Chap. 8). These responses include increased heart rate, blood pressure, and respiratory rate; dilated pupils; and sweating. Behavioral signs of acute pain may include restlessness, an inability to concentrate, apprehension, and overall distress (Table 9–2).

Acute pain is usually temporary, of sudden onset, and easily localized. The client can frequently describe the pain, which may subside with or without treatment. Acute pain frequently results from sudden, accidental trauma, such as fractures, burns, and lacerations, or from surgery, ischemia, and acute inflammation. Acute pain is often the result of trauma involving superficial or cutaneous structures. This pain is confined to the affected area. As the painful area heals, the quality or sensation of the pain changes. Acute pain, although possibly severe, is limited over time and generally can be managed successfully. Both the caregiver and the client can see an end to the pain, which makes coping somewhat easier.

TABLE 9-2

Physiologic and Behavioral Responses to Acute and Chronic Pain

Pain Type	Physiologic Response	Behavioral Response
Acute	• Increased blood pressure initially • Increased pulse rate • Increased respiratory rate • Dilated pupils • Perspiration	• Restlessness • Inability to concentrate • Apprehension • Distress
Chronic	• Normal blood pressure • Normal pulse rate • Normal respiratory rate • Normal pupils • Dry skin	• Immobility or physical inactivity • Withdrawal • Despair

Postoperative Pain

Pain accompanying surgery is one of the most common examples of acute pain, but it is poorly understood and not always well managed. It is conservatively estimated that 20% of all clients who undergo surgery experience mild pain, 20% to 40% experience moderate pain, and 40% to 70% experience severe pain (Bonica, 1983). According to some authorities, the alarmingly high number of clients who experience pain after surgery can be attributed to inadequate analgesia (Acute Pain Management Guideline Panel, 1992). As discussed earlier, others believe that inadequate pain control stems from societal attitudes and believe that people in pain should "grin and bear it." Still others identify the fear of addiction as a major factor in physician-prescribing practices such as administering less than optimal amounts of analgesics after surgery. Whatever the reason, some people undergoing surgery suffer needlessly.

Pain is an expected outcome of surgery. Not only is there a sensory component arising from the area of tissue destruction, there is also a major psychosocial component.

RELATIONSHIP TO TYPE OF SURGICAL APPROACH. According to several studies, the type and site of the operation are the most important predictors in determining the incidence, severity, and duration of postoperative pain. Similarly, the extent of the operation, the degree of tissue trauma, and the positioning of the client during surgery contribute to the overall incidence and severity of postoperative pain.

Intrathoracic and upper intra-abdominal surgical approaches are generally associated with more severe, steady wound pain, as well as pain on movement in the postoperative period. Conversely, many clients who undergo superficial surgery of the head and neck, chest wall, or limbs report minimal or no pain postoperatively. Muscle-splitting procedures are far more painful than muscle-stretching procedures. On the basis of this information, surgeons have modified their techniques over the years in an attempt to reduce or minimize the components of this type of pain.

INFLUENCE OF PSYCHOSOCIAL VARIABLES. A person's postoperative pain experience is not limited to the level of tissue trauma. Postoperative pain is also influenced by many psychosocial variables. Personal factors, such as age and sociocultural group, may be important determinants for predicting patterns of expressing and coping with postoperative pain.

Anxiety is perhaps the best-explored psychological determinant in predicting postoperative pain. A highly anxious client may appear to be more distressed and affected by pain. Numerous studies have been done in an attempt to correlate preoperative information with postoperative pain (Acute Pain Management Guideline Panel, 1992). Some nursing studies, such as that of Johnson et al. (1978), indicate that clients who receive preoperative procedural or sensory information (i.e., a description of the expected sensation, as well as techniques to enhance relaxation) seem to cope better with postoperative pain. In addition, these clients recover more quickly than clients given only factual information about the anticipated postoperative experience.

Highly anxious clients, however, may be given minimal procedural information, such as the location of the incision, the sequence of events before surgery (e.g., preoperative sedation and visits from perioperative personnel), and postoperative care regimens. For these clients, too much information can exacerbate fear and pain (Acute Pain Management Guideline Panel, 1992).

The nurse stresses to the client the importance of requesting analgesia when he or she perceives pain. The nurse should repeat these instructions at regular intervals if the client is anxious, because anxiety interferes with the ability to process information. The nurse also uses non-pharmacologic interventions, such as distraction and relaxation, to help the highly anxious client (see later).

Chronic Pain
Characteristics of Chronic Pain

Chronic pain is a major health problem. It has been estimated that in the United States alone, 25% of people, many of them older than 65 years, are affected with a chronic illness and chronic pain. In contrast to acute pain, chronic pain serves no biological purpose. After the pain's initial warning signal, the body must learn to adapt to the persistent pain impulses by blocking or adjusting to the activation of the sympathetic nervous system, which causes the fight-or-flight reaction in acute pain. Because of this adaptation, many of the obvious symptoms that are associated with physiologic responses to pain are absent or less obvious in the client with chronic pain.

Chronic pain is defined as pain that persists or recurs for indefinite periods, usually for more than 2 months.

Onset is gradual, and the character and quality of the pain change over time. Because chronic pain frequently involves deep somatic and visceral structures, it is usually diffuse, poorly localized, and often difficult to describe. If the underlying cause of the chronic pain cannot be treated medically, controlling the long-term effects of chronic pain may be a difficult clinical challenge.

Chronic pain is associated with a variety of health problems, such as cancer, connective tissue diseases, peripheral vascular diseases, and musculoskeletal disorders. It is also seen in post-traumatic problems, such as phantom limb pain and low back pain. The degree of chronic pain varies, depending on the type of problem and whether it is progressive, stable, or capable of resolution. Unless the disease process is arrested or reversed, the severity of chronic pain may worsen to the point that the client is physically and emotionally debilitated. Even when the physiologic pain stimuli are eliminated or tissue damage has resolved, the client's perception of pain may linger. This is sometimes called the "chronic pain syndrome." A client's response to chronic pain is influenced by his or her ability to cope, the availability of family support and social resources, and the severity of the physiologic and emotional consequences (see Table 9–2).

Because chronic pain persists for extended periods, it can interfere with activities of daily living and personal relationships. It can also result in emotional and financial burdens. Thus, the efforts of an interdisciplinary health care team are needed to manage the situation effectively. If pain is inadequately managed, it is an overwhelming, frustrating experience for both sufferer and caregiver. Although many of the characteristics of chronic pain are similar in different clients, the nurse should be aware that each chronic pain situation is unique and requires a highly specialized plan of care.

Chronic Nonmalignant Pain

Chronic nonmalignant pain may be caused by chronic diseases such as rheumatoid arthritis, lupus, sickle cell anemia, diabetic neuropathy, and peripheral vascular disease. It may also be related to painful conditions such as fibromyalgia, low back pain, chronic headaches, osteoporosis, and facial pain. Whenever possible, the source(s) of the chronic nonmalignant pain should be targeted and managed with nonopioid analgesics and nondrug measures. However, chronic opioid therapy has gained wide acceptance in selected populations when other therapies have failed to provide optimal pain relief.

In the past, physicians were reluctant to consider opioid therapy in clients who did not have cancer. Clients experiencing nonmalignant pain were traditionally managed with nonopioid analgesics or adjuvant drugs, and nondrug measures. However, today some clients with chronic nonmalignant pain are managed with long-term opioid therapy. This type of therapy is generally reserved for clients who have a documented physiologic source for the pain—more specifically, those with chronic diseases. Structured regimens using long-acting or extended-release opioids with occasional short-acting analgesics, if necessary, are preferred.

There is enough evidence to suggest that the benefits of alleviating pain and suffering with chronic opioid therapy far outweigh any risks. Several published reports in selected client populations have documented favorable clinical outcomes such as improved function, better quality of life, less psychological distress, and less dependence on the health care system when opioids have been used (Schofferman et al., 1993; Vallerand, 1991). Moreover, the risk of addiction remains exceedingly low. Even when chronic opioids are given to clients with nonmalignant pain having a known history of substance abuse, drug-seeking behavior is seldom a significant problem (Dunbar & Katz, 1996).

Only those clients who have demonstrated measurable benefits from opioids should be considered for long-term use of these medications for nonmalignant pain. Compassionate use of opioids may be considered for the elderly with debilitating pain (i.e., compression fractures of the spine) both at home and in extended care facilities. The nurse recognizes that the elderly may be more prone to side effects of opioids (i.e., sedation, constipation, mental status changes) and implements measures to reduce the risk of opioid-induced adverse effects.

Chronic Pain Syndrome

Clients sometimes have chronic pain associated with a physical problem. Eventually, the physiologic alterations resolve or become less detectable, and the etiology for the pain is unclear. Sometimes these painful conditions are referred to as idiopathic pain, pain of unknown etiology, or chronic pain syndrome. However, the perception or sensation of pain persists. The degree of pain appears to be out of proportion to the physical findings, yet the pain is real to the person experiencing it. Clients in this situation often subject themselves to a variety of medical tests and frequent hospitalization while searching for a cause for or explanation of their pain. So-called doctor shopping is common in this group of clients. Some clients invest an incredible amount of time and energy in the health care system in the hope of uncovering a solution for their pain. As a result, clients with chronic pain syndrome focus on what they cannot do rather than what they can to do. Clients often demonstrate learned helplessness, powerlessness, dependency, and sick role behaviors. They may experience loss of confidence, disuse of their bodies, risks of losing income, and difficulty in adapting to social and work situations. When pain persists for long periods, family members are often emotionally drained, frustrated, and in need of help in dealing with the client.

Interdisciplinary pain centers, like pain clinics or programs, are best equipped to handle the complex psychosocial pain issues associated with chronic pain syndromes. Published data show that comprehensive pain centers have demonstrated modest success in eliminating the need for prescription analgesics, reducing dependence on the health care system, and reintegrating clients into social and occupational networks (Flor et al., 1992). Behavioral and cognitive approaches, which focus on family-centered care, are useful strategies for these clients.

Chronic Malignant (Cancer-Related) Pain

Although many clients with advanced malignant disease experience severe pain, adequate pain control could be achieved for most of them. Even when the best pain management techniques are used, however, the complexity and progressive nature of this type of pain often limit the success of pain management efforts.

Cancer-related pain arises from a variety of mechanisms. For example, as a malignant tumor invades the bone, chemicals known as prostaglandins are released. These substances sensitize nerve receptors in the bone and increase their sensitivity to painful stimuli. In part, this explains the extreme degree of pain associated with bony metastases. Other causes of cancer-related pain include arterial ischemia, venous engorgement, nerve compression, infection, inflammation, necrosis, and ulcerations. In addition, the sources of these problems are usually in deep somatic and visceral structures. These types of painful sensations, coupled with the diffuse nature of the pain, hamper the client's ability to describe and localize cancer pain.

The psychological impact of cancer can be devastating, especially if clients must contend with unrelieved pain (see Research Applications for Nursing). Investigators have documented marked psychological distress among clients with higher pain intensities and poorer relief of pain. (Polomano, 1995; Zimmerman et al., 1996).

▷ Research Applications for Nursing

Psychological Variables and Their Effect on Cancer Pain

Zimmerman, L., Turner Story, K., Gaston-Johansson, F., & Rowles, J. (1996). Psychological variables and cancer pain. Cancer Nursing, 19(1), 44–53.

The purpose of this study was to determine whether cancer clients with pain had higher scores of depression, anxiety, somatization, and hostility than did cancer clients without pain. Thirty clients in each group were given the Brief Symptom Inventory (BSI), the McGill Pain Questionnaire (MPQ), and a visual analogue scale for pain. Clients with pain scored higher on all four subscales of the BSI, meaning that they were experiencing more depression, anxiety, somatization, and hostility. However, these differences were only significant for somatization and hostility. For all subjects, there were significant positive relationships between the scores on the MPQ and all four subscales. Higher MPQ scores, indicative of more pain, were associated with higher BSI subscale scores, which reflect poorer outcomes

Critique. This study was an attempt to further clarify the nature of affective, cognitive, and behavioral components of pain. The small convenience sample limits the ability to generalize these findings to other clients with cancer but points the way to further research.

Possible Implications for Nursing. The findings suggest a relationship between psychological status and dimensions of the pain experience. Nursing interventions for the client in pain should be directed at assessing and modifying both pain level and psychological status.

Most clients with advanced cancer have more than one location of and physiologic source of pain. Approximately one third of these clients experience a component of neuropathic pain or nerve injury pain (Polomano, 1995). Because the pharmacologic approaches may vary depending on whether clients have somatic, visceral, and/or neuropathic pain, it is important for the nurse to identify the cause or causes of the pain in each location. (For additional information on this type of pain, see Chapter 26 and consult Management of Cancer Pain Clinical Practice Guidelines, 1994.)

Collaborative Management

 Assessment

➤ *History*

The nurse asks the client about the pain experience, including the sequence of events (precipitating and relieving factors); the nature of adjustments, if any, in the client's life or in the family; and beliefs about the cause of the pain and what should be done about it (client's expectations). Personal characteristics, such as the client's age and culture, influence attitudes about reporting a pain history. Families and significant others are included in this information-gathering process.

Clients may report pain in the absence of any observable or documented physiologic changes in the body. The nurse keeps in mind that all pain is real and operates from the premise that pain is "whatever the person experiencing it says it is." The nurse respects the client's verbal and nonverbal expressions of pain without making judgments or inferences about the reality of the pain. If clients perceive that health professionals doubt the existence of their pain, mistrust and other negative feelings can arise and interfere with a therapeutic nurse-client relationship.

The nurse also assesses the length of time the client has experienced pain. Clients who experience acute pain may welcome an opportunity to discuss their pain with the nurse, because acute pain is a relatively short-term experience and is easily described by clients. However, clients with chronic pain can be frustrated when they are unable to adequately describe their vague, diffuse pain experience. Structured interviews using assessment aids, such as pain scales and descriptors, often help clients to express their pain.

ELDERLY CONSIDERATIONS

The elderly client's complaints of pain may be ignored by caregivers. Herr and Mobily (1991) found that some elderly clients in a residential center stopped expressing their discomfort because they were treated as "chronic complainers." Other elders stated that the response to their complaints was "What do you expect at your age?" Older adults do not typically have age-related pain.

Nurses should also consider that when they take a history from elderly clients, the clients may be anxious or temporarily disoriented as a result of pain or because they

Chart 9–1

Nursing Focus on the Elderly: The Elderly Client Experiencing Pain

When taking a client history

- Realize that the prevalence of pain is estimated to be double those younger than 60 years and well over 70% among elders in care facilities.
- Consider the elderly at risk for the undertreatment of pain, especially cancer pain, because of inappropriate beliefs about pain sensitivity, tolerance, and ability to use opioids.
- Recognize that cognitive impairment in the elderly may pose barriers to pain assessment, but the elderly with mild to moderate cognitive impairment may be able to accurately report pain at the moment or when prompted.
- Cognitively impaired elderly may require more frequent assessments of pain than clients who are not impaired.
- Use visual representations of pain meases rather than mental images of pain rating scales. Be sure that the client is wearing glasses and hearing aid(s), if needed and available.
- Alter a written pain scale to include large lettering, adequate space between lines, nonglossy paper, and color for increased visualization.
- Provide adequate lighting and privacy to avoid distracting background noise.

If the client cannot verbally communicate

- Assess for nonverbal indicators of pain, such as grimacing or crying.
- Observe for changes in the client's behavior, such as increased confusion or combativeness.
- Respond to complaints of pain promptly—they are typically not age-related complaints.
- Administer the prescribed amount of analgesics for postoperative pain in a timely manner. If pain is not relieved, evaluate the effectiveness of the analgesic regimen and immediately notify the physician.
- Use nondrug pain relief measures.

Data from the Acute Pain Management Guideline Panel. (1994). *Acute pain management: Operative or medical procedures and trauma. Clinical practice guideline.* AHCPR Pub. No. 92-0032. Rockville, MD: Agency for Health Care Policy and Research, Public Health Service, U.S. Department of Health and Human Services.

are in an unusual environment. The nurse observes for nonverbal indicators of pain, such as grimacing, and checks for changes in behavior. For example, if a client becomes restless, hostile, or combative, the nurse considers pain as a possible underlying reason. Too often a client who behaves in this manner is labeled with a diagnosis of dementia or other cognitive impairment or is categorized by the nursing staff as "difficult." Chart 9–1 highlights key points for assessing an elderly client in pain.

➤ Essential Data for a Complete Pain History

Information about a client's pain can be helpful in understanding the factors that are associated with the client's present pain or previous episodes of pain. If the client is in pain when the nurse is taking the history, the nurse should keep the session reasonably short or continue at a later time. Data to obtain include

- *Precipitating factors.* Does the client associate any activities, ingestion of food, or other environmental factors with the onset of pain? What does the client think causes the present pain? Was the onset of pain sudden or insidious? Has the client done anything or taken anything to relieve the pain? What were the results of the intervention?
- *Aggravating factors.* What factors make the pain worse? What influence has this pain had on the client's activity? What changes in life activity have been affected (e.g., diet, job, sleep)?
- *Localization of pain.* Can the client localize the pain or describe where it travels or radiates?
- *Character and quality of pain.* What words does the client use to describe the pain, its character, quality, or intensity?
- *Duration of pain.* How long has the client experienced this pain?

➤ Physical Assessment/Clinical Manifestations

The overt or observable clinical manifestations of pain include physiologic responses, motor or body movements, and affective behaviors such as crying. Although physiologic changes occur in response to acute noxious stimuli, these changes are usually *not* reliable indicators of chronic pain. Acute pain, with its property of warning an individual about harm, elicits several physiologic signs and symptoms. These signs and symptoms are largely a function of sympathetic nervous system stimulation. Clients with acute pain often manifest pronounced changes in vital body functions, such as tachycardia and blood pressure changes. The blood pressure is usually elevated initially and is then decreased. In addition, clients with acute pain may become diaphoretic, restless, and apprehensive.

Physiologic changes in response to chronic pain are usually masked as the body attempts to compensate for and adapt to the noxious stimuli. The pain no longer serves as a necessary warning. Changes in vital signs related to chronic pain may be evident only when pre-existing pain occurs or as new sites of painful stimuli arise.

Certain motor or body movements may be associated with acute or chronic pain. Some may be more exaggerated or obvious than others. Clients in pain may support or shield ("splint"), holding painful body parts while moving, or lie listlessly because they are afraid to move. The nurse assesses the functional status and degree of impairment in the client with pain.

Location of Pain

The nurse assesses the location of pain from two dimensions: the level of pain, either deep or superficial, and the position or location of pain. Most clients, whether they are experiencing acute or chronic pain, can usually describe the depth of pain perceived. However, the actual area or location of the pain may not be as easily identified.

The nurse asks the client whether the pain is superficial or deep. In general, clients who have pain involving superficial or cutaneous structures describe their pain as superficial and can often localize the pain to a specific area. These structures have an abundant nerve supply, which contributes to the ease and accuracy of the client localizing the pain. In contrast, clients who perceive pain from deeper somatic or visceral structures within the body may have difficulty localizing their pain (a result of the poor innervation of this area).

Pain may be described as belonging to one of four categories, related to its location:

- Localized pain—pain confined to the site of origin
- Projected pain—pain along a specific nerve or nerves
- Radiating pain—diffuse pain around the site of origin that is not well localized
- Referred pain—pain perceived in an area distant from the site of painful stimuli

A client who has difficulty specifying the exact location of pain can be asked to point to the painful areas on his or her own body or on another person. Sometimes having the client point to or shade in the painful areas on a diagram of the front and back of the human body is helpful (see Fig. 9–2). When clients cannot identify the painful areas and state that they just "hurt all over," the nurse encourages the client to focus on parts of the body that are not painful. The nurse asks the client to concentrate on different body parts, beginning with the hand and fingers of one extremity, while asking him or her to identify the presence or absence of pain. As the nurse focuses attention on selected areas of the body, the client is assisted in localizing painful areas. Often clients who state that they hurt everywhere begin to realize that some parts of the body are not painful.

Clients may present with more than one discrete painful site. In fact, about one half of clients with advanced cancer report having pain in more than one location. As painful areas are identified, the nurse helps the client to understand the origin of the pain. This understanding is particularly important for clients with cancer because every new pain often raises the suspicion of metastasis (spread of disease). The pain may be caused by other reasons, such as immobility or constipation.

Character and Quality of Pain

After asking the client to locate the pain, the nurse asks him or her to describe how the pain feels. Clients may use a word or group of words to convey the sensations or feelings of the pain. The nurse avoids suggesting descriptive words for the pain. Some clients who are frustrated and are having difficulty describing their pain may benefit from using the McGill-Melzack Pain Questionnaire (see Fig. 9–3). With this measurement tool, the nurse asks the client to circle descriptive terms in the appropriate categories to best describe the pain. This questionnaire may be too difficult for clients with poor reading or verbal skills. The Short-Form McGill Pain Questionnaire (SF-MPQ) provides a simpler way of describing the sensory and affective components of pain (Melzack, 1987) (see Fig. 9–5). Its use is of particular value in measuring

changes in sensations of the pain when adjuvant or non-opioid analgesics such as tricylcic antidepressants and anticonvulsants are tried.

Another useful strategy is to ask the client to describe the sensation by comparing it to a situation or event that may be comparable to the feeling of pain. For example, a man with excruciating diffuse abdominal pain from advanced cancer once said that his pain felt as if a soldier were walking around inside his abdomen, with no set path or destination, stepping on mines. For this man, pain was unpredictable and never-ending and produced "blowing-up" sensations.

Pattern of Pain

Pain is rarely the same at all times. It is perceived differently over time and is subjected to various precipitating and aggravating factors (see earlier discussion under History).

Intensity of Pain

Subjective measurements of pain intensity are more reliable and accurate than the overt or observable parameters of pain. Only the client can determine the amount or severity of pain experienced. Various visual analog scales, numeric rating scales (NRS), descriptive word scales, and other measures have been designed to help clients communicate the magnitude or severity of pain and to help nurses quantify the pain.

The nurse uses pain intensity scales to measure pain in the clinical setting and to assess and determine the effectiveness of relief-oriented interventions. The client is presented with an appropriate pain scale and asked to rate the amount of painful stimuli. Clients with more than one discrete painful site may wish to specify their pain levels by location. Clinicians have recently been encouraged to elicit self-report measures of pain that reflect not only present pain levels but also the average or general pain level and least and worst pain intensities.

When describing varied levels of pain, the client is asked to recall the pain over a specified time interval.

A variety of scales can be used to measure pain intensity, and some also assess the emotional aspects of pain. Verbal descriptive scales typically group words such as "none," "moderate," or "severe" and permit an intensity rating of pain. Visual analog scales (VAS) usually use a 10-cm line to represent a continuum of pain intensity and include verbal anchors that describe the intensity of the stimuli. Numeric rating scales (0–10) (NRS) are commonly employed in clinical practice because they are easily communicated and interpreted. Studies have shown strong correlations between the NRS and the VAS (Puntillo & Weiss, 1994). For examples of such pain intensity rating scales, see Figure 9–4.

Variations in the scales are important determinants for selecting the appropriate measurement tool. Clients with chronic, nagging, diffuse pain may have difficulty using broad numeric ranges such as the NRS. Some clients are better able to use word associations and prefer measurements that contain descriptive words or phrases rather than just numbers. The Faces Rating Scale is particularly useful for assessing pain in culturally diverse populations

PAIN INTENSITY SCALES

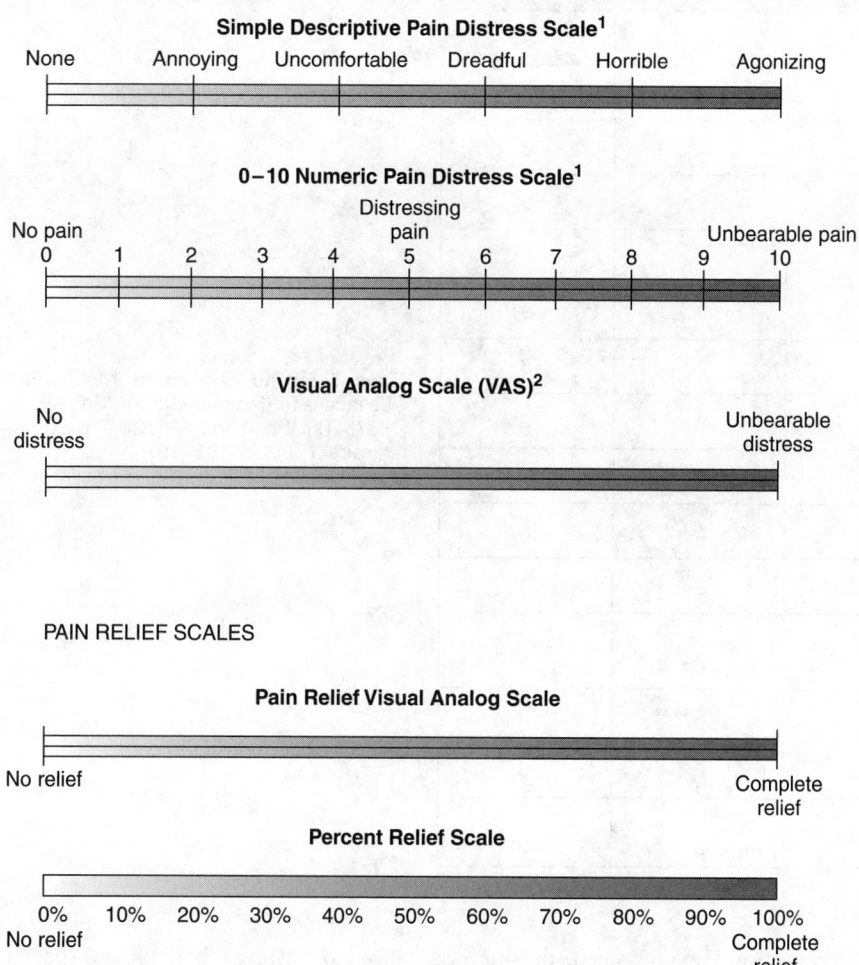

Figure 9–4. Pain rating scales and pain relief scales. (Simple Descriptive Pain Distress Scale, 0–10 Numeric Pain Distress Scale, and Visual Analog Scale redrawn from Acute Pain Management Guideline Panel. [1992]. *Acute pain management: Operative or medical procedures and trauma. Clinical practice guideline.* AHCPR Pub. No. 92-0032. Rockville, MD: Agency for Health Care Policy and Research, Public Health Service, U.S. Department of Health and Human Services; Pain Relief Visual Analog Scale redrawn from Fishman, B., Pasternak, S., Wallenstein, S. L., Houde, R. W., Holland, J. C., & Foley, K. M. [1987]. The Memorial Pain Assessment Card: A valid instrument for the evaluation of cancer pain. *Cancer, 60*[5], 1151–1158; Percent Relief Scale redrawn from the Brief Pain Inventory. Pain Research Group, Department of Neurology, University of Wisconsin-Madison.)

[1]If used as a graphic rating scale, a 10-cm baseline is recommended.

[2]A 10-cm baseline is recommended for VAS scales.

who encounter language barriers in expressing their pain.

Perception of Pain Relief

Pain relief is a dimension separate from pain intensity. Therefore, the amount of relief that is achieved from pain therapies, in addition to the amount or level of pain experienced, should be assessed. Valid measures of pain relief can be obtained by using relief scales. As with pain intensity measures, it is critical to provide a time frame for evaluating the pain therapy. Evaluation of pain relief can be accomplished with either a pain relief analogue scale or a percent rating scale (see Figure 9–4).

Issues in Pain Measurement

It is critical that reliable and valid measures be used to evaluate dimensions of pain. Nurses should avoid using self-report scales that have not been adequately tested in clinical practice settings. Pain measures should be appropriate for the client's cognitive level and issues with pain.

ELDERLY CONSIDERATIONS

When using tools to measure pain in elderly clients, the nurse considers possible visual or hearing limitations. The client should wear glasses and one or two hearing aids, if appropriate. Increased lighting with nonglare bulbs may improve visual perception. The tools may be altered to include large lettering, adequate spacing between lines, and color on a white background (Herr & Mobily, 1991). Pasero and McCaffery (1994) provide additional strategies for assessing pain in the elderly.

► Psychosocial Assessment

Acute Pain

All pain holds significant meaning for the person experiencing it. For clients experiencing acute pain from sur-

Type	None	Mild	Moderate	Severe
Throbbing	0	1	2	3
Shooting	0	1	2	3
Stabbing	0	1	2	3
Sharp	0	1	2	3
Cramping	0	1	2	3
Gnawing	0	1	2	3
Hot-burning	0	1	2	3
Aching	0	1	2	3
Heavy	0	1	2	3
Tender	0	1	2	3
Splitting	0	1	2	3
Tiring/exhausting	0	1	2	3
Sickening	0	1	2	3
Fearful	0	1	2	3
Punishing/cruel	0	1	2	3

Figure 9–5. The Short-Form McGill Pain Questionnaire (Recreated from Melzack, R. [1987]. The Short-Form McGill Pain Questionnaire. *Pain, 30,* 191–197.)

gery, the pain may be interpreted as necessary and expected. The pain may be viewed with relief as a sign that some greater problem has been resolved or alleviated by the surgery. Knowledge that the duration of the pain is limited may allow the client to deal with unpleasant sensations without too much difficulty. In contrast, acute chest pain associated with angina may mark the beginning of a life of fear and uncertainty for the client.

Chronic Pain

Psychosocial factors that influence chronic pain vary. Some are similar to those found in the acute pain experience, such as anxiety or fear related to the meaning of the pain for each client. Because pain persists in the chronic situation or is perhaps only partially relieved, the client may feel powerless, angry, hostile, or desperate. The client with chronic pain is also vulnerable to labels such as "chronic complainer" or "fake." Because many of the behavioral manifestations of acute pain (e.g., sweating, writhing, increased blood pressure) are absent in the client with chronic pain, the caregiver might doubt the existence of the pain. In some chronic pain conditions (e.g., myofacial pain disorders), there may be an absence of objective physical findings that corroborate the report of pain. This may produce problems of depression, difficulties socializing, and conflicts with others. Clients may need outside assistance to resolve their illness-specific controversies with others.

The status of family and other close relationships, along with the breadth of social resources available to the chronic pain client, must be assessed. The existence of pain-specific conflict with a spouse or significant other may affect or limit pain coping strategies (Faucett, 1994). Other people may react to chronic pain with depression, social withdrawal, and preoccupation with physical symptoms.

If the pain is chronic and associated with a progressive disease, such as cancer, rheumatoid arthritis, or peripheral vascular disease, the client may have worries and concerns about the consequences of the illness. Clients suffering from cancer-related pain may fear death or body mutilation. Some may think that they are being punished for some wrongdoing in life. Others may attach a religious or spiritual significance to lingering pain and may think that suffering on earth exemplifies the experience of pain so often associated with those in the Bible.

The nurse asks open-ended questions (e.g., "Tell me how your pain has affected your job or role as a mother") to allow the client to describe personal attitudes about pain and its influence on his or her life. This opportunity can help a client whose life has been changed by pain. However, some clients choose not to share private information or fears related to the meaning of their pain readily, and this decision should be respected by the nurse.

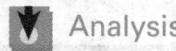 Analysis

➤ Common Nursing Diagnoses and Collaborative Problems

The actual diagnoses for a client with pain are divided into two main categories:

- Pain
- Chronic Pain

The etiologic factors are not included here because they vary, depending on the cause of the pain and each client's response.

➤ Additional Nursing Diagnoses and Collaborative Problems

In addition to the common nursing diagnoses, the client experiencing acute or chronic pain may have one or more of the following nursing diagnoses:

- Anxiety related to loss of control
- Fear related to pain
- Powerlessness related to illness-related regimen
- Altered Role Performance related to a change in health status and impaired coping
- Altered Sexuality Patterns related to illness and pain
- Impaired Physical Mobility related to pain and discomfort
- Activity Intolerance related to pain and/or depression
- Sleep Pattern Disturbance related to pain
- Self-Care Deficit (total or partial) related to pain
- Altered Health Maintenance related to a feeling of hopelessness

➤ Pain

 Planning and Implementation

Pharmacologic measures are the major means used to relieve acute pain. Nonpharmacologic measures, such as the use of a pillow for splinting an incision and complementary therapies, are also effective, but these measures are usually used in conjunction with drug therapy.

Drug Therapy. Clients who achieve adequate analgesia during the postoperative phase experience fewer complications and have shorter recovery periods than clients who have a significant degree of pain (Acute Pain Management Guideline Panel, 1992). Nurses must ensure that clients receive adequate interventions to manage their pain.

Nonopioid Analgesics. Many people underestimate the effectiveness of nonopioid analgesics, also referred to as peripheral-acting analgesics. Acetylsalicylic acid (ASA; aspirin, Ancasal✦), 650 mg, and acetaminophen (Datril, Tylenol, Ace-Tabs✦), 650 mg (which are nonopioids), produce pain relief comparable to that of codeine, 32 mg orally, and meperidine (Demerol), 50 mg orally, which are opioids, for mild pain. Aspirin has direct analgesic effects because it inhibits prostaglandin synthesis in the presence of inflammation.

Over-the-counter (OTC) medications are not given alone for the treatment of severe pain. They are usually administered in conjunction with opioid analgesics. Aspirin or aspirin-containing compounds must be used with caution after surgery because they can irritate the gastrointestinal tract and interfere with platelet aggregation. The nurse monitors the client carefully for bleeding and bruising.

Nonsteroidal anti-inflammatory drugs (NSAIDs) are also popular nonopioids that possess anti-inflammatory properties, largely by inhibiting prostaglandins. Ketoprofen (Orudis), also an NSAID, seems to block the synthesis of leukotrienes, which also sensitize the nociceptors. These drugs are particularly useful in the management of acute inflammation caused by tissue destruction. Parenteral ketorolac (Toradol) is one of the most popular NSAIDs prescribed by physicians for short-term use in cases of acute pain. Unlike other NSAIDs, this drug is available in both oral and parenteral form. Table 9–3 outlines the NSAIDs most commonly prescribed for acute pain.

The side effects of NSAIDs are similar to those of aspirin—gastric irritation and upset, renal toxicity and effects on coagulation. They can also cause sodium and water retention, which is of special concern in elderly clients, who can easily develop congestive heart failure from fluid retention. The elderly may also be more at risk for renal toxicity and should be monitored closely with renal function blood values. The nurse observes for and teaches the client and family to observe for these untoward effects of medication.

Opioid Analgesics. Opioid analgesics (also called opioids or narcotics) are central-acting analgesics that are the cornerstone of pharmacologic acute pain management (Acute Pain Management Guideline Panel, 1992). These drugs work by binding with opioid receptors, both within and outside of the central nervous system. For acute pain, they may be administered by the oral, rectal, intramuscular, intraspinal, intravenous, or subcutaneous route.

Classification of Opioids. Opioid analgesics are classified as full agonists, partial agonists, or mixed agonist-antagonists. "Full agonists produce a maximal response within the cells to which they bind; partial agonists produce a lesser response; and mixed agonist-antagonists activate one type of opioid receptor while simultaneously blocking another type" (Acute Pain Management Guideline Panel, 1992, p. 17).

The most important type of opioid receptor is the mu receptor. Commonly used opioids that bind with mu (mu opioids) are short-acting morphine (Roxanol, MSIR, Statex✦); controlled-released morphine (MS Contin, Oramorph); hydromorphone (Dilaudid); codeine; short-acting oxycodone (Roxicodone) and in combination with acetaminophen (Percocet, Roxicet, Tylox), controlled-released oxycodone (OxyContin), meperidine (Demerol), and fentanyl (Sublimaze). Clients receiving these agonists should not receive mixed agonist-antagonists, such as pentazocine (Talwin), nalbuphine (Nubain), butorphanol (Stadol), or tramadol (Ultram), or partial agonists like buprenorphine because they may negate the effect of the agonists. Table 9–4 lists common opioid agonists with dosing guidelines and additional information.

Meperidine (Demerol) used to be routinely prescribed by physicians after surgery because it was mistakenly

TABLE 9-3

Nonsteroidal Anti-Inflammatory Drugs for the Treatment of Acute Pain		
Drug	**Usual Adult Dose**	**Comments**
Oral NSAIDs		
Acetaminophen	650–975 mg q 4 hr	Acetaminophen lacks the peripheral anti-inflammatory activity of other NSAIDs
Aspirin	650–975 mg q 4 hr	The standard against which other NSAIDs are compared. Inhibits platelet aggregation; may cause postoperative bleeding
Choline magnesium trisalicylate (Trilisate)	1000–1500 mg bid	May have minimal antiplatelet activity; also available as oral liquid
Diflunisal (Dolobid)	1000 mg initial dose followed by 500 mg q 12 hr	
Etodolac (Lodine)	200–400 mg q 6–8 hr	
Fenoprofen calcium (Nalfon)	200 mg q 4–6 hr	
Ibuprofen (Motrin, others)	400 mg q 4–6 hr	Available as several brand names and as generic; also available as oral suspension
Ketoprofen (Orudis)	25–75 mg q 6–8 hr	
Magnesium salicylate	650 mg q 4 hr	Many brands and generic forms available
Meclofenamate sodium (Meclomen)	50 mg q 4–6 hr	
Mefenamic acid (Ponstel)	250 mg q 6 hr	
Naproxen (Naprosyn)	500 mg initial dose followed by 250 mg q 6–8 hr	Also available as oral liquid
Naproxen sodium (Anaprox)	550 mg initial dose followed by 275 mg q 6–8 hr	
Salsalate (Disalcid, others)	500 mg q 4 hr	May have minimal antiplatelet activity
Sodium salicylate	325–650 mg q 3–4 hr	Available in generic form from several distributors
Parenteral NSAID		
Ketorolac	30 or 60 mg IM initial dose followed by 15 or 30 mg q 6 hr Oral dose following IM dosage: 10 mg q 6–8 hr	Intramuscular dose not to exceed 5 days

Acute Pain Management Guideline Panel. (1992). *Acute pain management: Operative or medical procedures and trauma. Clinical practice guideline* (pp. 110–111). AHCPR Pub. No. 92–0032. Rockville, MD: Agency for Health Care Policy and Research, Public Health Service, U.S. Department of Health and Human Services.

thought to possess certain advantages over morphine and other opioids. Often, an insufficient amount was prescribed, resulting in less than optimal pain control. Meperidine is only effective for 2.5 to 3.5 hours, and a dose of 75 mg is equivalent to only 5 to 7.5 mg of morphine.

ELDERLY CONSIDERATIONS

Elderly clients and those with renal disease should not take meperidine because of the prolonged half-life of its drug metabolite normeperidine (Acute Pain Management Guideline Panel, 1992). Normeperidine, an excitotoxin, accumulates with repeated dosing and can lead to life-threatening seizures. The drug is also contraindicated in elderly clients, as they may excrete the metabolite more slowly, making them more at risk for cerebral irritation, which leads to seizures, memory loss, hallucinations, paranoia, and depression (Hofland, 1992). Some

institutions have established guidelines to restrict the use of meperidine, monitor the duration of therapy, and offer alternative choices for the use of other opioids.

All mu opioids may cause urinary retention, constipation, sedation, respiratory depression, and nausea and vomiting. Urinary retention and respiratory depression are less common among opioid-dependent clients or those who take opioids for extended periods. Opioid-induced side effects generally correlate with the blood level of the medication. The nurse observes for these problems and reports their occurrence to the physician. The nurse remembers that pain and the stress and anxiety that accompany it are potent respiratory *stimulants* that may negate the respiratory depressive action of the drugs. The nurse also keeps in mind that the effect of all opioid analgesics may be potentiated in a client who is elderly, has reduced blood volume or renal disease, or has received anesthetic agents or other central nervous system depressants.

TABLE 9-4

Dosing Guidelines for Opioids in the Treatment of Acute Pain*†

Drug	Approximate Equianalgesic Oral Dose	Approximate Equianalgesic Parenteral Dose	Recommended Starting Dose (Adults More Than 50 kg Body Weight)		Recommended Starting Dose (Children and Adults Less Than 50 kg Body Weight)‡	
Opioid Agonist			Oral	Parenteral	Oral	Parenteral
Morphine§	30 mg q 3–4 hr (around-the-clock dosing) 60 mg q 3–4 hr (single dose or intermittent dosing)	10 mg q 3–4 hr	30 mg q 3–4 hr	10 mg q 3–4 hr	0.3 mg/kg q 3–4 hr	0.1 mg/kg q 3–4 hr
Codeine¶	130 mg q 3–4 hr	75 mg q 3–4 hr	60 mg q 3–4 hr	60 mg q 2 hr (intramuscular/subcutaneous)	1 mg/kg q 3–4 hr**	Not recommended
Hydromophone§ (Dilaudid)	7.5 mg q 3–4 hr	1.5 mg q 3–4 hr	6 mg q 3–4 hr	1.5 mg q 3–4 hr	0.06 mg/kg q 3–4 hr	0.015 mg/kg q 3–4 hr
Hydrocodone (in Lorcet, Lortab, Vicodin, others)	30 mg q 3–4 hr	Not available	10 mg q 3–4 hr	Not available	0.2 mg/kg q 3–4 hr**	Not available
Levorphanol (Levo-Dromoran)	4 mg q 6–8 hr	2 mg q 6–8 hr	4 mg q 6–8 hr	2 mg q 6–8 hr	0.04 mg/kg q 6–8 hr	0.02 mg/kg q 6–8 hr
Meperidine (Demerol)	300 mg q 2–3 hr	100 mg q 3 hr	Not recommended	100 mg q 3 hr	Not recommended	0.75 mg/kg q 2–3 hr
Methadone (Dolophine, others)	20 mg q 6–8 hr	10 mg q 6–8 hr	20 mg q 6–8 hr	10 mg q 6–8 hr	0.2 mg/kg q 6–8 hr	0.1 mg/kg q 6–8 hr
Oxycodone (Roxicodone, also in Percocet, Percodan, Tylox, others)	30 mg q 3–4 hr	Not available	10 mg q 3–4 hr	Not available	0.2 mg/kg q 3–4 hr**	Not available
Oxymorphone§ (Numorphan)	Not available	1 mg q 3–4 hr	Not available	1 mg q 3–4 hr	Not recommended**	Not recommended
Opioid Agonist-Antagonist and Partial Agonist						
Buprenorphine (Buprenex)	Not available	0.3–0.4 mg q 6–8 hr	Not available	0.4 mg q 6–8 hr	Not available	0.004 mg/kg q 6–8 hr
Butorphanol (Stadol)	Not available	2 mg q 3–4 hr	Not available	2 mg q 3–4 hr	Not available	Not recommended
Nalbuphine (Nubian)	Not available	10 mg q 3–4 hr	Not available	10 mg q 3–4 hr	Not available	0.1 mg/kg q 3–4 hr
Pentazocine (Talwin, others)	150 mg q 3–4 hr	60 mg q 3–4 hr	50 mg q 4–6 hr	Not recommended	Not recommended	Not recommended

*Note: Published tables vary in the suggested doses that are equianalgesic to morphine. Clinical response is the criterion that must be applied for each client; titration to clinical response is necessary. Because there is not complete cross tolerance among these drugs, it is usually necessary to use a lower than equianalgesic dose when changing drugs and to retitrate to response.

†**Caution:** Recommended doses do not apply to clients with renal or hepatic insufficiency or other conditions affecting drug metabolism and kinetics.

‡**Caution:** Doses listed for clients with body weight less than 50 kg cannot be used as initial starting doses in babies less than 6 months of age. Consult the *Clinical Practice Guideline for Acute Pain Management: Operative or Medical Procedures and Trauma* section on management of pain in neonates for recommendations.

§For morphine, hydromorphone, and oxymorphone, rectal administration is an alternate route for clients unable to take oral medications, but equianalgesic doses may differ from oral and parenteral doses because of pharmacokinetic differences.

¶**Caution:** Codeine doses above 65 mg often are not appropriate due to diminishing incremental analgesia with increasing doses but continually increasing constipation and other side effects.

Caution: Doses of aspirin and acetaminophen in combination opioid/NSAID preparations must also be adjusted to the client's body weight.

Acute Pain Management Guideline Panel. (1992). *Acute pain management: Operative or medical procedures and trauma. Clinical practice guideline* (pp. 112–113). AHCPR Pub. No. 92-0032. Rockville, MD: Agency for Health Care Policy and Research, Public Health Service, U.S. Department of Health and Human Services.

When respirations fall below 10, the nurse should rouse the client. If respirations do not increase, the health care provider typically orders naloxone (Narcan), an opioid antagonist, to reverse the respiratory depression. Naloxone can potentially reverse the effects of the opioid analgesic. Doses of more than 0.2 mgs generally reverse analgesia and precipitate acute physiologic withdrawal in clients who are opioid dependent. Smaller doses (< 0.2 mg) can be given and titrated slowly to reduce the respiratory depressant effects of opioid agonist drugs. Naloxone is always given with caution to clients who are physically dependent on opioids and only in life-threatening situations. In the hospital or nursing home setting, this drug is kept in an emergency drug box or cabinet on each unit for use as necessary.

Opioid Analgesic Regimens. Immediately after surgery or traumatic injury, the health care provider typically prescribes oral or parenteral opioid analgesics on a continuous time schedule or on an intermittent as needed (PRN) schedule. Round-the-clock dosing schedules should be used during the first 24 to 36 hours following surgery (Acute Pain Management Guideline Panel, 1992). Oral drugs are the most convenient and least expensive but should be prescribed in doses equianalgesic to parenteral ones.

When the health care provider orders an intermittent schedule, the client depends on the nurse to give the medication when requested. Not all clients will ask for medication. It is imperative for the nurse to offer the medication at the prescribed intervals and to anticipate the need for medication based on behavioral and nonverbal cues.

Use of Opioids for Substance Abusers. Acute pain management for clients who are known or suspected substance abusers is a difficult but increasingly common problem. Some hospitals have pain management teams that assist with this type of problem in managing a client's pain. The team members usually represent several disciplines, including, but not limited to, nurses, physicians, clinical pharmacists, and social workers.

Clients who are substance abusers often have traumatic injuries and other health problems that cause acute pain. Chart 9–2 lists some recommendations that the nurse can follow when planning and implementing pain management for a client who is a substance abuser. It is important for the nurse to recognize that substance abusers, typically those abusing opioids, are often tolerant to the pain-relieving effects of opioid analgesics and generally require increase doses. There is always the danger of abrupt physiologic withdrawal when recreational users of opioid agonists are given mixed agonist-antagonists and partial *agonists.*

Adjuvant Drugs for Acute Opioid Analgesia. A relatively common practice in the treatment of acute pain is the administration of adjuvant drugs—drugs that add to the action or effects of opioids. The ones most frequently used are hydroxyzine pamoate (Vistaril) and promethazine (Phenergan, Histanil✣). These drugs were once thought to potentiate the action of opioids, but evidence has shown that they enhance the sedating effects of the opioid and not the actual pain-relieving effects. They do help to relieve the anxiety and nausea that frequently follow general anesthesia and accompany acute pain. Some analgesic effects have been demonstrated with hydroxyzine alone in the treatment of postoperative pain. The nurse observes clients receiving promethazine or hydroxyzine in addition to opioid analgesics for the side effect of sedation.

Anxiolytic agents such as the benzodiazepines may be helpful in reducing the anxiety that accompanies acute pain. However, these agents do cause sedation and should be cautiously administered along with opioids.

Patient-Controlled Analgesia. Patient-controlled analgesia (PCA) is one way to combat the problem of inadequate analgesia in the management of acute and chronic pain. This method allows the client to control the dosage of opioid analgesia received. This approach to pain control can improve pain relief and increase client satisfaction. It can also decrease the amount of opioid consumption per day when compared with intermittent dosing methods.

Clients receiving medication on an as needed basis for postoperative pain must sense the pain, report it to the nurse, and wait until the nurse is aware of the client's need and has the time to administer the analgesic. Considerable time may pass in this sequence because the client may wait too long before asking for the medication. Alternatively, the nurse may not understand the need to respond promptly to the request, or the nurse may have other equally pressing responsibilities. Whatever the reasons, the client's pain may be more severe or out of control by the time the analgesic is received. More medication is then required to relieve the pain adequately.

However, clients who have ready access to an analgesic are more likely to medicate themselves before the pain becomes severe, and thus they may require a reduced

---

Chart 9–2

Nursing Care Highlight: Pain Management for the Substance Abuser

- Define the exact source(s) of pain and treat them; e.g., heat for muscle spasms, antibiotics for infection.
- Follow the principles of opioid use, such as not giving agonist-antagonists to clients receiving opioid agonists.
- Use nonopioid therapies, including medication, cutaneous stimulation techniques, and cognitive and behavioral strategies.
- Monitor the client for drug abuse while in the health care agency to ensure that drugs are not being stolen or hoarded.
- Set limits and negotiate with the client about drug choices and dosing.
- Provide clear instructions about drug use and dosing schedules.
- Consult with other members of the health care team, such as physicians, psychiatrists, psychologists, pharmacists, and social workers.

Data from the Acute Pain Management Guideline Panel. (1992). *Acute pain management: Operative or medical procedures and trauma. Clinical practice guideline.* AHCPR Pub. No. 92-0032. Rockville, MD: Agency for Health Care Policy and Research, Public Health Service, U.S. Department of Health and Human Services.

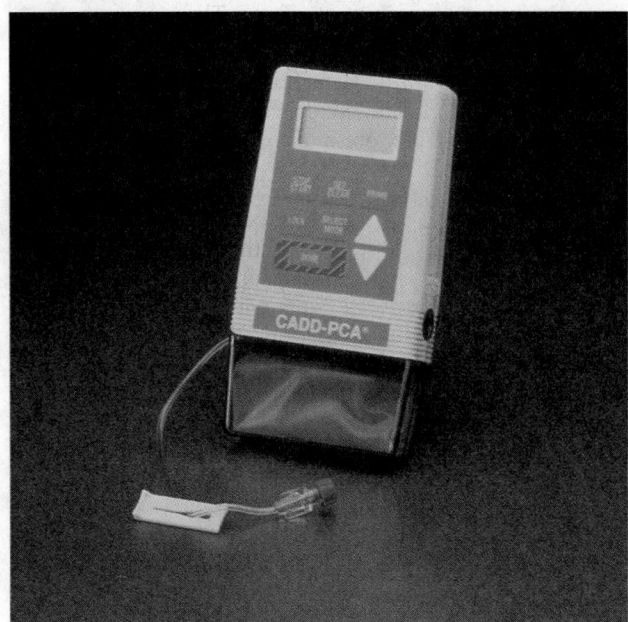

Figure 9–6. An ambulatory patient-controlled analgesia (PCA) infusion pump. (CADD-PCA is a registered trademark of Pharmacia Deltec.)

amount. Having control over when the drug can be administered also reduces the client's anxiety, which helps relieve pain.

Patient-controlled analgesia is achieved through the use of a PCA infusion pump (Fig. 9–6). Both stationary pole pumps for hospital use and ambulatory pumps for nursing home or home use are available. The infusion pump delivers the desired amount of medication through a conventional intravenous route for acute pain. The most commonly used drug for PCA is morphine. However, the use of PCA hydromorphone (Dilaudid) and fentanyl (Sublimaze) is gaining popularity. Meperidine (Demerol) is still reserved for short-term use, usually less than 48–72 hours, because its toxic metabolite, normeperidine, which is capable of inducing confusion and seizures, may accumulate in the blood.

Drug security to avoid overdosing is achieved through a locked syringe pump system or locked drug reservoir system. The device is programmed to deliver a certain amount of drug within a specific interval known as a lockout interval. The physician specifies the amount of the demand dose. Morphine doses typically range from 1 to 2 mg; hydromorphone, 0.15 to 0.4 mg; fentanyl, 12.5 to 25.0 μg; and meperidine, 10 to 15 mg. Doses may vary according to the client's degree of pain and tolerance for opioids. The lockout interval is usually 5 to 15 minutes.

The nurse programs the dosing parameters into the PCA delivery device. When the client presses the button or pendant (on ambulatory pumps), the appropriate bolus or demand dose is delivered. If the client attempts access to the drug before the designated time interval between doses has elapsed, no drug will be administered. With this technique, there is little chance of clients overmedicating themselves.

The PCA regimen may consist of a demand-dosing-only schedule or a continuous infusion or basal rate and demand dosing. With demand or self-administered dosing only, the client relies soley on a push of the pendant or bolus feature of the device to seek pain relief. Continuous or basal infusions of the opioid in addition to demand dosing provide more consistent analgesia and allow the client to sleep without fear of missing pain medication. The usual morphine dose prescribed by the health care provider for postoperative pain is 1 to 2 mg per hour; hydromorphone, 0.15 to 0.4 mg per hour; and fentanyl, 12.5 to 25.0 μg. A continuous infusion of meperidine is not recommended. When a continuous infusion is added to the regimen, clients may be at greater risk for opioid-induced side effects (i.e., nausea and vomiting, sedation, respiratory depression), especially if the hourly dose is too much for the client.

The nurse's role in caring for clients using PCA is to teach them how to use the device and to report side effects, such as dizziness, nausea and vomiting, and inability to void. As with all opioids, the nurse monitors the client's vital signs frequently—at least every 4 hours. In some cases, the nurse may need to anticipate the client's need for pain medication and administer doses of the drug if the client is unable to do so. For example, the client who is confused or cannot move may need the nurse to push the pump button to administer the drug. The physician specifies the PCA demand doses, or bolus amounts, along with the lockout interval.

Epidural Analgesia. *Epidural* analgesia, also known as peridural or extradural analgesia, refers to the instillation of a pain-blocking agent, usually an opioid analgesic alone or in combination with a local anesthetic into the epidural space (the space between the dura mater and the vertebral column). Epidural analgesia is far more popular for management of acute pain, such as postoperative pain. It has been used since the 1950s, but it has become more popular as newer and more innovative approaches to acute pain control are explored. Epidural analgesia is used with clients who are predisposed to respiratory complications, including those undergoing thoracic surgery, those with pre-existing respiratory disease, and those who are obese.

Morphine (preservative free) and fentanyl (Sublimaze) are the most commonly used opioids for epidural administration. A local anesthetic such as bupivacaine, which affects both sensory and motor nerves, may be given alone or in combination with an opioid. Low concentrations of local anesthetics are used to avoid significant sensory and motor deficits that can accompany epidural anesthesia. With the introduction of ropivacaine, a new local anesthetic that is selective for sensory nerves, the incidence of lower motor weakness is far less (Cederholm, 1997).

A temporary externalized epidural catheter is used for acute pain control. This device is not sutured to the skin and is easily dislodged. The nurse tapes the catheter in two places to anchor it properly. Some clinicians do not recommend transparent dressings, because the catheter may be dislodged when the dressing is removed. The catheter is generally placed in either the lumbar or thoracic region. Rarely is the catheter placed above the level of sixth thoracic vertebra, as the diaphragmatic muscle may be affected by the analgesia.

Complications of Epidural Analgesia. In caring for a client with epidural analgesia, the nurse helps to prevent associated complications, monitors the client for them, and implements prescribed medical therapies for managing side effects (Polomano et al., 1993). Complications that occur with epidural analgesia are directly related to catheter placement, catheter maintenance, and the type of analgesic used.

Pruritus (itching) and nausea and vomiting are common side effects of epidural opioids. Pruritus is treated with a small amount of naloxone (Narcan) first. Because epidural-induced pruritus does not appear to be mediated by histamine release, diphenhydramine (Benadryl, Allerdryl✦) may not be effective in relieving itching and may only work via its sedating effects. The physician usually prescribes an antiemetic for nausea and vomiting.

Infection results from failure to maintain aseptic technique during catheter placement, direct drug instillation, and infusion solution and tubing changes. Infection also results from failure to maintain aseptic conditions for indwelling catheters at the site of insertion or at the site of tube junctions. To prevent infections, the nurse ensures that all catheter line connections are secure and that an occlusive sterile dressing is maintained over the catheter site.

ELDERLY CONSIDERATIONS

The nurse also observes the elderly or restless client carefully for possible dislodgement of the catheter. The older client may become confused or disoriented as a result of surgery and try to pull out the temporary catheter. The catheter usually stays in place for about 48–72 hours, depending on the reason for the analgesia and the hospital policy.

Clients who receive epidural opioids are also at risk for respiratory depression resulting from high plasma and/or cerebrospinal fluid concentrations of the instilled drug. Clients receiving just epidural therapy with local anesthetic are not at risk for respiratory depression. Morphine, because of its potential for greater rostral or vertical spread up the spinal cord, is more likely to cause respiratory depression than fentanyl. When a larger distribution of analgesia is required, such as for the relief of pain from extensive abdominal wounds, morphine is preferred to fentanyl.

The nurse monitors respirations frequently and immediately reports to the physician respiratory rates below 10 per minute during and after the administration of epidural opioids. Opioid-induced respiratory depression usually occurs within the first few hours after the administration of fentanyl but may not be seen for 12 hours or more when morphine is given. This complication is managed by the administration of low doses (<0.2 mg) of naloxone (Narcan), either intravenously or intramuscularly.

Urinary retention is another common problem associated with epidural analgesia, but it occurs no more frequently than postoperative urinary retention in clients not receiving epidural analgesia. Although the cause is not clear, this problem usually occurs during the first or second day of analgesia administration and may be treated with bethanecol chloride (Urecholine) or intermittent urinary catheterization. The incidence of this complication is less than 25% and is more likely to occur in men than in women (Wild & Coyne, 1992).

Lower motor weakness is more common when an epidural local anesthetic is used. Clients who get out of bed for the first time should be assisted by the nurse to determine the degree, if any, of leg weakness.

Intrapleural Opioid Analgesia. While not commonly used, local anesthetics may be administered via the intrapleural route to achieve pain control. This method is sometimes used postoperatively for clients who have had a videothoracoscopy and less frequently for open thoracotomy (chest surgery) (Polomano et al., 1993).

Placebos. The clinical use of placebos in non–research-based therapies has not been shown to have a sustained effect on pain relief. McCaffery's definition of a placebo is "any medical treatment (medication or procedure, including surgery) or nursing care that produces an effect in a patient because of its implicit or explicit or nursing care therapeutic intent and not because of its specific nature (physical or chemical properties)" (1979, p. 160). Placebos are substances or actions that produce an effect regardless of their intrinsic known value. When a client responds favorably to a placebo, it is known as the *placebo effect.*

Some clients who receive placebos report pain relief. Evidence has shown that these clients release endogenous opiates, such as endorphins, because of the power of suggestion, trust in the caregiver's interventions, or belief that something, regardless of what it is, will help the pain. A client's favorable response to a placebo does not mean that the pain was not real or was imaginary. Placebos should never be used to determine whether a client's pain is real. Even clients with documented physiologic causes for pain can respond favorably to placebos.

Placebos are sometimes used incorrectly and unethically. For example, placebos such as intramuscular saline may be administered and the client informed that the injection contains a pain medication. This practice deceives the client and perpetuates mistrust in caregivers and the health care system. Some health care providers are concerned that placebos may not be legal; therefore, they are not used in many settings.

Physical Measures. Physical measures may be used instead of or in addition to drug therapy for the relief of acute pain. Cutaneous stimulation strategies to relieve pain have been in use for many years. Various types of stimulation to the skin and subcutaneous tissue produce pain relief. Mobily et al. (1994) have identified areas of nursing practice that are critical to the successful implementation of cutaneous stimulation. Nurses play an important role in educating clients about these techniques. Methods of cutaneous stimulation include techniques such as

- Transcutaneous electrical nerve stimulation (TENS)
- Application of heat, cold, and pressure
- Therapeutic touch

- Massage
- Vibration

Whatever the method, several characteristics of cutaneous stimulation must be considered:

- The benefits of these techniques are highly unpredictable and may vary from application to application.
- Pain relief is generally sustained only as long as the stimulation continues.
- Multiple trials may be necessary to establish the desired effects.
- Stimulation itself may aggravate pre-existing pain or may produce new pain.

Despite these drawbacks to cutaneous stimulation, these methods are effective in the management of both acute and chronic pain. These techniques have physiologic as well as psychological effects on the client. The use of cutaneous stimulation techniques also gives clients an opportunity to participate actively in the management of their pain.

Transcutaneous Electrical Nerve Stimulation. Transcutaneous electrical nerve stimulation (TENS) involves the use of a battery-operated device capable of delivering small electrical currents to the skin and underlying tissues. The first-generation, or conventional, TENS unit is used most frequently. Electrodes connected to a small box are placed over the painful sites. The voltage or current is regulated by adjusting a dial to the point at which the client perceives a prickly, "pins and needles" sensation. The current is adjusted on the basis of the client's degree of pain relief and level of comfort.

The physician, nurse, or physical therapist (depending on the health care setting) assists the client in applying the electrodes either on the painful area or above or below it (Fig. 9–7). A conducting substance (usually a gel) is placed between the electrode and the client's skin.

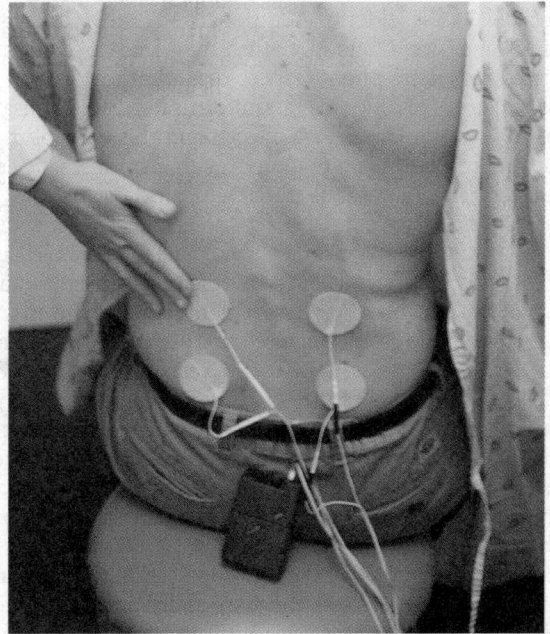

Figure 9–7. Application of a TENS unit.

The advantages of these units are that the client can wear the unit and achieve a level of pain relief while participating in activities of daily living. The unit is easy to use and can be worn for several hours. However, the skin at the site of the electrode placement may become irritated. To prevent this, the nurse teaches the client to rotate electrode sites.

In general, clients use TENS units for the management of both acute and chronic pain. This type of therapy is indicated for localized pain, such as postoperative or local chronic pain, particularly low back pain (Fishbain et al., (1996).

Other Cutaneous Techniques. Additional cutaneous stimulation techniques, such as the use of touch, pressure, massage, and vibration, as well as the application of heat and cold, stimulate the skin and somehow interrupt the pain pathway. These interventions are relatively easy for the client to learn and are fairly economical. Table 9–5 summarizes these techniques.

Cognitive and Behavioral Strategies. Cognitive and behavioral strategies to relieve pain, such as distraction, have also been popular for years, either as adjuncts to drug therapy or as alternative interventions. Theoretical explanations for the effectiveness of these measures reflect the premises of the gate control theory.

Distraction can be an effective method of acute pain relief. Simple measures such as holding a client's hand, taking the client for a walk, or encouraging deep breathing exercises can divert attention from the pain. Nurses often observe that clients request less pain medication when family members are present. After visiting hours are over, many clients request something for pain. Instead of viewing distraction as a therapeutic pain relief measure, some nurses may question the presence or severity of the pain if a client is easily distracted from it.

Distraction alters the perception of pain, but it does not influence the cause or peripheral mechanism of pain. It is a transient method of pain relief and is probably best used with other pain control measures.

Nurses can provide several methods of distraction. Visual distractors, such as pictures or television, can divert the client's attention to something pleasant or interesting. Auditory distractors, which include music or relaxation tapes, can have a calming effect. Changing the environment can remove unpleasant stressors or reminders that may enhance the client's pain. Physical distractions, such as deep breathing exercises, help the client concentrate on other physiologic sensations.

Distraction is used for

- Exacerbations of pain
- Painful procedures (e.g., dressing changes or invasive procedures)
- Interrupting the client's constant perception of pain

➤ *Chronic Pain*

 Planning and Implementation

The client is expected to experience a reduction in or relief of the pain, modification of the pain, or prevention of the recurrence or worsening of the pain.

TABLE 9–5

Cutaneous Stimulation Techniques Used to Interrupt the Pain Pathway

Technique	Method of Application	Comments
Therapeutic touch or "laying on of hands"	• The hands of the caregiver are placed on or close to the client's body.	• The intent to help on the part of the caregiver may contribute to the success of this technique. This technique may extend the nurse-client relationship.
Pressure	• A hand or other object is placed firmly over or around the painful area.	• Pressure seems to relieve pain, decrease bleeding, and prevent swelling. Release of pressure is associated with increased blood flow and return of pain.
Massage	• The hands or fingers are moved slowly or briskly over a body part. A lubricant or other substance is sometimes used.	• Effects include muscle relaxation and sedation.
Vibration	• Electrical and battery-operated vibrators produce a massage effect.	• Vibration may decrease the intensity of the noxious (pain) stimuli.
Application of heat and cold	• Heat may be applied in a variety of ways, including short-wave diathermy, microwave diathermy, sonography, use of melted paraffin and Hubbard tank, use of hot water bottle or heating pad, use of heat cradle and lamp, application of moist pads or towels, use of hot tub or shower, or use of gel packs. • Cold may be applied in a dry or moist way, similar to heat applications. Ice chips, cold towels and packs, and chilled gel packs are commonly used.	• Both heat and cold may reduce muscle spasm and decrease pain. Cold probably slows the conduction velocity of nerves. Heat increases the tendency for bleeding and therefore should not be used after trauma. Heat may also increased edema and is not indicated if circulation is poor. Both heat and cold should be used cautiously if clients have impaired sensation or cannot communicate.

Data from McCaffery, M. (1979). *Nursing management of the patient with pain* (2nd ed., pp. 117–126). Philadelphia: J. B. Lippincott.

The goals for chronic pain management are accomplished by interrupting the relentless cycle of pain, anxiety, and sometimes depression. Nonsurgical methods of pain reduction are generally used before surgical techniques are tried. The client may eventually need a combination of nonsurgical and surgical measures.

Nonsurgical Management. A pharmacologic approach to the treatment of chronic pain is the most effective and reliable method of pain management. Other measures may be used in combination with drug therapy.

Drug Therapy. Although a number of drugs have been used in the management of chronic pain, the physician most commonly prescribes nonopioid and opioid analgesics.

Nonopioid Analgesics. Acetylsalicylic acid (aspirin, Ancasal✦), acetaminophen (Tylenol, Ace-Tabs✦), and nonsteroidal anti-inflammatory drugs (NSAIDs) such as ibuprofen (Motrin, Amersol✦) are effective in the management of mild chronic pain. They are also effective in combination with opioid analgesics. Aspirin and NSAIDs possess anti-inflammatory properties, in that they peripherally inhibit prostaglandins. This property makes them particularly useful in treating the inflammation associated with arthritis and cancer. The requirements for opioid analgesics in the client with chronic pain can be reduced by aspirin and NSAIDs. However, both aspirin and NSAIDs can cause gastric disturbances and can have an effect on platelets, which results in a tendency toward bleeding. The nurse observes the client for gastric discomfort or vomiting and bleeding or bruising and reports these problems to the physician immediately. NSAIDs can cause renal toxicity; therefore, renal function blood tests should be routinely monitored with long-term therapy, especially in the elderly. Additionally, NSAIDs can cause sodium and water retention that may lead to congestive heart failure, more often in the older client.

Salicylates (choline magnesium trisalicylate [Trilisate]) also have anti-inflammatory effects, and this class of drugs has certain benefits. Compared with aspirin, salicylates cause less gastrointestinal upset and are less toxic to the kidneys and have little effect on platelet aggregation. These advantages make salicylates a more favorable alternative to NSAIDs in clients undergoing cancer therapy, those at risk for bleeding, and elderly clients who may be more susceptible to the renal effects of NSAIDs (see Table 9–6).

The health care provider also commonly prescribes acetaminophen for chronic pain. Acetaminophen exerts its analgesic action by blocking peripheral pain receptors, thus increasing the threshold of these receptors to painful stimuli. Reports of liver toxicity have been associated with higher doses of this drug (1000 mg) taken more frequently than every 4 hours for long-term use. Current recommendations restrict the total daily amount of acetaminophen to no more than 4000 mg or 4 g. Therefore, nurses must check all combination analgesic products for

TABLE 9–6

Nonopioid Analgesics for Chronic Pain

Drug	Usual Dose for Adults and Children ≥50 kg Body Weight	Usual Dose for Children* and Adults† ≤50 kg Body Weight
Acetaminophen and Over-the-Counter NSAIDs		
Acetaminophen‡	650 mg q 4 h 975 mg q 6 h	10–15 mg/kg q 4 h 15–20 mg/kg q 4 h (rectal)
Aspirin§	650 mg q 4 h 975 mg q 6 h	10–15 mg/kg q 4 h 15–20 mg/kg q 4 h (rectal)
Ibuprofen (Motrin, others)	400–600 mg q 6 h	10 mg/kg q 6–8 h¶
Prescription NSAIDs		
Carprofen (Rimadyl)	100 mg tid	
Choline magnesium trisalicylate (Trilisate)**	1,000–1,500 mg tid	25 mg/kg tid
Choline salicylate (Arthropan)**	870 mg q 3–4 h	
Diflunisal (Dolobid)††	500 mg q 12 h	
Etodolac (Lodine)	200–400 mg q 6–8 h	
Fenoprofen calcium (Nalfon)	300–600 mg q 6 h	
Ketoprofen (Orudis)	25–60 mg q 6–8 h	
Ketorolac tromethamine (Toradol)‡‡	10 mg q 4–6 h to a maximum of 40 mg/day	
Magnesium salicylate (Doan's, Magan, Mobidin, others)	650 mg q 4 h	
Meclofenamate sodium (Meclomen)§§	50–100 mg q 6 h	
Mefenamic acid (Ponstel)	250 mg q 6 h	
Naproxen (Naprosyn)	250–275 mg q 6–8 h	5 mg/kg q 8 h
Naproxen sodium (Anaprox)	275 mg q 6–8 h	
Sodium salicylate (Generic)	325–650 mg q 3–4 h	
Parenteral NSAIDs		
Ketorolac tromethamine (Toradol)‡‡,¶¶	60 mg initially, then 30 mg q 6 h intramuscular dose not to exceed 5 days	

Management of Cancer Pain Guideline Panel. (1994). *Management of cancer pain: Clinical practice guidelines* (pp. 48 and 49). AHCPR Pub. No. 94-0592. Rockville, MD: Agency for Health Care Policy and Research, Public Health Service, U.S. Department of Health and Human Services.
*Only drugs that are FDA approved as an analgesic for use in children are included.
†Acetaminophen and NSAID dosage for adults weighing less than 50 kg should be adjusted for weight.
‡APAP lacks the peripheral anti-inflammatory and antiplatelet activities of the other NSAIDs.
§The standard against which other NSAIDs are compared. May inhibit platelet aggregation ≥1 week and may cause bleeding. Aspirin is contraindicated in children with fever or other viral disease because of its association with Reye's syndrome.
¶Not FDA approved for use in children as an over-the-counter drug; has FDA approval for use in children as a prescription drug for fever. However, clinicians have experience in prescribing ibuprofen for pain in children.
**May have minimal antiplatelet activity.
††Administration with antacids may decrease absorption.
‡‡For short-term use only.
§§Coombs-positive autoimmune hemolytic anemia has been associated with prolonged use.
¶¶Has the same GI toxicities as oral NSAIDs.
NOTE: Only the above NSAIDs have FDA approval for use as simple analgesics, but clinical experience has been gained with other drugs as well.

their acetaminophen content and caution the client regarding maximum dosing.

Capsaicin (Zostrix), an over-the-counter cream, can be applied to the skin in painful areas. Its pain-relieving qualities lie in its ability to deplete the painful site of substance P, a pain mediator. The preparation is marketed for painful arthritis, diabetic neuropathy, and other chronic pain conditions. For the first few applications, the cream produces noticeable pain as the release of substance P is intensified, but, this can be alleviated with the addition of a local anesthetic cream or ointment. Regular applications are recommended to sustain its pain-relieving properties.

Adjuvant Drugs. Other nonopioid drugs that are used to control the pain of certain neuralgias (pain along the distribution of nerves) or nerve injury pain include carbamazepine (Tegretol, Mazepine♦), phenytoin (Dilantin), and valproic acid (Depakene). The exact mechanism of action of these drugs is unknown, but it is believed that they inhibit or reduce the paroxysmal firing of nerve impulses. Both carbamazepine and phenytoin are associated with a wide variety of side effects (hematopoietic, hepatic, and pulmonary effects and central nervous system toxicity). Therefore, these drugs are used with extreme caution.

Tricyclic antidepressants, such as amitriptyline (Elavil), nortriptyline (Pamelor), imipramine (Tofranil), desipramine, and doxepin (Sinequan) may be beneficial in the treatment of chronic neuropathic pain. Both tricyclic antidepressants and other antidepressants like trazodone (Desyrel), fluoxitine (Prozac), paroxitine (Paxil), and sertraline (Zoloft) help treat the depression that can accompany chronic pain. They also stimulate the activity of endogenous opiates (endorphins and enkephalins) by increasing levels of serotonin, a neurotransmitter. Perhaps the greatest advantage of this group of drugs, particularly the tricyclic antidepressants, is the sedative effect, which can be helpful in promoting sleep when administered at bedtime.

In some cases, antianxiety agents help relax the client and thus help relieve pain. The physician selects the drugs that have the fewest side effects, because many of these drugs cause confusion, drowsiness, and hypotension. Examples of drugs that may be ordered include alprazolam (Xanax), clorazepate (Tranxene, Novoclopate♦), lorazepam (Ativan), and oxazepam (Serax, Zapex♦). Clonazepam (Klonopin), also used for anxiety, has been shown to be particularly helpful for certain types of nerve injury pain.

Oral local anesthetics such as mexilitine (Mexitil) act by suppressing aberrant electrical activity of both peripheral nerves and neurons in the CNS. They are useful for lancinating, electric shock-like pain, and continuous pains. Mexilitine is contraindicated for clients who have cardiac conduction defects or arrhythmias or are currently taking cardiac antiarrhythmic medications.

Opioid Analgesics. Opioid analgesics are drugs capable of relieving pain by binding to various opiate receptors located in the central nervous system (see the discussion under Nursing Interventions for Pain). For chronic pain, opioids are more commonly administered by the oral route; however, other acceptable routes include trans-

dermal, rectal, sublingual, subcutaneous, intravenous, or intraspinal.

An equianalgesic guide (Table 9–7) can help determine the appropriate dose conversions when switching routes of a drug or from one drug to another. Equianalgesic refers to the dose and route of administration of one drug that produces approximately the same degree of analgesia as the given dose and route of another drug. Most commonly, 10 mg of morphine is the standard dose against which other opioids are measured. Equianalgesic opioid drug guides only provide the comparative analgesic potencies among these drugs. Dose modifications may be necessary according to each client's response to the drugs. When converting from one opioid to another in clients on higher than usual opioid amounts, the new opioid should be started at one half of the equianalgesic dose. This is because incomplete cross-tolerance between opioids may occur.

Considerations with Long-Term Use of Opioids. The side effects of opioid analgesics are discussed under Nursing Interventions for Pain. The long-term use of these agents is associated with some concerns.

Physical Dependency. Physical dependency is associated with the administration of opioids on a long-term basis. Physical dependency is *not* the same as addiction. However, it is sometimes confused with addiction. Nursing textbooks and resource materials often fail to make the appropriate distinctions (Ferrell et al., 1992a). Physical dependency is a physiologic adaptation of the body tissues that requires continued administration of the drug for normal tissue function. When a client who has become physically dependent on opioids abruptly ceases using them, so-called withdrawal symptoms result. These symptoms result from autonomic nervous system responses, which include nausea and vomiting, abdominal cramping, muscle twitching, profuse perspiration, delirium, and convulsions. When it is necessary to discontinue opioid analgesia for a client who is opioid dependent, a slow tapering, or weaning, of the drug dosage lessens or alleviates physical withdrawal symptoms.

Addiction. Addiction is a common fear of health professionals who administer or prescribe opioids and of clients who receive them. Addiction is a term used to describe persistent craving and abuse of a drug for recreational purposes. Addiction is a psychologic phenomenon, not a physical one. Physical dependence does occur in many people who become addicted; however, it does not define the problem of addiction. Although addiction rarely occurs in clients who use opioids for medicinal relief of pain, the fear of addiction is a major factor contributing to the inadequate prescription and administration of opioid analgesics.

Clients also worry about becoming addicted to analgesics (Champlin, 1992). They may be concerned about the possibility of drug withdrawal symptoms, which are often associated with the "street addict." The nurse clarifies the term addiction with clients while stressing the concept of physical dependency.

Drug Tolerance. The client may also experience drug tolerance from opioid analgesic therapy. Tolerance is

TABLE 9–7

Dose Equivalents for Opioid Analgesics in Opioid-Naive Adults*

Drug	Approximate Equianalgesic Dose		Usual Starting Dose for Moderate to Severe Pain	
	Oral	Parenteral	Oral	Parenteral
Opioid Agonist†				
Morphine‡	30 mg q 3–4 h (repeat around-the-clock dosing) 60 mg q 3–4 h (single dose or intermittent dosing)	10 mg q 3–4 h	30 mg q 3–4 h	10 mg q 3–4 h
Morphine, controlled-release†§ (MS Contin, Oramorph)	90–120 mg q 12 h	N/A	90–120 mg q 12 h	N/A
Hydromorphone§ (Dilaudid)	7.5 mg q 3–4 h	1.5 mg q 3–4 h	6 mg q 3–4 h	1.5 mg q 3–4 h
Levorphanol (Levo-Dromoran)	4 mg q 6–8 h	2 mg q 6–8 h	4 mg q 6–8 h	2 mg q 6–8 h
Meperidine (Demerol)	300 mg q 2–3 h	100 mg q 3 h	N/R	100 mg q 3 h
Methadone (Dolophine, other)	20 mg q 6–8 h	10 mg q 6–8 h	20 mg q 6–8 h	10 mg q 6–8 h
Oxymorphone‡ (Numorphan)	N/A	1 mg q 3–4 h	N/A	1 mg q 3–4 h
Combination Opioid/NSAID Preparations¶				
Codeine** (with aspirin or acetaminophen)	180-200 mg q 3–4 h	130 mg q 3–4 h	60 mg q 3–4 h	60 mg q 2 h (IM/SC)
Hydrocodone (in Lorcet, Lortab, Vicodin, others)	30 mg q 3–4 h	N/A	10 mg q 3–4 h	N/A
Oxycodone (Roxicodone, also in Percocet, Percodan, Tylox, others)	30 mg q 3–4 h	N/A	10 mg q 3–4 h	N/A

*Caution: Recommended doses do not apply for adult patients with body weight less than 50 kg. For recommended starting doses for children and adults <50 kg body weight, see Table 9–4.

†Caution: Recommended doses do not apply to patients with renal or hepatic insufficiency or other conditions affecting drug metabolism and kinetics.

‡Caution: For morphine, hydromorphone, and oxymorphone, rectal administration is an alternate route for patients unable to take oral medications. Equianalgesic doses may differ from oral and parenteral doses because of pharmokinetic differences.

§Transdermal fentanyl (Duragesic) is an alternative option. Transdermal fentanyl dosage is not calculated as equianalgesic to a single morphine dosage. See the package insert for dosing calculations. Doses above 25 μg/hr should not be used in opioid-naive patients.

¶Caution: Doses of aspirin and acetaminophen in combination opioid-NSAID preparations must also be adjusted to the patient's body weight. Aspirin is contraindicated in children in the presence of fever or other viral disease because of its association with Reye's syndrome.

**Caution: Codeine doses above 65 mg often are not appropriate because of diminishing incremental analgesia with increasing doses but increasing nausea, constipation, and other side effects.

NOTE: Published tables vary in the suggested doses that are equianalgesic to morphine. Clinical response is the criterion that must be applied for each patient; titration to clinical responses is necessary. Because there is not complete cross-tolerance among these drugs, it is usually necessary to use a lower-than-equianalgesic dose when changing drugs and to retitrate to response.

N/A = not available; N/R = not recommended.

Management of Cancer Pain Guideline Panel. (1994). *Management of cancer pain: Clinical practice guidelines* (pp. 52 and 53). AHCPR Pub. No. 94-0592. Rockville, MD: Agency for Health Care Policy and Research, Public Health Service, U.S. Department of Health and Human Services.

characterized by a gradual resistance of the body to the effects of an opioid, including its pain-relieving properties. When tolerance occurs, clients usually require more of the drug to achieve the same analgesic effects. Tolerance should be recognized, and appropriate analgesic plans should be designed to account for increased opioid requirements at times of acute exacerbations of chronic or procedural-related pain. Issues with sedation and analgesia for clients with cancer can be especially difficult (Polomano, et al., 1997).

Tolerance to opioid analgesics is particularly a problem in clients who are substance abusers (see Chart 9–2). Keep in mind that tolerance is measured not only by the analgesic effects but also by the body's ability to adjust to the adverse reactions.

Continuous Intravenous Opioid Analgesia. For chronic cancer pain management, hourly doses of continuous opioid infusions vary, depending on the severity of the pain and the client's tolerance to the opioid. If the hourly dose needs to be increased, the physician usually increases it no more than 10% to 20% of the hourly rate and no sooner than every 3 to 4 hours. It may be necessary for the nurse to monitor the client's vital signs frequently (at least every hour) until an adequate and safe level of drug is achieved.

Patient-controlled analgesia (PCA) can provide effective relief of chronic pain. Although the principles of how PCA works are the same for both and acute and chronic pain, dosing guidelines and methods of administration differ. PCA for chronic pain, typically cancer pain, can be administered either by intravenous or subcutaneous routes. The idea is to provide most of the analgesia in a continuous rate. The physician calculates demand doses based on the amount of continuous hourly opioid administration. Usually the PCA demand dose is a minimum of 33% of the basal or continuous rate, but sometimes it may be as high as 100% of the hourly rate. The lockout interval, unlike in PCA for acute pain, is usually longer, between 20 and 30 minutes. Longer lock-out intervals with higher demand doses keep the client from having to work hard at managing the pain.

Continuous Subcutaneous Opioid Analgesia. Continuous subcutaneous opioid analgesia is best for clients who have compromised venous access or for those whose central venous lines are being used for other fluids (Haviley et al., 1992). Subcutaneous infusion is accomplished through the use of a small (25- or 27-gauge) butterfly-type catheter or a special subcutaneous needle device placed under the skin into the subcutaneous tissue.

Typically, the subclavicular tissue underneath the clavicle or the abdomen is used. Placing the catheter in the extremities should be avoided, if possible, especially in terminally ill clients, because peripheral circulation may be impaired or edema may be present, possibly affecting absorption of the drug. The nurse applies an occlusive dressing over the site and rotates the site every 3 to 7 days, depending on the drug and the volume delivered. The physician usually orders no more than 3 to 6 mL per hour.

Morphine is the most common drug given by this route. Occasionally, hydromorphone (Dilaudid) is used; however, this drug is more irritating to the tissues, requiring more site changes. If the physician orders a PCA demand-dosing schedule in addition to the continuous infusion, the volume of the bolus dose does not usually exceed 1 mL. In addition, the lockout interval, or time between doses that the client may access more opioids, is usually no more frequent than 30 to 60 minutes. Clients receiving continuous narcotic infusions with a PCA feature may require dose adjustments in their continuous rates if more than 6 to 12 bolus doses per day are used.

The nurse observes for and reports complications of subcutaneous infusion, which include leakage of fluid around the insertion site, inadequate pain relief, and edema around the site (Haviley et al., 1992).

Neuraxial Delivery of Analgesia. Neuraxial drug delivery involves the epidural, subarachnoid or intrathecal, and intraventricular routes. Neuraxial administration is sometimes referred to as the intraspinal route. There are two major methods for administering intraspinal analge-

sia: epidural and intrathecal. Intraspinal therapy is particularly useful for intractable pain that is refractory to systemic opioids (Rauck, 1997) or patients who may not be able to tolerate the effects of systemic opioid analgesics.

Long-term epidural analgesia, also known as peridural or extradural analgesia, refers to the instillation of a pain-blocking agent, usually an opioid analgesic alone or in combination with a local anesthetic, into the epidural space (the space between the dura mater and the vertebral column) through an externalized catheter (Fig. 9–8), an implantable port, or an implantable drug delivery system. *Intrathecal* (subarachnoid) analgesia, in which a pain-blocking agent is introduced into the space between the arachnoid mater and pia mater of the spinal cord where cerebrospinal fluid is located, is the route of choice for long-term management (>3 months) of intractable pain.

Action of Intraspinal Analgesia. The goal of both types of intraspinal analgesia is to interrupt the conduction of pain at the point that the sensory fibers exit from the spinal cord. Morphine (preservative free) is the opioid of choice for long-term intraspinal administration; however, fentanyl (Sublimaze) and hydromorphone (Dilaudid) may also be used. The addition of a local anesthetic, such as bopivacaine or ropivacaine, may provide an opioid-sparing effect and is often considered for many intractable neuropathic pain syndromes. For intraspinal analgesia, lower concentrations of local anesthetics are used to minimize significant sensory and motor deficits that often accompany intraspinal anesthesia. Similar to opioids, tolerance may also develop to local anesthetics, necessitating increasing doses over time.

Long-Term Intraspinal Analgesia. Long-term intraspinal opioid administration may be used for the management of chronic, intractable (uncontrollable or unyielding) pain, usually from cancer. A permanent *epidural catheter* may be inserted. Several catheter devices are available for this purpose. The DuPen Silastic catheter (Davol) is the most commonly used *external* catheter. A portion of the catheter exits the skin, where drugs can be intermittently injected, or the catheter can be attached to an infusion device for continuous drug administration.

Implantable devices are also used. The epidural Port-A-Cath (SIMS Deltec, Inc.) is implanted under the skin, and the catheter portion is inserted into the epidural space. Like the DuPen catheter, this device can be injected with drugs intermittently or can be connected to an infusion device for continuous opioid delivery. Injectable ports have been shown to reduce the incidence of catheter dislodgement and early infection. (de Jong & Kansen, 1994). Systems that consist of either an externalized catheter or a drug delivery device are rarely used for intrathecal or subarachnoid drug administration. The SynchroMed pump (Medtronic, Inc.) is a totally implantable system that contains a drug reservoir, which is filled on a routine basis and is capable of continuously administering a certain volume of drug each day (Fig. 9–8).

Side effects of intraspinal opioids are more common in clients who have had little exposure to opioids in the past. Clients who receive intraspinal therapy are usually

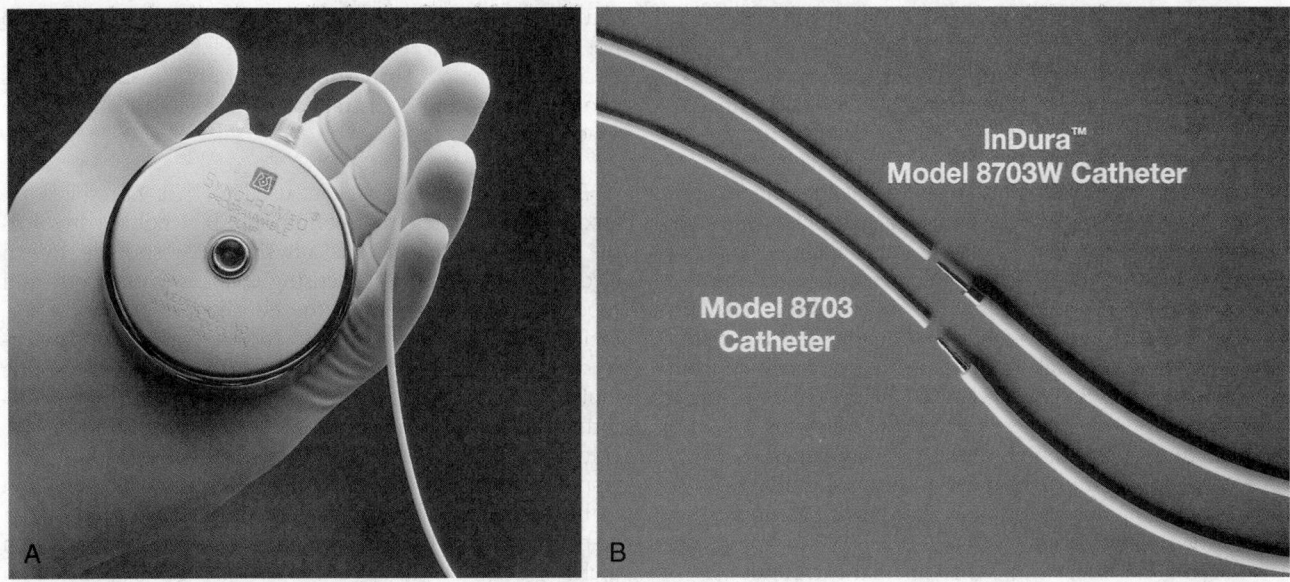

Figure 9–8. A SynchroMed implantable pump (*A*) and spinal catheters (*B*) for delivery of a precise volume of long-term intraspinal analgesia each day. (Courtesy of Medtronic, Inc., Columbia Heights, MN.)

more tolerant of the effects of opioids and may not require the rigorous monitoring needed for postoperative analgesia. Some male clients on long-term spinal opioids may complain of sexual dysfunction, decreased libido, and difficulty maintaining an erection, whereas female clients may experience amenorrhea (Paice et al., 1994). If sexual problems occur in male clients, testosterone injections seem to help improving sexual function.

Transdermal Opioid Administration. Transdermal opioid administration is now possible with the transdermal fentanyl system (Duragesic). Duragesic is available in patch dose strengths of 25 mcg/hr, 50 mcg/hr, 75 mcg/hr, and 100 mcg/hr. This system is used for clients who can take nothing by mouth, have difficulty taking pills, or cannot comply with their analgesic regimen. Duragesic is reserved for those with continuous and relatively stable pain. Because of the extended length of time needed to achieve steady state optimal serum concentrations of the opioid, the application of a Duragesic patch is supplemented with intermittent opioid administration of short-acting opioids. Intermittent "rescue" dosing should continue if the client has periods of episodic pain requiring an increased need for opioid analgesia. Duragesic should be used for clients with a known opioid requirement that is effective in relieving pain as it is difficult to titrate quickly to pain relief.

The system is applied by removing the adhesive backing and placing it on the skin of the client's chest, either front or back, preferably on an area without hair. If hair is present on the chest, the nurse clips it. Once the patch is applied, it delivers a specified amount of drug into the skin. The drug absorbs over 72 hours. The physician calculates the appropriate dosage from the client's previous opioid requirement; if the requirement is known, the lowest patch strength is used initially. Transdermal administration should be used cautiously when the requirement is *not* known.

The nurse teaches the client and family how to apply the patch and to report side effects, such as dizziness, sedation, nausea, or a decrease in respiratory rate, to the physician or nurse. The nurse also explains that when the patch is first applied, it may take up to 24 hours before pain relief is apparent. Supplemental analgesia with short-acting opioids is usually ordered until adequate blood levels of the transdermal drug are reached. The absorption of transdermal analgesics is affected by the client's body temperature. The nurse teaches the client and family that a fever of 102° F (38.9° C) or greater might accelerate absorption of the drug from the skin and increase side effects. Clients should be monitored closely for increased effects of the medication, such as sedation when fever is present. Once the system is removed, the client is monitored for about 24 hours, as the drug may still be released into the bloodstream from the site of application.

Complementary Therapies. Cognitive and behavioral strategies including imagery, relaxation, hypnosis, and biofeedback, are often effective in the relief of chronic pain. Analgesic therapy is an essential component of pain management, but cognitive and behavioral strategies may be effectively used in addition to and sometimes instead of drug therapy. A recent study provided support for the value of progressive muscle relaxation and guided imagery for the attenuation of cancer pain (Sloman, 1995). Subjects in this study reported a significant reduction in pain sensation, present pain intensity, overall pain severity, and the consumption of nonopioid analgesic medication. However, these interventions failed to reduce the affect or worry associated with pain, suggesting that knowledge of the potential threat to life that can accompany a cancer diagnosis was not relieved by these techniques.

Imagery. Imagery is a form of distraction in which the client is encouraged to visualize or think about some pleasant or desirable feeling, sensation, or event. Guided imagery takes place when a person, frequently a nurse, assists the client in sustaining a sequence of thoughts aimed at diverting the client's attention away from pain. Clients require intense concentration to visualize images. Clients who are extremely anxious, agitated, or unable to concentrate may benefit first from mild distraction.

Imagery is particularly useful with clients who experience chronic pain. Clients who practice this technique can mentally experience sights, sounds, smells, events, or other sensations vividly. First, the nurse assesses the client's level of concentration to determine if he or she can sustain a particular thought or thoughts for a desired time. The time interval for mental imagery can vary from 5 to 60 minutes. Behaviors that are helpful in assessing a client's capacity for imagery include the following:

- Reading and comprehending the newspaper
- Listening to music or other auditory stimuli
- Having the ability to follow and participate in sustained conversation
- Having an interest in environmental surroundings

When the client has demonstrated some ability to concentrate, the nurse assists the client in identifying a pleasant or favorable thought. The client is then encouraged to focus on this thought to divert attention away from painful stimuli. Audiotapes may help clients form and maintain images. The nurse, client, or family may wish to create such tapes for the client's use, or commercially available tapes may be used. An example of guided imagery instructions follows: "Imagine yourself on the beach on some deserted island. You can hear the sound of waves rushing onto the shore, the cry of sea gulls flying high above, and the rustling of trees as they are brushed gently by the wind. You can feel the warmth of the sun over your body and the cooling breeze."

Relaxation Techniques. Clients may use relaxation techniques to reduce anxiety, tension, and emotional stress, which may exacerbate pain. Techniques to help clients relax can be both physical and psychological. Physical techniques include

- The client receiving a body massage, back rub, or warm or hot bath
- Modifications in the client's environment to reduce distractions
- The client moving into a comfortable position.

Psychological techniques include

- The use of pleasant conversation
- The use of music
- The use of relaxation tapes

There are relaxation tapes that assist the client with progressive relaxation of the muscles. Relaxation exercises can be effectively coupled with guided imagery, distraction, and hypnosis. Chapter 8 describes relaxation techniques in detail.

Hypnosis. Hypnosis is defined as an altered state of consciousness in which a person enters a trance and loses an overall sense of reality. Although the person is in a trance, he or she has some sense of awareness and contact with reality and an understanding of what is actually happening. Hypnosis is used to treat a variety of pain syndromes, particularly chronic pain. It is used to help clients overcome the emotional consequences of pain and

can promote a positive state of mind. Although nurses do not usually teach clients hypnosis, they are in a key position to help clarify misconceptions, instruct clients about relaxation and distraction, and encourage clients to practice self-hypnosis.

Biofeedback. Biofeedback is used to treat chronic pain, anxiety, and other stress conditions. Biofeedback involves the monitoring of various physiologic responses by an electric device capable of sensing changes in the body and reporting this information to the client. Certain physiologic signals are transmitted to the feedback unit by electrode sensors, which are placed on the client's skin. The biofeedback unit amplifies and transforms physiologic information into visual signals (usually meter readings or colored lights). Clients are first alerted to stress-related responses, such as increased muscle tension or elevation in blood pressure. Then they are taught to regulate these responses through a combination of techniques, which include deep breathing exercises, progressive relaxation exercises, distraction, and visual imagery.

Biofeedback units vary. Some measure muscle contraction via electromyography and brain activity via electroencephalography. Galvanic skin response and skin temperature, which can reflect changes in blood flow, heart rate, or blood pressure, are also measured. Whatever the technique, physiologic responses that tend to worsen or prolong the client's pain are voluntarily controlled.

The client who is interested in learning biofeedback techniques to control pain is usually trained by a skilled therapist. The client is taught to observe the feedback information, report sensations or feelings that become apparent, and practice stress-reducing or pain-reducing techniques. Clients may need several sessions before they can recognize and control these responses. The client eventually becomes aware of even the most subtle changes in body function that indicate the onset or worsening of pain and automatically responds without the help of the biofeedback unit.

Biofeedback training helps the client gain control over pain. Clients require training and self-discipline if biofeedback and all other cognitive therapy strategies are to be used effectively.

Invasive Pain Management Techniques for Chronic Pain. Invasive techniques are used to interrupt the pain pathways when pain is intractable or severely debilitating. Depending on the technique, some degree of nerve destruction and neurologic deficits is expected. When chronic or persistent pain can no longer be adequately controlled with drugs or other pain-reducing methods, various invasive techniques are used (Fig. 9–9).

Nerve Blocks. Nerve blocks can be used for both diagnostic and treatment purposes. These procedures are usually indicated for pain that is confined to a specific area or nerve distribution. The technique involves localizing a nerve root (or roots) and injecting either a local anesthetic for temporary relief or diagnostic evaluations or a chemical agent (e.g., phenol or alcohol) to achieve permanent neurolysis or destruction of the nerve(s). Nerve areas where temporary blocks or permanent destruction (neu-

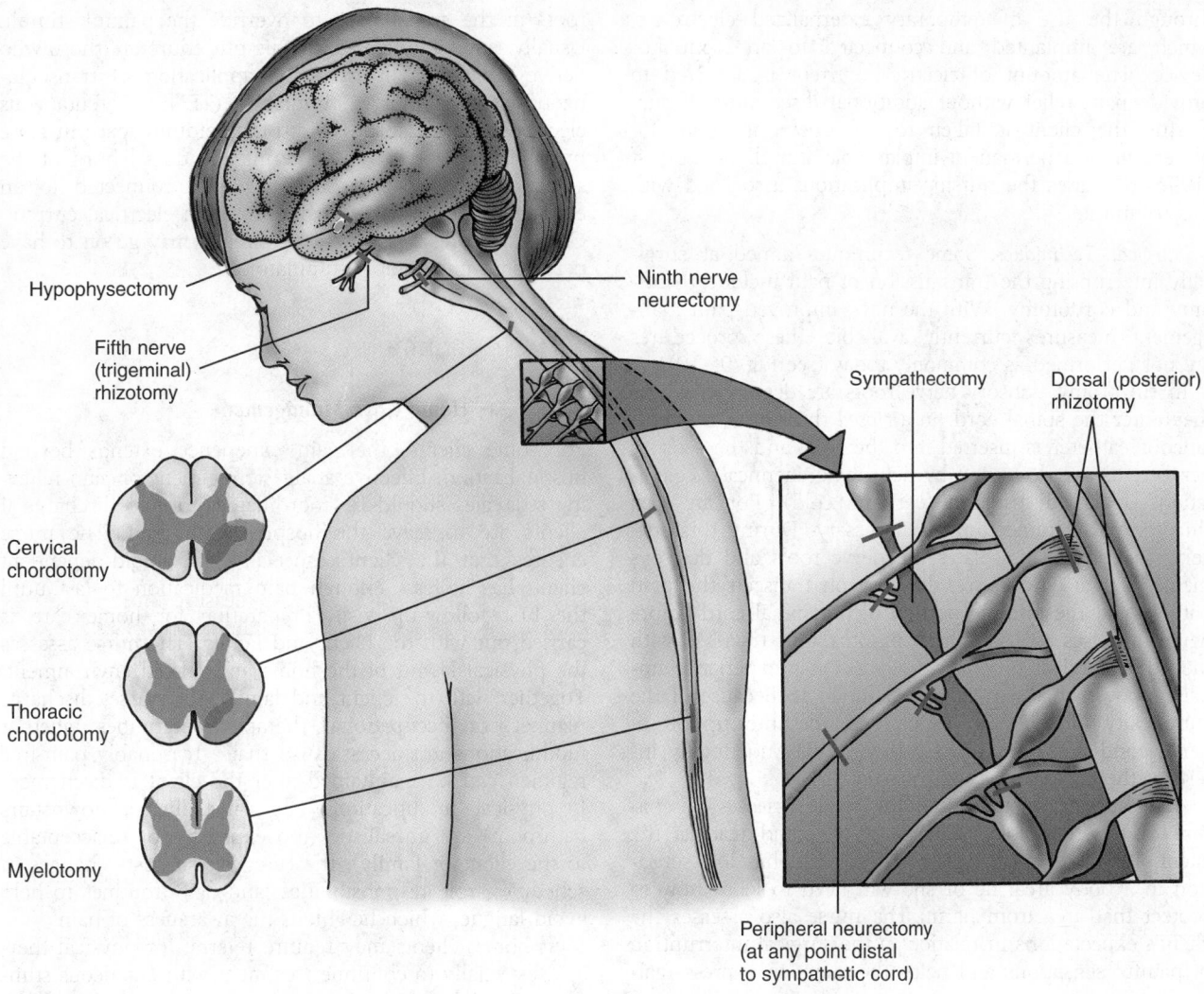

Hypophysectomy

Fifth nerve
(trigeminal)
rhizotomy

Cervical
chordotomy

Thoracic
chordotomy

Myelotomy

Ninth nerve
neurectomy

Sympathectomy

Dorsal (posterior)
rhizotomy

Peripheral neurectomy
(at any point distal
to sympathetic cord)

Figure 9–9. Surgical procedures designed to alleviate pain.

roablation) might be considered include intercostal nerves, celiac plexus, superior hypogastric block, or craniofacial nerves.

Complications associated with this technique vary. Injections into peripheral nerve root with local anesthetic or chemical agents generally lead to decreased sensation in the area, with no effect on motor function. Injections into the lumbosacral area of the spinal cord area with local anesthetic may cause transient motor and bowel and bladder dysfunction. However, neurolysis of lumbosacral nerves can damage motor nerve roots, resulting in lost or impaired bowel, bladder, or sexual function. This procedure is generally reserved for clients who have intractable cancer-related pain. Before permanent neurolysis is considered, a temporary nerve block may be given to determine the degree of relief if nerve impulses are disrupted. Although the intent of neurolysis is to permanently destroy nerve transmission, clients may only experience short-term pain relief because of nerve cell regeneration or the development of alternative pathways capable of transmitting pain. Although relatively new, permanent ablation of nerve roots can be done with thermal techniques

such as radiofrequency ablation, which uses heat, or cyroanalgesia, which involves cold.

Because a nerve block is an invasive procedure performed by anesthesiologists, neurosurgeons, surgeons, and neurologists, the physician is responsible for informing the client about the procedure, its risks, and alternative treatments. The nurse reinforces this information with the client and family.

Epidural steroids may also be used for pain; however, their use in certain pain conditions is controversial. Some investigators have looked at the evidence for use of epidural steroids in clients with low back pain (Koes et al., 1995). Their review of 12 randomized clinical trials found this treatment to be effective in only half of the published studies. They concluded that the benefits of epidural injection, if any, are of short duration.

Spinal Cord Stimulation. Spinal cord stimulator therapy offers a more invasive method of nerve stimulation. This technique involves the use of electrodes implanted under the skin into the area of nerve(s) responsible for the pain. At first, a trial of spinal cord stimulation is attempted through the use of temporary externalized electrodes, which are implanted and connected to an stimulator device. The amount of electrical current is adjusted to provide pain relief without additional discomfort. If successful, the client is taken to the operating room for placement of a permanent implantable stimulator. Forrest (1996) discusses the nursing implications associated with this technique.

Surgical Techniques. Some techniques aimed at surgically interrupting the transmission of pain include rhizotomy and cordotomy. With the new, improved pain management measures currently available, these procedures are not performed as commonly today (see Fig. 9–10).

In rhizotomy, sensory nerve roots are destroyed where they enter the spinal cord. In a *closed* rhizotomy, a percutaneous catheter is inserted into the area, and the sensory nerve roots are destroyed by neurolytic chemicals, coagulation, or cryodestruction (extreme cold). For an *open* rhizotomy, a laminectomy is necessary. During this surgery, the physician isolates the nerve roots and destroys them. With a cordotomy, the surgeon transects the pain pathways at the midline portion of the spinal cord before nerve impulses ascend to the spinothalamic tract. As with the other surgical procedures, clients may experience impaired bowel, bladder, or sexual function. Because of the complexity of the pain experience, the interruption of nerve conduction and pain pathways may not totally interrupt the client's sensation of pain.

After surgical intervention, the nurse assesses the nature of the neurologic deficits, if any, and teaches the client how to adapt to them. If the client has lost sensation in a body area, he or she will need to learn how to protect that area from harm. The nurse also assesses the client's expectations in relation to the surgical interruption of painful sensations and helps the client to express realistic expectations.

Stimulation Techniques. Acupuncture and dorsal column stimulation are means of achieving pain control through stimulating certain parts of the nervous system.

Acupuncture. The practice of acupuncture originated in China. According to ancient beliefs, the body is divided into 10 hypothetic sections by parasagittal lines, or meridians. Specific acupuncture points are located within these meridians. The acupuncturist inserts tiny needles into the skin and subcutaneous tissues at these points, and manual vibration or electrical stimulation is delivered. This technique is used to relieve pain and is thought to cure certain diseases.

Acupuncture is still widely acclaimed in China, but it is less popular in the West. Because the physiologic basis for this technique is unclear, many Western health professionals are skeptical about its usefulness. Nonetheless, acupuncture is practiced for anesthetic purposes during diagnostic procedures, during labor and delivery, during surgery, and for the treatment of pain. It is also used to help clients change behavior, for example, to stop smoking. More than 1000 acupuncture sites have been identified, and 14 "lines" exist as *meridians* (Fig. 9–10).

Dorsal Column Stimulation. Dorsal column stimulation is a temporary or permanent way of stimulating nerve

roots in the spinal cord to override the painful stimuli. Usually, good candidates for this procedure are those who derive some benefit from the application of transcutaneous electrical nerve stimulation (TENS). Percutaneous electrodes can be inserted into the epidural space in close proximity to nerve roots entering the dorsal horn of the spinal cord. The electrodes are then connected to an external device capable of delivering an electrical current. Clients who respond to this technique may go on to have permanent implantable stimulators.

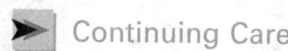

Continuing Care

➤ *Home Care Management*

For some clients, the pain experience extends beyond hospitalization. Effective analgesic regimens or pain-relieving strategies should be coordinated prior to discharge if clients are to leave the hospital with pain. The nurse ensures that the client, especially the opioid-dependent client, has at least enough pain medication to last until the first follow-up visit. Preparation for home care is carried out with the client and family. The nurse assesses the physical layout of the home and related environment. Together with the client and family, the nurse, discharge planner, or occupational therapist determines whether modifications are necessary so that a reasonably pain-free regimen can be maintained after the client is discharged. If physical modifications (e.g., installing a downstairs bathroom) are unrealistic (too expensive or unacceptable to the client or family), the caregiver suggests changes in schedules, role responsibilities, and daily routines to help avoid fatigue, which heightens the awareness of pain.

At home, clients may require referral for physical therapy, especially to continue treatment with cutaneous stimulation, TENS, or heat or cold techniques. Clients may need a psychiatric clinical nurse specialist or social worker to help them develop coping strategies or maintain adequate family dynamics. In the management of terminally ill clients, hospice referral (hospital based or within the community) can help maintain continuity of care. Clients with cancer may be at risk for developing uncontrolled pain that, if not managed at home, will result in hospitalization (Plaisance, 1997). Importantly, nurses knowledgeable about palliative care and end-of-life issues are better able to manage pain crises.

The growing number of home infusion therapy programs provides a wide variety of services to clients who require technology-supported pain care at home. Many of these services depend on insurance-carrier approval generally before analgesic options are considered and placement of technology is performed. Well-defined home agency practices and professional support at home are key if clients are required to leave the hospital with infusional pain therapy (Gorski & Grothman, 1996).

➤ *Health Teaching*

The nurse directs educational efforts toward involving clients and their families in continuing health care behaviors that will relieve pain and improve psychological well-being and overall functional status. The nurse teaches the

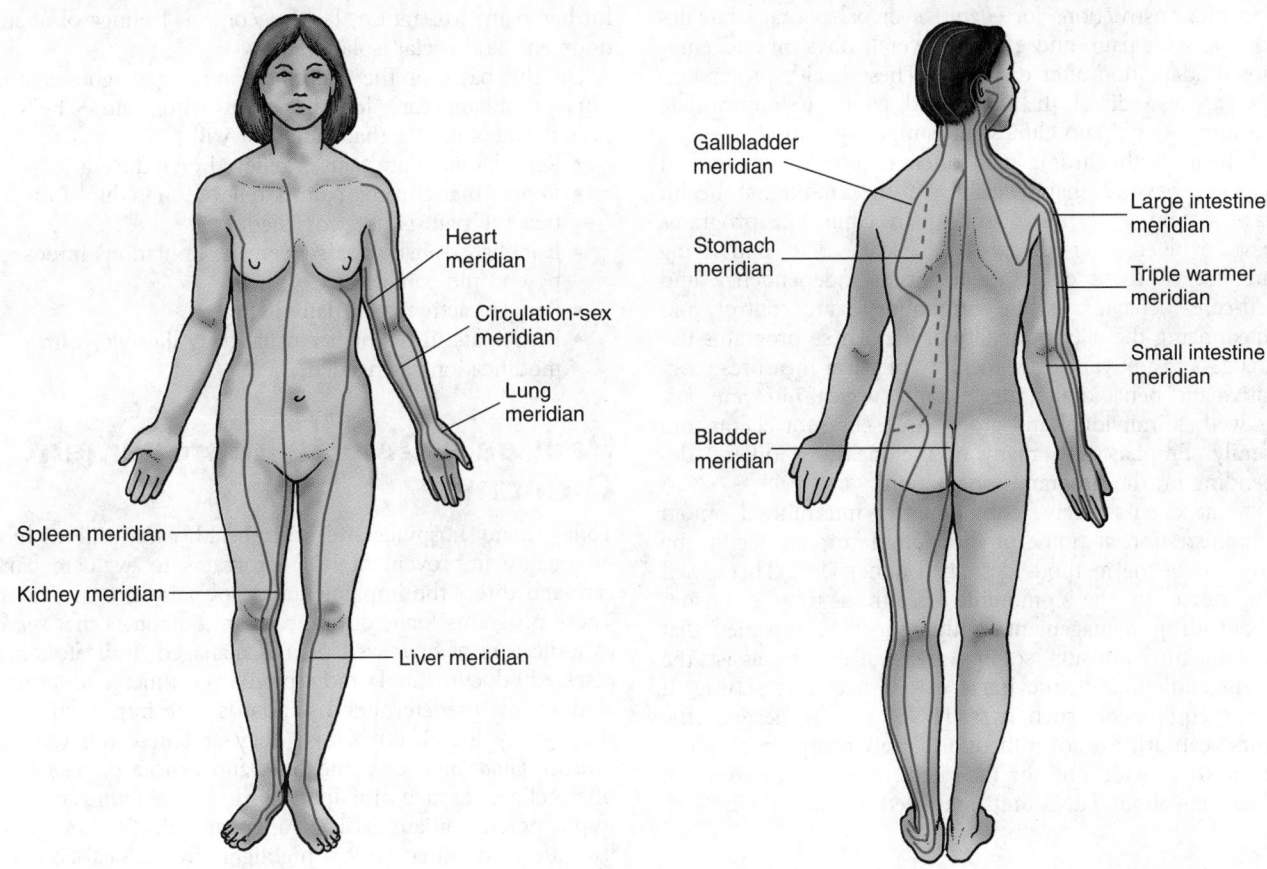

Figure 9–10. Acupuncture meridians.

client and family about analgesic regimens, the purpose and action of medications, their side effects or adverse reactions, and the importance of dosage intervals.

The nurse explains that ideally the analgesic regimen should not interfere with the client's sleep, rest, appetite, or level of physical mobility. If such interference occurs, the nurse encourages the family or significant other to consult with the physician or the visiting nurse.

In clients with pain from advanced cancer, all efforts should be directed toward maximizing pain relief and symptom control at home to eliminate unnecessary readmissions. This may mean that the physician prescribes a flexible analgesic schedule that allows the client to titrate analgesics based on the amount of pain. The nurse teaches the client and family how to safely increase the medication within the prescribed dosing guidelines.

The nurse evaluates family support systems to assist the client in adhering to and continuing the proposed medical and nursing plans. Family members are informed about and included in activities during and after hospitalization.

To achieve a reasonable level of expectation for the client, the nurse suggests ways to continue participation in household, social, sexual, and work-oriented activities after discharge. The nurse can help the client identify important activities and plan them around adequate rest schedules.

The client with chronic pain needs continued support to cope with the anxiety, fear, and powerlessness that often accompany this type of pain. The nurse helps the client and family or significant others to identify coping strategies that have worked in the past. Outside support systems are also identified. Chapter 8 discusses stress and coping in detail.

➤ Health Care Resources

A home health nurse referral is made when it is anticipated that clients will require assistance or supervision with their pain relief regimen at home. This referral should include specific information from the hospital-based staff nurse about the client's overall physical condition, general level of sedation, weakness or fatigue, possible constipation or nutritional problems, and sleep patterns.

In addition to explaining the client's physical status to the home health nurse, the staff nurse also describes the client's levels of anxiety and depression and general expectations about pain status after discharge. The nurse describes family interactions and determines whether the client or family anticipates any altered role functions at home. The client's close relationships and available support network are important factors in providing ongoing support for effective pain intervention strategies.

Referrals to the clinical nurse pain specialist, social worker, or psychologist are appropriate ways to continue to provide emotional support to the client and family, reinforce instructions for cognitive or behavioral strategies to deal with pain, and evaluate overall physical and emotional adaptation after discharge. These health professionals can also direct the client and family to appropriate resources (e.g., pain clinics and support groups).

Clients with chronic pain often require treatment and support beyond that available in the traditional health care system. For this reason, pain clinics or programs have evolved over the past 25 years. The underlying premise of these clinics is to foster independence and self-care behaviors while promoting pain control and maximizing the client's quality of life. These programs use analgesics, adjuvant drug therapy, physical measures, cognitive and behavioral strategies, and surgical interventions, as well as individual and group counseling for clients and family. Emphasis on many of the measures differs, depending on the program's orientation.

Some clients receive continuous or intermittent opioid administration at home or in a long-term care facility by any one of the methods described under Drug Therapy. If the nurse in the community health setting is unsure about drug management, a number of companies that manufacture infusion set-ups are available to assist the client and nurse in the home or alternate care setting. If other equipment, such as a TENS unit, is needed, the nurse can arrange for a medical supply company or pharmacy to provide one for the client. Answers to common questions about TENS units are listed in Chart 9–3.

 Evaluation

Historically, inadequate attention has been given to evaluating the effects of pain interventions. Caregivers may not assess the degree of pain relief and intensity accurately or often enough. Furthermore, nurses may not establish pain relief goals that are consistent with the client and families' expectations. Because of this, the client is at risk for further pain, frustration, lack of control, feelings of abandonment, and social isolation.

On the basis of the identified nursing diagnoses, the nurse evaluates care for the client with pain. The expected outcomes are that the client will

- Report that acute pain is relieved or reduced.
- Report that chronic pain is relieved or reduced or that the pain is not worsened.
- Establish realistic goals given the limitations imposed by chronic pain.
- Perform activities of daily living.
- Participate in his or her usual daily lifestyle, with modifications as needed.

Pain as a Quality Improvement Outcome

Today, many hospitals and other health care facilities rely on quality improvement (QI) programs to evaluate pain care and direct the implementation of pain care strategies. These programs focus on critical pain outcomes that serve as indicators of how well pain is managed. Indicators are assessed, documented, monitored over time, and evaluated against predetermined standards. The introduction of the Agency for Health Care Policy and Research *Clinical Practice Guidelines* for acute pain and cancer pain (1992) offers clinicians a useful framework for designing quality improvement initiatives. The American Pain Society Quality Care Committee (1995) highlights five critical components of a QI program for pain. Programs should be based on the following tenets: 1) unrelieved pain should attract clinicians' attention; 2) information about analgesics should be accessible where orders are written; 3) clients should be assured of responsive analgesic care and urged to communicate pain; 4) policies and safeguards should be implemented for the use of technology-supported pain care; and 5) implementation of these measures should be assessed and coordinated.

Some investigators have used self-report measures of pain and assessments of analgesic therapy as a QI initiative to gauge the level of compliance with the Agency for Health Care Policy and Research Clinical Practice Guidelines for Acute Pain (1992) (Dietrick-Gallagher et al., 1994). Others have identified systems and caregivers' barriers to pain control through QI monitoring (Bookbinder et al., 1996).

Costs of Pain Care

When caring for clients with pain, the nurse appreciates the financial aspects of pain care, especially in the current climate of managed care. Kolassa (1994) identifies several factors associated with medication costs. First, costs differ depending on the location of administration. Parenteral drug therapy administered in a hospital setting may be more costly than at home. Second, the commercial success of the agent influences the price of a pharmaceutical product. Third, the type of manufacturer and history of drug development and testing influences the market price of a drug. Drug innovations like extended-release or controlled-release products may be more costly per tablet

---

Chart 9–3

Education Guide: TENS Units

- The cost of using your TENS unit should be comparable to that for a regimen of prescription drugs or surgery.
- Insurance usually covers the cost of buying or leasing a TENS unit.
- You can get a TENS unit only through the physician who prescribed it.
- Whether a TENS unit works for you will depend on your type of pain. These units have been used successfully on back pain, arm and leg pain, pain from neuralgia, arthritis pain, and other types of pain. A trial period under a physician's care is generally advised.
- TENS units are relatively simple to operate. You simply attach color-coded electrodes to your skin over the painful area. You then turn the unit on and, depending on your level of pain, you make day-to-day adjustments.

TABLE 9–8

Economics of Pain Care: Cost Analysis Framework

Costs associated with oral alternative route medications
Costs associated with parenteral/neuraxial administration
Unreimbursed charges of medication therapy
Costs of surgical interventions
Costs of specialized pain care
Costs of nondrug measures
Expenditures to justify costs
Reimbursement issues
Expenditures by various health care settings and home
   costs associated with preventing and treating
   complications of pain/pain therapy

Adapted from Agency for Health Care Policy and Research. (1994). *Clinical Practice Guidelines for Cancer Pain.* From: Ferrell, B. R., Griffith, H. (1994). Cost issues related to pain management: Report from the Cancer Pain Panel of the Agency for Health Care Policy and Research. *Journal of Pain and Symptom Management, 9*(4), 221–234.

than short-acting agents. However, the cost of the overall therapy (dose per day) may be similar or only slightly more. A cost-analysis framework for evaluating the economic implications for pain care is provided in Table 9–8).

Technology-supported pain care is always associated with increased costs, but the financial expenditures in selected populations may be worth it in terms of improved clinical outcomes. Epidural analgesia and patient-controlled analgesia in the immediate postoperative period have shown significant benefits in improving pain control and recovery, compared with intermittent nurse-administered analgesics. The use of technology in delivering analgesia may also be cost-efficient for certain clients with intractable chronic nonmalignant and cancer-related pain. Despite the inflated costs of extended-release or controlled-release preparations, clients report better compliance and achieve better pain control.

For long-term management of pain, the oral route is preferred. The nurse considers the cost of both opioid and nonopioid analgesics to ensure that the cost expenditures for drug therapy are within the client's financial budget. Knowledge of the client's prescription plan aids the nurse in assessing "out of pocket" expenses by the client. Certainly, the nurse must factor in any other health care expenditures for the client and/or family. Some pharmaceutical companies, usually manufacturers of opioid analgesics, supply indigent clients with free medication if they meet certain eligibility criteria.

Significant health care costs are associated with hospitalizations for pain control (Grant et al., 1995). The nurse recognizes the importance of aggressive pain care to facilitate discharge and prevent subsequent hospitalizations for pain.

SELECTED BIBLIOGRAPHY

*Acute Pain Management Guideline Panel. (1992). *Acute pain management: Operative or medical procedures and trauma. Clinical practice guideline.* AHCPR Pub. No. 92-0032. Rockville, MD: Agency for Health Care Policy and Research, Public Health Service, U.S. Department of Health and Human Services.

Allock, N. (1996). The use of different research methodologies to evaluate the effectiveness of programmes to improve the care of patients in postoperative pain. *Journal of Advanced Nursing, 23*(1), 32–38.

Altman, G. B., & Lee, C. A. (1996). Strontium-89 for treatment of painful bone metastasis from prostate cancer. *Oncology Nursing Forum, 23*(3), 523–527.

*American Pain Society. (1989). *Principles of analgesic use in the treatment of acute pain and chronic cancer pain: A concise guide to medical practice.* Washington, D.C.: American Pain Society.

American Pain Society Quality of Care Committee. (1995). Quality improvement guidelines for the treatment of acute pain and cancer pain. *Journal of American Medical Association, 274*(23), 1874–1880.

*Arathuzik, M. D. (1991). The appraisal of pain and coping in cancer clients. *Western Journal of Nursing Research, 13*(6), 714–731.

*Barker, E. (1987). Pain. *Journal of Neurosurgical Nursing, 19,* 233–234.

*Bonica, J. (1983). The importance of education and training in pain diagnosis and therapy. In R. Rizzi & M. Visentin (Eds.), *Pain therapy* (pp. 1–10). Amsterdam: Elsevier Biomedical.

Bookbinder, M., Coyle, N., Kiss M., Goldstein, M. L., Holritz, K., Thaler, H., Gianella, A., Derby, S., Brown, M., Racolin, A., Ho, M.-N., & Portenoy, R. K. (1996). Implementing national standards for cancer pain management: Program model and evaluation. *Journal of Pain & Symptom Management, 12*(6), 334–347.

*Burckhardt, C. S. (1990). Chronic pain. *Nursing Clinics of North America, 25,* 868–870.

*Burke, S. O., & Jerrett, M. (1989). Pain management across age groups. *Western Journal of Nursing Research, 11,* 164–178.

*Calvillo, E. R., & Flaskerud, J. H. (1991). Review of literature on culture and pain of adults with focus of Mexican-Americans. *Journal of Transcultural Nursing, 2,* 16–23.

*Calvillo, E. R., & Flaskerud, J. H. (1993). Evaluation of the pain response by Mexican-American and Anglo-American women and their nurses. *Journal of Advanced Nursing, 18,* 451–459.

*Carroll, K. C., & Magruder, C. C. (1993). The role of analgesics and sedatives in the management of pain and agitation during weaning from mechanical ventilation. *Critical Care Nursing Quarterly, 15*(4), 68–77.

Cederholm, I. (1997). Preliminary risk-benefit analysis of ropivacaine in labour and following surgery. *Drug Safety, 16*(6), 391–402.

*Champlin, L. (1992). Inadequate analgesia: Clients endure pain, fear addiction. *Geriatrics, 47*(8), 71–74.

*Clark, I. M. (1993). Management of postoperative pain. *Lancet, 341,* 27.

Clarke, E. B., French, B., Bilodeau, M. L., Capasso, V. C., & Empoliti, J. (1996). Pain management knowledge, attitudes and clinical practice: The impact of nurses' characteristics and education. *Journal of Pain & Symptom Management, 11*(1), 18–31.

Cleeland, C. S., Gonin, R., Hatfield, A. K., Edmonson, J. H., Blum, R. H., Stewart, J. A., & Pandya, K. J. (1994). Pain and pain treatment in outclients with metastatic cancer: The Eastern Cooperative Oncology Group's outpatient pain study. *The New England Journal of Medicine, 330,* 592–596.

Cleeland, C. S., & Ryan, K. M. (1994). Pain assessment: Global use of the Brief Pain Inventory. *Annals of the Academy of Medicine, Singapore, 23*(2), 129–138.

Cleeland, C. S., Nakamura, Y., Mendoza, T. R., Edwards, K. R., Douglas, J., & Serlin, R. C. (1996). Dimensions of the impact of cancer pain in a four-country sample: New information from multidimensional scaling. *Pain, 67*(2–3), 267–273.

Cobb, S. C. & Mindel, S. A. (1996). Creating a cost-effective pain management task force in a community hospital. *MEDSURG Nursing, 5*(6), 445–448.

*Deikmann, J. M., & Wassem, R. A. (1991). A survey of nursing students' knowledge of cancer pain control. *Cancer Nursing, 14,* 314–320.

deJong, P. C., & Kansen, P. J. (1994). A comparison of epidural catheters with or without subcutaneous injection ports for treatment of cancer pain. *Anesthesia and Analgesia, 78*(1), 94–100.

Dietrick-Gallagher, M., Polomano, R. C., & Carrick, L. (1994). Pain as a quality management initiative. *J Nurs Care Qual 9*(1), 30–42.

*Dobkin de Rios, M., & Achauer, B. M. (1991). Pain relief for the Hispanic burn patient using cultural metaphors. *Plastic and Reconstructive Surgery, 88*(1), 160–164.

*Donovan, M. W. (1990). Acute pain relief. *Nursing Clinics of North America, 25,* 851–861.

Dunbar, S. A., & Katz, N. P. (1996). Chronic opioid therapy for nonmalignant pain in clients with a history of substance abuse: Report of 20 cases. *Journal of Pain and Symptom Management, 11*(3), 163–171.

Eckes Peck, S. D. (1997). The effectiveness of therapeutic touch for decreasing pain in elders with degenerative arthritis. *Journal of Holistic Nursing, 15*(2), 176–198.

*Egbert, A. M. (1991). Help for the hurting elderly: Safe use of drugs to relieve pain. *Postgraduate Medicine, 89*(4), 217–228.

Faucett, J. A. (1994). Depression in painful chronic disorders: The role of pain and conflict about pain. *Journal of Pain and Symptom Management, 9*(8), 520–526.

*Ferrell, B. A., Ferrell, B. R., & Osterweil, D. (1990). Pain in the nursing home. *Journal of the American Geriatrics Society, 38,* 409–414.

Ferrell, B. R., & Griffith, H. (1994). Cost issues related to pain management: Report from the Cancer Pain Panel of the Agency for Health Care Policy and Research. *Journal of Pain and Symptom Management, 9*(4), 221–234.

*Ferrell, B. R., McCaffery, M., & Grant, M. (1991). Clinical decision making and pain. *Cancer Nursing, 14,* 289–297.

*Ferrell, B. R., McCaffery, M., & Rhiner, M. (1992a). Pain and education: An urgent need for change in nursing education. *Journal of Pain and Symptom Management, 7*(2), 117–124.

*Ferrell, B. R., McCaffery, M., & Ropchan, R. (1992b). Pain management as a clinical challenge for nursing administration. *Nursing Outlook, 40,* 263–268.

*Ferrell, B. R., McGuire, D. B., & Donovan, M. I. (1993). Knowledge and beliefs regarding pain in a sample of nursing faculty. *Journal of Professional Nursing, 9*(2), 79–88.

Ferrell, B., Whedon, M., & Rollins, B. (1995). Pain and quality assessment/improvement. *Journal of Nursing Care Quality, 9*(3), 69–85.

*Ferrell-Torry, A. T., & Glick, O. J. (1993). The use of therapeutic massage as a nursing intervention to modify anxiety and the perception of cancer pain. *Cancer Nursing, 16,* 93–101.

*Fife, B. L., Irick, N., & Painter, J. D. (1993). A comparative study of the attitudes of physicians and nurses toward the management of pain. *Journal of Pain and Symptom Management, 8*(3), 132–139.

Fishbain, D. A., Chabal, C., Abbott, A., Heine, L. W., & Cutler R. (1996). Transcutaneous electrical nerve stimulation (TENS) treatment outcome in long-term users. *Clinical Journal of Pain, 12*(3), 201–214.

*Flor, H., Fydrich, T., & Turk, D. C. (1992). Efficacy of multidisciplinary pain treatment centers: A meta analytic review. *Pain, 49,* 221–230.

Forrest, D. M. (1996). Spinal cord stimulator therapy. *Journal of Perianesthesia Nursing, 11*(5), 349–352.

*Gaston-Johansson, F., Albert, M., Fagan, E., & Zimmerman, L. (1990). Similarities in pain descriptions of four different ethnic-culture groups. *Journal of Pain and Symptom Management, 5*(2), 94–100.

Gorski, L. A., & Grothman L. (1996). Home infusion therapy. *Seminars in Oncology Nursing, 12*(3), 193–201.

Grant, M., Ferrell, B. R., Rivera, L. M., & Lee, J. (1995). Unscheduled readmissions for uncontrolled symptoms. *Nursing Clinics of North America, 30*(4), 673–682.

*Greenwald, H. P. (1991). Interethnic differences in pain perception. *Pain, 44*(2), 157–163.

*Greipp, M. (1992). Undermedication for pain: An ethical model. *Advances in Nursing Science, 15*(1), 44–53.

Guyton, A. C. (1996). *Textbook of medical physiology* (9th ed.) Philadelphia: W. B. Saunders.

Harkins, S. W. (1996). Geriatric pain. Pain perceptions in the old. *Clinics of Geriatric Medicine, 12*(3), 435–459.

*Haviley, C., et al. (1992). Pharmacological management of cancer pain: A guide for the health professional. *Cancer Nursing, 15,* 331–346.

Heiser, R. M., Chiles, K., Fudge, M., & Gray, S. E. (1997). The use of music during the immediate postoperative recovery period. *AORN Journal, 65*(4), 777–785.

*Herr, K. A., & Mobily, P. R. (1991). Complexities of pain assessment in the elderly. *Journal of Gerontological Nursing, 17*(4), 12–19.

*Herr, K. A., & Mobily, P. R. (1992). Interventions related to pain. *Nursing Clinics of North America, 27,* 347–370.

Hitchcook, L. S., Ferrell, B. R., & McCaffery, M. (1994). The experience of chronic nonmalignant pain. *Journal of Pain and Symptom Management, 9*(5), 312–318.

*Hofland, S. L. (1992). Elder beliefs: Blocks to pain management. *Journal of Gerontological Nursing, 18*(6), 19–40.

*Hyman, R. B., Feldman, H. R., Harris, R. B., et al. (1989). The effects of relaxation training on clinical symptoms: A meta-analysis. *Nursing Research, 38*(4), 216–220.

*International Association on Pain, Subcommittee of Taxonomy. (1979). Pain terms: A list with definitions and notes on usage. *Pain, 6,* 249.

*Jacox, A. K. (Ed.) (1977). *Pain: A source book for nurses and other health care professionals.* Boston: Little, Brown.

*Johnson, J., Rice, V., Fuller, S., et al. (1978). Sensory information, information in a coping strategy, and recovery from surgery. *Research in Nursing and Health, 1,* 4–17.

*Keeney, S. A. (1993). Nursing care of the postoperative patient receiving epidural analgesia. *MEDSURG Nursing, 2*(3), 191–196.

*Keller, E., & Bzdek, V. (1986). Effects of therapeutic touch on tension headache pain. *Nursing Research, 35,* 101–105.

Koes, B. W., Scholten, R. J., Mens, J. M., & Bouter, L. M. (1995). Efficacy of epidural steroid injections for low back pain and sciatica: A systematic review of randomized clinical trials. *Pain, 63,* 279–288.

Kolassa, E. M. (1994). Guidance for clinicians in discerning and comparing the price of pharmaceutical agents. *Journal of Pain and Symptom Management, 9*(4), 221–234.

*Kreiger, D. (1975). Therapeutic touch: The imprimatur of nursing. *American Journal of Nursing, 75,* 784–787.

Malek, C. J., & Olivieri, R. J. (1996). Pain management—Documenting the decision making process. *Nursing Case Management, 1*(2), 64–74.

Management of Cancer Pain Guideline Panel. (1994). *Management of cancer pain: Clinical practice guidelines.* AHCPR Pub. No. 94-0592. Rockville, MD: Agency for Health Care Policy and Research, Public Health Service, U.S. Department of Health and Human Services.

*McCaffery, M. (1979). *Nursing management of the patient with pain.* (2nd ed.) Philadelphia: J. B. Lippincott.

*McCaffery, M. (1980). Relieving pain with noninvasive techniques. *Nursing '80, 10*(12), 54–57.

*McCaffery, M. (1990). Pain management: Nurses lead the way to new priorities. *American Journal of Nursing, 90,* 45–50.

*McCaffery, M., & Beebe, A. (1989). *Pain: Clinical manual for nursing practice.* St. Louis: C. V. Mosby.

*McCaffery, M., Ferrell, B., O'Neil-Page E., Lester, M., & Ferrell, B. (1990). Nurses' knowledge of opioid analgesic drugs and psychological dependence. *Cancer Nursing, 13*(1), 21–27.

*McGuire, D. B. (1984). The measurement of clinical pain. *Nursing Research, 33,* 152–156.

McGuire, L. (1994). The nurse's role in pain relief. *MEDSURG Nursing, 3*(2), 94–107.

*Melzack, R. (1973). *The puzzle of pain.* New York: Basic Books.

*Melzack, R. (1975). The McGill Pain Questionnaire: Major properties and scoring methods. *Pain, 1,* 277–299.

*Melzack, R. (1983). The McGill Pain Questionnaire. In R. Melzack (Ed.), *Pain assessment and management* (pp. 41–47). New York: Raven Press.

*Melzack, R. (1987). The short form McGill Pain Questionnaire. *Pain, 30,* 191–197.

*Melzack, R., & Wall, P. D. (1982). *The challenge of pain.* New York: Basic Books.

Miller, J., Neelon, V., Dalton, J., Ng'andu, N., Bailey, D., Layman, E., & Hosfeld, A. (1996). The assessment of discomfort in elderly confused patients: A preliminary study. *Journal of Neuroscience Nursing, 28*(3), 175–182.

Mobily, P. R., Herr, K. A., & Nicholson, A. C. (1994). Validation of cutaneous stimulation interventions for pain management. *International Journal of Nursing Studies, 31*(6), 533–544.

Mulloney, S. S., & Wells-Federman, C. (1996). Therapeutic touch: A healing modality. *Journal of Cardiovascular Nursing, 10*(30), 27–82.

*National Institutes of Health. (1986). *The integrated approach to the management of pain: Consensus Development Conference statement.* Washington, D. C.: U.S. Government Printing Office.

*Neeley, M. A. (1993). Pain management in elderly clients. *MEDSURG Nursing Quarterly, 1*(4), 32–51.

*Neill, K. M. (1993). Ethnic pain styles in acute myocardial infarction. *Western Journal of Nursing Research, 15*(5), 531–547.

Paice, J. A., Penn, R. D., & Ryan, W. G. (1994). Altered sexual function and decreased testosterone in clients receiving intraspinal opioids. *Journal of Pain and Symptom Management, 9,* 126–131.

*Pasero, C. L. (1994). Pain control. *American Journal of Nursing, 94*(2), 22–23.

Pasero, C. L., & McCaffery, M. (1994). Avoiding opioid-induced respiratory depression. *American Journal of Nursing, 94*(4), 25–30.

Plaisance, L. (1997). Managing cancer pain crisis effectively in the home. *Home Health Nurse, 15*(6), 411–413.

Polomano, R. C. (1995). *The relationship of pain characteristics, type of cancer, and opioid consumption to quality of life, psychological distress and pain outcomes* [Unpublished doctoral dissertation]. University of Maryland, Baltimore, MD.

*Polomano, R. C., Blumenthal, N., Schiavonne-Gatto, P., & O'Brien, J. (1993). Recommendations for developing policies and procedures for the administration of continuous epidural narcotics/local anesthetics with or without patient controlled epidural analgesia. *MEDSURG Nursing, 2*(3), 195–196.

*Polomano, R. C., Blumenthal, N. P., & Riegler, F. X. (1993). Intrapleural analgesia for the management of postoperative pain. *MEDSURG Nursing, 2*(3), 185–190.

Polomano, R. C., Soulen, M., & McDaniel, C. (1997). Sedation and analgesia with interventional radiology for oncology patients. *Critical Care Nursing Clinics of North America, 9*(3), 335–353.

*Poniatowski, B. C. (1991). Continuous subcutaneous infusions for pain control. *Journal of Intravenous Nursing, 14,* 30–35.

Puntillo, K., & Weiss, S. J. (1994). Pain: Its mediators and associated morbidity in critically ill cardiovascular surgical clients. *Nursing Research, 43*(1), 31–36.

Rauck, R. L. (1997). Intraspinal therapy in the management of refractory cancer pain. *Techniques in Regional Anesthesia and Pain Management, 1*(1), 38–48.

*Ruda, M. A. (1993). Gender and pain. *Pain, 53,* 1–2.

Sloman, R. (1995). Relaxation and the relief of cancer pain. *Nursing Clinics of North America, 30*(4), 697–709.

*Sternbach, R. A. (1968). *Pain: A psychophysiological analysis.* New York: Academic Press.

*Stevens, K. (1990). Clients' perceptions of music during surgery. *Journal of Advanced Nursing, 15,* 1045–1051.

*Thomas, B. L. (1990). Pain management for the elderly: Alternative interventions (Part 1). *AORN Journal, 52,* 1268–1272.

*Vallerand, A. H., (1991). The use of narcotic analgesics in chronic nonmalignant pain. *Holistic Nursing Practice, 6*(1), 17–23.

Vallerand, A. H., (1994). Street addicts and clients with pain: Similarities and differences. *Clinical Nurse Specialist, 8*(1), 11–12.

Vallerand, A. H. (1995). Gender differences in pain. *Image: Journal of Nursing Scholarship, 27*(3), 235–237.

*Von Roenn, J. H., Cleeland, C. S., Gonin, R., Hatfield, A. K., & Pandya, K. J. (1993). Physician attitudes and practices in cancer pain management: A survey from the Eastern Cooperative Oncology Group. *Annals of Internal Medicine, 119,* 121–126.

*Walding, M. F. (1991). Pain, anxiety, and powerlessness. *Journal of Advanced Nursing, 16,* 388–397.

Wallace, K. G., Reed, B. A., Pasero, C., & Olsson, G. L. (1995). Staff nurses' perceptions of barriers to effective pain management. *Journal of Pain and Symptom Management, 10*(3), 205–213.

Ward, S., & Gatwood, J. (1994). Concerns about reporting pain and using analgesics. *Cancer Nursing, 17*(3), 200–206.

Weber, S. E. (1996). Cultural aspects of pain in childbearing women. *Journal of Obstetric, Gynecologic, & Neonatal Nursing, 25*(1), 67–72.

*Wells, N. (1982). The effect of relaxation on postoperative pain. *Nursing Research, 31,* 236–238.

*Wild, L., & Coyne, C. (1992). The basics and beyond: Epidural analgesia. *American Journal of Nursing, 92*(4), 26–34.

Wilke, D. J. (1995). Neural mechanisms of pain: A foundation for cancer pain assessment and management. In D. B. McGuire, C. H. Yarbro, & B. R. Ferrell (Eds.) *Cancer pain management* (2nd ed.; pp. 61–87). Boston: Jones and Bartlett Publishers.

Willens, J. S. (1994). Giving fentanyl for pain outside the OR. *American Journal of Nursing, 94*(2) 24–28.

*Zatzick, D. F., & Dimsdale, J. E. (1990). Cultural variations in response to painful stimuli. *Psychosomatic Medicine, 52,* 544–557.

Zimmerman, L., Nieveen, J., Barnason, S., & Schmaderer, M. (1996). The effects of music therapy on postoperative pain and sleep in coronary artery bypass graft (CABG) patients. *Scholarly Inquiry for Nursing Practice, 10*(2), 153–170.

Zimmerman L., Story, K. T., Gaston-Johansson, F., & Rowles, J. R. (1996). Psychological variables and cancer pain. *Cancer Nursing, 19*(1), 44–53.

SUGGESTED READINGS

Heiser, R. M., Chiles, K., Fudge, M., & Gray, S. E. (1997). The use of music during the immediate postoperative recovery period. *AORN Journal, 65*(4), 777–784.

This study examined the effect of music therapy on pain management in the post-anesthesia care unit (PACU). Two groups of clients were compared—one group listened to music during the last 30 minutes of their surgery and during the first hour in the PACU. No differences were found in pain management between the treatment group and the control group, but the clients who heard music stated that it helped them relax and functioned as a distractor.

Malek, C. J. & Olivieri, R. J. (1996). Pain management—Documenting the decision making process. *Nursing Case Management, 1*(2), 64–74.

The authors examined hospital nurses' clinical decisions regarding pain management and found that they did not adequately document pain assessments or pain relief and that they undertreated pain by not administering the amount of analgesia that was ordered. Additionally, there was minimal documentation of cognitive, behavioral, or physical interventions for pain.

BODY IMAGE

Self-concept is the sum of self-esteem, role performance, and body image (Fig. 10–1). Body image involves both conscious and unconscious information, perceptions, and feelings about one's body. Many illnesses, diseases, and disabilities affect a person's body image.

OVERVIEW

If someone's body image is definite and consistent with reality, the person is likely to feel satisfied with himself or herself. When illness or chronic disability is present, it is a challenge for someone to integrate the physical changes into his or her body image. Nurses, by diagnosing and treating responses to health problems in a holistic manner, are concerned about the total experience of body image development. Therefore, to assess client responses accurately, medical-surgical nurses must understand how illness can change the body image.

Definition of Body Image

Body image includes perceptions of shape, size, mass, function, structure, and significance of the physical, living body in relation to its parts. It also may include inanimate objects that are part of a person's daily contact with the body (e.g., make-up, jewelry, eyeglasses, clothing, wheelchair, crutches, or other appliances). Body image is a complex concept that is difficult to assess in nursing practice and is influenced by many factors.

Factors Affecting Body Image

Body image is influenced by several factors, including aging, culture, gender roles, and technology.

AGING. The Western World continues to place a major emphasis on the "ideal body," which represents youth, an ideal body weight, beauty, and agility. If a person does not fit this social image, as the middle-aged and older adult *may* not, he or she may receive negative messages about his or her value as a human being. Therefore, the normal aging process can influence body image.

CULTURE. The role of culture in the formation of body image can also be significant. People learn to judge themselves by how well they live up to the expectations and demands of their culture. The Western World places a high value on physical appearance and popularity with peers. If a person does not meet these expectations, the culture may perceive him or her less favorably. For example, the adult with anorexia nervosa or obesity may be the brunt of cruel jokes. Therefore, the negative attitudes of a person's culture can contribute to the creation of a poor body image.

GENDER ROLES. Gender roles play a major role in body image and the way in which it develops. The women's movement in the Western World has emphasized that although women and men are different, they

147

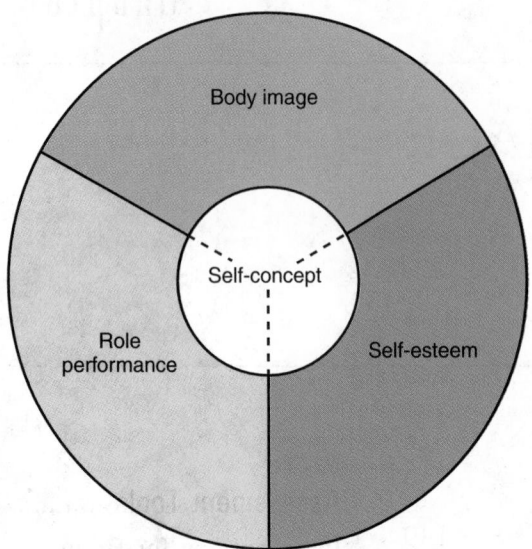

Figure 10–1. Relationship of self-concept to its components. Self-concept is the sum of self-esteem, role performance, and body image.

are of equal *value*. Nevertheless, boys and girls learn at an early age that society's expectations of them may differ greatly.

Body image and sexuality tend to go hand in hand. However, a positive body image does not necessarily predict positive feelings about sexuality or sexual satisfaction. (For more information on human sexuality, see Chapter 11.)

TECHNOLOGY. In the past decade, there have been many technological developments in health care. For example, joint replacements with artificial materials are now very common. Kidney and liver transplants are also common. Never before has so much replacement of human body parts been possible. However, these advances have an impact on body image, although this impact is not clearly understood.

The Life Cycle of Body Image

The body attempts to achieve consistency throughout the life cycle. A person's body image does readjust and adapt through interaction with significant others and the environment; that is, body image development is an ongoing process of learning and maturation through the cycle of life.

Most developmental theorists say that development of body image does not begin until after birth. The newborn is unable to distinguish clear boundaries between itself and the environment: Therefore, the newborn has no perceived body image. Table 10–1 summarizes body image development from infancy through adolescence. Body image development during adulthood is described here.

Young Adulthood (Ages 18–35 Years)

RELATIONSHIPS. Young adults are normally very concerned with developing intimate relationships with others.

Over time, body image becomes more stable and positive as a young adult develops these relationships. Without these relationships, the young adult experiences feelings of isolation. A healthy and realistic body image requires positive social reinforcement because people tend to become what others tell them they are. Unfortunately, stereotyping is common during this stage of development. For example, a young, overweight woman may be stereotyped as undisciplined and inactive when she may be just the opposite. This social reinforcement can strongly influence body image development.

PERSONAL CHARACTERISTICS. Body image develops and changes as the physical body changes. However, certain personal characteristics seem to be more crucial to body image than others. Sexual identification is central to body image, and any circumstance that alters or threatens this identification can affect it. For example, the woman who experiences a mastectomy (breast removal) may begin to question her sexuality and femininity and wonder "Am I still desirable and attractive?" "Am I still a woman?" "Who am I?"

WORK. The kind of work in which the young adult engages is another characteristic that influences body image. A person's identity may center on a career or occu-

TABLE 10–1

Development of Body Image from Infancy Through Adolescence	
Period of the Life Cycle	**Body Image Development Task**
Infancy (birth to age 1 year)	• Develops and uses touch • Perceives the differentiation between self and environment
Toddlerhood (age 1–3 years)	• Learns about body parts • Begins to trust feelings
Preschool (age 3–6 years)	• Develops a sexual identity • Begins to understand the concepts of normal and different, pretty and not pretty
Middle childhood (age 6–12 years)	• Recognizes differences in body types and structures • Focuses on physical appearance, peer relationships, and adherence to social group norms
Adolescence (age 12–18 years)	• Undergoes many internal and external physical changes • Makes comparisons with others and strives for the "perfect" body • Is confused by sexual feelings

pation, such as nurse, artist, farmer, or homemaker. Injury, illness, or change in career may require a total readjustment of body image. A musician who is no longer able to play an instrument because of amputation must readjust and adapt to the changes in his or her body. A painter who is affected by macular degeneration, which causes blindness, also faces the developmental task of body image readjustment.

Women usually have clearer and more accurate images of their bodies than men. Women tend to equate body more with self and are more aware of physical changes, especially around the face. Perhaps these images have related to the historical roles of woman as nurturer and mother, which are closely identified with the body. On the contrary, men have tended to be much less specific in how they view their bodies, perhaps because their roles have traditionally related more toward life accomplishments and attaining power and position in their careers than to their bodies.

Middle Adulthood (Ages 35–65 Years)

The body image of the middle-aged adult (the "middlescent") continues to develop as his or her interaction with the environment becomes more complex. During this period, the middlescent must readjust his or her body image to adapt to the psychological and physical changes of normal aging. This readjustment can be adaptive or maladaptive.

An example of *maladaptive* readjustment of body image is the middlescent who attempts to recapture or mimic youth by applying excessive cosmetics, wearing extremely youthful clothes, or adopting youthful hairstyles. If such an adult continues to perceive his or her physical appearance negatively, the negative body image may result in depression, irritability, and anxiety. The tendency to use maladaptive readjustment strategies depends on a person's personality and level of satisfaction with life up to middlescence.

An example of *adaptive* readjustment is the middle-aged adult who views the changes of this period as evidence of maturity, experience, and knowledge. Such an adult might participate in regular exercise programs, which may slow the normal physical aging process. The middle-aged adult who has successfully developed a realistic body image accepts the self and the body while realizing that acceptance from others cannot be expected unless self-acceptance is present.

Late Adulthood (Older Than 65 Years)

No matter when older adults begin to consider themselves as "elderly," they tend to undergo a marked change in body image. For example, sensory deficits resulting from normal aging are common in the older adult and may decrease the ability to enjoy hobbies, such as reading or listening to music. Decreased strength and increased fatigue may reduce the ability to remain a productive, active worker. These reduced abilities may lead to feelings of worthlessness and despair, which influence body image. Other events that can affect both body image and self-concept as a whole are retirement, loss of a spouse,

and loss of other close family members and friends (see Chap. 5).

Body Image Disturbance

Illness, whether chronic or acute, can change both external and internal body appearance and function. Changes in *external* body appearance and function can be devastating to body image. Chronic illness is usually more disabling than acute illness because it requires continuous body image reintegration as the disease process continues. For example, a client who has had a stroke is aware each day of the mobility or communication deficits that the illness has caused. As a result, the client continuously attempts to reintegrate not only the current body changes into the body image but also the ever-present fear of future immobility or communication losses that can result from further strokes.

Illness can also affect a person's *internal* function. For instance, a woman who has had a hysterectomy appears physically unchanged but has lost organs that contribute to her image as a woman. The medical-surgical nurse must be aware of these less obvious causes of body image disturbance.

The Theory of Readjustment to Body Image Disturbance

Body image readjustment is a lengthy process. Stages of this adaptation process include (1) psychological shock, (2) withdrawal, (3) acknowledgment, and (4) integration (Fig. 10–2).

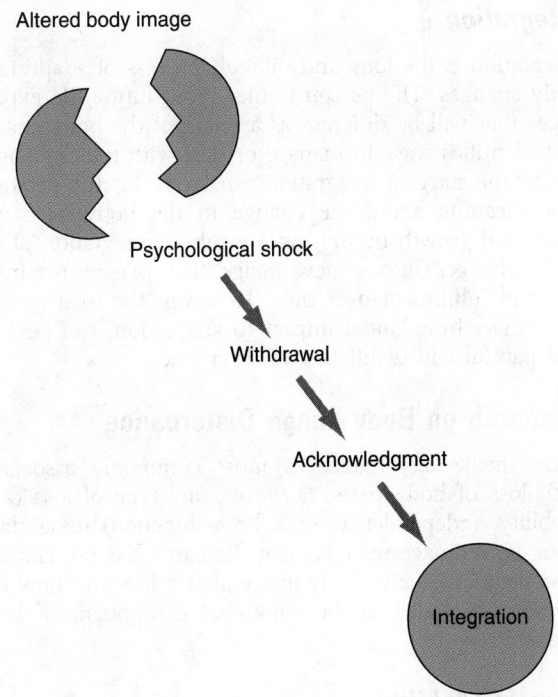

Figure 10–2. Readjustment to altered body image. Stages of the adaptation process include psychological shock, withdrawal, acknowledgment, and integration.

Psychological Shock

Psychological shock is often the initial emotional reaction to the impact of the life change that occurs when a person first becomes aware of a problem. This shock may occur at the time of an injury, illness, or developmental change, or it may occur later, when body changes are seen or experienced more acutely. Psychological shock is a defense mechanism that people use in reaction to anxiety. Denial and anger are common reactions during this stage.

Withdrawal

Withdrawal is the next stage of readjustment. Once the person becomes aware of an injury, illness, or developmental change and begins to think about the future, he or she may feel an overwhelming desire to run away from the reality of the situation. Because this is not physically possible, emotional retreat serves as a coping mechanism. This withdrawal provides an opportunity for the person to replenish physical and psychological energies used during the emotional shock phase. The person may become passive and dependent and lack motivation.

Acknowledgment

Acknowledgment occurs gradually, as the person recognizes the change in body image. Once the loss or change is acknowledged, the person can begin mourning (see Chapter 12 on grieving, death, and dying). The person may contemplate the meaning of the change and its implications for the future. This acknowledgment allows the person to view the body change itself and to begin reintegration of the body image.

Integration

Integration is the long and difficult process of adapting to body changes. The person thinks about future life experiences that will be different as a result of the body change and identifies ways to manage or deal with these changes. Often, the stage of integration can create for the person a new meaning about the change in the body part, and emotional growth occurs. As a result of integration of the body changes into a new image, the person regains a sense of fulfillment over time. However, the total process of change, from initial impact to adaptation, can be long and painful and is different for everyone.

Research on Body Image Disturbance

Body image disturbance is most commonly associated with loss of body parts. However, any type of loss (e.g., mobility, independence, or a body function) necessitates some body image readjustment. Research has not clarified how people perceive body image after a loss and how this perception relates to the emotional component of body image.

Loss of Mobility

People value the drive and ability to be mobile. Mobility is of such fundamental importance that healthy adults, even during resting periods, turn or change position frequently. Mobility enables people to exert control or influence over their environment. This control is threatened when mobility is restricted or lost (Hanna, 1996).

People view immobility, whether temporary or permanent, as a loss that can influence body image. This loss and the lifestyle changes that result can threaten the survival of the immobilized person. In this respect, body image in relation to immobility can have a considerable impact on nursing practice.

Pain

Pain can play a role in body image development. The impact of illness and pain on body image can be overwhelming. If severe pain continues, the painful body part can become isolated from the rest of the body to the point that it becomes alienated from the body image.

Cancer

Cancer often changes the way people feel about their personal appearance (Burt, 1995). Alopecia (hair loss) that occurs during the treatment of disease is one important factor. Cancer clients with alopecia have a lower self-image than cancer clients without alopecia. For these clients, alopecia is seen as a constant reminder of their disease. With or without hair loss, the experience of cancer can affect the body image.

Chronic Illness

Certain chronic illnesses can affect body image, whether or not pain is involved. For example, people with deforming arthritis, such as the rheumatoid type, are usually very self-conscious about their appearance. Some of these people refuse to socialize or be seen in public. The presence of chronic pain further affects the body image of these people.

Nicholas and Leuner (1992) studied people with another type of chronic illness—chronic obstructive pulmonary disease (COPD). They found that the body image of these people decreased as the disease became more severe.

Surgery

For any client, the anticipation of surgery can create anxiety, a fear of mutilation, and an unrealistic body image (see the Research Applications for Nursing box). Facial disfigurement resulting from surgical treatment of head and neck cancer, in particular, can cause severe body image disturbances. Likewise, the deformity that may result from burns or burn surgery can seriously affect a person's body image.

Another procedure that can cause body image disturbances is mastectomy. For most women, a mastectomy results in the loss of a body part that is viewed as essential for maintaining femininity, attractiveness, and self-esteem. This loss is based on the historical (or traditional) belief that the female breast is a symbol of femininity and maternity.

▶ Research Applications for Nursing

Does Body Image Perception Change After Lumbar Laminectomy?

Neatherlin, J. S., & Brillhart, B. (1995). Body image in preoperative and postoperative lumbar laminectomy patients. Journal of Neuroscience Nursing, 27(1), 43–46.

This study was conducted to determine whether patients undergoing lumbar laminectomy had a change in body image perception between the preoperative and postoperative phases. Twenty-four middle-aged and elderly clients were assessed using the Body-Cathexis Scale. Scores on the tool were higher postoperatively, indicating that body image perception changed. In addition, the subjects rated a difference in energy level and sexual activity.

Critique. This was a comparative study using a small convenience sample. The researchers stated that a larger sample and more time are needed to see if the perceptions remain the same after surgery.

Possible Nursing Implications. Although nurses may not categorize a laminectomy as a deforming surgery that changes external appearance, this study shows that any type of surgery is a threat to body image. Therefore, nurses need to help all surgical clients cope with body image changes.

Body image disturbances are also common after the surgical creation of an ostomy (Giese & Terrell, 1996). These disturbances can result from the person's perception of the appearance of the stoma and from the reaction to the stoma by significant others. The person and significant others may equate the stoma with the genital region. Thus, exposure and direct handling of the stoma can be especially damaging to body image.

For body image to remain healthy, it must accurately incorporate the actual physical changes of surgery. That is, the person must accept the body as it has become. For example, the client with an ostomy must recognize that the stoma is probably lifesaving and that it serves the same purpose as the bowel tract and rectum. This recognition is realistic.

Amputation, Paralysis, and Deformity

For a person with a limb amputation or any type of paralysis, body image reintegration is required. In clients with an amputation, phantom limb pain, in which the limb is gone but pain continues, creates different body perceptions that necessitate body image reintegration.

Limb amputation, paralysis, and deformity can all limit mobility. For example, the client with a spinal cord injury also experiences serious changes in mobility. These changes in mobility can, in turn, affect body image.

Eating Disorders

Obesity, anorexia nervosa, and bulimia nervosa commonly reflect body image disturbances (Amara & Cerrato, 1996; Segal-Isaacson, 1996). People with these conditions have a tendency to overestimate their body size, both during and after weight loss. This overestimation results in a feeling of having lost no weight even after dieting has produced a significant weight loss. (Also see Chapters 63 and 64 for more information on body image and eating disorders.)

Collaborative Management

 Assessment

▶ History

The North American Nursing Diagnosis Association (NANDA) (1992) states that to justify a diagnosis of Body Image Disturbance, the client must have a verbal or nonverbal response to an actual or perceived change in body structure and/or function. To assess and understand a body image disturbance, the nurse collects data about how the client perceives and has adapted to a body change (Chart 10–1).

View of Self

The nurse begins the nursing assessment by obtaining data that identify the client's view of self. As the client shares information about body image, the nurse can better diagnose Body Image Disturbance and its cause. The nurse gathers data by inquiring about the client's recent physical body change. Is this perceived positively or negatively? What feelings does this change create? Are current feelings a change from feelings before this illness? Does the client describe herself or himself as hopeful or helpless?

Perception of Body Change

After assessing the client's view of self, the nurse identifies the body change as perceived by the client and his or her family or significant others. The nurse must assess both client and family perceptions because they may conflict and/or lend insight into further assessment and interven-

---

Chart 10–1

Nursing Care Highlight

Specific Factors to Consider When Taking a History of the Client with Body Image Disturbance

- What is the client's view of himself or herself? (e.g., "How would you describe your body to another person?")
- What is the client's or family's perceived body change?
- What is the client's developmental level?
- What are the client's or family's past successful coping strategies?
- What is the client's current occupation or work history?
- What was the client's past experience with pain?
- What is the client's environment?

tion. For example, do the client and family understand the actual physiologic surgical alteration? Is the body change perceived a certain way (e.g., lifesaving, positive, or negative)? What does this mean to them?

Developmental Level

When assessing body image disturbance, the nurse should take into account the client's developmental level. A young adult client may be functioning only as an adolescent. Therefore, the client's body image may not be developed to the level of an adult, and certain expectations will not be appropriate. The nurse assesses the developmental level of a client by evaluating responses of the client to questions and by noticing the way he or she is affected during an interview. Body language and maturity of responses are important clues to the developmental level of a client. For example, does the client give inconsistent verbal responses to questions? Does he or she have poor eye contact? Is the client unable to answer some questions because he or she does not understand?

Coping Strategies

To establish baseline data regarding coping behaviors, nurses should identify the client's and/or family's past successful coping strategies. The nurse can assess these strategies by asking
- "How have you dealt with hard times in your life in the past?"
- "What did you do in the past that helped you get through them?"
- "Have you been doing some of these same things this time?"
- "Do you think that these things might help you now?"
Chapter 8 discusses the assessment of coping in detail.

Occupation or Work History

The client's current occupation or work history can lend further insight into his or her self-image and body image. For example, is the client currently employed, laid off, fired, or retired? Does this work situation create any negative feelings or problems? Does the client anticipate return to work, or is he or she not currently working? Does the client feel useful?

Experience with Pain

Body image assessment must also include data about the client's past experience with pain. Has the client ever experienced pain before? Was this pain chronic or acute? Did this pain control the client's life? What caused the pain? How did the client deal with the pain? Were friends or family supportive about the pain? Did the pain change the client's life in any way? The nurse assesses the client's pain experience regardless of whether it is a past or current problem.

Environment

As well as assessing the client and family, the nurse also collects data about the client's immediate environment. The environment includes the immediate physical area at

home, social supports, and community. Does the client have easy access to follow-up care? Is the home environment conducive to self-care needs (e.g., one-level versus two-level home, steps into home, bathroom and bedroom locations)? Is the community supportive of this client's needs (e.g., presence of wheelchair ramps, easy transportation)? By collecting all of this information, the nurse can assess body image disturbances more accurately.

➤ Physical Assessment/Clinical Manifestations

The nurse completes a collection of data concerning body changes. NANDA identifies the following *objective* clinical manifestations, or defining characteristics, for assessment of Body Image Disturbance. Although these defining characteristics have not been clinically validated by research, they provide direction for nursing assessment. NANDA's definition and defining characteristics have not been revised or refined since 1986:
- Missing body part
- Actual change in structure or function
- Not looking at body part
- Not touching body part
- Hiding or overexposing body part (intentional or unintentional)
- Trauma to nonfunctioning body part
- Change in social involvement
- Change in ability to estimate spatial relationship of body to environment

➤ Psychosocial Assessment
Personalization of a Body Part

The North American Nursing Diagnosis Association (NANDA) has also identified as indicative of a body image disturbance client extension of the body boundary to incorporate environmental objects and personalization of the body part or loss by name. However, research has not established these characteristics as unhealthy behavior. For example, could it be that the client who envisions the body and wheelchair as one has successfully adapted to the new body image? Has the client who calls the colostomy "Sam" successfully incorporated this body change into a healthy image of the body? Future research may clarify these questions.

The client who depersonalizes the body part or loss by the use of impersonal pronouns (e.g., "it") may exhibit difficulty in adapting to the body change. The use of an impersonal pronoun to refer to a mastectomy, colostomy, or stump demonstrates one's inability to perceive the body change as part of the self. Such a reference keeps the body change impersonal and may facilitate denial of the change. By using denial, the client may demonstrate a refusal to verify the actual body change. This refusal then prolongs the grieving and coping process and can interrupt body image reintegration.

Coping and Support Systems

The nurse assesses the client's current coping behaviors and the client's attempts at body image adaptation to the change. Current coping behaviors can also be compared with past coping behaviors to assist the client with body

Subjective Interview

Points

____ 1. I will be undergoing a major change in my job status as a result of this experience.
____SA ____A ____U ____D ____SD
If so, what?
____Decrease in job status   ____Job loss
____Change in job   ____Other (specify)
_____

____ 2. I do not have someone available to help me or talk to.
____SA ____A ____U ____D ____SD
If someone is available, who?
____Spouse   ____Parents
____Close friend   ____Children
____Significant other ____Nurse
(relative)

____ 3. I think of myself differently as a result of this experience.
____SA ____A ____U ____D ____SD
If so, how?
____Negatively   ____Other (specify)
____Increased physical _____
complaints

____ 4. My ability to move around by myself has changed as a result of this experience.
____SA ____A ____U ____D ____SD
If so, how?
____Less mobile   ____Other (specify)
____No change   _____

____ 5. I have definite feelings about specific parts of my body.
____SA ____A ____U ____D ____SD
If so, what?
____Hate   ____Fear

____Disgust   ____Other (specify)

____ 6. I am more fearful now than before this experience.
____SA ____A ____U ____D ____SD
If so, why?
____Fear of falling   ____Fear of pain
____Fear of recurrence   ____Fear of inability
of problem   to care for self
____Fear of others'   ____Other (specify)
reactions   _____

Objective Interview

7. Does the patient display any prominent body feature?
____Obesity   ____Disfigurement
____Limb loss   ____Other (specify)_____
____Paralysis

8. Does the patient exhibit evidence of or complain of pain?
____Facial expression
____Physical strain or fatigue
____Body language (immobile, purposeless, protective, rubbing)
____Sleep disturbances
____Other (specify)_____

9. Does the patient exhibit any major change in affect?
____Withdrawal ____Crying
____Hostility   ____Other (specify)_____

10. Is there any equipment present?
____Foley's catheter   ____Traction
____NG or other tubes   ____Tracheotomy
____Walker or crutches   ____Cardiac monitor
____Cast   ____Side rails up
____Other (specify)_____

SA, strongly agree; A, agree; U, undecided; D, disagree; SD, strongly disagree, IV, intravenous; NG, nasogastric.

Figure 10–3. The Baird Body Image Assessment Tool. (Courtesy of Susan Baird Holmes.)

image changes. The client who has used anger to cope with past stressful life events may need to demonstrate anger in response to body changes. With the knowledge of these data, the nurse is better prepared to treat a body image disturbance. (Also see Chapter 8.)

Nurses also evaluate the client's current family role to gain an understanding about communication patterns, support systems, and family dynamics. The client's role in the family may be a significant part of the client's identity. If this image of self is interrupted by a body change, major problems with body image may occur. In addition, family members may be significantly influenced by the client's body change and inability to perform previous family roles.

The nurse assesses client and family support systems. The success or failure of a client and family to deal with physical body changes can depend greatly on the existence of support systems. Support systems may consist of specific people, groups, communities, financial plans, or assistive devices. The nurse initiates this assessment on first contact with the client. However, much of this data collection is ongoing. To develop an effective plan of care, the nurse should know the client and family support systems.

➤ Assessment Tools

Various written tools have been developed, primarily through the efforts of psychology researchers who study self-concept and body image. However, these tools are time-consuming for clients to complete and difficult to evaluate. To assist the nurse in identifying body image disturbances, a clinically useful nursing assessment tool is needed. The Baird Body Image Assessment Tool (BBIAT) attempts to clarify potential versus actual body image disturbances (Fig. 10–3). The client completes the subjective portion, answering each question with "strongly agree" (SA), "agree" (A), "undecided" (U), "disagree" (D), or "strongly disagree" (SD). The nurse asks clients to respond to questions 1 through 6. Points are then assigned to each answer as follows: SA = 5, A = 4, U = 3, D = 2, SD = 1. The total possible score for the subjective portion of the BBIAT is 30. Reliability and validity of this nursing tool have been established. A score of 23 to 30 points may indicate a serious need for nursing intervention; 19 to 22 points, a potential need that requires nursing intervention; and 18 or lower, no need for nursing intervention or the client has adapted to body changes.

The BBIAT is meant to be used only as a guide or tool to clarify for nurses, in daily practice, the assessment of body image alterations. The nurse uses the objective portion to identify other physical evidence that may have an impact on body image reintegration. No score is given for this portion. However, if so many objective variables exist that the nurse is unsure whether the client has a body image disturbance, this portion of the tool may help the nurse clarify the nursing diagnosis, etiology, or both. Further research and tool refinement are needed before one can draw any conclusions.

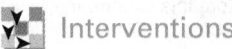 Interventions

Research has established the role of teaching in providing reassurance to clients who are about to undergo surgical body alterations. For example, preoperative teaching can decrease anxiety before and after surgery (see Chap. 20). Visits to clients by people who have had the same health problems have also been effective in assisting the client to adjust to the body image alteration.

If accepted by the client's culture, light touch to an extremity may be used by the nurse during discussion to help clients in re-establishing changed body boundaries. This practice can convey to the client a sense of being valued and that the physical body is still present. Talking to clients at equal eye level can be especially helpful in establishing an open, trusting relationship with those who may be feeling anxious or fearful.

The nurse encourages client verbalization and active thinking by providing for client participation in planning for the client's own needs. A client's sense of independence and responsibility is also enhanced by self-initiated activity. For example, a client with a spinal cord injury usually requires extra time for self-care. The nurse asks the client to suggest the best time for physical therapy appointments according to the client's need to have sufficient time to prepare for the appointment.

Nursing interventions for body image disturbance also focus on helping clients cope with alterations in body structure function.

➤ *Understanding the Grieving Process*

The nurse teaches the client and family or significant other the components of the healthy grieving process. Teaching begins by increasing client and family awareness of the various stages of grieving as well as understanding coping behaviors that are used in response to loss. For example, the client, family member, or significant other who responds with anger or denies the body change that has occurred may not be aware of his or her response. The nurse specifically helps the person to discuss feelings, recognize current behaviors, and possibly identify other therapeutic coping strategies. The nurse should also teach an understanding of healthy body image development throughout the life span. Clients and families should be better prepared to understand their fears and concerns and should be more effective in coping by developing an awareness about body image development.

➤ *Goal Setting*

Nursing interventions also focus on setting small, achievable goals; the nurse does this together with the client, family, or both. Goals are established during hospitalization to provide positive reinforcement about remaining strengths as well as effective coping strategies. For example, a client may be convinced that a burn site is noticeable, even under clothing, and may refuse to leave the hospital room. The nurse helps the client set a goal to dress in personal clothes of his or her choice and visit the gift shop in the hospital. The client meets the goal within 3 days and by the end of the week is in the visitors' lounge every afternoon, meeting new people and enjoying social interaction. Meeting the public for the first time after surgery can be threatening, and clients may become progressively desensitized to physical body changes. The nurse helps the client to be aware of his or her feelings about being stared at in public and to plan coping strategies to deal with these feelings.

Clients need to realize their remaining strengths and capabilities. In addition, the nurse can assist the client and/or family with identification of long-term effective coping mechanisms by validating realistic concerns and fears. For example, the amputee who in the past coped with life events by jogging every day needs assistance to identify and practice new coping behaviors. In addition, the nurse may arrange for another client who has experienced similar body changes and has successfully reintegrated these changes into a new body image to visit the client and to discuss concerns.

➤ *Family Support*

Family members and significant others need the same kind of assistance as the client in coping with body changes. Family members need support so that they in turn can be supportive to the client. The family must be able to deal with both any feelings about previous problems concerning the client and new feelings related to the kind and extent of body changes incurred by the client. For example, family members may feel guilty about a belief that their mother's leg might have been saved if they had gotten her to the doctor sooner. The nurse serves as the client's and family's most consistent health caregiver. This consistency establishes a caring rapport, which increases comfort in discussing these sensitive issues.

Providing empathy, *not* sympathy, can be the single most important intervention when treating body image disturbance. For example, an empathic supporting statement to a client might be, "This must be very difficult for you." A sympathetic statement to a client might be, "I'm so sorry for you." The nurse may convey sensitivity and empathy more clearly to the client and family by the use of a light touch to the arm or hand during these discussions. In addition, the nurse should sit at eye level with the client and family or significant others to facilitate even more open verbalization of concerns.

The nurse may also actively attempt to involve the family in the client's care during hospitalization, but only as they desire. This intervention may increase both the client's and family's sense of control over the situation and may decrease feelings of powerlessness. In addition, with this involvement in care, family members are impressed with the importance for the client to gradually increase responsibility for self-care and other activities. For example, teaching family members how to care for a stump at home after an amputation provides the client with positive reinforcement about the physical change and assists the family in recognizing that the client is still their loved one.

The client and family may need to restructure their relationships, depending on the extent and impact of the body change. The nurse can assist with this restructuring by serving as a buffer between client and family, if necessary. The nurse may also provide knowledge about community or hospital resources if family roles have changed as a result of the body alteration. For example, if the client is unable to maintain the family role as breadwinner, community resources may assist with financial needs. By helping the client and family share concerns or fears and solve problems together, the nurse can alleviate miscommunication problems and can enhance existing support systems.

SELECTED BIBLIOGRAPHY

Amara, A., & Cerrato, P. L. (1996). Eating disorders—Still a threat. *RN, 59*(6), 30–35.

*Baird, S. E. (1985). Development of a nursing assessment tool to diagnose altered body image in immobilized patients. *Orthopaedic Nursing, 4,* 47–54.

Beer, J. (1995). Body image of patients with ESRD and following renal transplantation. *British Journal of Nursing, 4*(10), 591–598.

Burt, K. (1995). The effects of cancer on body image and sexuality. *Nursing Times, 91*(7), 36–37.

Carpenter, J. S., & Brockopp, D. Y. (1994). Evaluation of self-esteem of women with cancer receiving chemotherapy. *Oncology Nursing Forum, 21*(4), 751–757.

Cowen, L., Clark, C., MacGillivary, C., Harper, R., & Wilson, L. (1995). Positive images of aging. *Elder Care, 7*(1), 14–15.

*Fischer, S. (1964). Sex differences in body perception. *Psychological Monographs,* 1–22.

Giese, L. A., & Terrell, L. (1996). Sexual health issues in inflammatory bowel disease. *Gastroenterology Nursing, 19*(1), 12–17.

Hanna, B. (1996). Sexuality, body image, and self-esteem: The future after trauma. *Journal of Trauma Nursing, 3*(1), 13–17, 19–20.

*Leonard, B. J. (1972). Body image changes in chronic illness. *Nursing Clinics of North America, 7,* 687–695.

Lisanti, P., & Verdisco, L. A. (1994). Perceived body space and self-esteem in adult females with chronic low back pain. *Orthopaedic Nursing, 13*(2), 55–63.

*Morris, C. A. (1985). Self-concept as altered by the diagnosis of cancer. *Nursing Clinics of North America, 20,* 611–630.

Neatherlin, J. S., & Brillhart, B. (1995). Body image in preoperative and postoperative lumbar laminectomy patients. *Journal of Neuroscience Nursing, 27*(1), 43–46.

*Nicholas, P. K., & Leuner, J. D. (1992). Relationship between body image and chronic obstructive pulmonary disease. *Applied Nursing Research, 5,* 83–84.

Paier, G. S. (1996). Specter of the crone: The experience of vertebral fracture. *Advances in Nursing Science, 18*(3), 27–36.

Price, B. (1994). The asthma experience: Altered body image and noncompliance. *Journal of Clinical Nursing, 3*(3), 139–145.

Segal-Isaacson, C. J. (1996). American attitudes toward body fatness. *Nurse Practitioner, 21*(3), 9–10, 12–13.

Walsh, B. A., Grunert, B. K., Telford, G. L., & Otterson, M. F. (1995). Multidisciplinary management of altered body image in the patient with an ostomy. *Journal of Wound, Ostomy, and Continence Nursing, 22*(5), 227–236.

SUGGESTED READINGS

Beer, J. (1995). Body image of patients with ESRD and following renal transplantation. *British Journal of Nursing, 4*(10), 591–598.

This study examines the need for nurses and other health care professionals to understand the social consequences and emotional aspects of clients living with a long-term illness, such as end stage renal disease (ESRD). Although the clients in the study accepted dialysis and other treatment options, they had difficulty adjusting to the disfiguring changes that occurred to their bodies.

Burt, K. (1995). The effects of cancer on body image. *Nursing Times, 91*(7), 36–37.

Nurses often dismiss the changes in body image experienced by clients who have cancer and cancer treatments. This article emphasizes the need for nurses to counsel clients and help them adjust to these changes.

Walsh, B. A., Grunert, B. K., Telford, G. L., & Otterson, M. F. (1995). Multidisciplinary management of altered body image in the patient with an ostomy. *Journal of Wound, Ostomy, and Continence Nursing, 22*(5), 227–236.

This article presents selected cases in which a multidisciplinary approach was successful in facilitating adaptation to an altered body image caused by an ostomy. The team included an enterostomal therapist, a nurse, and a psychologist. Clients with ostomies also have difficulty with personal acceptance, sexual concerns, and reduced self-care skills.

HUMAN SEXUALITY

A person's sexual health and well-being are created by the relationships among various factors. Sexual health can be described as a person's freedom from physical and psychological impairment that would compromise expression of one's sexuality. Sexual well-being includes the individual's awareness of open and positive attitudes toward one's body and sexual functioning, accurate knowledge about sexual anatomy and physiology, and acceptance of sexual arousal and responsibility for sexual behaviors.

OVERVIEW

Medical-surgical nurses are concerned with issues of sexual health and well-being. In providing nursing care, the nurse recognizes the importance of sexuality and encourages the growth and development of clients as sexual beings. The nurse also intervenes in a variety of situations to promote sexual health and to prevent sexual dysfunctions related to illness and injury throughout a client's life cycle.

Conceptual Model of Sexual Health and Well-Being

Throughout the life cycle, various factors determine an individual's optimal status of sexual health and well-be-

ing. Sexual health and well-being are holistic concepts that suggest the interrelationships among biological, psychological, social, and spiritual aspects of being human:

- Physical factors are associated with maturational changes in one's body; these include age, reproductive history, level of sexual functioning, past and present illnesses and injuries, the use of medications, and specific sexual behaviors.
- Psychological factors are associated with the mind; these include both emotional and cognitive processes. These factors include body image, self-esteem, gender identity, knowledge of sexuality, attitudes toward gender roles, beliefs about sexuality, and preference for sexual partners.
- Sociocultural factors include race, ethnicity, social status, marital status, family and social connectedness, occupation, and level of education.

External threats to the individual—in the form of physical illness, injury, or medical and surgical interventions—may lead to alterations in these factors and can reduce a person's level of sexual health and well-being. Similarly, threats to a person's psychological and sociocultural domains, such as family violence or changes in family composition, may result in changes that diminish sexual health and well-being.

To promote optimal sexual health in clients, the medical-surgical nurse assesses these factors and compares current findings with past patterns that clients have reported. The nurse evaluates the impact of external threats on these dimensions and provides nursing interventions that reduce or prevent the negative effects of the threats. The nurse also anticipates potential threats to optimal sexual health and well-being and provides guidance congruent with health-promoting goals.

Effect of Anatomy and Physiology on Sexual Health and Well-Being

The physical structure and function of the body affect a person's sexual health. Internal reproductive organs, such as the ovaries and uterus in a woman and the testes in a man, constitute one aspect of the anatomy that influences sexual health. In addition, external structures, such as the breasts and external genitalia, affect sexual health. A deformity, injury, disease, or surgical alteration of any of these internal or external structures poses a threat to one's sexual health. The endocrine system also maintains both structure and function of the reproductive organs.

Psychosexual Development

A person's psychosexual and physiologic development begin at the moment of conception and continue throughout young adulthood. Females are generally physically mature by the late teen years, whereas males may continue to develop mature secondary sexual characteristics into their early to late 20s. Overt sexual behaviors are observed in adults of all ages. Age, illness or injury, and life experiences have major impacts on an adult's sexuality. Attitudes and values are generally more firmly established in the adult than in the adolescent and influence overt sexual behavior. Although a man may reach his peak of sexual urgency in his 20s, a woman may not reach her peak until her 30s or 40s. This "mismatch" may lead to conflicts within marriage or other intimate heterosexual relationships.

Research on Human Sexuality

The history of research in human sexuality is fairly short. Before Alfred Kinsey's surveys of human sexual behavior in the 1930s, most research had addressed people with deviant or criminal behavior and little was known about average or typical sexual behavior. Kinsey trained interviewers who questioned more than 18,000 people in the United States about their sexual histories. Some of these findings led to new understandings about the sexual activities of women and of people with a homosexual orientation. In addition, the findings enabled the U.S. public to redefine the social code of acceptable sexual activities and to acknowledge more openly the reality of human sexual characteristics.

In the late 1950s and 1960s, the team of Masters and Johnson (1970) began to observe couples engaging in sexual activity and used various instruments to measure the responses of both men and women. In addition to using case studies and clinical and experimental research designs to increase the knowledge base of human sexual response and behavior, this team developed and tested interventions for use with couples who had recognizable sexual dysfunctions. The contributions of Masters and Johnson to the field of sexology as well as to the knowledge of the general public are well documented.

Sexual Response Cycle of the Adult

In the 1960s, Masters and Johnson described and measured in detail the sexual response cycle of both male and female adults. This cycle consists of four phases: excitement, plateau, orgasm, and resolution (Table 11–1). The underlying physiology of this cycle consists of vasocongestion and myotonia. *Vasocongestion* refers to blood trapped in tissues of the breast, vulva, and penis. This congestion results in erection of the nipples, clitoris, and penis. *Myotonia* refers to the tension of both voluntary and involuntary muscles that occurs during sexual excitement and orgasm. The differences in male and female sexual response cycles are illustrated in Figure 11–1. The problems of sexual dysfunction in adults are categorized according to the different phases of these cycles.

Sexual Preferences
Homosexuality

Sexual behavior and preference for partners may change over one's life span. Although most children and many adolescents engage in some types of overt homosexual activities as a normal part of sexual play, only a small percentage of adults identify themselves as homosexual. *Homosexuality* is defined as a person's attraction to one or more persons of the same sex. This preference is the most common of the sexual minorities.

Many stereotypic myths remain about homosexual (gay) men and lesbian women. Many such myths are based on homophobia, an irrational fear of homosexuality. However, the nurse who is equipped with an appropriate knowledge base and positive attitude toward human sexuality can help to dispel these myths and provide nursing care that includes attention to the person's sexual preference or orientation.

Although nursing care of homosexual clients does not differ from care of heterosexual ones and these groups have much in common, they also have some different concerns. For example, lesbians may experience the same concerns about gynecologic and breast problems as heterosexual women but may not have the same needs for contraception. Furthermore, lesbians are less likely to become pregnant than women who are sexually active with heterosexual partners. However, there is an increasing interest in parenting among homosexual couples, and artificial insemination followed by pregnancy is becoming more frequent in this population. Moreover, there is evi-

TABLE 11–1

The Adult Sexual Response Cycle

Phase	Male Response	Female Response
Excitement	• Skin flushing begins on the abdomen, then spreads to the neck and face. • The nipples become erect. • Myotonia of the legs and arms occurs. • Erection of the penis may subside and return. • The testes become elevated. • Pulse and blood pressure increase.	• Skin flushing begins on the abdomen and throat, then spreads to the breasts. • The nipples become erect, the veins distend, areolae darken, and the breasts enlarge by 25%. • Myotonia of the entire body occurs. • The clitoris becomes erect. • The vagina is lubricated. • Pulse and blood pressure increase.
Plateau	• Myotonia increases, with carpopedal spasms and facial grimaces. • The penis remains erect and darkens. • The testes continue to swell and elevate toward the perineum. • Pulse, respirations, and blood pressure increase.	• Myotonia increases, with carpopedal spasms, flared nostrils, and an arched back. • The clitoris retracts under its hood. • The vaginal barrel distends, and contractions begin. • Pulse, respirations, and blood pressure increase.
Orgasm	• The skin flush is maximal. • Myotonia of the entire body occurs, and the rectal sphincter contracts. • Semen is ejaculated through the penis. • Pulse and blood pressure increase. • The respiratory rate doubles.	• The skin flush is maximal. • Myotonia of the entire body occurs. • The clitoris remains retracted. • Pulse and blood pressure increase. • The respiratory rate doubles.
Resolution	• The skin flush disappears within 5 minutes in most men, followed by perspiration. • The muscles relax. • The nipples return to normal. • The penis returns to its normal size in two stages. • The testes return to their normal size and position. • Pulse, respirations, and blood pressure return to normal.	• The skin flush disappears and may be followed by perspiration. • The muscles relax. • The nipples and breasts return to their normal color and size. • The clitoris returns to its normal position within 10 seconds. • The vagina collapses and loses its dark color. • Pulse, respirations, and blood pressure return to normal.

dence that some pregnant teenagers are lesbians who want to be mothers.

Many lesbians approach the health care system cautiously because of widespread homophobia among health professionals. Because of the lesbian's fear and suspicions about the type of care that she may receive, she may pay incomplete attention to minor problems that have the potential to become serious.

Similarly, gay men may avoid the traditional health care system and thus may receive inadequate preventive or primary health care. Nonetheless, gay men have many of the same concerns about genitourinary problems as heterosexual men. However, because of the high incidence of anal intercourse among gay men, these clients seek treatment more frequently for injuries of the rectum and for gastrointestinal infections known as the "gay bowel syndrome." Gay men with this syndrome are infected and reinfected with microorganisms that cause one or more gastrointestinal infections. The incidence of sexually transmitted diseases (STDs) is also higher among gay men. At this time, gay men also represent the group with the highest incidence of acquired immunodeficiency syndrome (AIDS) (see Chap. 25).

Other Sexual Variations

The nurse should be familiar with other sexual variations, such as the following:

BISEXUALITY. *Bisexuality* refers to a person's preference for intimate relationships with members of either sex.

INTERSEXUALITY. *Intersexuality* refers to a person having been born with either ambiguous genitalia (i.e., it is not clearly apparent whether the baby is male or female) or with internal and external genitalia of both sexes (e.g., penis, scrotum, and uterus).

TRANSSEXUALITY. *Transsexuality* refers to a person being dissatisfied with his or her gender assignment and being convinced that he or she is trapped within the wrong body. Sex reassignment surgery for the man who has a strong urge to live as a woman includes orchiectomy (removal of the testes), penectomy (removal of the penis), and vaginoplasty (construction of a vagina). Hormone replacement treatment is also given. A woman who

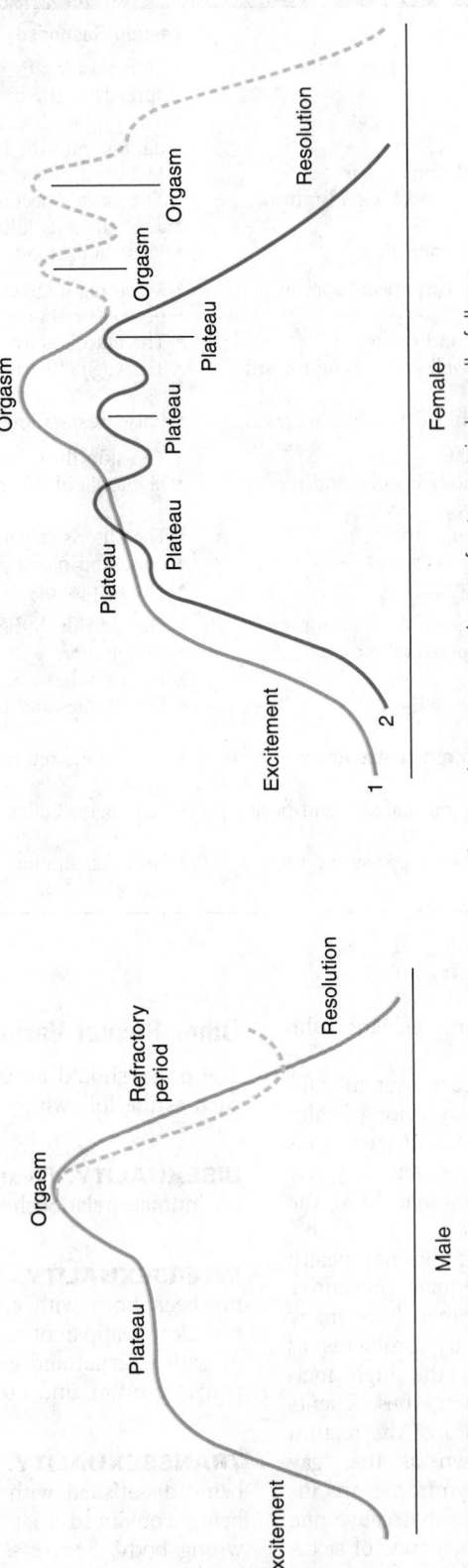

Figure 11-1. The male and female adult sexual response cycles. In the male sexual response cycle, a refractory period usually follows orgasm before another erection occurs. Women respond in various ways to sexual stimulation: Pattern 1 depicts single or multiple orgasms; pattern 2 shows some peaks but no orgasm.

is reassigned as a man undergoes hysterectomy (uterus removal), oophorectomy (ovary removal), and mastectomy (breast removal) along with hormone replacement therapy.

TRANSVESTISM. Also known as cross-dressing, *transvestism* refers to a person liking to wear clothes associated with the opposite sex for the sake of his or her sexual arousal. Transvestism is more common in men than in women. Unlike the transsexual, the transvestite does not have a conflict about his or her gender; some transvestites are married, and most engage in transvestism in private.

PEDOPHILIA. Pedophilia is a sexual preference for children. It is a psychiatric disorder (not discussed in this chapter).

Changes in Sexual Function Associated with Aging

Physical, social, and psychological changes affect sexual functioning throughout the life cycle. Chart 11–1 summarizes the major changes in the older adult. For more information on sexuality during each phase of adult development, see Chapter 5.

Effects of Illness on Sexuality

Many illnesses and injuries can have a negative effect on sexual health and well-being. In some cases, sexual dysfunctions may result that can be temporary or permanent (Table 11–2).

Chart 11–1

Nursing Focus on the Elderly

Changes Affecting Sexuality
Physical Changes
- In women, vaginal tissue gradually atrophies.
- Women become infertile; male fertility varies.
- Sexual arousal takes longer, and sperm count and the force of ejaculation in men decrease.

Social Changes
- Men and women experience increased losses in social networks.
- Men and women experience a heightened need for human contact and intimacy.
- Society views the elderly as asexual, having no sexual desires or needs.
- Health care providers often ignore the sexual needs and desires of the elderly.

Psychological Changes
- Men and women engage in life review and desire to be useful.
- The elderly may experience negative body image and lowered self-esteem.

Hospitalization

People often perceive the process of hospitalization as impersonal. Elements of sexual identity and behaviors associated with gender roles are frequently denied or seriously curtailed by the social milieu in most hospitals. Hospitals provide little privacy; in addition, symbols of sexual identity, such as certain clothing and jewelry, are usually removed. Behaviors that express sexual arousal and satisfaction are discouraged.

Acute Illness

When a person is hospitalized for acute illness or injury, sexual health may be impaired. Not only is the social climate not conducive to sexual expression for the reasons just identified, but a client's physical and psychological conditions may not be congruent with optimal sexual health and well-being. Acute medical conditions for which a client may be hospitalized can render the person physically unable to engage in sexual activity because of anxiety, fatigue, pain, malaise, or direct tissue damage or surgery that interferes with sexual arousal.

Specific acute disorders, such as sexually transmitted diseases (STDs), or complications associated with these disorders may affect the sexuality of the hospitalized person (see Chap. 80). Nurses should consider care that includes assessment of risk factors and sexual contacts when caring for the client with an acute condition requiring hospitalization. Because of the social stigma associated with the diagnosis of STDs, the hospitalized client may also suffer from guilt, embarrassment, and low self-esteem, which may impair his or her pursuit of behaviors that would lead to sexual health.

Specific acute bacterial or viral infections, such as pneumonia, hepatitis, gastroenteritis, and prostatitis, affect sexual health. In addition to the fatigue and malaise that are associated with these conditions, specific changes in body function may threaten an ill person's body image and self-esteem. These physical problems are closely related to psychological aspects of sexual well-being.

Chronic Illness

The sexual health of the client with a chronic illness or impairment may be threatened in various ways. For example, clients with hypertension, connective tissue disease, cancer, cardiovascular disease, diabetes, end-stage renal disease (ESRD), chronic respiratory disease, chronic liver disease, or spinal cord injury face limitations in sexual behavior patterns. These clients must deal with changes in body structure, function, or both in addition to psychological factors, such as uncertainty, fear, and depression. The client's body image is threatened, and tissue damage may disrupt the sexual response cycle or may render the client unable to engage in preferred sexual activities. (See also Chapter 10 on Body Image.)

HYPERTENSION. Adults who experience hypertension are at risk for problems in sexual functioning. Centrally acting adrenergic inhibitor drugs, such as methyldopa (Aldomet and Amodopa) and beta-adrenergic blockers such

TABLE 11-2

Effects of Illness on Adult Sexuality

Illness	Effects on Men	Effects on Women
Arthritis	• Decreased libido • Low self-esteem • Altered body image • Depression, anxiety	• Dyspareunia • Low self-esteem • Altered body image • Depression, anxiety
Cancer	• Altered body image • Erectile dysfunction • Decreased libido • Depression, anxiety • Low self-esteem	• Altered body image • Dyspareunia • Decreased libido • Depression, anxiety • Low self-esteem
Cardiovascular disease	• Erectile dysfunction • Low self-esteem • Depression, anxiety	• Decreased libido • Low self-esteem • Depression, anxiety
Diabetes	• Erectile dysfunction • Retrograde ejaculation • Decreased fertility	• Decreased libido • Orgasmic dysfunction • Decreased fertility • Dyspareunia • Chronic vaginitis • Decreased vaginal lubrication
Hepatic disease	• Loss of libido • Sexual unresponsiveness • Erectile dysfunction	• Decreased libido • Orgasmic dysfunction • Amenorrhea
Hypertension	• Decreased libido • Erectile failure • Ejaculatory failure • Gynecomastia	• Decreased libido • Galactorrhea
Renal disease	• Low self-esteem • Altered body image • Loss of libido • Erectile dysfunction • Decreased fertility • Depression, fatigue	• Low self-esteem • Altered body image • Loss of libido • Orgasmic dysfunction • Decreased fertility • Depression, fatigue
Respiratory disease	• Low self-esteem • Decreased libido • Erectile dysfunction	• Low self-esteem • Decreased libido • Orgasmic dysfunction
Spinal cord injury	• Erectile dysfunction • Possible infertility • Retrograde ejaculation • Ejaculatory dysfunction • Orgasmic dysfunction • Low self-esteem • Impaired body image • Loss of libido	• Orgasmic dysfunction • Amenorrhea • Low self-esteem • Impaired body image • Loss of libido

as propranolol (Inderal, Novopranol✚), have been associated with decreased libido (sexual desire) in both men and women. In addition, men may experience erectile and ejaculatory failure, whereas women may experience galactorrhea (the presence of milk in the breasts) and an inability to have an orgasm. These adverse effects usually disappear within 2 weeks after medication is discontinued.

Clonidine hydrochloride (Catapres), another antihypertensive agent, may lead to urinary retention, impotence, and gynecomastia (breast enlargement in men), thus affecting the sexual response cycle. Calcium-channel—blocking drugs such as nifedipine (Procardia, Adalat) and amlodipine besylate (Norvasc) reportedly have fewer sexual side effects. Metoprolol tartrate (Lopressor) also contributes to impotence in men. The nurse should assess the effects of such drugs in both men and women so that the physician may consider changes in dosages or types of medication if needed.

CONNECTIVE TISSUE DISEASE. Clients with connective tissue diseases, such as rheumatoid arthritis and systemic lupus erythematosus, face a chronic disabling condition characterized by problems with mobility, pain, and weakness. Although research on the specific incidence of sexual dysfunction among people with arthritis is lacking, obvious physical barriers exist to the usual sexual activities of such clients. Limited joint movement, weakness, fatigue, pain, swelling, and stiffness of extremities make activities of daily living, including sexual activity, difficult.

In addition to the often deforming nature of some forms of arthritis, large dosages of corticosteroid drugs may alter an arthritic person's physical appearance, which can result in lowered self-esteem and altered body image. Depression and anxiety about the unrelenting course of arthritic conditions may interfere with interpersonal communication and result in decreased sexual desire. Dyspareunia (painful intercourse) may result from changes in secretory function of the vagina, as seen in clients with Sjögren's syndrome.

CANCER. Various types of cancer directly affect sexual functioning and body image. Cervical or uterine cancer that results in hysterectomy and breast cancer that results in mastectomy are among the obvious malignancies affecting both sexual functioning and body image in women. In men, testicular and prostatic cancer may result in radical surgery that alters both sexual functioning and body image.

Other primary malignant tumors also contribute to the decline of a person's sexual health. These include cancers of the gastrointestinal tract, urinary system, and larynx, often necessitating surgical diversion or radical neck dissection. In addition to the damaging effects of malignant growths and surgical procedures, radiation and chemotherapy affect the sexual response cycle, appearance, and self-esteem of a client with cancer. Clients may experience alopecia (loss of hair), fatigue, anorexia, malaise, decline in libido, and secondary ovarian or testicular failure as a result of these therapies.

CARDIOVASCULAR DISEASE. Cardiovascular disease affects a person's sexual health and well-being because sexual activity makes demands on the cardiopulmonary system. Cardiovascular disease also affects the client's self-concept, self-esteem, and role function. When a person is resuming sexual activity after a myocardial infarction, for example, the activity should be planned and implemented on an individual basis. The conditions under which sexual activity is pursued (e.g., relaxing versus anxiety-provoking conditions) and the amount of physical stress that the heart can handle must be considered. The severity of tissue damage and the effects of medications may limit the degree to which people with chronic cardiovascular disease can pursue sexual activity. With physical conditioning programs, regulation of drug therapy, and adequate teaching and support, a client may continue to resume previous patterns of sexual activity or develop new and satisfying ones (see Research Applications for Nursing).

DIABETES MELLITUS. Diabetes has long been associated with sexual problems. Secondary erectile dysfunction (impotence) in men is often associated with microvascular

▷ Research Applications for Nursing

Clients May Want to Talk About Sexual Functioning and Cardiovascular Disease

Quadagno, D., Nation, A. J., Johnson, D., Waitley, C., Waitley, N., Epstein, D., & Satterwhite, A. (1995). Cardiovascular disease and sexual functioning. Applied Nursing Research, 8(3), 143–146.

Researchers studied 29 married men (mean age = 56.1 years) and 8 married women (mean age = 59.2 years) who had experienced cardiovascular problems, including heart transplant, myocardial infarction, bypass surgery, and hypertension. A questionnaire was distributed to the subjects at their cardiologist's office and included questions about general health, sexual activity, and sexual concerns. The subjects were also asked if health care workers had discussed resuming sexual activity and had provided them with adequate information about resuming normal activities following their cardiovascular health problem.

The majority of men and women in the sample reported having received no information from their health care providers about resuming sexual activities. Older subjects were less likely to receive this information than younger subjects, and they were also less likely to resume previous levels of sexual activity. Health care providers were also less likely to discuss sexual activity with women than with men.

These findings indicate that health care providers continue to perpetuate the myth that elderly clients have less sexual desire or fewer sexual needs than younger clients. Similarly, they suggest that women with cardiovascular disease do not receive information about resuming sexual activity. Nurses could fill an important gap in providing preliminary information to these clients.

Critique. The results of this study are limited by the small sample size, self-reported data, and use of questionnaires rather than interviews. However, the topic is important to nurses who care for these clients.

Possible Nursing Implications. Any nurse caring for clients undergoing surgery or receiving medical treatment for cardiovascular disease should be aware of the importance of sexuality. The nurse can provide preliminary information about resuming sexual activity and should be available to answer questions and provide emotional support to these clients. Moreover, nurses can be client advocates and assist such clients in requesting information from their physicians.

changes and neuropathy and occurs in more than half of men who have diabetes. A small percentage of diabetic men may experience retrograde ejaculation (the ejaculate is released into the urinary bladder instead of through the urinary meatus). This difficulty and the presence of disease of long duration may contribute to problems with fertility in diabetic men. Comparable changes in women lead to decreased libido, orgasmic dysfunctions, and infertility. A decrease in vaginal lubrication and increased risk of infection contribute to chronic vaginitis in diabetic women. The incidence of sexual problems in people who have had diabetes for longer periods is increased.

END-STAGE RENAL DISEASE. The effects of end-stage renal disease (ESRD) are monumental. Every system in the body is affected by impairment of the metabolism and regulation of electrolytes. In addition to the physical limitations resulting from fatigue, pruritus (itching), anorexia, lethargy, and muscle cramping, the client with ESRD faces overwhelming psychosocial changes. The client's self-concept, body image, and self-esteem suffer as a result of the gradual deterioration of body functions and structures. Role functions and issues of dependency are altered if the client is forced to stop working or cannot manage usual responsibilities in the home and community. The financial burdens of lost income and expensive treatments add to the stressors for the person with chronic renal disease. As a result of these multiple factors, the person may experience depression, loss of libido, decreased frequency of sexual activity, impotence, and sterility. New patterns of sexual expression must be explored to promote sexual well-being.

CHRONIC RESPIRATORY DISEASE. A person with chronic respiratory disease may experience increased levels of fatigue with accompanying threats to self-esteem. For example, people with chronic airflow limitation often report difficulty in continuing sexual intercourse. A review of the adult sexual response cycle indicates that respiratory rates double during plateau and orgasmic phases, which makes coitus difficult for both men and women with respiratory disease. Clients may need to learn alternative methods and positions for satisfying sexual activity.

LIVER DYSFUNCTION. Chronic conditions affecting the liver and immune system frequently lead to impaired sexual health. Clients experiencing anorexia, fatigue, joint pain, nausea, fever, and jaundice associated with chronic hepatitis may become uninterested in sexually overt behavior. In addition, the client may experience complications such as erectile dysfunction or sexual unresponsiveness. Similarly, many clients with cirrhosis of the liver related to malnutrition, infection with parasites, or alcohol abuse experience a loss of libido and specific pathologic conditions, including gynecomastia and erectile dysfunction in men and amenorrhea in women.

SPINAL CORD INJURY. Clients with spinal cord injury experience various sexual dysfunctions as a result of altered physical functioning and psychosocial changes. The dysfunctions depend on the extent and location of the injury, and they differ for men and women. Men with injury to the cervical spinal cord usually continue to have reflexive erections of the penis. Men whose injury occurred at lower levels of the spine experience erectile dysfunction because the neural pathways from the spinal cord are damaged or destroyed.

Incomplete injury to the spinal cord permits some sensation and motor function of the genitalia; complete injury results in loss of libido in both men and women, loss of erection and ejaculation in men, and orgasmic dysfunction in women. Men in whom the lumbosacral cord has been completely cut are infertile because of retrograde ejaculation or damaged sperm. Women, however, may experience temporary amenorrhea, may retain fertility, and may be capable of a full-term pregnancy. Each person's injury must be addressed individually.

Psychosocial problems may contribute to a decline in sexual health for spine-injured clients because of the accompanying change in body image and decrease in self-esteem. However, many people with spinal cord injuries continue to have satisfying sexual activity when their physical, psychological, and social problems are addressed. Many resources are available to assist them in promoting satisfying sexual expression. Women with spinal cord disabilities are often overlooked by health care providers concerning their needs for specialized menstrual products, contraception, and pregnancy. Many have suffered from the oppressive attitudes and behaviors of others who fail to appreciate their struggle for reproductive freedom (Waxman, 1994). Nurses can be strong advocates for these women in helping to design feminine hygiene products and obtaining optimal sexual health care services.

Effects of Drug and Alcohol Abuse

Nurses should not overlook the possibility of drug abuse or alcoholism as a central factor when suspecting or validating sexual problems in men and women. As middle adulthood approaches, some people turn to alcohol or other drugs to ease their anxieties, including anxiety specifically related to diminished sexual functioning (Table 11–3). The primary effects of limited alcohol intake are often initially stimulating, and both men and women may experience release of inhibitions, relief of anxiety, and an increase in libido. However, as the amount or frequency of alcohol intake increases, clients experience several negative effects. In women, for example, the desire for sexual activity may gradually decrease until there is no interest. Women in the stages of late alcoholism also experience a gradual decrease in vaginal lubrication and sensitivity. It takes more time for such women to have an orgasm, and they experience fewer orgasms.

Men in the late stage of alcoholism experience decreased desire, often accompanied by an increase in aggression and, finally, a total loss of desire and profound aggression. A delay in penile erection leads to an inability to attain an erection even with maximum stimulation, and the man's orgasm may be tentative or may not occur under any circumstances. The man may also experience diminished pleasurable sensations associated with sexual arousal. Although erection is still possible, the resolution stage is prolonged, and the man experiences a loss of sexual satisfaction.

Alcohol and drug use have also been implicated in risky sexual behaviors among adolescents and young adults, sometimes leading to unplanned pregnancies, sexually transmitted diseases, and personal violence. The role of alcohol and drug abuse as a factor in family violence is beyond the scope of this chapter, but the nurse should be aware of the increased risk to young pregnant women and to both males and females who may be raped when a sexual partner is a substance abuser.

TABLE 11–3

Effects of Alcohol and Other Drugs on Sexual Functioning

Drug	Effects on Men	Effects on Women
Alcohol	• Decreased libido • Increased aggression, possibly leading to sexual abuse • Erectile dysfunction • Decreased fertility • Low sexual satisfaction	• Decreased libido • Increased passivity, possibly leading to sexual abuse from partner • Orgasmic dysfunction • Amenorrhea, sterility • Low sexual satisfaction
Antidepressants	• Erectile dysfunction • Delayed ejaculation	• Delayed orgasm
Antihypertensives	• Decreased libido • Erectile dysfunction • Ejaculatory dysfunction • Retrograde ejaculation	• Decreased libido • Anovulation, amenorrhea • Galactorrhea • Impaired orgasm
Cocaine and amphetamines	• Delayed orgasm • Delayed ejaculation	• Orgasmic dysfunction • Decreased libido
Opioids	• Decreased libido • Erectile dysfunction • Delayed ejaculation	• Decreased libido • Spontaneous abortion • Amenorrhea
Tranquilizers	• Retrograde ejaculation • Erectile dysfunction	• Galactorrhea • Amenorrhea, anovulation

TRANSCULTURAL CONSIDERATIONS

Many factors affect a person's sexual health and his or her willingness to discuss this very private part of life. Spanish-speaking clients and Native Americans tend to be hesitant to talk about sexually related matters. In some cases, people from these groups may talk more freely to a nurse or other health care professional of the same sex or from the same culture (Giger & Davidhizar, 1995).

Cultural or religious background can also influence one's willingness to discuss sexual matters. This background may permit certain practices and prohibit others. The teachings of the Roman Catholic Church, for instance, prohibit the use of artificial contraception.

The decision to circumcise a male is also culturally based. In the United States, for example, 80% to 90% of males are circumcised, although fewer boys today are being circumcised than 20 years ago. In other countries of the world, such as Canada, England, Sweden, and China, circumcision is thought to be unnecessary. Some religious groups, such as Jews and Muslims, include circumcision as part of their religious practice. Other groups, like Hispanics and Native Americans, do not traditionally practice male circumcision (Jarvis, 1996). There is scant scientific evidence that circumcision is necessary, although penile carcinoma occurs more frequently in men who are not circumcised.

Female circumcision is not traditionally performed in the United States. However, immigrants from central Africa and India may enter the formal health care system with complications directly related to this practice. Female circumcision varies from minor procedures such as removal of the prepuce of the clitoris to infibulation, which is complete excision of the clitoris, labia minora, and parts of the labia majora and partial closure of the vaginal opening. Most of these procedures are done as tribal rituals associated with coming of age and often are performed without sterile conditions and anesthetics. Incisions are rarely sutured: A small piece of wood or some other hard object may be inserted into the vagina to permit flow of menstrual blood, and often the girl's legs are bound together to facilitate healing. Some young women hemorrhage or suffer from urinary retention and infection. Others face delayed complications such as vaginal stenosis, chronic urinary tract infections, and chronic pelvic inflammatory disease (Walker & Morgan, 1995). The culturally sensitive nurse provides care without judging the morality of cultural customs that promote these practices.

Nurses' Comfort with Sexuality

Our increased knowledge and awareness of human sexuality throughout the life cycle have led to an increased demand for solutions to problems in sexual functioning. Nursing, as a major provider of health care services, has responded to this demand by developing strategies to prevent the development of sexual problems and to promote sexual health.

In addition to having an adequate knowledge base in human sexuality, the nurse should feel comfortable in addressing the sexual health needs of clients. To help clients achieve optimal sexual health and well-being, nurses should have an attitude of openness and willingness to approach the subject. Nurses must first be aware of their personal attitudes toward sexuality and their ability to promote the sexual health and well-being of others

TABLE 11–4

Values Clarification Exercise

Situation: Mary is a 26-year-old single woman hospitalized for a radical hysterectomy. She has a malignancy. Which of the following responses by nurses is most like your response to assessing, diagnosing, and intervening with regard to her actual and potential sexual problems?

Nurse A: "I hope she doesn't ask about having sexual relations or I'll just die of embarrassment!"

Nurse B: "I know how I'll handle any questions about sex. I'll just refer her to the head nurse. She can handle that stuff."

Nurse C: "It's OK if she asks about sex, but I'm not sure I know all the answers. I know I can listen and try to help her find answers if I don't know them."

Nurse D: "It's just fine if she asks about how this will affect her sexually. In fact, even if she doesn't bring it up, I will. I really believe it's an important aspect of her health."

Clarification of values in responses: If you answered that you feel most like one of the nurses above, check below to clarify what this means.

Nurse A: This nurse feels uncomfortable handling concerns about sexual health and needs to do more reading and talking about her feelings with other health professionals.

Nurse B: This nurse also feels uncomfortable and is willing to shirk responsibility, passing it on to one with more authority. Again, more learning and exploration of his or her attitudes are needed.

Nurse C: This nurse feels comfortable. Being able and willing to look for additional information is essential to helping the client.

Nurse D: This nurse also feels comfortable and is willing to take more responsibility for including sexual health in client care.

(Table 11–4). If inquiring about sexual functioning or behavior is embarrassing to the nurse, he or she must be willing to acknowledge this and refer the client to another nurse with more experience. This nurse should also attempt to learn more about human sexuality and its relationship to health and well-being.

Sexual Harassment

There has been an increased realization of and discussion about sexual harassment in the workplace and other settings. Because most nurses are women, it is possible that they will be harassed at some point while caring for their clients. Sexual harassment by a client can interfere with the nurse's ability to complete a sexual health assessment and effectively intervene for specific sexual problems.

In addition to the possibility of being sexually harassed by clients, the nurse may encounter harassment from other members of the health care team or the client's family members or visitors. Several court cases have determined that people should be protected from harassment and the offenders legally punished.

Collaborative Management

 Assessment

> *History*

In managing the sexual health of hospitalized clients, the nurse takes a brief sexual history that is integrated with the general health history. Nurses need to be sensitive to clients' willingness to discuss this private part of their lives. Factors such as the age of both the client and the nurse may affect the client's willingness to disclose such personal information. For example, elderly clients may be reluctant to discuss sexual health, especially if they were taught that sex should not be discussed openly. An equally embarrassing situation might be one in which a young female nurse interviews a young heterosexual male; both people may feel hesitant about discussing this topic.

Nurses address three areas in taking the sexual health history:
- Physical development and situational changes in sexual functioning
- Alterations in body image, gender identity, sex role, and self-esteem
- Sociocultural factors, such as ritualistic practices and beliefs

Here are some examples of questions that the nurse can ask while obtaining a history:
- "Have you ever experienced any injury or disease of the genitourinary system? Is there any history of sexually transmitted diseases?"
- "What was the pattern of development of secondary sexual characteristics (e.g., onset of menstruation)? Have there been any changes in these characteristics (e.g., hirsutism [excessive hair growth in females] or gynecomastia)? What changes do you attribute to your age?"
- "Have you ever experienced any unwanted or traumatic sexual events such as incest, rape, or sexual harassment?"
- "Have you noticed any changes in sexual functioning in the past related to the use of alcohol or other drugs?"
- "Have you experienced any changes in sexual functioning or desire for sexual activity since your current illness, injury, or surgery?"
- "Has this physical problem (illness, injury, or surgical treatment) changed the way you view your body or feel about yourself as a woman or man?"
- "As a result of this physical problem, have you noticed changes in your usual activities as a woman or man, or changes in your usual roles, such as those of wife or mother, or husband or father?"
- "What are some of your beliefs and practices about sexual behavior? Have any of these been affected by your current illness, injury, or surgery?"

Although some of these questions may be answered easily with "yes" or "no," the nurse should pose them in such a way as to invite the client to discuss his or her sexual identity, roles, or activity. The nurse should phrase questions in language that the client understands, according to his or her educational level and sociocultural background. Beginning each phrase with "Tell me how" may encourage further information. Taking a sexual history is one way to identify misinformation that should be corrected as part of the nursing intervention. Chart 11–2 summarizes the information contained in a brief sexual history and assessment.

Chart 11–2

Nursing Care Highlights

Brief Sexual History and Assessment Guide
History: Current Assessment
Physical
- Note development of secondary sexual characteristics (onset and pattern of menses in woman): Observe and palpate. Note changes over time.
- Note use of contraceptives; problems with fertility or pregnancy. Assess.
- Note current use and problems with contraception; issues of fertility or pregnancy.
- Note episodes of sexually transmitted diseases.
- Note recent changes in sexual activity level or pattern.
- Ask about past genitourinary disease, injury, or surgery.
- Note thickening or discharge from the breast or genitalia.
- Ask about past use of alcohol or other drugs.
- Note current drug use.
- Ask about past patterns of sexual function.
- Note changes in levels of sexual arousal or function.

Psychological
- Ask about past sexual dysfunction.
- Identify knowledge of sexual function.
- Ask about past problems with body image, gender role, or self-esteem.
- Note current values and current feelings about body parts and functions and self-esteem.
- Take history of incest, rape, or other unwanted sexual experiences.
- Identify recent unwanted sexual experiences.

Social
- Ask about cultural rituals, beliefs, and inhibitions (e.g., circumcision, menses, marriage).
- Note cultural expectations for sexual behavior.
- Note family composition and roles.
- Note changes in composition of family or peers.
- Ask about pattern of marital or sexual status and living arrangements.
- Note change in living arrangements or marital status.
- Ask about past sexual orientation and preference (e.g., homosexuality, bisexuality, heterosexuality, transsexuality).
- Identify current sexual preference and patterns of sexual activity.

➤ *Physical Assessment/Clinical Manifestations*

The nurse incorporates the sexual health assessment into a general physical assessment. Subjective data concerning body image may be gathered as the nurse palpates various parts of the body, moving from relatively neutral areas, such as the face and extremities, to the breasts and external genitalia. Nurses should always have concern for the client's dignity when assessing these more private areas. The nurse explains what is to be examined, in what manner, and for what reason. As in other physical assessments, the nurse pays attention to external appearance, palpation of internal structures, and any discharges (which may also need to be further assessed in the laboratory) as well as the client's subjective response to this examination.

While assessing the client's genitalia and breasts, the nurse may elicit additional information about sexual activity, knowledge, and attitudes. For example, when inspecting the external genitalia, the nurse might ask the client to describe his or her usual pattern of sexual activities and ask whether there is any discomfort or anxiety related to these behaviors.

Chapter 76 includes a detailed description of the physical assessment of genitalia and breasts. The clinical manifestations described in this chapter relate specifically to sexual functioning.

Dyspareunia

Dyspareunia (painful intercourse) in women may be related to several factors, such as
- An intact hymen
- Scarring from an episiotomy or infibulation
- Infections of the vagina or vulva, including venereal warts or other sexually transmitted diseases (STDs)
- Insufficient vaginal lubrication
- Irritation from chemical products, such as contraceptives, douches, and feminine deodorants

Pathologic conditions of the uterus, cervix, ovaries, and fallopian tubes may also result in dyspareunia. Such conditions should be ruled out through referral to a gynecologist or other physician. In a classic study by Gloeckner (1991), dyspareunia was the major complaint of women who had undergone a proctocolectomy (surgical removal of the colon and rectum). Dyspareunia may also be related to psychogenic factors, such as trauma from rape, incest, or other unwanted sexual experiences, or to previous experience with an inconsiderate partner.

In men, dyspareunia may be associated with inflammation or infection of the penis, prostate, urinary bladder, urethra, or testes. Men infrequently experience pain related to exposure to vaginal contraceptive creams or foams or lubricants on condoms or from irritation from the partner's intrauterine device (IUD). An increase in latex allergies must be considered as a possible cause of painful inflammatory responses in both men and women where condoms are routinely used.

Hypoactive Sexual Desire

Hypoactive sexual desire is a loss of interest in sexual activity or a decline in libido. In women it may be related to several factors, including

- Hormonal replacement therapy
- Use of oral contraceptives
- Eating disorders (e.g., anorexia nervosa or bulimia nervosa)
- Weight gain or loss
- Substance abuse
- Chronic illness (e.g., cancer or end-stage renal disease)

Psychosocial factors, such as abuse, marital or partner discord, family violence, depression, anxiety, fear, or other environmental stressors, may be major contributing factors.

In men, hypoactive sexual desire may be related to
- The use of antihypertensive drugs
- Substance abuse
- A chronic illness that affects energy levels

The psychosocial factors that affect men are the same as those affecting women.

Vaginismus

In a woman with vaginismus, the muscles of the outer third of the vaginal barrel contract powerfully and prevent insertion of a tampon or other object. This condition may be related to physical factors, such as sexual activity during the healing phase after childbirth, infections of the vagina and vulva, abnormalities of the hymen, and atrophy of the vagina. Other contributing factors include the person's lack of information, anxiety, and fear. Vaginismus is more likely to be related to psychogenic causes, including strong religious teachings, rape trauma, physical or psychosocial abuse, or homosexual experimentation about which the individual has conflicting feelings.

For an accurate assessment of vaginismus, the physician or nurse practitioner or nurse specialist must perform a direct pelvic examination.

Vaginitis

Vaginitis may be either acute or chronic. Because the vulva perspires more than other parts of the body, wearing restrictive clothing that is nonabsorbent places the woman at risk for irritation and infection. Strenuous exercising such as bike riding or horse-back riding in tight clothing can cause such irritation. Heterosexual intercourse without condoms changes the pH balance of the vagina, making it more alkaline and thus vulnerable to infection in the presence of other contributing factors. Other factors that contribute to vaginitis include stress, chemical irritants such as tampons containing deodorants and scented douches, and the use of antibiotics to treat other infections (Northouse, 1995).

Orgasmic Dysfunction

Orgasmic dysfunction is defined as the inability to achieve orgasm (primary dysfunction) or as the inability to achieve orgasm with intercourse or at an appropriate time during intercourse (secondary dysfunction). These dysfunctions are the most common sexual complaints of adult women. Orgasmic dysfunctions are related to physical factors, such as adhesions of the clitoris that interfere with stimulation, lack of strength in the pubococcygeal

muscles, and diminished contractions of the uterus. The nurse should refer women with these conditions to a nurse practitioner or physician for confirmation.

Other factors contributing to orgasmic dysfunction are psychogenic and may include
- Feelings of anxiety or guilt
- Lack of knowledge
- Poor communication skills
- Marital or partner discord/family violence

Fear of rejection and conscious withholding of orgasm may lead to secondary orgasmic dysfunctions. General expectations of the culture or society may also be contributing factors.

Erectile Dysfunction

Erectile dysfunction (impotence) is the inability of a man to attain or maintain an erection of the penis of sufficient firmness to permit penetration. This problem can be primary (the man has never been able to sustain an erection) or secondary (he has experienced at least one erection of sufficient firmness to permit penetration). The term *erectile dysfunction* is preferred to *impotence*.

Organic causes include spinal cord injury, diabetes mellitus, alcoholism, neurologic disease (such as multiple sclerosis), endocrine disorders, various infections or surgical procedures involving the genitourinary system, and specific drug use and abuse. Psychosocial factors contributing to erectile dysfunction include marital or partner discord, anxiety, depression, excessive weight gain or loss, insomnia, and fatigue.

Premature Ejaculatory Dysfunction

A man with a premature ejaculatory dysfunction ejaculates after penetration but sooner than either partner desires. Although there are no established norms for the timing of ejaculation during intercourse, this timing is important to the satisfaction of both partners involved in sexual activity. If the man is unable to exercise any voluntary control over the timing of this learned response, premature ejaculation may become a problem.

Organic causes are rare, if they exist at all; psychosocial factors contribute to the learning of this response. A man's feelings of anxiety, guilt, and fear, along with situations in which he may hurry toward a climax, may result in this type of dysfunction.

Retrograde Ejaculation

Retrograde ejaculation, or "dry orgasm," may sometimes be confused with ejaculatory incompetence because there is no external evidence of the ejaculate. Men experiencing retrograde ejaculation discharge semen in a reverse manner—into the urinary bladder rather than forward through the penis. This may result from prostatic surgery, diabetes, multiple sclerosis, structural defects of the urethra and bladder neck, or the use of tranquilizers. During orgasm, the bladder neck does not close and the semen is forced directly into it. The man experiences the sensation of orgasm but is infertile. In some cases, live sperm have been harvested from the urinary bladder and used for in vitro fertilization.

➤ *Psychosocial Assessment*

Once a sexual problem is identified or suspected, the nurse completes a more comprehensive and specific sexual health history. Although the general sexual history described earlier is an essential part of a nursing assessment, the nurse should obtain additional information about the psychological and social factors related to past and present sexual functioning when making a nursing diagnosis of sexual dysfunction. Subjective responses include the way in which the client perceives the problem as well as how he or she feels, thinks, and acts. The following questions may guide the nurse in making a more complete assessment of past and present factors related to sexual dysfunctions:

- How does the client describe the problem? What specific behaviors, thoughts, feelings, or attitudes are problematic?
- What is the client's perception of what caused the problem or what continues to contribute to the problem?
- What environmental or situational factors were present at the onset of the problem? Do these factors continue to interfere with sexual health and well-being?
- How has the problem changed over time? Has it become more severe or less severe? Does it occur in more than one setting?
- What has the client previously done to seek help from others, both professionals and peers? What forms of self-help has he or she tried? Have they been effective or ineffective and in what ways?
- What are the client's expectations and goals, both realistic and ideal, for therapeutic intervention and resolution of the problem?

In addition to this direct assessment of the client's sexual health, the nurse may notice problems of sexuality as a result of the client's "acting-out" behaviors. An example would be a client who exhibits inappropriate behaviors, such as exposing genitalia or overtly soliciting sexual favors from the nurse. The nurse should realize that such behavior may represent a coping mechanism on the part of the client, who may be overwhelmed by actual or potential threats to body image, gender identity, gender role, and sexual functioning. This pattern of behaviors may also indicate unresolved issues related to early sexual abuse or trauma.

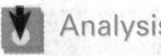

Analysis

➤ *Common Nursing Diagnoses and Collaborative Problems*

The major sexual problems addressed through the nursing process are sexual dysfunctions. Common problems related to sexual dysfunctions may affect either men or women or both and include

1. Sexual Dysfunction related to dyspareunia or hypoactive sexual desire
2. Sexual Dysfunction related to vaginismus or orgasmic dysfunction

3. Sexual Dysfunction related to erectile dysfunction, premature ejaculatory dysfunction, or retrograde ejaculation

➤ *Additional Nursing Diagnoses and Collaborative Problems*

In addition to the common nursing diagnoses, some clients may experience one or more of the following diagnoses:

- Ineffective Individual Coping related to loss of control over body part or body function
- Anxiety related to feelings of failure or loss of control
- Pain related to infectious process, inflammation, or muscle spasm
- Self Esteem Disturbance related to loss of function or physical appearance
- Body Image Disturbance related to change in physical appearance

 Planning and Implementation

➤ *Sexual Dysfunction Related to Dyspareunia or Hypoactive Sexual Desire*

Planning: Expected Outcomes

The outcomes, determined with the client, are that the client is expected to be free from pain or discomfort during sexual intercourse and resume interest in sexual activity.

Interventions

The nursing care for the man or woman who experiences dyspareunia depends in part on the cause of the problem.

Interventions for Dyspareunia in Women. Nursing interventions for the woman with dyspareunia depend on the contributing factors. When pain results from physical factors (e.g., an intact hymen, scarring from an episiotomy or infibulation, or pathologic conditions of the reproductive organs), the nurse refers the client to a gynecologist. Infections of the vagina or vulva also require medical diagnosis and treatment. If infection is present, the nurse administers prescribed antibiotics, provides increased fluid intake, and encourages the client to rest and avoid sexual activity. The nurse can use therapeutic communication and education to reduce further episodes of infection by listening with a nonjudgmental attitude and explaining about the risk of multiple partners, if this is a factor. The nurse also explains the risks associated with the client's usual sexual activities. For example, chronic irritations may result from foreign objects placed into the vagina without adequate lubrication, the use of chemical irritants, or wearing restrictive clothing.

When the major contributing factors include inadequate vaginal lubrication or irritation from excessive use of chemical contraceptives, douches, or feminine deodorants, clients need accurate information and specific suggestions for behavioral changes. The nurse reviews anatomy and physiology and emphasizes the ability of the vagina to clean itself. The nurse describes alternative methods of contraception and encourages the client to use unscented feminine products, including tampons or sanitary pads. Increasing vaginal lubrication through the use of over-the-counter water-soluble gels or a vaginal dilator may also be suggested.

Interventions for Dyspareunia in Men. When dyspareunia results from inflammation or infection of organs within the man's genitourinary system, the nurse administers prescribed antibiotics and encourages the client to drink fluids and to rest. The nurse encourages the man with acute inflammation or infection to avoid sexual intercourse with his partner until the acute condition is resolved. Alternative sexual activities that avoid intercourse are suggested and explored with both partners. Much literature is available to assist clients in trying alternative behaviors.

When the major contributing factor for dyspareunia in the man is exposure to vaginal contraceptive creams and foams or an intrauterine device (IUD) in the sexual partner, the nurse may suggest alternatives to both partners, such as mutual body massage and caressing until the infection clears.

Interventions for Hypoactive Sexual Desire. If hypoactive sexual desire in the woman is related to hormonal replacement therapy or oral contraceptive use, the nurse may present alternatives or refer the client to a gynecologist. For example, contraceptive foams, creams, or patches may be used in place of oral contraceptives. To increase the client's interest and sexual arousal, the nurse may suggest that the client use erotic reading or video materials or change the time and setting of usual sexual activities.

When drug or alcohol abuse or chronic illness is the major contributing factor in clients with hypoactive sexual desire, medical management of the underlying factor is required before other interventions can be tried. Certain hypothalamopituitary disorders result in loss of desire as well as problems with vaginal lubrication and orgasm (Hulter & Lundberg, 1994). If the prognosis for any of these conditions is poor, the outcome for the sexual problem is often poor. The nurse informs the client about the relationship between the underlying causes and the resulting sexual dysfunction.

Psychosocial factors that affect the development of hypoactive sexual desire are similar in both men and women. Marital or partner discord, depression, anxiety, and fear may be sufficiently severe to require the specialized education and experience of a nurse specialist or clinician with expertise in the area of psychology or psychiatry. Other psychiatric diagnoses such as depression may be associated with hypoactive sexual desire (American Psychiatric Association, 1994). Nursing interventions include therapeutic communication, encouraging the client to pursue intensive therapy with a qualified sex therapist, and referring the client to a competent professional. Often the process involves either the client or his or her sexual partner or partners or all of these people.

➤ *Sexual Dysfunction Related to Vaginismus and Orgasmic Dysfunction*

Planning: Expected Outcomes

The outcomes are that the client is expected to (1) relieve or prevent the involuntary spasms of the vagina and (2) experience an orgasm by any personally satisfying means.

Interventions

Interventions are often focused toward relieving the cause of the problem.

Interventions for Vaginismus. The nursing interventions for an actual problem of vaginismus aim to relieve the underlying contributing factors. The interventions for a potential problem of vaginismus are directed at educating the woman who is at risk for this response, thus preventing its occurrence.

If the major contributing factor is psychogenic, such as trauma from rape, conflicts surrounding homosexual experimentation, or strong religious teachings, the interventions are similar to those already discussed and range from giving permission to express anxiety and conflict to providing intensive therapy. If the major contributing factor is a physical one, such as sexual activity too soon after birth trauma, infection, abnormality of the hymen, or atrophy of the vagina, referral to a gynecologist may be indicated. Nursing interventions include encouraging the client to explore alternatives to vaginal intercourse during the healing process. The nurse also educates the woman and her sexual partner about the relationship between physical factors and involuntary muscular response.

Interventions for Orgasmic Dysfunction. When the major contributing factors in primary or secondary orgasmic dysfunction are psychogenic, the nurse provides opportunities for the client to talk about this situation. The nurse teaches the client about the relationship between stressors and the physical response of orgasm. The nurse also explains Kegel exercises, which strengthen the pubococcygeal muscles, and encourages general exercise to strengthen the pelvic musculature. Instructions for Kegel exercises are provided in Chart 11–3.

The client may need more intensive therapy, such as marriage counseling or in-depth counseling, for issues of anxiety and guilt. The nurse might refer the client to a nurse specialist or other professional in one or both of these specialties.

Chart 11–3

Education Guide

Kegel Exercises
1. Tighten the muscles as you would when stopping the flow of urine.
2. Hold for 2 to 3 seconds, then release.
3. Contract and relax these muscles 10 to 12 times and repeat this series several times daily.

If adhesions of the clitoris result in orgasmic dysfunction, the nurse refers the client to a physician for possible surgical intervention and provides encouragement that the condition may be corrected.

➤ Sexual Dysfunction Related to Erectile Dysfunction, Premature Ejaculatory Dysfunction, or Retrograde Ejaculation

Planning: Expected Outcomes

The outcomes are that the client is expected to (1) attain or maintain an erection, (2) delay ejaculation until he and his sexual partner are satisfied, and (3) accept the alteration of retrograde ejaculation and adjust to the resulting possibility of sterility.

Interventions

Interventions usually include treatment of the underlying cause of the problem(s).

Interventions for Erectile Dysfunction. For nursing interventions to influence the client's symptoms of erectile dysfunction, underlying diseases (e.g., diabetes mellitus, alcoholism, multiple sclerosis, endocrine disorders, and infections of the genitourinary system) must be under medical supervision. Appropriate nursing interventions include education; specific suggestions, such as the "sensate focus" technique; and alternatives for satisfying sexual activities. The sensate focus technique may also be used when the underlying factors are psychogenic. The nurse instructs the client and his partner in the following steps:

1. Mutual body touching and pleasuring without contact in the area of the genitalia
2. Genital stimulation, resulting in penile erection but not followed by intercourse
3. Orgasm and ejaculation through manual or oral stimulation (not vaginal penetration)
4. Vaginal penetration without orgasm or ejaculation (simple containment)
5. Vaginal penetration with orgasm and ejaculation
6. Dialogue between partners throughout steps

As with all sexual problems in which the major contributing factors are psychogenic, therapeutic communication and intensive therapy are indicated. The nurse makes the appropriate referrals, and the nurse specialist, psychotherapist, or psychiatrist provides therapy directed at alleviating underlying marital or partner discord, anxiety, or depression.

In the absence of underlying disease or obvious psychological factors, the use or abuse of various drugs may be the major etiologic factor in erectile dysfunction. The nurse explains the effects of such drugs as antihypertensives, barbiturates, sedatives, and amphetamines on the sexual response cycle. The nurse refers the client to a physician to evaluate the drug regimen so that an alternative drug, dosage, or therapy may be considered.

The client may also need referral to a urologist who treats men by self-injection of papaverine (Pavatine) and phentolamine (Regitine, Rogitine✲). These drugs are vasodilators that allow more blood to flow to the penis and facilitate erection. Many men have found these drugs to be successful. The nurse explains about possible side effects, including prolonged erection, bruising, and liver abnormalities. Another drug, prostaglandin E_1, has been found effective with intracavernosal self-injection (into the shaft of the penis) for use in elderly males (Godschalk et al., 1994).

Interventions for Premature Ejaculation. Nursing interventions for premature ejaculation include educating the client and sexual partner about the relationship between emotions and the sexual response cycle. The nurse may teach the client, partner, or both systematic relaxation exercises to alleviate anxiety as a major contributing factor. The nurse should be sure to include the client's sexual partner in the treatment, because the partner's communication of desires and expressions of distress may be instrumental in maintaining the dysfunction.

With appropriate preparation, the nurse may instruct the client and his partner in the "squeeze technique" for learning voluntary control for premature ejaculatory dysfunction. The man's partner can provide two types of squeezes.

In the traditional method, the partner places the thumb and first and second fingers just above and below the head of the penis and applies a squeezing pressure. In the basilar method, the thumb and fingers are placed at the base of the penis rather than at the head. Either position is held firmly for approximately 4 seconds, then released. The partner is instructed to always apply the pressure from the front to back of the shaft of the penis and never from side to side because this may result in tissue injury. The nurse should stress the importance of avoiding injury from the fingernails. The partner applies the squeeze shortly after erection occurs, and periodically thereafter, until both partners are ready for penetration to take place. Once the man has been aroused to the point of ejaculatory inevitability, this squeeze technique should not be used; instead, ejaculation should be allowed to continue.

Interventions for Retrograde Ejaculation. When the man's problem is retrograde ejaculation, the underlying cause is physiologic. Men who have diabetes, prostatic disease, multiple sclerosis, or abnormalities of the bladder and urethra must be referred to a urologist for further evaluation and medical or surgical intervention. With the exception of a physical abnormality, clients with diabetes, multiple sclerosis, or prostatic disease have an irreversible condition, and nursing interventions are thus directed at assisting them with coping skills. These men have an altered sensation from previous ejaculations and may be rendered sterile.

Education and counseling of the client and his sexual partner are important nursing interventions. The nurse reassures both partners that there are no harmful effects to the ejaculate being deposited in the bladder. Some clients who wish to have children are referred to an infertility clinic. It is possible for semen to be centrifuged from the urine and prepared for in vitro fertilization.

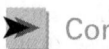 Continuing Care

When preparing clients to return home after hospitalization for illness, injury, or surgery, the nurse should anticipate plans for follow-up care and sexual counseling.

The nurse teaches the client and sexual partner, when appropriate, about the relationship of the illness, injury, or surgery to sexual functioning. For example, when clients have surgery or chemotherapy for cancer, they may experience temporary alterations in sexual desire. It is appropriate for the nurse to explain this situation and offer suggestions for less strenuous expressions of intimacy. Similarly, the nurse should counsel the client who has had a myocardial infarction about his or her anxiety related to resuming sexual intercourse.

The nurse teaches clients to report any adverse effects of medications on their sexual functioning. Nurses must be aware of how specific drugs affect sexual functioning and provide appropriate information to clients who will continue to receive these medications after discharge.

When clients are discharged to home health care, additional follow-up may be directed at the family caregiver. The caregiver who takes primary responsibility for care of a client in the absence of professional home health caregivers is often a spouse whose own health needs must also be considered.

Providing nursing care and being a sexual partner of the client may present conflicts for a spouse who accepts the role of family caregiver. Nurses should anticipate and prevent such conflict by discussing these roles with the family caregiver. The home health nurse can offer counseling or seek more expert assistance as the situation warrants.

 Evaluation

The expected outcomes are that the client
- Does not experience pain or discomfort associated with intercourse
- Describes restored levels of interest in sexual activity
- States that sexual activity is no longer accompanied by painful involuntary spasms of the vaginal wall
- Experiences orgasm as desired
- Reports satisfaction and enjoyment of orgasm
- Attains or maintains erections of the penis of sufficient firmness to permit vaginal penetration in at least 50% of attempts
- Learns voluntary control over the ejaculatory response

SELECTED BIBLIOGRAPHY

American Psychiatric Association. (1994). *Diagnostic and statistical manual of mental disorders (4th ed.).* Washington, D. C.: American Psychiatric Association.

*Cholewinski, J. T., & Burge, J. M. (1990). Sexual harassment of nursing students. *Image: Journal of Nursing Scholarship, 22,* 106–110.

Giger, J. N., & Davidhizar, R. E. (1995). *Transcultural nursing: Assessment and intervention* (2nd ed.). St. Louis: Mosby–Year Book.

Gloeckner, M. (1991). Perception of sexuality after ostomy surgery. *Journal of Enterostomal Therapy, 18*(1), 36–38.

Godschalk, M. F., Chen, J., Katz, P. G., & Mulligan, T. (1994). Prostaglandin E1 as treatment for erectile failure in elderly men. *Journal of the American Geriatric Society, 42,* 1263–1265.

Hulter, B., & Lundberg, P. O. (1994). Sexual function in women with hypothalamo-pituitary disorders. *Archives of Sexual Behavior, 23,* 171–183.

Jarvis, C. (1996). *Physical examination and health assessment* (2nd ed.). Philadelphia: W. B. Saunders.

Kendall, J. (1996). Human association as a factor influencing wellness in homosexual men with human immunodeficiency virus disease. *Applied Nursing Research, 9,* 195–203.

*Masters, W. M., Johnson, V. E., & Kolodny, R. C. (1985). *Human sexuality* (2nd ed.). Boston: Little, Brown.

Northouse, C. (1995). *Women's bodies, women's wisdom.* New York: Bantam Books.

Quadagno, D., Nation, A. J., Johnson, D., Waitley, C., Waitley, N., Epstein, D., & Satterwhite, A. (1995). Cardiovascular disease and sexual functioning. *Applied Nursing Research, 8*(3), 143–146.

*Roth, S., & Newman, E. (1991). The process of coping with sexual trauma. *Journal of Traumatic Stress, 4,* 279–297.

*Schiavi, R. C. (1992). Normal aging and the evaluation of sexual dysfunction. *Psychiatric Medicine, 10,* 217–225.

Skidmore-Roth, L. (1995). *Mosby's 1995 nursing drug reference.* St. Louis: Mosby.

Walker, L. R. & Morgan, M. C. (1995). Female circumcision: A report of four adolescents. *Journal of Adolescent Health, 17,* 128–132.

Waxman, B. F. (1994). Up against eugenics: Disabled women's challenge to receive reproductive health services. *Sexuality and Disability, 12,* 155–171.

SUGGESTED READINGS

Aloni, R., Schwartz, J., & Ring, H. (1994). Sexual function in post-stroke female patients. *Sexuality and Disability, 12,* 191–199.
These researchers studied the sexual functioning in female patients 26 to 59 years of age who experienced strokes. They found their sexual functioning, including sexual desire, to be related to the severity of neurologic impairment. The article has good implications for nurses caring for young and middle-aged women with neurologic impairment.

Kendall, J. (1996). Human association as a factor influencing wellness in homosexual men with human immunodeficiency virus disease. *Applied Nursing Research, 9,* 195–203.
This nursing study presents findings from in-depth interviews with 29 gay men with human immunodeficiency virus infection. The subjects stated that the need for intimacy and community were crucial to their well-being. The authors suggested that nurses should help clients connect and interact with others to enhance their wellness.

LOSS, DEATH, AND DYING

CHAPTER

HIGHLIGHTS

Loss, dying, and death are integral parts of living that accompany the developmental stages of late adulthood and are frequently associated with illness. Because nurses frequently face loss and death in their work, knowledge of responses to loss is essential in assisting clients and families to cope with these experiences.

LOSS
Overview

Loss is being deprived of or being without something valued that one once had. We begin life with loss, cast from the womb, and we experience losses throughout life. Although death may be considered the ultimate loss, it is not the only loss worthy of attention. There are various types of loss, each of which gives rise to grief reactions. Even minor losses give rise to grief, and insufficient attention to such losses could have a more profound impact on an individual in the long run than a loss through death.

Mitchell and Anderson (1983) have identified six major types of loss. The first is material loss, loss of a physical object to which one has important attachment. The second type is relationship loss, the ending of opportunities to relate to another human being. Although death is one example of this type of loss, any temporary or permanent separation of two human beings can be a relationship loss. Intrapsychic loss, the third type of loss, occurs when a person loses an emotionally important image of herself or himself. This experience often involves a vision or

dream of how things might have been; a change in one's perception of another; loss of emotions such as faith, hope, or courage; or emotions that occur on successful completion of a major task.

Functional loss, the fourth type of loss, involves the loss of a functional ability, as in the bodily decline of illness or aging. Role loss, the fifth type of loss, is loss of one's accustomed place in a social network. Role loss can occur through retirement or promotion, when one goes from being single to being married or vice versa, or when a person becomes a client.

Systemic loss, the sixth type of loss, occurs when one loses contact with certain interactional behaviors within a system. An employee leaving the workplace or a child leaving home affects the interactional behaviors within the workplace or the family.

Responses to Loss
Grief

Grieving is the psychologic, social, and physical reaction to the perception of significant loss. It is a natural response to loss and varies from one person to another, manifested as thoughts, feelings, and behaviors associated with often overwhelming distress or sorrow. Although a grief reaction can result from the loss of any precious element in a person's life, loss through death is used as the major example of grief for the remainder of this chapter.

Mourning is the process of doing the grief work. There

are numerous conceptualizations of mourning (or grieving), which use different labels to describe stages or phases. Conceptualizations differ in their focus or names. All were developed to describe reaction to loss, and all cover similar basic feelings. A major limitation of conceptualizations is that they describe only part of the grieving process.

Kübler-Ross's (1969) stages of coping with imminent death was one of the first conceptualizations to describe grieving after loss and included shock and disbelief, denial, anger, bargaining, depression, and acceptance.

SHOCK AND DISBELIEF. During this phase, the person has a desire to avoid the acknowledgment of loss because it is too overwhelming to deal with. Numbness and disbelief are prominent, and people are often confused, dazed, and unable to comprehend what has happened.

DENIAL. When a person is faced with an overwhelming loss, denial often buffers reality, allowing him or her to absorb the loss a little at a time. Denial is often therapeutic.

ANGER. At several times after news of an actual or anticipated loss, the client or family members feel and possibly express anger. Family members may be angry at the client or the deceased for leaving them and at God or fate for allowing the illness or death. Survivors of deceased people may be angry at family, friends, or caregivers for not saving the person's life. A person who is dying might ask, "Why me?"

BARGAINING. In this stage, people bargain with fate, physicians, the disease, or a deity for a short-term or long-term postponement of the loss. Characteristic responses are "I'll do anything as long as he lives . . ." and "Just let me live until my daughter gets married."

DEPRESSION. Crying and tearfulness are common during this stage. People lose interest in life and its meaning. Some isolate themselves socially, withdrawing from any conversation. Survivors may avoid discussions or activities, such as hobbies, that they had shared with the lost loved one. Many see life as a weighty burden and describe a lack of pleasure. They cannot believe that life will ever hold meaning and joy again. They may talk of suicide during the first year of bereavement and express a strong desire for reunion with the deceased.

The intensity of these negative feelings can be frightening. People who have had relatively stable or calm personalities may have a horror of losing emotional control. Their fears can be intensified by memory lapses and difficulty in concentrating. To gain control, they center on themselves, which can be interpreted as selfishness by themselves as well as by others.

Depression contributes to the bereaved's difficulty in concentrating and fuels excesses of anger, guilt, and extreme sadness. The bereaved may focus exclusively on the deceased and reject all offers of comfort.

ACCEPTANCE. The feelings and symptoms of grief do not simply stop completely one day. Sadness decreases only gradually, and a new life, based on the acceptance of a new reality, emerges slowly as time passes. With time, the bereaved may experience a new awareness of the precious gift each day brings.

Although Kübler-Ross and other theorists described grief in stages, it is now believed that these stages are not necessarily sequential, nor must each person go through each stage. More recent grief theorists describe reactions as opposed to stages, which include, but are not limited to, reactions described previously. These include guilt ("I should have done more;" or "It's my fault she died"), identification with the deceased (taking up one of his or her hobbies), "grief attacks" manifested as waves and pangs of emotional or physical pain, and visual or auditory hallucinations.

Manifestations of grief vary widely; people may take one step forward and two steps back, then half steps from side to side as they cycle through healing. Many people achieve healthy accommodation to a loss by doing the grief work or mourning rapidly, with very little disruption in their lives. Others' response may involve great life disruption.

Although estimates of a "normal" duration for grieving have been made, it is now believed that there is no fixed timetable by which a person passes through grieving. Normal grief is now viewed as a long-term process that may require long-term bereavement follow-up at critical points in the mourner's life. Because such a wide range of normal responses exist, nurses may need to consult with bereavement experts before labeling a reaction abnormal.

Rando (1993) identified six processes of mourning necessary for healthy accommodation to any loss:

- Recognizing the loss through acknowledgment and understanding
- Reacting to the separation by experiencing the pain and some form of expression of all the psychological reactions
- Realistically recollecting and reviewing the relationship with the lost object or person
- Relinquishing old attachments to the lost object or person and the old assumptive world
- Readjusting and adapting to the new world, developing a new relationship with the lost object or person, and adopting new ways of being in the new world (forming a new identity)
- Reinvesting in the new world

Complicated Mourning

Complicated mourning describes a state of compromise, distortion, or failure of one of the six processes of mourning (given a realistic amount of time since the loss). In all forms of complicated mourning, there are attempts to deny, repress, or avoid aspects of the loss and to hold onto and avoid relinquishing the loss. High-risk factors for complicated mourning are either associated with the specific loss (e.g., death) or are antecedent and subsequent variables (see Chart 12–1).

Chart 12–1

Nursing Care Highlight: High-Risk Factors for Complicated Mourning

Factors Associated with Death
- Sudden, unanticipated death (especially when traumatic, violent, mutilating, or random)
- Death from an overly lengthy illness
- Loss of a child
- Mourner's perception that the death was preventable

Antecedent and Subsequent Variables
- A premorbid relationship with deceased that was markedly angry, ambivalent, or dependent
- Prior or concurrent mourner liabilities of unaccommodated losses and/or stresses or mental health problems
- The mourner's perceived lack of social support

Collaborative Management

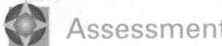 Assessment

➤ History

In assessing a person who is grieving a death, the nurse obtains information on the relationship to and age of the deceased, cause of death and length of illness (if appropriate), length of preparation for the death, and degree of intimacy or intensity of the relationship. The nurse also obtains information on the bereaved person's age, education, employment, economic status, history of losses, history of depressions, personality or mental health problems, substance abuse, ethnic background, family structure, social support, coping strategies, and spiritual aspects (sense of meaning and purpose). Nurses must understand that the process of eliciting the material for a thorough assessment from the bereaved also can be a therapeutic encounter.

In all likelihood, the grieving client will not be able to supply all information in a business-like and straightforward manner. There will be pauses at certain questions for either the control or expression of feelings. Because it is difficult to predict which parts of the assessment will affect individual clients and in what ways, the nurse moves from topic to topic, not necessarily in order but guided by the client's response. The key is to keep the information flowing while comforting the person as much as possible.

➤ Review of Loss

Because most newly bereaved people have a need to repeat the circumstances of the terminal episode and the death, questions related to this need are asked at the beginning of the assessment. Often, by retelling the story to an empathic listener and possibly discharging tears, guilt, or anger, the client feels accepted and understood and does not react to the more factual and sensitive assessment items as intrusive or callous.

➤ Physical Assessment/Clinical Manifestations

Grief can cause physiologic distress in addition to emotional pain, which may lead to serious illness. Recent studies indicate that the physical health of caregivers often deteriorates while caring for a loved one, and caregivers often delay contact with health providers because they are preoccupied with their loved one's needs. The nurse should always assess survivors for any physical signs and symptoms of serious disease.

TRANSCULTURAL CONSIDERATIONS

 Most of the research on loss, grieving, and death has focused on Caucasian, English-speaking populations. The grieving responses of other cultural groups have not been widely studied, except in relation to religious origin. Table 12–1 lists specific beliefs and customs about death and dying of various religious groups.

 Analysis

➤ Common Nursing Diagnoses and Collaborative Problems

The nursing diagnoses given the highest priority when caring for a client reacting to potential death are
- Potential for Ineffective Individual Coping related to loss of significant other
- Anticipatory Grieving related to an actual or perceived loss

➤ Additional Nursing Diagnoses and Collaborative Problems

One or more of the following common diagnoses and collaborative problems may apply:
- Avoidance Coping related to support system deficit
- Compromised Family Coping related to knowledge deficit, emotional conflicts, role changes, or exhaustion of supportive capacity
- Disabling Family Coping related to unexpressed guilt, hostility, or anxiety of family member
- Spiritual Distress related to challenged belief and value system due to the loss
- Social Isolation related to others' intolerance to loss

Planning and Implementation

➤ Potential for Ineffective Individual Coping

Planning: Expected Outcomes. The client and family or significant others are expected to readjust, adapt, and be able to reinvest in the new world.

Interventions. Interventions are largely psychosocial and aim to provide sensitive support.

Offering Physical and Emotional Support. The nurse intervenes with those mourning a death by "being with" as opposed to "being there." "Being with" implies that the nurse is physically and psychologically with the grieving client, empathizing to provide emotional support. Listen-

TABLE 12–1

Major Religious Groups in the United States: Concepts and Practices Related to Death				
Religious Group	**Afterlife**	**Rituals**	**Handling of the Body After Death**	**"Extraordinary" Life-Prolonging Measures**
Eastern Orthodoxy (including Greek and Russian Orthodoxy)	• Yes; the soul blends into the spiritual cosmos	• The client's arms are crossed after death, with the fingers set in the shape of a cross • Special prayers are said for those who have been baptized to bless the sick and dying • Last Rites must be delivered while the person is still conscious • Holy Communion is obligatory	• Autopsy and embalming are discouraged • Organ and body donation are discouraged • Cremation is discouraged	• Encouraged
Judaism	• The dead will be resurrected with the coming of the Messiah • A person lives on in the memories of his or her survivors • For Reform Jews, no concept of eternal punishment	• The dying and dead are never left unattended before burial because the soul should depart in the presence of people • The body is ritually washed, sometimes by members of a ritual burial society • Burial is in a wooden casket within 24 hours or as soon as possible after death • Five stages of mourning extend over a year • Funerals are very simple, with no flowers (flowers are a symbol of life)	• Orthodox Jews prohibit autopsy and allow no removal of body parts Conservative and Reform Jews permit autopsy For Orthodox Jews, no embalming is allowed • Beliefs about organ and body donation vary Orthodox Jews generally prohibit both but may agree, with rabbinical consent • Cremation is largely prohibited, but beliefs vary Reform Jews allow cremation but recommend burial of ashes in a Jewish cemetery	• Generally discouraged after irreversible brain damage is determined Orthodox Jews advocate life support without "heroic measures"

ing and somehow acknowledging the legitimacy of the client's pain are often more therapeutic than speaking. Physical support such as gentle touching, holding hands, and hugging are especially important during the first phases of grief. When necessary, nurses facilitate the expression of grief by giving the person mourning permission to express herself or himself. The nurse's manner and words show that the expression of grief is not only acceptable and expected but also healthy. Nurses can say something like "Just let the tears come. Don't hold back."

Being Realistic. The pain of loss cannot be, nor should it be, taken away no matter how committed the nurse may be to the client's comfort. The nurse avoids trite assurances such as "Things will be fine. Don't cry" or

"Don't be upset. She wouldn't want it that way" or "In a year you will have forgotten." Such comments comfort the nurse—not the client. The nurse accepts whatever the griever says about the situation and remains present, ready to listen attentively and guide gently. In this way, nurses help the bereaved prepare for the necessary reminiscence and integration of the loss.

Avoiding Explanations of the Loss. The nurse should not try soon after the death to explain the loss in philosophical or religious terms. Statements such as "Everything happens for the best" or "God sends us only as much as we can bear" are not helpful when the bereaved person has yet to express feelings of anguish or anger. Telling someone too soon that they have other children to

TABLE 12–1

Major Religious Groups in the United States: Concepts and Practices Related to Death *Continued*				
Religious Group	Afterlife	Rituals	Handling of the Body After Death	"Extraordinary" Life-Prolonging Measures
Roman Catholicism	• The faithful go to Heaven, but those who reject God's grace go to Hell • The soul goes to Purgatory for a time and is released by prayers and Masses • Resurrection occurs at the second coming of Christ	• The family and priest choose prayers • Holy Communion and rites for anointing the sick are mandatory • Confession may be desired but is not mandatory; however, repentance is recommended	• Autopsy is permitted, but all body parts must be buried appropriately • Organ and body donation are unrestricted provided that the donor is not harmed • Cremation is not restricted	• Discouraged
Protestantism	• Varies; Episcopalians, Presbyterians, and Lutherans strongly believe in an afterlife, Quakers strongly do not	• Varies; anointing rites, confession, and communion may be available but are not mandatory • Healing services may be available, but there are no official sacraments • The client and family may have a large role in planning services and prayer; services range from traditional funerals to memorial services • Clergy may minister through prayer, scripture reading, and counseling	• Beliefs about autopsy, organ and body donation, and cremation vary by group from no restriction to individual choice to preferred	• Discouraged
Nonaffiliated	• Varies	• Spontaneous and individualized, possibly including reading of original or traditional prayers or songs such as Psalm 23 • Traditional secular funeral or memorial services are used	• Autopsy, organ and body donation, and cremation are by individual preference	• Individual preference

rely on or that there are other family members who need them does not diminish the intensity of the grief. In fact, doing so can create feelings of anger and resentment toward the nurse because it reflects an insensitivity to the acute initial pain.

"Being with" remains important as the weeks or months pass and the funeral crisis supports dissipate. The out-of-town relatives return home, and friends and local relatives resume their own lives. The nurse offers physical and emotional support by encouraging the bereaved to eat, drink, rest, and stay as physically active as possible. Exercise to tolerance levels is a wonderful psychic as well as physical energizer.

Referral to Bereavement Counselors. The nurse informs the family about bereavement counselors and groups for persons who have experienced the death of a loved one. This process can be especially effective if the nurse can help locate a group to meet the family's special needs. Many survivors experience uncomfortable feelings during the grief work, which they often don't discuss. They question their own mental stability and worry about what others will think of them. Seeing a counselor or being a part of a support group can help people discover that others have gone through a similar sequence and intensity of emotion, making them more likely to share their feelings and thus gain some comfort from others.

Chart 12-2

Education Guide: Common Physical Signs and Symptoms of Approaching Death

Coolness of Extremities

- Circulation to the extremities is decreased; the skin may become mottled or discolored
  - Cover the client with a blanket
  - Do not use an electric blanket, hot water bottle, electric heating pad, or hair dryer to warm the client

Increased Sleeping

- Metabolism is decreased
  - Spend time sitting quietly with the person
  - Do not force the person to stay awake
  - Talk to the person as you normally would, even if he or she does not respond

Fluid and Food Decrease

- Metabolic needs have decreased
  - Do not force the person to eat or drink
  - Offer ice chips or small sips of liquids frequently if the person is alert
  - Use glycerine swabs to keep the mouth moist and comfortable
  - Coat the lips with lip balm or petroleum jelly

Incontinence

- Perineal muscles relax
  - Keep the area clean and dry
  - If the person would be more comfortable, use urine catheters

Congestion and Gurgling

- The person is unable to cough up secretions effectively
  - Suctioning can be used to remove secretions, but this may cause the person discomfort
  - Medications can decrease the production of secretions

Breathing Pattern Change

- Slowed circulation to the brain may cause the breathing pattern to become irregular, with brief periods of no or shallow breathing
  - Elevate the person's head
  - Position the person on his or her side

Disorientation

- Decreased metabolism and slowed circulation to the brain may occur
  - Identify yourself whenever you communicate with the person
  - Speak softly, clearly, and truthfully

Restlessness

- Decreased metabolism and slowed circulation to the brain may occur
  - Play soothing music
  - Do not restrain the person
  - Massage the person's forehead
  - Reduce the number of people in the room

Adapted from the Hospice of North Central Florida, Inc.

➤ Anticipatory Grieving

Anticipatory grieving refers to accomplishing part of the grief work before the actual loss. Although dying clients experience anticipatory grieving, the term most often describes the process undergone by the families of clients with terminal illness. Anticipatory grieving can be beneficial if it helps people progress to a healthier state after the loss.

Planning: Expected Outcomes. The family or significant others should be able to accept the reality of the loss and share grief with others.

Interventions. Interventions aim to provide the family members of the dying client with appropriate information and emotional support.

Teaching About the Physical Signs of Death. Witnessing the death of a loved one is one of the most effective experiences in helping the family accept the reality of the loss. If death is anticipated, the nurse gives the client and family or significant others information about the signs of death, using nontechnical language. The nurse describes the physical signs in detail, realistic enough to be unmistakable, yet not so graphic as to alarm the listeners. Chart 12–2 describes common signs and symptoms of approaching death in lay terms. Such charts are often shared with family and friends anticipating a loved one's death.

Ensuring Palliative Care. When family and friends anticipate the death of a loved one, they may fear that the death will be characterized by pain and suffering. The nurse reassures families that clients will be monitored closely for any sign or symptom of distress and that appropriate medications will be administered as needed until pain is controlled. The nurse also reassures families that significant advances have been made in pain and symptom control. (See Interventions under Active Dying.)

 Evaluation

The nurse evaluates the care of the client and family anticipating or grieving loss on the basis of identified nursing diagnoses. Expected outcomes include that the client and family

- State acceptance and adaptation to the loss
- Share their grief with others

ACTIVE DYING
Overview
Death

Death is manifested as cessation of respiration and heartbeat caused by physiologic dysfunction, generally related to an illness or trauma that overwhelms the body's compensatory mechanisms. Direct causes of death include respiratory failure (PCO_2 accumulation and PO_2 deficit) and hypovolemic, septic, or cardiogenic shock, manifested as inadequate blood flow to meet the demands of vital organs. Inadequate blood flow to tissues deprives cells of their source of oxygen and biochemical exchange, the ultimate factor in their death. *Clinical death* refers to the short interval after cessation of heartbeat and cessation of breathing when no evidence of brain function is present. If this termination of function occurs suddenly, as in cardiac arrest or massive hemorrhage, a brief time remains before vital organs lose their viability, and cardiopulmonary resuscitation (CPR) may succeed. People with healthy organs are most likely to survive resuscitation. CPR is likely to be futile, and therefore inappropriate in resuscitating those with terminal disease. However, legal and ethical standards of care must be followed.

Most agencies require that CPR be initiated on clients when breathing or heartbeat ceases unless a doctor's order of "do not resuscitate" (DNR) is obtained. Because CPR is generally futile (and often inappropriate) in terminal illness, nurses need to address advance directives and DNR status with all clients who are actively dying.

Dying

Death is the termination of life. Dying is a process. Emotional responses of dying patients are similar to those described previously in responses to loss. Chart 12–3 lists some of the common emotional symptoms that the dying client may express. However, as death nears, clients

---

Chart 12–3

Education Guide: Common Emotional Signs of Approaching Death

Withdrawal

- The person is preparing to "let go" from surroundings and relationships.

Vision-like Experiences

- The person may talk to people you cannot see or hear and see objects and places not visible to you. These are not hallucinations or drug reactions.
  - Do not deny or argue with what the person claims
  - Affirm the experience

Letting Go

- The person may become agitated or continue to perform repetitive tasks. Often, this indicates that something is unresolved or preventing the person from letting go. As difficult as it may be to do or say, when loved ones are able to say such things as "It's okay to go. We'll be all right," the dying person takes on a more peaceful demeanor.

Saying Goodbye

- When the person is ready to die and you are ready to let go, saying "Goodbye" is important for you both. Touching, hugging, crying, and saying "I love you," "Thank you," "I'm sorry," or "I'll miss you so much" are all natural expressions of your sadness and loss. Verbalizing these sentiments can bring comfort to the dying person as well as to those left behind.

Adapted from the Hospice of North Central Florida, Inc.

Chart 12–4

Nursing Care Highlight: Contents of Symptom Relief Kit

- For unrelieved pain: Morphine solution, 20 mg/mL, 1–2 mL (PO/SL) q2–3h PRN
- For unrelieved dyspnea: Morphine solution, 20 mg/mL, 0.25–0.5 mL (PO/SL) q2h PRN
- For nausea or vomiting: Prochlorperazine, 25 mg suppository, 1 PR q8h PRN
- For unrelieved nausea, vomiting, restlessness: ABR* suppository, 1 PR q8h PRN
- For severe agitation and restlessness:
  - Determine if client is in pain; treat accordingly
  - Determine if client is constipated or having urinary retention; take appropriate action
  - If agitation persists and safety of client or caregiver is at risk, administer pentobarbitol suppository 1 PR, q4–6h PRN
- For loud, wet respirations or excessive secretions: Levsin/SL tablets, 1–2 PO or SL q4–6h PRN
- For unrelieved respiratory fluid accumulation: Furosemide (Lasix) 40–80 mg PO, SC, IM, or IV q2h PRN

Printed with permission from VNA Hospice, Optima Health Visiting Nurse Services, Manchester, NH.

*Many hospice and palliative care organizations will use pharmacist-compounded suppositories for symptom relief. One such combination is ABR, which stands for Ativan, Benadryl, and Reglan (lorazepam, diphenhydramine, and metoclopramide).

---

may manifest fear, anxiety, and physical symptoms of distress, which require treatment and control. Although the majority of symptoms near death can be controlled, expert clinical judgment and knowledge of palliative care are often required. Even with optimal care, a certain percentage of clients have intractable symptoms that may require sedation until death. Providers on oncology units or in hospice services are often knowledgeable about palliative care. Chart 12–4 summarizes the contents of a symptom relief kit used by hospice nurses to provide immediate relief from uncomfortable or distressing symptoms. Palliative care nurses and physicians may be consulted if clients cannot be transferred to these services.

Hospice Services

Hospice care was developed in the United States in the 1970s in response to unmet needs of terminally ill clients. As both a philosophy and a system of care, hospice care seeks to facilitate quality of life and death with dignity for clients with terminal disease, using a multidisciplinary approach. Hospice programs are frequently affiliated with home care agencies, providing services to clients at home or in an extended care facility. Some communities also have hospice "houses," which admit clients in the terminal phase of their illness, allowing them to die there.

Not all hospices restrict their services to the terminally ill. Some hospice agencies divide their services into "supportive care" for clients with advanced disease not necessarily limited to a 6-month prognosis and "hospice" for clients with a documented prognosis of 6 months or less.

This facilitates the delivery of expert palliative care to clients whose exact prognosis might not be known, and/or when clients, families, and/or physicians referring clients are averse to the word "hospice." To many, *hospice* connotes only the negative aspects of death.

Collaborative Management

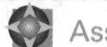 Assessment

➤ *History*

The nurse obtains information on the client's diagnosis, past medical history, and recent state of health to identify possible risks for symptoms near death. For example, clients with lung cancer, cardiac failure, or chronic respiratory disease are at high risk for respiratory distress near death. Clients with pain syndromes may continue with the same pain intensity or have more or less pain as death nears.

➤ *Physical Assessment/Clinical Manifestations*

The nurse assesses for signs and symptoms of impending death. Most research on symptoms near death has been conducted on clients with cancer. These studies have identified anywhere from 14 to 44 symptoms during the active phase of dying (see Charts 12–2 and 12–3), including pain, dyspnea, delirium, nausea, and vomiting, as the most distressing symptoms occurring near death in clients with terminal cancer.

The nurse assesses vital signs, respiratory rate, breath sounds, cough, bowel sounds, abdominal distention, last bowel movement, and urine output to determine any possible or potential symptom of distress. All clients or family members are subjectively assessed for pain or discomfort. Any discomfort is rated by the client, using a visual or verbal analog scale if possible. Information on pain is also elicited with regard to its location, character, level of intensity in the past, reaction to medication, effect on activities, and effect on sleep. Frequency and amount of medications to treat and control pain are documented at least daily, along with client satisfaction and goals regarding pain control. Chapter 9 provides detailed information regarding types of pain and methods of control.

TRANSCULTURAL CONSIDERATIONS

Mainstream United States values affect how middle-class, upper-middle-class, and upper-class people in the United States deal with "dying." These groups believe that an answer or solution is always possible and that choices should always be available. This is probably why the dying process in this country is so frequently oriented to a "high-tech" hospital setting and why family demands for testing and treatment are common, even when clients themselves prefer a palliative approach.

Hispanic-Americans tend to see dying as a family affair: One primary caregiver, usually a wife or daughter, tends to take responsibility for the majority of care. For Southeast Asians, discussing dying brings bad luck, and

hospitals and treatments are alien. Some Southeast Asians, especially if uneducated, are likely to avoid visiting terminally ill family members for fear of contracting the disease.

Various other values, religious beliefs, practices of healing (e.g., faith healing), and family structures can also affect dying in both positive challenging and negative ways. Nurses need to assess cultural beliefs of both clients and families to assess their potential effect on the process of dying and symptom control. (See Chapter 9 for transcultural pain considerations.)

Interventions

Interventions for the actively dying client are to prevent and control symptom distress until death.

Food and Fluids

Because of weakness and fatigue, clients should be restricted to bed during the active phase of dying, unless they express the desire to be up in a recliner. Because they are weak and fatigued, they commonly experience impaired swallowing. They may also lack desire to eat or drink. In either of these situations, caregivers should refrain from providing anything by mouth because of the risk of regurgitation and aspiration. Nurses need to reassure family that anorexia is frequently normal at the end of life. Families may have great difficulty accepting that their loved ones are not being fed and may request that intravenous fluids be initiated. With great sensitivity, nurses reinforce that cessation of food and liquids is thought to be a natural process and that hydration can actually increase discomfort in a person with multisystem slow-down. Discomfort from fluid replacement could lead to respiratory secretions (and distress), increased gastrointestinal secretions, nausea, vomiting, edema, and ascites.

With poor or no fluid intake, the client's mouth becomes uncomfortably dry. However, comfort can be provided by moistening the mouth and lips with applicators and saturated gauze and by applying emollient to the lips.

Nausea and vomiting can be controlled with a variety of antiemetic agents. Combinations of antiemetics often must be individualized for clients for maximal relief of nausea and vomiting (see Chart 12–4).

Pain Management

Pain is the symptom that dying clients fear the most; although not universal, pain is common. There are many possible causes for pain in dying clients. Diseases such as cancer often cause tumor pain due to infiltration of malignant cells into organs, nerves, and bones. Other causes of pain in dying clients include "disturbance" pain resulting from headaches, osteoarthritis, muscle spasms, and stiff joints caused by immobility.

Clients who have had their pain controlled by long-acting narcotics (e.g., clients with cancer or HIV) may or may not have an increase in pain near death. These clients must still continue scheduled doses of opioids to prevent any recurrence of pain. Increases in pain require immediate-relief analgesics (e.g., morphine sulfate immediate-release liquid) and possibly an increase in long-acting opioids. Long-acting opioids may be increased by an amount equal to the previous day's total opioid requirement as frequently as every 24 hours, with physician guidance. Clients who cannot safely swallow receive analgesics by rectum, sublingually, or by subcutaneous or intravenous infusion.

Nurses are often concerned that high doses of opioids may cause a client's death and are often reluctant to administer opioids, especially when death is near. Nurses should understand the importance of medicating clients when *any* symptoms of pain manifest, regardless of level of consciousness. According to the Agency for Health Care Policy and Research *Management of Cancer Pain Clinical Practice Guideline* (1994), "when death due to progressive cancer is imminent, a risk of earlier death counts little against the benefit of pain relief and a painless death" (p. 64). Nurses should be knowledgeable about equigesic doses and formulas to calculate bolus dosages for breakthrough pain (see Chap. 9).

Respiratory Distress

Accumulation of mucus in the large bronchi may cause loud, noisy respirations. This noise, known as the "death rattle," is very distressing to family members. The secretions can be reduced with sublingual administration of anticholinergic agents such as hyoscyamine (Levsin). If this is not effective, a diuretic such as furosemide (Lasix) may be tried. The client may be made more comfortable by a change of position onto his or her side with the head slightly elevated (supported on a pillow).

Dyspnea and/or labored respirations, which often require morphine, are common symptoms near death. The starting dose for treating dyspnea is 2.5 to 5.0 mg of oral morphine every 4 hours, which can be increased to 5 to 10 mg orally or subcutaneously every 2 hours (see Chart 12–4). Clients who are already receiving morphine for pain control usually require a 50% increase for relief of dyspnea. Other interventions to relieve dyspnea include opening a window, administering oxygen, and administering antianxiety drugs such as lorazepam (Ativan).

Anxiety and Agitation

The dying client may experience restlessness or agitation. When such symptoms are present, the client should be assessed for pain or urinary retention. If analgesia and catheterization do not relieve restlessness, sedation can be prescribed to promote a peaceful death. Once adequate sedation is achieved, sedatives should be continued around the clock to prevent further restlessness and terminal agitation.

Skin Changes

The client's skin may be damp with cold perspiration even though he or she complains of feeling overly warm. The nurse keeps the client dry by frequent sponging if a fever is present. Only a light covering is necessary.

As the peripheral circulation lessens, the client's hands, feet, ears, and nose become cold. The client's hands and feet may become mottled and cyanotic. If blood pressure has been monitored, the nurse will notice that it becomes lower and then disappears. The dying person's pulse may double in rate, weaken, gradually decrease, and stop. Meanwhile, respirations become shallow until they too stop. Death has taken place when respirations and heartbeat cease.

Sensory Perception

The family and health care professionals should be aware that the dying client's sense of hearing may remain intact even though it appears that he or she can perceive no other stimuli. Conversation in the room and near the client should be carried on as if the client were alert. Caregivers should be encouraged to talk softly to the client and to touch and gently stroke him or her. The dying person may not respond, but the family will feel better maintaining a normal interchange. This activity fosters a sense of active, reciprocal communication for everyone right up to the end. Soft music might also be played on a tape recorder.

Postmortem Care

The dying client may have such reduced physical activity that actual death can be difficult to ascertain. Chart 12–5 lists physical manifestations of death.

After a client's death, the nurse or the physician (depending on the state of death) pronounces death. He or she then completes a death certificate, which must accompany the body to the funeral home. The nurse or other member of the nursing staff prepares the body for immediate postmortem viewing. All tubes and linens are removed or cut according to agency policy, the eyes are closed, dentures are replaced, and the body is straightened. The nurse removes all pillows except for one supporting the head, kept in place to delay blood pooling and discoloration of the face. Pads are placed under the client's hips and around the perineum to absorb fecal material and fluid. Each health care agency has its own policies and procedures for postmortem care. Chart 12–6 lists typical postmortem nursing interventions.

Chart 12–5

Education Guide: Physical Manifestations of Death

- No breathing
- No heartbeat
- Release of bowel and bladder contents
- No response to name, environmental sounds, touch, or pain
- Eyelids slightly open
- Pupils enlarged and not constricting in response to light
- Eyes fixed on a certain spot
- No blinking in response to air moving over the eyes or to a light touch on the eye
- Jaw relaxed and mouth slightly open

Chart 12-6

Nursing Care Highlight: Postmortem Care

- Ensure that the nurse or physician has completed and signed the death certificate
- Ask the family or significant others if they wish to wash or help wash the client
- Remove or cut all tubes and lines according to health care agency policy
- Close the client's eyes
- Replace dentures or other dental appliances, if worn
- Straighten the client and lower the bed to a flat position
- Place a pillow under the client's head
- Wash the client as needed; comb and arrange the client's hair
- Place pads under the client's hips and around the perineum to absorb feces and urine
- Clean up the client's room or unit
- Allow the family or significant others to see the client in private and perform any religious or cultural customs they wish
- Notify the hospital chaplain or appropriate community religious leader if requested by the family or significant others
- Prepare the client for transfer to either a morgue or funeral home; wrap the client in a shroud and attach identification tags per agency policy (if the client is to be transferred to the morgue)

The family or significant others may then have privacy while they join the deceased in the room. They may perform religious or cultural customs, as described in Table 12-1. If the family wishes to see a member of the clergy, the nurse notifies the hospital chaplain or appropriate community religious leader.

After the family or significant others view the body, the nurse follows agency procedure for preparing the client for transfer to either the morgue or a funeral home. The necessary materials, such as a shroud and identification tags, are usually supplied in a packet.

Home Care

Most people who choose hospice care prefer the home to other caregiving environments during the final episodes of the illness. Although there are exceptions, being surrounded by familiar people and things and having ready access to friends and relatives and the freedom from institutional restriction often make the home setting more comfortable and give the client and family more control. Clients whose cases are being followed by home hospice agencies have access to nurses, social workers, spiritual and/or bereavement counselors, and volunteers to assist in dealing with multiple end-of-life issues. Multidisciplinary hospice team meetings are regularly scheduled to review client needs and solve problems.

Although home care is less costly than any sort of inpatient care, it generally requires that a friend or family member(s) take on the responsibility of providing most physical and emotional care. Some families may not be able to manage the physically and psychologically de-

manding schedule of 24-hour, 7-day-a-week care. Depending on insurance benefits, some families may be entitled to assistive personnel for personal client care in the home. Generally, health care aides are only allowed to assist in the home for 1 to 2 hours once a day, sometimes twice each day if clients are bedbound or incontinent. Families who require more assistance with personal (custodial) care are often referred to agencies that hire out private duty nursing assistants. However, the family must pay for these services, and many families cannot afford them. If families are exhausted from providing care, respite care of the client in a hospital or nursing home for a short time may be available to allow caregivers a few days of rest.

Some family members may have crippling anxiety about what to do when clients manifest symptoms such as pain, dyspnea, or difficulty breathing. Hospices generally provide 24-hour on-call services to facilitate client needs, and medications to control symptoms of distress should be readily available in the home. Because it is not always possible to predict the final phase of the terminal process, some hospices have arranged for pharmacies to supply clients (by prescription) with "symptom relief kits." These provide a limited amount of commonly used medications effective in treatment of symptoms near death. Chart 12-4 describes contents and directions for a "hospice symptom relief kit" to facilitate "safe passage" in the home.

End-of-Life Issues

Under some conditions, keeping someone alive through technological life support rather than actively and arbitrarily ending his or her life can provide time—time to try an experimental new therapy or perhaps for a remission. Unfortunately, an interval like this is not always "good" or "quality" time for peace and growth but is time fraught with pain, suffering, and confusion. The occurrence and fear of pain and suffering have stimulated movements that provide and support the controversial practice of euthanasia in our society.

Euthanasia, derived from a Greek word meaning "easy or pleasant death," implies that under some circumstances, death is preferable to life. *Active euthanasia* refers to an act of commission that directly and *intentionally* shortens a person's life. *Passive euthanasia* is an act of omission and usually refers to letting the person die by either withdrawing or withholding a treatment that might prolong life.

Although active euthanasia, or "mercy killing," is condemned by many professional organizations (e.g., the American Nurses' Association, the American Medical Association) and religious communities (e.g., the Catholic Church), the rights of clients or their surrogates to refuse or stop life-sustaining treatment (e.g., mechanical ventilation, tube feedings, antibiotics) are actually supported by these same communities. Advance directives (e.g., durable power of attorney for health care, living will) have allowed United States residents to make their wishes known about treatment at the end of life, helping surrogate decision-makers to make their own decisions when clients are unconscious or incompetent. The Patient Self-

▷ Research Applications for Nursing

Painful Deaths for Seriously Ill Hospitalized Patients Continue Despite a Physician Education Intervention

A controlled trial to improve care for seriously ill hospitalized patients. (1995). Journal of the American Medical Association, 274, 1591–1598.

The objectives of this two-phase study were to improve end-of-life decision-making and to reduce the frequency of mechanically supported, painful, prolonged dying in seriously ill hospitalized clients. The sample involved 9105 adults hospitalized with one or more of nine life-threatening diseases in one of five major teaching hospitals in the United States. Phase I, a 2-year prospective observational study, found that only 47% of physicians knew when their clients preferred to avoid cardiopulmonary resuscitation (CPR); 38% of clients who died spent at least 10 days in an intensive care unit; and family reports of moderate to severe pain occurred at least half the time in 50% of clients near death.

In phase II (intervention phase), physicians were provided with estimates of client 6-month survival (given their disease and condition), estimates of outcomes for CPR, and estimates on functional disability for clients at 2 months. This phase also included a specially trained nurse making multiple contacts with clients, families, physicians, and hospital staff to elicit preferences, improve understanding of outcomes, encourage attention to pain control, and facilitate advance directive planning and client-physician communication. Results of phase II were that clients experienced no improvement in client-physician communication, no improvement occurred in physicians' knowledge of client preferences not to be resuscitated, the number of days clients spent on mechanical ventilation or comatose in intensive care units did not decrease, and the level of pain reported by families of clients near death did not decrease.

Critique. This study was rigorous in its experimental design and large sample size. However, it does not explain why aggressive treatment was continued despite poor odds for recovery. For example, did clients change their minds? Did physicians simply ignore what clients and nurses communicated? Did they see the teaching hospital as one that assumes aggressive care, regardless of the odds? A qualitative component to the study might shed light on findings.

Possible Nursing Implications. The role of the nurse in discussing end-of-life issues in acute care may not be deemed appropriate by providers making treatment decisions. Despite this perception, nurses are generally guided by state nurse practice acts to obtain comprehensive assessment data on all clients, and nurses are often the best equipped to initiate discussions on end-of-life issues. Nurses working with clients with serious illnesses should identify and fulfill their educational needs regarding end-of-life issues and effectively communicate their knowledge and concerns to physicians, clients, and families when appropriate.

given information about the process and implications of having (or not having) these in place and should be assisted in drafting them.

Much confusion exists regarding euthanasia and treatment of dying clients. It is important that health care providers, clients, and families understand the distinctions of active and passive euthanasia and assisted suicide versus appropriate treatment of pain and symptoms of distress. Because nurses spend more time with clients than any other health providers, they should be competent in and committed to initiating discussions of end-of-life issues when appropriate. Recent research indicates that many hospitalized clients die undergoing aggressive treatment and pain, without regard for their wishes. Better communication between clients and health providers and more collaboration among physicians and nurses are needed if end-of-life decisions of clients in acute care are to be heeded (see Research Applications for Nursing).

SELECTED BIBLIOGRAPHY

*Amenta, M., & Bohnet, N. (1986). *Nursing care of the terminally ill.* Boston: Little, Brown.

*American Nurses' Association. (1987). *Standards and scope of hospice nursing practice.* Kansas City: American Nurses' Association.

Benzein, E., & Saveman, B. (1998). Nurses' perception of hope in patients with cancer: A palliative care perspective. *Cancer Nursing, 21*(1), 10–16.

Callanan, M. (1994). Farewell messages. *American Journal of Nursing, 94*(5), 19–20.

*Carmack, B. J. (1992). Balancing engagement/detachment in AIDS-related multiple losses. *Image: Journal of Nursing Scholarship, 24,* 9–14.

A controlled trial to improve care for seriously ill hospitalized patients. (1995). *Journal of the American Medical Association, 274,* 1591–1598.

*Cooley, M. E. (1992). Bereavement care: A role for nurses. *Cancer Nursing, 15*(2), 125–129.

Corless, I. B., Germino, B. B., & Pittman, M. (1994). *Dying, death, and bereavement: Theoretical perspectives and other ways of knowing.* Boston: Jones and Bartlett.

Dean, G. E. (1995). Symptom management for the dying patient. *Quality of Life—A Nursing Challenge 3*(3), 61–66.

Edwards, B. S. (1994). When the family can't let go. *American Journal of Nursing, 94*(1), 52–56.

*Farberow, N. L. (1992). Changes in grief and mental health of bereaved spouses of older suicides. *Journal of Gerontology, 47,* 357–366.

*Gardner, D. L. (1992). Presence. In G. M. Bulachek & J. C. McCloskey (Eds.), *Nursing interventions: Essential nursing treatments* (2nd ed., pp. 191–200). Philadelphia: W. B. Saunders.

Gavrin, J., & Chapman, C. R. (1995). Clinical management of dying patients. *Caring for patients at the end of life [Special Issue]. Western Journal of Medicine, 163,* 268–277.

Kazanowski, M. (1997). A commitment to palliative care—Could it impact assisted suicide? *Journal of Gerontological Nursing, 3*(3), 1–7.

Kemp, C. (1995). *Terminal illness.* Philadelphia: J. B. Lippincott.

*Kübler-Ross, E. (1969). *On death and dying.* New York: Macmillan.

*Lindemann, E. (1944). Symptomatology and management of acute grief. *American Journal of Psychiatry, 101,* 141–149.

*Lindley-Davis, B. (1991). Process of dying: Defining characteristics. *Cancer Nursing, 14,* 328–333.

Management of Cancer Pain Guideline Panel. (1994). *Management of cancer pain clinical practice guideline.* AHCPR Pub. No. 94-0592. Rockville, MD: Agency for Health Care Policy and Research.

Meares, C. (1994). Terminal dehydration: A review. *The American Journal of Hospice & Palliative Care, 11*(3), 10–14.

*Mitchell, K. R., & Anderson, H. (1983). *All our losses, all our griefs.* Philadelphia: Westminster Press.

*Nuland, S. B. (1993). *How we die.* New York: Vintage Books.

*Rando, T. A. (1984). *Grief, dying, and death.* Champaign, IL: Research Press.

Determination Act (1990) requires that all clients admitted to health care agencies be asked if they have drafted advance directives. The Act's intent was to facilitate end-of-life treatment decisions prior to a crisis situation. Clients who have not drafted advance directives should be

*Rando, T. A. (1993). *Treatment of complicated mourning.* Champaign, IL: Research Press.

Sheehan, D. C., & Forman, W. B. (1996). *Hospice and palliative care.* Sudbury, MA: Jones and Bartlett.

*United States Congress. (1990). *Omnibus Budget Reconciliation Act of 1990* (pp. 101–508). Pub L Washington, D. C.: United States Congress.

SUGGESTED READINGS

Dean, G. E. (1995). Symptom management for the dying patient. *Quality of Life—A Nursing Challenge* 3(3), 61–66.

This article provides a concise, valuable description of common symptoms of distress in patients with cancer near death. Causes and interventions are discussed for pain, dyspnea, restlessness, agitation, problems with elimination, and fatigue.

Kazanowski, M. (1997). A commitment to palliative care—Could it impact assisted suicide? *Journal of Gerontological Nursing, 3*(3), 1–7.

This is one of several articles on end-of-life issues published in a special issue of the *Journal of Gerontological Nursing.* In support of palliative care, the author describes how this philosophy differs from the acute care model and suggests that more widespread knowledge about both the existence and goals of palliative care might make assisted suicide less appealing.

Meares, C. (1994). Terminal dehydration: A review. *The American Journal of Hospice & Palliative Care, 11*(3), 10–14.

This article is based on a review of the literature on terminal dehydration near death. The author describes the physiology, patient symptoms, ethical and legal issues, and physician and nurse perceptions of withholding fluid near death. The author points out that the vast majority of hospice nurses studied believe that aggressive nutritional support in a dying patient does more harm than good.

Chapter 13

REHABILITATION OF CLIENTS WITH CHRONIC AND DISABLING CONDITIONS

A chronic illness or condition is one that has existed for at least 3 months. A disabling condition is any physical or mental health problem that can cause disability. This text focuses on physical health problems; mental health problems are discussed in textbooks on mental health nursing.

Clients with chronic and disabling conditions often participate in rehabilitation programs to prevent disability, maintain functional ability, and restore as much function as possible. The nurse is a vital rehabilitation team member.

OVERVIEW

Chronic illness is a major health problem in the United States. Approximately 50% of the population have one or more chronic illnesses. About 35 million people, or one in seven, experience activity limitations because of their chronic health problems. Most of these individuals are in residential settings.

In the United States, the annual cost of chronic and disabling conditions is more than $200 billion in medical care and lost productivity. Disability occurs slightly more often in men than in women and in families with lower incomes (Institute of Medicine, 1991).

Stroke is the leading cause of disability, costing more than $30 billion each year in medical costs and loss of productivity (Collins, 1997). Coronary artery disease, cancer, chronic airflow limitation (CAL), and arthritis are other common chronic conditions that may result in varying degrees of disability. Most of these conditions occur in people older than 65 years.

Chronic and disabling conditions are not always diseases such as cancer; they may also result from accidents. Accidents are the leading cause of death among young adults and the third leading cause of death in people 45 to 54 years old. Today, increasing numbers of people survive accidents because of advances in medical technology. These survivors are often faced with chronic or disabling conditions, such as head and spinal cord injuries (SCIs). Therefore, the need for rehabilitation is on the rise. Such survivors may need months to years of follow-up health care after returning to the community.

CONCEPTS RELATED TO REHABILITATION

Rehabilitation is the process of learning to live with chronic and disabling conditions, often those resulting from trauma. The goal of rehabilitation is to return the client to the fullest possible physical, mental, social, vocational, and economic capacity. However, rehabilitation is not limited to the return of function in post-traumatic situations. It includes education and therapy for any chronic illness characterized by a change in a body system function or body structure. Rehabilitation programs related to respiratory, cardiac, musculoskeletal, and oncologic disorders are common examples that do not involve trauma.

In any discussion of rehabilitation, it is important to define and distinguish the terms *impairment, disability,* and *handicap.* These terms have been used interchangeably in some settings; however, for this chapter, the terms are defined according to the classic, but still widely used, *International Classification of Impairments, Disabilities and Handicaps* (World Health Organization, 1980).

Impairment

Impairment is an abnormality of a body structure or structures or an alteration in a body system function resulting from any cause; it represents a disturbance at the organ level. Impairments can be temporary or permanent and may or may not be associated with an active pathologic condition.

Disability

Disability is the consequence of an impairment and is usually described in terms of a client's altered functional ability; it represents disturbance at the personal level. A variety of diseases or traumas impair mobility and may result in a decreased ability to function.

Handicap

A handicap is the disadvantage experienced by a person as a result of impairments and disabilities; it represents disturbance at the societal level. This disadvantage is based on interactions that the client experiences with the environment. Handicaps are associated with negative values that a person or society ascribes to the person's situation or experience. Handicaps are both preventable and reversible, although impairments caused by pathologic changes in a body organ and the resulting disabilities are often unpreventable or irreversible.

REHABILITATION AS PART OF CONTINUING CARE

After a client's acute condition or injury has been stabilized in a hospital, the client may be discharged to continue the healing process, generally under the follow-up care of a nonhospital health care provider, such as a family physician. The nurse provides home care prepara-

tion, health teaching, psychosocial preparation, and information about various health care resources to help the client resume their usual roles in society.

Some health problems, however, require the intermediate step of rehabilitation, which can take place in a number of settings. Rehabilitation starts in the acute care hospital (sometimes called acute rehabilitation) and continues after discharge from the hospital. The nurse's coordination of care from acute care through continuing care is critical to the success of rehabilitation.

Settings for Rehabilitation

For continuing rehabilitation services, the most common settings are freestanding rehabilitation hospitals, rehabilitation units within hospitals, and skilled nursing home units to which the client is typically admitted for 1 to 4 weeks (Fig. 13–1). Outpatient (ambulatory) rehabilitation departments and home rehabilitation programs may be needed to continue less intensive rehabilitative services after discharge from one of the inpatient settings or as an alternative to inpatient rehabilitation.

Some hospitals and nursing homes have converted one or more inpatient units into subacute care units or transitional care units (TCUs). The client can then stay in the same health care system for both acute and continuing rehabilitative care.

After disabled clients become more confident and independent in the inpatient setting, they may choose to live at home or in a group home. These living centers are facilities in which clients live independently while together with other disabled adults. Each client or group of clients has a care provider, such as a personal care aide,

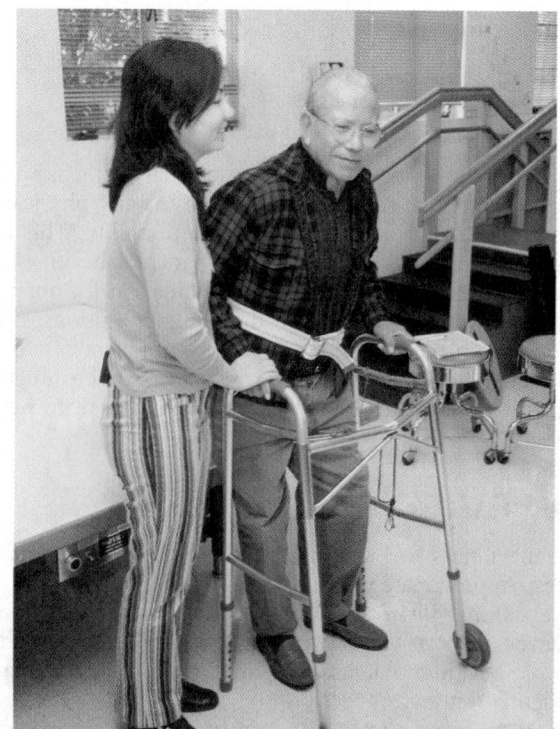

Figure 13–1. A physical therapist helping a client to ambulate.

to assist with the activities of daily living (ADLs) and decisions requiring accurate judgments. The clients may or may not be employed. The goal of these centers is to provide independent living arrangements outside an institution, especially for younger clients with head injury or spinal cord injury.

The Rehabilitation Team

Successful rehabilitation depends on the coordinated effort of a group of health care professionals—the interdisciplinary rehabilitation team—and the involvement of the client, family, and other support systems in planning and implementing care.

Goals of the Rehabilitation Team

The rehabilitation team has two basic goals: prevention of injury and restoration of function. The aim of prevention is to maintain the client's activity levels to avoid the deterioration of an unaffected organ or part and to eliminate possible hazards or factors that may contribute to further injury. Prevention is a continuous aspect of care for the chronically ill or disabled client. For example, meticulous skin care is necessary to prevent the formation of pressure ulcers. The other major goal of the rehabilitation team is restoration of as much function as possible to the injured or diseased body part or system to facilitate the client's independence.

Members of the Rehabilitation Team

The interdisciplinary health care team members in the rehabilitation setting include physicians, nurses, physical therapists, occupational therapists, speech-language pathologists, recreational therapists, cognitive therapists, aides, social workers, psychologists, vocational counselors, the clients themselves, and family members or significant others. Not all settings that offer rehabilitation services have all of these members on their team.

PHYSIATRISTS. The physician who specializes in rehabilitative medicine is called a physiatrist. Most inpatient rehabilitation settings, except for most freestanding skilled nursing facilities, employ physiatrists.

REHABILITATION NURSES. The rehabilitation nurse coordinates the efforts of the team members and is, therefore, usually designated as the clients' case manager. In clients undergoing rehabilitation, health problems are characterized by an altered functional ability and a diminished quality of life. The goal of rehabilitation nursing is to assist clients in restoring and maintaining optimal health. The rehabilitation nurse must be innovative and patient in helping clients regain independence.

THERAPISTS. Physical therapists (PTs) intervene to help the client achieve mobility (e.g., by facilitating ambulation and teaching the client to use a walker). They may also teach techniques for performing certain ADLs, such as transferring (e.g., moving into and out of bed), ambulating, and toileting.

Occupational therapists (OTs) work to develop the client's fine motor skills used for ADLs, such as those required for eating, maintaining hygiene, dressing, and driving. OTs may also teach the client skills related to coordination, such as hand movements (Fig. 13–2).

Speech-language pathologists (SLPs) evaluate and retrain clients with speech, language, or swallowing problems. Speech is roughly defined as the ability to say words, and language is the ability to understand and put words together in a meaningful way. Some clients, especially those with head injury or cerebrovascular accident (CVA, or stroke), have difficulty with both speech and language. Clients who have experienced CVAs also typically have dysphagia (difficulty with swallowing).

Recreational or activity therapists work to help clients continue or develop hobbies or interests. These therapists often coordinate their efforts with those of the OT.

Cognitive therapists, usually neuropsychologists, work primarily with clients with head injuries who have cognitive impairments. These therapists often use computers to assist with cognitive retraining.

Aides and health care assistants work in the nursing or therapy departments to assist in the care of clients. These rehabilitation team members are under the direct supervision of the nurse or therapist.

COUNSELORS. Various counselors are helpful in promoting community reintegration of the client and acceptance of the disability or chronic illness. Social workers help clients identify support services and resources, including financial assistance. They usually coordinate the clients' transfer to or discharge from the rehabilitation setting. Psychologists also counsel clients and families on their psychological problems and on strategies to cope with disability.

Vocational counselors assist the client with job placement, training, or further education. Work-related skills

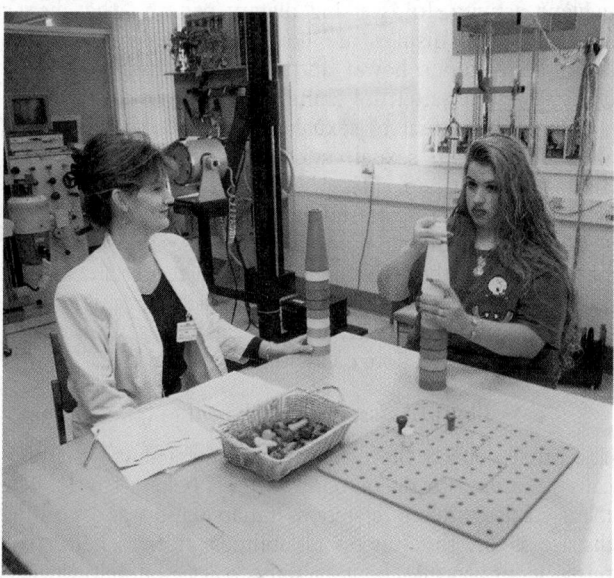

Figure 13–2. An occupational therapist working with a client.

are taught if the client needs to change careers because of the disability. If the client has not yet completed high school, educational tutors may help the client in the rehabilitation setting to complete the requirements for graduation.

Interdisciplinary team conferences for the exchange of ideas are held with the client, family members and significant others, and health care providers on a regular basis. Chart documentation is shared and read by all team members.

Collaborative Management

 Assessment

➤ History

As the case manager, the nurse collects the client's health history, including the history of the present condition, any current medications, and any treatment programs in progress.

General Background Data. The nurse obtains general background data about the client and family. These data include financial status, occupations, educational levels, cultural background, and home situation. In collaboration with the occupational therapist, the nurse addresses architectural features of the environment, such as the layout of the home. The nurse determines whether the physical layout at home, such as the presence of stairs or the width of doorways, will present a problem to the client. Data are gathered on the client's neighborhood, such as the location of shopping centers and available transportation. The nurse determines who will do the client's shopping, cooking, and housework. This information is essential for discharge planning.

Daily Schedule and Habits. The nurse also assesses the client's usual daily schedule and habits of everyday living. These include hygiene practices, eating, and elimination; sexual activity; and sleep. The nurse asks about the client's preferred method and time of bathing and hygiene activity. In assessing dietary patterns, the client's food likes and dislikes are noted. The nurse also elicits information about bowel and bladder function and the client's normal pattern of elimination.

In the assessment of sexuality patterns, the nurse asks about changes in sexual function since the onset of the disability (see Chap. 11). The client's current and previous sleep habits, patterns, usual number of hours of sleep, and use of hypnotics are also assessed. The nurse should ask whether the client feels well rested after sleep. Sleep patterns have a significant impact on activity patterns. Assessment of activity patterns focuses on work, exercise, and recreational activities.

➤ Physical Assessment/Clinical Manifestations

The nurse collects the physical assessment data systematically according to major body systems (Chart 13–1). The focus of assessment related to rehabilitation and chronic disease is on the functional abilities of the client. The nurse identifies the client's ability to use self-help devices during this portion of the assessment.

Cardiovascular System. An alteration in cardiac status may affect the client's cardiac output or cause activity intolerance. The nurse assesses the manifestations of decreased cardiac output, such as chest pain and fatigue, and determines when the client experiences these symptoms and what relieves them. The nurse seeks medical consultation before the client continues activities that provoke these symptoms. The physician may order a change in medications or may prescribe a prophylactic dose of nitroglycerin to be taken before the client resumes the activities. The nurse collaborates with the physician and appropriate therapists to determine whether activities can be modified to be accomplished without these symptoms.

For the client showing fatigue, the nurse and the client together plan methods of using the client's limited energy resources. For instance, the client could take frequent rest periods throughout the day, especially before undertaking activities. Major tasks could be performed in the morning because most people have the most energy at that time.

A great hindrance to rehabilitation for clients with cardiac disorders is fear. A client may have survived a life-threatening experience, such as a myocardial infarction, but now is so afraid of recurrence (and death) that he or she is unable, or unwilling, to resume any activity. The client with cardiac disorders experiencing fear usually benefits from participation in a structured cardiac rehabilitation program. The nurse discusses available programs with the client and the family (see Chapter 40 for a complete description of cardiac rehabilitation).

Respiratory System. The nurse asks the client whether he or she is experiencing shortness of breath during or after activity. It is important to determine the level of activity that the client can accomplish without experiencing shortness of breath. For example, can the client climb one flight of stairs without shortness of breath, or does shortness of breath occur after the client climbs only two steps?

The fear associated with any inability to breathe normally can render a person dependent in many facets of life. Some problems related to disorders of the respiratory system can be resolved or diminished, but some breathing difficulties must be endured (e.g., in emphysema).

Gastrointestinal System and Nutrition. The nurse assesses the client's oral intake and pattern of eating. The client is also assessed for the presence of anorexia, dysphagia, nausea, vomiting, or discomfort related to or interfering with oral intake. In collaboration with the physician and the dietitian, the nurse assesses the client's height; weight; hemoglobin, and hematocrit levels; and serum albumin, transferrin, and blood glucose concentrations (see Chapter 64 for complete nutritional assessment). Weight loss or gain is particularly significant and may be related to an associated disease or to the illness that caused disability.

Elimination habits vary from person to person; they are often related to daily job or activity schedules, dietary patterns, and family or cultural background. Elimination habits may be difficult to assess, because many nurses are hesitant to request—and many clients are afraid to volunteer—information pertaining to elimination. When assessing the client's elimination status, the nurse first asks

Chart 13-1

Nursing Care Highlight: Physical Assessment of Clients Undergoing Rehabilitation

Body System	Relevant Data
Cardiovascular system	• Chest pain • Fatigue • Fear of cardiac failure
Respiratory system	• Shortness of breath or dyspnea • Activity tolerance • Fear of inability to breathe
Gastrointestinal system and nutrition	• Oral intake, eating pattern • Anorexia, nausea, and vomiting • Dysphagia • Laboratory data (e.g., serum albumin level) • Weight loss or gain • Bowel elimination pattern or habits • Change in stool • Ability to get to toilet
Renal-urinary system	• Urinary pattern • Fluid intake • Urinary incontinence or retention • Urine culture or urinalysis
Neurologic system	• Motor function • Sensation • Cognitive abilities
Musculoskeletal system	• Functional ability • Range of motion • Endurance • Muscle strength
Integumentary system	• Risk of skin breakdown • Presence of skin lesions

what the usual elimination patterns were for that person before the injury or the illness.

The nurse is attuned to any changes in the client's bowel routine or the consistency of the stool. If the client is noticing any change in elimination pattern, the nurse tries to determine whether this alteration can be attributed to a change in diet, activity pattern, or use of medications that could cause increased or decreased motility of the gastrointestinal tract. Bowel habits are evaluated on the basis of what is normal for that person.

The nurse also determines whether the client can manage bowel functions independently. Independence in bowel elimination requires cognition, manual dexterity, sensation, muscle control, and mobility. If the client requires help, the nurse determines whether there is someone available at home to provide the assistance. The client's (and family's) ability to cope with any dependency in bowel elimination must be assessed as well.

Renal/Urinary System. When assessing the client's urinary system, the nurse determines the client's baseline urinary patterns, asking about the number of times the client usually voids and whether the client routinely awakens during the night to empty the bladder or has uninterrupted sleep. The client's fluid intake patterns and

volume are recorded, including the type of fluids ingested and the timing of fluid consumption throughout the day.

The nurse determines whether the client has experienced any problems with urinary incontinence or retention in the past. Laboratory reports, especially the results of urine culture and urinalysis, are also monitored.

Neurologic System. In rehabilitation, the neurologic assessment identifies the functional aspects of motor ability, sensation, and cognition. The nurse assesses the client's pre-existing problems, general physical condition, and communication abilities.

Motor Ability. The movement of an extremity is compared with the function of the opposite extremity to identify paresis (weakness) or paralysis (absence of movement).

Sensation. The identification of sensory-perceptual alterations is important in assessing the client's risk for injury. The nurse assesses the client's response to light touch, hot or cold temperature, and position change in each extremity and on the trunk. Levels of decreased sensation are identified. For a perceptual assessment, the nurse evaluates the client's ability to receive and understand what is heard and seen and the ability to express appropriate motor and verbal responses. During this portion of the assessment, the nurse can also begin assessing short- and long-term memory.

Cognitive Abilities. The nurse also assesses the client's cognitive abilities, especially if there is a head injury or stroke. Several tools are available to evaluate cognition. One of the most common is the Mini-Mental State Examination, which is described in detail in Chapter 44.

Musculoskeletal System. As is the case for other body systems, the rehabilitation nursing assessment of the musculoskeletal system focuses on function. The nurse assesses the client's musculoskeletal status, response to the impairment, and demands of the home, work, or school environment. The nurse determines the client's endurance level and measures both active and passive range of motion (ROM) of joints. The nurse reviews the results of manual muscle testing by physical therapy, which identifies the client's ROM and resistance against gravity. In this procedure, the therapist determines the degree of muscle strength present in each body segment. The grading system usually ranges from 0 (no evidence of muscle contractility) to 5 (normal muscle contractility) (see Chap. 52).

Integumentary System. In assessing a client's integumentary system, the nurse identifies actual or potential interruptions in the integrity of the skin.

Risk for Skin Breakdown. To maintain healthy skin, the body must have adequate food, water, and oxygen intake; intact waste removal mechanisms; sensation; and functional mobility. Changes in any of these variables can lead to rapid and extensive skin breakdown. If the client cannot protect or maintain the skin, the nurse must be able to assess and plan for the client's needs. The nurse monitors the client to determine the risk of skin breakdown before it occurs.

Some rehabilitation settings use special skin assessment tools to identify clients at risk for skin breakdown. For example, the classic Braden Scale for Predicting Pressure Sore Risk (see Chap. 70) assesses six areas: sensory perception, skin moisture, activity level, nutritional status, and potential for friction and shear.

Several other skin risk assessment tools are available. Some tools also include additional indicators of nutritional status, such as the serum albumin or transferrin level. When either of these levels is low, the client is at high risk for pressure sores. Some tools include incontinence and altered mental state as risk factors. Regardless of which tool is used, Braden and Bergstrom (1992) recommended the following schedule for skin assessment:
- For clients in critical care units: during every nursing shift when the client is unstable and at least daily when the client is stable
- For clients in medical-surgical units: every other day when the client's condition is stable and when the condition changes significantly (e.g., after surgery)
- For clients in nursing homes or rehabilitation units: weekly for 1 month and then monthly after the first month unless there is a significant change in the client's condition

Actual Skin Breakdown. If a pressure ulcer or other change in skin integrity develops, the nurse accurately assesses the problem and its possible causes. The nurse inspects the client's skin every 2 hours, or more often if needed, until the client has learned to inspect his or her own skin several times a day. The nurse documents the depth and diameter of the open skin area in centimeters or inches, depending on the facility's policy. The area around the open lesion must also be assessed to determine the presence of cellulitis or other tissue damage. Chapter 70 includes a widely used classification system for staging skin breakdown. The nurse also assesses the client's understanding of the cause and treatment of skin breakdown as well as his or her ability to inspect the skin and participate in maintaining skin integrity.

In many health care agencies, a skin assessment and documentation tool, or "skin sheet," is used to keep track of each area of skin breakdown. A baseline assessment is conducted on admission to the agency, and the form is updated periodically, depending on the agency's policy and the nurse's judgment. In some long-term care or rehabilitation settings, photographs of the client's skin are taken at various intervals with the client's permission to document the skin's condition.

➤ Functional Assessment

Functional ability refers to the client's ability to perform activities of daily living (ADLs), such as bathing, dressing, feeding, and ambulating, and instrumental activities of daily living (IADLs), such as using the telephone, shopping, preparing food, and housekeeping. Functional assessment tools are used to assess a person's abilities (Research Applications for Nursing). Rehabilitation nurses, physiatrists, or therapists complete one or more of these assessment tools on the basis of the client's abilities and the policy of the health care setting. Some of the commonly used tools are briefly described next. For further information, consult corresponding references in this chapter.

PULSES Profile. One of the earliest tools used was the PULSES profile. It was developed in 1957 and adapted in 1975 to evaluate and classify functional capacity in the chronically ill and aging client population. The six categories included for evaluation are
- *Physical condition (basic health status)*
- *Upper limb function (self-care)*
- *Lower limb function (mobility)*
- *Sensory components (sight, communication)*
- *Excretory function*
- *Support factors*

Scoring uses four numeric grades for each category; scores increase as functional ability is diminished. The maximum score is 24. High scores indicate greater levels of dependency for the client. The adapted form of the PULSES profile has been a useful tool in many rehabilitation programs. It indicates the level of independence in life-functioning skills necessary for a person to make adaptations to community living.

Katz Index of Activities of Daily Living. One of the best known and most widely used instruments was developed during the 1950s from observations of clients with

► Research Applications for Nursing

Do Spinal Cord–Injured (SCI) Clients Retain Their Self-Care Skills Learned in Acute Rehabilitation?

Boss, B. J., Pecanty, L., McFarland, S. M., & Sasser, L. (1995). Self-care competence among persons with spinal cord injury. SCI Nursing, 12(2), 48–53.

This study examined the self-care competence of 48 clients with SCI from two Veterans Affairs Medical Centers and a state university–affiliated rehabilitation program to determine the retention of cognitive and functional skills after discharge from these programs. The data collection tool was the Self-Care Assessment Tool, which measures eight functional areas, such as bathing and grooming, skin management, and bladder management. The score of the study participants was high, indicating that they retained both the cognitive information and functional skills that had been emphasized in their rehabilitation programs.

Critique. Although the sample was fairly small and purposefully selected, this study was an attempt to examine outcomes over an extended period of time. As the health care industry continues to move toward managed care, measurement of both quality and cost outcomes is critical.

Possible Nursing Implications. Additional studies to determine the long-term effect of nursing and interdisciplinary interventions are needed. Activities that promote self-care enable clients to be independent and maintain their highest level of wellness.

fractured hips. The Katz Index of Activities of Daily Living addresses six functional tasks: bathing, dressing, toileting, achieving transfers, level of continence, and feeding (Katz et al., 1963). Each of the six areas is scored as either "dependent" or "independent" on the basis of the client's need for help in performing the task (Table 13–1). The overall functional status is then assigned a grade from A (independent in feeding, being continent, transferring, toileting, dressing, and bathing) through G (dependent in all six functions) from total scores.

The Katz Index has been used for clients with many types of chronic illnesses. It is a valuable tool for evaluating care and developing data about the course of an illness over time.

Barthel Index. The Barthel Index was designed to measure functional levels and mobility in the physically impaired client. This tool consists of 10 variables according to which the clients are scored by their degree of independence in performance. Categories include feeding, bathing, and mobility. The scoring system consists of two descriptive areas: doing an activity with help and performing an activity independently. Scores range from 0, indicating total dependence, to 100, indicating complete independence. The Barthel Index was intended for use in both immediate and long-term care rehabilitation programs.

Level of Rehabilitation Scale. The Level of Rehabilitation Scale (LORS), developed by Carey and Posavec (1978), provides a general assessment of the client's functioning for program evaluation rather than clinical assessment. The LORS provides an overview through measurement of function regarding ADLs, cognition, home activities, activities outside the home, and social interactions. The LORS was then expanded to include 11 items related to activities of daily living, mobility, and communication (Posavec & Carey, 1982). These items receive a score of 0–4, determined through the use of a coding manual ascribing numeric values to behavioral terms.

Functional Independence Measure. Assessment tools have also been designed for use on a national level; thus, uniform outcome data can be obtained from numerous rehabilitation programs. An example of this kind of system—a uniform data system—is the Functional Independence Measure (FIM), developed by Granger and Gresham (1984). The FIM, as a basic indicator of the severity of a disability, attempts to quantify what the person actually does, whatever the diagnosis or impairment. It does not measure what a person should do or how the person would perform under a different set of circumstances. To eliminate the bias of a particular discipline, the assessment may be done by trained clinicians; the entire assessment may be done by one person, or certain categories may be performed by representatives of various disciplines.

Categories for assessment are self-care, sphincter control, mobility and locomotion, communication, and cognition. Scoring is done with numbers using predetermined criteria for measurement. The evaluation is performed when the client is admitted to and discharged from a rehabilitation institution and at a specified follow-up time. The FIM assessment system has also been adapted for use in other health care settings, including acute care and home care.

► Psychosocial Assessment

The nurse must understand the theories of body image and self-esteem to assess the client's psychosocial needs adequately. These concepts serve as a basis for understanding psychological responses to chronic illness and resulting disability. The client's self-esteem and body image are assessed through the client's verbal indicators and descriptions of self-care. Body image can also be assessed by tools such as the Baird Body Image Assessment Tool (BBIAT) (see Chap. 10).

The nurse assesses the client's use of defense mechanisms and manifestations of anxiety, such as those noted in facial expressions and communication patterns. To assess the client's response to loss, the nurse asks the client to describe feelings concerning the loss of a body part or function. The nurse also notes any stress-related physical problems. The client may experience symptoms of depression, such as fatigue, a change in appetite, or feelings of powerlessness.

The nurse assesses the availability of support systems for the client. The major support system is typically the family or significant others. The family interactions and coping patterns are assessed.

TABLE 13–1

Katz Index of Activities of Daily Living

Independence means without supervision, direction, or active personal assistance, except as specifically noted below. This is based on actual status and not ability. A patient who refuses to perform a function is considered as not performing the function, even though he or she is deemed able.

Bathing (sponge, shower, or tub)

Independent: assistance only in bathing a single part (back or disabled extremity) or bathes self completely

Dependent: Assistance in bathing more than one part of body; assistance in getting in or out of tub; does not bathe self

Dressing

Independent; gets clothes from closets and drawers; puts on clothes, outer garments, braces; manages fasteners; act of tying shoes is excluded.
Dependent: does not dress self or remains partly undressed

Going to Toilet

Independent: gets to toilet; gets on and off toilet; arranges clothes, cleans organs of excretion (may manage own bedpan used at night only and may or may not be using mechanical supports)
Dependent: uses bedpan or commode or receives assistance in getting to and using toilet

Transfer

Independent: moves in and out of bed and in and out of chair independently (may or may not be using mechanical supports)
Dependent: assistance in moving in or out of bed and/or chair; does not perform one or more transfers

Continence

Independent: urination and defecation entirely self-controlled
Dependent: partial or total incontinence in urination or defecation; partial or total control by enemas, catheters, or regulated use of urinals and/or bedpans

Feeding

Independent: gets food from plate or its equivalent into mouth (precutting of meat and preparation of food, as buttering bread, are excluded from evaluation)
Dependent: assistance in act of feeding (see above); does not eat at all or parenteral feeding

Evaluation Form

Name _____ Date of Evaluation _____

For each area of functioning listed below, circle description that applies (the word "assistance" means supervision, direction, or personal assistance).

Bathing—either sponge bath, tub bath, or shower

| Receives no assistance (gets in and out of tub by self if tub is usual means of bathing) | Receives assistance in bathing only one part of body (such as back or a leg) | Receives assistance in bathing more than one part of body (or does not bathe self) |

Dressing—gets clothes from closets and drawers; puts on clothes, including underclothes, outer garments; manages fasteners (including braces, if worn)

| Gets clothes and gets completely dressed without assistance | Gets clothes and gets dressed without assistance except for tying shoes | Receives assistance in getting clothes or in getting dressed or stays partly or completely undressed |

Toileting—going to the "toilet room" for bowel and urine elimination; cleaning self after elimination and arranging clothes

| Goes to "toilet room," cleans self, and arranges clothes without assistance (may use object for support such as cane, walker, or wheelchair and may manage night bedpan or commode, emptying same in morning) | Receives assistance in going to "toilet room" or in cleansing self or in arranging clothes after elimination or in use of night bedpan or commode | Does not go to room termed "toilet" for the elimination process |

Transfer

| Moves in and out of bed and in and out of chair without assistance (may use object for support such as cane or walker) | Moves in or out of bed or chair with assistance | Does not get out of bed |

Continence

| Controls urination and bowel movement completely by self | Has occasional "accidents" | Supervision helps keep urine or bowel control; catheter is used or is incontinent |

Feeding

| Feeds self without assistance | Feeds self except for getting assistance in cutting meat or buttering bread | Receives assistance in feeding or is fed partly or completely by tubes or intravenous fluids |

From Katz, S., et al. (1963). Studies of illness in the aged. The index of ADL: A standardized measure of biological and psychosocial function. *Journal of the American Medical Association, 185,* 914–919. Copyright 1963, American Medical Association.

➤ *Vocational Assessment*

The rehabilitation nurse assists the client in maximizing functional status, allowing the client to resume many usual activities. The nurse should be aware of appropriate resources for each client in compiling a vocational data base for the client. In collaboration with vocational counselors, the nurse helps the client find meaningful training, education, or employment after discharge from the rehabilitation setting. The nurse gathers data on the client's educational and employment history, including previous jobs held. The nurse also obtains employers' attitudes toward the disabled client and information on the client's performance on the job, such as absenteeism and work record.

The nurse informs clients who are United States residents about the 1991 Americans with Disabilities Act passed by Congress to prevent employer discrimination against disabled people. Within reason, the employer must offer assistance to the disabled to allow them to perform the job. For example, if a client has a severe hearing loss, the employer may need to hire an interpreter for sign language so that the client can work.

The nurse also notes the cognitive and physical demands of the jobs held and ascertains whether the client can return to the former job or whether retraining in another field will be needed. The physical demands of jobs range from light in sedentary occupations (0–10 pounds frequently lifted) to heavy (more than 100 pounds frequently lifted). The nurse must also consider other aspects of the job, such as strength, mobility, or senses required in the job (e.g., hearing).

Job analysis also involves assessing the work environment of the client's former job. The nurse works with the vocational counselor to determine whether the environment is conducive to the client's return. Union contracts must also be considered, and any job modifications must be noted. If the injured worker requires vocational rehabilitation, the nurse refers the client to vocational rehabilitation personnel and assists the client to work with the counselors on evaluating present skills and learning new skills for employment. The nurse may also help with job placement in the community.

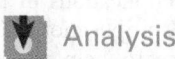 Analysis

➤ *Common Nursing Diagnoses and Collaborative Problems*

Regardless of the client's age or specific disability, the following nursing diagnoses are commonly applicable to the client with chronic illness or disability:

1. Impaired Physical Mobility related to neuromuscular impairment, sensory-perceptual impairment, pain, activity intolerance, fatigue, or the effects of trauma or surgery
2. Self-Care Deficit (total or partial) related to effects of trauma or chronic illness, muscular weakness, pain, immobility, or perceptual or cognitive impairment
3. Risk for Impaired Skin Integrity related to altered sensation or immobility

4. Altered Urinary Elimination related to sensorimotor impairment or immobility
5. Constipation related to neuromuscular or musculoskeletal impairment or immobility
6. Ineffective Individual Coping related to the effects of chronic illness, the loss of control over a body part or a body function, or major changes in lifestyle
7. Body Image Disturbance related to a change in body structure or function

➤ *Additional Nursing Diagnoses and Collaborative Problems*

Additional nursing diagnoses may apply, depending on the client's specific disability. For example, a client with rheumatoid arthritis also experiences chronic pain. The client with a spinal cord injury may also have sexual dysfunction.

 Planning and Implementation

➤ *Impaired Physical Mobility*

Planning: Expected Outcomes. The primary outcomes are that the client is expected to achieve the maximal physical mobility possible with the least restriction of activity and not experience complications resulting from immobility.

Interventions. Most problems requiring rehabilitation relate to impaired physical mobility. Clients with neurologic disease or injury, amputations, arthritis, severe burns, and cardiopulmonary disease experience some degree of impaired mobility. Physical and occupational therapists are the key rehabilitation team members who help clients meet mobility goals. Clients often spend several hours every day working in the physical therapy department to regain function and skills.

ELDERLY CONSIDERATIONS

Older clients may not be able to tolerate extensive therapy work-outs and may need shorter sessions to prevent extreme fatigue or physical complications. The nurse reinforces the physical therapist's instructions and must be aware of the client's progress and abilities.

Transfer Techniques. Clients with decreased mobility may require assistance with transfers, for example, from a bed to a chair, a commode, or a wheelchair. Because the degree of assistance required varies with the client and the specific disability, the nurse carefully assesses the client's mobility status before attempting a transfer. The physical or occupational therapist usually specifies how a particular client is to be transferred. For example, a quadriplegic client may use a sliding board for transfer. The client with an above-knee amputation may need a wheelchair with removable arms. In any case, the nurse always plans the transfer technique before initiating it. The desired outcome is that the client will eventually be able to transfer independently and safely.

Basic techniques for the nurse to use for assisting in the transfer of the client from a bed to a chair or a wheelchair, and vice versa, are identified in Chart 13–2. These techniques are also taught to the family member or other caregiver who will be caring for the client at home.

Alternative Transfer Techniques. Some clients cannot bear weight. For example, a client with a spinal cord injury resulting in quadriplegia either uses a sliding board (which requires balance skills) or, with the nurse or therapist, uses a "bear hug" technique. The sitting client places his or her arms around the nurse's neck while the nurse lifts the client from the bed to the chair, or vice versa. Another person assists with the transfer by stabilizing the wheelchair and holding onto the client's waist. Most physical therapists recommend that the client wear pants or a gait belt so that the assistant can hold on to the belt during the transfer.

Potential Problems with Transfers. Before any client transfer, the nurse carefully observes the client for potential problems. Orthostatic, or postural, hypotension is a common problem for the client in rehabilitation. If the client moves from a lying to a sitting or standing position too quickly, the client's blood pressure drops and he or she becomes dizzy or faints as a result. This complication contributes to falls, which are common in any client with

impaired mobility. The problem is worsened when the client, especially if elderly, is taking antihypertensive medications. The nurse helps the client change positions slowly with frequent rest periods to allow the blood pressure to stabilize. The nurse may take the client's blood pressure with the client in lying, sitting, and standing positions to examine the differences. More than a 20-mmHg drop in systolic pressure or a 10-mmHg drop in diastolic pressure between positions indicates orthostatic hypotension. The nurse notifies the physician about this change.

Another potential problem for the client who requires transfers is weight gain. Because the client undergoing rehabilitation has impaired mobility, he or she tends to gain weight. Excessive weight hinders transfers both for the nurse or the therapist who is assisting and for the client, who is learning to transfer independently. The client is usually weighed every week to check for weight gain or loss.

Gait Training. The physical therapist works with clients for gait training if they are able to ambulate. While regaining the ability to ambulate, clients may need to use canes or walkers (Fig. 13–3). When working with clients who are using such assistive devices, also known as ambulatory aids, the physical therapist ensures that the client has a level surface on which to walk. The nurse reinforces the physical therapist's instructions and encourages the client to practice. The goal is for the client to walk independently with or without an assistive device. Elderly clients typically use a walker for a broader base of support. Younger clients or clients with minimal impairment often progress to the use of a hemi-cane or straight cane. Chart 13–3 outlines how to use assistive devices for ambulation.

Some clients never regain the ability to walk because of their impairment, such as multiple sclerosis and spinal cord injury. These clients may become wheelchair dependent and need to learn wheelchair mobility skills. With the help of physical and occupational therapy, most clients can learn to move anywhere they want in the wheelchair.

Prevention of Complications. During the rehabilitation phase, clients are vulnerable to complications of immobility. Table 13–2 lists common complications and major strategies that the nurse can use to help prevent each complication. Implementing range-of-motion (ROM) routines, adhering to schedules for turning and repositioning, and maintaining skin care are constant components of rehabilitation nursing care to prevent the complications of immobility. The key is to increase the client's mobility.

One way to increase mobility, even with clients who are bedridden, is through ROM exercises. ROM techniques are beneficial for any client with decreased mobility (Table 13–3). Although basic ROM techniques are presented in basic nursing textbooks, a few key principles are pertinent for rehabilitation nursing care:

- The human body contains more joints than simply the knees, the hips, the elbows, and the shoulders. For ROM techniques to be effective in preventing musculoskeletal contractures, the client must exercise

---

Chart 13–2

Nursing Care Highlight: Transfer Techniques

Bed to Wheelchair or Chair
1. Place the chair at an angle to the bed on the client's strong side.
2. Lock the wheelchair brakes or secure the chair position.
3. Assist the client to stand and move his or her strong hand to the armrest.
4. Keep the client's body weight forward and pivot.
5. When the client's legs touch the chair edge, assist the client in sitting.

Wheelchair or Chair to Bed
1. Place the chair with the client's strong side next to the bed.
2. Lock the wheelchair brakes or secure.
3. Assist the client to stand and move the client's strong hand to the armrest.
4. Keep the client's body weight forward and pivot.
5. When the client's legs touch the bed edge, assist the client in sitting and then reclining.

Use of a Sliding Board
1. Place the chair or wheelchair as close to the bed as possible.
2. Remove the armrest from the chair or (if removable) wheelchair.
3. Powder the sliding board.
4. Place the sliding board under the client's buttocks.
5. Instruct the client to reach toward the client's side.
6. Assist the client in sliding gently to the bed.

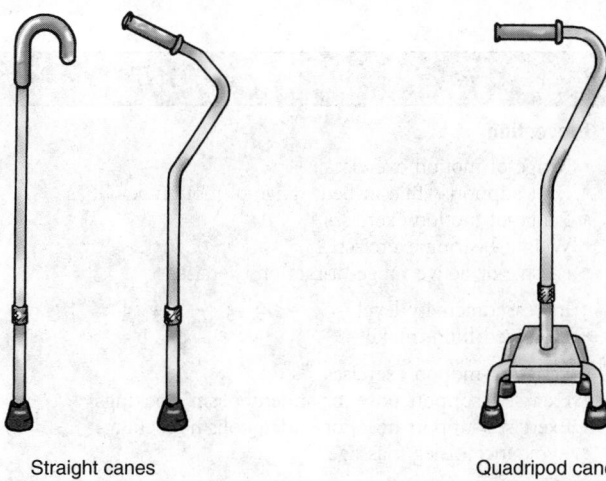

Straight canes   Quadripod cane
                                    ("quad" cane)

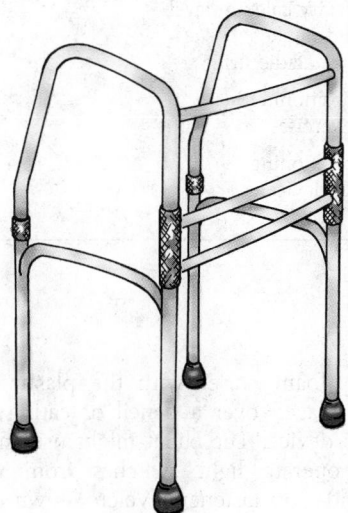

Standard walker

Figure 13–3. Assistive devices for ambulation. Assistive devices vary in the amount of support they provide. A straight cane provides less support than a quadripod cane or walker.

all joints, including each joint of the fingers, hands, toes, and so forth.

■ In performing ROM activities, the nurse or client completes full-range movement of each joint five times or more and completes the entire process at least three times daily.

■ The nurse does not move joints beyond points at which the client expresses pain or the nurse perceives stiffness or difficulty.

Clients with decreased mobility who are able to follow directions are taught by the nurse and the physical therapist to perform active or active-assisted ROM exercises.

▶ *Self-Care Deficit*

Planning: Expected Outcomes. The primary outcome is that the client is expected to become independent in

ADLs to the extent possible based on the client's disability.

Interventions. Activities of daily living, or self-care activities, include eating, bathing, dressing, grooming, and toileting. The nurse encourages clients to perform as much self-care as possible. The nurse and occupational therapist collaborate to identify ways in which self-care activities can be modified so that the client can perform them independently. For example, the occupational therapist teaches a hemiplegic client to put a shirt on by placing the affected arm in the sleeve first and putting the unaffected arm in the appropriate sleeve next. The nurse reinforces this dressing technique and encourages the client to practice.

Use of Assistive-Adaptive Devices. A variety of assistive-adaptive devices are available for clients with chronic illness and disability. An assistive-adaptive device, or self-care support device, is any item that enables the client to perform all or part of an activity independently. Table 13–4 identifies common devices and describes their use.

Many department stores carry clothing and assistive-adaptive devices designed for clients with disabilities. The occupational therapist works with the client to determine specific needs with regard to such equipment. In addition, the nurse and the occupational therapist help the client look for creative and inexpensive alternatives to meeting needs. For example, barbecue tongs may be used as "reachers" for pulling up pants or obtaining items on

---

Chart 13–3

Nursing Care Highlight: Gait Training Techniques

Walker Assisted

1. Apply a gait belt around the client's waist.
2. Assist the client to a standing position.
3. Assist the client in placing both hands on the walker.
4. Ensure that the client is well balanced.
5. Assist the client repeatedly to perform the following sequence:
    a. Lift the walker.
    b. Move the walker 2 ft forward and set it down on all legs.
    c. While resting on the walker, take small steps.
    d. Check balance.

Cane Assisted

1. Apply a gait belt around the client's waist.
2. Assist the client to a standing position.
3. Assist the client in placing his or her strong hand on the cane.
4. Ensure that the client is well balanced.
5. Assist the client repeatedly to perform the following sequence:
    a. Move the cane forward.
    b. Move the weaker leg one step forward.
    c. Move the stronger leg one step forward.
    d. Check balance.

TABLE 13–2

Prevention of Some Common Hazards of Immobility

Body System	Complication	Prevention
Musculoskeletal	• Contractures • Foot drop • Osteoporosis • Susceptibility to fractures • Muscular atrophy	• Range-of-motion exercises • Foot support while in bed, range-of-motion activities • Range-of-motion exercises • Weight-bearing exercises • Passive or active range-of-motion exercises
Gastrointestinal	• Constipation	• Increased activity level • Increased fluid intake
Cardiovascular	• Decreased cardiac output • Increased venous stasis • Thrombus formation • Embolism	• Range-of-motion exercises • Exercise, support hose, or antiembolism stockings • Exercise, support hose, or antiembolism stockings • Avoidance of leg massage
Neurologic	• Disorientation • Postural hypotension	• Sleep-wake schedule in accord with light-dark pattern • Reorientation (to person, place, and time) • Control of sensory stimulation • Avoidance of sudden position changes
Renal/urinary	• Calculi	• Decreased dietary calcium level • Increased fluid intake • Maintenance of acidic urine
Respiratory	• Pneumonia	• Frequent repositioning • Respiratory exercises
Integumentary	• Pressure ulcers	• Frequent repositioning • Pressure relief devices • Skin care

TABLE 13–3

Types of Range-of-Motion Exercises

Type	Description	Indications
Passive	• Exercises are performed by the nurse for the client.	• The client is too weak to participate actively.
Active	• Exercises are performed by the client.	• The client is able to complete range-of-motion movements.
Assisted, or active assisted	• Exercises are performed by the client but are guided by the nurse or the therapist.	• The client is weak and needs assistance.
Resistive	• The actions of the client are in opposition to those performed by the nurse or the therapist.	• The client has full range of motion, and an increase in strength is desired.

high shelves. A foam curler with the plastic insert removed may be placed over a pencil or eating utensil to make a built-up device. The client might use an extended shoe horn to operate light switches from wheelchair height. Hook-and-loop fasteners (Velcro) sewn on clothes can prevent the frustrations caused by buttons and zippers.

Energy Conservation. Nurses work with occupational therapists to assess the client's self-care abilities and to determine possible ways of conserving energy. Fatigue is commonly associated with chronic and disabling conditions. The nurse and the therapist develop strategies for energy conservation after evaluating the client's self-care routines. Preparation for ADLs can be helpful in reducing the client's effort and energy expenditure (e.g., the client gathers all needed equipment before starting grooming routines). The nurse can teach the client with high energy levels in the morning to schedule energy-intensive activities in the morning rather than later in the day or evening. Spacing activities is also helpful for saving energy. Additionally, allowing time to rest before and after eating and toileting decreases the strain on the client's energy level.

➤ Risk for Impaired Skin Integrity

Planning: Expected Outcomes. The primary outcome is that the client is expected to have intact skin.

TABLE 13-4

Uses of Assistive-Adaptive Devices	
Device	**Use**
Buttonhook	• Threaded through the buttonhole to enable clients with weak finger mobility to button shirts. • Alternative uses include serving as a pencil holder or a cigarette holder.
Extended shoe horn	• Assists in the application of shoes for clients with decreased mobility. • Alternative uses include turning light switches off or on while the client is in a wheelchair.
Plate guard	• Applied to a plate to assist clients with weak hand and arm mobility to feed themselves.
Gel pad	• Placed under a plate or a glass to prevent dishes from slipping and moving. • Alternative uses include placement under bathing and grooming items to prevent their moving.
Foam build-ups	• Applied to eating utensils to assist clients with weak handgrasps to feed themselves. • Alternative uses include the application to pens and pencils to assist with writing or over a buttonhook to assist with grasping the device.
Hook and loop fastener (Velcro) straps	• Applied to utensils, a buttonhook, or a pencil to slip over the hand and provide a method of stabilizing the device when the client's handgrasp is weak.
Long-handled reacher	• Assists in obtaining items located on high shelves or at ground level for clients who are not able to change positions easily.

Interventions. An enormous variety of topical and mechanical remedies have been used to prevent and treat pressure ulcers, with varying success. Pressure reduction is a nursing intervention that may be achieved when the nurse temporarily repositions the client or alters the physical properties of the mattress surface, such as adding a mattress overlay.

Turning and Repositioning. The best intervention to prevent skin impairment is frequent position changes in combination with adequate skin care and sufficient nutritional intake. In general, the nurse turns and repositions the client every 2 hours; however, this may not be sufficient for people who are frail and have thin skin, especially elderly people (Chart 13-4). Therefore, the nurse assesses the client's skin condition each time the client is turned and repositioned to determine the best turning schedule. For example, if the client has been sleeping for 2 hours and the nurse decides to postpone turning for 1 hour, reddened areas over the client's bony prominences may be present. If such reddened areas do not fade within 30 minutes after pressure relief or do not blanch, they may be classified as pre-ulcer areas, or stage I pressure areas (see Chap. 70). Some clients need to be turned and repositioned every hour to prevent the development of pressure sores; others may tolerate 2–3 hours between turnings.

For clients who sit for prolonged periods in a wheelchair, the nurse repositions them at least every 1–2 hours. Clients who are able are taught to perform "wheelchair pushups" by using their arms to lift their buttocks off the wheelchair seat for 10 seconds or longer every hour, or more often if needed. The physical therapist helps clients strengthen arm muscles in preparation for teaching wheelchair pushups.

Skin Care. Adequate skin care is an essential component of prevention. The nurse performs or assists clients in completing skin care each time they are turned, repositioned, or bathed. Skin care includes cleaning soiled areas, followed by careful drying and application of body lotion. For clients who are incontinent, topical barrier creams or ointments can help to protect the skin from moisture, which facilitates skin breakdown. If pre-ulcer (reddened) areas are noted, the nurse does not rub these areas because this causes more extensive damage to the already fragile capillary system. Instead, the nurse carefully observes the pre-ulcer areas for further breakdown and relieves pressure on the areas as much as possible. Bed pillows are often good pressure-relieving devices (see Chapter 70 for a complete discussion of skin care interventions).

Chart 13-4

Nursing Focus on the Elderly: Special Considerations in Rehabilitation

• When getting the client out of bed, move the client or instruct the client to move or sit up slowly to prevent orthostatic hypotension. This problem is most common in elderly clients who take antihypertensive medications.
• Turn the client more often than every 2 hours even if it is just a minor position change. Skin becomes thinner and more fragile with age.
• Determine whether the client had any problem with urinary patterns before the illness or rehabilitation. A client with a previous problem may not have a successful bladder training program.
• Be aware that intestinal motility decreases with age, which leads to constipation.
• Assess the client's support system of family and significant others. Many elderly clients have no spouse or close friends who would usually serve as a support network.

Nutrition. Clients need sufficient nutrition both to repair wounds and to prevent pressure ulcers. The nurse collaborates with the dietitian to assess the client's food selection and ensure that it contains adequate protein and carbohydrates. Both the nurse and the dietitian closely monitor the client's weight and serum albumin and transferrin levels. If either of these indexes decreases significantly, the client may be given high-protein, high-carbohydrate food supplements, such as milkshakes, or commercial preparations, such as Ensure Plus (also see Chap. 64).

Mechanical Devices. Pressure-relieving devices include waterbeds, foam (egg crate) or gel mattresses or pads, air mattresses, alternating-pressure mattresses, low air loss overlays or beds, and air-fluidized beds. Mattress overlays, such as foam, air, and gel types, are controversial because their effectiveness has not been proven. The nurse and the client usually decide the type of device. The use of any mechanical device (except air-fluidized beds) does not eliminate the need for turning and repositioning.

Specialty beds are categorized as either "low air loss" or "air fluidized." Air-fluidized therapy (e.g., Clinitron or FluidAir bed) provides the most effective pressure relief. The client is maintained in a nearly pressure-free environment (Fig. 13–4). These beds are generally not used for the prevention of skin breakdown, because most insurers will not reimburse the agency for the use of the bed. Special beds are, therefore, usually reserved for severe skin problems that have not healed with use of a conventional bed or other mechanical device. If optimal nutrition and healing conditions are maintained, skin breakdowns that have occurred should heal with continued use of air-fluidized therapy. The primary disadvantage is its expense, which may exceed several hundred dollars for each day of use. The cost of air-fluidized therapy may be reimbursed by some health insurance providers, such as Medicare.

► *Altered Urinary Elimination*

Planning: Expected Outcomes. The primary outcomes are that the client is expected to achieve a personally acceptable form of urinary elimination and be free from urinary complications, such as infection.

Interventions. Neurologic disabilities may interfere with successful bladder control in a client undergoing rehabilitation. These disabilities result in three basic functional types of neurogenic bladder: reflex (spastic) bladder, flaccid bladder, and uninhibited bladder.

A reflex or spastic (upper motor neuron) bladder causes incontinence characterized by sudden gushing voids. However, the bladder does not usually empty completely. A reflex bladder is also sometimes referred to as a "spastic" bladder. Neurologic problems affecting the upper motor neuron typically occur with high-level or mid-level spinal cord injuries, above the 12th thoracic vertebra (T-12). These injuries result in a failure of impulse transmission from the lower spinal cord areas to the cortex of the brain. When the bladder fills and transmits impulses to the spinal cord, the client is not conscious of the filling sensation. However, because there is no injury at the lower spinal cord level and the voiding reflex arc is intact, the efferent (motor) impulse is relayed and the bladder contracts.

A flaccid (lower motor neuron) bladder results in urinary retention and overflow (dribbling). Injuries that cause damage to the lower motor neuron at the spinal cord level of S2–4 (e.g., multiple sclerosis and spinal cord injury below T-12) may directly interfere with the reflex arc or may result in inappropriate interpretation of the impulses to the brain. The bladder fills, and afferent (sensory) impulses conduct the message via the spinal cord to the cortical region of the brain. Because of the injury, however, the impulse is not interpreted correctly by the cortical bladder center in the brain, and there is a failure to respond with a message for the bladder to contract.

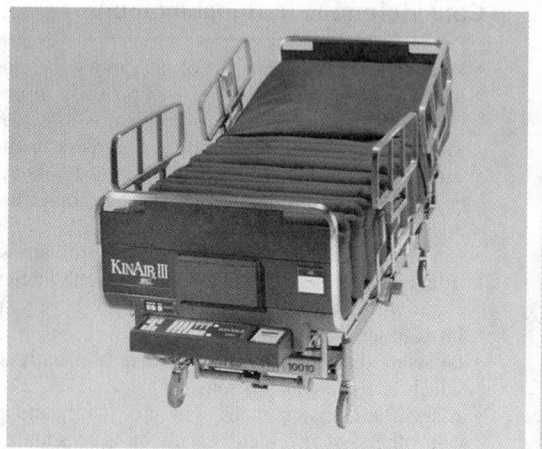 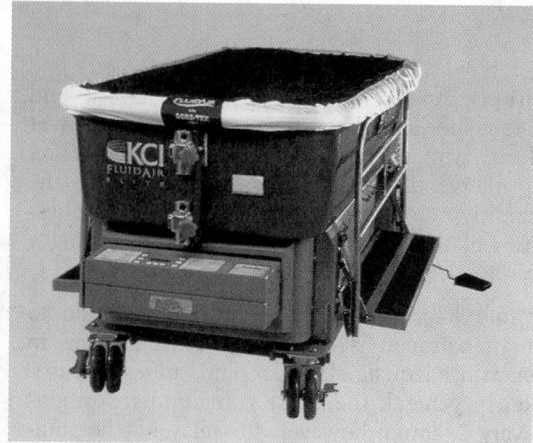

Figure 13–4. Pressure relief devices. *Left,* KinAirIII beds provide controlled air suspension to redistribute body weight away from bony prominences. *Right,* FluidAir Elite beds use airflow and bead fluidization. Both of these beds are covered with GORE-TEX fabric, which resists tearing. This fabric is also waterproof and acts as a barrier against bacteria. (Courtesy of Kinetic Concepts, Inc., San Antonio, TX.)

An uninhibited bladder may occur when the client has a neurologic problem that affects the cortical bladder center of the brain (frontal lobe), such as stroke or brain injury. When the bladder needs to empty, the client has little sensorimotor control and cannot wait until he or she is on the commode or bedpan before voiding. Therefore, the client is incontinent, but the bladder may not completely empty.

Bladder Training. The nurse can teach three techniques to assist the client in "repatterning" voiding, or bladder training:

- Facilitating, or triggering, techniques
- Intermittent catheterization
- Consistent scheduling of toileting routines

These techniques may not be as effective in a client with physiologic changes associated with aging.

Facilitating or Triggering Techniques. The nurse uses facilitating (triggering) techniques to stimulate voiding (Table 13–5). If there is an upper motor neuron problem, and the reflex arc is intact (reflex bladder pattern), any stimulus that sends the message to the spinal cord level S2–4 that the bladder might be full can initiate the voiding response. Such techniques include stroking the medial aspect of the thigh, pinching the area above the groin, pulling pubic hair, massaging the penoscrotal area, pinching the posterior aspect of the glans penis, and providing digital anal stimulation.

When the client has a lower motor neuron problem, the voiding reflex arc is not intact (flaccid bladder pattern) and additional stimulation may be needed to initiate voiding. Two techniques used to facilitate voiding are the Valsalva maneuver and Credé's maneuver. In teaching the client the Valsalva maneuver, the nurse instructs the client to hold his or her breath and bear down as if trying to defecate. The nurse assists the client in performing Credé's maneuver by placing the client's hand in a cupped position directly over the bladder area and instructing the client to push inward and downward as if massaging the bladder to empty.

Intermittent Catheterization. This is a method of bladder training frequently used for disorders involving a flaccid bladder, generally caused by a lower motor neuron problem. In assisting the client with intermittent catheterization, the nurse inserts a urinary catheter every 2–3 hours initially. Insertion is done after the client has attempted voiding and has used the Valsalva and Credé's maneuvers. If less than 150 mL of residual urine is obtained, the nurse increases the interval between catheterizations. The interval may be to 3–4 hours, according to the physician's order or health care agency protocol. The interval may be gradually increased to 4–6 hours, but the client should not go beyond 8 hours between catheterizations. The exception occurs when the residual urine volume is less than 150 mL each time with an adequate intake of fluids. If the client will be performing intermittent self-catheterization at home after discharge from the rehabilitation facility, the nurse instructs the client about clean (not sterile) technique.

Intermittent catheterizations may also be done to determine residual urine volumes for the client with a reflex (upper motor neuron) or uninhibited bladder. The client with this types of neurogenic bladder can void but often does not empty the bladder completely. The nurse catheterizes the client within 10 minutes after the client voids to determine the residual amount of urine in the bladder. For most clients, the desired amount is less than 100 mL of residual urine.

Toileting Schedule. Consistent toileting routines may be the best way of re-establishing voiding continence when the client displays an uninhibited bladder pattern (associated with brain damage or head injury). The nurse assesses the client's previous voiding pattern and determines the client's daily routine. At a minimum, the nurse assists the client with voiding in the morning after rising, before and after meals, before and after physical activity, and at bedtime. The nurse considers the client's bladder capacity, which may range from 100 to 500 mL, as well as the client's mobility limitations and clothing that may be restrictive. Bladder capacity is determined by measuring the client's urine output. The nurse ensures that the client is aware of nearby bathrooms at all times or has a call system to contact the nurse for assistance.

TABLE 13–5

Management of Altered Urinary Elimination

Functional Type	Neurologic Disability	Clinical Manifestations	Re-establishing Voiding Patterns
Reflex (spastic)	• Upper motor neuron spinal cord injury above T-12	• Urinary frequency, incontinence	• Triggering or facilitating techniques • Medications
Flaccid	• Lower motor neuron spinal cord injury below T-12 (affects S2–4 reflex arc)	• Urinary retention, overflow	• Valsalva and Credé maneuvers • Medications
Uninhibited	• Brain damage from injury or stroke	• Frequency, urgency, incontinence, voiding in small amounts	• Intermittent catheterization • Consistent toileting schedule • Regulation of fluid intake

Drug Therapy. Medications that may be used for urinary elimination problems include cholinergics (to promote bladder emptying), antispasmodics (to prevent incontinence), and skeletal muscle relaxants (to decrease spasticity, which promotes self-care) (Chart 13–5). Medications are not usually prescribed by the physician in the initial management of bladder problems but may be used to assist a bladder training program. The nurse reports the client's progress in bladder training to the health care provider so that he or she can make the best decision regarding drug therapy. In general, anticholinergics, antispasmodics, and skeletal muscle relaxants help to promote continence in clients with a reflex (upper motor neuron) bladder. Cholinergics, such as bethanechol chloride (Urecholine), may decrease urinary retention problems in the client with a flaccid bladder. This drug type may also facilitate complete bladder emptying in a client with a large residual volume, such as in reflex bladder problems. The client with an uninhibited bladder does not routinely require medications for bladder training programs unless urinary function is affected by additional pathologic changes.

Chart 13–5

Drug Therapy for Clients in Bladder-Training Programs

Drug	Usual Dosage	Nursing Interventions	Rationale
Cholinergics			
Bethanechol chloride (Urecholine)	• 10–50 mg bid-qid PO	• Give 1 hr before or 2 hr after meals. • Instruct clients to change positions slowly. • Give 1 hr before toileting or triggering or facilitating measure.	• This agent may cause nausea and vomiting. • Orthostatic hypotension is a possible side effect. • The drug is effective when using other measures for bladder training.
Antispasmodics			
Oxybutynin chloride (Ditropan)	• 5 mg bid or tid PO	• Instruct the client to avoid driving. • Instruct the client to avoid hot environmental temperatures. • Assess the client for urinary retention.	• Vertigo, drowsiness, and blurred vision may occur. • Sweating is suppressed. • Retention may be a side effect of the drug.
Flavoxate hydrochloride (Urispas)	• 100–200 mg tid or qid PO	• Instruct the client to avoid driving. • Instruct the client to avoid hot environmental temperatures. • Assess the client for urinary retention.	• Drowsiness, mental confusion, and blurred vision may occur. • Sweating is suppressed. • Retention may be a side effect of the drug.
Skeletal Muscle Relaxants			
Dantrolene (Dantrium)	• 25 mg once daily PO initially; increase to 25 mg bid–qid, then by 25-mg increments up to 100 mg	• Instruct the client to avoid driving. • Instruct the client to avoid prolonged sun exposure.	• Fatigue, dizziness, and muscular weakness are side effects. • Photosensitivity may occur.
Baclofen (Lioresal)	• 5 mg tid PO; may increase by 5 mg daily until desired effect attained to maximum of 80 mg	• Instruct the client to avoid alcohol. • Instruct the client to avoid driving.	• Alcohol potentiates the drug's effects. • Drowsiness and dizziness may occur.

Fluid Intake. The nurse instructs the client to maintain an adequate intake of fluids, at least 2000–2500 mL/day. The nurse encourages the client to drink fluids that promote an acidic urine, including large amounts of cranberry juice, prune juice, bouillon, tomato juice, and water. Fluids that promote an alkaline urine are discouraged, including citrus juices, excessive amounts of milk and milk products, and carbonated beverages. An acidic urine minimizes risks of urinary tract infection and calculus (stone) formation, although this belief is controversial. Some microorganisms, such as *Escherichia coli*, grow best in acidic environments.

In addition, the nurse discourages high-calorie fluids for overweight clients. Disabled clients have more difficulty with mobility and self-care if weight is not controlled.

ELDERLY CONSIDERATIONS

The nurse may decrease fluid intake to prevent complications in clients with congestive heart disease or renal problems, especially elderly clients. Some clients, especially those with flaccid bladder patterns, decrease fluid intake after 6 or 7 PM to avoid the need for catheterization during the night.

Prevention of Complications. The client with altered urinary elimination is at risk for skin breakdown from incontinence, urinary tract infection from urinary retention, and urinary calculi from urinary retention and stasis. The nurse keeps the client clean and dry and provides skin care as described under Risk for Impaired Skin Integrity earlier in this chapter. (See Chapter 73 for preventive measures for urinary tract infection and calculi.)

➤ **Constipation**

Planning: Expected Outcomes. The primary outcomes are that the client is expected to achieve a personally acceptable form of bowel elimination and be free from bowel elimination complications, such as impaction or diarrhea.

Interventions. Neurologic problems often affect the client's bowel pattern by causing a reflex (spastic) bowel, a flaccid bowel, or an uninhibited bowel.

Upper motor neuron diseases and injuries, such as a high-level or midlevel spinal cord injury, may result in a reflex (spastic) bowel pattern, with defecation occurring suddenly and without warning. With a reflex pattern, any facilitating or triggering mechanism may lead to defecation if the lower colon contains stool. Examples of facilitating or triggering techniques include providing anal stimulation (by inserting a finger, using either a finger cot or rubber glove and lubrication, to the first joint), gently pinching the anus, and pulling pubic hair. Digital stimulation should not be used for clients with cardiac disease because of the risk of inducing a vagal response (a rapid decrease in heart rate).

Lower motor neuron diseases and injuries interfere with transmission of the nervous impulse across the reflex arc and may result in a flaccid bowel pattern, with defecation occurring infrequently and in small amounts. The use of facilitating and triggering mechanisms in combination with a toileting schedule, suppository use, and disimpaction yields the best results. Clients may be able to self-administer the suppository or disimpact if necessary.

Neurologic injuries affecting the brain may cause an uninhibited bowel pattern, with frequent defecation, urgency, and complaints of hard stool. Clients may manage uninhibited bowel patterns through a consistent toileting schedule, a high-fiber diet, and the use of stool softeners.

Bowel Training. An overview of management techniques for bowel dysfunction is presented in Table 13–6. In many cases, clients are not able to regain control over their bowel function in the manner previously possible. The nurse assists clients in designing a bowel elimination program that accommodates the disability.

The nurse works with clients to schedule bowel elimi-

TABLE 13–6

Management of Bowel Dysfunction			
Functional Type	**Neurologic Disability**	**Dysfunction**	**Re-establishing Defecation Patterns**
Reflex (spastic)	• Upper motor neuron spinal cord injury above T-12	• Defecation without warning	• Triggering mechanisms • Facilitation techniques • High-fiber diet • Suppository use • Consistent toileting schedule
Flaccid	• Lower motor neuron spinal cord injury below T-12 (affects S2–4 reflex arc)	• Infrequent, small stools	• Triggering or facilitating techniques • High-fiber diet • Suppository use • Consistent toileting schedule • Manual disimpaction
Uninhibited	• Brain damage from injury or stroke	• Frequent, urgency, and constipation	• Consistent toileting schedule • High-fiber diet • Stool softener use

nation as close to their previous routine as possible. For example, a client who had stools at noon every other day before the illness or injury should have the bowel program scheduled in the same way. An exception is the client who prefers another time that best fits into his or her daily routine. If the client is employed during the day, a time-consuming bowel elimination program in the morning may not be reasonable. The client may prefer to change the bowel protocol until the evening, when there is more time.

Drug Therapy. Bowel training programs for clients with neurologic problems are often designed to include the combination of suppository use and a consistent toileting schedule. Although medications should not be a first choice when a bowel training program is being formulated, the nurse routinely considers the need for a suppository if clients do not re-establish defecation habits through consistent scheduling of toileting, dietary modification, anal stimulation, and disimpaction.

The most common agents prescribed by physicians as suppositories in bowel training programs are bisacodyl (Dulcolax) and glycerin. Suppositories must be placed against the bowel wall to stimulate the sacral reflex arc and promote rectal emptying. Both agents are equivalent in effect; results occur in 15–30 minutes. The suppository is administered by the nurse when the client expects to defecate. For example, if a client had a previous bowel habit of defecating every other day after breakfast, the suppository is administered every other day after breakfast. Ordinarily, administering the suppository every second or third day is effective in re-establishing defecation patterns. Depending on each client's need, other medications, such as laxatives, may be indicated for bowel training programs.

Nutrition. Bowel elimination is directly related to the type and quality of food and fluid ingested. A high-fiber diet is a mainstay of most bowel training programs and includes whole-grain foods, bran, and fresh and dried fruits. Increasing dietary fiber is effective in facilitating defecation only if the client reduces fat intake.

Prevention of Complications. Common complications of any bowel training program are constipation, diarrhea, and flatulence. The nurse assesses clients for these complications and modifies the bowel training program accordingly, in collaboration with the physician and the dietitian.

➤ Ineffective Individual Coping

Planning: Expected Outcomes. The major outcome is that the client is expected to learn to cope with the chronic illness or disability and participate in the rehabilitation program.

Interventions. The client with a disability often has a poor self-concept because of changes in body image from structural or functional changes. The use of an assistive device, such as a wheelchair, also differentiates the client from most other people, and the client may not want to accept the need for the device. The nurse encourages the client to discuss feelings and asks questions to elicit specific information that can help in assessing the client's acceptance of and coping with the disability.

A disability also affects a person's role in society. For instance, a young medical student may fall from a ladder and become a paraplegic, and plans for a career as a surgeon are altered. A middle-aged farmer may be burned severely when his tractor catches on fire. He can no longer care for his farm, and his wife takes over during his rehabilitation process. An elderly woman who cares for her grandchildren is crippled with rheumatoid arthritis and can no longer provide child care. Disability requires role changes and always involves losses in the lives of those affected.

In addition to role changes, relationships with people change. Socializing with friends and family may be a strain when a person feels "different." Intimate relationships are affected because sexual dysfunction may result from disability. The nurse should be sensitive to these issues and should not avoid discussing them.

The nurse assesses coping strategies and support systems that the client has used in the past so that they can be used during rehabilitation if needed. The nurse asks the client what strategies have been used in the past to cope successfully with life crises, if any. Spiritual and religious beliefs are important for some people and should not be overlooked as the nurse helps the client identify sources of support.

➤ Continuing Care

The nurse begins discharge planning at or before client admission. If the client is being transferred from a hospital to a rehabilitation unit or facility, the nurse orients the client to the change in routine and emphasizes the importance of self-care. When the client is admitted to the rehabilitation unit or facility, the nurse assesses the client's current living situation at home. The nurse determines, with the client and family members or significant others, the adequacy of the client's current situation and potential needs after discharge to the home. The client with chronic illness and disability may require home care, assistance with ADLs, nursing care, or physical or occupational therapy after discharge. The nurse case manager assesses these needs and plans with the client, family or significant other, social worker, physical or vocational therapist, and physician for the best ways to meet identified needs.

Other health care professionals may be necessary to meet the unique needs of special populations. For example, brain-injured clients benefit from life planning, a process that examines and plans to meet the lifelong needs of clients. Case managers specializing in life planning are often part of the interdisciplinary rehabilitation team.

➤ Home Care Management

Before the client returns home, the nurse assesses the client's readiness for discharge from the rehabilitation facility. The client's home may be assessed in multiple ways.

Predischarge Assessment. The case manager or occupational therapist may visit the home before discharge to assess the home's layout and accessibility. These professionals may be employed by the health care agency or third-party payer, such as a health maintenance organization (see Chapter 3 for a discussion of third-party payers). For example, because of the stress of hospitalization, a client with a fractured hip who is ambulating well with a walker may neglect to explain to the nurse that the home has three steps at the entrance and that the bathroom is accessible by stairway only. The client may not consider it important to mention to the nurse that throw rugs, which do not provide a completely level surface on which to use a cane, are scattered throughout the apartment.

During a predischarge visit to the home, the case manager assesses the accessibility of the home in general and of the bathrooms, bedrooms, and kitchen. If the client will be wheelchair dependent after discharge from the facility, ramps are needed to replace steps, and doorways should be checked for adequate width. Usually, a doorway width of 36–38 inches (slightly less than 1 m) is sufficient for a standard-sized wheelchair. Any room that the client needs to use is checked. The bedroom should have sufficient space for the client to maneuver transfers to and from the wheelchair and the bed.

Space requirements vary, depending on the client's need to use a wheelchair, a walker, or a cane. In the bathroom, grab bars may need to be installed before the client comes home. Bathtub benches can provide support for the client who has difficulty with mobility and, when used in combination with a hand-held showerhead, can provide easily accessible bathing facilities. Assessment of the kitchen may or may not be critical, depending on whether the client has help with cooking and preparing meals. If the client will be responsible for cooking after discharge from the hospital or facility, the kitchen is assessed for wheelchair or walker accessibility, appliance accessibility, and the need for adaptive equipment.

Leave-of-Absence Visit. A second method of assessing the client's home is through a brief home visit, also called a leave-of-absence (LOA) visit, by the client before discharge. The nurse prepares the client by explaining the need for the trial home visit and by assessing the client's comfort level with this idea. The client who has been hospitalized for a lengthy period may feel intense anxiety about returning home. The nurse may allay such anxieties with careful preparation. Before the visit, the nurse meets with the client and family members or significant others to set goals for the visit and to identify specific tasks that the client should attempt during the time at home. After the client has been home, the nurse interviews the client to determine the success of the visit and to assess additional education or training needs before final discharge.

Going home may not be an option for all clients. Some clients may not have a support network of family members or significant others. For example, many elderly clients have no spouse or close friends living nearby. Children may reside at a distance, which can make home care difficult. If there is no caregiver available, the family must decide whether care can be provided in the home by an outside resource or whether the client needs to be admitted to a 24-hour supervised health care setting, such as a

nursing home. Rehabilitation services are available in most long-term care settings (skilled nursing facilities) at least 5 days a week.

➤ Health Teaching

Education of the client and the family is the cornerstone of nursing care. The nurse assesses every component of the client's care to determine how the client can be taught to perform activities of daily living (ADLs) independently. The nurse assesses the client's learning potential and cognitive capacity. As care is provided, the nurse explains the procedure and its rationale. The client is encouraged to perform or direct the technique independently to verify understanding. The nurse gives written material explaining the steps in the procedure to the client and family members to reinforce learning and to provide support with the technique after discharge. However, before giving the client written material, the nurse assesses the reading level of the material and determines whether it is appropriate for the client's reading ability and language skills.

Any chronic illness or disability necessitates changes in a client's lifestyle and body image. The nurse assists the client in dealing with such changes by encouraging the client to verbalize feelings and emotions. The nurse also helps the client focus on existing capabilities instead of disabilities.

The client may fail to relate psychologically to the disability during hospitalization. For example, the client may display anger or frustration in attempting to perform self-care routines before discharge from the rehabilitation facility. The nurse encourages the client to be open about such feelings and to talk about ways to prevent worries from becoming realities after discharge.

The leave-of-absence home visit assists the client and family members or significant others in psychosocial preparation for discharge. It allows the client to experience the home situation while being able to return to the hospital environment after a few hours. Often the client finds that fears were not realized during the home visit, but frequently find new problems in the home that must be addressed before discharge. The nurse reviews this information with the client in preparation for discharge to the home.

➤ Health Care Resources

Various health care resources, such as physical therapy, home care nursing, and vocational counseling, are available to the client with chronic illness and disability after discharge to the home. The nurse assesses the client's need for additional care and support throughout the client's hospitalization and works with the case manager and physician in arranging for home services.

 Evaluation

On the basis of the identified nursing diagnoses and collaborative problems, the client and the nurse evaluate the rehabilitation interventions for the client with a disabling or chronic condition. Expected outcomes may include that the client will

- Ambulate independently, with or without assistive devices, or be independent in wheelchair mobility skills
- Perform ADLs independently with or without assistive-adaptive devices
- Have intact skin
- Demonstrate effective urinary elimination through an individualized bladder training program
- Demonstrate effective bowel elimination through an individualized bowel training program
- State acceptance of the disability and use coping strategies effectively

SELECTED BIBLIOGRAPHY

Badley, E. M. (1995). The impact of disabling arthritis. *Arthritis Care Research, 8*(4), 221–228.

Boss, B. J., Pecanty, L., McFarland, S. M., & Sasser, L. (1995). Self-care competence among persons with spinal cord injury. *SCI Nursing, 12*(2), 48–53.

*Boynton De Sepulveda, L. I., & Chang, B. (1994). Effective coping with stroke disability in a community setting: The development of a causal model. *Journal of Neuroscience Nursing, 26*(4), 193–203.

*Braden, B. J., & Bergstrom, N. (1992). Pressure reduction. In G. M. Bulachek & J. C. McCloskey (Eds.), *Nursing interventions: Essential nursing treatments* (2nd ed., pp. 94–108). Philadelphia: W. B. Saunders.

*Carey, R. G., & Posavec, E. J. (1978). Program evaluation of a physical medicine and rehabilitation unit: A new approach. *Archives of Physical Medicine and Rehabilitation, 59*, 330–337.

Collins, R. C. (1997). *Neurology*. Philadelphia: W. B. Saunders.

Donohoe, K. M., Wineman, N. M., & O'Brien, R. A. (1996). Are alternative long-term-care programs needed for adults with chronic progressive disability? *Journal of Neuroscience Nursing, 28*(6), 373–380.

Edwards, P. A. (1996). Health promotion through fitness for adolescents and young adults following spinal cord injury. *SCI Nursing, 13*(3), 69–73.

Evans, R. W. (1997). The role of the neuropsychologist in life care planning for brain-injured populations. *The Journal of Care Management, 3*(5), 46–47, 49.

Galindo-Ciocon, D., Ciocon, J. O., & Galindo, D. (1995). Functional impairment among elderly women with osteoporotic vertebral fractures. *Rehabilitation Nursing, 20*(2), 79–83.

*Granger, C. V., & Gresham, G. E. (1984). *Functional assessment in rehabilitation medicine*. Baltimore: Williams & Wilkins.

*Granger, C. V., Hamilton, B. B., Lenacre, J. M., Heinemann, A. W., & Wright, B. D. (1993). Performance profiles of the Functional Independence Measure. *Journal of Physical Medicine and Rehabilitation, 72*, 84–89.

Hamilton, L., & Lyon, P. S. (1995). A nursing-driven program to preserve and restore functional ability in hospitalized elderly patients. *Journal of Nursing Administration, 25*(4), 30–37.

*Hellman, E. A., & Williams, M. A. (1994). Outpatient cardiac rehabilitation in elderly patients. *Heart and Lung, 23*(6), 506–512.

Hickey, J. V. (1996). *The clinical practice of neurological and neurosurgical nursing* (4th ed.). Philadelphia: J. B. Lippincott.

Huntt, D. C., & Growick, B. S. (1997). Managed care for people with disabilities. *Journal of Rehabilitation*, July/August/September, 10–14.

Ignatavicius, D. D. (1998). *Introduction to long term care nursing*. Philadelphia: F. A. Davis.

*Institute of Medicine. (1991). *Disability in America*. Washington, DC: National Academy Press.

*Katz, S., et al. (1963). Studies of illness in the aged. The index of ADL: A standardized measure of biological and psychosocial function. *Journal of the American Medical Association, 185*, 914–919.

*Mason, M., & Bell, J. (1994). Functional outcomes of rehabilitation in the frail elderly: A two-year retrospective review. *Perspectives, 18*(2), 7–9.

*Miller, J. M. (1991). *Coping with chronic illness: Overcoming powerlessness* (2nd ed.). Philadelphia: F. A. Davis.

Neal, L. J. (1995). The rehabilitation nurse in the home care setting: Treating chronic wounds as a disability. *Rehabilitation Nursing, 20*(5), 261–264.

*Posavec, E. J., & Carey, R. G. (1982). Using a level of function scale (LORS-II) to evaluate the success of inpatient rehabilitation programs. *Rehabilitation Nursing, 7*(6), 17–19.

*Redeker, N. S., Mason, D. J., Wykpisz, E., Glica, B., & Miner, C. (1994). First postoperative week activity patterns and recovery in women after coronary artery bypass surgery. *Nursing Research, 43*(3), 168–173.

Somervill, B. A. (1997). Transitional and subacute care. *Case Review, 3*(3), 61–63.

Wojner, A. W. (1996). Optimizing ischemic stroke outcomes: An interdisciplinary approach to rehabilitation in acute care. *Critical Care Nursing Quarterly, 19*(2), 47–61.

*World Health Organization. (1980). *International classification of impairments, disabilities and handicaps*. Geneva: Author.

SUGGESTED READINGS

Hamilton, L., & Lyon, P. S. (1994). A nursing-driven program to preserve and restore functional ability in hospitalized elderly patients. *Journal of Nursing Administration, 25*(4), 30–37.

In this article, the authors discuss the hazards of hospitalization for the elderly and the successful implementation of a six-bed unit for geriatric assessment and rehabilitation in a community hospital. Although interdisciplinary in focus, the entire program was managed and evaluated by the nursing staff.

Hellman, E. A., & Williams, M. A. (1994). Outpatient cardiac rehabilitation in elderly patients. *Heart and Lung, 23*(6), 506–512.

The authors review available data regarding exercise training in elderly clients with heart disease. Both female and male clients improve in functional capacity and reduced myocardial work as a benefit of exercise. A quiz for continuing education contact hours follows this article.

Neal, L. J. (1995). The rehabilitation nurse in the home setting: Treating chronic wounds as a disability. *Rehabilitation Nursing, 20*(5), 261–264.

Rehabilitation nurses, along with other home care nurses, treat clients with chronic wounds, including a focus on lifestyle modification. Rehabilitation nurses also treat clients with other disabilities who are at risk for developing wounds and instruct them in wound prevention.

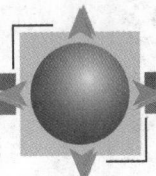

Management of Clients

with Fluid, Electrolyte,

and Acid-Base Imbalances

FLUID AND ELECTROLYTE BALANCE

Every body system is affected by the fluids in and around the tissues and cells. For proper physiologic function, body fluids must be regulated carefully. This regulation ensures adequate distribution, total volume, and concentrations of various substances, especially electrolytes, dissolved in body water. Excesses and deficiencies of body water or electrolytes can cause organ dysfunction that may lead to death. Therefore, all nurses must understand the processes involved in fluid and electrolyte balance to assess accurately each client's total health status.

ANATOMY AND PHYSIOLOGY REVIEW
Physical and Biological Influences on Fluid and Electrolyte Balance

Many physical and biological processes control the normal balance of body fluids and electrolytes. These processes work together to regulate homeostasis (equilibrium) so that even when the external environment undergoes dramatic changes, the body's internal environment remains stable.

Being familiar with the terminology related to solutions is necessary to understand the processes involved in fluid and electrolyte balance (Table 14–1). Body fluids are composed of water and particles dissolved or suspended in water. *Solvent* is the water portion of body fluids. *Solutes* are the particles dissolved in the water. Solutes vary in type and concentration from one body fluid compartment to another. Proper body function is highly dependent on maintaining the correct balance of fluid and specific electrolytes within each body fluid compartment.

Important processes involved in fluid and electrolyte balance include filtration, diffusion, osmosis, and active transport. Capillary dynamics also affect fluid and electrolyte balance. All of these processes or events influence the movement of fluids and particles across biological membranes.

Filtration
Definition

Filtration is the movement of fluid through a biological membrane because of hydrostatic pressure differences on both sides of the membrane. Because filtration depends on hydrostatic pressure, knowledge about the factors influencing hydrostatic pressure is necessary.

All fluid has weight. The overall weight of the fluid is related to the amount of fluid present in the confined space. Water molecules in a confined space constantly

TABLE 14-1

Terminology Associated with Fluid and Electrolyte Balance

Term	Definition
Active transport	• Assisted movement of a substance through a permeable membrane between two fluid compartments against a concentration, electrical, or pressure gradient; requires the expenditure of chemical energy
Adenosine triphosphate (ATP)	• A substance that is generated by the metabolism of glucose or fat within cells and that releases chemical energy for physiologic function when a high-energy phosphate bond ($\sim P$) is broken
Aldosterone	• A hormone secreted by the adrenal cortex that stimulates the renal reabsorption of sodium and water and the renal excretion of potassium
Anion	• A molecule (electrolyte) that carries an overall negative charge when dissolved in water
Antidiuretic hormone (ADH)	• A hormone secreted from the posterior pituitary gland that increases the renal reabsorption of pure water and decreases urinary output
Atrial natriuretic peptide (ANP)	• A hormone secreted by cardiac atrial cells that increases renal excretion of sodium and water
Brownian motion	• Inherent molecular motion
Capillary (plasma) hydrostatic pressure	• The force generated by fluid within a capillary that tends to move fluid out from the capillary and into the interstitial space
Capillary (plasma) osmotic pressure	• The force generated by the concentration of plasma solutes (osmotic and oncotic pressures) that tends to retain fluid within the capillary or move fluid from the interstitial space into the capillary
Cation	• A molecule (electrolyte) that carries an overall positive charge when dissolved in water
Cofactor	• A substance required to enhance the activity of an enzyme or a physiologic reaction
Colloidal oncotic pressure	• The osmotic pressure exerted by the concentration of colloids (proteins) within a solution
Diffusion	• Unimpeded movement of a substance through a permeable membrane between two fluid compartments down a concentration gradient; does not require the expenditure of chemical energy
Disequilibrium	• A state in which two fluid compartments are unequal in at least one characteristic
Electrolytes	• Substances that carry an electrical charge when dissolved in water
Electroneutrality	• A state in which a body fluid has an equal number of cations and anions, so that the fluid does not express an electrical charge
Equilibrium	• A state in which two fluid compartments are equal in one or more characteristics
Extracellular fluid (ECF)	• Body fluid present outside of cells; includes plasma, interstitial fluid, and transcellular fluid
Facilitated diffusion	• Assisted movement of a substance through a permeable membrane between two fluid compartments down a concentration gradient; does not require the expenditure of chemical energy
Filtration	• The movement of fluid through a biologic membrane as a result of hydrostatic pressure differences on the two sides of the membrane
Gradient	• A graded difference in some characteristic between two fluid compartments
Hydrostatic pressure	• The force of pressure exerted by static water in a confined space—"water-pushing" pressure

press outward against the confining boundaries. *Hydrostatic pressure* is the force water molecules exert against the confining walls of the space. This pressure is caused by the weight of fluid against the walls. Hydrostatic pressure may be thought of as "water-pushing" pressure, because it is a major force in moving water outward from a confined space through a membrane (Fig. 14–1).

Physiologic Activity

Water is the largest component of any body fluid. The amount of water in any body fluid compartment is a main factor in determining the hydrostatic pressure of that compartment. The proportion of water present in a fluid is inversely related to the *viscosity* (thickness) of that fluid. Viscosity is a property of fluid relating to its density, specific gravity, and surface tension. Blood, a viscous fluid (one that is thicker than water), is confined within the blood vessels of the vascular system. Blood has hydrostatic pressure because of its weight and volume and also because of cardiac contraction causing the ejection of blood into the arterial circulation.

Whenever a permeable (porous) membrane separates two fluid compartments, the hydrostatic pressures of the two compartments can be compared. If hydrostatic pressure is the same in both fluid compartments, then a state

TABLE 14–1

Terminology Associated with Fluid and Electrolyte Balance *Continued*	
Term	**Definition**
Hypertonic (hyperosmotic)	• Any solution with a solute concentration (osmolarity) greater than that of normal body fluids (>310 mOsm/L)
Hypotonic (hyposmotic)	• Any solution with a solute concentration (osmolarity) less than that of normal body fluids (<270 mOsm/L)
Impermeable membrane	• A membrane separating two fluid compartments that does not permit the movement of one or more substances through the membrane (by diffusion) from one compartment to the other
Insensible fluid loss	• Unregulated fluid losses from the skin, the gastrointestinal tract, wounds, and the pulmonary epithelium
Interstitial fluid	• Fluid present in tissues between cells
Intracellular fluid (ICF)	• Fluid found inside cells
Isotonic (isosmotic)	• Any solution with a solute concentration equal to the osmolarity of normal body fluids or normal saline (0.9% NaCl), ~300 mOsm/L
Obligatory urinary output	• The minimal amount of urinary output necessary to ensure the excretion of metabolic wastes (~400 mL/day)
Osmolality	• The concentration of solute within a solution as measured by the amount of solute osmoles per kilogram of solvent
Osmolarity	• The concentration of solute within a solution as measured by the amount of solute osmoles per liter of solution
Osmoreceptor	• Specialized sensory nerve cells in the thalamus or the hypothalamus that are sensitive to changes in the osmolarity of extracellular fluid
Osmosis	• Diffusion of water only through a selectively permeable membrane from an area of lower osmotic pressure to an area of greater osmotic pressure
Osmotic pressure	• The pressure exerted by a solution that contains a relatively high concentration of solute; this pressure draws water from areas or compartments with lower concentrations of solute into the areas or compartments with higher concentrations of solute—"water-pulling" pressure
Permeable membrane	• A membrane separating two fluid compartments that permits movement of one or more substances through the membrane (by diffusion) from one compartment to the other
Solubility	• The degree to which any given solute completely dissolves (dissociates) in water
Solute	• The solid particles dissolved in a solution
Solvent	• The fluid (water) portion of a solution
Tissue hydrostatic pressure (THP)	• The force generated by fluid within the interstitial spaces that tends to move fluid into the capillary from the interstitial space
Tissue osmotic pressure (TOP)	• The force generated by the concentration of interstitial fluid solutes that tend to retain fluid in the interstitial space or move fluid from the capillary into the interstitial space
Transcellular fluid	• Extracellular fluid confined to a specific area or region of the body (cerebrospinal fluid, pericardial fluid, visceral fluid, aqueous humor, peritoneal fluid, and pleural fluid)
Viscosity	• Gumminess or thickness of the molecules in a solution, causing friction within that solution

of *equilibrium* exists for hydrostatic pressure. If the hydrostatic pressure is not the same in both compartments, then a state of *disequilibrium* exists. This means that the two compartments have a *gradient*, or graded difference, of hydrostatic pressure: One compartment has a higher hydrostatic pressure than the other. Because the human body is a dynamic system and constantly seeks equilibrium, a gradient across a membrane causes forces to rearrange the distribution of substances on both sides of the membrane until an equilibrium is reached (Fig. 14–2).

In most instances, substances move or are rearranged in the direction from the greater amount of pressure or concentration to the lesser amount. Thus, when a hydrostatic pressure gradient exists between two fluid compartments, fluid from the compartment with the higher hydrostatic pressure moves (filters) through the membrane into the fluid compartment with the lower hydrostatic pressure. This filtration continues only as long as the hydrostatic pressure gradient exists. When enough fluid leaves the compartment that initially had the higher pressure and enters the compartment that initially had the lower pressure to make the hydrostatic pressure in both compartments equal, an equilibrium is reached.

When the two compartments are in equilibrium for hydrostatic pressure, a gradient no longer exists between them. Although water molecules may be exchanged

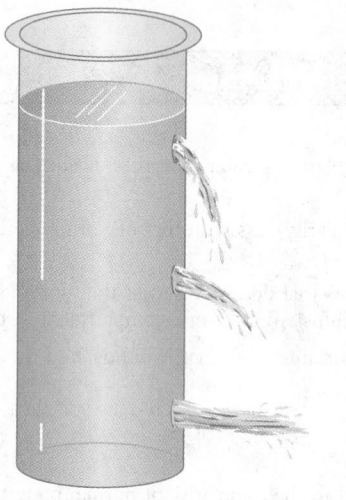

Figure 14–1. Hydrostatic pressure. The pressure water molecules exert against the sides of the container is highest where the weight of the water is greatest. (From Nave, C., & Nave, B. [1985]. Hydrostatic pressure. In *Physics for the health sciences* [3rd ed.]. Philadelphia: W. B. Saunders.)

evenly back and forth between two compartments in equilibrium, no net filtration of fluid occurs. In equilibrium, neither compartment gains or loses water molecules, and the hydrostatic pressure in both compartments remains the same.

Clinical Function and Significance

Blood pressure is a hydrostatic filtering force measured in millimeters of mercury (mmHg). It moves whole blood from the heart to tissue areas where filtration can occur. Filtration is important for the exchange of water, nutri-

ents, and waste products when blood arrives at the tissue capillaries. One factor that determines whether fluid leaves the vascular system and enters the tissue spaces (interstitial fluid) is the difference between the hydrostatic pressure of the fluid in the capillaries and that of the fluid in the interstitial tissue spaces.

The lining of capillaries is only one cell layer thick. Therefore, the wall holding blood in the capillaries is thin. In addition, large spaces, or *pores,* between the cells in the capillary membrane (Fig. 14–3) help water filter freely through capillary membranes in either direction if a hydrostatic pressure gradient is present. This concept is discussed later in this chapter under the heading Capillary Dynamics.

Edema (tissue swelling) can develop as a result of changes in normal hydrostatic pressure gradients, such as in clients with right-sided congestive heart failure. In this clinical situation, the volume of blood in the right side of the heart increases greatly because the right ventricle is too weak to efficiently pump blood into the pulmonary vascular system. As blood volume accumulates, blood backs up into the venous system, and the venous hydrostatic pressure rises. The increased venous pressure causes capillary hydrostatic pressure to increase until it is higher than the hydrostatic pressure in the interstitial spaces. Excess filtration of fluid from the capillaries into the interstitial tissue spaces then occurs, resulting in the formation of visible edema.

Diffusion
Definition

Diffusion is the free movement of particles across a permeable membrane down a *concentration gradient,* that is,

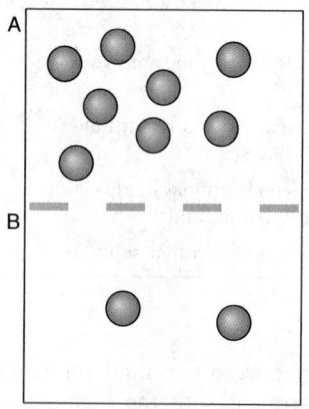

Compartment A has more water molecules and greater hydrostatic pressure than does compartment B.

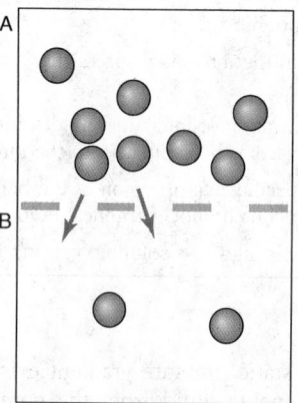

Water molecules move down the hydrostatic pressure gradient from compartment A through the permeable membrane into compartment B, which has a lower hydrostatic pressure.

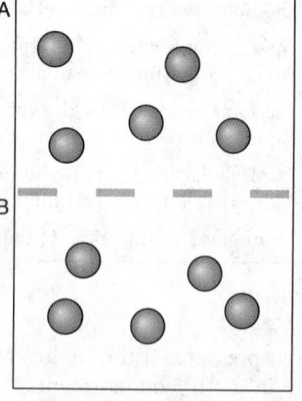

Enough water molecules have moved down the hydrostatic pressure gradient from compartment A into compartment B that both sides now have the same amount of water and the same amount of hydrostatic pressure. An equilibrium of hydrostatic pressure now exists between the two compartments, and no further *net* movement of water will occur.

Figure 14–2. The process of filtration. (© M. Linda Workman, 1992. All rights reserved.)

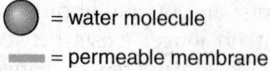

= water molecule

= permeable membrane

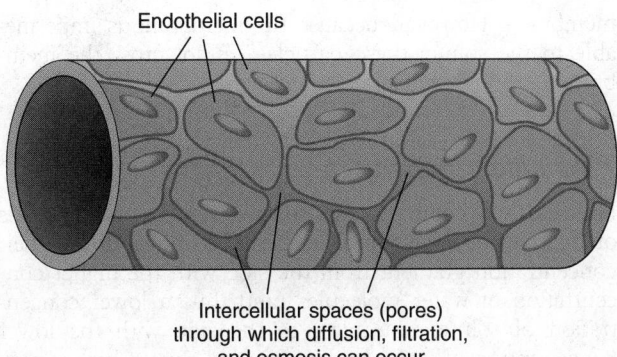

Endothelial cells

Intercellular spaces (pores)
through which diffusion, filtration,
and osmosis can occur

Figure 14–3. The basic structure of a capillary.

from an area of higher concentration to an area of lower concentration. Diffusion controls the movement of particles in solution across various body membranes.

Physiologic Activity

Diffusion of particles into and out of cells and fluid compartments occurs via *brownian motion,* the kinetic energy of molecular motion. Brownian motion is the vibration of individual molecules caused by electrons orbiting at the core of a molecule. It produces totally random movement of molecules. This random movement causes molecules to move and collide with each other within a confined space. The collisions usually cause a temporary increase in the speed of the movement after the molecules hit.

As a result of these collisions, molecules in a solution spread out evenly through whatever space is available. They move from an area of higher concentration of atoms and molecules to an area of lower concentration, until an equality of concentrations is achieved in all areas. The number of collisions is related to the concentration of molecules in a confined space. Spaces with many molecules have more collisions and faster molecular motion than spaces with fewer molecules.

A concentration gradient exists when two areas have different concentrations of the same type of molecules. Brownian motion of the molecules causes them to move down the concentration gradient. As a result of the brownian motion, any membrane that separates two areas is struck repeatedly by molecules. When the molecule strikes a pore in the membrane that is large enough for it to pass through, diffusion occurs (Fig. 14–4). The likelihood of any single molecule colliding with the membrane and going through a pore is much greater on the side of the membrane with a higher molecule concentration.

The speed of diffusion is directly related to the degree of concentration difference between the two sides of the membrane. The degree of concentration difference is usually referred to as the steepness of the gradient: The larger the concentration difference between the two sides, the steeper the gradient. Diffusion occurs more rapidly when the concentration gradient is steeper (just as a ball rolls downhill more rapidly when the hill is steep than when the hill is nearly flat). The greater the difference in concentration, the more rapidly diffusion occurs from the

area of higher concentration to the area of lower concentration.

Diffusion of solute particles continues through the membrane as long as a concentration gradient exists between the two sides of the membrane. When the concentration of solute is the same on both sides of the membrane, an equilibrium exists and an equal exchange—not a net movement—of solute continues.

Clinical Function and Significance

Diffusion is important in the transport of gases and in the movement of most electrolytes, atoms, and molecules through biological membranes. Unlike capillary membranes, which permit diffusion of most small-sized substances down a concentration gradient, cell membranes are *selective.* That is, they permit movement of some substances and inhibit movement of other substances. Some molecules cannot move across a cell membrane, even when a steep "downhill" gradient exists, because the membrane is impermeable (not porous) to that molecule. Thus, the concentration gradient is maintained across the membrane.

This impermeability, along with special transport mechanisms, accounts for differences in concentrations of specific substances from one fluid compartment to another. For example, under normal conditions the extracellular fluid (ECF) contains almost ten times more sodium ions than the fluid inside the cell, the intracellular fluid (ICF). The relative impermeability of the cell membrane to sodium and a special "sodium pump" that moves any extra sodium out of the cell "uphill" against its concentration gradient and back into the extracellular fluid account for this extreme concentration difference.

In some instances, diffusion cannot occur without assistance, even down steep concentration gradients, because of membrane selectivity. A clinical example is the fact that even though the concentration of glucose is much higher in the ECF than it is in the intracellular

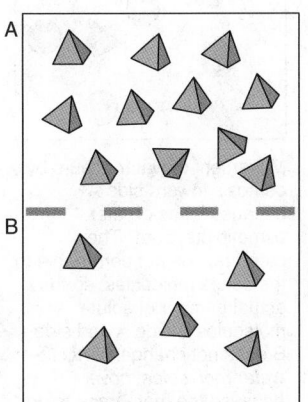 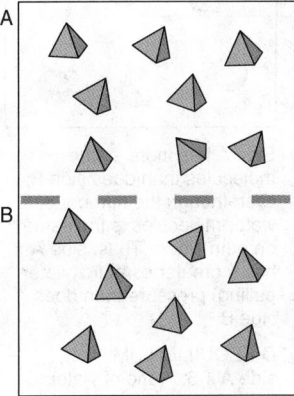

The concentration of solute is greater on side A than on side B, with a permeable membrane separating the two compartments.

Solute molecules have diffused from side A through the membrane into side B until an equilibrium of solute exists and the concentration of solute is the same on both sides.

Figure 14–4. Diffusion of a solute.

fluid (ICF), creating a steep gradient for glucose, glucose cannot cross most cell membranes without the assistance of insulin. When insulin is present in the ECF, it binds to insulin receptor sites on cell membranes. When insulin binds to the cell membranes, the membranes become much more permeable to glucose.

Glucose can then cross the cellular membrane down its concentration gradient until either an equilibrium of glucose concentration is created or insulin binding decreases. Diffusion across a cell membrane requiring the assistance of a transport system or membrane-altering system, such as insulin, is called *facilitated diffusion* or *facilitated transport*. Because this type of transport occurs down a concentration gradient and requires no energy expenditure by the cell, it is considered a form of diffusion.

Osmosis
Definition

Osmosis is the process by which only the water molecules (solvent) move through a selectively permeable membrane. A membrane must separate two fluid compartments for osmosis to occur. At least one of these fluid compartments must contain a solute that cannot move through the membrane. (The membrane is therefore impermeable to this solute.) A concentration gradient of this solute must also exist. If the membrane were permeable to this solute, then the solute would diffuse through the membrane down its concentration gradient until the concentrations of solute were equal on both sides of the membrane. However, because the membrane is impermeable to the solute, these particles cannot cross the membrane (although water molecules can).

Physiologic Activity

For the fluid compartments to have equal concentrations of solute, the water molecules must move down their concentration gradient from the side with the higher concentration of water molecules (and thus a lower concentration of solute molecules) to the side with the lower concentration of water molecules (and thus a higher concentration of solute molecules). This movement continues until both compartments contain the same proportions of solute to solvent. The less concentrated fluid contains proportionately fewer solute molecules and more water molecules than the more concentrated fluid. Water therefore moves by osmosis down its concentration gradient from the area of more dilute solute to the area of more concentrated solute until a new equilibrium is achieved (Fig. 14–5).

At this point, the concentrations of solute in the fluid compartments (the proportion of solute to solvent) on both sides of the membrane are equal, even though the total numbers of solute and volume of water may be different. This equilibrium is achieved by the movement of water molecules rather than the movement of solute molecules.

Factors that determine whether and how rapidly osmosis occurs include

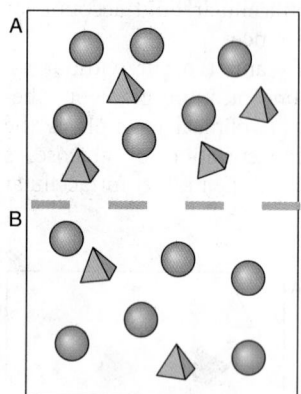

Side A has more solute molecules than does side B, even though the number of water molecules is the same on both sides. Thus, side A has a greater osmotic (water pulling) pressure than does side B.

DISEQUILIBRIUM
side A 1.5:1 ratio of water to solute
side B 3:1 ratio of water to solute

○ = water molecule

▬▬ = permeable membrane

△ = solute molecule

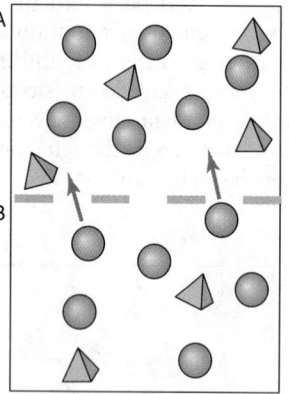

Movement of water occurs by osmosis toward side A because it has greater osmotic pressure. The membrane is *not* permeable to the solute molecules, so the actual number of solute molecules is side A and side B does not change. *Only the water molecules move because the membrane is not permeable to the solute molecules.*

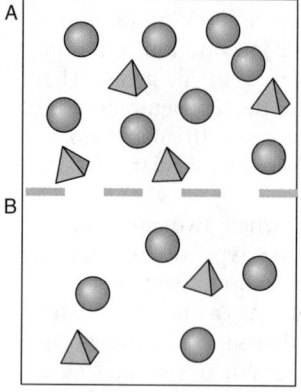

Enough water molecules have moved from side B into side A that the actual concentration of solute is now the same on both sides, with a ratio of water to solute of 2:1. An equilibrium of osmotic pressure now exists between the two compartments, and no further *net* movement of water molecules or solute molecules will occur.

EQUILIBRIUM
side A 2:1 ratio of water to solute
side B 2:1 ratio of water to solute

Figure 14–5. The process of osmosis.

- The overall concentration of osmotically active particles (solute) in solution
- The solubility of the solute (how easily the solute dissolves in water)
- The amount of membrane available for osmosis

Concentration of Solute. The concentration of particles in human body fluids is expressed in milliequivalents per liter (mEq/L), millimoles per liter (mmol/L), and milliosmoles per liter (mOsm/L). Osmoles and milliosmoles are used to express the total concentration of solute particles (including electrolytes) contained within a solution. The number of milliosmoles present in body fluids can be expressed as either osmolarity or osmolality.

Osmolarity is defined as the number of milliosmoles in a *liter* of solution; *osmolality* is defined as the number of milliosmoles in a *kilogram* of solution. The normal osmolarity value for plasma and other body fluids ranges from 270 to 300 mOsm/L (Guyton & Hall, 1996).

The body functions best when the osmolarity of the fluids in all compartments is about 300 mOsm/L. Many mechanisms function to maintain solute concentration homeostasis. When all body fluids have this solute concentration, the osmotic pressures (water-pulling) of the various fluid compartments are essentially equal and no *net* water movement occurs. In such a situation, the body fluids are said to be *isosmotic* to each other. Another term with essentially the same meaning is *isotonic* (sometimes called *normotonic*). Examples of specific intravenous solutions with overall concentrations of specific substances equaling 270 to 300 mOsm/L include 0.9% sodium chloride in water and the complex formula of Ringer's lactate in water (Trissel, 1994). Because these substances are isotonic, or isosmotic, to plasma, their addition to plasma does not change plasma osmolarity or plasma osmotic pressure.

Fluids with osmolarities (solute concentrations) greater than 300 mOsm/L are said to be hyperosmotic, or hypertonic, compared with isosmotic fluids. Hyperosmotic fluids have a greater osmotic pressure than do isosmotic fluids and tend to pull water from the isosmotic fluid compartment into the hyperosmotic fluid compartment until an osmotic balance is achieved.

Fluids with osmolarities of less than 270 mOsm/L are said to be hypo-osmotic, or hypotonic, compared with isosmotic fluids. Hyposmolar fluids have a lower or smaller osmotic pressure than isosmotic fluids. As a result, water tends to be pulled from the hypo-osmotic fluid compartment into the isosmotic fluid compartment until an osmotic balance is achieved (Metheny, 1996).

Solubility of Solute. *Solubility* refers to the degree to which a solute dissolves or dissociates completely in water. Solubility is directly related to osmotic pressure: The greater the solubility of the solutes in a fluid, the higher the osmotic pressure of that fluid.

Amount of Available Membrane. The greater the amount of membrane available for osmosis, the faster the rate of osmosis. More membrane increases the chances that water molecules will strike the membrane at a point where penetration is possible.

Clinical Function and Significance

The process of osmosis acts with the process of filtration in capillary fluid dynamics to regulate both extracellular and intracellular fluid volumes. The thirst mechanism is an excellent example of the importance of osmosis in maintaining homeostasis. Thirst results from activation of cells in the hypothalamus of the brain that respond to changes in extracellular fluid (ECF) osmolarity. These cells are so sensitive to changes in ECF osmolarity that they are called *osmoreceptors*. When a person loses body fluids, especially water, such as through excessive sweating during prolonged heavy exercise, the ECF volume is decreased and the osmolarity is increased (hypertonic conditions exist). The cells in the thirst center shrink as water moves from the cells into the hypertonic ECF. Shrinking of these cells stimulates a person's awareness of thirst and increases the urge to drink. The person will usually drink enough fluid to replace that lost through sweating and restore the ECF osmolarity to its normal value. After the ECF volume and osmolarity return to normal levels, the osmoreceptors return to their normal size and no longer send stimulatory messages.

Active Transport
Definition

A cell must expend energy to move a substance across the cell membrane against a concentration gradient (uphill). Such movement is called *active transport*, because the cell must make active efforts for the net movement to occur. Because of its energy demands and uphill movement, active transport is sometimes called "pumping," and the mechanisms are known as membrane pumps.

Physiologic Activity

Active transport systems, or pumps, are usually located in the cell membrane and act as "gatekeepers" to maintain special environments inside cells. Some active transport pumps can carry more than one substance across the membrane at the same time. In these instances, the pump usually moves one substance into a cell and a different substance out of the cell at the same time. This process is called *cotransport*. Both transports are uphill against individual concentration gradients and require energy. The sodium-potassium pump is an example of such a double active transport system.

Sodium tends to diffuse slightly down its concentration gradient into the intracellular fluid (ICF) because it has such a high extracellular fluid (ECF) concentration compared with its ICF concentration. Similarly, because potassium has such a high concentration inside the cells compared with its concentration in ECF, it tends to diffuse slightly down its concentration gradient into the ECF. The action of the sodium-potassium pump moves the extra sodium out of the cell, while returning the lost potassium back into the cell. The sodium-potassium pump requires cellular energy expenditure.

The cellular energy for this process usually comes from breaking a high-energy bond ($\sim$P) when a phosphate group is split off from an adenosine triphosphate (ATP) molecule. Functioning of active transport pumps depends on the presence of adequate cellular ATP.

Clinical Function and Significance

Cells use active transport to control the intracellular concentration of many substances and to regulate cell volume. All cells function best when their internal environments are maintained separately from the changes occurring in the extracellular fluid (ECF) environment.

A clinical example of the results of active transport failure is the series of events following hypoxia (decreased oxygen supply in the body). Without adequate oxygen, ATP cannot be produced in sufficient amounts. Without ATP, the sodium-potassium pump cannot remove the extra sodium ions that have diffused from the ECF into the cell. The increased sodium concentration inside the cell increases the osmolarity and the osmotic pressure of the fluid inside the cell. Water moves into the cell in response to the increased osmotic pressure, which causes the cell to swell and perhaps to lyse (break open) and die if oxygen is not provided.

Table 14-2 summarizes the membrane processes involved in fluid and electrolyte balance.

Capillary Dynamics

The circulatory system distributes nutrients and removes wastes at the tissue level. The most important blood vessels for nutrient-waste exchange are the thin-walled, porous capillaries. Nutrient distribution and waste removal depend on capillary fluid movement.

Fluid movement at the capillary level is dynamic not only because it is continuous but also because relative homeostasis of vascular and interstitial fluid volumes must be maintained. Opposing processes must occur for nutrients to move into tissue spaces, for wastes to move into circulation, and for the fluid volumes of both the vascular and tissue spaces to be maintained. In these processes, some fluid with nutrients must leave the capillary and enter the interstitial (tissue space) fluid compartment for a short period, which temporarily expands the interstitial fluid volume. The nutrients in the interstitial fluid are then taken up by the cells through various membrane transport processes. Water may be exchanged between the intracellular compartment and the interstitial compartment, but under normal circumstances, no net change in water volume occurs. Metabolic wastes created in the cells are moved into the interstitial fluid. Any extra fluid in the interstitial space, together with the waste products excreted from cells, must be returned via the capillary to the systemic circulation. Without a way to return the fluid originally lost into the interstitial compartment back to the blood, the vascular volume would become depleted to the point of circulatory failure and the interstitial fluid compartment would greatly expand.

Capillary Forces Influencing Fluid Movement

Forces at the capillary level permit capillary fluid loss to be followed by a return of fluid to the capillary so that a near-equilibrium of fluid distribution is maintained at the capillary-tissue level. These forces, known as *Starling's forces*, are outlined in Figure 14-6. The near equilibrium is based on the fact that forces tending to move fluid out from the capillary at the arterial end are nearly equal to the forces tending to move fluid from the interstitial compartment back into the capillary at the venous end.

Blood flowing from the arterial end of the capillary to the venous end is controlled by

TABLE 14-2

Summary of Membrane-Fluid Actions		
Action	**Definition**	**Specific Characteristics**
Filtration	• The movement of fluid through a biologic membrane as a result of hydrostatic pressure differences on both sides of the membrane	• Does not require energy • Is limited to solvent and low–molecular-weight solute • Usually occurs from capillaries to the interstitial fluid • Depends on hydrostatic pressure differences • Occurs more rapidly with steep gradients
Diffusion	• Free movement of substances across a permeable membrane down a concentration gradient	• Does not require energy • Is not pressure-dependent • Moves solute as well as solvent down their individual gradients • Occurs more rapidly with steep gradients • Is directly related in speed to the amount of membrane available • Occurs in both directions across capillary and cell membranes • Is responsible for maintaining tissue nutrition
Osmosis	• The process by which only the *solvent* diffuses through a selectively permeable membrane	• Does not require energy • Involves movement of water only • Depends on hydrostatic and osmotic pressures • Occurs more rapidly with steep gradients
Active transport	• The movement of a substance across a selectively permeable membrane against a concentration, electrical, or pressure gradient	• Requires energy • Requires a transport system (pump) • Helps maintain a special intracellular environment

Capillary blood normally flows from the arterial to the venous end:

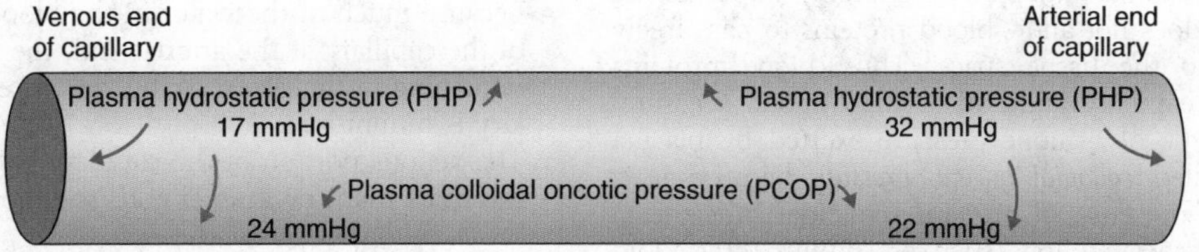

Venous end
of capillary

Arterial end
of capillary

Plasma hydrostatic pressure (PHP) ↗
17 mmHg

↖ Plasma hydrostatic pressure (PHP)
32 mmHg

↙ Plasma colloidal oncotic pressure (PCOP) ↘
24 mmHg

22 mmHg

Tissue hydrostatic pressure (THP) 8 mmHg
Tissue osmotic pressure (TOP) 6 mmHg

Tissue hydrostatic pressure (THP) 4 mmHg
Tissue osmotic pressure (TOP) 10 mmHg

At the arterial end, the forces that tend to move fluid from the capillary into the tissue space are
Plasma hydrostatic pressure 32 mmHg
+
Tissue osmotic pressure 10 mmHg
_____
Total forces moving fluid out = 42 mmHg
At the arterial end, the forces that tend to move fluid from the tissue spaces into the capillary are
Tissue hydrostatic pressure 4 mmHg
+
Plasma colloidal oncotic pressure 22 mmHg
_____
Total forces moving fluid in = 26 mmHg
The total forces tending to move fluid out at the arterial end are 16 mmHg higher than the total forces tending to move
fluid in at the arterial end (42 − 26 = 16). Thus, at the arterial end, fluid leaks out of the capillary into the tissue
(interstitial) spaces.
At the venous end of the same capillary, the forces that tend to move fluid from the capillary into the tissue space are
Plasma hydrostatic pressure 17 mmHg
+
Tissue osmotic pressure 6 mmHg
_____
Total forces moving fluid out = 23 mmHg
At the venous end of the capillary, the forces that tend to move fluid from the tissue spaces back into the capillary are
Tissue hydrostatic pressure 8 mmHg
+
Plasma colloidal oncotic pressure 24 mmHg
_____
Total forces moving fluid in = 32 mmHg
The total forces tending to move fluid out at the venous end are 9 mmHg lower than the total forces tending to move
fluid into the capillary at the venous end (32 − 23 = 9). Thus, at the venous end, fluid moves from the tissue spaces back
into the capillary.
Because the pressures tending to move fluid out of the capillary at the arterial end (16 mmHg) are greater than the pressures
that tend to move fluid back into the capillary at the venous end (9 mmHg), more fluid is lost from the capillary than is returned
to it. Lymph drainage eventually returns this extra lost fluid to systemic circulation.

Figure 14–6. Capillary dynamics.

- Hydrostatic pressure of blood
- Dynamic ejection of blood from the left ventricle of the heart
- Patency or openness of the capillaries

The blood entering the arterial end of the capillary has a blood pressure, or a capillary (plasma) hydrostatic pressure (PHP), of about 32 mmHg. The capillary membrane is thin and permeable. The usual tissue hydrostatic pressure is low. These factors create a natural tendency for filtration from the blood outward into the tissue spaces. The fluid portion of the blood, along with most of the smaller substances dissolved in the blood, filters through the capillary membrane into the tissue spaces. Through this process, nutrients and other essential substances can reach the cells.

If net filtration, as a result of plasma hydrostatic pres-

sure, were the only force or factor involved at this level, blood volume would be progressively lost from the vascular space and would appear in the tissues. Fortunately, other mechanisms that favor the reabsorption of tissue fluid into the capillaries are also part of capillary dynamics. These mechanisms are plasma osmotic pressure and tissue hydrostatic pressure.

Osmosis (of water) through the capillary membrane (in either direction) occurs in response to differences in the concentrations of osmotically active substances in the capillary blood and in the tissue fluid. Tissue osmotic pressure (TOP) tends to draw fluid out of the capillary. Plasma osmotic pressure (POP) in the capillary tends to keep fluid in the capillary and to draw fluid from the interstitial space into the capillary. Under normal conditions, capillary plasma osmotic pressure is greater than tissue osmotic pressure because of the higher concentration of proteins in the blood compared with the protein concentration in the interstitial fluid.

Because the capillary membrane is highly impermeable to proteins, it does not allow blood proteins to pass freely through it into the tissue space. Thus, blood proteins remain in the capillary and add to the osmotic pressure. The specific type of osmotic pressure exerted by plasma proteins is called *colloidal oncotic pressure* because it is caused by the presence of proteins (colloidal substances) rather than dissociated ions such as sodium (crystalloid substances). The average colloidal oncotic pressure in capillary blood is about 22 mmHg.

Blood pressure (hydrostatic pressure) is greater than colloidal oncotic pressure at the arterial end of the capillary. Capillary hydrostatic pressure favors the filtration of fluid from the capillary into the tissue spaces, and colloidal oncotic pressure favors the reabsorption of fluid from the interstitial space into the capillary. The difference between these two capillary pressures at the arterial end of the capillary indicates a greater filtering force outward than a reabsorbing force inward.

Tissue Forces Influencing Fluid Movement

Tissue forces also influence the movement of solutions at the capillary level. These forces are tissue hydrostatic pressure (THP) and tissue osmotic pressure (TOP). Usually, both are relatively small forces. However, in some diseases, these forces increase greatly and significantly alter capillary dynamics.

To determine the direction of fluid movement in any one area of the capillary, the forces that move fluid out of the capillary are compared with the forces that move fluid into the capillary. Two forces at the arterial end that move fluid out of the capillary are the plasma hydrostatic pressure (PHP) (normally about 32 mmHg) and the tissue osmotic pressure (TOP) (normally about 10 mmHg). The pressures at the arterial end that return fluid to the capillary are the plasma colloidal oncotic pressure (normally about 22 mmHg) and the tissue hydrostatic pressure (THP) (normally about 4 mmHg). Because the outward filtration force is 16 mmHg higher than the inward reabsorbing force, the overall result at the arterial end of the capillary is the outward filtration of fluid and small solute particles into the tissue spaces.

Plasma hydrostatic pressure (PHP) decreases along the length of the capillary as blood flows through it. As filtration proceeds along the capillary, water is lost from the capillary, and the PHP gradually decreases. Therefore, the pressures that create the outward filtration force (from the capillary into the interstitial fluid) decrease, while the pressures that create the inward reabsorption force (from the interstitial fluid into the capillary) remain the same. Eventually, the outward filtration pressures and the inward reabsorption pressures become equal.

Clinical Function and Significance

Finally, at the venous end of the capillary, the inward reabsorption forces exceed the outward filtration forces. The venous end of the capillary has a much lower hydro-static pressure than does the arterial end. This decreased hydrostatic pressure has two causes:

- Because much of the water in the blood was filtered out of the capillary at the arterial end, the volume of water remaining in the blood at the venous end of the capillary is diminished.
- The venous portion of the capillary is farther away from the heart than the arterial end, so blood pressure is lower in the venous end.

The hydrostatic pressure in the venous end of the capillary is low, and the interstitial fluid (tissue) hydrostatic pressure is high (because water moved from the arterial end of the capillary into the interstitial space). The colloidal osmotic pressure at the venous end of the capillary exceeds that at the arterial end because water was lost, increasing the concentration of proteins. The tissue osmotic pressure at the venous end of the capillary is lower than at the arterial end of the capillary because the water lost from the capillary has diluted the solute concentration of the tissue fluid. As a result, forces favoring the return of water from the tissues into the capillary are greater than the forces favoring filtration, and some water returns from the interstitial space back into the capillary at the venous end.

Lymph

Usually, not all the fluid that leaves the capillary at the arterial end and enters the interstitial space is returned to the capillary at the venous end. A small amount remains in the tissues. If this situation were not balanced by another mechanism to return the fluid to the systemic circulation, the circulating volume would become depleted and the interstitial areas would constantly be edematous. Instead, this extra fluid leaking out from the capillaries is returned to systemic circulation as *lymph*.

Lymph fluid is similar to blood plasma (from which it is formed) but contains far less protein. It is returned to systemic circulation by components of the auxiliary venous system known as lymph vessels, or *lymphatics*. Lymphatics begin as small, thin-walled, vein-like vessels that merge to form larger lymphatic vessels. Two large groups of lymphatic vessels connect the entire lymph system with the general circulatory system. The left thoracic lymph duct drains lymph from the abdomen, the gastrointestinal tract, the pelvis, the lower extremities, the left side of the thorax, the left arm, and the left side of the head and neck into the left subclavian vein at the point where it joins the left internal jugular vein (Fig. 14–7). Lymph from the right arm, the right side of the thorax, and right side of the head and neck drains into the right subclavian vein through three lymph ducts. Lymph nodes are situated along the lymphatic paths and act as lymph fluid filters.

Lymphatics carry lymph fluid in one direction— toward the heart. Lymph flow is slower than blood flow because lymph has no pump and no direct connection between the arterial blood circulation and the lymphatic system. The physical mechanisms that enhance lymph flow are skeletal muscle contractions, intrathoracic pres-

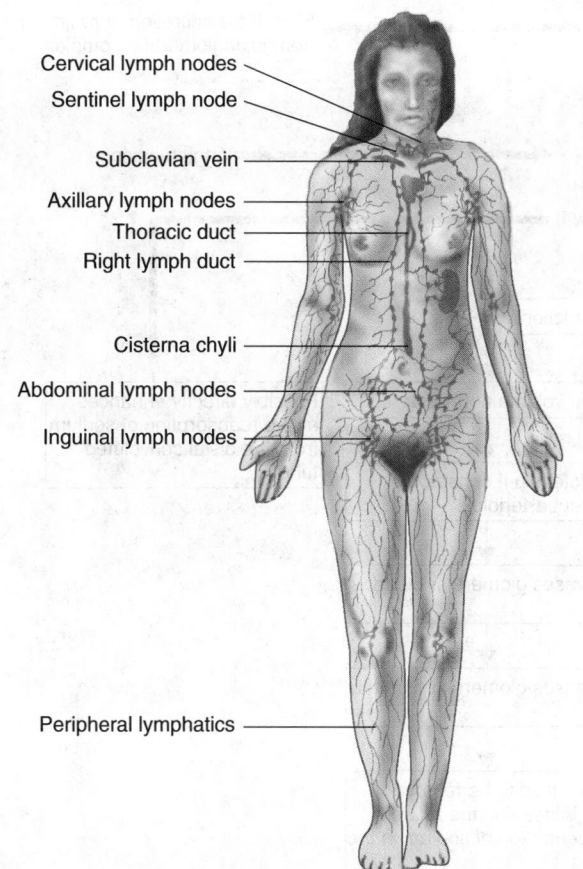

Cervical lymph nodes
Sentinel lymph node
Subclavian vein
Axillary lymph nodes
Thoracic duct
Right lymph duct
Cisterna chyli
Abdominal lymph nodes
Inguinal lymph nodes
Peripheral lymphatics

Figure 14–7. Patterns of lymph drainage. (From Lymph drainage. In Guyton, A., & Hall, J. [1996]. *Textbook of medical physiology* [9th ed., p. 194]. Philadelphia: W. B. Saunders.)

sure changes that occur during pulmonary ventilation, and an intrinsic peristalsis-like motion in lymph vessels.

Hormonal Influences on Fluid and Electrolyte Balance

Many endocrine mechanisms assist in the regulation of fluid and electrolyte balance. Three hormones that help control these critical balances are aldosterone, antidiuretic hormone (ADH), and atrial natriuretic peptide (ANP).

Aldosterone

Aldosterone is a *mineralocorticoid* (a naturally occurring steroid) secreted by the adrenal cortex. Aldosterone secretion is stimulated by either a decreased sodium level in the extracellular fluid (ECF) or an increased sodium level in urine. Aldosterone, angiotensinogen, and angiotensin secretion and function are outlined in Figure 14–8. Aldosterone directly influences sodium balance by preventing sodium loss. Because sodium in body fluids exerts osmotic (water-pulling) pressure, water attempts to follow sodium in physiologically proportionate amounts (Guyton

& Hall, 1996). As a result of this sodium-water relationship, aldosterone secretion also indirectly regulates water balance.

In the kidney, blood is supplied to the glomerulus of nephrons via the afferent arteriole. Specialized cells (juxtaglomerular cells) inside the afferent arteriole near the glomerulus are sensitive to changes in serum concentrations of sodium. This area of the afferent arteriole comes into direct contact with a specialized area of the distal convoluted tubule (the macula densa). Together, the juxtaglomerular cells and the macula densa form a functional group called the *juxtaglomerular complex*. When this complex senses that actual serum sodium concentrations are lower than normal or that the total blood volume is low, the macula densa stimulates juxtaglomerular cells to secrete renin.

Renin acts enzymatically on an inactive plasma protein called *angiotensinogen*, converting it to angiotensin I. Angiotensin I is immediately further degraded by an enzyme called angiotensin-converting enzyme into angiotensin II. Angiotensin II causes massive vasoconstriction of many blood vessels and stimulates increased secretion of aldosterone from the adrenal cortex.

Aldosterone acts on the distal convoluted tubules of the nephrons. When serum osmolarity is too low, aldosterone secretion stimulates these areas to reabsorb sodium (in exchange for potassium) from the filtrate (urine) back into systemic circulation, thus increasing serum osmolarity. Aldosterone secretion increases when blood osmolarity or serum sodium levels are low, and its presence is normally required to prevent excessive renal excretion of sodium. Aldosterone secretion also helps prevent serum potassium levels from becoming too high. Secretion of aldosterone is inhibited when serum sodium level or blood osmolarity is greater than normal.

Antidiuretic Hormone

Antidiuretic hormone (ADH), also known as *vasopressin*, is synthesized in specific areas of the brain and stored in the posterior pituitary gland. The release of ADH from the posterior pituitary gland is controlled by the hypothalamus in response to changes in blood osmolarity. The hypothalamus contains specialized cells, known as osmoreceptors, that are sensitive to changes in blood osmolarity. Increased blood osmolarity, especially an increase in plasma sodium concentration, results in slight shrinkage of these cells and triggers the hypothalamus to stimulate the posterior pituitary to release ADH.

Antidiuretic hormone acts directly on the renal tubules and collecting ducts, making them more permeable to water. As a result, more water is reabsorbed by these tubules and returned to the systemic circulation, causing the blood to have decreased osmolarity by becoming more dilute. When the blood osmolarity decreases, especially when the plasma sodium concentration is below normal, the osmoreceptors swell slightly and inhibit the release of ADH. Then, less water is reabsorbed and more is lost from the body in the urine. As a result, the amount of water in the extracellular fluid (ECF) decreases, bringing osmolarity to normal.

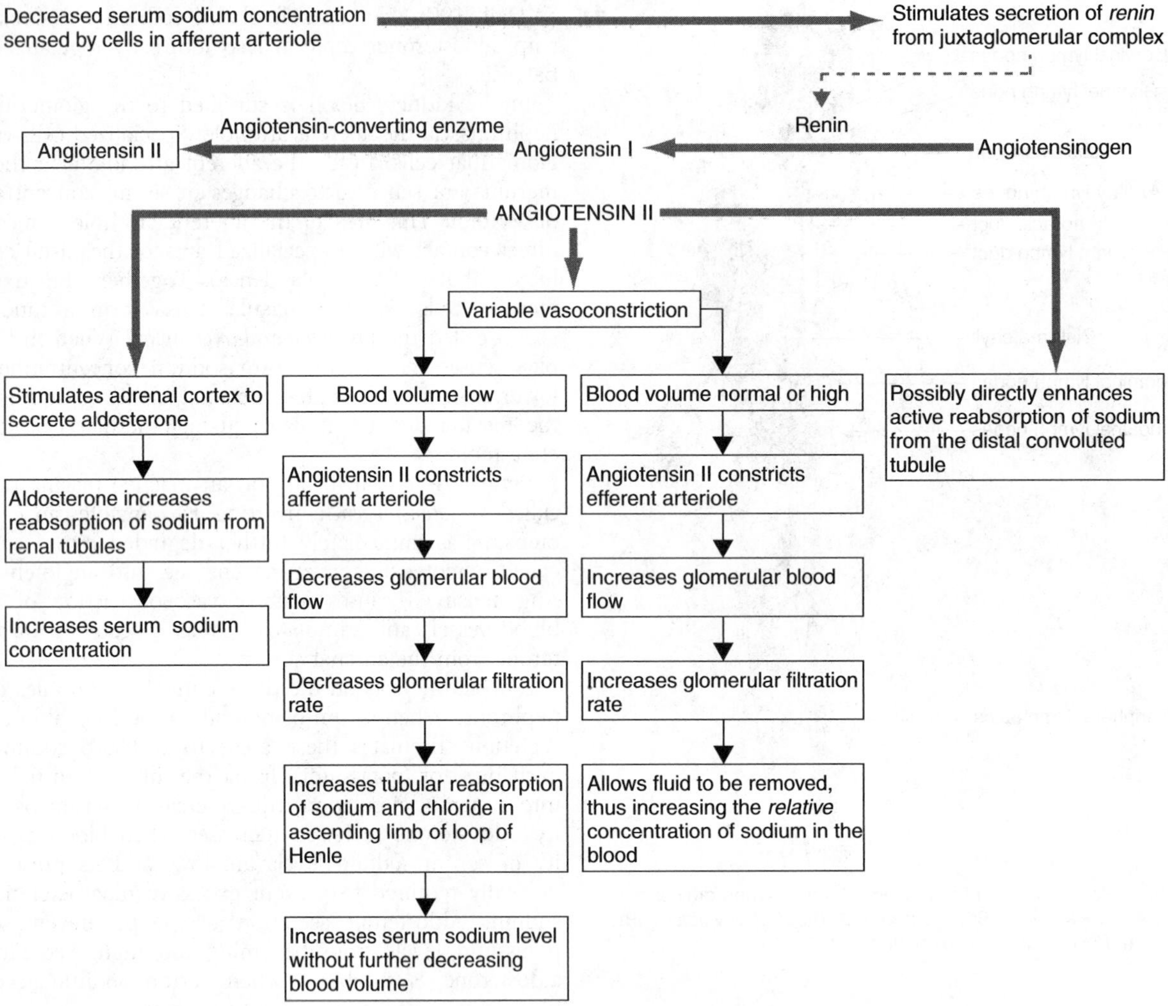

Decreased serum sodium concentration sensed by cells in afferent arteriole ⟶ Stimulates secretion of *renin* from juxtaglomerular complex

Angiotensin II ⟵ Angiotensin-converting enzyme ⟵ Angiotensin I ⟵ Renin ⟵ Angiotensinogen

ANGIOTENSIN II

Variable vasoconstriction

| Stimulates adrenal cortex to secrete aldosterone | Blood volume low | Blood volume normal or high | Possibly directly enhances active reabsorption of sodium from the distal convoluted tubule |

Aldosterone increases reabsorption of sodium from renal tubules

Increases serum sodium concentration

Angiotensin II constricts afferent arteriole

Decreases glomerular blood flow

Decreases glomerular filtration rate

Increases tubular reabsorption of sodium and chloride in ascending limb of loop of Henle

Increases serum sodium level without further decreasing blood volume

Angiotensin II constricts efferent arteriole

Increases glomerular blood flow

Increases glomerular filtration rate

Allows fluid to be removed, thus increasing the *relative* concentration of sodium in the blood

Figure 14–8. The role of aldosterone, angiotensinogen, angiotensin I, and angiotensin II in the renal regulation of water and sodium.

Atrial Natriuretic Peptide

Atrial natriuretic peptide (ANP) is secreted by special cells lining the atria of the heart in response to increased blood volume and blood pressure. ANP binds to receptor sites in the collecting ducts of the nephrons, creating effects opposite to those of aldosterone. Tubular reabsorption of sodium is inhibited at the same time that glomerular filtration is increased (Briggs et al., 1996). The outcome is increased output of urine with a high sodium content, which results in decreased circulating blood volume and decreased blood osmolarity.

Body Fluids

Fluids constitute approximately 55% to 60% of total adult body weight and consist of the extracellular fluid (ECF) and intracellular fluid (ICF). The ECF compartment is approximately 15 L (40%) of total body water and includes interstitial fluid, blood plasma, lymph, bone and connective tissue water, and the fluid within special spaces (called transcellular fluid), such as cerebrospinal

fluid, synovial fluid, peritoneal fluid, and pleural fluid. ICF composes the remaining 25 L (60%) of total body water. Figure 14–9 shows the normal distribution of total body water.

A person's age, gender, and lean mass to body fat ratio influence the amounts and distribution of body fluids. An elderly adult has less body water than a younger adult. Because fat cells contain practically no water compared with other cells, an obese person has less water than a lean person of the same body weight.

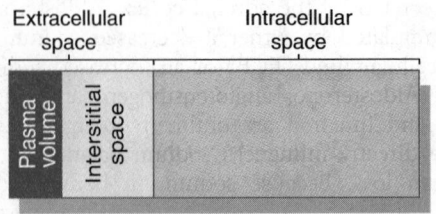

Figure 14–9. Normal distribution of total body water.

WOMEN'S HEALTH CONSIDERATIONS

A woman of any age usually has less total body water than does a man of similar stature of the same age. This difference is because men have greater muscle mass than women, and women have a higher percentage of fat body weight. Differences in muscle mass and percentage of fat body weight are partly due to the influence of sex hormones. This difference in fat to lean body weight may be responsible for some differences seen in women's and men's responses to drugs.

Body fluids are solvents and transport substances. They allow the nutrition of cells and transport biological molecules (such as hormones) important to the regulation of normal physiologic functions. Most physiologic processes occur only in a liquid environment. Body fluids are constantly renewed, purified, and replaced as fluid balance is maintained through intake and output. The total amount of water within each fluid compartment is stable, but water movement occurs continually among all compartments. Water in any compartment is not static but rather is exchanged constantly while maintaining a volume equilibrium. Table 14–3 summarizes key points regarding fluid and electrolyte balance.

Sources of Fluid Intake

Fluid intake is regulated through the thirst drive. Fluids enter the body primarily as liquids (Table 14–4). Because solid foods contain up to 85% water, some fluid also enters the body in ingested solid foods. In addition, water

TABLE 14–3

Summary of Key Points Regarding Fluid and Electrolyte Balance

- All plasma electrolyte values must remain within a narrow range for proper physiologic functioning
- The plasma is the entrance and exit site for all fluids and electrolytes
- The primary organs or tissues of fluid and electrolyte regulation are the hypothalamus, the kidney, the adrenal glands, the posterior pituitary gland, the thyroid gland, and the parathyroid glands
- The total number of positive charges within a solution must be balanced by an equal number of negative charges to maintain electroneutrality
- Although the specific types and concentrations of substances (solute) dissolved in body fluid vary from one fluid compartment to another, the total concentration of all solutes is the same in all fluid compartments (270–300 mOsm/L)
- Whenever possible, the body's regulatory mechanisms attempt to create or maintain an osmolar equilibrium in all body fluid compartments
- A fluid compartment that is hyposmolar (hypotonic) to normal body fluids will expel water from the compartment
- A fluid compartment that is hyperosmolar (hypertonic) to normal body fluids will draw water into it

TABLE 14–4

Routes of Fluid Ingestion and Excretion

Intake	Output
Measurable	
Oral fluids	Urine
Parenteral fluids	Emesis†
Enemas*	Feces†
Irrigation fluids*	Drainage from body cavities
Not Measurable	
Solid foods	Perspiration
Metabolism	Vaporization through the lungs

* Measured by subtracting the amount returned from the amount instilled.
† Measurement accurate only when these substances are excreted in liquid form.

is a byproduct of cellular metabolism. This byproduct is called the water of oxidation. Approximately 10% (300 mL) of daily water requirements is met by the water of oxidation. A rising plasma osmolarity or a decreasing plasma volume stimulates the sensation of thirst. Other sensory input to the hypothalamus, such as dryness of the oral mucosa or sensorimotor input from higher brain areas, can trigger the thirst drive. An adult consumes an average of 1500 mL of fluid per day and obtains an additional 800 mL of fluid from ingested foods.

Routes of Fluid Loss

The body has several routes by which excessive water and waste products are removed (Table 14–4). Of all the water loss pathways, the renal route is the most important and most sensitive. Fluid loss via the renal route is closely regulated and is adjustable. The volume of urine excreted daily varies, depending on the amount of fluid intake and the body's need to conserve fluids.

The minimum amount of urine per day needed to dissolve and excrete the toxic waste products of metabolism ranges from 400 to 600 mL. This minimal volume is called the *obligatory urinary output*. If the 24-hour urine volume falls below the obligatory output amount, metabolic wastes are retained and can cause lethal electrolyte imbalances, acidosis, and toxic build-up of nitrogen. This urine is maximally concentrated, with a specific gravity (weight of the liquid compared with weight of pure water) of 1.032 or higher, and an osmolarity of at least 1200 mOsm/L.

Urine can also become maximally dilute, with a specific gravity of 1.005 and an osmolarity of 200 mOsm/L. This dilution can result from a large fluid intake and is reflected in a large volume of urine output. The concentrating and diluting capacity of the renal tubules is a response to changes in the osmolarity of the extracellular fluid (ECF), the volumes and pressures of the ECF compartments, and variation in the secretion of aldosterone, antidiuretic hormone (ADH), and atrial natriuretic peptide (ANP).

Other normal water loss occurs through the skin, the lungs, and the gastrointestinal tract. Additional water losses can occur via salivation, drainage from fistulas and drains, and gastrointestinal suction.

Water loss from the skin, lungs, and stool, termed *insensible water loss,* can be significant. In a healthy adult, insensible water loss is about 15 to 20 mL/kg per day. Insensible water loss can increase dramatically in hypermetabolic states such as thyroid crisis, trauma, burns, states of extreme stress, and fever. For every degree Celsius of increase in body temperature, insensible water loss increases by 10%. When atmospheric conditions are hot and dry, insensible water loss also increases. Examples of clients at risk for increased insensible water loss include those undergoing mechanical ventilation and those with rapid respirations (tachypnea). Insensible water loss (not including sweat) is pure water and does not contain electrolytes. Therefore, excessive amounts of insensible water loss result in a more hypertonic extracellular fluid (ECF) of a smaller volume. If this loss is not balanced by intake, the hypertonic ECF and accompanying dehydration can lead to *hypernatremia* (elevated serum sodium level).

Loss by sweating is variable and can reach a maximal rate of about 2 L/hour. Sweat, although it contains electrolytes, is slightly hypotonic to plasma. The amount of sweating is regulated by the autonomic nervous system, body temperature, and the skin blood flow.

Water loss through stool is normally minimal. However, in severe diarrhea or excessive fistula drainage, this loss can increase significantly. Clients with ulcerative colitis can have diarrheal fluid loss of several liters per day. Diarrheal fluid contains water, potassium, sodium, bicarbonate, and chloride. Thus, with diarrhea, hypotonic fluid containing some electrolytes is lost.

Electrolytes

Electrolytes, or ions, are substances in body fluids that carry an electrical charge. *Cations* are positively charged ions; *anions* are negatively charged ions. The body fluids are electrochemically neutral: positive ions are balanced by negative ions. However, the composition and distribution of ions differ in the extracellular fluid (ECF) and the intracellular fluid (ICF) (Fig. 14–10).

Most electrolytes have different concentrations in the ICF and in the ECF. This concentration difference helps maintain membrane excitability and transmit impulses. The electrolyte concentration ranges in these fluid compartments are extremely narrow. Thus, even small changes in these concentrations can result in major pathologic alterations.

Table 14–5 lists the major body fluid electrolytes together with their normal serum concentrations and primary functions. Most electrolytes enter the body in the form of ingested food.

Electrolyte homeostasis is controlled by balancing the dietary intake of electrolytes with the renal excretion or reabsorption of electrolytes. For example, plasma potassium concentration is maintained between 3.5 and 5.1 mmol/L. Potassium in common foods could in theory dramatically increase the ECF potassium concentration and lead to major pathologic consequences. However, the renal excretion of potassium keeps pace with potassium intake and prevents major changes in the plasma potassium concentration.

Sodium

Sodium (Na^+) is the major cation in the extracellular fluid (ECF) and is the main factor responsible for maintaining ECF osmolarity. The activity of the sodium-potassium pump keeps the sodium concentration of the intracellular fluid (ICF) low (about 14 mmol/L) while maintaining high sodium concentrations in the plasma and other ECFs. Preserving this difference in sodium concentration is vital for these normal physiologic functions:

- Initiation of skeletal muscle contraction
- Initiation of cardiac contractility
- Transmission of neuronal impulses
- Maintenance of ECF osmolarity
- Maintenance of ECF volume
- Maintenance of the renal urine-concentrating system

The concentration of sodium in the ECF determines whether water is retained, excreted, or moved from one body compartment to another.

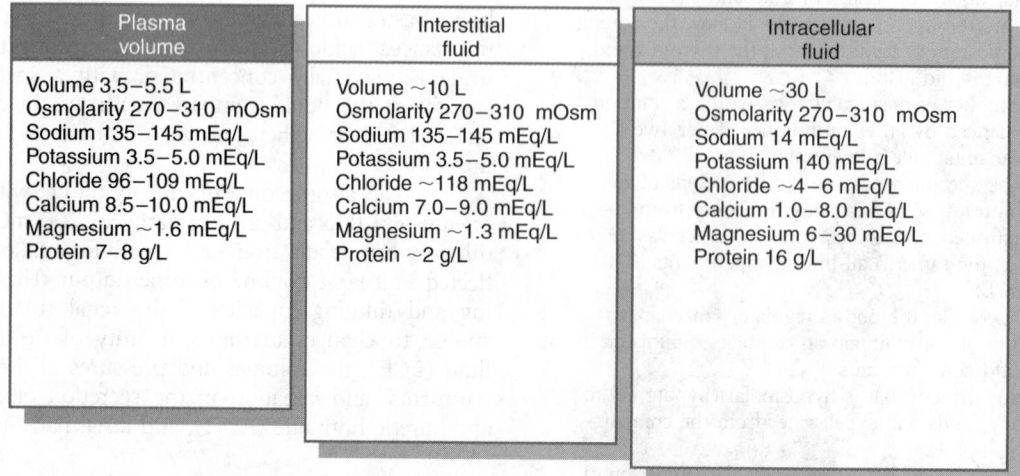

Plasma volume	Interstitial fluid	Intracellular fluid
Volume 3.5–5.5 L Osmolarity 270–310 mOsm Sodium 135–145 mEq/L Potassium 3.5–5.0 mEq/L Chloride 96–109 mEq/L Calcium 8.5–10.0 mEq/L Magnesium ~1.6 mEq/L Protein 7–8 g/L	Volume ~10 L Osmolarity 270–310 mOsm Sodium 135–145 mEq/L Potassium 3.5–5.0 mEq/L Chloride ~118 mEq/L Calcium 7.0–9.0 mEq/L Magnesium ~1.3 mEq/L Protein ~2 g/L	Volume ~30 L Osmolarity 270–310 mOsm Sodium 14 mEq/L Potassium 140 mEq/L Chloride ~4–6 mEq/L Calcium 1.0–8.0 mEq/L Magnesium 6–30 mEq/L Protein 16 g/L

Figure 14–10. The composition of various body fluids.

TABLE 14–5

Major Serum Electrolyte Concentrations and Functions

Electrolyte	Reference Range	International Recommended Units	Functions
Sodium (Na^+)	136–145 mEq/L	136–145 mmol/L	• Maintenance of plasma and interstitial osmolarity • Generation and transmission of action potentials • Maintenance of acid-base balance • Maintenance of electroneutrality
Potassium (K^+)	3.5–5.1 mEq/L	3.5–5.1 mmol/L	• Regulation of intracellular osmolarity • Maintenance of electrical membrane excitability • Maintenance of plasma acid-base balance
Calcium (Ca^{2+})	8.6–10.0 mg/dL	2.15–2.5 mmol/L	• Cofactor in blood clotting cascade • Excitable membrane stabilizer • Adds strength/density to bones and teeth • Essential element in cardiac, skeletal, and smooth muscle contraction
Chloride (Cl^-)	98–107 mEq/L	98–107 mmol/L	• Maintenance of plasma acid-base balance • Maintenance of plasma electroneutrality • Formation of hydrochloric acid
Magnesium (Mg^{2+})	1.6–2.6 mg/dL	0.66–1.07 mmol/L	• Excitable membrane stabilizer • Essential element in cardiac, skeletal, and smooth muscle contraction • Cofactor in blood clotting cascade • Cofactor in carbohydrate metabolism • Cofactor in DNA and protein synthesis
Phosphorus (Pi)	2.7–4.5 mg/dL	0.87–1.45 mmol/L	• Activation of B-complex vitamins • Formation of adenosine triphosphate and other high-energy substances • Cofactor in carbohydrate, protein, and lipid metabolism

Data from Tietz, N. (Ed.) (1995). *Clinical guide to laboratory tests* (3rd ed.). Philadelphia: W. B. Saunders.

The concentration of sodium, a cation, within a body fluid must be matched by an equal concentration of anions to maintain electrical balance. Each cation in the ECF must be balanced by an anion so that the fluid does not carry either an overall positive or an overall negative charge. When such a balance is maintained, a state of *electroneutrality* exists in that fluid. Changes in the plasma sodium concentration profoundly affect the fluid volume and the distribution of other electrolytes.

The normal concentration of plasma sodium ranges between 136 and 145 mEq/L or mmol/L (see Table 14–5). Sodium enters the body from ingestion of many foods and fluids (Table 14–6). The average dietary intake of sodium is about 6 to 12 g/day. Sodium is also stored in interstitial fluid areas deep within the renal tissues and can be released to ECF as needed. Despite great variations in sodium intake, serum sodium concentration usually remains within the normal range. Plasma sodium balance is regulated by the kidney under the influences of aldosterone, antidiuretic hormone (ADH), and atrial natriuretic peptide (ANP).

Low serum sodium levels inhibit ADH and ANP secretion while stimulating aldosterone secretion. These actions together increase serum sodium concentration by increas-

TABLE 14–6

Common Food Sources of Sodium*

Food Source	Amount (mg)
Table salt (1 tsp)	2000
Cheddar cheese (1 oz)	176
Cottage cheese (4 oz)	457
American cheese (1 oz)	439
Whole milk (8 oz)	120
Skim milk (8 oz)	126
Butter (1 tsp)	123
White bread (1 slice)	123
Whole-wheat bread (1 slice)	159
Soy sauce (1 tbsp)	1029
Ketchup (1 tbsp)	156
Mustard (1 tbsp)	188
Beef, lean (4 oz)	60
Pork, lean, fresh (4 oz)	60
Pork, cured (4 oz)	850
Chicken, light meat (4 oz)	70
Chicken, dark meat (4 oz)	70

Data from Pennington, J. (1994). *Bowe's and Church's food values of portions commonly used* (16th ed.). Philadelphia: J. B. Lippincott.

* U. S. Department of Agriculture recommended daily allowance for adults: 1100–3300 mg.

ing renal reabsorption of sodium and enhancing renal loss of water.

High serum sodium levels inhibit aldosterone secretion and directly stimulate ADH and ANP secretion. Together, these hormones cause an increase in the renal excretion of sodium and the renal reabsorption of water.

Potassium

In contrast to sodium, potassium (K^+) is the major cation of the intracellular fluid (ICF). The normal plasma concentration of potassium ranges from 3.5 to 5.1 mEq/L or mmol/L (see Table 14-5). The normal ICF concentration of potassium is about 140 mEq/L (mmol/L). Because of its high concentration inside cells, potassium exerts some control over intracellular osmolarity and volume. Maintaining this large difference in potassium concentration between ICF and the extracellular fluid (ECF) is critical for enabling excitable tissues to generate action potentials and to transmit impulses. Intracellular and extracellular functions of potassium include

- Regulation of protein synthesis
- Regulation of glucose use and storage
- Maintenance of action potentials in excitable membranes

Because ECF potassium levels are so low, any alteration in concentration is poorly tolerated by the body and profoundly affects physiologic activities. For example, a decrease in plasma potassium of only 1 mEq/L (from 4 mEq/L to 3 mEq/L) represents a significant difference (25%) in total ECF potassium concentration, whereas a decrease in plasma sodium of 1 mEq/L (from 140 mEq/L to 139 mEq/L) represents a much smaller change (less than 1%) in total ECF sodium concentration.

Potassium drifts out of cells down its concentration gradient into the ECF. In addition, almost all foods contain potassium (Table 14-7). Potassium intake averages about 2 to 20 g/day. Despite heavy potassium ingestion and the drifting of potassium from cellular storage sites into the ECF, the healthy body keeps plasma potassium levels within the narrow range of normal values required for physiologic function.

The primary controller of ECF potassium concentration is the sodium-potassium pump within the membranes of all body cells. The pump removes three sodium ions from the fluid inside the cell for every two potassium ions that it returns to the cell. In this way, the concentration differences for both ions are maintained.

Some potassium regulation also occurs through renal function. The kidney is the excretory route for ridding the body of ECF potassium (80% of potassium removed from the body occurs via the kidney). Unlike sodium, no hormone has been identified that directly controls renal reabsorption of potassium, and thus, the kidney does not conserve potassium directly.

Calcium

Calcium (Ca^{2+}) is a mineral whose presence and functions are closely related to those of phosphorus and magnesium. Calcium is a *divalent cation* (an ion expressing

TABLE 14-7

Common Food Sources of Potassium*	
Food Source	**Amount (mg)**
Corn flakes (1¼ c)	26
Cooked oatmeal (¾ c)	99
Egg (1 large)	66
Codfish, raw (4 oz)	400
Salmon, pink, raw (3½ oz)	306
Tuna fish (4 oz)	375
Apple, raw with skin (1 medium)	159
Banana (1 medium)	451
Cantaloupe (1 c pieces)	494
Grapefruit (½ medium)	175
Orange (1 medium)	250
Raisins (½ c)	700
Strawberries, raw (1 c)	247
Watermelon (1 c pieces)	186
White bread (1 slice)	27
Whole-wheat bread (1 slice)	44
Beef (4 oz)	480
Beef liver (3½ oz)	281
Pork, fresh (4 oz)	525
Pork, cured (4 oz)	325
Chicken (4 oz)	225
Veal cutlet (3½ oz)	448
Whole milk (8 oz)	370
Skim milk (8 oz)	406
Avocado (1 medium)	1097
Carrot (1 large)	341
Corn (4-inch ear)	196
Cauliflower (1 c pieces)	295
Celery (1 stalk)	170
Green beans (1 c)	189
Mushrooms (10 small)	410
Onion (1 medium)	157
Peas (¾ c)	316
Potato, white (1 medium)	407
Spinach, raw (3½ oz)	470
Tomato (1 medium)	366

Data from Pennington, J. (1994). *Bowe's and Church's food values of portions commonly used* (16th ed.). Philadelphia: J. B. Lippincott.
* U. S. Department of Agriculture recommended daily allowance for adults: 1875-5625 mg.

two positive charges) that exists in the body in two forms: bound and ionized (unbound or free).

Bound calcium is usually connected to specific serum proteins, especially albumin. Ionized calcium is present in blood and other extracellular fluids (ECFs) as free calcium. Free calcium is physiologically active and must be maintained within a narrow range in the ECF. The body functions best when plasma calcium concentrations are maintained between 8.6 and 10.0 mg/dL, or 2.15 and 2.5 mmol/L. Because the intracellular fluid (ICF) concentration of calcium is low, calcium has a steep gradient between ECF and ICF. Calcium functions in many ways and in many specialized body systems, including

- Biochemical cofactor (a substance required to enhance the activity of enzymes or reactions)
- Skeletal muscle contraction
- Cardiac contractility

TABLE 14-8

Common Food Sources of Calcium*

Food Source	Amount (mg)
Cheddar cheese (1 oz)	204
Cottage cheese (4 oz)	68
American cheese (1 oz)	174
Whole milk (8 oz)	288
Skim milk (8 oz)	302
Yogurt, low-fat (1 c)	415
Broccoli, raw (½ c)	75
Carrot (1 large)	37
Collard greens, raw (3 oz)	200
Green beans (1 c)	62
Rhubarb (1 c)	266
Spinach, raw (3½ oz)	93
Tofu (3 oz)	100

Data from Pennington, J. (1994). *Bowe's and Church's food values of portions commonly used* (16th ed.). Philadelphia: J. B. Lippincott.
* U. S. Department of Agriculture recommended daily allowance for adults: 800–1200 mg.

- Regulation of neural impulse transmission
- Blood clotting
- Bone strength and density

Calcium enters the body by dietary intake and subsequent absorption through the intestinal tract (Table 14–8). Absorption of dietary calcium requires the active form of vitamin D. Calcium is stored in the bones. When both plasma calcium levels and stored calcium levels are adequate, intestinal absorption of dietary calcium is inhibited and urinary excretion of excess calcium increases. When more plasma calcium is needed, parathyroid hormone (PTH, or parathormone) is secreted and released from the parathyroid glands (Table 14–9). PTH causes ECF calcium levels to increase through the following processes:

- Release of free calcium from bone storage sites directly into the ECF (*resorption*)

- Stimulation of vitamin D activation, thus increasing intestinal absorption of dietary calcium
- Inhibition of renal excretion of calcium and stimulation of renal tubular reabsorption of calcium

When excess calcium is present in plasma, secretion of PTH is inhibited and secretion of thyrocalcitonin (TCT), a hormone secreted by the thyroid gland, is increased. TCT causes the plasma calcium level to decrease through the following processes:

- Inhibition of bone resorption of calcium
- Inhibition of activation of vitamin D; decreased gastrointestinal uptake of calcium
- Increased renal excretion of calcium in the urine

Phosphorus

Phosphorus (P) is present in the body in both inorganic and organic forms. Normal plasma levels of phosphorus range from 2.7 to 4.5 mg/dL, or 0.87 to 1.45 mmol/L. The majority of phosphorus (80%) can be found in the bones. Phosphorus is the major anion in the intracellular fluid (ICF), and its concentration inside cells is much higher than that in extracellular fluid (ECF). Phosphorus is vital to the following intracellular activities:

- Activation of B-complex vitamins
- Formation and activation of high-energy substances, including adenosine triphosphate (ATP)
- Cell division
- Carbohydrate metabolism
- Protein metabolism
- Lipid (fat) metabolism

Extracellular fluid phosphorus functions include acid-base buffering and calcium homeostasis. Phosphorus is present in a variety of foods, such as nuts, legumes, dairy products, red meat, organ meat, bran, and whole grains (Table 14–10). The average diet is high in phosphorus (1–2 g/day).

Phosphorus balance and calcium balance are intertwined. Normally, plasma concentrations of calcium and

TABLE 14-9

Hormonal Regulation of Calcium

Hormone	Action
Parathyroid Hormone (PTH) Secreted in response to low or low-normal serum calcium levels Secretion results in a rise in serum calcium concentration	• Increases bone resorption of calcium (leaching of stored calcium) • Increases the absorption of ingested calcium from the gastrointestinal tract into extracellular fluid • Increases renal reabsorption of calcium at the proximal convoluted tubule
Thyrocalcitonin (TCT) Secreted by the thyroid gland in response to high or high-normal serum calcium levels Secretion results in a reduction of the serum calcium concentration	• Increases bone uptake of calcium • Inhibits the absorption of calcium from the gastrointestinal tract so that ingested calcium is excreted from the body in feces • Inhibits renal reabsorption of calcium at the proximal convoluted tubule so that more calcium is excreted in the urine

TABLE 14-10

TABLE 14-10

Common Food Sources of Phosphorus*	
Food Source	**Amount (mg)**
Rolled oats, cooked (¾ c)	133
Egg (1 large)	90
Codfish (3 oz)	175
Tuna fish, white, canned (6½ oz)	405
Raisins (½ c)	75
White bread (1 slice)	26
Whole-wheat bread (1 slice)	23
Cheddar cheese (1 oz)	145
American cheese (1 oz)	211
Whole milk (8 oz)	228
Skim milk (8 oz)	247
Yogurt, low-fat (8 oz)	326
Beef (4 oz)	215
Beef liver (4 oz)	375
Pork, fresh (4 oz)	325
Chicken (4 oz)	200
Almonds (1 oz)	141
Peanuts (1 oz)	110

Data from Pennington, J. (1994). *Bowe's and Church's food values of portions commonly used* (16th ed.). Philadelphia: J. B. Lippincott.
* U. S. Department of Agriculture recommended daily allowance for adults: 800 mg.

phosphorus exist in a reciprocal relationship, in that the product of the plasma concentrations remains constant. Therefore, a change in the concentration of phosphorus results in an equal and opposite change in the concentration of calcium (and vice versa).

The regulation of ECF phosphorus occurs through the activity of parathyroid hormone (PTH). Increased PTH secretion results in a net loss of phosphorus. Reduced PTH levels enhance renal reabsorption of phosphorus, resulting in increased ECF phosphorus concentrations.

Magnesium

Magnesium (Mg^{2+}) is another mineral that forms a cation when dissolved in water. The adult human body has an average of 25 g of magnesium, most of which (60%) is stored in bones and cartilage. Little magnesium is present in the extracellular fluid (ECF), and more than 25% of that is bound to albumin. Plasma levels of ionized magnesium range from 1.6 to 2.6 mg/dL, or 0.66 to 1.07 mmol/L. Much more magnesium is present in the intracellular fluid (ICF), and it has more functions inside the cells than in the plasma. Magnesium is critical for the following intracellular reactions or activities:

- Muscle contraction
- Carbohydrate metabolism
- Activation and use of adenosine triphosphate (ATP)
- Activation of many B-complex vitamins
- DNA synthesis
- Protein synthesis

Extracellular magnesium regulates blood coagulation and skeletal muscle contractility.

Magnesium is abundant in many foods, such as nuts, vegetables, fish, and whole grains (Table 14-11). The daily magnesium requirement for adults is about 300 mg.

Although magnesium is similar to calcium in many respects and its presence in plasma must be maintained within a narrow range of normal values, little is known about its regulation. Magnesium is absorbed from the intestinal tract at the same point as for calcium. The absorption of phosphorus inhibits magnesium absorption. Parathyroid hormone (PTH) stimulates the release of magnesium from bone in much the same way that it stimulates the release of calcium.

Chloride

Chloride (Cl^-) is the major anion of the extracellular fluid (ECF). It works with sodium in maintaining ECF osmotic pressure. Chloride is important in the formation of hydrochloric acid in the stomach. The normal plasma concentration of chloride ranges from 98 to 107 mEq/L, or 98 to 107 mmol/L.

Only a small quantity of chloride is present inside the cells because negatively charged particles on the cell membrane repel chloride and prevent it from crossing the cell membranes. However, extracellular chloride can enter cells when it is exchanged for another anion that is leaving the cell. This situation, a *chloride shift*, results in decreased plasma chloride concentration but no net body loss of chloride. Bicarbonate (HCO_3^-) is the anion most commonly exchanged for chloride. Chloride enters the body through dietary intake. Because chloride, with sodium, potassium, and many other minerals, is a part of a

TABLE 14-11

Common Food Sources of Magnesium*	
Food Source	**Amount (mg)**
Rolled oats, cooked (¾ c)	42
Tuna fish, white, canned (6½ oz)	59
Raisins (½ c)	25
Beef (4 oz)	24
Pork (4 oz)	30
Chicken (4 oz)	26
Whole milk (8 oz)	33
Skim milk (8 oz)	28
Yogurt, low-fat (8 oz)	40
Peanut butter (1 tbsp)	22
Avocado (1 medium)	70
Broccoli (1 stalk)	24
Cauliflower (1 c pieces)	24
Peas (¾ c)	35
Potato (1 medium)	34
Spinach, raw (3½ oz)	88

Data from Pennington, J. (1994). *Bowe's and Church's food values of portions commonly used* (16th ed.). Philadelphia: J. B. Lippincott.
* U. S. Department of Agriculture recommended daily allowance for adults: 300–350 mg.

Chart 14–1

Nursing Focus on the Elderly: Impact of Age-Related Changes on Fluid and Electrolyte Balance

System	Change	Result
Integumentary	• Loss of elasticity • Decreased turgor • Decreased oil production	• An unreliable indicator of fluid status • Dry, easily damaged skin
Renal	• Decreased glomerular filtration • Decreased concentrating capacity	• Poor excretion of waste products • Increased water loss
Muscular	• Decreased muscle mass	• Decreased total body water • Greater risk of dehydration
Neurologic	• Diminished thirst reflex	• Decreased fluid intake, increasing risk of dehydration
Endocrine	• Adrenal atrophy	• Poor regulation of sodium and potassium, predisposing the client to hyponatremia and hyperkalemia

---

salt, most diets contain enough chloride to meet the body's normal needs.

Fluid and Electrolyte Changes Associated with Aging

Only 45% to 50% of the body weight of elderly people is water, compared with 55% to 60% in younger adults. This decrease represents a net loss of muscle mass and a reduced ratio of lean body weight to total body weight. The decrease in total body water places elderly people at greater risk for water-deficit states. Multiple symptoms point to fluid volume deficit in the elderly person.

Skin *turgor* (the normal resiliency of a pinched fold of skin) is not always an accurate assessment of extracellular fluid (ECF) volume deficit in the elderly person because the natural aging process is associated with decreased

turgor (Chart 14–1). Furthermore, the elderly person may have a diminished thirst sensation and decreased renal function, both of which contribute to risk of fluid volume deficit and make assessment more difficult. Accurate documentation of intake and output and accurate weight measurement are extremely important when nurses work with elderly clients because these measurements reflect hydration status more accurately than does skin turgor.

The normal concentration of serum electrolytes also changes with the aging process. Chart 14–2 lists the normal electrolyte values for people older than 60 years.

Electrolyte balance may be more difficult to maintain in older people. Small changes in the concentrations of potassium and calcium in particular may produce unexpectedly profound results. Although plasma and intracellular fluid (ICF) electrolyte ranges may remain normal, the balance is fragile and more easily disturbed in an elderly

---

Chart 14–2

Nursing Focus on the Elderly: Normal Plasma Electrolyte Values for People Older than 60 Years

Electrolyte	Reference Range	International Recommended Units
Calcium (Ca^{2+})	8.8–10.2 mg/dL	2.2–2.55 mmol/L
> 90 years	8.2–9.6 mg/dL	2.05–2.40 mmol/L
Chloride (Cl^-)	98–107 mEq/L	98–107 mmol/L
> 90 years	98–111 mEq/L	98–111 mmol/L
Magnesium (Mg^{2+})	1.6–2.4 mg/dL	0.66–0.99 mmol/L
> 90 years	1.7–2.3 mg/dL	0.70–0.95 mmol/L
Phosphorus (Pi)	2.3–3.7 mg/dL (male) 2.8–4.1 mg/dL (female)	0.74–1.20 mmol/L 0.90–1.32 mmol/L
Potassium (K^+)	3.5–4.5 mEq/L (male) 3.4–4.4 mEq/L (female)	3.5–4.5 mmol/L 3.4–4.4 mmol/L
Sodium (Na^+)	136–145 mEq/L	136–145 mmol/L
> 90 years	132–146 mEq/L	132–146 mmol/L

Data compiled from: Tietz, N. (Ed.) (1995). *Clinical guide to laboratory tests* (3rd ed.). Philadelphia: W. B. Saunders.

person. Part of this fragility is related to decreased regulatory functions that occur with aging. Age-related renal changes include decreased renal blood flow, decreased glomerular filtration rate, and decreased numbers of functional nephrons. Renal and membrane changes associated with hypertension may also be present in the elderly person.

Assessment of Fluid and Electrolyte Balance

➤ History

A client's nutritional history can often reveal an underlying pathophysiologic process influencing fluid and electrolyte balance. The nurse directly elicits this information because the client may not understand the connection between dietary intake and the onset of fluid and electrolyte imbalances.

Guidelines for obtaining a thorough fluid and electrolyte history do not differ from those for assessing any other system; however, the information collected is more quantitative. For example, intake and output volumes are often extremely important, as are serial daily weights. The nurse may need to guide clients in accurately reporting the amount of fluid ingested and changes in voiding patterns. The nurse also assesses the types of fluids and foods ingested to determine osmolarity as well as amount. In addition, many clients do not consider solid food to contain liquid. Solid foods such as ice cream, gelatin, and ices are liquids at body temperature, and the nurse includes them when calculating fluid intake.

Output fluids include not only losses through urine but also those through significant diaphoresis and diarrhea and insensible loss during fevers. The nurse asks specific questions about prescribed and over-the-counter medications that the client has taken and ascertains the dosage, the length of time taken, and the client's compliance with the medication regimen. A client taking diuretics can have an imbalance of fluid, potassium, sodium, or hydrogen ions if additional threats to water balance, such as vomiting or excessive sweating, also occur.

Elderly people frequently use laxatives, which can disturb fluid and electrolyte balance. Misuse and overuse of these drugs can lead to serious imbalances.

Other pertinent areas of the client history include body weight changes, thirst or excessive drinking, exposure to environmental heat, and the presence of other preexisting disorders such as renal or endocrine diseases (e.g., Cushing's disease, Addison's disease, diabetes mellitus, and diabetes insipidus). The nurse makes a general assessment of the client's level of consciousness and mental status, because changes in mental status may further support findings of imbalance. In such cases, the nurse may need to verify with family members the accuracy of historical data.

➤ Physical Assessment

Hydration is the normal state of fluid balance. A normally hydrated adult is alert, has moist eyes and mucous mem-

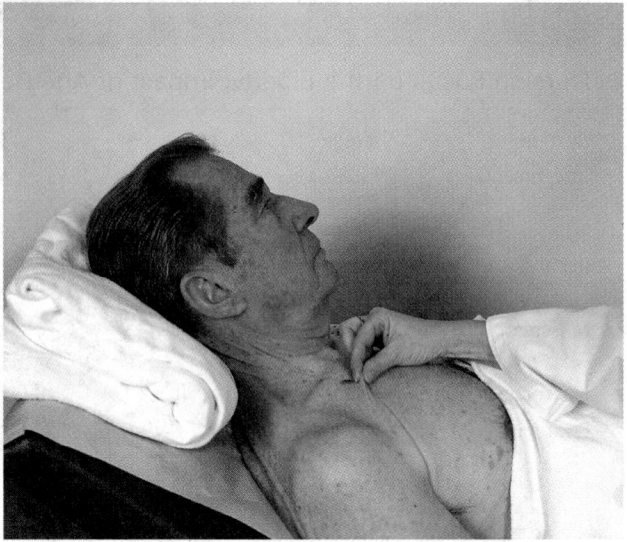

Figure 14–11. Examining the skin turgor of an elderly client.

branes, has a urinary output appropriate for the amount of fluid ingested (with a urine specific gravity of approximately 1.015), and has an adequate state of skin hydration as assessed by skin turgor.

The nurse assesses skin turgor by pinching a fold of skin. This pinched fold should return immediately to its original shape after release. Decreased turgor, a sign of dehydration, is present when the fold remains in a pinched shape after being released and rebounds slowly *(tenting)* (Fig. 14–11). The nurse can best assess skin turgor in body areas that contain little adipose tissue, such as over the sternum or on the back of the hand. An elderly person may have poor skin turgor because of the loss of tissue elasticity related to the aging process; thus, a true state of hydration may be more difficult to assess in an older adult than in a younger adult. The test areas for assessing turgor in the elderly are over the sternum and on the forehead.

Skin hydration assessment also includes an examination for dryness. The mucous membranes and the conjunctiva are normally moist. An assessment of fluid balance always includes an examination of the eyes, the nose, and oral mucous membranes. A dry, sticky, "cottony" mouth; the absence of tearing; the presence of weight loss; and decreased urinary output all indicate an actual fluid volume deficit.

A major criterion used in assessing fluid and electrolyte status is accurate measurement of fluid intake and output. Accurate assessment of actual fluid intake and output is the nurse's responsibility, and volumetric measuring devices must be used.

Behavioral and neurologic assessments are included in fluid assessment because changes in fluid balance can result in alteration of neurologic function. In hypertonic states, neuronal cell shrinkage may induce serious nervous system excitability and hyperactivity, and convulsions may occur. Another variable to assess is the degree of thirst. Thirst may be difficult to gauge in a confused elderly client.

The nurse approximates insensible water loss (e.g., sweat) in every client. Special situations also require an assessment of fluid loss from other routes, including

- Fluid losses from wounds
- Gastric or intestinal drainage
- Blood loss from hemorrhage
- Drainage of body secretions, such as bile and pancreatic juices, through surgical fistulas

Electrolytes control the activity of excitable membranes, and electrolyte imbalances are associated with altered function of these membranes. Electrolyte assessment includes a complete neuromuscular assessment of muscle tone and strength, movement, coordination, and tremors. Assessment of other systems, including cardiac (heart rate, the strength of contractions, and the presence of dysrhythmias) and gastrointestinal (peristalsis) systems, may indicate alterations of excitable membrane function.

Part of the nurse's assessment focuses on changes from previous findings (including mental status, physical examination data, and laboratory data). Fluid and electrolyte imbalances can occur quickly; therefore, the nurse must be familiar with the client's baseline assessment data to detect any changes.

➤ Psychosocial Assessment

Psychosocial assessment related to fluid and electrolyte status includes both psychologic and cultural factors that might influence balance. Depressed clients may refuse fluids or forget to drink adequate fluids. Clients with bulimia or anorexia nervosa (eating disorders) may use laxatives to excess or may induce vomiting, resulting in fluid and electrolyte imbalances. The nurse also assesses social practices. For example, excessive alcohol or drug use may lead to fluid or electrolyte imbalance.

➤ Diagnostic Assessment

Laboratory results are crucial in identifying specific fluid and electrolyte imbalances or disorders that alter fluid and electrolyte status. Normal serum electrolyte values are presented in Table 14–5, and normal values for people older than 60 years appear in Chart 14–2. Other laboratory values helpful in assessing fluid and electrolyte status include blood urea nitrogen level, glucose concentration, creatinine level, pH, bicarbonate level, osmolarity, hemoglobin, and hematocrit.

The urine test results may be helpful in assessing fluid status (Table 14–12). If a laboratory report is not avail-

TABLE 14–12

Normal Urine Electrolyte Values

Electrolyte/Characteristics	Normal Value*	Significance of Abnormal Value†
Calcium	2.5–7.5 mmol/day	Increased: Malignancy, thyrotoxicosis, hyperparathyroidism, osteoporosis, vitamin D intoxication Decreased: Hypoparathyroidism, rickets, kidney disease, hypothyroidism
Chloride	100–250 mEq/day 110–250 mmol/day	Increased: Increased salt intake, drug-induced diuresis, adrenocortical insufficiency Decreased: Reduced salt intake, water retention, vomiting, cerebral edema, adrenocortical hyperfunction
Magnesium	3.0–5.0 mmol/day	Increased: Alcohol intake, diuretics, corticosteroid therapy, cisplatin therapy Decreased: Dietary insufficiency
Phosphorus	12.9–42.0 mmol/day	Increased: Hyperparathyroidism, renal tubular damage, immobility, nonrenal acidosis Decreased: Hypoparathyroidism
Potassium	25–125 mmol/day (varies with diet)	Increased: Early starvation, hyperaldosteronism, metabolic acidosis Decreased: Addison's disease, renal disease
Sodium	40–220 mEq/day 40–220 mmol/day	Increased: Increased dietary intake, adrenal failure, diuretic therapy Decreased: Low sodium intake, sodium and water retention, adrenocortical hyperfunction, excessive diaphoresis, diarrhea
Osmolarity (osmolality)	300–900 mOsm/kg water	Increased: Dehydration, SIADH Decreased: Diabetes insipidus, primary polydipsia
Specific gravity	1.015–1.025	Increased: Dehydration, SIADH, diabetes mellitus, toxemia of pregnancy Decreased: Chronic renal insufficiency, diabetes insipidus, lithium toxicity, early renal disease

* Based on 24-hour total volume urine sample.
† Common conditions associated with abnormal values.
Data from Tietz, N. (Ed.) (1995). *Clinical guide to laboratory tests* (3rd ed.). Philadelphia: W. B. Saunders.

able, the nurse can perform various tests using a dipstick to help determine fluid and electrolyte status, including detecting substances that should not be present in the urine, such as glucose, acetone, protein, and blood. Urine measurements such as pH and specific gravity also can be determined in this way.

SELECTED BIBLIOGRAPHY

Bove, L. (1996). Restoring electrolyte balance: Sodium & chloride. *RN, 59*(1), 25–29.

Bove, L. (1996). Restoring electrolyte balance: Calcium & phosphorus. *RN, 59*(3), 47–52.

Braxmeyer, D., & Keyes, J. (1996). The pathophysiology of potassium balance. *Critical Care Nurse, 16*(5), 59–71.

Briggs, J., Singh, I., Sawaya, B., & Schnermann, J. (1996). Disorders of salt balance. In J. Kokko and R. Tannen (Eds.), *Fluid and electrolytes* (3rd ed., pp 3–62). Philadelphia: W. B. Saunders.

Ferrin, M. (1996). Restoring electrolyte balance: Magnesium. *RN, 59*(5), 31–35.

Frizzell, J. (1998). Avoiding lab test pitfalls. *American Journal of Nursing, 98*(2), 34–38.

Guyton, A., & Hall, J. (1996). *Textbook of medical physiology* (9th ed.). Philadelphia: W. B. Saunders.

Kokko, J., & Tannen, R. (1996). *Fluids and electrolytes* (3rd ed.). Philadelphia: W. B. Saunders.

Metheny, N. (1996). *Fluid and electrolyte balance: Nursing considerations* (3rd ed). Philadelphia: Lippincott-Raven.

Norris, M. K. (1994). Checking chloride levels. *Nursing94, 24*(3), 76.

O'Donnell, M. (1995). Assessing fluid and electrolyte balance needs in elders. *American Journal of Nursing, 95*(1), 41–46.

Pennington, J. (1994). *Bowe's and Church's food values of portions commonly used* (16th ed.). Philadelphia: J. B. Lippincott.

Terry, J. (1994). The major electrolytes: Sodium, potassium, and chloride. *Journal of Intravenous Nursing, 17*(5), 240–247.

Tietz, N. W. (ed.) (1995). *Clinical guide to laboratory tests* (3rd ed.). Philadelphia: W. B. Saunders.

Toto, K. (1994). Regulation of plasma osmolality. *Critical Care Nursing Clinics of North America, 6*(4), 661–674.

Toto, K., & Yucha, C. (1994). Magnesium: Homeostasis, imbalances, and therapeutic uses. *Critical Care Nursing Clinics of North America, 6*(4), 767–783.

Trissel, L. (1994). *Handbook on injectable drugs* (8th ed.). Bethesda, MD: American Society of Hospital Pharmacists.

Yu-Yahiro, J. (1994). Electrolytes and their relationship to normal and abnormal muscle function. *Orthopaedic Nursing, 13*(5), 38–40.

SUGGESTED READINGS

O'Donnell, M. (1995). Assessing fluid and electrolyte balance needs in elders. *American Journal of Nursing, 95*(1), 41–46.

This excellent article provides realistic cues to assist nurses in the differentiation between age-related skin changes and manifestations of actual fluid imbalances in the elderly. A case presentation approach is used to identify common signs and symptoms of fluid or electrolyte imbalances. Self-assessment questions are included at the end of the article.

Terry, J. (1994). The major electrolytes: Sodium, potassium, and chloride. *Journal of Intravenous Nursing, 17*(5), 240–247.

This article describes the sources, activities, and regulation of three common electrolytes. The information is presented in a user-friendly and practical format, highlighted with nursing considerations.

Toto, K. (1994). Regulation of plasma osmolality. *Critical Care Nursing Clinics of North America, 6*(4), 661–674.

A thorough explanation of the physiology of water balance is provided. The author describes the interaction of the thirst reflex and antidiuretic hormone in maintaining normal plasma osmolarity. Clinical examples and graphic artwork help the reader visualize the physiologic applications.

Chapter 15

INTERVENTIONS FOR CLIENTS WITH FLUID IMBALANCE

A proper balance of all body fluids is required for normal physiologic functioning. All clients are at risk for some degree of fluid imbalance because many health problems can disrupt fluid intake or output. This chapter focuses only on the problems surrounding fluid imbalances, although most fluid imbalances are accompanied by electrolyte imbalances.

Dehydration

Overview

In dehydration, the body's fluid intake is not sufficient to meet the body's fluid needs, resulting in a fluid volume deficit. Three basic types of dehydration are possible (Fig. 15–1):

- *Isotonic dehydration*, in which water and dissolved electrolytes are lost in equal proportions
- *Hypertonic dehydration*, in which water loss exceeds electrolyte loss
- *Hypotonic dehydration*, in which electrolyte loss exceeds water loss

Dehydration is a clinical state rather than a disease and can be caused by many factors. Dehydration may be an actual decrease in total body water caused by either inadequate fluid intake or excessive fluid loss. Dehydration also can occur without an actual decrease in total body water, such as when water shifts from the plasma into the interstitial space.

Pathophysiology
Isotonic Dehydration

Isotonic dehydration, or hypovolemia, is the most common type of dehydration. Problems associated with isotonic dehydration result from a reduction in plasma volume. Isotonic dehydration involves loss of isotonic fluids from the extracellular fluid (ECF) compartment (both the plasma and the interstitial space). Because isotonic fluid is lost, plasma osmolarity remains normal. This type of dehydration does not result in a shift of fluids between compartments; thus the intracellular fluid (ICF) volume remains normal. Isotonic dehydration results in decreased circulating blood volume and inadequate tissue perfusion. Compensatory mechanisms attempt to maintain adequate tissue perfusion to vital organs in spite of decreased vascular volume (Fig. 15–2).

Hypertonic Dehydration

Hypertonic dehydration is the second most common type of fluid volume deficit. The problems associated with hypertonic dehydration result from alterations in the concentrations of specific plasma electrolytes.

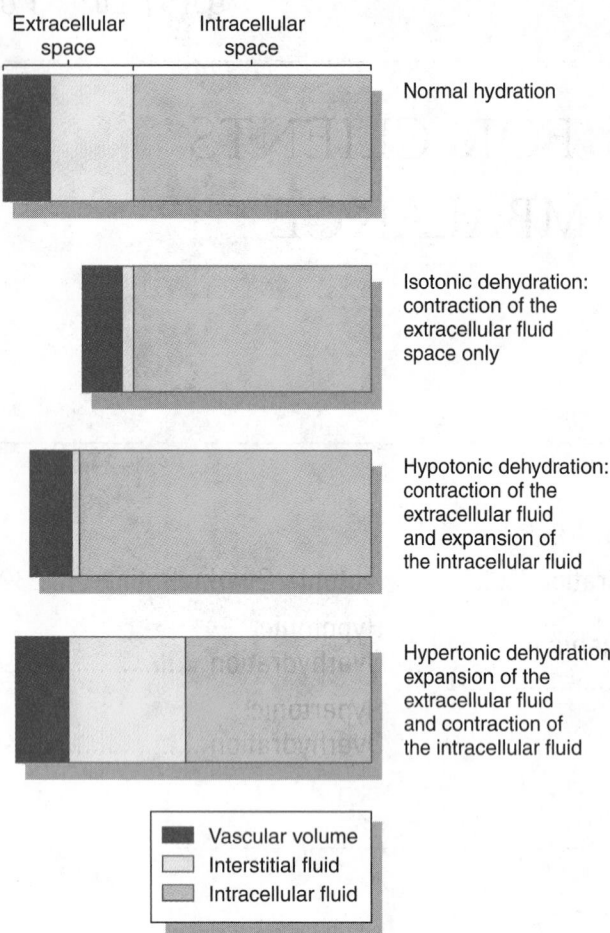

Figure 15–1. Three types of dehydration. (© 1992 M. Linda Workman. All rights reserved.)

Hypertonic dehydration occurs when water loss from the ECF exceeds electrolyte loss. This water loss increases the osmolarity of the remaining plasma, making it hypertonic or hyperosmolar compared with normal ECF. The hyperosmolar plasma has an increased osmotic pressure that causes fluid to move from the ICF into the plasma and interstitial fluid spaces. This fluid shift results in cellular dehydration and shrinkage. The fluid shift also causes the plasma volume to approach (or perhaps exceed) normal levels. Thus, the compensatory mechanisms and signs and symptoms of hypovolemic shock are not present. However, excitable membrane activity and cardiac contractility are affected by altered plasma levels of potassium and calcium. Compensatory mechanisms for hypertonic dehydration occur in response to the increased ECF osmolarity (Fig. 15–3).

Hypotonic Dehydration

Hypotonic dehydration is the least common type of dehydration. The problems associated with hypotonic dehydration result from fluid shifts between compartments, causing a decrease in plasma volume.

Hypotonic dehydration involves the excessive loss of sodium and potassium from the ECF. This loss results in decreased osmolarity of the remaining ECF, making it hypotonic compared with normal ECF. The decreased ECF osmolarity lowers the osmotic pressure of plasma and interstitial fluids to below that of the fluid inside the cells (the ICF). As a result of this difference in osmotic pressure, water moves from the plasma and interstitial spaces into the cells, creating a plasma volume deficit and causing the cells to swell.

Intracellular swelling causes widespread problems and symptoms. Because brain cells are more sensitive to cellular fluid changes than the cells of other tissues, neurologic dysfunction usually accompanies hypotonic dehydration. Hypotonic fluid also dilutes the normal electrolyte concentrations and causes sodium and potassium imbalances.

Etiology
Isotonic Dehydration

Isotonic dehydration has many causes (Table 15–1). These include inadequate intake of fluids and solutes, fluid shifts between compartments, and excessive losses of isotonic body fluids.

Hypertonic Dehydration

Hypertonic dehydration results from the loss of any body fluid that is hypotonic (low osmolarity, or decreased concentration of solute particles compared with isotonic body fluid). Common causes of hypertonic dehydration are conditions that increase insensible fluid loss. Such conditions include excessive perspiration, hyperventilation, ketoacidosis, prolonged fevers, diarrhea, early-stage renal failure, diabetes insipidus, and ketoacidosis in the diuretic phase (see Table 15–1).

Hypotonic Dehydration

Hypotonic dehydration is usually associated with chronic illness. Chronic renal failure, in which the kidneys waste sodium, leads to hypotonic dehydration. Chronic malnutrition and excessive ingestion of hypotonic fluids also cause hypotonic dehydration.

Incidence/Prevalence

Although the actual incidence of dehydration is not known, virtually every ill client is at risk. Elderly clients are at high risk because they have less total body water than younger adults. Conditions contributing to inadequate fluid intake in the elderly include diminished thirst sensation and possible difficulty with ambulation or other motor skills necessary for ingesting fluids. Nursing home residents older than 85 years appear to be at greatest risk for dehydration (see Research Applications for Nursing, p. 232).

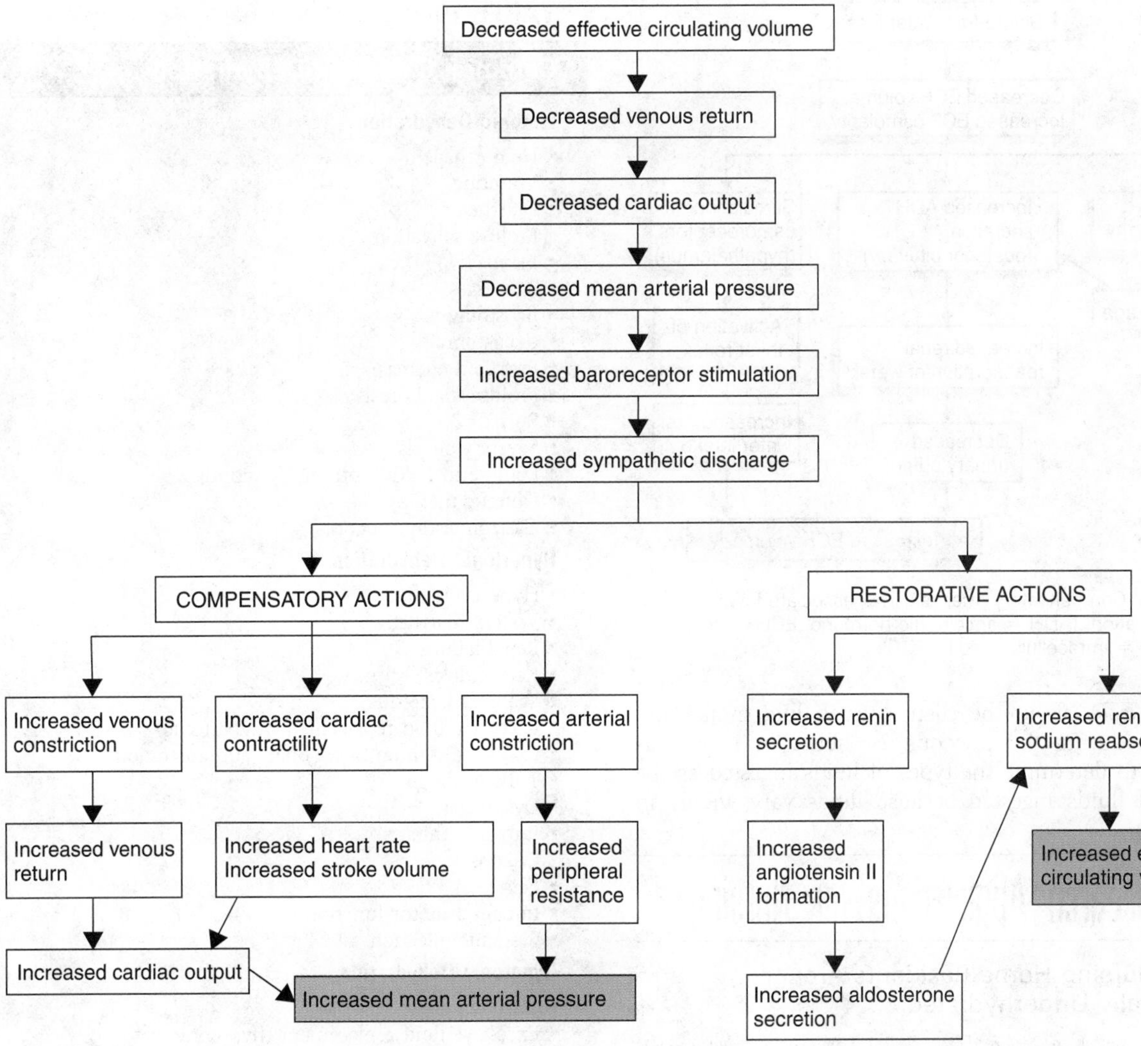

```
┌─────────────────────────────────────┐
│   Decreased effective circulating volume   │
└─────────────────────────────────────┘
                    │
                    ▼
         ┌──────────────────────┐
         │ Decreased venous return │
         └──────────────────────┘
                    │
                    ▼
         ┌──────────────────────┐
         │ Decreased cardiac output │
         └──────────────────────┘
                    │
                    ▼
      ┌────────────────────────────┐
      │ Decreased mean arterial pressure │
      └────────────────────────────┘
                    │
                    ▼
      ┌────────────────────────────┐
      │ Increased baroreceptor stimulation │
      └────────────────────────────┘
                    │
                    ▼
      ┌────────────────────────────┐
      │ Increased sympathetic discharge │
      └────────────────────────────┘
```

COMPENSATORY ACTIONS	RESTORATIVE ACTIONS

Compensatory Actions:

- Increased venous constriction → Increased venous return → Increased cardiac output
- Increased cardiac contractility → Increased heart rate / Increased stroke volume → Increased mean arterial pressure
- Increased arterial constriction → Increased peripheral resistance → Increased mean arterial pressure

Restorative Actions:

- Increased renin secretion → Increased angiotensin II formation → Increased aldosterone secretion → Increased renal sodium reabsorption → Increased effective circulating volume

Figure 15–2. Compensatory mechanisms associated with isotonic dehydration.

Collaborative Management

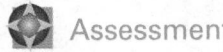 Assessment

➤ History

The nurse collects data on risk factors and factors causing dehydration (Table 15–2).

Age. This is an important consideration because dehydration in the elderly develops in response to relatively small fluid losses. In addition, elderly people are more likely to have chronic illnesses or to be taking medications that can lead to fluid and electrolyte imbalances (Anderson, 1996; O'Donnell, 1995).

Height and Weight. Measuring height and weight is important for calculating approximate fluid needs. If this information is not known or if the client is confused, the nurse obtains these measurements directly. Because weight and liquid measurements are related, changes in daily weights are good indicators of fluid losses or excesses. One liter of water weighs approximately 1 kg (2.2 pounds). Therefore, a weight change of 1 pound corresponds to a fluid volume change of about 500 mL.

Other Changes. The nurse questions the client about changes in the tightness of clothing, rings, and shoes. A sudden decrease in tightness may indicate dehydration; an increase may reflect a fluid shift to the interstitial space. Other relevant findings include the sensation of palpitations or lightheadedness on moving from a lying or a sitting position to a standing position (caused by orthostatic, or postural, hypotension).

The nurse further asks about any abnormal or excessive fluid losses, such as perspiration, diarrhea, bleeding, vomiting, urination, salivation, and wound drainage. Other important history information includes chronic illnesses, recent acute illnesses, recent surgery, and medications.

The nurse asks specific questions about urine output, including the frequency and amount of voidings. The

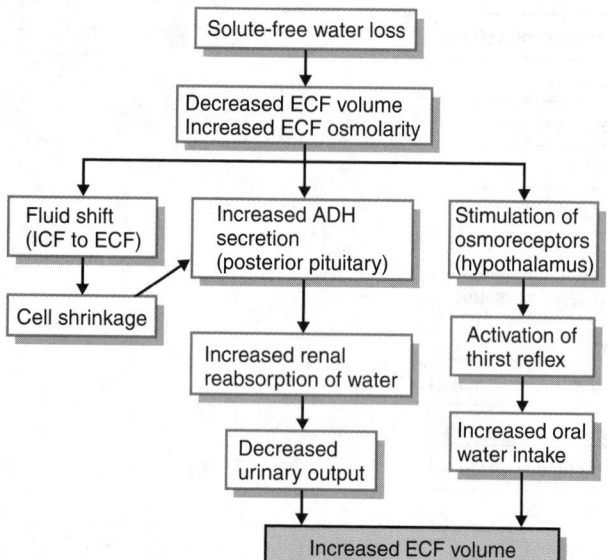

Figure 15–3. Compensatory mechanisms associated with hypertonic dehydration. (ADH = antidiuretic hormone; ECF = extracellular fluid; ICF = intracellular fluid.)

nurse also asks about the client's usual fluid intake and the intake during the previous 24 hours. It is just as important to determine the types of fluids ingested as the amount of fluids ingested because fluids vary widely in

▷ Research Applications for Nursing

Many Nursing Home Residents Are Chronically Underhydrated

Colling, J., Owen, T., & McCreedy, M. (1994). Urine volumes and voiding patterns among incontinent nursing home residents. Geriatric Nursing, 15(4), 188–192.

This prospective, descriptive clinical study observed 24-hour voiding patterns for 88 elderly nursing home residents a total of 14 times each over a 9-month period. Clients were mostly female and older than 85 years. Most clients had physical or mental impairments that limited their ability to obtain oral liquids independently. Oral intake was accurately measured. Liquid output was measured volumetrically when available and by weight when clients were incontinent.

Clients rarely exceeded a 1500-mL output for 24 hours, and more than 33% averaged less than 1000 mL total output for 24 hours. The two major findings of this study were that most clients were underhydrated and most experienced higher output at night.

Critique. The study was well designed. The conclusions were supported by the data obtained. The study could have been strengthened by the inclusion of additional objective data indicative of hydration status, however.

Possible Nursing Implications. Cognitively and physically impaired elders are dependent on caregivers to provide adequate oral hydration. Little attempt is made in nursing homes to assess accurately each resident's intake and output patterns, however. Implementing an action plan of regularly scheduling oral hydration breaks or offerings in a manner similar to medication administration could improve the hydration status of impaired elders.

TABLE 15–1

Common Causes of Dehydration

Isotonic Dehydration
- Hemorrhage
- Vomiting
- Diarrhea
- Profuse salivation
- Fistulas
- Abscesses
- Ileostomy
- Cecostomy
- Frequent enemas
- Profuse diaphoresis
- Burns
- Severe wounds
- Long-term NPO (nothing by mouth)
- Diuretic therapy
- Gastrointestinal suction

Hypertonic Dehydration
- Hyperventilation
- Watery diarrhea
- Renal failure
- Ketoacidosis
- Diabetes insipidus
- Excessive fluid replacement (hypertonic)
- Excessive sodium bicarbonate administration
- Tube feedings
- Dysphagia
- Impaired thirst
- Unconsciousness
- Fever
- Impaired motor function
- Systemic infection

Hypotonic Dehydration
- Chronic illness
- Excessive fluid replacement (hypotonic)
- Renal failure
- Chronic or severe malnutrition

osmolarity. The nurse also asks whether the client has recently engaged in strenuous physical activity and, if so, whether the activity took place in hot or dry environmental conditions.

TABLE 15–2

Risk Factors for Dehydration

Illnesses	**Other Situations**
• Vomiting	• Extremes of age: elderly, infants
• Diarrhea	• Unconsciousness
• Burns	• Motor limitations
• Large draining wounds	**Therapies**
• Liver dysfunction	• Surgery
• Diabetes mellitus	• Diuretics
• Diabetes insipidus	• Nothing by mouth
• Renal disease	• Excessive hypertonic enemas
• Hemorrhage	• Nasogastric suction
• Major venous obstruction	
• Prolonged febrile state	

➤ *Physical Assessment/Clinical Manifestations*

The clinical manifestations of dehydration depend on which fluid compartments lose fluid, although all body systems are affected to some degree (Chart 15–1). The most obvious and life-threatening clinical manifestations are seen when dehydration causes a decrease in the plasma volume.

Cardiovascular Manifestations. Cardiovascular changes are the most reliable indicators of changes in plasma volume. The heart rate increases with plasma volume deficits. Peripheral pulses are weaker, difficult to find, and easily blocked with light pressure. If interstitial edema accompanies the dehydration, the peripheral pulses may not be palpable. Blood pressure also decreases, as does the pulse pressure, with a greater decrease in the systolic blood pressure. Hypotension is more profound with the

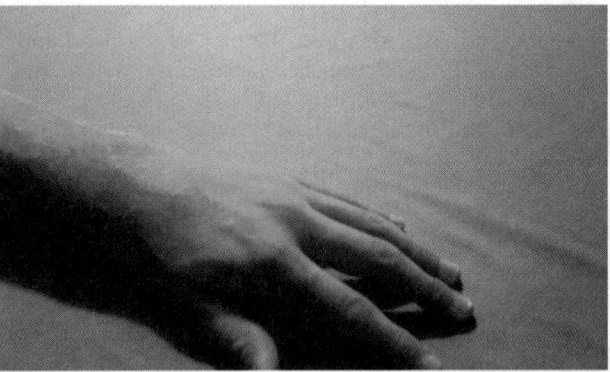
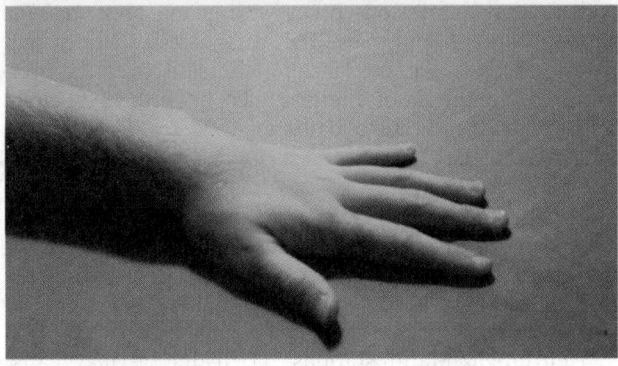

Figure 15–4. Hand veins full and bulging in the dependent position (*top*). Hand veins collapsed (*bottom*).

client in the standing position than in the sitting or the lying position. Because the blood pressure with the client standing may be much lower than in other positions, blood pressure is measured first with the client lying down, then sitting, and finally standing.

Another cardiovascular indicator of hydration status is the degree of neck and hand vein filling. Normally, hand veins fill and become engorged when the hands are lower than the level of the heart. As the hands are raised above the level of the heart, the veins flatten or collapse (Fig. 15–4). Neck veins are normally distended when a client is in the supine position. These veins flatten when the client moves to a sitting position. When dehydration involves a plasma volume deficit, neck and hand veins are flat, even when not raised above the level of the heart. These cardiovascular changes are not seen in hypertonic dehydration.

Respiratory Manifestations. Respiratory rate increases directly with the degree of fluid loss from plasma volume. When acidosis accompanies dehydration, respirations become deep and rapid. This type of respiratory pattern is called *Kussmaul breathing.*

Integumentary Manifestations. Integumentary changes may be useful indicators of hydration. The nurse assesses for changes in the skin and mucous membranes that may indicate dehydration, including skin color, moisture, skin turgor, and edema. In elderly clients, this information is less reliable because of poor skin turgor resulting from the loss of elastic tissue and the loss of tissue fluids with aging.

Chart 15–1

Key Features of Dehydration

Manifestations of Dehydration in General*

Cardiovascular

- Increased pulse rate
- Thready pulse quality
- Decreased blood pressure
- Postural hypotension
- Flat neck and hand veins in dependent positions
- Diminished peripheral pulses

Respiratory

- Increased respiratory rate
- Increased depth of respirations

Neuromuscular

- Decreased central nervous system activity (lethargy to coma)
- Fever

Renal

- Decreased urinary output
- Increased specific gravity

Integumentary

- Skin dry and scaly
- Turgor poor, tenting present
- Mouth dry and fissured, paste-like coating present

Gastrointestinal

- Decreased motility
- Diminished bowel sounds
- Constipation
- Thirst

Manifestations of Hypotonic Dehydration

- Skeletal muscle weakness

Manifestations of Hypertonic Dehydration

- Hyperactive deep tendon reflexes
- Increased sensation of thirst
- Pitting edema

*These manifestations are most severe with hypotonic dehydration.

The nurse assesses skin turgor by noting

- How easily the skin over the back of the hand and arm can be gently pinched between the thumb and the forefinger to form a "tent"
- How soon the pinched skin resumes its normal position after release
- Whether depressions (pits) remain in the skin after a finger is pressed firmly but gently (over the shin, over the sternum, and over the sacrum)
- How deep the depression is (in millimeters)
- How long the depression remains

In generalized dehydration, skin turgor is poor, with the tenting remaining for minutes after pinching the skin, and no skin depressions occur with gentle pressure. The skin appears dry and scaly. The nurse assesses skin turgor in an elderly client by pinching the skin over the sternum, the forehead, or the abdomen because these areas more reliably indicate hydration (see Fig. 14–11). As a person ages, the skin loses elasticity and tents on extremities even if the person is well hydrated.

In dehydration, oral mucous membranes are not moist. They may be covered with a thick, sticky, paste-like coating and may have cracks and fissures. The surface of the tongue may have deep furrows.

Neurologic Manifestations. Dehydration may cause changes in body temperature and mental status. The client with dehydration typically has a low-grade fever. A client with a temperature exceeding 39° C (102° F) for longer than 6 hours is especially at risk. Elderly clients who normally have a body temperature range of 35.4° to 36.6° C (96°–98° F) are at greater risk for dehydration during episodes of fever. Mental status changes are also common with dehydration. Chart 15–2 outlines how to assess mental status quickly.

Renal Manifestations. The volume and the composition of urine output indicate the hydration status of the renal system. The nurse closely monitors urine output, comparing total output to total fluid intake and daily weight. Accurate intake and output measurement is a major nursing responsibility. Urine output below 500 mL/day for any client without renal disease is cause for concern. A client with fluid imbalance is weighed each day at the same time and on the same scale. When possible, the client should be wearing the same amount and type of clothing for each weigh-in. Usually, metabolic tissue loss (even in starvation) accounts for only about 1/2 pound of weight loss per day. Any weight loss in excess of this amount is considered fluid loss.

➤ *Psychosocial Assessment*

The nurse observes the client for behavioral changes that accompany dehydration. Initially, a dehydrated client may have a flat affect and may seem unconcerned or indifferent about the state of health and possible treatment regimens. As dehydration worsens, the client's psychosocial activities reflect abnormal functioning of the central nervous system. The client may become apprehensive, rest-

Chart 15–2

Nursing Care Highlight: Brief Check of Mental Status

- Is the client awake?
- If the client is not awake, what type of stimulation is needed to waken the client?
  - Calling the client's name in a normal voice volume
  - Calling the client's name in a louder voice volume
  - Touching the client's arm or face while calling name
  - Gently tapping or shaking an arm
  - Vigorously shaking a hand or arm
  - Applying a painful stimulus
- If the client is awake, ask questions that require more than a "yes" or "no" response to establish orientation to time and place.
- Avoid the use of nonsense questions (such as "Do helicopters eat their young?").
- Ask questions that are reasonable and likely to be known by the client, such as "When is your birthday?" Avoid questions such as "Who was vice president under Truman?"
- Is it necessary to repeat questions to obtain a response?
- Does the response answer the question asked?
- Does the client have difficulty with word choices in forming responses?
- Is the client irritated or upset by the questions?
- Can the client concentrate on a question long enough to provide an appropriate response or is the attention span short?
- Can the client count by threes?
- Can the client count backward from 100 by threes?
- Does the client know the names of immediate family members?
- Does the client know who the questioner is (not necessarily the questioner's name but that person's role in the client's care such as nurse, doctor, chaplain, therapist)?
- Does the client know his or her immediate location (e.g., home, hospital, clinic)?
- Does the client know the year?

less, lethargic, and confused. These behavioral changes are more obvious in hypertonic and hypotonic dehydration because of intracellular fluid (ICF) shifts in brain cells, resulting in shrinkage or swelling of the cells. If the conditions causing the dehydration continue, circulation to cerebral tissues becomes so impaired that delirium and coma can occur.

➤ *Laboratory Assessment*

No single laboratory test result confirms or rules out dehydration. Instead, a diagnosis of dehydration must be based on laboratory findings along with presenting signs and symptoms. Such laboratory findings depend on the type of dehydration present (Chart 15–3). Isotonic and hypotonic dehydration states with accompanying plasma volume deficits are manifested as hemoconcentration, with elevated levels of hemoglobin and increased hematocrit, and as increased serum osmolarity, with increased levels of glucose, protein, blood urea nitrogen (BUN), and

---

Chart 15–3

Laboratory Profile: Dehydration

Values*	Isotonic Dehydration	Hypotonic Dehydration	Hypertonic Dehydration
Blood Values			
BUN	• Normal or increased	• Increased	• Increased
Creatinine	• Normal or increased	• Increased	• Increased
Sodium	• Normal	• <120 mEq/L (mmol)	• >150 mEq/L (mmol)
Osmolality	• Normal	• Decreased	• Increased
Hematocrit	• Increased	• Increased	• Normal or decreased
Hemoglobin	• Increased	• Increased	• Normal or decreased
WBCs	• Increased	• Increased	• Normal or decreased
Protein	• Increased	• Increased	• Increased
Urine Values			
Specific gravity	• >1.010	• <1.010	• >1.030
Osmolality	• Increased	• Increased	• Increased
Volume	• Decreased	• Decreased	• Decreased

*All values reflect dehydration states alone and not the underlying pathologic changes or disease states contributing to the dehydration.
BUN = blood urea nitrogen; WBC = white blood cell.

---

various electrolytes. Hemoconcentration is not evident when dehydration results from hemorrhage, because loss of all blood and plasma products occurs.

Specific urine laboratory values can help to determine dehydration if the client does not have renal dysfunction. Usually, the urine of clients with dehydration is highly concentrated, with a specific gravity exceeding 1.030. Volume is decreased, and osmolarity is greatly increased. Usually, the color is dark amber, and a strong odor is evident.

 Analysis

➤ Common Nursing Diagnoses and Collaborative Problems

The priority nursing diagnoses to consider when caring for a client with dehydration are as follows:
1. Fluid Volume Deficit related to excessive fluid loss or inadequate fluid intake
2. Decreased Cardiac Output related to insufficient plasma volume
3. Altered Oral Mucous Membranes related to inadequate oral secretions

The primary collaborative problem is Potential for Dysrhythmias.

➤ Additional Nursing Diagnoses and Collaborative Problems

In addition to the common nursing diagnoses and collaborative problems, one or more of the following may apply:
- Constipation related to decreased body fluids
- High Risk for Injury (fall) related to orthostatic (postural) hypotension

- Knowledge Deficit related to medication regimen and preventive measures
- High Risk for Impaired Skin Integrity related to deficiencies of interstitial fluid and inadequate tissue perfusion
- Ineffective Airway Clearance related to thick, tenacious secretions
- Potential for Hypovolemic Shock
- Potential for Electrolyte Imbalances

 Planning and Implementation

➤ Fluid Volume Deficit

Planning: Expected Outcomes. The expected outcome is that the client will have normal body fluid levels.

Interventions. Management of dehydration aims to prevent further fluid losses and increase fluid compartment volumes to normal ranges. Diet therapy, oral rehydration therapy, and drug therapy are the methods of choice.

Diet Therapy. Mild to moderate dehydration may be successfully treated with oral fluid replacement if the client is alert enough to swallow and can tolerate oral fluids. The nurse or assistive personnel encourages and measures all fluid intake. The specific type of fluid needed for replacement varies with the type of dehydration.

The client's compliance in ingesting oral replacement fluids can be enhanced by using fluids the client enjoys at temperatures with which the client is comfortable and by carefully timing the intake schedule. Dividing the total amount of fluids needed by nursing shifts helps to meet fluid needs more evenly with less danger of overhydration. The nurse or assistive personnel offers the conscious

TABLE 15–3

Commercial Solutions for Oral Rehydration Therapy

Brand Name	Na+ (mEq/L)	K+ (mEq/L)	Cl− (mEq/L)	Citrate (mEq/L)	Sugar or Starch	Calories (kcal/L)
Ricelyte (Mead-Johnson)	50	25	45	34	Rice syrup (30 g)	126
Resol (Wyeth-Ayerst)	50	20	50	34	Dextrose (20 g)	84
Rehydralyte (Ross Labs)	75	20	65	30	Dextrose (25 g)	100
Pedialyte (Ross Labs)	45	20	35	30	Dextrose (25 g)	100
Gastrolyte (Rorer)	60	20	60	10	Dextrose (17.8 g)	75
Rapolyte (Richmond)	90	20	80	30	Dextrose (20 g)	84
Lytren (Mead-Johnson)	50	25	45	30	Dextrose (20 g)	84
Naturalyte (United Beverages)	45	20	35	48	Dextrose (25 g)	100
Oralyte (Rugby)	45	20	25	48	Dextrose (25 g)	100

Data from United States Pharmacopeial Convention, Inc. (1998). USPDI Vol I, *Drug information for the health care professional*. Rockville, MD: United States Pharmacopeial Convention. Printed by Rand McNally, Taunton MA.

client small volumes of fluids every hour to increase compliance.

Oral Rehydration Therapy. Oral rehydration therapy (ORT) is the most cost-effective way to replace fluids and treat the client with diarrhea. Specifically formulated solutions containing glucose and electrolytes cause water to be absorbed even in the presence of diarrhea and vomiting. Fluid losses from diarrhea are usually 2 to 3 L/day and should be replaced liter for liter, especially in elderly clients. A typical physician's order might be "Resol 1 L every 8 hours." Table 15–3 lists commercially available ORT solutions.

Drug Therapy. Drug therapy for dehydration is directed at restoring fluid balance and controlling the conditions causing dehydration. Whenever possible, fluids are replaced by the oral route. When dehydration is severe or life-threatening, intravenous (IV) fluid replacement may be necessary. Calculation of the volume of replacement fluids needed is based on both the client's weight loss and presenting symptoms. The rate of fluid replacement depends on the client's degree of dehydration and the presence of pre-existing cardiac, pulmonary, or renal problems.

The type of fluid ordered by the physician varies with the type of dehydration and the client's cardiovascular status. The desired outcomes of therapy are appropriate fluid replacement and normal volumes in all body fluid compartments. Usually, the client receives IV infusions of water with whatever solutes (especially electrolytes) are determined necessary on the basis of laboratory values. Table 15–4 lists the osmolarity, caloric content, and tonicity of common IV fluids. Generally, isotonic dehydra-

tion is treated with isotonic fluid solutions; hypertonic dehydration, with hypotonic fluid solutions; and hypotonic dehydration, with hypertonic fluid solutions.

Drug therapy includes the use of medications to correct the underlying cause of the dehydration. Antidiarrheal medications are ordered when excessive diarrhea causes dehydration. Antimicrobial therapy may be used in clients with bacterial diarrhea. Antiemetics to control vomiting may be necessary when excessive vomiting produces dehydration. Antipyretics to reduce body temperature are helpful when fever contributes to dehydration.

► *Decreased Cardiac Output*

Planning: Expected Outcomes. The expected outcomes are that the client should

- Have cardiac output restored to normal levels
- Maintain adequate oxygenation to vital organs

Interventions. Interventions aim to increase circulating fluid volume, support compensatory mechanisms, and prevent ischemic complications mainly through drug therapy and oxygen therapy.

Drug Therapy. Drug therapy to increase body fluid volume and prevent excessive fluid loss is the same as that for the client with fluid volume deficit. Drugs to increase venous return or improve cardiac contractility are used only when a co-existing cardiac problem is present.

Oxygen Therapy. Oxygen can be delivered by mask, hood, nasal cannula, nasopharyngeal tube, endotracheal tube, or tracheostomy tube. Usually, masks and nasal cannulas are used to administer oxygen to clients with dehydration. The nurse administers water-nebulized oxy-

TABLE 15–4

Characteristics of Common Intravenous Therapy Solutions

Solution	Osmolarity (mOsm/L)	pH	Calories* (kcal)	Tonicity
0.9% saline	308	5	0	Isotonic
0.45% saline	154	5	0	Hypotonic
5% dextrose in water (D₅W)	272	3.5–6.5	170	Isotonic†
10% dextrose in water (D₁₀W)	500	3.5–6.5	340	Hypertonic†
5% dextrose in 0.9% saline	560	3.5–6.5	170	Hypertonic†
5% dextrose in 0.45% saline	406	4	170	Hypertonic†
5% dextrose in 0.225% saline	321	4	170	Isotonic†
Ringer's lactate	273	6.5	9	Isotonic
5% dextrose in Ringer's lactate	525	4.0–6.5	179	Hypertonic†

Data from Trissel, L. (1994). *Handbook on injectable drugs* (8th ed.). Bethesda, MD: American Society of Hospital Pharmacists.
*Calories are calculated on the basis of a volume of 1000 mL.
†*Solution tonicity at the time of administration.* Within a short time after administration, the dextrose is metabolized, and the tonicity of the infused solution decreases in proportion to the osmolarity or tonicity of the nondextrose components (electrolytes) within the water.

gen to the client at the rate or amount specified by the physician's order.

Monitoring. Monitoring vital signs and level of consciousness is an important responsibility of nurses caring for dehydrated clients. The nurse or assistive personnel monitors the client's pulse, blood pressure, pulse pressure, central venous pressure, respiratory rate, skin and mucous membrane color, and urinary output at least every hour until the fluid imbalance is resolved.

► Altered Oral Mucous Membranes

Planning: Expected Outcomes. The expected outcomes are that the client should experience less discomfort and remain free of complications.

Interventions. Interventions include drug therapy, fluid replacement, good oral hygiene, and the early diagnosis and prevention of complications. Diet therapy may also be used to resolve the dehydration.

Drug Therapy. Drug therapy to increase body fluid volume and prevent excessive fluid loss is the same as that discussed earlier for fluid volume deficit. Commercial preparations of artificial saliva can reduce the sensation of mouth dryness. The nurse avoids using such agents in an unconscious client, however, to prevent aspiration.

Oral Hygiene. Nursing actions to promote oral hygiene can increase the client's comfort. The nurse keeps the client's lips clean and moistens them with a petrolatum-based lubricant. The thick, sticky coating on the oral cavity during episodes of dehydration can be reduced with frequent oral hygiene measures.

Mouth care includes gentle tooth brushing several times a day and rinsing hourly. The nurse teaches the client to avoid commercial mouthwashes that contain alcohol and glycerin-containing washes and swabs, because these products dry the oral mucosa further and may cause increased discomfort by stinging or burning open fissures in the mucosa. Rinsing the mouth with dilute solutions of hydrogen peroxide two or three times per day is a good form of oral hygiene; however, when used more frequently, this treatment increases oral dryness. Tap water and normal saline rinses can be used safely as often as the client wishes.

Prevention of Complications. A dry mouth contributes to the development of sores and fissures in the mucosa, providing a portal of entry for many pathogens. The thick, sticky coating also is an excellent breeding ground for microorganisms. A major complication of mouth dryness is a wide variety of oral infections. Chart 15–4 summarizes nursing interventions for mouth care.

Chart 15–4

Nursing Care Highlight: Mouth Care for Clients with Dehydration

- Examine the client's mouth (including under the roof, on the tongue, and between the teeth and cheek) every 4 hours.
- Document the location, size, and character of fissures, blisters, sores, or drainage.
- Obtain an order to culture sores or drainage.
- Brush the client's teeth and tongue with a soft-bristled brush or sponges every 8 hours.
- Rinse the client's mouth with a 50:50 solution of ½ peroxide and ½ normal saline every 12 hours.
- Avoid the use of alcohol or glycerin-based mouthwashes.
- Assist the conscious client to swish and spit room-temperature tap water or normal saline PRN.
- Apply petrolatum jelly to the client's lips after each episode of mouth care and PRN.
- Assist the client in using artificial saliva.
- Assist the client in menu choices to avoid spicy or hard foods.
- Offer complete mouth care before and after every meal.

PRN = as necessary.

➤ *Potential for Dysrhythmias*

Planning: Expected Outcomes. The expected outcome is that the client will maintain his or her normal cardiac rhythm.

Interventions. Interventions are aimed at correcting the dehydration and recognizing dysrhythmias so appropriate drug therapy can be initiated.

Drug Therapy. Drug therapy to increase body fluid volume and prevent excessive fluid loss is the same as that discussed earlier for fluid volume deficit.

Elevated potassium or calcium level can cause life-threatening dysrhythmias. Drug therapy to reduce these electrolytes may be ordered. If potassium levels are elevated, a combination of 20 units of regular insulin in 100 mL of 20% dextrose may be administered to promote movement of potassium into the ICF. Drugs such as etidronate (Didronel) and plicamycin (Mithracin) may be administered to reduce an elevated serum calcium level.

Monitoring. The nurse monitors the client for signs and symptoms of cardiac dysrhythmias every 15 minutes until the client is fully rehydrated. The rate, rhythm, and quality of the apical pulse are assessed and compared with the client's baseline measurements. The nurse further assesses the client for fatigue, chest discomfort or pain, and shortness of breath. Hand grasps and deep tendon reflexes are assessed, and changes from baseline are noted.

Clients at risk for dysrhythmias are monitored using electrocardiography (ECG). The pattern may show tall T waves or a shortened ST segment. Any change from the client's baseline ECG is reported to the physician immediately.

 Continuing Care

No extensive home care preparations are necessary for clients with mild dehydration or for those with dehydration of sudden onset. The imbalance is corrected before discharge from the facility and, with minimal precautions, is unlikely to recur. Clients who are most likely to be discharged before the imbalance is completely corrected and who are susceptible to recurrent episodes are those with chronic pathologic conditions, such as renal insufficiency, diabetes, malignancy, adrenal insufficiency, and specific endocrine disorders. These clients often require long-term diet and drug therapy.

➤ *Health Teaching*

Education is important in the prevention and early detection of dehydration. The teaching plan for any client at risk for dehydration includes diet, drug regimens, and the signs and symptoms of dehydration.

➤ *Home Care Management*

The nurse, occupational therapist, or social worker evaluates the client's home environment with regard to precipitating factors for dehydration. Particular attention is paid to environmental temperature and humidification. Kitchen

and bathroom access are assessed, and suggestions for modifications made as necessary.

Home adjustments may be necessary for elderly clients or clients whose dehydration is caused by chronic illness. One contributing factor to dehydration in the elderly is the fear of incontinence. Clients may limit fluid intake to reduce their need to go to the bathroom. This tactic is used frequently among elderly women who do not have a toilet available on the same floor where they spend most of their time. A portable toilet on the living floor can remedy this situation if home remodeling is not an option.

The nurse instructs the family to keep appropriate fluids for the client in places that the client can access. Container modifications, such as opening zip-top cans and covering them with foil, can be made to ensure the client can easily open container lids. Sipper containers not only provide easy access but also are unbreakable and reduce spillage.

The nurse performs a focused assessment (Chart 15–5)

Chart 15–5

Focused Assessment for Home Care Clients at Risk for Dehydration

- Assess cardiovascular status.
  - Vital signs, including apical pulse, pulse pressure, presence or absence of orthostatic hypotension, and quality and rhythm of peripheral pulses
  - Presence or absence of peripheral edema
  - Hand vein filling in the dependent position
  - Neck vein filling in the recumbent and sitting positions
  - Weight gain or loss
- Assess cognition and mental status.
  - Level of consciousness
  - Orientation to time, place, and person
  - Can the client accurately read a seven-word sentence containing no words greater than three syllables?
- Assess condition of skin and mucous membranes.
  - Presence or absence of skin tenting over the sternum or the forehead
  - Moistness of skin, most reliable on chest and back
  - Presence or absence of coating on tongue or teeth
  - Can the client spit?
- Assess neuromuscular status.
  - Reactivity of patellar and biceps reflexes
  - Oral temperature
  - Handgrip strength
  - Steadiness of gait
- Assess renal system.
  - Observe urine specimen for color, odor, cloudiness, and amount
- Ask about the following:
  - 24-hour fluid intake and output
  - 24-hour diet recall
  - 24-hour activity recall
  - Over-the-counter and prescribed medications the client has taken
- Assess client's understanding of illness and compliance with treatment.
  - Signs and symptoms to report to health care provider
  - Medication plan (correct timing and dose)

and a mental status check at every home visit to a client at risk for dehydration. Medication regimens, signs and symptoms of dehydration, and health care resources are reviewed with the client and family.

> ### ► *Health Care Resources*

A client with severe chronic health problems may be discharged to a nursing home or extended-care facility on a permanent or a temporary basis. The hospital nurse uses the transfer chart to communicate all important information about the client's individual needs and special care problems. The nurse refers the client discharged to home to specific resources available for client education and family support. Two examples of such support agencies are the American Diabetes Association and the Kidney Foundation.

A home care nurse may be needed to assess the client's hydration status and adherence to drug and diet therapies. If the client lives alone, a daily visit by a home health aide to assist with activities of daily living and reinforce an oral intake plan may be helpful.

 ## Evaluation

On the basis of the identified nursing diagnoses, the nurse evaluates the care of clients with dehydration. Outcomes include that the client is expected to

- Ingest at least 1500 mL of hypotonic fluids each day
- Maintain a fluid output that is approximately equal to the fluid intake
- State that oral mucosal discomfort is relieved
- Experience no oral mucosal complication

Overhydration

Overview

Overhydration, also referred to as fluid overload, is an excess of body fluid. It is not an actual disease but rather a clinical manifestation of a physiologic problem in which fluid intake or retention exceeds the body's fluid needs. Overhydration may be characterized as either an actual excess of total body fluid or a relative fluid excess in one or more fluid compartments. The three basic types of fluid volume excess are isotonic overhydration, hypotonic overhydration, and hypertonic overhydration (Figure 15–5).

Pathophysiology

Most problems associated with overhydration are related to fluid volume excess in the vascular space or to dilution of specific electrolytes and blood components. Clinical manifestations vary with the type and degree of overhydration (Chart 15–6).

Isotonic Overhydration

Isotonic overhydration is also called *hypervolemia* because its associated problems result from excessive fluid in the

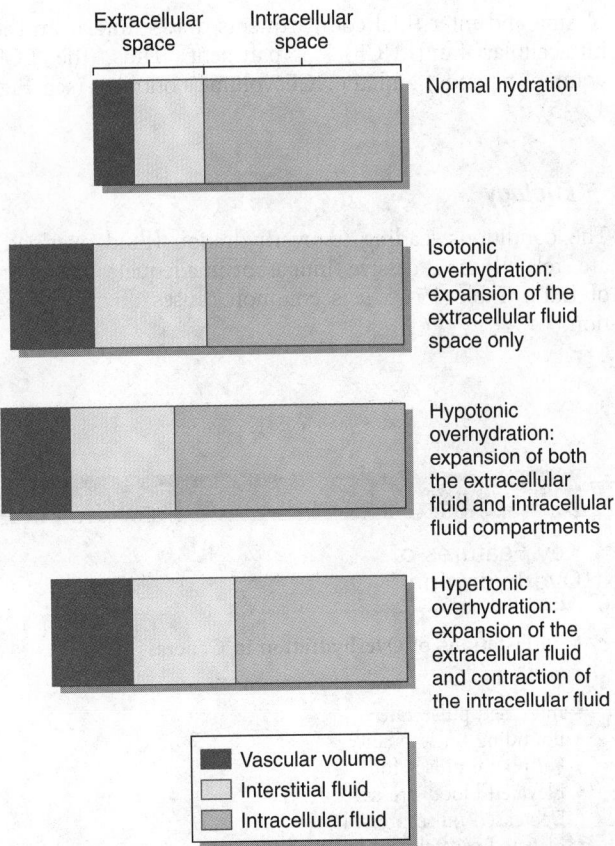

Figure 15–5. Three types of overhydration. (© 1992 M. Linda Workman. All rights reserved.)

extracellular fluid (ECF) compartment. In isotonic overhydration, isotonic fluids are ingested or retained, so that osmolarity remains normal. Only the ECF compartment is expanded, and fluid does not shift between the extracellular and intracellular compartments. The effects of severe isotonic overhydration are circulatory overload and the formation of interstitial edema. Figure 15–6 outlines the compensatory mechanisms associated with mild to moderate isotonic overhydration. When isotonic overhydration is severe or when it occurs in a person with poor cardiac status, overhydration results in congestive heart failure and pulmonary edema.

Hypotonic Overhydration

In hypotonic overhydration (water intoxication), the excess fluid is hypotonic to normal body fluids. Thus, the osmolarity of the ECF decreases, and hydrostatic pressure increases. The excessive fluid moves into the intracellular space because of the decreased vascular osmotic pressure, and all body fluid compartments expand (see Figure 15–5). Because the excessive fluid is hypotonic, electrolyte imbalances resulting from dilution accompany hypotonic overhydration.

Hypertonic Overhydration

Hypertonic overhydration is rare and is caused by an excessive sodium intake. The hyperosmolarity of the plasma and interstitial compartments draws fluid from the intracellular fluid (ICF) compartment. Thus, the ECF volume expands, and the ICF volume contracts (see Fig. 15–5).

Etiology

The conditions leading to overhydration (fluid overload) are related to excessive intake or inadequate excretion of fluid. Table 15–5 lists common causes of overhydration.

Chart 15–6

Key Features of Overhydration

Manifestations of Overhydration in General

Cardiovascular

- Increased pulse rate
- Bounding pulse quality
- Peripheral pulses full
- Elevated blood pressure
- Decreased pulse pressure
- Elevated central venous pressure
- Distended neck and hand veins
- Engorged venous varicosities

Respiratory

- Respiratory rate increased
- Shallow respirations
- Dyspnea increases with exertion or in the supine position
- Moist crackles present on auscultation

Integumentary

- Pitting edema in dependent areas
- Skin pale and cool to touch

Neuromuscular

- Altered level of consciousness
- Headache
- Visual disturbances
- Skeletal muscle weakness
- Paresthesias

Gastrointestinal

- Increased motility

Manifestations of Isotonic Overhydration

- Liver enlargement
- Ascites formation

Manifestations of Hypotonic Overhydration

- Polyuria
- Diarrhea
- Nonpitting edema
- Cardiac dysrhythmias associated with electrolyte dilution
- Projectile vomiting

TABLE 15–5

Common Causes of Overhydration

Isotonic Overhydration

- Poorly controlled intravenous therapy
- Renal failure
- Long-term corticosteroid therapy

Hypotonic Overhydration

- Early renal failure
- Congestive heart failure
- Syndrome of inappropriate antidiuretic hormone
- Poorly controlled intravenous therapy
- Replacement of isotonic fluid loss with hypotonic fluids
- Psychogenic polydipsia
- Irrigation of wounds and body cavities with hypotonic fluids

Hypertonic Overhydration

- Excessive sodium ingestion
- Rapid infusion of hypertonic saline
- Excessive sodium bicarbonate therapy

Collaborative Management

 Assessment

Clinical manifestations of overhydration vary with the specific type, the fluid compartments involved, and the degree of overhydration. Clients with isotonic overhydration or hypertonic overhydration have signs and symptoms associated with circulatory overload. Clients with hypotonic overhydration have problems associated with ICF increase and electrolyte dilution. Chart 15–6 summarizes the common clinical manifestations of overhydration.

A diagnosis of overhydration is based on physical assessment findings together with the results of several laboratory tests. In isotonic overhydration, serum electrolyte values are normal, but decreased hemoglobin, hematocrit, and serum protein levels may result from *hemodilution* (excessive water in the vascular compartment). Elevated levels of most electrolytes, along with increased BUN and creatinine levels, are associated with overhydration caused by renal failure. Hypotonic overhydration is accompanied by decreased complete blood count and decreased protein and electrolyte levels.

Interventions

Interventions for clients with fluid volume excess aim to restore normal fluid balance, provide supportive care until the imbalance is resolved, and prevent future fluid overload. Drug and diet therapies form the basis of intervention.

➤ Drug Therapy

The physician may order diuretics for clients with overhydration if renal failure is not the cause. Diuretics work on

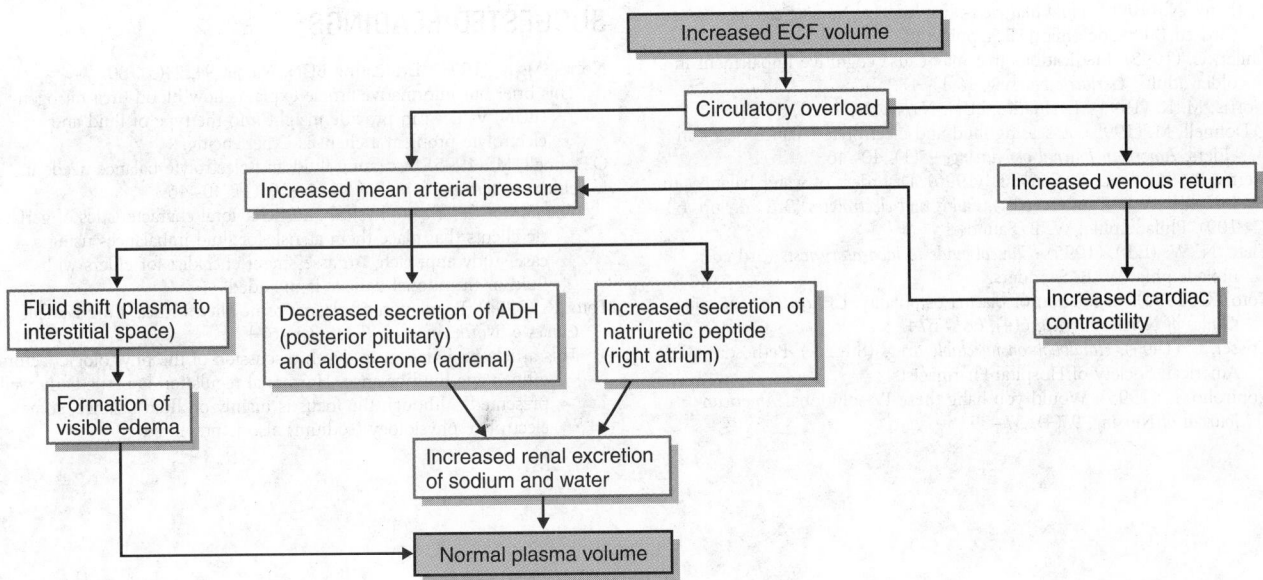

Figure 15–6. Compensatory mechanisms associated with hypervolemia. (ADH = antidiuretic hormone; ECF = extracellular fluid.)

the kidneys to increase the excretion of water or sodium from the body. Osmotic diuretics, such as mannitol, are typically prescribed first to prevent severe electrolyte imbalances. Osmotic diuretics primarily cause renal excretion of water rather than excretion of sodium or potassium. If osmotic diuretics are not effective, the physician may prescribe high-ceiling (loop) diuretics, such as furosemide (Lasix, Furoside✱).

The nurse monitors the client for response to medication, especially weight loss and increased urine output. The nurse also observes the client for signs and symptoms of electrolyte imbalance and assesses laboratory findings every 8 hours.

> ➤ *Diet Therapy*

For the client with mild or chronic overhydration, long-term diet therapy may be valuable in controlling fluid volume through restrictions of both fluid and sodium intake. The client's serum sodium concentration should be considered whenever overhydration is present.

> ➤ *Monitoring*

Intake and Output. The nurse or assistive personnel accurately measures fluid intake and output and explains the reason for any fluid restriction. In addition to regulating the total amount of fluid ingested in a 24-hour period, the nurse carefully schedules fluid offerings throughout the 24 hours. Urine also is monitored for color, character, and specific gravity.

If the client is receiving IV therapy, the nurse administers the exact amount ordered by the physician and monitors the client for increased fluid overload.

Weight. Fluid retention may not be visible. However, a sudden weight gain indicates fluid retention. The nurse weighs the client at the same time every day (before breakfast) using the same scale. Whenever possible, the client wears the same type of clothing for each weigh-in.

 CASE STUDY for the Client with Dehydration

■ You are making a home visit to an 86-year-old woman who underwent hip replacement 2 months ago. She lives alone. When the client answers the door, you find that she is confused. She says she is thirsty and that "it hurts when I piddle." You find a half-empty pan of soup on the stove and evidence of vomiting in the bathroom. Her vital signs are as follows: blood pressure, 102/80 mm Hg; pulse, 102 (thready); respirations, 32; and oral temperature, 38.6° C (101° F).

QUESTIONS:

1. What additional assessment techniques would you perform?
2. How would you assess hydration status?
3. What other data would you gather?
4. What are your action priorities?

SELECTED BIBLIOGRAPHY

Anderson, S. (1996). Fluid and electrolyte disorders in the elderly. In J. Kokko & R. Tannen (Eds.), *Fluids and electrolytes* (3rd ed., pp. 831–839). Philadelphia: W. B. Saunders.

Colling, J., Owen, T., & McCreedy, M. (1994). Urine volumes and voiding patterns among incontinent nursing home residents. *Geriatric Nursing, 15*(4), 188–192.

Frizzell, J. (1998). Avoiding lab test pitfalls. *American Journal of Nursing, 98*(2), 34–38.

Guyton, A., & Hall, J. (1996). *Textbook of medical physiology* (9th ed.). Philadelphia: W. B. Saunders.

Halperin, M., & Goldstein, M. (1994), *Fluid, electrolyte and acid-base physiology: A problem-based approach* (2nd ed) Philadelphia: W. B. Saunders.

Kokko, J., & Tannen, R. (1996). *Fluids and electrolytes* (3rd ed.). Philadelphia: W. B. Saunders.

Kuhn, M. (1996). Laboratory analysis. *Critical Care Nurse, 16*(5), 74–76.

Metheny, N. (1996). *Fluid and electrolyte balance: Nursing considerations* (3rd ed.). Philadelphia: J. B. Lippincott.

Miller, C. (1995). Medications that may cause cognitive impairment in older adults. *Geriatric Nursing, 16*(1), 47.

Norris, M. K. (1994). Evaluating BUN. *Nursing94, 24*(5), 80.

O'Donnell, M. (1995). Assessing fluid and electrolyte balance needs in elders. *American Journal of Nursing, 95*(1), 40–46.

Sterns, R., Spital, A., & Clark, E. (1996). Disorders of water balance. In J. Kokko & R. Tannen (eds.), *Fluids and electrolytes* (3rd ed., pp. 63–109). Philadelphia: W. B. Saunders.

Tietz, N. W. (Ed.). (1995). *Clinical guide to laboratory tests* (3rd ed.). Philadelphia: W. B. Saunders.

Toto, K. (1994). Regulation of plasma osmolality. *Critical Care Nursing Clinics of North America, 6*(4), 661–674.

Trissel, L. (1994). *Handbook on injectable drugs* (8th ed.). Bethesda, MD: American Society of Hospital Pharmacists.

Vonfrolio, L. (1995). Would you hang these IV solutions? *American Journal of Nursing, 95*(4), 37–39.

SUGGESTED READINGS

Norris, M. K. (1994). Evaluating BUN. *Nursing94, 24*(5), 80.

This brief but informative article explains how blood urea nitrogen (BUN) values can provide insight into the type of fluid and electrolyte problem a client is experiencing.

O'Donnell, M. (1995). Assessing fluid and electrolyte balance needs in elders. *American Journal of Nursing, 95*(1), 40–46.

The author describes physical and behavioral characteristics of geriatric clients that place them at risk for fluid imbalances using a case study approach. An assessment checklist for elders with fluid or nutritional deficits is included.

Toto, K. (1994). Regulation of plasma osmolality. *Critical Care Nursing Clinics of North America, 6*(4), 661–674.

This article provides an in-depth discussion of the physiologic factors influencing fluid balance. Hormonal regulation is particularly well presented. Although the focus is mainly on fluid balance, some electrolyte physiology (sodium) also is presented.

Chapter 16

INTERVENTIONS FOR CLIENTS WITH ELECTROLYTE IMBALANCES

Mild electrolyte imbalances occur frequently in healthy people as a result of variation in fluid intake and output. Such imbalances are of short duration and do not require interventions from health care professionals. Severe electrolyte imbalances, however, are life-threatening and can occur in any setting. Elderly clients and clients taking medications that alter fluid and electrolyte status are at greater risk for electrolyte imbalances.

POTASSIUM IMBALANCES

Hypokalemia

Overview

Because 98% of total body potassium (K$^+$) is intracellular, minor changes in extracellular potassium levels cause major changes in cell membrane excitability as well as in other cellular processes. Hypokalemia is indicated by a serum potassium level below 3.5 mEq/L (mmol/L). A relatively common electrolyte imbalance, hypokalemia is potentially life-threatening because every body system can be affected.

Pathophysiology

Decreased serum potassium level increases the difference in potassium concentration between the fluid inside the cells, or intracellular fluid (ICF), and the extracellular fluid (ECF). This increased difference reduces the excit-

ability of cells. Consequently, the cell membranes of all excitable tissues, such as nerve and muscle, are less responsive to normal stimuli.

The severity of problems caused by hypokalemia is directly related to how rapidly the serum potassium level decreases. When extracellular potassium loss is gradual, cells adjust and intracellular potassium decreases in proportion to the ECF potassium level. In this situation, the potassium concentration difference between the two fluid compartments remains unchanged, and symptoms of hypokalemia may not appear until the potassium loss is extreme. Rapid changes in extracellular potassium levels (representing a more rapid loss of potassium) cannot be compensated for quickly, and result in dramatic changes in body function.

Etiology

Hypokalemia may result either from actual total body potassium loss or from movement of potassium from the ECF to the ICF, causing a relative decrease in extracellular potassium level. Table 16–1 summarizes the common causes of hypokalemia.

Actual potassium depletion occurs when potassium loss is excessive or when potassium intake is not sufficient to match normal potassium loss. Relative hypokalemia occurs when total body potassium levels are normal but the potassium distribution between fluid compartments is abnormal. Conditions that increase the cellular uptake of

TABLE 16–1

Common Causes of Hypokalemia

Actual Potassium Deficits

Excessive Potassium Loss

- Inappropriate or excessive use of drugs
  - Diuretics
  - Digitalis
  - Corticosteroids
- Increased secretion of aldosterone
  - Cushing's syndrome
- Diarrhea
- Vomiting
- Wound drainage (especially gastrointestinal)
- Prolonged nasogastric suction
- Heat-induced excessive diaphoresis
- Renal disease impairing reabsorption of potassium

Inadequate Potassium Intake

- Nothing by mouth

Relative Potassium Deficits

Movement of Potassium from Extracellular Fluid to Intracellular Fluid

- Alkalosis
- Hyperinsulinism
- Hyperalimentation
- Total parenteral nutrition

Dilution of Serum Potassium

- Water intoxication
- Intravenous therapy with potassium-poor solutions

potassium, leading to hypokalemia, include metabolic alkalosis and insulin administration.

Incidence/Prevalence

Exact statistics about the incidence of hypokalemia are not available. This imbalance occurs frequently in both hospitalized clients and in those receiving ambulatory care. Hypokalemia may be associated with any illness (Braxmeyer & Keyes, 1996). Elderly clients are especially at high risk for hypokalemia resulting from chronic illness or prescribed medications.

Collaborative Management

 Assessment

➤ *History*

The nurse collects data from clients at risk as well as those with actual hypokalemia.

Age. This is an important consideration because renal capacity to concentrate urine decreases with aging, increasing potassium loss. Moreover, elderly clients are more likely to use medications that promote potassium loss.

Medication Use. The nurse questions the client about medication use, especially diuretics and corticosteroids. These drugs increase potassium loss through the kidneys.

One of the most common causes of hypokalemia is the use and misuse of diuretics. In clients taking digitalis preparations such as digoxin (Lanoxin, Novodigoxin✦), hypokalemia increases the sensitivity of the myocardium to the drug and may result in digitalis toxicity, even when the dosage is within the therapeutic range.

The nurse questions whether the client takes a prescribed potassium supplement, such as potassium chloride (KCl). The client may not be taking the potassium chloride as prescribed because of its unpleasant taste.

Other Factors. Any acute or chronic disease state may lead to hypokalemia. The nurse asks about recent illnesses and medical or surgical interventions. A thorough diet history, including a typical day's food and beverage intake, helps the nurse identify clients at risk for hypokalemia.

➤ *Physical Assessment/Clinical Manifestations*

Clinical manifestations of hypokalemia are associated with altered function of many systems (Chart 16–1).

Chart 16–1

Key Features of Hypokalemia

Cardiovascular

- Variable pulse rate, more often rapid
- Pulse quality thready and weak
- Peripheral pulses difficult to palpate
- Orthostatic (postural) hypotension
- Electrocardiographic abnormalities
  - ST depression
  - Inverted T wave
  - Prominent U wave
  - Heart block

Respiratory

- Shallow, ineffective respirations resulting from profound weakness of the skeletal muscles of respiration
- Diminished breath sounds

Neuromuscular

- Anxiety, lethargy, confusion, coma
- Loss of tactile discrimination
- General skeletal muscle weakness
- Deep tendon hyporeflexia
- Eventual flaccid paralysis

Gastrointestinal

- Decreased motility
- Hypoactive to absent bowel sounds
- Nausea
- Vomiting
- Abdominal distention
- Paralytic ileus
- Constipation

Renal

- Decreased ability to concentrate urine
- Polyuria
- Decreased specific gravity

Musculoskeletal Manifestations. Skeletal muscles become weak in response to hypokalemia, and a stronger stimulus is needed to begin muscle contraction. A client may be so weak as to be unable to stand. Handgrasps are weak, and hyporeflexia (a decreased response to deep tendon reflex stimulation) may be noted. Severe hypokalemia can lead to flaccid paralysis. The nurse assesses the degree of muscle weakness and determines the client's ability to perform activities of daily living (ADLs).

Respiratory Manifestations. The respiratory system can be profoundly affected by hypokalemia through depression of the nerves and muscles needed for breathing. Weakness of the skeletal muscles of respiration results in shallow respirations. The nurse assesses breath sounds, ease of respiratory effort, color of nail beds and mucous membranes, and rate and depth of respiration. The nurse assesses the client's respiratory status at least every 2 hours, because respiratory insufficiency frequently accompanies hypokalemia and is a major cause of death (Tannen, 1996).

Cardiovascular Manifestations. Cardiovascular changes often accompany hypokalemia. The nurse assesses the cardiovascular system by first palpating peripheral pulses. In the client with hypokalemia, the pulse is usually thready and weak. Palpation is difficult, and the pulse is easily blocked with light pressure. The pulse rate ranges from excessively slow to excessively rapid, depending on whether a dysrhythmia (irregular heartbeat) is present. The nurse measures blood pressure with the client in lying, sitting, and standing positions, because orthostatic (postural) hypotension accompanies hypokalemia.

Neurologic Manifestations. Neurologic manifestations of hypokalemia include changes in mental status. The client may experience short-term irritability and anxiety followed by lethargy progressing to confusion and coma as hypokalemia worsens. Severe hypokalemia affects sensory nerves by decreasing sensory awareness. For example, the client may not be able to identify mild sensations of pain, touch, heat, and cold.

Gastrointestinal Manifestations. Hypokalemia results in decreased smooth muscle contractility within the gastrointestinal system, leading to decreased peristalsis. The affected client has hypoactive bowel sounds and may experience nausea, vomiting, constipation, and abdominal distention. The nurse assesses distention by measuring abdominal girth. The nurse also assesses bowel sounds in all four abdominal quadrants to determine the extent of decreased peristalsis. Severe hypokalemia can cause paralytic ileus (the absence of peristalsis).

➤ Psychosocial Assessment

Because hypokalemia is seldom a long-term problem, any associated behavioral changes usually occur within a short period. Information about the client's behavior may need to be obtained from close family members or friends, depending on the client's condition.

The nurse collects data about the onset and duration of behavioral changes as well as their association with any other physical signs and symptoms. These data are impor-

tant and need to be as accurate as possible. The client may be lethargic and unable to perform simple problem-solving tasks that require concentration, such as counting backward from 100 by threes. As hypokalemia progresses, the client may become increasingly confused, in particular being disoriented to time and place. In severe hypokalemia, coma may develop.

➤ Laboratory Assessment

Hypokalemia is confirmed by a serum potassium value below 3.5 mEq/L (mmol/L). However, this value does not indicate whether a true potassium deficit exists or whether a shift of potassium from the blood to the intracellular fluid (ICF) has occurred.

➤ Other Diagnostic Assessment

The physician usually orders a baseline electrocardiogram (ECG) followed by continuous cardiac monitoring for a client with severe hypokalemia. Hypokalemia causes electrical conduction abnormalities, including ST-segment depression, flat or inverted T waves, and increased U waves. Dysrhythmias can result in death, particularly in elderly clients taking digitalis.

 Analysis

➤ Common Nursing Diagnoses and Collaborative Problems

The priority nursing diagnoses for clients with hypokalemia are as follows:
1. High Risk for Injury related to skeletal muscle weakness
2. Constipation related to smooth muscle atony.

The primary collaborative problem is High Risk for Ineffective Breathing Pattern Related to Neuromuscular Impairment.

➤ Additional Nursing Diagnoses and Collaborative Problems

In addition to the common nursing diagnoses and collaborative problems, clients with hypokalemia may have one or more of the following:
- Impaired Mobility related to skeletal muscle weakness
- Total Self-Care Deficit related to skeletal muscle weakness
- Decreased Cardiac Output related to dysrhythmia.

 Planning and Implementation

➤ High Risk for Injury

Planning: Expected Outcomes. The client is expected to avoid injury and show a return to a normal serum potassium level.

Interventions. These aim to prevent potassium loss, increase serum potassium levels, and provide a safe environment for the client. Drug and diet therapies help restore normal serum potassium levels.

Drug Therapy. Potassium supplements (oral or intravenous [IV]) are commonly given for the treatment and prevention of hypokalemia.

Potassium Supplements. Most potassium supplements (replacements) consist of potassium chloride. The amount and the route of potassium replacement depend on the degree of potassium loss. A client with a serum potassium level of 3 mEq/L needs 100 to 200 mEq of potassium supplement, for example, and one with a serum potassium level of 2.0 mEq/L needs 500 to 600 mEq (Tannen, 1996).

Potassium is given IV for severe hypokalemia. A dilution of no more than 1 mEq/10 mL of solution is recommended. The maximum recommended infusion rate is 5 to 10 mEq/hour, *never to exceed 20 mEq/hour under any circumstances.* Elderly clients may not be able to handle this rate. Because rapid infusion of potassium can cause cardiac arrest, the nurse never gives potassium by IV push.

Potassium is a severe tissue irritant and is never administered as an intramuscular or subcutaneous injection. Tissues damaged by potassium can become necrotic and slough, leading to loss of function and requiring reconstructive surgery. IV potassium solutions irritate veins and can cause phlebitis. The nurse checks the physician's orders carefully to ensure that the client receives the correct amount of potassium. The nurse assesses the IV site every 2 hours and asks the client whether he or she feels burning or pain at the site. The IV solution is stopped immediately if infiltration occurs.

Oral potassium preparations may be administered as liquids or solids. Potassium chloride has a strong, unpleasant taste that is difficult to mask. Because potassium chloride can cause nausea and vomiting, it should not be taken on an empty stomach.

Potassium-Sparing Diuretics. Diuretics that increase renal excretion of potassium commonly cause hypokalemia. These classes of diuretics include high-ceiling, or loop, diuretics, such as furosemide (Lasix, Furoside✦), bumetanide (Bumex), and ethacrynic acid (Edecrin), and the thiazide diuretics, such as chlorothiazide (Diuril), hydrochlorothiazide (Esidrix, Nefrol✦), and quinethazone (Hydromox, Aquamox✦). Thus, these drugs are avoided in clients with actual hypokalemia and in those who are susceptible to hypokalemia. For a client with hypokalemia who requires diuretic therapy, a potassium-sparing diuretic may be appropriate. Potassium-sparing diuretics cause diuresis without increasing potassium excretion. Diuretics with this action include spironolactone (Aldactone, Novospiroton✦), triamterene (Dyrenium), and amiloride (Midamor).

Diet Therapy. The nurse consults with the dietitian in teaching the client how to increase dietary potassium intake. Eating food naturally rich in potassium helps restore normal potassium levels and prevent further loss. Table 14–7 lists foods with a high potassium content.

Safety Measures. For a client experiencing muscle weakness, the nurse uses safety measures and eliminates hazards. The nurse or assistive personnel assists the client with ambulation. Obstacles or slippery areas are removed from the ambulation path, and the client wears nonslip footgear. When ambulating with assistance, the client wears a gait belt around the waist.

➤ Constipation

Planning: Expected Outcomes. The client's normal bowel elimination pattern is expected to be restored.

Interventions. These aim to restore normal serum potassium levels and induce gastric motility. Specific interventions include drug and diet therapies to restore serum potassium levels to normal values (discussed earlier under drug and diet therapies for High Risk for Injury) and stimulate intestinal peristalsis as well as interventions designed to prevent constipation.

Drug Therapy. Laxatives that add bulk or fiber may be used to stimulate peristalsis. Other drugs that enhance gastric emptying and stimulate gastrointestinal motility, such as metoclopramide (Reglan, Maxeran✦), are used to treat constipation associated with hypokalemia.

Diet Therapy. The nurse provides high-fiber foods and plenty of liquids for the client who is not on fluid restrictions. To ensure client cooperation, the nurse prepares a list of foods that contain high concentrations of fiber and asks the client to select favorite items from that list.

Comfort Measures. The nurse or assistive personnel can help the client maintain normal bowel elimination patterns in several ways. When the client is using the toilet or bedpan, privacy is provided. The door is closed, privacy curtains are drawn, and visitors are asked to step out of the room. Physical activity and exercise promote gastric motility. The client is encouraged to ambulate whenever his or her condition permits. A bedridden client benefits from frequent position changes and mild bed exercises.

➤ Ineffective Breathing Pattern

Planning: Expected Outcomes. The client is expected to have a breathing pattern adequate to maintain gas exchange.

Interventions. The nurse monitors the client's rate and depth of respiration at least once per hour, noting particularly increased rate and decreased depth. The effectiveness of respiratory muscles can also be determined by assessing the client's ability to cough. The nurse also examines the client's face, oral mucosa, and nail beds for pallor or cyanosis. The nurse evaluates arterial blood gas values for *hypoxemia* (decreased blood oxygen concentration) and *hypercapnia* (increased arterial carbon dioxide concentration). (Chapters 29 and 30 discuss respiratory assessment and interventions in more detail.)

▶ Continuing Care

No extensive home care preparations are necessary for clients with mild hypokalemia and those with sudden-onset hypokalemia. The imbalance is corrected before discharge and, with minimal precautions, is unlikely to recur. Clients who are most likely to be discharged before the imbalance is completely corrected and who are susceptible to recurrent episodes of imbalance have chronic pathologic conditions or diseases. These clients often require long-term diet and drug therapy.

▶ Health Teaching

The nurse instructs the at-risk client (especially one receiving diuretics or corticosteroids) regarding the proper use of medications, the signs and symptoms of hypokalemia, when to seek medical help, and foods rich in potassium. The nurse also teaches the client to assess the rate, rhythm, and quality of peripheral pulses at least once each day and whenever any signs or symptoms of hypokalemia are present. The nurse discusses with a chronically ill client how potassium is lost from the body so that the client can act to reduce potassium loss before actual deficits occur. The nurse reinforces how often the client should have serum potassium levels assessed.

▶ Home Care Management

When hypokalemia is resolved and the underlying cause is controlled, home care management techniques are individualized to the client's baseline physical and mental functioning. The home environment is assessed for the client's ability to perform ADLs safely.

A client with a chronic condition that increases his or her risk for hypokalemia and other electrolyte imbalances may not be able to live alone. The nurse assesses the ability and willingness of family members to share in the client's care. The nurse also determines whether and what type of home care assistance may be needed.

A home health aide may be needed to assist with hygiene and ensure a safe environment. Weekly visits by a nurse may also be needed to assess changes and ensure compliance with the medication regimen. At every home visit to a client at risk for hypokalemia, the nurse performs a focused assessment (Chart 16–2). Medication regimens, signs and symptoms of hypokalemia, and health care resources are reviewed with the client and family.

▶ Health Care Resources

Because hypokalemia is a manifestation of other health problems rather than a distinct disease, needed health care resources vary with the client's underlying health problem. For the client with chronic health problems that increase the risk for hypokalemia, appropriate health care resources include the physician, home care nurse, pharmacist, and nutritionist or dietitian. When special equipment needs or financial problems interfere with the client's ability to obtain necessary food or medications, the nurse contacts the social services department of the facil-

Chart 16–2

Focused Assessment for Home Care Clients at Risk for Hypokalemia

- Assess respiratory status.
  - Rate, depth, rhythm of respiration
  - Color of lips, tongue, nail beds
  - Can the client complete a sentence without taking a breath?
- Assess cardiovascular status.
  - Vital signs, including apical pulse, pulse pressure, presence or absence of orthostatic hypotension, and quality and rhythm of peripheral pulses
  - Presence or absence of peripheral edema
  - Hand vein filling in the dependent position
  - Neck vein filling in the recumbent and sitting positions
  - Weight gain or loss
- Assess cognition and mental status.
  - Level of consciousness
  - Orientation to time, place, and person
  - Can the client accurately read a seven-word sentence containing no words greater than three syllables?
- Assess condition of skin and mucous membranes.
  - Presence or absence of skin tenting over the sternum or the forehead
  - Moistness of skin, most reliable on chest and back
  - Presence or absence of coating on tongue or teeth
  - Can the client spit?
- Assess neuromuscular status.
  - Reactivity of patellar and biceps reflexes
  - Oral temperature
  - Handgrip strength
  - Steadiness of gait
- Assess renal system.
  - Observe urine specimen for color, odor, cloudiness, and amount
- Ask about the following:
  - 24-hour fluid intake and output
  - 24-hour diet recall
  - 24-hour activity recall
  - What over-the-counter and prescribed medications has the client taken?
  - Has the client experienced any dizziness or lightheadedness?
  - Does the client have a headache (what time of day, associated with what activities)?
  - Muscle twitches, cramps, pain, or spasms
- Assess client's understanding of illness and compliance with treatment.
  - Signs and symptoms to report to health care provider
  - Medication plan (correct timing and dose)

ity. The client with chronic health problems frequently requires assistance with self-care. If no one is available to perform these functions, home care nursing may be necessary or the client may have to be placed in an extended-care facility. Specific organizations related to the chronic disease or organ problem causing the hypokalemia may be helpful. Such organizations include the Kidney Foundation and the American Diabetes Association.

 Evaluation

On the basis of the identified nursing diagnoses and collaborative problems, the nurse evaluates the care of the client with hypokalemia. The client is expected to
- Return to and maintain a normal serum potassium level (between 3.5 and 5.1 mEq/L)
- Comply with drug and diet therapies as prescribed
- State the early signs and symptoms of hypokalemia
- Avoid injury
- Have normal bowel elimination patterns
- Maintain adequate gas exchange
- Maintain regular cardiac rate and rhythm

Hyperkalemia

Overview

Hyperkalemia occurs when the serum potassium level exceeds 5.1 mEq/L (mmol/L). Because the range of normal serum potassium values is narrow, even slight increases above normal values can have serious adverse effects on the physiologic function of excitable tissues, especially the myocardium.

Pathophysiology

An elevated serum potassium level produces a decreased potassium concentration difference between the intracellular fluid (ICF) and the extracellular fluid (ECF). This decreased difference increases cell excitability, so excitable tissues respond to less intense stimuli and may even discharge spontaneously.

Hyperkalemia alters the function of all excitable membranes to some degree. The myocardium is the excitable membrane most sensitive to serum potassium increases; thus, the more serious complications of hyperkalemia are associated with altered cardiac function.

Pathologic changes associated with hyperkalemia are directly related to how rapidly ECF potassium levels increase. Sudden increases in serum potassium levels cause profound functional changes at potassium levels between 6 and 7 mEq/L. When serum potassium levels increase slowly, problems with excitable membrane function may not be obvious until potassium levels reach 8 mEq/L.

Etiology

Hyperkalemia may result from an actual increase in the amount of total body potassium. It also may result from abnormal movement of potassium from the cells to the ECF. Table 16-2 summarizes common causes of hyperkalemia.

Hyperkalemia is rare in persons with normally functioning kidneys. Most cases of hyperkalemia occur in hospitalized clients and those undergoing medical treatment. Clients at greatest risk for hyperkalemia are the chronically ill, debilitated, and elderly.

TABLE 16–2

Common Causes of Hyperkalemia

Actual Potassium Excesses

Excessive Potassium Intake
- Overingestion of potassium-containing foods or medications
  - Salt substitutes
  - Potassium chloride
- Rapid infusion of potassium-containing intravenous solution
- Bolus intravenous potassium injections

Decreased Potassium Excretion
- Adrenal insufficiency (Addison's disease, adrenalectomy)
- Renal failure
- Potassium-sparing diuretics

Relative Potassium Excesses

Movement of Potassium from Intracellular Fluid to Extracellular Fluid
- Tissue damage
- Acidosis
- Hyperuricemia
- Hypercatabolism

Collaborative Management

 Assessment

➤ *History*

The client's age is an important factor because renal function decreases with aging. The nurse asks about chronic illnesses, particularly renal disease and diabetes mellitus, and recent medical or surgical interventions. The client is questioned about urine output, including the frequency and amount of voidings. The nurse also inquires about medication use, particularly potassium-sparing diuretics. The nurse obtains a diet history to pinpoint possible causative factors, such as the intake of potassium-rich foods. The client is specifically asked about the use of salt substitutes, many of which contain potassium salts.

The nurse collects data pointing to symptoms related to hyperkalemia. The client is asked whether he or she has experienced palpitations, skipped heartbeats, or other cardiac irregularities as well as muscle twitching, weakness in leg muscles, and unusual tingling or numbness in the hands, feet, or face. The nurse inquires about recent changes in bowel habits, especially diarrhea, colic, and explosive bowel movements.

➤ *Physical Assessment/Clinical Manifestations*

The clinical manifestations of hyperkalemia are summarized in Chart 16–3.

Cardiovascular Manifestations. Cardiovascular changes are the most severe results of hyperkalemia and are the most common cause of death in clients with hyperkalemia (Tannen, 1996). The nurse, therefore, carefully assesses the cardiac status of all clients with hyperkalemia through careful observation and cardiac monitoring. Con-

Key Features of Hyperkalemia

Cardiovascular

- Irregular heat rate, usually slow
- Decreased blood pressure
- Electrocardiographic abnormalities
  - Tall T waves
  - Widened QRS complexes
  - Prolonged PR intervals
  - Flat P waves
- Ectopic beats
- Late: dysrhythmias, ventricular fibrillation, cardiac arrest in diastole

Respiratory

- Unaffected until late, when profound weakness of the skeletal muscles causes respiratory failure

Neuromuscular

- Early phase, or mild, hyperkalemia
  - Muscle twitches, cramps
  - Paresthesias
- Late phase, or severe, hyperkalemia
  - Profound weakness
  - Ascending flaccid paralysis in distal to proximal direction involving the arms and the legs

Gastrointestinal

- Increased motility
- Hyperactive bowel sounds
- Diarrhea

duction changes indicating hyperkalemia include gradual worsening of bradycardia; heart block; tall, peaked T waves; prolonged PR intervals; flattened or absent P waves; and widened QRS complexes (Fig. 16–1).

As serum potassium levels rise, impulse conduction through the cardiac Purkinje system slows and may be blocked at the atrioventricular (AV) node. The heart muscle dilates and becomes flaccid. As electrical conduction is blocked at the AV node, ectopic beats (beats generated outside the normal conduction system in the ventricles) may appear. Complete heart block, ventricular standstill, and ventricular fibrillation are major life-threatening complications of severe hyperkalemia.

Besides noting specific ECG changes, the nurse also assesses cardiac status through peripheral pulse and blood pressure measurements. The client with hyperkalemia usually has a slow, weak pulse and low blood pressure.

Neuromuscular Manifestations. The neuromuscular response to hyperkalemia has two phases. In the early stages of hyperkalemia, skeletal muscles twitch, and the client may be aware of unusual nerve sensations, such as tingling and burning, followed by numbness in the hands and feet and around the mouth. As hyperkalemia progresses, muscle twitching changes to weakness followed

by flaccid paralysis. The weakness ascends from distal to proximal areas and initially affects the muscles of the arms and the legs. Trunk, head, and respiratory muscles are not affected until serum potassium levels reach lethal levels.

Gastrointestinal Manifestations. The smooth muscle of the gastrointestinal tract responds to hyperkalemia by increasing peristalsis. The nurse assesses the gastrointestinal system by listening to bowel sounds and observing stools. The client may experience diarrhea and spastic colonic activity. Bowel sounds are hyperactive, with frequent audible rushes and gurgles. Bowel movements may be frequent, watery, and explosive.

► *Laboratory Assessment*

A serum potassium value exceeding 5.1 mEq/L confirms hyperkalemia. If hyperkalemia results from dehydration, levels of other serum electrolytes, hematocrit, and hemoglobin may be elevated. Hyperkalemia associated with renal failure is usually accompanied by elevated serum creatinine and blood urea nitrogen levels, decreased blood pH, and normal or low hematocrit and hemoglobin levels.

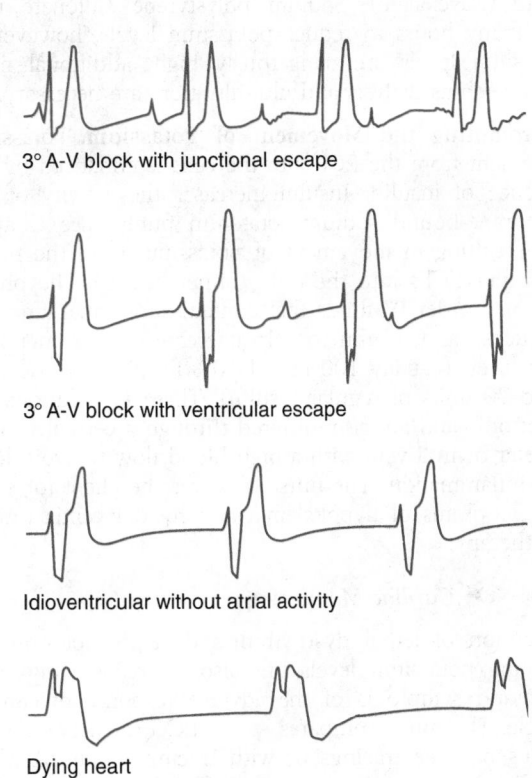

Figure 16–1. Electrocardiographic (ECG) changes associated with hyperkalemia. (Modified with permission from John M. Clochesy.)

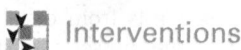
Interventions

Although identifying the causes of hyperkalemia is important, interventions are aimed at immediately reducing the serum potassium level. Drug therapy is useful for restoring normal potassium balance.

➤ *Drug Therapy*

The aims of drug therapy are to prevent further increases in serum potassium level by eliminating potassium administration, enhancing potassium excretion, and promoting the movement of potassium from the extracellular fluid (ECF) into the cells.

Eliminating Potassium Administration. When hyperkalemia occurs, the nurse stops infusions of potassium-containing IV solutions, but keeps the IV catheter open. Oral potassium supplements are withheld, and a potassium-restricted diet is ordered.

Increasing Potassium Excretion. If renal function is not impaired, the physician orders administration of potassium-excreting diuretics, such as furosemide (Mendyka, 1992). For a client with renal problems, drug therapy to increase potassium excretion includes cation exchange resins that promote gastrointestinal sodium absorption and potassium excretion, such as sodium polystyrene sulfonate (Kayexalate). Sodium polystyrene sulfonate may take many hours to reduce potassium levels, however. If potassium levels are dangerously high, additional measures, such as dialysis and ultrafiltration, are necessary.

Promoting the Movement of Potassium. Potassium movement from the ECF into the cells is enhanced by the presence of insulin. Insulin increases the activity of the membrane-bound sodium-potassium pump (see Chapter 14), resulting in movement of potassium from the blood and other ECFs into the cell (Tannen, 1996). The physician may order IV fluids that contain substantial amounts of glucose and insulin to help decrease the serum potassium levels (usually 100 mL of 10% to 20% glucose with 10 to 20 units of regular insulin). These IV solutions are hypertonic and are administered through a central venous catheter or in a vein with a high blood flow to avoid local vein inflammation. The nurse observes the client for signs and symptoms of hypokalemia and hypoglycemia during this therapy.

➤ *Cardiac Monitoring*

Prevention of lethal dysrhythmias depends not only on reducing potassium levels but also on recognizing early signs and symptoms of the adverse response of cardiac muscle. The nurse compares recent ECG tracings with the client's baseline tracings or with tracings obtained when the client's serum potassium level was close to normal.

➤ *Health Teaching*

Education is a key factor in the prevention of hyperkalemia and in the early detection of its life-threatening complications. The teaching plan for the client at risk for hyperkalemia includes diet, medications, and recognition of the signs and symptoms of hyperkalemia. Diet educa-

---

Chart 16–4

Education Guide: Dietary Management of Hyperkalemia

You Should Avoid	You May Eat
• Organ meats	• Eggs
• Fish	• Breads
• Fresh fruits	• Cereals
• Dried fruits	• Butter
• Beef	• Sugar
• Chicken	
• Pork	
• Milk	
• Vegetables	

---

tion includes knowledge of foods to avoid (those high in potassium) and permissible foods containing little potassium (Chart 16–4). The nurse instructs the client to examine medication and food package labels to determine the potassium content and to avoid salt substitutes, because these preparations usually contain potassium.

SODIUM IMBALANCES

Hyponatremia

Overview

Hyponatremia is a serum sodium (Na^+) level below 135 mEq/L (mmol/L). Because sodium is the major cation of the blood and interstitial fluid and is primarily used for maintaining the osmolarity of these fluids, sodium imbalances are usually associated with fluid volume imbalances.

Pathophysiology

The pathophysiologic changes underlying hyponatremia involve two mechanisms. The first mechanism is a change in cell excitability or activity. As the concentration of sodium in the blood and other extracellular fluid decreases, the sodium concentration gradient between the extracellular fluid (ECF) and the intracellular fluid (ICF) also decreases. Less sodium is available to move across the excitable membrane, causing delayed and slower membrane depolarization. The second mechanism is the movement of water from the ECF space into the ICF space. Cells swell and their functions are impaired.

Etiology

Various conditions can lead to hyponatremia by causing either an actual or a relative decrease in sodium content (Table 16–3). Hyponatremia can represent a loss of total body sodium, movement of sodium from the blood to other fluid spaces, or dilution of serum sodium as a result of excessive water in the plasma.

WOMEN'S HEALTH CONSIDERATIONS

 Hyponatremia as a complication during early postoperative recovery has a relatively high occurrence

TABLE 16-3

Common Causes of Hyponatremia

Actual Sodium Deficits

Increased Sodium Excretion

- Excessive diaphoresis
- Diuretics (high-ceiling diuretics)
- Wound drainage (especially gastrointestinal)
- Decreased secretion of aldosterone
- Hyperlipidemia
- Renal disease (scarred distal convoluted tubule)

Inadequate Sodium Intake

- Nothing by mouth
- Low-salt diet

Relative Sodium Deficits

Dilution of Serum Sodium

- Excessive ingestion of hypotonic fluids
- Psychogenic polydipsia
- Freshwater drowning
- Renal failure (nephrotic syndrome)
- Irrigation with hypotonic fluids
- Syndrome of inappropriate antidiuretic hormone secretion
- Hyperglycemia
- Congestive heart failure

in the United States, ranging from 1% to 5%. Although this complication occurs as often among men as women, more women develop brain damage and die from coma or seizure activity. The accompanying Research Applications for Nursing feature suggests a physiologic basis for this gender difference in response to hyponatremia.

Collaborative Management

 Assessment

The clinical manifestations of hyponatremia are associated with its effects on excitable cellular activity. The cells especially affected are involved in cerebral, neuromuscular, and gastric smooth muscle functions (Chart 16–5).

➤ Cerebral Manifestations

Changes in cerebral function are the most obvious signs and symptoms of hyponatremia. Because these changes may be seen as either depressed activity or excessive activity (and sometimes both), establishing the client's usual cerebral function and behavioral patterns is essential to detecting changes associated with hyponatremia. Behavioral changes result from cerebral edema and increased intracranial pressure. The nurse closely observes and documents the client's behavior. The nurse assesses the client's current mental status, starting with the level of consciousness, in the same manner described under neurologic manifestations of dehydration (p. 000).

➤ Neuromuscular Manifestations

The nurse assesses the client's neuromuscular status during each nursing shift for changes from baseline values. The neuromuscular response to hyponatremia is generalized muscle weakness. Muscle tone and deep tendon reflex responses diminish.

Muscle weakness associated with hyponatremia occurs bilaterally and is worse in the extremities. The nurse assesses deep tendon reflexes by lightly tapping the patellar (knee) tendons and Achilles (heel) tendons with a reflex hammer and documenting the degree of reflex movement. The technique for assessing motor strength and reflexes is described in depth in Chapter 43.

⊳ Research Applications for Nursing

Men and Women Differ in Their Ability to Recover from Postoperative Hyponatremia

Ayus, J. C., & Arieff, A. (1996). Brain damage and postoperative hyponatremia: The role of gender. Neurology, 46(2), 323–328.

This article is a meta-analysis of the incidence and treatment of postoperative hyponatremia in the United States from 1935 to 1990. This analysis determined that postoperative hyponatremia occurred at a minimum frequency of 1% in 25 million inpatient surgical procedures. Hyponatremia induces cerebral encephalopathy with neuronal swelling and hypoxia. The incidence of postoperative hyponatremia is nearly equal among men and women; however, more women than men suffer severe complications of encephalopathy, permanent brain damage, or death.

The investigators explored an animal model for gender differences in hyponatremic encephalopathy. In female rats, the hypoxic effects of hyponatremia were compounded by estrogen and vasopressin interacting to decrease cerebral perfusion. Male rats, without the interactive effect of estrogen on vasopressin activity, did not experience cerebral hypoxia.

The investigators found that the hyponatremia in both male and female animal models could be reversed with the administration of intravenous (IV) hypertonic saline. The literature review confirmed that patients who were treated with hypertonic saline, water restriction, and loop diuretics had better outcomes than those who received standard isotonic or hypotonic fluid therapy.

Critique. This study blended prospective experimental bench research with retrospective clinical research in an attempt to explain a life-threatening phenomenon. Although the results are not absolute, the findings are compelling enough to call into question the practice of supporting postoperative clients with IV hypotonic fluids.

Possible Nursing Implications. Increasing the IV fluid rate in clients whose urine output is below 20 mL/hour is common in postoperative recovery. When the client is a woman aged 18 to 55 years, and the urine output remains decreased for 2 consecutive hours with no other indications of hemorrhage or hypovolemia, the nurse should consider the possibility of surgically induced hyponatremia before aggressively administering IV fluids. Serum electrolytes showing a dilutional pattern (decreased sodium, potassium, chloride, hematocrit, and hemoglobin) can alert the nurse to the possibility of hyponatremia leading to encephalopathy.

Chart 16–5

Key Features of Hyponatremia

Cardiovascular*

- Normovolemic
  - Rapid pulse rate
  - Normal blood pressure
- Hypovolemic
  - Rapid pulse rate
  - Pulse quality thready and weak
  - Hypotensive
  - Central venous pressure normal or low
  - Flat neck veins
- Hypervolemic
  - Rapid, bounding pulse
  - Central venous pressure normal or elevated
  - Blood pressure normal or elevated

Respiratory

- Late manifestations related to skeletal muscle weakness
  - Shallow, ineffective respiratory movements
- Hypervolemia
- Pulmonary edema
  - Rapid, shallow respiration
  - Moist rales

Neuromuscular

- Generalized skeletal muscle weakness
- Diminished deep tendon reflexes

Cerebral

- Personality changes
- Headache

Renal

- Increased urinary output
- Decreased specific gravity

Gastrointestinal

- Increased motility
- Nausea
- Hyperactive bowel sounds
- Diarrhea

*Symptoms vary with changes in vascular volume.

➤ Gastrointestinal Manifestations

The smooth muscle of the gastrointestinal system responds to decreased serum sodium levels with increased gastrointestinal motility, causing nausea, diarrhea, and abdominal cramping. The nurse assesses the gastrointestinal system by listening to bowel sounds and observing stools. Bowel sounds are hyperactive, with frequent rushes and gurgles, especially over the splenic flexure and in the lower left quadrant. Bowel movements are frequent, watery, and explosive. Peristaltic movements may be palpated through the abdominal wall and may even be visible on the abdominal surface.

➤ Cardiovascular Manifestations

Hyponatremia has little direct effect on cardiac muscle contractility; however, alterations in cardiac output are associated with hyponatremia. When hyponatremia is accompanied by changes in the plasma volume, these fluid changes alter cardiac function. Generally, cardiac responses to hyponatremia with accompanying hypovolemia (decreased plasma volume) are manifested as a rapid, weak, thready pulse. Peripheral pulses are difficult to palpate and are easily blocked with light pressure. Neck veins are flat with the client in the upright position and possibly also in the supine position. Blood pressure, especially diastolic pressure, is decreased. The client may have severe hypotension when moving from a lying or sitting position to a standing position. The central venous pressure is low.

When hyponatremia is accompanied by plasma hypervolemia (increased plasma volume), cardiac manifestations include a rapid, full pulse. Blood pressure is normal or elevated. Central venous pressure is normal or elevated depending on how well the left ventricle handles the extra fluid. Peripheral pulses are full and difficult to block; however, if edema is present, peripheral pulses may not be palpable.

 Interventions

Interventions aim to restore serum sodium levels to normal values and prevent further decreases in serum sodium levels. Primary treatment modalities are drug therapy and diet therapy.

➤ Drug Therapy

Drug therapy attempts to restore the serum sodium level to normal. Drug therapy regimens vary depending on whether fluid imbalance accompanies hyponatremia.

When hyponatremia occurs with a fluid deficit (hypovolemia), the physician orders IV saline infusions to restore both sodium content and fluid volume. The nurse monitors the infusion rate and the client's response. The infusions are delivered through a controller or a pump to prevent accidental alterations in infusion rate.

When hyponatremia is accompanied by fluid excess, drug therapy includes administration of diuretics that primarily promote the excretion of water rather than sodium. These drugs are osmotic diuretics, such as mannitol (Osmitrol✦). The nurse assesses the client hourly for signs of excessive losses of fluids and potassium and dramatic increases in sodium levels.

Drug therapy for hyponatremia as a result of inappropriate or excessive secretion of antidiuretic hormone (ADH) includes agents that antagonize ADH, such as lithium and demeclocycline (Declomycin).

➤ Diet Therapy

Diet therapy can help restore normal sodium balance in mild hyponatremia. Table 14–6 lists the sodium content of common foods. The nurse collaborates with the dietitian in teaching the client about which foods to increase in the diet. Therapy consists of increasing oral sodium intake and restricting oral fluid intake to some degree. When overhydration with oral hypotonic fluids is the underlying cause of the hyponatremia or when renal fluid excretion is impaired, fluid restriction may be a long-term regimen. The nurse or assistive personnel measures fluid intake and output. The nurse also verbally reinforces the purpose of the fluid restriction.

Hypernatremia

Overview

Hypernatremia is a serum sodium level exceeding 145 mEq/L. Increased serum sodium level can be caused by or can cause changes in fluid volumes. Table 16–4 lists common causes of hypernatremia.

As the extracellular sodium level rises, a larger sodium concentration difference occurs between the extracellular fluid (ECF) and the intracellular fluid (ICF). More sodium is available to move rapidly across cell membranes. With mild hypernatremia, almost all excitable tissues are excited more easily, a condition called *irritability*. This irritability causes excitable tissues to overrespond to stimuli. As the extracellular sodium concentration increases, however, the osmolarity of the ECF also increases. This situation causes water to move from the cells into the ECF as a compensatory action to dilute the hyperosmolar ECF. When hypernatremia persists or worsens, the compensatory action causes severe intracellular dehydration, and excitable tissues may no longer be able to respond to stimuli.

Collaborative Management

 Assessment

The clinical manifestations of hypernatremia vary with the degree of imbalance and whether a fluid imbalance is also present. Rapid increases in serum sodium level generally produce more obvious and severe symptoms. Gradual in-

TABLE 16–4

Common Causes of Hypernatremia

Actual Sodium Excesses

Decreased Sodium Excretion

- Hyperaldosteronism
- Renal failure
- Corticosteroids
- Cushing's syndrome

Increased Sodium Intake

- Excessive oral sodium ingestion
- Excessive administration of sodium-containing intravenous fluids

Relative Sodium Excesses

Decreased Water Intake

- Nothing by mouth

Increased Water Loss

- Increased rate of metabolism
- Fever
- Hyperventilation
- Infection
- Excessive diaphoresis
- Watery diarrhea
- Dehydration

Chart 16–6

Key Features of Hypernatremia

Cardiovascular

- Decreased myocardial contractility
- Diminished cardiac output
- Heart rate and blood pressure respond to vascular volume

Respiratory

- Problems associated with pulmonary edema when hypernatremia is accompanied by hypervolemia

Central Nervous System*

- Hypernatremia and normovolemia or hypovolemia
  - Increased neural activity
  - Agitation, confusion, seizures
- Hypernatremia and hypervolemia
  - Decreased neural activity
  - Lethargy, stupor, coma

Neuromuscular

- Mild or early hypernatremia
  - Spontaneous muscle twitches
  - Irregular contractions
- Severe or late hypernatremia
  - Skeletal muscle weakness
  - Deep tendon reflexes diminished or absent

Renal

- Decreased urinary output
- Increased specific gravity

Integumentary

- Dry, flaky skin
- Presence or absence of edema related to accompanying fluid volume changes

*Upper neural function changes are related to volume changes as well as sodium increases.

creases in serum sodium levels may produce no observable physical changes, however, even when sodium levels increase to well above normal ranges. Clinical manifestations of hypernatremia are primarily associated with changes in cell membrane activity, especially among excitable tissues involved in cerebral, neuromuscular, and cardiac functions (Chart 16–6).

▶ *Central Nervous System Manifestations*

Altered cerebral function is the most common manifestation of hypernatremia. The nurse assesses the client's mental status in terms of attention span, recall of recent events, and ability to perform cognitive functions. In hypernatremia with normal or decreased fluid volumes, the client may have a short attention span and be agitated or confused about the sequence of recent events. If serum sodium concentration continues to increase, the client may become manic or experience convulsions. When hypernatremia is accompanied by an extracellular volume overload, the client may exhibit lethargy, drowsiness, stupor, and even coma.

➤ Neuromuscular Manifestations

Skeletal muscles respond differently to various degrees of hypernatremia. Mild hypernatremia causes muscle twitching and irregular muscle contractions. As hypernatremia worsens, the ability of skeletal muscle and nerves to respond to a stimulus diminishes. Muscles become progressively weaker and demonstrate rigid paralysis. Deep tendon reflexes are diminished or absent. The nurse assesses neuromuscular status by observing for twitching in muscle groups. The nurse also assesses muscle strength by having the client perform handgrip and arm flexion against resistance. Muscle weakness associated with hypernatremia occurs bilaterally and has no specific progressive pattern. The nurse assesses peripheral nerve response by lightly tapping the patellar (knee) tendons and Achilles (heel) tendons with a reflex hammer and measuring the degree of movement. (For an in-depth description of nursing assessment of mental status, deep tendon reflexes, and muscle strength, see Chapter 43.)

➤ Cardiovascular Manifestations

Increased serum sodium level prevents movement of calcium into the myocardium, thus decreasing the ability of the myocardium to contract. The nurse assesses cardiovascular status by taking blood pressure and measuring the rate and quality of apical and peripheral pulses. Pulse rate and blood pressure may be normal, above normal, or below normal during hypernatremic episodes, depending on the fluid volume and the speed with which the imbalance occurs.

In clients with hypernatremia and hypovolemia, the pulse rate is increased. Peripheral pulses may be difficult to palpate and are easily blocked with light pressure. The client is hypotensive, with severe orthostatic (postural) hypotension, and pulse pressure is greatly diminished.

Clients with hypernatremia and hypervolemia have slow to normal bounding pulses. Peripheral pulses are full and difficult to block. Neck veins are distended, even with the client in the upright position. Blood pressure, especially diastolic, is increased.

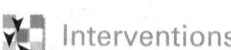 Interventions

Interventions aim to prevent further increases in serum sodium levels and decrease elevated serum sodium levels. Drug administration and diet therapy play important roles in restoring normal sodium balance. Other interventions used when hypernatremia becomes life-threatening include hemodialysis, peritoneal dialysis, and blood ultrafiltration.

➤ Drug Therapy

When hypernatremia is caused by fluid loss, drug therapy focuses on restoring fluid balance. The physician orders IV infusions of glucose and water (e.g., 5% dextrose in water). When hypernatremia is caused by fluid and sodium losses, it may be necessary to replace the fluid with IV administration of isotonic sodium chloride (NaCl) solutions. When hypernatremia is caused by inadequate renal excretion of sodium, drug therapy with diuretics promoting sodium loss, such as furosemide (Lasix, Furoside✦), bumetanide (Bumex), and ethacrynic acid (Edecrin), is ordered. The nurse assesses the client hourly for symptoms indicating excessive loss of fluids, sodium, or potassium.

➤ Diet Therapy

Dietary sodium restriction is useful in preventing hypernatremia. Often fluids must be restricted as well. The nurse collaborates with the dietitian in helping the client understand how to determine the sodium content of foods, beverages, and medications and the importance of complying with the diet.

CALCIUM IMBALANCES
Hypocalcemia
Overview

Hypocalcemia is a total serum calcium (Ca^{2+}) level below 8.6 mg/dL or 2.15 mmol/L. Calcium is stored in bone, and only a small fraction of the total body calcium is present in ECF. Because the normal serum level of calcium is so low, small changes in serum calcium levels have major effects on body function.

Pathophysiology

Calcium ions decrease excitable membrane permeability to sodium ions, preventing spontaneous depolarization. Calcium is considered a membrane stabilizer, regulating depolarization and the generation of action potentials. Low serum calcium levels increase the permeability of excitable membranes to sodium, so that depolarization occurs more easily and at inappropriate times.

Excitable tissues vary in their sensitivity to low serum calcium levels. Peripheral nerves, skeletal muscles, cardiac muscle, and the smooth muscle of the gastrointestinal system demonstrate the most obvious responses to decreased serum calcium levels. The severity of the manifestations associated with hypocalcemia depends on the degree of the calcium imbalance.

Hypocalcemia can also cause pathologic effects on bone. Bone is the primary storage site for calcium and can release calcium into the bloodstream when needed. Excessive calcium loss from bone can cause bone to weaken its supporting structure. Chronic hypocalcemia leads to progressive osteoporosis, resulting in bones that are less dense and more susceptible to fracture or deformity. (See Chapter 53 for a discussion of osteoporosis.)

Etiology

Hypocalcemia can result from various chronic and acute pathologic states as well as specific medical or surgical treatments. Table 16–5 lists common causes of hypocalcemia.

Actual calcium loss (a reduction in total body calcium) occurs in response to conditions that either inhibit calcium absorption from the gastrointestinal tract or increase the loss of calcium from the body.

TABLE 16-5

Common Causes of Hypocalcemia

Actual Calcium Deficits

Inhibition of Calcium Absorption from the Gastrointestinal Tract

- Inadequate oral intake of calcium
- Lactose intolerance
- Malabsorption syndromes
  - Celiac sprue
  - Crohn's disease
- Inadequate intake of vitamin D
- End-stage renal disease

Increased Calcium Excretion

- Renal failure—polyuric phase
- Diarrhea
- Steatorrhea
- Wound drainage (especially gastrointestinal)

Relative Calcium Deficits

Conditions That Decrease the Ionized Fraction of Calcium

- Hyperproteinemia
- Alkalosis
- Calcium chelators or binders
  - Citrate
  - Mithramycin
  - Penicillamine
  - Sodium cellulose phosphate (Calcibind)
  - Aredia
- Acute pancreatitis
- Hyperphosphatemia
- Immobility

Endocrine Disturbances

- Removal or destruction of parathyroid glands
  - Thyroidectomy
  - Radiation to thyroid
  - Strangulation
  - Neck injuries

Relative calcium loss causes the total body calcium concentration to remain normal while serum calcium levels are too low. This type of hypocalcemia occurs in response to conditions that either decrease the free, or ionized (unbound), calcium in the body or decrease parathyroid gland function.

TRANSCULTURAL CONSIDERATIONS

Many African-American clients have a lactose intolerance related to a genetic deficiency of the enzyme lactase. These clients cannot use the nutrients present in milk, and they experience cramping, diarrhea, and abdominal pain after ingesting dairy products. Dairy products, especially milk, are a common and rich source of both calcium and vitamin D. Clients with lactose intolerance may, therefore, experience difficulty obtaining enough calcium and vitamin D from other sources to maintain normal calcium levels in the blood and bones.

WOMEN'S HEALTH CONSIDERATIONS

Postmenopausal women are susceptible to hypocalcemia. This occurrence appears to be related to reduced weight-bearing activities and a decrease in sex hormone (estrogen) levels. Osteoporosis occurs when weight-bearing activity decreases or is limited. Because women generally are smaller framed than men, the female skeleton does not experience as much weight-bearing as the male skeleton. In addition, as they age, many women decrease weight-bearing activities, such as running and walking. Also, the estrogen secretion that protects against osteoporosis diminishes. All of these factors increase the risk of hypocalcemia in women, particularly the elderly.

Hypocalcemia and the Elderly

Elderly people are at risk for most electrolyte imbalances. Major organs and body systems undergo changes with aging. For example, an older adult has a smaller fluid volume per body weight than a younger adult, so that any variation in fluid volumes or electrolyte levels leads to imbalances more quickly. The elderly client is also more likely to be taking prescription or over-the-counter medications that affect fluid or electrolyte balance. Some elderly clients have dietary calcium or vitamin D deficits because of economic conditions or general problems with obtaining, preparing, or eating food.

Collaborative Management

 Assessment

The most critical factor in assessing for the risk of actual or potential hypocalcemia is the diet history. The nurse questions clients regarding the intake of calcium-containing foods (see Table 14–8). The nurse also identifies whether the client uses a calcium supplement on a regular basis.

One indicator of hypocalcemia is a report of frequent, painful muscle spasms (charley horses) in the calf or foot during periods of inactivity or sleep. Other information that can alert the nurse to a possible risk of hypocalcemia is a history of recent orthopedic surgery or bone healing. Disorders and treatments related to endocrine disturbances are significant for hypocalcemia. History of thyroid surgery, therapeutic radiation to the upper middle chest and neck area, or a recent anterior neck injury predisposes the client to hypocalcemia.

The most common clinical manifestations of hypocalcemia are related to overstimulation of nerves and muscles (see Chart 16–7).

> *Neuromuscular Manifestations*

Although all nerves and muscles are affected by hypocalcemia to some degree, the client usually notices symptoms first in the limbs, with distal to proximal movement from the hands and feet. At first, paresthesias may be noted, with sensations of tingling alternating with sensations of numbness. If hypocalcemia continues or worsens, these sensations may progress to actual muscle twitching or painful cramps and spasms. Paresthesias may also af-

---

Chart 16-7

Key Features of Hypocalcemia

Cardiovascular

- Decreased heart rate
- Decreased myocardial contractility
- Diminished peripheral pulses
- Hypotension
- Electrocardiographic abnormalities
  - Prolonged ST interval
  - Prolonged QT interval

Respiratory

- Not directly affected
- Respiratory failure or arrest can result from decreased respiratory movement because of muscle tetany or seizure activity

Neuromuscular*

- Anxiety, irritability, psychosis
- Paresthesias followed by numbness
- Irritable skeletal muscles—twitches, cramps, tetany, seizures
- Hyperactive deep tendon reflexes
- Positive Trousseau's sign
- Positive Chvostek's sign

Gastrointestinal

- Increased gastric motility
- Hyperactive bowel sounds
- Abdominal cramping
- Diarrhea

---

*The neuromuscular system is most profoundly affected by hypocalcemia.

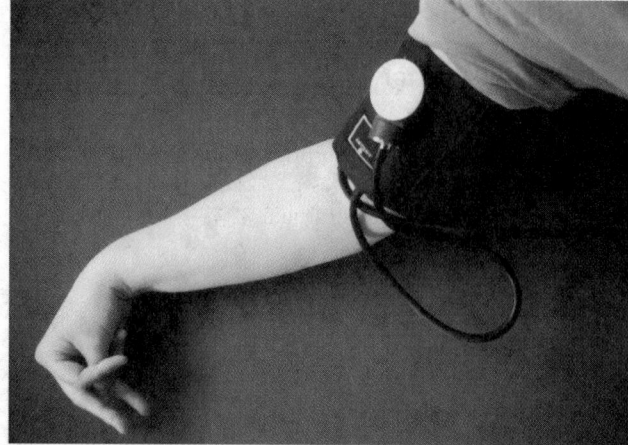

Figure 16-2. Palmar flexion—positive Trousseau's sign in hypocalcemia.

hyperactive bowel sounds. The client may report painful abdominal cramping and diarrhea.

 Interventions

Interventions aim to prevent further decreases in serum calcium levels, restore normal serum calcium levels, and prevent complications. Appropriate interventions may include drug therapy, diet therapy, reduction of environmental stimuli, and injury prevention.

➤ Drug Therapy

Drug therapy for hypocalcemia consists of direct calcium supplements or replacements, drugs that enhance absorption of calcium, and drugs that decrease nerve and muscle responsiveness to overstimulation. Chart 16-8 lists different drug types used to manage hypocalcemia.

fect the lips, nose, and ears. These symptoms signal the approach of serious neuromuscular overstimulation and tetany.

The nurse assesses for hypocalcemia by testing for Trousseau's and Chvostek's signs. To test for Trousseau's sign, the nurse places a blood pressure cuff around the upper arm, inflating the cuff to greater than the client's systolic pressure and keeping it inflated for 1 to 4 minutes. Under these hypoxic conditions, a positive Trousseau's sign occurs if the hand and fingers go into spasm in palmar flexion (Fig. 16-2). To test for Chvostek's sign, the nurse taps on the face just below and anterior to the ear (over the facial nerve) to trigger facial twitching of one side of the mouth, nose, and cheek (Fig. 16-3).

➤ Cardiovascular Manifestations

The heart rate may be slower or slightly faster than normal, but myocardial contractility is weaker, resulting in a diminished pulse quality. Severe hypocalcemia causes profound hypotension and ECG changes, including a prolonged ST interval leading to a prolonged QT interval.

➤ Gastrointestinal Manifestations

Overstimulation associated with hypocalcemia increases peristaltic activity. The nurse auscultates the abdomen for

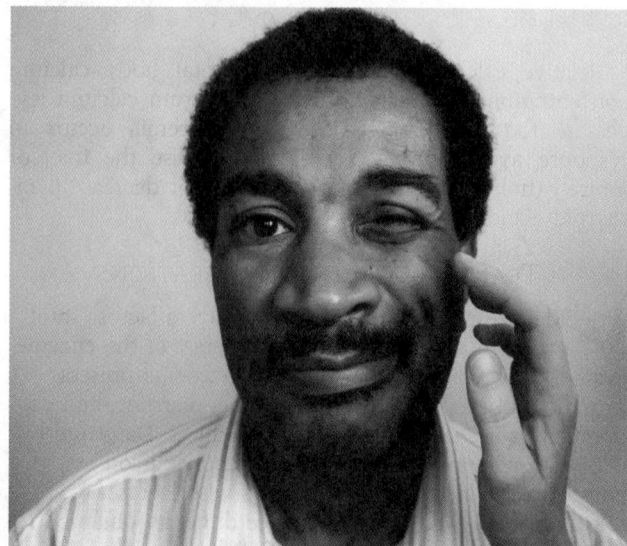

Figure 16-3. Facial muscle response—positive Chvostek's sign in hypocalcemia.

Chart 16–8

Drug Therapy for Hypocalcemia

Drug	Precautions
Oral Calcium Supplements	
Calcium carbonate	Dose must be increased in elderly clients because of decreased intestinal absorption.
Calcium citrate	Use with thiazide diuretics can increase the risk for hypercalcemia.
Calcium gluconate	Use with phenytoin decreases the bioavailability of both drugs; phenytoin should not be
Calcium lactate	given within 3 hours of calcium administration.
Intravenous Calcium	
Calcium acetate	All must be administered slowly, not to exceed 27 g/min.
Calcium chloride	Clients should be monitored for electrocardiographic changes during administration.
Calcium gluconate	Observe client for infiltration; calcium is a severe tissue irritant/vesicant.
	Potential for hypercalcemia and hypomagnesemia.
	Injection should be warmed to body temperature before administration.
Agents That Increase Calcium Absorption	
Aluminum hydroxide	Reduces serum phosphorus levels, causing the countereffect of increasing calcium levels; potential for hypophosphatemia. Signs and symptoms include bradycardia, decreased deep tendon reflexes, shortness of breath, confusion.
Vitamin D	Increases the intestinal absorption of calcium; potential for hypercalcemia.
Alfacalcidol	This is a fat-soluble vitamin and is stored to some degree; risk for vitamin D toxicity
Calcifediol	resulting in renal failure and/or cardiac failure.
Calcitriol	
Dihydrotachysterol	
Agents That Reduce Nerve and Skeletal Muscle Excitability	
Magnesium sulfate	Tissue irritant; the preferred route of administration is intravenous.
	Potential for hypermagnesemia; signs and symptoms of toxicity include bradycardia, flushing, headache, nausea, vomiting, shortness of breath, hypotension.
Methocarbamol	These agents act at the level of the central nervous system to decrease skeletal muscle
Robaxin	activity.
Carbacot	All have some sedative effect.
Metaxalone	All have some risk for psychological dependency and abuse.
Skelaxin	
Orphenadrine	
Banflex	
Flexoject	
Myolin	
Diazepam	
Valium	
Rival	
Epam✦	
Carisoprodol	
Soma	
Vanadom	

➤ Diet Therapy

A high-calcium diet is indicated for clients with mild hypocalcemia and for those with chronic conditions that cause them to be at continuous risk for hypocalcemia. The nurse consults with the dietitian to assist the client in selecting calcium-rich foods. Common sources of calcium are listed in Table 14–8.

➤ Reduction of Environmental Stimuli

The excitable membranes of both the nervous and the skeletal systems are overstimulated in hypocalcemia. The nurse, therefore, provides an environment that reduces extraneous stimulation of these systems.

➤ Prevention of Injury

The nurse places the client on seizure precautions, which include padding the side rails of the bed and keeping emergency equipment, such as oxygen and suction, at the bedside. An emergency cart equipped with emergency drugs and an endotracheal tray is positioned just outside the client's room.

The client with long-standing calcium loss may have brittle, fragile bones that fracture at only slight provocation and cause little pain. When lifting or moving a client with fragile bones, the nurse and assistive personnel use a lift sheet rather than pull or grasp the client directly. The nurse also observes the client for any unusual surface projections or depressions over bony areas as well as for normal range of joint motion.

Hypercalcemia

Overview

Hypercalcemia occurs when the total serum calcium level exceeds 10 mg/dL or 2.5 mmol/L. Because the normal range for serum calcium is extremely narrow, even small increases can have severe effects on body function. Although the effects of hypercalcemia are most noticeable in body systems that depend on cell excitability, all body systems are affected to some degree.

Pathophysiology

Hypercalcemia indicates either that the amount of serum calcium is so great that the normal calcium-regulating mechanisms are overburdened or that at least one calcium-regulating mechanism is not functioning properly. Because extracellular calcium ions function as stabilizers of excitable cell membranes, hypercalcemia causes excitable tissues to be less sensitive to normal stimuli and require a stronger stimulus to function. Excitable tissues that demonstrate obvious and serious immediate responses to hypercalcemia are cardiac muscle tissue, nerve tissue, skeletal muscle, and gastrointestinal smooth muscle.

Calcium is also a critical cofactor for many of the enzymes involved in the blood-clotting process. Hypercalcemia usually results in faster clotting times. This condition may cause clots to form at inappropriate times and places. Excessive clotting related to hypercalcemia is more likely in vessels or organs in which blood flow is slow or blocked.

Etiology

Underlying causes of hypercalcemia include increased absorption of calcium, decreased excretion of calcium, and increased bone resorption of calcium (Table 16–6).

Collaborative Management

 Assessment

Clinical manifestations of hypercalcemia are related to both the severity of the imbalance and how quickly the imbalance occurred. The client with mild excess of serum calcium level that occurred rapidly usually experiences more severe signs and symptoms than the client whose hypercalcemic state is severe but developed slowly. The clinical manifestations of hypercalcemia are primarily associated with alterations of excitable membrane activity (Chart 16–9). Thus, the body systems most affected by hypercalcemia include the cardiovascular, neuromuscular, gastrointestinal, and renal–urinary systems.

TABLE 16–6

Common Causes of Hypercalcemia

Actual Calcium Excesses

Increased Calcium Absorption

- Excessive oral intake of calcium
- Excessive oral intake of vitamin D

Decreased Calcium Excretion

- Renal failure
- Use of thiazide diuretics

Relative Calcium Excesses

Increased Bone Resorption of Calcium

- Hyperparathyroidism
- Malignancy
  - Direct invasion (cancers of breast, lung, prostate, and osteoclastic bone and multiple myeloma)
  - Indirect resorption (liver cancer, small cell lung cancer, and cancer of the adrenal gland)
- Hyperthyroidism
- Immobility
- Use of glucocorticoids

Hemoconcentration

- Dehydration
- Use of lithium
- Adrenal insufficiency

➤ Cardiovascular Manifestations

The most serious and life-threatening clinical manifestations of hypercalcemia involve alterations in cardiac function. Mild hypercalcemia initially causes increased heart rate and blood pressure. Severe or prolonged hypercalcemia affects electrical conduction.

The nurse assesses cardiac status by measuring pulse and blood pressure and observing for indications of inadequate tissue perfusion such as cyanosis and pallor. The nurse also observes ECG tracings for indications of dysrhythmias, especially a shortened QT interval.

Although hypercalcemia does not directly cause formation of blood clots, increased calcium levels produce clot formation more easily whenever abnormal conditions are present. Thus, the client with hypercalcemia may be at an increased risk for clot formation in locations where blood vessel or tissue damage have occurred and in vessels or organs in which blood flow is blocked. Blood clotting is more likely in the lower legs, the pelvic region, areas where blood flow is blocked by internal or external constrictions, and regions where internal blood vessel obstruction occurs.

The nurse assesses each client at risk for hypercalcemia for indications of slowed or impaired blood flow. Calf circumferences are measured with a soft tape measure and recorded. The nurse asks the client to alternately dorsiflex and plantar flex the ankles and state whether calf pain occurs in either position. The nurse assesses the lower legs for temperature, color, and capillary refill to determine the adequacy of blood flow to and from the area.

Chart 16-9

Key Features of Hypercalcemia

Cardiovascular

- Increased heart rate (early phase)
- Increased blood pressure
- Bounding, full peripheral pulses
- Electrocardiographic abnormalities
  - Shortened ST segment
  - Widened T wave
- Potentiation of digitalis-associated toxicities
- Decreased clotting time
- Late phase
  - Bradycardia
  - Cardiac arrest, sinus arrest

Respiratory

- Ineffective respiratory movement related to profound skeletal muscle weakness

Neuromuscular

- Disorientation, lethargy, coma
- Profound muscle weakness
- Diminished or absent deep tendon reflexes

Renal

- Increased urinary output
- Dehydration
- Formation of renal calculi

Gastrointestinal

- Decreased motility
- Hypoactive bowel sounds
- Anorexia, nausea
- Abdominal distention
- Constipation

➤ Neuromuscular Manifestations

The neuromuscular manifestations of hypercalcemia include severe muscle weakness without accompanying paresthesia and greatly diminished deep tendon reflexes. Central nervous system manifestations include altered level of consciousness ranging from disorientation and lethargy to coma.

➤ Gastrointestinal Manifestations

Decreased peristalsis is an early manifestation of hypercalcemia. The nurse assesses the gastrointestinal tract by auscultating for bowel sounds in all four abdominal quadrants. Bowel sounds are hypoactive or absent. The abdomen increases in size because intestinal contents remain in the gastrointestinal tract instead of being propelled to the outside. The nurse assesses abdominal size by measuring abdominal girth with a soft tape measure in a line circling the abdomen at the level of the umbilicus. The client may report constipation, anorexia, nausea, vomiting, and abdominal pain.

➤ Renal Manifestations

Hypercalcemia causes increased urinary output and leads to serious dehydration. Chronic hypercalcemia results in the formation of renal calculi (stones) in the kidney tubular system, because the excessive calcium precipitates out of solution in a solid form. The nurse or assistive personnel measures intake and output, assesses voided urine for blood or cloudiness, and strains the urine for the presence of renal calculi.

 Interventions

Interventions for hypercalcemia aim to prevent further increases in serum calcium levels and decrease excessive serum calcium levels through drug therapy and dialysis.

➤ Drug Therapy

Drug therapy for the treatment of hypercalcemia restores normal calcium balance by preventing additional calcium administration and promoting calcium excretion. IV infusions of solutions containing calcium are stopped. In addition, administration of oral drugs containing calcium or vitamin D, such as calcium-based antacids, is discontinued.

Fluid volume replacement alone can help restore normal serum calcium levels. The physician usually orders IV normal saline (isotonic sodium chloride) because it does not contain calcium.

Thiazide diuretic administration is discontinued for clients with hypercalcemia. Diuretics that enhance the excretion of calcium such as furosemide (Lasix, Furoside✤) are prescribed instead.

Agents that act as calcium chelators (calcium binders) can be useful in lowering serum calcium levels. Such drugs include plicamycin (Mithracin) and penicillamine (Cuprimine, Pendramine✤).

Other drugs that may be useful in treating hypercalcemia include agents that inhibit calcium resorption from bone, such as phosphorus, calcitonin (Calcimar), bisphosphonates (etidronate), and prostaglandin synthesis inhibitors (aspirin, nonsteroidal anti-inflammatory drugs).

➤ Dialysis

In severe hypercalcemia that causes life-threatening cardiac problems, drug therapy may not reduce serum calcium levels quickly enough to prevent death. Dialysis (either hemodialysis or peritoneal dialysis) or blood ultrafiltration may be necessary.

➤ Cardiac Monitoring

Clients with hypercalcemia usually undergo continuous cardiac monitoring to identify possible dysrhythmias and decreased cardiac output. The nurse compares recently obtained ECG tracings with the client's baseline tracings or those obtained when the client's serum calcium level was normal. The nurse observes the ECG for changes in the T waves and the QT interval as well as changes in rate and rhythm.

PHOSPHORUS IMBALANCES

Hypophosphatemia

Overview

Hypophosphatemia is a serum phosphorus level below 2.7 mg/dL. Even though the serum concentration of phosphorus has a narrow range of normal values (2.7–4.5 mg/dL), body functions are not significantly impaired as a result of rapid, wide changes in serum phosphorus levels. Alterations in function are more obvious when hypophosphatemia is chronic.

Pathophysiology

Most of the pathophysiologic effects of hypophosphatemia are related to decreased energy metabolism and altered levels of other electrolytes and body fluids. Because of the reciprocal relationship between phosphorus and calcium, decreases in serum phosphorus levels are accompanied by increases in serum calcium levels.

Etiology

Three main processes underlie decreased serum phosphorus levels: decreased absorption of phosphorus, increased excretion of phosphorus, and intracellular phosphorus shift (Table 16–7).

Collaborative Management

 Assessment

Clinical manifestations of hypophosphatemia occur when the decrease in serum phosphorus levels is severe or pro-

---

TABLE 16–7

Common Causes of Phosphorus Imbalance

Hypophosphatemia

Insufficient Phosphorus Intake
- Malnutrition
- Starvation
- Use of aluminum hydroxide–based antacids
- Use of magnesium-based antacids

Increased Phosphorus Excretion
- Hyperparathyroidism
- Hypocalcemia
- Renal failure
- Malignancy

Intracellular Shift
- Hyperglycemia
- Hyperalimentation
- Respiratory alkalosis

Hyperphosphatemia
- Decreased renal excretion resulting from renal insufficiency
- Tumor lysis syndrome
- Increased intake of phosphorus
- Hypoparathyroidism

Chart 16–10

Key Features of Hypophosphatemia

Cardiovascular
- Decreased contractility
- Cardiomyopathy (reversible)

Respiratory
- Shallow respirations

Musculoskeletal
- Weakness
- Rhabdomyolysis
- Decreased deep tendon reflexes

Central Nervous
- Irritability
- Confusion
- Seizures

Hematologic
- Increased bleeding
- Decreased platelet aggregation
- Immunosuppression

---

longed. Acute manifestations of hypophosphatemia are related to the decreased availability of high-energy compounds (such as adenosine triphosphate [ATP]) necessary to perform normal cellular metabolic functions. These clinical manifestations include alterations in cardiac, musculoskeletal, hematologic, and central nervous system functions (Chart 16–10).

➤ *Cardiovascular Manifestations*

The cardiac manifestations of hypophosphatemia include decreased stroke volume and decreased cardiac output. Peripheral pulses are slow, difficult to find, and easy to block. Myocardial depression is caused by low intracellular energy stores. Without sufficient quantities of energy in myocardial cells, contractions are weak and ineffective. Prolonged hypophosphatemia can lead to progressive, but reversible, myocardial damage.

➤ *Musculoskeletal Manifestations*

The mechanism of hypophosphatemia that weakens cardiac muscles also appears to be responsible for weakening skeletal muscles. The weakness is generalized, and paresthesias usually are not present. When the skeletal muscle weakness becomes profound, respiratory movements are ineffective, which can lead to respiratory failure. The nurse assesses for muscle strength and observes respiratory ability.

The clinical manifestations of chronic hypophosphatemia are most evident in the skeletal system. Bone density is decreased, possibly causing fractures and alterations in bone shape. These changes result from the calcium resorption that often accompanies hypophosphatemia. The nurse assesses the client for unusual lumps, projections, or depressions over bony areas indicating fracture of demineralized bone.

➤ Central Nervous System Manifestations

Central nervous system manifestations are not apparent until hypophosphatemia is severe. These first appear as increased irritability and may progress to seizure activity followed by coma.

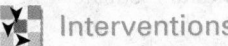 Interventions

➤ Drug Therapy

Administration of drugs that contribute to the development of hypophosphatemia, such as antacids, osmotic diuretics, and calcium supplements, is discontinued. Generally, oral replacement of phosphorus along with a vitamin D supplement is sufficient to correct hypophosphatemia. IV phosphorus administration is initiated only when serum phosphorus levels fall below 1 mg/dL and the client has serious clinical manifestations. IV phosphorus is administered slowly because problems associated with hyperphosphatemia are equally serious.

➤ Diet Therapy

Diet therapy for hypophosphatemia consists primarily of increasing the intake of phosphorus-rich foods while decreasing the intake of calcium-rich foods (Chart 16–11).

Hyperphosphatemia

Overview

Hyperphosphatemia occurs when the serum phosphorus level exceeds 4.5 mg/dL. Elevated serum phosphorus levels above normal are tolerated well by most body systems.

The health problems associated with hyperphosphatemia center on the hypocalcemia that results when serum phosphorus levels increase. These problems include increased sensitivity of excitable membranes to the extent that they may depolarize spontaneously and inappropriately.

Underlying causes of increased serum phosphorus levels include renal insufficiency, some cancer treatments,

increased phosphorus intake, and hypoparathyroidism. Table 16–7 lists specific common causes of hyperphosphatemia.

Collaborative Management

Hyperphosphatemia produces few direct problems with body function. However, hypocalcemia is usually present as well because the calcium and phosphorus ions exist in the blood in a balanced reciprocal relationship: when one increases, the other decreases. The accompanying hypocalcemia dramatically alters the physiologic functioning of many body systems and has the potential for causing serious and life-threatening side effects. Thus, the management of hyperphosphatemia entails the management of hypocalcemia.

MAGNESIUM IMBALANCES

Hypomagnesemia

Overview

Hypomagnesemia occurs when the serum magnesium (Mg^{2+}) level decreases below 1.6 mg/dL. Because most conditions resulting in hypomagnesemia are related either to decreased magnesium intake or to increased magnesium loss, measurable hypomagnesemia reflects a decrease in total body magnesium concentration.

The direct pathophysiologic effects of hypomagnesemia are related to alterations in the function of excitable membranes and accompanying imbalances of serum calcium and potassium. These problems include increased sensitivity of excitable membranes, especially nerve cell membranes, to the extent that they may depolarize spontaneously and inappropriately.

Hypomagnesemia results from either decreased absorption of dietary magnesium or increased renal excretion of magnesium. Table 16–8 lists specific causes of hypomagnesemia.

Collaborative Management

 Assessment

Most clinical manifestations of hypomagnesemia result from alterations in the activity of excitable cell membranes. The most common manifestations are seen in the neuromuscular, central nervous, and gastrointestinal systems (Chart 16–12).

➤ Neuromuscular Manifestations

The neuromuscular manifestations of hypomagnesemia result from increased nerve impulse transmission at some synaptic areas. Normally, magnesium inhibits the release of the neurotransmitter acetylcholine from the presynaptic cell. Decreased magnesium levels allow greater release of acetylcholine, which increases the transmission of impulses from nerve to nerve or from nerve to skeletal muscle. The client with hypomagnesemia has hyperactive deep tendon reflexes (+4) accompanied by painful paresthesia (numbness and tingling) and tetanic muscle contractions. Positive Chvostek's and Trousseau's signs may

---

Chart 16–11

Education Guide: Dietary Management of Hypophosphatemia

You Should Avoid	You May Eat
• Milk	• Fish
• Cheese	• Beef
• Yogurt	• Chicken
• Collard greens	• Pork
• Rhubarb	• Organ meats
	• Nuts
	• Whole-grain breads and cereals

TABLE 16–8

Common Causes of Magnesium Imbalance

Hypomagnesemia

Insufficient Magnesium Intake
- Malnutrition
- Starvation
- Diarrhea
- Steatorrhea
- Celiac disease
- Crohn's disease

Increased Magnesium Excretion
- Drugs (diuretics, aminoglycoside antibiotics, cisplatin, amphotericin B, cyclosporine)
- Citrate (blood products)
- Ethanol ingestion

Intracellular Movement of Magnesium
- Hyperglycemia
- Insulin administration
- Sepsis
- Alkalosis

Hypermagnesemia
- Increased magnesium intake
  - Magnesium-containing antacids and laxatives
  - Intravenous magnesium replacement
- Decreased renal excretion of magnesium resulting from renal insufficiency

be present because hypomagnesemia may be accompanied by hypocalcemia (see prior discussion of these assessment signs under Hypocalcemia). Skeletal muscle weakness may be present if intracellular magnesium levels are also decreased in an attempt to restore normal magnesium balance. As hypomagnesemia progresses, the client may experience tetany and seizures.

➤ Central Nervous System Manifestations

The central nervous system manifestations of hypomagnesemia are related to a general increase in the transmission of nerve impulses. Increased central nervous system irritability may manifest as psychological depression, psychosis, and confusion.

➤ Gastrointestinal Manifestations

Gastrointestinal manifestations are associated with decreased contractility of intestinal smooth muscle. Clients have decreased gastric motility with anorexia, nausea, and abdominal distention. If the hypomagnesemia is severe, a paralytic ileus may occur.

 Interventions

Interventions for hypomagnesemia aim to correct the electrolyte imbalance and manage the specific condition that caused the hypomagnesemia. In addition, because hypocalcemia frequently accompanies hypomagnesemia, some

interventions also aim to restore normal serum calcium levels.

➤ Drug Therapy

The administration of drugs that contribute to the development of hypomagnesemia, such as high-ceiling (loop) diuretics, osmotic diuretics, aminoglycosides, and drugs containing phosphorus, is discontinued. Magnesium is replaced IV in the form of magnesium sulfate ($MgSO_4$) when hypomagnesemia is severe. The IV route is used because $MgSO_4$ causes pain and tissue damage when injected intramuscularly. Oral preparations of magnesium frequently cause diarrhea and increase magnesium loss. If hypocalcemia is also present, the physician prescribes drug therapy to increase serum calcium concentration.

➤ Diet Therapy

Diet therapy for hypomagnesemia consists of increasing the intake of foods that contain high concentrations of magnesium (see Table 14–11).

Chart 16–12

Key Features of Hypomagnesemia

Cardiovascular
- Electrocardiographic changes
  - Tall T waves
  - Depressed ST segments
- Dysrhythmias
  - Ectopic beats
  - Ventricular tachycardia
  - Ventricular fibrillation
- Hypertension

Gastrointestinal
- Decreased motility
- Anorexia
- Nausea
- Abdominal distention
- Decreased bowel sounds

Respiratory
- Shallow respirations

Neuromuscular
- Fasciculations
- Twitches
- Paresthesias
- Positive Trousseau's sign
- Positive Chvostek's sign
- Hyperreflexia
- Tetany
- Seizures

Central Nervous
- Irritability
- Confusion
- Psychosis

Hypermagnesemia

Overview

Hypermagnesemia occurs when the serum magnesium level exceeds 2.6 mg/dL. Magnesium is a membrane stabilizer. When excesses of magnesium occur, excitable membranes require a stronger-than-normal stimulus to respond and thus are less sensitive or less excitable. If hypermagnesemia is severe, excitable membranes may not respond to any stimulus.

Hypermagnesemia results from increased intake of magnesium coupled with decreased renal excretion of magnesium. Table 16–8 lists specific causes of hypermagnesemia.

Collaborative Management

 Assessment

Most clinical manifestations of hypermagnesemia occur as a result of alterations in the activity of excitable cell membranes. Usually, manifestations are not apparent until serum magnesium levels exceed 4 mg/dL. The most common manifestations are seen in the cardiac, central nervous, and neuromuscular systems.

➤ *Cardiovascular Manifestations*

Cardiac manifestations of hypermagnesemia are related to bradycardia, peripheral vasodilation, and hypotension. These become more severe as serum magnesium concentration increases. ECG changes include a prolonged PR interval with a widened QRS complex. Bradycardia can be severe; cardiac arrest is possible during diastole of the cardiac cycle. Hypotension with a wide pulse pressure is also severe; the diastolic pressure is much lower than normal. Clients with severe hypermagnesemia are in grave danger of cardiac arrest.

➤ *Central Nervous System Manifestations*

Central nervous system manifestations of hypermagnesemia are related to depressed transmission of nerve impulses at specific synaptic points. Clients may be drowsy to the point of lethargy. Coma may occur if the hypermagnesemia is prolonged or becomes severe.

➤ *Neuromuscular Manifestations*

Neuromuscular manifestations of hypermagnesemia are related to decreased transmission of impulses from nerves to skeletal muscles. Deep tendon reflexes are greatly diminished or even absent. Voluntary skeletal muscle contractions become progressively weaker and finally stop.

➤ *Respiratory Manifestations*

Hypermagnesemia has no direct effect on the organs of respiration. However, when the skeletal muscles of respiration are involved, respiratory insufficiency may occur, leading to respiratory failure and death from anoxia.

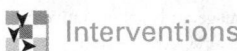 Interventions

Interventions for hypermagnesemia aim to reduce the serum magnesium level and correct the underlying pathologic change that initiated or contributed to the development of hypermagnesemia.

➤ *Drug Therapy*

All oral and parenteral administration of magnesium is discontinued. When renal failure is not a contributing factor, administration of magnesium-free IV fluids can assist in reducing serum magnesium levels. Administration of high-ceiling (loop) diuretics such as furosemide (Lasix, Furoside✦) can further reduce serum magnesium levels. When cardiac manifestations are severe, administration of calcium may reverse the cardiac effects of hypermagnesemia.

➤ *Diet Therapy*

Diet therapy is most effective in preventing hypermagnesemia when other chronic pathologic conditions predispose the client to the development of excess serum magnesium levels. Dietary restrictions involve limiting the ingestion of meat, nuts, legumes, fish, vegetables, and whole-grain cereal products.

 CASE STUDY for the Client with Hypokalemia

■ An 89-year-old woman is one of your nursing home residents. She has a history of myocardial infarction, congestive heart failure, and adult-onset diabetes mellitus. Her medication orders include Lasix, 80 mg qd, Digoxin, 0.125 mg qd, potassium chloride, 40 mEq qd, and Orinase, 500 mg.

Today the resident seems confused when you bring her morning medications. She says she feels "sick to her stomach" and does not want breakfast. The nursing assistant reports that the client's pulse is weak and slightly irregular at 62 bpm and her blood pressure is 102/68 mm Hg.

Q U E S T I O N S :

1. When taking a history from this resident, what important questions should you ask?
2. What additional physical assessment techniques would you perform?
3. During respiratory assessment, you find that the client's respirations are rapid and shallow. Breath sounds are present in both lungs with no crackles or wheezes audible on auscultation. Given these assessment findings, what should you do first?

SELECTED BIBLIOGRAPHY

Anderson, S. (1996). Fluid and electrolyte disorders in the elderly. In J. Kokko & R. Tannen (Eds.), *Fluids and electrolytes* (3rd ed., pp. 831–839). Philadelphia: W. B. Saunders.

Ayus, J. C., & Arieff, A. (1996). Brain damage and postoperative hyponatremia: The role of gender. *Neurology, 46*(2), 323–328.

Bove, L. (1996). Restoring electrolyte balance: Calcium and phosphorus. *RN, 59*(3), 47–52.

Bove, L. (1996). Restoring electrolyte balance: Sodium & chloride. *RN, 59*(1), 25–29.

Braxmeyer, D., & Keyes, J. (1996). The pathophysiology of potassium balance. *Critical Care Nurse, 16*(5), 59–71.

Bryce, J. (1994). S.I.A.D.H. *Nursing94, 24*(4), 33.

*Chenevey, B. (1987). Overview of fluids and electrolytes. *Nursing Clinics of North America, 22*(4), 749.

Dennis, V. (1996). Phosphate disorders. In J. Kokko & R. Tannen (Eds.), *Fluids and electrolytes* (3rd ed., pp. 359–390). Philadelphia: W. B. Saunders.

Ellis, S. (1995). Severe hyponatremia: Complications and treatment. *Quarterly Journal of Medicine, 88*(12), 905–909.

Fenves, A., Thomas, S., & Knochel, J. (1996). Beer potomania: Two cases and review of the literature. *Clinical Nephrology, 45*(1), 61–64.

Ferrin, M. (1996). Restoring electrolyte balance: Magnesium. *RN, 59*(5), 31–34.

Guyton, A., & Hall, J. (1996). *Textbook of medical physiology* (9th ed.). Philadelphia: W. B. Saunders.

Halperin, M., & Goldstein, M. (1994), *Fluid, electrolyte and acid-base physiology: A problem-based approach* (2nd ed.). Philadelphia: W. B. Saunders.

Held, J. (1995). Correcting fluid and electrolyte imbalances. *Nursing95, 25*(4), 71.

Kaplan, R. (1994). Hypercalcemia of malignancy. *Oncology Nursing Forum, 21*(6), 1039–1046.

Kokko, J., & Tannen, R. (1996). *Fluids and electrolytes* (3rd ed.). Philadelphia: W. B. Saunders.

Kuhn, M. (1996). Laboratory analysis. *Critical Care Nurse, 16*(5), 74–76.

Kumar, R. (1996). Calcium disorders. In J. Kokko & R. Tannen (Eds.), *Fluids and electrolytes* (3rd ed., pp. 391–419). Philadelphia: W. B. Saunders.

McConnell, E. (1994). What's wrong with this patient? *Nursing94, 24*(5), 92–93.

McConnell, E. (1995). What's wrong with this patient? *Nursing95, 24*(4), 73–74.

*Mendyka, B. (1992). Fluid and electrolyte disorders caused by diuretic therapy. *AACN Clinical Issues in Critical Care Nursing, 3*(3), 672–680.

Metheny, N. (1996). *Fluid and electrolyte balance: Nursing considerations* (3rd ed.). Philadelphia: J. B. Lippincott.

Miller, C. (1995). Medications that may cause cognitive impairment in older adults. *Geriatric Nursing, 16*(1), 47.

Norris, M. K. (1994). Checking chloride levels. *Nursing94, 24*(3), 76.

O'Donnell, M. (1995). Assessing fluid and electrolyte balance needs in elders. *American Journal of Nursing, 95*(1), 40–46.

Rude, R. (1996). Magnesium disorders. In J. Kokko & R. Tannen (Eds.), *Fluids and electrolytes* (3rd ed., pp. 421–445). Philadelphia: W. B. Saunders.

Sica, D. (1994). Renal disease, electrolyte abnormalities, and acid-base imbalance in the elderly. *Clinics in Geriatric Medicine, 10*(1), 197–211.

Tannen, R. (1996). Potassium disorders. In J. Kokko & R. Tannen (Eds.), *Fluids and electrolytes* (3rd ed., pp. 111–199). Philadelphia: W. B. Saunders.

Tietz, N. W. (Ed.). (1995). *Clinical guide to laboratory tests* (3rd ed.). Philadelphia: W. B. Saunders.

Toto, K., & Yucha, C. (1994). Magnesium: Homeostasis, imbalances, and therapeutic uses. *Critical Care Nursing Clinics of North America, 6*(4), 767–783.

Trissel, L. (1994). *Handbook on injectable drugs* (8th ed.). Bethesda, MD: American Society of Hospital Pharmacists.

Vonfrolio, L. (1995). Would you hang these IV solutions? *American Journal of Nursing, 95*(4), 37–39.

Yucha, C., & Toto, K. (1994). Calcium and phosphorus derangements. *Critical Care Nursing Clinics of North America, 6*(4), 747–766.

Zelingher, J., Putterman, C., Ilan, Y., Dann, E., Zveibil, F., Shvil, Y., & Galun, E. (1996). Case series: Hyponatremia associated with moderate exercise. *American Journal of the Medical Sciences, 311*(2), 86–91.

SUGGESTED READINGS

Braxmeyer, D., & Keyes, J. (1996). The pathophysiology of potassium balance. *Critical Care Nurse, 16*(5), 59–71.
This outstanding article presents potassium physiology, deficits, and excesses in a comprehensive, yet user-friendly manner. The article is enhanced by flow charts, clear discussions of nursing actions and implications, and associated self-assessment questions.

Mendyka, B. (1992). Fluid and electrolyte disorders caused by diuretic therapy. *AACN Clinical Issues in Critical Care Nursing, 3*(3), 672–680.
This article presents in text and tables the mechanisms of action and electrolyte effects of the major diuretic categories. Normal nephron function is reviewed. Nursing care considerations for specific electrolyte disturbances are summarized.

O'Donnell, M. (1995). Assessing fluid and electrolyte balance needs in elders. *American Journal of Nursing, 95*(1), 40–46.
The author describes physical and behavioral characteristics of geriatric clients that place them at risk for electrolyte imbalances, using a case study approach. An assessment checklist for elders with nutritional deficits is included.

INFUSION THERAPY

The term "infusion therapy" refers to a wide variety of techniques and procedures health care professionals utilize to deliver parenteral medications and fluids to their clients. The delivery of these medications and fluids may be into clients' vascular systems, such as in intravenous therapy or arterial therapy. Some clients require administration of fluids and medications into their tissue (subcutaneous therapy) or into their epidural or intrathecal spaces as in central nervous system therapies. Infusion of fluids or medications into a client's body cavity is intraperitoneal therapy; into a client's bones is intraosseous therapy.

INTRODUCTION TO INFUSION THERAPY

Approximately 90% of hospitalized clients receive some type of infusion therapy. Health care providers prescribe infusion therapy for their clients for a variety of reasons or therapeutic goals, including maintenance, replacement, treatment, diagnosis, monitoring, palliation, or a combination of these.

Not long ago, most clients received their infusion therapies as inpatients in acute care facilities. With the advent of computerized ambulatory and implantable infusion control devices, as well as long-term infusion access devices, clients now receive infusion therapy in virtually any setting—from their homes to long-term care facilities.

Some agencies have specialized teams that focus on all of the procedures associated with infusion therapy. These infusion or intravenous (IV) teams develop infusion policies and procedures, initiate peripheral intravenous and peripherally inserted central catheters, administer parenteral fluids and medications, administer parenteral nutrition and blood products, maintain infusion devices, provide input to agency purchasing departments regarding infusion devices and equipment, monitor infusion-related complications, provide consultation to health care providers and clients regarding device selection and placement, and engage in quality improvement activities.

The continued use of IV teams in health care settings is a controversial issue. In this time of "downsizing," "rightsizing," and "re-engineering," many agencies have disbanded their IV teams, leaving these responsibilities to nurse generalists or unlicensed technicians. The Veteran's Affairs Medical Center in Pittsburgh, Pennsylvania, however, founded its IV team in 1992. As a result of its IV team, the hospital reported a decrease in IV-related bacteremia to 1.5 per 1000 patient discharges from 4.6 per 1000 client discharges on the medical-surgical units of its 330-bed acute care facility. In the critical care areas, where house staff and general staff nurses continued to care for IV lines, there was no change in the rate of IV-related bacteremia. The study demonstrated a significant decrease in morbidity and mortality in the medical surgical clients at this institution, and the authors estimate that the IV team saved $124,906 during the year, considering the decrease in the treatment of bacteremias (Miller et al., 1996).

The Intravenous Nurses Society (INS), the professional nursing organization for infusion therapy nurses, publishes standards of care that provide the basis for the practice of infusion nursing. Its affiliate organization, the Intravenous Nurses Certification Corporation (INCC), offers a written certifying examination. Nurses who successfully complete this examination may use the initials "CRNI," which stand for "certified registered nurse infusion." The INS is currently the only organization offering certification in infusion therapy. Many agencies offer basic and advanced instruction in infusion therapy.

INFUSION SYSTEMS

Nurses administering infusion therapies need to understand the way in which infusion systems work. This knowledge ensures that the nurse can optimize a particular system's advantages while minimizing any potential complications.

Containers

Infusion containers are generally made of glass or plastic. Each of these systems has advantages as well as disadvantages (Table 17–1).

Glass infusion systems are of two types—the separate airway design and the integral airway system. The separate airway design has a plastic tube or "straw" attached to the inside of the thick, hard cork-type stopper. This tube extends almost the entire length of the bottle to above the fluid level of a full bottle. Unfiltered air enters through the straw and exerts pressure on the surface of the fluid, allowing the fluid to pass through the administration set. The integral airway design glass system is also an "open" system. In this system, air enters through a

side port filter on the administration set. This type of set is often referred to as "vented" tubing.

Plastic containers may be soft and totally collapsible or semirigid. Both of these systems are considered "closed" systems as they do not rely on outside air to allow the fluid to infuse. Instead, atmospheric pressure pushes against the flexible sides of the container, allowing the fluid to flow by gravity. For this reason, plastic containers use "nonvented" or "unvented" tubing.

The totally collapsible variety of plastic containers is usually made of PVC (polyvinyl chloride). Some PVC materials cause container-medication compatibility problems with nitroglycerin, insulin, and fat emulsions. Nitroglycerin and insulin adhere to the walls of the PVC container, making it impossible to know exactly how much medication the client is receiving. Fat emulsions leach the plasticizer diethylhexylphthalate (DEHP), a component of some PVC containers, thereby unintentionally making this substance part of the client's infusion.

Although they are plastic, semirigid containers do not have the same compatibility problems associated with containers made of PVC. This container, as its name indicates, is less flexible than totally collapsible plastic containers.

Administration Sets

The administration set is the connection between the client's access device and the solution container. Numerous administration sets are available in many different configurations. The type and purpose of the infusion assists in determining the type of administration set the nurse should choose. Many sets are generic, meaning that they are appropriate for most infusions. Some sets are specialty sets to be used for specific types of infusions; still other sets are dedicated, meaning that they must be used with a specific manufacturer's infusion control device. Nurses

TABLE 17–1

Advantages and Disadvantages of Infusion Containers		
Container Type	**Advantages**	**Disadvantages**
Glass	Able to withstand trauma and varying pressures during sterilization process	Difficult to see small cracks, which alter the integrity of the system
	Clarity allows the nurse to inspect the container for any particulate matter	Rigid sides make storage and disposal bulky
	Rigid sides allow nurse to accurately determine the container's volume	Requires a source of air to allow fluid to drip, thereby making it an "open" system
	Glass is an inert product and will not react with solutions or medications	
Plastic	Not likely to break when dropped or bumped	Not clear, making it difficult to visualize particulate matter
	Some designs may be stored on top of one another for ease	May be pierced by needle when making additions to the bag
	Because they collapse when empty, disposal is easier and less bulky than glass	Difficult to accurately measure volumes because sides collapse as the bag empties
	Able to withstand freezing and thawing	Compatibility problems with some medications
	Can be manufactured to hold any volume and still be manageable for most nurses	

From Booker, M. F., & Ignatavicius, D. D. (1996). *Infusion therapy: Techniques and medications.* Philadelphia: W. B. Saunders.

can usually find information on the packaging that describes the proper use of the administration set inside. Table 17–2 and Charts 17–1 and 17–2 describe some of the standard and miscellaneous components of administration sets and the factors determining their use.

Filters remove particulate matter suspended in the infusion solution while allowing the fluid to pass through to the client. The nurse may see filters of two types: membrane filters and depth filters. Either of these filters may be "in-line" (an integral part of the administration set) or "add-on" (a filter set that is separate and must be added to the administration set).

A membrane filter has tiny pores or holes sized to prevent the passage of particles into the filter. These pores capture any particles that may be in the solution and trap them on the surface of the filter. One problem associated with membrane filters is that they are prone to "loading," a phenomenon that occurs when the filter's surface is completely coated with particulate matter, rendering it inoperable and therefore of no value. It is for this reason that membrane filters are best suited as final filters rather than the primary or singular filtering mechanism.

A depth filter has a maze-like configuration. Any particles suspended in the fluid pass through the surface and become trapped in the multitude of passages as they travel through the labyrinth. Additionally, depth filters also have adsorption properties that cause any particles to adhere to the filter material itself. The size of the particle does not influence the adsorption of the filter material.

Both membrane and depth filters are rated by the size

Chart 17–1

Nursing Care Highlight: Piggybacking an Intermittent Medication

1. Verify the order from the health care provider.
2. Check the compatibility between the medication and the large-volume parenteral (LVP) and its additives.
3. Spike the medication mini-bag with the secondary set.
4. Prime the secondary set, close the roller clamp, and hang the mini-bag on the other arm of the intravenous (IV) pole.
5. Place the hanger that comes with the secondary set on the IV pole with the LVP.
6. Cleanse the lowest "Y-site" injection port on the LVP administration set.
7. Attach the secondary set to the "Y-site."
8. Lower the level of the LVP by hanging it from the hanger. Do not adjust the LVP roller clamp. (The rate will decrease and then stop when the secondary set is opened.)
9. Open the roller clamp on the secondary set and regulate the flow to the desired rate.
10. When the intermittent infusion completes, the LVP will automatically begin again. Hang the LVP from the IV pole and adjust the roller clamp to deliver the prescribed rate.

Chart 17–2

Nursing Care Highlight: How to Use a Burette

1. To fill the burette, close the main clamp below the burette.
2. Open the clamp between the solution container and the burette, allowing the fluid to flow into the burette.
3. When the burette contains the amount of fluid desired, close the clamp between the solution container and the burette.
4. If using the burette for administration of intermittent medications, add the prescribed medication now and gently swirl the burette.
5. Regulate the rate of the infusion from the burette with the lower clamp.

---

of the smallest particles they hold back. A 0.22-micron filter retains any particles 0.22 micron and larger. These particles may be particulate matter or organisms such as *Escherichia coli* and *Pseudomonas.*

Needleless Systems

In July 1992, the Occupational Safety and Health Administration published its guidelines entitled *Occupational Exposure to Bloodborne Pathogens, Final Rule.* This document requires health care organizations to initiate engineering controls "that isolate or remove the bloodborne pathogen hazard from the workplace." Currently, there are a number of products available and more entering the market every day designed to minimize health care workers' exposure to contaminated needles. Some of these products include devices that use blunt metal cannulae or needles recessed into a plastic housing; others use a blunt plastic cannula, and still others include valves. It is estimated that needleless systems can eliminate up to 80% of the traditional metal needles used in a hospital setting (Beason et al., 1993). Figure 17–1 displays some of the common needleless systems currently available.

Infusion Regulation Devices

The ability to regulate the rate and volume of infusions is critical to the safe and accurate administration of medications and fluids to clients. Nurses have a choice of numerous devices designed to regulate infusions. Most are classified as either controllers or pumps and require either AC (alternating current) or a battery as a power source.

Nurses and clients who use infusion pumps and controllers reap the benefits of some of the latest computer technology. Infusion regulation devices can save nursing time and prevent runaway infusions, as well as reduce the incidence of infiltration and keep infusion access devices patent. However, the nurse must remember that the use of these devices does not decrease the practitioner's responsibility to carefully monitor the client's infusion site and the infusion rate.

Not every regulation device is appropriate for every

TABLE 17–2

Components of Administration Sets

Component	Description or Characteristics	Purpose or Function
Standard Components		
Spike	Hard plastic tube with a sharp point; plastic cover or sheath over spike must be removed before use	Sharp point penetrates the solution container; sheath maintains sterility of spike
Shield	Hard plastic disk below the spike	Prevents the nurse's hands from slipping onto the spike when inserting it into the fluid container
Drip chamber	Plastic tube between the shield and the tubing; the bottom of the spike extends into this chamber	Used to prime the administration set and to verify continued flow
Bottom of spike	Plastic or metal piece that extends into the drip chamber	Size controls the volume of fluid in each drop; may be macrodrip or mini- or microdrip. Volume of a macrodrip varies among manufacturer from 10 to 20 drops/mL (gtt/mL); micro- or minidrip is 60 gtt/mL
Tubing	May be of varying lengths and diameters	Connects the drip chamber to the connector device
Clamps	May be screw clamp or roller clamp	Controls the rate of fluid flow through the administration
Flashball	A piece of latex with small circles on the surface that highlight areas reinforced with self-sealing material	Connects the tubing to the connector; reinforced areas used for needle access to infusion to administer intravenous push medications
Connectors	At the end of the tubing, may be slip tip, luer lock, or slip luer	Connects the administration set to the client's access device
Y-site	Set may have one or more; may be called injection site or side-arm; hard plastic tube; upper end has either a self-sealing injection port or a valve; the bottom of the Y-site is an integral part of the administration set tubing	Used for piggybacking intermittent medications into the client's primary infusion (Chart 17–1)
Miscellaneous Components		
On-off clamps	May be slide or clip; not appropriate for regulating rate of flow	Used to open or close the administration set to flow
Burettes	Reservoir that is either incorporated into the administration set or an add-on device; the reservoir holds between 100 and 150 mL of fluid; the burette is calibrated on the side to assist with accurate measurement; at the top or bottom of the burette is a rubber cap that looks like the end of a "Y site"; through this self-sealing cap, the nurse can add any medications or additives ordered for the client	The burette is useful for mixing intravenous medications for administration or for controlling the amount of fluid available for administration, a critical consideration in the care of the young child or the elderly client (Chart 17–2)
Back-check valves	When present, a back-check valve is built into the administration set; the device is a hard plastic one-way valve	Back-check valves allow fluid to travel away from the solution container but prevent fluid from flowing upstream toward the container
Passive flow control devices	Usually an add-on device that looks like an extension set with a dial	Regulates the rate of infusion in mL/hr; all other clamps are left open, and the passive flow control device regulates the administrations at the prescribed rate

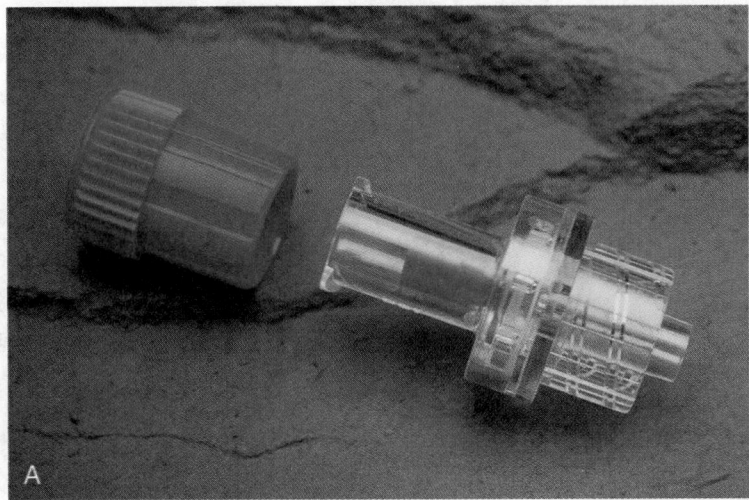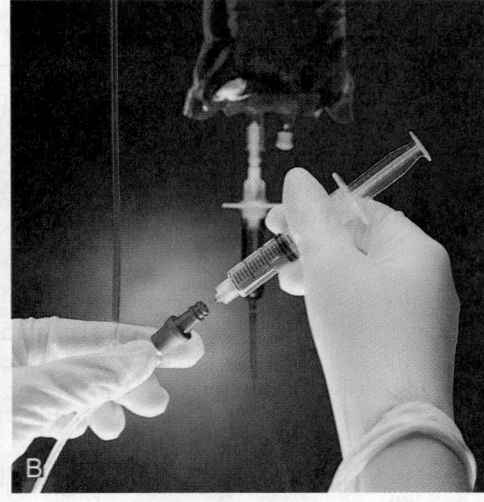

Figure 17-1. Needleless infusion systems. *A,* Burron Safesite IV System valve and "deadhead." *B,* Clave system in use. (*A,* courtesy of B. Braun Medical, Inc., Bethlehem, PA; *B,* courtesy of ICU Medical, Inc., San Clemente, CA.)

situation. It is important for the nurse to consider the purpose of the infusion, the drug or solution, the client, the client care setting, and the type of access device the client has before deciding on a particular type of infusion regulation device.

A controller is a stationary (pole-mounted) electronic device that can be classified as either nonvolumetric or volumetric. Nonvolumetric controllers rely completely on gravity for flow. A drop sensor attached to the drip chamber of the administration set regulates flow. Volumetric controllers also count drops and electronically convert the drops to mL/hr. Because controllers rely on counting drops, which may and do vary in size and therefore volume, controllers are not as accurate as pumps.

Pumps may be either stationary (pole mounted or tabletop), ambulatory (portable), or implantable (surgically implanted into the client). As their name indicates, these devices actually pump medications or solutions under pressure. Stationary pumps may be nonvolumetric or volumetric. Nonvolumetric pumps count drops and, as with controllers, are inherently inaccurate because of the variation in drop size. Three types of volumetric pumps are available: syringe, cassette, and peristaltic.

Syringe pumps use a mechanism that continuously closes the plunger at a selected mL/h rate. The use of syringe pumps is limited for small-volume continuous infusions or for administration of intermittent medications such as antiinfectives. Syringe pumps are generally not appropriate for use in the continuous administration of larger volumes, as they require very frequent syringe changes.

Cassette pumps use special sets (dedicated sets) that include a pumping chamber of exact volume. This volume is displaced by means of either a piston or a diaphragm at the selected mL/hr rate. Cassette pumps usually require special techniques to prime the administration set but are appropriate for use when delivering large volume infusions.

Peristaltic pumps are also appropriate for large-volume infusions. They control the rate of the infusion by squeez-

ing the tubing with finger-like projections intermittently walking across the administration set tubing.

Ambulatory pumps are generally used for home care clients and allow clients to return to their usual activities while receiving infusion therapy.

Implantable pumps usually include a catheter as part of the pump. The physician places the catheter in a vessel feeding the "target organ," or structure. Implantable pumps also have a chamber that holds the medication and at least one self-sealing septum that the clinician uses to access the medication chamber for (re)filling and emptying the medication chamber. Implantable pumps are placed in the client's trunk via a laparotomy. Usual implant sites are the lower abdomen, the subclavicular area, and the subscapular area. Common uses for these pumps include regional chemotherapy and continuous intraspinal pain management.

TYPES OF INFUSION THERAPY
Intravenous Therapy

Intravenous (IV) therapy involves infusing medications and/or solutions into a client's veins through a venous access device (VAD). The tip placement of the IV cannula determines whether the therapy is considered peripheral or central venous therapy. In peripheral venous therapy the tip of the cannula remains in the client's peripheral veins. Central venous therapy involves placing the tip of the cannula or catheter into the client's superior vena cava (SVC).

Peripheral Intravenous Therapy
Description

Peripheral IV therapy is the most common *method* of gaining access to the client's venous system. Nurses competent in venipuncture insert the needle or flexible cannula percutaneously (through the skin) into a client's veins. Under most circumstances, the peripheral veins offer the quickest and easiest approach to establishing a route for administering IV solutions and medications. These solutions and medications may be administered for therapeutic or diagnostic purposes. Replacement of fluid, electrolyte, and nutrient losses; administration of anti-infectives; blood and blood product transfusions; and medication administration can be accomplished via the peripheral venous system. Enhancing agents for diagnostic imaging may also be administered via the peripheral veins.

An order from a health care provider is necessary before the nurse initiates IV therapy. The order usually includes the specific type of solution to be given; the rate of the administration written in mL/hr, mg/hr, μg/hr, or u/hr; the total volume of the infusion; and the number of hours for infusion. If the health care provider orders medication for IV administration, the dose, volume, solution or diluent, rate, and frequency of administration are usually included in the order. In many agencies, the infusion pharmacist determines the solution and volume for the medication admixture.

When determining which site to use to initiate the client's peripheral intravenous therapy, the nurse considers the client's age, history, and diagnosis; the type and duration of the prescribed therapy; and, whenever possible, the client's preference. Chart 17-3 lists some criteria for the placement of peripheral venous access devices.

The veins considered the most appropriate for most peripheral IV therapy are in the upper extremities and include the metacarpal, basilic, cephalic, and median veins, as well as their branches (Fig. 17-2). Veins that are resilient, long, and straight are the best choices for cannula placement. Veins that are hard, knotty, or sclerotic are difficult to encannulate and are likely to infiltrate. For short-term therapy, it is recommended that the

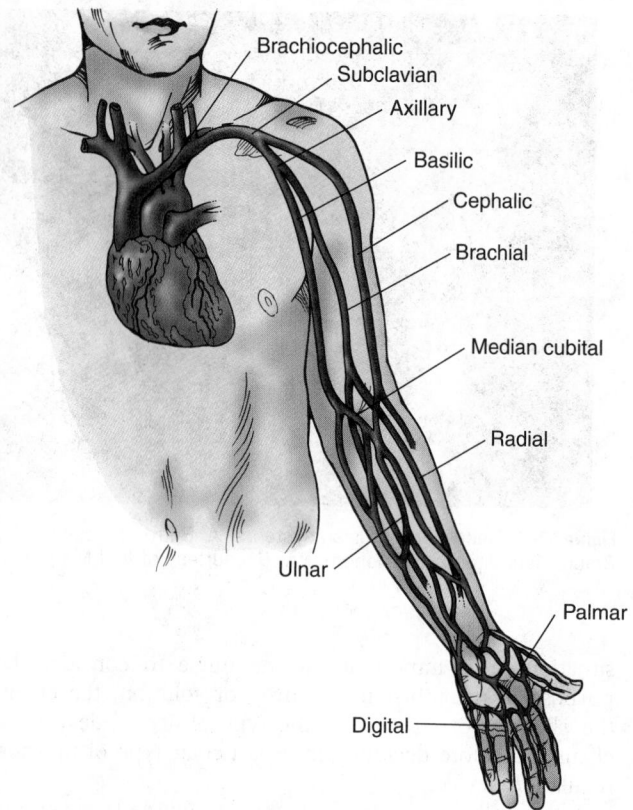

Figure 17–2. The superficial veins of the arm.

nurse place the initial IV catheter in the most distal site of the client's arm and use more proximal sites for subsequent IV cannula insertions.

The product to be infused requires the nurse's consideration when determining which vein and which type of peripheral access device to use. The administration of an isotonic solution, such as D5W, does not require any specific precautions related to the size of the vein or type of catheter the nurse uses for the infusion. However, the administration of medications or solutions that are viscous or those with a high osmolality or a high or low pH can be harsh and cause vein irritation. Medications or solutions with these properties require that the nurse consider the use of a larger vein to increase hemodilution and thereby decrease the potential for complications. Additionally, a midline or midclavicular catheter provides more reliable and longer-term access for solutions that are potentially irritating to veins.

Intravenous administrations that are of short duration, such as a one-time dose of an IV push medication that does not have vein-irritating properties, may be given into most veins. An infusion of a medication or solution with vein-irritating properties requires a larger vessel to reduce the probability of complications.

Devices

The nurse considers the age and condition of the client; the size, location, and condition of the available veins;

Chart 17–3

Nursing Care Highlight: Criteria for Placement of Peripheral Venous Access Devices

- Obtain a health care provider's order for placing a peripheral intravenous (IV) cannula.
- For adults, place a peripheral IV catheter only in the upper extremities.
- Use the client's nondominant hand when possible.
- Do not use the arm on the side where the client has a mastectomy, a lymph node dissection, an arteriovenous shunt or fistula, or venous revision.
- Use the most distal area of the client's arm above the wrist for the initial insertion and work your way up the client's arm to more proximal sites for subsequent insertions.
- Avoid placing a peripheral IV catheter over a joint.
- Avoid placing a peripheral IV cannula in a vein that is bruised, has puncture wounds from other venipunctures, is streaked, is hard, has a palpable cord, or is tender to touch.

and the type and duration of the infusion. The shortest, smallest-gauge device that accommodates the vein, type of infusion, and duration of therapy is the nurse's best choice when selecting an IV catheter.

Intravenous access devices may be categorized in a variety of ways. For the purpose of this discussion, peripheral IV catheters are categorized by dwell time (the amount of time the catheter may stay in the vein before being replaced)—either short-term dwell or long-term dwell.

SHORT-TERM DWELL CATHETERS. Winged metal sets and most over-the-needle catheters are short-term dwell catheters. Most short-term dwell peripheral catheters have a dwell time of 48–72 hours (Pearson et al., 1996).

A metal winged IV set is commonly known as a butterfly. Many practitioners consider these catheters easy to insert, but they may contribute to practitioner needlesticks. The practitioner holds the wings between the thumb and forefinger to insert the device. After insertion, the wings lie flat against the client's skin.

The standard over-the-needle catheter is between ¾ and 3 inches long and ranges in gauge size from 14 G to 26 G. The over-the-needle catheter consists of a needle inside a polyethylene or plastic catheter. The practitioner removes the needle after making the venipuncture, and the plastic catheter remains inside the vessel. Some manufacturers make over-the-needle winged sets. The nurse inserts these catheters in the same manner as a metal-winged set. However, after the insertion, the needle-stylet is removed, leaving only the catheter in the vessel.

LONG-TERM DWELL CATHETERS. Longer dwell time peripheral catheters, such as the midline or midclavicular catheters, are usually through-the-needle catheters. Through-the-needle catheters have either a break-away needle or a plastic peel-away sheath to encase the needle after the catheter is advanced through it. Some controversy exists over the amount of time these longer-dwell catheters may stay in place. Some believe that the midline and mid-clavicular catheters may remain in place for as long as the client exhibits no complications, or until the client no longer requires venous access (Pearson et al., 1996). In a position paper, the Intravenous Nurses Society (INS) recommends that maximum dwell time for midline catheters be limited to 2–4 weeks and to 2–3 months dwell time for midclavicular catheters (INS, 1997). Blood specimens may be drawn from indwelling peripheral catheters (see Research Applications for Nursing).

A midline catheter is a through-the-needle catheter that the nurse usually inserts at the antecubital fossa into the basilic, cephalic, or median cubital veins. The tip of the midline rests in the vein about 6–8 inches above the insertion site.

A mid-clavicular catheter is a through-the-needle catheter that is longer than the midline catheter. The tip of the mid-clavicular catheter usually rests at the mid-clavicular line. This area is the approximate junction of the axillary and subclavian veins.

► Research Applications for Nursing

What Is the Proper Discard Volume When Drawing Blood Through an Indwelling Catheter?

Yucha, C. B., & DeAngelo, E. (1996). The minimum discard volume. Journal of Intravenous Nursing, 19(3), 141–146.

Nurses frequently use indwelling central venous catheters for acquiring venous blood samples from their clients in both inpatient and outpatient settings. Most protocols involve withdrawing some blood to clear the catheter dead space and to remove the impact of the catheter's flushing solution on the test results. How does the nurse know how much blood should be withdrawn before acquiring the test sample? Does the appropriate amount vary with the test to be completed? The type of flush? Or the type of catheter?

Yucha and DeAngelo conducted a study to quantify the minimum amount of blood to be discarded from an indwelling peripheral intravenous catheter to obtain an accurate hematocrit reading. Using a study sample of nine subjects, repeat blood sampling was used to develop a mathematical model (Michaelis-Menton curve) describing the mixing of the flush solution and blood. This model was used to estimate the hematocrit when different volumes of blood are discarded. The differences between the computed hematocrit and true hematocrit were determined for each subject. When 1.5 mL (three times the deadspace volume) is discarded, the 95% confidence interval is within 0.6% of the true hematocrit.

Critique. This study was performed on nine young, healthy subjects with peripheral intravenous catheters. Only hematocrit readings were quantified in this study. For these reasons, the conclusions cannot be generalized to include other types of catheters, other types of laboratory determinations, ill clients, or those in other age groups. Further studies are therefore indicated.

Possible Nursing Implications. The nurse's ability to know the amount of discard required to ensure accurate laboratory testing has direct implications on client care and treatment, as well as on costs. Spurious laboratory results can cause the client to receive inappropriate doses of medication or unnecessary treatments. Having to repeat laboratory tests to get accurate results places the client at risk and adds to the cost of client care.

ELDERLY CONSIDERATIONS

Elderly clients receiving intravenous (IV) therapy have special needs. The normal aging process presents changes in the skin and vessels that require the nurse's attention.

The elderly person's skin may be described as loose, thin, and transparent. As people age, they lose subcutaneous fat, the dermis thins, and the density and amount of collagen lessen. Elastin fibers just below the dermis become more abundant but less effectively organized. The fine elastin fibers in the dermis disappear. All of these changes account for the decreased elasticity found in the elderly client's skin.

The elderly client's veins appear tortuous and large because of inadequate venous pressure. The veins are likely to roll, as there is little connective tissue to hold them, and the veins themselves become more fragile. These changes may require the nurse to alter the IV insertion technique in the elderly. Chart 17–4 outlines special considerations for the elderly client receiving peripheral IV therapy.

Central Intravenous Therapy

Description

Central venous therapy involves the placement of a flexible catheter into one of the client's central veins. The tip of the catheter is situated in the superior vena cava. Drugs, fluids, nutrients, enhancing agents, and blood and blood products may be infused through a central IV line. At times a central venous catheter (CVC) is placed be-

cause the client's peripheral venous access is inadequate for the duration or type of IV therapy required. In some clients, a CVC allows the nurse to measure and monitor central venous pressure (CVP). In other cases, a CVC is inserted to ensure venous access when IV therapy is prescribed.

There are a number of criteria to consider when determining the type of CVC a client will have. The type and duration of therapy, the setting in which the client is to receive the therapy, and the client's lifestyle, activity, and personal preference all play a role in determining the type of catheter the client will receive.

Each of the devices discussed here, with the exception of the peripherally inserted central catheter (PICC), requires a physician to insert the catheter.

Devices

Nontunneled catheters may be placed at the client's bedside. The physician places the catheter percutaneously (through the skin) in a manner similar to a through-the-needle peripheral IV catheter. The site of placement may be into the client's chest or neck veins (usually the subclavian, or internal or external jugular veins). The catheters are made of polyurethane or silastic and may be single lumen or multiple lumen. The chest and neck vein sites are generally used for short-term therapy for clients who will remain as inpatients in a facility or who are outpatients. After placement and before it is used for infusions, the catheter's placement is checked by x-ray.

The PICC is another type of nontunneled catheter (Fig. 17–3). The PICC is currently the only type of central venous catheter that falls within the realm of nursing practice. Boards of nursing in every state now recognize the specially trained nurse's ability to safely and efficiently access the client's central venous system with a PICC. Many agencies and regulating boards agree that before a nurse be considered "PICC competent," he or she must complete a minimum of 8 hours of didactic (classroom) training and perform at least three successful PICC placements under the guidance of a preceptor or clinical trainer.

The PICC is appropriate for any setting and for administration of any IV therapy. As with other direct insertion catheters, PICCs are available in single or multiple lumen and require an x-ray to verify placement before use. According to the INS's position paper, a PICC that is functioning well may remain in place for up to 12 months (INS, 1997).

Tunneled CVCs include the Broviac, Hickman, Leonard, and Groshong catheters. These catheters, named for their developers, are made from silicone or polyurethane. Some of the differences among these catheters have to do with their inside diameters or gauge of lumen and the catheter tips. Before the nurse uses these catheters, the physician will confirm the placement of the catheter tip by radiography.

The Broviac catheter is usually a smaller-bore catheter than the Hickman, Leonard, or Groshong. Like the Hickman and Leonard, the Broviac is an open-ended catheter, meaning that it has a tip that is open, similar to that of peripheral venous catheters. The external portions of the

---

Chart 17–4

Focus on the Elderly: Special Considerations for the Elderly Client Receiving Peripheral Intravenous Therapy

- If the client's veins appear large and tortuous, do not use a tourniquet. Having the client hold the arm in a dependent position may fill the veins sufficiently for venipuncture.
- Do not use hand veins for starting an IV line. These veins are too small and limit the elderly client's ability to perform activities of daily living.
- Use the smallest-gauge intravenous (IV) catheter possible, preferably 21 G or smaller. (Most 24-G catheters allow the delivery of 100 mL/h.)
- Do not use a traditional tourniquet. A blood pressure cuff is easier on the elderly client's skin.
- Take time to find the most suitable vein.
- Use strict aseptic technique, because the elderly client is typically immunocompromised.
- Do not slap the arm to visualize the client's veins.
- Use a decreased angle for insertion—usually between 5 and 15 degrees.
- Set the flow rate of IV medications, especially antibiotics, to no more than 100 mL/h; for clients with congestive heart failure or renal failure set the rate at 50 mL/h.
- Use a protective skin preparation before applying a transparent dressing over the IV insertion site; dry gauze pads may be best for clients with tissue-thin skin.
- Cover the IV dressing with flexible netting. If netting is unavailable, use minimal tape or an elastic bandage to secure the dressing and protect the site; keep the insertion site visible at all times.
- Do not use circumferential restraints on the extremity with the IV catheter.
- Do not use the client's lower extremities for IV insertion, because the circulation may be impaired in the client's legs and feet.
- Assess the client's mental status at least every 4 hours.
- Use pumps, controllers, or burettes to control infusion volume and rate.

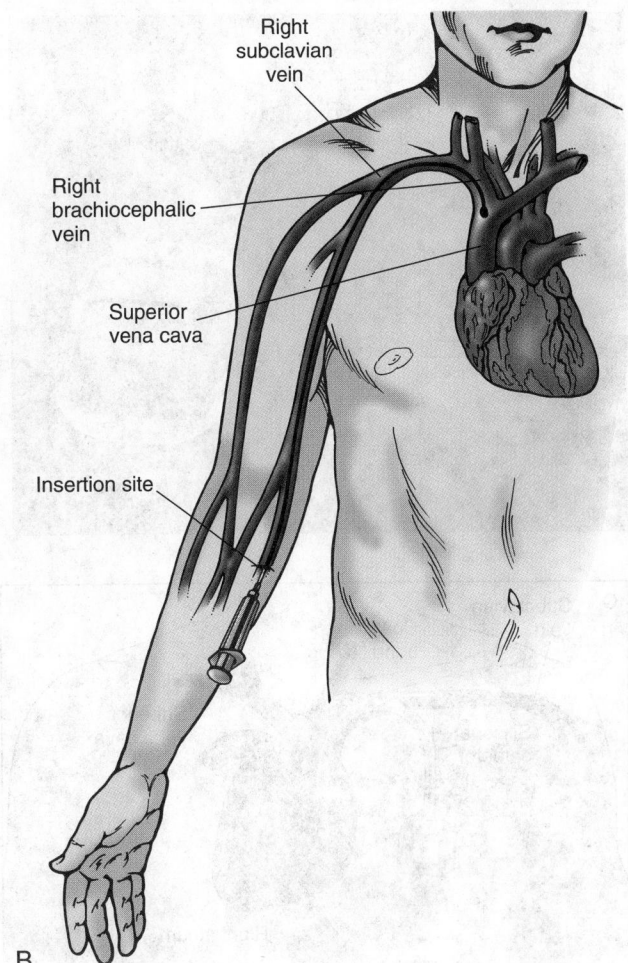

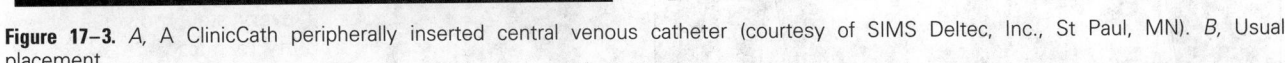

Figure 17–3. *A,* A ClinicCath peripherally inserted central venous catheter (courtesy of SIMS Deltec, Inc., St Paul, MN). *B,* Usual placement.

Hickman and Broviac catheters have a reinforced area on each lumen. When the catheter is not being used for infusions, the lumens are clamped at the reinforced area to avoid air embolism.

The Groshong catheter is a closed-end catheter. Toward the tip of the Groshong catheter on the side there is a slit-valve that opens out and allows fluid to infuse if there is positive pressure in the catheter and opens in and allows blood to be aspirated if there is negative pressure in the catheter. When the pressure in the catheter is neutral, the valve is closed. The Groshong catheter is not supplied with clamps, and the manufacturer's instructions state that the catheter should not be clamped to maintain the integrity of the valve. The Groshong tip is available on PICC catheters as well as tunneled catheters.

The rest of the features of the Broviac, Hickman, and Groshong catheters are similar in design. Each of these catheters is available in single, double, triple, and quadruple lumen. The catheters are usually 42–90 cm in length until the physician trims them during insertion. Each has a cuff positioned inside the subcutaneous tunnel. This cuff is designed to rest just inside the tunnel, under the skin. Fibrous tissue develops around it after insertion to

secure the catheter in place and produce a physical barrier to the migration of organisms up the tunnel into the client's bloodstream.

Implanted ports consist of a portal body, a central septum, a reservoir, and a catheter (Fig. 17–4). The port is surgically placed in a subcutaneous pocket in the client's trunk. The surgeon threads the catheter into the central vascular system and positions the tip in the superior vena cava. The catheter is attached to the portal body. The distal tip of the catheter is either open end or closed end. The septum is made of self-sealing silicone, located in either the center or on the side of the portal body. The nurse uses a noncoring device to access the system by piercing the skin over the portal body and puncturing the septum.

Complications of Intravenous Therapy

Vigilant nursing care is the key to decreasing the incidence of complications associated with all infusion therapy. A major nursing responsibility when caring for clients receiving infusion therapies is prevention, assessment, and management of complications. Table 17–3 de-

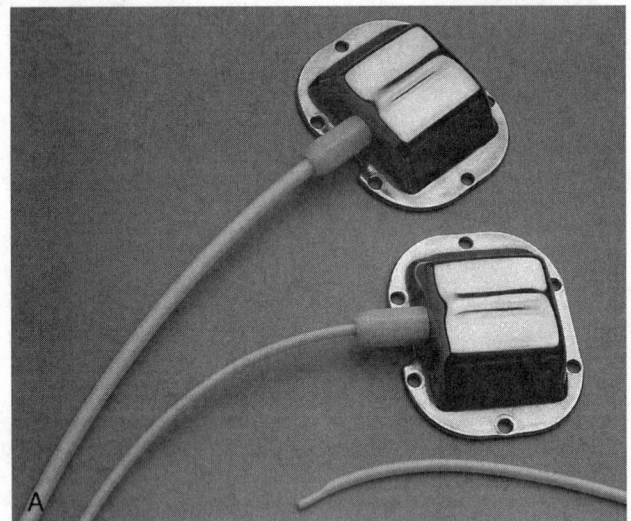

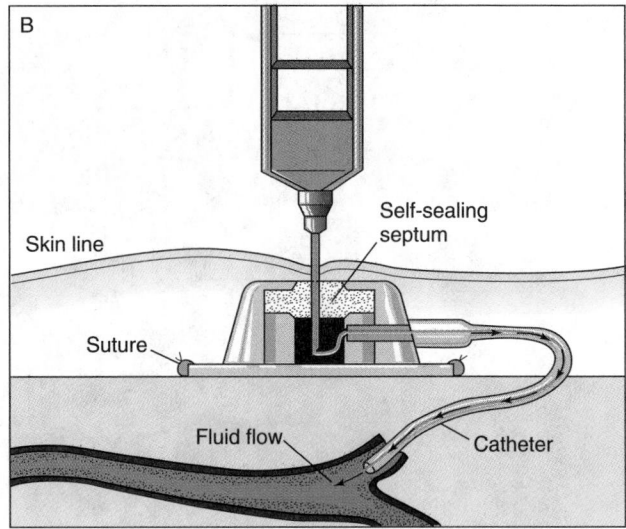

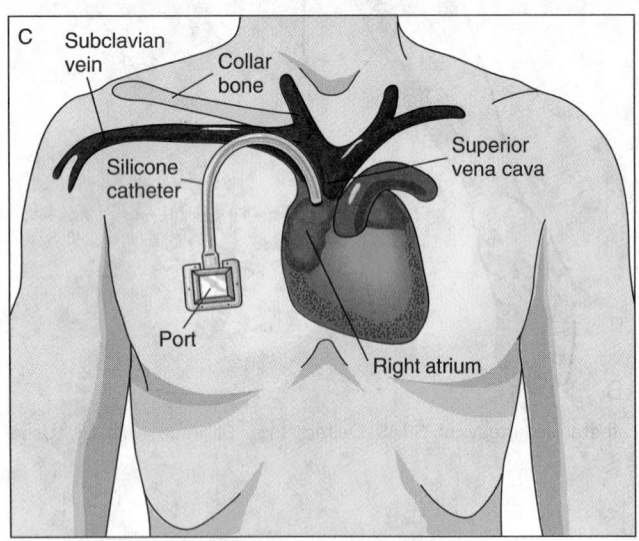

Figure 17–4. *A,* A dual-access implantable port for venous access. *B,* A needle puncture through the skin into the port allows drugs, fluids, and blood to be administered. *C,* For systemic drug and fluid delivery, the catheter is placed in the subclavian vein. (*A,* courtesy of Harbor Medical Devices, Inc., Boston, MA. *B* and *C,* redrawn from Winters, B. [1984]. Implantable vascular access devices. *Oncology Nursing Forum, 11*[6], 25–30.)

scribes local and systemic complications of peripheral intravenous (IV) therapy.

Arterial Therapy

Description

The use of a client's arteries for infusion therapy is usually to provide the client with intra-arterial chemotherapy (IAC). Chemotherapy administered arterially allows the administration of a high concentration of drug to the tumor site before it is diluted in the circulatory system or metabolized in the liver or kidneys. A high drug concentration at the tumor site optimizes tumor site cell kill while minimizing systemic side effects. This action is important to clients who are receiving chemotherapy because frequently debilitating systemic side effects may lead to discontinuation of some therapeutic regimens or alteration of others. Additionally, enough drug is available systematically to treat undetected micrometastases.

The physician is responsible for initiating the arterial catheter because the catheter placement is usually a surgical procedure or completed as an interventional radiologic procedure. The nurse's responsibility is the monitoring and maintenance of IAC.

The artery selected for encannulation (placement of a catheter) is specific to the diseased organ or structure to be treated. The physician usually prescribes IAC to treat a client's localized inoperable tumor in the liver, head, neck, or bones. Liver tumors are usually treated through the hepatic artery or branches of the celiac artery. The nurse may see the external carotid artery used in the treatment of head and neck tumors and the internal carotid artery used for the treatment of brain tumors.

Generally, the length of the therapy regimen and number of treatments determine which type of catheter the client will have. If the client is going to have intermittently scheduled therapy for a limited number of times, the physician will likely place a nonpermanent catheter using a radiologic procedure in the x-ray department. If the client is prescribed continuous therapy over a period of weeks or months, the physician will likely elect to place a permanent arterial catheter and a surgically implanted port. In either case, the physician places the catheter in a main artery that feeds the target organ or structure.

Devices

Catheters placed under radiography are usually made of polymer or Teflon. The catheters inserted surgically are usually ports. These ports are similar to those discussed in the central venous therapy section of this chapter, but the lumen of the catheter is generally smaller.

Whether the physician is placing the catheter surgically or radiologically, the catheter is threaded into the main artery feeding the tumor site. Some clients may have several vessels supplying the tumor site or the target vessel cannot be infused without infusing other adjacent vessels. When this occurs, the physician may elect to occlude these other vessels by injecting Gelfoam or metal coils through the catheter. Embolizing the arteries in this way may cause the tumor to shrink without the chemotherapy. The body absorbs the Gelfoam within a few days, re-establishing circulation. Metal coils provide permanent vascular occlusion. Until the client's body establishes collateral circulation, the client may complain of general malaise and pain in the area occluded.

Complications

Catheter displacement is the most common problem associated with temporary arterial catheters. Clients whose catheters become displaced may exhibit dyspepsia, excessive nausea and vomiting or diarrhea, gastric pain from peptic ulcers, or abdominal pain from pancreatitis. Treatment may include discontinuation of the chemotherapy infusion temporarily until the client can be treated with antiemetics and antacids.

A subintimal tear is the separation of the intima and media of the arterial wall, resulting from manipulation during placement. The client may complain of pain near the target organ during the infusion. Subintimal tears can delay therapy for weeks until the tear heals.

Arterial occlusion may occur with either a temporary radiologically placed catheter or a surgically placed catheter. The physician may order heparin in the chemotherapy infusion or have the client take 650 mg of aspirin twice daily to avoid catheter occlusion. Even with this prophylactic therapy, the nurse may observe transient or permanent loss or decrease in the client's pulse distal to the insertion site. The nurse must report these symptoms immediately. If the physician diagnoses the client with an embolism, the physician will either remove the catheter or use the fibrolytic agent urokinase (Abbokinase) in an attempt to lyse the clot.

Intraperitoneal Therapy
Description

Intraperitoneal (IP) therapy is the administration of therapeutic agents (cytotoxic drugs and biological response modifiers [BRMs]) into the peritoneal cavity. Intraperito-

neal therapy is usually prescribed for the treatment of tumors that are confined to the peritoneal cavity. Carcinomas of the ovaries and fallopian tubes generally meet this criterion.

Devices

There are three categories of IP catheters generally available: temporary indwelling catheters, semipermanent indwelling external catheters, and implantable IP ports. The initiation of an IP catheter is a physician responsibility, but the administration and monitoring of the therapeutic agent is generally a nursing responsibility.

Administration of the IP therapy includes three phases: the instillation phase, the dwell phase, and the drain phase. The peritoneal cavity generally acts as a tumor refuge, separated from the bloodstream by a cellular enclosure similar to the blood-brain barrier. This enclosure protects IP tumors from systemically infused chemotherapeutic agents. IP therapy, like intraarterial therapy allows for the administration of antineoplastic agents directly to the tumor sites. This enhances the drug's penetration and cell kill while restricting systemic effects.

Temporary indwelling catheters include the temporary peritoneal dialysis catheter, paracentesis catheters, and a 16- or 18-gauge over-the-needle IV catheter. Semipermanent indwelling external catheters include the Tenckhoff catheter, the Gore-tex catheter, and the column-disk catheter. IP implanted ports are similar to intravenous and arterial ports, but the portal body and the catheter diameter are larger.

Temporary indwelling catheters may be inserted and removed at the bedside. Clients receiving a temporary indwelling catheter benefit from having a new catheter inserted at the time of each therapy. Complications such as the development of fibrous sheaths and infection do not plague these clients.

Semipermanent indwelling external catheters and IP implanted ports are inserted in the operating room. Both of these catheters are appropriate for longer-term therapy.

Complications

Exit site infection, indicated by redness, tenderness, and warmth of the tissue around the catheter, is more often seen in clients who have Tenckhoff catheters. Frequent dressing changes to the exit site using sterile technique can help prevent this complication.

Microbial peritonitis is the inflammation of the peritoneal membranes from the invasion of microorganisms. The client may experience a fever and complain of abdominal pain. There may be abdominal rigidity and rebound tenderness. This condition is preventable with strict aseptic technique in the handling of all equipment and infusion supplies. Treatment includes antimicrobial therapy either intravenously or intraperitoneally.

Chemical peritonitis is the irritation of the peritoneal membranes by the chemotherapeutic agent. The client may complain of symptoms similar to those experienced with microbial peritonitis. If severe, chemical peritonitis may delay further treatment.

Occlusion is the inability to administer fluids into the

TABLE 17–3

Complications of Peripheral Intravenous Therapy

Local Complications

Complication	Definition	Cause	Signs and Symptoms	Treatment	Prevention
Infiltration	Infusion or seepage of intravenous (IV) solution or medication into the extravascular tissue	Access device either partially or completely dislodges from the vein	IV rate slows down; increasing edema above IV insertion site; client may complain of burning and tightness at IV site	If recent, ice may prevent any further seepage into the surrounding tissue; if older, warm moist compresses will assist with reabsorption of the fluid	Stabilize the IV catheter well; use the smallest catheter than will accomplish the infusion, avoid placement over area of flexion; monitor site frequently
Phlebitis	Inflammation of the vein	May be mechanical due to insertion technique or not stabilizing catheter well; may be chemical due to the pH or osmolality of the solution or medication	Client may complain of pain at IV site; nurse may observe that vein appears red and inflamed along the length; client may spike temperature; vein may become hard and cord-like	Remove the catheter; warm compresses to relieve pain; adjustment of infusion solution or admixture to prevent further injury	Change short-term IV catheter every 72 hours; when infusing medications or solutions with high osmolality, choose large veins; anchor catheters well to avoid movement in vein
Hematoma	Leaking of blood into the surrounding tissue	May be caused by piercing the back of the vein during insertion of the catheter; client may have faulty coagulation ability or be on anticoagulants	Discolored area of bruising around IV site; client may complain of pain; area may be swollen	Remove IV device and apply pressure; see treatment for infiltration	Carefully advance catheter, staying parallel with the client's skin; select the smallest catheter that will accomplish the task
Local infection	Bacterial contamination at the IV site	Break in aseptic technique during insertion or the handling of sterile equipment	Site appears red, swollen, and warm; client may complain of tenderness at the site; may observe purulent or malodorous exudate	Remove IV catheter and allow site to bleed for a few seconds and use 2 × 2 to express discharge; send catheter tip for culture; clean site with antibacterial solution and cover with dry sterile dressing; physician to evaluate for septic phlebitis and need for surgical intervention	Use careful technique when inserting IV; change site every 72 hours
Catheter embolism	A shaving or piece of catheter breaks off and floats freely in the vessel	May occur if needle of an over-the-needle catheter is reinserted into the catheter or if the catheter of a through-the-needle catheter is inadvertently pulled back through the catheter	Client will experience a decrease in blood pressure and complain of pain along the vein; pulse becomes weak, rapid, and thready, and the nurse may note cyanosis of the nail beds and circumorally; client may lapse into unconsciousness	Discontinue the catheter and apply a tourniquet high on the limb of the catheter site; inspect the catheter for any rough edges; an x-ray is taken to determine the presence of any catheter piece; surgical intervention may be necessary	When inserting over-the-needle catheters, never reinsert the needle into the catheter; avoid pulling a through-the-needle catheter back through the needle during insertion

Systemic Complications

Bloodstream infection	Pathogenic organisms enter the client's circulation	Early symptoms include fever, chills, headache, and general malaise; if left untreated, the client may experience severe infection, which may lead to vascular collapse and death	Same as for local infection above
			Change the entire infusion system from solution to IV device; notify physician, obtain cultures, and administer antibiotics as ordered; if the infusate is the suspected cause, send a specimen to the laboratory for evaluation
Circulatory overload	The disruption of fluid homeostasis with excess fluid in the circulatory system	Client may complain of shortness of breath and cough; client's blood pressure is elevated, and there is puffiness around the eyes and edema in dependent areas; the client's neck veins may be engorged, and the nurse may hear moist breath sounds	Monitor intake and output carefully and notify the physician as soon as an imbalance is noticed between the client's intake and output
	The infusion of fluids at a rate greater than the client's system can accommodate		Slow the IV rate and notify the physician; raise the client to an upright position; monitor vital signs and administer oxygen as ordered; administer diuretics as ordered
Speed shock	A systemic reaction to the rapid infusion of a substance unfamiliar to the client's circulatory system	Client may complain of lightheadedness or dizziness and chest tightness; the nurse may note that the client has a flushed face and an irregular pulse; without intervention, the client may lose consciousness and go into shock and cardiac arrest	The nurse is aware of the appropriate infusion rate of medications and adheres to them; use of infusion control devices assists in prevention of speed shock
	Rapid infusion of drugs or bolus infusion, which causes the drug to reach toxic levels quickly		Immediately discontinue the drug infusion and hang D5W to keep the vein open; monitor the client's vital signs carefully and notify the physician for further treatment orders
Allergic reaction	A local or general response to an allergen	The client having a local reaction may exhibit a wheal, redness, or itching at the IV site; in the case of a general reaction, the client may complain of itching, running nose, and tearing; the nurse may note bronchospasm, wheezing, and a truncal rash; without treatment, the client may experience anaphylaxis	
	May be the response to tape, cleansing agent, drug, solution, or IV device		

peritoneum or withdraw fluid from the peritoneum. Occlusion is caused by formation of fibrous sheaths or fibrin clots or plugs inside the catheter or around the tip or by compartmentalization of fluid due to adhesions or twisting, kinking, or displacement of the catheter. Management may include the infusion of a lysing agent such as urokinase. If the catheter is an indwelling external catheter, the physician may attempt to dislodge the clot by using a push-pull method with a syringe and 0.9% normal satire solution (NSS). Sometimes, the physician may insert a sterile stylet through an external catheter to dislodge the catheter.

Subcutaneous Therapy

Description

Subcutaneous (SC) therapy involves the insertion of a small-gauge needle into the client's subcutaneous space and the continuous administration of isotonic fluids or medications at a slow rate—usually 1 mL/min. Continuous subcutaneous infusion (CSQI) has been used as an alternative to intravenous therapy for maintenance, treatment, and palliation.

Devices

The nurse implements CSQI by cleansing any area on the client's body that has sufficient SC tissue. The nurse primes the attached tubing and, gently pinching an area of approximately 2 inches, inserts a small-gauge needle. Appropriate needle choices for CSQI include a 25- to 27-gauge butterfly needle or a Sub-Q-Set (Baxter). If using a butterfly needle, the nurse inserts the device at a 35- to 45-degree angle. The Sub-Q-Set is inserted at a 90-degree angle. After anchoring the needle, the nurse covers the site with a transparent dressing.

Clients who benefit from CSQI are those who

- Are unable to take oral medications (e.g., have dysphagia, gastrointestinal obstruction, or malabsorption)
- Have intractable nausea and vomiting
- Require parenteral medication but have poor venous access
- Require subcutaneous injections for longer than 48 hours
- Have a need for prolonged use of parenteral medication
- Need a continuous level of medication to control pain
- Cannot cope with the expense of intravenous therapy
- Are confused or depressed

Complications

Insertion site irritation, evidenced by erythema, heat, or swelling, is a local complication of CSQI. Rotation of the SC site approximately every 5–7 days usually helps prevent this problem.

Central Nervous System Therapy

Central nervous system therapy involves the infusion of medications into the epidural space or intrathecally.

Epidural Therapy

In epidural therapy, the physician or specially trained nurse administers medication into the epidural space of the spinal column. Located between the wall of the vertebral canal and the dura mater, the epidural space consists of fat, connective tissue, and blood vessels that protect the spinal cord. The most common uses of epidural therapy are to relieve postoperative or chronic pain and the pain associated with labor and delivery. The physician, usually an anesthesiologist or neurosurgeon, initiates epidural therapy. There are four different categories of catheters used for epidural therapy. The choice of one over the other depends on the purpose and duration of therapy. Table 17–4 describes each type and lists their indications.

Opioids administered epidurally slowly diffuse across the dura mater to the dorsal horn of the spinal cord and lock onto receptors and block pain impulses from ascending to the brain. The client receives pain relief from the level of the injection caudally (toward the toes). Local anesthetics administered epidurally work on the sensory nerve roots in the epidural space to block pain impulses. After the physician administers the first dose of medication, depending on state law, the type of medication, and facility policies, nurses trained in epidural therapy administer subsequent doses. In all cases, it is a nursing responsibility to monitor the client receiving epidural therapy for any signs of complications.

Complications associated with epidural therapy are usually caused by the medications administered. Table 17–5 outlines medication-related complications seen in the administration of epidural opiates and local anesthetics.

Intrathecal Therapy

Intrathecal therapy provides a means of administering chemotherapy, pain medication, or antibiotics directly into the ventricular cerebral spinal fluid (CSF) of clients who suffer from CSF malignancies or metastases, chronic cancer pain, or CSF infections. Some medications used to treat CSF neoplasms, such as methotrexate and cytarabine, cannot be administered intravenously because they cannot cross the blood-brain barrier. Others must be administered in very large doses to cross this natural protective mechanism. Large doses of chemotherapy may not be possible due to the severe systemic side effects associated with them. Administration of medications via the intrathecal route eliminates this problem, as the medication is administered directly into the CSF.

The Ommaya reservoir is the catheter commonly used for intrathecal therapy. A neurosurgeon is usually responsible for the placement of the catheter in the operating room under strict asepsis. The Ommaya reservoir consists of two pieces: a mushroom-shaped self-sealing dome made of silicone and a catheter that attaches to the dome. The tip of the catheter is placed in one of the lateral ventricles. The reservoir is attached and placed beneath a flap in the client's scalp. Some models of the reservoir have a side outlet tube that can be used as a shunt to remove excess CSF in the client with increased intracra-

TABLE 17–4

Catheters Used for Epidural Therapy

Type of Device	Description	Indications
Percutaneous catheter	Flexible nylon catheter threaded through a spinal needle into the epidural space. The external end has a standard female Luer-Lok hub, which accepts an intermittent injection cap.	Temporary pain relief post-operatively or during labor and delivery. For pain control in clients with end-stage cancer or a temporary measure to determine if the chronic pain client will receive relief with epidural therapy.
Subcutaneous tunneled catheter	A Silastic catheter tunneled from the point where it exits the spine to a point on the client's trunk, usually on the side just above the waist. Like a tunneled central venous catheter, the catheter has a Dacron cuff that prevents the migration of micro-organisms along the catheter into the epidural space.	A more permanent catheter indicated for clients in whom epidural therapy has proved to be effective and who have a life expectancy of weeks to months.
Totally implantable reservoir or port	Appears identical to a venous or arterial port. The surgeon places the portal body over a bony prominence, such as the spine itself, or one of the client's lower ribs.	Indicated for clients who respond to epidural therapy and have a life expectancy of months to years. Another indication is the client who is confused and repeatedly pulls out his or her subcutaneous tunneled catheter.
Totally implantable infusion pump	Consists of a catheter whose tip sits in the epidural space at the appropriate level. The catheter is tunneled subcutaneously and attached to the pump, which is usually implanted in a pocket in the abdominal region of chest wall. As described earlier, the medication is in the pump's reservoir.	The most expensive method of administering epidural therapy. Indicated for clients who will require therapy for a long period (chronic pain) and who have a life expectancy of months to years.

nial pressure. The physician or, in some cases, the chemotherapy nurse administers the medication by inserting a needle through the client's skin into the Ommaya dome. After removing the amount of CSF equal to the volume of the medication to be administered, the physician slowly injects the medication. The physician removes the needle and pumps the dome of the reservoir to release the medication into the catheter for delivery to the

TABLE 17–5

Medication-Related Complications of Epidural Therapy

System	Epidural Opiates	Epidural Local Anesthetics
Cardiovascular	No postural hypotension Minor changes in heart rate	Postural hypotension Decrease in heart rate
Respiratory	If occurs, may be early at 1–2 hours due to systemic absorption or late after dose at 6–24 hours due to migration to brain	Usually unimpaired
Central nervous system	Sedation may be marked Convulsions absent	Sedation absent to mild Convulsions possible due to rapid vascular absorption Sensory losses Motor weakness
Genitourinary	Urinary retention	Urinary retention
Integumentary	Pruritis	Pruritis rarely occurs
Gastrointestinal	Nausea and vomiting	Nausea and vomiting rarely occurs

From Booker, M. F., & Ignatavicius, D. D. (1996). *Infusion therapy: Techniques and medications.* Philadelphia: W. B. Saunders.

CSF. The nurse is responsible for monitoring the client for any complications.

Complications of Central Nervous System Therapy

Infection in the client receiving either epidural or intrathecal therapy is the result of a lack of asepsis when handling the medication or during the administration. There may be local evidence of infection, such as redness or swelling at the catheter exit site or over the Ommaya reservoir. The client may also exhibit neurological and systemic signs of infection, such as headache, stiff neck, or temperature higher than 101° F (38.3° C). The nurse may observe cloudy CSF, indicating a proliferation of white blood cells in clients undergoing intrathecal therapy.

Misplacement or migration of the catheter may occur at the time of placement, or the catheter can move or become kinked after placement. In clients with epidural catheters, when the nurse aspirates to check placement, he or she may observe clear free-flowing fluid (CSF), indicating that the catheter has migrated into the subarachnoid space, or the nurse may withdraw blood, indicating that the catheter has migrated into a blood vessel. An inadvertent administration of local anesthetics directly into the subarachnoid space may lead to high or total spinal block and convulsions or cardiovascular depression. Clients who mistakenly receive local anesthetics intravenously may experience toxic reactions with convulsions. In the client receiving intrathecal therapy via an Ommaya reservoir, the physician may observe no or very slow filling when "pumping" the dome. The client may exhibit new neurologic symptoms if the catheter has migrated.

Intraosseous Therapy

Description

Intraosseous (IO) therapy is a previously used and re-emerging method of gaining access to a client's vascular system. Primarily utilized in critically injured clients with vascular collapse, IO therapy is the topic of a number of research studies that confirm that it is a viable option for other clients requiring infusion therapy as well. In some states, prehospital providers such as emergency medical technicians (EMTs) and paramedics, as well as trained clinicians in trauma centers and emergency departments, initiate IO therapy.

Intraosseous therapy allows access to the rich vascular network located in the client's long bones. This vascular network is more prominent in children younger than 6 years. Victims of trauma, burns, cardiac arrest, and other life-threatening conditions benefit from IO therapy, because frequently clinicians are unable to access these clients' vascular systems using traditional methods such as intravenous therapy. Research indicates that absorption rates of large volume peripheral infusions (LVPs) and medications administered via the IO route are similar to those achieved with peripheral or central venous administration.

Devices

Theoretically, any needle may be used to provide IO therapy and access the medullary space. However, there are criteria that make some needles superior to others for IO therapy. A needle that has a removable stylet that screws into the cannula to keep the needle from retracting during insertion, a short shaft to eliminate accidental dislodgment after placement, an adjustable guard to stabilize the needle at skin level, and graduations along the needle to guide the practitioner during the insertion are features that make a needle well suited for IO therapy.

Complications

Improper needle placement is the most common complication of IO therapy. An accumulation of fluid under the skin at either the insertion site or on the other side of the limb indicates that the needle is either not far enough in to penetrate the bone marrow or is too far into the limb and has protruded through the other side of the shaft.

Needle obstruction occurs when the puncture has been accomplished but there has been delay in flushing. This delay may cause the needle to become clotted with bone marrow.

Osteomyelitis is a very serious complication of IO therapy. This infection in the bone tissue is unusual, but when it occurs it is generally due to leaving the cannula in place too long or the client having had a source of infection prior to the needle's insertion.

Embolus is a complication of any orthopedic procedure, and IO therapy is no exception. Embolus occurs when a bone fragment or fat enters the peripheral circulation. The client exhibits classic symptoms of respiratory distress, tachycardia, hypertension, tachypnea, fever, and petechiae. Laboratory data indicate an increased sedimentation rate and decreased red blood cell and platelet counts.

Compartment syndrome is a condition in which increased tissue pressure in a confined anatomic space causes decreased blood flow to the area. The decreased circulation to the area leads to hypoxia and pain in the area. This is very rare in IO therapy, but the nurse should monitor the site of the IO therapy carefully and alert the physician promptly should the client exhibit any signs of decreased circulation to the limb, such as coolness, swelling, mottling, and discoloration. Without improvement in perfusion to the limb, the client may require amputation of the limb.

SELECTED BIBLIOGRAPHY

*Beason, R., Bourguignon, J., Fowle, D., et al. (1993). Evaluation of a needle-free intravenous access system. *Journal of Intravenous Nursing, 15*(1), 11–15.

Booker, M. F., & Ignatavicius, D. D. (1996). *Infusion therapy: Techniques and medications.* Philadelphia; W. B. Saunders.

Clemence, M. A., Walker, D., & Farr, B. M. (1995). Central venous catheter practices: Results of a survey. *American Journal of Infection Control, 23*(1), 5–12.

Hunt, M. L., & Rapp, R. P. (1996). Intravenous medication errors. *Journal of Intravenous Nursing, 19*(3S), S9–S15.

Intravenous Nurses Society. (1997) Position paper: Midline and midclavicular catheters. *Journal of Intravenous Nursing, 20*(4), 175–178.

Intravenous Nurses Society. (1997). Position paper: Peripherally inserted central catheters. *Journal of Intravenous Nursing, 20*(4), 172–174.

Miller, J. M., Goetz, A., et al. (1996). Reduction in nosocomial intravenous device-related bacteremias after institution of an intravenous therapy team. *Journal of Intravenous Nursing, 19*(2), 103–106.

Pearson, M. L., et al. (1996). Guideline for prevention of intravascular-device–related infections. *Infection Control and Hospital Epidemiology, 17*(7), 438–473.

Treston-Aurand, J., Olmsted, R. N., et al. (1997). Impact of dressing materials on central venous catheter infection rates. *Journal of Intravenous Nursing, 20*(4), 201–206.

SUGGESTED READINGS

Clemence, M. A., Walker, D., & Farr, B. M. (1995). Central venous catheter practices: Results of a survey. *American Journal of Infection Control, 23*(1), 5–12.

This article describes the significant diversity among health care agencies in the care of central venous catheters. Certain protocols, still in use, that have been linked to an increase in bloodstream infections are presented, as well as suggestions for further research.

Treston-Aurand, J., Olmsted, R. N., et al. (1997). Impact of dressing materials on central venous catheter infection rates. *Journal of Intravenous Nursing, 20*(4), 201–206.

In the mid-1980s, many health care organizations changed their central venous catheter dressing regimens from gauze to transparent semipermeable polyurethane dressings. However, some studies have linked these dressings with microbial growth under the dressing and, consequently, an increase in catheter-related infections (CRIs). This article discusses the positive impact that the use of a highly permeable transparent dressing had on CRIs in one facility.

Hunt, M. L., & Rapp, R. P. (1996). Intravenous medication errors. *Journal of Intravenous Nursing, 19*(3S), S9–S15.

This article provides a brief history of modern hospital pharmacy practices, as well as a thorough discussion of the factors related to intravenous medication errors and strategies for physicians, pharmacists, and nurses to avoid them.

ACID-BASE BALANCE

Acids and bases regulate the body's hydrogen ion (H^+) production and elimination. Body fluid pH is a measure of its hydrogen ion concentrations. Even small changes in the hydrogen ion concentration, or *pH,* of body fluids can cause major problems in bodily function. Body fluid pH has the narrowest range of normal and the tightest control mechanisms of all electrolytes. Acids and bases perform the processes that release or bind hydrogen ions.

The normal hydrogen ion concentration of blood and other body fluids is quite low (< 0.0001 mEq/L) compared with the body fluid concentrations of other electrolytes (see Chapters 14 and 16). Because it is so low, hydrogen ion concentration is measured in pH units, calculated as the negative logarithm of the concentration in milliequivalents per liter (Fig. 18–1). Normal pH ranges from 7.35 to 7.45 for arterial blood and from 7.32 to 7.42 for venous blood.

Because pH is calculated in negative logarithm units, the value of pH is inversely related to the concentration of hydrogen ions. In other words, the lower the pH value of a fluid, the higher is the concentration of hydrogen ions in that fluid. In the 14-point pH scale, *a change of 1 pH unit actually represents a 10-fold change in hydrogen ion concentration.* Therefore, even a pH unit change of one tenth (e.g., a change from 7.4 to 7.3) represents a large increase in the hydrogen ion concentration of a given

solution. Table 18–1 lists terms used to describe acid-base balance.

Changes in pH interfere with many normal physiologic functions, including

- Altering the shape or position of hormones and enzymes to the extent that they can no longer perform their designated functions
- Changing the distribution of other electrolytes, causing fluid and electrolyte imbalances
- Altering the responses of excitable membranes, so that the heart, nerves, skeletal muscles, and gastrointestinal tract are either less or more active than normal
- Decreasing the uptake, activity, and distribution of many hormones and drugs, possibly reducing their effectiveness

Fortunately, the body has many well-regulated mechanisms to ensure minimal changes in hydrogen ion concentration. Table 18–2 lists the key concepts of acid-base balance.

ACID-BASE BALANCE

As discussed in Chapters 14 and 16, body fluids are electrically neutral even though they contain ions with an overall positive charge (cations or protons) and ions with

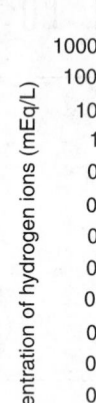
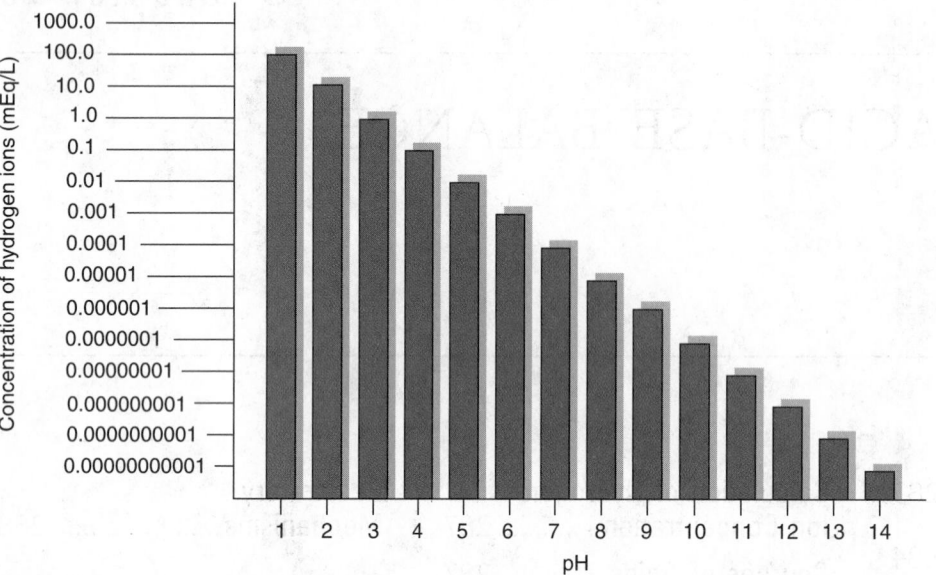

Figure 18–1. Relationship between pH and concentration of hydrogen ions.

an overall negative charge (anions). When fluids contain an equal number of positive and negative charges, the electrical charge remains neutral. The system maintains a body fluid pH between 7.35 and 7.45 in a similar manner; however, this value is not strictly neutral (7.0 is neutral) but rather is slightly alkaline. Normal body fluid pH remains at a near-neutral value when the acid components and base components are in relative balance, thus limiting the total number of free hydrogen ions. That is, acid-base balance occurs by matching the rate of hydro-

gen ion production with the activity of mechanisms for hydrogen ion removal and uptake.

Acid-Base Chemistry

Acids

Acids are substances that donate, or release, a hydrogen ion when the substance is dissolved in water (H_2O). An

TABLE 18–1

Pertinent Acid-Base Balance Terminology	
Term	**Definition**
Acid	• Any substance releasing a hydrogen ion when dissolved in water
Anaerobic metabolism	• Cellular metabolism occurring without the presence of oxygen
Base	• Any substance binding a hydrogen ion when dissolved in water
Buffer	• A substance capable of binding a hydrogen ion from body fluids (acting as a base) or releasing a hydrogen ion into body fluids (acting as an acid)
Chemoreceptors	• Special cells in the respiratory center of the brain sensitive to changes in the carbon dioxide concentration of extracellular fluid
pH	• The concentration of hydrogen ions in a solution, calculated as the negative logarithm of the milliequivalent concentration per liter

TABLE 18–2

Key Concepts of Acid-Base Balance
• The normal pH of the body's extracellular fluids (including blood) is 7.35–7.45.
• The pH in the body can be described as the relationship of bicarbonate to carbonic acid, or a 20:1 ratio.
• Carbon dioxide is the most changeable component of carbonic acid.
• The concentration of carbon dioxide is directly related to the concentration of hydrogen ions.
• An acid gives up hydrogen ions in solution; a base binds hydrogen ions in solution.
• Acids are formed in the body as a result of metabolism and incomplete oxidation of glucose and fats.
• Acid-base balance is regulated by chemical, respiratory, and renal mechanisms.
• Chemical buffers are the immediate way that acid-base imbalances are corrected.
• The lungs control the amount of carbon dioxide that is retained or exhaled.
• The kidneys regulate the amount of hydrogen and bicarbonate ions that are retained or excreted by the body.
• Compensation is the process in which the body uses its three regulatory mechanisms to correct for changes in the pH of body fluids.

acid in solution thus increases the concentration of free hydrogen ions in that solution. The strength of an acid is determined by how easily it releases a hydrogen ion in solution. A strong acid, such as hydrochloric acid (HCl), dissociates (separates) completely in water and readily releases all its hydrogen ions:

$$HCl + H_2O \longrightarrow H^+ + Cl^- + H_2O$$

hydrochloric acid   water   hydrogen ion   chloride ion   water

A weak acid does not completely dissociate in water; it releases only some of its total hydrogen ions. In the following example, each molecule of acetic acid (CH_3COOH), a weak acid, contains a total of four hydrogen molecules. When acetic acid combines with water, it releases only one of its four hydrogen molecules. The other three hydrogen molecules remain bound to the acetic acid molecule:

$$CH_3COOH + H_2O \longrightarrow H^+ + CH_3COO^- + H_2O$$

Bases

A base is a substance that binds free hydrogen ions in solution. Thus, bases are hydrogen acceptors: they reduce the concentration of free hydrogen ions in solution. Strong bases bind hydrogen ions easily. Some may bind more than one hydrogen ion to one base molecule. Examples of strong bases include sodium hydroxide (NaOH) and ammonia (NH_3); weak bases include aluminum hydroxide ($Al(OH)_3$) and bicarbonate (HCO_3^-).

Weak bases bind hydrogen ions less readily. Although bicarbonate is a relatively weak base, bicarbonate ions in the body are crucial in preventing major disturbances in body fluid pH.

Buffers

Buffers are substances that either release a hydrogen ion into a fluid or bind a hydrogen ion from a fluid. Most substances, when dissolved in water, react by either releasing a hydrogen ion (an acidic substance) or binding a free hydrogen ion (a basic substance). Buffers dissolved in water can react in two ways: either as an acid, releasing a hydrogen ion, or as a base, binding a hydrogen ion.

How a buffer reacts when dissolved in water or other fluid depends on the existing acid-base balance of that fluid. Buffers always try to bring the fluid as close as possible to a normal body fluid pH of 7.35 to 7.45. Thus, if the fluid is basic (with few free hydrogen ions), the buffer will release hydrogen ions into the fluid (Fig. 18–2). If the fluid is acidic (with many free hydrogen ions), the buffer will act as a base, binding some hydrogen ions. In a sense, buffers are hydrogen ion "sponges," soaking up hydrogen ions when too many are present in a fluid and squeezing out hydrogen ions when too few are present in a fluid. Because of this flexibility, buffers are important regulators of body fluid pH or hydrogen ion concentration (acid-base balance).

Solutions with a pH of 7.0 are considered neutral; they contain a set concentration of hydrogen ions whose number and strength of acid and base components are in equilibrium. Figure 18–3 is an artificial yet concrete representation of the concept of neutral pH. This repre-

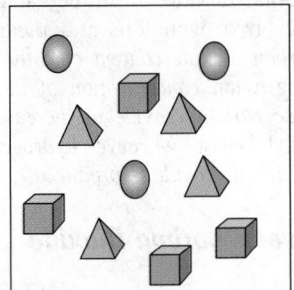
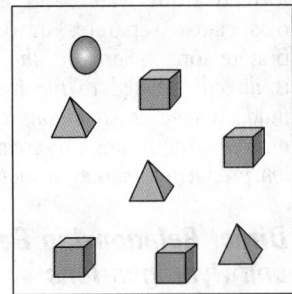
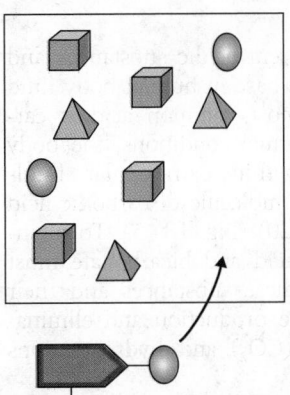
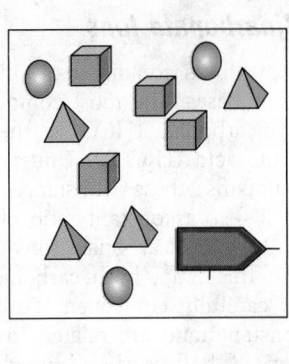

Fluid pH 7.38 (normal). The number and strength of acid components are equal to the number and strength of base components. Hydrogen ion concentration is limited and constant.

Fluid pH 7.51 (alkaline). The number and strength of base components are greater than the number and strength of acid components. Hydrogen ion concentration is below normal.

Buffer is added to the alkaline fluid.

The buffer acts as an acid, releasing a hydrogen ion.

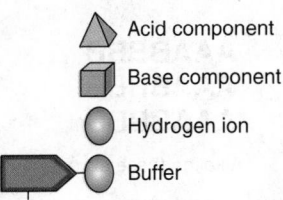

△ Acid component

▢ Base component

○ Hydrogen ion

⬠ Buffer

Figure 18–2. Action of buffer in solution. (© 1992 by M. Linda Workman. All rights reserved.)

AAABBB   AAAABBB   AAABB
AAABBB   AAAABBB   AAABB
AAABBB   AAAABBB   AAABB

Neutral   Acidic (acid excess)   Acidic (base deficit)

Figure 18–3. Concept of acidic versus normal pH. (A = acid; B = base.)

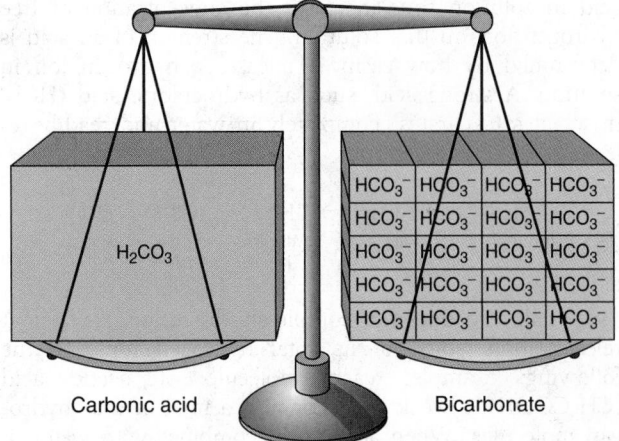

Figure 18–5. Normal ratio of carbonic acid to bicarbonate is 1:20.

sentation indicates that the strength as well as the amount of all acid components is equal to the strength as well as the amount of all the base components in a given solution. Although this is never the actual case in human physiology, in acid-base homeostasis, the relative amounts and strengths of acids and bases are approximately equal, so the overall hydrogen ion concentration remains constant.

Solutions with a pH from 1.0 to 6.99 contain an excessive amount or strength (or both) of the acid components compared with the amount or strength (or both) of the base components. Such solutions are considered *acidic* (see Fig. 18–3). This results in more hydrogen ions being released than bound, greatly increasing the number of free hydrogen ions.

Solutions with a pH ranging from 7.01 to 14.0 have an excessive amount or strength (or both) of the base components compared with the amount or strength (or both) of the acid components. These solutions are considered *basic*. This results in more hydrogen ions being bound than released, causing a deficit in the number of free hydrogen ions (Fig. 18–4).

Body Fluid Chemistry
Bicarbonate Ions

Body fluids contain many different acidic substances and a few bases. The most common base in human body fluid is bicarbonate (HCO_3^-); the most common acid is carbonic acid (H_2CO_3). Under normal conditions, the body maintains these substances within extracellular fluids (ECFs) at a constant ratio of 1 molecule of carbonic acid to 20 free bicarbonate ions (1:20) (Fig. 18–5). To maintain this ratio, both carbonic acid and bicarbonate must be carefully controlled. Both these substances and their constant ratio are related to the production and elimination of both carbon dioxide (CO_2) and hydrogen ions (H^+).

A key concept that aids understanding acid-base balance is the *carbonic anhydrase equation* (shown next). This

equation, driven by the enzyme carbonic anhydrase, demonstrates how hydrogen ion concentration and carbon dioxide concentration are directly related to one another, so that an increase in one causes a corresponding increase in the other:

$$CO_2 + H_2O \longleftrightarrow H_2CO_3 \longleftrightarrow H^+ + HCO_3^-$$

carbon   water   carbonic   hydrogen   bicarbonate
dioxide   acid   ion   ion

Carbon dioxide is a gas that, when combined with water, forms carbonic acid. Carbon dioxide thus is a changeable part of carbonic acid. Because carbonic acid is not stable and the body needs to maintain a 1:20 ratio of carbonic acid to bicarbonate, as soon as carbonic acid is formed from water and carbon dioxide, it immediately dissociates (separates) into free hydrogen ions and bicarbonate ions. *Therefore, the carbon dioxide content of a fluid is directly related to the hydrogen ion concentration of that fluid. Whenever conditions cause carbon dioxide to increase, more hydrogen ions are created. Likewise, whenever hydrogen ion production increases, more carbon dioxide is produced.*

Direct Relationship Between Carbon Dioxide and Hydrogen Ions

When excess carbon dioxide is produced, the concentration of carbon dioxide increases and the carbonic anhydrase equation shifts to the right, demonstrating an increase in the hydrogen ion concentration (and a decrease in pH):

$$CO_2 + H_2O \Longleftrightarrow H_2CO_3 \Longleftrightarrow H^+ + HCO_3^-$$

When very little carbon dioxide is produced, no hydrogen ions are generated by the carbonic anhydrase equation.

When excess hydrogen ions are produced or brought into the body, the carbonic anhydrase equation shifts to the left, demonstrating the creation of more carbon dioxide:

AAABBB   AAABBBB   AABBB
AAABBB   AAABBBB   AABBB
AAABBB   AAABBBB   AABBB

Neutral   Alkaline (base excess)   Alkaline (acid deficit)

Figure 18–4. Concept of alkaline versus normal pH. (A = acid; B = base.)

$$CO_2 + H_2O \rightleftharpoons H_2CO_3 \rightleftharpoons H^+ + HCO_3^-$$

When the body fluids are low on hydrogen ions, no extra carbon dioxide is produced.

Calculation of Hydrogen Ion Concentration

The pH is a calculated measurement of hydrogen ion concentration in body fluids, because the actual number or percentage of hydrogen ions in these fluids is not easily measured. The pH calculations are derived from the Henderson-Hasselbalch equation, a mathematical formula that expresses the interrelatedness of three factors: the concentration of free hydrogen ions, the concentration of bases, and the concentration of acids in a solution. When other influences (such as temperature and pressure) remain constant, if two of the three factors are known, then the third factor can be calculated.

$$pH = 6.1 + \log \frac{[HCO_3^-]}{[H_2CO_3 + CO_2]}$$

Because the ratio of carbonic acid and bicarbonate concentration in ECF is 1:20 under normal physiologic conditions, the major factor in the equation that tends to change is the carbon dioxide concentration. Whenever the carbon dioxide concentration changes, pH changes correspondingly.

In the Henderson-Hasselbalch formula, carbon dioxide concentration is on the bottom of the equation, making it inversely related to pH while it is directly related to the hydrogen ion concentration. Thus, when the carbon dioxide concentration of a solution increases, the pH drops, indicating an increase in the hydrogen ion concentration. Conversely, when the carbon dioxide concentration of a solution decreases, the pH rises, indicating a decrease in the hydrogen ion concentration.

An increase in the bicarbonate concentration causes the hydrogen ion concentration to decrease and the pH to increase, or become more alkaline (basic). Conversely, an increase in the carbon dioxide concentration causes the hydrogen ion concentration to increase and the pH to decrease, or become more acidic. In either case, the normal 1:20 ratio is changed and the pH of the blood is also changed.

Because the kidneys control bicarbonate concentration and the lungs control carbon dioxide concentration in the body, pH can also be described as the function of the kidneys divided by the function of the lungs, or

$$pH = \frac{\text{Kidneys (bicarbonate)}}{\text{Lungs (carbon dioxide)}}$$

Sources of Acids

Acids are formed in the body as byproducts of normal metabolism. Common sources of hydrogen ions are carbon dioxide production, metabolism of proteins and fats, anaerobic metabolism of glucose or fats, and destruction of cells.

Production of Carbon Dioxide

Carbon dioxide is a byproduct of glucose breakdown and many other metabolic reactions. (The complete breakdown of 1 molecule of glucose results in the formation of 36 molecules of adenosine triphosphate, 6 molecules of water, and 6 molecules of carbon dioxide.) Because of the relationship between carbon dioxide and hydrogen ions through the carbonic anhydrase equation, any increase in carbon dioxide concentration in body fluids always leads to the formation of increased amounts of hydrogen ions in those fluids, with a resulting decrease in pH.

Carbon dioxide is exhaled by the lungs during breathing. Therefore, one determinant of blood pH is how much carbon dioxide is produced by body cells during metabolism versus how rapidly carbon dioxide is removed by respiration.

Metabolism of Fats and Proteins

The catabolism (breakdown) of food for energy results in the formation of *fixed acids*. Protein catabolism creates sulfuric acid. Fat catabolism creates fatty acids.

Anaerobic Metabolism of Glucose and Fats

Incomplete oxidation—as occurs whenever cells continue to metabolize substances under anaerobic, or no oxygen, conditions—of glucose leads to the formation of lactic acid. Incomplete breakdown of fatty acids, either because excessive amounts of fatty acids are being metabolized or because insufficient oxygen is present during any fatty acid breakdown, results in the formation of ketoacids (Guyton & Hall, 1996).

Destruction of Cells

Whenever cells are damaged or destroyed, plasma membranes are broken and intracellular contents are released. Some cell structures contain acids that are released into the extracellular fluid (ECF) when this occurs.

Sources of Bicarbonate Ions

Bicarbonate is the principal buffer of the ECF. Sources of bicarbonate in the ECF include the breakdown of carbonic acid, gastrointestinal absorption of ingested bicarbonate, pancreatic synthesis and secretion of bicarbonate, movement of intracellular bicarbonate into the ECF, and renal reabsorption of filtered bicarbonate. Once bicarbonate is in the ECF, it is maintained at a concentration 20 times greater than that of carbonic acid.

Homeostasis

As long as body cells are capable of metabolism, the production of various acids, carbon dioxide, and hydrogen ions is a normal and continuous process. Despite this production, homeostasis of body fluids in terms of hydrogen ion, bicarbonate, oxygen, and carbon dioxide concentrations is maintained under normal physiologic conditions. Chart 18–1 lists normal values for these substances

Laboratory Profile: Acid-Base Assessment

Test	Arterial	Venous	Significance of Abnormal Findings
		Normal Range for Adults	
pH	7.35–7.45	7.32–7.43	Increased: metabolic alkalosis, loss of gastric fluids, decreased potassium intake, diuretic therapy, fever, salicylate toxicity
>90 years	7.25–7.45		Decreased: metabolic or respiratory acidosis, ketosis, renal failure, starvation, diarrhea, hyperthyroidism
PaO_2 (mm Hg)	83–108		Increased: increased ventilation, oxygen therapy, exercise
>90 years	>50		Decreased: respiratory depression, high altitude, carbon monoxide poisoning, decreased cardiac output
$PaCO_2$ (mm Hg)	35–48	41–55	Increased: respiratory acidosis, emphysema, pneumonia, cardiac failure, respiratory depression
			Decreased: respiratory alkalosis, excessive ventilation, diarrhea
Bicarbonate (mEq/L or mmol/L)	22–26	24–29	Increased: bicarbonate therapy, metabolic alkalosis
			Decreased: metabolic acidosis, diarrhea, pancreatitis
Lactate (mg/dL)	<11.3	8.1–15.3	Increased: hypoxia, exercise, insulin infusion, alcoholism, pregnancy
			Decreased: fluid overload

PaO_2 = partial pressure of arterial oxygen; $PaCO_2$ = partial pressure of arterial carbon dioxide.

in arterial and venous blood. This homeostasis depends on three factors:

- Hydrogen ion production must be consistent and not excessive.
- Carbon dioxide loss from the body through breathing must occur at a rate that keeps pace with hydrogen ion production.
- The ratio between carbonic acid and bicarbonate must be maintained at 1:20.

Acid-Base Regulatory Mechanisms

To maintain the hydrogen ion concentration (pH) of the extracellular fluid (ECF) within the narrow ranges of normal, the body has three well-regulated mechanisms for acid-base balance: chemical, respiratory, and renal (Table 18–3).

Chemical Mechanisms

Buffers are the first line of defense against changes in hydrogen ion concentration. Because they are constantly present in body fluids, buffers can take immediate action to reduce or raise the hydrogen ion concentration to normal. By acting as hydrogen ion "sponges," buffers can bind hydrogen ions when the concentration is too high or release hydrogen ions when the concentration is too low. Fluid buffers are composed of chemicals or proteins.

CHEMICAL BUFFERS. Chemical buffers are paired mixtures, usually consisting of a weak base and the conjugated salt of an acid. The two most common chemical buffer systems are bicarbonate buffers (which are active in both the ECF and intracellular fluid [ICF]) and phosphate buffers (which are active in the ICF).

PROTEIN BUFFERS. Proteins are the largest source of buffers. Proteins in body fluids can either bind or release hydrogen ions as needed. Both intracellular and extracellular proteins serve as buffers.

The major intracellular protein buffer is hemoglobin. Hemoglobin buffers hydrogen ions directly, and also buffers whole acids formed during the synthesis and transport of carbon dioxide. When the hydrogen ion concentration of the blood increases, some of the excess hydrogen ions cross the plasma membrane of red blood cells and bind to the large numbers of hemoglobin molecules in each red blood cell.

Extracellular buffering proteins include albumins and globulins. These proteins buffer both carbonic acid and the fixed acids present in the ECF as a result of catabolism.

Respiratory Mechanisms

When chemical buffers alone cannot prevent changes in body fluid pH, the respiratory system is the second line of defense against changes. Breathing controls hydrogen ion concentration by regulating the carbon dioxide concentration in arterial blood. Carbon dioxide is converted into hydrogen ions through the carbonic anhydrase reaction; therefore, the carbon dioxide concentration is directly related to the hydrogen ion concentration. Breathing is a major mechanism for ridding the body of

TABLE 18-3

Acid-Base Regulatory Mechanisms

Chemical Mechanisms

Protein buffers
  Extracellular
    Albumin
    Globulins
  Intracellular
    Hemoglobin
Chemical buffers
  Extracellular
    Bicarbonate
  Intracellular
    Phosphate
    Bicarbonate
	• Very rapid
	• Provide immediate response to changing conditions
	• Can handle relatively small fluctuations in hydrogen ion production and elimination encountered under normal metabolic and health conditions

Respiratory Mechanisms

Increased hydrogen ions
Increased carbon dioxide
  Stimulates central respiratory neurons, leading to increased rate and depth of breathing, causing more carbon dioxide to be lost and decreasing the hydrogen ion concentration
Decreased hydrogen ions
Decreased carbon dioxide
  Inhibition of central respiratory neurons, leading to decreased rate and depth of breathing, causing normally produced carbon dioxide to be retained, increasing the hydrogen ion concentration
	• Primarily assist buffering systems when the fluctuation of hydrogen ion concentration is acute

Renal Mechanisms

Mechanisms to decrease pH
  Increased renal excretion of bicarbonate
  Increased renal reabsorption of hydrogen ions
Mechanisms to increase pH
  Decreased renal excretion of bicarbonate
  Decreased renal reabsorption of hydrogen ions
	• The most powerful regulator of acid-base balance
	• Respond to large or chronic fluctuations in hydrogen ion production or elimination

carbon dioxide, which is created as a byproduct of metabolism.

The carbon dioxide concentration in venous blood increases during normal metabolism. This carbon dioxide is transported to the capillaries of the lungs. Because the partial pressure (concentration) of carbon dioxide is far higher in capillary blood than in the atmospheric air in the alveoli, carbon dioxide diffuses freely from the blood into the alveolar air. Once in the alveoli, carbon dioxide

is exhaled during breathing and is lost from the body. Because the partial pressure (concentration) of carbon dioxide in atmospheric air is nearly zero, carbon dioxide usually continues to be exhaled at an appropriate rate even when breathing is impaired to some degree.

HYPERVENTILATION. Respiratory regulation of acid-base balance is under the control of the nervous system (Fig. 18-6). Special chemoreceptors in the areas of the brain that directly regulate the rate and depth of respiration are sensitive to changes in the carbon dioxide concentration in the cerebral extracellular fluid (ECF). As the carbon dioxide concentration begins to rise in cerebral blood and tissues, these central chemoreceptors stimulate the neurons that control the rate and depth of respiration. Under this stimulation, both the rate and the depth of respiration increase, so that more carbon dioxide is exhaled ("blown off") from the alveoli and the carbon dioxide concentration of the ECF decreases. When the arterial carbon dioxide concentration returns to normal, the rate and depth of respiration return to levels normal for the individual.

HYPOVENTILATION. If the ECF hydrogen ion concentration is too low, then the carbon dioxide concentration is also too low. Central chemoreceptors sense these low carbon dioxide levels and inhibit stimulation of neurons in the respiratory control centers. As a result of this lack of stimulation, the rate and depth of respiration dramatically diminish, so that less carbon dioxide is lost through the lungs and more carbon dioxide is retained in arterial blood. This retention, coupled with the normal carbon dioxide–generating metabolic reactions, results in a rapid return of the arterial carbon dioxide concentration (and hydrogen ion concentration) to normal levels. When these levels are normal, the rate and depth of respiration also return to basal levels.

The respiratory system's response in regulating acid-base balance is rapid. Changes in the rate and depth of respiration occur within minutes after changes in the hydrogen ion concentration or carbon dioxide concentration of the ECF occur.

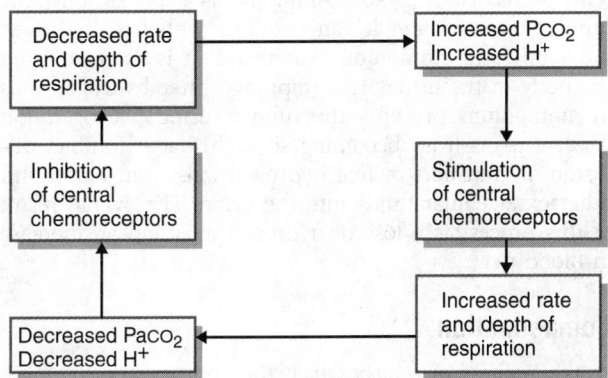

Figure 18-6. Neural regulation of respiration and hydrogen ion concentration. (PaCO$_2$ = partial pressure of arterial carbon dioxide; H$^+$ = hydrogen ion.)

Renal Mechanisms

The kidneys are the third line of defense against fluctuations in body fluid pH. Renal mechanisms are the most powerful mechanism for regulating acid-base balance, but take longer to start than the chemical and respiratory mechanisms. When changes in body fluid pH are persistent, renal mechanisms that increase excretion and reabsorption rates of acids or bases (depending on the direction of the pH changes) begin to operate (Fig. 18–7). These mechanisms include renal tubular movement of bicarbonate, formation of acids, and formation of ammonium.

TUBULAR MOVEMENT OF BICARBONATE. This first renal mechanism occurs in the kidney tubules in two ways: (1) renal movement of bicarbonate produced elsewhere in the body and (2) renal movement of bicarbonate produced in the kidneys. Much of the bicarbonate made in other body areas is absorbed into the blood and filtered from the blood into early urine in the nephron. When blood hydrogen ion levels are high, this filtered bicarbonate is reabsorbed from the tubules back into systemic circulation, where it can help buffer excess hydrogen ions. When blood hydrogen ion levels are low, the filtered bicarbonate remains in the urine and is excreted. When a hydrogen ion excess is evident, the kidney tubules can respond by making additional bicarbonate that will be reabsorbed.

FORMATION OF ACIDS. The second renal mechanism occurs through the phosphate-buffering mechanism inside the cells of the kidney tubules. When the newly created bicarbonate made in the tubule cells is reabsorbed into systemic circulation along with the sodium, the urine has an excess of anions, including phosphate (HPO_4^{2-}). This negatively charged environment draws hydrogen ions into the urine. Once the hydrogen ion is in the urine, it combines with the phosphate ion, forming an acid, H_2PO_4, which is then excreted from the body in the urine.

FORMATION OF AMMONIUM. In the third renal mechanism, ammonium (NH_4^+) is formed from ammonia, which is a byproduct of normal amino acid catabolism (Guyton & Hall, 1996). Ammonia is excreted into the tubular urine, where it can combine with free hydrogen ions and form ammonium. Afterward, it is excreted from the body in the urine. This trapping of free hydrogen ions in ammonium prevents the tubular urine hydrogen ion concentration from becoming so high that it inhibits diffusion or transport of free hydrogen ions from blood and other extracellular fluids into the urine. The overall result of this process is a loss of hydrogen ions and an increase in blood pH.

Compensation

In the process of *compensation*, the body attempts to correct for changes in body fluid (blood) pH. A pH below 6.9 or above 7.8 is usually fatal. The normal pH range for human extracellular fluids is 7.35 to 7.45.

Renal Compensation

A healthy renal system can correct or compensate for changes in pH when the respiratory system is either overwhelmed or is actually a cause of the imbalance. For example, in a person with chronic airflow limitation (CAL), the respiratory system cannot exchange gases adequately. Carbon dioxide is thus retained, and the pH of the extracellular fluid (ECF) falls, or becomes more acidic. To counteract this process, the renal system increases its excretion of hydrogen ions and increases the reabsorption of bicarbonate back into the body. As a result, the pH of body fluids remains either within or closer to the normal range. When these back-up mechanisms are completely effective, respiratory problems are fully compensated and the pH of the blood returns to normal, even though the concentration of other substances (such as oxygen and bicarbonate) may be abnormal.

Sometimes, however, the respiratory factors contributing to the acid-base imbalance are so severe that renal actions can only partially compensate, and thus the pH is not normal. Even partial compensation is critically important to acid-base balance because it prevents the imbalance from becoming severe (and possibly life-threatening).

Respiratory Compensation

The respiratory system can compensate for acid-base imbalances of a metabolic origin. For example, when prolonged running causes excess build-up of lactic acid, hydrogen ion concentration in the ECF increases and the pH drops. To bring the pH back to normal, the healthy respiratory system is stimulated by the increased carbon dioxide concentration to increase both the rate and depth of respiration. These respiratory efforts cause the blood to lose carbon dioxide with each exhalation, so ECF levels of carbon dioxide and hydrogen ions gradually decrease. When the respiratory system can fully compensate, the pH returns to normal.

Both the renal and respiratory systems can compensate for acid-base imbalances but are not equal in their compensatory actions and reactions. The respiratory system is much more sensitive to acid-base changes and can begin compensation efforts within seconds to minutes after a change in pH. These efforts are limited and can be overwhelmed easily, however. The renal compensatory mechanisms are much more powerful and result in dramatic changes in ECF composition. However, these more powerful mechanisms are not fully stimulated until the acid-base imbalance has been sustained for a period ranging from several hours to several days.

AGE-RELATED CHANGES IN ACID-BASE BALANCE

The elderly are more susceptible to pH disturbances than younger people because their normal physiologic mechanisms are less able to respond to minor fluctuations in hydrogen ion production or elimination. In addition, an elderly person may be taking medications that alter the activity of normal pH-compensating mechanisms (Chart 18–2).

1. TUBULAR MOVEMENT OF BICARBONATE

METHOD A: Movement of Pre-existing Bicarbonate   **METHOD B:** Movement of New Bicarbonate

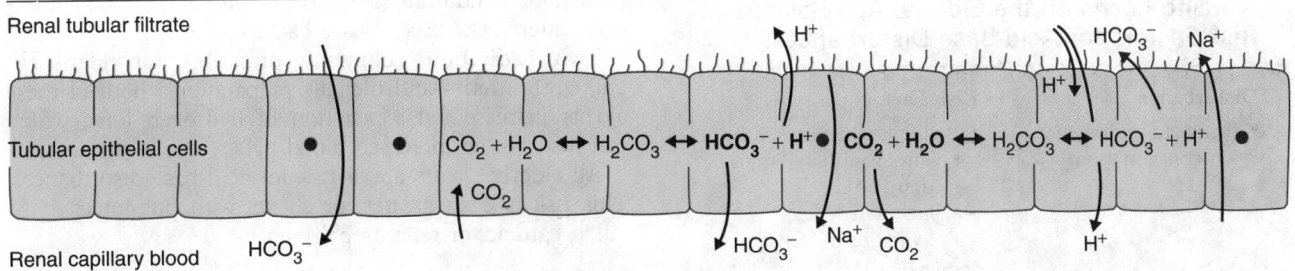

Renal tubular filtrate

Tubular epithelial cells

Renal capillary blood

Bicarbonate filtered at the glomerulus into the filtrate ("early urine") is reabsorbed across the renal tubular epithelium into the renal capillaries and returned to the systemic circulation. This movement of bicarbonate into the systemic circulation increases blood pH (makes blood less acidic).

If Blood CO_2 Levels Are High
Carbon dioxide enters the tubular epithelium, shifting the carbonic anhydrase equation to the right to form bicarbonate and hydrogen ions. Bicarbonate moves into the renal capillaries. Hydrogen moves into the tubular filtrate in exchange for sodium. The loss of hydrogen ions from blood increases its pH (makes it less acidic).

To prevent excess hydrogen in the renal tubular filtrate, hydrogen ions must combine with other substances. The second and third renal mechanisms of acid-base balance now come into play.

If Blood CO_2 Levels Are Low
Hydrogen ions from the tubular filtrate are reabsorbed into the renal capillaries in exchange for sodium. This flow of hydrogen may be direct, or it may shift the carbonic anhydrase equation to the left so that carbon dioxide is reabsorbed into the systemic circulation and bicarbonate moves into the renal tubular filtrate. Retention of acids and excretion of bases reduce blood pH (makes blood more acidic).

2. FORMATION OF TITRATABLE ACIDS

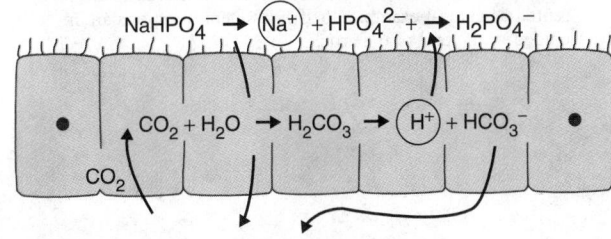

After the newly generated bicarbonate and the cation sodium are passed into the systemic circulation, the renal tubular filtrate has an excess of anions, including phoshate. The cation hydrogen is attracted to the negatively charged environment of the renal tubular filtrate. There, hydrogen binds with phosphate to form the titratable acid H_2PO_4, which is excreted in urine.

3. FORMATION OF AMMONIUM

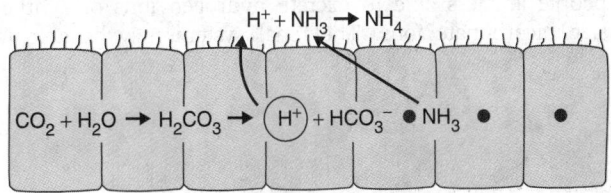

Ammonia produced by amino acid (glutamine) catabolism is excreted into the renal tubular filtrate. There, ammonia combines with hydrogen cations to form ammonium, which is excreted in urine.

Figure 18–7. Renal mechanisms of acid-base balance. (CO_2 = carbon dioxide.)

Nursing Focus on the Elderly: Age-Related Risk Factors for Acid-Base Disturbances

Disturbance	Risk Factors
• Increased hydrogen ion concentration	• Pulmonary diseases • Chronic airflow limitation (CAL) • Pneumonia • Dehydration • Infection • Renal disease • Vascular disease • Atherosclerosis • Arteriosclerosis • Angiitis
• Decreased hydrogen ion concentration	• Overhydration • Congestive heart failure • Drugs • Diuretics (loop and thiazide) • Digitalis preparations • Insulin • Antibiotics • Chemotherapeutic agents

handle ordinary changes resulting from normal metabolism, but it cannot compensate adequately when other pathologic conditions (such as pneumonia, fever, or infection) interfere with acid-base balance.

Two medications commonly prescribed for elderly clients are diuretics and digitalis preparations. Both of these agents increase renal excretion of hydrogen ions, which can result in an increased blood pH.

All elderly clients are at risk for acid-base disturbances. This risk is even greater for clients with pulmonary, vascular, cardiac, or renal impairments.

SELECTED BIBLIOGRAPHY

Cornock, M. (1996). Making sense of arterial blood gases and their interpretation. *Nursing Times, 92*(6), 30–31.
Guyton, A., & Hall, J. (1996). *Textbook of medical physiology* (9th ed.). Philadelphia: W. B. Saunders.
Halperin, M., & Goldstein, M. (1994), *Fluid, electrolyte and acid-base physiology: A problem-based approach* (2nd ed.). Philadelphia: W. B. Saunders.
Kuhn, M. (1996). Laboratory analysis. *Critical Care Nurse, 16*(5), 74–76.
Mays, D. (1995). Turn ABGs into child's play. *RN, 58*(1), 36–40.
Metheny, N. (1996). *Fluid and electrolyte balance: Nursing considerations* (3rd ed.). Philadelphia: J. B. Lippincott.
O'Donnell, J. (1995). Can you prevent respiratory depression? *Nursing95, 25*(4), 32JJ.
Tasota, F., & Wesmiller, S. (1994). Assessing A.B.G.s: Maintaining the delicate balance. *Nursing94, 24*(5), 34–46.
Tietz, N. W. (Ed.). (1995). *Clinical guide to laboratory tests* (3rd ed.). Philadelphia: W. B. Saunders.

SUGGESTED READINGS

Mays, D. (1995). Turn ABGs into child's play. *RN, 58*(1), 36-40.
 The author uses a game approach to describe a simple method of determining the pH status for an individual client. Practice opportunity is provided through the use of several case presentations.
Tasota, F., & Wesmiller, S. (1994). Assessing A.B.G.s: Maintaining the delicate balance. *Nursing94, 24*(5), 34–46.
 This well-written article describes the interaction among oxygenation, ventilation and acid-base balance. Several case studies are presented as clinical examples. Self-assessment questions are included at the end of the article.

The effectiveness of gas exchange during breathing is also reduced as a person ages. There is less alveolar membrane for gas exchange in older people, and many also have some degree of blood vessel thickening, which further impairs gas diffusion through capillaries. These conditions can cause carbon dioxide retention, increasing the concentration of hydrogen ions.

Because renal function diminishes with age, elderly people are less able to excrete hydrogen ions or synthesize bicarbonate ions. The renal system may be able to

Chapter 19

INTERVENTIONS FOR CLIENTS WITH ACID-BASE IMBALANCE

Acid-base balance, or hydrogen ion concentration as measured by pH, is the most carefully regulated body parameter. The normal pH range of body fluids is 7.35 to 7.45. Changes in the pH of blood indicate either problems with the body's acid-base regulatory mechanisms or exposure of the body to dangerous conditions. Severe impairment of normal physiology accompanies acid-base imbalances and can be life-threatening. Table 19–1 lists key points associated with acid-base imbalance.

ACIDOSIS

Overview

In acidosis, the acid-base balance of the blood and other extracellular fluid (ECF) is disturbed. Acidosis is characterized by an excess of hydrogen ions (H^+), or an arterial blood pH below 7.35. The concentration or strength, or both, of acid components is greater than normal compared with the concentration or strength of the base components.

Acidosis is not a disease but rather a condition caused by a disease or pathologic process. Acidosis can be caused by metabolic problems, respiratory problems, or both.

Pathophysiology

Acidosis can result from an actual or relative increase in the concentration or strength of acid components. In an actual acid excess, acidosis results from processes that cause either an overproduction of acids (and release of hydrogen ions) or an underelimination of normally produced acids (retention of hydrogen ions).

In *relative* acidosis, the actual amount or strength of acid components does not increase. Instead, the concentration or strength (or both) of the base components decreases (to create a *base deficit*), which makes the fluid relatively more acidic than basic. A relative acid-excess acidosis (or *actual base deficit*) results from processes that cause either an overelimination (usually in the form of bicarbonate ions [HCO_3^-]) or an underproduction of base components (Fig. 19–1).

Regardless of its origin, acidosis causes major changes in physiologic function. Its primary pathologic effects are related to the fact that hydrogen ions are cations (positively charged electrolytes). An increase in hydrogen ion concentration creates imbalances of other electrolytes, especially potassium, the principal cation in intracellular fluid, which then disrupts functions of excitable membranes, such as nerve and cardiac tissue. Many of the early signs and symptoms associated with acidosis thus appear in the neuromuscular, cardiac, respiratory, and central nervous systems (Metheny, 1996). Even slight increases in hydrogen ion concentration cause many body hormones and enzymes, as well as medications, to become inactive and may lead to death.

TABLE 19–1

Key Points Related to Acid-Base Imbalances

- Acidemia is defined as an increase in the hydrogen ion concentration (pH) of the blood, and is reflected by an arterial blood pH below 7.35.
- Acidemia can result from an actual acid excess or a relative base deficit.
- Metabolic acidosis usually results from a lack of bicarbonate or an excess acid production in the body.
- Respiratory acidosis results from retention of carbon dioxide in the body, causing increased carbonic acid production.
- Manifestations of acidemia are related to fluid and electrolyte imbalances that accompany acid-base imbalance, such as hyperkalemia.
- Chronic respiratory acidosis is common in the medical-surgical setting as a result of chronic obstructive pulmonary disease, such as emphysema.
- Alkalemia is defined as a decrease in the hydrogen ion concentration of the blood, reflected by an arterial blood pH above 7.45.
- Alkalemia can result from an actual base excess or an acid deficit.
- Metabolic alkalosis most often occurs when body acids are lost, such as in prolonged vomiting or nasogastric suctioning.
- Respiratory alkalosis most often occurs when hyperventilation causes excessive carbon dioxide loss.
- Dehydration and hypokalemia are associated with metabolic alkalosis, and account for most of the clinical manifestations seen in this acid-base imbalance.
- The goal of management for any type of acid-base imbalance is to restore fluid, electrolyte, and acid-base balance to normal or near normal.

Etiology

Acidosis can be caused by metabolic disturbances, respiratory disturbances, or combined metabolic and respiratory disturbances. The causes of metabolic and respiratory acidosis are summarized in Table 19–2.

Metabolic Acidosis

Four processes can result in metabolic acidosis: overproduction of hydrogen ions, underelimination of hydrogen ions, underproduction of bicarbonate ions, and overelimination of bicarbonate ions.

OVERPRODUCTION OF HYDROGEN IONS. Three metabolic processes that can increase body fluid hydrogen

AAABBB	AAAABBB	AAABB
AAABBB	AAAABBB	AAABB
AAABBB	AAAABBB	AAABB
Acid-base balance	Actual acidosis (acid excess)	Relative acidosis (base deficit)

Figure 19–1. Concepts of actual and relative acidosis. (A = acid; B = base.)

TABLE 19–2

Common Causes of Acidosis

Pathology	Condition
Metabolic Acidosis	
Overproduction of Hydrogen Ions	• Excessive oxidation of fatty acids • Diabetic ketoacidosis • Starvation • Hypermetabolism • Heavy exercise • Seizure activity • Fever • Hypoxia, ischemia • Excessive ingestion of acids • Ethanol intoxication • Methanol ingestion • Salicylate intoxication
Underelimination of Hydrogen Ions	• Renal failure
Underproduction of Bicarbonate	• Renal failure • Pancreatitis • Liver failure • Dehydration
Overelimination of Bicarbonate	• Diarrhea • Buffering of organic acids
Respiratory Acidosis	
Underelimination of Hydrogen Ions	• Respiratory depression • Anesthetics • Drugs (especially opioids) • Poisons • Electrolyte imbalance • Trauma Cerebral edema Spinal cord injuries • Neuritic diseases Guillain-Barré Polio Myasthenia gravis • Inadequate chest expansion • Skeletal deformities • Muscle weakness • Nonpulmonary restriction Obesity Fluid Tumor • Airway obstruction • Asthma • Cancer • Bronchiolitis • Alveolar-capillary block • Thrombus or embolus • Vascular occlusive disease • Pneumonia • Pulmonary edema • Tuberculosis • Cystic fibrosis • Atelectasis • Adult respiratory distress syndrome (ARDS) • Emphysema • Cancer

ion concentration are excessive breakdown of fatty acids, hypermetabolism (anaerobic lactic acidosis), and excessive ingestion of acidic substances.

Excessive Breakdown of Fatty Acids. Excessive breakdown of fatty acids is usually a result of diabetic ketoacidosis or starvation. When glucose is not readily available for metabolic fuel, the body metabolizes fats (lipids) instead. The metabolites from fatty acid breakdown form strong acids called *ketoacids,* which release large amounts of hydrogen ions.

Hypermetabolism (Anaerobic Lactic Acidosis). When cells are forced to use glucose without adequate oxygen (anaerobic metabolism), glucose is incompletely metabolized and forms lactic acid. Lactic acid molecules leave the cell, enter the extracellular fluid (ECF), and release hydrogen ions, causing acidosis. Anaerobic metabolism that results in lactic acidosis occurs whenever the body has insufficient oxygen. Some conditions leading to lactic acidosis include strenuous exercise, seizure activity, fever, and presence of tissue hypoxia.

Excessive Intake of Acidic Substances. Excessive ingestion of acidic substances floods the body directly with hydrogen ions. Some of the most common substances that cause acidosis when ingested in excess include ethyl (for drinking) alcohol, methyl alcohol (a poison), and acetylsalicylic acid (aspirin).

UNDERELIMINATION OF HYDROGEN IONS. The major routes for hydrogen ion elimination are respiratory (via the lungs) and renal (via the kidneys). Renal failure causes acidosis when the renal tubules cannot secrete hydrogen ions into the urine. As a result, too many hydrogen ions are retained.

UNDERPRODUCTION OF BICARBONATE IONS. As discussed in Chapter 18, bicarbonate is the most common base in the fluid outside the cells and is responsible for buffering carbonic acid (H_2CO_3). When body fluid levels of bicarbonate are too low, a base-deficit state exists. Base-deficit acidosis occurs when hydrogen ion production and elimination are normal, but too few molecules of bicarbonate ions are present to balance the hydrogen ions. Such base deficits occur when bicarbonate ions are not produced at the normal rate. Because bicarbonate is made in the kidney tubules and in the pancreas, renal failure and diminished hepatic or pancreatic function can result in a base-deficit acidosis (Guyton & Hall, 1996).

OVERELIMINATION OF BICARBONATE IONS. Base-deficit acidosis can also occur when hydrogen ion production and elimination are normal but too many bicarbonate ions have been eliminated (overelimination). The most common example of overelimination is diarrhea.

Respiratory Acidosis

Respiratory acidosis results from an impairment in any area of respiratory function, causing an inadequate exchange of oxygen (O_2) and carbon dioxide (CO_2). This impairment causes carbon dioxide retention. Because any increase in carbon dioxide concentration causes a corresponding increase in hydrogen ion concentration, carbon dioxide retention leads to acidosis, as demonstrated in the carbonic anhydrase equation:

$$CO_2 + H_2O \longleftrightarrow H_2CO_3 \longleftrightarrow H^+ + HCO_3^-$$

An excess of carbon dioxide forces the equation to the right, first increasing the production of carbonic acid. The carbonic acid then rapidly dissociates (separates) into hydrogen ions and bicarbonate ions. This increase in the free hydrogen ion concentration of the blood is acidosis.

Unlike metabolic acidosis, respiratory acidosis results from only one primary mechanism: retention of carbon dioxide, causing an underelimination of hydrogen ions. Virtually all causes of respiratory acidosis result in an acid-excess acidosis. Four types of respiratory problems can cause respiratory acidosis: respiratory depression, inadequate chest expansion, airway obstruction, and interference with alveolar-capillary diffusion.

RESPIRATORY DEPRESSION. Respiratory depression involves a change in the function of brain stem neurons stimulating inhalation and exhalation. The overall result is a reduced rate and depth of respiration, causing inadequate gas exchange and a retention of carbon dioxide. Respiratory depression may be chemical or physical in origin.

Chemical Depression. Chemical depression of respiratory neurons in the brain can result from the action of anesthetic agents, drugs (especially opioids), and poisons that cross the blood-brain barrier. Specific electrolyte imbalances (see Chapter 16 for hyponatremia, hypercalcemia, and hyperkalemia) also slow or inhibit respiratory neurons.

Physical Depression. Physical depression of respiratory neurons can occur in response to many conditions. Respiratory neurons can be damaged or destroyed by trauma or when problems in other areas of the brain cause an increase in intracranial pressure. Such an increase causes edema of brain tissues, which then presses into the respiratory centers located in the brain stem. Conditions causing cerebral edema with resultant respiratory depression include brain tumors, cerebral aneurysm, cerebrovascular accidents, overhydration, and hyponatremia.

INADEQUATE CHEST EXPANSION. Any condition that restricts or limits chest expansion can result in inadequate gas exchange. Inadequate chest expansion can result from skeletal trauma or deformities, respiratory muscle weakness, or non–respiratory-associated movement restrictions.

Skeletal Problems. Respiratory movement of the chest wall will be restricted if broken or malformed bones distort the shape of the chest. Broken ribs restrict chest movement because they cannot provide the rigid structure needed for thoracic pressure changes (as in flail chest).

Pain from broken ribs may also cause voluntary restriction of chest movement.

Respiratory Muscle Weakness. Conditions causing respiratory muscle weakness that can make chest expansion inadequate include electrolyte imbalances (especially hyperkalemia and hyponatremia), fatigue, muscular dystrophy, rhabdomyosarcoma, and inflammatory myositis.

Nonrespiratory Conditions. Nonrespiratory conditions also can restrict the chest movement necessary for full lung expansion. Causes of restricted chest movement include body cast enclosure of the thoracic cavity, tight scar tissue formation around the chest, severe obesity, abdominal masses, ascites, and hemothorax (blood in the thoracic cavity).

AIRWAY OBSTRUCTION. Prevention of air movement in and out of the lungs through airway obstruction can lead to ineffective gas exchange, carbon dioxide retention, and acidosis. The upper airway can be obstructed externally by restrictive clothing, neck edema, and regional lymph node enlargement. Internal obstruction of the upper airway can be caused by aspiration of foreign objects, constriction of bronchial smooth muscles, and edema. Internal obstruction of the lower airways is caused by constriction of smooth muscle, edema, and excessive mucus, which occurs in asthma, bronchiolitis, and emphysema.

INTERFERENCE WITH ALVEOLAR-CAPILLARY DIFFUSION. Most pulmonary gas exchanges occur by diffusion where the alveolar membrane and the capillary membranes meet. Any condition that prevents or slows this diffusion process can cause retention of carbon dioxide and acidosis. Conditions or disease that can prevent alveolar-capillary diffusion include pneumonia, pulmonary edema, aspiration of fluids, pneumonitis, tuberculosis, emphysema, adult respiratory distress syndrome, chest trauma, pulmonary emboli, and pulmonary edema.

Combined Metabolic and Respiratory Acidosis

Metabolic and respiratory acidosis can occur simultaneously. Uncorrected acute respiratory acidosis always leads to anaerobic (lacking molecular oxygen) metabolism and lactic acidosis (Metheny, 1996). The resulting acidosis is more profound than that caused by either metabolic acidosis or respiratory acidosis alone. Cardiac arrest is an example of a condition leading to combined metabolic and respiratory acidosis. Another example is the development of severe diarrhea in a client with chronic obstructive lung disease.

Incidence/Prevalence

Because acidosis is a manifestation of many pathologic conditions rather than a separate disease state, its actual incidence is not known. Mild metabolic acidosis resulting from lactic acidosis is common even among healthy people, however. Normal respiratory compensation usually prevents this acidosis from becoming severe or prolonged, and no intervention is necessary. Clients at particular risk

---

Chart 19–1

Nursing Focus on the Elderly: The Elderly Client Experiencing Acid-Base Imbalance

When Taking a Client's History

- Assess risk factors for acid-base imbalance, including medications, chronic health problems (especially renal disease, pulmonary disease), and acute health problems.
- Take the history when the client is awake and more familiar with surroundings.
- Ask the client to list all prescribed and over-the-counter medications (especially diuretics and antacids). If the client cannot recall this information or seems confused, ask the significant other to bring medications from home to show the nurse.
- Ask the client to recall what liquids she or he has taken in the past 24 hours and whether the client has urinated as much as usual.

When Assessing the Client

- Compare the client's mental status with what the family, significant other, or health record states is the client's baseline.
- Observe the rate and depth of respiration.
  - Can the client complete a sentence without stopping to take a breath?
  - Examine the color of the client's nail beds and mucous membranes.
- Obtain a specimen of urine and observe for color and character. Test for specific gravity and pH.
- Examine skin turgor for dehydration. Attempt to pinch the skin up to form a tent over the sternum and on the forehead. If a tent forms, record how long it remains.
- Measure the rate and quality of the pulse.

Observe the client's clinical responses and laboratory values carefully while the acid-base imbalance is being corrected.
Administer intravenous therapy by pump or controller.

---

for acidosis are those with conditions that impair any aspect of respiratory function to any degree, as in the elderly (see Chart 19–1).

Collaborative Management

 Assessment

➤ *History*

When obtaining a history from any client, the nurse collects data related to risk factors as well as causative factors related to the development of acidosis, specifically age, nutrition, and presenting symptoms.

Age. The elderly are more vulnerable to conditions that may cause an acid-base imbalance. Such conditions include impairments of cardiac, renal, and pulmonary functions. In addition, elderly persons are more likely to be taking prescribed or over-the-counter medications that interfere with acid-base, fluid, and electrolyte balance, especially diuretics, aspirin, and products containing alcohol. The nurse asks about specific risk factors, such as any type of respiratory problem, renal failure, diabetes mellitus, diarrhea, pancreatitis, and fever.

Nutrition. The nurse obtains a detailed diet history to determine total caloric intake as well as approximate proportions of carbohydrates, fats, and proteins ingested. The nurse specifically asks the client whether he or she has fasted or followed a strict diet during the preceding week.

Symptoms. Because the client's central nervous system is frequently depressed in acidosis, the nurse may question a close family member or the client's significant other. The nurse asks the client whether he or she has experienced headaches, behavior changes, increased drowsiness, reduced alertness, reduced attention span, lethargy, anorexia, abdominal distention, nausea or vomiting, muscle weakness, or increased fatigue. Having the client relate activities of the previous 24 hours may disclose additional information about activity intolerance, changes in behavior, and unexplained fatigue.

➤ *Physical Assessment/Clinical Manifestations*

The key clinical manifestations of acidosis are similar whether the cause is metabolic or respiratory (Chart 19–2). Clinical manifestations are associated primarily with changes in activity of excitable membranes involved in cerebral, neuromuscular, and gastric smooth muscle functions.

Central Nervous System Manifestations. Depression of central nervous system function is common in acidosis

---

Chart 19–2

Key Features of Acidosis

Central Nervous System Manifestations
• Depressed activity (lethargy, confusion, stupor, and coma)

Neuromuscular Manifestations
• Hyporeflexia
• Skeletal muscle weakness
• Flaccid paralysis

Cardiovascular Manifestations
• Delayed electrical conduction
  • Bradycardia to block
  • Tall T waves
  • Widened QRS complex
  • Prolonged PR interval
• Hypotension
• Thready peripheral pulses

Respiratory Manifestations
• Kussmaul respirations (in metabolic acidosis with respiratory compensation)
• Variable respirations (generally ineffective in respiratory acidosis)

Integumentary Manifestations
• Warm, flushed, dry skin in metabolic acidosis
• Pale to cyanotic and dry skin in respiratory acidosis

---

and may be manifested as lethargy that progresses to confusion, especially in elderly clients. As acidosis worsens or if it is accompanied by hyperkalemia, the client may become stuporous and unresponsive. The nurse assesses the client's level of consciousness (see Chap. 43).

Neuromuscular Manifestations. An increase in serum hydrogen ion concentration, along with any accompanying hyperkalemia, causes a decrease in muscle tone and deep tendon reflexes. The nurse assesses muscle strength by having the client

• Squeeze the nurse's hand
• Attempt to keep arms flexed while the nurse pulls downward on the lower arms
• Push both feet against a flat surface while the nurse applies resistance

Muscle weakness associated with acidosis is bilateral and can progress to flaccid paralysis. Respiratory efforts are reduced when skeletal muscles become weak.

Cardiovascular Manifestations. Early cardiac manifestations of acidosis include increased heart rate and cardiac output. As acidosis worsens or if it is accompanied by hyperkalemia, electrical conduction through the myocardium is reduced and the heart rate decreases. The nurse monitors for clinical as well as electrocardiographic changes. Peripheral pulses may be hard to find and are easily blocked with light pressure. The client may experience hypotension as a result of vasodilation.

Respiratory Manifestations. The nurse assesses the client's respiratory system by observing the rate, depth, and ease of respirations. Pulse oximetry is performed to determine the effectiveness of oxygen delivery to peripheral tissues. Some agencies are using protective shields for pulse oximetry sensors, reducing costs by allowing the sensors to be reused. This manipulation of the sensor does not appear to alter its accuracy (see Research Applications for Nursing).

Metabolic Causes. If acidosis is metabolic in origin, the rate and depth of respiration increase in proportion to the increase in the hydrogen ion concentration. Respirations are deep, rapid, and not under voluntary control. This pattern is called *Kussmaul respiration.*

Respiratory Causes. If acidosis is respiratory in origin, the effectiveness of respiratory efforts is greatly reduced. Respirations are usually shallow and quite rapid.

Integumentary Manifestations. Respiration is unimpaired and respiratory rate increased in metabolic acidosis. The increased gas exchange, coupled with a vasodilation, makes the client's skin and mucous membranes warm, dry, and pink. Because respirations are ineffective in respiratory acidosis, skin and mucous membranes are pale to cyanotic.

➤ *Psychosocial Assessment*

It is vital that the nurse complete a psychosocial assessment, because behavioral changes resulting from central nervous system effects may be the first observable clinical manifestations of acidosis. The nurse observes and docu-

Research Applications for Nursing

Save Money on Pulse Oximetry Without Sacrificing Accuracy

Russell, G., & Graybeal, J. (1995). Accuracy of laminated disposable pulse-oximetry sensors. Respiratory Care, 40(7), 728–733.

The purpose of this study was to determine whether pulse-oximetry sensors protected with a disposable, plastic-laminated shield were as sensitive and accurate at measuring oxygen saturation (SPO_2) as unshielded sensors. Pulse-oximeter accuracy reported by the manufacturers is ± 2 percentage points for values in the 70 to 100% range and ± 3 percentage points for values below 70%. Five healthy adult male volunteers had arterial blood gases measured at the same time pulse oximetry was measured using both shielded and unshielded sensors. All subjects were subjected to hypoxemic episodes by exposure to a hypoxic gas mixture of 8 to 10% oxygen in balance with helium. A total of 20 hypoxemic episodes were measured. Desaturation was measured every 10 seconds during each hypoxemic episode for a total of 907 pulse oximetry pairs. For SPO_2 measurements above 70% saturation, both the shielded and unshielded sensors were within the manufacturer's reported accuracy. Response times to reductions in SPO_2 were also unaffected. Both shielded and unshielded sensors were less consistently accurate below 70% saturation.

Critique. The study was well controlled and answered the question with a high degree of confidence. These studies were performed over a relatively short period of time, however (each hypoxemic episode lasted only 10 minutes). No data are available to determine whether lamination affects sensor accuracy with multiple uses over a longer period (such as 24 hours).

Possible Nursing Implications. It may be possible to re-use disposable sensors labeled "single use only" without sacrificing accuracy. Cross-contamination is a danger in reusing any equipment, however. Until such reuse has been demonstrated to not increase the risk for cross-contamination and infection, use should be limited to high-volume areas with immunocompetent clients only.

ments the client's presenting behavior by description (objectively) rather than by interpretation (subjectively). For example, the nurse may state that "the client is unable to recognize close family members" rather than "the client is confused" or "the client spit out the oral medication" rather than "the client is uncooperative." The nurse questions family members and significant others further to determine whether the client's presenting behavior and mental status are typical.

➤ Laboratory Assessment

Arterial blood pH is the laboratory value used to confirm acidosis. When arterial blood pH is less than 7.35, acidosis is present. This test alone does not indicate the underlying pathologic condition or the origin of the acidosis, however. Because the clinical manifestations of metabolic acidosis and respiratory acidosis are similar but their effective treatments are different, it is critical that the nurse obtain and interpret additional laboratory data, such as arterial blood gas (ABG) values and measurements of certain serum electrolytes (Chart 19–3).

Metabolic Acidosis. Pure metabolic acidosis is indicated by a low pH, a low bicarbonate level, a normal partial pressure of arterial carbon dioxide ($PaCO_2$), and an elevated serum potassium level.

pH. The pH is low because buffering and respiratory compensation are not adequate to maintain the hydrogen ion concentration at a normal level.

Bicarbonate. Decreased bicarbonate level, coupled with the normal carbon dioxide level, indicates metabolic acidosis. The bicarbonate level is below normal for any one (or all) of the following reasons:
- Bicarbonate has been lost from the body, creating actual base-deficit acidosis.
- Bicarbonate has not been produced in sufficient quantities, creating actual base-deficit acidosis.
- Bicarbonate may be bound to other substances during the buffering of organic acid–stimulated acidosis.

Carbon Dioxide and Oxygen. The carbon dioxide level is normal or even slightly decreased because gas

---

Chart 19–3

Laboratory Profile: Acid-Base Imbalances

Imbalance	Laboratory Value Changes						
	pH	HCO_3^-	PaO_2	$PaCO_2$	K^+	Ca^{2+}	Cl^-
• Metabolic acidosis	↓	↓	Ø	Ø	↑	Ø	↑
• Respiratory acidosis	↓	↑	↓	↑	↑	Ø	↕
• Combined acidosis	↓	↑	↓	↑	↑	Ø	↕
• Metabolic alkalosis	↑	↑	Ø	↑	↓	↓	↓
• Respiratory alkalosis	↑	↓	Ø	↓	↓	↓	↑
• Combined alkalosis	↑	↑	Ø	↓	↓	↓	↓

↑ = above normal; ↓ = below normal; Ø = normal; HCO_3^- = bicarbonate ions; PaO_2 = partial pressure of arterial oxygen; $PaCO_2$ = partial pressure of arterial carbon dioxide; K^+ = potassium ions; Ca^{2+} = calcium ions; Cl^- = chloride ions.

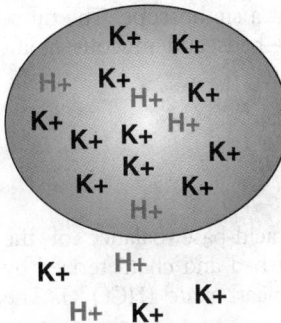

Under normal conditions, the intracellular potassium content is much greater than that of the extracellular fluid. The concentration of hydrogen ions is low in both compartments.

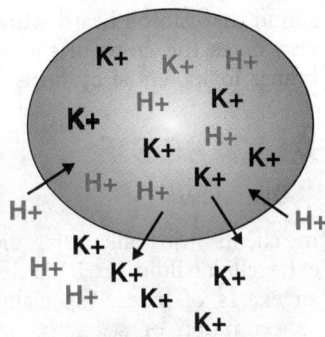

In acidemia, the extracellular hydrogen ion content increases, and the hydrogen ions move into the intracellular fluid. To keep the intracellular fluid electrically neutral, an equal number of potassium ions leave the cell, creating a relative hyperkalemia.

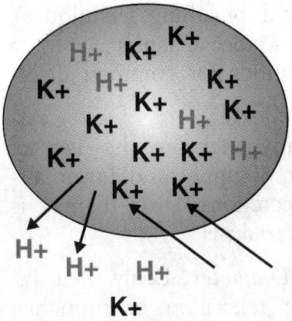

In alkalemia, more hydrogen ions are present in the intracellular fluid than in the extracellular fluid. Hydrogen ions move from the intracellular fluid into the extracellular fluid. To keep the intracellular fluid electrically neutral, potassium ions move from the extracellular fluid into the intracellular fluid, creating a relative hyperkalemia.

Figure 19–2. Movement of potassium in response to changes in the extracellular fluid hydrogen ion concentration. (© 1992 M. Linda Workman. All rights reserved.)

exchange is adequate and carbon dioxide retention is not a factor. The oxygen level is normal because gas exchange is adequate.

Potassium. The serum potassium level is frequently elevated in metabolic acidosis as a result of the body's attempt to maintain electroneutrality during buffering. In some cases, prolonged elevation of potassium in the blood may contribute to the development of metabolic acidosis.

Figure 19–2 demonstrates movement of potassium ions associated with changes in serum pH. As the hydrogen ion concentration of the blood increases, some of the excess hydrogen ions enter cells (especially red blood cells), the site of intracellular buffering mechanisms. The movement of hydrogen ions into the cells creates an intracellular excess of positive ions. To prevent intracellular charge imbalances, an equal number of potassium ions then move from the cells into the blood. This increases the extracellular potassium concentration, causing hyperkalemia.

Respiratory Acidosis. Low pH, elevated $PaCO_2$, and decreased partial pressure of arterial oxygen (PaO_2) indicate respiratory acidosis. Changes in bicarbonate and serum potassium levels vary with the duration of the acidosis and the degree of renal compensation (see Chap. 18).

pH. The increase in the ECF hydrogen ion concentration lowers pH. If the renal system partially compensates for this acidosis, then pH is low but not as abnormal as could be expected, considering the degree of derangement apparent in the retention of carbon dioxide.

Bicarbonate. Rapid onset of respiratory acidosis is characterized by a normal bicarbonate level. When respiratory acidosis persists for 24 hours or longer, renal compensation for the acidosis results in increased generation and reabsorption of bicarbonate. An elevated bicarbonate

level, coupled with increased $PaCO_2$, indicates chronic respiratory acidosis.

Carbon Dioxide and Oxygen. $PaCO_2$ is elevated and PaO_2 is decreased because the cause of this acid-base disturbance is impaired gas exchange. The impairment causes carbon dioxide retention, and the client cannot inhale adequate amounts of oxygen.

Potassium. Serum potassium levels are elevated in acute respiratory acidosis. Serum potassium levels are normal or low in chronic respiratory acidosis when renal compensation is present.

 Interventions

Interventions for acidosis focus on correcting the underlying problem and supporting aerobic metabolism. To ensure appropriate interventions, the specific type of acidosis must first be identified.

> ***Metabolic Acidosis***

Interventions for metabolic acidosis include hydration therapy and specific drugs or treatments to control or eliminate the condition causing the acidosis. For example, if the acidosis is a result of diabetic ketoacidosis, insulin is given to correct the hyperglycemia and production of ketone bodies. If the acidosis is a result of prolonged diarrhea, rehydration and antidiarrheal drugs are administered. Bicarbonate is administered only if serum bicarbonate levels are low.

> ***Respiratory Acidosis***

Interventions for respiratory acidosis aim at maintaining a patent airway and enhancing gas exchange. Such interventions can include drug therapy, oxygen therapy, pulmonary hygiene (positioning and breathing techniques), and prevention of complications. (See Chapter 32 for a complete discussion of interventions for common disorders causing respiratory acidosis.)

Drug Therapy. Drug therapy includes the use of agents to increase the diameter of upper and lower airways and to thin pulmonary secretions. Drug therapy is not aimed directly at altering arterial pH.

Drugs to Increase Airway Diameter. Drugs that increase airway diameter induce relaxation of bronchial smooth muscle. Many of these agents are adrenergic agonists, sympathomimetic agents, antimuscarinic drugs, and methylxanthines. These drugs include albuterol (Novo-Salmol✦, Proventil, Ventolin), ephedrine, fenoterol (Berotec), isoproterenol (Isuprel), metaproterenol (Alupent), pirbuterol (Maxair), terbutaline (Brethine, Bricanyl), ipratropium (Atrovent), atropine, aminophylline (Phyllocontin, Truphylline), and theophylline (Bronkodyl, Theo-Dur✦).

Clients may take agents that increase bronchodilation by reducing inflammation of bronchial luminal tissues. These agents are primarily cortisol (steroid) based, such as beclomethasone (Vanceril, Beclovent), dexamethasone (Decadron Respihaler, Dexasone✦), flunisolide (AeroBid, Bronalide✦), and triamcinolone (Azmacort).

Drugs to Thin Bronchial Secretions. Some drugs can break up mucus when thick, tenacious pulmonary secretions contribute to airway obstruction. These agents are classified as mucolytic; an example is acetylcysteine (Mucomyst, Mucosil). (For a discussion of drugs used for clients with chronic obstructive pulmonary disease or chronic airflow limitation [CAL], see Chapter 32.)

Oxygen Therapy. Oxygen therapy can help promote gas exchange for clients with respiratory acidosis. However, the nurse must use caution when administering oxygen to clients with CAL and carbon dioxide retention, as evidenced by a high $PaCO_2$ level in arterial blood. The only respiratory trigger for these clients is a decreased arterial oxygen level. Administration of too much oxygen to these clients decreases their respiratory efforts and increases carbon dioxide retention.

Pulmonary Hygiene. To promote effective gas exchange, the nurse considers client positioning, techniques to enhance excretion of pulmonary secretions, and specific breathing techniques to change airway resistance and maintain inflated alveoli. The nurse helps clients assume a Fowler's or semi-Fowler's position to help increase lung expansion. Increasing clients' fluid intake also may reduce the thickness of pulmonary secretions and assist in their excretion.

Prevention of Complications. Monitoring clients' respiratory status is critical in preventing pulmonary complications. At least every 2 hours, the nurse assesses the respiratory status of clients experiencing chronic respiratory acidosis. In addition to assessing the rate and depth of respiration, the nurse auscultates breath sounds. The nurse notes the ease with which air moves in and out of the lungs, including any muscle retractions, use of accessory muscles, and whether respiratory effort produces a

sound that can be heard without a stethoscope. The nurse also notes the color of the nail beds and mucous membranes for potential cyanosis.

ALKALOSIS

Overview

In clients with alkalosis, the acid-base balance of the extracellular fluid (ECF) is disturbed and characterized by an excess of bases, especially bicarbonate (HCO_3^-). The concentration or strength, or both, of the base components is greater than normal compared with the concentration or strength of acid components. Alkalosis is defined as a decrease in the hydrogen ion concentration of the blood, reflected by an arterial blood pH above 7.45. Like acidosis, alkalosis is not a disease but rather a manifestation of a disease or pathologic process. Alkalosis can be caused by metabolic problems, respiratory problems, or both.

Pathophysiology

Alkalosis can result from an actual or relative increase in the concentration or strength, or both, of base components. In an actual base excess, alkalosis is the result of processes that cause either an overproduction of base components or an underelimination of normally produced base components (usually bicarbonate).

In *relative* alkalosis, the actual amount or strength of base components does not increase. Instead, the concentration or strength (or both) of the acid components decreases (creating an *acid deficit*), which makes the fluid relatively more basic than acidic. A relative base-excess alkalosis (or *actual acid deficit*) results from processes that cause either an overelimination or an underproduction of acid components (Fig. 19–3).

Alkalosis can cause serious and life-threatening disturbances in metabolism and in pulmonary respiration. Because alkalosis is the manifestation of another abnormal process (or processes), treatment is most effective when directed at the underlying abnormal processes. Treatment that is effective for metabolic alkalosis is different from treatment that is effective for respiratory alkalosis. Therefore, one must be able to distinguish between metabolic and respiratory alkalosis to prevent and manage this condition.

Whether its origin is metabolic, respiratory, or both, alkalosis greatly affects specific physiologic functions. Its pathologic effects are related to the accompanying electrolyte imbalances that occur in response to decreased blood cation concentration. The most common manifestations of

AAABBB	AAABBBB	AABBB
AAABBB	AAABBBB	AABBB
AAABBB	AAABBBB	AABBB
Acid-base balance	Actual alkalosis (base excess)	Relative alkalosis (acid deficit)

Figure 19–3. Concepts of actual and relative alkalosis. (A = acid; B = base.)

alkalosis are associated with increased stimulation of the central nervous, neuromuscular, and cardiovascular systems.

Etiology

Alkalosis can be caused by metabolic disturbances, respiratory disturbances, or combined metabolic and respiratory disturbances. The causes of alkalosis are listed in Table 19–3.

Metabolic Alkalosis

Most conditions that result in metabolic alkalosis create the acid-base disturbance through either of two mechanisms: an actual increase of base components or an actual decrease of acid components.

INCREASE IN BASE COMPONENTS. Increases in base components (base excesses) occur as a result of oral or parenteral ingestion of bicarbonates, carbonates, acetates, citrates, and lactates. Excessive use of oral antacids

TABLE 19–3

Common Causes of Alkalosis	
Pathology	**Condition**
Metabolic Alkalosis	

Increase of base components	• Oral ingestion of bases
	  • Antacids
	  • Milk-alkali syndrome
	• Parenteral base administration
	  • Blood transfusion
	  • Sodium bicarbonate
	  • Total parenteral nutrition

Decrease of acid components	• Prolonged vomiting • Nasogastric suctioning • Cushing's syndrome (hypercortisolism) • Hyperaldosteronism • Thiazide diuretics
Respiratory Alkalosis	

Excessive loss of carbon dioxide	• Hyperventilation
	  • Fear
	  • Anxiety
	  • Mechanical ventilation
	  • Central nervous system stimulation
	    • Salicylates
	    • Catecholamines
	    • Progesterone
	• Hypoxemia
	  • Asphyxiation
	  • High altitudes
	  • Shock
	  • Early-stage pulmonary problems
	    • Pneumonia
	    • Asthma
	    • Pulmonary emboli

containing sodium bicarbonate or calcium carbonate can also cause a metabolic alkalosis. Other base excesses can occur as a result of medical treatments, such as citrate excesses during rapid or massive blood transfusions, acetate and lactate excesses during hyperalimentation, and intravenous sodium bicarbonate administration to correct lactic acidosis or ketoacidosis.

DECREASE IN ACID COMPONENTS. Decreases in acid components (acid deficit) can occur in response to disease processes or medical treatment. Contributing conditions include prolonged vomiting, Cushing's syndrome (hypercortisolism), and hyperaldosteronism. Medical treatments that promote acid loss and can cause metabolic alkalosis include the use of thiazide diuretics and prolonged nasogastric suctioning.

Respiratory Alkalosis

The primary mechanism responsible for respiratory alkalosis is the excessive loss of carbon dioxide through hyperventilation (rapid respirations). Clients may hyperventilate in response to anxiety, fear, or improper settings on mechanical ventilators. Hyperventilation can also result from direct stimulation of central respiratory centers. Conditions that directly stimulate these centers include fever, respiratory compensation for metabolic acidosis, central nervous system lesions, and certain drugs (e.g., salicylates, catecholamines, and progesterone).

Collaborative Management

 Assessment

➤ *Physical Assessment/Clinical Manifestations*

Clinical manifestations of alkalosis are consistent whether metabolic or respiratory in origin. Many symptoms are the result of the hypocalcemia (low calcium levels) and hypokalemia (low potassium levels) that usually accompany alkalosis. These key manifestations are associated with changes in central nervous system, neuromuscular, and cardiovascular functions (Chart 19–4).

Central Nervous System Manifestations. Overexcitement of the central and peripheral nervous systems is the major cause of symptoms associated with alkalosis. Clients experience lightheadedness, agitation, confusion, and hyperreflexia, which may progress to seizure activity. Paresthesias may be present as tingling or numbness around the mouth and in the toes. Other reliable indicators of alkalosis with accompanying hypocalcemia are positive Chvostek's and Trousseau's signs (see Chap. 16).

Neuromuscular Manifestations. Alkalosis with hypocalcemia or hypokalemia increases nervous system activity. This nerve stimulation, in turn, causes nonvoluntary skeletal muscle contractions manifested as cramps, twitches, and charley horses. Deep tendon reflexes are hyperactive. *Tetany* (continuous spasms) of isolated muscle groups also may be present. Tetany is painful and indicates a rapidly worsening condition.

Although skeletal muscles may contract as a result of

Key Features of Alkalosis

Central Nervous System Manifestations
- Increased activity
- Anxiety, irritability, tetany, seizures
- Positive Chvostek's sign
- Positive Trousseau's sign
- Paresthesias

Neuromuscular Manifestations
- Hyperreflexia
- Muscle cramping and twitching
- Skeletal muscle weakness

Cardiovascular Manifestations
- Increased heart rate
- Normal or low blood pressure
- Increased digitalis toxicity

Respiratory Manifestations
- Increased rate and depth of ventilation in respiratory alkalosis
- Decreased respiratory effort associated with skeletal muscle weakness in metabolic alkalosis

nerve overstimulation, the skeletal muscles themselves become weaker because of the alkalosis and hypokalemia. Handgrip strength diminishes, and the client may be unable to walk or support his or her own weight. Respiratory efforts also become less effective as the skeletal muscles of respiration weaken.

Cardiovascular Manifestations. Alkalosis causes increased irritability of the myocardium, especially when accompanied by hypokalemia. The heart rate increases, and the pulse is thready. When hypovolemia (decreased blood volume) is also present, the client may experience profound hypotension. Alkalosis also increases myocardial sensitivity to digitalis derivatives, resulting in increased risk for digitalis toxicity.

Respiratory Manifestations. Alterations in the rate and depth of respiration are the underlying causes of respiratory alkalosis. Tidal volume (the volume of air inhaled and exhaled with each breath) is nearly normal, but minute respiratory volume (the total volume of air inhaled and exhaled in 1 minute) rises in proportion to the increase in respiratory rate. The increase in minute respiratory volume may result from other physiologic changes or from anxiety.

➤ Laboratory Assessment

As in acidosis, arterial blood pH confirms alkalosis. When arterial blood pH is above 7.45, alkalosis is present. This test alone does not identify the underlying pathologic condition or the origin of the alkalosis, however. Because the clinical manifestations of metabolic alkalosis are similar to those of respiratory alkalosis, it is critical that the nurse obtain additional laboratory data, especially arterial

blood gas (ABG) values and specific serum electrolytes levels (see Chart 19-3).

Metabolic Alkalosis. Metabolic alkalosis is indicated by
- High pH (>7.45)
- Elevated bicarbonate level (>28 mEq/L)
- Normal PaO_2
- Rising $PaCO_2$
- Decreased serum potassium levels
- Decreased serum calcium levels

The pH is high because buffering and respiratory compensation are not adequate to maintain the hydrogen ion concentration at a normal level.

The increased bicarbonate level, coupled with a rising $PaCO_2$, is the hallmark of metabolic alkalosis. The rising $PaCO_2$ compensates for the decreased hydrogen ion concentration. The serum potassium level decreases as the body attempts to maintain electroneutrality (see Fig. 19-2). As the pH increases, calcium binding increases and the serum calcium concentration decreases, creating an accompanying state of hypocalcemia. Most of the serious clinical manifestations of alkalosis are attributed to this accompanying hypocalcemia.

Respiratory Alkalosis. Arterial blood data that demonstrate respiratory alkalosis are
- High pH
- Low bicarbonate level
- Low $PaCO_2$
- Low serum potassium level
- Low serum calcium level

The pH is high because buffering and renal compensation cannot maintain the hydrogen ion concentration at a normal level.

The classic respiratory alkalosis profile is a reduced bicarbonate level (not usually <15 mEq/L) coupled with a very low $PaCO_2$. The carbon dioxide level is so low because it is being exhaled through hyperventilation more rapidly than it is being produced. The bicarbonate level is reduced in response to the pH increase. Various blood and intracellular buffers generate hydrogen ions, which immediately combine with the serum bicarbonate ions and form carbonic acid, thus reducing the serum concentration of bicarbonate.

As in metabolic alkalosis, the serum potassium level is reduced as the body attempts to maintain electroneutrality. Again, as the pH increases, calcium binding increases and the concentration of serum calcium decreases, resulting in hypocalcemia.

 Interventions

Interventions aim to prevent further losses of hydrogen, potassium, calcium, and chloride ions and to restore fluid balance.

Drug therapy is the intervention of choice for alkalosis. Drugs are prescribed to resolve the underlying causes of alkalosis and to restore normal fluid, electrolyte, and acid-base balance. For example, the client with metabolic alkalosis caused by diuretic therapy receives fluid and electrolyte replacement and is then re-evaluated by the physician for the need to resume a diuretic. The physician may prescribe a potassium-sparing diuretic to prevent potassium loss. The physician orders antiemetic medications to halt vomiting in the client experiencing emesis. Fluids and electrolytes are replaced orally or parenterally. The nurse carefully monitors the client's progress and titrates fluid and electrolyte therapy. Serum electrolyte values are monitored daily until they return to normal or near normal.

SELECTED BIBLIOGRAPHY

Ahern, J. (1995). A guide to blood gases. *Nursing Standard, 10*(49), 50–52.

Anderson, S. (1996). Fluid and electrolyte disorders in the elderly. In J. Kokko & R. Tannen (Eds.), *Fluids and electrolytes* (3rd ed., pp. 831–839). Philadelphia: W. B. Saunders.

Cornock, M. (1996). Making sense of arterial blood gases and their interpretation. *Nursing Times, 92*(6), 30–31.

Guyton, A. C., & Hall, J. (1996). *Textbook of medical physiology* (9th ed.). Philadelphia: W. B. Saunders.

Halperin, M., & Goldstein, M. (1994), *Fluid, electrolyte and acid-base physiology: A problem-based approach* (2nd ed.). Philadelphia: W. B. Saunders.

Kelly, M. (1996). Acute respiratory failure. *American Journal of Nursing, 96*(12), 46.

Kokko, J., & Tannen, R. (1996). *Fluids and electrolytes* (3rd ed.). Philadelphia: W. B. Saunders.

Mays, D. (1995). Turn ABGs into child's play. *RN, 58*(1), 36–40.

Metheny, N. (1996). *Fluid and electrolyte balance: Nursing considerations* (3rd ed.). Philadelphia: J. B. Lippincott.

Molony, D., Schiess, M., & Dosekum, A. (1996). Respiratory acid-base disorders. In J. Kokko & R. Tannen (Eds.), *Fluids and electrolytes* (3rd ed., pp. 267–342). Philadelphia: W. B. Saunders.

O'Donnell, J. (1995). Can you prevent respiratory depression? *Nursing95, 25*(4), 32JJ.

Russell, G., & Graybeal, J. (1995). Accuracy of laminated disposable pulse-oximetry sensors. *Respiratory Care, 40*(7), 728–733.

Schwartz-Goldstein, B., Malik, A., Sarwar, A., & Brandstetter, R. (1996). Lactic acidosis associated with a deceptively normal anion gap. *Heart & Lung, 25*(1), 79–80.

Sica, D. (1994). Renal disease, electrolyte abnormalities, and acid-base imbalance in the elderly. *Clinics in Geriatric Medicine, 10*(1), 197–211.

Tasota, F., & Wesmiller, S. (1994). Assessing A.B.G.s: Maintaining the delicate balance. *Nursing94, 24*(5), 34–46.

Tietz, N. W. (Ed.). (1995). *Clinical guide to laboratory tests* (3rd ed.). Philadelphia: W. B. Saunders.

Toto, R., & Alpern, R. (1996). Metabolic acid-base disorders. In J. Kokko & R. Tannen (Eds.), *Fluids and electrolytes* (3rd ed., pp. 201–266). Philadelphia: W. B. Saunders.

White, V. (1997). Hyperkalemia. *American Journal of Nursing, 97*(6), 35.

SUGGESTED READINGS

Kelly, M. (1996). Acute respiratory failure. *American Journal of Nursing, 96*(12), 46.

This brief but informative article uses a case presentation approach to help readers identify the key indicators of acute respiratory failure. The pathophysiology is explained in understandable terms, and the reader directed toward appropriate interventions.

O'Donnell, J. (1995). Can you prevent respiratory depression? *Nursing95, 25*(4), 32JJ.

This brief article can assist the nurse in preventing respiratory depression when administering opioids and benzodiazepines, two classes of agents commonly implicated in causing respiratory depression among clients in acute care settings. Assessment and intervention tips are presented in a logical, easy-to-remember format.

Sica, D. (1994). Renal disease, electrolyte abnormalities, and acid-base imbalance in the elderly. *Clinics in Geriatric Medicine, 10*(1), 197–211.

This comprehensive article includes a detailed section on acid-base abnormalities commonly seen among elderly clients. Although written for a medical audience, the article is clear and concise and outlines realistic therapy and medical interventions.

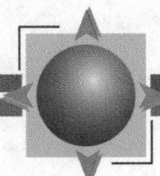

Management of

Perioperative Clients

Chapter 20

INTERVENTIONS FOR PREOPERATIVE CLIENTS

With cost reduction as a driving force over the past decade, new or re-engineered policies and procedures have changed the way a surgical client is handled by the health care community. Outpatient surgical services have expanded, more clients are being admitted as inpatients *after* a procedure (rather than before), and the length of hospital stay after a procedure has been shortened. Perioperative, or surgical, nursing focuses on client care before (preoperative), during (intraoperative), and after (postoperative) surgery, regardless of setting.

Overview

The preoperative period begins when the client is scheduled for surgery and ends at the time of transfer to the surgical suite. The nurse acts as an educator, an advocate, and a promoter of health. Perioperative nursing places special emphasis on safety.

After a thorough assessment, the nurse develops an individualized teaching care plan to help the client and family through the surgical experience. Preoperative care mainly consists of education to reduce anxiety and postoperative complications and to promote cooperation in postoperative procedures. In preoperative teaching, the nurse uses adult teaching and learning principles and

validates and clarifies information that the physician has provided.

Categories and Purposes of Surgery

The nurse understands the terminology for surgical procedures to provide the client and family members with comprehensive information. Procedures are usually categorized according to

- The reason for the surgery
- The urgency of the procedure
- The degree of risk
- The anatomic location
- The extent of surgery required

The primary purposes, or reasons, for surgery can be divided into five general subcategories: diagnostic, curative, restorative, palliative, and cosmetic. Palliative surgery makes the client more comfortable, and cosmetic surgery reconstructs the skin and underlying structures. The urgency of the procedure can be divided into three subcategories: elective, urgent, and emergent. The degree of risk is classified as minor or major. Classification by location

TABLE 20–1

Selected Categories of Surgical Procedures

Category	Description	Condition or Surgical Procedure
Reasons for Surgery		
Diagnostic	• Performed to determine the origin and cause of a disorder or the cell type for cancer	• Breast biopsy • Exploratory laparotomy
Curative	• Performed to resolve a health problem by repairing or removing the cause	• Cholelithiasis • Mastectomy • Hysterectomy
Restorative	• Performed to improve a client's functional ability	• Total knee replacement • Finger reimplantation
Palliative	• Performed to relieve symptoms of a disease process, but does not cure	• Colostomy • Nerve root resection • Tumor debulking • Ileostomy
Cosmetic	• Performed primarily to alter or enhance personal appearance	• Liposuction • Revision of scars • Rhinoplasty • Blepharoplasty
Urgency of Surgery		
Elective	• Planned for correction of a nonacute problem	• Cataract removal • Hernia repair • Hemorrhoidectomy • Total joint replacement
Urgent	• Requires prompt intervention; or may be life-threatening if treatment delayed more than 24–48 hr	• Intestinal obstruction • Bladder obstruction • Kidney or ureteral stones • Bone fracture • Eye injury • Acute cholecystitis
Emergent	• Requires immediate intervention because of life-threatening consequences	• Gunshot or stab wound • Severe bleeding • Abdominal aortic aneurysm • Compound fracture • Appendectomy
Degree of Risk of Surgery		
Minor	• Procedure without significant risk, often done with local anesthesia	• Incision and drainage (I&D) • Implantation of a venous access device (VAD) • Muscle biopsy
Major	• Procedure of greater risk, usually longer and more extensive than a minor procedure	• Mitral valve replacement • Pancreas transplant • Lymph node dissection
Extent of Surgery		
Simple	• Only the most overtly affected areas involved in the surgery	• Simple/partial mastectomy
Radical	• Extensive surgery beyond the area obviously involved; is directed at finding a root cause	• Radical prostatectomy • Radical hysterectomy

is based on the area of the body on which surgery occurs: for example, abdominal surgery, intracranial surgery, and heart surgery. The extent can be simple, modified, or radical. Table 20–1 explains the categories and gives examples of surgical procedures.

Surgical Settings

The term *inpatient* refers to a client who is admitted to a hospital. The client may be admitted the day before or the day of surgery (often termed same-day admission

[SDA]) or may already be an inpatient when the need for surgical intervention is identified. In contrast, the term *outpatient* refers to a client who goes to the surgical area the day of the surgery and returns home on the same day (i.e., same-day surgery [SDS]). Hospital-based ambulatory surgical centers, freestanding surgical centers, physicians' offices, and ambulatory care centers are becoming increasingly more common.

One of the many advantages of outpatient surgery is that clients are not separated from the comfort and security of their home and family. With continuous improvements in surgical techniques and anesthesia, more procedures are being safely performed on an outpatient basis. However, changes in the surgical experience present particular challenges for the client without an adequate or available support system. An elderly spouse may be unable to assist in the preoperative and postoperative care of the client. A client who is primarily responsible for others may be unable to perform his or her usual tasks within the family. Clients may try to continue their family role but jeopardize their own health by doing so. As a result, the client's stress, fears, and anxieties about the surgical experience and about returning home immediately after surgery may be increased.

Collaborative Management

 Assessment

➤ History

Collection of data about the client before surgery begins in various settings (e.g., the surgeon's office, the preadmission or admission office, the inpatient unit, and over the telephone). The nurse provides privacy to increase the client's comfort with the interview process. Anesthesia and surgery are both physical and emotional stressors for the client. The nurse collects the following data:

- Age
- Tobacco, alcohol, and illicit substance use, including marijuana
- Current medications
- Medical history
- Prior surgical procedures and experiences
- Prior experience with anesthesia
- Autologous or directed blood donations
- Allergies
- General health
- Family history
- Type of surgery planned
- Knowledge and understanding about events during the perioperative period
- Support system adequacy and availability

When taking a history, the nurse screens the preoperative client for risks that may contribute to complications during the perioperative period. Some conditions that could either increase the surgical risk or increase the possibility of postoperative complications are outlined in Table 20–2.

Age. Elderly clients are at increased risk. The normal aging process decreases immune system functioning and delays wound healing. Frequency of chronic illness increases in elderly clients. See Chart 20-1 for other physiologic changes in elderly clients.

Medication and Substance Use. The use of tobacco products increases the risk of pulmonary complications because of changes they cause to the lungs and thoracic cavity. Excessive alcohol and illicit substance use can alter the effects of anesthesia and response to pain medication. Withdrawal of alcohol in preparation for surgery may precipitate delirium tremens. Prescription and over-the-

TABLE 20–2

Selected Factors That Increase Surgical Risk or Increase the Risk of Postoperative Complications

Age
- Older than 65 yr

Medications
- Antihypertensives
- Tricyclic antidepressants
- Anticoagulants
- Nonsteroidal anti-inflammatory drugs (NSAIDs)

Medical History
- Decreased immunity
- Diabetes
- Pulmonary disease
- Cardiac disease
- Hemodynamic instability
- Multisystem disease
- Coagulation defect or disorder
- Anemia
- Dehydration
- Infection
- Hypertension
- Hypotension
- Any chronic disease

Prior Surgical Experiences
- Less-than-optimal emotional reaction
- Anesthesia reactions or complications
- Postoperative complications

Health History
- Malnutrition or obesity
- Medication, tobacco, alcohol, or illicit substance use or abuse
- Altered coping ability

Family History
- Malignant hyperthermia
- Cancer
- Bleeding disorder

Type of Surgical Procedure Planned
- Neck, oral, or facial procedures (airway complications)
- Chest or high abdominal procedures (pulmonary complications)
- Abdominal surgery (paralytic ileus, deep vein thrombosis)

Chart 20–1

Nursing Focus on the Elderly

Changes of Aging as Surgical Risk Factors

Physiologic Change	Nursing Interventions	Rationale
Cardiovascular system Decreased cardiac output Increased blood pressure Decreased peripheral circulation	• Determine normal activity levels and note when the client tires. • Monitor vital signs, peripheral pulses, and capillary refill.	• Knowing limits helps prevent fatigue. • Having baseline data helps detect deviations.
Respiratory system Reduced vital capacity Loss of lung elasticity Decreased oxygenation of blood	• Teach coughing and deep breathing exercises. • Monitor respirations and breathing effort.	• Pulmonary exercises help prevent pulmonary complications. • Having baseline data helps detect deviations.
Renal/urinary system Decreased blood flow to kidneys Reduced ability to excrete waste products Decline in glomerular filtration rate Nocturia common	• Monitor intake and output. • Assess overall hydration. • Monitor electrolyte status. • Assist frequently with toileting needs, especially at night.	• Ongoing assessment helps detect fluid and electrolyte imbalances and decreased renal function. • Frequent toileting helps prevent incontinence and falls.
Neurologic system Sensory deficits Slower reaction time Decreased ability to adjust to changes in the surroundings	• Orient the client to the surroundings. • Allow extra time for teaching the client. • Provide for the client's safety.	• An individualized preoperative teaching plan is developed on the basis of the client's orientation and any neurologic deficits. • Safety measures help prevent falls and injury.
Musculoskeletal system Increased incidence of deformities related to osteoporosis or arthritis	• Assess the client's mobility. • Teach turning and positioning. • Encourage ambulation. • Place on fall precautions, if indicated.	• Interventions help prevent complications of immobility. • Safety measures help prevent injury.

---

counter medications may also affect how the client reacts to the perioperative experience. The potential effects of specific medications are noted in Table 20–3.

Medical History. The nurse asks the client about his or her medical history. The presence of certain chronic illnesses increases perioperative risks and is considered when planning care. For example, a client with systemic lupus erythematosus may need additional medication to offset the physical and emotional stress of the surgery. A diabetic client may need a more extensive preoperative bowel preparation because of decreased gastrointestinal motility. An infection may need to be treated before surgery.

Prior Cardiac History. The nurse obtains a history of cardiac disease because complications from anesthesia could occur in clients with cardiac problems. Cardiac disorders that increase risks associated with surgery include coronary artery disease, angina pectoris, myocardial infarction (MI) within 6 months before surgery, congestive heart failure, hypertension, and dysrhythmias. These disorders impair the client's ability to withstand and re-

spond to both anesthesia and the hemodynamic changes during surgery. The risk of intraoperative MI is also higher in clients with pre-existing heart problems.

Pulmonary History. Adults with chronic respiratory problems, elderly people, and smokers are at risk for pulmonary complications because of physiologic pulmonary changes. Increased rigidity of the thoracic cavity and loss of lung elasticity reduce the efficiency of anesthesia excretion. Smoking increases the level of circulating carboxyhemoglobin (carbon monoxide in the oxygen-binding sites of the hemoglobin molecule), which in turn decreases oxygen delivery to organs. Concurrently, mucociliary transport decreases, which leads to increased secretions and predisposes the client to infection (pneumonia) and atelectasis (collapse of alveoli). Atelectasis prevents the exchange of oxygen and carbon dioxide and causes intolerance of anesthesia. Chronic conditions such as asthma, emphysema, and chronic bronchitis also reduce the elasticity of the lungs, which causes an ineffective exchange of carbon dioxide and oxygen. As a result, clients with these conditions have decreased oxygen diffusion and decreased oxygenation of the tissues.

TABLE 20–3

Effects of Routine Medications Taken Preoperatively

Drug	Implications for the Perioperative Experience	Nursing Interventions	Rationale
Antiarrhythmics Quinidine gluconate (Quinate✦, Quinaglute Dura-Tabs) Procainamide hydrochloride (Pronestyl, Procan-SR)	• Antiarrhythmic medications affect the client's tolerance of anesthesia and potentiate anesthetics that are neuromuscular blockers. • Antiarrhythmics depress cardiac function by decreasing cardiac output and slowing the pulse rate. • Antiarrhythmics may cause peripheral vasodilation.	• Communicate the use and type of antiarrhythmics to the anesthesia personnel. • Monitor vital signs. • Obtain a baseline electrocardiogram, as ordered. • Assess the client's peripheral circulation.	• Cardiac complications during surgery can be life-threatening. • Ongoing monitoring helps to detect deviations and potential complications.
Antihypertensives Methyldopa (Aldomet, Novomedopa✦) Captopril (Capoten) Clonidine hydrochloride (Catapres)	• Antihypertensive agents alter the client's response to muscle relaxants and opioid analgesics by inhibiting synthesis and storage of norepinephrine. • Antihypertensives may cause a hypotensive crisis intraoperatively and postoperatively.	• Monitor blood pressure and pulse frequently. • Assess for hypotension during transfer and turning.	• Ongoing monitoring helps to detect deviations and potential complications. • Hypotensive crisis can occur and may be prevented through timely assessments.
Corticosteroids Dexamethasone (Decadron, Dexasone✦) Hydrocortisone sodium (Solu-Cortef) Prednisone (Deltasone, Winpred✦)	• Surgery increases the demand for corticosteroids in the client with no adrenal function. • Steroids delay wound healing because of blockage of collagen formation. • Steroids increase the serum glucose level and block fibroblast formation. • Steroids increase the risk of hemorrhage. • Steroids mask the signs and symptoms of infection.	• Continue steroid therapy during surgery. • Monitor vital signs. • Assess for signs of hyperglycemia. • Assess for subtle signs of infection and bleeding. • Monitor wound healing, support the incision area with binders, and splint the wound when the client is turning, coughing, and deep breathing.	• Continuation of steroid therapy avoids problems associated with abrupt withdrawal. • Ongoing monitoring helps to detect deviations and potential complications. • It is important to detect early signs and symptoms of infection. • Specific wound and incision care helps to prevent complications.
Anticoagulants Warfarin sodium (Coumadin, Warfilone sodium✦) Heparin sodium (Lipo-Hepin, Hepalean✦) Aspirin (acetylsalicylic acid, Ancasal✦, Astin✦, Coryphen✦)	• Anticoagulant therapy increases the risk of hemorrhage intraoperatively and postoperatively.	• Monitor coagulation studies (APTT, PT). • Monitor for signs of bleeding. • Gradually discontinue anticoagulants 24–48 hr before surgery, as ordered. • Have an antidote (protamine sulfate for heparin and vitamin K [Mephyton] for warfarin sodium) available to reverse the effects of the anticoagulant.	• Coagulation studies help detect bleeding disorders. • Anticoagulant administration is discontinued to avoid hemorrhage. • An antidote needs to be available to prevent complications of bleeding in an emergency situation.

Previous Surgery and Anesthesia. The number and type of previous surgeries and previous surgical experiences affect the preoperative client's readiness for surgery. Previous perioperative complications may contribute to the client's fears and concerns about the scheduled surgery. The nurse asks about the client's experience with anesthetic agents and all allergies. These data provide the nurse with information about tolerance of and possible fears about the use of anesthesia. The client's sensitivity or allergy to certain substances alerts the nurse to a possi-

TABLE 20-3

Effects of Routine Medications Taken Preoperatively *Continued*

Drug	Implications for the Perioperative Experience	Nursing Interventions	Rationale
Antiseizure Medications			
Phenobarbital (Luminal✤, Gardenal✤)	• Seizure activity can cause injury to the surgical wound. • Antiseizure medications alter the metabolism of anesthetic agents.	• Maintain use of the drug. • Inform the anesthesiologist or anesthetist to allow for adjustment of the dosage of the anesthetic. • Assess for seizure activity. • Pad the side rails of the bed. • Place suction equipment at the bedside.	• Antiseizure medications prevent seizures. • Safety measures prevent injury.
Glaucoma Medications			
Demecarium bromide (Humorsol) Echothiophate (Phospholine iodide) Pilocarpine hydrochloride (Isopto-Carpine, Pilocar, Miocarpine✤) Timolol maleate (Timoptic)	• Glaucoma medications have cumulative systemic effects and can cause respiratory and cardiovascular collapse, especially during surgery.	• Consult the physician about stopping Humorsol at least 2 weeks before surgery. • Monitor respiratory status and cardiac output. • Assess for increased intraocular pressure.	• Collaboration with the physician helps prevent complications. • Ongoing monitoring helps to detect complications.
Antidiabetic Agent			
Insulin	• Insulin needs decrease preoperatively when the client is on NPO status. • Postoperative insulin demands increase because of IV administration of dextrose. • Insulin levels may fluctuate during healing because of dietary and activity restrictions and the physical stress of surgery.	• Monitor serum glucose levels. • Administer antibiotics and other intermittent medications in normal saline instead of dextrose when possible, as ordered, or as per facility policy.	• Monitoring will detect an increased or a decreased need for insulin. • The use of normal saline prevents complications.

ble reaction to anesthetic agents or to substances that are used for preoperative skin preparation. For example, povidone-iodine used for skin preparation contains some of the same components found in shellfish. The family medical history and problems with anesthetics may indicate possible intraoperative needs and reactions to anesthesia, such as malignant hyperthermia.

Autologous or Directed Blood Donations. Clients may donate their own blood (autologous donations) in the few weeks immediately before the scheduled surgery date. If clients then need blood because of their surgery, an autologous blood transfusion can be given. This practice eliminates the possibility of transfusion reactions and the transmission of disease.

Clients may be candidates for autologous blood donations up to 5 weeks preoperatively if they are afebrile, have a hemoglobin level greater than 11 g/dL (110 g/L), and have a physician's recommendation. The physician usually orders supplemental iron beginning before the first donation. Autologous donations can be made as fre-

quently as every 3 days if the other criteria can be met. Usually, a total of 2 to 4 units is donated. The last donation cannot be less than 72 hours before surgery.

A special tag is affixed to the transfusion bag when an autologous blood donation has been made. The blood donor center gives the client a matching tag that he or she brings to the surgical area preoperatively. This procedure helps to ensure that the client receives only his or her own blood. If the client does not use the blood, the blood goes to the blood bank to be used as would any other unit of donated blood.

Clients may wish to have family and friends donate blood exclusively for their use, if needed. This practice of *directed* blood donation is possible only if the blood types are compatible and the donor's blood is acceptable. Clients may fear disease transmission from unknown blood and feel more comfortable knowing who gave the blood. Some blood collection centers and other health care personnel are discouraging the practice, stating that it gives the client a false sense of security. As with autologous blood donations, a special tag is affixed to the blood. This tag notes the names of the client and the donor and has the client's signature.

The nurse asks whether autologous or directed blood donations have been made and documents this information in the chart. It may be important to know the specific blood collection center and whether the blood has arrived before the client goes into surgery.

Planning for Bloodless Surgery. Growth in bloodless surgery programs is helping to provide another alternative for clients with religious or medical contradications to blood transfusions. These programs reduce or eliminate the need for transfusion during and after surgery. Some techniques employed include limiting preoperative blood samples (the number of samples as well as the volume of blood drawn per sample) and stimulating the client's own red cell production with epoetin alfa (EPO) before, during, and after surgery. The physician may prescribe supplemental iron, folic acid, vitamin B_{12}, and vitamin C preoperatively to further stimulate erythropoiesis. Special equipment and techniques used during the surgical procedure allows less blood loss than usually expected. The nurse assesses, monitors, teaches, and supports the client during the bloodless surgery process (Vernon & Pfeifer, 1997).

Discharge Planning. The nurse also assesses the client's home environment, self-care capabilities, and support systems. The nurse anticipates the client's postoperative needs during the preoperative period. All clients should have discharge planning. Elderly people and dependent adults may need referrals for transportation to and from the physician's office. They may need a home care nurse to monitor their postoperative recovery and to provide instruction on wound care. All clients with inadequate support systems may need follow-up care at home.

➤ *Physical Assessment/Clinical Manifestations*

The preoperative client may be of any age, with a health status that varies from well to debilitated. The nurse performs a complete preoperative physical assessment to obtain baseline data. During physical assessment, the nurse also identifies current health problems, potential complications related to the administration of anesthesia, and potential postoperative complications.

When beginning the assessment, the nurse obtains a complete set of vital signs. The nurse may need to obtain vital signs several times for accurate baseline values. Abnormal vital signs may cause the postponement of surgery until the underlying problem is treated and the client's condition is stable. The nurse also assesses for anxiety, which could increase the client's blood pressure, pulse, and respiratory rate, and documents this in the client's chart as part of the overall assessment.

Throughout the physical assessment, the nurse focuses on problem areas identified from the client's history and on all body systems affected directly or indirectly by the surgical procedure. The elderly (Chart 20–2; see also Chapter 6) or chronically ill client is at increased risk for intraoperative and postoperative complications. Perioperative morbidity and mortality are higher in elderly and chronically ill clients owing to their preoperative physical condition.

The nurse reports any abnormalities found on physical assessment to the physician and anesthesiology personnel. In this manner, the nurse functions as a proactive client advocate and is exercising his or her legal responsibility.

Cardiovascular System. Alterations in cardiac status are responsible for as many as 30% of perioperative deaths. The nurse evaluates the client for hypertension, which is common, often undiagnosed, and can affect surgery. Cardiovascular assessment also includes auscultation of heart sounds for rate, regularity, and abnormalities. The nurse evaluates the client's extremities for temperature, color, peripheral pulses, capillary refill, and edema. Any physical alterations, such as absent peripheral pulses and pitting edema, or cardiac symptoms, such as chest pain, shortness of breath, and dyspnea, are reported to the physician for further assessment and evaluation. (Chapter 35 further discusses cardiovascular assessment.)

Respiratory System. In assessing the client's respiratory status, the nurse considers the client's age and history of smoking and the presence of chronic illness. The nurse observes the client's posture; respiratory rate, rhythm, and depth; overall respiratory effort; and lung expansion. Clubbing of the fingertips (swelling at the base of the nailbeds caused by a chronic lack of oxygen) or any cyanosis is noted. The nurse auscultates the lungs to determine the quality and presence of any adventitious (crackles, wheezes, rubs) or abnormal breath sounds. (More information is found in Chapter 29.)

Renal/Urinary System. Renal and urinary function affects the filtration and eventual excretion of waste products. If renal and urinary function is not optimal, fluid and electrolyte balance can be altered, especially in the elderly client. The nurse asks the client about the presence or absence of symptoms such as urinary frequency, dysuria (painful urination), nocturia (awakening during nighttime sleep because of a need to void), difficulty

---

Chart 20–2

Nursing Focus on the Elderly

Specific Considerations When Planning Care for the Elderly Preoperative Client

- Greater incidence of chronic illness
- Greater incidence of malnutrition
- More allergies
- Increased incidence of impaired self-care abilities
- Inadequate support systems
- Decreased ability to withstand the stress of surgery and anesthesia
- Increased risk of postoperative cardiopulmonary complications
- Risk of a change in mental status when admitted (related to unfamiliar surroundings, change in routine, medications administered, and so forth)
- Increased risk of a fall and resultant injury

starting urine flow, and oliguria (scant amount of urine). The nurse also asks about the appearance and odor of the urine. Equally important is an assessment of the client's usual fluid intake and degree of continence. If the client is suspected of having underlying renal or urinary problems, the nurse consults with the physician about further client work-up. (Chapter 72 further discusses renal/urinary assessment.)

Abnormal renal function can decrease the excretion rate of preoperative medications and anesthetic agents. As a result, the drug's effectiveness may be altered. Scopolamine (Buscospan❋), morphine, meperidine (Demerol), and barbiturates frequently cause confusion, disorientation, apprehension, and restlessness when administered to clients with decreased renal function.

Neurologic System. The nurse assesses the client's overall mental status, including level of consciousness, orientation, and ability to follow commands, before planning preoperative teaching and postoperative care. A deficit in any of these areas affects the type of care required during the perioperative experience. The nurse determines the client's baseline neurologic status to be able to identify changes that may occur later. The nurse also assesses for any motor or sensory deficits. (See Chapter 43 for complete nervous system assessment.)

The usual neurologic status of a mentally impaired or elderly client may be difficult to assess. The client who has been independent and oriented while in the home environment may become disoriented in an unfamiliar hospital setting. Family members and significant others can often provide information about what the client was like at home.

Often, as part of the neurologic assessment, the nurse assesses the client's risk of falling, especially for elderly clients. Factors such as mental status, muscle strength, steadiness of gait, and sense of independence are evaluated to determine the client's risk. The client's ability to ambulate and his or her steadiness of gait are noted preoperatively as baseline data.

Musculoskeletal System. Deformities of the musculoskeletal system may interfere with intraoperative and postoperative positioning of the client. For example, clients with arthritis may be able to assume conventional intraoperative positions but then have unnecessary discomfort postoperatively from prolonged immobilization of joints. Other anatomic characteristics, such as the shape and length of the client's neck and the shape of the thoracic cavity, may interfere with respiratory and cardiac function and positioning during surgery.

The nurse asks about a history of joint replacements. During surgery, the nurse ensures that electrocautery pads, which could cause an electrical burn, are not placed near the area of the prosthesis.

Nutritional Status. Malnutrition and obesity can increase surgical risks. Surgery usually increases the body's metabolic rate and consequently depletes potassium, ascorbic acid, and B vitamins, all of which are needed for wound healing and fibrin formation. In malnourished clients, hypoproteinemia retards postoperative recovery.

Negative nitrogen balance may result from depleted protein stores. This situation increases the risk of perioperative morbidity and mortality from delayed wound healing, possible dehiscence or evisceration (see Chap. 22), fluid volume deficit, and sepsis.

Some elderly clients are susceptible to nutritional imbalances because of chronic illness, diuretic or laxative use, poor dietary planning or habits, anorexia, lack of motivation, and financial limitations. Clinical indications of alterations in the fluid and nutritional status of the client preoperatively include brittle nails, muscle wasting, dry or flaky skin, hair alterations (e.g., dull, sparse, dry), decreased skin turgor, orthostatic (postural) hypotension, decreased serum albumin levels, and abnormal serum electrolyte values.

The obese client is often malnourished because of poor eating habits and an imbalanced diet and has an increased chance of poor or incomplete wound healing because of excessive adipose tissue. Fatty tissue lacks nutrients, is not as vascular, and has little collagen, and nutrients, vascularity, and collagen are important for wound healing. Obesity causes increased stress on the heart and reduces the available lung volumes, which can affect the client's intraoperative experience and postoperative recovery.

➤ Psychosocial Assessment

The nurse performs a psychosocial assessment and preparation of the client to determine the client's level of anxiety, coping ability, and support systems; provide information; and offer support.

A client scheduled for surgery experiences some preoperative anxiety and fear. The extent and type of these reactions vary for each client according to the kind of surgery, the perceived effects of the surgery and its potential outcome, and the client's basic personality. Surgery may be seen as a threat to the client's biological integrity, body image, self-esteem, self-concept, or lifestyle. Clients may fear death, pain, helplessness, decreased socioeconomic status, a diagnosis of life-threatening conditions, possible disabling or crippling effects, and the unknown.

The client's anxiety and fear affect his or her ability to learn, cope, and cooperate with preoperative teaching and perioperative procedures. Anxiety and fear may also influence the amount and type of anesthesia needed and may retard postoperative recovery. The nurse is aware of potential fears and anxieties when interviewing the client and planning preoperative teaching.

The nurse assesses coping mechanisms used by the client under similar situations or in the past when the client had been confronted with a stressful situation. The nurse asks open-ended questions pertaining to the client's feelings about the entire perioperative experience. The nurse assesses factors that influence coping, including age, previous surgical and sick-role experiences, emotional and physical signs of fear, anxiety, and discomfort. Signs of fear and anxiety include anger, crying, restlessness, diaphoresis (sweating, usually profusely), increased pulse rate, palpitations, sleeplessness, diarrhea, and urinary frequency. (For more information on stress and coping, see Chapter 8.)

➤ Laboratory Assessment

Preoperative laboratory tests provide baseline data about the client's health and help predict potential complications. The client scheduled for surgery in a surgical center or admitted to the hospital on the morning of or day before surgery may have preadmission testing performed 48 hours to 21 days before the scheduled surgery, depending on the facility's policy. The results of prior tests are usually valid unless there has been a change in the client's condition that warrants repeated testing. Depending on the test or tests needed, the hospitalized client has testing done under similar time guidelines.

The choice of routine preoperative laboratory tests varies among facilities and depends on the client's age and medical history and type of anesthesia planned. The most common tests are

- Urinalysis
- Blood type and cross-match
- Complete blood count or hemoglobin level and hematocrit
- Coagulation studies (prothrombin time [PT], activated partial thromboplastin time [APTT], and platelet count)
- Electrolyte levels
- Serum creatinine

Depending on a female client's age, a pregnancy test may also be ordered.

A preoperative urinalysis is performed to assess for the presence of protein, glucose, blood, and bacteria, all of which are abnormal constituents of the urine. If renal disease is suspected or the client is elderly, the physician may order other tests to determine the type and degree of disease present.

The nurse reports electrolyte imbalances or other abnormal results to the surgeon before surgery. Hypokalemia (decreased serum potassium level) increases the risk of digitalis toxicity (if the client is receiving a digitalis preparation), slows recovery from anesthesia, and increases cardiac irritability. Hyperkalemia (increased serum potassium level) increases the risk of cardiac dysrhythmias, especially with the use of anesthesia. Both hypokalemia and hyperkalemia should be treated before the surgery.

The physician may order other studies, depending on the client's medical history. For example, baseline arterial blood gas (ABG) values are assessed before surgery for clients with chronic pulmonary problems. Chart 20–3 presents abnormal laboratory findings and their possible causes.

➤ Radiographic Assessment

A chest radiograph, when ordered by the physician or anesthesiologist, is commonly obtained to determine size and contour of the heart, lungs, and major vessels and to determine the presence of any infiltrates that could indicate pneumonia or tuberculosis. A chest radiograph also provides baseline data in the event of postoperative complications. Abnormal radiograph results alert the physician to potential cardiac or pulmonary complications. The presence of congestive heart failure, cardiomyopathy, pneumonia, or infiltrates may cause cancellation or delay of elective surgery. For emergency surgery, radiograph results assist the anesthesiologist in the selection of anesthesia. In many facilities, chest radiograph results are valid when done within 6 months before surgery, provided that there has not been a change in the client's condition.

Other radiographic studies are based on individual client need, medical history, and nature of the surgical procedure. For example, a client with back pain may have computed tomography (CT) or magnetic resonance imaging (MRI) done before a laminectomy to identify the exact location of the abnormality.

➤ Other Diagnostic Assessment

An electrocardiogram (ECG) may routinely be required for all clients older than a specific age who are to have general anesthesia. The age varies among facilities but is often 40–45 years. An ECG may also be ordered for clients with a history of cardiac disease or those at risk for cardiovascular complications. An ECG provides baseline information on new or pre-existing cardiac conditions, such as an old anterior wall myocardial infarction. A client with a known cardiac condition may require a preoperative consultation with a cardiologist. Prophylactic medication, such as nitroglycerin and antibiotics, may be needed during the perioperative period to reduce or prevent stress on the cardiovascular system. Abnormal or potentially life-threatening ECG results may cause the cancellation of surgery until the client's cardiac status is stable.

A focused assessment of the preoperative client is shown in Chart 20–4.

 Analysis

➤ Common Nursing Diagnoses

Two nursing diagnoses are common to the preoperative client:
1. Knowledge Deficit related to a lack of education and lack of exposure to the specific perioperative experience
2. Anxiety related to the threat of a change in health status or fear of the unknown

➤ Additional Nursing Diagnoses

In addition to the common diagnoses, other nursing diagnoses may apply:
- Sleep Pattern Disturbance related to internal sensory alterations (e.g., illness and anxiety)
- Ineffective Individual Coping related to the impending surgery
- Anticipatory Grieving related to the effects of surgery
- Body Image Disturbance related to anticipated changes in the body's appearance or function
- Ineffective Family Coping: Compromised related to temporary family disorganization and role changes
- Powerlessness related to the health care environment, loss of independence, and loss of control of one's body
- Altered Family Processes related to situational crisis

Chart 20–3

Laboratory Profile

Perioperative Assessment

Test	Normal Range for Adults	Significance of Abnormal Findings	
		Increased in	**Decreased in**
Potassium (K⁺) level	• 3.5–4.5 mEq/L, or 3.5–4.5 mmol/L	• Dehydration • Renal failure • Acidosis • Cellular/tissue damage • Hemolysis of the specimen	• NPO states when K⁺ replacement is inadequate • Excessive use of non–K⁺-sparing diuretics • Vomiting • Malnutrition • Diarrhea • Alkalosis
Sodium (Na⁺)	• Up to 90 yo: 136–145 mEq/L, or 136–145 mmol/L • >90 yo: 132–146 mEq/L, or 132–146 mmol/L	• Cardiac or renal failure • Hypertension • Excessive amounts of IV fluids containing normal saline • Edema • Dehydration (hemoconcentration)	• Nasogastric drainage • Vomiting or diarrhea • Excessive use of laxatives or diuretics • Excessive amounts of IV fluids containing water • Syndrome of inappropriate antidiuretic hormone secretion (SIADH)
Chloride (Cl⁻)	• Up to 90 yo: 98–107 mEq/L, or 98–107 mmol/L • >90 yo: 98–111 m Eq/L, or 98–111 mmol/L	• Respiratory alkalosis • Dehydration • Renal failure • Excessive amounts of IV fluids containing sodium chloride (NaCl)	• Excessive nasogastric drainage • Vomiting • Excessive use of diuretics • Diarrhea
Carbon dioxide (CO₂)	• Up to 60 yo: 23–29 mEq/L, or 23–29 mmol/L • 60–90 yo: 23–31 mEq/L, or 23–31 mmol/L • >90 yo: 20–29 mEq/L, or 20–29 mmol/L	• Chronic pulmonary disease • Intestinal obstruction • Vomiting or nasogastric suctioning • Metabolic alkalosis	• Hyperventilation • Diabetic ketoacidosis • Diarrhea • Lactic acidosis • Renal failure • Salicylate toxicity
Glucose (fasting)	• Up to 60 yo: 74–106 mg/dL, or 4.1–5.9 mmol/L • 60–90 yo: 82–115 mg/dL, or 4.6–6.4 mmol/L • >90 yo: 75–121 mg/dL, or 4.2–6.7 mmol/L	• Hyperglycemia • Excess amounts of IV fluids containing glucose • Stress • Steroid use • Pancreatic or hepatic disease	• Hypoglycemia • Excess insulin

Creatinine	• Females:
	  • Up to 60 yo: 0.6–1.1 mg/dL, or 53–97 μmol/L
	  • 60–90 yo: 0.6–1.2 mg/dL, or 53–106 μmol/L
	  • >90 yo: 0.6–1.3 mg/dL, or 53–115 μmol/L
	• Males:
	  • Up to 60 yo: 0.9–1.3 mg/dL, or 80–115 μmol/L
	  • 60–90 yo: 0.8–1.3 mg/dL, or 71–115 μmol/L
	  • >90 yo: 1.0–1.7 mg/dL, or 88–150 μmol/L
		• Renal damage with destruction of large number of nephrons
		• Renal insufficiency
		• Acute renal failure
		• Chronic renal failure
		• End-stage renal disease (ESRD)
			• Atrophy of muscle tissue

Continued

CHART 20-3. Laboratory Profile   Continued

Perioperative Assessment

Test	Normal Range for Adults	Significance of Abnormal Findings	
		Increased in	Decreased in
Blood urea nitrogen (BUN)	• Up to 60 yo: 6–20 mg/dL, or 2.1–7.1 mmol/L • 60–90 yo: 8–23 mg/dL, or 2.9–8.2 mmol/L • >90 yo: 10–31 mg/dL, or 3.6–11.1 mmol/L	• Dehydration • Renal failure • Excessive protein in diet • Liver failure	• Overhydration • Malnutrition
Prothrombin time (Pro Time, PT)	• 11–15 sec, 85%–100%, or 1–1.1 client/control ratio	• Coagulation defect (bleeding disorder) • Liver disease • Anticoagulant therapy (aspirin, warfarin)	• Coagulation (clotting) disorder such as thrombophlebitis or pulmonary embolus • Extensive cancer
Partial thromboplastin time, activated (APTT)	• Less than 35 sec	• Coagulation defect (bleeding disorder) • Anticoagulant therapy (heparin) • Liver disease	• Coagulation (clotting) disorder such as thrombophlebitis or pulmonary embolus • Extensive cancer
White blood cell (WBC) count (leukocyte count)	• Total: $4.5–11.0 \times 10^3$ cells/μL, or 7.4 IRU • African Americans: $3.6–10.2 \times 10^3$ cells/μL	• Infection • Inflammation • Stress • Tissue necrosis	• Immune disorder • Immunosuppressant therapy
Hemoglobin, total	• Females: • 18–44 yo: 11.7–15.5 g/dL, or 117–155 g/L • 45–64 yo: 11.7–16.0 g/dL, or 117–160 g/L • 65–74 yo: 11.7–16.1 g/dL, or 117–161 g/L • Males: • 18–44 yo: 13.2–17.3 g/dL, or 132–173 g/L • 45–64 yo: 13.1–17.2 g/dL, or 131–172 g/L • 65–74 yo: 12.6–17.4 g/dL, or 126–174 g/L	• Dehydration • Polycythemia • Chronic pulmonary disease • Congestive heart failure	• Blood loss • Anemia • Renal failure
Hematocrit	• Females: • 18–44 yo: 35%–45% • 45–74 yo: 35%–47% • Males: • 18–44 yo: 39%–49% • 45–64 yo: 39%–50% • 65–74 yo: 37%–51%	• Dehydration • Polycythemia • High altitude	• Blood loss • Anemia • Renal failure

IRU = international recommended unit; yo = years of age; NPO = nothing by mouth.

 Planning and Implementation

➤ *Knowledge Deficit*

Planning: Expected Outcomes. Two outcomes are that the client will
- Verbalize and comply with preoperative procedures
- Demonstrate techniques to prevent postoperative complications

Interventions. Because the perioperative experience is foreign to many people, the nurse focuses on preoperative education of the client and family members. Preoperative teaching typically begins in the surgeon's office for planned or elective surgery. Pamphlets and written instructions may be given and sent to the client as well. More teaching may occur when the client has preadmission testing. Some facilities conduct preoperative classes for groups of clients who are having the same or similar

Focused Assessment of the Preoperative Client

As part of the cardiopulmonary assessment, take and record vital signs; report the following:

- Hypotension or hypertension
- Heart rate of less than 60 or more than 120 beats/min
- Irregular heart rate
- Chest pain
- Shortness of breath or dyspnea
- Tachypnea
- Pulse oximetry reading of <94%

Assess for and report any signs or symptoms of infection, including

- Fever
- Purulent sputum
- Dysuria or cloudy, foul-smelling urine
- Any red, swollen, draining intravenous or wound site
- Increased white blood cell count

Assess for and report signs or symptoms that could contraindicate surgery, including

- Increased Pro Time or activated partial thromboplastin time
- Hypokalemia or hyperkalemia
- Client report of possible pregnancy or positive pregnancy test

Assess for and report other clinical conditions that may need to be evaluated by a physician or advanced nurse practitioner before proceeding with the surgical plans, including

- Change in mental status
- Vomiting
- Rash
- Recent administration of an anticoagulant medication

---

surgical procedures. A tour of the operating suite and the postanesthesia care unit (PACU) may be included.

Information about informed consent, dietary restrictions, preoperative preparation (bowel and skin preparations), and postoperative exercises and procedures promotes the client's participation in health care. A sample preoperative educational checklist is shown in Table 20–4. Because education of the client takes place in a variety of settings, coordination of client teaching efforts is particularly challenging. The nurse who cares for the client immediately before surgery (same-day, ambulatory surgery outpatient or inpatient hospital unit) assesses the client's knowledge and provides additional information as needed.

Ensuring Informed Consent. Surgery of any type involves invasion of the body and requires informed consent from the client or legal guardian (Fig. 20–1). Consent implies that one has been provided with information necessary to understand the following:

- The nature of and reason for surgery
- All available options and the risks associated with each option

- The risks of the surgical procedure and its potential outcomes
- The risks associated with the administration of anesthesia

Signed permission helps protect the client from any unwanted procedures and the physician and the facility from lawsuit claims related to unauthorized surgery or uninformed clients.

The physician is usually responsible for having the consent form signed before preoperative sedation is given and before surgery is performed. The nurse is not responsible for providing detailed information about the surgical procedure. Rather, the nurse clarifies facts that have been presented by the physician and dispels myths that the client and family may have about the perioperative experience. The nurse ensures that the consent form is signed and serves as a witness to the signature, not to the fact that the client is informed. The surgeon is contacted and requested to see the client for clarification of information if the nurse believes that the client has not been adequately informed. The nurse documents this action in the client's chart.

Clients who cannot write may sign with an **X**, which must be witnessed by two people. In an emergency, telephone or telegram authorization is acceptable and should be followed with written consent as soon as possible. The number of witnesses (usually two) and the type of documentation vary according to the facility's policy. In a life-threatening situation in which every effort has been made to contact the person with medical power of attorney, consent is desired but not essential. In lieu of written or oral consent, written consultation by at least two physicians who are not associated with the case may be requested by the physician. This formal consultation legally supports the decision for surgery until the appropriate person can sign a consent form. If the client is not capable of giving consent and has no family, the court can appoint a legal guardian to represent the client's best interests.

TABLE 20–4

Preoperative Teaching Checklist
Consider the following items when planning individualized preoperative teaching for clients and families:
Fears and anxieties
Surgical procedure
Preoperative routines (e.g., NPO, enemas, blood samples, showering)
Invasive procedures (e.g., lines, catheters)
Coughing, turning, deep breathing
Incentive spirometer
How to use
How to tell when used correctly
Lower extremity exercises
Stockings and pneumatic compression devices
Early ambulation
Splinting
Pain management

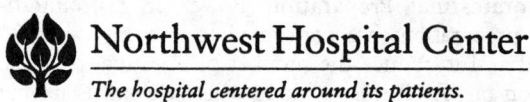

Northwest Hospital Center
The hospital centered around its patients.

**REQUEST AND AUTHORIZATION FOR
MEDICAL AND/OR SURGICAL TREATMENT,
BLOOD PRODUCTS ADMINISTRATION**

1. I hereby request and authorize Dr._____ and/or his/her associates and whomever they may designate as their assistants, to administer such treatment as is necessary and to perform the following operation_____
_____
and such additional operations or procedures as are considered necessary on the basis of conditions that may be revealed during the course of said operation or treatment.

2. The reasons why the above named surgery and/or treatment is considered necessary, its advantages, probability of success, possible complications, and risks, as well as possible alternative modes of treatment were explained to me by
Dr._____.

3. I request and authorize the administration of such anesthetics and/or other medications as are necessary.

4. Final disposition of any tissues or parts surgically removed is to be handled in accordance with the customary practices of the hospital.

5. I am aware that the practice of medicine and surgery is not an exact science and I acknowledge that no guarantees have been made to me concerning the results of the operation or procedure.

6. I hereby acknowledge that I have read and fully understand the above request and authorization for medical and/or surgical treatment.

7. I consent to the admittance of permitted observers, the use of closed-circuit television, taking of photographs (including motion pictures), and the preparation of drawings and similar illustrative material, and I also consent to the use of such photographs and other material for scientific purposes, provided my identity is not revealed by the pictures or by the descriptive text accompanying them.

8. I consent to release of my social security number in accordance with the Safe Medical Device Act.

_____ _____ _____
Date   Time   Signature of Patient or Patient Surrogate

_____ _____
Witness   Signature of Physician

CONSENT TO BLOOD/BLOOD PRODUCTS TRANSFUSION

After discussing the risks, benefits and alternatives to transfusion of blood (donor/autologous) (circle one or both) or blood products with my physician or his designee, I consent to the administration of these products.

_____ _____ _____
Date   Time   Signature of Patient or Patient Surrogate

_____ _____
Witness   Signature of Physician

703/1019-3-R-8/97   (40-1331)

Figure 20–1. A surgical consent form. (Courtesy of Northwest Hospital Center, Randallstown, MD.)

A blind client is capable of signing his or her own consent form, which usually needs to be witnessed by two people. Clients who speak a language other than the general language in the agency require a translator and a second witness. Some facilities have consent forms written in more than one language.

Some surgical procedures require a special permit in addition to the standard consent. National and local governing bodies and the individual surgical facility determine which procedures require a separate permit. Intraocular lens implants, sterilization, and experimental procedures are examples of procedures for which the extra form is usually required. Separate consents for anesthesia and the administration of blood products may be required as well.

Implementing Dietary Restrictions. Regardless of the type of surgery and anesthesia planned, the client is restricted to nothing by mouth (NPO) for 6 to 8 hours before surgery. *NPO* means no eating of food, drinking (including water), or smoking (nicotine stimulates gastric secretions). It is common practice to begin NPO status for all preoperative clients at midnight on the night before surgery. This extra precaution ensures that the stomach contains a limited volume of gastric secretions, which helps decrease the possibility of aspiration. Outpatients and clients who are scheduled for admission to the hospital on the same day that surgery is performed must receive written and oral instructions about remaining NPO after midnight. The nurse emphasizes the importance of compliance; failure to comply can result in cancellation of surgery or an increased risk of intraoperative or postoperative aspiration.

Administering Regularly Scheduled Medications. On the day of surgery, the client's usual medication schedule may need to be altered. The nurse consults the client's medical physician for instructions about administration of medications, such as those used for diabetes mellitus, cardiac disease, and glaucoma, as well as regularly scheduled anticonvulsants, antihypertensives, anticoagulants, antidepressants, and corticosteroids. The physician may order some medications to be stopped until after surgery. The physician may order other medications to be administered by the intravenous (IV) route to maintain the client's blood level of the medication. Medications for cardiac disease and hypertension are commonly allowed with a sip of water if taken at least 2 hours before surgery. Some antihypertensive or antidepressant medications may be withheld on the day of surgery because of a possible adverse affect on the blood pressure intraoperatively.

The diabetic client who is taking insulin may be given a reduced dose of intermediate- or long-acting insulin on the basis of the serum glucose level, or the client may be given regular (fast-acting) insulin subcutaneously in divided doses on the day of surgery. An alternative method of diabetes management is an IV infusion of 5% dextrose in water given with the insulin to prevent hypoglycemia intraoperatively. Because of numerous treatment approaches to diabetes, the nurse clarifies medication and IV orders with the physician. (More information about the surgical client with diabetes is found in Chapter 68.)

Gastrointestinal Preparation. Bowel or gastrointestinal (GI) preparations are performed to prevent injury to the colon and to reduce the number of intestinal bacteria. Evacuation of the GI tract is done when a client is having major abdominal, pelvic, perineal, or perianal surgery. The surgeon's preference and type of surgical procedure determine the type of bowel preparation. Table 20–5 shows typical GI preparation regimens for common surgical procedures and complications of the regimens. An enema ordered to be given until return flow is clear is a physically stressful procedure for anyone but especially for the elderly client. Repeated enemas can cause electrolyte imbalance (especially potassium depletion), fluid volume deficit, vagal stimulation, and postural (orthostatic) hypotension. Enemas also cause severe anorectal discomfort in clients with hemorrhoids. To prevent complications, some physicians prescribe potent laxatives (e.g., polyethylene glycol–electrolyte solution [GoLYTELY]) instead of enemas, especially for elderly clients. Bowel preparation procedures can be exhausting, and the nurse takes safety precautions to prevent client falls.

Skin Preparation. The skin preparation may be embarrassing or uncomfortable for the client, especially if the surgical site is in a sensitive or generally private area. The nurse provides a warm, comfortable, and private environment for the client during the procedure.

The skin is the body's first line of defense against infection. A break in this protective mechanism increases the risk of infection, especially for elderly clients. Preoperative skin preparation is the initial step in the prevention of wound infection. One or two days before the scheduled surgery, the surgeon may require the client to shower using an antiseptic solution such as povidone-iodine (Betadine) or hexachlorophene. The physician may want the client to be especially attentive to cleaning around the proposed surgical site. If the patient is hospitalized before surgery, the showering and cleaning is often repeated the night before surgery or in the morning before the client is transferred to the surgical suite. This cleaning reduces contamination of and the number of microorganisms on the surgical field. After the final cleaning procedure, especially for an orthopedic surgery, the area may be covered with sterile towels or drapes to prevent contamination.

A controversial step in preoperative skin preparation after the cleaning or showering is the shave. Many health care practitioners believe that the shaving procedure itself is a possible source of contamination of the surgical area and traumatizes the skin around the area where the incision will be made. Those factors believed to predispose the client to wound contamination include bacteria found in hair follicles, disruption of the normal protective mechanisms of the skin, and nicks in the skin (e.g., from shaving). Shaving of hair creates the potential for infection. Clipping of the hair with electrical surgical clippers is becoming increasingly popular to decrease the complications associated with traditional razors. In the United States, the Centers for Disease Control and Prevention recommend that if shaving is necessary, the hair should be removed using disposable sterile supplies and aseptic principles *immediately* before the start of the surgical pro-

TABLE 20–5

Complications of Common Bowel Preparations for the Surgical Client		
Surgical Site	**Preparation**	**Complications**
Stomach, duodenum, and proximal jejunum	• Oral laxative (e.g., castor oil preparation or bisacodyl [Dulcolax, Laxit✱]) • Clear liquid diet the evening before surgery • NPO after midnight	• Abdominal cramping • Dehydration • Electrolyte imbalance • Fatigue
Small intestine	• Oral laxative (e.g., magnesium citrate) • Clear liquid diet the evening before surgery • Multiple-position enema the evening before surgery • NPO after midnight	• Abdominal cramping • Dehydration • Electrolyte imbalance • Fatigue
Large intestine to rectum	• Multiple or combination of oral laxatives 12–24 hr before surgery • Multiple-position tap water or antibiotic (neomycin) enemas (three times or until the return flow is clear) the evening and morning before surgery • Oral antibiotics to sterilize the bowel (e.g., neomycin and erythromycin) 24 hr before surgery • Clear liquid diet the day before surgery • NPO after midnight	• Abdominal cramping • Fatigue and weakness • Fluid excess or deficit • Potassium or sodium deficit • Decreased cardiac output from vagal stimulation • Irritation of bowel and rectal mucosa from enemas

cedure. Thus, shave preparations are performed in the treatment room, the holding area of the operating suite, or the operating room. Figure 20–2 shows areas shaved for various surgical procedures. Shaving of hair, especially from the head or genital area, can be emotionally upsetting to the client, and regrowth of this hair can be uncomfortable.

Preparing the Client for Tubes, Drains, and Intravenous Access. The nurse prepares the client for possible insertion of tubes, drains, and IV access devices. Preparation reduces the client's postoperative anxiety and fear. The nurse is careful not to scare the client while providing information about the purpose of each tube.

Tubes. The client may require an indwelling urinary catheter (Foley) before, during, or after surgery to keep the bladder empty and to enable monitoring of renal function. The client having major abdominal or genitourinary surgery usually has a Foley catheter.

A nasogastric tube may be inserted before emergency surgery or major abdominal surgery for decompressing or emptying the stomach and the upper bowel. However, it is more often inserted after the induction of anesthesia, when insertion is less disturbing to the client and is easier to perform.

Drains. Drains are frequently inserted during surgery to promote the evacuation of fluid from the surgical site. Some drains are under the dressing, whereas others are visible and require emptying. Drains come in various shapes and sizes (see Chapter 22). The nurse informs the client that drains are often used routinely and that generally they are not painful. The nurse further discusses with

clients the reasons why they should not kink or pull on the drain.

Intravenous Access. An IV access (line) is placed by the nurse or anesthesia personnel for all clients receiving general anesthesia and some clients receiving other types of anesthesia. An access is needed to administer medication and fluids before, during, and after surgery. Clients who are dehydrated or who are at risk for dehydration, such as elderly clients, may receive fluids before surgery. Elderly clients are more susceptible to dehydration because their fluid reserves are lower than those of young or middle-aged adults. Careful monitoring is required for the elderly and for clients with cardiac disease receiving IV fluids. (See Chapter 17 for more information on IV therapy.)

The IV access is usually placed in the arm or the posterior aspect of the hand using a large, short catheter (e.g., 18 gauge, 1 inch). This type of catheter provides the least resistance to fluid or blood infusion, especially in an emergency when rapid infusions may be necessary. Depending on the individual client's needs and the facility's policies and practices, the IV can be placed before surgery when the client is in the hospital room, in the holding or admission area of the surgical suite, or in the operating room.

Teaching About Postoperative Procedures and Exercises. The nurse instructs the client and family members about postoperative exercises and procedures, e.g., checking dressings and obtaining vital signs frequently (see the Client Care Plan). Preoperative teaching reduces the client's apprehension and fear, increases the client's cooperation and participation in postoperative care, and decreases

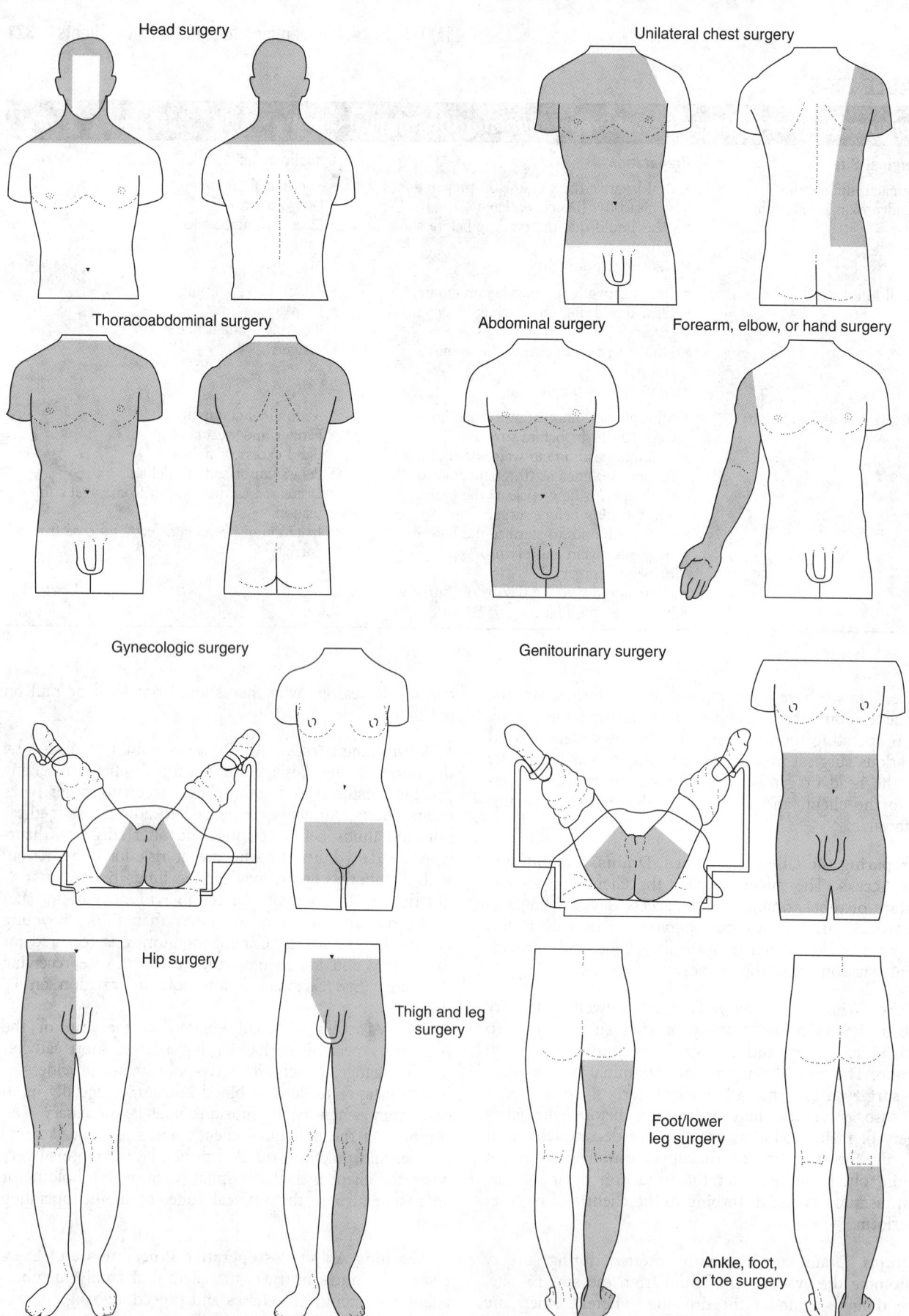

Head surgery

Unilateral chest surgery

Thoracoabdominal surgery

Abdominal surgery

Forearm, elbow, or hand surgery

Gynecologic surgery

Genitourinary surgery

Hip surgery

Thigh and leg surgery

Foot/lower leg surgery

Ankle, foot, or toe surgery

Figure 20–2. Skin preparation of common surgical sites. Shaded areas indicate areas of hair removal.

Client Care Plan

The Preoperative Client

Nursing Diagnosis No. 1: Knowledge Deficit related to lack of exposure to the specific perioperative experience

Expected Outcomes	Nursing Interventions	Rationale
The client will Verbalize an understanding of the perioperative routine.	■ Assess the client's current level of knowledge and provide information about the perioperative routine, as necessary.	■ By assessing the client's knowledge base, the nurse is able to individualize the preoperative teaching.
State reasons for and expected frequency of the postoperative exercises.	■ Discuss with the client and significant others the reasons for the postoperative exercises. ■ Discuss and demonstrate correct breathing and leg exercises.	■ Clients are more likely to comply when they understand the reasons for the activities. ■ Significant others are able to reinforce instructions and encourage the client postoperatively.
Demonstrate correct use of an incentive spirometer (IS). State the goals to achieve with the IS.	■ Encourage the client to practice the exercises. ■ Supplement instructions with written materials, videos, and so on, as available.	■ Repetition helps the learning process. ■ Reinforcement of instructions in more than one format facilitates learning.
Demonstrate splinting of the anticipated surgical area.	■ Discuss and demonstrate the technique for splinting.	■ Client demonstration preoperatively will make it easier to perform postoperatively.

Nursing Diagnosis No. 2. Anxiety related to the threat of a change in health status or fear of the unknown

Expected Outcomes	Nursing Interventions	Rationale
The client will Verbalize the reasons for anxieties or fears, if possible.	■ Assess the client's level of anxiety. ■ Encourage the client to verbalize concerns and fears. ■ Review perioperative events and routines.	■ By assessing the client's anxiety level, support systems, and coping mechanisms, the nurse is able to individualize the plan for anxiety reduction. ■ Familiarity with the usual perioperative events decreases the unknown, which is often a source of anxiety.
Demonstrate relaxation breathing exercises. Identify available diversional activities. Use successful coping mechanisms.	■ Teach relaxation breathing. ■ Provide distractions such as music and television. ■ Assess the client's support systems and coping mechanisms. ■ Incorporate the client's methods of reducing stress, as indicated.	■ Focused thoughts and distractions help to decrease anxiety. ■ Focused thoughts and distractions help to decrease anxiety. ■ When the client is able to continue familiar activities and actions, anxiety is reduced.
State that anxiety is reduced or manageable.	■ Encourage the client to identify which specific interventions reduce anxiety.	■ When client is aware of successful interventions, outcomes can be met in a more timely fashion.

the incidence and severity of postoperative complications. However, when the client's fear or anxiety level is high, the nurse explores the client's attitudes and feelings before discussing procedures (Cipperley et al., 1995). Discussion, demonstration, and return demonstration and practice by the client aid in the ability to perform various breathing (Chart 20–5) and leg (Chart 20–6) exercises during postoperative recovery. The nurse emphasizes the need to begin exercises early in the recovery phase and to continue them, with five to ten repetitions each, every 1 to 2 hours after surgery for at least the first 48 hours. The nurse also explains that the client may need to be awakened for these activities.

Breathing Exercises. In deep, or diaphragmatic, breathing, the diaphragm flattens during inspiration, enlarging the upper abdominal cavity. During expiration, the abdominal muscles and diaphragm contract, which completely expands the lungs. After the nurse demonstrates and explains the technique, the client is encouraged to practice the five steps of deep breathing.

For clients with chronic pulmonary disease or limited upper chest expansion, as seen in elderly clients because of the aging process, expansion breathing exercises are useful. For the client having thoracic surgery, expansion breathing exercises strengthen accessory muscles and should be initiated preoperatively. Expansion breathing may be used postoperatively during chest physiotherapy (percussion, vibration, and postural drainage) to assist with loosening secretions and maintaining an adequate air exchange.

Incentive Spirometry. Incentive spirometry is another way to encourage the client to take deep breaths. Its purpose is to promote complete lung expansion and to prevent respiratory complications. Various types of incentive spirometers are available; some examples are shown in Figure 20–3. With all types, the client must be able to seal his or her lips tightly around the mouthpiece, inhale spontaneously, and hold his or her breath for 3 to 5 seconds to achieve effective lung expansion. Goals (e.g., attaining specific volumes) can be set according to the client's ability and the type of incentive spirometer. Visualization by seeing a light move up a column or a bellows expanding often reinforces and motivates the client to continue performance.

Coughing and Splinting. Coughing may be performed in conjunction with deep breathing every 1 to 2 hours postoperatively. The purposes of coughing are to promote expectoration of secretions, keep the lungs clear, allow full aeration, and prevent pneumonia and atelectasis. Coughing may be uncomfortable for the client, but when performed correctly, it should not harm the surgical area. Splinting (e.g., holding) the incision area provides support, promotes a feeling of security, and reduces pain during coughing. The proper technique for splinting the incision site and coughing was described in Chart 20–5. A folded bath blanket is helpful to use as a splint.

Some practitioners think that coughing exercises should no longer be encouraged routinely. Their belief is that coughing has the potential to harm the surgical wound and that it would be better to emphasize other, safer

---

Chart 20–5

Education Guide: Perioperative Respiratory Care

Deep (diaphragmatic) breathing

1. Sit upright on the edge of the bed or in a chair, being sure that your feet are placed firmly on the floor or a stool. [After surgery, deep breathing is done with the client in Fowler's position or in semi-Fowler's position.]
2. Take a gentle breath through your mouth.
3. Breathe out gently and completely.
4. Then take a deep breath through your nose and mouth, and hold this breath to the count of five.
5. Exhale through your nose and mouth.

Expansion breathing

1. Find a comfortable upright position, with your knees slightly bent. [Bending the knees decreases tension on the abdominal muscles and decreases respiratory resistance and discomfort.]
2. Place your hands on each side of your lower rib cage, just above your waist.
3. Take a deep breath through your nose, using your shoulder muscles to expand your lower rib cage outward during inhalation.
4. Exhale, concentrating first on moving your chest, then on moving your lower ribs inward, while gently squeezing the rib cage and forcing air out of the base of your lungs.

Splinting of the surgical incision

1. Unless coughing is contraindicated, place a pillow, towel, or folded blanket over your surgical incision and hold the item firmly in place.
2. Take three slow, deep breaths to stimulate your cough reflex.
3. Inhale through your nose, then exhale through your mouth.
4. On your third deep breath, cough to clear secretions from your lungs while firmly holding the pillow, towel, or folded blanket against your incision.

---

measures for pulmonary hygiene, such as the deep breathing and incentive spirometer exercises. When routine coughing exercises are contraindicated for a client, such as after a hernia repair, the physician usually writes a "do not cough" order.

Leg Procedures and Exercises. Antiembolism stockings (TED stockings or Jobst hose), elastic (Ace) wraps, or pneumatic compression devices (e.g., "sequentials" and "boots") may be used perioperatively in combination with leg exercises and early ambulation to promote venous return. Venous stasis can lead to deep vein (venous) thrombosis (DVT) or a pulmonary embolus (PE) if the blood clot breaks off and travels to the lungs. Interventions depend on the client's risk factors. Clients at greater risk for deep vein thrombosis

■ Are obese
■ Are older than 40 years of age
■ Have a concurrent cancer diagnosis

Chart 20–6

Education Guide: Postoperative Leg Exercises

Exercise No. 1

1. Lie in bed with the head of your bed elevated to about 45 degrees. [Using semi-Fowler's position during postoperative leg exercises improves peripheral circulation, prevents thrombus formation, and strengthens muscles.]
2. Beginning with your right leg, bend your knee, raise your foot off the bed, and hold this position for a few seconds.
3. Extend your leg by unbending your knee, and lower the leg to the bed.
4. Repeat this sequence four more times with your right leg, then perform this same exercise five times with your left leg.

Exercise No. 2

1. Beginning with your right leg, point your toes toward the bottom of the bed.
2. With the same leg, point your toes up toward your face.
3. Repeat this exercise several times with your right leg, then perform this same exercise with your left leg.

Exercise No. 3

1. Beginning with your right leg, make circles with your ankles, first to the left, then to the right.
2. Repeat this exercise several times with your right leg, then perform this same exercise with your left leg.

Exercise No. 4

1. Beginning with your right leg, bend your knee and *push* the ball of your foot into the bed or floor until you feel your calf and thigh muscles contracting.
2. Repeat this exercise several times with your right leg, then perform this same exercise with your left leg.

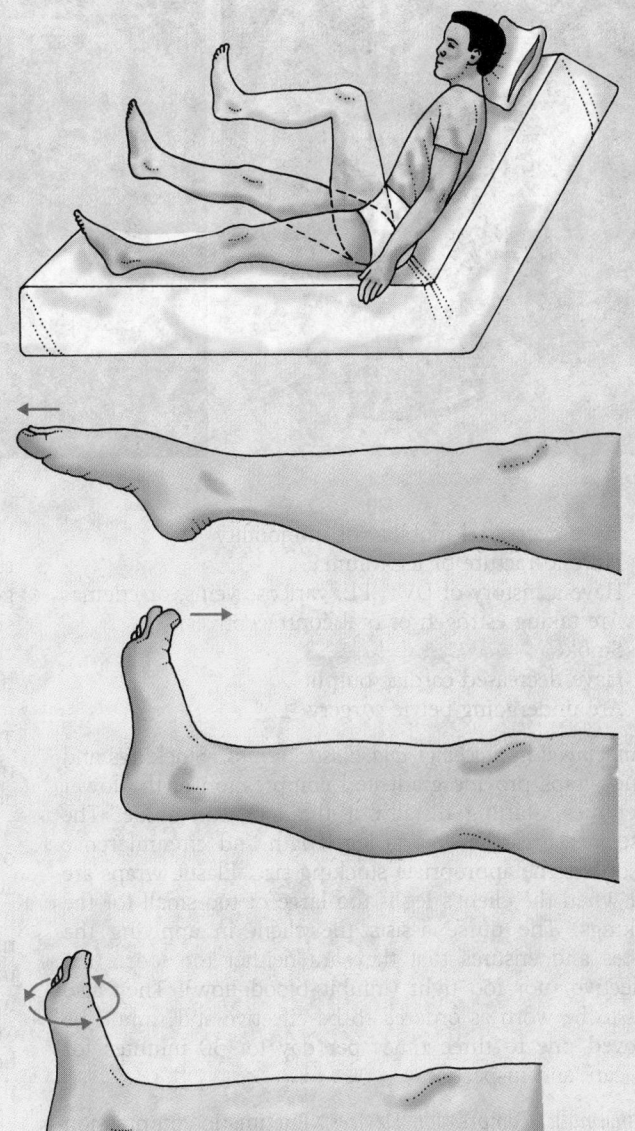
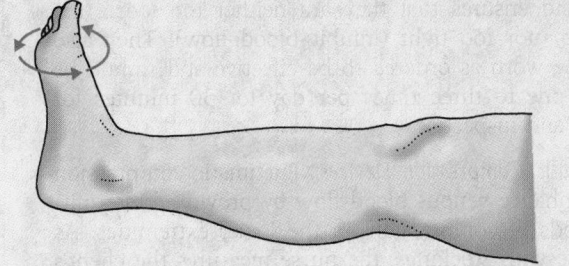
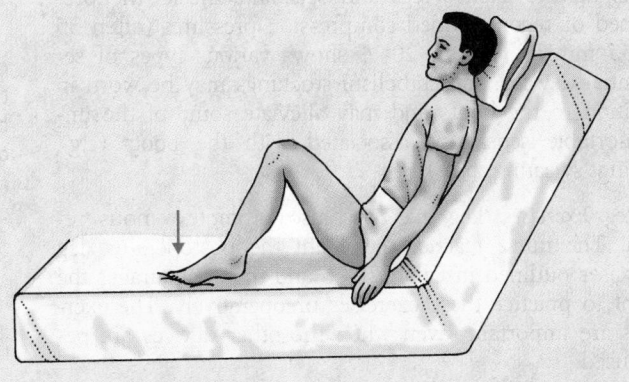

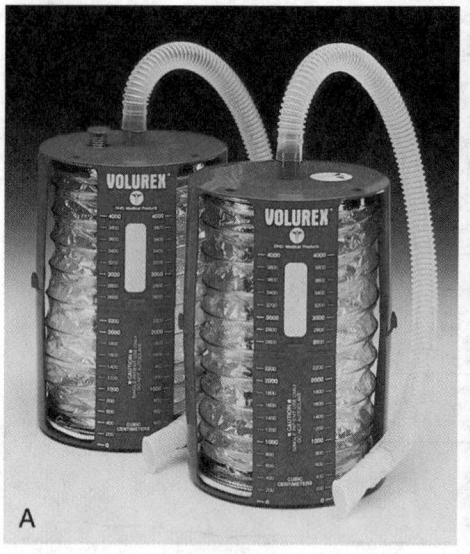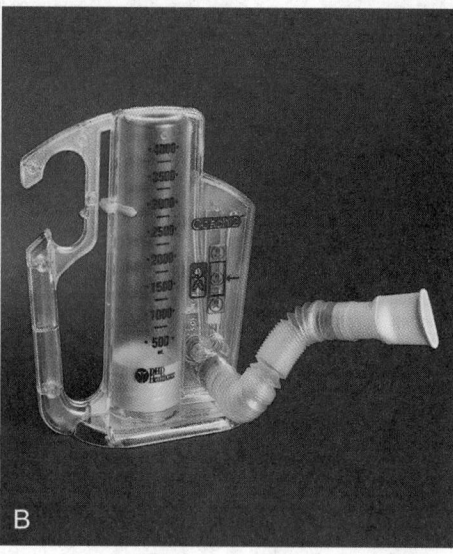

Figure 20–3. Examples of volume incentive spirometers for lung expansion. *A.* A volume displacement incentive spirometer. *B,* A volumetric incentive spirometer. (Courtesy of DHD Healthcare, Canastota, NY.)

- Have decreased mobility or immobility
- Have a fracture or leg trauma
- Have a history of DVT, PE, varicose veins, or edema
- Are taking estrogen or oral contraceptives
- Smoke
- Have decreased cardiac output
- Are undergoing pelvic surgery

Antiembolism Stockings and Elastic Wraps. Stockings and elastic wraps provide graduated compression of the lower extremities, starting distally at the foot and ankle. The nurse measures the client's leg length and circumference and orders the appropriate stocking size. Elastic wraps are used when the client's leg is too large or too small for the stockings. The nurse assists the client in applying the devices and ensures that they are neither too loose (are ineffective) nor too tight (inhibit blood flow). They also need to be worn as ordered to be effective and should be removed one to three times per day for 30 minutes for skin care and inspection.

Pneumatic Compression Devices. Pneumatic compression devices enhance venous blood flow by providing intermittent periods of compression on the lower extremities. As is the case with stockings, the nurse measures the client's leg and orders the appropriate size. The nurse places the boots on the client's legs and sets and checks the prescribed or recommended compression pressures (often 35 to 55 mmHg). Figure 20–4 shows various types of sequential devices. Antiembolism stockings may be worn in addition to the boots and may alleviate some of the uncomfortable sensations associated with the boots (e.g., itching, sweating, heat).

Leg Exercises. Leg exercises also promote venous return. The nurse teaches the client the postoperative leg exercises outlined in Chart 20–6 and then encourages the client to practice these exercises preoperatively. The exercises are important, even when the other devices are being used.

Early Ambulation. Mobility soon after surgery (early ambulation) stimulates gastrointestinal motility, enhances

lung expansion, mobilizes secretions, promotes venous return, prevents rigidity of joints, and relieves pressure. In general, the nurse instructs the client that he or she should turn at least every 2 hours after surgery while confined to bed. To aid clients, the nurse teaches them how to use the bed side rails safely for turning and how to protect the surgical wound (splinting) when turning. The nurse assures clients that assistance will be given as needed to alleviate any anxiety they may have about this activity.

For certain surgeries, such as some brain, spinal, and orthopedic surgeries, the physician may order turning restrictions. The nurse discusses with the physician other interventions to prevent complications associated with immobility in clients with turning restrictions. The nurse informs the client of anticipated turning restrictions during preoperative teaching.

Many clients are allowed and encouraged to get out of bed the day of or the day after surgery. The nurse assists the client into a chair or with ambulation the evening after the surgery or the next day, depending on the type and time of surgery and the physician's preference. If a client must remain in bed, he or she must turn, deep breathe, and perform leg exercises at least every 2 hours to prevent the complications of postoperative immobility.

Range-of-Motion Exercises. Passive or active range-of-motion (ROM) exercises help prevent joint rigidity and muscle contracture. The client should do these exercises three to five times each, three to four times a day while bedridden. The nurse instructs the client in these procedures and informs the client that he or she will receive assistance as needed postoperatively. (Guidelines for ROM exercises are found in Chapter 24.)

➤ *Anxiety*

Planning: Expected Outcomes. The outcomes are that the client will

- Verbalize decreased or manageable preoperative anxiety
- Demonstrate evidence of relaxation when at rest

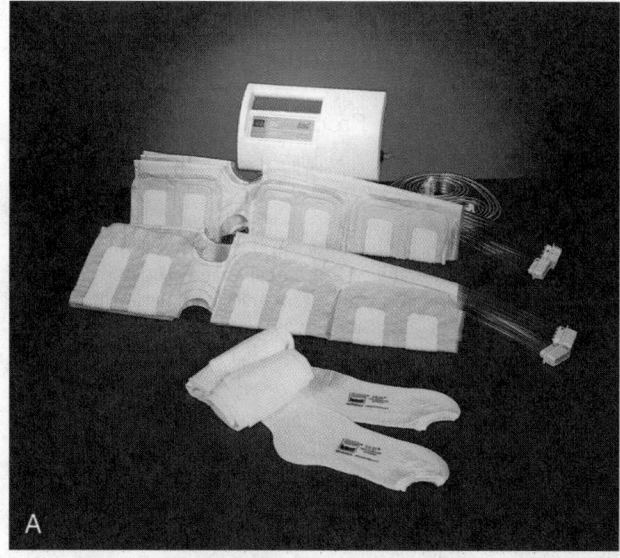
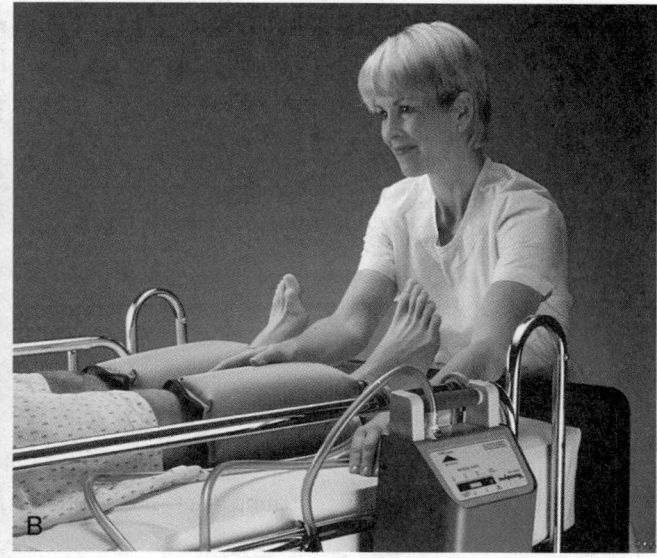
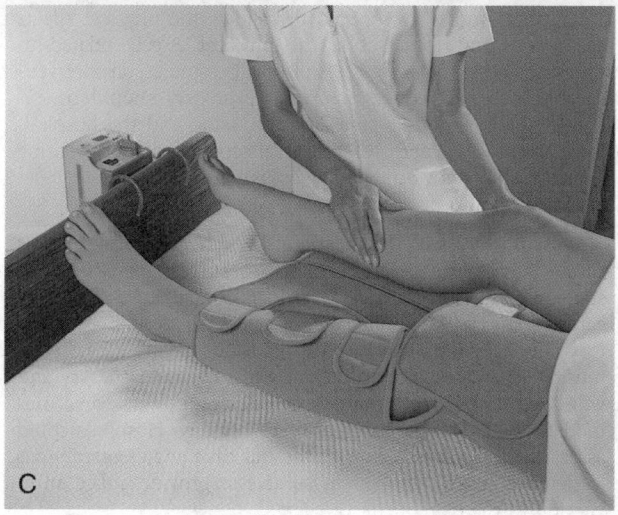

Figure 20–4. Examples of external pneumatic compression devices used to promote venous return and prevent deep vein thrombosis (DVT). *A.* Kendall SCD machine, sleeves, and TED stockings (Courtesy of Kendall Healthcare Company). *B,* Venodyne pneumatic compression system (Courtesy of Venodyne, Inc.). *C,* Flowtron DVT calf garments (Courtesy of Huntleigh Healthcare).

Interventions. Preoperative anxiety frequently causes the client to exhibit physical symptoms such as restlessness and sleeplessness. The surgical client perceives the perioperative experience as a threat to biopsychosocial integrity. The nurse first assesses the client's level of anxiety, as discussed earlier in this chapter. Interventions such as teaching and communicating with the client preoperatively, enabling the client to utilize previously successful coping mechanisms, and administering antianxiety agents help to reduce the anxiety and subsequent complications. The nurse incorporates appropriate and available support systems into the plan of care.

Preoperative Teaching. The nurse assesses the client's knowledge about the perioperative experience that he or she has acquired from prior surgical experiences and procedures and from other sources (see Knowledge Deficit earlier in this chapter). The nurse provides factual information about the surgery and the perioperative experience

to promote the client's understanding. The nurse allows ample time for the client's questions. The nurse responds to the client's questions appropriately and accurately and refers unanswered questions to the proper person. During the discussion between the client and the nurse, the nurse continually assesses the client's responses and anxiety level. The nurse must be careful not to provide information that might increase anxiety. Clients have ranked psychosocial support as the most important component during preoperative teaching. The informed, educated client is better able to anticipate events and maintain self-control and is thus less anxious.

Encouraging Communication. Stating feelings, fears, and concerns is an appropriate way to reduce anxiety. The nurse develops a trusting relationship with the client so he or she can express feelings freely without fear of ridicule or judgment. The nurse keeps the client informed, clarifies information, answers questions, and allays some of the client's apprehensions about surgery.

Promoting Rest. The stress and anxiety of impending surgery frequently interfere with the client's ability to sleep and rest the night before surgery. The preoperative experience is physically and emotionally stressful. To assist the client in relaxing, the nurse determines what the client usually does to relax and fall asleep. If permitted and able, the client is encouraged to continue these methods of relaxation. A back rub is a relaxing and therapeutic measure and can be performed by a nurse or family member. The physician may prescribe a sedative or short-acting hypnotic to ensure that the client is well rested for surgery.

Using Distraction. The nurse may plan distraction as an intervention for anxiety. Especially in the 24 hours immediately before surgery, listening to music (see Research Applications For Nursing) or comedy audiotapes may decrease anxiety, as may watching television, reading, or visiting with family members.

Teaching Family and Significant Others. The nurse assesses the readiness and desire of the family or significant others to take an active part in the client's care. The involved family provides support for the client and helps reduce anxiety. A positive sign of family interest is members' initiation of questions about the perioperative experience. After family readiness is determined, the nurse keeps family members informed and encourages their involvement in all aspects of preoperative education with the client. The nurse emphasizes the important role of the family preoperatively but guides discussions and practice sessions so that family members do not dominate the sessions. Family members can encourage and help the client practice postoperative exercises.

The nurse informs the family of the time for surgery, if known, and of any schedule changes. If the client is an outpatient, he or she and the family need clear directions regarding any specific night-before procedures, what time and where to report, and what to bring with them. The family is encouraged to stay with the client preoperatively for support.

Most families are anxious about the surgery planned for their loved one. To reduce their anxiety, the nurse explains the intraoperative and postoperative routine to them. The nurse explains that after the client leaves the hospital room or admission area, there is usually a 30- to 60-minute preparation period in the operating area (holding room, treatment area, and so on) before the surgery actually begins. After surgery, the client is taken to the postanesthesia care unit (PACU) for 1 to 2 hours before returning to the hospital room or discharge area. The nurse instructs the family about the best place to wait for the client or surgeon according to the facility's policy and the physician's preference. Many hospitals and surgical centers have designated surgical waiting areas so families can wait in comfortable surroundings and be easily located when the procedure is completed.

► *Preoperative Chart Review*

The nurse reviews the client's chart to ensure all documentation, preoperative procedures, and orders are completed. The nurse checks the surgical informed consent

► Research Applications for Nursing

Music May Reduce Preoperative Anxiety

Augustin, P., & Haines, A. A. (1996). Effect of music on ambulatory surgery patients' preoperative anxiety. AORN Journal, 63(4), 750, 753–758.

In this study, 42 ambulatory surgical clients were assigned to either an experimental or a control group to determine the effect music had on reducing preoperative anxiety. Vital signs and client self-reports of anxiety, using the State-Trait Anxiety Inventory, were measured. All clients received preoperative instruction.

Critique. This sample was limited to 42 ambulatory patients. Anxiety is generally believed to have an effect on heart and respiratory rates and blood pressure. In this study, heart rates were found to be significantly lower in the experimental group, but the effect on blood pressure and respiratory rate approached significance only.

Further studies are needed to validate the physical effects of anxiety and to describe the physical effects related to different causes of anxiety. Additionally, studies on interventions that could reduce preoperative anxiety should be expanded to include the same-day admission and the hospitalized client. The study of music effects on clients awaiting consultation, diagnostic tests, or other, nonsurgical procedures could also be studied.

Possible Nursing Implications. Health care professionals caring for clients before ambulatory surgery may need to start interventions aimed at reducing preoperative anxiety earlier than in the immediate preoperative period. Ambulatory surgical suites may need to consider having a variety of music for clients to choose from while awaiting surgery and will need an adequate number of listening devices to accommodate their usual number of cases per day. Hospitals could assess their physical environment and their inpatient routines to determine how they might be able to provide music intervention to their preoperative clients.

form and, if indicated, any other special consent forms to see that they are signed, dated, and contain the witnesses' signatures. Allergies should be noted according to facility policy. Accurate documentation of height and weight is important for proper dosage calculation of the anesthetic agents. The results of all laboratory, radiographic, and diagnostic tests should be on the chart; any abnormal results are documented and reported to the physician and the anesthesiologist or anesthetist. If the client was an autologous blood donor or had directed blood donations made, those special slips must be included in the chart. The nurse records a current set of vital signs (within 1–2 hours of the scheduled surgery time) and documents any significant physical or psychosocial observations. The nurse reports special needs and concerns of the client to the surgical team. For example, the nurse advises the surgical team whether the client is a member of Jehovah's Witnesses and does not accept blood products or whether the client is hard of hearing and does not have his or her hearing aid. This information assists the surgical team in providing continuity of care while the client is in the surgical area.

➤ Preoperative Client Preparation

Facilities generally require that the client remove most clothing and wear a hospital gown into the operating room. Underwear may be permitted for surgery above the waist; socks may be worn, except for foot or leg surgery. If ordered by the surgeon, antiembolism stockings are applied preoperatively.

The client's valuables, including jewelry, money, and clothes, are locked in a safe place, according to the facility's policy. The nurse tapes in place rings that cannot be removed. Religious emblems may be pinned or fastened securely to the client's gown; in some facilities, paper emblems are available from a religious leader.

The client wears an identification band that clearly gives first and last names and hospital number. A bracelet designating that a blood sample for type and crossmatch has been drawn may be worn, depending on the facility's policy.

Dentures, including partial dental plates, are removed and placed in a labeled denture cup. The removal of dentures is a safety measure to prevent aspiration and obstruction of the airway. If a client has any capped teeth, the nurse documents this finding on the preoperative checklist.

All prosthetic devices, such as artificial eyes and limbs, are removed and safely stored, as are contact lenses, wigs, and toupees. The nurse checks for hairpins and clips, which, if not removed, can conduct electrical current used during surgery and cause scalp burns.

Some facilities allow hearing aids in the surgical suite to facilitate communication before and after surgery. If the client is sent to surgery with a hearing aid, the nurse communicates this to the surgical nurse to prevent accidental loss of or damage to the aid. Some facilities allow dentures, wigs, glasses, and so on to be worn by the client into the operating suite to prevent embarrassment to the client. These items can then be removed when absolutely necessary.

The removal of fingernail polish or artificial nails is controversial. Polish is flammable, and artificial nails may affect the accuracy of pulse oximetry readings. In some facilities, at least one artificial nail must be removed for this reason.

After the client is prepared for surgery and the operating suite is ready to receive the client, the nurse asks the client to empty his or her bladder to prevent incontinence or overdistention and to provide a starting point for intake and output measurement. An overly full bladder may hinder access to the surgical site. The nurse answers any final questions the client has, offers reassurance as needed, and administers any ordered preoperative medication.

➤ Preoperative Medications

Preoperative medication may be ordered for clients, regardless of the type of planned anesthesia. Various preoperative medications reduce anxiety, promote relaxation, reduce pharyngeal secretions, prevent laryngospasm, inhibit gastric secretions, and decrease the amount of anesthetic required for the induction and maintenance of anesthesia. The selection of medication is based on the client's age, physical and psychological condition, medical history, and height and weight; the medications that the client takes routinely; the results of preoperative tests; and the type and extensiveness of the surgical procedure. If more than one pharmacologic response is required, combination therapy is usually ordered. A typical combination consists of a sedative or tranquilizer, an opioid analgesic, and an anticholinergic agent.

The preoperative medication is often ordered when the client is "on call" to the surgical suite. After the nurse positively identifies the client (using the arm band) and makes sure the operative permit is signed, he or she administers the correct medication. Then the nurse raises the side rails, places the call system within easy reach of the client while reminding him or her not to try to get out of bed, and places the bed in a low position. The nurse tells the client that he or she may become drowsy and have a dry mouth owing to the medication.

An increasingly common practice is for the premedication to be given *after* the client is transferred to the operating area. This practice permits the operating and anesthesia personnel to make more accurate assessments and have last-minute discussions with a client not yet affected by medication. In addition, after the client is in the operating area, medications can be given via the IV route. The oral (PO) or intramuscular (IM) route is less desirable because of unpredictable absorption rates.

➤ Client Transfer to the Surgical Suite

In the immediate preoperative preparation, the nurse reviews and updates the client's chart, reinforces preoperative teaching, ensures that the client is appropriately dressed for surgery, and administers preoperative medication, if ordered. The nurse uses a preoperative checklist to assist in the smooth, efficient transfer of the client to the surgical suite (Fig. 20–5). The client, along with the signed consent form, the completed preoperative checklist, the chart, and the addressograph plate, is transported to the surgical suite.

Most clients in the hospital setting are transferred to the surgical suite on a stretcher with the side rails up. In special circumstances (e.g., clients requiring traction, those having orthopedic surgery, and those who should be moved as little as possible immediately after surgery), the client is transferred in his or her hospital bed. Other factors that influence the nurse's decision to transfer the client in a bed are the client's age, size, and physical condition.

 Evaluation

The nurse evaluates the care of the preoperative client according to the identified nursing diagnoses. The outcomes for the client in the preoperative phase of the perioperative experience include that the client

- States that he or she understands informed consent as it applies to surgery
- Complies with the nothing by mouth requirement before surgery

NORTHWEST HOSPITAL CENTER
PRE-OPERATIVE CHECKLIST

Date of Surgery_____

Addressograph Plate

<u>**ALLERGIES**</u>

CLINICAL DATA:	YES	NO	COMMENTS
Authorization for Surgical Treatment Completed			
Height & Weight Charted			
History and Physical			
Chest X-Ray			
EKG Report			
Urine Report			
Blood Sugar Within Range of (75-250mg%)			
Hematocrit Within Range of (27-55%)			
Potassium Within Range of (3.2-5.5mEq/L)			
Results Out of Range Reported to Dept. of Anesthesia			
Anesthesiologist Time:		By:	

PATIENT PREPARATION:	YES	NO	COMMENTS
Jewelry Removed			
Hair Piece, Wig, Hairpin, Barrettes, Beads, Rubberbands Removed			
Loose Teeth or Caps Noted			
Dentures Removed			
Artificial Eye, Contact Lenses, Glasses Removed			
Any Prosthetic Appliance Removed			
Voided or Catheterized - I&O Sheet on Chart			
Identification Bracelet in Place			
Parenteral Fluids Patent & Infusing at cc/hr			
B/P, T.P.R. Charted			
Premedication Given As Ordered			
Side Rails Up-Pt. Care Data & Care Plan on Chart			
Is Patient on Isolation - If Yes, What Type			

COMMUNICATION ASSESSMENT:	Normal	Abnormal	COMMENTS
Vision			
Hearing			
Mental			
Speech			
Other			
Patient's Preferred Name:			
Limb For Burial ☐ Yes ☐ No Funeral Home:			

R.N. Completing Checklist

702/1091-3-R-4/95 (40-1471)   (O V E R)   pl/3133N

Figure 20–5. A preoperative checklist. (Courtesy of Northwest Hospital Center, Randallstown, MD.)

- Verbalizes an understanding of and the reason for a bowel preparation, if applicable
- States the purpose of the skin preparation
- Verbalizes an understanding of how tubes, drains, and IV lines and catheters may be used during and after surgery
- Demonstrates postoperative exercises: turning, deep breathing, splinting, coughing, and performing specific leg exercises
- Demonstrates the use of an incentive spirometer
- States that preoperative anxiety is lessened after preoperative teaching

CASE STUDY For the Preoperative Client

■ Mrs. James, a 68-year-old diabetic woman, is scheduled for a left below-the-knee amputation. You get a report from the off-going nurse who tells you that her preoperative checklist is completed. Three hours later, the operating room calls for Mrs. James. You have her void, take and record a set of vital signs, note that no premedication is ordered, and send her to the operating suite. Five minutes later, an angry holding room nurse calls you and says, "You sent this patient to the operating suite without a signed consent, without an armband, and with her wedding ring on!"

QUESTIONS:

1. How should you respond to the holding room nurse?
2. The holding room nurse continues to be quite angry for this situation, causing delays within the operating room and blames you personally—even threatens to report you to your supervisor. On what should your response focus?
3. How could you prevent this situation from reoccurring?

SELECTED BIBLIOGRAPHY

Augustin, P., & Haines, A. A. (1996). Effect of music on ambulatory surgery patients' preoperative anxiety. *AORN Journal, 63*(4), 750, 753–758.

Balcom, C. (1994). The new code of ethics: Implications for perioperative nurses. *Canadian Operating Room Nursing Journal, 12*(1), 6–8.

Blake, G. J. (1994). Administering prophylactic antibiotics before surgery: Consult this chart for the regime your patient will need. *Nursing94, 24*(12), 18.

Brick, J. (1996). OR nursing law. Informed consent and perioperative nursing. *AORN Journal, 63*(1), 258, 261.

Bright, L. D. (1994). How to protect your patient from DVT. *American Journal of Nursing, 94*(12), 28–32.

Brumfield, V. C., Kee, C. D., & Johnson, J. Y. (1997). Preoperative patient teaching in ambulatory surgery settings. *AORN Journal, 64*(6), 941, 943–946, 948, 951–952.

Burden, N. (1994). Patient and family education in the ambulatory surgery setting. *Seminars in Perioperative Nursing, 3*(3), 145–151.

*Caldwell, L. M. (1991). The influence of preference for information on preoperative stress and coping in surgical outpatients. *Applied Nursing Research 4*(4), 177–183.

Chalfin, D. B., et al. (1994). Preoperative evaluation and postoperative care of the elderly patient undergoing major surgery. *Clinics in Geriatric Medicine, 10*(1), 51–70.

Chapman, A. (1996). Current theory and practice: a study of preoperative fasting. *Nursing Standard, 10*(18), 33–36.

Chiarella, M. (1995). The consent form: Perils and possibilities. *Australian Confederation of Operating Room Nurses Journal, 8*(4), 21–22.

Chiarella, M. (1996). The consent form: Perils and possibilities—part 2. *Australian Confederation of Operating Room Nurses Journal, 9*(1), 29–30.

Cipperley, J. A., Butcher, L. A., & Hayes, J. E. (1995). Research utilization: The development of a preoperative teaching protocol. *MEDSURG Nursing, 4*(3), 199–206.

Cirina, C. L. (1994). Effects of sedative music on patient preoperative anxiety. *Today's OR Nurse, 16*(3), 15–18.

DeFazio-Quinn, D. M. (1997). Ambulatory surgery. *Nursing Clinics of North America, 32*(2), 375–488.

*Dellasega, C., & Burgunder, C. (1991). Perioperative nursing care for the elderly surgical patient. *Today's OR Nurse, 13*(6), 12–17, 30–31.

Diabetic patients require special care in same-day surgery. (1994). *Same-Day Surgery, 18*(3), 33–36.

*Drago, S. S. (1992). Banking on your own blood. *American Journal of Nursing, 92*(3), 61–64.

Droogan, J., et al. (1996). Pre-operative patient instruction: Is it effective? *Nursing Standard, 10*(35), 32–33.

Etchason, J., Petz, L., Keeler, E., et al. (1995). The cost effectiveness of preoperative autologous blood donations. *New England Journal of Medicine, 332*(11), 719–724.

Evans, M. M., et al. (1994). Music: A diversionary therapy. *Today's OR Nurse, 16*(4), 17–22.

*Friedman, S. B., Fitzpatrick, S., & Badere, B. (1992). The effects of television viewing on preoperative anxiety. *Journal of Post Anesthesia Nursing, 7*(4), 243–250.

*Gaberson, K. B. (1991). The effect of humorous and musical distraction on preoperative anxiety. *AORN Journal, 62*(5), 784–788+.

Giordano, B. P. (1996). Clinical exemplars demonstrate perioperative nurses' courage and commitment to quality patient care. *AORN Journal, 63*(1), 15, 18.

Giordano, B. P. (1996). Ensuring the readability of patient education materials is one way to demonstrate perioperative nurses' value. *AORN Journal, 63*(4), 699–700.

Green, D. (1995). Patient assessment for surgery. *British Journal of Theatre Nursing, 5*(1), 10–12.

Groves, H. (1994). Preoperative patient fasting regimes. *British Journal of Theatre Nursing, 4*(2), 14–16.

Hnatiuk, O. W., Dillard, T. A., & Torrington, K. G. (1995). Adherence to established guidelines for preoperative pulmonary function testing. *Chest, 107*(5), 1294–1297.

*Johnson, G. M., & Bowman, R. J. (1992). Autologous blood transfusion: Current trends, nursing implications. *AORN Journal, 56*(2), 281–285, 288–293, 296–298.

*Kapp, M. B. (1990). Informed, assisted, delegated consent for elderly patients. *AORN Journal, 52*(4), 857–862.

*Keene, A. (1991). Perioperative assessment and nursing implications for the elderly. *Plastic Surgical Nursing, 11*(4), 143–150, 163–167.

Kendrick, J. M., & Powers, P. H. (1994). Perioperative care of the pregnant surgical patient. *AORN Journal, 60*(2), 203–219.

*Leckrone, L. (1991). Preparing your patient for surgery. *Nursing91, 21*(7), 46–49.

*Leske, J. S. (1992). Practice-based perioperative research. *AORN Journal, 55*(2), 581–590.

*Litwak, K. (1991). What you need to know about administering preoperative medications. *Nursing91, 21*(8), 44–47.

Marshall, W. J. (1994). Perioperative nutritional support. *Care of the Critically Ill, 10*(4), 163–167.

Martin, D. (1996). Pre-operative visits to reduce patient anxiety: A study. *Nursing Standard, 10*(23), 33–38.

McGaughey, J., et al. (1994). Understanding the pre-operative information needs of patients and their relatives in intensive care units. *Intensive & Critical Care Nursing, 10*(3), 186–194.

Meckes, P. F. (1995). Geriatric surgery. In M. H. Meeker & J. C. Rothrock (Eds.), *Alexander's care of the patient in surgery* (10th ed., pp. 1195–1209). St. Louis: Mosby–Year Book.

Meeker, M. H., & Rothrock, J. C. (Eds.). (1995). *Alexander's care of the patient in surgery* (10th ed.). St. Louis: Mosby–Year Book.

*Moore, L. W., et al. (1993). Communicating effectively with elderly surgical patients. *AORN Journal, 58*(2), 345, 347, 349–350+.

Moran, S., et al. (1995). Quality indicators for patient information in short-stay units. *Nursing Times, 91*(4), 37–40.

Moss, V. A. (1994). Assessing learning abilities, readiness for education. *Seminars in Perioperative Nursing, 3*(3), 113–120.

Nash, C. A., & Jensen, P. L. (1994). When your surgical patient has hypertension. *American Journal of Nursing, 94*(12), 39–45.

Null, S. L. (1994). Preadmission testing: A coordinator can be the answer. *AORN Journal, 59*(5), 1051–1056, 1059–1060.

Oberle, K., Allen, M., & Lynkowski, P. (1994). Follow-up of same day surgery patients. *AORN Journal, 59*(5), 1016–1025.

*Oetker-Black, S. L., Hart, F., Hoffman, J., et al. (1992). Preoperative self-efficacy and postoperative behaviors. *Applied Nursing Research, 5*(3), 134–139.

*Persson, A. V., Davis, R. J., & Villavicencio, J. L. (1991). Deep vein thrombosis and pulmonary embolism. *Surgical Clinics of North America, 71*(6), 1195–1209.

*Peterson, K. J. (1992). Nursing management of autologous blood transfusion. *Journal of Intravenous Nursing, 15*(3), 128–134.

Planchock, N. Y., et al. (1994). Preoperative assessment and teaching: Physiological and psychological preparation. *Seminars in Perioperative Nursing, 3*(2), 61–69.

Proposed recommended practices for surgical skin preparation (1996). *AORN Journal, 63*(1), 221–224, 227.

Redmond, C. (1994). Postoperative instructions: Is your timing right? . . . postoperative instructions should be given prior to the day of surgery. *Breathline, 14*(3), 1, 8.

Salzbach, R. (1995). Presurgical testing improves patient care. *AORN Journal, 61*(1), 210–212, 215–216, 218.

Schwartz-Barcott, D., et al. (1994). Client-nurse interaction: Testing for its impact in preoperative instruction. *International Journal of Nursing Studies, 31*(1), 23–35.

SDS program streamlines pre-admit assessment . . . same-day surgery program (1995). *Same-Day Surgery, 19*(2), 18–20.

*Shea, S. I. (1992). Our patients face recovery with confidence. *RN, 55*(6), 17–18, 20.

Small, S. P. (1996). Preoperative hair removal: A case report with implications for nursing. *Journal of Clinical Nursing, 5*(2), 79–84.

Stewart, B. (1994). Teaching culturally diverse populations. *Seminars in Perioperative Nursing, 3*(3), 160–167.

Sutherland, R. (1994). Is this the way forward? . . . the role of the nurse in day surgery. *British Journal of Theatre Nursing, 4*(1), 12–13.

Swan, B. A. (1994). A collaborative ambulatory preoperative evaluation model: Implementation, implications, evaluation. *AORN Journal, 59*(2), 430–437.

Take a close look at pre-op visits: How much is too much? (1995). *Same-Day Surgery, 19*(2), 13–17.

Thomas, D. R., & Ritchie, C. (1995). Preoperative assessment of older adults. *Journal of the American Geriatrics Society, 43*(7), 811–821.

Tietz, N. W. (1995). *Clinical guide to laboratory tests* (3rd ed.). Philadelphia: W. B. Saunders.

Toy, P. T. C., & Kerr, K. (1996). Preoperative autologous blood donation. *AACN Clinical Issues: Advanced Practice in Acute and Critical Care, 7*(2), 221–228.

Vernon, S., & Pfeifer, G. M. (1997). Are you ready for bloodless surgery? *American Journal of Nursing, 97*(9), 40–47.

Watson, D. S., & Sangermano, C. A. (1995). Ambulatory surgery. In M. H. Meeker & J. C. Rothrock (Eds.), *Alexander's care of the patient in surgery* (10th ed., pp. 1125–1144). St. Louis: Mosby–Year Book.

Webb, R. A. (1995). Preoperative visiting from the perspective of the theatre nurse. *British Journal of Theatre Nursing, 4*(16), 919–925.

West, B. J. M., et al. (1995). Day surgery: Cheap option or challenge to care? *British Journal of Theatre Nursing, 5*(1), 5–8.

When the fast track isn't the best track (1995). *Same-Day Surgery, 19*(9), 104–105.

*Which presurgical tests are worthwhile? (1992). *Emergency Medicine, 24*(14), 88–90.

Wicker, P. (1995). Pre-operative visiting—making it work. *British Journal of Theatre Nursing, 5*(7), 16–19.

Young, R., et al. (1994). Effect of preadmission brochures on surgical patients' behavioral outcomes. *AORN Journal, 60*(2), 232–236, 239–241.

SUGGESTED READINGS

Brick, J. (1996). OR nursing law. Informed consent and perioperative nursing. *AORN Journal, 63*(1), 258, 261.

    This two-page article gives a brief but informative review of battery and negligence as may arise from lack of consent. Specific examples involving nurses are included. Consent terminology, such as implied consent and informed consent, is explained.

Bright, L. D. (1994). How to protect your patient from DVT. *American Journal of Nursing, 94*(12), 28–32.

    This easy-to-read article first identifies risk factors for deep vein thrombosis and then discusses interventions for the low-, medium-, and high-risk patient. The article reviews the physiologic principles of graduated compression stockings, how to apply them, and what complications to assess for. In discussing pneumatic compression devices, the authors differentiate the intermittent from the sequential device and provide much nursing detail, including cost factors.

Cipperley, J. A., Butcher, L. A., & Hayes, J. E. (1995). Research utilization: The development of a preoperative teaching protocol. *MED-SURG Nursing, 4*(3), 199–206.

    These authors wanted to develop a preoperative teaching tool that would enhance patient outcomes; e.g., reduced pain, complications and length of stay. First they describe findings from their literature search, which focused on preoperative instruction in two main areas: educational content and instructional methods. Then a protocol was developed, which includes content in the procedural, behavioral, and sensory domains. The authors explain that after the nurse assesses the client's level of fear and anxiety, a pathway is decided on for teaching. Both the protocol and a surgical teaching flow sheet are reprinted in the article.

INTERVENTIONS FOR INTRAOPERATIVE CLIENTS

As the client enters the surgical suite, the intraoperative phase of the perioperative experience begins. This is an anxious time for the client, as he or she enters into unfamiliar experiences involving unknown outcomes. Nursing care during the intraoperative period addresses all of the client's physical needs, as well as his or her comfort, safety, dignity, and psychological status. Specific procedures and policies may differ among agencies, but similarities are evident and reflect the standards and recommended practices for perioperative nursing, as published by the Association of Operating Room Nurses.

OVERVIEW
Members of the Surgical Team

The surgical team consists of the surgeon, one or more surgical assistants, the anesthesiologist and/or nurse anesthetist, and operating room nurses.

Operating room nurses include the holding area nurse, circulating nurse, scrub nurse, and any specialty nurses. The number of assistants, circulating nurses, and scrub nurses depends on the complexity and projected length of the surgical procedure. For some minor diagnostic or outpatient procedures, only a scrub nurse or a circulating nurse may be required in addition to the surgeon.

Surgeon and Surgical Assistant

The surgeon is a physician who assumes responsibility for the surgical procedure and any surgical judgments about the client. The surgical assistant might be another surgeon (or physician, such as a resident or intern) or a physician's assistant, nurse, or surgical technologist. Under the direction of the surgeon, the assistant may hold retractors, suction the wound (to allow visualization of the operative site), cut tissue, suture, and dress wounds. Regulating agencies determine who may qualify to be a surgical assistant and usually delineate the functions of the surgical assistant.

Anesthesiologist and Nurse Anesthetist

The anesthesiologist is a physician who specializes in the administration of anesthetic agents. A certified registered

Our Lady of Lourdes Medical Center
1600 Haddon Avenue Camden, N.J. 08103

PRE-OPERATIVE RECORD

PRE-OPERATIVE

Patient Name _____ Surgeon _____ Date _____

Procedure _____

Arrival _____ **ID** ☐ Verbal ☐ Nameband **Pt Verbalizes** ☐ Procedure Site ☐ Surgeon **NPO** Since _____

Allergies: ☐ NDA ☐ Latex ☐ Other _____ ☐ Drugs _____

Lab Data: ☐ CBC   Reports: Consents: Blood Products - # of units
         ☐ Urinalysis   ☐ EKG   ☐ Surgical   In OR _____
         ☐ Chemistry   ☐ Chest   ☐ Blood   Blood Bank _____   ☐ Autologus _____
         ☐ Coag Studies   ☐ H & P   ☐ Anesthesia   ☐ Type and Screen _____ ☐ Directed _____
   _____ ☐ Pregnancy Test   ☐ Other   ☐ Type and Cross _____ ☐ Homologus _____

Equipment: ☐ IV's ☐ Foley ☐ Ventilator ☐ Cardiac Monitor ☐ IABP ☐ Other _____

Prosthesis: ☐ None ☐ Opthalmic ☐ Otic ☐ Dental ☐ Jewelry   Disposition of Prosthesis _____

Orientation: ☐ Awake ☐ Oriented ☐ Sedated ☐ Confused ☐ Agitated ☐ Crying

Implants / Other Comments: _____

_____ RN SIGNATURE _____

INTRA OPERATIVE

Identification: ☐ Verbal ☐ Nameband   Scrub Nurse: ☐ Sees Permits ☐ Aware of Allergies

Skin Condition: ☐ Intact ☐ Presence of Lesions - Type / Location _____

Skin Prep: ☐ Betadine ☐ Hibiclens ☐ Other _____

Position: ☐ Supine ☐ Prone ☐ Lithotomy ☐ Lateral ☐ Jackknife ☐ Fracture Table

☐ Other _____ Positioned by _____

Equipment Codes: **Supports:**

= - Safety Strap   applied by _____ ☐ Kidney Rest _____

X - Grounding Pad applied by _____ ☐ Stirrups _____

T - Tourniquet   applied by _____ ☐ Arms @ Side _____

Δ - Pressure Pads applied by _____ ☐ Arms on Armboard _____

S - Sandbag   applied by _____ ☐ Action Pads _____

R - Roll   applied by _____ ☐ Black Leg Positioner _____

A - Action Donut   applied by _____ ☐ Bean Bag _____

Z - Zoll Defib Pad applied by _____

Tourniquet Unit # _____ mm/Hg _____ Inflated _____ Deflated _____

Warming Blanket Unit # _____ Temp _____ On _____ Off _____

Electrocautery Unit # _____ Coag @ _____ Cut @ _____

Pad # _____ Exp. Date _____ ESU Pad Skin Site _____

Defibrillator # _____ Time / Joules _____

BiPolar Unit # _____ Setting _____ Other Equipment _____

Comments _____

_____ RN SIGNATURE _____

FORM #PO1 (REV. 4/96)

Figure 21–1. A perioperative nursing record with areas for charting preoperatively upon the client's arrival in the operating room (OR) suite and upon initial preparation intraoperatively. (Courtesy of Our Lady of Lourdes Medical Center, Camden, NJ.)

nurse anesthetist (CRNA) is a specially trained registered nurse with additional credentials who administers anesthetics under the supervision of an anesthesiologist, surgeon, dentist, or podiatrist. The anesthesiologist or CRNA administers anesthetic drugs to induce and maintain anesthesia and administers other medications as indicated to support the client's physical status during surgery.

The anesthesiologist or nurse anesthetist usually monitors the client intraoperatively by measuring, assessing, and monitoring the following:

- The level of anesthesia (i.e., by using a peripheral nerve stimulator)
- Cardiopulmonary function (via electrocardiographic [ECG] monitoring, pulse oximetry, end-tidal CO_2 monitoring, arterial blood gases, and hemodynamic monitoring via arterial lines and/or pulmonary artery catheters)
- Vital signs
- Intake and output

Depending on the client's needs, anesthesia personnel administer intravenous (IV) fluids, including blood and blood components, to maintain the client's physiologic homeostasis.

(See Units 3, 6, and 7 for further discussion on fluid balance and acid-base balance; oxygenation; and cardiac monitoring, assessment, and function.)

Operating Room Nurses

Operating room (OR) nurses assume several roles within the operating suite, depending on their education, experience, skill, and job responsibilities.

HOLDING AREA NURSE. Some operating suites feature a presurgical holding area adjacent to the main ORs. The client waits in this area until the OR is ready. The holding room nurse manages the client's care while the client is in this area. This nurse greets the client on arrival, reviews the chart and preoperative checklist, and ensures the operative consent forms are signed. The nurse assesses the client's physical and emotional status, lends emotional support, answers questions, and provides additional education as needed. The nurse initiates documentation on a perioperative nursing record (Fig. 21–1).

The holding area can be very busy, with many staff members performing a number of preoperative procedures (e.g., establishing IV lines or inserting nasogastric tubes). The holding area nurse maintains an atmosphere conducive to the client's overall well-being and intervenes on behalf of the client to maintain comfort, privacy, and confidentiality.

CIRCULATING NURSE. The circulating nurse (who must be a registered nurse) coordinates, oversees, and participates in the client's nursing care while the client is in the OR. The circulating nurse's actions are vital to the smooth flow of events before, during, and after the operation. The circulator sets up the OR, ensures that necessary supplies and equipment are readily available, and checks that all equipment is safe and functional before the surgery. The circulating nurse makes the operating bed (formerly called the OR table) with gel pads (to prevent pressure sores) and heating pads (to prevent hypothermia) under the sheets as indicated.

If there is no holding room nurse, the circulator assumes the responsibilities of that nursing role as well. Even when there is a holding room nurse, the circulator also greets the client and reviews findings with the holding area nurse because the circulator is responsible for continuity of client care.

Once the client is ready to move into the OR, the circulating nurse assists the OR team in transferring the client onto the operating bed. The nurse then positions the client, protecting bony prominences with extra padding as indicated while comforting and reassuring the client. The circulating nurse also assists the anesthesiologist or CRNA with the induction of anesthesia and then may "prep" (scrub) the surgical site before the client is draped with sterile drapes.

Throughout the surgery, the circulating nurse

- Monitors traffic in the room
- Assesses the amount of urine and blood loss
- Reports findings to the surgeon and anesthesia personnel
- Ensures that the surgical team maintains sterile technique and a sterile field
- Documents care, events, interventions and findings

Depending on facility policy, the circulating nurse may obtain and record medications, blood, and blood components. (This may partially be a function of anesthesia personnel.) Before the surgical procedure is over, the circulating nurse completes documentation (Fig. 21–2; see also Fig. 21–1). The nurse notes drains or catheters in place, length of surgery, and a count of all sponges, "sharps" (needles, blades), and instruments. The nurse notifies the postanesthesia care unit (PACU) of the client's estimated time of arrival and any special needs of the client.

SCRUB NURSE AND SURGICAL TECHNOLOGIST. The scrub nurse sets up the sterile field (Fig. 21–3), assists with draping the client, and hands sterile supplies and instruments to the surgeon and the assistant. Knowledge of anatomy and physiology and familiarity with the surgical procedure allow the scrub nurse to anticipate which instruments and types of sutures the surgeon will need; the nurse's ability to anticipate these needs reduces the duration of anesthesia for the client. Throughout the surgical procedure, the scrub nurse (with the circulating nurse) maintains an accurate account of sponges, sharps, and instruments and the amounts of irrigation fluid used.

The scrub role may be performed by a specially trained person who is not a nurse. Such people are called operating room technicians (ORTs) or surgical technologists. (The term *CST* may be used for those who are certified surgical technologists.)

SPECIALTY NURSES. The specialty coordinator nurse is educated in a particular type of surgery (e.g., orthopedic, cardiac, ophthalmologic) and is responsible for intraoperative nursing care specific to clients needing that type of surgery. The specialty coordinator nurse also cares for and maintains equipment and instruments used in the specialty and maintains needed supplies. During surgery, the specialty nurse may function as the scrub or circulating nurse.

If the facility has laser technology, nurses specially trained in the use, care, and maintenance of the laser should be on hand. Such a nurse may be called a laser specialty nurse or a laser nurse coordinator. *Laser* is an

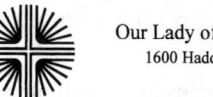

Our Lady of Lourdes Medical Center
1600 Haddon Avenue Camden, N.J. 08103

INTRA-OPERATIVE RECORD

Patient Name _____ Date _____ Suite _____

☐ Scheduled ☐ Emergency ☐ Add On   In Room _____ Began _____ End _____ Out _____

Surgeon _____ Assistant _____

Anesthesia _____ Perfusion/Other _____

Type of Anesthesia: ☐ General   ☐ Spinal   ☐ Epidural   ☐ Regional Block   ☐ Local ASB   ☐ Local

Scrub _____ Circulator _____

Relief _____ Relief _____

Preoperative Diagnosis _____
_____

Postoperative Diagnosis _____
_____

Procedure _____
_____
_____

Clamp/Bypass on _____ off_____   EBL _____

Specimens: Cultures ☐ **Aerobic** ☐ **Anerobic** _____   Implant Log# _____

_____   **Irrigation:** _____

_____   Wound Classification:

_____   Pre-Op   I   II   III   IV

_____   Post-Op   I   II   III   IV

                                                      ASA Classification   I   II   III   IV

Medication Dispensed to OR Table (Include time, drug, amt used, site/route should be prepared by and given by)
_____
_____
_____
_____
_____
_____

Counts: ☐ Correct _____ ☐ Incorrect _____ Comments: _____
_____

Intra operative X-ray   ☐ Yes   ☐ No   Type _____

Drains / Packing: ☐ None ☐ Foley   Inserted by _____ ☐ Immediate urine output

☐ Jackson Pratt / Davol _____ ☐ Hemovac_____ ☐ Penrose _____ ☐ Packing _____ Other _____

☐ Chest Tubes # and size _____ ☐ Pleuravac   ☐ Auto transfusion pleuravac

Post Op Skin Condition: _____

ESU Pad Skin Site _____ Dressing Site _____

Receiving Unit ☐ PACU ☐ CVU ☐ ICU / CCU ☐ SDS ☐ Nursing Unit _____ Report given to _____

RN Signature _____ Surgeon Signature _____

FORM #PO2 (REV. 7/96)   White - Original Copy   Yellow - O.R. Copy   Pink - Surgeon Copy   Goldenrod - Pharmacy Copy

Figure 21–2. An interdisciplinary intra-operative record. Names of all personnel involved are listed, and both the circulating nurse's and surgeon's signatures are required for completion. (Courtesy of Our Lady of Lourdes Medical Center, Camden, NJ.)

acronym for light amplification by the stimulated emission of radiation. A laser emits a high-powered beam of light that cuts tissue more cleanly than scalpel blades do. This process produces intense heat for rapid coagulation of blood vessels or tissue and can turn tissue (such as a tumor) into vapor. It is essential for all personnel to observe safety measures (e.g., eye shields, door signs) during laser procedures.

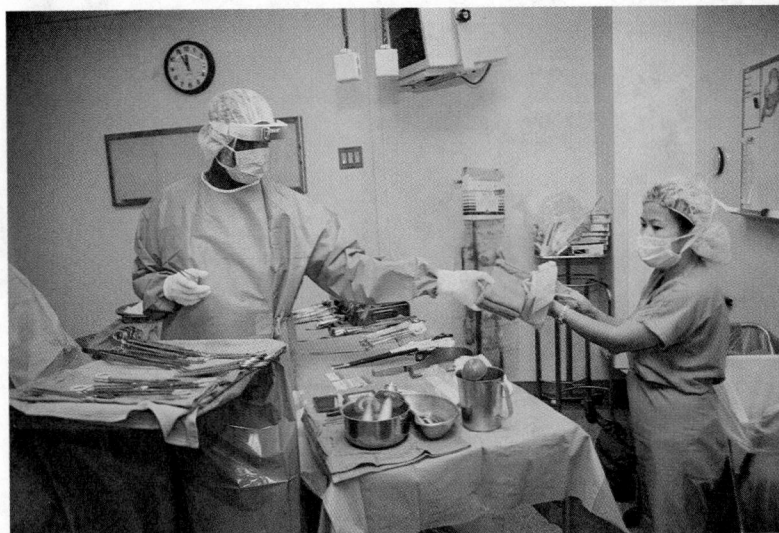

Figure 21–3. Setting up the sterile table.

Preparation of the Surgical Suite and Team Safety

During the intraoperative phase, safety of the client is a primary concern of all members of the surgical team. The operating room (OR) layout is designed to prevent infection by limiting the source of contaminants. The staff uses safety straps for the client and securely locks the operating bed in place. Heating pads are used to prevent hypothermia, and interventions are instituted to prevent skin breakdown.

The nurse ensures electrical safety through proper placement of grounding pads and use of electrical equipment that meets safety standards. All equipment that might be used during surgery must be appropriately cleaned and sterilized and in proper working condition. The nurse ensures a correct count of surgical instruments and sponges before, during, and after surgery.

Fire prevention is of utmost concern to OR personnel, as is prevention of complications associated with the use of hazardous and potentially toxic substances. A cool room temperature and low humidity are optimal, and staff and clients must be protected against thermal or chemical burns caused by fire or spills. The nurse is aware of appropriate emergency measures to take in the event of a fire or spill.

Layout

The surgical suite should be located out of the mainstream of the hospital or facility and adjacent to the postanesthesia unit (PACU) and support services (e.g., blood bank, pathology and laboratory departments). Traffic flow should be such that contamination from outside the suite is minimal. Within the suite, clean and contaminated areas must be separate. Traffic flow is controlled by designating areas as unrestricted, semirestricted, and restricted.

The size of a surgical suite depends on the size and surgical capabilities of the facility. The average suite contains staff changing rooms (staff locker rooms) and staff lounges, an admission (or preoperative holding) area, a scrub area (for staff), a number of ORs, designated cabinets for sterile supplies, separate utility rooms for clean and soiled equipment, and a clean linen room.

Figure 21–4 shows a typical OR. The exact number of tables and specialized equipment used in the room is based on the needs of each client. A reliable communication system provides the vital link between the OR and the main desk of the surgical unit or suite. The system should include an intercom and the capability to differentiate between routine and emergency calls.

Health and Hygiene of the Surgical Team

Everyone has a large number of potentially pathogenic bacteria on the skin and hair and in the respiratory tract. Because these pathogens can be transmitted to the client, special health requirements and dress are required. Health standards require that all members of the surgical team and other support personnel in the surgical suite be free from communicable diseases. Anyone who has an open wound, cold, or other infection should not participate in surgery.

Good personal hygiene aids in the control of infection, as does frequent and appropriate hand washing. Shedding of microorganisms and skin debris is greatest immediately after showering, so surgical staff should bathe a few hours before changing into OR attire. Jewelry, which can carry multiple microorganisms, should be minimal.

In preparing for surgery, all personnel must wash their hands between procedures and more frequently when indicated. Specimens from the hands of surgical personnel may be obtained for culture periodically to maintain an awareness of the potential for nosocomial (hospital-acquired) infections and to identify the source of pathogenic invasion. Further interventions or cultures are necessary if quality reports (e.g., through the Quality Improvement Program or Quality Reviews) indicate a problem. The average time between routine cultures is 3 to 6 months. Surgical attire and the surgical scrub are additional interventions that help to prevent contaminations.

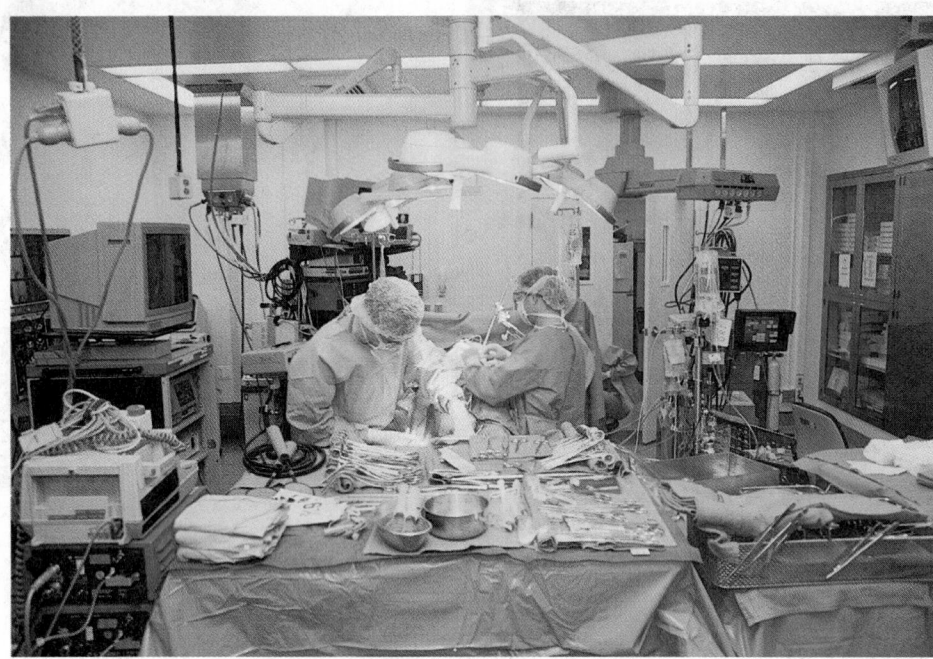

A

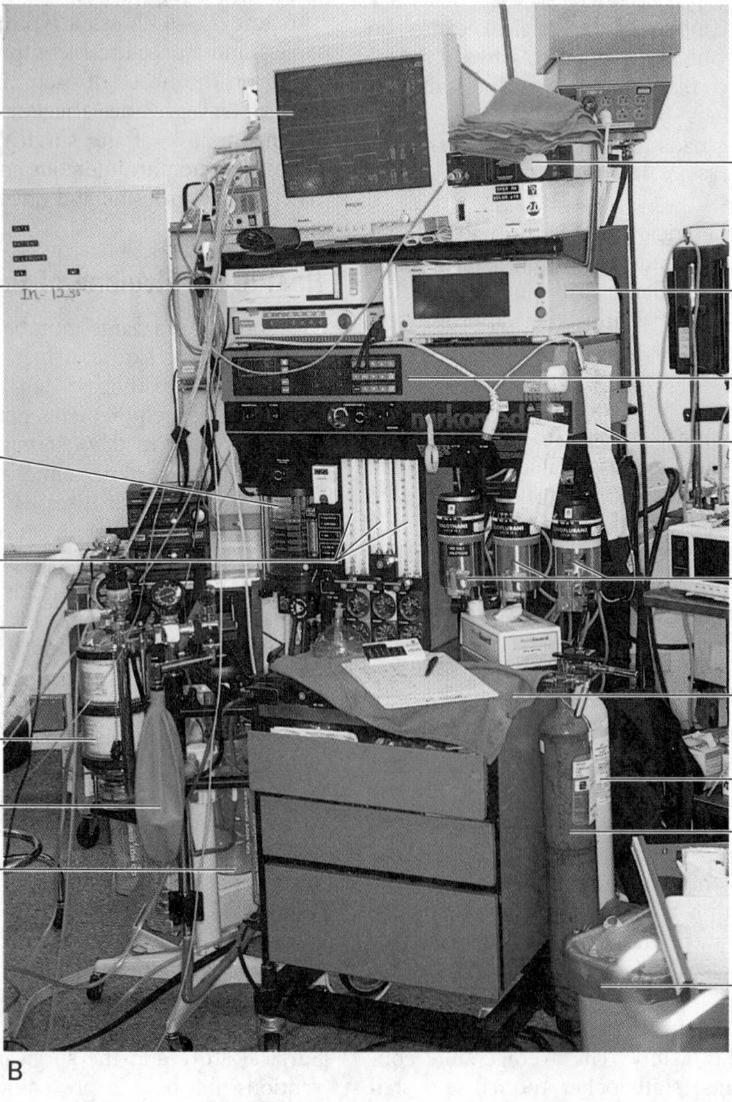

B

Monitor screen displaying client's heart rate and rhythm, blood pressure and other hemodynamic parameters

Printer to accompany the monitor

Ventilator bellows

Nitrous oxide, air, and oxygen flow meters

Anesthesia circuit

Carbon dioxide absorber

Anesthesia breathing bag

Suction canister

Pulse oximeter

Blood pressure monitor

Ventilator

Laboratory results

Vaporizers

Airway equipment (under sterile towel)

Extra supply of air (yellow) and oxygen (green)

Hazardous waste ("red bag" trash)

Figure 21–4. *A,* A typical operating room. *B,* A typical anesthesia station with an anesthesia machine.

Surgical Attire

All members of the surgical team and all OR personnel must wear scrub attire. Scrub attire is clean, not sterile. It is worn to decrease contamination from microorganisms. As one enters the operating *suite,* the basic attire consists of a shirt and pants, a cap or hood (Fig. 21–5), and shoe coverings. Staff change into clean surgical attire in the operating suite locker rooms, not at home. All members of the surgical team must cover their hair.

In addition to basic attire, anyone who enters an OR must wear a mask. Members of the surgical team who are scrubbed to be at the bedside of the client during the surgical procedure must also be in a sterile gown, with sterile gloves and eye protectors (Fig. 21–6). Members of the surgical team in the OR who are *not* scrubbed (e.g., anesthesiologist and circulating nurse) usually wear cover scrub jackets to prevent shedding of organisms from bare arms.

Surgical Scrub

The surgeon, all assistants, and the scrub nurse perform the surgical scrub after putting on a mask and before putting on the sterile gown and gloves (Fig. 21–7). The scrub does not make the hands and forearms sterile; however, when it is effectively carried out, it reduces the number of microorganisms.

A disposable scrub brush or sponge, impregnated with an antimicrobial solution, and a nail cleaner are used. As with hand washing, the effectiveness of the scrub depends on the application of friction from the fingertips to the elbow. The surgical scrub usually continues for 3 to 5 minutes (see Research Applications for Nursing), followed by a rinse. During the rinse, surgical personnel position their hands and arms in such a way that water runs off, rather than up or down, their arms. After scrubbing,

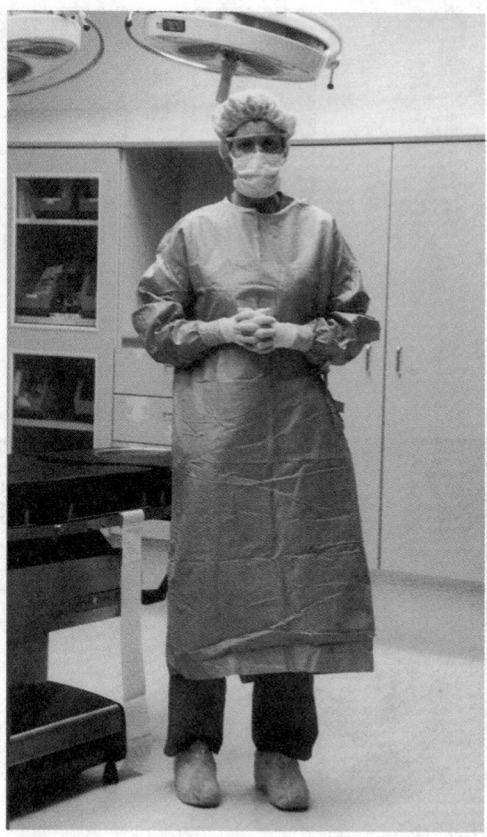

Figure 21–6. Typical attire for all scrubbed personnel. Note complete hair covering, eye shields, mask, sterile gloves over the sleeves of the sterile gown, and shoe coverings. Note that when not in use, the hands are typically folded in front of the body, never below the waist.

personnel enter the OR with their hands held higher than the elbows and thoroughly dry their hands and forearms with a sterile towel. After drying, the scrubbed staff member is assisted into a sterile gown ("gowning") and puts on sterile gloves ("gloving").

Gowns, gloves, and materials used at the operative field must be sterile and are changed between surgical procedures. The areas of the surgical gown considered sterile are the front of the gown from 2 inches below the neck to the waist area, and the elbow to wrist area. Only when they are properly scrubbed and attired should members of the surgical team handle sterile drapes and other equipment.

Anesthesia

The word *anesthesia* comes from the Greek word *anesthesis,* meaning "negative sensation." Administration of anesthesia is an exact and sophisticated science requiring the skill of a licensed anesthesiologist or a certified registered nurse anesthetist (CRNA).

Anesthesia is an artificially induced state of partial or total loss of sensation, occurring with or without loss of consciousness. The purpose of anesthesia is to block the transmission of nerve impulses, suppress reflexes, promote muscular relaxation, and, in some cases, achieve a

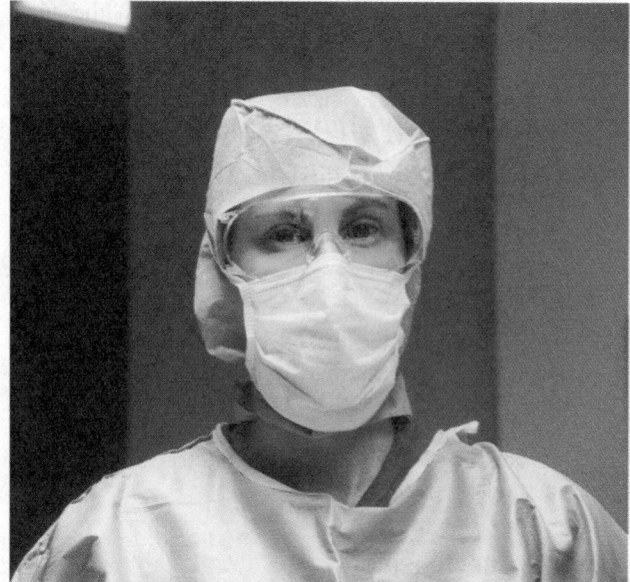

Figure 21–5. An example of a hood-type hair covering that adequately covers facial and scalp hair.

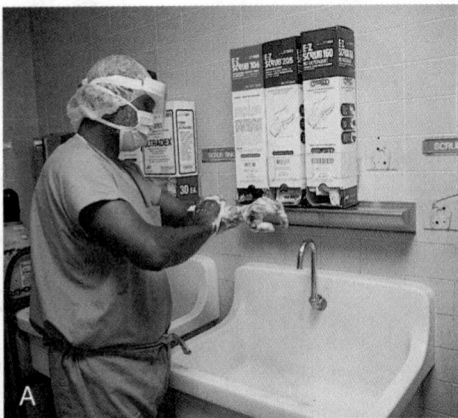
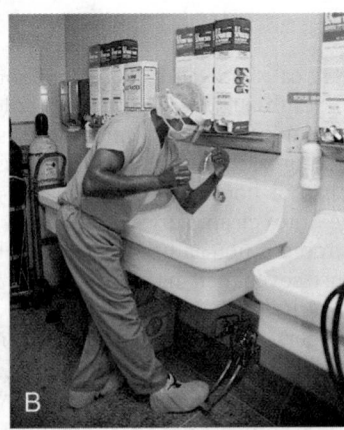
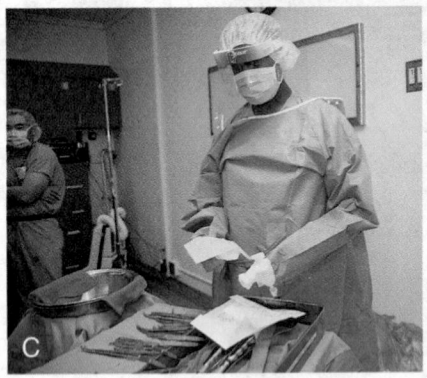
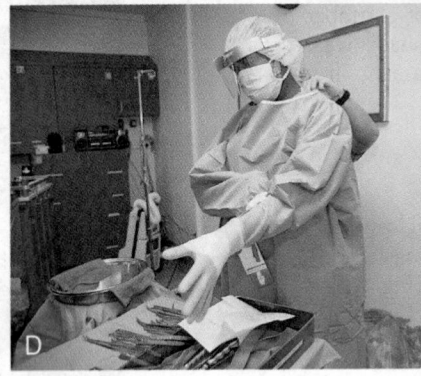
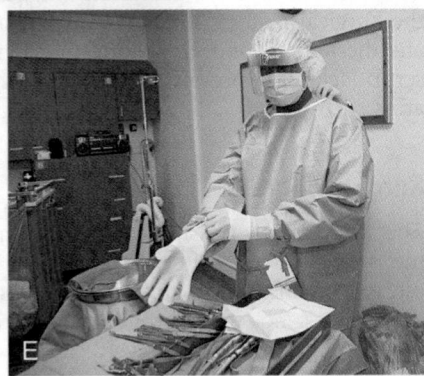

Figure 21–7. The scrubbing, gowning, and gloving process. *A,* The surgical scrub. *B,* Rinsing. Note the water falling off the hands and arms. Also note the foot-operated handle that controls the water flow. (After scrubbing and rinsing, the scrub nurse dries his hands and arms with a sterile towel inside the operating room, then is assisted into a sterile gown.) *C,* The scrub nurse prepares sterile gloves. Note that the scrub nurse's hands are *inside* the sleeve of the gown and that he is touching the sterile gloves only with the sterile sleeve. *D,* The scrub nurse puts on his first sterile glove while the sterile gown is being tied in the back. Note again that his hand never emerges from under the sterile sleeve. *E,* The scrub nurse puts on his second sterile glove.

controlled level of unconsciousness. Anesthesia personnel use a separate anesthesia record for documentation (Fig. 21–8).

The choice of anesthesia is determined primarily by the anesthesiologist or CRNA after consultation with the surgeon and consideration of specific client-related factors. The nurse or client or both communicate the client's preference and fears related to a particular type of anesthesia to the anesthesiologist or CRNA. Specific problems noted in the client's history or preoperative physical examination are major factors in the selection and dosage of anesthesia. Selection is also influenced by the following factors:

- Type and duration of the procedure
- Area of body being operated on
- Whether the procedure is an emergency
- How long it has been since the client ate
- The client position indicated for the surgical procedure

The administration of anesthesia begins with the selection and administration of preoperative medication, if any (see Chap. 20).

The nurse should know the pharmacologic characteristics of commonly used agents and their effects on the client during and after surgery. Anesthesia produces multiple systemic effects, which can affect the client's care

and can compound other coexisting problems. For example, most anesthetics are metabolized by the liver and excreted by the kidneys. Hepatic or renal dysfunction can significantly enhance anesthetic effects and toxicity. In addition, drug interactions may occur between the anesthetic agents and other medications the client has been receiving.

The state of anesthesia may be produced in a number of ways (Table 21–1):

- General or balanced anesthesia
- Local or regional anesthesia
- Hypnosis or hypnoanesthesia
- Cryothermia
- Acupuncture

Hypnosis or hypnoanesthesia (which induces a passive trance-like state), cryothermia (use of cold—for example, with ice—to lower the surface temperature of the surgical site), and acupuncture are not commonly used in the United States or Canada. However, interest in the use of these methods is growing.

General Anesthesia

General anesthesia is a reversible state in which the client loses consciousness as a result of the inhibition of neuro-

Research Applications for Nursing

A 2-Minute Scrub May Be as Effective as a 3-Minute Scrub

Wheelock, S. M., & Lookinland, S. (1997). Effect of surgical hand scrub time on subsequent bacterial growth. AORN Journal, 65(6), 1087–1090, 1092, 1094–1098.

The researchers note that the effectiveness of the surgical hand scrub, which is supposed to reduce surgical wound infections, has not been confirmed by study. They review the history of handwashing and gloving during surgery and note that today, scrub times vary facility to facility from 2 to 10 minutes. They cite studies that have shown a 5-minute scrub to be as effective as a 10-minute scrub and report on a study that concluded that 3 minutes was an effective scrub time.

In this study, 25 surgical nurses and technologists performed either a 2- or 3-minute scrub. Then, using a cross-over sampling scheme after a minimum of 7 days in between, the same subject scrubbed a second time for the alternate amount of time. After the scrub, the subject wore sterile gloves and went about his or her regular duties, but without contact with patients or any of the sterile fields. After 1 hour, samples of the subject's glove juice were taken.

On average, the bacteria count after the 2-minute scrub was higher than that after the 3-minute scrub. In 11 instances, however, the 2-minute scrub performed better than the 3-minute scrub. Both the 2- and 3-minute scrubs resulted in bacteria counts of less than 0.5 log, which is the threshold for practical and clinical significance. This finding suggests that 2-minute scrubs are as effective as 3-minute scrubs. The incidence of glove perforation was 4%.

Critique. Not all subjects in the study used the same surgical scrub agent, although one of the three most popular agents was used in all cases.

Possible Nursing Implications. If surgical scrub times can be reduced without untoward effects, the operating staff will have more time to devote to other aspects of patient care, increasing the cost-effectiveness of their care. Cost savings would be achieved from using less water. Further, because of a possible decrease in hand irritations, staff may not lose as much time from work.

---

nal impulses in the brain. This state is achieved by the administration of a single agent or a combination of chemical agents. The anesthetic agents used induce depression of the central nervous system (CNS), a depression characterized by analgesia (pain relief or pain suppression), amnesia (memory loss of the surgery), and unconsciousness, with loss of muscle tone and reflexes. The client is unconscious, unaware, and anesthetized. Some indications for general anesthesia include surgery of the head, neck, and upper torso; extensive abdominal surgery; and situations in which clients are unable to cooperate.

STAGES OF GENERAL ANESTHESIA. Four stages of general anesthesia are classically described. Table 21–2 presents the client's physiologic responses and nursing interventions for each stage.

The speed of *emergence,* or recovery from the anesthesia, depends on the type of anesthetic agent, the length of time the client is anesthetized, and whether a reversal agent for the neuromuscular blocking agent has been administered. Although not as common as they once were (because of advances made in the pharmacology of anesthesia), retching, vomiting, and restlessness may occur during emergence; the nurse has suction equipment available to prevent aspiration. During recovery, shivering, rigidity, and slight cyanosis are not uncommon; these phenomena may reflect a temporary disturbance in the body's temperature control. The nurse provides the client with warm blankets, radiant light, and oxygen to decrease the undesirable effects of emergence.

ADMINISTRATION OF GENERAL ANESTHESIA. The two methods of administering general anesthesia are inhalation and intravenous (IV) injection.

Inhalation. Inhalation is the most controllable method of administering general anesthesia because intake and elimination of the anesthetic are accomplished primarily by respiration. The lungs act as a passageway for entrance and exit of the anesthetic agent. The client inhales the anesthetic vapor of a volatile liquid or the anesthetic gas via mask; the anesthetic then passes across the alveolar membrane to the general circulation. It is transported, via the bloodstream, to the various tissues, where it is metabolized.

To improve ventilation and control the anesthesia, respiration may be assisted or controlled. With *assisted* respiration, an endotracheal (ET) tube is inserted. It is then connected to a reservoir (breathing) bag of the anesthesia machine (see Fig. 21–4). The anesthesiologist overrides, or "assists," the client's own respiratory effort to initiate the respiratory cycle by manually compressing the reservoir bag.

Controlled respiration can be accomplished with the use of a mechanical device (such as a mechanical ventilator) that automatically and rhythmically inflates the lungs with intermittent positive pressure; the client is not required to participate. Controlled ventilation is initiated after the anesthesiologist has produced apnea either through hyperventilation or by administering respiratory depressant or neuromuscular blocker drugs.

The anesthesiologist or CRNA inserts the ET tube, with the assistance of the circulating nurse. A laryngoscope is used to visualize the vocal cords, and the tube is placed in the trachea (Fig. 21–9). With the ET tube safely in place, the client has an open airway (through the tube) and an avenue for the safe administration of the inhaled anesthetic and oxygen.

Inhalation anesthetic agents are divided into two categories: gases and volatile agents. Table 21–3 lists the advantages, disadvantages, and related nursing implications of various inhalation anesthetic agents.

GASEOUS AGENTS. In the past, gaseous agents included ether and cyclopropane gas. *Nitrous oxide* (N_2O) is now the most commonly used gaseous anesthetic agent and is usually administered with oxygen. It is a colorless, odor-

OUR LADY OF LOURDES MEDICAL CENTER
CAMDEN, NEW JERSEY

ANESTHESIA RECORD

DATE	ANESTHESIA RECORD NUMBER
CONSENT	PHYS. STATUS 1 2 3 4 E1 E2 E3 E4 5
PREMEDICATION (DRUG, DOSE, TIME, EFFECT)	

NAME
ADDRESS
ROOM
MEDICAL RECORDS NUMBER
SEX
AGE
BUSINESS DATA PLATE

15 30 45 15 30 45 15 30 45 15 30 45 15 30

N_2O
O_2
AGENTS
FLUIDS

B.P. ∨ ∧	°C	
		240
	38	220
PULSE •	36	200
START ANES X	34	180
	32	160
START OP ⊙	30	140
END ANES ⊗		120
		100
TEMP △		80
SUCTION S		60
		40
REC. ROOM R		20
RESP. O	SPON ASST. CONT. VENT.	10

SYMBOLS

PREOPERATIVE DIAGNOSIS

AGENTS	TECHNIQUES	DOSAGE
A.		
B.		
C.		
D.		
E.		
F.		
G.		

REMARKS (INDUCTION, MAINTENANCE, EMERGENCE)

FLUID SUMMARY	RECOVERY (OR)
DEXTROSE - H_2O	REFLEX IN OR YES______NO ___
RING - LAC	CONSC. IN OR YES______NO ___
SALINE	NAUSEA ______EMESIS ______
PLASMA	HYPOTENSION
BLOOD	
OTHER	
BLO. LOSS, HOW MEASURED	

POST OPERATIVE DIAGNOSIS

OPERATION

SURGEON	ANESTHETIST

1. OP NP OT NT (D - B)
2. CUFF-PACK TUBE SIZE________
3. TECHNICAL DIFFICULTY
4. MACHINE
   VAPORIZER
   MONITOR

OLLH FORM F20 (12/81)

Figure 21–8. An anesthesia record. (Courtesy of Our Lady of Lourdes Medical Center, Camden, NJ.)

TABLE 21–1

Advantages and Disadvantages of Various Types of Anesthesia

Type	Advantages	Disadvantages
General		
Inhalation	• Most controllable method • Induction and reversal accomplished with pulmonary ventilation • Few side effects	• Must be used in combination with other agents for painful or prolonged procedures • Limited muscle relaxant effects • Postoperative nausea and shivering common • Explosive
Intravenous	• Rapid and pleasant induction • Low incidence of postoperative nausea and vomiting • Requires little equipment	• Must be metabolized and excreted from the body for complete reversal • Contraindicated in presence of hepatic or renal disease • Increased cardiac and respiratory depression • Retained by fat cells
Balanced	• Minimal disturbance to physiologic function • Minimal side effects • Can be used with elderly and high-risk clients	• Drug interactions can occur • Pharmacological effects on the body may be unpredictable
Regional or Local	• Gag and cough reflexes stay intact • Allows participation and cooperation by the client • Less disruption of physical and emotional body functions • Decreased chance of sensitivity to the agent • Decreased intraoperative stress	• Difficult to administer to an uncooperative or upset client • No way to control agent after administration • Absorbs rapidly into the blood and causes cardiac depression (hypotension) or overdose • Increased nervous system stimulation (overdose) • Not practical for extensive procedures because of the amount of drug that would be required to maintain anesthesia

less, nonirritating gas and provides analgesia equivalent to 10 mg of morphine sulfate.

VOLATILE AGENTS. Liquids vaporized for inhalation are considered volatile agents. Oxygen acts as a carrier, flowing over or bubbling through the liquid in the vaporizer system on the anesthesia machine. All volatile agents can produce postoperative shivering in the client because of an effect on the hypothalamus. Awakening is usually rapid, within 15 to 20 minutes.

Halothane (Fluothane). Halothane is a halogenated hydrocarbon that depresses the cardiovascular system. The intraoperative use of epinephrine to control bleeding may exacerbate or precipitate a dysrhythmia when halothane is used. Clients can have memory impairment for up to 24 hours later.

Enflurane (Ethrane). Enflurane is an inhalation anesthetic agent that reduces the client's ventilations and decreases blood pressure as the depth of anesthesia increases.

Isoflurane (Forane). Isoflurane is another halogenated compound and appears to be a preferred inhalation agent.

Desflurane (Suprane). Desflurane produces a rapid induction of anesthesia but can cause coughing and excitation during the process. The rapid elimination of desflurane produces awakening in 8 to 10 minutes. Cardiopulmonary depressant effects and malignant hyperthermia are the most common adverse effects.

Sevoflurane (Sevoflurane). Sevoflurane is like desflurane, except less coughing and laryngospasm occur with sevoflurane. Adverse effects are similar to those associated with desflurane.

Intravenous (IV) Injection. Intravenous anesthetic agents are injected, usually via a peripheral IV line, into the circulation. A pleasant, rapid, and smooth dissipation of the agent occurs. The drug is diluted by the blood, but it travels in high concentration to the organs of high

TABLE 21-2

The Four Stages of General Anesthesia and Related Nursing Interventions

Stage	Description	Nursing Interventions	Rationale
Stage 1 (Analgesia and Sedation, Relaxation)	• Begins with induction and ends with loss of consciousness. • Client feels drowsy and dizzy, has a reduced sensation to pain, and is amnesic. • Hearing is exaggerated.	• Close operating room doors, dim the lights, and control traffic in the operating room. • Position client securely with safety belts. • Keep discussions about the client to a minimum.	• Avoiding external stimuli in the environment promotes relaxation. • Using safety measures in stage 1 prepares for stage 2. • Being sensitive to the client maintains his or her dignity.
Stage 2 (Excitement, Delirium)	• Begins with loss of consciousness and ends with relaxation, regular breathing, and loss of the eyelid reflex. • Client may have irregular breathing, increased muscle tone, and involuntary movement of the extremities during this stage. • Laryngospasm or vomiting may occur. • Client is susceptible to external stimuli.	• Avoid auditory and physical stimuli. • Protect the extremities. • Assist the anesthesiologist or CRNA with suctioning as needed. • Stay with client.	• Sensory stimuli can contribute to the client's response. • Safety measures help to prevent injury. • Staying with the client is emotionally supportive.
Stage 3 (Operative Anesthesia, Surgical Anesthesia)	• Begins with generalized muscle relaxation and ends with loss of reflexes and depression of vital functions. • The jaw is relaxed, and there is quiet, regular breathing. • The client cannot hear. • Sensations are lost (i.e., to pain).	• Assist the anesthesiologist or CRNA with intubation. • Place client into operative position. • Prep (scrub) the client's skin over the operative site as directed.	• Providing assistance helps promote smooth intubation and prevent injury. • Performing procedures as soon as possible promotes time management to minimize total anesthesia time for the client.
Stage 4 (Danger)	• Begins with depression of vital functions and ends with respiratory failure, cardiac arrest, and possible death. • Respiratory muscles are paralyzed, apnea occurs. • Pupils fixed and dilated.	• Prepare for and assist in treatment of cardiac and/or pulmonary arrest. • Document occurrence in the client's chart.	• Teamwork and preparedness help decrease injuries and complications, and promote the possibility of a desired outcome for the client.

blood flow (brain, liver, and kidneys). The reversal and removal of the agent from circulation are not possible with IV injection, and the recovery from the agent is directly related to the client's metabolism. Table 21-4 lists advantages, disadvantages, and related nursing implications of various intravenous anesthetic agents.

BARBITURATES. Barbiturates are often used for IV induction of anesthesia. These drugs act directly on the central nervous system, producing a reaction ranging from mild sedation to unconsciousness. The principal barbiturate used is thiopental sodium (Pentothal), which can also be used for rectal induction. Intravenously, it acts rapidly, resulting in unconsciousness in 30 seconds. Because thiopental is a potent respiratory and cardiovascular system depressant, the client's vital signs must be monitored continuously during administration.

KETAMINE (KETALAR). Ketamine is a dissociative anesthetic agent (one that promotes a feeling of dissociation from the environment). It acts by selectively interrupting various pathways in the brain. Rapid onset of a trance-like, analgesic state occurs. It is commonly used for diagnostic and short surgical procedures or to supplement weaker agents, such as nitrous oxide.

During the client's recovery from ketamine, emergence reactions are expected. The OR nurse reports the use of the drug to the postanesthesia nurse so that safety precautions can be implemented. If the client is combative or restless, the nurse pads the side rails of the bed to prevent injury. The nurse minimizes external stimuli until the client awakens naturally. For severe reactions during the recovery phase, small doses of diazepam (Valium, Vivol✦, Novodipam✦) may be given as needed. The medical-surgical nurse continues interventions until the effects of the drug have worn off.

PROPOFOL (DIPRIVAN). Propofol is in a newer classification of IV anesthetic agents, the alkylphenols. Its short action makes it desirable as an anesthetic agent. Hypnosis occurs

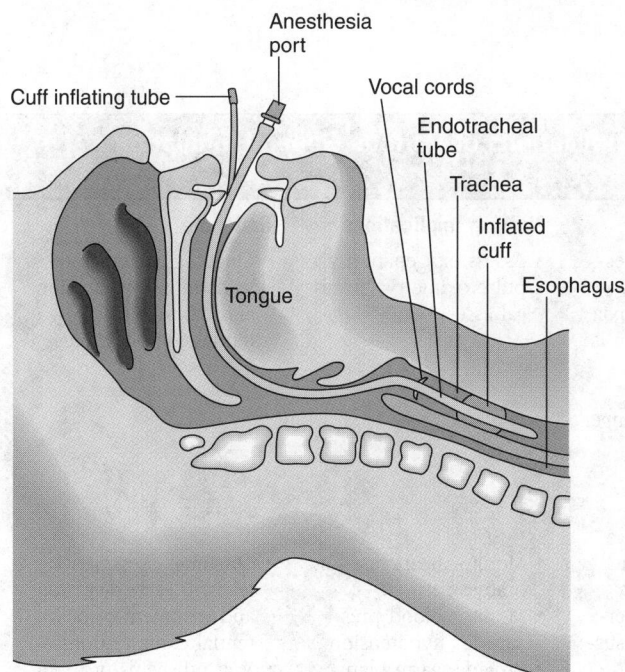

Figure 21–9. An oral endotracheal tube in position. The cuff of the tube was placed just below the vocal cords, then inflated to seal off the airway.

in less than 1 minute from the time of injection, and because the drug is so rapidly metabolized, it does not accumulate during maintenance of the anesthesia. The client becomes responsive quickly after the infusion is ended (within 8 minutes). Propofol is also used to supplement nitrous oxide during short procedures and is used as a hypnotic agent with regional anesthesia.

ADJUNCTS TO THE GENERAL ANESTHESIA AGENTS. Other drugs, such as hypnotics, opioid analgesics, and neuromuscular blocking agents, may be used as part of the anesthesia regimen.

Hypnotics. The benzodiazepines may be used for various effects. Common drugs in this classification include midazolam (Versed), lorazepam (Ativan, Novolorazem♣), and diazepam (Valium, Vivol♣, Novodipam♣). All have hypnotic, sedative, antianxiety, muscle relaxant, and amnesic effects. Generally, lower doses are ordered for preoperative sedation. Each may be used as part of an IV conscious sedation regimen for diagnostic or endoscopic procedures. Higher doses of midazolam may be used to induce general anesthesia. The benzodiazepines may also be used intraoperatively in conjunction with regional or local anesthesia. Adverse reactions include respiratory depression, apnea, and oversedation.

Opioid Analgesics. Common opioid analgesics used to supplement inhalation anesthesia include morphine sulfate (Statex♣), meperidine hydrochloride (Demerol), fentanyl citrate (Sublimaze), and sufentanil (Sufenta). The

use of opioids during surgery contributes to postoperative analgesia. All opioid analgesics decrease alveolar ventilation and are respiratory depressants. The nurse monitors respirations and maintains an open airway. Reduced dosages are prescribed for the elderly, the client with a circulatory problem (such as heart failure), and the debilitated client.

Fentanyl and sufentanil provide analgesia in lower doses, but at higher doses, they can be used as the anesthetic agent. Fentanyl has a potency 75 to 125 times greater than that of morphine (Omoigui, 1995). Sufentanil has five to seven times the analgesic potency of fentanyl (Omoigui, 1995) and produces a more rapid onset of central nervous system effects than does fentanyl. It is often used in open heart surgery when the sternum must be opened. The nurse monitors the client who has received sufentanil for bradycardia and decreased cardiac output.

Neuromuscular Blocking Agents. The neuromuscular blockers are used to relax the jaw and vocal cords immediately after induction so the anesthesiologist or certified registered nurse anesthetist (CRNA) can pass the endotracheal tube. These drugs are also used throughout the surgical procedure to provide continued overall muscle relaxation. Neuromuscular blocking agents act on the striated muscles of the body by interfering with impulse transmission at the neuromuscular junction. The drugs are administered intravenously in small amounts and may cause circulatory alterations and decreased respirations or apnea from muscle paralysis. The nurse ensures the client's safety by securing the client on the operating bed with safety straps and assists the anesthesiologist or CRNA with intubation. Throughout the surgery, the anesthesiologist or CRNA checks the effectiveness of the blocker agent by using a peripheral nerve stimulator. There are two types of neuromuscular blocking agents: non-depolarizing and depolarizing.

NON-DEPOLARIZING BLOCKER AGENTS. The non-depolarizing blockers block acetylcholine at the neuromuscular junction. Only skeletal muscles are blocked, and the drug is easily reversed with an antidote of neostigmine and atropine. Examples of non-depolarizing blockers include pancuronium (Pavulon), atracurium (Tracrium), vecuronium (Norcuron), doxacurium (Nuromax), tubocurarine (Tubarine♣), and mivacurium (Mivacron). Pancuronium has has a relatively long effect (45–60 minutes) compared with vecuronium (25–30 minutes) or mivacurium (6–16 minutes). The longer the effect of the drug, the longer it takes for the client to recover.

DEPOLARIZING BLOCKER AGENTS. The depolarizing blocker agents, also called "noncompetitive" blockers, depolarize the motor end plate at the neuromuscular junction. In the process, potassium is forced out of the muscle cells and into general circulation, which can cause hyperkalemia. Clients often experience transient intraoperative muscle twitching, which can result in generalized muscle aches after awakening. There is no specific antidote. Other side effects include increased salivation, which puts the client

TABLE 21–3

Advantages, Disadvantages, and Related Nursing Implications of Various General Inhalation Anesthetic Agents				
Agent	**Advantages**	**Disadvantages**	**Nursing Implications**	**Rationale**
Nitrous oxide (N₂O)	• Rapid induction and recovery • Useful for short procedures • When used with other agents, reduces the required concentration of the other agents • Minimal cardiovascular and respiratory depression	• Relatively weak anesthetic agent • May produce hypoxia if the concentration is high • Needs addition of other agents for longer procedures	• Assess oxygenation via pulse oximetry, physical assessment.	• Ongoing assessment leads to early detection and treatment of potential complications.
Halothane (Fluothane)	• Rapid and smooth induction • Low incidence of postoperative nausea and vomiting • Less irritating to the respiratory tract than other inhalation agents • Sweet smell makes it easy to use in children • Tolerated well by children	• Shivering common postoperatively • Malignant hyperthermia is possible in susceptible clients. • Metabolized by the liver • Hypotension and bradycardia may occur. • Can sensitize the myocardium to dysrhythmias	• Monitor heart rate for bradycardia. • Monitor blood pressure for hypotension. • Provide warm blankets, radiant heat.	• Ongoing assessment leads to early detection and treatment of potential complications. • Warmth helps promote client comfort and decrease shivering.
Enflurane (Ethrane)	• Rapid induction and recovery • Does not alter heart rate or rhythm	• Respiratory depression and hypotension may occur. • Malignant hyperthermia is possible in susceptible clients. • Lowers seizure threshold	• Monitor respiratory rate and depth for hypoventilation. • Assess oxygenation via pulse oximetry, physical assessment. • Monitor blood pressure for hypotension.	• Ongoing assessment leads to early detection and treatment of potential complications.
Isoflurane (Forane)	• Rapid induction and recovery • Has some muscle relaxant properties • Stimulates heart, which helps keep a stable heart rate • Is not significantly metabolized; no renal or hepatic damage	• Respiratory depression may occur. • Malignant hyperthermia is possible in susceptible clients.	• Monitor respiratory rate and depth for hypoventilation.	• Ongoing assessment leads to early detection and treatment of potential complications.
Desflurane (Suprane)	• Rapid induction, recovery and awakening	• May cause coughing and excitement during induction. • Deep levels of anesthesia may increase heart rate and blood pressure. • Malignant hyperthermia is possible in susceptible clients. • May cause changes in mental function.	• Monitor heart rate and blood pressure. • Caution client and family that client should not drive or operate hazardous machinery until mental status has returned to preoperative baseline.	• Ongoing assessment leads to early detection and treatment of potential complications. • Specific instructions will help prevent other injuries or accidents.

TABLE 21–4

Advantages, Disadvantages, and Related Nursing Implications of Various General Intravenous Anesthetic Agents

Agent	Advantages	Disadvantages	Nursing Implications	Rationale
Barbiturates				
Thiopental sodium (Pentothal), methohexital sodium (Brevital), thiamylal sodium (Surital)	• Rapid, pleasant induction and recovery • Acts directly on the central nervous system • Short-acting • Low incidence of postoperative nausea and vomiting	• Strong respiratory and cardiovascular depressant effect • No antagonist medication available • Mild to severe local tissue reaction with extravasation • Poor analgesic, muscle relaxant effects	• Monitor respiratory rate and depth for hypoventilation. • Monitor heart rate for bradycardia. • Monitor blood pressure for hypotension. • Assess IV site.	• Ongoing assessment leads to early detection and treatment of potential complications.
Nonbarbiturates				
Ketamine hydrochloride (Ketalar)	• Rapid induction • Short-acting • Can be given IM or IV • No respiratory depression or loss of muscle tone (protects the airway) • Protective reflexes remain intact • Stimulates the cardiovascular system • Can use for clients with respiratory or cardiac disorders • Good amnesic effect • Postop emergence reactions generally last only 24 hr	• Emergence reactions are common: hallucinations, irrational behaviors, distorted images, unpleasant dreams, restlessness • Increased heart rate • Increased blood pressure • Increased cardiac output • Poor muscle relaxant effect • Nausea, vomiting, and aspiration can occur	• Minimize external stimuli: noise, light, touch, movement. • Speak in a calm, soothing voice. • Reassure client and family that emergence reactions are common and temporary. • Have suction equipment near. • Monitor blood pressure for hypertension. • Monitor heart rate for tachycardia.	• Stimuli increase the severity of the emergence reaction. • Quiet promotes comfort, decreases anxiety. • Reassurance decreases anxiety. • Suction may be needed in the event of vomiting to prevent aspiration. • Ongoing assessment leads to early detection and treatment of potential complications.
Propofol (Diprivan)	• Short-acting • Rapidly metabolized • Client becomes responsive quickly postoperatively • Minimal postoperative nausea, vomiting, or sedation	• Allergic skin reactions have occurred • Client becomes aware of postoperative pain and discomfort sooner than with other anesthetics	• Be prepared to administer analgesic medications as ordered early in the postoperative period. • Plan for nonpharmacologic pain interventions (see Chapter 9).	• Awareness of pain very early in the postoperative period can be frightening. • Pain can increase blood pressure and increase anxiety.
Opioids (as adjunct)				
Fentanyl (Sublimaze)	• Excellent postoperative analgesia • Long-acting analgesia	• Significant respiratory depression can occur several hours after administration • Cardiovascular depression can occur	• Monitor respiratory rate and depth for hypoventilation. • Monitor blood pressure for hypotension. • Have atropine, naloxone (Narcan), vasopressors, and resuscitative equipment nearby.	• Ongoing assessment leads to early detection and treatment of potential complications. • Having necessary supplies and equipment available provides for prompt response to an emergency.

at risk for aspiration, and increased intraocular pressure, which may be contraindicated with glaucoma. An example of a depolarizing blocker is succinylcholine (Anectine).

BALANCED ANESTHESIA. Balanced anesthesia is widely used. It provides a safe and controlled anesthetic experience, especially for elderly and high-risk clients. A combination of agents is used to provide hypnosis, amnesia, analgesia, muscle relaxation, and relaxation of reflexes with minimal disturbance of the client's physiologic function. An example of balanced anesthesia is the use of a barbiturate (such as thiopental) administered intravenously for induction, nitrous oxide for amnesia, morphine for analgesia, and a muscle relaxant (such as pancuronium) to provide additional relaxation of the muscles.

A second example of balanced anesthesia is the use of 70% nitrous oxide for induction and maintenance (to prevent awareness throughout the procedure and to prevent recall afterward), 30% oxygen to maintain the client's oxygenation saturation greater than 90%, along with an opioid and a muscle relaxant. Many combinations are possible, and selection reflects assessment of the individual client and the specific surgical procedure.

COMPLICATIONS FROM GENERAL ANESTHESIA OR ANESTHESIA MANAGEMENT. Complications can range from minor and annoying to the most severe—death.

Malignant Hyperthermia. Malignant hyperthermia (MH) is an acute, life-threatening complication of general anesthesia. The client with a genetic predisposition for MH is at risk for this complication from certain MH-triggering general anesthetic agents, including halothane, enflurane, isoflurane, desflurane, sevoflurane, and succinylcholine. Stressors, such as severe fatigue, strenuous exercise, muscle injury, and emotional stress, may also trigger this crisis. A biochemical reaction occurs as a result of a defect in the muscle cell membrane, causing a rise in the circulating calcium level, an increase in metabolic rate, hyperkalemia, and metabolic and respiratory acidosis.

Signs of malignant hypothermia include tachycardia or other dysrhythmia; muscle rigidity, especially of the jaw (masseter muscle rigidity) and upper chest; hypotension; tachypnea; and skin mottling, cyanosis, and myoglobinuria (cola-colored urine). The first indication is an unexpected rise in the end-tidal CO_2 level with a decrease in oxygen saturation (Dunn, 1997). The second indication may be unexplained sinus tachycardia. Extremely elevated temperature, perhaps as high as 44° C (111.2° F), is a late sign of MH. Treatment and survival of the client depend on early diagnosis and cooperation of the entire surgical team.

Once a client or family history of MH is known, close family members can undergo a muscle biopsy to determine whether they are at risk. In the case of a known history or predetermination, the client can be treated preoperatively, intraoperatively, and postoperatively with dantrolene to prevent this complication. Chart 21–1 summarizes the nursing care of the client with malignant hyperthermia.

Overdose. An anesthesia overdose can occur if the client's pharmacokinetics do not react or respond as expected. Drugs (e.g., antihypertensive medications) also alter the pharmacokinetics, and drug interactions can occur between the anesthetic agents and other regularly administered medications. Accurate, accessible information about the client, such as height, weight, and history, is

---

Chart 21–1

Nursing Care Highlight: Malignant Hyperthermia

The Susceptible Client

- Assess client and family history preoperatively for signs and symptoms of malignant hyperthermia (MH) or of muscular dystrophy.
- Counsel client regarding quadriceps femoris muscle biopsy to determine his or her predisposition to MH.
- Assist client in finding a muscle biopsy testing center.
- Provide information about MH and the MH Association of the United States (MHAUS).
- Reassure the client that surgery can still be performed safely.

The Client in Malignant Hyperthermia Crisis

- Call for help!
- Assist the physician and anesthesiologist and/or certified registered nurse anesthetist with the immediate discontinuation of surgery.
- Hyperventilate with 100% oxygen (15–20 L/min).
- Call the malignant hyperthermia hotline at 800-644-9737.
- Reconstitute dantrolene (Dantrium) with sterile *distilled* water.
- Give 2.5–10.0 mg/kg of dantrolene (Dantrium) intravenously as ordered.
- With increasing body temperature, or if temperature is greater than 40° C (104° F), cool the client with external ice packs, iced intravenous (IV) saline; iced lavages of the rectum, stomach, and wound; and hypothermia blankets for over and under the client as ordered. Discontinue cooling when the client's body temperature is less than 38° C (100.4° F).
- Collect urine and blood specimens as ordered.
- Have sodium bicarbonate, mannitol (Osmitrol♣), procainamide (Pronestyl), hydrocortisone (Solu-Cortef), furosemide (Lasix, Furoside♣), regular insulin, 50% dextrose, 10% calcium chloride, 2% lidocaine, and heparin (Hepalean♣) available to treat acidosis, hyperkalemia, dysrhythmias and DIC, and to maintain urinary output.
- Assist with monitoring urinary output (insert Foley catheter), serum potassium and calcium levels, ABGs, clotting studies, and cardiac rhythms as indicated.
- Document the event, detailing times, interventions, and client response. Submit an adverse metabolic reaction to anesthesia report to the North American Malignant Hyperthermia Registry at 717-531-6936.

ABGs = arterial blood gases; DIC = disseminated intravascular coagulation.

---

vital in determining anesthetic type and dosage. Intraoperative death, however, is more often related to the client's premorbid condition, rather than overdosage of anesthetics.

Unrecognized Hypoventilation. The respiratory system is most frequently involved when the client experiences a damaging event related to anesthesia. Failure to ventilate can lead to cardiac arrest, central nervous system

TABLE 21–5

Advantages, Disadvantages, and Related Nursing Implications of Local or Regional Anesthetic Agents

Agent	Advantages	Disadvantages	Nursing Implications	Rationale
Procaine (Novocain) Tetracaine (Pontocaine) Lidocaine (Xylocaine) Mepivacaine (Carbocaine, Polocaine) Bupivacaine (Marcaine, Sensorcaine)	• Easily administered • Rapid onset (4–17 min) • Can be administered topically or by injection • Excellent muscle relaxant effects • Protective reflexes (cough, gag) remain intact • Client does not lose consciousness • Many are available with epinephrine added	• Absorbs into the bloodstream • Can cause cardiac depression and dysrhythmias with absorption • Difficult to control dosage • Drug interactions with monoamine oxidase (MAO) inhibitors can cause hypertension • Tremors, twitching shivering, respiratory arrest can occur with absorption	• Assess for return of movement and sensation in the area anesthetized. • Monitor blood pressure and pulse. • Assess administration site for pallor, drainage. • Protect area anesthetized until full sensation has returned.	• Movement returns first, then sense of touch, pain, warmth, and cold, in that order. • Ongoing assessment leads to early detection and treatment of potential complications. • Protection prevents injury to the area. • Duration of the anesthetic is 3–6 hr.

damage (e.g., permanent brain damage), and death. Monitoring standards include the use of an end-tidal carbon dioxide monitor to confirm carbon dioxide in the client's expired gas and a breathing system disconnect monitor to detect any break in the breathing circuit equipment.

Complications Related to Specific Anesthetic Agents. Specific complications were discussed earlier in the chapter. The elderly or debilitated client may be more susceptible to complications of anesthesia because of an intolerance to the agent, decreased metabolism, or general physical condition. (For preoperative risk factors, see Chapter 20.)

Complications of Intubation. Many complications can occur from intubation; for example, broken or injured teeth and caps, swollen lip, or vocal cord trauma. Intubation may be difficult because of the individual client's anatomy or disease process (e.g., small oral cavity, tight mandibular joint, tumor). Improper extension of the client's neck during intubation may cause injury. The surgeon should be in the operating room (OR) in case an emergency arises (e.g., a tracheostomy is needed) when the endotracheal tube is placed. Placement of the endotracheal tube causes some degree of irritation and edema of the trachea and accounts for the client's sore throat postoperatively.

Local or Regional Anesthesia

Local or regional anesthesia temporarily interrupts the transmission of sensory nerve impulses from a specific area or region. Motor function may or may not be affected, and the client does not lose consciousness. Thus, the client is able to follow instructions throughout the procedure. Because the gag and cough reflexes remain intact, there is little risk of aspiration or other respiratory complications. Local or regional anesthesia is typically

supplemented with sedatives, opioid analgesics, and/or hypnotics.

The OR nurse provides the client with information, directions, and emotional support before, during, and after the procedure. Table 21–5 describes various anesthetic agents and related nursing interventions.

LOCAL ANESTHESIA. Techniques used to administer local anesthesia include topical anesthesia and local infiltration. Sometimes when the term *local* is used, it means *any* form of anesthesia that is not general anesthesia. The client could be receiving regional anesthesia, but local anesthetic agents are used.

Topical Anesthesia. Topical anesthesia refers to an anesthetic applied *directly* to the surface of the area to be anesthetized. Often the anesthetic is in the form of an ointment or spray. This method is often used for respiratory intubation or for diagnostic procedures, such as laryngoscopy, bronchoscopy, or cystoscopy. The onset of action is 1 minute, and the duration is 20 to 30 minutes. Collapse or depression of the cardiovascular system may occur after the topical anesthetic is applied to the respiratory tract.

Local Infiltration. Local infiltration is the injection of an anesthetic agent intracutaneously and subcutaneously *into* the tissue surrounding an incision, wound, or lesion. The anesthetic blocks peripheral nerve stimulation at its origin. Local infiltration is commonly used during the suturing of superficial lacerations.

REGIONAL ANESTHESIA. Regional anesthesia—a type of local anesthesia—may be used as follows:

■ When general anesthesia is contraindicated because of the presence of medical problems (e.g., dysrhythmias and respiratory disease)

- When the client has experienced previous adverse reactions to general anesthetic agents
- When the client has a preference and a choice is possible

If the client has eaten and the surgery is an emergency, it may be possible to perform the procedure with the client under regional anesthesia (depending on the procedure) to decrease the risks associated with gastric contents (e.g., aspiration). Types of regional anesthesia include field block, nerve block, spinal, and epidural.

Field Block. A field block is produced by a series of injections *around* the operative field. Injecting around a specific nerve or group of nerves depresses the entire sensory nervous system of a localized area. This type of blocking is used for thoracic procedures, herniorrhaphy (hernia repair), dental procedures, and plastic surgery.

Nerve Block. A nerve block is achieved by injection of the local anesthetic agent *into or around* a nerve or nerves supplying the involved area. Nerve blocks interrupt sensory, motor, or sympathetic transmission. They are used surgically to prevent pain during a procedure, diagnostically to identify the cause of pain, and therapeutically to relieve chronic pain and increase circulation in some vascular diseases.

Figure 21–10 shows common nerve block sites. Lidocaine (Xylocaine) or bupivacaine (Marcaine) is frequently the agent used. A nerve block takes effect within minutes after the injection, and the anesthesia lasts longer than is achieved with local infiltration. Epinephrine added to the anesthetic agent potentiates the drug, causing a prolonged effect. Seizures, cardiac depression, dysrhythmias, and/or respiratory depression may occur if the nerve-blocking agent is injected into the bloodstream. The nurse observes for signs of systemic absorption, sensitivity, or overdose.

Spinal Anesthesia. Spinal anesthesia—intrathecal block—is achieved by injection of the anesthetic agent into the subarachnoid space (Fig. 21–11). The drug acts on the nerves as they emerge from the spinal cord and before they leave the spinal canal through the intervertebral foramen, thereby inhibiting conduction in the autonomic, sensory, and motor systems. The drug is rapidly absorbed into the nerve fibers and produces analgesia with relaxation, which is effective for lower abdominal and pelvic surgical procedures.

Epidural Anesthesia. The anesthetic is injected into the epidural space so that the protective coverings of the spinal cord (dura mater and arachnoid mater) are never entered. Because the anesthetic can diffuse or float up the vertebral column, the client can achieve anesthetic effects as high as the T-4 level; however, potential respiratory complications may make injection at this high a level undesirable.

Epidural anesthesia is used for anorectal, vaginal, and perineal procedures, as well as for hip and lower extremity operations, such as total hip or knee replacements. Two important advantages are associated with this type of anesthesia:

- Decreased cardiopulmonary complications—particularly important for the elderly client
- Ability to retain the epidural catheter for postoperative analgesic administration (see Chap. 9)

COMPLICATIONS OF LOCAL OR REGIONAL ANESTHESIA. Major intraoperative complications are usually attributable to client sensitization to the anesthetic agent (anaphylaxis), incorrect administration technique, systemic absorption, and overdosage. The nurse observes for signs of a systemic toxic reaction, which is manifested by central nervous system (CNS) stimulation followed by CNS

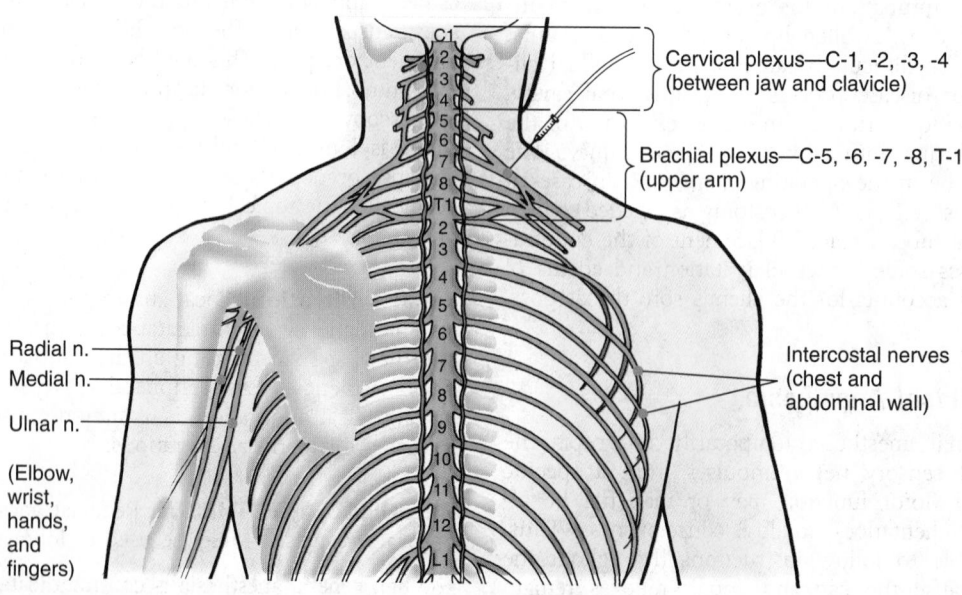

Cervical plexus—C-1, -2, -3, -4 (between jaw and clavicle)

Brachial plexus—C-5, -6, -7, -8, T-1 (upper arm)

Radial n.
Medial n.
Ulnar n.

(Elbow, wrist, hands, and fingers)

Intercostal nerves (chest and abdominal wall)

Figure 21–10. Nerve block sites.

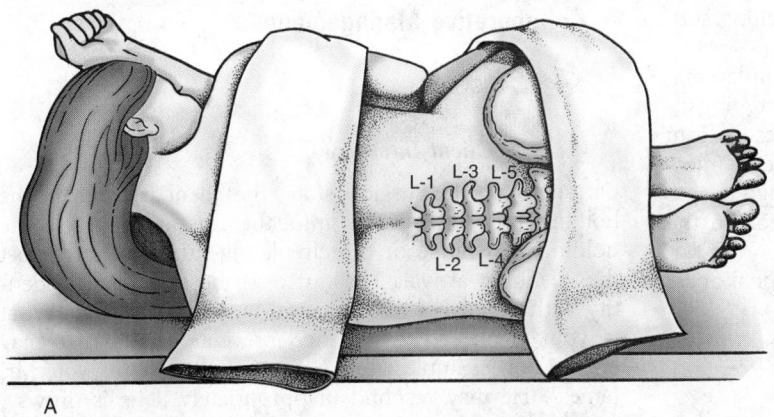

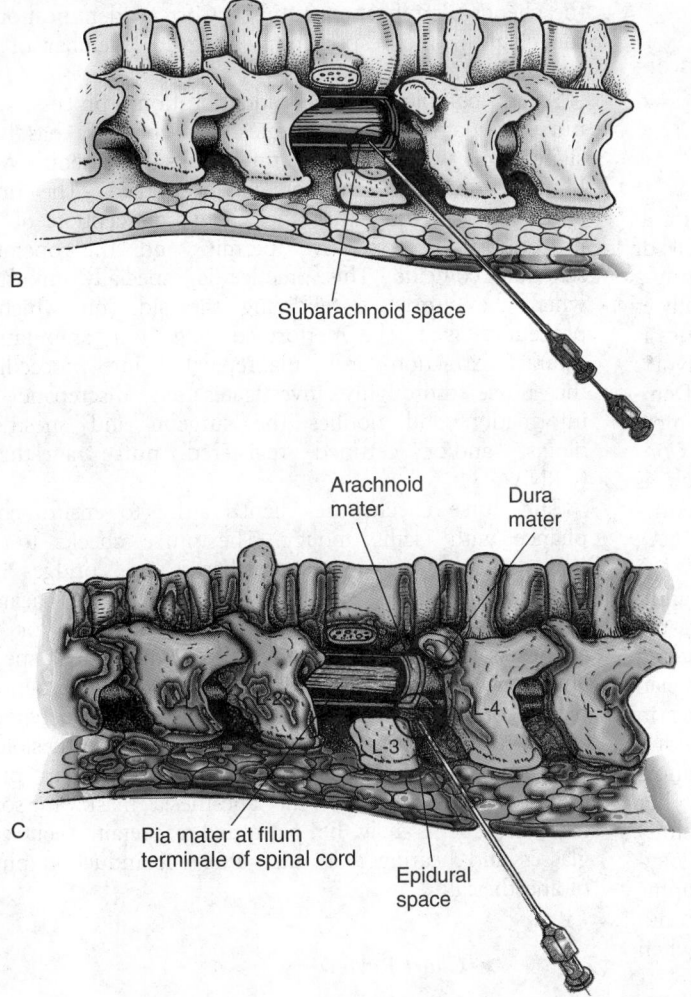

Subarachnoid space

Arachnoid mater

Dura mater

Pia mater at filum terminale of spinal cord

Epidural space

Figure 21–11. Administration of spinal and epidural anesthesia. *A,* Spinal or epidural anesthesia is administered by inserting a spinal needle between the second and third or the third and fourth lumbar vertebrae (L2–3 or L3–4). The client is placed in the flexed lateral (fetal) position (shown here) or seated on the edge of the operating bed with the back arched and the chin tucked to the chest. *B,* Spinal anesthesia (viewed from the side). A large needle is inserted to the surface of the dura mater, and a second, smaller needle is passed through the first to penetrate the dura mater and arachnoid mater. An anesthetic is injected, sometimes through an indwelling catheter, directly into the cerebrospinal fluid in the subarachnoid space. *C,* Epidural anesthesia (viewed from the side). The needle is inserted to the surface of the dura mater, and the anesthetic is injected, usually through an indwelling catheter, into the epidural space.

and cardiovascular depression. The nurse assesses for such initial behaviors as restlessness; excitement; incoherent speech; headache; blurred vision; metallic taste; nausea; vomiting; tremors; seizures; and increased pulse, respirations, and blood pressure. Nursing interventions include establishing and maintaining an open airway, administering oxygen, and notifying the surgeon. It is usu-

ally necessary to administer a fast-acting and short-acting barbiturate. If the client's toxic reaction remains untreated, unconsciousness, hypotension, apnea, cardiac arrest, and death may result.

A cardiac arrest may rarely occur as a complication of spinal anesthesia, possibly related to unknown autonomic nervous system effects. Epinephrine may prevent the arrest when administered to the client who develops sudden, unexplained bradycardia (Biddle, 1994).

Localized complications include edema and inflammation initially, with possible abscess, necrosis, and/or gangrene later. Inflammation and abscess usually result from a break in sterile technique occurring at the time of injection of the anesthetic agent. Necrosis and gangrene are rare but may occur as a result of vasoconstriction in the area of the injection.

The nurse's role in the administration of regional anesthesia consists of

- Assisting the anesthesiologist or certified registered nurse anesthetist (CRNA)
- Observing for breaks in sterile technique
- Providing physical and emotional support for the client
- Staying with the client
- Providing the client a chance to verbalize feelings
- Offering information, encouragement, and reassurance
- Positioning the client comfortably and safely

Conscious Sedation

Conscious sedation, usually administered by direct intravenous (IV) injection ("IV push"), is given to dull or reduce the intensity of pain or awareness of pain during a procedure without loss of defensive reflexes. Usually a combination of opioid analgesics and sedative-hypnotics is used (Berkowitz, 1997). Diazepam (Valium, Vivol✦, Novodipam✦), midazolam (Versed), meperidine (Demerol), fentanyl (Sublimaze), alfentanil (Alfenta), and morphine sulfate are the most commonly used drugs. Conscious sedation is typically used for procedures such as endoscopy, cardiac catheterization, closed fracture reduction, percutaneous transluminal cardiac angiography (PTCA), cardioversion, and other special procedures.

The physician determines whether the client is a candidate for IV conscious sedation and often administers the first dosages. In most states, a credentialed registered nurse may administer conscious sedation under physician supervision. Credentialing involves advanced training in IV medication administration, airway management, and advanced cardic life support (ACLS). The nurse monitors the client during and after the procedure for his or her response to drug administration. The nurse carefully monitors the client's airway, level of consciousness, oxygen saturation via pulse oximetry, electrocardiographic (ECG) status, and vital signs every 15 to 30 minutes until the client is fully awake, alert, and oriented and when vital signs have returned to preprocedural levels.

Clients receiving IV conscious sedation may be discharged to go home with a responsible adult. If the client returns to the general medical-surgical nursing unit, the unit staff nurses continue to monitor the client. The client is expected to be sleepy but arousable for several hours after the procedure. The nurse usually does not permit oral intake until 30 minutes after the client has received medication or, in other cases, according to physician order. When fluids are permitted, the nurse makes sure that the client is awake and positioned to avoid aspiration.

Collaborative Management

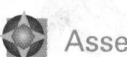 Assessment

➤ *Client Interview*

On arrival in the surgical suite, the client is taken to the holding area or directly into the operating suite. The holding area nurse or the circulating nurse or both greet the client on arrival. The nurse verifies the client's identity with his or her identification bracelet and asks, "What is your name?" This practice prevents errors that may occur. For example, if a client is asked, "Are you Mr. James?" He may respond inappropriately if he is drowsy, anxious, or sedated. The nurse always validates the identification obtained using the chart, the client's name, and the client's identification number. Correct identification of the client is the responsibility of every member of the health care team.

After completing the identification process, the nurse validates that the surgical consent form has been signed and witnessed. The nurse asks the client, "What kind of operation are you having today?" The nurse checks to ascertain that the client's perception of the procedure, the operative permit, and the operative schedule coincide. This practice is especially important when the nurse is validating the side on which a procedure is to be performed (e.g., for amputation, cataract extraction, or hernia repair). Before proceeding, the nurse thoroughly investigates *any* discrepancy in information and notifies the surgeon and anesthesiologist and/or certified registered nurse anesthetist (CRNA).

The nurse checks the client's attire to ensure compliance with facility policy. The nurse checks to see that dentures and dental prostheses (e.g., bridges and retainers), jewelry, eyeglasses, contact lenses, hearing aids, wigs, and other prostheses are removed for the client's safety during surgery. The nurse pays special attention to the removal of dentures, because the denture plate could become loose and obstruct the client's airway during surgery. Occasionally, the anesthesiology team may request that the dentures be left in place to ensure a snug fit of the anesthesia mask. In some facilities, clients may be permitted to retain their eyeglasses and hearing aids until after the induction phase of anesthesia.

➤ *Chart Review*

The circulating nurse and anesthesia personnel review the client's chart in the holding area (or in the operating room if there is no holding area). The chart provides information needed to identify potential and actual needs of the client during the intraoperative period and allows the circulating nurse to assess and plan for the client's needs during and after surgery. The client's chart is a primary source of information on the type and location of the planned surgical procedure. A check of the chart ensures that all required data are present before the procedure is begun.

Allergies and Previous Reactions to Anesthesia or Transfusions

In reviewing the chart, the nurse asks the client about allergies and previous reactions to anesthesia or blood transfusions. Allergies or sensitivity to iodine products or shellfish may indicate the potential for a reaction to the antimicrobial agents used to clean the surgical area. The nurse clearly indicates the allergies on the chart and notifies the operating room (OR) team. The client's previous experience with anesthesia helps the nurse and anesthesiologist or CRNA plan and anticipate the client's needs. For example, if a client is restless or agitated as a reaction to anesthesia, the nurse can have padding for the stretcher side rails and protective restraints available. The use of blood and blood products during surgery may be influenced by the client's history, religious beliefs or preferences, and type of transfusion reaction in the past.

Autologous Blood Transfusion

Increasingly, autologous blood transfusion (reinfusing the client's own blood) is being used for surgery. This method of blood transfusion eliminates the risk of acquiring blood-borne infections, such as hepatitis B and human immunodeficiency virus (HIV), from another person. Chapter 20 discusses autologous blood transfusion in more detail, and Chart 21–2 outlines key points of intraoperative autologous blood transfusion.

Laboratory and Diagnostic Test Results

The OR nurse reviews preoperative laboratory and diagnostic test results. The nurse assesses most recent laboratory results to inform the surgical team about the client's medical condition and to alert them to potential intraoperative and postoperative interventions. The most recent results are usually obtained within 24 to 28 hours before surgery for hospitalized clients and within 2 weeks for ambulatory surgery clients. The nurse reports all abnormalities to the surgeon and anesthesiologist or CRNA. Laboratory values significantly greater than or less than the normal range are potentially life-threatening for any client, but especially for the client undergoing surgery (see Chap. 20). For example, if the hemoglobin concentration is less than 10 g/dL, the client's oxygen transport capacity is lessened; this condition affects the amount and type of anesthesia used and the potential impact of blood loss during surgery.

Medical History and Physical Examination Findings

The OR nurse checks that the client's medical history and examination findings, including usual pulse and blood pressure, are recorded. This information provides the circulating nurse, surgeon, anesthesiologist and/or CRNA, and postanesthesia care unit (PACU) nurse with baseline data to assess the client's reaction to the surgical procedure and anesthesia. Medications the client has routinely taken preoperatively may affect the client's reaction to surgery and wound healing. For example, aspirin has an anticoagulant effect and can cause increased clotting time and danger of hemorrhage.

Knowing the client's medical history and age (Chart 21–3) allows the nurse to take special precautions and plan appropriate interventions for the care and safety of high-risk clients. The nurse carefully monitors elderly clients and those with cardiac disease for potential fluid overload, which can be life-threatening.

After completing the chart review, the nurse may insert an intravenous catheter and perform a surgical shave. The circulating nurse provides additional emotional support and explains procedures to the client. The client is never left unattended. If the client is in the holding area, he or she is transferred to the OR after the preoperative routine is completed.

Chart 21–2

Nursing Care Highlight: Intraoperative Autologous Blood Salvage and Transfusion

- Be aware of the cell-processing method to be used.
- Make sure that collection containers are labeled for the client.
- Assist with sterile set-up as necessary.
- Assist with processing and reinfusing procedures as needed.
- Document the transfusion process.
- Monitor the client's vital signs during the transfusion procedure.

Chart 21–3

Nursing Focus on the Elderly: Intraoperative Nursing Interventions

- Allow clients to retain eyeglasses and hearing aids until anesthesia has been administered.
- Use a small pillow under the client's head if his or her head and neck are normally bent slightly forward.
- Lift clients into position to prevent shearing forces on fragile skin.
- Position arthritic and artificial joints carefully to prevent postoperative pain and discomfort from strain on those joints.
- Pad bony prominences to prevent pressure sores.
- Provide extra padding for those clients with decreased peripheral circulation.
- Use head caps to prevent heat loss through the scalp.
- Place stockinette on extremities to conserve body heat.
- Warm prepping solutions and intravenous and irrigation fluids as indicated.
- Follow strict aseptic technique.
- Carefully monitor intake and output, including blood loss.

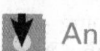 Analysis

➤ *Common Nursing Diagnoses and Collaborative Problems*

Common nursing diagnoses for intraoperative clients include

1. Risk for Perioperative Positioning Injury related to immobilization and effects of anesthesia
2. Impaired Skin Integrity and Impaired Tissue Integrity related to the surgical incision

A common collaborative problem for the intraoperative client is Potential for Hypoventilation.

➤ *Additional Nursing Diagnoses and Collaborative Problems*

Additional nursing diagnoses and collaborative problems may apply to intraoperative clients:

- Risk for Infection related to break in skin integrity, i.e., incision, invasive lines
- Risk for Injury related to fire and electrical hazards within the operating environment
- Risk for Disuse Syndrome related to decreased level of consciousness or to immobilization
- Hypothermia related to evaporation from skin and exposed tissue in a cool environment, body heat loss, alteration in the hypothalamus from anesthetic agents, inadequate body covering, or aging
- Ineffective Thermoregulation related to sedation, fluctuating environmental temperature, medications, or age extremes
- Fear related to threat of death, actual or perceived, or to anticipation of events posing a threat to self-esteem
- Anxiety related to loss of control or threat of death
- Fluid Volume Deficit related to decreased intake, evaporative fluid loss through the skin and exposed tissue, or blood loss
- Potential for Peripheral Nerve Damage related to intraoperative positioning

 Planning and Implementation

➤ *Risk for Perioperative Positioning Injury*

Planning: Expected Outcomes. The primary goal is for the client to be free of injury.

Interventions. Interventions are directed toward preventing injury resulting from intraoperative positioning.

Because of preoperative medication, anesthetic agents, and the narrowness of the bed, the client's normal defense mechanisms cannot guard against nerve or joint damage and muscle stretch and strain. Proper positioning, therefore, is important. The circulating nurse pads the operating bed with foam and/or silicone gel pads, properly places the grounding pads, coordinates the transfer of the client to the operating bed, and helps the client obtain a comfortable position. The circulating nurse assesses

the skin, especially of the elderly, for bruising or injury, placing extra padding as indicated.

The client is usually in a dorsal recumbent (supine) position after transfer to the operating bed. Anesthesia may be administered with the client supine, and the client may be repositioned for surgery. When general anesthesia is used, the nurse repositions the client after he or she is in stage 3 (see Table 21–2).

The circulating nurse coordinates repositioning of the client for surgery and modifies the position according to the client's safety and special needs. Factors influencing the *timing* of repositioning include

- The surgical site
- The age and size of client
- Anesthetic administration technique
- Pain experienced by the conscious client on movement

Factors influencing the actual *position* include

- The specific procedure being performed
- The surgeon's request
- The client's age, size, and weight
- Any respiratory, skeletal, or neuromuscular limitations, such as rheumatoid arthritis, joint replacements, or emphysema

Table 21–6 presents possible complications related to prolonged surgical immobility and preventive nursing actions.

The dorsal recumbent, prone, lithotomy, and lateral positions are frequently used for surgery. Figure 21–12 illustrates common surgical positions and the use of protective padding. When general anesthesia is used, the nurse positions the client slowly to prevent vasogenic hypotension. The nurse ensures proper positioning by assessing for

- Physiologic alignment
- Minimal interference with circulation and respiration
- Protection of skeletal and neuromuscular structures
- Optimal exposure of the operative site and intravenous line
- Adequate access to the client for the anesthesiologist or CRNA
- The client's comfort and safety
- Preservation of the client's dignity

The nurse must be aware of potential complications related to specific positions and modifies care as indicated. For example, clients in lithotomy position may develop leg swelling, pain in the legs or back, and diminished sensation or pulses. The nurse ensures proper padding and position changes at regular intervals. Throughout the intraoperative period, the nurse assists in preventing obstruction of circulatory, respiratory, or neurologic systems caused by tight straps, improperly placed pads and pillows, or position of the bed.

➤ *Impaired Skin Integrity and Impaired Tissue Integrity*

Planning: Expected Outcomes. The primary goal is that the client will experience minimal skin and tissue impairment and contamination as a result of surgery.

TABLE 21-6

Interventions to Prevent Neuromuscular Complications Related to Intraoperative Positioning

Anatomic Area	Complications	Interventions
Brachial plexus	• Paralysis • Loss of sensation in the arm and shoulder	• Pad the elbow. • Avoid excessive abduction. • Secure the arm firmly on an arm board, positioned at shoulder level.
Radial nerve	• Wrist drop	• Support the wrist with padding. • Do not overtighten wrist straps.
Medial or ulnar nerves	• Hand deformities	• Place a safety strap above or below area.
Peroneal nerve	• Foot drop	• Place pillow or padding under knees. • Support lower extremities. • Do not overtighten leg straps.
Tibial nerve	• Loss of sensation on the plantar surface of the foot	• Place a safety strap above the ankle. • Do not place equipment on lower extremities.
Joints	• Stiffness • Pain • Inflammation	• Place pillow or foam padding under bony prominences. • Maintain good body alignment. • Slightly flex joints and support with pillows, trochanter rolls, or pads.

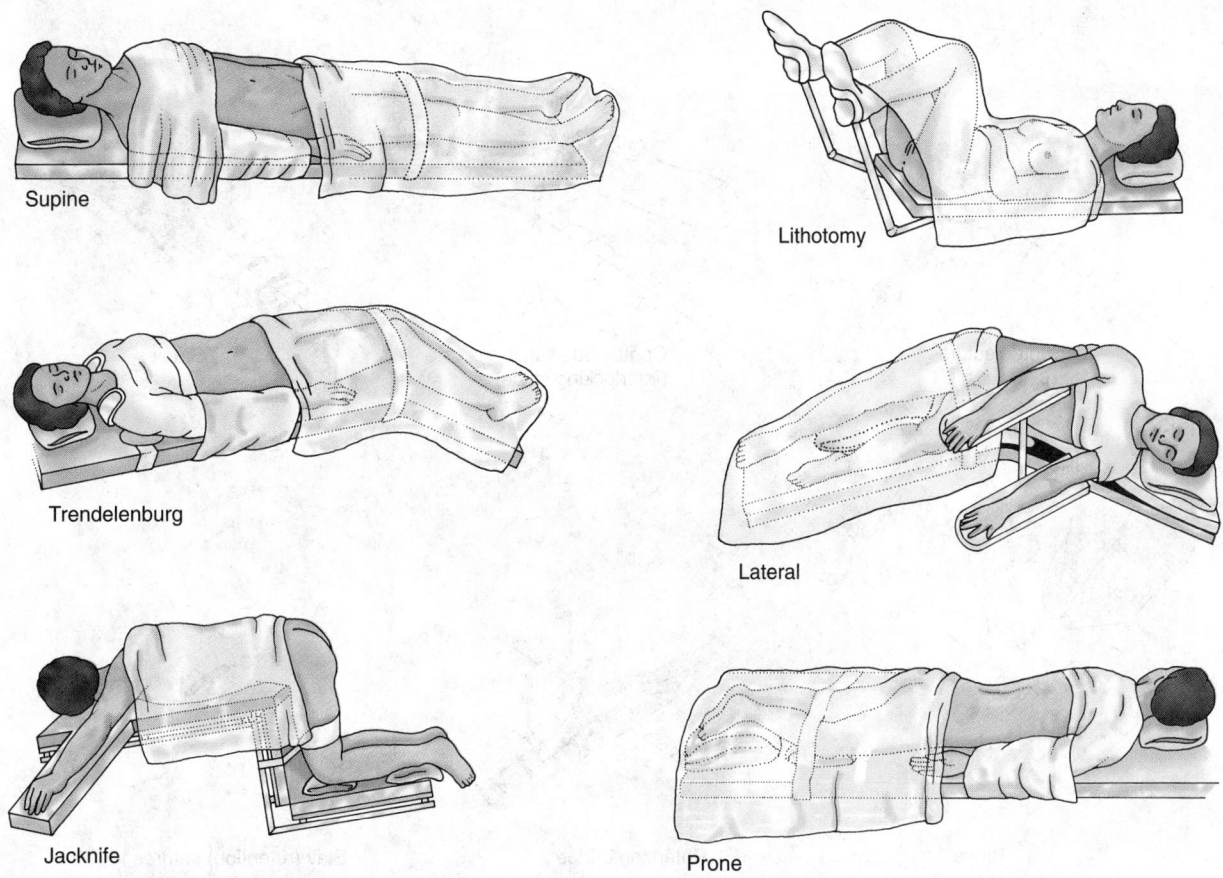

Figure 21-12. Common surgical positions.

Interventions. Surgery is an invasive procedure that places the client at risk for complications related to the surgical wound (such as incisional tears and lacerations), bacterial contamination, and loss of body fluids from the wound during and after surgery. Sterile surgical technique and the use of protective drapes, skin closures, and dressings help to minimize complications and promote wound healing.

Plastic Adhesive Drapes. If a sterile plastic adhesive drape is used, the scrub nurse helps the surgical assistant apply the drape after the surgical site has been cleaned and dried. The plastic drape is applied directly to the client's skin to prevent shifting and exposure of skin edges. The surgeon makes the incision through the plastic drape. The cut edge remains adherent to the skin and keeps the surgical incision sealed from the migration of bacteria into the wound. The scrub nurse and surgical assistant *gently* remove the drape after closure of the surgical incision. The nurse pays special attention to the elderly and to clients with fragile skin to prevent skin tearing when the adhesive drape is removed.

Skin Closures. Skin and tissue closures, such as sutures and staples, are used for several reasons:

- To approximate wound edges until wound healing is complete
- To occlude the lumen of blood vessels, preventing hemorrhage and loss of body fluids
- To prevent wound contamination

The quality of the approximated tissue and the type of closure material are two factors that determine the strength and integrity of the closure. The wound is usually closed in layers to maintain tissue integrity and promote healing with minimal scarring. The surgeon selects the method and type of closures to be used on the basis of the surgical site, the tissue involved, the size and depth of the surgical wound, and the age and medical history of the client. A combination of sutures and clips is commonly used for closure of internal layers of the wound. Staples, stay and retention sutures, and skin closure tapes (Steri-Strips) are used for closure of superficial wounds of the epidermis. Figure 21–13 illustrates commonly used wound closures.

A suture consists of one or more strands of material and is designated by its size, or gauge. The size designation sequence, from largest diameter to smallest, is 5, 4, 3, 2, 1, 0, 2-0, 3-0, 4-0, and so forth, to 11-0. Size 5 may be used to close the deep layers of an abdominal wound; 11-0 is the smallest-diameter suture and is used in plastic surgery and ophthalmology. Other characteristics of the suture material, such as type (nylon, silk, Vicryl), color (e.g., green, blue, black, white, violet), and structure (twisted, braided), are often listed on the package.

Suture material can be absorbable or nonabsorbable. *Absorbable* sutures are digested over time by body enzymes. These sutures first lose strength and then gradually disappear from the tissue. Catgut suture, such as "plain gut" and "chromic gut," was a common type of

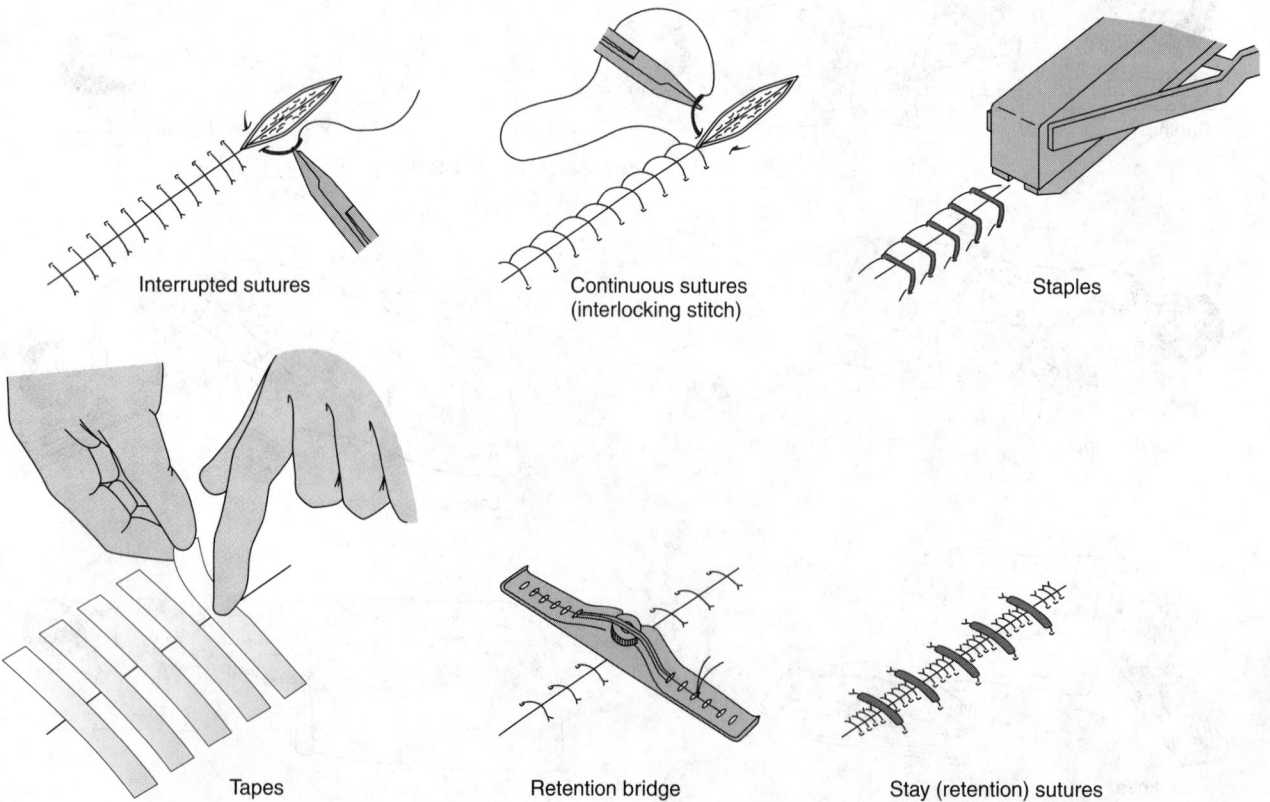

Figure 21–13. Common skin closures.

absorbable suture material that is still in use today, although not as frequently as it once was. Other absorbable sutures are made of synthetics and are labeled as such on the package. The client's physical status, the presence of inflammation, and the type of suture used all influence the rate of absorption, which is usually up to about 2 weeks.

Nonabsorbable sutures are not affected by body enzymes. Nonabsorbable sutures become encapsulated in the tissue during the healing process and remain embedded in the tissue unless they are removed. These sutures are made of silk, cotton, steel, nylon, polyester, or other synthetic material. Nonabsorbable sutures are used for vascular anastamosis, "wiring" the sternum together after open heart surgery, and closing external wounds. The surgeon may use a double or interlocking stitch to increase the integrity of the closure. Retention and stay sutures (see Fig. 21–13) may be used in addition to standard suture material for high-risk clients (those having major abdominal surgery, obese clients, diabetic clients, and clients taking steroids, which inhibit wound healing).

After the incision is closed, the physician may inject a local anesthetic or instill an antibiotic into the wound. A gauze or spray dressing may be applied to protect it from contamination. A variety of dressings may also be used to absorb drainage and provide support to the incision. A pressure dressing may be applied to prevent or stop a vascular area from bleeding postoperatively. One or more drains (see Chap. 22) may be inserted to prevent the accumulation of secretions within tissues around the surgical area. These secretions, if not drained, impede healing and serve as a medium for bacterial growth, which could result in wound infection.

After the dressing is secure, the nurse coordinates the surgical team in repositioning and transferring the client as indicated. A roller board or a lift sheet is used to transfer the client safely from the operating bed to a stretcher or bed. The circulating nurse and anesthesiologist or certified registered nurse anesthetist (CRNA) accompany the client to the postanesthesia care unit (PACU) and give a report of the client's intraoperative experience to the PACU nurse (see Chap. 22).

➤ *Potential for Hypoventilation*

Planning: Expected Outcomes. The primary goal is for the client to be free of damaging events related to hypoventilation.

Interventions. Interventions are directed toward preventing injury resulting from anesthesia (see earlier). The nurse, physician, and anesthesiologist or CRNA monitor the client according to official standards. These standards, which have been adopted by both the American Society of Anesthesiologists and the American Association of Nurse Anesthetists, include continuous monitoring of ventilation, circulation, and cardiac rhythms; blood pressure and heart rate recordings every 5 minutes; and the continuous presence of an anesthesiology practitioner during the case (Biddle, 1994).

 Evaluation

On the basis of identified nursing diagnoses, collaborative problems, and desired outcomes, the nurse evaluates the care of the intraoperative client and ensures that the client

- Is safely anesthetized without complications
- Does not experience any injury related to intraoperative positioning or equipment
- Is free of skin or tissue contamination during surgery
- Is free of skin tears, bruises, redness, abrasion, or maceration over pressure points and elsewhere

---

 CASE STUDY for the Intraoperative Client

■ You are an operating room nurse having lunch in the hospital cafeteria with one of your friends who works in the open-heart surgery unit. He says to you, "Boy, we seem to get a lot of patients out of the OR with skin breakdown on the back of their heads." On further discussion, he tells you that most often the breakdown is black eschar.

QUESTIONS:

1. Is it possible that these patients developed the skin breakdown while in the operating suite? Why or why not?
2. What should you do with the information your friend passed on to you and why?
3. How could this situation have been prevented?

SELECTED BIBLIOGRAPHY

Atkinson, L. J. (1996). *Berry & Kohn's operating room technique* (8th ed.). St. Louis: Mosby–Year Book.

Ball, K. A. (1995). *Lasers: The perioperative challenge* (2nd ed.). St. Louis: C. V. Mosby.

*Ball, K. A. (1990). The basics of laser technology. *Nursing Clinics of North America, 25*(3), 619–634.

Ballantyne, G. H., Leahy, P. F., & Modlin, I. M. (1994). *Laparoscopic surgery*. Philadelphia: W. B. Saunders Co.

Beck, C. F. (1994). Malignant hyperthermia: Are you prepared? *AORN Journal, 59*(2), 367, 370–372, 374–378+.

Berkowitz, C. M. (1997). Conscious sedation: A primer. *RN. 60*(2), 32–36.

Biddle, C. (1994). AANA journal course: Update for nurse anesthetists—outcome measures in anesthesiology: Are we going in the right direction? *American Association of Nurse Anesthetists Journal, 62*(2), 117–124.

Boike, L., et al. (1995). Development of an outpatient perioperative care record. *Journal of Post Anesthesia Nursing, 10*(3), 140–150.

Brown, K. A. (1997). Malignant hyperthermia. *American Journal of Nursing, 97*(10), 33.

*Bruton-Maree, N. (1990). Anesthesia and the aging population. *CRNA, 1*(1), 25–31.

*Burden, N. (1988). Post-anesthesia: While the patient is unconscious. *RN, 51*(4), 34–44.

Clinch, C. (1996). Pressure area care in one operating theatre. *British Journal Theatre Nursing, 6*(3), 25–27.

Corey-Plett, P. (1994). Fluid replacement therapy and perioperative management. *Canadian Operating Room Nursing Journal, 12*(4), 18–21.

*Cruz, L. D. (1991). A history of the RN first assistant. *AORN Journal,* 53(6), 1536–1537.

Curry, M. (1994). Perioperative nursing care of the elderly patient: A case study. *ACORN Journal,* 7(2), 23–26.

*Davidhizar, R. (1992). When patients die in the operating room. *Today's OR Nurse,* 14(1), 4.

*Davidson, J. E. (1991). Neuromuscular blockade. *Focus on Critical Care—AACN,* 18(6), 512–520.

*Dellasega, C., & Burgunder, C. (1991). Perioperative nursing care of the elderly surgical patient. *Today's OR Nurse,* 13(6), 12–17.

Dougherty, J. (1996). Same-day surgery: The nurse's role. *Orthopedic Nursing,* 15(4), 15–18.

Dunn, D. (1997). Malignant hyperthermia. *AORN Journal,* 65(4), 728–762.

*Entrup, M. H. (1991). Perioperative complications of anesthesia. *Surgical Clinics of North America,* 71(6), 1151–1173.

Fawcett, D. L., et al. (1996). A pilot study appraising the climate for perioperative research. *AORN Journal,* 63(1), 205–208.

*Fiesta, J. (1992). Anesthesia-related liability. *Nursing Management,* 23(10), 28–30.

Fogg, D. M. (1996). Clinical issues. Length of sterile drapes; counts; alcohol skin preps; food and drink in ORs; houseplants in OR lounges. *AORN Journal,* 63(1), 262–264, 267.

*Gallagher, M. T., & Kahn, C. (1990). Lasers: Scalpels of light. *RN,* 53(5), 46–53.

Gerber, D. E., et al. (1995). Death in the operating room and postanesthesia care unit: Helping nurses to cope. *Journal of Post Anesthesia Nursing,* 10(2), 84–88.

Gillette, V. A. (1996). Applying nursing theory to perioperative nursing practice. *AORN Journal,* 64(2), 261–264, 267–268, 270.

Golanowski, M. (1995). Do not resuscitate: Informed consent in the operating room and postanesthesia care unit. *Journal of Post Anesthesia Nursing,* 10(1), 9–11.

Green, S. (1996). Positioning the patient for surgery. *British Journal Theatre Nursing,* 6(5), 35–38.

Gruendemann, B. J., & Fernsebner, B. (1995). *Comprehensive perioperative nursing.* Sudbury, MA: Jones & Bartlett.

Haney, P. E., Raymond, B. A., Hernandez, J. M., et al. (1996). Tuberculosis makes a comeback. *AORN Journal,* 63(4), 705, 707, 709, 713–715.

Hankela, S., et al. (1996). Intraoperative nursing care as experienced by surgical patients. *AORN Journal,* 63(2), 435–442.

Hussar, D. A. (1997). New drugs (ropivacaine HCl). *Nursing97,* 27(6), 38.

*Hussar, D. A. (1992). New drugs (mivacurium chloride). *Nursing92,* 22(12), 61.

*Jackson, M. F. (1989). Implications of surgery in very elderly patients. *AORN Journal,* 50(4), 859–869.

*Jarpe, M. B. (1992). Nursing care of patients receiving long-term infusion of neuromuscular blocking agents. *Critical Care Nurse,* 12(7), 58–63.

*Johnson, G. M., & Bowman, R. J. (1992). Autologous blood transfusion. *AORN Journal,* 56(2), 282–298.

Jonasen, A. M. (1994). Therapeutic touch: A holistic approach to perioperative nursing. *Today's OR Nurse,* 16(1), 7–12, 50–51.

*Keene, A. (1991). Perioperative assessment and nursing implications for the elderly. *Plastic Surgical Nursing,* 11(4), 143–167.

Keffer, M. J. & Keffer, H. L. (1994). The do-not-resuscitate order: Moral responsibilities of the perioperative nurse. *AORN Journal,* 59(3), 641–650.

Kobs, A. (1997). Conscious sedation: Questions about the anesthesia continuum. *Nursing Management,* 28(4), 14, 17.

Leske, J. S. (1995). Effects of intraoperative progress reports on anxiety levels of surgical patients' family members. *Applied Nursing Research,* 8(4), 169–173.

Leske, J. S. (1996). Intraoperative progress reports decrease family members' anxiety. *AORN Journal,* 64(3), 424–436.

Ley, S. J. (1996). Intraoperative and postoperative blood salvage. *AACN Clinical Issues in Advanced Practice of Acute Critical Care,* 7(2), 238–248.

McCraine, J. (1994). Fire safety in the operating room. *Today's OR Nurse,* 16(1), 33–37.

McEwen, D. R. (1996). Intraoperative positioning of surgical patients. *AORN Journal,* 63(6), 1059–1063, 1066–1075, 1077–1082, 1084–1085.

Meckes, P. F. (1995). Geriatric surgery. In M. H. Meeker & J. Rothrock (Eds.), *Alexander's care of the patient in surgery* (10th ed., pp. 1195–1209). St. Louis: Mosby–Year Book.

Meeker, M. H., & Rothrock, J. (1995). *Alexander's care of the patient in surgery* (10th ed.). St. Louis: Mosby–Year Book.

Miller, R. D. (1994). *Anesthesia* (Vols. 1 & 2, 4th ed.). New York: Churchill Livingstone.

*Moore, J. L., & Rice, E. L. (1992). Malignant hyperthermia. *American Family Physician,* 45(5), 2245–2251.

Moss, M. T. (1995). Perioperative nursing in the managed care era. Collaborative relationships in the operating room part II—hospitals and nurses: Strategies of partnership. *Nursing Economics,* 13(5), 310, 313.

*Murphy, E. K. (1991). Liability for injury resulting from poor patient positioning. *AORN Journal,* 53(6), 1361–1365.

Null, S., et al. (1995). Development of a perioperative nursing diagnoses flow sheet. *AORN Journal,* 61(3), 547–550.

Nussbaum, W., et al. (1994). Perioperative challenges in the care of the Jehovah's Witness: A case report. *American Association of Nurse Anesthetists Journal,* 62(2), 160–164.

Omoigui, S. (1995). *The anesthesia drugs handbook* (2nd ed.). St. Louis: Mosby–Year Book.

Ouellette, R. G. (1994). Perioperative hypothermia. *Current Reviews For Nurse Anesthetists,* 16(22), 195–200.

Palmerini, J. (1996). Practical innovations. Developing a comprehensive perioperative nursing documentation form. *AORN Journal,* 63(1), 239–242, 245–247.

Patient outcomes: Standards of perioperative care (1997). *AORN Journal,* 65(2), 408–416.

Paulson, D. S. (1994). Comparative evaluation of five surgical hand scrub preparations. *AORN Journal,* 60(2), 249, 251–256.

Pearlman, R. C., et al. (1994). Intraoperative neural monitoring: An introduction for perioperative nurses . . . to determine whether nerve impulses are being conducted at normal levels. *AORN Journal,* 60(4), 648, 650–651.

*Pereira, L. J., Lee, S. M., & Wade, K. J. (1990). The effect of surgical handwashing routines on the microbial counts of operating room nurses. *American Journal of Infection Control,* 18(6), 354–364.

*Peterson, K. J. (1992). Nursing management of autologous blood transfusion. *Journal of Intravenous Nursing,* 15(3), 128–134.

*Polis, S. L. (1992). Competency-based laser education: Its implementation in the OR. *AORN Journal,* 55(2), 567–572.

Position statement: AORN position statement on perioperative care of patients with do-not-resuscitate (DNR) orders (1995). *AORN Journal,* 61(6), 954–955.

Position statement: AORN recommended education standards for RN first assistant programs (1995). *AORN Journal,* 61(3), 476–478.

Prior, L. (1996). Caring for patients from ethnic minority groups. *British Journal Theatre Nursing,* 6(3), 28–30.

*Proposed recommended practices—disinfection (1991). *AORN Journal,* 54(1), 75–80.

Proposed recommended practices for establishing and maintaining a sterile field (1996). *AORN Journal,* 63(1), 211, 213–218.

Proposed recommended practices for sterilization in the practice setting (1994). *AORN Journal,* 60(1), 109–110, 112–117, 119–120.

Proposed recommended practices for surgical attire (1994). *AORN Journal,* 60(1), 282, 284–286, 289–290+.

Proposed recommended practices for surgical hand scrubs (1994). *AORN Journal,* 60(2), 270, 273–274, 276, 279.

Proposed recommended practices for surgical skin preparation (1996). *AORN Journal,* 63(1), 221–224, 227–228.

Pursell, S. (1996). The role of the OR nurse in relation to HIV. *ACORN Journal,* 9(1), 23–24, 26–28.

*Ratner, L. E., & Smith, G. W. (1993). Intraoperative fluid management. *Surgical Clinics of North America,* 73(2), 229–241.

*Recommended practices: Aseptic technique (1991). *AORN Journal,* 54(4), 819–824.

Recommended practices: Documentation of perioperative nursing care (1996). *AORN Journal,* 63(6), 1145, 1148.

Recommended practices: Environmental cleaning for the surgical practice setting (1996). *AORN Journal,* 64(4), 611–615.

Recommended practices for the care and cleaning of surgical instruments and powered equipment (1997). *AORN Journal,* 65(1), 124–128.

Recommended practices for managing the patient receiving conscious sedation/analgesia (1997). *AORN Journal,* 65(1), 129–134.

*Recommended practices: Laser safety in the practice setting (1993). *AORN Journal, 58*(5), 1027–1031.

Recommended practices: Positioning the patient in the perioperative practice setting (1996). *AORN Journal, 64*(2), 278, 281–284.

Recommended practices: Safe care through identification of potential hazards in the surgical environment (1996). *AORN Journal, 63*(4), 802–806.

Recommended practices: Sponge, sharp, and instrument counts (1996). *AORN Journal, 64*(4), 616, 618–622.

Recommended practices: Traffic patterns in the perioperative practice setting (1996). *AORN Journal, 63*(3), 655–656, 658.

*Recommended practices: Universal precautions in the perioperative practice setting (1993). *AORN Journal, 57*(2), 554–558.

Recommended practices: Use and selection of barrier materials for surgical gowns and drapes (1996). *AORN Journal, 63*(3), 650, 653–654.

*Reeder, J. M. (1993). Do-not-resuscitate orders in the operating room. *AORN Journal, 57*(4), 947–951.

*Revised AORN official statement on RN first assistants (1993). *AORN Journal, 57*(1), 47–51.

Ringler, J. D. (1995). The use of diazepam and ketamine for IV conscious sedation in outpatient surgery settings. *AORN Journal, 62*(4), 638–645.

Roth, R. A. (1995). *Perioperative nursing core curriculum: Achieving competency in clinical practice.* Philadelphia: W. B. Saunders.

Rothrock, J. C. (1996). *Perioperative nursing care planning* (2nd ed.). St. Louis: Mosby–Year Book.

*Rowell, C. C. (1990). The nosocomial wound infection report: Its impact in the OR. *Today's OR Nurse, 12*(10), 21–23, 50–51.

*Rivelli, D. (1993). Local and regional anesthesia: Nursing implications. *Nursing Clinics of North America, 28*(3), 547–572.

*Scott, S. M., Mayhew, P. A., & Harris, E. A. (1992). Pressure ulcer development in the operating room: Nursing implications. *AORN Journal, 56*(2), 242–250.

*Smalley, P. J. (1992). Laser nursing—a perioperative challenge. *Canadian Operating Room Nursing Journal, 10*(1), 18–22+.

Smith, C. J. (1994). Preparing nurses to monitor patients receiving local anesthesia: Using the decision-making process. *AORN Journal, 59*(5), 1033, 1036–1041.

*Smith, K. A. (1990). Positioning principles: An anatomical review. *AORN Journal, 52*(6), 1196, 1198, 1200–1202+.

Somerson, S. J., et al. (1995). Insights into conscious sedation. *American Journal of Nursing, 95*(6), 26–33.

Standards and recommended practices for perioperative nursing (1996). Denver, CO: Association of Operating Room Nurses.

Standards: Perioperative nursing care. The function of the nurse as first assistant (1995). *Canadian Operating Room Nursing Journal, 13*(2), 25–28.

Stein, R. H. (1995). The perioperative nurse's role in anesthesia management. *AORN Journal, 62*(5), 794–795, 797–797, 801+.

*Stephens, G. (1992). Technology and its effect on OR nursing. *Canadian Operating Room Nursing Journal, 10*(1), 6–7.

*Takes, K. L. (1992). Cost-effective practice: Do OR nurses care? *Nursing Management, 23*(4), 96Q–R, V–X.

*Tappen, R. M. (1991). Alzheimer's disease: Communication techniques to facilitate perioperative care. *AORN Journal, 54*(6), 1279–1286.

Tappen, R. M., et al. (1996). Inadvertent hypothermia in elderly surgical patients. *AORN Journal, 63*(3), 639–644.

*Thomas, S. D. (1989). Malignant hyperthermia. *Critical Care Nurse, 3*(6), 58–69.

Thompson, J. (1996). AORN's multisite clinical study of bloodborne exposures in OR personnel. *AORN Journal, 63*(2), 428–430, 433.

*Treat, M. R., Oz, Mehmet C., & Bass, L. S. (1992). New technologies and future applications of surgical lasers: The right tool for the right job. *Surgical Clinics of North America, 72*(3), 705–742.

Walsh, J. (1994). AANA journal course: Update for nurse anesthetists—patient positioning. *American Association of Nurse Anesthetists Journal, 62*(3), 289–298.

*Walsh, J. (1993). Postop effects of OR positioning. *RN, 56*(2), 50–57.

*Watson, D. S. (1991). Safe nursing practices involving the patient receiving local anesthesia. *AORN Journal, 53*(4), 1055, 1058–1059.

Watson, D. S., & Sangermano, C. A. (1995). Ambulatory surgery. In M. H. Meeker & J. Rothrock (Eds.), *Alexander's care of the patient in surgery* (10th ed., pp. 1125–1144). St. Louis: Mosby–Year Book.

Wheelock, S. M., & Lookinland, S. (1997). Effect of surgical hand scrub time on subsequent bacterial growth. *AORN Journal, 65*(6), 1087–1090, 1092, 1094–1098.

Williams, M. (1996). The expanding role of the nurse in laparoscopic surgery. *British Journal Theatre Nursing, 6*(4), 34–35.

Wilson, L. (1995). Continuous quality improvement: A staff nurse perspective. *Canadian Operating Room Nursing Journal, 13*(1), 29–33.

Winter, M. J. (1994). Music reduces stress and anxiety of patients in the surgical holding area. *Journal of Post Anesthesia Nursing, 9*(6), 340–343.

Woodin, L. M. (1996). Resting easy. How to care for patients receiving I.V. conscious sedation. *Nursing96, 26*(6), 33–41.

Wound closure manual (1994). Somerville, NJ: Ethicon. (Pub. No. EPB010).

Wynd, C. A., et al. (1994). Bacterial carriage on the fingernails of OR nurses. *AORN Journal, 60*(5), 796, 799–805.

*Young, M. A., Meyers, M., McCulloch, L. D., et al. (1992). Latex allergy: A guideline for perioperative nurses. *AORN Journal, 56*(3), 485–497.

SUGGESTED READINGS

Dunn, D. (1997). Malignant hyperthermia. *AORN Journal, 65*(4), 728–762.

This very comprehensive and current article on malignant hyperthermia discusses pathophysiology, incidence, triggering agents, signs and symptoms, crisis management, testing for susceptibility, preparedness for an episode of malignant hyperthermia, and future research considerations. Numerous tables and charts help the reader comprehend the topic. A case study, numerous references, and a continuing education test are included.

McEwen, D. R. (1996). Intraoperative positioning of surgical patients. *AORN Journal, 63*(6), 1059–1063, 1066–1075, 1077–1082, 1084–1085.

The positioning injuries of pressure ulcers (occiput), alopecia, nerve injuries, and respiratory and cardiovascular compromise are discussed in this article. An extensive table outlining upper and lower extremity neuropathies associated with intraoperative positioning and how to correctly position to prevent these injuries is included. Risk factors, positioning considerations, and positioning devices are all addressed. Positioning devices needed to prevent specific injuries in the supine, prone, lateral, sitting, and lithotomy positions are detailed. The article concludes with a 38-item reference list and a 40-question CEU test.

Woodin, L. M. (1996). Resting easy. How to care for patients receiving I.V. conscious sedation. *Nursing96, 26*(6), 33–41.

This comprehensive article on intravenous conscious sedation follows an outpatient having an esophageal gastric dilation and biopsy. General indications for conscious sedation, as well as specific preprocedural nursing assessments, are included. The opioids and benzodiazepines and their antagonists and monitoring related to these medications are discussed in detail. Appropriate emergency responses to potential complications are addressed. A 13-item CEU test is included.

Chapter 22

INTERVENTIONS FOR POSTOPERATIVE CLIENTS

CHAPTER HIGHLIGHTS

The postoperative period begins with completion of the surgical procedure. Ambulatory surgery clients who had local anesthesia may be able to be discharged home. Clients who received conscious sedation will move to a quiet area where they can be observed and monitored until discharge criteria are met. Other clients move from the operating room (OR) to another area for specialized nursing care (often a postanesthesia care unit [PACU]), until their condition stabilizes. The postoperative period continues after the client's condition is stabilized and after the client is discharged from the ambulatory surgery facility or hospital. The actual time spent away from home after surgery varies according to the client's age, physical health, self-care ability, support systems, type and length of surgical procedure, anesthesia, complications (if any), and community resources.

Overview

The postanesthesia care unit is usually located close to the operating department. The unit is usually a large and open room to provide maximal visibility of clients, appropriate ventilation and lighting, and easy access to supplies and emergency equipment. The client area in the unit is often divided into individual cubicles. Curtains or screens for privacy are available but are usually closed only during bedside procedures. Each cubicle is stocked with equipment and supplies commonly used by the nurse to monitor and care for the client, such as oxygen, suction equipment, cardiac monitors, airway equipment, and emergency medications.

After the surgical procedure is completed, the circulating nurse and the anesthesiologist or nurse anesthetist (certified registered nurse anesthetist, or CRNA) accompany the client to the PACU. In some situations, such as when the client is in critical condition, he or she may go directly from the operating department to the intensive (critical) care unit. On arrival, anesthesiology personnel and the circulating nurse give the postanesthesia nurse a verbal report (Table 22–1).

The postanesthesia nurse is skilled in the care of clients of all ages with multiple medical and surgical problems immediately after surgery. This nurse has in-depth knowledge of anesthetic agents, analgesics, pain management, and surgical procedures; is skilled in physical and psychosocial assessment; and can make quick decisions if emergencies or complications occur. The postanesthesia nurse monitors the client closely and consults with the anesthesiology personnel and the surgeons as needed.

TABLE 22-1

Report Guidelines on Arrival in the Postanesthesia Care Unit

Anesthesiology personnel explain the following:
- Type and extent of the surgical procedure
- Type of anesthesia
- Client's tolerance of anesthesia and the surgical procedure
- Client's allergies
- Pathologic condition
- Status of vital signs
- Type and amount of intravenous fluids and medications administered
- Estimated blood loss (EBL)
- Any intraoperative complications, such as a traumatic intubation

The circulating nurse adds information related to
- Client's primary language spoken and any sensory impairments
- Client's anxiety level before receiving anesthesia
- Special requests that were verbalized by the client preoperatively
- Client's preoperative and intraoperative respiratory function and dysfunction
- Pertinent medical history
- Location and type of incisions, dressings, catheters, tubes, drains, or packing
- Intake and output, including current intravenous fluid administration and estimated blood loss
- Joint or limb immobility while in the operating room, especially in the elderly client
- Other intraoperative positioning that may be relevant in the postoperative phase
- Any other important intraoperative occurrences

Collaborative Management

 Assessment

➤ History

The postanesthesia nurse uses the information from the surgical team's report in planning care for the client. After receiving the report and assessing the client, the PACU nurse reviews the chart for information about the client's history and his or her presurgical physical and emotional status. In ideal situations, the postanesthesia nurse reviews pertinent information before the client arrives in the unit. If the client is remaining as an inpatient, the nurse on the medical-surgical unit later incorporates all of the surgical and postanesthesia information into the client's postoperative plan of care. Chapter 20 identifies clinical situations that put a client at risk for the following postoperative complications:
- Allergic reactions
- Hypothermia
- Hyperthermia
- Hypertension
- Hypotension

- Hypovolemic shock
- Renal failure
- Electrolyte imbalances
- Dysrhythmias
- Congestive heart failure
- Paralytic ileus
- Acute urinary retention
- Deep venous thrombosis
- Pulmonary embolism
- Atelectasis or pneumonia
- Laryngeal edema
- Ventilator dependence
- Gastrointestinal (GI) bleeding
- Disseminated intravascular coagulation (DIC)
- Anemia
- Wound evisceration

➤ Physical Assessment/Clinical Manifestations

The postanesthesia nurse assesses the client and compiles data on a PACU record form (Fig. 22–1). Assessment data include the client's temperature, pulse, respiration, and blood pressure. The nurse examines the surgical area for bleeding. The postanesthesia nurse initiates assessments, and the intensive care or medical-surgical nurse continues assessments when the client is discharged to the inpatient unit. The frequency of vital signs measurement is based on the facility's policy and the surgeon's orders. Vital signs are often recorded every 15 minutes for four times, every 30 minutes for four times, every 2 hours for four times, and then every 4 hours for 24 to 48 hours if the client's condition is stable. Thereafter, vital signs are assessed according to the facility's policy, the client's condition, and the nurse's judgment.

The health care team determines the client's readiness for discharge from the postanesthesia area by noting a postanesthesia recovery score on the postanesthesia recovery scale of at least 10 (see Figure 22–1). In addition, the facility may have specific criteria for discharge (e.g., stable vital signs, normothermia, no overt bleeding, and return of gag, cough, and swallow reflexes). After the nurse determines that all criteria have been met, the client is discharged by the anesthesiologist to the hospital unit or to home. When an anesthesiologist has not been involved, such as may be the case with local anesthesia or conscious sedation, the surgeon or nurse discharges the client once the discharge criteria have been met.

Physical assessment continues from the PACU to the intensive care or medical-surgical nursing unit. If the client is to be discharged from the PACU to the home, physical assessment is continued by home care nurses or by the client or family members themselves after adequate instruction.

Respiratory System

Airway Assessment. When the client is admitted to PACU, the nurse immediately assesses for a patent airway and adequate respiratory exchange. An artificial airway, such as an endotracheal (ET) tube, a nasal trumpet, or an oral airway, may be in place. If the client is receiving supplemental oxygen, the nurse notes the type of delivery device and the concentration or liter flow of the oxygen.

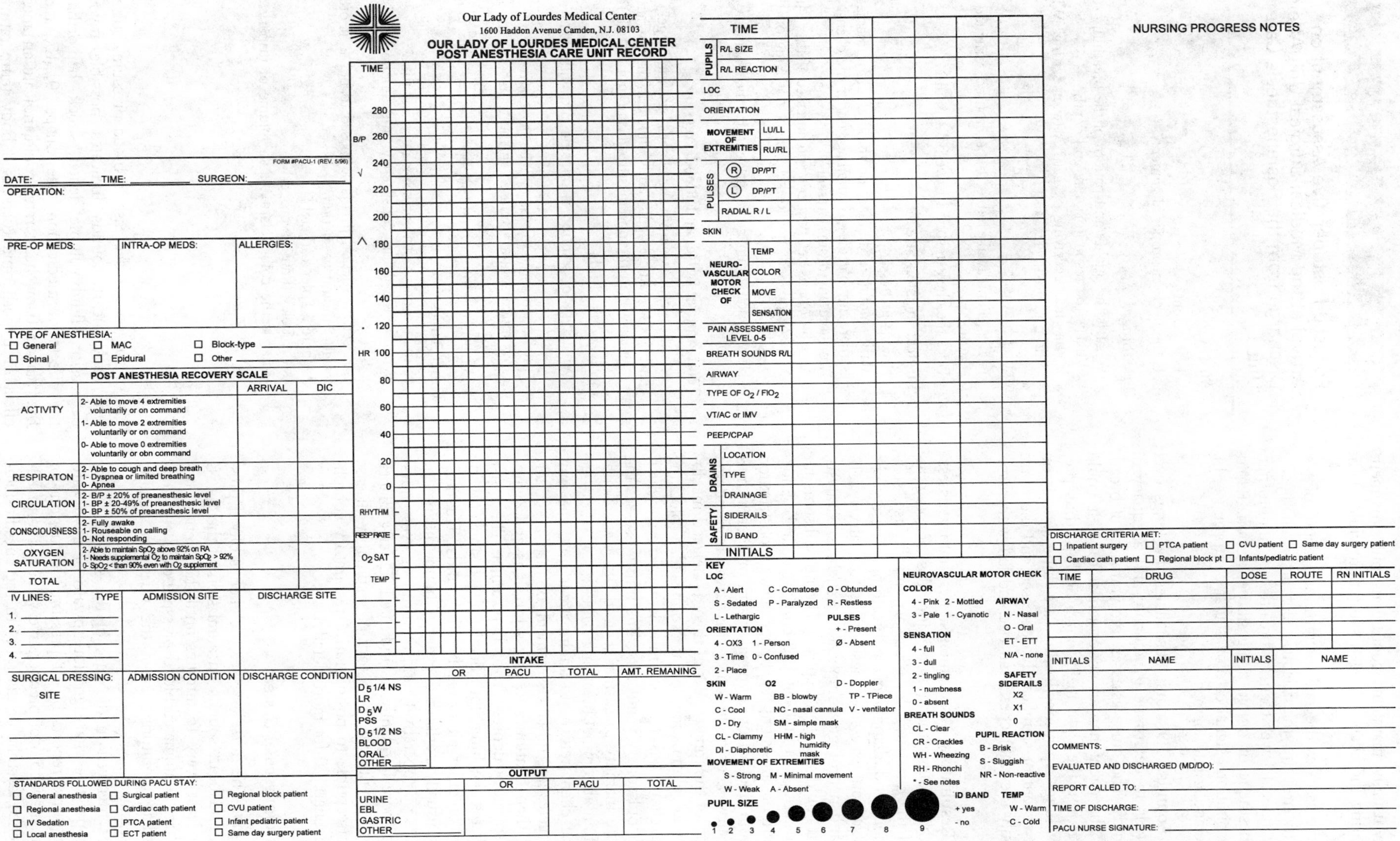
Our Lady of Lourdes Medical Center
1600 Haddon Avenue Camden, N.J. 08103
OUR LADY OF LOURDES MEDICAL CENTER
POST ANESTHESIA CARE UNIT RECORD

FORM #PACU-1 (REV. 5/96)

DATE: ________ TIME: ________ SURGEON: ________
OPERATION:

PRE-OP MEDS: | INTRA-OP MEDS: | ALLERGIES:

TYPE OF ANESTHESIA:
☐ General ☐ MAC ☐ Block-type ________
☐ Spinal ☐ Epidural ☐ Other ________

POST ANESTHESIA RECOVERY SCALE		ARRIVAL	DIC
ACTIVITY	2- Able to move 4 extremities voluntarily or on command 1- Able to move 2 extremities voluntarily or on command 0- Able to move 0 extremities voluntarily or obn command		
RESPIRATON	2- Able to cough and deep breath 1- Dyspnea or limited breathing 0- Apnea		
CIRCULATION	2- B/P ± 20% of preanesthesic level 1- BP ± 20-49% of preanesthesic level 0- BP ± 50% of preanesthesic level		
CONSCIOUSNESS	2- Fully awake 1- Rouseable on calling 0- Not responding		
OXYGEN SATURATION	2- Able to maintain SpO_2 above 92% on RA 1- Needs supplemental O_2 to maintain SpO_2 > 92% 0- SpO_2 < than 90% even with O_2 supplement		
TOTAL			

IV LINES:	TYPE	ADMISSION SITE	DISCHARGE SITE
1.			
2.			
3.			
4.			

SURGICAL DRESSING:	ADMISSION CONDITION	DISCHARGE CONDITION
SITE		

STANDARDS FOLLOWED DURING PACU STAY:
☐ General anesthesia ☐ Surgical patient ☐ Regional block patient
☐ Regional anesthesia ☐ Cardiac cath patient ☐ CVU patient
☐ IV Sedation ☐ PTCA patient ☐ Infant pediatric patient
☐ Local anesthesia ☐ ECT patient ☐ Same day surgery patient

TIME
B/P 280 260 240 √ 220 200 ^ 180 160 140 · 120 HR 100 80 60 40 20 0
RHYTHM
RESP RATE
O_2 SAT
TEMP

	INTAKE			
	OR	PACU	TOTAL	AMT. REMANING
$D_5$1/4 NS LR D_5W PSS $D_5$1/2 NS BLOOD ORAL OTHER ______				

	OUTPUT		
	OR	PACU	TOTAL
URINE EBL GASTRIC OTHER ______			

TIME						
PUPILS R/L SIZE						
PUPILS R/L REACTION						
LOC						
ORIENTATION						
MOVEMENT OF EXTREMITIES LU/LL						
MOVEMENT OF EXTREMITIES RU/RL						
PULSES Ⓡ DP/PT						
PULSES Ⓛ DP/PT						
PULSES RADIAL R / L						
SKIN						
NEUROVASCULAR MOTOR CHECK OF TEMP						
NEUROVASCULAR MOTOR CHECK OF COLOR						
NEUROVASCULAR MOTOR CHECK OF MOVE						
NEUROVASCULAR MOTOR CHECK OF SENSATION						
PAIN ASSESSMENT LEVEL 0-5						
BREATH SOUNDS R/L						
AIRWAY						
TYPE OF O_2 / FIO_2						
VT/AC or IMV						
PEEP/CPAP						
DRAINS LOCATION						
DRAINS TYPE						
DRAINS DRAINAGE						
SAFETY SIDERAILS						
SAFETY ID BAND						
INITIALS						

KEY
LOC: A - Alert, C - Comatose, O - Obtunded, S - Sedated, P - Paralyzed, R - Restless, L - Lethargic
PULSES: + - Present, Ø - Absent
ORIENTATION: 4 - OX3, 1 - Person, 3 - Time, 0 - Confused, 2 - Place
SKIN: W - Warm, C - Cool, D - Dry, CL - Clammy, DI - Diaphoretic
O2: BB - blowby, NC - nasal cannula, SM - simple mask, HHM - high humidity mask, D - Doppler, TP - TPiece, V - ventilator
MOVEMENT OF EXTREMITIES: S - Strong, M - Minimal movement, W - Weak, A - Absent
PUPIL SIZE: 1 2 3 4 5 6 7 8 9

NEUROVASCULAR MOTOR CHECK
COLOR: 4 - Pink, 2 - Mottled, 3 - Pale, 1 - Cyanotic
AIRWAY: N - Nasal, O - Oral, ET - ETT, N/A - none
SENSATION: 4 - full, 3 - dull, 2 - tingling, 1 - numbness, 0 - absent
SAFETY SIDERAILS: X2, X1, 0
BREATH SOUNDS: CL - Clear, CR - Crackles, WH - Wheezing, RH - Rhonchi, * - See notes
PUPIL REACTION: B - Brisk, S - Sluggish, NR - Non-reactive
ID BAND: + yes, - no
TEMP: W - Warm, C - Cold

NURSING PROGRESS NOTES

DISCHARGE CRITERIA MET:
☐ Inpatient surgery ☐ PTCA patient ☐ CVU patient ☐ Same day surgery patient
☐ Cardiac cath patient ☐ Regional block pt ☐ Infants/pediatric patient

TIME	DRUG	DOSE	ROUTE	RN INITIALS

INITIALS	NAME	INITIALS	NAME

COMMENTS: ________
EVALUATED AND DISCHARGED (MD/DO): ________
REPORT CALLED TO: ________
TIME OF DISCHARGE: ________
PACU NURSE SIGNATURE: ________

Figure 22–1. Example of a postanesthesia care unit record. (Courtesy of Our Lady of Lourdes Medical Center, Camden, NJ.)

The nurse usually maintains continuous pulse oximetry for monitoring the client's oxygen saturation while in the PACU.

The nurse assesses the rate, pattern, and depth of respirations to measure the adequacy of air exchange. A respiratory rate of fewer than 10 breaths per minute may indicate anesthetic or opioid analgesic depression. Rapid, shallow respirations signal cardiovascular compromise, increased metabolic rate, or pain.

Breath Sounds. The nurse auscultates the lungs over all lung fields to determine the quality and adequacy of breath sounds. The nurse assesses for symmetry of breath sounds. If the client has an endotracheal tube, it could move down into the right mainstem bronchus, thus preventing left lung expansion. In this case, lung sounds on the left are absent or significantly decreased and the nurse observes only the right chest wall rise and fall with respirations.

Other Respiratory Assessments. Respiratory assessment by the postanesthesia nurse includes ongoing inspection of the chest wall for accessory muscle use, sternal retraction, and diaphragmatic breathing. These signs could indicate an excessive anesthetic effect, airway obstruction, and neurologic complications such as paralysis, all of which could result in hypoxia. The nurse listens for snoring and stridor (a high-pitched crowing sound). Snoring and stridor are signs of upper airway obstruction resulting from tracheal or laryngeal spasm or edema, mucus in the airway, or occlusion of the airway from edema or relaxation of the tongue. When there is delayed metabolism of and elimination of neuromuscular blocking agents, the client has residual muscle weakness, which could affect pulmonary ventilation. The nurse assesses the client for the inability to sustain a head lift, weak handgrasps, and an abdominal breathing pattern.

When the client returns to an inpatient unit, the unit nurse completes an initial assessment on arrival (Chart 22–1) and then continues to assess for signs and symptoms of respiratory depression or hypoxemia. The nurse also auscultates the lungs for effective expansion and for adventitious or other abnormal breath sounds. This auscultation is usually performed every 4 hours during the first 24 hours postoperatively and then during every nursing shift, or more frequently, as indicated. Elderly clients, smokers, and clients with a history of respiratory disease are more susceptible to postoperative respiratory complications (see Chap. 20 for more details).

Cardiovascular System

Vital Signs. The nurse assesses the client's blood pressure, pulse, and heart sounds on admission to the PACU and then at least every 15 minutes until the client's condition stabilizes. Automated blood pressure cuffs and continuous cardiac monitoring assist the nurse in making frequent assessments.

All nurses involved in the care of the surgical client review postoperative vital signs for upward or downward trends. The nurse reports blood pressure fluctuations of more or less than 25% of preoperative values (15- to 20-point difference, systolic or diastolic) to the anesthesiolo-

gist or surgeon. A decrease in blood pressure, pulse pressure, and heart sounds indicates possible myocardial depression, fluid volume deficit, shock, hemorrhage, or the effects of medication (see Chaps. 9, 15, and 39). Bradycardia (slow heart rate) could indicate an anesthesia effect or hypothermia (decreased body temperature). El-

Chart 22–1

Focused Postoperative Assessment on Arrival at the Medical-Surgical Unit After Discharge from the Postanesthesia Care Unit

Airway
Is it patent?
Is the neck in proper alignment?

Breathing
What is the quality and pattern of the breathing?
What is the respiratory rate and depth?
Is the client receiving oxygen? At what setting? What is the pulse oximetry result?

Mental Status
Is the client awake, able to be aroused, oriented, and aware?
Does the client respond to verbal stimuli?

Surgical Incision Site
How is it dressed?
Mark amount of drainage on the dressing immediately.
Is there any bleeding or drainage under the client?
Are there any drains present?
Are the drains set properly (compressed if they should be compressed, not kinked, client not lying on them, etc.)?
How much drainage is present in the drainage container?

Temperature, Pulse, and Blood Pressure
Are these values within the client's baseline range?
Are these values significantly different than when the client was in the postanesthesia care unit (PACU)?

Intravenous Fluids
What type of solution is infusing and with what additives?
How much solution was remaining on arrival?
How much solution infused in the transport time from PACU?
What is the infusion rate supposed to be set at? Is it?

Other Tubes
Is there a nasogastric or other intestinal tube?
What is the color, consistency, and amount of drainage?
Is it set on suction if it is supposed to be? Is it on the right amount of suction?
Is there a Foley catheter?
Is the Foley draining properly?
What is the color, clarity, and volume of urinary output?

derly clients are especially predisposed to hypothermia because of aging changes in the hypothalamus (the temperature regulation center), loss of subcutaneous tissue, and coolness of the operating suite. An increased pulse rate could indicate hemorrhage, shock, or pain.

Cardiac Monitoring. Cardiac monitoring is routinely maintained until the client is discharged from the PACU. For clients at risk for dysrhythmias, monitoring may continue on either specialized telemetry units or on general medical-surgical units. In assessing the vital signs of a client who is not undergoing continuous monitoring, the nurse determines the rate, rhythm, and quality of the client's apical pulse compared with those of a peripheral pulse such as the radial pulse. A pulse deficit (a difference between the apical and peripheral pulses) could indicate a dysrhythmia.

Peripheral Vascular Assessment. Anesthesia and positioning during surgery (e.g., the lithotomy position for genitourinary procedures) may compromise the client's peripheral circulation. The nurse assesses the client's peripheral circulation by comparing distal pulses bilaterally for the presence and quality of pulsation, noting the color and temperature of extremities, evaluating sensation, and determining the speed of capillary refill. Palpable dorsalis pedis pulses indicate adequate circulation and tissue perfusion of the distal lower extremities.

As part of the ongoing assessment, the nurse assesses the lower extremities for redness, pain, warmth, swelling, and the presence of Homan's sign, any of which could indicate the presence of deep venous thrombosis (DVT), a life-threatening condition. Assessment of the lower extremities may be performed once during a nursing shift, once daily, or once per visit, depending on the risk of complications and the facility's or agency's policy. (Chapters 20, 38, and 54 have further information on deep venous thrombosis.)

Neurologic System

General Cerebral Functioning. Regardless of the type of surgical procedure, the postanesthesia nurse assesses cerebral function and the level of consciousness or awareness of all clients who have received general anesthesia (Table 22-2) or any type of sedation. To assess the client's level of consciousness, the nurse observes for lethargy, restlessness, or irritability and tests coherence and orientation. The nurse determines awareness by observing responses to calling the client's name, touching the client, and giving simple commands such as "Open your eyes" and "Take a deep breath." Eye opening in response to a command indicates wakefulness or arousability but not necessarily awareness. The nurse determines the degree of orientation to person, place, and time by asking the conscious client to answer simple questions, such as "What is your name?" (person), "Where are you?" (place), and "What day is it?" (time).

For an elderly client, a rapid return to his or her prior level of orientation may not be realistic. The preoperative, intraoperative, and postoperative medications and anesthetic agents often affect the elderly client's reorientation ability (see Chaps. 20 and 21).

TABLE 22-2

Immediate Postoperative Neurologic Assessment: Return to Preoperative Level
Order of Return to Consciousness After General Anesthesia
1. Muscular irritability
2. Restlessness and delirium
3. Recognition of pain
4. Ability to reason and control behavior
Order of Return of Motor and Sensory Functioning After Local or Regional Anesthesia
1. Sense of touch
2. Sense of pain
3. Sense of warmth
4. Sense of cold
5. Ability to move

The nurse compares the client's preoperative baseline neurologic status with the postoperative assessment findings. Clients with altered cerebral functioning preoperatively as a result of a pre-existing condition continue to have that alteration postoperatively. After the client has returned to a satisfactory consciousness level (and all other criteria have been met), he or she is discharged from the PACU. Assessment of the client's level of consciousness continues every 4 to 8 hours or as indicated by the client's condition and the facility's policy.

Motor/Sensory Assessment. For all clients receiving general and regional anesthesia, motor and sensory function is assessed. General anesthesia renders clients unconscious and depresses voluntary motor function; regional anesthesia alters the motor and sensory function of only part of the body. (See Chapter 21 for more information on anesthesia.) Motor and sensory assessment is especially important after the client has had epidural or spinal anesthesia. The postanesthesia nurse evaluates motor function by instructing the client to move each extremity. The client who had epidural or spinal anesthesia remains in the PACU until sensory function (feeling) and voluntary motor movement of the lower extremities have returned (see Table 22-2). In addition, the nurse assesses the strength of each limb and compares the results bilaterally.

The postanesthesia nurse also tests for the return of sympathetic nervous system tone by gradually elevating the client's head and monitoring for hypotension. This evaluation begins after the client's sensation has returned to at least the spinal dermatome level of T-10. (See Chapter 43 for further neurologic assessment.) After the client is transferred to the nursing unit, the medical-surgical nurse continues neurologic assessment as indicated.

Fluid and Electrolyte Balance

Fasting before and during surgery, the loss of fluid during the procedure, and the type and amount of blood or IV fluid administered affect the client's postoperative fluid and electrolyte balance. Either fluid volume deficit or fluid volume overload may occur after surgery. Sodium, potassium, chloride, and calcium imbalances also may result, as may alterations in other electrolyte levels. Complications of fluid and electrolyte imbalances occur more often in elderly or debilitated clients and in clients with medical problems such as diabetes mellitus, Crohn's disease (especially after major intestinal surgery), and heart failure.

Intake and Output. Intraoperative intake and output measurement is part of the operative record and part of the circulating nurse's report to the postanesthesia nurse. The postanesthesia nurse records any intake or output, including intravenous (IV) fluid intake, vomitus, urine, and nasogastric (NG) tube drainage. When he or she gives report, the medical-surgical nurse needs to know the total intake and output from both the OR and the PACU to assess fluid balance accurately and to complete the 24-hour intake and output record.

Hydration Assessment. The medical-surgical nurse continues to assess the client's hydration. The nurse inspects the color and moist appearance of mucous membranes; the turgor, texture, and "tenting" of the skin (test over the sternum or forehead of an elderly client); the amount of drainage on dressings; and the presence of axillary sweat, which indicates adequate hydration. The nurse measures total output (e.g., NG tube drainage, urinary output, and wound drainage) and compares it with total intake to identify a possible fluid imbalance. The nurse considers insensible fluid loss when reviewing total output. The nurse continues to assess the client's intake and output while the client is at risk for fluid imbalances. Some facilities have policies that require intake and output to be measured if the client receives IV fluids or has a catheter, drains, or an NG tube.

Intravenous Fluids. The nurse administers and closely monitors IV fluids to promote fluid and electrolyte balance. Standard isotonic solutions such as lactated Ringer's (LR) and 5% dextrose with lactated Ringer's (D5/LR) are used for IV fluid replacement and maintenance in the PACU. After the client returns to the medical-surgical unit, the type and rate of administration of IV solutions are based on the individual client's need. A typical IV solution for the client when admitted to the nursing unit is 5% dextrose with 0.45% normal saline (D5/½ NSS). (See Chapters 15 and 17 for further discussion of IV fluid administration, electrolyte balance, and assessment of hydration.)

Acid-Base Balance

Acid-base balance may be affected by preoperative, intraoperative, and postoperative respiratory status, intraoperative metabolic changes, and losses of acids or bases in drainage. For example, NG tube drainage or vomitus represents a loss of hydrochloric acid. The nurse assesses acid-base status mostly through arterial blood gas measurement and other laboratory values. (See Chapter 19 for more detailed information on acid-base imbalances.)

Renal/Urinary System

Voluntary control of urinary function may return immediately after surgery or may not return for 6 to 8 hours or longer after inhalation, IV, and epidural or spinal anesthe-

sia. The effects of preoperative medications and anesthetic agents and manipulation during surgery, in combination or alone, can cause urinary retention. The nurse assesses for this complication by inspection, palpation, and percussion of the client's lower abdomen for bladder distention. Assessment may be difficult to perform when the client has had lower abdominal surgery. Urinary retention is common in the early postoperative period and requires appropriate intervention, often one or more intermittent (straight) catheterizations to empty the bladder.

When the client has an indwelling urinary (Foley) catheter, the nurse assesses the urine for color, clarity, and amount. If the client is voiding, the nurse also assesses the urinary frequency, associated amount per void, and any symptoms. Urinary output should correlate with total input for a 24-hour period, but other sources of output need to be considered. The nurse reports a urinary output of less than 30 mL/hour (240 mL/8-hour nursing shift) to the physician. Decreased urinary output may indicate hypovolemia or renal complications. (Refer to Chapter 72 for complete information on the assessment of renal/urinary function, including the interpretation of specific gravity, electrolyte values, and osmolality of urine.)

Gastrointestinal System

Nausea and Vomiting. One of the most common postoperative reactions is nausea and vomiting. Approximately 30% of clients receiving general anesthesia have some form of gastrointestinal upset within the first 24 hours after surgery. Clients with a history of motion sickness are more likely to develop postoperative nausea and vomiting. Obese individuals may be at risk because many anesthetics are retained by fat cells and, therefore, have a lingering effect. Abdominal surgery and the use of opioid analgesics reduce intestinal peristalsis after surgery. These situations predispose the client to nausea and vomiting for longer than the first 24 hours after surgery.

Postoperative nausea and vomiting can cause stress and irritation of abdominal and gastrointestinal (GI) wounds, increase intracranial pressure in clients who had head and neck surgery, elevate intraocular pressure in clients who had eye surgery, and increase the risk of aspiration and aspiration pneumonia. The nurse assesses for nausea and vomiting continuously. Often a client experiences nausea as the head of the bed is raised in the early postoperative period. This symptom may occur with or without associated dizziness. The nurse has the client in side-lying position before raising his or her head slowly.

Gastrointestinal Peristalsis. The nurse in the postanesthesia care unit and later on the medical-surgical unit assesses for the return of peristaltic function. Peristalsis may be delayed because of the length of time under anesthesia, the amount of bowel handling intraoperatively, and opioid analgesic use.

Assessment. The nurse auscultates for bowel sounds in all four abdominal quadrants and at the umbilicus. If the client is undergoing nasogastric (NG) suctioning, the suction must be turned off before auscultation of the abdomen. Otherwise, the nurse could mistake the sound of the suction for bowel sounds. In addition, the nurse asks the client whether flatus has been passed. Both bowel sounds and flatus passage indicate peristalsis, but abdominal cramping denotes trapped, nonmoving gas and not peristalsis.

Complications. Decreased peristalsis can occur in clients with paralytic ileus. The intestine wall is distended and there is no movement of the intestinal wall (aperistalsis). The nurse assesses for the clinical manifestations of paralytic ileus. These include few or absent bowel sounds, distended abdomen, diffuse abdominal discomfort (as a result of the distention), vomiting, lack of flatus, and no passage of stool.

The client may also experience constipation postoperatively owing to anesthesia, analgesia (especially codeine [Paveral✳] and other opioid analgesics), decreased activity, and decreased oral intake. The nurse assesses the client's abdomen by inspection, palpation, percussion, and auscultation and records the client's elimination pattern to determine whether interventions are needed. Increased dietary fiber intake, the administration of mild laxatives or bulk-forming agents, or the use of enemas may be necessary.

Nasogastric Tube Drainage. An NG tube may be inserted intraoperatively to decompress and drain the stomach, to promote gastrointestinal rest, to allow the lower gastrointestinal tract to heal, and to provide an enteral feeding route. It may also be used to monitor the occurrence of bleeding and prevent intestinal obstruction. The Levin tube and the Salem sump tube are the two most common tubes used. The Salem tube is a double-lumen tube with an air vent to keep the tube from adhering to the gastric mucosa. This feature allows easy drainage of the stomach and prevents gastric mucosal damage. The Levin tube is a single-lumen tube with no air vent. To promote drainage, varying degrees of suction (high, medium, or low) are applied to the nasogastric tube. Suction is either continuous (recommended for the Salem tube) or intermittent on the basis of the surgeon's preference and the tube type.

Assessment. The nurse records the color, consistency, and amount of the drained material every 8 hours (Table 22–3). In some instances, the results of an occult blood test (Gastroccult) may also be recorded. Normal NG drainage fluid is greenish-yellow; red drainage fluid indicates active bleeding, and brown liquid or coffee-ground drainage indicates the possibility of old bleeding.

Complications. The nurse assesses the client for possible complications related to NG tube use, including fluid and electrolyte imbalances, aspiration, and nares discomfort. To prevent aspiration, the nurse checks the tube placement every 4 to 8 hours and before the instillation of irrigation solution into the tube (see Chapter 58 for information on tube placement and care). After gastric surgery, the tube should not be manipulated or irrigated without an order from the physician. Fluid and electrolyte imbalances can result from NG drainage and tube irrigation with water instead of saline. Imbalances include fluid volume deficit (see Chap. 15), hypokalemia and hyponatremia (see Chap. 16), hypochloremia, and metabolic alkalosis (see Chap. 19).

TABLE 22–3

Calculating Nasogastric Tube Drainage

Formula

$$\text{drainage in collection device} - \text{amount of irrigant} = \text{true (actual) amount of drainage}$$

Example

A client's drainage container was marked at 150 mL at 7 AM. At 3 PM, there was 525 mL in the container. During the nursing shift, the nurse instilled 30 mL of saline as an irrigant into the tube four times, as ordered by the physician.

$$525 \text{ mL} - 150 \text{ mL} = 375 \text{ mL of drainage}$$

$$30 \text{ mL} \times 4 = 120 \text{ mL of irrigant}$$

$$375 \text{ mL} - 120 \text{ mL} = 255 \text{ mL of actual drainage}$$

Integumentary System

The clean surgical wound heals itself at skin level in approximately 2 weeks in the absence of trauma, connective tissue disease, malnutrition, and the use of some medications such as steroids. Smokers, elderly clients, obese clients, and those with diseases that decrease immunity have delayed wound healing. Complete healing of underlying tissue and return to presurgical integrity may take 6 months to 2 years. The physical condition and age of the client, size and location of the wound, and stress on the surgical wound also affect the length of time for wound healing. Because of rich blood supply, wounds of the face and head heal more quickly than abdominal and leg wounds.

Normal Wound Healing. During the first few days of normal wound healing, the incised tissue regains blood supply and begins to bind together. Fibrin from the clotting process and a thin layer of epithelial cells seal the incision. After 1 to 4 days, epithelial cells continue to grow along the fibrin while growing strands of collagen begin to fill in the gaps in the wound (Strimike et al., 1997). This process continues for 2 to 3 weeks when the wound appears to be healed; however, healing is not complete for up to 2 years until the scar is strengthened. (See Chapter 70 for discussion of wound healing and wound infection.)

When the client is an inpatient, the surgeon usually removes the original postoperative dressing the first or second postoperative day. The nurse assesses the incision on a regular basis, usually every 8 hours, for redness, increased warmth, swelling, tenderness or pain, and the type and amount of drainage. Some drainage is normal during the first few days, changing from sanguineous (bloody) to serosanguineous to serous (serum-like or yellow). Serosanguineous drainage continuing beyond the fifth postoperative day should alert the nurse to the possibility of dehiscence, and the surgeon should be notified. Slight crusting on the incision line is normal, as is a pink color to the line itself owing to inflammation from the surgical procedure. Slight swelling under the sutures or staples is also normal. Redness or swelling of or around the incision line, excessive tenderness or pain on palpation, and purulent or odorous drainage could indicate wound infection and is reported to the surgeon.

Ineffective Wound Healing. Ineffective wound healing may be caused by wound infection, distention from edema or paralytic ileus, stress at the surgical site, and pre-existing conditions that cause delayed wound healing. Wound *dehiscence* is a partial or complete separation of the outer layers of the wound, sometimes described as a "splitting open of the wound". *Evisceration* is the total separation of the layers and extrusion of internal organs or viscera (usually abdominal) through the open wound (Fig. 22–2). Both of these alterations in wound healing are more often seen between the 5th and 10th postoperative days and occur more frequently in obese clients or others predisposed to delayed wound healing. Wound dehiscence or evisceration may be preceded by excessive coughing, not splinting the surgical site, vomiting, or straining. The client may state, "Something gave way" or "I feel as if I just split open."

Dressings and Drains. All dressings, including casts and elastic (Ace) bandages, are assessed for bleeding or other drainage on admission to the PACU and then frequently until the client is discharged to home or transferred to the inpatient unit. The medical-surgical nurse assesses the client's dressing each time vital signs are taken. When inspecting the dressing, the nurse checks for drainage and notes the amount, color, consistency, and odor of the drainage fluid. The nurse also checks underneath the client, because drainage (often blood from hemorrhage) may leak from the side of the dressing and yet

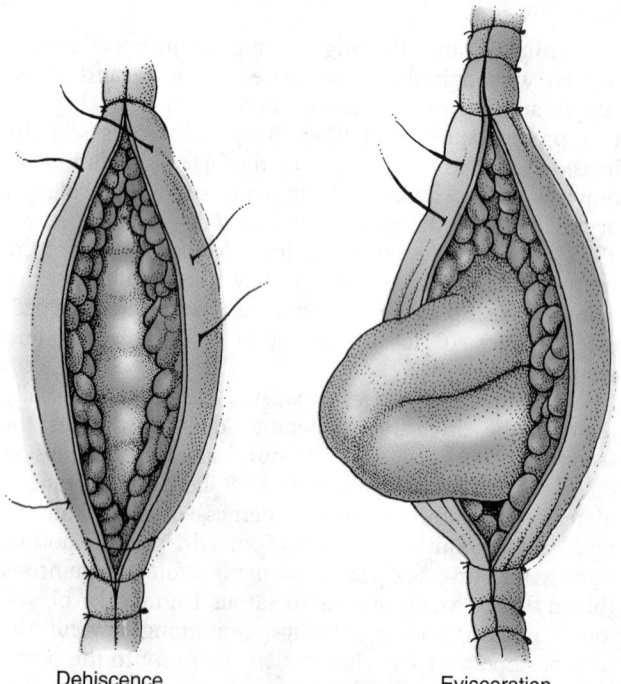

Dehiscence   Evisceration

Figure 22–2. Complications of wound healing.

not appear on the dressing itself. The dressing should not restrict circulation or sensation.

To confine or contain drainage, the surgeon inserts a drain into or close to the wound if more than a minimal amount of drainage is expected. A Penrose drain (a single-lumen, soft latex tube) is a gravity-type drain under the dressing. The nurse assesses closed-suction drains such as Hemovac, VacuDrain, and Jackson-Pratt drains to ensure maintenance of compression and thus suction. The surgeon may place a T tube after abdominal cholecystectomy to drain bile. Figure 22–3 shows commonly used drains.

The nurse assesses all drains for patency when the client is admitted to the PACU and every time vital signs are taken during the postoperative period. The nurse monitors the amount, color, and consistency of the drainage while the client is in the PACU and at least every 8 hours after the client is transferred to the medical-surgical nursing unit. For example, large amounts of sanguineous drainage may indicate internal bleeding.

Discomfort/Pain Assessment

The surgical client almost always reports pain. Postoperative pain is related to the surgical wound, tissue manipulation, presence of drains, and intraoperative positioning. In assessing the client's discomfort or pain and need for medication, the nurse considers the type, extent, and length of the surgical procedure. The nurse assesses for physical and emotional signs of pain such as increased pulse and blood pressure, increased respiratory rate or hyperventilation, diaphoresis (profuse perspiration), restlessness, increased confusion (in the elderly), wincing, moaning, and crying. When possible, the nurse asks the client to quantify or rate the discomfort or pain before and after medication is given (e.g., on a scale of 1 to 10, with 1 being least intense and 10 being extreme pain). In addition, the nurse observes for a return of the client's normal (baseline) physical behaviors. (See Chapter 9 for further discussion of pain assessment.)

Discomfort or pain assessment is initiated by the postanesthesia nurse. After the client is transferred from the PACU, the medical-surgical nurse continues to assess the client's comfort level. Postoperative pain generally reaches its peak on the second postoperative day, when the client is more awake and the anesthetics and analgesics given intraoperatively have been metabolized and excreted.

➤ Psychosocial Assessment

As the nurse completes the physical aspects of postoperative assessment, the psychological, social, and cultural characteristics of the client are considered. This assessment may be delayed or difficult to perform in the PACU when the client is drowsy or incoherent. The nurse considers the client's age and medical history, surgical procedure, and impact of the procedure on the client's recovery, body image, roles, and lifestyle.

Physical signs indicating anxiety include restlessness; increased pulse, blood pressure, and respiratory rate; and crying. The client may be anxious and ask questions about the results or findings of the surgical procedure.

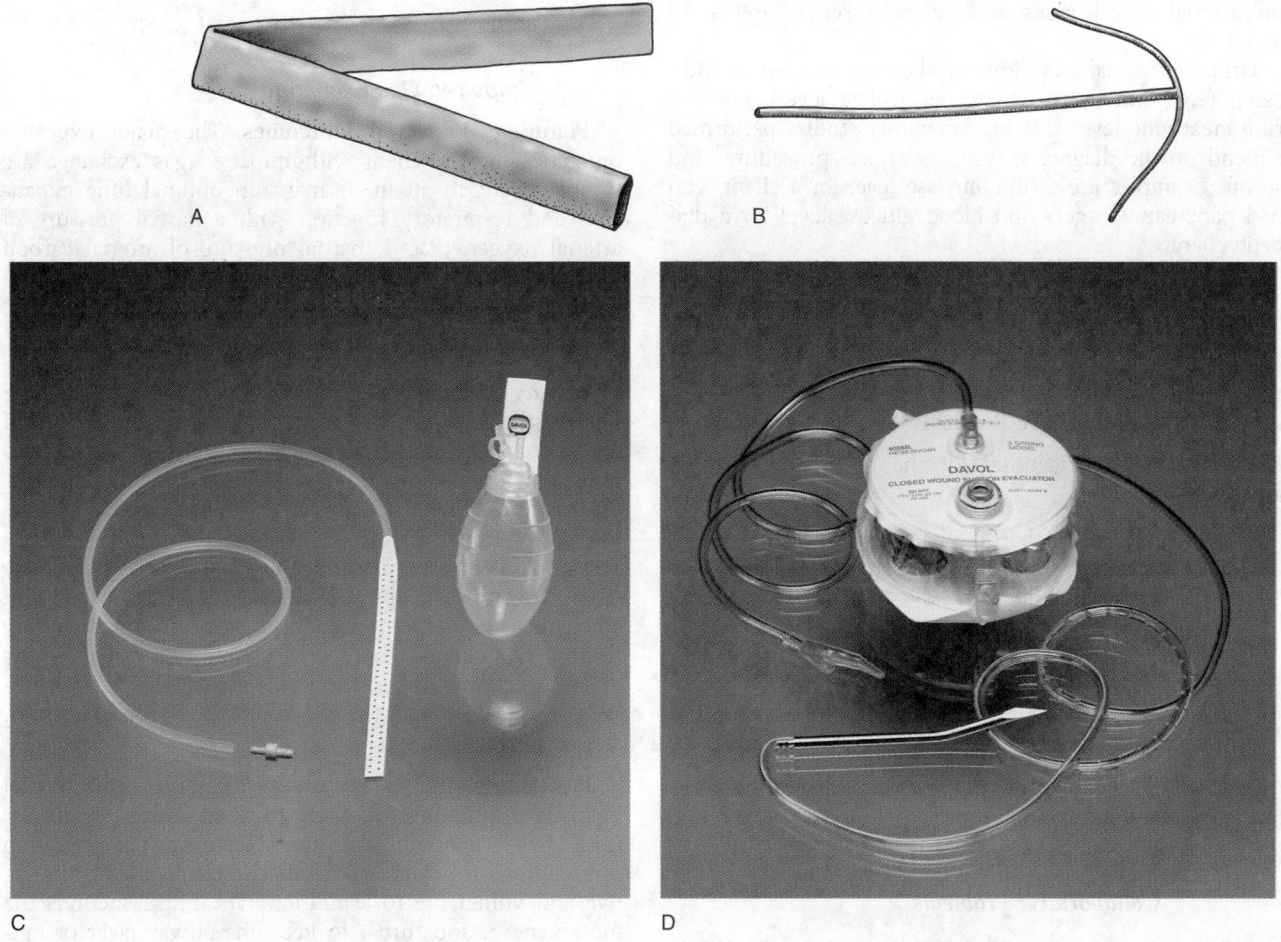

Figure 22–3. Types of surgical drains. Gravity drains, such as the Penrose (A) and the T tube (B) drain directly through a tube from the surgical area. In closed wound drainage systems, such as the Jackson-Pratt (C) and Hemovac (D), drainage collects in a collecting vessel by means of compression and reexpansion of the system. (C and D, courtesy of C. R. Bard, Inc., Covington, GA.)

The nurse reassures the client that the surgeon will speak with him or her after the client is fully awake. If the surgeon has already spoken with the client, the nurse reinforces what was said. (Chapter 8 has further information on stress.)

After the client returns to the medical-surgical unit, the medical-surgical nurse continues the psychosocial assessment of the client and assesses significant others as well.

➤ *Laboratory Assessment*

Postoperative laboratory tests are performed to monitor the client for complications. Tests are based on the surgical procedure and the client's medical history and postoperative clinical manifestations. Common postoperative serum tests include analysis of electrolytes and a complete blood count (see Chart 20–3). A change in laboratory test results (e.g., electrolyte levels, hematocrit, and hemoglobin levels) commonly occurs during the first 24 to 48 hours postoperatively because of blood and fluid loss and the body's reaction to the surgical process. Fluid loss without significant blood loss may result in hemoconcentrated laboratory values (decreased fluid in the blood with resultant increased concentration). The laboratory test re-

sult is reported as increased, but actually represents a concentrated normal value.

A subtle early indication of infection is an increase in the band cells (immature neutrophils) in the white cell differential count. This increase is termed a *shift to the left.* The source of infection may be the respiratory system, urinary tract, wound, or IV site. The nurse obtains appropriate specimens for culture and sensitivity testing and monitors the culture results reported from the microbiology laboratory at 24, 48, and 72 hours. The nurse notifies the physician of positive culture results. (See Chapter 28 for more information on infection.)

Arterial blood gas (ABG) determinations may be indicated for clients with a history of respiratory or cardiac disease, those undergoing prolonged mechanical ventilation postoperatively, and those having had surgery involving the thoracic cavity. The nurse interprets ABG results and notifies the surgeon of any deviation from the expected norm for that client (acid-base imbalance or hypoxemia). The anion gap can be calculated from serum electrolyte values or recorded by the chemistry laboratory. An increase in the anion gap alerts the nurse to the possibility of metabolic acidosis. (For more discussion on arterial blood gases and acidosis, see Chapters 18 and 19.)

Urine and renal laboratory studies are ordered as indicated (e.g., urinalysis, urinary electrolyte levels, and serum creatinine levels). Other laboratory studies performed depend on the diagnosis, type of surgical procedure, and so on. Examples are serum amylase level for a client who had pancreatic surgery and blood glucose level for a diabetic client.

 Analysis

➤ *Common Nursing Diagnoses and Collaborative Problems*

Common nursing diagnoses for the postoperative client are

1. Impaired Gas Exchange related to the residual effects of anesthesia, pain, the use of opioid analgesics, and immobility
2. Impaired Skin Integrity related to surgical wounds, inflammatory processes, drains and drainage, and tubes
3. Pain related to the surgical incision and positioning during surgery

A common collaborative problem for the postoperative client is potential for hypoxemia.

➤ *Additional Nursing Diagnoses and Collaborative Problems*

Depending on the type and extent of surgery, the family structure, and so on, there may be additional nursing diagnoses or collaborative problems for the postoperative client (see the discussion of surgical management in other chapters as appropriate), such as

▪ Risk for Aspiration related to decreased mobility, anesthesia, and opioid analgesic use
▪ Ineffective Airway Clearance related to ineffective or absent cough
▪ Fluid Volume Deficit related to decreased oral intake and abnormal fluid loss
▪ Potential for Hypovolemic Shock
▪ Potential for Deep Venous Thrombosis and Pulmonary Embolism
▪ Constipation related to decreased mobility, anesthesia, and opioid analgesic use
▪ Risk for Infection related to surgery and invasive lines, catheters, and tubes
▪ Urinary Retention related to anesthesia, surgical procedures, and decreased mobility
▪ Sleep Pattern Disturbance related to the use of medications and hospitalization
▪ Self-Care Deficit related to surgical procedures and decreased mobility
▪ Body Image Disturbance related to surgical procedures, loss of a body part or function, and pain
▪ Altered Family Processes related to the impact of surgery and illness on the family system
▪ Altered Sexuality Patterns related to surgery, pain, and hospitalization

 Planning and Implementation

Impaired Gas Exchange

Planning: Expected Outcomes. The major expected outcomes for the client with impaired gas exchange are for the client to attain or maintain optimal lung expansion and respiratory function with a partial pressure of arterial oxygen (PaO_2), partial pressure of arterial carbon dioxide ($PaCO_2$), and oxygen saturation values within baseline range.

Interventions

Airway Maintenance. After assessing the airway, the postanesthesia nurse may need to insert an oral airway if the client does not already have one. The oral airway pulls the tongue forward and holds it down to prevent obstruction. If the client has clenched teeth, a large tongue, or upper airway obstruction, the nurse could insert a nasal airway (nasal trumpet) to keep the airway open. The nurse keeps the manual resuscitation bag and emergency equipment for intubation or tracheostomy nearby. For clients whose only airway is a tracheostomy or laryngectomy stoma, the nurse alerts other staff members by posting signs in the room, notes on the chart, and so forth.

Positioning. Immediate care by the nurse in the PACU includes positioning the client in a side-lying position or turning the client's head to the side to prevent aspiration of secretions (or vomitus) while the client is still unreactive and vulnerable to aspiration. The nurse suctions the mouth, nose, and throat to keep the airway clear of mucus or vomitus as necessary.

The postanesthesia nurse keeps the client's head flat to prevent hypotension and possible shock, unless this position is contraindicated by the client's condition or surgical procedure. (For example, after intracranial surgery, the head of the bed or stretcher is elevated to promote respiratory function and prevent postoperative cerebral edema.) The nurse administers oxygen via face tent, nasal cannula, or mask to facilitate the excretion of inhalation anesthetic agents, to increase arterial oxygen levels, and to raise the level of consciousness. After the client is fully reactive and stable, the postanesthesia nurse raises the head of the bed to promote respiratory function.

Breathing Exercises. After the client regains the gag and cough reflex and meets the agency's criteria for extubation (if intubated), the airway or endotracheal (ET) tube is removed. Examples of extubation criteria are the client's ability to raise and hold the head up and evidence of thoracic breathing. The nurse encourages the client to cough (with the incision splinted) and deep breathe to expand the lungs, promote gas exchange, and hasten the elimination of inhalation anesthetic agents. Chart 20–5 reviews the teaching of postoperative breathing exercises and splinting of the surgical wound area to the client. As soon as the client is awake enough to follow commands, and throughout the postoperative period, the nurse encourages the client to cough, use the incentive spirometer, and take deep breaths. The client who is unable to expectorate mucus or sputum voluntarily may require oral or nasal suctioning. Meticulous mouth care is important after the removal of secretions.

Mobilization. The client is out of bed and ambulating as soon as possible to help mobilize secretions and promote lung expansion. Even for the hospitalized client with extensive surgery, the goal may be to get the client out of bed the same day as or the first day after surgery. If this is not possible, given the individual client's situation, the nurse turns the client at least every 2 hours (side to side) and ensures that the client performs his or her respiratory exercises and leg exercises (see Chart 20–6). Early ambulation minimizes the risk of pulmonary complications, including a pulmonary embolism, which could arise from impaired venous circulation in the legs. The client may report pain and resist getting up, but the nurse stresses the importance of activity to prevent postoperative complications. When indicated, the nurse offers pain medication 30 to 45 minutes before the client gets out of bed.

Impaired Skin Integrity

Planning: Expected Outcomes. The expected outcome for the client with impaired skin integrity is for the client to have incision healing without postoperative wound complications.

Interventions. Nursing assessment of the surgical area postoperatively is critical (see the discussion of integumentary system assessment earlier in this chapter). Although most wound complications can be treated without additional surgical intervention, emergency surgical procedures may be necessary.

Nonsurgical Management. Postoperative nonsurgical wound care usually includes changing and care of the dressing, assessment of the wound for signs of infection, and care of drains, including emptying, measuring, and documenting characteristics of the drainage. The nurse emphasizes to the client the importance of early deep-breathing exercises (see Chap. 20) to prevent respiratory complications that could cause forceful coughing. The nurse encourages hip flexion when the client is in the supine position to reduce tension on a chest or abdominal wound. The nurse also reminds the client always to splint the incision when coughing. The nurse promotes an atmosphere conducive to wound healing and protective of the skin in general, especially for the elderly client (Chart 22–2).

Dressings. The surgeon usually performs the first dressing change to assess the wound, remove any packing, and advance (pull partially out) or remove drains as indicated. Before the first dressing change, the nurse reinforces the dressing if it becomes wet from drainage. The nurse documents the reinforcement as well as the color, type, amount, and odor of drainage fluid and time of observation in the client's chart. The nurse assesses the surgical area frequently and reports any unexpected findings to the surgeon.

After removal of the surgical dressing, the surgeon may wish to leave the suture or staple line open to the air, which allows easy assessment of the wound and early

---

Chart 22–2

Nursing Focus on the Elderly: Postoperative Skin Care

- Improve perfusion to the wound to promote wound healing:
  - Keep the client adequately hydrated to maintain cardiac output.
  - Keep the airway patent and provide adequate oxygenation.
  - Keep the client's oxygen saturation on pulse oximetry at greater than 93%.
- Conserve the client's energy:
  - Allow the client to sleep in darkened, quiet room.
  - Administer medication to combat pain and sleeplessness, as ordered.
  - Provide rest periods throughout the day.
  - Control the client's room temperature.
  - Assist in activities of daily living.
- Place the client on a safety program to prevent falls, if indicated.
- Maintain strict aseptic technique in caring for breaks in the integument (intravenous or other catheters, indwelling urethral catheter, wound).
- Maintain the client's psychosocial health:
  - Prevent unnecessary stressors.
  - Allow the client liberal visitation of supportive others.
  - Enable the client to use individual successful coping mechanisms.
  - Keep the client well groomed and bathed.
- Protect fragile skin:
  - Minimize the use of tape on the skin.
  - Use hypoallergenic tape or Montgomery straps.
  - Change dressings as soon as they become wet.
  - Lift the client during transfer or repositioning.

Data from Jones, P. L., & Millman, A. (1990). Wound healing and the aged patient. *Nursing Clinics of North America, 25*(1), 263–277.

detection of poor approximation, drainage, swelling, or redness. Some surgeons believe that air-drying promotes healing. A draining wound, however, is always covered with a dressing.

Dressing changes are generally ordered by the surgeon, but the facility or unit may have standards or policies that dictate specific protocols for postoperative dressing changes and incision care. An unchanged wet or damp dressing becomes a source of infection. The nurse performs dressing changes under aseptic conditions until the sutures or staples are removed.

Dressings vary depending on the surgical procedure and the surgeon's preference. The standard postoperative dressing for a large incision consists of gauze or nonadherent pads covered with a larger absorbent pad held in place by tape or by Montgomery straps (Fig. 22–4). In other cases, the incision may be covered with a transparent plastic surgical dressing (such as Op-Site) or a spray in the operating room. This type of dressing stays intact for 3 to 6 days and allows visualization (observation) of the wound while preventing contamination and eliminating the need for dressing changes.

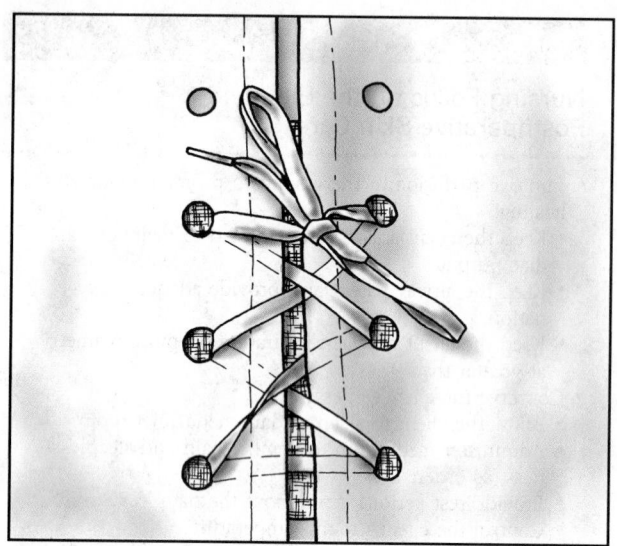

Figure 22–4. Montgomery straps may be used when frequent dressing changes are anticipated. They help to prevent skin irritation from frequent tape removal.

Wound or suture line care generally consists of changing gauze dressings at least once during a nursing shift or daily and may include cleaning the area with sterile saline or some other solution. The hospital's policy, the unit's standards, and the surgeon's preference determine what solution, if any, is used on the wound and also the frequency of the dressing changes. For extensive dressing changes or drain removal, the nurse offers the client an ordered analgesic before the procedure.

Skin sutures or staples are usually removed 6 to 8 days postoperatively, and the incision is secured with Steri-Strips. Either the surgeon or the nurse removes the sutures or staples, depending on the agency's policy. Before removing sutures, the nurse notes the condition and healing stage of the wound. If the wound does not appear to be healing well, the nurse notifies the surgeon before proceeding with suture removal.

Drains. Drains (see Figure 22–3) may be inserted into the wound or through a separate small incision (known as a stab wound) close to the operative site during surgery. The drain provides an exit through which air and fluids, such as blood and bile, can be evacuated. Drains also help prevent deep infections and abscess formation within the wound during healing.

The Penrose drain is a superficial device placed into the external aspect of the incision and that drains directly onto the client's dressing and perisurgical area (the skin around the incision). The nurse changes a damp or soiled dressing by carefully cleaning under and around the Penrose drain. The nurse then pads the area distal to the drain with absorbent pads to prevent skin irritation and contamination of the surgical wound. Whether sutured in place or not, the drain can easily be dislodged or accidentally pulled out during a dressing change. As the wound heals, the surgeon shortens (advances) the drain by pulling it out and removing the excess external portion until drainage stops.

Jackson-Pratt and Hemovac drains are two commonly used self-contained drainage systems by which the wound drains directly through a tube via gravity, suction, or vacuum. These drains are commonly sutured in place with a pursestring suture that seals the area when the drain is removed. The nurse empties the reservoir of the drain and records the amount and color of drainage during every nursing shift or more frequently if ordered by the surgeon. After emptying and compressing the reservoir, the nurse secures the drain to the client's gown or pajamas (never to the sheet or mattress) to prevent pulling and stress on the surgical wound.

Drug Therapy. Wound infection is a major postoperative complication. It usually results from contamination during surgery, preoperative infection, debilitation, or immunosuppression. A client at risk for wound infection may receive prophylactic antibiotic therapy with a broad-spectrum antibiotic or one that is effective in fighting organisms common to the specific surgical site. These antibiotics are usually continued for 24 to 72 hours postoperatively to ensure that adequate antibiotic levels are reached in this critical time period. The first dose may be administered IV before or during the surgery.

Wounds that become infected and open (without intact sutures) are usually treated with specific dressing changes and prolonged systemic antibiotic administration. Depending on physician order, the nurse irrigates the wound (e.g., with sterile saline, hydrogen peroxide, povidone-iodine, or acetic acid), loosely packs it with solution-soaked gauze (e.g., with neomycin, gentamicin, iodoform, povidone-iodine, saline, or acetic acid), and covers the wound with dry, sterile dressings. This procedure (wet-to-dry dressings) may be ordered one to three times daily. The packing promotes healing from within the wound and debridement (removal) of the infected tissue as the wound heals.

Surgical Management

Management of Dehiscence. If dehiscence (wound opening) occurs, the nurse applies a sterile nonadherent (such as Telfa) or saline dressing to the wound and notifies the surgeon. A wound that becomes infected dehisces by itself, or it may be opened by the surgeon through an incision and drainage (I&D) procedure. In either case, the wound is left open rather than resutured and is treated as described previously.

Management of Evisceration. An evisceration (a wound opening with the protrusion of internal organs or viscera) is considered a surgical emergency. One nurse tends to the client while another nurse immediately notifies the surgeon. Chart 22–3 outlines emergency care. The nurse provides emotional support by explaining what happened and reassuring the client that the emergency can, and will, be handled by competent, capable individuals.

The surgeon may order an NG tube to decompress the stomach and relieve some of the pressure internally or to remove the stomach's contents if the client has been eating and general anesthesia is planned. The nurse prepares the client for surgery (see Chap. 20) to close the wound. Regional or local anesthesia may be used, depending on the location of the wound and the surgeon's or the anes-

Chart 22-3

Nursing Care Highlight: Surgical Wound Evisceration

1. Call for help! Instruct the person who responds to notify the surgeon immediately and to bring any needed supplies into the client's room.
2. Stay with the client.
3. Cover the wound with a nonadherent dressing premoistened with warmed sterile normal saline. Note: The supplies needed for this emergency should be in the client's room, especially if the client is at high risk.
4. If premoistened dressings are not available, moisten sterile gauze or sterile towels in a sterile irrigation tray with sterile saline, then cover the wound.
5. If saline is not immediately available, cover the wound with gauze, and then moisten with sterile saline using a sterile irrigation tray as soon as someone brings saline.
6. Do not attempt to reinsert the protruding organ or viscera.
7. While covering the wound, note the client's response and assess for signs and symptoms of shock.
8. Place the client in a supine position with the hips and knees bent.
9. Take and document vital signs. Note: If the person who answered the call for help is back in the room before this, instruct that individual to take vital signs while you focus on covering the wound and repositioning the client.
10. Provide support and reassurance to the client.
11. Continue assessing the client, including vital signs assessment, every 5 to 10 min, until the surgeon arrives.
12. Keep dressings continuously moist by adding warmed sterile saline to the dressing as often as necessary. Do not let the dressing become dry.
13. When the surgeon arrives, report your findings and your interventions. Then follow the surgeon's directions.
14. Document the incident, the activity the client was engaged in at the time of the incident, your actions, and your assessments.

thesiologist's preference. Postoperative nausea and vomiting, which place undue stress on the already fragile incision, are minimized when regional or local anesthesia is used. To increase the incision's integrity, stay or retention sutures of wire or nylon are used over the standard suture or staple line (see Figure 21–13).

Pain

Planning: Expected Outcomes. The expected outcome for the client with pain is for the client to attain or maintain optimal comfort levels throughout the postoperative phase. This outcome entails the alleviation or reduction of pain or discomfort associated with the surgical wound and positioning during surgery.

Interventions. Postoperative pain management usually includes drug therapy and other methods such as positioning, massage, relaxation techniques, and diversion. Often the client achieves greater benefit from a combination of approaches. The nurse assesses the client's comfort level and the effectiveness of the therapies. (Chapter 9 provides a comprehensive discussion of pain assessment and management for the postoperative client.) The client who has optimal pain control is better able to cooperate with the therapies and exercises designed to prevent postoperative complications and to promote the postoperative rehabilitation process.

Drug Therapy. The use of opioids or other analgesics for the management of pain may mask or increase the amount and severity of symptoms of an anesthesia reaction. Therefore, these drugs must be administered with caution, especially in the PACU when the client's condition is not stabilized. Pain medication, when administered in the PACU, is usually given IV in small doses. After the nurse administers medication for pain, the client remains in the PACU for a defined period (often 30–45 minutes). The postanesthesia nurse assesses for hypotension, respiratory depression, and other side effects. Approximately 5 to 10 minutes after an IV injection, the nurse assesses the effectiveness of the medication (i.e., on a rating scale) in relieving the client's pain.

Opioid analgesics are routinely given during the first 24 to 48 hours after surgery to control acute pain. Around-the-clock administration is generally more effective than medicating on client demand because more constant blood levels can be obtained. Drugs commonly used include meperidine hydrochloride (Demerol), morphine sulfate (Statex✦), hydromorphone hydrochloride (Dilaudid), ketorolac (Toradol), codeine sulfate, butorphanol tartrate (Stadol), and oxycodone hydrochloride with aspirin (Percodan), or oxycodone hydrochloride with acetaminophen (Tylox, Percocet). The nurse assesses the type, location, and intensity of the pain before and after the administration of medication (see also Discomfort/Pain Assessment earlier in this chapter). The nurse monitors the client's vital signs closely, especially for hypotension and hypoventilation, after the administration of opioid analgesics. Chart 22–4 contains further information on various analgesics used during the postoperative period.

Patient-controlled analgesia (PCA) via IV or internal pump (the catheter is sutured into or proximal to the surgical area) and epidural analgesia are becoming more common to achieve better pain control. In PCA, the client adjusts the rate or dosage of infusion of an opioid analgesic on the basis of the pain level and physical response to the drug. This method allows more consistent pain relief and more control by the client. The maximal dose per hour is "locked in" to the pump so the client cannot accidentally overdose. Drugs commonly used by the PCA method include morphine, meperidine, and hydromorphone.

Epidural analgesia can be administered intermittently by the anesthesiologist or via continuous drip with or without PCA through an epidural catheter left in place after epidural anesthesia. Drugs commonly given by epidural catheter include the opioids fentanyl citrate (Subli-

Chart 22–4

Drug Therapy for Management of Postoperative Pain

Drug	Usual Dosage	Nursing Interventions	Rationale
Meperidine hydrochloride (Demerol)	• 50–150 mg q3–4h PO or IM • 12.5–25 mg IV • Maximum 6–8 doses	• Monitor blood pressure. • Move and ambulate the client slowly. • Monitor pulse rate. • Assess for decreased GI motility or GI upset.	• Common side effects include decreased blood pressure, orthostatic (postural) hypotension, and bradycardia. • Constipation, nausea, and vomiting can occur.
Morphine sulfate (Epimorph✦, Statex✦)	• 2–15 mg IM or IV incrementally • 10–30 mg q4h PO • Maximum 6 doses	• Monitor respiratory status. • Monitor blood pressure. • Assess for GI motility and urinary output.	• Respiratory depression can be severe and need medical intervention. • Hypotension, constipation, and urinary retention can occur.
Hydromorphone hydrochloride (Dilaudid)	• 1–4 mg q3–4h IV or IM • 2–4 mg q3–4h PO	• Monitor respirations. • Monitor blood pressure. • Monitor for food intolerance. • Monitor fluid and electrolyte balance. • Assess GI motility.	• Respiratory depression, hypotension, anorexia, nausea, vomiting, and constipation can occur.
Codeine sulfate, codeine phosphate (Paveral✦)	• 15–60 mg q4h IM or PO • Maximum 6 doses	• Monitor respiratory status. • Monitor for food intolerance. • Monitor fluid and electrolyte balance. • Assess GI motility.	• Respiratory depression, nausea, and vomiting can occur. • Constipation is common; prophylactic interventions may be indicated.
Butorphanol tartrate (Stadol)	• 1–4 mg q3–4h IM • 0.5–2 mg IV • Maximum 6–8 doses	• Monitor neurologic status and changes in level of consciousness. • Monitor respiratory status.	• Butorphanol can cause increased intracranial pressure and respiratory depression.
Oxycodone hydrochloride and aspirin (Percodan, Endocan✦, Oxycodan✦)	• 1–2 tablets (5–10 mg) q3–4h PO • Maximum 80 mg	• Assess GI tolerance of medication. • Assess for GI bleeding. • Monitor GI motility. • Monitor coagulation respiratory studies (PT, APTT). • Monitor respiratory status.	• The aspirin component can irritate the stomach and could cause GI bleeding. • Bleeding times and other coagulation study results may be increased because of the aspirin component. • Respiratory depression and constipation can be caused by the oxycodone component.
Oxycodone hydrochloride and acetaminophen (Tylox, Percocet, Endocet✦, Oxycocet✦)	• 1–2 tablets q3–4h PO • Maximum 12 tablets	• Monitor blood pressure and respiratory status. • Assess for GI motility.	• Respiratory depression, hypotension, and constipation can occur.

Continued

Chart 22–4. Drug Therapy for Management of Postoperative Pain   Continued

Drug	Usual Dosage	Nursing Interventions	Rationale
Ketorolac tromethamine (Toradol)	• 15–60 mg IM or IV q6h • Maximum 120 mg • 5 day administration maximum	• Monitor for GI bleeding. • Monitor for renal effects, especially in the elderly.	• GI bleeding, ulceration, and perforation can occur. • Decreased urinary output, increased serum creatinine, hematuria, and proteinuria can occur. • Ketorolac is cleared more slowly in the elderly. • The elderly are more sensitive to the renal effects of NSAIDs.
Ibuprofen (Motrin, Amersol♣, Novoprofen♣)	• 300–800 mg q4–6h PO • Maximum 2400 mg daily	• Monitor upper GI tolerance of medication. • Give with food or milk. • Monitor coagulation studies (PT, APTT). • Assess for signs of bleeding or delayed clotting.	• Food or milk helps decrease irritation of the stomach. • Bleeding times and other coagulation study results may be increased. • Monitoring leads to early detection of complications.

PT = prothrombin time; PTT = partial thromboplastin time; NSAID = nonsteroidal antiinflammatory drug; GI = gastrointestinal; PO = orally; IM = intramuscularly; IV = intravenously.

maze) and preservative-free morphine (Duramorph), and the local anesthetic bupivacaine (Marcaine).

The nurse uses care not to overmedicate or undermedicate the client, especially the elderly client. In assessing for overmedication, the nurse monitors the client's vital signs, especially blood pressure and respiratory rate, and level of consciousness. Complications from the use of opioid analgesics include respiratory depression, hypotension, nausea, vomiting, and constipation. An opioid antagonist such as naloxone hydrochloride (Narcan) may be administered to reverse the acute effects of opioid depression. Because of the short effect of the opioid antagonist, the nurse monitors the blood pressure and respirations closely (i.e., every 15–30 minutes) until the full effect of the opioid analgesic has passed. The nurse may need to give more doses of the opioid antagonist during this time. See Chart 22–5 for more information on the opioid antagonists. In addition, the client has breakthrough pain after the opioid antagonist is administered, so the nurse initiates other interventions to promote comfort.

The nurse assesses for undermedication by questioning the client about the effects of the medication and observing for nonverbal cues that indicate pain (e.g., restlessness, increased confusion, "picking" at bedcovers, and aggressive behaviors). The nurse offers pain medication after checking for hypotension and respiratory depression.

As the client's recovery progresses, the nurse administers pain medications in reduced doses and frequency. The medications are changed from injectable or PCA to oral as soon as the client can tolerate oral administration. Nonopioid analgesics, such as acetaminophen (Tylenol, Atasol♣), and nonsteroidal antiinflammatory drugs (NSAIDs), such as ibuprofen (Motrin, Novoprofen♣, Amersol♣) and ketorolac (Toradol), are used during convalescence or can be given with an opioid analgesic as an adjunct. Antianxiety drugs, such as hydroxyzine (Vistaril, Novohydroxyzin♣), may be given in combination with an opioid analgesic. This combination decreases pain-related anxiety, alleviates muscle tension that could contribute to the client's pain or discomfort, and controls nausea.

Other Methods of Pain Control. The nurse provides comfort measures that may lower the amount of pain medication needed. These measures reduce anxiety and allow the client to relax and rest.

Positioning. In positioning the client, the nurse considers the client's position during surgery, the location of the surgical incision and drains, and medical problems such as arthritis and chronic pulmonary disease. The nurse assists the client in achieving a position of comfort, while enabling the client to maintain optimal function. The client's extremities are supported with pillows. No pillows are placed under the client's knees, and the knee gatch of the bed is not raised because this position could restrict circulation and increase the risk of thrombophlebitis. The nurse turns or helps the client turn at least every 2 hours while the client is bedridden to prevent pulmonary and other complications sometimes caused by immobility.

On the basis of the surgeon's orders and the nurse's assessment of the client's tolerance, the nurse encourages the client progressively to increase activity. Activity decreases stiffness, promotes lung expansion, and promotes

---

Chart 22–5

Drug Therapy for Management of Opioid Overdose

Drug	Usual Dosage	Nursing Interventions	Rationales
Naloxone hydrochloride (Narcan)	• 0.1–2 mg IV, SC, and IM; repeat every 2–3 minutes PRN on the basis of the client's response up to 10 mg	• Maintain an open airway. • Administer oxygen as ordered. • Have suction available. • Closely monitor vital signs and pulse oximetry readings until the client responds. • Do not leave the client unattended until he or she is fully responsive. • Observe for significant reversal of analgesia. • Continue to monitor the client for effects of the naloxone for at least 1 hour.	• A patent airway maximizes respiratory effort. • Oxygen helps to prevent hypoxemia. • Vomiting can occur with administration of naloxone; suction prevents aspiration. • The threat of hypoxemia and respiratory depression or arrest is a concern until the naloxone becomes effective. • Staying with the client promotes safety. • With reversal of the narcotic's respiratory-depressive effects, analgesic effects will also be reversed. • Continued monitoring leads to early detection of hypertension, hypotension, tachycardia, and dysrhythmias, which can be effects of naloxone.

---

venous circulation. When the client is initially allowed out of bed, the nurse assists him or her to the side of the bed and into a chair. The client splints the surgical wound for support and comfort during the transfer.

Massage. The nurse uses gentle massage of stiff joints or a sore back to decrease postoperative discomfort. The nurse positions the client in a side-lying position and applies lotion with smooth, gentle strokes to increase blood flow to the area and promote general relaxation. The legs, especially the calves, are not massaged because of the increased risk of loosening a thrombus and causing a pulmonary embolus, which can be life threatening.

Other Interventions. Relaxation and diversion are also used to control acute episodes of pain, such as during painful procedures such as dressing changes and injections. Chapters 8 and 9 discuss how the nurse instructs and guides the client through these pain control methods. Music and noise reduction have been shown to decrease awareness of discomfort. Chart 22–6 lists examples of other interventions that may help to reduce pain and promote comfort.

Potential for Hypoxemia

Planning: Expected Outcomes. The expected outcome for the client with hypoxemia is for the client to attain or maintain preoperative baseline PaO_2 values.

Interventions. The key to preventing hypoxemia is to follow the interventions appropriate to the nursing diagnoses of impaired gas exchange (discussed earlier), ineffective airway clearance, and ineffective breathing pattern. Postoperatively, the nurse and physician monitor the client's arterial blood gas and pulse oximetry results. A client who received conscious sedation with midazolam (Versed) or lorazepam (Ativan, Nu-Loraz✢) may be overly sedated or have cardiopulmonary depression sufficient to require reversal with flumazenil (Romazicon) (Chart 22–7). Postoperative hypothermia and its associated shivering causes increased oxygen demands and can contribute to hypoxemia. Various rewarming methods are used in PACUs, although prevention may be more important (see Research Applications for Nursing). The highest incidence of postoperative hypoxemia, however, is on the second postoperative day. Those clients who have a low normal PaO_2, such as those with underlying pulmonary disease or the elderly, are at higher risk for hypoxemia.

The physician treats the potential for hypoxemia with oxygen administration. Depending on the surgeon's preference and established guidelines, the physician may continue oxygen administration until after the second postoperative day. When hypoxemia occurs despite preventive care, the physician orders treatment to manage the cause of the hypoxemia and prescribes oxygen therapy, respiratory treatments, and mechanical ventilation as indicated.

Chart 22–6

Nursing Care Highlight: Examples of Nonpharmacologic Interventions to Reduce Postoperative Pain and Promote Comfort

- Control or remove noxious stimuli.
- Cushion and elevate painful areas; avoid tension or pressure on those areas.
- Provide adequate rest to increase pain tolerance.
- Encourage the client's participation in diversional activities.
- Instruct the client in relaxation techniques; use audiotapes and breathing exercises.
- Provide opportunities for meditation.
- Help the client to stimulate sensory nerve endings near the painful areas to inhibit ascending pain impulses.
- Use ice to reduce and prevent swelling, as indicated.
- Find a general position of comfort for the client.
- Help the client to stimulate the area contralateral (opposite) to the painful area.

 Continuing Care

Many clients are discharged after a brief hospital stay or directly from the PACU to home. Because of the shortened length of hospitalization, discharge planning, teaching, and referral begin preoperatively and continue postoperatively.

➤ *Health Teaching*

The teaching plan for the postoperative client and appropriate others includes

- Prevention of infection
- Care and assessment of the surgical wound
- Diet therapy
- Pain management
- Drug therapy
- Progressive increase in activity

If dressing changes are needed, the client and family members are instructed on the importance of proper hand washing to prevent infection. The nurse thoroughly explains and demonstrates wound care to the client and family. The client or a family member performs a return demonstration of that care. During teaching sessions, the nurse evaluates learning and promotes compliance after discharge. At the same time, the nurse teaches signs and symptoms of complications such as wound infection. The nurse also discusses with the client and family members appropriate measures to take if complications occur.

A diet high in protein, calories, and vitamin C promotes wound healing. A dietary consultation before the client is discharged helps him or her to select a balanced diet to promote healing. Supplemental vitamin C, iron, and multivitamins are often prescribed after surgery to aid in wound healing and in the formation of red blood cells. Often these supplements are prescribed for 10 to 14 days postoperatively. The nurse instructs the client with prior dietary restrictions about the importance of following the prescribed diet during convalescence. The elderly or debilitated client is encouraged to continue using dietary supplements, if ordered, between meals until the wound is completely healed and energy level restored.

Chart 22–7

Drug Therapy for Management of Benzodiazepine Overdose

Drug	Usual Dosage	Nursing Interventions	Rationales
Flumazenil (Romazicon)	• 0.2–1 mg IV at rate of 0.2 mg/min; repeat every 2–3 minutes PRN up to 3 mg in any 1 hour	• Maintain an open airway.	• A patent airway maximizes respiratory effort.
		• Administer oxygen as ordered.	• Oxygen helps to prevent hypoxemia.
		• Have suction available.	• Vomiting can occur with administration of flumazenil; suction prevents aspiration.
		• Closely monitor the client's level of sedation, vital signs and pulse oximetry readings until the client responds.	• Hypoventilation may not be fully reversed with flumazenil; sedation, amnesia, and psychomotor effects of the benzodiazepines should be reversed.
		• Do not leave the client unattended until fully responsive.	• Seizures have occurred with reversal.
		• Observe for significant reversal of sedation.	• With reversal of the benzodiazepine's sedative and amnesia effect, the client will become more aware of pain/discomfort.
		• Observe for up to 2 hours for re-sedation and respiratory depression.	• The duration of action of the benzodiazepines is longer than that of flumazenil.

▷ Research Applications for Nursing

Hypothermia Still a Problem in Postanesthesia Care Units

Hershey, J., Valenciano, C., & Bookbinder, M. (1997). Comparison of three rewarming methods in a postanesthesia care unit. AORN Journal, 65(3), 597–601.

These researchers noted how frequently clients enter the postanesthesia care unit (PACU) with temperatures less than 36° C (98.6° F). With hypothermia comes shivering, a finding that they and other researchers have concluded is a normal homeostatic response, because the temperatures of clients who shiver will return to normal more quickly than those who do not shiver. They report, however, that shivering increases oxygen demands by as much as 400%, which puts the elderly and those with cardiac conditions at risk.

The nurses studied three rewarming approaches common in PACUs. All clients received two warmed thermal blankets, but each of the study groups also received either a hospital bedspread; a reflective blanket and a bedspread; or a reflective blanket, a bedspread, and a reflective head covering. There were 48 clients in each study group. There were no significant differences among the three nursing interventions and duration of hypothermia.

Critique. All clients in the study were women between the ages of 20 and 60 years; all were having diagnostic laparotomy procedures. These factors may limit the interpretation of the findings.

Possible Nursing Implications. Warming interventions may need to be initiated earlier in the surgical client's experience to prevent hypothermia. For example, nurses can place head coverings on in the holding area, and circulating nurses can be sure to cover any exposed skin of the client while in the operating room. Irrigation and intravenous fluids could be warmed before use in the operating room. Further research is needed to determine whether interventions can be identified that will be effective in either preventing hypothermia in surgical clients or reducing the effects of hypothermia.

The nurse instructs the client about taking pain medication, with special attention to the proper dosage and frequency of administration. The nurse instructs the client to notify the surgeon if the medication does not control the pain or if the pain suddenly increases. If antibiotics or other medications are prescribed, the client is instructed to finish the entire prescription as ordered by the surgeon.

Surgery places physical and emotional stress on the body, and time and rest are required for healing. The nurse instructs the client to increase activity level slowly, balance rest with activity (e.g., plan rest periods), and avoid straining the surgical wound or the surrounding area. Depending on the type of surgery and the client's occupation and usual activities, the surgeon decides when the client may climb stairs, return to work, drive, and resume other usual activities such as sexual intercourse. The amount of weight a client may safely lift after dis-

charge from the facility needs to be specifically defined by the surgeon (i.e., in pounds or kilograms, as appropriate) and interpreted and reinforced as necessary by the nurse (grocery bags, laundry baskets, children, books, and so on).

The nurse also instructs the client in the use of proper body mechanics. A client whose work involves a moderate amount of physical labor may be allowed back to work 6 weeks after nonlaser abdominal surgery. The client may be eager to return to work or to other activities and may not follow activity restrictions. The nurse emphasizes the importance of compliance to prevent complications or disability. It is imperative that the client receive written discharge instructions for reinforcement at home. A visiting nurse may be necessary for follow-up.

➤ Home Care Management

If the client is discharged directly home, the nurse reviews data to help assess the home environment for safety, cleanliness, and availability of caregivers. The nurse uses the data base that was completed when the client was admitted to the hospital or the ambulatory surgical unit to ascertain the client's needs. For example, if the client is unable or not allowed to climb stairs and lives in a two-story house with only one bathroom, the nurse advises the client to rent a bedside commode. The social worker or discharge planner, in collaboration with the nurse, helps the client identify needs related to postoperative care, including meal preparation, dressing changes, and personal hygiene. A referral to a home care nursing agency may be indicated.

The client is usually apprehensive about postoperative complications, pain, and changes in the usual activity level; thus, the nurse must allay fears. The more extensive the surgical procedure is, the more fearful the client is of assuming self-care. The nurse supports the client and family members as they make discharge plans. The client whose surgical procedure has left visible scars may require more emotional support from his or her family for acceptance. (See Chapter 10 for further discussion of body image.) The client may express anger about the surgical outcome or temporary or permanent role changes and concern about financial matters and work. The surgical outcome may not have met the client's expectations, and further interventions may be necessary to assist the client in resolving his or her feelings. Referrals are made for additional counseling as indicated.

➤ Health Care Resources

After returning home, the client may need equipment and assistance with dressing changes, activities of daily living (ADL), and meal preparation. Referral to a home care agency is made and may be paid for by third-party insurance payers, including Medicare, if the client is homebound and requires skilled care. The home care nurse provides skilled nursing assessments, dressing supplies, education in self-care, and referrals for services as needed by the client. Such referrals include Meals on Wheels, support groups, and homemaker services (e.g., for housecleaning and food shopping).

Evaluation

On the basis of the identified nursing diagnoses, collaborative problems, and desired outcomes, the nurse evaluates the care of the postoperative client. The outcomes include that the client

- Maintains a patent airway
- Maintains adequate lung expansion and respiratory function as evidenced by clear breath sounds
- Has stable vital signs
- Returns to baseline arterial blood gas values
- Returns to preoperative mental state
- Has complete wound healing without complications
- States that postoperative pain is reduced or alleviated by interventions

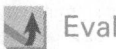 **CASE STUDY** for the Postoperative Client

■ You are a nurse working on a medical-surgical unit. Midway through your shift you are notified that a postoperative client was just placed in one of your rooms. You had not received any notice that you were receiving *any* patient in that room, nor did you get any report.

QUESTIONS:

1. What do you do first?
2. What do you say to the client?
3. What action should you take regarding not being notified of the admission and not receiving a report?

SELECTED BIBLIOGRAPHY

Acute pain management in adults: Operative procedures (AHCPR Pub. No. 92–0019). (1992). Rockville, MD: Agency for Health Care Policy and Research, U.S. Department of Health and Human Services.

*Aker, J. (1994). Immediate care in the postoperative period. *Current Review of Post Anesthesia Care Nurses, 16*(17), 147–154, 156.

Atsberger, D. B. (1995). Relaxation therapy: Its potential as an intervention for acute postoperative pain. *Journal of Post Anesthesia Nursing, 19*(1), 2–8.

Bach, D. M. (1995). Implementation of the Agency for Health Care Policy and Research postoperative pain management guideline. *Nursing Clinics of North America, 30*(3), 515–527.

Black, J. M. (1996). Surgical options in wound healing. *Critical Care Nursing Clinics of North America, 8*(2), 169–182.

Blinkhorne, K. (1995). Prepared for a smooth recovery?...Post-operative nausea and vomiting. *Nursing Times, 91*(28), 42–47.

Boike, L., et al. (1995). Development of an outpatient perioperative care record. *Journal of Post Anesthesia Nursing, 10*(3), 140–150.

*Bowman, A. M. (1992). The relationship of anxiety to development of postoperative delirium. *Journal of Gerontological Nursing, 18*(1), 24–30.

*Brockopp, D. Y., Warden, S., Colclough, G., et al. (1994). Postoperative pain: Getting a grip on the facts. *Nursing94, 24*(6), 49–50.

Brooks-Brunn, J. A. (1995). Consult stat. What accounts for pulmonary problems in these cases? *RN, 58*(11), 66.

Brooks-Brunn, J. A. (1995). Postoperative atelectasis and pneumonia: Risk factors. *American Journal of Critical Care, 4*(5), 340–351.

Brooks-Brunn, J. A. (1995). Postoperative atelectasis and pneumonia. *Heart Lung, 24*(2), 94–115.

Burden, N. (1995). Ambulatory approach. A case study: Identification and treatment of narcotic depression in the ambulatory surgical patient. *Journal of Post Anesthesia Nursing, 10*(2), 94–99.

*Chalfin, D. B., et al. (1994). Preoperative evaluation and postoperative care of the elderly patient undergoing major surgery. *Clinics in Geriatric Medicine, 10*(1), 51–70.

*Dean, B. E. (1994). Overcoming sedation...Your postoperative patient refuses to take analgesics. *Nursing94, 24*(12), 28.

Dennison, R. D. (1997). Nurses' guide to common postoperative complications. *Nursing97, 27* (11), 56–57.

Dickinson, G. M., et al. (1995). Antimicrobial prophylaxis of infection. *Infectious Disease Clinics of North America, 9*(3), 783–804.

*Ehrlichman, R. J., Seckel, B. R., Bryan, D. J., & Moschella, C. J. (1991). Common complications of wound healing. *Surgical Clinics of North America, 71*(6), 1323–1351.

*Elmquist, L. (1992). Decision making for extubation of the post-anesthesia patient. *Critical Care Nursing Quarterly, 15*(1), 82–86.

Ferrara-Love, R., Sekeres, L., & Bircher, N. G. (1996). Nonpharmacologic treatment of postoperative nausea. *Journal of Perianesthesia Nursing, 11*(6), 378–383.

Ferrell, B. R. (1995). Controlling pain in the elderly. *Nursing95, 25*(7), 73.

Gerber, D. E., et al. (1995). Death in the operating room and postanesthesia care unit: Helping nurses to cope. *Journal of Post Anesthesia Nursing, 10*(2), 84–88.

Good, M. (1995a). A comparison of the effects of jaw relaxation and music on postoperative pain. *Nursing Research, 44*(1), 52–57.

Good, M. (1995b). Complementary modalities/part 2: Relaxation techniques for surgical patients. *American Journal of Nursing, 95*(5), 38–43.

Gordon, D. B., et al. (1995). Correcting patient misconceptions about pain. *American Journal of Nursing, 95*(7), 43–45.

*Heffline, M. S. (1992). Managing PACU emergencies. *Journal of Post Anesthesia Nursing, 7*(3), 215.

Hershey, J., Valenciano, C., & Bookbinder, M. (1997). Comparison of three rewarming methods in a postanesthesia care unit. *AORN Journal, 65*(3), 597–601.

*Hinojosa, R. J. (1992). Nursing interventions to prevent or relieve postoperative nausea and vomiting. *Journal of Post Anesthesia Nursing, 7*(1), 3–14.

Hinojosa, R. J. (1995). Postoperative nausea and vomiting: How nurses can help. *Plastic Surgery Nursing, 15*(2), 85–88, 98–100.

Holden, U. (1995). Dementia in acute units: Confusion. *Nursing Standards, 9*(17), 37–39.

Hunt, K. (1995). Perceptions of patient's pain: A study assessing nurses' attitudes. *Nursing Standards, 10*(4), 32–35.

*Hypoxemia on the general care floor. (1992). Newport Beach, CA: Communicore.

Jackson, A. (1995). Acupressure for post-operative nausea. *Nursing Times, 91*(26), 58.

*Jones, P. L., & Millman, A. (1990). Wound healing and the aged patient. *Nursing Clinics of North America, 25*(1), 263–277.

Kaempfe, G., & Goralski, V. J. (1996). Monitoring postop patients. *RN, 59*(7), 30–35.

*Kane, A. M., et al. (1994). Improving the postoperative care of acutely-confused older adults. *MedSurg Nursing, 3*(6), 453–458.

*Kearns, P. C. (1986). Exercises to ease pain after abdominal surgery. *RN, 49*(7), 45–48.

Komara, J. J., et al. (1995). The impact of a postoperative oxygen therapy protocol on use of pulse oximetry and oxygen therapy. *Respiratory Care, 40*(11), 1125–1129.

*Lawler, M. (1991). Preventing postop complications: Managing other complications. *Nursing91, 21*(11), 33, 40–48.

*Litwak, K. (1991). Managing postanesthesia emergencies. *Nursing91, 21*(9), 49–51.

*Litwak-Saleh, K. (1993). The elderly patient in the post anesthesia care unit. *The Nursing Clinics of North America, 28*(3), 507–518.

Lusis, S. A. (1996). The challenges of nursing elderly surgical patients. *AORN Journal, 64*(6), 954–955, 957–962.

Maklebust, J., & Palleschi, M. (1996). Promoting surgical wound healing. *Nursing96, 26*(6), 24c–24h.

Marley, R. A., et al. (1996). Patient discharge from the ambulatory setting. *Journal of Post Anesthesia Nursing, 11*(1), 39–49.

*Marshall, M. (1993). Postoperative confusion: Helping your patient emerge from the shadows. *Nursing93, 23*(1), 44–47.

*McConnell, E. A. (1990). Determining the cause of post-operative fever. *Nursing90, 20*(8), 82–83.

*McConnell, E. A. (1991). Preventing postop complications: Minimizing respiratory problems. *Nursing91, 21*(11), 33–39.

*McConnell, E. A. (1992a). Assessing postoperative chills and tremors. *Nursing92, 22*(4), 110–114.

*McConnell, E. A. (1992b). Assessing wound drainage. *Nursing92, 22*(7), 66.

*McConnell, E. A. (1992c). Diagnosing postoperative fatigue. *Nursing92, 22*(3), 70–74.

McConnell, E. A. (1995). What's wrong with this patient? When your patient's urine output decreases. *Nursing95, 25*(4), 73–74.

*Metzler, D. J., & Fromm, C. G. (1993). Laying out a care plan for the elderly postoperative patient. *Nursing93, 23*(4), 67–74.

Minnick, A., Roberts, M. J., Young, W. B. et al. (1995). An analysis of posthospitalization telephone survey data. *Nursing Research, 44*(6), 371–375.

Modderman, G. R. (1995). Barriers to pain management in elderly surgical patients. *AORN Journal, 61*(6), 1073–1075.

Morris, J. (1995). Monitoring post-operative effects in day-surgery patients. *Nursing Times, 91*(10), 32–34.

*Nash, C. A., & Jensen, P. L. (1994). When your surgical patient has hypertension. *American Journal of Nursing, 94*(12), 38–45.

*Neal, J. M. (1992). Management of postdural puncture headache. *Anesthesiology Clinics of North America, 10*(1), 163–178.

O'Donnell, M. E. (1995). Assessing fluid and electrolyte balance in elders. *American Journal of Nursing, 95*(11), 40–46.

O'Rourke, K. (1995). Epidural analgesia: Postoperative pain management. *CACCN, 6*(4), 12–15.

Ouellette, S. M. (1995). Postoperative myocardial ischemia: Etiology, recognition and management. *Current Review of Nurse Anesthetists, 18*(5), 38–44.

Paice, J., Mahon, S. M., & Faut-Callahan, M. (1995). Pain control in hospitalized postsurgical patients. *MedSurg Nursing, 4*(5), 367–372.

Pasero, C. L. (1996). Managing postoperative pain in the elderly. *American Journal of Nursing, 96*(10), 38–46.

*Pasero, C. L., & McCaffery, M. (1994). Avoiding opioid-induced respiratory depression. *American Journal of Nursing, 94*(4), 24–31.

*Peden, L. (1992). Helping postop patients to sleep. *RN, 55*(4), 24–26.

*Pediani, R. (1994). Recent developments in the control of surgical wound pain. *Journal of Wound Care, 3*(8), 394–396.

Rowbotham, D. (1995). Recognizing risk factors...Post-operative nausea and vomiting. *Nursing Times, 91*(28), 44–46.

*Rowland, M. A. (1990). Myths—and facts—about postop discomfort. *American Journal of Nursing, 90*(5), 60–64.

Schumacher, S. B. (1995). Monitoring vital signs to identify postoperative complications. *MedSurg Nursing, 4*(2), 142–145.

Sherman, D. W. (1997). Developing quality assurance programs in ambulatory surgery. *Nursing Management, 28*(9), 44–48.

Springhouse Corp. (1996). Controlling pain. Avoiding the I.M. route for analgesic administration. *Nursing96, 26*(1), 67.

Strimike, C. L., Wojcik, J. M., & Stark, B. A. (1997). Incision care that really cuts it. *RN, 60*(7), 22–26.

Swan, B. A. (1996). Assessing symptom distress in ambulatory surgery patients. *MedSurg Nursing, 5*(5), 348–354.

*Thomas, J. A., & McIntosh, J. M. (1994). Are incentive spirometry, intermittent positive pressure breathing, and deep breathing exercises effective in the prevention of postoperative pulmonary complication after upper abdominal surgery? A systematic overview and meta-analysis. *Physical Therapy, 74*(1), 3–16.

*Treloar, D. M. (1984). When a surgical wound bursts. *RN, 47*(6), 20–30, 78.

Wall, M. P. (1995). Dimensions of clinical practice. Postoperative respiratory complications. *Perspectives in Respiratory Nursing, 6*(4), 1, 3–4.

Weant, C. A. (1995). Soundwaves. What floor nurses want to hear from you. *Journal of Post Anesthesia Nursing, 10*(2), 100–101.

*Whitman, G. R. (1991). Hypertension and hypothermia in the acute postoperative period. *Critical Care Nursing Clinics of North America, 3*(4), 661–673.

*Wild, L., & Coyne, C. (1992). The basics and beyond: Epidural analgesia. *American Journal of Nursing, 92*(4), 26–35.

Wilkinson, R. (1996). A non-pharmacological approach to pain relief. *Professional Nurse, 11*(4), 222–224.

*Willens, J. S. (1994). Giving fentanyl for pain outside the OR. *American Journal of Nursing, 94*(2), 24–28.

Winslow, E. H., et al. (1995). Research for practice. Well-timed antibiotics prevent postop infection. *American Journal of Nursing, 95*(3), 60.

Wren, K. R., et al. (1996). Postsurgical urinary retention. *Urological Nursing, 16*(2), 45–49.

Zalon, M. L. (1997). Pain in frail, elderly women after surgery. *Image: Journal of Nursing Scholarship, 29*(1), 21–26.

SUGGESTED READINGS

Pasero, C. L. (1996). Managing postoperative pain in the elderly. *American Journal of Nursing, 96*(10), 38–46.

This article first addresses reasons why traditional pain management in the elderly may be less than optimal. The authors then introduce, define, and describe the multimodal approach to pain management, balanced analgesia, and preemptive analgesia, all of which have been found to be benefical in the elderly. Specific interventions for managing pain in the elderly and for administering pain medication to the elderly are covered as are details related to different classifications of analgesic medication. Tips on minimizing adverse effects and situations to avoid are discussed. The article concludes with a section on planning for discharge. A continuing education test is included.

Strimike, C. L., Wojcik, J. M., & Stark, B. A. (1997). Incision care that really cuts it. *RN, 60*(7), 22–26.

The article begins with a physiologic description of the various stages of incisional healing. The authors then identify and discuss risk factors for wound complications. The remainder of the article addresses two factors to facilitate wound healing. The first is to perform wound care appropriate to the type of wound, and guidelines are included in the article. The second factor is adequate nutrition; an explanation of various nutrients and their role in wound healing is included in chart form.

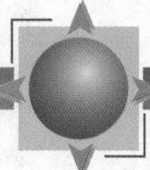

Problems of Protection:

Management of Clients

with Problems of the

Immune System

Chapter 23

CONCEPTS OF INFLAMMATION AND THE IMMUNE RESPONSE

Humans are susceptible to diseases caused by the invasion of microorganisms. Two major defenses, inflammation and immunity, protect the immunocompetent person against diseases and other problems when the body is invaded by microorganisms. These defenses also help the body to recover after injury or tissue damage. Therefore, inflammation and immunity have critical roles in maintaining health and preventing disease. Many diseases, injuries, and medical therapies alter immune function to some degree. These alterations in immune function may be temporary or permanent, but they always endanger the health of the client. Nurses need to understand the processes involved in inflammation and immunity to protect clients and minimize complications.

BASIC CONCEPTS OF INFLAMMATION AND IMMUNITY

Immunity encompasses a variety of functions that protect people against the effects accompanying injury or invasion of the body. People interact with many other living organisms in the environment. The size of these organisms varies from large (other humans and animals) to microscopic (bacteria, viruses, molds, spores, pollens, protozoa, and cells from other people or animals). As long as microorganisms do not enter the body's internal environment, they pose no threat to health. The body has some defenses to prevent microorganisms from gaining access to the internal environment. However, these defenses are not perfect, and invasion of the body's internal environment by microorganisms occurs often. Invasion occurs much more frequently than does an actual disease or illness because of proper immune functioning.

Purpose

The purpose of the immune system is to neutralize, eliminate, or destroy microorganisms that invade the internal environment. To accomplish this purpose without harming the body, immune system cells use defensive actions only against non-self proteins and cells. Therefore, immune system cells can differentiate between the body's own healthy self cells and other non-self proteins and cells.

Self Versus Non-Self

Non-self proteins and cells include infected or debilitated body cells, self cells that have become cancerous, and all invading cells and microorganisms. This ability to recognize self versus non-self, which is necessary to prevent healthy body cells from being destroyed along with the invaders, is called *self-tolerance*. The immune system cells are the only body cells capable of recognizing self from non-self. The process of self-tolerance is possible because of the different kinds of proteins present on cell membranes.

All organisms are made up of cells. Each cell is surrounded by a plasma membrane (Fig. 23–1). With any cell, many different proteins protrude through the plasma membrane. For example, in liver cells, many different proteins are present on the cell surface (protruding through the membrane). The amino acid sequence of each protein type differs from that of all other protein types. Some of these proteins are found on the liver cells of all animals (including humans) that have livers because these protein types are specific to the liver and actually serve as a marker for liver tissues. Other protein types are found only on the liver cells of humans, because these protein types are specific markers for humans. Still other protein types are found only on the liver cells of humans with a specific blood type. In addition, each person's liver cells have surface protein types that are specific to that individual. These proteins are unique to the person and would be identical only to the proteins of an identical twin. These unique proteins, found on the surface of all body cells of that individual, serve as a "universal product

code" or a "cellular fingerprint" for that person (Workman et al., 1993). The proteins that make up the universal product code for one person are recognized as "foreign" by the immune system of another person. Because the cell-surface proteins would be recognized as foreign by another person's immune system, they are antigens, proteins capable of stimulating an immune response.

This unique universal product code for each person is composed of the human leukocyte antigens (HLAs). "Leukocyte" antigen is actually an incorrect term, because these antigens are also present on the surfaces of nearly all body cells, not just on leukocytes. HLAs are a normal part of the person and act as antigens only if they enter another person's body. These antigens specify the tissue type of a person. Other names for these personal cellular fingerprints are human transplantation antigens, human histocompatibility antigens, and class I antigens.

Humans have about 40 major HLAs (known as *histocompatibility antigens*) that are determined by a series of genes collectively called the major histocompatibility complex (MHC). However, the exact number of minor HLAs that any person has is not known. The specific antigens that any person has (of a large number of possible antigens) are genetically determined by which MHC genes were inherited from his or her parents.

This universal product code (HLA) is a key feature for recognition and self-tolerance. The immune system cells constantly come into contact with other body cells and with any invader that happens to enter the body's internal environment. At each encounter, the immune system cells compare the surface protein universal product codes (HLAs) to determine whether or not the encountered cell

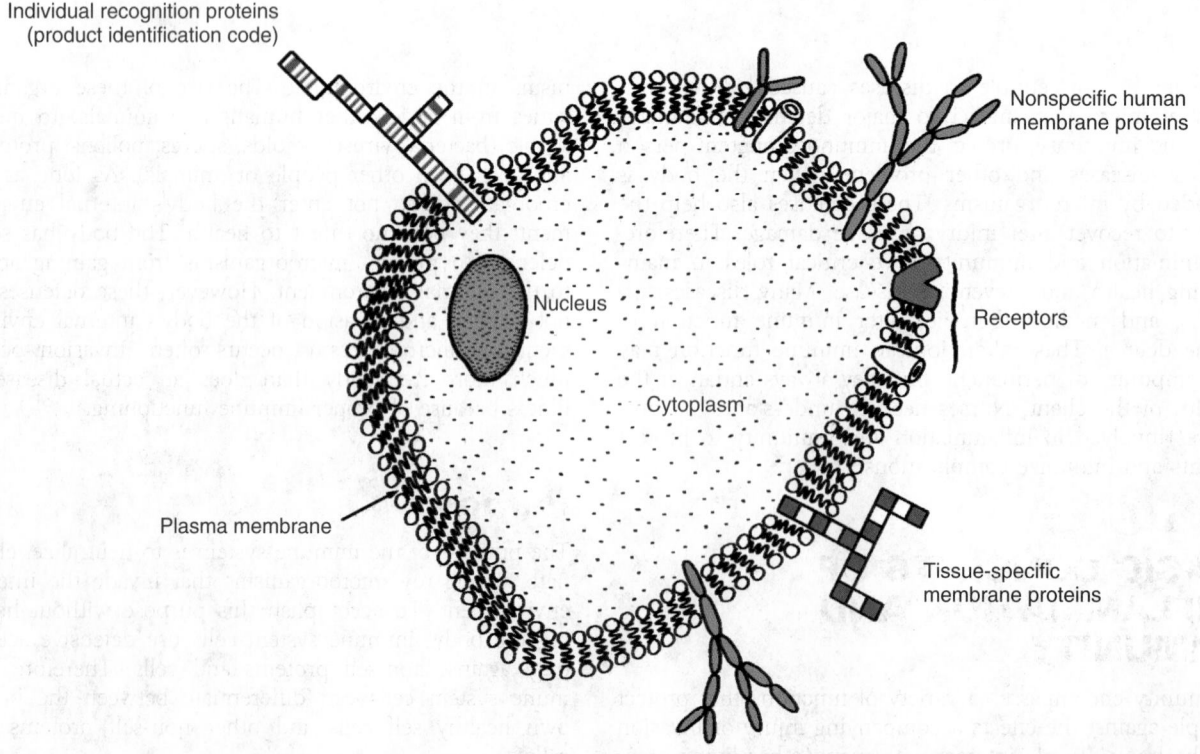

Figure 23–1. Properties of human cell membranes.

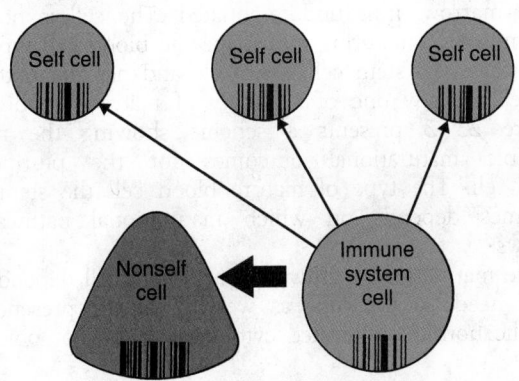

Figure 23–2. Determination of self versus non-self cells.

belongs in the body's internal environment (Fig. 23–2). If the encountered cell's universal product code (HLA) perfectly matches the HLA of the immune system cell, the encountered cell is considered self and is not further molested by the immune system cell. If the encountered cell's universal product code (HLA) does not perfectly match the HLA of the immune system cell, the encountered cell is considered non-self or foreign. The immune system cell takes actions to neutralize, destroy, or eliminate the foreign invader.

Immune function changes during a person's life, according to nutritional status, environmental conditions, medications, the presence of disease, and age. Immune function is most efficient when people are in their 20s and 30s and slowly declines with increasing age. The elderly have decreased immune function, causing greater susceptibility to a variety of pathologic conditions (Chart 23–1).

Organization of the Immune System

The immune system does not reside in any one organ or area of the body. The cells of the immune system originate in the bone marrow. Some of these cells mature in

Chart 23–1

Nursing Focus on the Elderly: Changes in Immune Function Related to Aging

Immune Component	Functional Change	Nursing Implications
Inflammation	• Probable defect in neutrophil function	• Neutrophil counts may be normal, but activity is reduced or impaired.
	• Leukocytosis does not occur during episodes of acute infection	• Clients may have an infection but not show standard changes in white blood cell counts.
	• Elderly persons may not have a fever during inflammatory or infectious episodes	• Not only is there potential loss of protection through inflammation, but minor infections may be overlooked until the client becomes severely infected or septic.
Antibody-mediated immunity	• The total number of colony-forming B lymphocytes and the ability of these cells to mature into antibody-secreting cells are diminished	• The elderly are less able to make new antibodies in response to the presence of new antigens. Thus, the elderly should receive immunizations, such as "flu shots" and the pneumococcal vaccination.
	• There is a decline in natural antibodies, decreased response to antigens, and reduction in the amount of time the antibody response is maintained	• Elderly people may not have sufficient antibodies present to provide protection when they are re-exposed to microorganisms against which they have already generated antibodies. Thus, elderly clients need to avoid people with viral infections and to receive "booster" shots for old vaccinations and immunizations.
Cell-mediated immunity	• Thymic activity decreases with aging, and the number of circulating T lymphocytes decreases	• Skin tests for tuberculosis may be falsely negative.
		• Elderly clients are more at risk for bacterial and fungal infections, especially on the skin and mucous membranes, in the respiratory tract, and in the genitourinary tract.

the bone marrow; others leave the bone marrow and mature in different specific body sites. After maturation, most immune system cells are released into the blood, where they circulate to most areas of the body and exert specific effects.

The bone marrow is the source of all blood cells, including immune system cells. The bone marrow produces an immature, undifferentiated cell called a stem cell (Abbas et al., 1997). This immature stem cell is also described as pluripotent, multipotent, totipotent, and even omnipotent. These adjectives describe the potential future of the stem cell. When the stem cell is first created in the bone marrow, it is undifferentiated. The cell is not yet committed to maturing into a specific blood cell type. At this stage, the stem cell is flexible and has the potential to become any one of a variety of mature blood cells. Figure 23–3 presents a scheme showing the major possible maturational outcomes for the pluripotent stem cell. The type of mature blood cell the stem cell becomes depends on which maturational pathway it follows.

The maturational pathway of any stem cell depends on body needs at the time as well as on the presence of specific hormones (termed cytokines, factors, or poietins)

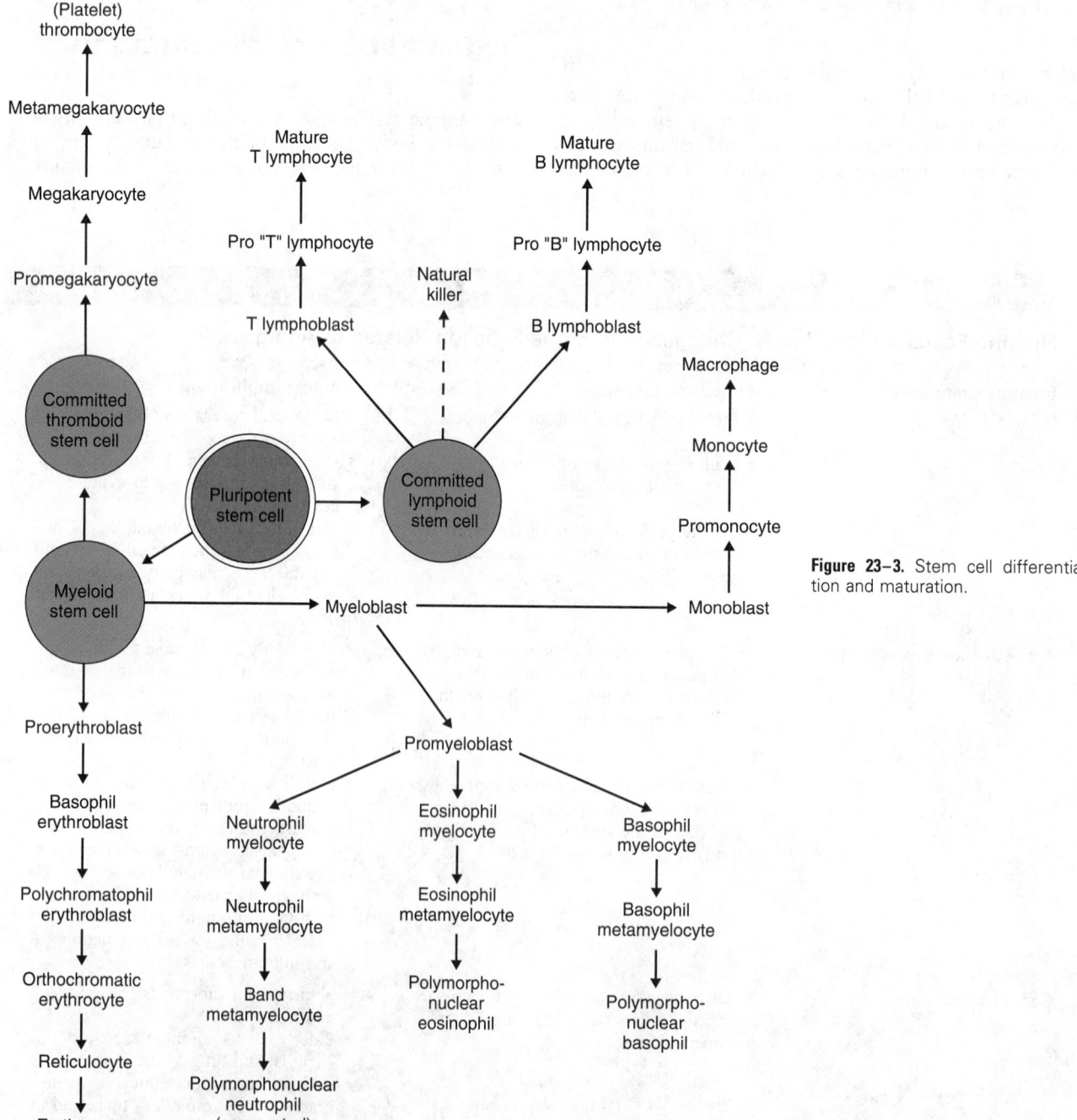

Figure 23–3. Stem cell differentiation and maturation.

TABLE 23–1

Immune Functions of Specific Leukocytes

Variable	Leukocyte	Function
Inflammation	Neutrophil	• Nonspecific ingestion and phagocytosis of microorganisms and foreign protein
	Macrophage	• Nonspecific recognition of foreign proteins and microorganisms; ingestion and phagocytosis
	Monocyte	• Destruction of bacteria and cellular debris; matures into macrophage
	Eosinophil	• Weak phagocytic action; releases vasoactive amines during allergic reactions
	Basophil	• Releases histamine and heparin in areas of tissue damage
Antibody-mediated immunity	B lymphocyte Plasma cell	• Becomes sensitized to foreign cells and proteins • Secretes immunoglobulins in response to the presence of a specific antigen
	Memory cell	• Remains sensitized to a specific antigen and can secrete increased amounts of immunoglobulins specific to the antigen
Cell-mediated immunity	T lymphocyte helper–inducer T cell	• Enhances immune activity through secretion of various factors, cytokines, and lymphokines
	Cytotoxic–cytolytic T cell	• Selectively attacks and destroys non-self cells, including virally infected cells, grafts, and transplanted organs
	Natural killer cell	• Nonselectively attacks non-self cells, especially body cells that have undergone mutation and become malignant; also attacks grafts and transplanted organs

that direct commitment and induce maturation. For example, erythropoietin is made in the kidney. When immature stem cells are exposed to erythropoietin, the immature stem cells commit to the erythrocyte maturational pathway and become mature red blood cells.

White blood cells (leukocytes) are cells that protect the body from the effects of invasion by foreign microorganisms. These cells are the immune system cells. Table 23–1 summarizes the functions of different immune system cells. The leukocytes can provide protection through a variety of defensive actions (Abbas et al., 1997). These actions include

- Recognition of self versus non-self
- Phagocytic destruction of foreign invaders, cellular debris, and unhealthy or abnormal self cells
- Lytic destruction of foreign invaders and unhealthy self cells
- Production of antibodies directed against invaders
- Activation of complement
- Production of hormones that stimulate increased formation of leukocytes in bone marrow
- Production of hormones that increase specific leukocyte growth and activity

The three processes necessary for immunity and the cells involved in these responses can be categorized as inflammation, antibody-mediated immunity (AMI) (humoral immunity), and cell-mediated immunity (CMI).

These three processes represent different defensive actions (Fig. 23–4). Full immunity, or immunocompetence, requires the function and interaction of all three processes.

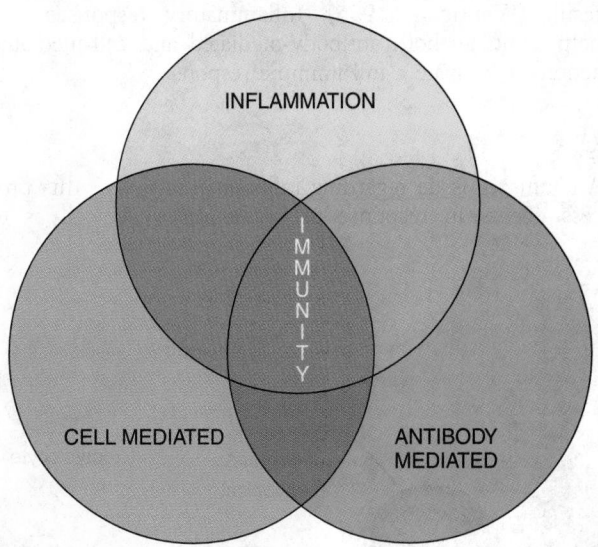

Figure 23–4. The three divisions of immunity. Each division (inflammation, antibody-mediated immunity, and cell-mediated immunity) has an important independent function. In addition, the function of each division of immunity is profoundly influenced by the other two divisions. Most important, optimal function of all three divisions is necessary for complete immunity.

INFLAMMATION

Inflammation provides immediate protection against the effects of tissue injury and invading foreign proteins. The ability to produce an inflammatory response is critical to health and well-being. Inflammation differs from AMI and CMI in two important ways:

1. Inflammatory responses provide immediate but short-term protection against the effects of injury or foreign invaders rather than sustained, long-term immunity on repeated exposure to the same foreign invaders.
2. Inflammation is a nonspecific body defense to invasion or injury.

Inflammation is nonspecific because the same tissue responses occur with any type of injury or invasion, regardless of the location on the body or the specific initiating agent. Therefore, the inflammatory processes stimulated by a scald burn to the hand are the same as the inflammatory processes stimulated by excessive acid in the stomach or the presence of bacteria in the middle ear. How widespread the symptoms of inflammation are in the body depends on the intensity, severity, duration, and extent of exposure to the initiating injury or invasion. For example, a splinter in the finger triggers an inflammatory response only at the splinter site, whereas a burn injuring 60% of the skin surface results in an inflammatory response involving the entire body.

Purpose

Inflammatory responses result in tissue actions that cause visible and uncomfortable symptoms. Despite the discomfort, these inflammatory actions are important in ridding the body of harmful microorganisms. However, if the inflammatory response is excessive, tissue damage may result (Workman, 1995). Inflammatory responses also help stimulate both antibody-mediated and cell-mediated actions to activate a full immune response.

Infection

A confusing issue regarding inflammation is that this process occurs in response to tissue injury as well as to invasion by microorganisms or other foreign proteins. Infection is usually accompanied by inflammation; however, inflammation can occur without invasion by microorganisms. For example, inflammatory responses not associated with infection occur with sprain injuries to joints, myocardial infarction, sterile surgical incisions, thrombophlebitis, and blister formation caused by temperature extremes. Examples of inflammatory responses associated with noninfectious invasion by foreign proteins include allergic rhinitis, contact dermatitis, and other immediate-type allergic reactions. Inflammatory responses associated with invasion by disease-causing microorganisms include otitis media, appendicitis, bacterial peritonitis, viral hepatitis, and bacterial myocarditis, among others. Thus, inflammation does not always mean that an infection is present.

Cell Types Involved in Inflammation

The leukocytes associated with inflammatory responses are neutrophils, macrophages, eosinophils, and basophils. Neutrophils and macrophages participate in phagocytosis, destroying and eliminating foreign invaders. Basophils and eosinophils act on blood vessels to cause tissue-level responses.

Neutrophils
Description and Origin

Mature neutrophils usually compose between 55% and 70% of the total white blood cell count. Neutrophils arise from the stem cells and complete the maturation process in the bone marrow (Fig. 23–5). They belong to the class of leukocytes known as granulocytes because of the large number of granules present inside each cell. Other names for neutrophils are based on their physical characteristics and degree of maturation. Mature neutrophils are also called segmented neutrophils ("segs") or polymorphonuclear cells ("polys") because of their segmented nucleus. Less mature neutrophils are called band neutrophils ("bands" or "stabs") because of their nuclear appearance.

Usually, maturation from the undifferentiated stem cell

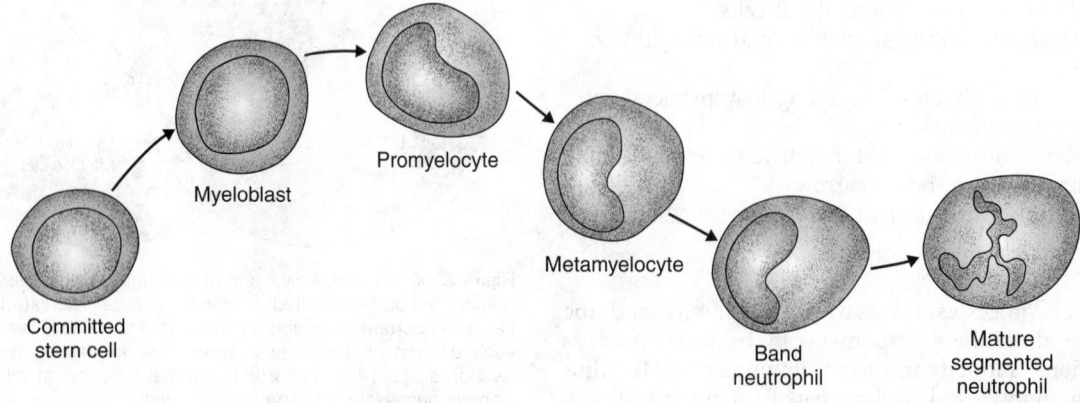

Committed stem cell

Myeloblast

Promyelocyte

Metamyelocyte

Band neutrophil

Mature segmented neutrophil

Figure 23–5. Neutrophil maturation.

to the functional segmented neutrophil requires 12 to 14 days. This time can be shortened by certain conditions that stimulate the body to produce specific cytokines such as granulocyte-macrophage colony–stimulating factor and granulocyte colony–stimulating factor. The purpose and action of cytokines are described later in this chapter under Cytokines.

In the immunocompetent, healthy person, more than 100 billion fresh, mature neutrophils are released from the bone marrow into the systemic circulation daily (Abbas et al., 1997). This massive production of neutrophils is necessary because the life span of a circulating neutrophil is extremely short, averaging only about 12 to 18 hours.

Function

Although the neutrophils are the largest group of circulating leukocytes, each individual cell is small. This army of powerful small cells provides the first internal line of defense, via phagocytosis, against foreign invaders (especially bacteria) in blood and extracellular fluid. It is the granules inside the neutrophils that cause the phagocytic destruction of foreign invaders. The mature neutrophil is filled with large numbers of granules containing various enzymes that can degrade different parts of foreign invaders.

Neutrophils have a small energy supply and no way of replenishing either that energy supply or the enzymes used in degradation. Thus, each neutrophil can participate in only one episode of phagocytic destruction before supplies are exhausted.

The mature, segmented neutrophil is the only neutrophil stage capable of effective phagocytosis. Because this cell type is responsible for continuous, instant, nonspecific protection against microorganisms, the percentage and actual number of circulating white blood cells that are mature neutrophils reliably measure a client's susceptibility to infection: the higher the numbers, the greater is the resistance to infection. This measurement is the *absolute neutrophil count* (sometimes called the absolute granulocyte count or total granulocyte count).

The differential of a normal white blood cell count indicates that most of the neutrophils released into the blood from the bone marrow are segmented neutrophils; only a small percentage are composed of band neutrophils (Fig. 23–6). The less mature neutrophil forms should not be present in the blood. Some conditions cause the major population of neutrophils in the blood to change from mostly segmented neutrophils to less mature forms. This situation is termed a *left shift* because the segmented neutrophil, which is seen at the far right of the neutrophil maturational pathway (see Fig. 23–5), no longer represents the greatest number of circulating neutrophils. Instead, the major population is made up of one of the cell types found farther left on the neutrophil maturational pathway.

A left shift is a clinical sign indicating that the client's bone marrow cannot produce enough mature neutrophils to keep pace with the continuing presence of microorganisms and is releasing immature neutrophils into the blood. Unfortunately, most of these immature neutrophils

Differential	%	/mm^3
Total WBC	100	10,000
segs	62	6200
bands	5	500
monos	3	300
lymphs	28	2800
eosin	1.5	150
baso	0.5	50

Figure 23–6. Example of a laboratory slip showing the differential of a normal white blood cell (WBC) count.

are of no benefit to the client, because they are not capable of phagocytosis.

Macrophages
Description and Origin

Macrophages arise from the committed myeloid stem cell in the bone marrow and form the mononuclear phagocyte system. This cell first begins to differentiate into a monocyte and is released into the blood at this stage. Until they mature, monocytes have only limited activity. Most monocytes move into various tissues, where they complete the maturation process into macrophages. Some macrophages become "fixed" in position within the tissues, whereas others remain mobile in the tissue's interstitial fluid. Macrophages in various tissues have slightly different appearances and different names. Table 23–2 lists the names of the different tissue macrophages. Figure 23–7 shows the distribution of tissue macrophages throughout the body. The liver and spleen contain the greatest concentration of these cells.

Tissue macrophages have relatively long life spans, lasting from months to years. Macrophages are the largest of all the leukocytes and have granules containing many lytic enzymes.

TABLE 23–2

Tissue Macrophages

Tissue	Macrophage
Lung	• Alveolar macrophage
Connective tissue	• Histiocyte
Brain	• Microglial cell
Liver	• Kupffer cell
Peritoneum	• Peritoneal macrophage
Bone	• Osteoclast
Joints	• Synovial type A cell
Kidney	• Mesangial cell

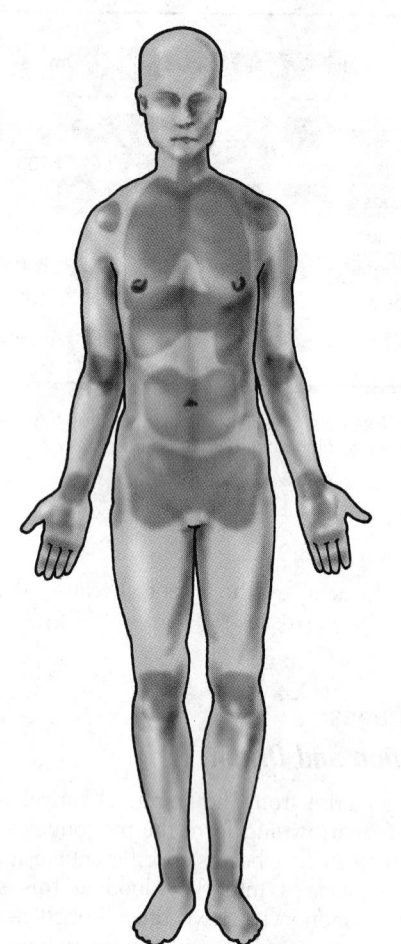

Figure 23–7. Areas of highest concentration of tissue macrophages.

Function

Macrophages play more than one role in protecting against invasion and tissue injury. These cells are important in immediate inflammatory responses and can also stimulate the longer lasting immune responses associated with antibody-mediated immunity (AMI) and cell-mediated immunity (CMI). Specific macrophage functions include phagocytosis, repair of injured tissues, antigen processing, and secretion of cytokines that help control the immune system.

The inflammation-associated macrophage function is phagocytosis. Macrophages are efficient at distinguishing between self and non-self and are especially effective at trapping invading cells. Unlike neutrophils, macrophages are able to regenerate the energy supplies and enzymes needed to degrade foreign protein. Therefore, each macrophage can participate in many phagocytic events during its life span.

Basophils
Description and Origin

The rarest leukocytes, basophils, arise from myeloid stem cells and are released from the bone marrow after a short maturation period. Basophils cause the obvious signs and symptoms accompanying inflammation.

Function

Basophilic granules contain many vasoactive chemicals that act on blood vessels, including heparin, histamine, serotonin, kinins, and leukotrienes. When released into the blood, most of these chemicals act on smooth muscle and blood vessel walls. Heparin inhibits coagulation of blood and other protein-containing extracellular fluids. Histamine constricts the smooth muscles of the respiratory system and small veins. Constriction of respiratory smooth muscle narrows the lumen of airways and restricts breathing. Constriction of venular smooth muscle inhibits blood flow through small veins and decreases venous return. This effect causes blood to collect in capillaries and small arterioles. Kinins cause vasodilation of arterioles and, together with serotonin, increased capillary permeability. These actions permit the plasma portion of the blood to leak into the interstitial space. This chemical-induced process is called *vascular leak syndrome*.

Eosinophils
Description and Origin

Eosinophils arise from the myeloid line and contain more vasoactive chemicals. Usually only 1% to 2% of the total white blood cell count is composed of eosinophils.

Function

Eosinophils are not efficient phagocytes, although they can act against infestations of parasitic larvae. Eosinophil granules contain many substances with vastly different actions. Some of these substances are vasoactive chemicals that produce inflammatory reactions when released. In addition, certain enzymes from eosinophils degrade vasoactive chemicals and in this way may control or modulate the extent of inflammatory reactions.

Phagocytosis

The key mechanism for the successful outcome of inflammation is *phagocytosis*, or the destruction of non-self cells. Phagocytosis is the process by which leukocytes engulf invaders and destroy them by enzymatic degradation. Phagocytosis rids the body of debris after tissue injury and destroys foreign invaders. Of all the leukocytes, neutrophils and macrophages perform phagocytosis most efficiently. Phagocytosis occurs in a predictable manner and involves the seven steps depicted in Figure 23–8.

Exposure and Invasion

Leukocytes that engage in phagocytosis and stimulate inflammation are present in the blood and most other extracellular fluids. For phagocytosis to be initiated, these leukocytes must first be exposed to debris from damaged tissues or foreign proteins (antigens). Therefore, the initiating event for phagocytosis is injury or invasion.

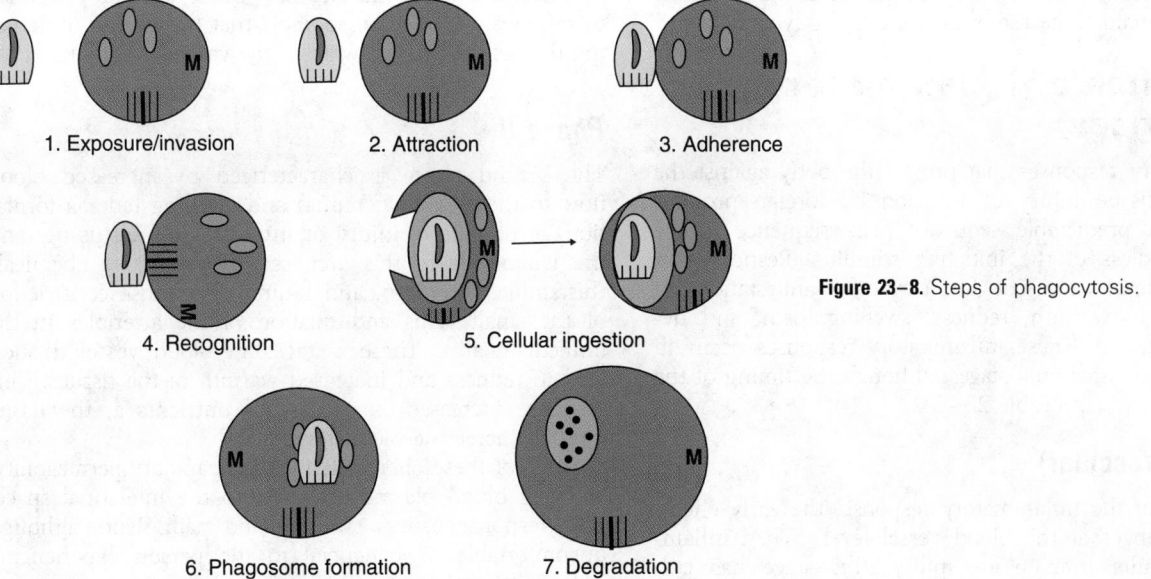

Figure 23–8. Steps of phagocytosis.

Attraction

Phagocytosis is effective only when the phagocytic cell comes into direct contact with the target (antigen, invader, or foreign protein). Special chemical substances can act as chemical magnets that attract neutrophils and macrophages. These substances are called chemotaxins, or leukotaxins. Damaged tissues and blood vessels secrete chemotaxins. In addition, substances that combine with surface components of invading foreign proteins serve as chemotaxins. This combining (and attracting) mechanism is described next.

Adherence

Because phagocytosis requires direct contact of the phagocyte with its intended target, the phagocytic cell must first bind to the surface of the target. A special process called *opsonization* helps provide direct contact of the phagocyte with its target.

Opsonization

The word *opsonin* is derived from the Greek and literally means "to cover food with a sauce in preparation for eating." In biological processes, opsonins coat a target cell (antigen or foreign protein); this changes the target cell's surface charge and makes it easier for phagocytic cells to stick to it. Many substances can act as opsonins. Some of these substances are particles from dead neutrophils, antibodies, and activated (fixated) complement components.

Complement Activation and Fixation

One mechanism of opsonization and phagocytic adherence to target cells is complement activation and fixation. Twenty different inactive protein components of the complement system are present in the blood. These components are made by the liver. With proper stimulation, individual complement proteins become activated and to-

gether cause dramatic actions as a result of fixation (adherence) to specific tissues. Complement fixation must occur quickly, but consequences can be devastating if its effects are exerted at the wrong time or in the wrong place. Therefore, the complement system works as a cascade reaction (chain reaction), with many sites of activation and control.

Recognition

When the phagocytic cell sticks to the surface of the target cell, recognition of non-self occurs. The body's phagocytic cells examine the universal product codes (HLAs) of whatever they encounter. Recognition of non-self is enhanced by opsonins on the surface of the target cell. Phagocytic cells proceed with phagocytosis only if the target cell is recognized either as foreign or as debris from damaged self cells.

Cellular Ingestion

Because phagocytic destruction is an intracellular process, the target cell or foreign protein must be brought inside the phagocytic cell. The phagocytic cell changes its shape and bends its membrane around to enclose (engulf) the target cell. Once the target is enclosed in the phagocytic cells, a vacuole is formed.

Phagosome Formation

When the phagocyte's granules are inside the vacuole, the structure is called a *phagosome* (or phagolysosome). These granules break open and release enzymes into the fluid of the phagosome and destroy the ingested target.

Degradation

The enzymes within the phagosome exert their specific effects on different parts of the ingested target. The target is broken down into smaller pieces until only minute particles remain to be removed from the body as debris.

Sequence of Inflammatory Responses

Inflammatory responses that protect the body against the effects of tissue injury or invasion by foreign proteins occur in a predictable sequence. The sequence is the same regardless of the initiating stimulus. Responses at the tissue level cause the five cardinal manifestations of inflammation: warmth, redness, swelling, pain, and decreased function. These inflammatory responses occur in three distinct functional stages, although the timing of the stages may overlap (Table 23–3).

Stage I (Vascular)

In stage I of the inflammatory response, the early effects involve changes at the blood vessel level. When inflammation results from tissue injury, this stage has two phases.

Phase I

The first phase is an immediate, short-term constriction of arterioles and venules as a direct result of physical trauma to vascular smooth muscle. This phase lasts only seconds to minutes and may be so short that the person undergoing the response is unaware of the vasoconstriction.

Phase II

The second phase is characterized by increased blood flow to the area (hyperemia) and swelling (edema formation) at the site of injury or invasion. Injured tissues and the leukocytes in this area secrete vasoactive chemicals (histamine, serotonin, and kinins) that cause constriction of the small veins and dilation of the arterioles in the immediate area. These changes in blood vessel dilation lead to redness and increased warmth of the tissues. This response increases the supply of nutrients at the tissue level by increasing blood flow.

Some of these chemicals increase capillary permeability, allowing blood plasma to leak into the interstitial space. This response causes swelling and pain. Pain, although uncomfortable, is beneficial to the person experiencing inflammation. Pain increases the person's awareness that a problem exists and encourages action to avoid further injury or inflammation. Edema formation at the site of injury or invasion is also a helpful event. This swelling protects the area from further injury by creating a cushion of fluid. The extra fluid can dilute the concentration

TABLE 23–3

Stages of Inflammation

Stage	Onset	Cells Involved	Actions
Stage I: vascular	• Minutes after injury or invasion	• Tissue macrophages	• Limited phagocytosis of invading microorganisms or cell debris from injured tissues • Secretion of vasoactive amines (histamine, bradykinin, serotonin) to dilate blood vessels and increase capillary leak; this action results in redness, warmth, swelling, and pain at the site but also increases blood flow to the area; more nutrients are available to the tissues; plasma proteins moved into the tissues clot and "wall off" microorganisms, limiting their spread • Secretion of chemotaxins to draw more leukocytes into the area to sustain the inflammatory response • Secretion of cytokines to increase bone marrow production of granulocytes
Stage II: cellular exudate	• Hours after injury or invasion	• Granular myeloid cells • Neutrophils • Basophils • Eosinophils	• Increased phagocytosis • Secretion of slow-acting vasoactive amines to ensure a sustained inflammatory response • Secretion of substances to increase the rate of neutrophil maturation and macrophage maturation
Stage III: tissue repair and replacement	• Begins at initial injury and continues until new tissues are formed and mature or are functional	• Neutrophils • Macrophages	• Stimulation of mitotically active cells to divide; stimulation of fibroblasts in blood vessels to grow and release collagen to form scaffold on which to build scar tissue

of any toxins or microorganisms that have entered the area. The duration of these responses depends on the severity of the initiating event.

The major leukocyte involved in stage I of the inflammatory response is the tissue macrophage. The response of tissue macrophages is immediate, because they are already in place at the site of injury or invasion. However, this response is limited, because the number of such macrophages is so small. In addition to functioning in phagocytosis, the tissue macrophages secrete several cytokines to enhance the inflammatory response. One cytokine is colony-stimulating factor, which stimulates the bone marrow to reduce the time of leukocyte production from 14 days to a matter of hours. Tissue macrophages also secrete substances that increase the release of neutrophils from the bone marrow and attract them to the site of injury or invasion, which leads to the next stage of inflammation.

Stage II (Cellular Exudate)

Stage II of inflammation is characterized by neutrophilia (increased number of circulating neutrophils), secretion of many factors into the interstitial fluid, and formation of exudate.

The most active leukocyte in this stage is the neutrophil. Under the influence of chemotactic agents and cytokines, the neutrophil count can increase up to five times within 12 hours after the onset of inflammation. At the site of inflammation, neutrophils attack and destroy foreign materials and remove dead tissue through phagocytosis.

During acute inflammatory responses, the healthy person can produce enough mature neutrophils to keep pace with the effects of injury or invasion and to prevent the invaders from multiplying. At the same time, the leukocytes secrete cytokines, which increase reproduction of tissue macrophages and bone marrow production of monocytes. Although this reaction begins slowly, its effects are long lasting.

When infectious processes stimulating inflammation are longer or chronic, the bone marrow cannot produce and release enough mature neutrophils into the blood to keep pace with the ability of microorganisms to multiply. In this situation, the bone marrow begins to release only immature neutrophils. Such a reduction in the number of functional phagocytic neutrophils limits the effectiveness of the inflammatory response and increases the susceptibility to microbial infections.

Stage III (Tissue Repair and Replacement)

Although stage III is completed last, it begins at the time of injury and is critical to the ultimate function of the inflamed area.

Some of the leukocytes involved in inflammation start the replacement and repair of lost or damaged tissues by inducing the remaining healthy tissue to divide. In tissues that are nondividing, leukocytes stimulate new blood vessel growth and scar tissue formation. Because scar tissue does not behave like normal tissue, functional loss occurs where damaged tissues are replaced with scar tissue. The extent of the functional loss is determined by the percentage of tissue replaced by scar tissue.

Inflammation alone cannot confer immunity; however, the interaction of inflammatory cells with lymphocytes helps provide long-lasting immunity against re-exposure to the same microorganisms. Long-lasting immune actions are those generated by antibody-mediated immunity (AMI) and cell-mediated immunity (CMI).

ANTIBODY-MEDIATED IMMUNITY

Antibody-mediated immunity (AMI), also known as humoral immunity, involves antigen-antibody actions to neutralize, eliminate, or destroy foreign proteins. Antibodies for these actions are produced by populations of B lymphocytes.

Purpose

The primary functions of B lymphocytes are to become sensitized to a specific foreign protein (antigen) and to synthesize an antibody directed specifically against that protein. The antibody (rather than the actual B lymphocyte) then participates in one of several actions to neutralize, eliminate, or destroy that antigen.

Cell Types Involved in Antibody-Mediated Immunity

The leukocytes with the most direct role in AMI are the B lymphocytes. Macrophages and T lymphocytes (discussed later under Cell-Mediated Immunity) cooperate with B lymphocytes to start and complete antigen–antibody actions. Therefore, for optimal AMI, the entire immune system must function adequately.

B lymphocytes start life as pluripotent stem cells in the bone marrow, the primary lymphoid tissue. The pluripotent stem cells destined to become B lymphocytes commit early to the lymphocyte maturational pathway (see Fig. 23–3). At the point of commitment, these stem cells are no longer pluripotent but are limited to differentiation into lymphocytes. The committed lymphocyte stem cells are released from the bone marrow into the blood. They then migrate into various secondary lymphoid tissues, where maturation is completed.

In humans, the secondary lymphoid tissues for B lymphocyte maturation are the spleen, germinal centers of lymph nodes, tonsils, and Peyer's patches of the intestinal tract.

Antigen-Antibody Interactions

The body learns to make enough of any specific antibody to provide long-lasting immunity against specific microorganisms or toxins. Seven steps in a series of special interactions are required for the production of a unique and specific antibody directed against a unique and specific antigen whenever the person is exposed to that antigen: exposure and invasion, antigen recognition, lymphocyte sensitization, antibody production and release, antigen-antibody binding, antibody-binding reactions, and sustained immunity—memory (Fig. 23–9).

Exposure and Invasion

Antigen–antibody interactions occur in the body's internal environment. For the body to make an antibody that can exert its effects on a specific antigen, the antigen must first enter the body. Not all exposures result in the stimulation of antibody production, even when exposure includes penetration. Invasion by the antigen must occur in such large numbers that some of the antigen either evades detection by the normal nonspecific defenses or overwhelms the ability of the inflammatory response to neutralize, eliminate, or destroy the invader.

Take, for example, a person who has never contracted or even been exposed to the childhood viral disease chickenpox. This person baby-sits for three children who show chickenpox lesions within the next 10 hours. These children, in the pre-eruption stage, shed many millions of live chickenpox virus particles via the droplets from the upper respiratory tract. Because small children are often unconcerned about the finer points of infection control, they drink out of the baby-sitter's soft drink can, kiss the sitter directly (and wetly) on the lips, and sneeze and cough directly into the sitter's face. After spending 5 hours with the children at close range, the baby-sitter has been overwhelmingly invaded by the chickenpox virus (varicella zoster) and will become sick with this disease within 14 to 21 days. While the virus is incubating and the disease is developing, the sitter's leukocytes are partic-

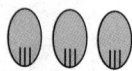

1. Invasion of the body by new antigens in sufficient numbers to stimulate an immune response.

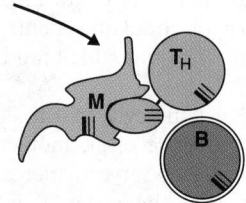

2. Interaction of macrophage (M) and T helper (T_H) cell in the processing and presenting of the antigen to the unsensitized "virgin" B lymphocyte (B).

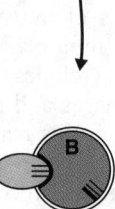

3. Sensitization of the virgin B lymphocyte to the new antigen.

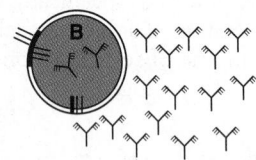

7. On reexposure to the same antigen, the sensitized lymphocytes and their progeny produce large quantities of the antibody specific to the antigen. In addition, new "virgin" B lymphocytes become sensitized to the antigen and also begin antibody production.

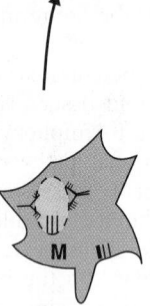

6. Antibody binding causes cellular events and attracts other leukocytes to the complex. The interaction of other leukocytes along with the cellular events results in the neutralization, destruction, or elimination of the antigen.

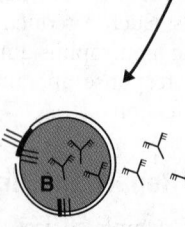

4. Antibody production by the B lymphocyte. These antibodies are directed specifically against the initiating antigen. The antibodies are released from the B lymphocyte and float freely in the blood and some other fluids.

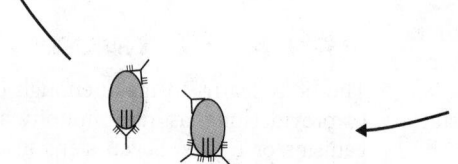

5. Antibodies bind to the antigen, forming an immune complex.

Figure 23–9. Sequence of events stimulating antibody-mediated immunity.

ipating in the next steps in the series of antibody-antigen interactions to prevent the development of chickenpox more than once.

Antigen Recognition

To begin to make antibodies against an antigen, the "virgin" or previously unsensitized B lymphocyte must first recognize the antigen as non-self. B lymphocytes cannot carry out this important function alone; they require the assistance of macrophages and helper/inducer T cells.

This cooperative effort is initiated by the macrophages. After the membrane of the antigen has been altered somewhat by opsonization (previously discussed under Adherence), the macrophage recognizes the invading foreign protein (antigen) as non-self and physically attaches itself to the antigen. This particular macrophage attachment to the antigen does not result in phagocytosis or in immediate destruction of the antigen. Instead, the macrophage brings the attached antigen in contact with a helper/inducer T cell. At this time, the helper/inducer T cell and the macrophage process the antigen in such a way as to expose the antigen's recognition sites (universal product code). After processing the antigen, the helper/inducer T cell brings the antigen into contact with the B lymphocyte

so that the B lymphocyte can recognize the antigen as non-self.

Lymphocyte Sensitization

Once the B lymphocyte recognizes the antigen as non-self, the B lymphocyte becomes sensitized to this antigen. An individual virgin B lymphocyte can undergo sensitization only once. Therefore, each B lymphocyte can be sensitized to only one antigen.

As a result of sensitization, this B lymphocyte can respond to any substance that carries the same antigens (codes) as the original antigen. Once it is sensitized to a specific antigen, the B lymphocyte always remains sensitized to that specific antigen. In addition, all daughter cells of that sensitized B lymphocyte are sensitized to that same specific antigen.

Immediately after it is sensitized, the B lymphocyte (or B blast) divides and forms two different types of lymphocytes, each one remaining sensitized to that specific antigen (Fig. 23–10). One new cell becomes a *plasma cell* and immediately starts to produce antibody directed specifically against the antigen that originally sensitized the B lymphocyte. The other new cell becomes a *memory cell*. The plasma cell functions immediately and has a short life span. The memory cell remains sensitized but functionally

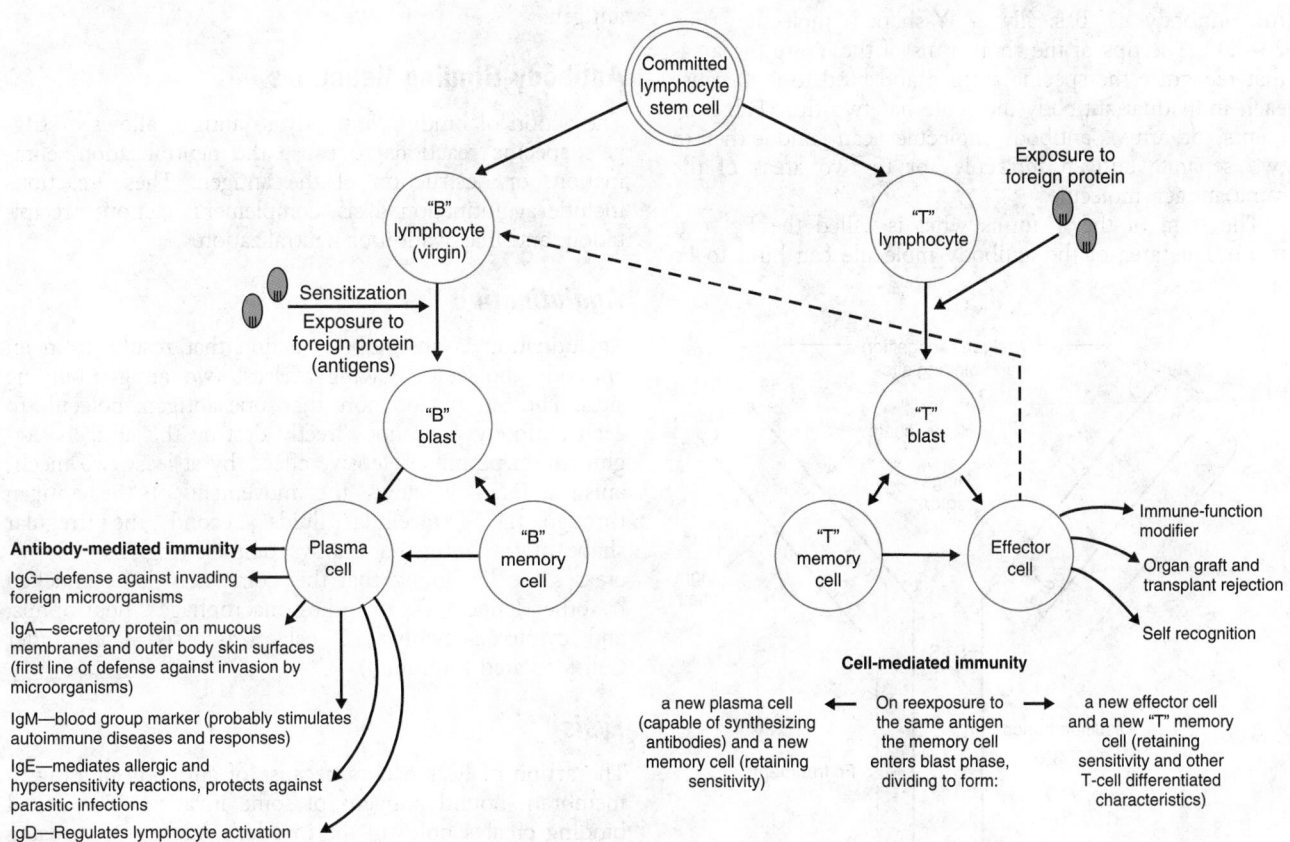

Figure 23–10. Differentiated functions of lymphocytes.

dormant until the next exposure to the same antigen (discussed later under Sustained Immunity–Memory).

Antibody Production and Release

Antibodies are produced by the plasma cell. When fully stimulated, each plasma cell can produce as much as 300 molecules of antibody per second. Each plasma cell produces antibody specific only to the antigen that originally sensitized the parent B lymphocyte. For example, in the case of the baby-sitter who was exposed to and invaded by chickenpox virus, the plasma cells derived from the B lymphocytes sensitized to the chickenpox virus can produce only antichickenpox antibodies. The exact antibody type (e.g., immunoglobulin G [IgG] or immunoglobulin M [IgM]) that the plasma cell can produce may vary, but the specificity of that antibody remains forever directed against chickenpox virus.

Antibody molecules produced by the plasma cells are secreted into the blood and other extracellular fluids as free antibody. Individual molecules of free antibody remain in the blood 3 to 30 days. Because the antibody circulates in body fluids (or body "humors") and is separate from the B lymphocytes, the immunity provided is sometimes called *humoral immunity*. Circulating antibodies can be transferred from one person to another to provide the receiving person with immediate immunity of short duration.

Antigen-Antibody Binding

An antibody is basically a Y-shaped molecule (Fig. 23–11). The tips of the short arms of the Y are the areas that recognize the specific antigen and bind to it. Because each individual antibody molecule has two tips (Fab fragments, or arms), antibody molecules can bind either to two separate antigen molecules or to two areas of the same antigen molecule.

The stem of the Y forms what is called the Fc fragment. This area of the antibody molecule can bind to Fc

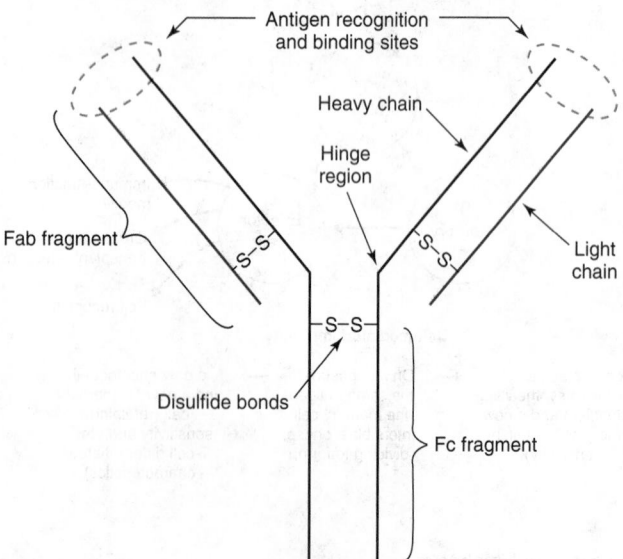

Figure 23–11. Basic antibody structure.

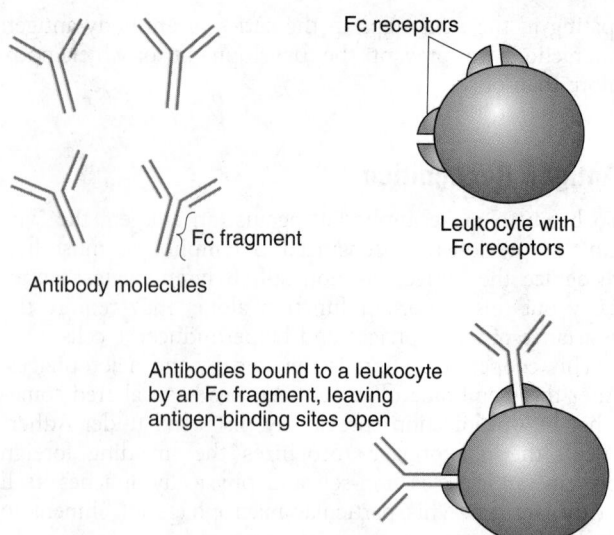

Figure 23–12. Antibody Fc receptors on leukocytes.

receptor sites on leukocytes, so that the leukocyte then has not only its own mechanisms of attacking antigens but also the added power of having antibodies on its surface that stick to antigens (Fig. 23–12).

The actual binding of antibody to antigen is not usually lethal to the antigen. Instead, the physical binding of the antibody to the antigen initiates other actions that result in the neutralization, elimination, or destruction of the antigen.

Antibody-Binding Reactions

The action of binding antibody to antigen allows or triggers specific reactions to cause the neutralization, elimination, or destruction of the antigen. These reactions include agglutination, lysis, complement fixation, precipitation, and inactivation or neutralization.

Agglutination

Agglutination is an antibody action that results from an antibody molecule's having at least two antigen-binding sites. The binding of more than one antigen molecule to each antibody does not directly destroy the antigen. Agglutination permits defensive effects by at least two mechanisms. First, it slows the movement of the antigen through the extracellular fluids. Second, the irregular shape of the antigen-antibody complex (Fig. 23–13) increases the likelihood that this complex will be attacked by other leukocytes, including macrophages, neutrophils, and cytotoxic–cytolytic T cells (discussed later under Cell-Mediated Immunity).

Lysis

The action of lysis occurs because of antibody binding to membrane-bound antigens of some invaders. The actual binding creates holes in the invader's membrane, causing lethal changes in its intracellular environment. This response usually requires that complement be involved in the antigen-antibody action. Bacteria and viruses are the

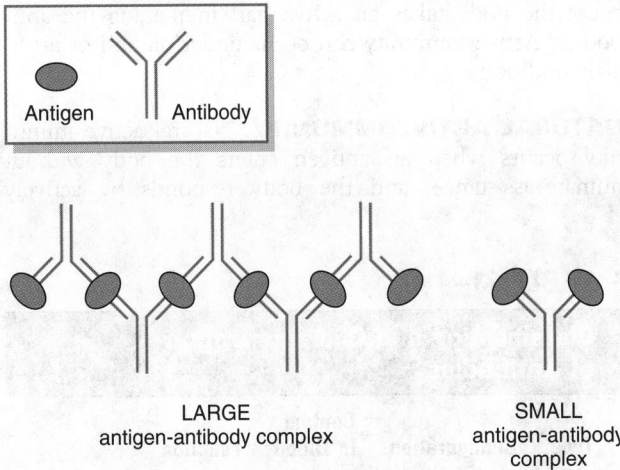

Figure 23–13. Antibody–antigen complexes.

non-self cells most susceptible to damage through lysis caused by the binding of antibody to membrane-surface antigens.

Complement Fixation

Specific classes of antibodies can cause the neutralization, elimination, or destruction of non-self antigen through activation of the complement cascade and complement fixation. (The mechanism by which complement assists in immunity was discussed earlier under Adherence.)

The two classes of antibody commonly associated with stimulating the complement system are IgG and IgM. Binding of antibody from either of these classes to an appropriate antigen provides a binding site for the first component of complement (C1q). Once C1q is activated, other components of the complement system are activated in a cascade.

Precipitation

Precipitation is similar to agglutination. However, in precipitation, antibody molecules bind so much antigen that large, insoluble antigen-antibody complexes are formed. These complexes cannot stay in suspension in the blood. Instead, they form a large, stationary precipitate, which can be acted on and removed by other nonspecific leukocytes.

Inactivation-Neutralization

Inactivation-neutralization is unique in that it does not result in the immediate destruction of the antigen. Usually, a relatively small area of the antigen is actually responsible for exerting harmful effects. The remainder of the antigen is not harmful to the host. Binding of antibody can interfere with the function of the active site by covering it up or changing its shape. Either mechanism inhibits the activity of the antigen and renders it harmless without destroying or eliminating it.

Sustained Immunity–Memory

The sustained immunity–memory function of AMI provides humans with long-lasting immunity to a specific antigen. Sustained immunity is provided by the action of the B-lymphocyte memory cells generated during the lymphocyte sensitization stage. These memory cells remain sensitized to the specific antigen to which they were originally exposed. On re-exposure to the same antigen, the memory cells are stimulated into rapid response. First, the cells divide and form new sensitized blast cells and new sensitized plasma cells. The blast cells continue to divide to generate even more sensitized plasma cells. The sensitized plasma cells begin to rapidly make and secrete large amounts of the antibody specific for the sensitizing antigen.

This ability of the sensitized memory cells to initiate events on re-exposure to the antigen that originally sensitized the B lymphocyte allows a rapid and widespread immune (*anamnestic*) response to the antigen. This response usually eliminates the invading antigen completely so that the person does not become ill. Because of this process, most people do not become ill with chickenpox or other viral diseases more than once, even though they are exposed many times to the causative organism. Without the process or action of memory, people would remain susceptible to specific diseases on subsequent exposure to the antigen, and no sustained immunity would be generated.

General Antibody Classification

All antibodies are referred to as immunoglobulins and gamma globulins. These names are based on the structure, location, and function of antibodies. A globulin is a type of protein structure that is globular rather than straight. Because antibodies are composed of this type of protein, they are globulins. The name immunoglobulin is appropriate for antibodies because they are globular proteins that assist in immune function. Antibodies are called gamma globulins because, during the process of electrophoresis, different groups of proteins in blood plasma separate out at different times, depending on how they move in response to electrical charge (Fig. 23–14). The protein groups are named according to when they emerge. The first group to emerge are the plasma albumins, which make up a large group. Three smaller groups emerge at specific times after the albumins. The fourth group, or protein fraction (gamma fraction), contains all five different types of antibody proteins. The five antibody types are classified by differences in antibody structure, molecular weight, and patterns of association (Table 23–4).

Acquiring Antibody-Mediated Immunity

Two broad categories of immunity are innate immunity and acquired immunity.

SEPARATION OF PLASMA PROTEINS BY ELECTROPHORESIS

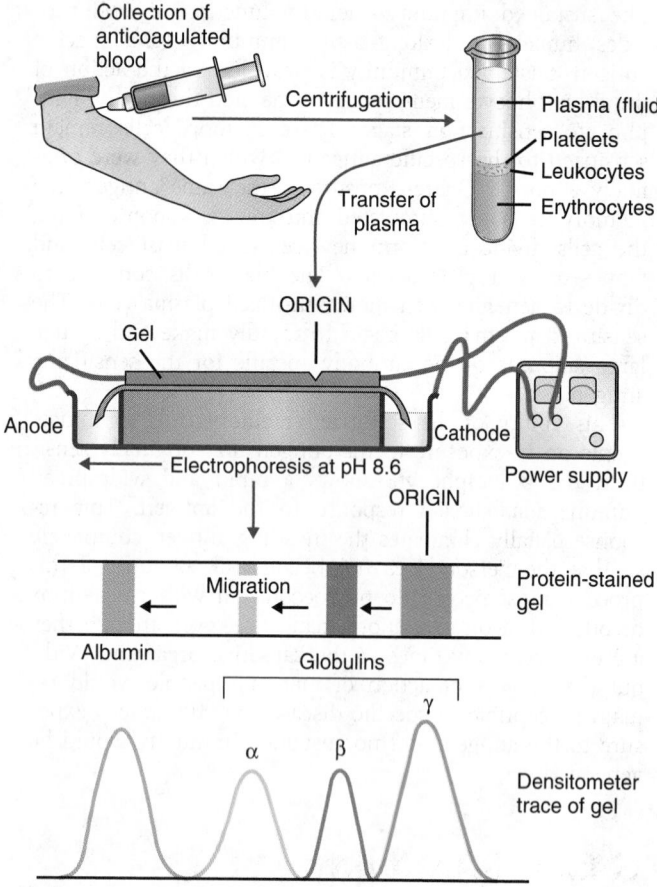

Figure 23–14. Electrophoresis of plasma proteins, including gamma globulin.

Innate Immunity

Innate immunity is a genetically determined characteristic of an individual, group, or species. A person either has or does not have innate immunity. For example, humans have many innate immunities to viruses and other microorganisms that cause specific diseases in animals. As a result, humans are not susceptible to such diseases as mange, distemper, hog cholera, or any of a variety of animal afflictions. This type of immunity cannot be developed or transferred from one person to another and is not an adaptive response to exposure or invasion by foreign proteins.

Acquired Immunity

Acquired immunity is the immunity that every person's body makes (or can receive) as an adaptive response to invasion by foreign proteins. AMI is an acquired immunity. Acquired immunity occurs either naturally or artificially and can be either active or passive.

Active Immunity

Active immunity occurs when antigens enter the body and the body responds by making specific antibodies against the antigen. This type of immunity is active be-

cause the body takes an active part in making the antibodies. Active immunity can occur under natural or artificial conditions.

NATURAL ACTIVE IMMUNITY. Natural active immunity occurs when an antigen enters the body without human assistance, and the body responds by actively

TABLE 23–4

Classification and Characterization of Antibodies

Type	Configuration	Content in Blood	Function
IgA	• Dimer	• <15%	• "Secretory"; present in body secretions, such as tears, mucus, saliva • Inhibits bacteria and viruses from adhering to skin and mucous membranes, making penetration into the internal environment more difficult
IgD	• Monomer	• <1%	• Modification of IgM activity
IgE	• Monomer	• <1%	• Degranulation of basophils and mast cells during inflammatory responses • Assists in clearance of parasites and prevention of pulmonary infections • Mediates many types of allergic reactions
IgG	• Monomer	• 75%	• Activates complement • Neutralizes toxins • Enhances phagocytosis • Provides significant sustained immunity against viral and bacterial infections
IgM	• Pentomer	• 10%	• Activates complement • Clears antigens through precipitation • Possibly mediates autoimmune reactions • Mediates ABO incompatibility reactions in blood transfusions

Ig = immunoglobulin.

making antibodies against that antigen (e.g., chickenpox virus). Most of the time, the first invasion of the body by the antigen results in manifestations of disease. However, processes occurring in the body at the same time confer immunity to that antigen, so that the person will not become ill after a second exposure to the same antigen. This type of immunity is the most effective and the longest lasting.

ARTIFICIAL ACTIVE IMMUNITY. Artificial active immunity is a type of protection developed against serious illnesses for which total avoidance is most desirable. Examples of diseases for which artificially acquired active immunity can be obtained include tetanus, diphtheria, measles, smallpox, mumps, and rubella. Small amounts of specific antigens are deliberately placed (as a vaccination) in the body, so that the body responds by actively making antibodies against the antigen. Because antigens used for this procedure have been specially processed to make them less likely to proliferate within the body, this exposure does not in itself cause the disease. Artificial active immunity lasts many years, although repeated but smaller doses of the original antigen are required as a "booster" for maintaining complete protection against the antigen.

Passive Immunity

Passive immunity occurs when antibodies against a specific antigen are in a person's body but were not created there. Rather, these antibodies are made in the body of one person or animal and then transferred to the body of another person. Because these antibodies are foreign to the individual, the body recognizes the antibodies as non-self and takes steps to eliminate them relatively quickly. For this reason, passive immunity can provide only immediate, short-term protection against a specific antigen.

Natural passive immunity occurs when antibodies are passed from the mother to the fetus via the placenta or to the infant through colostrum and breast milk.

Artificial passive immunity involves deliberately injecting one person with antibodies that were produced in another person or animal. This type of immunity is used when a person is exposed to a serious disease or illness for which he or she has little or no known actively acquired immunity. Instead, the injected antibodies are expected to inactivate the antigen. This type of immunity provides only temporary protection lasting for days to a few weeks. Some of the conditions or diseases for which artificial passive immunity may be used include exposure to rabies, tetanus, and poisonous snake bites.

Antibody-mediated immunity works with the inflammatory responses in providing protection against infection. However, AMI can provide the most effective, long-lasting immunity only when its actions are combined with the processes of cell-mediated immunity.

CELL-MEDIATED IMMUNITY

Cell-mediated immunity (CMI), or cellular immunity, involves many leukocyte actions, reactions, and interactions ranging from simple to complex. This type of immunity is provided by committed lymphocyte stem cells that mature in the secondary lymphoid tissues of the thymus and pericortical areas of lymph nodes. Certain CMI responses influence and regulate the activities of AMI and inflammation by producing and releasing cytokines. Therefore, for total immunocompetence, CMI must function optimally.

Cell Types Involved in Cell-Mediated Immunity

The leukocytes playing the most important roles in CMI include several specific T-lymphocyte subsets along with a special population of cells known as natural killer (NK) cells. T lymphocytes further differentiate into a variety of subsets, each of which has a specific function.

One way of identifying different T-lymphocyte subsets is to determine the presence or absence of certain "marker proteins" (antigens) on the cell membrane's surface. More than 50 different T-lymphocyte proteins have been identified on the cell membrane, and 11 of these (named T1 through T11) are commonly used in clinical situations to identify various immune system components. Antibodies have been made against each of these 11 proteins so that each T-lymphocyte subset can be identified by how the T lymphocyte reacts to the commercial antibodies. Most T lymphocytes have more than one antigen on their cell membranes. For example, all mature T lymphocytes contain T1, T3, T10, and T11 proteins. Certain subsets of T lymphocytes also contain other specific T-lymphocyte membrane antigens.

The names used to identify specific T-lymphocyte subsets include the specific membrane antigen and the overall functional activities of the cells in a subset. The three T-lymphocyte subsets critically important for the development and continuation of CMI are helper/inducer T cells, suppressor T cells, and cytotoxic–cytolytic T cells.

Helper/Inducer T Cells
Description

The cell membranes of these T cells contain the T4 protein. Usually, these cells are called T4+ cells or T_H cells. A newer name for helper/inducer T cells is CD4+ (cluster of differentiation 4). Several companies have made antibodies to the T4 cell membrane protein. These antibodies include OKT4 and Leu-3; thus, the helper/inducer T cells may also be referred to as cells that are OKT4 positive or Leu-3 positive.

Function

Helper/inducer T cells act efficiently in the recognition of self versus non-self. These important cells indirectly participate in CMI by stimulating the activity of many other leukocytes. In response to the recognition of non-self (antigen), helper/inducer T cells secrete lymphokines that can regulate the activity of other leukocytes.

In general, the lymphokines secreted by the helper/inducer T cells have overall stimulating effects on immune function. These lymphokines increase bone marrow production of stem cells and speed up the maturation of cells of myeloid and lymphoid origin. In effect, the helper/inducer T cells act as organizers in "calling to arms" various squads of leukocytes involved in inflammatory, antibody, and cellular defensive actions to destroy, eliminate, or neutralize antigens.

Suppressor T Cells

Description

The cell membranes of suppressor T cells contain the T8 lymphocyte antigen, and these cells are commonly called T8 cells, or T_S cells. Suppressor T cells participate in the regulation of CMI.

Function

Suppressor T cells prevent continuous overreaction or hypersensitivity reactions to exposure to non-self cells or proteins. This function is important in preventing the formation of autoantibodies directed against normal, healthy self cells, the basis for many autoimmune diseases.

The suppressor T cells secrete cytokines that have an overall inhibitory action on most and perhaps all cells of the immune system. These cytokines inhibit both the proliferation of immune system cells and the activation of immune system cells.

In general, suppressor T cells directly oppose the activity of helper/inducer T cells. Therefore, for optimal function of CMI, a balance between helper/inducer T-cell activity and suppressor T-cell activity must be maintained. This balance is usually provided when the helper/inducer T cells outnumber the suppressor T cells by a ratio of 2:1. When this ratio increases, overreactions can be expected, some of which are tissue-damaging as well as unpleasant. When the helper–suppressor ratio decreases, immune function is suppressed profoundly, and the body is much more vulnerable to invasion by non-self cells and infections of all types.

Cytotoxic–Cytolytic T Cells

Description

Cytotoxic–cytolytic T cells are also called T_C cells. Because they have the T8 protein present on their surfaces, they are a subset of suppressor cells. Cytotoxic–cytolytic T cells function in CMI by lysing (destroying) cells that contain a processed antigen–MHC complex. This activity is most effective against self cells infected by parasitic organisms, such as viruses or protozoa.

Function

Parasite-infected self cells have both self MHC proteins (universal product code) and the parasite's antigens on the cell surface. This allows the person's immune system cells to recognize the infected self cell as abnormal, and the cytotoxic–cytolytic T cell can bind to it.

The binding of the cytotoxic–cytolytic T cell to the infected cell's antigen–MHC complex stimulates activities that result in the death of the infected cell. The cyto-

toxic–cytolytic T cell bores a hole in the membrane of the infected cell and delivers a "lethal hit" of enzymes to the infected cell, causing it to lyse and die. Once the lethal hit has been administered to the infected cell, the cytotoxic–cytolytic T cell releases the dying infected cell and can attack and destroy other infected cells that carry the same antigen–MHC complex.

Natural Killer Cells

Description

Natural killer cells are extremely important in providing CMI. The actual site of differentiation and maturation of NK cells is unknown. Although this cell population has some T-cell characteristics, it is not considered a true T-cell subset (Abbas et al., 1997).

Function

NK cells direct cytotoxic–cytolytic effects on target non-self cells. Unlike cytotoxic–cytolytic T cells, NK cells can exert these cytotoxic effects without first undergoing a period of sensitization to non-self cell membrane antigens. Moreover, NK cells do not need to share any of the MHC proteins in common with the non-self cell to initiate defensive actions against the non-self cell. The defensive actions of NK cells appear to be totally unrelated to either antigen sensitivity or the interactions of other leukocytes. NK cells conduct "seek and destroy" missions in the body to eliminate invaders and unhealthy self cells.

NK cells are most effective in destroying unhealthy or abnormal self cells. The non-self cells most susceptible to defensive actions of NK cells are self cells that are virally infected and cancer cells.

Cytokines

The inducing and regulatory aspects of CMI are controlled through the selected production and activity of cytokines. Cytokines are small protein hormones produced by the various leukocytes. Cytokines made by the mononuclear phagocytes (macrophages, neutrophils, eosinophils, and monocytes) are termed *monokines*; cytokines produced by T lymphocytes are *lymphokines*.

Cytokine activity is similar to the action of any other kind of hormone: one cell produces and secretes a cytokine, which in turn exerts its effects on other cells of the immune system. The cells responding to the cytokine may be located close to or remote from the cytokine-secreting cell. The cells that change their activity in response to the cytokine are known as "responder" cells. For a responder cell to respond to the presence of a cytokine, the membrane of the responder cell must have a specific receptor for the cytokine to bind to and initiate changes in the responder cell's activity (Fig. 23–15).

Cytokines regulate a variety of inflammatory and immune responses. Most cytokines are produced as needed, and they are not stored to any great extent. The actions of some cytokines are pleiotropic in that the effects are widespread within the immune system, setting into motion various immunomodulating actions. Other cytokines have specific actions limited to only one type of cell.

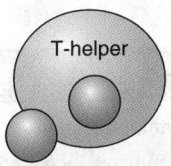

T-helper cell making and releasing a cytokine
(MAF—macrophage activating factor)

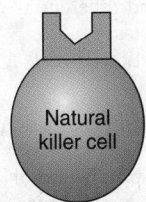

Leukocyte with one type
of surface receptor

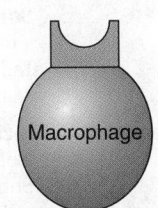

Leukocyte with a surface receptor
specific for the cytokine released
by the T-helper cell

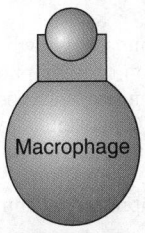

Cytokine binding to a cytokine-specific
receptor on the leukocyte (macrophage)

Figure 23–15. Cytokine receptors on leukocytes.

Table 23–5 summarizes the origins and activities of the currently known cytokines.

Protection Provided by Cell-Mediated Immunity

Cell-mediated immunity helps provide protection to the body through its highly developed ability to differentiate self from non-self. The non-self cells most easily recognized by CMI are those self cells infected by organisms that live within host cells and cancer cells. CMI provides a surveillance system for ridding the body of self cells that might potentially harm the body. CMI is important in preventing the development of cancer and metastasis after exposure to carcinogens.

Transplantation Rejection

Natural killer cells and cytotoxic–cytolytic T cells also destroy cells from other people or animals. Although this action is generally helpful, it is also responsible for rejection of grafts and transplanted organs. Because the solid organ transplanted into the host is seldom a perfectly identical match of universal product codes (HLAs) between the donated organ and the recipient host, the client's immune system cells recognize a newly transplanted organ as non-self. Without intervention, the host's im-

mune system initiates standard inflammatory and immunologic actions to destroy, eliminate, or neutralize these non-self cells. This activity causes rejection of the transplanted organ. Graft rejection is the result of a complex series of responses that change over time and involve different components of the immune system. Graft rejection can be hyperacute, acute, or chronic.

Hyperacute Rejection

Hyperacute graft rejection begins immediately on transplantation and is an antibody-mediated response. Antigen–antibody complexes form within the blood vessels of the transplanted organ. The host's blood has pre-existing antibodies to one or more of the antigens (including blood group antigens) present in the donated organ. The antigen–antibody complexes adhere to the lining of blood vessels and stimulate complement activation. The activated-fixated complement in the blood vessel linings initiates the blood clotting cascade; microcoagulation occurs throughout the organ vasculature. Widespread coagulation and occlusion lead to ischemic necrosis, inflammation with phagocytosis of the necrotic blood vessels, and release of lytic enzymes into the transplanted organ. These enzymes cause massive cellular destruction and graft loss.

Hyperacute rejection occurs primarily in transplanted kidneys. People at greatest risk for hyperacute rejection are

1. Those who have received donated organs of an ABO blood type different from their own
2. Those who have received multiple blood transfusions at any time in life before transplantation
3. Those who have a history of multiple pregnancies
4. Those who have received a previous transplant

The manifestations of hyperacute rejection become apparent within minutes of attachment of the donated organ to the host's blood supply. *The process cannot be stopped once it has started, and the rejected organ must be removed as soon as hyperacute rejection is diagnosed.*

Acute Rejection

Acute graft rejection occurs within 1 week to 3 months after transplantation. Two mechanisms are responsible. The first mechanism is antibody-mediated and results in vasculitis within the transplanted organ. This reaction differs from that of hyperacute rejection in that blood vessel necrosis (rather than thrombotic occlusion) leads to the organ's destruction.

The second mechanism is cellular. Host cytotoxic–cytolytic T cells and NK cells enter the transplanted organ through the blood, infiltrate the organ cells (rather than the blood vessel cells), and cause lysis of the organ cells.

Diagnosis of acute rejection is made by laboratory tests indicating impaired function of the specific organ, along with biopsy of the grafted organ. Manifestations of acute rejection vary with each client and with the specific organ transplanted. For example, when acute rejection occurs in a transplanted kidney, the client usually experiences some tenderness in the kidney area and may experience other general symptoms of inflammation.

TABLE 23–5

Summary of Cytokine Activity

Cytokine	Cellular Origin	Inducing Event	Cytokine Action
IL-1	Macrophages Monocytes Natural killer cells	Contact with gram-negative bacterial products Contact with CD4+ cell Presence of TNF	Stimulates increased production of prostaglandins Induces fever Increases proliferation of CD4+ cells Stimulates growth and differentiation of B lymphocytes Induces further secretion of IL-1 and IL-6
IL-2	Helper T cells (CD4+ T cells) CD8+ T cells	T-cell activation by antigens	Increases growth and differentiation of T lymphocytes Stimulates increased production of IL-2 from activated lymphocytes Enhances NK activity and activity of tumor-infiltrating lymphocytes
IL-3 (multilineage colony-stimulating factor)	Helper T cells (CD4+ T cells)	Infection or antigen invasion	Pluripotent (pleiotropic) stimulation of bone marrow stem cells
IL-4 (B-cell stimulatory factor)	Helper T cells (CD4+ T cells) Activated mast cells	Presence of anti-Ig antibody	Stimulates growth and differentiation of B lymphocytes Stimulates increased production of IgG and IgE Induces further secretion of IL-4, IL-5, and IL-6 Suppresses inflammation
IL-5 (B-cell growth factor)	Helper T cells (CD4+ T cells) Activated mast cells	Helminth infection Pulmonary infection	Stimulates growth and differentiation of eosinophils Stimulates increased production of IgA and IgE
IL-6	Activated T cells Fibroblasts Vascular endothelial cells Macrophages Monocytes	Infection or inflammation Presence of IL-1 TNF	Stimulates liver to produce fibrinogen, macroglobulin, protein C Stimulates growth of activated B lymphocytes Increases production of bone marrow stem cells
IL-7 (B-cell growth factor)	Bone marrow stromal cells	Presence of antigens	Stimulates growth and differentiation of committed B-lymphocyte stem cells Stimulates T-cell production of IL-2
IL-8 (monocyte chemotactic factor)	Activated T cells Macrophages Platelets Fibroblasts Endothelial cells	Infection or inflammation	Chemotactic factor for neutrophils, basophils, and eosinophils Stimulates neutrophil activation
IL-9	Helper T cells (CD4+ T cells)	Infection or inflammation	Stimulates mast cell growth Induces IL-4 production Stimulates lymphocyte activation
IL-10	Mature lymphocytes Macrophages Monocytes	Infection or inflammation	Enhances activity of cytotoxic–cytolytic T cells Suppresses inflammatory response
IL-11	Bone marrow stromal cells	Viral infection or inflammation	Enhances B-lymphocyte activity Stimulates platelet proliferation and maturation
IL-12	Macrophages Activated B cells	Infection or inflammation	Induces production of interferon Enhances NK activity and activity cytotoxic–cytolytic T cells Induces production of IL-2 and IL-4

TABLE 23-5

Summary of Cytokine Activity *Continued*

Cytokine	Cellular Origin	Inducing Event	Cytokine Action
IL-13	Activated T cells (CD4+ T cells and CD8+ T cells)	Infection	Induces B-lymphocyte proliferation Increases platelet and erythrocyte production Increases IL-6 production Decreases neutrophil activity
IL-14	Activated T cells	Infection, plasma cell malignancies	Induces B-lymphocyte proliferation Decreases Ig secretion Enhances B-cell differentiation
INF-α	Macrophages	Viral infection	Decreases viral proliferation
INF-β	Fibroblasts	Viral infection	Decreases viral proliferation
INF-γ	Helper T cells (CD4+ T cells) Suppressor T cells (CD8+ T cells) NK cells	Viral infection	Decreases viral proliferation Activates macrophages Induces differentiation of committed lymphoid stem cells Activates neutrophils Activates NK cells
TNF	Activated macrophages Activated mast cells Activated NK cells Activated T cells	Infection or inflammation (especially infection with gram-negative microorganisms)	Increases leukocyte adhesion Induces fever Stimulates production of CSF Induces cytolysis of virally infected cells Induces secretion of IL-1 and IL-6
GM-CSF	Activated T cells Macrophages Fibroblasts Vascular endothelial cells	Infection or inflammation	Increases growth and differentiation of committed myeloid stem cells Slightly activates macrophages
M-CSF	Fibroblasts Vascular endothelial cells	Infection or inflammation	Increases growth and differentiation of committed monocyte-macrophage progenitor cells
G-CSF	Macrophages Vascular endothelial cells Fibroblasts	Infection or inflammation	Increases proliferation and maturation of neutrophils

IL = interleukin; TNF = tumor necrosis factor; NK = natural killer; Ig = immunoglobulin; INF = interferon; G = granulocyte; M = macrophage; CSF = colony-stimulating factor.

An episode of acute rejection after solid organ transplantation does not automatically mean that the client will lose the transplant. Pharmacologic manipulation of host immune responses at this time may limit the damage to the organ and allow the graft to be maintained.

Chronic Rejection

The origin of chronic rejection is not clear, but it resembles the aftermath of chronic inflammation and scarring. Functional tissue of the transplanted organ is replaced with fibrotic, scar-like tissue. Because this fibrotic tissue does not resemble the organ tissue in either structure or function, the ability of the transplanted organ to perform differentiated tasks diminishes in proportion to the percentage of normal tissue replaced by fibrotic tissue. This type of reaction is long-standing and occurs continuously

as a response to chronic ischemia caused by blood vessel injury.

Although good control over host immune function can delay the manifestations of this type of rejection, the process probably occurs to some degree with all solid organ transplants. Because the fibrotic changes are permanent, there is no cure for chronic graft rejection. When the fibrosis increases to the extent that it significantly interferes with the functional capacity of the transplanted organ, the only recourse is retransplantation.

Treatment of Transplant Rejection

Rejection of transplanted solid organs involves all three components of immunity, although cell-mediated immune responses are most significant in the rejection process.

Maintenance Therapy

Three pharmacologic agents are generally used for routine immunosuppressive therapy after solid organ transplantation. These agents are azathioprine (Imuran); cyclosporine (Sandimmune); and one of the corticosteroids, such as prednisone (Apo-Prednisone✲, Deltasone) or prednisolone (Delta-Cortef). Drug dosage is adjusted for the immune response of each client. Treatment with these agents increases the client's risk for bacterial and fungal infections.

Rescue Therapy

Certain agents are used not to maintain the graft within the host but rather to reduce the host's immunologic responses during rejection episodes, especially acute rejection. These agents may be used in addition to or in place of any of the maintenance drugs in the host's post-transplantation treatment regimen.

Antilymphocyte Globulin

Antilymphocyte globulin (ALG) is an antibody (or group of antibodies) generated in an animal after the animal has been exposed to human lymphocytes. The globulin can be made more specific by exposing the animal to human T cells instead of mixed lymphocytes. When these antihuman lymphocyte antibodies are administered to humans, the antibodies selectively attack and clear lymphocytes from the blood, extracellular fluids, and tissues into which they have infiltrated (such as the transplanted organ). This agent is given only for a short time to combat the acute rejection episode.

Most clients receiving ALG have some associated immunologic response, ranging from low-grade fever and malaise to serum sickness and anaphylaxis. The response usually increases in intensity on repeated exposure to ALG.

OKT3

OKT3 is an antibody directed specifically against the human T-cell cell-surface antigen CD3. OKT3 is generated with a murine (mouse) model rather than an equine (horse) model. Because the agent is generated in mice, the humans receiving it rapidly develop antimouse antibodies. These antimouse antibodies attack the OKT3 and prevent its anti–T-cell activities. Thus, OKT3 is most effective against rejection during the first episode for which it is used. Its utility in combating graft rejection decreases with each subsequent use.

FK 506

FK 506 is used in maintenance therapy and rescue therapy, primarily after liver transplantation. It is similar in chemical composition to erythromycin and specifically suppresses T-cell actions, including synthesis of interleukin-2 (IL-2). These effects are achieved through various mechanisms. In the presence of FK 506, receptor sites for IL-2 are inhibited on helper/inducer T cells and cyto-

toxic–cytolytic T cells. Without continuous stimulation by IL-2, these lymphocytes are slow to reproduce and do not perform their usual functions. In addition, FK 506 is able to prevent activation of immature or unsensitized cytotoxic–cytolytic T cells. Because cytotoxic–cytolytic T cells are primarily responsible for immunologic destruction of transplanted cells and tissues, and because helper/inducer T cells boost the activity of cytotoxic–cytolytic T cells, selective suppression of the activity of these two cell populations allows the transplanted organ to remain free from immunologic destruction, yet does not result in so profound an immunosuppressive state as to put the host at great risk for infection.

SELECTED BIBLIOGRAPHY

Abbas, A., Lichtman, A., & Pober, J. (1997). *Cellular and molecular immunology* (3rd ed.). Philadelphia: W. B. Saunders.
Beck, G., & Habicht, G. (1996). Immunity and the invertebrates. *Scientific American, 275*(5), 60–66.
DeLaPena, L., Tomaszewski, J., Bernato, D. L., Kryk, J., Molenda, J., & Gantz, S. (1996). Programmed instruction: Biotherapy module IV. Interleukins. *Cancer Nursing, 19*(1), 60–74.
DeLaPena, L., Woolery-Antill, M., Tomaszewski, J., Gantz, S., Bernato, D. L., DiLorenzo, K., Molenda, J., & Kryk, J. (1996). Programmed instruction: Biotherapy module V. Hematopoietic growth factors. *Cancer Nursing, 19*(2), 135–150.
Ford, R., Tomayo, A., Martin, B., Niu, K., Claypool, K., Cabaniilas, F., & Ambrus, J. (1995). Identification of B-cell growth factors (interleukin-14; high molecular weight–B-cell growth factors) in effusion fluids from patients with aggressive B-cell lymphomas. *Blood, 86*(1), 283–293.
Gantz, S., Tomaszewski, J., DeLaPena, L., Molenda, J., Bernato, D. L., & Kryk, J. (1995). Programmed instruction: Biotherapy module III. Interferons. *Cancer Nursing, 18*(6), 479–494.
Guyton, A. C., & Hall, J. (1996). *Textbook of medical physiology* (9th ed.). Philadelphia: W. B. Saunders.
Krenitsky, J. (1996). Nutrition and the immune system. *AACN Clinical Issues: Advanced Practice in Acute and Critical Care, 7*(3), 359–369.
Lai, Y., Heslan, J., Poppema, S., Elliot, J., & Mosmann, T. (1996). Continuous administration of IL-13 to mice induces extramedullary hemopoiesis and monocytosis. *Journal of Immunology, 156*(9), 3166–3173.
Post-White, J. (1996). The immune system. *Seminars in Oncology Nursing, 12*(2), 89–96.
Roitt, I. (1994). *Essential immunology* (8th ed.). London: Blackwell Scientific.
Secor, V. (1994). The inflammatory/immune response in critical illness. *Critical Care Clinics of North America, 6*(2), 251–262.
Workman, M. L. (1995). Essential concepts of inflammation and immunity. *Critical Care Clinics of North America, 7*(4), 601–615.
*Workman, M. L., Ellerhorst-Ryan, J., & Koertge, V. (1993). *Nursing care of the immunocompromised patient.* Philadelphia: W. B. Saunders.
Workman, M. L. (1998). The lymphoid system and its role in immunocompetence. *Seminars in Oncology Nursing* (In press).

SUGGESTED READINGS

Secor, V. (1994). The inflammatory/immune response in critical illness. *Critical Care Clinics of North America, 6*(2), 251–262.
The physiology of inflammatory and immune responses is presented, with mechanisms clearly depicted in line drawings. The article also discusses sepsis and systemic inflammatory response syndrome.
Workman, M. L. (1995). Essential concepts of inflammation and immunity. *Critical Care Clinics of North America, 7*(4), 601–615.
This article reviews the normal immune and inflammatory responses. Clinical situations leading to altered immune function are presented. Traditional and new treatment modalities also are discussed.

Chapter 24

INTERVENTIONS FOR CLIENTS WITH CONNECTIVE TISSUE DISEASE

A *rheumatic disease* is any disease or condition involving the musculoskeletal system. Connective tissue disease (CTD) is the major focus of *rheumatology,* the study of rheumatic disease. In this text, CTDs are discussed separately from other musculoskeletal conditions because most CTDs are classified as probably autoimmune.

More than 37 million people in the United States, or 1 in 7, have one or more of over 100 CTDs. The primary clinical manifestation of many of these diseases is *arthritis,* the inflammation of one or more joints. Some CTDs present with additional localized clinical manifestations, whereas others are systemic. Management of clients with CTDs requires an interdisciplinary approach, including medicine, surgery, nursing, and physical and occupational therapy.

DEGENERATIVE JOINT DISEASE (OSTEOARTHRITIS)

Overview

Several terms describe degenerative joint disease (DJD), the most common connective tissue disease. *Osteoarthritis* (OA) and *osteoarthrosis* are used interchangeably with DJD; however, this condition is not a primary inflamma-

tory disease, and thus osteoarthritis may not be the best term.

Pathophysiology

Degenerative joint disease is characterized by the progressive deterioration of and loss of articular cartilage in peripheral and axial joints. It is caused by prolonged or excessive use of these joints. Weight-bearing joints (hips and knees), the vertebral column, and hands are primarily affected because they are used most often and bear the stress of body weight. Therefore, DJD is also known as the "wear and tear disease." Most clients have the primary (idiopathic) form of the disease, but secondary DJD can result from other musculoskeletal conditions or from trauma.

In the affected joints, the normal bluish, translucent cartilage becomes soft, opaque, and yellow. Fissures, pitting, and ulcerations develop, and the cartilage thins. As cartilage and bone beneath the cartilage begin to erode, the joint space narrows and osteophyte (bone spur) formation occurs (Fig. 24–1). Inflammatory enzymes enhance tissue deterioration as a result of the alteration in cartilage metabolism. As a result, the repair process is unable to overcome the rapid process of degeneration.

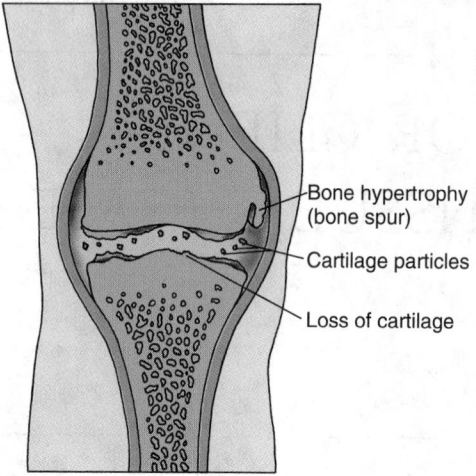

Figure 24–1. Joint changes in degenerative joint disease.

Bone cysts and secondary synovitis are common in advanced disease. Eventually, subluxation and joint deformities cause marked immobility, pain, and muscle spasm.

Etiology

Although the causative mechanisms of primary DJD at the cellular level have not been well identified, the risk factors for DJD are known. Age is the strongest risk factor, but research does not support that aging alone is the cause of DJD (Mankin & Brandt, 1997). Joints that are used most often are typically affected. Obesity also contributes to the likelihood of degeneration, particularly in the hips and knees, the weight-bearing joints. Overuse or abuse of certain joints causes chronic pain and degeneration. Joint hyperextensibility, as seen in gymnasts, also predisposes the person to DJD. Certain heavy manual occupations, such as carpet installation, construction, and farming, cause increased mechanical stress to joints. The risk of hip and knee DJD is significantly increased in former athletes.

Congenital anomalies, trauma, and joint sepsis can result in secondary DJD. Certain metabolic diseases (such as diabetes mellitus and Paget's disease) and blood disorders (such as hemophilia) can also cause joint degeneration. Inflammatory joint diseases, such as rheumatoid arthritis, can also lead to secondary DJD.

Incidence/Prevalence

More than 20 million people in the United States have symptomatic DJD, but probably more than 40 million have degenerative joint changes that can be seen on x-ray examinations. Generalized disease is seen more often in women than in men.

ELDERLY CONSIDERATIONS

Prevalence increases with age; almost everyone older than 60 years has some degree of symptomatic joint degeneration. DJD of the hands is especially common in the elderly, affecting more than 70% of those older than 70 years (Solomon, 1997).

TRANSCULTURAL CONSIDERATIONS

 Native Americans are affected more often than non–Native American groups, but the reason is unknown (Giger & Davidhizar, 1995).

Collaborative Management

Assessment

➤ History

At the initial interview, the nurse collects information from the client that is specifically related to DJD. Because this disease is observed more often in older women, age and sex are important factors for the nursing history. The nurse asks about the client's occupation, nature of work, history of trauma, and current or previous involvement in sports. Even if the client appears to be within the ideal range for body weight, the nurse asks the client about a possible history of obesity. The nurse should also note a family history of "arthritis" because many CTDs seem to have familial tendencies.

Finally, the nurse determines whether the client has a current or previous medical condition that may cause joint manifestations. As with all musculoskeletal disorders, the nurse asks questions about the course of the disease.

➤ Physical Assessment/Clinical Manifestations

In the early stage of the disease, the clinical manifestations of degenerative joint disease (DJD) may appear similar to those of rheumatoid arthritis (RA). As the disease progresses, the distinction between DJD and RA becomes more evident. Table 24–1 differentiates the major characteristics of both diseases and their treatments.

Joint Pain. The major complaint of the client with DJD is typically nagging joint pain, which early in the course of the disease diminishes after rest and intensifies after activity. Later the pain occurs with slight motion or even when the person is at rest. Because cartilage has no nerve supply, the pain is probably due to joint and soft-tissue involvement and to spasms of surrounding muscles. During examination of the joints, the nurse can often elicit pain or tenderness by palpation or by putting the joint through range of motion. Crepitus, a continuous grating sensation, may be felt or heard as the joint is put through range of motion. One or more joints are affected. The client may also complain of joint stiffness that usually lasts less than 30 minutes after a period of inactivity.

Joint Changes. On inspection, the nurse notes that the joint is frequently enlarged because of bony hypertrophy; rarely does a joint appear to be hot and inflamed. The presence of inflammation in clients with DJD usually indicates a secondary synovitis. Approximately 50% of clients with hand involvement display the characteristic Heberden's nodes (at the distal interphalangeal joints) and

TABLE 24–1

Differential Features of Rheumatoid Arthritis and Degenerative Disease

Characteristic	Rheumatoid Arthritis	Degenerative Joint Disease
Typical onset	• At 35–45 yr	• At >60 yr
Sex affected	• Female (3:1)	• Female (2:1)
Risk factors or cause	• Probably autoimmune • Emotional stress	• Aging • Obesity • Trauma • Occupation
Disease process	• Inflammatory	• Degenerative
Disease pattern	• Bilateral, symmetric, multiple joints • Usually affects upper extremities first • Distal interphalangeal joints of hands spared • Systemic	• May be unilateral, single joint • Affects weight-bearing joints and hands, spine • Metacarpophalangeal joints spared • Nonsystemic
Laboratory findings	• Elevated rheumatoid factor, antinuclear antibody, ESR	• Normal or slightly elevated ESR
Drug therapy	• Salicylates • NSAIDs • Methotrexate • Gold or penicillamine • Corticosteroids • Other immunosuppressive agents • Other analgesics	• NSAIDs • Acetaminophen • Other analgesics

ESR = erythrocyte sedimentation rate; NSAIDs = nonsteroidal antiinflammatory drugs.

Bouchard's nodes (at the proximal interphalangeal joints). Although DJD is not a bilateral, symmetric disease, these large bony nodes appear in that pattern, especially in women. The nodes may be painful and red, but some clients do not experience discomfort from their presence. The nodes have a familial tendency and are usually a cosmetic concern to clients. The nodes feel hard when the nurse palpates them; clients may complain of tenderness on palpation.

Other Clinical Manifestations. Joint effusions are common when the knees are involved. When trying to differentiate the presence of fluid from subcutaneous tissue, the nurse is able to move fluid from the infrapatellar notch (the area directly below the knee) into the suprapatellar notch (the area directly above the knee). Subcutaneous tissue cannot be relocated.

The nurse also observes skeletal muscle atrophy from disuse. The vicious pain cycle of the disease discourages movement of painful joints, which then results in contractures, muscle atrophy, and further pain. Loss of function may result, depending on which joints are involved, Hip pain may cause the client to limp and restrict walking distance.

Degenerative joint disease can frequently affect the spine, especially the lumbar region at the L3-4 level or the cervical region at C4-6. Compression of spinal nerve roots may occur as a result of vertebral facet bone spurs. The client typically complains of radiating pain, stiffness, and muscle spasms in one or both extremities. Spinal and vertebral arteries may also become compressed.

In addition to performing a musculoskeletal assessment, the nurse performs a functional assessment of the client with DJD to determine mobility and ability to perform activities of daily living (ADLs). Severe pain and deformity interfere with ambulation and self-care. (Chapter 13 describes ADLs and functional assessment in depth.)

➤ Psychosocial Assessment

Degenerative joint disease is a chronic condition that may cause permanent changes in the client's lifestyle. A person's inability to care for oneself in advanced disease prevents socialization and results in role changes and other losses. Therefore, the client may exhibit a variety of behaviors indicative of the grieving process, such as anger and depression.

The client may experience a role change in the family, workplace, or both. The nurse asks the client about his or her roles before the disease developed to identify changes that have been or need to be made. The nurse and client mutually determine problem areas and adjustment in lifestyle that may still be needed as a result of the disease.

In addition to role change, joint deformities and bony nodules often cause an alteration in body image and self-esteem. The nurse observes the client's response to body changes. Does the client ignore them or seem overly occupied with them? How does the client refer to the changes—with anger, degradation, or humor? These clues help the nurse assess the client's acceptance of body alterations.

➤ Laboratory Assessment

There are no significant laboratory tests for DJD. The erythrocyte sedimentation rate (ESR) may be slightly elevated when secondary synovitis occurs.

➤ Radiographic Assessment

Routine x-rays are useful in determining structural joint changes. Specialized views are obtained when the disease cannot be visualized on standard x-ray but is suspected. A computed tomography (CT) scan may be used to determine vertebral involvement.

➤ Other Diagnostic Assessment

The health care provider may order magnetic resonance imaging (MRI) studies of the vertebral column to detect degenerative bony changes in the spine. A bone scan using technetium (Tc) 99m can often show early DJD years before typical x-ray changes appear.

 Analysis

➤ Common Nursing Diagnoses and Collaborative Problems

The priority for nursing diagnoses when the nurse is caring for a client with degenerative joint disease (DJD) is
1. Chronic Pain related to muscle spasm and/or inflammation
2. Impaired Physical Mobility related to pain and muscle atrophy

➤ Additional Nursing Diagnoses and Collaborative Problems

In addition to the common diagnoses, the client may have secondary problems caused by the pain and immobility common in DJD. These include
- Activity Intolerance related to pain and fatigue
- Self-Care Deficit (partial) related to pain, fatigue, and immobility
- Body Image Disturbance related to effects of loss of body function

 Planning and Implementation

Chronic Pain

Planning: Expected Outcomes. The major concern of the client with DJD is pain control. Therefore, the desired outcome is that the client is expected to experience a reduction in chronic pain.

Interventions. Pain control may be accomplished by drug and nondrug measures at home. If these measures become ineffective, surgery may be performed to reduce pain.

Nonsurgical Management. Management of chronic joint pain is difficult for both the client and the health care professional. A combination of modalities is often used, including medication, diet, physical therapy, and rest. Chapter 9 elaborates on methods of pain control for chronic pain.

Drug Therapy. The purpose of drug therapy is to reduce pain, relieve muscle spasm, and reduce secondary inflammation if present. The drug class of choice is usually nonsteroidal anti-inflammatory drugs (NSAIDs) (Chart 24–1). Acetaminophen (Tylenol, Atasol✤) may also be used. For temporary relief of pain in a single joint, the physician may inject the joint with a corticosteroid, such as cortisone, or a newer drug, Hyalgan (sodium hyaluronate). Muscle relaxants, such as cyclobenzaprine HCl (Flexeril), are sometimes given for severe muscle spasms, especially those occurring in the back. Potent analgesics are not usually appropriate for the client with DJD because of the chronic nature of the pain.

Rest. Several types of rest are used to treat clients with DJD:
- Local rest involves the immobilization of a joint with a splint or brace. If a joint becomes acutely inflamed, the joint is rested until inflammation subsides. The nurse or physician consults the occupational therapist (OT), who fits the client for the appropriate device and explains its use.
- Systemic rest refers to the immobilization of the entire body, such as a nap. The nurse teaches the client about the importance of sleeping about 10 hours and, if possible, resting an additional 1–2 hours each day.
- *Psychological* rest is equally important because it allows relief from daily stresses that can enhance pain.

Chapter 8 describes methods for relaxation and strategies for coping that the nurse can use to teach clients.

Positioning. Joints should be placed in their functional position, which may not be the position of comfort. When the client is in a supine position (recumbent), the nurse or assistive nursing personnel places a small pillow under the client's head or neck but avoids the use of other pillows. The client may quickly experience flexion contractures from the use of large pillows under the knees or head. If needed, the client's legs may be elevated 8–12 inches (20.3–30.5 cm) to reduce back discomfort. Lying prone twice a day is recommended if the client can tolerate that position. The nurse also reminds the client to use proper posture when standing and sitting to reduce undue strain on the vertebral column.

Heat. The client with DJD generally uses heat instead of cold to reduce pain. Cold application is usually reserved for acutely inflamed joints. The nurse suggests hot showers and baths, hot packs or compresses, and moist heating pads. Regardless of treatment, the nurse teaches the client to check that the heat source is not too heavy or so hot as to cause burns. A temperature just above the body's temperature is adequate to promote comfort.

A physical therapist may provide special heat treatments, such as paraffin dips, diathermy (use of electrical current), and ultrasonography (use of sound waves). Usually a 15- to 20-minute heat application is sufficient to temporarily reduce pain, spasm, and stiffness.

Diet Therapy. There is no "arthritis diet," as has been proposed by the media and uninformed authors. In collaboration with the dietitian, the nurse explains which foods are high in protein and vitamin C to promote tissue healing. In addition, the nurse encourages obese clients to lose weight to lessen stress on weight-bearing joints. Less weight reduces pain and slows the disease process in

Chart 24–1

Drug Therapy for Connective Tissue Disease

Drug	Usual Dosage	Nursing Interventions	Rationale
Salicylates (e.g., aspirin, buffered aspirin) (Ecotrin, Ascriptin, Ancasal✤)	12–18 tablets/d (4–6 g) are given in divided doses to achieve therapeutic effect.	• Give with meals or snacks. • Instruct client to observe for tinnitus, bleeding, or bruising (especially seen in elderly clients). Teach client to use soft-bristled toothbrush.	• Aspirin products can cause gastrointestinal problems, including bleeding and ulcers, because of increased stomach acid production. Drugs can damage eighth cranial nerve and prevent platelet aggregation, which causes clotting. • Gums may bleed easily because of decreased clotting.
NSAIDs, e.g., naproxen (Naprosyn, Apo-Naproxen✤), sulindac (Clinoril), indomethacin (Indocin, Apo-Indomethacin✤), ibuprofen (Motrin, Advil, Amersol✤), mefenamic acid (Ponstel, Ponstan✤), phenylbutazone (Butazolidin, Novobutazone✤), piroxicam (Feldene, Apo-Piroxicam✤), diclofenac sodium (Voltaren), flurbiprofen (Ansaid)	Dose varies depending on which drug is used. Piroxicam and naproxen are given in fewer doses because of longer half-life. Indomethacin and phenylbutazone are not as commonly used because of tendencies to cause peptic ulcer and CNS changes.	• Same as for salicylates above. • In addition, observe for fluid retention, increased blood pressure, and changes in renal function. • Monitor electrolyte and complete blood count values. • Observe for CNS changes, e.g., dizziness or confusion. • If a client is taking aspirin and an NSAID or is taking two NSAIDs, observe carefully for side effects or toxic effects.	• Same as for salicylates above. • Most NSAIDs cause sodium retention, which can lead to edema, hypertension, renal damage, and/or congestive heart failure. Drugs should be used with caution in elderly population. • Most NSAIDs cause increased sodium levels and can cause bone marrow suppression. • Most NSAIDs can cause CNS effects especially in the elderly. • Drugs are often used in combination, especially in clients with rheumatoid arthritis. Additive effects can cause serious complications.
Gold Auranofin (Ridaura)	Dose is 3 mg bid PO.	• Observe for and instruct client to report gastrointestinal problems, such as diarrhea, nausea/vomiting, abdominal cramping.	• This side effect causes discomfort and can lead to electrolyte imbalance.
Gold sodium thiomalate (water-based gold) (Myochrysine)	After a 10-mg test dose, 25 mg and then 50 mg is given every week until monthly maintenance of 50 mg IM is reached.	• Observe for rash or other skin change and for mouth ulceration (stomatitis).	• Drug may be discontinued for a short period, then restarted.

Continued

Chart 24–1. Drug Therapy for Connective Tissue Disease   Continued

Drug	Usual Dosage	Nursing Interventions	Rationale
Aurothioglucose (oil-based gold) (Solganal)	Same as for gold sodium thiomalate. If total of 1000 mg is used and no clinical change is seen, gold is discontinued.	• Instruct client to expect metallic taste in mouth; teach importance of proper mouth care. • Monitor urine for protein and serum for CBC. If CBC is markedly decreased or if proteinuria is present, discontinue drug. • Give *deep* IM, preferably by Z-track technique. • After IM administration, observe for nitroid crisis, a form of anaphylactic reaction.	• Proper, frequent mouth care reduces risk of stomatitis and metallic taste. • These changes indicate serious toxic effects, and drug needs to be discontinued. • Drug is locally irritating to soft tissue. • Flushing, dyspnea, and anxiety may occur shortly after drug administration.
Hydroxychloroquine sulfate (Plaquenil)	200 mg PO each day is given.	• Instruct client to have frequent (every 3–6 mo) ophthalmologic examination.	• Drug can cause retinal damage.
Penicillamine (Cuprimine)	125–250 mg PO each day is used (may be given in two divided doses).	• Same as for IM gold, except no nitroid crisis occurs.	• Same as for IM gold.
Immunosuppressive agents, e.g., azathioprine (Imuran), cyclophosphamide (Cytoxan, Procytox♣), methotrexate (Mexate)	Dose varies depending on disease activity and route of drug administration.	• Observe for side effects and toxic effects, including, but not limited to, nausea/vomiting, bone marrow suppression, and alopecia. • Instruct client to avoid crowds and people with infections such as influenza.	• Side effects and toxic effects of these drugs can be devastating. Drugs are reserved for severe forms of CTDs in which organ involvement is potentially life threatening. • Bone marrow suppression or immune suppression increases risk of infection.
Prednisone (Deltasone, Apo-Prednisone♣)	Dose is 10–150 mg PO each day. For maintenance, attempt to give dose every other day (to allow client's adrenal glands to function).	• Observe for cushiongoid changes, e.g., moon-face, buffalo hump, striae, acne, thin skin, bruising, fluid retention, and increased blood pressure. • Monitor electrolyte and glucose levels. • Observe for long-term effects of chronic steroid therapy, such as osteoporosis, cataracts, hypertension, diabetes, and impaired healing. • Instruct client to avoid crowds and individuals with infections such as influenza.	• These changes are expected and tend to be dose related. Changes diminish as dose decreases. • Chronic steroid therapy can cause sodium or fluid retention, potassium depletion, and elevated glucose level. • These complications may need to be treated with other drugs or modalities. • Drug suppresses immune system (lymphocytes) and increases risk of infection or decreased healing.

NSAIDs = nonsteroidal anti-inflammatory drugs; CNS = central nervous system; CBC = complete blood count; CTDs = connective tissue diseases.

affected joints. If needed, the nurse collaborates with the dietitian to provide more in-depth client teaching about nutrition and meal planning.

Other Pain Relief Measures. Additional measures may be used for pain reduction. A transcutaneous electrical nerve stimulator (TENS) may be particularly helpful for vertebral involvement. The health care provider collaborates with the nurse and physical therapist to determine whether the client might benefit from this pain management modality. The client must be able to control the TENS unit for pain relief.

Complementary Therapies. Clients may also use acupuncture, hypnosis, music therapy, and imagery for pain relief (see Chaps. 4 and 9).

Surgical Management. When all other measures are inadequate to provide pain control for clients with DJD, surgery may be indicated. The most common surgical procedure performed for these clients is the total joint replacement (TJR). An osteotomy may be done to correct joint deformity instead, but this procedure is rare owing to the success rate of TJR.

Any synovial joint of the body can be replaced with a prosthetic system consisting of at least two parts, one for each joint surface. A TJR is the major type of arthroplasty (surgical creation of a joint) that is performed.

Indications. Total joint replacement is a procedure of last resort for pain management; it is used when all other methods of pain relief have been unsuccessful. Hips and knees are most commonly replaced, but replacements of finger and wrist joints, elbows, shoulders, and toe joints and ankles have become more popular in the past 20 years.

Although TJRs are performed most often for clients with degenerative joint disease (DJD), other conditions causing joint damage may also require surgery. These disorders include rheumatoid arthritis (RA), congenital anomalies, trauma, and avascular necrosis—bony necrosis secondary to lack of blood flow, usually from trauma or chronic steroid therapy.

Contraindications. The primary contraindications for TJR are infection anywhere in the body, advanced osteoporosis, and severe inflammation. An infection from a source in the body or from the joint being replaced can result in an infected TJR and subsequent prosthetic failure. If a client has a urinary tract infection, for example, the physician treats the infection before surgery. Advanced osteoporosis can cause bone shattering during replacement when the prosthetic device is inserted. Acute joint inflammation is treated before surgery because the mechanical stress of the procedure may promote further inflammation and prosthetic failure.

As a group, TJRs are quite successful. Many clients who have lived with chronic, unbearable pain for years and who could not function independently at home or in the workplace no longer experience pain in the diseased joint. The pain relief and psychological benefit may outweigh the perioperative risks, but the surgeon and client must make that decision. When the client is of advanced age, this decision may become an ethical issue in addition to a physical risk−versus−benefit decision.

Total Hip Replacement (THR). The most commonly replaced joint is the hip. Clients of any age have the surgery, but the procedure is done most often for clients older than 60. The special needs and normal physiologic changes of elderly clients often complicate the perioperative period and may result in additional postoperative complications. (See Chapters 20–22 for routine perioperative care and the special considerations needed for care of the elderly client.)

Preoperative Care. Some insurance companies assign TJR candidates to their case managers (CMs). During the assessment process, the CM determines whether the client will have support and caregiving services postoperatively. If none are available, the client's surgery is not approved until arrangements can be made for care in a nursing home or alternative placement.

As with any surgical procedure, preoperative care begins with assessment of the client's level of understanding about the impending replacement. The physician explains the procedure and postoperative care expectations during the office visit, but this explanation may have occurred weeks or months before the surgery was scheduled. Elderly clients, in particular, may forget some of the information or may not know what questions to ask. Many orthopedic surgeons employ nurses in the office who can follow up and address any of the client's special concerns. A clinical pathway outlining expectations during prehospitalization, hospitalization, and posthospitalization phases of care can be reviewed with the client and family.

In addition, nurse educators or orthopedic nurses may lead formal classes in the hospital several weeks before surgery to answer questions and clarify information. During class, the client is shown the prosthesis or a picture of the device and receives written instructions or teaching booklets to reinforce the information.

In some hospitals or orthopedic office practices, the physical therapist can meet the surgical candidate before surgery to explain ambulation and postoperative exercises.

Clients are admitted on the morning of surgery and do not come to the orthopedic, surgical, or medical-surgical unit until after surgery.

Operative Procedure. Before the start of the procedure, the operating room may be specially cleaned to reduce the risk of infection. Laminar airflow surgical suites and body exhaust systems ("spacesuits") may also be used. The surgery is usually scheduled early in the morning, if possible, and movement into and out of the room is kept to a minimum. The client is given a dose of intravenous antibiotics, usually a cephalosporin, such as cefazolin (Ancef), at least 1 hour before the initial surgical incision is made. Vancomycin (Vancocin) or clindamycin (Cleocin) may be used for clients allergic to cephalosporins.

The anesthesiologist or nurse anesthetist places the client under general or epidural anesthesia. Epidural induction reduces blood loss and the incidence of deep venous thrombosis. Intraoperative blood loss with hypotensive epidural anesthesia is usually less than 300 mL, which decreases the need for postoperative blood transfusions (Ranawat et al., 1997).

The 8- to 10-inch (20.3–24.5 cm) incision is usually longitudinal on the anterolateral thigh. A posterior incision may be used instead to preserve muscle, depending on surgeon preference.

If the prosthesis is cemented, polymethyl methacrylate (an acrylic fixating substance) is used. During the surgical procedure, the operative area is irrigated with a cool solution. To help prevent infection, the surgeon may mix an antibiotic with the cement or may use antibiotic-impregnated beads to plant deep into the wound. The surgeon also inserts one or two wound drains to remove exudate from the tissues that might serve as a medium for pathogenic growth and cause wound infection.

A major advance in joint replacement surgery is the increased use of noncemented prostheses, especially for hip replacements. Although polymethyl methacrylate is an excellent initial fixator, it has a finite life span and deteriorates over time, which causes loosening of the implant and pain. The average life span of a cemented hip is 10 years. When a prosthesis eventually loosens and causes pain, it is replaced; this procedure is called a *revision arthroplasty*. To prevent repeated replacements, several devices that do not require a fixating substance have been designed.

The most common mechanism that is used to avoid polymethyl methacrylate is a porous metal coating on the shaft of the femoral component and the back of the acetabular cap. By using a tight fit, known as a "press fit," the surgeon places the implant (prosthesis) snugly against the client's bone tissue. Most of the prostheses used today are custom designed by computers to match the size of the prosthesis with the size of the client's own joint. Figure 24–2 illustrates a typical noncemented hip replacement system.

New bone tissue grows between the pores of the prosthesis and "grafts" to the device within 6–12 weeks. The older the client, the longer the bone grafting may take. This bony ingrowth serves as the fixating mechanism and, ideally, lasts a lifetime. However, the earliest noncemented total joint systems, which were inserted in the 1970s and 1980s, have needed revisions, primarily because of undersizing of the prosthesis. As a result, the device loosens and is replaced with a new noncemented

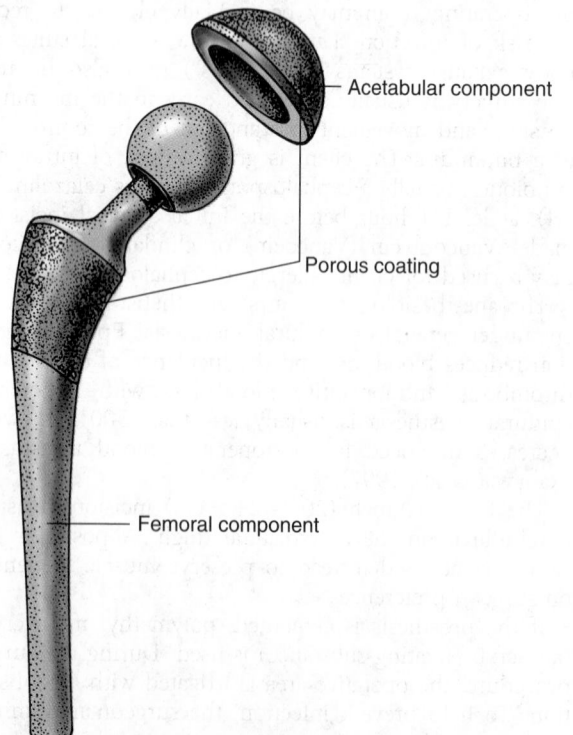

Figure 24–2. Noncemented, porous-coated hip replacement system.

TABLE 24–2

Nursing Interventions to Prevent Complications of Total Joint Replacement Surgery

Complication	Prevention/Intervention
Dislocation	• Position correctly. • For hip, keep legs slightly abducted. • For hip, prevent hip flexion beyond 90 degrees. • Assess for pain, rotation, and/or extremity shortening. • Keep client in bed. • Report immediately to physician.
Infection	• Use aseptic technique for wound care and emptying of drains. • Wash hands thoroughly when caring for client. • Culture drainage fluid. • Monitor temperature. • Report excessive inflammation and/or drainage to physician.
Deep venous thrombosis/pulmonary embolism	• Have client wear elastic stockings and/or sequential compression stockings. • Teach leg exercises to client. • Encourage fluid intake. • Observe for signs of thrombosis (redness, swelling, or pain). • Observe client for changes in mental status. • Keep client in bed. • Do not massage legs. • Do not use knee gatch on bed.
Hypotension, bleeding, or infection	• Take vital signs at least every 4 hr. • Observe client for bleeding. • Report excessively low blood pressure or bleeding to physician.

device. Freeze-dried bone grafts (*allografts*) are used to fill in bony defects that result from removing the old prosthesis. During the healing process, the essentially dead bone revascularizes and grafts with the client's own bone. Clients older than 75 and those who do not have sufficient bone mass are often not candidates for the noncemented hip.

Postoperative Care. In addition to providing the routine postoperative care discussed in Chapter 22, the nurse assesses for and assists in the prevention of postoperative complications that could occur after a joint replacement. Table 24–2 summarizes common postoperative complications of total hip replacement surgery, including nursing measures for prevention, assessment, and intervention.

Chart 24–2 highlights special concerns for the care of the elderly in the postoperative period.

Prevention of Dislocation. A common complication of total hip replacement is subluxation (partial dislocation) or total dislocation. Therefore, correct positioning is maintained at all times. When the client returns from the postanesthesia care unit (PACU), the nurse places the client in a supine position with the head slightly elevated. The nurse may place a trapezoid-shaped abduction pillow, wedge, sling, or splint, with or without straps, between the client's legs to prevent adduction beyond the body's midline. In some hospitals, this device is no longer used because it is uncomfortable for the client and not necessary in most cases. Abduction devices are usually reserved for clients who are very restless or who are unable to follow instructions, especially the elderly. One or two regular bed pillows are used instead for most clients.

The nurse may place and support the affected leg in neutral rotation by using a device such as the cradle boot. The cradle boot not only prevents rotation but also elevates the leg to the desired functional position and keeps the client's heel off the bed linen to prevent heel tissue breakdown. Keeping the heels off the bed is particularly important for the elderly client who is at high risk for pressure sores.

The nurse turns the client toward either side as long as the abduction or other pillow is in place. Some surgeons only allow turning directly onto one side or the other. This policy varies, depending on the surgeon's preference and the policy of the hospital unit.

The nurse observes the client for possible signs of hip dislocation, which include increased hip pain, shortening of the affected leg, and leg rotation. If any of these clinical manifestations occurs, the nurse keeps the client in bed and notifies the surgeon immediately. The surgeon manipulates and relocates the affected hip after the client receives analgesia or is anesthetized. The hip is then immobilized by an abduction splint or other device until healing occurs, usually in about 6 weeks.

Prevention of Infection. Another common potential complication of hip replacement is infection. As soon as the client's bowel sounds return and the client is voiding in sufficient quantity, the nurse discontinues intravenous therapy unless otherwise contraindicated.

The nurse also monitors the surgical incision and vital signs carefully: every 4 hours for the first several days and every 8 hours thereafter. The nurse observes for signs of infection, such as elevated temperature and excessive or foul-smelling drainage from the incision. An elderly client may not have a fever with infection but may experience an altered mental state instead. The nurse obtains a sample of the drainage for culture and sensitivity to determine the offending organisms and the antibiotics that may be needed for treatment.

An infection that occurs within 1 year of surgery is referred to as an early infection. It is most often due to contamination during surgery. In addition to antibiotics, laminar airflow operating rooms, body exhaust systems, ultraviolet light, and double gloving help reduce the incidence of infection. If an early infection occurs, the surgeon usually prescribes IV antibiotic therapy. Late infection can occur anywhere after 1 year postoperatively. If the late infection does not resolve with treatment, the surgeon may replace the prosthesis.

The clinical manifestations of infection are variable. The erythrocyte sedimentation rate (ESR) is elevated, and the client typically complains of incisional pain, swelling, erythema, and wound drainage.

Assessment of Bleeding and Prevention of Anemia. The nurse observes the surgical hip dressing for bleeding or other type of drainage at least every 4 hours or when vital signs are taken. The nurse empties and measures the fluid in the drain every shift. The nurse also observes and records the characteristics of the drainage, which is typically bloody. The total amount of drainage is usually less than 50 mL every 8 hours. If the client has received a plasma expander (such as dextran), this amount may be increased. The surgeon removes the drains and operative dressing 48–72 hours postoperatively. Care must be taken to prevent tape burns when the surgical dressing is removed, especially in an elderly client.

The surgeon also orders periodic hemoglobin and hematocrit assessments to determine whether the client is anemic and requires blood transfusions. Although some clients receive several units of blood during surgery, the hematocrit and hemoglobin may fall below the normal level so that additional blood is needed 2 or 3 days postoperatively. The client's blood pressure may be lower than usual because of blood loss during surgery or the use of cement, which tends to dilate blood vessels and cause hypotension.

Because total joint replacements (TJRs) are elective procedures, autologous blood transfusions are common. The

---

Chart 24–2

Nursing Focus on the Elderly: Total Hip Replacement

- Use an abduction pillow or splint to prevent adduction after surgery if the client is very restless or has an altered mental state.
- Keep the client's heels off the bed to prevent pressure sores.
- Do not rely on fever as a sign of infection; elderly clients often have infection without fever. Decreasing mental status typically occurs when the client has an infection.
- When assisting the client out of bed, move the client slowly to prevent orthostatic (postural) hypotension.
- Encourage the client to deep breathe and cough, and use the incentive spirometer every 2 hours to prevent atelectasis and pneumonia.
- As soon as permitted, get the client out of bed to prevent complications of immobility.
- Anticipate the client's need for pain medication, especially if the client is unable to verbalize the need for pain control.
- Expect a temporary change in mental state immediately after surgery as a result of the anesthesia and unfamiliar sensory stimuli. Reorient the client frequently.

414 UNIT 5 ■ Problems of Protection: Management of Clients with Problems of the Immune System

client donates blood before surgery to be used as needed during and after surgery. This predeposit autologous blood donation is a cost-effective blood replacement alternative in clients with elective surgeries.

Another method for blood replacement is intraoperative or postoperative blood salvage. Intraoperatively, the shed blood is collected via aspiration from the surgical site. Using a cell saver, about 50% of the red blood cells are saved for reinfusion. This procedure is used most commonly for bilateral joint replacements or for revision surgeries. Postoperatively, blood can be replaced by collecting shed blood via suction into a reservoir, filtering the blood, and then reinfusing it. The American Association of Blood Banks recommends that the blood be reinfused within 6 hours of collection (Maher et al., 1994).

Assessment for Neurovascular Compromise. As with other bone surgery, frequent neurovascular assessments, which are performed at the same time as vital signs are checked, are necessary to monitor for possible compromise in circulation to the distal extremity.

Management of Incisional Pain. Although hip replacement is performed to relieve joint pain, the client experiences pain related to the surgical procedure. Many clients state that they have pain after surgery but that it is a different type and less excruciating than the pain before surgery. Pain control may be achieved by epidural analgesia, patient-controlled analgesia (PCA), intramuscular opioid analgesia, or a combination of techniques. (Chapter 9 contains a chart of commonly used opioid analgesics and related nursing interventions.)

The nurse anticipates the elderly client's need for pain medication if he or she cannot verbalize the need. Many elderly clients experience several days of increased disorientation or delirium as a result of surgery and anesthesia.

Regardless of the pain management method used, most clients do not require parenteral analgesia after the first two days. Oral opioids, such as oxycodone (Supeudol♦) or oxycodone plus acetaminophen (Percocet, Tylox), are then commonly prescribed until the client's pain can be controlled by NSAIDs, such as ibuprofen (Motrin, Apo-Ibuprofen♦).

Progression of Activity. The client with a total hip replacement is usually allowed to get out of bed the day after surgery, and physical therapy is initiated. Activities that are permitted differ among surgeons and hospitals, but prolonged bed rest can cause numerous complications, such as atelectasis and pneumonia, especially in the elderly. When getting the client out of bed, the nurse stands on the same side of the bed as the client's affected leg. After achieving a sitting position, the client stands on the unaffected leg and pivots to the chair with assistance. To prevent hip dislocation (Fig. 24–3), the nurse at all times ensures that the client does not flex the hips beyond 90 degrees. Raised toilet seats, straight-back chairs, and reclining wheelchairs help prevent hyperflexion.

The surgeon, the type of prosthesis, and the surgical approach all determine the resumption of weight-bearing on the affected leg. A client with a cemented implant is usually allowed partial weight-bearing (PWB) or full weight-bearing (FWB) to tolerance immediately. A client with an uncemented prosthesis cannot tolerate FWB until bony ingrowth occurs. PWB typically is only permitted for the first 6 weeks or until there is x-ray evidence of bony ingrowth.

The physical therapist (PT) teaches the client how to follow these weight-bearing restrictions and helps the client progress to full-weight-bearing (FWB) status, if possible. Most clients generally use a walker, although young clients may use crutches. Clients are usually advanced to a single cane or crutch if they can walk without a severe limp 1 month after surgery. When the limp disappears, they no longer need an ambulatory assistive device and are permitted to sit in normal-height chairs, use regular toilets, and drive a car.

Prevention of Thromboembolic Complications. The risk of developing deep venous thrombosis postoperatively is high. Fatal pulmonary embolism syndrome occurs in 0.5% to 2% of cases (Ranawat et al., 1997). Elderly clients are especially at increased risk for thrombi because of age and compromised circulation before surgery. Obese clients and those with a history of deep venous thrombi are also at high risk for thrombi. In clients with total hip replacement, thrombi usually develop in the thigh; these thrombi become life-threatening emboli more readily than calf and other thrombi. For this reason, thigh-high stockings, elastic bandages, and sequential compression devices (SCDs) are used during the hospital stay (see Chap. 20).

Anticoagulants, such as aspirin (Ecotrin or buffered aspirin), warfarin (Coumadin, Warfilone♦), or subcutaneous low-molecular-weight (LMW) heparin (Lovenox), are prescribed in maintenance doses. Warfarin is the most commonly used anticoagulant. If the client takes warfarin, the dosage is adjusted to maintain an international normalized ratio (INR) of 2.0.

The PT teaches leg exercises, which are begun in the immediate postoperative period and continue until the client is fully ambulatory. These exercises include plantar flexion and dorsiflexion (heel pumping), circumduction (circles) of the feet, gluteal and quadriceps muscle setting, and straight-leg raises (SLRs). The client performs gluteal exercises by pushing the heels into the bed. The client achieves quadriceps-setting exercises ("quad sets") by straightening the legs and pushing the back of the knees into the bed. In addition to preventing clots, these exercises improve muscle tone, which aids in restoration of function of the extremity.

Promotion of Self-Care. The hospital's occupational therapy department often supplies assistive-adaptive devices to help with activities of daily living (ADLs). Particularly important for clients are devices designed for reaching to prevent them from bending or stooping and flexing at the hips more than 90 degrees. Extended handles on shoehorns and dressing sticks are particularly useful for helping clients achieve independence in ADLs.

Clients typically stay in the hospital for 3–5 days, but elderly clients or those experiencing postoperative complications may stay longer. Discharge may be to the home, a rehabilitation unit, transitional care unit (subacute unit), or a long-term care facility for rehabilitation or custodial care. The nurse provides written instructions for posthospital care and reviews them with clients and their family

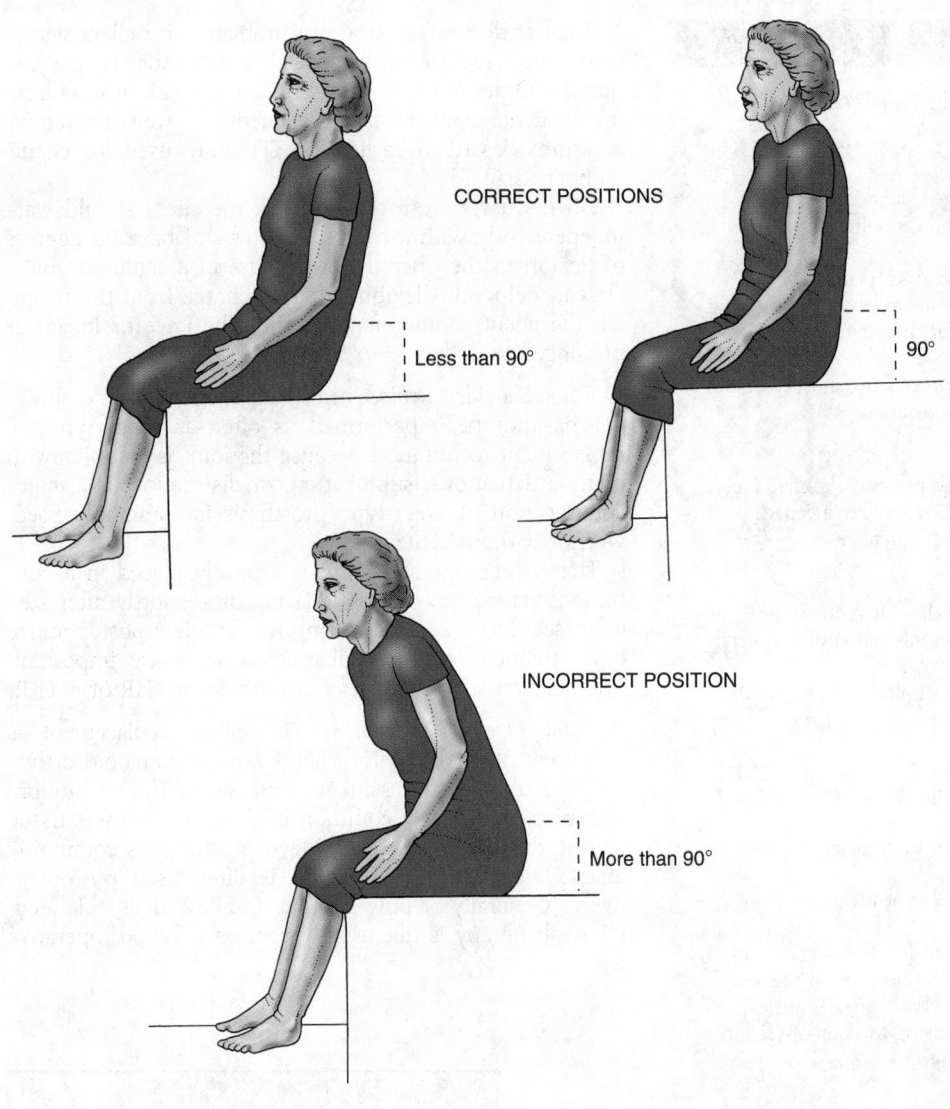

CORRECT POSITIONS

Less than 90°

90°

INCORRECT POSITION

More than 90°

Figure 24–3. Correct and incorrect hip flexion after a total hip replacement.

members (Chart 24–3). If the client is transferred to a facility, a copy of the posthospital instructions is sent with the client to the facility.

Total Knee Replacement (TKR). After total hip replacement, the second most common total joint replacement (TJR) procedure is for the knee. Before 1980, attempts at knee replacement were not successful, and most of the prostheses inserted before then have been removed. The knee is not a simple, hinged joint; it is a condylar joint that rotates slightly when flexed and extended. As seen in Figure 24–4, the typical total knee prosthesis is a three-part system: a femoral component, a tibial plate, and a patellar button. For some clients, only one surface is replaced.

Preoperative Care. Only severe symptoms and disability justify TKR in clients with DJD. TKRs are avoided in people younger than 60 years (Windsor & Insall, 1997). The preoperative care for clients undergoing a TKR is similar to that for total hip replacement. The major difference is the teaching, which depends on the postoperative protocol used by the orthopedic surgeon. After surgery,

clients may not be allowed to bend the operative knee for several days until a large, bulky pressure dressing is removed. Most surgeons have abandoned this traditional approach for the continuous passive motion (CPM) machine (see later in this chapter).

Operative Procedure. As with the hip, the knee can be replaced with the client under general or epidural anesthesia. The surgeon typically makes a central longitudinal incision, approximately 8–10 inches (20.3–25.4 cm) long. Osteotomies of the femoral and tibial condyles and of the posterior patella are performed; the surfaces are prepared for the prostheses. Noncemented implants, once popular in the 1980s, are used less for the knee than they are for the hip. The surgeon inserts one or two surgical drains and applies a pressure dressing to prevent bleeding.

Postoperative Care. Postoperative nursing care of the client with a total knee replacement is similar to that for the client with a total hip replacement, but maintaining abduction is not necessary. The surgeon usually orders a

---

Chart 24–3

Education Guide: Total Hip Replacement

Hip Precautions

- Do not sit or stand for prolonged periods.
- Do not cross your legs beyond the midline of your body.
- Do not bend your hips more than 90 degrees.
- Use an ambulatory aid, such as a walker, when walking.
- Use assistive-adaptive devices for dressing, such as for putting on shoes and socks.
- You can resume sexual intercourse as usual, but use the hip precautions learned in the hospital.

Pain Management

- Report increased hip pain to the physician immediately.
- Take oral analgesics, as prescribed, only as needed.
- Do not overexert yourself; take frequent rests.

Incisional Care

- Inspect your hip incision every day for redness, heat, or drainage; if any of these are present, call your physician immediately.
- Cleanse your hip incision with a mild soap and water every day; be sure to dry it thoroughly.

Other Care

- Continue walking and performing the leg exercises as you learned in the hospital.
- Report pain, redness, or swelling in your legs to your physician immediately.
- Report chest pain and/or shortness of breath to your physician immediately.
- If you are taking an anticoagulant for 4–6 weeks, follow the precautions learned in the hospital to prevent bleeding: avoid using a straight razor, avoid injuries, report bleeding or excessive bruising to your physician immediately.

Because dislocation is a rare problem for a client with a total knee replacement, special positioning is not required. Other complications affecting total hip replacement clients may affect these clients as well. Preventive measures described earlier for THRs are used for clients with TKRs.

On discharge from the hospital, the client should walk independently with a cane or walker and have 90 degrees of flexion in the operative knee. Use of a stationary bicycle can help gain flexion. After discharge from the hospital, the client should not hyperflex the knee or kneel for prolonged periods.

Total Shoulder Replacement. Replacement of the shoulder has not been performed as often as other types of replacement techniques. Because the joint is complex with many articulations, subluxation, or dislocation, is a major complication. A Neer-type prosthesis is commonly used, with or without cement.

The client's operative arm is typically placed in a continuous passive motion (CPM) machine shortly after surgery (see Chart 24–4). During the first few postoperative days, frequent neurovascular assessments are important. The hospital stay is shorter than that for a THR or a TKR.

Total Elbow Replacement. The elbow replacement is performed most often for clients with rheumatoid arthritis. It is usually successful in increasing range of motion, but infection is fairly common because of extensive tissue cutting during surgery. The Mayo prosthesis is commonly inserted, and the CPM device is often used postoperatively. Generally, elbow motion is allowed as tolerated. Physical therapy is not usually necessary for postoperative

---

CPM machine, which is can be applied in the postanesthesia care unit (PACU) or not used until 1–2 days after surgery (Fig. 24–5). The CPM keeps the prosthetic knee in motion and prevents scar tissue formation, which could impede mobility of the knee and exacerbate postoperative pain.

The surgeon, physical therapist, or technician presets the CPM machine for the appropriate range of motion and cycles per minute. A typical initial setting is 20–30 degrees range of motion at 2 cycles/minute, but this setting varies according to surgeon preference. The machine is generally used for 8–12 hours/day, and the range of motion is increased gradually. The current trend is intermittent use for several hours at a time. Each day the nurse notes the client's response to the use of the device.

Some machines do not allow the leg to achieve full extension, thus promoting flexion contractures; however, one solution is for the client to use the CPM machine during the day and sleep in a knee immobilizer at night to achieve the desired extension. Chart 24–4 outlines the nurse's responsibility when caring for a client using the CPM machine.

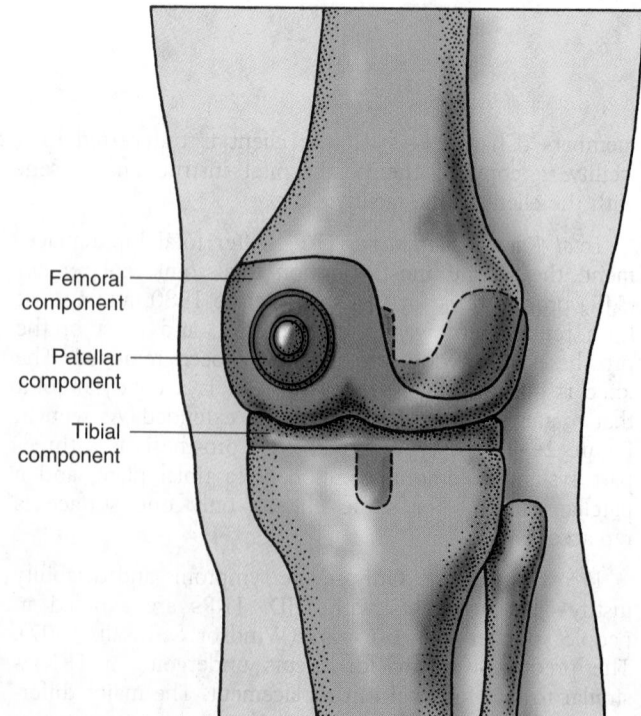

Femoral component

Patellar component

Tibial component

Figure 24–4. Typical three-part condylar knee replacement system.

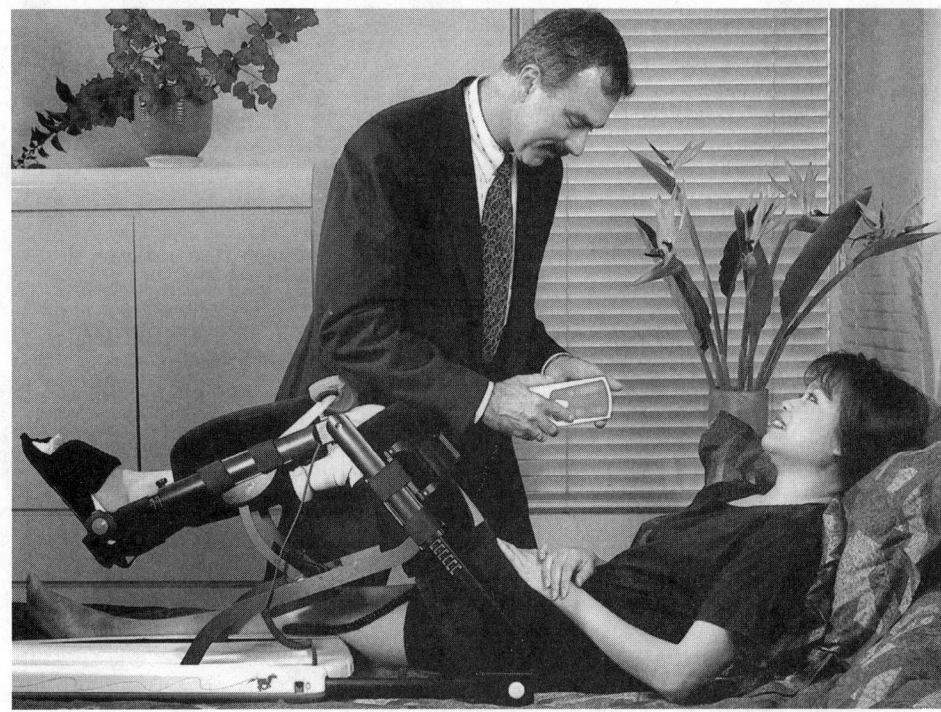

Figure 24–5. A continuous passive motion machine in use. (Courtesy of Orthologic, Tempe, AZ.)

clients with a total elbow replacement. Generalized swelling usually resolves in 3–6 months.

Finger and Wrist Replacements. Any joint of the hand can be replaced, often for clients with rheumatoid arthritis. The flexible, silicone prostheses are implanted without the use of polymethyl methacrylate because no weight-bearing is required for the prostheses.

Postoperatively, a bulky dressing is used temporarily and then replaced by a dynamic splint, brace, or cast or by a very small CPM machine. Edema formation is controlled if the client elevates the arm as much as possible. The rehabilitation program for finger arthroplasties may

last for weeks, until normal function and strength return. These procedures are typically performed in specialized hand centers.

Any bone of the wrist can be replaced, including the heads of the radius and ulna. The postoperative pressure dressing is removed in 2–3 days, and a splint or short arm cast is applied. The client usually regains full function within 6–12 weeks, but lifting may be restricted for a longer period. Occupational therapists are usually involved with upper extremity rehabilitation.

Ankle and Toe Replacements. Because the ankles support approximately 25% of the body's weight, developing an implant that is both small and strong enough to withstand the weight of the body has been difficult. When the ankle is replaced, usually an arthrodesis, or bone fusion, is performed for added stability. Replacing the ankle is not a common procedure.

The metatarsal implants are made of silicone and cannot bear excessive weight. Typically, the client has one or more osteotomies and fusions, which are immobilized by wires and a cast while healing occurs. Chapter 53 discusses foot osteotomies and their associated nursing care.

Impaired Physical Mobility

Planning: Expected Outcomes. The primary outcome for the client with DJD is that the client is expected to function independently in performing activities of daily living (ADLs) and ambulation.

Interventions. Management of the client with DJD is an interdisciplinary effort. The nurse collaborates with the physical and occupational therapists to meet the goal of independent function. The major interventions include therapeutic exercise and promotion of ADLs and ambula-

---

Chart 24–4

Nursing Care Highlight: The Client Using a Continuous Passive Motion (CPM) Machine

- Ensure that the machine is well padded with sheepskin or other similar material.
- Check the cycle and range-of-motion settings at least once per shift (every 8 hours).
- Ensure that the joint being moved is properly positioned on the machine.
- If the client is confused, place the controls to the machine out of the client's reach.
- Assess the client's response to the machine.
- Turn off the machine while the client is having a meal in bed.
- When the machine is not in use, do not store it on the floor.

tion through teaching about health and use of assistive-adaptive devices.

Exercise. Two types of exercise are recommended for the client with DJD: recreational and therapeutic. Recreational exercise includes hobbies and sports, with no planned purpose other than relaxation. Therapeutic exercise includes carefully planned activities that are designed to improve muscle strength and tone and joint ROM. Therapeutic exercise can also reduce pain and improve the client's psychological health.

Certain recreational activities may also be therapeutic, such as doing the breast stroke during swimming to enhance chest and arm muscles. Aerobic exercises, such as walking, biking, swimming, and aerobic dance, are recommended. Usually the physical therapist prescribes exercises for the client with DJD, but the nurse reinforces their techniques and principles. The ideal time for exercise is immediately after the application of heat. To prevent further joint damage, clients should rigorously follow the instructions for exercise outlined in Chart 24-5.

Use of Assistive-Adaptive Devices. The physical therapist evaluates the client's need for ambulatory aids, such as canes, walkers, or platform crutches. Although many clients do not like to use these aids or may forget how to use them, these aids help prevent further joint deterioration and pain. An occupational therapist evaluates the client's ability to perform ADLs and can provide ideas and devices for assistance.

 Continuing Care

The client with degenerative joint disease (DJD) is not usually hospitalized for the disease itself but for surgical management. However, the client may be admitted for

---

Chart 24-5

Education Guide: Exercises for Clients with Degenerative Joint Disease or Rheumatoid Arthritis

- Follow the exercise instructions that have been specifically prescribed for you. There are no universal exercises; your exercises have been specifically tailored to your own needs.
- Do your exercises on both "good" and "bad" days. Consistency is important.
- Respect pain. If pain increases as you exercise, stop and report this to your physician.
- Use active rather than active-assist or passive exercise whenever possible.
- Reduce the number of repetitions when the inflammation is severe and you have more pain.
- Do not substitute your normal activities or household tasks for the prescribed exercises.
- Avoid resistive exercises when your joints are severely inflamed.

Chart 24-6

Education Guide: Instructions for Joint Protection

- Use large joints instead of small ones; for example, place your purse strap over your shoulder instead of grasping the purse with your hand.
- Do not turn a doorknob clockwise. Turn it counter-clockwise to avoid twisting your arm and promoting ulnar deviation.
- Use two hands instead of one to hold objects.
- Sit in a chair with a high, straight back.
- When getting out of bed, do not push off with your fingers; use the entire palm of both hands.
- Do not bend at your waist; bend your knees instead, while keeping your back straight.
- Use long-handled devices, such as a hairbrush with an extended handle.
- Use assistive-adaptive devices, such as Velcro closures and built-up utensil handles, to protect your joints.
- Do not use pillows in bed, except a small one under your head.
- Avoid twisting or wringing your hands.

---

another medical or surgical reason. The nurse considers the problems that are present as a result of arthritis before the client is discharged home.

➤ Home Care Management

If weight-bearing joints are markedly involved, the client may have difficulty going up or down stairs. Making arrangements to live on one floor with accessibility to all rooms is often the best solution. A home care nurse, physical therapist, or occupational therapist assesses the need for structural alterations to the home to accommodate ambulatory aids and to enable the client to perform activities. For example, a kitchen counter may need to be lowered or a seat and hand rails to be installed in the shower. If the client has a total hip replacement, an elevated toilet seat is necessary for several weeks postoperatively to prevent excessive hip flexion.

➤ Health Teaching

Learning how to protect the joint is the most important feature of client education. Preventing further damage to joints slows the progression of DJD and minimizes pain. The nurse explains general rules of joint protection and cites examples, as in Chart 24-6.

As with other diseases in which drugs and diet therapy are used, the nurse teaches the drug protocol, side effects, and toxic effects to the client and family. The nurse also emphasizes the importance of reducing weight and eating a well-balanced diet to promote tissue healing.

Many clients with "arthritis" become frustrated and desperate about the course of the disease and treatment, and they look for a cure. Unfortunately, there is no cure for these joint diseases, even though tabloids, books, and the media frequently cite "curative" remedies. People spend billions of dollars each year on quackery, including liniments, special diets, and copper bracelets. More hazardous substances, such as snake venom and industrial cleaners, are also advertised as remedies. The nurse instructs the client to always check with The Arthritis Foundation about new "cures." For example, if a client believes that wearing a copper bracelet or eating more foods with a high vitamin C content is helpful, the nurse may encourage the continuation of the practice as long as it is not harmful. If there is a potential for harm, the nurse instructs the client to avoid the modality and provides the rationale for doing so.

With most types of CTD, clients must live with a chronic, unpredictable, and painful disorder. Their roles, self-esteem, and body image may be affected by these diseases. Body image is often not as devastating in DJD as in the inflammatory arthritic diseases, such as rheumatoid arthritis. The psychosocial component is discussed in more detail under Rheumatoid Arthritis.

➤ Health Care Resources

The client who has undergone surgery is most likely to need help from community resources. After a joint replacement, the client needs extensive assistance with mobility. The client may be discharged to home, a long-term care facility, a subacute unit (transitional care unit), or a rehabilitation unit. The nurse collaborates with the social worker, discharge planner, case manager, and physician to find the best placement for each client. If the client is discharged to home, home care nurses visit for the first 2–3 weeks, depending on the client's concurrent systemic diseases. A nursing assistant may visit the home to help with hygiene-related needs; a physical therapist may work with the client on ambulatory and mobility skills. In addition, a client who has had a total hip or knee replacement should not be discharged to home alone. A family member or significant other must be in the home at all times for at least the first 4–6 weeks, when the client needs the most assistance.

The nurse provides written instructions about the care that is required, regardless of whether the client goes home or to another inpatient facility. For continuity of care, communication with the new care provider is ideal. Arrangements are made so that the client can return to the same acute care hospital if needed.

The Arthritis Foundation is an important community resource for all clients with CTD. This organization provides information to laypeople and health professionals and refers clients and their families to other resources as needed. Local support groups can help clients and their families cope with these diseases.

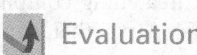 Evaluation

The nurse evaluates the care provided by determining whether the client

- States that chronic pain is reduced as a result of interdisciplinary interventions

- Ambulates without personal assistance (although a mechanical aid such as a walker may be used)
- Is independent in ADLs (may use assistive-adaptive devices)

RHEUMATOID ARTHRITIS
Overview

Rheumatoid arthritis (RA) is the second most commonly occurring connective tissue disease but is the most destructive to joints. It is a chronic, progressive, systemic inflammatory process that affects primarily synovial joints.

The onset of RA is characterized by synovitis, or inflammation of the synovial tissue in joints. Inflammatory mediators, such as cytokines, chemokines, and proteases, attract and activate neutrophils and other cells (see Chapter 23 for a complete discussion of the inflammatory response). The synovium thickens and becomes hyperemic, fluid accumulates in the joint space, and a pannus forms. The pannus is vascular granulation tissue, composed of inflammatory cells, that erodes articular cartilage and eventually destroys bone. As a result, fibrous adhesions, bony ankylosis, and calcifications occur; bone loses density and secondary osteoporosis occurs.

If the disease is diagnosed early, permanent joint changes may be avoided. Early, aggressive treatment to suppress synovitis may cause a remission; about 25% of clients experience a remission, which may last as long as 20 years. Some clients also experience spontaneous remissions and exacerbations without treatment.

Rheumatoid arthritis is a systemic disease; that is, areas of the body—in addition to synovial joints—can be affected. Inflammatory responses similar to those occurring in synovial tissue may be seen in any organ or body system in which connective tissue is prevalent. If blood vessel involvement (*vasculitis*) occurs, the organ that is supplied by that vessel can be affected. The result is malfunction and eventual failure of the organ or system. These pathologic changes occur late in the disease process and cause life-threatening problems.

The etiology of RA remains a mystery, but research suggests a combination of environmental and genetic factors. The most popular theory to date—the immune complex hypothesis—states that unusual antibodies of the immunoglobulin (Ig) G or IgM type (rheumatoid factor) develop against IgG antigenic determinants to form complexes that lodge in synovium and other connective tissues. Local and systemic inflammatory responses result. RA has been found to be strongly associated with the human leukocyte antigen (HLA) DRw4. Other antigens have been identified but are observed less frequently. (See Chapter 23 on inflammation and the immune response.)

Although RA is probably an autoimmune disease, the origin of rheumatoid factor is unclear. A genetic predisposition for RA is most likely because the disease affects people with a family history of RA two to three times more often than the rest of the population.

Some researchers suspect that female reproductive hormones influence the development of RA because it affects women more often than men. Others suspect that a virus, such as Epstein-Barr virus, may trigger the autoimmune process. Physical and emotional stresses have been linked to exacerbations of the disorder and may be contributing factors in its development.

WOMEN'S HEALTH CONSIDERATIONS

 Rheumatoid arthritis affects 1% of the world's population, women three times more often than men. Women who are taking or who have taken oral contraceptives are less likely to have RA. The onset of the disease is typically between ages 35 and 45 years, but it can occur at any age.

There are no significant differences among geographic locations, despite the common lay belief that warmer, drier climates can be beneficial to people with RA. The incidence of RA in China is somewhat lower than elsewhere in the world (about 0.3%) and substantially higher among the Pima Indians in North America (about 5%) (Harris, 1997).

TRANSCULTURAL CONSIDERATIONS

With the exception of Native Americans, there are no major differences among races or ethnic groups. Studies of several northern Native American groups revealed RA prevalence rates that were three to seven times higher that those in non–Native American groups (Giger & Davidhizar, 1995).

Collaborative Management

Assessment

The onset of RA may be acute and severe or slow and insidious; clients may have vague complaints lasting for several months before diagnosis. The manifestations of RA can be categorized as early or late disease and as articular or extra-articular (Chart 24–7).

➤ Physical Assessment/Clinical Manifestations

Early Disease Manifestations. The client with RA typically complains of fatigue, generalized weakness, anorexia, and a weight loss of about 2 or 3 pounds (1 kg) early in the disease process. Persistent low-grade fever may accompany these complaints because RA is an inflammatory disease. In clients with early disease, the nurse notes that the upper extremity joints are involved initially, typically the proximal interphalangeal (PIP) and metacarpophalangeal (MCP) joints of the hands. These joints may be slightly reddened, warm, stiff, swollen, and tender or painful, particularly on palpation. The typical pattern of joint involvement in RA is bilateral and symmetric (e.g., both wrists), and the number of joints involved usually increases as the disease progresses.

ELDERLY CONSIDERATIONS

Rheumatoid arthritis developing in the elderly affects men more often than women. The client typically complains of stiffness; swelling of the hands, wrists, and forearms; and limb girdle pain (Harris, 1997).

Chart 24–7

Focused Assessment of the Client with Rheumatoid Arthritis

Early Manifestations
Joint
• Inflammation

Systemic
• Low-grade fever
• Fatigue
• Weakness
• Anorexia
• Paresthesias

Late Manifestations
Joint
• Deformities (e.g., swan neck or ulnar deviation)
• Moderate to severe pain and morning stiffness

Systemic
• Osteoporosis
• Severe fatigue
• Anemia
• Weight loss
• Subcutaneous nodules
• Peripheral neuropathy
• Vasculitis
• Pericarditis
• Fibrotic lung disease
• Sjögren's syndrome
• Renal disease

Late Disease Manifestations. As the disease worsens, the joints become progressively inflamed and quite painful. The client complains of morning stiffness (also called the gel phenomenon), which lasts between 30 minutes and several hours after awakening. On palpation, the nurse notes that the joints feel soft because of synovitis and effusions. The fingers often appear spindle like. The nurse may observe muscle atrophy, which can result from disuse secondary to joint pain, and a decreased range of motion in affected joints.

Eventually, most or all synovial joints are affected. In severe disease, the temporomandibular joint (TMJ) may be involved, but this involvement is infrequent. When the TMJ is affected, the client typically complains of pain when chewing or opening the mouth.

When the spinal column is involved, the cervical joints are most likely to be affected. The nurse palpates the posterior cervical spine to elicit pain or tenderness. Cervical disease may result in subluxation, especially the first and second vertebrae. This is a life-threatening complication because branches of the phrenic nerve that supply the diaphragm can be compressed and respiratory function may be subsequently compromised. The client is also in danger of becoming quadriparetic or quadriplegic.

Joint Manifestations. Joint deformity occurs as a late, articular manifestation, and secondary osteoporosis can cause bone fractures. The nurse observes common defor-

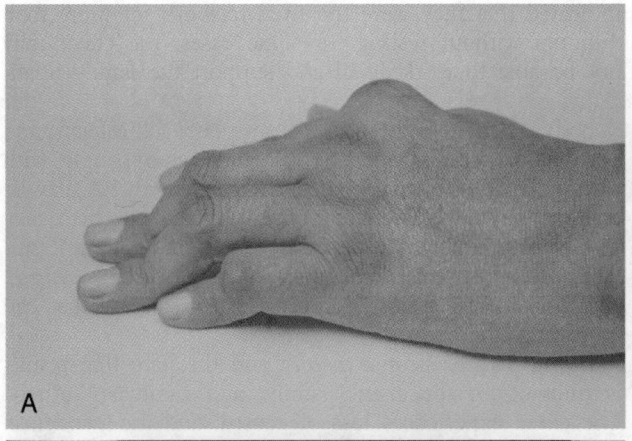

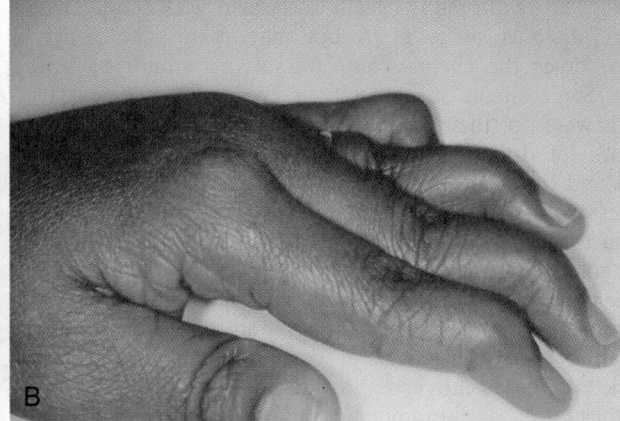

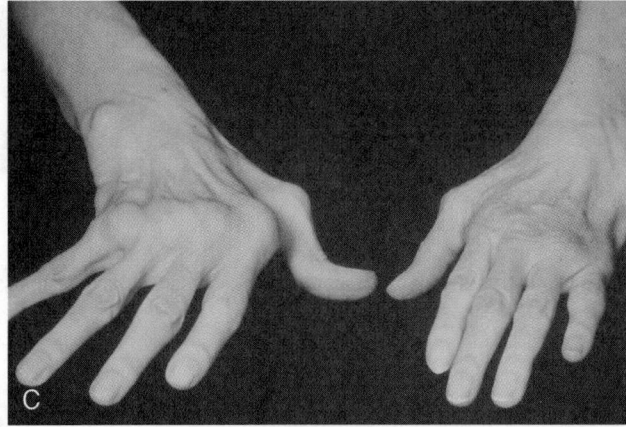

Figure 24–6. Common joint deformities seen in rheumatoid arthritis. *A,* Boutonniére, or buttonhole. *B,* Swan neck. *C,* Ulnar deviation (on left). (From the Arthritis Teaching Slide Collection, copyright 1980. Used by permission of the Arthritis Foundation.)

mities, especially in the hands and feet (Fig. 24–6). Extensive wrist involvement can result in carpal tunnel syndrome (see Chapter 54 for assessment and management).

The nurse palpates the tissues around the joints to elicit pain or tenderness associated with other rheumatoid complications. For example, Baker's cysts (enlarged popliteal bursae) may occur and cause tissue compression and pain. Tendon rupture is also common, particularly rupture of the Achilles tendon.

Systemic Manifestations. Numerous extra-articular clinical manifestations are associated with advanced disease. Consequently, the nurse assesses other body systems to ascertain systemic involvement. Moderate to severe weight loss, fever, and extreme fatigue are common in late disease exacerbations, often called "flares." Approximately 25% of clients have the characteristic round, movable, nontender subcutaneous nodules, which most often appear on the ulnar surface of the arm. These nodules disappear and reappear at any time and are associated with severe, destructive disease. They occasionally open and become infected, but otherwise they do not usually cause a problem.

Inflammation of the blood vessels results in vasculitis, particularly of small to medium-sized vessels. When arterial involvement (RA) occurs, major organs and body systems become ischemic and malfunction. Ischemic skin lesions appear in groups as small, brownish spots, most commonly around the nail bed (periungual lesions). The nurse and health care provider monitor the number of lesions and note their location each day. An increased number of lesions indicates increased vasculitis; a decreased number indicates decreased vasculitis. The nurse also carefully assesses any larger lesions that appear on the lower extremities; they often lead to ulcerations, which heal slowly as a result of decreased circulation. Peripheral neuropathy associated with decreased circulation can cause foot drop and paresthesias (burning and tingling sensations), most often in the elderly.

Respiratory complications manifest as pleurisy, pneumonitis, diffuse interstitial fibrosis, and pulmonary hypertension. Cardiac complications include pericarditis and myocarditis. The nurse also assesses for ocular involvement, which typically manifests as iritis and scleritis. If either of these complications is present, the nurse notes that the sclera of one or both eyes is reddened and the pupils have an irregular shape.

Associated Syndromes. Several syndromes are seen in clients with advanced RA. The most common is Sjögren's syndrome, which includes a triad of
- Dry eyes (keratoconjunctivitis sicca [KCS], or the sicca syndrome)
- Dry mouth (xerostomia)
- Dry vagina (in some cases)

In Sjögren's syndrome, immune complexes and inflammatory cells are thought to obstruct secretory glands and ducts. The syndrome is usually associated with connective tissue diseases such as RA but may occur alone. The nurse notes the client's complaint of dry mouth or dry eyes. Some clients state that their eyes feel "gritty," as if sand were in their eyes. The nurse also inspects the mouth for dry, sticky membranes and the eyes for redness and lack of tearing.

Less commonly observed is Felty's syndrome, which is characterized by RA, hepatosplenomegaly (enlarged liver and spleen), and leukopenia.

Caplan's syndrome is characterized by the presence of rheumatoid nodules in the lungs and pneumoconiosis, which is noted primarily in coal miners and asbestos workers. The health care provider diagnoses these syndromes by physical examination and diagnostic testing.

➤ Psychosocial Assessment

Rheumatoid arthritis can be a crippling disease. After 10–15 years of having the disease, fewer than 50% of clients are totally independent in ADLs. These physical limitations result in role changes in the family and society. For example, the person may not be able to cook for the family or be an active sexual partner. In addition, extreme fatigue often causes clients to desire an early bedtime and may result in a reluctance to socialize. In a classic nursing study by Crosby (1991), 52% of 101 people with RA indicated that they were too tired to work for more than 4 hours without resting. In some cases, the client may not be able to work at all and support the family financially.

Body changes may also cause poor self-esteem and body image. Because many societies value people with physically fit, attractive bodies, the client with RA may be embarrassed to be seen in public places. The client may grieve, may experience depression, and may attempt suicide. The client may experience a feeling of helplessness, accompanied by a loss of control over a disease that can "consume" the body.

Living with a chronic disease and the pain that results is difficult for the client, family, and significant others. The client experiences loss of control and independence. Chronic suffering affects quality of life (Dildy, 1996). The nurse assesses the client's emotional and mental status in relation to the disease and its problems and evaluates the client's support systems and resources.

➤ Laboratory Assessment

Laboratory tests help to support a diagnosis of rheumatoid arthritis, but no single test or group of tests can confirm it. Chart 24–8 summarizes the common laboratory tests that the health care provider uses for diagnosis of connective tissue disease.

Chart 24–8

Laboratory Profile: Connective Tissue Disease

Test	Normal Range for Adults	Significance of Abnormal Findings
Rheumatoid factor Rose-Waaler	• Negative	• Elevations of either titer (increase in number at right of colon) indicative of possible CTD • Increased Rose's titer indicative of RA (seropositive); not a sensitive test
Latex agglutination	• <1:16	• Latex titer not as specific to one disease, but quite sensitive test
ANA (total)	• Negative (if positive, types of ANA identified, e.g., anti-DNA, anti-DNP, anti-RNA, to indicate what part of cells involved)	• Elevations common in SLE, PSS, RA, and other inflammatory CTDs (5% of healthy adults have positive ANA results)
Serum complement (C' or CH_{50})	• Varies greatly among laboratories	• Decreased value indicative of active autoimmune disease such as SLE
LE preparation	• Negative	• A type of ANA (anti-DNP); not reliable because negative result does not rule out SLE; can be used as screening test
SPEP Albumin	• 3.5–5.0 g/dL	• Increased levels of gamma globulins indicative of CTD (inflammatory type)
Globulin		• Increased level of alpha globulins possible in RA
Alpha$_1$ globulin	• 0.1–0.3 g/dL	
Alpha$_2$ globulin	• 0.6–1.0 g/dL	
Beta globulin	• 0.7–1.1 g/dL	
Gamma globulin	• 0.8–1.6 g/dL	
HLA testing (HLA-B27)	• None	• Presence of HLA-B27 indicative of Reiter's syndrome or ankylosing spondylitis

ANA = antinuclear antibody; CTD = connective tissue disease; DNP = dinitrophenol; SLE = systemic lupus erythematosus; PSS = progressive systemic sclerosis; LE = lupus erythematosus; SPEP = serum protein electrophoresis; RA = rheumatoid arthritis; HLA = human leukocyte antigen; ESR = erythrocyte sedimentation rate.

Rheumatoid Factor. The test for rheumatoid factor (RF) measures the presence of unusual antibodies of the IgG and IgM type that develop in a number of connective tissue diseases. Two methods may be used to ascertain the degree to which these antibodies are present in the body: Rose-Waaler and latex agglutination. In both procedures, values are reported as titers.

The Rose-Waaler test is more specific for a diagnosis of RA than the latex but is not as sensitive. A client with a positive Rose-Waaler result probably has RA and is seropositive; a client with a negative test result may or may not have the disease and is seronegative. About 60% of RA clients are seropositive and have a positive titer.

The latex agglutination test is sensitive but is not as specific for RA. Its normal value is less than 1:16 (Tietz, 1995). Generally, the higher the titer, the more active is the disease process.

Antinuclear Antibody Titer. The antinuclear antibody (ANA) test measures the titer of unusual antibodies that destroy the nuclei of cells and cause tissue death. When the fluorescent method is used, the test is sometimes referred to as FANA. If this test result is positive (a value higher than 1:8), various subtypes of this antibody are identified and measured. As with the RF, the higher the titer, the more active is the disease process. ANA is often negative until later in the disease process.

Erythrocyte Sedimentation Rate. The "sed rate," as the ESR is sometimes called, can confirm inflammation or infection anywhere in the body. It is particularly useful in connective tissue disease because the value directly correlates with the degree of inflammation and, later, with the severity of the disease.

Because several laboratory procedures are used to measure ESR, normal values vary; women have higher normal values than men. Generally, a value of 30–40 mm/hour indicates mild inflammation; 40–70 mm/hour, moderate inflammation; and 70–150 mm/hour, severe inflammation.

The ESR is also used to monitor a client's response to anti-inflammatory drug therapy. The value should decrease if the drug dosage is effective.

Serum Complement. In an attempt to destroy the immune complexes, complement (C′) attaches to the complex. If a large amount of complement is used in this lytic process, the concentration of free-floating complement in the blood diminishes. Normal values vary considerably, depending on the laboratory technique used. An abnormal finding is indicated by a decrease in serum complement and is seen primarily in clients with vasculitis.

Serum Protein Electrophoresis. In serum protein electrophoresis, the protein fractions of the plasma are measured using electrical current to separate them. In acute inflammation, the level of alpha globulin is raised, but in chronic inflammatory conditions such as RA, the level of gamma globulin is increased because of the increase in immunoglobulins.

Immunoglobulins. The serum immunoglobulins can be separated into subtypes. In chronic inflammation, IgG

is needed to combine with RF. Thus, in RA the IgG value is typically elevated.

Other Laboratory Tests. The presence of most chronic diseases usually causes mild to moderate anemia, which contributes to the client's fatigue. Therefore, the client's complete blood count (CBC) is monitored for a low hemoglobin, hematocrit, and red blood cell (RBC) count. An increase in white blood cell (WBC) count is consistent with an inflammatory response. A decrease in the WBC count may indicate Felty's syndrome. Thrombocytosis (increased platelets) is common in clients with RA. Additional laboratory tests may be performed, depending on the body systems and organs that may be affected by the disease. For example, if heart involvement is suspected, the health care provider may order cardiac enzymes.

➤ Radiographic Assessment

The standard x-ray is used to visualize the joint changes and deformities that are typical of RA. The computed tomography (CT) scan may help to determine the presence and degree of cervical spine involvement.

➤ Other Diagnostic Assessment

An *arthrocentesis* is a diagnostic procedure that may be used for clients with joint involvement. It may be done at the bedside or in a physician's office or clinic. After administering a local anesthetic, the physician inserts a large-gauge needle into the joint, usually the knee, to aspirate a sample of synovial fluid, which may also relieve pressure. The fluid is analyzed by use of tests described in Chart 24–8. After the procedure, the nurse monitors the insertion site for bleeding or leakage of synovial fluid. If either of these problems occur, the nurse notifies the physician.

A bone scan or joint scan can also assess the extent of joint involvement. Magnetic resonance imaging (MRI) may be performed to assess spinal column disease.

Because RA can affect multiple body systems, tests to diagnose specific systemic manifestations are performed as necessary. For example, electromyography helps to confirm peripheral neuropathy. Pulmonary function tests help to determine the presence of lung involvement.

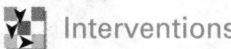 Interventions

As in other types of arthritis, the health care team manages pain by using a combination of drug and nondrug measures. When these measures are no longer effective, surgery may be indicated. The accompanying Client Care Plan highlights the most important nursing interventions for the client with RA.

Nonsurgical Management. Although numerous pain relief modalities are available, the client with RA often needs a variety of medications to relieve pain or slow the progression of the disease.

Drug Therapy. Medications that are prescribed for clients with RA have analgesic, antipyretic, and/or anti-inflammatory actions.

Client Care Plan

The Client with Rheumatoid Arthritis

Nursing Diagnosis No. 1: Chronic Pain related to joint inflammation

Expected Outcomes	Nursing Interventions	Rationale
The client will experience a reduction in joint pain.	■ Give prescribed drugs, as ordered, on time.	■ Giving drugs on time ensures a consistent blood level (e.g., salicylates).
	■ Give analgesic drugs as needed, if ordered, and periods of rest, especially after periods of increased activity (e.g., physical therapy).	■ Supplemental analgesics may be needed to control chronic pain; rest is necessary to prevent overuse of joints and help decreased inflammation.
	■ Provide a warm shower, tub bath, and/or hot compresses after periods of decreased activity or rest.	■ Heat application increases blood flow to the joints to decrease pain and increase joint mobility.
	■ Provide nonpharmacologic pain relief measures, such as imagery, massage, and music therapy. (Determine which of these measures are effective for each client.)	■ Independent nursing interventions help reduce pain and decrease the amount of analgesics needed for pain relief.
	■ Evaluate the effectiveness of all pain relief interventions and document/communicate the outcome to the physician and other involved health care team members. (Also see Chapter 9 for additional interventions and pain assessment tools.)	■ Evaluation of the effectiveness of pain relief interventions helps the health care team plan care for the client. Changes may be necessary if the plan is not effective in meeting the expected outcome.

Nursing Diagnosis No. 2: Impaired Physical Mobility related to fatigue, inflammation, and pain

Expected Outcomes	Nursing Interventions	Rationale
The client will ambulate independently, with or without ambulatory aids.	■ Reinforce the importance of and techniques for therapeutic joint and muscle exercises as taught by the physical therapist.	■ Therapeutic joint and muscle exercises increase joint mobility, decrease pain, and increase muscle strength.
	■ Teach the importance of recreational exercises, such as walking and swimming.	■ Walking and swimming increase muscle tone and enhance psychological well-being.
	■ Reinforce the importance of and techniques for use of ambulatory aids, such as a cane or walker; allow rest periods during ambulation.	■ Ambulatory aids help reduce stress on affected joints and, therefore, reduce pain and inflammation.
	■ Emphasize the client's abilities and strengths in mobility skills.	■ Focusing on the client's abilities rather than deficits builds the client's self-esteem and confidence.

Client Care Plan

Nursing Diagnosis No. 3: Self-Care Deficit (Partial) related to fatigue, pain, stiffness, and joint deformity

Expected Outcomes	Nursing Interventions	Rationale
The client will independently perform activities of daily living (ADLs) with or without the use of assistive-adaptive devices.	■ In collaboration with the occupational therapist, assess the client's abilities in ADLs.	■ The nurse allows the client to perform all ADLs independently. If the client needs assistance, the nurse plans ways to promote independence in these areas.
	■ Set up the client's try, if needed, by opening packages and cartons and cutting food; assess the need for assistive-adaptive devices.	■ The client may be able to self-feed if the tray is set up and/or if assistive devices, such as plate guard, are obtained.
	■ For dressing activities, assess the need for long-handled assistive-adaptive devices and other mechanical aids.	■ The client may be able to dress independently if assistive-adaptive devices are available.
	■ Encourage the client to use large muscle groups and joints instead of smaller ones, if possible.	■ Using larger joints helps prevent stress and pain in small joints (joint protection).
	■ Emphasize the client's abilities in performing ADLs.	■ Focusing on the client's abilities builds self-esteem and confidence.
	■ Teach the client to allow rest periods during ADLs.	■ Rest reduces fatigue that contributes to a decreased ability to perform ADLs.
	■ Assess the client's pain level, and intervene appropriately (see Nursing Diagnosis No. 1).	■ Pain and stiffness contribute to a decreased ability to perform ADLs.

Salicylates. A common drug of choice is salicylates, a type of nonsteroidal anti-inflammatory drugs (NSAIDs), although the selection of drugs varies by health care provider and geographic area. As seen in Chart 24–1, any one of several agents may be used. Large doses of aspirin (ASA, Ancasal✦) may be prescribed unless gastrointestinal distress (nausea, vomiting, or ulcers) occurs or the client has a history of one or more of these symptoms.

The initial dosage of aspirin is typically 12 to 18 tablets each day in divided doses (usually four times a day) until a therapeutic serum salicylate level of 20 to 25 mg/100 mL (25 mg/dL) is achieved, usually in 3 to 6 weeks. The health care provider regulates the dosage so that side effects are minimized and the serum level is less than 30 mg/100 mL. A level higher that this often results in signs of toxicity, such as tinnitus. The nurse asks the client whether he or she has experienced this symptom. If so, the health care provider usually reduces the daily dosage of the drug. Once the client's pain and other clinical manifestations are alleviated or reduced, the dosage can

be adjusted to a maintenance level, which usually falls between 15 and 20 mg/100 mL (not > 1.45 mmol/L).

Nonsteroidal Anti-Inflammatory Drugs. These are often the drug of choice for inflammatory arthritis. The choice of which drug to administer depends on the client's needs and the physician's preference. To minimize gastrointestinal problems, the NSAID may be given with misoprostol (Cytotec), 100 to 200 μg/day. If after 6 weeks or so there is no clinical change, the health care provider may discontinue the NSAID, and another NSAID may be tried instead. This process may be repeated until the appropriate drug is found to be effective for that client.

ELDERLY CONSIDERATIONS

Adverse effects of NSAIDs include gastrointestinal distress and central nervous system changes, especially in the elderly. Many of these agents also cause retention of sodium and water, which poses a life-threatening risk to clients with hypertension, renal disease, or congestive heart failure. Elderly clients are especially vulnerable to these problems. The nurse carefully monitors these clients and reports problems as early as possible to the health care provider.

Gold Salts. When pain and inflammation are not reduced by NSAIDs, gold therapy may be added to the drug regimen as a second-line drug. Unlike the former drugs, gold can induce disease remission as well as reduce pain and inflammation. The most commonly used parenteral preparation is gold sodium thiomalate (Myochrysine). After a small test dose of 10 mg intramuscularly to detect an allergy to the drug, weekly gold injections are given. The dosage increases from 25–50 mg/week until improvement is evident or until a cumulative total of 1000 mg is administered.

If the client responds to gold without having toxic effects, such as rash, blood dyscrasias, or renal involvement, the injections are slowly tapered to every 2 weeks, then every 3 weeks, and then once a month. Before each drug administration, the client's urine is tested for protein level and a complete blood count is taken. If remission does not occur after a total of 1000 mg has been given, the drug is usually discontinued.

Because intramuscular administration of gold preparations is painful, auranofin (Ridaura), an oral gold product, is used more commonly. The client must take this drug daily to achieve a therapeutic serum level. Its major side effect is gastrointestinal symptoms, especially diarrhea, nausea, and vomiting. The nurse teaches the client to report any gastrointestinal problems to the health care provider.

Other Remittive Agents. Other remittive agents may be prescribed, such as the antimalarial drug hydroxychloroquine (Plaquenil) and penicillamine (Cuprimine). These drugs are not used as often as gold in rheumatoid disease because they produce numerous side effects and toxic effects and are often not as effective. The health care provider recommends that clients receiving hydroxychloroquine have an eye examination every 3–6 months to detect changes in vision, because retinal toxicity may occur. Retinal toxicity results in decreased visual acuity. If this complication occurs, the physician discontinues the drug. The side and toxic effects of penicillamine are similar to those of gold.

Cytotoxic Drugs. Methotrexate (MTX) in a low once-a-week dosage, has become the mainstay of therapy for advancing and sustaining RA because it is inexpensive, less toxic than other cytotoxic drugs, and effective. Because any cytotoxic drug can cause *Pneumocystis carinii* pneumonia, some rheumatologists advocate giving pentamidine to clients receiving MTX (Harris, 1997).

The nurse observes for the side and toxic effects of MTX, which include mouth sores, acute dyspnea from pneumonitis, chronic liver inflammation, and bone marrow suppression.

Other cytotoxic agents that may be used are azathioprine (Imuran) and cyclophosphamide (Cytoxan, Procytox✦). In addition to these adverse drug effects, lymphoma and bone marrow suppression may occur with azathioprine administration. Cyclophosphamide (Cytoxan, Procytox✦) is sometimes given to control RA vasculitis; however, this drug may cause leukemia or other types of malignancy.

Chronic Steroid Therapy. For clients who do not experience relief of symptoms from the commonly administered medications, steroids, usually prednisone (Deltasone, Winpred✦, Apo-Prednisone✦), are given for their anti-inflammatory and immunosuppressive effects. Prednisone may also be used short term as bridge therapy when NSAIDs are insufficient and other second-line drugs (remittive agents) have not yet had an effect.

Unfortunately, chronic steroid therapy can result in devastating complications, such as diabetes mellitus, infection, fluid and electrolyte imbalances, hypertension, osteoporosis, and glaucoma. As shown in Chart 24–1, some drug effects are dose related, whereas others are not. The nurse observes the client for complications associated with chronic steroid therapy and reports them to the health care provider. For example, if the client's blood pressure becomes elevated or significant laboratory values change, the nurse notifies the physician.

Analgesic Drugs. Other analgesic drugs may be prescribed to supplement the anti-inflammatory drugs that are specific for RA. Some analgesics include acetaminophen (Tylenol, Exdol✦), propoxyphene (Darvon, Novopropoxyn✦), and propoxyphene napsylate (Darvocet-N). Propoxyphene and its associated products can cause headache, dizziness, and drowsiness. Over a long period, in clients with decreased metabolic rates, this slow-excreting drug may accumulate in the body and may cause death. The nurse teaches the client about the side and toxic effects of these drugs and advises the client to report any unusual symptom or complaint to the physician.

Rest, Positioning, Ice, and Heat. Adequate rest, proper positioning, and ice and heat application are important in pain management (see Chronic Pain in the discussion of degenerative joint disease). If acute inflammation is present, the physical therapist (PT) or assistive nursing personnel applies ice to the "hot" joints for pain relief until the inflammation lessens. The ice pack should not be too heavy.

To relieve morning stiffness or the pain of late-stage disease, the nurse recommends a hot shower for the client rather than a sponge bath or a tub bath. It is often difficult for the client with RA to get into and out of the bathtub, although special hydraulic lifts and tub chairs may be available. Hot packs applied directly to involved joints are also beneficial. Most physical therapy departments have hydrocollators that keep hot packs ready any time they are needed (Fig. 24–7).

Complementary Therapies. As in any client with arthritis, other nonpharmacologic pain relief techniques are available. For example, some clients may achieve relief with transcutaneous electrical nerve stimulation (TENS), hypnosis, acupuncture, imagery, or music therapy. Stress management is also becoming more popular as a pain relief intervention. Chapters 8 and 9 describe these interventions in detail.

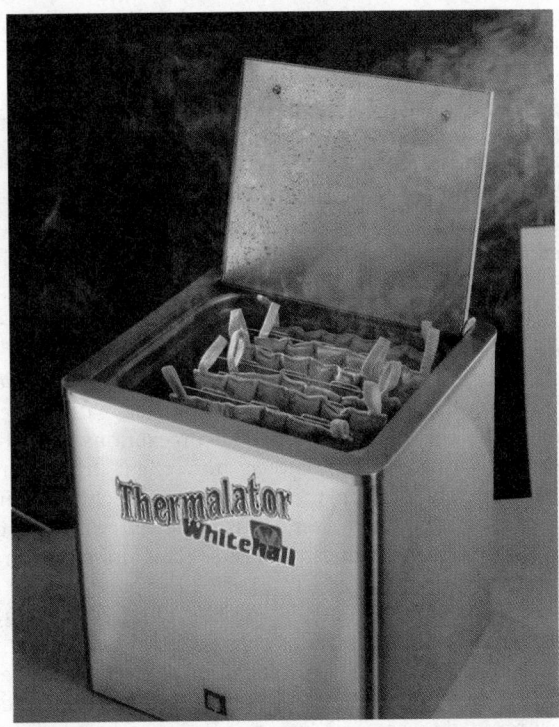

Figure 24–7. Heating units used for keeping hot packs warm. (Courtesy of Whitehall Manufacturing, City of Industry, CA.)

Experimental Therapies. In addition to the drug regimens described earlier, two techniques—pulse therapy and plasmapheresis—are being tried and evaluated to treat severe RA. In pulse therapy, the client receives rapid infusions of high-dose steroids or chemotherapeutic agents, usually over a period of several days. Plasmapheresis is a procedure in which the client's plasma is treated to remove the antibodies that are causing the disease. Sometimes called a plasma exchange, this procedure may be combined with pulse therapy for clients with severe life-threatening disease.

Promotion of Self-Care. Although the physical appearance of a client with severe RA may lead the nurse to believe that independence in ADLs is not possible, the client can use a number of alternative methods to perform these activities. The nurse should not automatically perform activities for the client; clients with RA do not want to be dependent. For example, hand deformities frequently prevent a client from opening packages of food, such as a box of crackers. The client may prefer to use his or her teeth to open the crackers rather than depend on someone else.

In the hospital or long-term care facility, a client may not eat because of the barriers of heavy plate covers, milk in cartons, small packages of condiments, and heavy containers. Styrofoam or paper cups may bend and collapse as the client attempts to hold them. A china or heavy plastic cup with handles may be easier to manipulate. The nurse and client collaborate with the dietitian to allow the client access to food and total independence in eating activity.

When fine motor activities (such as squeezing a tube of toothpaste) become impossible, larger joints or body surfaces can substitute for smaller ones. In this case, the nurse teaches the client to use the palm of the hand to press the paste onto the brush. Devices such as long-handled brushes can allow clients to brush their hair; dressing sticks can facilitate putting on pants. These examples illustrate the need for the nurse to assess the problem area, suggest alternative methods, and refer the client to an occupational or physical therapist for special assistive and adaptive devices if necessary.

Management of Fatigue. Nursing interventions depend, in part, on identifying the factors contributing to fatigue. For example, in a classic nursing study, Crosby (1991) found that increases in pain, sleep disturbance, and weakness were positively associated with increased fatigue. Anemia may also be a contributing factor and may be treated with iron (if an iron deficiency anemia is present), folic acid, or vitamin supplements, prescribed by the health care provider. Chronic normochromic or chronic hypochromic anemia frequently occurs in most chronic, systemic diseases. The nurse also assesses for drug-related blood loss, such as that caused by salicylate therapy or other NSAIDs, by checking the stool for gross or occult blood. Elderly Caucasian women are the most likely clients to experience gastrointestinal bleeding from these medications.

When a client's fatigue results from muscle atrophy, the physician prescribes an aggressive physical therapy program to strengthen muscles and to prevent further atrophy. Clients experience increased fatigue when pain prevents them from getting adequate rest and sleep. Measures to facilitate sleep include promoting a quiet environment, giving warm beverages, and administering hypnotics or relaxants as prescribed, if necessary. Pain relief measures have been discussed.

In addition to identifying and managing specific reasons for fatigue, the nurse assesses the client's daily activities and teaches principles of energy conservation, including

■ Pacing activities
■ Allowing rest periods
■ Setting priorities
■ Obtaining assistance when needed

Chart 24–9 lists specific suggestions for conserving the client's energy and thus increasing activity tolerance.

Enhancement of Body Image. A client's body image may be affected by the disease process and drug therapy as well. Steroids, for instance, can cause a moon-faced appearance, acne, striae, "buffalo humps," and weight gain. The nurse determines the client's perception of these changes and the impact of family and significant others' reactions to them. The most important intervention for the nurse is communicating acceptance of the client. When a trusting relationship is established, the nurse encourages the client to express his or her feelings.

Another way to improve body image while the client is in the hospital or nursing home is the use of personal items. The client's use of a hospital gown reinforces the sick role. The nurse encourages clients to wear their own

---

Chart 24-9

Education Guide: Energy Conservation for the Client with Arthritis

- Balance activity with rest. Take one or two naps each day.
- Pace yourself; do not plan too much for one day.
- Set priorities. Determine which activities are most important, and do them first.
- Delegate responsibility and tasks to your family and friends.
- Plan ahead to prevent last-minute rushing and stress.
- Learn your own activity tolerance and do not exceed it.

---

clothes, to brush their hair, and to use make-up if desired. The nurse assists in making the client as presentable as possible. The use of colored bows for hair, nail polish, and perfume may improve the female client's image and self-concept. Chapter 10 identifies additional strategies for care of a client with an altered body image.

As a reaction to body image disturbance and the presence of a chronic, painful disease, clients may display behaviors indicative of loss. They may use coping strategies ranging from denial or fear to anger or depression. In an attempt to regain control over the effects of the disease process, clients may appear to be manipulative and demanding and may sometimes be referred to as having an "arthritis personality." This personality, which has negative connotations, is a myth. Clients are trying to cope with the effects of their illness and should be treated with patience and understanding. The nurse continually assesses and accepts these behaviors but remains realistic in discussing goals to improve self-esteem. Clients' strengths are emphasized, and previously successful coping strategies are identified.

Nurses need to assess and intervene appropriately for clients who experience pain and suffering. A qualitative nursing study by Dildy (1996) found that clients with RA benefit from nurses who are empathetic, gentle, caring, and cheerful. Additionally, clients want nurses to decrease their suffering and provide comfort (Research Applications for Nursing).

 Continuing Care

Clients with RA are usually managed at home but may be institutionalized in a long-term care setting if they become restricted to bed or a wheelchair. Some clients may be discharged to a rehabilitation facility for several weeks to aid in developing strategies, techniques, and skills for independent living at home.

➤ Home Care Management

The amount of home care preparation depends on the severity of the disease. Structural changes may be necessary if there are deficits in ADLs or mobility. Doors must be wide enough to accommodate a wheelchair or a walker if one is used. Ramps are needed to prevent the client in a wheelchair from being homebound. If the client cannot negotiate stairs, the client must have access to facilities for all ADLs on one floor.

To promote continued homemaking functions, structural changes of countertops and appliances may be needed. The client may also require hand rails and elevated chairs and toilet seats, which facilitate transfers (Fig. 24-8).

➤ Health Teaching

Health teaching is the most important nursing intervention for promoting the client's compliance with a treatment plan. The nurse should take precautions regarding myths and quackery to protect the client from harm. Information about drug therapy, joint protection, energy conservation, rest, and exercise is reviewed with the client, family, and significant others. This information is summarized in Charts 24-1, 24-5, 24-7, and 24-9.

The client with rheumatoid disease often complains of being on an "emotional roller coaster" from coping with a chronic illness every day of life. Control over one's life is an important human need. The client with an unpredictable chronic disease may lose this control, which lowers self-esteem. Health providers must allow the client to make decisions about care. Families and significant others must also include the client in decision making. Although the client's behavior may be perceived as demanding or manipulative, the client's self-esteem cannot be improved

---

➤ Research Applications for Nursing

Nurses Can Have an Impact on Client Suffering

Dildy, S. P. (1996). Suffering in people with rheumatoid arthritis. Applied Nursing Research, 9, 177–183.

This qualitative study attempted to describe the concept of suffering in clients with rheumatoid arthritis (RA). Fourteen people with RA were interviewed; all were Caucasian and well educated. Some clients were in remission, whereas others had active disease. The clients described the changes in their lives as a result of RA and the impact of their suffering. They also shared anecdotes regarding their experiences with nurses and other health care professionals. The general feeling was that nurses need to show empathy, be caring and gentle, and provide comfort, including the administration of medications as needed.

Critique. The study sample was small, and the group was homogeneous. However, the advantage of the interview technique for a qualitative study may outweigh this limitation. An enormous amount of information was collected and analyzed, which provides insight into the life of people with RA.

Possible Nursing Implications. The implications identified by the study were that nurses and other health care professionals need to be more empathetic when caring for clients with RA. Providing comfort is also a major nursing intervention, including touch, receptivity, and gentleness.

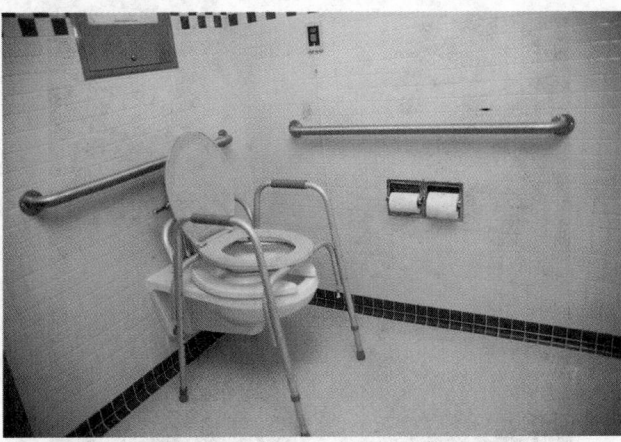

Figure 24–8. Handrails and an elevated toilet seat make transfers easier for the client.

without this important aspect of interpersonal relationships.

Increased dependency also affects the client's sense of control and self-esteem. Some clients ignore their health needs and portray a tough image for others by insisting that they need no assistance. The nurse emphasizes to the client and family that asking for help may be the best decision at times to prevent further joint damage and disease progression.

Social and work roles are dramatically affected by RA. The client may find new friends among others who have the same problem to be a support system to cope with these changes. Becoming an active member of and volunteering for The Arthritis Foundation can help the client to meet social and work needs. Loss of income from being unable to be gainfully employed can also be a major source of stress. The client may qualify for disability benefits through the federal Social Security program. If possible, the client can learn new skills for a less stressful career.

In addition to the interventions just described for self-esteem disturbance, the nurse may need to refer the client to a counselor or to a religious or spiritual leader for emotional support and guidance during times of crisis. The nurse should identify and recommend other support systems within the family and community when necessary.

> ➤ *Health Care Resources*

The need for health care resources for the client with RA is similar to that for the client with degenerative joint disease. A home health nurse or aide, physical therapist, or occupational therapist may be indicated. In collaboration with the discharge planner, the nurse in the hospital or nursing home identifies these resources and makes sure that they are available before the client is discharged.

 Evaluation

The nurse evaluates the care provided for the client with RA. The desired outcomes are that the client

- States that pain and stiffness are reduced after intervention
- Ambulates without personal assistance (may use an ambulatory aid such as a walker)
- Is independent in all ADLs (may use assistive-adaptive devices)
- States that fatigue is decreased
- Participates in daily activities at his or her own pace
- Demonstrates a positive self-esteem as evidenced by participation in daily activities and decision making

LUPUS ERYTHEMATOSUS

Overview

The word lupus is the Latin term for "wolf." In the mid-19th century, the facial rash that was seen in clients with the disease was thought to look like bites caused by a wolf. The rash was usually red, and thus the term *erythematosus*, a Latin word meaning reddened, was added to describe the disease.

There are two main classifications of lupus: discoid lupus erythematosus (DLE) and systemic lupus erythematosus (SLE). A small percentage of clients with lupus have the DLE type, which affects only the skin.

The systemic disorder is a chronic, progressive, inflammatory connective tissue disorder that can cause major body organs and systems to fail. It is characterized by spontaneous remissions and exacerbations, and the onset may be acute or insidious. The condition is potentially fatal, although the survival rate has dramatically improved over the past 20 years. Today more than 85% of clients with systemic lupus are alive 5 years after diagnosis (Hahn, 1997). Improvements in determining the cause, diagnosis, and treatment of lupus account for the prolonged survival of these clients.

Lupus is thought to be an autoimmune process; that is, abnormal antibodies are produced that react with the client's tissues. These antinuclear antibodies (ANAs) primarily affect the deoxyribonucleic acid (DNA) within the cell nuclei. As a result, immune complexes form in the serum and organ tissues, which causes inflammation and damage. The complexes invade organs directly or cause vasculitis (vessel inflammation), which deprives the organs of arterial blood and oxygen.

Many clients with SLE have some degree of kidney involvement, the leading cause of death. Other causes of death from SLE are cardiac and central nervous system involvement.

In kidney disease, renal biopsies show progressive changes within the glomeruli:

- In minimal lupus nephritis, the glomeruli are slightly irregular; immunoglobulins and complement are seen by electron microscopy.
- Focal, or mild, lupus nephritis is characterized by further glomerular changes, and immune complex deposits are common. In this type of lupus, the client begins to show clinical signs of renal impairment.
- In diffuse, severe proliferative nephritis, more than 50% of the glomeruli are affected, and the client is in renal failure.

Lupus affects women between the ages of 15 and 40 years at a rate 8–10 times more often than men. The onset of the disease is most often during the childbearing years, but it has been reported in young children and the elderly.

TRANSCULTURAL CONSIDERATIONS

 Although incidence and prevalence data vary, about 1 in 700 women between the ages of 15 and 64 years have the disease; 1 in 250 African-American women of this age group are affected.

Collaborative Management

 Assessment

It is impossible to describe a typical textbook picture of a client with lupus because of the extreme variability of symptoms among affected clients. When the disease is in remission, the client may appear healthy with no activity limitations. When the disease flares, the client may be so ill that admission to a critical care unit is required. Chart 24–10 highlights the clinical manifestations that occur in clients with systemic lupus.

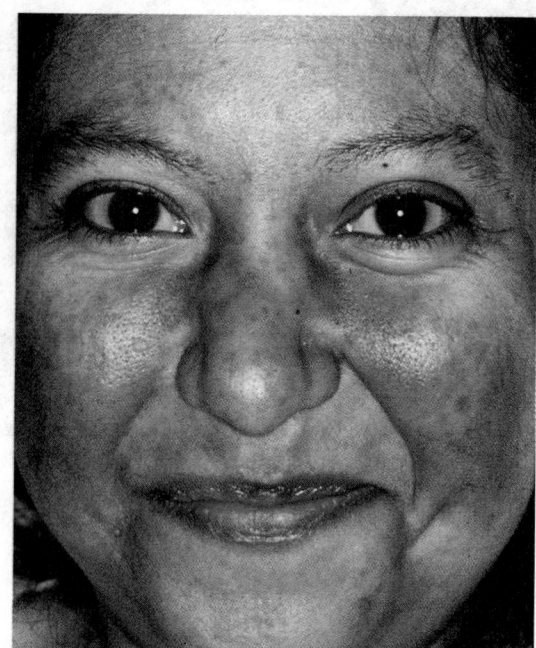

Figure 24–9. The characteristic "butterfly" rash of SLE.

Chart 24–10

Key Features of Systemic Lupus Erythematosus (SLE) and Progressive Systemic Sclerosis (PSS)

SLE	PSS
Skin Manifestations	
• Inflamed, red rash	• Inflamed
• Discoid lesions	• Fibrotic
	• Sclerotic
	• Edematous
Renal Manifestations	
• Nephritis	• Renal failure
Cardiovascular Manifestations	
• Pericarditis	• Myocardial fibrosis
• Raynaud's phenomenon	• Raynaud's phenomenon
Pulmonary Manifestations	
• Pleural effusions	• Interstitial fibrosis
Neurologic Manifestations	
• CNS lupus	• Not common
Gastrointestinal Manifestations	
• Abdominal pain	• Esophagitis
	• Ulcers
Musculoskeletal Manifestations	
• Joint inflammation	• Joint inflammation
• Myositis	• Myositis
Other Manifestations	
• Fever	• Fever
• Fatigue	• Fatigue
• Anorexia	• Anorexia
• Vasculitis	• Vasculitis

CNS = central nervous system.

➤ Physical Assessment/Clinical Manifestations

Skin Involvement. The major and usually only manifestation of discoid lupus is a dry, scaly, raised rash appearing on the face ("butterfly" rash) or upper body or individual round lesions, sometimes referred to as discoid (coin-like) lesions (Fig. 24–9). The nurse observes all skin changes and monitors changes daily while the client is in an acute care setting.

Musculoskeletal Changes. In addition to skin changes, articular involvement occurs in most clients with systemic lupus erythematosus (SLE). The initial joint changes are similar to those seen in rheumatoid arthritis (RA), but severe deformities are not common. Avascular necrosis (bone necrosis from lack of oxygen) is often seen in clients with SLE who have been treated for at least 5 years, usually with steroids. Chronic steroid therapy may cause constriction of small blood vessels supplying the joint causing the tissue to die. The hip is most commonly affected, and the client complains of pain and decreased mobility as a result.

The nurse observes for muscle atrophy, which can result from disuse or from skeletal muscle invasion by the immune complexes (myositis). Myalgia (muscle pain) may also occur. The nurse inspects and palpates major muscles, especially those in the extremities.

Systemic Manifestations. Because SLE is an inflammatory condition, fever is a common finding. The presence of fever is the classic sign of a flare, or exacerbation. Various degrees of generalized weakness, fatigue, anorexia, and weight loss occur. These signs may be the only evidence of impending disease, which makes diagnosis by the health care provider difficult. Consequently, some clients have a diagnosis of "probable SLE."

Any or all body systems may be affected by SLE. Because lupus nephritis is the leading cause of death, the nurse carefully assesses for signs of renal involvement (e.g., changes in urinary output, proteinuria, hematuria, and fluid retention). About 50% of clients with systemic lupus have some type of nephritis.

Pleural effusions are found in almost half of clients with SLE, but this complication is usually not life threatening. Pulmonary restrictive or obstructive changes may not result in overt clinical signs. However, progressive involvement can lead to dyspnea and arterial blood gas abnormalities. The nurse performs a complete respiratory assessment to determine any abnormalities in respiratory pattern or breath sounds.

Pericarditis is the most common cardiovascular manifestation and causes tachycardia, chest pain, and myocardial ischemia. The nurse monitors the client's vital signs at least every 4 hours while the client is in the hospital and reports chest pain immediately to the physician.

Raynaud's phenomenon is noted in 15% of clients with lupus. On exposure to cold or extreme stress, the client complains of the characteristic red, white, and blue color changes and severe pain in the digits caused by arteriolar vasospasm. The nurse may not observe these episodes but should ask clients whether color changes occur when their hands or feet are exposed to cold or when these clients are extremely stressed.

Neurologic manifestations are varied. Central nervous system effects include psychoses, paresis, seizures, migraine headaches, and cranial nerve palsies. Peripheral neuropathies are also common. The nurse performs a neurologic assessment as described in Chapter 43.

The nurse also monitors for reports of abdominal pain. Recurrent abdominal pain occurs frequently, but its cause may not be identified. Mesenteric arteritis, pancreatitis from arteritis of the pancreatic artery, and colonic ulcers can cause abdominal pain in the client with lupus. The nurse may note liver enlargement on assessment of the abdomen, but jaundice is rare. More than 50% of clients have lymph enlargement, and 10% have splenomegaly. The nurse palpates lymph nodes and documents findings.

➤ Psychosocial Assessment

The psychosocial results from lupus can be devastating. In either discoid or systemic disease, the rash can be disfiguring and embarrassing to the client. Young adult women who never had a blemish are confronted with a rash that cannot be completely covered with make-up. If chronic steroid therapy is used, side effects such as acne, striae, fat pads, and weight gain intensify the problem of an already altered body image.

Chronic fatigue and generalized weakness may prevent the client from being as active as in the past. The client may avoid social gatherings and may withdraw from family activities. The unpredictability and chronicity of SLE can cause fear and anxiety. Fear may heighten if the client knows another person with the disease, particularly if the other person has more advanced, severe disease. The myth that lupus is always a fatal condition is still common.

The nurse assesses the client's feelings about the illness to identify areas that require intervention. The nurse should assess the person's usual coping mechanisms and support systems before developing a plan of care.

(For additional information about psychosocial assessment of clients with chronic illness, see Rheumatoid Arthritis in this chapter.)

➤ Laboratory Assessment

Because discoid lupus is not a systemic condition, the only test that is significant is a skin biopsy. The physician gently scrapes skin cells from the rash for microscopic evaluation. The characteristic lupus cell and a number of inflammatory cells confirm the diagnosis.

The immunologic-based laboratory tests that are used to diagnose systemic lupus are the same as those performed for rheumatoid arthritis (RA): rheumatoid factor, antinuclear antibody, erythrocyte sedimentation rate, serum protein electrophoresis, serum complement, and immunoglobulins. The lupus cell preparation (LE cell prep) may also be performed, but this assay is a poor indicator of disease; rather, the test is best used for screening. (See the corresponding section under Rheumatoid Arthritis as well as Chart 24–8.)

In addition to immunologic testing, several tests are performed to evaluate possible involvement of major organs and body systems. A complete blood count (CBC) commonly shows pancytopenia (a decrease of all cell types), probably caused by direct attack of the blood cells or bone marrow by immune complexes. Serum electrolyte levels, renal function, cardiac and liver enzymes, and clotting factors are also routinely assessed to determine other body system functioning.

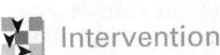 Interventions

The health care provider often prescribes potent drugs that are used topically and systemically. In addition, the client takes precautions to prevent further skin impairment and exacerbations (flare-ups) of the disease. Many of the skin lesions do not disappear, even with treatment, but they usually fade when the disease is in remission.

Drug Therapy. In discoid lupus, the client's major concern is the rash or discoid lesions. Clients with systemic lupus may also have concern about skin changes. Topical cortisone preparations help reduce inflammation and promote fading of the skin lesions. In addition, the health care provider may prescribe the antimalarial hydroxychloroquine (Plaquenil) for some clients to decrease the inflammatory response, but other systemic medications are usually not used (see Chart 24–1).

For clients with systemic lupus, the aim of management is to treat the disease aggressively until remission. In addition to medications for skin lesions, the health care provider often prescribes chronic steroid therapy to treat the systemic disease process. For clients with renal or central nervous system lupus, the health care provider may also order immunosuppressive agents, which are sometimes used for clients with rheumatoid arthritis (see Chart 24–1). Although clinical manifestations improve during remission, maintenance doses of these drugs are usually continued to prevent further exacerbations of disease. The nurse observes for side and toxic effects of these medications and reports their occurrence to the physician.

Skin Protection. Clients with lupus should avoid prolonged exposure to sunlight and other forms of ultraviolet lighting, including certain types of fluorescent light. The nurse instructs clients that, when outdoors, they may need to wear long sleeves and a large-brimmed hat. They should use sun-blocking agents with an SPF (sun protection factor) of 30 or higher on exposed skin surfaces.

In addition, the nurse teaches the client to clean the skin with mild soap (such as Ivory) and to avoid harsh, perfumed substances. The client rinses and dries the skin well and applies lotion. Excess powder and other drying substances are avoided. The client carefully selects cosmetics and should include moisturizers and sun protectors. The nurse may refer the client to a medical cosmetologist who specializes in applying make-up for clients with skin lesions of all types.

The client's hair should receive special attention because alopecia (hair loss) is common. The nurse recommends mild protein shampoos and avoidance of harsh treatments, such as permanents or frostings, until the hair regrows during remission.

 Continuing Care

Continuing care for the client with lupus is similar to that for rheumatoid arthritis. The client is generally managed at home but may need repeated hospitalizations during exacerbations of disease. Usually, however, the client does not need rehabilitation or a long-term care facility, because severe joint deformity and prolonged immobility are not common.

Two major differences exist between SLE and rheumatoid arthritis in terms of education of the client and family or significant others. First, the nurse teaches the client with SLE how to protect the skin (Chart 24–11).

Chart 24–11

Education Guide: Skin Protection and Care for Clients with Lupus Erythematosus

- Cleanse your skin with a mild soap like Ivory.
- Dry your skin thoroughly by patting rather than rubbing.
- Apply lotion liberally to dry skin areas.
- Avoid powder and other drying agents, such as rubbing alcohol.
- Use cosmetics that contain moisturizers.
- Avoid direct sunlight and any other type of ultraviolet lighting (including tanning beds).
- Wear a large-brimmed hat, long sleeves, and long pants when in the sun.
- Use a sun-blocking agent with a sun protection factor (SPF) of at least 30.
- Inspect your skin daily for open areas and rashes.

Second, body temperature is monitored carefully in SLE. Fever is the major sign of an exacerbation, during which the client can become seriously ill. The nurse teaches the client to report any other unusual or new clinical manifestation to the health care provider immediately.

Many clients become frustrated that family members, significant others, and the laypeople do not have a good understanding of lupus. When lupus is in complete remission, the client appears to be healthy. However, an exacerbation can necessitate rapid admission to a critical care unit. This unpredictability disrupts the client's life and can cause fear and anxiety. The nurse helps the client identify coping strategies and support systems that can help the client function in the community.

Although The Arthritis Foundation is a general resource for all clients with connective tissue disease, the Lupus Foundation is a national organization, with chapters in every state, that provides information and assistance for clients with lupus. Local support groups and services are offered without charge to the client.

PROGRESSIVE SYSTEMIC SCLEROSIS

Overview

Progressive systemic sclerosis (PSS), one of a family of diseases, is often referred to as systemic scleroderma. "Scleroderma" means hardening of the skin, which is only one clinical manifestation of PSS. As the name implies, PSS is a systemic disease. It is less common than systemic lupus erythematosus (SLE) but is associated with a higher mortality rate. Chart 24–10 shows a comparison of the clinical manifestations of these two diseases.

Progressive systemic sclerosis is a chronic connective tissue disease that is characterized by inflammation, fibrosis, and sclerosis of the skin and vital organs. The inflammatory process is so similar to that of lupus that clients are often diagnosed as having probable SLE until the disease progresses. The inflamed tissue undergoes fibrotic and then sclerotic changes. The most obvious tissue affected is the skin, but renal involvement is the leading cause of death. Unfortunately, clients with PSS do not respond well to steroids and immunosuppressants that are used for lupus, and the mortality rate is, therefore, higher.

The prognosis seems to be worse when the client presents with a group of manifestations that occur at the same time, the CREST syndrome:

- *C*alcinosis (calcium deposits)
- *R*aynaud's phenomenon
- *E*sophageal dysmotility
- *S*clerodactyly (scleroderma of the digits)
- *T*elangiectasia (spider-like hemangiomas)

The disease tends to progress rapidly, but spontaneous remissions and exacerbations can occur.

Little is known about the cause of PSS, but autoimmunity is suspected. The occurrence of more than one case per family is uncommon, although other connective tissue diseases may be noted in the family history.

Progressive systemic sclerosis has been described in

people of all races and in all geographic areas. Women are affected three to four times more often than men. The onset of the disease is usually between the ages of 30 and 50 years. The incidence is higher in coal miners, who have a high incidence of silicosis, which may be a predisposing or contributing factor to PSS.

Collaborative Management

 Assessment

➤ Physical Assessment/Clinical Manifestations

Arthralgia (joint pain) and stiffness are common manifestations that the nurse can elicit during the musculoskeletal examination. The acute inflammation that occurs in people with rheumatoid arthritis (RA) is not common, and deformities are rare.

Findings on inspection of the skin depend on the stage of the scleroderma. Typically, there is a painless, symmetric, pitting edema of the hands and fingers, which may progress to include the entire upper and lower extremities and face. In this edematous phase, the fingers are described as sausage like. The skin is taut, shiny, and free from wrinkles. If diffuse scleroderma occurs, swelling is replaced by tightening, hardening, and thickening of skin tissue; this phase is sometimes called the *indurative phase* (Fig. 24–10). The skin loses its elasticity, and range of motion is markedly decreased; ulcerations may occur. Joint contractures may develop, and the client may be unable to perform ADLs independently.

Major organ damage is likely to develop in clients with diffuse scleroderma, specifically affecting
- The gastrointestinal tract
- The cardiovascular system
- The pulmonary system
- The renal system

Gastrointestinal tract involvement, particularly of the esophagus, is common. The esophagus loses its motility, and dysphagia and esophageal reflux result. A small, slid-

ing hiatal hernia may be present, and swallowing may be difficult. Reflux of gastric contents can cause esophagitis and subsequent ulceration, particularly in the lower two thirds of the esophagus. Intestinal changes are similar to those of the esophagus. Peristalsis is diminished, which causes clinical manifestations similar to a partial bowel obstruction; malabsorption is a frequent complication.

In addition to assessing problems of the digestive tract, the nurse observes for cardiovascular manifestations. Raynaud's phenomenon occurs in various degrees in most clients with progressive systemic sclerosis. On exposure to cold or emotional stress, the small arterioles in the digits of both hands and feet rapidly constrict, which causes decreased blood flow. In severe cases, the client experiences digit necrosis, excruciating pain, and autoamputation of distal digits (the tips of digits fall off spontaneously). (See Chapter 38 for a complete discussion of this disorder.) The nurse notes vasculitic lesions, often around the nail beds (periungual lesions), in many clients. Myocardial fibrosis, another common problem, is evidenced by electrocardiographic (ECG) changes, cardiac dysrhythmias, and chest pain.

Lung involvement in the client with PSS may go undetected until autopsy. Fibrosis of the alveoli and interstitial tissues is present in almost all clients with the disease, but clinical manifestations may not be present.

Renal involvement is an important aspect of the overall disease process and frequently causes malignant hypertension and death. The nurse assesses for signs of impending organ failure, such as changes in urinary output.

➤ Laboratory Assessment

The laboratory findings in a client with PSS are similar to those in a client with systemic lupus. Clinical findings and the client's response to drug therapy help the health care provider differentiate the two diseases. Additional tests ordered for the client depend on which organs seem to be affected. Upper and lower gastrointestinal series are commonly performed because of the frequency of gastrointestinal clinical manifestations.

 Interventions

The aim of medical management of PSS is to force the disease into remission and thus slow disease progression. The health care provider uses drug therapy primarily for this purpose, but it is often unsuccessful. Systemic steroids and immunosuppressants are used in large doses and often in combination.

Local skin protective measures can help to maintain the client's skin integrity. The nurse teaches the client to use mild soap and lotions and gentle cleaning techniques. The skin should be inspected daily for further changes or open lesions. Skin ulcers are treated according to their type and location.

In addition to drug therapy to control the overall disease process, specific measures can provide comfort. The client with PSS not only experiences chronic joint pain but also has severe, acute pain during episodes of Raynaud's phenomenon. A bed cradle and footboard keep

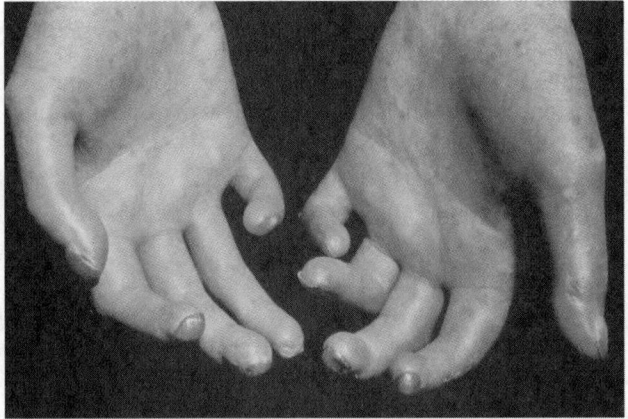

Figure 24–10. Late-stage skin changes seen in clients with progressive systemic sclerosis. (From the Arthritis Teaching Slide Collection, copyright 1980. Used by permission of the Arthritis Foundation.)

Chart 24–12

Nursing Care Highlight: The Client with Progressive Systemic Sclerosis and Esophagitis

- Keep the client's head elevated at least 60 degrees during meals and for at least 1 hour after each meal.
- Provide small, frequent meals rather than three large meals each day.
- Give the client small amounts of food for each bite, and explain the importance of chewing each bite carefully before swallowing.
- Provide semisoft foods, such as mashed potatoes and pudding or custard; liquids are most likely to cause choking.
- Collaborate with the dietitian about the client's diet.
- Teach the client to avoid foods that increase gastric secretion, for instance, caffeine, pepper, and other spices.
- Give antacids if the physician prescribes them.

---

bed covers away from the skin in severe cases. The nurse adjusts the room temperature to prevent chilling, which can precipitate digit vasospasm. The client who can tolerate touching of the affected areas can wear gloves and socks to increase warmth. Because cigarette smoking and extreme emotional stress can also cause recurrence of symptoms, the client should try to avoid or minimize these factors as much as possible.

The client with esophageal involvement may need small, frequent meals rather than the traditional three meals daily. The client should minimize the intake of foods and liquids that stimulate gastric secretion (e.g., spicy foods, caffeine, and alcohol). The nurse instructs the client to keep his or her head elevated for 1–2 hours after meals. The client may need to be in this position continuously. Histamine antagonists and antacids help to reduce and neutralize gastric acid. To help the client avoid choking, the nurse collaborates with the dietitian for dietary changes (Chart 24–12).

Nursing care for the client with joint pain and decreased mobility is very similar to that for the client with rheumatoid arthritis (see Rheumatoid Arthritis earlier).

 Continuing Care

Continuing care for the client with PSS is similar to that for the client with lupus. The client is treated at home but may need frequent hospitalizations if major organ involvement occurs during exacerbations.

GOUT

Overview

Gout, or gouty arthritis, is a systemic disease in which urate crystals deposit in joints and other body tissues, causing inflammation. The cause and treatment of gout have been firmly established. The classic case of well-

advanced disease is seldom seen today unless the client does not comply with the therapeutic regimen. There are two major types of gout: primary and secondary.

Primary gout is the most common type and results from one of several inborn errors of purine metabolism. An end-product of purine metabolism is uric acid, which is usually excreted by the kidneys. In primary gout, uric acid production exceeds the excretion capability of the kidneys, and sodium urate is deposited in synovium and other tissues, which results in inflammation. Primary gout is inherited as an X-linked trait; males are affected through female carriers. About 25% of clients have a family history of gout. Primary gout affects middle-aged and older men (85–90% of clients with gout) and postmenopausal women. The peak time of onset is during a person's 30s and 40s.

Secondary gout involves hyperuricemia (excessive uric acid in the blood) that is caused by another disease. Secondary gout affects people of all ages. Renal insufficiency, diuretic therapy, and certain chemotherapeutic agents decrease the normal excretion of waste products, including uric acid. Disorders such as multiple myeloma and certain carcinomas bring about increased uric acid production because of greater turnover of cellular nucleic acids. Treatment involves management of the underlying disorder.

There are four phases of the primary disease process: asymptomatic hyperuricemic, acute, intercritical (intercurrent), and chronic. The client is usually unaware of the asymptomatic hyperuricemic phase unless he or she has had a serum uric acid level determination. The client's serum level is elevated, but no overt signs of the disease are present.

The first "attack" of gouty arthritis begins the acute phase. The client experiences excruciating pain and inflammation in one or more small joints, usually the metatarsophalangeal joint of the great toe. Of all clients with gout, 75% have inflammation of this joint (podagra) as the initial manifestation.

Months or perhaps years can pass before additional attacks occur; this is the intercritical, or intercurrent, phase of the disease. The client is asymptomatic, and no abnormalities are found on examination of the joints.

After repeated episodes of acute gout, deposits of urate crystals develop under the person's skin and within major organs, particularly in the renal system. The client is then classified as having chronic tophaceous gout. Urate kidney stone formation is more common than renal insufficiency in chronic gout.

Collaborative Management

 Assessment

The historical data that the nurse collects include age, sex, and a family history of gout. Gout affects men, particularly those who have relatives with gout. A complete medical history is needed to determine whether gout has been caused by another problem. In women, especially, there is a tendency to overuse diuretics, which can lead to secondary gout.

Acute Gout. Overt manifestations are present in the acute and chronic phases of gout. The nurse encounters a client with acute gout most often because chronic gout is not common today in the United States. Joint inflammation is the most frequent finding and is usually so painful that the client seeks medical care. The nurse uses inspection skills only; the inflamed area is usually too painful and swollen to be touched or moved.

Chronic Gout. When the client has chronic gout, the nurse inspects the skin for tophi, or deposits of sodium urate crystals (Fig. 24–11). Common sites for tophi are the ear, arms, and fingers near joints. The tophi are hard on palpation and are irregular in shape. When the skin over the tophi is irritated, it may break open, and a yellow, gritty substance is discharged. Infection may result. Although tophi may occur anywhere, they commonly appear on the outer ear.

Other manifestations of chronic gout include signs of renal calculi (stones) or renal dysfunction. Stones develop in about 20% of clients with gout. In some cases, urate kidney stones occur before the arthritis is present.

The health care provider orders determinations of serum uric acid levels to validate hyperuricemia. Because the serum uric acid level can be altered by food intake, serial measurements are usually taken. A consistent level of more than 8 mg/100 mL is generally considered abnormal. Urinary uric acid levels are also measured; an overproduction of uric acid is confirmed by an excretion of more than 600 mg per 24 hours after a 5-day restriction of purine intake.

The health care provider may order renal function tests, such as blood urea nitrogen (BUN) and serum creatinine level, to monitor possible kidney involvement. A definitive diagnostic test for the disease is synovial fluid aspiration (arthrocentesis) to detect the needle-like crystals that are characteristic of the disorder (see Other Diagnostic Assessment under Rheumatoid Arthritis.)

 Interventions

Gout is one of the easiest diseases for the health care provider to diagnose and treat in its early phases. If the client receives treatment and complies with drug therapy, the client should experience no further symptoms and no change in body image or lifestyle. The client with gout is usually treated on an outpatient basis.

Drug Therapy. Drug therapy is the primary component of management for clients with gout. In acute gouty "attacks," the inflammation subsides spontaneously within 3–5 days, but most clients cannot tolerate the pain for that long. The drugs used in acute gout are different from those used in chronic gout. The physician typically prescribes a combination of colchicine (Colsalide, Novocolchicine✦) and a nonsteroidal anti-inflammatory drug, such as indomethacin (Indocin, Novomethacin✦) or ibuprofen (Motrin, Amersol✦), for acute gout. The client takes these medications until the inflammation subsides, usually for 4–7 days, or until severe diarrhea occurs (a side effect of colchicine).

For clients with chronic gout, the health care provider prescribes drugs to promote uric acid excretion or to reduce its production on a continuous, maintenance basis. Allopurinol (Zyloprim) is the drug of choice. As a xanthine oxidase inhibitor, it prevents the conversion of xanthine to uric acid. Probenecid (Benemid, Benuryl✦) is also effective as a uricosuric drug in gout (it promotes excretion of excess uric acid). Combination drugs, such as ColBenemid, that contain probenecid and colchicine are also available. The health care provider and nurse monitor serum uric acid levels to determine the effectiveness of these medications.

Diet Therapy. Whether to recommend special dietary restrictions for clients with gout is controversial. Some physicians advocate a strict low-purine diet, advising the clients to avoid such foods as organ meats, shellfish, and oily fish with bones, such as sardines. Some health care providers and dietitians believe that limiting protein foods, especially red and organ meats, is sufficient. Still others do not believe that diet restrictions affect treatment. It is well known, however, that excessive alcohol intake and fad "starvation" diets can cause a gouty attack. The nurse helps clients determine which foods may precipitate a gout attack.

In addition to food and beverage restrictions, clients with gout should avoid all forms of aspirin and diuretics because they may precipitate an attack. Likewise, excessive physical or emotional stress can exacerbate the dis-

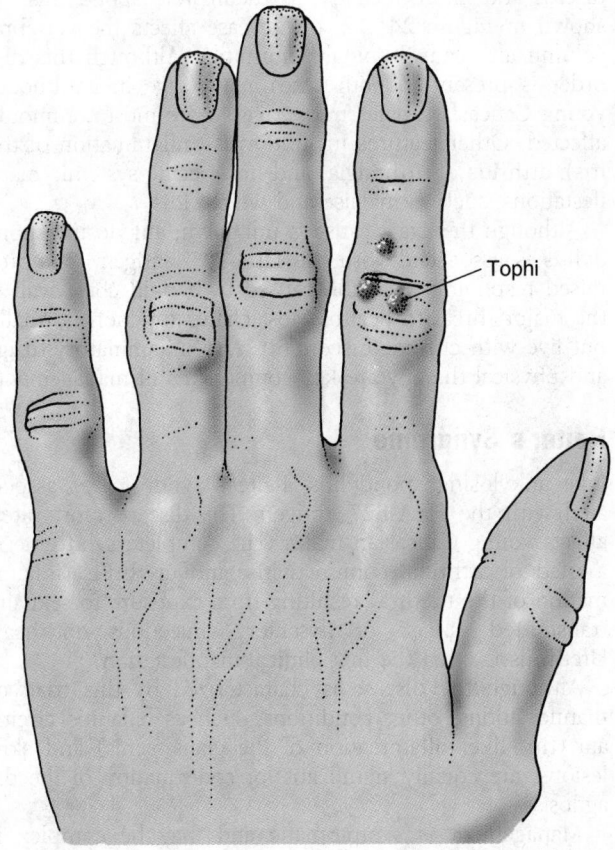

Figure 24–11. Typical appearance of tophi, which may occur in chronic gout, on an index finger.

Tophi

ease. The nurse may need to teach stress management techniques (see Chap. 8).

Having the client drink more fluids is one of the best measures to prevent urinary stone formation. Such a measure helps to dilute the urine and prevent sediment formation. Uric acid is less likely to form urinary stones in urine that has a high pH because it is more soluble in that environment. The client's urinary pH can be increased by intake of alkaline ash foods, such as citrus fruits and juices, and milk and certain dairy products. However, the value of adhering to a strict diet that is rich in these foods is questionable.

The client with a diagnosis of gout is seldom hospitalized unless renal complications develop. If the client follows the prescribed interventions, chronic tophaceous gout should not develop.

OTHER CONNECTIVE TISSUE DISEASES

The care of clients with connective tissue diseases (CTDs) is often similar regardless of the specific diagnosis. This section describes other fairly common diseases that are classified as CTDs.

Polymyositis/Dermatomyositis

Polymyositis is a diffuse, inflammatory disease of striated muscle that causes symmetric weakness and atrophy. When a rash accompanies polymyositis, the disease is called *dermatomyositis*. Both diseases vary in their mode of onset and progression and are characterized by spontaneous remissions and exacerbations. Women are affected twice as often as men, and 30- to 60-year-olds are most susceptible to either disease.

In addition to proximal muscle and possible skin involvement, clients typically have polyarthritis, polyarthralgia (pain around multiple joints), and Raynaud's phenomenon (see Chap. 38). Clients with dermatomyositis have the characteristic heliotrope (lilac) rash and periorbital edema. Malignant neoplasms occur more frequently in these clients than in the rest of the population; as many as 30% of clients older than 55 have internal malignancies. Many clients have difficulty in swallowing or talking because of severe muscle weakness.

Clients are treated with high-dose steroids, immunosuppressive agents, and supportive care, with particular attention to nutrition.

Systemic Necrotizing Vasculitis

Necrotizing vasculitis is a term for a group of diseases whose primary manifestation is arteritis (inflammation of arterial walls), which causes ischemia in tissues usually supplied by the involved vessels.

Polyarteritis nodosa affects middle-aged men and involves every body system. Treatment is similar to that for clients with systemic lupus, but the prognosis is not as promising. Renal disorders and cardiac involvement are the most frequent causes of death.

Hypersensitivity vasculitis is the most common form of vasculitis and primarily causes skin lesions as an allergic response to drugs, infections, or tumors.

Takayasu's arteritis, or the aortic arch syndrome, is also called the "pulseless" disease. Women in their 20s, particularly those of Japanese descent, are affected most often. Cerebral ischemia is manifested by visual changes, syncope, and vertigo.

The drug of choice for most types of vasculitis is chronic steroid therapy.

Polymyalgia Rheumatica

Polymyalgia rheumatica (PMR) is a clinical syndrome characterized by stiffness, weakness, and aching of the proximal musculature (i.e., the shoulder and pelvic girdles). Systemic manifestations, such as fever, arthralgias (pain around joints), and weight loss, occur in the majority of cases. The disease commonly occurs in women older than 50 years and typically responds to steroid therapy in 3–5 days.

Giant cell (temporal) arteritis is frequently associated with PMR. The branches of the aorta are vasculitic, which causes headaches and changes in vision. This disorder is easy to miss because most clients with PMR are elderly women who complain of declining vision (also an age-related change). Corticosteroids are highly effective in controlling giant cell arteritis.

Ankylosing Spondylitis

Ankylosing spondylitis is also known as Marie-Strümpell disease and, more recently, as rheumatoid spondylitis. As shown in Figure 24–12, the disease affects the vertebral column and causes spinal deformities. Although this disorder is present in both sexes at any age in adulthood, young Caucasian males under age 40 are most commonly affected. Other features include iritis (inflammation of the iris), arthritis or arthralgia, and nonspecific systemic manifestations, such as malaise and weight loss.

Although the exact cause is unknown, ankylosing spondylitis is associated with the HLA-B27 antigen. Compromised respiratory function caused by a rigid chest wall is the major threat to health. Most clients function normally but live with chronic discomfort. Anti-inflammatory drugs and physical therapy are key components of management.

Reiter's Syndrome

Like ankylosing spondylitis, Reiter's syndrome is associated with the HLA-B27 antigen. The disease most often affects young Caucasian males. The complete syndrome is a triad of arthritis, conjunctivitis, and urethritis (inflammation of the urethra) resulting from exposure to sexually transmitted disease or dysentery (infectious diarrhea). Urethritis is often the first clinical manifestation.

Although the disease is characterized by this triad of manifestations, other conditions, such as balanitis circinata (ring-like inflammation of the glans penis) and skin lesions, are equally significant for confirmation of the diagnosis.

Management is symptomatic and may be complex if there is organ involvement. Nonsteroidal anti-inflammatory drugs and physical therapy are generally prescribed.

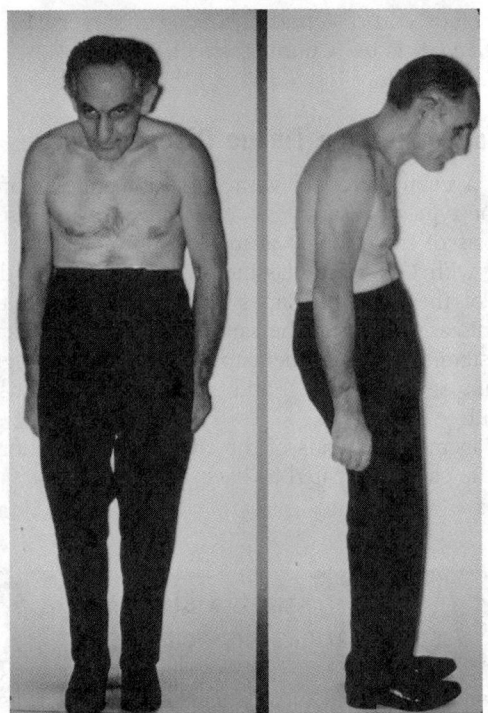

Figure 24–12. Spinal deformity and posture that are often seen in clients with advanced spondylitis. (From the Arthritis Teaching Slide Collection, copyright 1980. Used by permission of the Arthritis Foundation.)

Sjögren's Syndrome

In clients with Sjögren's syndrome, inflammatory cells and immune complexes obstruct secretory ducts and glands. As a result, the client has dry eyes (sicca syndrome), dry mouth (xerostomia), and dry vagina. In severe cases, swelling of the parotid and lacrimal areas and systemic manifestations, such as fever and fatigue, occur. Of clients with the syndrome, 50% have an associated disease, such as rheumatoid arthritis (RA).

Local management includes meticulous mouth, eye, and perineal care and the use of artificial tears and saliva. Systemic steroids may also be administered. Without treatment, the client can lose vision, and oral ulcerations, dental caries, and difficulty in swallowing or talking may ensue.

Infectious Arthritis

Any infectious agent can invade the joint space and cause inflammation and tissue destruction. Certain pathogens, such as *Staphylococcus aureus,* destroy tissue rapidly; others, especially viruses, do not cause irreversible damage. The cornerstone of management is local or systemic antibiotic therapy.

Lyme Disease

Lyme disease has been added to the list of connective tissue diseases (CTDs). Unlike many CTDs, however, the cause has been identified. The infected deer tick (*Ixodes dammini*) transmits a bacterium (a spirochete) that causes a circular rash, malaise, fever, headache, and muscle or joint aches.

If Lyme disease is not diagnosed and treated, later complications, such as arthritis, enlarged lymph nodes, and neurologic and cardiac problems, can result. Prompt treatment with antibiotics, such as tetracycline, is usually effective. A new vaccine to prevent Lyme disease, Lymrex, is being tested for use in humans. Chart 24–13 lists ways to avoid Lyme disease.

Pseudogout

Pseudogout is a disease that mimics the clinical manifestations of gout. The crystals that deposit in joints, however, are calcium pyrophosphate, not sodium urate. Most often, these crystals migrate to cartilage, but they can also deposit in tendons, ligaments, and synovium.

The client most susceptible to pseudogout is an elderly male who is hospitalized. Although the cause is not certain, the incidence is highest in men who have metastatic cancer or endocrine imbalances, such as hypothyroidism. Nonsteroidal anti-inflammatory drugs usually control the manifestations of the disease.

Disease-Associated Arthritis

A number of diseases can cause secondary arthritis. Tuberculosis, Crohn's disease, ulcerative colitis, hemophilia, psoriasis, and sickle cell anemia are typical examples. To manage joint involvement, the primary disease is treated. For example, when a client with Crohn's disease has a remission, joint manifestations also subside. Conditions in which joint involvement can occur are presented in Table 24–3.

Chart 24–13

Health Promotion Guide: Prevention and Early Detection of Lyme Disease

- Avoid heavily wooded areas or areas with thick underbrush.
- Walk in the center of the trail.
- Avoid dark clothing. Lighter-colored clothing makes spotting ticks easier.
- Use an insect repellent on your skin and clothes in an area where ticks are likely to be found.
- Wear long-sleeved tops and long pants.
- Wear closed shoes and a hat or cap.
- Bathe immediately after being in an infested area, and inspect your body for ticks (about the size of a pinhead), paying special attention to your arms, legs, and hairline.
- Gently remove with tweezers or fingers any tick that you find. Dispose of the tick by flushing it down the toilet (burning a tick could spread infection).
- Wait 4 to 6 weeks after being bitten by a tick before being tested for Lyme disease (testing before this time is not reliable).
- Report symptoms, such as a rash or influenza-like illness, to your physician.

TABLE 24–3

Common Disorders Associated with Arthritis

- Crohn's disease
- Ulcerative colitis
- Tuberculosis
- Hemophilia
- Whipple's disease
- Intestinal bypass surgery
- Hyperparathyroidism
- Hyperthyroidism
- Diabetes mellitus
- Sickle cell anemia crisis
- Psoriasis
- Infection

Fibromyalgia

The term *fibromyalgia,* also called fibrositis, describes a syndrome characterized by trunk, extremity, and facial pain and tenderness without other objective findings. The primary manifestations are pain, muscle stiffness and spasm, sensory changes, and exhaustion, which may be attributable to severe sleep disturbances. Tender areas, known as trigger points, typically can be palpated to elicit pain in a predictable, reproducible pattern. Physical therapy, nonsteroidal anti-inflammatory drugs, and muscle relaxants usually provide temporary relief.

In most clients, fibrositis is the result of deep sleep deprivation. Clients may need hypnotics and other sleep-inducing methods to overcome this sleep disturbance. Antidepressive agents, such as amitriptyline (Elavil, Apo-Amitriptyline✦) or nortriptyline (Pamelor), may promote sleep and reduce muscle spasm. These drugs should be used with caution in the elderly because they can cause confusion and orthostatic hypotension. Trazodone (Desyrel) is the preferred drug for this population. The nurse observes the client for side effects and monitors for postural blood pressure changes.

Secondary fibrosis syndromes can accompany any connective tissue disease, particularly lupus and rheumatoid disease, and may not necessarily be related to sleep patterns.

Local Inflammatory Disorders

Two of the most common inflammatory conditions are localized to specific connective tissues: bursitis and tendinitis. Both problems are caused by repetitive motion and overuse related to aging, sports, or work injuries. Bursitis is an irritation of subcutaneous tissues and inflammation of the underlying bursae. Tendinitis is inflammation of one or more tendon sheaths.

Tight shoes often irritate the heel and cause bursitis. Diseases, such as rheumatoid arthritis (RA) and gout, and aerobic exercise can lead to bursitis and tendinitis.

The conservative management for both inflammatory conditions includes rest, ice, and nonsteroidal anti-inflammatory agents to relieve pain. More aggressive treatment may include corticosteroid injections or surgery to remove the inflamed tissue (Cunningham, 1994).

Mixed Connective Tissue Disease

When a client presents with clinical manifestations that are not typical of any one connective tissue disease, a diagnosis of mixed CTD is made. Approximately 10% of clients with CTDs are classified as having mixed disease. Some of these are overlap syndromes, in which two or more diseases occur at the same time. Common examples are systemic lupus erythematosus (SLE) plus progressive systemic sclerosis (PSS) and rheumatoid arthritis (RA) plus SLE.

Management depends of the clinical manifestations, but often the client is treated as having SLE.

 CASE STUDY for the Client with **Systemic Lupus Erythematosus**

■ Susan, a 32-year-old Caucasian female, presents at her physician's office where you are a nurse with complaints of a facial rash. On further questioning, you find that she has been more fatigued than usual and has an achy left ankle. Her infant son is 4 months old, and she has just stopped bleeding from her traumatic vaginal delivery (the baby weighed 10 pounds, and she was in labor for 18 hours).

QUESTIONS:

1. When taking a complete history, what other questions should you ask Susan at this time?
2. If Susan has systemic lupus erythematosus (SLE), what other clinical manifestations might she have?
3. What risk factors does she have for SLE?
4. What laboratory tests will the physician most likely order?

SELECTED BIBLIOGRAPHY

Arcury, T. A., Bernard, S. L., Jordan, J. M., & Cook, H. L. (1996). Gender and ethnic differences in alternative and conventional arthritis remedy use among community-dwelling rural adults with arthritis. *Arthritis Care Research, 9*(5), 384–390.

*Crosby, L. (1991). Factors which contribute to fatigue associated with rheumatoid arthritis. *Journal of Advanced Nursing, 16,* 974–981.

Crutchfield, J., Zimmerman, L., Nieveen, J., et al. (1996). Preoperative and postoperative pain in total knee replacement patients. *Orthopaedic Nursing, 15*(2), 65–72.

Cunningham, M. (1996). Becoming familiar with fibromyalgia. *Orthopaedic Nursing, 15*(2), 33–38.

*Cunningham, M. E. (1994). Bursitis and tendinitis. *Orthopaedic Nursing, 13*(5), 13–16, 70.

Dildy, S. P. (1996). Suffering in people with rheumatoid arthritis. *Applied Nursing Research, 9,* 177–183.

Failla, S., Kuper, B. C., Nick, T. G., & Lee, F. A. (1996). Adjustment of women with lupus erythematosus. *Applied Nursing Research, 9*(2), 87–92.

Giger, J. N., & Davidhizar, R. E. (1995). *Transcultural nursing: Assessment and intervention* (2nd ed.). St. Louis, MO: Mosby Year Book.

Gio-Fitman, J. (1996). The role of psychological stress in rheumatoid arthritis. *MedSurg Nursing, 5,* 422–426.

Hahn, B. H. (1997). Management of systemic lupus erythematosus. In W. N. Kelley, S. Ruddy, E. D. Harris, & C. B. Sledge (Eds.), *Textbook of rheumatology* (5th ed., pp. 1040–1056). Philadelphia: W. B. Saunders.

Harris, E. D. (1997). Treatment of rheumatoid arthritis. In W. N. Kelley, S. Ruddy, E. D. Harris, & C. B. Sledge (Eds.), *Textbook of rheumatology* (5th ed., pp. 933–950). Philadelphia: W. B. Saunders.

*Maher, A. B., Salmond, S. W., & Pellino, T. A. (1994). *Orthopedic nursing*. Philadelphia: W. B. Saunders.

Mankin, H. J., & Brandt, K. D. (1997). Pathogenesis of osteo-arthritis. In W. N. Kelley, S. Ruddy, E. D. Harris, & C. B. Sledge (Eds.), *Textbook of rheumatology* (5th ed., pp. 1369–1382). Philadelphia: W. B. Saunders.

McGrath, A. (1997). Clinical snapshot: Raynaud's syndrome. *American Journal of Nursing, 97*(1), 34–35.

Ranawat, C. S., Miyasaka, K. C., Umlas, M. E., & Rodriguez, J. A. (1997). The hip. In W. N. Kelley, S. Ruddy, E. D. Harris, & C. B. Sledge (Eds.), *Textbook of rheumatology* (5th ed., pp. 1723–1738). Philadelphia: W. B. Saunders.

Schumacher, H. R., Jr. (1988). *Primer on the rheumatic diseases*. Atlanta: The Arthritis Foundation.

Solomon, L. (1997). Clinical features of osteoarthritis. In W. N. Kelley, S. Ruddy, E. D. Harris, & C. B. Sledge (Eds.), *Textbook of rheumatology* (5th ed., pp. 1383–1393). Philadelphia: W. B. Saunders.

Tietz, N. W. (1995). *Clinical guide to laboratory tests* (3rd ed.). Philadelphia: W. B. Saunders.

*Wetherbee, L. L. (1994). Caring for the client with rheumatoid arthritis. *Home Healthcare Nurse, 12*(1), 13–18.

Windsor, R. E. M., & Insall, J. N. (1997). The knee. In W. N. Kelley, S. Ruddy, E. D. Harris, & C. B. Sledge (Eds.), *Textbook of rheumatology* (5th ed., pp. 1739–1758). Philadelphia: W. B. Saunders.

Ulak, L. J. (1995). Special considerations for SLE patients. *MedSurg Nursing, 4*(2), 146–148.

SUGGESTED READINGS

Crutchfield, J., Zimmerman, L., Nieveen, J., et al. (1996). Preoperative and postoperative pain in total knee replacement patients. *Orthopaedic Nursing, 15*(2), 65–72.

  The authors report the findings of their descriptive study, which compared pain levels in clients before and after total knee replacement. Participants in the study reported less pain after the surgery (on days 1 and 3) than before the surgery. The researchers also found that different words were used to describe the nature of acute and chronic pain.

*Cunningham, M. E. (1994). Bursitis and tendinitis. *Orthopaedic Nursing, 13*(5), 13–16, 70.

  This article presents a thorough discussion of the pathophysiology, etiology, clinical manifestations, and treatment of two common local inflammatory conditions: bursitis and tendinitis. Nursing care of clients with these conditions is also described.

Gio-Fitman, J. (1996). The role of psychological stress in rheumatoid arthritis. *MedSurg Nursing, 5*, 422–426.

  The author explores the relationship of rheumatoid arthritis (RA) and stress in this article. Studies that show a correlation between stress and RA are summarized. Nursing interventions that can help clients cope with their stress are also discussed.

Chapter 25

INTERVENTIONS FOR CLIENTS WITH HIV AND OTHER IMMUNOLOGIC DISORDERS

The purpose of immune function is to protect the body from disease and stimulate repair when tissue damage occurs. Problems of the immune system can result in inadequate function, excessive function, or inappropriate function. Clients who have inadequate immune function are at increased risk for infection and cancer. Clients who have excessive or inappropriate immune function are at increased risk for tissue damage. For some clients, malfunction of the immune system is the cause of disease; for others, it is the result. All clients with immunologic disorders are at high risk for development of other problems. Therefore, coordination of care through case management, which provides comprehensive, interdisciplinary care, can optimize client health outcomes.

IMMUNODEFICIENCIES

A deficient response of the immune system that is due to a missing or damaged immune component is an *immuno-*deficiency. The immunodeficient person cannot defend adequately against potentially harmful substances that an immunocompetent person can. An immunodeficient person's immune system cannot recognize or eliminate antigens normally, and the person is, therefore, susceptible to infection, malignancy, and other disease.

A *primary* or *congenital* immunodeficiency is one in which the immune malfunction is present from birth. An *acquired* or *secondary* immunodeficiency is one that occurs in a person who has a normally functioning immune system at birth but later becomes immunodeficient as a consequence of disease, injury, exposure to toxins, medical therapy, or unknown cause. These people are referred to as *immunocompromised* because their immune systems have been compromised, resulting in an impaired ability to neutralize, destroy, or eliminate antigens (see Chap. 23).

The immunodeficient client manifests clinical symptoms that vary in severity and occur in multiple body systems. For many immunodeficiencies, the cause is unknown or uncontrollable, the pathophysiology is not well understood, and effective treatment may not be available. The complications, not the actual immune defect, can be treated. Most immunodeficiencies are chronic conditions, and periods of wellness are interspersed with clinical problems.

Regardless of the cause, the immunodeficient person constantly faces the possibility that the next infection might be fatal. Normal environmental exposures to people, objects, and microorganisms may pose significant danger. The nurse is instrumental in teaching the immunodeficient person how to avoid infection and the signs and symptoms of infection. The nurse assesses the client for subtle changes related to early infection and treats the client quickly according to physician's orders. Supporting the client and family is an essential part of nursing care.

Acquired (Secondary) Immunodeficiencies

Acquired Immunodeficiency Syndrome

Overview

Acquired immunodeficiency syndrome (AIDS) is the late stage of a continuum of symptoms that result from infection with the human immunodeficiency virus (HIV). AIDS is not the same as HIV infection, and not everyone infected with HIV has AIDS. Persons with AIDS are profoundly immunosuppressed and usually have lived with HIV for several years before AIDS develops. The nurse provides education, physical care, and psychological support for the person living with AIDS.

AIDS is a serious, debilitating, and eventually fatal disease. To date, 84% of those with AIDS have been between the ages of 25 and 49 years (Table 25–1). To be diagnosed as having AIDS, a person must be infected with HIV and have a clinical disease that indicates cellular

TABLE 25–1

AIDS Cases Among Adults and Adolescents in the United States June 1, 1981–June 1997	
Age (years)	**No. Cases**
13–19	2,953
20–24	22,070
25–29	85,211
30–34	140,559
35–39	136,814
40–44	98,393
45–49	55,302
50–54	29,148
55–59	16,399
60–64	9,214
65+	8,113
Total	604,176 (374,656 deaths)

Data from the Centers for Disease Control and Prevention.
HIV/AIDS Surveillance Report, Mid-year 1997 Edition, 9(1). Atlanta: Author.

▷ Research Applications for Nursing

AIDS Fears and Concerns Among Registered Nurses

Wang, J. F. (1997). Attitudes, concerns, and fear of acquired immune deficiency syndrome among registered nurses in the United States. Holistic Nursing Practice, 11(2), 36–49.

The purpose of this descriptive, correlational study was to explore the attitudes of registered nurses from different educational levels, work settings, and ages with regard to people with AIDS (PWAs). The study used a questionnaire that incorporated the Fear of AIDS (FOA) Scale II along with other questions related to demographics, working conditions, and HIV transmission knowledge. Participants (anonymous volunteers) were 376 registered nurses employed in a variety of settings within one mid-Atlantic state.

The results of this study indicate that, even though the health care profession does not carry a greater risk than the rest of the U.S. population for contracting AIDS, many registered nurses perceive the risk to be high and the stigma great. Not only do many of these nurses fear AIDS, but they have negative attitudes toward gays and IV drug abusers. Younger participants and those more involved with direct patient care likely to have blood contact had greater fear and more negative attitudes.

Critique. The study design was appropriate for the purpose. Reliability and validity data for the instruments used were not presented. The study could have been strengthened by obtaining information about the participants' knowledge level of HIV–AIDS, use of Standard Precautions, and personal experience with people who are HIV-positive.

Implications for Nursing. The study points out that, more than a decade after the cause and transmission paths of AIDS have been elucidated, registered nurses continue to harbor unjustified fear of AIDS and of people with AIDS. Accurate information regarding HIV–AIDS transmission should be integrated into all basic nursing education and agency orientation programs. Yearly updates in the workplace are advisable as are sensitivity training sessions to assist nurses in providing safe, compassionate, individualized nursing care to all clients.

immunodeficiency or CD4+ T-lymphocyte (T4) count below 200/mm^3 or a CD4+ T-lymphocyte total percentage below 14.

The care of the person with AIDS can evoke complex personal issues for nurses. Nurses must acknowledge their own fear of acquiring HIV and any negative attitudes regarding possible client lifestyles contributing to HIV infection, such as intravenous (IV) drug use or homosexual behaviors (see Research Applications for Nursing). Knowledge and practice of appropriate infection control techniques can reduce nurses' fears about becoming infected. To provide competent, compassionate nursing care to the person with AIDS, nurses must suspend judgment.

Pathophysiology

The Centers for Disease Control and Prevention (CDC) classification scheme for HIV infection is based on clinical

TABLE 25–2

Centers for Disease Control and Prevention (CDC) Classification System for HIV Infection and AIDS Case Definition

Clinical Categories	Criteria	CD4+ T-Cell Categories
A1	Asymptomatic, acute (primary HIV or persistent generalized) Lymphadenopathy	≥ 500/μL
A2	Same as A1	200–400/μL
A3	Same as A1	< 200/μL*
B1	Symptomatic, not category A or C	≥ 500/μL
B2	Same as B1	200–400/μL
B3	Same as B1	< 200/μL*
C1	AIDS indicator conditions†	≥ 500/μL
C2	Same as C1	200–400/μL
C3	Same as C1	< 200/μL*

From U.S. Department of Health and Human Services, 1992.
* AIDS indicator T-cell count.
† Candidiasis (bronchi, trachea, lungs, or esophagus)
  Cervical cancer, invasive
  Coccidioidomycosis (disseminated or extrapulmonary)
  Cryptosporidiosis (chronic intestinal)
  Cytomegalovirus disease (other than liver, spleen, or nodes)
  Cytomegalovirus retinitis (with vision loss)
  Encephalopathy (HIV-related)
  Herpes simplex (chronic, or bronchitis, pneumonitis, or esophagitis)
  Histoplasmosis (disseminated or extrapulmonary)
  Isosporiasis (chronic intestinal)
  Kaposi's sarcoma
  Lymphoma (Burkitt's, immunoblastic, or primary brain)
  Mycobacterium avium-intracellulare complex or *M. kansasii* (disseminated or extrapulmonary)
  Mycobacterium tuberculosis
  Mycobacterium
  Pneumocystis carinii pneumonia
  Pneumonia, recurrent
  Progressive multifocal leukoencephalopathy
  Salmonella septicemia
  Toxoplasmosis (brain)
  Wasting syndrome resulting from HIV

conditions associated with HIV infection and three ranges of CD4+ T-lymphocyte counts (Table 25–2). The classification begins with acute infection and spans a continuum that culminates with AIDS. The person with HIV can transmit the virus to others at all stages of disease.

Acute infection (CDC group I) can occur within 1 to 8 weeks after infection with HIV and is characterized by a flu-like syndrome that resolves completely. The next stage is asymptomatic infection (CDC group II), in which the infected person has no signs or symptoms. The first symptomatic stage occurs with the appearance of persistent generalized lymphadenopathy (lymph node enlargement lasting more than 3 months) (CDC group III).

The next stage includes constitutional disease, which can include persistent fever or diarrhea (more than 1 month) or involuntary loss of more than 10% of body weight (CDC group IV-A). Neurologic disease, including dementia, neuropathy, and myelopathy, is an indicator for

CDC group IV-B classification. CDC groups IV-C and IV-D include a CD4 T-lymphocyte (see Chap. 23) count below 200/mm³ and such clinical conditions as opportunistic infections (infection by organisms that take advantage of a defective immune system), recurrent pneumonia, invasive cervical cancer, pulmonary tuberculosis, and other cancers.

The time from initial HIV infection to development of AIDS ranges from 18 months to more than 10 years. The range depends how HIV was acquired and a variety of personal factors. For people who have been transfused with HIV-contaminated blood, for instance, AIDS develops more quickly; for those who become HIV-positive as a result of a single sexual encounter, there is a longer latency period before the condition progresses to AIDS. Other personal factors that may influence progression to AIDS include frequency of re-exposures to HIV, presence of other sexually transmitted diseases (STDs), nutritional status, pregnancy, and stress.

Etiology

AIDS is caused by the profound suppression of immune responses resulting from infection with HIV. Two subtypes of the virus have been identified: type 1 (HIV-1) and type 2 (HIV-2). Type 1 is the form most frequently isolated from infected persons in the Western Hemisphere, Europe, and Asia. Type 2 is endemic to West Africa. Although they differ in viral surface molecules, both subtypes can cause AIDS.

HIV belongs to a special class of viruses known as *retroviruses,* which differ from other viruses in their efficiency of cellular infection. Retroviruses have only ribonucleic acid (RNA) as their genetic material. The most important difference between retroviruses and other viruses is a special complex of enzymes within the retrovirus called *reverse transcriptase* (RT). This enzyme complex increases the efficiency of viral replication once the retrovirus enters a human cell.

Once a retrovirus gains entry into the body and infects a human cell, the RT enzymes force the human cell's deoxyribonucleic acid (DNA) synthesis machinery to use the viral RNA as a pattern and make a piece of human DNA complementary to the viral RNA. This new piece of DNA is then incorporated successfully into the person's cellular DNA, where it acts as a template for viral production. HIV then spreads quickly throughout the lymphoid system, sequestering in macrophages and in the germinal centers of lymph nodes (Volberding, 1994). Throughout the course of infection, HIV is actively replicated by infected T lymphocytes, synthesizing up to 2 billion viral particles daily (Fig. 25–1). After many rounds of replication, these viral particles exhaust the immune system.

The HIV retrovirus attaches to, infects, and ultimately destroys immune system cells with a CD4 surface receptor. These cells include T4 lymphocytes (CD4+ cells) and macrophages. The T4 lymphocyte, also called the helper or inducer lymphocyte, regulates the activity of all immune system cells (see Chap. 23). When infected by HIV, the T4 cell does not function normally, causing general malfunction of the whole immune system. The results of HIV infection are

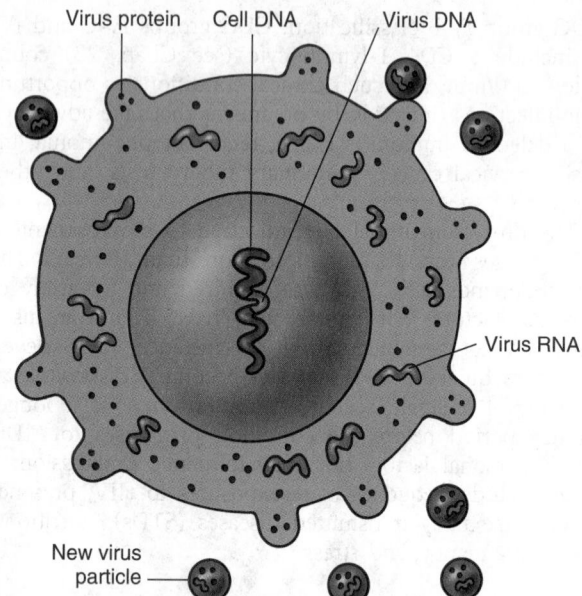

Figure 25–1. A T lymphocyte infected with human immunodeficiency virus. The virus can be seen budding from the infected T cell.

- Lymphocytopenia with selective T4 cell depletion
- Abnormal T-cell function
- Increased production of incomplete and nonfunctional antibodies
- Abnormally functioning macrophages

As a result of these immune dysfunctions, the client with HIV is susceptible to opportunistic infections and cancer. Macrophages infected by HIV are not destroyed by infection; they act as a reservoir for the virus.

Incidence/Prevalence

The incidence of AIDS in the United States has grown exponentially from the early 1980s. In 1981, 291 new cases of AIDS were reported; in 1995, 74,180 new cases were reported. From June 1981 through June 1997, there have been 604,176 reported cases and 374,656 AIDS-related deaths in the United States (Centers for Disease Control and Prevention, 1997). The Public Health Service (PHS) estimates that 1 million persons in the United States are infected with HIV. This includes those living with AIDS, those who have tested positive for HIV, and those who are positive but have not been tested.

Epidemiologic and demographic data have shown that most people with AIDS in the United States are (1) men who have had sex with other men (47%) or (2) persons of both sexes who have used IV drugs (22%) (Table 25–3). The fastest growing infected groups are women and minorities, with a disproportionate number of cases reported in racial and ethnic minority groups. Approximately 52% of all AIDS cases in North America have occurred in African-Americans and Hispanics, who constitute only 18.5% of the population. Between 1985 and 1995, the demographics of the disease changed dramatically. The rates for women increased 8.2%, and the inci-

dence of AIDS in minority groups increased 41.7% (Table 25–4).

AIDS is a disease with high mortality. The overall fatality rate is about 65% for adults (Centers for Disease Control and Prevention, 1997), and to date there have been no reports of a cure. Currently, there are 31 persons with AIDS identified as *nonprogressors,* individuals infected with HIV for at least 10 years who remain asymptomatic and have maintained CD4+ T-lymphocyte counts within a normal range. Researchers are studying nonprogressors to determine whether they resist disease because of differences in viral factors, such as infection with a weak HIV strain, or because they have an unusually strong immune response (Barnes, 1995).

TRANSCULTURAL CONSIDERATIONS

AIDS has been reported in 162 countries and in each of the United States (World Health Organization [WHO], 1991). In 1991, a total of 418,403 cases were reported worldwide (WHO, 1991), but reporting of AIDS cases to the WHO is generally incomplete. The pattern of HIV infection and manifestations of AIDS differ in countries such as West Africa, where HIV-2 is the predominant viral strain.

The main difference in HIV-2 infection is that it occurs primarily in the heterosexual population, with equal numbers of men and women infected. The modes of transmission are the same as those of HIV-1. The large number of infected females results in a high rate of perinatal transmission and large numbers of HIV-infected children.

WOMEN'S HEALTH CONSIDERATIONS

Women comprise the fastest growing group with HIV infection and AIDS (CDC, 1996). Women with HIV appear to have a poorer outcome with shorter survival than men. This outcome may be the result of late

TABLE 25–3

AIDS Cases Among Adults and Adolescents in the United States by Exposure Category: June 1, 1981–June 30, 1997		
Category	**No. Cases**	**%**
Men who have sex with men	298,699	49
Injecting drug users (female and male heterosexual)	154,664	26
Men who have sex with men and inject drugs	38,923	6
Hemophilia	4,567	1
Heterosexual contact	54,571	9
Recipients of blood transfusion, blood components, or tissue	8,075	2
Other and unidentified risk	44,677	7
Total	604,176	100

Data from the Centers for Disease Control and Prevention.
HIV/AIDS Surveillance Report, Mid-year 1997 Edition, Vol. 9, No. 1. Atlanta: Author.

TABLE 25–4

Distribution of Adult/Adolescent AIDS Cases in the United States by Race and Ethnic Group, June 1, 1981–June 30, 1997	
Category	**No. Cases**
Caucasian, not Hispanic	277,672
African-American, not Hispanic	212,394
Hispanic	107,419
Asian/Pacific Islander	4,329
Native American	1,651
Unknown	711
Total	604,176

Data from the Centers for Disease Control and Prevention, 1997.

diagnosis and social and economic factors that reduce access to medical care rather than any viral pathology.

Gynecologic symptoms, particularly persistent or recurrent vaginal candidiasis, may be the first signs of HIV in women (Sabo & Carwein, 1994). Additional symptoms include genital herpes, pelvic inflammatory disease, and cervical neoplasia.

Most women with HIV are of childbearing age. The effect of pregnancy on the course of HIV infection is not known. There is conflicting evidence that it may or may not speed up the progression of disease.

ELDERLY CONSIDERATIONS

 Infection with HIV can occur at any age. The nurse or assistive nursing personnel should assess the elderly client for risk behaviors, including a sexual and drug use history. Decline in immune function may increase susceptibility to HIV infection in this population. In the older woman, changes in vaginal tissue as a result of aging may increase susceptibility to sexually transmitted HIV infection (Whipple & Scura, 1996).

Collaborative Management

⬥ Assessment

Continuous, careful, comprehensive assessment of the client with AIDS is crucial, because he or she may have signs and symptoms related to disease in multiple organ systems. Subtle changes must be assessed so infections and other clinical problems can be found early and treated effectively.

► *History*

Information relevant to HIV and AIDS from the general history includes age, gender, occupation, and residence. The nurse thoroughly assesses the current complaint or current illness, including its nature, when it started, severity of symptoms, associated problems, and any interventions to date. The nurse questions the client about when AIDS was diagnosed and what clinical symptoms led to that diagnosis. The client is asked to give a chro-

nology of infections and clinical problems since the diagnosis. The nurse assesses health history, including whether the client received a blood transfusion between 1978 and 1985.

The client also is questioned about sexual practices, history of STDs, and history of major infectious diseases, including tuberculosis and hepatitis. If the client is a hemophiliac, the nurse asks about treatment with clotting factors. The client is asked about past or present drug use, including needle exposure and sharing. The nurse assesses the client's level of knowledge regarding the diagnosis, symptom management, diagnostic tests, treatments, community resources, and modes of transmission of the virus. The nurse also assesses the client's understanding of, familiarity with, and use of safer sex practices.

► *Physical Assessment/Clinical Manifestations*

The nurse or assistive personnel looks for many possible signs and symptoms. These include shortness of breath or cough, fever, night sweats, fatigue, nausea and vomiting, weight loss, lymphadenopathy, diarrhea, visual changes, headache, memory loss, confusion, seizures, personality changes, dry skin, rashes, skin lesions, pain, and discomfort (Chart 25–1).

Opportunistic Infections. Opportunistic infections occur because of the profound immune suppression of the person with AIDS (see Chart 25–1). They may result from primary infection or reactivation of a latent infection. Opportunistic infections account for most of the clinical manifestations observed in AIDS, and can be protozoan, fungal, bacterial, or viral. The nurse may note more than one infection in a client with AIDS.

Protozoal Infections. *Pneumocystis carinii* pneumonia (PCP) is the most common opportunistic infection in persons with HIV; its incidence ranges from 75% to 80% (Henry & Holzemer, 1992). The nurse notes dyspnea on exertion, tachypnea, a persistent dry cough, and fever. The client with PCP complains of fatigue and weight loss. On auscultation of the lungs, the nurse notes crackles.

Toxoplasmosis encephalitis, caused by *Toxoplasma gondii,* is acquired through contact with contaminated cat feces or ingesting infected, undercooked meat. The client may experience subtle changes in mental status, neurologic deficits, headaches, and fever. Other symptoms include difficulties with speech, gait, and vision, seizures, lethargy, and confusion. The nurse performs a comprehensive baseline mental status examination and monitors the client to detect subtle changes.

Cryptosporidiosis is a gastroenteritis caused by *Cryptosporidium.* In AIDS, this illness ranges from a mild diarrhea to a cholera-like syndrome with wasting and electrolyte imbalance. The nurse notes voluminous diarrhea, with a volume loss of up to 15 to 20 L/day.

Fungal Infections. *Candida albicans* is part of the natural flora of the gastrointestinal tract. In the person with AIDS, candidiasis occurs because the regulatory mechanisms of the immune system can no longer control fungal overgrowth. *Candida* stomatitis or esophagitis is a frequent finding in AIDS; clients complain of food tasting "funny,"

Chart 25-1

Key Features of AIDS

Immunologic Manifestations
- Low white blood cell counts:
  - T_4:T_8 ratio < 2
  - T_4 count < 200/mm^3
- Hypergammaglobulinemia
- Opportunistic infections
- Lymphadenopathy
- Fatigue

Integumentary Manifestations
- Dry skin
- Poor wound healing
- Skin lesions
- Night sweats

Respiratory Manifestations
- Cough
- Shortness of breath

Gastrointestinal Manifestations
- Diarrhea
- Weight loss
- Nausea and vomiting

Central Nervous System Manifestations
- Confusion
- Dementia
- Headache
- Fever
- Visual changes
- Memory loss
- Personality changes
- Pain
- Seizures

Opportunistic Infections
- Protozoal Infections
  - *Pneumocystis carinii* pneumonia
  - Toxoplasmosis
  - Cryptosporidiosis
  - Isosporiasis
  - Microsporidiosis
  - Strongyloidiasis
  - Giardiasis
- Fungal Infections
  - Candidiasis
  - Cryptococcosis
  - Histoplasmosis
  - Coccidioidomycosis
- Bacterial Infections
  - *Mycobacterium avium-intracellulare* complex infection
  - Tuberculosis
  - Nocardiosis
- Viral Infections
  - Cytomegalovirus infection
  - Herpes simplex virus infection
  - Varicella-zoster virus infection

Malignancies
- Kaposi's sarcoma
- Non-Hodgkin's lymphoma
- Hodgkin's lymphoma
- Invasive cervical carcinoma

---

mouth pain, difficulty in swallowing, and retrosternal pain (pain behind the ribs). On examination of the mouth and the back of the throat, the nurse sees the characteristic "cottage cheese"–like, yellow-white plaques and inflammation. Esophagitis is diagnosed by endoscopic biopsy and culture. Women with AIDS may have vaginal candidiasis, characterized by severe pruritus (itching), perineal irritation, and a thick, white vaginal discharge.

Cryptococcosis is a severe, debilitating meningitis and occasionally a disseminated disease in AIDS. It is caused by *Cryptococcus neoformans.* Clinical manifestations of meningitis include fever, headache, blurred vision, nausea and vomiting, nuchal rigidity (stiff neck), mild confusion, and other mental status changes. The client sometimes experiences seizures and other focal neurologic abnormalities, or may present with mild symptoms and complain only of malaise and fever with or without headaches.

Histoplasmosis, caused by *Histoplasma capsulatum,* begins as a respiratory infection and progresses to disseminated infection in the person with AIDS. The nurse may note dyspnea, fever, cough, and weight loss. The client's spleen, liver, and lymph nodes may be enlarged.

Bacterial Infections. Mycobacterium avium-intracellulare complex (MAC) is the most common bacterial infection associated with AIDS. This complex is caused by *Mycobacterium intracellulare* or *Mycobacterium avium,* which infects the respiratory or gastrointestinal tract. MAC is a disseminated infection. Positive cultures may be obtained from lymph nodes, bone marrow, and blood. Clinical manifestations include fever, debility, weight loss, malaise, and sometimes lymphadenopathy or organ disease.

Tuberculosis, caused by *Mycobacterium tuberculosis,* occurs in 2% to 10% of persons with AIDS. People with HIV are at increased risk for active tuberculosis. More than 50% of all clients who have AIDS and tuberculosis have extrapulmonary disease sites, including the central nervous system, bones, liver, spleen, skin, and gastrointestinal tract. The client's systemic symptoms include fever, chills, night sweats, weight loss, and anorexia; pulmonary involvement causes cough, dyspnea, and chest pain. Symptoms of extrapulmonary infection vary with the site. The person with tuberculosis and a CD4+ count below 200/mm^3 may not have a positive purified protein derivative (PPD) skin test because of an inability to mount an immune response to the antigen, a condition known as *anergy*. Other diagnostic measures should include chest x-ray film, acid-fast sputum smear, and sputum culture.

The nurse giving aerosol treatments such as pentamidine isethionate prophylaxis that induce coughing to clients with AIDS should be screened with a PPD skin test every 6 months.

Recurrent pneumonia from bacterial infections occurs frequently among immunocompromised clients. Under the 1993 revised CDC classification system for AIDS, two or more episodes of pneumonia in a 12-month period was added as an AIDS case definition. Symptoms include chest pain, productive cough, fever, and dyspnea.

Viral Infections. Cytomegalovirus (CMV) can infect multiple sites in people with AIDS, including the eye (CMV retinitis), respiratory and gastrointestinal tracts, and central nervous system. CMV infection can also result in many nonspecific symptoms associated with AIDS, such as fever, malaise, weight loss, fatigue, and lymphadenopathy. CMV retinitis causes visual impairment ranging from slight to total bilateral blindness.

Cytomegalovirus infection also causes colitis, with diarrhea, abdominal bloating and discomfort, and weight loss. In addition, CMV can cause encephalitis, pneumonitis, adrenalitis, hepatitis, and disseminated infection.

Herpes simplex virus (HSV) infections in people with AIDS occur in the perirectal, oral, and genital areas. Clients describe numbness or tingling at the site of infection up to 24 hours before vesicle formation. Vesicular lesions are painful, with chronic ulcerative lesions after vesicle rupture. The nurse notes fever, pain, bleeding, and lymph node enlargement in the affected area. Systemic symptoms include headache, myalgia, and malaise.

Varicella-zoster virus (VZV) infection usually does not represent a new infection for people with AIDS. This virus, present in nerve ganglia of many people, causes chickenpox. When these people are immunocompromised, VZV leave the nerve ganglia, enter body fluids and other tissue areas, causing *shingles*. Symptoms begin with pain and burning along dermatome nerve tracts. Large fluid-filled vesicles form and eventually crust over. Systemic symptoms include headache and low-grade fever.

Malignancies. The altered immunocompetence of AIDS increases the risk for cancer in this group. Cancers associated with AIDS include Kaposi's sarcoma (KS), Hodgkin's lymphoma, and non-Hodgkin's lymphoma.

Kaposi's Sarcoma. This is the most common malignancy associated with AIDS, occurring in 1% to 21% of clients with AIDS. Hemophiliacs with HIV have the lowest incidence of KS, and men infected through homosexual contact the highest.

Kaposi's sarcoma presents as small, purplish-brown, palpable discrete lesions that are usually not painful or pruritic; they can occur anywhere on the body. Most clients with KS present with mucocutaneous (skin or mucous membrane) lesions. In some, extracutaneous lesions develop, especially in the lymph nodes, gastrointestinal tract, or lungs. The nurse assesses KS lesions for number, size, and location and monitors their progression. KS is diagnosed by biopsy and histologic examination of the lesion.

Malignant Lymphomas. Malignant lymphomas associated with AIDS are primarily non-Hodgkin's B-cell lymphomas. Systemic symptoms include weight loss, fever, and night sweats. (See Chapter 42 on clinical course and care relevant to malignant lymphomas.)

Other Clinical Manifestations. All body systems are affected to some degree in AIDS; however, manifestations most consistently appear as changes in cognitive function, weight, and the skin.

AIDS Dementia Complex. HIV-associated dementia complex, or AIDS dementia complex (ADC), refers to the signs and symptoms of central nervous system involvement. ADC occurs in up to 70% of persons with AIDS. It is probably the result of direct infection of cells within the central nervous system by HIV. ADC is characterized by three components: cognitive, motor, and behavioral impairments (Chart 25–2). Symptoms range from subclinical to severe dementia.

Other neurologic complications may be due to HIV infection or drug side effects, including peripheral neuropathies and myopathies. Symptoms of peripheral neuropathies include paresthesias and burning sensations, pain, and gait changes. Myopathies are accompanied by leg weakness, ataxia, and muscle pain.

Wasting Syndrome. AIDS wasting syndrome is not due to any single factor. It may be the result of altered metabolism from malignancy or opportunistic infection. Diarrhea, malabsorption, anorexia, and oral and esophageal lesions can all contribute to persistent and sometimes

---

Chart 25–2

Key Features of AIDS Dementia Complex

Cognitive Impairment
- Slowed thinking
- Slowed reaction time to external stimuli
- Loss of concentration while thinking or speaking
- Memory loss
- Forgetfulness
- Wandering attention

Motor Impairment
- Loss of coordination
- Loss of balance
- Increased minor accidents such as tripping, bumping into things, or dropping things
- Slowed motor performance
- Leg weakness

Behavioral Impairment
- Apathy
- Withdrawal

or
- Irritability
- Hyperactivity

extreme weight loss, and the client may appear quite emaciated.

Integumentary Changes. Many clients complain of dry, itchy, irritated skin and diffuse rashes of seborrheic dermatitis. The nurse may also observe folliculitis, eczema, or psoriasis; petechiae or bleeding gums may present as a result of a low platelet count.

➤ Psychosocial Assessment

Psychosocial data collection for a client with AIDS is extremely important. The nurse asks about the client's social support system, including family, significant others, and friends. To protect the client's confidentiality, the nurse assesses who in this support system is aware of the client's diagnosis so that the nurse does not inadvertently mention it. Some clients, because of real or threatened discrimination, are quite selective about whom they tell. Health care providers should respect the client's choices as much as possible without compromising care. The nurse can offer resources to help the client with disclosure to sexual partners or significant others.

The client may be closest to a lover or a friend who is not legally recognized as next of kin. The nurse obtains the name and telephone number of that person and learns whether a durable power of attorney document has been executed.

The nurse elicits information about the client's activities of daily living as well as any changes that may have occurred since diagnosis. The nurse assesses the client's employment status and occupation, social activities and hobbies, living arrangements, and financial resources, including health insurance.

To plan care and monitor changes, the nurse assesses the client's anxiety level, mood, and cognitive ability. The nurse also asks the client about any experiences with discrimination and how they were handled. After the nurse assesses the client's level of self-esteem and changes in body image, together the nurse and client identify the client's strengths and coping strategies. The nurse gathers information about any suicidal ideation, depression, or other psychological problems. The nurse also obtains information about the client's involvement with support groups or other community resources.

➤ Laboratory Assessment

Lymphocyte Counts. A lymphocyte count is generally performed as part of a complete blood count (CBC) with differential (see Chap. 23). The normal white blood cell count (WBC) is between 4500 and 11,000 cells/mm^3, with a differential of approximately 30% to 40% lymphocytes (an absolute number of 1500–4500). Clients with AIDS are often leukopenic, with a WBC count of less than 3500 cells/mm^3 and usually lymphopenic (less than 1500 cells/mm^3).

T4-T8 Ratio. The percentage and number of T4 and T8 cells are an important part of an immune profile. People with HIV infection usually have a lower than normal number of T4 cells. Some clients with AIDS have fewer than 100 cells/mm^3 (normal: between 800 and 1200 cells/mm^3), whereas the number of T8 cells is usually normal. The normal ratio of T4 to T8 cells is approximately 2:1. In AIDS, because of a low number of T4 cells, this ratio is low. Low T4 cell counts and a low T4–T8 ratio are associated with increased clinical manifestations of disease.

Antibody Tests. Antibody tests measure the client's response to the presence of the virus (the antigen) rather than to the virus itself. HIV antibody can be measured by enzyme-linked immunosorbent assay (ELISA) and Western blot analysis. After infection with the virus, it usually takes from 3 weeks to 3 months for a person to test positive for HIV antibodies. However, in some infected people, it can take up to 36 months for antibodies to be detectable (Imagawa et al., 1989). False-negative results (incorrectly indicating the absence of HIV infection) have been reported: early in the infection, in people with cancer, and in people on long-term immunosuppressive therapies.

Enzyme-Linked Immunosorbent Assay. The client's serum is mixed with HIV grown in culture. If the client has antibodies to HIV, they will bind to the HIV antigens and can be detected (a positive test). Two considerations in HIV antibody testing are sensitivity and specificity. False-positive test results (incorrectly indicating HIV infection) occur in approximately 0.1% of those tested with the ELISA. False-positive results (McMahon, 1988) have been reported in multiparous or pregnant women, intravenous drug users, people with a history of malaria, clients with lymphomas, and those with reactivity to the HLA-DR4 leukocyte antigen.

Western Blot. If the results of an ELISA are positive, they are confirmed by Western blot analysis. This test is not as widely available as ELISA because of its cost and complexity. The Western blot analysis is a more specific test to detect serum antibodies to four specific major HIV antigens. A positive Western blot is based on the presence of antibodies to two of the major HIV antigens.

The result is considered indeterminate if two of the major antibodies are not detected but other antibodies to HIV are. The person should then be retested. In people whose tests are positive, conversion from an indeterminate to a positive Western blot usually occurs within 6 months. If a person has a positive test result for HIV antibodies, it does not mean that he or she has AIDS, only that he or she has been infected with the virus.

Viral Culture. Virus culture techniques also can determine the presence of HIV. One method involves placing the infected client's blood cells in a culture medium and measuring the amount of reverse transcriptase (RT) activity over a 28-day period. The more RT present, the more actively the virus is thought to be replicating.

Viral Load Testing. Viral load testing (also called viral burden testing) measures the presence of HIV viral genetic material (RNA) or another actual viral protein in the client's blood rather than the body's response to the presence of the virus. These test types are quantitative and more directly indicate the level of viral burden or viral load. Such tests are very useful in monitoring disease progression or treatment effectiveness.

p24 Antigen Assay. The p24 antigen assay quantifies the amount of p24 (HIV viral core protein) in the client's serum. Antibodies to p24 are mixed with the serum and can detect even low levels of viral antigen present in serum. However, the assay is not as sensitive as antibody tests or assays of viral genetic material. Because this test is less expensive than measure of viral RNA, it is most frequently used to chart a client's disease progression rather than make an initial diagnosis.

Quantitative RNA Assays. Currently, three quantitative assays are available in some areas for viral load testing: RT-polymerase chain reaction (RT-PCR), branched DNA method (bDNA), and the nucleic acid sequence-based assay (NASBA). All three assays use gene amplification processes to determine the amount of HIV RNA present in a client's serum, and all have a specificity of 100% (Coste et al., 1996). Even if only a few infected cells are present in a serum sample, minute amounts of the HIV RNA are amplified by these methods in sufficient quantities to be detected. Such tests are useful in the clinical management of disease and in diagnosing HIV infection in people who have no other indication of infection. Limitations of viral load testing include cost and local availability of the gene amplification assays.

Other Laboratory Tests. Other laboratory tests establish and monitor the overall condition of the client and detect or diagnose any infections or secondary clinical processes. Standard tests include blood chemistries, CBC with differential and platelets, prothrombin time and partial thromboplastin time, serologic test for syphilis (STS), hepatitis B surface antigen, and immunoglobulin levels. Tests to evaluate further the immune profile of a client include skin testing for delayed hypersensitivity and bone marrow aspiration with biopsy and cultures.

➤ *Other Diagnostic Assessment*

On the basis of the clinical symptoms with which the client presents, other diagnostic tests are chosen, including stool for ova and parasites; biopsies of skin, lymph nodes, lungs, liver, gastrointestinal tract, or brain; chest x-ray film; gallium scans; bronchoscopy, endoscopy, or colonoscopy; liver and spleen scans; computed tomography scans; pulmonary function tests; and arterial blood gas analysis.

 Analysis

➤ *Common Nursing Diagnoses and Collaborative Problems*

The most common nursing diagnoses relevant to the client with AIDS are
1. Impaired Gas Exchange related to anemia, respiratory infection or malignancy (PCP, CMV pneumonitis, pulmonary KS, and/or *Mycobacteria* infection), anemia, fatigue, or pain

2. Altered Nutrition: Less than Body Requirements related to high metabolic need, nausea/vomiting, diarrhea, difficulty chewing or swallowing, anorexia
3. Diarrhea related to infection, food intolerance, medications
4. Impaired Skin Integrity related to KS, infection, altered nutritional state, incontinence, immobility, hyperthermia, malignancy
5. Risk for Infection related to immune deficiency
6. Altered Thought Processes related to ADC, central nervous system infection, or malignancy
7. Self-Esteem Disturbance related to changes in body image changes, decreased self-esteem, and helplessness
8. Social Isolation related to stigma, virus transmissibility, infection control practices, and fear

The primary collaborative problem is Potential for Infection.

➤ *Additional Nursing Diagnoses and Collaborative Problems*

Clients with AIDS also may present with one or more of the following additional diagnoses:
- Activity Intolerance related to fatigue, discomfort, central nervous system defect, weakness, or anemia
- Risk for Injury related to central nervous system deficit, mental status changes, depression, and thrombocytopenia
- Pain related to neuropathy, myelopathy, malignancy, or infection
- Sensory/Perceptual Alterations (Visual) related to CMV retinitis and blindness
- Sleep Pattern Disturbance related to pain, discomfort, anxiety, or depression
- Ineffective Individual Coping related to the diagnosis of AIDS
- Ineffective Family/Significant Other Coping related to the diagnosis of AIDS
- Anticipatory Grieving related to potential loss of role and function and impending death

 Planning and Implementation

➤ *Impaired Gas Exchange*

Planning: Expected Outcomes. The client is expected to
- Maintain adequate oxygenation and perfusion
- Experience minimal dyspnea and discomfort

Interventions. As outlined in the clinical pathway, the nurse, respiratory therapist, or assistive personnel provides interventions, including drug therapy, respiratory support and maintenance, comfort, and rest.

Drug Therapy. Appropriate drug therapy is initiated after identification of an infectious or neoplastic cause for respiratory difficulty (Chart 25–3). One of the two treatments of choice for PCP is trimethoprim-sulfamethoxazole (Apo-sulfatrim♣, Bactrim, Protrin♣, Septra), given IV or orally, depending on the severity of infection. A high percentage of clients with AIDS experience adverse reac-

Chart 25–3

Drug Therapy for AIDS-Related Opportunistic Infections and Malignancies

Drug	Indication	Usual Dosage	Nursing Interventions	Rationale
Trimethoprim (TMP) and sulfamethoxazole (SMX) (Apo-sulfatrim✳, Bactrim, Protrin✳, Septra)	• *Pneumocystis carinii* pneumonia	• PO 160 mg TMP and 800 mg SMX every 12 hours	• Monitor I&O • Encourage fluids • Monitor CBC, urinalysis, bilirubin, creatinine, alkaline phosphatase. • Assess for sore throat, pallor, purpura, jaundice, weakness.	• I&O are monitored because TMP-SMX is nephrotoxic. • These values are monitored because TMP-SMX suppresses the immune system. • These signs are assessed for because TMP-SMX is hepatotoxic.
Pentamidine isethionate (Lomidine✳, Pentam)	• *P. carinii* pneumonia	• IM or IV 4 mg/kg once daily for 14–21 days	• Monitor blood pressure, heart rate, and rhythm. • Administer with client lying down. • Monitor for hypoglycemia. • Administer IV over 1 hour. • Monitor liver function, CBC.	• BP and heart rate are monitored because pentamidine causes hypotension when administered rapidly. • Monitoring is necessary because pentamidine causes severe hypoglycemia that may be fatal. • Liver function and CBC are monitored because pentamidine is hepatotoxic and immunosuppressive.
Pentamidine isethionate (Pentam, Pentarcarinate)	• *P. carinii* pneumonia	• Inhalant 300 mg every 4 weeks via nebulizer	• See above.	• See above.
Pyrimethamine (with sulfadiazine) (Daraprim)	• Toxoplasmosis	• PO 50–75 mg/day for 1–3 weeks, then 25 mg/day for 4–5 weeks	• Administer with food or milk. • Monitor CBC and platelets.	• Pyrimethamine irritates the GI tract. • The CBC and platelets are monitored because pyrimethamine suppresses bone marrow activity.
Sulfadiazine	• Toxoplasmosis • Nocardiasis	• PO 500–2000 mg daily every 6 hours for 3–4 weeks	• Monitor urine output, CBC. • Encourage fluids. • Advise client to avoid sun. • Assess for sore throat, pallor, purpura, jaundice, weakness.	• Urine output and the CBC are monitored because sulfadiazine causes renal toxicity. • Fluids are necessary because sulfadiazine suppresses bone marrow activity. • Clients should avoid the sun because sulfadiazine increases photosensitivity.
Dapsone (Avlosulfon✳, DDS)	• Toxoplasmosis	• PO 50–100 mg daily	• Monitor CBC. • Assess for fever, sore throat, purpura, jaundice.	• The CBC is monitored because dapsone suppresses bone marrow activity.

Continued

CHART 25-3. Drug Therapy for AIDS-Related Opportunistic Infections and Malignancies Continued

Drug	Indicaton	Usual Dosage	Nursing Interventions	Rationale
Metronidazole (Flagyl, Novonidazol✤)	• Cryptosporidiosis • Giardiasis	• PO 7.5 mg/kg every 6 hours, IV 15 mg/kg initial dose, then 7.5 mg/kg every 6 hours	• Administer with food or milk. • Teach client to avoid alcohol during treatment. • Assess for dry mouth, dizziness, fungal infection.	• Food or milk is recommended because metronidazole irritates the GI tract. • Alcohol causes formation of acetaldehyde and headache, nausea, vomiting, and diarrhea.
Ketoconazole (Nizoral)	• Candidiasis • Coccidioidomycosis • Histoplasmosis	• PO 200–400 mg/day, single dose	• Administer with food or milk. • Avoid antacids for 2 hours. • Teach client to avoid sun and alcohol during treatment. • Monitor hepatic function.	• Ketoconazole irritates the GI tract. • Gastric acid is needed to activate drug. • Ketoconazole increases photosensitivity. • Hepatic function is monitored because ketoconazole is hepatotoxic.
Fluconazole (Diflucan)	• Candidiasis • Cryptococcal meningitis	• PO, IV 200–400 mg initially, then 100–200 mg daily for 2–4 weeks	• Monitor hepatic function. • Assess for abdominal pain, fever, diarrhea.	• Hepatic function is monitored because fluconazole is hepatotoxic.
Rifampin (Rifadin, Rofact✤)	• *Mycobacterium avium* complex • Tuberculosis	• PO 10 mg/kg/day	• Assess breath sounds, sputum. • Monitor hepatic function, CBC. • May turn body secretions orange.	• Assessment of breath sounds and sputum determines treatment effectiveness. • Rifampin is hepatotoxic.
Ethambutol (Myambutol, Etibi✤)	• *Mycobacterium avium-intracellulare* complex • Tuberculosis	• PO 25–30 mg/kg 2–3 times a week	• Assess vision changes. • Assess hepatic and renal function, CBC, urinalysis.	• Vision changes are assessed because ethambutol causes retrobulbar neuritis and decreased visual acuity (reversible). • This assessment is necessary because ethambutol increases uric acid concentrations. • Ethambutol suppresses bone marrow activity.
Amphotericin B (Fungizone)	• Candidiasis • Other fungal infections	• IV 0.3–1 mg/kg/day, maximum 50 mg/day	• Assess renal function. • Assess infusion site. • Assess CBC.	• Renal function is assessed because amphotericin B is nephrotoxic. • Amphotericin B causes thrombophlebitis. • The CBC is checked because amphotericin B suppresses bone marrow activity. • Amphotericin B is *very* toxic.

Continued

CHART 25-3. Drug Therapy for AIDS-Related Opportunistic Infections and Malignancies Continued

Drug	Indicaton	Usual Dosage	Nursing Interventions	Rationale
Ciprofloxacin (Cipro)	• *Mycobacterium avium-intracellulare* complex • Urinary tract infections	• PO 250–750 mg every 12 hours, IV 200–400 mg every 12 hours	• Monitor I&O. • Encourage fluids. • Administer on empty stomach (1 hour before or 2 hours after meals) if tolerated. • Teach client to avoid sun. • Assess for dizziness, fungal infection. • Infuse over 1 hour.	• An empty stomach is recommended for best absorption. • Clients should avoid the sun because ciprofloxacin increases photosensitivity.
Clofazimine (Lamprene)	• *Mycobacterium avium-intracellulare* complex	• PO 50–300 mg every day	• Assess vision changes, dizziness, drowsiness. • Instruct client to avoid sun. • Use lotions for dry skin. • Monitor hepatic and renal function.	• Vision changes and dizziness are assessed because clofazimine increases sedation. • Clofazimine increases photosensitivity (especially of eyes). • Clients should use lotions because clofazimine causes dry, scaly skin.
Pyrazinamide (Tebrazid✦)	• Tuberculosis	• PO 20–30 mg/kg/day	• Monitor hepatic function, uric acid. • Assess temperature every 4 hours.	• Pyrazinamide is hepatotoxic and increases uric acid concentration. • The client's temperature is assessed because pyrazinamide stimulates fever.
Isoniazid (Laniazid, Isotamine)	• Tuberculosis	• PO, IM 5–10 mg/kg/day or 15 mg/kg 2–3 times a week	• Administer on empty stomach. • Monitor hepatic function. • Assess for vision changes. • Instruct client to avoid alcohol and tyramine-containing foods.	• Taking isoniazid on an empty stomach enhances absorption. • Isoniazid is hepatotoxic. • Vision changes are assessed because isoniazid is neurotoxic. • Isoniazid is an MAO inhibitor.
Ganciclovir (Cytovene)	• Cytomegalovirus retinitis • PO 1000 mg every 8 hr	• IV 5 mg/kg every 12 hours for 14–21 days	• Monitor neutrophil and platelet count. • Infuse over 1 hour. • Give with food.	• Neutrophil and platelet counts are monitored because ganciclovir suppresses bone marrow activity.
Acyclovir (Zovirax)	• Herpes simplex • Herpes zoster • Varicella zoster	• PO 200–800 mg 5 times a day, IV 5–10 mg/kg every 8 hours for 7–10 days	• Monitor renal function. • Encourage fluids. • Rotate infusion site.	• Acyclovir is nephrotoxic. • Various infusion sites are used because acyclovir is a blood vessel irritant.

Continued

CHART 25-3. Drug Therapy for AIDS-Related Opportunistic Infections and Malignancies   Continued

Drug	Indication	Usual Dosage	Nursing Interventions	Rationale
Zidovudine (Retrovir)	• HIV seropositivity	• PO 100–200 mg every 4 hours	• Must be administered around the clock. • Assess for dizziness. • Monitor CBC, hepatic and renal function.	• Zidovudine is given around the clock for maximum antiviral effect. • Dizziness is assessed because zidovudine crosses the blood-brain barrier. • Zidovudine suppresses bone marrow activity. • Zidovudine is hepatotoxic. • Zidovudine is nephrotoxic.
Didanosine (Videx)	• HIV seropositivity	• PO 125–300 mg every 12 hours	• Administer on empty stomach. • Instruct client to chew tablet or crush. • Monitor for dizziness, neuropathy, pancreatitis.	• Taking didanosine on an empty stomach enhances absorption. • Didanosine crosses the blood-brain barrier.
Zalcitabine (ddC)	• HIV seropositivity	• PO 0.75 mg every 8 hours (with AZT)	• Monitor liver function. • Given with AZT.	• This can cause serious liver damage. • Combination of ddC and AZT acts synergistically.
Lamivudine (Epivir, 3TC✽)	• HIV seropositivity • Prophylaxis—occupational exposure	• PO 150 mg tid	• Teach client to avoid fatty foods.	• This can cause severe pancreatitis.
Stavudine (d4T, Zerit)	• HIV seropositivity	• PO 40 mg bid	• Observe client's gait. Ask about paresthesia.	• This can cause severe peripheral neuropathy.
Ritonavir (Norvir)	• HIV seropositivity	• PO 600 mg bid	• Administer 1 hour before or 2 hours after meals. • Monitor triglyceride levels.	• Ritonavir is absorbed best in fasting state. • This can increase triglyceride levels.
Saquinavir (Invirase)	• HIV seropositivity	• PO 600 mg every 8 hours	• Administer with meals. • Warn client to avoid sun exposure.	• Saquinavir is absorbed best with a high-calorie, high-fat meal. • Saquinavir increases photosensitivity.
Interferon-alpha$_{2b}$	• Kaposi's sarcoma	• IM, SC 30 million IU/m^2 three times weekly	• Monitor vital signs, cardiac status. • Assess for bleeding, low-grade fever, malaise, muscle aches, headache, chills, infection, nausea.	• Vital signs and cardiac status are monitored because interferon-alpha$_{2b}$ poses a danger of hyperviscosity. • Interferon-alpha$_{2b}$ causes malaise and flu-like symptoms.

AIDS = acquired immunodeficiency syndrome; I&O = input and output; HIV = human immunodeficiency virus; CBC = complete blood count; MAO = monoamine oxidase; GI = gastrointestinal.

tions to this medication, including nausea, vomiting, hyponatremia, rashes, fever, leukopenia, thrombocytopenia, and hepatitis.

The second drug of choice is pentamidine isethionate (Lomidine✽, Pentam), usually given IV or intramuscularly (IM). Aerosolized pentamidine isethionate is used prophylactically in those with T4 counts below 200 and in those who have already had PCP.

Respiratory Support and Maintenance. The client also needs appropriate care to maintain respiratory function and avoid complications. The nurse, respiratory therapist, or assistive personnel assesses the client's respiratory rate, rhythm, and depth, breath sounds, and vital signs and monitors for cyanosis at least every 8 hours. The nurse applies and maintains oxygen therapy and room humidification, as ordered. In addition, the nurse monitors mechanical ventilation, performs suctioning and chest physical therapy as needed, and evaluates blood gas results.

Comfort. The nurse or assistive nursing personnel assesses the client's comfort. The client with respiratory difficulties often is more comfortable with the head of the bed elevated. The nurse helps the client pace activities to minimize shortness of breath and exhaustion. The nurse provides the patient with psychological support during periods of respiratory distress.

Rest and Activity. The nurse consults with the client to pace client activities to conserve energy. The nurse guides the client in active and passive range of motion (ROM) exercises, scheduling them and activities such as bathing so the client is not fatigued at mealtime.

➤ Altered Nutrition: Less Than Body Requirements

Many clients with AIDS have difficulty maintaining their weight and nutritional status. This problem may be associated with fatigue, anorexia, nausea and vomiting, difficult or painful swallowing, diarrhea, or wasting syndrome.

Planning: Expected Outcomes. The client is expected to maintain optimum weight through adequate nutrition and hydration.

Interventions. Because there are multiple factors for alterations in nutrition in AIDS, diagnostic procedures are undertaken to determine the cause. Once the cause is determined, appropriate therapy is initiated. For example, in the client who has candidal esophagitis, nutrition is affected because of the client's difficulty in swallowing.

Drug Therapy. Therapy can include ketoconazole (Nizoral) or fluconazole (Diflucan) orally, or IV amphotericin B (Fungizone). The nurse administers the medication as ordered and monitors the client for side effects such as nausea and vomiting, which further compromise nutritional status. The nurse provides mouth care and ice chips, and keeps unpleasant odors out of the client's environment. Antiemetics are used as ordered.

Diet Therapy. The nurse monitors the client's weight, intake and output, and calorie count. The nurse assesses the client's food preferences and any dietary cultural or religious practices. The nurse also instructs the client in a high-calorie, high-protein, low-microbial, nutritionally sound diet (see Chap. 42). In collaboration with the dietitian, the nurse provides an appropriate diet for the client, including small, frequent meals (better tolerated than large meals). Supplemental vitamins and fluids are indicated in some cases. For the client who cannot achieve adequate nutrition through food, tube feedings or total parenteral nutrition may be needed.

Mouth Care. For clients susceptible to oral ulceration or infection, the nurse or nursing staff member provides meticulous mouth care. Rinses of sodium bicarbonate with normal saline every 2 hours or several times a day are helpful. The client is given a soft toothbrush and advised to drink plenty of fluids. For oral pain that interferes with the client's ability to eat, analgesics or viscous lidocaine may be necessary.

➤ Diarrhea

Clients with AIDS frequently suffer from diarrhea. Sometimes an infectious cause (e.g., *Giardia* or *Amoeba*) can be determined and treated, or the cause is determined but no effective therapy is available, as in cryptosporidiosis or CMV colitis. In some cases, clients with AIDS have diarrhea and no infectious cause can be identified.

Planning: Expected Outcomes. The client is expected to
- Experience decreased diarrhea
- Maintain fluid, electrolyte, and nutritional status
- Minimize incontinence

Interventions. For most clients with AIDS and diarrhea, symptomatic management is all that is available. Antidiarrheals, such as diphenoxylate hydrochloride (Diarsed✦, Lomotil), given on a regular schedule, provide the client some degree of relief. In collaboration with the dietitian, the nurse offers dietary counseling and appropriate foods. Recommended dietary changes include less roughage; less fatty, spicy, and sweet foods; and no alcohol or caffeine. Some clients experience symptomatic relief if they eliminate dairy products from the diet or eat smaller amounts of food more often and drink plenty of fluids, especially between meals.

The nurse or assistive personnel provides the client a bedside commode or a bedpan if needed. Some clients cannot reach the bathroom in time because of immobility or anal sphincter weakness, others because of the urgency to defecate. The nurse provides privacy, support, and understanding.

➤ Impaired Skin Integrity

The most common skin lesion in AIDS is Kaposi's sarcoma (KS). Cutaneous involvement may be localized or disseminated. Large lesions can cause pain and restrict movement or ambulation. They can impede circulation, causing open, weeping, painful lesions. Another cause of impaired skin integrity is HSV infection.

Planning: Expected Outcomes. The client is expected to
- Experience healing of any existing lesions
- Avoid increased skin breakdown or secondary infection

Interventions. KS can be treated locally with radiotherapy, intralesional chemotherapy, or cryotherapy. KS responds to local radiation therapy but only transiently. Systemic therapy is used in clients with rapidly progressive disease or with significant involvement of the gastrointestinal tract, lungs, or other organs. These therapies include chemotherapy (single agent or combination), interferon-alpha, and interferon-alpha–zidovudine combinations.

Treatment of painful KS lesions includes the use of analgesics and comfort measures. Open, weeping KS lesions must be kept clean and dressed to minimize the risk of secondary infection. Many clients with cutaneous KS are concerned about their appearance and the risk of being identified as HIV-positive. Make-up (if open lesions are not present), long-sleeved shirts, and hats may help the client maintain a normal appearance.

For the client with an HSV abscess, the nurse provides meticulous skin care. The nurse or assistive personnel cleans the abscess regularly with a diluted solution of povidone-iodine (Betadine) and leaves it to air-dry or exposes it to a heat lamp. This infection can be painful and necessitates analgesics, assistance with position, and other comfort measures. Modified Burow's solution (Domeboro) soaks help to promote healing for some clients. HSV infection is treated with acyclovir (Zovirax) given IV, orally, or, in some cases, topically, depending on the severity of the infection.

➤ Risk for Infection

The client with AIDS is susceptible to opportunistic infections because of immunodeficiency secondary to HIV infection.

Planning: Expected Outcomes. The client is expected to remain free of opportunistic diseases.

Interventions. Several strategies can help the client minimize the chances of acquiring an infection. Some strategies are investigational, including drug therapy and immune function enhancement.

Drug Therapy. Chart 25–3 lists treatments for opportunistic infections and neoplasms. Several experimental medications have demonstrated antiretroviral effects in vitro and in animal studies. New regimens, called "cocktails," consisting of combinations of antiretroviral agents and protease inhibitors, are showing good results in reducing viral load and improving T4 lymphocyte counts.

Nucleoside Analogs. Zidovudine, or AZT (Retrovir), is an antiviral medication given orally or IV; the usual dose is 200 mg orally every 4 hours. Side effects include a potentially severe macrocytic anemia that often necessitates regular transfusions, mild headache, nausea, abdominal pain, diarrhea, and, less commonly, changes in WBC count or liver function tests. Didanosine, or ddI (Videx), is an antiviral used for persons who are unable to tolerate zidovudine or who have had continued loss of immune function despite AZT therapy. Two potential side effects are pancreatitis and peripheral neuropathy. Zalcitabine (ddC) is used in combination with AZT for those whose CD4+ count drops below 300 despite AZT treatment. Stavudine (d4T, Zerit) is used for those with CD4+ counts below 300 who are unable to tolerate AZT or ddI or for whom these drugs are ineffective. Lamivudine (3TC✲, Epivir) is used prophylactically after occupational exposure to HIV. It also is used in combination with either AZT or a

protease inhibitor for treatment of AIDS. The most common side effect for zalcitabine, stavudine, and lamivudine is peripheral neuropathy.

Protease Inhibitors. The newest drugs against HIV are the protease inhibitors, which block the HIV protease enzyme, preventing viral replication and release of viral particles. In recent studies, ritonavir (Norvir) reduced the viral load, slowed disease progression, and reduced the death rate in persons with AIDS. Potential side effects include diarrhea, nausea, vomiting, fatigue, and tingling around the mouth. Clinical benefits of other protease inhibitors, including indinavir (Crixivan) and saquinavir (Invirase), are under investigation. All three current protease inhibitors have fewer side effects than the nucleoside analogs but have shown rapid resistance (Bechtel-Boenning, 1996). Additionally, the protease inhibitors are extremely expensive; costs average more than $15,000 per client per year (McKinnon, 1996).

Immune Enhancement. Research is also being conducted to evaluate modalities that may enhance or reconstitute the immune system of clients who are made immunodeficient by HIV infection. Some of these methods include bone marrow transplantation, lymphocyte transfusion, and administration of lymphokines, particularly interleukin-2, and other biologic response modifiers (Ungvarsky, 1997).

Complementary Therapies. Complementary therapies to increase immune function are frequently used by people with HIV/AIDS (see Research Applications for Nursing). Such therapies include vitamins, shark cartilage, and botanical products available at health food stores. The clinical usefulness of these products has yet to be established through well-controlled clinical trials.

Health Promotion. HIV can remain latent inside a cell for long periods and cause active infection when the cell is stimulated. The specific signals for the cell to become activated are not known, but concurrent viral or parasitic infections are suspected. The nurse teaches the client to avoid exposure to infection.

➤ Altered Thought Processes

Neurologic changes and alterations in thought processes are major areas of concern for clients with AIDS. These changes may be due to psychological stressors accompanying the disease or to organic disorders caused by opportunistic infections, cancer, or HIV encephalitis.

Planning: Expected Outcomes. The client is expected to
- Demonstrate improved mental status
- Sustain no injury

Interventions. Clients with AIDS suffer from enormous loss and psychological stress, which complicate the assessment of any changes in behavior or affect. The nurse or assistive personnel establishes baseline neurologic and mental status by using neurologic assessment tools (see Chap. 43) to compare any changes. Subtle changes in memory, ability to concentrate, affect, and behavior are evaluated. Differential diagnosis is important

▷ Research Applications for Nursing

People with HIV Use Alternative Therapies

Nokes, K. M., Kendrew, J., & Longo, M. (1995). Alternative/complementary therapies used by persons with HIV disease. Journal of the Association of Nurses in AIDS Care, 6(4), 19–24.

The purpose of this descriptive study was to determine the types and frequency of use of alternative or complementary therapies by persons with HIV. The investigators developed an instrument that consisted of 55 alternative therapies based on a review of the literature and interviews with persons with HIV and experts in alternative therapies. Participants were asked to identify their familiarity with each therapy and how often they used it, if at all. A convenience sample of 145 persons with HIV, recruited from both inpatient and outpatient settings in two major cities, participated in the study. Participants were primarily young, Caucasian men whose HIV-related risk behavior was either male-to-male sex or bisexual sex. Each of the identified therapies on the questionnaire was used by at least one respondent. The five most frequently used alternative therapies were vitamins, relaxation, humor, spirituality, and meditation.

Critique. Content validity for the instrument was established through the literature, the input of content experts, and the population of interest. Reliability was established in this sample, with a Cronbach's alpha of .74. The use of a convenience sample and the demographics of the participants limit the generalizability of findings.

Possible Nursing Implications. Nurses caring for persons with HIV should include questions about alternative or complementary therapies in their assessments. They should also be familiar with the types of alternative therapies and understand each. This is necessary to teach the client about potential interactions between standard treatments and alternative therapies and to incorporate appropriate alternative therapies into the client's plan of care.

to determine whether the cause of the neurologic changes is treatable.

Orientation. The nurse reorients the confused client to person, time, and place as needed, reminding the client of the nurse's identity and explaining what is to be done at any given time. Using calendars, clocks, and radios and putting the bed close to a window also may help keep the client oriented. The nurse gives simple directions; uses short, uncomplicated sentences; explains activities in simple language; and involves the client in planning the daily schedule. Relatives or significant others are asked to bring in familiar items from home, and all items in the client's environment are arranged in the same location as at home.

Drug Therapy. Chart 25–3 lists agents appropriate for different conditions contributing to altered thought processes in the person with AIDS.

Safety Measures. Attention to safety is crucial to the well-being of the neurologically impaired client with AIDS. The client may not be aware of activities or surroundings, and may need assistance with bathing, dressing, eating, ambulating, and other activities of daily living. The environment, whether a hospital room, long-term care facility, or home, is made safe and comfortable. Some clients are prone to seizures. The nurse or assistive nursing personnel institutes seizure precautions, including using padded side rails and having an airway available. Anticonvulsants may be added to the client's medications.

The nurse assesses the client with neurologic disease for signs and symptoms of increased intracranial pressure. The nurse immediately reports any changes in level of consciousness, vital signs, pupil size or reactivity, or limb strength to the physician for appropriate intervention. Some clients are given corticosteroids to reduce intracranial pressure.

Support. The nurse and assistive personnel work closely with the family and significant others of the neurologically impaired client. There is great trauma in seeing a loved one unable to care for him- or herself or demonstrating unusual or child-like behavior. The nurse answers questions honestly and sensitively and teaches the family and significant others how to reorient the client. They are encouraged to continue to provide the client with news of family happenings or current events. The nurse, in collaboration with the social worker, identifies community resources for the client and family.

▶ Self-Esteem Disturbance

The client with AIDS is susceptible to changes in self-esteem and self-concept. Contributing to this are real and often dramatic changes in appearance that alter the person's body image. Many clients also experience abrupt, significant changes in their relationships with others and in day-to-day activities, including a job or other productive activities. All changes can disrupt the client's self-concept.

Planning: Expected Outcomes. The client is expected to

- Identify positive aspects of him- or herself
- Accept him- or herself

Interventions. The nurse and other members of the health care team provide a climate of acceptance for clients with AIDS by promoting a trusting relationship and helping clients express feelings and identify positive aspects of themselves. The nurse allows for client privacy but does not avoid or isolate the client. The nurse encourages the client's self-care, independence, control, and decision making, helping the client formulate short-term, attainable goals and offering encouragement and praise when achieved.

Complementary therapy in the form of guided imagery is used by many clients to increase their sense of control and enhance self-esteem. Imagery can focus on helping clients cope with distressing side effects or painful procedures. Other uses of imagery include picturing battle scenes in which the virus is killed by immune system cells.

▶ Social Isolation

Many clients with AIDS face discrimination, rejection, and isolation. Friends or health care workers sometimes avoid or refuse to have anything to do with these clients. Misunderstanding and fear lead to misuse of proper infection control procedures, and clients are inappropriately isolated.

Planning: Expected Outcomes. The client is expected to
- Identify behaviors that cause social isolation
- Demonstrate behaviors that reduce social isolation

Interventions. Interventions for social isolation focus on promoting interactions and on education to reduce fear of AIDS transmission.

Promotion of Interaction. The nurse does not isolate the client but establishes a therapeutic nurse–client relationship. The nurse shows understanding and concern while helping the client find ways to minimize feelings of rejection and isolation. The nurse reduces barriers to social contact for the client. Client social support resources are assessed. Family and significant others are taught about HIV transmission and use of Standard Precautions to reduce anxiety and increase contact with the client (see Chap. 28).

The nurse encourages the client to verbalize feelings about self, coping skills, and sense of ability to control the situation. The nurse helps the client identify support systems, including those already in place and those that need to be arranged.

Education. The most important aspect for prevention of HIV transmission is education. All people, regardless of age, sex, ethnicity, or sexual orientation, are susceptible to HIV infection. Because of the mode of viral transmission and the fragile nature of the virus, AIDS is a preventable disease.

HIV has been isolated from multiple body secretions and tissues, including blood, semen, vaginal secretions, breast milk, amniotic fluid, urine, feces, saliva, tears, cerebrospinal fluid, lymph nodes, cervical cells, Langerhans' cells, corneal tissue, and brain tissue. HIV is primarily transmitted in three ways:
- Sexual: genital, anal, or oral sexual contact with exposure of mucous membranes to infected semen or vaginal secretions
- Parenteral: sharing needles contaminated with infected blood or receiving contaminated blood products
- Perinatal: from the placenta, from contact with maternal blood and body fluids during birth, or from breast milk from an infected mother to child

HIV infection is not transmitted by casual contact in the home, school, or workplace. Studies of persons sharing household utensils, towels and linens, and toilet facilities in crowded households showed no evidence of HIV transmission (Friedland et al., 1990). Transmission by insect vectors is "highly improbable" (Gershon et al., 1990).

Sexual Transmission. Abstinence and mutually monogamous sex with a noninfected partner are the only absolutely safe methods of preventing HIV infection through sexual contact. However, this may not be feasible for personal, cultural, and economic factors.

Safer sex practices are those that reduce the risk of

Chart 25–4

Health Promotion Guide: Condom Use to Prevent Sexually Transmitted Diseases

- Use latex condoms rather than natural membrane condoms.
- Store condoms in a cool, dry place.
- Do not use condoms that were in damaged packages or those that show signs of age, such as those that are brittle, sticky, or discolored.
- Handle condoms carefully to avoid puncturing them.
- Put a condom on before making any genital contact. Hold the tip of the condom and unroll it onto the erect penis, making sure that no air is trapped in the tip. Leave space at the tip to collect semen.
- Use adequate lubrication. Use water-based lubricants only. Petroleum or oil-based lubricants such as petroleum jelly, cooking oil, shortening, and lotions can damage the condom.
- Using a spermicide-lubricated condom or additional spermicide can provide additional protection against sexually transmitted diseases.
- Replace a broken condom immediately. If ejaculation occurs after the condom breaks, there may be some protection in the immediate use of a spermicide.
- After ejaculation, the condom must remain on until the penis is withdrawn. While the penis is still erect, hold the condom against the base of the penis while withdrawing.
- Never reuse condoms.

From Centers for Disease Control. (1988). Condoms for prevention of sexually transmitted diseases. *Morbidity and Mortality Weekly Report, 37*(9), 133–137.

nonintact skin or mucous membranes coming in contact with potentially infected body fluids and blood (Chart 25–4). Such practices include using
- A latex condom and spermicide containing nonoxynol 9 for genital and anal intercourse
- A condom or latex barrier (dental dam) over the genitals or anus during oral-genital or oral-anal sexual contact
- Latex gloves for finger or hand contact with the vagina or rectum

Parenteral Transmission. Preventive practices to reduce parenteral transmission among IV drug users include the use of proper cleaning of "works" (needles, syringes, and other drug paraphernalia). Clients are instructed to clean a used needle and syringe by first filling and flushing with clear water. Next, the syringe should be filled with ordinary household bleach. The bleach-filled syringe should be shaken for 30 to 60 seconds. Drug users are advised to carry a small container with this solution whenever sharing needles. Some communities have a needle exchange program, in which needles and syringes are used only once and exchanged for clean ones.

The risk of AIDS transmission through blood and blood products has been reduced to a national average of 0.02%. Several measures have been implemented to protect the nation's blood supply. All donated blood in

North America is screened for the HIV antibody, and blood that reacts positively is discarded. However, current tests detect the antibody, not the virus itself. Because of time lag in antibody production (seroconversion) after exposure to HIV, infected blood can test negative for HIV antibodies. False-negative results also can occur. The small but real possibility of HIV transmission through blood and blood products has resulted in more stringent indications for transfusion and an increase in autologous transfusion.

Perinatal Transmission. The risk of perinatal transmission in pregnant clients with AIDS has been reported at 14% to 45% for each pregnancy. Studies have shown that pregnant women who received zidovudine had an 8.3% perinatal transmission rate compared with 25.5% in women who received a placebo (National Institute of Allergy and Infectious Disease, 1994). HIV transmission is thought to occur transplacentally in utero, intrapartally during exposure to blood and vaginal secretions during birth, or postpartally through breast milk. Women of childbearing age with HIV infection should be fully informed of the risks of perinatal transmission.

Transmission and Health Care Workers. Needlestick injuries are the primary means of HIV infection for health care workers. In addition, health care workers can be infected through exposure of nonintact skin and mucous membranes to blood and body fluids. Because there is a time lag between the time of infection with HIV and the pro-

---

Chart 25–5

Health Promotion Guide: CDC Recommendations for Human Immunodeficiency Virus (HIV) Testing

You should be tested for AIDS if you fall within one or more of the following groups:

- People with sexually transmitted disease
- Intravenous drug abusers
- People who consider themselves at risk
- Women of childbearing age with identifiable risks, including
  - Having used IV drugs
  - Having engaged in prostitution
  - Having had sexual partners who were infected or at risk
  - Having had contact with men from countries with high HIV prevalence
  - Having received a transfusion between 1978 and 1985
- People planning to get married
- People undergoing medical evaluation or treatment for signs and symptoms that may be HIV-related
- People admitted to hospitals
- People in correctional institutions such as jails and prisons
- Prostitutes and their customers

Modified from Centers for Disease Control. (1987). Public Health Service guidelines for counseling and antibody testing to prevent HIV infection and AIDS. *Morbidity and Mortality Weekly Report, 36*(31), 509–515.

TABLE 25–5

Recommendations for Preventing Human Immunodeficiency Virus by Health Care Workers

- Workers should adhere to Standard Precautions.
- Workers with exudative lesions or weeping dermatitis should not perform direct patient care or handle patient care equipment and devices used in invasive procedures.
- Workers must follow guidelines for disinfection and sterilization of reusable equipment used in invasive procedures.
- Workers infected with HIV are not restricted from practice of non-exposure–prone procedures, provided that they comply with Standard Precautions and sterilization/ disinfection recommendations.
- Workers should identify exposure-prone procedures by institutions where they are performed.
- Workers who perform exposure-prone procedures should know their HIV antibody status.
- Workers who are infected with HIV should seek advice from an expert review panel before performing exposure-prone procedures to determine under what circumstances they may continue to practice these procedures. These circumstances would include notification of prospective clients of HIV positivity.

Adapted from Centers for Disease Control. (1991b). Recommendations for preventing transmission of human immunodeficiency virus and hepatitis B virus to patients during exposure-prone invasive procedures. *Morbidity and Mortality Weekly Report, 40*(RR-8), 1–9.

---

duction of serum antibodies (seroconversion), infected people can test negative for HIV and yet still transmit the virus. Therefore, the best prevention for health care providers is the scrupulous and consistent application of Standard Precautions for all clients as recommended by the Centers for Disease Control and Prevention (CDC) (see Chap. 28).

Reports of possible HIV transmission by a dentist during invasive dental procedures have alarmed the public about HIV transmission by health care workers. It is recommended that HIV-infected health care workers wear gloves when in contact with clients' nonintact skin or mucous membranes. Infected workers with weeping dermatitis or exudative lesions should not perform direct care activities. The CDC (1991) also has issued recommendations for preventing HIV transmission by health care workers during exposure-prone invasive procedures. These include any procedure in which there is a risk of percutaneous injury to the health care worker and the worker's blood is likely to make contact with the patient's body cavity, subcutaneous tissues, or mucous membranes. These recommendations aim to reduce the risk of HIV transmission to clients (Table 25–5).

Testing. Testing plays a role in prevention, because those who test positive can be educated and encouraged to modify their behaviors to prevent transmission to others. The CDC has issued recommendations describing who should be advised to seek HIV antibody testing (Chart 25–5). Pre- and post-test counseling must be performed

Chart 25-6

Education Guide: Recommendations for HIV-Positive People

- Seek regular medical evaluation and follow-up.
- Either avoid sexual activity or inform your prospective partner of your antibody test results and protect him or her from contact with your body fluids during sex. "Body fluids" include blood, semen, urine, feces, saliva, and women's genital secretions. Use a condom and avoid practices that may injure body tissues (e.g., anal intercourse). Avoid oral-genital contact and open-mouthed, intimate kissing.
- Inform your present and previous sex partners, and any persons with whom needles may have been shared, of their potential exposure to HIV and encourage them to seek counseling and antibody testing from their physicians or at appropriate health clinics.
- Don't share toothbrushes, razors, or other items that could become contaminated with blood.
- If you use drugs, enroll in a drug treatment program. Needles and other drug equipment must never be shared.
- Do not donate blood, plasma, body organs, other body tissue, or sperm.
- Clean blood or other body fluid spills on household or other surfaces with freshly diluted household bleach: 1 part bleach to 10 parts water. (Do not use bleach on wounds.)
- Inform your physician, dentist, and eye doctor of your positive HIV status so that proper precautions can be taken to protect you and others.
- Women with a positive antibody test should avoid pregnancy until more is known about the risks of transmitting HIV from mother to infant.

by appropriately trained personnel. Counseling helps the client make an informed decision about testing and provides an opportunity to teach the client risk-reduction behaviors. Post-test counseling is needed to interpret the results, discuss risk reduction, and provide psychological support and health promotion information for the client with a positive test result.

Recommendations for people who have had positive test results for antibody to HIV are presented in Chart 25-6. People who test positive should also be counseled on how to inform sexual partners and those with whom they have shared needles.

 Continuing Care

The usual course of illness is one of intermittent acute infections interspersed with periods of relative wellness over months or years and, ultimately, a chronic, progressive debilitation. Because of the fluctuating nature of HIV infection, the client often spends long periods at home between hospital admissions or clinic visits. In some instances, especially as the illness becomes more severe, the client may need referral to a long-term care facility, home health care agency, or hospice.

The nurse, in collaboration with the social worker, di-

etitian, and other available resources, works with clients to plan what will be needed and how they will manage at home with self-care and activities of daily living.

➤ Health Teaching

Educating the client, family, and significant others is a high priority, especially when preparing the client for discharge. The nurse instructs the client about modes of transmission and preventive behaviors (safer sex guidelines; not sharing toothbrushes, razors, and other potentially blood-contaminated articles). Caregivers also need instruction about infection control precautions to prevent transmission while caring for the client in the home (Chart 25-7), nursing techniques to use in the home, and coping and support strategies.

Chart 25-7

Education Guide: Infection Control for Home Care of the Person with AIDS

Direct Care
- Follow Standard Precautions and good handwashing techniques.
- Do not share razors or toothbrushes.

Housekeeping
- Wipe up feces, vomitus, sputum, urine, or blood or other body fluids and the area with soap and water. Dispose of solid wastes and solutions used for cleaning by flushing them down the toilet. Disinfect the area by wiping with a 1:10 solution of household bleach (1 part bleach to 10 parts water). Wear gloves during cleaning.
- Soak rags, mops, and sponges used for cleaning in a 1:10 bleach solution for 5 minutes to disinfect them.
- Wash dishes and eating utensils in hot water and dishwashing soap or detergent.
- Clean bathroom surfaces with regular household cleaners, then disinfect them with a 1:10 solution of household bleach.

Laundry
- Rinse clothes, towels, or bedclothes if they become soiled with feces, vomitus, sputum, urine, or blood. Then dispose of the soiled water by flushing it down the toilet. Launder these clothes with hot water and detergent with one cup of bleach added per load of laundry.
- Keep soiled clothes in a plastic bag.

Waste Disposal
- Dispose of needles and other "sharps" in a labeled puncture-proof container such as a coffee can with a lid, using Standard Precautions to avoid needlestick injuries. Decontaminate full containers by adding a 1:10 bleach solution. Then seal the container with tape and place it in a paper bag. Dispose of the container in the regular trash.
- Remove solid waste from contaminated trash such as paper towels or tissues, dressings, disposable incontinence pads, and disposable gloves, then flush the waste down the toilet. Place these items in tied plastic bags and dispose of them in the regular trash.

The nurse teaches the client, family, and significant others how to protect the client from infection, how to identify signs and symptoms of potential infections, and what to do if these appear. The nurse instructs the client about the importance of self-care strategies, such as good hygiene, balanced rest and exercise, skin care, mouth care, and safe administration of any ordered medications (including potential side effects). Dietary teaching stresses

- Good nutrition
- Avoidance of raw or rare fish, fowl, or meat
- Thorough washing of fruits and vegetables
- Proper food handling
- Refrigeration practices

The nurse also teaches the client about preventing infections by avoiding large crowds, especially in enclosed areas, not traveling to countries with poor sanitation, and not cleaning pet litter boxes.

➤ Home Care Management

If the client is discharged to home, the nurse carefully assesses the client's status, ability to function, and actual or potential needs for care. Some clients do not need home care but do need to maintain a link with the physician or primary care providers. Home care can range from assistance with activities of daily living for clients with weakness, debility, or limited function to around-the-clock nursing care, medications, and nutritional support for severely or terminally ill clients. The nurse assesses available resources, including family members and significant others willing and able to be caregivers. The nurse helps to make arrangements for outside caregivers or respite care, if needed. Clients may need referrals or help in planning housing, finances, insurance, legal services, funeral arrangements, and spiritual counseling.

Home health aids may be involved in daily or weekly care of the client with AIDS in the home. Usually a home care nurse makes routine visits for assessment purposes, especially as the client becomes increasingly debilitated. Chart 25–8 lists assessment areas for the client with AIDS at home.

➤ Psychosocial Preparation

Clients with AIDS are often concerned about the possible social stigma and rejection that they may experience. The nurse is aware that this fear is realistic, and helps the client to identify ways to avoid problems as well as coping strategies for difficult situations.

Family and significant others are supported in efforts to help the client and provide protection from discrimination.

The nurse encourages clients to continue as many usual activities as possible. Except when clients are too ill or too weak, they can continue to work and participate in most social activities. Because of potential stigma and discrimination, clients are supported in their selection of friends and relatives with whom to discuss the diagnosis. Sexual partners and care providers should be informed; beyond that, it is up to the client. Some clients experience severe depression or anxiety about the future. Almost all feel the burden of having a fatal disease widely

---

Chart 25–8

Focused Assessment for the Home Care Client with AIDS

Assess cardiovascular and respiratory status:

- Vital signs
- Presence of acute chest pain or dyspnea
- Presence of cough
- Presence of fever
- Activity tolerance

Assess nutritional status:

- Food intake
- Weight loss or gain
- General condition of skin
- Financial resources

Assess neurologic status:

- Cognitive changes
- Motor changes
- Sensory disturbances

Assess gastrointestinal status:

- Mouth and oropharynx
- Presence of dysphagia
- Presence of abdominal pain
- Presence of nausea, vomiting, diarrhea

Assess psychological status:

- Presence of anxiety
- Presence of depression

Assess activity and rest:

- Activities of daily living
- Mobility and ambulation
- Fatigue
- Sleep pattern
- Presence of pain

Assess home environment:

- Safety hazards
- Structural barriers affecting functional ability

Assess client's and caregiver's compliance and understanding of illness and treatment, including

- Signs and symptoms to report to nurse
- Medication schedule and side or toxic effects

Assess client's and caregiver's coping skills

---

considered unacceptable, and feel compelled to maintain some secrecy about the illness. Referrals to community resources, mental health professionals, and support groups can help the client verbalize fears and frustrations and cope with the illness.

➤ Health Care Resources

In many cities, community organizations have been set up to assist persons with AIDS. Often composed of volunteers, they offer excellent services to the community. The types and number of services vary by agency and city, but many include HIV testing and counseling, clinic services, buddy systems, support groups, respite care, education and outreach, referral services, and even housing. Clients may also need referrals to other local resources, such as home care agencies, companies that provide home IV therapy, community mental health agencies, Meals on Wheels, and others.

 Evaluation

The overall goals for care of clients with AIDS are to maintain the maximum possible level of function for as long as possible, minimize infections, and maintain quality of life and dignity during the course of progressive illness. On the basis of the identified nursing diagnoses, the nurse evaluates care for the client with AIDS. Expected outcomes include that the client should be able to

- Demonstrate adequate respiratory function
- Attain adequate weight, nutritional, and fluid status
- Maintain skin integrity
- Not develop opportunistic infections
- Remain oriented and/or in a safe environment
- Maintain self-esteem
- Maintain a support system and involvement with others
- Comply with the appropriate and available therapy

Nutrition-Related Deficiencies

Adequate and balanced nutrition is necessary for the proper functioning of the immune system. For example, lymphocytes are highly active metabolic cells that constantly shed surface components (such as immunoglobulin and marker antigens) and need nutrients to resynthesize these components. Immunodeficiency related to nutrition is an acquired abnormality and results from multiple factors—biologic, political, economic, and cultural. Acquired immunodeficiencies from inadequate or inappropriate nutrition are potentially preventable and treatable.

Malnutrition is a major cause of global immunodeficiency, seen with the greatest frequency in developing countries, in the urban and rural poor of developed countries, and in the chronically ill. Hospitalized adult medical-surgical clients also are at high risk for malnutrition. Four points should be kept in mind:

- Anorexia associated with chronic disease, acute infection, or treatment often leads to reduced oral intake.
- Absorption, assimilation, or utilization of nutrients is sometimes impaired because of gastrointestinal diseases or absorption problems.
- Host defense mechanisms mobilized in infection result in increased demand for nutrients, met at the expense of the body's stores.
- Hospitalized clients often receive a semistarvation regimen with many hours of nothing by mouth because of procedures that will be performed or because of IV fluid administration lacking essential nutrients.

Malnutrition can impair any or all aspects of the immune system; the degree of impairment is related to the severity of the malnutrition. An excess of nutrients, especially fats and certain carbohydrates, can also have a detrimental effect on immune function. Nutritional problems are almost never simple but a complex of deficiency or excess of one or multiple nutrients.

Protein-Calorie Malnutrition

Overview

Protein-calorie malnutrition (PCM) affects all aspects of the immune system. The greatest impairment is noted in cell-mediated immunity, with a decreased number of T lymphocytes, reduced delayed hypersensitivity, and thymic changes. The result is *anergy* (no cutaneous delayed hypersensitivity response to common antigens) and an increased incidence of infection. The incidence of PCM is unknown, but estimates range from 25% to 50% of hospitalized adult medical-surgical clients. PCM causes a deficiency in energy and protein synthesis, requiring that other body stores (if available) be used.

The usual manifestations of PCM in adults include

- Leanness and cachexia
- Decreased effort tolerance
- Lethargy
- Intolerance to cold
- Ankle edema
- Dry, flaking skin and various types of dermatitis
- Poor wound healing
- A higher than usual incidence of postoperative infection

Collaborative Management

The management strategy for clients with PCM is to treat the precipitating event and supply protein and calories, sometimes with nutrient supplements. In clients with severe PCM, any infection is first treated and fluid and electrolyte imbalances corrected. Then a gradual but steady repletion of protein and energy is undertaken. Often this refeeding begins parenterally, because a severely malnourished gut undergoes atrophy of the mucosa and depletion of gastric enzymes, resulting in an inability to tolerate food. Replenishment of protein and calories is accompanied by vitamin supplementation as appropriate, nutrition education, psychosocial stimulation, and a progressive increase in physical activity.

Protein-calorie malnutrition is easier to prevent than to treat. The nurse is aware of hospitalized clients at risk for PCM. To reduce this risk, the nurse

- Measures height and weight when the client is admitted to the agency, reweighing at least weekly
- Monitors the client's ability to eat the ordered diet and the amounts eaten
- Obtains dietary consultation when needed
- Evaluates whether nutrients consumed are sufficient to meet basal and stress-related energy needs
- Avoids prolonged use of standard IV fluids that provide less than 200 calories/L.
- Assesses and monitors laboratory values for serum albumin, prealbumin, and leukocyte counts
- Schedules tests and procedures so that the client spends minimal time fasting

Obesity

Overview

The incidence and severity of infectious disease increase among obese people. Impaired cell-mediated immunity and decreased intracellular killing by neutrophils are associated with obesity, making obese people more susceptible to infection. Excess dietary fats have a generalized suppressive action on all aspects of immune function. In addition, the obese client may have a co-existing PCM.

Often the obese client is not recognized as malnourished because of the excessive weight. For these clients, nutritional status must be assessed by laboratory measurements and diet history.

Collaborative Management

Although more research is needed regarding the interaction between obesity and specific immune functions, appropriate nutrition is an important factor in maintaining and improving host immunologic defenses. The nurse, in consultation with the physician and dietitian, provides a diet that has sufficient calories and protein but is low in fat.

Because the obese client is somewhat immunodeficient, the nurse protects the client by maintaining a safe environment. Good hand washing is practiced before all contact with the client. All invasive procedures are conducted using strict aseptic technique. The nurse assesses the client every shift for signs and symptoms of local or systemic infection and notifies the physician of any suspected infection.

Therapy-Induced Immunodeficiencies

Overview

Some secondary immunodeficiencies may be related to other conditions that cause the loss of immunoglobulins or destruction of lymphocytes (T and B cells). The most common cause of secondary immunodeficiency is iatrogenesis, drugs, and other treatment modalities used for various diseases. Sometimes this is a desired effect, as in organ transplantation or the treatment of certain autoimmune disorders. At other times, immunosuppression is an undesirable, complicating side effect of therapy that is used for another intent, such as cancer chemotherapy, and may even necessitate altering the therapeutic regimen. Various therapies cause different types and degrees of immunosuppression. The challenge is deriving maximal therapeutic effect without leaving the client overly immunosuppressed and, therefore, susceptible to potentially serious complications.

Drug-Induced Immunodeficiencies

Several classes of drugs have powerful and significant immunosuppressive effects. Some induce general immunosuppression; others are more specific and target one part of the immune system more than another.

Cytotoxic Drugs

Cytotoxic drugs are usually not selective but interfere with all rapidly proliferating cells. White blood cells, including immunocompetent lymphocytes and phagocytes, rapidly proliferate and are, therefore, susceptible to this type of destruction (see Chaps. 23 and 27). The result is a decrease in the number of lymphocytes and phagocytic cells. Cytotoxic agents also interfere with the ability of lymphocytes to synthesize and release products such as lymphokines and antibodies, thereby causing a general immunosuppression. Most cytotoxic drugs are used to treat cancer (see Chap. 27) and autoimmune disorders.

Corticosteroids

Corticosteroids are adrenocortical hormones used to treat many immunologically mediated diseases, neoplasms, and several neurologic and endocrine disorders. Corticosteroids have both anti-inflammatory and immunosuppressive effects. They inhibit inflammation by stabilizing the vascular membrane and decreasing permeability, thereby blocking the migration and mobilization of neutrophils and monocytes. Corticosteroids disrupt the synthesis of arachidonic acid, the main precursor for a variety of vasoactive amines.

Corticosteroids sequester T cells in the bone marrow, reducing the number of circulating T cells and resulting in lymphopenia and suppressed cell-mediated immunity.

Corticosteroids appear to interfere with immunoglobulin G (IgG) synthesis and immunoglobulin binding to antigen. These drugs have many physiologic and immunologic effects, which can alter disease activity, and numerous side effects, including

- Central nervous system changes, such as euphoria, insomnia, or psychosis
- Cardiovascular changes, such as hypertension and edema
- Gastrointestinal tract effects, such as gastric irritation, ulcers, and increased appetite (with weight gain)
- Other changes, such as cataracts, hyperglycemia and glucose intolerance, muscle weakness, osteoporosis, delayed wound healing, redistribution of body fat

Cyclosporine

Cyclosporine (Sandimmune) is a specific immunosuppressant that selectively suppresses the helper subset of T lymphocytes by blocking proliferation and development (see Chap. 23). Cyclosporine has been used primarily to prevent organ transplant rejection and graft-versus-host disease (see Chaps. 42 and 75). The drug is undergoing clinical trials for use in other disorders, such as uveitis, rheumatoid arthritis, and other autoimmune diseases.

Radiation-Induced Immunodeficiency

Radiation is cytotoxic to proliferating and resting cells. Because most lymphocytes are sensitive to radiation, exposure can induce profound lymphopenia in lymphoid organs and in the circulation, causing general immunosuppression. Whether or not immunodeficiency occurs after radiation therapy depends on the location and dose of radiation. Exposure to the iliac and femur in adults can cause generalized immunosuppression because these medullary areas are the primary blood cell–producing sites. Total nodal irradiation is used in certain diseases, such as Hodgkin's disease, to induce immunosuppression, causing lymphopenia and decreased T-cell function.

Collaborative Management

Management of the client with treatment-induced immunodeficiency aims to improve immune function and protect the client from infection. The most severe immunosuppression occurs while the client is receiving the immunosuppressive drugs or during radiation treatment. The severity and duration of the immunosuppression are related directly to the dosage of specific drugs. Although this impairment is usually temporary, with good recovery of immune and inflammatory responses evident within weeks or months of therapy completion, the seriousness of the potential infection complications makes this problem a major treatment concern. The infectious processes most commonly observed during this period include those of fungal origin, yeast, some residual viral breakthrough, and a wide variety of bacteria.

The nurse works closely with the client and other health care professionals to provide safe care to clients at risk for infection. Chart 27–6 lists specific nursing care actions to prevent infection among clients with drug-induced immunosuppression. Good hand washing by the all health care professionals and unlicensed assistive personnel before contact with the client is the cornerstone for prevention of infection. Health care professionals must practice asepsis (prevention of contact with microorganisms) when any invasive technique or procedure must be done.

In some instances, drug-induced immunosuppression can be managed medically by the administration of biologic response modifiers (BRMs) to stimulate bone marrow production of immune system cells. Although not appropriate for all types of disorders, this supportive treatment can reduce the client's risk for infection during drug therapy. However, BRMs are expensive and not consistently covered by insurance. Further discussion of this treatment is presented in Chapters 27 and 42.

Many clients remain at home during periods of immunosuppression. The nurse teaches the client and family precautions to take to reduce the client's chances of developing an infection (see Chart 27–7).

For clients receiving chronic therapy with immunosuppressive drugs, drug dosages are regulated according to the client's responses. The aim is to give the lowest dose that will achieve the desired effect.

Congenital (Primary) Immunodeficiencies

Congenital, or primary, immunodeficiencies are disorders in which the immunodeficient person is born with a defect in the development or function of one or more of the

TABLE 25–6

Congenital Immunodeficiencies

Antibody-Mediated Immunodeficiencies
- X-linked agammaglobulinemia (Bruton's)
- Acquired hypogammaglobulinemia (common variable immunodeficiency)
- Selective IgA deficiency

Cell-Mediated Immunodeficiencies
- Congenital thymic aplasia (DiGeorge syndrome)
- Chronic mucocutaneous candidiasis

Combined Immunodeficiencies
- Severe combined immunodeficiencies
- Wiskott-Aldrich syndrome
- Immunodeficiency with ataxia-telangiectasia
- Nezelof syndrome

immune components. As a result, the immune response does not adequately protect the client from infection, cancer, or other disease. Fortunately, most congenital immunodeficiencies are rare.

Some congenital immunodeficiencies are inherited as an X-linked trait (such as Bruton's disease or Wiskott-Aldrich syndrome), and some are autosomal-recessive (such as immunodeficiency with ataxia-telangiectasia). For many congenital immunodeficiencies, however, the genetic defect and inheritance pattern have not been clearly identified. Examples of congenital immunodeficiencies are listed in Table 25–6.

Congenital immunodeficiencies are classified according to the type of immune function that is impaired: antibody-mediated, cell-mediated, and combined. Because cell-mediated and combined immunodeficiencies are so severe that the affected person usually does not survive infancy or childhood, only antibody-mediated immunodeficiencies (seen in adults) are discussed in this chapter.

Bruton's Agammaglobulinemia

Overview

A prototypic congenital antibody-mediated immunodeficiency is Bruton's or X-linked agammaglobulinemia. Boys born with this disease present at about 6 months of age, after the loss of maternal antibodies, with recurrent sinusitis, pneumonia, otitis, furunculosis, meningitis, and septicemia with extracellular pyogenic organisms, such as *Pneumococcus, Streptococcus,* and *Haemophilus.* Laboratory evaluation of the client with Bruton's agammaglobulinemia reveals an absence of circulating immunoglobulin.

Collaborative Management

Except for clients with poliomyelitis, chronic echovirus infection, or a lymphoreticular malignancy, the overall prognosis is fairly good if antibody replacement is begun early. IV or IM immune serum globulin is regularly given to these clients, usually about 100 to 400 mg/kg every 3 to 4 weeks (Chart 25–9). The dosage and schedule are

---

Chart 25–9

Nursing Care Highlight: Administration of Intravenous Immune Serum Globulin

Indications	Dosage	Interventions	Rationale

B cell or humoral immunodeficiencies
  Bruton's hypogammaglobulinemia
  Common variable immunodeficiency
  Combined immunodeficiencies: severe combined immunodeficiencies
Pediatric AIDS
	• Gamimune, 100–200 mg/kg or 2–4 mL/kg, IV once monthly
	or
	• Sandoglobulin, 0.2–0.3 g/kg, IV once monthly
	• Gammagard 200–400 mg/kg, IV once monthly
	• Iveegam 200–800 mg/kg, IV once monthly
		• Observe client closely and monitor vital signs during infusion and for 30–60 minutes thereafter.
		
		• Slow the rate of infusion or stop it temporarily if side effects occur.
			• Monitoring detects signs of anaphylaxis and routine side effects. Side effects occur in 10% of clients and include skeletal pain, back pain, nausea, chills, headache, chest tightness, and abdominal cramps.
			
			• Side effects appear to be related to the rate of infusion.

---

individualized. Intermittent courses of antibiotics are used for specific infections. Long-term prophylactic antibiotic therapy may also be used. Despite therapy, severe sinopulmonary disease later develops in some clients.

Common Variable Immunodeficiency

Overview

Common variable immunodeficiency, or acquired hypogammaglobulinemia, is characterized by recurrent bacterial infections similar to those seen in clients with Bruton's disease. The client has low levels of circulating immunoglobulins of all classes.

Acquired hypogammaglobulinemia differs from Bruton's disease in that it usually first appears later (in adolescence or young adulthood), occurs almost equally in males and females, and is associated with a less severe susceptibility to infection. Frequent complications include giardiasis (intestinal infection with the protozoon *Giardia lamblia*), bronchiectasis, gastric carcinoma, lymphoreticular malignancy, and cholelithiasis (gallbladder stones).

Collaborative Management

Treatment is similar to that for Bruton's disease. Regular administration of IV or IM immune serum globulin and regular or intermittent use of antibiotics protect the affected person against infection.

Selective Immunoglobulin A Deficiency

Overview

Selective immunoglobulin A (IgA) deficiency is the most common congenital immunodeficiency, occurring in 1 per 600 to 800 individuals (Cotran et al., 1994). The client may be asymptomatic or have chronic recurrent respiratory tract infections, atopic diseases, or collagen-vascular diseases. Usually, clients with selective IgA deficiency have a normal life span. Because IgA is the major immunoglobulin in secretions, bacterial infections are seen primarily in the respiratory, gastrointestinal, and urogenital tracts. Some adults with IgA deficiency also have a malabsorption syndrome.

Collaborative Management

Therapy for selective IgA deficiency is limited to appropriate and vigorous treatment of infections. Unlike other immunoglobulin deficiencies, selective IgA deficiency should never be treated with exogenous immune globulin for two reasons. First, exogenous immune globulin contains very little IgA. Second, because clients with selective IgA deficiency make normal amounts of all other classes of immunoglobulins, they are at high risk for severe allergic reactions to exogenous immune globulin. If malabsorption syndrome accompanies the selective IgA deficiency, the client will need nutritional supplementation (such as total parenteral nutrition).

HYPERSENSITIVITIES

Hypersensitivity is a state of altered reactivity in which a previously sensitized immune system reacts excessively or inappropriately, with resultant tissue damage and pathology. The primary function of the immune system is to protect the host from harm. However, the same protective mechanisms, if prolonged or excessive, have a deleterious effect and may produce tissue damage (Workman, 1995).

Immune mechanisms resulting in tissue damage to the host are classified into five basic types of hypersensitivity (Table 25–7) (Roitt, 1994):

- Type I: rapid hypersensitivity (anaphylactic) reactions
- Type II: (cytotoxic) reactions
- Type III: (immune complex–mediated) reactions
- Type IV: (delayed) hypersensitivity reactions
- Type V: (stimulatory) reactions

Clinical manifestations may be the consequence of one or any combination of these mechanisms of tissue injury.

TABLE 25–7

Mechanisms and Examples of Types of Hypersensitivities	
Mechanism	**Clinical Examples**
Type I: Immediate	
Reaction of IgE antibody on mast cells with antigen, which results in release of mediators	• Hay fever • Allergic asthma • Anaphylaxis
Type II: Cytotoxic	
Reaction of IgG with host cell membrane or antigen adsorbed by host cell membrane	• Autoimmune hemolytic anemia • Goodpasture's syndrome • Myasthenia gravis
Type III: Immune Complex–Mediated	
Formation of immune complex of antigen and antibody, which deposits in walls of blood vessels and results in complement release and inflammation	• Serum sickness • Vasculitis • Systemic lupus erythematosus • Rheumatoid arthritis
Type IV: Delayed	
Reaction of sensitized T cells with antigen and release of lymphokines, which activate macrophages and induce inflammation	• Poison ivy • Graft rejection • Tuberculosis • Sarcoidosis
Type V: Stimulated	
Reaction of autoantibodies with normal cell-surface receptors, stimulating a continual overreaction of the target cell	• Graves' disease • B-cell gammopathies

Type I: Rapid Hypersensitivity Reactions

Type I, or rapid, hypersensitivity occurs when IgE responds to an otherwise harmless antigen, such as pollen, and causes the release of histamine and other vasoactive amines from basophils, eosinophils and mast cells (see Chap. 23). This response results in an acute inflammatory reaction and symptoms such as bronchospasm, wheezing, and rhinorrhea.

On first exposure to an allergen (an antigen that provokes allergic sensitization with IgE), the host responds by making antigen-specific IgE. This antigen-specific IgE then binds to the surface of basophils and mast cells. These cells have large numbers of granules containing vasoactive amines (including histamine) that are released when stimulated (see Chap. 23). Once the antigen-specific IgE is formed, the host is sensitized to that allergen.

In a type I hypersensitivity reaction, the previously sensitized person is re-exposed to the provoking allergen. The allergen binds to two adjacent IgE molecules on the surface of a basophil or mast cell, distorting the cell

membrane. This distortion initiates a series of biochemical events causing the cell granules to swell, migrate, and fuse with the cell membrane. The granular contents (vasoactive amines) are then expelled and released into the extravascular space, a process called *degranulation.*

The most important mediator is *histamine,* a short-acting vasoactive amine. Histamine causes increased capillary permeability, mucous secretion (both nasal and bronchial), smooth muscle contractions (especially of bronchioles and small blood vessels), and itching (pruritus), sometimes accompanied by redness. These symptoms last for approximately 10 minutes; the maximum reaction occurs 1 to 2 minutes after histamine release.

Clinical examples of type I reactions include systemic anaphylaxis, allergic asthma, and atopic (genetic tendency) allergies such as hay fever, allergic rhinitis, and allergies to specific allergens. Allergens can be

■ Inhaled (plant pollens, fungal spores, animal dander, house dust, grass, ragweed)
■ Ingested (foods, food additives, drugs)
■ Injected (bee venom, drugs, biological substances such as contrast dyes and adrenocorticotropic hormone)
■ Contacted (pollens, foods, environmental proteins)

Chapter 69 describes methods of allergy testing.

Anaphylaxis

Overview

Anaphylaxis, the most dramatic example of a type I hypersensitivity reaction, occurs rapidly, systemically, and affects multiple organs simultaneously within seconds to minutes after exposure to an allergen. Anaphylaxis is not common, but it can be fatal. Many substances can trigger anaphylaxis in a susceptible person (see Table 25–8).

Collaborative Management

 Assessment

Typically, a client experiencing an anaphylactic reaction first complains of feelings of uneasiness, apprehension, weakness, and impending doom. The nurse notes that the client is anxious and frightened. These feelings are followed, often quickly, by a generalized pruritus and urticaria. The nurse sees erythema and sometimes angioedema of the eyes, lips, or tongue. Frequently, discrete cutaneous wheals or urticarial eruptions appear that are intensely pruritic and sometimes merge together in a large, red blotch.

Histamine and other chemical mediators cause bronchoconstriction, mucosal edema, and excess mucus. On respiratory assessment, the nurse notes congestion, rhinorrhea, dyspnea, and increasing respiratory distress with audible wheezing.

On auscultation, the nurse detects crackles, wheezing, and diminished breath sounds. Clients may experience laryngeal edema as a "lump in the throat," hoarseness, and stridor (a crowing sound). Distress increases as the tongue and larynx become more edematous and excess mucous secretion continues. The nurse may note increas-

TABLE 25-8

Common Agents That Cause Anaphylaxis

Drugs/Foreign Proteins

- Antibiotics (penicillin, cephalosporins, tetracycline, sulfonamides, streptomycin, vancomycin, chloramphenicol, amphotericin B, others)
- Adrenocorticotropic hormone, insulin, vasopressin, protamine*
- Allergen extracts, muscle relaxants, hydrocortisone, vaccines, local anesthetics (lidocaine, procaine)*
- Whole blood, cryoprecipitate, immune serum globulin*
- Radiocontrast media*
- Opiates

Foods

- Shellfish
- Eggs
- Legumes, nuts
- Grains
- Berries
- Preservatives

Other Agents

- Pollens
- Exercise
- Heat/cold
- Other

Insects/Animals

- Hymenoptera: bees, wasps, hornets
- Fire ants
- Snake venom

* Anaphylaxis caused by these substances is probably a result of direct mast cell degranulation rather than an IgE-mediated hypersensitivity event.

ing stridor and anxiety as the airway begins to close. Respiratory failure may follow quickly as a complication of laryngeal edema, suffocation, or lower airway bronchoconstriction causing hypoxemia (insufficient oxygenation of blood) and hypercapnia (increased carbon dioxide in blood).

In performing the cardiovascular assessment, the nurse usually finds hypotension and a rapid, weak, possibly irregular pulse. These findings are due to chemical mediators causing vasodilation and increased capillary permeability with resultant leakage of intravascular fluids. The nurse notes faintness and diaphoresis, increasing anxiety, confusion, and, if the client is not treated immediately, loss of consciousness. Dysrhythmias, shock, and cardiac arrest may occur within minutes as intravascular volume is lost. Less often, the client may have abdominal cramping, diarrhea, or vomiting. Seventy percent of deaths are caused by respiratory failure or by shock and cardiac dysrhythmias.

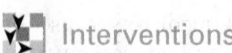 Interventions

➤ Emergency Respiratory Management

Emergency respiratory management is critical for the client having an anaphylactic reaction, because the severity of the reaction and gravity of the consequences increase with time. An airway must be established or stabilized immediately. The nurse may need to initiate cardiopulmonary resuscitation. Epinephrine (1:1000), 0.2 to 0.5 mL, should be given subcutaneously as soon as possible after

a person displays symptoms of systemic anaphylaxis. This agent constricts blood vessels, increases myocardial contraction, and dilates the bronchioles. The same dose may be repeated every 15 to 20 minutes if needed. Other commonly administered drugs are listed in Chart 25-10.

Antihistamines, such as diphenhydramine (Allerdryl❖, Benadryl), 25 to 100 mg, are usually given IV, IM, or orally to treat angioedema and urticaria. This agent blocks the histamine receptor site (H_1) in vascular and bronchiolar smooth muscle. If the extent of upper airway narrowing requires it, the physician may insert a small endotracheal tube or perform an emergency tracheostomy.

If the client can breathe independently, the nurse administers oxygen, as ordered, to minimize hypoxemia. Oxygen should be started via nasal cannula at 5 to 10 L/minute or via face mask at 40% to 60% before arterial blood gas results are obtained. The nurse monitors tissue oxygen saturation using pulse oximetry. Arterial blood gas concentrations are monitored to determine oxygenation adequacy, with the goal of maintaining partial pressure of oxygen between 80 and 100 mm Hg. The nurse uses suction to remove excess mucous secretions, if indicated. The client's rate, rhythm, and depth of respirations as well as the presence of bronchospasm and abnormal breath sounds are assessed continually. The nurse or other assistive personnel elevates the client's bed to 45 degrees unless contraindicated because of hypotension.

For severe bronchospasm, the client is given aminophylline (Truphylline), 6 mg/kg IV, over 20 to 30 minutes. If the client is taking aminophylline regularly, no more than 3 mg/kg is given. Maintenance aminophylline (0.3-0.5 mg/kg/hour) is initiated. The client may be given an inhaled beta-adrenergic agonist such as metaproterenol (Alupent) or albuterol (Proventil) every 2 to 4 hours. For persistent symptoms (after 1-2 hours), corticosteroids are added to prevent the late recurrence of symptoms.

The nurse's primary role in caring for the client with anaphylaxis is to assess changes in any body system or adverse effects of drug therapy. For severe anaphylaxis, the client is admitted to a critical care unit for cardiac, pulmonary arterial, and capillary wedge pressure monitoring. The nurse carefully observes the client for fluid overload from the rapid administration of medications and IV fluids and reports changes to the physician immediately. The client may be discharged from the hospital when respiratory and cardiovascular systems have returned to baseline.

➤ Prevention

Because of the rapid onset of life-threatening symptoms and the potential for a fatal outcome, sometimes even with appropriate medical intervention, preventing anaphylaxis is paramount. The nurse teaches the client with a history of allergic reactions to avoid allergens whenever possible, to wear a medical alert bracelet, and to alert health care personnel about specific allergies. Some clients must carry an emergency anaphylaxis kit, such as a bee sting kit with injectable epinephrine, or an epinephrine injector, such as the EpiPen automatic injector (Center Laboratories). The EpiPen device is an easy-to-use, spring-

Chart 25–10

Drug Therapy for Anaphylaxis

Drug	Mechanism	Side Effects
Sympathomimetics		
• Epinephrine (Adrenalin)	• Rapidly stimulates alpha- and beta-adrenergic receptors of autonomic nervous system (alpha: vasoconstriction; beta: bronchodilation)	• Pallor, tachycardia and palpitations, nervousness, muscle twitching, sweating, anxiety, insomnia, hypertension, headache, hyperglycemia
• Isoproterenol (Isuprel)	• Stimulated beta-adrenergic receptors, relaxing bronchial muscle and dilating vessels	• Same as for epinephrine
• Ephedrine sulfate (Vatronol)	• Similar to isoproterenol, but with longer duration of action	• Same as for epinephrine
Antihistamines		
• Diphenhydramine HCl (Allerdryl✦, Benadryl)	• Competes with histamine for H_1 receptors on effector cells, thus blocking effects of histamine on bronchioles, gastrointestinal tract, and blood vessels	• Drowsiness, confusion, insomnia, headache, vertigo, photosensitivity, diplopia, nausea, vomiting, dry mouth
Corticosteroids		
• Prednisone (PO)	• Anti-inflammatory; inhibits mast cell degranulation	• Fluid and sodium retention, hypertension, cushingoid state, gastric distress, adrenal suppression, psychosis, osteoporosis, susceptibility to infection
• Hydrocortisone sodium succinate (Solu-Cortef) (IV/IM)		
• Methylprednisolone sodium succinate (Solu-Medrol) (IV/IM)		
• Beclomethasone (inhalant)		
Methylxanthines		
• Aminophylline (Truphylline)	• Relaxes bronchial smooth muscle	• Restlessness, dizziness, palpitations, tachycardia, nausea, vomiting, epigastric distress, headache, convulsions
Vasopressors		
• Norepinephrine (Levophed)	• Raises blood pressure and cardiac output in severely decompensated states	• Headache, tachycardia, fibrillation, decreased urinary output, hypertension, metabolic acidosis
• Dopamine (Intropin)		• Arrhythmias, tachycardia, hypertension, dyspnea, nausea and vomiting, azotemia, headache
Inhaled Beta-Adrenergic Agonists		
• Metaproterenol (Alupent, Metaprel)	• Rapidly stimulates $beta_2$-receptor sites in pulmonary smooth muscle, causing bronchodilation	• Palpitations, tachycardia, dysrhythmias, hypokalemia
• Albuterol (Proventil, Ventolin)	• Same as for metaproterenol	• Same as for metaproterenol, plus painful urination, flushing of the face

loaded injector that delivers 0.3 mg of epinephrine per 2 mL dose.

The medical record of a client with a history of anaphylactic symptoms should prominently display the list of allergens to which the client is sensitive. A careful history is taken before any drug or therapeutic agent is given. Skin tests should be performed before any substance with a highly associated incidence of anaphylactic reactions, such as allergenic extract or horse serums, is administered. Physicians and nurses must be aware of common cross-reacting agents. For example, a client with a history of sensitivity to penicillin is also likely to react to cephalosporins because both have a similar biochemical structure.

If an agent must be used despite a history of allergenic reactions, precautionary measures should be taken. IV solution should be started, and intubation equipment and a tracheostomy set placed at the bedside. The substance should be given first intradermally, then subcutaneously, and then intramuscularly in increasing doses at 20- to 30-minute intervals so the initial dose by the next route does not exceed the final dose by the previous route. When carefully done, this procedure is fairly safe.

Atopic Allergy

Atopic reactions are allergic manifestations that occur in people who are genetically predisposed to respond to a variety of environmental allergens by forming immunoglobulin E (IgE). Once the person has sensitized IgE, allergic symptoms occur on re-exposure to the allergen via degranulation of mast cells. Conditions such as allergic asthma, allergic rhinitis, urticaria (hives), and eczematous dermatitis are manifested alone or in combination. Dermatitis and urticaria are described in Chapter 70 as types of skin inflammation. Asthma is discussed in Chapter 32. Allergic rhinitis is discussed in Chapter 31.

Type II: Cytotoxic Reactions
Overview

In a type II (cytotoxic) reaction, the body makes special autoantibodies directed against self cells or tissues that have some form of foreign protein attached to them. The autoantibody binds to the self cell and forms an antigen–antibody complex, or immune complex. The self cell is then destroyed by phagocytosis or complement-mediated lysis (see Chap. 23). Clinical examples of type II reactions include Coombs'-positive hemolytic anemias, thrombocytopenic purpura, hemolytic transfusion reactions (when an individual receives the wrong blood type during a transfusion), hemolytic disease of the newborn, Goodpasture's syndrome, and drug-induced hemolytic anemia.

Collaborative Management

Treatment of type II cytotoxic reactions begins with discontinuation of the offending drug or blood product. Plasmapheresis to remove autoantibodies may be beneficial. Otherwise, treatment is symptomatic. Complications such as hemolytic crisis and renal failure can be life threatening.

Type III: Immune Complex Reactions
Overview

In a type III reaction, soluble immune complexes are formed, usually with antigen excess (Fig. 25–2). These circulating immune complexes are then usually deposited in small blood vessel walls. Common sites include the kidneys, skin, joints, and other small blood vessels. The deposited immune complex activates complement, and tissue or vessel damage results.

There are many immune complex disorders (mostly connective tissue disorders) in which the type III reaction is the major mechanism of disease. For example, the clinical manifestations of rheumatoid arthritis are caused by immune complexes that lodge in joint spaces followed by destruction of tissue and, later, scarring and fibrous changes. Similarly, the clinical manifestations of systemic lupus erythematosus result from immune complex deposition in the vessels (vasculitis), the glomeruli (nephritis), the joints (arthralgia, arthritis), and other organs and tissues. In this disorder, the immune complex is composed of cellular DNA and anti-DNA antibodies. (For a detailed discussion of these and other connective tissue disorders, see Chapter 24.)

Serum sickness is a complex of symptoms that occurs after administration of a foreign serum or certain drugs, caused by collection of immune complexes deposited in blood vessel walls of the skin, joints, and kidney. The most common causes of serum sickness today are penicillin and related drugs and some animal serum antitoxins. Serum sickness used to be quite common when vaccines were made with horse or rabbit serum, but now most vaccines are made with human serum or antigen fragments. Relatively new agents that can cause serum sickness are antilymphocyte globulin and antithymocyte globulin, used to suppress the immune response in organ transplantation.

Collaborative Management

The client with serum sickness has symptoms of fever, arthralgia (achy joints), rash, lymphadenopathy (enlarged lymph nodes), malaise, and possibly polyarthritis and nephritis, usually about 7 to 12 days after administration of the causative agent. The nurse alerts the client to the possibility of serum sickness and what symptoms to look for. When administering a foreign serum to a client, the nurse is also prepared for a type I anaphylactic reaction and has emergency equipment and medications close at hand.

Serum sickness is usually self-limiting, and symptoms subside after several days. Treatment is usually symptomatic; antihistamines are given for pruritus and aspirin for arthralgias. Prednisone is given if symptoms are severe.

Type IV: Delayed Hypersensitivity Reactions
Overview

In a type IV reaction, the reactive cell is the T lymphocyte. Antibodies and complement are not involved. Sensitized T lymphocytes (from a previous exposure) respond to an antigen by producing and releasing certain lymphokines (chemical mediators) and recruit, retain, and activate macrophages to destroy the antigen. A type IV response typically occurs hours to days after exposure rather than immediately, as in a type I hypersensitivity reaction. A type IV reaction is characterized by an accu-

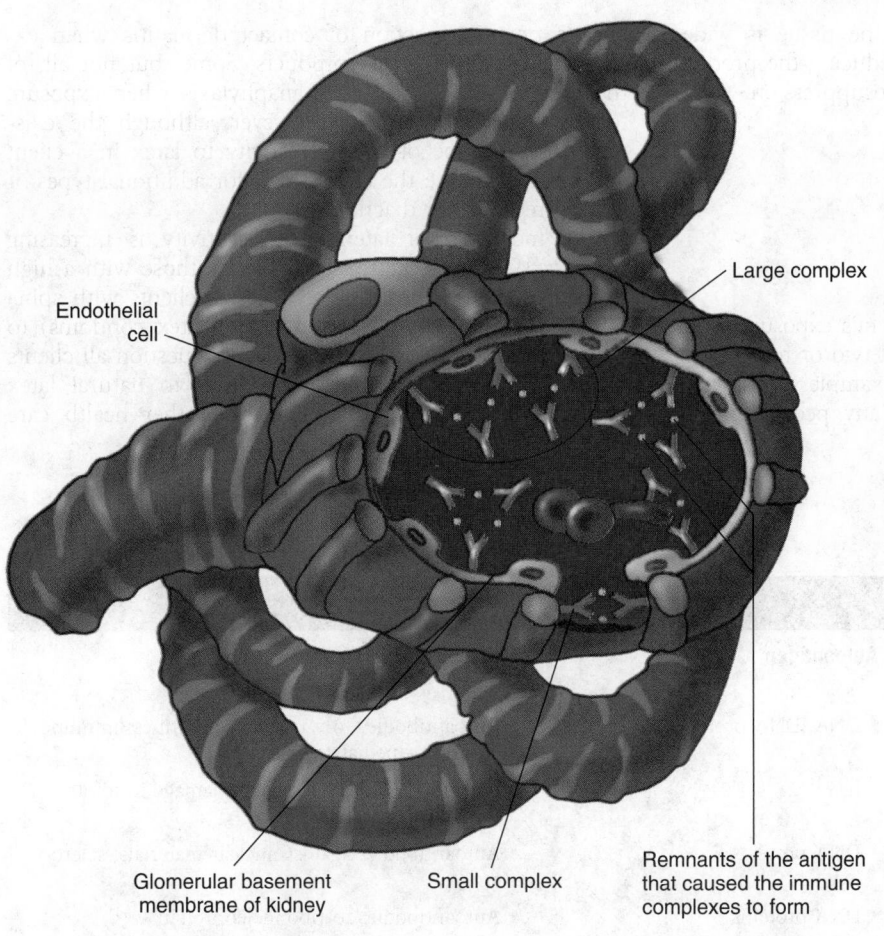

Figure 25–2. An immune complex in a type III hypersensitivity reaction.

mulation of lymphocytes and macrophages, causing edema, ischemia, and tissue destruction at the site.

An example of a type IV reaction is a positive purified protein derivative (PPD) test. In a client who had previously been exposed to tuberculosis, an intradermal injection of this agent causes sensitized T cells to accumulate at the injection site, release lymphokines, and recruit and activate macrophages. Induration and erythema at the site of the injection appear approximately 24 to 48 hours later.

Clinical examples of type IV hypersensitivity reactions include contact dermatitis, poison ivy skin rashes, local response to insect stings, allograft (tissue transplant) rejections, and granulomatous diseases in which the antigen is unknown (e.g., sarcoidosis).

Collaborative Management

Removal of the offending antigen is the major focus of management. The reaction is self-limiting in 5 to 7 days, and the client is treated symptomatically. Nursing responsibilities include monitoring the reaction site and sites distal to the reaction for circulation adequacy. Diphenhydramine is of minimal benefit for type IV reactions because histamine is not the main mediator. Corticosteroids or other anti-inflammatory agents can reduce the discomfort and resolve the reaction more quickly.

Type V: Stimulatory Reactions
Overview

This relatively new category of hypersensitivity reactions involves inappropriate stimulation of a normal cell surface receptor by an autoantibody, resulting in a continuous "turned-on" state for the cell. The classic example of a stimulatory reaction is Graves' disease, in which an autoantibody binds to the thyroid-stimulating hormone (TSH) receptor sites on the thyroid gland. This binding continually stimulates the thyroid cells to produce thyroid hormones, causing the client to have symptoms of severe hyperthyroidism (see Chap. 67), although the thyroid gland is completely normal. In a sense, the tissue responding to the autoantibody is "out of control" from the body's normal feedback system of checks and balances.

Collaborative Management

For type V reactions involving only one organ, the management focuses on removing enough of the responding (stimulated) tissue to return the function to normal. In the case of Graves' disease, thyroid tissue usually is either surgically removed or destroyed with radiation. For type V reactions in which either more than one tissue is being

Labels on figure:
Endothelial cell
Large complex
Glomerular basement membrane of kidney
Small complex
Remnants of the antigen that caused the immune complexes to form

stimulated by the autoantibodies or the tissue is widespread, the focus of treatment is on reducing the production of autoantibodies through immunosuppression.

Mixed Hypersensitivity Reactions: Latex Hypersensitivity

It is important to remember that a client's exposure to an allergen can result in a combination of two or more types of hypersensitivity reactions. One example of such a mixed reaction is latex sensitivity. Many people experi-

ence a type IV reaction of contact dermatitis when exposed externally to latex products. Some, but not all, of these people also experience anaphylaxis when exposure to latex occurs internally. However, although the existence of one type of hypersensitivity to latex in a client appears to increase the client's risk for additional types, it is not predictive or diagnostic.

The incidence of latex hypersensitivity is increasing (Kellett, 1997). People most at risk are those with a high exposure (such as health care workers, clients with spina bifida, and people who routinely use latex condoms) to natural latex products. The nurse must question all clients regarding use of and known reactions to natural latex products. In addition, the nurse and other health care

TABLE 25-9

Autoimmune Disorders*		
Disorder	**Autoantigen**	**Comments**
Systemic or Non–Organ-Specific		
Systemic lupus erythematosus	• DNA, DNA proteins	• Autoantibodies to a number of entities; immune complex–mediated damage
Rheumatoid arthritis	• IgG	• Immune complex–mediated damage in joints (arthritis, fibrosis)
Progressive systemic sclerosis	• DNA proteins	• Autoantibodies against nuclear materials; sclerosis
Mixed connective tissue disease	• DNA proteins	• Autoantibodies to ribonucleoprotein
Organ-Specific		
Autoimmune hemolytic anemia	• Erythrocytes	• Killing of antibody-coated erythrocytes
Autoimmune thrombocytopenic purpura	• Platelets	• Killing of antibody-coated platelets or innocent bystander effect
Myasthenia gravis	• Acetylcholine receptor	• Blocking of impulse transmission by autoantibody to acetylcholine receptor on muscle
Graves' disease	• Thyroid-stimulating hormone receptor	• Stimulation by autoantibody to thyroid-stimulating hormone receptor
Rheumatic fever	• Myocardial cells	• Cross-reaction of antibody with myocardial cells
Idiopathic Addison's disease	• Adrenal cell	• Antibody- and cell-mediated adrenal cytotoxicity
Hashimoto's thyroiditis	• Thyroid cell surface	• Antibody- and cell-mediated thyroid cytotoxicity
Pernicious anemia	• Intrinsic factor/parietal cell	• Autoantibodies to intrinsic factor, intrinsic factor/B_{12} complexes, and parietal canalicula cells
Goodpasture's syndrome	• Basement membrane	• Antiglomerular basement membrane antibodies, which also cross-react with pulmonary basement membrane
Glomerulonephritis	• Glomerular basement membrane	• Autoantibodies and/or immune complex–mediated damage
Uveitis	• Uvea	• Cell-mediated and humoral damage
Vasculitis	• Unknown	• Probably primarily immune complex–mediated damage

* Other inflammatory, granulomatous, degenerative, and atrophic disorders are thought to be autoimmune because there is no more reasonable alternative explanation.

workers need to consider their own exposure and risk for hypersensitivities to natural latex products.

Autoimmunities

Overview

Autoimmunity is a process whereby a person develops and expresses immunologic reactivity, especially in the form of antibodies, against self components. For unknown reasons, certain cells or tissues of the body are recognized as non-self or no longer tolerated as self, and immune reactions occur. The responses, both antibody- and cell-mediated, are similar to normal immune responses against non-self, although inappropriate and sometimes excessive. Reasons for alterations in self-tolerance are not known, but there are multiple theories.

Autoimmunity research is ongoing, and there are few confirmed, established data. Not only is the cause of autoimmunity uncertain, but there is also a lack of consensus as to which diseases are truly autoimmune. Diseases that are generally believed to be autoimmune include systemic lupus erythematosus, polyarteritis nodosa, rheumatoid arthritis, autoimmune hemolytic anemia, rheumatic fever, and Hashimoto's thyroiditis (Table 25–9).

Connective tissue disorders, sometimes referred to as collagen disorders, are characterized by changes in connective tissue. Many of these diseases are considered autoimmune, and for most, autoantibodies have been detected. Connective tissue disorders include systemic lupus erythematosus, rheumatoid arthritis, scleroderma, and polyarteritis nodosa. Most of these tissue disorders are characterized as organ-nonspecific autoimmunities, which means that the autoantibodies and the tissue damage are not limited to a specific organ. In organ-specific autoimmunities, tissue damage occurs in a specific organ (see Chap. 24).

Collaborative Management

Treatment of autoimmunities depends on the organ or organs affected. Anti-inflammatory drugs and immunosuppressive drugs are commonly used.

Gammopathies: Multiple Myeloma

Overview

Gammopathies are relatively rare disorders involving abnormal reproduction of the lymphoid cells that produce immunoglobulins. More specifically, gammopathies are associated with increased production of an abnormal clone of immunoglobulin-secreting plasma cells derived from B lymphocytes (see Chap. 23). Several terms other than gammopathies are used to describe this group of diseases: monoclonal gammopathies, plasma cell dyscrasias, paraproteinemias, dysproteinemias, and immunoglobulinopathies.

The most common example of disease in this group is multiple myeloma. Other gammopathies are plasmacytoma, Waldenström's macroglobulinemia, heavy chain disease, and histiocytoses.

Multiple myeloma is a malignant condition in which a clone of transformed (cancer-like) plasma cells multiplies in bone marrow. The result is disruption of normal bone marrow function and eventual invasion and destruction of adjacent bone. The ability of plasma cells to make functional antibodies decreases, leaving the client immunocompromised. The cause of multiple myeloma is unknown, but genetic predisposition, oncogenic viruses, inflammatory stimuli, and chronic antigenic stimulation have all been identified as possible etiologic factors.

Essentially, an excess number of abnormal plasma cells invade the bone marrow, develop into tumors, and ultimately destroy bone. They then invade lymph nodes, liver, spleen, and kidneys. These plasma cells produce an abnormal antibody often referred to as a myeloma protein, or the *Bence Jones protein,* found in the blood and urine of people with multiple myeloma. Multiple myeloma occurs in middle-aged and elderly clients and in men more often than in women.

The onset of multiple myeloma is insidious, and most people remain asymptomatic until the disease is advanced. Some people are diagnosed without symptoms by Bence Jones proteinuria and an elevated total serum protein level. The major complaint is usually skeletal pain—especially in the pelvis, spine, and ribs—weakness, fatigue, and recurrent infection. Other clinical manifestations include osteoporosis (bone loss) and hypercalcemia (increased serum calcium) related to destruction of bone. If there is vertebral involvement and destruction, spinal cord compression and paraplegia may occur. Pathologic fractures are also common.

Anemia is a major problem for these clients. Anemia is due to invasion of the bone marrow by plasma cells and, therefore, a failure of normal marrow function. Thrombocytopenia (decreased serum platelets) and granulocytopenia (decreased serum granulocytes) also occur. Renal failure occurs in approximately 20% of clients as a result of increased calcium levels, severe proteinuria, and hyperuricemia (increased serum uric acid).

Collaborative Management

The diagnostic work-up shows pancytopenia (a decrease of all serum blood cells), a high total serum protein level, hyperuricemia, hypercalcemia, an elevated serum creatinine level, and Bence Jones proteinuria. Radiograph and isotope scans show the extent of bony destruction. X-ray films show bones with multiple dark lesions—a "Swiss cheese" appearance.

Treatment includes systemic chemotherapy and supportive care of complications. The chemotherapeutic agent most commonly used is melphalan (Alkeran), often with corticosteroids and cyclophosphamide (Cytoxan). Therapy with cytokines is under investigation for multiple myeloma. Supportive care is important to control symptoms and prevent complications, especially bone fractures, renal failure, and infections.

Clients need fluids (approximately 3–4 L/day) to offset the potential problems of hypercalcemia and proteinuria.

(See Chapters 16 and 27 for additional interventions in reducing the serum calcium level.)

The nurse is alert for back pain and the development of neurologic symptoms in the lower extremities. These symptoms may indicate impending spinal cord compression and should be diagnosed and treated (with surgery or radiation) as soon as possible to prevent paraplegia. The nurse teaches the client to recognize signs and symptoms of infection so infections can be diagnosed and treated early and efficiently. Blood transfusions are often required for anemia. Pain control is essential. Analgesics, orthopedic supports, local radiation, and relaxation techniques are all helpful.

CASE STUDY for the Client with AIDS

■ A 32-year-old woman is one of your home care clients with AIDS. Her medication orders include TMP 160 mg BID, SMX 800 mg BID, Ketoconazole, 200 mg QD, Didanosine, 200 mg BID.

■ Today, she complains that she is short of breath, and has sharp pains in her chest. She appears anxious. During the respiratory assessment, you find that she is dyspneic and tachypneic at rest, with a respiratory rate of 30. On auscultation, you hear crackles in her right lower lobe.

QUESTIONS:

1. When taking the client's history, what important questions should you ask?
2. What physical assessment techniques should you perform?
3. Given the respiratory findings, what should you do first?

SELECTED BIBLIOGRAPHY

Abbas, A., Lichtman, A., & Pober, J. (1997). *Cellular and molecular immunology* (3rd ed). Philadelphia: W. B. Saunders.

Anastasi, J., & Lee, V. (1994). HIV wasting: How to stop the cycle. *American Journal of Nursing, 94*(6), 18–25.

Anastasi, J., & Rivera, J. (1994). Understanding prophylactic therapy for HIV. *American Journal of Nursing, 94*(2), 36–41.

Barnes, D. (1995). HIV-1-infected long-term non-progressors: A distinct group or part of a continuum? *Journal of NIH Research, 7*(2), 19–21.

Bechtel-Boenning, C. (1996). State of the art: Antiviral treatment of HIV infection. *Nursing Clinics of North America, 31*(1), 1–13.

Bjorgen, S. (1998). Clinical snapshot: Herpes zoster. *American Journal of Nursing, 98*(2), 46–47.

*Centers for Disease Control. (1987). Public Health Service guidelines for counseling and antibody testing to prevent HIV infection and AIDS. *MMWR. Morbidity and Mortality Weekly Report, 36*(31), 509–515.

*Centers for Disease Control. (1991). Recommendations for preventing transmission of human immunodeficiency virus and hepatitis B virus to patients during exposure-prone invasive procedures. *MMWR. Morbidity and Mortality Weekly Review, 40*(RR-8), 1–9.

Centers for Disease Control and Prevention. (1997). *HIV/AIDS surveillance report*. Atlanta, GA: Author.

Coste, J., Montes, B., Reynes, J., Peeters, M., Segarra, C., Vendrell, J., Delaporte, E., & Segondy, M. (1996). Comparative evaluation of three assays for the quantitation of human immunodeficiency virus type 1 RNA in plasma. *Journal of Medical Virology, 50*(4), 293–302.

Cotran, R., Kumar, V., & Robbins, S. (1994). *Robbins' pathologic basis of disease* (5th ed). Philadelphia: W. B. Saunders.

Dowling, M. (1997). Multiple myeloma. *Professional Nurse, 12*(5), 354–357.

Emlet, C. (1997). HIV/AIDS in the elderly. *Home Care Provider, 2*(2), 69–75.

*Friedland, G., Kahl, P., Saltzman, B., Rogers, M., Feiner, C., Mayers, M., Schable, C., & Klein, R. (1990). Additional evidence for lack of transmission of HIV infection by close interpersonal (casual) contact. *AIDS, 4*, 639–644.

*Gershon, R., Vlahov, D., & Nelson, K. (1990). The risk of transmission of HIV-1 through non-percutaneous, non-sexual modes: A review. *AIDS, 4*, 645–650.

Greening, J. G. (1994). Intravenous foscarnet administration for treatment of cytomegalovirus retinitis. *Journal of Intravenous Nursing, 17*(2), 74–77.

Guyton, A., & Hall, J (1991). *Textbook of medical physiology* (9th ed.). Philadelphia: W. B. Saunders.

Hellmann, D. (1995). Vasculitis: When should you suspect it? *Emergency Medicine, 27*(2), 22–36.

*Henry, S., & Holzemer, W. (1992). Critical care management of the patient with HIV infection who has *Pneumocystis carinii* pneumonia. *Heart & Lung, 21*(3), 243–249.

Howard, B. A. (1994) Guiding allergy sufferers through the medication maze. *RN, 57*(4), 26–30.

*Imagawa, D. T., Lee, M. H., Wolinsky, S. M., Sano, K., Morales, F., Kwok, S., Shinsky, J. J., Nishanian, P. G., Giorgi, J., Fahey, J. L., Dudley, J., Visscher, B. R., & Detels, R. (1989). Human immunodeficiency virus type 1 infection in homosexual men who remain seronegative for prolonged periods. *New England Journal of Medicine, 320*(22), 1458–1489.

Kelly, A. (1994). Human immunodeficiency virus: Current trends in assessment, diagnosis, and treatment. *Journal of Intravenous Nursing, 17*(2), 83–92.

Kellett, P. (1997). Latex allergy: A review. *Journal of Emergency Nursing, 23*(1), 27–36.

Lewis, J., Doyle, K., & Sampson, D. (1995). Self-test: Caring for AIDS patients. *Nursing95, 25*(4), 76–78.

Lisanti, P. (1996). Anaphylaxis. *American Journal of Nursing, 96*(11), 51.

Lisanti, P., & Zwolski, K. (1997). Understanding the devastation of AIDS. *American Journal of Nursing, 97*(1), 26–35.

McKinnon, B. (1996). New AIDS drugs offer hope, but bring even higher costs. *Continuing Care, 15*(7), 12–14.

*McMahon, K. (1988). The integration of HIV testing and counseling into nursing practice. *Nursing Clinics of North America, 23*(4), 803–821.

Meisenhelder, J. B. (1994). Contributing factors to fear of HIV contagion in registered nurses. *Image, 26*(1), 65–69.

National Institute of Allergy and Infectious Disease. (1994, February 21). AZT reduces rate of maternal transmission of HIV. *NIAID News*. Bethesda, MD: National Institutes of Health, U.S. Public Health Service.

Nokes, K., Kendrew, J., & Longo, M. (1995). Alternative/complementary therapies used by persons with HIV disease. *Journal of the Association of Nurses in AIDS Care, 6*(4), 19–24.

Nowak, M., & McMichael, A. (1995). How HIV defeats the immune system. *Scientific American, 273*(2), 58–65.

Roitt, I. (1994). *Essential immunology* (8th ed). Boston: Blackwell Scientific Publications.

Sabo, C. E., & Carwein, V. L. (1994). Women and AIDS. *Journal of the Association of Nurses in AIDS Care, 5*(3), 15–21.

Sande, M. A., & Volberding, P. A. (1997). *The medical management of AIDS* (5th ed.). Philadelphia: W. B. Saunders.

Tierney, A. (1995). HIV/AIDS: Knowledge, attitudes and education of nurses: A review of the research. *Journal of Clinical Nursing, 4*(1), 13–21.

Ungvarski, P. (1995). Adults and HIV/AIDS: Clinical considerations for care management. *The Journal of Care Management, 1*(3), 40–55.

Ungvarski, P. (1997). Update on HIV infection. *American Journal of Nursing, 97*(1), 44–52.

Volberding, P. A. (1994). Treatment dilemmas in HIV infection. *Hospital Practice, 29*(4), 49–60.

Wang, J. F. (1997). Attitudes, concerns, and fear of acquired immune deficiency syndrome among registered nurses in the United States. *Holistic Nursing Practice, 11*(2), 36–49.

Whipple, B., & Scura, K. (1996). The overlooked epidemic: HIV in older adults. *American Journal of Nursing, 96*(2), 23–29.

Workman, M. L. (1995). Essential concepts of inflammation and immunity. *Critical Care Clinics of North America, 7*(4), 601–615.

*World Health Organization. (1991). Statistics from the World Health Organization and the Centers for Disease Control. *AIDS, 5, 1399–1403.*

SUGGESTED READINGS

Anastasi, J. K., & Lee, V. S. (1994). HIV wasting: How to stop the cycle. *American Journal of Nursing, 94*(6), 18–25.
This article describes factors underlying HIV wasting syndrome. Suggestions regarding how to conduct a nutritional assessment are presented, and interventions for nutritional support are outlined.

Sabo, C. E., & Carwein, V. L. (1994). Women and AIDS. *Journal of the Association of Nurses in AIDS Care, 5*(3), 15–21.
This article describes the issues specific to women with HIV. These include psychosocial, sociocultural factors, and female-specific clinical conditions associated with HIV infection.

Ungvarski, P. J. (1995). Adults and HIV/AIDS: Clinical considerations for care management. *The Journal of Care Management, 1*(3), 40–55.
This article describes a comprehensive model of care for persons at risk for or with HIV that includes primary, secondary, and tertiary prevention. Strategies for screening, prevention of complications, and minimization of disability are outlined.

ALTERED CELL GROWTH AND CANCER DEVELOPMENT

All people experience some form of altered cell growth. The most common forms are harmless (benign) and do not require intervention. Cancer, or malignant cell growth, is the most serious type and, without intervention, leads to death. Approximately 1.5 million people in the United States and Canada are newly diagnosed with cancer each year (American Cancer Society, 1998), making cancer a very common health problem. Some types of cancer can be prevented, and others have better cure rates if diagnosed early. The nurse is crucial in educating the public about cancer prevention and early detection methods. A strong knowledge base of the causes and consequences of cancer development can assist nurses in this role.

HISTORICAL PERSPECTIVE

Cancer is not a new disorder. There is evidence that even prehistoric humans experienced cancer. Some types of cancer are more prevalent today, especially among industrialized societies, than in centuries past. Two reasons are the increasing longevity of people in industrialized countries and increased environmental exposure to substances that stimulate cancer development.

Cancer will occur in approximately one of every three people currently living in North America (American Cancer Society, 1998), although cancer risk differs for each person. More than 10 million Americans with a history of cancer are alive today, nearly 5 million of whom can be considered cured (American Cancer Society, 1998). Terms used to describe abnormal cell growth and cancer are presented in Table 26–1.

OVERVIEW

The continuous growth of cells and tissues is expected during infancy and childhood, and many human body cells continue to "grow" by cell division (mitosis) long after development and maturation are complete. Such cells are located in tissues where constant damage or wear is likely and where continued cell growth is necessary to replace dead tissues. Cells of the skin, hair, mucous membranes, bone marrow, and linings of glandular organs (lungs, stomach, intestines, bladder, uterus) and support cells of the brain (glial cells), among others, keep the ability to divide through a person's life span. The growth of these cells is well controlled, so only the

TABLE 26-1

Terminology Commonly Associated with Abnormal Cell Growth

Term	Definition
Anaplastic	• Without shape or definition
Benign	• New cell growth not needed for normal growth or replacement that is not malignant
Carcinogenesis	• The transformation of a normal cell into a cancer cell
Doubling time	• The amount of time it takes for a tumor to double in size by mitotic cell divisions
Fibronectin	• A large, extracellular, transformation-sensitive cell-surface protein present on normal cells that allows normal cells to adhere tightly together
Gene expression	• The activation, or "turning on," of a specific gene to the extent that it synthesizes a specific protein that influences the activity of a cell or group of cells
Gene repression	• The deactivation, or "turning off," of a specific gene so that it is silent and does not synthesize a protein
Generation time	• The period of time necessary for one cell to enter and complete one round of cell division by mitosis
Initiation	• The damage of a normal cell's DNA by a carcinogen
Latency	• The period of time between when a carcinogenic agent or substance damaged the DNA of a normal cell (initiated it) and when an overt cancer is present
Malignant	• Cancerous, new growth of cells by invasion that is not needed for normal development or tissue replacement
Metastasis	• Invasive growth of cancer cells from the original tumor into distant areas
Mitosis	• Cell division by exact duplication
Morphology	• Appearance or shape
Multipotent	• An undifferentiated cell that has multiple potentials for maturation and differentiation (also called totipotent and pluripotent)
Neoplasia	• New cell growth not needed for normal body growth or replacement of dead or missing tissue
Oncogene	• Developmental gene (proto-oncogene) expressed at an inappropriate time, capable of transforming a normal cell into a cancer cell
Ploidy	• The chromosome content of a cell
Aneuploid	• Chromosome content of a cell that is greater or lesser than the normal chromosomal number for the species
Diploid (euploid)	• Normal chromosome content of a cell for the species (e.g., human cells have 46 chromosomes [23 pairs] per cell)
Primary tumor	• A tumor formed in a specific tissue as a result of a carcinogenic agent or event
Promotion	• Enhancement of cell division in a cell initiated by a carcinogen
Proto-oncogene	• A developmental gene expressed during early embryonic development
Secondary tumor	• A tumor formed as a result of breaking off from a primary tumor and spreading to distant sites (metastasis)
Transformation	• The changing of a normal cell into a cancer cell by a carcinogenic agent or event

right number of cells is always present in any tissue or organ.

Some tissues and organs stop growing by cell division after development is complete. For example, heart muscle cells no longer divide after fetal life; the number of heart muscle cells is fixed at birth. The size of the heart increases as the person grows because each of the cells gets larger, but the number of muscle cells in the heart does not. Growth that causes an organ or tissue to increase in size by enlarging individual cells is called *hypertrophy.* Growth that causes an organ or tissue to increase in size by increasing the number of cells is called *hyperplasia* (Fig. 26–1).

Any new or continued cell growth not needed for normal development or replacement of dead and damaged tissues is called *neoplasia* and is always considered abnormal even if it causes no harm. Whether the new cells are benign or malignant, neoplastic cells develop from normal cells (parent tissues or cells). Thus, cancer or any neoplastic cells were once normal cells but changed to no longer look, grow, or function normally. The strict processes controlling normal growth and function have been lost or suppressed. To understand how cancer cells grow, it is first necessary to understand the regulation and function of normal cells.

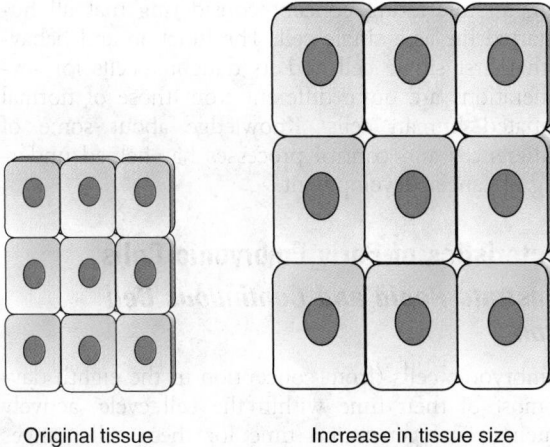

Original tissue

Increase in tissue size
by hypertrophy

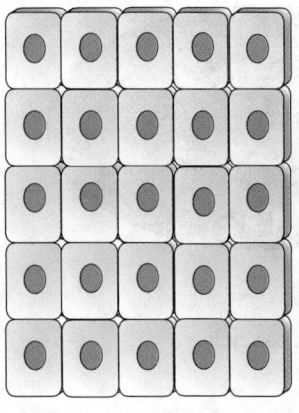

Increase in tissue size
by hyperplasia

Figure 26–1. Tissue growth by hypertrophy and hyperplasia.

Biology of Normal Cells

Different types of normal cells work together to make the whole person function at an optimal level. To achieve optimal function, each individual cell must perform in a predictable manner.

Characteristics of Normal Cells

Have Limited Cell Division

Normal cells divide (undergo mitosis) for one of two reasons: (1) to develop normal tissue or (2) to replace lost or damaged normal tissue. Even when capable of mitosis, normal cells divide only when all internal body conditions and nutrition are just right to promote cell division.

Show Specific Morphology

Each normal cell type has a distinct and recognizable appearance, size, and shape, as shown in Figure 26–2.

Have a Small Nuclear–Cytoplasmic Ratio

As shown in Figure 26–2, the space that the nucleus occupies inside a normal cell is small compared with the size of the cell. The nuclear space is small in proportion to the cytoplasmic space.

Perform Specific Differentiated Functions

Every normal cell must perform at least one special function to contribute to whole body homeostasis. For example, skin cells make keratin, liver cells make bile, cardiac muscle cells contract rhythmically, nerve cells generate and conduct impulses, and red blood cells make hemoglobin to carry oxygen.

Adhere Tightly Together

Normal cells make and secrete cell-surface proteins that protrude from the cell surface, allowing cells to bind closely and tightly together. In the presence of a protein

called fibronectin, normal cells composing any normal tissue are bound tightly to each other.

Are Nonmigratory

Because normal cells are tightly bound together, they do not wander from one tissue to the next (with the exception of erythrocytes and leukocytes).

Grow in an Orderly and Well-Regulated Manner

Normal cells capable of mitosis do not divide unless all internal body conditions are optimal for cell division. These conditions include the need for more cells, adequate space, and sufficient nutrients and other resources. Cell division, occurring in a well-recognized pattern, is described by the cell cycle. Figure 26–3 shows the phases of the cell cycle.

Living cells not actively reproducing are not in the cell cycle but in a reproductive resting state termed G_0. During the G_0 period, cells actively carry out specific functions but do not divide. Most normal cells spend most of their existence in the G_0 state, just like most humans spend the majority of their lives in a nonpregnant state.

Mitotic cell division makes a cell divide into two cells. These two cells are identical to each other and to the original cell that started the mitotic cell division. The

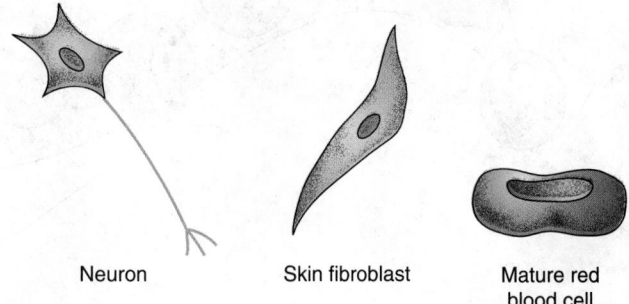

Neuron   Skin fibroblast   Mature red
                                          blood cell

Figure 26–2. Distinctive morphology of some normal cells.

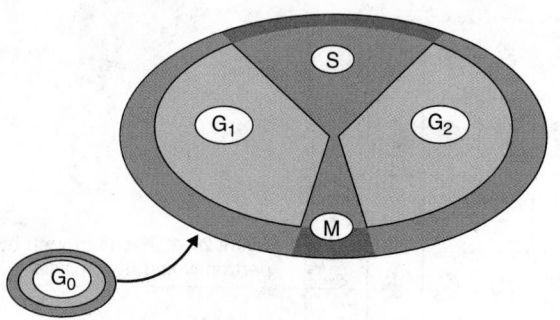

Figure 26–3. The cell cycle.

processes of entering and completing the cell cycle are rigidly controlled. Figure 26–4 shows the activities occurring during the phases of the cell cycle:

- G_1. The cell is preparing for division by taking on extra nutrients, generating more energy, and making extra membrane. The amount of cell fluid (cytoplasm) also increases.
- S. Because making one cell into two cells requires twice as much of everything, including deoxyribonucleic acid (DNA), the cell doubles its DNA content through DNA synthesis.
- G_2. The cell makes important proteins that will be used in actual cell division and in normal physiologic function after cell division is complete.
- M. The single cell splits apart into two cells (actual mitosis).

Are Contact Inhibited

Among normal cells capable of cell division, each individual cell will divide only as long as it has some surface not in direct contact with another cell. Once a normal cell is in direct contact on all surface areas with other cell membranes, it no longer undergoes mitosis. Thus, normal cell division is *contact inhibited*.

Each normal, mature cell has a specific structure and

function, an interesting concept considering that all humans started life as a single cell. The function and behavior of that first single cell and its daughter cells for several generations are quite different from those of normal differentiated human cells. Knowledge about some of their differences and control processes has helped understanding of cancer development.

Characteristics of Early Embryonic Cells
Demonstrate Rapid and Continuous Cell Division

Early embryonic cells (from conception to the eighth day) spend most of their time within the cell cycle, actively reproducing. The generation time for these cells ranges from 2 to 8 hours.

Show Anaplastic Morphology

The term *anaplasia* means "without structural shape or differentiation." Early embryonic cells do not look like the mature cells they will eventually become. They all have the same anaplastic appearance, small and round (Fig. 26–5).

Have a Large Nuclear–Cytoplasmic Ratio

The nucleus of an early embryonic cell takes up most of the space inside the cell. The ratio of nuclear space to cytoplasmic space is larger than that of a normal differentiated cell.

Perform No Differentiated Functions

In the early embryonic period, cells do not have any differentiated functions. They have not yet committed to a specific maturity. Each early embryonic cell is totally flexible and can mature to become any body cell. This flexibility is called *pluripotency*, *multipotency*, or *totipotency* because each cell has an unlimited potential for maturation.

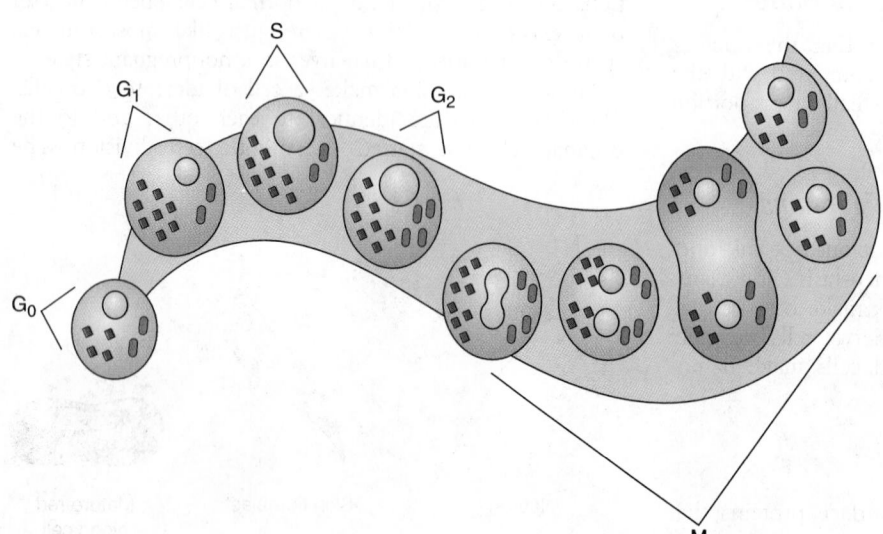

Figure 26–4. Cellular events during mitotic cell division.

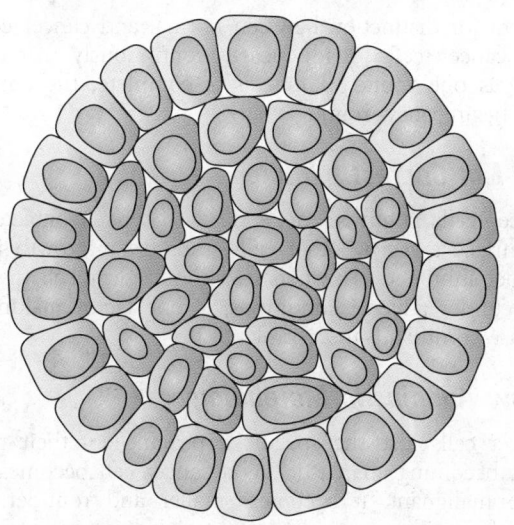

Figure 26–5. Embryonic cells at about 5 days after conception.

Adhere Loosely Together

Early embryonic cells do not make fibronectin and are not tightly bound together.

Are Able to Migrate

Because early embryonic cells are not tightly bound together, they do not remain in one place within the embryo but migrate throughout the early embryo.

Are Not Contact Inhibited

Having all sides or areas of an early embryonic cell in continuous contact with the membrane surfaces of other cells does not inhibit embryonic cell division.

Commitment

At some point in early embryonic development, cells become differentiated. In response to an unknown signal, each cell commits itself to a specific differentiated maturational outcome. The cell has not yet taken on any differentiated features or functions; rather, it positions itself within a group of cells that will eventually become only one specific organ or tissue.

Commitment involves turning off specific early embryonic genes that controlled or regulated early rapid growth, called *proto-oncogenes*. These genes have no apparent normal function at any other point in life.

After the early embryonic regulatory genes are "turned off" (repressed), other specific genes that control the expression of specific differentiated functions must be "turned on" (expressed) selectively in different cell types. For example, the gene for insulin is actively expressed only in fetal pancreatic beta cells and repressed in all other cells. This selective gene expression directs the normal growth and differentiation of specific body cells.

Biology of Abnormal Cells

Body cells do not exist in isolation but are exposed to personal and environmental changes, which can alter how the cells grow or function. When either cell growth or cell function is changed, the cells are considered abnormal. Table 26–2 compares characteristics of normal, embryonic, benign tumor, and cancer cells.

Characteristics of Benign Cells

Benign tumor cells are normal cells growing in the wrong place, at the wrong time, or at the wrong rate. Examples include moles, uterine fibroid tumors, skin tags, endometriosis, and nasal polyps.

TABLE 26–2

Characteristics of Normal and Abnormal Cells				
Characteristic	**Normal Cell**	**Embryonic Cell**	**Benign Tumor Cell**	**Malignant Cell**
Cell division	• None or slow	• Rapid, continuous	• Continuous or inappropriate	• Rapid or continuous
Appearance	• Specific morphologic features	• Anaplastic	• Specific morphologic features	• Anaplastic
Nuclear–cytoplasmic ratio	• Small	• Large	• Small	• Large
Differentiated functions	• Many	• None	• Many	• Some-none
Adherence	• Tight	• Loose	• Tight	• Loose
Migratory	• No	• Yes	• No	• Yes
Growth	• Well regulated	• Well regulated	• Expansion	• Invasion
Chromosomes	• Diploid (euploid)	• Diploid (euploid)	• Diploid (euploid)	• Aneuploid*
Mitotic index	• Low	• High	• Low	• High*

*Depends on the degree of malignant transformation.

Demonstrate Continuous or Inappropriate Cell Growth

Benign tumors are tissues unnecessary for normal function, growing too much or in the wrong place.

Show Specific Morphology

Benign tumors strongly resemble their parent tissues, retaining the specific morphologic features of parent tissue.

Have a Small Nuclear–Cytoplasmic Ratio

Just like completely normal cells, benign tumor cells have a small nucleus compared with the rest of the cell.

Perform Differentiated Functions

Not only do benign tumors look like their parent tissues, but they also perform the same differentiated functions. For example, in endometriosis, one type of benign tumor, the normal lining of the uterus (endometrium) grows in an abnormal place (such as on an ovary, on the peritoneum, or in the chest cavity). This displaced endometrium acts just like normal endometrium by increasing vascularity and tissue thickness each month under the influence of estrogen and progesterone. When these hormone levels drop and the normal endometrium sheds from the uterus, the displaced endometrium—wherever it is—also sheds.

Adhere Tightly Together

Benign tumor cells make and secrete fibronectin, and benign tumor cells bind tightly to one another. In addition, many benign tissues are "encapsulated," or surrounded with fibrous connective tissue, helping to hold the benign tissue together.

Are Nonmigratory

Benign tissues do not wander but remain tightly bound and do not invade other body tissues.

Grow in an Orderly Manner

Benign tumor cells follow normal cell growth patterns even though their growth is not needed. Growth may continue beyond an appropriate time, but the rate of growth is normal for the parent tissue. The benign tumor grows by hyperplastic expansion.

Characteristics of Malignant Cells

Cancer (malignant) cells are abnormal, serve no useful function, and are harmful to normal body tissues. The following characteristics are common in malignant tumors.

Demonstrate Rapid or Continuous Cell Division

Some cancer cells have a short generation time (2–4 hours); others have a generation time even longer than that of normal cells. Most cancer cells have a generation time similar to that of the parent tissue.

A major distinction between normal and cancer cells is that cancer cells divide nearly continuously. Almost as soon as one round of mitosis is complete, the daughter cells begin a new round.

Are Not Contact Inhibited

Cancer cells continue to divide even when contacted on all surface areas by other cells; thus, their growth is not contact inhibited. The persistence of cancer cell division, even under adverse conditions, is one factor making the disease so difficult to control.

Show Anaplastic Morphology

Cancer cells lose the specific appearance of their parent cells, becoming anaplastic. As a cancer cell becomes even more malignant, it becomes smaller and rounder. This loss of specific appearance can make diagnosis of cancer type difficult, because many types of cancer cells look alike.

Have a Large Nuclear–Cytoplasmic Ratio

The nucleus of a cancer cell is larger than that of a normal cell, and the cancer cell is small. The nucleus occupies much of the space within the cancer cell, creating a large nuclear–cytoplasmic ratio.

Lose Some or All Differentiated Functions

Along with losing the appearance of the parent cell, cancer cells lose some differentiated functions the parent tissue performed. Cancer cells serve no useful purpose.

Adhere Loosely Together

Cancer cells make little, if any, fibronectin. As a result, they adhere poorly to each other, and little pressure is needed to allow some cancer cells to break off from the primary tumor.

Are Able to Migrate

Because cancer cells do not bind tightly together and have many enzymes on their cell surfaces, they are able to slip through blood vessels and tissues and spread from the original tumor site to many other body sites. This ability to spread (metastasize) is a key characteristic of cancer cells.

Grow by Invasion

Cancer cells expand and extend into other tissues, both close by and more remote from the original tumor, by invasion or *metastasis*. Together with persistent growth, metastasis makes untreated cancer deadly.

CANCER DEVELOPMENT
Carcinogenesis/Oncogenesis

Carcinogenesis and *oncogenesis* are synonyms for cancer development. Table 26–3 summarizes key concepts about cancer development. The process of changing a cell with

TABLE 26–3

Key Concepts Related to Cancer Development

- Neoplastic cells originate from normal body cells.
- Transformation of a normal cell into a cancer cell involves mutation of the genes (DNA) of the normal cell.
- Early embryonic genes activated at an inappropriate time can cause a cell to develop into a tumor.
- Only one cell has to undergo malignant transformation for cancer to begin.
- Benign tumors grow by expansion, whereas malignant tumors grow by invasion.
- Most tumors arise from cells that are capable of cell division.
- Primary prevention of cancer involves avoiding exposure to known causes of cancer.
- Secondary prevention of cancer involves screening for early detection.
- Tobacco use is a causative or permissive factor in 30% of all malignant neoplasms.
- Tumors that metastasize from the primary site into another organ are still designated as tumors of the originating tissue.

a normal appearance and function into a cell with malignant characteristics is called *malignant transformation*. Malignant transformation occurs through the steps of *initiation*, *promotion*, *progression*, and *metastasis* (Caudell et al., 1996).

Initiation

The first step in carcinogenesis is initiation. Normal cells can become cancer cells if their proto-oncogenes are turned back on any time after early embryonic development is complete. Anything that can penetrate a cell, get into the nucleus, and damage the DNA can damage the genes, turning on genes that should remain repressed and turning off normal genes (Cooper, 1995). Substances that can change the activity of a cell's genes so the cell has malignant characteristics are called *carcinogens*. Carcinogens may be chemicals, physical agents, or viruses. Table 26–4 lists common carcinogens and the types of cancers they cause. Chapters presenting the care of clients with specific cancers discuss specific carcinogens (when known) under the heading "Etiology."

Pure carcinogens initiate mutational changes in a cell's genes and are thus called *initiators*. Initiation is an irreversible event that can lead to cancer development if it does not interfere with the cell's ability to divide.

Once a cell has been initiated, it can become a cancer cell if the cellular changes that occurred during initiation are enhanced by *promotion*. One cancer cell is not significant, however, unless it can divide. If it cannot divide, it cannot form a tumor. *If growth conditions are right, however, widespread metastatic disease can develop from just one cancer cell.*

Promotion

Once a normal cell has been initiated by a carcinogen and has cancer cell characteristics, it can become a tumor if its growth is enhanced. The time between a cell's initiation and development of an overt tumor is called the *latency period*, which can range from months to years and depends on the type of cell initiated and the presence of promoters.

Promoters are substances that promote or enhance initiated cell growth (Weinberg, 1996). They can also shorten the latency period. Promoters may be hormones, drugs, and a wide variety of industrial chemicals.

Progression

After cancer cells have grown to the point that a detectable tumor is formed (a 1-cm tumor has at least 1 billion cells in it), other events must occur for this tumor to become a health problem. First, the tumor must establish its own blood supply. In the early stages, the center cells of the tumor receive nutrition only by diffusion from the surrounding fluids. However, after the tumor reaches 1 cm, diffusion is not efficient, and cells in the center of the tumor become hypoxic and start to die. To continue

TABLE 26–4

Known Environmental Carcinogens

Carcinogen	Associated Cancer Site or Neoplasm
Alcoholic beverages	• Liver, esophagus, mouth, pharynx, breast, colon, and rectum
Anabolic steroids	• Liver
Arsenic	• Lung, skin
Asbestos	• Lung, pleura, peritoneum, pericardium
Benzene	• Myelogenous leukemia
Chemotherapy drugs Alkylating agents Anthracycline antibiotics Antimetabolites	• Acute leukemia, lymphoma
Cyclosporine	• Non-Hodgkin's lymphoma
Diesel exhaust	• Lung
Formaldehyde	• Nasopharynx
Hair dyes	• Bladder
Ionizing radiation	• Bone marrow, thyroid, many organs
Mineral oils	• Skin
Pesticides	• Lung
Polycyclic hydrocarbons	• Lung, skin, scrotum
Polychlorinated biphenyls	• Liver, skin
Sunlight	• Skin, eyes
Tobacco	• Lung, esophagus, mouth, pharynx, larynx, pancreas, bladder, kidney, liver, stomach, colon, rectum, leukemia

to grow and survive, the tumor makes *tumor angiogenesis factor* (TAF). TAF stimulates capillaries and other blood vessels in the area to grow new branches into the tumor (Pitot, 1986). These blood vessels ensure the tumor's continued nourishment.

As tumor cells continue to divide, some of the new cells experience more change from the original initiated cancer cell. Actual colonies or subpopulations within the tumor begin to appear. These subpopulations differ from the original cancer cell. Some of the differences provide these subpopulations with advantages that allow them to live and divide no matter how the environmental conditions around them change, and are thus called "selection advantages" (Fidler & Hart, 1982). Changes that a tumor undergoes at this time allow it to become more malignant. Over time the tumor cells come to have fewer and fewer normal cell characteristics.

The original tumor formed from transformed normal cells is called the *primary* tumor. It is usually identified by the tissue from which it arose (parent tissue), such as in breast cancer or lung cancer. When primary tumors are located in vital organs, such as the brain or lungs, they can grow to such an extent that they either lethally damage the vital organ or "crowd out" healthy organ tissue and interfere with that organ's ability to perform its vital function. At other times, the primary tumor is located in soft tissue that can expand without damage as the tumor grows. One such site is the breast. The breast is not a vital organ, and even if it had a large tumor in it, the primary tumor would not cause the client's death. When the tumor spreads from the original site into vital areas, life functions can be disrupted.

Metastasis

In metastasis, cancer cells move from their original location by breaking off from the original group and establishing remote colonies. These additional tumors are called *metastatic* or *secondary tumors*. Even though the tumor is now in another organ, it is still a cancer from the original altered tissue. For example, when breast cancer spreads to the lung and the bone, it is breast cancer in the lung and bone, not lung cancer and not bone cancer. Metastasis occurs through several progressive steps, shown in Figure 26–6 (Liotta, 1992; Nicolson, 1979).

Extension into Surrounding Tissues

Tumors secrete enzymes that open up areas of surrounding tissue. Mechanical pressure, created as the tumor increases in size, forces tumor cells to invade new territory.

Penetration into Blood Vessels

The same enzymes that open up areas of surrounding tissue make large pores in the client's blood vessels, allowing tumor cells to enter blood vessels.

Release of Tumor Cells

Because tumor cells are loosely held together, clumps of cells break off the primary tumor into blood vessels for transport.

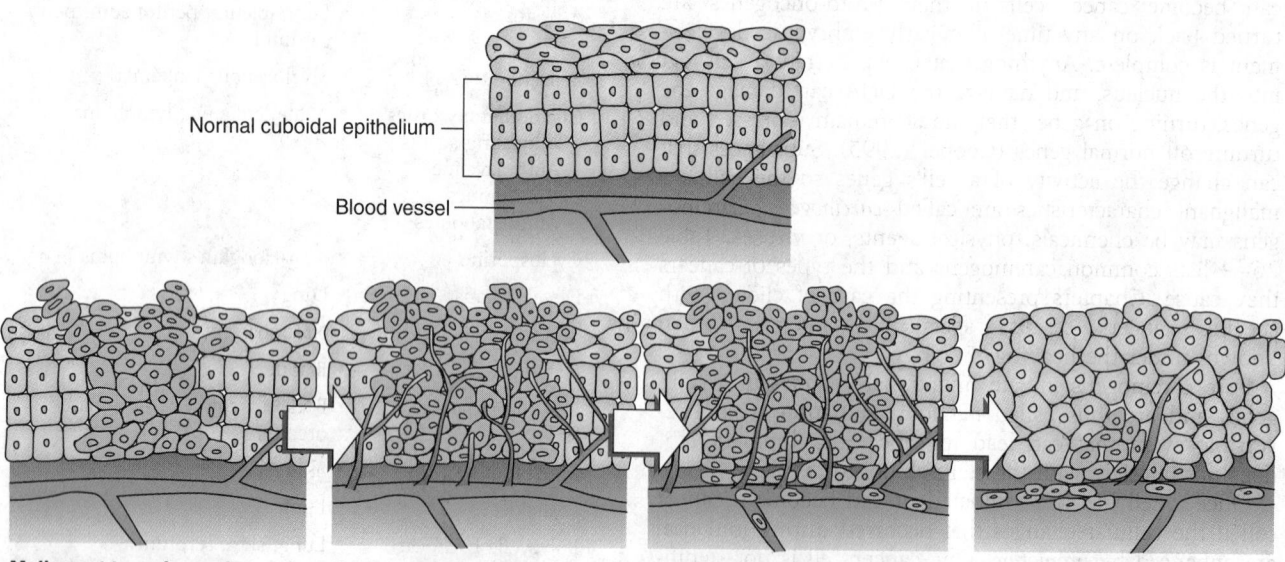

Normal cuboidal epithelium

Blood vessel

Malignant transformation
Some normal cuboidal cells have undergone malignant transformation and have divided enough times to form a tumorous area within the cuboidal epithelium.

Tumor vascularization
Cancer cells secrete tumor angiogenesis factor (TAF), stimulating the blood vessels to bud and form new channels growing into the tumor.

Blood vessel penetration
Cancer cells have broken off from the main tumor. Enzymes on the surface of the tumor cells make holes in the blood vessels, allowing cancer cells to enter blood vessels and travel around the body.

Arrest and invasion
Cancer cells clump up in blood vessel walls and invade new tissue areas. If the new tissue areas have the right conditions to support continued growth of cancer cells, new tumors (metastatic tumors) will form at this site.

Figure 26–6. The steps of metastasis.

TABLE 26-5

Common Sites of Metastasis for Different Cancer Types

Cancer Type	Sites of Metastasis
Breast cancer	• Bone* • Lung* • Liver • Brain
Lung cancer	• Brain* • Bone • Liver • Lymph nodes • Pancreas
Colorectal cancer	• Liver* • Lymph nodes • Adjacent structures
Prostate cancer	• Bone (especially spine and legs)* • Pelvic nodes
Melanoma	• Gastrointestinal tract • Lymph nodes • Lung • Brain
Primary brain cancer	• Central nervous system

*Most common site of metastasis for the specific malignant neoplasm.

Invasion of Tissue at Site of Arrest

Tumor cells circulate through the blood and enter tissues at remote sites. When conditions in the remote site are appropriate for the tumor, the cells stop circulating (arrest) and invade the surrounding tissues, creating secondary tumors. Table 26–5 lists the common sites of metastasis for specific tumor types. Three routes responsible for metastatic spread are local seeding, blood-borne metastasis, and lymphatic spread.

LOCAL SEEDING. Local seeding involves distribution of shed cancer cells in the local area of the primary tumor. In ovarian cancer, for example, cells often spill from the primary tumor into the peritoneal cavity and set up multiple seeding sites.

BLOOD-BORNE METASTASIS. Blood-borne metastasis (tumor cell release into the blood) is the most common cause of cancer spread. Combined with seeding, distribution via the bloodstream determines the area of metastases.

Many circulating tumor cells are destroyed by factors in the circulation, immune responses, or unsuitable environments in the organs in which the cells stop. Clumps of tumor cells can become trapped in capillaries. These clumps damage the capillary wall and allow tumor cells to enter the surrounding tissue.

LYMPHATIC SPREAD. Lymphatic spread is related to the number, structure, and location of lymph nodes and vessels. Primary sites rich in lymphatics are more susceptible to early metastatic spread than are areas with few lymphatics.

Cancer Classification

Terms that describe neoplasia by tissue origin and classify the tumor as benign or malignant are listed in Table 26–6. Other terms describe the tumor's biologic behavior, anatomic site, and degree of differentiation.

Approximately 100 different types of cancer arise from various tissues or organs. Figure 26–7 compares cancer

TABLE 26-6

Classification of Tumors by Tissue Type

Tissue of Origin	Benign Tumors	Malignant Tumors
Epithelial	Adenoma	Adenocarcinoma
Glandular	Polyp,	Carcinoma
Epithelial	papilloma	
Connective		
Bone	Osteoma	Osteosarcoma
Fibrous	Fibroma	Fibrosarcoma
Fat	Lipoma	Liposarcoma
Smooth muscle	Leiomyoma	Leiomyosarcoma
Striated muscle	Rhabdomyoma	Rhabdomyosarcoma
Hematopoietic		
Erythrocytes		Erythroleukemia
Lymphocytes		Lymphocytic leukemia
Lymphatic tissue		Malignant lymphoma, Hodgkin's disease
Plasma cell		Multiple myeloma
Pigmented cells	Nevus	Melanoma
Neural	Neuroma	Glioblastoma

Modified from Caudell, K., Cuaron, L., & Gallucci, B. (1996). Cancer biology: Molecular and cellular aspects. In R. McCorkle, M. Grant, M. Frank-Stromborg, & S. Baird (Eds.), *Cancer nursing: A comprehensive textbook* (2nd ed., p. 154). Philadelphia: W. B. Saunders.

LEADING SITES OF CANCER INCIDENCE AND DEATH–1998 ESTIMATES

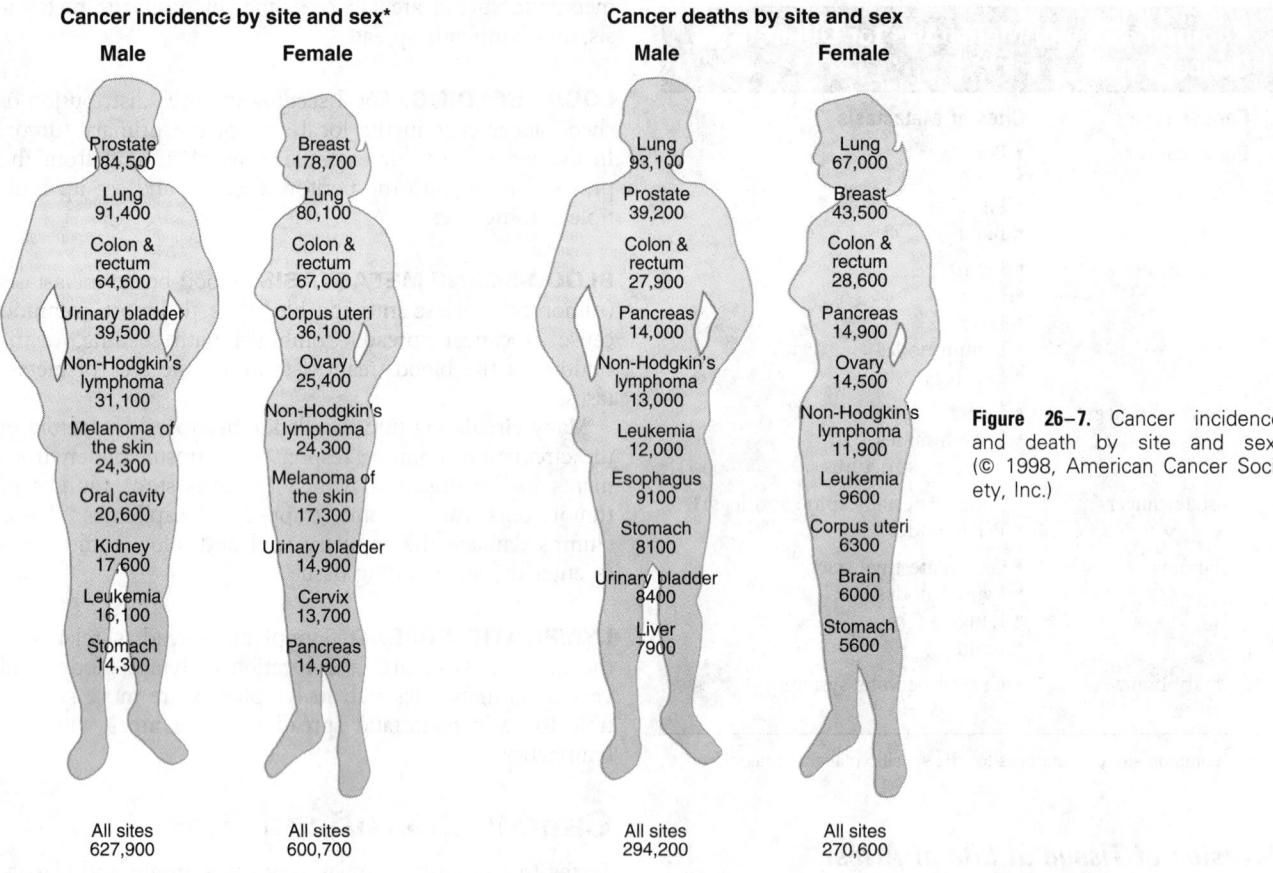

Figure 26–7. Cancer incidence and death by site and sex. (© 1998, American Cancer Society, Inc.)

*Excluding basal and squamous cell skin cancer and in situ carcinomas except bladder.

distribution by site and gender. Cancers are divided into two major categories: solid and hematologic.

Solid tumors are associated with the organs from which they develop, for example, breast cancer and lung cancer. Hematologic cancers (e.g., leukemias and lymphomas) originate from blood cell–forming tissues, which communicate with all organs.

Cancer Grade and Stage

To help standardize cancer diagnosis, prognosis, and treatment, classification systems of grading and staging were developed. Grading a tumor classifies cellular aspects of the cancer. Staging of the client classifies clinical aspects of the cancer.

Grading

Some cancer cells are "more malignant" than others, varying in their aggressiveness and sensitivity to treatment. Some cancer cells barely resemble the tissue from which they arose, are aggressive, and rapidly metastasize. These cells are considered more malignant, a "high-grade tumor." On the basis of cell appearance and activity, grading compares the cancer cell with the normal parent tissue from which it arose (Caudell et al., 1996).

Different groups have established different grading systems for different kinds of cancer cells, but overall they resemble the standard system listed in Table 26–7. This system rates tumor cells; the lowest rating is given to those tumors that closely resemble normal cells and the highest to those that little resemble normal cells.

Grading the cells is the first step in confirming cancer. Grading provides one means of evaluating the client with cancer for prognosis and appropriate therapy. It also allows health care professionals to evaluate the results of management and compare local, regional, national, and international statistics.

Ploidy

Another biological feature describing cancer cells is chromosome number and appearance. Normal human cells have 46 chromosomes (23 pairs), the normal diploid number. When malignant transformation occurs, changes in the genes and chromosomes also occur. Some tumor cells gain or lose whole chromosomes and may have structural abnormalities of the remaining chromosomes. When a tumor cell has more or less than the normal diploid number, it is said to be *aneuploid*. The degree of aneuploidy generally increases with the degree of malignant transformation.

TABLE 26–7

Grading of Malignant Tumors

Grade Cellular Characteristics

GX • Grade cannot be determined.

G1 • Tumor cells are well differentiated and closely resemble the normal cells from which they arose.
    • This grade is considered a low grade of malignant change.
    • These tumors are malignant but are relatively slow-growing.

G2 • Tumor cells are moderately differentiated; they still retain some of the characteristics of normal cells but also have more malignant characteristics than do G1 tumor cells.

G3 • Tumor cells are poorly differentiated, but the tissue of origin can usually be established.
    • The cells have few normal cell characteristics.

G4 • Tumor cells are poorly differentiated and retain no normal cell characteristics.
    • Determination of the tissue of origin is difficult and perhaps impossible.

Staging

Staging determines the cancer's exact location and degree of metastasis present at diagnosis. Staging is important because, for most cancers, the smaller the tumor is at diagnosis and the less it has spread, the greater the chances are that treatment will result in a cure. Tumor stage also influences selection of therapy. Staging is done in three different ways:

1. Clinical Staging. This assesses the client's clinical manifestations and evaluates clinical signs for the tumor size and degree of metastasis. Clinical tests are used, and tumor cells may be obtained for biopsy, but clinical staging does not include major surgery.
2. Surgical Staging. This determines the tumor size, number, sites, and degree of metastasis by inspection at surgery.
3. Pathologic Staging. This is the most definitive type of staging. Tumor size, number, sites, and degree of metastasis are determined by pathologic examination of tissues obtained at surgery.

Some site-specific staging systems exist, such as Dukes' staging of colon and rectal cancer and Clark's levels method of staging skin cancer. The American Joint Committee on Cancer (AJCC) developed the TNM (tumor, node, metastasis) system to describe the anatomic extent of cancers. The stages guide treatment and are useful for prognosis and comparison of the end results of treatment. The TNM staging system is based on the concept that similar cancers share similar patterns of growth and extension. TNM staging systems are specific to each solid tumor site. Table 26–8 gives basic definitions for the TNM staging system. TNM staging is not useful for can-

cers that arise in the bone marrow or lymphoid tissues. Staging for these cancers is discussed in Chapter 42.

Tumor growth is discussed in terms of doubling time (the amount of time it takes for a tumor to double in size) and mitotic index (the percentage of actively dividing cells within a tumor). The smallest tumor likely to be detected by a physical examination or diagnostic test is 1 cm in diameter and contains 1 billion cells. To reach this size, a tumor will have undergone at least 30 doublings. A tumor with a mitotic index of less than 10% is a relatively slow-growing tumor; a tumor with one of 85% is fast growing. Tumors have a wide range of growth rates. Fast-growing tumors, such as lymphomas, may double in 4 weeks; an adenocarcinoma of the lung may double in 21 to 40 weeks.

Causes of Cancer Development

Carcinogenesis or oncogenesis takes years and depends on several tumor and client factors. Essentially, three interacting primary factors influence the development of cancer: environmental exposure to carcinogens, genetic predisposition, and immune function. These interactions account for variation in cancer development from one person to another, even when each person is exposed to the same hazards.

For some types of cancers, specific causes have been identified, and people at risk can avoid contact with specific agents associated with the development of that cancer type. This is called *primary prevention of cancer* and is effective in minimizing the risk for some types of cancers. For many types of cancer, however, absolute causes remain unknown. For other cancer types, even though the cause may be known, exposure cannot be avoided. These problems make primary prevention of some types of can-

TABLE 26–8

Staging of Cancer: TNM Classification

Primary Tumor (T)	
TX	• Primary tumor cannot be assessed
T0	• No evidence of primary tumor
Tis	• Carcinoma in situ
T1, T2, T3, T4	• Increasing size and/or local extent of the primary tumor
Regional Lymph Nodes (N)	
NX	• Regional lymph nodes cannot be assessed
N0	• No regional lymph node metastasis
N1, N2, N3	• Increasing involvement of regional lymph nodes
Distant Metastasis (M)	
MX	• Presence of distant metastasis cannot be assessed
M0	• No distant metastasis
M1	• Distant metastasis

Modified from American Joint Committee on Cancer. (1988). In O. H. Beahrs, D. E. Henson, R. V. Hutter, & M. H. Myers (Eds.), *Manual for staging of cancer* (3rd ed., p. 7). Philadelphia: J. B. Lippincott.

cers impossible (Mettlin & Michalek, 1996). For people with these cancers, early detection, or *secondary prevention*, can be helpful because treatment outcome is usually better with diagnosis of small tumors that have not metastasized.

Oncogene Activation

Regardless of specific cause, the mechanism of carcinogenesis appears to be the same: the activation of proto-oncogenes into oncogenes. When a normal cell is exposed to any carcinogen (initiator), the normal cell's DNA can be damaged or mutated. The mutations can cause the early embryonic genes (proto-oncogenes), which should be repressed forever, to be turned on or activated again. These genes are then oncogenes and can cause the cell to change from normal to malignant (Cooper, 1995).

About 50 different proto-oncogenes that can be activated into oncogenes have been identified so far, and scientists estimate that at least 50 more exist (Cooper, 1995; Weinberg, 1994). *These oncogenes are not abnormal genes* but are part of every cell's normal make-up and were critically important in early development. Oncogenes become a problem only if they are activated (derepressed) after development is complete, as a result of exposure to carcinogenic agents or events. Activation of some specific oncogenes causes specific cancers. Table 26–9 lists known oncogenes and the malignancies they have been found to cause. Extrinsic and intrinsic factors are associated with oncogene activation.

Extrinsic Factors Influencing Cancer Development

Up to 80% of cancer in North America may be the result of environmental, or extrinsic, factors (Trichopoulos et al., 1996). Environmental carcinogens are chemical, physical, or viral agents that cause cancer. Table 26–4 lists known environmental causes of human cancer.

Chemical Carcinogenesis

Many chemicals capable of causing malignant transformation appear to have similar chemical structures. More than 20 organic and inorganic industrial chemicals, drugs, and other products used in everyday life are known to be carcinogenic, and hundreds are suspected of being so.

Some chemicals are complete carcinogens that can both initiate and promote cancer. Others are pure initiating agents, or incomplete carcinogens. Still others are only promoting agents. Some substances, such as tobacco and alcohol, appear to be only mildly carcinogenic; it takes chronic exposure to large amounts before a cancer develops. However, these two substances can act as cocarcinogens; when taken together, they enhance the carcinogenic activity of each other or other carcinogens.

Cells are not equally susceptible to chemically induced malignant transformation. Normal cells that retain the capacity for mitotic cell division are at greater risk for cancer development than are normal cells not capable of cell division. Cancers commonly arise in bone marrow, skin, lining of the gastrointestinal tract, ductal cells of the breast, and lining of the lungs. All of these cells normally undergo mitotic cell division. Cancers of nerve tissue, cardiac muscle, and skeletal muscle are rare. These cells do not normally undergo mitotic cell division.

Approximately 30% of cancers diagnosed in North America are related to tobacco use (American Cancer Society, 1998). It is the single most important source of preventable chemical carcinogenesis. Tobacco contains many different chemical compounds, including complete carcinogens and cocarcinogens. Tobacco use or ingestion can initiate and promote cancer. The risk of cancer development for a person who uses tobacco depends on his or her immune function; amount, depth, and mode of exposure; and tobacco tar content. The type of cancer that develops depends on the susceptibility of specific sites to various concentrations of tobacco and its metabolites.

Tissues associated with the greatest risk for cancer are those with direct contact with tobacco smoke. Cigarette smoking and tobacco use are also implicated in the development of cancers remote from tissues with direct contact with tobacco. Table 26–10 summarizes the association of tobacco and development of specific cancers.

Physical Carcinogenesis

Physical agents or events may cause cancer by the same mechanism as for chemical carcinogens, that is, by in-

TABLE 26–9

Malignancies Associated with Altered Oncogene Activity

Oncogene	Malignancies
abl	Chronic myelogenous leukemia, other leukemias
c-myc	Burkitt's lymphoma; T-cell and B-cell neoplasms; breast, stomach, and lung carcinomas
erb B	Glioblastomas, squamous cell carcinoma
erb B-2	Breast, salivary gland, ovarian carcinomas
ets	Lymphoma
hst	Breast carcinoma, squamous cell cancers
int-2	Breast carcinoma, squamous cell cancers
L-myc	Lung carcinomas
met	Osteosarcoma
myb	Colorectal carcinomas, leukemia
PRAD-1	Breast carcinoma, squamous cell cancers
H-ras *K-ras* *N-ras*	Carcinomas, sarcomas, neuroblastoma, leukemias, lymphomas
ret	Thyroid carcinomas
trk	Colorectal and thyroid carcinomas

Data from Cooper, G. (1995). *Oncogenes* (2nd ed.). Boston: Jones and Bartlett.

TABLE 26–10

Malignancies Associated with Tobacco Use

Lung	Oral cavity
Pharyngeal	Laryngeal
Esophagus	Pancreatic
Cervical	Kidney
Bladder	

Data from American Cancer Society. (1998). *Cancer Facts & Figures—1998* (Report No. 98-300M-No. 5008.98). Atlanta, GA: Author.

duction of DNA damage. Two types of physical agents suspected of causing cancer are radiation and chronic irritation (Pitot, 1986).

Radiation

Radiation is a physical agent capable of carcinogenesis. Even small doses of radiation affect cells. Some effects are temporary and reparable; others are irreversible and may be lethal to the damaged cell. The two types of radiation associated with carcinogenesis are ionizing and ultraviolet. Ionizing radiation occurs naturally in such minerals as radon, uranium, and radium. Most rocks and soil contain various concentrations of uranium and radium. Other sources of ionizing radiation include diagnostic and therapeutic x-rays and cosmic radiation. Ultraviolet (UV) radiation is the most common type of solar radiation. Other sources of UV radiation include tanning beds and germicidal lights. UV rays do not penetrate deeply, and the most common type of cancer associated with UV exposure is skin cancer.

Both ionizing and ultraviolet radiation produce gene mutations and chromosomal damage. Although radiation exposure induces cancers more frequently among cells that can divide, it can also cause cancer among nondividing cells as well.

Chronic Irritation

Chronic irritation and tissue trauma have been suspected as predisposing physical agents to cancer development, but this theory has not yet been supported directly. The incidence of skin cancer is higher in people with burn scars and other tissues that have sustained severe injury. Chronically irritated tissues may undergo frequent mitosis and, thus, are at an increased risk for spontaneous DNA mutation (Pitot, 1986).

Viral Carcinogenesis

Relatively few viruses have yet been proved to be carcinogenic to humans, although suspected to play major roles in cancer development. When viruses infect body cells, they break the DNA chain and insert their own genetic material into the human DNA chain. Breaking the DNA along with viral gene insertion mutates the normal cell's DNA and can either activate an oncogene or repress a

TABLE 26–11

Malignancies Associated with a Known Viral Origin

Virus	Malignancies
Epstein-Barr virus	Burkitt's lymphoma, B-cell lymphomas, naso-pharyngeal carcinoma
Hepatitis B virus	Primary liver carcinoma
Human papillomavirus	Cervical carcinoma, vulvar carcinoma, and other anogenital carcinomas
Human lymphotrophic virus type I	Adult T-cell leukemia
Human lymphotrophic virus type II	Hairy cell leukemia

Data from Cooper, G. (1995). *Oncogenes* (2nd ed.). Boston: Jones and Bartlett.

suppressor gene. Viruses capable of causing cancer are known as oncoviruses. Table 26–11 lists specific cancers of known viral origin.

Dietary Factors Related to Carcinogenesis

Epidemiologic data relate cancer development to many dietary practices or combinations of dietary practices and environmental exposures. However, the relationship of diet to carcinogenesis is poorly understood. Because dietary considerations are rarely independent of other possible carcinogenic agents, evidence of dietary contributions to cancer development is clouded. Suspected dietary factors include low crude fiber intake, high intake of red meat, and high animal fat intake. Preservatives, contaminants, preparation methods, and additives (dyes, flavorings, and sweeteners) are being assessed for possible carcinogenic effects. Chart 26–1 identifies foods considered to have high carcinogenic potential.

Chart 26–1

Health Promotion Guide: Dietary Habits to Reduce Cancer Risk

- Avoid excessive intake of animal fat.
- Avoid nitrites (prepared lunch meats, sausage, bacon).
- Minimize your intake of red meat.
- Keep your alcohol consumption to no more than one or two drinks per day.
- Eat more bran.
- Eat more cruciferous vegetables, such as broccoli, cauliflower, Brussels sprouts, and cabbage.
- Eat foods high in vitamin A (such as apricots, carrots, and leafy green and yellow vegetables) and vitamin C (such as fresh fruits and vegetables, especially citrus fruits).

> ### Chart 26–2
>
> ## Nursing Focus on the Elderly: Cancer Assessment Considerations
>
> | Cancer Type | Assessment Consideration | Cancer Type | Assessment Consideration |
> |---|---|---|---|
> | Colorectal cancer | • Ask the client whether bowel habits have changed over the past year (e.g., in consistency, frequency, or color).
• Is there any obvious blood in the stool?
• Test at least one stool specimen for occult blood during the client's hospitalization.
• Encourage the client to have a baseline colonoscopy.
• Encourage the client to reduce dietary intake of animal fats, red meat, and smoked meats.
• Encourage the client to increase dietary intake of bran, vegetables, and fruit. | Skin cancer | • Examine skin areas for moles or warts.
• Ask the client about changes in moles (e.g., color, edges, or sensation). |
> | | | Leukemia | • Observe the skin for color, petechiae, or ecchymosis.
• Ask the client about
  Fatigue
  Bruising
  Bleeding tendency
  History of infections and illnesses
  Night sweats
  Unexplained fevers |
> | Bladder cancer | • Ask the client about the presence of
  Pain on urination
  Blood in the urine
  Cloudy urine
  Increased frequency or urgency | Lung cancer | • Observe the skin and mucous membranes for color.
• How many words can the client say between breaths?
• Ask the client about
  Cough
  Hoarseness
  Smoking history |
> | Prostate cancer | • Ask the client about
  Hesitancy
  Change in the size of the urine stream
  Pain in back or legs
  History of urinary tract infections | | Exposure to inhalation irritants
  Shortness of breath
  Activity tolerance
  Frothy or bloody sputum
  Pain in the arms or chest
  Difficulty swallowing |

Intrinsic Factors Influencing Cancer Development

Other intrinsic factors affect whether a person is likely to develop cancer, including immune function, age, and genetic predisposition.

Immune Function

The immune system protects the body from foreign invaders and non-self cells (see Chap. 23). Non-self cells include cells made in the body that are no longer normal, such as cancer cells. The part of the immune system responsible for cancer protection is cell-mediated immunity. Natural killer (NK) and helper T cells are most important to immune surveillance (Applebaum, 1992).

The instrumental role of the immune system in protecting the body from cancer is supported by cancer incidence statistics in immunosuppressed people. Children younger than 2 years and adults older than 60 years have immune systems that function at less than optimal levels, and both groups have a higher incidence of cancer compared with that of the general population. Organ transplant recipients taking immunosuppressive drugs to re-

duce the risk of organ rejection also have a higher incidence of cancer. In clients with AIDS, incidence may be as high as 70% (Pitot, 1986).

Age

Advancing age is probably the single most significant risk factor related to the development of cancer (American Cancer Society, 1991). Of all cancers, 50% occur in people older than 65 years (American Cancer Society, 1998). The higher cancer incidence in this age group may reflect

TABLE 26–12

> ### The Seven Warning Signs of Cancer
>
> • C Changes in bowel or bladder habits
> • A A sore that does not heal
> • U Unusual bleeding or discharge
> • T Thickening or lump in the breast or elsewhere
> • I Indigestion or difficulty swallowing
> • O Obvious change in a wart or mole
> • N Nagging cough or hoarseness

TABLE 26-13

Malignancies Associated with Altered Suppressor Gene Activity

Suppressor Gene	Malignancies
APC	Colorectal, stomach, and pancreatic carcinomas
DCC	Colorectal carcinomas
MTS1	Melanoma; brain tumors; leukemias; sarcomas; breast, bladder, ovarian, lung, and kidney carcinomas
NF1	Neurofibroma, colon, astrocytoma
NF2	Neurofibroma, meningioma, schwannoma
p53	Breast, bladder, colorectal, esophageal, liver, lung, and ovarian carcinomas; brain tumors; sarcomas; leukemias and lymphomas
Rb	Retinoblastomas; sarcomas; breast, bladder, esophageal, and lung carcinomas
VHL	Renal cell carcinoma, pheochromocytoma, hemangioblastoma
WT1	Wilms' tumor

Data from Cooper, G. (1995). *Oncogenes* (2nd ed.). Boston: Jones and Bartlett.

lifelong accumulation of DNA mutations that result in cell transformation and cancer. The body may no longer be able to repair these mutations as it once did. The effectiveness of the immune system, especially cell-mediated immunity, is also reduced in the elderly, resulting in a limited ability to recognize and eliminate altered self cells. Cancer assessment considerations for the elderly are given in Chart 26–2.

Manifestations of cancer in elderly clients may be overlooked and attributed to changes that coincide with normal aging. Elders must be aware of and report symptoms, such as the seven warning signs of cancer (Table 26–12), to health care providers. Health care providers must treat these reports with respect and thoroughly investigate all manifestations suggestive of disease.

Genetic Predisposition

As previously discussed, oncogenes are primarily intrinsic factors related to carcinogenesis. Proto-oncogenes, precursors of oncogenes, are passed on from generation to generation. The development of cancer, however, depends on more than these genes. The proto-oncogene needs to be damaged or altered to allow expression of the oncogene. In some people, the location of specific proto-oncogenes is different and may allow them to be activated more easily (Cooper, 1995). In other people, the position of the oncogene may be normal, but the gene controlling the oncogene's activity, the *suppressor gene*, may be abnormal or out of place. These variations in gene location are

inheritable. Table 26–9 lists specific malignancies associated with altered oncogene activity; Table 26–13 lists specific malignancies associated with altered suppressor gene activity.

Patterns of genetic predisposition for cancer other than oncogenes have also been identified, including

- Inherited predisposition for specific cancers
- Inherited conditions associated with cancer
- Familial clustering
- Chromosomal aberrations

Table 26–14 lists different conditions associated with a genetic predisposition for cancer development.

TRANSCULTURAL CONSIDERATIONS

The incidence of cancer varies among races. American Cancer Society data, as reported by Wingo et al. (1996), show that African-Americans have a higher incidence of cancer than Caucasians do, and the death rate is higher for African-Americans. Since 1960, the overall incidence among African-Americans has increased 27%, whereas for Caucasians it has increased 12%. Cancer sites and cancer-related mortality vary along racial lines as well. Table 26–15 summarizes common cancers among Caucasian, African-American, Asian, and Hispanic populations.

When risks for cancer development are assessed, however, race and genetic predisposition cannot be considered alone. Behavior related to culture or ethnic group, geographic location, diet, and socioeconomic factors must also be assessed (Olsen & Frank-Stromborg, 1994; Palos, 1994). The American Cancer Society (1998) has reported that cancer incidence and survival are often related to socioeconomic factors, such as the availability of health care services or the belief that seeking early health care

TABLE 26-14

Conditions Associated with a Genetic Predisposition for Cancer

Condition	Specific Cancer Type
Inherited cancers*	• Retinoblastoma • Wilms' tumor
Familial clustering	• Breast cancer • Melanoma
Bloom's syndrome	• Leukemia
Familial polyposis	• Colorectal cancer
Chromosomal aberrations Down syndrome (47 chromosomes)	• Leukemia
Klinefelter's syndrome (47, XXY)	• Breast cancer
Turner's syndrome (45, XO)	• Leukemia • Gonadal carcinoma • Meningioma • Colorectal cancer

*Not all retinoblastomas or Wilms' tumors are inherited.

TABLE 26–15

Racial Differences in Cancer Development	
Race	**Common Cancer Types**
Caucasian	1. Lung
	2. Breast
	3. Colorectal
	4. Prostate
African-American	1. Lung
	2. Prostate
	3. Breast
	4. Colorectal
	5. Uterine
Asian	1. Breast
	2. Colorectal
	3. Prostate
	4. Lung
	5. Stomach
Hispanic	1. Prostate
	2. Breast
	3. Colorectal
	4. Lung

Data from American Cancer Society. (1994). *Cancer facts and figures— 1994.* Atlanta, GA: Author.

has a positive effect on the outcome of cancer diagnosis (see Research Applications for Nursing).

CANCER PREVENTION
Avoidance of Known or Potential Carcinogens

A very effective means of preventing cancer development is avoidance of known or potential carcinogens. This method of prevention is appropriate when the cause of a specific cancer is known or strongly implicated and avoidance is easily accomplished. Examples of effective avoidance are using skin protection during sun exposure, avoiding tobacco, and eliminating environmental asbestos. As more causes of cancer are identified, the prevention method of avoidance will likely become even more effective.

Avoidance or Modification of Associated Factors

Absolute causes are not known for many cancers, but specific conditions or exposures appear to have an associated risk. Some examples are the increased incidence of some cancer types among people who consume alcohol; the association of a diet high in fat and low in fiber with colon cancer, breast cancer, and ovarian cancer; and the greater incidence of cervical cancer among women with many sexual partners. It is thought that avoidance or reduction of exposure to the associated condition or factor might result in decreased risks for cancer development.

Chemoprevention

A new form of cancer prevention, chemoprevention, is currently under study to determine its effectiveness. This strategy uses exogenous chemicals, such as synthetic chemicals, natural nutrients, or other substances found in plant food sources, to disrupt one or more steps important to cancer development. Such agents may be able to reverse existing damage or halt the progression of the transformation process. Chemoprevention agents have a variety of actions that disrupt at least one important step in the process of cancer development, including

- Blocking an inactive compound from becoming an active carcinogen
- Blocking the direct action of a carcinogen on DNA

▷ Research Applications for Nursing

Elderly African-American and Caucasian Women's Attitudes Toward a Cancer Diagnosis

Powe, B. (1995). Cancer fatalism among elderly Caucasians and African Americans. Oncology Nursing Forum, 22(9), 1355–1359.

The investigator of this prospective descriptive study surveyed the beliefs of elderly Caucasian and African-American women in senior citizen centers in a southern state. The majority of women were older than 70 years, and their average education was at the 8th-grade level. The survey questionnaire was developed by the investigator after an extensive literature review. Testing of the instrument revealed an alpha coefficient for reliability ranging from 0.84 to 0.87. Because the overall education level was relatively low, the questionnaire was read to the participants.

The results indicated that African-American participants had higher fatalism scores than did their Caucasian counterparts. It is suggested that people who are fatalistic about any diagnosis are less likely to seek screening or appropriate medical care and thus would reduce their chances for cure or long-term survival. The investigator suggests that educational interventions targeted to African-Americans could dispel myths and reduce fatalism, contributing to greater compliance with recommended cancer screening regimens.

Critique. Although the results showed a greater degree of fatalism among African-Americans as compared with Caucasians, educational and income levels were also predictors of fatalism. Replication of this study among people of different ethnicities but with higher educational backgrounds and socioeconomic resources could be conducted to determine whether ethnic differences in fatalistic outlook hold when other variables diminish. The survey questions were all "forced-choice" questions. Including open-ended questions may address the origin of fatalistic beliefs.

Possible Nursing Implications. Much of fatalism toward cancer is based on inaccurate information. Many people with fatalistic beliefs either have had negative experiences with cancer or are basing their opinions on out-of-date cancer statistics. Nurses must take responsibility in determining each client's beliefs regarding cancer prognosis and provide accurate, culturally sensitive information about the potential for improved cancer outcomes with different types of treatment.

TABLE 26-16

Agents Under Investigation for Chemoprevention of Cancer

Category of Prevention	Specific Agents
Prevention of carcinogen formation	Ascorbic acid (vitamin C) Tocopherol (type of vitamin E) Selenium Caffeic acid
Blocking the action of a carcinogen on DNA ("antimutagens")	Carotenoids (vitamin A derivative) Retinoids (vitamin A derivative) Ellagic acid Flavones Oltipraz Butylated hydroxyanisole
Enhancing the elimination of a carcinogen	Isothiocyanate Indole-3-carbinol
Suppression of carcinogenic action	Aspirin Retinoids Indomethacin Selenium Steroidal anti-inflammatory agents Protease inhibitors

Antipromotion activity	Carotenoids
	Retinoids
	Selenium
	Coumarin
	Piroxicam
	Indomethacin
	Calciferol (vitamin D)
	Hormone antagonists
	  Tamoxifen
	  Fenasteride

Suppression of progression	Danazol Interferon Cysteamine Vorozole

- Enhancing the rate of elimination of a carcinogen from the body
- Suppressing the activity of a carcinogen
- Suppressing the promoting activity of a carcinogen
- Suppressing the progression of a premalignant or early-stage malignancy into a more malignant state

Table 26–16 lists agents under current investigation for effectiveness in chemoprevention.

The ultimate goal of chemopreventive strategies is prevention of cancer development. Target populations for whom chemoprevention might be effective include

- Healthy people with no known specific cancer risk
- People at greater than normal risk because of increased environmental exposure or decreased immune function
- People with precancerous lesions
- People with a history of cancer

Gene Alteration as a Potential Form of Cancer Prevention

Because cancer development clearly involves gene changes, either congenital genetic abnormalities or acquired gene damage, researchers have suggested that altering damaged genes could prevent cancer development. At the present state of science, people can be screened for some gene alterations that will eventually lead to cancer. Such screening can help a genetically susceptible person either alter lifestyle factors or participate in early detection methods to identify a malignancy when cure is more likely. Although it is not yet possible to "fix" or remove an abnormal gene in humans, "gene therapy" in the future is not out of the realm of possibility.

SELECTED BIBLIOGRAPHY

*American Cancer Society. (1991). *Proceedings of the National Workshop on Cancer Control and the Older Person* (Report No. 91–3M–No. 3043). Atlanta, GA: Author.

American Cancer Society. (1998). *Cancer facts & figures—1997* (Report No. 98–300M–No. 5008.98). Atlanta, GA: Author.

Ames, B., Gold, L., & Willett. (1995). The causes and prevention of cancer. *Proceedings of the National Academy of Sciences, 92*(12), 5258–5265.

*Applebaum, J. (1992). The role of the immune system in the pathogenesis of cancer. *Seminars in Oncology Nursing, 8*(1), 51–62.

Appling, S. (1996). One in nine: Risks and prevention strategies for breast cancer. *Medical-Surgical Nursing, 5*(1), 62–64.

Baron, R., & Borgen, P. (1997). Genetic susceptibility for breast cancer: Testing and primary prevention options. *Oncology Nursing Forum, 24*(3), 461–468.

*Bishop, J. (1982). Oncogenes. *Scientific American, 246*(3), 80–92.

Bishop, J. (1995). Cancer: The rise of the genetic paradigm. *Genes and Development, 9*(11), 1309–1315.

Calzone, K. (1997). Genetic predisposition testing: Clinical implications for oncology nurses. *Oncology Nursing Forum, 24*(4), 712–718.

Caudell, K., Cuaron, L., & Gallucci, B. (1996). Cancer biology: Molecular and cellular aspects. In R. McCorkle, M. Grant, M. Frank-Stromborg, & S. Baird (Eds.), *Cancer nursing: A comprehensive textbook* (2nd ed., pp. 150–170). Philadelphia: W. B. Saunders.

Cooper, G. (1995). *Oncogenes* (2nd ed). Boston: Jones & Bartlett.

Cox, B. (1995). Cancer update 95. *Nursing 95, 25*(4), 47–49.

Daley, E. (1998). Clinical update on the role of HPV and cervical cancer. *Cancer Nursing, 21*(1), 31–35.

Dimond, E., Calzone, K., Davis, J., & Jenkins, J. (1998). Programmed instruction: The role of the nurse in cancer genetics. *Cancer Nursing, 21*(1), 57–74.

Erdos, D., & Mowad, L. (1995). Resources for helping patients to quit smoking. *Cancer Practice, 3*(4), 254–257.

Fidler, I., & Hart, I. (1982). Biologic diversity in metastatic neoplasia: Origins and implications. *Science, 217*(4564), 998.

Foltz, A., & Culhane, B. (1994). Cancer resources in the United States. *Oncology Nursing Forum, 21*(9), 1583–1593.

Frank-Stromborg, M., Heusinkveld, K., & Rohan, K. (1996). Evaluating cancer risks and preventive oncology. In R. McCorkle, M. Grant, M. Frank-Stromborg, & S. Baird (Eds.), *Cancer nursing: A comprehensive textbook* (2nd ed., pp. 213–264). Philadelphia: W. B. Saunders.

*Frank-Stromborg, M., & Olsen, S. (1993). *Cancer prevention in minority populations: Cultural implications for health care professionals.* St. Louis: C. V. Mosby.

Greco, K., & Kulawiak, L. (1994). Prostate cancer prevention: Risk reduction through life-style, diet, and chemoprevention. *Oncology Nursing Forum, 21*(9), 1504–1511.

Greenwald, P. (1996). Chemoprevention of cancer. *Scientific American, 275*(3), 96–99.

Greenwald, P., Kelloff, G., Burch-Whitman, C., & Kramer, B. (1995). Chemoprevention. *CA: A Cancer Journal for Clinicians, 45*(1), 31–49.

Grenier, L. M. (1995). Cancer information and resources for Hispanic populations. *Cancer Practice, 3*(5), 317–319.

Harrison, K., & Tempero, M. (1995). Diagnostic use of radiolabeled antibodies for cancer. *Oncology, 9*(7), 625–631.

*Liotta, L. (1992). Cancer cell invasion and metastasis. *Scientific American, 266*(2), 54–62.

McCorkle, R., Grant, M., Frank-Stromborg, M., & Baird, S. (1996). *Cancer nursing: A comprehensive textbook* (2nd ed.). Philadelphia: W. B. Saunders.

Mettlin, C., & Michalek, A. (1996). The causes of cancer. In R. McCorkle, M. Grant, M. Frank-Stromborg, & S. Baird (Eds.), *Cancer nursing: A comprehensive textbook* (2nd ed., pp. 138–149). Philadelphia: W. B. Saunders.

Misner, T., & Fuller, S. (1995). Testicular versus breast and colorectal cancer screening. *Cancer Practice, 3*(5), 310–316.

Mitelman, F. (1994). Chromosomes, genes, and cancer. *CA: A Cancer Journal for Clinicians, 44*(3), 133–135.

Morrison, C. (1996). Determining crucial correlates of breast self-examination in older women with low incomes. *Oncology Nursing Forum, 23*(1), 83–93.

*Nicolson, G. (1979). Cancer metastasis. *Scientific American, 240,* 66–79.

Olsen, S., & Frank-Stromborg, M. (1994). Cancer prevention and screening activities reported by African American nurses. *Oncology Nursing Forum, 21*(3), 487–494.

Olsen, S., & Frank-Stromborg, M. (1996). Cancer screening and early detection. In R. McCorkle, M. Grant, M. Frank-Stromborg, & S. Baird (Eds.), *Cancer nursing: A comprehensive textbook* (2nd ed., pp. 265–297). Philadelphia: W. B. Saunders.

Palos, G. (1994). Cultural heritage: Cancer screening and early detection. *Seminars in Oncology Nursing, 10*(2), 104–113.

*Pitot, H. (1986). *Fundamentals of Oncology* (2nd ed.). New York: Marcel Dekker.

Poe, M., & DeVore, L. (1996). Using the telephone for cancer information. *Cancer Practice, 4*(1), 47–49.

Powe, B. (1996). Cancer fatalism among African-Americans: A review of the literature. *Nursing Outlook, 44*(1), 18–21.

Powe, B. (1995). Cancer fatalism among elderly Caucasians and African-Americans. *Oncology Nursing Forum, 22*(9), 1355–1359.

Ruoslahti, E. (1996). How cancer spreads. *Scientific American, 275*(3), 72–77.

Soltis, M., Hubbard, S., & Kohn, E. (1996). The biology of invasion and metastasis. In R. McCorkle, M. Grant, M. Frank-Stromborg, & S. Baird (Eds.), *Cancer nursing: A comprehensive textbook* (2nd ed., pp. 190–212). Philadelphia: W. B. Saunders.

Stellman, J., & Stellman, S. (1996). Cancer and the workplace. *CA: A Cancer Journal for Clinicians, 46*(2), 70–92.

Swan, D., & Ford, B. (1997). Chemoprevention of cancer: Review of the literature. *Oncology Nursing Forum, 24*(4), 719–727.

Tomaino-Brunner, C., Freda, M., & Runowicz, C. (1996). "I hope I don't have cancer": Colposcopy and minority women. *Oncology Nursing Forum, 23*(1), 39–44.

Trichopoulos, D., Li, F., & Hunter, D. (1996). What causes cancer? *Scientific American, 275*(3), 80–87

Weinberg, R. (1996). How cancer arises. *Scientific American, 275*(3), 62–70.

Weinberg, R. (1994). Oncogenes and tumor suppressor genes. *CA: A Cancer Journal for Clinicians, 44*(3), 160–170.

Willett, W., Colditz, G., & Mueller, N. (1996). Strategies for minimizing cancer risk. *Scientific American, 275*(3), 88–95.

Wingo, P., Bolden, S., Tong, T., Parker, S., Martin, L., & Heath, C. (1996). Cancer statistics for African Americans, 1996. *CA: A Cancer Journal for Clinicans, 46*(2), 113–125.

SUGGESTED READINGS

Erdos, D., & Mowad, L. (1995). Resources for helping patients to quit smoking. *Cancer Practice, 3*(4), 254–257.

Cigarette smoking has been implicated as a cause of or major contributing factor to cancer development. This article suggests additional counseling and personal-contact interventions to be combined with alternative nicotine sources to help clients stop smoking through behavior modification.

Palos, G. (1994). Cultural heritage: Cancer screening and early detection. *Seminars in Oncology Nursing, 10*(2), 104–113.

This excellent article reviews the literature regarding culture, compliance, and cancer screening interventions. The author includes the cultures of poverty and aging as separate from the mainstream or dominant culture of the United States. A model for developing culturally appropriate cancer screening and early detection programs is also presented.

Ruoslahti, E. (1996). How cancer spreads. *Scientific American, 275*(3), 72–77.

The author makes excellent use of color diagrams and common language to describe what is known currently about metastasis. Scientific jargon is avoided when explaining the research that supports theories of cancer spread. A great article to give to clients and families.

INTERVENTIONS FOR CLIENTS WITH CANCER

Cancer, discussed in Chapter 26, is a broad term for a variety of malignant diseases originating in many different tissues and organs. The purpose of this chapter is to provide a general overview of common client problems and care issues related to the diagnosis and treatment of cancer. Specific risk factors, treatments, and side effects for each cancer type are presented in the chapters associated with the body system in which the cancer first developed. For example, melanoma is presented in Chapter 70, and breast cancer is presented in Chapter 77. Table 27–1 provides a guide to the text location of discussions of specific cancer types.

Cancer is a diagnosis that people fear and equate with death in spite of the fact that many types of cancer can be cured or controlled. A diagnosis of cancer causes psychological distress and has the potential to disrupt personal and professional relationships, finances, role identity, self-esteem, body image, and normal physiologic function. Providing care to clients and families experiencing cancer is challenging and complex. Table 27–2 lists key concepts about living with cancer.

GENERAL DISEASE-RELATED CONSEQUENCES OF CANCER
Pathophysiology

Cancer can develop in any organ or tissue, but tends to occur in some much more frequently than in others. Cancer destroys normal tissue, resulting in decreased function in that tissue or organ. Even when cancers occur in nonvital tissues or organs, they can cause death by metastasizing (spreading) into vital organs and disrupting critical physiologic processes (see Chap. 26). Left untreated, cancers produce serious health problems, such as

- Impaired immune and hematopoietic (blood-producing) function
- Altered gastrointestinal (GI) tract structure and function
- Motor and sensory deficits
- Decreased respiratory function

Not only do these impairments cause great physical and emotional distress to the client, but, without inter-

Table 27–1

Text Location of Specific Cancer Content				
Cancer Type	Chapter	Pathology/Etiology	Treatment	Nursing Care
Breast	77	1962	1963–1978	1963–1978
Lung	32	640–644	645–659	647–656
Prostate	79	2031	2032–2036	2032–2036
Colorectal	59	1410–1411	1411–1412	1412–1420
Skin	70	1743	1744–1746	1744–1746
Leukemia	42	961–963	963–978	967–978
Lymphoma	42	978–980	978–980	978–980
Ovarian	78	2013	2014–2015	2015

vention, persistent cancer invasion of normal tissues leads to death.

Impaired Immune and Hematopoietic Function

Impaired immune and hematopoietic function occurs most often in clients who have leukemia and lymphoma, but such impairment can occur with any cancer that invades the bone marrow. Tumor cells enter the bone marrow, causing decreased production of healthy white blood cells needed for normal immune function (see Chap. 23). Thus, clients who have cancer, especially leukemia, are at an increased risk for infection.

When cancer invades the bone marrow, it also decreases the number of red blood cells and platelets. These changes may be caused by the cancer itself, such as in leukemia, or by cancer treatment. In either case, the client becomes anemic and has an increased tendency to bleed.

Altered Gastrointestinal Structure and Function

Cancer can alter GI function and disturb the client's nutritional status. For example, tumors may cause obstruc-

Table 27–2

Key Points About Cancer Treatment
• With multiapproach to cancer treatment, 50% of clients with cancer can be cured.
• Surgery is most effective for cancer therapy when tumors are small and well localized.
• Radiation therapy is only effective on the tissues directly within the radiation path.
• Side effects of radiation therapy are confined to the tissues within the radiation path.
• The most common side effects of radiation therapy are skin irritation, fatigue, and altered taste sensation.
• Chemotherapy is systemic therapy for cancer and affects all body tissues.
• The most common side effects of chemotherapy are alopecia, nausea and vomiting, mucositis, skin changes, and bone marrow suppression.
• The most life-threatening side effect of chemotherapy is bone marrow suppression.

tion or compression anywhere along the GI tract, interfering with the client's ability to ingest or digest adequate nutrients and eliminate waste products. In addition, tumors can affect a person's basal metabolic rate and increase requirements for protein, carbohydrates, and fat at the same time the person has less energy available to prepare food and eat.

Many tumors spread to the liver, causing profound damage. The liver has many important metabolic functions and helps digest and utilize proteins and fats. Altered liver function contributes to malnutrition and death among clients with cancer.

The anorexia experienced by clients with cancer often interferes with the client's ability to meet energy requirements. Cachexia (extreme body wasting and malnutrition) develops from the imbalance between food intake and energy use, and may occur in spite of what appears to be adequate nutritional intake. Changes in a client's taste can result from the cancer or the treatment and cause a decrease in appetite. A complete list of cancer-related factors that can contribute to malnutrition is presented in Table 27–3.

Nutritional support for the client with cancer, especially one undergoing cancer therapy, is complex and controversial. Often a diet high in protein and carbohydrates is ordered to assist the client to maintain his or her weight and provide nutrients needed for energy and cellular repair. However, some scientists believe that excessive intake of protein, carbohydrates, and vitamins increases the nutrition of the cancer cells and contributes to cancer progression. Clients often believe that by eating more food, especially a diet low in fat and high in fiber, grains, fruit, and vegetables, their cancer can be cured more easily. At present, no one nutritional plan meets the needs of all clients with cancer.

Motor and Sensory Deficits

Motor (movement) and sensory deficits can occur when cancers invade bone or the brain or compress nerves. In most clients with bone metastases, the primary cancer is in the prostate, breast, or lung. Bone sites most affected include the vertebrae, ribs, pelvis, and femur. The humerus, scapula, sternum, skull, and clavicle are also common metastatic sites. Bone metastases can cause fractures, spinal cord compression, and hypercalcemia,

Table 27–3

Causes of Malnutrition in Clients with Cancer

Anorexia
- Local causes
  - Pelvic or abdominal tumors
  - Hepatic metastases
  - Intestinal compression or obstruction
  - Others
- Remote causes
  - Food aversions
  - Early satiety
- Treatment-related causes
  - Postsurgical small stomach or stasis
  - Drugs, including chemotherapy
  - Radiation—local and systemic effects
- Systemic illness
  - Infection
  - Hepatitis or pancreatitis
  - Endocrinopathies
- Taste disorders
  - Drugs (e.g., metronidazole)
  - Remote effects of neoplasm and its treatment
  - Local disease and its treatment (e.g., stomatitis, naso-pharyngeal tumor, radiation, and surgery)
  - Nausea and vomiting
- Psychogenic causes
  - Depression
  - Anxiety
  - Conditioned aversions
- Intolerance of institutional food

Difficulty in Eating
- Head and neck tumors and their treatment
- Xerostomia

- Stomatitis
- Loss of teeth and dental problems
- Dysphagia and odynophagia

Maldigestion or Malabsorption
- Pancreatic insufficiency
- Bile salt deficiency
- Hypersecretory states
  - Zollinger-Ellison syndrome
  - Pancreatic cholera
  - Bowel infiltration
  - Diffuse invasion (e.g., lymphoma)
  - Local blockage
  - Fistula
- Postsurgical causes
  - Esophageal surgery (with vagotomy, gastric stasis diarrhea, and steatorrhea)
  - Gastrectomy—dumping, achlorhydria, or afferent loop syndrome
  - Small intestine resections
- Postirradiation causes
  - Enteritis (may occur as late sequela)
  - Fistula
  - Stenosis
  - Obstruction

Protein-Losing Enteropathy
Malutilization
- Cancer cachexia
- Steroids
  - Nitrogen wasting
  - Hyperglycemia
  - Calcium loss

each of which results in decreased mobility for the client.

The client may also experience sensory changes if the spinal cord is damaged by tumor compression or if nerve ganglia are compressed. When tumors metastasize to the brain, sensory, motor, and cognitive functions are severely disrupted.

The client with cancer may also experience pain. Pain does not always accompany cancer, but can be a significant problem for clients with terminal cancer. Chapter 9 provides an in-depth discussion of cancer pain causes and management.

Decreased Respiratory Function

Cancer can disrupt a client's respiratory function in several ways and often results in death. Tumors involving the airways can cause airway obstruction, for instance. If lung tissue is involved, lung capacity is decreased. Tumor growth can also press on vascular and lymphatic structures in the chest, blocking blood flow through the chest and lungs, resulting in pulmonary edema and dyspnea. Tumors also can thicken the alveolar membrane

and damage pulmonary blood vessels, reducing gas exchange.

TREATMENT-RELATED CONSEQUENCES OF CANCER

The purpose of any cancer treatment is to prolong clients' survival time or improve quality of life. Although a few spontaneous regressions of malignant tumors have been reported, most clients with cancer would die within months of diagnosis without appropriate cancer therapy. Therapies for cancer include surgery, radiation, chemotherapy, hormonal manipulation, immunotherapy, and gene therapy. These therapies may be used individually or in combination to kill tumor cells. The type and amount of therapy are determined by the

- Specific type of cancer present
- Extent of the disease
- Overall health of the client

For most types of cancer, one or more regimens of therapy (protocols) have been established, based on ex-

Table 27—4

Diagnostic/Biopsy Surgeries for Cancer		
Biopsy Type	**Description**	**Problem/Limitations**
Needle	• Aspiration of cells in a fluid or in very soft tissue • Bore a "core" of solid tissue by using a long needle or making a punch, scrape, or bite.	• Sample error—may biopsy only noncancerous cells in a tissue or organ • Sample size may not be adequate for accurate testing • Procedure may spread cancer by seeding it into surrounding tissues • Procedure may damage healthy tissue
Incisional	• Wedge of suspected tissue is removed from a larger tissue mass, leaving some tumor cells remaining in the tissue.	• Sample error • Tumor seeding • Damage to healthy tissue
Excisional	• Complete removal of an entire lesion without removing any adjacent normal tissues	• Tumor seeding • Leaving micrometastasis • Damage to healthy tissue
Staging	• Multiple needle or incisional biopsies in tissues where metastasis is suspected or likely	• Tumor seeding • Sample error • Damage to healthy tissue

periments with cancer cells, animals, and other clients with cancer.

Surgery

Rationale for Cancer Treatment

Surgery for cancer involves removal of diseased tissue. If cancer is confined to the tissue removed, surgery alone can result in "cure" for that cancer. Although many cancers have spread too far at the time of diagnosis for surgery alone to be curative, surgery may still be a useful part of diagnosis, treatment, follow-up, and rehabilitation.

Mechanism of Action

Surgery is the oldest form of cancer treatment and the first method to cure cancer. Cancer surgery may be prescribed for any of the following purposes: prophylaxis, diagnosis, cure, control, palliation, determination of therapy effectiveness, and reconstruction.

Prophylaxis

Prophylactic surgery is performed when a client has either an existing "premalignant" condition or a known family history that strongly predisposes the person to the development of cancer. An attempt is made to remove the tissue or organ "at risk" and thus prevent the development of cancer. An example of prophylactic surgery for a premalignant condition is removal of a benign mole from a location where it would receive continuous irritation or exposure to sunlight.

Diagnosis (Biopsy)

Diagnostic surgery can provide histologic proof of malignancy. Usually, all or part of a suspected lesion is removed for microscopic examination and testing. Specific types of biopsies are summarized in Table 27–4.

Cure

Surgery for cure can, without additional therapy, result in a cure rate of 25% to 30%. All gross and microscopic tumor is either removed or destroyed. Types of curative surgeries are described in Table 27–5.

Control (Cytoreductive Surgery)

Cancer control, or cytoreductive surgery, is a "debulking" procedure that consists of removing part of the tumor while known gross tumor is left. This type of surgery alone cannot result in a cure, but it does decrease the number of cancer cells and increase the chances that other therapies can be successful.

Palliation

Palliative surgery aims not to cure (or even increase survival time in many instances) but to improve quality of life during the survival time. The surgeon removes tumor tissue that is causing pain, intestinal obstruction, or difficulty swallowing. What is done specifically during palliative surgery depends on the client's specific problem.

Determination of Therapy Effectiveness ("Second Look")

Second-look surgery is essentially a "rediagnosis" after treatment, performed to assess the disease status in clients who have been treated and have no symptoms of remaining or recurrent tumor. The results of this surgery serve as a basis for discontinuing or continuing specific therapy.

Reconstructive or Rehabilitative Surgery

Reconstructive-rehabilitative surgery is relatively new. People with cancer are surviving long enough to need reconstruction. This type of surgery increases function, en-

Table 27-5

Curative Surgeries for Cancer		
Surgery Type	**Description**	**Purpose/Use**
Local excision	• Removal of all identifiable tumor along with a small margin of normal tissues	• Small, localized tumors
Wide local excision (radical)	• Removal of identifiable tumor plus immediate tissue or adjacent tissue	• Small tumors with only local tissue invasion
Wide excision	• Removal of tumor, surrounding tissue, adjacent structures, and usual lymph channels draining the area	• Small to moderate-size tumors with known local invasion
Extended radical excision	• Removal of tumor, lymphatics, adjacent organs, and all tissues in the region	• Tumor infiltrate in a wide area but with no known distant metastasis

hances cosmetic appearance, or both. Examples include breast reconstruction after mastectomy, replacement of the esophagus after radiation damage, bowel reconstruction, revision of scars, release of contractures, and placement of penile implants.

Side Effects of Surgical Therapy

Unlike surgery performed for many other reasons, cancer surgery often involves the loss or loss of function of a specific body part. Sometimes whole organs are removed, such as the kidney, lung, breast, testes, arm, or tongue. Any organ loss results in reduced function. The amount of function that is lost and the degree to which the loss physically affects clients depend on the location and extent of the surgery. Some surgical procedures for cancer also may result in significant scarring or disfigurement. In addition to actual body part loss and anxiety about the chances of surviving, clients may be grieving about a loss of body image or a change in lifestyle imposed by the cancer or its treatment.

Nursing Care Needs of Clients Undergoing Surgical Therapy

Nursing care associated with surgery for cancer is not vastly different from that related to surgery for other reasons (see Chaps. 20–22). The nurse considers all the physical and psychosocial factors related to the client's ability (or that of family and significant others) to cope with the uncertainty of cancer and its treatment, along with changes in body image and role. For example, surgery involving the genitals, urinary tract, colon, and rectum may permanently damage these organs. Surgical procedures that create a urinary or fecal diversion (such as a colostomy) may disturb innervation, causing erectile impotence or ejaculatory dysfunction in men and painful intercourse (dyspareunia) in women.

Radiation

Rationale for Cancer Treatment

The purpose of all types of radiation therapy for cancer is to destroy cancer cells with minimal exposure of the normal cells to damaging actions of the radiation. The effects of radiation are seen only in those tissues in the path of the radiation beam. Some effects are apparent within days or weeks after radiation treatment; others may not be apparent for months to years after radiation therapy is completed.

Mechanism of Action

Most of the radiation used to treat malignant tumors is *ionizing* radiation. When cells are exposed to this type of radiation, atoms within the cell are "kicked out" of orbit, resulting in a tremendous release of intracellular energy. Ionizing radiation is given off naturally by some substances, such as radium and cobalt, and can also be generated by machines called linear accelerators. Naturally occurring radiation is called *gamma* radiation; radiation that is generated by machine is called *roentgen* radiation. Their effect on cells is exactly the same.

Cells damaged by radiation either die outright or become unable to divide. Cellular damage, caused by a combination of intracellular oxidation and tight binding of deoxyribonucleic acid (DNA) strands, inhibits cells' capacity to divide.

Radiation damage can occur any time a cell is exposed to radiation; it is not confined to cells actively in the cell cycle. However, cells in the cell cycle experience more damage when exposed to radiation than do nondividing cells.

Three different types of energy, or rays, are produced by gamma radiation: gamma, beta, and alpha rays (Hilderley & Dow, 1996). These rays vary in their ability to penetrate tissues and damage cells. Table 27–6 summarizes the features of these three types of gamma radiation, and Figure 27–1 shows the penetrating ability of each.

The intensity of the radiation emitted decreases with the distance from the radiation source (Fig. 27–2), the *inverse square law*. In practice, this means that the dose of radiation received at a distance of 2 inches from the radiation source is only 25% of the dose received at a distance of 1 inch from the radiation source; the dose of radiation received at 3 inches is only one-ninth the dose received at a distance of 1 inch (Hassey, 1987).

The amount of radiation aimed at or delivered to a tissue is called *exposure*, and the amount of radiation absorbed by the recipient tissue is called the *dose*. The

Table 27–6

Characteristics of Different Types of Gamma Radiation	
Type of Ray	**Characteristics**
Gamma	• Gamma rays are very light with a low energy-transfer potential and travel at the speed of light allowing them to be concentrated and penetrate deeply into tissues. • This is the most common type of radiation used for the treatment of cancer. • This type of radiation can also cause serious, irreversible harm to tissues. • Exposure to this type of radiation must be avoided or severely limited.
Beta	• Beta rays are heavier with moderate to high speed. They have a high linear energy-transfer potential and do not penetrate tissues or other substances well. • Some beta rays are used inside the body for specific radiation therapy. • Beta rays are used in some diagnostic tests. • Beta rays pose health hazards to humans exposed to them, but exposure must be considerable for damage to occur.
Alpha	• Alpha rays are very heavy and slow. They easily transfer energy to surroundings and quickly lose their ability to penetrate tissues (0.04 mm into tissue). • Currently, alpha rays are used in laboratory tests rather than as treatment for cancer. • This type of radiation is harmful to humans only if it is ingested chronically.

dose is always somewhat less than the exposure. Three major factors determine the absorbed dose: intensity of the radiation exposure, proximity of the radiation source to the cells, and duration of exposure.

Killing Effects of Radiation

If the dose of radiation is high enough, all cells will be killed immediately, but this does not usually happen. Instead, radiation damage to the DNA is not usually apparent until the cell attempts to divide. In a population of tumor cells treated with a single exposure of radiation, all cells within the tumor absorb the radiation slightly differently; thus, their overall response to the radiation is slightly different. A few cells die immediately on exposure, and more die within the next 24 hours as they attempt to divide. Some cells become sterile as a result of this single treatment; still others repair the radiation-induced damage and continue to reproduce for many cell generations.

Because of the varying responses of all cancer cells within a given tumor, radiation for cancer therapy is administered as a series of divided doses. Small doses of radiation are delivered on a daily basis for a set period of time. Giving radiation treatment serially rather than as a single dose allows multiple opportunities to catch and destroy cancer cells that survived the initial hit of radiation while minimizing damage to normal tissues. This dose division is called *fractionation*. Standard radiotherapy is usually fractionated between 180 and 250 rad/day, multiplied by as many days as needed to achieve the total prescribed dose.

The total therapeutic dose of radiation to a tumor varies according to the size of the tumor, location of the tumor, radiation sensitivity of the tumor, and radiation sensitivity of the surrounding normal tissues. Some normal tissues are more sensitive to radiation than other normal tissues. For example, a total dose of 1200 rad might be prescribed for a primary liver tumor, but a total dose of 5000 to 6000 rad for a breast carcinoma (delivered over 25–30 separate days). If a 6000-rad dose were delivered to the liver, such extensive damage would occur to liver tissue that the client would experience liver failure and die even if the tumor were destroyed.

Two types of radiation delivery are most commonly used for cancer therapy: teletherapy and brachytherapy. The type used depends on the site of the tumor, stage of the tumor (including size and depth of the lesion), radiosensitivity of the tumor, and the client's general condition and state of health. Regardless of how administered, the optimum dose of radiation is one that cures or pro-

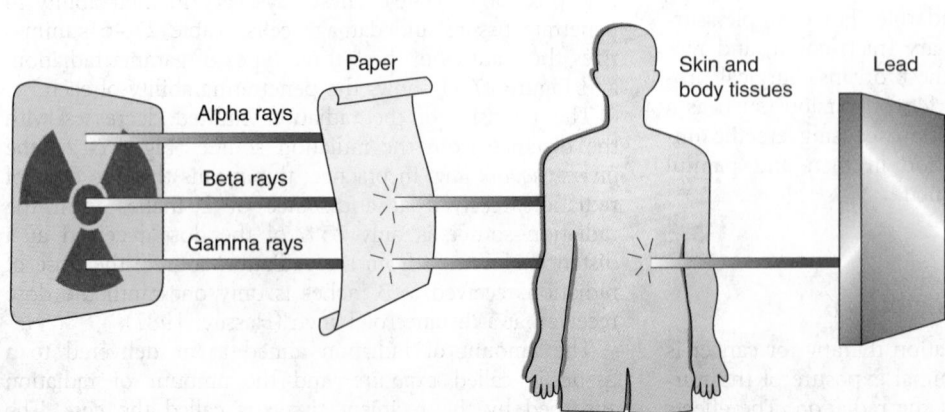

Figure 27–1. Penetrating capacity of different types of radiation.

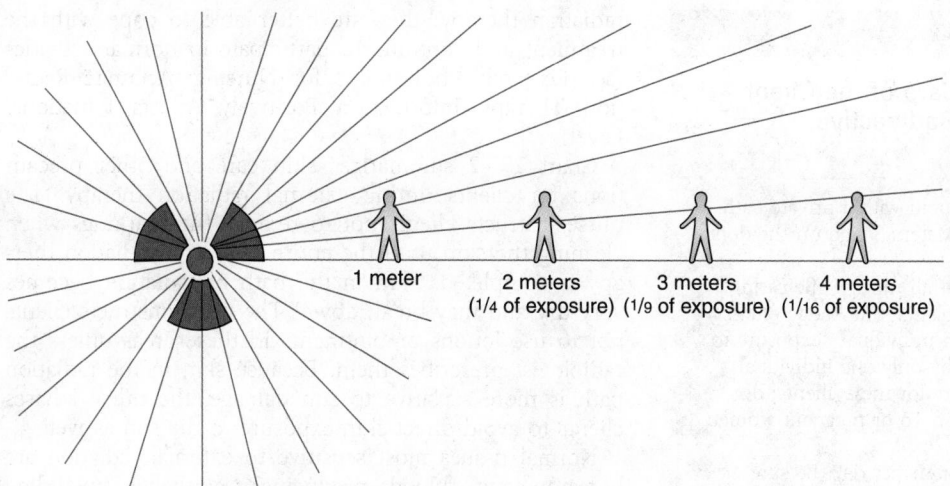

Figure 27-2. The inverse square law of radiation exposure.

1 meter   2 meters   3 meters   4 meters
(1/4 of exposure) (1/9 of exposure) (1/16 of exposure)

duces the desired killing effect on the cancer cells with an acceptable level of damage to normal tissues (some damage to normal tissues cannot be avoided).

Teletherapy

Teletherapy is derived from the Greek prefix "tele," meaning distant. In teletherapy, the actual radiation source is external to the client and remote from the tumor site. Because the source is external, the client never emits radiation and poses no hazard to anyone else. This type of therapy is also called *beam* radiation.

To increase the accuracy of radiation delivery to cancer cells, exact localization of the tumor is determined first. Once the pattern of radiation delivery has been established, the client must always be in exactly the same position for all treatments. The nurse makes sure that the client can get into and maintain this position with relative ease. Position-fixing devices and markings, either on the client's body or on the devices, ensure that the client assumes the proper position each day of treatment.

Brachytherapy

Brachytherapy is derived from the Greek word "brach," meaning short. In brachytherapy, the radiation source must come into direct, continuous contact with the tumor tissues for a specific period of time. The rationale is to provide a high absorbed dose of radiation in tumor tissues and a very limited absorbed low dose in surrounding normal tissues. The radiation delivered by brachytherapy has the same tissue effects as ionizing radiation delivered by external sources.

Brachytherapy involves the use of radioactive isotopes, either in solid form or within body fluids. Isotopes can be delivered to the tumor tissues in several ways. *With all types of brachytherapy, the radiation source is within the client; thus, for a period of time, the client emits radiation and can pose a hazard to others.*

UNSEALED RADIATION SOURCES. Soluble isotopes are unsealed radioactive sources administered via the oral or intravenous (IV) routes, or as an instillation into body cavities such as the peritoneal cavity and the spinal fluid space. Because the isotopes are unsealed, they are not completely confined to any one body area, although they may concentrate more in some body tissues than in others. These soluble isotopes enter body fluids, and eventually are eliminated from the body in various excreta (waste products), which are radioactive and can be harmful to other people.

An example of brachytherapy with soluble isotopes is the ingestion or injection of the radionuclide iodine 131 (an iodine base with a half-life of 8.05 days) to treat hyperthyroidism and some thyroid malignancies. The radioactive iodine concentrates in the thyroid gland, destroying the thyroid cancer cells. Most of this isotope is eliminated from the body within 48 hours. Once eliminated, neither the client nor the excreta are radioactive.

SEALED RADIATION SOURCES. The solid forms of brachytherapy involve sealed, temporary or permanent radiation sources implanted within the tumor target tissues. Most of the implants emit lower energy radiation continuously to tumor tissues. Some devices, such as seeds or needles, can be placed into the tissues and will stay in place alone. Other solid radiation sources must be held in place within the tissue or cavity by special applicators. The needles and seeds are radioactive at the time of insertion or implantation, and have already been preloaded with the radioactive isotope ("hot implantation"). Some of these devices are so small and the half-life of the isotope so short that the device is permanently left in place (most often for clients with prostate cancer). Other devices are removed and are reused in other clients.

In afterloading, the implant, without the radioactive isotope, is placed within the cavity, with special applicators that hold it in position. When placement has been ascertained and the client is in the proper environment, the implants are loaded with the radioisotope. After the prescribed dose has been delivered, the implant, radioisotopes, and position-holding applicators are removed. *With solid implants, the client emits radiation while the implant is in place, but the excreta are not radioactive* (Chart 27-1).

Chart 27-1

Nursing Care Highlight: Care of the Client with Sealed Implants of Radioactive Sources

- Assign the client to a private room with a private bath.
- Place a "Caution: Radioactive Material" sign on the door of the client's room.
- Wear a dosimeter film badge at all times while caring for clients with radioactive implants. The badge offers no protection, but measures an individual's exposure to radiation and should be used by only one individual.
- Pregnant nurses should not care for these clients; do not allow children younger than 16 or pregnant women to visit.
- Limit each visitor to one-half hour per day. Be sure visitors are at least 6 feet from the source.
- Never touch the radioactive source with bare hands. In the rare instance that it is dislodged, use a long-handled forceps to retrieve it. Deposit the radioactive source in the lead container kept in the client's room.
- Save all dressings and bed linens until after the radioactive source is removed. After the source is removed, dispose of dressings and linens in the usual manner. Other equipment can be removed from the room at any time.

Side Effects of Radiation Therapy

Because the immediate and long-term side effects for all types of radiation are limited to the tissues exposed to the radiation, side effects vary according to the site. Skin changes and hair loss (alopecia) are local but likely to be permanent, depending on total absorbed dose (Hilderley & Dow, 1996).

Depending on the dose, altered taste sensations and fatigue are two systemic side effects often noted by clients receiving external beam radiation, regardless of radiation site. Change in taste is thought to be caused by metabolites released from dead and dying cells. In particular, many clients experience an aversion to the taste of red meats. Fatigue may be related to the increased energy demands needed to repair radiation-damaged cells (Hilderley & Dow, 1996).

Radiation damage to normal tissues during cancer therapy can initiate inflammatory responses that cause tissue fibrosis and scarring. Their effects may not be apparent for many years after radiation treatment. For example, women who receive high-dose radiation therapy for uterine cancer may experience radiation-induced changes in the colon years later, resulting in constipation and obstruction.

Nursing Care of Clients Undergoing Radiation Therapy

Most clients are anxious about radiation. The nurse must be knowledgeable about its nature and be able to explain its purpose and side effects to clients and families. When clients receive concrete objective information regarding

radiation therapy, they are better able to cope with the treatment and continue to participate in normal activities (see Research Applications for Nursing: Accurate Radiation Therapy Information Positively Affects Functional Level).

Chart 27-2 summarizes skin care and other precautions for clients during external radiation therapy. The nurse instructs clients not to remove the markings when cleaning the skin until the entire course of radiation therapy is completed. Skin in the path of radiation becomes very dry and may break down. The nurse instructs clients not to use lotions or ointments in these areas unless the radiologist prescribes them. Because skin in the radiation path is more sensitive to sun damage, the nurse advises clients to avoid direct skin exposure to the sun as well.

Normal tissues most sensitive to external radiation are hematopoietic (blood producing), epithelial (including

---

▷ Research Applications for Nursing

Accurate Radiation Therapy Information Positively Affects Functional Level

Johnson, J. (1996). Coping with radiation therapy: Optimism and the effect of preparatory interventions. Research in Nursing & Health, 19(1), 3–12.

The investigator of this prospective experimental study hypothesized that pessimistic clients undergoing radiation therapy for cancer might benefit from concrete information on self-regulation theory and that optimistic clients would benefit from instruction in self-care and coping. The interventions were audiotaped messages. The control group's tape recordings focused on radiation therapy topics not specific to the client's situation. The coping experimental group's tape recordings focused on specific strategies to deal with particular side effects of radiation therapy. The concrete objective group's tape recordings focused on exactly what would happen during radiation therapy and what types of side effects could be expected. Mood, outcome expectancies, disruption of usual activities, and clinical data were measured during and after radiation therapy.

Neither the self-care instruction nor the coping strategy intervention affected the outcome variables. The concrete objective intervention had a positive effect on function for both pessimists and optimists. The findings of this study are not consistent with similar studies conducted one and two decades ago.

Critique. The article did not indicate whether the clients were tested for their coping skills, knowledge of radiation therapy, or previous experience with cancer (their own or a close contact's) before the interventions. No pretreatment data on activity disruption were obtained. Such information could be useful in determining homogeneity of the participant groups.

Possible Nursing Implications. Although research in the area of coping indicates that some clients do not actively seek information as a coping strategy, most clients appear to benefit from honest and accurate objective information. Nurses need to provide objective concrete information regarding procedures and treatments to all clients and family members.

Education Guide: Radiation Therapy for Cancer

- Wash the irradiated area gently each day with either water alone or a mild soap and water.
- Use your hand rather than a washcloth to be more gentle.
- Rinse soap thoroughly from your skin.
- Take care not to remove the markings that indicate exactly where the beam of radiation is to be focused.
- Dry the irradiated area with patting motions rather than rubbing motions, using a clean, soft towel or cloth.
- Use no powders, ointments, lotions, or creams on your skin at the radiation site unless they are prescribed by your *radiologist*.
- Wear soft clothing over the skin at the radiation site.
- Avoid wearing belts, buckles, straps, or any type of clothing that binds or rubs the skin at the radiation site.
- Avoid exposure of the irradiated area to the sun.
- Avoid heat exposure.

skin, mucous membranes, and hair follicles), and gonadal (reproductive) tissues. Some changes caused by radiation are permanent. Long-term problems experienced by clients vary with the location and dose of radiation administered. For example, radiation to the throat and upper chest can cause the client difficulty in swallowing. Head and neck radiation may damage the salivary glands and cause dry mouth. The nurse teaches clients about the types of symptoms that might be expected from the location and dose of radiation delivered.

Chemotherapy

Chemotherapy, the treatment of disease through chemical agents, has assumed a major role in managing clients with cancer. Chemotherapy as a cancer treatment is used to cure, increase mean survival time, and decrease the risk for specific life-threatening complications.

Rationale for Cancer Treatment

As described in Chapter 26, a characteristic of cancer growth is the ability of cancer cells to separate from the original tumor, spread to new areas, and establish new cancers at distant sites (metastasize). Clients with metastatic disease will die of their cancers unless treatment focuses on the metastatic cancer cells as well as the original cancer cells. Chemotherapy is useful in treating cancer because its effects are systemic and thus provide the opportunity to kill metastatic cancer cells that may have escaped local treatment. Table 27–7 indicates general responsiveness of specific cancers for chemotherapy.

Mechanism of Action

Chemotherapy can be successful in treating cancer because it has some demonstrated selectivity for cancer cells

over normal cells. The killing effect of chemotherapy on cancer cells appears to be related to its ability to damage DNA and interfere with cell division. Because of this, the tumors most sensitive to chemotherapy are those that have rapid growth.

Unfortunately, chemotherapeutic agents usually are administered systemically and exert their cell-damaging (cytotoxic) effects against both healthy and cancerous cells. Normal cells most profoundly affected by systemic chemotherapy are those that undergo frequent cell division, including skin, hair, epithelial lining of the gastrointestinal (GI) tract, spermatocytes, and hematopoietic cells.

Chemotherapy includes many drugs or chemical compounds that are effective in killing cancer cells, and are classified by the specific

- Types of biologic action they exert in the cancer cell
- Period in the life of a cell during which the chemotherapeutic agent is most likely to succeed in disrupting vital cell processes

Table 27–8 lists categories and specific chemotherapeutic agents.

Antimetabolites

Antimetabolites are chemicals similar to normal metabolites (cofactors, vitamins, and nucleotides—purines and

Table 27–7

General Tumor Responsiveness to Standard Chemotherapy

Malignancies Usually Very Responsive to Chemotherapy
- Acute lymphocytic leukemia (ALL)
- Chronic lymphocytic leukemia (CLL)
- Lymphoma (Hodgkin's)
- Choriocarcinoma
- Small cell lung cancer

Malignancies Often Responsive to Chemotherapy
- Breast carcinoma
- Testicular carcinoma
- Prostatic carcinoma
- Head and neck carcinoma
- Acute myelocytic leukemia (AML)
- Chronic myelocytic leukemia (CML)

Malignancies Occasionally Responsive to Chemotherapy
- Colorectal carcinomas
- Central nervous system tumors
- Multiple myeloma
- Ovarian carcinoma
- Uterine carcinoma

Malignancies Usually Nonresponsive to Chemotherapy
- Renal cell carcinoma
- Pancreatic carcinoma
- Bladder carcinoma
- Liver carcinoma (primary)
- Non–small cell carcinomas of the lung

From Guy, J. (1991). Medical oncology—The agents. In S. Baird, R. McCorkle, & M. Grant (Eds.), *Cancer nursing: A comprehensive textbook* (pp. 266–290). Philadelphia: W. B. Saunders. Used with permission.

Table 27–8

Categories of Chemotherapeutic Agents

Generic Name	Trade Name	Usual Dose	Nadir
Antimetabolites			
Methotrexate	Mexate, Folex	3.3 mg/m^2	10–14 days
6-Mercaptopurine	Purinethol	80–100 mg/m^2	5–40 days
6-Thioguanine	Lanvis	2–3 mg/kg	1–4 weeks
5-Fluorouracil	Adrucil, Efudex, Fluoroplex	300–750 mg/m^2	9–14 days
Fludarabine	Fludara	25 mg/m^2	3–25 days
Floxuridine	FUDR	0.1–0.6 mg/kg	4–7 days
Cytarabine	Cytosar, ara-C	100–300 mg/m^2	4–7 days
Pentostatin	Nipent	4 mg/m^2	3–10 days
Gemcitabine	Gemzar	800 mg/m^2	7–12 days
Antibiotics			
Bleomycin	Blenoxane	10–20 U/m^2	7–14 days
Dactinomycin	Cosmegen	0.4–0.6 mg/m^2	14–21 days
Doxorubicin	Adriamycin, Rubex	50–80 mg/m^2	10–15 days
Daunorubicin	Cerubidine	30–60 mg/m^2	10–14 days
Idarubicin	Idamycin	12–25 mg/m^2	10–14 days
Plicamycin	Mithracin	0.025–0.030 mg/m^2	10–12 days
Mitomycin C	Mutamycin	10–20 mg/m^2	21–50 days
Mitoxantrone	Novantrone	12–14 mg/m^2	7–10 days
Alkylating Agents			
Cyclophosphamide	Cytoxan, Procytox	50–500 mg/m^2	7–14 days
Cisplatin	Platinol	25–120 mg/m^2	10–20 days
Carboplatin	Paraplatin	360 mg/m^2	21–28 days
Ifosfamide	IFEX	1.2 g/m^2	10 days
Mechlorethamine	Mustargen	0.2–0.3 mg/kg	10–14 days
Busulfan	Myleran	1–8 mg	14–21 days
Chlorambucil	Leukeran	1–4 mg/m^2	> 28 days
Melphalan	Alkeran	1–6 mg/m^2	14–21 days
Carmustine	BiCNU	200–250 mg/m^2	4–6 weeks
Lomustine	CCNU, CeeNU	130 mg/m^2	4–6 weeks
Thiotepa		0.3–0.8 mg/kg	15–30 days
Streptozocin	Zanosar	500–1500 mg/m^2	14 days
Antimitotics			
Vincristine	Oncovin, leurocristine, VCR	0.5–2.0 mg/m^2	7 days
Vinblastine	Velban, Velbe, Velsar	5–10 mg/m^2	5–11 days
Vindesine	DAVA, Eldisine	2 mg/m^2	2–7 days
Vinorelbine	Navelbine	30 mg/m^2	7–10 days
Etoposide	VP16, VePesid	50–100 mg/m^2	8–10 days
Paclitaxel	Taxol	100–250 mg/m^2	8–11 days
Teniposide	Vumon, VM-26	100–180 mg/m^2	8–10 days
Docetaxel	Taxotere	60–100 mg/m^2	8–10 days
Topoisomerase Inhibitors			
Irinotecan	Camptosar	125–150 mg/m^2	18–25 days
Topotecan	Hycamtin	1.5 mg/m^2	7–14 days
Other Agents			
Procarbazine	Matulane, Natulan	100–300 mg	14–28 days
Dacarbazine	DTIC	75–250 mg/m^2	10–14 days
Hydroxyurea	Hydrea	25 mg/kg	4–7 days
Asparaginase	Elspar	200–1000 IU/kg	4–10 days

United States Pharmacopeia (1998). Drug information for the health care professional (Vol. I, 18th ed.). Taunton, MA: World Color Book Services.

pyrimidines) that play critical roles in essential cell processes. Most cellular reactions require metabolites to begin or continue the reaction. Antimetabolites closely resemble normal metabolites, and can be considered "counterfeit" metabolites that literally fool cancer cells into using the antimetabolites in cellular reactions. Because antimetabolites cannot function as proper metabolites, their presence impairs or prevents cell division.

Antitumor Antibiotics

Antitumor antibiotics are a class of anticancer drugs initially developed to combat bacterial infections by causing major damage on the cell's DNA and interrupting DNA or ribonucleic acid (RNA) synthesis. Exactly how the interruptions occur varies with each antibiotic.

Alkylating Agents

All alkylating agents cross-link DNA by various means. Whatever the mechanism, the double strands of DNA become more tightly bound together. This tight binding prevents proper DNA and RNA synthesis, thus resulting in inhibition of cell division.

Antimitotic Agents

Antimitotic agents are alkaloid substances made from plant sources. Their primary mechanism of action is to interfere with the proper formation of microtubules, so cells cannot complete mitosis during cell division. As a result, the cell either does not divide at all or divides only once, resulting in two daughter cells with unequal amounts of DNA that cannot continue to divide.

Miscellaneous Chemotherapeutic Agents

The actions of other chemotherapeutic agents do not fit any of the broad categories of chemotherapeutic agents and include

- Inhibition of important enzyme systems
- Competition for important substances in metabolic pathways

Combination Chemotherapy

Chemotherapy for cancer usually involves the timed administration of more than one specific anticancer drug, called *combination chemotherapy*. Using more than one drug is much more effective in killing cancer cells than using a single agent. Unfortunately, the damage caused to normal tissues also is increased with combination chemotherapy.

Table 27–9 presents one protocol (among many) of combination chemotherapy for breast cancer. The selection of drugs is based on known tumor sensitivity to the

Table 27-9

Example of One Chemotherapy Protocol for Breast Cancer

Agent	Dose	Route
Cyclophosphamide	250–400 mg/m²	Intravenous
Methotrexate	3–5 mg/m²	Intravenous
5-Fluorouracil	500 mg/m²	Intravenous

This combination is administered every 3–4 weeks (depending on severity of immunosuppression) × six rounds.

drugs and the degree of side effects expected. For example, most chemotherapeutic drugs suppress bone marrow activity and immune function to some degree, but some agents are more profoundly immunosuppressive than others. These include busulfan, cyclophosphamide, etoposide, dactinomycin, doxorubicin, and mechlorethamine. There is also variation in the timing of drug-induced immunosuppression.

The time during which bone marrow activity and peripheral white blood cell counts are at their lowest levels after chemotherapy is the *nadir*. The nadir occurs at different times for different chemotherapeutic agents (see Table 27–8). For instance, the expected nadir after cytosine arabinoside administration is 5 to 7 days; after methotrexate, 10 to 14 days, and after mitomycin C, about 4 weeks. Combination chemotherapy is planned to avoid prescribing different drugs with nadirs at or near the same time to minimize immunosuppression.

Drug Dosage

Doses of most chemotherapeutic agents are calculated according to the type of cancer and the client's size. A few drug dosages are calculated in terms of milligrams per kilogram of body weight. More frequently, calculations are based on milligrams per square meter of total body surface area (TBSA). This parameter also takes into account the client's height and weight and is calculated as follows: the height of the client (in centimeters) divided by his or her weight (in kilograms), and the result divided by 10,000 (moving the decimal point four spaces to the left). For example, a woman who is 68 inches tall (173 cm) and weighs 143 pounds (65 kg) would have a TBSA of 11,245 cm², or 1.12 m².

Drug Schedule

Chemotherapeutic agents are administered on a regular basis, timed to maximize cancer cell kill and minimize damage to normal cells. The schedule may vary somewhat to accommodate individual client response to therapy, but usually chemotherapy is scheduled every 3 to 4 weeks for a specified number of times (on average, 6–12 times). The entire planned schedule is the *course* of chemotherapy; the individual days of administration are the *rounds*.

Drug Administration

Most chemotherapeutic drugs are administered intravenously, although other routes may be used for specific cancers (Table 27–10). Techniques and nursing care considerations for different routes are described with the specific cancer type most commonly associated with the special administration route. Chapter 17 describes various types of venous access devices, many of which are used to administer chemotherapy.

Intravenous is the most preferred route for chemotherapy because the therapeutic effects of the drugs are rapid and many of these agents are irritating or damaging to tissues. A major complication of IV administration is extravasation, or movement of the IV needle so that the

Table 27-10

Routes of Chemotherapy Administration

Route	Typical Cancer
Oral	• Hodgkin's lymphoma • Leukemia (maintenance phase) • Small cell lung cancer
Intravenous	• Most solid tumors, leukemias • Lymphomas
Intra-arterial	• Hepatic tumors (primary and metastatic) • Head and neck cancers

Isolated limb perfusion	• Cancers confined to a limb
	  • Osteogenic sarcoma
	  • Ewing's sarcoma
	  • Rhabdomyosarcoma
	  • Regional melanoma

Intracavitary • Intraperitoneal • Intraventricular • Intrathecal • Intravesical	 • Ovarian cancer • Brain tumors • Brain tumors • Prophylaxis for acute lymphocytic leukemia • Bladder tumors

drug leaks into the surrounding skin and subcutaneous tissues. The results of extravasation when the administered agents are vesicants (chemicals that cause tissue damage on direct contact) can include pain, infection, and tissue loss, sometimes necessitating surgical intervention. (See Table 27-11 for known vesicant or irritant chemotherapeutic agents.)

The most important nursing intervention for extravasation is prevention (Wood & Gullo, 1993). Most extravasations resolve without extensive treatment if less than 0.5 mL of the irritating drug has infiltrated into the tissues; if a larger amount has leaked, extensive tissue damage occurs and surgical intervention may be necessary. Immediate treatment depends on the specific agent extravasated. With some agents, cold compresses to the area are appropriate and for others, warm compresses. Antidotes may be injected into the site of extravasation. The nurse consults with the oncologist and pharmacist to determine the specific antidote needed for the agent extravasated. Chart 27-3 outlines appropriate documentation of an extravasation event.

Most chemotherapeutic agents are readily absorbed through the skin and mucous membranes. As a result, health care workers, especially nurses and pharmacists, who prepare or administer chemotherapeutic agents are at risk for absorbing these agents. Even at low doses, chronic exposure to chemotherapeutic agents can seriously affect health. Nurses and other health care professionals must use extreme caution and wear protective clothing whenever preparing, administering, or disposing of chemotherapeutic agents. The Occupational Safety and Health Administration (OSHA) and the Oncology Nursing Society have established practice guidelines and protective standards.

Side Effects of Chemotherapy

Serious side effects are associated with aggressive chemotherapy, including alopecia (hair loss), nausea and vomiting, open sores on mucous membranes (mucositis), and various skin changes. Common side effects of chemotherapy on the hematopoietic (blood-producing) system can be life threatening and are the most common reason for altering the dosage or schedule. Chemotoxic effects on the blood-forming cells of the bone marrow also produce specific side effects, including immunosuppression, anemia, and thrombocytopenia (decreased numbers of platelets).

Nursing Care of Clients Undergoing Chemotherapy

The major nursing care issue during chemotherapy is managing clients' therapy-associated distressing symptoms. For some clients, the symptoms are so disagreeable that they discontinue treatment.

Alopecia

OVERVIEW. Clients receiving chemotherapy for cancer frequently experience whole body hair loss. Some drugs, such as methotrexate, may cause only thinning of scalp hair. Others, such as doxorubicin, vincristine, and cisplatin, cause a more complete hair loss.

COLLABORATIVE MANAGEMENT. The nurse reassures clients that hair loss is temporary. Usually, hair regrowth begins about 1 month after chemotherapy is completed. The nurse cautions clients that the new hair may differ from the original hair in color, texture, and thickness.

No known treatment totally prevents alopecia. Techniques to reduce the amount of chemotherapeutic agents reaching the hair follicles during treatment have been somewhat effective in reducing it, however. These tech-

Table 27-11

Chemotherapy Tissue Vesicants and Irritants

Vesicants	Irritants
Amsacrine	Bleomycin
Dactinomycin	Carmustine
Daunorubicin	Cisplatin
Doxorubicin	Dacarbazine
Epirubicin	Etoposide
Esorubicin	Fluorouracil
Idarubicin	Mitoxantrone
Mechlorethamine	Paclitaxel
Menogaril	Plicamycin
Mitomycin C	Streptozocin
Pyrazofurin	Teniposide
Vinblastine	
Vincristine	
Vindesine	
Vinorelbine	

Chart 27-3

Nursing Care Highlight: Documentation of Extravasation

- Document the date and time when extravasation was suspected or identified.
- Note the date and time when the infusion was started.
- Record the time when the infusion was stopped.
- Note the exact contents of the infusion fluid and the volume of fluid infused.
- Document the estimated amount of fluid extravasated.
- Note the needle type and size.
- Diagram the exact insertion site.
- Indicate on the diagram the location and number of venipuncture attempts.
- Record the time between the extravasation and the last full blood return.
- Identify all agents administered in the previous 24 hours through this site (list agent administered, dosage and volume, and order of administration).
- Note the client's vital signs.
- Take a photograph of the site.
- Document the administration of neutralizing or antidote agents.
- Note the application of compresses.
- Note other nursing interventions.
- Record the client's responses to nursing interventions.
- Document the physician notification (including the time).
- Document the written and oral instructions given to the client about follow-up care.
- Note any consultation request.
- Sign the documentation.

niques include applying ice packs and caps to the scalp or applying a scalp tourniquet during chemotherapy administration and for a few hours immediately afterward. These techniques are not endorsed by oncologists or oncology nurses because it is believed that some circulating cancer cells may escape chemotherapy, resulting in a less favorable treatment outcome.

Nurses can assist clients in selecting a type of head covering that suits their financial means and lifestyle. High-quality wigs are expensive but can look very much like the client's own hair. Many local units of the American Cancer Society offer wigs that other clients have used temporarily and have donated to be lent to other clients with cancer. Clients can disguise hair loss relatively inexpensively by the creative use of scarves and turbans, available in many fabrics, styles, and prices, or with caps.

Nausea and Vomiting

OVERVIEW. Chemotherapy-induced nausea and vomiting arises from a variety of local and central nervous system mechanisms (Fessele, 1996). Most chemotherapeutic agents are emetogenic (vomiting inducing) to some degree, depending on the dose, but agents producing the most severe nausea and vomiting include cisplatin, doxorubicin, mithramycin, nitrogen mustard, vinblastine, and

etoposide. Most of these agents induce nausea and vomiting during drug administration and for 1 to 2 days afterward. Some agents, such as cisplatin, induce delayed nausea and vomiting that can continue as long as 5 to 7 days after administration. Clients who have experienced chemotherapy-related nausea and vomiting during one round of chemotherapy may begin having the same symptoms before the next round as a result of sheer anticipation.

ELDERLY CONSIDERATIONS

E It has long been thought that older clients do not tolerate chemotherapy, especially the side effects of nausea and vomiting, as well as younger clients do. At times, older clients have received lower doses of chemotherapy agents in anticipation of these side effects. More recent research indicates that older clients do not have greater nausea and vomiting than do younger clients, and should not have their chemotherapy regimens altered on this basis alone. See the accompanying Research Applications for Nursing: Older Versus Younger Clients and Chemotherapy-Induced Nausea, Vomiting, and Retching.

▷ Research Applications for Nursing

Older Versus Younger Clients and Chemotherapy-Induced Nausea, Vomiting, and Retching

Dodd, M., Onishi, K., Dibble, S., & Larson, P. (1996). Differences in nausea, vomiting, and retching between younger and older outpatients receiving cancer chemotherapy. Cancer Nursing, 19(3), 155–161.

The purpose of this descriptive, prospective study was to determine the rates of nausea, vomiting, and retching among 127 clients undergoing outpatient chemotherapy with some combination of five specific chemotherapeutic agents. Demographic, treatment, and response to treatment data were collected using the Disease and Treatment Questionnaire. Twenty-five clients were older than 65 years, and 102 were younger than 65 years. The younger clients had higher incomes and had more years of education than did older clients. The questionnaires were distributed to the clients before each cycle of chemotherapy, and were completed 24 and 48 hours after chemotherapy.

The younger clients consistently reported more difficulty with nausea, vomiting, and retching than did the older ones. Younger clients also participated in more distractive behaviors to ignore their symptoms.

Critique. There were four times as many subjects in the younger group than the older group. Cancer types experienced also differed by group. Repeating this study with more homogeneous groups of clients in terms of cancer type and number and type and dosage of chemotherapy could increase the credibility of the findings.

Possible Nursing Implications. In the belief that older clients would not be able to tolerate chemotherapy side effects, many may not be offered the same treatment options as younger clients. This limitation could have serious adverse effects on overall cancer treatment outcome.

Chart 27–4

Drug Therapy for Chemotherapy-Induced Nausea and Vomiting

Drug	Usual Dosage	Side Effects
Serotonin Antagonists		
Ondansetron (Zofran)	8 mg q8h	Constipation, diarrhea, fever, lightheadedness, drowsiness
Granisetron (Kytril)	1 mg q12h	Fever, dysrhythmias, chest pain, fainting
CNS Depressants		
Trimethobenzamide (Tigan, Benzacot, Arrestin, T-Gen)	200 mg tid or qid	Drowsiness, blurred vision, dizziness, diarrhea, headache, mental depression, tremors
Benzodiazepines		
Lorazepam (Ativan)	1–3 mg bid or tid	Amnesia, bradycardia, hypotension, muscle weakness, anemia
Phenothiazines		
Prochlorperazine (Compazine, Stemetil)	10–20 mg qid	Hypotension, CNS depression, extrapyramidal reactions, dry mouth, blurred vision
Chlorpromazine (Thorazine, Ormazine)	25–50 mg qid	Hypotension, CNS depression, extrapyramidal reactions, dry mouth, blurred vision
Antihistamines		
Diphenhydramine (Benadryl)	25–50 mg qid	Drowsiness, dry mouth, hypotension
Corticosteroids		
Dexamethasone (Decadron)	5–10 mg qd	Fluid and electrolyte imbalances, immunosuppression, GI bleeding, bruising, cushingoid symptoms

CNS = central nervous system; GI = gastrointestinal.

COLLABORATIVE MANAGEMENT. Many oral and parenteral antiemetics (agents that alleviate nausea and vomiting) are available. These agents vary in their production of side effects as well as their effectiveness in controlling chemotherapy-induced nausea and vomiting. Usually, one or more antiemetics are administered before and after chemotherapy. Drugs commonly used to control chemotherapy-induced nausea and vomiting are presented in Chart 27–4. Client response to antiemetic therapy is highly variable, and the drug combinations must be individualized for best effect.

The nurse also assists the client with chemotherapy-induced nausea and vomiting to achieve comfort through nonpharmacologic means. Progressive muscle relaxation, guided imagery, or distraction may help reduce anxiety and relieve some nausea and vomiting. The nurse also assesses the client for complications associated with excessive vomiting, such as dehydration and electrolyte imbalances.

Some facilities have created clinical pathways for clients with nausea, vomiting, and dehydration related to cancer and its treatment (see Oncology Clinical Pathway).

Mucositis

OVERVIEW. Clients undergoing chemotherapy for cancer frequently have mucositis (sores in mucous membranes) of the entire GI tract, especially in the mouth (stomatitis). Normally, the mucous membrane of the GI tract undergoes rapid cell division and replaces dead or damaged cells quickly. In chemotherapy, mucous membrane cells are killed more rapidly than they are replaced, resulting in sore formation. Mouth sores are painful and interfere with clients' desire and ability to eat. (Chart 27–5 lists nursing care highlights for clients with mucositis.)

COLLABORATIVE MANAGEMENT. Frequent mouth assessment is key in managing stomatitis and mucositis. A variety of assessment tools have been developed with varying degrees of utility. In the Research Applications for Nursing: Reliability of One Mouth Assessment Instrument for Mucositis, the efficacy of one such tool is described.

A major component in managing oral mucositis is oral hygiene. The nurse stresses the importance of good and frequent oral hygiene, including tooth cleaning and mouth rinsing. Because most clients with chemotherapy-induced mucositis also have bone marrow suppression, they must take care to avoid traumatizing the oral mucosa. The nurse instructs clients to use a soft-bristled toothbrush or disposable mouth sponges and to avoid using dental floss and water pressure gum cleaners (such as a water pick). The nurse encourages clients to rinse the mouth every hour while awake with plain water or saline. The nurse warns them against using commercial mouth-

1 - 7-3
2 - 3-11
3 - 11-7

LAST ☐ Chemotherapy Date _____
     ☐ Radiation Date _____

CARE NEED	DAY 1 ADMIT DAY date ___	DAY 2 date ___	DAY 3 date ___	DAY 4 date ___
ASSESSMENTS/ TREATMENTS	Postural BP on admission & prn Weight documented I&O Baseline vital signs documented Vital signs q shift and prn Review old chart Previous admit for n/v/d date: ___ Safety/fall assessment	AM weight I&O Vital signs q shift — stable Evaluate lab results	AM weight I&O Vital signs ONLY 7-3 and 3-11 if stable	
FLUIDS/ NUTRITIONS	Start IV hydration @ admit 1000cc D₅ ½ NS 20 KCL @ 100 IV antiemetics Adjust IV fluids based on lab results within 8° of admit Clear liquids as tolerated	IV fluids continue Start PO or PR antiemetics q 6° around-the-clock Cont. IV antiemetics for BREAKTHROUGH Clear liquids-Intake: 7-3 500; 3-11 400; 11-7 100 Advance to full liquid dinner or as tolerated	DC or HL IV by noon Antiemetics AC and HS PO only Advance to regular diet for lunch Fluid Intake: 7-3 600; 3-11 500; 11-7 100	
LAB/ DIAGNOSTICS	CBC—if not available from MD office SMA 20-SMA 7 stat	SMA-7		
ACTIVITY	Up to BR Ambulate in room 1x day/evenings	Up to BR Ambulate ½ length of hallway TID	Ambulate full length of hallway TID	
SELF-CARE	Mouth care Face/hand washing Feeding	Mouth care Self bath @ bedside Feeding	Mouth care Shower	
DISCHARGE PLANNING	Evaluate home care support Refer to Social Services if: Social Work intervention needed	Document discharge plan: Social Services or Nursing	Finalize home care needs	Discharge by 11:00 AM
TEACHING	___ Assess current knowledge of antiemetics; document on kardex	___ Medication instruction ___ Dietary consult evaluate need for diet counseling	___ Review/reinforce med instruction ___ Review/reinforce diet instruction	___ Verbalizes understanding of meds for home care and diet

RN	D	E	N		RN	D	E	N		RN	D	E	N		RN	D	E	N
Initial		Signature			Initial		Signature			Initial		Signature			Initial		Signature	

Good Samaritan Hospital
A division of Good Samaritan Community Healthcare
407-14th Ave SE, PO Box 1247, Puyallup, WA 98371-0192 (206) 848-6661

Oncology
Clinical Pathway

Nausea/Vomiting/Dehydration

Chart 27–5

Nursing Care Highlight: Mouth Care for Clients with Mucositis

- Examine the client's mouth (including the roof, under the tongue, and between the teeth and cheek) every 4 hours.
- Document the location, size, and character of fissures, blisters, sores, or drainage.
- Get an order to obtain specimens of sores or drainage for culture.
- Brush the teeth and tongue with a soft-bristled brush or sponges every 8 hours.
- Rinse the mouth with solution of ½ peroxide and ½ normal saline every 12 hours.
- Avoid use of alcohol or glycerin-based mouthwashes.
- Administer antimicrobial medications as prescribed.
- Administer topical analgesic medications as prescribed or as needed.
- Help the conscious client to "swish and spit" room-temperature tap water or normal saline as needed.
- Apply petrolatum jelly to the client's lips after each episode of mouth care and as needed.
- Assist the client in using "artificial saliva" as needed, if ordered.
- Assist the client in menu choices to avoid spicy or hard food.
- Offer complete mouth care before and after every meal.

---

washes that contain alcohol or other drying agents that may further irritate the mucosa.

Clients must keep oral hygiene equipment clean. The nurse reminds clients not to share toothbrushes with anyone. Clients can clean toothbrushes daily by running them through a home dishwasher or rinsing them with either a concentrated solution of liquid bleach or hydrogen peroxide.

Many compounds are available for pain relief from stomatitis or mucositis. Many hospitals offer their own special "swish and spit" mixtures, which usually contain a local anesthetic combined with anti-inflammatory agents. The nurse stresses that these mixtures are not to be swallowed.

Bone Marrow Suppression

OVERVIEW. Bone marrow suppression results in decreased numbers of circulating leukocytes, erythrocytes, and platelets. Decreased leukocyte numbers cause immunosuppression. Decreased erythrocytes and platelets cause hypoxia, fatigue, and increased bleeding tendency.

Immunosuppression, which places the client at extreme risk for infection, is the major dose-limiting side effect of cancer chemotherapy. Most chemotherapeutic agents suppress bone marrow function to some degree. The agents associated with severe bone marrow suppression include busulfan, cyclophosphamide, cytosine arabinoside, dactinomycin, doxorubicin, daunorubicin, etoposide, mitomycin C, nitrogen mustard, and triethylenethiophosphor-

amide. *Suppression of immune function is the most life-threatening side effect and presents the nurse with the serious challenge of providing the client with the understanding, environment, and support to withstand this potentially devastating complication.*

The clinical problems associated with immunosuppression are related primarily to a temporary reduction of circulating neutrophils and tissue macrophages, causing a decrease in the body's protective inflammatory responses to microorganism invasion. The severity and duration of the impairment are related directly to the dosage of specific chemotherapeutic agents. Although this impairment is usually temporary, with good recovery of inflammatory responses evident within weeks or months of therapy completion, the seriousness of potential infection complications makes this a major treatment concern. The infectious processes most commonly observed include those of

---

▷ Research Applications for Nursing

Reliability of One Mouth Assessment Instrument for Mucositis

Dibble, S., Shiba, G., MacPhail, L., & Dodd, M. (1996). MacDibbs mouth assessment. Cancer Practice, 4(3), 135–140.

The purpose of this descriptive, longitudinal study was to evaluate the ease of use and accuracy of the MacDibbs Mouth Assessment instrument in determining mouth changes among clients receiving radiation therapy for head and neck cancer. The MacDibbs instrument consists of a one-page check list with clients rating pain, dryness, eating, talking, swallowing, tasting, and amount of saliva; report of examination by a health care professional regarding observations and measurements of lesions and areas of color change; and results of potassium hydroxide (KOH) smears or herpes simplex virus (HSV) cultures.

Client symptom reports correlated with health care professional observations. Interrater reliability for observable signs was 100%, except for lesion size, which was thought to vary because the measuring probe was of insufficient length. Information regarding KOH smear and HSV cultures was not provided in the study. The investigators deemed the instrument to be useful in measuring radiation-induced mucositis.

Critique. Symptoms and signs total scores could be calculated separately. Although the instrument appears reliable in determining mucositis, the investigators did not offer clear-cut guidelines regarding the point at which to initiate specific treatments. Although developed for clients undergoing radiation therapy, the instrument may also have value in assessing mouth problems for clients undergoing chemotherapy. Further research is necessary to determine generalizability.

Possible Nursing Implications. The main value of this article is in pointing out the importance of having a specific mouth assessment tool to accurately document changes in oral status among clients undergoing therapy for cancer. A user-friendly assessment tool should be concise and should incorporate both client subjective symptoms and health care provider objective assessment data. The MacDibbs Mouth Assessment appears to meet these criteria.

fungal origin, yeast, some residual viral breakthrough, and a wide variety of bacteria.

Decreased numbers of circulating erythrocytes (anemia) and platelets (thrombocytopenia) result from the generalized bone marrow suppression caused by some chemotherapeutic agents. The anemia causes clients to feel fatigued, and some tissues must operate under hypoxic conditions. The cardiac and respiratory systems may be overtaxed in their effort to maintain adequate oxygenation. Thrombocytopenia increases the risk for uncontrolled bleeding. When the platelets are less than 50,000/mm³, any small trauma can lead to episodes of prolonged bleeding. When less than 20,000/mm³, clients may experience spontaneous and uncontrollable bleeding, requiring extensive transfusion therapy and other interventions to resolve.

COLLABORATIVE MANAGEMENT. Management of clients with immunosuppression aims to improve immune function and protect them from infection.

In some instances, immunosuppression can be managed medically by the administration of biological response modifiers (BRMs) to stimulate bone marrow production of immune system cells. Although not appropriate for all types of cancer, this supportive treatment can reduce clients' risk for infection during chemotherapy. However, BRMs are expensive and not consistently covered by insurance. Further discussion of this treatment is presented under Immunotherapy.

The nurse works closely with clients and other health care professionals to provide safe care to clients at risk for infection. Chart 27–6 lists specific nursing care actions to prevent infection among immunosuppressed clients. Good hand washing by all health care professionals and unlicensed assistive personnel before contact with clients is the cornerstone for prevention of infection. Health care professionals must practice asepsis (prevention of contact with microorganisms) when performing any invasive technique or procedure.

Many clients remain at home during periods of immunosuppression. The nurse teaches clients and family members precautions to take to reduce clients' chances of developing an infection (Chart 27–7).

The nurse provides a safe hospital environment for clients with thrombocytopenia, and teaches them how to avoid excessive bleeding when they are discharged before the platelet count has returned to normal. Chart 27–8 lists nursing actions to reduce clients' risk for bleeding during hospitalization. The nurse teaches clients how to prevent bleeding and what to do if bleeding should occur after discharge (Chart 27–9).

Hormonal Manipulation
Rationale for Cancer Treatment

Hormones are naturally occurring chemicals secreted by endocrine (ductless) glands and picked up by capillaries. Once in the bloodstream, hormones circulate to all body areas but exert their effects only on their specific target tissues. Some hormones make hormone-sensitive tumors

---

> **Chart 27–6**
>
> ### Nursing Care Highlight: Care of the Client with Immunosuppression
>
> - Place the client in a private room whenever possible.
> - Use good hand washing technique before touching the client or any of the client's belongings.
> - Ensure that the client's room and bathroom are cleaned at least once each day.
> - Do not use supplies from common areas for immunosuppressed clients. For example, keep a sleeve or box of paper cups in the client's room and do not share this box with any other client. Other articles include drinking straws, plastic knives and forks, dressing materials, gloves, and bandages.
> - Limit the number of care personnel entering the client's room.
> - Monitor vital signs every 4 hours; note minor temperature elevation, which may suggest early sepsis.
> - Inspect the client's mouth at least every 8 hours.
> - Inspect the client's skin and mucous membranes (especially the anal area) for the presence of fissures and abscesses at least every 8 hours.
> - Inspect open areas, such as IV sites, every 4 hours for manifestations of infection.
> - Change wound dressings daily.
> - Obtain specimens of all suspicious areas for culture, and promptly notify physician.
> - Assist the client in performing coughing and deep-breathing exercises.
> - Encourage activity at appropriate level for the client's current health status.
> - Change IV tubing daily.
> - Keep frequently used equipment in the room for use by the client only (e.g., blood pressure cuff, stethoscope, thermometer).
> - Limit visitors to healthy adults.
> - Use strict aseptic technique for all invasive procedures.
> - Monitor the white blood cell count, especially the absolute neutrophil count (ANC), daily.
> - Avoid the use of indwelling urinary catheters.
> - Keep fresh flowers and potted plants out of the client's room.
> - Teach the client to eat a low-bacteria diet (see Chart 27–7).

grow more rapidly. Some tumors actually require specific hormones to divide. Therefore, altering the availability of these hormones to hormonally sensitive tumors can directly alter tumor growth rate.

Mechanism of Action
Hormones

Hormonal manipulation can help control some types of cancer for many years; however, this therapy does not lead to cure. The endocrine system usually keeps hormones within narrow ranges, and a balance is maintained. When a large amount of one hormone is administered, it

---

Chart 27–7

Education Guide: Prevention of Infection

- Avoid crowds and other large gatherings of people who might be ill.
- Do not share personal toilet articles, such as toothbrushes, toothpaste, washcloths, or deodorant sticks, with others.
- If possible, bathe daily.
- Wash the armpits, groin, genitals, and anal area at least twice a day with an antimicrobial soap.
- Clean your toothbrush daily by either running it through the dishwasher or rinsing it in liquid laundry bleach.
- Wash your hands thoroughly with an antimicrobial soap before you eat or drink, after touching a pet, after shaking hands with anyone, as soon as you come home from any outing, and after using the toilet.
- Eat a low-bacteria diet, and avoid salads, raw fruit and vegetables, undercooked meat, pepper, and paprika.
- Wash dishes between use with hot, sudsy water or use a dishwasher.
- Do not drink water that has been standing for longer than 15 minutes.
- Do not reuse cups and glasses without washing.
- Do not change pet litter boxes.
- Take your temperature at least once a day.
- Report any of the following signs or symptoms of infection to your physician immediately:
  - Temperature greater than 100°F (38°C)
  - Persistent cough (with or without sputum)
  - Pus or foul-smelling drainage from any open skin area or normal body opening
  - Presence of a boil or abscess
  - Urine that is cloudy or foul smelling or that causes burning on urination
- Take all prescribed medications as ordered.
- Do not dig in the garden or work with houseplants.

---

upsets the balance and disturbs the uptake of some other hormones. If a tumor depends on hormone A for growth and a large quantity of hormone B (structurally but not functionally related to A) is given to the client, hormone B will interfere with the tumor's uptake of hormone A or will limit the amount of hormone A produced (through competition or feedback inhibition), and tumor growth is slowed. Thus, hormonal therapy may increase survival time. Table 27–12 lists drugs commonly used in hormonal manipulation for cancer therapy.

Hormone Antagonists

Hormone antagonists, competitors for the hormones at the receptor sites, may be antibodies specific to the receptor. When hormone antagonists are administered, they bind to the specific hormone receptor of the tumor cell and prevent the needed hormone from binding to the receptor. Therefore, if a tumor requires a certain hormone to grow and the hormone can enter or activate the cell

only through a receptor, hormone antagonists can slow down tumor growth.

Side Effects of Hormonal Manipulation

In women, androgens and the antiestrogen receptor drugs cause masculinizing manifestations. Chest and facial hair may develop, menstrual periods stop, and breast tissue shrinks. Women usually experience some fluid retention. For men and women receiving androgens, acne may develop, hypercalcemia is common, and liver dysfunction may occur with prolonged therapy. Women receiving estrogens or progestins have irregular but heavy menses, fluid retention, and breast tenderness. Male and female clients taking estrogen or progestins are at an increased risk for thrombus formation.

When men take estrogens, progestins, or antiandrogen receptor drugs, some feminine clinical manifestations usually develop. Facial hair thins or disappears, facial skin becomes smoother, body fat is redistributed, and gynecomastia (breast development in men) can occur. Testicular and penile atrophy occurs to some degree as well. Although sexual function may continue, achieving and maintaining an erection are much more difficult.

Chart 27–8

Nursing Care Highlight: Care of the Client with Thrombocytopenia

- Handle the client gently.
- Use a lift sheet when moving and positioning the client in bed.
- Avoid intramuscular injections and venipunctures.
- When injections or venipunctures are necessary, use the smallest-gauge needle for the task.
- Apply firm pressure to the needlestick site for 10 minutes or until site no longer oozes blood.
- Apply ice to areas of trauma.
- Test all urine and stool for the presence of occult blood.
- Observe intravenous sites every 2 hours for bleeding.
- Avoid trauma to rectal tissues:
  - Do not take temperatures rectally.
  - Do not administer enemas.
  - Administer well-lubricated suppositories and with caution.
  - Advise the client not to have anal intercourse.
- Measure the client's abdominal girth daily.
- Use an electric razor.
- Teach the client to avoid mouth trauma by
  - Using soft-bristled toothbrush or tooth sponges
  - Not flossing
  - Avoiding dental work, especially extractions
  - Avoiding hard foods
  - Making certain that dentures fit and do not rub
- Encourage the client not to blow the nose or insert objects into the nose.
- Instruct the client to avoid contact sports.
- Advise the client to wear shoes with firm soles whenever he or she is ambulating.

Education Guide: The Client at Risk for Bleeding

- Use an electric razor.
- Use a soft-bristled toothbrush, and do not floss.
- Do not have dental work done without consulting your doctor.
- Do not take aspirin or any aspirin-containing products. Read the label to be sure that the product does not contain aspirin or salicylates.
- Do not participate in contact sports or any activity likely to result in your being bumped, scratched, or scraped.
- If you are bumped, apply ice to the site for at least 1 hour.
- Notify your doctor if you
  - Experience an injury and persistent bleeding results
  - Have excessive menstrual bleeding
  - See blood in your urine or bowel movement
- Avoid anal intercourse.
- Take a stool softener to prevent straining during a bowel movement.
- Do not use enemas or rectal suppositories.
- Avoid bending over at the waist.
- Do not wear clothing or shoes that are tight or that rub.
- Avoid blowing your nose or placing objects in your nose. If you must blow your nose, do so gently without blocking either nasal passage.

Immunotherapy: Biological Response Modifiers

Biological response modifiers (BRMs) are agents or approaches that modify the client's biologic responses to tumor cells with a beneficial result (Clark & Longo, 1986). BRMs in current use or under investigation for use as cancer therapy are cytokines, small protein hormones synthesized by the various leukocytes. Cytokines synthesized by the mononuclear phagocytes (macrophages, neutrophils, eosinophils, and monocytes) are monokines; cytokines produced by lymphocytes (especially the T lymphocytes) are lymphokines. Essentially, cytokines make the immune system work better (see Chap. 23, especially Table 23–5).

Rationale for Cancer Treatment

Cytokines enhance immune system effectiveness. Immune function plays an important role in cancer prevention (see Chaps. 23 and 26). Cytokines and other BRMs are potentially therapeutic as a cancer treatment by stimulating the immune system to recognize cancer cells and take actions to eliminate or destroy them. Some BRMs may also be useful in a supporting role. Other BRMs (colony-stimulating factors) stimulate faster recovery of bone marrow function after treatment-induced suppression.

Mechanism of Action

Cytokine activity is similar to that of any other kind of peptide hormone in that one cell produces and secretes a cytokine, which then exerts its effects on other cells of the immune system. The cells responding to the cytokine may be right next to the cytokine-secreting cell or quite remote from it. The cells that change their activity in response to the cytokine are *responder* cells. For a responder cell to be able to respond to a cytokine, the membrane of the responder cell must have a specific receptor for the cytokine to bind to and initiate changes in the responder cell's activity.

Biological Response Modifiers for Cancer Therapy

Two categories of BRMs are being used as cytotoxic therapy for cancer: interleukins and interferons. These agents can stimulate some immune system cells to attack and destroy cancer cells.

INTERLEUKINS. Sixteen interleukins (ILs) have been identified (see Table 23–5), many now synthetically produced through recombinant DNA technology. Interleukins help different immune system cells recognize and destroy abnormal body cells. In particular, IL-1, -2, and -6 appear

Table 27–12

Common Agents Used for Hormonal Manipulation of Cancer	
Type of Agent	**Example**
Hormone Agonists	
Androgen	• Calusterone
	• Danocrine
	• Fluoxymesterone
	• Testosterone
	• Testolactone
Estrogen	• Conjugated estrogens
	• Diethylstilbestrol
	• Ethinyl estradiol
Progestin	• Medroxyprogesterone
	• Megestrol
Luteinizing-hormone releasing hormone (LHRH)	• Leuprolide
	• Goserelin
Hormone Antagonists	
Antiandrogens	• Flutamide
	• Cyproterone acetate
Antiprogestins	• Mifepristone
Antiestrogens	• Droloxifen
	• Idoxifene
	• Tamoxifen
	• Toremifene
	• Trioxifene mesylate
	• Zindoxifene

to "charge up" the immune system and enhance attacks on cancer cells by macrophages, natural killer (NK) cells, lymphokine-activated killer (LAK) cells, and tumor-infiltrating lymphocytes. At present, cancer treatment with interleukins is experimental, but good responses have occurred in clients with renal cell carcinoma, colorectal cancer, and melanoma.

INTERFERONS. Interferons are substances produced by cells that can protect noninfected cells from viral infection and replication. There are many types of interferons, and, although they all have similar functions, each type has unique properties and functions. The most completely characterized interferon is interferon-alpha$_{2b}$.

Although different body cells can produce interferon, leukocytes produce the most. Today, interferons are mass produced synthetically by recombinant DNA technology. Cancer-related functions of interferon include the ability to

- Slow down tumor cell division
- Stimulate the proliferation and activation of NK cells
- Help cancer cells resume a more normal appearance and revert to their previous characteristics
- Inhibit expression of oncogenes

Although interferons are approved for limited use as a cancer treatment, they have been effective to some degree in the treatment of hairy cell leukemia, renal cell carcinoma, ovarian cancer, and cutaneous T-cell lymphoma.

Biological Response Modifiers for Cancer Support

Biological response modifiers approved for use as supportive therapy during cancer treatment are the colony-stimulating factors (Table 27–13). Essentially, these factors induce more rapid recovery of the bone marrow after suppression by chemotherapy.

This effect may have two benefits. First, when bone marrow suppression is less severe or of shorter duration, clients are less at risk for life-threatening infections and anemia. Second, because the colony-stimulating factors allow more rapid bone marrow recovery, clients can re-

Table 27–13

Colony-Stimulating Factors			
Variable	**Granulocyte/Macrophage Colony-Stimulating Factor (GM-CSF)**	**Granulocyte Colony-Stimulating Factor (G-CSF)**	**Erythropoietin (EPO)**
Generic name	• Sargramostim	• Filgrastim	• Epoetin alfa
Brand name	• Leukine (Immunex) • Prokine (Hoechst/Roussel)	• Neupogen (Amgen)	• Epogen (Amgen) • Procrit (Ortho Biotech)
Source	• T cells (lymphokine)	• Monocytes • Fibroblasts • Endothelial epithelial cells	• Renal
Cell type affected	• All granulocytes • Neutrophils • Eosinophils • Monocytes/macrophages	• Neutrophil	• Red blood cells
Indications	• To accelerate myeloid recovery in patients with non-Hodgkin's lymphoma, ALL, and Hodgkin's disease who are undergoing autologous bone marrow transplantation	• To decrease the incidence of infection, manifested by febrile neutropenia, in patients with nonmyeloid malignancies receiving myelosuppressive anti-cancer drugs associated with a significant incidence of severe neutropenia with fever	• Anemia of chronic renal failure patients • Anemia in AZT-treated HIV patients
Dosage	• 250 $\mu g/m^2$/day × 21 days as a 2-hour IV infusion beginning 2–4 hours after autologous bone marrow transplantation and not < 24 hours after the last dose of chemotherapy and 12 hours after the last dose of radiotherapy	• 5 $\mu g/kg$/day, SC or IV, as a single daily injection not < 24 hours after cytotoxic chemotherapy or in the 24 hours preceding chemotherapy • Give for up to 2 weeks, until the absolute neutrophil count has reached 10,000 mm^3 after the expected chemotherapy-induced neutrophil nadir	• Starting dose 50–100 $\mu g/kg$ TIW • IV for dialysis patients • IV or SC for nondialysis CRF patients • Individualize dose to reach the HCT target range of 30–33%

IV = intravenous; SC = subcutaneous; ALL = acute lymphocytic leukemia; AZT = zidovudine; HIV = human immunodeficiency virus; CRF = chronic renal failure; HCT = hematocrit.
Modified from Susan M. Schneider. © 1992, Susan M. Schneider, All Rights Reserved.

ceive their chemotherapy on time and may even be able to tolerate higher doses, potentially improving the curative outcome of chemotherapy. These agents must be used cautiously for malignancies in which the cancer cells may also have a BRM receptor, such as the leukemias and lymphomas.

Side Effects of Biological Response Modifier Therapy

Clients receiving interleukins at therapeutic doses experience generalized and sometimes severe inflammatory reactions. Fluid shifts and capillary leak are widespread. Tissue swelling affects the function of all major organs and can be life threatening. Clients receiving high-dose BRM therapy should be cared for in intensive care or monitoring units. These effects are limited to the period of acute drug administration and resolve spontaneously when treatment is completed.

Many of the BRMs induce general symptoms of mild inflammatory reactions during and immediately after administration, including fever, chills, rigors, and flu-like general malaise. Symptoms are worse when higher doses are given and seem to become less severe over time. Fever is treated with acetaminophen. Clients with rigors, if severe, are managed with meperidine (Demerol, pethidine).

Gene Therapy

Gene therapy as a primary or adjunct cancer treatment modality has only investigational status currently. Although response rates to date are limited, experimental successes indicate potential for gene therapy as a form of cancer treatment.

Increased Tumor Cell Susceptibility

One method of using gene therapy for cancer is to render the tumor cells more susceptible to damage or death by other treatments. Insertion of a viral enzyme gene into brain tumor cells makes the cancer cells more susceptible to being killed by antiviral agents. Other techniques involve inserting human leukocyte antigen (HLA) genes different from the client's own HLAs into the client's tumor cells. This technique makes the client's immune system cells better able to recognize the cancer cells as foreign and take steps to eliminate or destroy them. Both methods of gene therapy for cancer have shown some success in early-phase clinical trials.

Increased Immune System Cell Activity

Some immune system cells are capable of attacking and killing cancer cells (see Chap. 23). This ability is increased when more of certain cytokines, like IL-2, is present. Some gene therapy for cancer involves inserting additional genes for cytokines into the client's own immune system cells. These "charged-up" cancer-fighting immune system cells remain active in the client for up to

6 months and can participate in cancer cell–killing episodes.

Potential Uses of Gene Therapy for Cancer

Because cancer is caused by one or more changes in the genes of a normal cell, it is not unreasonable to think that gene alterations could influence a cancer cell to become normal. Areas under current research for gene therapy against cancer include

- Insertion of additional or healthy suppressor genes into cancer cells
- Insertion of chemotherapy resistance genes into normal cells so higher doses of chemotherapy can be given without affecting normal cells
- Removing damaged, mutated, or activated oncogenes
- Inserting multiple genes into cancer cells to make them more easily recognized by immune system cells and more susceptible to other treatment modalities

ONCOLOGIC EMERGENCIES

Cancer is considered a chronic disease; however, a number of acute conditions associated with cancer and its treatment can occur. These conditions, or complications, often require immediate medical intervention and are thus considered *oncologic emergencies*. Early diagnosis of such conditions is essential to avoid life-threatening situations.

Sepsis and Disseminated Intravascular Coagulation
Overview

Sepsis, or septicemia, is a condition in which microorganisms enter the bloodstream. Septic shock is a life-threatening result of sepsis and a frequent cause of death in clients with cancer. These clients are at increased risk for infection and sepsis because their white blood cell counts are often low and their immune function is usually impaired. (Chapter 39 describes the pathophysiology of sepsis and septic shock.)

Disseminated intravascular coagulation (DIC) is a condition indicating a problem with a person's blood-clotting process, triggered by many severe illnesses, including cancer. In clients with cancer, DIC is caused by sepsis (usually gram-negative infection), by release of thrombin or thromboplastin (clotting factors) from cancer cells, or by blood transfusions. DIC is most often associated with leukemia and with adenocarcinomas of the lung, pancreas, stomach, and prostate.

In clients with DIC, extensive, abnormal clot formation occurs throughout small blood vessels. The widespread clotting consumes all circulating clotting factors and platelets. This process is followed by extensive bleeding. Bleeding from many sites is the most common problem and ranges from minimal to fatal hemorrhage. Blockage of blood vessels from clots decreases blood flow to major body organs and results in pain, stroke-like signs and symptoms, dyspnea, tachycardia, oliguria (decreased urine output), and bowel necrosis (tissue death). (Chapter 39 describes the pathophysiology and collaborative management of sepsis-induced DIC.)

Collaborative Management

DIC is a life-threatening problem; the mortality rate is 70% even when appropriate therapies are instituted. Therefore, the best treatment plan for sepsis and DIC is prevention. The nurse identifies those clients at greatest risk for development of sepsis and DIC. Strict adherence to aseptic technique is practiced during invasive procedures and during manipulation of nonintact skin and mucous membranes in immunocompromised clients. The nurse teaches clients and family members the early clinical manifestations of infection and sepsis and when to seek medical assistance.

When sepsis is present and DIC is likely, treatment focuses on reducing the infection and halting the DIC process. Appropriate IV antibiotic therapy is initiated. During the early phase of DIC, anticoagulants (especially heparin) are administered to limit unnecessary clotting and prevent the rapid consumption of circulating clotting factors. When DIC has progressed to the later phase and hemorrhage is the primary problem, cryoprecipitated clotting factors are administered.

Syndrome of Inappropriate Antidiuretic Hormone
Overview

In healthy people, antidiuretic hormone (ADH) is secreted by the posterior pituitary gland only when more fluid (water) is needed in the body, such as when plasma volume is decreased (see Chap. 14). In people with certain health problems, however, ADH is secreted when not needed by the body or it is secreted inappropriately.

Cancer is the most common cause of the syndrome of inappropriate ADH (SIADH). The type of cancer most frequently associated with SIADH is carcinoma of the lung (especially small cell lung cancer), but SIADH may occur in other types of cancer as well, especially when tumors are present in the brain. Some tumors actually make and secrete ADH; others stimulate the brain to synthesize and secrete ADH. In addition, certain drugs frequently used in clients with cancer can cause the problem (most notably morphine sulfate and cyclophosphamide).

In SIADH, excessive amounts of water are reabsorbed by the kidney and put into systemic circulation. The increased water causes hyponatremia (decreased serum sodium levels) and some degree of fluid retention. Mild symptoms, including weakness, muscle cramps, loss of appetite, and fatigue, occur; serum sodium levels range from 115 to 120 mEq/L (normal range: 135–145 mEq/L). More serious signs and symptoms are related to water intoxication, including weight gain, nervous system changes (especially personality changes), confusion, and extreme muscle weakness. As the sodium level approaches 110 mEq/L, seizures, coma, and eventually death may follow unless the condition is rapidly treated.

Collaborative Management

The syndrome of inappropriate antidiuretic hormone is managed by treating the condition and the cause.

Treatment regimens for SIADH usually include fluid restriction (sometimes total fluid intake is reduced to 1 L/day), increased sodium intake, and drug therapy. A commonly used drug for this condition is demeclocycline, a form of tetracycline antibiotic, taken orally. The mechanism of action appears to be antagonistic to ADH. Because hypernatremia can develop suddenly as a result of this treatment, serum sodium levels should be monitored closely with this regimen.

The second method is to reduce or eliminate the underlying cause. The immediate institution of appropriate cancer therapy, usually either radiation or chemotherapy, can cause such tumor regression that ADH synthesis and release processes return to normal.

Spinal Cord Compression
Overview

Spinal cord compression and damage occur when a tumor directly enters the spinal cord or when the vertebral column collapses from tumor entry. Tumors may begin in the spinal cord but more commonly spread from other areas of the body, such as the lung, prostate, breast, and colon. Spinal cord compression causes back pain, usually before neurologic deficits occur. These are related to the spinal level of compression and include numbness; tingling; loss of urethral, vaginal, and rectal sensation; and muscle weakness. If paralysis occurs, it is usually permanent.

Collaborative Management

Nurses caring for clients with spinal cord compression must recognize the condition early. The nurse assesses the client for neurologic changes consistent with spinal cord compression. The nurse also teaches clients and families to recognize symptoms of early spinal cord compression and to seek medical assistance as soon as symptoms are apparent.

Treatment is largely palliative. Usually, high-dose radiation is administered to reduce the size of the tumor in the area and to relieve compression. Radiation may be given in conjunction with chemotherapy to treat the total disease. Occasionally, surgery is performed to remove the tumor from the area and rearrange the bony tissue so that less pressure is placed on the spinal cord. External back or neck braces may be prescribed to reduce the weight borne by the spinal column and reduce pressure on the spinal cord or spinal nerves.

Hypercalcemia
Overview

Hypercalcemia (increased serum calcium level), a late manifestation of extensive malignancy, occurs most often in clients with bone metastasis. Cancer in bone causes the bone to release calcium into the bloodstream. In clients with cancer in other parts of the body, especially the lung, head and neck, kidney, or lymph nodes, the tumor secretes parathyroid hormone (parathormone), causing bone to release calcium. Decreased physical mobility also contributes to or worsens hypercalcemia.

Early signs and symptoms of hypercalcemia include fatigue, loss of appetite, nausea, vomiting, constipation, and polyuria (increased urine output). More serious signs and symptoms include severe muscle weakness, diminished deep tendon reflexes, paralytic ileus, dehydration, and electrocardiographic (ECG) changes. The severity of signs and symptoms depends on how high the serum calcium level is and how quickly it developed (see also Chapter 16).

Collaborative Management

Hypercalcemia as a consequence of cancer develops very slowly for many clients, allowing the body time to adapt to this electrolyte change. As a result, the symptoms of hypercalcemia may not be evident until the serum calcium level is greatly elevated. Because adaptation does occur, treatment of hypercalcemia associated with cancer is instituted only when clinical manifestations are present.

Conservative management, such as oral hydration alone, may be enough to reduce the serum calcium to an acceptable level. When parenteral hydration is needed, normal saline is the fluid of choice.

Many drugs lower serum calcium levels, some quite dramatically (e.g., oral glucocorticoids, calcitonin, diphosphonate, gallium nitrate, mithramycin). These agents do not cure hypercalcemia but reduce the serum calcium levels temporarily. In addition, when cancer-induced hypercalcemia is life threatening or accompanied by renal impairment, dialysis can temporarily reduce serum calcium levels.

Superior Vena Cava Syndrome
Overview

Superior vena cava (SVC) syndrome occurs when the SVC is compressed or obstructed by tumor growth (Figure 27–3). SVC compression can lead to a painful and life-threatening emergency, most often in clients with lymphomas and bronchogenic carcinoma. Clients with cancer of the breast, esophagus, colon, and testes may also be affected.

The signs and symptoms associated with SVC syndrome result from blockage of blood flow in the venous system of the head, neck, and upper trunk. Early signs and symptoms generally occur in the early morning and include edema of the face, especially around the eyes (periorbital edema), and tightness of the shirt or blouse collar (Stokes' sign). As the compression worsens, the

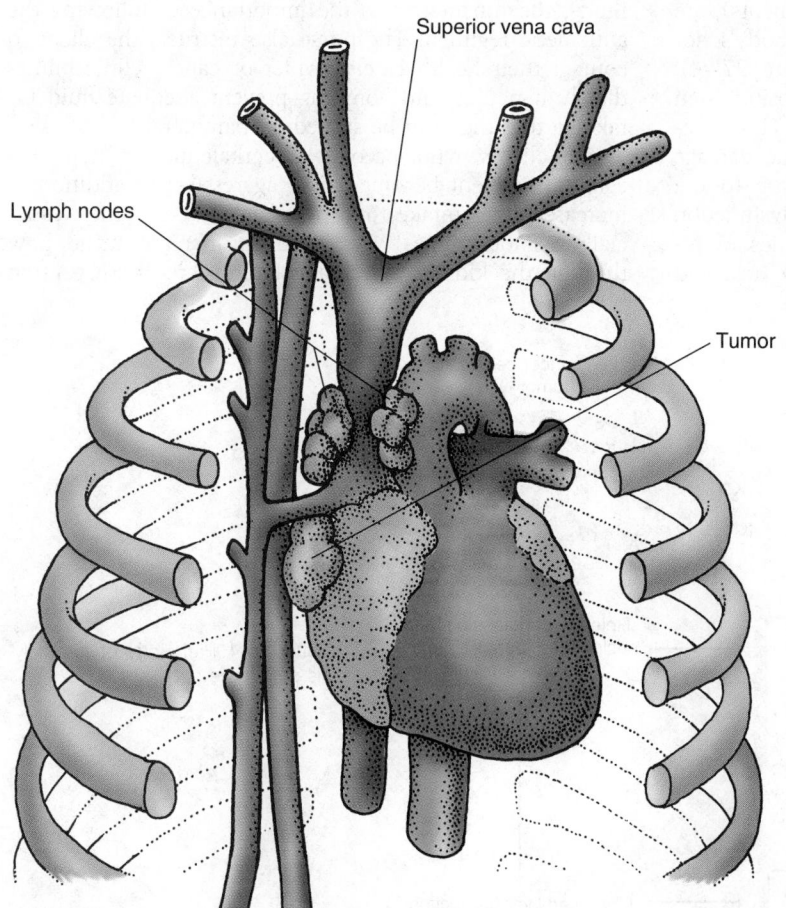

Superior vena cava

Lymph nodes

Tumor

Figure 27–3. Compression of the superior vena cava in SVC syndrome.

client typically experiences edema in the arms and hands, dyspnea, erythema of the upper body, and epistaxis (nosebleeds). Late life-threatening signs and symptoms include hemorrhage, cyanosis, mental status changes from lack of blood to the brain, decreased cardiac output, and hypotension (low blood pressure). Death can result if compression is not relieved.

Collaborative Management

Superior vena cava syndrome is a late-stage manifestation; the tumor is usually widespread. High-dose radiation therapy to the mediastinal area is most frequently the treatment of choice and can provide temporary relief in about 70% of clients. Surgery is not performed for this condition because the tumor may have increased the intrathoracic pressure so high it may not be possible to close the chest after the procedure.

The best therapeutic and palliative results occur when SVC syndrome is in the early stages. The nurse assesses each client for signs and symptoms of SVC syndrome and notifies the physician.

Tumor Lysis Syndrome

Overview

In tumor lysis syndrome (TLS), large quantities of tumor cells are destroyed rapidly; their intracellular contents, including potassium and purines (DNA components), are released into the bloodstream faster than the body's homeostatic mechanisms can handle them (Figure 27–4). Unlike other oncologic emergencies, TLS is a positive sign that cancer treatment is effective. However, if TLS is severe or left untreated, it can cause severe tissue damage and death. Serum potassium levels can increase to the point of hyperkalemia, causing severe cardiac dysfunction (see Chap. 16). In addition, the large quantities of released purines are converted in the liver to uric acid and

released into systemic circulation, causing hyperuricemia. These uric acid molecules precipitate in the kidney, forming a sludge in the kidney tubules, blocking them, and leading to acute renal failure.

TLS is most commonly seen in clients receiving radiation or cancer drug therapy for cancers initially very sensitive to these therapies, including leukemia, lymphoma, small cell lung cancer, and multiple myeloma.

Collaborative Management

Prevention through hydration is the best management for TLS. Hydration alone can dilute the serum potassium level and increases the glomerular filtration rate. As a result, urine flows through the kidney at a greatly increased rate, preventing precipitation of uric acid crystals, enhancing renal excretion of potassium, and mechanically flushing out any renal tubular sludge.

For clients with tumors known to be very sensitive to cancer therapy, the nurse instructs them to drink at least 3000 mL (5000 mL is more desirable) of fluid each day on the day before, the day of, and for 3 days after the treatment. Some fluids should be alkaline to help prevent crystallization of uric acid. The nurse stresses the importance of keeping fluid intake relatively consistent throughout the 24-hour day and helps clients draw up a schedule of fluid intake.

Because some clients experience nausea and vomiting after cancer therapy and may not feel like taking oral fluids, the nurse stresses the importance of following the antiemetic regimen. The nurse also instructs the client to contact their health care provider or cancer clinic immediately if nausea and vomiting prevent adequate fluid intake so that they can be started on parenteral fluids.

For clients who become hyperkalemic or hyperuricemic, treatment becomes more aggressive. In addition to increased fluid intake (oral or parenteral), diuretics (especially osmotic types) are given to increase urine flow through the kidney. These are administered with caution

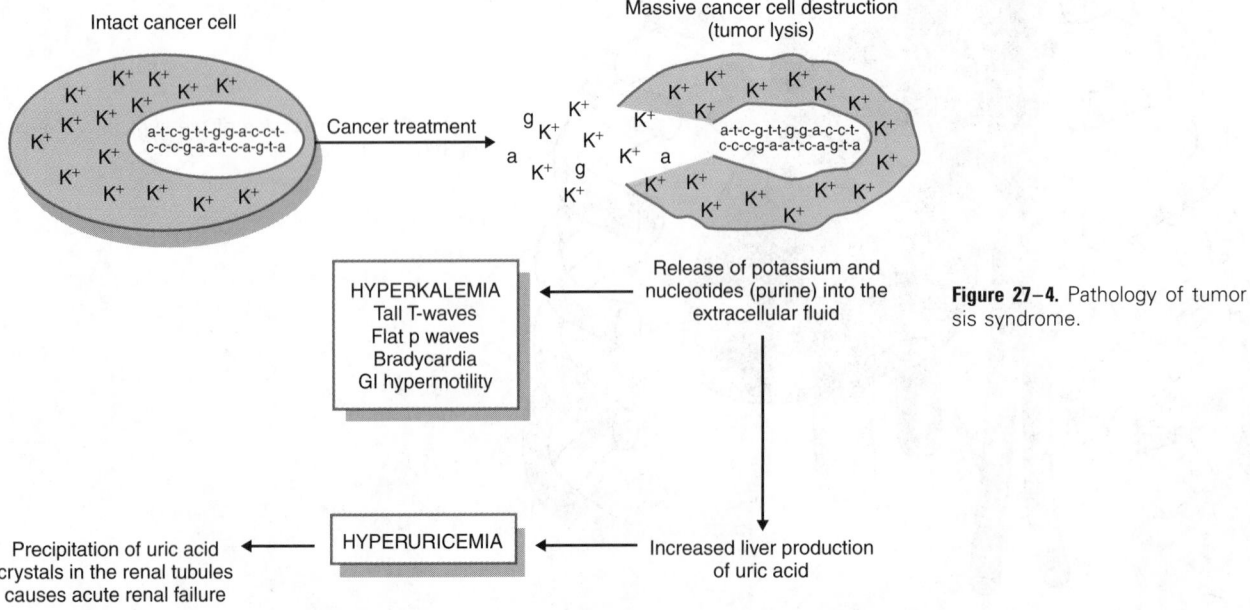

Figure 27–4. Pathology of tumor lysis syndrome.

because clients must not become dehydrated. Drugs that increase the excretion of purines, such as allopurinol (Alloprin, Zyloprim), are administered. To reduce serum potassium levels, clients may be given IV infusions containing glucose and insulin. Those clients who experience more severe and persistent hyperkalemia and hyperuricemia may require dialysis.

CANCER TREATMENT FAILURE

Although more than 50% of people diagnosed with cancer in North America this year will be cured of their disease and many others will live 2 years or longer, some clients will experience cancer treatment failure and die. The process of dying with cancer is usually long, lasting weeks or months. Clients and families require special support and assistance during this time. Chapter 12 addresses hospice care and other important physical, emotional, social, and spiritual needs of clients and families during and after the dying process.

SELECTED BIBLIOGRAPHY

*American Cancer Society. (1991). *Proceedings of the National Workshop on Cancer Control and the Older Person.* Atlanta: American Cancer Society.

American Cancer Society. (1998). Cancer facts and figures—1998 (Report No. 98-300M-No.5008.98). Atlanta: American Cancer Society.

Angel, F. E. (1995). Current controversies in chemotherapy administration. *Journal of Intravenous Nursing, 18*(1), 16–23.

Armstrong, T. S. (1994). Stomatitis. *Cancer Nursing, 17,* 403–410.

Aulas, J. (1996). Alternative cancer treatments. *Scientific American, 275*(3), 162–163.

Bender, C. (1995). Cognitive dysfunction associated with cancer and cancer treatment. *Medsurg Nursing, 4*(5), 398–400.

Bociek, R. G., & Armitage, J. (1996). Hematopoietic growth factors. *CA: A Cancer Journal for Clinicians, 46*(3), 165–184.

Boyle, D., & Engelking, C. (1995). Vesicant extravasation: Myths and realities. *Oncology Nursing Forum, 22*(1), 57–67.

Boyle, N., Bertin-Matson, K., & Bratschi, A. (1994). A patient's guide to Taxol. *Oncology Nursing Forum, 21*(9), 1569–1572.

Bryce, J. (1994). S.I.A.D.H. *Nursing 94, 24*(4), 33.

Campbell, M., & Pruitt, J. (1996). Radiation therapy: Protecting your patient's skin. *RN, 59*(1), 46–47.

Chan, B., & Ignoffo, J. (1995). Vinorelbine tartrate. *Cancer Practice, 3*(5), 320–323.

*Clark, J., & Longo, D. (1986). Biologic response modifiers. *Mediguide to Oncology, 6,* 1–10.

Clayton, K. (1997). Cancer-related hypercalcemia: How to spot it, how to manage it. *American Journal of Nursing, 97*(5), 42–49.

*Cooper, G. (1992). *Elements of human cancer.* Boston: Jones & Bartlett.

Daley, E. (1998). Clinical update on the role of HPV and cervical cancer. *Cancer Nursing, 21*(1), 31–35.

Davis, M., DeSantis, D., & Klemm, K. (1995). A flow sheet for follow-up after chemotherapy extravasation. *Oncology Nursing Forum, 22*(6), 979–983.

Dibble, S., Shiba, G., MacPhail, L., & Dodd, M. (1996). MacDibbs mouth assessment. *Cancer Practice, 4*(3), 135–140.

DiSipio, L. (1995). Relieving xerostomia from radiation therapy. *Oncology Nursing Forum, 22*(8), 1287.

*Doane, L., Fisher, L., & McDonald, T. (1990). How to give peritoneal chemotherapy. *American Journal of Nursing, 90*(4), 58–65.

Dodd, M., Onishi, K., Dibble, S., & Larson, P. (1996). Differences in nausea, vomiting, and retching between younger and older outpatients receiving cancer chemotherapy. *Cancer Nursing, 19*(3), 155–161.

Dumas, M. A. (1996). What it's like to belong to the cancer club. *American Journal of Nursing, 96*(4), 40–42.

Eckardt, J., Eckhardt, G., Villalona-Calero, M., Drengler, R., & Von

Hoff, D. (1995). New anticancer agents in clinical development. *Oncology, 9*(11), 1191–1200.

Ferrell, B., & Dow, K. H. (1996). Portraits of cancer survivorship. *Cancer Practice, 4*(2), 76–80.

Fessele, K. (1996). Managing the multiple causes of nausea and vomiting in the patient with cancer. *Oncology Nursing Forum, 23*(9), 1409–1417.

Folkman, J. (1996). Fighting cancer by attacking its blood supply. *Scientific American, 275*(3), 150–154.

*Fraser, M., & Tucker, M. (1989). Second malignancies following cancer therapy. *Seminars in Oncology Nursing, 5*(1), 43.

Gates, M., Lackey, N., & White, M. (1995). Needs of hospice and clinic patients with cancer. *Cancer Practice, 3*(4), 226–232.

Grindel, C. (1994). Fatigue and nutrition. *Medsurg Nursing, 3*(6), 475–481.

Gullo, S. (1995). Safe handling of cytotoxic agents. *Oncology Nursing Forum, 22*(3), 517–601.

Guy, J., & Ingram, B. (1996). Medical oncology—The agents. In R. McCorkle, M. Grant, M. Frank-Stromborg, & S. Baird (Eds.), *Cancer nursing: A comprehensive textbook* (2nd ed., pp. 359–394). Philadelphia: W. B. Saunders.

*Hassey, K. (1987). Principles of radiation therapy and protection. *Seminars in Oncology Nursing, 3,* 23–29.

*Hawthorne, J., Schneider, S., & Workman, M. (1992). Common electrolyte imbalances associated with malignancy. *AACN Clinical Issues in Critical Care, 3*(3), 714–723.

Hedges, C. (1994). Recognizing the patient at risk for opportunistic infections. *Medsurg Nursing, 3*(6), 445–452.

Held, J. (1995). Preventing and treating constipation. *Nursing 95, 25*(3), 28–30.

Hellman, S., & Vokes, E. (1996). Advancing current treatments for cancer. *Scientific American, 275*(3), 118–123.

Henry, D. (1996). Recombinant human erythropoietin treatment of anemic cancer patients. *Cancer Practice, 4*(4), 180–184.

Hilderley, L., & Dow, K. H. (1996). Radiation oncology. In R. McCorkle, M. Grant, M. Frank-Stromborg, & S. Baird (Eds.), *Cancer nursing: A comprehensive textbook* (2nd ed., pp. 331–358). Philadelphia: W. B. Saunders.

Hoffman, V. (1996). Tumor lysis syndrome: Implications for nursing. *Home Healthcare Nurse, 14*(8), 595–602.

Hood, L., & Abernathy, E. (1996). Biologic response modifiers. In R. McCorkle, M. Grant, M. Frank-Stromborg, & S. Baird (Eds.), *Cancer nursing: A comprehensive textbook* (2nd ed., pp. 434–457). Philadelphia: W. B. Saunders.

Houldin, A., & Wasserbauer, N. (1996). Psychosocial needs of older cancer patients. *MedSurg Nursing, 5*(4), 253–256.

Jain, R. (1994). Barriers to drug delivery in solid tumors. *Scientific American, 271*(1), 58–65.

*Jassak, P., & Sticklin, L. (1986). Interleukin-2: An overview. *Oncology Nursing Forum, 13*(6), 17–22.

Johnson, J. (1996). Coping with radiation therapy: Optimism and the effect of preparatory interventions. *Research in Nursing & Health, 19*(1), 3–12.

Johnson, M., Moroney, C., & Gay, C. (1997). Relieving nausea and vomiting in patients with cancer: A treatment algorithm. *Oncology Nursing Forum, 24*(1), 51–57.

Jones, S., & Burris, H. (1996). Topoisomerase I inhibitors: Topotecan and irinotecan. *Cancer Practice, 4*(1), 51–53.

Kaplan, R. (1994). Hypercalcemia of malignancy. *Oncology Nursing Forum, 21*(6), 1039–1046.

Karius, D., & Marriott, M. (1997). Immunologic advances in monoclonal antibody therapy: Implications for oncology nursing. *Oncology Nursing Forum, 24*(3), 483–494.

Kimmick, G., & Muss, H. (1995). Current status of endocrine therapy for metastatic breast cancer. *Oncology, 9*(9), 877–886.

Krakoff, I. (1996). Systemic treatment of cancer. *CA: A Cancer Journal for Clinicians, 46*(3), 136–141.

*Maddock, P. (1987). Brachytherapy sources and applicators. *Seminars in Oncology Nursing, 3*(1), 15.

Madeya, M. L. (1996). Oral complications from cancer therapy: Part 1. Pathophysiology and secondary complications. *Oncology Nursing Forum, 23*(5), 801–807.

Madeya, M. L. (1996). Oral complications from cancer therapy: Part 2. Nursing implications for assessment and treatment. *Oncology Nursing Forum, 23*(5), 808–821.

Martin, V., Walker, F., & Goodman, M. (1996). Delivery of cancer chemotherapy. In R. McCorkle, M. Grant, M. Frank-Stromborg, & S. Baird (Eds.), *Cancer nursing: A comprehensive textbook* (2nd ed., pp. 395–433). Philadelphia: W. B. Saunders.

Mayo, D., & Pearson, D. (1995). Chemotherapy extravasation: A consequence of fibrin sheath formation around venous access devices. *Oncology Nursing Forum, 22*(4), 675–680.

McCorkle, R., Grant, M., Frank-Stromborg, M., & Baird, S. (Eds.). (1996). *Cancer nursing: A comprehensive textbook* (2nd ed.). Philadelphia: W. B. Saunders.

McMenamin, E., McCorkle, R., Barg, F., Abrahm, J., & Jepson, C. (1995). Implementing a multidisciplinary cancer pain education program. *Cancer Practice, 3*(5), 303–309.

Miaskowski, C. (1996). Oncologic emergencies. In R. McCorkle, M. Grant, M. Frank-Stromborg, & S. Baird (Eds.), *Cancer nursing: A comprehensive textbook* (2nd ed., pp. 1183–1192). Philadelphia: W. B. Saunders.

Morse, J., & Doberneck, B. (1995). Delineating the concept of hope. *Image, 27*(4), 277–285.

Old, L. (1996). Immunotherapy for cancer. *Scientific American, 275*(3), 136–143.

Oliff, A., Gibbs, J., & McCormick, F. (1996), New molecular targets for cancer therapy. *Scientific American, 275*(3), 144–149.

Pitler, L. (1996). Hematopoietic growth factors in clinical practice. *Seminars in Oncology Nursing, 12*(2), 115–129.

Pu, A., Robertson, J., & Lawrence, T. (1995). Current status of radiation sensitization by fluoropyrimidines. *Oncology, 9*(8), 707–714.

Rhodes, V., McDaniel, R., Simms, S., & Johnson, M. (1995). Nurses' perceptions of antiemetic effectiveness. *Oncology Nursing Forum, 22*(8), 1243–1252.

Rhodes, V., Watson, P., McDaniel, R., Hanson, B., & Johnson, M. (1995). Expectation and occurrence of postchemotherapy side effects. *Cancer Practice, 3*(4), 247–253.

Richardson, A., Ream, E., & Wilson-Barnett, J. (1998). Fatigue in patients receiving chemotherapy: Patterns of change. *Cancer Nursing, 21*(1), 17–30.

Rieger, P., & Haeuber, D. (1995). A new approach to managing chemotherapy-related anemia: Nursing implications of epoetin alfa. *Oncology Nursing Forum, 22*(1), 71–81.

Rose, M., Shrader-Bogen, C., Korlath, G., Priem, J., & Larson, L. (1996). Identifying patient symptoms after radiotherapy using a nurse-managed telephone interview. *Oncology Nursing Forum, 23*(1), 99–102.

Russell, S. (1994). Septic shock: Can you recognize the clues? *Nursing 94, 24*(4), 40–48.

Schneider, S. (1994). Clinical implications for the administration of colony stimulating factors. *Journal of Orthopaedic Nursing, 13*(1), 56–62, 64.

*Strohl, R. (1992). The elderly patient receiving radiation treatment: Sequelae and nursing care. *Geriatric Nursing, 13*(3), 152–156.

Sweet, V., Servy, E., & Karow, A. (1996). Reproductive issues for men with cancer: Technology and nursing management. *Oncology Nursing Forum, 23*(1), 51–58.

Toth, B., Chambers, M., Fleming, T., Lemon, J., & Martin, J. (1995). Minimizing oral complications of cancer treatment. *Oncology, 9*(9), 851–858.

Ward, U. (1995). Biological therapy in the treatment of cancer. *British Journal of Nursing, 4*(15), 869–899.

Weintraub, F., & Neumark, D. (1996). Surgical oncology. In R. McCorkle, M. Grant, M. Frank-Stromborg, & S. Baird (Eds.), *Cancer nursing: A comprehensive textbook* (2nd ed., pp. 315–330). Philadelphia: W. B. Saunders.

Wilmoth, M., & Townsend, J. (1995). A comparison of the effects of lumpectomy versus mastectomy on sexual behaviors. *Cancer Practice, 3*(5), 279–285.

*Wood, L., & Gullo, S. (1993). IV vesicants: How to avoid extravasation. *American Journal of Nursing, 93*(4), 42–46.

Workman, M. L. (1996). Gene therapy. In R. McCorkle, M. Grant, M. Frank-Stromborg, & S. Baird (Eds.), *Cancer nursing: A comprehensive textbook* (2nd ed., pp. 458–469). Philadelphia: W. B. Saunders.

*Workman, M. L., Ellerhorst-Ryan, J., & Koertge, V. (1993). *Nursing care of the immunocompromised patient*. Philadelphia: W. B. Saunders.

Yost, L. (1995). Cancer patients and home care. *Cancer Practice, 3*(2), 83–87.

SUGGESTED READINGS

Gullo, S. (1995). Safe handling of cytotoxic agents. *Oncology Nursing Forum, 22*(3), 517–601.

Originally published in 1988, this updated article provides gold-standard information regarding the safe handling of chemotherapeutic agents.

Madeya, M. L. (1996). Oral complications from cancer therapy: Part 1. Pathophysiology and secondary complications. *Oncology Nursing Forum, 23*(5), 801–807.

This excellent article provides a comprehensive explanation of mucositis, stomatitis, and other oral complications of cancer therapy. The text is enhanced by color photographs of oral mucous membranes with different types of infections.

Madeya, M. L. (1996). Oral complications from cancer therapy: Part 2. Nursing implications for assessment and treatment. *Oncology Nursing Forum, 23*(5), 808–821.

In a follow-up to the previous article, the author stresses assessment techniques and nursing interventions for mucositis, stomatitis, and other oral complications. The table on agents used to treat primary and secondary oral complications is particularly useful.

Pitler, L. (1996). Hematopoietic growth factors in clinical practice. *Seminars in Oncology Nursing, 12*(2), 115–129.

This article provides a comprehensive, current description of how hematopoietic growth factors are being used in clinical practice. Although targeted specifically to oncology nurses, students would particularly benefit from the tables addressing monitoring and other nursing care issues.

INTERVENTIONS FOR CLIENTS WITH INFECTION

Many infections and infectious diseases are easily preventable and treatable with vaccines or appropriately used antibiotics; nevertheless, infectious diseases remain a major cause of illness and death worldwide. New, re-emerging, and drug-resistant infections are significant health threats now and into the new century. Changes in the way people live, eat, and travel have made them more vulnerable to infectious diseases. Advancing technology and invasive procedures introduce previously harmless microorganisms into the body with resulting infection. The nurse's understanding of the infectious process can help prevent or minimize the effects of infection.

INFECTIOUS PROCESS

Overview

Definitions

An infection is caused by microorganisms when they invade the body. Infections can be communicable (e.g., hepatitis and influenza) or noncommunicable (e.g., pancreatitis and cellulitis).

The process of infection requires a pathogen, or causative agent, and a susceptible host, or recipient of infection. A pathogen is any microorganism capable of producing disease in a person. People are surrounded by countless microorganisms with differing degrees of pathogenicity (ability to cause disease). *Virulence* is a term often used as a synonym for *pathogenicity*. However, virulence is related more to the frequency that a pathogen causes disease in exposed people (degree of communicability) and its ability to invade and damage a host. Virulence can also indicate the severity of the disease. Another important characteristic is invasiveness: the ability of pathogens to spread and grow in the tissues of a host after entrance.

Most microorganisms commonly live in or on the human host without causing disease. Some microbes are actually beneficial. For example, each body location harbors its own characteristic bacteria, or *normal flora*. One important function of normal flora is to compete with and prevent infection by unfamiliar microorganisms attempting to invade a body site. In some instances, microorganisms may be present in the tissues of the host and yet not cause symptomatic disease; this process is called *colonization*.

In many instances, microorganisms behave as parasites; that is, the microorganisms live at the expense of their human hosts. In this interaction with its host, the microbe gains some advantage and infection occurs. Infection is the establishment of a host-parasite interaction.

TABLE 28-1

Infectious Diseases that Must Be Reported to the CDC

Acquired immunodeficiency syndrome (AIDS)	*Haemophilus influenzae,* invasive disease	Psittacosis
Anthrax	Hansen's disease (leprosy)	Rabies, animal
Botulism†	Hantavirus pulmonary syndrome	Rabies, human
Brucellosis	Hemolytic-uremic syndrome, postdiarrhea†	Rocky Mountain spotted fever
Chancroid	Hepatitis A	Rubella
Chlamydia trachomatis, genital infection	Hepatitis B	Salmonellosis†
Cholera	Hepatitis C	Shigellosis†
Coccidioidomycosis†	Human immunodeficiency virus infection, pediatric (i.e., in persons ages <13 years)	Streptococcal disease, invasive, group A†
Congenital rubella syndrome		*Streptococcus pneumoniae,* drug resistant†
Congenital syphilis	Legionellosis	Streptococcal toxic-shock syndrome†
Cryptosporidiosis	Lyme disease	Syphilis
Diphtheria	Malaria	Tetanus
Encephalitis, California	Measles	Toxic-shock syndrome
Encephalitis, eastern equine	Meningococcal disease	Trichinosis
Encephalitis, St. Louis	Mumps	Tuberculosis
Encephalitis, western equine	Pertussis	Typhoid fever
Escherichia coli O157:H7	Plague	Yellow fever†
Gonorrhea	Poliomyelitis, paralytic	Varicella (chicken pox)*

* Although varicella is not a nationally notifiable disease, the Council of State and Territorial Epidemiologists recommends reporting of cases of this disease to CDC.
† Not currently published in the weekly tables.
Data from Centers for Disease Control and Prevention (1997). Summary of notifiable diseases, United States, 1996. *Morbidity and Mortality Weekly,* 45(53), iv.

Subclinical infection causes no apparent reaction in the host and thus elicits no detectable symptoms. Most often, subclinical infection can be identified only by the immune response of the host. This is demonstrated by a rise in the titer of antibody directed against the infecting agent. Clinically apparent infection in which the host-parasite interaction causes obvious injury is accompanied by one or more clinical manifestations and is known as infectious disease. Disease caused by an infectious agent may range from mild to fatal.

The Centers for Disease Control and Prevention (CDC) collects information about the occurrence and nature of infectious diseases. The CDC then makes recommendations to health care agencies for infection control and prevention. Certain diseases must be reported to health departments and the CDC (Table 28–1).

Chain of Infection

Infectious disease development depends on the chain of infection (Fig. 28–1). Transmission of infection requires the following factors:

Reservoir
Pathogen
Susceptible host
Portal of entry
Mode of transmission
Portal of exit

Preventing the spread of infection depends on breaking the chain of infection at any point. Eliminating the microorganism, providing the host with immunity, or, most often, interrupting the mode of transmission breaks the

chain of infection. In health care settings, nurses and other personnel interrupt the transmission of pathogens by scrupulous hand washing, implementing barrier precautions, and using antimicrobial agents.

Reservoir

Reservoirs, or sources of infectious agents, are numerous. A reservoir is any place where the pathogen is found; it can be animate (living) or inanimate (not living). Animate reservoirs include people, animals, and insects. Inanimate reservoirs include soil, water, other environmental sources, and medical equipment, such as intravenous (IV) solutions and urine collection devices. The host's own body can be a reservoir; pathogens can colonize in skin and body substances, such as feces, sputum, saliva, and wound drainage. A person with an active infection or an asymptomatic carrier (a person who does not have a disease but harbors the infectious agent) can be a reservoir. A carrier can be incubating the pathogen before signs and symptoms develop, have a subclinical infection, be convalescing from an infection, or be a chronic carrier of the pathogen. Examples of community reservoirs are sewage or stagnant water and certain improperly cooked foods.

Pathogen

Several different classes of microorganisms produce infection (Table 28–2). Survival and continued multiplication of a pathogen are often accompanied by the production of *toxins.* Toxins are protein molecules released by bacteria to affect host cells at a distant site. *Exotoxins* are produced and released by certain bacteria into the sur-

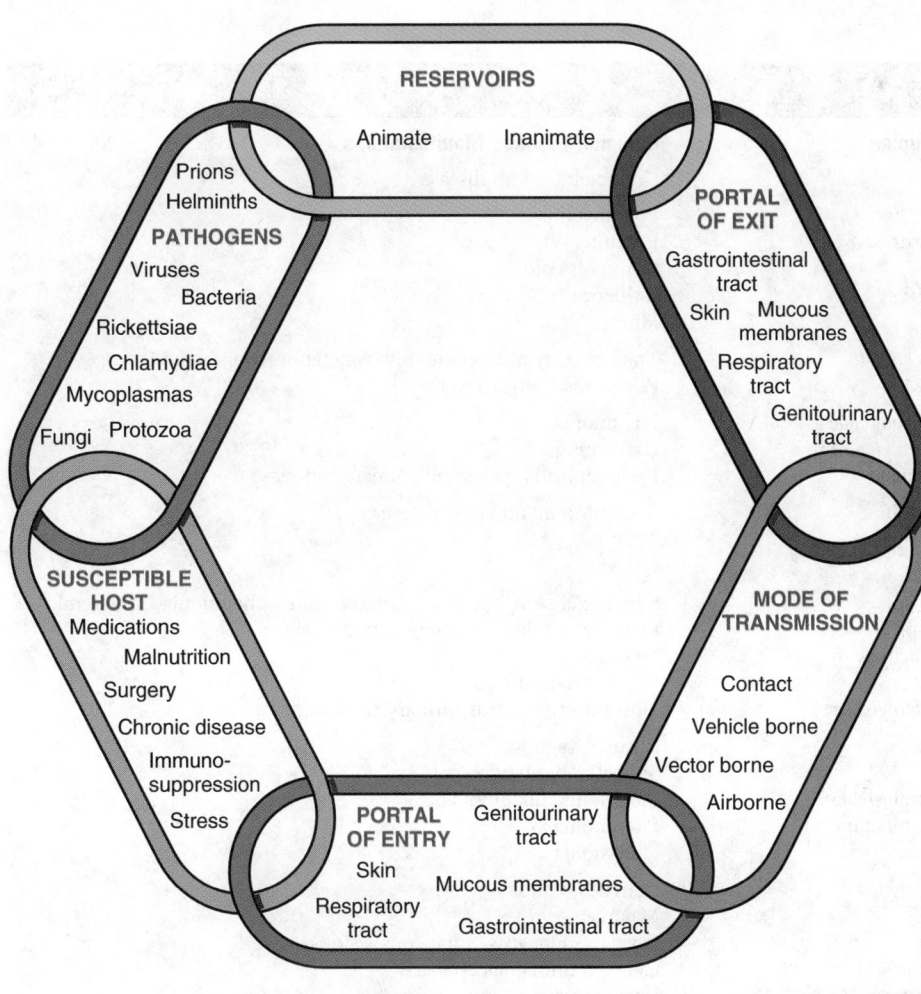

Figure 28–1. The chain of infection: the process by which pathogens are transmitted from the environment to a host, invade the host, and cause infection.

rounding environment. Botulism, tetanus, and diphtheria are attributed to exotoxins. *Endotoxins* are produced in the cell walls of certain bacteria and released only with cell lysis. Typhoid and meningococcal diseases are caused by endotoxins.

Host

Several host factors influence the development of infection (Table 28–3). The human body has an efficient system for self-protection against pathogens known as host defense (see later discussion). Breakdown of any of these defense mechanisms may increase the susceptibility of the host to infection.

Clients' immune status plays the largest role in determining their risk for infection. Congenital abnormalities as well as acquired health problems, such as acquired immunodeficiency syndrome (AIDS), can result in numerous immunologic deficiencies. Such depression of the immune system may render the host particularly susceptible to infection or cripple the host's ability to combat organisms that have gained entry.

IMMUNITY. Immunity is resistance to infection usually associated with the presence of antibodies or cells that act on specific microorganisms. *Passive immunity* is of short duration (days or months) and either natural by transpla-

cental transfer from the mother or artificial by injection of antibodies (e.g., immune globulin). *Active immunity* lasts for years and is either natural by infection or artificial by injection of the agent itself or a modified form of the agent.

ELDERLY CONSIDERATIONS

Host factors such as age may influence immunity. Because of their decreased ability to produce an adequate immune response, elderly clients are at increased risk for infection. Immunity declines in the elderly, as evidenced by decreasing T-cell and primary antibody responses (also see Chap. 23).

OTHER FACTORS. Hormonal factors play a role in the incidence and mortality rate of many infectious diseases. People with diabetes mellitus and adrenal insufficiency experience increased numbers of acute and chronic bacterial infections.

Certain environmental factors may influence clients' immune status and thus their susceptibility to or ability to fight infection. Examples include alcohol consumption, inhalation of toxic chemicals that may suppress bone marrow function, and certain vitamin deficiencies. Malnutrition, especially protein-calorie malnutrition, places clients at increased risk for infection.

TABLE 28–2

Infectious Organisms*

Organism Class	Common Examples	Common Disease Manifestations
Prions		Creutzfeldt-Jakob disease
Viruses	Poliovirus	Poliomyelitis
	Hepatitis A virus	Hepatitis
	Rhinovirus	Common cold
	Influenza A virus	Influenza
	Mumps virus	Mumps
Chlamydiae	*Chlamydia trachomatis*	Trachoma, lymphogranuloma venereum, conjunctivitis
	C. psittaci	Psittacosis (parrot fever)
Mycoplasmas	*Mycoplasma pneumoniae*	Pneumonia
	Ureaplasma urealyticum	Urethritis
	Mycoplasma hominis	Pyelonephritis, pelvic inflammatory disease
Rickettsiae	*Rickettsia rickettsii*	Rocky Mountain spotted fever
	R. prowazekii	Typhus
	Coxiella burnetii	Q fever
Bacteria	*Staphylococcus* sp.	Superficial skin infections, osteomyelitis, pneumonia, bacteremia
	Streptococcus sp.	Pharyngitis, skin infections, pneumonia
	Neisseria meningitidis	Meningitis
	Escherichia coli	Urinary tract infection
	Pseudomonas aeruginosa	Skin infection, otitis, urinary tract infection
Fungi	*Candida albicans*	Thrush, vaginitis
	Aspergillus sp.	Sinusitis, brain abscess
	Cryptococcus neoformans	Meningitis, pneumonia
	Histoplasma capsulatum	Pneumonia
	Coccidioides immitis	Pneumonia
Protozoa	*Entamoeba histolytica*	Diarrhea, colitis
	Plasmodium sp.	Malaria
	Leishmania sp.	Fever, weight loss, cutaneous lesions
	Toxoplasma gondii	Chorioretinitis, encephalitis
	Pneumocystis carinii	Pneumonia
Helminths	*Ancylostoma duodenale* (hookworm)	Anemia
	Ascaris lumbricoides (roundworm)	Intestinal obstruction
	Enterobius vermicularis (pinworm)	Anal pruritus
	Schistosoma sp. (blood flukes)	Hydronephrosis
	Taenia solium (pork tapeworm)	Epilepsy from cysticercosis

* Organisms are presented in order of increasing complexity.

Finally, certain types of medical interventions may suppress or impair the normal immune response. Corticosteroid therapy, chemotherapy for malignant neoplasms, and cytotoxic therapy specifically intended to suppress the immune response (e.g., cyclophosphamide [Cytoxan] for lupus nephritis and cyclosporine in organ transplant recipients) increase the risk of infection. Medical devices, such as percutaneous intravascular catheters, urethral catheters, and endotracheal tubes, also impair or violate normal host defense mechanisms.

Portal of Entry

Microorganisms may enter the body in a variety of ways (Table 28–4).

RESPIRATORY TRACT. A number of pathogens enter the body through the respiratory tract. Microbes in con-

taminated droplets are sprayed into the air when people with infected oral, nasal, or throat tissues talk, cough, or sneeze. These droplets are then inhaled by a susceptible host and either localize in the lung or are distributed via the lymphatic system or the bloodstream to other areas of the body. Microorganisms that enter the body by the respiratory tract but produce distant infection include *Mycobacterium tuberculosis,* influenza virus, and *Neisseria meningitidis* (the organism most commonly responsible for epidemic meningitis).

GASTROINTESTINAL TRACT. Some pathogens enter the body through the gastrointestinal (GI) tract. Of these, some stay in the GI tract and produce disease (e.g., enteroviruses, *Giardia,* and the organisms that cause self-limited food poisoning). Others invade the GI tract to produce local and then distant infection (e.g., *Salmonella enteritidis*). Still others produce limited GI symptoms,

TABLE 28-3

Host Factors that Influence the Development of Infection	
Host Factor	**Increased Risk of Infection**
Natural immunity	Congenital or acquired immuno-deficiencies
Normal flora	Alteration of normal flora by antibiotic therapy
Age	Infants and elderly clients
Hormonal factors	Pregnancy, diabetes, corticosteroid therapy, and adrenal insufficiency
Phagocytosis	Defective phagocytic function, circulatory disturbances, and neutropenia
Skin/mucous membranes/normal excretory secretions	Break in skin or mucous membrane integrity; interference with flow of urine, tears, or saliva; interference with cough reflex or ciliary action; changes in gastric secretions
Nutrition	Malnutrition or dehydration
Environmental factors	Smoking, alcohol consumption, and inhalation of toxic chemicals
Medical interventions	Invasive therapy, chemotherapy, radiation therapy, and steroid therapy; surgery

causing either a systemic infection (e.g., *Salmonella typhi*) or profound involvement of another organ (e.g., hepatitis A virus).

ELDERLY CONSIDERATIONS

Clostridium difficile can cause diarrhea, especially in the elderly, and occurs when antibiotic therapy destroys the normal flora of the bowel. When diarrhea subsides, stool cultures may still be positive for the microbe.

GENITOURINARY TRACT. A third portal of entry for microorganisms is the genitourinary tract. Urinary tract infection is one of the most common infectious diseases treated each year.

WOMEN'S HEALTH CONSIDERATIONS

Microorganisms (often normal colonic bacterial flora) colonize the perineal area, the urethral meatus, and the bladder, especially in women. The elderly woman is at an even greater risk because of decreased resistance to infection, stress incontinence, or, possibly, inability to practice proper hygiene.

SKIN/MUCOUS MEMBRANES. Some pathogens, such as *Treponema pallidum,* can enter the body through intact skin or mucous membranes. Most enter through breaks in these normally effective surface barriers. Sometimes a medical procedure creates a break in the normal cutaneous (skin) or mucocutaneous (mucous membrane) barriers, as in catheter-acquired bacteremia (bacteria in the bloodstream) and surgical wound infections. Fragile skin of the elderly and of those on prolonged steroid therapy increases infection risk.

BLOODSTREAM. Microorganisms can gain direct access to the bloodstream. Normal skin bacteria introduced by vascular devices cause more than 31% of hospital-acquired (nosocomial) bloodstream infections (NNIS, 1996). Insects can inject organisms into the bloodstream by biting the host, causing such infections as malaria, Lyme disease, and Rocky Mountain spotted fever.

Mode of Transmission

For infection to be transmitted, a mechanism must transport the invading organism from the infected source to a susceptible host. Microorganisms are transmitted by several routes, and the same microorganism may be transmitted by more than one route. The four common routes are

> Contact transmission
> Airborne transmission
> Vehicle transmission
> Vectorborne transmission

CONTACT TRANSMISSION. Many infections are spread by contact, which may be direct or indirect. With direct contact, the source and host come into physical contact; microorganisms are transferred directly, usually through skin to skin or mucous membrane to mucous membrane. Often called person-to-person transmission, direct contact is best illustrated by the spread of sexually transmitted diseases.

Indirect contact leading to transmission of infectious agents involves transfer of microorganisms from a source to a host by passive transfer from an inanimate (not living) intermediate object (also called a fomite). Contaminated articles, especially those that may contact nonintact skin or mucous membranes, may serve as sources of infection. One example of transmission through indirect contact is transfer of hepatitis B virus from a contaminated source to a susceptible host by a contaminated needlestick.

Another method of indirect contact, *droplet spread,* involves transmission of infection through contact with infective secretions. Droplets are relatively large, usually greater than 5 μm in size. These droplets are produced when a person talks or sneezes, and they travel through the air only a short distance (usually less than 3 feet, or 1 m). Susceptible hosts may acquire infection by contact with droplets deposited on the membranes of the nose, mouth, or conjunctivae. A common example of droplet-spread infection is influenzae. Susceptible people who are closest to the infected source have the highest risk for infection with a droplet-spread organism.

TABLE 28–4

Portals of Entry of Selected Disease-Producing Organisms

Portal of Entry	Infecting Organisms	Resultant Diseases
Respiratory tract	*Neisseria meningitidis*	Meningococcal pneumonia, meningococcal meningitis, meningococcemia
	Cryptococcus neoformans	Cryptococcal meningitis, cryptococcal pneumonia
	Mycobacterium tuberculosis	Tuberculosis
	Influenza A virus	Influenza
	Streptococcus pneumoniae	Pneumococcal pneumonia
	Measles virus (rubeola)	Measles
	Legionella pneumophila	Legionnaires' disease
	Varicella-zoster virus	Chickenpox
Gastrointestinal tract	*Salmonella enteritidis*	Gastroenteritis
	Salmonella typhi	Typhoid fever
	Giardia lamblia	Diarrhea
	Clostridium botulinum	Botulism
	Poliovirus	Poliomyelitis
	Hepatitis A virus	Hepatitis A
Genitourinary tract	*Neisseria gonorrhoeae*	Gonorrhea
	Chlamydia trachomatis	Lymphogranuloma venereum, cervicitis, urethritis, endometritis
	Enterobacteriaceae (*Escherichia coli, Klebsiella* sp., *Serratia* sp., *Proteus* sp.)	Urinary tract infections
Intact skin or mucous membranes	Rhinovirus	Common cold
	Respiratory syncytial virus	Pneumonia, bronchiolitis, tracheobronchitis
	Schistosoma sp.	Schistosome dermatitis (swimmer's disease)
	Herpes simplex virus	Oral or genital herpes
Bloodstream	Hepatitis B virus	Hepatitis B
	Plasmodium	Malaria
	Clostridium tetani	Tetanus
	Human immunodeficiency virus	Acquired immunodeficiency syndrome

Oral-fecal transmission is another example of indirect contact for the spread of infection. Ingestion of enteric pathogens (e.g., eating food prepared by a person with hepatitis A infection who does not wash his or her hands) can cause transmission of the virus.

AIRBORNE TRANSMISSION. Airborne transmission occurs when small, airborne, infected particles leave the infected source and travel farther than 3 feet (approximately 1 m) in the air. These particles are usually contained in droplet nuclei or dust; they are most often propelled from the respiratory tract by coughing or sneezing. A susceptible person then inhales the particles directly into the respiratory tract. Tuberculosis, chickenpox, and rubeola measles are transmitted by the airborne route.

VEHICLE TRANSMISSION. Vehicle transmission occurs when infectious agents are transmitted through a common source, such as contaminated food, water, or IV fluid. Salmonellosis is an example of a frequently vehicle-transmitted disease.

VECTORBORNE TRANSMISSION. Vectorborne transmission of infection involves insects and animals that act as intermediaries between two or more hosts. For example, ticks can transmit Rocky Mountain spotted fever and mosquitoes can spread malaria.

Portal of Exit

The portal of exit completes the chain of infection. An infecting organism exits from the once-susceptible person who has become a reservoir for infection. Exit from the host most often occurs through the portal of entry. An organism, such as *Mycobacterium tuberculosis,* enters the susceptible client's respiratory tract and exits the respiratory tract as the infected host coughs into the air. However, some organisms may exit from the infected host by several routes. For example, varicella-zoster virus can spread through direct contact with infective fluid in the chickenpox vesicles and by droplet contact.

Defense Against Infection

Several host factors influence the development of infection. Strong and intact host defenses can prevent a microbe from entering the body, or they can destroy a pathogen that has gained entry. Conversely, impaired host defenses may be unable to defend against microbial invasion, allowing entry of microorganisms that can destroy host cells and cause infection.

Host defense mechanisms may be classified as nonspecific or specific.

TABLE 28-5

Nonspecific Defenses Against Infection

Body Tissue	Type of Action	Defense Action
Intact skin	Physical	Provides a barrier
	Chemical	Normal flora and acid pH create a hostile environment
Mucous membranes	Mechanical	Mucociliary action clears bacteria
	Chemical	Lysosomes dissolve bacterial wall
Respiratory tract	Mechanical	Mucociliary action Cough
	Chemical	Lysosome action Humidification
Gastrointestinal tract	Mechanical	Peristalsis
	Chemical	Enzymes Acid pH Normal bowel flora
Genitourinary tract	Mechanical	Flushing action of urine
	Chemical	Acid pH

Nonspecific Defenses

Nonspecific mechanisms, most often representing the first encounter an invading pathogen has with its human host, include body tissues, such as the skin and mucous membranes; phagocytosis; and inflammation (Table 28–5).

BODY TISSUES. Intact skin forms the first and most important physical barrier to the entry of microorganisms into the body. In addition to providing a mechanical barrier, the skin's slightly acidic pH (resulting from the breakdown of lipids into fatty acids), together with the normal skin flora, creates an unfriendly environment for pathogenic bacteria.

Mucous membranes, by their mucociliary action, provide some mechanical protection against pathogenic invasion. More important, however, mucous membranes are bathed in secretions that inactivate many microorganisms. Lysozymes, which are enzymes that dissolve the cell walls of some bacteria, are present in large quantities in many body secretions, particularly in nasal mucus and tears.

Other body systems provide natural barriers to infection. The respiratory tract can clear about 90% of all inhaled material by filtration in the upper airways, humidification, mucociliary transport, and expulsion by coughing. Peristaltic action mechanically empties the gastrointestinal tract of pathogenic organisms. In addition, the acid pH of the stomach, intestinal secretions, pancreatic enzymes, and bile, together with the competition from normal bowel flora, provides an environment that protects the gastrointestinal tract from invasion by harmful organisms. In the genitourinary tract, the flushing action of urine eliminates pathogenic organisms. The low pH of urine also maintains a sterile environment, although certain microorganisms, like *Escherichia coli*, can thrive in an acid medium.

PHAGOCYTOSIS. Phagocytosis occurs when a foreign substance evades the first-line mechanical barriers and enters the body. Various types of leukocytes function differently in the immune reaction, but neutrophils bear the primary responsibility for phagocytosis. This process of engulfing, ingesting, killing, and disposing of an invading organism is an essential mechanism in host defense. Phagocytic dysfunction dramatically increases a client's risk for infection and recurrent infections.

INFLAMMATION. Inflammation is another important nonspecific defense mechanism in preventing the spread of infection. Inflammation occurs when tissue becomes damaged. The damaged cells release enzymes, and polymorphonuclear leukocytes are attracted to the infected site from the bloodstream. One important enzyme, histamine, increases the permeability of the capillaries in the inflamed tissues, thus allowing fluid, proteins, and white blood cells to enter the inflamed area. Still other enzymes activate fibrinogen, which causes the leaked fluid to clot and prevents its flow away from the damaged site into unaffected tissue, essentially "walling off" the inflamed tissue. The process of phagocytosis then disposes of the invading microorganism and often the dead tissue. If the inflammation is caused by infection, the end products of inflammation form the substance commonly known as pus, which is subsequently absorbed or exits the body through a break in the skin. (See also Chapter 23 for a discussion of the inflammatory response.)

Specific Defenses

Specific defenses against infection, that is, specific responses to specific microorganisms, are provided by the antibody-mediated and cell-mediated immune systems. The antibody-mediated immune system produces antibodies directed against certain pathogens. These antibodies inactivate or destroy the invading microorganism as well as protect against future infection with that microorganism. Resistance to other microorganisms is mediated by the action of specifically sensitized T lymphocytes and is called cell-mediated immunity. The components of the immune system work both independently and together to protect against infection (see Chap. 23).

Infection Control in Health Care Agencies
Inpatient Facilities

Infection acquired in the hospital, nursing home, or other inpatient setting (not present or incubating at the time of admission) is termed *nosocomial.* Nosocomial infections can be endogenous (from the client's own flora) or exogenous (from outside the client, usually from the health care facility environment or hands of health care workers). Nosocomial infections are acquired by about 2 million inpatients annually with a cost of approximately $4.5

billion annually (NNIS, 1996). The costs associated with the additional morbidity and mortality cannot be measured. Infection control within a health care facility is designed to reduce the risk of nosocomial infection in clients or personnel and thus reduce morbidity and mortality and their associated costs. A program for infection control and prevention includes facility- and department-specific infection control policies and procedures, surveillance and analysis, client and staff education, and product evaluation and an overall emphasis on cost and quality. The program is coordinated and implemented by an infection control practitioner who is usually a nurse certified in infection control (CIC) and who also has varied experience in the clinical setting with administrative skills.

Home Care Settings

Guidelines on infection control in home care are beginning to be published. Currently, the Joint Commission on Accreditation of Healthcare Organizations (JCAHO) does not require a designated infection control practitioner or committee. Commonsense approaches to infection control in the home are used. For example, the nurse is not required to place a barrier under the nursing bag, but the bag should be placed on a clean surface. Closed sharps containers may be hand carried or hooked to the outside of the nursing bag. Home care nurses should follow CDC guidelines for protection when caring for a client with an infection (Friedman, 1997).

Methods of Infection Control

Infection or the spread of infection can be prevented or controlled in at least five ways:

> Hand washing
> Hygiene
> Sanitation
> Disinfection/sterilization
> Barriers (such as gloves)

Every health care agency employee who comes in contact with clients or client care areas is involved in some aspect of the infection control program of the agency.

Hand Washing

Hand washing is the single most effective mechanism for preventing the spread of infection. Effective hand washing takes 10 to 15 seconds and consists of wetting, soaping, lathering, applying friction under running water, rinsing, and drying adequately. Friction may be supplied by soft brushes or simply by rubbing the skin surfaces together. Friction is essential to emulsify the oils on the skin and to disperse transient bacteria and soil from the skin surface. To minimize chapped or cracked skin, nurses should rinse and dry their hands thoroughly.

A recent study found that 27% of nurses had irritant dermatitis from frequent hand washing. Lotions and other products that do not contain iodophor may help protect the skin. The most promising skin-protecting lotions apply a film to the skin for 3 or 4 hours during multiple hand washings, acting like invisible gloves. Examples of

these new products include DermaMed, HealthSafe, and Viragard (Beaumont, 1997).

Health care personnel should always wash their hands before and after direct contact with a client and immediately after contact with blood, secretions, and excretions. The use of gloves does not eliminate the need for hand washing. Some studies have shown that 20% to 34% of gloves allow bacterial penetration, and as many as 53% leak or allow bacterial penetration during use (Beaumont, 1997).

The Centers for Disease Control and Prevention (CDC) recommend the use of antiseptic solutions, such as chlorhexidine or povidone-iodine, for hand washing in the care of clients who are at high risk (e.g., immunocompromised clients). The use of these solutions is also recommended after caring for clients who are colonized or infected with multiply-resistant or other virulent organisms.

Other Infection Control Measures

Potentially harmful microorganisms are eliminated or greatly reduced through various methods. Meticulous hand washing and proper hygiene, including bathing, are important in preventing infection for both clients and health care personnel. Strict attention to health care facility sanitation and infectious waste disposal (e.g., soiled dressings) and incineration must be followed in keeping with CDC guidelines. Sterilization and disinfection procedures keep equipment and the physical environment clean. Housekeeping personnel use strong but safe cleaning disinfectants that eliminate or minimize microbes.

The nurse must try to keep infectious clients apart from those who are highly susceptible to infection. Clients who are immunocompromised or who have just had surgery will be more susceptible to infections. Keeping these clients separate helps prevent client-to-client transmission of infection.

BARRIER PRECAUTIONS. *Barriers* are items placed between the client and the health care provider. Gloves, masks, and gowns are examples. Barrier precautions, also called isolation precautions, are designed to prevent the spread of infection. These precautions have changed dramatically over the past 20 years as transmission of infections has become better understood and new infections have emerged. Additional guidelines from the CDC continue to be distributed periodically to health care facilities. The latest guidelines are reviewed by each health care facility's infection control committee and then tailored to meet the specific needs of that facility. Policies and procedures for types of barriers and precautions may vary among facilities, but the principles are the same.

UNIVERSAL PRECAUTIONS GUIDELINES. In 1987 the CDC published Universal Precautions guidelines. The guidelines address the prevention of bloodborne disease transmission. All clients' blood and certain body fluids are considered potentially infected with bloodborne disease. Feces, urine, and perspiration are not considered potential routes of bloodborne disease, unless there is visible blood. Most of the focus is on the human immunodeficiency

TABLE 28–6

Universal Precautions

These precautions are to be used with all clients to protect health care providers from bloodborne communicable diseases.

- *Gloves* should be worn for contact with blood and body fluids, nonintact skin, and mucous membranes of all clients; for handling surfaces or items soiled with blood and body fluids; and for performing venipuncture and other vascular access procedures. Gloves should be changed after each client contact.
- *Masks or protective goggles* should be worn during procedures that are likely to cause splashes of blood or body fluids.
- *Gowns or aprons* should be worn during procedures likely to result in splashes of blood or body fluids.
- *Hand washing* should be done immediately on contact with blood or other body fluids. Wash hands as soon as gloves are removed.
- *Needles and sharp instruments* should be placed in puncture-resistant containers for disposal to prevent injuries from needles or other sharp items. Needles should not be recapped, bent, or removed from the syringe.
- *Mouth-to-mouth resuscitation* should be performed with use of mouthpieces or other ventilation devices.

Data from Centers for Disease Control, (1987). Recommendations for prevention of HIV transmission in health-care settings. *Morbidity and Mortality Weekly Report, 36*(25), 3–17.

virus (HIV), which causes acquired immunodeficiency syndrome (AIDS), and hepatitis B virus (HBV). HBV is more contagious and more commonly transmitted and affects health care workers more often than HIV. Table 28–6 outlines the guidelines for Universal Precautions, and Table 28–7 notes which body fluids are the highest risk for transmission of any bloodborne disease and which are not.

The increased glove use required by universal precautions has at times promoted hand irritation problems to specific gloves and sometimes latex allergy. Hand irritation is most often due to development of sensitivity to the powder or the chemicals used in the manufacture of gloves. Switching to another brand of gloves may resolve hand irritation. The use of vinyl or other nonlatex gloves or cotton glove liners may be required. Masks not made with latex ear loops should be used for those with latex allergy. When latex allergy is suspected, medical evaluation and treatment are necessary.

BODY SUBSTANCE PRECAUTIONS. Universal Precautions were expanded by infection control experts to include other body fluids and materials rather than only those that caused bloodborne diseases. These expanded guidelines are called body substance precautions or body substance isolation (BSI). With the increased occurrence of GI microorganisms, like *Clostridium difficile,* any client's feces is considered a potential source of infection. Therefore, in addition to wearing barriers as for universal precautions, the nurse and other health care personnel should always wear gloves when coming in contact with

feces or anything contaminated with feces, like soiled linen and underpads. Gowns may also be necessary to protect the staff's uniform.

Another trend in infection control practice discourages the term *isolation,* which implies that the client is removed from everyone else. Nonprofessional health care facility employees are often afraid of isolation and fear that they will "catch" an infection from the isolated client. The terms *barrier* and *precautions* are preferred.

Whichever system for precautions is used, the nurse must be careful to prevent forced client solitude and to promote quality care. In some cases, initiating barrier precautions may be associated with untoward psychosocial effects. For the few clients who must be confined to their rooms, the constant environment of the hospital room may be difficult to tolerate. Family members may also express fear or anxiety because the client is isolated.

CDC TRANSMISSION-BASED GUIDELINES. The CDC published new isolation guidelines for hospitals in 1997 (Table 28–8) to replace the 1983 disease- and category-specific precautions. The new CDC guidelines apply available knowledge, focus on mechanisms of transmission, and combine the best aspects of previous guidelines. Included in these guidelines are standard, airborne, droplet, and contact precautions. Standard precautions, or the equivalent, should be used in the care of all clients. Airborne, droplet, and contact precautions are used in addition to standard precautions.

Standard Precautions acknowledge that all body excretions, secretions, and moist membranes and tissues, excluding perspiration, are potentially infectious. The exten-

TABLE 28–7

Transmission of Bloodborne Disease by Various Body Fluids

Body Fluids Likely to Transmit Bloodborne Disease (Universal Precautions apply)

- Blood and other body fluids containing visible blood
- Semen and vaginal/cervical secretions
- Tissues
- Cerebrospinal fluid
- Amniotic fluid
- Synovial fluid
- Pleural fluid
- Peritoneal fluid
- Pericardial fluid
- Breast milk

Body Fluids Not Likely to Transmit Bloodborne Disease (Universal Precautions do not apply unless the fluids contain visible blood)

- Feces
- Nasal secretions
- Sputum
- Vomitus
- Sweat
- Tears
- Urine
- Saliva, except in dentistry

TABLE 28–8

Transmission-Based Infection Control Precautions

Category	Precautions* In addition to Standard Precautions	Examples of Diseases in Category†
Airborne Precautions	1. Private room with monitored negative airflow (with appropriate # air exchanges & air discharge to outside or through HEPA). Keep door(s) closed 2. Special respiratory protection: • N-95† or HEPA† respirator mask for known or suspected TB • Susceptible persons not to enter room of client with known or suspected measles or varicella unless immune caregivers are not available; Susceptible persons who must enter room must wear N-95 or HEPA 3. Transport: client to leave room only for essential clinical reasons wearing surgical mask	Diseases that are known or suspected to be: Measles (rubeola) *M. tuberculosis,* including multi-drug-resistant TB (MDRTB) Varicella (chickenpox)‡ Zoster, disseminated (shingles)‡
Droplet Precautions	1. Private room: if not available, may cohort with client with same active infection with same microorganisms if no other infection present; maintain at least 3 feet distance from other clients if private room not available 2. Mask: required when working within 3 feet of client 3. Transport: as above	Diseases that are known or suspected to be: Diphtheria (pharyngeal) Strep. pharyngitis, pneumonia, scarlet fever (in infants or young children) Influenza Rubella Invasive disease (meningitis, pneumonia, sepsis) caused by *H influenzae* type b or *Neisseria meningitidis* Mumps Pertussis
Contact Precautions	1. Private room: if not available, may cohort with client with same active infection with same microorganisms if no other infection present 2. Wear gloves when entering room. 3. Wash hands with antimicrobial soap before leaving client's room 4. Wear gown to prevent contact with client or client contaminated items or if client has uncontrolled body fluids; remove gown before leaving room 5. Transport: client to leave room only for essential clinical reasons; during transport use needed precautions to prevent disease transmission 6. Dedicated equipment for this client only (or disinfect after use before taking from room)	Diseases that are known or suspected to be: *Clostridium difficile* Colonization or infection caused by multi-drug-resistant organisms (e.g., MRSA or VRE) Pediculosis Respiratory syncytial virus Scabies Viral hemorrhagic infections (Ebola, Lassa, or Marburg)

Modification by facilities: CDC encourages individual facilities to adapt these guidelines, still following sound epidemiologic principles (e.g., some have removed TB transmission prevention guidelines from the airborne precautions category and added the category of AFB precautions).
HEPA = high-efficiency particulate air filter; TB = tuberculosis; MRSA = methicillin-resistant *Staphylococcus aureus;* VRE = vancomycin-resistant *Enterococcus.*
* In addition to standard precautions.
† Before use: training and fit testing required for personnel.
‡ Add contact precautions for draining lesions.
(CDC, 1997)

sive protective safety measures and controls from Universal Precautions and from Body Substance Isolation are combined.

Airborne Precautions are used for clients known or suspected to have serious infections transmitted by small droplet nuclei. These nuclei can be suspended in the air for a prolonged time and are usually expelled into the air during coughing or sneezing. To prevent microbes from being spread through the ventilation system, negative airflow ventilation rooms are required. Special enclosed booths with high-efficiency particulate air (HEPA) filtration and/or ultraviolet (UV) light may be used for sputum-induction procedures. Tuberculosis, measles (rubeola), and chickenpox (varicella) are examples of airborne diseases.

Health care workers must wear HEPA respirators or

N-95 respirators to filter inspired air when entering the room of a client with known or suspected pulmonary tuberculosis. The client wears a surgical mask when leaving his or her room to filter expired air.

Droplet Precautions are used for clients known or suspected to have serious infections transmitted by large-particle droplets. These droplet-spread microbes are transmitted in the air for about 3 feet. Examples of infectious conditions requiring droplet precautions include influenza, mumps, pertussis, mycoplasma pneumonia, and meningitis caused by either *Neisseria meningitidis* or *Haemophilus influenzae* type B.

Contact Precautions are used for clients known or suspected to have serious infections transmitted by direct contact with the infected client or items in the client's environment. Clients with significant multi-drug–resistant organism infection or colonization (e.g., methicillin-resistant *Staphylococcus aureus* [MRSA] or vancomycin-resistant *Enterococcus* [VRE]), are placed on contact precautions. Some of the other infections needing contact precautions include scabies, pediculosis, respiratory syncytial virus (RSV), and *Clostridium difficile*. Information about drug-resistant infections is found in Chart 28–1.

Occupational Exposure to Sources of Infection

The Occupational Safety and Health Administration (OSHA) is a federal agency that protects all workers from injury or illness at their place of employment. Unlike the voluntary guidelines developed by the CDC, OSHA regulations are law. Employers can be disciplined or fined for noncompliance with OSHA regulations.

In 1991, Congress passed the Bloodborne Pathogens Standard prepared by OSHA (Table 28–9). Effective March 6, 1992, this legislation eliminates or minimizes occupational exposure to hepatitis B virus (HBV), human immunodeficiency virus (HIV), and other bloodborne pathogens. The standard defines whether a health care employee is at risk for occupational exposure to blood or body fluids and requires administrators to provide HBV vaccine for those employees. Engineering and work controls to reduce exposure risk are mandated. A written agency plan, annual education, and record keeping of education and vaccine are also required.

Bloodborne Pathogens

Reduction of percutaneous injuries (e.g., needlesticks) is of utmost importance to reduce transmission of bloodborne pathogens to health care personnel. OSHA mandates that sharps and needles be handled with care. Availability and consistency in the use of protective devices are vital (e.g., needleless systems). In a national survey involving 56 diversified U.S. hospitals, the rate of percutaneous injuries was 32 per 100 occupied beds for 1993 and 1994 and 22 in 1995 (Jagger & Bently, 1996). In a case-control study among health care workers occupationally exposed to HIV, CDC reported a 79% decrease in the risk for HIV seroconversion for those who took zidovudine (ZDV) after exposure, compared with exposed health care workers who did *not* take ZDV. In 1996, CDC issued provisional guidelines for postexposure prophylaxis (PEP)

Chart 28–1

Nursing Care Highlight: Drug-Resistant Infections

Prevalent Resistant Organisms:

- Aminoglycoside*-resistant *Pseudomonas*
- Methicillin-resistant *Staphylococcus aureus* (MRSA)
- Penicillin-resistant *Neisseria gonorrhoeae*
- Vancomycin-resistant *Enterococcus* (VRE)

Enabling and Contributing Factors:

- Long-term antibiotic use and misuse
- Fewer new antibiotics are being developed
- Invasive devices or procedures, especially
  - Gastric/endotracheal tubes
  - Catheters
  - Surgical drains or wounds
  - Vascular devices
- Increased exposure risk through prolonged or repeated hospital stays
- Compromised or weakened defenses
- Inadequate health care hand washing facilities or practices
- Inconsistent cleaning and decontamination of health care equipment or environment
- Food preparation or handling inconsistencies
- Delayed identification and institution of infection control precautions

CDC Control Plan Emphasizes Four Goals:

- Rapid national and international detection and response
- Applied research in disease diagnosis and prevention
- Better communication and implementation of prevention strategies
- Stronger connections among local, state, and federal public health providers to support tracking, prevention, and control programs.

Nursing Implications:

- Early identification is important. Look for
  - Signs of new or spreading infection
  - Culture and sensitivity (C&S) result that shows resistance (e.g., MRSA, VRE)
  - C&S result that matches another client's drug sensitivity pattern (possibly indicating a cluster of infections from the same source)
- Implementation of infection control measures should be done in a timely manner:
  - Consistent use of Standard or Universal Precautions.
  - Implement special additional precautions promptly (Contact Precautions).
  - Post signs and labels to notify others as per hospital policy.
  - Educate the client and family about infection control measures.
  - Notify the physician and infection control practitioner about infection.
- Appropriately administer antibiotics and teach discharged client and family about appropriate antibiotic use.

*Gentamicin, tobramycin, amikacin.
CDC = Centers for Disease Control and Prevention.

TABLE 28-9

OSHA Bloodborne Pathogens Standard

- Employers whose workers are at risk of "occupational exposure" must establish a written exposure control plan that is updated annually and available to all employees.
- Employers must implement and enforce procedures that reduce the risk of occupational exposure, including, but not limited to, Universal Precautions, hand washing, and providing supplies for avoidance of blood or other infectious materials.
- Employers must provide and launder protective garments and other equipment, such as gloves, gowns, masks, face shields, goggles, and ventilation devices. Gloves must be hypoallergenic or powderless for employees allergic to glove material.
- Employers must provide the hepatitis B vaccine to all employees at no cost to the employee within 10 days of employment. If the employee refuses the vaccine, the employer must obtain a signed statement indicating this refusal.
- Employers must provide postexposure evaluation for all employees who are exposed to blood or other infectious material.
- Employers must train employees about the hazards of blood and other infectious materials, and the bloodborne pathogens standard; this training must be done annually.

Adapted from the Occupational Safety and Health Administration, (1991)

after occupational exposure to HIV and requested that health care providers in the United States enroll all workers who receive PEP in an anonymous registry (see Research Applications for Nursing).

Tuberculosis

In addition to standards protecting workers from bloodborne diseases, OSHA is developing regulations that address protection from tuberculosis and the newer resistant strains of tuberculosis. Some states have already implemented legislation for this purpose. To prevent occupational exposure, each agency will be required to provide employee education and counseling, tuberculosis screening at the appropriate frequency, specially designed client isolation rooms, and special respirators (N-95 or HEPA) with fit testing to protect the health care worker.

Complications of Infection

Most complications of infection relate to inadequate treatment. This may range from an incorrect choice of antibiotics to poor client compliance. Some infections relapse in a subtle fashion when a client thinks he or she is slowly getting better. Noncompliance with the drug regimen (e.g., taking the medicine when the client feels like it) prevents contact of the harmful microorganism with sufficient concentrations of the antibiotic and contributes to the development of resistant organisms.

Local Complications

Serious complications of infection may result from incomplete antibiotic therapy. Local infections that could be cured without complications, such as cellulitis and pneumonia, may progress to abscess formation if appropriate drug therapy is not continued. Although adequate antibiotic therapy does not always prevent abscess, early therapy may prevent or at least limit the size of an abscess.

Systemic Complications

In addition to abscess formation, systemic complications may develop as a result of inadequate therapy. If a client's infection is not completely resolved or if it is being treated with drugs that are not effective against the offending microorganism, the pathogen may enter the bloodstream. Systemic sepsis or septicemia results. Even small local infections, if left untreated or treated inadequately, may spread locally or via the bloodstream to produce significant complications, such as leukocytosis (increased white blood cell count) or leukopenia (decreased white blood cell count) and disseminated intravascular coagulation (DIC) (see Chap. 27). After pathogens invade the bloodstream, no site is protected from invasion.

Sepsis may progress to sepsis-induced distributive shock, also known as septic shock. In septic shock, insufficient cardiac output is compounded by hypovolemia; inadequate blood supply to vital organs leads to hypoxia (lack of oxygen) and metabolic failure (see Chap. 39).

▷ Research Applications for Nursing

Hospital-wide Infections Reduced with the Implementation of a Bloodborne Pathogens Control Plan

Malone, N., & Larson, E. (1996). Factors associated with a significant reduction in hospital-wide infection rates. American Journal of Infection Control, *24(3), 180–185.*

A 500-bed northwestern Arkansas hospital noted a significant reduction in total hospital nosocomial infection rates over the past 10 years from 3.6% to 2.6% in 1993. Factors that were statistically associated with this decrease were implementation of an OSHA bloodborne pathogens control plan with body substance isolation, increased glove use, and a barrier hand foam. Fewer inpatient surgeries and shorter length of stays may also have had some impact.

Critique. The authors controlled for other variables that could have had an impact on decreased infection rates. They noted that care practices, policies, and procedures in general had not changed. Client demographics and the top five causative nosocomial organisms had also not changed.

Possible Nursing Implications. Compliance with a bloodborne pathogens control plan and the new CDC transmission-based precautions should help reduce infections for both personnel and clients. Barrier hand foams are new products with potential to reduce infections and need further study.

Collaborative Management

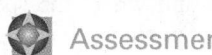 Assessment

➤ History

Careful attention to the history of a client with a possible infectious disease helps the nurse determine risk factors for infection. The age of a client, history of cigarette smoking or alcohol use, current illness or disease (such as diabetes), past and current medication use (such as steroids), familial predisposition, and poor nutritional status may place the client at increased risk for a number of infectious diseases.

The nurse also determines whether the client has been exposed to infectious agents. A history of recent exposure to someone with similar clinical symptoms (does a family member have the same symptoms?) or to contaminated food or water, as well as the time of exposure, assists in identifying a possible source for infection. Nurses may find this information helpful for determining the incubation period for the disease and thus for providing a clue to its cause.

Contact with animals, including pets, may facilitate exposure to infection. The nurse asks the client about recent contact with animals at home, at work, or in the course of leisure activities, such as hunting. The nurse also asks about recent contact with insects.

The nurse obtains a travel history from the client. Travel to areas both within and outside the client's home country may expose a susceptible client to infectious organisms not encountered in the local community.

A thorough sexual history may reveal sexual behavior associated with increased risk of sexually transmitted diseases. The nurse should obtain a history of IV drug use and a transfusion history to assess the client's risk for hepatitis B, hepatitis C, and HIV infections.

Ascertaining the type and location of symptoms may provide a key to the affected organ system. The order of onset of symptoms may also provide clues to the client's specific problem.

➤ Physical Assessment/Clinical Manifestations

Disorders caused by pathogens vary, depending on the cause and the site of infection. Common clinical manifestations are associated with specific sites of infection (Chart 28–2). Symptoms of local infection at any site include pain, swelling, heat, redness, and possibly pus. The nurse carefully inspects the skin for these symptoms.

Fever (generally a body temperature above 38° C [101° F]), chills, and malaise are primary indicators of a systemic infection. Fever may also accompany other noninfectious disorders, and infection can be present without fever. The elderly client whose normal body temperature may be 1° to 2° lower than in younger adults may manifest fever at 37° C (99° F). The nurse assesses the client for these symptoms and carefully questions the client about the history and patterns of symptoms.

Lymphadenopathy, photophobia, pharyngitis, and gastrointestinal disturbance (usually diarrhea or vomiting) are

---

Chart 28–2

Key Features of Infection of Specific Sites

Gastrointestinal Infections

Fever
Nausea and vomiting
Diarrhea
Abdominal distention

Genitourinary Infections

Dysuria
Frequency
Urgency
Hematuria
Fever
Purulent discharge
Pelvic or flank pain

Respiratory Infections

Cough
Congestion
Rhinitis
Sore throat
Sputum
Fever
Chest pain

Skin Infections

Redness
Warmth
Swelling
Drainage
Pain

Generalized Infections

Fever
Malaise
Fatigue
Muscle aches
Joint pain

---

often associated with infection. The nurse palpates the cervical and axillary lymph nodes to detect enlargement and examines the throat for redness. Other lymph nodes are also palpated for enlargement.

ELDERLY CONSIDERATIONS

In the elderly, a change in mental status may be the first, if not the only, presenting symptom. The nurse determines the client's baseline mental status for comparison. The client typically becomes increasingly confused and disoriented (Chart 28–3).

➤ Psychosocial Assessment

The client with an infectious disease often has psychosocial concerns. Typically, several diagnostic tests must be performed, and definitive identification of the microorganism responsible for the client's symptoms may be prolonged. This delay produces frustration and anxiety for

---

Chart 28–3

Nursing Focus on the Elderly: Infection

- Assess for atypical clinical manifestations of infection, such as confusion and unusual behavior. Typical manifestations, such as fever and pain, may not be present.
- Monitor renal function carefully when the client receives antibiotic therapy, especially aminoglycosides.
- Observe for and report adverse effects of antibiotic therapy because they may cause serious complications or death in an elderly client.
- Monitor for diarrhea from *Clostridium difficile* infection; obtain a specimen for culture if diarrhea occurs.
- Keep the client well hydrated because the elderly client is at high risk for dehydration.

---

the client. The nurse assesses the client's level of understanding about various diagnostic procedures and the time that may be required to obtain accurate results.

Frequently noted symptoms of infection are prolonged feelings of malaise and fatigue. The nurse assesses the client's psychological and sociologic adjustment to a decreased energy level. The nurse evaluates the client's current level of activity and the impact of these symptoms on usual family, occupational, and recreational activities.

An additional stress associated with the diagnosis of an infection is the potential spread of infection to others. The client may curtail family and social interactions for fear of spreading the illness. The nurse assesses the client's and family's levels of understanding of the infection, its mode of transmission, and mechanisms that may limit or prevent transmission. The nurse assesses the effects of the client's illness on usual interpersonal interactions.

Finally, a number of transmissible infectious diseases, especially those associated with socially unacceptable lifestyles (such as IV drug abuse), are associated with some degree of social labeling. The client may feel socially isolated and may experience guilt related to behavior that increases the risk for infection. The nurse observes carefully for signs of the client's reaction to social labels and how these feelings further affect socialization.

➤ Laboratory Assessment

The definitive diagnosis of an infectious disease requires identification of a microorganism in the tissues of an infected client. Direct examination of blood, body fluids, and tissues under a microscope in the laboratory may not yield positive identification of an organism. However, laboratory assessment usually provides helpful information about the microorganism, such as its shape, motility, and reaction to various staining agents. Even when direct microscopy does not prove diagnostic, enough information is often gathered for initiating appropriate antibiotic therapy.

Culture and Sensitivity. The most definitive procedure for identification of a microorganism is *culture,* or isolation of the pathogen by cultivation in tissue cultures or various artificial media. Specimens for culture may be obtained from almost any body fluid or tissue. The health care provider usually decides when and where the specimen for culture is taken. The nurse often obtains the specimen when ordered.

Proper collection and handling of specimens for culture are essential for obtaining accurate results. The specimen collected by the nurse must be appropriate for the suspected infection. Material must be in sufficient quantity, freshly obtained, placed in a sterile container that adequately preserves the specimen and microorganism to be examined, and properly labeled. Chart 28–4 suggests techniques for collecting specimens for culture. The nurse always checks with the laboratory or laboratory manual for the specific procedure to be followed in a particular facility, but uses Standard Precautions for collecting and handling specimens.

After isolation of a microorganism in culture, antibiotic sensitivity testing is usually performed to determine the effects of various antibiotics on that particular microorganism. A microorganism that is killed by acceptable levels of an antibiotic is considered sensitive to that drug. An organism that is not killed by tolerable levels of an antibiotic is considered resistant to that drug. If sensitivity testing is desired, the nurse ensures that the laboratory slip is marked for a "C & S," indicating that both culture and sensitivity testing are to be performed on the specimen. Preliminary results are usually available in 24 to 48 hours, but the final results generally take 72 hours.

Serology. A less specific laboratory test for determining the presence of an infectious microorganism is a serologic test, a blood test to look for antibodies that react with a certain antigen. Serologic tests are available for virtually all classes of microorganisms. Examples of diseases for which serologic studies commonly aid diagnosis include syphilis, mononucleosis, Rocky Mountain spotted fever, Lyme disease, and cryptococcosis.

A positive serologic result does not necessarily indicate active infection but merely signifies that the client has had previous exposure to the antigen in question. Two serum specimens are typically obtained from a client: the first during the acute phase of illness, and the second 7 to 10 days later. A fourfold or greater rise in antibody titer in the second specimen indicates a recent infection.

Complete Blood Count. A complete blood count (CBC) is nearly always performed on the client with a suspected infectious disease. Five types of leukocytes (white blood cells) have been identified: neutrophils, lymphocytes, monocytes, eosinophils, and basophils. In most active infections, especially those caused by bacteria, the total leukocyte count is elevated. Various diseases are characterized by changes in the percentages of the different types of leukocytes. The differential count most often shows an increased number of immature neutrophils, or a shift to the left. A few infectious diseases, however, are associated with neutropenia (decreased neutrophils), such as malaria and infectious mononucleosis.

Erythrocyte Sedimentation Rate. The erythrocyte sedimentation rate (ESR) measures the rate at which red blood cells fall through plasma. This rate is most significantly affected by an increased number of acute phase

Chart 28–4

Nursing Care Highlight: Collection Techniques for Commonly Cultured Specimens

Specimen	Collection Method	Comments
Blood	1. Decontaminate the skin with 70% alcohol followed by 2% tincture of iodine, allowed to dry. 2. Perform venipuncture and collect 10 mL of blood (2 mL in infants). 3. Inject into sterile culture bottles—usually one vented and one unvented for anaerobic culture.	Three separate specimens are usually collected over a 24-hr period to ensure isolation of the causative organism. Avoid use of intravenous catheters because of contamination and possible false bacteremia report.
Urine Clean void	1. Clean the urethral meatus with tincture of iodine or other antiseptic solution. 2. Have the client void small amount and then collect approximately 2 mL of midstream urine specimen into a sterile container.	The specimen may be refrigerated. If not, the specimen must be delivered to the laboratory within 30 min to be useful for quantitative studies.
Indwelling catheter	1. Clean the aspiration site on catheter drainage tubing with iodine. 2. Collect a 2-mL specimen into a sterile container.	
Wound	1. Decontaminate the skin with 70% alcohol. 2. Swab an active margin of the wound with a sterile swab and place the swab into a sterile tube.	
Throat	1. Swab an inflamed area of the throat, especially areas of exudate. 2. Place the swab into sterile medium for transport.	Inform the laboratory of any suspected organism other than group A streptococcus.
Sputum	1. Collect first-morning expectorated sputum into a sterile container.	Production of an adequate specimen may be aided by saline aerosol administration or by postural drainage. Sputum specimens may also be collected via tracheal or transtracheal aspiration.
Pus (abscesses)	1. Decontaminate the skin with alcohol. 2. Coat a sterile swab rapidly with pus. 3. Insert the swab immediately into a specially prepared anaerobic transport tube.	Deliver the specimen to the laboratory immediately.
Vagina	1. Wipe the vagina clean of secretions with dry gauze. 2. Swab the exudate with a sterile swab. 3. Insert into a sterile container or into specially prepared medium.	If trichomoniasis is suspected, place the swab in a small amount of sterile saline and send to the laboratory immediately.
Rectal swab	1. Insert the swab into the rectum approximately 1 inch (2.5 cm) and rotate once. 2. Place into transport medium.	The specimen is usually sent on 3 consecutive days. The swab should show obvious soiling.
Stool	1. Collect stool in a clean waxed cardboard container.	Deliver to the laboratory immediately. The specimen is often collected on 3 consecutive days.
Intravenous catheters	1. Clean the catheter insertion site with alcohol. 2. Withdraw the catheter and cut off approximately a 5-cm tip with sterile scissors. 3. Place into a sterile container.	In general, catheter tips that are contaminated during removal will grow only a few colonies, whereas infected catheters usually show heavy growth.

reactants, which occurs with inflammation. Thus, an elevated ESR (>20 mm/hr) indicates inflammation or infection somewhere in the body. Chronic infection, most notably osteomyelitis, and chronic abscesses are commonly associated with an elevated ESR. The effectiveness of therapy is often monitored by a fall in this value.

➤ Radiographic Assessment

X-rays are often obtained to determine activity or destruction by an infectious microorganism. Radiologic studies (such as chest films, sinus films, joint films, gastrointestinal studies, and renal films) are typically obtained for diagnosis of infection in a specific body site.

A more sophisticated technique for diagnosis of an infection is computed tomography. This method is particularly helpful in assessing the presence and location of abscesses.

➤ Other Diagnostic Assessment

Another diagnostic tool for the evaluation of a client with an infectious disease is *ultrasonography*. This noninvasive procedure is particularly helpful in detecting infection that has affected the heart valves.

Scanning techniques using radioactive substances, such as gallium, can determine the presence of inflammation. Inflammatory tissue is identified by its increased uptake of the injected radioactive material.

To obtain tissue for culture, biopsy of the infected site may be necessary. Biopsy sites may include the liver, bone marrow, skin, pleura, lymph nodes, kidney, bone, or even the brain. To obtain specimens for examination, invasive procedures (such as bronchoscopy or endoscopy) or even surgery (such as open lung biopsy or laparotomy) may be necessary. These procedures are described in detail elsewhere in this text.

 Analysis

➤ Common Nursing Diagnoses and Collaborative Problems

The most common nursing diagnoses for clients with an infection or infectious disease include
1. Hyperthermia related to increased metabolic state
2. Fatigue related to increased metabolic energy production
3. Social Isolation related to effects of illness

The inclusion of other nursing diagnoses depends on the type and extent of the infection. For example, a client with pneumonia might experience ineffective airway clearance; a client with a sexually transmitted disease may have altered sexuality patterns.

➤ Additional Nursing Diagnoses and Collaborative Problems

The major collaborative problem is a client's risk for sepsis, septic shock, and disseminated intravascular coagulation (DIC).

 Planning and Implementation

➤ *Hyperthermia*

Planning: Expected Outcomes. The primary outcome is that the client's body temperature is expected to return to baseline.

Interventions. Fever (hyperthermia) is one way in which the body attempts to destroy pathogens. The primary concern is to provide measures to eliminate the underlying cause of hyperthermia, to destroy the causative microorganism. Interventions are implemented to reduce fever, such as antimicrobial therapy, antipyretic therapy, external cooling, and fluid administration.

Antimicrobial Therapy. The cornerstone of therapy for infectious diseases is antimicrobial drug therapy, also called antiinfective therapy. Antibiotics, antiviral agents, and antifungals are types of antimicrobials. The sulfonamides, the first antibiotic group, were used in the mid-1930s. Shortly thereafter, in the 1940s, penicillin became the primary antibiotic used systemically. Since these early days, a wide variety of antimicrobial drugs have been developed for treatment as well as prevention of infection associated with virtually every class of microorganism. Effective antibiotics are available to treat nearly all bacterial infections, but misuse of antibiotics has contributed to the development of antibiotic-resistant bacteria. A few effective antifungal agents have been developed, but these drugs generally exhibit more toxicity than do antibacterial agents. Few effective chemotherapeutic agents are currently available for treatment of infections caused by viruses.

Effective antimicrobial therapy requires delivery of the appropriate agent, sufficient dosage, proper route of administration, and sufficient duration of therapy. Fulfilling these four requirements ensures that a concentration of drug is delivered in excess of that needed to inhibit or kill the infecting microorganism. The health care provider, often in consultation with the pharmacist, decides about each requirement. The nurse needs to know the drug actions, side effects, and toxic effects and teach them to the client.

Antimicrobials act on susceptible pathogens by
- Inhibiting cell wall synthesis (penicillins and cephalosporins)
- Injuring the cytoplasmic membrane (antifungal agents)
- Inhibiting biosynthesis (reproduction) (erythromycin, tetracycline, and gentamicin)
- Inhibiting nucleic acid synthesis (actinomycin)

The nurse observes and reports side effects and toxic effects, which vary according to the specific classification of the drug. Most antibiotics can cause nausea, vomiting, and rashes along with a long list of other problems. The nurse ensures that the prescribed drug is not one to which the client is allergic. An accurate allergy history before drug therapy begins is essential.

Antipyretic Therapy. The health care provider prescribes antipyretic drugs, such as aspirin (Ancasal✦) and acetaminophen (Tylenol, AceTabs✦) to reduce hyperthermia. However, because antipyretics mask fever, monitoring the course of the client's disease may be difficult. Therefore, unless the client is extremely uncomfortable or if hyperthermia presents a significant risk (e.g., in the client with heart failure, febrile seizures, or head injury), antipyretics are not always ordered.

The nurse must be alert for waves of sweating after each dose. Sweating may be accompanied by a fall in blood pressure and subsequent return of fever. These unpleasant side effects of antipyretic therapy can often be alleviated by liberal administration of fluids and by regular scheduling of drug administration.

External Cooling. Cooling or hypothermia blankets, or ice bags and packs, are highly effective external mechanisms for reducing fever. For convenience, cooling blankets are used extensively in the hospital setting, yet there are no universal guidelines for their use.

Alternatives to cooling blankets may be used, particularly in settings other than hospitals. The nurse may sponge the client's body with tepid water or saline solution or apply cool compresses to the skin and pulse points to reduce body temperature. The nurse observes the client for shivering during any form of external cooling. Shivering indicates that the client is possibly being cooled too quickly.

Fluid Administration. In clients with fever, there is increased fluid volume loss from rapid evaporation of body fluids as well as increased perspiration. As body temperature increases, fluid volume loss increases. The nurse carefully monitors for signs of dehydration, such as increased thirst, decreased skin turgor, and dry mucous membranes, especially in the elderly. The nurse encourages increased oral fluid intake and administers IV fluids as prescribed by the health care provider (see Chapter 15 for additional information on fluid volume deficit).

➤ Fatigue

Planning: Expected Outcomes. The desired outcome is that the client is expected to progress from previous level of activity.

Interventions. Whether a client achieves the outcome depends on recognition and correction of factors that contribute to activity intolerance. Malaise and easy fatigability are classic clinical manifestations of an infectious process. Fever accelerates many metabolic processes, which accentuates weight loss and nitrogen wasting. The heart rate increases, and water loss may be excessive; both factors contribute to a feeling of general malaise.

Nutrition. The nurse observes the client for causative factors of malaise and easy fatigability, such as nutritional deficiencies or fluid and electrolyte imbalances. The nurse collaborates with the client and dietitian to establish a dietary program that is tolerable for the client and meets calorie and protein requirements.

Activity Management. The nurse encourages bed rest during the acute phase of the client's illness while treatment for the underlying infection is initiated. The nurse

works closely with the client to develop a progressive program for return to his or her normal level of activity. The program depends on the client's response to antibiotic therapy, as evidenced by diminished clinical manifestations of infection. Frequent rest periods are encouraged. Throughout the course of the client's illness, the nurse encourages the client to verbalize feelings of frustration and discouragement related to chronic fatigue and decreased ability to perform activities of daily living.

➤ Social Isolation

Planning: Expected Outcomes. The desired outcome is that the client is expected to be free of feelings of social isolation.

Interventions. Education is the major intervention for meeting this goal. The nurse develops an educational program to instruct the client and the family about the mode of transmission of infection and mechanisms that prevent its spread to others. The nurse also initiates appropriate barrier precautions.

The nurse ensures that the client and family understand the client's disease process and its cause. The nurse specifically explains the mode of transmission of the infecting microorganism, the risk for transmission to others, and mechanisms that may prevent transmission. If necessary, the nurse ensures that the client and family can state specific ways in which precautions will be instituted in the home after discharge from the hospital.

Because the client requiring precautions may feel secluded, the nurse encourages health care personnel as well as family members and friends to maintain contact with the client. The nurse reminds all personnel caring for the client that the disease—not the client—requires isolation. Family members and friends are encouraged to visit the client and to use the appropriate barrier precautions when necessary. Communication by telephone is often effective for continuing contact with loved ones. Television and radio help bring the outside world into the life of the client confined to the room.

In the nursing home setting, an outbreak of respiratory or GI infection usually requires a limit on visitors, activities, and admissions to the facility. The nurse working in a nursing home needs to be familiar with state regulations regarding handling infections in nursing homes.

 ## Continuing Care

Clients with infections may be cared for in the home, hospital, nursing home, or ambulatory care setting, depending on the type and severity of the infectious process. Infections among the elderly in nursing homes are very common (Table 28-10).

➤ Health Teaching

Infection Control

The nurse explains the disease and makes certain that the client understands what is causing the illness. The nurse also explains whether the pathogen causing the client's

TABLE 28-10

Factors that May Promote Infection in the Elderly Client	
Factor	**Aging-Associated Changes or Conditions**
Immune system	Decreased antibody production, lymphocytes, and fever response
Integumentary system	Thinning skin, decreased subcutaneous tissue, decreased vascularity, slower wound healing
Respiratory system	Decreased cough and gag reflexes
Gastrointestinal system	Decreased gastric acid and intestinal motility
Chronic illness	Diabetes mellitus, chronic airflow limitation, neurologic impairments
Functional/cognitive impairments	Immobility, incontinence, dementia
Invasive devices	Urinary catheters, feeding tubes, intravenous devices, tracheostomies
Institutionalization	Increased person-to-person contact and transmission

infection can be spread to family members, social contacts, or other community contacts. If the client has an infectious disease caused by a transmissible agent, the nurse describes how the pathogen causing the client's infection is transmitted.

If the client has an infectious disease that is potentially transmissible, the nurse teaches the client, family, or home caregivers the precautions for preventing transmission of infection. General household cleaning measures are often sufficient (e.g., a dishwasher for dishes, a washer and dryer for laundry). If these are not available, dishes can be sanitized with weak bleach solution (100 parts per million [ppm] available chlorine) attained by adding 30 mL (1 ounce) of bleach to 4 gallons of water. Clothing soiled with blood or other body fluids can be washed with bleach or disinfectant (e.g., Lysol). Recommended cleaning measures should be based on actual available equipment or facilities.

Drug Therapy

For the client who is discharged to the home setting to complete a course of antibiotic therapy, the nurse also explains the importance of compliance with the planned drug regimen. The nurse emphasizes the importance of both the timing of doses and the completion of the planned number of days of therapy. The nurse also teaches the client how the agents should be taken (e.g., before meals, with meals, and without other agents), and explains to the client and family the possible side effects. Side effects include those that are expected (such as gas-

tric distress after the oral administration of erythromycin) as well as more severe adverse reactions (such as rash, fever, or other systemic signs and symptoms of an acute adverse drug reaction). The nurse also teaches the client about allergic manifestations (Table 28-11) and the need for the client and family or significant other to notify the health care provider if adverse or allergic reactions occur.

In the past, many clients with severe infection were hospitalized for several weeks or more simply to receive intravenous (IV) antibiotic therapy. Since the implementation of managed care, many clients have been discharged with an IV device in place and continue to receive IV antibiotics at home or in the nursing home. Clients, a family member, or a nurse administers the drugs. When clients are discharged with an indwelling intravascular device in place, the nurse teaches them or their assisting family members how to care for it. The nurse also instructs clients to be alert for malfunction of the device as well as for signs of inflammation resulting from infection at the catheter insertion site (e.g., redness, heat, pain, swelling, and purulent discharge). Chapter 17 discusses infusion therapy in detail.

Psychosocial Support

The client with an infection is often anxious and fearful that the infection will be transmitted to family members or friends. The nurse allays these fears by teaching the client and the family ways of preventing the spread of disease. Careful attention is paid to the client's concerns. The nurse makes concrete suggestions (e.g., "Your wife can wear gloves when changing your dressing") to address specific concerns.

The client with an infectious disease associated with lifestyle behaviors, such as sexual activity or IV drug abuse, may experience guilt related to the disease. The nurse encourages the client to verbalize feelings associated with the illness and assists the client in locating support systems that may help alleviate these problems. Supportive family members, friends, or groups can help in easing the client's adjustment to illness.

TABLE 28-11

Allergic Reactions to Antibiotic Therapy
Flushing
Wheezing
Sneezing
Pruritus
Urticaria
Rashes
Maculopapular to exfoliative dermatitis
Vascular eruptions
Erythema multiforme (Stevens-Johnson syndrome)
Angioneurotic edema
Serum sickness (headache, fever, chills, hives, malaise, and conjunctivitis)
Anaphylaxis (laryngeal edema, bronchospasm, hypotension, vascular collapse, and cardiac arrest)
Death

➤ Home Care Management

The client with an infectious disease, such as osteomyelitis, who is discharged from the hospital to home may require continued, long-term antibiotic therapy. The nurse emphasizes the importance of a clean home environment, especially for the client who continues to be immunocompromised or who is uniquely susceptible to superinfection (i.e., reinfection or second infection of the same kind) because of antimicrobial drug therapy. Medications often need to be refrigerated. The nurse ensures that the client has access to proper storage facilities and instructs the client to check for signs of improper storage, such as discoloration of the medication.

The nurse questions the client to be sure that hand washing facilities are available in the home and provides supplies and instructions as needed.

➤ Health Care Resources

In unusual instances, a client who has been hospitalized for an infectious disease may not be able to return to the home setting immediately. In such circumstances, temporary placement in a long-term care facility may be advantageous. The staff nurse carefully notes the client's care requirements, medication schedules, and personal needs and preferences on the transfer documents. When possible, the staff nurse communicates directly with a nurse at the receiving facility to facilitate a smooth transition from the hospital to the intermediate care setting.

Because of the early discharge trend from hospitals, the client with severe or chronic infections may be discharged to home before completing long-term antibiotic therapy. The client may continue to receive IV antibiotic therapy at home. The ambulatory client may be asked to return to an outpatient facility every third day to have a new peripheral venous catheter placed for use as a heparin lock. Implanted ports may be used for convenience and to decrease the chance of infection at the skin site. The client's primary nurse communicates with the outpatient facility staff to effect a smooth transition from the hospital to the outpatient setting.

Home health care services are frequently used to ensure appropriate administration of antibiotics at the client's home. These home care services have proved efficient, effective, and much less expensive than hospitalization or intermediate care facilities. Occasional visits from a home care nurse may also facilitate detection of early antimicrobial failures, toxic reactions, or other side effects of therapy.

 Evaluation

On the basis of the identified common nursing diagnoses, the nurse evaluates the care of the client with an infectious disease. Expected outcomes for the client with an infection include that the client

- Describes and complies with the antibiotic regimen as ordered
- Maintains baseline body temperature
- Returns to his or her usual level of activity
- Describes and implements precautions so that infection is not transmitted to others
- Exhibits no clinical manifestations of recurrence, relapse, or reinfection

SELECTED BIBLIOGRAPHY

Baker, O. G., et al. (1996). ICPs show power of prevention in efficacy efforts cost-saving projects. *Hospital Infection Control, 23*(10), 121–124.

Beaumont, E. (1997). Technology scorecard: Focus on infection control. *American Journal of Nursing, 97*(12), 51–54.

Beneson, A. S. (Ed.). (1995). *Control of Communicable Diseases Manual* (16th ed., pp. 533–545). Washington, DC: American Public Health Association.

Carter, L. W. (1994). Bacterial translocation: Nursing implications in the care of patients with neutropenia. *Oncology Nursing Forum, 21*(5), 857–867.

*Centers for Disease Control. (1987). Recommendations for prevention of HIV transmission in health care settings. *Morbidity and Mortality Weekly Report, 36*(2S), 3–17.

Centers for Disease Control and Prevention. (1994). Guidelines for preventing the transmission of *Mycobacterium tuberculosis* in health-care facilities, 1994. *Morbidity and Mortality Weekly Report, 43,* RR–13.

Centers for Disease Control and Prevention. (1996a). Update: Provisional Public Health Service recommendations for chemoprophylaxis after occupational exposure to HIV. *Morbidity and Mortality Weekly Report, 45*(22), 468–472.

Centers for Disease Control and Prevention. (1997). Summary of notifiable diseases, United States, 1996. *Morbidity and Mortality Weekly Report, 45*(53), 6.

Centers for Disease Control and Prevention and Hospital Infections Advisory Committee. (1994). Recommendations for prevention of nosocomial pneumonia. *American Journal of Infection Control, 22*(4), 267–277.

Centers for Disease Control and Prevention and HICPAC. (1994). Recommendations for preventing the spread of vancomycin resistance. *Infection Control and Hospital Epidemiology, 16*(2), 105–113.

Chiarello, L., Feinstein, S. A., Irwin, W., Murtha, K., Stanley, A. H., & Stricof, R. L. (1995). Antibiotic resistance B an emerging trend. *Practice—Infection Control & Prevention in Home Care, 2*(2), 3–4.

Cohen, F. L., & Larson, E. (1996). Emerging infectious diseases: Nursing responses. *Nursing Outlook, 44*(4), 164–168.

Emerging Infections Information Network. (1997). *Emerging/reemerging infections.* New Haven, CT: Department of Epidemiology and Public Health, Yale University.

Friedman, M. M. (1997). Joint Commission on Accreditation of Healthcare Organizations infection control requirements. *Home Healthcare Nurse, 15*(4), 236–238.

Garner, J. S., & HICPAC. (1996). *Guidelines for isolation precautions in hospitals.* Atlanta: Centers for Disease Control and Prevention.

Gould, D., & Chamberlanine, A. (1995). *Staphylococcus aureus:* A review of the literature. *Journal of Clinical Nursing, 4*(1), 5–12.

Herwaldt, L. A., Smith, S. D., & Carter, C. D. (1998). Infection control in the outpatient setting. *Infection Control and Hospital Epidemiology, 19*(1), 41–73.

Jagger, J. J., & Bently, M. (1996). Substantial nationwide drop in percutaneous injury rates detected for 1995. *Advances in Exposure Prevention, 2*(4), 1–12.

Larson, E. L. (1995). APIC guidelines for handwashing and hand antisepsis in health care settings. *American Journal of Infection Control, 23*(4), 251–269.

Malone, N., & Larson, E. (1996). Factors associated with a significant reduction in hospital wide infection rates. *American Journal of Infection Control, 24*(3), 180–185.

Mayone-Ziomek, J. M. (1997). Handwashing in critical care. *MedSurg Nursing, 6*(6), 364–369.

National Nosocomial Infections Surveillance System. (1996). *NNIS report, data summary from October 1986—April 1996, issued May 1996.* Atlanta: Hospital Infection Program, National Center for Infectious Diseases, Centers for Infectious Diseases and Prevention.

Nicolle, L. E., & Garibaldi, R. A. (1995). Infection control in long term care facilities. *Infection Control and Hospital Epidemiology, 16*(6), 348–353.

Reiss, P. J. (1996). Battling the super bug. *RN Magazine, 59*(3), 36–41.

Schumann, D. (1996). *Reducing post critical care infection. MedSurg Nursing, 5*(3), 169–176.

Sheff, B. (1998). VRE & MRSA—Putting bad bugs out of business. *Nursing 98, 28*(3), 40–44.

Shoup, A. (1995). Risk factors related to the use of latex gloves: Taking measures to minimize risk and hidden costs while maintaining quality outcomes. *QRC Advisor, 11*(9).

Smith, P. W., & Rusnak, P. G. (1997). Infection prevention and control in the long-term-care facility. *American Journal of Infection Control, 25*(6), 488–512.

Strausbaugh, L. J., Crossley, K. B., Nurse, B. A., & Thrupp, L. D. (1996). SHEA position paper: Antimicrobial resistance in long-term care facilities. *Infection Control and Hospital Epidemiology, 17*(2), 129–140.

Sutterly, L. (1995). Winning the war against antibiotic resistant infections. *Nursing Spectrum, XX,* 12–14.

Workman, M. L. (1995). Essential concepts of inflammation and immunity. *Critical Care Clinics of North America, 7*(4), 601–615.

SUGGESTED READINGS

Beneson, A. S. (Ed.). (1995). *Control of communicable diseases manual* (16th ed.). Washington, DC: American Public Health Association.

This reference book details information about specific infectious diseases. It is frequently used by infection control practitioners, epidemiologists, physicians, and nurse practitioners in all health care settings and is an excellent resource for nurses as well.

Cohen, F. L., & Larson, E. (1996). Emerging infectious diseases: Nursing responses. *Nursing Outlook, 44*(4), 164–168.

This article describes the problem of emerging and re-emerging infectious disease and the needed role of nurses in prevention of infections.

Workman, M. L. (1995). Essential concepts of inflammation and immunity. *Critical Care Clinics of North America, 7*(4), 601–615.

This article reviews the physiology of inflammation and immunity, concepts that need to be understood to provide appropriate client assessments and interventions.

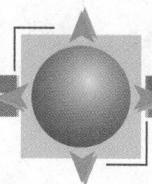

Problems of Oxygenation:

Management of Clients

with Problems of the

Respiratory Tract

ASSESSMENT OF THE RESPIRATORY SYSTEM

To assess the client with respiratory problems accurately, the nurse needs an adequate knowledge of anatomy, physiology, pathophysiology, and various diagnostic tests. Respiratory disease currently ranks as the fifth leading cause of death in the United States (Parker et al., 1997). As clients with chronic respiratory impairments live longer because of advances in diagnosis, treatment, and management, the nurse is confronted with the need for expert assessment skills to plan and implement care for increasing numbers of clients with various respiratory disorders.

ANATOMY AND PHYSIOLOGY REVIEW

The two major purposes of the respiratory system are to provide oxygen for metabolism in the tissues and to remove carbon dioxide, the waste product of metabolism. The respiratory system performs several secondary functions:

Maintaining acid-base balance
Producing speech
Facilitating the sense of smell
Maintaining body water levels
Ensuring heat balance

Upper Respiratory Tract

The upper airways consist of the nose, the sinuses, the pharynx, and the larynx (Fig. 29–1).

Nose and Sinuses

The nose, a rigid structure that is bony in the upper third and cartilaginous in the lower two thirds, contains two passages separated in the middle by the septum. The septum and interior walls of the nasal cavity are lined with mucous membranes, as is the rest of the respiratory tract. The nostrils (anterior nares), or external openings into the nasal cavities, are lined with skin and hair follicles (vibrissae). Vibrissae are the first defense mechanisms of the respiratory system, keeping foreign particles or organisms from entering the lungs. The posterior nares are openings from the nasal cavity into the nasopharynx.

Three major bony projections called *turbinates*, or conchae, arise from the lateral walls of the internal portion of the nose (Fig. 29–1). Turbinates increase the total surface area for filtering, heating, and humidifying inspired air before it passes into the nasopharynx. Inspired air entering the nose is filtered first by vibrissae in the nares. Particles not filtered out in the nares are trapped in the mucous layer of the turbinates. These particles are passed

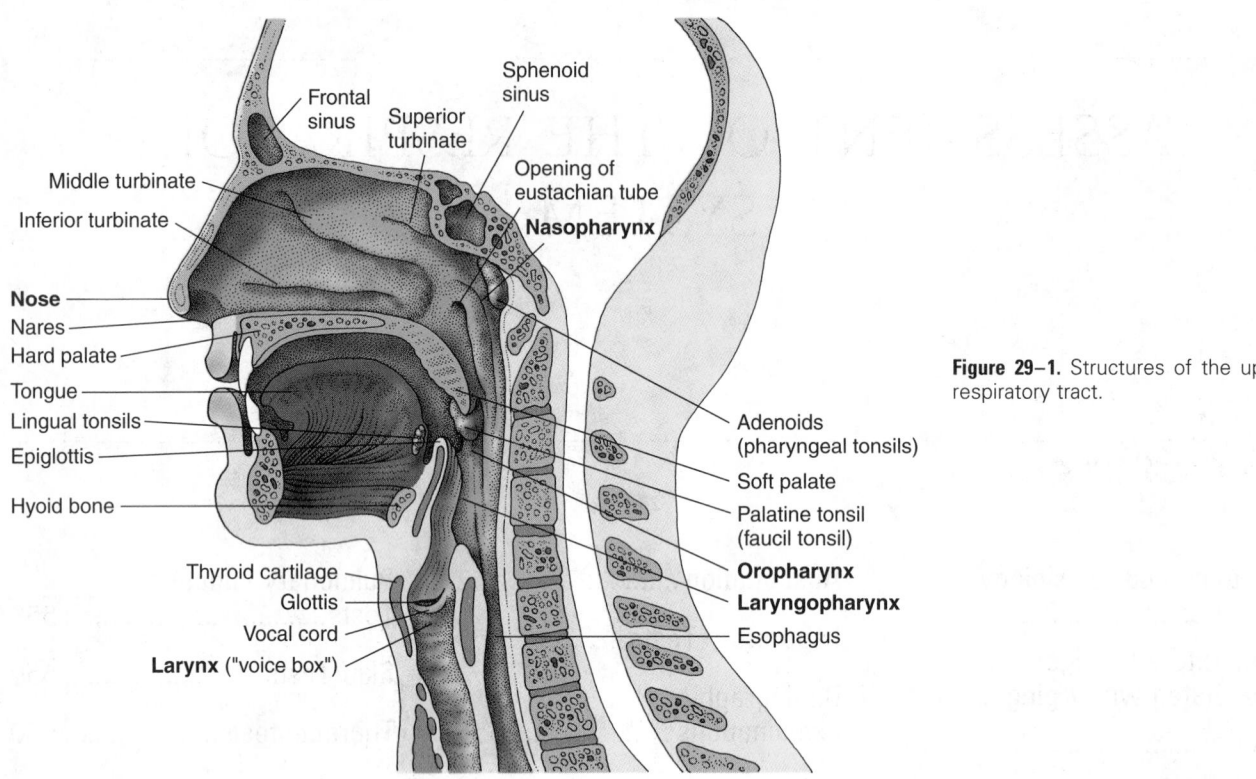

Figure 29–1. Structures of the upper respiratory tract.

posteriorly by cilia (hair-like projections) to the oropharynx, where they are swallowed or expectorated. Inspired air is humidified by contact with the mucous membrane and is warmed by exposure to heat from the vascular network. The nose is the organ of smell; olfactory receptors from cranial nerve I are located in the roof of the nose and in the superior turbinate.

The paranasal sinuses are air-filled cavities within the bones that surround the nasal passages. They are lined with ciliated epithelium. The four paranasal sinuses are shown in Figure 29–2. The sinuses provide resonance during speech.

Pharynx

The pharynx, or throat, serves as a passageway for both the respiratory and digestive tracts and is located behind the oral and nasal cavities. It is divided into the nasopharynx, the oropharynx, and the laryngopharynx (see Fig. 29–1).

Located behind the nose, the nasopharynx lies above the soft palate and contains the adenoids and the distal opening of the eustachian tube. The adenoids (pharyngeal tonsils) act as an important defense mechanism by trapping organisms entering the nose and the mouth. The eustachian tube connects the nasopharynx with the middle chamber of the ear and opens during swallowing to equalize the pressure within the middle ear.

The oropharynx is located behind the mouth below the nasopharynx. It extends from the soft palate to the base of the tongue. The palatine tonsils (also known as faucial tonsils) are located on the anterolateral borders of the

oropharynx. These tonsils also guard the body against invading organisms.

Located behind the larynx, the laryngopharynx extends from the base of the tongue to the esophagus. The laryngopharynx is the critical dividing point where solid foods and fluids are separated from air. At this point, the passageway bifurcates into the larynx and the esophagus.

Larynx

The larynx, or voice box, is located above the trachea, just below the pharynx at the root of the tongue. It is

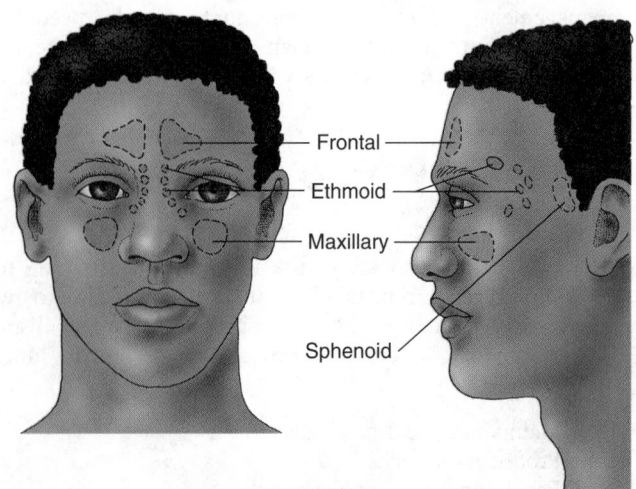

Figure 29–2. The paranasal sinuses.

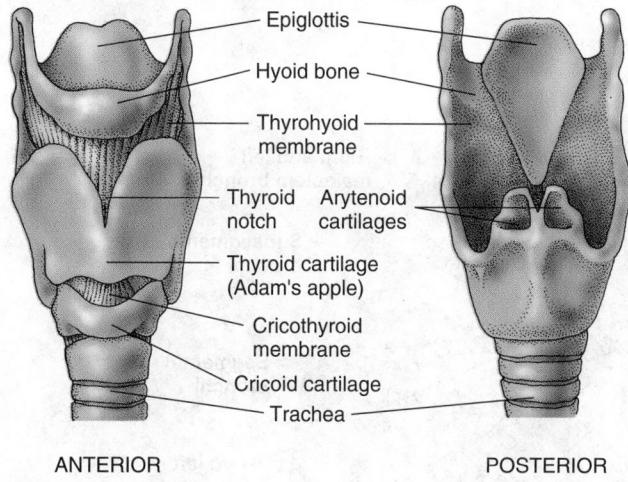

Epiglottis

Hyoid bone

Thyrohyoid membrane

Thyroid notch   Arytenoid cartilages

Thyroid cartilage (Adam's apple)

Cricothyroid membrane

Cricoid cartilage

Trachea

ANTERIOR   POSTERIOR

Figure 29–3. Structures of the larynx.

innervated by the recurrent laryngeal nerves. The larynx is composed of several cartilages (Fig. 29–3). The thyroid cartilage is the largest and is commonly referred to as the Adam's apple. The cricoid cartilage, which contains the vocal cords, lies below the thyroid cartilage. The cricoid cartilage is the only complete ring of cartilage in the airway. The cricothyroid membrane is below the level of the vocal cords and joins the thyroid and cricoid cartilages. This site is used in an emergency for access to the lower airways. The procedure, a cricothyroidotomy (an opening made between the thyroid and cricoid cartilage), is also called a cricothyrotomy and results in a tracheostomy. The two arytenoid cartilages, to which the posterior ends of the vocal cords are attached, are used together with the thyroid cartilage in vocal cord movement.

Inside the larynx are two pairs of vocal cords: the false and true cords. The opening between the true vocal cords is the *glottis* (Fig. 29–4). The glottis plays an important role in coughing, which is the most fundamental defense mechanism of the lungs. The *epiglottis* is a leaf-shaped, elastic structure that is attached along one edge to the top of the larynx. Its hinge-like action prevents food from entering the tracheobronchial tree (aspiration) by closing over the glottis during swallowing.

Lower Respiratory Tract

The lower airways consist of the trachea; two mainstem bronchi; lobar, segmental, and subsegmental bronchi; bronchioles; alveolar ducts; and alveoli (Fig. 29–5). The tracheobronchial tree is an inverted tree-like structure consisting of muscular, cartilaginous, and elastic tissues. This system of bifurcating tubes, which decrease in size from the trachea to the respiratory bronchioles, allows the passage of gases to and from the pulmonary parenchyma. Gas exchange takes place in the pulmonary parenchyma between the alveoli and the pulmonary capillaries.

Trachea

The trachea, commonly referred to as the windpipe, is located in front of (anterior to) the esophagus. It begins

at the lower border of the cricoid cartilage of the larynx and extends to the level of the fourth or fifth thoracic vertebra. The trachea branches into the right and left mainstem bronchi at the carina. The carina is located at the sternal angle where the manubrium joins the sternum.

The trachea is composed of 6 to 10 C-shaped cartilaginous rings. The open portion of the C is the back (posterior) portion of the trachea; it contains smooth muscle that is shared with the esophagus. Low pressure must be maintained in endotracheal and tracheostomy tube cuffs so as not to cause erosion of this posterior wall and create a tracheoesophageal fistula.

Mainstem Bronchi

The mainstem, or primary, bronchi begin at the carina. The structure of a bronchus resembles that of the trachea. The right bronchus is slightly wider, shorter, and more vertical than the left bronchus. Because of the more vertical line of the right bronchus, accidental intubation of the right bronchus is possible when an endotracheal tube is passed. Also if a foreign object is aspirated from the pharynx, it most likely enters the right bronchus.

Lobar, Segmental, and Subsegmental Bronchi

The mainstem bronchi further divide into the five secondary, or lobar, bronchi that enter each of the five lobes of the lung. Each lobar bronchus is surrounded by connective tissue, blood vessels, nerves, and lymphatics, and each branches into segmental and subsegmental divisions. The cartilage of these lobar bronchi is nearly circumferential and resists collapse. The bronchi are lined with ciliated, mucus-secreting epithelium. The cilia propel mucus up and away from the lower airway to the trachea, where it can be expectorated or swallowed.

Bronchioles

The bronchioles, branching from the secondary bronchi, subdivide into smaller and smaller tubes: the terminal and respiratory bronchioles (Fig. 29–6). These terminal and respiratory tubes are less than 1 mm in diameter. They have no cartilage and, therefore, depend entirely on the elastic recoil of the lung for patency. The terminal bronchioles contain no cilia and do not participate in gas exchange.

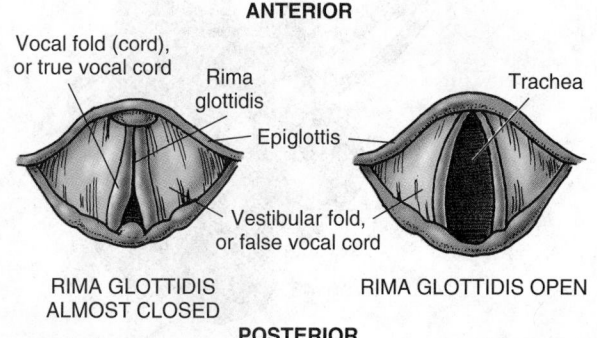

ANTERIOR

Vocal fold (cord), or true vocal cord

Rima glottidis

Epiglottis

Trachea

Vestibular fold, or false vocal cord

RIMA GLOTTIDIS ALMOST CLOSED

RIMA GLOTTIDIS OPEN

POSTERIOR

Figure 29–4. Detail of the glottis (two vocal folds and the intervening space, the rima glottidis).

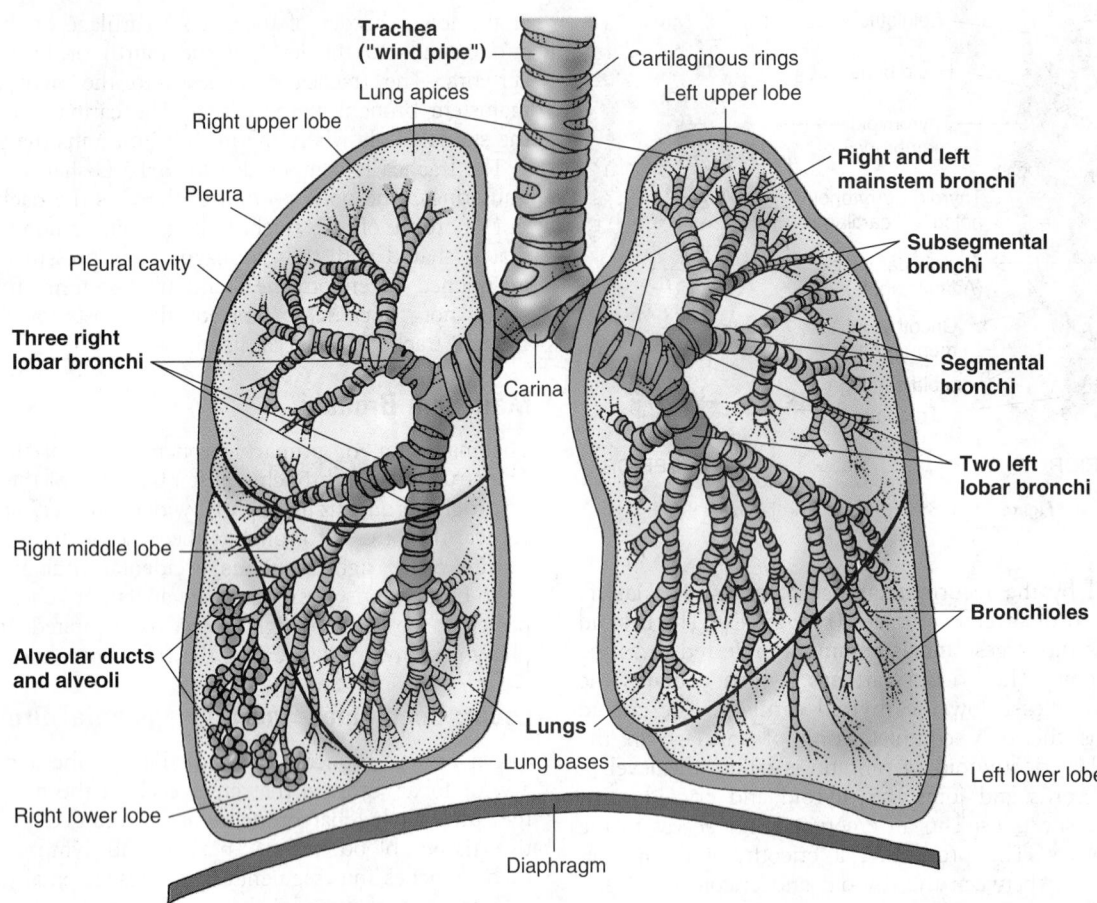

Figure 29–5. Structures of the lower respiratory tract (structural size and proportions not drawn to scale).

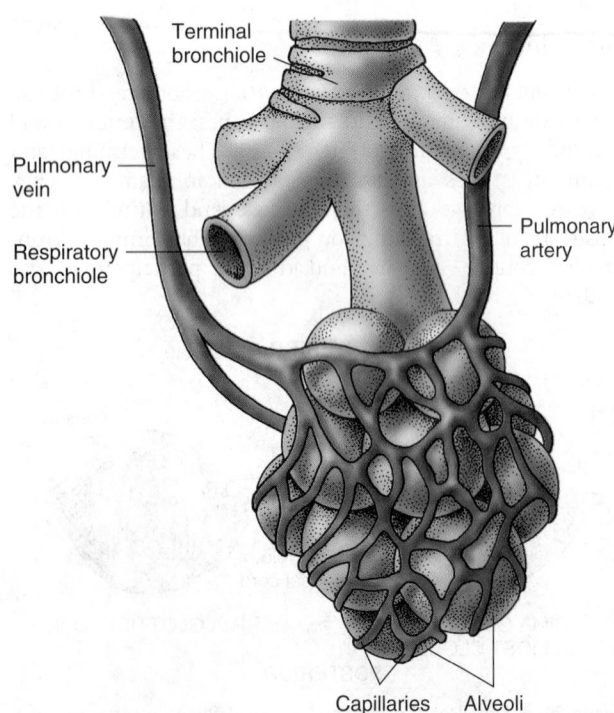

Figure 29–6. The terminal bronchioles and the acinus.

TABLE 29–1

Age Distributions and Partial Pressure of Arterial Oxygen (PaO$_2$) Values (Mean)	
Age (years)	**PaO$_2$**
40–44	95
45–49	88.6
50–54	87.1
55–59	85.1
60–64	84.8
65–69	82.3
70–74	79.1
75–79	82.9
80–84	83.4
85–90	83.2

Modified with permission from Cerveri, I., Zoia, M. C., Fanfulla, F., et al. (1995). Reference values of arterial oxygen tension in the middle-aged and elderly. *American Journal of Respiratory and Critical Care Medicine, 152,* 934–941.

Alveolar Ducts and Alveoli

Alveolar ducts, which resemble a bunch of grapes, branch from the respiratory bronchioles. Alveolar sacs arise from these ducts. The alveolar sacs contain clusters of alveoli, which are the basic units of gas exchange (see Fig. 29–6). It is estimated that the lungs contain about 300 million alveoli, surrounded by pulmonary capillaries. Because these microscopic alveoli are so numerous and share common walls, the surface area for gas exchange in the lungs is extensive. In a healthy adult, this surface area is approximately the size of a tennis court. *Acinus* is a term used to indicate all structures distal to the terminal bronchiole (e.g., respiratory bronchiole, alveolar duct, and alveolar sac).

Certain cells located in the walls of the alveoli secrete *surfactant,* a phospholipid protein that reduces the surface tension in the alveoli. Without sufficient surfactant, atelectasis (collapse of the alveoli) ultimately occurs. In atelectasis, gas exchange is reduced because the surface area is reduced.

Lungs

The lungs are sponge-like, elastic, cone-shaped organs located in the pleural cavity in the thorax. The apex of each lung extends above the clavicle; the base of each lung lies just above the diaphragm (the major muscle of inspiration). The lungs are composed of millions of alveoli and their related ducts, bronchioles, and bronchi. The right lung, which is larger than the left, is divided into three lobes: upper, middle, and lower. The left lung, which is somewhat narrower than the right lung to accommodate the heart, is divided into two lobes.

The hilum is the point at which the primary bronchus, pulmonary blood vessels, nerves, and lymphatics enter each lung. Innervation of the chest wall is via the phrenic (pleura) and intercostal (diaphragm, ribs, and muscles) nerves; innervation of the bronchi is via the vagus nerve.

Composed of two surfaces, the pleura, a continuous smooth membrane, totally encloses the lung. The parietal pleura lines the inside of the thoracic cavity, including the upper surface of the diaphragm. The visceral pleura covers the pulmonary surfaces, including the major fissures between the lobes. A thin fluid (surfactant) produced by the cells lining the pleura lubricates these two surfaces, thereby allowing them to glide smoothly and painlessly during respirations.

Blood flow through the lungs occurs via two separate systems: the pulmonary system and the bronchial system. The bronchial arteries, arising from the thoracic aorta, are part of the systemic circulation and do not participate in gas exchange. This system carries the blood necessary to meet the metabolic demands of the lungs. The pulmonary circulation is composed of a highly vascular capillary network. Oxygen-depleted blood travels from the right ventricle of the heart into the pulmonary artery, which eventually branches into arterioles that form the capillary networks. The capillaries are enmeshed around and through the alveoli, the site of gas exchange (see Fig. 29–6). Freshly oxygenated blood then travels through the venules to the pulmonary vein and on to the left atrium, where it is pumped throughout the systemic circulation.

Accessory Muscles of Respiration

Accessory muscles of respiration include the scalene muscles, which elevate the first two ribs; the sternocleidomastoid muscles, which raise the sternum; and the trapezius and pectoralis muscles, which fix the shoulders. Additionally, various back and abdominal muscles are used in disease states.

Respiratory Changes Associated with Aging

Respiratory changes that occur with aging are described in Chart 29–1. Many changes associated with elderly clients are due to a lifetime of exposure to environmental stimuli (e.g., cigarette smoke, bacteria, air pollutants, and industrial fumes and irritants) and heredity. Table 29–1 shows the results of one study demonstrating that partial pressure of arterial oxygen (PaO_2) decreases with age up to age 75 years and then increases. Partial pressure of arterial carbon dioxide ($PaCO_2$) did not increase with age.

Chart 29–1

Nursing Focus on the Elderly: Changes in the Respiratory System Related to Aging

Physiologic Change	Nursing Implications	Rationales
Chest Wall		
Anteroposterior diameter increases. Thorax becomes shorter.	Discuss the normal changes of aging.	Clients may be anxious because they must work harder to breathe.
Progressive kyphoscoliosis occurs. Chest wall compliance (elasticity) decreases.	Discuss the need for increased rest periods during exercise.	Older clients have less tolerance for exercise.
Mobility may decrease. Osteoporosis is possible.	Encourage adequate calcium intake (especially during a woman's premenopause phase).	Calcium intake helps prevent osteoporosis by building bone in younger clients.

Continued

Chart 29–1. Nursing Focus on the Elderly: Changes in the Respiratory System Related to Aging   Continued

Physiologic Change	Nursing Implications	Rationales
Alveoli		
Alveolar surface area decreases. Diffusion capacity decreases. Elastic recoil decreases. Bronchioles and alveolar ducts dilate. Ability to cough decreases. Airways close early.	Encourage vigorous pulmonary hygiene (i.e., encourage the client to turn, cough, and deep breathe), especially if the client is confined to bed or has had surgery. Encourage upright position.	There is increased potential for mechanical or infectious respiratory complications in these situations. The upright position minimizes ventilation-perfusion mismatching.
Lungs		
Residual volume increases. Vital capacity decreases. Efficiency of oxygen and carbon dioxide exchange decreases. Elasticity decreases.	Include inspection, palpation, percussion, and auscultation in lung assessments. Help client in actively maintaining health and fitness. Assess the client's respirations for abnormal breathing patterns. Encourage frequent oral hygiene.	Inspection, palpation, percussion, and auscultation are needed to detect normal age-related changes. Health and fitness helps to keep losses in respiratory functioning to a minimum. Periodic breathing patterns (e.g., Cheyne-Stokes) can occur. Oral hygiene aids in the removal of secretions.
Pharynx and Larynx		
Muscles atrophy. Vocal cords become slack. Laryngeal muscles lose elasticity and cartilage.	Have face-to-face conversations with client when possible.	Client's voices may be soft and difficult to understand.
Pulmonary Vasculature		
Increased vascular resistance to blood flow through pulmonary vascular system occurs. Pulmonary capillary blood volume decreases. Risk of hypoxia increases.	Assess the client's level of consciousness.	Clients can become confused during acute respiratory conditions.
Exercise Tolerance		
Body's response to hypoxia and hypercarbia decreases.	Assess for subtle signs and symptoms of hypoxia.	Early assessment helps to prevent complications.
Muscle Strength		
Respiratory muscle strength, especially the diaphragm and the intercostals, decreases.	Encourage pulmonary hygiene and help the client in actively maintaining health and fitness.	Regular pulmonary hygiene and overall fitness help maintain maximal functioning of the respiratory system and prevent illness.
Proneness to Infection		
Effectiveness of the cilia decreases. Immunoglobulin A decreases. Alveolar macrophages are altered.	Encourage pulmonary hygiene and help the client in actively maintaining health and fitness.	Regular pulmonary hygiene and overall fitness help maintain maximal functioning of the respiratory system and prevent illness.

Respiratory disease is a major cause of acute illness and chronic disability in elderly clients. Although respiratory function normally declines with age, there is usually little difficulty with the demands of ordinary activity. However, the sedentary elderly client often reports feeling breathless during exercise.

It is difficult to differentiate the normal changes related to aging from the pathologic changes associated with respiratory disease or exposure to pollutants. In addition, disorders of the neuromuscular and cardiovascular systems that occur with aging may cause abnormal respiration even if the lungs are normal.

HISTORY
Demographic Data

Age, sex, and race can affect the physical and diagnostic findings. Many of the diagnostic studies relevant to respiratory disorders (e.g., pulmonary function tests) use these data for determining predicted normal values.

WOMEN'S HEALTH CONSIDERATIONS

 Women have greater bronchial responsiveness (i.e., bronchial hyperreactivity) than men, especially

women smokers. Women also have larger airways than men (Paoletti et al., 1995, p. 1775–1776). Increased bronchial responsiveness is a risk factor for a more rapid decline in lung function in the elderly, particularly in former and current smokers (Villar et al., 1995).

TRANSCULTURAL CONSIDERATIONS

The largest chest volumes are found in Caucasians; the smallest volumes are found in Native Americans. The chest volumes of African-Americans are significantly larger than those of Asian-Americans but not as large as those of Caucasians (Jarvis, 1996, p. 468).

Personal and Family History
Medical and Family History

The nurse questions clients about their respiratory history (Table 29–2). The client's history as well as that of family members could be significant. The nurse obtains a family history to consider respiratory disorders with a genetic component, such as cystic fibrosis, some lung cancers, and alpha$_1$-antitrypsin deficiency (one cause of emphysema). Clients with asthma often have a family history of allergic symptoms and reactive airways. The nurse assesses for a family history of infectious disease such as tuberculosis and considers that family members may have similar environmental or occupational exposures.

Smoking History

The nurse questions the client about the use of cigarettes, cigars, pipe tobacco, and marijuana and other controlled substances, and notes whether the client has passive exposure to smoke in the home or workplace. If the client smokes, the nurse asks how long the client has smoked, how many packs a day, whether the client has quit, and how long ago the client stopped smoking. The smoking history is documented in pack-years (number of packs smoked per day multiplied by number of years). Because the client may harbor guilt or denial about this habit, the nurse assumes a nonjudgmental attitude when questioning the client.

Smoking induces anatomical changes in the large and peripheral airways, which lead to varying degrees of airway obstruction (Paoletti et al., 1995). Men who continue to smoke have a more rapid decline in their pulmonary function than do nonsmokers. After quitting for 2 years, however, the decline in function has been found to be similar to that of a nonsmoker (Burchfiel et al., 1995).

Medication Use

The nurse questions the client about medications taken for breathing problems and also about drugs taken for other conditions. Cough, for example, can be a side effect of the angiotensin-converting enzyme (ACE) inhibitors. The nurse determines which over-the-counter medications, such as cough syrups, antihistamines, decongestants, inhalants, and nasal sprays, the client is using. The nurse also assesses home remedies. The nurse asks about past medication use and why it was discontinued. For

---

TABLE 29–2

Important Aspects to Assess in a Respiratory System History

- Smoking history
- Childhood illnesses
  - Asthma
  - Pneumonia
  - Communicable diseases
  - Hay fever
  - Allergies
  - Eczema
  - Frequent colds
  - Croup
  - Cystic fibrosis
- Adult illnesses
  - Pneumonia
  - Sinusitis
  - Tuberculosis
  - HIV and AIDS
  - Lung disease such as emphysema and sarcoidosis
  - Diabetes
  - Hypertension
  - Heart disease
- Influenza, pneumococcal (Pneumovax) and BCG vaccinations
- Surgeries of the upper or lower respiratory system
- Injuries to the upper or lower respiratory system
- Hospitalizations
- Date of last chest x-ray, pulmonary function test, tuberculin test, or other diagnostic tests and results
- Recent weight loss
- Night sweats
- Sleep disturbances
- Lung disease and condition of family members

HIV = human immunodeficiency virus; AIDS = acquired immunodeficiency syndrome; BCG = bacille Calmette-Guérin.

---

example, a client may have used numerous bronchodilator metered-dose inhalers but may prefer one particular drug for relieving breathlessness.

Allergies

Data about allergies are extremely important and relevant to the respiratory history. The nurse determines whether the client has any known allergies to foods, dust, molds, pollen, bee stings, trees, grass, animal dander and saliva, or medications. The nurse asks the client to explain a specific allergic response. For example, does the client wheeze, have trouble breathing, cough, sneeze, or experience rhinitis after exposure to the allergen? Has the client ever been treated for an allergic response? If the client has received treatment, the nurse asks about the circumstances leading up to the need for treatment, the type of treatment, and the client's response to treatment.

ELDERLY CONSIDERATIONS

Allergy is a risk factor for a more rapid decline in lung function in the elderly (Villar et al., 1995).

Travel and Area of Residence

Travel and area of residence may be relevant for a history of exposure to certain diseases. For example, histoplasmosis, a fungal disease caused by inhalation of contaminated dust, is found in the central United States, the Mississippi and Missouri river valleys, and Central America. Coccidioidomycosis, another fungal disease, is found predominantly in the western and southwestern United States, Mexico, and portions of Central America.

Diet History

An evaluation of the client's diet history may reveal allergic reactions after ingestion of certain foods or preservatives. Signs and symptoms range from rhinitis, chest tightness, weakness, shortness of breath, urticaria, and severe wheezing to loss of consciousness. The nurse notes allergies and the allergic response in a prominent location of the client's record. The nurse asks about the client's usual food intake and ascertains whether any symptoms occur with eating. Malnutrition may occur when the client has difficulty breathing during the food preparation process or during eating.

Occupational History and Socioeconomic Status

The nurse considers the home, community, and workplace for environmental factors possibly causing or contributing to the client's lung disease. Occupational pulmonary diseases include pneumoconiosis (resulting from the inhalation of dust such as coal dust, stone dust, and silicone dust), toxic lung injury, and hypersensitivity disease (as from latex). The occupational history includes exact dates of employment and a brief job description. Exposure to industrial dusts (both organic and inorganic) or noxious chemicals found in smoke and fumes may cause respiratory disease. Some of the most susceptible clients include coal miners, stonemasons, cotton handlers, welders, potters, plastic and rubber manufacturers, printers, farm workers, and steel foundry workers.

The nurse obtains information about the client's home and living conditions, such as the type of heat used (e.g., gas heater, wood-burning stove, fireplace, and kerosene heater) and exposure to environmental irritants (e.g., noxious fumes, chemicals, animals, birds, and air pollutants). The nurse also asks about the client's hobbies and leisure activities. Pastimes such as painting, working with ceramics, model airplane building, furniture refinishing, or woodworking may have exposed the client to harmful chemical irritants.

Current Health Problem

Whether the pulmonary problem is acute or chronic, the client's chief complaint is likely to include cough, sputum production, chest pain, and shortness of breath at rest or on exertion. During the interview, the nurse explores the history of the present illness, preferably in a chronological order. This analysis includes the following:

Onset
Duration
Location
Frequency
Progressing and radiating patterns
Quality and number of symptoms
Aggravating and relieving factors
Associated signs and symptoms
Treatments

Cough

Cough is the cardinal sign of respiratory disease. The nurse asks the client how long the cough has persisted (e.g., 1 week, 3 months). The nurse also asks whether it occurs at a specific time of day (e.g., on awakening in the morning, as is common in smokers) or in relation to any physical activity. The nurse determines whether the cough is productive or nonproductive, congested, dry, tickling, or hacking.

Sputum Production

An important symptom associated with coughing is sputum production. The nurse notes the duration, color, consistency, odor, and amount of sputum. Sputum may be clear, white, tan, gray, or, if infection is present, yellow or green.

The nurse describes sputum consistency as thin, thick, watery, or frothy. Smokers with chronic bronchitis have mucoid sputum because of chronic stimulation and hypertrophy of the bronchial glands (George et al., 1995). Voluminous, pink, frothy sputum is characteristic of pulmonary edema. Pneumococcal pneumonia is often associated with rust-colored sputum, and foul-smelling sputum is often found in anaerobic infections such as lung abscess. Blood in the sputum (hemoptysis) is most commonly noted in clients with chronic bronchitis or bronchogenic carcinoma. Clients with tuberculosis, pulmonary infarction, bronchial adenoma, or lung abscess may expectorate grossly bloody sputum.

Sputum can be quantified by describing its production in terms of measurements such as teaspoon, tablespoon, and cups or fractions of cups. Normally, the tracheobronchial tree can produce up to 3 ounces (90 mL) of sputum per day. The nurse determines whether sputum production is increasing, possibly from external stimuli (such as an irritant in the work setting) or from an internal cause (such as chronic bronchitis or a pulmonary abscess).

Chest Pain

A detailed description of chest pain helps the nurse differentiate pleural, musculoskeletal, cardiac, and gastrointestinal pain. Because perception of pain is purely subjective, the nurse analyzes pain in relation to the characteristics described in the history of the present illness. Coughing, deep breathing, or swallowing usually makes chest wall pain worse. (Chapter 9 discusses pain in detail.)

TABLE 29–3

Correlation of Dyspnea Classification with Performance of Activities of Daily Living (ADLs)

Classification	Activities of Daily Living Key
Class I: No significant restrictions in normal activity. Employable. Dyspnea occurs only on more than normal or strenuous exertion.	• *4:* No breathlessness, normal.
Class II: Independent in essential ADLs but restricted in some other activities. Dyspneic on climbing stairs or on walking on an incline but not on level walking. Employable for only sedentary job or under special circumstances.	• *3:* Satisfactory, mild breathlessness. Complete performance is possible without pause or assistance, but not entirely normal.
Class III: Dyspnea commonly occurs during usual activities, such as showering or dressing, but the client can manage without assistance from others. Not dyspneic at rest; can walk for more than a city block at own pace but cannot keep up with others of own age. May stop to catch breath partway up a flight of stairs. Is probably not employable in any occupation.	• *2:* Fair, moderate breathlessness. Must stop during activity. Complete performance is possible without assistance, but performance may be too debilitating or time consuming.
Class IV: Dyspnea produces dependence on help in some essential ADLs such as dressing and bathing. Not usually dyspneic at rest. Dyspneic on minimal exertion; must pause on climbing one flight, walking more than 100 yards, or dressing. Often restricted to home if lives alone. Has minimal or no activities out of home.	• *1:* Poor, marked breathlessness. Incomplete performance; assistance is necessary.
Class V: Entirely restricted to home and often limited to bed or chair. Dyspneic at rest. Dependent on help for most needs.	• *0:* Performance not indicated or recommended; too difficult.

Dyspnea

The perception of difficulty in breathing (breathlessness) is subjective and varies among clients, and a client's perception may not be consistent with the severity of the presenting problem. For that reason, the nurse determines the type of onset (slow or abrupt), the duration (number of hours, time of day), relieving factors (changes of position, medication use, activity cessation), and evidence of audible sounds (wheezing, crackles, stridor).

The nurse tries to quantify dyspnea by determining whether this symptom interferes with activities of daily living (ADLs) and, if so, how severely. For example, is the client breathless while dressing, showering, shaving, or eating? Does dyspnea on exertion occur after the client walks one block or climbs one flight of stairs? Table 29–3 correlates dyspnea classifications with ADL performance. The nurse also may use a dyspnea assessment scale to assess dyspnea (see Chap. 32).

The nurse inquires about paroxysmal nocturnal dyspnea (PND) and orthopnea, which are commonly associated with chronic pulmonary disease and left ventricular failure. In PND, the client has a sudden onset of difficulty breathing that is severe enough to awaken the client from sleep. The term *orthopnea* is used when the client needs to be in an upright position to have easier breathing.

PHYSICAL ASSESSMENT
Nose and Sinuses

The nurse inspects the client's external nose for deformities or tumors and the nostrils for symmetry of size and shape. Nasal flaring may indicate increased respiratory effort. To observe the interior nose, the nurse asks the client to tilt the head back for a penlight examination. The nurse may use a nasal speculum and nasopharyngeal mirror for a more thorough examination of the nasal cavity.

The nurse inspects for color, swelling, drainage, and bleeding. The mucous membrane of the nose normally appears redder than the oral mucosa, but it may appear pale, engorged, and bluish gray in clients with allergic rhinitis. The nurse checks the nasal septum for evidence of bleeding, perforation, or deviation. Some degree of septal deviation is common in most adults and appears as an S shape, inclining toward one side or the other. A perforated septum is noted if the light shines through the perforation into the opposite nostril; it is often found in cocaine users. Nasal polyps, a frequent cause of obstruction, appear as pale, shiny, gelatinous structures attached to the turbinates (see also Chap. 31).

The nurse occludes one nare at a time to check whether air moves through the nonoccluded nare easily. The nurse also palpates the nose and the paranasal sinuses to detect tenderness or swelling. Only the frontal and maxillary sinuses are readily accessible to clinical examination because the ethmoid and sphenoid sinuses lie deep within the skull (see Fig. 29–2). Using the thumbs, the nurse checks for sinus tenderness by pressing upward on the frontal and maxillary areas; both sides are assessed simultaneously. Tenderness in these areas suggests inflammation or acute sinusitis. Slight tapping with the plexor over the sinuses also will elicit tenderness if inflamed.

The nurse may use transillumination of the sinuses to detect sinusitis. A darkened room and a penlight are needed for this procedure. Normally, the nurse sees a faint glow of light through the bone outlining the sinus. Transillumination is absent or decreased in sinusitis. Computed tomographic (CT) scans and x-rays of the sinuses are more definitive tools for detecting inflammation or sinusitis.

Pharynx, Trachea, and Larynx

Examination of the pharynx begins with inspection of the external structures of the mouth. Chapter 55 describes a complete physical assessment of the oral cavity, and Chapter 56 discusses disorders of the oral cavity.

Using a tongue depressor, the nurse presses down one side of the tongue at a time (to avoid stimulating the client's gag reflex) to examine the structures of the posterior pharynx. As the client says "ah," the nurse notes the rise and fall of the soft palate and uvula and observes for color and symmetry, evidence of mucopurulent discharge (postnasal drainage), edema or ulceration, and tonsillar enlargement or inflammation.

The nurse inspects the neck for symmetry, alignment, masses, swelling, bruises, and the use of accessory neck muscles in breathing. The nurse palpates lymph nodes for size, shape, mobility, consistency, and tenderness. Tender nodes are usually movable and suggest inflammation. Malignant nodes are often hard and fixed to the surrounding tissue.

The nurse gently palpates the trachea for deviation, mobility, tenderness, and masses. Firm palpation may elicit coughing or gagging. The space on either side of the trachea should be equal. Many pulmonary disorders cause the trachea to deviate from the midline. Tension pneumothorax, large pleural effusion, mediastinal mass, and neck tumor push the trachea away from the affected area, whereas pneumonectomy, fibrosis, and atelectasis cause a pull toward the affected area. Decreased tracheal mobility may occur with carcinoma or fibrosis of the mediastinum.

The larynx is usually examined by a specialist with a laryngoscope. The nurse may observe an abnormal voice, especially hoarseness, when there are abnormalities of the larynx.

Lungs and Thorax

Before examining the thorax, the nurse becomes familiar with anatomic landmarks. Identifying the location of physical assessment findings depends on accurate numbering of the ribs, intercostal spaces, and vertebrae and on accurate use of imaginary lines drawn on the chest (Fig. 29–7).

Inspection

Inspection of the chest begins with assessment of the anterior and posterior thorax, with the client in a sitting position, if possible. The client should be undressed to the waist and draped for privacy and warmth. The chest is observed by comparing one side with the other. The nurse works from the top (apex) and moves downward toward the base. The nurse inspects for discoloration, scars, lesions, masses, and spinal deformities such as kyphosis, scoliosis, and lordosis.

The nurse notes the rate, rhythm, and depth of inspirations as well as symmetry of chest movement. An im-

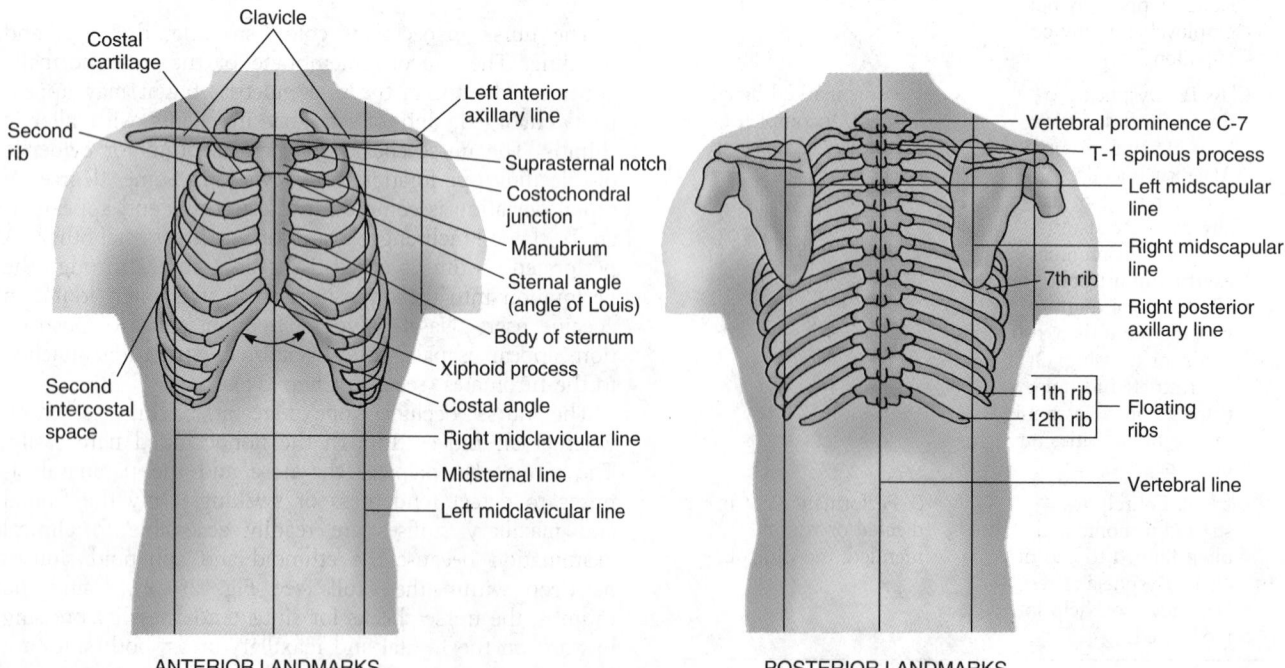

ANTERIOR LANDMARKS   POSTERIOR LANDMARKS

Figure 29–7. Anterior and posterior thoracic landmarks.

paired movement or unequal expansion may indicate underlying disease of the lung or the pleura. The nurse observes the type of breathing, such as pursed-lip or diaphragmatic breathing, and the use of accessory muscles. In observing respiration, the nurse notes the duration of the inspiratory (I) and expiratory (E) phases. The ratio of these phases (the I/E ratio) is normally 1:2. A prolonged expiratory phase indicates obstruction of air outflow and is frequently seen in clients with chronic airflow limitation (CAL).

The nurse notes the client's chest configuration and compares the anteroposterior (AP) diameter with the lateral diameter. This ratio normally ranges from 1:2 to about 5:7, depending on the client's body build. The ratio approximates 1:1 in the client with emphysema, thus giving the client the typical barrel chest appearance (see Fig. 32–5).

Normally, the ribs slope downward. However, clients with air trapping in the lungs caused by chronic asthma or emphysema have little or no slope to the ribs (i.e., the ribs are more horizontal).

The nurse also checks for abnormal retractions of the intercostal spaces during inspiration, which indicate airflow obstruction. These retractions may be due to fibrosis of the underlying lung, severe acute asthma, emphysema, or tracheal or laryngeal obstruction.

Palpation

After inspection, the nurse palpates the chest. Palpation enables the nurse to assess symmetry of respiratory movement and observable abnormalities, to identify areas of tenderness, and to elicit vocal or tactile fremitus (vibration).

In palpation, the nurse assesses thoracic expansion by placing the thumbs posteriorly on the spine at the level of the ninth ribs; the fingers are extended laterally around the rib cage. As the client inhales, both sides of the chest should move upward and outward together in one symmetric movement; the nurse's thumbs thus move apart. On exhalation, the thumbs should come back together as they return to the midline. Splinting or decreased movement on one side (unilateral or unequal expansion) may be due to pleuritic pain, trauma, or pneumothorax (air in the pleural cavity). Respiratory lag or impairment of thoracic movement may also indicate the presence of a pulmonary mass, pleural fibrosis, atelectasis, pneumonia, or a lung abscess.

The nurse palpates the thorax for any abnormalities found on inspection (e.g., masses, lesions, bruises, and swelling). The nurse also palpates for tenderness, particularly if the client has reported pain. *Crepitus,* or subcutaneous emphysema, is a crackling sensation felt beneath the fingertips and should be noted, especially around a wound site or if a pneumothorax is suspected. Crepitus indicates that air is trapped within the tissues.

Vocal fremitus is a vibration of the chest wall produced when the client speaks; when palpated, it is termed *tactile fremitus*. To elicit tactile fremitus, the nurse places the palm or the base of the fingers against the client's chest wall and instructs the client to say the number *99*. The nurse compares vibrations (with the same hand) from one side of the chest with those from the other side, moving from the apices to the bases. Palpable vibrations are transmitted from the tracheobronchial tree, along the solid surface of chest wall, to the nurse's hand.

The nurse notes symmetry of the vibrations and areas of enhanced, diminished, or absent fremitus. Fremitus is decreased if the transmission of sound waves from the larynx to the chest wall is slowed. This situation can occur when the pleural space is filled with air (pneumothorax), fluid (pleural effusion), or solid tissue (pleural thickening). Fremitus is increased over large bronchi because of their proximity to the chest wall. Disease processes such as pneumonia and abscesses decrease the distance vibrations must travel to reach the chest wall, also resulting in increased tactile fremitus.

Percussion

The nurse uses percussion to assess for pulmonary resonance, the boundaries of organs, and diaphragmatic excursion. Percussion involves tapping the chest wall, which sets the underlying tissues into motion and produces audible sounds. The nurse places the distal joint of the middle finger of the less dominant hand firmly on the surface over the intercostal space to be percussed. No other part of the nurse's hand touches the client's chest wall because it absorbs the vibrations. The nurse uses the middle finger of the dominant hand to deliver quick, sharp strikes to the distal joint of the positioned finger (Fig. 29–8). The nurse maintains a loose, relaxed wrist while delivering the taps with the tip of the finger, not the finger pad. The nurse repeats this technique two or three times and listens to the intensity, pitch, quality, and duration of the sound produced. Long fingernails may limit the ability to percuss.

Percussion produces five distinguishable notes as described in Table 29–4. These sounds assist the nurse in determining the density of the underlying structures (i.e., whether the lung tissue contains air or fluid or is solid). Percussion of the thorax is performed over the rib intercostal spaces because percussing the sternum, ribs, or scapulae yields sound indicating solid bone. Percussion penetrates only 2 to 3 inches (5–7 cm), so deeper lesions are not detected with this technique.

The percussion technique begins with the client sitting in an upright position. The nurse assesses the posterior thorax first and proceeds systematically, beginning at the apex and working toward the base. The apex of the lung extends about ¾ to 1½ inches (2–4 cm) above the clavicle anteriorly. Posteriorly, there is approximately a 2-inch (5 cm) width of lung tissue at the apex.

The nurse assesses diaphragmatic excursion by instructing the client to "take a deep breath and hold it" while percussing downward until dullness is noted at the lower border of the lung. Normal resonance of the lung stops at the diaphragm, where the sound becomes dull, and this site is marked. The nurse repeats the process after instructing the client to "let out all your breath and hold." The difference between the two markings or sounds is the diaphragmatic excursion, which may range from 1 to 2 inches (3–5 cm). The diaphragm is normally higher on the right because of the location of the liver. Diaphrag-

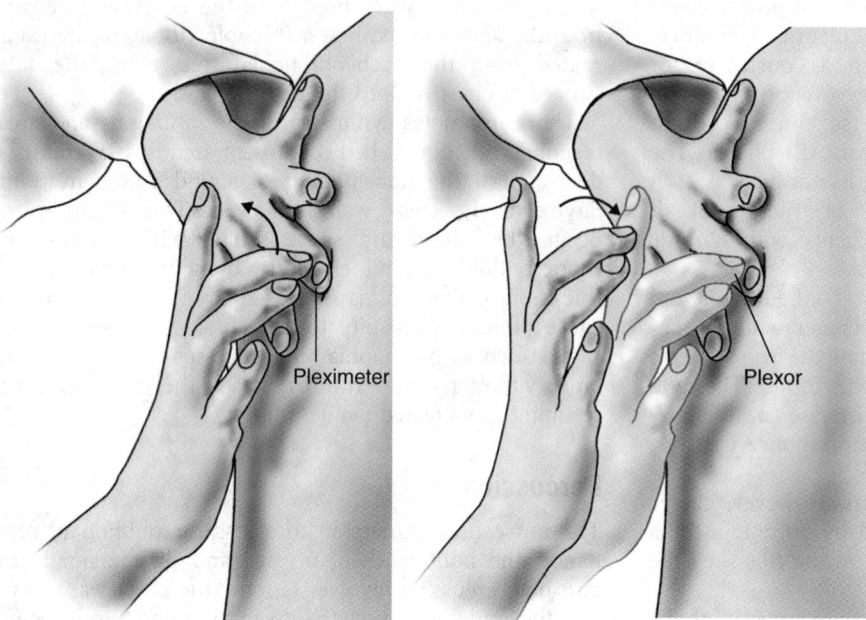

Figure 29–8. Percussion technique.

Pleximeter

Plexor

matic excursion may be decreased or absent in clients with pleurisy, diaphragm paralysis, or emphysema.

The nurse continues assessment of the thorax with percussion of the anterior and lateral chest. The percussion note changes from resonance of the normal lung to dullness at the borders of the heart and the liver. If a dull percussion note is found over lung tissue, the nurse expects that fluid or solid material is replacing the normal air-containing lung (as occurs in pneumonia, pleural effusion, fibrosis, atelectasis, and tumor).

Auscultation

Auscultation includes listening for normal breath sounds, adventitious sounds, and voice sounds. Auscultation provides information about the flow of air through the tracheobronchial tree and helps the listener identify fluid, mucus, or obstruction in the respiratory system. The diaphragm of the stethoscope is designed to detect high-pitched sounds.

The auscultation procedure begins with the client sit-

TABLE 29–4

Characteristic Features of the Five Percussion Notes

Note	Pitch	Intensity	Quality	Duration	Findings
Resonance	• Low	• Moderate to loud	• Hollow	• Long	• Resonance is characteristic of normal lung tissue.
Hyperresonance	• Higher than resonance	• Very loud	• Booming	• Longer than resonance	• Hyperresonance indicates the presence of trapped air, so it is commonly heard over an emphysematous or asthmatic lung and occasionally over a pneumothorax.
Flatness	• High	• Soft	• Extreme dullness	• Short	• An example location is the sternum. Flatness percussed over the lung fields may indicate a massive pleural effusion.
Dullness	• Medium	• Medium	• Thud-like	• Medium	• An example location is over the liver and the kidneys. Dullness can be percussed over atelectatic lung or consolidated lung.
Tympany	• High	• Loud	• Musical, drum-like	• Short	• Examples are the cheek filled with air and the abdomen distended with air. Over the lung, a tympanic note usually indicates a large pneumothorax.

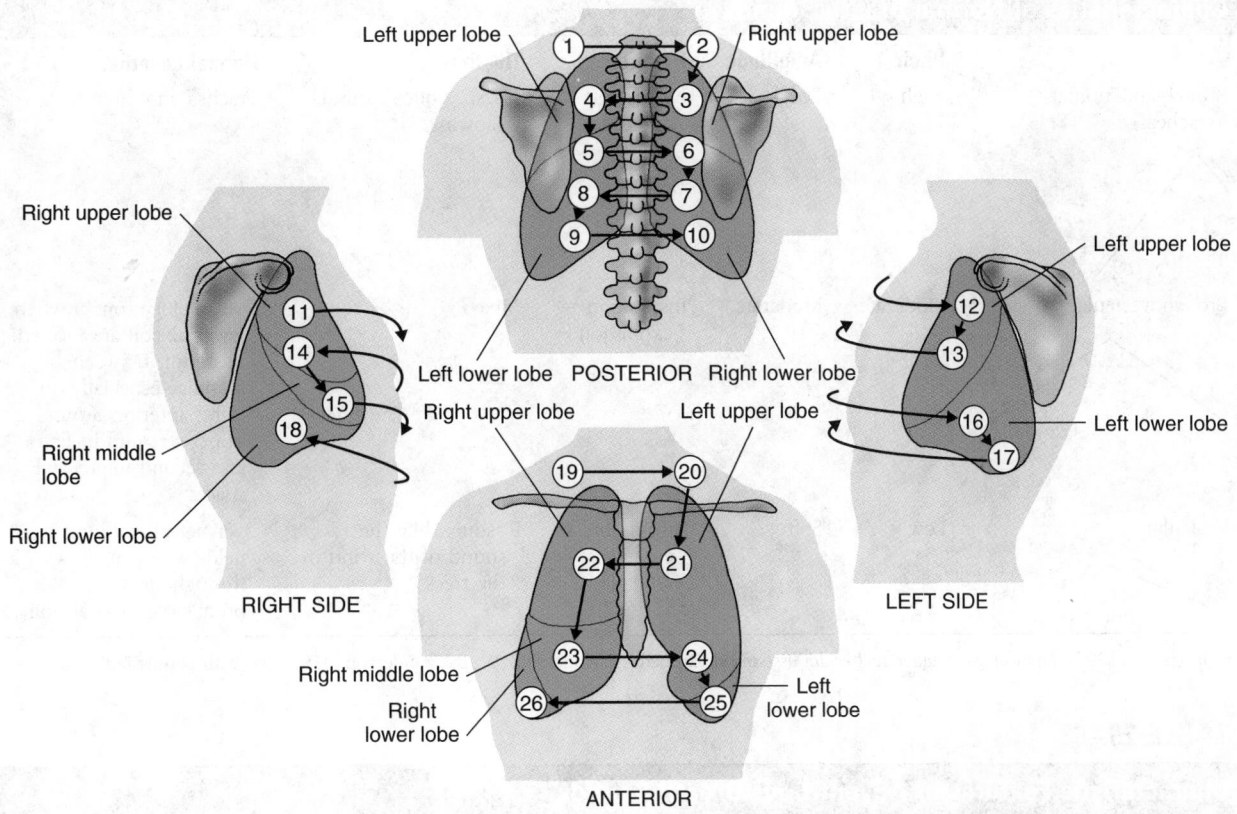

Figure 29–9. Sequence for percussion and auscultation.

ting in an upright position. With the stethoscope pressed firmly against the chest wall (clothing can distort or muffle sounds), the nurse instructs the client to breathe slowly and deeply through an open mouth. Breathing through the nose would set up turbulent sounds that are transmitted to the lungs. The nurse uses a systematic approach beginning at the apices and moving down through the intercostal spaces to the bases (Fig. 29–9). The nurse avoids listening over bony structures while auscultating the thorax posteriorly, laterally, and anteriorly. The nurse listens to a full respiratory cycle, noting the quality and intensity of the breath sounds. The nurse observes the client for signs of lightheadedness or dizziness caused by hyperventilation during auscultation and allows the client to breathe normally for a few minutes if these symptoms occur.

Normal Breath Sounds

Normal breath sounds are produced as air vibrates while passing through the respiratory passages from the larynx to the alveoli. Breath sounds are identified by their location, intensity, pitch, and duration within the respiratory cycle (e.g., early or late inspiration and expiration). Normal breath sounds are known as bronchial (or tubular), bronchovesicular, and vesicular (Table 29–5). The nurse describes these sounds as normal, increased, decreased (diminished), or absent.

When bronchial breath sounds are heard peripherally, they are abnormal. This increased sound occurs when there is transmission of centrally generated bronchial sounds to an area of increased density such as in clients with atelectasis, tumor, or pneumonia. Bronchovesicular breath sounds, when audible in an abnormal location, may indicate normal aging or an abnormality such as pulmonary consolidation and chronic airway disease.

Adventitious Breath Sounds

Adventitious sounds are additional breath sounds superimposed on normal sounds and indicate pathologic changes in the tracheobronchial tree. Table 29–6 classifies and describes the adventitious sounds: crackle, wheeze, rhonchus, and pleural friction rub (American College of Chest Physicians and the American Thoracic Society Joint Committee on Pulmonary Nomenclature, 1975; Mikami et al., 1987). Various subclassifications of these categories exist. Adventitious sounds vary in pitch, intensity, duration, and the phase of the respiratory cycle in which they occur. The terms for adventitious sounds vary among respiratory care practitioners. The nurse is encouraged to document exactly what is heard on auscultation instead of relying on numerous labels.

Voice Sounds

If the nurse discovers abnormalities during the physical assessment of the lungs and thorax, the client is assessed for vocal resonance. Auscultation of voice sounds through the normally air-filled lung produces a muffled, unclear sound because sound vibrations travel poorly through air. Vocal resonance is increased when the sound must travel

TABLE 29–5

Characteristics of Normal Breath Sounds

	Pitch	Amplitude	Duration	Quality	Normal Location
Bronchial (Tubular, tracheal)	High	Loud	Inspiration < expiration	Harsh, hollow, tubular, blowing	Trachea and larynx
Bronchovesicular	Moderate	Moderate	Inspiration = expiration	Mixed	Over major bronchi where fewer alveoli are located: posterior, between scapulae especially on right; anterior, around upper sternum in first and second intercostal spaces
Vesicular	Low	Soft	Inspiration > expiration	Rustling, like the sound of the wind in the trees	Over peripheral lung fields where air flows through smaller bronchioles and alveoli

From Jarvis, C. (1996). *Physical examination and health assessment* (2nd ed.). Philadelphia: W. B. Saunders, p. 479. Used with permission.

TABLE 29–6

Characteristic Features of Adventitious Breath Sounds

Adventitious Sound	Occurrence in the Respiratory Cycle	Character	Association
Discontinuous			
Fine crackles Fine rales High-pitched rales	• Either early or late inspiration	• Popping, discontinuous sounds caused by air moving into previously deflated airways; sounds like hair being rolled between fingers near the ear • "Velcro" sounds late in inspiration usually associated with restrictive disorders	Asbestosis Atelectasis Interstitial fibrosis Bronchitis Pneumonia Chronic pulmonary diseases
Coarse crackles Low-pitched crackles	• More common on expiration, but may be present early in inspiration	• Lower pitched, coarse, discontinuous rattling sounds caused by fluid or secretions in large airways; likely to change with coughing or suctioning	Bronchitis Pneumonia Tumors Pulmonary edema
Continuous			
Wheeze	• Audible during either inspiration or expiration, or both	• Squeaky, musical, continuous sounds associated with air rushing through narrowed airways; may be heard without a stethoscope • Arise from the small airways • Usually do not clear with coughing	Inflammation Bronchospasm Edema Secretions Pulmonary vessel engorgement (as in cardiac "asthma")
Rhonchus (rhonchi)	• Audible during both inspiration and expiration, but commonly more prominent on expiration	• Lower-pitched, coarse, continuous snoring sounds • Arise from the large airways	Thick tenacious secretions Sputum production Obstruction by foreign body Tumors
Pleural Friction Rub	• Heard during both inspiration and expiration, generally at the end of inspiration and the beginning of expiration	• Loud, rough, grating, scratching sounds caused by the inflamed surfaces of the pleura rubbing together; often associated with pain on deep inspirations • Heard in lateral lung fields	Pleurisy Tuberculosis Pulmonary infarction Pneumonia Lung cancer

through a solid or liquid medium, as it does in clients with a consolidated area of the lung, pneumonia, atelectasis, pleural effusion, tumor, or abscess.

BRONCHOPHONY. This is the abnormally loud and clear transmission of voice sounds through an area of increased density. For assessment of bronchophony, the client repeats the number *99* while the nurse systematically auscultates the thorax.

WHISPERED PECTORILOQUY. This is much more sensitive than bronchophony and is perceived by having the client whisper the number sequence *one, two, three.* Normally, whispered words sound faint and indistinct; if they are heard loudly and distinctly, the nurse suspects consolidation of lung tissue.

EGOPHONY. This is another form of abnormal vocal resonance and has a high-pitched, bleating, nasal quality. The nurse instructs the client to repeat the letter *E* and auscultates the thorax. Egophony exists when this letter is heard as a flat, nasal sound of *A* through the stethoscope. This abnormal sound indicates an area of consolidation, pleural effusion, or abscess.

PSYCHOSOCIAL ASSESSMENT

The nurse assesses aspects of the client's lifestyle that may significantly affect respiratory function. Some respiratory conditions may be exacerbated by stress. The nurse questions the client about present life stresses and usual coping mechanisms.

Chronic respiratory illnesses may cause changes in family roles and relationships, social isolation, financial problems, and unemployment or disability. By discussing coping mechanisms, the nurse assesses the client's reaction to these psychosocial stressors and discovers strengths as well as ineffective behaviors. For example, the client may react to stress with dependence on family members, withdrawal, or noncompliance with interventions. After completing the psychosocial assessment, the nurse assists the client in determining the support systems available to help cope with respiratory impairment.

DIAGNOSTIC ASSESSMENT
Laboratory Tests
Blood Tests

Several laboratory tests (Chart 29–2) are relevant to the care of clients with respiratory disorders. A red blood cell count (also see Chap. 41) provides data regarding the transport of oxygen from the lungs. A hemoglobin deficiency directly affects tissue oxygenation because hemoglobin transports oxygen to the cells and could cause hypoxemia.

Arterial blood gas (ABG) analysis assesses oxygenation (arterial oxygen pressure [PaO_2]), alveolar ventilation (arterial carbon dioxide pressure [$PaCO_2$]), and acid-base balance. Blood gas studies (also see Chap. 18) provide valuable information for monitoring treatment results, adjusting oxygen therapy, and evaluating the client's responses to treatment and therapy as during weaning from mechanical ventilation.

Sputum Tests

Sputum specimens obtained by expectoration or tracheal suctioning assist in the identification of pathogenic organisms or abnormal cells such as in a malignancy or a hypersensitivity state. Sputum culture and sensitivity analyses identify bacterial infection with either gram-negative or gram-positive organisms and determine the vulnerability to specific antibiotics. Cytologic examination is performed on sputum to help diagnose and specify malignant lesions by identifying cancer cells. Benign conditions, such as a hypersensitivity state, may also be identified by cytologic testing. Eosinophils and Curschmann's spirals (a mucous form) are often found by cytologic study in clients with allergic asthma.

Radiographic Examinations
Standard Radiography

Chest x-rays are taken for clients with respiratory tract disorders to evaluate the present status of the chest and to provide a baseline for comparison with future changes. Standard chest x-rays are taken from posteroanterior (PA; back to front) and left lateral (LL) projections. Portable chest x-rays (taken anteroposterior, or AP, front to back) cost more, and the films produced are of lower quality and are more difficult for the radiologist to interpret.

Chest x-rays can be used to assess pathologic changes in the lung such as those occurring in clients with pneumonia, atelectasis, pneumothorax, and tumor. The presence of pleural fluid and the position and placement of an endotracheal tube or other invasive catheters also can be detected by chest radiography. However, these films have limitations; they may appear normal even in a severe form of certain diseases, such as chronic bronchitis, asthma, and emphysema.

Sinus and facial x-rays are taken to assess the fluid levels in the sinus cavities to assist in the diagnosis of acute or chronic sinusitis.

Digital Chest Radiography

By using a computer, bone images can be eliminated from the chest x-ray, thereby creating better views of nonbone images. The test is useful in detecting lung lesions.

Tomography

Tomography is valuable in the assessment of the client with a respiratory disorder because pulmonary densities, tumors, and lesions can be seen. Positron emission tomography (PET) is useful for studying ventilation-perfusion relationships in the lung. Computed tomography (CT) provides consecutive 10-mm cross-sectional views of the thorax and produces a three-dimensional assessment of the lungs and the thorax.

Chart 29–2

Laboratory Profile: Respiratory Assessment

Test	Normal Range for Adults	Significance of Abnormal Findings
Blood Studies		
Complete blood count		
Red blood cells	Females: 18–44 years: 3.8–5.1 million/mm³ 45–64 years: 3.8–5.3 million/mm³ 65–74 years: 3.8–5.2 million/mm³ Males: 18–44 years: 4.3–5.7 million/mm³ 45–64 years: 4.2–5.6 million/mm³ 65–74 years: 3.8–5.8 million/mm³	*Elevated levels* (polycythemia) may be due to the excessive production of erythropoietin, which occurs in response to a hypoxic stimulus, as in CAL and from living at high altitude. *Decreased levels* indicate possible anemia, hemorrhage, or hemolysis.
Hemoglobin, total	Females: 18–44 years: 11.7–15.5 g/dL, or 117–155 g/L 45–64 years: 11.7–16 g/dL, or 117–160 g/L 65–74 years: 11.7–16.1 g/dL, or 117–161 g/L Males: 18–44 years: 13.2–17.3 g/dL, or 132–173 g/L 45–64 years: 13.1–17.2 g/dL, or 131–172 g/L	Same as for red blood cells
Hematocrit	Females: 18–44 years: 35%–45% 45–74 years: 35%–47% Males: 18–44 years: 39%–49% 45–64 years: 39%–50% 65–74 years: 37%–51%	Same as for red blood cells
White blood cell count (leukocyte count, WBC count)	Total: 4.5–11.0 × 10³ cells/μL, or 7.4 IRU African-Americans: 3.6–10.2 × 10³ cells/μL	*Elevations* indicate possible acute infections or inflammations, pneumonia, meningitis, tonsillitis, or emphysema. *Decreased levels* may indicate an overwhelming infection, an autoimmune disorder, or immunosuppressant therapy.
Differential white blood cell (leukocyte) count		
Neutrophils	1.8–7.7 × 10³ cells/μL; 18%–77% of total African-Americans: slightly lower	*Elevations* indicate possible acute bacterial infection (pneumonia), CAL, or inflammatory conditions (smoking). *Decreased levels* indicate possible viral disease (influenza).
Eosinophils	0–0.7 × 10³ cells/μL; 0%–7% of total	*Elevations* indicate possible CAL, asthma, or allergies. *Decreased levels* in pyogenic infections
Basophils	0–0.15 × 10³ cells/μL; 0%–1.5% of total	*Elevations* indicate possible inflammation; seen in chronic sinusitis, hypersensitivity reactions. *Decreased levels* may be seen in an acute infection.

Continued

Fat, cystic, and solid tissue can be distinguished with CT. By adding an intravenously (IV) injected contrast agent, vessels and other soft tissue structures can be identified. CT is especially valuable in studying the mediastinum, the hilar region, and the pleural space. The newer high-resolution CT (HRCT) uses 1.5-mm to 2-mm "slices" to assist in the assessment of bronchial abnormalities, interstitial disease, and emphysema. Nursing interventions for clients undergoing CT include education about the procedure and determination of the client's sensitivity to the contrast medium.

Ventilation and Perfusion Scanning

A ventilation and perfusion scan (also known as a $\dot{V}/\dot{Q}$ scan) identifies the areas of the lung being ventilated and the distribution of pulmonary blood. It is used primarily to confirm or rule out a diagnosis of pulmonary embolism.

Chart 29–2. Laboratory Profile: Respiratory Assessment   Continued

Test	Normal Range for Adults	Significance of Abnormal Findings
Lymphocytes	$1.5–4.0 \times 10^3$ cells/μL; 15%–40% of total	*Elevations* indicate possible viral infection, pertussis, and infectious mononucleosis. *Decreased levels* may be seen during corticosteroid
Monocytes	$0–0.8 \times 10^3$ cells/μL; 0%–8% of total	*Elevations*: see Lymphocytes; also may indicate active tuberculosis. *Decreased levels*: see Lymphocytes.
Arterial blood gases		
PaO$_2$	83–100 mmHg Elderly: values may be lower	*Elevations* indicate possible excessive oxygen administration. *Decreased levels* indicate possible CAL, chronic bronchitis, cancer of the bronchi and lungs, cystic fibrosis, respiratory distress syndrome, anemias, atelectasis, or any other cause of hypoxia.
PaCO$_2$	Females: 32–45 mmHg Males: 35–48 mmHg	*Elevations* indicate possible CAL, pneumonia, anesthesia effects, or use of opioids (respiratory acidosis). *Decreased levels* indicate hyperventilation/respiratory alkalosis.
pH	Up to 60 years: 7.35–7.45 60–90 years: 7.31–7.42 >90 years: 7.26–7.43	*Elevations* indicate metabolic or respiratory alkalosis. *Decreased levels* indicate metabolic or respiratory acidosis.
HCO$_3^-$	22–26 mEq/L	*Elevations* indicate possible respiratory acidosis as compensation for a primary metabolic alkalosis. *Decreased levels* indicate possible respiratory alkalosis as compensation for a primary metabolic acidosis.
SaO$_2$	94%–98% Elderly: values may be slightly lower	*Decreased levels* indicate possible impaired ability of hemoglobin to release oxygen to tissues.
Sputum studies		
Gram's stain	Negative	Presence of gram-positive or gram-negative bacteria indicates the type of microorganism that is causing the respiratory infection.
Culture and sensitivity	Negative	Presence of microorganisms indicates possible respiratory infections (e.g., pneumonia or bronchitis).
Acid-fast stain	No acid-fast bacilli	Presence of bacilli indicates possible tuberculosis.
Cytologic tests	Negative	Presence of abnormal cells indicates possible malignancy.

CAL = Chronic airflow limitation (formerly referred to as chronic obstructive pulmonary disease [COPD]); IRU = international recommended unit; PaO$_2$ = partial pressure of arterial oxygen; PaCO$_2$ = partial pressure of arterial carbon dioxide; HCO$_3^-$ = bicarbonate ion; SaO$_2$ = arterial oxygen saturation.

To perform the study, the physician first injects a radionuclide with the client in a supine position and then takes six perfusion views: anterior, posterior, right and left lateral, and two obliques. If the perfusion scan is normal, there is no reason to continue with the ventilation scan. Otherwise, the client inhales a radioactive gas or a radioaerosol and the lung is scanned continuously as the substance is making its way into the lungs (the wash-in phase), once the substance has reached equilibrium within the lungs, and then during the time the substance is leaving the lungs (the wash-out phase).

The nurse teaches the client about the procedure and explains that the radioactive substance will clear from the body in approximately 8 hours.

Bronchography

Bronchography is now considered an archaic technique for evaluation of the bronchial tree (Bordow & Moser, 1996, p. 7).

Other Noninvasive Diagnostic Tests

Pulse Oximetry

Pulse oximetry identifies hemoglobin saturation. Usually, hemoglobin is almost 100% saturated with oxygen. The pulse oximeter uses a wave of infrared light and a sensor placed on the client's finger, toe, nose, earlobe, or forehead. Ideal normal pulse oximetry values are 95% to 100%; in elderly clients, values may be a little lower. So as not to be confused with the PaO_2 values from arterial blood gases, the pulse oximetry reading is recorded as the SaO_2, or SpO_2.

A pulse oximetry reading can alert the nurse to desaturation before clinical signs occur (e.g., dusky skin, pale mucosa, and nail beds). The nurse, however, considers client movement, hypothermia, decreased peripheral blood flow, ambient light (sunlight, infrared lamps), decreased hemoglobin, and edema as possible causes for low readings. Positioning or covering of the sensor could yield better accuracy if ambient light was present.

The nurse may consider results lower than 91% (and certainly below 86%) an emergency, necessitating immediate treatment. If the SaO_2 is below 85%, the body's tissues have a difficult time becoming oxygenated. An SaO_2 of less than 70% is certainly life threatening in the typical person, but values below 80% may be life threatening in others. Pulse oximetry readings are the least accurate at the lower values.

Pulmonary Function Tests

Pulmonary function tests (PFTs) evaluate lung function and dysfunction and include studies such as lung volumes and capacities, flow rates, diffusion capacity, gas exchange, airway resistance, and distribution of ventilation. The physician interprets the results by comparing the client's data with normal findings predicted according to age, sex, race, height, and weight. Smoking has a definite effect on PFTs, but studies have shown that smoking cessation is beneficial to the lungs (see Research Applications for Nursing).

PFTs are useful in screening clients for pulmonary disease even before the onset of signs or symptoms. Serial testing gives objective data that may be used as a guide to treatment (e.g., changes in pulmonary function can support a decision to continue, change, or discontinue a specific therapy). Preoperative evaluation with pulmonary function tests may identify the client at risk for postoperative pulmonary complications. One of the most common reasons for performing such tests is to determine the cause of breathlessness. When performed while the client exercises, PFTs help to determine whether dyspnea is caused by a pulmonary or a cardiac dysfunction or by muscle deconditioning. These tests are also useful for determining the effect of the client's occupation on pulmonary function and evaluating any related disability for legal purposes.

CLIENT PREPARATION. The nurse prepares the client for PFTs by explaining the purpose and value of the tests for planning the client's care. The client is advised not to smoke for 6 to 8 hours before testing. According to institutional policy and procedure, the nurse withholds bronchodilator medication for 4 to 6 hours before the test. Frequently, the client with respiratory impairment fears further breathlessness and is usually anxious before these so-called "breathing" tests. The nurse helps to alleviate apprehension by describing what the client will experience during and after the testing.

PROCEDURE. PFTs can be performed at the client's bedside or in the respiratory laboratory. The client is asked to breathe through the mouth only. A nose clip may be used to prevent air from escaping. The client performs different breathing maneuvers while measurements (Fig. 29–10) are obtained. Table 29–7 describes the most frequently used PFTs and their purpose.

FOLLOW-UP CARE. Because numerous breathing maneuvers are performed during pulmonary function tests, the nurse observes the client for increased dyspnea or bronchospasm after such studies. The nurse notes whether bronchodilator medication was administered during testing and alters the client's medication schedule as indicated.

Exercise Testing

Exercise, or activity in general, increases metabolism and gas transport as energy is generated. Five reasons for exercise testing are listed in Table 29–8. The tests are performed on a treadmill or bicycle or by a self-paced 12-minute walking test. The normal client's exercise is limited by hemodynamic factors, whereas the pulmonary client's limitation is ventilatory capacity or pulmonary

---

▷ Research Applications for Nursing

Cessation of Smoking Has an Effect on Pulmonary Function

Burchfiel, C. M., Marcus, E. B., Curb, J. D., et al. (1995). Effects of smoking and smoking cessation on longitudinal decline in pulmonary function. American Journal of Respiratory and Critical Care Medicine (151), 1778–1785.

In this study the effects of smoking and smoking cessation on the rate of FEV_1 decline over 6 years were examined in 4451 men between the ages of 45 and 68 years.

The researchers found that the men who continued to smoke had steeper rates of decline than those who had never smoked. The duration of their smoking habit was significantly associated with the rate of decline, but pack-years was of only borderline significance.

In the first 2 years for men who had quit smoking, the rate of decline was the same as those who continued to smoke, but after those 2 years, the rate of decline was similar to those who had never smoked. Even the men who were smokers and had impaired pulmonary function showed a slower rate of decline after smoking cessation.

Critique. Only men from a limited geographic area were studied, which could limit the generalization of these results to the broader population.

Possible Nursing Implications. With knowledge from this and other research studies, the nurse can become more involved with public education regarding smoking and smoking cessation at the community and national levels. The nurse can lobby for more research funds to be devoted to duplicating studies such as this one in women.

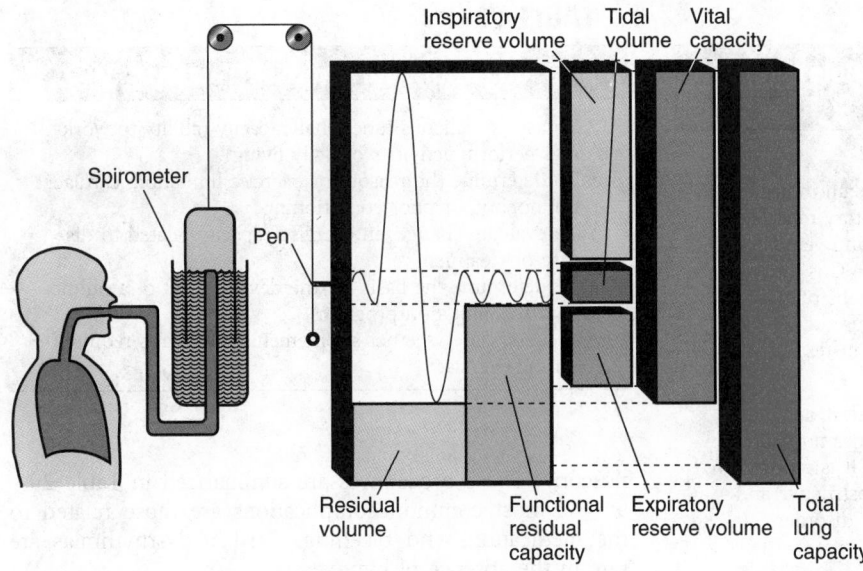

Figure 29–10. Common measurements in pulmonary function testing. Adapted from Luce, J. M., Pierson, D. J., & Tyler, M. L. (1993). *Intensive respiratory care* (2nd ed.). Philadelphia: W. B. Saunders).

gas exchange compromise, or both. The nurse explains exercise testing to the client and assures the client of close monitoring by trained professionals throughout the testing.

Skin Tests

Skin tests are used in combination with other diagnostic data to identify various infectious diseases (such as tuberculosis), viral diseases (such as mononucleosis and mumps), and fungal diseases (such as coccidioidomycosis and histoplasmosis). The presence of allergic hypersensitivity and the status of the immune system can be demonstrated through skin testing. Exposure to the allergen or organism used in testing produces a specific reaction (delayed hypersensitivity reaction) of the client's immune system. (For further discussion, see Chapters 23 and 25.)

CLIENT PREPARATION. To ensure cooperation and to alleviate anxiety, the nurse explains the purpose of skin testing and the procedure to the client. The client is questioned about a history of hypersensitivity to any of the local antigens used or a previous reaction to skin tests. The nurse also informs the client what is expected after testing is completed; for example, to prevent infection or abscess formation, the client is warned not to scratch the testing site. The client is also instructed to refrain from washing test or injection sites that have been circled with a marking pen for identification.

PROCEDURE. The actual procedure depends on the specific purpose of the test and the institution's policy. An intradermal injection technique causes a wheal to form after injection of the antigen. It is vital that the nurse perform the procedure correctly because incorrect antigen administration is responsible for erroneous results. The nurse ensures that the chosen test site is free from excessive body hair, dermatitis, and blemishes. A severe anaphylactic response can occur in clients who are hypersensitive to the test antigens. The nurse must recognize

and be prepared to treat reactions as described in Chapter 25.

FOLLOW-UP CARE. The reaction at injection sites is interpreted 24 to 72 hours after administration of the test antigen. If the testing is done as an outpatient procedure, the nurse instructs the client when to return to have the results read. The nurse documents the amount of induration (hard swelling) in millimeters and the presence of erythema and vesiculation (formation of small blister-like elevations).

Magnetic Resonance Imaging

Magnetic resonance imaging (MRI) assists in the diagnosis of respiratory system disorders by providing information about the type and condition of the tissues being imaged along any plane inside the body: vertically, horizontally, and diagonally. This costly procedure requires little client preparation other than the removal of all metal objects. Because of the powerful magnets used in MRI, clients with pacemakers, aneurysm clips, inner-ear implants, cardiac valves, or metallic foreign objects in the body are not candidates for MRI. The nurse informs the client of possible claustrophobia and discomfort from lying inside the magnet's small cylinder on a hard, cool table. The nurse instructs the client in the use of relaxation techniques and imagery to help decrease these sensations. In some cases, however, sedation may be necessary. In addition, the nurse informs the client that the noises heard during the examination are the natural, rhythmic sounds of radiofrequency pulses, which may range from barely audible to noticeable.

Other Invasive Diagnostic Tests

Endoscopic Examinations

Endoscopic diagnostic studies to assess respiratory disorders include bronchoscopy, laryngoscopy, and mediasti-

TABLE 29-7

Characteristics and Purposes of Pulmonary Function Tests

Test	Purpose
FVC (forced vital capacity) records the maximal amount of air that can be exhaled as quickly as possible after maximal inspiration.	• FVC gives an indication of respiratory muscle strength and ventilatory reserve. FVC is often reduced in obstructive disease because of air trapping and in restrictive disease.
FEV_1 (forced expiratory volume in 1 sec) records the maximal amount of air that can be exhaled in the first second of expiration.	• FEV_1 is effort dependent and declines normally with age. It is reduced in certain obstructive and restrictive disorders.
FEV_1/FVC is the ratio of expiratory volume in 1 sec to FVC.	• This ratio provides a much more sensitive indication of obstruction to airflow. This ratio is the hallmark of obstructive pulmonary disease. It is normal or increased in restrictive disease.
$FEF_{25\%-75\%}$ records the forced expiratory flow over the 25%–75% volume (middle half) of the FVC.	• This measure provides a more sensitive index of obstruction in the smaller airways.
FRC (functional residual capacity) is the amount of air remaining in the lungs after normal expiration. FRC requires use of the helium dilution technique.	• Increased FRC indicates hyperinflation of air trapping, which may result from obstructive pulmonary disease. FRC is normal or decreased in restrictive pulmonary diseases.
TLC (total lung capacity) is the amount of air in the lungs at the end of maximal inhalation.	• Increased TLC indicates air trapping associated with obstructive pulmonary disease. Decreased TLC indicates restrictive disease.
RV (residual volume) is the amount of air remaining in the lungs at the end of a full, forced exhalation.	• RV is increased in obstructive pulmonary disease such as emphysema.
DLCO (diffusion capacity of carbon monoxide) reflects the surface area of the alveolocapillary membrane. The client inhales a small amount of CO, holds for 10 sec, then exhales. The amount inhaled is compared with the amount exhaled.	• DLCO is reduced whenever the alveolocapillary membrane is diminished, as occurs in emphysema, pulmonary hypertension, and pulmonary fibrosis. It is increased with exercise and in conditions such as polycythemia and congestive heart disease.

TABLE 29-8

Five Indications for Exercise Testing

• To assess a client's functional capacity (ability to work and perform activities of daily living)
• To determine the reason for exercise limitation: cardiac, pulmonary, or poor conditioning
• To evaluate changes in exercise capacity related to disease or treatment
• To determine the basis for the development of a pulmonary rehabilitation program
• To determine whether supplemental oxygen is required during exercise

noscopy. These procedures are summarized in Table 29-9. The most common complications are those related to the medications and bleeding. Cardiac dysrhythmias are rare in the absence of hypoxemia.

Thoracentesis

Thoracentesis is the aspiration of pleural fluid or air from the pleural space. This procedure is used for diagnosis or treatment. Microscopic examination of the pleural fluid helps make a diagnosis. Pleural fluid may be drained to relieve pulmonary compression and the resultant respiratory distress caused by cancer, empyema, pleurisy, or tuberculosis. To assist in further assessment of the parietal pleura, thoracentesis is often followed by pleural biopsy. Thoracentesis also allows the instillation of medications into the pleural space, which may be necessary to prevent further fluid formation in certain cases of pleural effusion caused by lung cancer.

CLIENT PREPARATION. Adequate client preparation is essential before thoracentesis to ensure the client's cooperation during the procedure and to prevent complications. The nurse tells the client to expect a stinging sensation from the local anesthetic agent and a feeling of pressure when the needle is inserted. The nurse reinforces the importance of the client's not moving (avoiding coughing, deep breathing, or sudden movement) during the procedure to avoid puncture of the visceral pleura or lung.

Figure 29-11 illustrates appropriate positions for thoracentesis. These positions widen the intercostal spaces and permit the physician to have easy access to where the pleural fluid gravitates. The nurse properly positions and physically supports the client. Pillows are used to make the client comfortable and to provide physical support.

Before the procedure, the nurse checks the client's history for hypersensitivity to local anesthetic agents and checks to make sure the client has signed an informed consent. The entire chest or back is exposed, and the aspiration site is shaved if necessary. The actual site depends on the volume and location of the effusion, which are determined by radiography and physical examination procedures such as percussion.

PROCEDURE. Thoracentesis is usually done at the bedside, although ultrasonography or computed tomography

TABLE 29-9

Care of the Client Undergoing Endoscopic Tests for Respiratory Disorders

Procedure	Purpose and Description	Nursing Interventions	Rationale
Bronchoscopy	• To assess airway anatomy for tumors, obstruction, and atelectasis • To assist in the diagnosis of infection or cancer by biopsy of lesions; biopsy techniques include the brush biopsy and needle aspiration • To remove thick secretions, mucus plugs, or foreign bodies • A flexible fiberoptic bronchoscope is inserted through the mouth, nose, endotracheal tube, or tracheostomy tube. The procedure may be done in the operating room or the radiology department. Oxygen administration and blood pressure monitoring are standard procedures.	• Allow the client nothing by mouth for several hours before the test. • Assess for allergies to iodine, local anesthetics, or pretest medications. • Place pulse oximeter • Administer pretest medications (atropine, diazepam) as ordered. • Prepare the client for topical anesthetic administration into the oropharynx. • Remove the client's dentures if present. • After the procedure, monitor the client's vital signs for 15 min until stable and monitor for hemoptysis. • After the procedure, allow the client nothing by mouth until the gag reflex returns. • Discourage smoking, talking, and coughing for several hours.	• The client may aspirate gastric contents if vomiting occurs. • A knowledge of allergies helps prevent allergic reactions. • For continuous monitoring throughout the procedure. • Pretest medications help decrease secretions and reduce anxiety. • Explanations about the effects of the anesthetic agent (numbness and gagging) help to decrease anxiety. • Injury may occur if dentures are left in place. • Assessment helps the nurse detect respiratory distress and signs of complications related to the procedure. • Allowing the client nothing by mouth reduces the possibility of aspiration. • Throat irritation is decreased by avoiding these activities.
Laryngoscopy	• *Direct:* To detect or remove lesions or foreign bodies in the larynx or to diagnose cancer by removing tissue for biopsy or samples for culture. A fiberoptic laryngoscope is used. • *Indirect:* To assess the function of the vocal cords or to obtain tissue for biopsy. Observations are made during rest and phonation by using a laryngeal mirror, head mirror, and light source.	• Allow the client nothing by mouth for several hours before the test. • Assess the client for allergies to iodine, contrast media, or local anesthetics. • Administer pretest medications (atropine, diazepam) as ordered. • Assess the client for fears concerning the procedure. Assure the client that he or she will be monitored for any respiratory problems. • For indirect laryngoscopy, assist the client to sit in an upright position and encourage normal breathing. • After the procedure, allow the client nothing by mouth until the gag reflex returns. • Encourage coughing and fluid intake. • Assess vital signs frequently for 24 hr. Assess the client for bleeding. • After the procedure, administer lozenges or gargles as ordered.	• Aspiration is possible if vomiting occurs. • A knowledge of allergies helps prevent allergic reactions. • Pretest medications help decrease secretions and reduce anxiety. • Reassurance helps decrease fears about not being able to breathe during the procedure. • An upright sitting position facilitates the passage of the laryngeal mirror into the mouth. • The client may aspirate gastric contents if vomiting occurs. • Hydration and coughing promote the expectoration of secretions. • Frequent monitoring of vital signs enables the nurse to detect changes such as dyspnea. • Lozenges and gargles help to relieve sore throat.

Table continued on following page

TABLE 29–9

	Care of the Client Undergoing Endoscopic Tests for Respiratory Disorders *Continued*		
Procedure	**Purpose and Description**	**Nursing Interventions**	**Rationale**
Mediastinoscopy	• To inspect and remove samples for biopsy of lymph nodes that drain the lung • To detect metastasis of lung cancer • To obtain tissue for biopsy for diagnosis of tuberculosis or sarcoidosis • The procedure is done in the operating room with the client given local or general anesthesia; a suprasternal incision is used.	• Explain preoperative measures and the procedure to the client. • Postoperatively, assess the client for bleeding, pneumothorax, and vocal cord paralysis. • Assess the client for pain, and administer analgesics as ordered.	• Explanations about the anticipated procedure help to decrease anxiety. • Ongoing assessment for complications helps to ensure prompt treatment. • Medication decreases discomfort associated with the procedure.

may be used to guide it. After draping the client and cleaning the skin with a germicidal solution, the physician uses aseptic technique and injects a local anesthetic agent into the selected intercostal space. The nurse keeps the client informed of the procedure while observing for shock, pain, nausea, pallor, diaphoresis, cyanosis, tachypnea, and dyspnea. The physician advances the short 18- to 25-gauge thoracentesis needle with a syringe attached into the pleural space. Gentle suction is applied as the fluid in the pleural space is slowly aspirated. A vacuum collection bottle is sometimes necessary to remove larger volumes of fluid. To prevent reexpansion pulmonary edema, no more than 1000 mL of fluid is removed at one time (Bordow & Moser, 1996, p. 57). If a pleural biopsy is to be performed, a second, larger needle with a cutting edge and collection chamber is used (Luce et al., 1993, p. 95). After the physician withdraws the needle, pressure is applied to the puncture site, followed by the application of a small sterile dressing.

FOLLOW-UP CARE. After thoracentesis, the physician orders a chest x-ray to rule out possible pneumothorax and subsequent mediastinal shift. The nurse monitors the client's vital signs and auscultates breath sounds while

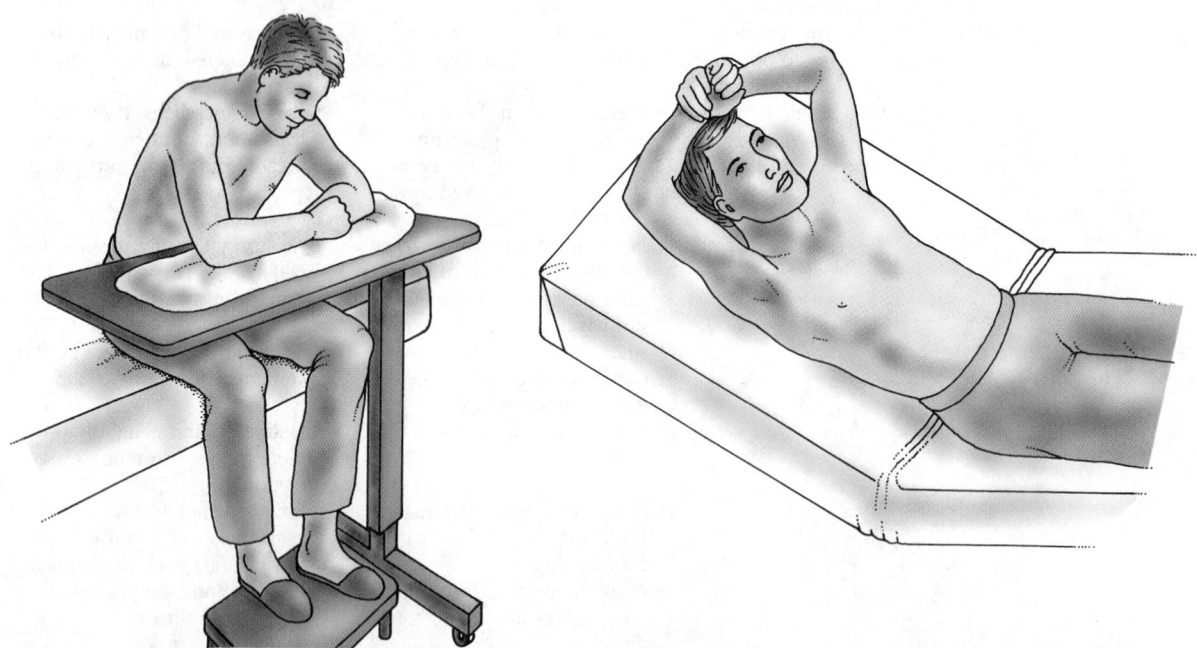

Sitting on the edge of a bed with the feet supported. The arms and shoulders are elevated, and the head is resting on the overbed table, which is padded with pillows or bath blankets.

Sitting in bed in semi-Fowler's position with the arm on the side on which the procedure will be performed raised above the head. The other arm may be used to hold the one arm as still as possible.

Figure 29–11. Positions for thoracentesis.

noting absent or diminished sounds on the affected side. The nurse observes the puncture site and dressing for leakage or bleeding. The nurse also assesses for other complications after thoracentesis, such as reaccumulation of fluid in the pleural space, subcutaneous emphysema, pyrogenic infection, and tension pneumothorax. The client is encouraged to breathe deeply to promote reexpansion of the lung. The nurse documents the procedure in the client's chart and notes the client's tolerance, the volume and character of the fluid removed, any specimens sent to the laboratory, the location of the puncture site, and respiratory assessment findings before, during, and after the procedure.

Lung Biopsy

Lung biopsy is performed to obtain tissue for histologic analysis, culture, or cytologic examination. The physician uses tissue samples to make a definite diagnosis regarding the type of malignancy, infection, inflammation, or other type of lung disease. Biopsy procedures include transbronchial biopsy (TBB) and transbronchial needle aspiration (TBNA), both performed in conjunction with bronchoscopy; transthoracic needle aspiration (percutaneous approach for areas not accessible by bronchoscopy); and open lung biopsy (in the operating room).

CLIENT PREPARATION. The nurse prepares the client by explaining what the client can expect before and after the biopsy. The client may have predetermined ideas about the outcome. The terms *biopsy* and *cancer* may be closely associated in the client's mind, so the nurse explores the client's feelings and fears before and after the procedure. To reduce discomfort and anxiety, the physician may prescribe an analgesic or sedative before the procedure. The nurse informs the client undergoing percutaneous biopsy that discomfort is minimized by the administration of a local anesthetic agent, but that the client may experience a sensation of pressure during insertion of the needle and aspiration of the tissue. For an open lung biopsy, the usual preoperative preparations apply.

PROCEDURE. Percutaneous lung biopsy may be performed in the client's room or in the radiology department after an informed consent has been obtained. Fluoroscopy, CT, or ultrasonography is frequently used to better visualize the area undergoing biopsy and to guide the procedure. Positioning of the client is similar to that for thoracentesis. The physician cleans the skin with an antibacterial agent and then administers a local anesthetic agent. Under sterile conditions, the physician inserts a spinal-type 18- to 22-gauge needle through the skin into the desired area (e.g., tissue, nodule, or lymph node) and obtains the tissue needed for microscopic examination. The nurse then applies a dressing.

Open lung biopsy is performed in the operating room. The client undergoes thoracotomy where lung tissue is exposed. At least two tissue specimens are taken (usually from an upper lobe and a lower lobe site). The surgeon places a chest tube to remove air and fluid so the lung can reinflate and then closes the chest.

FOLLOW-UP CARE. The nurse monitors the client's vital signs and breath sounds every 4 hours for 24 hours and assesses for signs of respiratory distress (e.g., dyspnea, pallor, diaphoresis, and tachypnea). Pneumothorax is the major complication after needle biopsy and open lung biopsy, so it is important for the nurse to report untoward signs and symptoms promptly. The nurse also monitors for hemoptysis, which may be scant and transient, or, in rare cases, for frank bleeding from vascular or lung trauma during the procedure.

SELECTED BIBLIOGRAPHY

*American College of Chest Physicians and the American Thoracic Society Joint Committee on Pulmonary Nomenclature. (1975). Pulmonary terms and symbols. *Chest, 67,* 583–593.

*Avalos-Bock, S. (1994). Getting a rise out of tuberculosis with the P.P.D. skin test. *Nursing, 24*(8), 51–53.

Bates, B. (1995). *A guide to physical examination and history taking* (6th ed.). Philadelphia: J. B. Lippincott.

Bordow, R. A., & Moser, K. M. (1996). *Manual of clinical problems in pulmonary medicine* (4th ed.). Boston: Little, Brown.

Burchfiel, C. M., Marcus, E. B., Curb, J. D., et al. (1995). Effects of smoking and smoking cessation on longitudinal decline in pulmonary function. *American Journal of Respiratory and Critical Care Medicine, 151,* 1778–1785.

*Carrieri-Kohlman, V., Douglas, M., Gormley, J., & Stulborg, M. (1993). Desensitization and guided mastery: Treatment approaches for the management of dyspnea. *Heart & Lung, 22*(3), 226–234.

Carroll, P. (1997). Pulose oximetry at your fingertips. *RN, 60*(2), 22–27.

Cerveri, I., Zoia, M. C., Fanfulla, F., et al. (1995). Reference values of arterial oxygen tension in the middle-aged and elderly. *American Journal of Respiratory and Critical Care Medicine, 152,* 934–941.

*Clemente, C. D. (Ed.). (1985). *Gray's anatomy of the human body* (30th ed.). Philadelphia: Lea & Febiger.

*Davis, D., & Scarpa, N. (1991). Transbronchial needle aspiration. *Gastroenterology Nursing, 14*(2), 80–84.

George, R. B., Light, R. W., Matthay, M. A., & Matthay, R. A. (1995). *Chest medicine: Essentials of pulmonary and critical care medicine* (3rd ed.). Baltimore: Williams & Wilkins.

*Gift, A. G. (1990). Dyspnea. *Nursing Clinics of North America, 25*(4), 955–965.

Guyton, A. C. (1996). *Textbook of medical physiology* (9th ed.). Philadelphia: W. B. Saunders.

Jarvis, C. (1996). *Physical examination and health assessment* (2nd ed.). Philadelphia: W. B. Saunders.

*Kernicki, J. G. (1993). Differentiating chest pain: Advanced assessment techniques. *Dimensions of Critical Care Nursing, 12*(2), 66–76.

*Kersten, L. D. (1989). *Comprehensive respiratory nursing: A decision making approach.* Philadelphia: W. B. Saunders.

Kirton, C. A. (1996). Assessing breath sounds. *Nursing, 26*(6), 50–51.

*Kuhn, J. K., & McGovern, M. (1992). Respiratory assessment of the elderly. *Journal of Gerontological Nursing, 18*(5), 40–43.

*Lehrer, S. (1993). *Understanding lung sounds* (2nd ed.). Philadelphia: W. B. Saunders.

Levitzky, M. G. (1995). *Pulmonary physiology* (4th ed.). New York: McGraw-Hill.

*Luce, J. M., Pierson, D. J., & Tyler, M. L. (1993). *Intensive respiratory care* (2nd ed.). Philadelphia: W. B. Saunders.

Matteson, M. A., McConnell, E. S., & Linton, A. D. (1997). *Gerontological nursing: Concepts and practice* (2nd ed.). Philadelphia: W. B. Saunders.

*Mikami, R., Murao, M., Cugell, D. W., et al. (1987). International Symposium on Lung Sounds: Synopsis of proceedings. *Chest, 92,* 342–345.

*Nield, M., & Kim, M. J. (1991). The reliability of magnitude estimation for dyspnea measurement. *Nursing Research, 40*(1), 17–19.

Paoletti, P., Carrozzi, L., Viegi, G., et al. (1995). Distribution of bronchial responsiveness in a general population: Effect of sex, age, smoking, and level of pulmonary function. *American Journal of Respiratory and Critical Care Medicine, 151,* 1770–1777.

Parker, S. L., Tong, T., Bolden, S., & Wingo, P. A. (1997). Cancer statistics, 1997. *CA-A Cancer Journal for Clinicians, 47*(1), 5–27.

*Report of the American College of Chest Physicians and the American Thoracic Society Ad Hoc Subcommittee on Pulmonary Nomenclature. (1977). *ATS News, 3,* 5–6.

Springhouse Corp. (1995). A quick look at common respiratory patterns. *Nursing, 25*(1), 32L.

Tietz, N. W. (1995). *Clinical guide to laboratory tests* (3rd ed.). Philadelphia: W. B. Saunders.

Villar, M. T. A., Dow, L., Coggon, D., et al. (1995). The influence of increased bronchial responsiveness, atopy, and serum IgE on decline in FEV1. *American Journal of Respiratory and Critical Care Medicine, 151,* 656–662.

*Wilkins, R., Hodghin, J., & Lopez, B. (1988). *Lung sounds: A practical approach.* St. Louis: C. V. Mosby.

*Williams, T. F. (Ed.). (1984). *Rehabilitation in the aging.* New York: Raven.

SUGGESTED READINGS

Avalos-Bock, S. (1994). Getting a rise out of tuberculosis with the P.P.D. skin test. *Nursing, 24*(8), 51–53.

The article includes clear photographs showing the steps to take in placing a P.P.D. Interpretation of results, even for high-risk groups, is included. Proper documentation of the test and results is addressed.

Carroll, P. (1997). Pulse oximetry at your fingertips. *RN, 60*(2), 22–27.

This clear and concise article covers a number of items related to determining a client's state of oxygenation, including dissolved oxygen versus bound oxygen, the importance of knowing the client's hemoglobin to interpret the pulse oximetry reading accurately, and an explanation of technical factors such as motion and ambient light that can affect readings. The formula for calculating a client's overall oxygen-carrying capacity is included, as is an explanation of the graphic relationship between the PaO_2 and the oxygen saturation.

Springhouse Corp. (1995). A quick look at common respiratory patterns. *Nursing, 25*(1), 32L.

This one-page chart identifies the characteristics of eight different respiration patterns, including Cheyne-Stokes respirations, cluster breathing, and apneustic breathing. A drawing accompanies each pattern.

Chapter 30

INTERVENTIONS FOR CLIENTS WITH OXYGEN OR TRACHEOSTOMY

Oxygen Therapy

Overview

Oxygen (O_2) is a potent drug prescribed by the physician for relief of symptoms of hypoxemia (low levels of oxygen in the blood) and its resultant hypoxia (decreased tissue oxygenation). The usual oxygen content of atmospheric air is approximately 21%; supplemental oxygen is prescribed when oxygen needs of the body cannot be met on "room air" alone. Oxygen is used for both episodic (acute) and subacute or chronic respiratory conditions associated with decreased partial pressure of arterial oxygen (PaO_2) levels. Oxygen therapy is indicated in conditions outside the respiratory system such as increased oxygen demand, decreased oxygen-carrying capability of the blood, and decreased cardiac output. Conditions that increase oxygen demand include sepsis, fever, and the increased workload of dyspnea. Insufficient amounts of hemoglobin or altered hemoglobin quality result in the inability of the hemoglobin to carry enough oxygen to the tissues.

The goal of oxygen therapy is to use the lowest fraction of inspired oxygen (FIO_2) to produce the most acceptable oxygenation without causing the development of harmful side effects. Although oxygen improves the PaO_2 level, it does not cure the condition or stop the disease process.

The average client requires an oxygen flow of 2–4 L/minute via nasal cannula or up to 40% via Venturi mask. The client who is hypoxemic and also has chronic hypercarbia requires lower levels of oxygen delivery, usually 1–2 L/minute via nasal cannula. A low arterial oxygen level is this client's primary drive for breathing.

Collaborative Management

 Assessment

Arterial blood gas (ABG) analysis is the best tool for determining the need for oxygen therapy and for evaluating its effects. Oxygen need can also be determined by noninvasive monitoring, such as pulse oximetry.

 Interventions

The nurse administers oxygen as per physician order or approved protocol. Before initiating oxygen therapy and while caring for a client receiving oxygen therapy, the nurse is knowledgeable about associated hazards and complications. For a particular client, the nurse also knows the rationale and the expected outcome related to oxygen therapy.

> *Hazards and Complications of Oxygen Therapy*

Oxygen therapy is associated with several hazards and complications. Understanding these hazards and complications, the nurse can detect early signs and symptoms.

Combustion. Oxygen itself does not burn, but it supports combustion. Therefore, a fire burns more readily in the presence of oxygen. The nurse takes special precautions, including posting a sign on the door of the client's room. During the administration of oxygen, smoking is prohibited in the client's room, including at home. All electrical equipment must be grounded (i.e., with three prongs having a green or red dot on the plate). Frayed cords must be repaired because they can cause a spark that can ignite a flame. Any type of flammable solution containing alcohol or oil is prohibited from the room when oxygen is in use.

Oxygen-Induced Hypoventilation. The nurse assesses for oxygen-induced hypoventilation in the client whose principal respiratory drive is hypoxia (hypoxic drive), as in the client with chronic lung disease who also has hypercarbia. Arterial carbon dioxide level ($PaCO_2$) for these clients gradually rises over time. The central chemoreceptors in the brain (medulla) are normally sensitive to high $PaCO_2$ levels, which stimulate breathing and cause an increased respiratory rate. When the $PaCO_2$ increases above 60–65 mmHg, however, this normal mechanism shuts off. At that point, peripheral chemoreceptors found in the carotid and aortic arch bodies become the major stimulus for breathing. These peripheral receptors are sensitive to low PaO_2 levels. When PaO_2 drops below 55–60 mmHg, these receptors signal the brain to increase the respiratory rate or depth, which results in a hypoxic drive to breathe (Fig. 30–1).

The hypoxic drive occurs only in the presence of severely elevated $PaCO_2$ levels (i.e., in the client who has hypoxemia *and* hypercarbia). When the client with PaO_2 levels less than 55–60 mmHg (and $PaCO_2$ levels greater than 60–65 mmHg) receives oxygen therapy, the PaO_2 level increases. The hypoxic drive, however, the only stimulation for breathing, is eliminated. As a result, the client experiences respiratory depression that could lead to apnea or respiratory arrest. (The client being ventilated mechanically will not be at risk for this complication.)

The physician prescribes oxygen therapy at the lowest liter flow (usually 1–2 or 3 L/minute) necessary to treat the hypoxemia without raising the $PaCO_2$. A system that delivers precise oxygen concentrations in low amounts, such as a nasal cannula or Venturi mask, is preferred for this client.

The nurse closely monitors the respiratory rate and depth while the client is receiving oxygen. This monitoring is especially important when it is the first time the client has received oxygen or when the $PaCO_2$ levels are not known. Signs and symptoms of hypoventilation are seen during the first 30 minutes of oxygen administration; the client's color improves (from ashen or gray to pink) related to an increase in the PaO_2 level before the apnea or respiratory arrest occurs from the loss of the hypoxic drive. The nurse, therefore, questions oxygen orders for clients at risk for oxygen-induced hypoventilation, apnea, and respiratory arrest.

Oxygen Toxicity. Oxygen toxicity is related to the concentration of oxygen delivered, duration of oxygen therapy, and degree of lung disease present before oxygen therapy is started. In general, an oxygen concentration greater than 50% administered continuously for more than 24–48 hours may damage the lungs.

The pathophysiologic mechanism and clinical manifestations of lung injury associated with oxygen toxicity are the same as those for adult respiratory distress syndrome (ARDS) (see Chap. 34). The nurse observes for initial symptoms, which include nonproductive cough, substernal chest pain, gastrointestinal (GI) upset, and dyspnea. As exposure to high concentrations of oxygen continues, the symptoms become more severe and are accompanied by decreased vital capacity, decreased compliance (which results in more dyspnea), crackles, and hypoxemia. Prolonged exposure to high concentrations of oxygen causes structural damage to the lungs. Atelectasis, pulmonary edema, pulmonary hemorrhages, and hyaline membrane formation result. Mortality depends on the ability of the health care team to correct the underlying disease process and to decrease the oxygen amount delivered.

The toxic effects of oxygen are difficult to treat; hence, the physician orders the lowest concentration of oxygen required by the client to prevent oxygen toxicity. The nurse closely monitors arterial blood gases during oxygen administration and notifies the physician of PaO_2 levels greater than 100 mmHg. The nurse also monitors the prescribed oxygen concentration and length of time of administration to identify the client at higher risk. High concentrations of oxygen are avoided unless absolutely necessary. The addition of continuous positive airway pressure (CPAP) with an oxygen mask, bilevel positive airway pressure (Bi-Pap) or positive end-expiratory pres-

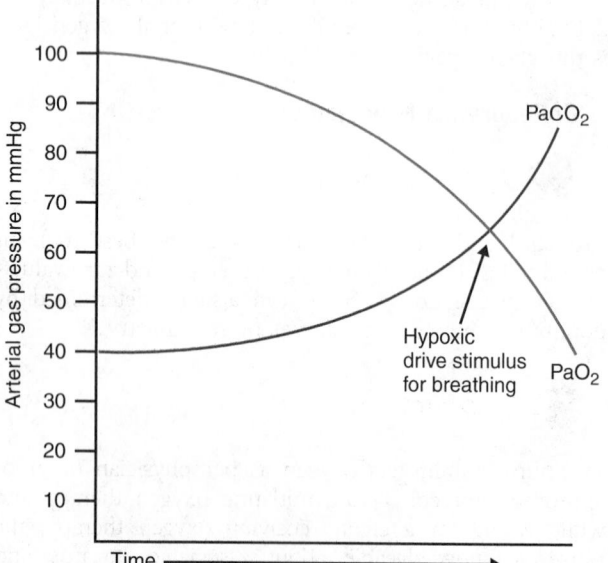

Figure 30–1. Arterial gas changes in chronic lung disease, showing the point at which the hypoxic drive becomes the stimulus for breathing.

sure (PEEP) on the mechanical ventilator (see Chap. 34) may reduce the amount of oxygen needed. As soon as the client's clinical condition allows, the physician decreases the prescribed amount of oxygen.

Absorption Atelectasis. Nitrogen normally plays a large role in the maintenance of patent airways and alveoli. Making up 79% of room air, it prevents alveolar collapse. When high concentrations of oxygen are delivered, nitrogen is washed out, oxygen diffuses from the alveoli into the pulmonary circulation, and the alveoli collapse. Collapsed alveoli cause atelectasis, called absorption atelectasis, which the nurse detects by auscultation. The nurse monitors the client closely for crackles and decreased breath sounds every 1–2 hours when the client is initially placed on oxygen therapy and frequently thereafter.

Drying of the Mucous Membranes. When an oxygen flow rate higher than 2 L/minute is needed, the nurse adds humidification upon order (Fig. 30–2). The nurse ensures that a constant mist of humidification escapes from the vents of the delivery system during inspiration and expiration. A sufficient amount of sterile water must be in the humidification container, and an adequate flow rate must be maintained so that proper humidification is delivered to the client. Condensation often forms in the tubing and is removed as needed by disconnecting the tubing and emptying the water into an appropriate receptacle. Some manufacturers place a water trap that hangs from the tubing so the nurse can drain the condensation without disconnecting. For prevention of bacterial contamination, the nurse never drains the fluid back into the humidification container. The nurse checks the water level and changes the humidifier as needed.

Oxygen can also be humidified via a nebulizer in mist form (aerosol). A heated nebulizer raises the humidity even more and is used when oxygen is administered via an artificial airway. Usually the upper airway passages have sufficient warming ability, but these passages are bypassed when an artificial airway is in use.

Infection. As mentioned, the humidification system may be a source of bacteria. *Pseudomonas aeruginosa* is frequently the organism involved. Oxygen delivery equipment such as cannulas and masks can also harbor organisms. The nurse changes equipment as per policy or protocol, which can range from 24 hours for humidification systems to every 7 days or whenever necessary for cannulas and masks.

Oxygen Delivery Systems. Oxygen can be delivered by numerous systems. Regardless of the type of delivery system used, the nurse needs to understand its indications, advantages, and disadvantages. Knowing the rationale for the oxygen delivery system used for a particular client, the nurse uses the equipment properly and ensures appropriate equipment maintenance. The type of delivery system depends on the following:

- Oxygen concentration required by the client
- Oxygen concentration achieved by a delivery system
- Importance of accuracy and control of the oxygen concentration
- Client comfort
- Expense to the client
- Importance of humidity
- Client mobility

Oxygen delivery systems are classified according to the rate at which oxygen is delivered. There are two systems: low-flow systems and high-flow systems. Low-flow systems do not provide enough oxygen to meet the total inspiratory effort of the client. Part of the tidal volume is supplied by the client's inspiring room air. The total concentration of oxygen received depends on respiratory rate and tidal volume. In contrast, high-flow systems provide a flow rate that is adequate to meet the entire inspiratory effort and tidal volume of the client regardless of the respiratory pattern. High-flow systems are used for critically ill clients and when it is particularly important to know the precise concentration of oxygen being delivered.

If the client requires a mask but is able to eat, the nurse requests an order for a nasal cannula at an appropriate liter flow for mealtimes only. The nurse replaces the mask after the meal is completed. To increase the client's mobility, up to 50 feet of connecting tubing can be used with proper connecting pieces. Other nursing interventions are listed in Chart 30–1.

Low-Flow Oxygen Delivery Systems

Low-flow delivery systems include the nasal cannula, simple face mask, partial rebreather mask, and non-rebreather mask (Table 30–1). These systems are inexpensive, easy to use, and fairly comfortable for the client. A major disadvantage is that the actual amount of oxygen obtained per liter is variable and depends on the client's breathing pattern. The oxygen delivered by the system is diluted with room air (21%), which lowers the amount of oxygen the client actually receives.

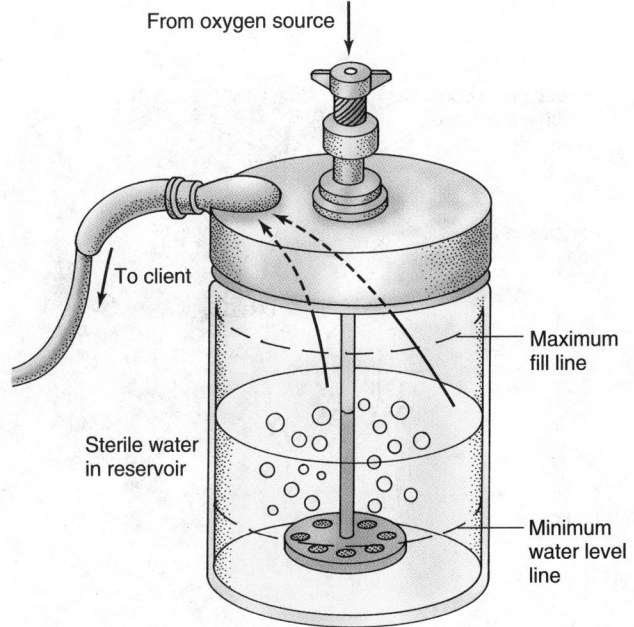

From oxygen source

To client

Sterile water in reservoir

Maximum fill line

Minimum water level line

Figure 30–2. A bubble humidifier bottle used with oxygen therapy.

Chart 30-1

Nursing Care Highlight: The Client Receiving Oxygen Therapy

- Check the physician's order with the type of delivery system and liter flow or percentage of oxygen actually in use.
- Obtain an order for humidification if oxygen is being delivered at 2 L/minute or more.
- Be sure the oxygen and humidification equipment is functioning properly.
- Check the skin around the client's ears, back of the neck, and face every 4 to 8 hours for pressure points and signs of irritation.
- Provide mouth care every 8 hours and as needed; assess nasal and oral mucous membranes for cracks or other signs of dryness.
- Pad the elastic band and change its position frequently to prevent skin breakdown.
- Cleanse cannula or mask by rinsing with clear warm water every 4 to 8 hours or as needed.
- Cleanse skin under tubing, straps, and mask every 4 to 8 hours or as needed.
- Lubricate the client's nostrils, face, and lips with water-soluble jelly to relieve the drying effects of oxygen.
- Position the tubing so it does not pull on the client's face, nose, or artificial airway.
- Ensure that there is no smoking and that no candles or matches are lit in the immediate area.
- Assess and document the client's response to oxygen therapy.
- Provide the client with ongoing teaching and reassurance to enhance the client's compliance with oxygen therapy.

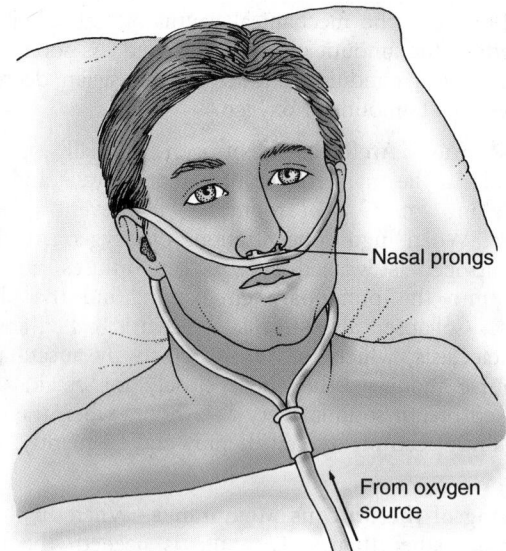

Figure 30-3. A nasal cannula (prongs).

Nasal Cannula. The nasal cannula, or nasal prongs (Fig. 30-3), is used at flow rates of 1-6 L/minute. Approximate oxygen concentrations of 24% (at 1 L/minute) to 44% (at 6 L/minute) can be achieved. Flow rates greater than 6 L/minute do not significantly increase oxygenation because the anatomic reserve or dead space (oral and nasal cavities) is full. In addition, high flow rates increase mucosal irritation. With the use of a nasal cannula, an effective oxygen concentration can be delivered to both nose breathers and mouth breathers.

The nasal cannula is frequently used for the client with chronic lung disease and for long-term maintenance of clients with other illnesses. The client who retains carbon dioxide rarely receives oxygen at a rate higher than 2-3 L/minute because of the concern of apnea or respiratory arrest. The nurse places the nasal prongs in the nostrils, with the openings facing the client.

Simple Face Mask. A simple face mask is used to deliver oxygen concentrations of 40% to 60% for short-term oxygen therapy or in an emergency (Fig. 30-4). A minimal flow rate of 5 L/minute is needed to prevent the rebreathing of exhaled air. The nurse gives special attention to skin care and to the proper fitting of the mask so that inspired oxygen concentration is maintained.

Partial Rebreather Mask. A partial rebreather mask provides oxygen concentrations of 60% to 75%, with flow rates of 6-11 L/minute. It consists of a mask with a reservoir bag but no flaps (Fig. 30-5). The client first rebreathes one third of the exhaled tidal volume, which is high in oxygen, thus providing a high FIO_2. The nurse ensures that the bag remains slightly inflated at the end of inspiration; otherwise, the client will not be getting the desired oxygen prescription. If needed, the nurse calls the respiratory therapist for assistance.

Non-Rebreather Mask. A non-rebreather mask provides the highest concentration of the low-flow systems and can deliver an FIO_2 greater than 90%, depending on the client's ventilatory pattern. The non-rebreather mask

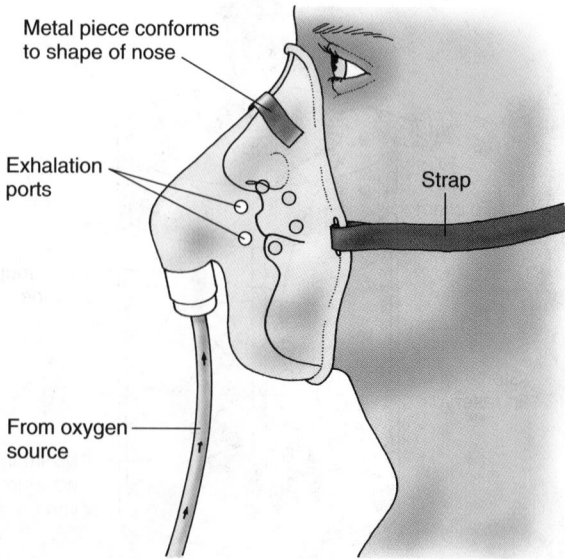

Figure 30-4. A simple face mask used to deliver oxygen.

TABLE 30-1

Comparison of Low-Flow Oxygen Delivery Systems

System	FIO$_2$ Delivered	Nursing Interventions	Rationale
Nasal cannula	24%–40% FIO$_2$ at 1–6 L/min ≈24% at 1 L/min ≈28% at 2 L/min ≈32% at 3 L/min ≈36% at 4 L/min ≈40% at 5 L/min ≈44% at 6 L/min	• Ensure that prongs are in the nares properly. • Provide water-soluble jelly to nares PRN. • Assess the patency of the nostrils. • Assess the client for changes in respiratory rate or depth.	• A poorly fitting nasal cannula leads to hypoxemia and skin breakdown. • This substance prevents mucosal irritation related to the drying effect of oxygen; promotes comfort. • Congestion or a deviated septum prevents effective delivery of oxygen through the nares. • The respiratory pattern affects the amount of oxygen delivered. A different delivery system may be needed.
Simple face mask	40%–60% FIO$_2$ at 5–8 L/min; flow rate must be set at least 5 L/min to flush mask of carbon dioxide ≈40% at 5 L/min ≈45%–50% at 6 L/min ≈55%–60% at 8 L/min	• Be sure mask fits securely over nose and mouth. • Assess skin and provide skin care to the area covered by the mask. • Monitor the client closely for risk of aspiration. • Provide emotional support to the client who feels claustrophobic. • Suggest to physician to switch the client from a mask to the nasal cannula during eating.	• A poorly fitting mask reduces the FIO$_2$ delivered. • Pressure and moisture under the mask may cause skin breakdown. • The mask limits the client's ability to clear the mouth, especially if vomiting occurs. • Emotional support decreases anxiety, which contributes to a claustrophobic feeling. • Use of the cannula prevents hypoxemia during eating.
Partial rebreather mask	60%–75% at 6–11 L/min, a liter flow rate high enough to maintain reservoir bag two thirds full during inspiration and expiration	• Make sure that the reservoir does not twist or kink, which results in a deflated bag. • Adjust the flow rate to keep the reservoir bag inflated.	• Deflation results in decreased oxygen delivered and rebreathing of exhaled air. • The flow rate is adjusted to meet the pattern of the client.
Non-rebreather mask	80%–95% FIO$_2$ at liter flow to maintain reservoir bag two thirds full	• Interventions as for partial rebreather mask; this client requires close monitoring. • Make sure that valves and rubber flaps are patent, functional, and not stuck. Remove mucus or saliva. • Closely assess the client on increased FIO$_2$ via non-rebreather mask. Intubation is the only way to provide more precise FIO$_2$.	• Rationales as for partial rebreather mask. • Monitoring ensures proper functioning and prevents harm. • Valves should open during expiration and close during inhalation to prevent dramatic decrease in FIO$_2$. Suffocation can occur if the reservoir bag kinks or if the oxygen source disconnects. • The client may require intubation.

is most frequently used for a client with deteriorating respiratory status who might soon require intubation.

The non-rebreather mask has a one-way valve between the mask and the reservoir and two flaps over the exhalation ports (Fig. 30–6). The valve allows the client to draw all needed oxygen from the reservoir bag, and the flaps prevent room air from entering through the exhalation ports. During exhalation, air leaves through these

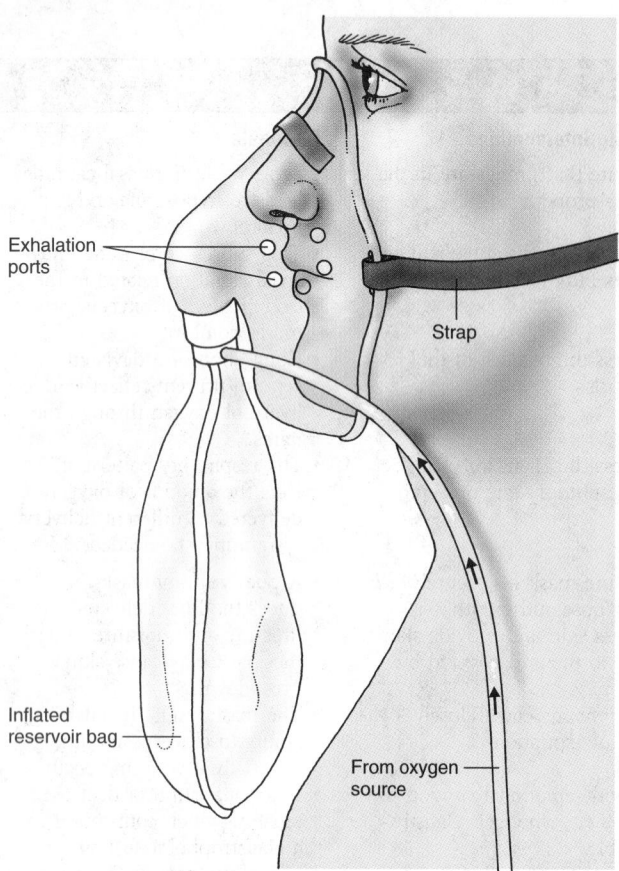

Figure 30–5. A partial rebreather mask.

exhalation ports while the one-way valve prevents exhaled air from re-entering the reservoir bag. It is crucial for the nurse to ensure that the valve and flaps are intact and functional during each breath. Some manufacturers include only one flap on the mask, or one of the exhalation flaps may be removed for safety purposes. If the oxygen source should fail or be depleted when both flaps are in place, the client would not be able to breathe in room air. The nurse assesses for this safety feature.

High-Flow Oxygen Delivery Systems

High-flow systems (Table 30–2) include the Venturi mask, aerosol mask, face tent, tracheostomy collar, and T-piece. These devices deliver a consistent and accurate oxygen concentration that meets the client's inspiratory effort when properly fitted. A high-flow system provides oxygen concentrations of 24% to 100% at 8–15 L/minute.

Venturi Mask. The Venturi mask (commonly called Venti mask) delivers the most accurate oxygen concentration. Its operation is based on a mechanism that pulls in a specific proportional amount of room air for each liter flow of oxygen. An adaptor is located between the bottom of the mask and the oxygen source (Fig. 30–7). Adaptors with holes of different sizes allow only specific amounts of air to mix with the oxygen. Precise delivery of oxygen results. Each adaptor also specifies the flow rate with which it is to be used; for example, to deliver 24% of oxygen, the flow rate must be 4 L/minute. Another type

of Venturi mask has one adaptor with a dial the nurse uses to select the amount of oxygen desired. Humidification is not necessary with the Venturi mask. The Venturi system is the best one for the client with chronic lung disease because it delivers a precise oxygen concentration.

Other High-Flow Systems. The face tent, aerosol mask, tracheostomy collar, and T-piece are often used to administer high humidity. A dial on the humidification source regulates the oxygen concentration being delivered. A face tent fits over the client's chin, with the top extending halfway across the face. The oxygen concentration varies, but the face tent is useful instead of a tight-fitting mask for the client who has facial trauma and burns. An aerosol mask is used for the client who requires high humidity after extubation or upper airway surgery or for the client who has thick secretions. The tracheostomy collar can be used to deliver high humidity and the desired oxygen to the client with a tracheostomy. A special adaptor, called the T-*piece,* can be used to deliver any desired FIO_2 to the client with a tracheostomy, laryngectomy, or endotracheal tube (Fig. 30–8). The flow rate is regulated so that the aerosol does not disappear on the exhalation side of the T-piece.

Transtracheal Oxygen Therapy

Transtracheal oxygen (TTO) is a long-term method of delivering oxygen directly into the lungs. The physician

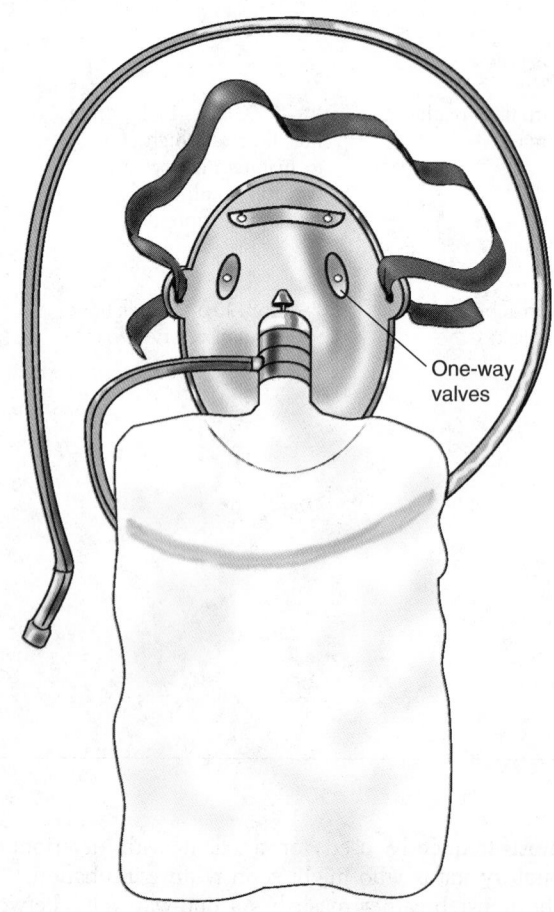

Figure 30–6. A non-rebreather mask.

TABLE 30–2

Comparison of High-Flow Oxygen Delivery Systems

System	FIO₂ Delivered	Nursing Interventions	Rationale
Venturi mask (Venti mask)	24%–55% FIO$_2$ with flow rates as recommended by the manufacturer, usually 4–10 L/min; provides high humidity	• Perform constant surveillance to ensure accurate flow rate for specific FIO$_2$. • Keep the orifice for the Venturi adaptor open and uncovered. • Provide a mask that fits snugly and tubing that is free of kinks. • Assess the client for dry mucous membranes. • Change to a nasal cannula during mealtimes.	• An accurate flow rate ensures FIO$_2$ delivery. • If the Venturi orifice is covered, the adaptor does not function and oxygen delivery varies. • FIO$_2$ is altered if kinking occurs or if the mask fits poorly. • Comfort measures may be indicated • Oxygen is a drug that needs to be given continuously.
Aerosol mask, face tent, tracheostomy collar	24%–100% FIO$_2$ with flow rates of at least 10 L/min; provides high humidity	• Assess that aerosol mist escapes from the vents of the delivery system during inspiration and expiration. • Empty condensation from the tubing. • Change the aerosol water container as needed.	• Humidification should be delivered to the client. • Emptying prevents the client from being lavaged with water and promotes an adequate flow rate. • Adequate humidification is ensured only when there is sufficient water in the canister.
T-piece	24%–100% FIO$_2$ with flow rates of at least 10 L/min; provides high humidity	• Empty condensation from the tubing. • Keep the exhalation port open and uncovered. • Position the T-piece so that it does not pull on the tracheostomy or endotracheal tube. • Make sure the humidifier creates enough mist. A mist should be seen during inspiration and expiration.	• Condensation interferes with flow rate and may drain into the tracheostomy if not emptied. • If the port is occluded, the client can suffocate. • The weight of the T-piece pulls on the tracheostomy and causes pain or erosion of skin at the insertion site. • An adequate flow rate is needed to meet the inspiration effort of the client. If not, FIO$_2$ is decreased.

passes a small, flexible catheter into the trachea via a small incision (Fig. 30–9A) with use of local anesthesia. TTO allows better compliance and avoids the irritation that nasal prongs cause. Clients also report it to be more cosmetically acceptable. A TTO team provides formal client education, including the purpose of TTO and care of the catheter. The physician prescribes a TTO flow rate for rest and for activity and a flow rate for the nasal cannula. The average client will have a 55% reduction of required oxygen flow at rest and a 30% decrease with activity.

SCOOP is one brand of catheter made by Transtracheal Systems. All SCOOP oxygen catheters (Fig. 30–9B) are made of kink-resistant thermoplastic polyurethane. Two opposing barium stripes provide x-ray visibility on the otherwise clear catheter. The outside diameter is 9 French (Fr). Overall length is 20 cm with a standard internal length of 11 cm. Nonstandard catheter lengths are also available. The physician determines proper length after viewing the postprocedure x-ray with an 11-cm Pre-SCOOP stent in place. Oxygen is attached to the catheter using a SCOOP oxygen hose with a Luer taper connection. Catheters are sterilely packaged individually or in pairs and contain a cleaning rod(s), lubricating jelly, physician and client instructions, and a registration card.

 Continuing Care

➤ Criteria for Home Oxygen Therapy

The client must be clinically stable and optimally treated before the need for home oxygen is considered. For Medicare to cover the cost of continuous oxygen therapy, the client must have severe hypoxemia. For reimbursement purposes, severe hypoxemia is generally defined as a PaO₂

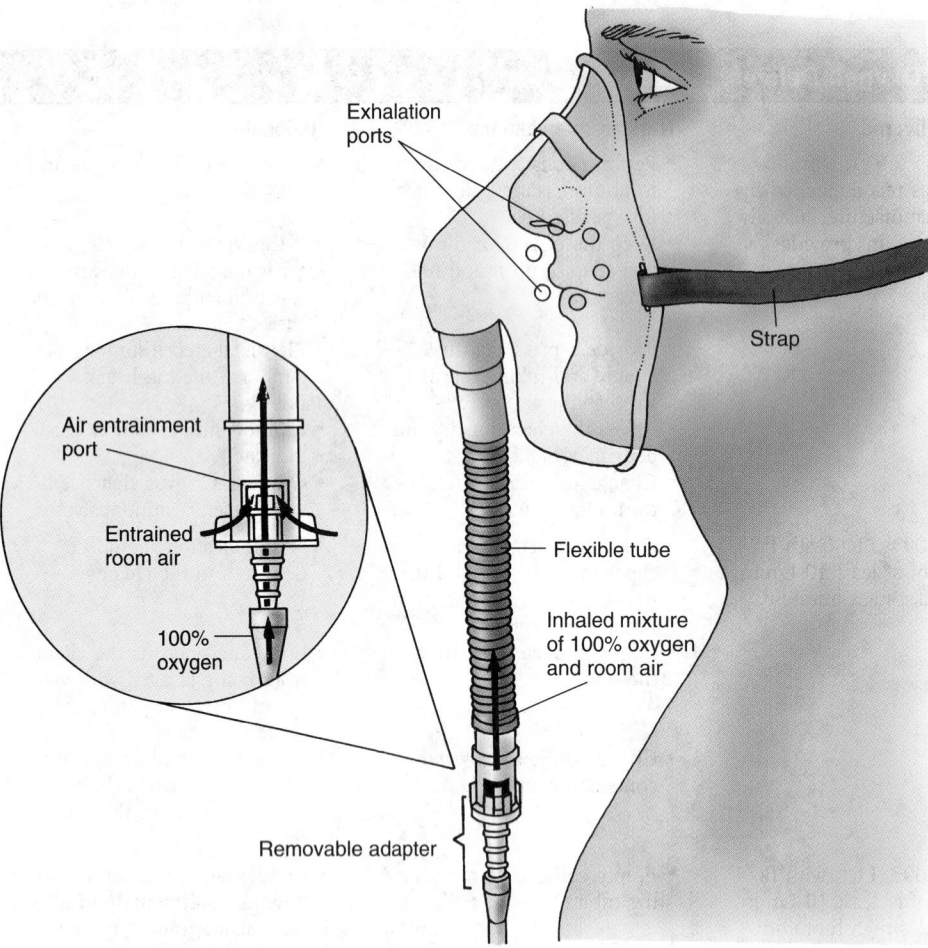

Figure 30–7. A Venturi mask for precise oxygen delivery.

level of less than 55 mmHg or an arterial oxygen saturation of less than 85% on room air and at rest. A variation of this criterion is a PaO_2 value of 56–59 mmHg or an arterial oxygen saturation value of 86% to 89% with a secondary diagnosis of symptomatic congestive heart failure, cor pulmonale as seen on an electrocardiogram, or erythrocytosis with a hematocrit of 56%. Specific criteria are also established for coverage of nocturnal oxygen and portable oxygen therapy. Medicare guidelines are continually changing; therefore, it is important for the nurse to be aware of these criteria and the documentation required to meet the standards.

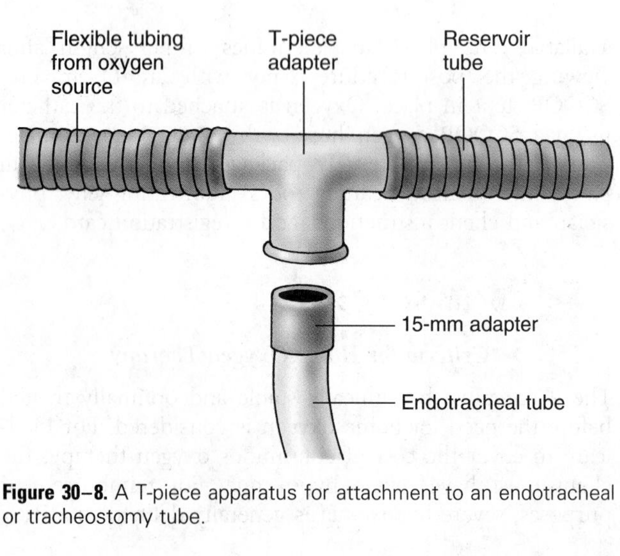

➤ Teaching About Home Oxygen Therapy

After the need for home oxygen therapy is verified, the nurse begins a teaching plan about oxygen therapy. The client, with the nurse's assistance, selects a durable medical equipment (DME) company to deliver oxygen equipment and a community health nursing agency for follow-up care in the home. The physician re-evaluates the client's need for oxygen therapy approximately 6 months after discharge from the health care facility and yearly thereafter.

While providing discharge planning and teaching, the nurse is sensitive to the client's psychological adjustment to oxygen therapy. The nurse encourages the client to share feelings and concerns. The client may be concerned about social acceptance and misconceptions of friends. The nurse helps the client realize that compliance with oxygen therapy is important so that normal activities of daily living (ADLs) and events that bring enjoyment can be continued.

Figure 30–8. A T-piece apparatus for attachment to an endotracheal or tracheostomy tube.

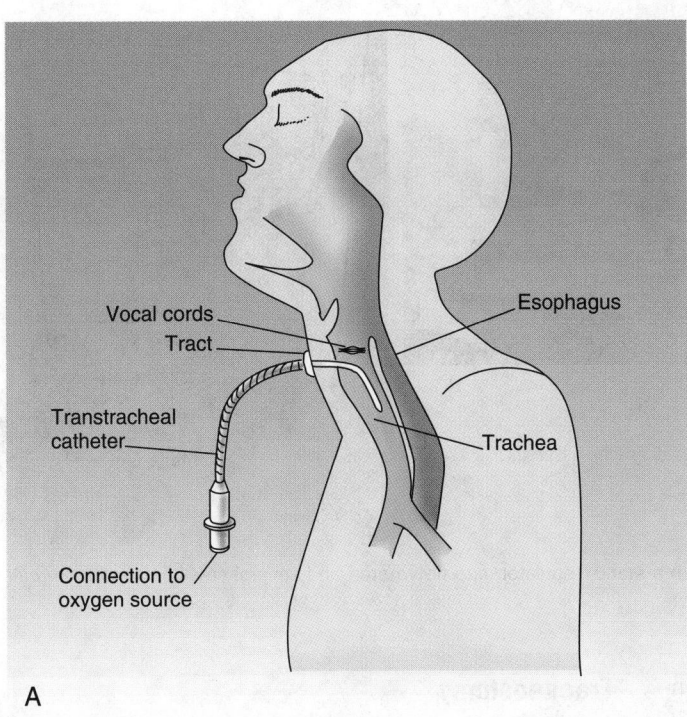

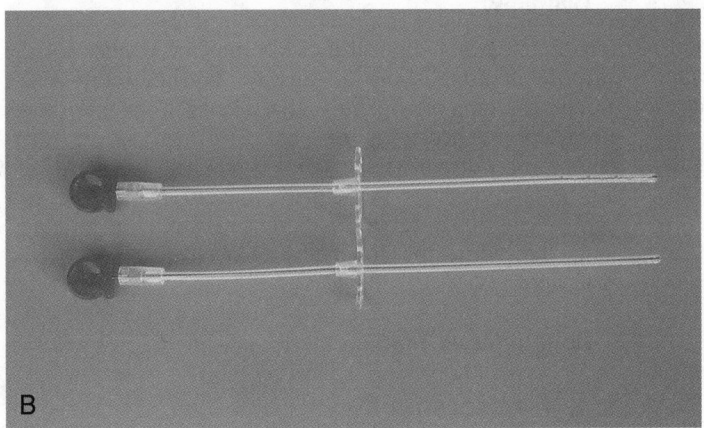

Figure 30–9. *A,* Example of transtracheal oxygen delivery. *B,* SCOOP-2 (*top*) and SCOOP-1 (*bottom*) transtracheal oxygen catheters. (*B,* Courtesy of Transtracheal Systems, Inc., Englewood, Co.)

➤ Equipment for Home Oxygen Therapy

The nurse or respiratory therapist teaches the client about the equipment needed for home oxygen therapy:

- Oxygen source
- Oxygen delivery device
- Humidification source
- Safety aspects of using and maintaining the equipment

Home oxygen is provided in one of three ways:

- Compressed gas in a tank or a cylinder
- Liquid oxygen in a reservoir
- An oxygen concentrator

Compressed gas in an oxygen tank (green) is the most common oxygen source. The large H cylinder is used as a stationary source; the small E tank is available for transporting the client (Fig. 30–10). As a safety precaution, the tanks must always be in a stand or rack. A tank that is accidentally knocked over could explode. Even smaller (and lighter) D or C cylinders are available for the client to carry. An oxygen tank is economical, and pure oxygen can be delivered at a wide range of flow rates.

The second type of home oxygen, liquid oxygen, is oxygen gas that has been liquefied by cooling to −300° F (−147° C); thus, a concentrated amount of oxygen is available in a lightweight and easy-to-carry container similar to a Thermos bottle (Fig. 30–11). This type of oxygen lasts longer than oxygen in a conventional tank of the same size; however, it is expensive, and the oxygen evaporates if it is not used continuously.

The last type of home oxygen source is the oxygen concentrator, which is a machine that removes nitrogen, water vapor, and hydrocarbons from room air. It is sometimes referred to as an oxygen extractor. Oxygen is concentrated from room air and is delivered at more than 90%. The concentrator is the least expensive of the systems but is not portable and is often noisy.

Humidification is rarely needed for any of these oxygen systems. Nevertheless, humidification may help when the physician prescribes a flow rate higher than 2 L/minute.

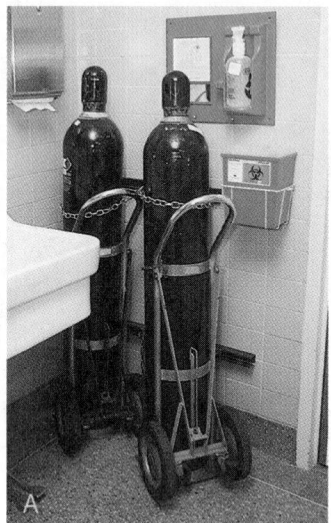
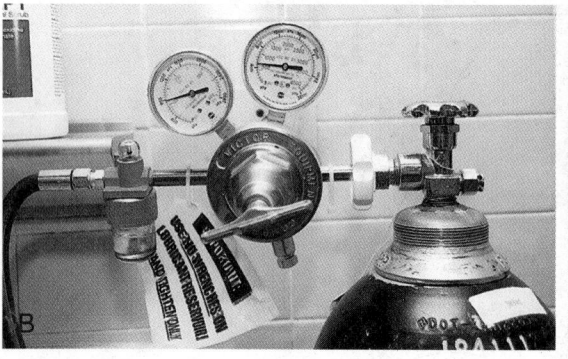
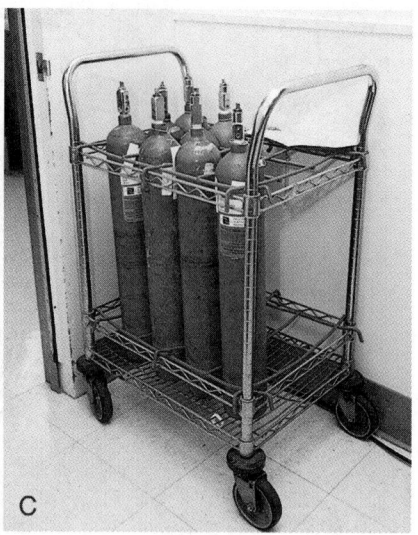

Figure 30–10. Comparison of a large H oxygen cylinder (*left*), with a stand, regulator, and flowmeter, and several small E cylinders (*right*).

In any of the three home oxygen systems, an oxygen-conserving reservoir-type nasal cannula can be used to reduce oxygen flow requirements by approximately 50%. Two types currently available are the mustache type and the pendant type. Attached to the tubing is a reservoir where exhaled oxygen is stored and then redelivered back to the client on the next inhalation. The reservoir sits on top of the upper lip (mustache type) or hangs around the neck (pendant type).

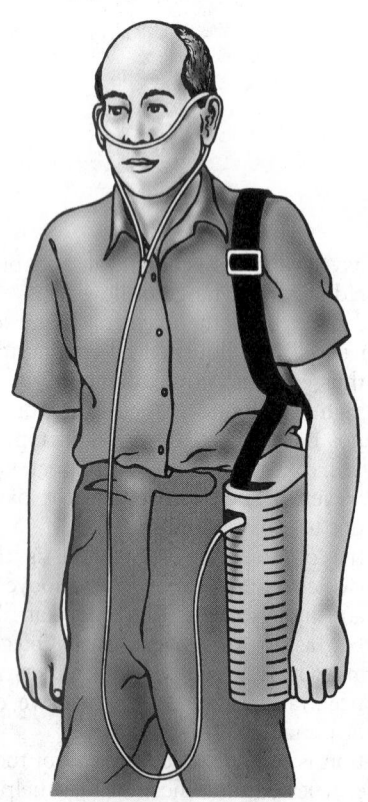

Figure 30–11. Liquid oxygen.

Tracheostomy

Overview

Tracheotomy is a surgical incision into the trachea for the purpose of establishing an airway. Tracheostomy is the (tracheal) stoma, or opening, that results from the tracheotomy. A tracheostomy can be performed as an emergency procedure or as a scheduled surgical procedure and can be temporary or permanent. Indications for tracheostomy are listed in Table 30–3. Tracheostomy as an emergency procedure for upper airway obstruction is covered in Chapter 31.

Collaborative Management

 Assessment

Assessment of the natural airway is covered in Chapter 31, as is assessment for upper airway obstruction. Assessment of a client with a tracheostomy is related to interventions that comprise nursing care for that client.

TABLE 30–3

Indications for Tracheostomy
• Acute airway obstruction when oral or nasal intubation is not feasible
• Airway protection (e.g., after head and neck cancer surgery)
• Prolonged intubation or need for mechanical ventilation
• Decreased airway dead space in combination with other indicators
• Control of pulmonary secretions refractory to conventional methods
• Airway reconstruction after laryngeal trauma or laryngeal cancer surgery
• Obstructive sleep apnea refractory to conventional therapy

Interventions

Once the determination of need for tracheostomy has been established, the nurse prepares the client for surgery.

Preoperative Care. The preoperative care for the client undergoing a tracheostomy is similar to that for a client scheduled for a laryngectomy (see Chap. 31). The nurse focuses on the client's knowledge deficits through teaching and discusses tracheostomy care, communication, and speech.

Operative Procedures. Initially, the anesthesiologist or nurse anesthetist extends the neck and places an endotracheal (ET) tube to maintain the airway. The surgeon then makes an incision through the anterior skin of the neck, dissects the subcutaneous tissue for exposure, separates the thyroid, and identifies the thyroid artery and tracheal rings. Another incision is made through the second and third or third and fourth tracheal rings to enter the trachea (Fig. 30–12). The types of incisions and specific techniques vary, depending on the surgeon's preference and the reason for the surgery.

After the surgeon enters the trachea, the ET tube is carefully removed while the tracheostomy tube is inserted. The surgeon secures the tracheostomy tube in place with sutures and tracheostomy ties and orders a chest x-ray to ensure proper placement of the tube. In clients who cannot be intubated, tracheostomy can be done with the client awake under local anesthesia.

Postoperative Care. Immediate postoperative nursing care focuses on ensuring a patent airway, confirming the presence of bilateral breath sounds, recovering the client from anesthesia, and assessing for complications from the procedure.

Complications. Six major complications may arise in the postoperative period: tube obstruction with secretions, tube dislodgment or accidental decannulation, pneumo-thorax, subcutaneous emphysema, bleeding, and infection. Table 30–4 summarizes signs and symptoms, management, and prevention of other serious complications of tracheostomy.

Tube Obstruction. By helping the client with coughing and deep breathing, providing inner cannula care, humidifying the oxygen source, and suctioning, the nurse prevents secretions from obstructing the tube. If tube obstruction occurs as a result of cuff prolapse over the end of the tracheostomy tube, the physician repositions or replaces the tube. Specific signs and symptoms of obstruction include difficulty in breathing; noisy respirations from the tracheostomy; difficulty in inserting a suction catheter; thick, dry secretions; and unexplained peak pressures if a mechanical ventilator is in use.

Tube Dislodgment or Accidental Decannulation. The nurse prevents tube dislodgment and decannulation by securing the tube in place, thus minimizing manipulation and traction on the tube from oxygen or ventilator tubing or accidental pulling by the client. Tube dislodgment in the first 72 hours after surgery is a medical emergency because the tracheostomy tract has not matured and tissue planes are not well defined. Attempts at replacement of a fresh tracheostomy in this time frame can lead to cannulation of subcutaneous tissue planes instead of the trachea itself. In this situation, the nurse attempts to ventilate the client using a manual resuscitation bag while another nurse calls the resuscitation team for help.

The nurse ensures that a tracheostomy tube of the same type (including an obturator) and size (or one size smaller) is at the client's bedside at all times, along with a tracheostomy insertion tray. If decannulation occurs after 72 hours, the nurse extends the client's neck and opens the tissues of the stoma to secure the airway. With the obturator inserted into the tracheostomy tube, the nurse quickly and gently replaces the tube and removes the obturator. The nurse checks for airflow through the tube and for bilateral breath sounds. If unable to secure the airway, the nurse notifies a more experienced nurse or physician for assistance. The nurse attempts to ventilate via a bag-valve mask. If the client is in distress and further attempts to secure the airway fail, the nurse calls the resuscitation team, including an anesthesiologist, for assistance.

Pneumothorax. Pneumothorax (air in the chest cavity) can develop during the tracheostomy procedure if the thoracic cavity is accidentally entered. When pneumothorax occurs, it does so medially and superiorly at the apex of the lung. Chest x-ray after placement is used to assess for pneumothorax.

Subcutaneous Emphysema. When there is an opening (rent) in the trachea, air escapes into fresh tissue planes of the neck, causing subcutaneous emphysema. Air can also progress throughout the chest and axilla into the face. The nurse inspects and palpates for air under the skin of a client with a new tracheostomy.

Bleeding. A small amount of bleeding from the tracheostomy incision can be expected for the first few days,

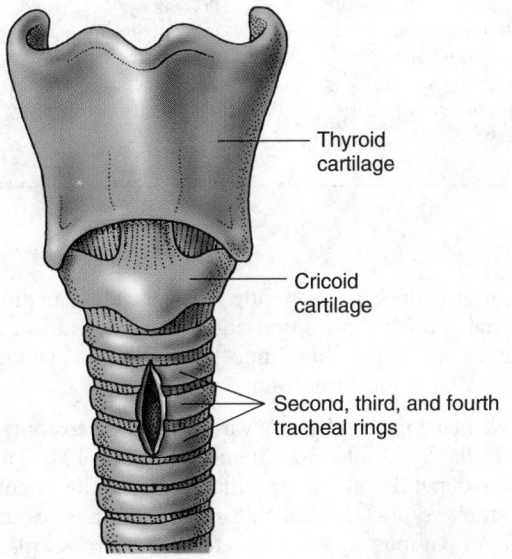

Figure 30–12. A vertical tracheal incision for a tracheostomy.

Thyroid cartilage

Cricoid cartilage

Second, third, and fourth tracheal rings

TABLE 30–4

Complications of Tracheostomy

Complications and Description	Signs and Symptoms	Management	Prevention
Tracheomalacia: constant pressure exerted by the cuff causes tracheal dilation and erosion of cartilage.	• An increased amount of air is required in the cuff to maintain the seal. • A larger tracheostomy tube is required to prevent an air leak at the stoma. • Food particles are seen in tracheal secretions. • The client does not receive tidal volume on the ventilator.	• No special management is needed unless bleeding occurs.	• Use an uncuffed tube as soon as possible. • Monitor cuff pressure and air volumes closely and detect changes.
Tracheal stenosis: narrowed tracheal lumen is due to scar formation from irritation of tracheal mucosa by the cuff.	• Stenosis usually seen after the cuff is deflated or the tracheostomy tube is removed. • The client has increased coughing; inability to expectorate secretions; or difficulty in breathing or talking.	• Tracheal dilation or surgical intervention is used.	• Prevent pulling of and traction on the tracheostomy tube. • Properly secure the tube in the midline position. • Maintain proper cuff pressure. • Minimize oronasal intubation time.

Tracheoesophageal fistula (TEF): excessive cuff pressure causes erosion of the posterior wall of the trachea. A hole is created between the trachea and the anterior esophagus. The client at highest risk also has a nasogastric tube present.	• Similar to tracheomalacia:
	  • Food particles are seen in tracheal secretions.
	  • Increased air in cuff is needed to achieve a seal.
	  • The client has increased coughing and choking while eating.
	  • The client does not receive the set tidal volume on the ventilator.
		• Manually administer oxygen by mask to prevent hypoxemia.
		• A small soft feeding tube is used instead of a nasogastric tube for tube feedings. A gastrostomy or jejunostomy may be performed.
		• Monitor the client with a nasogastric tube closely; assess for TEF and aspiration.
			• Maintain cuff pressure
			• Monitor the amount of air needed for inflation and detect changes.
			• Progress to deflated cuff or cuffless tube as soon as possible.

Trachea-innominate artery fistula: a malpositioned tube causes its distal tip to push against the lateral wall of the tracheostomy. Continued pressure causes necrosis and erosion of the innominate artery. **This is a medical emergency.**	• The tracheostomy tube pulsates in synchrony with the heart beat. • There is exsanguination from the stoma. • This is a life-threatening complication.	• Remove the tracheostomy tube immediately. • Apply direct pressure to the innominate artery at the stoma site. • Prepare the client for immediate repair surgery.	• Correct the tube size, length, and midline position. • Prevent pulling or tugging on the tracheostomy tube. • Immediately notify the physician of pulsating tube.

but constant oozing warrants surgical intervention, cauterization, or ligation of vessels. With physician order, the nurse wraps petroleum (Vaseline)-covered gauze around the tube and packs it gently into the wound to apply pressure to the bleeding sites.

Infection. While in the hospital, the nurse uses sterile technique to prevent infection during suctioning and tracheostomy care and assesses the stoma site for purulent drainage, redness, pain, swelling, or cellulitis. Tracheostomy dressings may be used to keep the stoma clean and dry; moist dressings provide an excellent medium for bacterial growth. Prevention and early detection of a local infection are, therefore, important. Diligent wound care prevents most local infections.

Tracheostomy Tubes. A variety of tracheostomy tubes are available (Table 30–5 and Fig. 30–13). The one chosen depends on the specific needs of the client. Tracheostomy tubes are available in numerous sizes and are made of various types of materials, such as plastic or metal. The tubes may be disposable or reusable. A tra-

TABLE 30–5

Types of Tracheostomy Tubes

Type	Description	Type	Description
Double-lumen tube	• The double-lumen tube has three major parts: • Outer cannula—fits into the stoma and keeps the airway open. The face plate indicates the size and type of tube and has small holes on both sides for securing the tube with tracheostomy ties. • Inner cannula—fits snugly into the outer cannula and locks into place. Provides the universal adaptor for use with the ventilator and other respiratory therapy equipment. Some may be removed, cleaned, and reused; others are disposable. • Obturator—is a stylet with a blunt end used to facilitate direction of the tube when inserting or changing a tracheostomy tube. It is removed immediately after tube placement and is always kept with the client and at the bedside in case of accidental decannulation.	Fenestrated tube	• The fenestrated tube has a precut opening (fenestration) in the upper posterior wall of the outer cannula. It is used to wean the client from a tracheostomy by ensuring that the client can tolerate breathing through his or her natural airway before the entire tube is removed. This tube allows the client to speak.
		Cuffed fenestrated tube	• The cuffed fenestrated tube facilitates mechanical ventilation and speech. It is often used for clients with spinal cord paralysis or neuromuscular disease who do not require ventilation all the time. When not on the ventilator, the client can have the cuff deflated and the tube capped for speech. A cuffed fenestrated tube is never used in weaning from a tracheostomy because the cuff, even fully deflated, may partially obstruct the airway.
Single-lumen tube	• The single-lumen tube is a long tube used for clients with long or extra thick necks. Often called a "bull neck trach" because of the long distance from the skin to the trachea or the longer length of the trachea in large people. More intensive nursing care is required with this tube because there is no inner cannula to ensure a patent lumen.	Metal tracheostomy tube	• The metal tracheostomy tube is used for permanent tracheostomy. It is a cuffless double-lumen tube and can be cleaned and reused indefinitely. A special adaptor attaches a manual resuscitation bag. Popular types are the Jackson and Holinger tubes.
Cuffed tube	• A cuff, when inflated, seals the airway. Used with mechanical ventilation, in preventing aspiration of oral or gastric secretions, or for tube feeding. A pilot balloon attached to the outside of the tube indicates the presence or absence of air in the cuff.	Talking tracheostomy tube	• The talking tracheostomy tube provides a means of communication for the client who is using a ventilator on a long-term basis. An extra air channel allows air to flow up through the vocal cords so that the client can speak with the cuff inflated. The air can cause drying of the vocal cords from constant dry airflow. Examples are the Pitt Trach Speaking Tube (National Catheter Corporation) and Communitrach (Implant Technologies, Inc.).
Cuffless tube	• The cuffless tube is a plastic, silicone-like (Silastic), or metal tube, usually double lumen. Used for long-term airway management in those clients who require a tracheostomy, who can protect themselves from aspiration, and who do not require mechanical ventilation. Many people can speak with this tube in place.		

cheostomy tube may or may not have a cuff. It also may have an inner cannula that can be either disposable or reusable. For clients receiving mechanical ventilation, a cuffed tube is used in acute care settings. A noncuffed tube is used for airway maintenance when mechanical ventilation is not required or when the client is being discharged.

For tubes with an inner cannula, the nurse inspects, suctions, and cleans the inner cannula. During the immediate postoperative period, the nurse may provide cannula care frequently as needed, perhaps every 30–60 minutes. Thereafter, care is usually determined by the client's needs and agency policy. In planning for self-care, the nurse teaches the client to remove the inner cannula and

Slots for
attachment
of tube ties   Face   Outer   Disposable
                plate   cannula   inner cannula

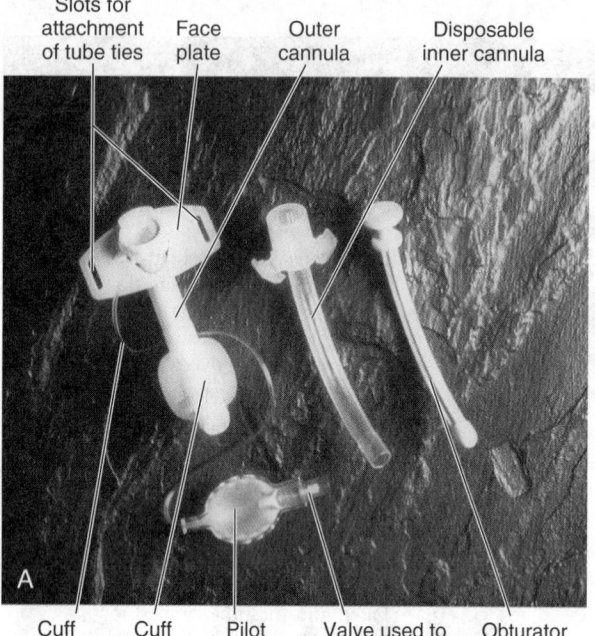

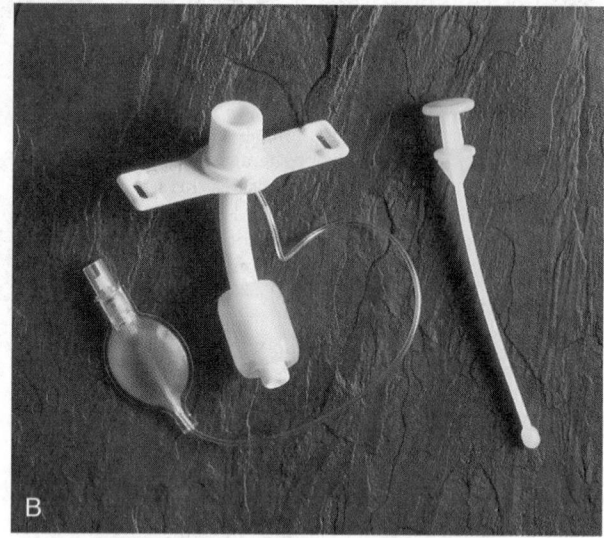

Cuff   Cuff   Pilot   Valve used to   Obturator
infaltion (inflated) balloon   inflate and deflate
tube   cuff and measure
                                cuff pressure

Fenestration

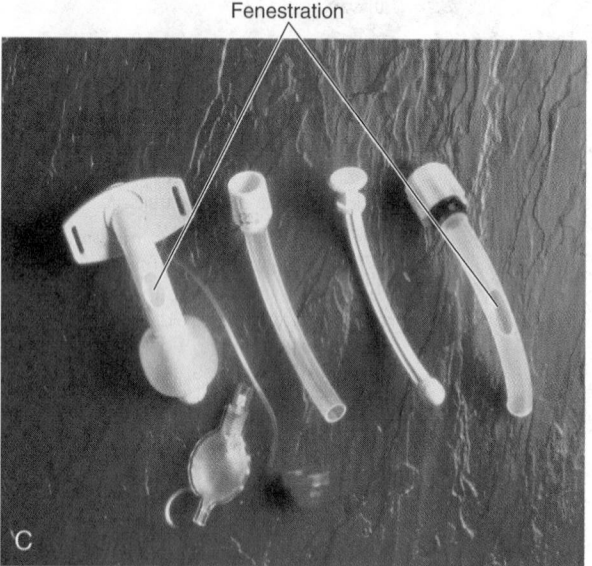

Figure 30–13. Tracheostomy tubes. *A,* Dual-lumen cuffed tracheostomy tube with disposable inner cannula. *B,* Single-lumen cannula cuffed tracheostomy tube. *C,* Dual-lumen cuffed fenestrated tracheostomy tube. (Courtesy of Mallinckrodt, Inc., Shiley Tracheostomy Products, St. Louis, MO.)

check for cleanliness. As teaching progresses, the nurse also instructs the client about suctioning and tracheostomy cleaning.

Because movement of breathing and swallowing moves the tube, a cuffed tube may not always be entirely protective against aspiration. Additionally, the pilot balloon does not reflect whether the correct amount of air is present in the cuff.

A fenestrated tube can function in many different ways. When the inner cannula is in place, the fenestration is covered over (closed), and the tube functions as a double-lumen tube. With the inner cannula removed and the plug or red decannulation stopper locked in place, air can then pass through the fenestration as well as around

the tube and up through the natural airway. The client can cough and speak, becoming reaccustomed to breathing through the upper air passages. If the client has trouble with any of these maneuvers, the nurse and physician evaluate the client for proper tube placement, patency, size, and fenestration. The nurse does not cap the tube until the problem is identified and corrected. A fenestrated tube may or may not have a cuff.

With a cuffed fenestrated tube, some air flows through the natural airway when the client is not depending on mechanical ventilation. The nurse always deflates the cuff before capping the tube with the decannulation cannula; otherwise, the client has no airway (Fig. 30–14).

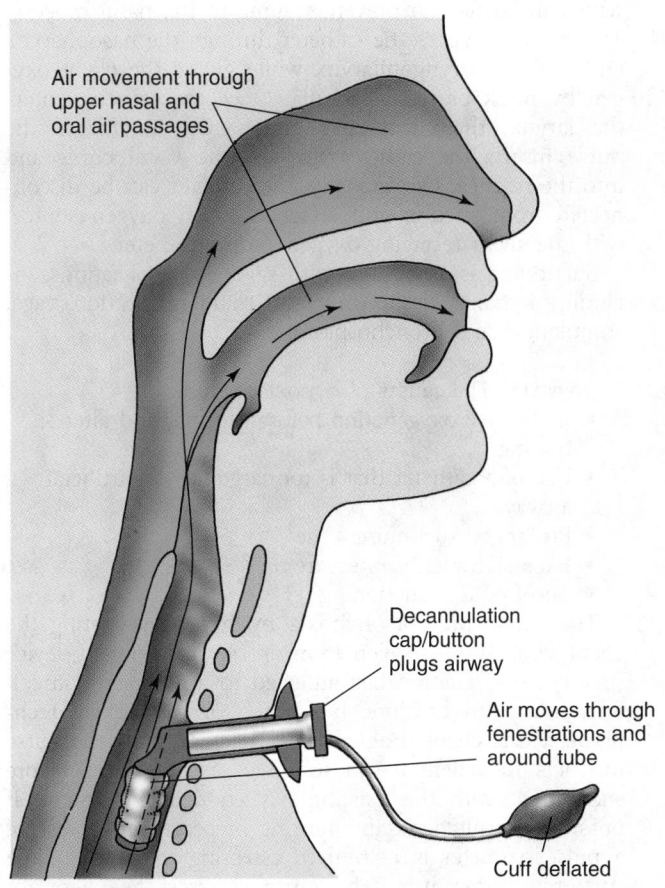

Air movement through upper nasal and oral air passages

Decannulation cap/button plugs airway

Air moves through fenestrations and around tube

Cuff deflated

Figure 30–14. Breathing through a fenestrated tracheostomy tube with a cap in place and the cuff deflated.

Prevention of Tissue Damage. Tissue damage can occur at the point where the inflated cuff presses against the tracheal mucosa. Mucosal ischemia occurs when the pressure of the cuff exerted on the mucosa exceeds the capillary perfusion pressure. Arterial capillary perfusion pressure is 30 mmHg; venous capillary perfusion pressure is 18 mmHg; and lymphatic perfusion pressure is 5 mmHg. To reduce the incidence of tracheal damage, the nurse ensures a cuff pressure between 14 and 20 mmHg.

Most cuffs are designed to use a high volume of air while maintaining a low pressure on the tracheal mucosa. The nurse inflates the cuff to provide an adequate seal between the trachea and the cuff while creating the least amount of pressure. There are two methods of cuff inflation: the minimal leak technique (for cuffs without pressure relief valves) and the occlusive technique (for cuffs with pressure relief valves).

The nurse checks cuff pressures each shift, especially with the minimal leak technique, and maintains it at 14–20 mmHg. In rare situations, cuff pressure is increased to maintain ventilator volumes when peak pressures are greater than 50 mmHg and positive end-expiratory pressure (PEEP) is greater than 10 mmHg. Manufacturers provide guidelines for the approximate recommended volumes allowed for each tracheostomy cuff size. Most cuffs are sufficiently inflated with less than 10 mL of air.

Although a high cuff pressure causes tracheal damage, other factors contribute to the severity of damage. The client's condition determines, to a degree, susceptibility to tissue damage. The client who is malnourished, hypoten-

sive, dehydrated, hypoxic, elderly, or receiving corticosteroids is unable to promote adequate tissue healing and is vulnerable to further tissue damage. Duration of intubation, extent and technique of suctioning, and stabilization of the tube against friction and movement are important factors that determine the extent of tracheal mucosa damage. The nurse minimizes local airway damage through the maintenance of proper cuff pressures, stabilization of the tube, judicious suctioning, and prevention and treatment of malnutrition, hemodynamic instability, or hypoxia.

Humidification and Warming of Air. The tracheostomy tube bypasses the upper air passages of the nose and mouth, which normally humidify, warm, and filter the air before it reaches the lower part of the respiratory tract. If humidification and warming are not adequate, tracheal damage can result from extremes in humidity and air temperature. In addition, thick, dried secretions can occlude the proximal and distal airway.

To prevent these complications, the nurse provides a humidification source, as ordered. The nurse then assesses, on an ongoing basis, for a fine mist emerging from the tracheostomy collar or T-piece during inspiration and expiration. To increase the amount of humidification delivered, the respiratory therapist attaches a warming device to the humidification source. At the same time, a temperature probe is placed in the tubing circuit. Temperature is constantly monitored and is generally maintained between 37° and 38° C (98.6° F–100.4° F), but no greater than 40° C (104° F). The nurse monitors the client's temperature by feeling the tubing during client care and by checking the temperature probe. In addition, the nurse ensures adequate hydration, which also helps to liquefy secretions.

Suctioning. Suctioning (Chart 30–2) maintains a patent airway and promotes gas exchange by removing secretions from the client who cannot adequately cough. The nurse assesses the client's need for suction, indicated by audible or noisy secretions, crackles or rhonchi on auscultation, restlessness, increased pulse or respiratory rates, presence of mucus in the artificial airway, client requests for suctioning, or an increase in the peak airway pressure on the ventilator.

Suctioning is most often through an artificial airway but can be accomplished either through the nose or mouth. Suctioning of both routes is considered routine for the client with retained secretions.

The technique of suctioning through the nose is associated with similar complications as suctioning through an artificial airway. Entry through the nasal vault into the nasopharynx can be painful. Slow, careful placement of the catheter, with a good understanding of the nasopharyngeal anatomy, can make the procedure less traumatic. The nurse may place a nasopharyngeal airway through which to suction to prevent trauma to the nasal mucosa. The nurse advances the catheter through the nasopharynx and into the laryngopharynx while giving the client oxygen by mask or nasal cannula. Once the catheter enters the larynx, the client may cough. On inhalation, the nurse inserts the catheter through the vocal cords and into the trachea. Occasionally, the catheter can be disconnected from suction and attached to an oxygen source, with the client receiving oxygen via the catheter.

Suctioning is associated with several complications, including hypoxia, tissue (mucosal) trauma, infection, vagal stimulation, and bronchospasm.

Hypoxia. The causes of hypoxia include
- Ineffective oxygenation before, during, and after suctioning
- Use of a catheter that is too large for the artificial airway
- Prolonged suctioning time
- Excessive suction pressure
- Too-frequent suctioning

The nurse prevents hypoxia by hyperoxygenating the client with 100% oxygen from an oxygen-delivery device (manual resuscitation bag attached to an oxygen source). Suctioning can be done by a one- or two-person technique. If the client is able to take deep breaths, the nurse instructs the client to do so three or four times before suctioning, with the existing oxygen delivery system. If possible, simultaneous monitoring of heart rate or use of a pulse oximeter is helpful in assessing tolerance of the suctioning procedure. The nurse assesses the client for signs and symptoms of hypoxia (e.g., increased heart rate and blood pressure, oxygen desaturation, cyanosis, restlessness, anxiety, and cardiac dysrhythmias). Oxygen desaturation below 90% as determined by pulse oximetry indicates hypoxemia. If hypoxia occurs, the nurse terminates the suctioning procedure. Using the 100% oxygen-delivery system, the nurse reoxygenates the client until baseline parameters are achieved.

The nurse prevents hypoxia by using a catheter of the correct size. The size should not exceed half of the size of the tracheal lumen. In adults, the standard catheter size is 12 or 14 Fr. Adequate catheter size facilitates efficient removal of secretions without causing hypoxemia.

Tissue Trauma. The mucosa of the respiratory tract is extremely fragile, and frequent suctioning, prolonged suctioning time, excessive suction pressure, and nonrotation of the catheter cause damage. The nurse prevents tissue trauma by suctioning only when indicated. The nurse lubricates the catheter with sterile water or saline before insertion and suctions only during the withdrawal of the catheter. Use of a twirling motion during withdrawal prevents excessive grabbing of the mucosa.

In addition, the nurse applies suction intermittently for only 10–15 seconds. The nurse can estimate this time frame by holding his or her own breath and counting to 10 or 15 during suctioning. At the end of the 15 seconds, the suctioning procedure is finished. Fifteen seconds does not seem long to a healthy person, but most clients requiring suctioning have respiratory compromise and cannot tolerate more than 15 seconds of suctioning.

Chart 30–2

Nursing Care Highlight: Suctioning the Artificial Airway

1. Assess the need for suctioning (routine unnecessary suctioning causes mucosal damage, bleeding, and bronchospasm).
2. Wash hands. Don protective eyewear. Maintain Standard Precautions or body substance precautions.
3. Explain to the client that sensations such as shortness of breath and coughing are to be expected but that any discomfort will be very short in duration.
4. Check the suction source. Occlude the suction source, and adjust the pressure dial to between 80 and 120 mmHg to prevent hypoxemia and trauma to the mucosa.
5. Set up a sterile field.
6. Preoxygenate the client with 100% oxygen for 30 seconds to 3 minutes (at least three hyperinflations) to prevent hypoxemia. Keep hyperinflations synchronized with inhalation.
7. Quickly insert the suction catheter until resistance is met. Do not apply suction during insertion.
8. Withdraw the catheter 0.4 to 0.8 inch (1–2 cm), and begin to apply suction. Use intermittent suction and a twirling motion of the catheter during withdrawal. Never suction longer than 10 to 15 seconds.
9. Hyperoxygenate for 1 to 5 minutes or until the client's baseline heart rate and oxygen saturation are within normal limits.
10. Repeat as needed for up to three total suction passes.
11. Suction mouth as needed, and provide mouth care.
12. Describe secretions, and document client's responses.

Infection. Each catheter pass introduces bacteria into the trachea. In the hospital, the nurse uses sterile technique for suctioning and for all suctioning equipment, including suction catheters, gloves, and saline or water. After suctioning the artificial airway, the nurse then suctions the client's mouth. Oral suction equipment is never used for suctioning an artificial airway because the mouth is contaminated with bacteria, which are necessary for digestion, but could be introduced into the lungs. Home suctioning procedures emphasize clean technique because the number of virulent organisms in the home environment is lower than in the hospital.

Vagal Stimulation and Bronchospasm. Vagal stimulation results in severe bradycardia, hypotension, heart block, ventricular tachycardia, or asystole. If vagal stimulation occurs, the nurse stops suctioning immediately and oxygenates the client manually with 100% oxygen. Bronchospasm sometimes occurs when the catheter passes into the airway. The client may require a bronchodilator to relieve the bronchospasm and respiratory distress.

Tracheostomy Care. Tracheostomy care (Chart 30–3) keeps the tracheostomy tube free of obstructing secretions, maintains a patent airway, and provides wound care. This procedure is performed whether or not the client is able to clear secretions. The nurse performs tracheostomy care according to agency policy, usually every shift and as needed.

Before proceeding with tracheostomy care, the nurse assesses the client as shown in Chart 30–4. The extent of both suctioning and tracheostomy care depends entirely

---

Chart 30–4

Focused Assessment of the Client with a Tracheostomy

- Note the quality, pattern, and rate of breathing:
  - Within client's baseline?
    Tachypnea can indicate hypoxia.
    Dyspnea can indicate secretions in airway.
- Assess for any cyanosis, especially around the lips, which could indicate hypoxia.
- Check the client's pulse oximetry reading.
- If oxygen is ordered, is the client receiving the correct amount, with the correct equipment and humidification?
- Assess the tracheostomy site:
  - Note the color, consistency, and amount of secretions in the tube or externally.
  - If the tracheostomy is sutured in place, is there any redness, swelling, or drainage from suture sites?
  - If the tracheostomy is secured with ties, what is the condition of the ties? Are they moist with secretions or perspiration? Are the secretions dried on the ties? Is the tie secure?
  - Assess the condition of the skin around the tracheostomy and neck. Be sure to check underneath the neck for secretions that may have drained to the back. Check for any breakdown related to pressure from the ties or from excess secretions.
  - Assess behind the face plate for the size of the space between the outer cannula and the client's tissue. Are any secretions collected in this area?
- If the tube is cuffed, check cuff pressure.
- Auscultate the lungs.
- Is a second (emergency) tracheostomy tube and obturator available?

Chart 30–3

Nursing Care Highlight: Tracheostomy Care

1. Assemble the necessary equipment.
2. Wash your hands. Maintain Standard Precautions or body substance precautions.
3. Suction the tracheostomy tube if necessary.
4. Remove old dressings and excess secretions.
5. Set up a sterile field.
6. Remove and clean the inner cannula. Use half-strength hydrogen peroxide to clean the cannula, and sterile saline to rinse it. If the inner cannula is disposable, remove the cannula and replace it with a new one.
7. Clean the stoma site and then the tracheostomy plate with half-strength hydrogen peroxide followed by sterile saline. Ensure that none of the solutions enters the tracheostomy.
8. Change tracheostomy ties if they are soiled. Secure new ties in place before removing soiled ones to prevent accidental decannulation. If a knot is needed, tie a square knot that is visible on the side of the neck. One or two fingers should be able to be placed between the tie tape and the neck.
9. Document the type and amount of secretions and the general condition of the stoma and surrounding skin. Document the client's response to the procedure and any teaching or learning that occurred.

---

on the needs of the client. The need for suctioning and tracheostomy care is determined by the amount and consistency of secretions, medical diagnosis (specifically pulmonary diseases), ability of the client to cough and deep breathe, need for mechanical ventilation, and wound care required. The nurse inspects the inner lumen of a single-lumen tube with a flashlight or penlight to assess for the presence of secretions.

The nurse changes tracheostomy ties once a day to keep them clean and to avoid having them act as a medium for infection. A properly secured tie allows space for only one or two fingers to be placed between the tie and the neck. Tube movement causes irritation and coughing, which, in turn, may cause decannulation. Keeping the tube secure while changing the ties to prevent accidental decannulation is imperative. One way to accomplish this safely is to keep the old ties on the tube while changing ties, but a secure hand on the tube is the most reliable method of tube stabilization. The nurse includes the client in this process as a step toward self-care. Figure 30–15 demonstrates a correct technique for applying a tracheostomy dressing.

Bronchial and Oral Hygiene. Bronchial hygiene promotes a patent airway, prevents pulmonary infections,

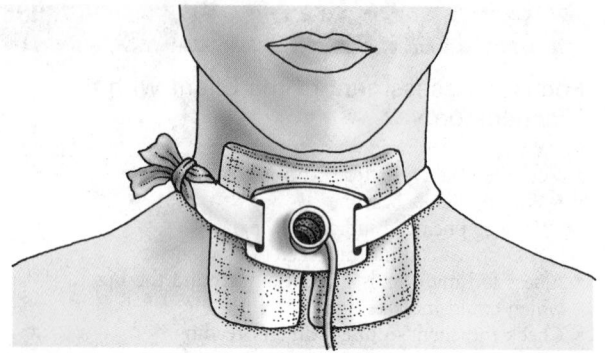

Figure 30–15. Placement of precut gauze and tie around a tracheostomy tube.

and stimulates the pulmonary system. The nurse turns and repositions the client every 1–2 hours, supports out-of-bed activities, and encourages ambulation. These interventions promote lung expansion and gas exchange and facilitate the mobilization of secretions. Coughing and deep breathing, combined with the chest physical therapy techniques of percussion, vibration, and postural drainage, are powerful measures in promoting pulmonary care (see Chap. 32).

Frequent oral hygiene is important not only to ensure a patent airway but also to prevent bacterial overgrowth and dental caries and to promote client comfort. The nurse maintains standard or body substance precautions during the procedure. Cleansing the mouth with glycerin swabs and mouthwash, which contains significant amounts of alcohol, are contraindicated because these interventions dry the oral mucosa, change its pH, and promote bacterial growth. The nurse instead uses a toothette or soft-bristle brush moistened in water for mouth care. Hydrogen peroxide solutions can help to remove crusted materials but may break down granulating tissue and are used only with a physician's order.

During oral care, the nurse examines the mouth for any alterations in mucosal integrity, dental abnormalities, and alterations in tissue integrity. Ulcers (aphthous or herpes simplex), bacterial or fungal (Candida) growth, or other infections are treated medically. Application of lip balms or water-soluble jelly can prevent cracked lips and further skin breakdown and can help keep the client comfortable. Providing mouth care is a simple but very effective method of promoting oral health, comfort, and aesthetic appearance. Offering an opportunity for the client or family member to perform mouth care encourages participation in care and increases the client's self-esteem.

Nutrition. Swallowing can be a major problem for the client with a tracheostomy tube in place. In a normal swallow, the larynx elevates and moves forward to protect itself from the passing stream of food and saliva. Laryngeal elevation also assists in the opening of the cricopharyngeal muscle, the upper esophageal sphincter. The tracheostomy tube sometimes tethers the larynx in place, rendering it unable to execute this motion efficiently. The result is difficulty in swallowing. Likewise, when the tracheostomy tube cuff is inflated, it can balloon posteriorly and interfere with the passage of food through the

esophagus. The common wall of the posterior trachea (trachealis muscle) and the anterior esophagus is very thin, allowing this pushing phenomenon.

Provided that the tracheostomy tube is not capped, the nurse usually inflates the cuff during feeding to prevent aspiration. The nurse then instructs the client to keep the head of the bed elevated for at least 30 minutes after feeding and keeps the cuff inflated for the same period. Clients who are cognitively intact, however, may adapt to eating normal food when the tracheostomy tube is small and the cuff is not inflated.

Speech and Communication. The client will be able to speak when there is a cuffless tube, when a fenestrated tracheostomy tube is in place, and when the fenestrated tube is capped or covered. Until one of the methods for natural vocalization is feasible, the nurse establishes and teaches alternative communication methods that are easy for the client to use. A writing tablet, "magic slate," communication board with pictures and letters, hand signals, or a computer, as well as a call light within reach, is essential to promote communication and decrease the client's frustration from not being able to speak or be understood. The nurse moves the client closer to the nurses' station and marks the central call light system with indicators to communicate that the client cannot speak. Questions phrased for "yes" or "no" answers help the client respond efficiently.

The inability to talk is a major stressor for the client. Every effort to facilitate communication and speech is important. When the client can tolerate cuff deflation, the client places a finger over the tracheostomy tube on exhalation. This forces air up through the larynx, vocal cords, and mouth and allows for articulation. During the process of decannulation, when the fenestrated tube is "capped," the client experiences a very positive but secondary benefit of speech without the need to cover the tube.

Emotional Care. Addressing psychologic concerns is an important aspect of nursing care of clients recovering from a tracheostomy. While providing physical care to the client, the nurse keeps in mind the emotional impact of an artificial airway. Acknowledging the client's frustration in communication and allowing sufficient time for communication are critically important. When speaking to the client, the nurse uses a normal tone of voice. The tracheostomy tube has not altered the client's ability to hear or understand.

Body Image. The client experiences a change in body image because of deformity, the presence of a stoma or artificial airway, speech changes, a change in the method of eating, and possibly difficulty with speech. The nurse helps the client to set realistic goals, starting with involvement in self-care.

The nurse and family must make all attempts to ease the client into a more normal social environment. The nurse provides encouragement and positive reinforcement while demonstrating acceptance and caring behaviors. The family may benefit from counseling sessions that the nurse initiates in the hospital.

After surgery, the client may feel reserved and socially isolated. To cover the tracheostomy tube the client can wear loose-fitting shirts or scarves. (See Chapter 10 for a detailed discussion of body image, including additional nursing interventions.)

Weaning. Weaning the client from a tracheostomy tube entails a gradual decrease in the tube size and ultimate removal of the tube. The nurse carefully monitors this process, especially after each change. The physician or a specially trained nurse performs the steps in the process.

First, the cuff is deflated as soon as the client can manage secretions and does not require mechanical ventilation. This change allows the client to breathe through the tube and also through the upper airway. Next, the tube is changed to an uncuffed tube; then the size of the tube is gradually decreased. When a small fenestrated tube is placed (No. 4 or No. 6, depending on the size of the airway), the tube is capped so that all air passes through the upper airway and the fenestra, with none passing through the tube. The tube is removed after the client tolerates more than 24 hours of capping. The nurse places a dry dressing over the stoma, which then gradually heals on its own. A small scar remains.

Another device used for the transition from tracheostomy to natural breathing is a tracheostomy button. The button maintains patency of the stoma and facilitates spontaneous breathing. The Kistner tracheostomy tube and Olympic tracheostomy button are examples of this type of device. To function, they must fit properly. A disadvantage of these buttons is the possibility of decannulation: the tube dislodges from the trachea but remains in the anterior subcutaneous tissues of the neck.

▶ Continuing Care

By the time of discharge from the hospital, the client should be able to provide self-care, which may include tracheostomy care, nutritional care, suctioning, and methods of communication. Although education begins during preoperative teaching sessions, most self-care is taught in the hospital. The nurse teaches the client and family how to care for the tracheostomy tube. The nurse reviews airway care, including cleaning and inspecting for signs of infection. The nurse teaches clean suction technique and reviews the client's plan of care.

The nurse instructs the client to use a shower shield over the tracheostomy tube when bathing to prevent water from entering the airway. To shield the airway during the day, the client may wear a protective cover. Covering the permanent opening has several benefits: filtering the air entering the stoma, keeping humidity in the airway, and enhancing aesthetic appearance. To protect the airway and increase humidity, the nurse instructs the client to cover the airway with cotton or foam. Attractive coverings are available in the form of cotton scarves, crocheted bibs, and jewelry. Using colored seam binding for tracheostomy ties after the stoma has matured may enhance the client's overall body image. The client's shirt or dress color can be matched or coordinated with seam bindings of various colors. The nurse also teaches the client to increase humidity in the home.

The nurse may teach the client to instill normal saline into the artificial airway 10–15 times a day as ordered. The client continues the selected method of alternative communication that began in the hospital and wears a medical alert (Medic-Alert) bracelet.

The client should feel safe and secure with the extended plan of care. The multidisciplinary care team assesses the client's specific discharge needs and makes appropriate referrals to home care agencies and durable medical equipment companies (for suction equipment and tracheostomy supplies). Clinic or physician follow-up visits occur early after discharge, but the home care nurse also becomes a very important resource for the client and family. The home care nurse initiates, with physician order, and coordinates the services of professionals such as nutritionists, nurses, speech pathologists, and social workers. The home care or hospital nurse informs the client and family of community organizations that can offer support and friendships. When the client has problems paying for health care services, equipment supply, and prescriptions, the visiting nurse agency may be helpful in directing the client to available resources.

SELECTED BIBLIOGRAPHY

*Albarren, J. W. (1991). A review of communication with intubated patients and those with tracheostomies within an intensive care environment. *Intensive Care Nursing, 7*(3), 179–186.

*American Association of Respiratory Care. (1991). Clinical practice guideline: Oxygen therapy in the acute care hospital. *Respiratory Care, 36*(12), 1410–1413.

*Ball, R. A. (1994). Review. Liquid oxygen: A new look for an old companion. *JEMS: Journal of Emergency Medical Services, 19*(3), 85–86.

*Bolgiano, C. S., Bunting, K., & Shoenberger, M. M. (1990). Administering oxygen therapy: What you need to know. *Nursing90, 20*(6), 47–51.

Celia, L. M. (1995). Consultation stat. Supplying oxygen when a trach tube is dislodged. *RN, 58*(4), 61.

Crimlisk, J. T., Horn, M. H., Wilson, D. J., et al. (1996). Artificial airways: A survey of cuff management practices. *Heart and Lung: Journal of Acute and Critical Care, 25*(3), 225–235.

Eisenhauer, B. (1996). Action stat. Dislodged tracheostomy tube. *Nursing96, 26*(6), 25.

Hatfield, B. O. (1997). Cost effective trache teaching. *RN, 60*(3), 48–49.

*Kersten, L. D. (1989). *Comprehensive respiratory nursing: A decision making approach.* Philadelphia: W. B. Saunders.

Ladyshewsky, A., & Gousseau, A. (1996). Successful tracheal weaning. *Canadian Nurse, 92*(2), 35–38.

*Mapp, C. (1988). Trach care: Are you aware of all the dangers? *Nursing88, 18*(7), 34–43.

Mathews, P. J. (1995). Safely delivering a breath of fresh air. *Nursing95, 25*(5), 66–69.

McConnell, E. A. (1997). Administering oxygen by mask. *Nursing97, 21*(9), 26.

*Montanari, J., & Spearing, C. (1986). The fine art of measuring tracheal cuff pressure. *Nursing86, 16*(7), 46–49.

*Openbrier, D. R., Fuoss, C., & Mall, C. (1988). What patients on home oxygen therapy want to know. *American Journal of Nursing, 88*(2), 198–202.

*Openbrier, D. R., Hoffman, L., & Wesmiller, S. (1988). Home oxygen therapy. *American Journal of Nursing, 88*(2), 192–197.

Pfister, S. M. (1995). Home oxygen therapy: Indications, administration, recertification, and patient education. *Nurse Practitioner: American Journal of Primary Health Care, 20*(7), 44, 47–52, 54–56.

Provine, B. (1996). Consultation corner. Education about tracheostomy care. *Perspectives in Respiratory Nursing, 7*(2), 6.

*Schuring, L. T., Pollock, K., Cyr, M., et al. (1994). Otorhinolaryngology–head and neck nursing practice guidelines: Tracheostomy. *Otorhinolaryngology—Head and Neck Nursing, 12*(4), 26–29.

Somerson, S. J., Husted, C. W., Somerson, S. W., et al. (1996). Mastering emergency airway management. *American Journal of Nursing, 96*(5), 24–31.

*Tayal, V. S. (1994). Tracheostomies. *Emergency Medicine Clinics of North America, 12*(3), 707–727.

*Weiletz, P. B., & Dettenmeier, P. A. (1994). Test your knowledge of tracheostomy tubes. *American Journal of Nursing, 94*(2), 46–50.

SUGGESTED READINGS

Eisenhauer, B. (1996). Action stat. Dislodged tracheostomy tube. *Nursing96, 26*(6), 25.

This brief article reviews emergency measures for the nurse to take when a client's new tracheostomy tube visually appears to be in place but is actually dislodged. Assessment and rationale for interventions are included.

Mathews, P. J. (1995). Safely delivering a breath of fresh air. *Nursing95, 25*(5), 66–69.

This photoguide addresses specific steps to follow when using a portable "E" cylinder for transport. Included are safety measures, determining the amount of oxygen in the tank, using the wrench key, and bleeding the tank. Also included is a calculation the nurse can use to determine how many minutes the oxygen in the tank will last.

Chapter 31

INTERVENTIONS FOR CLIENTS WITH NONINFECTIOUS PROBLEMS OF THE UPPER RESPIRATORY TRACT

The upper respiratory tract includes the structures of the nose, sinuses, oropharynx, larynx, and trachea. Many common acute and chronic disorders affect the upper airways. The nurse encounters clients with diseases of the upper respiratory system across the health care continuum, in homes, clinics, primary care practitioners' offices, emergency departments, and hospitals and nursing homes. The major nursing priority for clients with disorders of the upper respiratory tract is to maintain a patent and functioning airway.

NONINFECTIOUS DISORDERS OF THE NOSE AND SINUSES
Fracture of the Nose

Overview

Nasal fractures commonly occur from injuries received during falls, participation in sports, or trauma related to violence or motor vehicle accidents. Usually, if the bone or cartilage is not displaced, no serious complications result from the fracture, and treatment may not be necessary. Displacement, however, can cause airway obstruc-

tion or cosmetic deformity and is a potential source of infection.

Collaborative Management

 Assessment

The nurse notes and documents nasal deviation, misaligned nasal bridge, change in nasal breathing, crepitus on palpation, midface ecchymosis, and pain. Blood or clear (cerebrospinal) fluid rarely drains from one or both nares, but such drainage could indicate a skull fracture. Radiographic examination is not always useful in nasal fractures, but is very important in evaluating the client for other concurrent facial fractures.

 Interventions

The physician performs a simple closed reduction of the fracture using local or general anesthesia within the first 24 hours after injury. After 24 hours, the fracture is more difficult to reduce because of edema and scar formation.

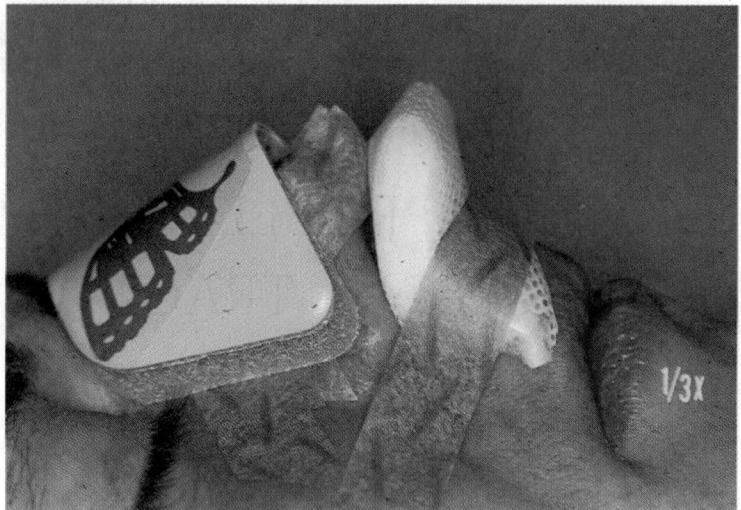

Figure 31–1. Immediate postoperative appearance of a client who has undergone rhinoplasty. Note the splint and gauze drip pad. From Tardy, M. E. (1997). *Rhinoplasty: The art and the science* (p. 207). Philadelphia: W. B. Saunders. Used with permission.

Simple closed fractures need not be surgically treated; treatment focuses on pain relief and local cold compresses to decrease swelling.

➤ Rhinoplasty

For severe fractures or those that do not heal properly, a reduction and rhinoplasty may be required. Rhinoplasty is a surgical reconstruction of the nose for cosmetic purposes and for functional improvement of airflow. The client returns from surgery with packing in both nostrils to prevent bleeding and to provide a *stent* (object that provides support and structure) for the reconstructed nose. The ½-inch gauze packing is typically treated with an antibiotic ointment, such as bacitracin (Bacitrin) to reduce the risk of infection. The client typically has a "mustache" dressing, or drip pad, usually a folded 2 × 2-inch gauze pad, placed under the nose. A splint or cast may cover the nose for additional alignment and protection (Fig. 31–1). The nurse or client changes the drip pad as necessary.

Postoperatively, the nurse observes the client for edema and bleeding and takes vital signs every 4 hours until discharge. The nurse assesses how often the client swallows. Repeated swallowing may indicate posterior nasal bleeding. The nurse examines the pharynx with a penlight for bleeding and, if bleeding is present, notifies the physician. The client with uncomplicated rhinoplasty with or without related surgical procedures (brow-lifts, blepharoplasties, face-lifts) is usually sent home the day of surgery. The client and family or significant other are instructed in routine care.

The nurse or family member places the client in a semi-Fowler's position and instructs the client to move slowly and to rest as much as possible. Cool compresses are applied to the nose, eyes, or face to reduce swelling and prevent excessive discoloration. Once the effects of anesthesia are eliminated and the physician has so ordered, the client may eat soft foods. An oral fluid intake of at least 2500 mL/day is encouraged. To prevent bleeding, the nurse also instructs the client to limit the Val-salva maneuver, such as forceful coughing or straining at stool, for the first few days after removal of the nasal packing. Laxatives or stool softeners may be appropriate to facilitate defecation. The client is instructed to avoid aspirin and nonsteroidal antiinflammatory drugs during this time to prevent the possibility of bleeding. The physician may order prophylactic antibiotics to prevent postoperative infection and pain medication to relieve discomfort. The nurse explains to the client that edema and discoloration usually last for several weeks and that the final surgical result will be evident in 6–12 months.

➤ Nasoseptoplasty

Nasoseptoplasty, or submucous resection (SMR), may be necessary to straighten a deviated septum when chronic symptoms (e.g., a "stuffy" nose) or discomfort occurs. A slight deviation of the nasal septum is present in most adults and causes no symptoms. Major deviations may obstruct the nasal passages or interfere with airflow and sinus drainage. The surgeon removes the deviated section of the cartilage and bone. The amount resected depends on the type and degree of deformity.

Nursing care is similar to that for the client with a rhinoplasty. Nasoseptoplasty is often an outpatient procedure; the nurse reviews written instructions with the client on discharge.

Epistaxis

Overview

Because of the rich capillary network within the nose, epistaxis (nosebleed) is a common problem. Nosebleeds may occur as a result of trauma, hypertension, blood dyscrasia (e.g., leukemias), inflammation, tumor, decreased humidity, excessive nose blowing, and nose picking. Men are usually affected more than women, and the elderly tend to bleed most often from the posterior portion of the nose.

Chart 31-1

Nursing Care Highlight: Emergency Care of a Nosebleed

1. Position the client in an upright position, leaning forward, to prevent blood from entering the stomach and possible aspiration.
2. Reassure the client and attempt to keep him or her quiet to reduce anxiety and blood pressure.
3. Apply direct lateral pressure to the nose for 5 minutes, and apply ice or cool compresses to the nose and face if possible.
4. Maintain standard or body substance precautions.
5. If nasal packing is necessary, loosely pack both nares with gauze or nasal tampons.
6. To prevent rebleeding from dislodging clots, instruct the client not to blow the nose for several hours after the bleeding stops.
7. Seek medical assistance if these measures are ineffective or if the bleeding occurs frequently.

Collaborative Management

 ### Assessment

The client may be holding a tissue or gauze pad up to the nares while explaining to the nurse what happened. Often the client will report that the bleeding started after sneezing or blowing the nose. The nurse notes the amount and color of the blood and takes vital signs. The nurse also assesses and documents the number, duration, and causes of previous bleeding episodes.

 ### Interventions

Chart 31-1 summarizes first aid for the client with a nosebleed. If the nosebleed does not respond to these interventions, medical attention is needed. The physician cauterizes the affected capillaries with silver nitrate or electrocautery, followed by anterior packing. Anterior packing is very effective in controlling bleeding from the anterior nasal cavity.

When bleeding originates in the posterior nasal region, the physician uses a posterior pack to stop the bleeding. A string is attached to a large gauze pack and then threaded through the nose and out the mouth. The physician positions the pack in the posterior nasal cavity above the pharynx, and then tapes the string to the client's cheek to prevent movement of the pack. This procedure is uncomfortable and may cause airway obstruction if the pack slips.

The nurse observes the client for respiratory distress and for tolerance of the packing. The physician may prescribe humidification and oxygen as well as bed rest and antibiotics. To maintain gag and cough reflexes and optimal level of consciousness, the client should not receive any sedatives and only limited pain medication. The nurse provides oral care and ensures adequate hydration, which is important because of mouth breathing. The nurse uses pulse oximetry or a cardiac monitor to observe for hypoxemia and hypercapnia. After 2–5 days, the physician removes the packing. Petroleum jelly can be applied to the nares for lubrication and comfort. Nasal saline solution and humidification may be helpful to add moisture and prevent crusting and rebleeding. At discharge the client should continue gentle saline irrigations and lubrication to the nasal cavity to prevent further crusting and subsequent rebleeding.

Nasal Polyps

Overview

Nasal polyps are benign, grape-like clusters of mucous membrane and loose connective tissue. Polyps typically occur bilaterally and are often caused by irritation to the nasal mucosa or sinuses, allergies, or infection (chronic sinusitis). If polyps become too large, airway obstruction may result.

Collaborative Management

Benign nasal polyps are treated medically with nasally inhaled steroids in conjunction with removal of the polyps. Surgical removal (polypectomy) can be accomplished with either local or general anesthesia. The nurse observes the client for postoperative bleeding. The nostrils are usually packed with gauze for 24 hours postoperatively. Nasal polyps tend to recur if not completely resected.

Inverting papilloma is a rare, histologically benign condition consisting of a space-occupying lesion that erodes nasal and maxillary skeletal structures. Often initially diagnosed as benign polyps, inverting papillomas grow by pressure into other adjacent structures. Extensive sinus and nasal surgery is necessary for complete removal. If these papillomas are completely resected, they do not recur.

Juvenile angiofibromas are similar in growth pattern but histologically different from other polyps. These tumors usually occur in adolescent males and may undergo resolution when the client reaches adulthood. These may be resected by traditional nasal surgery; more invasive tumors may require skull base resections.

Cancer of the Nose and Sinuses

Overview

Tumors of the nasal cavities and sinuses are relatively uncommon and may be benign or malignant. Malignant lesions of these areas can occur at all ages, but the peak incidence is 40 to 45 years in males and 60 to 65 years in females. There is a higher incidence of nasopharyngeal cancer in Asian-Americans.

Collaborative Management

 Assessment

The onset of sinus malignancies is insidious, and symptoms resemble sinusitis. Therefore, clients may have relatively advanced disease at diagnosis. Persistent nasal obstruction, drainage, bloody discharge, and pain that does not improve after treatment of sinusitis suggest nasal or sinus malignancy. Cervical lymph node enlargement usually occurs on the side with greater tumor mass.

 Interventions

Radiation therapy is the primary treatment for nasopharyngeal cancers. Surgical resection may be indicated in radiation therapy failures. Chemotherapy has not proved to be effective. The specific surgical procedure depends on the amount of tumor, its anatomic location, and degree of tissue invasion. The primary deficit is change in body image, speech, and alteration in nutrition, especially when the maxilla and floor of the nose are involved in the resection.

The nurse provides general postoperative care (see Chap. 22), including maintenance of a patent airway, wound care, strict attention to nutrition, and tracheostomy care (if necessary). (Tracheostomy care is covered in Chapter 30.) The nurse provides meticulous mouth and maxillary cavity care with saline irrigations for the client, using a water pick (e.g., Water Pik) or a syringe. The nurse also assesses for alterations in comfort and for infection. Optimal nutrition is essential during the perioperative period for adequate healing.

Facial Trauma

Overview

Facial trauma is defined by the specific bones (i.e., mandibular, maxillary, zygomatic, orbital, or nasal fractures) and the side of the face involved. Mandibular (lower jaw) fractures can occur at any location of the mandible and make up the majority of facial fractures. Le Fort I is a nasoethmoid complex fracture. Le Fort II is a transverse maxillary and nasoethmoid complex fracture. Le Fort III is a combination of I and II plus an orbital zygoma fracture, often called "craniofacial disjunction" because it leaves the midface with no connection to the skull. Because the face is very vascular, there is often much bleeding with facial trauma.

Collaborative Management

 Assessment

The priority in the management of facial trauma is assessment for a patent airway. Signs and symptoms of an upper airway obstruction include stridor, shortness of breath, dyspnea, anxiety, restlessness, hypoxia, hypercarbia, decreased oxygen saturation, cyanosis, and loss of consciousness. After establishing the airway, the nurse assesses the amount and site of soft-tissue trauma, bleeding, and palpable fractures. Additional findings on assessment include edema of soft tissue, asymmetry, pain, or leakage of cerebrospinal fluid through the ears or nose, or both, indicating temporal bone or basilar skull fracture. Because orbital and maxillary fractures can entrap the eye, the nurse assesses vision and extraocular movement (EOM) and also observes for neurologic changes (see Chap. 43). Because spinal cord trauma and skull fractures often occur in conjunction with facial trauma, cranial computed tomography, facial series, and cervical spine films are then obtained.

 Interventions

The nurse's priority is to establish and maintain a patent airway. The nurse must anticipate the need for emergent intubation, tracheotomy, or cricothyroidotomy. When the client arrives at a trauma center, care focuses on controlling hemorrhage, establishing an airway, and assessing for the extent of injury. If signs and symptoms of shock are present (see Chap. 39), fluid resuscitation and identification of bleeding sites must be initiated immediately.

In head and neck trauma, the nurse must be astute in trauma and critical care nursing. Time is paramount in stabilizing the client. Early treatment and response of the appropriate services, including the trauma team, maxillofacial surgeon, general surgeon, otolaryngologist, plastic surgeon, and dentist, optimize the client's posttrauma recovery. (Consult a specialized trauma book for more information about trauma care.)

Stabilization of the fractured segment of a mandibular fracture allows the teeth to heal in proper alignment or occlusion. The client remains in fixed centric occlusion for 6–10 weeks. Antibiotic therapy may be prescribed because of oral wound contamination. Delay in treatment, infection of the adjacent tooth, and poor oral care may result in infection in the mandibular segment. The client may then require surgical debridement, intravenous (IV) antibiotic therapy, and an extended period in fixation.

Facial fractures are now most often repaired with microplating surgical systems. These shaping plates fix the bone fragments in place until osteoneogenesis occurs. Large areas of skull can be replaced with BoneSource. The osteoblasts and osteoclasts grow into the BoneSource and rematrix into a stabilized bone support. In the United States, the plates remain in place permanently; in Europe the plates are removed after healing has occurred.

Intermaxillary fixation (IMF) is a common method of securing a mandibular fracture. The physician can repair nondisplaced aligned fractures in a clinic or office using local dental anesthesia. General anesthesia is used for repair of displaced or complex fractures or fractures that occur with other facial bone fractures.

If the mandibular fracture is repaired with titanium plates, the nurse teaches the client oral care, soft-diet restrictions, and follow-up care with a dentist. The plates are permanent and do not interfere with magnetic resonance imaging (MRI) studies.

Postoperatively, the nurse teaches oral care with an irrigating device, such as a Water Pik. If the client is in inner maxillary fixation, the nurse teaches self-care with wires in place, including a dental liquid diet. The nurse also explains the proper method of cutting the wires if emesis occurs. The client keeps wire cutters nearby at all times in preparation for this emergency. The nurse instructs the client to return to the physician for rewiring as soon as possible to reinstitute fixation.

Nutrition is important for any client with fractures. Because of oral fixation, pain, and surgery, clients may not attend to their nutritional needs. Dietary consultations are important for teaching and support.

NONINFECTIOUS DISORDERS OF THE ORAL PHARYNX AND TONSILS
Obstructive Sleep Apnea

Overview

Sleep apnea is breathing disruption during sleep lasting at least 10 seconds and occurring a minimum of five times in an hour. Although sleep apnea can have a neurologic or central origin, the most common form of adult sleep apnea occurs as a result of upper airway obstruction. Factors that contribute to sleep apnea include obesity, a large uvula, short neck, smoking, enlarged tonsils or adenoids, and oropharyngeal edema. Men are more commonly affected than women, and the incidence increases with age.

During sleep, with relaxation of skeletal muscles and displacement of the tongue and neck structures, the upper airway is obstructed even though chest wall movement is unimpaired. The apnea increases the arterial carbon dioxide level and decreases the pH. These blood gas changes stimulate neural activity. The sleeper is aroused spontaneously after 10 or more seconds of apnea and corrects the obstruction, resulting in a resumption of respiration. Upon resumption of sleep, the cycle begins again, sometimes as often as every 5 minutes.

This cyclic pattern of disrupted sleep prevents the person from reaching the prolonged state of deep sleep necessary for maximum rest. As a result, the person may have excessive daytime sleepiness, an inability to concentrate, and irritability. Some people experience *narcolepsy*, an uncontrollable and dangerous state of unintentional daytime sleep, while performing daytime activities.

Collaborative Management

 Assessment

Clients who have excessive daytime sleepiness or complaints of "waking up tired," particularly if they are known to snore heavily, may have sleep apnea. Sleep apnea can be diagnosed in some clients through the observation of family members while the client sleeps in a supine position. A complete health assessment should be performed on any client for whom excessive daytime sleepiness is a problem.

 Interventions

For mild sleep apnea, a change in sleeping position or weight loss may be all that is required to reduce or correct the problem. Simple position-fixing devices that prevent subluxation of the tongue and neck structures also may be effective in preventing obstruction. For more severe sleep apnea, nonsurgical or surgical methods to prevent obstruction may be necessary.

A common nonsurgical method to prevent airway collapse is the use of continuous positive airway pressure (CPAP) ventilation through a face mask during sleep. A small electric compressor delivers positive pressure at an individually determined setting. Proper fit of the mask over the nose and mouth is key to successful treatment. Although intrusive, this method is well accepted by clients after an initial adjustment period.

Surgical intervention for sleep apnea may involve a simple adenoidectomy or uvulectomy, or it may require remodeling of the entire posterior oropharynx (uvulopalatopharyngoplasty). Both conventional and laser surgeries are applied for this purpose.

Oropharyngeal Cancer

Clients with cancer of the mouth, tongue, tonsils, and pharynx present special nursing needs related to airway maintenance, communication, nutrition, and self-image. (Chapter 56 provides an in-depth discussion of the collaborative management of clients with oropharyngeal cancer.)

NONINFECTIOUS DISORDERS OF THE LARYNX
Vocal Cord Paralysis

Overview

Vocal fold (cord) paralysis may result from injury, trauma, or disease affecting the larynx, the laryngeal nerves, or the vagus nerve. Prolonged intubation with an endotracheal (ET) tube may cause temporary or, rarely, permanent paralysis. Laryngeal paralysis may occur in clients with central neurologic disorders. Damage to the vagus nerve (by chest injury) or brain stem may lead to nerve dysfunction. The superior and recurrent laryngeal nerves may be damaged in disorders or trauma involving the chest, esophagus, or thyroid. Paralysis of both vocal cords may result from direct traumatic injury or bilateral cerebrovascular accident (CVA), especially involving the brain stem or after total thyroidectomy.

Collaborative Management

 Assessment

Vocal fold paralysis may be unilateral or bilateral. When only one vocal cord is involved, as is commonly the case,

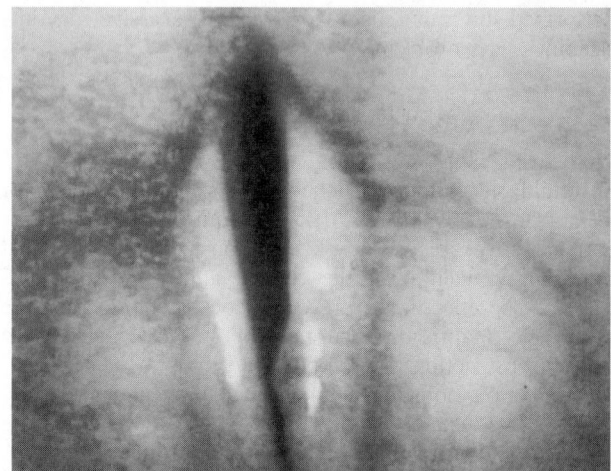

Figure 31–2. Unilateral left vocal cord nodule caused by contact and voice abuse, often seen after viral illnesses. Differential diagnosis includes cancer and trauma. The origin of the nodule may be scar tissue, bacteria, or viruses.

the airway usually remains patent, but voice use may be affected. Symptoms of abducted bilateral vocal cord paralysis include hoarseness; a breathy, weak voice; and aspiration of food. Bilateral adducted vocal cord paralysis presents with airway obstruction and dyspnea and is a medical emergency if the symptoms are severe and the client is unable to compensate. Stridor is the major presenting symptom. The client with vocal cord dysfunction is at risk for aspiration because of the inability to protect the airway by normal vocal cord closure.

✖ Interventions

The nurse assesses for airway compromise and symptoms of upper airway obstruction. Securing a patent airway is the primary intervention. The nurse positions the client in a high Fowler's position to aid in breathing and proper alignment of airway structures. Dyspnea with stridor indicates an inadequate airway, and the nurse immediately notifies the physician. Emergent endotracheal intubation, cricothyroidotomy, or tracheostomy may be necessary.

Many surgical procedures have been used to improve the voice. In one procedure for abducted vocal cord paresis, polytef (Teflon) is injected into the affected cord so that it will enlarge toward the unaffected cord, improving approximation.

Additional nursing interventions include teaching clients to hold their breath during swallowing. This intervention allows the larynx to elevate, close, and divert the food stream posteriorly into the esophagus during swallowing. The nurse evaluates clients for aspiration of liquids and saliva related to vocal cord dysfunction. Signs and symptoms include immediate coughing on swallowing of liquids, a "wet"-sounding voice, and fever. Chest x-rays and laryngeal and chest auscultation are also useful

to diagnose the signs and symptoms of aspiration pneumonia.

Nodules and Polyps of the Vocal Cords

Overview

Nodules often appear at the point where the vocal cords touch during voicing. Nodules are hypertrophied fibrous tissue (Fig. 31–2) resulting from overuse of the voice or after an infectious process. The populations most affected are teachers, coaches, sports fans, singers, and people who use their voices in noisy environments.

Vocal cord polyps (Fig. 31–3) are chronic edematous masses. Polyps occur most commonly in adults who smoke, have many allergies, or live in dry climates. Vocal cysts also may occur.

Collaborative Management

Both nodules and polyps are painless, but they produce hoarseness because of the loss of coordinated approximation of the vocal cords and vocal wave (Fig. 31–4).

Nursing management of the client with vocal cord nodules or polyps is aimed at client and family education. The nurse teaches the client about the hazards of tobacco use, smoking cessation programs, and the importance of voice rest. Conservative treatment includes not whispering and avoiding heavy lifting. Stool softeners are used to avoid excessive Valsalva maneuvers to close the glottis.

Humidification and specialized speech therapy help to reduce the intensity of speech. Speech therapy is a primary treatment for behavioral voice changes. A conservative approach using speech therapy may make surgery unnecessary.

If hoarseness or the presenting voice disturbance is not relieved by voice rest or speech therapy, the physician may excise the nodules or polyps under direct laryngos-

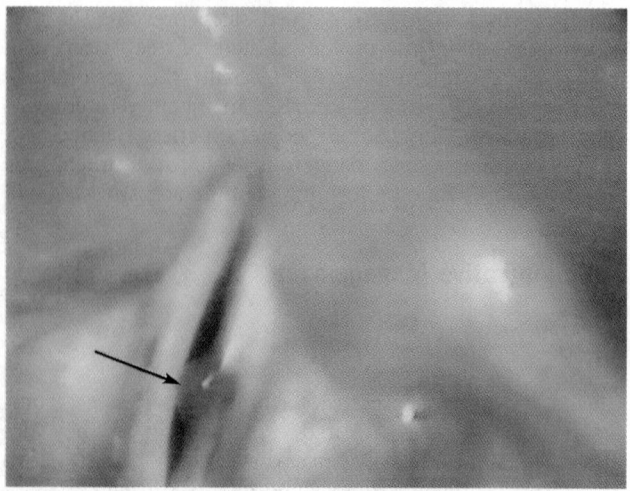

Figure 31–3. A hemorrhagic vocal cord polyp.

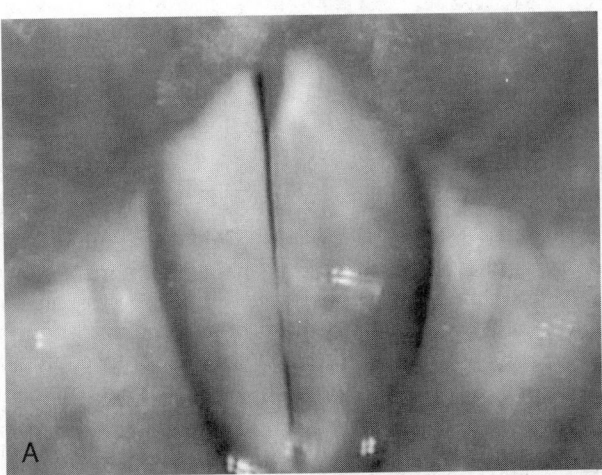 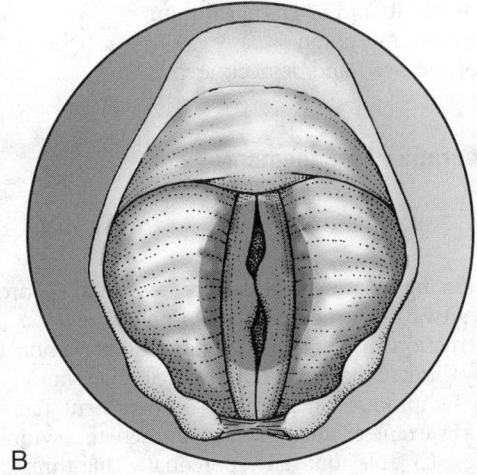

Figure 31–4. *A,* Close-up view of normal vocal folds in phonation. Saying the letter *E* in a high pitch allows the examiner to evaluate the total movement of the cords in all pitch ranges and evaluate membrane contact. *B,* Vocal cord nodules and polyps prevent approximation of the vocal cords. Hoarseness results.

copy. Laser and surgical resection are used to excise or strip the mucous membrane of the affected cord. If both cords are involved, one cord is usually allowed to heal before surgery is performed on the other cord.

After surgery, the client must maintain complete voice rest for about 14 days to promote healing. Alternative methods of communication, such as a slate board, pen and paper, "magic slate," or alphabet board are used. The nurse places a sign on the client's door, over the bed, and on the intercom system to help implement this important nursing intervention. Education is imperative before the operation and before the client returns home because these procedures are often performed in an outpatient setting.

Laryngeal Trauma

Overview

Laryngeal trauma is a result of crushing or direct blow injury, fracture, or intrinsic injury such as that induced by prolonged endotracheal intubation.

Collaborative Management

Symptoms of laryngeal trauma include dyspnea, aphonia, hoarseness, and subcutaneous emphysema. Bleeding from the airway (hemoptysis) may occur, depending on the location of the trauma. The physician performs a direct visual examination by laryngoscopy or fiberoptic laryngoscopy, of the larynx to determine the exact nature of the injury.

Management of clients with laryngeal injuries consists of assessing and frequent monitoring of vital signs (every 15–30 minutes), including respiratory status and pulse oximetry. The nursing priority is to maintain a patent airway. The nurse places oxygen and humidification as ordered to maintain adequate oxygen saturation. If the client has respiratory difficulty, as evidenced by signs such as increasing tachypnea, anxiety, sternal retraction, shortness of breath, dyspnea, restlessness, decreased oxygen saturation, decreased level of consciousness, nasal flaring, and stridor, the nurse stays with the client and instructs other trauma team members to prepare for emergency cricothyroidotomy (cricothyrotomy) or tracheostomy.

For lacerations of the mucous membranes, cartilage exposure, and paralysis of the cords, surgical intervention is necessary. Laryngeal repair is performed as soon as possible to prevent laryngeal stenosis and to cover any exposed cartilage. An artificial airway may be indicated. Maintenance of a patent airway is the utmost priority.

OTHER UPPER AIRWAY DISORDERS
Upper Airway Obstruction

Overview

Upper airway obstruction is a life-threatening emergency defined as any significant interruption in airflow through the nose, mouth, pharynx, or larynx. Early recognition is essential to prevent further complications, including respiratory arrest. Some potential causes of upper airway obstruction are

- Tongue edema (surgery, trauma)
- Occlusion by the tongue (e.g., with loss of protective reflexes, loss of pharyngeal muscle tone, unconsciousness, and coma)
- Laryngeal edema
- Peritonsillar and pharyngeal abscess
- Head and neck carcinoma
- Thick secretions in the airway
- Cerebral disorders (i.e., cerebrovascular accident [CVA])
- Smoke inhalation edema

- Facial, tracheal, and/or laryngeal trauma
- Foreign body aspiration
- Burns of the head and/or neck area
- Anaphylaxis

Collaborative Management

 Assessment

Prompt nursing and medical care are essential to prevent a partial airway obstruction from progressing to a complete obstruction. A client with a partial obstruction (e.g., caused by limited edema or a small foreign body) may have few symptoms. Unexplained or persistent recurrent symptoms warrant evaluation even though the symptoms are vague. To rule out any potentially life-threatening condition, such as a tumor, foreign body, or infection, the physician orders diagnostic procedures, such as chest x-ray, lateral neck films, direct laryngoscopic examination, and computed tomography. Upper airway obstruction can be a frightening experience for the client and family.

The nurse observes for signs of hypoxia and hypercapnia, restlessness, increasing anxiety, sternal retractions, "seesawing" chest, abdominal movements, or a feeling of impending doom related to actual air hunger. The nurse performs pulse oximetry for the ongoing monitoring of oxygen saturation and assesses for stridor, cyanosis, and changes in level of consciousness.

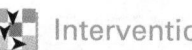 Interventions

The nurse assesses for the cause of the obstruction. When obstruction is due to the tongue falling back or to the accumulation of secretions, the nurse places the client's head and neck in a slightly extended position, inserts an oral airway, and may use suction to remove obstructing secretions. If the airway obstruction results from a foreign body, the nurse performs abdominal thrusts (Fig. 31–5).

Upper airway obstruction may necessitate emergency procedures, such as a cricothyroidotomy, endotracheal intubation, or tracheostomy. These procedures are often preceded or followed by direct laryngoscopy to evaluate the cause of obstruction. The physician uses direct laryngoscopy in a controlled situation as the treatment of choice for removal of foreign bodies.

➤ *Cricothyroidotomy*

Cricothyroidotomy is a life-saving emergency procedure and is usually performed outside the hospital by emergency medical personnel or in the emergency department by a physician. A cricothyroidotomy is a stab wound at the cricothyroid membrane between the thyroid cartilage and the cricoid cartilage ring (see Fig. 29–3). Any hollow tube—but preferably a tracheostomy tube—can be placed through this opening to keep the new airway open until a formal tracheotomy can be performed. This proce-

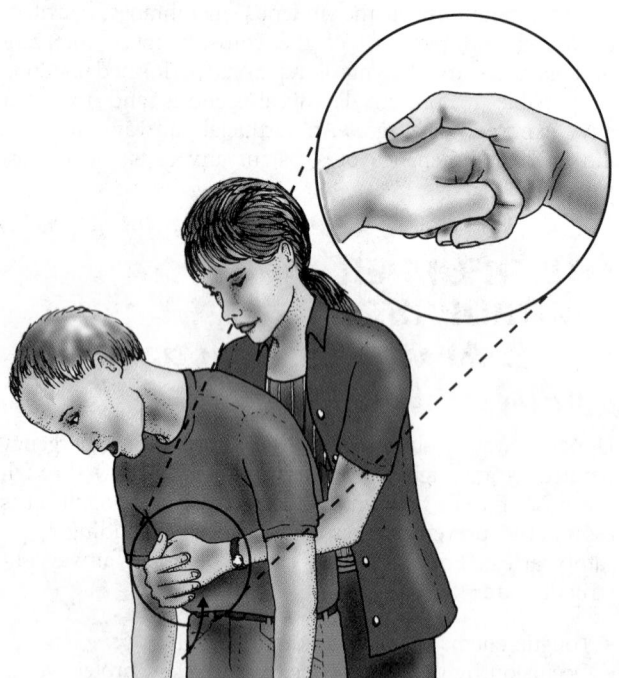

With the **conscious victim standing or sitting,** place your fist between the victim's lower rib cage and navel. Wrap the palm of your other hand around your fist. A quick inward, upward thrust expels the air remaining in the victim's lungs and with it the foreign body. If the first thrust is unsuccessful, repeat several thrusts in rapid succession until the foreign body is expelled or until the victim loses consciousness.

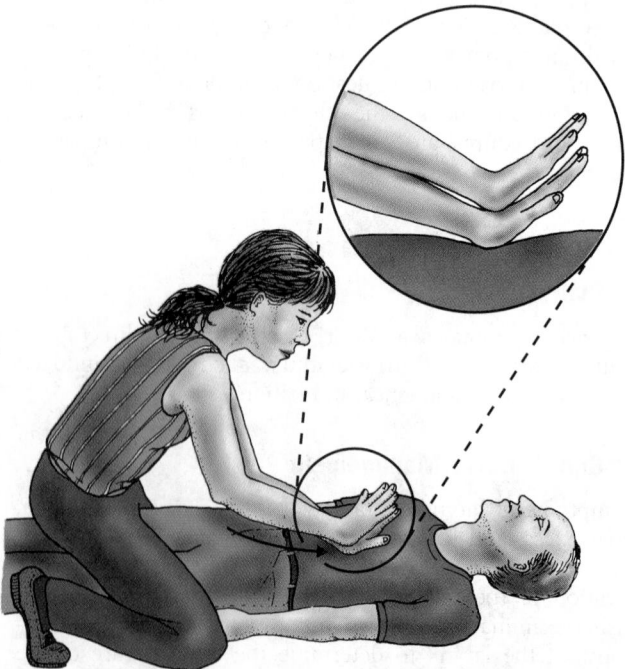

With the **unconscious victim lying supine,** straddle the victim's thighs. Place your hands one over the other as shown, with the heel of the bottom hand just above the victim's navel. Quickly thrust inward and upward, toward the victim's head.

Figure 31–5. The abdominal thrust maneuver (formerly referred to as the Heimlich maneuver) for relief of upper airway obstruction caused by a foreign body.

dure is warranted when it is the only way to secure an airway for the client. Alternatively, the physician can make an incision by inserting a 14-gauge needle immediately into the cricoid space to allow air into and out of the lungs, thus bypassing the obstruction.

➤ Endotracheal Intubation

To accomplish endotracheal intubation, a tube is inserted into the trachea via the nose (nasotracheal) or mouth (orotracheal) by a physician, a nurse anesthetist, or another specially trained nurse.

➤ Tracheostomy

Tracheostomy is usually an elective procedure that takes about 5–10 minutes to perform. The procedure takes place in the operating room (preferably) with the client under local or general anesthesia, or it can be done at the bedside. Infrequently, an awake tracheostomy with local anesthesia is done if the concern is losing the airway during induction of anesthesia. An emergency tracheostomy is reserved for the client who cannot be immediately intubated with an oral or nasal endotracheal tube. The airway can be established in less than 2 minutes in an emergency situation. (Care of the client with a tracheostomy is discussed in detail in Chapter 30.)

The client receiving mechanical ventilation as part of the treatment for upper airway obstruction or respiratory failure may require elective tracheostomy after 7 or more days of continuous oral or nasal intubation. The procedure is then performed to prevent laryngeal injury by the endotracheal tube (ET).

Neck Trauma

Overview

Injuries to the neck are most often caused by a knife, gunshot, or traumatic accident. Clients with neck trauma may have multiple injuries, including cardiovascular, respiratory, gastrointestinal, and neurologic damage. The final outcome of this type of injury depends on the initial assessment and management. (Consult a critical care or emergency textbook as well as Chapter 47 for more indepth information. Advanced cardiac life support courses are also valuable.)

Collaborative Management

 Assessment

The priority in the management of neck trauma is assessment for a patent airway. The nurse then assesses the cardiovascular system for signs of internal or external bleeding or impending shock.

The nurse performs a baseline neurologic assessment for mental status, sensory level, and motor function. Injury to the carotid artery may result in death, stroke, or paralysis related to interruption of blood to the brain. The physician may order a carotid angiogram (see Chap. 35) to rule out vascular injuries.

Injuries involving the esophagus also may occur with neck trauma. The nurse assesses for chest pain and tenderness, oral bleeding, and crepitus. The physician may order a barium or meglumine diatrizoate (Gastrografin) swallow to rule out esophageal perforation injury.

 Interventions

Cervical spine injuries often occur at the same time as a neck injury (see Chap. 45). The nurse and emergency personnel must take great care not to exacerbate these injuries by causing neck movement while establishing the airway. The nurse prepares to assist in emergency intubation, cricothyrotomy, or tracheostomy to establish a patent airway. (Interventions for clients in shock are detailed in Chapter 39.)

Head and Neck Cancer

Overview

Head and neck cancer interferes with breathing, eating, facial appearance, self-image, speech, and communication. This form of cancer can be a devastating disease even if it is successfully treated. The nurse is challenged in caring for the client with these complex problems. The client can receive appropriate care only through accurate identification of the location and size of the original tumor. An interdisciplinary health care team approach is essential to address the entire spectrum of needs for these clients.

Head and neck cancer can be a curable disease when treated early. The prognosis for those who have more advanced disease at diagnosis depends on the extent and location of the tumor. Untreated cancer of the head and neck is a fatal disease, and the untreated client will usually die within 2 years of diagnosis.

Pathophysiology

Most head and neck cancers (80%) are squamous cell (mucosal epithelial) carcinomas (Fig. 31–6), usually requiring several years to develop. Many head and neck tumors present as malignant ulcerations with underlying infiltration.

Initially, the mucosa is subjected to an irritating substance and transforms itself into a tougher mucosa (squamous metaplasia) by increasing the mucosal thickness (acanthosis or hyperplasia) or by developing a keratin layer (keratosis). At the same time, cellular gene changes lead to the proliferation of atypical or dysplastic epithelial cells that eventually become malignant. These atypical lesions may then take the form of white, patchy lesions or red, velvety patches. Head and neck carcinoma is often diagnosed on the basis of white, patchy mucosal lesions called *leukoplakia*, or red patches called *erythroplasia*.

Growth and spread of the carcinoma depend on the site of the primary tumor. Spread is predominantly to adjacent anatomic areas like mucosa, muscle, and bone. Systemic dissemination through the circulatory and lymphatic systems may also occur. When metastasis occurs, it is most commonly to the lungs or liver.

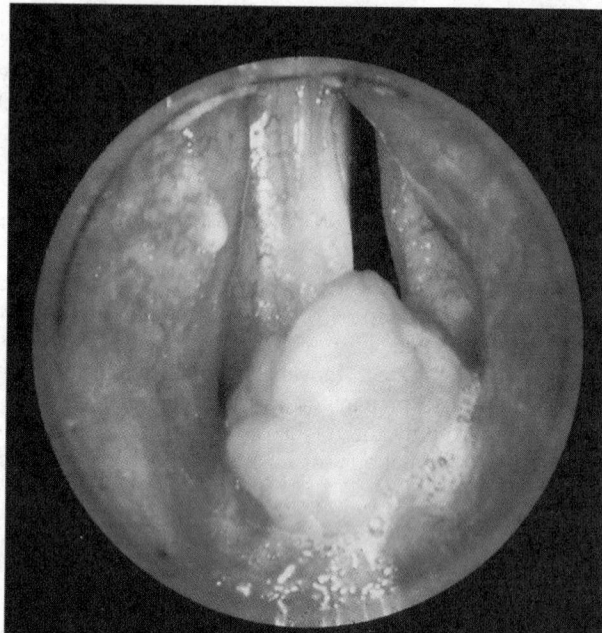

Figure 31–6. Laryngeal cancer is frequently caused by the combination of alcohol and tobacco. This laryngoscopic photograph shows a large granular cell tumor of the true vocal cord. From Wenig, B. M. (1993). *Atlas of head and neck pathology.* Philadelphia: W. B. Saunders. Used with permission.

The histologic description of squamous cell cancers includes carcinoma in situ, well-differentiated carcinoma, moderately differentiated carcinoma, or poorly differentiated carcinoma. Most head and neck cancers are of squamous origin, but they also can be of salivary gland or thyroid (papillary or follicular) origin. They can also be epidermoid, adenoid cystic, malignant melanoma, or adenocarcinoma. These tumors are treated by various methods directed by the type of tumor and its known response to therapies.

Etiology

Numerous risk factors have been identified as contributing to the development of head and neck cancer. The two most important risk factors are tobacco and alcohol use and especially the combination of the two. Other risk factors include chewing tobacco, pipe smoking, marijuana, voice abuse, chronic laryngitis, exposure to industrial chemicals or hardwood dust, and complete neglect of oral hygiene.

Incidence/Prevalence

The frequency of occurrence of head and neck carcinoma is increasing. The American Cancer Society (ACS) estimates 42,100 newly diagnosed cases of oral and laryngeal cancers per year, accounting for more than 4% of all carcinomas and more than 11,000 deaths per year (American Cancer Society, 1998). About three times more males are affected than females, and most head and neck cancers occur in people older than 60 years.

 The rate of death for men of all races from cancer of the larynx has not changed over three decades, but there has been a 110% increase in the non-Caucasian population, up from 2.3 to 4.9 cases. Death rates for women with oral or laryngeal cancers have increased for all races over the past three decades.

Collaborative Management

Assessment

➤ *History*

The client with head and neck cancer may have difficulty speaking because of hoarseness, shortness of breath, tumor bulk, and pain. The nurse is sensitive to these difficulties during the interview.

The nurse questions the client about tobacco and alcohol use, history of recurrent acute or chronic laryngitis or pharyngitis, oral sores, and lumps in the neck. The client's smoking history is calculated in *pack-years* (the number of packs smoked per day times the number of years the client has smoked). The nurse asks about alcohol intake (how many drinks per day and for how many years). Questions of this nature may be uncomfortable for both the client and the nurse but are an important part of the history. The nurse also asks whether the client has been exposed to any environmental or occupational pollutants.

The nurse assesses problems related to risk factors. For example, nutrition may be poor because of alcohol intake and impairment of liver function. The nurse assesses dietary habits and any reported weight loss. The nurse notes a history of chronic lung disease, which has an impact on the client's breathing pattern and is an important operative risk factor.

➤ *Physical Assessment/Clinical Manifestations*

Table 31–1 summarizes the warning signs of head and neck cancer. With laryngeal cancer, hoarseness may occur because of tumor bulk and a lack of ability to approximate vocal cords in a normal fashion during phonation (see Fig. 31–7 for common sites of laryngeal cancer). Lesions of the true vocal cords are the earliest form of laryngeal cancer. A careful evaluation is important for anyone who has a history of hoarseness, sores in the mouth, or a lump in the neck for a period of 3–4 weeks or longer.

The techniques of inspection and palpation of the head and neck are an important part of the physical examination. A nurse who is specially trained may perform a laryngeal examination, which includes the use of the laryngeal mirror or fiberoptic laryngoscope. Lesions may be visible on direct inspection, and the nurse palpates the neck for tumor nodal involvement. A cranial nerve assessment (see Chap. 43) is also valuable because some tumors have an affinity for dissemination along these nerves as well as direct tumor invasion.

TABLE 31-1

Warning Signs of Head and Neck Cancer

- Pain
- A lump in the mouth, throat, or neck
- Difficulty in swallowing
- Color changes in the mouth or tongue to red, white, gray, dark brown, or black
- An oral lesion or sore that does not heal in 2 weeks
- Persistent or unexplained oral bleeding
- Numbness of the mouth, lips, or face
- Change in the fit of dentures
- Burning sensation when drinking citrus juices or hot liquids
- Persistent, unilateral ear pain
- Hoarseness or change in voice quality
- Persistent or recurrent sore throat
- Shortness of breath
- Anorexia and weight loss

➤ Psychosocial Assessment

The typical client with head and neck carcinoma has a long-standing history of cigarette or alcohol use, or both. The client or family may experience denial, guilt, blame, or shame once the diagnosis is suspected. The nurse assesses the availability and adequacy of support systems and coping mechanisms. Because the client frequently requires extensive assistance at home after treatment, assessment and documentation of social and family support are essential. The nurse consults the social worker for assistance as needed. Because of the importance of preoperative and postoperative teaching, the nurse also evaluates cognitive functioning (see Chap. 43), level of education, and literacy of the client and family.

The nurse notes any family history of cancer as well as the client's age, gender, occupation, interests, and ability to perform the activities of daily living. The nurse investigates whether the client's occupation requires continual oral communication, whether the client will need retraining in other vocational areas, or whether the client will be able to resume the same job after treatment.

➤ Laboratory Assessment

Routine diagnostic laboratory tests include a complete blood count, bleeding times, urinalysis, and SMA-20. The nurse is alert to decreased hemoglobin or hematocrit values and an increased alkaline phosphatase level. Decreased protein and albumin levels indicate a loss of protein stores and define nutritional risks often seen in the alcoholic client. Renal and liver function tests are performed to rule out metastatic disease and to evaluate the client's ability to metabolize medications and chemotherapeutic agents.

➤ Radiographic Assessment

Many types of radiographic studies, including x-rays of the skull, sinuses, neck, and chest, are useful in diagnosing metastases, second primary tumors, and the extent of tumor invasion. Computed tomography (CT) of the head and neck, with or without contrast media, helps evaluate the tumor's exact location.

➤ Other Diagnostic Assessment

Magnetic resonance imaging (MRI) can differentiate normal from diseased tissue. MRI is more sensitive than CT in defining the extent of soft-tissue invasion.

The brain, bone, and liver may also be evaluated with nuclear imaging, bone scans, SPECT (single photon emission computed tomography) and PET (positron emission tomography) scans. These tests help locate additional tumor sites.

Other diagnostic tests include direct and indirect laryngoscopy, tumor mapping, and biopsy. Panendoscopy is performed with general anesthesia to define the extent of the tumor. This procedure includes laryngoscopy, nasopharyngoscopy, esophagoscopy, and bronchoscopy. Anatomic tumor mapping uses biopsy to outline and identify tumor location. At the time of the panendoscopy, the biopsy confirms the diagnosis and determines the tumor type, histologic presentation, and defined location. Tumor staging by the TNM classification (see Chap. 26 and Table 26-8) is done at this time.

 Analysis

➤ Common Nursing Diagnoses and Collaborative Problems

The primary collaborative problem is High Risk for Ineffective Breathing Pattern related to impaired airway from

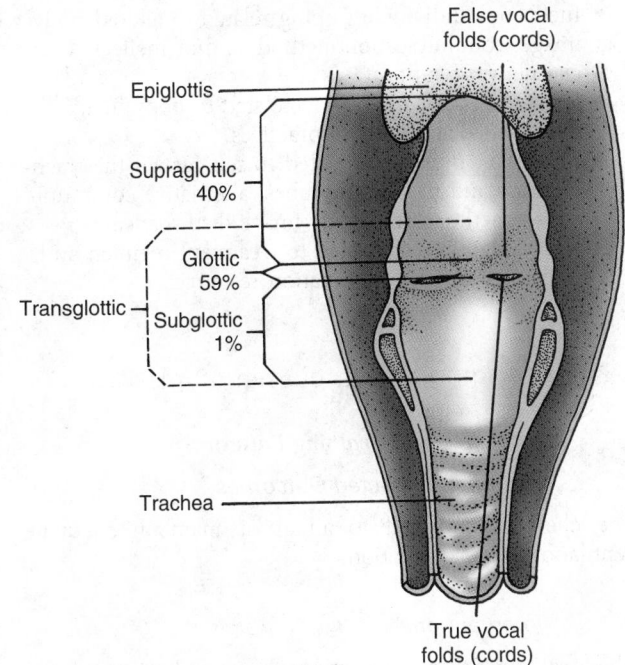

Figure 31-7. Sites and incidence of primary laryngeal tumors.

the disease process (i.e., tumor invasion or obstruction, edema, and chronic lung disease).

The priority nursing diagnoses for clients with head and neck carcinomas are

1. Risk for Aspiration related to edema, anatomic changes, or alteration of protective oropharyngeal reflexes
2. Anxiety related to fear of the unknown
3. Body Image Disturbance related to tumor and treatment modalities

➤ Additional Nursing Diagnoses and Collaborative Problems

In addition to the common nursing diagnoses and collaborative problems, the client may present with one or more of the following:

- Pain related to tumor invasion of tissues and nerves and surgical intervention
- Altered Nutrition: Less than Body Requirements related to dysphagia, anxiety, tumor process, surgical resection, or chronic alcohol intake
- Impaired Verbal Communication related to tumor invasion, associated aphonia, hoarseness, pain, and/or surgical resection
- Altered Cerebral Tissue Perfusion related to wound breakdown, recurrent tumor, and resultant interruption of arterial blood flow from carotid rupture
- Impaired Tissue Integrity related to altered circulation, nutritional deficit, tumor invasion, radiation, chemical factors (body secretions or substances), or surgical wound
- Impaired Skin Integrity related to altered circulation, nutritional deficit, tumor invasion, radiation, chemical factors (body secretions or substances), or surgical wound
- Ineffective Individual Coping related to altered body image, communication method, and/or ineffective social network support
- Impaired Social Interaction related to body image disturbance and lifestyle practices
- Impaired Adjustment related to self-care of the tracheostomy and nasogastric tubes, alternative communication methods, and body image disturbance
- Knowledge Deficit related to treatment regimen and unfamiliarity with information resources

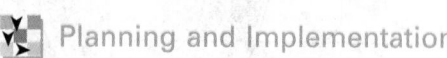

Planning and Implementation

➤ Ineffective Breathing Pattern

Planning: Expected Outcomes

The client is expected to attain or maintain adequate ventilation and oxygenation.

Interventions

The goal of treatment is removal or eradication of the cancer with preservation of as much normal function as possible. The physician presents available treatment op-

tions to the client. Modalities may be used alone or in combination. When planning treatment options, the physician considers general physical condition, nutritional status, age, effects of the tumor on body function, and, most importantly, the client's personal choice. Before recommending extensive surgery, the physician considers the client's ability to manage his or her own care postoperatively.

The treatment of laryngeal cancer may range from radiation therapy, for a small specific area or tumor, to total laryngopharyngectomy, with bilateral neck dissections followed by radiation therapy. The specific treatment depends on the extent and location of the lesion. Voice conservation procedures are elected only if they can be accomplished without risking incomplete removal of the tumor. The nurse focuses on the client's total needs, including preoperative preparation, competent in-hospital care, discharge planning and teaching, and extensive outpatient rehabilitation.

Nonsurgical Management. The nurse monitors the client's respiratory system by assessing respiratory rate, breath sounds, pulse oximetry, arterial blood gas values, and results of pulmonary function tests. Signs of respiratory distress may indicate narrowing of the airway related to tumor growth, edema, or both. The nurse positions the client for optimal air exchange. The nurse educates the client and family about the use of Fowler's and semi-Fowler's positions. The client may breathe more comfortably by sitting upright in a reclining chair. Chapters 9 and 12 and texts on hospice care can provide additional information on palliation and pain control for the client who elects no therapy and for the client whose therapy has not been effective.

Radiation Therapy. Radiation treatment of small cancers in specific locations offers a cure rate of 80% and greater. Treatment of larger cancers offers a lower cure rate when radiation is used as a single-modality therapy. Standard therapy uses 5000–7500 rad usually over 6 weeks in daily or twice-daily doses. The physician may recommend radiation alone or in combination with surgery. Because radiation therapy causes alterations in tissue healing, it might not be recommended preoperatively. Radiation therapy is commonly an outpatient procedure (see Chap. 27). During and for a few weeks after radiation therapy, the client will have uncomfortable side effects.

Hoarseness becomes worse. The nurse reassures the client and family that vocalization will improve to at least pretreatment levels within 4–6 weeks after completion of radiation therapy. The client is encouraged to use voice rest and alternative means of communication until the effects of radiation have subsided.

Most clients have a sore throat and difficulty swallowing during radiation therapy. Gargling with saline or sucking ice may decrease discomfort. Pain medication is ordered as needed.

The skin at the site of radiation becomes red and tender, and it may peel during therapy. The client must avoid exposing this area to sun, heat, cold, and abrasive treatments such as shaving. The nurse instructs the client to wear protective clothing made of soft cotton and to wash this area gently with a mild soap, such as Dove. The client should use only lotions or powders prescribed by the radiologist until the area has healed.

If the salivary glands are in the path of radiation, the client will have a dry mouth. This side effect is long term and may be permanent. Heavy fluid intake, particularly of water, and a humidified atmosphere can help relieve the discomfort. Some clients benefit from the use of artificial saliva.

Chemotherapy. Chemotherapy is not usually used alone for cancers of the head and neck. At times, it is an adjuvant to surgery or radiation. The most commonly used chemotherapeutic agents for cancer of the neck include methotrexate (Mexate), vincristine (Oncovin), bleomycin (Blenoxane), and cisplatin (Platinol). Methotrexate may be used for patients who cannot undergo rigorous surgery, radiation, or chemotherapy. Often terminal patients receive methotrexate for control (not cure) of the disease, and for assistance in pain control. (Chapter 27 includes general care needs of clients receiving chemotherapy.)

Surgical Management. Tumor size and location (TNM classification) defines the extent of surgical intervention for cancer of the head and neck. The method of reconstruction is also determined by the tumor size and amount of tissue to be resected and reconstructed. Surgical procedures for head and neck cancers include laryngectomy (total and partial), tracheostomy, and oropharyngeal cancer resections.

Laryngectomy and Related Surgical Procedures. The major types of resections for laryngeal cancer include cordal stripping, *cordectomy* (excision of a vocal cord), partial laryngectomy, and total laryngectomy. If neck lymph nodes are involved or if the tumor carries with it a known high rate of nodal spread, the surgeon performs a nodal neck dissection in conjunction with removal of the primary tumor. A pathologist evaluates the resected lymph nodes for tumor invasion.

Preoperative Care. As the client advocate, the nurse teaches the client and family about the tumor. The physician explains the surgical procedure and obtains the client's informed consent. The nurse discusses and interprets the implications of such consent.

The nurse explains about self-care of the airway, compensatory methods of communication, suctioning, pain control methods, the critical care environment (including ventilators and critical care routines), nutritional support, feeding tubes, and goals for discharge. The client must learn new methods of speech postoperatively. The nurse prepares the client for this change through preoperative teaching and establishes with the client an alternative form of communication (e.g., pen and pencil, "magic slate," picture or alphabet board) before surgery.

The explanations of routines and outcomes of care are very important because these discussions are used to plan the hospitalization and rehabilitation. Multidisciplinary teams of speech pathologists, social workers, dietitians, and occupational and physical therapists, along with the nurses and physicians, are vitally important in the preop-

TABLE 31-2

Surgical Procedures for Laryngeal Cancer and Their Effect on Voice Quality

Procedure	Description	Resulting Voice Quality
Laser surgery	• Tumor reduced or destroyed by laser beam through laryngoscope	• Normal/ hoarse
Transoral cordectomy	• Tumor (early lesion) resected through laryngoscope	• Normal (high cure rate)/ hoarse
Laryngofissure	• No cord removed (early lesion)	• Normal (high cure rate)
Supraglottic partial laryngectomy	• Hyoid bone, false cords, and epiglottis removed • Neck dissection on affected side performed if nodes involved	• Normal/ hoarse
Hemilaryngectomy or vertical laryngectomy	• One true cord, one false cord, and one half of thyroid cartilage removed	• Hoarse voice
Total laryngectomy	• Entire larynx, hyoid bone, strap muscles, one or two tracheal rings removed • Nodal neck dissection if nodes involved	• No natural voice

erative evaluation and preparation of clients with cancer. (Chapter 20 describes general preoperative assessment and education in detail.)

Operative Procedures. Hemilaryngectomy (vertical or horizontal) and supraglottic laryngectomy are types of partial voice conservation laryngectomies. Table 31–2 presents more specific information on the various surgical procedures.

To protect the airway, a temporary or permanent tracheostomy is usually performed with a partial laryngectomy. With a total laryngectomy, the upper airway is separated from the pharynx and esophagus, and the trachea is brought out through the skin in the neck and sutured in place, creating a stoma. This airway opening is *always* permanent and is referred to as a laryngectomy stoma.

Neck dissection includes removal of tumor-involved lymph nodes, the sternocleidomastoid muscle, the jugular vein, the 11th cranial nerve, and surrounding involved soft tissue. Because the 11th cranial nerve—the spinal accessory nerve—is resected during the nodal dissection, shoulder drop will be present postoperatively. Physical therapy exercises are imperative and help the client ease the shoulder drop by increasing the use of other muscle groups.

Postoperative Care. Head and neck surgical procedures often last 8 hours or longer. Because of the duration of anesthesia and the amount of resection and reconstruction, the client may spend the immediate postoperative period in the surgical intensive care unit. The nurse monitors the client's airway patency, vital signs, hemodynamic status, and comfort level. The nurse is also alert to the possibility of postoperative hemorrhage and other general complications of anesthesia and surgery (see Chap. 22). Vital signs are monitored every hour for the first 24 hours and then every 2 hours until the client is stable. After the client is transferred from the critical care unit, vital signs can be monitored every 4 hours or according to agency policy. The client is generally out of bed by the second postoperative day.

Complications after a head and neck cancer resection include airway obstruction, hemorrhage, wound breakdown, and tumor recurrence. The priorities in postoperative head and neck cancer care include airway maintenance and ventilation; wound, flap, and reconstructive tissue care (see Client Care Plan); pain management; nutrition; and psychological adjustment, including speech therapy.

Airway Maintenance and Ventilation. In the immediate postoperative period, clients may need ventilatory assistance because of a long-term smoking history, chronic lung disease, or long duration of anesthesia. Although many clients also have chronic lung disease, weaning usually is not difficult because the thoracic and abdominal cavities are not entered during the surgical procedure and because the cough mechanism is intact. When weaned from the ventilator, clients typically use a tracheostomy collar (over the artificial airway or open stoma) with oxygen and humidification to help mobilize mucous secretions. Secretions may remain blood tinged for 1–2 days. The nurse maintains body substance precautions and reports any increase in bleeding to the physician. Humidification helps to remove crusts and prevent obstruction of the tube with secretions. Sterile saline instillation of 5–10 mL every 2 hours or as needed may also be ordered.

Clients who have had a total laryngectomy and need an appliance to prevent scar tissue contracture at the skin tracheal border use a laryngectomy tube. This tube is similar to a conventional tracheostomy tube but is shorter and fatter with a larger lumen and a more acute angle (Fig. 31–8). Laryngectomy tube care is similar to tracheostomy tube care (see Chap. 30), except that clients can change the laryngectomy tube on a daily or an as-needed basis. A laryngectomy button is similar to a laryngectomy tube but is made of a silicone-like substance (Silastic), has a single lumen, and is very short. A button is very comfortable for laryngectomy patients, is easily removed for cleaning, and is available in various sizes and lengths for a custom fit. The nurse provides a "magic slate" or paper and pencil for communication because clients have no immediate oral communication capabilities other than mouthing words.

Coughing, deep breathing, and saline instillation are often totally effective in clearing secretions. The lack of

surgical interruption in the thoracic cavity or abdomen improves the ability to cough. The nurse instructs clients in the proper techniques for coughing and deep breathing (see Chap. 20) to clear secretions.

Oral secretions can be suctioned with a Yankauer or tonsillar suction. The nurse teaches clients to suction away from the side of an oral cavity cancer resection to preserve continuity of the wounds immediately after surgery. The nurse teaches clients self-care by providing this catheter for suctioning oral airway secretions. Using a table mirror for visibility, clients can participate in their own care. The nurse provides a clean environment for the catheter.

Stoma care after total laryngectomy is a combination of wound care and airway care. Careful inspection of the stoma with a flashlight is routine. The nurse cleans the suture line with half-strength hydrogen peroxide to prevent secretions from forming crusts and obstructing the airway. Suture line care is performed every 1–2 hours initially, advancing to every 4 hours by the fifth postoperative day. The mucosa of the stoma and trachea should be bright and shiny without crusts, similar to the appearance of the buccal mucosa.

Wound, Flap, and Reconstructive Tissue Care. Commonly used reconstructive flaps are pectoralis major myocutaneous flaps, island flaps, rotation flaps, trapezius flaps, split-thickness skin grafts (STSGs), and free flaps with microvascular anastomosis (scapula, fibula, or radial forearm free flaps). These flaps may be used for reconstruction

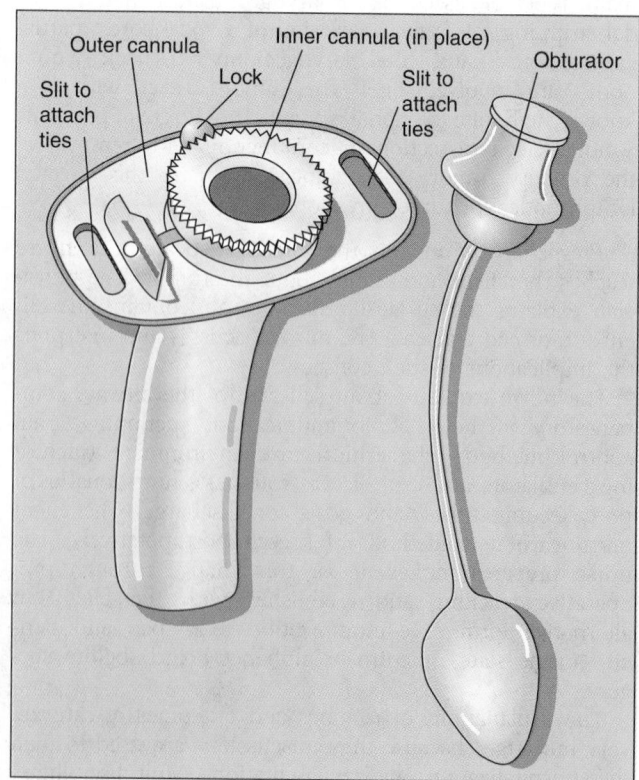

Figure 31-8. A laryngectomy tube. Note that the outer cannula is shorter and has a diameter wider than that of a tracheostomy tube.

Client Care Plan

The Client Who Has Had Head and Neck Surgery

Nursing Diagnosis No. 1: Ineffective Airway Clearance related to impaired airway from disease process (i.e., tumor invasion/obstruction, edema, chronic lung disease) and surgical intervention

Expected Outcomes	Nursing Interventions	Rationale
The client is expected to attain and/or maintain a patent airway. Lung sounds are expected to be maintained at the client's baseline or improved. Breathing efforts are expected to be without distress.	■ Monitor airway patency. ■ Assess for signs and symptoms of respiratory distress. ■ Place client in semi-Fowler's or Fowler's position as soon as possible postoperatively. ■ Suction client via the artificial airway frequently postoperatively (q30–60 minutes and advance to q2h and as needed). ■ Suction oral cavity as ordered using a Yankauer tonsillar tip catheter. ■ Inspect and clean laryngectomy stoma q2h and as needed. Use cotton-tipped applicators with peroxide and saline. ■ Perform laryngectomy tube care q4h, and advance to q shift, as needed, if ordered. ■ Have the client cough and deep breathe; if ordered, instill saline as needed. ■ Place an appropriate-sized laryngectomy set at bedside. ■ Document assessment findings and the client's response to interventions.	■ Ongoing assessment promotes early detection and treatment of complications. ■ Positioning makes breathing easier and facilitates oxygenation, secretion removal, and airway patency. ■ Suctioning and tube (if present) care promote removal of secretions that could obstruct airway. ■ A laryngectomy tube prevents scar tissue contracture and maintains airway. ■ Peroxide removes crusts and secretions. ■ Suction and cleaning procedures help to prevent obstruction and infection and promote healing. ■ Pulmonary hygiene exercises prevent pooling of secretions and promote oxygenation and ventilation. ■ Having duplicate equipment readily available enables prompt response in the event of distress or if urgent replacement of the tube is required (i.e., if the tube accidentally comes out). ■ Documentation provides an ongoing, permanent record of the client's progress and care requirements.

Nursing Diagnosis No. 2: Impaired Tissue Integrity and Impaired Skin Integrity related to the surgical wound

Expected Outcomes	Nursing Interventions	Rationale
The client's surgical wound area is expected to remain intact and heal without complications.	■ Assess wound integrity, capillary refill, and color q1–2 h for 48 hr. ■ Strip surgical drains q1–2h to ensure correct functioning. ■ Record each drain amount separately at least q shift.	■ Ongoing assessment promotes early detection and treatment of complications. ■ An accumulation of drainage beneath the skin or reconstructive flaps impairs tissue nutrition, resulting in vascular insufficiency and tissue breakdown.

(Continued)

Client Care Plan

Expected Outcomes	Nursing Interventions	Rationale
	▪ Avoid constricting dressings, ties, or oxygen tubing around the suture lines or reconstructive flaps.	▪ Pressure on altered or operated skin and tissue causes alteration in circulation.
	▪ Keep wound clean and dry; perform routine care as ordered.	▪ Appropriate wound care promotes healing and prevents complications.
	▪ Ensure adequate nutrition by the enteral or parenteral feeding method.	▪ Nutrition is imperative for tissue nutrition and healing.
	▪ Document assessment findings and the client's response to interventions.	▪ Documentation provides an ongoing, permanent record of care.

Nursing Diagnosis No. 3: Risk for Impaired Tissue Integrity and Impaired Skin Integrity related to tumor resection, wound breakdown, altered circulation, nutritional deficit, and chemical factors (body secretions or substances)

Expected Outcomes	Nursing Interventions	Rationale
The client's wound is expected to remain intact without complications of infection, bleeding, dehiscence, or fistula.	▪ Monitor for signs of infection (e.g., redness, pus, suture line separation, increasing white blood cell count, fever, malaise).	▪ Ongoing assessment promotes early detection and treatment of complications.
	▪ Assess for saliva or refluxed enteral feeding in wound secretions.	▪ Feedings or saliva in the wound represents a pharyngocutaneous fistula and wound infection.
	▪ Provide wound care, as ordered, q2–4h	▪ Aggressive nursing care keeps the wounds clean and free of cellular debris and promotes granulation tissue formation and healing.
	▪ Maintain adequate nutrition via enteral or parenteral route, as ordered.	▪ Adequate nutrition helps to prevent wound breakdown and promotes healing.

Nursing Diagnosis No. 4: Risk for Altered (Cerebral) Tissue Perfusion related to wound breakdown, recurrent tumor, and resultant interruption of arterial blood flow from carotid rupture

Expected Outcomes	Nursing Interventions	Rationale
The client's carotid artery is expected to remain intact without bleeding complications. If bleeding occurs, the client is expected to suffer minimal or no residual complications (i.e., stroke, cerebral insufficiency, cardiac damage).	▪ Maintain carotid precautions if the carotid artery is exposed: ▪ Keep the carotid artery and dressing wet with *sterile* saline at all times, as ordered by the physician. ▪ Change dressings q2h to maintain a wet-to-wet dressing.	▪ Keeping the carotid dressing clean and moist prevents drying and infection, which could cause bleeding, and promotes granulation of tissue over the carotid artery.

(Continued)

Client Care Plan

Expected Outcomes	Nursing Interventions	Rationale
	■ Move client to room closest to the nursing station or to the intensive care unit. ■ Place two large-gauge IV catheters, as ordered. ■ Keep dressing supplies, sterile saline, gloves, and IV solution (lactated Ringer's) at the bedside. ■ Be sure client has had a type and cross-match for blood ordered. ■ Alert operating room of any client receiving carotid precautions. ■ Monitor for and report any bleeding to the physician.	■ Being prepared for a carotid bleed may result in a more positive outcome. ■ Ongoing assessment promotes early detection and treatment of complications. ■ A small amount of bright red bleeding that stops spontaneously may herald a true carotid bleed.
	■ Discuss with client and family the potential for carotid rupture along with prevention, precautions, preparations, and goals of care. ■ If carotid bleeding occurs: ■ Apply immediate direct pressure to the artery and **do not remove pressure.** ■ Call for assistance! ■ Direct another nurse to call the physician **immediately.** ■ Secure the client's airway. ■ Institute intravenous hydration as per standing order. ■ If possible, talk to the client during emergency care. ■ Transport to the operating room and **do not remove pressure** during transport.	■ Client and family education helps promote understanding, acceptance, and participation in the plan of care. ■ Direct pressure applied to the arterial bleeding site prevents rapid blood loss. ■ Assistance will be needed for this emergency situation. ■ A patent airway will help to ensure oxygenation. ■ Talking to the client provides reassurance.

after any type of head and neck resection. After neck dissection, the surgeon places an STSG over the exposed carotid artery before covering it with skin flaps or reconstructive flaps.

The first 24 hours are critical. The nurse evaluates all flaps every hour for the first 72 hours, monitoring capillary refill, color, and Doppler activity of the major feeding vessel. Any changes are reported to the surgeon immediately because surgical intervention may be indicated. The nurse positions the client to protect the vascular supply of the reconstructed flaps.

Hemorrhage. Hemorrhage is a possible postoperative complication for all clients undergoing surgery, but it is uncommon in clients with laryngectomy. The physician often places a closed surgical drain (see Chap. 22) in the neck area to collect blood and drainage for approximately 72 hours postoperatively. The drain also helps to maintain the position of the reconstructed skin flaps. Any drain obstruction or equipment malfunction may cause a build-up of blood or serum under the flaps. This accumulation jeopardizes the blood supply of the flaps by interfering with both arterial supply and venous drainage.

Malfunction of the drains may necessitate a surgical procedure to remove accumulated clots.

Wound Breakdown. Wound breakdown is a frequent complication because of poor nutrition, wound contamination from the oral cavity, and previous radiation therapy. A history of alcohol use further complicates the nutritional status.

The nurse treats such wound breakdown with packing and local care as ordered to keep the wound clean and stimulate the growth of healthy granulation tissue. Wounds may be extensive, and the carotid artery may be exposed under the dehisced wounds. At the initial surgical resection, STSGs are placed over the carotid for protection in the event of such a wound dehiscence. As the wound heals, granulation tissue covers the artery and prevents rupture. If granulation is slow and the carotid artery is at risk, another surgical flap may be raised to cover the carotid artery and close the wound.

If the carotid artery ruptures because of drying or infection, the nurse places *immediate constant pressure* over the site and secures the airway. The client, still with direct manual pressure on the carotid artery, is *immediately* transported to the operating room for carotid resection. Carotid artery rupture has a high risk of stroke and death. Immediate nursing response can save the client's life.

Pain Management. After cancer surgery, the client's pain should be controlled, and the client should still be able to participate in care. Morphine (Statex✲) often is given by intravenous (IV) bolus and continuously for the first days after surgery. As the client progresses, acetaminophen with codeine and then acetaminophen alone can be given, all by feeding tube. Oral medications for pain and discomfort are started only after the client can tolerate oral nutrition. After discharge, the client still requires pain medication, especially if he or she is receiving radiation therapy. An adjunct to the pain regimen may be liquid nonsteroidal antiinflammatory drugs (NSAIDs); these drugs provide excellent pain relief and can be used in conjunction with opioid analgesics (see also Chap. 9). Amitriptyline (Elavil) or similar medications may also be used as an adjunct to pain medication administration for the lancinating pain of nerve root involvement.

Nutrition. A nasogastric, gastrostomy, or jejunostomy tube is placed intraoperatively for nutritional support while the aerodigestive tract heals. Initially, however, the client receives IV fluids (see Chap. 17) or parenteral nutrition (see Chap. 64) until the gastrointestinal tract has recovered from the effects of anesthesia. After that, nutrients may be administered via the feeding tube. The nutritional support team or dietitian assesses the client preoperatively and is available for consultations after surgery. A standard postoperative therapeutic goal is 35–40 kcal/kg of body weight. Protein and insensible water loss must also be very carefully calculated.

The nasogastric tube (the most commonly used tube type) usually remains in place for about 10 days after surgery. Before removing the tube, the nurse assesses the client's ability to swallow if the client is to receive nutrition by mouth. A client cannot aspirate after an uncomplicated total laryngectomy because the airway and esophagus are separated completely. The nurse reassures the client that aspiration will not occur and stays with the client during the first few swallowing attempts. The nurse anticipates that swallowing may be uncomfortable at first and may administer analgesics as ordered.

Speech Rehabilitation. Because the client's voice and speech can be expected to be altered after surgery, the speech pathologist and nurse discuss the principles of speech therapy with the client and family early in the course of the treatment plan. The differences will depend on the type of surgical resection (see Table 31–2). Speech production varies with client practice, amount of resection, and radiation effects, but the client's speech can be very understandable.

The speech rehabilitation plan for the client undergoing total laryngectomy consists initially of writing, then using an artificial larynx, and then learning esophageal speech. The client needs support and encouragement from the speech pathologist, hospital team, and family while relearning to speak. This process can be time consuming and necessitates concentration each time the client speaks. Having a laryngectomee from one of the local self-help organizations visit the client and family is often beneficial. The International Association of Laryngectomees is very active and supportive, as is the American Cancer Society Visitor Program.

Esophageal Speech. Most total laryngectomees attempt esophageal speech. Clients produce esophageal speech by "burping" the air swallowed or injected through the pharyngoesophageal (P-E) segment and articulate words in the mouth. The voice produced is a monotone; it cannot be raised or lowered and carries no pitch. Clients must have adequate hearing, or esophageal speech will be difficult because they use the mouth to shape the words as they hear them. Hearing-impaired clients may require hearing aids. In the English language, the vocal cords are necessary for 15 consonants; the remaining 10 consonants can be formed by shaping the mouth.

Initially, gastrointestinal bloating occurs as a result of swallowing air for esophageal speech. Antacids may help to diminish bloating sensations. Esophageal speech also helps to strengthen the respiratory and abdominal musculature, which aids the client in expectorating secretions and in breathing.

Mechanical Devices. Clients who cannot attain esophageal speech can use mechanical devices called electrolarynges. Most are battery-powered devices placed against the side of the neck or cheek. The air inside the mouth and pharynx is vibrated, and the client articulates as usual. Another external device (Cooper Rand), also battery powered, consists of a plastic tube, placed within the client's mouth, that vibrates on articulation.

Tracheoesophageal Fistula. A tracheoesophageal fistula (TEF) may be used if esophageal speech is insufficient for communication and if the client meets strict criteria. A surgical fistula is created between the trachea and the esophagus either at the time of the laryngectomy or in the postoperative period (Fig. 31–9). The surgeon places a

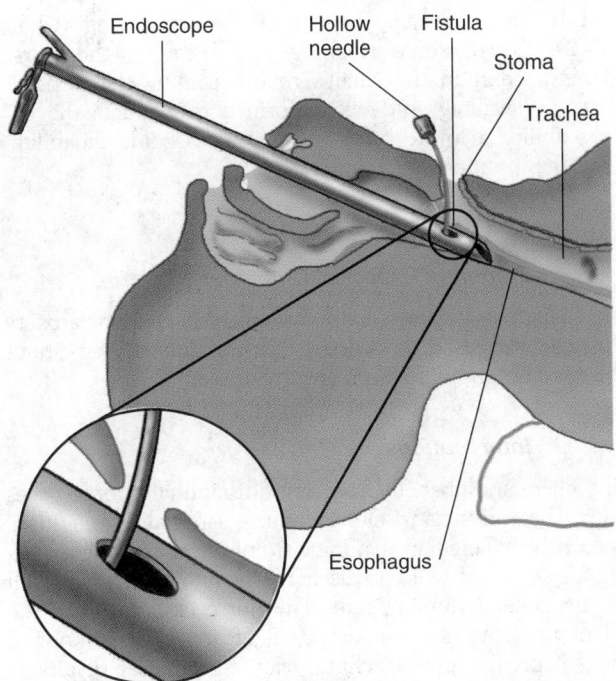

Figure 31–9. One method of creating a tracheoesophageal fistula.

catheter into the laryngectomy stoma and surgically creates a fistula into the esophagus. Usually, the catheter is then sutured to the neck to prevent accidental dislodgment. After the fistula heals, a silicone prosthesis, such as the Blom-Singer prosthesis (Fig. 31–10), is inserted in place of the catheter. The client covers the stoma and the opening of the prosthesis with a finger or opens and closes the opening with a special valve to divert air from the lungs, through the trachea, into the esophagus, and out of the mouth. Lip and tongue movement, not the prosthesis itself, produces speech.

Surgical Procedures for Other Head and Neck Cancers. The major types of resections, defined by the tumor location of the oropharyngeal cancer, are called composite resections. Composite resections are a combination of surgical procedures that include partial or total glossectomies, partial mandibulectomies, and, if required, nodal neck dissections. Tracheostomy may be planned to provide an adequate airway. (More information on oral cancer is found in Chapter 56.)

Tracheostomy. A tracheostomy can be performed as an emergency procedure or as a scheduled surgical procedure. A tracheotomy is a surgical incision into the trachea for the purpose of establishing an airway. Tracheostomy is the (tracheal) stoma, or opening, that results from the tracheotomy. The tracheostomy can be temporary or permanent. (Chapter 30 presents in detail the nursing care requirements of a client with a tracheostomy.)

➤ *High Risk for Aspiration*

Planning: Expected Outcomes

The client is expected not to aspirate food, gastrointestinal contents, or oral secretions into the lungs.

Interventions

Depending on tumor size and location or type of tumor resection, the client may aspirate during eating. This inci-

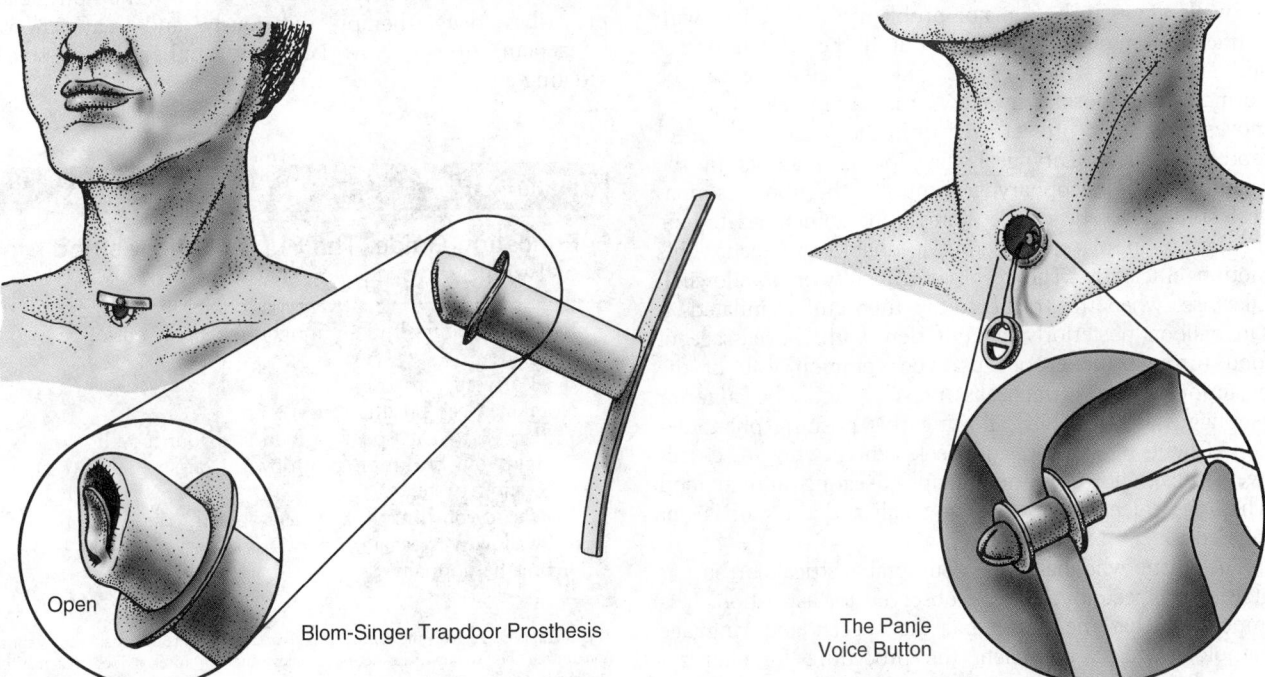

Figure 31–10. Examples of tracheoesophageal prostheses.

dent can result in life-threatening pneumonia, weight loss, further hospitalization, and increased costs.

Because of anatomic or surgical changes in the upper respiratory tract and altered swallowing mechanisms, the client with head and neck cancer is at risk for aspiration. The presence of a nasogastric (NG) feeding tube may further increase the potential for aspiration because of the incompetent lower esophageal sphincter (LES). The one exception is the client who has had a total laryngectomy; because the airway is separated from the esophagus, making aspiration impossible, such a person is not at risk.

A dynamic swallow study evaluates a client's ability to protect the airway from aspiration and helps to determine the appropriate method of swallow rehabilitation. Bedside clinical assessment of swallowing is important but carries with it a high rate of inaccuracy. In many cases, the physician must institute enteral feedings either because of the client's inability to swallow or because of continued aspiration potential.

When an NG tube is in place, the nurse helps to prevent aspiration through routine reflux precautions, including elevating the head of the bed and strictly adhering to tube feeding regimens, including no bolus feedings at night. The nurse checks residual feeding amounts before each bolus feeding (or every 4–6 hours with continuous feeding) and evaluates the client's tolerance of the tube feeding. If the residual volume is too high (<100 mL), the nurse withholds the feeding and notifies the physician. The nurse adds food coloring to the tube feeding and observes tracheal secretions. If aspiration occurs, secretions may be the color of the food coloring. Methylene blue is not used today as an additive to tube feedings because it is systemically excreted through the lungs and can appear in pulmonary secretions. (See Chapter 64 for other interventions related to NG tubes and tube feedings.)

Swallowing can be a major problem for the client with a tracheostomy tube in place, but if the cranial nerves and anatomical structures are intact, swallowing can be normal. In a normal swallow, the larynx elevates and moves forward to protect itself from the passing stream of food and saliva. Laryngeal elevation also assists in the opening of the cricopharyngeal muscle, the upper esophageal sphincter. The tracheostomy tube sometimes tethers the larynx in place, rendering it unable to execute this motion efficiently. The result is difficulty in swallowing. Likewise, when the tracheostomy tube cuff is inflated, it can balloon posteriorly and interfere with the passage of food through the esophagus. The common wall of the posterior trachea (trachealis muscle) and the anterior esophagus is very thin, allowing this pushing phenomenon. Clients with head and neck cancer who are cognitively intact, however, may adapt to eating normal food when the tracheostomy tube is small and the cuff is not inflated.

The client who has had a subtotal, vertical, or supraglottic laryngectomy, *must* be observed for aspiration. It is imperative that the nurse and the speech and language pathologist teach the client the procedure for alternate methods of swallowing without aspirating. Especially effective after partial laryngectomy or base-of-tongue resec-

tion is the "supraglottic method" of swallowing (Chart 31–2). To reinforce teaching and learning, the nurse places a chart in the client's room detailing the steps. A dynamic swallow study is performed to evaluate the client's ability to protect the airway and to guide rehabilitation therapy for swallowing.

► Anxiety

Planning: Expected Outcomes

The client is expected to verbalize decreased anxiety through increased knowledge and understanding about the specific, individualized treatment plan.

Interventions

The client may benefit from multidisciplinary conferences with the physician, clinical nurse specialist, dietitian, speech and language pathologist, physical therapist, psychologist, social worker, discharge planning nurse, as well as the general nursing staff. The nurse explores with the client the reason for anxiety (e.g., fear of the unknown, lack of preoperative teaching, fear of pain, fear of airway compromise, fear of hospitalization, and loss of control). Many times the client and family can benefit from further information. Before the client is scheduled for surgery and while the client is still at home, home care nurses or community-sponsored associations, such as the American Cancer Society, may be able to alleviate the fears of the client and family about the disease process and surgical interventions.

The nurse administers antianxiety agents, such as diazepam (Valium), with caution because of the possibility of hypercarbia and hypoxia in an already compromised client. The location of the tumor and any other concurrent lung disease may be causing some degree of airway obstruction. For anxiety in this client, the physician prescribes drug therapy judiciously and may choose lorazepam (Ativan, Novo-Lorazem♣) rather than a solely sedating agent.

Chart 31–2

Education Guide: The Supraglottic Method of Swallowing

1. Position yourself in an upright, preferably out-of-bed, position.
2. Clear your throat.
3. Take a deep breath.
4. Place ½ to 1 teaspoon of food into your mouth.
5. Hold your breath or "bear down" (Valsalva maneuver).
6. Swallow twice.
7. Release your breath, and clear your throat.
8. Swallow twice again.
9. Breathe normally.

This method exaggerates the normal protective mechanisms of cessation of respiration during the swallow. The double swallow attempts to clear food that may be pooling in the pharynx, vallecula, and piriform sinuses. This method is used only after a dynamic radiographic swallow study has demonstrated that it is appropriate and safe for the client.

➤ *Body Image Disturbance*

Planning: Expected Outcomes

The client is expected to state understanding and, in time, acceptance of body image changes and returns to the previous lifestyle within the limits of the disease.

Interventions

The client with head and neck cancer experiences a permanent change in body image because of deformity, the presence of a stoma or artificial airway, speech changes, and a change in the method of eating. The client may be aphonic (unable to speak) or may have permanent hoarseness or speech deficits. The nurse helps the client to set realistic goals, starting with involvement in self-care. The nurse teaches alternative communication methods so that the client can functionally communicate in the hospital and after discharge.

The nurse and family must make all attempts to ease the client into a more normal social environment. The nurse provides encouragement and positive reinforcement while demonstrating acceptance and caring behaviors. The family may benefit from counseling sessions that the nurse initiates in the hospital.

After surgery, the client may feel reserved and socially isolated because of the change in voice and facial appearance. To cover the laryngectomy stoma, the tracheostomy tube, and postoperative changes related to surgery, the client can wear loose-fitting, high-collar shirts or sweaters (e.g., turtleneck), scarves, and jewelry. Cosmetics may aid in covering any disfigurement. Most surgeons try to place the surgical incisions in the client's natural skin fold lines if doing so does not pose a risk for cancer recurrence. (See Chapter 10 for a detailed discussion of body image, including additional nursing interventions.)

 Continuing Care

If no complications occur, the client is usually ready to be discharged home or to an extended care facility within 2 weeks. At the time of discharge, the client should be able to provide self-care, which may include tracheostomy or stoma care, nutrition, wound care, and methods of communication.

The client and family may feel more secure about discharge if they receive a referral to a community health agency familiar with the care of the client recovering from head and neck cancer. The multidisciplinary team assesses the client's specific discharge needs and makes the appropriate referrals to home care agencies, including such professionals as nutritionists, nurses, physical therapists, speech pathologists, and social workers. The nurse coordinates the scheduling for chemotherapy or radiation therapy with the client and family.

➤ *Health Teaching*

Although education begins during preoperative teaching sessions, most self-care is taught in the hospital. The nurse teaches the client and family how to care for the stoma or tracheostomy or laryngectomy tube, depending

---

Chart 31–3

Education Guide: Home Laryngectomy Care

- Avoid swimming, and use care when showering or shaving.
- Lean slightly forward and cover the stoma when coughing or sneezing.
- Wear a stoma guard or loose clothing to cover the stoma.
- Clean the stoma with mild soap and water. Lubricate the stoma with non-oil-based ointment as needed.
- Increase humidity by using saline in the stoma as instructed, a bedside humidifier, pans of water, and houseplants.
- Obtain and wear a Medic-Alert bracelet and emergency care for life-threatening situations.

---

on the type of surgery performed. The nurse reviews incision and airway care, including cleaning and inspecting for signs of infection. The nurse teaches clean suction technique and reviews the client's plan of care.

Chart 31–3 summarizes the highlights of self-care for the client discharged after laryngeal cancer surgery. Many of the highlights are also applicable to someone discharged after any resection for head and neck cancer.

Stoma Care. To prevent water from entering the airway, the nurse instructs the client to use a shower shield over the tracheostomy tube or laryngectomy stoma when bathing. To shield the airway during the day, the client may wear a protective cover or stoma guard.

For the client with a permanent stoma after laryngectomy or for the client with a permanent tracheostomy, covering the permanent opening has a double benefit: filtering the air entering the stoma while keeping humidity in the airway and enhancing aesthetic appearance. To protect the airway and increase humidity, the nurse instructs the client to cover the airway with cotton or foam. Attractive coverings are available in the form of cotton scarves, crocheted bibs, and jewelry. Using colored seam binding for tracheostomy ties after the stoma has matured may enhance the client's overall body image. The client's shirt or dress color can be matched or coordinated with seam bindings of various colors. The nurse also teaches the client how to increase humidity in the home. The nurse may teach the client to instill normal saline into the artificial airway 10–15 times a day as ordered.

Communication. The client continues the selected method of alternative communication that began in the hospital. The client wears a medical alert (Medic-Alert) bracelet and carries a special identification card (Fig. 31–11). For the client who had a laryngectomy, this card is available from the local chapter of the International Association of Laryngectomees. The card instructs the reader in providing an emergency airway or resuscitating the client who has a stoma.

Smoking Cessation. A difficult but important issue for the client after head and neck cancer surgery is smok-

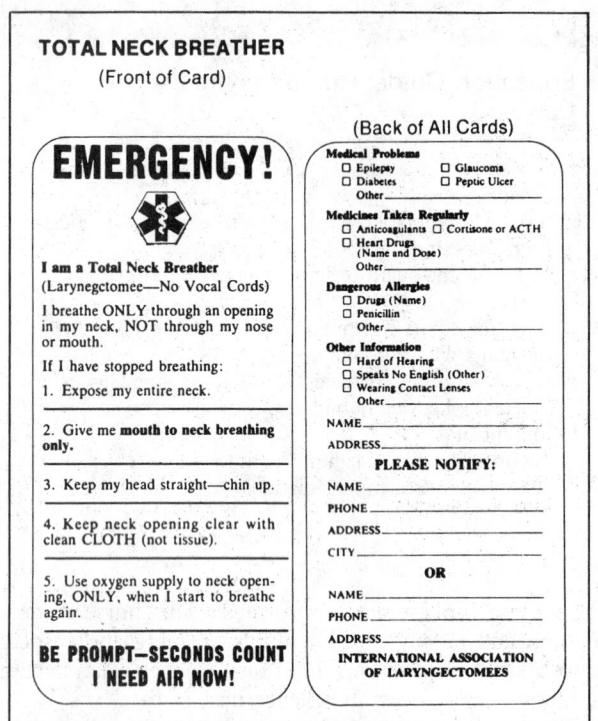

TOTAL NECK BREATHER
(Front of Card)

EMERGENCY!

I am a Total Neck Breather
(Larynegctomee—No Vocal Cords)

I breathe ONLY through an opening in my neck, NOT through my nose or mouth.

If I have stopped breathing:

1. Expose my entire neck.

2. Give me **mouth to neck breathing only.**

3. Keep my head straight—chin up.

4. Keep neck opening clear with clean CLOTH (not tissue).

5. Use oxygen supply to neck opening. ONLY, when I start to breathe again.

**BE PROMPT—SECONDS COUNT
I NEED AIR NOW!**

(Back of All Cards)

Medical Problems
☐ Epilepsy ☐ Glaucoma
☐ Diabetes ☐ Peptic Ulcer
Other_____

Medicines Taken Regularly
☐ Anticoagulants ☐ Cortisone or ACTH
☐ Heart Drugs
(Name and Dose)
Other_____

Dangerous Allergies
☐ Drugs (Name)
☐ Penicillin
Other_____

Other Information
☐ Hard of Hearing
☐ Speaks No English (Other)
☐ Wearing Contact Lenses
Other_____

NAME_____

ADDRESS_____

PLEASE NOTIFY:

NAME_____

PHONE_____

ADDRESS_____

CITY_____

OR

NAME_____

PHONE_____

ADDRESS_____

**INTERNATIONAL ASSOCIATION
OF LARYNGECTOMEES**

Figure 31–11. Emergency wallet card for identification of laryngectomy.

ing cessation. Smoking plays a major role in the development of head and neck cancer. The nurse stresses to the client that smoking cessation can reduce the risk for developing additional malignancies and increase the rate of healing from surgery. Chemical and psychological assistance is available for smoking cessation.

➤ Psychosocial Preparation

The many physical changes resulting from a laryngectomy influence clients' physical, social, and emotional functioning. Many clients perceive changes in their quality of life (the Research Application for Nursing examines the effectiveness of a quality of life assessment tool among people undergoing head and neck surgery for cancer). The nurse begins to prepare the client and family for these changes, but another client who has adjusted to these changes is usually more effective in helping clients adjust.

Clients who are discharged with a permanent stoma, tracheostomy tube, nasogastric tube, and wounds experience an alteration in body image. The nurse stresses the importance of returning to a normal lifestyle as much as possible. About half of these clients return to full-time employment. The remainder work part time or apply for disability income. Most clients can resume many of their usual activities within 4–6 weeks after surgery or longer after a combination of radiation therapy and surgery. Clients may be frustrated at times while trying to adjust to changes in smell, taste, and communication during this time.

The client with a total laryngectomy cannot produce sounds during laughing and crying, and mucous secre-

tions may appear unexpectedly when these emotions or coughing or sneezing occurs. The mucus can be embarrassing, and the client needs to be prepared to cover the stoma with a handkerchief or gauze. The client who has undergone composite resections will have difficulty with speech and swallowing. This client may have tracheostomy and feeding tubes to deal with in public places.

➤ Home Care Management

Extensive home care preparation is required for the client with a laryngectomy for cancer. The convalescent period is long, and airway management is complicated. The client or family must be able to take an active role in client care.

General cleanliness of the home is assessed. If the client has severe or long-standing respiratory problems, adjustments in the home to allow for one-floor living may be necessary. Increased humidification is needed. A hu-

▷ Research Applications for Nursing

A New Functional Status/Quality of Life Scale

Baker, C. A. (1995). Functional status scale for measuring quality of life outcomes in head and neck cancer patients. Cancer Nursing, 18(6), 458–466.

The purpose of this study was to determine the validity and reliability of a newly developed functional status scale measuring quality of life among clients with head and neck cancer. The scale was initially developed with the input of 115 clients with head and neck cancer and reflects the concerns and terminology used by this population. Forced choices included 10 physical activities and 5 subjective symptom areas (such as pain, fatigue, appearance). An open-ended question concluded the questionnaire. The scale was tested with 172 clients with head and neck cancer and 30 clients with other types of cancer.

Psychometric testing indicates excellent discriminate validity and moderate to strong convergent validity with other measures of performance. Reliability was established at 0.88 (Cronbach's α). The scale was sensitive to the population for which it was developed.

Critique. The study was well designed and involved a sufficient number of participants. Incorporation of an open-ended question increased the sensitivity and specificity of the instrument. Longitudinal studies with this scale are needed to determine its usefulness in identifying within-participant changes in functional status over time.

Implications for Nursing. Clients with different types of cancer have different residual problems and concerns. Many functional status/quality of life measures, although designed and tested with one client population, are regarded generally as appropriate for clients with any cancer type. Client concerns, however, have probably been misunderstood and not addressed because instruments and scales have not been sufficiently sensitive to the target population. To identify and meet the needs of clients with special problems, nurses must use instruments appropriate to the population in need.

Chart 31–4

Focused Assessment for Home Care Clients After Laryngectomy

- Assess respiratory status.
  - Observe rate and depth of respiration.
  - Auscultate lungs.
  - Check patency of airway.
  - Examine the tracheostomy exudate for amount, color, and character.
  - Examine nail beds and mucous membranes for evidence of cyanosis.
  - Take a pulse oximetry reading.
- Assess condition of wound.
  - Remove dressings (noting condition of dressings).
  - Cleanse the wound.
  - Compare with previous notations of wound condition:
    Presence, amount, and nature of exudate
    Presence/absence of cellulitis
    Presence/absence of odor
- Assess client's psychosocial functioning.
  - Ask the client about passing the time, visitors, and trips outside the house.
  - Observe whether the client communicates responses directly or whether a family member speaks for the client.
  - Observe client and family member interactions.
  - Determine what method of communication the client has selected and observe the client's skill with it.
  - Is the client wearing pajamas or the client dressed?
- Take the client's temperature.
- Assess client's understanding of illness and compliance with treatment.
  - Signs and symptoms to report to health care provider
  - Medication plan (correct timing and dose)
  - Ambulation or positioning schedule
  - Dressing changes/skin care
  - Diet modifications (24-hr diet recall)
  - Skill in tracheostomy or dressing care
- Assess client's nutritional status.
  - Change in muscle mass
  - Lackluster nails/sparse hair
  - Recent weight loss >10% of usual weight
  - Impaired oral intake
  - Difficulty swallowing
  - Generalized edema

midifier add-on to a forced-air furnace can be obtained. If the cost is not manageable or if the home is heated by radiators, a room humidifier or vaporizer may be appropriate.

A home care nurse is involved with the client's care after discharge and becomes a very important resource for the client and family. The home care nurse assesses the client and home situation for problems in self-care, complications, adjustment, and adherence to medical regimen. Chart 31–4 lists assessment areas for the client in the home after laryngectomy. The nurse reinforces health care teaching, self-care teaching, and smoking cessation regimens.

► *Health Care Resources*

The home care or hospital nurse informs the client and family of community organizations, such as the American Cancer Society, and local laryngectomee clubs, which can offer support, accurate information, and friendships. When the client has problems paying for health care services, equipment supply and prescriptions, a visiting nurse agency may be helpful in directing the client to available resources.

In many areas, the local unit of American Cancer Society or the Canadian Cancer Society can help provide dressing materials and nutritional supplements to the client in need. This organization may also provide transportation to and from follow-up visits or radiation therapy.

 Evaluation

On the basis of the identified nursing diagnoses, the nurse evaluates the entire plan of care for the client with head and neck cancer. The expected outcomes are that the client

- Maintains a patent airway
- Attains or maintains clear lung sounds in all lung fields
- Demonstrates an understanding of head and neck cancer and its treatment
- Performs self-care of the artificial airway and wound
- Performs the activities of daily living (ADLs) independently or with minimal assistance
- States that levels of anxiety are reduced
- Resumes as normal a lifestyle as possible through rehabilitation
- States understanding of and adapts to body image changes
- Attains or maintains adequate nutrition
- Does not aspirate gastric contents or food
- Complies with smoking and alcohol cessation

CASE STUDY for the Client with Vocal Cord Paralysis

■ You are making a home visit to a 64-year-old man with terminal lung cancer who is receiving hospice services at home. When you arrive, the client's wife tells you that she thinks he has a cold because his voice is hoarse and he has been coughing ever since breakfast 20 minutes ago. On initial assessment, you find the client to be able to talk, but his voice is raspy and does not get louder with increased effort. He is somewhat anxious and says he is coughing because "some crumbs went down the wrong way." The color of his lips and nail beds is good. His respiratory rate and depth are within the range found at the last visit 2 days ago.

QUESTIONS:

1. What assessment information do you need to document?
2. What additional assessment data do you need to document?
3. What priority nursing actions do you need to implement?
4. What expected outcomes would be specific to this situation?

SELECTED BIBLIOGRAPHY

*American Cancer Society. (1990). Cancer of the larynx. *Ca: A Cancer Journal for Clinicians, 40*(3), 133–183.

American Cancer Society. (1998). *Cancer facts and figures, 1998.* Atlanta: American Cancer Society. (98–300M, No. 5008.98)

*Baker, C. A. (1992). Factors associated with rehabilitation in head and neck cancer. *Cancer Nursing, 15*(6), 395–400.

Baker, C. A. (1995). Functional status scale for measuring quality of life outcomes in head and neck cancer patients. *Cancer Nursing, 18*(6), 458–466.

*Bartkiw, T. P., & Pynn, B. R. (1993). Close-up on mandible fracture. *Nursing 93, 23*(12), 45.

Boucher, M. (1996). When laryngectomy complicates care. *RN, 59*(8), 40–45.

Clark, L. (1995). A critical event in tracheostomy care. *British Journal of Nursing, 4*(12), 676, 678–681.

Dropkin, M. L. (1997). Coping with disfigurement/dysfunction and length of hospital stay after head and neck cancer surgery. *ORL Head and Neck Nursing, 15*(1), 22–26.

Fetzer, S. (1998). Laryngeal mask airway: Indications and management for critical-care. *Critical Care Nurse, 18*(1), 83–87.

Friedman, C. D., & Costantino, P. (1994). General concepts in craniofacial skeletal augmentation and replacement. *Otolaryngologic Clinics of North America, 27*(5), 847–857.

Garp, M. (1998). Pulse oximetry. *Critical Care Nurse, 18*(1), 94–99.

*Grant, M., Rhiner, M., & Padilla, G. (1989). Nutritional management in the head and neck cancer patient. *Seminars in Oncology Nursing, 5*(3), 195–204.

Hecht, J., Emmons, K., Brown, R., Everett, K., Farrell, N., Hitchcock, P., & Sales, S. (1994). Smoking interventions for patients with cancer: Guidelines for nursing practice. *Oncology Nursing Forum, 21*(10), 1657–1666.

Hooper, M. (1996). Nursing care of the patient with a tracheostomy. *Nursing Standard, 10*(34), 40–43.

Madeya, M. (1996a). Oral complications from cancer therapy: Part 1. Pathophysiology and secondary complications. *Oncology Nursing Forum, 23*(5), 801–807.

Madeya, M. (1996b). Oral complications from cancer therapy: Part 2. Nursing implications for assessment and treatment. *Oncology Nursing Forum, 23*(5), 808–819.

Perera, F. P. (1996). Uncovering new clues to cancer risk. *Scientific American, 275*(3), 54–62.

Phillips, S. (1997). Obstructive sleep apnea: Diagnosis and management. *Nursing Standard, 11*(17), 43–46.

Reese, J. (1996). Head and neck cancers. In R. McCorkle, M. Grant, M. Frank-Stromborg, & S. Baird (Eds.). *Cancer nursing: A comprehensive textbook* (2nd ed., pp. 773–795). Philadelphia: W. B. Saunders.

Shellenbarger, T., & Narielwala, S. (1996). Caring for the patient with laryngeal cancer at home. *Home Healthcare Nurse, 14*(2), 80–90.

*Weber, M., & Reimer, M. (1993). Laryngectomy: Grieving disfigurement and dysfunction. *The Canadian Nurse, 89*(3), 31–34.

*Weimert, T. A. (1992). Common ENT emergencies: The acute nose and throat, part 2. *Emergency Medicine, 24*(6), 26–28, 31–32, 34–36.

SUGGESTED READINGS

Hecht, J., Emmons, K., Brown, R., Everett, K., Farrell, N., Hitchcock, P., & Sales, S. (1994). Smoking interventions for patients with cancer: Guidelines for nursing practice. *Oncology Nursing Forum, 21*(10), 1657–1666.

This excellent article describes the physiologic benefits of smoking cessation on different body systems. The information is research based and includes a discussion of the health impact of continued smoking during cancer treatment. Nursing interventions include pharmacologic and nonpharmacologic strategies for assisting the client with smoking cessation.

Madeya, M. (1996). Oral complications from cancer therapy: Part 2. Nursing implications for assessment and treatment. *Oncology Nursing Forum, 23*(5), 808–819.

The author describes the most common oral complications from cancer therapy and presents them as nursing diagnoses. Clear and detailed interventions are listed in outline form for each diagnosis. Questions for self-assessment or continuing education credit follow the article.

Shellenbarger, T., & Narielwala, S. (1996). Caring for the patient with laryngeal cancer at home. *Home Healthcare Nurse, 14*(2), 80–90.

Clients with laryngeal cancer have many needs and complicated care regimens. This article presents organized assessment tips and intervention strategies for assisting these clients and families in the home.

Chapter 32

INTERVENTIONS FOR CLIENTS WITH NONINFECTIOUS PROBLEMS OF THE LOWER RESPIRATORY TRACT

Lower airway disorders account for much morbidity and mortality. Some disorders may be aggravated by environmental irritants; others have a familial tendency. The major nursing diagnoses include impaired gas exchange, ineffective breathing pattern, and ineffective airway clearance. For the elderly client with a respiratory disorder, some general nursing considerations are listed in Chart 32-1.

CHRONIC AIRFLOW LIMITATION

Overview

Chronic airflow limitation is the term for a group of chronic lung diseases, including pulmonary emphysema, chronic bronchitis, and bronchial asthma. Emphysema and chronic bronchitis are characterized by bronchoconstriction and dyspnea; these conditions have little reversibility. Unlike emphysema and chronic bronchitis, asthma is primarily an inflammatory process characterized by *re-*versible airflow obstruction and wheezing. The terms chronic obstructive pulmonary disease (COPD) and chronic airflow limitation (CAL) are often used interchangeably.

More than 1 million people between the ages of 40 and 65 are sufficiently disabled from COPD to receive regular disability income from Social Security (Bordow & Moser, 1996). Better prevention and rehabilitation will help maintain optimal functioning and improve overall health.

The onset of respiratory failure is a major event in the life of a client with CAL. More than half of the clients diagnosed with CAL will die within 10 years of diagnosis. Health care professionals have an obligation to assist clients in formulating directives before respiratory decompensation. Advanced directives provide clients with the opportunity to specify their health care wishes.

Pathophysiology

Most clients with respiratory problems present with two or more diseases (e.g., emphysema and chronic bronchi-

---

Chart 32-1

Nursing Focus on the Elderly: Respiratory Disorders

- Provide rest periods between such activities as bathing, meals, and ambulation.
- Place the client in an upright position for meals to prevent aspiration.
- Encourage nutritional fluid intake after the meal to promote increased calorie intake.
- Schedule medications around routine activities to increase medication compliance.
- Arrange chairs in strategic locations to allow the client with dyspnea to walk and rest as needed.
- Encourage prompt access to a health care facility for any sign or symptom of infection.
- Ensure that the client has received the pneumococcal vaccine.
- Encourage the client to have an annual flu vaccination.

---

tis) simultaneously, but each condition has its own pathophysiologic process (Fig. 32–1).

Pulmonary Emphysema

Pulmonary emphysema is characterized by the destruction of alveoli, loss of elastic recoil, and narrowing of small airways (bronchioles), resulting in increased resting lung volumes, increased airflow resistance, alveolar hyperinflation, and diaphragm flattening. These changes are reflected in the client by increased respiratory rate and dyspnea.

Specific Pathologic Changes

Four pathologic changes occur in the client (see Fig. 32–1):

- Loss of lung elasticity. Proteases (lung enzymes) alter or destroy the alveoli and the small airways by breaking down elastin. As a result, the alveolar sacs lose their elasticity, and the small airways collapse or narrow. Some alveoli are destroyed, whereas others remain enlarged.
- Hyperinflation of the lung. The enlarged alveoli prevent the lung from returning to its normal resting state during expiration.
- Formation of bullae. The alveolar walls deteriorate and connect to form bullae (air-filled spaces) that can be seen on x-ray examination.
- Small airway collapse and air trapping. As the client forcibly attempts to exhale air trapped in the enlarged alveoli, positive intrathoracic pressures collapse the small airways.

EFFECTS OF PATHOLOGIC CHANGES ON BREATHING. Emphysema, like other CAL diseases, increases the work of breathing. In moderate to severe emphysema, the work of breathing is increased because the hyperinflated lung causes the diaphragm to flatten (Fig.

32–2). The flattened diaphragm requires the use of accessory respiratory muscles, such as neck and abdominal muscles, during expiration when the diaphragm must rise against gravity. A healthy person uses about 65% diaphragm and 35% accessory muscles to breathe; the client with emphysema uses about 30% diaphragm and 70% accessory muscles to breathe. The client needs more oxygen for more muscle use and so may experience an "air hunger" sensation. The client usually starts inspiration before expiration is completed, resulting in dyspnea with an inefficient and uncoordinated pattern of breathing.

EFFECTS OF PATHOLOGIC CHANGES ON GAS EXCHANGE. The increased work of breathing may affect gas exchange, although arterial blood gas (ABG) values are not usually affected until the client has advanced disease. Then carbon dioxide is often produced faster than the body can eliminate it, which causes carbon dioxide retention and chronic respiratory acidosis (see Chap. 19). The client with late-stage emphysema has a low arterial blood oxygen concentration (PaO_2) as well because it is difficult for oxygen to move from diseased lung tissue into the bloodstream.

CLASSIFICATION OF EMPHYSEMA. Emphysema is classified according to the pattern of destruction and dilation of the gas-exchanging units (acini) of the lung. Emphysema can be divided into panlobular, centrilobular, and paraseptal types (see Fig. 32–1). Each type can occur alone or in combination in the same lung.

Panlobular (panacinar) emphysema (PLE) involves destruction of the entire alveolus uniformly. Panacinar emphysema is a diffuse disease that is usually more severe in the lower lung area. This type of emphysema is seen with homozygous alpha₁-antitrypsin (ATT) deficiency.

In centrilobular (centriacinar) emphysema (CLE), openings develop in the respiratory bronchioles and allow spaces to develop as tissue walls disintegrate. Although this is a diffuse disease, the upper lung sections are most severely affected. This type of emphysema is often seen in long-standing cigarette smokers.

In paraseptal, distal acinar emphysema, the disease is confined to the distal portion of the acinus; only alveolar ducts and alveoli are involved. This disease type tends to be localized and is associated with the formation of bullae. Spontaneous pneumothorax, with the formation of blebs, can result in the diseased lung area. Spontaneous pneumothorax is a collapse of a portion of the lung because of an opening from the lung side into the pleural space. A bleb is a collection of air within the pleura that is generally less than 1–2 cm.

Alpha₁-antitrypsin deficiency is a genetic abnormality that leads to emphysema. Less than 1% of clients with emphysema have this type. The physician or Nurse Practitioner suspects ATT in the client who presents with an onset of dyspnea, cough, wheeze, and increased mucus production at an early age (younger than 50 years). ATT, a serum protein produced by the liver, is found in the lungs. Its primary function is to inhibit neutrophil elastase. Diagnosis is made by analysis of the serum ATT levels and Pi typing (serum protease inhibitor phenotyping).

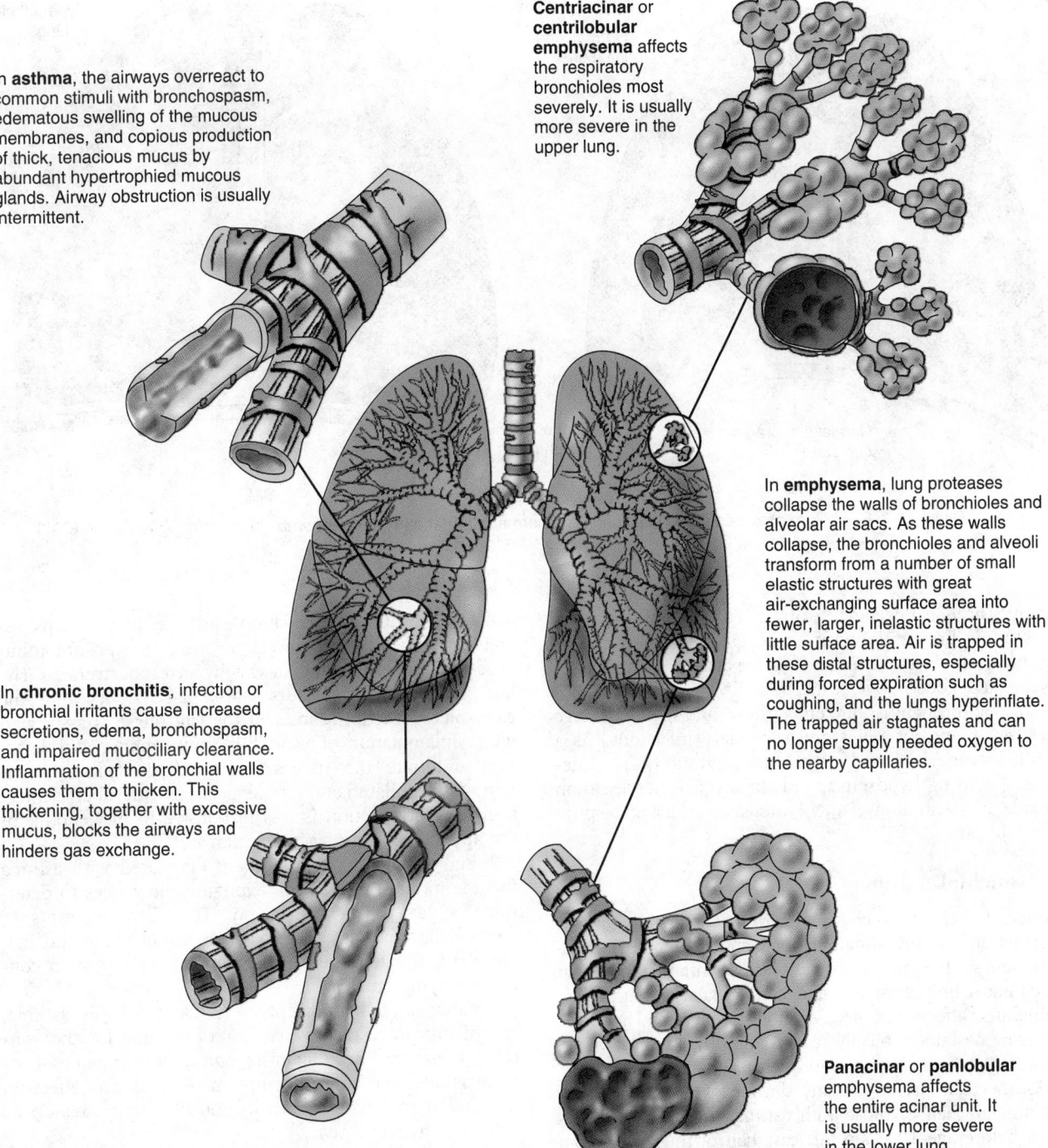

In **asthma**, the airways overreact to common stimuli with bronchospasm, edematous swelling of the mucous membranes, and copious production of thick, tenacious mucus by abundant hypertrophied mucous glands. Airway obstruction is usually intermittent.

Centriacinar or **centrilobular emphysema** affects the respiratory bronchioles most severely. It is usually more severe in the upper lung.

In **emphysema**, lung proteases collapse the walls of bronchioles and alveolar air sacs. As these walls collapse, the bronchioles and alveoli transform from a number of small elastic structures with great air-exchanging surface area into fewer, larger, inelastic structures with little surface area. Air is trapped in these distal structures, especially during forced expiration such as coughing, and the lungs hyperinflate. The trapped air stagnates and can no longer supply needed oxygen to the nearby capillaries.

In **chronic bronchitis**, infection or bronchial irritants cause increased secretions, edema, bronchospasm, and impaired mucociliary clearance. Inflammation of the bronchial walls causes them to thicken. This thickening, together with excessive mucus, blocks the airways and hinders gas exchange.

Panacinar or **panlobular** emphysema affects the entire acinar unit. It is usually more severe in the lower lung.

Figure 32–1. The pathophysiology of chronic airflow limitation (CAL).

Acute and Chronic Bronchitis

Bronchitis results from exposure to infectious or noninfectious irritants, especially tobacco smoke. The irritant produces an inflammatory response, which causes vasodilation, congestion, mucosal edema, and bronchospasm. Unlike emphysema, bronchitis affects the small and large airways rather than the alveoli. Airflow may or may not be limited.

Acute bronchitis can occur as a single episode or can represent an acute exacerbation of chronic bronchitis. An upper respiratory infection, usually viral, often precedes the acute bronchitis episode.

Chronic bronchitis is chronic inflammation of the airways. Chronic inflammation results in mucous gland hypertrophy and hyperplasia, which produce increased viscid mucus. The bronchial walls thicken (often to twice the normal thickness) and impair airflow. This thickening, together with production of excessive mucus, blocks some of the smaller airways and narrows larger ones. Small airways (bronchioles) are often affected before the large

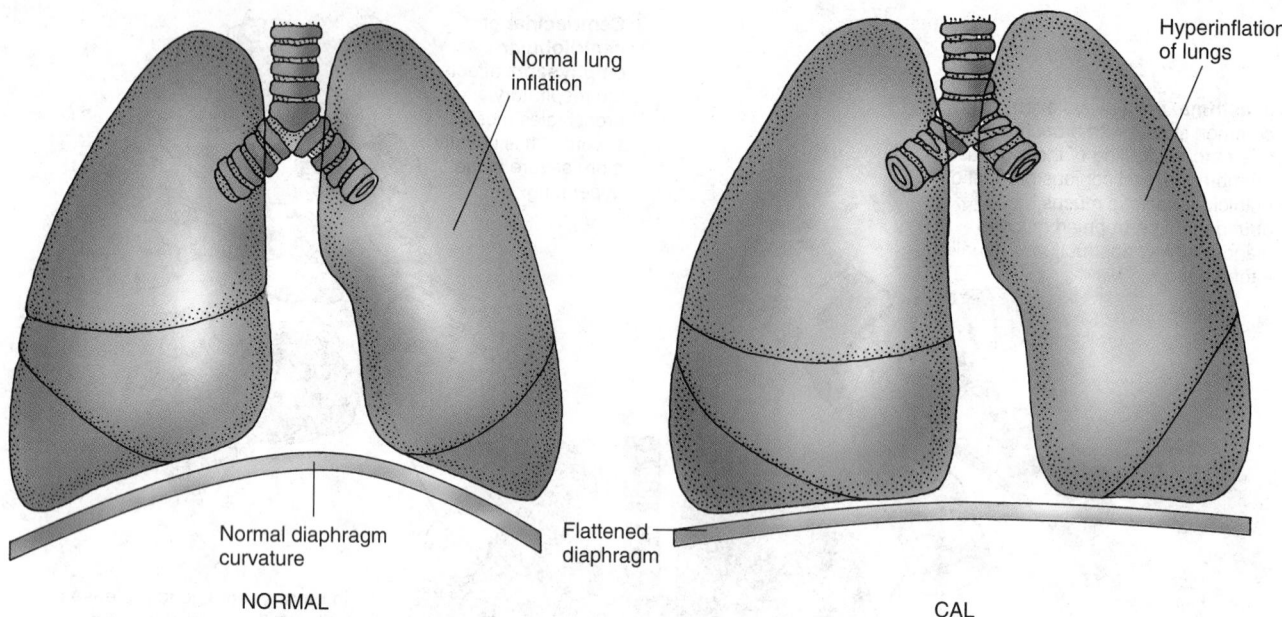

Figure 32-2. Diaphragm shape and lung inflation in the normal client and in the client with chronic airflow limitation (CAL).

airways (bronchi) become involved. The physician diagnoses chronic bronchitis when a client has had a cough or sputum production on most days for at least 3 months of a year for 2 consecutive years.

Chronic bronchitis hinders airflow and gas exchange because of mucous plugs and secondary infections. As a result, the arterial blood oxygen concentration (PaO_2) decreases, causing hypoxemia, and the arterial blood carbon dioxide concentration ($PaCO_2$) increases, causing respiratory acidosis.

Bronchial Asthma

Bronchial asthma is characterized by reversible airflow obstruction, airway inflammation, and airway hyperresponsiveness. It is primarily a disease of inflammation that precipitates bronchospasm and can be fatal. Asthma, like bronchitis, affects the airways, not the alveoli. Therefore, asthma does not typically lead to emphysema; however, asthma may coexist with emphysema and bronchitis.

Asthma can present in any decade of life, but in approximately half of those with asthma, the disease developed before age 10 years. At least half of those in whom asthma develops in childhood will have remission as adults. Asthma is more common in urban than in rural settings and appears to be higher in minority populations (Bordow & Moser, 1996).

Bronchial hyperresponsiveness is a cardinal feature of asthma. Once the client is exposed to the stimulus, chemical mediators are immediately released. Within minutes of being exposed, the client experiences dyspnea, wheezing, cough, and mucus production.

Asthma is the result of acute- and late-phase reactions. The acute-phase reaction is the result of an immediate hypersensitivity to the allergen, which stimulates the mast cell to release histamine and other cell mediators. This reaction results in smooth muscle contraction, vascular leakage, flushing (vasodilation), hypotension, mucus secretion, and pruritus. Levels of allergen exposure influence the prevalence of airway hyperresponsiveness. The late-phase response occurs within 2–8 hours after the early-phase reaction. Onset of the late phase is associated with inflammation. Eosinophils, neutrophils, and basophils infiltrate the tissues and result in inflammation. Long-term inflammation is associated with fiber deposition. The obstruction is less responsive to bronchodilator therapy, and airway reactivity increases.

Initial approaches to the client diagnosed with asthma include monitoring of peak expiratory flow rates to determine a pattern of obstruction. The client attempts to control the environmental exposure to allergens and irritants and is established on a pharmacologic plan to control the symptoms.

Because inflammation plays the key role in asthma, antiinflammatory therapy is the cornerstone for the control of asthma. Beta agonists and other bronchodilator medications help control symptoms but have no effect on the underlying disease and do not alter inflammation or bronchial hyperreactivity.

TYPES OF ASTHMA. Asthma can be divided into extrinsic and intrinsic types. Extrinsic asthma (immunoglobulin E [IgE]–mediated), the allergic form of bronchial asthma, is seen more in children than in adults. By contrast, intrinsic asthma is the nonallergic form of the disease. Many factors, often a viral upper respiratory infection, can cause an attack. Some researchers believe intrinsic asthma develops from a hypersensitivity to the viruses causing the infection.

Nocturnal asthma is associated with circadian rhythms. The client often awakens with the worst symptoms between 3 and 5 AM. It is believed that half of all asthma deaths are due to this form of the disease.

PATTERNS OF DISEASE. In adults, asthma attacks are usually separated by symptom-free intervals but may also occur on a continuous basis. The airways of the person with asthma are overreactive and ready to respond to various stimuli. In those people with intrinsic asthma, changes in the environment may precipitate a wheezing episode. Common agents or stimuli include exercise, fog, smog, smoke (both first- and second-hand smoke), odors, aerosols, and upper respiratory tract infections. Pollen, mold spores, animal dander, and arthropods such as house dust mites and cockroaches usually produce bronchoconstriction only in the client with extrinsic (allergic) asthma. Certain foods or medications may be involved in the allergic form of asthma as well (Chart 32–2). Emotional excitement, anxiety, hormonal changes, and fatigue are not causes of asthma but may aggravate, initiate, or accompany an episode of wheezing or dyspnea.

PATHOLOGY OF BRONCHOCONSTRICTION. Inhaled agents stimulate the contraction of airway smooth muscle by different mechanisms. Some agents cause bronchoconstriction by directly stimulating the smooth muscle, and some cause smooth muscle contraction indirectly by affecting neural pathways. Three neural pathways have been studied in environmentally produced bronchoconstriction: muscarinic, alpha-adrenergic, and neuropeptide.

Chart 32–2

Education Guide: Asthma

- Avoid potential environmental asthma triggers, such as smoke, fireplaces, dust, mold, and weather changes (especially warm to cold, or sudden barometric changes).
- Avoid medications that could trigger asthma, for example, aspirin, nonsteroidal anti-inflammatory drugs (NSAIDs), and beta-blockers.
- Avoid food that has been prepared with monosodium glutamate (MSG) or metabisulfite.
- If you experience symptoms of exercise-induced asthma, use your bronchodilator inhaler 30 minutes before exercise to prevent or reduce bronchospasm.
- Be sure you know the proper technique and correct sequence when you use metered-dose inhalers.
- Be sure to get adequate rest and sleep.
- Reduce stress and anxiety; learn relaxation techniques; adopt coping mechanisms that have worked for you in the past.
- Wash all bedding with hot water to destroy the dust mite.
- Monitor your peak expiratory flow rates as you were instructed.
- Seek immediate emergency care if you experience any of the following:
  - Gray or blue fingertips or lips
  - Difficulty breathing, walking, or talking
  - Retractions of the neck, chest, or ribs
  - Nasal flaring
  - Failure of medications to control worsening symptoms
  - Peak expiratory flow rates declining steadily after treatment, or a flow rate 50% below your usual flow rate

---

The non-neural mechanisms of bronchoconstriction involve humoral cells: macrophages, eosinophils, and mast cells. Macrophages are present throughout the tracheobronchial tree. Eosinophils are the principal inflammatory cell in the pathophysiologic process of asthma. The extent of eosinophils in the sputum, peripheral circulation, and airway tissues correlates with severity of the disease. Mast cells in the lung release histamine and slow-reacting substance of anaphylaxis during allergic reactions, especially those caused by pollen.

Complications of Chronic Airflow Limitation

HYPOXEMIA. The client experiences subtle changes as hypoxemia ensues. Initially, the client may experience mood changes, be unable to concentrate, and be forgetful. Restlessness is common. Tachycardia and cyanosis are later signs of hypoxemia.

RESPIRATORY ACIDOSIS. Rising carbon dioxide levels in the arterial blood ($PaCO_2$) result in respiratory acidosis. Common signs of carbon dioxide retention (hypercapnia) include increased drowsiness and lethargy, headache, fatigue, dizziness, and tachypnea with hyperventilation.

RESPIRATORY INFECTIONS. The client with chronic airflow limitation (CAL) is susceptible to respiratory infections. The organisms frequently associated with bacteria infections include *Streptococcus pneumoniae*, *Haemophilus influenzae*, and *Moraxella catarrhalis*. Acute respiratory infections cause increased production of mucus, increased irritability of bronchial smooth muscle, and edema of the involved mucosa. Airflow is limited; the work of breathing increases; and dyspnea results. A bacterial cause cannot be identified in most acute respiratory illnesses. However, severely compromised and debilitated clients with CAL are treated with antibiotics even when an organism has not been isolated (called empirical therapy). Some physicians prescribe antibiotics on an as-needed basis; the client self-administers the antibiotic according to changes in sputum appearance, which may indicate infection.

CARDIAC FAILURE. Cardiac failure, especially cor pulmonale (right-sided ventricular heart failure caused by pulmonary disease), must be considered in a client with worsening dyspnea. This complication is most frequently associated with chronic bronchitis, but the client with advanced emphysema is also likely to develop this problem. Detection of cor pulmonale (also called pulmonary heart disease) is difficult because its clinical signs are generally masked by those of the underlying lung disease. Signs and symptoms are listed in Chart 32–3.

Chronic airflow limitation (CAL) places a heavy workload on the right side of the heart, which is responsible for pumping blood into the lungs. As the disease progresses, the amount of oxygen in the blood decreases, causing major blood vessels in the lung to constrict. To pump blood through these narrowed vessels, the right side of the heart must generate high pressures. In re-

---

Chart 32–3

Key Features of Pulmonary Heart Disease (Cor Pulmonale)

- Hypoxia and hypoxemia
- Increasing dyspnea
- Fatigue
- Weakness
- Enlarged and tender liver
- Warm cyanotic extremities with bounding pulses
- Cyanotic lips
- Distended neck veins
- Right ventricular enlargement (hypertrophy)
- Lower sternal or epigastric pulsations
- Gastrointestinal disturbances, such as nausea or anorexia
- Dependent edema
- Metabolic and respiratory acidosis
- Pulmonary hypertension

---

sponse to this heavy workload, the right chambers of the heart enlarge and thicken, causing right-sided heart failure, or cor pulmonale. Heart failure is frequently a cause of death in clients with CAL. (Treatment for right-sided heart failure is discussed in Chapter 37.)

CARDIAC DYSRHYTHMIAS. Clients with CAL frequently experience cardiac dysrhythmias. These dysrhythmias may be a result of hypoxemia (from decreased oxygen to the heart muscle), other cardiac disease, the effect of drugs, or respiratory acidosis. Treatment for dysrhythmias is described in Chapter 36.

STATUS ASTHMATICUS. Status asthmaticus is a major complication associated with bronchial asthma. It is a severe, potentially life-threatening acute episode of airway obstruction that tends to intensify once it begins and often does not respond to common therapy. The client arrives in the emergency department of the hospital with extremely labored breathing and wheezing. Use of accessory muscles for breathing and distention of neck veins are commonly noted. If the condition is not reversed, the client can experience cor pulmonale, pneumothorax, and eventual cardiac or respiratory arrest. The physician immediately orders intravenous (IV) fluids, potent bronchodilators, steroids (to decrease inflammation), epinephrine, and oxygen in an attempt to reverse the acute condition. The nurse also prepares for emergency intubation. When wheezing diminishes, management is similar to that for any client with CAL.

Etiology

Cigarette Smoking

Smoking is the most important risk factor for CAL. The client with an 8 pack-year history usually has obstructive lung changes but no signs and symptoms of disease. The client with a 20 pack-year history or longer typically has

CAL. Pulmonary function studies reveal a forced expiratory volume in 1 second/forced vital capacity ratio (FEV_1/FVC) lower than 70% of predicted.

TRANSCULTURAL CONSIDERATIONS

The prevalence of smoking remains higher among African-Americans, blue-collar workers, and less educated people than in the overall population of the United States. Approximations of smoking prevalence range from 37% among the least educated people to 14% among the most educated. Smoking prevalence is highest among Northern Plains Native Americans (42%–70%) and Alaskan Natives (56%). The overall prevalence of smoking for both men and women has decreased over the past two decades, but the decrease for women has been proportionately less than for men. The prevalence of smoking is approximately 28% for men and 23% to 25% for women (National Center for Health Statistics, 1996).

The harmful effects of tobacco result in part because inhaled smoke stimulates excess release of the enzyme elastase protease from cells normally found in the lung. The elastase protease breaks down elastin, the major component in alveoli. By impairing the action of cilia, smoking also inhibits the cilia from clearing the tracheobronchial tree of mucus, cellular debris, and fluid.

In addition to the increased risk of CAL from active smoking, much attention has been given to passive smoking, or second-hand smoke. Although a person may not smoke, exposure to smoke, particularly in a small or confined space, may contribute to the development of upper and lower respiratory tract problems, including CAL. As a result of this finding, cigarette smoking is often considered an environmental hazard.

Family History

Emphysema and chronic bronchitis occur in families more often than would be expected by chance. This finding may be related to family smoking habits. However, in some people, a genetic defect results in decreased levels of the substance alpha$_1$-antitrypsin (ATT), which normally works to inhibit or prevent proteases from breaking down the elastic tissue (alveoli) of the lungs. When the amount of ATT is decreased, more damage can be done by the proteases.

Asthma and cystic fibrosis also have a strong familial association. Asthma, especially extrinsic asthma, tends to occur in families. Intrinsic asthma may occur in clients with a family or personal history of allergies. Cystic fibrosis, an inherited autosomal recessive disease, is often discussed in relation to CAL.

Although cystic fibrosis involves many organs besides the lungs (sweat glands and the pancreas), it is the main cause of chronic lung disease in children. Disease in these clients is now being diagnosed earlier, and they are living into their 30s and even 40s. Cystic fibrosis is no longer just a disease affecting children. Treatment is aimed at clearing secretions, preventing airway obstruction, and preventing and treating infection. (More information on cystic fibrosis can be found in current pediatric textbooks.)

ELDERLY CONSIDERATIONS

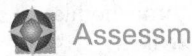 Asthma in the aged is believed to be associated with a beta-adrenergic receptor dysfunction. This hypothesis may explain the decreased response to beta-adrenergic medications in treating bronchospasm. Older asthmatics who were former smokers are found to have higher IgE levels than their nonsmoking peers.

Air Pollution

The effect of air pollution appears now to be additive to tobacco exposure. Air pollution alone plays only a relatively small role in the client with emphysema and chronic bronchitis. For the client with asthma, however, increased air pollution can cause an asthma attack.

Incidence/Prevalence

The prevalence of chronic bronchitis and emphysema has been estimated at about 13.5 million and 2 million, respectively, in the United States. Another 12 million suffer from asthma, and 10 million have acute bronchitis (Benson & Marano, 1994). Since 1979, the number of people, especially elderly women, who suffer from these conditions has rapidly increased. In 1995 alone, 102,899 deaths were caused by COPD/CAL and its associated conditions. COPD/CAL is ranked as the fourth leading cause of death for females of all ages and the fifth for males (Parker et al., 1997). More than 30,000 children and young adults are affected by cystic fibrosis.

WOMEN'S HEALTH CONSIDERATIONS

In 1993, for women between the ages of 35 and 54, COPD/CAL was the ninth leading cause of death. It was the third leading cause of death in women between the ages of 55 and 74 and the fifth leading cause after age 74 (Parker et al., 1997).

Chronic airflow limitation (CAL) is responsible for a greater restriction of activity than is any other major disease category. For example, nearly 20% of people with asthma have some limitation in their daily activities. Although CAL is seen more in men, the incidence among women is increasing. The highest incidence of bronchitis is seen after age 40, and for emphysema, after age 50. Asthma is seen in the young adult as well.

Collaborative Management

◆ Assessment

➤ History

Risk Factors. The nurse considers age, sex, occupational history and ethnic-cultural background when taking a history from a client who has, or is suspected of having, chronic airflow limitation (CAL). Each of these factors can place the client at risk for CAL. For example, CAL is seen more often in the elderly male client. The nurse also reviews family history because certain types of CAL diseases, especially extrinsic asthma and panlobular emphysema, occur in families.

The nurse obtains a thorough smoking history, if appropriate. Tobacco abuse tends to be the greatest risk factor, but the effects of cigarette smoking vary from person to person. The nurse takes a careful smoking history, which includes

- Length of time the client has smoked
- Number of packs or amount of tobacco smoked daily
- Type of cigarette or other tobacco smoked (for tar and nicotine content)
- Family history of lung disease

The nurse then quantifies this information into pack-years (for cigarette smokers) as follows:

$$\text{Years of smoking} \times \text{packs smoked per day} = \text{pack-years}$$

Nature of Disease Presentation. The nurse asks the client to discuss the chief complaint and pays particular attention to the client's ability to answer questions. Can the client give clear answers and state them in complete sentences? Or is breathlessness so severe that the client gives one- or two-word answers to the questions?

Cough, dyspnea, and wheezing are the three classic signs and symptoms of CAL, although they occur in various combinations and intensity. The nurse questions the client about each of these symptoms. Early signs and symptoms of CAL include mild shortness of breath, especially on exertion (also known as dyspnea on exertion, or DOE), and a slight cough in the morning. A long-term cough is associated most often with chronic bronchitis. The nurse determines the coughing pattern by asking the client

- When, if ever, are you troubled by coughing?
- How does the cough sound? Is it dry? Hacking? Loose?
- Is the cough worse in the morning or at night?
- Is the cough worse after you smoke or are exposed to irritants?

The client's cough may be productive or nonproductive of sputum. If the cough is productive, the nurse asks whether sputum is clear or colored and how much is expectorated each day. The sputum should be clear. The nurse also asks the client to recall the time of day when most sputum is expectorated. Smokers typically have a productive cough when they get up in the morning; non-smokers generally do not. The nurse asks whether sputum production has increased or changed.

Shortness of breath and coughing may be much worse when the client with CAL experiences an acute respiratory tract infection. The sputum usually turns from clear to yellow or green as a result of the infection, and wheezing is likely to occur. Wheezing is more commonly associated with asthma.

The nurse determines how long any of the signs and symptoms have been present, whether they are intermittent or continuous, and whether they have become progressively worse over time. The nurse realizes the client usually has an accurate perception of the severity of the symptoms; the client with asthma describes signs and symptoms as intermittent; the client with chronic bronchitis and emphysema describes signs and symptoms as continuous and worsening.

In addition to determining the onset, duration, and severity of the classic symptoms of CAL, the nurse always asks the client about the relationship between activity tolerance and dyspnea. The client is asked to compare activity level and shortness of breath with those of a month ago and a year ago. Likewise, the nurse asks about any difficulty with eating and sleeping. Many clients sleep in a semisitting position because breathlessness prevents them from lying down (thereby causing orthopnea).

The nurse or assistive personnel weighs the client on admission and compares this weight with previous weights in collaboration with the nutritionist. The client with CAL has increased metabolic requirements associated with the increased work of breathing. The increased metabolic requirements plus bothersome dyspnea and mucus production often result in poor food intake and inadequate nutrition. The nurse and nutritionist ask the client to recall a typical day's meals and fluid intake. The nurse determines whether the client uses any breathing exercises (such as pursed-lip breathing) during dyspneic episodes to help make eating easier and asks for a demonstration. The nurse, physical therapist, and occupational therapist obtain additional information about the client's usual daily activities and any difficulty with sleeping, bathing, dressing, or sexual activities.

➤ Physical Assessment/Clinical Manifestations

Regardless of the client's specific chronic airflow limitation (CAL) disease, the nurse observes the client's general appearance. Is the client calm or extremely anxious? The chest is inspected to determine the breathing rate and pattern. The client with respiratory muscle fatigue typically breathes with rapid, shallow respirations and may have paradoxical respirations or use accessory muscles in the abdomen or neck. The respiratory rate could be as high as 40–50 breaths per minute. Three breathing patterns commonly seen in the client with respiratory muscle fatigue are abdominal paradox, respiratory alternans, and asynchronous breathing (Table 32–1).

The nurse systematically palpates the client's anterior chest, feeling for areas of tenderness and abnormal retractions and for symmetric chest expansion. In the client with emphysema, the nurse expects to find limited excur-

sion (movement) of the diaphragm because it is typically flattened and below its usual resting state. In palpating the posterior chest for tactile fremitus (vibrations felt while the client speaks), the nurse notes decreased fremitus when the client says "99" because vibrations are not transmitted through obstructed airways.

The nurse percusses the chest, anteriorly and posteriorly, for hyperresonance in the client with emphysema related to trapped air in the alveoli. On percussion of the anterior chest, hyperresonance is often easily identified over the area of usual cardiac dullness.

The nurse then auscultates the chest to determine the depth of inspiration and to listen for adventitious breath sounds. Crackles are associated with emphysema and chronic bronchitis; wheezes are most commonly heard in a client with asthma. The nurse notes the pitch and location of the sound as well as the point in the respiratory cycle at which the sound is heard. A silent chest may indicate airflow obstruction or pneumothorax.

In addition to assessing breathing patterns and breath sounds, the nurse assesses for signs and symptoms of CAL complications. The nurse can detect early signs of hypoxemia by assessing the client's level of consciousness every 8 hours. With a concurrent respiratory infection, the client may have fever and sputum changes. Because cardiac complications are likely, the nurse determines heart rate and rhythm. The nurse assesses for swelling of the feet and ankles (dependent edema) or other signs and symptoms of right-sided heart failure (see Chart 32–3 and Chap. 37). The nurse also assesses for signs and symptoms of specific CAL diseases.

Emphysema. The most common clinical manifestation experienced by the client with emphysema is dyspnea. As the disease progresses, dyspnea worsens. Although the focus of discussions among health care professionals about dyspnea is varied, most agree there is both a subjective and an objective component to dyspnea.

The nurse assesses the degree of dyspnea by questioning the client, but this may aggravate the problem. Another approach the nurse can use is an assessment tool called a Visual Analog Dyspnea Scale (VADS). The VADS is a straight line with verbal anchors at the beginning and end of a 100-mm line. The nurse asks the client to place a mark on the line to indicate breathing difficulty. The Modified Borg Scale, a 10-point scale that rates breathlessness from nothing at all to maximal, is also used to rate perceived breathlessness. Figure 32–3 illustrates an assessment guide that combines subjective and objective assessments. The nurse uses these scales to assess dyspnea, determine the effectiveness of bronchodilator and other therapy, and pace the client's activities.

In advanced disease, the client becomes orthopneic; that is, the client must be in a sitting position, often leaning forward with arms over several pillows or an overbed table (Fig. 32–4) to breathe easier. The nurse observes for orthopnea.

The nurse also assesses for cough, which may produce only minimal sputum, and examines the client's chest, which usually has an altered shape known as a barrel chest (Fig. 32–5). In a client with a barrel chest, the ratio between the anteroposterior (AP) diameter of the chest

TABLE 32–1

Three Breathing Patterns Commonly Seen in Clients with Respiratory Muscle Fatigue

- Abdominal paradox: the diaphragm is nonfunctional; inspiration is accomplished by the intercostal and abdominal accessory muscles
- Respiratory alternans: diaphragmatic breathing alternates with abdominal paradox; may serve to rest the diaphragm
- Asynchronous breathing: the chest wall motion is unorganized; reflects the uncoordinated activity of fatigued muscles

---

Dyspnea Assessment Guide

Direct Measure of Dyspnea

Indicate the amount of shortness of breath you are having at this time by marking the line.

shortness of breath as bad as can be

no shortness of breath

Subjective Symptoms

On a scale of 0–4 with 0 indicating no distress and 4 indicating much distress, how much are you presently distressed by: *(circle answer)*.

poor appetite	0	1	2	3	4
worn out or weak	0	1	2	3	4
suffocation	0	1	2	3	4
tightness	0	1	2	3	4
congestion	0	1	2	3	4
a feeling of panic or anxiety	0	1	2	3	4

Objective Sign

Rise of the clavicle during inspiration:
ABSENT = not detected
MILD = seen but not pronounced
SEVERE = pronounced

Figure 32–3. A dyspnea assessment tool. (Redrawn from Gift, A. G. [1989]. A dyspnea assessment guide. *Critical Care Nurse,* *9*[8], 79.)

and its lateral (transverse) diameter is 2:2 rather than the normal ratio of 1:2. This change in shape results from hyperinflation of alveoli and flattening of the diaphragm, which are typical of emphysema.

Because arterial oxygen levels do not change remarkably until the terminal stage, the client with emphysema is not usually cyanotic until then. Instead, the nurse observes a pinkish skin color (most easily observed if the client has light-colored skin). The client also appears cachectic, is typically malnourished, and complains of a chronic cough and worsening dyspnea. Hypercarbia (increased $PaCO_2$ levels) usually becomes a concern in advanced disease.

Inadequate nutrition in clients with CAL, particularly elderly clients with emphysema, has been documented since the early 1960s. Malnutrition in the elderly client with CAL is a vicious cycle. The dyspnea, fatigue, abdominal bloating, and sputum production prevent the client from wanting to prepare or eat a meal. However, in malnutrition, lung tissue and respiratory muscle further deteriorate, which makes breathing even more difficult.

In addition to promoting structural changes, malnutrition impairs the immune system. The client is then more likely to experience a respiratory infection, which can be life threatening in the presence of CAL. This problem is particularly critical for the elderly client, who typically has a compromised immune system as a normal change associated with aging.

Chronic Bronchitis. The bronchitic client typically has a cyanotic, or blue-tinged, dusky appearance and complains of excessive sputum production. The nurse observes the client for cyanosis, delayed capillary refill, and clubbing of the fingers (Fig. 32–6), which indicate chronically decreased arterial oxygen levels. Clubbing is most often associated with a compensatory polycythemia. There is less hypercarbia than would be expected for the degree of hypoxemia present.

Bronchial Asthma. During an asthma attack, the nurse assesses the client for dyspnea, audible wheezing, and coughing. Breath sounds reveal inspiratory and expiratory wheezes. The cough is usually productive if the client also has an upper respiratory tract infection. The client complains of chest tightness and a feeling of suffocation. Between attacks, the client's signs and symptoms usually disappear.

➤ *Psychosocial Assessment*

Like any chronic disease, chronic airflow limitation (CAL) affects all aspects of a person's life: social, economic, and psychological.

Social Effects. CAL can affect socialization in two ways:
1. Friends may avoid the client because of annoying coughs, excessive sputum, or dyspnea.
2. The client may choose to be isolated because dyspnea interferes with the ability to socialize with friends.

The nurse questions the client about interests and hobbies but cautions the client to avoid exposure to irritants, such as aerosols, smoke, the harsh chemicals used to build or refinish furniture, and occupational exposures.

The client is questioned about home conditions. The nurse determines whether the client lives near a constant source of air pollution, such as a chemical factory or a freeway. Crowded living conditions promote the transmission of communicable respiratory diseases. Exposure to such animals as cats, dogs, and hamsters may cause allergic responses or asthma attacks.

Economic Effects. The client's economic status may be affected by the disease if both income and health insurance coverage are concerns. If the client is the head of the household, severe CAL may require a role reversal with the spouse or mate. This change may have a negative impact on the client's self-image. When the client is employed, the nurse asks about on-the-job exposure to cigarette smoke or to other substances that may irritate the respiratory system. Pulmonary medications, especially the metered-dose inhalers, are expensive, and many clients on limited incomes may use these medications only during exacerbations of the disease and not on a scheduled basis.

Psychological Effects. The nurse assesses the psychological impact of CAL and the client's ability to cope with chronic disease. Anxiety and fear related to episodes of

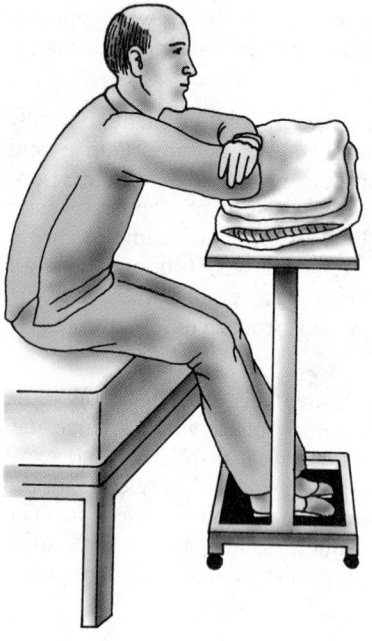

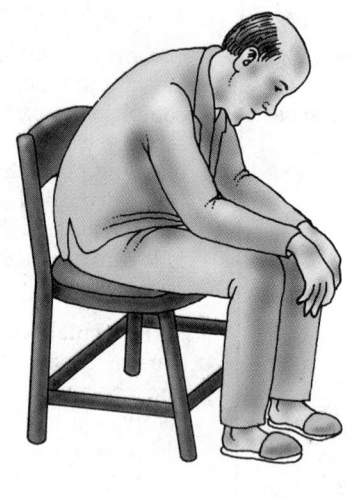

Figure 32–4. Orthopnea positions that clients with chronic airflow limitation (CAL) can assume to ease the work of breathing.

Sitting on the edge of a bed with the arms folded and placed on two or three pillows positioned over a nightstand.

Sitting in a chair with the feet spread a shoulder-width apart and leaning forward with the elbows on the knees. Arms and hands are relaxed.

dyspnea and feelings of breathlessness directly influence the client's ability to participate in a full life. Work, family, social, and sexual roles can be affected. The nurse asks whether the client is aware of support groups sponsored by the American Lung Association (ALA). Various hospitals and physicians' offices also offer group support. Those clients with access to the Internet will find many consumer-oriented educational programs.

➤ Laboratory Assessment

Arterial blood gas (ABG) values identify abnormalities of oxygenation, ventilation, and acid-base status. To assess

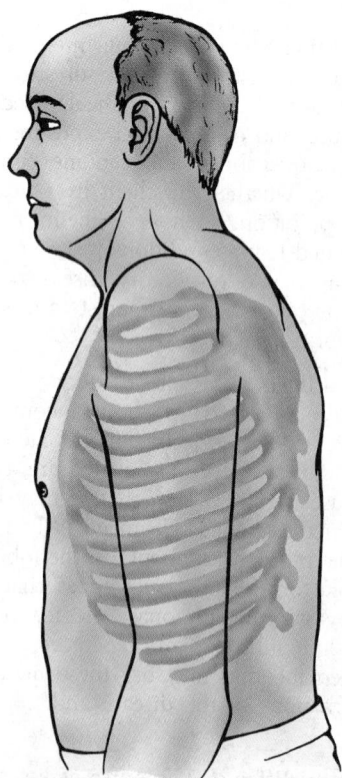

Figure 32–5. Typical barrel chest in a client with chronic airflow limitation (CAL).

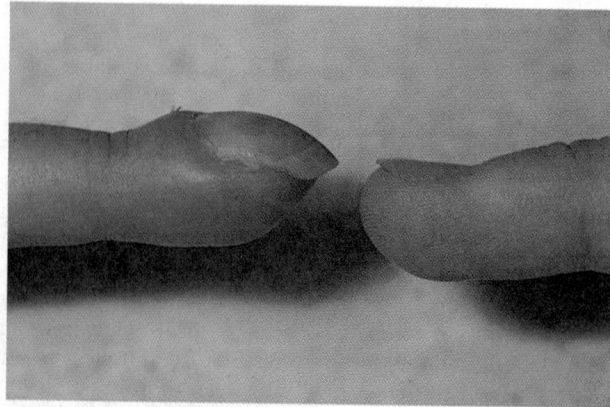

Figure 32–6. Late digital clubbing (on left) compared to a normal digit (on right). (From Swartz, M. H. [1998]. *Textbook of physical diagnosis: History and examination*. Philadelphia: W. B. Saunders Co.)

changes in the client's status over time, the nurse and respiratory therapist compare serial, or repeated, ABG values. Once baseline ABGs are obtained, pulse oximetry can gauge the client's response to treatment. In general, as CAL progresses, the amount of oxygen in the blood decreases (causing hypoxemia) and the amount of carbon dioxide in the blood increases (causing hypercarbia). Chronic respiratory acidosis (increased $PaCO_2$) then results; metabolic alkalosis (increased arterial bicarbonate) occurs as compensation. Not all clients with CAL are carbon dioxide retainers, even when hypoxemia is present. Carbon dioxide is more easily diffused across the alveolar membrane than oxygen. Hypercarbia is mostly a problem in advanced emphysema (because the alveoli are affected) and during exacerbations of emphysema rather than bronchitis (where airways are affected).

Sputum samples are collected for culture from clients who exhibit signs of an acute respiratory tract infection while hospitalized. When in the ambulatory care setting, sputum cultures are rarely obtained; the client is treated on the basis of signs and symptoms and the usual cause of bacterial organisms. A bacterial cause cannot be identified in most acute respiratory illnesses. A white blood cell count may help identify leukocytosis present in a bacterial infection.

Other blood tests that may be indicated in clients with CAL include hemoglobin and hematocrit to determine polycythemia (a compensatory increase in red blood cells in the chronically hypoxic client). The eosinophil count on the white blood cell differential is often increased in the client with extrinsic (allergic) asthma.

Initial screens for hypophosphatemia, hyperkalemia, hypocalcemia, and hypomagnesemia are important because they are associated with diminished diaphragmatic function. In clients suspected of alpha$_1$-antitrypsin (ATT) deficiency, a serum AAT and Pi typing should be performed.

► Radiographic Assessment

The physician orders PA and lateral chest x-rays to rule out other chest diseases and to determine the progress of clients with respiratory tract infections and chronic disease. In clients with advanced emphysema, chest x-rays usually show marked hyperinflation and flattened diaphragms. Chest x-rays, however, may not be helpful in the diagnosis of early or moderate disease.

► Other Diagnostic Assessment

Chronic airflow limitation is classified from mild to severe on the basis of results of pulmonary function tests (PFTs). Airflow rates and lung volume measurements help distinguish airway disease from restrictive patterns typical of interstitial lung disease. The three major components of PFTs are measurements that determine lung volumes, flow volume curves, and diffusion capacity. Each test is performed before and after the client inhales a bronchodilator agent. In the client with asthma, an improvement in abnormal results is usually observed after inhalation of a bronchodilator. If no reversibility is seen after bronchodilator treatment, however, the diagnosis of asthma cannot be excluded.

Lung volume measurements most relevant to CAL are vital capacity (VC), residual volume (RV), and total lung capacity (TLC). Although most of the measured lung volumes or capacities change to some degree with chronic lung disease, RV usually increases markedly. This increase reflects the trapped, stagnant air remaining in the lungs.

Flow volume curves measure the client's ability to move air into and out of the lung. The rate of airflow out of the lungs during a rapid, forceful, and complete expiration from TLC to RV (forced expiratory volume, or FEV) indirectly measures the flow-resistive properties of the lung. A diagnosis of chronic lung disease is based primarily on the FEV_1 (the FEV in the first second of expiration). FEV_1 can also be expressed as a percentage of the forced vital capacity (FVC). As the disease progresses, the ratio of FEV_1 to FVC becomes smaller.

The third part of pulmonary function testing is diffusion, formerly called the "diffusing" capacity of the lung. This test measures how well a test gas (carbon monoxide) diffuses across the alveolar-capillary membrane and combines with the hemoglobin of red blood cells. In emphysema, the decrease in diffusion ability results from the destruction of alveolar walls, leading to a significant decrease in surface area for diffusion of gas into the blood. In asthma and bronchitis, even though lung volumes are increased, the diffusion capacity is usually normal.

Pulmonary function tests are further discussed in Chapter 29 and outlined in Table 29–7. Typical pulmonary function findings in CAL are given in Table 32–2.

Clients with CAL may have a decreased oxygen saturation, often as low as 91%. Pulse oximetry results lower than 90% (and certainly below 86%) may be considered an emergency necessitating immediate treatment. Chapter 29 contains more information on pulse oximetry.

Peak expiratory flow meters are monitors used by the client, nurse, and respiratory therapist to determine the effectiveness of the prescribed treatment to alleviate obstruction. Peak flow rates will increase as the client's obstruction resolves. The client is often taught to continue to self-monitor the peak expiratory flow rates at home and adjust medications accordingly.

 Analysis

► Common Nursing Diagnoses and Collaborative Problems

The most common nursing diagnoses for clients with chronic airflow limitation (CAL) are

1. Impaired Gas Exchange related to alveolar membrane changes, diminished airway size, airflow limitation, respiratory muscle fatigue, excess mucus production
2. Ineffective Breathing Pattern related to airflow obstruction (narrowed airways), diaphragm flattening, fatigue, and decreased energy
3. Ineffective Airway Clearance related to excessive secretions, fatigue, and decreased energy, ineffective cough
4. Altered Nutrition: Less than Body Requirements related to dyspnea, excessive secretions, anorexia, and fatigue

TABLE 32-2

Pulmonary Function Findings in Chronic Airflow Limitation	
Test	**Findings**
Residual volume (RV): the volume of gas remaining in the lungs after a maximal expiration	• Loss of elastic recoil causes RV to be increased in emphysema and chronic bronchitis because of the narrowing and obstruction of airways.
Total lung capacity (TLC): the total amount of gas in the lungs at the end of a maximal inspiration	• TLC is increased in emphysematous clients because of loss of elastic recoil. TLC is normal in clients with chronic bronchitis.
Vital capacity (VC): the maximal amount of gas that can be expired after a maximal inspiration	• VC may be normal or decreased in the client with CAL.
Forced vital capacity (FVC): VC that is produced from a maximal forced expiratory effort	• FVC is often increased in CAL clients secondary to air trapping.
Forced expiratory volume (FEV_1, FEV_2): volume of air that is exhaled during a specified time (in seconds) while measuring FVC	• FEV mainly reflects resistance in large airways and is usually reduced in the client with CAL.
Functional residual capacity (FRC): the amount of gas remaining in the lungs at the end of a tidal expiration	• FRC is increased in clients with chronic bronchitis if obstruction is severe.
Diffusion: measure of carbon monoxide uptake across the alveolar-capillary membrane	• The diffusion value is decreased in severe emphysema. Chronic bronchitis has little effect on diffusion.

5. Anxiety related to loss of control during dyspneic episodes or asthma attacks, dyspnea, change in health status, and situational crisis
6. Activity Intolerance related to fatigue, dyspnea, and an imbalance between oxygen supply and demand

A common collaborative problem for clients with COPD/CAL is potential for pneumonia or other respiratory infections.

> ➤ *Additional Nursing Diagnoses and Collaborative Problems*

In addition to the common diagnoses, the client with CAL may also have other associated problems, which may include

- Fatigue related to change in metabolic energy, hypoxemia
- Knowledge Deficit (disease process, prescribed treatments, activity limitations) related to unfamiliarity with information resources
- Altered Sexuality Patterns related to extreme fatigue
- Inability to Sustain Spontaneous Ventilation related to respiratory muscle fatigue
- Ineffective Management of Therapeutic Regimen related to knowledge deficits, decreased support systems, or economics.
- Sleep Pattern Disturbance related to dyspnea, unfamiliar environment (hospitalization)
- Altered Thought Processes related to hypoxemia, sleep deprivation
- Powerlessness related to difficulty in performing self-care, illness-related regimen
- Ineffective Individual Coping related to effects of chronic illness, loss of control over body function, major changes in lifestyle, situational crisis, knowledge deficit regarding therapeutic regimen/disease process/prognosis

- Altered Role Performance related to change in health status, role loss

Other collaborative problems for clients with COPD/CAL include potential for status asthmaticus, potential for acute exacerbation of disease, potential for respiratory failure, and potential for right heart failure.

 Planning and Implementation

> ➤ *Impaired Gas Exchange*

The client should attain and maintain PaO_2 (or oxygen saturation) and $PaCO_2$ levels within normal ranges or within the client's chronic baseline values. The *minimum* goal for most clients is a PaO_2 of 55–60 mmHg and an oxygen saturation between 91% and 95%, but this goal varies according to the client's age and disease process.

Also expected is that the client will

- Demonstrate a decrease in tachypnea, dyspnea, and confusion (from the hypoxemia)
- State that fatigue is reduced
- Demonstrate techniques and methods that support improved oxygenation without carbon dioxide retention

Some facilities have created clinical pathways to guide the planning of care for the client with asthma or for the client with an exacerbation of COPD/CAL.

 Interventions

The nurse assesses the client at frequent intervals (every 2 hours), especially during the acute phase of the illness. The nurse provides the prescribed oxygen, assesses the client's response to treatment, and intervenes to prevent complications. Additional interventions can be found in the Client Care Plan regarding CAL.

Client Care Plan

The Client with Chronic Airflow Limitation

Nursing Diagnosis No. 1: Impaired Gas Exchange related to alveolar membrane changes, airflow limitation, respiratory muscle fatigue, excess production of mucus, and intrapulmonary shunting

Expected Outcomes	Nursing Interventions	Rationale

The client demonstrates correct use of techniques and methods that support improved oxygenation.	■ Assess oxygenation of the client, including
	  a. Level of consciousness
	  b. Pulse oximetry
	  c. Breathing pattern, rate, and depth; chest expansion; dyspnea, nasal flaring; pursed-lip breathing; prolonged expiratory phase; and use of accessory muscles
	  d. Peak expiratory flow rate
	■ Instruct client and monitor proper placement of oxygen devices (e.g., nasal cannula).
	■ Teach energy conservation techniques:
	  a. Encourage sitting for most activities, such as peeling potatoes or talking on the telephone.
	  b. Teach the client never to hold his or her breath while performing activities.
	  c. Be aware that activities involving the arms may increase dyspnea.
	  d. Plan rest between periods of activity.
	■ Instruct the client in the following:
	  a. Pursed-lip breathing
	  b. Diaphragmatic breathing
	  c. Relaxation therapy
	  d. Controlled cough techniques
	■ Formulate a plan with the client and family for pacing activities of daily living.
		■ Information will provide answers to questions of hypoxemia.
		
		■ Clients with hypoxemia will desaturate rapidly within minutes once oxygen is removed.
		■ Increased activity and work of breathing will increase oxygen consumption. These techniques assist the client in oxygen conservation.
		
		■ These techniques assist the client with better ventilation.
		
		■ Planned activities are better controlled and provide better data for evaluation.

The client demonstrates correct technique to normalize $PaCO_2$.	■ Assess the quality and quantity of sputum: color, consistency, amount, and odor. ■ Maximize the effect of medical interventions by proper sequence of respiratory treatments and by judicious use of bronchodilators and steroids.	■ Increased mucus and inflammation can cause airflow limitation. ■ These interventions result in decreased airflow limitation.

(Continued)

Client Care Plan

Expected Outcomes	Nursing Interventions	Rationale
	■ Instruct and monitor client's technique with metered-dose inhalers. ■ Teach potential hazard of excessive inspired oxygen to clients and family. ■ Teach signs and symptoms of hypercapnia: a. Headache b. Drowsiness and fatigue	■ Correct technique, sequence, and use are key to effective treatment. ■ Clients with chronic hypercapnia have blunted CO_2 drives to breathe. ■ Acute hypercapnia can result in respiratory failure.

Nursing Diagnosis No. 2: Ineffective Breathing Pattern related to airflow obstruction (narrowed airways), fatigue, and decreased energy from respiratory muscle fatigue

Expected Outcomes	Nursing Interventions	Rationale
The client will demonstrate a breathing pattern that decreases the work of breathing.	■ Assess respiratory rate, depth, and rhythm at least every shift. ■ Assist the client in maintaining proper positioning during dyspneic episodes: a. Sitting up and leaning on overbed table b. Sitting up and resting with elbows on knees c. Standing and leaning against the wall ■ Teach pursed-lip and diaphragmatic breathing techniques. ■ Teach energy conservation techniques. ■ Initiate respiratory muscle training, if appropriate. ■ Identify in writing various factors that elicit an anxious response. ■ Help the client to formulate a plan for coping with dyspneic and wheezing episodes. ■ Allow the client to verbalize feelings. ■ Teach the client various interventions for anxiety: a. Relaxation techniques b. Biofeedback ■ Refer the client for professional counseling if necessary.	■ Assessment provides the nurse with baseline information. ■ These positions can decrease the work of breathing. ■ These breathing techniques facilitate increased expiratory flow. ■ Respiratory muscles fatigue easily in CAL clients. ■ Inspiratory muscle training can assist in strengthening the diaphragm. ■ This process gives the client control of his or her situation. ■ A plan prepares the client for episodes of anxiety. ■ Verbalization tends to prevent or decrease anxiety. ■ Interventions decrease stress. ■ Counseling assists the client with self-analysis and coping techniques.

Client Care Plan

Nursing Diagnosis No. 3: Ineffective Airway Clearance related to excessive secretions, fatigue and decreased energy, and ineffective cough

Expected Outcomes	Nursing Interventions	Rationale

The client will demonstrate effective airway clearance techniques and will attain optimal lung sounds.	■ Assess sputum for color, amount, consistency, and odor.
	■ Assess the client's ability to expectorate sputum with ease.
	
	■ Assess breath sounds at least every 8 hours.
	■ Monitor and encourage adequate fluid intake daily.
	
	■ Position the client to prevent aspiration.
	■ Teach a method of controlled cough.
	
	■ Suction as necessary to remove secretions.
	■ Teach postural drainage and chest physiotherapy techniques, if ordered:
	  a. Assess level of consciousness.
	  b. Observe for hypoxemia.
	  c. Assess breath sounds for wheezes caused by bronchospasm.
		■ Secretions can obstruct airways.
		■ Observe the client's cough efforts to determine best technique.
		■ Assessment provides vital information of respiratory status.
		■ Dehydration impairs ciliary action; hydration helps to liquify secretions.
		■ Aspiration is the leading cause of pneumonia in the elderly.
		■ This technique will produce the best results with the least effort.
		■ Suctioning is based on breath sound assessment.
		■ Chest physiotherapy can cause hypoxemia and bronchospasm.

If the client's condition continues to deteriorate despite treatment, more aggressive therapy is required. Intubation and mechanical ventilation may be necessary for clients in respiratory failure, including those who are unable to sustain spontaneous ventilation. Chapter 34 discusses mechanical ventilation in detail.

Maintaining Airway Patency. The nurse's first intervention to improve gas exchange is to maintain a patent airway. The nurse maintains the client's head, neck, and chest in alignment, assists the client in liquefying secretions, and clears the airway of secretions. (More information on airway obstruction can be found in Chapter 31.)

Oxygen Therapy. Oxygen (O_2) is a potent drug prescribed by the physician for relief of symptoms of hypoxemia (low levels of oxygen in the blood) and its resultant hypoxia (decreased tissue oxygenation). Arterial blood gas (ABG) analysis is the best tool for determining the need for oxygen therapy and for evaluating its effects. Oxygen need can also be determined by noninvasive monitoring, such as pulse oximetry.

The average client requires an oxygen flow of 2–4 L/minute via nasal cannula or up to 40% via Venturi mask.

The client who is hypoxemic and also has chronic hypercarbia requires lower levels of oxygen delivery, usually 1–2 L/minute via nasal cannula. A low arterial oxygen level is this client's primary drive for breathing. More information on oxygen therapy can be found in Chapter 30.

Drug Therapy. The physician or Nurse Practitioner uses six main classes of drugs in managing a client with COPD/CAL:

- Bronchodilators
- Anticholinergics
- Corticosteroids
- Cromolyn sodium/nedocromil
- Mucolytics
- Leukotriene modifiers

Chart 32–4 summarizes these drugs.

Stepped therapies have been recommended for clients with asthma and chronic bronchitis or emphysema (Tables 32–3 and 32–4). The key elements of stepped therapy include pharmacologic therapy, monitoring (i.e., peak expiratory flow rates in the client with asthma), and control of environmental irritants and allergens. The expected outcomes of stepped therapy are for the client to have more awareness of the disease and to increase participa-

Chart 32–4

Drug Therapy for Chronic Airflow Limitation (CAL)

Drug	Usual Dosage	Nursing Interventions	Rationale
Bronchodilators			
Sympathomimetics (adrenergics, beta stimulants)			
Metaproterenol (Meta-prel, Alupent)	• MDI: 2–4 puffs q4–6hr • PO: 20 mg tid • Aerosol: 0.2–0.3 mL q4–6hr	• Instruct the client to use the bronchodilator inhaler before the steroid inhaler (if ordered). • Teach the client the correct method of using the inhaler and observe the client's technique.	• Use of the beta-2 agent inhaler first opens the airways and facilitates deeper penetration of the steroid. • Correct technique ensures proper inhalation. Sequencing the steps in using an inhaler can be tricky for children and the elderly. Two critical variables are the speed of inhalation and the duration of breath holding.
Albuterol (salbutamol, Proventil, Ventolin)	• MDI: 2–4 puffs q4–6hr • PO: 2–4 mg q6–8hr • Aerosol: 0.5 mL q4–6hr	• Observe the client for fine finger tremors.	• The nurse observes the client to detect side effects of this selective beta-2 agent.
Pirbuterol (Maxair)	• MDI: 1–2 puffs q4–6hr	• Observe the client for tremors, nervousness, insomnia, headache, nausea, tachycardia, and palpitations.	• The nurse observes the client to detect side effects. The drug stimulates beta-adrenergic receptors in the heart and lungs.
Salmeterol xinafoate (Serevent)	• MDI: 2 puffs q12hr	• Do not use to relieve acute symptoms. • Give 30 min before exercise or HS	• The drug is a long-acting bronchodilator. • Serevent is used to prevent exercise-induced or nocturnal symptoms.
Isoetharine (Bronkosol)	• MDI: 2–4 puffs q3–6hr • Nebulizer: 0.5 mL diluted 1:3 with saline	• Observe the client for tachycardia, palpitations, headache, and blood pressure alterations.	• Same as for pirbuterol.
Epinephrine (Adrenalin, Primatene Mist, Bronkaid Mist-ometer♣, Dysne-Inhal♣)	• MDI: 2–3 puffs q2–4hr • SC or IM: 0.2–0.5 mL of 1:1000 solution; may repeat in 10–15 min • IV: 0.1–0.25 mL of 1:1000 solution	• Observe the client for anxiety, tremors, and palpitations. • Assess the client for a history of hyperthyroidism and ischemic heart disease.	• The nurse observes the client to detect side effects. The drug is fast acting, with an onset of about 20 min. • The nurse observes the client to detect possible contraindications.
Isoproterenol (Isuprel, Medihaler-Iso)	• MDI: 1–2 puffs 4–6 times/day	• Monitor the client for palpitations.	• The nurse monitors the client to detect severe cardiac dysrhythmias, especially with IV administration.
Terbutaline (Brethine, Brethaire, Bricanyl)	• MDI: 2–4 puffs q4–8hr • PO: 5 mg q8hr • SC: 0.25 mg, not to exceed 0.5 mg q4hr	• Monitor the client for palpitations and tachycardia.	• The nurse monitors the client to detect these infrequent side effects. The drug has a more selective beta-2 action, slower onset, and longer duration than do other sympathomimetics.
Methylxanthines			
Aminophylline (contains 80% theophylline; Corophyllin♣)	• IV loading dose: 5–7 mg/kg over 20–40 min • IV maintenance dose: 0.5–1.2 mg/kg/hr	• Monitor drug levels.	• Monitoring blood levels detects possible toxicity. The drug has a narrow therapeutic range of 10–20 μg/mL. (Some clients do well at levels of 5–12 μg/mL.)

Chart 32–4. Drug Therapy for Chronic Airflow Limitation (CAL)   Continued

Drug	Usual Dosage	Nursing Interventions	Rationale
		• Observe the client for nausea and vomiting, diarrhea, tachycardia, palpitations, dizziness, and restlessness. • Space doses equally throughout a 24-hr period. • Give in saline or 5% dextrose/water by infusion pump. • Avoid caffeine intake.	• The nurse observes the client to detect side effects and potential toxic effects, most of which are dose related. • Spacing of doses ensures even coverage throughout the day. • Infusion is constant, steady, and controlled. • Avoidance of caffeine reduces other sources of sympathetic stimulation.
Theophylline (Slo-Phyllin, Theo-Dur, Theobid, Uniphyl, Uni-Dur, Slo-bid Gyrocaps, Acet-Am✦)	• PO: initially: 10–12 mg/kg/day, increased by 25% at 3-day intervals until a maximal oral dose of 13 mg/kg/day in 2–4 divided doses (usually 400–800 mg/day) is reached; Uni-Dur is once a day.	• Same as for aminophylline. • Administer with food, such as milk and crackers. • Instruct client to take medication even when feeling good. • Know whether the medication is the immediate-release form or the timed-release form.	• Taking the drug with food prevents gastrointestinal irritation. • A therapeutic blood level is maintained. • Sustained-release preparations give better coverage than regular preparations, which makes them ideal for clients who awaken at night with shortness of breath.
Anticholinergics (give 5 min after the sympathomimetic)			
Ipratropium bromide (Atrovent)	• MDI: 2–3 puffs qid, up to 6–8 puffs 3–4 times per day in acute exacerbation	• Instruct the client to close eyes while activating inhaler if not using spacer. • Monitor the client for cough, dry mouth, headache, nausea, blurred vision, nervousness, palpitations.	• Medication in the eyes will cause temporary blurring of vision. • The nurse monitors the client to detect side effects.
Atropine	• Aerosol: 0.2% (1 mg) 0.5% (2.5 mg) 5–10 mg q6–8hr (long-term maintenance) 2.5–5 mg q4–6hr (acute severe asthma)	• Monitor for troublesome anticholinergic side effects (i.e., drying of mucous secretions, decreased mucociliary transport tachycardia, glaucoma, prostatism, and urinary retention).	• The nurse monitors the client to detect side effects.
Corticosteroids (give 5 minutes after the anticholinergic)			
Prednisone (Deltasone, Apo-Prednisone✦, Winpred✦) Methyl-prednisolone (Solu-Medrol, Medrol✦)	• PO, IV: dosage varies	• Instruct the client about the side effects of long-term steroid use, such as hyperglycemia, osteoporosis, increased fat production and weight gain, immunologic impairment, reduced inflammatory response, increased gastric acidity • Monitor serum potassium levels for hypokalemia. • Instruct the client to take medication with food. • Instruct the client never to discontinue steroid use suddenly.	• The nurse warns the client of possible side effects, many of which are irreversible but must be treated. • Systemic steroids cause potassium loss with sodium and water retention. • Food minimizes gastric irritation. • Sudden discontinuation of steroids precipitates adrenal crisis and shock.
Beclomethasone (Vanceril, Beclovent, Rotacaps✦)	• MDI: 2–4 puffs tid–qid	• Observe the client's mouth daily for the bright, fire red or cherry color of oral candidiasis.	• Oral candidiasis is a complication of inhaled steroids.

Continued

Chart 32–4. Drug Therapy for Chronic Airflow Limitation (CAL) Continued

Drug	Usual Dosage	Nursing Interventions	Rationale
		• Instruct the client in the proper sequencing of sympathomimetic and steroid inhalers, if appropriate, and observe the client's technique.	• Proper sequencing and technique promote optimal distribution of the steroid.
		• Instruct the client to drink 8 ounces of water after inhaling steroids or gargle and rinse mouth after use.	• Drinking water washes away excess medication from the back of the throat and thus minimizes the growth of *Candida*.
		• Provide reservoir spacer.	• A spacer decreases oropharyngeal deposition of the drug.
Triamcinolone (Azmacort)	• MDI: 2–6 puffs tid–qid • Maximum: 16 puffs/day	• Same as for beclomethasone.	
Flunisolide (AeroBid)	• MDI: 2–4 puffs bid	• Same as for beclomethasone.	
Fluticasone (Flovent)	• MDI: 2–4 puffs bid	• Same as for beclomethasone.	
Cromolyn and nedocromil			
Nedocromil (Tilade)	• MDI: 2 puffs q6–12hr	• Monitor for headache, unpleasant taste in the mouth, runny nose, and nausea.	• The nurse observes the client for side effects.
		• Instruct client to stop medication and call physician if bronchospasm or continued coughing occurs.	• The client may be sensitive to propellants in the MDI.
		• Instruct the client that the drug must be used even when symptom free.	• The medication is not effective during acute episodes.
Cromolyn Sodium (Intal, Gastrocrom, Rynacrom✤) (Intal, Rynacrom✤)	• MDI: 1 or 2 puffs qid • Aerosol • PO: 200 mg qid before meals and HS	• Observe the client for maculopapular rash and urticaria. • Instruct the client that cromolyn is a prophylactic drug.	• The nurse observes the client to detect rare side effects. • Encourage the client to seek other treatment during an acute attack.
		• Inform the client that an optimal response may not occur before 2 months of daily use.	• Continued use is promoted until the drug takes effect.
Mucolytics			
Acetylcysteine (Mucomyst, Airbron✤)	• Aerosol (nebulizer): 3–5 mL (20%) 3–4 times daily 6–10 mL (10%) 3–4 times daily	• Observe the client for nausea and bronchospasm.	• The nurse observes the client to detect common side effects.
Dornase alfa (Pulmozyme)	• Aerosol (nebulizer): 2.5 mg once daily	• Observe the client for pharyngitis, voice alterations, laryngitis, conjunctivitis, rash, urticaria.	• The nurse observes the client to detect common side effects.
Iodinated glycerol (Organidin)	• PO: 60 mg qid	• Instruct the client to have T$_3$ and T$_4$ tests done before starting therapy and then at the 3-month follow-up examination.	• The iodine content can cause hypothyroidism.
Leukotriene Modifiers			
Zafirlukast (Accolate)	• PO: 20 mg bid 1 hr before or 2 hr after meals	• Do not use to relieve acute symptoms	• Accolate will not reverse acute bronchospasm.
Zileuton (Zyflo)	• PO: 600 mg qid	• Monitor liver enzymes.	• A serious side effect is the elevation of liver enzymes.

MDI = metered-dose inhaler; T$_3$ = triiodothyronine; T$_4$ = thyroxine.

TABLE 32-3

Pharmacologic Stepped Approach to Treating Asthma Symptoms

Asthma Symptoms	Treatment
Step 1: mild intermittent	• Beta-2 agonist (short acting), 1–2 puffs prn rescue treatment < 3×/wk
Step 2: mild persistent	• Add inhaled, cromolyn sodium or nedocromil, or leukotriene antagonist • May add long-acting beta-2 agonist (client >12 years) • Client adjusts doses according to peak expiratory flow rates
Step 3: moderate persistent	• Daily inhaled corticosteroid • May add nedocromil or theophyllin
Step 4: severe persistent	• Add corticosteroids PO or IV PO dose: 40–60 mg/day for up to 2 weeks. • Wean to low dose or inhaled corticosteroid

tion symptom management. When adequate symptom control has been achieved for a few months, "stepping down" may be attempted.

Bronchodilators. The preferred technique for administration of bronchodilators is via the metered-dose inhaler (MDI) because it delivers the drug directly to the lung. Side effects are reduced because only a limited amount of the drug gets into the general circulation. The bronchodilators are divided into sympathomimetics and methylxanthines.

Sympathomimetics. The sympathomimetic drugs, or adrenergic bronchodilators, are drugs that mimic, or act like, the sympathetic nervous system. These drugs cause bronchodilation through activation of the enzyme adenylate cyclase, which converts adenosine triphosphate (ATP) to adenosine $3',5'$-cyclic monophosphate (cAMP), the body's own natural bronchodilator.

In choosing a specific drug, the physician considers the beta-adrenergic activity of each drug. $Beta_1$-receptors are located in the heart, whereas $beta_2$-receptors are located in the lung. The more selective $beta_2$-adrenergic drugs (e.g., metaproterenol [Alupent], albuterol [Proventil, Ven-

tolin], and terbutaline [Brethine]) generally do not stimulate the heart directly, have a faster onset of action, and are longer in duration. The long-acting form is preferred for the client with symptoms of nocturnal asthma or requiring step 2 therapy for asthma. Many of the sympathomimetics can be administered in an inhaled form (Chart 32–5).

The rapidly metabolized, short-acting sympathomimetic drugs are first line for acute exacerbations of asthma and for prevention of exercise-induced bronchospasm. Their effect, however, is often minimized in the elderly. The nurse teaches the client with asthma to use the $beta_2$-adrenergic inhaler (rather than the anticholinergic) at the onset of symptoms because of the more rapid onset of action.

Methylxanthines. Methylxanthines act to increase the levels of cAMP. Other actions include the antagonism of adenosine and prostaglandins, both natural bronchoconstrictors.

Aminophylline. In an acute flare-up of asthma or severe bronchospasm caused by any type of CAL, the physician may prescribe a loading dose of intravenous (IV) amino-

TABLE 32-4

Pharmacologic Stepped Approach to Treating Chronic Bronchitis and Emphysema

Step 1: mild symptoms	• Beta-2 agonist, 1–2 puffs q2–6 hr, prn (not to exceed 8–12 puffs in 24 hr)
Step 2: mild to moderate symptoms daily	• Ipratropium bromide 2–6 puffs q6–8 hr • Beta-2 agonist, 1–4 puffs for rescue treatment or as regular supplement
Step 3: unsatisfactory response to step 2	• Add theophylline 200–400 mg, bid or 400–800 mg HS (nocturnal bronchospasms) or albuterol SR 4–8 mg bid or HS only
Step 4: unsatisfactory response to step 3	• Add prednisone 40 mg/day for 10–14 days *Wean when improvement noted to low daily or QOD dose *Place on steroid metered-dose inhaler if has bronchial hyperreactivity *Stop steroids if no improvement noted
Step 5: severe exacerbation	• Beta-2 agonist with spacer, 6–8 puffs q½–2hr • Ipratropium bromide with spacer, 6–8 puffs q3–4hr • Theophylline IV • Methylprednisolone 50–100 mg IV STAT, then q6–8hr. Wean as soon as possible. • Antibiotics if indicated • Mucokinetic agents if sputum tenacious

Chart 32–5

Education Guide: How to Use an Inhaler Correctly*

Without a Spacer (Preferred Technique)

1. Before each use, remove the cap and shake the inhaler according to the instructions in the package insert.
2. Tilt your head back slightly and breathe out fully.
3. Open your mouth and place the mouthpiece 1 to 2 inches away.
4. As you begin to breathe in deeply through your mouth, press down firmly on the canister of the inhaler to release one dose of medication.
5. Continue to breathe in slowly and deeply (usually over 3 to 5 seconds).
6. Hold your breath for at least 10 seconds to allow the medication to reach deep into the lungs, then breathe out slowly.
7. Wait at least 1 minute between puffs.
8. Replace the cap on the inhaler.
9. At least once a day, remove the canister and clean the plastic case and cap of the inhaler by thoroughly rinsing in warm, running tap water.

Without a Spacer (Alternative Method)

1. Follow steps 1 and 2 above.
2. Place the mouthpiece into your mouth, over your tongue, and seal your lips tightly around it.
3. Follow steps 4 to 9 above.

With a Spacer

1. Before each use, remove the caps from the inhaler and the spacer.
2. Insert the mouthpiece of the inhaler into the non-mouthpiece end of the spacer.
3. Shake the whole unit vigorously 3 or 4 times.
4. Place the mouthpiece into your mouth, over your tongue, and seal your lips tightly around it.
5. Press down firmly on the canister of the inhaler to release one dose of medication into the spacer.
6. Breathe in slowly and deeply. If the spacer makes a whistling sound, you are breathing in too rapidly.
7. Remove the mouthpiece from your mouth and, keeping your lips closed, hold your breath for at least 10 seconds, then breathe out slowly.
8. Wait at least 1 minute between puffs.
9. Replace the caps on the inhaler and the spacer.
10. At least once a day, clean the plastic case and cap of the inhaler by thoroughly rinsing in warm, running tap water; at least once a week, clean the spacer in the same manner.

*Avoid spraying in the direction of the eyes.

phylline. Maintenance doses may need to be higher for heavy smokers.

Theophylline. Theophylline is useful in managing severe bronchospasms and in treating nocturnal symptoms. It is usually given orally in immediate- or sustained-release preparations. The drug is well absorbed orally, with peak serum concentrations occurring in 1–2 hours. Achieving a therapeutic level can be challenging because various conditions influence the serum concentration (Table 32–5). The physician or Nurse Practitioner makes adjustments in dosage based on the client's clinical response to therapy.

Over-the-Counter (OTC) Bronchodilators. The Food and Drug Administration (FDA) believes people should have ready access to certain bronchodilator drug products. A potential for abuse exists, particularly when these preparations are taken with prescription drugs. The nurse teaches clients that OTC preparations contain active ingredients, usually epinephrine, ephedrine, and theophylline, and are to be respected. The nurse asks whether the client routinely uses OTC preparations and cautions the client about potential abuse.

Anticholinergics. Most of the autonomic nerves in the airways are branches of the vagus nerve. They are predominantly located in the large and medium-sized airways. Release of acetylcholine at these sites results in smooth muscle contraction. An anticholinergic agent, then, acts as a bronchodilator. It is most useful in the elderly and those clients with chronic bronchitis and emphysema, whereas beta-2 agonists are more useful in the treatment of asthma.

Corticosteroids. Steroid preparations reduce inflammation in the throat and lungs but also act to stimulate cAMP production and cause bronchodilation. They are known to decrease the production of cysteinyl leukotrienes, which are involved in the early- and late-phase asthmatic response, thus reducing the levels of preinflam-

TABLE 32–5

Factors that Influence Theophylline Clearance

Factors that Decrease Clearance (Resulting in Increased Drug Levels)	Factors that Increase Clearance (Resulting in Decreased Drug Levels)
Diseases	
• Renal failure	• Hyperthyroidism
• Cirrhosis or other liver abnormalities	
• Congestive heart failure	
• Alcoholism	
• Upper respiratory tract infections	
• Hypothyroidism	
Drugs	
• Caffeine	• Isoproterenol (Isuprel)
• Allopurinol (Zyloprim)	• Rifampin (Rifadin, Rofact✽)
• Erythromycin (E-Mycin, Apo-Erythro✽)	• Phenobarbital (Luminal✽)
• Cimetidine (Tagamet)	• Phenytoin (Dilantin)
• Ciprofloxacin (Cipro)	
• Calcium channel blockers	
Other factors	
• Older age, elderly	• Cigarette smoking

matory cytokines. When long-term oral use is necessary, alternate-day therapy minimizes adrenal suppression and other side effects. See Chapter 66 for more information on steroids and steroid side effects.

An advantage of the aerosol route of administration is equivalent or greater bronchodilation and protection with fewer systemic side effects. However, at doses greater than 1000 μg of inhaled steroid, systemic symptoms have been seen, including bone loss, thinning skin, and purpura.

If the physician has prescribed both an inhaled bronchodilator and an inhaled steroid for administration at the same time, the nurse instructs the client to use the bronchodilator first. With dilation of the large airways, a greater portion of the steroid preparation reaches the peripheral airways.

The client with asthma who is using stepped therapy will monitor peak expiratory flow rates in the early morning and in the evening. If the difference in the expiratory flow rates exceeds 20%, the client adjusts the treatment dosage of oral or inhaled corticosteroid to that recommended by the health care provider.

Cromolyn Sodium and Nedocromil. Cromolyn sodium (Intal) or nedocromil (Tilade) can be used prophylactically in clients with asthma whose symptoms are not controlled adequately by bronchodilators or as a first-line treatment before bronchodilators are given. It is not useful during acute attacks. The desired effects of cromolyn are to reduce the severity and frequency of asthma attacks and to reduce the need for bronchodilators and steroids. Cromolyn probably acts by strengthening the mast cell membrane to prevent release of histamine and thereby decreases bronchospasm in the allergic asthmatic. Nedocromil sodium works much like cromolyn but may have additional anti-inflammatory effects. It is thought to be more useful in the elderly and reduces the airway response in the nonallergic asthmatic. Cromolyn is administered via metered-dose inhaler (MDI) or as solution in a nebulizer, usually four times a day.

Cromolyn, nedocromil, and beta-2 agonists are the preferred treatment for exercise-induced bronchospasm. Although corticosteroids can reduce or prevent exercised induced bronchospasm, they may take several weeks to become effective.

Mucolytics. The physician orders mucolytic agents for clients with thick, tenacious (sticky) mucous secretions. Nebulizer treatments with normal saline or with a mucolytic agent like acetylcysteine (Mucomyst) and normal saline help to thin secretions and facilitate expectoration.

Leukotriene Modifiers. This new therapy is indicated as adjunct therapy for the prophylaxis and chronic treatment of early- and late-phase asthmatic response. These drugs either block the leukotrienes released in response to the allergen (zafirlukast), or inhibit leukotriene formation (zileuton). They are not bronchodilators and should not be used to treat acute asthma episodes.

Lung Volume Reduction. Lung volume reduction (LVR) is used in the treatment of end-stage emphysema. LVR was first introduced in 1957 and again reintroduced in 1990. Currently, it is considered most appropriate for those clients with pure emphysema.

Criteria used for selection of patients include evidence of bullous or nonbullous emphysema, disabling dyspnea, postbronchodilator FEV$_1$ less than 35% predicted, residual volumes greater than 200% predicted, total lung capacity greater than 120% predicted, and an ability to perform in a preoperative pulmonary rehabilitation program (Naunheim & Ferguson, 1996). The purpose of LVR is to resect the dysfunctional areas of the lung, thus reducing the amount of trapped air. The results are reduced dyspnea and improved functional status, spirometric indexes, and oxygen saturation. Additional interventions introduced in 1989 include single lung transplantation. Although this option is available, its actual use is limited.

➤ *Ineffective Breathing Pattern*

Planning: Expected Outcomes. The client should achieve an effective breathing pattern that decreases the work of breathing. Specific outcomes may be for the client to have
- A respiratory rate, depth, and timing within normal limits
- A respiratory rhythm within normal limits for the client's age
- Synchronous thoracoabdominal movement
- Use of accessory muscles appropriate to activity level
- Increased activity tolerance

Interventions. Before any interventions can be implemented, the nurse, physician, physical therapist, and respiratory therapist assess the client to determine the breathing pattern, especially the rate, rhythm, depth, and use of accessory muscles. The client with chronic airflow limitation (CAL) relies more on accessory muscles than on the diaphragm for ventilation. However, these muscles are less efficient than the diaphragm; consequently, the client experiences increased work of breathing. The nurse determines whether there are any contributing factors to the increased work of breathing, such as respiratory tract infection. Interventions are aimed at improving the client's breathing efforts and decreasing the work of breathing (see Client Care Plan addressing CAL).

Breathing Techniques. Diaphragmatic or abdominal and pursed-lip breathing maneuvers may be beneficial interventions for managing dyspneic episodes. The client uses these techniques, shown in Chart 32–6, during all activities. The amount of stagnant air in the lung is minimized, and the client gains confidence and control in managing dyspnea.

Diaphragmatic or Abdominal Breathing. In diaphragmatic breathing, the client attempts consciously to increase diaphragmatic movement. Lying on the back allows the abdomen to relax.

Pursed-Lip Breathing. The technique of pursed-lip breathing uses the mild resistance of partially opposed lips to prolong exhalation and to increase airway pressure, thereby delaying dynamic compression of airways and minimizing the effects of air trapping. Many clients with CAL learn this technique on their own. Pursed-lip breathing can be used during diaphragmatic or abdominal

Chart 32–6

Education Guide: Breathing Exercises

Diaphragmatic or Abdominal Breathing

- Lie on your back with your knees bent.
- Place your hands or a book on your abdomen to create resistance.
- Begin breathing from your abdomen while keeping your chest still. You can tell if you are breathing correctly if your hands or the book rises and falls accordingly.

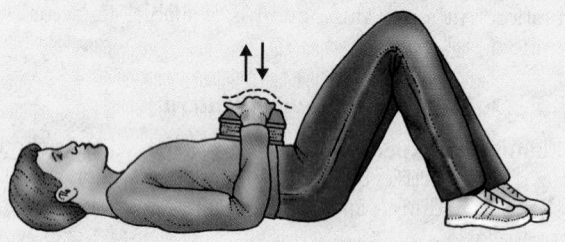

Pursed-Lip Breathing

- Close your mouth and breathe in through your nose.
- Purse your lips as you would to whistle. Breathe out slowly through your mouth, without puffing your cheeks. Spend at least twice the amount of time it took you to breathe in. Use your abdominal muscles to squeeze out every bit of air you can.
- Remember to use pursed-lip breathing during any physical activity. Always inhale before beginning the activity and exhale while performing the activity. Never hold your breath.

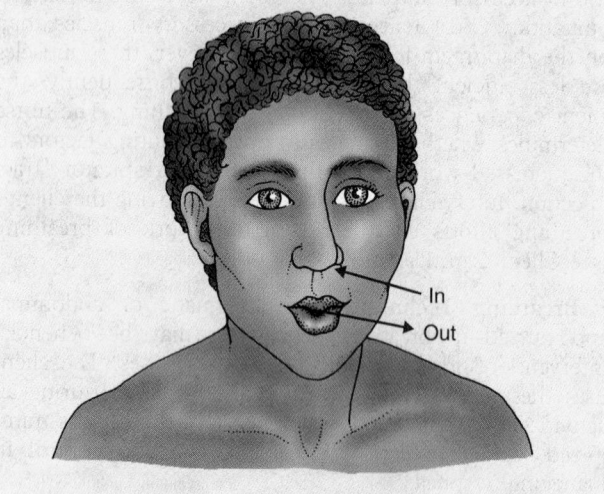

breathing. The nurse teaches both of these breathing techniques when the client is free from dyspnea.

Positioning. The nurse assists the client to an upright position, with the head of the bed elevated to promote easier breathing patterns. The client uses various positions to assist in alleviating dyspnea (see Fig. 32–4). In one position, the client sits on the edge of the bed with the arms resting on two or three pillows on an overbed table. If extra pillows are not available, the client may lean on a table or rest on the elbows. These positions promote increased chest expansion, relax the chest muscles, and place the diaphragm in the proper position to contract while conserving energy by supporting the client's arms and upper body. The client may also find this position particularly helpful during an acute attack when tired but too short of breath to lie back.

The client uses the standing position (Fig. 32–7) when there is no place to sit. Clients with CAL use a greater proportion of their accessory muscles for breathing. Supporting the thorax, therefore, allows these muscles to work better.

Exercise Conditioning. Clients suffering from exercise-induced shortness of breath respond to dyspnea by limiting their activity, even basic activities of daily living (ADLs). Over time, the muscles of respiration and the general large muscle groups weaken, becoming less efficient in their use of oxygen. The result is increased dyspnea with lower activity levels. (Table 29–3 summarizes the relationship between dyspnea and the performance of daily activities.)

Exercise conditioning is part of a complete pulmonary rehabilitation program. Conditioning of the large muscle groups (indirect) or retraining of the respiratory muscles (direct) can be done. The indirect approach is accomplished through any general exercise program.

Two direct techniques currently used are isocapneic hyperventilation and resistive breathing. Isocapneic hyperventilation is designed to increase endurance. The client hyperventilates into a machine that controls the concen-

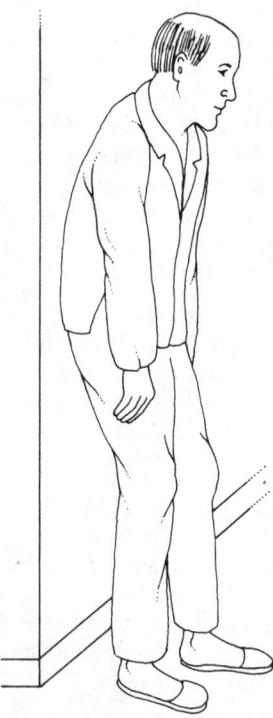

Figure 32–7. The standing position that is used to help clients with chronic airflow limitation (CAL) to breathe. The client stands with the back and hips against a wall and with the feet about 30 cm (12 inches) from the wall. The shoulders are relaxed and bent slightly forward.

trations of oxygen and carbon dioxide. In resistive breathing, the client breathes against a set resistance. Resistive breathing theoretically trains respiratory muscles for both strength and endurance. Retraining of the respiratory muscles is currently done predominantly in research settings.

Energy Conservation. Energy conservation is the planning and placing of activities for maximal tolerance and minimal discomfort. Once the FEV_1 falls below 50% predicted, the client's ability to perform ADLs is disturbed. The nurse or therapist (physical or occupational) begins by asking the client to describe a typical daily schedule. Then each activity is divided into its smaller parts to determine whether that task can be performed in a different way or at a different time of the day. The nurse assists the client in planning and pacing activities for the day. Rest periods are paced between activities. It is helpful for the nurse and the client to develop a chart outlining the day's activities and planned rest periods. Once a day, the nurse and client review the previous day's plan and make adjustments as indicated to promote energy conservation and yet provide activity.

The nurse reminds the client to avoid working with the arms raised. Activities involving the arms decrease exercise tolerance because the accessory muscles of respiration are then used to stabilize the shoulders. Many activities involving the arms can be done sitting at a table leaning on the elbows.

The nurse reminds the client to adjust work heights. Improper working height causes back strain and fatigue. The best work height for a table top is 5 cm (2 inches) below the bent elbow. Rapid, jerky arm motions cause shortness of breath and fatigue and put an extra strain on the heart. Clients should be reminded to keep arm motions smooth and flowing. Long-handled dustpans, sponges, and feather dusters minimize bending and reaching.

The nurse gives suggestions to the client about the organization of work spaces so that items used most often are within easy reach. Measures like dividing laundry or groceries into small parcels that can be handled easily, using disposable plates to save washing time, and letting dishes dry in the rack also conserve energy. The nurse suggests that clients straighten bed covers before getting out of bed for easier bed making. Talking requires energy and use of the lungs; therefore, the nurse instructs the client not to talk when engaged in other activities that require energy, such as walking. In addition, the nurse instructs the client that the key to any activity is to remember to avoid holding the breath and always to exhale while performing any activity.

Ineffective Airway Clearance

Planning: Expected Outcomes. The client should attain optimal lung sounds. Additional outcomes include that the client will
- Maintain a patent airway
- Demonstrate an effective cough
- Remain free from aspiration
- Implement the stepped therapy approach to control of symptoms

Interventions. The client with chronic bronchitis and advanced emphysema often has difficulty with removal of secretions, which results in compromised breathing and inadequate oxygenation. In addition to impairing breathing, excessive mucus predisposes the client to respiratory infections. The nurse auscultates breath sounds routinely as part of physical assessment but also before and after interventions as part of the evaluation for ineffective airway clearance. Careful use of drugs combined with controlled coughing, hydration, and postural drainage may help in airway clearance. If these measures fail, a tracheostomy may be required on a temporary or permanent basis.

Controlled Coughing. Because clients with chronic airflow limitation (CAL) produce more mucus than healthy people, they may benefit from specific coughing at certain times of the day. The nurse teaches the client to cough on arising early in the morning to eliminate mucus that collected during the night. Coughing to expectorate mucus before mealtimes may facilitate a more pleasant meal, and coughing before bedtime may ensure clear lungs for an uninterrupted night's sleep.

To cough effectively, the client sits in a chair or on the side of a bed with feet placed firmly on the floor. The nurse instructs the client to turn the shoulders inward and to bend the head slightly downward, hugging a pillow against the stomach. The pillow helps decrease chest discomfort.

The nurse then instructs the client to take a few diaphragmatic breaths (see Charts 20-5 and 32-6). After the third to fifth deep breath (in through the nose, out through pursed lips), the nurse instructs the client to bend forward slowly while producing two or three strong coughs from the same breath. The first cough moves the secretions; the second and third coughs facilitate expectoration. The nurse notes the color, consistency, odor, and amount of secretions. On return to a sitting position, the client takes a comfortable deep breath. The entire coughing procedure is repeated at least twice. After coughing exercises, the nurse allows the client to rest and then assists in providing mouth care.

Chest Physiotherapy and Postural Drainage. Chest physiotherapy (PT) with postural drainage (Fig. 32-8) is a technique that assists in mobilizing secretions from peripheral to central airways, in re-expanding lung tissue, and in promoting efficient use of the respiratory muscles. Chest PT combines chest percussion with vibration to loosen secretions. Postural drainage uses specific positions and gravity to assist in removing bronchial secretions. Postural drainage with chest PT may be helpful for select CAL clients with excessive secretions and airway clearance problems but should not be used routinely on all CAL clients.

Suctioning. Suctioning is based on the auscultation of adventitious breath sounds and is not performed on a routine schedule. For the client with a weak cough, weak pulmonary musculature, and inability to expectorate effectively, the nurse or respiratory therapist performs nasotracheal suctioning. The nurse assesses the client for dyspnea and tachycardia or other dysrhythmias during the

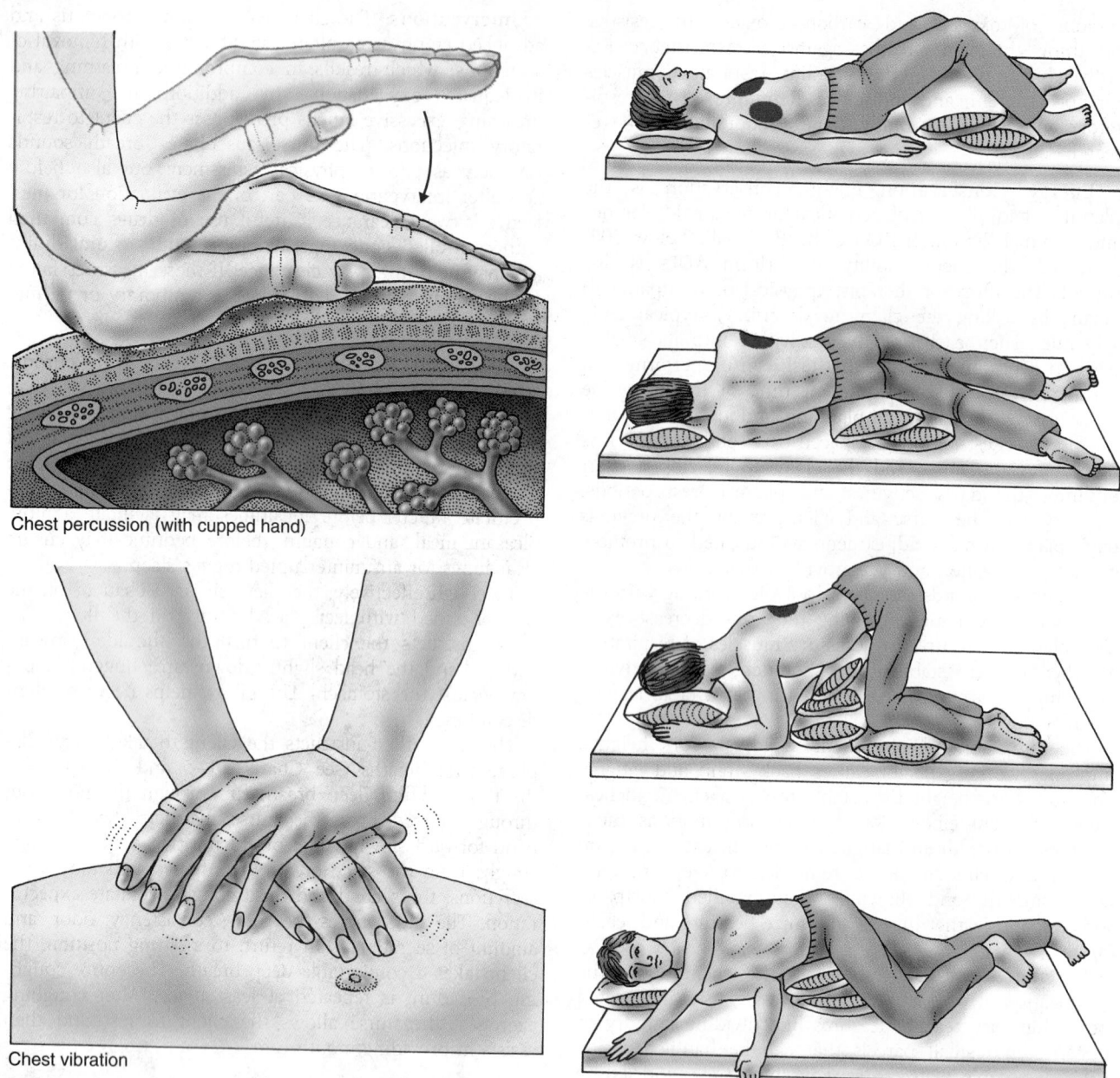

Chest percussion (with cupped hand)

Chest vibration

Figure 32–8. Chest physiotherapy (chest PT) and postural drainage. *Left,* Percussion and vibration techniques. The nurse may use one or two hands with vibration, which is performed when the client exhales or coughs. *Right,* Positions for postural drainage of respiratory secretions.

suctioning procedure and for improved breath sounds afterward. (Chapter 30 discusses suctioning in detail.)

Positioning. When the client can tolerate sitting in a chair, the nurse assists the client out of bed for 1-hour periods two to three times a day. This intervention helps mobilize secretions and also places the diaphragm in a position to provide more effective ventilation of the lungs.

Hydration. Unless hydration is medically contraindicated, the nurse teaches clients with CAL to drink 2–3 L/ day to maintain adequate hydration, which helps liquefy secretions. Humidifiers may be useful for clients living in a dry climate or who complain of dry heat during the winter. The nurse instructs the client to clean the humidifier daily to prevent the growth of mold spores.

> ➤ *Altered Nutrition: Less than Body Requirements*

Planning: Expected Outcomes. The client should achieve and then maintain a body weight within 10% of ideal.

Interventions. Clients with acute or chronic lung disease often complain of food intolerance, nausea, early satiety, loss of appetite, and meal-related dyspnea. In addition, the increased work of breathing raises calorie and protein requirements. These situations lead to protein-calorie malnutrition for many clients with chronic airflow limitation (CAL). Malnourished clients lose total body mass, respiratory muscle mass, respiratory muscle strength, lung elasticity, and alveolocapillary surface area, which contributes to an ineffective breathing pattern.

The nurse identifies clients at risk or those experiencing this complication and initiates dietary consultation. The nurse and nutritionist monitor the client's weight and other indicators of nutrition, such as skin condition and serum pre-albumin levels.

Dyspnea Management. Shortness of breath is the most common complaint related to eating. The nurse teaches the client that shortness of breath during mealtimes can be minimized by resting before meals. The biggest meal of the day is planned for the time when the client is most hungry. Four to six small meals a day may be preferred. The nurse suggests the use of pursed-lip and abdominal breathing to alleviate dyspnea. A bronchodilator used 30 minutes before the meal may be helpful if the meal-related dyspnea is due to bronchospasm or secretions.

Food Selection. Abdominal bloating and a feeling of fullness often prevent the client from eating a complete meal. In the acute care setting, the client may need assistance in choosing menus; the nurse reminds the client to choose foods that are easy to chew and not gas forming. Dry foods stimulate coughing, and foods like milk and chocolate may increase the thickness of saliva and secretions. The nurse advises avoidance of these foods in the symptomatic client. The nurse also teaches the client to avoid caffeinated beverages; they promote diuresis and contribute to dehydration and increased nervousness.

The nurse and nutritionist explore the types of high-calorie foods that the client likes. Dietary supplements such as Pulmocare are specifically designed to provide nutritional supplementation with reduced CO_2 production. If the client has early satiety, the nurse recommends that the client avoid drinking fluids before and during the meal.

Assistance with Feeding. The nurse assists in feeding of the client who tires easily. Most clients do not have the energy to feed themselves when they are working hard to breathe. Many times, clients do not have the urge to eat. The nurse tries various interventions to deal with the anorexia. Sucking on hard candy or chewing gum before meals to begin salivation and stimulate taste buds may help. The nurse also offers to assist the client with oral hygiene before meals.

➤ Anxiety

Planning: Expected Outcomes. The client should demonstrate decreased anxiety, be able to identify factors that contribute to anxious behaviors, and identify activities that tend to decrease anxious behaviors.

Interventions. Anxiety plays a major role in clients with CAL. Emotional upset can trigger or aggravate wheezing episodes in clients with asthma. The resultant dyspnea increases anxiety even more. Clients with emphysema and chronic bronchitis typically experience increased anxiety during acute dyspneic episodes, especially if they feel they are choking on excess secretions. Anxiety has been shown to cause dyspnea, which then affects

clients' functional status (see Research Applications for Nursing).

Psychological Interventions. If a client's symptoms are worsened because of anxiety, it is important that the client understand this effect and have a clear plan prepared in advance for dealing with anxiety. The nurse and the client together develop a written plan that states exactly what the client should do if symptoms flare. Having a plan gives the client confidence and control in knowing exactly what to do, which often helps reduce anxiety.

For example, the nurse helps clients to think of themselves not as asthmatics but as people who have asthma. The client is encouraged to discuss feelings and concerns with the nursing staff and other members of the health care team. The nurse explores other alternative psychological approaches to help the client control dyspneic episodes and panic attacks. Examples include relaxation techniques (see Chap. 8), hypnosis therapy, and biofeedback. Biofeedback helps the client determine the impact of various stimuli on symptoms. The client ultimately learns to relax and control these stimuli to avoid the aggravating symptoms.

The client uses pursed-lip and diaphragmatic breathing techniques in conjunction with relaxation therapy. The nurse instructs the client in the various techniques and assesses the client's understanding and performance of the

---

▷ Research Applications for Nursing

Psychologic Factors Influence Functional Status in COPD

Weaver, T. E., Richmond, T. S., & Narsavage, G. L. (1997). An explanatory model of functional status in chronic obstructive pulmonary disease. Nursing Research, 46(1), 26–32.

This study examined which variables influenced the functional status of 104 clients with chronic obstructive pulmonary disease (COPD). All clients were diagnosed with emphysema, bronchitis, or COPD; 82% were male; 70% were married; the mean age was 65.6 years; and the mean duration of illness was 11.6 years. Functional status was measured using the Pulmonary Functional Status Scale (PFSS), which defines functional status in terms of physical, mental, and social functioning in everyday life. Exercise capacity, dyspnea, and depressed mood were found to influence functional status directly. Dyspnea, depression, and pulmonary function indirectly influenced functional status through exercise capacity. Self-esteem and anxiety indirectly influenced functional status through depressed mood.

Critique. This well-designed study has few limitations. The majority of the subjects were males, and no data were included to address whether any differences exist between men and women. The PFSS tool includes the "everyday tasks" of grocery shopping, household tasks, and meal preparation and would be more common to women than men.

Possible Nursing Implications. To improve functional status of clients with COPD, the nurse should focus on interventions that will improve exercise capacity, reduce dyspnea and anxiety, and elevate the client's depressed mood.

techniques. The client practices the techniques daily and uses the techniques during panic attacks or episodes of dyspnea.

Family, friends, and support groups can be quite helpful. Professional counseling, if recommended, should be viewed as a positive suggestion; in no way should the client view this need as a failure to cope. The nurse helps the client understand that talking with a professional counselor can assist in identifying potential techniques that can help in maintaining control over the dyspnea and feelings of panic.

Drug Therapy. Some clients may benefit from drugs that reduce anxiety. These drugs are particularly helpful for some clients with asthma during an attack.

➤ *Activity Intolerance*

Planning: Expected Outcomes. The client should
- Perform activities of daily living (ADLs) without assistance or with limited assistance
- Adjust the daily schedule, making minimal changes in usual routine or lifestyle
- Perform activities, including walking for short distances, without experiencing dyspnea or tachycardia
- Participate in family or social activities as desired

Interventions. The client with emphysema and chronic bronchitis typically experiences chronic fatigue. While in the acute phases of the illness, the client may require extensive assistance with ADLs, like bathing and grooming. As the client's acute episode resolves, the nurse encourages the client to pace activities and provide as much self-care as possible. The nurse instructs the client not to rush through morning activities because rushing is likely to increase dyspnea, fatigue, and also, potentially, hypoxemia in the client requiring oxygen. As the client gradually increases activity, the nurse continually assesses the physiologic response by noting skin color changes, pulse rate and regularity, and blood pressure and work of breathing. If the physician has ordered supplemental oxygen, it should be used continually, particularly during periods of increased energy use such as bathing or walking for short periods. (Other interventions, such as energy conservation, are discussed under Ineffective Breathing Pattern.)

➤ *Potential for Pneumonia or Other Respiratory Infection*

Planning: Expected Outcomes. The client should not experience secondary respiratory infection and should recognize early signs and symptoms of infection. The client should then seek prompt treatment.

Interventions. Pneumonia is one of the most common complications of COPD/CAL. Clients who have excessive secretions or have artificial airways are at increased risk for respiratory infections. The risk is greatly increased in the elderly. The nurse teaches clients to avoid large crowds of people, such as in a shopping center. The nurse also teaches clients the importance of receiving an annual influenza vaccine ("flu shots") and a pneumococcal vaccination (as frequently as recommended by the physi-

cian or Nurse Practitioner) to prevent these potentially deadly diseases. The highest mortality from these diseases is in elderly clients with CAL. (See Chapter 33 for more information on pneumonia and influenza.)

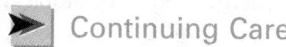

➤ Continuing Care

➤ *Health Teaching*

Clients with a chronic, disabling disease like CAL need to know as much about the disease as possible so they can better manage it and themselves. Specifically, clients and family members or significant others should be able to discuss medications, signs and symptoms of infection, avoidance of respiratory irritants, diet therapy regimen, and activity progression. They need to identify and avoid stressors that can exacerbate the disease. The nurse stresses the importance of communication between clients and their family. Spouses or family members frequently avoid any communication they believe will upset the client. Family therapy may be needed to facilitate communication techniques.

The nurse instructs clients in techniques of breathing, including pursed-lip breathing, diaphragmatic breathing, positioning, relaxation therapy, energy conservation, and coughing and deep breathing. Figure 32–9 is a sample CAL client education checklist used for discharge teaching. Education related to specific interventions has been discussed under the various nursing diagnoses. Two factors may interfere with teaching hospitalized clients: the shortened length of stay coupled with a multitude of topics to discuss and clients' level of tolerance and dyspnea. It may be unrealistic to cover all of the topics in the education checklist during a single hospitalization. The primary nurse or case manager will coordinate teaching with the home health or clinic staff.

Hypoxemic clients can benefit from long-term use of oxygen at home. As with other therapies, the physician's decision to prescribe home oxygen is made with calculated analysis. The physician may prescribe oxygen only during periods of exercise or sleep if hypoxemia occurs only during these times. Continuous, long-term administration of oxygen can reverse tissue hypoxia and decrease pulmonary vascular resistance; it can also improve cognitive ability and well-being. (More information on oxygen therapy is found in Chapter 30.)

➤ *Home Care Management*

Most clients are treated in the ambulatory care setting and cared for at home. The client with chronic airflow limitation (CAL) in whom pneumonia or a severe exacerbation of the disease develops is usually treated and discharged from the hospital to a previous home setting. For clients with advanced disease, however, 24-hour care may be needed for ADLs and for monitoring clients for acute episodes or progression of the illness. Clients may not be able to enjoy work or recreational activities because of spending all available energy on the work of breathing. If arrangements for home care are not possible, clients may need to be transferred to a long-term care setting.

Most clients can benefit from a structured pulmonary

Checklist for CAL Client Education

The Client Has Received the Following Education: Date   Signature

A. Basic anatomy and physiology of the respiratory system   _____   _____
    1. Structures composing the respiratory system
    2. Functions of the respiratory passageways
B. Pathophysiology related to condition   _____   _____
    1. Name of lung disease
    2. Generalized physiologic effects
    3. Generalized psychosocial effects
C. Medications   _____   _____
    1. Medication safety
    2. Name of each medication
    3. Action of each medication
    4. Dosage
    5. How to take each medication
    6. How to use a metered dose inhaler with or without a "spacer"
    7. Recognition of side effects
    8. Importance of carrying a medication list and a medical alert
       (Medic Alert) bracelet or card
D. Respiratory therapy interventions and bronchial hygiene   _____   _____
    1. Proper care and cleaning of home equipment, i.e., oxygen, cannulas, nebulizers
    2. Sequence of treatments
    3. Adequate hydration
    4. Postural drainage and chest physiotherapy (optional and only with excessive secretions)
    5. Prevention of respiratory tract infection:
       a. Avoid exposure to crowds and people with respiratory tract infections
       b. Signs and symptoms of respiratory tract infection
       c. Use of prescribed antibiotics with as needed (prn) schedule
       d. Influenza immunization; pneumococcal immunization
       e. Use of measures to promote oronasal hygiene
E. Management of dyspnea   _____   _____
    1. Controlled cough maneuver
    2. Pursed-lip breathing
    3. Diaphragmatic breathing
    4. Positioning techniques
    5. Stress management and relaxation techniques
F. Adaptation of a daily routine   _____   _____
    1. Daily schedule of graded exercises
    2. Walking exercise on level ground
    3. Stair climbing
    4. Activities of daily living: adjust activities according to individual fatigue patterns
G. Nutrition   _____   _____
    1. Type of diet prescribed
    2. Balanced diet: meat, dairy, grain, fruit and vegetables: 2:2:4:4 ratio
    3. Low salt intake
H. Control of environment   _____   _____
    1. Environmental problems related to pulmonary disease
    2. Ways to make the environment conducive to living with pulmonary disease
       a. Avoid irritants and use air purification system
       b. Use mask when exposed to dusts and cold air
       c. Stay indoors with air conditioning operating when air quality is poor
       d. Check air quality telephone recording
I. Smoking   _____   _____
    1. Rationale for smoking cessation
    2. Suggest ways to stop smoking
J. Body image and human sexuality   _____   _____
    1. Alterations in self-esteem and body image related to pulmonary disease
    2. Communication in human relationships.
    3. Alterations in sexual relationships related to pulmonary disease
K. Available community resources   _____   _____
    1. Discharge planning; referral to home care professionals
    2. Available community services: Meals on Wheels; American Lung Association;
       American Heart Association; American Cancer Society

Figure 32–9. A checklist for education of the client with chronic airflow limitation (CAL).

TABLE 32-6

Areas of Focus in a Pulmonary Rehabilitation Program

- Education
- Exercise conditioning
- Energy conservation
- Breathing retraining
- Bronchial hygiene
- Dietary counseling
- Vocational training
- Psychological counseling

rehabilitation program (Table 32–6). Pulmonary rehabilitation programs vary, but the overall goal of these multidisciplinary programs is to increase a person's ability to compensate for and live with CAL. In collaboration with the physician, the nurse refers clients with CAL to a pulmonary rehabilitation program before illness becomes severe. Clients with the least severe functional abnormality benefit the most.

The nurse works with the hospital discharge-planning nurse or case manager to obtain the necessary equipment for care at home. Often the case manager coordinates the necessary resources to facilitate a smooth transition back to the community and ensures appropriate follow-up in the community. Client needs may include oxygen therapy, a hospital-type bed, a nebulizer, a tub transfer bench, and arrangements for a home health nurse to continue monitoring the health status, review medication compliance, and evaluate home care needs.

The client with CAL faces a lifelong disease with remissions and exacerbations. The nurse explains to both the client and the family that the client may experience periods of anxiety, depression, and ineffective coping. The client who was a smoker also may have self-directed anger, particularly if the client recognizes that smoking contributed to the disease.

Financial concerns often increase the client's and family's anxiety and interfere with disease management. The client's condition may worsen to the point that the client cannot work. Disability benefits through Social Security or private disability insurance plans can help ease the financial burden. Medicare or other health insurers may assist with payment for home oxygen therapy and nebulizer treatments. The nurse collaborates closely with the social worker or discharge-planning nurse to help the client make the necessary arrangements.

➤ Health Care Resources

The nurse provides appropriate referrals as necessary. Home care visits may be warranted, particularly if the client must use home oxygen therapy for the first time. Referral to assistance programs, such as Meals on Wheels, can be extremely helpful. The nurse provides the client with a list of various support groups and Better Breathing groups sponsored by the American Lung Association. If the client is having difficulty with smoking cessation and

indicates the need for assistance, the nurse makes the appropriate referrals.

 Evaluation

The nurse evaluates the care of the client with CAL on the basis of the identified nursing diagnoses. The expected outcomes are that the client

- Attains and maintains ventilation parameters (PaO_2, $PaCO_2$) within the normal range for the client
- Adheres to the prescribed pharmacologic therapy
- Demonstrates lung sounds optimal for the client
- Demonstrates breathing techniques of pursed-lip breathing and abdominal or diaphragmatic breathing
- Demonstrates positioning techniques to use during dyspneic episodes
- Identifies various methods of conserving energy
- Maintains a patent airway by removing excessive secretions
- Demonstrates controlled coughing
- Increases or maintains fluid intake
- Attains and maintains body weight within 10% of ideal
- States methods of reducing anxiety
- Identifies personal strengths rather than focusing on limitations
- Performs self-care independently or with minimal assistance for as long as possible
- States the need to avoid irritants and sources of infection
- Participates in social and family activities as desired
- Maintains employment or same level of activity
- Decreases exacerbations of symptoms
- Decreases use of emergency room treatment
- Decreases hospitalizations

SARCOIDOSIS

Overview

Sarcoidosis is a multisystem granulomatous disorder of unknown cause that can affect virtually any organ. It is one of a group of diseases within a broader classification of pulmonary diseases called interstitial lung disease. Interstitial lung disease is used interchangeably with the term *fibrotic lung disease*. The hallmark of sarcoidosis is noncaseating granuloma. The granulomas of sarcoidosis can occur in almost any organ or tissue of the body but most frequently affected are the lung, liver, spleen, lymph nodes, eyes, small bones of the hands and feet, and skin.

The disease often presents in young adults. It peaks between age 20 and 30 years and again between 45 and 65 years. Physical findings include bilateral hilar adenopathy, pulmonary infiltrates, skin lesions, and eye lesions. The first presentation may be an abnormal chest radiograph in an asymptomatic client. The most common symptoms include nonproductive cough, dyspnea, and chest discomfort. Fortunately, in most clients, the illness resolves spontaneously. Others may experience pulmonary fibrosis and severe systemic disease.

The organ most frequently involved is the lung. More than 90% of the clients affected will have lung or intra-thoracic lymph node involvement. Pulmonary sarcoidosis is a chronic disorder of the alveolar structure that develops over time in a step-by-step manner. Growths called granulomas characterize the disease. Granulomas are composed of lymphocytes, macrophages, epithelioid cells, and giant cells.

It is currently believed that the development of pulmonary sarcoidosis involves the activation of T lymphocytes; the stimulus for this activation is unknown. However, normal resident immune cells (the T lymphocytes) recruit additional immune cells, probably by releasing chemotactic factor. Monocytes are then attracted to the T lymphocytes. Monocytes are precursors of macrophages, epithelioid cells, and the multinucleated giant cells that compose the granuloma. *Alveolitis* is the term that describes this process of accumulation of inflammatory immune cells in the alveoli.

It is believed that the T lymphocytes are primarily responsible for granuloma formation and that the activated macrophages are primarily responsible for interstitial fibrosis because of their ability to recruit and increase the number of fibroblasts. The fibrosis results in a loss of lung compliance (elasticity) and a loss of functional ability to exchange gases. Cor pulmonale (right-sided cardiac failure) is often present because the heart can no longer pump against the noncompliant, fibrotic lung.

Collaborative Management

 ### Assessment

A diagnosis of sarcoidosis is suspected in clients who present with symptoms of cough and dyspnea and have incidental abnormal chest radiograph findings but are otherwise asymptomatic. Sarcoidosis is considered a disease of exclusion. The most important diseases to exclude are infections and neoplasms.

Sarcoidosis is staged on the basis of radiograph criteria:
- Stage 0: normal chest x-ray
- Stage 1: bilateral hilar adenopathy
- Stage 2: bilateral hilar adenopathy with diffuse parenchymal infiltrates
- Stage 3: diffuse infiltrates with adenopathy
- Stage 4: lung fibrosis

Stage 2 radiograph findings are considered a reliable sign of sarcoidosis. A client who presents with a stage 0 or 1 radiograph may have a high-resolution computed tomographic (CT) scan to detect any parenchymal involvement. For all those diagnosed with sarcoidosis, two thirds will have resolution of the disease.

Pulmonary function studies often show a restrictive pattern of decreased lung volumes and impaired diffusing capacity. Irreversible lung changes develop in 10% to 15% of clients. In those in whom severe restrictive disease develops, pulmonary hypertension may develop in response to the severe disease.

Fiberoptic bronchoscopy (see Chap. 29) allows researchers to sample the epithelial fluid of the lower respiratory tract to investigate the alveolitis of clients with active disease. This test confirms that pulmonary sarcoidosis is a disease associated with an intense cellular immune response in the alveolar structure.

TRANSCULTURAL CONSIDERATIONS

 In the United States, sarcoidosis affects African-Americans 10 times more frequently than Caucasians. The overall prevalence is similar in women and men, but it is twice as common in women of childbearing age as in women of other ages. A distinctive feature of sarcoidosis is its age distribution: most cases develop in people between 20 and 40 years of age. Other countries with high prevalence include Scandinavian countries, England, and Japan.

Interventions

The goal of therapy is to lessen symptoms and prevent fibrosis. Indications for treatment vary. If the client is asymptomatic and has no abnormal pulmonary function, no treatment is given. Indications for treatment include clinical symptoms; decrease in total lung capacity, diffusing capacity, or forced vital capacity; extrapulmonary involvement; and hypercalcemia.

Corticosteroids are the cornerstone of therapy. Protocols may vary from 40–60 mg/day with tapering doses over 6–8 weeks to a maintenance dose of 10–15 mg for 6 months. Further therapy will occur over 12 months. Follow-up and monitoring includes review of symptoms, pulmonary function studies, chest x-rays, complete blood count, serum creatinine, serum calcium, and urinalysis. The nurse and pharmacist teach the client and family about side effects of steroid therapy and other aspects of the client's physical care as indicated and appropriate.

IDIOPATHIC PULMONARY FIBROSIS

Overview

Idiopathic pulmonary fibrosis is the second major form of the interstitial pulmonary disease. Unlike sarcoidosis, it is a highly lethal interstitial lung disease. Most clients have progressive disease with few remission periods. Remission in this disease is rare. Outcomes are fairly predictive at the end of 1 year.

Pulmonary fibrosis has been described as a model of excessive wound healing. Once lung injury occurs, an inflammatory process ensues. The initial response is predominantly neutrophilic followed by a predominance of lymphocytes and macrophages. There is an exudation of serum proteins into the alveolar space, resulting in collapse of alveolar units and healing by fibrosis. Normal lung tissue can be found interspersed between areas of fibrosis.

Although the cause of pulmonary fibrosis is unknown, factors such as cigarette smoking and exposure to metal dust, organic dust, and wood fires has been shown to be predictors of the disease.

TRANSCULTURAL CONSIDERATIONS

Between 1979 and 1991, there was an increase in mortality rates for both men and women with pulmonary fibrosis. Mortality rates were lowest in the Midwest and Northeast and highest in the West and Southeast. Rates were also higher for the older aged. The age-adjusted rate for the period 1979 through 1991 was 33.0 per 1,000,000.

Collaborative Management

Assessment

The onset of symptoms can be insidious, with initial symptoms of dyspnea. Pulmonary function studies reveal decreased forced vital capacities. As the fibrosis progresses, the client becomes more dyspneic, and hypoxemia becomes severe. These clients will eventually require high levels of oxygen and often remain hypoxemic on these high oxygen levels.

The nurse obtains a complete history and performs a complete respiratory assessment. Dyspnea is measured, and hypoxemia is assessed. Particular attention is paid to any recent exposure to an occupational or environmental agent. (More details as to occupational causes of fibrosis are described under Occupational Pulmonary Disease.)

Interventions

The physician usually prescribes corticosteroids for treatment. Most clients are also treated with a cytotoxic drug such as cyclophosphamide (Cytoxan, Neosar, Procytox✦), azathioprine, chlorambucil (Leukeran), or methotrexate (Folex), which by themselves can cause lung injury. Of the clients who respond to therapy, initiation of therapy early in the disease process is critical. Current therapy and research are aimed at agents that inhibit cytokines, growth factors, and oxidant injury in the lung. Gene therapy is also being explored. Single-lung transplantation is considered an option. However, the selection criteria, cost, and availability of organs make this option unlikely for most candidates.

The client and family will require support and assistance with community resources once the diagnosis is made. The goal of therapy is to minimize the fibrotic process and control symptoms. The nurse and health care team begins by assisting the client and family in understanding the disease process and yet maintaining hope for control of the fibrosis. It is important to prevent further lung insult from respiratory infections. The client and family are educated regarding the signs and symptoms of infection and encouraged to avoid respiratory irritants, crowds, and those with known infections.

Home oxygen is often required once the diagnosis is made because by the time the client becomes symptomatic significant fibrosis has already occurred. The nurse and respiratory therapist begin education regarding oxygen use and stress the importance of using the oxygen as a continuous therapy. The occupational therapist is most helpful in assessing ADL limitations and recommending adaptive equipment to assist in energy conservation, which will minimize oxygen consumption and decrease work of breathing. As with other restrictive lung diseases, these clients have rapid respirations associated with decreased lung compliance. The nurse supports the client's need to be as independent as possible and yet encourages the client to pace activities and accept assistance as needed.

The social worker meets with the family to answer questions regarding community resources and provide assistance with applications regarding disability, if applicable. The disease can be economically devastating to a family because the client is often unable to continue work. Home health nurses may be arranged to assist in continued monitoring of the client's health status and oxygen needs.

In the later stages of the disease, the focus is to minimize the sensation of shortness of breath, which is often accomplished with the use of morphine, either oral or intravenous. The home health nurse can assist the physician in regulating the medication to control the symptoms.

The physician and Nurse Practitioner keep the client informed of the disease process and assist the client with identification of advanced health care wishes. The client and family are provided information regarding hospice, which provides support and coordination of resources to meet the needs of the client and family when the prognosis is less than 6 months.

OCCUPATIONAL PULMONARY DISEASE

Overview

Exposure to occupational or environmental fumes, dust, vapors, gases, bacterial or fungal antigens, and allergens can result in a variety of respiratory disorders. Depending on the degree, frequency, and intensity of exposure, the smoking history, and underlying pulmonary disease, clients may experience acute reversible effects or chronic pulmonary disease.

With a greater focus on ambulatory care, nurses and other health care providers are refocusing and retooling their education to care of the client outside the hospital setting. Many occupational diseases have an onset of symptoms long after their initial exposure to the offending agent. Through skilled history taking, the nurse investigates the many nuances of respiratory symptoms associated with the work environment over a lifetime.

OCCUPATIONAL ASTHMA. Occupational asthma (OA) is the most common form of occupational lung disease in the United States. OA differs from other forms of asthma in that it is associated with variable airway narrowing related to an exposure in the working environment and not to stimuli outside the workplace. These clients usually have no childhood or family history of the disease. In some cases, symptoms may develop after several years of exposure. OA may be difficult to recognize because the client may continue to experience respiratory distress when away from the work setting.

With the rapid development of the chemical industry, large numbers of inorganic and organic substances have been found to cause asthma by direct bronchial irritation. Aside from chemical irritants, enzymes used in food processing, detergent, and pharmaceutical industries may be asthma-inducing agents. Plant- and animal-derived materials also may be sources of irritation.

Occupational asthma is divided into two types, which are differentiated by onset of symptoms. The most common type is OA with a latency period. The disease develops after a period of exposure, which can vary from a few weeks to several years. Included are all instances induced by immunoglobulin E (IgE)–dependent agents. These agents are classified as high molecular weight and low molecular weight.

The IgE-dependent agents with high molecular weights include cereals, animal-derived allergens, enzymes such as those in detergents, gums used in carpets, latex found in gloves, seafoods, and pharmaceuticals. The low-molecular-weight agents act as haptens and induce specific IgE antibodies by combining with a body protein. The most commonly occurring low-molecular-weight agent is toluene diisocyanate, which is used in the manufacture of polyurethane foam and coatings. Other agents that cause OA include wood dust, anhydrides used in plastic and epoxy resins, amines found in shellacs, flux, chloramine-T found in janitors' cleaners, dyes used in textiles, persulfate used by hairdressers, formaldehyde and glutaraldehyde used by hospital staff, acrylate found in adhesives, metal, and drugs.

Clients diagnosed with latency OA related to a specific allergen will have a permanent impairment or disability, which is observed when performing pulmonary function testing using a bronchial provocation test to stimulate hyperresponsiveness. These clients will demonstrate airflow limitation.

The second type of OA does not have a latency period. In the past it was referred to as reactive airways dysfunction syndrome (RADS), but it is more frequently referred to as *irritant-induced asthma*. This terminology recognizes that similar effects and outcomes also occur in clients with multiple exposures but with lower levels of concentration of the offending agent. The client who experiences this type of OA may have been near a chemical spill. Onset of symptoms occurs within 24 hours. The most commonly occurring precipitating agents include chlorine, ammonia, and phosgene. Exposure to massive concentrations of the chemical can result in pulmonary edema, adult respiratory distress syndrome (ARDS), and death.

Pathologic changes associated with irritant-induced asthma include desquamation of the epithelial layer, thickening of the basement membrane, and inflammation of cells of the bronchial mucosa. T lymphocytes and activated eosinophils can be found in the bronchial mucosa.

Symptoms often persist for 3 months but can occur for years or even permanently after the exposure. These symptoms frequently include cough, wheeze, and dyspnea. Some clients report a burning sensation in the throat and nose and chest discomfort.

PNEUMOCONIOSIS. Pneumoconiosis is the lodging of any inhaled dust in the lungs. Two types of pneumoconiosis are silicosis and coal miners' pneumoconiosis.

Silicosis, a chronic fibrosing disease of the lungs, is produced by excessive inhalation of free crystalline silica dust. Mining and quarrying are associated with a high incidence of silicosis. Hazardous exposure to silica dust also occurs in foundry work, tunneling, sandblasting, pottery making, stone masonry, and manufacture of glass, tile, and bricks. The finely ground silica used in soaps, polishes, and filters is especially dangerous.

Chronic silicosis results from exposure to low concentrations of silica dust for 20 years or more. The formation of selective nodules in the pulmonary parenchyma is characteristic. This process may be accompanied by progressive massive fibrosis.

Uncomplicated, or simple, silicosis is often entirely asymptomatic and causes only mild ventilating restriction and evidence of fibrosis on an x-ray. Clients with chronic complicated disease experience significant dyspnea on exertion, marked reduction in lung volume, and massive fibrosis of the upper lobes. Malaise, anorexia, and weight loss may be present with an outcome of respiratory failure.

Coal Miners' Pneumoconiosis. Chronic pneumoconiosis of coal miners also results in massive pulmonary fibrosis as a result of deposition of coal dust in the lung. There is an additive effect of cigarette smoking to inhalation of coal dust. Symptoms are related to the amount and frequency of exposure. Initial symptoms are similar to bronchitis with eventual development of centrilobular emphysema.

DIFFUSE INTERSTITIAL FIBROSIS. *Asbestosis* refers to diffuse interstitial fibrosis caused by exposure to asbestos. There is generally a considerable latency period between the initial exposure and the onset of clinical manifestations of fibrosis, often 10–20 years. People who are at risk for asbestosis are asbestos miners and millers and those employed in the building trades and shipyards, carpenters and electricians, loggers, insulation workers, pipe fitters, steamfitters, sheet metal workers, and welders.

Asbestos causes a diffuse pleural thickening with diaphragmatic calcification. Presence of calcified pleural plaques on a chest radiograph is the most common manifestation of asbestos exposure. Pulmonary function abnormalities usually indicate a restrictive ventilatory defect. Removal of the worker from exposure does not necessarily prevent the effects of the disease. The chances of arresting the disease are best in its early stages. Clients with this disease frequently have respiratory infections.

Malignant asbestosis includes bronchial cancers and malignant mesotheliomas of the pleura and peritoneum.

Talcosis is a pulmonary fibrosis that occurs after years of exposure to high concentrations of talc dust. Significant exposures can occur during the manufacture of paints, ceramics, asphalt, roofing materials, cosmetics, and rubber goods. The clinical picture of the client closely resembles that of asbestosis.

Berylliosis is a chronic granulomatous disorder of the lungs caused by inhalation of beryllium. The typical exposure history includes involvement in an operation in which metals are heated to fumes (e.g., welding, burning, or casting) or are machined to dust. Clients with berylliosis exposure may be screened with a peripheral blood lymphocyte proliferation test. Results will be elevated in those with chronic beryllium disease or with exposure to beryllium, who are more likely to progress to advanced irreversible disease than are those with sarcoidosis of unknown cause.

EXTRINSIC ALLERGIC ALVEOLITIS. A granulomatous inflammatory reaction, extrinsic allergic alveolitis is a hypersensitivity pneumonitis caused by an immunologic response to inhaled organic dust or chemicals containing bacteria or fungal antigens. Three of the most common forms of this disease include farmer's lung, bird fancier's lung, and machine operator's lung.

Farmer's lung is caused by the inhalation of fungal antigens found in molding hay and straw. The client will complain of a dry cough and experience minimal wheezing, if any.

Bird fancier's lung results from inhalation of antigens found in bird excreta. The nurse suspects this condition if the client presents with flu-like symptoms after exposure to the antigen and recovers within 48 hours after removal from the source. The chest radiograph may show a ground-glass pattern. Pulmonary function studies reveal reduced lung volumes and impaired gas transfer.

Machine operator's lung is caused by exposure to metal working fluid. The fluid, which is recirculated at a high pressure, creates an aerosol, which may contain a bacterial antigen. Once inhaled, a hypersensitivity pneumonitis ensues. The client may report dyspnea, cough, fatigue, fever, or weight loss. Chest radiograph may show interstitial infiltrates.

Collaborative Management

 Assessment

An occupational cause should be investigated for all clients with new-onset asthma. The health care team screens the client for all known causes of occupational asthma. Because there may or may not be a latency period between exposure and onset of symptoms, the nurse obtains a thorough history of occupational exposure, onset of symptoms associated with the work environment, symptoms while away from work, dose exposure, frequency of exposure, history of smoking, history of lung disease, and use of a protective device. The client with occupational asthma with a latency period should be removed from the site of exposure, transferred to a job without exposure, and treated with medications for asthma.

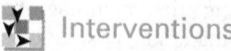 Interventions

Prevention is extremely important for avoiding pulmonary disability caused by occupationally related disease. The nurse or other public health advocate stresses the importance of using special respirators and ensuring adequate ventilation when working in potentially harmful environ-

ments. When assessing the client with respiratory distress, the nurse ascertains whether symptoms are acute or chronic. If the client is having an allergic reaction, the nurse stresses avoidance of the allergen. Nursing care is similar to care of the client with asthma not caused by the workplace environment. The nurse refers the client to a social worker, who provides information regarding compensation and pension.

Nursing interventions for clients experiencing occupational pulmonary restrictive disease are related to the effects of decreased chest wall compliance, vital capacity, and total lung volume. These deficits are related to the fibrotic process, which restricts lung expansion. Most nursing diagnoses appropriate for clients with chronic airflow limitation (CAL) apply to these clients. Hypoxemic clients require supplemental oxygen. In addition, respiratory therapies to promote sputum clearance are essential.

LUNG CANCER

Overview

Lung cancer is the leading cause of cancer-related deaths worldwide. Lung cancer accounts for 25% of all cancer deaths. The overall 5-year survival rate for all clients with lung cancer is 12.5%. Metastatic disease is often present, and only 14% of clients have localized disease at the time of diagnosis (Parker et al., 1997). The prognosis for lung cancer remains poor. Cancer of the lung is essentially incurable unless surgical resection can be accomplished. Treatment of lung cancer is often aimed toward relieving symptoms (palliation) rather than cure because of the presence of metastasis. It has been estimated that 85% of lung cancers might be prevented through the elimination of cigarette smoking. (Chapter 26 further discusses causes of cancer development.) Therefore, the nurse plays a major role in public education to prevent the initiation of smoking. The nurse also uses interventions that improve the quality of life for clients with lung cancer.

Pathophysiology

More than 90% of all primary lung cancers arise from the bronchial epithelium. These cancers are collectively called bronchogenic carcinomas. Lung cancers are classified according to their histologic cell type as

- Small cell or oat cell
- Epidermoid or squamous cell
- Adenocarcinoma
- Large cell

The last three types are often referred to as non–small cell lung cancers (NSCLC). All of the bronchogenic carcinomas can be further divided into more specific subtypes, such as a variant of adenocarcinoma known as bronchioloalveolar carcinoma (Travis et al., 1996). Approximately 60% of clients with NSCLC will have metastasis at the time of diagnosis, which eliminates surgery as a curative treatment modality (Carney, 1996). Major tumor cell types are summarized in Table 32–7.

TABLE 32-7

Differential Features of the Major Types of Lung Cancer

Type	Approximate Incidence	Characteristics	Treatment
Small cell (oat cell)	• 20%	• Centrally located tumors (80%), rapidly growing, most malignant type • High rate of metastasis via the lymph and circulatory systems with early extra-thoracic involvement • Associated with paraneoplastic syndromes • Prognosis poor; survival usually not more than 2 yr with treatment	• Combination chemotherapy is the initial treatment of choice • Surgical resectability poor • Palliative endobronchial laser therapy to relieve obstruction • Radiation not recommended for metastatic disease
Non-small cell Epidermoid (squamous cell)	• 30%	• Frequently originates in a central or hilar location and at the bifurcation points of segmental bronchi • In a peripheral location, cavities may form in lung tissue • Strong association with cigarette smoking • Slower growing, less invasive; metastasis often limited to the thorax, including regional nodes, pleura, and chest wall • Commonly associated with obstructive symptoms and pneumonias; client presents with chest pain, cough, dyspnea, and hemoptysis	• Surgical resectability good if stage I or stage II • Chemotherapy and radiation therapy may be used to palliate symptoms
Adenocarci-noma	• 30%–35%	• Tumors are located peripherally • Slow growing • Hematogenous spread occurs frequently and usually early in the course of the disease • High frequency of metastasis to brain; other sites include adrenals, liver, bone, and kidneys • Predominant type in nonsmokers; most frequent type of lung cancer found in women • Often arises in previously scarred or fibrotic lungs	• Surgical resectability good if stage I or stage II • Moderately good response to chemotherapy • Radiation therapy used to palliate pulmonary and metastatic disease
Large cell	• 11%	• Peripheral, subpleural lesions with necrotic surfaces or cavities • Often form larger tumor masses than adenocarcinoma • Slow growing • Metastasis is similar to that for adenocarcinoma with addition of gastrointestinal tract • Prognosis poor	• Surgical resectability good if stage I or stage II • Chemotherapy has limited benefit • Palliative radiation therapy

Metastasis

Lung cancers metastasize (spread) by direct extension, lymphatic invasion, and blood-borne avenues. Bronchial tumors can spread by direct invasion and grow to occlude the bronchus partially or completely. Invasion of the bronchial wall and encircling or obstruction of the airway can also occur. Pulmonary spread can compress lung structures other than the airway, including the alveoli, nerves, blood vessels, and lymph vessels.

The patterns of metastasis depend on the type of tumor cell and the anatomic location of the tumor. Lymphatic spread is usually associated with embolization and invasion by tumor. The mediastinal, paratracheal, and central hilar lymph nodes are most commonly involved. Lower lobe tumors tend to metastasize diffusely more often by lymph channels than do tumors located in other portions of the lung.

Hematogenous (blood-borne) metastasis of lung cancer is due to invasion of the pulmonary venous system. Tumor emboli spread to other, distant areas of the body. Distant sites of metastasis include the bone (lower thoracic and upper lumbar vertebrae and long bones; 19%–33%), adrenal glands (18%–38%), abdominal lymph

TABLE 32–8

Endocrine Paraneoplastic Syndromes Associated with Lung Cancer	
Ectopic Hormone	**Manifestation**
Adrenocorticotropic hormone (ACTH)	• Cushing's syndrome
Antidiuretic hormone	• Syndrome of inappropriate antidiuretic hormone (SIADH)
Follicle-stimulating hormone (FSH)	• Gynecomastia
Parathyroid hormone	• Hypercalcemia
Ectopic insulin	• Hypoglycemia

TABLE 32–9

Nonendocrine Paraneoplastic Syndromes Associated with Lung Cancer	
Tissue/System	**Manifestation**
Connective tissue	• Arthralgia • Digital clubbing
Hematologic system	• Anemia • Leukocytosis • Thrombocytopenia purpura • Polycythemia • Thrombocytosis
Neuromuscular system	• Peripheral neuropathy • Carcinomatous myopathy • Cortical cerebellar degeneration • Seizure • Polymyositis • Myasthenia-like syndrome
Integumentary system	• Dermatomyositis • Scleroderma • Acanthosis nigricans
Vascular system	• Thrombophlebitis • Nonbacterial endocarditis
Renal system	• Arterial thrombosis • Nephrotic syndrome • Proteinuria

nodes (29%), brain (15%–43%), kidney (16%–23%), and liver (33%–40%).

Additional pathophysiologic manifestations, known as paraneoplastic syndromes, complicate certain lung cancers. The paraneoplastic syndromes are caused by various hormones, antigens, or enzymes. Small cell carcinomas are most commonly associated with paraneoplastic syndromes. Tables 32–8 and 32–9 list the endocrine and nonendocrine paraneoplastic syndromes, respectively, that may be associated with lung cancer.

Staging

The staging of lung cancer is based on the TNM system (T, primary *tumor*; N, regional lymph *nodes*; M, distant *metastasis*). The TNM staging system determines the anatomic extent of the disease and predicts prognosis. The TMN system is further described in Chapter 26.

Staging groups are used clinically because of the significant relationship between the extent of the disease and survival rates. Table 32–10 describes stage grouping for lung cancers. Figure 32–10 shows the various anatomic stages of lung cancer (Mountain et al., 1991).

Etiology

Exposure

Lung cancers have been associated with repeated exposure to substances that cause chronic tissue irritation or inflammation. Cigarette smoking is the major risk factor and is responsible for 85% of all lung cancer deaths (Shottenfeld, 1996).

TABLE 32–10

TMN Stage Grouping for Lung Cancer			
Occult carcinoma	TX	N0	M0
Stage 0	Tis	Carcinoma in situ	
Stage I	T1	N0	M0
	T2	N0	M0
Stage II	T1	N1	M0
	T2	N1	M0
Stage IIIa	T3	N0	M0
	T3	N1	M0
	T1–3	N2	M0
Stage IIIb	Any T	N3	M0
	T4	Any N	M0
Stage IV	Any T	Any N	M1

From Mountain, C. F., Greenberg, M. D., & Fraire, A. E. (1991). Tumor stages in non-small cell carcinoma of the lung. *Chest, 99*(5), 1258.

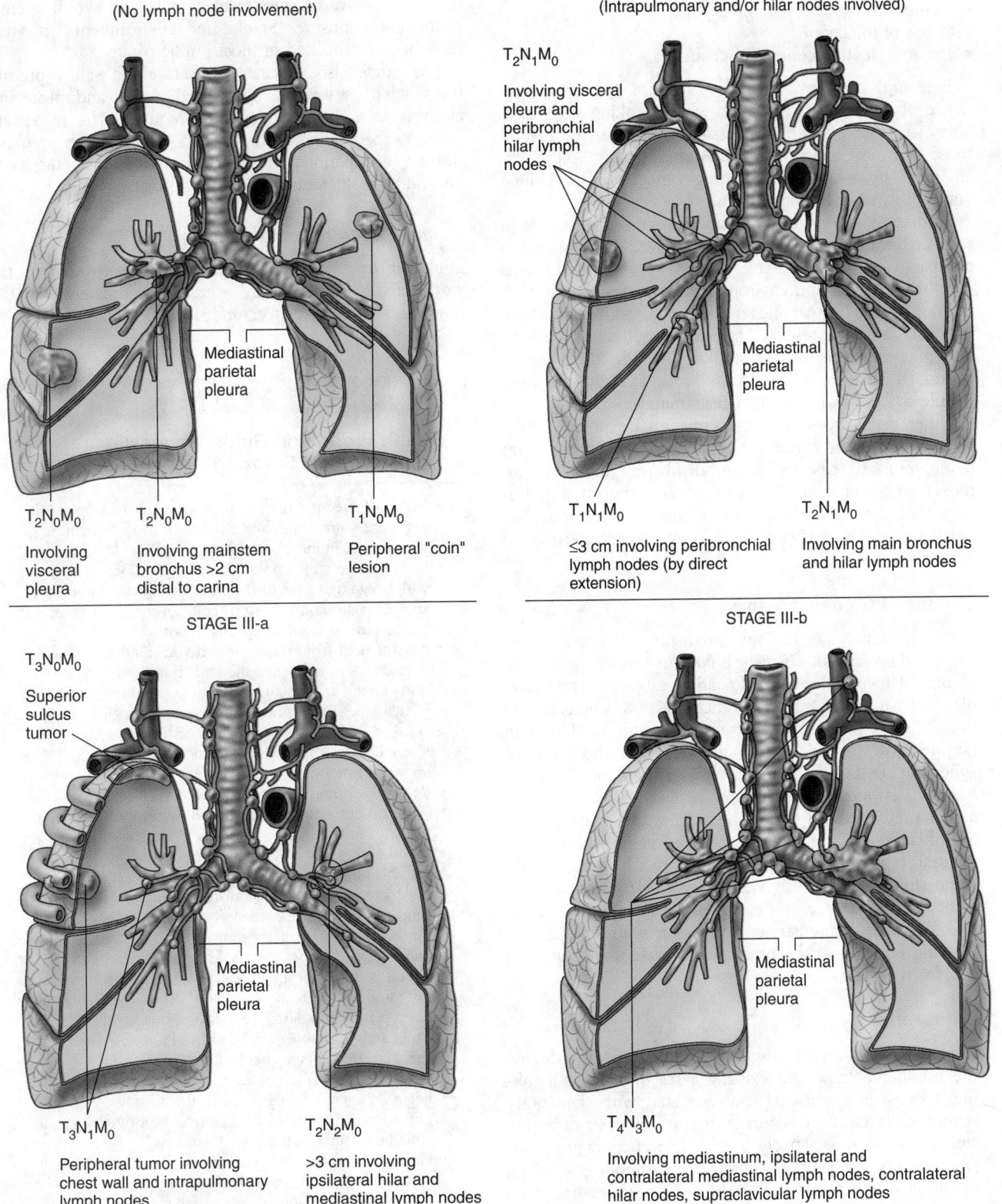

STAGE I
(No lymph node involvement)

$T_2N_0M_0$

Involving
visceral
pleura

$T_2N_0M_0$

Involving mainstem
bronchus >2 cm
distal to carina

$T_1N_0M_0$

Peripheral "coin"
lesion

Mediastinal
parietal
pleura

STAGE II
(Intrapulmonary and/or hilar nodes involved)

$T_2N_1M_0$

Involving visceral
pleura and
peribronchial
hilar lymph
nodes

$T_1N_1M_0$

≤3 cm involving peribronchial
lymph nodes (by direct
extension)

$T_2N_1M_0$

Involving main bronchus
and hilar lymph nodes

Mediastinal
parietal
pleura

STAGE III-a

$T_3N_0M_0$

Superior
sulcus
tumor

$T_3N_1M_0$

Peripheral tumor involving
chest wall and intrapulmonary
lymph nodes

$T_2N_2M_0$

>3 cm involving
ipsilateral hilar and
mediastinal lymph nodes

Mediastinal
parietal
pleura

STAGE III-b

$T_4N_3M_0$

Involving mediastinum, ipsilateral and
contralateral mediastinal lymph nodes, contralateral
hilar nodes, supraclavicular lymph nodes

Mediastinal
parietal
pleura

Figure 32–10. Anatomic staging of lung cancer. (Redrawn from Mountain, C. F., Greenberg, M. D., & Fraire, A. E. [1991]. Tumor stages in non-small cell carcinoma of the lung. *Chest, 99*[5], 1258.)

Increased risk for lung cancer is directly related to

- Total exposure to cigarette smoke as determined by the number of years of smoking
- Number of cigarettes smoked per day
- Depth of inhalation
- Tar and nicotine content of cigarettes

Pipe and cigar smoking also increase risk. The incidence of lung cancer decreases when smoking stops and, after 15 years of smoking cessation, approaches that of those who have never smoked. Approximately 48,000 ex-smokers, however, develop lung cancer in the United States each year (Minna, 1996).

Studies demonstrate that nonsmoking spouses of a smoker have a higher risk for lung cancer from inhalation of "passive" smoke. Passive smoke, also referred to as sidestream smoke and environmental tobacco smoke, contains many of the carcinogens found in actively inhaled, or "mainstream," tobacco smoke (Schottenfeld, 1996). Others at risk from passive smoking include those heavily exposed to passive smoke in the workplace, among them people who work in bars and restaurants.

Other risk factors include occupational exposure to asbestos, beryllium, chromium, coal distillates, cobalt, iron oxide, mustard gas, petroleum distillates, radiation, tar, nickel, and uranium. Atmospheric and industrial pollution that contains benzopyrenes and hydrocarbons has also been associated with an increased incidence of lung cancer.

Other Etiologic Factors

Some hereditary conditions predispose to cancer, although they are not strongly linked to bronchogenic carcinoma. However, evidence for adenocarcinoma and alveolar cell carcinoma suggests genetic factors. These factors do not seem to be related to smoking and are found in families with other tumors, acquired immunodeficiency syndrome (AIDS), or inheritable disorders of the lung. Research supports a correlation between a specific gene and a predisposition to lung cancer, which may thus be an inherited trait (Shell et al., 1996). Clients with chronic respiratory diseases are also at higher risk for lung cancer. A possible link between vitamin A and β-carotene deficiency in the diet and the development of lung cancer also has been demonstrated. A person who smokes and has one or more of the predisposing factors is at greatest risk for the disease.

Prevention

Primary prevention for lung cancer is directed at reducing the number of new and existing cases of tobacco smoking. Extensive educational strategies start with elementary school children to discourage them from beginning to smoke. Nurses are actively involved in encouraging nonsmokers not to begin to smoke, in promoting smoking cessation programs, and in establishing a smoke-free environment. For example, nurses from the Canadian Cancer Society's Industrial Education Program visit places of employment to educate workers about the dangers of smoking. This avenue of education has also been successfully used in the United States. Smoking cessation programs

for assisting those who smoke are available in most geographic areas. Chart 32–7 reviews interventions to help a person stop smoking. The nurse encourages nonsmokers to avoid passive or sidestream smoking by avoiding environmental exposure. Smoke-free environments or areas have been established in most public places.

The nurse also educates workers about safety precautions, such as wearing specialized masks and protective clothing to reduce occupational hazards. The nurse encourages people who are at high risk through smoking history, occupational hazards, or possible genetic background to seek frequent health examinations.

Incidence/Prevalence

Lung cancer is a major health problem throughout the world. Estimates for 1997 were approximately 178,100 new cases of lung cancer and 160,400 deaths from this

---

Chart 32–7

Health Promotion Guide: Suggestions to Help You Stop Smoking

- Make a list of the reasons that you want to stop smoking (e.g., your health and the health of those around you, saving money, social reasons).
- Set a date to stop smoking and keep it. Decide whether you are going to begin to cut down on the amount you smoke or are going to stop "cold turkey." Whatever way you decide to do it, keep this important date!
- Ask for help from those around you. Find someone who wants to quit smoking and "buddy up" for support. Look for assistance in your community, such as formal smoking cessation programs, counselors, and certified acupuncture specialists or hypnotists.
- Consult your physician about nicotine replacement therapy (i.e., patches or gum).
- Remove ashtrays and lighters from view.
- Talk to yourself! Remind yourself of all the reasons you want to quit.
- Avoid places that might tempt you to smoke. If you are used to having a cigarette after meals, get up from the table as soon as you are finished eating. Think of new things to do at times when you used to smoke.
- Find activities that keep your hands busy: needlework, painting, gardening, even holding a pencil.
- Take five deep breaths of clean, fresh air through your nose and out your mouth if you feel the urge to smoke.
- Keep plenty of healthy, low-calorie snacks, such as fruits and vegetables, on hand to nibble on. Try sugarless gum or mints as a substitute for tobacco.
- Drink at least eight glasses of water a day.
- Begin an exercise program with the approval of your physician. Be aware of the positive, healthy changes in your body since you stopped smoking.
- Plan a special way to reward yourself with the money that you save from not smoking.
- List the many reasons why you are glad that you quit. Keep that list handy as a reminder of the positive things you are doing for yourself.
- Think of each day without tobacco as a major accomplishment. It is!

disease in the United States. Lung cancer represents 13% of new cancers in both men and women. Deaths from lung cancer account for 32% of cancer deaths in men and 25% of cancer deaths in women (Parker et al., 1997). In 1986, deaths from lung cancer in women began to exceed deaths from all other cancers, including breast cancer. Researchers attribute this change to a causal relationship with cigarette smoking.

TRANSCULTURAL CONSIDERATIONS

 Lung cancer occurs more frequently and with higher mortality in non-Caucasians. Lung cancer is the most common newly diagnosed cancer in African-Americans (Parker et al., 1997). The impact of industrial factors on the geographic variation in lung cancer rates is pronounced. Mortality rates are higher in countries with significant paper and petroleum industries.

Collaborative Management

Assessment

➤ History

Risk Factors. The nurse extensively questions the client about risk factors, including smoking and occupational hazards in the workplace, and warning signals (Table 32–11). A detailed history of the duration, frequency, and intensity of exposure is elicited. Cigarette smoking history is described in terms of *pack-years*. For example, a person who has smoked two packs per day for 22 years has a 44 pack-year smoking history.

Hoarseness and Cough. When obtaining the history, the nurse notes vague but persistent subjective complaints. Hoarseness, caused by laryngeal nerve invasion, is an early sign of lung cancer. In addition, the nurse asks whether changes in position affect hoarseness, because a recumbent position often exacerbates this sign. The nurse questions the client about any persistent cough or change

in cough and whether the cough is productive of sputum. The nurse also notes a history of any change in respiratory pattern, shortness of breath, or hemoptysis.

Pain. The nurse assesses for chest pain or discomfort, which can occur at any stage of tumor development. Chest pain may be localized or unilateral and can range from mild to severe. The nurse assesses for any vague sensation of fullness, tightness, or pressure in the chest, which may suggest obstruction. A piercing chest pain or pleuritic pain may accompany inspiration. Subscapular pain radiating to the arm commonly results from tumor invasion in advanced disease.

➤ Physical Assessment/Clinical Manifestations

Clinical manifestations associated with lung cancer are often nonspecific and noted late in the disease process. Clinical signs and symptoms depend on the type of primary tumor. Persistent chills, fever, and cough may be related to persistent pneumonitis, indicating obstruction of the bronchi.

Sputum. The nurse assesses sputum quantity and quality. Blood-tinged sputum may be associated with bleeding from a malignant tumor. Hemoptysis is a later finding in the course of the disease. If infection or necrosis is present, sputum may be purulent and copious. The nurse also elicits any history of fever indicative of infection.

Breathing Patterns. The nurse assesses breathing patterns, which may be labored or painful. An obstructive breathing pattern may be evident; expiration is prolonged and labored and alternates with periods of shallow breathing. Rapid, shallow breathing suggests pleuritic chest pain and an elevated diaphragm. Inspiratory efforts may be diminished in advanced disease. The nurse assesses for abnormal retractions, the use of accessory muscles, flared nares (which could be signs of hypoxemia), and stridor (which can indicate obstruction by tumor). The nurse also observes for asymmetry of diaphragmatic movement on inspiration. Bronchial obstruction or pressure in the carina, mediastinum, or trachea may produce dyspnea or wheezing. The nurse assesses the client's level of dyspnea at rest and with activity. The nurse also notes the compensatory mechanisms the client uses to overcome this difficulty. Pursed-lip breathing and orthopnea are common compensatory mechanisms.

Fremitus. On palpation of the chest wall, the nurse may find areas of tenderness or masses. Changes in tactile fremitus (vibrations felt on the chest wall) indicate areas of consolidation (the process whereby air spaces in the lung are replaced with solid material, such as tumor or fluid). Fremitus is decreased or absent when the bronchus is obstructed or the pleural space is occupied by a tumor. Palpation of the trachea may reveal deviation from midline, or "shifting," related to a thoracic mass.

Masses. By percussion of the chest wall, the nurse examines for areas of dullness or obvious masses. With diaphragmatic excursion, resonance usually occurs around the 10th rib.

TABLE 32–11

Warning Signals Associated with Lung Cancer

- Hoarseness
- Change in respiratory pattern
- Persistent cough or change in cough
- Blood-streaked sputum
- Rust-colored or purulent sputum
- Frank hemoptysis
- Chest pain or chest tightness
- Shoulder, arm, or chest wall pain
- Recurring episodes of pleural effusion, pneumonia, or bronchitis
- Dyspnea
- Fever associated with one or two other signs
- Wheezing
- Weight loss
- Clubbing

Breath Sounds. The nurse auscultates the chest to determine changes in breath sounds directly related to the presence of a tumor. Wheezes indicate partial obstruction of airflow in passages narrowed by tumors. Decreased or absent breath sounds are an ominous sign. Absent breath sounds indicate impairment of air passages from obstruction by a tumor or replacement of lung tissue with a solid tumor or fluid. Auscultation of vocal fremitus (i.e., bronchophony, pectoriloquy, and egophony [see Chap. 29]) reveals changes in the sound normally heard. Increased loudness or sound intensity indicates consolidation or compression of the pleural tissue by tumor. Auscultation of a pleural friction rub suggests an inflammatory response to an invading tumor.

Cardiac Status. The nurse notes distant heart sounds, which may indicate cardiac tamponade related to an extended tumor. Dysrhythmias may be present as a result of hypoxemia. The nurse may also observe cyanosis of the lips and fingertips or clubbing (see Fig. 32–6).

Late Signs and Symptoms. Late manifestations of lung cancer may include nonspecific systemic symptoms, such as fatigue, recent weight loss, anorexia, dysphagia, and nausea and vomiting. Superior vena cava syndrome may result from intrathoracic spread of the malignant tumor; this syndrome constitutes an emergency (see Chap. 27). Lethargy and somnolence may develop; therefore, the nurse performs a baseline neurologic assessment. Bowel and bladder tone and function may be affected by tumor spread to the spine and spinal cord.

➤ Psychosocial Assessment

To complete the psychosocial assessment of the client with lung cancer, the nurse evaluates various parameters, including

- Age
- Occupation
- Previous experience with illness
- Marital status
- Dependents
- Support systems
- Usual coping mechanisms

Symptoms associated with lung cancer, especially dyspnea, often add to the client's fear and anxiety. Clients with a history of cigarette smoking may experience guilt and shame. The nurse conveys acceptance of the client and interacts in a nonjudgmental way.

Societal awareness of the poor prognosis of lung cancer poses many challenges for the client and family. Few clients with the diagnosis of lung cancer are candidates for curative therapy. Most are given palliative treatment limited to relief of symptoms. Overall survival time is only moderately lengthened. Fear of abandonment and separation is common in clients with lung cancer.

The client and family will undergo a rapid course in which the nurse

- Supports the client and family through the diagnosis and treatment phases
- Assesses the client's emotional response to the diagnosis of lung cancer
- Listens carefully to the client's and family's concerns

Family members play an important role in the physical and psychosocial care of the client. Family members and significant others can help alleviate the client's anxiety, anticipate needs, and act as liaisons between the staff and the client. The nurse recognizes that the family and significant others also have unmet psychosocial needs and assists them in expressing their needs and concerns.

The nurse identifies resources to assist the client and family in the treatment phase, through the progression of illness, and during anticipatory and actual bereavement. The nurse assesses the grief response as the client and family react to their situation and adjusts care accordingly. A holistic approach includes spiritual counseling and crisis intervention, which are incorporated into the multidisciplinary treatment plan as needed (Georgesen & Dungan, 1996). (Chapter 12 covers grief and loss in detail.)

➤ Laboratory Assessment

A definitive diagnosis of lung cancer is made by isolation of malignant cells. Cytologic examination of early morning sputum specimens may identify tumor cells. However, even with a lung tumor, malignant cells may not be obtained in sputum. With pleural effusion, fluid can be obtained for cytologic examination by thoracentesis.

➤ Radiographic Assessment

Pulmonary lesions are frequently seen on chest x-ray, but tomograms and computed tomography (CT) are used to identify the lesions clearly. CT scan identifies and localizes the extent of masses in the chest, including mediastinal and lymph node involvement.

➤ Other Diagnostic Assessment

Fiberoptic bronchoscopy is extremely important in the diagnosis of lung cancer. It provides direct visibility of the tracheobronchial tree. Specimens and bronchial brushings can thus be obtained, especially when lesions are located endobronchially or are close to an airway. Transthoracic and transbronchial needle biopsy also may be used in an attempt to obtain malignant cells.

A thoroscopy may be performed for diagnostic and therapeutic indications through a video-assisted thorascope entering the chest cavity via small incisions through the chest wall. This procedure allows direct visibility of the pulmonary tissue and leads to a definitive diagnosis (Davidson & Colt, 1997).

To identify metastasis in mediastinal lymph nodes, the physician may perform mediastinoscopy by inserting a scope through a small anterior chest incision at the suprasternal notch. Mediastinoscopy is an important staging tool for determining the extent of the lung cancer and formulating a treatment plan. If scalene (near the first rib) or supraclavicular lymph nodes are palpable, biopsy of these nodes also may be performed.

To determine a definitive diagnosis and assess overall pulmonary status, other diagnostic studies may be needed, including percutaneous needle biopsy, direct surgical biopsy, and thoracentesis with pleural biopsy. A magnetic resonance imaging (MRI) study may be ordered to identify possible invasion or compression of vascular structures by tumor. Radionuclide scans of the liver, spleen, brain, and bone may be used to assess metastasis of lung cancer. Pulmonary function studies and arterial blood gas analysis may be included to determine the client's overall respiratory status.

 Analysis

➤ *Common Nursing Diagnoses*

Three nursing diagnoses are common in clients with lung cancer:

1. Impaired Gas Exchange related to decreased lung capacity secondary to tissue destruction
2. Ineffective Airway Clearance related to tumor obstruction and increased tracheobronchial secretions
3. Pain related to tumor pressure on surrounding tissues and erosion of tissues

➤ *Additional Nursing Diagnoses and Collaborative Problems*

In addition to the common diagnoses, the client may present with one or more of the following diagnoses:

- Ineffective Breathing Pattern related to decreased energy, fatigue, pain, tracheobronchial obstruction, anxiety
- Activity Intolerance related to imbalance between oxygen supply and demand, dyspnea, fatigue, generalized weakness, weight loss, malnourishment, pain, depression
- Fluid Volume Excess related to compromised antidiuretic hormone regulating mechanism
- Risk for Injury related to metabolic imbalances (e.g., hypercalcemia)
- Fatigue related to increased metabolic energy production, overwhelming emotional demands, states of discomfort, altered body chemistry (e.g., chemotherapy)
- Risk for Trauma related to weakness
- Altered Nutrition, Less than Body Requirements related to the active disease process (increased metabolism), anorexia, nausea, vomiting
- Decreased Cardiac Output related to electrical malfunction secondary to hypoxic dysrhythmias
- Impaired Physical Mobility related to decreased strength and endurance, fatigue, intolerance to activity, dyspnea
- Anticipatory Grieving related to actual or potential loss of health status
- Anxiety related to change in health status, situational crisis, threat of death, loss of control
- Fear related to pain, threat of death, effects of loss of body part or function
- Altered Role Performance related to change in health status, role loss
- Ineffective Family Coping related to effects of major life events, effects of impending death of family member, temporary family disorganization and role changes, effects of acute or chronic illness

- Ineffective Individual Coping related to effects of acute or chronic illness, loss of control over body part or function, major changes in lifestyle, situational crisis, knowledge deficit regarding therapeutic regimen/disease process/prognosis
- Potential for Superior Vena Cava Syndrome

➤ *Impaired Gas Exchange*

Planning and Implementation. The major goal is that the client will be adequately oxygenated, as evidenced by decreased symptoms of hypoxia (such as dyspnea) and decreased signs of hypoxemia (i.e., acceptable blood gas or pulse oximetry results).

Interventions. The nurse evaluates the hypoxemic client's respiratory status as often as indicated, perhaps every 2–4 hours. Color of the skin, lips, ear lobes, and nail beds is noted. The nurse also assesses for signs of respiratory distress, such as dyspnea and use of accessory muscles for breathing. The client in obvious distress is further evaluated by pulse oximetry and arterial blood gas studies.

Nonsurgical Management

Oxygen Therapy. If the client is hypoxemic, the nurse provides supplemental oxygen via mask or nasal cannula as ordered. Even if the client is not overtly hypoxemic, the physician may order oxygen as needed to relieve dyspnea (difficulty breathing) and anxiety in the lung cancer client. (See Chapter 30 for nursing care associated with oxygen therapy.)

Drug Therapy. If the client is experiencing bronchospasm, the physician may prescribe bronchodilators (as for clients with asthma) and corticosteroids to decrease bronchospasm, inflammation, and edema.

Chemotherapy. Chemotherapy is frequently the treatment of choice for lung cancers, especially small cell lung cancer, and as adjuvant therapy in combinations with surgery or in the presence of metastasis for non–small cell lung cancer. Chemotherapy may also be used in conjunction with surgical treatment modalities. Chemotherapeutic agents commonly administered for the treatment of lung cancer include combinations such as

- Cyclosphamide, doxorubicin, and vincristine or etoposide
- Etoposide and cisplatin or carboplatin
- Ifosfamide, carboplatin, and etoposide
- Mitomycin, vinblastine, and cisplatin

Recent combination drug regimens using paclitaxel (Taxol) or vinorelbine (Navelbine) with some of these agents are yielding promising results in the treatment of lung cancer (Le Chevalier, 1996). New drug regimens containing taxines, gemcitabine, and topoisomerase 1 inhibitors are on the front line of lung cancer research (McVie, 1996).

The nurse understands the mode of action for each chemotherapeutic agent and takes measures to control common side effects (Table 32–12). The nurse supports the client and family throughout the course of chemotherapy. The nurse educates the client and family about this

TABLE 32-12

Side Effects of Chemotherapeutic Agents Used in the Treatment of Lung Cancer

Drug	Side Effects				Specific Toxic Effects
	Alopecia	Nausea and Vomiting	Bone Marrow Suppression	Diarrhea	
Cisplatin (Platinol)	+	++++	+++	–	• Constipation • Nephrotoxic effects • Ototoxic effects • Hypophosphatemia
Cyclophosphamide (Cytoxan, Procytox✦)	++	++	++	+	• Hemorrhagic cystitis • Syndrome of inappropriate antidiuretic hormone (SIADH) • Hyperpigmentation
Doxorubicin (Adriamycin)	+++	++	+++	+	• Tissue vesicant • Cardiotoxic effects • Mucositis • Hyperpigmentation
Etoposide (VP-16, Vepesid)	+++	+++	++++	–	• Constipation • Postural hypotension
Methotrexate (MTX)	+	++	+++	+	• Mucositis
Mitomycin-C (Mutamycin)	+++	++	+++	+	• Tissue vesicant • Pulmonary injury
Procarbazine (Matulane)	+	+++	+++	+++	• Postural hypotension • Myalgia • Arthralgia
Vinblastine (VLB, Velban)	+	+++	+	–	• Tissue vesicant • Pain at tumor site • Jaw pain • Neurotoxic effects • Loss of deep tendon reflexes

treatment modality and explains how to prevent and manage potential side effects. (See Chapter 27 for further discussion of chemotherapeutic agents and associated nursing care.)

Immunotherapy. Many clients with lung cancer are immunocompromised (unable to defend adequately against potentially harmful substances). Treatment is directed at enhancing an effective immune response, which favorably affects the course of the disease. Immunotherapeutic agents (cytokines) that are "growth factors" are most commonly administered. Cytokines decrease the time that the client is neutropenic (has a low white-blood-cell count) and allow continuation of chemotherapy (also see Chaps. 23 and 27).

Radiation Therapy. Radiation therapy can be an effective primary treatment for localized, unresectable, intrathoracic lung tumors. Radiation therapy also can be helpful for palliation of hemoptysis, obstruction of the bronchi and great veins (superior vena cava syndrome), dysphagia related to esophageal compression, and pain resulting from bone metastasis. Preoperative irradiation

may be attempted to shrink a tumor and promote resectability. After surgical resection of primary tumors, radiation has successfully reduced residual pleural or mediastinal disease. Because of the high frequency of brain metastasis with small cell carcinoma and adenocarcinoma, prophylactic brain radiation may be recommended for clients with these types of lung cancer.

Laser Therapy. Neodymium-yttrium aluminum garnet (YAG) lasers and (rarely) carbon dioxide lasers have been used for palliation of endobronchial obstruction in clients with benign or malignant tumors that are accessible by bronchoscopy. The surgeon debulks the obstructive portion of the tumor, and the airway is reopened. Laser therapy does not produce systemic or toxic effects and is well tolerated by most clients.

Thoracentesis and Pleurodesis. Malignant pleural effusions can be a common problem for clients with lung cancer. Effusions can be caused by involvement of the visceral or parietal pleura by tumor and also by mediastinal lymphatic obstruction or obstructive pneumonitis. The goal of treatment is to remove pleural fluid and prevent its accumulation (Fox, 1994). Thoracentesis (see Chap. 29) removes fluid from the intrapleural space and relieves immediate signs and symptoms of hypoxia.

Fluid can rapidly reaccumulate in the pleural space, and the client may again experience respiratory compromise within a few days. Repeated thoracentesis can create pain and anxiety and can place the client at risk for further complications. As an alternative to repeated thoracentesis, the physician inserts a chest tube to drain the fluid and instills a sclerosing agent, an irritant that causes inflammation and results in fibrosis of tissue. Doxycycline, thiotepa, bleomycin, minocycline, nitrogen mustard, and 5-fluorouracil as well as talc have been used for this treatment. Clinical studies have demonstrated talc to be the most effective and cost-effective sclerosing agent (Sahn, 1996). The aim of thoracentesis and intrapleural administration of one of these agents is to create a *pleurodesis,* which causes adherence of the pleura to the chest wall. Thus, the potential space is eliminated, and reaccumulation of effusion is prevented.

Before pleurodesis, the nurse medicates the client with an analgesic or sedative, as ordered. The physician anesthetizes the pleural surfaces by injecting 1% lidocaine through the chest tube. The physician instills the sclerosing agent; then the nurse or physician clamps the chest tube to prevent drainage of the agent. The physician may order that the client be rotated through various positions at 15- to 30-minute intervals. However, limited research has demonstrated that dispersion of the sclerosing agent is not enhanced by rotation of the client's position (Scott et al., 1993). Chart 32–8 reviews nursing care of the client undergoing pleurodesis.

Surgical Management

Surgery is the treatment of choice for stage I and stage II non–small cell lung cancer (see Fig. 32–10). Total resection of a non–small cell primary bronchogenic tumor is undertaken in hope of achieving a cure. If complete resectability is not possible, the surgeon removes the bulk of the tumor and decreases the possibility of metastatic extension. The choice of surgical procedure depends on the findings of the staging process and the client's overall health and functional status.

Thoracotomy. A thoracotomy is an opening into the thoracic cavity to locate tumors, perform a biopsy, or identify sites of bleeding or injury. Thoracotomy is most often performed to remove all or a portion of the lung.

Preoperative Care. The goals of preoperative care are to relieve anxiety and promote the client's participation (see Chap. 20 for routine preoperative care). The nurse uses interventions to relieve the client's anxiety related to the diagnosis of lung cancer, postoperative management, and loss of a portion or all of a lung. The nurse encourages the client to express fears and concerns, reinforces the physician's explanation of the surgical procedure, and provides education related to the postoperative course. The nurse teaches the client the anticipated location of the surgical incision, if known; shoulder exercises; and about the chest tube and drainage system (except after pneumonectomy).

Chart 32–8

Nursing Care Highlight: The Client Undergoing Pleurodesis

- Reinforce explanation of the pleurodesis and inform the client that medication will be provided to promote comfort before the procedure. (The physician may administer IV analgesia/sedation immediately before the procedure.)
- Ensure that the chest tube is clamped after instillation of the sclerosing agent.
- Monitor vital signs and respiratory status at the completion of the procedure and then at least every 30 min until the effects of the IV medication have dissipated.
- Thereafter, monitor vital signs every 4 hr for 24 hr. (The client may experience a low-grade fever. Pleurodesis creates pleuritis between the visceral and parietal layers, thus preventing reaccumulation of fluid.)
- If a rotation schedule is ordered, assist the client to the correct position for appropriate time frames and provide reassurance.
- Unclamp the chest tube after completion of the rotation schedule or at the specified time ordered by the physician.
- Assess chest tube drainage and document the amount and character of the drainage.
- Perform a complete respiratory assessment every 8 hr and observe for signs and symptoms of distress, including those of pneumothorax.
- Analgesics may be administered as needed to promote the client's comfort.
- When drainage has decreased (<150 mL in 12–24 hr), the physician may remove the chest tube. Maintain an occlusive dressing at the insertion site for a minimum of 48 hr.

Operative Procedures. Three types of incisions can be made:
- Posterolateral thoracotomy
- Anterolateral thoracotomy
- Median sternotomy

A posterolateral thoracotomy incision begins in the submammary fold of the anterior chest, is drawn down below the scapular tip and along the course of the ribs, and then curves posteriorly and upward as far as the spine of the scapula. An anterolateral thoracotomy involves an incision below the breast and above the costal margins. This incision extends from the anterior axillary line and then turns downward to avoid the axillary apex. A median sternotomy is a straight incision from the suprasternal notch to the area below the xyphoid process. The sternum must be transected with an electric or air-driven saw.

Postoperative Care. General care of the client after thoracotomy is reviewed in the Client Care Plan concerning lung cancer. Postoperative management of clients who have undergone thoracotomy requires closed-chest drainage to drain air and blood that may accumulate in the pleural space. A chest tube, a drain placed in the pleural

Text continued on page 654

Client Care Plan

The Client Who Has Had a Thoracotomy for Lung Cancer

Nursing Diagnosis No. 1: Impaired Gas Exchange related to ventilation-perfusion imbalance secondary to removal of all or part of a lung and ineffective airway clearance

Expected Outcomes	Nursing Interventions	Rationale
The client will have adequate lung expansion and mobilization of secretions.	• Perform complete respiratory assessment every 2 hr. Assess breath sounds; rate, depth, and pattern of respirations; signs and symptoms of hypoxia, including restlessness and irritability; and position of mediastinum.	• Ongoing astute assessments alert the nurse to subtle and early signs and symptoms of changes in respiratory status.
The client's blood gases and pulse oximetry will be within normal range.	• Monitor vital signs, pulse oximetry, and arterial blood gases as ordered. Report abnormalities to the physician.	• Prompt reporting of abnormalities enable the physician to institute early treatment and prevent further complications.
	• Administer oxygen therapy as ordered.	• Supplemental oxygen will help correct hypoxemia.
	• Maintain patency and integrity of the chest tube and drainage system, if present.	• A properly functioning chest drainage system promotes adequate drainage of blood and air that may accumulate in the pleural space, allowing re-expansion of the lung.
	• Assess for and report signs and symptoms of air leak from the chest tube or hemorrhage.	• Prompt reporting of abnormalities helps prevent further complications.
	• Perform pain assessment and administer analgesics as ordered. (Observe for signs and symptoms of respiratory depression related to opioids.)	• Effective pain management promotes the client's participation in deep breathing and mobility, thus fostering optimal respiratory effort.
	• Reposition the client every 2 hr. Check order for positioning carefully and seek clarification if necessary. (Do not place the client on the operative side after pneumonectomy.)	• Repositioning promotes lung expansion.
	• Encourage the client to perform deep-breathing exercises every 2 hr and to use incentive spirometry devices as soon as he or she is physically able.	• Breathing exercises promote lung expansion and help prevent atelectasis and pneumonia.
	• Coach in effective coughing technique if secretions are present. Assist to high-Fowler's position with knees bent and feet flat on bed. Instruct the client to obtain maximal inspiration and to hold the breath for 2 sec; follow by having the client cough twice with the mouth open, pause, and then inhale through the nose and rest.	• Effective coughing improves airway clearance and prevents stasis of secretions.

Client Care Plan

Expected Outcomes	Nursing Interventions	Rationale
	■ Assist the client to remove and properly dispose of secretions. ■ Assist the client to sit in a chair, when ordered, and monitor tolerance.	■ Proper disposal of secretions is required for infection control purposes. ■ Lung expansion is enhanced when the client is able to be out of bed.

Nursing Diagnosis No. 2: Pain related to tissue trauma as a result of surgery, inflammation of incised muscles, and presence of chest tubes

Expected Outcomes	Nursing Interventions	Rationale
The client will be as pain-free and alert as possible.	■ Perform a complete pain assessment using designed pain level scale (i.e., 0 = no pain, 5 = severe pain). ■ Assist with incisional splinting during deep-breathing exercises, with turning, and in anticipation of cough stimulation. ■ Secure the chest tube to prevent excessive discomfort resulting from movement of the tube. ■ Promote optimal comfort through proper positioning, hygiene, gentle massage, and relaxation techniques. ■ Administer analgesics as ordered. Plan activities to coincide with peak of analgesic effectiveness. Observe for signs and symptoms of respiratory depression associated with opioids. ■ Use diversional activities as appropriate. ■ Document the client's response to the pain control regimen and seek adjustment as needed.	■ Obtain the baseline pain assessment rating and use it for comparison with the routine pain assessment score to determine the effectiveness of pain management interventions. ■ Splinting promotes the client's comfort and participation in measures that promote respiratory function. ■ Nonpharmacologic nursing interventions are instrumental in helping the client to achieve optimal comfort. ■ The client's participation in respiratory excursion activities will be increased with effective pain management. ■ Ongoing assessment and evaluation of the effectiveness of the pain control regimen are essential to the client's optimal comfort.

(Continued)

Client Care Plan

Nursing Diagnosis No. 3: Activity Intolerance related to restricted arm and shoulder movement

Expected Outcomes	Nursing Interventions	Rationale
The client will maintain normal arm and shoulder movement and function as evidenced by the ability to perform range-of-motion exercises on the operative side.	■ Educate the client about the possible complication and prevention of "frozen shoulder syndrome." ■ Monitor and report restricted arm and shoulder movement postoperatively. ■ Perform passive range-of-motion exercises to the affected arm and shoulder 2 times every 4 hr during the first 24 hr postoperatively and then 10 times every 2 hr. ■ Instruct the client in active range-of-motion exercises beginning the second day after surgery. ■ Encourage the client to use the affected arm for activities of daily living and place frequently used items on the same side of the bed as the operative side to facilitate reaching and gentle stretching. ■ Administer analgesic as needed to promote active participation in exercises. ■ Offer encouragement and support for the client's progress.	■ The client is more likely to actively participate in preventive measures when he or she is knowledgeable about this potential postoperative complication. ■ Ongoing assessments help detect early signs of complications. ■ Exercising maintains strength, facilitates mobility, and prevents fixation. ■ Active participation by the client promotes well-being, autonomy, and independence. ■ Effective levels of analgesia allow the client to perform prescribed exercises and prevent complications. ■ Positive reinforcement enables the client to continue the rehabilitation process.

Nursing Diagnosis No. 4: Body Image Disturbance related to actual change in body structure and function

Expected Outcomes	Nursing Interventions	Rationale
The client will verbalize feelings about loss of all or part of a lung and identify ways in which to compensate for altered lung capacity.	■ Establish a therapeutic nurse-client relationship by building trust and confidence. ■ Encourage expression of feelings and concerns related to lung cancer diagnosis, grief about loss of lung, and effects on lifestyle. ■ Support a realistic hope of regaining aspects of usual activities.	■ Sincere behaviors that display concern and caring enable the client to feel comfortable and at ease with the nurse. ■ Ventilation of feelings and concerns can serve as an effective coping strategy and assist the client to express needs. ■ Hope is a universal coping mechanism and can enable the client to attain activity potential within the present physical limitations.

Client Care Plan

Expected Outcomes	Nursing Interventions	Rationale
	■ Assist the client to identify activities that can be performed with present lung capacity.	■ Identification of activities that can be performed by the client encourages independence and increased self-esteem.
	■ Identify measures to promote increased endurance and participation in activities (i.e., carefully schedule activities, ensure rest periods and proper nutrition).	■ Energy conservation and health promotion activities assist the client to achieve optimal physical activity.
	■ Provide support for accomplishments and encourage the concept of slow progression without compromising respiratory status.	■ Positive reinforcement of achievements enhances body image and self-esteem.

Nursing Diagnosis No. 5: Knowledge Deficit related to care after hospitalization

Expected Outcomes	Nursing Interventions	Rationale
The client will verbalize follow-up care and signs and symptoms to report to the primary care provider.	■ Review the discharge instructions with the client, including follow-up visit, medications, permitted activities, and arm and shoulder exercises.	■ Ensuring that the client understands required information before discharge promotes the client's participation in the treatment plan and minimizes anxiety after discharge.
	■ Instruct the client to report signs and symptoms of fever, cough and sputum production, increased discomfort, or dyspnea to the primary care provider (physician or nurse).	■ Early detection and treatment of possible respiratory infection or other respiratory complications can reduce the extent of the complication.
	■ Encourage the client to pace tolerable activities and rest periods.	
	■ Reinforce that heavy lifting is to be avoided for 6 months and to stop any activity that provokes excessive dyspnea or discomfort.	■ When the client understands how to balance and limit activities, complications can be prevented.
	■ Review and educate the client about additional proposed treatment as indicated (chemotherapy, radiation therapy).	■ Education related to further treatment modalities fosters the client's understanding of and compliance with the treatment plan and can reduce anxiety and possible misconceptions.
	■ Refer the client to appropriate community resources, if indicated (e.g., home health agency, American Cancer Society, American Lung Association).	■ Community resources are an additional avenue for information and support.

space to restore intrapleural pressure, allows re-expansion of the lung. The chest tube also prevents air and fluid from returning to the chest. The drainage system consists of

- One or more chest tubes or drains
- A collection container placed below the chest level
- A water seal to keep air from entering the chest

The tip of the tube used to drain air is usually placed anteriorly near the lung apex. The tube that drains liquid is placed laterally near the base of the lung. After lung resection, two tubes, anterior and posterior, are used. The puncture wounds are covered with airtight dressings.

The chest tube is connected to approximately 6 feet of tubing that leads to a collection device placed several feet below the chest. The tubing allows the client to turn and move easily. Positioning the collection device below the chest allows gravity to drain the pleural space. When two chest tubes are inserted, they are usually joined by a Y-connector near the client's body; the 6 feet of tubing are attached to the Y-connector.

The chest drainage system has a separate water seal mechanism that acts as a one-way valve. In setting up current chest drainage systems, the nurse adds a specified amount of sterile saline to the water seal chamber. (In older systems, the end of the tubing was placed beneath the surface of a sterile saline solution to create the water seal.) The water seal closes the open end of the system (or the end of the tubing) from the atmosphere. When the positive pressure in the lungs during exhalation pushes air out of the pleural space through the tubing, the air bubbles into the saline and cannot re-enter the chest.

Earlier chest drainage consisted of one-, two-, and three-bottle systems. Technology has greatly improved these bulky glass bottle systems through the availability of one-piece disposable chest drainage devices. The Pleur-Evac system, one of the most widely distributed, uses a one-piece disposable, molded plastic unit with three chambers. This system duplicates the older three-bottle system. From right to left, the system contains chambers for drainage, a water seal, and suction control (Fig. 32–11). The plastic devices reduce the risk of breakage or contamination of the drainage system and allow the client increased mobility. All systems are vented so that incoming pleural air cannot build up, thereby preventing further air entry into the chest. Suction may be added, as ordered.

In one system, a knob on the collection device can be set to the ordered amount of suction. The wall suction source dial is then turned until a small orange floater valve appears in a certain window (Fig. 32–12). When the orange valve is in the window, the right amount of suction has been applied. With this system, the nurse notes the absence of bubbling in the chamber, which is normal for this so-called dry suction system.

The nurse routinely checks to ensure the sterility and patency of the system. The nurse tapes the tubing junctions to prevent accidental disconnections and maintains an occlusive dressing at the chest tube insertion site. To cover the insertion site immediately if the chest tube becomes accidentally dislodged, sterile gauze is kept at the bedside. The nurse keeps heavily padded clamps at the bedside for use if the drainage system is inadvertently interrupted or to facilitate changing of the drainage system when necessary. The nurse carefully positions the drainage tubing to prevent kinks and large loops of tubing, which can impede drainage and lung re-expansion. Vigorous stripping of the chest tube should be avoided. Gentle milking of the tube, however, may prevent obstruction by moving any blood clots.

The nurse assesses the client's respiratory status and notes the amount and type of drainage. Immediately after surgery, the nurse records hourly the amount of drainage. Drainage of more than 100 mL/hr is considered excessive, and the physician is notified. After the first 24 hours, the nurse usually assesses drainage and the drainage system minimally every 8 hours.

The nurse checks the water seal chamber for unexpected bubbling created by an air leak in the system. Bubbling is anticipated during forceful expiration or coughing because air in the chest is being expelled. Continuous bubbling indicates an air leak and requires an effort to identify its source. On the physician's order, the nurse gently applies a padded clamp on the drainage tubing close to the occlusive dressing. If the bubbling stops, the air leak may be at the chest tube insertion site or within the chest. Further assessment of the insertion site and chest tube position is necessary, and the nurse consults the physician for identified problems. Air bubbling that does not cease when the nurse applies a padded clamp indicates that the air leak is between the clamp and the drainage system. For ensuring patency and sterility of the system, this tubing and drainage device should be replaced, as ordered.

The nurse also checks for rising and falling of fluid in the water seal as the client breathes in and out. These fluctuations act like a manometer by representing the pressure changes in the pleural space, and they reliably indicate overall respiratory effort. Fluctuations of 5–10 cm (2–4 inches) during normal breathing are common. The absence of fluctuations could mean the tubing is obstructed by a kink, the client is lying on the tubing, or dependent fluid has filled a loop of tubing. Expanded lung tissue can also block the chest tube eyelets during expiration, or no more air may be leaking into the pleural space.

Suction can be added to current collection systems on physician's order. Suction enhances the pressure difference between the pleural space and the drainage system, causing the pressure to drop inside the system by 15–20 cm. In some systems, the ordered amount of suction, often a negative 20 cm, is determined by the height of the saline in the water seal chamber. When suction is added, air is pulled down into the water seal chamber. When the depth of the saline solution is 20 cm, 20 cm of water creates the negative pressure required to pull air to the bottom of the chamber, where it bubbles out into the solution. While suction is applied, the nurse notes gentle bubbling in the chamber. The depth of the saline determines the maximal suction level for the system. Increasing the suction source causes more bubbling, but it cannot increase the effective suction because the outside air offsets any further air removal. When vigorous bubbling is noted, an air leak may be present. Bubbling also en-

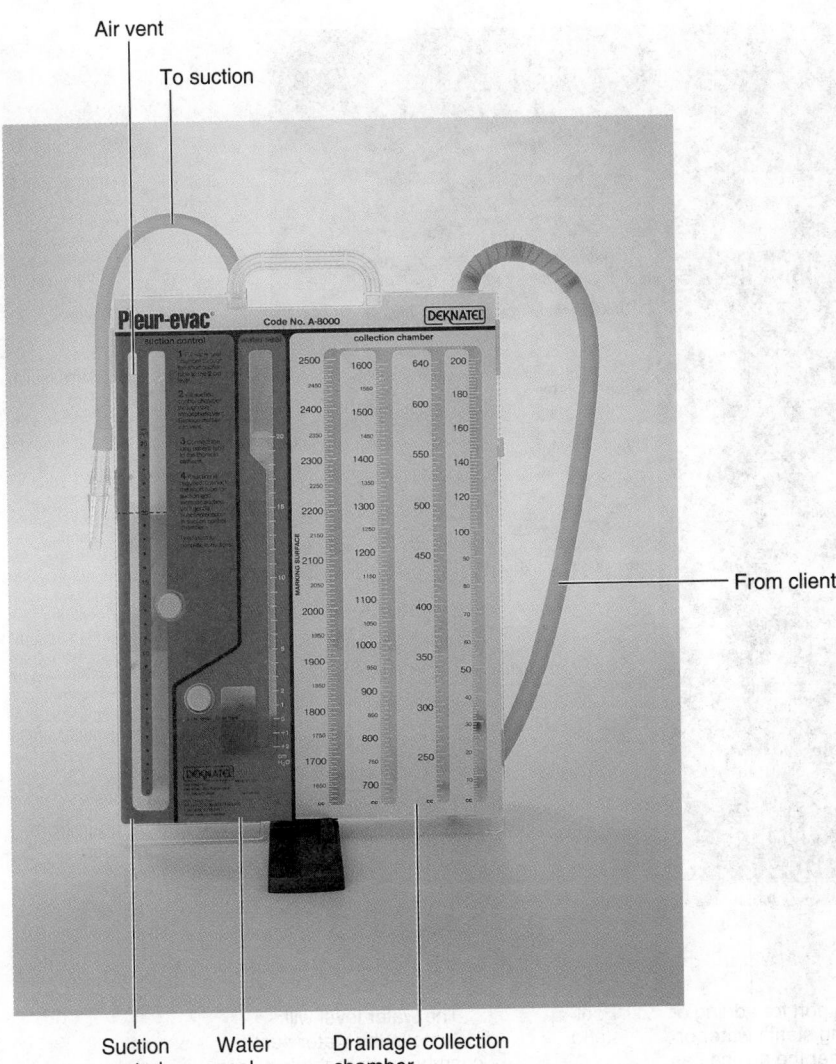

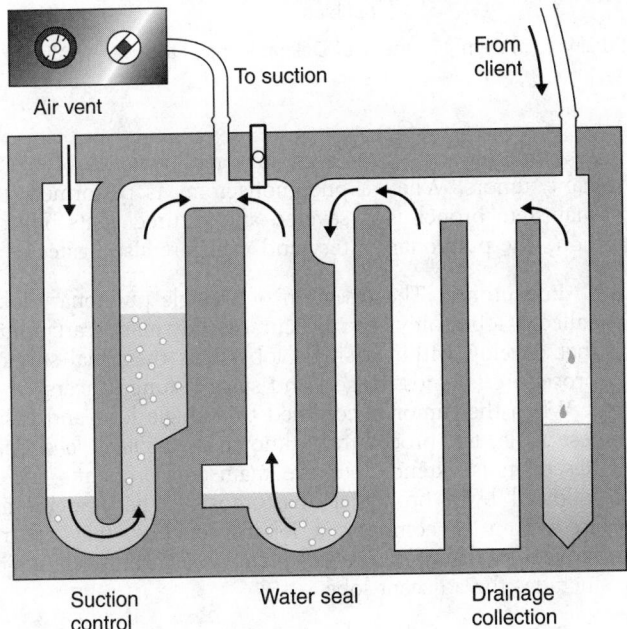

Figure 32–11. *Top,* The Pleur-Evac drainage system, a commercial three-bottle chest drainage device. *Bottom,* Schematic of the drainage device.

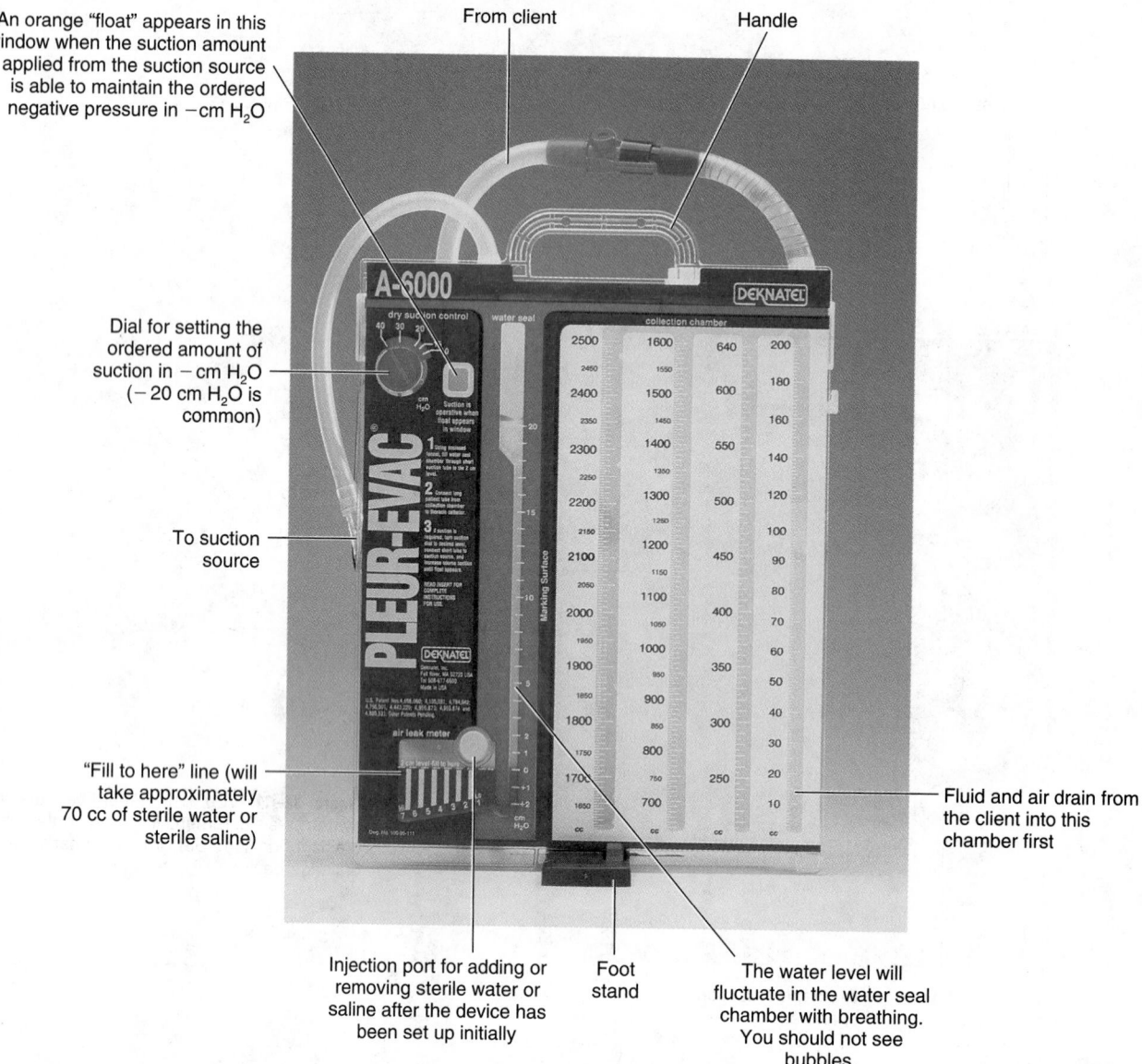

An orange "float" appears in this window when the suction amount applied from the suction source is able to maintain the ordered negative pressure in −cm H₂O

From client

Handle

Dial for setting the ordered amount of suction in −cm H₂O (−20 cm H₂O is common)

To suction source

"Fill to here" line (will take approximately 70 cc of sterile water or sterile saline)

Fluid and air drain from the client into this chamber first

Injection port for adding or removing sterile water or saline after the device has been set up initially

Foot stand

The water level will fluctuate in the water seal chamber with breathing. You should not see bubbles.

Figure 32–12. The A-6000 dry suction control Pleur-Evac chest drainage system. (Courtesy of Deknatel, Inc., Fall River, MA.)

hances evaporation, so that the nurse adds more sterile saline in the chamber as needed.

Other Procedures

Preoperative Care. The preoperative care for the client undergoing these surgical procedures is the same as for the client having a thoracotomy.

Operative Procedures

Pneumonectomy. Pneumonectomy, removal of an entire lung, is required for

- Large, centrally located bronchogenic tumors
- Involvement of a mainstem bronchus
- Invasion of the main pulmonary artery

Less frequent indications for pneumonectomy include extensive unilateral tuberculosis (TB), extensive bronchiecta-

sis, multiple lung abscesses, and rare varieties of malignant tumors. When a pneumonectomy is performed, the mainstem bronchus is severed and sutured at its bifurcation. The pulmonary artery and veins are also ligated.

Lobectomy. The resection of a single pulmonary lobe, called a lobectomy, can be curative for many carcinomas that develop within a single lobe. It is the usual surgical procedure for most stage I and stage II lung cancers.

When the tumor is confined to a single lobe and easily resectable, the procedure is known as a *simple lobectomy*. Resection is extended to the mainstem bronchus and is followed by a bronchial anastomosis. When carcinomas are within or compress a lobar bronchus, they are removed by using a *sleeve lobectomy (bilobectomy)*, which includes the adjacent lobe.

Resection. A limited pulmonary resection is any surgical resection of the lung that does not involve a complete lobectomy. A *limited resection* is considered only when the lung tumor is in stage I, the tumor size is 3 cm or less, and the client's pulmonary status is compromised. A lung resection may be used if the client cannot tolerate a lobectomy or pneumonectomy.

A *segmental resection (segmentectomy)* is a pulmonary resection that includes the bronchus, pulmonary artery and vein, and lung parenchyma of the involved lung segment or segments, which are divisions of lobes. A *wedge resection* is removal of the peripheral portion of small localized areas of disease.

Postoperative Care. After pneumonectomy, the pleural cavity on the affected side is an empty space. The physician sometimes inserts a clamped chest tube for only a day because serous fluid may then accumulate in the empty space and create adhesions, which reduce mediastinal shift toward the affected side. Closed-chest drainage is not usually used.

Possible complications of a pneumonectomy can include empyema and the development of a bronchopleural fistula. The nurse is careful not to turn the client onto the operative side immediately after a pneumonectomy. Positioning on the operative side can place increased stress on the bronchial stump incision and risk disruption of the suture line.

After lobectomy, the remaining lung tissue expands to fill in the portion of lung space previously occupied by the removed lung tissue. A chest tube is usually inserted for postoperative closed drainage. Nursing care after lobectomy or lung resection is the same as for the client undergoing thoracotomy (see the Client Care Plan concerning lung cancer). The nurse continues to assess respiratory status and observes for general postoperative complications (see Chap. 22).

➤ Ineffective Airway Clearance

Planning: Expected Outcomes. The client should
- Breathe without dyspnea or discomfort
- Maintain a patent airway

Interventions. The client who produces copious secretions may benefit from the use of a humidifier and a vaporizer, which provide moisture to loosen the secretions. The nurse suctions the client, as indicated and as ordered, to clear secretions from the airway. If the client also has an underlying chronic lung disease, beta agonists and inhaled steroids may relieve symptoms. In moderately advanced disease, postural drainage and chest physiotherapy may help.

The client with lung cancer fatigues easily and is often most comfortable resting in a semi-Fowler's position. Dyspnea can be reduced with supplemental oxygen, use of a morphine drip, and positioning for comfort and to facilitate drainage of secretions. The severely dyspneic client may be most comfortable sitting in a lounge or a reclining chair. The nurse monitors the amount of blood loss in the client with hemoptysis. Because blood is an excellent medium for bacterial growth, the nurse is alert for signs and symptoms of infection. The nurse and phy-

sician work closely together to provide a regimen effective in relieving pain, discomfort, and dyspnea.

➤ Pain

Planning: Expected Outcomes. The client should experience relief or reduction of pain and discomfort.

Interventions. The client with lung cancer may experience chest pain and possibly subscapular pain radiating to the arm. With bone metastasis, the client may also experience bone pain. The nurse performs a complete pain assessment with attention to
- Onset, intensity, quality, duration, and client's description of the pain
- Discomfort
- Accompanying symptoms
- Factors that alleviate the pain
- Factors that increase the intensity of the pain

The nurse needs to identify ways in which to correlate the nursing assessment of pain with the client's self-reporting. Accurate interpretation of the client's perception of the pain experience leads to improved pain management, minimized suffering, and optimal functioning of the client with lung cancer (Wilkie et al., 1995). The nurse intervenes with nonpharmacologic measures, such as positioning, hot or cold compresses, distractions, and guided imagery. The nurse administers prescribed analgesic medications, as ordered, to foster pain relief. Oral, parenteral, transdermal opioid analgesics or an intravenous opioid infusion may be used for more severe pain in clients with advanced disease. The nurse observes the clients' respiratory status for changes when administering potentially respiration-depressing medications. Clients experiencing pain usually have advanced disease and a limited prognosis. Ongoing assessment and evaluation of the effectiveness of the pain control regimen is a primary nursing responsibility (Kodiath & Kodiath, 1995). The nurse's goal is to assist the client to be as pain free and as comfortable as possible.

 Continuing Care

➤ Health Teaching

Symptom Management

The nurse reviews any limitations of physical activity with the client and family and prescribes an acceptable activity level. Nurses provide instruction on dealing with dyspnea and explain positions that facilitate easier breathing, such as leaning forward and sitting in a chair. The nurse emphasizes the need to prevent exposure to others with infections and outlines signs and symptoms that should be reported to health care professionals. The nurse instructs the family to call the physician when the prescribed pain medications or respiratory therapy is not providing comfort and when the client is not receiving adequate relief from dyspnea. The nurse also provides specific information about medications as well as safety precautions for the use of oxygen.

Psychosocial Preparation

Psychosocial interventions differ, depending on the prognosis. The client with resectable carcinoma of the lung can be encouraged to have an optimistic outlook and gradually to resume normal activities. The nurse continues to help the client and family with their fear of death and their anxiety related to the cancer diagnosis as well as the client's uncertain future health.

The client whose prognosis is poor is one who, with the family, is facing death. The nurse facilitates the expression of fears and concerns, encourages the client and family to maintain open lines of communication, and stresses the quality of life defined by the client. The nurse's continued support and understanding can help the client and family through this difficult time. The nurse, case manager, or social worker makes referrals to community hospice and home care agencies as indicated. (Chapter 12 presents nursing interventions for people experiencing loss and grief.)

Home Care Management

Clients and their families usually have significant needs upon the client's discharge from the acute care setting. The nurse works with the client and family before discharge to identify their expected needs. Appropriate referrals are made to community agencies, including home health nursing or hospice programs as indicated. The nurse coordinates arrangements for oxygen and other respiratory therapy to be available if needed by the client at home.

Health Care Resources

For the client in the terminal phase of lung cancer, a referral to a hospice program can be beneficial. The discharge-planning nurse, case manager, or social worker can assist in making these arrangements. Hospice programs provide support to the terminally ill client and the family by meeting physical and psychosocial needs, adjusting the palliative care regimen as needed, making home visits, and providing volunteers for errands and respite care. The American Cancer Society may also be able to provide assistance through support groups for clients and families or through the use of equipment, such as a hospital bed.

 Evaluation

In evaluating the care of the client with lung cancer, the nurse expects that the client will
- Maintain a patent airway
- State that pain or discomfort is reduced or alleviated
- Breathe without severe dyspnea
- Maintain acceptable arterial blood gas levels
- Resolve the reality of the diagnosis and prognosis
- State an understanding of the treatment plan
- Experience no major complications from radiation therapy, chemotherapy, or surgery

---

 CASE STUDY for the Client with Lung Cancer

■ G.F. is a 62-year-old married man with three independent children. He was initially seen by his family physician and treated for an upper respiratory tract infection. His symptoms did not resolve, and further diagnostic tests were initiated. G.F. presents now with a 6-week history of right shoulder pain and dyspnea on exertion, cough productive of yellow sputum, a 7-pound weight loss over the last 4 weeks, and intermittent diaphoresis.

MEDICAL HISTORY

No chronic illness
Pneumonia: 1992
Bronchitis: "every year or so"
No current medications
Alcohol: social
Tobacco: quit smoking 4 years ago, prior 40-pack-year history

FAMILY HISTORY

Father: deceased, age 68, emphysema
Mother: deceased, age 72, myocardial infarction
Brother: alive, age 64, hypertension
Sisters: alive, ages 59, 66; no chronic illness

PHYSICAL EXAMINATION

■ Well-developed, alert, and oriented male in no acute distress. Vital signs: afebrile; pulse, 124; respirations, 24; blood pressure, 138/72. Neck exam revealed three right-sided supraclavicular lymph nodes measuring approximately 1–2 cm in diameter. Auscultation of the chest: lungs clear on the left and rhonchi on the right. The abdomen was soft, nondistended with positive bowel sounds in all quadrants, and no hepatosplenomegaly. The extremities were without clubbing, cyanosis, or edema. Right shoulder and axilla tenderness was noted.

DIAGNOSTIC STUDIES

■ Chest computed tomography (CT) revealed a 3-cm mass in the apex of the right lung with invasion into the right axilla. Additionally, tracheobronchial and mediastinal lymph node enlargement was noted. Bone scan: normal. CT of head: mild atrophy without lesions. CT-guided fine needle biopsy: Tissue samples revealed adenocarcinoma of the lung, classified as non–small cell lung carcinoma. Staging bronchoscopy and mediastinoscopy: Bronchoscopy demonstrated no evidence of endobronchial lesions, and mediastinoscopy showed additional mediastinal lymph node involvement measuring greater than 1.5 cm. Histologic staging: stage IIIb T2, N3, M0.

QUESTIONS:

1. On the basis of G.F.'s staging, what treatment is most likely to be recommended?
2. In preparing G.F. for treatment, what areas does the nurse need to include in the teaching plan?
3. To what resources can the nurse direct G.F.?

CASE STUDY for the Client with Chronic Airflow Limitation

■ A 55-year-old man arrives at your primary care clinic with complaints of persistent cough, shortness of breath, and occasional wheezing. His symptoms have become progressively worse over the past 2 weeks. The client's medical history includes hypertension. Social history includes tobacco abuse for 15 years, and the client currently smokes one pack of cigarettes per day.

Current medications include daily vitamins and atenolol, 50 mg per day. Vital signs are blood pressure, 130/78; pulse, 96; and respirations, 26. The client denies any sputum production, fever, and chills.

QUESTIONS:

1. While obtaining a history from your client, what important questions do you want to ask?
2. What initial physical assessments do you want to perform?
3. What are some possible diagnoses related to the symptoms?
4. What interventions may be ordered or implemented to minimize or treat the client's symptoms?
5. What are some key educational interventions related to health promotion or disease prevention that you will consider and or implement?

SELECTED BIBLIOGRAPHY

Aboussouan, L. S. (1996). Acute exacerbations of chronic bronchitis. *Postgraduate Medicine, 99*(4), 89–102.

Alberts, W. M., & Brooks, S. M. (1995). Occupational asthma. *Postgraduate Medicine, 97*(6), 93–104.

*American Thoracic Society. (1991). Standards of nursing care for adult patients with pulmonary dysfunction. *American Review of Respiratory Disease, 144*(1), 231–236.

American Thoracic Society. (1995). Standards for the diagnosis and care of patients with chronic obstructive pulmonary disease. *American Journal of Respiratory and Critical Care Medicine, 152*(5), S78–S121.

Baldini, E. H. (1997). Palliative radiation therapy for non–small cell lung cancer. *Hematology/Oncology Clinics of North America, 11*(20), 303–319.

Ball, P. (1995). Epidemiology and treatment of chronic bronchitis and its exacerbations. *Chest, 108*(2), 43S–52S.

Benson, V., & Marano, M. A. (1994). *Current estimates from the National Health Interview Survey* (DHHS Pub. No. [PHS] 94–1517). Hyattsville, MD: National Center for Health Statistics.

Berg, D. T. (1997). New chemotherapy treatment options and implications for nursing care. *Oncology Nursing Forum Suppl, 24*(1), 5–12.

Blackmon, G. M., & Raghu, G. (1995). Pulmonary sarcoidosis: A mimic of respiratory infection. *Seminars of Respiratory Infections, 10*(3), 176–186.

Bone, R. C. (1996). Goals of asthma management. A step care approach. *Chest, 109*(4), 1056–1065.

Bordow, R. A., Moser, K. M. (1996). Manual of clinical problems in pulmonary medicine (4th ed.). Philadelphia, PA: Lippincott-Raven.

Bunn, P. A. (1996a). Combination paclitaxel and platinum in the treatment of lung cancer: U.S. experience. *Seminars in Oncology Suppl, 23*(6), 9–16.

Bunn, P. A. (1996b). Current therapy for small cell lung cancer. *Seminars in Oncology Suppl, 23*(6), 1–5.

Busse, W. W. (1996). Long and short acting beta$_2$-adrenergic agonists. *Archives of Internal Medicine, 156*, 1514–1520.

*Busse, W. W., Lemanske, R. F., & Dick, E. C. (1992). The relationship of viral respiratory infections and asthma. *Chest, 101*(6), 385s–388s.

Carney, D. N. (1996). Non–small cell lung cancer: Slow but definite progress. *Seminars in Oncology, 23*(6), 5–6.

*Carrieri-Kohlman, V., Douglas, M. K., Gormley, J. M., & Stulbarg, M. S. (1993). Desensitization and guided mastery: Treatment approaches for the management of dyspnea. *Heart and Lung, 22*(3), 226–234.

Carroll, P. (1995). Chest tubes made easier. *RN, 58*(12), 46–55.

Celli, B. R. (1995). Pulmonary rehabilitation in patients with COPD. *American Journal of Respiratory and Critical Care Medicine, 152*, 861–864.

Celli, B. R. (1996). Current thoughts regarding treatment of chronic obstructive pulmonary disease. *Medical Clinics of North America, 80*(3), 589–609.

Chan-Yeung, M. (1995). Assessment of asthma in the workplace. *Chest, 108*(4), 1084–1117.

Chang, J. T., Moran, M. B., Cugell, D. W., & Webster, J. R. (1995). COPD in the elderly. *Chest, 108*(3), 736–740.

Chapman, K. R. (1996). Therapeutic approaches to chronic obstructive pulmonary disease: An emerging consensus. *American Journal of Medicine, 100*(Suppl. 1A), 1A-5S–1A-10S.

Chestnutt, A. N. (1995). Enigmas in sarcoidosis. *Western Journal of Medicine, 162*(6), 519–526.

Chiocca, E., & Russo, L. (1997). Action stat: Acute asthma attack. *Nursing97, 26*(7), 43.

Cockcroft, D. W., & Dosman, J. A. (1996). Obstructive lung diseases, part II. *The Medical Clinics of North America.*

Cockcroft, D. W., & Kalra, S. (1996). Outpatient asthma management. *Medical Clinics of North America, 80*(4), 701–718.

Couser, J. I., Guthmann, B. A., Hamadeh, M. A., & Kane, C. S. (1995). Pulmonary rehabilitation improves exercise capacity in older elderly patients with COPD. *Chest, 107*(3), 730–734.

Davidson, J. E,. & Colt, H. G. (1997). Thoracoscopy: Nursing implications for optimal patient outcomes. *Dimensions of Critical Care Nursing, 16*(1), 20–28.

*DeLetter, M. C. (1991). Nutritional implications for chronic airflow limitation patients. *Journal of Gerontological Nursing, 17*(5), 21–26.

DeRemee, R. (1995). Concise review for primary-care physicians. *Mayo Clinic Procedures, 70*, 177–181.

Dosman, J. A., & Cockcroft, D. W. (1996). Obstructive lung diseases, part I. *The Medical Clinics of North America.*

Dow, J. S., & Mest, C. G. (1997). Psychosocial interventions for patients with chronic obstructive pulmonary disease. *Home Healthcare Nurse, 15*(6), 414–420.

Emmons, K. M., & Kawachi, I. Tobacco control: A brief relief of its history and prospects for the future. *Hematology/Oncology Clinics of North America, 11*(2), 177–195.

*Faryniarz, K., & Mahler, D. (1990). Writing an exercise prescription for patients with COPD. *Journal of Respiratory Diseases, 11*(7), 638–648.

Fieler, V. K., Wlasowicz, G. S., Mitchell, M. L., Jones, L. S., & Johnson, J. E. (1996). Information preferences of patients undergoing radiation therapy. *Oncology Nursing Forum, 23*(10), 1603–1608.

Fiocco, M., & Krasna, M. J. (1997). The management of pleural and pericardial effusions. *Hematology/Oncology Clinics of North America, 11*(20), 253–265.

Fishman, A. P. (1994). Pulmonary rehabilitation research. *American Journal of Respiratory and Critical Care Medicine, 149*, 825–833.

Fox, J. M. (1994). Malignant pleural effusion. *MEDSURG Nursing, 3*(5), 353–360.

*Frank-Stromborg, M., & Rohan, K. (1992). Nursing's involvement in primary and secondary prevention of cancer: Nationally and internationally. *Cancer Nursing, 15*(2), 79–108.

Garshick, E., Schenker, M., & Dosman, J. (1996). Occupationally induced airways obstruction. *Medical Clinics of North America, 80*(4), 851–878.

Gazarian, P. K. (1997). Teaching your patient to use a metered-dose inhaler: The direct route for asthma therapy. *Nursing97, 27*(10), 52–54.

Georgesen, J., & Dungan, J. M. (1996). Managing spiritual distress in patients with advanced cancer pain. *Cancer Nursing, 19*(5), 376–383.

Gianaris, P. G., & Golish, J. A. (1994). Changing strategies in the management of asthma. *Postgraduate Medicine, 95*(5), 105–110.

Gibbons, M. (1996). Rx for asthma: Are providers following the NHLBI strategy? *ADVANCE for Nurse Practitioners, 4*(7), 45–47.

*Gift, A. G., & Cahill, C. (1990). Psychophysiologic aspects of dyspnea in chronic obstructive pulmonary disease: A pilot study. *Heart and Lung, 19*(3), 252–257.

*Gift, A. G., Moore, T., & Soeken, K. (1992). Relaxation to reduce dyspnea and anxiety in COPD patients. *Nursing Research, 41*(4), 242–246.

Glover, J., & Miaskowski, C. (1994). Small cell lung cancer: Pathophysiologic mechanisms and nursing implications. *Oncology Nursing Forum, 21*(1), 87–97.

Goldstein, R. H., & Fine, A. (1995). Potential therapeutic initiatives for fibrogenic lung disease. *Chest, 108*(3), 848–855.

Gray-Donald, K., Gibbons, L., Shapiro, S. H., Macklem, P. T., & Martin, J. G. (1996). Nutritional status and mortality in chronic obstructive pulmonary disease. *American Journal of Respiratory and Critical Care Medicine, 153*, 961–966.

Hanson, M. J. S. (1997). The theory of planned behavior applied to cigarette smoking in African-American, Puerto Rican, and non-Hispanic white teenage females. *Nursing Research, 46*(3), 155–162.

*Houston, S. J., & Kendall, J. A. (1992). Psychosocial implications of lung cancer. *Nursing Clinics of North America, 27*(3), 681–690.

Hunninghake, G. W., & Kalica, A. R. (1995). Approaches to the treatment of pulmonary fibrosis. *American Journal of Respiratory and Critical Care Medicine, 151*, 915–918.

Imbruce, R. P., & Selevan, J. (1997). Pharmacoeconomics and the quality of life in the diagnosis and management of asthma: What is your FEEVY? *The Journal of Care Management, 3*(Suppl., 3), 1–10.

Kanner, R. E. (1996). Early intervention in chronic obstructive pulmonary disease. *Medical Clinics of North America, 80*(3), 523–544.

*Kersten, L. D. (1989). *Comprehensive respiratory nursing: A decision making approach.* Philadelphia: W. B. Saunders.

Knoell, D. L., & Wewers, M. D. (1995). Clinical implications of gene therapy for alpha$_1$-antitrypsin deficiency. *Chest, 107*(2), 535–545.

Kodiath, M. F., & Kodiath, A. (1995). A comparative study of patients who experience chronic malignant pain in India and the United States. *Cancer Nursing, 18*(3), 189–196.

*Kronenberg, R. S., & Griffith, D. E. (1993). Chronic bronchitis: Key points in evaluation. *Postgraduate Medicine, 94*(8), 93–100.

Langhorne, M. (1996). Chemotherapy. In S. E. Otto (Ed.), *Oncology nursing* (pp. 530–572). St. Louis, MO: C. V. Mosby.

Lareau, S. C. (1996). Functional status instruments: Outcome measure in the evaluation of patients with chronic obstructive pulmonary disease. *Heart and Lung, 25*(3), 212–224.

Lazarus, S. C., & Lofholm, P. W. (1996). *Asthma management: Optimizing the healthcare team.* Laguana, CA: The Institute of Medical Studies.

Le Chevalier, T. (1996). New directions in anticancer chemotherapy. *Seminars in Oncology, 23*(6), 1–2.

Lee, J. D., & Ginsberg, R. J. (1997). The multimodality treatment of stage III a/b non-small cell lung cancer. *Hematology/Oncology Clinics of North America, 11*(20), 279–299.

Lemiere, C., Malo, J., & Gautrin, D. (1996). Nonsensitizing causes of occupational asthma. *Medical Clinics of North America, 80*(4), 749–774.

*Lordi, G. M., & Reichman, L. B. (1993). Pulmonary complications of asbestos exposure. *American Family Physician, 48*(8), 1471–1477.

*Make, B. (1991). COPD: Management and rehabilitation. *American Family Physician, 43*(4), 1315–1324.

Manning, D., Etzel, R., & Parrish, G. (1996). Pulmonary fibrosis deaths in the United States, 1979–1991. *American Journal of Respiratory and Critical Care Medicine, 153*, 1548–1552.

Mathews, P. J. (1997). Using a peak flowmeter. *Nursing97, 27*(6), 57–59.

*McDowell, K. (1993). Drugs for acute bronchitis: An up-to-date guide. *Nursing93, 23*(5), 32I–32L.

McGregor, R. J., & Schakenbach, L. H. (1996). Lung volume reduction surgery: A new breath of life for emphysema patients. *MEDSURG Nursing, 5*(4), 245–252.

McMillian, S. C. (1996). Pain and pain relief experienced by hospice patients with cancer. *Cancer Nursing, 19*(4), 298–307.

McVie, J. G. (1996). Non-small cell lung cancer: Meta-analysis of efficacy of chemotherapy. *Seminars in Oncology, 23*(3), 12–14.

Middleton, A. D. (1997). Managing asthma: It takes team work. *American Journal of Nursing, 97*(1), 39–43.

Minna, J. A. (1996). Molecular biology overview. In H. I. Pass, J. B. Mitchell, D. H. Johnson, & A. T. Turrisi (Eds.), *Lung cancer* (pp. 143–148). Philadelphia, PA: Lippincott-Raven.

Miracle, V., & Miller, D. (1997). Lung volume reduction surgery: Making room for easier breathing. *Nursing97, 27*(6), 65–68.

*Mountain, C. F., Greenberg, S. D., & Fraire, A. E. (1991). Tumor stage in non-small cell carcinoma of the lung. *Chest, 99*(5), 1258–1259.

Nagai, S., & Izumi, T. (1995). Pulmonary sarcoidosis: Population differences and pathophysiology. *Southern Medical Journal, 88*(10), 1001–1010.

*National Center for Health Statistics. (1993). *Health United States, 1992 and healthy people 2000 review* (DHHS Pub. No. [PHS] 93–1232). Hyattsville, MD: Public Health Service.

National Center for Health Statistics. (1996). *Health, United States, 1995* (DHHS Pub. No. [PHS] 96–1232). Hyattsville, MD: Public Health Service.

*National Institute of Health. (1997). *Guidelines for the diagnosis and management of asthma. Expert panel report 2*(97–4051). Bethesda, MD: U.S. Department of Health and Human Services.

Naunheim, K. S., & Ferguson, M. K. (1996). The current status of lung volume reduction operations for emphysema. *Annals of Thoracic Surgery, 62*, 601–612.

Nally, A. T. (1996). Critical care of the patient with lung cancer. *AACN Clinical Issues, 7*(1), 79–94.

*Nelson, D. M. (1992). Interventions related to respiratory care. *The Nursing Clinics of North America, 27*(2), 301–323.

Nelson, H. S. (1995). Beta adrenergic bronchodilators. *New England Journal of Medicine, 333*(8), 499–506.

*O'Donnell, D. E., Webb, K. A., & McGuire, M. A. (1993). COPD: Benefits of exercise training. *Geriatrics, 48*(1), 59–69.

Parker, S. L., Tong, T., Bolden, S., & Wingo, P. A. (1997). Cancer statistics, 1997. *CA: A Cancer Journal for Clinicians, 47*(1), 5–27.

*Petty, T. (1990). *Treatment of asthma in the 1990's.* Princeton, NJ: Excerpta Medica.

*Piirila, P. (1992). Changes in crackle characteristics during the clinical course of pneumonia. *Chest, 102*(1), 176–183.

*Reed, P. G. (1991). Preferences for spiritually related nursing interventions among terminally ill and nonterminally ill hospitalized adults and well adults. *Applied Nursing Research, 4*(3), 122–128.

Reid, D. W., & Samrai, B. (1995). Respiratory muscle training for patients with chronic obstructive pulmonary disease. *Physical Therapy, 75*(11), 996–1005.

*Reinke, L. F., & Hoffman, L. A. (1992). Breathing space: How to teach asthma co-management. *American Journal of Nursing, 92*(10), 40–51.

Rogers, R. M., Sciurba, F. C., & Keenan, R. J. (1996). Lung reduction surgery in chronic obstructive lung disease. *Medical Clinics of North America, 80*(3), 623–644.

Sahn, S. (1996). Chemical pleurodesis for malignant effusions: What is the best agent? *Pulmonary Perspectives, 13*(1), 1–3.

Sarna, L., & Ganley, J. (1995). A survey of lung cancer patient-education. *Oncology Nursing Forum, 22*(10), 1545–1550.

Schottenfeld, D. (1996). Epidemiology of lung cancer. In H. I. Pass, J. B. Mitchell, D. H. Johnson, & A. T. Turrisi (Eds.), *Lung cancer* (pp. 305–321). Philadelphia, PA: Lippincott-Raven.

*Scott, R., Dryzer, M. D., Strange, C., & Sahn, S. A. (1993). A comparison of rotation and non-rotation in tetracycline pleurodesis. *Chest, 104*(6), 1763–1766.

Shell, J. A., Bulson, K. R., & Vanderlugt, L. F. (1996). Lung cancers. In S. E. Otto (Ed.), *Oncology nursing* (pp. 312–346). St. Louis, MO: C. V. Mosby.

Sherman, C. B. (1995). Late-onset asthma: Making the diagnosis, choosing drug therapy. *Geriatrics, 50*(12), 24–33.

Silverman, E. K., & Speizer, F. E. (1996). Risk factors for the development of chronic obstructive pulmonary disease. *Medical Clinics of North America, 80*(3), 501–522.

Snider, G. L. (1996). Reduction pneumoplasty for giant bullous emphysema. *Chest, 109*(2), 540–548.

Taylor, D. R., Sears, M. R., & Crockcroft, D. W. (1996). The beta-agonist controversy. *Medical Clinics of North America, 80*(4), 719–748.

Travis, W. D., Linder, J., & Mackay, B. (1996). Classification, histology, cytology, and electron microscopy. In H. I. Pass, J. B. Mitchell, D. H.

Johnson, & A. T. Turrisi (Eds.), *Lung cancer* (pp. 359–395). Philadelphia, PA: Lippincott-Raven.

*Vork, K. L., & Olson, D. K.(1990). Asbestos review and update. *American Association of Occupational Health Nurses, 38*(4), 160–164.

Walker-Coleman, S. (1996). Oncologic pharmacology: Selected topics for critic care. *AACN Clinical Issues, 7*(1), 46–64.

*Weaver, T. E., & Narsavage, G. L. (1992). Physiological and psychological variables related to functional status in chronic obstructive pulmonary disease. *Nursing Research, 41*(5), 286–291.

Weaver, T. E., Richmond, T. S., & Narsavage, G. L. (1997). An explanatory model of functional status in chronic obstructive pulmonary disease. *Nursing Research, 46*(1), 26–31.

*Webster, J. R., & Kadah, H. (1991). Unique aspects of respiratory disease in the aged. *Geriatrics, 46*(7), 31–43.

Weinberger, M., & Hendeles, L. (1996). Theophylline in asthma. *New England Journal of Medicine, 334*(21), 1380–1388.

Weinmann, G. G., & Hyatt, R. (1996). Evaluation and research in lung volume reduction surgery. *American Journal of Respiratory and Critical Care Medicine, 154*, 1913–1918.

Wilkie, D. J., Williams, A. R., Grevstad, P., & Mekwa, J. (1995). Coaching persons with lung cancer to report sensory pain. *Cancer Nursing, 18*(1), 7–15.

Wilson, R. (1995). Outcome predictors in bronchitis. *Chest, 108*(2), 53S–57S.

Witta, K. (1997). COPD in the elderly. *ADVANCE for Nurse Practitioners, 5*(7), 18–20, 22–23, 27, 72.

Wright, L., & Martin, R. (1995). Nocturnal asthma and exercise-induced bronchospasm. *Postgraduate Medicine, 97*(6), 83–90.

*Yeaw, E. M. J. (1992). Good lung down? *American Journal of Nursing, 92*(3), 27–32.

SUGGESTED READINGS

Dow, J. S., & Mest, C. G. (1997). Psychosocial interventions for patients with chronic obstructive pulmonary disease. *Home Healthcare Nurse, 15*(6), 414–420.

This article focuses on the emotional impact of chronic obstructive pulmonary disease (COPD). Levin's theoretical framework for promoting wholeness is applied to the client with COPD. Personal and social integrity is discussed, as are client and family assessments. The article concludes with a discussion of specific nursing interventions and various obstacles to coping.

Mathews, P. J. (1997). Using a peak flowmeter. *Nursing97, 27*(6), 57–59.

This brief article includes information on the different types of flowmeters and has step-by-step directions on how to use a flowmeter. Baseline parameters as well as the green, yellow, and red zones are defined. Photographs enhance the article.

Middleton, A. D. (1997). Managing asthma: It takes team work. *American Journal of Nursing, 97*(1), 39–43.

The article begins with a review of the pathologic process involved in the early- and late-phase responses to an allergen or irritant in asthma. Exacerbations of the disease; peak-flow monitoring and management; and bronchodilator and antiinflammatory medications are discussed. A chart outlining the stepwise approach to asthma management from the National Heart, Lung, and Blood Institute is included.

Chapter 33

INTERVENTIONS FOR CLIENTS WITH INFECTIONS OF THE RESPIRATORY SYSTEM

DISORDERS OF THE NOSE AND SINUSES

Rhinitis

Overview

Rhinitis is an inflammation of the nasal mucosa and is the most common disorder to affect the nose and sinuses of adults. The cause of rhinitis often involves an interplay of viruses, bacteria, and allergens.

Acute rhinitis may be caused by allergens, bacteria, or viruses. Allergic rhinitis, frequently called "hay fever" or "allergies," is commonly initiated by sensitivity reactions to allergens, especially plant pollens or molds. Acute episodes tend to be seasonal; that is, they disappear after a few weeks and recur at the same time the following year. Chronic rhinitis, or perennial rhinitis, presents intermittently or continuously when a person is exposed to certain allergens, such as dust, animal dander, wool, and foods (e.g., seafood). Rhinitis also can occur after excessive use of nose drops or sprays (rhinitis medicamentosa) as a rebound effect causing nasal congestion or after nasal inhalation of cocaine.

Acute viral rhinitis (coryza, or the common cold) is caused by any one of at least 200 viruses. It usually spreads from one person to another via droplet nuclei from sneezing or coughing and is most contagious in the first 2–3 days after symptoms appear. The condition is self-limiting unless a complication such as otitis media, sinusitis, bronchitis, or pneumonia occurs. Complications are most likely seen in young, elderly, or immunosuppressed people, especially if they live or work in crowded conditions or in group settings such as a long-term care facility.

Collaborative Management

 Assessment

In both acute and chronic allergic rhinitis, the offending substance causes a release of vasoactive mediators (e.g., histamine, serotonin, bradykinin, and prostaglandin), which induce vasodilation and increased capillary permeability. Edema and swelling of the nasal mucosa result, and the client complains of headache, nasal irritation, sneezing, nasal congestion, rhinorrhea (watery drainage from the nose), and itchy, watery eyes. (Chapter 23 further describes the physiologic mechanisms that occur in allergic reactions of the hypersensitivity type.)

In addition to the clinical manifestations observed in clients with allergic rhinitis, clients with viral infections often present with fatigue; a sore, dry throat; and, at times, a low-grade fever with chills.

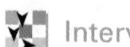 Interventions

Management of the client with any type of rhinitis includes symptomatic relief and client education. The physician prescribes appropriate drug therapy, and the nurse instructs the client as indicated. Drugs, including antihistamines and decongestants, are commonly given but must be used with caution in the elderly because of side effects such as vertigo, hypertension, urinary retention, and insomnia. These medications work by causing vasoconstriction and, subsequently, by decreasing edema. Antipyretics are administered if fever is present in the client with viral rhinitis. Antibiotics are not usually prescribed because these agents do not kill the offending virus. Decreasing or discontinuing the offending drug is the treatment for rhinitis medicamentosa.

The nurse instructs the client about the importance of rest (8–10 hours a day), and fluid intake of at least 2000 mL/day (about eight glasses) unless otherwise contraindicated (e.g., as with congestive heart failure, chronic renal failure). Humidification of air helps to relieve congestion; the nurse suggests inhaling steam from a pan of boiled water after removing it from the heat. Hot shower water produces the same effect. The nurse also instructs the client to avoid people who are susceptible to infection for 2–3 days after symptoms begin. Thorough hand washing is another important precaution, especially after the client cleans the nose or sneezes. An uncomplicated cold typically subsides within 7 days.

The client with recurrent allergic rhinitis can undergo allergy testing to determine the cause, and desensitization may help to prevent future episodes. The client may be able to avoid the offending substance. (Chapter 23 further discusses allergies.)

Sinusitis

Overview

Sinusitis is an inflammation of the mucous membranes of one or more of the sinuses. Acute sinusitis results in the obstruction of the flow of secretions from the sinuses, which may subsequently become infected. The disorder frequently accompanies or follows acute or chronic allergic rhinitis. It can also occur in conjunction with other influencing factors, including a deviated nasal septum, polyps, tumors, chronically inhaled air pollutants or cocaine, facial trauma, nasotracheal intubation, dental infection, or cystic fibrosis. In chronic sinusitis, the mucous membrane becomes permanently thickened from prolonged or repeated inflammation or infection.

The causative organism in sinus infection is usually *Streptococcus pneumoniae, Haemophilus influenzae, Diplococ-*

cus, or *Bacteroides*. Anaerobic infections also can cause sinusitis. Sinusitis most often develops in the maxillary and frontal sinuses. Complications include cellulitis, abscess, and meningitis.

Diagnosis is made on the basis of the client's history, signs and symptoms. Endoscopic examination and computed tomography (CT) of the client's sinuses may be performed.

Collaborative Management

 Assessment

The clinical manifestations of sinusitis include nasal swelling and congestion, headache, facial pressure, pain (usually aggravated by movement of the head to a dependent position), tenderness on percussion over involved area, low-grade fever, cough, and purulent or bloody nasal drainage.

 Interventions

➤ Nonsurgical Management

The treatment for sinusitis includes the use of broad-spectrum antibiotics (e.g., amoxicillin), analgesics for pain and fever (e.g., acetaminophen [Tylenol, Atasol✦]), decongestants (e.g., phenylephrine [Neo-Synephrine], astemizole [Hismanal]), steam humidification, hot, wet packs over the sinus area, and nasal saline irrigations. The nurse instructs the client to increase free water intake to more than ten glasses of water or juice per day unless medically contraindicated. When this treatment plan is not successful, the physician orders additional evaluation with sinus films and CT. Surgical intervention may be necessary.

➤ Surgical Management

Antral Irrigation. Antral irrigation, also known as maxillary antral puncture and lavage, is an outpatient surgical procedure. After local anesthesia, a large-gauge needle is inserted under the inferior turbinate of the nose and into the maxillary sinus on the affected side. Fluid or purulent material from the sinus is withdrawn. The sinus is then irrigated with saline solution, an antibiotic solution, or both.

Other Surgical Procedures. If antral irrigation is not successful, other surgical procedures may be used to open the sinus cavities in clients with chronic sinusitis. In the Caldwell-Luc procedure, the surgeon makes an incision in the anterior wall of the maxillary sinus under the upper lip. The infected mucosa in the maxillary sinus is removed. With the nasal antral window procedure, the surgeon creates an opening in the anterior portion of the inferior turbinate to allow for unobstructed drainage through the nares. With either procedure, the client may have difficulty eating for a few days postoperatively because of pain and swelling. Chart 33–1 covers nursing care for clients undergoing these procedures.

When the ethmoid sinuses need to be opened, the surgeon uses an external approach for better visibility and

Nursing Care Highlight: Postoperative Care for Clients with Sinus Surgery

- Position the client in the semi-Fowler's position to promote drainage and prevent swelling.
- Perform gentle oral hygiene to promote healing and prevent injury to the surgical incision.
- Use ice compresses as ordered for 24 hours.
- Change the "mustache" dressing under the nose as needed, and record the type and amount of drainage.
- Instruct the client to eat soft foods and increase fluid intake.
- Instruct the client to limit the Valsalva maneuver (no coughing, blowing the nose, or straining at stool) for at least 2 weeks postoperatively to prevent bleeding and tissue damage.

preservation of structures. The surgical incision is made along the side of the nose from the middle of the eyebrow (Weber-Ferguson incision).

Endoscopic Sinus Surgery. Endoscopic sinus surgery has become a revolutionary method of diagnosing and treating sinus disorders. Direct inspection of the sinuses through a sinus endoscope is an improved surgical procedure for refractory sinus disorders. Completed with the client under general anesthesia in an outpatient surgical center, the procedure takes only minutes. The client goes home the same day and can return to work in 4-5 days. Nasal mucosa may take up to 4-6 weeks to heal. The nurse instructs the client in frequent use of saline nasal sprays to prevent intranasal and sinus crusting and promote healing.

DISORDERS OF THE ORAL PHARYNX AND TONSILS

Pharyngitis

Overview

Pharyngitis is an inflammation of the mucous membranes of the pharynx. It may precede acute rhinitis or sinusitis, or these conditions may occur simultaneously with pharyngitis.

Acute pharyngitis has multiple causes (Table 33-1). The most common bacterial organism causing pharyngitis is group A beta-hemolytic *Streptococcus*, but most adult cases are caused by a virus. The incidence of streptococcal infection rises between late fall and spring, especially in the colder climates.

Collaborative Management

 Assessment

Pharyngitis is characterized by soreness and dryness in the throat, pain, pain on swallowing (odynophagia), difficulty in swallowing (dysphagia), and fever. Viral and bacterial pharyngitis is often difficult to differentiate on physical assessment. When inspecting the mucous membranes of a throat infected with either virus or bacteria, the nurse may note a mild to severe hyperemia (redness) with or without enlarged erythematous tonsils and with or without exudate. The nurse asks about nasal discharge, which can vary from thin and watery to thick and purulent. Cervical lymphadenopathy may be present in either viral or bacterial pharyngitis. With a parapharyngeal (or tonsillar) abscess, the client may have a characteristic "hot potato" voice, a thickened voice of poor quality.

Clinical studies indicate that streptococcal or other bacterial infections are more often associated with enlarged erythematous tonsils with exudate, purulent nasal discharge, and cervical lymphadenopathy. Chart 33-2 outlines the clinical manifestations of viral versus bacterial pharyngitis. Viral pharyngitis is communicable for 2-3 days; symptoms usually subside within 3-10 days after onset. The disease is usually self-limiting.

Bacterial pharyngitis, such as group A streptococcal infection, however, can lead to dangerous medical complications (Table 33-2). The two most serious complications, acute glomerulonephritis (Chap. 74) and rheumatic fever carditis (Chap. 37), occur in 1% to 3% of cases. Acute glomerulonephritis generally occurs 7-10 days after the acute infection, and rheumatic fever may develop 3-5 weeks after an acute streptococcal infection.

Throat cultures are important to diagnosing viral from

TABLE 33-1

Causes of Pharyngitis

Bacterial Causes
- *Streptococcus*
- *Staphylococcus*
- *Haemophilus influenzae*
- Pneumococcus
- *Corynebacterium diphtheriae*
- *Neisseria gonorrhoeae*

Viral Causes
- Adenovirus
- Rhinovirus
- Epstein-Barr virus
- Cytomegalovirus (CMV)
- Influenza virus
- Parainfluenza virus
- Herpesvirus
- Coxsackievirus A
- Echovirus

Other Causes
- *Chlamydia*
- *Mycoplasma pneumoniae*
- *Candida*
- Physical and chemical causes
  - Alcohol
  - Tobacco
  - Heat
  - Irritants
  - Dehydration
  - Trauma

Chart 33–2

Key Features of Acute Viral and Bacterial Pharyngitis

Feature	Viral Pharyngitis	Bacterial Pharyngitis
Temperature	• Low-grade or no fever	• High temperature (above 101° F [38° C], and usually 102°–104° F [38.5°–40° C])
Ear manifestations	• Retracted and/or dull tympanic membrane	• Retracted and/or dull tympanic membrane
Throat manifestations	• Scant or no tonsillar exudate	• Severe hyperemia of pharyngeal mucosa, tonsils, and uvula
	• Slight erythema of pharynx and tonsils	• Erythema of tonsils with yellow exudate
Neck manifestations	• Possible lymphadenopathy	• Anterior cervical lymphadenopathy and tenderness
Skin manifestations	• No rash	• Possible scarlatiniform rash
		• Possible petechiae on chest and/or abdomen
Dysphagia, odynophagia	• Present	• Present
Other symptoms	• No cough	• No cough
	• Rhinitis	
	• Mild hoarseness	
		• Voice characterized by pain on voicing and slurred speech
	• Headache	• Arthralgia
		• Myalgia
Laboratory data	• Complete blood count usually normal	• Complete blood count abnormal
	• White blood cell count usually lower than 10,000/mm³	• White blood cell count usually higher than 12,000/mm³
	• Negative throat culture results	• Throat culture results positive for beta-hemolytic streptococcus
Onset	• Gradual	• Abrupt

---

group A beta-hemolytic streptococcal infection, but results are not entirely accurate; both false-negative and false-positive results occur. To obtain a specimen, the nurse or physician rubs a cotton swab over each tonsillar area and over the posterior pharynx. The cotton swab is then

TABLE 33–2

Complications of Group A Streptococcal Infection

- Rheumatic fever
- Acute glomerulonephritis
- Peritonsillar abscess
- Retropharyngeal abscess
- Otitis media
- Sinusitis
- Mastoiditis
- Bronchitis
- Pneumonia
- Scarlet fever

streaked on a blood agar plate, which is incubated for 24 hours. An easier and faster method for determining the type of infection is a test using latex agglutination for group A streptococcal antigen; results are ready in 10 minutes, allowing rapid initiation of treatment. The incidence of sequelae of streptococcal infection should decrease with faster testing and treatment.

A complete blood count is performed when the client's condition is severe or not improving. The client may exhibit extremely high temperatures, lethargy, or signs and symptoms of complications. A complete blood count may indicate other causes of pharyngitis.

When taking a history, the nurse inquires about the client's recent contacts (within the last 10 days) with people who have been ill. Of particular importance is whether the client has been ill with symptoms of a cold or upper respiratory tract infection recently or in the past. Documenting previous streptococcal infections is essential. The nurse also notes a history of rheumatic fever, valvular heart disease, streptococcal infections, or penicillin allergy. Because diphtheria (*Corynebacterium diphtheriae*) can cause pharyngitis, the nurse questions and documents whether the client has had a diphtheria immunization.

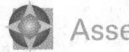 Interventions

Most sore throats in adults are viral and do not warrant the use of antibiotics. The treatment plan includes rest, increased fluid intake, humidification of the air, analgesics for pain, warm saline throat gargles, and throat lozenges containing mild anesthetics.

The management of bacterial pharyngitis involves the use of antibiotics and the same supportive care provided for viral pharyngitis. For streptococcal infection, the physician typically prescribes an oral penicillin preparation. If the client is allergic to penicillin, erythromycin is the alternative. The nurse counsels the client on the importance of completing the entire antibiotic prescription, even if symptoms subside. If the client cannot tolerate the medication, the nurse notifies the physician so that a change in the antibiotic regimen can be made. If compliance is a concern or the client cannot swallow pills, long-acting benzathine penicillin, 1.2 million units, can be administered intramuscularly in a single dose to eradicate the organism. The client should be re-evaluated if there is no improvement in 3 days or if the symptoms are still present after completion of the antibiotic course.

The nurse instructs the client in the proper procedure for taking an oral temperature reading. This reading should be taken in the morning and in the evening until convalescence is complete. The client is not contagious after 24 hours of treatment. Family members or significant others who experience a sore throat should be evaluated, and a throat culture may be indicated.

Tonsillitis

Overview

Tonsillitis is an inflammation and infection of the tonsils and the lymphatic tissue located on each lateral side of the oropharynx (where the palatine, or faucial, tonsils are located). The tonsils consist of lymphatic tissue shaped like a small almond. Each tonsil is covered by a mucous membrane. These lymphatic tissues filter microorganisms, thus functioning as a protective mechanism for the respiratory and gastrointestinal tracts.

Tonsillitis is a contagious airborne infection. Acute or chronic tonsillitis can occur in any age group, but 5- to 10-year-old children are affected most often. The infection is usually more severe when it occurs in adolescents or adults.

The acute form usually lasts 7–10 days and is most often caused by a bacterial organism. The most common organism is *Streptococcus*. Other bacterial pathogens include *Staphylococcus aureus*, *H. influenzae*, and *Pneumococcus*. Viruses may also cause tonsillitis. Chronic tonsillitis usually results from either an acute infection that did not resolve or from recurrent infections.

Collaborative Management

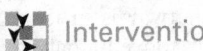 Assessment

Chart 33–3 summarizes the signs and symptoms of acute tonsillitis. Diagnostic studies are performed to rule out

---

Chart 33–3

Key Features of Acute Tonsillitis

- Sudden onset of a mild to severe sore throat
- Fever
- Muscle aches
- Chills
- Dysphagia, odynophagia (painful swallowing of food)
- Pain in the ears
- Headache
- Anorexia
- Malaise
- "Hot potato" voice (thickened voice of poor quality)
- Tonsils visually swollen and red with pus
- Tonsils may be covered with a white or yellow exudate
- Purulent drainage may be expressed upon pressing a tonsil
- Uvula visually edematous or inflamed
- Cervical lymph nodes usually tender and enlarged

---

other causes of the sore throat and fever (such as acute pharyngitis). A complete blood count, throat culture and sensitivity (C & S) studies, monospot test, and chest x-ray (if respiratory symptoms are present) may be ordered for a client with suspected tonsillitis. In bacterial infections, the white blood cell count is elevated. Throat culture and sensitivity studies identify the causative bacterial organism and direct the choice of regimen.

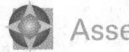 Interventions

The physician orders systemic antibiotics (usually penicillin or erythromycin) for 7–10 days. Warm saline throat gargles, analgesics, antipyretics, and lozenges with topical anesthetic ingredients may provide symptomatic relief.

Indications for surgical intervention include
- Recurrent acute infections or chronic infections that have not responded to antibiotic therapy
- Peritonsillar abscess
- Infected hypertrophy of the tonsils or adenoids that obstructs the airway

The indication for surgery becomes stronger with evidence of repeated group A beta-hemolytic streptococcal infections. Surgery is generally not indicated if the client is experiencing an acute tonsillar infection (except with an acute peritonsillar abscess) or has a blood dyscrasia such as aplastic anemia, hemophilia, or leukemia.

The most common surgical procedure to remove the tonsils is dissection and snare. The adenoids are removed with an adenoid curette or adenotome. A tonsillectomy and adenoidectomy (T&A) is usually performed with the client under general anesthesia but is performed infrequently in adults. Postoperatively, the nurse focuses care on the following nursing diagnoses:
- Risk for Injury related to ineffective airway clearance
- Pain related to surgery and edema
- Fluid Volume Deficit related to bleeding

Peritonsillar Abscess

Overview

Peritonsillar abscess (PTA), or *quinsy*, is a complication of acute tonsillitis. The acute infection spreads from the tonsil to the surrounding peritonsillar tissue, which forms an abscess. It is one of the most common abscesses of the head and neck area. The common cause of PTA is group A beta-hemolytic streptococcus. Anaerobic organisms also may be the cause.

Collaborative Management

 Assessment

At physical examination, signs of infection are pronounced. Pus forms behind the tonsil and causes a marked asymmetric swelling and deviation of the uvula. Because of the swelling, the client may experience drooling, severe throat pain that may radiate to the ear, a voice change, and difficulty swallowing. The client may also exhibit a tonic contraction of the muscles of mastication (trismus) and complain of difficulty breathing.

 Interventions

The nurse instructs the client about comfort measures such as warm saline gargles or irrigations, an ice collar, analgesics, and the importance of completing the antibiotic regimen. The client should improve in 24–48 hours. Outpatient management using percutaneous needle aspiration and antibiotic therapy may be indicated. Hospitalization is required when the client's airway is in jeopardy or when the infection is refractory to conventional antibiotic therapy. Incision and drainage (I&D) of the abscess, plus additional antibiotic therapy, may be indicated. A tonsillectomy may be performed to prevent recurrence.

DISORDERS OF THE LARYNX AND LUNGS

Laryngitis

Overview

Laryngitis is an inflammation of the mucous membranes lining the larynx and may or may not include edema of the vocal cords. It is commonly associated with upper respiratory tract infections, and can be an entity itself or a symptom of a related disease process. Etiologic factors include exposure to irritating inhalants and pollutants, including chemical agents, tobacco, alcohol, and smoke; overuse of the voice; inhalation of volatile gases such as glue, paint thinner, and butane; or intubation.

Collaborative Management

 Assessment

The nurse assesses the client for acute hoarseness, dry cough, and dysphagia. Complete but temporary voice loss (*aphonia*) also may occur. The physician performs a laryngeal examination to assist in the diagnosis. A laryngeal mirror is used to examine the larynx and to differentiate inflammation, polyps, edema, or tumor. The physician may further order radiography and CT and fiberoptic laryngoscopic examination. Most clients are referred to an ear, nose, and throat (ENT) specialist for any suspected disorder other than acute laryngitis.

 Interventions

Nursing management is aimed toward relief of presenting symptoms and the introduction of further preventive measures. Treatment consists of voice rest, steam inhalations, increased fluid intake, and topical throat lozenges. The physician may order antibiotic therapy and bronchodilators when sinusitis, bronchitis, or a bacterial upper respiratory tract infection is also present. The nurse informs the client and family about immediate acute care therapies, infection prevention, and avoidance of alcohol, tobacco, and pollutants.

Preventive therapy is aimed toward increasing the client's and family's awareness of the hazards of tobacco and alcohol use. The nurse also emphasizes the activities that place an added strain on the larynx, such as singing, cheering, public speaking, heavy lifting, and whispering. Speech therapy is often the treatment of choice for vocal cord injuries and should be implemented for any voice disorder. For recurrent bouts of laryngitis, further medical and speech therapy evaluation are necessary.

Influenza

Influenza, or "flu," is an acute viral respiratory infection that can occur in adults of all ages. Because influenza is highly contagious, epidemics are common and can lead to complications like pneumonia or death, especially in elderly and immunocompromised clients. Hospitalization may be required. Influenza may be caused by one of several viruses, usually referred to as A, B, and C. The client with this disorder typically complains of severe headache, muscle aches, fever, chills, fatigue, weakness, and anorexia. Clinical manifestations associated with the respiratory system, such as a sore throat, cough, and rhinorrhea (watery discharge from the nose), generally follow the initial symptoms for a week or more. Most clients continue to complain of general malaise for 1–2 weeks after the acute episode has resolved.

Treatment of influenza is symptomatic because antibiotics are ineffective against viral infections. The nurse recommends that the client remain in bed for several days and drink copious amounts of fluids unless contraindicated by some other physical condition, such as chronic renal failure or congestive heart failure. Saline gargles may ease sore throat pain; when ordered, antihistamines may reduce the rhinorrhea. Other palliative measures are the same as those for acute rhinitis.

During the past two decades, vaccinations for the prevention of influenza have been developed and widely administered. With advanced refinement of the vaccine, allergic reaction is rare. The vaccine is altered every year on the basis of specific viral strains that are likely to pose a problem during the influenza season, that is, late fall and winter. It is highly recommended that persons older than 65 years, those with chronic illness or immune compromise, those living in institutions, and health care personnel in direct care of clients receive the vaccine each year, typically during October or November.

Pneumonia

Overview

Pneumonia is an inflammatory process that results in edema of interstitial lung tissue and extravasation of fluid into alveoli, causing hypoxemia. It can be caused by infectious or noninfectious irritating agents, such as inhaled fumes or aspirated food or fluids. Pneumonias are classified as community acquired (which includes the community proper and extended care facilities) or nosocomial (hospital acquired). In the past, antibiotics have reduced the mortality of pneumonia, but the recent emergence of new pathogens and resistant organisms has the health care community concerned.

Pathophysiology

The inflammation in pneumonia occurs in the interstitial spaces, the alveoli, and often the bronchioles. The pneumonic process begins in infectious pneumonia when pathogens successfully penetrate the airway mucus and multiply in the alveolar spaces. To do this, they must survive the lung's many defenses against microbial invasion. As the pathogenic organisms multiply, edematous fluid forms, and other evidence of inflammation becomes apparent. White blood cells migrate into the alveoli and cause thickening of the alveolar wall. Red blood cells and fibrin extravasate into the alveoli. Fluid fills the alveoli, which protects the organisms from phagocytosis and facilitates the movement of organisms to other alveoli. In this way, the infection spreads. If the invading organisms obtain access to the bloodstream, septicemia results; if the infection extends into the pleural cavity, an empyema results. (Chapter 23 discusses inflammation in detail and Chapter 28 has more on the infectious process.)

The fibrin and edema of inflammation stiffen the lung, thus causing decreased lung compliance and a decline in the vital capacity (VC) of the lung. Decreased production of surfactant further reduces compliance and leads to atelectasis. Some of the venous blood coming into the lungs passes through the underventilated area. This unoxygenated blood then travels to the left side of the heart. As a result, arterial oxygen tension falls, causing hypoxemia (insufficient oxygen in the blood).

Systemically, fever results from the infection. The client may develop shaking chills in an attempt to increase heat production and raise the metabolic rate. Hypoxemia and an increase in metabolic demand cause secondary tachypnea with tachycardia. Blood pressure may fall as a result of peripheral vasodilation and decreased circulating blood volume secondary to dehydration. Cardiac function may be compromised by hypoxemia and enhanced metabolism. Congestive heart failure or shock may result, and

cardiac irritability may be enhanced because of inadequate tissue oxygenation, thus causing dysrhythmias.

Pneumonia may occur as lobar pneumonia with consolidation (solidification, lack of air spaces) in a segment or an entire lobe of the lung, or as bronchopneumonia, with diffuse patches around the bronchi. The extent of pulmonary involvement after the microbial invasion depends on the defenses of the host. In an immunocompromised host, bacteria can multiply. Tissue necrosis results when multiplying anaerobic organisms form an abscess that perforates the bronchial wall.

Etiology

In general, individuals develop pneumonia when their defense mechanisms are unable to combat the virulence of the invading organisms. Organisms from the environment, invasive devices, equipment and supplies, staff, or other people can invade the body. Risk factors are listed in Table 33–3. Bacteria, viruses, mycoplasmas, fungi, rickettsiae, protozoa, and helminths (worms) can all cause pneumonia; the most common organisms are listed in Table 33–4. Noninfectious causes of pneumonia include inhalation of toxic gases, chemicals, smoke, and aspiration of water, food, fluid, and vomitus.

Prevention is aimed at immunizing against the causative agent when possible and reducing the other risks of infection or exposure.

There are different serotypes of the pneumoniae organism, the most common being 6B, 23F, 14, 9V, 19A and 19F. All of these serotypes are included in the 23-valent pneumococcal vaccine that has been available since 1983. Client education is an important factor in the prevention of pneumonia (Chart 33–4), as is making the vaccines readily available to those most at risk.

TABLE 33–3

Risk Factors Associated with Pneumonia

Community-Acquired Pneumonias

Elderly
No history of pneumococcal vaccination
No history of having received the influenza vaccine in the previous year
Chronic or other co-existing condition
Recent history of, or exposure to, viral or influenza infections
History of tobacco or alcohol use

Nosocomial Pneumonias

Elderly
Chronic lung disease
Gram-negative colonization of the oropharynx and stomach
Altered level of consciousness
Aspiration
Endotracheal, tracheostomy, or nasogastric tube
Poor nutritional status
Immunocompromised status (from disease, medications)
Medications that increase gastric pH (H_2 blockers, antacids) or alkaline tube feedings
Mechanical ventilation

TABLE 33–4

Common Organisms Causing Pneumonia*

Community-Acquired Pneumonias
- *Streptococcus pneumoniae* (Gram positive)
- *Staphylococcus aureus* (Gram positive)
- *Haemophilus influenzae* (Gram negative)
- *Legionella pneumophila* (Gram negative)
- *Mycoplasma pneumoniae* (smallest free-living organism)
- *Chlamydia pneumoniae* (parasite)

Nosocomial Pneumonias
- *Staphylococcus aureus* (Gram positive)
- *Pseudomonas aeruginosa* (Gram negative)
- *Enterobacter* (Gram negative)
- *Klebsiella* (Gram negative)
- *Haemophilus influenzae* (Gram negative)
- *Acinetobacter* (Gram negative)
- *Candida albicans* (fungus)

*Because of various factors influencing the incidence of the pathogenic causes of pneumonia, these organisms are listed loosely in order of incidence.

The nurse follows strict hand washing and aseptic techniques to avoid the spread of organisms. Respiratory therapy equipment is well maintained and is decontaminated or changed as recommended. Sterile water rather than tap water is used in gastrointestinal tubes, and aspiration precautions are initiated as indicated. Specific interventions to prevent aspiration are discussed in Chapters 31 and 47.

Chart 33–4

Health Promotion Guide: Preventing Pneumonia

- Know whether you are at risk for pneumonia.
- Have the annual influenza vaccine after discussing appropriate timing of the vaccination with your primary health care provider.
- Discuss the usually once-in-a-lifetime pneumococcal vaccine with your primary health care provider and have the vaccination as recommended.
- Avoid crowded public areas during flu and holiday seasons.
- Cough, turn, move about, and perform deep-breathing exercises as directed by your nurse or other health care professional.
- If you are using respiratory equipment at home, clean the equipment as you have been taught.
- Avoid indoor pollutants, such as dust, secondhand (passive) smoke, and aerosols.
- If you don't smoke, don't start.
- If you smoke, seek professional help on how to stop, or at least decrease, your habit.
- Be sure to get enough rest and sleep on a daily basis.
- Eat a healthy, balanced diet and take in a sufficient amount of nonalcoholic fluids each day.

TRANSCULTURAL CONSIDERATIONS

A national health objective for the year 2000 is to vaccinate 60% of those at risk for pneumococcal disease and influenza; yet in 1995, only 35% of those older than 64 reported ever having received the pneumococcal vaccine, whereas 58% reported having received the influenza vaccine in the previous year. These percentages represent substantial increases since 1993. Of those older than 64, the highest levels of vaccination were found in women and Caucasians (Centers for Disease Control and Prevention [CDC], 1997a).

Incidence/Prevalence

There are 2–4 million cases of pneumonia per year in the United States; highest incidence occurs in those younger than 5 years, the elderly, nursing home residents, hospitalized clients, and those being mechanically ventilated (Craven & Steger, 1995; Mandell, 1995). During late fall and winter, a higher incidence of community-acquired pneumonia is likely because this illness frequently follows viral or influenza infection. Hospital-acquired pneumonia is the second most common nosocomial infection (Craven & Steger, 1995; Calianno, 1996).

Pneumonia and influenza as a combined cause of death rank sixth in the United States, and the combination is the number one cause of death from infection (King & Pippin, 1997). Nosocomial pneumonia has a 20% to 50% mortality; the highest incidence is in those with *Pseudomonas aeruginosa*, *Acinetobacter*, other "high-risk" organisms, or secondary bacteremia. Mortality also is higher in individuals who experience complications (Table 33–5). Over the past few years, interventions for pneumonia have become more aggressive in order to try to reduce the high incidence of death from this disorder.

ELDERLY CONSIDERATIONS

Pneumonia and influenza constitute the third leading cause of death for clients older than 85 years. For clients older than 64 years, the death rate between 1979 and 1992 increased 44%, from 145.6 deaths per 100,000 population to 209.1 (CDC, 1995c).

TABLE 33–5

Common Complications of Pneumonia

Hypoxemia	• Arterial oxygen <55 mmHg
Ventilatory failure	• Lungs unable to move gas in and out of lungs mechanically, resulting in hypoxemia and hypercapnia
Atelectasis	• Collapse of the affected alveoli and associated lobes of the lungs
Pleural effusion	• Collection of fluid in the pleural space (usually sterile fluid that resolves)
Pleurisy	• Pain caused by friction between layers of pleura

Collaborative Management

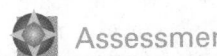 Assessment

➤ History

In preparing to take the history from the client who may have pneumonia, the nurse considers risk factors consistent with infection (see Table 33–3). The nurse collects essential data from the client or a family member if the client is too dyspneic. The nurse documents data on the following:

- Age
- Living, work, or school environment
- Diet, exercise, and sleep routines
- Swallowing problems
- Nasogastrointestinal tube
- Tobacco and alcohol use
- Past and current use of medications
- History of drug addiction or intravenous (IV) drug use

The nurse lists the client's past illnesses, particularly those with a respiratory origin, and determines whether the client has been exposed to influenza or pneumonia or has experienced a recent viral episode. In addition, the nurse notes a history of any rashes, insect bites, or exposure to animals.

If the client has chronic respiratory problems, the nurse asks whether respiratory equipment is used in the home. It is essential to determine whether the client's cleaning regimen is adequate to prevent infection. The nurse also notes prior inoculations with influenza or pneumococcal vaccine.

➤ Physical Assessment/Clinical Manifestations

The nurse first observes the general appearance of the client, who may present with flushed cheeks, bright eyes, and an anxious expression. The client may have chest or pleuritic pain or discomfort, myalgia, headache, chills, fever, cough, tachycardia, dyspnea, tachypnea, and sputum production. Severe chest muscle weakness also may be present from sustained coughing.

The nurse observes the client's breathing pattern, position, and use of accessory muscles. The acutely compromised client is uncomfortable in a lying position and sits upright, balancing with the hands. The nurse assesses the client's cough and the amount, color, consistency, and odor of sputum produced for diagnostic clues about the offending pathogen.

Upon auscultation, the nurse hears crackles when there is fluid in interstitial and alveolar areas. Wheezing may be heard as a result of inflammation and exudate in the airways. Bronchial breath sounds are heard over areas of density or consolidation. Tactile fremitus is increased over areas of pneumonia, and percussion is dulled in these areas. Chest expansion may be diminished or unequal on inspiration. (Chapter 29 discusses respiratory assessment in more detail.)

In evaluating vital signs, the nurse compares the results with baseline values. The client who has pneumonia is likely to be hypotensive with orthostatic changes. A rapid, weak pulse may indicate hypoxemia, dehydration, or impending shock.

The nurse also inspects the skin for a rash, which may occur with *Mycoplasma* infection, cytomegalovirus infection (CMV), or Rocky Mountain spotted fever. The pathophysiology of selected clinical manifestations of pneumonia is summarized in Table 33–6.

ELDERLY CONSIDERATIONS

The nurse is aware of risk and predisposing factors (see Table 33–3). The elderly often have weakness, fatigue, lethargy, confusion, and poor appetite. Fever and cough may be absent, but hypoxemia is usually present.

➤ Psychosocial Assessment

The client with pneumonia experiences pain, fatigue, and dyspnea, which promote anxiety. The nurse assesses anxiety by looking at the client's facial expression and general tenseness of facial and shoulder muscles. The nurse listens to the client carefully and uses a calm, slow approach to assessment. Because of airway obstruction and muscle fatigue, the client with dyspnea speaks in broken sentences. The nurse gauges the length of the interview on the degree of dyspnea or breathing discomfort the client experiences.

TABLE 33–6

Pathophysiology of Selected Clinical Manifestations of Pneumonia

Clinical Manifestation	Pathophysiology
Increased respiratory rate/dyspnea	• Stimulation of chemoreceptors • Increased work of breathing as a result of decreased lung compliance • Stimulation of J receptors • Anxiety • Pain
Hypoxemia	• Alveolar consolidation • Capillary shunting
Cough	• Fluid accumulation in the subepithelial mechanoreceptors in the trachea, bronchi, and bronchioles
Purulent, blood-tinged, or rust-colored sputum	• A result of the inflammatory process in which fluid from the pulmonary capillaries and red blood cells moves into the alveoli
Fever	• Phagocytes release endogenous pyrogens that cause the hypothalamus to increase body temperature
Pleuritic chest discomfort	• Inflammation of the parietal pleura causes pain on inspiration

➤ *Laboratory Assessment*

Sputum is obtained from the client and examined by Gram's stain, culture, and sensitivity testing. A sputum sample is easily obtained from the client who can cough into a specimen container. Extremely ill clients may require nasotracheal suctioning by the nurse or suctioning via a tracheostomy or endotracheal tube. In these situations, the nurse obtains a sputum specimen via sputum trap (Fig. 33–1) while suctioning. The responsible organism, however, may not be identified in as many as 50% of the cases. Sensitivity testing determines how resistant or sensitive the organism is to various anti-infective agents.

A complete blood count (CBC) is obtained to identify leukocytosis, which is a common finding, except in the elderly. Blood cultures may be performed to determine whether the organism has invaded the bloodstream. Assessment for human immunodeficiency virus (HIV) may be performed. Urine may be examined for hematuria, pyuria, and the presence of protein, which may occur in the septic client with pneumonia.

Arterial blood gases (ABGs) determine baseline arterial oxygen and carbon dioxide levels and help identify a need for supplemental oxygen. Serum electrolyte, blood urea nitrogen (BUN), and creatinine levels also are assessed. An increased BUN value may occur as a result of increased catabolism and a diminished glomerular filtration rate. Electrolyte changes occur with dehydration, a result of fever and malaise.

➤ *Radiographic Assessment*

In general, pneumonia appears on chest x-ray as an area of increased density. It may involve a lung segment, a lobe, one lung, or both lungs. In the elderly, the chest x-ray is essential for early diagnosis of pneumonia because their symptoms are often vague.

➤ *Other Diagnostic Assessment*

The nurse obtains oxygen saturation values by using pulse oximetry. This noninvasive test (see Chap. 29) helps detect hypoxemia. The physician may order invasive tests such as transtracheal aspiration, bronchoscopy, or direct needle aspiration of the lung to obtain lower airway specimens in selected clients; thoracentesis is most often used in those clients with pleural effusion.

 Analysis

➤ *Common Nursing Diagnoses and Collaborative Problems*

Two of the nursing diagnoses commonly identified for the client with pneumonia include
1. Impaired Gas Exchange related to effects of alveolo-capillary membrane changes
2. Ineffective Airway Clearance related to effects of infection, excessive tracheobronchial secretions, fatigue and decreased energy, chest discomfort, and muscle weakness

A common collaborative problem for the client with pneumonia is potential for sepsis related to an infectious organism.

➤ *Additional Nursing Diagnoses and Collaborative Problems*

In addition to the common diagnoses, the client may present with associated problems, which could include those listed for the client with chronic airflow limitation (see Chap. 32). Other nursing diagnoses include
- Pain related to effects of inflammation of parietal pleura, coughing
- Hyperthermia related to an increased metabolic rate, dehydration
- Fluid Volume Deficit related to fever, infection, increased metabolic rate
- Ineffective Breathing Pattern related to fatigue, decreased energy, pain, the inflammatory process, and anxiety
- Sleep Pattern Disturbance related to pain, dyspnea, unfamiliar environment (hospitalization)

An additional collaborative problem is potential for pleural effusion related to spread of the infection.

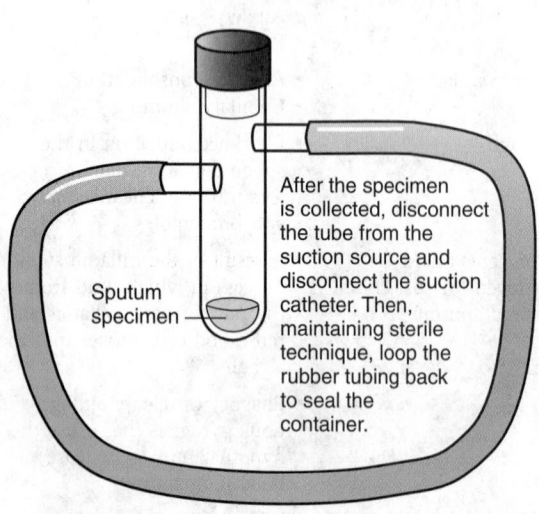

Cap

Attach to suction source (machine)

Attach to sterile suction catheter

To collect a sterile sputum specimen, attach a Lukens tube to a suction source; attach a sterile suction catheter; then suction. The sputum will get "caught" in the container.

A

After the specimen is collected, disconnect the tube from the suction source and disconnect the suction catheter. Then, maintaining sterile technique, loop the rubber tubing back to seal the container.

Sputum specimen

B

Figure 33–1. Method of collecting a sterile sputum specimen using a Lukens tube.

➤ Impaired Gas Exchange

Planning: Expected Outcomes. For the client with impaired gas exchange, the major expected outcome is to attain or maintain partial pressure of arterial oxygen and carbon dioxide (PaO_2 and $PaCO_2$, respectively) and oxygen saturation values within baseline ranges. Other expected outcomes are similar to those for the client with chronic airflow limitation (CAL).

Interventions. For the client with pneumonia, interventions to treat and manage impaired gas exchange are similar to those for the client with CAL (see Chap. 32). In pneumonia, the gas exchange affected most is oxygen; therefore, hypoxemia is the primary problem. Carbon dioxide retention is not as common in pneumonia as it is, for example, in chronic emphysema.

Incentive spirometry, also referred to as sustained maximal inspiration, is a type of bronchial hygiene used in pneumonia. The objective is to improve inspiratory muscle performance and to prevent or reverse atelectasis. The nurse obtains an incentive spirometer and instructs the client to exhale fully, then place the mouthpiece in the mouth, and take a long, slow, deep breath for 3–5 seconds. The nurse evaluates the client's technique and records the volume of air inspired. The client performs 5–10 breaths per session every hour while awake. Chapter 20 has more information on incentive spirometry.

➤ Ineffective Airway Clearance

Planning: Expected Outcomes. For the client with ineffective airway clearance, the major expected outcome is that the client will have optimal breath sounds. The goal may be to have clear lungs in all lobes upon auscultation or to have, minimally, improved breath sounds. Other goals are similar to those for the client with chronic airflow limitation (CAL).

Interventions. For the client with pneumonia, interventions for the treatment and management of ineffective airway clearance are similar to those for the client with CAL. Because of fatigue, muscle weakness, chest discomfort, and excessive secretions, the client with pneumonia often has difficulty clearing secretions. The nurse helps the client to cough and deep breathe at least every 2 hours. The alert client may use an incentive spirometer to facilitate deep breathing and stimulate coughing. Chest physiotherapy (CPT or chest PT), which was once thought to be useful for clearing secretions in the client with pneumonia, is no longer recommended in uncomplicated pneumonia. Whereas dehydration should be avoided, there is no evidence that hydration helps to clear secretions. Adequate hydration may help in thinning secretions and making them easier to remove. To ensure adequate hydration when fever and tachypnea are present, the nurse monitors intake and output.

The physician prescribes bronchodilators, especially beta-2 agonists (see Chart 32–4), when bronchospasm is part of the disease process. They are usually administered initially by aerosol nebulizer and then by metered-dose inhaler (see Chart 32–5). The use of mucolytic agents and expectorants has been found to be of marginal value in the treatment of pneumonia. Inhaled steroid preparations are generally not used with acute pneumonia except when the client also has bronchial asthma or respiratory failure.

➤ Potential for Sepsis

Planning: Expected Outcomes. For the client with sepsis, the major expected outcome is to be free of the invading organism and to return to a prepneumonia health status.

Interventions. The key to effective treatment of pneumonia is identification and eradication of the organism causing the infection. Anti-infectives are given for all types of pneumonias except those caused by viruses. The physician prescribes anti-infective therapy depending on the organism suspected or identified, whether the pneumonia is community acquired or hospital acquired, and whether the client has other contributing factors (Table 33–7). Treatment is often initiated empirically (based on prior experience) and may be continued empirically if the specific organism is not identified.

Aerosolized pentamidine may be used in the treatment and prevention of *Pneumocystis carinii* pneumonia (PCP). Pentamidine has antiprotozoal activity and is administered via a specialized nebulizer (Respirgard II), which nebulizes the medication into particles small enough to be delivered to the alveoli. When penicillin-resistant strains of *S. pneumoniae* have been identified, treatment consists of high-dose penicillin, a third-generation cephalosporin, meropenem (Merrem) or vancomycin (Vancocin) (King & Pippin, 1997).

The client may be able to be switched from intravenous to oral therapy in 2 or 3 days depending on the response (e.g., stable clinical condition, afebrile). The course of anti-infective therapy varies with the pharmacodynamics of the drug and the organism(s) involved but generally ranges from a low of 5 days for a client with uncomplicated community-acquired pneumonia to up to 21 days for the immunocompromised client.

➤ Continuing Care

The client needs to continue the anti-infective medications as prescribed by the physician or primary care provider. The nurse reinforces, clarifies, and provides additional information to the client and family as indicated. In addition, the nurse assists the client in overcoming any barriers to completing the medication prescription. The nurse also recognizes the importance of preventing further episodes of pneumonia and initiates applicable interventions.

➤ Health Teaching

The most important aspect of education for the client and family is the avoidance of upper respiratory tract infections and viruses. The client must avoid crowds, especially in the fall and winter when viruses are prevalent; persons who have a cold or flu; and exposure to irritants such as smoke. The influenza vaccine is recommended

TABLE 33–7

Drug Therapy for Pneumonia	
Community-Acquired Pneumonias*	**Nosocomial Pneumonias ‖**
Without comorbidity and client age <61 years	**Gram-negative infections**
Macrolide† or tetracylcine (doxycycline [Vibramycin])	Ceftazidime
With comorbidity and/or client age >59 years	Cefoperazone
Second- or third-generation cephalosporin or trimethoprim-sulfamethoxazole (Bactrim, Septra) or beta-lactam/beta-lactamase inhibitor§ with the possible addition of erythromycin (or other macrolide) or doxycycline	Aztreonam
	Amoxicillin/clavulanic acid
	Ciprofloxacin
	For *Pseudomonas* coverage:
	Ticarcillin
	Azlocillin
Less severe, requiring hospitalization or for those who are moderately ill	Ceftazidime
	Cefoperazone
Second- or third-generation cephalosporin or beta-lactam/beta-lactamase inhibitor with the possible addition of erythromycin (or other macrolide) or doxycycline	**Gram-positive infections**
	Ticarcillin/clavulanate
	Vancomycin
	Imipenem-cilastatin
Severe, requiring hospitalization	
Third-generation cephalosporin with anti-*Pseudomonas* activity or other antipseudomonal agents such as imipenem/cilastatin (Primaxin) or ciprofloxacin (Cipro), with the possible addition of an aminoglycoside and erythromycin (or other macrolide)	

*Modified from Niederman, 1993, and King, 1997.
†Macrolides include erythromycin, azithromycin (Zithromax), clarithromycin (Biaxin), dirithromycin (Dynabac).
‖ Modified from Bergone-Be're'zen, 1995.
§Such as amoxicillin-clavulanate (Augmentin).

annually, and the pneumococcal vaccine currently once in a lifetime (may be more often in some high-risk cases). A balanced diet and adequate fluid intake are essential. The nurse reviews all medication with the client and family and emphasizes completing anti-infective therapy. The nurse instructs the client to notify the physician if chills, fever, persistent cough, dyspnea, wheezing, hemoptysis, increased sputum production, chest discomfort, or increasing fatigue reoccurs or if symptoms fail to resolve. The client is instructed to get plenty of rest and gradually to increase exercise.

➤ Home Care Management

No special structural changes are needed in the home. If the home consists of more than one story, the client may prefer to stay on the first floor for a few weeks because stair climbing may increase fatigue and dyspnea. Bath and hygiene needs may be met by using a bedside commode if a bathroom is not located on the first level. Home care needs will depend on the client's level of fatigue, dyspnea, and family and social support.

The prolonged convalescent phase of the disease process, particularly in the elderly client, can be frustrating and perhaps depressing. Fatigue, weakness, and a residual cough can last for weeks. Some clients fear that they will never return to a "normal" level of functioning. It is important that the nurse prepare the client for the course of the disease and offer reassurance so that complete

recovery will occur. Initially after discharge, the client may benefit from a home health nursing assessment as outlined in Chart 33–5.

➤ Health Care Resources

Clients who smoke are taught that smoking is a risk factor for pneumonia. The nurse provides information on smoking cessation classes through the American Lung Association (ALA) and American Cancer Society. The physician or nurse practitioner may prescribe nicotine patches. The physician and nurse warn the client of the danger of myocardial infarction if smoking is continued while using the patches. The client should be enrolled in a smoking cessation program to assist in the nicotine withdrawal process in conjunction with using nicotine patches. The nurse also can give the client information booklets on pneumonia provided by the ALA. A client who has not already been vaccinated against influenza or pneumococcal pneumonia should be encouraged to take this preventive measure when the pneumonia has resolved.

 Evaluation

On the basis of the identified nursing diagnoses and collaborative problems, the nurse evaluates the care of the client with pneumonia. The expected outcomes are that the client

Nursing Care Highlight: Focused Assessment for the Client Recovering from Pneumonia

Ascertain whether the client has had any of the following:

- Chills
- Fever
- Persistent cough
- Dyspnea
- Wheezing
- Hemoptysis
- Increased sputum production
- Chest discomfort
- Increasing fatigue
- Any other symptoms that have failed to resolve

Assess the client for the following:

- Fever
- Diaphoresis
- Cyanosis, especially around the mouth or conjunctiva
- Dyspnea, tachypnea, or tachycardia
- Adventitious or abnormal breath sounds
- Weakness

- Attains and/or maintains a PaO_2, $PaCO_2$, and oxygen saturation values within baseline ranges
- Has optimal breath sounds, either clear lungs in all lobes on auscultation, or, minimally, improved breath sounds
- Is free of the invading organism
- Returns to his or her prepneumonia health status

Pulmonary Tuberculosis

Overview

In 1900, tuberculosis (TB) was the leading cause of death in the United States and Europe. After significant reduction in its incidence, TB has been on the rise, especially in clients with HIV and acquired immunodeficiency syndrome (AIDS), but it may be stabilizing currently. Continuous assessment and intervention to prevent and treat the disease must continue. Increasing poverty, numbers of homeless people and people with AIDS, and resistant strains of the TB organism (multi–drug-resistant TB [MDR-TB]) present new challenges to the control and eradication of TB.

Pathophysiology

Tuberculosis is a highly communicable disease caused by *Mycobacterium tuberculosis*. The tubercle bacillus is transmitted via aerosolization (i.e., an airborne route). When an infected person coughs, laughs, sneezes, or sings, droplet nuclei are produced, become airborne, and may be inhaled by others. When the tubercle bacillus reaches a susceptible site (bronchi or alveoli), it multiplies freely. An exudative response occurs, causing a nonspecific pneumonitis. With the development of acquired immunity, further multiplication of bacilli is controlled in most

initial lesions. The lesions typically resolve and leave little or no residual. However, a small percentage of individuals who are initially infected will acquire the disease (5% to 15%). The greatest risk of acquiring the disease for the non–HIV-infected person is in the first 2 years after infection.

Cell-mediated, or type IV, immunity develops 2–10 weeks after infection and is manifested by a significant reaction to a tuberculin test. A primary infection may be microscopic in size and may never appear on an x-ray. The process of infection occurs as follows:

- The granulomatous inflammation created by the tubercle bacillus in the lung becomes surrounded by collagen, fibroblasts, and lymphocytes.
- Caseation necrosis (necrotic tissue being turned into a granular mass) occurs in the center of the lesion. If this area becomes evident on x-ray, it is called Ghon tubercle, or the primary lesion.

Areas of caseation then undergo resorption, hyaline degeneration, and fibrosis. These necrotic areas may calcify (calcification) or may liquefy (liquefaction). If liquefaction occurs, the liquid material then empties into a bronchus, and the evacuated area becomes a cavity (cavitation). Bacilli continue to proliferate in the necrotic cavity wall and spread via the tracheobronchial lymph nodes into new areas of the lung.

A lesion also may progress by direct extension if bacilli multiply rapidly with marked exudative response to the inflammation. These lesions may extend through the pleura, which results in tuberculous pleural effusion with a small number of organisms. Pericardial effusions also may occur.

Miliary, or hematogenous, TB occurs when a large number of organisms enter the bloodstream and the disease becomes disseminated. Many tiny, discrete nodules scattered throughout the lung are typically seen on chest x-ray. The brain, meninges, liver, and kidney (see Chap. 74), or bone marrow are commonly involved as a result of dissemination.

Initial infection is seen more often in the middle or lower lobes of the lung. The regional lymph nodes, particularly the hilar and paratracheal nodes, are commonly involved. There is usually an asymptomatic interval after the primary infection that lasts for years, or less commonly, decades, before clinical symptoms develop. Although infected, an individual is not infectious to others until symptoms of disease occur.

Secondary TB occurs in a previously infected individual and most often represents reactivation (sometimes inaccurately termed reinfection) of the primary disease. Presumably, reactivation occurs whenever defenses are lowered, which may be part of the reason the elderly are susceptible to the development of TB. The upper lobes are the most common site of reactivation and are referred to as Simon's foci. The TB classification adopted and revised by the ALA is shown in Table 33–8.

Etiology

The organism *Mycobacterium tuberculosis* is a nonmotile, slow-growing, nonsporulating, acid-fast rod that secretes

TABLE 33-8

American Lung Association Classification of Tuberculosis (TB)
0 No TB exposure, not infected
1 TB exposure, no evidence of infection
2 TB infection, no disease
3 TB: clinically active (clients with completed diagnostic evidence of TB: both a significant reaction to tuberculin skin test and clinical or x-ray evidence of TB)
4 TB: not clinically active (clients with history of TB or with abnormal chest x-ray but no significant tuberculin skin test reaction or clinical evidence)
5 TB: suspect (diagnosis pending) (used during diagnostic testing of suspect clients, for no longer than a 3-month period)

niacin. The tubercle bacillus is transmitted via aerosolization.

People who are most commonly infected are those having repeated close contact with an infectious person who has not yet been diagnosed with TB. After the infectious person has received proper medication for 2–3 weeks, and clinical signs of improvement are seen (including reduction of acid-fast bacilli [AFB] in the sputum), the risk of transmission is greatly reduced.

Incidence/Prevalence

Figures for 1981 reveal that TB only accounted for 0.8% of deaths in the United States and that the incidence of TB was declining steadily. From 1985 on, however, the number of new TB cases have increased to more than 20,000 annually, largely thought to be related to the onset of the new disease of the time, HIV infection. Ten million persons are estimated to be infected with TB in the United States. The World Health Organization estimates that there are 10 million new cases each year with 2–3 million deaths per year worldwide. The highest at-risk populations currently include

- Those in constant, frequent contact with an untreated individual
- Those with immune dysfunction or HIV
- Those living in crowded areas such as long-term care facilities, prisons, mental health facilities
- The elderly, the homeless, and minorities
- Those who abuse intravenous drugs or alcohol
- Those from a lower socioeconomic group

TRANSCULTURAL CONSIDERATIONS

Groups known to have higher incidence of TB include African-Americans, Asians and Pacific Islanders, Native Americans and Alaskan Natives, Hispanics, and foreign-born persons from Asia, Africa, the Caribbean, and Latin America.

Collaborative Management

 Assessment

Early detection of TB depends on subjective findings rather than presentation of symptoms. TB has an insidious onset, and many clients are not aware of symptoms until the disease is well advanced. A diagnosis of TB should be considered for any client with a persistent cough or other symptoms compatible with TB such as weight loss, anorexia, night sweats, hemoptysis, shortness of breath, fever, or chills.

➤ History

A thorough history includes assessment of past exposure to TB. The nurse inquires about the client's country of origin and travel to foreign countries in which there is a high incidence of TB. It is important to note whether the client has had previous tests for TB and what the results were. In addition, the nurse asks whether the client has had bacille Calmette-Guérin (BCG) vaccine, a vaccine containing attenuated tubercle bacilli that is given routinely in many foreign countries to produce increased resistance to TB. Anyone who has received BCG will have a positive skin test and should be evaluated for TB with a chest x-ray. The BCG vaccine has minimal effectiveness and is not recommended by the CDC.

➤ Physical Assessment/Clinical Manifestations

The client with TB typically has progressive fatigue, lethargy, nausea, anorexia, weight loss, irregular menses, and a low-grade fever, which may have been present for weeks or months. Fever also may be accompanied by night sweats. The client finally notices a cough and the production of mucoid and mucopurulent sputum, which is occasionally streaked with blood. Chest tightness and a dull, aching chest pain may accompany the cough. Physical examination of the chest does not provide conclusive evidence of TB. The nurse may hear dullness with percussion over involved parenchymal areas, bronchial breath sounds, crackles, and increased transmission of spoken or whispered sounds. Partial obstruction of a bronchus because of endobronchial disease or compression by lymph nodes may produce localized wheezing.

➤ Diagnostic Assessment

Sputum culture of *M. tuberculosis* confirms the diagnosis. Three samples are usually obtained for an acid-fast smear. After medications are started, sputum samples are obtained again to determine the effectiveness of therapy. Most clients have negative cultures after 3 months, perhaps even earlier.

In the future, we can expect to see polymerase chain reaction (PCR) assays performed for rapid identification of mycobacteria. This process allows amplification of mycobacterial deoxyribonuclease acid and identification of the mycobacteria within hours instead of days to weeks. This test will allow for earlier diagnosis and treatment of the client with TB.

The tuberculin test (Mantoux's test) result is the most

reliable determinant of infection with TB. A small amount (0.1 mL) of intermediate-strength purified protein derivative (PPD) containing 5 tuberculin units is given intradermally in the forearm. An area of induration (not redness) measuring 10 mm or more in diameter 48–72 hours after injection indicates the person has been exposed to and infected with TB. A positive reaction does not mean that active disease is present but indicates exposure to TB or the presence of inactive (dormant) disease. For persons with HIV infection, a reaction of 5 mm or greater is considered positive. A negative skin test does not rule out TB disease or infection. People with HIV infection are more likely to have false-negative results as a result of an impaired immune system.

Once a person's skin test is positive, chest x-ray is essential to rule out clinically active TB or to detect old, healed lesions. Caseation and inflammation may be seen on the x-ray if the disease is active.

Routine, repeat skin tests and chest x-rays are no longer recommended in these clients. They should be instructed to seek medical attention if they experience symptoms suggestive of TB. The radiographic presentation in HIV-infected clients, however, may be unusual. Such clients may have infiltrates in any lung zone, often associated with hilar adenopathy, or may have a normal chest x-ray.

Interventions

Combination drug therapy is the most effective method of treating the disease and preventing transmission. Active TB is treated with a combination of drugs to which the organism is susceptible. Therapy is continued until the disease is under control. The use of multiple-drug regimens destroys organisms as quickly as possible and minimizes the emergence of drug-resistant organisms. Current therapy (Chart 33–6) uses isoniazid (INH) and rifampin throughout the therapy; pyrazinamide is added for the first 2 months. This protocol permits shortening of the therapy from 6–12 months to 6 months for most clients. Ethambutol and streptomycin are frequently added as the fourth drug to the treatment regimen. An early report using aerosolized interferon-gamma shows promise as additional treatment for multi–drug-resistant TB (see Research Applications for Nursing).

The nurse's major role is teaching clients about drug therapy. The nurse recognizes that the anxious client may not absorb information well. The nurse repeats the information and obtains the assistance of family members if they are available. In instructing, the nurse uses teaching aids such as those available through the ALA. The client should be able to describe the treatment regimen and major side effects for which to call the health care agency and physician.

Tuberculosis is frequently treated outside the acute care setting, so the client convalesces in the home setting. In this setting, airborne precautions are not necessary because family members have already been exposed; all members of the household need to undergo TB testing, however. The nurse instructs the client to cover the mouth and nose when coughing or sneezing, to confine used tissues to plastic bags, and to wear a mask when in contact with crowds until medication is effective in suppressing the infection.

The nurse informs the client that examinations of sputum are needed every 2–4 weeks once drug therapy is initiated. When results of three sputum cultures are negative, the client is considered to be no longer infectious and can usually return to former employment. The nurse reminds the client to avoid excessive exposure to silicone or dust because these substances can cause further lung damage.

The nurse places a hospitalized client with active TB in Airborne Precautions (see Chap. 28) in a well-ventilated room that exhausts to the outside. The room should have at least six exchanges of fresh air per minute and should be ventilated to the outside if possible. The nurse wears a N95 or HEPA respirator (Fig. 33–2) when caring for the client. Standard Precautions are implemented when there is risk of hand and clothing contamination, by using appropriate barrier protection (i.e., gowns and gloves). The nurse performs thorough hand washing before and after caring for the client. Precautions are discontinued when the client is no longer considered infectious.

Clients may prevent nausea related to the medications by taking the daily dose at bedtime. Antinausea drugs may also prevent this symptom. The nurse instructs the client about the need for adequate nutrition and a well-balanced diet to promote healing. The nurse recommends an increased intake of foods that are rich in iron, protein, and vitamin C. The nurse consults the nutritionist for specialized needs. The nurse should know the client's ideal body weight so that progress toward the goal can be evaluated. (See Chapter 64 for further discussion of nutrition.)

The client with TB notices changes in physical stamina, which may be frightening. The client also faces concerns about the prognosis of the disease. The nurse is realistic in offering a positive outlook for the client who complies with the medication regimen and suggests that fatigue will diminish as the treatment progresses. With current resistant strains of TB, however, the nurse must emphasize that noncompliance with medication could lead to an infection that is difficult to treat or has total drug resistance. The nurse listens carefully to the client's concerns throughout the treatment and responds in a supportive manner. The client's return to work and usual daily routines is likely to reduce anxiety.

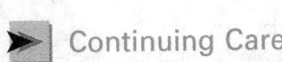

Continuing Care

➤ Health Teaching

The nurse instructs the client to follow the drug regimen exactly as prescribed and always to have a supply of medication on hand. The nurse stresses side effects and ways of minimizing them to ensure compliance. The nurse reminds the client with TB that the disease is usually no longer communicable after medication has been taken for 2–3 consecutive weeks and clinical improvement is seen. However, the client must continue with the prescribed medication for 6 months or longer as ordered.

Chart 33–6

Drug Therapy for Tuberculosis

Drug	Usual Dosage	Nursing Interventions	Drug Action/Rationale for Use
Isoniazid (INH)	• 5 mg/kg PO, IM (max 300 mg) daily; 15 mg/kg (max 900 mg) biweekly	• Observe for drug interactions. It may inhibit drug metabolism of phenytoin, carbamazepine, primidone, and warfarin. • Instruct the client to take on empty stomach and avoid antacids. • Monitor for signs of hepatitis and neurotoxicity effects.	• Isoniazid inhibits synthesis of mycolic acids and acts to kill actively growing organisms in the extracellular environment and inhibits growth of dormant organisms in the macrophages and caseating granulomas.
Rifampin (RIF)	• 10 mg/kg PO (max 600 mg) daily or biweekly	• Instruct the client that secretions, including urine, will be orange in color and will permanently discolor soft contact lenses. • Observe for drug interactions. It may enhance elimination of theophylline, steroids, opioids, oral hypoglycemics, warfarin, and occasionally vitamin D. • Observe for hepatotoxic effects. • RIF decreases effectiveness of oral contraceptives.	• Rifampin has the unique ability to kill slower growing organisms that reside in the caseating granuloma and macrophage.
Pyrazinamide (PZA)	• 15–30 mg/kg PO (max 2000 mg) daily; 50 mg/kg biweekly	• Observe for hepatotoxic effects.	• Pyrazinamide is the most active drug at killing mycobacteria present in macrophages. The acidic environment in the macrophage inhibits most agents.
Ethambutol (EMB)	• 15 mg/kg daily PO; 50 mg/kg biweekly	• Obtain baseline visual acuity and color discrimination, especially to the color green. Repeat testing q1–2 months.	• Ethambutol inhibits bacterial RNA synthesis. It is slow acting and must be used in combination with other bactericidal agents.
Streptomycin (SM)	• 1000 mg IM, or IV over 1 hr, daily for 2 months followed by biweekly injections until treatment is completed	• Obtain baseline audiometric test q1–2 months. It can impair the 8th cranial nerve. Elderly clients are especially susceptible.	• Streptomycin is an aminoglycoside antibiotic that is active against extracellular organisms only.
Amikacin	• 15 mg/kg daily IM, IV (usual dose 1 g)	• Ensure adequate hydration, monitor renal function, and hearing. Amikacin can lead to renal toxicity and ototoxicity.	• Amikacin is an aminoglycoside antibiotic that can be used if streptomycin is not available.

Current treatment recommendations:

INH + RIF + PZA + EMB or SM (induction phase)—2 months. Daily dosing. Ethambutol or streptomycin is included in the initial phase until drug susceptibility is determined.

INH + RIF (continuation phase)—4 months. Daily or 2–3 times/week dosing.

Continue treatment for at least 6 months, and 3 months beyond the time when the result of sputum culture converts to negative.

Clients with a drug resistance, co-existing HIV infection, or inability to take certain antituberculosis drugs require longer duration therapy (i.e., 9 total months, and at least 6 months after culture conversion).

Current treatment information and data from the official ATS statement. A joint statement of the ATS, American Academy of Pediatrics, the Centers for Disease Control, and the Infectious Disease Society of America. (1992). Control of tuberculosis in the United States. *American Review of Respiratory Disease, 146*(6), 1623–1633; U. S. Department of Health and Human Services, Recommendations of the Advisory Council for the Elimination of Tuberculosis. (1993). Initial therapy for tuberculosis in the era of multidrug resistance. *Morbidity and Mortality Weekly Report, 42*(RR-7), 1–8.

► Research Applications for Nursing

Aerosolized Interferon May Be of Benefit in Treating Multi–Drug-Resistant Tuberculosis

Condos, R., Rom, W. N., & Schluger, N. W. (1997). Treatment of multi–drug-resistant pulmonary tuberculosis with interferon-gamma via aerosol. Lancet, 349, 1513–1515.

Because interferon-gamma is a cytokine that can activate alveolar macrophages, cells important to immunity against *M. tuberculosis,* these researchers wanted to study its efficacy on severe, advanced multi–drug-resistant TB (MDR-TB). They selected five persons who had been receiving conventional directly observed TB drug therapy between 5 and 24 months and whose sputum smears and cultures were still positive. Each participant received 500 μg of recombinant human interferon-gamma three times a week for 4 weeks. Each person continued on their conventional therapy during the 4-week study period.

At the end of the study period, four of the five participants had become sputum-smear negative. The fifth had a significant reduction in the grade of the sputum smear and became negative 1 month later. Poststudy computed tomography results showed improvement compared with prestudy results. Body weight stabilized or increased in all participants during the study phase. All participants except one became sputum-smear positive after therapy with interferon was stopped.

Critique. Only five persons were studied, which limits the applicability of this treatment modality. One participant had diabetes and was HIV positive, which makes the group of five less homogeneous.

Possible Nursing Implications. The nurse who is aware of the latest research is able to contribute to the collaborative process in determining therapy for clients. The nurse communicates that muscle aches and cough were the minor adverse effects observed in this study. The nurse explains new therapies to clients and their families.

may be indicated. In addition, certain high-risk contacts receive prophylactic therapy, usually with isoniazid (INH).

► Home Care Management

Most clients with TB are managed outside the hospital. However, clients may be diagnosed with TB while in the hospital if pneumonia is suspected or other possible complications exist. Discharge may be delayed if the living situation is considered high risk or if the client is likely to be noncompliant. The nurse may consult with the social service worker in the hospital or the community health nursing agency to ensure the client's discharge to the appropriate environment with continued supervision. The home health nurse follows potentially infected people in the home environment because treating and then returning the client to the same environment only to become reinfected would be futile.

► Health Care Resources

The nurse instructs the client to receive follow-up care by a physician for at least 1 year during active treatment. In addition, the ALA, an organization that uses volunteers, can provide free information to the client about the disease and its treatment. Alcoholics Anonymous and other health care resources for clients with alcoholism are available as well, if needed. The nurse assists the client who uses drugs to locate an appropriate drug treatment program.

Lung Abscess

Overview

A lung abscess is a localized area of lung destruction caused by liquefaction necrosis, which is usually related

Directly observed therapy (DOT), where the nurse watches the client swallow the medications, may be indicated in some situations. This practice contributes to more treatment successes, less relapses, and less drug resistance.

The client who has experienced weight loss and severe lethargy should gradually resume usual activities. The client must maintain proper nutrition to prevent recurrence of infection.

To help the client encountering others with concerns about the contagious aspect of the infection, the nurse provides the client with information about TB. A key to preventing the transmission of TB is the identification of those in close contact with the infected person so that they can be tested and treated as necessary. Public health professionals have an important role in this aspect of care. When contacts have been identified, these people are assessed with a tuberculin test and possibly a chest x-ray to determine infection with TB. Multidrug therapy

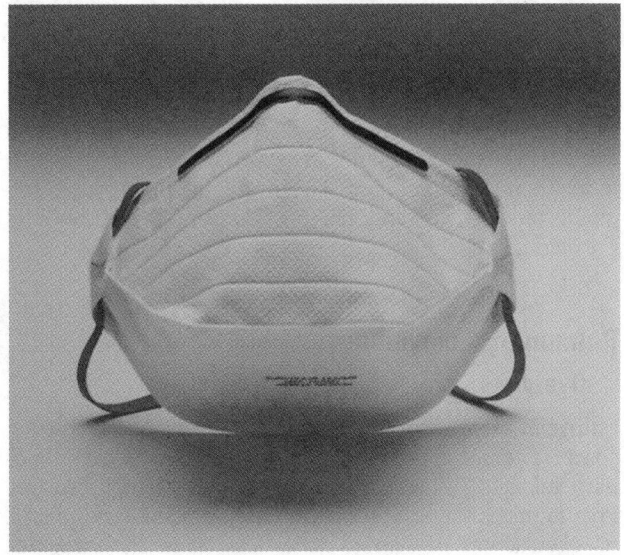

Figure 33–2. A HEPA respirator used in the care of clients with active or "rule-out" tuberculosis. (Courtesy of Uvex Safety, Smithfield, RI.)

to pyogenic bacteria. Clients who have this problem often have a history of pneumonia, possibly complicated by aspiration of oropharyngeal contents or proximal obstruction as a result of tumor or foreign body. Other causes of aspiration leading to abscess include alcoholism that causes loss of consciousness, seizure disorders or other neurologic deficits, and swallowing disorders. An obstruction of a bronchus may cause a necrotizing process in the distal lung that eventually becomes an abscess. Multiple abscesses and cavities commonly form in clients with TB or fungal infections of the lung. Immunosuppressed clients, such as those receiving chemotherapy, or those with a disease like leukemia or AIDS, are particularly susceptible to fungal infections. Most common organisms are anaerobic bacteria, *Staphylococcus* or other gram-positive organism, or gram-negative or opportunistic infections such as fungi.

Collaborative Management

 Assessment

The nurse notes a client's recent history of influenza, pneumonia, febrile illness, cough, and foul-smelling sputum production. In addition, the nurse inquires about the sputum color and odor, and about any pleuritic chest pain (a stabbing pain, especially when taking a deep breath). The client is often febrile, pale, fatigued, and cachectic. The nurse may note decreased breath sounds on auscultation and dullness on percussion in the involved area. Bronchial breath sounds and crackles are frequently heard over the site of the lesion. The physician orders a chest x-ray and sputum samples to assist in the diagnosis.

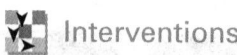 Interventions

Nursing diagnoses and interventions identified for the client with pneumonia also apply to the client with a lung abscess. Medical treatment is directed toward drainage of the abscess and antibiotics. The physician may prescribe more than one antibiotic. The nurse, then, provides frequent mouth care and observes for oral overgrowth of *Candida albicans*.

Pulmonary Empyema

Overview

Empyema refers to a collection of pus in the pleural space. The most common cause of empyema is pulmonary infection, lung abscess, or infected pleural effusion. Pneumonia or lung abscess can spread across the pleura, or obstruction of lymph nodes can cause a retrograde flood of infected lymph into the pleural space. In addition, an intrahepatic or subphrenic abscess can spread through the diaphragm's lymphatic system. Thoracic sur-

gery and chest trauma are common predisposing conditions in which bacteria are introduced directly into the pleural space. Blood from trauma may accumulate in the pleural space. Incomplete evacuation of this blood presents a culture medium for bacterial growth.

Collaborative Management

 Assessment

Important history findings include recent febrile illness (including pneumonia), chest pain, dyspnea, cough, and trauma. The nurse notes the characteristics of the sputum. On physical assessment, the nurse may observe diminished chest wall motion. If a pleural effusion is present, the nurse notes decreased or absent fremitus on palpation, a flat percussion note on percussion, and decreased breath sounds on auscultation. With compression of lung tissue adjacent to the effusion, the nurse auscultates bronchial breath sounds, egophony, and whispered pectoriloquy.

Some clients have fever, chills, night sweats, and weight loss. If there is cardiorespiratory compromise, the client may be hypotensive because of a mediastinal deviation; the nurse may note a displacement of the PMI (point of maximal impulse) on auscultation of the heart.

The physician orders a chest x-ray and obtains a sample of the pleural fluid via thoracentesis (see Chap. 29) for help in making the diagnosis. Empyema fluid is thick, opaque, exudative, and intensely foul smelling. The pleural fluid is sent to the laboratory and is analyzed for color, red blood cell count, white blood cell count and differential, glucose and protein levels, lactate dehydrogenase (LDH), and pH. Gram and acid-fast stains of the smears and cytology studies also are done. A protein concentration higher than 3 g/100 mL of pleural fluid indicates an exudative process.

 Interventions

Therapy for empyema is based on emptying the empyema cavity, reexpanding the lung, and controlling the infection. The physician usually treats the client with antibiotics appropriate for the isolated pathogen. In addition, closed-chest drainage (see Chap. 32) is used to promote lung expansion. The physician places one or more chest tubes in the inferior parts of the empyema sac. Underwater seal drainage is used without suction initially, but negative pressure may be added if the lung fails to expand. The physician removes the tube when the lung is fully expanded; and the infectious process is under control. Open thoracotomy and decortication (removal) of a portion of the pleura may be needed for thick pus or marked pleural thickening. Nursing considerations are the same as those for clients with a pleural effusion, pneumothorax, or infection.

CASE STUDY **for the Client with Tuberculosis**

▪ Ms. Chapel is a 25-year-old inner-city woman with AIDS. She is hospitalized now for active TB. She has four young children at home who are currently being cared for by her mother, a 42-year-old unemployed woman with diabetes.

Q U E S T I O N S :

1. In what kind of isolation must Ms. Chapel be placed and why?
2. Sputum cultures for acid-fast bacilli (AFB) are ordered. When is the best time to collect sputum? Can you still send sputum to the laboratory that contains saliva?
3. Before Ms. Chapel is discharged to home, what interventions need to be done at home in preparation for her return?

SELECTED BIBLIOGRAPHY

Afessa, B., Greaves, W. L., & Frederick, W. R. (1995). Pneumococcal bacteremia in adults: A 14-year experience in an inner-city university hospital. *Clinical Infectious Diseases, 21,* 345–351.

American College of Chest Physicians. (1995). Institutional control measures for tuberculosis in an era of multiple drug resistance (consumers statement). *Chest, 108,* 1690–1710.

*American Thoracic Society. (1990). Diagnostic standards and classification of tuberculosis. *American Review of Respiratory Disease, 142*(3), 725–735.

*American Thoracic Society. (1992). Control of tuberculosis in the United States (the official ATS statement). *American Review of Respiratory Disease, 146*(6), 1623–1633.

*Badhwar, A. K., & Druce, H. M. (1992). Allergic rhinitis. *Medical Clinics of North America, 76*(4), 789–804.

*Benson, V., & Marano, M. A. (1994). *Current estimates from the National Health Interview Survey* (DHHS Pub. No. [PHS] 94-1517). Hyattsville, MD: National Center for Health Statistics.

Bergone-Be're'zen, E. (1995). Treatment and prevention of nosocomial pneumonia. *Chest, 108*(2), 26S–34S.

Blumberg, H. M., Watkins, D. L., & Berschling, J. D. (1995). Preventing the nosocomial transmission of tuberculosis. *Annals of Internal Medicine, 122*(9), 658–663.

*Boutotte, J. (1993). TB the second time around. *Nursing93, 23*(5), 42–50.

*Brown, R. (1993). Community-acquired pneumonia: Diagnosis and therapy of older adults. *Geriatrics, 48*(2), 43–50.

Calianno, C. (1996). Nosocomial pneumonia. *Nursing96, 26*(5), 34–40.

*Campbell, G. D. (1994). Overview of community-acquired pneumonia: Prognosis and clinical features. *Medical Clinics of North America, 78,* 1035–1048.

*Cantwell, M. F., Snider, D. E., Cauthen, G. M., et al. (1994). Epidemiology of tuberculosis in the United States, 1985 through 1992. *Journal of the American Medical Association, 272*(7), 535–539.

*Caruthers, D. (1990). Infectious pneumonia in the elderly. *American Journal of Nursing, 90*(2), 56–60.

*Centers for Disease Control. (1993a). Estimates of future global tuberculosis morbidity and mortality. *Morbidity and Mortality Weekly Report, 42*(NO–49), 961–965.

*Centers for Disease Control. (1993b). Recommendations of the Advisory Council for the elimination of tuberculosis: Initial therapy for tuberculosis in the era of multidrug resistance. *Morbidity and Mortality Weekly Report, 42*(RR–7), 1–8.

*Centers for Disease Control. (1994). Guidelines for preventing the transmission of tuberculosis in health care settings. *Morbidity and Mortality Weekly Report, 43*(RR–13), 1–32.

Centers for Disease Control. (1995a). Increasing pneumonoccal vaccination rates—United States, 1993. *Morbidity and Mortality Weekly Report, 44*(40), 741–744.

Centers for Disease Control. (1995b). Influenza and pneumonoccal vaccination coverage levels among adults aged > 64 years—United States, 1973–1993. *Morbidity and Mortality Weekly Report, 44*(27), 506–507, 513–515.

Centers for Disease Control. (1995c). Pneumonia and influenza death rates—United States, 1979–1994. *Morbidity and Mortality Weekly Report, 44*(28), 535–537.

Centers for Disease Control and Prevention. (1996). Tuberculosis morbidity—United States, 1995. *Morbidity and Mortality Weekly Report, 45*(NO–18), 365–370.

Centers for Disease Control and Prevention. (1997a). Pneumonoccal and influenza vaccination among adults aged ≥ 65 years—United States, 1995. *Morbidity and Mortality Weekly Report, 46*(39), 913–919.

Centers for Disease Control and Prevention. (1997b). Recommendations of the Advisory Committee on immunization practices: Prevention of influenza. *Morbidity and Mortality Weekly Report, 46*(RR–9), 1–24.

Centers for Disease Control and Prevention. (1997c). Recommendations of the Advisory Committee on immunization practices: Prevention of pneumococcal disease. *Morbidity and Mortality Weekly Report, 46*(RR–8), 1–24.

Centers for Disease Control and Prevention. (1997d). Tuberculosis morbidity—United States, 1996. *Morbidity and Mortality Weekly Report, 46*(30), 695–700.

Cohen, M. L., Doeman, N. J., Kauffman, C. A., et al. (1995). Antimicrobial resistance: Are the pathogens winning? *Patient Care, 29*(9), 56–60, 63–64, 67–69.

Condos, R., Rom, W. N., & Schluger, N. W. (1997). Treatment of multidrug-resistant pulmonary tuberculosis with interferon-gamma via aerosol. *Lancet, 349,* 1513–1515.

Craven, D. E., & Steger, K. A. (1995). Epidemiology of nosocomial pneumonia: New perspectives on an old disease. *Chest, 108*(2), 1S–16S.

Crespo, J. (1995). Cost considerations of implementing OSHA tuberculosis regulations. *MEDSURG Nursing, 4*(5), 353–357.

Douville, L. (1995). Pharmacologic highlights: Management of acute sinusitis. *Journal of the American Academy of Nurse Practitioners, 7*(8), 407–411.

*Elpern, E. H., & Girzadas, A. M. (1993). Tuberculosis update: New challenges of an old disease. *MEDSURG Nursing, 2*(3), 176–183.

*Esler, R., Bentz, P., Sorensen, M., & Van Orsow, T. (1994). Patient-centered pneumonia care: A case management success story. *American Journal of Nursing, 94*(11), 34–38.

*Fedson, D. (1992). Clinical practice and public policy for influenza and pneumococcal vaccination of the elderly. *Clinics in Geriatric Medicine, 8*(1), 183–199.

Felmingham, D. (1995). Antibiotic resistance: Do we need new therapeutic approaches? *Chest, 108*(2), 70S–78S.

Finklestein, L., & Petrec, C. A. (1996). Sputum testing for TB: Getting good specimens. *American Journal of Nursing, 96*(2), 14.

*Gantz, N. M., & Sogg, A. J. (1992). An update on sinusitis. *Patient Care, 26*(8), 141–143, 147–148, 157–163.

Grimes, D. E., & Grimes, R. M. (1995). Tuberculosis: What nurses need to know to help control the epidemic. *Nursing Outlook, 43*(4), 164–173.

Hahn, M. S. (1995). Tuberculosis today. *ADVANCE for Nurse Practitioners, 3*(10), 19–23.

Haney, P. E., Raymond, B. A., Hernandez, J. M., et al. (1996). Tuberculosis makes a comeback. *AORN Journal, 63*(4), 705, 707, 709.

Hect, A. (1995). Diagnosis and treatment of pneumonia in the nursing home. *Nurse Practitioner, 20*(5), 24, 27–28, 35–39.

Hopkins, M. L., & Schoener, L. (1996). Tuberculosis and the elderly living in long-term care facilities. *Geriatric Nursing, 17*(1), 27–32.

*Howard, B. A. (1994). Guiding allergy sufferers through the medication maze. *RN, 57*(4), 26–30.

Howse, E. (1996). Pharmacy practice. *Mycobacterium tuberculosis:* Implications for home health care. *Home Health Care Management & Practice, 8*(3), 69–74.

*Jacobs, R. F. (1994). Multiple-drug-resistant tuberculosis. *Clinical Infectious Diseases, 19*(1), 1–8.

*Janzen, V. D. (1987). Rhinological disorders in the elderly. *Journal of Otolaryngology, 15,* 228–230.

*Josephson, J. S., & Rosenberg, S. I. (1994). Sinusitis. *Clinical Symposia, 46*(2), 2–32.

Jovell, R. J., & Salfinger, M. (1996). Molecular fingerprinting of myco-bacterium tuberculosis: A new diagnostic tool enhances TB control programs. *RT: Journal for Respiratory Care Practitioners, 9*(3), 66, 68, 70.

King, D. E., & Pippin, H. J. (1997). Community-acquired pneumonia in adults: Initial antibiotic therapy. *American Family Physician, 56*(2), 544–550.

Krouse, H. J., Parker, C. M., Purcell, R., et al. (1997). Powered func-tional endoscopic sinus surgery. *AORN Journal, 66*(3), 405, 408, 410–411, 413–414.

Lancaster, E., & Grimes, D. E. (1996). Tuberculosis: What nurses need to know to help control the epidemic (letter). *Nursing Outlook, 44*(2), 103–104.

Leibowitz, R. E. (1995). Critical care and tuberculosis. *Critical Care Nursing Clinics of North America, 7*(4), 661–666.

Leiner, S., & Mays, M. (1996). Diagnosing latent and active pulmonary tuberculosis: A review for clinicians. *Nurse Practitioner, 21*(2), 86, 88, 91–92.

Mandell, L. A. (1995). Community-acquired pneumonia. *Chest, 108*(2), 35S–42S.

Mayer, S. (1995). A sensitive issue . . . Detecting rhinitis. *Nursing Times, 91*(5), 23.

McAnulty, J. M., Fleming, D. W., et al. (1995). Missed opportunities for tuberculosis prevention. *Archives of Internal Medicine, 155*(7), 713–716.

*McCall, M. (1993). It killed George, or managing the peritonsillar abscess patient effectively. *ORL Head and Neck Nursing, 11*(1), 10–12.

*McCue, J. D. (1993). Pneumonia in the elderly. *Postgraduate Medicine, 94*(95), 39–40, 43–48, 51.

Mead, M. (1996). A guide to acute and chronic sinusitis. *Practice Nurse, 11*(10), 732–733.

Menzies, D., Fanning, A., & Yuan, G. (1995). Tuberculosis among health care workers. *New England Journal of Medicine, 332*(2), 92–98.

*Messner, R. L., & Zink, K. (1992). Nosocomial pneumonia: Combating a hospital menace. *RN, 55*(6), 48–53.

*Moran, G. J. (1994). Recognizing and minimizing the risks: Part 1. Multidrug-resistant TB. *Emergency Medicine, 26*(14), 36–42.

*Nadell, E. A. (1993). Environmental control of tuberculosis. *Medical Clinics of North America, 77*(6), 1315–1333.

*National Center for Health Statistics. (1993). *Health United States, 1992 and healthy people 2000 review* (DHHS Pub. No. [PHS] 93–1232). Hyattsville, MD: Public Health Service.

*Niederman, M. S., Bass, J. B., Campbell, G. D., et al. (1993). Guide-lines for the initial mamagement of adults with community-acquired pneumonia: Diagnosis, assessment of severity, and initial antimicro-bial therapy. Official American Thoracic Society statement. *American Review of Respiratory Disease, 148*, 1418–1426.

*Niederman, M. S., Sarosi, G. A., & Glassroth, J. (1994). *Respiratory infections: A scientific basis for management*. Philadelphia: W. B. Saun-ders Co.

*Norman, P. S. (1991). Allergic rhinitis: Combined therapy improves control. *Consultant, 31*(8), 25–29.

*Pattern, B. C., & Holt, J. (1992). When your patient is allergic. *Ameri-can Journal of Nursing, 92*(9), 58–61.

Petroff, P. F. (1997). Computer assisted endoscopic sinus surgery. *AORN Journal, 66*(3), 416, 418–420, 422–425.

*Piirila, P. (1992). Changes in crackle characteristics during the clinical course of pneumonia. *Chest, 102*(1), 176–183.

*Rubin, F. L. (1993). Viral pneumonias: The increasing importance of a high index of suspicion. *Postgraduate Medicine, 93*(7), 57–60, 63–64.

*Sanford, J. P. (1994). Combating drug-resistant pneumococcal infec-tions. *Hospital Practice, 29*(10), 31–37.

*Schwartz, R. (1994). The diagnosis and management of sinusitis. *Nurse Practitioner, 19*(12), 58–63.

Shehata, M. A. (1996). Atrophic rhinitis. *Medical Journal of Otolaryngol-ogy, 17*(2), 81–86.

Shulkin, D. J., & Brennan, P. J. (1995). The cost of caring for patients with tuberculosis: Planning for a disease on the rise. *American Jour-nal of Infection Control, 23*(1), 1–4.

*Slavin, R. G. (1991). Management of sinusitis. *Journal of the American Geriatrics Society, 39*(2), 212–217.

Stamp, D., & Arnold, M. S. (1995). Tuberculosis in home care: Comply-ing with OSHA. *Caring, 14*(2), 16–18, 20–22.

*Stead, W. W., Senner, J. W., Reddick, W. T., et al. (1990). Racial differences in susceptibility to infection by *Mycobacterium tuberculosis*. *New England Journal of Medicine, 322*(7), 422–427.

*Strolley, J. M., & Buckwalter, K. C. (1991). Iatrogenesis in the elderly. Nosocomial infections. *Journal of Gerontological Nursing, 17*(9), 30–34.

Telzak, E., & Sepkowitz, K. (1995). Multidrug-resistant tuberculosis in patients without HIV infection. *New England Journal of Medicine, 333*(14), 907–911.

*Walsh, K. (1994). Guidelines for the prevention and control of tuber-culosis in the elderly. *Nurse Practitioner, 19*(11), 79–84.

Wiseman, K. C. (1995). Tuberculosis: An old disease with a new face. *American Nephrology Nurses' Association Journal, 22*(6), 541–556.

*Wisinger, D. (1993). Bacterial pneumonia: *S. pneumoniae* and *H. in-fluenzae* are the villains. *Postgraduate Medicine, 93*(7), 43–46, 49–50, 52.

Wolf, L. (1995). A tuberculosis control plan for ambulatory care centers. *Nurse Practitioner, 20*(6), 34, 36, 39–40.

Wurtz, R., Lee, C., Lama, J., et al. (1996). A new class of close contacts: Home health care workers and occupational exposure to tuberculo-sis. *Home Health Care Management & Practice, 8*(2), 28–31.

*Yoshikawa, T. T. (1992). Tuberculosis in aging adults. *Journal of the American Geriatrics Society, 40*(2), 178–187.

SUGGESTED READINGS

Calianno, C. (1996). Nosocomial pneumonia. *Nursing96, 26*(5), 34–40.
The article begins with data regarding the incidence, severity, and increased length of hospital stay related to nosocomial pneumo-nia. The CDC criteria for definition of nosocomial pneumonia are listed. Specifics related to the elderly are emphasized. The au-thors then review the organisms associated with aspiration and inhalation, followed by preventive measures for bacterial, viral, and fungal causes of nosocomial pneumonia.

Hopkins, M. L., & Schoener, L. (1996). Tuberculosis and the elderly living in long-term care facilities. *Geriatric Nursing, 17*(1), 27–32.
This article begins with reporting the incidence of tuberculosis in the elderly and discusses reasons why the elderly are at risk for TB. The article then focuses on TB identification, diagnosis, and in-tervention for those in long-term care settings. Screening proto-cols, prevention, and disease control are covered. Differences in skin testing for the elderly are explained.

Petroff, P. F. (1997). Computer assisted endoscopic sinus surgery. *AORN Journal, 66*(3), 416, 418–420, 422–425.
This article explains how applying advanced computer imaging mo-dalities has increased the accuracy of endoscopic surgery on the sinuses and has decreased complications. As an ambulatory sur-gery procedure, the author proceeds to outline, step by step, the sequence of events from 1 day preoperatively to postoperative recovery and discharge. Of particular interest is the coordination of care aspects from all team members in all involved depart-ments.

Chapter 34

INTERVENTIONS FOR CRITICALLY ILL CLIENTS WITH RESPIRATORY PROBLEMS

Acute or chronic respiratory problems can progress rapidly and become life-threatening emergencies. Even with prompt treatment, such problems often lead to death. Although the elderly experience critical respiratory problems or complications more frequently, any person can sustain an acute injury or disorder resulting in severe respiratory impairment. The client who has difficulty breathing is anxious and fearful. The nurse must be prepared to manage the client's physical and emotional needs during respiratory emergencies.

Pulmonary Embolism

Overview

A pulmonary embolism is a collection of particulate matter (solids, liquids, or gaseous substances) that enters systemic venous circulation and lodges in the pulmonary vasculature. Large emboli obstruct pulmonary circulation, leading to decreased systemic oxygenation, pulmonary tissue hypoxia, and potential death. Any substance can cause an embolism, but a blood clot is the most common.

Pathophysiology

Pulmonary embolism (PE) is the most common acute pulmonary disease (90%) among hospitalized clients. In most people with a PE, a blood clot from a deep venous thrombosis (DVT) breaks loose from one of the veins in the lower extremities or the pelvis. The thrombus detaches, travels through the vena cava and right side of the heart, and then lodges in a smaller blood vessel off the pulmonary artery. Platelets accumulate behind the embolus, triggering the release of serotonin and thromboxane A_2, which causes vasoconstriction. Widespread pulmonary vasoconstriction and pulmonary hypertension impair ventilation and perfusion. Deoxygenated blood shunts into the arterial circulation to produce hypoxemia. Approximately 12% of clients with PE do *not,* however, have hypoxemia.

Etiology

Major risk factors for DVT leading to pulmonary embolism include

- Prolonged immobilization
- Surgery
- Obesity
- Advancing age
- Hypercoagulability
- History of thromboembolism

In addition, smoking, pregnancy, estrogen therapy, congestive heart failure, stroke, malignant neoplasms (particularly of the lung or prostate), Trousseau's syndrome, and major trauma increase the risk for DVT and pulmonary embolism.

Fat, oil, air, tumor cells, amniotic fluid, foreign objects (like broken intravenous [IV] catheters), injected particles, and infected fibrin clots or pus can gain access to the venous system and cause pulmonary embolism. Fat emboli from fracture of a long bone and oil emboli from lymphangiography do not impede blood flow; rather, they result in vascular injury and adult respiratory distress syndrome (ARDS). Amniotic fluid embolus is associated with a mortality rate of 80% to 90%; it occurs in 1 per 20,000 to 30,000 deliveries and can be a complication of abortion or amniocentesis. Septic emboli commonly arise from a pelvic abscess, an infected IV catheter, and non-sterile injections of illegal drugs. The problem with septic emboli lies in the toxic effects of the infection more than in the vascular occlusion.

Incidence/Prevalence

Pulmonary embolism affects at least 500,000 people a year in the United States, approximately 10% of whom die. Many die within 1 hour of onset of symptoms or before the diagnosis has even been suspected.

Collaborative Management

 Assessment

➤ History

The nurse questions any client with sudden onset of respiratory difficulty about the risk factors for pulmonary embolism, especially a history of deep venous thrombosis, recent surgery, or prolonged immobilization.

➤ Physical Assessment/Clinical Manifestations

Respiratory Manifestations. Chart 34–1 outlines the key features of PE. The nurse assesses the client for dyspnea accompanied by tachypnea, tachycardia, and pleuritic chest pain (sharp, stabbing-type pain on inspiration). These symptoms are found in 80% of clients diagnosed with PE. Other symptoms vary considerably depending on the severity and the type of embolism. Breath sounds may be normal, but crackles occur in 50% of clients with PE. The nurse typically notes a dry cough. Hemoptysis may result from pulmonary infarction.

Cardiovascular Manifestations. The nurse assesses for distended neck veins, syncope, cyanosis, and hypotension. Hypotension associated with massive emboli indicates acute pulmonary hypertension. Auscultation of heart

---

Chart 34–1

Key Features of Pulmonary Embolism

Symptoms
- Dyspnea, sudden onset
- Pleuritic chest pain
- Apprehension
- Feeling of impending doom
- Cough
- Hemoptysis

Signs
- Tachypnea
- Crackles
- Pleural friction rub
- Tachycardia
- S_3 or S_4 heart sound
- Diaphoresis
- Fever, low grade
- Petechiae over chest and axillae

---

sounds may reveal an S_3 or S_4 sound with an altered pulmonic component of S_2.

Electrocardiogram findings are abnormal, nonspecific, and transient. T-wave changes and ST-segment abnormalities develop in 50% of clients, but left- and right-axis deviations occur with equal frequency.

Miscellaneous Manifestations. A low-grade fever may be present. Petechiae may be present on the skin over the chest and in the axillae. Some clients have more vague symptoms resembling the flu, such as nausea, vomiting, and general malaise.

➤ Laboratory Assessment

The hyperventilation from hypoxia and pain initially leads to respiratory alkalosis, which the nurse confirms with low partial pressure of arterial carbon dioxide ($PaCO_2$) values on arterial blood gas (ABG) analysis. The alveolar-arterial (A-a) gradient is increased. As blood continues to be shunted without picking up oxygen from the lungs, the $PaCO_2$ level starts to rise, leading to respiratory acidosis. Later, metabolic acidosis results from tissue hypoxia.

Arterial blood gas studies and pulse oximetry may reveal hypoxemia, but these results alone are not sufficient for the diagnosis of PE. A client with a small embolus may not be hypoxemic, and PE is not the only cause of hypoxemia.

➤ Radiographic Assessment

Radiographic assessment alone is never diagnostic of a pulmonary embolism. Chest x-ray may show some pulmonary infiltration around the embolism site; however, the chest x-ray most frequently is normal.

➤ Other Diagnostic Assessment

One of the most important studies to determine PE is the ventilation-perfusion ($\dot{V}/\dot{Q}$) lung scan. A negative perfusion scan rules out PE. If the $\dot{V}/\dot{Q}$ scan is inconclusive, pulmonary angiography, the most definitive and specific test for PE, may be done.

In a few clients, the physician performs thoracentesis (see Chap. 29) or transesophageal echocardiography (TEE; see Chap. 35) for help in detecting PE. The physician often orders Doppler ultrasound studies or impedance plethysmography (IPG) to document the presence of DVT and to support a diagnosis of PE.

➤ Psychosocial Assessment

Because the onset of symptoms is usually abrupt, the client with PE generally is extremely anxious and fearful. Hypoxemia may cause the client to have a sense of impending doom and increased restlessness. The emergent nature of the disorder and the subsequent admission to an intensive care unit (ICU) may increase the client's anxiety and fear of death.

 Analysis

➤ Prevention

Although pulmonary embolism (PE) can occur in apparently healthy people and may have no warning, it occurs more frequently in some situations. Thus, prevention of conditions contributing to PE is a major nursing concern. Preventive actions for PE are those that also prevent venous stasis and DVT. These actions are listed in Chart 34–2.

The physician may order small doses of prophylactic heparin administered subcutaneously every 8 hours. Heparin prevents hypercoagulation in clients immobilized for a prolonged period after surgery or restricted to bed rest. Adequate fluid intake and avoidance of oral contraceptives are also preventive. (Further information on the prevention of DVT is found in Chapter 20.)

When a client complains of the acute onset of dyspnea with associated pleuritic chest pain, the nurse notifies the physician immediately. The nurse attempts to reassure the client and assists the client to a position of comfort with the head of the bed elevated. The nurse prepares for oxygen administration and blood gas analysis while con-

---

Chart 34–2

Nursing Care Highlight: Prevention of Pulmonary Embolism

- Initiating passive and active range-of-motion exercises for the extremities of immobilized and postoperative clients
- Ambulating postoperative clients soon after surgery
- Using antiembolism and pneumatic compression stockings and devices postoperatively
- Avoiding the use of tight garters, girdles, and constricting clothing
- Preventing pressure under the popliteal space (such as with a pillow)

---

tinuing to monitor and assess the client for additional signs and symptoms.

➤ Common Nursing Diagnoses and Collaborative Problems

The primary collaborative problem for the client with pulmonary embolism is Hypoxemia related to imbalanced ventilation-perfusion.

The priority nursing diagnoses to consider when caring for a client with pulmonary embolism are
1. Decreased Cardiac Output related to acute pulmonary hypertension
2. Anxiety related to hypoxemia and life-threatening illness
3. Risk for Injury (bleeding) related to anticoagulation–thrombolytic therapy

➤ Additional Nursing Diagnoses and Collaborative Problems

In addition to the common nursing diagnoses and collaborative problems, one or more of the following may apply:
- Activity Intolerance related to hypoxemia
- Ineffective Gas Exchange related to disrupted pulmonary perfusion
- Fatigue related to ineffective gas exchange
- Altered Oral Mucous Membrane related to oxygen therapy
- Acute Confusion related to hypoxemia
- Sleep Pattern Disturbance related to ICU environment

 Planning and Implementation

Hypoxemia

Planning: Expected Outcomes. As a result of interventions, the client is expected to have adequate oxygenation in all major organs.

Interventions. Nonsurgical approaches to management of PE are most common. In some cases, surgical approaches may be needed in addition to drug therapy.

Nonsurgical Management. Management of pulmonary embolism aims to increase alveolar gas exchange, improve pulmonary perfusion, eliminate the embolism, and prevent complications. Interventions include oxygen therapy, monitoring, and anticoagulation–antithrombolytic therapy.

Oxygen Therapy. Oxygen therapy is important for the client with PE (see Chap. 30). The severely hypoxemic client may require mechanical ventilation and close monitoring with ABGs. In less severe cases, oxygen may be administered by nasal cannula or mask. Pulse oximetry is useful in monitoring arterial oxygen saturation, which reflects the degree of hypoxemia.

Monitoring. The nurse assesses the client continually for any changes in status. The nurse assesses vital signs, lung sounds, and cardiac and respiratory status at least every 1 to 2 hours, noting increasing dyspnea, dysrhyth-

Chart 34–3

Drug Therapy for Pulmonary Embolism

Drug	Usual Dosage	Nursing Interventions	Rationale
Heparin sodium (Hepalean♣)	• 5000–10,000 units IVP initially; then dose adjustment is based on PTT, 1300 units/hr on continuous drip or, less preferably, intermittent infusion	• Monitor PTT. • Know expected therapeutic PTT range for each client. • Report PTT results. • Monitor client for bleeding or bruising. • Rebolus every time infusion is increased. • Do not use with salicylates. • Monitor platelets daily for thrombocytopenia. • Have the antidote, protamine sulfate, available. • Avoid puncture sites and apply pressure to venipuncture and IM injection sites. • Avoid use of firm toothbrushes, straight razors, and rectal thermometers.	• Ongoing assessment helps detect side effects and prevent complications. • Reporting enables the physician to begin early treatment of a prolonged PTT. • An increased anticoagulation effect can occur with salicylates. • White clot syndrome, a type of arterial thrombosis, can occur. • Being prepared for an emergency helps prevent further complications. • Pressure at puncture sites helps promote clotting. • Safety measures help prevent bleeding.
Warfarin sodium (Coumadin, Warfilone sodium♣)	• 10–15 mg PO for 3 days initially; then dose adjustment is based on INR, usually 5–10 mg PO daily	• Monitor INR. • Know expected therapeutic INR range for each client. • Report INR results. • Monitor the client for bleeding or bruising. • Monitor for fever and skin rash. • Consult the pharmacist about potential drug interactions. • Have the antidote, vitamin K, available. • Apply pressure to venipuncture and IM injection sites. • Avoid use of firm toothbrushes, straight razors, and rectal thermometers. • Teach the client which foods are high in vitamin K.	• Ongoing assessment helps detect side effects and prevent complications. • Reporting enables the physician to begin early treatment of a prolonged INR. • Adverse drug reaction can occur. • There are many drug interactions with warfarin. • Being prepared for an emergency helps prevent further complications. • Pressure at puncture sites helps promote clotting. • Safety measures help prevent bleeding. • Food sources of vitamin K will alter INR.

Continued

mias, distended neck veins, and pedal or sacral edema. The nurse also notes the presence of crackles and adventitious sounds on auscultation of the lungs along with cyanosis of the lips, conjunctiva, oral mucous membranes, and nail beds.

Anticoagulation–Thrombolytic Therapy. The physician usually orders anticoagulation to keep the embolus from enlarging and prevent the formation of new clots. Active bleeding, stroke, and recent trauma are some contraindications to the use of anticoagulants. Before proceeding,

the physician evaluates each client for risks and determines the risk versus the benefit of therapy.

Heparin is commonly used unless the PE is massive or is accompanied by hemodynamic instability. A thrombolytic enzyme agent may then be used to break up the existing clot. The physician and nurse review the client's partial thromboplastin time (aPTT; also called PTT) before therapy is initiated, every 4 hours when therapy is initiated, and then usually daily thereafter. Therapeutic PTT values usually range between 1½ and 2½ times the control value.

CHART 34–3. Drug Therapy for Pulmonary Embolism   Continued

Drug	Usual Dosage	Nursing Interventions	Rationale
Alteplase (tissue plasminogen activator, recombinant; tPA; Activase)	• 100 mg IV infusion over 2 hr	• Assess for internal and external bleeding. • Reconstitute with sterile water without preservative immediately before use. • Administer with caution to clients who had been receiving aspirin, dipyridamole, heparin, or other anticoagulants.	• Bleeding is the most common adverse effect. • Recommended preparation ensures drug stability. • Other drugs with anticoagulation effects increase the risk of bleeding.
Streptokinase	• 250,000–1,500,000 IU by IV infusion over 30 min as loading dose, then 100,000 IU/hr over 24–72 hr via continuous IV infusion pump	• Draw blood samples for PTT and INR before starting infusion. • Reconstitute and further dilute with sterile normal saline; roll to mix— do not shake. • Monitor the client for internal and external bleeding. • Avoid IM injections, venipunctures, other invasive procedures, or excessive handling of the client during therapy.	• The rate of infusion depends on blood studies. • Recommended preparation ensures drug stability. • Bleeding is a common adverse effect. • Safety measures help prevent bleeding. • Bruising is common.
Urokinase	• 4400–6000 IU/kg by IV infusion as a priming dose, then 4400 IU/kg/hr for 12–24 hr via continuous IV infusion pump	• Reconstitute with sterile water, then further dilute; total volume should not exceed 200 mL. • Monitor the client for internal and external bleeding. • Avoid IM injections, venipunctures, other invasive procedures, or excessive handling of the client during therapy.	• Recommended preparation ensures drug stability. • Bleeding is a common adverse effect. • Safety measures help prevent bleeding. • Bruising is common.

IVP = intravenous push, or bolus; PTT = partial thromboplastin time; IU = international units; INR = international normalized ratio; IV = intravenous; IM = intramuscular; PO = orally.

Heparin therapy usually continues for 5 to 10 days. The physician starts most clients on oral anticoagulants, such as warfarin (Coumadin, Warfilone✦), on the third day of heparin use. Therapy with both heparin and warfarin continues until the client has an international normalized ratio (INR) of 2.0 to 3.0. Heparin is then discontinued. The nurse and physician monitor the client's INR daily. The physician usually continues warfarin for 3 to 6 weeks, but particular clients at high risk may take warfarin indefinitely. Charts 34–3 and 34–4 present the drugs used and laboratory tests monitored. (Anticoagulants and associated nursing care are also discussed in Chapter 38.)

Surgical Management. Two surgical procedures for the management of pulmonary embolism are embolectomy and inferior vena caval interruption.

Embolectomy. When thrombolytic enzyme therapy is contraindicated in a client with massive or multiple large pulmonary emboli with shock, surgical embolectomy may be necessary. Embolectomy removes the embolus or emboli from the pulmonary arteries.

Inferior Vena Caval Interruption. The physician considers placing a vena caval filter as a lifesaving measure and to prevent further emboli formation for some clients. Candidates for this procedure include clients with an absolute contraindication to anticoagulation, recurrent or major bleeding while receiving anticoagulants, septic PE, and those undergoing pulmonary embolectomy. The physician orders a pulmonary angiogram before placing the filter. (Placement of a vena caval filter is detailed in Chapter 38.)

Decreased Cardiac Output

Planning: Expected Outcomes. As a result of intervention, the client is expected to have adequate circulation.

Interventions. In addition to the interventions used for hypoxemia induced by pulmonary embolism, IV fluid therapy and drug therapy aim to increase cardiac output.

Intravenous Fluid Therapy. Intravenous access is initiated and maintained for fluid and drug therapy. Fluid therapy involves administration of crystalloid solutions to restore plasma volume and prevent shock (see Chap. 39). Clients with pulmonary embolism receiving IV fluids should undergo continuous cardiac monitoring and monitoring of pulmonary wedge pressures because the increased fluids can worsen pulmonary hypertension and contribute to right-sided heart failure.

Drug Therapy. When IV therapy alone is not effective in improving cardiac output, drug therapy with agents that increase myocardial contractility (positive inotropic

---

Chart 34–4

Laboratory Profile: Blood Tests Used to Monitor Anticoagulation Therapy

Test	Normal Range for Adults	Significance of Abnormal Findings
Partial thromboplastin time (PTT, aPTT [APTT])	• Normal values for each local laboratory may vary. • When activator reagents are used by the laboratory, the normal clotting time is shortened. • Common normal ranges are 20–30 sec in some laboratories, or 30–40 sec in others. • Therapeutic range for PE is 1.5–2.5 times the normal value (e.g., if normal is 20–30 sec, then therapeutic range is 40–75 sec).	*Subtherapeutic times* may signify that the client is not receiving enough heparin to prevent extension of the blood clot. An increase in the dosage or rate of infusion is usually indicated. *Therapeutic times* mean that the clotting time is increased from normal, but this increase is indicated in the case of PE. *Prolonged times* in clients with PE (i.e., >75 sec) indicate that the client is at risk of serious spontaneous bleeding. Heparin is usually held or decreased until the PTT drops back into the therapeutic range.
Prothrombin time (protime, PT)	• 11–12.5 sec • Therapeutic range for anticoagulant therapy in PE is 1.5–2 times the normal or control value in seconds. • Control values can vary day to day because reagents used may vary. • If INR values are reported with the PT, therapeutic range for PE is 2.5–3.0, or 3.0–4.5 for recurrent PE.	*Subtherapeutic values* may signify that the client is not receiving enough warfarin. An increase in the dosage is usually indicated. *Therapeutic values* mean that the protime is increased from normal, but this increase is indicated in the case of PE. *Prolonged values* in the treatment of PE indicate that the client is at risk for bleeding. The warfarin dose is usually decreased or held, the client is instructed to eat foods high in vitamin K, or an injection of vitamin K may be given.

PE = pulmonary embolism; INR = international normalized ratio; aPTT or APTT = activated partial thromboplastin time.

---

agents) may be prescribed. Such agents include amrinone (Inocor) and dobutamine (Dobutrex). The nurse assesses the client's cardiac status hourly during therapy with inotropic agents.

Anxiety

Planning: Expected Outcomes. The client is expected to express a reduction in level of anxiety.

Interventions. The client with PE is anxious and fearful for a variety of physiologic and psychological reasons. Interventions for reducing anxiety in clients with PE include oxygen therapy (see interventions for hypoxemia), communication, and drug therapy.

Communication. The nurse acknowledges the anxiety and the client's perception of a life-threatening situation. Speaking calmly and clearly, the nurse assures the client that appropriate measures are being taken. When administering a drug, changing the client's position, taking vital signs, or obtaining assessment data, the nurse explains the rationale to the client and shares information appropriately.

Drug Therapy. If the client's anxiety increases or prevents adequate rest, an antianxiety drug may be prescribed. Unless the client is intubated and mechanically ventilated, agents that have a sedating effect are avoided.

Risk for Injury (Bleeding)

Planning: Expected Outcomes. The client is expected to remain free from bleeding.

Interventions. As a result of anticoagulation or thrombolytic therapy, the client's ability to initiate and continue the blood-clotting cascade when injured is seriously impaired and the client is at great risk for bleeding. The nurse's major objectives are to protect the client from situations that could lead to bleeding and to monitor closely the amount of bleeding that is occurring.

The nurse assesses the client frequently for evidence of bleeding in the form of oozing, confluent ecchymoses, petechiae, or purpura. All stools, urine, nasogastric drainage, and vomitus are examined visually for the appearance of blood and are tested for occult blood. The nurse measures any blood loss as accurately as possible. The nurse measures the client's abdominal girth every 8 hours. Increases in abdominal girth can indicate internal hemorrhage. Bleeding precautions are instituted (Chart 34–5).

The nurse monitors laboratory values daily. The complete blood count (CBC) results are reviewed daily to determine the client's risk for bleeding as well as to determine whether actual blood loss has occurred. If the client sustains a severe blood loss, packed red blood cells may be ordered (see transfusion therapy in Chapter 42).

Chart 34–5

Nursing Care Highlight: Bleeding Precautions

- Handle the client gently.
- Use a lift sheet when moving or positioning the client in bed.
- Avoid intramuscular injections and venipunctures.
- When injections are necessary, use the smallest gauge needle appropriate for the task.
- Apply firm pressure to the needlestick site for 10 minutes or until the site no longer oozes blood.
- Apply ice to areas of trauma.
- Test all urine and stool for the presence of occult blood.
- Check intravenous sites every 2 hours for bleeding.
- Avoid trauma to rectal tissue:
  - Do not take temperatures rectally.
  - Do not give enemas.
  - Administer well-lubricated suppositories with caution.
- Measure abdominal girth daily.
- If the client is to be shaved, use an electric razor.
- Use a soft-bristled toothbrush or tooth sponge for oral care.
- Inspect the mouth and gums for bleeding every 4 hours.
- Pad the side rails of the bed.
- Encourage the client not to blow the nose or insert objects into the nose.
- If the client is to ambulate, ensure that the footwear has a firm sole.

 Continuing Care

The client with a PE usually is discharged after the embolism has been resolved but may continue anticoagulation therapy.

➤ Health Teaching

The client with PE may continue anticoagulation therapy for weeks, months, or years after discharge, depending on the contributing factors. The nurse teaches the client and family about bleeding precautions, activities to reduce the risk for deep venous thrombosis and recurrence of PE, signs and symptoms of complications, and the importance of follow-up care (Chart 34–6).

➤ Home Care Management

Some clients will be discharged home with minimal risk for recurrence and no permanent physiologic changes. Other clients may have extensive lung damage and require lifestyle modifications.

Clients with extensive lung damage may have activity intolerance and become fatigued easily. The living arrangements may need to be modified so that clients can spend all or most of the time on one floor and avoid stair climbing. Depending on the degree of impairment, clients

may require some or much assistance with activities of daily living.

➤ Health Care Resources

For clients continuing with anticoagulation therapy, a home care nurse usually visits at least once per week to draw blood and perform an assessment (see Chart 34–7 for a focused assessment guide). Clients with severe dyspnea may require intermittent or continual home oxygen therapy. Respiratory therapy treatments can be performed in the home. The nurse or case manager coordinates arrangements for oxygen and other respiratory therapy to be available if needed by clients at home.

 Evaluation

On the basis of the identified nursing diagnoses and collaborative problems, the nurse evaluates the entire plan of

Chart 34–6

Education Guide: The Client After Pulmonary Embolism

- Use an electric razor.
- Use a soft-bristled toothbrush and do not floss.
- Do not have dental work done without consulting your health care provider.
- Do not take aspirin or aspirin-containing products. Read the labels of all over-the-counter medications to be sure that the product does not contain aspirin or salicylates.
- Do not participate in contact sports or in any activity in which you might be bumped, scraped, or scratched.
- Apply ice immediately to any site of injury.
- Avoid anal intercourse.
- Take a stool softener to prevent straining during a bowel movement.
- Do not use enemas or rectal suppositories.
- Do not wear clothing that is tight or rubs.
- Avoid bending over at the waist.
- Avoid positions in which your knees are bent for any length of time.
- Wear elastic stockings as prescribed.
- Avoid prolonged sitting or standing.
- Avoid blowing your nose or placing objects in your nose. If you must blow your nose, do so gently without blocking either nasal passage.
- Take the prescribed dosage of medication at the precise time it was ordered to be given.
- Do not stop taking the medication abruptly or without a physician's order.
- Notify your doctor if you
  - Have an injury and persistent bleeding results.
  - Have excessive menstrual bleeding.
  - See blood in your urine or bowel movement.
  - Notice large bruises or areas of small red or purple marks over the skin.

care for the client with PE. The expected outcomes are that the client

- Attains and maintains adequate gas exchange and oxygenation
- Does not experience hypovolemia and shock
- Remains free from bleeding episodes
- States that levels of anxiety are reduced

Chart 34–7

Focused Assessment for Home Care Clients After Pulmonary Embolism

- Assess respiratory status.
  - Observe rate and depth of respiration.
  - Auscultate lungs.
  - Examine nail beds and mucous membranes for evidence of cyanosis.
  - Take a pulse oximetry reading.
  - Ask the client if chest pain or shortness of breath is experienced in any position.
  - Ask the client about the presence of sputum and its color and character.
- Assess cardiovascular status.
  - Take vital signs; including apical pulse, pulse pressure; assess presence or absence of orthostatic hypotension and quality and rhythm of peripheral pulses.
  - Take blood pressure in both arms.
  - Note presence or absence of peripheral edema.
  - Examine hand vein filling in the dependent position.
  - Examine neck vein filling in the recumbent and sitting positions.
- Assess lower extremities for deep venous thrombosis.
  - Examine lower legs and compare with each other for
    General edema
    Calf swelling
    Surface temperature
    Presence of red streaks or cord-like palpable structure
  - Measure calf circumference.
  - Ask the client to dorsiflex and plantarflex each foot. Note the ease with which the client can do this and ask whether pain is experienced in either position.
  - Gently squeeze the calf of each leg laterally and from front to back. Ask the client whether pain or tenderness is experienced with either maneuver.
- Assess for evidence of bleeding.
  - Examine the mouth and gums for oozing or frank bleeding.
  - Examine all skin areas for bruising or petechiae.
  - If the client voids during the visit, test the urine for occult blood.
- Assess cognition and mental status.
  - Level of consciousness
  - Orientation to time, place, and person
  - Can the client accurately read a seven-word sentence containing no words greater than three syllables?
- Assess client's understanding of illness and compliance with treatment.
  - Signs and symptoms to report to health care provider
  - Medication plan (correct timing and dose)
  - Bleeding precautions
  - Prevention of deep venous thrombosis

Acute Respiratory Failure

Overview

Pathophysiology

Acute respiratory failure is categorized according to abnormal blood gases. The critical values are partial pressure of arterial oxygen (PaO_2) less than 60 mmHg, arterial oxygen saturation, (SaO_2) less than 90%, or $PaCO_2$ greater than 50 mmHg with accompanying acidemia (pH < 7.30). Acute respiratory failure is further classified as ventilatory failure, oxygenation failure, or combination of both ventilatory and oxygenation failure. Whatever the underlying disorder, the client in acute respiratory failure is always hypoxemic.

Ventilatory Failure

Ventilatory failure is the type of ventilation-perfusion ($\dot{V}/\dot{Q}$) mismatching in which perfusion is normal but ventilation is inadequate. Ventilatory failure occurs when the thoracic pressure cannot be changed sufficiently to permit appropriate air movement in and out of the lungs. As a result, insufficient oxygen reaches the alveoli and carbon dioxide is retained. Both problems lead to hypoxemia.

Ventilatory failure is usually the result of one or more of the following three mechanisms: a mechanical abnormality of the lungs or chest wall, a defect in the respiratory control center in the brain, or an impairment in the function of the respiratory muscles. Ventilatory failure is usually defined by a $PaCO_2$ level above 45 mmHg in clients who have otherwise healthy lungs.

Oxygenation Failure

In oxygenation failure, thoracic pressure changes are normal, and the lungs can move air sufficiently but cannot oxygenate the pulmonary blood properly. Oxygenation failure can result from the type of $\dot{V}/\dot{Q}$ mismatch in which ventilation is normal but perfusion is decreased.

Combined Ventilatory and Oxygenation Failure

Combined ventilatory and oxygenation failure involves insufficient respiratory movements (hypoventilation). Gas exchange at the alveolar-capillary membrane is inadequate, so that too little oxygen reaches the blood and carbon dioxide is retained. The condition may or may not include poor pulmonary circulation. When pulmonary circulation is not adequate, $\dot{V}/\dot{Q}$ mismatching occurs and both ventilation and perfusion are inadequate. This type of respiratory failure results in a more profound hypoxemia than either ventilatory failure or oxygenation failure alone.

Etiology

Ventilatory Failure

Numerous diseases and conditions can result in ventilatory failure. Causes of ventilatory failure are categorized

TABLE 34-1

Common Causes of Ventilatory Failure

Category	Disorder

Extrapulmonary	• Neuromuscular disorders
	  • Multiple sclerosis
	  • Myasthenia gravis
	  • Guillain-Barré syndrome
	  • Poliomyelitis
	• Spinal cord injuries affecting nerves to intercostal muscles
	• Central nervous system dysfunction
	  • Cerebrovascular accident (CVA)
	  • Cerebral edema
	  • Increased intracranial pressure
	  • Meningitis
	• Chemical depression
	  • Opioid analgesics
	  • Sedatives
	  • Anesthetic agents
	• Kyphoscoliosis
	• Massive obesity
	• Sleep apnea
	• External obstruction/constriction

Intrapulmonary	• Airway disease
	  • Chronic obstructive pulmonary disease
	  • Asthma
	• Ventilation-perfusion ($\dot{V}/\dot{Q}$) mismatching
	  • Pulmonary embolism
	  • Pneumothorax
	  • Adult respiratory distress syndrome (ARDS)
	• Amyloidosis
	• Pulmonary edema
	• Interstitial fibrosis

as either *extrapulmonary* (involving nonpulmonary tissues but affecting respiratory function) or *intrapulmonary* (disorders of the respiratory tract). Table 34–1 lists common extrapulmonary and intrapulmonary causes of ventilatory failure.

Oxygenation Failure

Many diseases and disorders of the lung can cause oxygenation failure. Mechanisms include impaired diffusion of oxygen at the alveolar level, right-to-left shunting of blood in the pulmonary vessels, ventilation-perfusion mismatching, breathing air with a low partial pressure of oxygen (a rare problem), and abnormal hemoglobin that fails to absorb the oxygen. In one type of ventilation-perfusion ($\dot{V}/\dot{Q}$) mismatching, areas of the lungs are still being perfused, but gas exchange is not able to occur, which leads to hypoxemia. An extreme example of $\dot{V}/\dot{Q}$ mismatching is a right-to-left shunt. A normal shunt is less than 5% of cardiac output. With right-to-left shunt, increased amounts of venous blood are not oxygenated, and 100% oxygen does not correct the deficiency. A clas-

sic cause of such a $\dot{V}/\dot{Q}$ mismatch is ARDS. Table 34–2 lists specific causes of oxygenation failure.

Combined Ventilatory and Oxygenation Failure

A combination of ventilatory failure and oxygenation failure occurs in clients who have abnormal lungs, as in all forms of chronic airflow limitation (CAL; i.e., chronic bronchitis, emphysema, and asthma). The bronchioles and alveoli are diseased (causing oxygenation failure), and the work of breathing increases until the respiratory muscles are unable to continue (causing ventilatory failure). Acute respiratory failure results. This process can also occur in clients who have cardiac failure as well as respiratory failure. This is a very dangerous situation because the cardiac system cannot compensate for the decreased oxygen by increasing the cardiac output.

Collaborative Management

 Assessment

The nurse assesses for dyspnea, the hallmark of respiratory failure. With use of a dyspnea assessment guide (Fig. 34–1), if one is available, the nurse objectively evaluates the dyspnea. Depending on the process, nature, and course of the underlying condition, the client may or may not be aware of dyspnea. In addition, the client needs to be alert enough to perceive the sensation of difficult breathing.

Dyspnea tends to be more intense when it develops rapidly. Slowly progressive respiratory failure may first manifest as dyspnea on exertion (DOE) or when lying down. The client notes orthopnea, finding it is easier to breathe in an upright position. In the client with CAL, a minor increase in dyspnea from the baseline condition may represent severe gas exchange abnormalities.

The nurse assesses for a change in the client's respiratory rate or pattern, a change in lung sounds, and the signs and symptoms of hypoxemia and hypercapnia (see Chap. 33). Pulse oximetry may indicate decreased oxygen

TABLE 34-2

Common Causes of Oxygenation Failure

• Low atmospheric oxygen concentration
  • High altitudes
  • Smoke inhalation
  • Carbon monoxide poisoning
• Pneumonia
• Abnormal hemoglobin
• Pulmonary embolism
• Pulmonary edema
• Interstitial pneumonitis-fibrosis
• Adult respiratory distress syndrome (ARDS)
• Mechanical obstruction
• Congestive heart failure
• Hypovolemic shock
• Hypoventilation

Dyspnea Assessment Guide

Indicate the amount of shortness of breath you
are having at this time by marking the line.

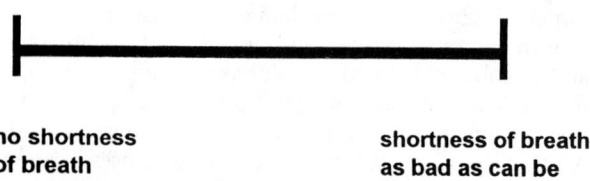

**no shortness
of breath**   **shortness of breath
                                as bad as can be**

Figure 34–1. A dyspnea assessment tool. Modified from Gift, A.
(1989). A dyspnea assessment guide. *Critical Care Nurse,* 9(8), 79.
Used with permission.

saturation, but an arterial blood gas (ABG) analysis is
needed for adequate assessment of oxygenation status.
The health care provider reviews the ABG studies to identify the degree of hypercapnia and hypoxemia.

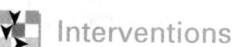 Interventions

The physician orders oxygen therapy for the client with
acute respiratory failure to keep the PaO_2 level above
60 mmHg while treating the underlying cause of the respiratory failure. (Oxygen therapy is discussed in detail in
Chapter 30.) If supplemental oxygen cannot maintain acceptable PaO_2 levels, the physician may order mechanical
ventilation.

The nurse or assistive nursing personnel helps the client find a position of comfort that allows easier breathing.
To decrease the anxiety commonly associated with dyspnea, the nurse assists the client with interventions such as
relaxation, guided imagery, and diversion. Energy-con-
serving measures, such as minimal self-care and no unnecessary procedures, are instituted. The physician may
order pulmonary medications administered systemically or
by metered-dose inhaler (MDI) to open the bronchioles
and promote gas exchange. The nurse instructs the client
about the use of the inhaler and about the medications.
Deep breathing and other breathing exercises are encouraged. (See Chapter 33 for further discussion of interventions for dyspnea and hypoxemia.)

Adult Respiratory Distress Syndrome
Overview

Adult respiratory distress syndrome (ARDS) is a form of
acute respiratory failure characterized by

- Refractory hypoxemia
- Decreased pulmonary compliance
- Dyspnea
- Noncardiogenic bilateral pulmonary edema
- Dense pulmonary infiltrates (ground-glass appearance)

Adult respiratory distress syndrome usually occurs after
an acute catastrophic event in people with no previous
pulmonary disease. The mortality rate is 50% to 60%.
Terminology for ARDS includes the current term *noncardiogenic pulmonary edema* and the former term *shock lung*.

Pathophysiology

Despite diverse causes leading to injury of the lung in
ARDS, no common pathway has been found in its development, although the principal clinical manifestations are
similar. In some forms of ARDS, the pathophysiologic
mechanism is understood; in many others, it is not. The
major site of injury in the lung is the alveolar-capillary
membrane, which is normally permeable to only small
molecules. The alveolar-capillary membrane can be injured intrinsically (causing sepsis, pulmonary embolism,
or shock) or extrinsically (causing aspiration or inhalation
injury). The interstitium of the lung normally remains
relatively dry, but in clients with ARDS, increased extravascular lung fluid contains a high concentration of proteins.

Other significant changes occur in the alveoli and respiratory bronchioles. The type II pneumocyte is responsible for producing surfactant, a substance that maintains
the elasticity of lung tissue and prevents alveolar collapse
on expiration. Surfactant activity is reduced in ARDS either because of destruction of the type II pneumocyte or
inactivation or dilution of surfactant. Consequently, the
alveoli become unstable and tend to collapse unless they
are filled with fluid from the interstitial space. These alveoli can no longer participate in gas exchange. As a result,
interstitial edema forms around terminal airways, which
are compressed and obliterated. Lung volume is further
reduced, and there is even less compliance (elasticity). As
the leak expands, fluid, protein, and blood cells collect in
the interstitium and alveoli. Lymph channels are compressed and ineffective. Poorly ventilated alveoli receive
blood. Thus, the shunt fraction increases, and hypoxemia
and ventilation-perfusion ($\dot{V}/\dot{Q}$) mismatching result.

Etiology

Adult respiratory distress syndrome is associated with a
number of causative factors (Table 34–3). Some causes
involve direct injury to lung tissue; others do not directly
involve the respiratory system. Serious nervous system
injury, such as trauma, cerebrovascular accidents, tumors,
and sudden increases in cerebrospinal fluid pressure, may
cause massive sympathetic discharge. Systemic vasoconstriction results with redistribution of large volumes of
blood into the pulmonary circuit. The marked elevation
of hydrostatic pressure, then, probably causes lung injury.
Processes that produce cerebral hypoxia, such as shock
and ascent to high altitudes, may operate by a similar
mechanism.

Some factors produce ARDS by direct injury to the
lung. For example, aspiration of gastric contents leads to
mechanical obstruction or produces an acid burn to the
airway when the pH of the gastric contents is less than
2.5. In such a direct injury, rapid necrosis of the alveolar
type I pneumocyte occurs. The injured capillary endothe-

TABLE 34-3

Common Causes of Adult Respiratory Distress Syndrome (ARDS)

- Shock
- Trauma
- Serious nervous system injury
- Pancreatitis
- Fat and amniotic fluid emboli
- Pulmonary infections
- Sepsis
- Inhalation of toxic gases (smoke, oxygen)
- Pulmonary aspiration
- Drug ingestion (e.g., heroin, opioids, aspirin)
- Hemolytic disorders
- Multiple blood transfusions
- Cardiopulmonary bypass
- Near-drowning (especially in fresh water)

lium allows protein and cellular elements to escape from the intravascular space. Radiation, near-drowning, and inhalation of toxic gases similarly injure the alveolar and capillary endothelium. In addition, trauma, sepsis, drowning, and burns cause the release of thromboplastins, which form fibrin clots in the peripheral blood. The clots, together with platelets and leukocytes, are filtered out in the lung. In many cases of ARDS, especially after trauma, production of plasminogen activation inhibitors by the liver is enhanced. Fibrinolysis is prevented, and microemboli remain in the lung. Disseminated intravascular coagulation (DIC) plays a role in some clients.

Incidence/Prevalence

Because of varying definitions, the incidence of ARDS is unknown, although a 1993 estimate suggested that more than 100,000 cases of ARDS occur yearly in the United States. Its high rank on the list of common diseases may be a result of the improved treatment of other catastrophic illnesses.

A major goal in the prevention of ARDS is early recognition of clients at high risk for the syndrome. Because clients with aspiration of gastric contents are at great risk, the nurse closely assesses and monitors elderly clients receiving tube feeding and clients with neurologic deficits and altered swallowing and gag reflexes. The nurse and assistive personnel meticulously follow all infection control guidelines, including hand washing, invasive catheter and wound care, and body substance precautions. In addition, the nurse carefully observes clients who are being treated for any of the diseases or disorders associated with ARDS.

Collaborative Management

 Assessment

The nurse assesses the client's respirations and notes whether increased work of breathing is evident, as indicated by hyperpnea, grunting respiration, cyanosis, pallor,

and retraction intercostally (between the ribs) or suprasternally (above the ribs). The nurse notes the presence of diaphoresis and any change in mental status. No abnormal lung sounds are present on auscultation because the edema of ARDS occurs first in the interstitial spaces and not in the airways. To assess for hypotension, tachycardia, and dysrhythmias, the nurse monitors vital signs frequently.

The primary laboratory study for establishing the diagnosis of ARDS is a lowered PaO_2 value, determined by arterial blood gas (ABG) measurements. The client with ARDS is poorly responsive to high concentrations of oxygen (*refractory hypoxemia*). Because a widening alveolar oxygen gradient (increased fraction of inspired oxygen [FIO_2] does not yield corresponding increased PaO_2 levels) develops with increased shunting of blood, the client has a progressive need for higher concentrations of oxygen. A large difference between the predicted and actual alveolar oxygen tension indicates shunting. The physician orders sputum cultures to isolate any organisms causing an infection that must be treated. Because decreased mortality depends on aggressive therapy, sputum may be obtained through bronchoscopy with protective brushings and by transtracheal aspiration.

The chest x-ray shows the diagnostic diffuse haziness or "whited-out" (ground-glass) appearance of the lung. An electrocardiogram rules out cardiac abnormalities and usually reveals no specific changes. The placement of a Swan-Ganz hemodynamic monitoring catheter is a diagnostic tool: in the client with ARDS, the pulmonary capillary wedge pressure (PCWP) is usually low to normal. This pressure differs from the client with cardiogenic pulmonary edema in whom the PCWP is higher than 15 mmHg.

 Interventions

Clients with adult respiratory distress syndrome (ARDS) usually require endotracheal intubation and mechanical ventilation with positive end-expiratory pressure (PEEP) or continuous positive airway pressure (CPAP). Sedation and paralysis may be necessary for adequate ventilation and for reducing oxygen requirements. Because one of the side effects of PEEP is tension pneumothorax, the nurse assesses lung sounds frequently and maintains a patent airway with suctioning. Positioning may be important in promoting gas exchange. (See the Research Applications for Nursing for a discussion of the prone position.)

► Drug and Fluid Therapy

Corticosteroids are seldom used in the treatment of ARDS, although they may impair neutrophil mobilization and stabilize the capillary membrane. Their efficacy, however, has not been determined. Antibiotics are used to treat infections with organisms identified by culture.

Many interventions are under investigation, but none have been shown to be effective in decreasing mortality. Some of these interventions include mediators (vitamins C and E, interleukin, prostacycline, aspirin), nitric oxide, surfactant replacement, and prone positioning.

▷ Research Applications for Nursing

Prone Position Improves Oxygenation in Clients with ARDS

Vollman, K. M., & Bander, J. (1996). Improved oxygenation in patients with acute respiratory distress syndrome. Intensive Care Medicine, 22(10), 1105–1111.

In clients with adult respiratory distress syndrome (ARDS) on mechanical ventilation, high tidal volumes, increased levels of inspired oxygen (O_2), and positive end-expiratory pressure (PEEP) are instituted to decrease shunt and improve oxygenation. More studies are indicating that the prone position improves oxygen and allows fraction of inspired oxygen (FIO_2) and pressures to be decreased. Contraindications to prone positioning include skin trauma from the turning maneuver and accidental disconnection or removal of tubes and catheters.

In this study, the primary author, a nurse, evaluated a device she developed to facilitate proning. Fifteen clients with ARDS were studied in this prospective controlled trial conducted in two medical intensive care units (ICUs). Oxygenation was better with clients in the prone position than in the supine position. Overall, there was a decrease in the alveolar-arterial (A–a) gradient of 21 mmHg when clients were prone. Responders were classified as those showing at least a 7-mmHg improvement in partial pressure of arterial oxygen (PaO_2). There were significant differences between responders and nonresponders (but not in positions) between PaO_2, partial pressure of arterial carbon dioxide ($PaCO_2$), baseline data, pulmonary artery pressures, peak inspiratory pressures on the ventilator, ICU length of stay, and time on mechanical support. No client suffered adverse hemodynamic effects, airway dislodgment, or loss of intravascular catheters during position changes. An important aspect of the turning frame is that the abdomen is not restricted.

Critique. The study sample was small and limited to a medical ICU population. The turning maneuvers were randomly assigned, and clients were used as their own controls. This study represents an important beginning to evaluate the effects of proning as well as the use of a positioning device to facilitate the maneuver.

Possible Nursing Implications. Oxygenation was found to increase in the prone position. Prone-positioned clients with ARDS may be treated with lower levels of O_2 and PEEP to maintain adequate gas exchange. Nurses have been reluctant to place clients in the prone position because of the difficulty entailed. Physicians are reluctant to request proning because of the complications that can arise, including unplanned extubation. If turning is achieved relatively easily, nurses and physicians may perform the maneuver more frequently. Use of the turning device may facilitate this nursing action and improve client outcome.

The optimal type of fluid therapy for the client with ARDS remains unknown. A colloidal solution may be effective for intravascular volume expansion. However, the value of colloid therapy is unknown. Fluid volume should be titrated to maintain adequate cardiac output and tissue perfusion. Judicious diuresis may help decrease extravascular lung fluid, but care should be taken to prevent overall dehydration and hypotension.

▷ Nutrition Therapy

Clients with ARDS are at risk for malnutrition, which further compromises the respiratory system. An altered immune response as well as an altered ventilatory response to hypoxemia may occur with undernourished clients. Diaphragmatic functioning is also altered. Therefore, enteral nutrition in the form of tube feeding or parenteral nutrition in the form of hyperalimentation is instituted as soon as possible.

▷ Case Management

Case management of the client with ARDS focuses on the phases of ARDS rather than day-to-day care. The course of ARDS and its management are divided into four phases.

- Phase 1: includes early changes with the client exhibiting dyspnea and tachypnea. Early interventions focus on supporting the client and providing oxygen.
- Phase 2: patchy infiltrates from increasing pulmonary edema. Interventions include mechanical ventilation and prevention of complications.
- Phase 3: occurs over days 2 to 10, and the client exhibits progressive refractory hypoxemia. Interventions focus on maintaining adequate oxygen transport, preventing complications, and supporting the failing lung until it has had time to heal.
- Phase 4: pulmonary fibrosis–pneumonia with progression; occurs after 10 days. This phase is irreversible and is frequently referred to as "late" or "chronic" ARDS. Interventions focus on preventing sepsis, pneumonia, and multiple organ failure (multiple organ dysfunction syndrome [MODS]) as well as weaning the client from the ventilator. Clients in this phase may be ventilator dependent for weeks to months. Clients may be cared for in specialized units or facilities that focus on rehabilitation and long-term weaning. Some clients may not be weanable and go home ventilator dependent (see Clinical Pathway).

Client Requiring Intubation and Ventilation

Overview

Through the use of mechanical ventilation, clients who have severe derangements of gas exchange may be supported until the underlying process has resolved or has been adequately treated. Thus, mechanical ventilation is nearly always a temporary life-support technique. The need for ventilatory support may, however, be lifelong, especially for those with chronic, progressive neuromuscular diseases that preclude effective spontaneous ventilation.

Mechanical ventilation is most commonly used for clients with hypoxemia and progressive alveolar hypoventilation with respiratory acidosis. The hypoxemia is usually due to intrapulmonary shunting of blood when external devices cannot provide sufficiently high FIO_2. Mechanical ventilation is also indicated

- For clients who need respiratory support after surgery
- For clients who are barely maintaining adequate gas

exchange at the cost of expending energy with high work of breathing
- For clients who require general anesthesia or heavy sedation to allow diagnostic or therapeutic interventions

Collaborative Management

 Assessment

The nurse assesses the client about to undergo intubation in the same way as for other clients with respiratory problems. Once mechanical ventilation has been initiated, the nurse assesses the respiratory system on an ongoing basis. The nurse monitors and assesses for complications related to the artificial airway or ventilator as well as for those related to mechanical ventilation.

 Interventions

> *Endotracheal Intubation*

Clients who need mechanical ventilation require an artificial airway. The most common type of artificial airway for establishing and maintaining the airway on a short-term basis is the endotracheal (ET) tube. If the client requires an artificial airway for longer than a specified period, usually longer than 10 to 14 days, the physician considers a tracheostomy (see Chap. 30) to avoid mucosal and vocal cord damage.

The goals of intubation include maintaining a patent airway, reducing the work of breathing, providing a means to remove secretions, and providing ventilation and oxygen. Major indications for intubation are listed in Table 34–4.

Endotracheal Tube. An ET tube is a long polyvinyl chloride tube that is passed through the mouth or nose and into the trachea (Fig. 34–2). When properly positioned, the tip of the ET tube rests approximately 2 to 3 cm (0.8 to 1.2 inches) above the carina (where the trachea divides into the right and left mainstem bronchi).

TABLE 34–4

Major Indications for Intubation

- Airway protection when the client loses reflexes because of anesthesia, medications, disease, or decreased level of consciousness
- To provide positive pressure or high oxygen concentration
- Bypass airway obstruction
- Facilitating pulmonary hygiene
- Suctioning of secretions when the client cannot handle secretions (as in diseases of chronic airflow limitation)

Oral intubation is the easiest and quickest method of establishing of an airway; therefore, it is also performed as an emergency procedure. The nasal route is reserved for elective intubation, for some facial or oral traumas and surgeries, and when oral intubation is not possible. This route is contraindicated if the client has a blood dyscrasia. An experienced, specially trained professional, such as an anesthesiologist, nurse anesthetist, or pulmonologist (MD), performs the intubation.

An ET tube has several parts (see Fig. 34–2). The shaft of the tube contains a radiopaque vertical line for the length of the tube, which permits demonstration of correct placement by chest x-ray. Short horizontal lines (depth markings) are used to designate correct placement of the tube at the nares or mouth (at the incisor tooth) and to identify how far the tube has been inserted.

The cuff at the distal end of the tube, with proper inflation, produces a seal between the trachea and the cuff. The seal prevents aspiration and ensures delivery of a set tidal volume when mechanical ventilation is used. When the cuff is inflated to an adequate sealing volume, no air can pass through the cuff to the vocal cords, nose, or mouth; therefore, the client is not able to talk when the cuff is inflated. The cuff should be inflated to a

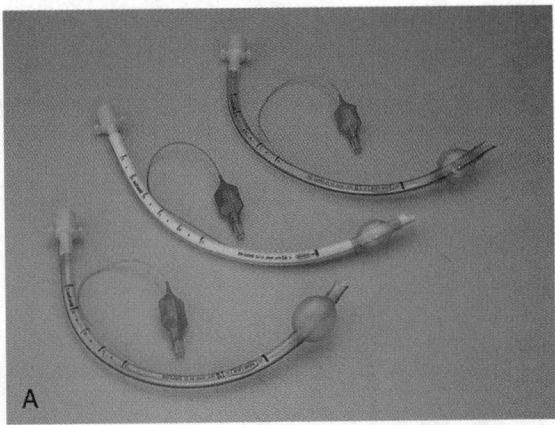
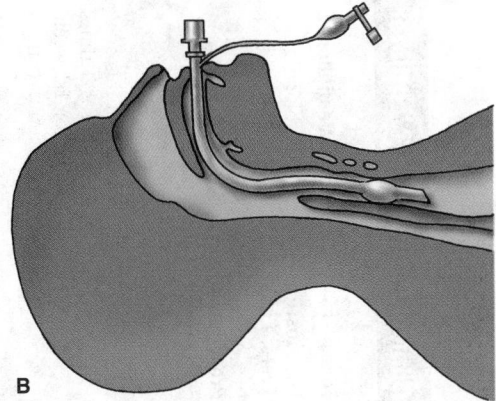

Figure 34–2. *A*, Endotracheal tubes. (Courtesy of Sims Porter, Inc.) *B*, Correct placement of an oral endotracheal tube.

Clinical Pathway for Ventilator Dependent Clients with Tracheostomy or Endotracheal Tube

Focus	Phase I Acute Ventilatory Support	Phase II Ventilatory Support	Phase III Weaning	Phase IV Resolution
Diagnostic Tests, Labs & Procedures	Arterial blood gas (ABG) Pulse oximetry CXR Complete blood count (CBC) SMA-7 SAM-12 ECG Sputum culture & sens after 72 hrs ETT Blood cultures as needed Phosphorus 4 times daily if on TF or TPN for 1st week Pre-albumin prn	Pulmonary mechanics ECG prn CBC CXR SMA-7 SMA-12 weekly ABG prn Pulse oximetry 24-hr urine urea nitrogen prn (if no renal failure) Pre-albumin prn	Pulmonary mechanics ECG prn CBC CXR SMA-7 SMA-12 weekly ABG prn Pulse oximetry 24-hr urine urea nitrogen prn (if no renal failure) Pre-albumin prn	Pulmonary mechanics Pulse oximetry prn
Consuls	Pulmonologist consultation if intubated after 72 hours or if re-intubation is required Assess need for swallow/speech consultation Nutritional support dietitian Respiratory care clinician Social worker: Supportive counseling/crisis intervention	Physical medicine and rehabilitation Physical therapy Occupational therapy Swallow/speech consultation Social worker: Supportive counseling/crisis intervention Social worker assesses client's and family's resource needs.	Physical medicine and rehabilitation Social worker: Supportive counseling Social worker to evaluate client for placement options	
Treatments	SVO$_2$ prn Mechanical ventilation Respiratory treatments Secretion management Tracheostomy after ETT in place × 7 days GI protection (histamine blockers/carafate) Sedation prn IV medications Diuretics prn Packed cells prn Vasopressors Antibiotics prn Vasoactive infusions Paralytics prn Daily weight I & O hourly Special bed prn Suction prn Foley Swallow/dysphagia assessment	Respiratory treatments Packed cells prn Secretion management Antibiotic prn Sedation prn Diuretics prn Tracheostomy care Daily weight Suction prn I & O Foley Evaluate need for permanent IV access	Respiratory treatments Packed cells prn Secretion management Antibiotic prn Diuretics prn Tracheostomy care Daily weight Suction prn I & O D/C Foley prn If prolonged TFs, evaluate need for PEG Evaluate continued need for IV access	Tracheostomy collar Decannulator Extubator Continue vent & slow wean Daily weight I & O every 8 hours Suction prn

Diet	Nutritional assessment TPN/TF TF preferred	If on TPN, transition to TF Reassess nutritional status every 10 days	Transition to PO diet if no dysphagia Reassess nutritional status every 10 days	Continue PO diet or TF
Activity	Bedrest Passive range of motion every 4 hours Increase activity as tolerated	Up on side of bed with assistance Foot support Up in chair if tolerated Active range of motion	Up in chair 3× daily Increase ambulation	Up in chair 3× daily for increased time Increased ambulation Increased client involvement in self-care activities
Treatment	Establish a communication mode with the client. Orient client to environment. Orient family to environment, procedures, client's current condition and prognosis, care needs, and hospital policy.	Keep client and family updated about the client's condition, new and continuing procedures, treatment plans, and changes in care needs.	Teach the client and family about weaning procedures and expected responses.	Keep the client and family informed re progress, changes in treatment plan, expected responses, new equipment or personnel.
Discharge Planning	Family members and social worker: Assessment of resources and a discharge plan appropriate and individualized to the expected outcomes for the ventilator-dependent client.	Inform social worker of client's progress. Social worker to assess client's and family's resource needs; explore rehabilitation and long-term insurance coverage.	Keep social worker updated about client progress. Social worker to evaluate client for placement options. Social worker to initiate referrals.	Social worker to finalize client's transportation and disposition. Social worker to finalize arrangements for needed equipment, home health services, and follow-up care.

CBC = complete blood count, CXR = chest x-ray, ECG = electrocardiogram, ETT = endotracheal tube, I & O = intake and output, O = oral, TF = tube feeding, TPN = total parenteral nutrition, PEG = percutaneous endoscopic gastronomy, prn = as needed.

pressure of 20 to 25 cm H$_2$O using minimal-leak or no-leak techniques.

The pilot balloon with a one-way valve permits air to be inserted into the cuff and yet prevents air from escaping. This balloon is used as a general guideline for determining the absence or presence of air in the cuff; it will not tell how much or how little air is present.

The universal adaptor, which is 15 mm in diameter, enables attachment to ventilator tubing or other types of oxygen delivery systems. The tubing size is indicated on the adaptor or the shaft of the tube. Adult tube sizes range from 5 to 10 mm. Sizes used are 8.0 to 9.0 for large adults, 7.0 to 8.0 for medium-size adults, and 6.0 to 7.0 for small adults.

Preparing for Intubation. The nurse and assistive nursing personnel know the proper procedure for summoning intubation personnel to the bedside in an emergency situation. The nurse explains the procedure to the client as clearly as possible under the circumstances. Basic life-support measures, such as the establishment of a patent airway and the administration of 100% oxygen via a resuscitation (Ambu) bag with a face mask, are crucial to the client's survival until help arrives. The coordination for resuscitation with a bag and mask device can be cumbersome; therefore, practice is necessary.

In an emergency, the nurse or assistive personnel brings the code (or "crash") cart, respiratory equipment box, and suction equipment (which is often already on the code cart) to the bedside. The nurse maintains a patent airway through positioning and the insertion of an oral airway until the client is intubated. During intubation, the nurse continuously monitors for changes in the client's vital signs, signs of hypoxia or hypoxemia, dysrhythmias, and aspiration. The nurse also ensures that each intubation attempt lasts no longer than 30 seconds, preferably less than 15 seconds. After 30 seconds, oxygen via mask and manual resuscitation bag is provided to prevent hypoxia and potential cardiac arrest. The nurse suctions as necessary.

Verifying Tube Placement. Immediately after an ET tube is inserted, its placement must be verified. The most accurate way of verifying placement is by checking end-tidal CO$_2$ concentration, if available. The nurse assesses for bilateral equal breath sounds, bilateral equal chest excursion, and air emerging from the ET tube. If breath sounds and chest wall movement are absent on the left side, the tube may be in the right mainstem bronchus. The person intubating the client should be able to reposition the tube without repeating the entire intubation procedure.

The nurse auscultates over the stomach to rule out esophageal intubation. If the tube is in the stomach, the nurse hears louder breath sounds over the stomach than over the chest and notes abdominal distention. The nurse continuously monitors chest wall movement and breath sounds until tube placement is verified by chest x-ray.

Stabilizing the Tube. The nurse, respiratory therapist, or anesthesia personnel stabilize the ET tube at the mouth or nose. The tube is marked at the level at which it touches the incisor tooth or naris. Two persons working together use a head halter technique to secure the tube. Chart 34–8 outlines the steps in the procedure.

An oral airway may also need to be inserted to keep the client from biting an oral tube. Ongoing nursing care requires an oral tube to be moved to the opposite side of the mouth daily. This common maneuver is thought to help prevent pressure and necrosis of the lip and mouth area, prevent nerve damage, and facilitate a thorough inspection and cleaning of the mouth. One person stabilizes the tube at the correct position and prevents head movement while a second person applies the tape. After the procedure is completed, the nurse verifies the presence of bilateral and equal breath sounds and the level of the tube.

Nursing Care. The nurse assesses tube placement, cuff pressure, breath sounds, and chest wall movement regularly. The nurse prevents pulling or tugging on the tube by the client to prevent dislodgment or "slipping" of the tube and checks the pilot balloon to ensure the cuff is inflated. Suctioning, coughing, and speaking attempts by the client place extra stress on the tube and also can cause dislodgment. Head flexion moves the tube away from the carina; head extension moves the tube closer to the carina. Rotation of the head also causes the tube to move. Mouth secretions and tongue movement can loosen the tape and allow malposition of the tube. When other measures fail, the nurse applies soft wrist restraints, as ordered, for the client who is voluntarily or involuntarily pulling on the tube. This intervention is a last resort to prevent accidental extubation. Adequate sedation (chemical restraint) may be necessary to decrease agitation or extubation. The nurse obtains permission for restraints from the client or family after explaining the rationale. More information on management of the artificial airway is found in Chapter 30.

Complications of an ET or nasotracheal tube can occur at each stage of the process: during placement, while in place, during extubation, or after extubation (either early or late). Trauma and complications can occur to the face; eye; nasal and paranasal areas; oral, pharyngeal, bronchial, tracheal, and pulmonary areas; esophageal and gastric areas; and cardiovascular, musculoskeletal, and neurologic systems.

➤ Mechanical Ventilation

Mechanical ventilation to support and maintain a client's respiratory function is widely used on medical-surgical units, in nursing homes, and in the home setting as well as in critical care units. The nurse plays a pivotal role in the coordination of care and the prevention of complications. Chart 34–9 reviews nursing care of the client during mechanical ventilation.

The goals of mechanical ventilation are to improve oxygenation and ventilation and decrease the amount of oxygen and work needed to accomplish an effective breathing pattern. Mechanical ventilation is used to support the client until lung function is adequate or until the acute episode has passed. A ventilator does not cure diseased lungs; it provides ventilation until the lungs are able to resume the process of breathing. Therefore, the nurse must remember why the client is using the ventilator so

Chart 34–8

Nursing Care Highlight: Taping an Oral and Nasal Endotracheal Tube

Little evidence is available to provide clinical direction on the best method to secure endotracheal (ET) and nasotracheal tubes. However, adhesive tape is the easiest, cheapest, and most frequently used.

Adhesive tape may be irritating to the skin, and frequent tape changes may disrupt the skin integrity. An additional reported complication is nosocomial cutaneous mucormycosis occurring around the surgical tape securing the ET tube. Protecting the skin, especially on the face, is a high priority for patients and nurses. This must be balanced against making sure the ET tube is not dislodged. A simple yet effective method of securing the oral and nasotracheal tube is demonstrated here.

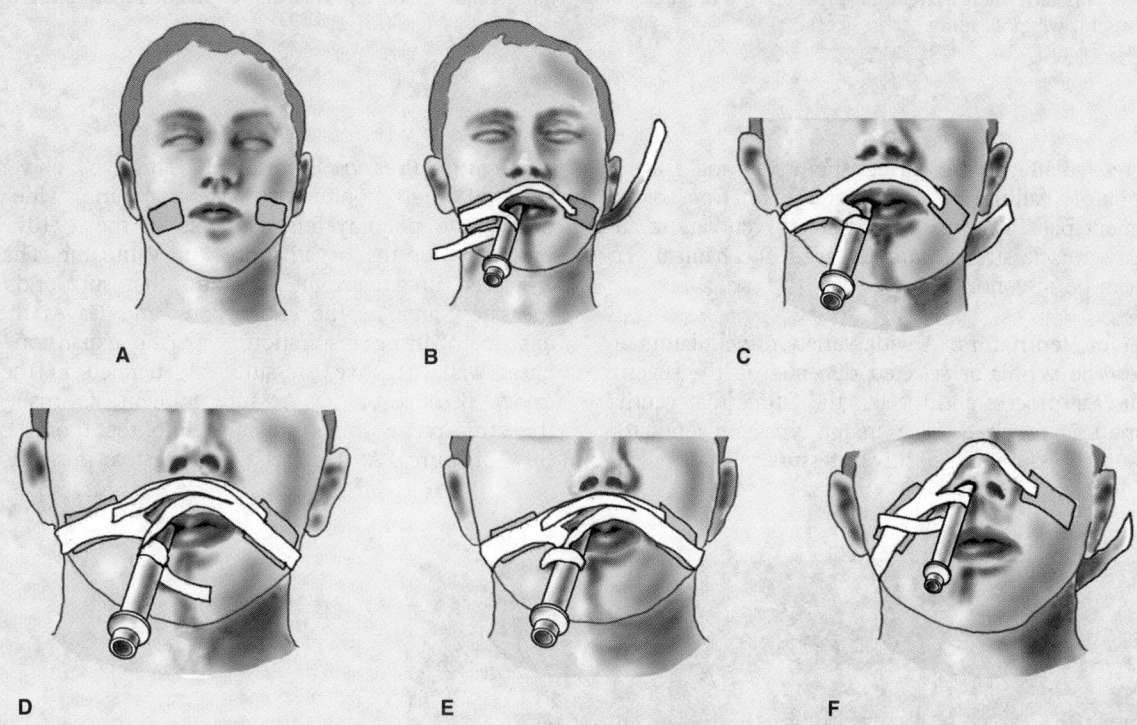

1. Prepare the skin by shaving the cheeks and upper lip, if possible.
2. Protect the skin by applying tincture of benzoin to the skin and ET tube and allow to dry (Mastisol may also be used, but Detachol **must** be used before removing the tape); then apply a 1 × 3-inch long piece of thin DuoDerm or other protective or hydrocolloid membrane to the skin on the cheeks (*A*).
3. Take a 30-inch (about 2 ½-foot) piece of adhesive tape and lay it on a flat surface, sticky side up. Take another piece of tape (about 10 inches) and cover the middle portion of the tape (sticky side to sticky side) to protect the back of the patient's neck. A tongue blade on each end folded over can keep it from getting tangled or sticking prematurely.
4. Place the tape behind the patient's neck. Remove the tongue blades, and place the tape on the protective membrane up to the end of the mouth on each side. Trim the tape as needed, and split each end of the tape.
5. Take the upper part of one end of the tape and place it on the upper lip. Take the lower part of the tape and wrap it securely around the tube (*B, C*). Take the upper part of the other end of the tape, place it on the upper lip, and wrap the lower part securely around the tube (*D, E*). Do not have the tube too far to either side of the mouth, or it can cause skin breakdown in the corner of the mouth or lips.
6. The same method can be used for nasal tubes, but do not tape the tube too tightly to the nose or skin breakdown will occur on the nares (*F*).
7. Always tape the tube to the upper lip, never the lower. The lower jaw moves too much with attempts to speak or oral care, which will move the tube and cause irritation and discomfort for the patient. The tape should be inspected at least every shift for signs of loosening or skin irritation or breakdown, especially with increased oral secretions. Tightness of the tape should also be checked each shift if swelling in the face and neck occurs or if there is an increase in fluid retention (as in anasarca, sepsis, or adult respiratory distress syndrome).

Continued

CHART 34–8. Nursing Care Highlight: Taping an Oral and Nasal Endotracheal Tube   Continued

An additional technique for securing tubing that can decrease ET tube movement and provide a fulcrum for pulling on ventilator tubing is to attach a 6-inch (50-mL) piece of flexible ventilator tubing between the ET tube adaptor and the **Y** connector of the ventilator tubing. The procedure for this technique is as follows:

1. Shave the chest or clean with alcohol a portion of the chest at right angles to the angle of Louis. Apply tincture of benzoin and allow to dry.
2. Prepare Montgomery straps by taking two 6-inch pieces of 2-inch wide adhesive tape. Double-back one end of each piece of tape, and cut a small hole in the ends that are doubled over.
3. Apply the tape to the prepared chest with the ends with the hole over each other. Take a 12-inch piece of twill (trach) tape and thread through both holes. Position the tubing with the **Y** connector over the holes and tie into place. This procedure allows all pulling on the tubing to place strain on the tape (straps) and not on the face or the tube. Caution should be taken if patients have increased partial pressure of arterial carbon dioxide retention, and end-tidal carbon dioxide monitoring may be useful when weaning.

that aggressive attempts to correct the underlying cause of the respiratory failure are always at the forefront of the management plan. If normal oxygenation, ventilation, and respiratory muscle strength are achieved, mechanical ventilation can be discontinued.

Types of Ventilators. A wide variety of ventilators are available. The ventilator selected depends on the severity of the disease process and the length of time that ventilator support is required. Two major types of ventilators are negative pressure and positive pressure.

Negative-Pressure Ventilators. This type of ventilator (Fig. 34–3) is noninvasive. The iron lung, widely used during the poliomyelitis epidemic in the 1940s, is the prototype for the negative-pressure ventilator. The client is placed in an airtight apparatus that surrounds either the chest area or the entire body and leaves the head exposed. During inspiration, with the expansion of the chest wall, negative pressure is generated in the chest cavity. Because of the pressure gradient, air rushes from the atmosphere (high pressure) into the thoracic cavity (low pressure). At a preset time, negative pressure ceases

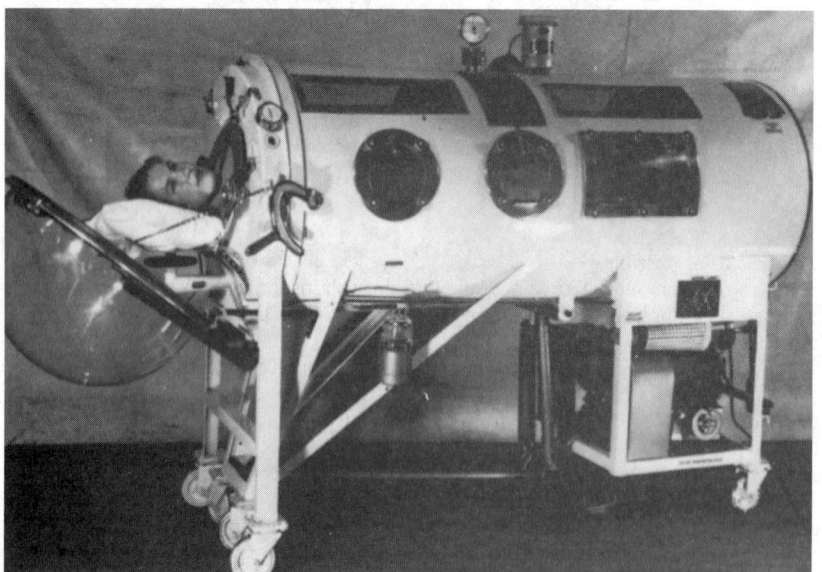

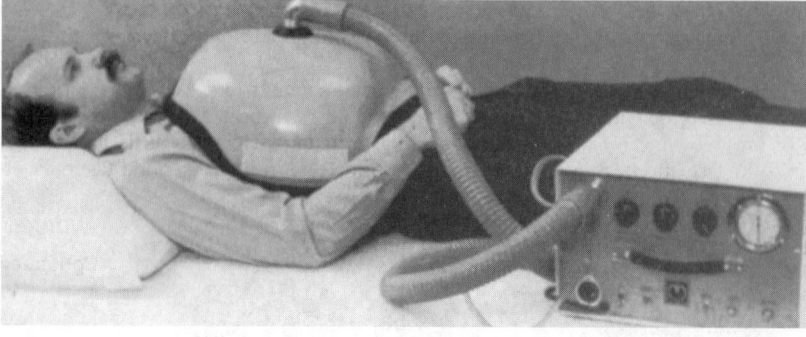

Figure 34–3. Two negative-pressure ventilators. *Top,* The Emerson iron lung. (Courtesy of J. H. Emerson Co., Cambridge, MA.) *Bottom,* Life-care Chest Shell. (From Hill, N. [1986]. Clinical application of body ventilators. *Chest,* 90[6], 900. Used with permission.)

Chart 34-9

Nursing Care Highlight: The Client on Mechanical Ventilation

- At least once every shift check to be sure the ventilator settings are set as ordered.
- Check to be sure alarms are set (especially low pressure and low exhaled volume).
- Observe the exhaled volume digital display to be sure the client is receiving the prescribed tidal volume.
- Empty ventilator tubings when moisture collects. Never empty fluid in the tubing back into the cascade.
- Ensure adequate humidity by keeping delivered air temperature maintained at body temperature.
- If the client is on PEEP, observe the peak airway pressure dial to determine the proper level of PEEP.
- Assess the client's respiratory status each shift and as needed:
  a. Observe the client's color (especially lips and nail beds).
  b. Observe the client's chest for bilateral expansion.
  c. Auscultate the lungs for rales, rhonchi, wheezes, equal breath sounds, and decreased or absent breath sounds.
  d. Obtain pulse oximetry reading.
  e. Evaluate ABGs as ordered.
- Take vital signs at least every 4 hr.
- Be sure the tracheostomy cuff (or the endotracheal cuff) is adequately inflated to ensure tidal volume.
- Administer mouth care *at least* twice per shift.
- Observe the client's need for tracheal/oral/nasal suctioning every 2 hr. Provide adequate suctioning as needed.
- Provide tracheostomy care every shift.
- Change tracheostomy tape or endotracheal tube tape as needed. Observe the client's mouth around the endotracheal tube for pressure sores.
- Move the oral endotracheal tube to the opposite side of the mouth once every 24 hr to prevent ulcers.
- Maintain accurate intake and output records to monitor fluid balance.
- Turn the client at least every 2 hr and get the client out of bed as ordered to promote pulmonary hygiene and prevent complications of immobility.
- Schedule treatments and nursing care at intervals to provide rest.
- Explain all procedures and treatments; provide access to a call bell; visit the client frequently.
- Include the client and his or her family in care whenever possible (especially suctioning and tracheostomy care).
- Provide a letter board or pencil and paper for communication. Request consultation with a speech therapist for assistance, if necessary.
- Observe ventilated clients for gastrointestinal distress (diarrhea, constipation, tarry stools).
- Document pertinent observations in the client's medical record (chart).

PEEP = positive end-expiratory pressure; ABGs = arterial blood gases.
Courtesy of Our Lady of Lourdes Medical Center, Camden, NJ.

and expiration occurs. Thus, negative-pressure ventilators create pressure gradients that mimic normal physiologic ventilation.

Newer negative-pressure ventilators include the cuirass, poncho, and body wrap. These ventilators are used for clients with neuromuscular disease, central nervous system disorders, spinal cord injuries, and chronic airflow limitation (CAL). Clients may use negative-pressure ventilation for home nighttime ventilatory support so that their muscles can rest. Advantages are that an artificial airway is not required and the newer models are lightweight and easy to use. The enclosing ventilator makes some direct nursing care more difficult. The client must be able to clear oral secretions and must have compliant (elastic) lungs to benefit from this mode of ventilation.

Positive-Pressure Ventilators. This is the most widely used type of ventilator in the acute care setting. During inspiration, pressure is generated that pushes air into the lungs and expands the chest. In most instances, an ET tube or tracheostomy is needed. Positive-pressure ventilators are classified according to the mechanism that ends inspiration and starts expiration. Inspiration is terminated or cycled in three major ways: pressure cycled, time cycled, or volume cycled.

Pressure-Cycled Ventilators. This type of rarely used ventilator pushes air into the lungs until a preset airway pressure is reached. Tidal volumes and inspiratory time are variable. Pressure-cycled ventilators are often used for short periods, such as in the postanesthesia care unit and for respiratory therapy.

Time-Cycled Ventilators. These push air into the lungs until a preset time has elapsed. Tidal volume and pressure are variable, depending on the characteristics of the client and the ventilator. The time-cycled ventilator is used primarily in pediatric and neonatal populations.

Volume-Cycled Ventilators. This type of ventilator pushes gas into the lungs until a preset volume is delivered. A constant tidal volume is delivered regardless of the pressure needed to deliver the tidal volume. However, a pressure limit is set to prevent excessive pressure from being exerted on the lungs. The advantage of the volume-cycled ventilator is that a constant tidal volume is delivered regardless of the changing compliance of the lungs and chest wall or the airway resistance found in the client or ventilator. Examples include the Bear I, II (Fig. 34–4), and III; Puritan-Bennett MA-1, MA-2, and MA-3; and Monaghan 225/SIMV.

Microprocessor Ventilators. These are the most sophisticated of the positive-pressure ventilators. A computer or microprocessor is built into the ventilator to allow ongoing monitoring of ventilatory functions, alarms, and client parameters. The ventilator often has components of volume-, time-, and pressure-cycled ventilators. The microprocessor ventilator is more responsive to clients who have severe lung disease, who require prolonged weaning trials, and who may not be able to be ventilated on older volume-cycled ventilators. Examples include the Bear IV and V, Puritan-Bennett 7200, Erisa, and Siemens Servo C and Servo D.

Modes of Ventilation. The mode of ventilation describes the way in which the client receives breaths from the ventilator.

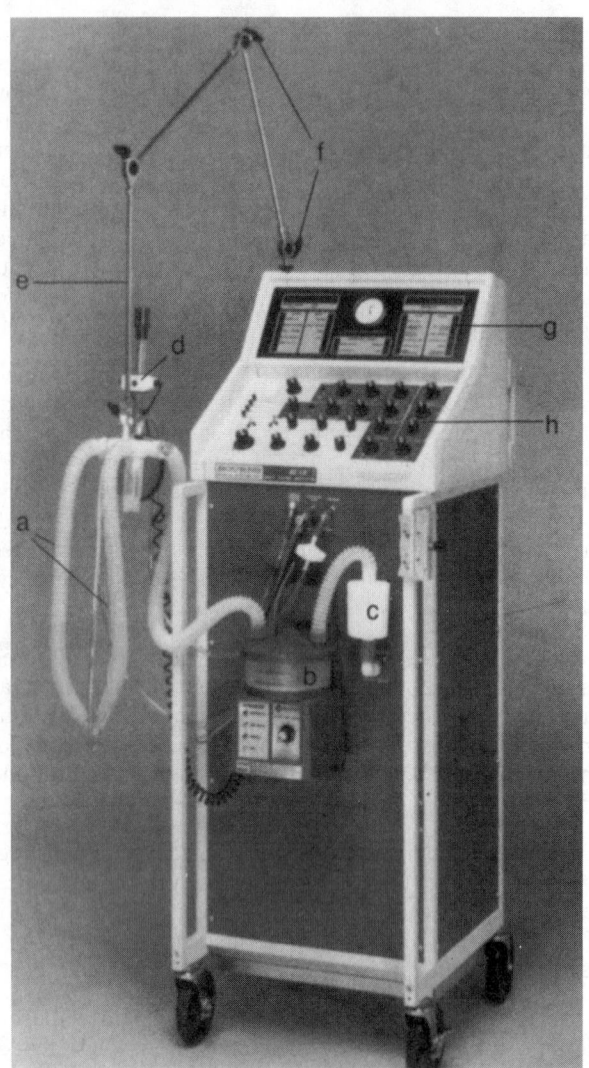

Figure 34–4. Bear II Adult Volume Ventilator. (Courtesy of Bear Medical Systems, Inc., Riverside, CA.)

Controlled Ventilation. This is the least used mode. The client receives a set tidal volume at a set rate. This mode may be used for clients who cannot initiate respiratory effort (e.g., those with polio or Guillain-Barré syndrome). It may be used for clients who are "paralyzed" as part of their medical management, such as those in status epilepticus or those with severely elevated intracranial pressure. If a client on controlled ventilation attempts to initiate a breath, the efforts are blocked by the ventilator. This maneuver may result in the client's "fighting" the ventilator.

Assist-Control Ventilation. Assist-control (AC) ventilation is the most commonly used mode. It is used mainly as a resting mode. The ventilator takes over the work of breathing for the client. Tidal volume and ventilatory rate are preset on the ventilator. If the client does not trigger spontaneous breaths, a minimal ventilatory pattern is established. The ventilator is also programmed to respond to the client's inspiratory effort if the client does initiate a breath. In this case, the ventilator delivers the preset tidal volume while allowing the client to control the rate of breathing.

One disadvantage of the AC mode is that if the client's spontaneous ventilatory rate increases, the ventilator continues to deliver a preset tidal volume with each breath. The client may then hyperventilate, and respiratory alkalosis occurs. Causes of hyperventilation, such as pain, anxiety, or acid-base imbalances, must be corrected.

Synchronized Intermittent Mandatory Ventilation. Synchronized intermittent mandatory ventilation (SIMV) is similar to AC ventilation in that tidal volume and ventilatory rate are preset on the ventilator. Therefore, if the client does not breathe, a minimal ventilatory pattern is established. In contrast to the AC mode, SIMV allows breathing spontaneously at the client's own rate and tidal volume between the ventilator breaths. SIMV can be used as a primary ventilatory mode or as a weaning modality. When SIMV is used as a weaning mode, the number of mechanical breaths (SIMV breaths) is gradually decreased (i.e., from 12 to 2), and the client gradually resumes spontaneous breathing. The mandatory ventilator breaths are delivered when the client is ready to inspire, promoting synchrony between the ventilator and the client.

Other Modes of Ventilation. Newer modes of ventilation, such as pressure support and continuous flow (flow-by), are available only in microprocessor ventilators. Both modalities decrease the work of breathing and are often used for weaning clients from mechanical ventilation. Other modes are maximum mandatory ventilation (MMV), inverse I:E ratio, permissive hypercapnia, airway pressure release ventilation, proportional assist ventilation, high-frequency ventilation, jet ventilation, and high-frequency oscillation. Many of these modes need specialized ventilators, tubing, or airways.

Ventilator Controls and Settings. The volume-cycled ventilator is the most widely used ventilator in the acute care setting. Regardless of the type of volume-cycled ventilator used, the controls and types of settings are universal (Fig. 34–5). The physician prescribes the ventilator settings, and usually the ventilator is readied or set up by the respiratory department. The nurse assists in connecting the client to the ventilator. The nurse understands and monitors the ventilator settings as part of the nursing care for the client.

Tidal Volume. Tidal volume (V_T) is the volume of air that the client receives with each breath; it can be measured on either inspiration or expiration. The average prescribed tidal volume ranges between 7 and 15 mL/kg of body weight. Adding a zero to the weight of clients in kilograms gives an estimate of tidal volume.

Rate, or Breaths per Minute. Rate, or breaths per minute (BPM), is the number of ventilator breaths delivered per minute. The rate is usually set between 10 and 14 breaths per minute.

Fraction of Inspired Oxygen. The fraction of inspired oxygen (FIO_2) is the oxygen concentration delivered to the client. The prescribed FIO_2 is determined by the arterial blood gas value and the client's condition. Ventilators

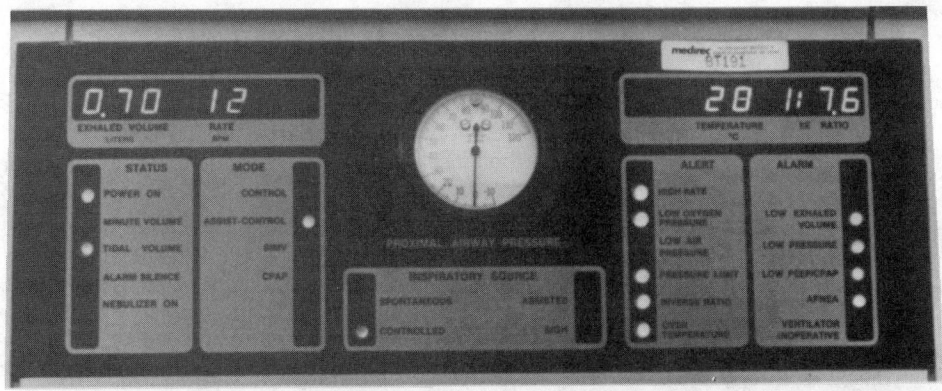

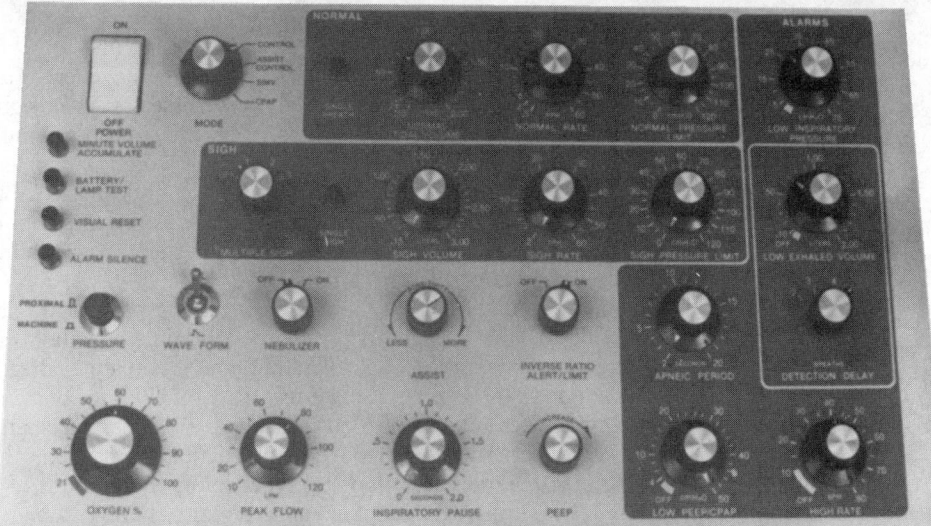

Figure 34–5. Display signals and alarms *(top)* and control panel *(bottom)* of a typical volume-cycled ventilator. (From Kersten, L. D. [1989]. *Comprehensive respiratory nursing: A decision-making approach.* Philadelphia: W. B. Saunders. Used with permission.)

can provide 21 to 100% oxygen, depending on the client's needs.

The oxygen delivered to the client is warmed to body temperature (37° C [98.6° F]) and humidified to 100%. Humidification and warming are necessary because upper air passages of the respiratory tree, which normally warm, humidify, and filter air, are bypassed by the endotracheal tube (ET) or tracheostomy tube. Humidification and warming prevent mucosal damage and facilitate clearance of secretions.

Sighs. These may be used to prevent atelectasis in special circumstances. Sighs are volumes of air that are 1½ to 2 times the set tidal volume, delivered 6 to 10 times per hour. Sighs are rarely used, however, because they can cause barotrauma (lung damage from excessive pressure) and have not been shown to be useful.

Peak Airway (Inspiratory) Pressure. Peak airway (inspiratory) pressure (PIP) indicates the pressure needed by the ventilator to deliver a set tidal volume at a given dynamic compliance. The peak airway pressure measurement appears on the digital readout or display on the front or top of the ventilator (labeled proximal airway pressure in Figure 34–5). Peak pressure is the highest pressure indicated during inspiration. Monitoring trends in PIP reflect changes in resistance of the lungs and resistance in the ventilator. An increased PIP reading means

increased airway resistance (bronchospasm, or pinched tubing), increased amount of secretions, pulmonary edema, or decreased pulmonary compliance (the lungs or chest wall are "stiffer" or harder to inflate). An upper pressure limit is set on the ventilator to prevent barotrauma. When the limit is reached, the high-pressure alarm sounds, and the remaining volume is not given.

Continuous Positive Airway Pressure. Continuous positive airway pressure (CPAP) is the application of positive airway pressure throughout the entire respiratory cycle for spontaneously breathing clients. Sedating medications should be given cautiously or not at all when a client is receiving CPAP so that respiratory effort is not suppressed. CPAP keeps the alveoli open during inspiration and prevents alveolar collapse during expiration. This process results in increased functional residual capacity (FRC), improved gas exchange, and improved oxygenation.

Continuous positive airway pressure is used primarily as a weaning modality. During CPAP, no ventilator breaths are delivered; the ventilator delivers oxygen and provides monitoring and an alarm system. The respiratory pattern is determined by the client's efforts. Normal levels of CPAP are 5 to 15 cm H_2O, adjusted to promote adequate oxygenation. If no pressure is set on the ventilator, the client receives no positive pressure. The client is essentially using the ventilator as a T piece with alarms.

Newer modifications of CPAP include nasal CPAP and BiPAP. The physician uses these modifications for select indications.

Positive End-Expiratory Pressure. Positive end-expiratory pressure (PEEP) is positive pressure exerted during the expiratory phase of ventilation. PEEP improves oxygenation by enhancing gas exchange and preventing atelectasis. It is indicated for the treatment of persistent hypoxemia that does not improve with an acceptable oxygen concentration. PEEP is often added when the PaO_2 value remains low with an FIO_2 of 50% to 70% or greater.

The need for PEEP indicates a severe gas exchange disturbance. It is important to lower the FIO_2 delivered when possible. Prolonged use of a high FIO_2 can result in lung damage from the toxic effects of oxygen. PEEP prevents alveoli from collapsing; the lungs are kept partially inflated so that alveolar-capillary gas exchange is facilitated throughout the ventilatory cycle. The effect should be an increase in arterial blood oxygenation so that the FIO_2 can be decreased.

PEEP is "dialed in" with the PEEP dial on the control panel. The amount of PEEP is often 5 to 15 cm H_2O and is read (monitored) on the peak airway pressure dial, the same dial used to read the PIP. When PEEP is added, the dial does not return to zero at the end of exhalation; rather, it returns to a baseline that has been increased from zero by the amount of PEEP applied.

Flow. Flow is how fast the ventilator delivers each breath. It is usually set at 40 L/min. If a client is agitated, restless, or has a widely fluctuating pressure reading on inspiration, or other signs of air hunger, the flow may be set too low. Increasing the flow should be tried before restraining the client chemically.

Other Settings. Other settings may be used, depending on the type of ventilator and mode of ventilation. Examples of additional settings include inspiratory and expiratory cycle, waveform, expiratory resistance, and plateau.

Nursing Management. The institution of mechanical ventilation for a client involves a complex decision-making process for both the family and the health care professionals. Both physical and psychological concerns of the client and family must be addressed. The mechanical ventilator frequently causes anxiety for the client and family. Therefore, the nurse carefully explains the purpose of the ventilator and notes that the client might feel some different sensations. The client and family are encouraged to express their concerns. The nurse acts as the coach who both physically and psychologically helps and supports the client and family through this experience. In emergencies, these explanations may not be accomplished until the emergency has been controlled. Clients undergoing mechanical ventilation in ICUs frequently experience delirium, or "ICU psychosis." Such clients require frequent, repetitive explanations and reassurance.

When caring for a ventilated client, the nurse's responsibility is to the client first and the ventilator second. It is vital that the nurse understand the reason for which the client requires mechanical ventilation. Such causes as excessive amounts of secretions, sepsis, and trauma require different interventions to facilitate ventilator independence. In addition, an appreciation of the client's chronic health problems—particularly chronic airflow limitation (CAL), left-sided heart failure, anemia, and malnutrition—is essential. These problems may impede weaning from mechanical ventilation and, therefore, warrant close monitoring and intervention.

Three nursing goals in caring for the client with mechanical ventilation are to monitor and evaluate the client's response to the ventilator, manage the ventilator system safely, and prevent complications.

Monitoring the Client's Response. The first goal of nursing care is to monitor and evaluate the client's response to the ventilator. The nurse assesses vital signs and listens to breath sounds every 30 to 60 minutes initially, monitors noninvasive respiratory parameters (e.g., capnography and pulse oximetry), and checks ABG values. Vital signs change during episodes of hypercapnia and hypoxemia. The nurse should note any precipitating causes and correct them promptly.

The nurse assesses the client's breathing pattern in relation to the ventilatory cycle to determine whether the client is fighting or tolerating the ventilator. Breath sounds are assessed and recorded, including bilateral equal breath sounds to ensure proper ET tube placement. To determine the frequency of suctioning needed, the nurse observes secretions for type, color, and amount.

The nurse assesses the area around the ET tube or tracheostomy site at least every 4 hours for color, tenderness, skin irritation, and drainage. Continuous noninvasive monitoring provides the nurse with information to guide the client's activities, such as weaning, physical or occupational therapy, and self-care. These activities can be paced so that oxygenation and ventilation are adequate. The nurse interprets ABG values to evaluate ventilation and suggests ventilator settings that help the client.

Because the nurse spends the most time with the client, he or she is most likely to be the first person to recognize slight changes in vital signs or ABG values and fatigue or distress in the client. The nurse promptly confers with the physician and implements the appropriate interventions.

While monitoring and evaluating the client's clinical status, the nurse also serves as a resource for addressing the psychological needs of the client and family. Anxiety can play a major role in the client's tolerance of mechanical ventilation. Therefore, skilled and sensitive nursing care promotes psychological well-being and facilitates synchrony with the ventilator. Because the client cannot speak, communication can be frustrating and anxiety producing. The client and family may panic because they believe the client has lost his or her voice. They must be reassured that the ET tube prevents speech but that it is temporary.

Alternative, creative methods of communication must be individualized to meet the client's needs. Magic slates, writing paper, computers, and tracheostomy tubes that permit talking are potential means of facilitating communication. Finding a successful means for communication is important because the client often feels isolated as a result of the inability to speak. Anticipation of the client's needs; easy access to frequently used belongings; visits from family, friends, and pets; and a nursing call light within reach are effective ways of giving the client a sense of control over the environment. In addition, the client can participate in self-care.

Managing the Ventilator System. The second goal of nursing care is directed toward safe management of the ventilator system. Ventilator settings are ordered by the physician and include tidal volume, respiratory rate, FiO_2, mode of ventilation (AC, SIMV), and any adjunctive modes, such as positive end-expiratory pressure (PEEP), pressure support, or continuous flow.

Nurses perform and document ventilator checks according to the standards of the unit or facility and respond promptly to emergencies as indicated by alarms. During a ventilator check, the nurse compares the ventilator settings ordered by the physician with the actual settings. The nurse checks the level of water in the humidifier and the temperature of the humidification system to ensure that they are within normal limits. Extremes in temperature cause damage to the mucosa of the airways. Any condensation in the ventilator tubing is removed by draining water into drainage collection receptacles, which should be emptied frequently. For prevention of bacterial contamination, moisture and water from the tubings are never allowed to enter the humidifier.

Mechanical ventilators have alarm systems that warn the nurse of a problem with either the client or the ventilator. Alarm systems must be activated and functional at all times. The nurse must recognize an emergency and intervene promptly so that complications are prevented. If the cause of the alarm cannot be determined, the nurse ventilates the client manually with a resuscitation bag until the problem is corrected by a second nurse, the respiratory therapist, or a physician. The two major alarms on a ventilator indicate either a high pressure or a low exhaled volume. Table 34–5 presents nursing interventions for various causes of ventilator alarms.

Ensuring proper functioning of the ventilator also includes care of the endotracheal (ET) tube or tracheostomy tube. A patent airway is maintained through suctioning only as needed. Indications for suctioning in the ventilated client include
- Presence of secretions
- Increased PIP
- Presence of rhonchi (wheezes)
- Decreased breath sounds

Careful maintenance of the ET or tracheostomy tube also ensures a patent airway. The nurse frequently assesses the tube's position, especially for the client whose airway is attached to heavy ventilator tubing that may pull on the tracheostomy or ET tube. The nurse positions the ventilator tubing in such a way that the client can move without pulling on the ET or tracheostomy tube. The ET tube can move and slip into the right mainstem bronchus. To detect minimal changes in the tube's position, the nurse marks the level at which the tube touches the client's teeth or nose. The nurse gives mouth care

frequently to promote adequate oral hygiene and to prevent loosening of the tape that holds the tube.

Preventing Complications. The third goal in caring for the client receiving mechanical ventilation is to prevent complications. Most complications are due to the positive pressure from the ventilator. Nearly every body system is affected.

Cardiac Complications. Cardiac complications of mechanical ventilation include hypotension and fluid retention. Hypotension is caused by the application of positive pressure, which increases intrathoracic pressure and inhibits blood return to the heart. The decreased venous return to the right side of the heart decreases cardiac output and is clinically reflected as hypotension. Hypotension is most frequently seen in the client who is dehydrated or requires high peak airway (inspiratory) pressure (PIP) to be ventilated. The nurse instructs the client to avoid a Valsalva maneuver and plans care to prevent constipation, which could result in a Valsalva maneuver.

Fluid is retained because of decreased cardiac output. The kidneys receive less blood flow and stimulate the renin-angiotensin-aldosterone system to retain fluid. In addition, humidified air via the ventilator system can contribute to fluid retention. If humidification is not adequate, the airways become dehydrated, and the secretions solidify. The nurse monitors the client's fluid intake and output, weight, hydration, and signs of hypovolemia.

Lung Complications. The lungs experience barotrauma (damage to the lungs by positive pressure), *volutrauma* (damage to the lung by excess volume delivered to one lung over the other), and acid-base abnormalities. Barotrauma includes pneumothorax, subcutaneous emphysema, and pneumomediastinum. Clients at risk for barotrauma have diseases of chronic airflow limitation (CAL), have blebs, are on PEEP, have dynamic hyperinflation, or require high pressures to ventilate the lungs (because of decreased compliance or "stiff" lungs, as seen in ARDS). Blood gas abnormalities, another pulmonary complication of mechanical ventilation, can be corrected by appropriate ventilator changes and adjustment of fluid and electrolyte imbalances.

Gastrointestinal and Nutritional Complications. Gastrointestinal alterations result from the stress of mechanical ventilation. Stress ulcers occur in approximately 25% of clients receiving mechanical ventilation. Prophylactic antacids, sucralfate (Carafate, Sulcrate), and the histamine blockers cimetidine (Tagamet) and ranitidine (Zantac) are often instituted as soon as the client is intubated. The nurse administers these medications and suggests therapeutic strategies for stress management (see Chap. 8).

Malnutrition is a prevalent problem in clients receiving mechanical ventilation. Because many other acute or life-threatening events are occurring simultaneously, nutrition is often neglected. Malnutrition is an extreme problem for these clients and a major reason that clients cannot be weaned from the ventilator. In malnourished clients, the respiratory muscles lose their mass and strength. The diaphragm, which is the major organ of inspiration, is affected early in this process. When the diaphragm and other muscles of respiration are weakened, an ineffective

TABLE 34–5

Nursing Interventions for Various Causes of Ventilator Alarms

Cause	Interventions
High-Pressure Alarm (sounds when peak inspiratory pressure reaches the set alarm limit [usually set 10–20 mmHg above the client's baseline PIP])	
There is an increased amount of secretions in the airways or a mucous plug.	• Suction as needed.
The client coughs, gags, or bites on the oral ET.	• Insert oral airway to prevent biting on the ET tube.
The client is anxious or fights the ventilator.	• Provide emotional support to decrease anxiety. • Increase the flow rate. • Explain all procedures to the client. • Provide sedation or paralyzing agent per the physician's order.
Airway size decreases related to wheezing or bronchospasm.	• Auscultate breath sounds. • Consult with the physician for management of bronchospasm.
Pneumothorax occurs.	• Auscultate breath sounds. • Consult with the physician about a new onset of decreased breath sounds or unequal chest excursion, which may be due to pneumothorax.
The artificial airway is displaced; the ET tube may have slipped into the right mainstem bronchus.	• Assess the chest for unequal breath sounds and chest excursion. • Obtain a chest x-ray as ordered to evaluate the position of the ET tube. • After the proper position is verified, tape the tube securely in place.
Obstruction in tubing occurs because the client is lying on the tubing or there is water or a kink in the tubing.	• Assess the system, moving from the artificial airway toward the ventilator. • Empty water from the ventilator tubing and remove any kinks.
There is increased PIP associated with deliverance of a sigh.	• Consult with respiratory therapist or physician to adjust the pressure alarm.
Decreased compliance of the lung is noted; a trend of gradually increasing PIP is noted over several hours or a day.	• Evaluate the reasons for the decreased compliance of the lungs. Increased PIP occurs in ARDS, pneumonia, or any worsening of pulmonary disease.
Low Exhaled Volume (or Low-Pressure) Alarm (sounds when there is a disconnection or leak in the ventilator circuit or a leak in the client's artificial airway cuff)	
A leak in the ventilator circuit prevents breath from being delivered.	• Assess all connections and all ventilator tubings for disconnection.
The client stops spontaneous breathing in the SIMV or CPAP mode or on pressure support ventilation.	• Evaluate the client's tolerance of the mode.
A cuff leak occurs in the ET or tracheostomy tube.	• Evaluate the client for a cuff leak. A cuff leak is suspected when the client is able to talk (air escapes from the mouth) or when the pilot balloon on the artificial airway is flat (see section on tracheostomy tubes in Chapter 30).
The exhalation valve on Bear I or II is wet.	• Keep exhalation valve and flow tube vertical. • Unsnap and check the membrane for dampness. If the sensor is wet, gently dab dry and resnap.

PIP = peak inspiratory pressure; ET = endotracheal; ARDS = adult respiratory distress syndrome; CPAP = continuous positive airway pressure; SIMV = synchronized intermittent mandatory ventilation.

breathing pattern emerges, fatigue occurs, and the client cannot be weaned from the ventilator.

A balanced diet via the parenteral or enteral route is essential whenever a ventilator is used. Furthermore, nutrition for the client with CAL requires that special attention be given to the percentage of carbohydrates in the client's diet. During metabolism, carbohydrates are broken down to glucose to produce energy (adenosine triphosphate), carbon dioxide, and water. Excessive carbohydrate loads increase carbon dioxide production, which the CAL client may be unable to exhale. Hypercapnic respiratory failure results. Enteral and parenteral formulas with a higher fat content (e.g., Pulmocare, NutriVent, Intralipids) can be an alternative source of calories to combat this problem.

Another important aspect of nutritional support is electrolyte replacement. Electrolytes also have a major impact on the efficiency of respiratory muscle function. Specifically, the nurse and physician closely monitor potassium, calcium, magnesium, and phosphate levels, and the nurse replenishes deficiencies as ordered. All four electrolytes are important in respiratory muscle contraction and function and can easily be added to the nutritional regimen.

Infection. Infections are always a potential threat for the client requiring a ventilator. The ET or tracheostomy tube bypasses the body's normal process of filtering and warming air and provides bacteria direct access to the lower parts of the respiratory system. Within 48 hours, the artificial airway is usually colonized with bacteria, and an environment is established in which pneumonia can develop. In addition, aspiration of colonized fluid from the mouth or the stomach can occur and be a source of pathogens. Pneumonia is associated with prolonged hospitalization and increased morbidity. Therefore, the focus must be on prevention of infections through strict adherence to infection control, especially hand washing, during suctioning and care of the tracheostomy or ET tube. To prevent pneumonia, the nurse implements ongoing oral care and pulmonary hygiene, including chest physiotherapy, postural drainage, and turning and positioning. More information on pneumonia can be found in Chapter 33.

Muscular Complications. Overall muscle deconditioning can occur because of immobility. Getting out of bed, ambulating with assistance, and performing exercises with the nurse, physical therapist, and occupational therapist not only improve muscle tone and strength but also boost the client's morale, facilitate gas exchange, and promote oxygen delivery to all muscles.

Ventilator Dependence. The final complication of mechanical ventilation is ventilator dependence, or inability to wean. Ventilator dependence can be psychological or physiologic but more often has a physiologic basis. The longer a client uses a ventilator, the more difficult is the weaning process because the respiratory muscles fatigue and cannot assume breathing. The health care team attempts to optimize all major body systems and to exhaust every method of weaning before a client is declared unweanable.

The physician and nurse, often with a social worker or psychologist and a member of the clergy, discuss with the family and the client, as able, the client's quality of life, goals, and values. In accordance with this discussion, arrangements are made for home ventilation, nursing home placement, or withdrawal of life support (in terminal cases). Special units and facilities are available to maximize the rehabilitation and weaning of ventilator-dependent clients.

Weaning. This is the process of going from ventilatory dependence to spontaneous breathing. The weaning process can be prolonged if complications develop. Many of these complications can be avoided by skillful nursing care. For example, turning and positioning the client not only promote comfort and prevent skin breakdown but also facilitate gas exchange and prevent pulmonary complications, such as pneumonia and atelectasis. Table 34–6 summarizes various weaning techniques.

Implications for the Elderly. The older client, especially one who has smoked or who has an underlying lung dysfunction such as CAL, is at risk for ventilator dependence and failure to wean. Age-related changes that de-

TABLE 34–6

Weaning Methods

Synchronous Intermittent Mandatory Ventilation
- The client breathes between the machine's present breaths per minute rate.
- The client is initially set on a SIMV rate of 12, meaning the client receives a minimum of 12 breaths per minute by the ventilator.
- The client's respiratory rate will be a combination of ventilator breaths and spontaneous breaths.
- As the weaning process ensues, the physician orders gradual decreases in the SIMV rate, usually at a decrease of 1 to 2 breaths per minute.

T-Piece Technique
- The client is taken off the ventilator for short periods (initially 5–10 min) and allowed to breathe spontaneously.
- The ventilator is replaced with a T piece (see Chap. 30) or CPAP, which delivers humidified oxygen.
- The ordered FIO_2 may be higher for the client on the T piece than on the ventilator.
- Weaning progresses as the client is able to tolerate progressively longer periods off the ventilator.
- Nighttime weaning is not usually attempted until the client is able to maintain spontaneous respirations most of the day.

Pressure Support Ventilation
- PSV allows the client's respiratory effort to be augmented by a predetermined pressure assist from the ventilator.
- As the weaning process ensues, the amount of pressure applied to inspiration is gradually decreased.
- Another method of weaning with PSV is to maintain the pressure but gradually decrease the ventilator's preset breaths per minute rate.

SIMV = synchronized intermittent mandatory ventilation; CPAP = continuous positive airway pressure; FIO_2 = fraction of inspired oxygen; PSV = pressure support ventilation.

crease the likelihood of weaning result in ventilatory failure and include increased chest wall stiffness, reduced respiratory muscle strength, and decreased lung elasticity. Because the usual manifestations of ventilatory failure, hypoxemia and hypercapnia, may be blunted in the elderly, the nurse must use other clinical measures of oxygenation, such as a change in mental status (Thompson, 1996).

Extubation. Removal of the ET tube is termed *extubation*. The tube is removed when the indication for intubation has been resolved. Before removal, the nurse explains the procedure to the client. The nurse or respiratory therapist sets up the prescribed oxygen delivery system at the bedside and brings in the equipment for emergency reintubation. The nurse or respiratory therapist hyperoxygenates the client and thoroughly suctions the ET tube as well as the oral cavity. The cuff of the ET tube is then rapidly deflated, and the tube is removed at peak inspiration. The nurse instructs the client to take deep breaths and to cough. It is normal for large amounts of oral secretions to have accumulated in the back of the throat. The nurse or respiratory therapist administers oxygen, usually ordered to be by face mask or nasal cannula. The FIO_2 is usually ordered at 10% higher than the level that was maintained while the ET tube was in place.

Monitoring after extubation is essential. The nurse monitors the client's vital signs every hour initially, assesses the client's ventilatory pattern, and assesses for any signs or symptoms of respiratory distress. It is common for the client to experience hoarseness and a sore throat for a few days after extubation. The nurse instructs the client to

- Sit in a semi-Fowler's position
- Take deep breaths every ½ hour
- Use an incentive spirometer (see Chap. 20) every 2 hours
- Limit speaking in the immediate period after extubation

These measures facilitate gas exchange and decrease laryngeal edema and vocal cord irritation. The nurse also closely observes the client for signs or symptoms of upper airway obstruction (see Chap. 31). Early signs are mild dyspnea, coughing, and the inability to expectorate secretions. With the onset of these signs, the nurse notifies the physician, who evaluates the need for reintubation. The nurse is especially concerned if the client develops stridor, a late sign of a narrowed airway. Stridor is a high-pitched, crowing noise during inspiration caused by laryngospasm or edema above or below the glottis. Racemic epinephrine, a topical aerosol vasoconstrictor, is given, and reintubation may be performed.

Chest Trauma

Thoracic injuries are directly responsible for approximately 25% of all civilian traumatic deaths; 50% of the injured succumb before arriving at health care facilities. Only 5% to 15% of all thoracic injuries require thoracotomy. The remainder can be treated with basic resuscitation, intubation, or chest tube placement. Emergency personnel's basic and initial approach to all chest injuries is

ABC (*Airway*, *Breathing*, *Circulation*) followed by rapid assessment and treatment of potentially life-threatening conditions.

Pulmonary Contusion
Overview

Pulmonary contusion, a potentially lethal injury, is the most common chest injury seen in the United States. After a contusion, respiratory failure can develop over time rather than instantaneously. This condition most frequently follows injuries caused by rapid deceleration during vehicular accidents. Interstitial hemorrhage, which is almost invariably associated with intra-alveolar hemorrhage, is characteristic of pulmonary contusion. The resultant interstitial edema causes a decrease in pulmonary compliance and a decreased area for gas exchange. The client usually becomes hypoxemic and dyspneic. The bronchial mucosa becomes irritated, and the client has increased bronchial secretions.

Collaborative Management

 Assessment

Clients who may initially be asymptomatic can develop respiratory failure. The client presents with hemoptysis, decreased breath sounds, crackles, and wheezes. The chest x-ray of pulmonary contusion may show a hazy opacity in the lobes or parenchyma. If there is no disruption of the parenchyma, resorption of the lesion often occurs without treatment.

 Interventions

Treatment includes maintenance of ventilation and oxygenation. Central venous pressure is monitored closely, and fluid intake is restricted accordingly. The client in obvious respiratory distress may require mechanical ventilation with positive end-expiratory pressure (PEEP) to inflate the lungs and provide positive-pressure ventilation.

A vicious circle occurs in which more muscle effort is required for ventilation, and the client becomes progressively hypoxemic. Attempting to compensate causes the client to tire easily, become less efficient in breathing, and become more fatigued and hypoxemic. Flail chest may also be associated with a pulmonary contusion accompanied by parenchymal damage. The sequela to this situation is the probable development of ARDS.

Rib Fracture
Overview

After chest wall contusion, rib fractures are the next most common injury to the chest wall. Rib fractures most frequently result from direct blunt trauma to the chest, usually with involvement of the fifth through ninth ribs. Direct force applied to the ribs tends to fracture them and drive the bone ends into the thorax. Thus, there is a potential for intrathoracic injury, such as pneumothorax or pulmonary contusion. Pneumothorax is almost invariably present if ribs one through four are fractured.

Collaborative Management

The client usually experiences pain with movement and splints the chest defensively. Thoracic splinting results in impaired ventilation and inadequate clearance of tracheobronchial secretions. If the client has pre-existing pulmonary disease, the likelihood of atelectasis and pneumonia related to the rib fracture is increased. Clients with injuries to the first or second ribs, flail chest, seven or more fractured ribs, or expired volumes less than 15 mL/kg have a poor prognosis; intrathoracic injury occurs in 50% of these cases.

Treatment for uncomplicated rib fractures is nonspecific because the fractured ribs unite spontaneously. The chest is usually not splinted by tape or other materials. The primary consideration for the client is to decrease pain so that adequate ventilatory status is maintained. Intercostal nerve block may be used if pain is severe. Potent analgesia that causes respiratory depression is avoided.

Flail Chest

Overview

Flail chest (paradoxic respiration) is the inward movement of the thorax during inspiration, with outward movement during expiration. It usually involves one hemithorax (one side of the chest) and results from multiple rib fractures caused by blunt chest trauma. Flail chest is frequently associated with high-speed vehicular accidents. It is more common in older clients. It is associated with a high mortality rate (40%) and is one of the most critical chest injuries.

Flail chest occurs when a loose segment of chest wall is left because of a fracture of two or more adjacent ribs. The movement of this segment becomes paradoxic to the expansion and contraction of the rest of the chest wall. Flail chest can also occur from bilateral fracture of multiple costochondral junctions (without rib fracture) anteriorly, such as might occur during cardiopulmonary resuscitation on an elderly person. There may be associated injury to the lung tissue under the flail segment. Gas exchange is significantly impaired, as is the ability to cough and clear secretions. Defensive splinting because of the rib fracture further reduces the client's ability to exert the extra effort required for breathing, which may contribute later to failure to wean.

Collaborative Management

 Assessment

The nurse assesses the client with a flail chest for paradoxic chest movement, dyspnea, cyanosis, tachycardia, and hypotension. Anxiety is often associated with pain and dyspnea.

 Interventions

Interventions for flail chest include
- Administration of humidified oxygen
- Pain management
- Promotion of lung expansion through deep breathing and positioning
- Secretion clearance by coughing and tracheal aspiration

The nurse gives psychosocial support to the extremely anxious client by explaining all procedures, talking slowly, and allowing the client time to verbalize feelings and concerns.

The client with a flail chest may be treated conservatively with vigilant respiratory care. The physician may prescribe mechanical ventilation if such complications as respiratory failure or shock ensue. The physician and the nurse monitor ABG values closely along with vital capacity. With severe hypoxemia and hypercapnia, the client is intubated and mechanically ventilated with PEEP. With pulmonary contusion or an underlying pulmonary disease, the potential for respiratory failure increases. Flail chest is best stabilized by positive-pressure ventilation rather than surgical intervention. Operative stabilization is reserved for extreme cases of flail chest.

The nurse monitors the client's vital signs and fluid and electrolyte balance closely so that hypovolemia or shock can be treated immediately. If the client has a pulmonary contusion, the nurse monitors central venous pressure and administers fluids as ordered. The nurse assesses the client for pain and intervenes to relieve the client's pain. The physician may order analgesic medication by the intravenous, epidural, or nerve block routes.

Pneumothorax

Overview

Any thoracic injury that allows accumulation of atmospheric air in the pleural space results in a rise in intrathoracic pressure and a reduction in vital capacity, depending on the amount of pulmonary collapse produced. Pneumothorax is often caused by blunt chest trauma and is associated with some degree of hemothorax. The pneumothorax can be open (when the pleural cavity has become exposed to the outside air, as through an open wound in the chest wall) or closed.

Collaborative Management

Assessment findings include

- Diminished breath sounds on auscultation
- Hyperresonance on percussion
- Prominence of the involved hemithorax, which moves poorly with respirations
- Deviation of the trachea away from (closed) or toward (open) the affected side

In addition, the client may have pleuritic pain, tachypnea, and subcutaneous emphysema (air under the skin in the subcutaneous tissues). A chest x-ray is used for diagnosis. Chest tubes may be indicated to allow the air to escape and the lung segment to reinflate.

Tension Pneumothorax

Overview

Tension pneumothorax, one of the most rapidly developing and life-threatening complications of blunt chest trauma, results from an air leak in the lung or chest wall. Air forced into the thoracic cavity causes complete collapse of the affected lung. Air that enters the pleural space during expiration does not exit during inspiration. As a result, air progressively accumulates under pressure, compresses the mediastinal vessels, and interferes with venous return. Because this process leads to decreased diastolic filling of the heart, cardiac output is compromised. If not promptly detected and treated, tension pneumothorax is quickly fatal. Typical causes of tension pneumothorax are

- Blunt chest trauma in which the parenchymal injury has failed to seal
- Mechanical ventilation with PEEP
- Closed chest drainage (chest tubes)
- Insertion of central venous access catheters

Collaborative Management

 Assessment

Assessment findings with tension pneumothorax include
- Asymmetry of the thorax
- Tracheal deviation to the unaffected side
- Respiratory distress
- Unilateral absence of breath sounds
- Distended neck veins
- Cyanosis

On percussion, there is a hypertympanic sound over the affected hemithorax. Pneumothorax is detectable on a chest x-ray. ABG assays demonstrate hypoxia and respiratory alkalosis.

 Interventions

The physician inserts a large-bore needle into the second intercostal space in the midclavicular line of the affected side as initial treatment for tension pneumothorax. After this lifesaving measure is completed, the physician places a chest tube into the fourth intercostal space of the midaxillary line and attaches the tube to a water seal drainage system until the lung reinflates.

Hemothorax

Overview

Hemothorax is one of the most common problems encountered after blunt chest trauma or penetrating injuries. A *simple* hemothorax is a blood loss of less than 1500 mL into the thoracic cavity; a *massive* hemothorax is a blood loss of more than 1500 mL.

Bleeding is frequently caused by injuries to the lung parenchyma, such as pulmonary contusions or lacerations, which are often associated with rib and sternal fractures. Massive intrathoracic bleeding in blunt chest trauma generally stems from the heart, great vessels, or major systemic arteries, such as the intercostal arteries.

Collaborative Management

 Assessment

Physical assessment findings vary with the size of the hemothorax. If the hemothorax is small, the client may be asymptomatic. If the hemothorax is larger, the client experiences respiratory distress. In addition, breath sounds are diminished on auscultation. The percussion note on the involved side is dull. Blood in the pleural space is visible on a chest x-ray and confirmed by diagnostic thoracentesis.

 Interventions

Interventions are aimed at evacuating the blood in the pleural space to normalize pulmonary function and to prevent infection related to blood accumulation. The physician inserts anterior and posterolateral chest tubes to evacuate the pleural space and to reduce the rush of clotted blood. The physician and the nurse carefully monitor the chest tube drainage, and chest x-rays are evaluated serially.

The physician considers open thoracotomy when there is initial evacuation of 1500 to 2000 mL of blood or persistent bleeding at the rate of 200 mL/hr over 3 hours. The nurse monitors the client's vital signs, blood loss, and overall intake and output; assesses the client's response to the chest tubes; and administers IV fluids and blood as ordered. Autotransfusion of the blood lost through chest drainage should be considered.

Tracheobronchial Trauma

Overview

Most tears of the tracheobronchial tree result from severe blunt trauma primarily involving the mainstem bronchi. Injuries to the cervical trachea usually occur at the junction of the trachea and cricoid cartilage. These injuries are frequently caused by striking the anterior neck against the dashboard or steering wheel during a vehicular accident. Clients with lacerations of the trachea develop massive air leaks, which produce pneumomediastinum (air in the mediastinum) and extensive subcutaneous emphysema. Upper airway obstruction may also occur and produce severe respiratory distress and inspiratory stridor. Major cervical tears are managed by cricothyroidotomy or tracheostomy below the level of injury.

Collaborative Management

The nurse assesses the client for hypoxemia by ABG assays. The nurse administers oxygen appropriately. Depending on the degree of injury, the client may require mechanical ventilation or surgical repair. Frequent assessment of vital signs is essential because the client is likely to be hypotensive and in shock. the nurse continues to assess for subcutaneous emphysema and auscultates lungs to assess for further complications every 1 to 2 hours initially. Decreased breath sounds or wheezing may indicate further obstruction, atelectasis, or pneumothorax. Care of the client with a tracheostomy is discussed in Chapter 30.

CASE STUDY for the Client with ARDS

■ H. B. is a 40-year-old man who was exposed to contents of a manure bin during a farming accident that killed three other men. He inhaled carbon dioxide, ammonia gas, hydrogen sulfide, and methane gas, and he aspirated manure. H. B. was in the bin for an unknown period and, when rescued, had no apparent respirations. A faint carotid pulse was palpated, so he was resuscitated, intubated, and transported to the hospital by helicopter, where x-ray showed bilateral diffuse infiltrates. His ABGs on 100% FIO_2 were pH 7.25; $PaCO_2$, 40 mmHg; and PaO_2, 40 mmHg. His pulmonary shunt was calculated to be 35%.

QUESTIONS:

1. What do the ABGs indicate about his oxygenation status?
2. For what treatment should you prepare?
3. He had large amounts of frothy, bloody secretions suctioned from his endotracheal tube. The colloid osmotic pressure of the secretions was 19.0 and of his serum was 14.9. What does this indicate?

BIBLIOGRAPHY

Aherns, T. S., Beattie, S., & Nienhaus, T. (1996). Experimental therapies to support the failing lung. *AACN Clinical Issues, 7*(4), 507–518.

Anderson, R. (1998). Another way to open an airway. *RN, 61*(3), 42–44.

*Arbour, R. (1993). Weaning a patient from a ventilator. *Nursing93, 23*(2), 52–56.

Baldwin-Myers, A., Geiger-Bronsky, M., Chacona, A., Ewing, L., Huiskes, B., Shiroma, J., & Gold, P. (1994). *Standards of care for the ventilator-assisted individual: A comprehensive management plan from hospital to home.* Loma Linda, CA: Loma Linda University/Respiratory Nursing Society.

Brandstetter, R., Sharma, K., DellaBadia, M., Cabreros, L., & Kabinoff, G. (1997). Adult respiratory distress syndrome: A disorder in need of improved outcome. *Heart & Lung, 26*(1), 3–14.

*Burns, S. M. (1992). A computerized assessment program for weaning patients from long-term mechanical ventilation. *Perspectives in Respiratory Nursing, 3*(6), 1, 6–8.

*Burns, S. M. (1991). Preventing diaphragm fatigue in the ventilated patient. *Dimensions of Critical Care Nursing, 10*(1), 13–20.

Burns, S. (1996). Understanding, applying, and evaluating pressure modes of ventilation. *AACN Clinical Issues: Advanced Practice in Acute Care and Critical Care, 7*(4), 495–506.

Burns, S., Clochesy, J., Goodnough-Hanneman, S., Ingersoll, G., Knebel, A., & Shekleton, M. (1995). Weaning from long-term mechanical ventilation. *American Journal of Critical Care, 4*(1), 4–22.

Carroll, P. (1997). When you WANT humidity. *RN, 60*(5), 30–35.

Carroll, P., & Milikowski, K. (1996). Getting your patient off a ventilator. *RN, 59*(6), 42–48.

Clochesy, J., Daily, B., & Montenegro, H. (1995). Weaning chronically critically ill adults from mechanical ventilatory support: A descriptive study. *American Journal of Critical Care, 4*(2), 93–99.

*Connolly, M. A., & Shekleton, M. E. (1991). Communicating with ventilator dependent patients. *Dimensions of Critical Care Nursing, 10*(2), 115–121.

*Curry, K., & Casday, L. (1992). Managing spontaneous pneumothorax. *The Nursing Spectrum, 1*(7), 12–13.

Cushinotto, N. (1997). Pharmacology update: Clinical considerations of heparinization. *Journal of the American Academy of Nurse Practitioners, 9*(6), 273–276.

Cutler, L. R. (1996). Acute respiratory distress syndrome: An overview. *Intensive and Critical Care Nursing, 12,* 316–326.

Dalen, J., & Hirsh, J. (Eds.). (1995). Fourth ACCP Consensus Conference on Antithrombotic Therapy. *Chest, 108*(3 Suppl).

*Dellenger, R. (Ed.). (1993). Adult respiratory distress syndrome: Current considerations in future directions. *New Horizons: The Science and Practice of Acute Medicine, 1*(4), 463.

*Demling, R. (1993). Acute respiratory failure. *New Horizons: The Science and Practice of Acute Medicine, 1*(3), 361.

*Demling, R. (1993). Adult respiratory distress syndrome: Current concepts. *New Horizons: The Science and Practice of Acute Medicine, 1*(3), 388–401.

*Dettenmeier, P. A., & Johnson, T. M. (1991). The art and science of mechanical ventilator adjustments. *Critical Care Nursing Clinics of North America, 3*(4), 575–583.

Ellstrom, K. (1997). Procedure for taping oral and nasal endotracheal tubes. *Perspectives in Respiratory Nursing, 8*(1), 7–8.

Enger, E. (1996). Patients with adult respiratory distress syndrome. In J. Clochesy, C. Breu, S. Cardin, A. Whittaker, & E. Rudy (Eds.), *Critical care nursing* (2nd ed., pp. 656–688). Philadelphia: W. B. Saunders

Fetzer, S. (1998). Laryngeal mask airway: Indications and management for critical-care. *Critical Care Nurse, 18*(1), 83–87.

Frederick, C. (1994). Noninvasive mechanical ventilation with the iron lung. *Critical Care Nursing Clinics of North America, 6*(4), 831–840.

Glass, C., Boling, P., & Gammon, S. (1996). Collaborative support for caregivers of individuals beginning mechanical ventilation at home. *Critical Care Nurse, 16*(4), 67–72.

Goodwin, R. S. (1996). Prevention of aspiration pneumonia: A research-based protocol. *Dimensions of Critical Care Nursing, 15*(2), 58–71.

Henneman, E. (1996). Patients with acute respiratory failure. In J. Clochesy, C. Breu, S. Cardin, A. Whittaker, & E. Rudy (Eds.), *Critical care nursing* (2nd ed., pp. 630–655). Philadelphia: W. B. Saunders.

Henneman, E., & Ellstrom, K. (1998). *Protocols for practice: Airway management.* Aliso Viejo, CA: American Association of Critical-Care Nurses.

*Hunter, F. C., & Mitchell, S. (1993). Managing ARDS. *RN, 56*(7), 52–58.

Jenny, J., & Logan, J. (1994). Promoting ventilator independence: A grounded theory perspective. *Dimensions of Critical Care Nursing, 13*(1), 29–37.

*Kelleghan, S. I., Salemi, C., & Padilla, S., et al. (1993). An effective continuous quality improvement approach to the prevention of ventilator-associated pneumonia. *American Journal of Infection Control, 21*(6), 322–330.

Kelly, M. (1996). Emergency! Acute respiratory failure. *American Journal of Nursing, 96*(12), 46.

Kite-Powell, D., Sabau, D., Ideno, K., Hargraves, D., & Dahlberg, C. (1996). Optimizing outcomes in ventilator-dependent patients: Challenging critical care practice. *Critical Care Nursing Quarterly, 19*(3), 77–90.

Knebel, A., Strider, V., & Wood, C. (1994). The art and science of caring for ventilator-assisted patients: Learning from our clinical practice. *Critical Care Nursing Clinics of North America, 6*(4), 819–830.

*Mason, S. G. (1992). When a ventilator patient is going home. *RN, 55*(10), 60–64.

Misasi, R., & Keyes, J. (1996). Matching and mismatching ventilation and perfusion in the lung. *Critical Care Nurse, 16*(3), 23–38.

Pahor, M., Guralnik, J., Havlik, R., Carbonin, P., Salive, M., Ferrucci, L.,

Corti, M., & Hennekens, C. (1996). Alcohol consumption and risk of deep vein thrombosis and pulmonary embolism in older persons. *Journal of the American Geriatrics Society, 44*(9), 1030–1037.

*Pierce, J. D., Wiggins, S. A., Plaskon, C., & Glass, C. (1993). Pressure support ventilation: Reducing the work of breathing during weaning. *Dimensions of Critical Care Nursing, 12*(6), 282–290.

Respiratory Nursing Society. (1994). *Standards and scope of respiratory nursing practice.* Washington, DC: American Nurses Publishing.

*Roberts, S. L. (1990). High-permeability pulmonary edema: Nursing assessment, diagnosis, and interventions. *Heart & Lung, 19,* 287–300.

*Roberts, S., & White, B. (1992). Common nursing diagnoses for pulmonary alveolar edema patients. *Dimensions of Critical Care Nursing, 11*(1), 13–27.

*Saul, L. (Ed.). (1991). *Activase therapy in acute myocardial infarction and acute massive pulmonary embolism.* Califon, NJ: Gardiner-Caldwell SynerMed.

Severson, A., Baldwin, L., & DeLoughery, T. (1997). International normalized ratio in anticoagulation therapy: Understanding the issues. *American Journal of Critical Care, 6*(2), 88–92.

Taggart, J. A., & Lind, M. A. (1994). Evaluating unplanned endotracheal extubations. *Dimensions of Critical Care Nursing, 13*(3), 114–122.

Thompson, L. F. (1996). Failure to wean: Exploration of the influence of age-related pulmonary changes. *Critical Care Nursing Clinics of North America, 8*(1), 7–16.

Tobin, M. J. (Ed). (1994). *Principles and practice of mechanical ventilation.* New York: McGraw-Hill.

Vollman, K. M., & Bander, J. (1996). Improved oxygenation in patients with acute respiratory distress syndrome. *Intensive Care Medicine, 22*(10), 1105–1111.

*West, J. B. (1992). *Pulmonary pathophysiology—The essentials* (4th ed.). Baltimore, MD: Williams & Wilkins.

West, J. B. (1995). *Respiratory physiology—The essentials* (5th ed.). Baltimore, MD: Williams & Wilkins.

*White, B., & Roberts, S. (1993). Powerlessness and the pulmonary alveolar edema patient. *Dimensions of Critical Care Nursing, 12*(3), 127–137.

Wilson, D. (1996). Care of the chronic mechanically ventilated patient. In J. Clochesy, C. Breu, S. Cardin, A. Whittaker, & E. Rudy (Eds.), *Critical care nursing* (2nd ed., pp. 689–713). Philadelphia: W. B. Saunders.

SUGGESTED READINGS

Burns, S. (1996). Understanding, applying, and evaluating pressure modes of ventilation. *AACN Clinical Issues: Advanced Practice in Acute Care and Critical Care, 7*(4), 495–506.

Earlier methods of positive-pressure mechanical ventilation involving pressure-cycled machines have been shown to increase the risk of baratrauma and other complications. Thus, their use has largely been discontinued. Newer methods of pressure ventilation are now being used successfully and show some superiority over volume-cycled ventilation. This excellent article describes and compares current pressure ventilation modes, including pressure support, pressure-controlled inverse ratio, and volume-guaranteed pressure ventilation.

Carroll, P. (1997). When you WANT humidity. *RN, 60*(5), 30–35.

The issue of humidity and the importance of maintaining adequate humidity in clients who have artificial airways (endotracheal tube, tracheostomy tube) are discussed in clear terms. Ensuring adequate humidity in ventilated clients with artificial airways is essential to prevent complications. Different systems of humidification and their cost effectiveness are described.

Thompson, L. F. (1996). Failure to wean: Exploration of the influence of age-related pulmonary changes. *Critical Care Nursing Clinics of North America, 8*(1), 7–16.

This excellent article discusses the age-related physiologic and anatomic changes that decrease the likelihood to wean from mechanical ventilation in the elderly. Nursing implications for evaluation of effective ventilation in the elderly are presented.

UNIT 7

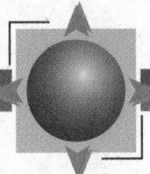

Problems of Cardiac

Output and Tissue

Perfusion: Management of

Clients with Problems of

the Cardiovascular System

ASSESSMENT OF THE CARDIOVASCULAR SYSTEM

Since 1979, there has been a 23.4% decline in the death rate from cardiovascular disease in the United States. Despite this dramatic reduction, cardiovascular disease remains the major cause of mortality, resulting in 42% of all deaths or nearly 1 million deaths each year in the United States. Additionally, the American Heart Association (AHA) estimates that approximately one in five people has experienced, and is living with, some form of cardiovascular disease (AHA, 1996).

ANATOMY AND PHYSIOLOGY REVIEW
Heart
Structure

The human heart is a cone-shaped, hollow, muscular organ located between the lungs (Fig. 35–1). It is approximately the size of an adult fist. The heart rests on the diaphragm, tilting forward and to the left in the client's chest. This small organ must pump continuously. Each beat of the heart pumps approximately 60 mL of blood, which is about 5 L/minute. During strenuous physical activity, the heart can double the amount of blood pumped to meet the increased oxygen needs of the peripheral tissues.

The heart is encapsulated by a protective covering called the *pericardium* (Fig. 35–2). The cardiac muscle tissue is composed of three layers: epicardium, myocardium, and endocardium. The epicardium, the outer surface, is a thin transparent tissue. The myocardium, the middle layer, is composed of striated muscle fibers interlaced into bundles. This layer is responsible for the heart's contractile force. The innermost layer, the endocardium, is composed of endothelial tissue. This tissue lines the inside of the chambers of the heart and covers the four heart valves.

Chambers of the Heart

A muscular wall, known as the septum, separates the heart into two halves: right and left. Each half has an upper chamber called an *atrium* and a lower chamber called a *ventricle* (Fig. 35–3).

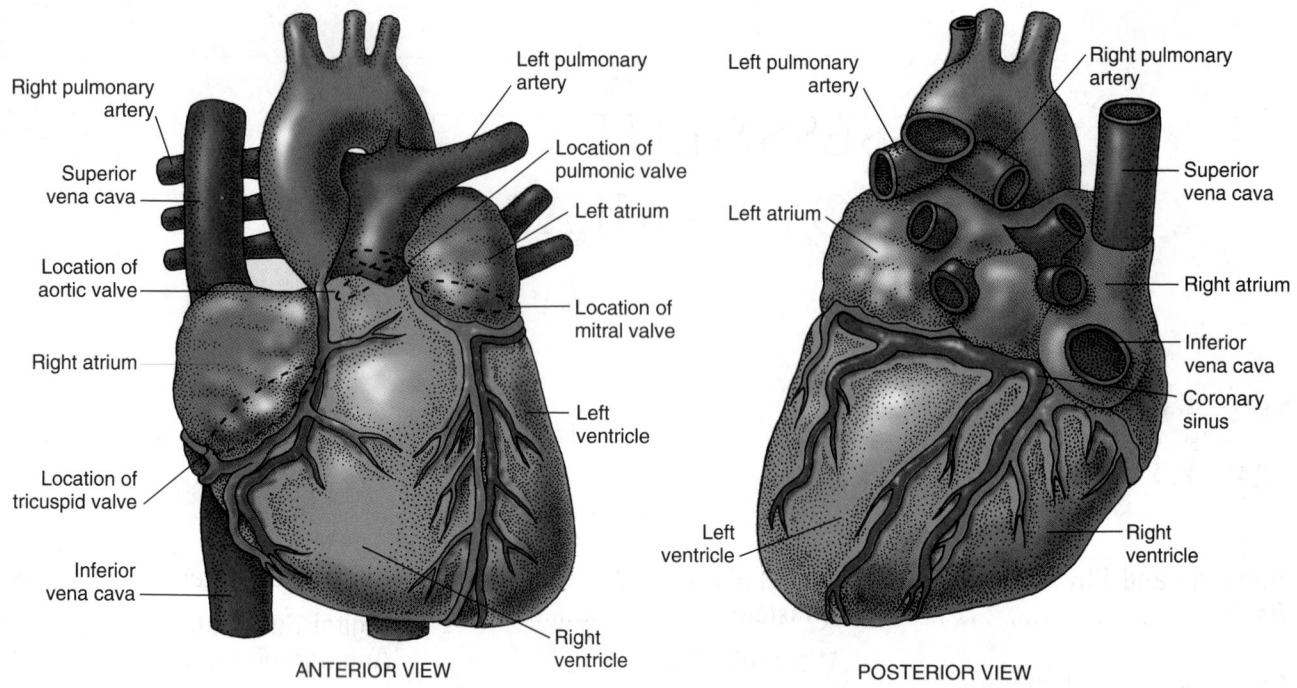

Figure 35–1. Surface anatomy of the heart.

Right Side

The right atrium is a thin-walled structure that receives deoxygenated venous blood (venous return) from all the peripheral tissues by way of the superior and inferior venae cavae and from the heart muscle by way of the coronary sinus. Most of this venous return flows passively from the right atrium through the opened tricuspid valve to the right ventricle during ventricular diastole, or filling. The remaining venous return is actively propelled by the right atrium into the right ventricle during atrial systole, or contraction.

The right ventricle is a flat muscular pump located behind the sternum. The right ventricle generates enough pressure (about 25 mmHg) to close the tricuspid valve, open the pulmonic valve, and propel blood into the pulmonary artery and the lungs. The workload of the right ventricle is light compared with that of the left ventricle because the pulmonary system is a low-pressure system, which imposes less resistance to flow.

Left Side

After blood is reoxygenated in the lungs, it flows freely from the four pulmonary veins into the left atrium. Blood then flows through an opened mitral valve into the left ventricle during ventricular diastole. When the left ventricle is almost full, the left atrium contracts, pumping the remaining blood volume into the left ventricle. Finally, with systolic contraction, the left ventricle generates enough pressure (about 120 mmHg) to close the mitral valve and open the aortic valve. Blood is propelled into the aorta and into the systemic arterial circulation. Blood flow through the heart is shown in Figure 35–2.

The left ventricle is ellipsoid and is the largest and most muscular chamber of the heart. Its wall is two to three times the thickness of the right ventricular wall. The left ventricle must generate a higher pressure than the right ventricle because it must contract against a high-pressure systemic circulation, which imposes a greater resistance to flow.

Blood is propelled from the aorta throughout the systemic circulation to the various tissues of the body; blood returns to the right atrium because of pressure differences. The pressure of blood in the aorta in a young adult averages about 100–120 mmHg, whereas the pressure of blood in the right atrium averages about 0–5 mmHg. These differences in pressure produce a pressure gradient and blood flows from an area of higher pressure to an area of lower pressure. The heart and vascular structures are responsible for maintaining these pressures.

Heart Valves

The four cardiac valves are responsible for maintaining the forward flow of blood through the chambers of the heart (see Fig. 35–2). These valves open and close passively in response to pressure and volume changes within the cardiac chambers. The cardiac valves are classified into two types: atrioventricular (AV) valves and semilunar valves.

Atrioventricular Valves

The AV valves separate the atria from the ventricles. The tricuspid valve is composed of three leaflets and separates the right atrium from the right ventricle. The mitral (bicuspid) valve is composed of two leaflets and separates the left atrium from the left ventricle.

During ventricular diastole, the valves act as funnels,

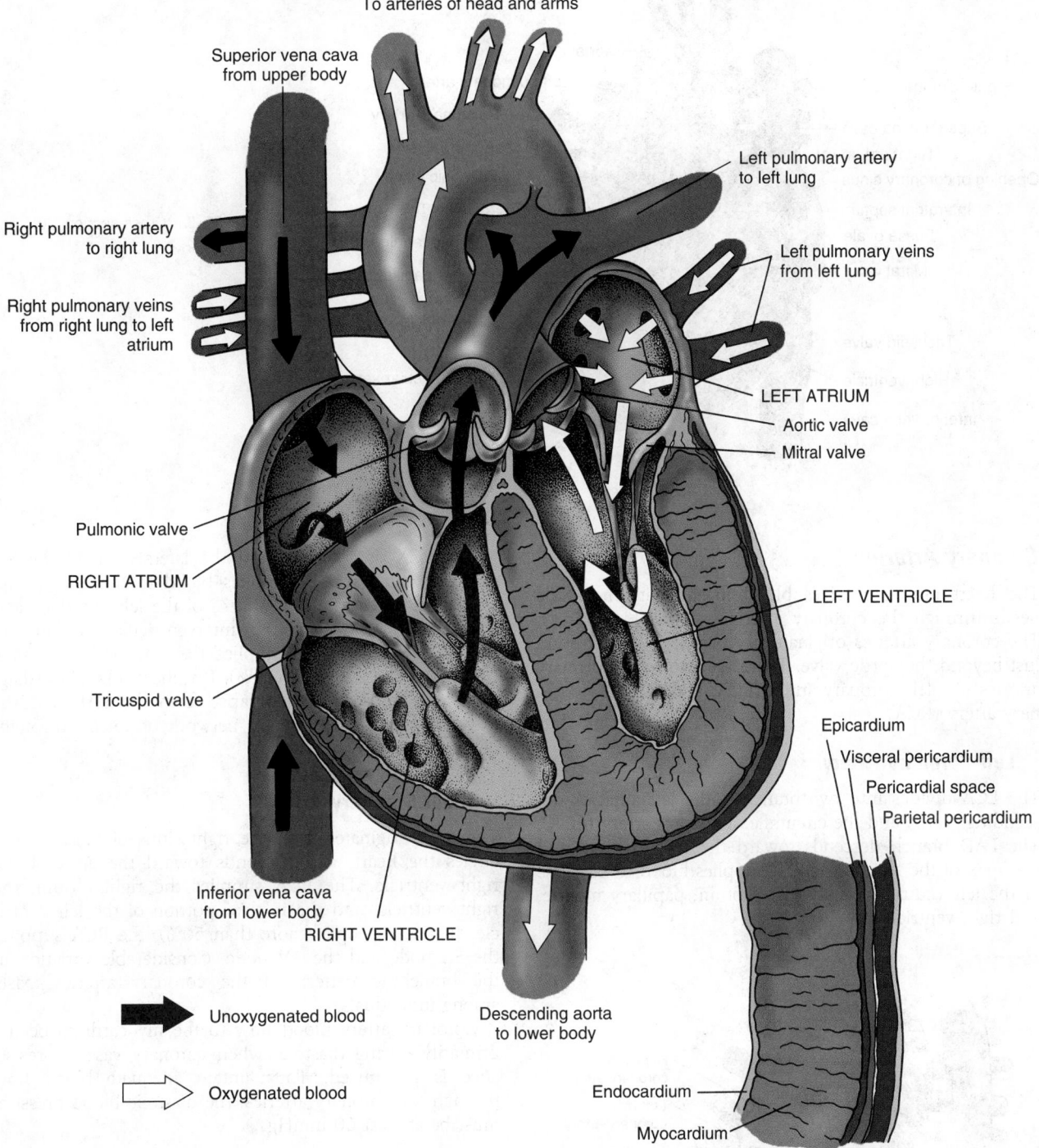

To arteries of head and arms

Superior vena cava
from upper body

Right pulmonary artery
to right lung

Right pulmonary veins
from right lung to left
atrium

Left pulmonary artery
to left lung

Left pulmonary veins
from left lung

LEFT ATRIUM

Aortic valve

Mitral valve

Pulmonic valve

RIGHT ATRIUM

LEFT VENTRICLE

Tricuspid valve

Epicardium

Visceral pericardium

Pericardial space

Parietal pericardium

Inferior vena cava
from lower body

RIGHT VENTRICLE

Unoxygenated blood

Descending aorta
to lower body

Oxygenated blood

Endocardium

Myocardium

Figure 35–2. Blood flow through the heart.

facilitating the flow of blood from the atria to the ventricles. During systole, the valves close to prevent the backflow (regurgitation) of blood into the atria.

Semilunar Valves

There are two semilunar valves: the pulmonic and the aortic valve. The pulmonic valve separates the right ven-

tricle from the pulmonary artery. The aortic valve separates the left ventricle from the aorta. Each semilunar valve consists of three cup-like cusps, or pockets, around the inside wall of the artery. These cusps prevent blood from flowing back into the ventricles during ventricular diastole. During ventricular systole, these valves are open to permit blood flow into the pulmonary artery and the aorta.

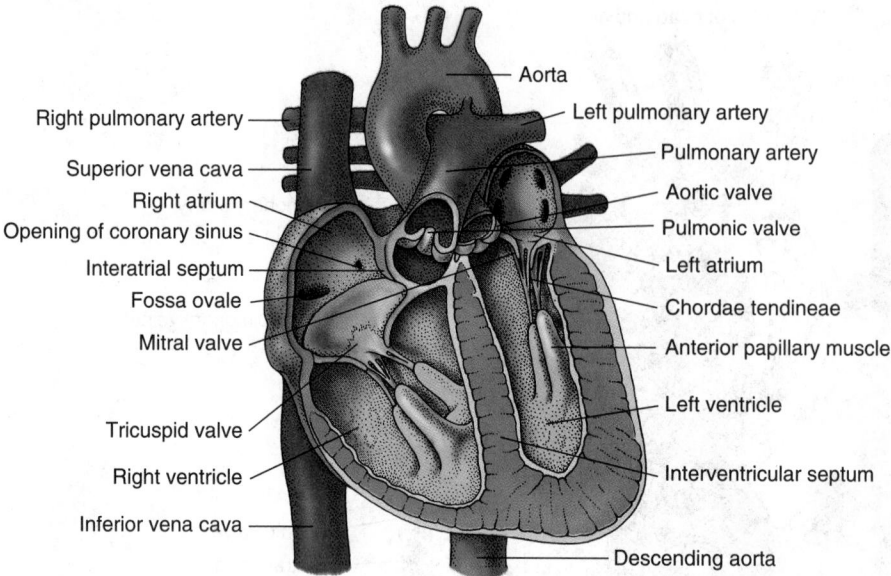

Figure 35-3. Cross-section of the heart.

Coronary Arteries

The heart muscle receives blood to meet its metabolic needs through the coronary arterial system (Fig. 35–4). The coronary arteries originate from an area on the aorta just beyond the aortic valve. There are two main coronary arteries: the left coronary artery (LCA) and the right coronary artery (RCA).

Left Coronary Artery

The LCA divides into two branches: the left anterior descending (LAD) and the circumflex coronary artery (LCX). The LAD branch descends toward the anterior wall and the apex of the left ventricle. It supplies blood to portions of the left ventricle, ventricular septum, papillary muscle, and right ventricle.

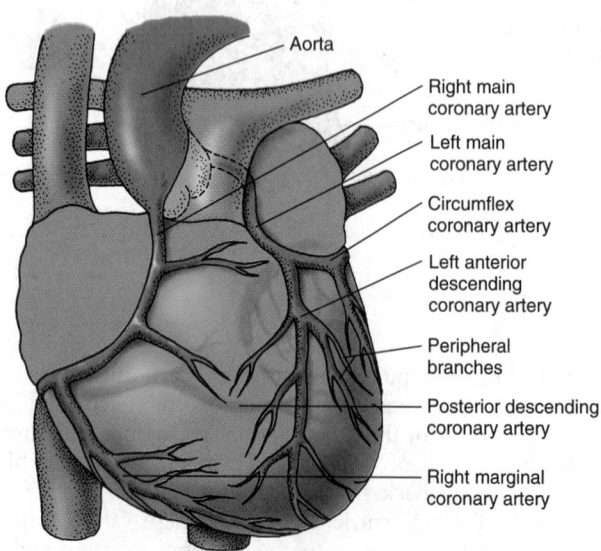

Figure 35-4. Coronary arterial system.

The LCX descends toward the lateral wall of the left ventricle and apex. It supplies blood to the left atrium, the lateral and posterior surfaces of the left ventricle, and sometimes portions of the interventricular septum. In some people, the LCX supplies the sinoatrial (SA) node (45%) and the AV node (10%). Peripheral branches (diagonal and obtuse marginal) arise from the LAD and the LCX and form an abundant network of vessels throughout the entire myocardium.

Right Coronary Artery

The RCA originates from the right sinus of Valsalva, encircles the heart, and descends toward the apex of the right ventricle. The RCA supplies the right atrium, the right ventricle, and the inferior portion of the left ventricle. In many people (more than 50%), the RCA supplies the SA node and the AV node. Considerable variation in the branching pattern of the coronary arteries exists among individuals.

Coronary artery blood flow to the myocardium occurs primarily during diastole, when coronary vascular resistance is minimized. To maintain adequate blood flow through the coronary arteries, the diastolic blood pressure must be at least 60 mmHg.

Function

Electrophysiologic Properties of the Heart

The electrophysiologic properties of heart muscle are responsible for regulating heart rate and rhythm. Cardiac muscle cells are unique and possess the special characteristics of automaticity, excitability, conductivity, contractility, and refractoriness.

Automaticity refers to the ability of all cardiac cells to initiate an impulse spontaneously and repetitively. Excitability is the ability of the cells to respond to a stimulus by initiating an impulse (depolarization). Conductivity means that cardiac cells transmit the electrical impulses they receive. Because the cells possess the property of contractility, they also contract in response to an impulse. Refractoriness means that cardiac cells are unable to respond to a stimulus until they have repolarized from the previous stimulus. These properties are more completely described in Chapter 36.

Conduction System of the Heart

The cardiac conduction system is composed of specialized tissue capable of rhythmic electrical impulse formation (Fig. 35–5). It can conduct impulses much more rapidly than other cells located in the myocardium. The SA node, located at the junction of the right atrium and the superior vena cava, is considered the main regulator of heart rate. The SA node is composed of pacemaker cells, which spontaneously initiate impulses at a rate of 60–100 per minute, and myocardial working cells, which transmit the impulses to surrounding atrial muscle.

An impulse from the SA node initiates the process of depolarization and hence the activation of all myocardial cells. The impulse travels through both atria to the atrioventricular (AV) node located in the junctional area. After the impulse reaches the AV node, conduction of the impulse is delayed briefly. This delay allows the atria to contract completely before the ventricles are stimulated to contract. The intrinsic rate of the AV node is 40–60 beats per minute.

The bundle of His is a continuation of the AV node located in the interventricular septum. It divides into the right and left bundle branches. The bundle branches extend downward through the ventricular septum and fuse with the Purkinje fiber system. The Purkinje fibers are the terminal branches of the conduction system and are responsible for carrying the wave of depolarization to both ventricular walls. The Purkinje fibers can act as an intrinsic pacemaker, but their discharge rate is only 20–40 beats per minute. Thus, these intrinsic pacemakers seldom initiate an electrical impulse.

Sequence of Events During the Cardiac Cycle

The phases of the cardiac cycle are generally described in relation to changes in pressure and volume in the left ventricle during filling (diastole) and ventricular contraction (systole) (Fig. 35–6). Diastole, normally about two thirds of the cardiac cycle, consists of relaxation and filling of the atria and ventricles, whereas systole consists of the contraction and emptying of the atria and ventricles.

Cardiac muscle contraction results from the release of large numbers of calcium ions from the sarcoplasmic reticulum. These ions diffuse into the myofibril sarcomere (the basic contractile unit of the myocardial cell). Calcium ions promote the interaction of actin and myosin protein filaments, causing a linking and overlapping of these filaments. As the protein filaments slide over or overlap each other, cross-bridges, or linkages, are formed. These cross-bridges act as force-generating sites. The sliding of these protein filaments of multiple myofibril sarcomeres causes shortening of the sarcomeres, producing myocardial contraction.

Relaxation of the cardiac muscle occurs when calcium ions are pumped back into the sarcoplasmic reticulum, causing a decrease in the number of calcium ions around the myofibrils. This reduced number of ions causes the protein filaments to disengage or dissociate, the sarcomere to lengthen, and the muscle to relax.

Mechanical Properties of the Heart

The electrical and mechanical properties of cardiac muscle determine the function of the cardiovascular system. The heart is able to adapt to various pathophysiologic conditions (e.g., stress, infections, and hemorrhage) to maintain

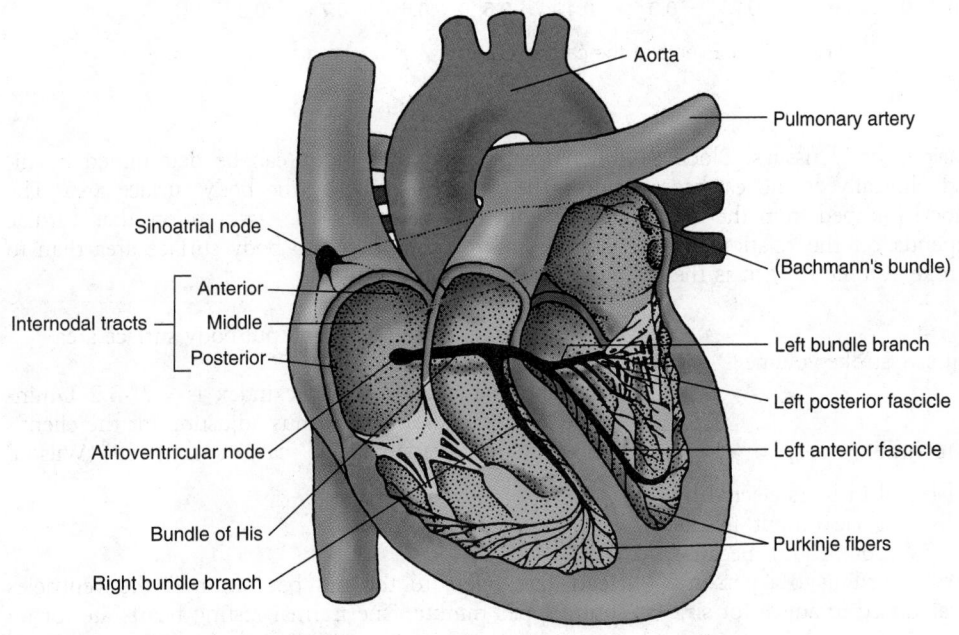

Figure 35–5. Conduction system of the heart.

Aorta

Pulmonary artery

Sinoatrial node

(Bachmann's bundle)

Internodal tracts — Anterior / Middle / Posterior

Left bundle branch

Left posterior fascicle

Atrioventricular node

Left anterior fascicle

Bundle of His

Purkinje fibers

Right bundle branch

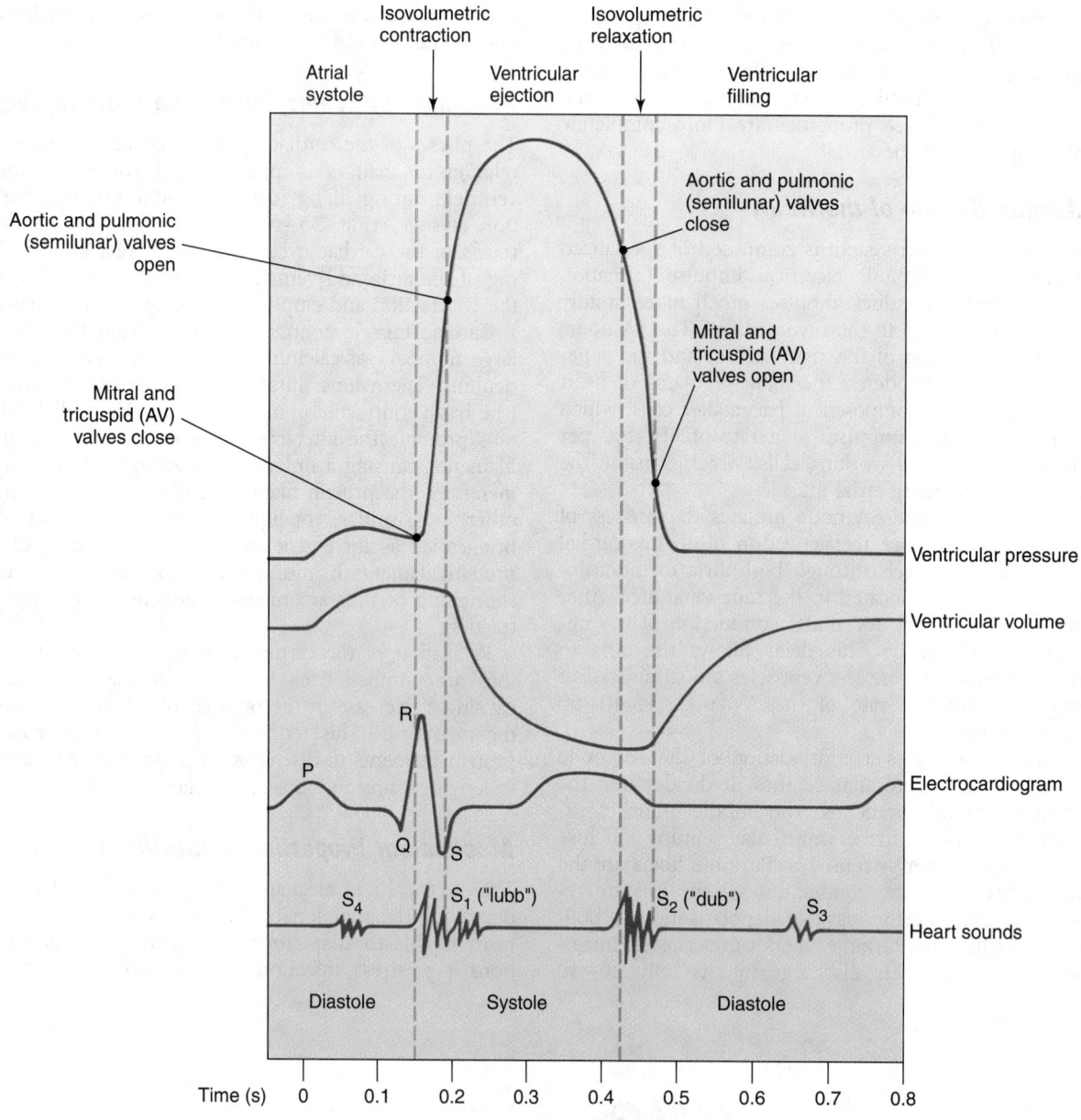

Figure 35–6. Events of the cardiac cycle.

adequate blood flow to the various body tissues. Blood flow to the tissues is measured clinically as the cardiac output (CO), the amount of blood pumped from the left ventricle each minute. CO depends on the relationship between heart rate (HR) and stroke volume (SV); it is the product of these two variables.

$$\text{Cardiac output} = \text{heart rate} \times \text{stroke volume}$$

Cardiac Output and Cardiac Index

Cardiac output is the volume of blood in liters ejected by the heart each minute. Normally, cardiac output in the adult ranges from 4–7 L/minute (Wilson, 1992). Because cardiac output requirements vary according to a person's body size, the cardiac index is calculated to adjust for size

differences. The cardiac index can be determined by dividing the cardiac output by the body surface area. The cardiac index is based on the assumption that cardiac output is more proportional to body surface area than to body mass. Therefore,

$$\text{Cardiac index} = \text{cardiac output/body surface area}$$

The normal range of cardiac index is 2.7–3.2 L/minute/m^2 of body surface area, thus adjusting for the client's body size and variability in cardiac function (Wilson, 1992).

Heart Rate

Heart rate refers to the number of times the ventricles contract per minute. The normal resting heart rate for an adult is between 60 and 100 beats per minute. Increases in heart rate increase myocardial oxygen demand. Rate is extrinsically controlled by the autonomic nervous system, which adjusts rapidly when necessary to regulate cardiac output. The parasympathetic system slows the heart rate, whereas sympathetic stimulation has an excitatory effect. An increase in circulating endogenous catecholamine, such as epinephrine and norepinephrine, usually causes an increase in heart rate, and vice versa.

Other factors, such as the central nervous system (CNS) and baroreceptor (pressoreceptor) reflexes, influence the effects of the autonomic nervous system on the heart rate. Pain, fear, and anxiety can cause an increase in heart rate. The baroreceptor reflex acts as a negative-feedback system. If a client experiences hypotension, the baroreceptors in the aortic arch sense a lessened pressure in the blood vessels. A signal is relayed to the parasympathetic system to have less inhibitory effect on the sino-atrial (SA) node, which results in a reflex increase in heart rate.

Stroke Volume

Stroke volume is the amount of blood ejected by the left ventricle during each systole. Several variables influence stroke volume and, ultimately, cardiac output (CO). These variables include heart rate, preload, afterload, and contractility.

PRELOAD. Preload refers to the degree of myocardial fiber stretch at the end of diastole just before contraction. The stretch imposed on the muscle fibers results from the volume contained within the ventricle at the end of diastole. Preload is determined by left ventricular end-diastolic (LVED) volume.

An increase in ventricular volume increases muscle fiber length and tension, thereby enhancing contraction and improving stroke volume. This statement is derived from Starling's law of the heart: the more the heart is filled during diastole (within limits), the more forcefully it contracts. However, excessive filling of the ventricles results in excessive LVED volume and pressure and decreased CO (Fig. 35–7).

AFTERLOAD. Another determinant of stroke volume is afterload. Afterload is the pressure or resistance that the ventricles must overcome to eject blood through the semilunar valves and into the peripheral blood vessels. The amount of resistance is directly related to arterial blood pressure and the diameter of the blood vessels.

Impedance, the peripheral component of afterload, is the pressure that the heart must overcome to open the aortic valve. The amount of impedance depends on aortic compliance and total peripheral vascular resistance, a combination of blood viscosity and arteriolar constriction. A decrease in stroke volume can result from an increase in afterload without the benefit of compensatory mechanisms.

CONTRACTILITY. Contractility also affects stroke volume and CO. Myocardial contractility is the force of cardiac contraction independent of preload. Contractility is

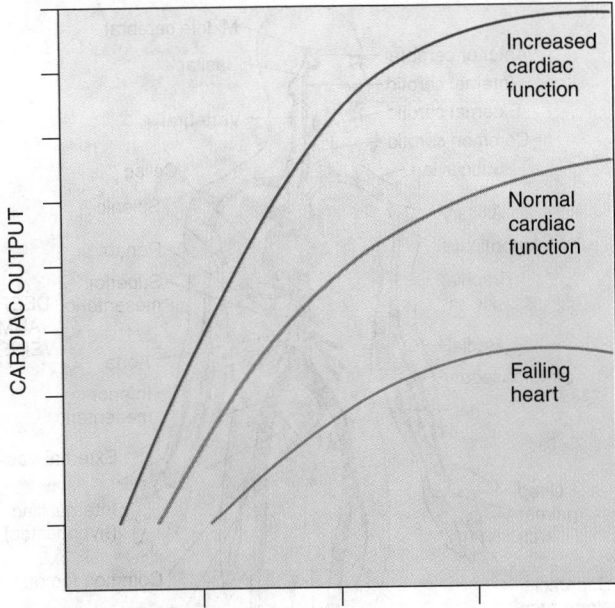

Figure 35–7. Length-tension ventricular function curves.

increased by such factors as sympathetic stimulation and calcium release. Factors such as hypoxia and acidemia decrease contractility.

Vascular System

The purpose of the vascular system is

- To provide conduits for blood to travel from the heart to nourish the various tissues of the body
- To carry away cellular wastes to the excretory organs
- To allow lymphatic flow to drain tissue fluid back into the circulation
- To return blood to the heart for recirculation

This system of conduits depends on an efficient heart and patent blood vessels to regulate and maintain systemic and regional blood flow and temperature.

The vascular system is divided into the arterial system and the venous system (Fig. 35–8). In the arterial system, blood moves from the larger conduits to a network of smaller blood vessels. In the venous system, blood travels from the capillaries to the venules and to the larger system of veins, eventually returning in the venae cavae to the heart for recirculation.

Arterial System
Structure

The high-pressure blood vessels of the arterial vascular system may be classified according to their size and wall structure. The large arteries, such as the aorta and femoral arteries, follow relatively straight routes and have few branches. Smaller arteries, such as the internal iliac and mesenteric arteries, divide from larger ones and have multiple branches.

Arteries may branch into arterioles or anastomose with

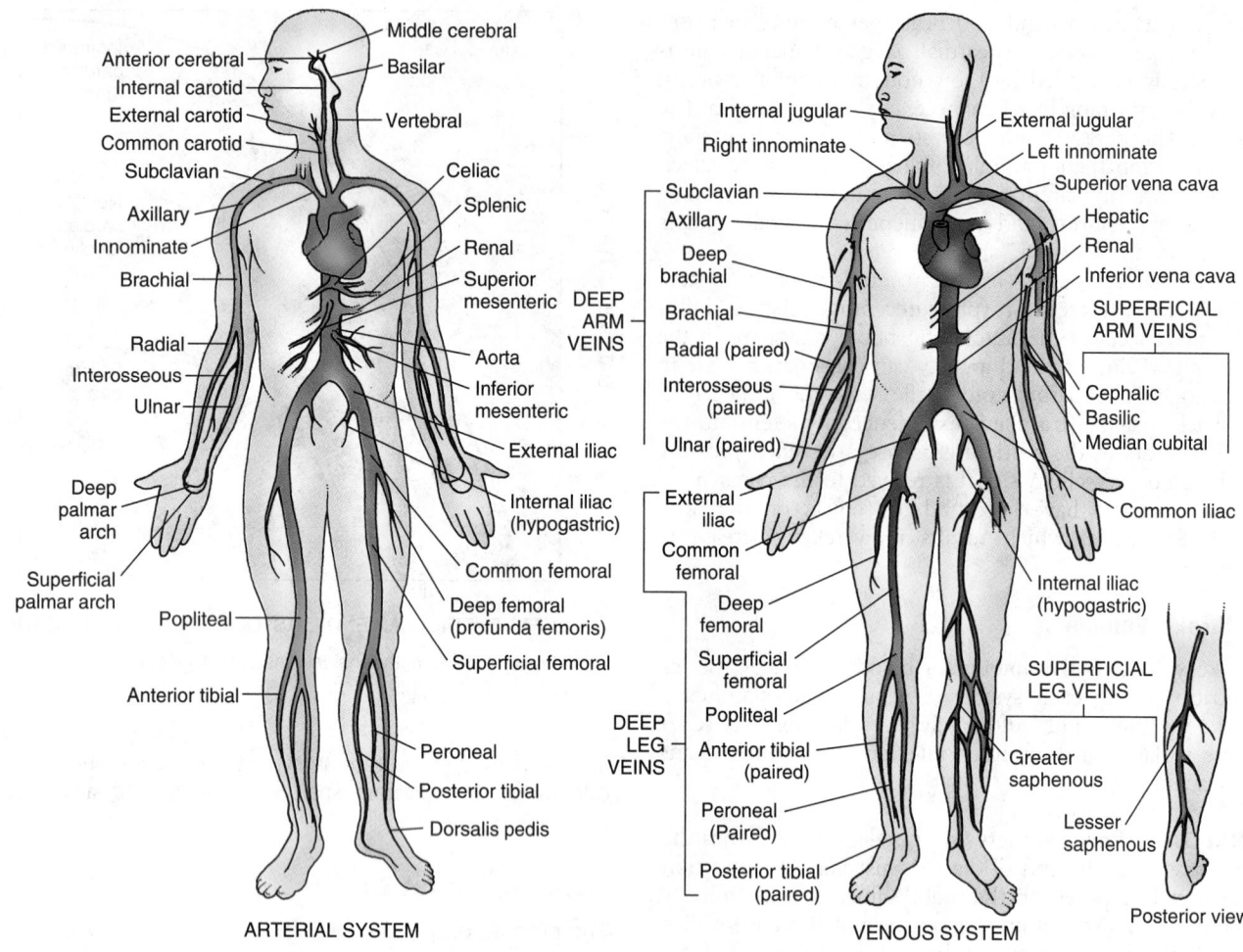

Figure 35–8. Anatomy of the arterial and venous systems.

other arteries. The arterioles branch into terminal arterioles, which join with the capillary or capillaries and ultimately with venules, forming the capillary network (Fig. 35–9). The exchange of nutrients across the capillary membrane occurs primarily by three processes: osmosis, filtration, and diffusion. (See Chapter 14 for detailed discussions of osmosis, filtration, and diffusion.)

Function

The arterial system delivers blood to various tissues for nourishment. At the tissue level, nutrients, chemicals, and body defense substances are distributed and exchanged for cellular waste products, depending on the needs of the particular tissue. The arteries transport the cellular wastes to the excretory organs, such as the kidneys and the lungs, to be reprocessed or removed. The arteries also contribute to the tissue's temperature regulation. Blood can be either directed toward the skin to promote heat loss or diverted away from the skin to conserve heat.

Blood Pressure

Blood pressure is the force of blood exerted against the vessel walls. Pressure in the larger blood vessels is greater

(about 80–100 mmHg) and decreases as blood flow reaches the capillaries (about 25 mmHg). By the time blood enters the right atrium, blood pressure is approximately 0–5 mmHg.

Indirect Measurement of Blood Pressure

The blood pressure in the arterial system is determined primarily by the quantity of blood flow or cardiac output (CO), and the resistance in the arterioles, so that

Blood pressure = CO × peripheral vascular resistance

Therefore, any factor that increases cardiac output or total peripheral vascular resistance increases blood pressure. In general, blood pressure is maintained at a relatively constant level, such that an increase or decrease in total peripheral vascular resistance is associated with a decrease or an increase in CO, respectively. Three mechanisms mediate and regulate blood pressure:

■ The autonomic nervous system, which, in responding to impulses from chemoreceptors and baroreceptors, excites or inhibits sympathetic nervous system activity

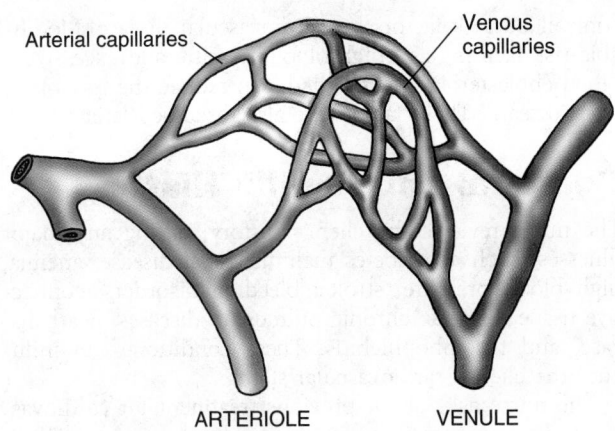

Arterial capillaries   Venous capillaries

ARTERIOLE   VENULE

Figure 35–9. Structure of the capillary bed.

- The kidneys, which sense a change in blood flow and activate the renin-angiotensin-aldosterone mechanism
- The endocrine system, which releases various hormones (e.g., catecholamine, kinins, serotonin, and histamine) to stimulate the sympathetic nervous system at the tissue level

Systolic blood pressure represents the highest pressure occurring in an artery with each contraction of the heart; diastolic blood pressure represents the lowest pressure during the relaxation phase of the heart. In the adult, systolic pressure is normally 90–135 mmHg, and diastolic pressure is normally 60–85 mmHg. Blood pressure is expressed as systolic/diastolic.

Systolic pressure is affected by a number of factors, including CO. When CO decreases, systolic pressure also decreases. Diastolic pressure is primarily determined by the amount of vasoconstriction in the periphery. An increase in peripheral vascular resistance increases diastolic pressure and cardiac workload.

Regulation of Blood Pressure

The autonomic nervous system (ANS) and the renal system are primarily responsible for regulating blood pressure, although external factors can also affect a person's blood pressure.

AUTONOMIC NERVOUS SYSTEM. Blood pressure is regulated by balancing the sympathetic and parasympathetic nervous systems of the autonomic nervous system. Changes in sympathetic and parasympathetic activity are responses to messages sent by the sensory receptors in the various tissues of the body. These receptors, including the baroreceptors, the chemoreceptors, and the stretch receptors, respond differently to biochemical and physiologic changes of the body.

Baroreceptors in the arch of the aorta and at the origin of the internal carotid arteries are stimulated when the arterial walls are stretched by an increased blood pressure. Impulses from these baroreceptors inhibit the vasomotor center, located in the pons and the medulla. Inhibition of this center results in a drop in blood pressure.

Several 1- to 2-mm collections of tissue have been identified in the bifurcations of the carotid arteries and along the aortic arch. Called the carotid and aortic bodies, respectively, they contain specialized chemoreceptors that are sensitive primarily to hypoxemia (a decrease in arterial oxygen pressure [PaO_2]). When stimulated, the carotid chemoreceptors send impulses along Hering's nerves, and the aortic chemoreceptors send impulses along the vagus nerves to activate a vasoconstrictor response.

The chemoreceptors are also stimulated by hypercapnia (an increase in arterial carbon dioxide pressure [$PaCO_2$]) and acidosis. However, the direct effect of carbon dioxide on the CNS is 10 times as strong as the effect it produces by stimulating the chemoreceptors.

Stretch receptors found in the venae cavae and the right atrium are sensitive to pressure or volume changes. When a client is hypovolemic, the stretch receptors in the blood vessels sense a reduced volume or pressure and send fewer impulses to the CNS. This reaction stimulates the sympathetic nervous system to increase heart rate and to constrict the peripheral blood vessels.

RENAL SYSTEM. The renal system also helps to regulate cardiovascular activity. When renal blood flow or pressure decreases, the kidneys retain sodium and water. Blood pressure tends to rise because of fluid retention and because of activation of the renin-angiotensin-aldosterone mechanism. Vascular volume is also regulated by the release of antidiuretic hormone (vasopressin) from the posterior pituitary gland (see Chap. 14).

EXTERNAL FACTORS. Other factors can influence the activity of the cardiovascular system. For example, emotional behaviors, such as excitement, pain, and anger, stimulate the sympathetic nervous system to increase blood pressure and heart rate. Increased physical activity such as exercise increases blood pressure and pulse rate as well. Body temperature can affect the metabolic needs of the tissues, thereby influencing the delivery of blood. In hypothermia, tissues require fewer nutrients and blood pressure falls. In hyperthermia, the metabolic requirement of the tissues is greater, and blood pressure and pulse rate rise.

Venous System

Structure

The venous system is composed of a series of veins that are located adjacent to the arterial system. In addition, a second superficial venous circulation runs parallel to the subcutaneous tissue of the extremity. These two venous systems are connected by communicating veins, which provide a means for blood to travel from the superficial veins to the deep veins. Blood flow is directed toward the deep venous circulation.

The venules collect blood from the capillaries and the terminal arterioles. Venules also serve as a location where white blood cells enter into and exit from the body tissues.

Venules branch into veins, which are low-pressure blood vessels. Veins have the ability to accommodate large shifts in volume with minimal changes in venous pressure. This flexibility allows the venous system to accommodate the administration of intravenous (IV) fluids and blood transfusions, blood loss, and dehydration. In both the superficial and deep venous systems, all veins, except for the smallest and the largest, have valves directing blood flow back to the heart, preventing retrograde flow (backflow).

Function

The primary function of the venous system is to complete the circulation of blood by returning blood from the capillaries to the right side of the heart. The venous system also acts as a reservoir for a large portion of the blood volume. In contrast to the arterial system, which consists of a high-pressure, continuous-flow system through relatively rigid conduits, the venous system consists of a low-pressure, intermittent flow system through collapsible tubes working against the effects of gravity.

Gravity exerts an increase in hydrostatic pressure (capillary blood pressure) when the client is in an upright position, which delays venous return. When the client is lying down, the hydrostatic pressure is lessened, and thus there is less hindrance of venous return to the heart.

Cardiovascular Changes Associated with Aging

A number of physiologic changes in the cardiovascular system occur with advancing age (Chart 35–1). Many of these changes result in loss of cardiac reserve. Thus, these changes are usually not evident when the older adult is resting. They become apparent only when the person is physically or emotionally stressed and the heart cannot meet the increased metabolic demands of the body.

HISTORY

The nurse obtains a thorough history, which includes demographic data, personal and family history, diet, socioeconomic status, and a functional assessment. Information relative to risk factors and symptoms of cardiovascular disease is the focus of the history.

Demographic Data

Demographic data include the client's age, sex, and ethnic origin. The incidence of conditions such as coronary artery disease (CAD) and valvular disease increases with age (Miller, 1995). The incidence of CAD also varies with the client's sex. Women who are premenopausal have a lower incidence of CAD than do men.

TRANSCULTURAL CONSIDERATIONS

Information about the client's ethnic or cultural background is important because some disease conditions may be more prevalent in specific ethnic groups. For example, African-Americans, Puerto Ricans, Cubans, and Mexican-Americans have a higher incidence of hypertension than do Caucasians (AHA, 1996; Jarvis, 1996).

Age, sex, ethnic background, and family history of cardiovascular disease are considered nonmodifiable or un-

controllable risk factors for cardiovascular disease. Modifiable risk factors (e.g., high blood pressure and excessive blood cholesterol), if controlled, can reduce the risk of heart disease. These factors are also discussed later.

Personal and Family History

The nurse reviews the client's history, noting any major illnesses, such as diabetes mellitus, renal disease, anemia, high blood pressure, stroke, bleeding disorders, connective tissue diseases, chronic pulmonary diseases, heart disease, and thrombophlebitis. These conditions can influence the client's cardiovascular status.

The nurse asks about previous treatment for cardiovascular disease, identifying previous diagnostic procedures (e.g., electrocardiography and cardiac catheterization) and requests information about any medical or invasive treatment of cardiovascular disease. It is important for the nurse to ask specifically about recurrent tonsillitis, streptococcal infections, and rheumatic fever, because these conditions may lead to valvular abnormalities of the heart. In addition, the nurse inquires about any known congenital heart defects.

The nurse questions clients in detail about their medication history beginning with any prescription or over-the-counter medications that the client is currently or has recently taken. The nurse questions clients about any known sensitivity to penicillin or any drugs that may be needed in an emergency, such as morphine. The nurse specifically asks clients whether they have recently used cocaine or any intravenous (IV) "street" drugs, because they may be associated with chest pain or endocarditis. The nurse also asks female clients whether they are taking oral contraceptives or estrogen replacement. There is an increased incidence of myocardial infarction (MI) and cerebrovascular accident (CVA) in older women who take oral contraceptives, but only if they smoke, have diabetes, or have hypertension (AHA, 1996). However, postmenopausal women who take estrogen replacement have a lower incidence of coronary artery disease (CAD).

The nurse reviews the family history, obtaining information about the age, health status, and cause of death of immediate family members. A family history of hypertension, obesity, diabetes, or sudden cardiac death is especially significant. The nurse may also ask about the extended family, including grandparents and grandchildren, and record this information in a narrative outline or as a diagram with the client's history.

Diet History

A diet history might include the client's recall of food and fluid intake during a 24-hour period, self-imposed or medically prescribed dietary restrictions or supplementations, and the amount and type of alcohol consumption. The nurse and the dietitian review the type of foods selected by the client for the amount of sodium, sugar, cholesterol, fiber, and fat. The nurse or dietitian also explores the client's attitudes toward food, knowledge level of essential and nonessential dietary elements, and willingness to make changes in the diet. Cultural beliefs and economic status can influence the client's choice of

Chart 35–1

Nursing Focus on the Elderly: Changes in the Cardiovascular System Related to Aging

Structure/Function	Change	Nursing Implications	Rationale
Cardiac valves	• Calcification and mucoid degeneration occur, especially in mitral and aortic valves.	• Assess heart sounds for murmurs. • Question clients about dyspnea.	• Murmurs may be detected before other symptoms.
Conduction system	• Pacemaker cells decrease in number. Fibrous tissue and fat in the sinoatrial node increase. • Few muscle fibers remain in the atrial myocardium and bundle of His. • Conduction time increases.	• Assess the electrocardiogram (ECG) and heart rhythm for dysrhythmias or a heart rate less than 60 beats per minute	• The SA node may lose its inherent rhythm. • Atrial dysrhythmias occur in 50–90% of elders, 80% of elders experience premature ventricular contractions (PVCs).
Left ventricle	• The size of the left ventricle increases. • The left ventricle becomes stiff and less distensible. • Fibrotic changes in the left ventricle decrease the speed of early diastolic filling by about 50%. • Conduction time increases.	• Assess the ECG for a widening QRS complex and a longer QT interval. • Assess for activity intolerance. • Assess the heart rate at rest and with activity. • Assess for activity intolerance.	• Ventricular changes result in decreased stroke volume, ejection fraction, and cardiac output during exercise; the heart is less able to meet increased oxygen demands. • Maximal heart rate with exercise is decreased. • The heart is less able to meet increased oxygen demands.
Aorta and other large arteries	• The aorta and other large arteries thicken and become stiffer and less distensible. Systolic blood pressure increases to compensate for the stiff arteries. • Systemic vascular resistance increases as a result of less distensible arteries, so the left ventricle pumps against greater resistance, contributing to left ventricular hypertrophy.	• Assess blood pressure. • Note increases in systolic, diastolic, and pulse pressures. • Assess for activity intolerance and shortness of breath. • Assess the peripheral pulses.	• Hypertension may occur, which must be treated to avoid target organ damage.
Baroreceptors	• Baroreceptors become less sensitive.	• Assess the client's blood pressure with the client lying and then sitting or standing. • Assess for dizziness when the client changes from a lying to a sitting or standing position. • Teach the client to change positions slowly.	• Orthostatic (postural) and postprandial changes occur because of ineffective baroreceptors. Changes may include decreases in blood pressure of 10 mmHg or more, dizziness, and fainting.

food items and, therefore, must be reviewed. Family members or significant others who are responsible for shopping and cooking are included in the discussion.

Socioeconomic Status

Social history includes information about the client's domestic situation, such as marital status, number of children, household members, living environment, and occupation. The nurse also identifies the client's support systems. It is especially important for the nurse to explore the possibility that the client might have difficulty paying for medications or treatment.

The nurse asks about the client's occupation, including the type of work performed and the requirements of the specific job. For instance, does the job involve lifting of heavy objects? Is the job emotionally stressful? What does a day's work entail? Does the client's job require him or her to be outside in extreme weather conditions?

Personal habits that are risk factors for heart disease

include cigarette smoking, physical inactivity, obesity, and type A behavior. These factors are considered modifiable or controllable risk factors. The nurse queries the client about each of the following modifiable risk factors.

Cigarette Smoking

Cigarette smoking is a major risk factor for cardiovascular disease, specifically CAD and peripheral vascular disease (PVD) (AHA, 1996). According to the U. S. Department of Health and Human Services (DHHS), cigarette smoking is directly responsible for 21% of all deaths from CAD (DHHS, 1990). Three compounds in cigarette smoke (tar, nicotine, and carbon monoxide) have been implicated in the development of CAD.

The risks to the cardiovascular system from cigarette smoking appear to be dose related, noncumulative, and transient. The smoking history should include the number of cigarettes smoked daily, duration of the smoking habit, and age of the client when smoking started. A person who smokes fewer than 4 cigarettes per day has twice the risk of cardiovascular disease of a person who does not smoke; a person who smokes more than 20 cigarettes per day has four times the risk. Typically, the nurse records the smoking history in pack-years, which is the number of packs per day multiplied by the number of years that the client smoked.

The nurse should also inquire about the client's desire to quit, past attempts to quit, and the methods used. Three to four years after a client has stopped smoking, his or her cardiovascular risk appears to be similar to that of a person who has never smoked. The nurse asks clients who do not currently smoke whether they have ever smoked and when they quit.

Physical Inactivity

Sedentary lifestyle is also considered a significant risk factor in the development of heart disease. Regular physical activity promotes cardiovascular fitness and produces beneficial changes in blood pressure and levels of blood lipids and clotting factors. Unfortunately, few people in the United States engage in the recommended exercise guidelines: 30 minutes daily of light-to-moderate exercise, equivalent to a 30-minute brisk walk. According to AHA (1996), only 22% of Americans engage in this much exercise five times a week and only 10% engage in vigorous physical activity, enough to promote cardiopulmonary fitness, three times a week. This puts more people at risk for CAD from physical inactivity than any other factor. The nurse questions clients concerning the type of exercise in which they engage, the period for which they have participated in the exercise, and the frequency and the intensity of the exercise.

Obesity

Approximately 61 million Americans are 20% or more above their desirable weight (AHA, 1996). Obesity in the American population has increased 36% in the last 30 years; it is particularly a problem for African-American females and native Hawaiians (AHA, 1996). Obesity is associated with hypertension, hyperlipidemia, and diabetes; all are known contributors to cardiovascular disease.

The nurse weighs and examines the client for the pattern of obesity, also known as waist:hip ratio.

WOMEN'S HEALTH CONSIDERATIONS

Caucasian women with abdominal obesity (greater waist than hip circumference) are more likely to experience cardiovascular disease than are Caucasian women with fat distributed in their buttocks, hips, and thighs (greater hip than waist circumference). Clients with an early onset of obesity (during adolescence) and an elevated waist:hip ratio appear to be at especially high risk for cardiovascular disease (Weigle, 1992).

Type A Personality

Researchers have identified people with type A personalities as being more vulnerable to the development of heart disease (Kottke et al., 1996). Type A personalities are highly competitive, overly concerned about meeting deadlines, and often hostile or angry. The chronic anger and hostility that type A people display appear to be most closely associated with cardiovascular disease. The constant arousal of the sympathetic nervous system resulting from the anger may influence blood pressure, serum fatty acids and lipids, and clotting mechanisms. The nurse observes the client and determines the response to stressful situations.

Current Health Problems

Inquiring about the client's major concerns helps the nurse to establish priorities in nursing care and management. The nurse asks the client to describe health concerns. Then the nurse expands on the client's description by obtaining information about the onset, duration, chronology, frequency, location, quality, intensity, associated symptoms, and precipitating, aggravating, and relieving factors. Major symptoms identified by clients with cardiovascular disease include chest pain or discomfort, dyspnea, fatigue, palpitations, weight gain, syncope, and extremity pain.

Chest Pain

Chest pain or discomfort, a cardinal symptom of heart disease, can result from ischemic heart disease, pericarditis, and aortic dissection. Chest pain can also be due to noncardiac conditions, such as pleurisy, pulmonary embolus, hiatal hernia, and anxiety. Nurses must thoroughly evaluate the nature and characteristics of the client's chest pain. Because chest pain resulting from myocardial ischemia is life threatening and can lead to serious complications, the cause of chest pain should be considered ischemic (reduced or obstructed blood flow to the myocardium) until proven otherwise.

When assessing for chest pain, the nurse uses alternative terms such as "discomfort," "heaviness," and "indigestion." Often clients do not experience a true pain in the chest but instead feel discomfort or indigestion. The client may also describe the sensation as aching, choking, strangling, tingling, squeezing, constricting, or vise-like.

The nurse asks the client to identify when the pain was first noticed (onset). Did the pain begin suddenly or develop gradually (manner of onset)? How long did the pain last (duration)? If the client has repeated chest pain episodes, the nurse assesses how frequently the pain occurs (frequency). The nurse asks whether this pain is different from any other episodes of pain. The nurse asks the client to describe what activities he or she was doing at the time it first occurred (e.g., sleeping, arguing, and running) (precipitating factors). The client can be asked to point to the area where the chest pain occurred (location) and to describe how the pain spread (radiation).

In addition, the client describes how the pain feels and whether it is sharp or dull (quality). To understand how severe the pain is, the nurse asks the client to grade the pain from 0 to 10, with 0 indicating the absence of pain and 10 indicating severe pain (intensity). The client may also report other signs and symptoms that occur at the same time (associated symptoms), such as dyspnea, diaphoresis, nausea, and vomiting. Other factors that need to be addressed are those that may have made the chest

pain worse (aggravating factors) or the pain less intense (relieving factors). Chest pain may arise from a variety of sources (Table 35–1). By obtaining appropriate information from the client, the nurse may assist in identifying the source of the client's chest discomfort.

Dyspnea

Dyspnea is a symptom that can occur from both cardiac and pulmonary disease. Dyspnea is objectively described as difficult or labored breathing and is subjectively experienced as uncomfortable breathing or shortness of breath. When obtaining the client's history, the nurse ascertains what factors precipitate and relieve dyspnea, what level of activity produces dyspnea, and the client's body position when dyspnea occurred.

There are several types of dyspnea. Dyspnea that is associated with activity, such as climbing stairs, is referred to as dyspnea on exertion (DOE). This is usually an early symptom of heart failure.

The client with advanced heart disease may experience orthopnea, dyspnea that appears when the client lies flat. The client may use several pillows at night to elevate the

TABLE 35–1

Assessment of Chest Discomfort: How Various Types of Chest Pain Differ

Source	Onset	Quality and Severity	Location and Radiation	Duration and Relieving Factors
Angina	• Sudden, usually in response to exertion, emotion, or extremes in temperature	• Squeezing, vise-like pain	• Substernal: may spread across the chest and the back and/or down the arms	• Usually lasts less than 15 min; relieved with rest, nitrate administration, or oxygen therapy
Myocardial infarction	• Sudden, without precipitating factors, often in early morning	• Intense stabbing, vise-like pain or pressure, severe	• Substernal; may spread throughout the anterior chest and to the arms, jaw, back, or neck	• Usually lasts 30 min or longer or is relieved with opioids
Pericarditis	• Sudden	• Sharp stabbing, moderate to severe	• Substernal; usually spreads to the left side or the back	• Intermittent; relieved with sitting upright, analgesia, or administration of antiinflammatory agents
Pleuropulmonary	• Variable	• Moderate ache, worse on inspiration	• Lung fields	• Continuous until the underlying condition is treated or the client has rested
Esophageal–gastric	• Variable	• Squeezing, heartburn, variable severity	• Substernal; may spread to the shoulders or the abdomen	• Variable; may be relieved with antacid administration or food intake
Anxiety	• Variable, may be in response to stress or fatigue	• Dull ache to sharp stabbing; may be associated with numbness in fingers	• Usually the left side of chest without radiation	• Usually lasts a few minutes

head and chest or sleep in a recliner to prevent nighttime breathlessness. The severity of orthopnea is measured by the number of pillows or the amount of head elevation needed to provide restful sleep. Orthopnea is usually relieved within a matter of minutes by sitting up or standing.

Paroxysmal nocturnal dyspnea occurs after the client has been recumbent for several hours. When the client is lying down, blood from the lower extremities is redistributed to the venous system, increasing venous return to the heart. A diseased heart is unable to compensate for the increased volume and is ineffective in pumping the additional fluid into the circulatory system. Therefore, pulmonary congestion results. The client awakens abruptly, often with a feeling of suffocation and panic. The client usually sits upright with the legs dangled over the bedside to relieve the dyspnea. A client may experience 20 minutes of distress before obtaining relief.

Fatigue

Fatigue may be described as the feeling of tiredness or weariness resulting from activity. The client may complain that a certain activity takes longer to complete or that he or she tires easily after activity. Although fatigue in itself is not diagnostic of heart disease, many people with heart failure are limited by leg fatigue during exercise (Sullivan, 1994). Fatigue that occurs after mild activity and exertion usually indicates an inadequate cardiac output (low stroke volume) and anaerobic metabolism in skeletal muscle.

The nurse questions the client to determine the time of day he or she experiences fatigue as well as the activities that can be performed. Fatigue resulting from decreased cardiac output is often worse in the evening. The nurse asks whether the client can perform the same activities as a year ago or the same activities as others of the same age. Often the client limits activities in response to fatigue without being aware how much less active he or she has become unless questioned.

Palpitations

A feeling of fluttering in the chest or an unpleasant awareness of the heartbeat is referred to as palpitations. Palpitations may result from a change in heart rate or rhythm or from an increase in the force of heart contractions. Rhythm disturbances that may cause palpitations include paroxysmal supraventricular tachycardia, premature contractions, and sinus tachycardia. Palpitations that occur during or after strenuous physical activity, such as running and swimming, may indicate overexertion or possibly heart disease. Some noncardiac factors that may precipitate palpitations include anxiety, stress, fatigue, insomnia, and the ingestion of caffeine, nicotine, or alcohol.

Weight Gain

A sudden increase in weight of 2.2 pounds (1 kg) can be the result of an accumulation of excessive fluid (1 L) in the interstitial spaces, commonly known as *edema*. It is possible, however, for weight gains of up to 10–15 pounds (4.5–6.8 kg, or 4–7 L of fluid) to occur before any associated edema is apparent. The nurse should inquire whether the client has experienced a tightness of shoes, noted indentations from socks, or noted tightness of rings.

Syncope

Syncope refers to a transient loss of consciousness. The most common cause is decreased perfusion to the brain. Any condition that suddenly reduces the cardiac output, resulting in decreased cerebral blood flow, could potentiate a syncopal episode. Conditions such as cardiac rhythm disturbances (ventricular dysrhythmias or Stokes-Adams attack) and valvular disorders (aortic stenosis) may potentiate this symptom.

ELDERLY CONSIDERATIONS

Syncope in the aging client may result from hypersensitivity of the carotid sinus bodies, located in the neck arteries. Pressure applied to the carotid arteries (e.g., during turning the head, shrugging the shoulders, shaving, or buttoning a shirt) stimulates a vagal response. A decrease in blood pressure and heart rate usually results, but an exaggerated response may produce syncope. Syncope in the older adult may also result from orthostatic (postural) or postprandial hypotension as a result of an age-affected baroreceptor response.

Near-syncope refers to dizziness with an inability to remain in an upright position. The nurse explores the circumstances that lead to dizziness or syncope.

Extremity Pain

Extremity pain may result from two conditions: ischemia from atherosclerosis and venous insufficiency of the peripheral blood vessels. Clients who report a moderate to severe cramping sensation in their legs or buttocks associated with an activity such as walking have intermittent claudication related to reduced arterial tissue perfusion. Claudication pain is usually relieved by resting or lowering the affected extremity to decrease tissue demands or to enhance arterial blood flow. Leg pain that results from prolonged standing or sitting is related to venous insufficiency from either incompetent valves or venous obstruction. This pain may be relieved by elevating the extremity.

Functional History

After obtaining the history of the client's cardiac status, the client may be classified according to the New York Heart Association's Functional Classification (Table 35-2). The four classifications (I, II, III, and IV) depend on the degree to which ordinary physical activities (routine activities of daily living [ADLs]) are affected by heart disease.

PHYSICAL ASSESSMENT

A thorough physical assessment is the foundation for the nursing data base and the formation of nursing diagnoses. Any changes noted during the client's hospital course can be compared with this initial data base. The nurse evalu-

TABLE 35-2

New York Heart Association Functional Classification of Cardiovascular Disability

Class I
- Clients with cardiac disease but without resulting limitations of physical activity
- Ordinary physical activity does not cause undue fatigue, palpitation, dyspnea, or anginal pain.

Class II
- Clients with cardiac disease resulting in slight limitation of physical activity
- They are comfortable at rest.
- Ordinary physical activity results in fatigue, palpitation, dyspnea, or anginal pain.

Class III
- Clients with cardiac disease resulting in marked limitation of physical activity
- They are comfortable at rest.
- Less than ordinary physical activity causes fatigue, palpitation, dyspnea, or anginal pain.

Class IV
- Clients with cardiac disease resulting in inability to carry on any physical activity without discomfort
- Symptoms of cardiac insufficiency or of the anginal syndrome may be present, even at rest.
- If any physical activity is undertaken, discomfort is increased.

Excerpted from *Diseases of the heart and blood vessels—nomenclature and criteria for diagnosis*, 6th edition. Boston, Little, Brown and Company, copyright 1964 by the New York Heart Association, Inc.

ates vital signs (blood pressure, pulse rate, and respiration rate) when the client is admitted to the hospital and at least every 4 hours until the client's condition improves.

General Appearance

Physical assessment begins with clients' general appearance. The nurse assesses the following areas: general build and appearance of the client as well as skin color; distress level; level of consciousness; presence of shortness of breath; position; and verbal responses.

Clients with chronic heart failure may appear malnourished, thin, and cachectic. Latent signs of severe heart failure are ascites, jaundice, and anasarca as a result of prolonged congestion of the liver. Heart failure may cause fluid retention, and clients may have engorged neck veins and generalized dependent edema.

Coronary artery disease is suspected in clients with yellow lipid-filled plaques on the upper eyelids (xanthelasma) or earlobe creases. Clients with poor cardiac output and decreased cerebral perfusion may have mental confusion, memory loss, and slowed verbal responses.

Integumentary System

Assessment and evaluation of the integumentary system are determined primarily by the color and temperature of the skin. The best areas for the nurse to assess circulation include the nail beds, the mucous membranes, and the conjunctival mucosa, because small blood vessels are located near the surface of the skin.

Skin Color

If there is normal blood flow or adequate perfusion of a given area in light-colored skin, it appears pink, perhaps rosy in color, and warm to the touch. Decreased flow is depicted as cool, pale-looking, and moist skin. Pallor is characteristic of anemia and can be seen in areas such as the nail beds, palms, and conjunctival mucous membranes.

A bluish or darkened discoloration of the skin and mucous membranes is referred to as cyanosis. Cyanosis results from an increased amount of deoxygenated hemoglobin.

In central cyanosis, there is decreased oxygenation of the arterial blood in the lungs, which manifests as a bluish tinge of the conjunctivae and the mucous membranes of the mouth and tongue. Central cyanosis may indicate impaired lung function or a right-to-left shunt found in congenital heart conditions. Because of impaired circulation, there is a marked desaturation of hemoglobin in the peripheral tissues, which produces a bluish or darkened discoloration of the nail beds, the earlobes, the lips, and the toes.

Peripheral cyanosis occurs when blood flow to the peripheral vessels is decreased by peripheral vasoconstriction. The clamping down of the peripheral blood vessels is the result of a low cardiac output or an increased extraction of oxygen from the peripheral tissues. Peripheral cyanosis localized in an extremity is usually a result of arterial or venous obstruction.

Skin Temperature

The temperature of the skin can be assessed for symmetry by touching different areas of the client's body (e.g., arms, hands, legs, and feet) with the dorsal surface of the hand or fingers. Decreased blood flow results in decreased skin temperature. The skin temperature is lowered in several clinical conditions, including heart failure, peripheral vascular disease, and shock.

Extremities

The nurse assesses the client's hands, arms, feet, and legs for skin changes, vascular changes, clubbing, capillary filling, and edema. Skin mobility and turgor are affected by the fluid status of the client. Dehydration and aging reduce skin turgor, and edema decreases skin mobility. Vascular changes of an affected extremity may include paresthesia, muscle fatigue and discomfort, numbness, pain, coolness, and loss of hair distribution from a reduced blood supply. Clubbing of the fingers and toes results from chronic oxygen deprivation in these tissue beds. Clubbing is characteristic in clients with advanced chronic pulmonary disease, congenital heart defects, and cor pulmonale. Clubbing can be identified by assessing the angle of the nail bed. The angle of the normal nail bed is 160 degrees; with clubbing, the angle of the nail bed increases to greater than 180 degrees and the base of the nail

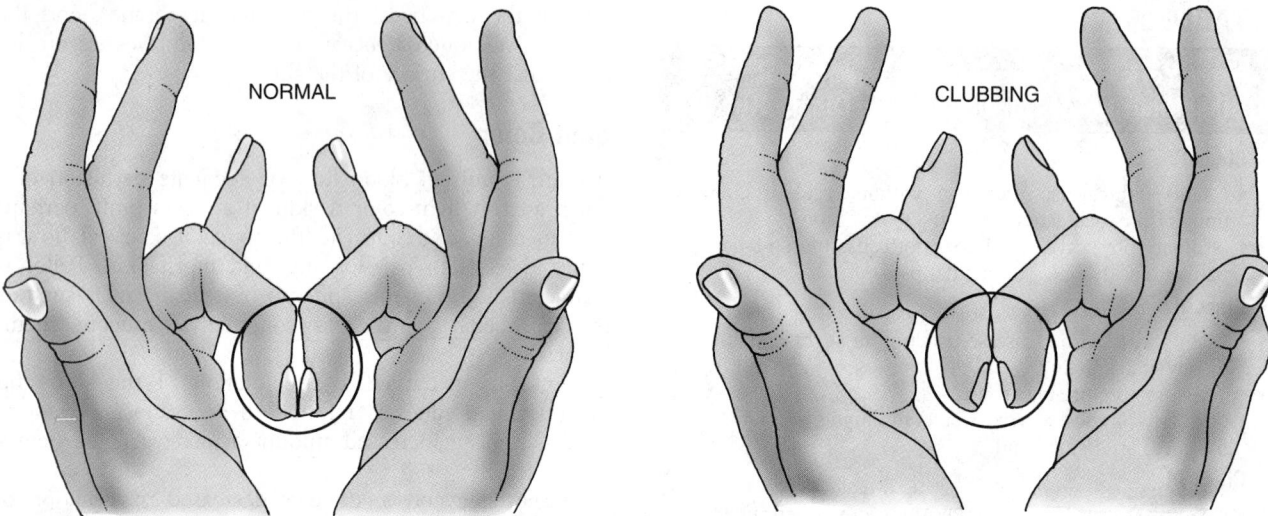

Figure 35–10. Assessment of clubbing by the Schamroth method. The client places the fingernails of the ring fingers together and holds them up to a light. If the examiner can see a diamond shape between the nails, there is no clubbing. Clubbing is identified by the absence of the diamond shape.

becomes spongy. Figure 35–10 describes the assessment of clubbing using the Schamroth method.

Capillary filling of the fingers and the toes is an indicator of peripheral circulation. Pressing or blanching the nail bed of a finger or a toe produces a whitening effect; when pressure is released, a brisk return of color should occur in the nail bed. If color returns within 3 seconds, peripheral circulation is considered intact. If the capillary refill time exceeds 3 seconds, the lack of circulation may be due to arterial insufficiency from atherosclerosis or spasm. Rubor (dusky redness) that replaces pallor in a dependent foot suggests arterial insufficiency.

Peripheral edema is a common finding in clients with cardiovascular problems. The location of edema helps the nurse to determine its potential cause. Bilateral edema of the legs may be seen in clients with heart failure or with chronic venous insufficiency. Abdominal and leg edema can be seen in clients with heart disease and cirrhosis of the liver. Localized edema in one extremity may be the result of venous obstruction (thrombosis) or lymphatic blockage of the extremity (lymphedema). Edema may also be noted in dependent areas, such as the sacrum, when a client is confined to bed.

The nurse documents the location of edema as precisely as possible (e.g., midtibial or sacral) and the number of centimeters from an anatomic landmark. Although some health care practitioners attempt to grade edema as mild, moderate, and severe or 1+, 2+, 3+, or 4+, no universal scale is used. In addition, these values are not precise and are subjective. Instead of using a grading scale, the nurse determines whether the edema is pitting (the skin can be indented) or nonpitting, the depth of the pit (in millimeters), and the amount of time the pit lasts (in seconds).

Blood Pressure Measurement

The indirect measurement of arterial blood pressure is done by sphygmomanometry (Chart 35–2). This technique of measurement is described in greater detail in nursing skills books.

The normal blood pressure in adults older than 45 years ranges from 90 to 140 mmHg for systolic pressure and from 60 to 90 mmHg for diastolic pressure (AHA, 1996). A blood pressure that exceeds 135/85 mmHg increases the workload of the left ventricle and oxygen consumption. A blood pressure less than 90/60 mmHg may be inadequate in providing proper and sufficient nutrition to the cells of the body.

In certain circumstances, such as shock, the Korotkoff sounds are less audible or absent. In such circumstances, the nurse might palpate the blood pressure, use an ultrasonic device (Doppler device), or obtain a direct measurement by arterial catheter. When a blood pressure is palpated, the diastolic pressure is usually not obtainable. More information on direct measurement of arterial pressure is available under Hemodynamic Monitoring in this chapter.

Postural Blood Pressure

Clients may report dizziness or lightheadedness when they move from a flat, supine position to a sitting or a standing position at the edge of the bed. Normally, these symptoms are transient and pass quickly; however, when these symptoms become pronounced, they may be due to orthostatic (postural) hypotension. Postural hypotension occurs when the client's blood pressure is not adequately maintained when moving from a lying to a sitting or standing position. It is defined as a decrease in blood pressure of more than 20 mmHg of the systolic pressure or a decrease of more than 10 mmHg of the diastolic pressure and a 10% to 20% increase in heart rate. The causes of postural hypotension include medications, depletion of blood volume, prolonged bed rest, and age-related changes or disorders of the autonomic nervous system.

To detect orthostatic changes in blood pressure, the

Nursing Care Highlight: Tips for Accurate Blood Pressure Measurement

- Select the proper cuff size.
  - Adult cuff size is 12- to 14-cm wide and 30-cm long.
  - Pediatric cuffs vary in width and length.
  - Larger adult cuff size is 18- to 20-cm wide.
- Ensure that equipment is properly assembled and calibrated.
  - The cuff bladder should be intact inside the cuff.
  - The sphygmomanometer should be calibrated to 0 mmHg every few months to ensure reliability.
- The cuff must be placed above the area to be auscultated (e.g., if the right arm is used, the cuff is placed above the brachial artery).
- Follow these steps to ensure correct blood pressure measurement and recording:
  - After palpating the brachial or radial pulse, inflate the cuff 30 mmHg above the level at which those pulses disappear. Release the cuff slowly to palpate the systolic pressure. Reinflate the cuff, and auscultate the systolic and diastolic pressures. The auscultated pulses are referred to as the Korotkoff sounds.
  - Record measurements on both arms to rule out dissecting aortic aneurysm, coarctation of the aorta, vascular obstruction, and possibly errors in measurement. Perform subsequent readings on the extremity with the highest pressure.
  - If the client's arms are inaccessible (after amputation or mastectomy), you can obtain readings using the client's thigh or calf. Auscultate the popliteal artery or the posterior tibial artery, respectively.
  - Obtain and record the client's blood pressure with the client in different positions, including supine, sitting, and standing positions.
  - Record the position of the client and the site used to obtain the blood pressure.

nurse first takes the client's blood pressure when the client is supine. After remaining supine for at least 3 minutes, the client changes position to sitting or standing. Normally, as the client rises, systolic pressure drops slightly or remains unchanged, whereas diastolic pressure rises slightly. After the client's change in position, a time delay of 1–5 minutes should be permitted before auscultating a blood pressure and palpating the radial pulse. The cuff should remain in the proper position on the client's arm. The nurse observes and records any signs or symptoms of distress in the client. If the client is unable to tolerate the position change, he or she is returned to the previous position of comfort.

ELDERLY CONSIDERATIONS

As a person ages, the autonomic nervous system may lose the ability to compensate rapidly for the gravitational effects of position change and may, therefore, cause postural hypotension. With autonomic insufficiency,

there is no increase in heart rate when the client moves to an upright position. Autonomic insufficiency can also occur from the effects of some cardiac drugs, including digoxin, calcium channel blockers, and beta-adrenergic blockers, that inhibit increases in heart rate. Antiparkinsonian drugs, such as levodopa (Dopar) or Sinemet, can cause severe postural hypotension as well. Some elders experience a similar phenomenon after a heavy meal (postprandial hypotension).

Paradoxical Blood Pressure

Paradoxical blood pressure is defined as an exaggerated decrease in systolic pressure by more than 10 mmHg (normal is 3–10 mmHg) during the inspiratory phase of the respiratory cycle. Certain clinical conditions, including pericardial tamponade, constrictive pericarditis, and pulmonary hypertension, that potentially alter the filling pressures in the right and left ventricles may produce a paradoxical blood pressure. During inspiration, the filling pressures normally decrease slightly. However, with decreased fluid volume in the ventricles because of these pathologic conditions, there is an exaggerated or marked reduction in cardiac output. The procedure for assessing a paradoxical blood pressure is found in Chart 37–10.

Pulse Pressure

The difference between the systolic and diastolic values is referred to as pulse pressure. A normal pulse pressure for an adult is 30–40 mmHg. This value can be used as an indirect measure of the client's cardiac output. Decreased pulse pressure is rarely normal and results from increased peripheral vascular resistance or decreased stroke volume in clients with heart failure, hypovolemia, or shock. Decreased pulse pressure can also be seen in clients who have mitral stenosis or regurgitation. An increased pulse pressure may be seen in clients with slow heart rates, aortic regurgitation, atherosclerosis, hypertension, and aging.

Ankle Brachial Index

The ankle brachial index (ABI) can be used to assess the vascular status of the lower extremities. The nurse applies a blood pressure cuff to the lower extremities just above the malleolli and measures the systolic pressure by Doppler ultrasound at both the dorsalis pedis and posterior tibial pulses. The higher of these two pressures is then divided by the higher of the two brachial pulses to obtain the ankle brachial index.

$$ABI = \frac{\text{higher systolic ankle pressure}}{\text{higher systolic brachial pressure}}$$

Normal values for ABI are 1 or higher, because blood pressure in the legs is usually higher than blood pressure in the arms. ABI values less then 0.80 usually indicate moderate vascular disease, whereas values less than 0.50 indicate severe vascular compromise.

Venous and Arterial Pulsations

Venous Pulsations

The nurse observes the venous pulsations in the neck to assess the adequacy of blood volume and central venous pressure (CVP). The nurse can assess jugular venous pressure (JVP) to estimate the filling volume and pressure on the right side of the heart (Chart 35–3). The right internal jugular vein is usually used to estimate JVP, because this vessel contains fewer valves than the left.

Jugular venous pressure is normally 3–10 cm. Increases in JVP are usually caused by right ventricular failure. Other causes include tricuspid regurgitation or stenosis, pulmonary hypertension, cardiac tamponade, constrictive pericarditis, hypervolemia, and superior vena cava obstruction.

The nurse determines hepatojugular reflux by positioning the client with the head of the bed elevated to 45 degrees and locating the internal jugular vein. The nurse compresses the right upper abdomen for 30–40 seconds. Sudden distention of the neck veins after abdominal compression is usually indicative of right-sided heart failure.

Arterial Pulsations

Assessment of arterial pulsations gives the nurse information about vascular integrity and circulation. All major peripheral pulses, including the temporal, carotid, brachial, radial, ulnar, femoral, popliteal, posterior tibial, and dorsalis pedis pulses, need to be assessed for presence or absence, amplitude, contour, rhythm, rate, and equality. The nurse examines the peripheral arteries in a head-to-toe approach with a side-to-side comparison (Fig. 35–11).

Chart 35–3

Nursing Care Highlight: Assessment of Jugular Venous Pressure and Central Venous Pressure

1. Place the client in a supine position.
2. Raise the head of the bed to approximately 30 to 45 degrees.
3. Shine a light across the client's neck (tangential lighting) to highlight the pulsations of the internal jugular vein.
4. To differentiate the internal jugular vein from the carotid artery, occlude the internal jugular vein with a fingertip at its base, then release. This maneuver easily eliminates the pulse wave in the internal jugular vein.

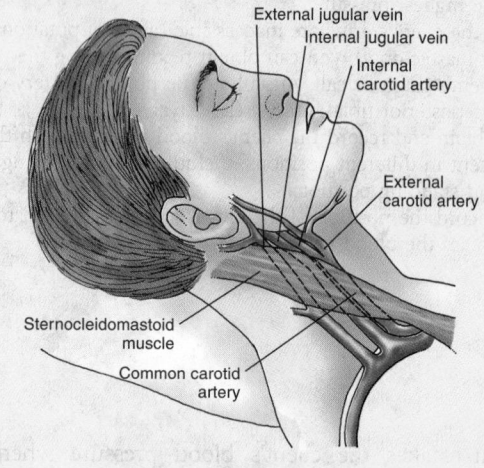

5. Locate the meniscus (the highest point at which pulsations of the internal jugular vein can be seen).
6. Locate the sternal angle (angle of Louis), which can be felt as a notch at the top of the sternum. It is roughly 4 cm above the right atrium.
7. With a centimeter rule, measure the vertical distance from the sternal angle to the meniscus of the internal jugular vein. The reading in centimeters equals the JVP, which generally does not exceed 4 cm.
8. To calculate CVP, add 4 cm to JVP.

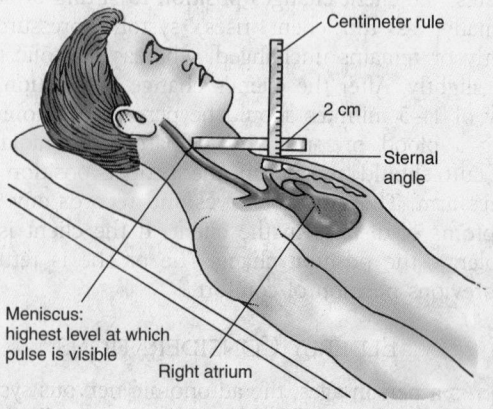

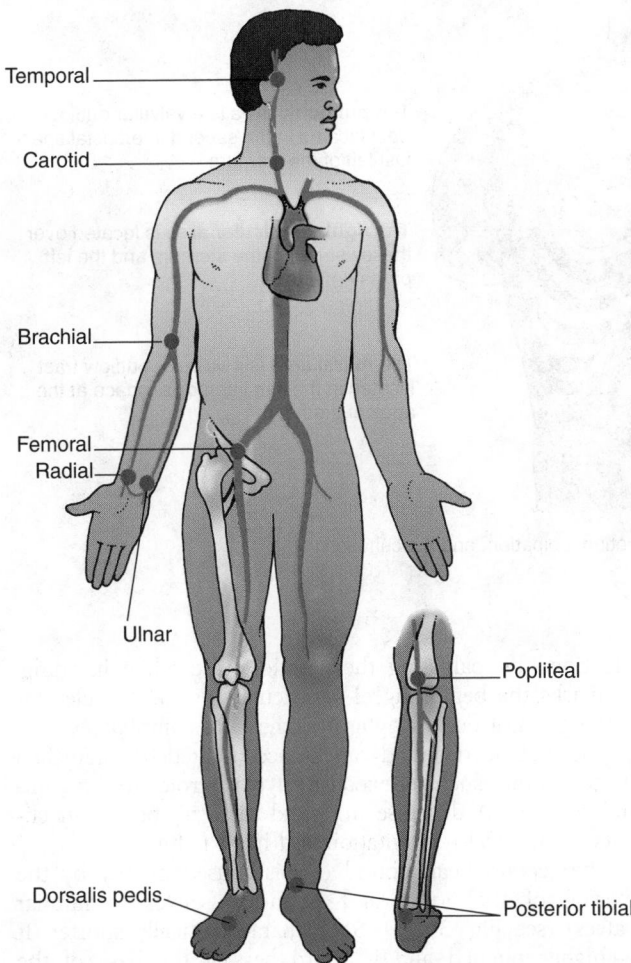

Figure 35–11. Pulse points for assessment of arterial pulses.

Temporal

Carotid

Brachial

Femoral
Radial

Ulnar

Popliteal

Dorsalis pedis

Posterior tibial

A hypokinetic pulse is a weak pulsation indicative of a narrow pulse pressure. It is seen in clients with hypovolemia, aortic stenosis, and decreased cardiac output.

A hyperkinetic pulse is a large, "bounding" pulse caused by an increased ejection of blood. It is seen in clients with a high cardiac output (with exercise or thyrotoxicosis) and in those with increased sympathetic system activity (with pain, fever, or anxiety).

In pulsus alternans, a weak pulse alternates with a strong pulse, despite a regular heart rhythm. It is seen in clients with severely depressed cardiac function. Clients may be asked to hold their breath to exclude any false readings. The nurse may palpate the brachial or radial arteries to assess this condition, but it is more accurately assessed by auscultation of blood pressure.

Auscultation of the carotid arteries is necessary to assess for bruits. Bruits are swishing sounds that may develop over narrowed carotid arteries. Using the bell of the stethoscope over the skin of the carotid artery with the client holding his or her breath, the nurse can assess for the absence or presence of sounds. Normally, there are no sounds if the carotid artery has uninterrupted blood

flow. A bruit may develop when the internal diameter of the vessel is narrowed by 50% or more. A bruit does not indicate the severity of disease in the carotid arteries. The severity of disease is determined by Doppler flow studies and arteriography.

Precordium

Assessment of the precordium (the area over the heart) is done by inspection, palpation, percussion, and auscultation. The nurse places the client in a supine position, with the head of the bed slightly elevated for the client's comfort. Some clients may require greater elevation of the head of the bed (to 45 degrees) for ease and comfort in breathing.

Inspection

Cardiac examination is usually done in a systematic order, beginning with inspection. The nurse inspects the chest from the side, at a right angle, and downward over areas of the precordium where vibrations are visible. Cardiac motion is of low amplitude, and sometimes the inward movements are more easily detected by the naked eye.

The nurse examines the entire precordium, focusing on the seven precordial areas (Fig. 35–12) and noting any prominent precordial pulsations. Movement over the aortic, pulmonic, and tricuspid areas is abnormal. Pulsations in the mitral area (the apex of the heart) are considered normal and are referred to as the apical impulse, or the point of maximal impulse (PMI). The PMI should be located at the left fifth intercostal space (ICS) in the midclavicular line. If the apical impulse appears in more than one intercostal space and has shifted lateral to the midclavicular line, it may indicate left ventricular hypertrophy.

Palpation

The nurse palpates with the fingers and the most sensitive part of the palm of the hand to detect precordial motion and thrills, respectively. The nurse palpates by inching his or her hand in a Z pattern along the chest, starting with the aortic area and passing through all seven areas. Turning the client on his or her left side brings the heart closer to the surface of the chest. This may be helpful for the nurse to achieve maximal tactile sensitivity.

An abnormal forceful thrust accompanied by a sustaining outward movement felt over the left anterior chest usually indicates left ventricular enlargement. An outward systolic lift along the left sternal border extending from the fourth to the fifth intercostal space represents right ventricular enlargement.

Heaves and lifts are terms found with pulsations associated with valvular diseases or pulmonary hypertension. Thrills are vibrations that are associated with abnormal heart valve function (mitral regurgitation, tricuspid regurgitation, and pulmonic stenosis). When palpating for heaves or thrills, the nurse should consider several factors, including location, amplitude, duration, distribution, and timing in relation to the cardiac cycle.

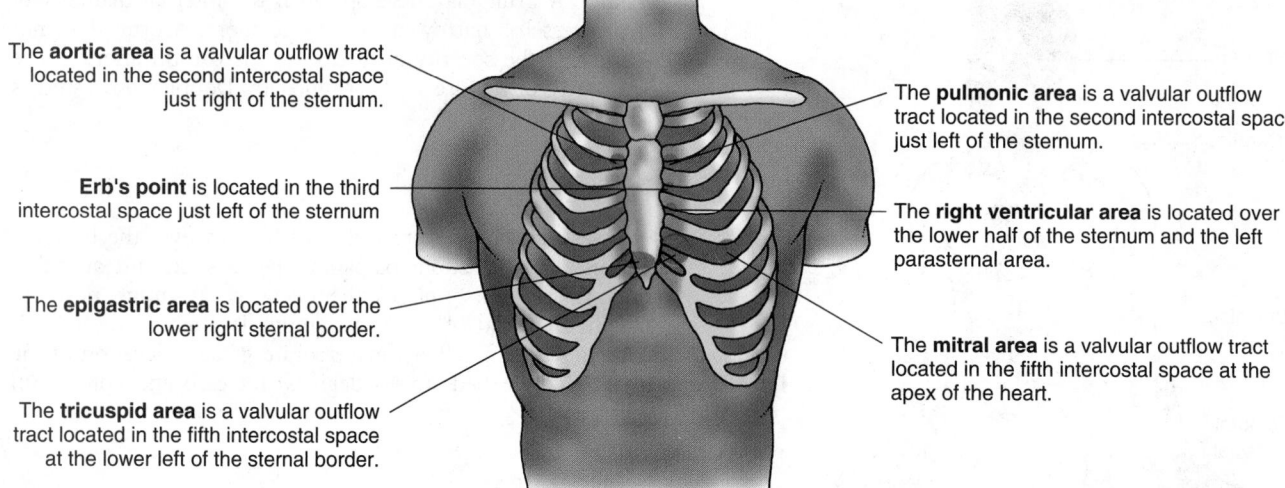

The **aortic area** is a valvular outflow tract located in the second intercostal space just right of the sternum.

Erb's point is located in the third intercostal space just left of the sternum

The **epigastric area** is located over the lower right sternal border.

The **tricuspid area** is a valvular outflow tract located in the fifth intercostal space at the lower left of the sternal border.

The **pulmonic area** is a valvular outflow tract located in the second intercostal space just left of the sternum.

The **right ventricular area** is located over the lower half of the sternum and the left parasternal area.

The **mitral area** is a valvular outflow tract located in the fifth intercostal space at the apex of the heart.

Figure 35–12. Areas for myocardial inspection, palpation, and auscultation.

Percussion

Cardiac size is determined most accurately by chest x-ray; percussion is rarely used now to determine the size of the heart. However, the size of the left ventricle should be estimated by locating the apical impulse by inspection and palpation.

Auscultation

Auscultation evaluates heart rate and rhythm, cardiac cycle (systole and diastole), and valvular function. The technique of auscultation requires a good-quality stethoscope and extensive clinical practice. The nurse evaluates heart sounds in a systematic order; examination usually begins at the aortic outflow tract area and progresses slowly to the apex of the heart, using the diaphragm of the stethoscope. The diaphragm of the stethoscope is pressed tightly against the chest to listen for high-frequency sounds and is useful in listening to the first and second heart sounds and high-frequency murmurs. The nurse then repeats the progression from the base to the apex of the heart using the bell of the stethoscope, which is held lightly against the chest. The bell is able to screen out high-frequency sounds and is useful in listening for low-frequency gallops (diastolic filling sounds) and murmurs.

The nurse auscultates by inching a stethoscope in a Z pattern across the base of the heart, down the left sternal border, then over to the apex, paying attention to the areas in Figure 35–12, except for the epigastric area. Auscultation is to check for heart rate and rhythm, murmurs, extrasystolic sounds, and rubs in the presence of a current or suspected cardiac problem.

Normal Heart Sounds

The first heart sound (S_1) is created by the closure of the mitral and tricuspid valves (AV valves) (see Fig. 35–6). When auscultated, the first heart sound is softer and longer; it is of a low pitch and is best heard at the lower left sternal border or the apex of the heart. It may be identified by palpating the carotid pulse while listening. S_1 marks the beginning of ventricular systole. On electrocardiogram, it occurs right after the QRS complex.

The first heart sound can be accentuated or intensified in conditions such as exercise, hyperthyroidism, and mitral stenosis. A decrease in sound intensity occurs in clients with mitral regurgitation and heart failure.

The second heart sound (S_2) is caused mainly by the closing of the aortic and pulmonic valves (semilunar valves) (see Fig. 35–6). S_2 is characteristically shorter. It is higher pitched and is heard best at the base of the heart at the end of ventricular systole.

Splitting of heart sounds is often difficult to differentiate from diastolic filling sounds (gallops). A splitting of S_1 (closure of the mitral valve followed by closure of the tricuspid valve) occurs physiologically because left ventricular contraction occurs slightly before right ventricular contraction. However, closure of the mitral valve is louder than closure of the tricuspid valve, so that splitting is often not heard. Normal splitting of S_2 occurs because of the longer systolic phase of the right ventricle. Splitting of S_1 and S_2 can be accentuated by inspiration (increased venous return) and narrows during expiration.

Abnormal Heart Sounds

Paradoxical Splitting

Abnormal splitting of S_2 is referred to as paradoxical splitting, which is characteristic of a wider split heard on expiration. Paradoxical splitting of S_2 is heard in clients with severe myocardial depression causing early closure of the pulmonic valve or a delay in aortic valve closure. Such conditions include myocardial infarction, left bundle branch block, aortic stenosis, aortic regurgitation, and right ventricular pacing.

Gallops and Murmurs

Gallops and murmurs are common abnormal heart sounds, which may occur when heart disease is present.

GALLOPS. Diastolic filling sounds (S_3) and (S_4) are produced when blood enters a noncompliant chamber during rapid ventricular filling. The third heart sound (S_3) is produced during the rapid passive filling phase of ventricular diastole when blood flows from the atrium to a noncompliant ventricle. The sound arises from vibrations of the valves and supporting structures. The fourth heart sound (S_4) occurs as blood enters the ventricles during the active filling phase at the end of ventricular diastole.

S_3 is termed *ventricular gallop,* and S_4 is referred to as *atrial gallop.* These sounds can be caused by decreased compliance of either or both ventricles. The nurse can best hear left ventricular diastolic filling sounds with the client on his or her left side, using the bell of the stethoscope at the apex and the left lower sternal border during expiration.

An S_3 heart sound is probably a normal finding in children or young adults up to 30 years of age. An S_3 gallop in clients older than 40 years is considered abnormal and represents a decrease in left ventricular compliance. S_3 can be detected as an early sign of heart failure, ventricular septal defect, or ruptured papillary muscle.

An atrial gallop (S_4) may be heard in clients with hypertension, anemia, ventricular hypertrophy, myocardial infarction, aortic or pulmonic stenosis, and pulmonary emboli. It may also be heard with advancing age because of a stiffened ventricle.

The auscultation of both S_3 and S_4, called a *summation,* or *quadruple gallop,* is an indication of severe heart failure. If the quadruple rhythm is present and the patient is tachycardiac (has a shortened diastole), the two sounds may actually fuse, producing a rhythm that sounds like a horse galloping.

MURMURS. Murmurs reflect turbulent blood flow through normal or abnormal valves. They are classified according to their timing in the cardiac cycle: systolic murmurs (such as aortic stenosis and mitral regurgitation) occur between S_1 and S_2, whereas diastolic murmurs (such as in mitral stenosis and aortic regurgitation) occur between S_2 and S_1. Murmurs can occur during presystole, midsystole, or late systole or diastole or last throughout both phases of the cardiac cycle. Murmurs are also graded according to their intensity, depending on their level of loudness (Table 35–3).

The nurse describes the location of a murmur by where it is best heard on auscultation. Some murmurs may transmit or radiate from their loudest point to other areas, including the neck, the back, and the axilla. The configuration of a murmur is described as crescendo (increases in intensity) or decrescendo (decreases in intensity). The quality of murmurs can be further characterized as harsh, blowing, whistling, rumbling, or squeaking. The murmur is also described by its pitch, usually high or low.

Pericardial Friction Rub

A pericardial friction rub originates from the pericardial sac and occurs with the movements of the heart during the cardiac cycle. Rubs are usually transient and are a sign of inflammation, infection, or infiltration. Pericardial friction rubs may be heard in clients with pericarditis resulting from myocardial infarction and cardiac tamponade.

The three phases of cardiac movement—atrial systole, ventricular diastole, and ventricular systole—can produce three components of a rub. Usually, only one or two components can be heard. With each movement, a short, high-pitched scratchy sound is produced; the loudest component is heard in systole. The nurse may be most able to auscultate the rubs when the client sits, leans forward, and exhales. The pericardial friction rub is better heard with the diaphragm of the stethoscope.

PSYCHOSOCIAL ASSESSMENT

To many people, the heart is the symbol of their existence and longevity. A client with a heart-related illness, whether acute or chronic, usually perceives it as a major life crisis. The client and families and significant others confront not only the possibility of death but also fears about pain, disability, lack of self-esteem, physical dependence, and changes in family role dynamics. The nurse may assess the meaning of the illness to the client and family members by asking, "What do you understand about what happened to you (or the client)?" and "What does that mean to you?" When the client or family members perceive the stressor as overwhelming, formerly adequate support systems may no longer be effective. In these circumstances, the client and family members attempt to cope to regain a sense or feeling of control.

Coping behaviors vary among clients. Those who feel helpless to meet the demands of the situation may exhibit behaviors such as disorganization, fear, and anxiety. The nurse may ask the client or family members, "Have you ever encountered such a situation before?", "How did you manage that situation?", and "To whom can you turn for help?" The answers to these questions often reassure the client that he or she has encountered difficult situations in the past and has the ability and resources to cope with them.

A common and normal response is *denial,* which is a defense mechanism to enable the client to cope with threatening circumstances. The client may deny that he or she has the current cardiovascular condition, may state that it was present but is now absent, or may be excessively cheerful. Denial of the seriousness of the illness while following the treatment regimen is a protective response. Denial becomes maladaptive only when the client

TABLE 35–3

Grading of Heart Murmurs

• Grade I	Very faint
• Grade II	Faint, but recognizable
• Grade III	Loud, but moderate in intensity
• Grade IV	Loud and accompanied by a palpable thrill
• Grade V	Very loud, accompanied by a palpable thrill, and audible with the stethoscope partially off the client's chest
• Grade VI	Extremely loud, may be heard with the stethoscope slightly above the client's chest

is noncompliant with significant portions of medical and nursing care (see Chapter 8 on coping).

Family members and significant others of the client with heart disease may be more anxious than the client. Often they recall all the events of the illness, are unprotected by denial, and are afraid of recurrence. Disagreements frequently occur between the client and family members over compliance with appropriate follow-up care.

DIAGNOSTIC ASSESSMENT
Laboratory Tests

Assessment of the client with cardiac dysfunction includes examination of the blood for abnormalities. This is done to establish a diagnosis, detect concurrent disease, assess risk factors, and monitor response to treatment. Normal values for serum cardiac enzymes and serum lipids are listed in Chart 35–4.

Serum Cardiac Enzymes

Events leading to cellular injury cause a release of enzymes from intracellular storage, and circulating levels of these enzymes are dramatically elevated. Acute myocardial infarction (MI) can be confirmed by abnormally high levels of enzymes or isoenzymes in the serum.

Creatine Kinase

Creatine kinase (CK) is an enzyme specific to cells of the brain, myocardium, and skeletal muscle. The appearance of CK in the blood indicates tissue necrosis or injury, and CK levels follow a predictable rise and fall during a specified period of time. Cardiac specificity must be determined by measuring isoenzyme activity. There are three isoenzymes of CK: CK-MM is the predominant isoenzyme of skeletal muscle; CK-MB is found in myocardial muscle; and CK-BB occurs in the brain. CK-MB activity is most specific for MI and shows a predictable rise and fall during 3 days; a peak level occurs approximately 24 hours after the onset of chest pain.

Newer treatment modalities and shorter hospital stays require more rapid diagnosis of myocardial infarction (MI). An assay using monoclonal anti–CK-MB antibodies (stat CK) is able to detect myocardial necrosis accurately at 3 hours after emergency department admission when examined with an electrogram (ECG). Two subforms of CK-MB (CK-MB$_1$, CK-MB$_2$) have also been identified. Abnormal elevations of these CK subforms may occur as early as 2 hours after MI. These CK subforms remain elevated for up to 12 hours after MI and appear to be very sensitive and specific early diagnostic markers of MI.

Other early markers of MI are myoglobin and troponin. Myoglobin, a low-molecular-weight protein found in skeletal muscle, is an early and sensitive but nonspecific marker for myocardial injury. Troponin T and I are specific markers of myocardial injury that have a wide diagnostic time frame, making them useful for clients who present several hours after the onset of chest pain. Table 35–4 describes the characteristics of these new serum assays for myocardial damage.

Lactate Dehydrogenase

Lactate dehydrogenase (LDH) is widely distributed in the body and is found in the heart, liver, kidney, brain, and erythrocytes. LDH elevation starts within 12–24 hours after an MI, peaks between 48 and 72 hours, and falls to normal in 7 days. Because LDH is not specific to the myocardial cell, assessment of isoenzymes and patterns of elevation is necessary for confirmation of MI. There are five isoenzymes for LDH, of which LDH$_1$ and LDH$_2$ are found in the heart. If the serum level of LDH$_1$ is higher than the concentration of LDH$_2$, the pattern is said to have flipped, signifying myocardial damage.

Serum Lipids

Elevated lipid levels are considered a coronary artery disease (CAD) risk factor. Cholesterol, triglycerides, and the protein components of high-density lipoproteins (HDL) and low-density lipoproteins (LDL) are evaluated to assess a client's degree of risk for CAD. A serum cholesterol level greater than 260 mg/dL gives a client a three times greater risk of CAD than a serum level of less than 200 mg/dL.

Each of the lipoproteins contains varying proportions of cholesterol, triglyceride, protein, and phospholipid. HDL contains mainly protein and 20% cholesterol, whereas LDL is predominantly cholesterol. Elevated LDL levels are positively correlated with CAD, whereas elevated HDL levels are negatively correlated and appear to be a protective factor.

A nonfasting blood sample for the measurement of serum cholesterol levels is acceptable. However, if triglycerides are to be evaluated, the physician requests the specimen after a 12-hour fast.

Blood Coagulation Tests

Blood coagulation tests evaluate the ability of the blood to clot and are important in clients with a greater tendency to form thrombi (e.g., clients with atrial fibrillation, prosthetic valves, or infective endocarditis). They are also important for clients receiving anticoagulant therapy (e.g., during cardiac surgery, after thrombolytic therapy, and during treatment of an established thrombus).

Prothrombin Time and International Normalized Ratio

Prothrombin time (PT) and international normalized ratio (INR) are used when initiating and maintaining therapy with oral anticoagulants, such as sodium warfarin (Coumadin, Warfilone❖). They measure the activity of prothrombin, fibrinogen, and factors V, VII, and X. INR is the most reliable way to monitor anticoagulant status in warfarin therapy. Therapeutic ranges for standard anticoagulant therapy are 2.0–3.0 INR.

Partial Thromboplastin Time

Partial thromboplastin time (PTT) is assessed in clients receiving heparin (Hepalean❖). It measures deficiencies in all coagulation factors, except factors VII and XIII.

Chart 35–4

Laboratory Profile: Cardiovascular Assessment

Normal Range	Significance of Abnormal Findings
Serum Cardiac Enzymes Creatine kinase (CK) • Females: 10–55 U/mL, or 26–140 U/L • Males: 12–70 U/mL, or 38–174 U/L • Values higher after exercise	• Elevations indicate possible brain, myocardial, and skeletal muscle necrosis or injury.
CK-MM (CK$_3$) • 95–100% of total CK	• Elevations occur with muscle injury
CK-MB (CK$_2$) • 0–5% of total CK	• Elevations occur with myocardial injury or after percutaneous transluminal angioplasty and intracoronary streptokinase infusion.
CK-BB (CK$_1$) • 0%	• Elevations occur with brain tissue injury.
Lactate dehydrogenase (LDH) • 140–280 U/L, or 0.4–1.7 mmol/L	• Elevation occurs with injury to heart, liver, kidney, brain, and erythrocytes.
LDH$_1$ • 18–33% of total LDH	• Elevation occurs higher than LDH$_2$ with myocardial damage
LDH$_2$ • 28–40% of total LDH	
LDH$_1$:LDH$_2$ ratio • <1	• Elevation occurs with myocardial damage.
Serum Lipids Total lipids • 400–1000 mg/dL	• Elevation indicates increased risk of CAD.
Cholesterol • 122–200 mg/dL, or 3.16–6.5 mmol/L • Elderly (>70 years): 144–280 mgdL, or 3.73–7.25 mmol/L	• Elevation indicates increased risk of CAD.
Triglycerides • Females: 39–262 mg/dL, or 0.44–2.96 mmol/L • Males: 37–286 mg/dL, or 0.42–3.23 mmol/L • Elderly (>65 years): 55–260 mg/dL, or 0.62–2.94 mmol/L	• Elevation indicates increased risk of CAD.
Plasma high-density lipoproteins (HDLs) • Females: mean, 55–60 mg/dL • Males: mean, 45–50 mg/dL • Elderly: range increases with age	• Elevations protect against CAD.
Plasma low-density lipoproteins (LDLs) • 57–197 mg/dL, or 1.48–5.10 mmol/L • Elderly (>65 years): 92–221 mg/dL, or 2.38–5.72 mmol/L	• Elevation indicates increased risk of CAD.
HDL:LDL ratio • 3:1	• Elevated ratios may protect against CAD.

CAD = coronary artery disease.

Arterial Blood Gases

Arterial blood gas (ABG) determinations are frequently obtained in the client with cardiovascular disease. Determination of tissue oxygenation, carbon dioxide removal, and the acid-base status is essential to appropriate intervention and treatment. Complete discussion of ABGs can be found in Chapter 18.

Serum Electrolytes

Fluid and electrolyte balance is essential for normal cardiovascular performance. Cardiac manifestations often occur when there is an imbalance in either fluids or electrolytes in the body. For example, the cardiac effects of hypokalemia (low serum potassium level) include increased electrical instability, ventricular dysrhythmias, the

TABLE 35-4

Characteristics of New Serum Assays for Myocardial Damage				
Test	**Time to Elevation (hr)**	**Time to Peak (hr)**	**Time to Normal**	**Assay Time (min)**
Stat CK-MB	3–8	12–24	2–3 days	8–34
CK-MB subforms	1–3	5–7	24 hours	25
Myoglobin	2–3	6–9	24 hours	10–20
Troponin T & I	4–6	10–24	10–14 days	10–90

appearance of U waves on the electrocardiogram, and an increased risk of digitalis toxicity. The effects of hyperkalemia on the myocardium include slowed ventricular conduction and contraction followed by asystole (cardiac standstill).

Cardiac manifestations of hypocalcemia are ventricular dysrhythmias, prolonged QT interval, and cardiac arrest. Hypercalcemia shortens the QT interval and causes AV block, digitalis hypersensitivity, and cardiac arrest.

Serum sodium values reflect fluid balance and may be decreased, indicating a fluid excess in clients with heart failure.

Because magnesium regulates some aspects of myocardial electrical activity, hypomagnesemia has been implicated in some forms of rapid ventricular dysrhythmias. Another manifestation of hypomagnesemia is hypokalemia that is unresponsive to potassium replacement.

Complete Blood Count

The erythrocyte count is usually decreased in rheumatic fever and infective endocarditis. It is increased in heart diseases characterized by inadequate tissue oxygenation.

Decreased hematocrit and hemoglobin levels (e.g., caused by hemorrhage or hemolysis from prosthetic valves) indicate anemia and can manifest as angina or can aggravate heart failure. Vascular volume depletion with hemoconcentration (e.g., hypovolemic shock and excessive diuresis) results in an elevated hematocrit.

The leukocyte count is typically elevated after MI and in the various infectious and inflammatory diseases of the heart (e.g., infective endocarditis and pericarditis). Chapter 41 discusses the complete blood count in detail.

Radiographic Examinations
Chest Radiography

Routinely, posteroanterior and left lateral x-ray views of the chest are taken to determine the size, silhouette, and position of the heart. In acutely ill clients, a simple anteroposterior view is taken at the bedside. Cardiac enlargement, pulmonary congestion, cardiac calcifications, and placement of central venous catheters, endotracheal tubes, and hemodynamic monitoring devices are all assessed by x-ray.

Cardiac Fluoroscopy

Fluoroscopy is a simple x-ray examination that reveals the action of the heart. Continuous visual observation of the heart, the lungs, and vessel movement on a luminescent x-ray screen in a darkened room is provided. Fluoroscopy is used to place and position intracardiac catheters and IV pacemaker wires and can be helpful in identifying abnormal structures, calcifications, and tumors of the heart. In critically ill clients, fluoroscopy can be performed at the bedside for the placement of intracardiac catheters of IV pacemaker wires. Client preparation and follow-up depend on the procedure. Commonly, fluoroscopy is used in conjunction with cardiac catheterization, and the client is taken to a special cardiac catheterization room (see later discussion of cardiac catheterization).

Angiography

Angiography of arterial vessels, or arteriography, is an invasive diagnostic procedure that involves fluoroscopy and x-ray studies. This procedure is performed when an arterial obstruction, narrowing, or aneurysm is suspected. The radiologist performs selective arteriography to evaluate specific areas of the arterial system. For example, coronary arteriography, which is performed during left-sided cardiac catheterization, assesses arterial circulation within the heart (see later in this chapter). Angiography can also be performed on arteries in the extremities, the mesentery, and the cerebrum.

CLIENT PREPARATION. The radiologist explains the procedure and the risks to the client before he or she or the designated responsible party signs a consent form. Because this procedure involves injection of contrast medium (sometimes called a dye) into the arterial system, the risks are serious. They include allergic reaction, hemorrhage, thrombosis, embolism, and death. The client is told to expect a warm sensation when dye is injected during the procedure. The nurse assesses the client for any allergies to contrast medium, iodine-containing substances such as seafood, or local anesthetics. The nurse prepares the area, usually the femoral area in the groin according to the health care agency's policy and procedure. The nurse documents vital signs and marks and describes pulses distal to the puncture site in the client's medical record.

PROCEDURE. The radiologist or the technician places the client in a supine position on an x-ray table in the radiology department. A radiologist usually performs this procedure and begins by injecting a local anesthetic into the tissue surrounding the artery being catheterized. Contrast medium is injected via this catheter, and fluoroscopy and x-ray studies are done.

FOLLOW-UP CARE. After the procedure, the client is typically restricted to bed rest in the supine position for 4–6 hours. The nurse ensures that the extremity that was catheterized is not flexed during this time. A pressure dressing or bandage is kept in place over the injection site; there may be a sandbag over the dressing.

The nurse assesses the insertion site for bloody drainage or hematoma formation, assesses distal pulses, and compares skin temperature in the affected extremity with that in the opposite extremity. Vital signs are assessed at every dressing, pulse, and temperature check; the first measurement is obtained immediately after the client is transferred from the radiology department. These assessments usually continue every 15 minutes for 1 hour, then every 30 minutes for 2 hours, followed by every 4 hours or as necessary per the health care agency's protocol. The nurse notifies the radiologist immediately if bleeding, loss of pulses, or changes in vital signs occur. The nurse carefully administers the prescribed IV or oral fluids after the procedure, because the contrast medium may damage the kidneys.

Cardiac Catheterization

The most definitive, but most invasive, test in the diagnosis of heart disease is cardiac catheterization. Cardiac catheterization may include studies of the right or left side of the heart and the coronary arteries. Some of the most common indications for cardiac catheterization are listed in Table 35–5.

CLIENT PREPARATION. Many clients express anxiety and fear regarding cardiac catheterization. The nurse assesses the client's physical and psychosocial readiness and knowledge level.

TABLE 35–5

Indications for Cardiac Catheterization

- To confirm suspected heart disease, including coronary artery disease, myocardial disease, valvular disease, and valvular dysfunction
- To determine the location and extent of the disease process
- To assess
  - Stable, severe angina unresponsive to medical management
  - Unstable angina pectoris
  - Uncontrolled heart failure, ventricular dysrhythmias, or cardiogenic shock associated with acute myocardial infarction, papillary muscle dysfunction, ventricular aneurysm, or septal perforation
  - Whether cardiac surgery is necessary
- To evaluate
  - Effects of medical treatment on cardiovascular function
  - Percutaneous transluminal coronary angioplasty or coronary artery bypass graft patency

TABLE 35–6

Complications of Cardiac Catheterization

Right-Sided Heart Catheterization
- Thrombophlebitis
- Pulmonary embolism
- Vagal response

Left-Sided Heart Catheterization and Coronary Arteriography
- Myocardial infarction
- Cerebrovascular accident
- Arterial bleeding or thromboembolism
- Dysrhythmias

Right- or Left-Sided Heart Catheterization*
- Cardiac tamponade
- Hypovolemia
- Pulmonary edema
- Hematoma or blood loss at insertion site
- Reaction to contrast medium

*In addition to those cited for each procedure.

The nurse reviews the purpose of the procedure. The nurse informs the client how long the procedure usually takes, states who will be present while it is going on, and describes the appearance of the catheterization laboratory. The client is also informed about the sensations that may be experienced during the procedure, such as palpitations (as the catheter is passed up to the left ventricle); a feeling of heat or hot flash (as the dye is injected into either side of the heart); and a desire to cough (as the dye is injected into the right side of the heart). The nurse may use written or illustrated materials or videotapes, if available, to assist the client's understanding (Houston et al., 1996).

The risks of cardiac catheterization are usually explained by the cardiologist. The risks vary with the procedures to be performed and the client's physical status (Table 35–6). Right-sided heart catheterization is less risky than left-sided catheterization. Several complications may follow coronary arteriography, such as

- Myocardial infarction (MI)
- Cerebrovascular accident (CVA)
- Arterial bleeding
- Thromboembolism
- Lethal dysrhythmias
- Death

The cardiologist or the radiologist obtains a written informed consent from the client or the responsible party.

The client may be admitted to the hospital before the catheterization procedure. Standard preoperative tests are performed, which usually include chest x-ray, complete blood count, coagulation studies, urinalysis, and 12-lead electrocardiogram. The client receives nothing by mouth after midnight or has only a liquid breakfast if the catheterization is to take place in the afternoon. The nurse shaves the catheterization site and antiseptically prepares the skin according to the hospital's policy.

Nursing assessment before the procedure includes measurement of the client's vital signs, auscultation of the heart and the lungs, and evaluation of peripheral pulses. The nurse questions the client as to any history of allergy to iodine-containing substances (e.g., seafood and contrast agents). An antihistamine may be given to a client with a positive history. A mild sedative is given before the procedure. If the client normally takes a digitalis preparation or diuretic, it is usually withheld before the catheterization.

PROCEDURE. The client is taken to the cardiac catheterization laboratory (sometimes referred to as the "cath lab") and is placed supine on an x-ray table. The client is securely strapped to the table. The nurse informs the client that this precaution is necessary because the table turns like a cradle during the procedure. The physician injects a local anesthetic at the insertion site. The nurse in the catheterization laboratory instructs the client to report any chest pain or other symptoms to the staff.

Right-Sided Heart Catheterization. The right side of the heart is catheterized first and may be the only side examined. The cardiologist inserts a catheter through the femoral vein to the inferior vena cava or through the basilic vein to the superior vena cava. The catheter is advanced through either the inferior or the superior vena cava and, guided by fluoroscopy, is advanced through the right atrium, through the right ventricle, and, at times, into the pulmonary artery (Fig. 35–13). Intracardiac pressures (right atrial, right ventricular, pulmonary artery, and pulmonary artery wedge pressures) are obtained, and blood samples are withdrawn. Contrast dye or medium is usually injected to detect any cardiac shunts or regurgitation from the pulmonic or tricuspid valves.

Left-Sided Heart Catheterization. Left-sided heart catheterization is more risky than right-sided heart catheterization. The cardiologist advances the catheter retrogradely from the femoral or brachial artery up the aorta, across the aortic valve, and into the left ventricle (Fig. 35–14). The cardiologist may pass the catheter from the right side of the heart through the atrial septum, using a special needle to puncture the septum. Intracardiac pressures and blood samples are obtained. The pressures of the left atrium, left ventricle, and aorta as well as mitral and aortic valve status are evaluated. In addition, the cardiologist injects contrast dye into the ventricle; cineangiograms (rapidly changing films) evaluate left ventricular motion. Calculations are made of end-systolic volume, end-diastolic volume, stroke volume, and ejection fraction.

Coronary Arteriography. The technique for coronary arteriography is the same as for left-sided heart catheterization. The catheter is advanced into the aortic arch and positioned selectively in the right or left coronary artery. Injection of contrast medium permits visualization of the coronary arteries. By assessing the flow of dye through the coronary arteries, information about the site and severity of coronary lesions is obtained.

Intravascular Ultrasonography. An alternative to injecting dye into coronary arteries is intravascular ultraso-

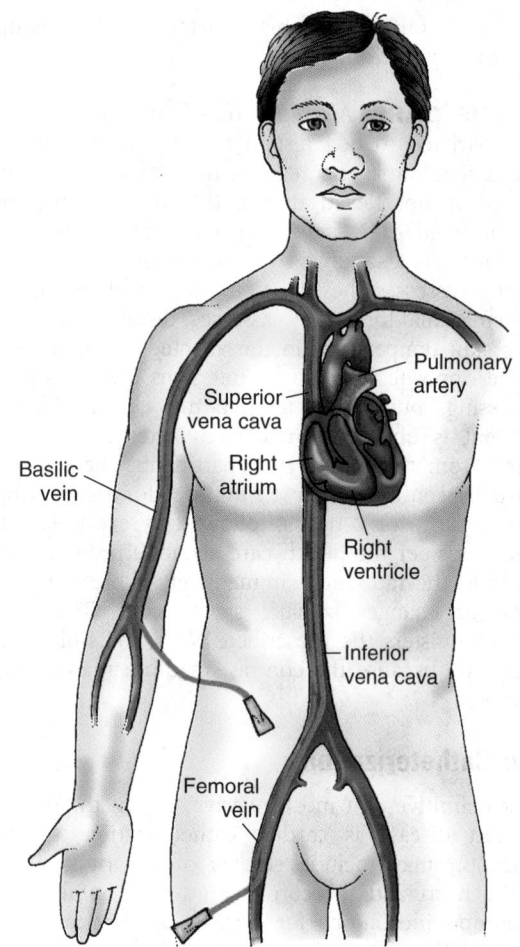

Figure 35–13. Right-sided heart catheterization. The catheter is inserted into the femoral vein and advanced through the inferior vena cava (or, if into an antecubital or basilic vein, through the superior vena cava), right atrium, and right ventricle and into the pulmonary artery.

nography (IVUS), which introduces a flexible catheter with a miniature transducer at the distal tip to visualize the coronary arteries. The transducer emits sound waves, which reflect off the plaque and the arterial wall, creating an image of the blood vessel (Strimike, 1996). IVUS is a more reliable indicator of plaque distribution and composition, arterial dissection, and degree of stenosis of the occluded artery than angiography (Strimike, 1996).

FOLLOW-UP CARE. After cardiac catheterization, the client is typically restricted to bed rest for 4–6 hours; the client is supine; the insertion site is kept extremity straight. Nursing researchers are evaluating bed rest protocols that might limit client discomfort while maintaining hemostasis (see Research Applications for Nursing).

A pressure dressing or bandage may be placed over the insertion site. A 5- or 10-pound sandbag or a C-clamp may be applied over the insertion site to ensure hemostasis. The nurse has many postcatheterization responsibilities. First, the nurse monitors vital signs every 15 minutes for 1 hour, then every 30 minutes for 2 hours or until vital signs are stable, and then every 4 hours or according

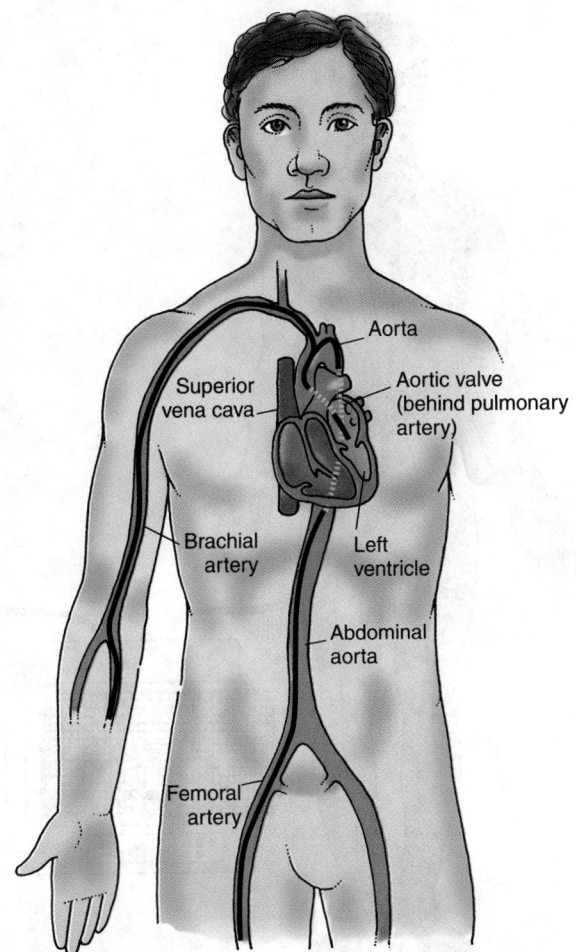

Figure 35–14. Left-sided heart catheterization. The catheter is inserted into the femoral artery or the antecubital artery. The catheter is passed through the ascending aorta, through the aortic valve, and into the left ventricle.

(labels in figure: Aorta; Superior vena cava; Aortic valve (behind pulmonary artery); Brachial artery; Left ventricle; Abdominal aorta; Femoral artery)

to the hospital's policy. The nurse observes the insertion site for bloody drainage or hematoma formation when taking vital signs. Peripheral pulses in the affected extremity as well as skin temperature and color are monitored with every vital sign check.

The nurse must be constantly vigilant for complications of cardiac catheterization (see Table 35–5). The nurse assesses the client's reports of pain and discomfort at the insertion site, chest pain, nausea, or feelings of lightheadedness. The client is often attached to a cardiac monitor. If not, the nurse auscultates the client's heart sounds, noting rhythm and rate to detect dysrhythmias. Because the contrast medium acts as an osmotic diuretic, the nurse monitors urinary output and ensures that the client receives sufficient oral and IV fluids for adequate excretion of the dye. The nurse may administer pain medication for insertion site or back discomfort, as ordered.

If the client experiences chest pain, dysrhythmias, bleeding, hematoma formation, or a dramatic change in peripheral pulses in the affected extremity, the nurse reports these findings to the physician immediately and provides prompt intervention. The nurse is also alert for

neurologic changes such as visual disturbances, slurred speech, difficulty in swallowing, and extremity weakness.

Digital Subtraction Angiography

Digital subtraction angiography (DSA) combines x-ray detection methods and a computerized subtraction technique with fluoroscopy for visualization of the cardiovascular system. There is no interference from adjacent structures, such as bone and soft tissue.

CLIENT PREPARATION. Digital subtraction angiography involves the injection of dye into the venous system. Therefore, before the procedure, the nurse assesses the client for a history of allergies to contrast medium (dye), iodine, or seafood.

▷ Research Applications for Nursing

Clients May Not Need to Remain Supine for 6–12 Hours After Cardiac Catheterization.

Pooler-Lunse, C., Barkman A., & Back, B. F. (1996). Effects of modified positioning and mobilization on back pain and delayed bleeding in patients who have received heparin and undergone angiography: A pilot study. Heart and Lung, 25(2), 117–122.

This study examined the effects of early head elevation (maximum 45 degrees) and early ambulation (after 4 hours) on client perception of pain and presence of delayed bleeding after cardiac catheterization. A small sample of clients (N = 29) were randomly assigned to either the control group (6 hours of supine bedrest) or the experimental group (head of bed elevated to 45 degrees after 15 minutes, out of bed for 2 minutes to stand or urinate after 4 hours). All clients were receiving heparin before angiography.

After the procedure, both pain and presence of delayed bleeding were assessed frequently. Femoral dressings and pedal pulses were evaluated by the staff nurses, and the research assistant palpated the site for presence and size of a hematoma. Pain was evaluated using the McGill Pain Questionnaire.

There was not a significant difference between the two groups in the presence of delayed bleeding. One client in each group had sanguineous drainage through the pressure dressing. However, there was a significant difference in the presence and intensity of pain; clients in the experimental group experienced less pain overall and less intense pain.

Critique. This is a very small sample involving clients from one institution. Delayed bleeding was considered significant only if a hematoma was larger than 5 cm and occluded a pedal pulse or if there was more than 100 mL of volume lost (enough to penetrate the pressure dressing).

Possible Nursing Implications. Since clients experience considerable back discomfort and difficulty urinating while lying supine for 6–12 hours after cardiac catheterization, interventions that would reduce these without causing complications would be highly beneficial. If this pilot study's findings—that head of bed elevation to 45 degrees and early ambulation at 4 hours reduce pain and do not increase bleeding—are replicated with a larger sample and varied populations, many clients might benefit.

PROCEDURE. For a DSA, the radiologist injects dye into the venous system via the superior vena cava. As the contrast medium circulates through the heart and the arterial system, a fluoroscopic image intensifier displays the vessels and focuses the image. A computer then converts the images to numbers. The first image obtained before the injection of the dye is subtracted from the postinjection images.

FOLLOW-UP CARE. Because DSA does not involve an arterial puncture and because little contrast dye is used, nursing care after the procedure is not as extensive as that after cardiac catheterization. The nurse monitors the client for vital signs and assesses the injection site for bleeding or discomfort.

Other Diagnostic Tests

Electrocardiography

The electrocardiogram (ECG) is a routine part of every cardiovascular evaluation and is one of the most valuable diagnostic tests. Various forms are available: resting ECG, continuous ambulatory ECG (Holter monitoring), exercise ECG (stress test), and signal averaged ECG. The resting ECG provides information about cardiac dysrhythmias, myocardial ischemia, the site and extent of myocardial infarction, cardiac hypertrophy, electrolyte imbalances, and the effectiveness of cardiac drugs. The normal ECG pattern of one cardiac cycle is illustrated in Figure 35–15. Further discussion of the interpretation and evaluation of normal and abnormal patterns is found in Chapter 36.

Resting Electrocardiography

The ECG graphically records electrical current generated by the heart. This current is measured by electrodes placed on the skin and connected to an amplifier and strip chart recorder (Fig. 35–16). In the standard 12-lead ECG, five electrodes attached to the arms, legs, and chest measure current from 12 different views or leads: three bipolar limb leads (Fig. 35–17), three unipolar augmented leads (Fig. 35–18), and six unipolar precordial leads (Fig. 35–19). Placement of the leads allows the

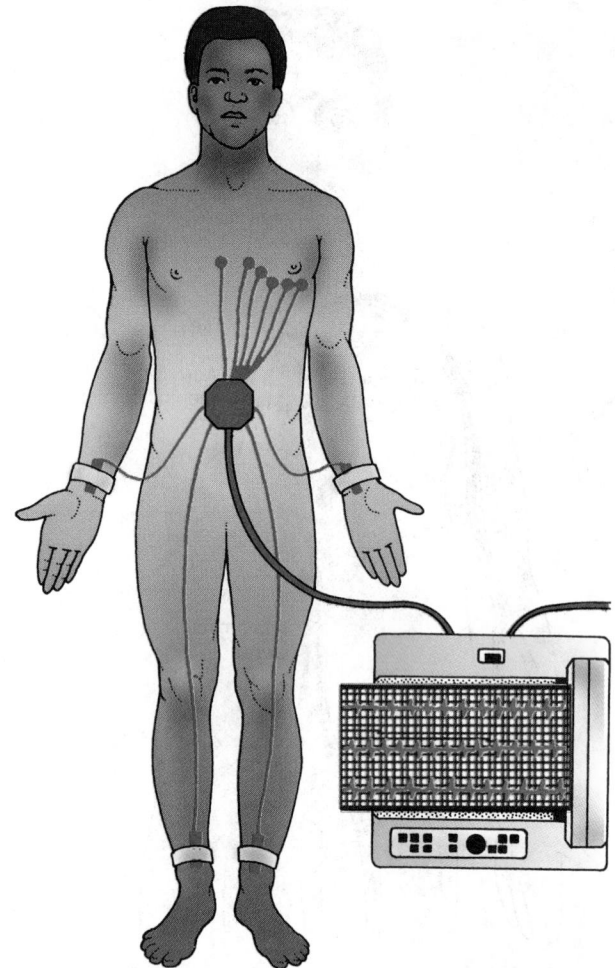

Figure 35–16. Electrode placement for a 12-lead ECG.

physician to view myocardial electrical conduction from different axes or positions, identifying sections of the heart in which electrical conduction is abnormal.

CLIENT PREPARATION. The nurse explains the purpose and procedure of the resting ECG and informs the client that the test is safe and painless. The nurse reminds the client to lie as still as possible during the test.

PROCEDURE. The ECG is performed with the client in a supine position with the chest exposed. Before applying the electrodes, the nurse or the technician washes the skin to reduce skin oils and to improve electrode contact. To ensure good contact between the skin and the electrodes for the limb leads, the electrodes should be placed on a flat surface above the wrists and the ankles. A total of 10 electrodes are used for a standard ECG and are attached to lead wires that connect to the ECG machine. The 12-lead ECG reading is obtained by selecting the indicators on the machine.

FOLLOW-UP CARE. No specific follow-up care is warranted.

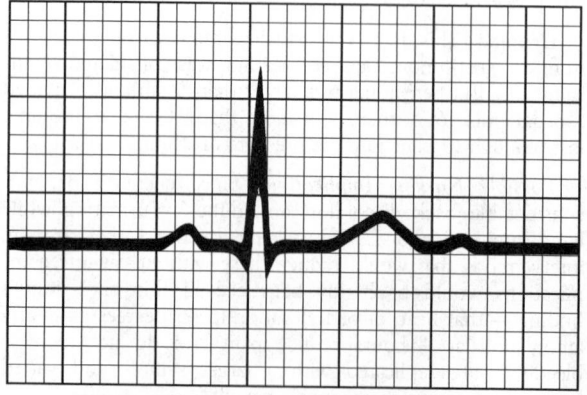

Figure 35–15. A normal ECG pattern in lead II.

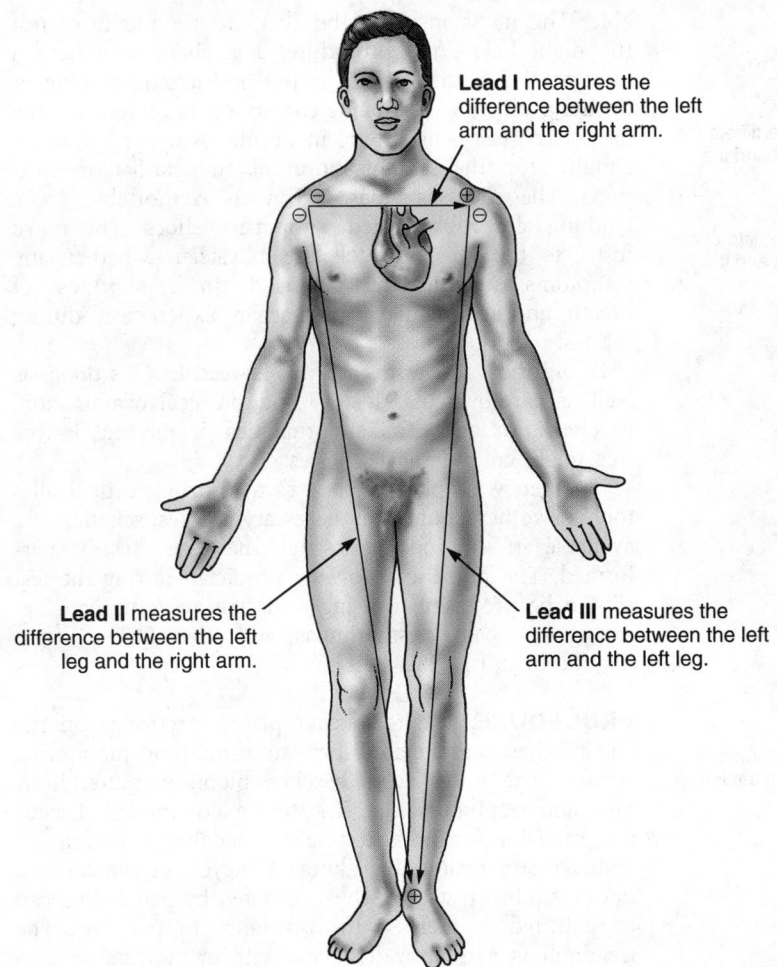

Lead I measures the difference between the left arm and the right arm.

Lead II measures the difference between the left leg and the right arm.

Lead III measures the difference between the left arm and the left leg.

Figure 35–17. Standard ECG limb leads.

Ambulatory Electrocardiography

Ambulatory ECG (also called Holter monitoring) allows continuous recording of cardiac activity during an extended period (usually 24 hours) while the client is performing the usual activities of daily living (ADLs). The ambulatory ECG allows assessment and correlation of dyspnea, chest pain, central nervous system symptoms (such as lightheadedness and syncope), and palpitations with actual cardiac events and the client's activities.

CLIENT PREPARATION. The nurse encourages the client to maintain a normal day's schedule. He or she is instructed to keep a diary, or log, in which to note the time of activities, such as eating, sleeping, walking, and working, and to record any symptoms, such as chest pain, lightheadedness, fainting, and palpitations. The nurse instructs the client to avoid operating heavy machinery, using electric shavers and hair dryers, and bathing or showering. These activities may interfere with the ECG recorder. If the client is hospitalized, the nurse may need to make the entries for the log.

PROCEDURE. The ECG technician places the electrodes on the client's chest and attaches them to the Holter monitor. The monitor is a small portable ECG tape recorder about the size of a transistor radio. The monitor is worn in a sling or holder around the client's chest or waist. After the prescribed monitoring period, the technician removes the electrodes and the monitor system. The ECG tape is analyzed by a microcomputer to allow correlation of the ECG findings with activities noted in the client's diary.

FOLLOW-UP CARE. No specific follow-up care is needed.

Exercise Electrocardiography (Stress Test)

The exercise ECG test (also known as exercise tolerance, or stress, test) assesses the cardiovascular response to an increased workload. The stress test helps to determine the heart's functional capacity and screens for asymptomatic coronary artery disease. Dysrhythmias that develop during exercise may be identified, and the effectiveness of antidysrhythmic drugs can be evaluated.

CLIENT PREPARATION. Because risks are associated with exercising, the client must be adequately informed about the purpose, procedure, and risks involved. A writ-

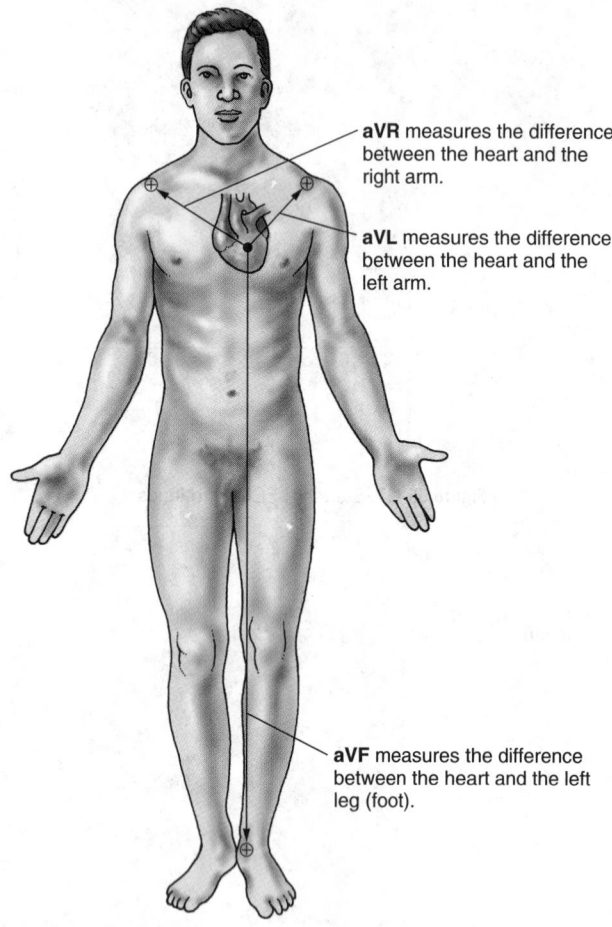

aVR measures the difference between the heart and the right arm.

aVL measures the difference between the heart and the left arm.

aVF measures the difference between the heart and the left leg (foot).

Figure 35–18. Unipolar augmented ECG leads.

able. The nurse instructs the client to get plenty of rest the night before the procedure. The client may have a light meal 2 hours before the test and avoid smoking or drinking alcohol or caffeine-containing beverages on the day of the test. The physician decides whether the client should stop the administration of any cardiac medications. The client is advised to wear comfortable, loose clothing and rubber-soled, supportive shoes. The nurse instructs the client to tell the physician whether any symptoms, such as chest pain, dizziness, shortness of breath, and an irregular heartbeat, are experienced during the test.

Before the stress test, a resting 12-lead ECG is done, as well as cardiovascular history and physical examination, to check for any ECG abnormalities or medical factors that might contraindicate the test.

Emergency supplies such as cardiac drugs, a defibrillator, and other equipment necessary for resuscitation are available in the room in which the stress test is performed. The nurse assisting the physician during the test should be proficient in using resuscitation equipment because chest pain, dysrhythmias, and other ECG changes may occur during this test.

PROCEDURE. The technician places electrodes on the client's chest and attaches them to a multilead monitoring system. The nurse notes baseline blood pressure, heart rate, and respiratory rate. The two major modes of exercise available for stress testing are pedaling a bicycle ergometer and treadmill walking. A bicycle ergometer is a device equipped with a wheel operated by pedals that can be adjusted to increase the resistance to pedaling. The treadmill is a motorized device with an adjustable conveyor belt; it can reach speeds of 1–10 miles/hour and can also be adjusted from a flat position to a 22-degree gradient.

After the nurse shows the client how to use the bicycle or how to walk on the treadmill, the client begins to exercise. During the test, the client's blood pressure and ECG are closely monitored as the speed and incline of

ten consent must be obtained. Anxiety and fear are common before stress testing. The nurse assures the client that the procedure is performed in a controlled environment with prompt nursing and medical attention avail-

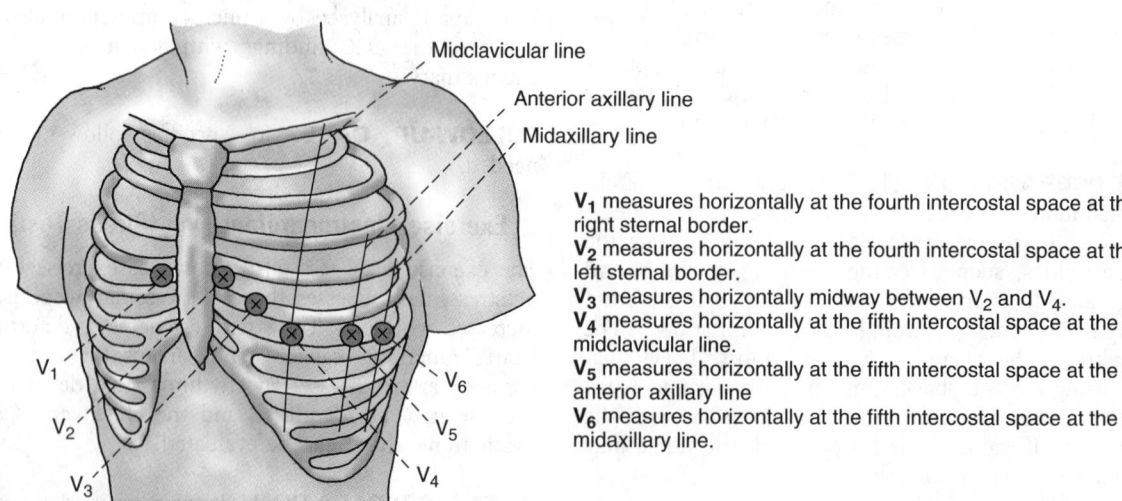

Midclavicular line

Anterior axillary line

Midaxillary line

V_1 measures horizontally at the fourth intercostal space at the right sternal border.
V_2 measures horizontally at the fourth intercostal space at the left sternal border.
V_3 measures horizontally midway between V_2 and V_4.
V_4 measures horizontally at the fifth intercostal space at the midclavicular line.
V_5 measures horizontally at the fifth intercostal space at the anterior axillary line
V_6 measures horizontally at the fifth intercostal space at the midaxillary line.

Figure 35–19. Unipolar precordial ECG leads.

the treadmill or the resistance to cycling are increased. The client exercises until one of the following occurs:

- A predetermined heart rate is reached and maintained.
- Signs and symptoms, such as chest pain, fatigue, extreme dyspnea, vertigo, hypotension, and ventricular dysrhythmias, appear.
- Significant ST-segment depression occurs.

FOLLOW-UP CARE. After the test, the nurse continues to monitor the ECG and blood pressure until the client has completely recovered. After the client has recovered, he or she can return home if the test was done on an outpatient basis. The nurse advises the client to avoid taking a hot shower for 1–2 hours after the test, because this may precipitate hypotension. If the client does not recover but continues to have chest pain or ventricular dysrhythmias or appears medically unstable, he or she is admitted to a coronary care unit for observation.

Echocardiography

As a noninvasive, risk-free test, echocardiography is easily performed at a client's bedside or on an outpatient basis. Echocardiography uses ultrasound waves to assess cardiac structure and mobility, particularly of the valves. ECGs help to assess and diagnose cardiomyopathy, valvular disorders, pericardial effusion, left ventricular function, ventricular aneurysms, and cardiac tumors.

CLIENT PREPARATION. There is no special preparation for echocardiography. The nurse informs the client that the test is painless and takes 30–60 minutes to complete. The nurse instructs the client to lie quietly during the test. The nurse assists the client to lie slightly on his or her left side with the head of the client elevated 15–20 degrees.

PROCEDURE. During an echocardiogram, a small transducer lubricated with gel to facilitate movement and conduction is placed on the client's chest at the level of the third or fourth intercostal space near the left sternal border. The transducer transmits high-frequency sound waves and receives them back from the client as they are reflected from different structures. These echoes are usually videotaped simultaneously with the client's echocardiogram and can be recorded on graph paper for a permanent copy.

Figure 35–20 is a representation of how echocardiograms examine the heart. After the images are taped, cardiac measurements that require several images can be obtained. Some routine measurements are chamber size, ejection fraction, and flow gradient across the valves.

FOLLOW-UP CARE. There is no specific follow-up care for a client having an echocardiogram.

Transesophageal Echocardiography

Echocardiograms may also be performed transesophageally. Transesophageal echocardiography examines cardiac structure and function with an ultrasound transducer placed immediately behind the heart in the esophagus or

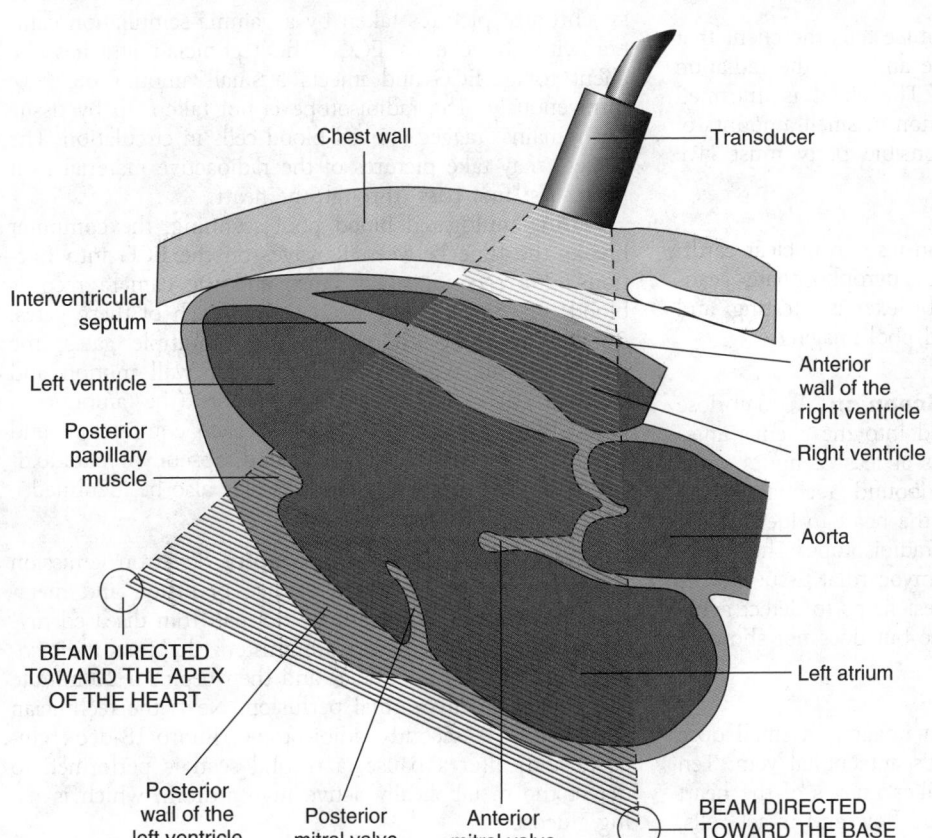

Figure 35–20. Echocardiographic imaging of the heart.

the stomach. The transducer provides especially detailed views of such posterior cardiac structures as the left atrium, the mitral valve, and the aortic arch. Preparation and follow-up are similar to those for the client having an upper gastrointestinal endoscopic examination (see Chap. 55).

Phonocardiography

Phonocardiography is the graphic recording of heart sounds during auscultation. It can be helpful in determining the exact timing and characteristics of extra heart sounds and murmurs.

A phonocardiography machine simultaneously records the pulse wave, ECG, and heart sounds. A pressure-sensitive transducer is applied to the selected pulse (e.g., apical or carotid artery), and the ECG is obtained through standard limb leads. A special microphone, used in the same manner as a stethoscope, is applied to the various areas for auscultation on the client's chest. Client preparation and follow-up care are similar to those for echocardiography (see earlier).

Nuclear Cardiography

The use of radionuclide techniques in cardiovascular assessment is called *nuclear cardiology*. Using radioactive tracer substances, cardiovascular abnormalities can be viewed, recorded, and evaluated. These studies are useful for detecting myocardial infarction (MI) and decreased myocardial blood flow and for evaluating left ventricular ejection.

CLIENT PREPARATION. The nurse tells the client that the tests are relatively noninvasive and that the radiation exposure and risks are minimal. The client is informed that the test involves the IV injection of small amounts of radioisotope. The client or responsible party must give written consent.

PROCEDURE. The most common tests in nuclear cardiology include technetium (^{99m}Tc) pyrophosphate scanning, thallium imaging, sestamibi exercise testing and scan, and multigated cardiac blood pool imaging.

Technetium Pyrophosphate Scanning. A small dose of ^{99m}Tc pyrophosphate is injected into the client's antecubital vein. The client then waits at least 2 hours while the renal system clears the unbound technetium. A gamma-scintillation camera scans the heart to identify the areas of increased uptake of the radioisotope. The radioisotope accumulates in damaged myocardial tissue and is referred to as a "hot spot." This test helps to detect acute MI and define its location and size but does not show an old infarction.

Thallium Imaging. For thallium imaging, a small dose of ^{201}Tl is injected into the client's antecubital vein. Ten minutes later, a nuclear camera takes images of the heart to detect the areas of normal blood flow and intact cells, which rapidly take up the thallium. Necrotic or ischemic tissue does not take up the radioisotope and appears as "cold spots" on the scan. Scanning is repeated in 2–4 hours to evaluate thallium clearance.

Thallium imaging may be performed with the client at rest or during an exercise test. In the Persantine thallium test, dipyridamole (Persantine, Apo-Dipyridamole✦) is administered before the test. Dobutamine hydrochloride (Dobutrex) or Adenosine (Adenocard) may be given instead. These drugs simulate the effects of exercise and are used for clients who are unable to exercise on a bike or treadmill.

Thallium imaging performed during an exercise test may demonstrate perfusion deficits not apparent at rest. First, the stress test procedure is performed (see earlier). After the client reaches maximal activity level, a small dose of ^{201}Tl is injected IV, and the client continues to exercise for approximately 1–2 minutes. The scanning is then done.

Thallium imaging is used to assess myocardial scarring and perfusion, detect the location and extent of an acute or chronic MI, evaluate graft patency after coronary bypass surgery, and evaluate antianginal therapy, thrombolytic therapy, or balloon angioplasty.

Sestamibi (technetium-99m pertechnetate) may be used rather than thallium for exercise testing with scanning. Sestamibi more accurately identifies ischemic areas in women, and high-quality images may be obtained on the first scan.

Cardiac Blood Pool Imaging. Cardiac blood pool imaging is a noninvasive test used to evaluate cardiac motion and calculate ejection fraction. It uses a computer to synchronize pictures taken by a gamma-scintillation camera with the client's ECG. The technician attaches the client to an ECG and injects a small amount of ^{99m}Tc intravenously. The radioisotope is not taken up by tissue but remains "tagged" to red blood cells in circulation. The camera may take pictures of the radioactive material as it makes its "first pass" through the heart.

During multigated blood pool scanning, the computer breaks the time between R waves on the ECG into fractions of a second called gates, and the camera records blood flow through the heart during each of these gates. By analyzing the information from multiple gates, the computer can evaluate the ventricular wall motion and calculate the client's ejection fraction (the amount of blood the left ventricle ejects with each contraction) and ejection velocity. Areas of decreased, absent, or paradoxical movement of the left ventricle may also be identified.

Positron Emission Tomography. Positron emission scans are used to compare cardiac perfusion and metabolic function and differentiate normal from diseased myocardium. The technician administers the first radioisotope (nitrogen-13-ammonia) and then begins a 20-minute scan to detect myocardial perfusion. Next, the technician administers a second radioisotope (fluoro-18-deoxyglucose) and, after a pause, a second scan is performed to detect the metabolically active myocardium, which is using glucose.

The two scans are compared; in a normal heart, performance and metabolic function will match. In an ische-mic heart, there will be a mismatch: a reduction in perfu-sion and increased glucose uptake by the ischemic myocardium. The scanning procedure takes 2–3 hours, and the client may be asked to use a treadmill or exercise bicycle in conjunction with the scan.

FOLLOW-UP CARE. The client may complain of fa-tigue, depending on which test is performed, or discom-fort at the antecubital injection site. If a stress test was paired with the study, the nurse needs to be aware of the same follow-up care as for the stress test (see earlier).

Magnetic Resonance Imaging

Magnetic resonance imaging (MRI) is a noninvasive diag-nostic option. An image of the heart or great vessels is produced through the interaction of magnetic fields, radio waves, and atomic nuclei showing hydrogen density. Sim-ply put, the radio waves "bounce off" the body tissue being examined. Because each tissue has its own density, the computer image clearly differentiates between different types of tissues. MRI permits determination of cardiac wall thickness, chamber dilation, and valve and ventricu-lar function as well as blood movement in the great ves-sels. Improved MRI techniques allow mapping of coro-nary artery blood flow with nearly the accuracy of a cardiac catheterization.

Before an MRI, the nurse determines that the client has removed all metallic objects, including watches, jewelry, clothing with metal fasteners, and hair clips. Clients with pacemakers should not have an MRI because the mag-netic fields can deactivate the pacemaker. Approximately 5% of clients experience claustrophobia during the 15–60 minutes required to complete the scan.

Hemodynamic Monitoring

Hemodynamic monitoring provides quantitative informa-tion about vascular capacity, blood volume, pump effec-tiveness, and tissue perfusion. Hemodynamic monitoring is often referred to as direct monitoring because it in-volves procedures that directly measure pressures in the heart and great vessels. Usually performed for more seri-ously ill clients, it can provide more accurate measure-ments of blood pressure as well as heart function and volume status.

Informed consent is required for hemodynamic moni-toring because there are significant risks, although com-plications are uncommon. After consent is obtained, the nurse prepares a pressure-monitoring system. The compo-nents of a pressure-monitoring system are a catheter with an infusion system, a transducer, and a monitor (Fig. 35–21). The catheter receives the pressure waves (mechanical energy) from the heart or the great vessels. The trans-ducer converts the mechanical energy into electrical en-ergy, which is displayed as waveforms or numbers on the monitor. To maintain patency of the catheter, the nurse prepares a heparinized solution. This solution is usually infused at 3–4 mL/hour under pressure to prevent back-up of blood and occlusion of the catheter.

To prepare the transducer, the nurse must balance and calibrate it according to the equipment manufacturer's specifications and the hospital's policy. Finally, the nurse must identify the phlebostatic axis (Chart 35–5) and level the transducer to it. When the monitoring system is pre-pared, the physician inserts the catheter.

Right Atrial, Pulmonary Artery, and Pulmonary Wedge Pressures

A pulmonary artery catheter is a triple- or quadruple-lumen catheter with the capacity to measure right atrial and indirect left atrial pressures or pulmonary artery wedge pressure (PAWP). A cardiac output measurement may also be obtained.

CLIENT PREPARATION. The physician explains the procedure and advises the client and family members or the significant other of the risks. Then the physician ob-tains a written consent for the procedure. The client and the family should understand that the hemodynamic monitoring system represents an assessment tool, and, although it is used to guide therapy, it is not itself a treatment. The nurse asks the client to remain still and supine for the insertion of the catheter.

PROCEDURE. The physician inserts a balloon-tipped catheter percutaneously through a large vein and directs it to the right atrium (RA). When the catheter tip reaches the RA, the physician inflates the balloon, and the cathe-ter advances with the flow of blood through the tricuspid valve, into the right ventricle, past the pulmonic valve, and into a branch of the pulmonary artery. The balloon is deflated after the catheter tip reaches the pulmonary ar-tery. Waveforms visualized on the oscilloscope as the pul-monary artery catheter is advanced (Fig. 35–22) and flu-oroscopy are used to determine the location of the catheter.

Right atrial pressure is measured by a pressure sensor on the catheter inside the right atrium. Normal RA pres-sure ranges from 1–8 mmHg. Increased RA pressures may occur with right ventricular failure, whereas low RA pressures are usually indicative of hypovolemia.

Normal pulmonary artery pressure (PAP) ranges from 15 to 28 mmHg/5 to 16 mmHg, with a mean of 15 (Daily & Kenner, 1992), and may be constantly visible on the monitor. When the balloon at the tip of the catheter is inflated, the catheter advances and wedges in a branch of the pulmonary artery. The tip of the catheter is able to sense pressures transmitted from the left atrium, which reflect left ventricular end-diastolic pressure (LVEDP). The pressure measured during balloon inflation is called the *pulmonary artery wedge pressure* (PAWP). PAWP closely approximates left atrial pressure and LVEDP in clients with normal left ventricular function, with normal heart rates, and without mitral valve disease. The PAWP is a mean pressure and is normally between 4 and 12 mmHg.

Elevated PAWP measurements may indicate left ventric-ular failure, hypervolemia, mitral regurgitation, or intra-cardiac shunt. A decreased PAWP is seen with hypovole-mia or afterload reduction. Individual values may be less important than the trend in values.

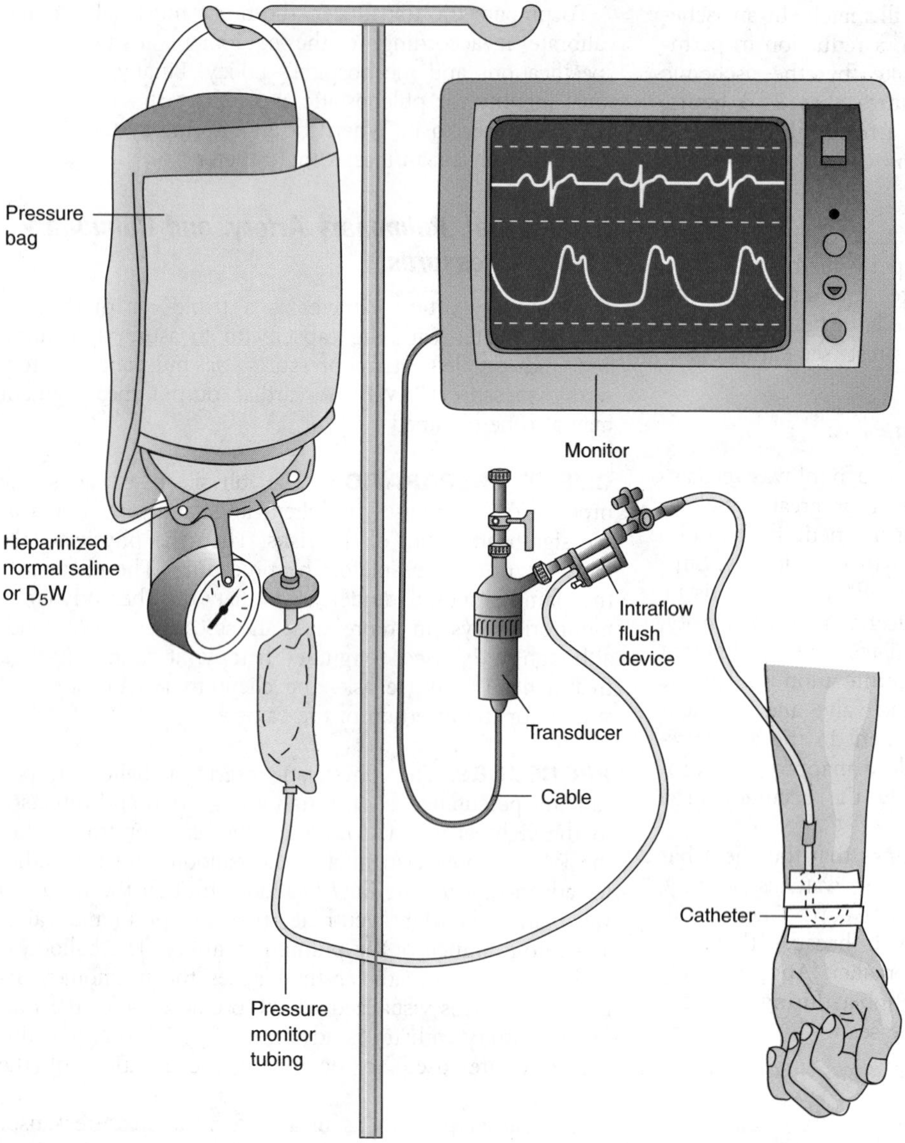

Figure 35–21. Components of a hemodynamic monitoring system.

FOLLOW-UP CARE. The patency of the catheter is maintained with infusion of a heparinized solution under pressure. The nurse obtains and records RA pressure, pulmonary artery pressure, and PAWP at appropriate intervals (usually every 1–4 hours). The trend of these pressures helps to guide medical therapy. During pressure recording, it is important that the transducer be at the level of the phlebostatic axis and the client's position be appropriate. While PAWPs are obtained, the client is usually supine with the head elevated up to 45 degrees or turned slightly to the side. If the balloon remains in the wedge position after PAWP measurement, the nurse attempts to change the catheter's position by asking the client to cough or changing the client's position. If these methods are not successful, the nurse notifies the physician immediately.

The nurse changes the occlusive dressing over the catheter aseptically according to the hospital's policy. The nurse inspects the insertion site for redness, heat, swelling, drainage, and intactness of the sutures. Detailed dis-

cussion of the management and care of clients with pulmonary artery catheters can be found in texts on critical care nursing.

The nurse assesses for a number of complications associated with pulmonary artery catheters. For example, pulmonary infarction or pulmonary rupture may occur if the catheter remains in the wedge position. Air embolism is possible if the balloon has ruptured and repeated attempts are made to inflate it. Ventricular dysrhythmias may occur if the catheter tip slips back into the right ventricle and irritates the myocardium. Thrombus and embolus formation may occur at the catheter site. Infection may result and bleeding may be pronounced if the infusion system becomes disconnected.

Cardiac Output

Cardiac output can be measured using the thermodilution method when the patient has a pulmonary artery catheter with a thermistor. The nurse injects a specified amount (5

Nursing Care Highlight: Identification of the Phlebostatic Axis

1. Position the client supine.
2. Palpate the fourth intercostal space at the sternum.

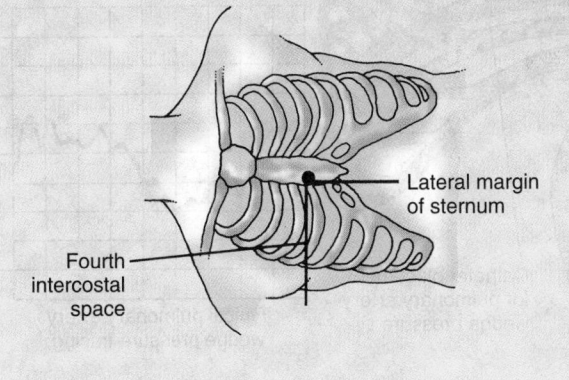

Lateral margin of sternum

Fourth intercostal space

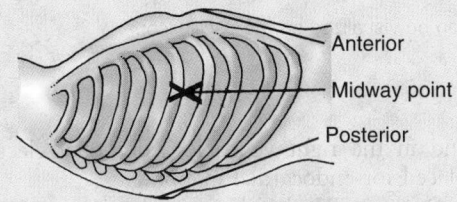

Anterior

Midway point

Posterior

3. Follow the fourth intercostal space to the side of the client's chest.
4. Determine the midway point between anterior and posterior.
5. Find the intersection between the midway point and the line from the fourth intercostal space, and mark it with an X in indelible ink. This is the phlebostatic axis.

or 10 mL) of iced or room-temperature IV solution (normal saline or dextrose in water) into the proximal port of the catheter. The solution mixes with the blood in the right atrium and travels with the flow of blood through the heart. A temperature-sensitive device located on the tip of the catheter in the pulmonary artery registers and senses the change in temperature of the blood. The information is transmitted to a cardiac output computer, which displays a digital value. The normal range of cardiac output in the adult client is 4–7 L/minute (Wilson, 1992). The cardiac index, the cardiac output adjusted for the person's size, may also be calculated.

Mixed Venous Oxygen Saturation Monitoring

Mixed venous oxygen saturation (SVO_2) reflects the balance between oxygen supply and demand. SVO_2 may be measured with a pulmonary artery catheter with fiberoptics. Light travels down one optical fiber, is reflected by the red blood cells according to the oxygen saturation of the hemoglobin, and returns to an optical module for interpretation and continuous display. Normal range for

SVO_2 is 60% to 80%. Using SVO_2 monitoring, the nurse can individualize the plan of care so the patient's SVO_2 remains in the normal range and the patient's oxygen supply and demand are in balance.

Central Venous Pressure Monitoring

If the physician desires measurement of pressures from the right atrium or central veins but a pulmonary artery catheter and pressure-monitoring system are not appropriate, pressures may be obtained with a water manometer attached to a conventional IV system. Central venous pressures (CVPs) are similar to right atrial pressures, but CVPs are measured in centimeters of water rather than millimeters of mercury. A normal CVP is 3–8 cm H_2O.

The physician inserts a catheter through the venous system into the right atrium. A chest x-ray is taken to assess placement. The nurse levels the manometer with the phlebostatic axis to ensure accurate pressure measurement (Chart 35–6).

Elevated CVPs may indicate right ventricular failure. Low CVPs may indicate hypovolemia. Caution must be used in predicting the function of the left side of the heart from a CVP reading.

Care of the site is similar to that for the pulmonary artery catheter site. Complications include pneumothorax during insertion, hemorrhage, infection, and catheter occlusion.

Systemic Intra-Arterial Monitoring

Direct measurement of arterial blood pressure is by invasive arterial catheter in critically ill clients. The physician usually inserts an intra-arterial catheter into the radial artery, but the femoral, brachial, or dorsalis pedis arteries may also be used. After the physician has inserted the catheter, the catheter is attached to pressure tubing and a heparinized solution is infused constantly under pressure to maintain the integrity of the system. A transducer attached to the tubing allows continuous direct monitoring of the arterial blood pressure. Direct measurements of blood pressure are usually 10–15 mmHg greater than indirect (cuff) measurements. The arterial catheter may also be used to obtain blood samples for arterial blood gas values and other blood tests.

Because the arterial vasculature is a high-pressure system, frequent assessment of the arterial site and infusion system is essential. The nurse notes any bleeding around the intra-arterial catheter or any loose connections and corrects the situation immediately. Collateral circulation is assessed by Doppler or Allen's tests before and during the time when an arterial catheter is in place. Color, pulse, and temperature at the insertion site should be scrupulously monitored for any early signs of circulatory compromise. Complications of systemic intra-arterial monitoring may include pain, infection, arteriospasm, obstruction at the site with potential for distal infarction, air embolism, and hemorrhage.

Electrophysiologic Studies

An electrophysiologic study (EPS) is an invasive procedure during which programmed electrical stimulation of

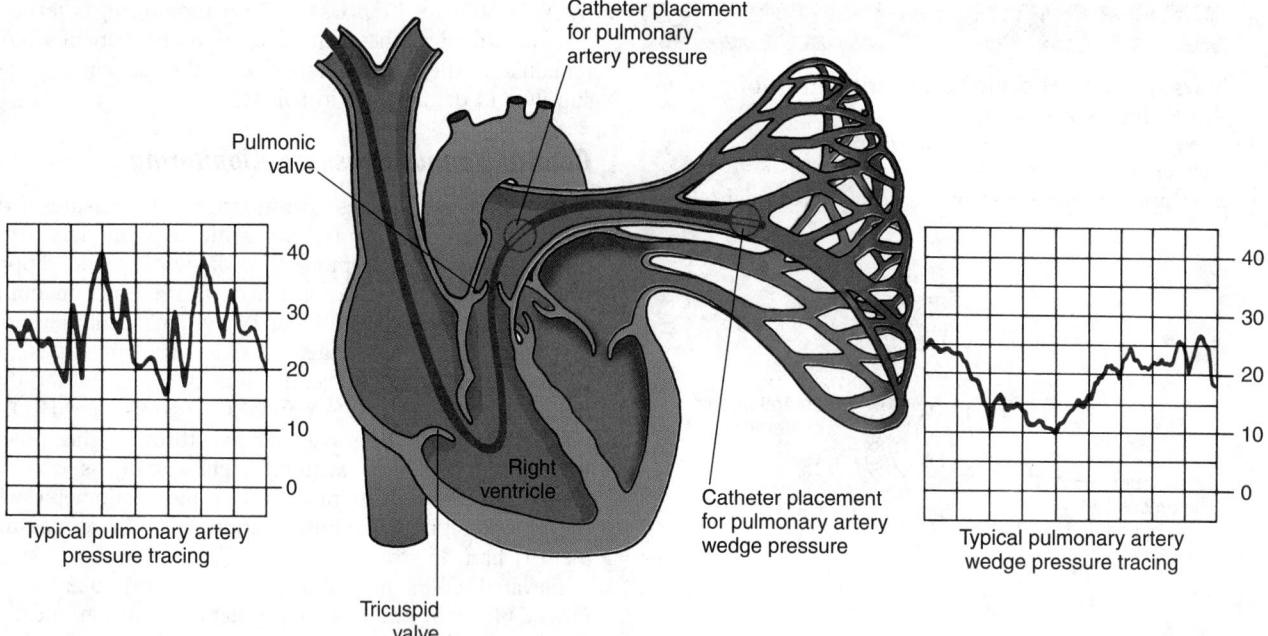

Figure 35–22. Cardiac pressure waveforms can be visualized on the oscilloscope.

the heart is used to induce and evaluate lethal dysrhythmias and conduction abnormalities. Clients who have survived cardiac arrest, have recurrent tachydysrhythmias, or experience unexplained syncopal episodes may be referred for EPS. Induction of the dysrhythmia during EPS permits accurate diagnosis of the dysrhythmia and aids in the search for an effective treatment. These procedures hold risks similar to those for cardiac catheterization and are performed in a special catheterization laboratory, where conditions are strictly controlled and immediate treatment is available for any adverse effects.

CLIENT PREPARATION. The preparation of clients for EPS parallels that of clients undergoing cardiac catheterization (see earlier). Clients may express fear or anxiety, because attempts are made to induce lethal dysrhythmias similar to those that led to the initial hospitalization or resuscitation. The nurse reassures clients that EPS is a planned, controlled event, and immediate treatment will be available for any dysrhythmia induced during the studies. An electrophysiologist (a physician who specializes in these studies) usually explains the purpose of the studies; describes the procedure, including benefits and risks; and obtains a written consent.

PROCEDURE. The client is taken to a cardiac catheterization laboratory or a similar laboratory where he or she is asked to assume a supine position on an x-ray table. Electrodes are attached for continuous ECG monitoring. Defibrillation pads are placed on the client's chest and back. After the nurse or the technician prepares the insertion site, the electrophysiologist injects a local anesthetic, and a multipolar electrode catheter is inserted. The catheter is advanced, guided by fluoroscopy, until electrodes rest in the right atrium, adjacent to the bundle of His,

and in the right ventricle. Additional electrodes may be placed for endocardial mapping.

During EPS, baseline conduction times can be measured: the AH interval (conduction time from the right atrium through the His bundle) and the HV interval (conduction time from the proximal His bundle to the ventricular myocardium). The catheter may be programmed to pace at varying rates to determine SA and AV node function, or it may be programmed to deliver premature paced stimuli in an effort to initiate and evaluate the client's tachydysrhythmia.

If the dysrhythmia is induced, it may terminate spontaneously or be treated by the physician. The physician might elect to use properly timed stimuli, rapid pacing, medications, or countershock to terminate the dysrhythmia.

The client is advised to tell the staff of any symptoms that he or she is experiencing. During rapid pacing, the client may be aware of the rapid heartbeat and state that he or she is experiencing palpitations. The client may also experience chest pain or loss of consciousness if he or she becomes hypotensive. The client often experiences back discomfort during the procedure, because he or she must remain supine for 2–6 hours. Pain may develop at the insertion site as the anesthetic wears off.

FOLLOW-UP CARE. The follow-up care is the same as that for the client who has undergone cardiac catheterization. The nurse may provide comfort measures to alleviate back discomfort, including massage and position changes. If the client lost consciousness during the procedure and received electrical cardioversion or defibrillation, the client may complain of chest discomfort over the area where the electrical current was applied. The nurse assesses the skin for any signs of redness, swelling, or burns. In addi-

Chart 35–6

Nursing Care Highlight: Obtaining a Central Venous Pressure Reading

1. Position the water manometer so that the zero mark or the air-fluid interface is at the same height as the phlebostatic axis.

2. Turn the stopcock as shown to fill the manometer with IV fluid.
3. Turn the stopcock as shown to record the CVP. With each respiration, the fluid level in the manometer should fluctuate. When the level has stabilized, read the highest level of the fluid column.
4. Return the stopcock to the position shown to resume the flow of IV fluid to the client.

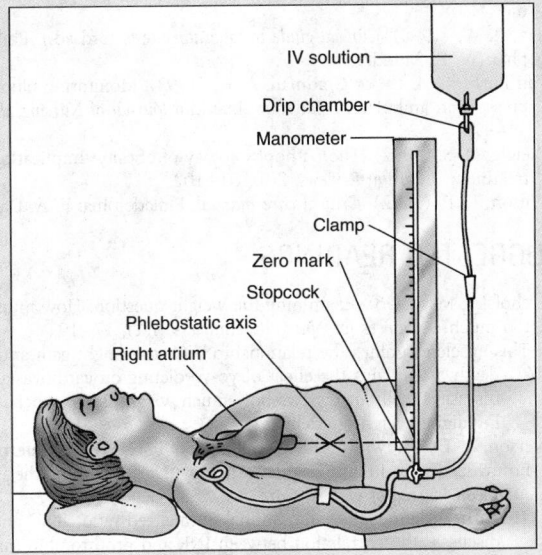

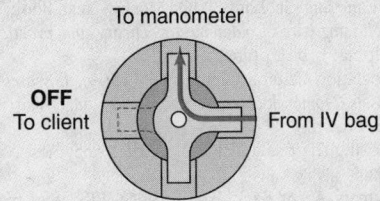

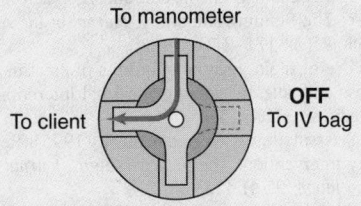

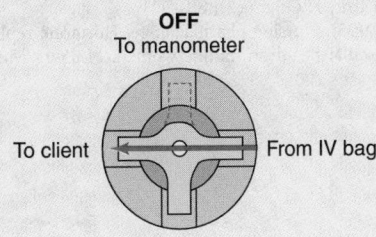

---

tion, the client might describe a loss of memory of the events during the procedure, and the nurse needs to provide reassurance and calmly explain the events of the procedure.

SELECTED BIBLIOGRAPHY

American Heart Association. (1996). *Heart and stroke facts: 1996 statistical supplement* (pp. 1–23). Dallas: Author.

*American Nurses' Association Division on Medical-Surgical Nursing Practice and American Heart Association Council on Cardiovascular Nursing. (1981). *Standards of cardiovascular nursing practice.* Kansas City, MO: American Nurses' Association.

Burke, M. M., & Walsh, M. B. (1997). *Gerontologic nursing: Wholistic care of the older adult* (2nd ed.). St. Louis, MO: C. V. Mosby

Chernecky, C. C., & Berger, B. J. (1997). *Laboratory tests and diagnostic procedures* (2nd ed.). Philadelphia: W. B. Saunders.

Corbett, J. V. (1996). *Laboratory tests and diagnostic procedures with nursing diagnoses* (4th ed.) Stamford, CT: Appleton & Lange.

Croft, J. B., Keenan, N. L., Sheridan, D. P., Wheeler, F., & Speers, M. (1995). Waist to hip ratio in biracial population: Measurement, implications, and cautions for using guidelines to define high risk for cardiovascular disease. *Journal of the American Dietetic Association, 95*(1), 60–64.

*Department of Health and Human Services. (1990). *Healthy people 2000: National health promotion and disease prevention objectives.* Washington, D.C.: U. S. Government Printing Office.

Gerchofsky, M. (1996). Examining the weight question: How much is too much? *Advances for Nurse Practitioners, 4*(1), 17–19.

*Hochrein, M., & Sohl, L. (1992). Heart smart: A guide to cardiac tests. *American Journal of Nursing, 92*(12), 22–25.

Hogsten, P. (1997). Hemodynamic monitoring. In P. S. Kidd (Ed.), *High acuity nursing* (pp. 227–256). Stamford, CT: Appleton & Lange.

Houston, S., Eagen, M., Freeborg, S., & Dougherty, D. (1996). A comparison of structured preheart catheterization information on mood states and coping resources. *Applied Nursing Research, 9*(4), 189–194.

Jarvis, C. (1996). *Physical examination and health assessment* (2nd ed.). Philadelphia: W. B. Saunders.

Keller, C., Fleury, J., & Bergstrom, D. L. (1995). Risk factors for coronary heart disease in African American women. *Cardiovascular Nursing, 31*(2), 9–14.

*Kirkendall, W. M., Feinleib, M. D., & Fries, E. D. (1988). *Recommendations for human blood pressure determination by sphygmomanometers.* Dallas: American Heart Association.

Kirton, C. A. (1995). Assessing normal heart sounds. *Nursing95, 25*(5), 34–35.

Kottke, T., Weidman, W., & Nguyon, Y. (1996). Prevention of coronary heart disease. In E. R. Guiliani (Ed.), *Mayo Clinic practice of cardiology* (3rd ed.). St. Louis, MO: C. V. Mosby.

Krenzer, M. E. (1995). Peripheral vascular assessment: Finding your ways through arteries and veins. *AACN Clinical Issues: Advanced Practice in Acute and Critical Care, 6*(4) 631–644.

Mahaffey, T. (1995). Cardiac catheterization. In N. Urban (Ed.), *Guidelines for critical care nursing.* St. Louis, MO: Mosby–Year Book.

Miller, C. A. (1995). *Nursing care of older adults: Theory and practice* (2nd ed.). Philadelphia: J. B. Lippincott.

*New York Heart Association Criteria Committee. (1964). *Diseases of the heart and blood vessels: Nomenclature and criteria for diagnosis* (6th ed.). Boston: Little, Brown.

Owen, A. (1995). Tracking the rise and fall of cardiac enzymes. *Nursing 95, 25*(5), 34–38.

Pooler-Lunse, C., Barkman, A., & Back, B. F. (1996). Effects of modified positioning and mobilization on back pain and delayed bleeding in patients who had received heparin and undergone angiography: A pilot study. *Heart and Lung, 25*(2), 117–122.

Posner, B. M., et al. (1995). Secular trends in diet and risk factors for cardiovascular disease: The Framingham study. *Journal of the American Dietetic Association, 95*(2), 171–179.

Puleo, P., et al. (1994). Use of rapid assay of subforms of creatine kinase MB to diagnose and rule out acute myocardial infarction. *New England Journal of Medicine, 331*(9), 561–566.

Robinson, J., Hoerr, S., Petersmark, K., & Anderson, J. (1995). Redefining success in obesity intervention: The new paradigm. *Journal of the American Dietetic Association, 95*(4) 422–423.

Scher, H. E. (1995). Chest pain: Developing rapid assessment skills. *Orthopedic Nursing, 14*(3), 30–34.

Severson, A. L., Baldwin, L. R., & Deloughty, T. G. (1996). International normalized ratio in anticoagulant therapy: Understanding the issues. *American Journal of Critical Care, 6*(2), 88–92.

Sharts-Hopro, N. C. (1995). Nursing pharmacology: Hormone replacement and cardiovascular health in midlife women. *MedSurg Nursing, 4*(4), 314–316.

Sims, L. K., D'Amico, D., Stiesmeyer, J. K., & Webster, J. A. (1995). *Health assessment in nursing.* Redwood City, CA: Addison-Wesley.

Strimike, C. (1996). New procedures: Understanding intravascular ultrasound. *American Journal of Nursing, 96*(6), 40–44.

Sullivan, M. J. (1994). New trends in cardiac rehabilitation in patients with chronic heart failure. *Progress in Cardiovascular Nursing, 9*(1), 13–21.

Swearingen, R. L., & Keen, J. L. (1995). *Manual of critical care* (3rd ed.). St. Louis, MO: Mosby Year Book.

*Thompson, E. J. (1993). Transesophageal echocardiography: A new window on the heart and great vessels. *Critical Care Nurse, 13*, 55–65.

Tietz, R. W. (1995). *Clinical guide to laboratory tests* (3rd ed.). Philadelphia: W. B. Saunders.

*Van Bushirk, M. C., & Gradman, A. H. (1993). Monitoring blood pressure in ambulatory patients. *American Journal of Nursing, 93*(6), 44–47.

*Weigle, D. S. (1992). The pathophysiology of obesity: Implications for treatment. *Clinician Reviews, 2*(5), 81–102.

*Wilson, R. F. (1992). *Critical care manual.* Philadelphia: F. A. Davis.

SUGGESTED READINGS

Gerchofsky, M. (1996). Examining the weight question: How much is too much? *Advances for Nurse Practitioners, 4*(1), 17–19.
This article examines the relationship between weight gain and early death. It explains the effect of yo-yo dieting on cardiovascular disease. Finally, it reviews how much weight is too much and highlights weight guidelines.

Severson, A. L., Baldwin, L. R., & Deloughty, T. G. (1997). International normalized ratio in anticoagulant therapy: Understanding the issues. *American Journal of Critical Care, 6*(2), 88–92.
This article defines the international normalized ratio (INR) and discusses the correlation between INR and prothrombin time (PT). It explains why it is beneficial to monitor the INR rather than the PT.

Tremko, L. (1997). Understanding diagnostic cardiac catheterization. *American Journal of Nursing, 97*(2), 16Q–16R.
This article describes the procedure of cardiac catheterization. After discussing preprocedure care and client education, it describes postprocedure care, including the prevention and control of hemorrhage.

Chapter 36

INTERVENTIONS FOR CLIENTS WITH DYSRHYTHMIAS

Cardiac dysrhythmias are disturbances of cardiac electrical impulse formation, conduction, or both. Many diseases can affect the electrical activity of the heart, causing dysrhythmias. Although more common in the elderly, dysrhythmias may occur in infants, children, and adults. Many dysrhythmias are benign. Some cause hemodynamic instability. A few result in cardiac arrest. To understand dysrhythmias and to interpret these disturbances correctly, the nurse must understand cardiac electrophysiology, the conduction system of the heart, and the principles of electrocardiography.

REVIEW OF CARDIAC ELECTROPHYSIOLOGY
Electrophysiologic Properties

The electrophysiologic properties of cardiac cells regulate heart rate and rhythm. Specialized cardiac muscle cells possess unique properties: automaticity, excitability, conductivity, and contractility.

Automaticity

Automaticity (spontaneous depolarization) is the ability of cardiac cells to generate an electrical impulse spontaneously and repetitively. Normally, only primary pacemaker cells possess this property. Under certain conditions, such

as myocardial ischemia and infarction, however, any cardiac cell may exhibit this property, generating electrical impulses independently and creating dysrhythmias.

Excitability

Excitability is the ability of nonpacemaker cardiac cells to respond to an electrical impulse generated from pacemaker cells and to depolarize. Depolarization occurs when the normally negatively charged cells develop a positive charge.

Conductivity

Conductivity is the ability to transmit an electrical stimulus from cell membrane to cell membrane. Consequently, excitable cells depolarize in rapid succession from cell to cell until all cells have depolarized. This wave of depolarization gives rise to the deflections of the electrocardiogram (ECG) waveforms that are recognized as the P wave and the QRS complex.

Contractility

Contractility is the ability of atrial and ventricular muscle cells to shorten their fiber length in response to electrical stimulation, generating sufficient pressure to propel blood forward. This is the mechanical activity of the heart.

Action Potential

The cardiac cell membrane (sarcolemma) exhibits selective permeability to ions. This creates an electrical imbalance, known as an *action potential,* across the cell membrane.

The cardiac cell at rest has an internal negative charge, whereas the charge outside the cell is positive. This state of electrical imbalance of the resting cell is called *resting membrane potential.* Two types of cardiac cells exist: fast-response cells (myocardial and Purkinje cells) and slow-response cells (nodal, or pacemaker, cells).

Fast-Response Cells

When myocardial and Purkinje cells are at rest, they have a negative internal charge that results from a small amount of potassium, a positive ion, leaving the cells. The outside of the cell, having gained potassium, has a positive charge. Positive charged cells are ready for action. The action potential of fast-response cells consists of several phases (Fig. 36–1).

Phase 0

Phase 0 is the phase of rapid depolarization. A stimulus from an impulse generated from pacemaker cells reaches the excitable myocardial and Purkinje cells. The stimulus causes sodium, a positive ion, to diffuse rapidly into the cells. The cells now develop an internal positive charge, while the outside of the cells becomes negative. This process is called *depolarization.* As depolarization occurs from cell to cell, a wave of positive current is created. The ECG lead system senses this current and inscribes a P wave during atrial depolarization or a QRS complex during ventricular depolarization.

Phase 1

Phase 1 is the phase of early rapid repolarization. Sodium channels are inactivated. As a small amount of positive potassium ions leaves the cells and a small amount of negative chloride ions enters the cells, the internal charge becomes nearly electrically equal with the outside of the cells.

Phase 2

Phase 2 is the plateau phase. Slow calcium channels allow calcium ions to enter the cells. Sodium may also enter via slow channels. These inward currents are balanced by an outward current of potassium ions leaving the cells, thus maintaining a membrane potential that is nearly equal electrically. The calcium influx into cells triggers the initiation of muscle contraction. Phases 1 and 2 in ventricular myocardial and Purkinje cells are reflected by the ST segment on the ECG.

Phase 3

Phase 3 is the phase of rapid repolarization. The cells regain their negative charge as potassium ions leave the cells while the other channels are inactivated, allowing the cells to become negatively charged again. This process of repolarization, or electrical recovery of cells, is reflected by the T wave on the ECG.

Phase 4

During the beginning of phase 4, a sodium-potassium pump is responsible for actively pumping sodium out of the cells and potassium back into the cells, against their concentration gradients. Adenosine triphosphate (ATP)

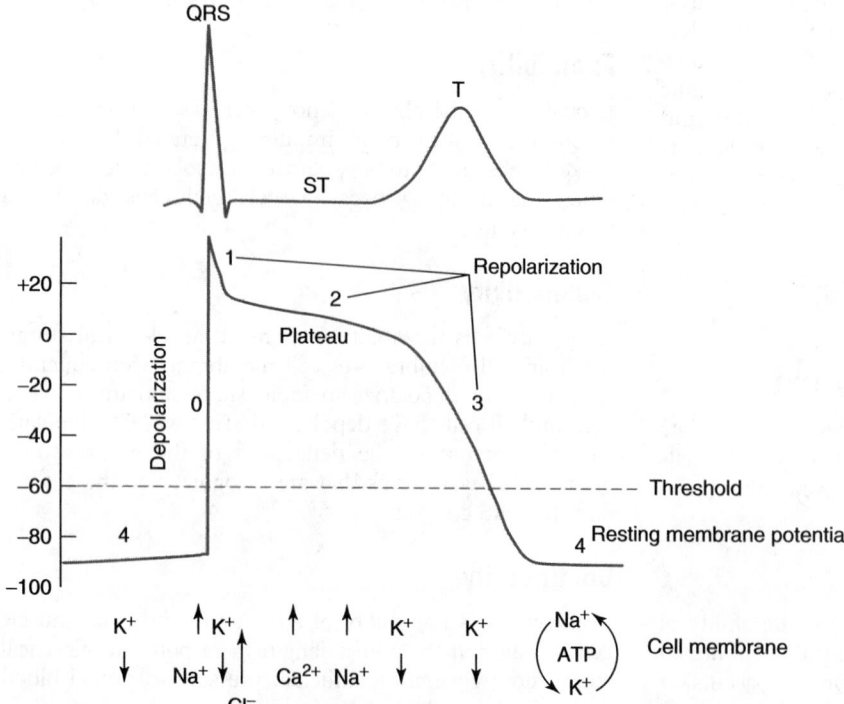

Figure 36–1. Action potential of a fast-response cell (muscle cell). Exchange of ions across the cell membrane occurs at different points of the action potential. At rest, the inside of the cardiac cell is more negatively charged than the outside of the cell, and the cell membrane is more permeable to potassium (K^+) than to sodium (Na^+) ions. With a sufficient electrical stimulus, the cell membrane becomes more permeable to Na^+. As Na^+ enters the cell, the inside becomes positively charged (Phase 0, depolarization). Sodium channels become inactivated. K^+ leaves the cell, and chloride (Cl^-) enters the cell, decreasing the positive charge (Phase 1, early repolarization). Calcium (Ca^{2+}) and Na^+ ions enter the cell while K^+ leaves the cell (Phase 2, plateau), allowing Ca^{2+} to initiate muscle contraction. K^+ leaves the cell (Phase 3, repolarization), returning the cell to its negative state. K^+ regains dominance over Na^+ diffusion and establishes equilibrium (Phase 4, resting membrane potential) before another stimulus is elicited.

provides energy. Resting membrane potential is then restored.

Slow-Response Cells

The action potential of slow-response cells (nodal, or pacemaker, cells) differs from that of fast-response cells (Fig. 36-2).

Phase 4

Phase 4 is the phase of spontaneous diastolic depolarization. It is an unstable phase, providing automaticity in pacemaker cells. This is accomplished through a slow inward current of calcium and sodium into the nodal cells. The cells thus decrease their negative charge and spontaneously reach their activation threshold, initiating an action potential. The faster the threshold is reached, the faster the heart rate becomes.

Phase 0

Phase 0, or depolarization, occurs after the cells reach their activation threshold. As calcium and sodium continue to enter the nodal cells, the electrical charge of the cells becomes less and less negative. The nodal cells then generate, or fire, an electrical impulse, which is again conducted to excitable fast-response cells.

Phase 3

Slow-response cells do not have phases 1 and 2. Slow repolarization begins (phase 3) as potassium leaves the nodal cells, causing the return of an internal negative charge (rapid repolarization). A sodium-potassium pump is then activated to return the electrolytes to their area of greatest concentration. This phase prepares the process again for the next cycle.

The sinoatrial (SA) node, which is the first structure in the heart's conduction system, is the primary pacemaker. It has the greatest number of nodal cells and conse-

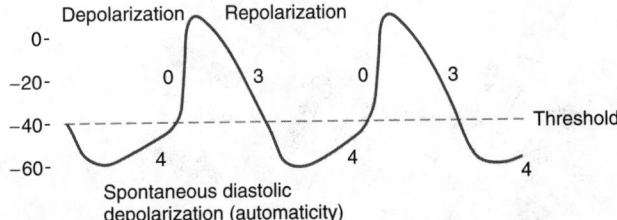

Figure 36-2. Action potential of a slow-response cell (pacemaker cell). At rest, this cell is less negative than the muscle cell. During Phase 4 (spontaneous diastolic depolarization), the pacemaker cell membrane is more permeable to Ca^{2+} and Na^+ ions than to K^+ ions. Ca^{2+} and Na^+ enter the cell, decreasing the negative charge (the property of automaticity) until threshold is reached. Ca^{2+} and Na^+ continue to enter the cell until the cell is no longer negatively charged (Phase 0, depolarization), and the cell fires an electrical stimulus. The cell is now more permeable to K^+ and less permeable to Ca^{2+} and Na^+. K^+ leaves the cell, returning the cell to its negative state (Phase 3, repolarization). The slow Ca^{2+} and Na^+ channels regain dominance over K^+, creating instability in the resting state (Phase 4), allowing the process to begin again for another cycle.

quently the fastest rate of automaticity. Secondary, or subsidiary, pacemakers have fewer nodal cells and therefore a slower rate of automaticity. Subsidiary pacemakers include atrioventricular (AV) junctional cells and ventricular Purkinje cells. They can serve as "escape," or latent, pacemakers when the primary pacemaker becomes dysfunctional.

CARDIAC CONDUCTION SYSTEM

The cardiac conduction system consists of specialized cells (Fig. 36-3). It is responsible for the generation and conduction of electrical impulses that cause atrial and ventricular depolarization. The conduction system consists of the sinoatrial node, atrioventricular (AV) junctional area, and bundle branch system.

Sinoatrial Node

The conduction system begins with the sinoatrial (SA) node (also called the sinus node), located close to the epicardial surface of the right atrium near its junction with the superior vena cava. The SA node is the heart's primary pacemaker. It can spontaneously and rhythmically generate electrical impulses at a rate of 60 to 100 per minute, possessing the greatest degree of automaticity.

The SA node is richly innervated by the sympathetic and parasympathetic nervous systems, which accelerate and decelerate the rate of discharge of the sinus node, respectively. This process results in changes in the heart rate.

It is now believed that impulses from the sinus node propagate directly through atrial muscle without specialized pathways. The impulses lead to atrial depolarization and are reflected by a P wave on the ECG trace. Atrial muscle contraction should follow. Within the atrial muscle are slow and fast pathways, leading to the AV node.

Atrioventricular Junctional Area

The AV junctional area consists of a transitional cell zone, the AV node itself, and the His bundle. The AV node lies just beneath the right atrial endocardium, between the tricuspid valve and the ostium of the coronary sinus. Here, T cells (transitional cells) cause impulses to slow down or be delayed in the AV node before proceeding to the ventricles. This delay is reflected by the PR segment on the ECG. This slow conduction provides a physiologic delay, allowing the atria to contract before ventricular stimulation and contraction. Atrial contraction, known as the "atrial kick," contributes 15% to 30% of additional blood volume for a greater cardiac output. Nodal cells in the AV junctional area may occasionally demonstrate automaticity, giving rise to junctional beats or rhythms. The AV node is innervated by both the sympathetic and the parasympathetic nervous systems. The His bundle connects with the distal portion of the AV node and continues on to perforate the interventricular septum.

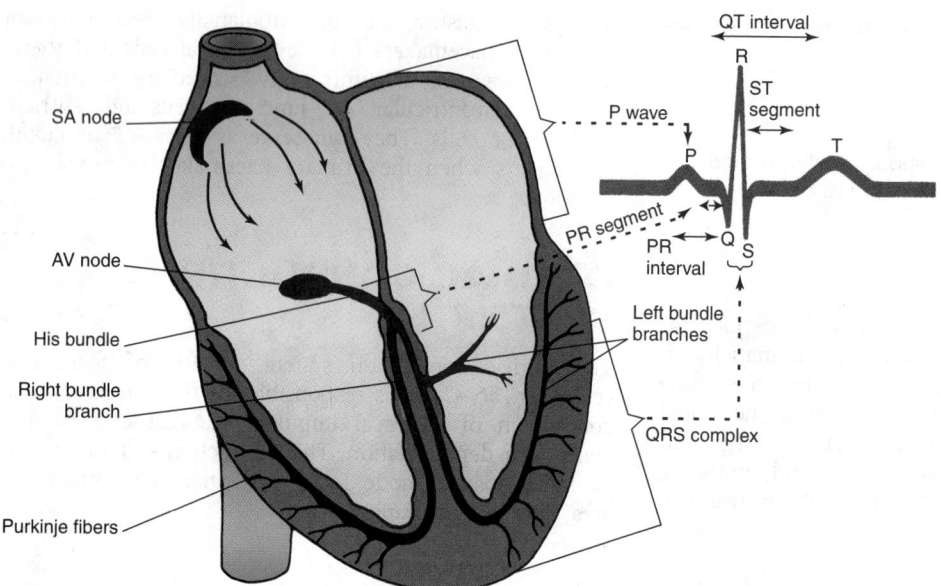

Figure 36–3. The cardiac conduction system.

Bundle Branch System

The His bundle extends as a right bundle branch down the right side of the interventricular septum to the apex of the right ventricle. On the left side, it extends as a left bundle branch, which further divides into two fascicles.

At the ends of both right and left bundle branch systems are the Purkinje fibers. These fibers are an interweaving network located on the endocardial surface of both ventricles, from apex to bases. The fibers then partially penetrate into the myocardium.

Purkinje cells make up the His bundle, bundle branches, and terminal Purkinje fibers. These cells are responsible for the rapid conduction of electrical impulses throughout the ventricles, leading to ventricular depolarization and the subsequent ventricular muscle contraction. A few nodal cells in the ventricles may also occasionally demonstrate automaticity, giving rise to ventricular beats or rhythms.

ELECTROCARDIOGRAPHY

The electrocardiogram (ECG) provides a graphic representation of cardiac electrical activity. The weak cardiac electrical currents are transmitted to the body surface. Electrodes, consisting of conductive medium on an adhesive pad, are placed on various sites on the body and attached to cables or wires connected to an ECG machine or to a monitor. The cardiac electrical current is transmitted via the electrodes and through the lead wires to the machine or monitor, which displays the cardiac electrical activity.

A lead provides one view of the heart's electrical activity. Multiple leads, or views, can be obtained. Electrode placement is the same for male and female clients.

Lead systems are made up of a positive pole and a negative pole. An imaginary line joining these two poles is called the *lead axis*. The direction of electrical current flow in the heart is the *cardiac axis*. The relationship between the cardiac axis and the lead axis is responsible for the deflections seen on the ECG pattern:

- The baseline is the isoelectric line. It occurs when there is no current flow in the heart after complete depolarization and also after complete repolarization. Positive deflections occur above this line, and negative deflections occur below it. Deflections represent depolarization and repolarization of cells.
- If the direction of electrical current flow in the heart (cardiac axis) is parallel to the lead axis with the current moving toward the positive pole, a monophasic (single-component) positive deflection is inscribed (Fig. 36–4A).
- If the cardiac axis is parallel to the lead axis but the current is moving away from the positive pole, toward

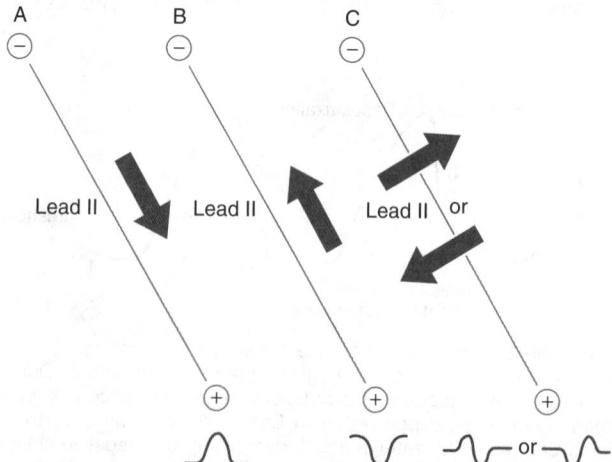

Figure 36–4. *A,* The cardiac axis (*bold arrow*) is parallel to the lead axis (the line between the negative and the positive electrodes), going toward the positive electrode; a positive deflection is inscribed. *B,* The cardiac axis is parallel to the lead axis, going toward the negative electrode; a negative deflection is inscribed. *C,* The cardiac axis is perpendicular to the lead axis, going neither toward the positive nor toward the negative electrode; a biphasic deflection is inscribed.

the negative pole, a monophasic negative deflection is inscribed (Fig. 36–4B).

- If the cardiac axis is exactly perpendicular to the lead axis, with the current crossing the lead axis, a biphasic (two-component) deflection is inscribed (Fig. 36–4C).

Lead Systems

The standard 12-lead ECG consists of 12 leads (or views) of the heart's electrical activity. Six of the leads are called limb leads because the electrodes are placed on the client's four limbs in the frontal plane. The remaining six leads are called chest (precordial) leads because the electrodes are placed on the client's chest in the horizontal plane (see Chap. 35).

Limb Leads

Standard bipolar limb leads consist of a positive and a negative electrode, which determine the lead axis, as well as a reference, or ground, electrode. Bipolar leads can be obtained by using a monitor with either three or five electrode cables, or a 12-lead ECG machine. Leads I, II, and III are bipolar leads (Table 36–1 and Chap. 35).

Unipolar limb leads consist of a positive electrode only. These leads can be obtained only by using a monitor with four or five electrode cables or a 12-lead ECG machine. The unipolar limb leads are leads aVR, aVL, and aVF, with "a" meaning augmented. "V" is a designation for a unipolar lead. The third letter denotes the positive electrode placement: "R" for right arm, "L" for left arm, and "F" for foot (left leg). The positive electrode is at one end of the lead axis. The other end is the center of the electrical field, at approximately the center of the heart (Table 36–1).

Chest Leads

Chest (precordial) leads are also unipolar, or V, leads and therefore can be obtained only from a monitor with five electrode cables or a 12-lead ECG machine, which usually has 10 electrode cables. There are six chest leads, determined by the placement of the chest electrode. The four limb electrodes are placed on the extremities, as designated on each electrode (right arm, left arm, right leg, and left leg). The fifth (chest) electrode on a monitor system is the positive, or exploring, electrode, and is placed in designated positions to obtain the desired chest lead (see Table 36–1).

TABLE 36–1

Electrode Placement for 12 Leads			
Lead	**Negative Electrode**	**Positive Electrode**	**Ground Electrode**
I	• Right arm, or under the right clavicle	• Left arm, or under the left clavicle	• Right leg, or lowest rib, left mid-clavicular line
II	• Right arm, or under the right clavicle	• Left leg, or lowest rib, left mid-clavicular line	• Right leg, or under the left clavicle
III	• Left arm, or under the left clavicle	• Left leg, or lowest rib, left mid-clavicular line	• Right leg, or under the right clavicle
aVR	• Average potential of left arm (or under the left clavicle) and left leg (or lowest rib, left mid-clavicular line)	• Right arm, or under the right clavicle	• Right leg, or lowest rib, right mid-clavicular line
aVL	• Average potential of right arm (or under the right clavicle) and left leg (or lowest rib, left mid-clavicular line)	• Left arm, or under the left clavicle	• Same as for aVR
aVF	• Average potential of right arm (or under the right clavicle) and left arm (or under the left clavicle)	• Left leg, or lowest rib, left mid-clavicular line	• Same as for aVR
V_1	• Average potential of right arm, left arm, and left leg	• Fourth intercostal space (ICS), right sternal border	• Same as for aVR
V_2	• Same as for V_1	• Fourth ICS, left sternal border	• Same as for aVR
V_3	• Same as for V_1	• Midway between V_2 and V_4	• Same as for aVR
V_4	• Same as for V_1	• Fifth ICS, left mid-clavicular line	• Same as for aVR
V_5	• Same as for V_1	• Horizontal to V_4, left anterior axillary line	• Same as for aVR
V_6	• Same as for V_1	• Horizontal to V_4, left mid-axillary line	• Same as for aVR

The nurse instructs the female client with large breasts to displace and hold the left breast so that electrode position can be accurate.

Technicians are commonly trained to take 12-lead ECGs in all health care settings. It is imperative that the technician bring any suspected abnormality to the attention of a nurse or physician. A nurse may direct a technician to take a 12-lead ECG on a client experiencing chest pain to observe for diagnostic changes, but it is ultimately the physician's responsibility to interpret the ECG.

Continuous Electrocardiographic Monitoring

For continuous ECG monitoring, the electrodes are not placed on the client's limbs because movement of the extremities causes "noise," or motion artifact, on the ECG signal. The nurse places the electrodes on the client's trunk, a more stable area, to minimize such artifacts and to obtain a clearer signal. If the monitoring system provides five electrode cables, the nurse places the electrodes as follows:

- Right arm electrode just below the right clavicle
- Left arm electrode just below the left clavicle
- Right leg electrode on the lowest palpable rib, on the right midclavicular line
- Left leg electrode on the lowest palpable rib, on the left midclavicular line
- The fifth electrode placed to obtain one of the six chest leads

With this placement, the monitor lead select control may be changed to provide lead I, II, III, aVR, aVL, or aVF or one chest lead. The monitor automatically alters the polarity of the electrodes to provide the lead selected.

If the monitoring system provides only three electrode cables, the nurse places the right arm, the left arm, and the left leg electrodes as described. In this case, the lead select provides only lead I, II, or III.

The popular MCL_1 lead is a modified (M) bipolar chest (C) lead. It approximates the V_1 lead without requiring a five-electrode cable monitoring system because it is a bipolar lead system. To obtain MCL_1, the nurse places the negative electrode just below the left (L) midclavicle and the positive electrode in the V_1 position. The ground electrode may be placed anywhere but is usually placed under the right clavicle. The nurse uses this lead for bedside or telemetry monitoring to differentiate left from right electrical activity, such as left from right bundle branch block or left from right premature ventricular complexes (PVCs), and to differentiate certain supraventricular beats from ventricular ectopic beats. The MCL_1 lead provides a right-sided view of cardiac electrical activity.

Another bipolar lead, MCL_6, is frequently used. It can be achieved by placing the negative and ground electrodes as for MCL_1 and moving the positive electrode to the V_6 position. This approximates the V_6 lead and pro-

vides a left-sided view of cardiac electrical activity. It is used for the same reasons as MCL_1.

The clarity of continuous ECG monitor recordings is affected by skin preparation and electrode quality. To optimize signal transmission, the nurse or assistive nursing personnel (ANP) decrease skin impedance by cleaning the skin with soap and water. The nurse or ANP then shaves the area if it is hairy, wipes the electrode sites with an alcohol or other skin preparation pad, and dries the sites well. The gel on each electrode must be moist and fresh. The nurse or ANP attaches the electrode to the lead cable, rubs the skin briskly with a gauze square or a washcloth (facecloth) until the skin is slightly reddened, and then rolls the electrode onto the site for proper contact. This action rubs off surface cells and increases capillary blood flow to the area to improve transmission of electrical activity. The nurse or ANP ensures that the contact site does not have any lotion, tincture, or other substance on it that increases skin impedance. Electrodes cannot be placed on abraded or irritated skin or over scar tissue. The application of electrodes may be done by a nursing assistant under the direction of the nurse, who must determine which lead to select. The nurse assesses the quality of the ECG rhythm transmission to the monitoring system and is responsible for assessment and management of the client.

ECG cables may be attached directly to a wall-mounted monitor (a hard-wired system) if the client's activity is restricted to bed rest and sitting in a chair, as in a critical care unit. For an ambulatory client, the ECG cable is attached to a battery-operated transmitter (a telemetry system) held in a pouch worn by the client. The client's ECG is transmitted via antennae located in strategic places, usually in the ceiling, to a remote monitor. This device allows the client freedom of movement within a certain radius without losing transmission of the ECG.

In the acute care setting, some institutions employ monitor technicians. These technicians are educated in ECG rhythm interpretation and are responsible for watching a bank of monitors on a unit, printing ECG rhythm strips routinely and PRN, interpreting rhythms, and communicating with the nurse to report the client's rhythm and significant changes. This technical support is particularly helpful on a telemetry unit that does not have monitors at the bedside. The nurse is reasonably assured that the client's ECG rhythm is being monitored "continuously," though human nature dictates that some rhythms would not be observed by the technician. The nurse remains ultimately responsible for accurate ECG rhythm interpretation, as well as client assessment and management.

Some units have full-disclosure monitors, which continuously store a client's ECG rhythms in memory up to a maximum amount of time, allowing nurses and physicians to access and print these rhythms for more thorough assessment and management of clients with dysrhythmias.

Pre-hospital personnel, such as paramedics and EMTs with advanced training, frequently monitor a client's ECG rhythm at the scene and enroute to a health care facility. They function under medical direction and protocols but may also be in communication with a nurse.

Electrocardiographic Complexes, Segments, and Intervals

Complexes that make up a normal ECG consist of a P wave, a QRS complex, a T wave, and possibly a U wave. Segments include the PR segment, the ST segment, and the TP segment. Intervals include the PR interval, QRS duration, and the QT interval (Fig. 36–5).

The P Wave

The P wave is a deflection representing atrial depolarization. The morphologic configuration (shape) of the P wave may be a positive, negative, or biphasic deflection,

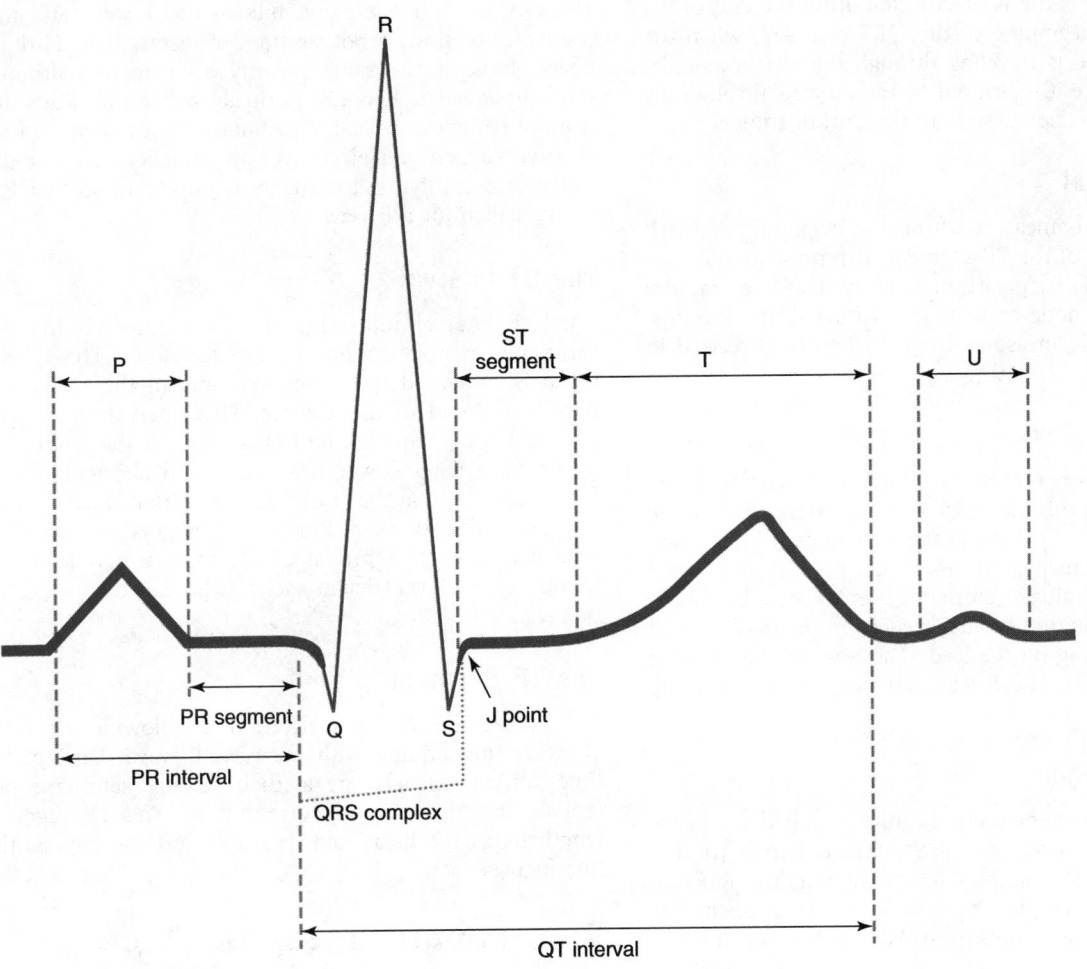

P wave:	Represents atrial depolarization.
PR segment:	Represents the time required for the impulse to travel through the AV node, where it is delayed, and through the bundle of His, bundle branches, and Purkinje fiber network, just before ventricular depolarization.
PR interval:	Represents the time required for atrial depolarization as well as impulse travel through the conduction system and Purkinje fiber network, inclusive of the P wave and PR segment. It is measured from the beginning of the P wave to the end of the PR segment.
QRS complex:	Represents ventricular depolarization and is measured from the beginning of the Q (or R) wave to the end of the S wave.
J point:	Represents the junction where the QRS complex ends and the ST segment begins.
ST segment:	Represents early ventricular repolarization.
T wave:	Represents ventricular repolarization.
U wave:	Represents late ventricular repolarization.
QT interval:	Represents the total time required for ventricular depolarization and repolarization and is measured from the beginning of the QRS complex to the end of the T wave.

Figure 36–5. The components of a normal electrocardiogram.

depending on the lead selected. When the electrical impulse is consistently generated from the SA node, the P waves have a consistent morphology in a given lead. If an impulse is then generated from a different (ectopic) focus, such as atrial tissue, the morphology of the P wave changes in that lead, indicating that an ectopic focus has fired.

The PR Segment

The PR segment is the isoelectric line from the end of the P wave to the beginning of the QRS complex, when the electrical impulse is traveling through the atrioventricular (AV) node, where it is delayed. It then travels through the ventricular conduction system to the Purkinje fibers.

The PR Interval

The PR interval is measured from the beginning of the P wave to the end of the PR segment. It represents the time required for atrial depolarization as well as the impulse delay in the AV node and the travel time to the Purkinje fibers. It normally measures from 0.12 to 0.20 second in duration.

The QRS Complex

The QRS complex represents ventricular depolarization. The morphology of the QRS complex depends on the lead selected. The Q wave is the first negative deflection and is not present in all leads. When present, it is small and represents initial ventricular septal depolarization. The R wave is the first positive deflection. It may be small or large, depending on the lead. The S wave is a negative deflection following the R wave and is not present in all leads.

The QRS Duration

The QRS duration represents the time required for depolarization of both ventricles. It is measured from the beginning of the QRS complex to the J-point (the junction where the QRS complex ends and the ST segment begins). It normally measures from 0.04 to 0.10 second.

The ST Segment

The ST segment is normally an isoelectric line and represents early ventricular repolarization. It occurs from the J-point to the beginning of the T wave. Its length varies with changes in the heart rate, the administration of medications, and electrolyte disturbances. It is normally not elevated more than 1 mm or depressed more than 0.5 mm from the isoelectric line as seen in the TP segment. Its amplitude is measured at a point 1.5 to 2 mm after the J-point. It is affected by myocardial ischemia or infarction, conduction abnormalities, and the administration of medications.

The T Wave

The T wave follows the ST segment and represents ventricular repolarization. It is usually positive, rounded, and slightly asymmetric. If an ectopic stimulus excites the ventricles during this time, it may cause ventricular irritability and possible cardiac arrest in the vulnerable heart. This is known as the *R-on-T phenomenon.* T waves may become tall and peaked, inverted (negative), or flat as a result of myocardial ischemia, potassium or calcium imbalances, administered medications, or autonomic nervous system effects.

The U Wave

The U wave, when present, follows the T wave and may result from slow repolarization of ventricular Purkinje fibers. It is of the same polarity as T waves, although generally smaller. It is not normally seen in all leads and is more common in lead V_3. Abnormal prominence of the U wave suggests an electrolyte abnormality or other disturbance. Identifying it correctly is important so that it is not mistaken for a P wave.

The QT Interval

The QT interval represents the total time required for ventricular depolarization and repolarization. The QT interval is measured from the beginning of the QRS complex to the end of the T wave. This interval varies with the client's age and sex and changes with the heart rate; lengthening with slower heart rates and shortening with faster rates. It may be prolonged by certain medications, electrolyte disturbances, Prinzmetal's angina, or subarachnoid hemorrhage. A prolonged QT interval may lead to a unique type of ventricular tachycardia called torsades de pointes.

The TP Segment

The TP segment is the isoelectric line following the T (or U) wave and ending with the next P wave. During this time, all cardiac cells are at their resting membrane potential, and there is no current flow. The TP segment lengthens as the heart rate decreases and shortens as the rate increases.

Electrocardiographic Paper

The ECG strip is printed on graph paper (Fig. 36–6), with each small block measuring 1 mm in height and width. ECG recorders and monitors are standardized at a speed of 25 mm/second. Time is measured on the horizontal axis. At this speed, each small block represents 0.04 second. Five small blocks make up one large block, defined by darker bold lines and representing 0.20 second. Five large blocks represent 1 second, whereas 30 large blocks represent 6 seconds. Vertical lines in the top margin of the graph paper are usually 15 large blocks apart, representing 3-second segments (Fig. 36–7).

Determination of Heart Rate

The heart rate may be estimated by counting the number of P-P intervals (atrial rate) or R-R intervals (ventricular rate) in 6 seconds and multiplying that number by 10 to calculate the rate for a full minute (Fig. 36–8). For accuracy, timing should begin on the P wave or the QRS

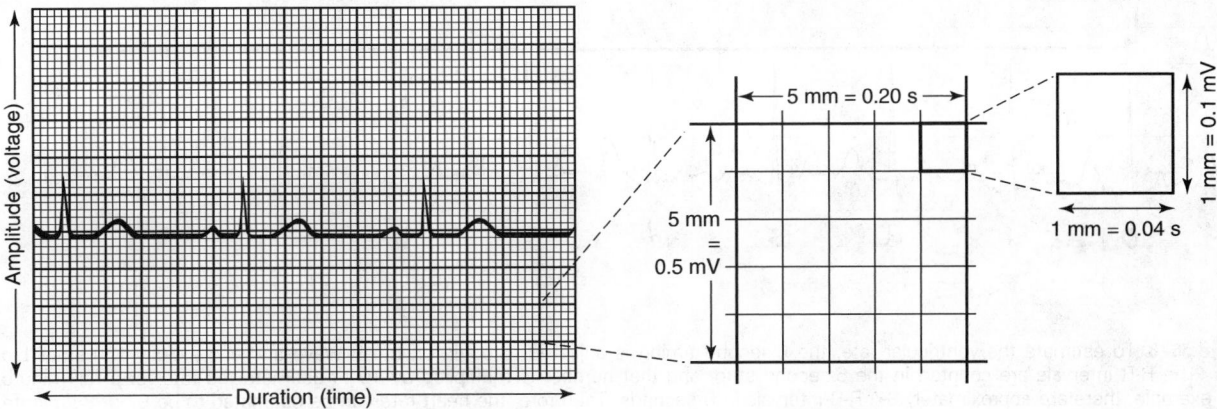

Figure 36–6. ECG waveforms are measured in amplitude (voltage) and duration (time).

complex and end exactly 30 large blocks (150 small blocks) later. The initial complex is the reference point and counts as zero. Subsequent complexes are counted until the end of 6 seconds, to include a fraction of the last interval: for example, if there are exactly seven R-R intervals, the heart rate is 70 beats per minute; if there are 9½ intervals, the heart rate is 95 beats per minute. This method may be used for both regular and irregular rhythms. It is called the 6-second strip method.

Another method, which may be used *only* if the rhythm is regular, relies on either of the following mathematic calculations:

- Count the number of small blocks in a P-P or R-R interval and divide into 1500 (the number of small blocks in 1 minute). For example, 20 small blocks equals a heart rate of 75 beats per minute (1500/20 = 75).
- Count the number of large blocks in an interval and divide into 300 (the number of large blocks in 1 minute). For example, three large blocks equals a heart rate of 100 beats per minute (300/3 = 100).

Commercially prepared ECG rate rulers are based on these calculations and may be used for regular rhythms.

Electrocardiographic Rhythm Analysis

Analysis of an ECG rhythm strip requires a systematic approach and is facilitated by the use of an ECG caliper (Chart 36–1):

1. *Analyze the P waves.* The nurse checks that the P wave morphology (shape) is consistent throughout the strip, indicating that atrial depolarization is occurring from impulses originating from one focus, normally the sinoatrial (SA) node. The nurse determines whether there is one P wave occurring before each QRS complex, establishing that a relationship exists between the P wave and the QRS complex. This relationship indicates that impulses from one focus are responsible for both atrial and ventricular depolarization. The nurse may observe more than one P wave shape, or more P waves than QRS

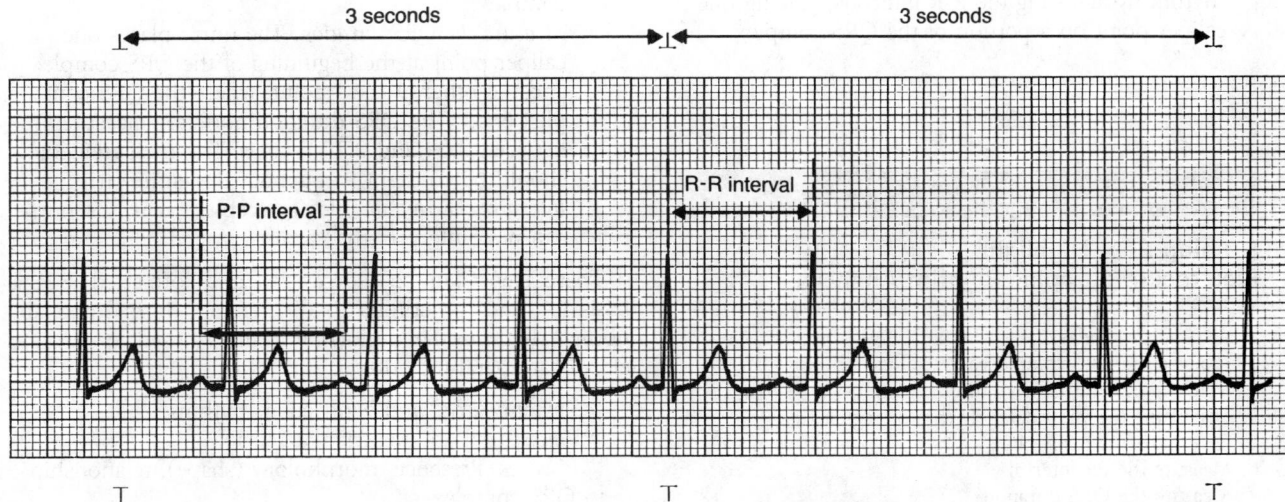

Figure 36–7. Each segment between the dark lines (above the monitor strip) represents 3 seconds, when the monitor is set at a speed of 25 mm/second.

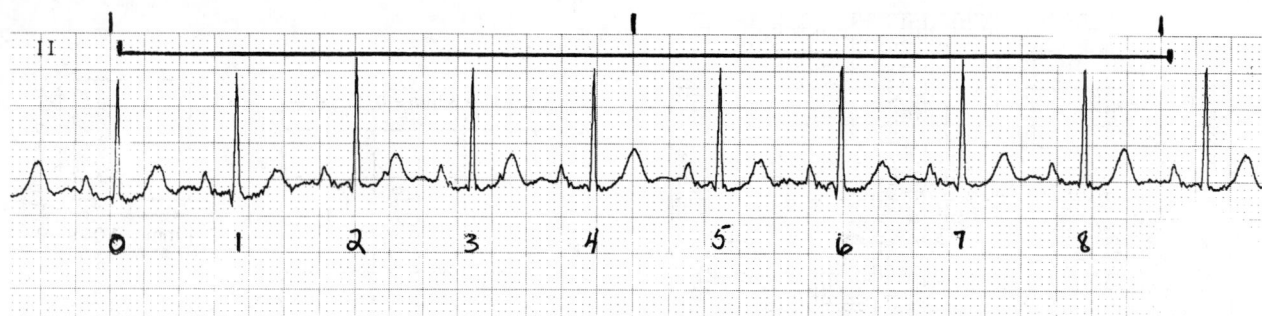

Figure 36–8. To estimate the ventricular rate, the 6-second timing is adjusted to begin on the R wave and end exactly 150 small blocks later. The R-R intervals are counted in the 6-second strip, and that number is multiplied by 10 to estimate the rate for a full minute. In this example, there are approximately 8¾ R-R intervals in 6 seconds. Therefore, the heart rate can be estimated to be 87 or 88/minute.

complexes, or absent P waves, or P waves coming after the QRS, each indicating that a dysrhythmia exists.

2. *Analyze the QRS complexes.* The nurse checks that the QRS complex morphology is consistent throughout the strip. The nurse may observe more than one QRS complex morphologic pattern or occasionally missing QRS complexes, indicating a dysrhythmia.

3. *Determine the atrial rhythm or regularity.* The nurse checks the regularity of the atrial rhythm by assessing the P-P intervals, placing one caliper point on a P wave and the other point on the next P wave. Then the caliper is moved from P wave to P wave along the entire strip ("walking out" the P waves) to determine the regularity of the rhythm. P waves of a different morphology (ectopic waves), if present, create an irregularity and do not walk out with the other P waves. A slight irregularity in the P-P intervals, varying no more than three small blocks, is considered essentially regular if the P waves are all of the same morphology.

4. *Determine the ventricular rhythm or regularity.* The nurse checks the regularity of the ventricular rhythm by assessing the R-R intervals, placing one caliper point on a portion of the QRS complex

(usually the most prominent portion of the deflection) and the other point on the same portion of the next QRS complex. The caliper is then moved from QRS complex to QRS complex along the entire strip (walking out the QRS complexes) to determine the regularity of the rhythm. QRS complexes of a different morphology (ectopic QRS complexes), if present, create an irregularity and do not walk out with the other QRS complexes. A slight irregularity of no more than three small blocks between intervals is considered essentially regular if the QRS complexes are all of the same morphology.

5. *Determine the heart rate.* If the atrial and ventricular rhythms are regular, the nurse may use any of the methods previously described to calculate the heart rate. If the rhythms are irregular, the nurse must use the 6-second strip method for accuracy.

6. *Measure the PR interval.* The nurse places one caliper point at the beginning of the P wave and the other point at the end of the PR segment. The PR interval normally measures between 0.12 and 0.20 second. The measurement should be constant throughout the strip. It cannot be measured if there are no P waves or if P waves occur after the QRS complex.

7. *Measure the QRS duration.* The nurse places one caliper point at the beginning of the QRS complex and the other at the J-point, where the QRS complex ends. The QRS duration normally measures between 0.04 and 0.10 second. The measurement should be constant throughout the entire strip.

8. *Interpret the rhythm.* Using accepted rules, the nurse can now interpret the cardiac rhythm.

These steps can be reorganized and formatted as the basis for rules or criteria to differentiate normal and abnormal rhythms. The following format is used to describe electrocardiographic criteria:

Rhythm: Atrial and ventricular rhythms
Rate: Atrial and ventricular rates
P waves: Presence, morphology (shape), relationship to QRS complexes
PR interval: Measurement and constancy
QRS duration: Measurement and constancy

Chart 36–1

Nursing Care Highlight:
Electrocardiographic Rhythm Analysis

1. Analyze the P waves.
2. Analyze the QRS complexes.
3. Determine the atrial rhythm or regularity.
4. Determine the ventricular rhythm or regularity.
5. Determine the heart rate.
6. Measure the PR interval.
7. Measure the QRS duration.
8. Interpret the rhythm.

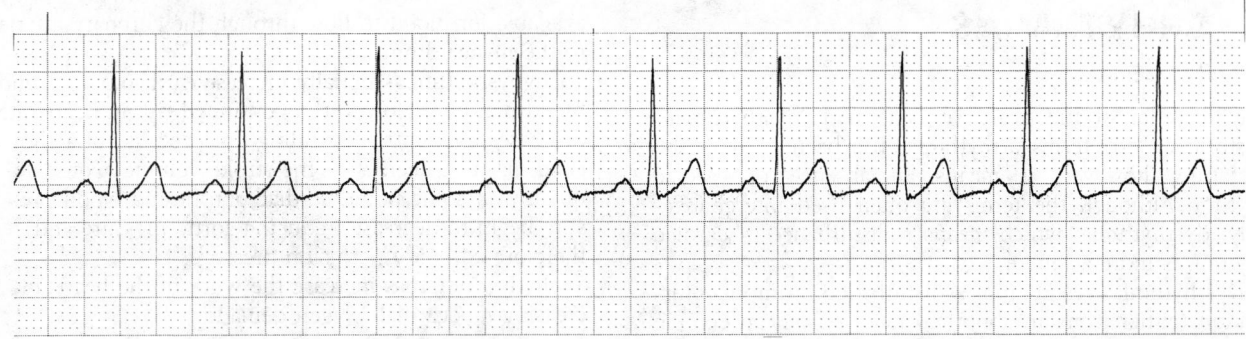

Figure 36–9. Normal sinus rhythm (NSR). Both atrial and ventricular rhythms are essentially regular (a slight variation in rhythm is normal). Atrial and ventricular rates are both 83/minute. There is one P wave before each QRS complex, and all the P waves are of a consistent morphology or shape. The PR interval measures 0.18 second and is constant; the QRS complex measures 0.06 second and is constant.

NORMAL RHYTHMS
Normal Sinus Rhythm

Normal sinus rhythm (NSR) is the rhythm originating from the sinoatrial node (dominant pacemaker) that meets the following electrocardiographic (ECG) criteria (Fig. 36–9):

> *Rhythm:* Atrial and ventricular rhythms regular
> *Rate:* Atrial and ventricular rates 60 to 100 beats per minute
> *P waves:* Present, consistent morphologic configuration, one P wave before each QRS complex
> *PR interval:* 0.12 to 0.20 second and constant
> *QRS duration:* 0.04 to 0.10 second and constant

Sinus Arrhythmia

Sinus arrhythmia is a variant of normal sinus rhythm. It results from changes in intrathoracic pressure during breathing. In this context, the term *arrhythmia* does not denote an absence of rhythm, as the term suggests. Instead, the heart rate increases slightly during inspiration and decreases slightly during expiration. This irregular rhythm is frequently observed in healthy children as well as adults.

Sinus arrhythmia has all the characteristics of normal sinus rhythm, except for its irregularity. The P-P and R-R intervals vary, with the difference between the shortest and the longest intervals greater than 0.12 second (three small blocks) (Fig. 36-10):

> *Rhythm:* Atrial and ventricular rhythms irregular, with the shortest P-P or R-R interval varying at least 0.12 second from the longest P-P or R-R interval
> *Rate:* Atrial and ventricular rates normal or less than 60 beats per minute
> *P waves:* One P wave before each QRS complex, consistent morphologic configuration
> *PR interval:* Normal, constant
> *QRS duration:* Normal, constant

Sinus arrhythmias may occasionally be due to nonrespiratory causes, such as the administration of digitalis or morphine. These drugs enhance vagal tone and cause decreased heart rate and irregularity unrelated to the respiratory cycle.

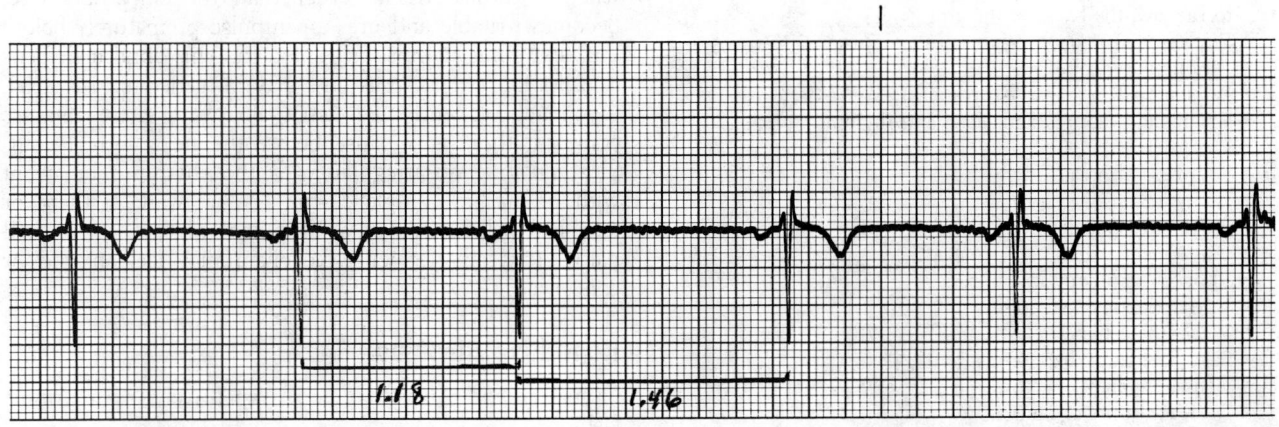

Figure 36–10. Sinus arrhythmia, considered normal, with sinus bradycardia, heart rate 46/minute. All the P waves have the same morphology, indicating that they are all from the sinus node. The rhythm is irregular, with the shortest RR interval (1.18 seconds) varying more than 0.12 second from the longest RR interval (1.46 seconds).

DYSRHYTHMIAS
Overview

Any disorder of the heartbeat is termed "dysrhythmia." Historically, the term "arrhythmia" has been used in the literature; however, it means an absence of cardiac rhythm. Although the terms are often used interchangeably, dysrhythmia, which means a disturbance in cardiac rhythm, is more accurate.

Dysrhythmias result from a disturbance in impulse formation (either from an abnormal rate or from an ectopic focus), from a disturbance in impulse conduction (delays and blocks), or from both mechanisms. Although many dysrhythmias have no clinical manifestations, many others have serious consequences. A summary is provided in Chart 36–2.

Dysrhythmia Terminology
Tachydysrhythmias

Tachydysrhythmias are heart rates greater than 100 beats per minute (BPM) in adults and older children or above the normal range for heart rates in infants and young children. These rhythms may have serious hemodynamic consequences in the adult client with coronary artery disease (CAD). Coronary artery blood flow occurs predominantly during diastole, when the aortic valve is closed, and is determined by diastolic time and blood pressure in the root of the aorta. The nurse must understand three important points to appreciate the seriousness of tachydysrhythmias in adults:

- Tachydysrhythmias shorten the diastolic time and therefore the coronary perfusion time (the amount of time available for blood to flow through the coronary arteries to the myocardium).
- Tachydysrhythmias initially increase cardiac output and blood pressure. However, a continued rise in heart rate decreases the ventricular filling time because of a shortened diastole, decreasing the stroke volume. Consequently, at some point, cardiac output and blood pressure begin to decrease, reducing aortic pressure and therefore coronary perfusion pressure.
- Tachydysrhythmias increase the work of the heart, increasing myocardial oxygen demand.

The adult client with a tachydysrhythmia could present with palpitations, chest discomfort, pressure or pain from myocardial ischemia or infarction, restlessness, anxiety, and syncope from hypotension, along with pale, cool skin. Tachydysrhythmias may also lead to heart failure in adults, children, or infants. The client may present with dyspnea, orthopnea, pulmonary crackles, distended neck veins, fatigue, and weakness.

Bradydysrhythmias

Bradydysrhythmias are heart rates less than 60 beats per minute in adults and older children or below the normal range for heart rates in infants and young children. These rhythms can have serious hemodynamic consequences. The nurse considers the following three points:

- Coronary perfusion time is adequate because of a prolonged diastole. This is desirable.
- Coronary perfusion pressure may decrease if the heart rate is too slow to provide adequate cardiac output and blood pressure. This is a serious consequence.
- Myocardial oxygen demand is reduced from the slow heart rate. This is beneficial.

Therefore, the client may tolerate the bradydysrhythmia well if the blood pressure is adequate. If the blood pressure is not adequate, symptomatic bradydysrhythmias may lead to myocardial ischemia or infarction, dysrhythmias, hypotension, and heart failure.

Premature Complexes

Premature complexes are early complexes. They occur when a cardiac tissue, other than the sinoatrial node, becomes irritable and fires an impulse prematurely before the next sinus impulse is generated. This abnormal focus is called an *ectopic focus* and may be generated by atrial, junctional, or ventricular tissue. Following the premature complex, there is a pause before the next normal complex, creating an irregularity in the rhythm. The client with premature complexes may be unaware of them or may feel palpitations or a "skipping" of the heartbeat. If palpitations are frequent, the client may feel anxious or concerned.

Repetitive Rhythms

Premature complexes may occur repetitively in a rhythmic fashion.

- *Bigeminy* exists when normal complexes and premature complexes occur alternately in a repetitive two-beat pat-

---

Chart 36–2

Key Features of Sustained Tachydysrhythmias and Bradydysrhythmias

- Chest discomfort, pressure, or pain, which may radiate to the jaw, the back, or the arm
- Restlessness, anxiety, nervousness, confusion
- Dizziness, syncope
- Palpitations (in tachydysrhythmias)
- Change in pulse strength, rate, and rhythm
- Pulse deficit
- Shortness of breath, dyspnea
- Tachypnea
- Pulmonary crackles
- Orthopnea
- S_2 or S_4 heart sounds
- Jugular venous distention
- Weakness, fatigue
- Pale, cool skin; diaphoresis
- Nausea, vomiting
- Decreased urinary output
- Delayed capillary refill
- Hypotension

tern, with a pause occurring after each premature complex so that complexes occur in pairs.

- *Trigeminy* is a repetitive three-beat pattern, usually occurring as two sequential normal complexes followed by a premature complex and a pause, with the same pattern repeating itself in triplets.
- *Quadrigeminy* is a repetitive four-beat pattern, usually occurring as three sequential normal complexes followed by a premature complex and a pause, with the same pattern repeating itself in a four-beat pattern.

Such patterns may occur with atrial, junctional, or ventricular premature complexes. Clients may be unaware of the premature beats or may feel palpitations.

Escape Complexes and Rhythms

Escape complexes or escape rhythms may occur when the sinoatrial (SA) node fails to discharge or is blocked or when a sinus impulse fails to depolarize the ventricles because of an atrioventricular (AV) nodal block. Escape complexes or rhythms serve as a subsidiary or escape pacemaker and are seen after a pause. Such impulses may originate from AV junctional or ventricular tissue. They cease when the SA node or the AV node regains the ability to function normally. If there are pauses followed by escape beats or rhythms, clients may feel lightheaded, dizzy, or faint during the pause.

Classification of Dysrhythmias

Dysrhythmias are classified according to their site of origin. The sites include sinus, atrial, junctional, ventricular, and AV nodal tissue. Dysrhythmias may be caused by a disturbance in impulse formation or by conduction delays or blocks. The incidence and the prevalence of dysrhythmias are not precisely known because they usually result from an underlying condition, such as heart disease. The incidence of dysrhythmias increases with age. A summary of the common dysrhythmias and their treatment is provided in Table 36–2.

Sinus Dysrhythmias

The sinus node is the pacemaker in all sinus dysrhythmias. Sympathetic and parasympathetic nerve fibers are distributed to the SA node. Innervation from these two systems is normally in balance to ensure a normal sinus rhythm. An imbalance increases or decreases the rate of SA node discharge either as a normal response to activity or physiologic changes or as a pathologic response to illness.

Sinus Tachycardia

Pathophysiology

Dominant sympathetic nervous system stimulation of the heart or vagal inhibition results in an increased rate of SA node discharge, which increases the heart rate (positive chronotropic effect).

When the rate of SA node discharge exceeds 100 beats per minute, the rhythm is called sinus tachycardia (Fig. 36–11A). Sinus tachycardia is normal in infants and chil-

dren, with the rate gradually decreasing until age 10 years. From 10 years to adulthood, the resting rate normally does not exceed 100 beats per minute except in response to activity and then usually does not exceed 160. Rarely, the resting rate may reach 180 beats per minute. Heart rates in infants and young children may reach 200 to 220 beats per minute. Sinus tachycardia initially enhances cardiac output and blood pressure. However, excessive increases in heart rate decrease coronary perfusion time and coronary perfusion pressure, while increasing myocardial oxygen demand.

Electrocardiographic criteria include

Rhythm: Atrial and ventricular rhythms regular
Rate: Atrial and ventricular rates 100 to 180 beats per minute in adults and up to 220 beats per minute in infants and young children
P waves: One P wave before each QRS complex, consistent morphologic configuration. P waves may encroach on preceding T waves
PR interval: Normal, constant
QRS duration: Normal, constant

Etiology

Increased sympathetic stimulation is a normal response to physical activity but may also be caused by anxiety, pain, stress, fear, fever, anemia, hypoxemia, hyperthyroidism, pulmonary embolus, and the administration of drugs such as catecholamines, atropine, caffeine, alcohol, nicotine, aminophylline, and thyroid drugs. Sinus tachycardia may also be a compensatory response to decreased cardiac output or blood pressure, as occurs in hypovolemia, shock, myocardial infarction, and heart failure. Common causes in infants and children include fever, anxiety, pain, anemia, and dehydration.

Physical Assessment/Clinical Manifestations

The client may be asymptomatic except for the increased pulse rate. However, if the rhythm is not well tolerated, the client may become symptomatic. The nurse assesses the client for fatigue, weakness, shortness of breath, orthopnea, neck vein distention, decreased oxygen saturation, and decreased blood pressure. The nurse also assesses for restlessness and anxiety from decreased cerebral perfusion and for decreased urinary output from decreased renal perfusion. The adult client may experience anginal pain. The electrocardiographic (ECG) pattern may show T-wave inversion or ST-segment elevation or depression in response to myocardial ischemia. During sinus tachycardia, the TP segment shortens.

Interventions

The nurse and the physician collaborate to identify the cause of sinus tachycardia and select the appropriate treatment. The goal is to decrease the heart rate to normal levels by treating the underlying cause. For example, if the client has angina, the nurse administers oxygen, assists the client to rest, and administers nitroglycerin or morphine as prescribed. The nurse administers diuretics and inotropic agents to the client in heart failure, initiates intravascular volume replacement for the hypovolemic cli-

TABLE 36–2

Common Dysrhythmias and Their Treatment

Dysrhythmia	Treatment*	Dysrhythmia	Treatment*
Sinus tachycardia	• Correction of the underlying problem (e.g., fever, hypovolemia, pain, anxiety, and CHF) • Beta-adrenergic blockade if increased catecholamine secretion is the underlying problem	**Premature Beats and Ectopic Rhythms** *Continued* 	 • Digitalis • Propranolol • Esmolol • Quinidine • Procainamide • Vagal stimulation with carotid massage • Valsalva maneuvers • Overdrive atrial pacing • Synchronized cardioversion if the above measures are unsuccessful
Sinus bradycardia	• Treatment necessary only if the client is symptomatic (has hypotension, diaphoresis, chest discomfort or pain, pulmonary congestion, or altered level of consciousness); • Atropine • Pacemaker • Avoidance of parasympathetic stimulation, such as prolonged suctioning and stimulation of the gag reflex	Premature ventricular complexes and ventricular tachycardia (not sustained)	• Correction of any underlying problem (e.g., infection, electrolyte imbalance, effects of drugs, myocardial infarction, CHF, stress, fatigue, and nicotine) • Medication administration • Lidocaine bolus and infusion • Procainamide bolus and infusion • Bretylium tosylate bolus and infusion • Magnesium sulfate infusion • Class I and II antidysrhythmics • Amiodarone • Restoration of electrolyte balance
Premature Beats and Ectopic Rhythms			
Supraventricular beats (PACs, PJCs)	• Correction of any underlying problem (e.g., anxiety, stress, caffeine and nicotine intake, CFH, effects of drugs, and CAL) • Medication administration • Quinidine • Procainamide • Digitalis • Propranolol • Sedatives		
Supraventricular rhythms	• Correction of any underlying problem (e.g., CHF, CAL, stress, and drugs) • Medication administration • Verapamil • Diltiazem • Adenosine	Atrial flutter	• Medication administration • Diltiazem • Verapamil • Digitalis • Propranolol

ent, administers antipyretics and antibiotics to the client with fever and infection, or provides comfort measures and administers analgesics or opioids to the client with noncardiac pain.

The nurse collaborates with the respiratory therapist when indicated to oxygenate and suction the client with hypoxemia from excessive airway secretions. The nurse administers beta-adrenergic–blocking agents when prescribed for the client with inappropriate sympathetic nervous system stimulation. The nurse provides emotional support and relevant teaching to the client and family and administers antianxiety agents for clients who are anxious.

Sinus Bradycardia

Pathophysiology

Dominance of the parasympathetic nervous system, with excessive vagal stimulation to the heart, causes a de-

creased rate of sinus node discharge. This slows the heart rate and decreases the speed of conduction through the AV node and conduction system. When the rate of sinus node discharge is less than 60 beats per minute in adults or below the normal range in infants and children, the rhythm is called *sinus bradycardia* (see Fig. 36–11B). Sinus bradycardia increases coronary perfusion time but may decrease coronary perfusion pressure. However, myocardial oxygen demand is decreased. Sinus bradycardia is not normal in infants and young children and may be an ominous sign.

Electrocardiographic criteria include

Rhythm: Atrial and ventricular rhythms regular
Rate: Atrial and ventricular rates less than 60 beats per minute in adults or less than the normal range in infants and children
P waves: One P wave before each QRS complex, consistent morphologic configuration

TABLE 36–2

Common Dysrhythmias and Their Treatment *Continued*

Dysrhythmia	Treatment*	Dysrhythmia	Treatment*
Premature Beats and Ectopic Rhythms *Continued*		**Conduction Delays** *Continued*	
	• Esmolol • Quinidine • Procainamide • Atrial overdrive pacing • Cardioversion • Catheter or surgical ablation	Second-degree AV block type II	• Pacemaker • Isoproterenol administration if pacemaker unavailable

Atrial fibrillation	• Medication administration
	  • Digitalis
	  • Diltiazem
	  • Verapamil
	  • Quinidine
	  • Procainamide
	• Anticoagulation
	• Atrial overdrive pacing
	• Cardioversion
	• Surgery
		Third-degree AV block	• Pacemaker
			• Isoproterenol administration if pacemaker unavailable

		Life-Threatening Dysrhythmias	

		Sustained ventricular tachycardia	• Medication administration
			  • Lidocaine bolus and infusion
			  • Procainamide bolus and infusion
			  • Bretylium tosylate bolus and infusion
			  • Magnesium sulfate infusion
			• If unstable: synchronized cardioversion
			• If pulseless: defibrillation, CPR

Escape beats and rhythms	• Correction of the underlying cause if the client is symptomatic
	• Atropine administration
	• Pacemaker
	• Isoproterenol administration if pacemaker unavailable
		Ventricular fibrillation	• Defibrillation
			• CPR
			• Medication administration
			  • Epinephrine
			  • Lidocaine
			  • Bretylium tosylate
			  • Procainamide
			  • Magnesium sulfate

Conduction Delays			

First-degree AV block	• Treatment necessary only if the client is symptomatic
	• Withhold digitalis (if the cause)
	• Atropine administration if block is associated with symptomatic bradycardia
		Ventricular asystole	• CPR
			• Medication administration
			  • Epinephrine
			  • Atropine
			  • Pacemaker

Second-degree AV block type I	• Same as for first-degree AV block		

*CHF, congestive heart failure; CAL, chronic airway limitation.

PR interval: Normal, constant
QRS duration: Normal, constant

Etiology

Increased parasympathetic stimulation of the heart by the vagus nerve is a normal response to decreased physical activity. It also often occurs in well-conditioned athletes because the strong heart muscle is extremely efficient in providing an adequate stroke volume while not requiring a higher heart rate for a normal cardiac output. Excessive vagal stimulation may result from carotid sinus massage, vomiting, suctioning, Valsalva maneuvers such as bearing down for a bowel movement or gagging, inferior myocardial infarction, ocular pressure, pain, and hypothyroidism. Sinus bradycardia may also result from the administration of drugs such as beta-adrenergic–blocking agents, calcium channel blockers, and digitalis. In infants and children, sinus bradycardia may be due to hypervagal tone but may also occur with cardiac disease or as a late response to hypoxia, acidosis, and hypotension, when it may be an ominous sign.

Physical Assessment/Clinical Manifestations

The client may be asymptomatic, except for the decreased pulse rate. However, at times the rhythm may not be well tolerated. The nurse assesses the client for dizziness, weakness, syncope, confusion, hypotension, diaphoresis, shortness of breath, and ventricular ectopy. Infants and children may become listless and lethargic. The adult client may experience anginal pain; T-wave inversion or ST-segment elevation or depression may occur in response to myocardial ischemia.

Interventions

In the adult, the treatment of choice for the client with a symptomatic sinus bradycardia is atropine administration. The nurse administers oxygen and atropine as prescribed to increase the client's heart rate to approximately 60 beats per minute. If the heart rate does not increase sufficiently, the nurse may apply a noninvasive pacemaker to increase the heart rate and notifies the physician. However, if atropine administration succeeds in achieving an

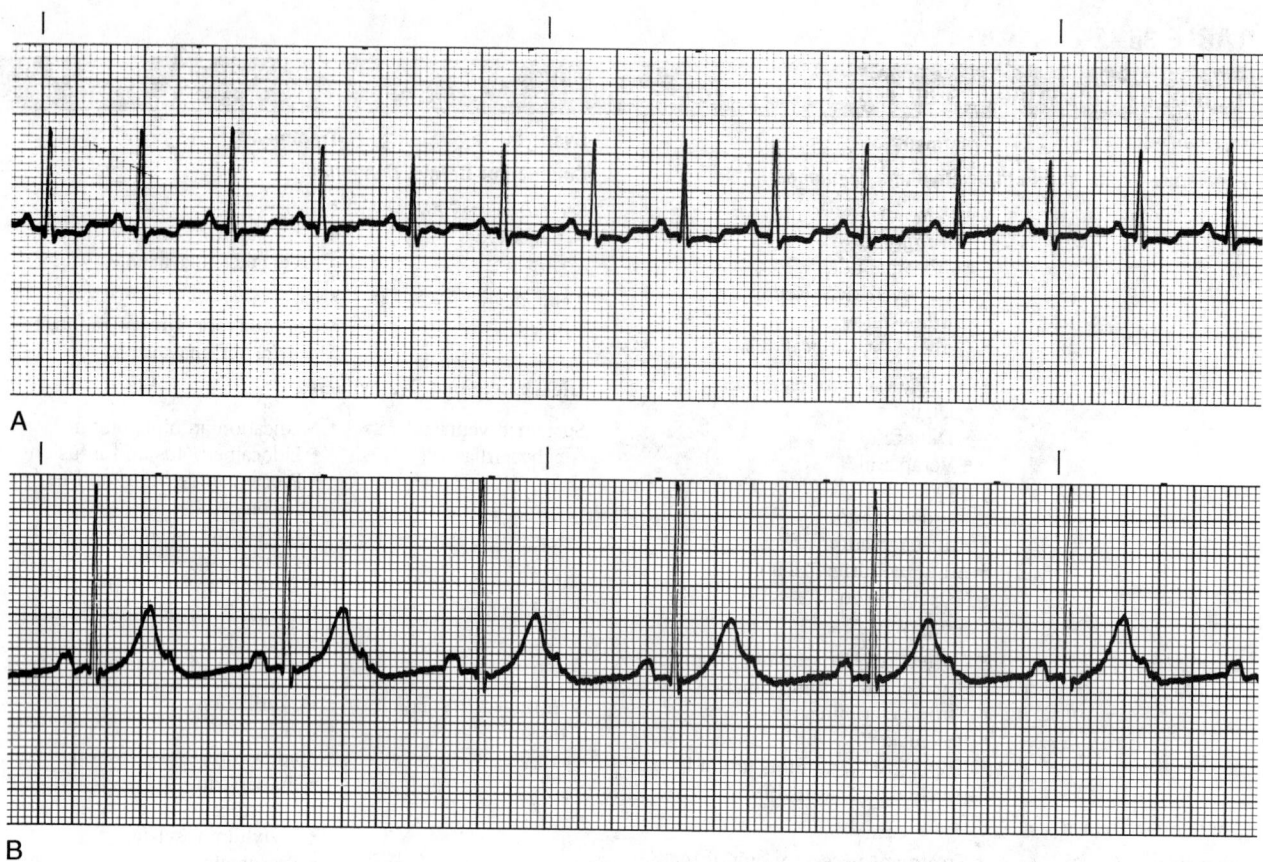

Figure 36–11. Sinus rhythms. *A,* Sinus tachycardia (HR = 110/minute, PR = 0.12 second, QRS = 0.08 second). *B,* Sinus bradycardia (HR = 52/minute, PR = 0.18 second, QRS = 0.08 second).

adequate heart rate but the client remains hypotensive, the nurse initiates intravascular volume replacement as ordered rather than administering another dose of atropine, because excessive atropine may induce tachycardia. If an offending drug is determined to be the cause, the nurse withholds the drug and notifies the physician for an order to discontinue the drug temporarily or permanently. Sinus bradycardia in infants and children may respond to oxygen administration and correction of acidosis and hypovolemia. Administration of atropine may be warranted for hypervagal tone.

Atrial Dysrhythmias

With atrial dysrhythmias, the focus of impulse generation has shifted away from the sinus node to the atrial tissue, which now acts as an ectopic pacemaker, for one or more beats. This shift changes the axis (direction) of atrial depolarization, resulting in a P-wave morphology that differs from that of P waves from sinus node origin.

Premature Atrial Complexes

Pathophysiology

A premature atrial complex (PAC or APC) occurs when atrial tissue becomes irritable, and this ectopic focus fires an impulse before the next sinus impulse is due, thus

usurping the sinus pacemaker (Fig. 36–12). The premature P wave from the atrial focus is early and has a morphology different from the P waves generated from the sinus focus. The premature P wave may not always be clearly visible, as it is often hidden in the preceding T wave. The T wave must be closely examined for any change in shape and compared with other T waves, to reveal a hidden P wave.

Electrocardiographic criteria include

Rhythm: The underlying sinus rhythm usually regular, unless sinus arrhythmia is present. Atrial and ventricular rhythms become irregular because of the early beat. There is a pause after the PAC

Rate: May be any rate, depending on underlying sinus rhythm. Atrial and ventricular rates are usually equal

P waves: One P wave before each QRS complex. Sinus P waves have one consistent morphologic pattern. The premature atrial P wave is early with a different morphologic configuration

PR interval: Normal and constant for sinus beats, normal or prolonged for PAC

QRS duration: Usually normal and constant

Etiology

The causes of atrial irritability include stress; fatigue; anxiety; inflammation; infection; intake of caffeine, nicotine,

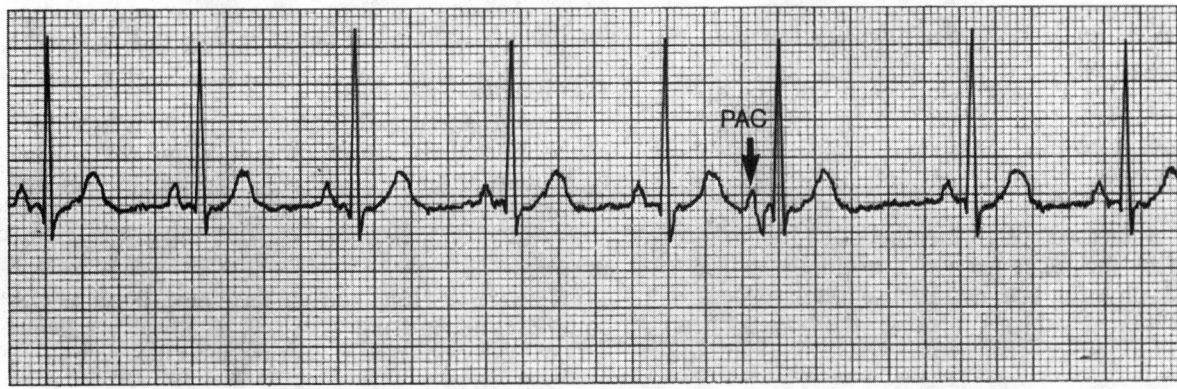

Figure 36–12. Atrial dysrhythmias. Normal sinus rhythm (NSR) with a premature atrial complex (PAC) at arrow.

and alcohol; and the administration of drugs such as digitalis, catecholamines, sympathomimetics, amphetamines, and anesthetic agents. PACs may also result from myocardial ischemia, hypermetabolic states, electrolyte imbalance, or atrial stretch, as may occur with congestive heart failure, valvular disease, and pulmonary hypertension with cor pulmonale.

Physical Assessment/Clinical Manifestations

The client is usually asymptomatic, except for possible heart palpitations, because PACs usually have no hemodynamic consequences.

Interventions

No intervention is usually needed except to treat the cause, such as heart failure or valvular disease. If PACs occur frequently, they may herald the onset of more serious atrial tachydysrhythmias and therefore may warrant treatment. The nurse administers prescribed type IA antidysrhythmics, such as quinidine and procainamide, or other drugs such as digitalis and propranolol. The nurse also initiates measures to reduce the client's stress and teaches the client to avoid substances known to increase atrial irritability.

Supraventricular Tachycardia

Pathophysiology

Supraventricular tachycardia (SVT) involves the rapid stimulation of atrial tissue at a rate of 100 to 280 beats per minute, with a mean of 170 beats per minute in adults (Fig. 36–13) and 200 to 300 beats per minute in children. SVT is most often due to a re-entry mechanism in which one impulse circulates repeatedly in a circuitous atrial pathway, restimulating the atrial tissue repetitively at a rapid rate. The term *paroxysmal supraventricular tachycardia* is used when the rhythm is intermittent, initiated suddenly by a premature complex such as a PAC, and terminated suddenly with or without intervention.

During SVT the P waves have a morphology different from that of sinus P waves. The P waves are usually not seen, however, if there is a 1:1 conduction with rapid rates because the P waves are obscured in the preceding T wave.

Electrocardiographic criteria include

Rhythm: Atrial and ventricular rhythms regular or nearly regular
Rate: Atrial and ventricular rates 100 to 280 beats per minute (mean 170 beats per minute) in adults and 200 to 300 beats per minute in children

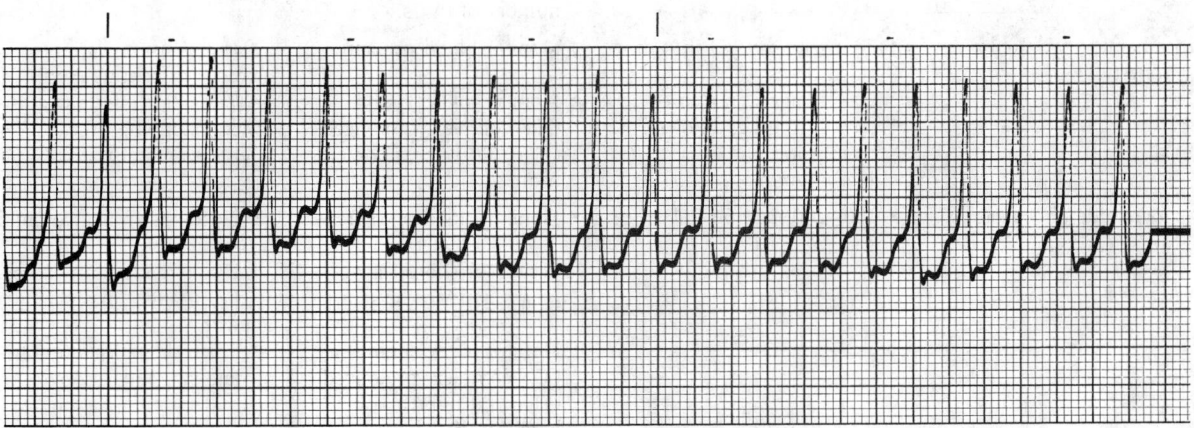

Figure 36–13. Atrial dysrhythmias. Sustained supraventricular tachycardia (SVT) in a client with Wolff-Parkinson-White syndrome. Heart rate is 200/minute.

P waves: Morphologic pattern of the first P (PAC) different from that of sinus P waves. Subsequent P waves are seldom visible, being buried in preceding T waves

PR interval: The PR interval prolonged with the first P (PAC); thereafter, not measurable

QRS duration: Usually normal and constant

Etiology

The causes of supraventricular tachycardia are the same as those for PACs. SVT may occur in healthy young people without evidence of heart disease, usually women under 40 years of age, and is also common in children. The condition commonly occurs in clients with a pre-excitation syndrome, such as Wolff-Parkinson-White syndrome.

Physical Assessment/Clinical Manifestations

The clinical manifestations depend on the duration of the SVT and the rate of the ventricular response. In clients with a sustained rapid ventricular response, the nurse assesses for palpitations, weakness, fatigue, shortness of breath, nervousness, anxiety, and syncope. Hemodynamic deterioration may occur in the client with cardiac disease, causing angina, heart failure, and shock. The infant or young child may demonstrate poor feeding, extreme irritability, and pallor. With a nonsustained or slower ventricular response, the client may be asymptomatic except for transient palpitations.

Interventions

If SVT occurs in a healthy person and terminates spontaneously, no intervention is necessary other than eliminating identified causative factors. If it is recurrent, the client should be studied in the electrophysiology laboratory. The preferred treatment for recurrent SVT is radiofrequency catheter ablation (Bubien et al., 1995). In sustained supraventricular tachycardia with a rapid ventricular response, the goals of treatment are to decrease the ventricular response, convert the dysrhythmia to a sinus rhythm, and treat the cause. Vagal stimulation may be successful, but often only transiently, and must be performed only by a physician.

The nurse administers oxygen and prescribed antidysrhythmic drugs, which slow the ventricular rate by increasing the AV block. These drugs include adenosine, verapamil, diltiazem, digitalis, esmolol, and propranolol (see Chart 36–3). Some may also succeed in converting the dysrhythmia.

Text continued on page 776

Chart 36–3

Drug Therapy for Dysrhythmias

Drug	Usual Dosage	Nursing Interventions	Rationale
Class I Drugs			
Type IA			
Quinidine sulfate (Quinidine, Apo-Quinidine✿)	• 300–600 mg q8–12h PO • 6–10 mg/kg IV slowly, may be given IM	• Monitor blood pressure. • Watch for diarrhea, nausea, or vomiting and administer with food if these occur. • Monitor for widening QRS complex, prolonged QT interval, heart block, and onset or increase in number of PVCs.	• Hypotension is a common side effect. • Diarrhea is common during early therapy. Diarrhea and other gastrointestinal symptoms often decrease when quinidine is administered with food. • Toxic side effects necessitate stopping quinidine administration.
Procainamide hydrochloride (Pronestyl)	• 50 mg/kg/day PO in 4 divided doses • 20–30 mg IV, not to exceed 17 mg/kg, followed by infusion of 1–4 mg/min	• Monitor blood pressure. • Monitor for widening QRS complex, prolonged QT or PR interval, or heart block.	• Hypotension warrants drug discontinuation. • Toxic side effects necessitate stopping procainamide administration.
Disopyramide phosphate (Norpace)	• 100–200 mg q6h PO	• Monitor blood pressure. • Watch for shortness of breath and weight gain. • Monitor for widening QRS complex, prolonged QT or PR interval, or heart block	• Hypotension is a common side effect. • Disopyramide can cause heart failure in a client with CAD. • Toxic side effects necessitate stopping disopyramide administration.

Chart 36-3. Drug Therapy for Dysrhythmias　Continued

Drug	Usual Dosage	Nursing Interventions	Rationale
Class I Drugs			
Type IB			
Lidocaine (Xylocaine)	• 1–1.5 mg/kg IV bolus, then 0.5–0.75 mg/kg IV boluses q5–10min to a loading dose of 3 mg/kg, followed by 2–4 mg/min infusion • For VF or pulseless VT: 1–1.5 mg/kg IV bolus q3–5 min to a loading dose of 3 mg/kg, followed by 2–4 mg/min infusion	• Watch for confusion, paresthesias, slurring of speech, drowsiness, or seizure activity.	• CNS adverse effects predominate; they may require a decrease in dosage or discontinuation of the infusion.
Mexiletine hydrochloride (Mexitil)	• 200–300 mg q8h PO with food • 125–250 mg IV bolus for 5–10 min • 0.5–1.5 mg/min infusion	• Monitor blood pressure and heart rate. • Assess for tremors, blurred vision, dizziness, ataxia, or confusion.	• Hypotension and bradycardia may occur. • CNS adverse reactions predominate.
Tocainide hydrochloride (Tonocard)	• 400 mg q8h PO initially • 400–800 mg q8h PO • Maximum of 2.4 g/day • Take with food.	• Watch for tremors. • Monitor heart rate and blood pressure. • Teach the client to report shortness of breath, wheezing, chest pain, or cough, as well as dyspnea and distended neck veins or swelling of the extremities	• Tremors indicate that the maximum dose is being approached. • Bradycardia and hypotension may occur. • Pulmonary fibrosis is a serious side effect, which necessitates discontinuation of the drug; the drug also may cause CHF.
Type IC			
Flecainide acetate (Tambocor)	• 100 mg bid PO • Maximum dose of 400 mg/day	• Monitor for an increase in frequency and severity of dysrhythmias. • Monitor heart rate and blood pressure. • Monitor for CHF, dizziness, visual disturbances, paresthesias, and tremors.	• Flecainide can induce dysrhythmias. • Bradycardia and hypotension may occur. • Side effects may require a decrease in dosage or discontinuation of the drug.
Propafenone hydrochloride (Rythmol)	• 150–300 mg q8h PO	• Monitor for an increase in dysrhythmias. • Monitor heart rate and blood pressure. • Monitor for CNS effects, dizziness, anxiety, ataxia, insomnia, confusion, and seizures, as well as CHF and gastrointestinal distress.	• Propafenone can induce dysrhythmias. • Bradycardia and hypotension may occur. • Side effects may require a decrease in dosage or discontinuation of the drug.
Moricizine hydrochloride (Ethmozine)	• 200–300 mg q8H PO	• Monitor for an increase in dysrhythmias. • Monitor heart rate and blood pressure. • Monitor for dizziness, hyperesthesias, anxiety, ataxia, insomnia, confusion, and seizures.	• Drug can induce dysrhythmias. • Bradycardia and hypotension may occur. • Side effects may require a decrease in dosage or discontinuation of the drug.

Continued

Chart 36–3. Drug Therapy for Dysrhythmias Continued

Drug	Usual Dosage	Nursing Interventions	Rationale
Class II Drugs			
Propranolol hydrochloride (Inderal, Apo-Propranolol✦)	• 10–80 mg qid PO before meals • 0.1 mg/kg slow IV bolus divided in 3 equal doses given at 2–3 min intervals, at rate of 1 mg/min	• Monitor heart rate and blood pressure. • Assess for shortness of breath or wheezing. • Assess for insomnia, fatigue, and dizziness.	• Bradycardia and decreased blood pressure are expected effects. • Beta$_2$-blocking effects on the lungs can cause bronchospasm. • Side effects may require decrease in dosage or discontinuation of the drug.
Acebutolol hydrochloride (Sectral)	• 600–1200 mg daily PO	• Monitor heart rate and blood pressure. • Assess for shortness of breath or wheezing. • Assess for insomnia, fatigue, and dizziness.	• Bradycardia and decreased blood pressure are expected effects. • Beta$_2$-blocking effects on the lungs can cause bronchospasm. • Side effects may require a decrease in dosage or discontinuation of the drug.
Esmolol hydrochloride (Brevibloc)	• Initially, 500 μg/kg/min for 1 min, then 50 μg/kg/min for 4 min IV • Titrate up, if necessary.	• Monitor heart rate and blood pressure. • Assess for shortness of breath or wheezing. • Assess for insomnia, fatigue, and seizures.	• Bradycardia and decreased blood pressure are expected effects. • Beta$_2$-blocking effects on the lungs can cause bronchospasm. • Side effects may require a decrease in dosage or discontinuation of the drug.
Sotalol hydrochloride (Betapace)	• Initial dose of 80 mg PO bid • Dosage may be increased every 2–3 days to 240–320 mg/day in 2–3 divided doses, if necessary	• Assess ECG rhythm for torsades de pointes and other serious new ventricular dysrhythmias. • Assess for fatigue, bradycardia, dyspnea, CHF, chest pain, hypotension, dizziness, hypoglycemia, nausea, and vomiting. • Sotalol should not be administered to clients with hypokalemia or hypomagnesemia before correction of these imbalances. • Sotalol is contraindicated in clients with bronchial asthma, sinus bradycardia, or second- and third-degree AV block (unless a functioning pacemaker is present), prolonged QT syndrome, cardiogenic shock, and CHF.	• Sotalol may have proarrhythmic effects. • Adverse reactions may warrant drug discontinuation. • Hypokalemia or hypomagnesemia may prolong the QT interval and cause torsades de pointes. • Sotalol has beta-blocking (class II) effects and class III effects.

Chart 36–3. Drug Therapy for Dysrhythmias   Continued

Drug	Usual Dosage	Nursing Interventions	Rationale
Class III Drugs			
Bretylium tosylate (Bretylol, Bretylate✱)	• 5–10 mg/kg, diluted in 50 mL IV, for 8–10 min, may repeat in 1–2 hr; maximum of 30–35 mg/kg • 1–2 mg/min infusion • For VF or pulseless VT: 5 mg/kg IV undiluted, IV bolus, followed by defibrillation; may give 10 mg/kg IV bolus, followed by defibrillation, and repeat q5min to maximum of 30–35 mg/kg	• Observe cardiac monitor for PVCs, increased heart rate, and other dysrhythmias. • Monitor blood pressure. • Maintain the client in a supine position for up to 8 hr. • When the client begins to sit up or get out of bed, raise the head of the bed slowly and advise the client to make position changes slowly. • Anticipate vomiting during drug administration. Except in cardiac arrest, the drug must be diluted and given slowly.	• PVCs and increased heart rate commonly occur within 30 min. • Hypertension may occur in the first hour, followed by significant hypotension. • Orthostatic hypotension is a significant problem until tolerance to the drug develops. • The client could become dizzy and faint. • Vomiting is a common side effect.
Amiodarone hydrochloride (Cordarone)	• 800–1600 mg qd PO in divided doses for 1–3 wk, then 600–800 mg qd for 1 mo, then 200–600 mg qd (average of 400 mg qd) • Rapid loading dose: 150 mg IV over first 10 min (15 mg/min); slow loading dose: 360 mg IV over next 6 hr (1 mg/min); maintenance infusion: 540 mg IV over next 18 hr (0.5 mg/min), then 720 mg/24 hr (0.5 mg/min)	• Administer IV dose diluted in D_5W in glass bottle; use volumetric infusion pump and PVC tubing with in-line filter and infuse via central line. • Rapid loading IV dose must not be administered faster than 10 min. Must stay with client and monitor heart rate and BP. • Continually monitor ECG rhythm during IV infusion; measure QT and QT_c. • Assess the client's knowledge of the treatment regimen and side effects. • Monitor heart rate, blood pressure, and cardiac rhythm when initiating therapy. • Teach clients to report any muscle weakness, tremors, or difficulty with ambulation.	• Drug is irritating to peripheral vasculature; drug is more stable in glass bottle. • Hypotension may occur. It should be treated by slowing the infusion and other standard therapy. Cordarone should not be discontinued unless necessary. • Bradycardia and AV block may occur and are treated by slowing the infusion rate and pacemaker therapy, if necessary. May cause a worsening of ventricular dysrhythmias. • Drug has major side effects, which make noncompliance a problem; clients may take the drug for 1½–3 mo before full clinical effects are apparent. • Bradycardia, hypotension, and worsening dysrhythmia can occur. • Muscle-related side effects usually develop during the first week of treatment.

Continued

Chart 36–3. Drug Therapy for Dysrhythmias Continued

Drug	Usual Dosage	Nursing Interventions	Rationale
Class III Drugs			
		• Teach clients to report shortness of breath, cough, pleuritic pain, or fever.	• Pulmonary side effects may indicate drug-induced pulmonary toxicity.
		• Teach clients to report any visual disturbances and to wear sunglasses outdoors in the daytime if they have photophobia.	• Corneal pigmentation occurs in most clients but generally does not interfere with vision; if it does, the dosage is decreased.
		• Teach clients to use barrier sunscreens.	• Photosensitivity reactions may occur.
		• Teach clients to report any signs of thyroid problems or hepatotoxicity.	• Thyroid problems or hepatotoxicity may occur, necessitating a decrease in dosage or discontinuation of the drug.
Ibutilide fumarate (Covert)	• 1 mg IV over 10 min for clients >60 kg; 0.01 mg/kg over 10 min for clients <60 kg • May repeat dose 10 min after completion of first infusion if necessary	• Stop infusion as soon as arrhythmia is terminated, or in event of sustained or nonsustained VT, or marked prolongation of QT or QT_c.	• Drug may cause potentially fatal dysrhythmias.
		• Observe clients with continuous ECG monitoring and measure QT or QT_c for at least 4 hr following infusion or until QT_c has returned to baseline.	• Acute ventricular dysrhythmias must be promptly identified and treated. Client may develop heart blocks.
		• Clients with atrial fibrillation of >2–3 days' duration must be adequately anticoagulated for at least 2 wk.	• Atrial fibrillation is associated with formation of thrombi in atrial chambers.
		• Hypokalemia and hypomagnesemia must be corrected before Covert infusion.	• This is important to reduce potential for proarrhythmia effects.
Class IV Drugs			
Verapamil hydrochloride (Calan, Isoptin♣)	• 2.5–5 mg IV, for 1–2 min for narrow-complex SVT or PSVT; after 15–30 min may give 5–10 mg IV for 1–2 min if necessary, and repeat to a maximum of 20 mg • 80–120 mg q6–8h PO	• Monitor heart rate and blood pressure.	• Bradycardia and hypotension are common side effects.
		• Teach clients to remain recumbent for at least 1 hr after IV administration.	• Hypotension may occur; may be reversed with calcium chloride ($CaCl_2$), 0.5–1 g slow IV.
		• Teach clients to change positions slowly when receiving oral therapy.	• Dizziness and orthostatic hypotension often occur until tolerance develops.
		• Teach clients to report dyspnea, orthopnea, distended neck veins, or swelling of the extremities.	• Heart failure may occur, necessitating a decrease in dosage or discontinuation of the drug.
Diltiazem hydrochloride (Cardizem)	• 0.25 mg/kg IV for 2 min • After 15 min, give 0.35 mg/kg IV for 2 min • 5–15 mg/hr IV infusion	• Monitor heart rate and blood pressure.	• Bradycardia and hypotension are common side effects.
		• Teach clients to remain recumbent for at least 1 hr after IV administration.	• Hypotension may occur.
		• Teach clients to report dyspnea, orthopnea, distended neck veins, or swelling of the extremities.	• Heart failure may occur, necessitating a decrease in dosage or discontinuation of the drug.

Chart 36–3. Drug Therapy for Dysrhythmias   Continued

Drug	Usual Dosage	Nursing Interventions	Rationale
Other Drugs			
Digoxin (Lanoxin, Novodigoxin✱)	• Rapid digitalization: 0.5–1 mg PO or IV initially; 0.125–0.5 mg PO or IV q6h until a total of 1–1.5 mg is reached • Maintenance: 0.125–0.25 mg qd or qod PO or IV (may be less for elderly)	• Assess apical heart rate for 1 min before each dose; withhold the dose if the heart rate is less than 60 beats per min. • Assess for sudden increase of heart rate and change of rhythm from regular to irregular, or irregular to regular. • Teach clients to report anorexia, nausea, vomiting, diarrhea, paresthesias, confusion, or visual disturbances. • Monitor serum potassium levels. • Monitor serum creatinine levels	• Decreased heart rate is an expected response, but bradycardia may indicate toxicity. • Changes in heart rate or rhythm may indicate toxicity. • Side effect can indicate toxicity. • Hypokalemia increases the risk of toxicity and ventricular dysrhythmias. • Impaired renal function can cause toxicity; the dosage is altered if this occurs.
Atropine sulfate	• 0.5–1 mg IV bolus may be repeated q3–5 min, if necessary, to a maximum of 0.04 mg/kg • For asystole, PEA, or EMD: 1 mg IV bolus q3–5min to a total of 0.04 mg/kg, if necessary	• Monitor heart rate and rhythm after administration. • Assess for chest pain after administration. • Assess for urinary retention and dry mouth after administration. • Avoid using in clients with angle-closure glaucoma.	• Increased heart rate is expected. • Increased heart rate may cause ischemia in client with CAD. • Atropine is an anticholinergic agent. • Atropine increases intraocular pressure.
Adenosine (Adenocard)	• 6 mg IV for 1–3 sec followed by 20-mL saline flush; may repeat in 1–2 min, if necessary, at 12 mg IV for 1–3 sec with 20-mL flush; may repeat 12 mg IV after 1–2 min, if necessary	• Monitor heart rate and rhythm after administration. • Assess clients for facial flushing, shortness of breath, dyspnea, and chest pain. • Assess clients for recurrence of PSVT or ventricular ectopy.	• A short period of asystole is common after administration; bradycardia and hypotension may occur. • These side effects commonly occur. • Recurrence of PSVT is common; PVCs may occur.
Magnesium sulfate	• 1–2 g diluted in 100 mL of D$_5$W administered for 1–2 min for VF or VT • 1–2 g in 50–100 mL of D$_5$W for 5–60 min for loading dose; 0.5–1 g/hr for 24 hr for supplementation	• Assess ECG rhythm for conversion to sinus rhythm. • Assess clients for facial flushing, hypotension, and respiratory and CNS depression.	• Hypomagnesemia may precipitate refractory VF. • Magnesium sulfate causes vasodilation and respiratory and CNS depression.

VF, ventricular fibrillation; VT, ventricular tachycardia; SVT, supraventricular tachycardia; PSVT, premature supraventricular tachycardia; PEA, pulseless electrical activity; EMD, electromechanical dissociation; PVC, premature ventricular contraction; CHF, congestive heart failure; CNS, central nervous system; CAD, coronary artery disease.

In the severely compromised client, the nurse may assist the physician to attempt atrial overdrive pacing or to deliver a synchronized electrical shock (cardioversion) to re-establish an organized rhythm and regain hemodynamic stability.

Atrial Flutter

Pathophysiology

Atrial flutter is rapid atrial depolarization occurring at a rate of 250 to 350 times per minute. The most common rate is approximately 300 times per minute. An AV block limits the number of impulses that reach the ventricles as a protective mechanism (Fig. 36–14A). When untreated, atrial flutter typically has a 2:1 block (Fig. 36–14B). In general, when a client's ventricular rate is 150 beats per minute, the nurse should suspect atrial flutter with 2:1 block and carefully scrutinize the ECG baseline for evidence of atrial flutter waves.

Electrocardiographic criteria include

Rhythm: Atrial rhythm regular. Ventricular rhythm regular if block is consistent; ventricular rhythm irregular if block is variable

Rate: Atrial rate 250 to 350 beats per minute. Ventricular rate variable, depending on block; usually rapid without treatment

P waves: Flutter (F) waves seen in a regular pattern, with a sawtooth or "picket fence" configuration and lack of an isoelectric segment between flutter waves. Some flutter waves may be partially hidden in QRS complexes

PR interval: Actually FR interval, may be constant or variable. Usually not measured

QRS duration: Usually normal and constant

Etiology

Atrial flutter may be caused by rheumatic or ischemic heart disease, congestive heart failure, AV valve disease, pre-excitation syndromes, septal defects, pulmonary emboli, thyrotoxicosis, alcoholism, or pericarditis. The condition commonly occurs after cardiac surgery.

Physical Assessment/Clinical Manifestations

The clinical manifestations depend on the rate of ventricular response. The nurse assesses the client for palpitations, weakness, fatigue, shortness of breath, nervousness, anxiety, syncope, and evidence of hemodynamic deterioration such as angina, heart failure, and shock. Carotid sinus massage transiently increases the AV block to facilitate rhythm interpretation but can be performed only by the physician. The client with a normal ventricular rate is usually asymptomatic.

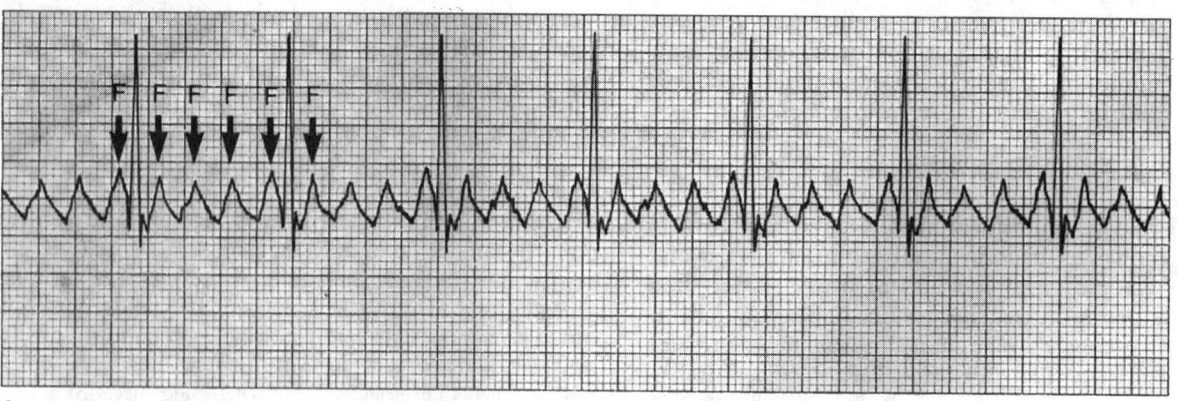

A

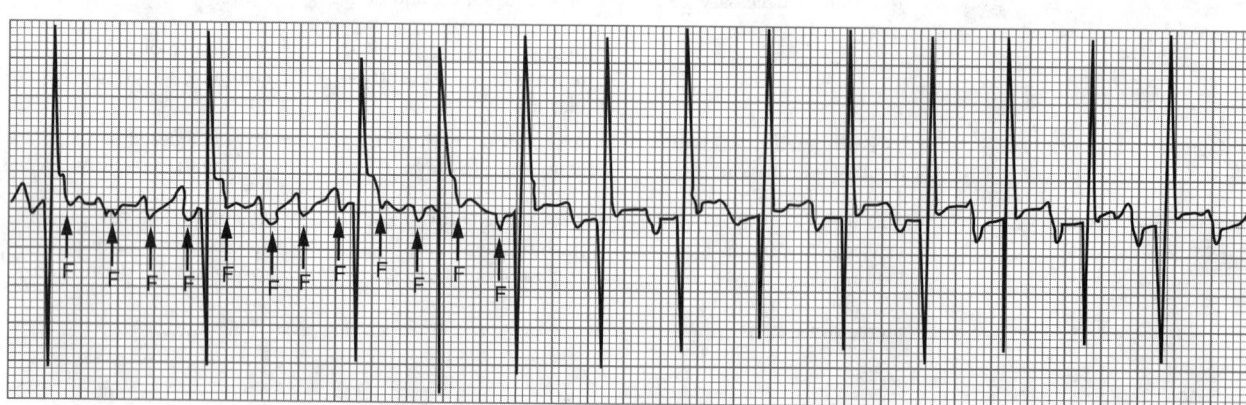

B

Figure 36–14. Atrial dysrhythmias. *A,* Atrial flutter (F) with 4:1 block. The atrial rate is 280/minute; the ventricular rate is 70/minute. *B,* Atrial flutter with 4:1 conduction, then an 11-beat run with 2:1 conduction.

Interventions

The treatment goals are the same as those for supraventricular tachycardia. The nurse administers oxygen and prescribed drugs, such as ibutilide, amiodarone, diltiazem, verapamil, propranolol, esmolol, and digoxin, to slow the rapid ventricular response. Quinidine or procainamide must not be administered unless one of the above agents has slowed the ventricular response. Both drugs slow the atrial rate and may increase AV conduction, which could cause a 1:1 conduction with an increase in ventricular rate and hemodynamic deterioration.

The nurse assists the physician to attempt rapid atrial overdrive pacing or to achieve cardioversion if the client is hemodynamically compromised. If the client is medically refractory, the physician may recommend radiofrequency catheter ablation to abolish the irritable focus in some types of atrial flutter. If the His bundle is ablated, the client is usually in a third-degree heart block and requires permanent pacemaker therapy.

Atrial Fibrillation

Pathophysiology

Multiple, rapid impulses from many foci, at a rate of 350–600 times per minute, depolarize the atria in a totally disorganized manner. The result is chaos, with no P waves, no atrial contractions, loss of the atrial kick, and an irregular ventricular response (Fig. 36–15). The atria merely quiver in fibrillation (commonly called "A fib"), which may lead to the formation of mural thrombi (within the cardiac wall) and potential embolic events.

Electrocardiographic criteria include

> *Rhythm:* Atrial rhythm consisting of an irregular undulating baseline. Ventricular rhythm totally irregular
> *Rate:* Atrial rate that cannot be counted because there are no P waves. The ventricular rate is usually 100 to 160 beats per minute or faster when untreated (uncontrolled "A fib"). The ventricular rate is 60 to 100 beats per minute when treated (controlled "A fib"). The ventricular rate may be less than 60 beats per minute when excessive AV nodal block occurs with drug treatment, such as with digoxin ("A fib" with high-grade AV block)

> *P waves:* P waves absent. Irregular fibrillatory (f) waves vary in amplitude and morphologic features in baseline
> *PR interval:* None
> *QRS duration:* Usually normal and constant

Etiology

Atrial fibrillation occurs most commonly in clients with systemic hypertension and is frequently seen in the elderly. It may also occur in clients with

- Myocardial infarction
- Rheumatic heart disease with mitral stenosis
- Atrial septal defect
- Congestive heart failure
- Cardiomyopathy
- Hyperthyroidism
- Pulmonary emboli
- Wolff-Parkinson-White syndrome
- Congenital heart disease
- Chronic constrictive pericarditis

Atrial fibrillation commonly occurs following cardiac surgery, in which case it is most often transient and usually responds well to treatment.

Physical Assessment/Clinical Manifestations

Atrial fibrillation may be intermittent or chronic. Symptoms depend on the ventricular rate. If the ventricular rate is rapid, the client may present as described for supraventricular tachycardia. Because of loss of the atrial kick, however, the client in uncontrolled atrial fibrillation is at greater risk for an inadequate cardiac output. The nurse assesses the client for the presence of a pulse deficit, fatigue, weakness, shortness of breath, distended neck veins, dizziness, decreased exercise tolerance, anxiety, syncope, palpitations, chest discomfort or pain, and hypotension.

In addition, the client is at risk for systemic emboli, particularly an embolic stroke, which may cause permanent severe neurologic impairment or death. Because approximately one-third of clients with atrial fibrillation have thromboemboli, the nurse must be astute in assessing the client for evidence of embolic events. The nurse

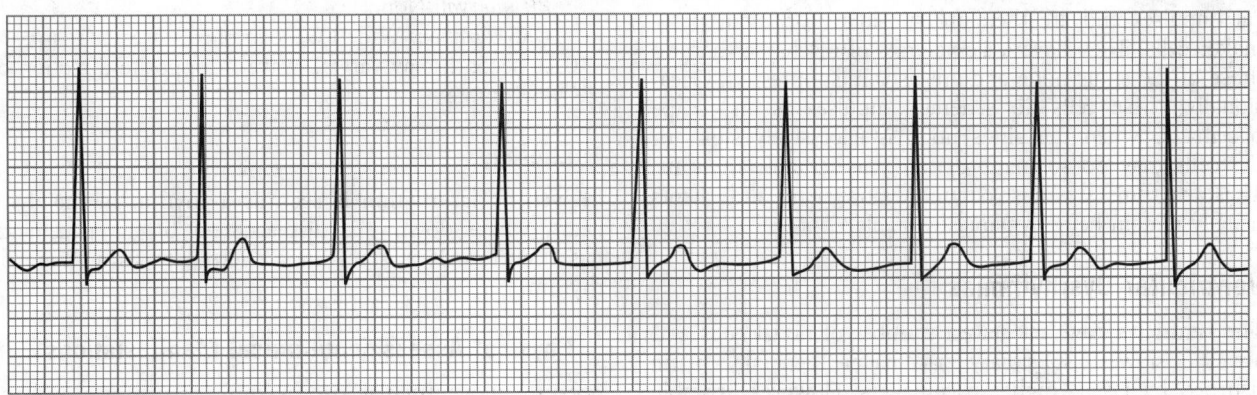

Figure 36–15. Atrial dysrhythmias. Atrial fibrillation, controlled, with a ventricular rate of approximately 80/minute.

particularly notes changes in mentation, speech, sensory function, and motor function and reports these to the physician immediately. Clients with atrial fibrillation who have valvular disease are particularly at risk for thromboemboli.

Interventions

Treatment is the same as for atrial flutter. In addition, the nurse may administer anticoagulants, such as heparin and sodium warfarin, as prescribed by the physician for clients considered to be at high risk for emboli. Prior to elective cardioversion, the nurse must initiate anticoagulation therapy for 4 to 5 weeks as prescribed to prevent a thromboembolic event if the rhythm is successfully converted. To assess for the presence of atrial clots, a contraindication for cardioversion in the hemodynamically compromised client, the physician may order a transesophageal echocardiogram prior to attempting emergency cardioversion. Atrial fibrillation of greater than 12 months duration is not likely to respond to attempts at conversion to sinus rhythm by drug therapies and may fail to respond to cardioversion.

Clients with recurring, symptomatic atrial fibrillation resistant to medical therapies may be treated with radiofrequency catheter ablation to the His bundle to interrupt all conduction between the atria and the ventricles. However, this requires implantation of a permanent ventricular pacemaker and does not stop the atria from fibrillating. The atrial kick is not restored, and patients remain at risk for embolic events.

Clients may benefit from the "maze" procedure, an open heart surgical technique (Futterman and Lemberg, 1994). In this procedure, the nurse first prepares the client for electrophysiologic mapping studies for confirmation of the diagnosis of atrial fibrillation. The nurse then prepares the client for surgery. The surgeon places a maze of sutures in strategic places in the atrial myocardium to prevent electrical circuits from developing and perpetuating atrial fibrillation. Sinus impulses can then depolarize the atria before reaching the AV node and preserve the atrial kick. The postoperative care of the client is similar to that after other open heart surgical procedures (see Chap. 40).

Junctional Dysrhythmias

Nodal cells in the AV junctional area can generate electrical impulses and are therefore subsidiary or latent pacemaker cells. They have a slower rate of discharge than do those of the sinus node and are usually suppressed. Occasionally, these cells do generate impulses as an escape pacemaker when the sinus node is excessively slow, or the cells may do so inappropriately as irritable rhythms. These rhythms are most commonly transient, and clients usually remain hemodynamically stable.

Ventricular Dysrhythmias

The ventricles have the fewest number of nodal cells and are the slowest subsidiary pacemaker, generally being usurped by faster, higher pacemakers. However, irritable ventricular cells may generate electrical impulses and fire prematurely. Because the impulse originates in and depolarizes one ventricle first, then spreads to depolarize the other, the resultant QRS complex is wide, usually measuring greater than 0.12 second. The QRS complex is bizarre or odd in shape, looking different from the normal QRS complexes. The repolarization sequence is also deranged so that the T wave is large and occurs in a direction opposite to the largest deflection of the QRS complex. The impulse most commonly is blocked in the AV node and cannot proceed further with retrograde conduction so that the atria and the SA node are usually not affected by the ventricular impulse. The atrial rhythm typically remains regular, unless the underlying rhythm is sinus arrhythmia.

A sinus P wave may sometimes be seen immediately preceding a wide QRS complex, or the sinus P wave may occur immediately after the QRS complex. Often, the sinus P wave is obscured by the QRS complex. In each case, the P-P interval remains regular in normal sinus rhythm but irregular in sinus arrhythmia. These P waves are not related to and are independent of the QRS complex; that is, the sinus impulse does not proceed forward to depolarize the ventricles. The ventricles are stimulated by an independent ventricular impulse. This is known as *AV dissociation,* meaning that a sinus impulse depolarizes the atria, and a separate ventricular impulse depolarizes the ventricles, so that the two impulses are not related.

Idioventricular Rhythm (Ventricular Escape Rhythm)

Pathophysiology

During idioventricular rhythm (ventricular escape rhythm), the ventricular nodal cells pace the ventricles. Because their inherent rate of firing is slow, the rate is usually less than 40 beats per minute (Fig. 36–16). If P waves are seen, they are independent of the QRS complexes and not related (AV dissociation).

Electrocardiographic criteria include

Rhythm: Atrial rhythm is usually absent because of downward displacement of the pacemaker with atrial standstill. Ventricular rhythm may be regular; often becomes irregular

Rate: No atrial rate. Ventricular rate usually less than 40 beats per minute

P waves: Usually absent

PR interval: None

QRS duration: Wide QRS complexes greater than 0.14 second, may vary; T wave in opposite direction of QRS complex

Etiology

Idioventricular rhythm is seen as a rhythm in the dying heart, where downward displacement of the pacemaker has occurred. It is sometimes referred to as an "agonal" rhythm.

Physical Assessment/Clinical Manifestations

Because idioventricular pacemakers are unstable and unreliable, the client is hypotensive and in shock or, most

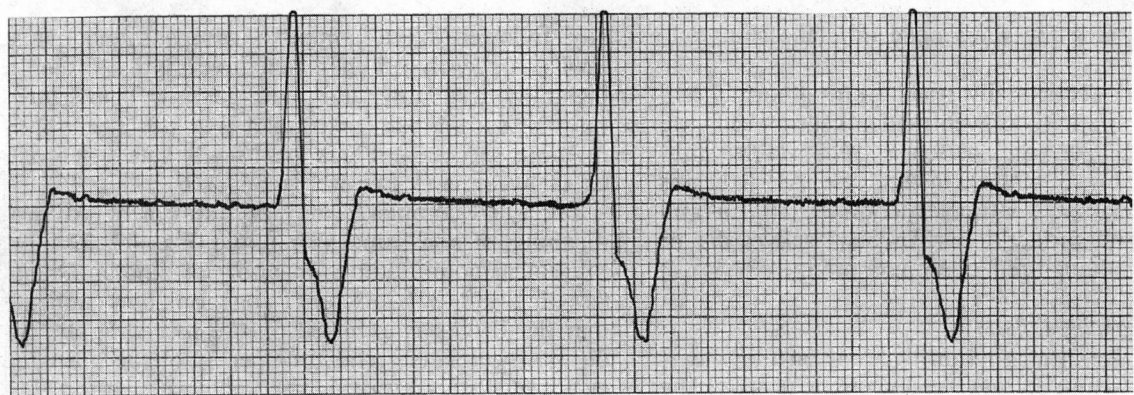

Figure 36–16. Ventricular dysrhythmias. Idioventricular rhythm with a rate of 35/minute.

typically, is pulseless and therefore in cardiac arrest. The nurse assesses the client's pulse, respirations, blood pressure, level of consciousness, and pupil response.

Interventions

Usually, idioventricular rhythms require immediate resuscitation measures, unless there is a DNR order. The nurse initiates cardiopulmonary resuscitation (CPR) and summons assistance. The team may initiate advanced cardiac life support (ACLS) measures, including epinephrine administration, intravascular volume replacement, and other measures, which tend to be unsuccessful. The physician may attempt pacemaker therapy or discontinue resuscitation efforts.

Premature Ventricular Complexes

Pathophysiology

Premature ventricular complexes (PVCs), also called ventricular premature beats (VPBs), result from increased irritability of ventricular cells. PVCs are early ventricular complexes, followed by a pause. When multiple PVCs are present, the QRS complexes may be unifocal or uniform, meaning of the same shape (Fig. 36–17A), or multifocal or multiform, meaning of different shapes (see Fig. 36–17B). PVCs frequently occur in repetitive rhythms, such as bigeminy, trigeminy, and quadrigeminy. Two sequential PVCs are a pair, or couplet. Three or more successive PVCs are usually called nonsustained ventricular tachycardia (NSVT) (see Fig. 36–17C).

R-on-T phenomenon indicates that the PVC has occurred on the preceding T wave, which is considered the vulnerable period. This may precipitate ventricular fibrillation.

Electrocardiographic criteria include

Rhythm: Underlying rhythm regular or irregular. PVC creates an irregularity, followed by a pause
Rate: Rate dependent on the underlying rhythm. PVCs can occur with any rate
P wave: With an underlying sinus rhythm, one P wave before each normal QRS complex. Sinus P waves are not related to PVC (AV dissociation); P waves may occur anywhere relative to PVCs. The underlying rhythm may be atrial flutter or atrial fibrillation
PR interval: PR interval not measured with the PVC because of AV dissociation
QRS duration: QRS duration normal in sinus rhythm. In PVC, it is wider than 0.14 second and may vary; the T wave condition occurs in the opposite direction

Etiology

PVCs are common, and their frequency increases with age. PVCs may be insignificant or may occur with myocardial ischemia or infarction; congestive heart failure; hypokalemia; hypomagnesemia; the administration of catecholamines, sympathomimetic drugs, and digitalis; acidosis; anesthesia; stress; nicotine intake; ingestion of caffeine and alcohol; infection; trauma; or surgery.

Physical Assessment/Clinical Manifestations

The client may be asymptomatic or may experience palpitations or chest discomfort caused by increased stroke volume of the normal beat after the pause. Peripheral pulses may be diminished or absent with the PVCs themselves because the decreased stroke volume of the premature beats may decrease peripheral perfusion. With acute myocardial infarction, PVCs may be considered warning dysrhythmias, possibly heralding the onset of VT or VF. For a client with chest discomfort or pain, the nurse reports to the physician whether PVCs increase in frequency, are multiform, are R-on-T phenomena, or occur in runs of VT.

Interventions

If there is no underlying heart disease, PVCs are not usually treated other than by eliminating any contributing cause (e.g., caffeine, stress). With acute myocardial ischemia or infarction, the nurse treats significant PVCs by administering oxygen and lidocaine as prescribed. Lidocaine is considered the drug of choice. The nurse may administer other drugs as ordered, including procainamide, bretylium, magnesium sulfate, propranolol, quinidine, mexiletine, tocainide, sotalol, and amiodarone (see

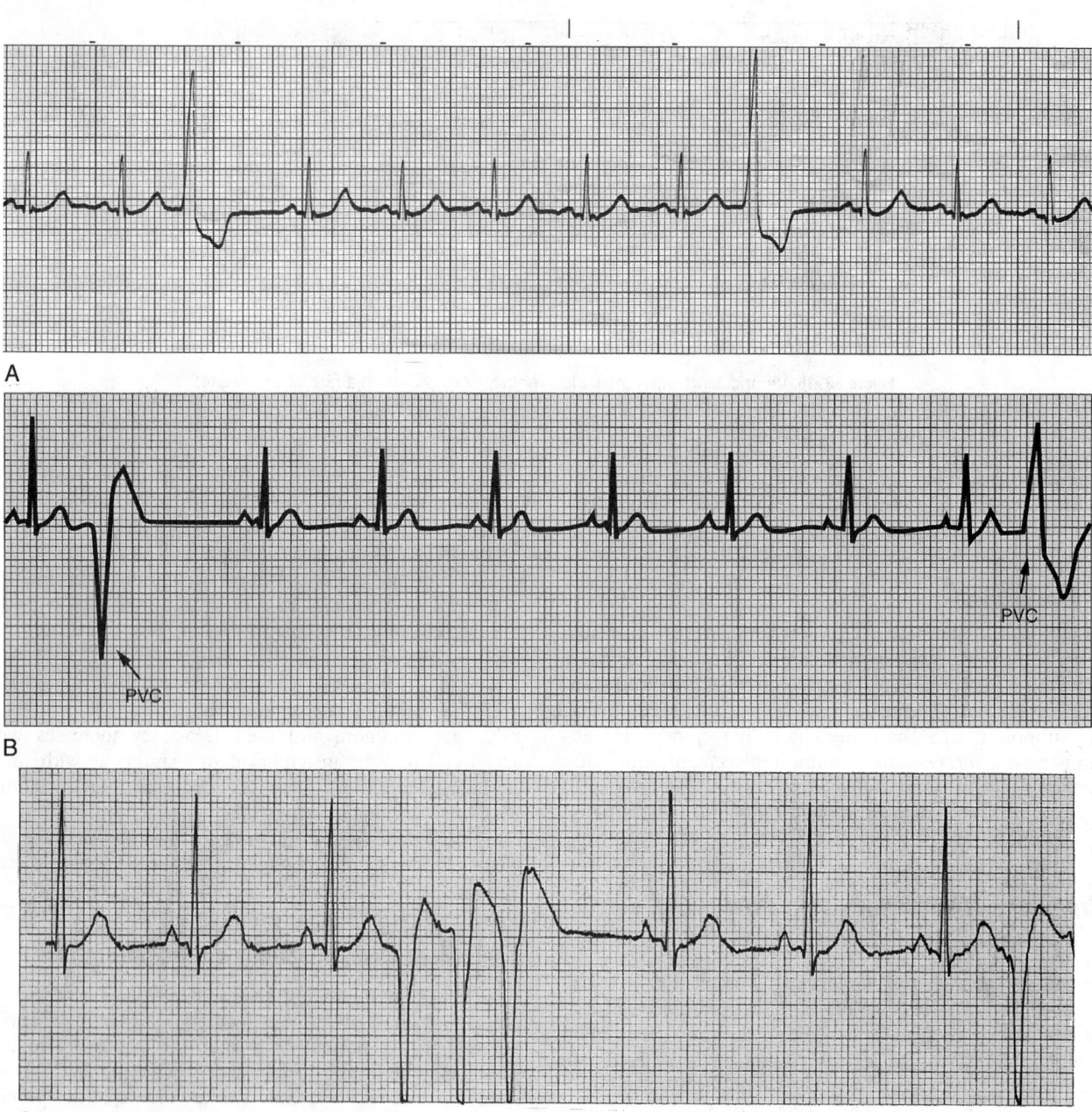

Figure 36–17. Ventricular dysrhythmias. *A,* Normal sinus rhythm (NSR) with unifocal premature ventricular complexes (PVCs). *B,* Normal sinus rhythm with multifocal PVCs (one negative and the other positive). *C,* Normal sinus rhythm with three consecutive PVCs (nonsustained ventricular tachycardia) and another unifocal PVC.

Chart 36–3). The nurse administers potassium as ordered for replacement therapy if hypokalemia is the cause.

Ventricular Tachycardia

Pathophysiology

Ventricular tachycardia (VT) (sometimes referred to as "V tach") occurs with repetitive firing of an irritable ventricular ectopic focus usually at a rate of 140 to 180 beats per minute or more (Fig. 36–18). VT may result from increased automaticity or a re-entry mechanism. VT may

present as a paroxysm of three or more self-limiting beats (nonsustained VT) or as a sustained rhythm (lasting longer than 15 to 30 seconds). The sinus node continues to discharge independently, depolarizing the atria but not the ventricles (AV dissociation), although P waves are seldom seen in sustained VT.

Electrocardiographic criteria include

Rhythm: Usually not possible to determine the atrial rhythm. Ventricular rhythm usually regular or nearly regular

Rate: Not possible to determine the atrial rate. Ven-

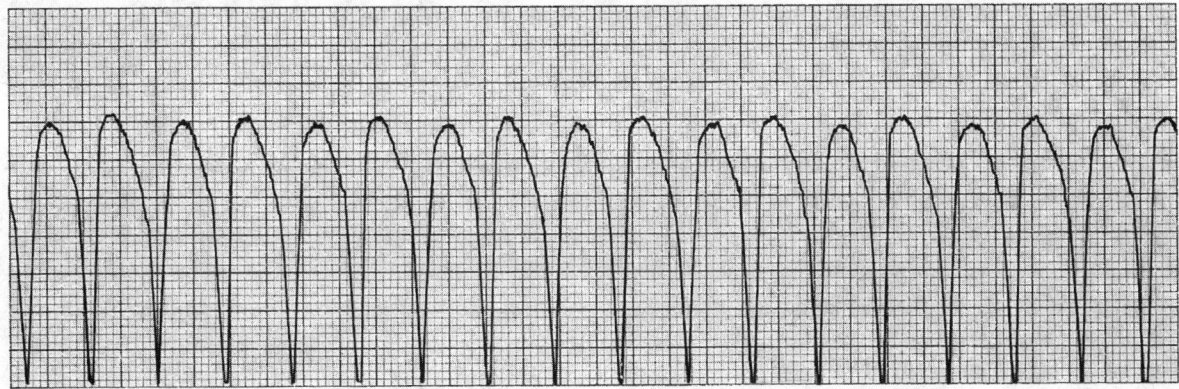

Figure 36–18. Ventricular dysrhythmias. Sustained ventricular tachycardia at a rate of 166/minute.

tricular rate can range from 100 to 250 beats per minute but most commonly 140 to 180 beats per minute

P waves: P waves usually not visible and obscured in QRS complexes. AV dissociation

PR interval: Not measured because of AV dissociation

QRS duration: Wide, greater than 0.14 second, may vary

Etiology

VT may occur in clients with ischemic heart disease, myocardial infarction, cardiomyopathy, hypokalemia, hypomagnesemia, valvular heart disease, heart failure, drug toxicity, hypotension, or ventricular aneurysm. In clients who go into cardiac arrest, VT is commonly the initial rhythm before deteriorating into ventricular fibrillation as the terminal rhythm. VT is not common in infants and children unless they have cardiac disease.

Physical Assessment/Clinical Manifestations

Clinical manifestations of sustained VT partially depend on the ventricular rate. Slower rates are better tolerated. Clients may be hemodynamically compromised if the cardiac output decreases because of the shortened ventricular filling time and loss of the atrial kick. In some clients, VT causes cardiac arrest. The nurse assesses the client's pulse, respirations, blood pressure, level of consciousness, and pupil response.

Interventions

For the stable client with sustained VT, the nurse administers oxygen and lidocaine as prescribed. If this is not successful, procainamide, bretylium, or magnesium sulfate may be given. The physician may prescribe an oral antidysrhythmic agent, such as procainamide, mexiletine, or sotalol.

For the client with unstable VT, the nurse assists the physician to attempt emergency cardioversion followed by oxygen and antidysrhythmic therapy (Chart 36–4). The nurse may instruct the client to perform cough CPR if prescribed, telling the client to inhale deeply and cough hard every 1 to 3 seconds. Cough CPR is sometimes successful in either terminating the VT or at least briefly sustaining cerebral and coronary perfusion until other measures can be initiated. The physician may attempt rapid atrial or ventricular overdrive pacing if the VT is related to a significant bradydysrhythmia.

A precordial thump is sometimes successful in terminating VT, at least transiently. The physician or the ACLS-qualified nurse may administer a precordial thump to a client with unstable VT only if a defibrillator and pacemaker are immediately available (Cummins et al., 1994).

For the client with pulseless VT, the physician or ACLS-qualified nurse or other health care provider must *immediately* defibrillate the client or initiate cardiopulmonary resuscitation (CPR) and defibrillate as soon as possible. A precordial thump may be administered initially, though it is frequently not successful in terminating VT. If the patient remains pulseless, the nurse or other health care provider must resume CPR and full resuscitative measures following defibrillation. This includes airway management and administration of oxygen, epinephrine, and antidysrhythmic therapy with lidocaine, bretylium, magnesium sulfate, and procainamide.

Chart 36–4

Nursing Care Highlight: The Client with Unstable Ventricular Tachycardia

- Assist the physician with cardioversion.
- Provide oxygen and antidysrhythmic drugs as ordered.
- Teach the client how to perform cough cardiopulmonary resuscitation (CPR), if ordered.
- Assist with or provide defibrillation (if you are qualified in advanced cardiac life support [ACLS]).
- Initiate CPR if the client does not respond to the above measures.
- Maintain a patent airway at all times.
- Monitor the client for premature ventricular complexes (PVCs) and the recurrence of VT.
- Assess for signs and symptoms of myocardial infarction, hypokalemia, or hypomagnesemia.

If the rhythm has been successfully converted, attention is given to treating reversible causes of VT, such as myocardial ischemia, hypokalemia, and hypomagnesemia. The nurse ensures that oxygen therapy and antidysrhythmic agent administration are continued, and the client is closely monitored for PVCs and the recurrence of VT. The client with recurrent, medically refractory VT should be studied in the electrophysiology lab and may benefit from radiofrequency catheter ablation. Some forms of VT may require surgical intervention, such as coronary artery bypass graft (CABG) surgery, implantation of a cardioverter/defibrillator, aneurysmectomy, encircling endocardial ventriculotomy, cryosurgery, or endocardial resection (see Chap. 40).

Ventricular Fibrillation

Pathophysiology

Ventricular fibrillation (VF) (sometimes called "V fib") is the result of electrical chaos in the ventricles. Impulses from many irritable foci fire in a totally disorganized manner so that ventricular contraction cannot occur. There are no recognizable deflections. Instead, there are irregular undulations of varying amplitudes, from coarse to fine (Fig. 36–19A). The ventricles merely quiver, consuming a tremendous amount of oxygen. There is no cardiac output, therefore no cerebral, myocardial, or systemic perfusion. This rhythm is *rapidly fatal* if not successfully terminated within 3 to 5 minutes.

Electrocardiographic criteria include

   Rhythm: Irregular, chaotic undulations of varying amplitudes in baseline
   Rate: Not measurable
   P waves: Not visible
   PR interval: Not measurable
   QRS duration: None. Fibrillatory waves may be coarse or fine

Etiology

VF may be the first manifestation of coronary artery disease. Clients with myocardial infarction are at great risk for VF. VF may also occur in clients with myocardial ischemia, hypokalemia, hypomagnesemia, antidysrhythmic therapy, rapid supraventricular tachydysrhythmias, shock, asynchronous pacing with competition, or severe metabolic derangements. VF also occurs following surgery or trauma.

Physical Assessment/Clinical Manifestations

On initiation of VF, the client becomes faint, immediately loses consciousness, and becomes pulseless and apneic. There is no blood pressure, and heart sounds are absent. Respiratory and metabolic acidosis develop. Seizures may occur. Within minutes, the pupils become fixed and dilated, and the skin becomes cold and mottled. Death

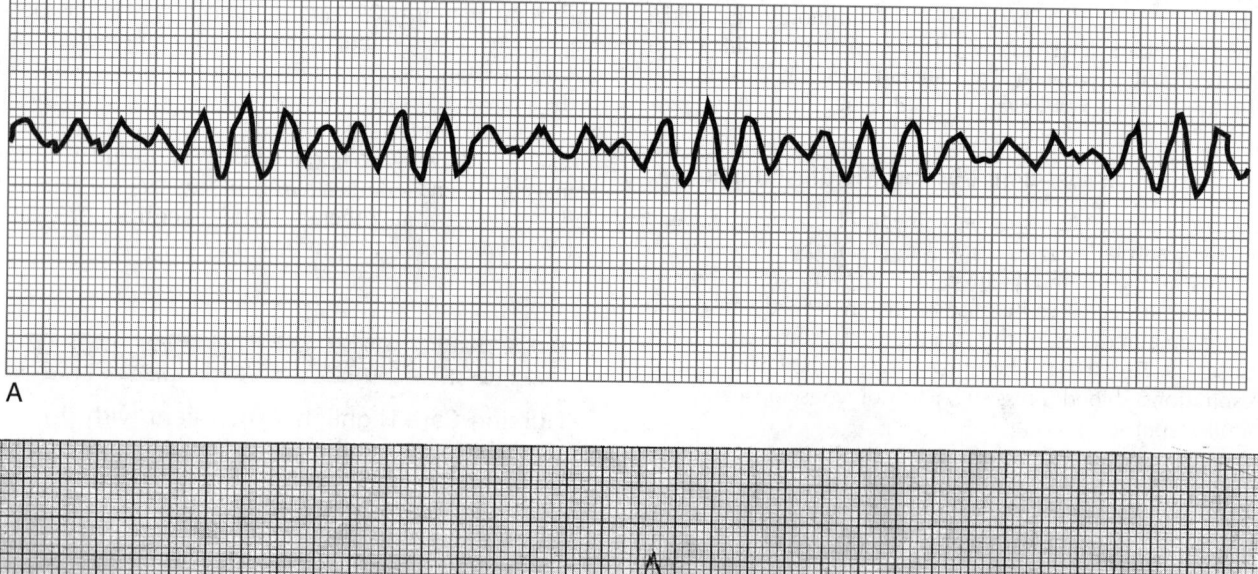

A

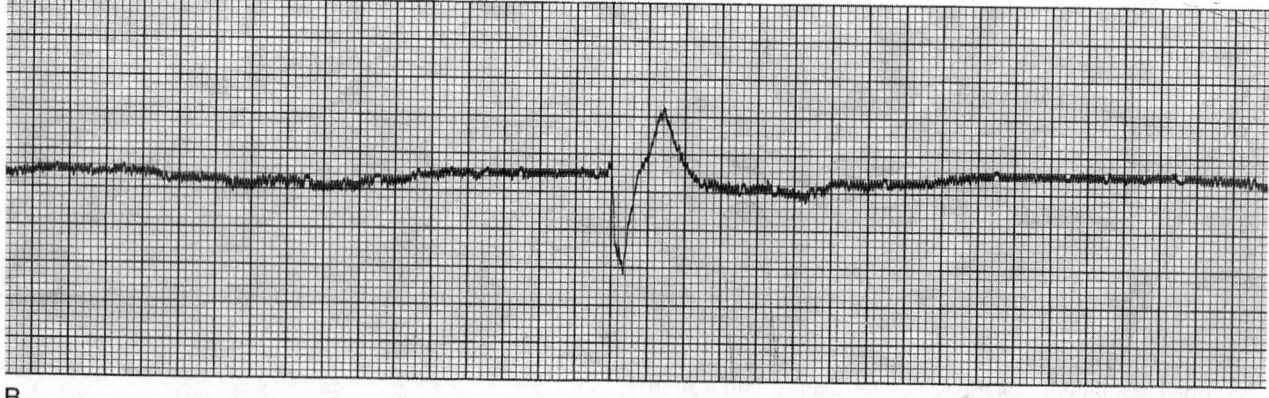

B

Figure 36–19. Ventricular dysrhythmias. *A*, Coarse ventricular fibrillation. *B*, Ventricular asystole with one idioventricular complex.

ensues without prompt restoration of an organized rhythm and cardiac output.

Interventions

The goals of treatment are to terminate VF promptly and to convert it to an organized rhythm. The physician or the advanced cardiac life support (ACLS)–qualified nurse or other health care provider must immediately defibrillate the client to accomplish this goal. This is the management priority. If a defibrillator is not readily available, a precordial thump may be delivered. CPR must be continued until the defibrillator arrives.

If the VF does not terminate after three rapid successive shocks of increasing energy, the nurse and resuscitation team resume CPR and provide airway management. They also administer oxygen, epinephrine, and antidysrhythmic therapy with lidocaine, bretylium, magnesium sulfate, and procainamide, along with attempting defibrillation frequently. Cough CPR may be successful in terminating the VF or at least in briefly sustaining cerebral and coronary perfusion until definitive treatment can be initiated if the client coughs vigorously before losing consciousness. If VF is successfully converted to an organized rhythm, the nurse continues supportive therapy and assists the physician to treat potential causes of VF and to prevent its recurrence.

Ventricular Asystole

Pathophysiology

Ventricular asystole, sometimes called *ventricular standstill,* is the complete absence of any ventricular rhythm (see Fig. 36–19B). There are no electrical impulses in the ventricles and therefore *no* ventricular depolarization, no QRS complex, no contraction, no cardiac output, and no pulse, respirations, or blood pressure. The client is in full cardiac arrest. The sinoatrial (SA) node, in some cases, may continue to fire and depolarize the atria, with only P waves seen on the electrocardiogram (ECG), but the sinus impulses do not conduct to the ventricles, and QRS complexes remain absent. In most cases, the entire conduction system is electrically silent, with no P waves seen on the ECG. There is only a mildly undulating line on the ECG. Fine VF may resemble asystole in some leads. Because treatment of these two rhythms differs significantly, the nurse must assess two ECG leads for an accurate rhythm interpretation.

Electrocardiographic criteria include

Rhythm: Atrial rhythm usually absent. If P waves present, atrial rhythm may be regular. Ventricular rhythm absent
Rate: No ventricular rate
P waves: P waves usually absent. Occasionally, regular P waves if the SA node continues to function
PR interval: None
QRS duration: QRS complexes absent

Etiology

Ventricular asystole usually results from myocardial hypoxia, which may be a consequence of advanced heart failure. It may also be caused by severe hyperkalemia and acidosis. If P waves are seen, asystole is likely because of severe ventricular conduction blocks. Rarely, excessive vagal stimulation may cause asystole.

Physical Assessment/Clinical Manifestations

Clients are in full cardiac arrest with loss of consciousness and absence of pulse, respirations, and blood pressure. Ventricular asystole is often fatal, unresponsive to resuscitation measures.

Interventions

The goal of treatment is to restore cardiac electrical activity. The nurse or other health care provider initiates CPR immediately and summons assistance. The nurse must assess another ECG lead to ensure that the rhythm is asystole and not fine VF, which warrants immediate defibrillation. When in doubt, the client should be defibrillated. The nurse and resuscitation team manage the airway and administer oxygen, epinephrine, and atropine. The nurse assists the physician with the initiation of noninvasive pacing or invasive transvenous or epicardial pacing, although pacemaker therapy is generally not effective. An isoproterenol infusion may also be tried. The prognosis for clients with asystole is poor.

Atrioventricular Blocks

Atrioventricular blocks (AV blocks) exist when supraventricular impulses are excessively delayed or totally blocked in the AV node or intraventricular conduction system. Conduction may be transiently or permanently abnormal for a number of reasons. The SA node continues to function normally, and atrial depolarizations and P waves occur regularly. Because of the conduction dysfunction, ventricular depolarizations and QRS complexes are either delayed or blocked.

There are different degrees of heart blocks, as follows:

- In first-degree AV block, all sinus impulses eventually reach the ventricles.
- In second-degree heart block, some sinus impulses reach the ventricles, but others do not because they are blocked.
- In third-degree heart block (complete heart block), none of the sinus impulses reach the ventricles. The ventricles, therefore, are depolarized by a second, independent pacemaker.

AV blocks are differentiated by their PR intervals.

First-Degree Atrioventricular Block

Pathophysiology

First-degree AV block is actually a conduction delay rather than a block. AV node conduction is slow, prolonging the PR interval to greater than 0.20 second. However, all sinus impulses eventually reach the ventricles. The underlying rhythm must still be identified (e.g., sinus tachycardia with first-degree AV block) (Fig. 36–20A).

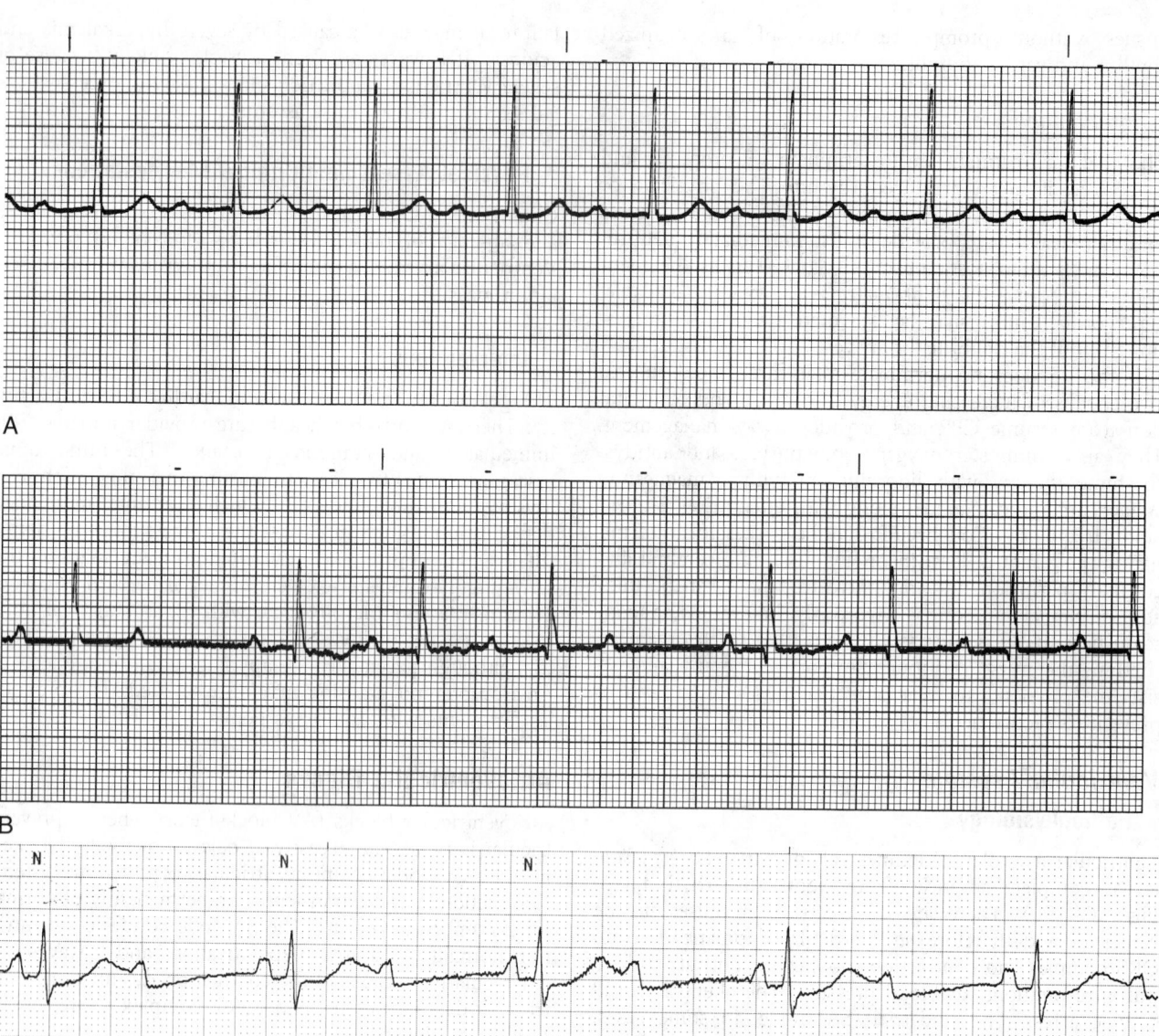

Figure 36–20. AV blocks. *A,* Normal sinus rhythm (NSR) with first-degree AV block (PR interval 0.36 second). *B,* Second-degree AV block type I (Wenckebach AV) with an irregular rhythm, grouped beating, and progressive prolongation of the PR interval until a P wave is completely blocked and not followed by a QRS complex. *C,* Second-degree AV block type II (Mobitz II) with 2:1 conduction, a constant PR interval, and wide QRS complex.

Electrocardiographic criteria include

Rhythm: Atrial and ventricular rhythms usually regular unless sinus arrhythmia is present

Rate: Depends on the underlying rhythm. Atrial and ventricular rates are equal

P waves: One P wave preceding each QRS complex. Constant morphologic pattern

PR interval: PR interval prolonged, greater than 0.20 second. It usually does not exceed 0.40 second

QRS duration: Normal, constant

Etiology

First-degree AV block may be due to AV nodal ischemia from occlusion of the right coronary artery, as with an inferior or posterior myocardial infarction. It may also result from hypokalemia or hyperkalemia; the administration of digitalis, beta-adrenergic blockers, calcium channel blockers; excessive vagal stimulation; or degenerative AV nodal disease. In children, it may occur following cardiac surgery as a result of edema in the AV nodal area and usually resolves without treatment.

Physical Assessment/Clinical Manifestations

First-degree AV block has no hemodynamic consequences and produces no symptoms. Any symptoms are the result of the underlying rhythm (e.g., sinus bradycardia). First-degree AV block may be insignificant and transient or may progress to more severe AV blocks, although this is uncommon.

Interventions

In the stable client, no treatment is needed. If the first-degree AV block is due to drug therapy, the nurse must withhold the offending drug and notify the physician. If the PR interval is particularly long or is getting progressively longer, the nurse must notify the physician. When first-degree AV block is associated with symptomatic bradycardia, the nurse administers oxygen and atropine as prescribed to accelerate AV conduction.

Second-Degree Atrioventricular Block Type I (AV Wenckebach or Mobitz Type I)
Pathophysiology

In second-degree AV block type I, each successive sinus impulse takes a little longer to conduct through the impaired AV node, until one impulse is completely blocked and fails to depolarize the ventricles because the AV node has become completely refractory. This block results in a nonconducted or dropped beat (missing QRS complex). There is progressive prolongation of the PR interval, followed by a dropped beat and a pause (the most characteristic feature of this rhythm). The pause allows sufficient time for the AV node to recover so that the next beat is conducted with a shorter PR interval and the Wenckebach sequence is repeated. Although the atrial rhythm is usually regular, the ventricular rhythm is irregular, with an appearance of grouped beats separated by pauses. Group size (conduction ratios) may be constant or may vary. Because of the dropped QRS complex, each group normally has one more P wave than QRS complexes (see Fig. 36–20B).

Electrocardiographic criteria include

Rhythm: Atrial rhythm usually regular. Ventricular rhythm irregular, with grouped beating and shortening R-R intervals in the group
Rate: Atrial rate dependent on the underlying sinus rhythm, which may be normal or slow. Because of dropped beats, ventricular rate always less than atrial rate
P waves: P waves normal, with constant morphologic pattern. Some P waves not conducted to the ventricles and not followed by a QRS complex
PR interval: Progressive lengthening of PR intervals until a dropped beat, which is followed by a pause. A new sequence then begins
QRS duration: QRS duration usually normal and constant. One QRS complex is missing in each grouped sequence

Etiology

The causes of AV Wenckebach are the same as for first-degree AV block. It is often a transient rhythm and may revert to first-degree AV block or even a normal sinus rhythm. Second-degree AV block type I is also seen with rheumatic fever and digitalis administration. AV Wenckebach may occur in a child following cardiac surgery and is usually transient.

Physical Assessment/Clinical Manifestations

The client is usually asymptomatic if the frequency of dropped beats and the overall ventricular rate do not decrease the cardiac output. If the ventricular rate is too slow, decreasing the cardiac output, the client presents with symptoms of a symptomatic bradydysrhythmia. This rhythm is usually transient and terminates spontaneously.

Interventions

No intervention is required in the stable client, because this rhythm rarely progresses to a more severe block. In the symptomatic client, the nurse administers oxygen and atropine as prescribed. If atropine is not successful in speeding AV nodal conduction time and increasing the heart rate, the nurse initiates pacemaker therapy as ordered and notifies the physician.

Second-Degree Heart Block Type II (Mobitz Type II)
Pathophysiology

In Mobitz type II block, the block is actually infranodal, occurring below the His bundle. It involves a constant block in one of the bundle branches, resulting in a wide QRS complex in conducted beats, and an intermittent block in the other bundle branch, resulting in dropped beats because both bundles are blocked. (P waves are not followed by a QRS complex.) Because the block is not in the AV node, sinus impulses that conduct to the ventricles always do so with a constant PR interval. Impulses may be blocked randomly, making the ventricular rhythm irregular. Alternatively, the impulses may be blocked at regular intervals, such as in 2:1 block, in which case the ventricular rhythm is regular (see Fig. 36–20C).

Electrocardiographic criteria include

Rhythm: Atrial rhythm usually regular. Ventricular rhythm regular or irregular, depending on the block
Rate: Atrial rate dependent on the underlying sinus rhythm. May be normal or slightly fast. Because of dropped beats, the ventricular rate is less than the atrial rate. This rate may be slow
P waves: P waves normal, with a constant morphologic pattern. One or more P waves not conducted to the ventricles
PR interval: Constant in conducted beats
QRS duration: Usually wide, indicating that the block is infranodal in one of the bundle branches, with missing QRS complexes because of intermittent block of the other bundle branch

Etiology

Second-degree AV block type II is less common than type I. It may occur in the adult with anterior myocardial infarctions and results from severe ischemic damage to the conduction system. It may also be caused by rheumatic heart disease or degenerative disease of the conduction system. It is a serious block that may progress suddenly to a third-degree AV block (complete heart block) and an ominous prognosis. Mobitz II may occur in children following cardiac surgery or, less frequently, children with congenital AV block.

Physical Assessment/Clinical Manifestations

Symptoms depend on the frequency of dropped beats and the overall ventricular rate. If the cardiac output is inadequate, the client presents with a symptomatic bradydysrhythmia.

Interventions

In the asymptomatic client, the nurse may assist the physician to initiate prophylactic pacing to avert the threat of sudden third-degree AV block. If slow ventricular rates are present, the nurse administers oxygen and atropine as prescribed. Atropine is usually ineffective because it does not reverse the infranodal block. An isoproterenol (Isuprel) infusion may be administered with caution but may be dangerous in adults with ischemic heart disease. Non-invasive or invasive pacing is preferred. A permanent pacemaker may be required in adults and children with recurrent or medically refractory Mobitz type II.

Third-Degree Heart Block (Complete Heart Block)

Pathophysiology

In third-degree heart block, none of the sinus impulses conducts to the ventricles. The SA node is usually the pacemaker for the atria, producing P waves at a normal or even accelerated rate. A separate, independent pacemaker paces the ventricles. Thus, AV dissociation exists. If the block is in the AV node, a junctional escape focus paces the ventricles, producing normal QRS complexes at a rate of 40 to 60 beats per minute (Fig. 36–21A). If the block is below the bundle of His (infranodal), a ventricular escape focus paces the ventricles, producing wide QRS complexes at a rate usually less than 40 beats per minute (see Fig. 36–21B). In either case, the atrial and ventricular rhythms are usually regular but independent of each other, with more P waves than QRS complexes.

Because the P waves and the QRS complexes are totally independent and bear no relationship to each other, the PR interval is inconstant, which is the most characteristic feature of this rhythm. The ventricular escape pacemaker is the least stable, least dependable pacemaker. It may abruptly fail, causing ventricular asystole, or it may predispose to irritability in the form of premature ventricular complexes (PVCs), ventricular tachycardia (VT), or ventricular fibrillation (VF).

Electrocardiographic criteria include

Rhythm: Atrial and ventricular rhythms usually regular, but independent of each other because of AV dissociation

Rate: Atrial rate dependent on the underlying sinus rhythm. May be normal or slightly fast. If paced by a junctional escape rhythm, the ventricular rate is 40 to 60 beats per minute. If paced by a ventricular escape rhythm, the ventricular rate is usually less than 40 beats per minute.

P waves: Normal, constant morphologic pattern, but not related to QRS complexes (AV dissociation); more P waves than QRS complexes

PR interval: Inconstant because of AV dissociation

QRS duration: With a junctional escape pacemaker, QRS complexes normal and constant. With a ventricular escape pacemaker, QRS complexes wide (greater than 0.14 second) and constant

Etiology

Third-degree heart block in the adult may occur from ischemic injury with coronary artery disease or myocardial infarction, degenerative disease of the conduction system, or calcific aortic stenosis. In adults and children, third-degree heart block may occur with congenital heart disease, the effects of drugs or electrolyte disturbances, or cardiac surgery.

Physical Assessment/Clinical Manifestations

Clinical manifestations depend on the overall ventricular rate and cardiac output. Transient third-degree heart block may be well tolerated, particularly when the block is in the AV node. If the block is infranodal, if may have serious hemodynamic consequences. If cerebral perfusion is inadequate, clients may be confused and lightheaded or may experience episodes of syncope with or without seizures (Stokes-Adams attacks). Inadequate cardiac output may cause myocardial ischemia or infarction, heart failure, and hypotension. Third-degree heart block may predispose to cardiac arrest, causing VT, VF, or asystole. Therefore, it is regarded as a dangerous rhythm.

Interventions

Third-degree AV block with a junctional escape pacemaker is often transient and well tolerated. If the client is symptomatic, the nurse administers oxygen and atropine as prescribed. Clients with third-degree heart block with a ventricular escape pacemaker are frequently symptomatic. The nurse administers oxygen and assists the physician to initiate prophylactic pacing to avert the threat of cardiac arrest. Atropine is usually not successful in infranodal blocks with wide QRS complexes. Cautious use of isoproterenol (Isuprel) infusions may be necessary as a temporary measure while awaiting pacemaker therapy but is dangerous in clients with acute myocardial infarction. Implantation of a permanent pacemaker may be required in patients with recurrent or medically refractory third-degree infranodal block.

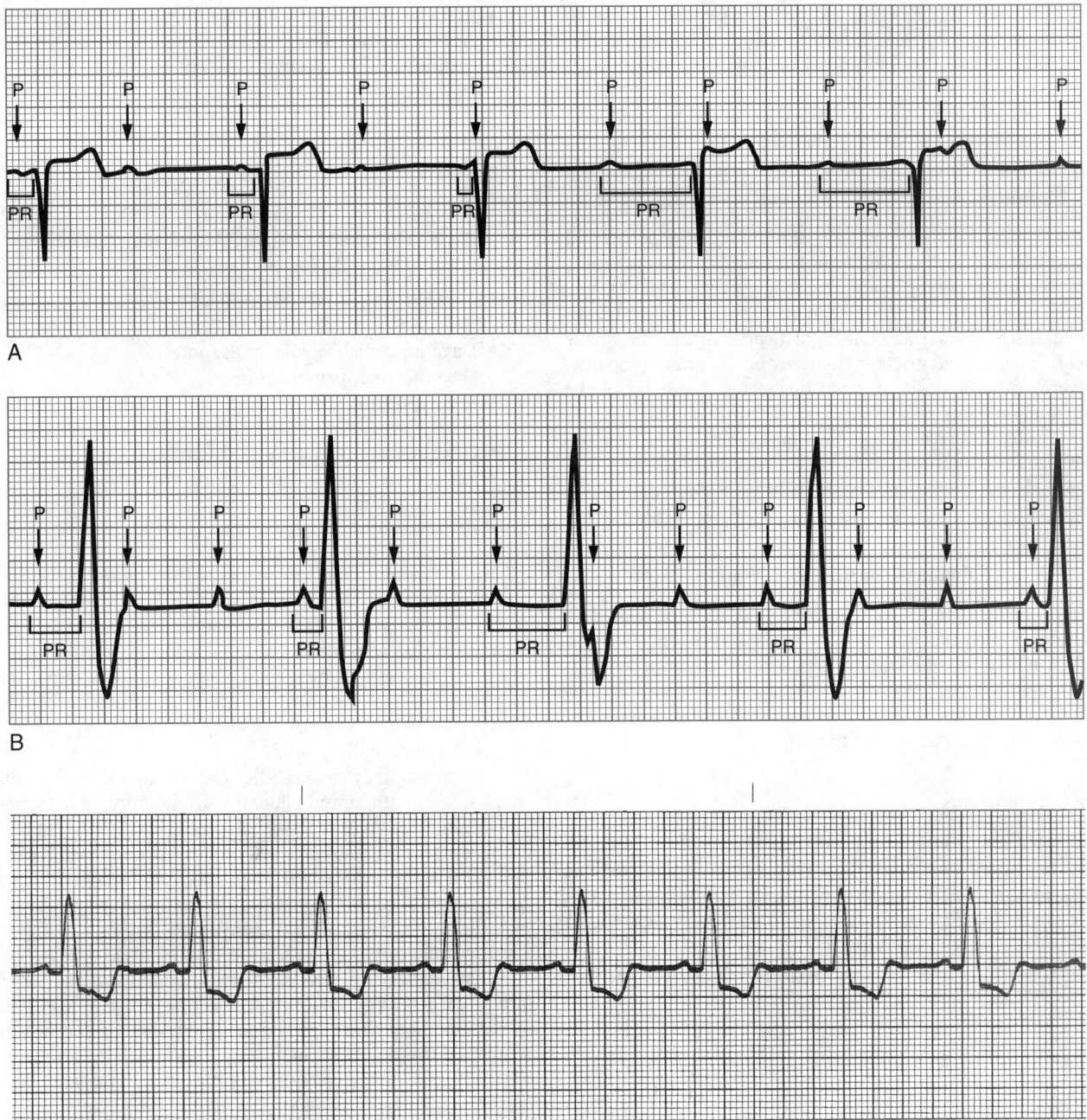

Figure 36-21. AV blocks. *A,* Third-degree AV block (complete heart block) with regular atrial and ventricular rhythms, inconstant PR intervals (AV dissociation), and a junctional escape focus (normal QRS complexes) pacing the ventricles at a rate of 44/minute. *B,* Third-degree AV block with regular atrial and ventricular rhythms, inconstant PR intervals (AV dissociation), and a ventricular escape focus pacing the ventricles at a rate of 38/minute, with wide QRS complexes. *C,* Normal sinus rhythm (NSR) with bundle branch block (wide QRS complexes measuring 0.12 second).

Bundle Branch Blocks

Pathophysiology

Bundle branch block is a conduction delay or block within one of the two main bundle branches below the bifurcation of the His bundle. When one bundle branch is blocked, the supraventricular impulse is able to descend only down the normal bundle branch and to depolarize that ventricle. The other ventricle is depolarized afterward, as the wave of depolarization from the first ventricle proceeds from cell to cell to the other ventricle. Such slow depolarization prolongs the QRS duration to 0.12 second or longer. The underlying rhythm is usually sinus in origin (e.g., sinus rhythm with bundle branch block) (see Fig. 36-21C).

Electrocardiographic criteria include

Rhythm: Atrial and ventricular rhythms usually regular

Rate: Atrial and ventricular rates equal. Bundle branch block may occur at any rate

P waves: One P wave before each QRS complex, with a constant morphologic pattern

PR interval: May be normal or may be prolonged (first-degree AV block)

QRS duration: Wide, usually 0.12 to 0.14 second and usually constant, but may vary slightly

Etiology

Bundle branch block may be a temporary or a permanent conduction disorder. Right or left bundle branch blocks may occasionally be seen in clients with normal hearts. More commonly, they are seen in clients with cardiovascular disease, such as congenital heart disease, rheumatic heart disease, ventricular hypertrophy, cardiomyopathy, severe aortic stenosis, chronic degenerative disease of the conduction system, and fibrotic scarring of the conduction system. Transient bundle branch block may be seen with acute conditions such as coronary insufficiency, myocardial infarction, and heart failure; during right-sided heart catheterization; or with rapid supraventricular rates.

Physical Assessment/Clinical Manifestations

There are no clinical manifestations specifically related to bundle branch block. The nurse must notify the physician when a new bundle branch block develops, especially in the client with an acute myocardial infarction. The conduction disorder may deteriorate to a more significant block requiring pacemaker therapy.

Interventions

No interventions are specifically related to bundle branch block. The nurse ensures that the client is resting and has adequate ventilation and oxygenation. The nurse assesses the client during alterations in heart rate for symptoms of hemodynamic compromise. The nurse reports symptoms to the physician and assists the physician in treating any underlying disorder.

Collaborative Management

 Analysis

> ### ➤ *Common Nursing Diagnoses and Collaborative Problems*

The most common nursing diagnoses pertinent to the client with dysrhythmias are

1. Decreased Cardiac Output related to electrical and mechanical dysfunction
2. Altered Tissue Perfusion related to decreased cardiac output

> ### ➤ *Additional Nursing Diagnoses and Collaborative Problems*

In addition to the common nursing diagnoses, some clients have one or more of the following:
- Impaired Gas Exchange related to altered oxygen supply

- Ineffective Individual Coping related to fear of death
- Activity Intolerance

The additional collaborative problem is Potential for Pulmonary Edema.

 Planning and Implementation

> ### ➤ *Decreased Cardiac Output and Altered Tissue Perfusion*

Planning: Expected Outcomes. The client is expected to
- Have a normal, regular pulse rate
- Have normal mental acuity
- Have a normal rate, rhythm, and depth of respiration
- Have normal skin color and temperature
- Perform activities of daily living without dyspnea or excess fatigue
- Be free of pulmonary edema

Interventions. The nurse or assistive nursing personnel monitors the client's ECG rhythm and/or assesses the client for signs and symptoms associated with dysrhythmias, such as abnormal pulse rate and rhythm, palpitations, chest pain, syncope, decreased oxygen saturation, decreased blood pressure, dyspnea, pulmonary congestion, neck vein distention, anxiety, restlessness, skin pallor, and poor capillary refill.

The nurse may assess the client's apical and radial pulses for a full minute for any irregularity, which may occur with premature beats, escape beats, atrial fibrillation, or second-degree heart blocks. If the apical pulse rate differs from the radial pulse rate, a pulse deficit exists and suggests that not all beats are perfusing. Clinical manifestations of sustained tachydysrhythmias and bradydysrhythmias are summarized in Chart 36–2.

In an acute care setting, if the client has a pulmonary artery catheter and an arterial line, the nurse assesses the client's hemodynamic profile to determine the physiologic effects of the dysrhythmia. The nurse must also assess the psychosocial impact of dysrhythmias on clients and families and the effectiveness of their coping mechanisms.

Assessment of the client's past and current history is essential because dysrhythmias are associated with both acute and chronic disorders and also with medical and surgical therapies. The nurse should also review the interpretation of the client's 12-lead ECG and other electrocardiographic diagnostic tests, such as the Holter monitor, event monitor, or signal-averaged ECG. The nurse must identify the client who is at risk for serious consequences from dysrhythmias.

Interventions are specific to the type of dysrhythmia, the cause, the effect it has on the client's cardiac output, and the risk it presents to the client. Interventions for specific dysrhythmias are summarized in Table 36–2.

Nonsurgical Management. Nonsurgical management of dysrhythmias includes drug therapy, vagal maneuvers, temporary pacing, cardioversion, cardiopulmonary resuscitation (CPR), defibrillation, and catheter ablation.

Drug Therapy. Pharmacologic therapy administered for the control of dysrhythmias often includes drugs from one or more classes of antidysrhythmic agents (see Chart 36–3). The Vaughn-Williams classification is commonly used to classify drugs according to their effects on the action potential of cardiac cells. Other drugs also have antidysrhythmic effects but do not fit the Vaughn-Williams classification.

Vaughn-Williams Classification. Class I antidysrhythmics are membrane-stabilizing agents, stabilizing phase 4 to decrease automaticity. There are three subclassifications in this group. Type IA drugs moderately slow conduction and prolong repolarization, prolonging the QT interval. These drugs are used to treat or to prevent supraventricular and ventricular premature beats and tachydysrhythmias. Examples include quinidine sulfate and procainamide hydrochloride (Pronestyl). Type IB drugs shorten repolarization. These drugs are used to treat or prevent ventricular premature beats, ventricular tachycardia (VT), and ventricular fibrillation (VF). Examples include lidocaine and mexiletine hydrochloride (Mexitil). Type IC drugs markedly slow conduction and widen the QRS complex. These drugs are used primarily to treat or to prevent recurrent, life-threatening ventricular premature beats, VT, and VF. Examples include flecainide acetate (Tambocor) and propafenone hydrochloride (Rythmol).

Class II antidysrhythmics control dysrhythmias associated with excessive beta-adrenergic stimulation by competing for receptor sites and thereby decreasing heart rate and conduction velocity. Beta-adrenergic–blocking agents, such as propranolol hydrochloride (Inderal) and esmolol hydrochloride (Brevibloc), are class II drugs. They are used to treat or to prevent supraventricular and ventricular premature beats and tachydysrhythmias. Sotalol hydrochloride (Betapace) is an antidysrhythmic agent with both noncardioselective beta-adrenergic–blocking effects (class II) and action potential duration prolongation properties (class III). It is an oral agent recommended for the treatment of documented ventricular dysrhythmias, such as VT, that are life-threatening.

Class III antidysrhythmics lengthen the absolute refractory period and prolong repolarization and the action potential duration of ischemic cells. They decrease the disparity with normal cells to prevent a re-entry response. Class III drugs include bretylium tosylate (Bretylol, Bretylate✳), amiodarone hydrochloride (Cordarone), and ibutilide fumarate (Corvert) and are used to treat or prevent ventricular premature beats, VT, and VF.

Class IV antidysrhythmics impede the flow of calcium into the cell during depolarization, thereby depressing automaticity of the sinoatrial (SA) and atrioventricular (AV) nodes, decreasing heart rate, and prolonging AV nodal refractoriness and conduction. Calcium channel blockers, such as verapamil hydrochloride (Calan, Isoptin✳) and diltiazem hydrochloride (Cardizem), are class IV drugs. They are used to treat supraventricular tachycardia (SVT), atrial flutter, and atrial fibrillation to slow down the ventricular response.

Other Antidysrhythmic Drugs. Other drugs, such as digoxin, atropine, adenosine, and magnesium sulfate, are frequently used to treat dysrhythmias. Digoxin increases vagal tone, slowing AV nodal conduction. It is useful in treating supraventricular tachydysrhythmias, particularly chronic atrial fibrillation, by controlling the rate of ventricular response. Atropine is a parasympatholytic or vagolytic agent. It is used to treat vagally induced symptomatic bradydysrhythmias. Adenosine is an endogenous nucleoside that slows AV nodal conduction to interrupt re-entry pathways. It is effective in terminating paroxysmal supraventricular tachycardia, a re-entrant tachydysrhythmia. Magnesium sulfate is an electrolyte administered to treat refractory VT or VF because these clients may be hypomagnesemic, with increased ventricular irritability.

Emergency Cardiac Drugs. In addition to antidysrhythmics, several other drugs are used during cardiac arrest (Chart 36–5). Epinephrine (Adrenalin) is a first-line agent in all cardiac arrests. It is given predominantly for its alpha-adrenergic effects to increase vasomotor tone for myocardial and cerebral perfusion. Its beta-adrenergic effects may stimulate the heart and increase myocardial contractility to improve cardiac output. Dopamine hydrochloride (Intropin) is generally used for its beta-adrenergic effects after cardiac arrest but may be used for its alpha-adrenergic effects during resuscitation. Dobutamine hydrochloride (Dobutrex) is a beta-adrenergic agent used to improve myocardial contractility and increase cardiac output.

Norepinephrine may be used for its alpha-adrenergic effects to increase vasomotor tone and increase perfusion pressure. Sodium bicarbonate is administered during cardiac arrest for clients who are hyperkalemic. It may also be used, if necessary, to treat a bicarbonate metabolic acidosis, as occurs in diabetic ketoacidosis or tricyclic antidepressant overdose. Isoproterenol (Isuprel), a beta-adrenergic agent, is rarely used to increase heart rate in an atropine-refractory, symptomatic bradydysrhythmia. Isoproterenol is indicated to increase the heart rate in heart transplant patients. Pacing is preferred. Calcium chloride, which increases myocardial contractility, is also rarely indicated. It is reserved for clients with hyperkalemia, hypocalcemia, or calcium channel–blocker toxicity because it may cause cell damage and cerebrovascular vasospasm.

Vagal Maneuvers. Vagal maneuvers induce vagal stimulation of the cardiac conduction system, specifically the SA and AV nodes. Vagal maneuvers are used to terminate supraventricular tachydysrhythmias. They include carotid sinus massage and Valsalva maneuvers.

Carotid Sinus Massage. The physician massages over the carotid artery for a few seconds, observing for a change in cardiac rhythm. Massaging the carotid sinus causes vagal stimulation, slowing SA nodal and AV nodal conduction. The nurse prepares the client for this procedure, instructs the client to turn the head slightly away from the side to be massaged, and observes the cardiac monitor for a change in rhythm. The nurse records an ECG rhythm strip before, during, and after the procedure. The nurse then assesses the client's vital signs and level of consciousness. Complications include bradydysrhythmias, asystole, ventricular fibrillation, and cerebral damage. Ca-

Chart 36–5

Drug Therapy for Cardiac Arrest

Drug	Usual Dosage	Nursing Interventions	Rationale
Epinephrine (Adrenalin)	• 1-mg IV bolus followed by 20-mL saline flush q3–5 min • If this fails, may consider: 2–5 mg IV bolus q3–5 min; 1-mg, 3-mg, and 5-mg IV bolus (3 min apart); or 0.1 mg/kg IV bolus q3–5 min • If necessary, may give endotracheally with dose at least 2–2½ times IV dose	• Monitor for return of rhythm and pulse when used for asystole or VF. • Assess for tachycardia, dysrhythmias, or hypertension. • Assess for the development of coarse VF when given during fine VF.	• Return of rhythm and pulse is the expected response. • Adverse reactions can occur with a dramatic response. • This may improve the response to defibrillation.
Dopamine hydrochloride (Intropin)	• 2.5–5 μg/kg/min IV infusion; titrate to desired clinical response • 1–2 μg/kg/min for renal and mesenteric vasodilation • 2–10 μg/kg/min for beta-adrenergic effects • 10–20 μg/kg/min for alpha-adrenergic effects	• Assess clients for increased blood pressure. • Monitor for tachycardia, dysrhythmias, or hypertension. • Monitor the IV site for infiltration. • Assess for urinary output <30 mL/hr, or pallor, cyanosis, pain, or numbness in the extremities.	• Increased blood pressure is the expected response. • Adverse reactions may occur. • Extravasation of drug can occur, causing necrosis. • Dosages >10 μg/kg/min cause vasoconstriction of renal and peripheral blood vessels; dosages of 2–5 μg/kg/min may improve urinary output by causing renal vasodilation and improving renal blood flow.
Dobutamine hydrochloride (Dobutrex)	• 2–20 μg/kg/min IV infusion	• Assess for increased blood pressure. • Assess for hypertension and dysrhythmias.	• Increased blood pressure is the expected response. • Adverse reactions may occur.
Norepinephrine (Levophed)	• 0.5–1 μg/min IV infusion, titrate to desired effect, up to 8–30 μg/min	• Assess for increased blood pressure. • Monitor for bradycardia.	• Increased blood pressure is the expected response. • Reflex bradycardia may occur with a rise in blood pressure.

rotid sinus massage is contraindicated in clients with cerebral arteriosclerosis and carotid bruits. A defibrillator and resuscitative equipment must be immediately available during the procedure.

Valsalva Maneuvers. To stimulate a vagal reflex, the health care provider instructs the client to bear down as if straining to have a bowel movement or induces the gag reflex in the client. The nurse prepares the client for the procedure; assesses the client's heart rate, heart rhythm, and blood pressure; observes the cardiac monitor; and records an ECG rhythm strip before, during, and after the procedure to determine the effect of therapy. If gagging is induced, the nurse provides an emesis basin and oral hygiene if the client vomits and takes measures to prevent aspiration.

Unintended vagal stimulation may sometimes occur, and the nurse must be cautious when performing procedures that may inadvertently cause vagal stimulation. For example, tracheal suctioning, enema administration, and rectal temperature checks can stimulate the vagus nerve and decrease the heart rate inappropriately. The nurse administers stool softeners as prescribed. The nurse instructs the client not to strain during bowel movements and to avoid constipation through proper diet and exercise. The client is also told to avoid inducing gagging during oral hygiene, which triggers a vagal response. The nurse assesses the heart rate and rhythm of a client who is vomiting, which may induce a vagal reflex. Some clients experience a vagal response when raising their arms above their head and must be instructed to avoid this movement.

Chart 36–5. Drug Therapy for Cardiac Arrest Continued

Drug	Usual Dosage	Nursing Interventions	Rationale
		• Monitor for hypertension and dysrhythmias.	• Adverse reactions may occur with a dramatic response.
		• Monitor the IV site for infiltration.	• Extravasation can occur, which necessitates immediate treatment with phentolamine injected at the site.
		• Assess for urinary output <30 mL/hr or pallor, cyanosis, pain, or numbness in the extremities.	• Norepinephrine is a powerful vasoconstrictor.
		• Assess for chest pain after resuscitation.	• Norepinephrine increases myocardial oxygen demand.
Sodium bicarbonate	• 1 mEq/kg IV bolus given after the first 10 min of cardiac arrest if necessary • 0.5 mEq/kg IV bolus q10min thereafter, if necessary	• Assess arterial blood gas values for metabolic acidosis.	• Administration without evidence of metabolic acidosis can result in alkalosis, which can hinder resuscitation efforts.
Isoproterenol (Isuprel)	• 2–10 μg/min IV infusion; titrate to desired clinical response	• Assess for increased heart rate. • Assess for tachycardia, hypotension, or hypertension. • Assess for chest pain after resuscitation. • Monitor for ventricular dysrhythmias.	• Increased heart rate is the expected response. • Adverse reactions may occur with a dramatic response. • Isoproterenol increases myocardial oxygen demand. • Isoproterenol increases ventricular irritability, especially in clients who are hypokalemic or who are receiving digitalis.
Calcium chloride (CaCl₂)	• 2–4 mg/kg IV slowly, may repeat, if necessary, q10min	• Calcium chloride is indicated only for cardiac arrest associated with hyperkalemia, hypocalcemia, or calcium channel blocker toxicity.	• Calcium chloride may cause cellular damage and cerebrovascular spasm.

VF, ventricular fibrillation.

Temporary Pacing. Temporary pacing is a nonsurgical intervention that provides a timed electrical stimulus to the heart when either the impulse initiation or the intrinsic conduction system of the heart is defective. The electrical stimulus then spreads throughout the heart to depolarize the cells, which should be followed by contraction and cardiac output. Electrical stimuli may be delivered to the right atrium or right ventricle (single-chamber pacemakers) or to both (dual-chamber pacemakers).

When a pacing stimulus is delivered to the heart, a spike (or pacemaker artifact) is seen on the monitor or ECG strip. The spike should be followed by evidence of depolarization (i.e., a P wave indicating atrial depolarization or a QRS complex indicating ventricular depolarization). This pattern is referred to as *capture*, indicating that the pacemaker successfully depolarized, or captured, the chamber.

Temporary pacing is generally initiated in clients with symptomatic, atropine-refractory bradydysrhythmias, particularly second-degree heart block type II and third-degree heart block, or in clients with asystole. Temporary pacing may also be initiated prophylactically in hemodynamically stable clients with left bundle branch block in certain situations, such as insertion of a pulmonary artery catheter.

A different type of pacing may be used to terminate symptomatic tachydysrhythmias. Occasionally, atrial overdrive pacing is attempted to terminate atrial tachydysrhythmias, such as atrial flutter or atrial fibrillation. Overdrive pacing is accomplished by rapidly pacing the atrium to capture the heart and control depolarization, followed by no pacing, in the hope that the sinus node will regain control of the heart. Ventricular overdrive pacing may be done to terminate ventricular tachydysrhythmias in much the same way. Overdrive pacing is usually performed by the physician or the physician's assistant. The nurse must

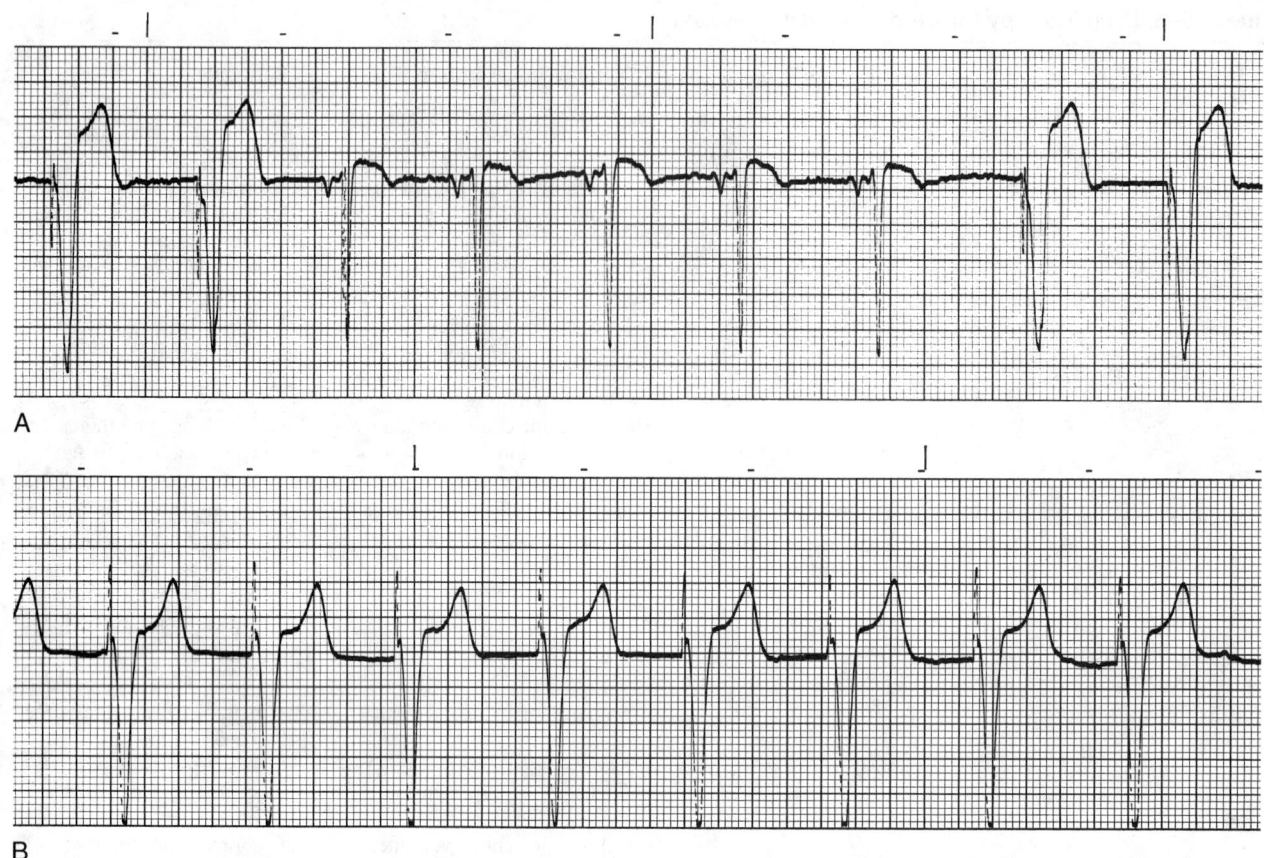

Figure 36–22. Modes of pacing. *A,* Synchronous (demand) ventricular pacing (VVI). *B,* Asynchronous (fixed-rate) ventricular pacing at a rate of 70 beats/minute (VOO).

have emergency equipment available in case the client becomes more unstable or goes into cardiac arrest.

Modes of Pacing. There are two basic modes of pacing: synchronous (demand) pacing and asynchronous (fixed-rate) pacing.

Synchronous (Demand) Pacing. Temporary pacing is most commonly done in the demand mode. The pacemaker's sensitivity is set to sense the client's own beats. When the client's intrinsic rate is above the rate set on the pulse generator, the pacemaker is inhibited from firing. When the client's rate is below that set on the generator, the pacemaker fires electrical impulses to stimulate depolarization (Fig. 36–22A).

Asynchronous (Fixed-Rate) Pacing. The asynchronous mode is used when the client is asystolic or profoundly bradycardiac, as may occur after open heart surgery. When the pulse generator is set in an asynchronous mode, it does not sense any intrinsic beats of the client. The pacemaker continues to fire at a fixed rate as set on the generator, regardless of the client's intrinsic rhythm. This continued firing is not a problem as long as the client remains asystolic or has a rate slower than the pacemaker rate, because all beats come from the pacemaker and there is no competition from the client's beats (see Fig. 36–22B). However, if the client's rate increases and equals or exceeds the pacemaker rate, competition (undersensing) is noted. The danger is that a pacemaker

stimulus may reach the heart during the vulnerable period of repolarization (R-on-T phenomenon, with the pacer spike falling on the T wave) and possibly induce ventricular fibrillation. The nurse must observe for pacemaker competition and set the pacemaker to a synchronous mode to avert potential problems.

Universal Pacemaker Code. In 1974, the Intersociety Commission for Heart Disease established a three-position pacemaker code (ICHD code) to standardize the description of pacemaker systems (Woods et al., 1995).

- The first letter of the code represents the chamber being paced: "A" for atrium, "V" for ventricle, "D" for dual (both atrium and ventricle), and "O" for none.
- The second letter represents the chamber being sensed, using the same three letters. This indicates a demand-pacing mode. If the pacemaker is asynchronous, the second letter is "O," because no chamber is sensed.
- The third letter represents the mode of response: "I" for inhibited, when the pacemaker senses an intrinsic depolarization and inhibits the pacemaker output; "T" for triggered, when the pacemaker senses an intrinsic depolarization and discharges an electrical stimulus along with the intrinsic one; "O" for no mode of response, when the pacemaker is asynchronous and therefore discharges electrical stimuli at a set rate; and "D" for dual mode of response, when sensed events may result in pacemaker inhibition or

TABLE 36–3

The Five-Position Pacemaker Code*

I Chamber(s) Paced	II Chamber(s) Sensed	III Mode of Response	IV Programmability, Rate Modulation	V Antitachycardia Function(s)
A = Atrium	A = Atrium	I = Inhibited	P = Simple programmable	P = Pacing
V = Ventricle	V = Ventricle	T = Triggered	M = Multiprogrammable	S = Shock
D = Dual (atrium and ventricle)	D = Dual (atrium and ventricle)	D = Atrial triggered and ventricular inhibited	C = Communicating R = Rate modulation	D = Dual (pacing and shock)
O = None	O = None	O = None	O = None	O = None

From Bernstein, A. D., et al. (1987). The NASPE/BPEG pacemaker code. *PACE, 10*(4), 794.
*The North American Society for Pacing and Electrophysiology (NASPE) and the British Pacing and Electrophysiology Group (BPEG) code (the NASPE/BPEG generic [NBG] code).

triggering so that a sensed atrial event initiates a pacemaker ventricular output unless an intrinsic ventricular event is sensed before a predetermined delay.

This code is used universally and makes it easier to identify quickly the primary functions of the pacemaker. AAI denotes an atrial demand pacemaker. AOO denotes an asynchronous atrial pacemaker. VVI denotes a ventricular demand pacemaker. VOO refers to an asynchronous ventricular pacemaker. DVI denotes a demand AV sequential pacemaker that can pace both chambers but senses only the ventricular chamber. DOO indicates an asynchronous dual-chamber pacemaker. DDD denotes a demand dual-chamber pacemaker that paces and senses both chambers and has a dual mode of response.

The code was expanded to five positions for standardization of multiprogrammable pacemakers and tachydysrhythmia functions, incorporating the original three-position code. This code was designed by the North American Society for Pacing and Electrophysiology (NASPE) and the British Pacing and Electrophysiology Group (BPEG). The code is referred to as the NASPE/BPEG generic (or NBG) code (Table 36–3).

There are two basic types of temporary pacing: noninvasive temporary pacing and invasive temporary pacing.

Noninvasive Temporary Pacing. Noninvasive temporary pacing (NTP) is accomplished through the application of two large patch electrodes. The electrodes are attached to

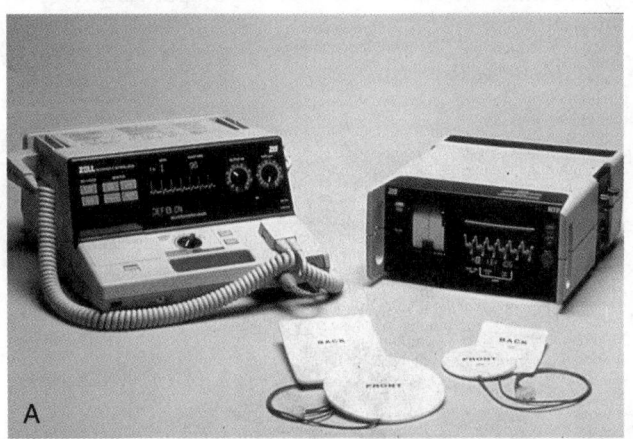
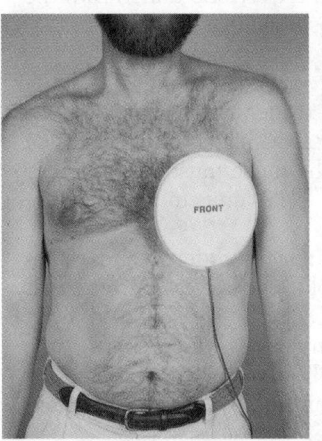
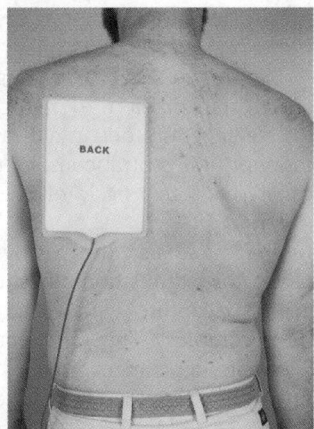
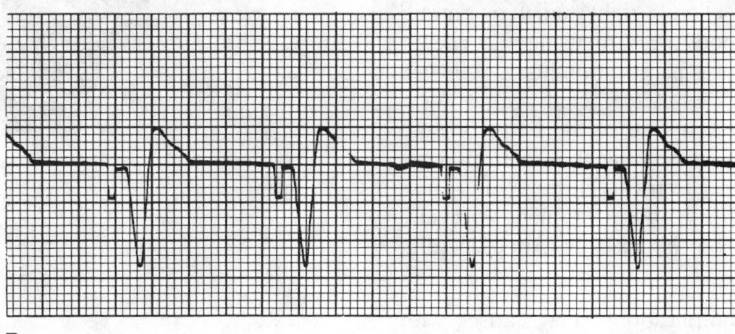

Figure 36–23. *A*, Equipment and electrode placement for transcutaneous external pacing. *B*, ECG rhythm strip showing wide pacing spikes. (*A*, courtesy of Zoll Medical Corporation, Burlington, MA.)

an external pulse generator, which can operate on alternating current (AC) or battery power (Fig. 36–23). The generator emits electrical pulses, which are transmitted through the cutaneous patches and then transcutaneously to stimulate ventricular depolarization when the client's heart rate is slower than the rate set on the pacemaker. Electrical currents of 60 milliamperes (mA) or more are usually required to achieve ventricular depolarization. The current is applied for 20 to 40 milliseconds (msec), producing a pacing stimulus, or spike, that occupies 0.02 to 0.04 second on the ECG paper.

NTP is used as an emergency measure to provide demand ventricular pacing in a profoundly bradycardiac or asystolic client until invasive pacing can be instituted or the client's intrinsic rate returns to normal. It may be used prophylactically when performing procedures or transporting clients at risk for bradydysrhythmias.

Procedure. The nurse explains NTP to the client and prepares the equipment. The nurse washes the client's skin with soap and water. To prevent skin abrasion, the skin must not be shaved. The nurse should not rub the skin or apply alcohol or tinctures on the skin, because electrical current flows from the patches through the skin and causes some discomfort. The nurse then applies the large posterior electrode on the client's back, between the spine and the left scapula, behind the heart. The electrode should not be placed higher over bone because bone is a poor conductor of electrical current. The anterior electrode is then applied on the client's chest, between the V_2 and the V_5 positions, over the heart. The electrode cannot be placed over female breast tissue. The nurse must displace the breast and position the electrode underneath the breast, avoiding a lower position that paces the diaphragm and causes discomfort and possible dyspnea.

The high electrical pacing current distorts the ECG signal transmission to the bedside monitor. To reduce interference and obtain a clear ECG signal on the bedside monitor and central console, the nurse must attach a filter cable from the back of the NTP unit to the bedside monitor.

The nurse sets the pacing rate as ordered and establishes the stimulation threshold, the lowest current that achieves capture with each pacing spike followed by a QRS complex. The QRS complex is wide because one ventricle depolarizes first, followed by the other. The nurse then sets the electrical current 10% above threshold levels.

The nurse palpates the client's right radial or carotid pulse and assesses the blood pressure using the client's right arm, ensuring that each paced stimulus is followed by a mechanical response (ventricular contraction). Vital signs are not taken on the left side of the body because they may not be accurate, particularly if a high milliamperage is used. This large electrical current can cause muscle twitching, which may stimulate blood pressure sounds or simulate a pulse on the left side (Appel-Hardin, 1992).

Complications. Three complications may arise with NTP. The first includes discomfort from cutaneous and muscle stimulation and skin irritation and diaphoresis from the patch electrodes. The nurse must ensure that the electrodes are in good contact with the skin and in the best location to achieve the lowest threshold for consistent capture. The nurse also administers prescribed analgesics or sedatives and provides comfort and support.

The second problem is loss of capture, when the pacing spike is not followed by a QRS complex. The nurse ensures that the electrodes are in good contact with the skin and, if necessary, increases the current until capture is regained; however, higher currents cause more discomfort for the client.

The third problem is inappropriate pacing, when the pacemaker does not sense the client's intrinsic QRS complex and therefore fires impulses at its preset rate, competing with the client's rhythm. The nurse must assess electrode contact and the effect of the client's position on pacemaker function. The client may have to avoid lying on the left side. If diaphoresis has caused poor contact and the electrodes must be replaced, the nurse must first turn the pacing function off to avoid receiving electrical shocks when touching the gel side of the electrodes.

Invasive Temporary Pacing. An invasive temporary pacemaker system consists of an external, battery-operated pulse generator (Fig. 36–24) and pacing electrodes, or lead wires. These wires attach to the generator on one end and are in contact with the heart on the other end. Electrical pulses, or stimuli, are emitted from the negative terminal of the generator, flow through a lead wire, and stimulate the myocardial cells to depolarize. The current seeks ground by returning through the other lead wire to the positive terminal of the generator, thus completing a circuitous route. The intensity of electrical current is set by selecting the appropriate current output, measured in milliamperes.

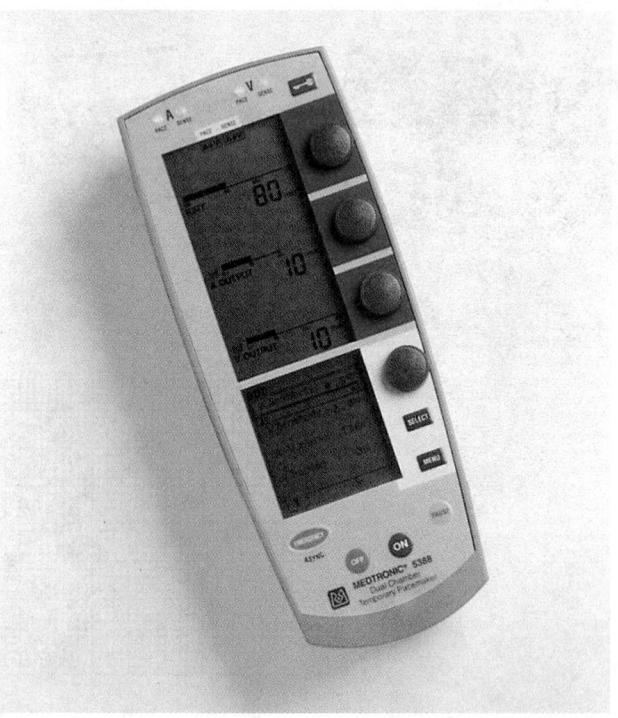

Figure 36–24. Temporary dual-chamber pacemaker. (Courtesy of Medtronic, Inc., Minneapolis, MN.)

The client does not usually feel invasive pacemaker stimuli; however, clients occasionally feel an uncomfortable sensation from the stimuli if strong electrical currents (high milliamperage) are delivered by the pacemaker. The discomfort may be alleviated by decreasing the current if possible.

The two types of invasive temporary pacing are transvenous pacing and epicardial pacing.

Transvenous Pacing. Transvenous ventricular pacing involves the use of fluoroscopy to thread a sterile catheter, containing two lead wires, percutaneously through a vein to the right ventricle for temporary pacing. The catheter electrode tip (negative electrode) is in contact with the endocardial surface of the ventricle, where it fixates for stability (Fig. 36–25A). The positive electrode is located just proximal to the tip of the catheter. The bifurcated

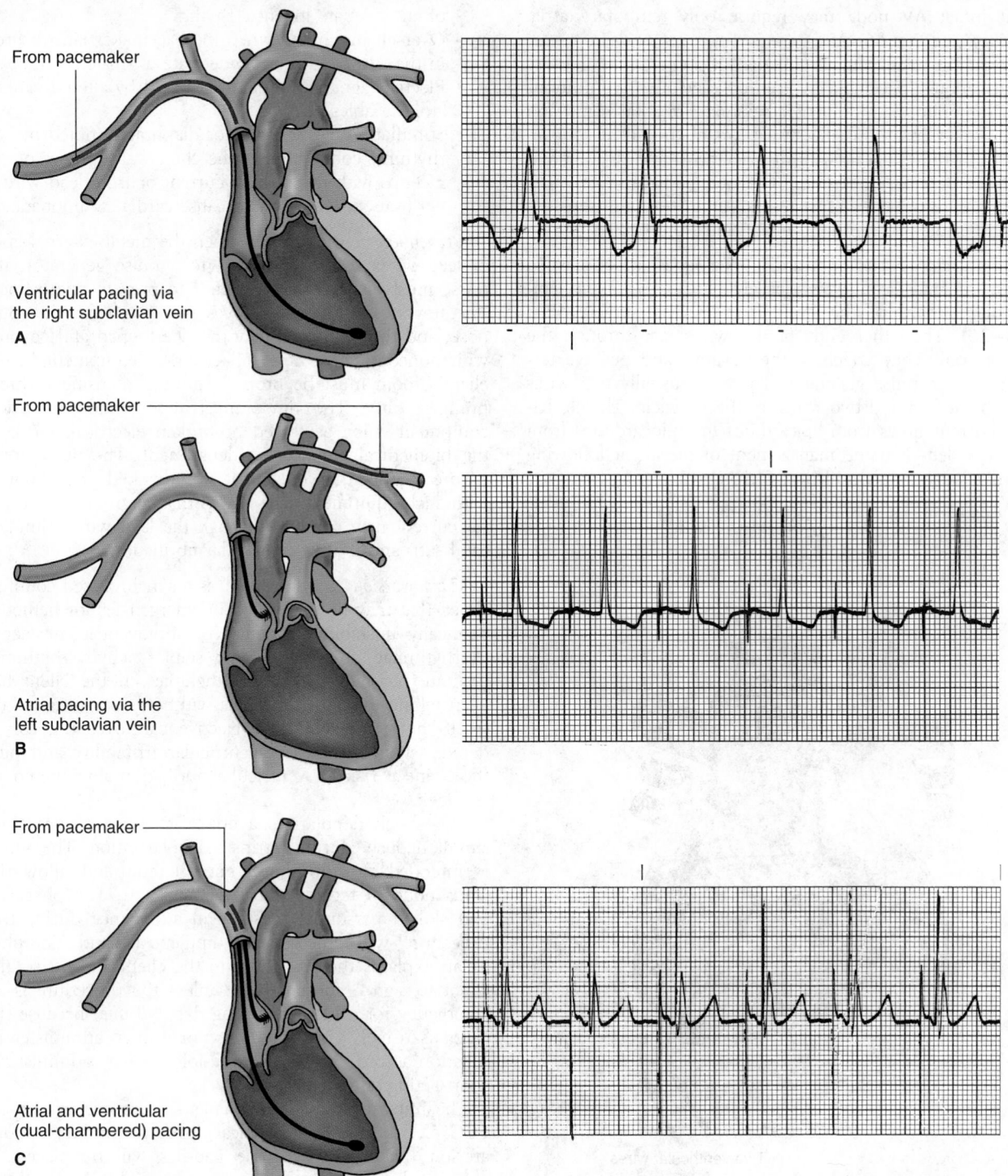

Figure 36–25. Pacemaker catheter electrode placement and corresponding ECG patterns in temporary transvenous pacing. *A,* Ventricular pacing at a rate of 72/minute. *B,* Atrial pacing at a rate of 88/minute, with intrinsic QRS complexes. *C,* AV pacing at a rate of 80/minute.

external end of the catheter is attached to the negative and positive terminals of a battery-operated pulse generator. The generator provides the electrical current to stimulate the myocardial cells to depolarize.

If the client needs the atrial kick from atrial contractions, a temporary dual-chamber pacemaker is used, with one catheter tip in the right atrium and the other in the right ventricle (see Fig. 36–25B). This preserves the normal synchrony of atrial contraction preceding ventricular contraction. Some clients with a dysfunctional sinus node but intact AV node may require only temporary atrial pacing (see Fig. 36–25C).

Nursing management of the client after temporary transvenous pacemaker insertion includes continuous ECG monitoring, frequent assessment of vital signs and pacemaker insertion site, restriction of the client's movement to prevent lead wire displacement, and documentation of pacemaker settings. The qualified nurse or other health care provider must assess stimulation and sensitivity thresholds according to institutional protocols.

Epicardial Pacing. Epicardial pacing is accomplished with separate lead wires loosely threaded on the epicardial surface of the heart after cardiac surgery (Fig. 36–26). The other ends of the wires exit through the chest wall. They attach to the negative and positive terminals of a pulse generator. There are usually two wires on the atrium and two wires on the ventricle. The electrical current flows from epicardium to endocardium, from right to left. Nursing management of the client following cardiac surgery is detailed in Chapter 40.

Complications. Complications of invasive temporary pacing may be serious and include

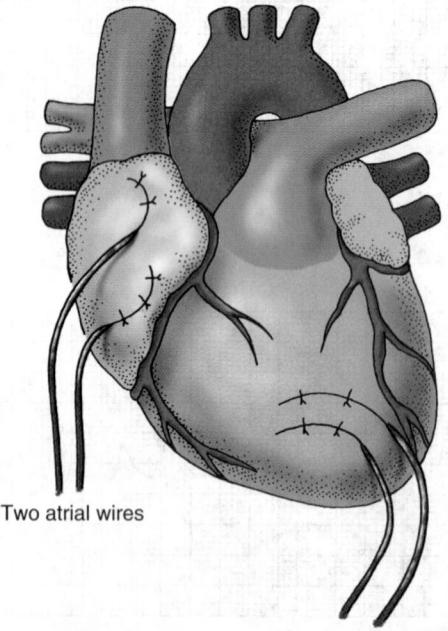

Two atrial wires

Two ventricular wires

Figure 36–26. Lead wire placement for epicardial pacing after cardiac surgery. Two wires are sutured on the right atrium and two on the right ventricle.

- Infection or hematoma at the pacemaker wire insertion site
- Ectopic complexes (usually premature ventricular complexes), caused by irritability from the pacing wire in the ventricle, use of high current, or undersensing with pacemaker competition
- Loss of capture, noted by the presence of a pacing stimulus or spike but no depolarization
- Undersensing or pacemaker competition, noted when pacing stimuli occur at a fixed rate in the presence of an adequate intrinsic rhythm
- Oversensing, noted when the pacemaker fails to fire in the presence of an inadequate intrinsic rhythm
- Electromagnetic interference, noted by altered generator variables
- Stimulation of chest wall or diaphragm, noted by rhythmic contraction of the chest wall muscles or hiccups with use of high current or from lead wire perforation, which could cause cardiac tamponade

Prevention of Microshock. When the metal external ends of lead wires are not attached to a pulse generator, the nurse must insulate the wire ends to prevent microshock. The fingertips of rubber gloves work well for this purpose, and the wire ends may then be looped and covered with nonconductive tape. All electrical equipment in the client's room must be properly grounded, using a three-pronged plug. The nurse must report faulty electrical equipment, such as frayed or broken electrical wires, to the biomedical engineering department. The nurse must ensure that neither the client nor the bed is in contact with such equipment. The risk is that ungrounded electrical current may conduct through the lead wire, stimulate the heart, and induce ventricular fibrillation.

Cardioversion. Cardioversion is a synchronized countershock that may be performed in emergencies for hemodynamically unstable ventricular or supraventricular tachydysrhythmias or electively for stable tachydysrhythmias that are resistant to medical therapies. If the client has been taking digitalis, the nurse withholds the drug for up to 48 hours preceding an elective cardioversion, as ordered. Digitalis increases ventricular irritability and puts the client at risk for ventricular fibrillation after the countershock.

The shock depolarizes a critical mass of myocardium simultaneously during intrinsic depolarization. The shock is intended to stop the re-entry circuit and allow the sinus node to regain control of the heart. The physician and skilled personnel must be in attendance during this procedure, with emergency equipment at hand. The physician explains the procedure to the client and assists the client to sign a consent form unless the procedure is an emergency for a life-threatening dysrhythmia. Because the client is usually conscious, the nurse must administer IV sedation as ordered. An anesthesiologist may administer a short-acting anesthetic agent.

The nurse examines the client's skin to ensure that no ECG electrodes and no topical nitroglycerin preparations are on the sites where the paddles will be placed. If present, they must be removed and the skin cleaned and dried. The physician or advanced cardiac life support (ACLS)–qualified nurse places conductive pads, one on

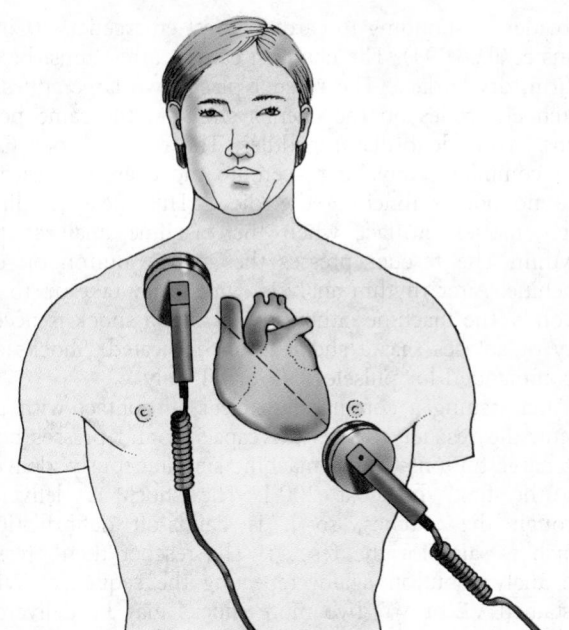

Figure 36–27. Standard electrode paddle placement for cardioversion or defibrillation.

the client's upper right chest below the clavicle and the other left of the nipple with the center in the mid–axillary line (Cummins et al., 1994). The nurse places the electrode paddles over the pads (Fig. 36–27), applying firm pressure.

The ECG electrodes from the monitor-defibrillator are applied for continuous monitoring. The nurse ensures that the defibrillator is synchronized to the client's R wave. This avoids discharging the shock during the vulnerable period (T wave), which may increase ventricular irritability, causing ventricular fibrillation. The nurse charges the capacitor on the defibrillator to the energy ordered by the physician, usually starting at 50–100 J. The nurse ensures that the oxygen delivery device has been removed and turned away from the client. Oxygen supports combustion, and a fire may result if there is arcing from the paddles. Arcing is usually due to improper paddle contact on the chest. The nurse then loudly and clearly commands all personnel to clear contact with the client and the bed, as required for electrical safety. The nurse ensures compliance of all personnel before delivering the shock. While the client is exhaling, the nurse discharges both paddles simultaneously to deliver the shock at end-expiration, when the heart is closer to the chest wall, so that more current flow can reach the heart for a better chance of success. This procedure may also be performed by a physician's assistant, paramedic, or other qualified health care provider following medical protocols.

After cardioversion, the nurse assesses the client's response and heart rhythm. Therapy is repeated as ordered, if necessary, until the desired result is obtained or alternative therapies are considered. If the client goes into ventricular fibrillation after cardioversion, the nurse must ensure that the synchronizer is turned off and then immediately defibrillate the client.

Nursing care after cardioversion includes
■ Maintaining a patent airway
■ Administering oxygen
■ Assessing the client's vital signs and level of consciousness
■ Administering antidysrhythmic drug therapy
■ Monitoring for dysrhythmias
■ Assessing for chest burns from paddle edges that may not have been on the conductive pad
■ Providing emotional support for the client

Cardiopulmonary Resuscitation. Management of the client in cardiac arrest depends on prompt recognition and therapeutic interventions for successful reversal of a potentially fatal event.

When cardiac arrest occurs, cardiac output ceases. The underlying rhythm is usually ventricular tachycardia, ventricular fibrillation, or asystole. In rare instances, cardiac arrest occurs in the presence of an organized electrocardiographic (ECG) rhythm, but with no effectual mechanical response, a condition referred to as PEA (pulseless electrical activity) (Cummins et al., 1994). Without a cardiac output, the client is pulseless and becomes unconscious because of inadequate cerebral perfusion. Shortly after cardiac arrest, respiratory arrest occurs.

CPR must be initiated immediately to help prevent brain damage and death. The nurse, finding an unresponsive client, calls out loudly for help while initiating CPR. The initial priorities are
■ Maintenance of a patent airway
■ Ventilation with a mouth-to-mask device
■ Chest compressions
As soon as help arrives, a board is placed under a client who is not on a firm surface. To make room for the resuscitation team and the crash cart, the nurse commands that the area be cleared of movable items and unnecessary personnel.

Complications of CPR include rib fractures, fracture of the sternum, costochondral separation, lacerations of the liver and spleen, pneumothorax, hemothorax, cardiac tamponade, lung contusions, and fat emboli. The goal of resuscitation is the rapid return of a pulse, blood pressure, and consciousness in the client. This is rarely achieved by CPR and basic measures alone. More definitive therapy must be initiated as soon as possible with ACLS measures, including defibrillation, if warranted.

Advanced Cardiac Life Support. When the crash cart arrives, the nurse applies ECG electrodes to the client's chest and turns on the monitor, directing the team to continue CPR. If the client is found to be in ventricular fibrillation or pulseless ventricular tachycardia, the immediate priority is to defibrillate the client. Following defibrillation, CPR is resumed. An oropharyngeal airway is inserted in the client to facilitate proper ventilation. A manual resuscitation bag (MRB) with mask is attached to an oxygen flowmeter, running at 10 to 15 L/minute. The nurse directs that the person managing the airway now ventilate the client with the MRB, maintaining the proper head-tilt, chin-lift position of the client. Nurses initiate two intravenous (IV) lines if the client does not have any, infusing normal saline. These lines provide access for emergency drug administration. Suction equipment is also set up, with a tonsillar suction tube for suctioning vomitus and a suction catheter for endotracheal suctioning. Carotid or femoral pulse checks, during chest compressions and without chest compressions, blood pressure measurements, and pupil assessments are done at frequent intervals. A nurse documents all assessments and findings, therapeutic measures, and the client's responses throughout the resuscitation.

Additional measures include endotracheal intubation with ventilation and oxygenation, IV administration of emergency cardiac drugs, and, occasionally, pacing. Chest compressions are continued as long as the client remains pulseless or until a physician decides to terminate resuscitation attempts.

Defibrillation. Defibrillation, an asynchronous countershock, depolarizes a critical mass of myocardium simultaneously to stop the re-entry circuit and to allow the sinus node to regain control of the heart. Early defibrillation is critical to terminate pulseless ventricular tachycardia (VT) or ventricular fibrillation (VF). It must not be delayed for any reason after the equipment and skilled personnel are present. The earlier defibrillation is performed, the greater the chance of survival.

If a defibrillator is not immediately available, an ACLS-qualified nurse may deliver a precordial thump to a pulseless client in VF. There is a slight chance that it may succeed in terminating the VF (Cummins et al., 1994). A precordial thump is performed by striking the lower half of the sternum with a closed fist from a height of 8 to 12 inches (12 to 30 cm) above the sternum. If the client remains in VF, CPR is resumed and the nurse prepares the client's chest for defibrillation.

The physician or the ACLS-qualified nurse places conductive gel pads, one on the client's upper right chest below the clavicle and the other to the left of the nipple with the center in the mid–axillary line (Cummins et al., 1994). The nurse places the electrode paddles over the pads (see Fig. 36–27), applies firm pressure, and charges the capacitor on the defibrillator to an initial energy of 200 J. The nurse ensures that the oxygen delivery device has been removed and turned away from the client. If the client is already intubated, the MRB may be left attached. The nurse loudly and clearly commands all personnel to clear contact with the client and the bed and ensures their compliance before delivering the shock.

After defibrillation, the nurse maintains paddle position while assessing the client's heart rhythm. If the first shock was unsuccessful, the nurse immediately delivers a second shock at 200 to 300 J, followed by a third shock at 360 J, if necessary. The shocks are given in rapid succession. Successive shocks decrease transthoracic impedance, allowing more current flow to reach the heart for a better chance of success. If defibrillation is successful, the nurse and team members maintain a patent airway, provide oxygen and ventilatory support, assess vital signs frequently, and continuously monitor the client for the recurrence of dysrhythmias. IV access, hemodynamic support, and antidysrhythmic medications are also essential.

Automatic External Defibrillation. The American Heart Association promotes the use of automatic external defibrillators (AEDs) for use by lay persons and health care providers responding to cardiac arrest emergencies (Cummins et al., 1994). The client in cardiac arrest must be on a firm, dry surface. The rescuer places two large adhesive patch electrodes on the client's chest, in the same positions as for defibrillator paddles. The rescuer stops CPR and commands anyone present to move away, ensuring that no one is touching the client. This measure eliminates motion artifact when the machine analyzes the rhythm. The rescuer presses the analyze button on the machine. After rhythm analysis, which may take up to 30 seconds, the machine either advises that a shock is necessary or advises that a shock is not indicated. Shocks are recommended for pulseless VF or VT only.

After issuing a command to clear all contact with the client, the rescuer charges the capacitor and presses both discharge buttons on the machine simultaneously, delivering the first shock at 200 J. The shock is delivered through the patches, so it is hands-off defibrillation, which is safer for the rescuer. The rescuer then presses the analyze button again, repeating the sequence. With sustained VF or VT, two more shocks may be delivered, with the third at 360 J. If the client remains in cardiac arrest, CPR is performed for 1 minute, and then another series of three shocks may be delivered, each at 360 J. It is imperative that ACLS be provided as soon as possible. Use of AEDs results in earlier defibrillation of clients and therefore a greater chance of successful rhythm conversion and survival.

Current-Based Defibrillation. Research is being conducted on the use of current-based defibrillation. Defibrillators in use deliver energy, measured in joules. It is not known what the optimal energy for defibrillation is or whether energy selected may be too low, which may be ineffective, or too high, which could result in myocardial damage. These problems would be avoided by the use of electrical current, measured in amperes, as it would take into account transthoracic impedance. Optimal defibrillation current has been found to be 30 to 40 mA (Cummins et al., 1994). Such defibrillators are under investigation.

Radiofrequency Catheter Ablation. Radiofrequency catheter ablation is an invasive procedure that may be used to abolish an irritable focus causing a supraventricular or ventricular tachydysrhythmia. The client must undergo electrophysiologic studies and mapping procedures to locate the focus. Then radiofrequency waves are delivered to abolish the irritable focus. When ablation is performed in the AV nodal or His bundle area, damage may also occur to the normal conduction system, causing heart blocks, requiring implantation of a permanent pacemaker.

Surgical Management. Clients who experience life-threatening dysrhythmias may require surgical treatment for long-term management. The type of treatment depends on the nature of the dysrhythmia. Procedures include permanent pacing, coronary artery bypass grafting, aneurysmectomy, insertion of an implantable cardioverter/defibrillator, and open-chest cardiac massage.

Permanent Pacing. Permanent pacemaker insertion is performed for the resolution of conduction disorders that are not temporary, including complete heart block and sick sinus syndrome. Permanent pacemakers are usually powered by a lithium battery and have an average life span of 10 years. After the battery power is depleted, the generator must be replaced, a procedure done under local anesthesia. Some pacemakers are nuclear powered and have a life span of 20 years or longer. Other pacemakers can be recharged externally.

Types of Pacemakers. Pacemakers may be single chambered or dual chambered. With single-chamber pacemakers, a lead wire is positioned in the chamber to be paced, most commonly the right ventricle. Occasionally, it is positioned in the right atrium for bradydysrhythmias originating from SA node disease with an intact atrioventricular (AV) conduction system.

Dual-chamber pacemakers have lead wires placed in the right atrium and the right ventricle (Fig. 36–28A,B) for a more physiologic effect, preserving the atrial kick. A programmed AV interval, which closely relates to the PR interval, ensures a ventricular response shortly after atrial depolarization. The DDD pacemaker is commonly implanted. It is able to sense both atrial and ventricular intrinsic activity and pace both the atrium and the ventricle. It allows sinus control of the ventricular rate to meet increased metabolic demands when the sinus node is functioning well. If the client's sinus rate drops below the lower rate set, the generator paces both the atrium and the ventricle.

Another feature of many pacemakers is rate responsiveness. To allow faster pacing rates to meet increased body demands, the generator changes pacing rate in response to a detected change in a physiologic variable, such as muscle movement within the client with impaired sinus or atrial function. Hysteresis, on the other hand, is a feature that allows the client's rate to slow to 10 to 20 beats lower than the generator's pre-set rate before the generator paces the client. The slower pace allows a more normal physiologic slowing response during rest or sleep.

Surgical Procedures. For both single-chamber and dual-chamber pacemakers, the surgeon most commonly implants the pulse generator in a surgically made subcutaneous pocket at the shoulder in the right or left subclavicular area. The leads are introduced transvenously via the cephalic or the subclavian vein to the endocardium on the right side of the heart. After the procedure, the nurse monitors the client's ECG rhythm to ensure that the pacemaker is functioning correctly. The nurse also assesses the implantation site for evidence of bleeding, swelling, redness, tenderness, and infection. The dressing over the site should remain clean and dry, and the client should be afebrile and have stable vital signs. The physician orders activity restrictions to enhance lead fixation. After 24 hours, activity is gradually increased. Complications of permanent pacemakers are similar to those for temporary invasive pacing.

Pacemaker checks are done on an outpatient basis at regular intervals. Reprogramming may be warranted if there are pacemaker problems. The pulse generator is interrogated using an electronic device to determine the pacemaker settings and battery life (Fig. 36–29).

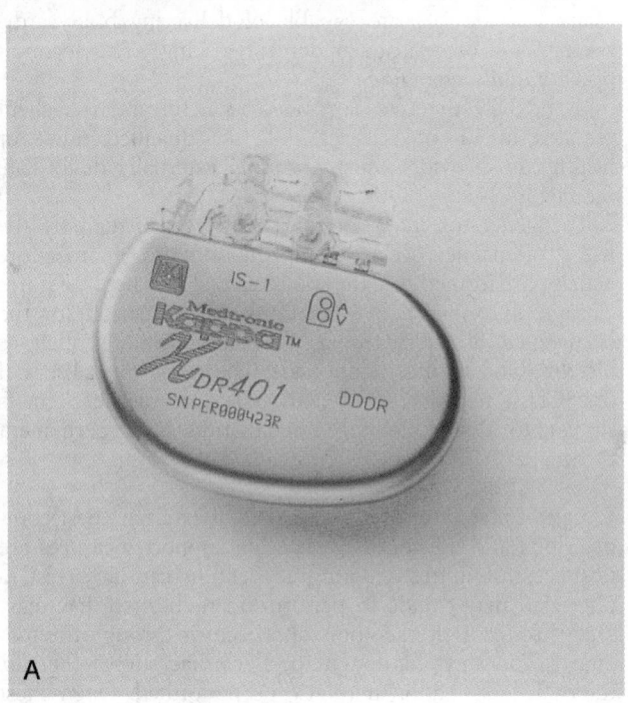

A

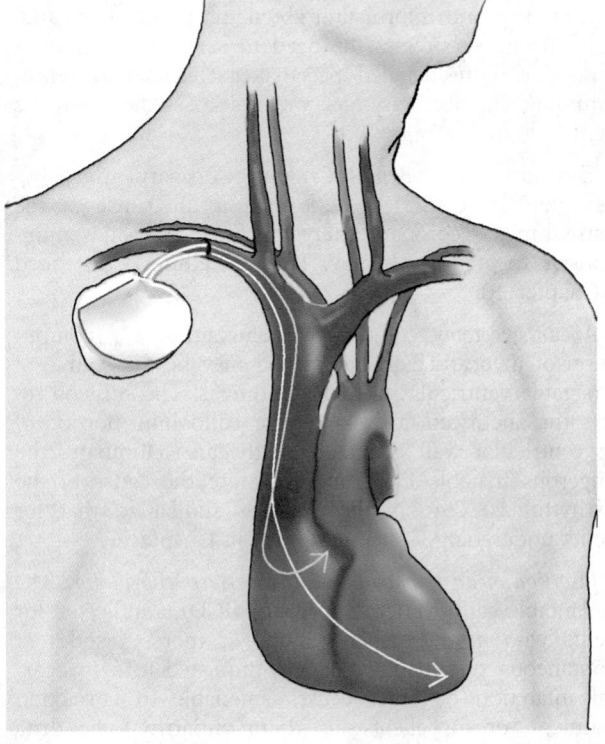

B

Figure 36–28. *A,* Permanent dual-chamber pacemaker. *B,* Implanted permanent dual-chamber pacemaker with endocardial leads introduced via the right subclavian vein into the right atrium and right ventricle. (Courtesy of Medtronic, Inc., Minneapolis, MN.)

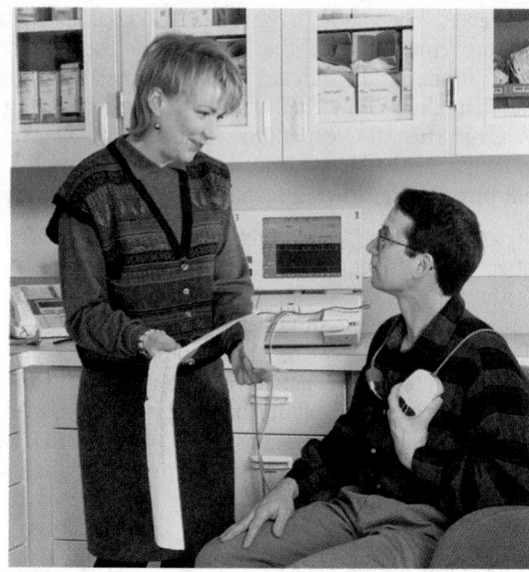

Figure 36–29. Permanent pacemaker check. The "head" of the device (shown being held in the client's left hand) is placed over the pulse generator to interrogate the pacemaker and reprogram it if necessary. (Courtesy of Medtronic, Inc., Minneapolis, MN.)

For clients who live far from the pacemaker clinic or physician's office, pacemaker information can be sent via transtelephonic transmission of data. The client attaches ECG electrodes to the wrists and places the telephone receiver in a transmitting unit. The sound signals are relayed via telephone lines to the clinic or office, where they are converted and recorded as the client's ECG rhythm strip and information about the pacemaker variables. The nurse stresses the need to keep clinic appointments for more detailed pacemaker checks and reprogramming, if necessary, as well as assessment of the client.

Coronary Artery Bypass Grafting. Coronary artery bypass grafting (CABG) is performed if the cause of the dysrhythmia is coronary artery insufficiency that is unresponsive to medical therapy. This procedure is described in Chapter 40.

Aneurysmectomy. Ventricular aneurysms are a complication of myocardial infarction and may be the source of intractable ventricular tachydysrhythmias. The surgeon resects the aneurysm, a dyskinetic or ballooning portion of the ventricular wall. Resection of the area eliminates the dangerous irritable focus and therefore the cause of the dysrhythmias. Care of the client is similar to that for clients undergoing CABG, described in Chapter 40.

Insertion of an Implantable Cardioverter/Defibrillator. The implantable cardioverter/defibrillator (ICD) is indicated for clients who have experienced one or more episodes of spontaneous sustained VT or VF, unrelated to a myocardial infarction or other causes amenable to correction treatment, or for clients in whom antiarrhythmic drug therapy to control life-threatening dysrhythmias has not been successful or is limited by drug intolerance or noncompliance. Clients undergo electrophysiologic studies to assess the inducibility of ventricular tachydysrhythmias and their response to medication. If the dysrhythmias can be induced despite medical therapy, the client is considered a candidate for ICD implantation. A psychological profile is done to determine whether the client will be able to cope with the discomfort and fear associated with internal defibrillation from the ICD.

In the past, a median sternotomy or left thoracotomy approach for implanting the leads of the device was used, and the generator was implanted in a paraumbilical pocket. This procedure was performed in an operating suite. Currently, the leads are introduced percutaneously, and the generator is implanted in the left pectoral area, similar to a permanent pacemaker insertion procedure. This procedure is performed in the electrophysiology laboratory.

The electronic pulse generator is designed to monitor and to deliver therapy for ventricular tachycardia or ventricular fibrillation. The generator is powered by a lithium battery and is connected to a transvenous endocardial lead. The ends of the lead are tunneled under the skin to attach to the generator. The sensing lead transmits electrical signals from the heart to the generator, which continuously monitors the heart rhythm. If the client's heart rate exceeds the generator's programmed rate (rate cutoff), such as with ventricular tachycardia, the generator takes a few seconds to sense the cardiac electrical activity and then delivers a burst of antitachycardia pacing (ATP) to overdrive pace the rhythm. A programmed number of ATP therapies may be delivered. If the client's rate continues to exceed the rate cutoff, the device can deliver a programmed number of low-energy and high-energy cardioversion shocks. In response to ventricular fibrillation, the device delivers defibrillation shocks. Following such therapy, the client may develop a transient bradycardia. Many ICD devices are capable of delivering bradycardia pacing (VVI or ventricular demand pacing). This technology is rapidly changing.

If the ICD therapies are not successful and the client remains in VF or pulseless VT, the qualified nurse or health care provider must promptly externally defibrillate the client.

The generator may be activated or deactivated by the use of a magnet over the implantation site, a procedure usually performed by the physician. The client requires close monitoring in the postimplantation period for the occurrence of dysrhythmias and complications such as bleeding and cardiac tamponade. The nurse must know if the ICD is activated or deactivated. Care of the client is similar to that following implantation of a permanent pacemaker.

Open-Chest Cardiac Massage. When external chest compressions and advanced cardiac life support measures are unsuccessful in resuscitating a client in cardiac arrest, a physician may decide to perform open-chest cardiac massage through a thoracotomy approach or through the median sternotomy incision in post–cardiac surgery clients. Internal defibrillation may also be performed. Open-chest cardiac massage is usually reserved for the cardiac surgical client who goes into cardiac arrest, often because of cardiac tamponade. It may also be beneficial but is rarely indicated for clients with hypothermia, crushing or penetrating chest injuries, penetrating abdominal trauma, or chest deformities prohibiting external chest compressions.

 Continuing Care

For many clients, dysrhythmias are a chronic disorder resulting from chronic cardiac and pulmonary diseases. Clients may be cared for in a variety of settings, including the acute care hospital, subacute unit, traditional nursing home, or their own homes. Clients are admitted to the hospital when they experience life-threatening or potentially life-threatening dysrhythmias, often associated with an acute disorder. Other clients can be managed with office or clinic visits or in other settings.

Clients discharged from the hospital may have considerable needs, often more related to their underlying chronic diseases than to their dysrhythmias, which should be essentially controlled by drug or device therapy. A case manager or care coordinator can assess the client's needs for health care resources and coordinate access to needed services.

➤ Health Teaching

Prevention of Recurrence. Clients who have experienced a dysrhythmia associated with an acute disorder, such as electrolyte imbalance or ischemia related to a myocardial infarction, are instructed in the prevention, early recognition, and management of that disorder. The nurse teaches the client and family about lifestyle modifications designed to prevent, decrease, or control the occurrence of dysrhythmias, as outlined in Chart 36–6. This teaching may be provided in the acute care setting, physician's office, health care clinic, or home setting.

Drug Therapy. Clients and the parents of children receiving antidysrhythmic drugs must have a thorough understanding of their medications. Pharmacies provide written instructions about antidysrhythmic agents prescribed for the client. The nurse teaches clients and families the generic and trade names of their drugs, as well as their purposes, using basic terms that are easily understood. The nurse must provide clear instructions on dosage schedules and common side effects (see Chart 36–3). The nurse emphasizes the importance of reporting these side effects and any dizziness, nausea, vomiting, chest discomfort, or shortness of breath to the health care provider. Chart 36–7 highlights special considerations for elderly clients receiving antidysrhythmic therapy.

Pulse Check. The nurse teaches all clients and their significant others or family members how to take the client's pulse. The nurse instructs them to report any signs of a change in heart rhythm, such as a significant decrease in pulse rate, a rate greater than 100 beats per minute, or increased irregularity.

Pacemaker. Clients and parents of children who have a permanent pacemaker are given written and verbal information about the type and settings of their pacemaker. The nurse teaches them to report any pulse rate lower than that set on the pacemaker or lower than the hystere-

---

Chart 36–6

Education Guide: How to Prevent or Decrease Dysrhythmias

For Clients at Risk for Vasovagal Attacks Causing Bradydysrhythmias
- Avoid doing things that stimulate the vagus nerve, such as raising your arms above your head, applying pressure over your carotid artery, applying pressure on your eyes, bearing down or straining during a bowel movement, and stimulating a gag reflex when brushing your teeth or putting objects in your mouth.

For Clients with Premature Beats and Ectopic Rhythms
- Take the medications that have been prescribed for you, and report any adverse effects to your physician.
- Stop smoking, avoid caffeinated beverages as much as possible, and drink alcohol only in moderation.
- Learn ways to manage stress and avoid getting too tired.

For Clients with Ischemic Heart Disease
- If you have an angina attack, treat it promptly with rest and nitroglycerin administration as prescribed by your physician. This decreases your chances of experiencing a dysrhythmia.
- If chest pain is not relieved after taking the amount of nitroglycerin that has been prescribed for you, seek medical attention promptly. Also, seek prompt medical attention if the pain becomes more severe or you experience other symptoms, such as sweating, nausea, weakness, and palpitations.

For Clients at Risk for Potassium Imbalance
- Know the symptoms of decreased potassium levels, such as muscle weakness and cardiac irregularity.
- Eat foods high in potassium, such as tomatoes, beans, prunes, avocados, bananas, strawberries, and lettuce.
- Take the potassium supplements that have been prescribed for you.

---

sis rate. The nurse teaches the client the proper care of the pacemaker insertion site and the importance of reporting any fever or any redness, swelling, or drainage at the pacemaker insertion site. If the surgical incision is near either shoulder, the nurse teaches and demonstrates range-of-motion exercises for the client to perform to prevent shoulder stiffness. The nurse instructs the client to keep hand-held cellular phones at least 6 inches away from the generator, with the handset on the ear opposite the side of the generator. The nurse also teaches clients with pacemakers to avoid sources of strong electromagnetic fields, such as magnets and telecommunications transmitters. These may cause interference and could change the pacemaker settings, causing a malfunction. Magnetic resonance imaging is contraindicated for clients with pacemakers. The nurse instructs the client to carry a pacemaker identification card and to wear a medical alert (Medic-Alert) bracelet. Chart 36–8 outlines the major points for client and family teaching after the insertion of a permanent pacemaker.

Chart 36–7

Nursing Focus on the Elderly: Dysrhythmias

Elderly clients are at increased risk for dysrhythmias because of changes in their cardiac conduction system. The sinoatrial node has fewer pacemaker cells. There is a loss of fibers in the bundle branch system. Therefore, elderly clients are at risk for sinus node dysfunction and may require pacemaker therapy. The most common dysrhythmias in the elderly are premature atrial contractions, premature ventricular contractions, and atrial fibrillation. Dysrhythmias tend to be more serious in elderly clients because of underlying heart disease, causing cardiac decompensation. Consequently, blood flow to organs, which may already be decreased because of the aging process, is further compromised, leading to multisystem organ dysfunction. The following are special nursing considerations for the elderly client with dysrhythmias:

- Evaluate the client with dysrhythmias immediately for the presence of a life-threatening dysrhythmia or hemodynamic deterioration.
- Assess the client with a dysrhythmia for angina, hypotension, heart failure, and decreased cerebral and renal perfusion.
- Consider the following causes of dysrhythmias when taking the client's history: hypoxia, drug toxicity, electrolyte imbalances, heart failure, and myocardial ischemia or infarction.
- Assess the client's level of education, hearing, learning style, and ability to understand and recall instructions to determine the best approaches for teaching.

- Assess the client's ability to read written instructions.
- Teach the client the generic and trade names of prescribed antidysrhythmic drugs, as well as their purposes, dosage, side effects, and special instructions for their use.
- Provide clear, written instructions in basic language and easy-to-read print.
- Provide a written drug dosage schedule for the client, taking into account all the medications the client is taking and possible drug interactions.
- Assess the client for possible side effects or adverse reactions to drugs, considering the client's age and health status.
- Teach the client to take his or her pulse and to report significant changes in heart rate or rhythm to the physician.
- Inform the client of available resources for blood pressure and pulse checks, such as blood pressure clinics, home health agencies, and cardiac rehabilitation programs.
- Instruct the client on the importance of keeping follow-up visit appointments with the physician and of reporting symptoms promptly.
- Include the client's family members or significant other in all teaching whenever possible.
- Instruct the client to avoid drinking caffeinated beverages, to stop smoking, to drink alcohol only in moderation, and to follow his or her prescribed diet.

Implantable Cardioverter/Defibrillator. Clients with an implantable cardioverter/defibrillator (ICD) usually continue to receive antidysrhythmic drugs after discharge from the hospital. The nurse stresses the importance of continuing to take these medications as prescribed. The nurse provides clear instructions about the purposes of the medications, the dosage schedules, special instructions for taking the medications, and side effects to report. The nurse teaches clients that if they experience an internal defibrillator shock, they must sit or lie down immediately and must notify the physician. Some clients describe the experience of a shock as a quick thud or kick in the chest, whereas other clients relate severe pain similar to that of external defibrillation. The nurse informs family members that they may feel an electrical shock if they are touching the client during delivery of the shock, but it is not harmful. The nurse provides instructions to the client and family members on how to access the emergency medical services (EMS) system in their community. The nurse also recommends resources for the family to learn how to perform CPR.

The nurse teaches clients with an ICD to avoid sources of strong electromagnetic fields, such as large electrical generators and radio or television transmitters. These may inhibit tachydysrhythmia detection and therapy or may cause inadvertent antitachycardia pacing or shocks. Mag-

netic resonance imaging is contraindicated for clients with ICDs. Hand-held cellular phones must be at least 6 inches away from the generator, with the handset to the ear opposite the side of the ICD. The nurse stresses that if the pulse generator emits a beeping sound or provides some other indicator, the client must move away from the area as quickly as possible to prevent deactivation of the device. The nurse instructs the client with an ICD to carry an ICD identification card and to wear a medical alert (Medic-Alert) bracelet. Chart 36–9 highlights the important points for teaching clients and family members and significant others.

▶ *Home Care Management*

The focus of the home care nurse's interventions is assessment and health teaching. Clients and families often fear recurrence of a life-threatening dysrhythmia. Clients with an ICD may dread or fear the activation of the ICD. The continuing care nurse provides the client and family members with the opportunity to verbalize their concerns and fears. The nurse provides emotional support, as well as information about support groups in the community, and makes appropriate referrals. The nurse assesses the client for possible side effects from antidysrhythmic agents or complications from a pacemaker or ICD and communicates concerns and problems to the client's

Chart 36–8

Education Guide: Permanent Pacemakers

- Follow the instructions for pacemaker site skin care that have been specifically prepared for you. Report any fever or redness, swelling, or drainage from the incision site to your physician.
- Keep your pacemaker identification card in your wallet and wear a medical alert (MedicAlert) bracelet.
- Take your pulse for one full minute at the same time each day and record the rate in your pacemaker diary. Take your pulse any time you feel symptoms of a possible pacemaker failure and report your heart rate and symptoms to your physician.
- Know the rate at which your pacemaker is set and the basic functioning of your pacemaker. Know what rate changes to report to your physician.
- Do not apply pressure over your generator. Avoid tight clothing or belts.
- You may take baths or showers without concern for your pacemaker.
- Inform other physicians and dentists that you have a pacemaker. Certain tests they may wish to perform (such as magnetic resonance imaging) could affect or damage your pacemaker.
- Know the indications of battery failure for your pacemaker as you were instructed, and report these findings to your physician if they occur.
- Do not operate electrical appliances directly over your pacemaker site, because this may cause your pacemaker to malfunction.
- Do not lean over electrical or gasoline engines or motors. Be sure that electrical appliances or motors are properly grounded.

- Avoid all transmitter towers for radio, television, and radar. Radio, television, other home appliances, and antennas do not pose a hazard.
- Be aware that antitheft devices in stores may cause temporary pacemaker malfunction. If symptoms develop, move away from the device.
- Inform airport personnel of your pacemaker before passing through a metal detector and show them your pacemaker identification card. The metal in your pacemaker will trigger the alarm in the metal detector device.
- Stay away from any arc welding equipment.
- Be aware that it is safe to operate a microwave oven unless it does not have proper shielding (old microwave ovens) or is defective.
- Report any of the following symptoms to your physician if you experience them: difficulty breathing, dizziness, fainting, prolonged weakness or fatigue, swelling of arms or legs, chest pain, weight gain, and prolonged hiccupping. If you have any of these symptoms, check your pulse rate and call your physician.
- If you feel symptoms when near any device, move 5 to 10 feet away from it and then check your pulse. Your pulse rate should return to normal.
- Keep all your physician and pacemaker clinic appointments.
- Take all medications prescribed for you as instructed.
- Follow your prescribed diet.
- Follow instructions on restrictions on physical activity, such as no sudden, jerky movement for 8 weeks to allow the pacemaker to settle in place.

---

health care provider or assists the client to access health care resources.

► Health Care Resources

The cardiac rehabilitation department nurse typically provides written and oral information about dysrhythmias, antidysrhythmic drugs, pacemakers, and ICDs, as well as information about cardiac exercise programs, educational classes, and support groups. The office or clinic nurse may also provide information about resources. The nurse instructs the client on how to contact the local affiliate of the American Heart Association or the provincial affiliate of the Heart and Stroke Foundation in Canada for information about dysrhythmias, pacemakers, and CPR training.

Manufacturers of pacemakers and ICDs provide helpful booklets and videotapes to assist clients and their families to better understand these therapies. Clients with pacemakers may have transtelephonic systems for transmission of their rhythms to a clinic or health care provider's office. The nurse teaches clients how to use these systems. The nurse stresses the importance of keeping ap-

pointments scheduled for office visits with the cardiologist and pacemaker or ICD clinic. The nurse instructs clients with an ICD to contact the local ambulance or paramedic services and emergency facilities to inform them that they have these devices implanted. The client and family are encouraged to attend pacemaker or ICD support groups.

 Evaluation

On the basis of the identified nursing diagnoses and collaborative problems, the nurse evaluates the care of the client with dysrhythmias. Outcomes include that the client is expected to

- Have a normal, regular pulse rate
- Have normal mental acuity
- Have a normal rate, rhythm, and depth of respiration
- Have normal skin color and temperature
- Perform activities of daily living without dyspnea or excess fatigue
- Be free of pulmonary edema

Chart 36-9

Education Guide: Implantable Cardioverter/Defibrillator (ICD)

- Follow the instructions for ICD site skin care that have been specifically prepared for you.
- Report to your physician any fever or redness, swelling, soreness, or drainage from your incision site.
- Do not wear tight clothing or belts that could cause irritation over the ICD generator.
- Avoid activities that involve rough contact with the ICD implantation site.
- Keep your ICD identification card in your wallet and consider wearing a medical alert (Medic-Alert) bracelet.
- Know the basic functioning of your ICD device and its rate cutoff, as well as the number of consecutive shocks it can deliver.
- Avoid magnets directly over your ICD because they can inactivate the device. If beeping tones are coming from the ICD, move away from the electromagnetic field immediately (within 30 sec) before the inactivation sequence is completed, and notify your physician.
- Inform all physicians and dentists caring for you that you have an ICD implanted, because certain diagnostic tests and procedures must be avoided to prevent ICD malfunction. These include diathermy, electrocautery, and nuclear magnetic resonance tests.
- Avoid other sources of electromagnetic interference, such as devices emitting microwaves (not microwave ovens); transformers; radio, television, and radar transmitters; large electrical generators; metal detectors, including hand-held security devices at airports; antitheft devices; arc welding equipment; and sources of 60-cycle (Hz) interference. Also avoid leaning directly over the alternator of a running motor of a car or boat.
- Report to your physician symptoms such as fainting, nausea, weakness, blackout, and rapid pulse rates.

- Take all medications prescribed for you as instructed.
- Follow instructions on restrictions on physical activity, such as not swimming, driving motor vehicles, or operating dangerous equipment.
- Follow your prescribed diet.
- Keep all physician and ICD clinic appointments.
- Sit or lie down immediately if you feel dizzy or faint to avoid falling if the ICD discharges.
- Post emergency telephone numbers.
- Know how to contact the local emergency medical services (EMS) systems in your community. Inform them in advance that you have an ICD so that they can be prepared if they need to respond to an emergency call for you.
- Know how to perform cough CPR as instructed.
- Encourage family members to learn how to perform CPR. Family members should know that, if they are touching you when the device discharges, they may feel a slight shock but that this is not harmful to them.
- Follow instructions on what to do if the ICD successfully discharges, after which you feel well. This may include maintaining a diary of the date, the time, activity preceding the shock, symptoms, the number of shocks delivered, and how you feel after the shock. The physician may wish to be notified each time the device discharges.
- Avoid strenuous activities that may cause your heart rate to meet or exceed the rate cutoff of your ICD, because this causes the device to discharge inappropriately.
- Notify your physician if you are leaving town or are relocating for information regarding access to health care.

CASE STUDY for the Client with a Dysrhythmia

■ A 78-year-old woman is a client admitted to a telemetry unit directly from a physician's office for evaluation and management of congestive heart failure. She has a history of systemic hypertension and chronic moderate mitral regurgitation. Her medication orders include Lasix 80 mg PO qid, digoxin 0.125 mg PO qd, and Cardizem 60 mg PO tid.

Your initial assessment of the client reveals a pulse rate that is rapid and very irregular. The client is restless, and her skin is pale and cool. Her blood pressure is 106/88. She is short of breath and anxious. Her ECG monitor pattern shows uncontrolled atrial fibrillation, with a rate ranging from 150 to 170 beats per minute. Her oxygen saturation level is 90%.

QUESTIONS:

1. Given the above assessment findings, what should you do first?
2. What additional physical assessment techniques would you perform?
3. Because it is not known how long she has been in atrial fibrillation, what potential problem should be evaluated before attempts to convert the rhythm are implemented?

SELECTED BIBLIOGRAPHY

Alton, R. (1994). Arrhythmias associated with cardiopulmonary arrest. *Nursing Times, 90*(19), 42–44.

*Appel-Hardin, S. (1992). The role of the critical care nurse in noninvasive temporary pacing. *Critical Care Nurse, 12*(3):10–16, 18–19.

Aronow, W. S. (1995). Treatment of ventricular arrhythmias in older adults. *Journal of the American Geriatrics Society, 43*(6), 688–695.

Bashford, C. W. (1994). When a patient survives sudden cardiac death. *RN, 57*(4), 34–37.

Boisvert, J. T., et al. (1995). Overview of pediatric arrhythmias. *Nursing Clinics of North America, 30*(2), 365–379.

Bubien, R. S., et al. (1995). Radiofrequency catheter ablation: Concepts and nursing implications. *Cardiovascular Nursing, 31*(3), 17–23.

Bush, D. E. (1994). Permanent cardiac pacemakers in the elderly. *Journal of the American Geriatrics Society, 42*(3), 326–334.

Cerrato, P. L. (1996). What's new in drugs. A new option for ventricular arrhythmias . . . amiodarone (Cordarone IV). *RN, 59*(2), 79.

Conover, M. B. (1996). *Understanding electrocardiography: Arrhythmias and the 12-lead ECG* (7th ed.). St. Louis: Mosby-Year Book.

Crowley, A. (1997). Emergency! Paroxysmal supraventricular tachycardia. *AJN, 97*(1), 53.

Cummins, R. O., et al. (1994). *Textbook of advanced cardiac life support.* Dallas, TX: American Heart Association.

Cunningham, C. A. (1995). Skills primer: ICD and AED defibrillation. *Emergency, 27*(2), 23–25.

Davenport, J. & Morton, P. G. (1997). Identifying nonischemic causes of life-threatening arrhythmias. *AJN, 97*(11), 50–56.

Dougherty, C. M. (1995). Psychological reactions and family adjustment in shock versus no shock groups after implantation of internal cardioverter defibrillator. *Heart & Lung, 24*(4), 282–292.

Dougherty, C. M., & Shaver, J. F. (1995). Psychophysiological responses after sudden cardiac arrest during hospitalization. *Applied Nursing Research, 8*(4), 160–168.

Dracup, K. (1995). *Meltzer's intensive coronary care* (5th ed.). Stamford, CT: Appleton & Lange.

Dunbar, S. B., et al. (1996). Mood disturbance in patients with recurrent ventricular dysrhythmia before insertion of implantable cardioverter defibrillator. *Heart & Lung: Journal of Acute and Critical Care, 25*(4), 253–261.

Elder, A. N. (1994a). Sinus bradycardia: Elevating a slow heart rate. *Nursing, 24*(11), 48–50.

Elder, A. N. (1994b). Sinus tachycardia: Lowering a high heart rate. *Nursing, 24*(12), 62–64.

Elder, A. N. (1996). Adenosine: Putting the brakes on SVT. *Nursing (Critical Care), 26*(10), 32aa–bb.

*Eorgan, P. A., & Greer, J. L. (1992). Cough CPR: A consideration for high-risk cardiac patient discharge teaching. *Critical Care Nurse, 12*(6), 21–27.

Fiore, L. D. (1996). Anticoagulation: Risks and benefits in atrial fibrillation. *Geriatrics, 51*(6), 22–24.

Flanders, A. (1994). A detailed explanation of defibrillation. *Nursing Times, 90*(18), 37–39.

Futterman, L. G., & Lemberg, L. (1994). An alternative to pharmacologic management of atrial fibrillation: The maze procedure. *American Journal of Critical Care, 3*(3), 238–242.

Goldberger, A. L. & Goldberger, E. (1994). *Clinical electrocardiography: A simplified approach* (5th ed.). St. Louis: Mosby-Year Book.

Gomes, J. A., et al. (1994). Atrial fibrillation: Common—and ominous. *Patient Care, 28*(16), 96–99.

Guaglianone, D. M., & Tyndall, A. (1995). Comfort issues in patients undergoing radiofrequency catheter ablation. *Critical Care Nurse, 15*(1), 47–50.

Hasemeier, C. S. (1996). Clinical snapshot. Permanent pacemaker. *American Journal of Nursing, 96*(2), 30–31.

Hayes, D. D. (1997). Bradycardia: Keeping the current flowing. *Nursing97, 27*(6), 50–56.

Hoffman, R. S. (1995). Lidocaine. *Emergency Medicine, 26*(4), 86, 88.

Holcomb, S. S. (1995). Sotalol. New weapon against ventricular tachycardia. *Nursing, 25*(12), 240–24P, 24R.

Holcomb, S. S. (1996). When beta-blockers aren't the drug of choice. *Nursing (Critical Care), 26*(10), 32dd, 32ff–gg.

Horwood, L., et al. (1995). Antitachycardia pacing: An overview. *American Journal of Critical Care, 4*(5), 397–404.

Huszar, R. J. (1994). *Basic dysrhythmias: Interpretation and management.* St. Louis: Mosby-Year Book.

Ide, B. (1995). Bedside electrocardiographic assessment. *Journal of Cardiovascular Nursing, 9*(4):10–23.

Karnes, N. (1995). Adenosine: A quick fix for PSVT . . . paroxysmal supraventricular tachycardia. *Nursing, 25*(7), 55–56.

Kastor, J. A. (1994). *Arrhythmias.* Philadelphia: W. B. Saunders.

Kishore, A. B., & Camm, A. J. (1995). Guidelines for the use of propafenone in treating supraventricular arrhythmias. *Drugs, 50*(2), 250–262.

Klein, L. S., & Miles, W. M. (1995). Ablative therapy for ventricular arrhythmias. *Progress in Cardiovascular Diseases, 37*(4), 225–242.

Lascelles, K. (1995). Permanent pacemakers. *Nursing Standard, 9*(20), 52–53.

Lenhart, R. C. (1995). Pacemaker assessment and care plans in long-term care. *Geriatric Nursing–American Journal of Care for the Aging, 16*(6):276–280.

Levine, J. H., et al. (1996). Implantable cardioverter defibrillator: Use in patients with no symptoms and at high risk. *American Heart Journal, 131*(1), 59–65.

Lewandowski, D. M., et al. (1995). AV blocks: Are you up to date? *American Journal of Nursing, 95*(12), 26–33.

Mancini, M. E., Richards, N., & Kaye, W. (1997). Saving lives with automated external defibrillators. *Nursing97, 27*(10), 42–43.

Nattel, S. (1995). Newer developments in the management of atrial fibrillation. *American Heart Journal, 130*(5), 1094–1106.

Nicolai, C. (1995). Ventricular dysrhythmias in ischemic heart disease. *AACN Clinical Issues: Advanced Practice in Acute & Critical Care, 6*(3), 452–463.

Norman, E. M. (1994). Identifying risks for atrial fibrillation. *American Journal of Nursing, 94*(10), 48N.

Perez, A. (1996). EKG electrode placement: A refresher course. *RN, 59*(9), 29–31.

Petrosky-Pacini, A. J. (1996). The automatic implantable cardioverter defibrillator in home care. *Home Healthcare Nurse, 14*(4), 238–243.

Pill, M. W., & McCloskey, W. W. (1995). Sotalol: What the emergency nurse needs to know. *Journal of Emergency Nursing, 21*(3), 229–231.

Robinson, B., et al. (1994). A primer on pediatric ECGs. *Contemporary Pediatrics, 11*(4), 69–72, 77–78, 80+.

Ruppert, S. D., et al. (1996). *Dolan's critical care nursing: Clinical management through the nursing process* (2nd ed.) Philadelphia: F. A. Davis.

Sbaih, L. (1995). Ventricular fibrillation in adults. *Emergency Nursing, 3*(2), 10–15.

Schneiderman, H., et al. (1995). What's your diagnosis . . . Wenckebach block (Mobitz type I second-degree atrioventricular block). *Consultant, 35*(4), 519–520, 522.

Searle, C., & Jeffrey, J. (1994). Uncertainty and quality of life of adults hospitalized with life-threatening ventricular arrhythmias. *Canadian Journal of Cardiovascular Nursing, 5*(3), 15–22.

Sims, J. M., & Miracle, V. (1997). Ventricular tachycardia. *Nursing97, 27*(11), 47.

Smith, L. F., & Fish, F. H. (1995). *Pure practice ECGs.* St. Louis: Mosby-Year Book.

Stahl, L. (1995). How to manage common arrhythmias in medical patients. *American Journal of Nursing, 95*(3), 36–41.

Vitale, M. B., & Funk, M. (1995). Quality of life in younger persons with an implantable cardioverter defibrillator. *Education Dimension, 14*(2):100–111.

Wagner, G. S. (1994). *Marriott's practical electrocardiography* (9th ed.). Baltimore: Williams & Wilkins.

Wood, K. (1995). Mechanisms and clinical manifestations of supraventricular tachycardias. *Progress in Cardiovascular Nursing, 10*(2):3–14.

Woods, S. L., et al. (1995). *Cardiac nursing* (3rd ed.). Philadelphia: J. B. Lippincott.

Yacone-Morton, L. A. (1995). Cardiovascular drugs: Antiarrhythmics. *RN, 58*(4):26–31, 33–36.

SUGGESTED READINGS

Aronow, W. S. (1995). Treatment of ventricular arrhythmias in older adults. *Journal of the American Geriatrics Society, 43*(6), 688–695.
This article summarizes the findings of studies and reports from available data in published articles on the treatment of ventricular arrhythmias in older adults. It provides guidelines for the use of class I antiarrhythmic agents, beta blockers, amiodarone, and angiotensin-converting enzyme inhibitors, all of which are commonly prescribed for elderly patients.

Davenport, J., & Morton, P. G. (1997). Identifying nonischemic causes of life-threatening arrhythmias. *AJN, 97*(11), 50–56.
This excellent article describes noncardiac health problems that can cause life-threatening dysrhythmias. The authors discuss electrolyte imbalances, metabolic disorders, drugs, and aging changes that can lead to cardiac irregularities. A CEU quiz follows the article.

Hayes, D. D. (1997). Bradycardia: Keeping the current flowing. *Nursing97, 27*(6), 50–56.
The author describes four categories of bradycardia and illustrates the electrocardiographic findings for each type. A case study is used to discuss treatment that focuses on drug therapy. The article concludes with a CEU quiz.

Chapter 37

INTERVENTIONS FOR CLIENTS WITH CARDIAC PROBLEMS

Primary cardiac dysfunction may have a number of causes, including impaired cardiac muscle function, structural cardiac defects, infections within the heart, and inflammatory conditions of the heart. Although most Americans do not consider heart disease an incurable illness, more people die of heart disease than of any other disorder. Five-year mortality rates range between 25% and 50% (Pratt, 1995). Moderately severe heart failure and dilated cardiomyopathy have 2-year survival rates of only 50%.

Long-term survival of clients with heart disease depends on a coordinated interdisciplinary approach to ensure the best management of the illness and the highest possible quality of life. Therefore, these high-risk clients are often targeted for case management to coordinate their care through the health care continuum, as described in Chapter 3.

HEART FAILURE

Overview

Heart failure, also called *cardiac failure* or *pump failure,* is the inability of the heart to pump sufficient blood to meet the demands of the body. Because fluid excess is not always present, the term *congestive heart failure* may not be applicable. Heart failure may be due to either increased cellular demands or, more commonly, impaired

pumping of the heart. When the heart fails, cardiac output is diminished, and peripheral tissue is not adequately perfused. Congestion of the lungs and periphery may also develop.

Pathophysiology

Compensatory Mechanisms

When cardiac output is insufficient to meet the demands of the body, compensatory mechanisms operate to improve cardiac output. Although the compensatory mechanisms may initially increase cardiac output, they eventually have a damaging effect on pump function. Compensatory mechanisms include

- Increased heart rate
- Improved stroke volume
- Arterial vasoconstriction
- Sodium and water retention
- Myocardial hypertrophy

In heart failure, stimulation of the sympathetic nervous system represents the most immediate compensatory mechanism. Stimulation of the adrenergic receptors causes an increase in heart rate and vasoconstriction.

INCREASED HEART RATE. Because cardiac output equals heart rate times stroke volume, an increase in heart rate results in an immediate increase in cardiac output. The increase in heart rate is limited in its ability to compensate for decreased cardiac output. If the heart rate becomes too rapid, diastolic filling time is limited and cardiac output may start to fall.

IMPROVED STROKE VOLUME. Stroke volume is also improved by sympathetic stimulation. With sympathetic stimulation, there is increased venous return to the heart, which stretches the myocardial fibers further. This increased stretch is referred to as *preload*. In accordance with Starling's law of the heart, increased myocardial stretch results in more forceful contraction, increasing stroke volume and cardiac output. However, after a critical point is reached, further volume and stretch reduce the force of contraction and cardiac output.

ARTERIAL VASOCONSTRICTION. Sympathetic stimulation also results in arterial vasoconstriction. Constriction of arteries has the beneficial effect of maintaining blood pressure and improving tissue perfusion in low-output states. However, constriction of arteries increases *afterload,* the resistance against which the heart must pump. Afterload is the major determinant of myocardial oxygen requirements. As afterload increases, the left ventricle requires more energy to eject its contents and stroke volume may decline.

RETENTION OF SODIUM AND WATER. Reduced blood flow to the kidneys, a common occurrence in low-output states, results in the activation of the renin-angiotensin-aldosterone mechanism. Vasoconstriction becomes more pronounced in response to angiotensin, while aldosterone secretion causes sodium and water retention. The volume of blood returning to the left ventricle is further increased by activation of this mechanism.

MYOCARDIAL HYPERTROPHY. Myocardial hypertrophy, with or without chamber dilation, is the final compensatory mechanism. A thickening of the walls of the heart occurs, providing more muscle mass, resulting in more forceful contractions, and further increasing cardiac output. However, cardiac muscle may hypertrophy more rapidly than collateral circulation can provide adequate blood supply to the muscle. Often, a hypertrophied heart is slightly oxygen deprived.

These mechanisms of compensation act primarily to restore cardiac output to near-normal levels. However, when these cardiac and peripheral circulatory adjustments become excessive, they may decrease pump function. All of them contribute to an increase in myocardial oxygen consumption. When this occurs and myocardial reserve has been exhausted, clinical manifestations of heart failure develop.

Classification of Heart Failure

Heart failure can be classified in many ways. Several important categories are discussed here.

Systolic Versus Diastolic Dysfunction

Systolic dysfunction results when the heart is unable to contract forcefully enough during systole to eject adequate amounts of blood into the circulation. The ejection fraction (the percentage of blood ejected from the heart during systole) drops from a normal of 50% to 70% to below 40%. As the ejection fraction decreases, tissue perfusion diminishes and the blood accumulates in the pulmonary vasculature. Symptoms of systolic dysfunction may be symptoms of inadequate tissue perfusion or pulmonary and systemic congestion.

In contrast, diastolic failure occurs when the left ventricle is unable to relax adequately during diastole. Inadequate relaxation prevents the ventricle from filling with sufficient blood to ensure an adequate cardiac output. Diastolic failure may represent 20% to 40% of all heart failure, primarily occurring in older adults and women following a myocardial infarction (Redfield, 1996). Symptoms of diastolic failure are similar to those of systolic. However, treatment is not clearly established and is not discussed in this text.

Left Versus Right Ventricular Failure

Because the two ventricles of the heart represent two separate pumping systems, it is possible for one to fail alone for a short period. Most heart failure begins with failure of the left ventricle and progresses to failure of both ventricles. Typical causes of left ventricular failure include hypertensive disease, coronary artery disease, and valvular disease (involving the mitral or aortic valve).

Decreased tissue perfusion from poor cardiac output and pulmonary congestion from increased pressure in the pulmonary vessels indicate left ventricular failure.

Right ventricular failure may be caused by left ventricular failure, right ventricular myocardial infarction, or pulmonary hypertension.

In right ventricular failure, the right ventricle is unable to empty completely, increased volume and pressure develop in the systemic veins, and systemic venous congestion and peripheral edema develop. Figure 37–1 illustrates the pathophysiology of heart failure.

Low-Output Versus High-Output Syndrome

Low-output syndrome, the more common type of heart failure, occurs when the heart fails as a pump, resulting in impaired peripheral circulation and peripheral vasoconstriction. When cardiac output remains normal or above normal but the metabolic needs of the body are not met, high-output syndrome is present. It may be caused by increased metabolic needs (hyperthyroidism, fever, pregnancy) or hyperkinetic conditions (arteriovenous fistulas, Paget's disease).

Functional Status

Heart failure may also be categorized by its effect on the client's functional status. Table 35–2 summarizes the New York Heart Association (NYHA) categories.

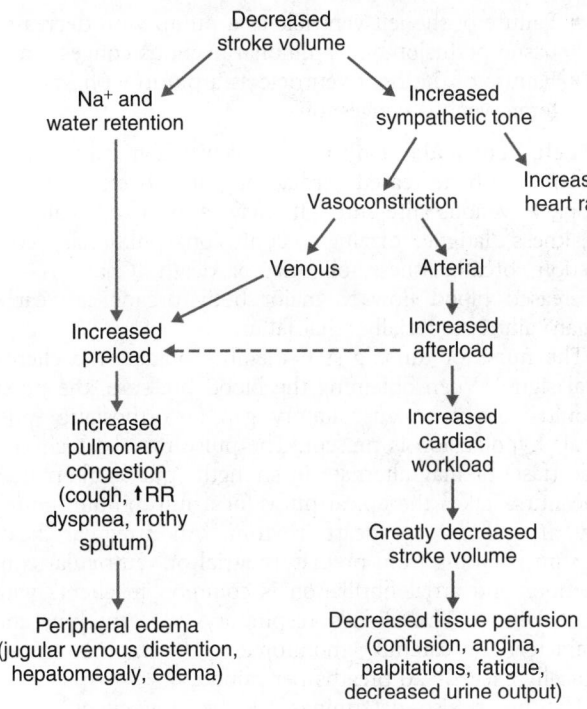

Figure 37–1. Pathophysiology of heart failure.

Etiology

The most common cause of heart failure is myocardial infarction. The next most common causes are conditions such as systemic hypertension and pulmonary stenosis, which cause pressure or volume overload on the heart. Other direct causes of heart failure are myocardial dysfunction, filling disorders, and increased metabolic demand. Some of the conditions capable of causing heart failure are listed in Table 37–1.

Incidence/Prevalence

More than 4.5 million people in the United States are living with heart failure (American Heart Association [AHA], 1996), with about 400,000 new cases occurring each year. Treatment and care for clients with heart failure costs over $10 billion every year (Konstam et al., 1994).

ELDERLY CONSIDERATIONS

Heart failure occurs most commonly in older adults, and its prevalence increases with age; 75% of clients with heart failure are older than 60 years. Heart failure is the most frequent cause of hospitalization for adults older than 65 (AHA, 1996). The prevalence of heart failure steadily increases with aging; heart failure occurs in 3% of people 45 to 64 years old, 6% of people 65 and older, and 10% of people older than 75 (Jensen and Miller, 1995). Heart failure is more common in men than women at all ages.

Collaborative Management

 Assessment

Manifestations of heart failure depend on the type of failure, the ventricle involved, and the underlying cause. Impaired tissue perfusion, pulmonary congestion, and edema dominate the picture of left ventricular failure. Systemic venous congestion and peripheral edema are associated with right ventricular failure.

➤ History

When taking a history, the nurse should keep in mind the many conditions that can lead to heart failure. The nurse carefully questions the client about past medical history, including a history of high blood pressure, angina, myocardial infarction, rheumatic heart disease, valvular disorders, endocarditis, and pericarditis.

The nurse asks about the client's perception of his or her activity tolerance, breathing pattern, urinary pattern, and fluid volume status and the client's knowledge about heart failure.

Left Ventricular Failure. With left ventricular systolic dysfunction, the cardiac output is diminished, impaired tissue perfusion results, anaerobic metabolism occurs, and the client often reports unusual fatigue. The nurse assesses the client's activity tolerance by asking if the client can perform normal activities of daily living (ADLs) or climb flights of stairs without fatigue or dyspnea. Many clients with heart failure experience weakness or fatigue with activity as a feeling of heaviness in their arms or legs. Clients should be asked about their ability to perform simultaneous arm and leg work (e.g., walking while carrying a bag of groceries). Such activity may place an unacceptable demand on the failing heart. The nurse should ask clients to name their most strenuous activity in the past week. Many clients unconsciously limit their activities in response to fatigue or dyspnea and may not realize how limited they have become.

Perfusion to the myocardium is often impaired, especially if cardiac muscle has hypertrophied. The client may report chest discomfort or may describe palpitations, skipped beats, or a fast heartbeat.

As the amount of blood ejected from the left ventricle diminishes, pressure builds in the pulmonary venous sys-

TABLE 37–1

Predisposing Factors to Systolic Heart Failure

Hypertension
Coronary artery disease
Cardiomyopathy
Alcohol
Valvular disease
Congenital defects

tem resulting in fluid-filled alveoli and pulmonary congestion. Thus, cough is often an early manifestation of heart failure. The client in early heart failure describes the *cough* as irritating, nocturnal, and usually nonproductive. As heart failure becomes more severe, the client may begin expectorating frothy pink-tinged sputum, a sign of pulmonary edema.

Dyspnea also results from rising pulmonary venous pressure and pulmonary congestion. The nurse carefully questions the client about the presence of dyspnea and when and how it developed. The client may refer to dyspnea as "trouble in catching one's breath," "breathlessness," or "difficulty in breathing."

As exertional dyspnea develops, the client often discontinues previously tolerated levels of activity owing to shortness of breath. Dyspnea at rest in the recumbent position is known as *orthopnea*. The nurse asks how many pillows the client usually uses to sleep or if the client sleeps in an upright position in a bed or a chair.

Clients who describe sudden awakening with a feeling of breathlessness 2 to 5 hours after falling asleep have paroxysmal nocturnal dyspnea (PND). Sitting upright, dangling their feet, or walking usually relieves this condition.

Elderly Considerations

Decreased cerebral perfusion resulting from low cardiac output leads to changes in mental status. Confusion may occur with even mild or moderate heart failure in the very old client. The nurse asks the client and his or her family members if any lapses in memory or periods of disorientation have occurred.

Right Ventricular Failure. Signs of systemic congestion occur as the right ventricle fails, fluid is retained, and pressure builds in the venous system. Edema develops in the lower legs and ascends to the thighs and the abdominal wall. Clients may note that shoes fit more tightly, or indentations may develop on their swollen feet from shoes or socks. Clients may indicate that they have removed their rings because of swelling in their fingers and hands. The nurse asks the client about weight gain. An adult may retain 4 to 7 L of fluid (10–15 pounds [4.5–6.8 kg]) before pitting edema occurs.

Gastrointestinal complaints of nausea and anorexia may be a direct consequence of the liver engorgement due to fluid retention. Another finding related to fluid retention is diuresis at rest. At rest, edema fluid is mobilized and excreted so the client describes frequent awakening at night to urinate.

The nurse or dietitian takes a careful nutritional history, questioning the client about the use of salt and the types of food consumed. The nurse also questions the client concerning daily fluid intake. Clients in heart failure may experience increased thirst and take in excessive fluid (4000–5000 mL) because of aldosterone secretion.

▶ Physical Assessment/Clinical Manifestations

The signs and symptoms of heart failure can be considered in the context of these components of the syndrome:

- Failure of the left ventricle as a pump with decreased tissue perfusion and pulmonary venous congestion
- Failure of the right ventricle as a pump with systemic venous congestion

Left Ventricular Failure. Left ventricular failure is associated with decreased cardiac output and elevated pulmonary venous pressure. It may appear clinically as weakness, fatigue, dizziness, confusion, pulmonary congestion, breathlessness, oliguria, or death (Chart 37–1). Decreased blood flow to major body organs can cause organ failure, especially renal failure.

The nurse or nursing staff member obtains the client's vital signs. When obtaining the blood pressure, the nurse should note if an auscultatory gap or orthostatic (postural) hypotension is present. The pulse may be tachycardiac (fast) or may alternate in strength (pulsus alternans). The nurse takes the apical pulse for a full minute, noting any irregularity in heart rhythm. An irregular heart rhythm resulting from premature atrial or ventricular contractions and atrial fibrillation is common in clients with heart failure. The client's respiratory rate, rhythm, and character are carefully monitored. The respiratory rate typically exceeds 20 breaths per minute.

The nurse also determines whether the client is oriented to person, place, and time. If there are concerns about orientation, a short mental status examination may be used (see Chap. 43). Objective data are important because many people are skillful at covering up memory losses in daily conversation.

The nurse palpates the precordium. Increased heart size is common, with a displacement of the apical impulse to the left. On auscultation, the nurse may hear a third heart sound (S_3) gallop, an early diastolic filling sound indicating an increase in left ventricular pressure. A fourth heart sound (S_4) can also occur, although it is not a sign of failure but a reflection of decreased ventricular compliance.

Chart 37–1

Key Features of Left-Sided Heart Failure

Decreased Cardiac Output

- Fatigue
- Weakness
- Oliguria during the day
- Angina
- Confusion, restlessness
- Dizziness
- Tachycardia, palpitations
- Pallor
- Weak peripheral pulses
- Cool extremities

Pulmonary Congestion

- Hacking cough, worse at night
- Dyspnea/breathlessness
- Crackles or wheezes in lungs
- Frothy pink-tinged sputum
- Tachypnea

When the nurse auscultates the lungs, crackles and wheezes may be present. Late inspiratory crackles and fine profuse crackles that repeat themselves from breath to breath and do not diminish with coughing indicate heart failure. Crackles are produced by intra-alveolar fluid and are frequently noted first in the dependent areas of the lungs. Usually, crackles develop in the bases and spread upward as the condition worsens. The nurse identifies precisely the location of the crackles. Wheezes indicate narrowing of the bronchial lumen caused by engorged pulmonary vessels.

Right Ventricular Failure. Right ventricular failure is associated with increased systemic venous pressures. Signs and symptoms are listed in Chart 37–2.

On inspection, the nurse assesses the neck veins for distention (see Chap. 35). The nurse also measures the client's abdominal girth and assesses for the presence of hepatomegaly (liver engorgement), hepatojugular reflux (see Chap. 35), and ascites. The collection of fluid in the abdomen (ascites) can reach volumes of more than 10 L.

In addition, the nurse examines the client for dependent edema. In the ambulatory client, edema is normally located in the ankles and legs. However, when the client is restricted to bed rest, the sacrum is dependent and edema accumulates there. Edema is an extremely unreliable sign of heart failure so accurate daily weights are needed to document fluid retention. Weight is the most reliable indicator of fluid gain or loss.

> *Psychosocial Assessment*

Acute episodes of heart failure may be precipitated in susceptible people by stressful life situations. Acute exacerbations of heart failure may result from feelings of rejection, insecurity, frustration, or rage. The nurse needs to question clients sensitively about any recent stressors in their lives. The nurse asks clients to rate their current level of stress and describe any significant recent life changes.

Many clients with heart failure have symptoms that are not well controlled. These clients may have anxiety and frustrations related to dealing with a chronic illness. The nurse assesses clients and their families for fears, anxieties, and frustrations and also assesses their usual methods of coping (see Chap. 8).

Hope is a major determinant of well-being for clients in heart failure. Clients who are hopeful tend to feel better and to be more socially involved. The nurse might ask clients what activities they engage in, who the significant people are in their life, and how often they are able to interact with them.

> *Laboratory Assessment*

Electrolyte imbalance in heart failure may occur from complications of failure or as side effects of drug therapy, especially diuretic therapy. It is essential that regular evaluations of a client's serum electrolytes be done, including sodium, potassium, magnesium, calcium, and chloride. Any impairment of renal function may be reflected by elevated blood urea nitrogen, serum creatinine, and creatinine clearance levels. Urinalysis may reveal proteinuria and high specific gravity. Hemoglobin and hematocrit tests should be performed to identify heart failure resulting from anemia.

Arterial blood gas values often reveal hypoxia (low oxygen level) because oxygen does not diffuse easily through fluid-filled alveoli. Respiratory alkalosis may occur because of hyperventilation; respiratory acidosis may occur because of carbon dioxide retention. Metabolic acidosis may indicate lactic acid accumulation.

ELDERLY CONSIDERATIONS

In clients who are over 65 years, have atrial fibrillation, or have evidence of thyroid disease, thyroxine (T_4) and thyroid-stimulating hormone (TSH) levels should be determined (Konstam et al., 1994). Heart failure may be due to or aggravated by hypo- or hyperthyroidism.

> *Radiographic Assessment*

Chest x-rays can be helpful in diagnosing left ventricular failure. Typically, the heart is enlarged (cardiomegaly), representing hypertrophy or dilation. Pleural effusions develop less often and generally reflect biventricular failure.

> *Other Diagnostic Assessment*

In addition to a chest x-ray, an electrocardiogram (ECG) is performed. The ECG may demonstrate ventricular hypertrophy, dysrhythmias, and any degree of myocardial ischemia, injury, or infarction. It is not helpful in determining the presence or extent of heart failure.

Echocardiography is useful in diagnosing cardiac valvular changes, pericardial effusion, chamber enlargement, and ventricular hypertrophy. Radionuclide studies (thallium imaging or technetium pyrophosphate scanning) can also indicate the presence and cause of heart failure. Multigated angiographic (MUGA) scans provide information about left ventricular ejection fraction and velocity, which is typically low in clients with heart failure.

Pulmonary artery catheters allow assessment of cardiac function and volume status in acutely ill clients. These measurements can confirm the diagnosis and guide the management of heart failure. The right atrial pressure may be normal or elevated in left ventricular failure and is elevated in right ventricular failure. Pulmonary artery pressure and pulmonary artery wedge pressure (PAWP)

Chart 37–2

Key Features of Right-Sided Heart Failure

- Jugular (neck vein) distention
- Enlarged liver and spleen
- Anorexia and nausea
- Dependent edema (legs and sacrum)
- Distended abdomen
- Swollen hands and fingers
- Polyuria at night
- Weight gain
- Increased blood pressure (from excess volume) or decreased blood pressure (from failure)

are elevated in left-sided heart failure because volumes and pressures are increased in the left ventricle. (See Chapter 35 for a more detailed description of the pulmonary artery catheter.)

 Analysis

➤ Common Nursing Diagnoses and Collaborative Problems

The most common nursing diagnoses pertinent to the client with heart failure are

1. Impaired Gas Exchange related to altered oxygen supply
2. Decreased Cardiac Output related to a reduction in stroke volume as a result of mechanical malfunctions
3. Activity Intolerance related to an imbalance between oxygen supply and demand, fatigue, or an electrolyte imbalance

The primary collaborative problem is Potential for Pulmonary Edema.

➤ Additional Nursing Diagnoses and Collaborative Problems

Some clients have one or more of the following:

- Ineffective Management of Therapeutic Regime related to failed social support systems, inadequate follow-up, inadequate discharge planning, or knowledge deficit
- Ineffective Individual Coping related to physical inactivity, major changes in lifestyle, loss of control over body function, or fear of death
- Altered Thought Processes related to impaired gas exchange or fear of the unknown
- Impaired Physical Mobility related to fatigue and activity intolerance

Some clients are also at risk for the following collaborative problems:

- Potential for Pneumonia
- Potential for Dysrhythmias

 Planning and Implementation

➤ Impaired Gas Exchange

Planning: Expected Outcomes. The client is expected to have a normal rate, rhythm, and depth of respiration and to have an O_2 saturation greater than 92%.

Interventions. The nurse or assistive nursing personnel monitors the client's respiratory rate, rhythm, and character every 1 to 4 hours and auscultates breath sounds. If clients are experiencing pulmonary congestion, the oxygen content of their blood is often markedly reduced. The nurse may titrate the amount of supplemental oxygen delivered to the client within a range prescribed by the health care provider to maintain the client's oxygen saturation at 92% or greater.

If the client experiences respiratory difficulty, the nurse or assistive nursing personnel places the client in a high Fowler's position with pillows under each arm to maximize chest expansion and improve oxygenation. Repositioning the client and having the client perform coughing and deep breathing exercises every 2 hours helps to improve oxygenation and to prevent atelectasis.

➤ Decreased Cardiac Output

Planning: Expected Outcomes. The primary outcome is that the client is expected to resume and maintain an adequate cardiac output.

Interventions. Interventions are aimed at improving cardiac output. A critical pathway for congestive heart failure that reflects an interdisciplinary approach to client care is included in this chapter. Therapy may be directed toward optimizing the two major components of cardiac output: stroke volume (determined by preload, afterload, and contractility) and heart rate.

Interventions to optimize stroke volume include reducing afterload, reducing preload, and improving cardiac muscle contractility.

Reducing Afterload. By relaxing arterioles, arterial vasodilators can reduce impedance to left ventricular ejection (afterload) and improve cardiac output. In the strictest sense, these drugs do not act as vasodilators but reverse some of the inappropriate or excessive vasoconstriction that is common in heart failure.

Clients with even mild heart failure due to left ventricular dysfunction should be given a trial of angiotensin-converting enzyme (ACE) inhibitors. ACE inhibitors, a group of arterial vasodilators such as enalapril (Vasotec), moexipril (Univasc), and captopril (Capoten), generally prolong and improve the quality of life of clients in heart failure (see Chart 37–3). Studies have shown that these drugs enhance functional status, with 40% to 80% of clients showing an improvement in NYHA class (Baker et al., 1994).

ACE inhibitors suppress the renin-angiotensin-aldosterone system, which is activated in response to decreased renal blood flow. ACE inhibitors benefit clients by reducing arterial resistance, decreasing pulmonary artery wedge pressure, and increasing stroke volume and cardiac output.

The health care provider usually starts ACE inhibitor doses slowly and cautiously. The first dose of an ACE inhibitor has been associated with a rapid drop in blood pressure in some clients. Clients at risk for hypotension following ACE inhibitor administration have initial systolic blood pressures less than 100, are older than 75 years, have a serum sodium level less than 135, or are volume depleted (Baker et al., 1994). After the initial dose and each increased dose, the nurse monitors the client's blood pressure for several hours.

The nurse clarifies with the health care provider the guidelines for administering the vasodilator. For example, many clinicians maintain clients in heart failure at systolic blood pressures ranging from 90 to 110 mmHg. When such a blood pressure is the client's maintenance level, the nurse assesses the client for orthostatic hypotension, confusion, poor peripheral perfusion, and reduced urinary output. While the client is receiving ACE inhibitors, the

OUR LADY OF LOURDES MEDICAL CENTER
CRITICAL PATHWAY
CONGESTIVE HEART FAILURE DUE TO LEFT VENTRICULAR DYSFUNCTION NOT REQUIRING ADMISSION TO A CRITICAL CARE UNIT

	DAY #1 DATE_____	DAY #2 DATE_____	DAY #3 DATE_____	DAY #4 DATE_____
LOCATION OF PATIENT	CARDIOLOGY FLOOR (PREFERRED) OR MED-SURG FLOOR	CARDIOLOGY FLOOR (PREFERRED) OR MED-SURG FLOOR	CARDIOLOGY FLOOR (PREFERRED) OR MED-SURG FLOOR	CARDIAC FLOOR (PREFERRED) OR MED-SURG FLOOR
RESPONSIBLE SERVICE	INTERNAL MEDICINE, FAMILY PRACTICE, OR CARDIOLOGY	INTERNAL MEDICINE, FAMILY PRACTICE, OR CARDIOLOGY	INTERNAL MEDICINE, FAMILY PRACTICE, OR CARDIOLOGY	INTERNAL MED, FAMILY PRACTICE, OR CARDIOLOGY
CONSULTS	CARDIOLOGY, DIETARY AND PATIENT EDUCATION, AS NECESSARY. CARDIAC REHAB	CARDIOLOGY, DIETARY AND PATIENT EDUCATION, AS NECESSARY. CARDIAC REHAB	CARDIOLOGY, DIETARY AND PATIENT EDUCATION, AS NECESSARY. CARDIAC REHAB	CARDIOLOGY, DIETARY AND PATIENT EDUCATION, AS NECESSARY. CARDIAC REHAB
LAB	BUN, CREATININE, LYTES, BLOOD GLUCOSE, ALBUMIN, URIC ACID, CBC, URINALYSIS. IF ACUTE MI IS BEING EXCLUDED, CK ON ADMISSION AND Q8H X3. CK-MB IF TOTAL CK ELEVATED	BUN, CREATININE, LYTES	BUN, CREATININE, LYTES, DIGOXIN LEVEL.	NONE
RADIOLOGY	CHEST X-RAY, PA AND LATERAL	NONE	CHEST X-RAY, PA AND LATERAL	NONE
OTHER TESTS	EKG ON ADMISSION AND FOR ANGINA AS PER PROTOCOL - CHEST LEAD LOCATIONS MARKED WITH PEN. CARDIAC ECHO - DOPPLER ORDERED FOR DAY 1 OR DAY 2. PULSE OXIMETRY.	ECHO - DOPPLER HEART IF NOT DONE DAY 1	NONE	NONE
ACTIVITY	BED REST, DANGLE TID, OR OUT OF BED, AS TOLERATED	AMBULATE AS TOLERATED	AMBULATE AD LIB	AMBULATE AD LIB
NURSING CARE	CHECK AND RECORD BP, HEART RATE, AND RESPIRATORY RATE ON ADMISSION, 1 HR AFTER ADMISSION AND Q 2 HRS UNTIL STABLE. AFTER STABLE, RECORD BP, HR, AND RR Q 4 H. CHECK AND RECORD TEMPERATURE ON ADMISSION AND Q 8 H THEREAFTER. WEIGH PATIENT ON ADMISSION (USE BED OR CHAIR SCALE IF NECESSARY: ESTIMATED WEIGHT NOT ALLOWED) I&O. ARRHYTHMIA AND ANGINA CARE PER PROTOCOLS.	RECORD I&O. MEASURE AND RECORD BP, HR, RR, AND TEMP EVERY 8 HOURS. RECORD AND EVALUATE RHYTHM STRIPS IF PATIENT ON TELEMETRY. WEIGH DAILY IN AM (POST-VOID, PRE-PRANDIAL). ARRHYTHMIA AND ANGINA CARE PER PROTOCOLS.	MEASURE AND RECORD BP, HEART RATE, RESP RATE Q 4 H. RECORD TEMP Q 8 H. WEIGH DAILY (POST-VOID), PRE-PRANDIAL.	ENCOURAGE AMBULATION
LINES, MONITORS, AND TUBES	TELEMETRIC MONITORING IF INDICATED. TEXAS OR FOLEY CATHETER AS INDICATED. PRN ADAPTER. SUPPLEMENTAL O2 PRN SOB, CHEST PAIN, OR O2 SAT<93%.	PRN ADAPTER. TELEMETRIC EKG MONITOR IF INDICATED. REMOVE TEXAS OR FOLEY CATHETER. O2, PRN SOB, CHEST PAIN, OR O2 SAT<93%.	DISCONTINUE TELEMETRIC MONITORING. REMOVE PRN ADAPTER AFTER TELEMETRY D/C'D. D/C O2 SUPPLEMENT.	NONE
MEDS	INTRAVENOUS DIURETICS. LOW DOSE ORAL ACE INHIBITOR. DIGOXIN LOAD, IF APPROPRIATE. ORAL OR CUTANEOUS NITRATES. MOM PRN. MAALOX, MYLANTA PRN. TYLENOL PRN. DAYTIME SEDATIVE PRN. HS SEDATIVE PRN. HEPARIN 5000 U SC Q 12 H WHILE PATIENT IS NON-AMBULATORY. COLACE 100 MG BID.	IV DIURETIC; SWITCH TO ORAL DIURETIC IF DIURESIS ADEQUATE. CONTINUE ORAL OR CUTANEOUS NITRATE AS INDICATED. ACE INHIBITOR; INCREASE DOSE AS TOLERATED. DIGOXIN, MAINTENANCE DOSE. MOM PRN. MAALOX, MYLANTA PRN. TYLENOL PRN. DAYTIME SEDATIVE PRN. HS SEDATIVE PRN. D/C S.C. HEPARIN WHEN PATIENT AMBULATORY.	ORAL DIURETIC; ADJUST DOSAGE AS INDICATED. ORAL OR CUTANEOUS NITRATE. ACE INHIBITOR; INCREASE DOSE AS TOLERATED. DIGOXIN. MOM PRN. MAALOX, MYLANTA PRN. TYLENOL PRN. DAYTIME SEDATIVE PRN. HS SEDATIVE PRN.	ORAL DIURETIC. ORAL OR CUTANEOUS NITRATE. ACE INHIBITOR. DIGOXIN. MOM PRN. MAALOX, MYLANTA PRN. TYLENOL PRN.
DIET	CARDIAC DIET (3 GM SODIUM, LOW CHOLESTEROL) AS TOLERATED.	CARDIAC DIET	CARDIAC DIET	CARDIAC DIET
PATIENT AND FAMILY EDUCATION	UNIT AND ROOM ORIENTATION. EXPLANATION OF MEDS. INTRODUCTION TO CRITICAL PATHWAY. EXPLAIN ADVANCED DIRECTIVES.	EXPLANATION OF MEDS TO PATIENT AND FAMILY. REHAB TEACHING AS PER PROTOCOL.	EXPLANATION OF MEDS TO PATIENT AND FAMILY. REHAB TEACHING AS PER PROTOCOL. DIET INSTRUCTIONS.	FINAL REVIEW OF MEDICATIONS, DIET, AND DISCHARGE INSTRUCTIONS.
DISCHARGE PLANNING	SOCIAL SERVICES CONSULT AS INDICATED. HOME HEALTH SERVICES CONSULT AS INDICATED.		REMIND PATIENT THAT DISCHARGE IS PLANNED FOR AM OF DAY 4. NOTIFY FAMILY OF PLANNED DISCHARGE AND MAKE TRANSPORTATION ARRANGEMENTS. SOCIAL SERVICES RE-EVALUATION. CONFIRM ARRANGEMENTS FOR HOME HEALTH.	ASSIST PATIENT IN PREPARING TO LEAVE HOSPITAL AND WITH TRANSPORTATION ARRANGEMENTS. PATIENT DISCHARGED TO HOME.

THIS CRITICAL PATHWAY HAS BEEN DEVELOPED TO SERVE AS A GUIDELINE FOR THE "OPTIMAL" MANAGEMENT OF PATIENTS HOSPITALIZED PRIMARILY FOR THE ABOVE NOTED DIAGNOSIS OR PROCEDURE WITHOUT COMPLICATING COMORBIDITIES.

Chart 37–3

Drug Therapy for Cardiac Failure

Drug	Usual Dosage	Nursing Interventions	Rationale
Drugs Used Primarily to Reduce Afterload			
Angiotensin-Converting Enzyme Inhibitors Captopril (Capoten)	• To start: 6.25–12.5 mg PO tid • May increase to 50–100 mg PO tid	• Monitor the client's blood pressure closely for several hours after the first dose. Consult with the physician to determine the desired range for blood pressure. • Monitor the serum creatinine and potassium levels carefully. • Report fever and sore throat to the physician. Monitor the results of the complete blood count. • Report cough to the health care provider	• Hypotension may occur as a first-dose effect. It is most common in Na^+- or volume-depleted clients. • Clients with impaired renal function may develop hyperkalemia. • Neutropenia, although rare, can be a hazardous complication. • Cough is a side effect of the drug.
Enalapril maleate (Vasotec)	• To start: 2.5–5 mg/day • May increase to 10–40 mg/day as a single dose or divided doses.	• Administer 1 hr before or 2 hr after meals. • Enalapril is similar to captopril but may be administered less frequently.	• Administration on an empty stomach enhances absorption. • Enalapril has a longer half-life than captopril.
Drugs Used Primarily To Reduce Preload			
Loop Diuretics Furosemide (Lasix, Furoside✽)	• 40 mg qd or bid PO • 40 mg qd IV push (may increase to 80 mg and repeat × 1 in 30 min in acute situations) • **Elderly:** Older adults may be more sensitive to the effects of the usual adult dose.	• Administer once daily when the client arises. • Assess the client for adequate diuresis. Obtain daily weights. Note changes in breath sounds and edema. • Monitor the client's serum electrolytes (especially K^+, Na^+, and Cl^-). Provide K^+ supplementation if prescribed. • Monitor the client for signs of dehydration (hypotension, dry mucous membranes, poor skin turgor, thirst, and oliguria). • Note any report of ringing in the ears.	• The volume and frequency of urination increase for 6–8 hr after an oral dose. • Weight is one of the most accurate noninvasive measurements of volume status. • Loop diuretics may produce excessive loss of these electrolytes. • Loop diuretics continue to cause diuresis even after the excessive fluid has been removed. • Tinnitus may indicate toxicity.
Nitrates Isosorbide dinitrate (Isodil, Sorbitrate, Coronex✽, Novosorbide✽)	• PO (tablet) 15–30 mg q6h • PO (sustained release) 40 mg q6–12h	• Observe the client for postural hypotension. Supervise ambulation until the dose response is determined.	• Relaxation of venous smooth muscle causes blood to pool in the veins when the client stands.
Nitroglycerin (Nitro-Dur)	• Transdermal ointment: starting dose of ½ inch q4–8h increasing to 2 inches q4–8h	• Assess the client for headache. Inform the physician and provide relief.	• Headache diminishes with tolerance. Mild analgesics and administration with food should provide relief until then.

Continued

CHART 37–3. Drug Therapy for Cardiac Failure Continued

Drug	Usual Dosage	Nursing Interventions	Rationale
Nitroglycerin (Nitrodisc)	• Transdermal patch: 2.5–15 mg/12–18 hr	• Administer PO dose 30 min before or 2 hr after meals. Make sure the client does not chew.	• Oral nitrates are most rapidly absorbed from an empty stomach.
		• Administer the ointment on a hairless part of the body in a uniform layer using an applicator.	• Proper administration ensures consistent dose administration.
		• If so prescribed, allow an 8–12-hr nitrate-free period at night.	• A nitrate-free period prevents the development of tolerance to the vasodilating effect of nitrates.
		• Rotate the skin sites of transdermal nitrate administration.	• Nitrates cause skin irritation.
		• Remove transdermal nitrates before defibrillation.	• Skin burns have occurred, and explosion is possible.
Cardiac Glycosides Digoxin (Lanoxin, Novodigoxin✦)	• Loading dose of 1 mg divided over 24 hr. • Then maintenance 0.125–0.5 mg PO qd • Usually 0.25–0.375 mg IV qd	• Ask the client about previous use of digitalis; provide the preparation previously taken. (Do not substitute one preparation for another.)	• Dosages, absorption rates, and duration of effects differ among drugs.
Digitoxin (Crystodigin) (infrequently used)	• Loading dose of 1.2–1.6 mg divided during 24 hr • Then 0.1 mg daily IV or PO	• Be alert for the following: • Myocardial infarction • Hypokalemia • Renal or hepatic disorders • Diuretic therapy • Diarrhea • Advanced age • Metabolic alkalosis	• Any of these factors may result in an increased sensitivity to digitalis and increase the risk of toxicity.
		• Monitor serum potassium levels and electrocardiograms.	• Hypokalemia is often associated with digitalis toxicity and dysrhythmias.
		• Take the apical pulse or check the cardiac monitor pattern before administering each dose of digitalis.	• Changes in pulse rate and rhythm may signify digitalis toxicity.
		• Monitor serum levels of digitalis. Therapeutic digoxin level is 0.9–1.2 ng/mL.	• There is a narrow margin between therapeutic and toxic doses of digitalis. Toxicity occurs in approximately 10%–20% of clients receiving digitalis.
		• Observe for signs of digitalis toxicity and notify the physician if any occur: • Confusion • Dysrhythmias • Anorexia • Fatigue • Muscle weakness	

nurse monitors serum potassium levels for hyperkalemia, serum creatinine for renal dysfunction, and the client for development of a cough. Table 37–2 compares the effects of selected agents that reduce the preload and the afterload. (Intravenous medications used to decrease preload and afterload are described in Chapter 40.)

Reducing Preload. When ventricular fibers are overstretched, as in the failing heart, they contract less forcefully. Interventions aimed at preload reduction attempt to decrease volume and pressure in the left ventricle, optimizing ventricular muscle stretch and contraction. Preload reduction is appropriate for clients in heart failure who

TABLE 37–2

Effects of Vasodilators*		
Drug	**Preload Reduction (Vasodilates Peripheral Veins)**	**Afterload Reduction (Vasodilates Arterioles)**
Nitrates (nitroglycerin, isosorbide dinitrate)	+ + +	+
Hydralazine hydrochloride (Apresoline)	0	+ + +
Nifedipine (Procardia)	0	+ +
Sodium nitroprusside (Nitropress)	+ + +	+ + +
Captopril (Capoten)	+	+ +
Prazosin (Minipress)	+ +	+

*0, no effect; +, mild effect; + +, moderate effect; + + +, maximal effect.

have congestion with total body sodium and water overload.

Diet Therapy. In heart failure, diet therapy is aimed at reducing sodium and water retention.

Sodium Restriction. In collaboration with the dietitian, the health care provider may restrict sodium intake in an attempt to decrease fluid retention. Many clients with heart failure need to omit only table salt (ingest no added salt) from their diet, thus reducing the sodium intake to 2 to 3 g/day. If salt intake must be reduced further, the client may need to eliminate all salt in cooking, thus reducing sodium intake to 1.2 to 2.0 g/day. The dietitian helps the client select foods that meet the prescribed therapeutic diet. Table 14–6 lists the sodium contents of some common foods.

Fluid Volume Restriction. Few clients are placed on severe fluid restrictions. However, because clients with excessive aldosterone secretion may experience thirst and drink 3 to 5 L of fluid each day, their fluid intake may be limited to a more normal 2 L/day. Compliance with these simple strategies may be high, especially if the client experiences relief of any of the symptoms of volume excess. When a fluid restriction is imposed on the hospitalized client, the nurse adjusts oral and intravenous therapy accordingly.

The nurse or assistive nursing personnel weighs the client daily (1 kg of weight gain or loss equals 1 L of retained or lost fluid, respectively) and keeps accurate records of fluid intake and output. The same scale should be used every morning before breakfast for the most accurate assessment of weight.

Drug Therapy. Common drugs prescribed to reduce preload are diuretics and venous vasodilators.

Diuretics. The health care provider adds diuretics to the regimen when diet and fluid restriction have not been effective in the management of symptoms of systemic or pulmonary congestion associated with heart failure. Diuretics enhance renal excretion of sodium and water

by reducing the circulating blood volume, decreasing preload, and reducing systemic and pulmonary congestion.

The type and dosage of diuretic prescribed depend on the degree of heart failure and renal function. The high-ceiling (loop) diuretics, such as furosemide (Lasix, Furoside♦), torsemide (Demadex), and ethacrynic acid (Edecrin), are most effective for treating fluid volume overload. However, the practitioner may initially use a thiazide diuretic, such as hydrochlorothiazide (Hydro-DIURIL, Urozide♦) and metolazone (Zaroxolyn), for elderly clients with mild volume overload. The action of thiazide diuretics is self-limiting (i.e., diuresis decreases after edema fluid is lost), so the excessive diuresis and dehydration that may occur with loop diuretics are uncommon. Clients often prefer thiazide diuretics because of the gradual onset of diuresis. However, for many clients in heart failure, loop diuretics are needed to ensure effective diuresis.

The nurse also needs to monitor for and prevent potassium deficiency (hypokalemia) from diuretic therapy. The signs of hypokalemia are nonspecific neurologic and muscular complaints, such as generalized weakness, depressed reflexes, and irregular heart rate. Therefore, to accurately identify hypokalemia, the physician, nurse, and dietitian monitor serum potassium levels.

If the client's serum potassium level is less than 4.0 mEq/L, the health care provider has several alternatives:

- Adding a potassium-sparing diuretic to the regimen
- Requesting that clients increase their dietary intake of potassium-rich foods
- Prescribing a potassium supplement

Clients being treated simultaneously with ACE inhibitors and diuretics may not experience hypokalemia. If their kidneys are not functioning well, they may develop hyperkalemia, an elevated serum potassium level. The nurse should review the client's serum creatinine level; if the creatinine is greater than 1.8, the nurse should notify the health care provider before administering supplemental potassium.

ELDERLY CONSIDERATIONS

Elderly clients receiving loop diuretics are very prone to dehydration, especially those with type 2 diabetes mellitus. The nurse must check orthostatic blood pressures in the elderly client receiving loop diuretics to detect volume depletion. The nurse also examines the client for flat neck veins when the client is supine, a loss of skin turgor, and a slow progressive weight loss despite an adequate diet. All of these signs, plus disorientation in the very old client, may indicate excessive diuresis and volume depletion (Chart 37–4).

Venous Vasodilators. The health care provider may prescribe venous vasodilators. (e.g., nitrates) for the client in heart failure with persistent dyspnea. To compensate for the client's reduced cardiac output, significant constriction of venous and arterial blood vessels occurs, reducing the volume of fluid that the vascular bed can hold and increasing the preload. Venous vasodilators may benefit clients by

- Returning the venous vasculature to a more normal capacity
- Decreasing the volume of blood returning to the heart
- Improving left ventricular function

Some of the most common vasodilators are summarized in Chart 37–3.

Nitrates may be administered intravenously, orally, or topically. These drugs cause primarily venous vasodilation but also a significant amount of arteriolar vasodilation. It is essential for the nurse to monitor the client's blood pressure when initiating nitrate therapy or increasing the dosage. Clients may initially report headache. The nurse should assure clients that they will develop a toler-

ance to this effect and that the headache will cease or diminish.

Unfortunately, when nitrates are uniformly administered during 24 hours, clients may develop tolerance to the vasodilating effects. To prevent such tolerance, the health care provider may order at least one 12-hour nitrate-free period out of every 24 hours, usually overnight. However, clients whose major complaint is nocturnal dyspnea may experience relief when nitroglycerine ointment is applied at bedtime and removed during the day.

Digitalis. Digoxin (Lanoxin), a cardiac glycoside, has been demonstrated to provide benefits for clients in heart failure with sinus rhythm and atrial fibrillation. "Dig" therapy reduces exacerbations of heart failure and hospitalizations, resulting in an estimated savings of $406 million annually. When added to a regimen of ACE inhibitors and diuretics, digoxin increases functional capacity and improves hemodynamic parameters in clients with NYHA class III and IV heart failure due to left systolic dysfunction (Redfield, 1996).

The potential benefits of digitalis derivatives include an increase in contractility, reduction in heart rate, slowing of conduction through the atrioventricular node, and inhibition of sympathetic activity while enhancing parasympathetic activity. Digitalis also may have a mild diuretic effect. At toxic digitalis levels, increased automaticity occurs, and ectopic beats (premature ventricular contractions [PVCs]) may result.

The most commonly prescribed cardiac glycoside is digoxin (Lanoxin, Novodigoxin✦). Digoxin is erratically absorbed from the gastrointestinal tract. Many medications, especially antacids, interfere with its absorption. It is eliminated primarily by renal excretion.

ELDERLY CONSIDERATIONS

The half-life of digoxin in middle-aged adults is 36 hours; in older adults, who typically have diminished renal function, the half-life may be 48 hours. Thus, elderly clients are particularly susceptible to digoxin toxicity. Toxicity occurs in 10% to 20% of all clients taking digoxin, more commonly in older clients and clients with hypokalemia. Toxicity in older, hypokalemic clients may be fatal.

Digitalis Toxicity. The presentation of digitalis toxicity may be vague and nonspecific. Toxicity may cause nearly any dysrhythmia, but PVCs are most commonly noted. The nurse or nursing staff member carefully monitors the apical pulse rate and heart rhythm of clients receiving digoxin. The nurse must identify and report to the health care provider when the resting heart rate is less than 60 beats per minute or greater than 100 beats per minute and when there is a significant change in rhythm or rate. It is equally important to report the development of an irregular rhythm in a client with a previously regular rhythm and a regular rhythm in a client with a previously irregular one. The nurse also monitors serum digoxin and potassium levels to identify toxicity. Chart 37–3 presents information about selected cardiac glycosides.

Any medication that increases the workload of the fail-

Chart 37–4

Nursing Focus on the Elderly: Heart Failure

- Assess older clients with confusion for indications of heart failure. People older than 80 years often present with restlessness or confusion as the initial manifestation of heart failure.
- Auscultate the lungs carefully, recognizing that dependent crackles may not be an indication of heart failure in the older adult.
- Do not expect crackles to clear rapidly after treatment. Crackles may persist in the lung bases of older adults for an extended period after pulmonary congestion has decreased.
- Be especially alert for the signs of digitalis toxicity in the elderly client because it occurs frequently.
- If loop diuretics are used for diuresis, monitor the client closely for signs of excessive diuresis, dehydration, and hypokalemia.
- In older clients receiving drug therapy for heart failure, monitor for orthostatic hypotension. Cardiovascular changes associated with aging make this likely to develop.

ing heart also increases its oxygen requirement. The nurse should be alert for the possibility that the client may experience angina (chest pain) in response to digoxin. Intravenous medications that increase contractility are described in Chapter 40.

➤ Activity Intolerance

Planning: Expected Outcomes. The client is expected to perform activities of daily living and walk at least two blocks without dyspnea or excessive fatigue.

Interventions. Initially, the client in severe heart failure requires physical and emotional rest. On the first day of hospitalization, clients may sit up in a chair for meals and do basic leg exercises while up. Nursing care should be organized to allow periods of rest. The interdisciplinary team observes and documents the client's physiologic response to activity.

As the client's condition improves, the nurse or physical therapist (PT) initiates ambulation, usually on hospital day 2. The nurse checks the client's blood pressure, pulse, and oxygen saturation before and after the activity. A blood pressure change of more than 20 mmHg or a pulse increase of more than 20 beats per minute may indicate that the activity is too stressful. Other indications that the client cannot tolerate the activity include dyspnea, fatigue, and chest pain. If a client displays any of these symptoms, he or she is asked to rate how hard he or she has been working on a scale of 1 to 20, with 20 being maximum perceived exertion. If the client rates the exertion higher then 12, the nurse counsels the client to slow down. If the client tolerates the activity, the nurse or PT steadily increases the client's activity level until the client is ambulating 200 to 400 feet several times a day.

If the client is able, the nurse or assistive nursing personnel might time the client for 6 minutes while walking at a comfortable pace. The distance the client can walk can be used to determine the client's functional level and activity plan.

➤ Potential for Pulmonary Edema

Planning: Expected Outcomes. The client is expected to be free of pulmonary edema.

Interventions. The nurse monitors clients for acute pulmonary edema, a life-threatening event that can result from severe heart failure. In pulmonary edema, the left ventricle fails to eject sufficient blood, and pressure increases in the lungs because of the accumulated blood. The increased pressure causes fluid to leak across the pulmonary capillaries and into the pulmonary interstitium.

The nurse assesses for early signs and symptoms of pulmonary edema, such as crackles in the lung bases, disorientation, and confusion, especially in the elderly client. Documentation of the precise location of the crackles is crucial, as the level of the fluid ascends as the pulmonary edema worsens. The client in pulmonary edema is also extremely anxious, tachycardiac, and struggling for air. He or she may have a moist cough productive of frothy, blood-tinged sputum, and the client's skin may be cold, clammy, or cyanotic.

The client diagnosed with pulmonary edema is admitted to the acute care hospital. The physician prescribes rapid-acting diuretics, such as furosemide (Lasix, Furoside✦). Furosemide is given intravenously over 1 to 2 minutes, usually at a starting dose of 40 mg and another 40 mg repeated if needed in 30 minutes (Booker & Ignatavicius, 1996).

Oxygen is always ordered, and the client is placed in a high-Fowler's position. IV morphine sulfate may be prescribed, 1 to 2 mg at a time, to reduce venous return (preload), but the nurse should monitor respiratory rate and blood pressure closely. Vasodilators, such as nitroglycerin (Tridil) and sodium nitroprusside (Nitropress), may be administered via continuous infusion pumps. Low dosages of these drugs must be given initially and increased slowly to avoid severe hypotension.

Once commonly used to decrease preload, rotating tourniquets and phlebotomy are now used rarely during the wait for these medications to be effective.

The nurse or assistive personnel inserts a Foley catheter, if ordered, to assess the client's urinary output after diuretic administration and to minimize exertion related to voiding. Diuresis normally begins within 5 minutes of the administration of IV furosemide and peaks at 30 minutes. Chart 37–5 summarizes the care of the client with acute pulmonary edema.

Clients often respond dramatically and quickly to these interventions, but their condition can also deteriorate rapidly because of pulmonary congestion and severe hypoxemia. Clients occasionally require Bipap or intubation and ventilation to survive the acute episode. A skilled nurse is needed to assist with intubation. (Management of the client who is critically ill with heart failure is detailed in Chapter 40.)

Chart 37–5

Nursing Care Highlight: Care of the Client with Pulmonary Edema

- Identify the client's chief complaint.
- If the client's blood pressure is adequate, place the client in a high-Fowler's position.
- Auscultate the client's lungs briefly (posterior assessment).
- Ensure that vascular access is present and check for patency.
- Provide oxygen as ordered.
- Provide IV diuretic (usually furosemide) as prescribed.
- Anticipate urinary output in 5–15 min after diuretic administration; catheterize if ordered.
- Monitor blood pressure, respiratory rate, pulse oximetry, pulse, and cardiac rhythm, and the client's subjective feelings of ability to breathe.
- Provide additional medications as prescribed (usually morphine sulfate or nitroglycerin).
- Provide comfort measures and reassurance.
- Notify the physician if the client does not have a rapid improvement and diuresis.

> ➤ Continuing Care

➤ *Case Management*

Clients who have not been adequately prepared for discharge or who do not have good community support and follow-up are at high risk for recurrent hospital admissions for heart failure (Dracup et al., 1995). In a case management system, the case manager or care coordinator assesses the client's needs for health care resources and facilitates appropriate placement. It is imperative that the case manager assess the available social supports because inability to obtain help in such activities as food shopping and obtaining medications is a major contributor to hospital readmission (Dracup et al., 1995). If home support is available, the client may be discharged home in the care of a family member or other caregiver. Home care nurses may direct the care, while aides may provide assistance with ADLs.

If the client has multiple health problems or has been severely compromised by heart disease, he or she may require admission to a subacute unit or traditional nursing home for either transitional or long-term care. Home care services cost about $125 per nursing visit compared with $150 to $300 per day in a traditional nursing home and up to $1,000 per day for hospital care.

➤ *Health Teaching*

Activity Schedule. Medicare usually provides reimbursement for client assessment and teaching so that a home care care nurse can continue teaching and assessment when the client returns home. The nurse encourages clients with heart failure to stay as active as possible and to develop a regular exercise regimen. Clients who are more active appear to have better outcomes (Dracup et al., 1995). The goal for clients with heart failure is development of a regular exercise routine, probably a home walking program, several times a week. Medicare and third-party payers do not reimburse for cardiac rehabilitation for heart failure clients, and paying for a cardiac rehabilitation program out of pocket would cost a client approximately $1,620 (Newkirk & Leeper, 1996).

Although most clients with heart failure appear to benefit from exercise programs, clients with persistent crackles and uncontrolled edema despite medical therapy are not encouraged to exercise until their heart failure is stabilized (Sullivan, 1994). When exercise is indicated, the nurse teaches the client to begin walking 200 to 400 ft/day. At home, the client should slowly increase the amount of time walked (perhaps 2 minutes a week) over several months, trying to walk at least three times a week. If the client experiences chest pain or pronounced dyspnea while exercising or fatigue the next day, he or she is probably advancing the activity too quickly and should slow down. The nurse encourages the client to keep an exercise diary that documents the time and duration of each exercise session as well as the client's heart rate and any symptoms occurring with exercise.

Twenty percent of clients who are readmitted to hospitals for treatment of heart failure fail to seek medical attention promptly when symptoms reoccur (Dracup et al., 1995). The nurse instructs the client and caregiver to immediately report the occurrence of any of the following symptoms of worsening heart failure to his or her health care provider:
- Rapid weight gain (3 pounds in a week)
- Decrease in exercise tolerance lasting 2 to 3 days
- Cold symptoms (cough) lasting more than 3 to 5 days
- Excessive awakening at night to urinate
- Development of dyspnea or angina at rest

Drug Therapy. The nurse or pharmacist provides oral and written instructions about the medication regimen. If the client is taking digoxin, the caregiver and the client are taught how to count a pulse rate. The nurse assesses the client's ability to accurately take and record his or her pulse rate. Chart 37–6 lists instructions for the client taking digoxin at home.

The nurse advises clients taking diuretics to take them in the morning to avoid waking during the night for voiding. After determining if the client has a weight scale and can use it, the nurse instructs the client to take his or her weight each morning. Daily weights indicate whether the client is losing or retaining fluid. Some motivated clients are taught to use a sliding scale to adjust their daily diuretic dose depending on their daily weight, similar to the way a diabetic adjusts an insulin dose based on the capillary glucose level. The home care nurse may reliably assess a client's volume status by checking the pattern of daily weights and noting jugular venous distention and hepatojugular reflux (see Chap. 35).

Clients receiving angiotensin-converting enzyme (ACE) inhibitors should be taught to move slowly when changing positions, especially from a lying to a sitting position. Dizziness, lightheadedness, and cough need to be reported to the health care provider.

Clients taking diuretics and ACE inhibitors require

Chart 37–6

Education Guide: Digoxin Therapy

- Noon is the best time of day to take this medication if you can remember to take it then.
- Continue administration of this medication unless you are told to stop it by your health care provider.
- Do not take digoxin at the same time as antacids or cathartics (laxatives).
- Take your pulse rate before taking each dose of digoxin. Notify your health care provider of a change in pulse rate (60–100 beats per minute is normal) or rhythm as well as increasing fatigue, muscle weakness, confusion, or loss of appetite (signs of digitalis toxicity).
- If you forget to take a dose, it may be delayed a few hours. However, if you do not remember it until the next day, you should take only your usual daily dose.
- Report for scheduled laboratory test (such as potassium and digoxin levels).
- If potassium supplements are prescribed, continue the dose until told to stop by your health care provider.

their serum potassium level and renal function to be monitored at least every few months. Diuretics, especially loop diuretics like furosemide, deplete potassium and often cause hypokalemia. Conversely, ACE inhibitors may result in potassium retention. If potassium levels drop below 4.0 mEq/L, the primary care physician may prescribe potassium supplementation or a potassium-sparing diuretic. A dietician may be consulted to provide the client with information about potassium-rich foods to include in the diet.

Diet Therapy. Clients with chronic heart failure are advised to restrict their dietary sodium. The dietitian provides written instructions on low- or restricted-sodium diets. For mild or moderate failure, a 3-g sodium diet is recommended. Clients usually find this diet palatable and fairly easy to follow. They are asked to avoid salty foods and table salt. For clients with severe heart failure, a 2-g sodium diet may be attempted. These clients are told not to add salt during or after meal preparation, to avoid milk and milk products, and to use few canned or prepared foods. The home care nurse or dietitian should assess the client for compliance with this diet because it is unpalatable and for many clients the cost of low-sodium foods can be a financial burden.

Clients are also instructed to confer with their health care provider if they want to use commercial salt substitutes. Most salt substitutes contain potassium, and the client's renal status and serum potassium level need to be considered before one can recommend these products. To enhance the flavor of low-salt foods, clients may use lemon, garlic, and herbs.

Advance Directives. Approximately 50% of deaths from heart failure are sudden, many without any warning or worsening of symptoms (Dracup et al., 1995). Because the majority of these deaths occur at home, it is important for the primary care provider or home care nurse to discuss advance directives with the client and family. The family should be prepared to act in accordance with the client's wishes in the event of cardiac arrest. If the client desires resuscitation to be attempted, the family should know how to activate the EMS system and how to provide CPR until an ambulance arrives. If the client does not wish to have CPR, the client, family, and nurse should plan how the family will respond.

➤ Home Care Management

The focus of the home care nurse's interventions is assessment and health teaching, which are reimbursable by Medicare and other third-party payers. Chart 37–7 lists major areas of assessment that the home care nurse performs.

Clients with chronic heart failure must make many adjustments in their lifestyles (Research Applications for Nursing). They must adhere to a medical regimen that includes dietary restrictions, activity prescriptions, and drug therapy. Clients need careful, concise explanations of the treatment plan. The continuing care nurse in any setting encourages the client to verbalize fears and concerns about his or her illness and assists the client

---

Chart 37–7

Focused Assessment for Home Care Clients with Heart Failure

- Assess for signs of heart failure, including
  - Changes in vital signs (heart rate >100 bpm at rest, new atrial fibrillation, BP <90 or >150 systolic)
  - Indications of poor tissue perfusion
    Fatigue
    Angina
    Activity intolerance
    Changes in mental status
    Pallor or cyanosis
  - Indications of congestion
    Presence of cough or dyspnea
    Weight gain
    Jugular venous distention and peripheral edema
- Assess functional ability, including
  - Performance of activities of daily living
  - Mobility and ambulation (review frequency and duration of walking, development of symptoms, and pulse rate)
  - Cognitive ability
- Assess nutritional status, including
  - Food and fluid intake
  - Intake of sodium-rich foods
  - Alcohol consumption
  - Skin turgor
- Assess home environment, including
  - Safety hazards, especially related to oxygen therapy
  - Structural barriers affecting functional ability
- Assess client's compliance and understanding of illness and its treatment, including
  - Signs and symptoms to report to health care provider
  - Dosages, effects, and side or toxic effects of medications
  - When to report for lab and health care provider visits
  - Ability to accurately weigh self on scale
  - Presence of advanced directive
  - Use of home oxygen, if appropriate
- Assess client and caregiver coping skills

---

in exploring appropriate coping skills. Clients' participation in treatment can help alleviate and control symptoms.

➤ Health Care Resources

A home care nurse may be needed to assess the client's adherence to medication and diet therapy and to monitor for worsening heart failure. Clients with activity limitations benefit from the services of a home care aide. A dietitian might be consulted to assist with menu planning and teaching. Although clients have been demonstrated to benefit from participation in structured cardiac rehabilitation programs, referral to such programs is not widespread because coverage is usually not provided by third-party payers.

In addition to home care support, other resources are available for client education and family support. The American Heart Association is an excellent community

- Have a normal rate, rhythm, and depth of respiration
- Have an O_2 saturation greater than 92%
- Resume and maintain an adequate cardiac output
- Perform activities of daily living without dyspnea or excessive fatigue
- Be free of pulmonary edema

VALVULAR HEART DISEASE

Valvular heart disease occurs when the heart valves cannot open fully (valvular stenosis) or close completely (valvular insufficiency or regurgitation). Acquired valvular dysfunctions most often involve the left side of the heart, especially the mitral valve. Acquired valvular dysfunctions, in rank order of occurrence, are mitral stenosis, mitral regurgitation, mitral valve prolapse, aortic stenosis, and aortic regurgitation.

The tricuspid valve is involved infrequently, and the pulmonic valve is affected rarely. Often, stenosis and regurgitation occur simultaneously in a defect called a mixed lesion.

Mitral Stenosis

Mitral stenosis usually results from rheumatic carditis, which can cause valve thickening by fibrosis and calcification. The valve leaflets fuse and become stiff, while the chordae tendineae contract and shorten. The valvular orifice narrows, preventing normal blood flow from the left atrium to the left ventricle. As a result of these changes, the left atrial pressure rises, the left atrium dilates, pulmonary artery pressures increase, and the right ventricle hypertrophies.

Initially, pulmonary congestion and right-sided heart failure occur. Later, when the left ventricle receives insufficient blood volume, the preload is decreased, and the cardiac output falls.

Clients with mild mitral stenosis are usually asymptomatic. As the valvular orifice narrows, and pressure in the lungs increases, the client experiences dyspnea on exertion, orthopnea, paroxysmal nocturnal dyspnea (sudden dyspnea at night), and dry cough. As the pulmonary hypertension and congestion progress, hemoptysis and pulmonary edema appear. Right-sided heart failure can cause hepatomegaly, neck vein distention, and pitting edema late in the disorder.

The pulse may be normal on palpation, tachycardiac, or irregularly irregular, as in atrial fibrillation. Because the development of atrial fibrillation indicates that the client may decompensate, the physician should be notified immediately. On auscultation, the nurse notes a rumbling, apical diastolic murmur.

Rheumatic fever is the most common cause of mitral stenosis. Nonrheumatic causes include atrial myxoma (tumor), calcium accumulation, and thrombus formation.

WOMEN'S HEALTH CONSIDERATIONS

 Two-thirds to three-fourths of all clients with mitral stenosis are women. About two-thirds of the women with rheumatic mitral stenosis are younger than 45 years.

Martensson, J., Karlsson, J. E., & Fridlund, B. (1997). *Male patients with congestive heart failure and their conception of the life situation.* Journal of Advanced Nursing, 25, 579–586.

Research Applications for Nursing

This qualitative study examined the experiences of 12 male Swedish clients with heart failure during the first 2 months to 2 years following diagnosis. Clients ranged from NYHA classification II (5) to IV (2), and most were married.

Six categories emerged that described how clients with heart failure perceived of their situation. Six men described feeling a belief in the future. These more hopeful men were more engaged in daily activities, possibly ignoring certain aspects of their illness. Eight men mentioned gaining awareness of their bodies' signals, changing their lifestyles, and adapting to heart failure. All of the men indicated that support from their environment affected their ability to function. Unfortunately, all of them expressed negative feelings about their relationship with their family and friends. Ten men identified feeling physically restricted by heart failure. Seven men identified a lack of physical and emotional energy or no energy at all. Finally, four men described being resigned, accepting that nothing could be done for them and passively awaiting death.

Critique. This is a qualitative study done on a small sample of 12 Swedish men; the size might limit its generalizability to others with heart failure. Because a saturation of the concepts was reached before data collection was completed, the results may be more trustworthy. In addition, a comparative study with women is currently in progress.

The study is a phenomenographic study that attempts to describe how people conceive of something. These conceptions are thought to be the basis on which opinions rest. It is different from a phenomenologic study, which attempts to explore what the person is experiencing.

Possible Nursing Implications. Additional studies to validate these six categories and relate them to other variables (such as NYHA classification or duration of heart failure) could assist nurses to further understand heart failure. Nursing interventions that focus on helping clients feel more positive are needed to prevent the negative feelings that these male subjects experienced.

resource for pamphlets, books, cookbooks, and videotapes related to heart failure and heart disease. The organization also provides referrals to various local support groups for clients and their caregivers in the community.

For equipment needs, such as home oxygen therapy or a hospital bed, medical supply companies provide set-up and maintenance services. A detailed description of home oxygen therapy is found in Chapter 30.

Evaluation

On the basis of the identified nursing diagnoses and collaborative problems, the nurse evaluates the care of the client with heart failure. Outcomes include that the client will

Mitral Regurgitation (Insufficiency)

The fibrotic and calcific changes occurring in mitral regurgitation prevent the mitral valve from closing completely during *systole*. Incomplete closure of the valve allows backflow of blood into the left atrium when the left ventricle contracts. During *diastole*, regurgitant output is returned with the normal blood flow from the left atrium to the left ventricle, increasing the volume that must be ejected during the next systole. To compensate for the increased volume and pressure, the left atrium and ventricle dilate and hypertrophy.

Mitral insufficiency usually progresses slowly; clients may remain symptom free for decades. Symptoms begin to occur when the left ventricle fails in response to increased blood volumes. The client most often reports fatigue and chronic weakness as a result of reduced cardiac output. Dyspnea on exertion and orthopnea develop later. A significant number of clients complain of anxiety, atypical chest pains, and palpitations.

Nursing assessment may reveal normal blood pressure, atrial fibrillation (an irregularly irregular rhythm occurring in 75% of clients), or changes in respirations characteristic of left ventricular failure.

When right-sided heart failure develops, the neck veins become distended, the liver enlarges (hepatomegaly), and pitting edema is noted. On auscultation, the nurse hears a high-pitched systolic murmur at the apex, with radiation to the left axilla. Severe regurgitation often exhibits a third heart sound.

Rheumatic heart disease is the predominant cause of mitral insufficiency. When mitral insufficiency results from rheumatic heart disease, it usually co-exists with some degree of mitral stenosis. Nonrheumatic causes include papillary muscle dysfunction or rupture due to ischemic heart disease, infective endocarditis, and a congenital anomaly.

Mitral regurgitation resulting from rheumatic heart disease is more common in women than in men. Mitral regurgitation of a nonrheumatic etiology occurs more often in men.

Mitral Valve Prolapse

Mitral valve prolapse occurs because the valvular leaflets enlarge and prolapse into the left atrium during systole. Usually this is a benign abnormality, but it may progress to pronounced mitral regurgitation.

Most clients with mitral valve prolapse are asymptomatic. However, clients may report chest pain, palpitations, or exercise intolerance. Chest pain is usually atypical, with clients describing a sharp pain localized to the left side of the chest. Dizziness, syncope, and palpitations may be associated with atrial or ventricular dysrhythmias.

On physical examination, the nurse usually finds a normal heart rate and blood pressure. A midsystolic click and a late systolic murmur may be audible at the apex.

The etiology of mitral valve prolapse is variable; it has been associated with such conditions as Marfan's syndrome and other cardiac defects. However, most of the time no other cardiac abnormality is found. A familial occurrence is well established.

Mitral valve prolapse affects 5% to 10% of people. Although it is present in all age groups, it is most common in women between the ages of 20 and 54 years.

Aortic Stenosis

In people with aortic stenosis, the aortic valve orifice narrows, obstructing left ventricular outflow during systole. This increased resistance to ejection or afterload results in ventricular hypertrophy. As the stenosis progresses, the cardiac output becomes fixed, unable to increase to meet the demands of the body during exertion, and symptoms develop. Eventually the left ventricle fails, volume backs up in the left atrium, and the pulmonary system becomes congested. Late in the disease process, right-sided heart failure can occur.

The classic symptoms of aortic stenosis result from the fixed cardiac output. They are dyspnea, angina, and syncope occurring on exertion. When cardiac output falls in the late stages of the disease, the client has marked fatigue, debilitation, and peripheral cyanosis. A narrow pulse pressure is noted when the blood pressure is examined. A diamond-shaped systolic crescendo-decrescendo murmur is usually noted on auscultation.

Congenital valvular disease or malformation is the predominant etiologic factor in aortic stenosis. Bicuspid or unicuspid aortic valves are the primary reason for aortic stenosis in clients younger than 30 years and account for about 50% of the disease in clients 30 to 70 years. Rheumatic aortic stenosis is always concomitant with rheumatic disease of the mitral valve. It develops in clients between the ages of 30 and 70. Atherosclerosis and degenerative calcification of the aortic valve are the predominant factors in people older than age 70. Aortic stenosis has become the most common valvular disorder in countries with aging populations. Of clients with aortic stenosis, 80% are men.

Aortic Regurgitation (Insufficiency)

In clients with aortic regurgitation, the aortic valve leaflets do not close properly during diastole, and the annulus (the valve ring that attaches to the leaflets) may be dilated, loose, or deformed. This allows regurgitation of blood from the aorta back into the left ventricle during diastole. The left ventricle, in compensation, dilates to accommodate the greater blood volume and eventually hypertrophies.

Clients with aortic regurgitation remain asymptomatic for many years because of the compensatory mechanisms of the left ventricle. As the disease progresses and left ventricular failure occurs, the principal concerns of the client are exertional dyspnea, orthopnea, and paroxysmal nocturnal dyspnea. The client with severe disease may note palpitations, especially while lying on the left side. Many clients with aortic regurgitation experience nocturnal angina with diaphoresis.

On palpation, the nurse notes a "bounding" arterial pulse. The pulse pressure is usually widened, with an elevated systolic pressure and diminished diastolic pressure. The classic auscultatory finding is a high-pitched, blowing, decrescendo diastolic murmur.

Aortic insufficiency is usual in nonrheumatic conditions such as infective endocarditis, congenital anatomic aortic valvular abnormalities, hypertension, and Marfan's syndrome (a rare, generalized, systemic disease of connective tissue). Approximately 75% of clients with aortic regurgitation are men.

Collaborative Management

 Assessment

A client with valvular disease may suddenly become ill or may slowly develop symptoms over the course of many years. The nurse collects information on the client's family health history, including valvular or other forms of heart disease to which the client may be genetically predisposed. The nurse questions the client about attacks of rheumatic fever, the specific dates when these occurred, and the use of antibiotic prophylaxis against recurrence of rheumatic fever. The client's fatigue level, the level of activity that is tolerated, the presence of angina or dyspnea, and the occurrence of palpitations, if present, are also discussed.

As part of physical assessment, the nurse obtains the client's vital signs, inspects the client for signs of edema, palpates and auscultates the client's heart and lungs, and palpates the client's peripheral pulses. Findings consistent with valvular malformation are summarized in Chart 37–8.

In clients with mitral stenosis, the chest x-ray shows left atrial enlargement, prominent pulmonary arteries, and an enlarged right ventricle. In those with mitral regurgitation, the chest x-ray reveals an increased cardiac shadow, indicating left ventricular and left atrial enlargement.

In the later stages of aortic stenosis, the chest x-ray may show left ventricular enlargement and pulmonary congestion. In clients with aortic *insufficiency,* left atrial and left ventricular dilation appear on the chest x-ray. If heart failure is present, pulmonary venous congestion is also evident.

For clients with valvular heart disease, echocardiography is usually indicated because it is an excellent noninvasive tool for defining cardiac structure, movement of the valve leaflets, and size and function of the cardiac chambers. Exercise tolerance testing (ETT) is sometimes performed to evaluate symptomatic response, to assess functional capacity, and to enhance auscultatory findings. In clients with either mitral or aortic stenosis, cardiac catheterization is frequently indicated to assess the severity of the stenosis and its other effects on the heart.

The health care provider also orders an electrocardiogram (ECG) to assess abnormalities such as left ventricular hypertrophy, as seen with mitral regurgitation and aortic regurgitation, or right ventricular hypertrophy, as seen in severe mitral stenosis. Atrial fibrillation is a common finding in both mitral stenosis and mitral regurgitation.

 Interventions

Management of valvular heart disease depends on which valve is affected and the degree of valve impairment. Some clients can be managed with yearly monitoring and medications, but other clients require invasive procedures or heart surgery.

> ► *Nonsurgical Management*

Nonsurgical management focuses on drug therapy and rest. During the course of valvular disease, clients may

---

Chart 37–8

Key Features of Valvular Heart Disease

Mitral Stenosis	Mitral Insufficiency	Mitral Valve Prolapse	Aortic Stenosis	Aortic Insufficiency
• Fatigue • Dyspnea on exertion • Orthopnea • Paroxysmal nocturnal dyspnea • Hemoptysis • Hepatomegaly • Neck vein distention • Pitting edema • Atrial fibrillation • Rumbling, apical diastolic murmur	• Fatigue • Dyspnea on exertion • Orthopnea • Palpitations • Atrial fibrillation • Neck vein distention • Pitting edema • High-pitched holosystolic murmur	• Atypical chest pain • Dizziness, syncope • Palpitations • Atrial tachycardia • Ventricular tachycardia • Systolic click	• Dyspnea on exertion • Angina • Syncope on exertion • Fatigue • Orthopnea • Paroxysmal nocturnal dyspnea • Harsh, systolic crescendo-decrescendo murmur	• Palpitations • Dyspnea • Orthopnea • Paroxysmal nocturnal dyspnea • Fatigue • Angina • Sinus tachycardia • Blowing, decrescendo diastolic murmur

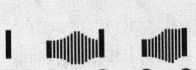

S_1 S_2 S_1 S_2 S_1

S_1 S_2S_3 S_1 S_2S_3	click click 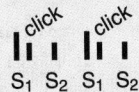 S_1 S_2 S_1 S_2	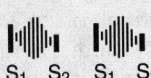 S_1 S_2 S_1 S_2	S_1 S_2 S_1 S_2 S_1

develop left ventricular failure with pulmonary or systemic congestion. Diuretics, digoxin, and oxygen are often administered to improve the symptoms of heart failure (see earlier). Nitrates are administered cautiously to clients with aortic stenosis because of the potential for syncope associated with a reduction in left ventricular volume (preload). Vasodilators such as nifedipine (Adalat, Procardia) may be used to reduce the regurgitant flow for clients with aortic or mitral stenosis.

Prophylactic antibiotic therapy is required for all clients with valve disease before any invasive procedure. Procedures for which clients require antibiotic coverage include bronchoscopy, endoscopy, sigmoidoscopy, colonoscopy, genitourinary instrumentations, surgery, and dental procedures of any type.

A major concern in valvular heart disease is maintaining cardiac output should atrial fibrillation develop. Atrial fibrillation occurs frequently in both mitral stenosis and mitral regurgitation because of distention of the atria. With mitral valvular disease, left ventricular filling is especially dependent on atrial contraction. When atrial fibrillation develops, there is no longer a single, coordinated atrial contraction. Cardiac output can decrease by 25% to 30%, and heart failure may occur. Ineffective atrial contraction may also lead to stasis of blood and thrombosis in the left atrium. The nurse monitors the client for the development of an irregularly irregular rhythm and notifies the primary care provider should it develop.

The primary care provider will usually institute therapy to restore normal sinus rhythm or, if that is unsuccessful, to slow the ventricular rate. The physician might elect to convert a client from atrial fibrillation to sinus rhythm using intravenous diltiazem (Cardiazem). The client should be on a unit where nurses are able to monitor the client's cardiac rhythm and blood pressure closely. If atrial fibrillation is rapid and the client is unresponsive to medical treatment, synchronized countershock (cardioversion) may be attempted (see Chap. 36).

Whether the client is converted to sinus rhythm or remains in an atrial fibrillation, digoxin is often prescribed to slow the ventricular rate and increase the force of contraction. If atrial fibrillation does not resolve, quinidine gluconate (Quinaglute, Quinate♣) or procainamide hydrochloride (Pronestyl hydrochloride, Procanbid) may be added to the regimen. A beta-blocking agent, such as propranolol hydrochloride (Inderal, Apo-Propranolol♣), or a calcium channel blocker, such as verapamil hydrochloride (Calan), may also be considered.

When a client has valvular heart disease and chronic atrial fibrillation, anticoagulation with sodium warfarin (Coumadin, Warfilone♣) is usually a part of the medical treatment plan to prevent thrombus formation. Thrombi may form in the atria or on defective valve segments, resulting in systemic emboli. As a result, clients may experience one or more cerebrovascular accidents (CVAs). Therefore, the nurse assesses the client's baseline neurologic status and regularly reassesses the client for neurologic changes.

Rest is often an important part of treatment. Activity may be limited because the client's cardiac output cannot meet the increased metabolic demands, and angina or heart failure can result.

> ### Surgical Management

Surgical repair or replacement of heart valves has a major effect on the prognosis of valvular heart disease. Correct timing is crucial. Repair or replacement of the valve is usually performed after symptoms of left ventricular failure have developed but before irreversible dysfunction occurs. Surgical therapy is the only definitive treatment of aortic stenosis and is recommended when angina, syncope, or dyspnea on exertion develop.

Reparative Procedures. Reparative procedures are gaining in popularity because of continuing problems with thrombi, endocarditis, and left ventricular dysfunction after valvular replacement. Reparative procedures do not result in a normal valve, but they usually "turn back the clock," resulting in a more functional valve and an improvement in cardiac output. Turbulent blood flow through the valve may persist, and degeneration of the repaired valve is possible.

Balloon Valvuloplasty. Balloon valvuloplasty, an invasive nonsurgical procedure, is possible for stenotic mitral and aortic valves. Careful selection of clients is necessary. For people with noncalcified, mobile, mitral valves, valvuloplasty may be the initial treatment of choice. Many clients selected for aortic valvuloplasty are older and are at high risk for surgical complications or have refused operative treatment. However, young adults with noncalcified congenital aortic stenosis may also benefit.

When performing mitral valvuloplasty, the physician passes a balloon catheter from the femoral vein through the atrial septum and to the mitral valve. The balloon is inflated, enlarging the mitral orifice. For aortic valvuloplasty, the physician inserts the catheter through the femoral artery and advances it to the aortic valve, where it is inflated, enlarging the orifice. Valvuloplasty usually offers immediate relief of symptoms because the balloon has dilated the orifice and improved leaflet mobility. The results are comparable with those of surgical commissurotomy for appropriately selected clients.

After the procedure, the nurse observes the client closely for bleeding from the catheter insertion site and institutes precautions for arterial puncture if appropriate. Bleeding is likely after valvuloplasty because of the large size of the catheter. The nurse also observes the client for signs of a regurgitant valve by closely monitoring the client's heart sounds, cardiac output, and heart rhythm. Because vegetations (thrombi) may have been dislodged from the valve, the nurse observes for any indication of systemic emboli (see Infective Endocarditis later in this chapter).

Direct, or Open, Commissurotomy. Direct commissurotomy is accomplished with cardiopulmonary bypass during open heart surgery. The surgeon visualizes the valve, removes thrombi from the atria, incises the fused commissures (leaflets), and debrides calcium from the leaflets, widening the orifice.

Mitral Valve Reconstruction. Mitral valve reconstruction is the reparative procedure of choice for most clients with acquired mitral insufficiency. To make the annulus (the valve ring that attaches to and supports the leaflets)

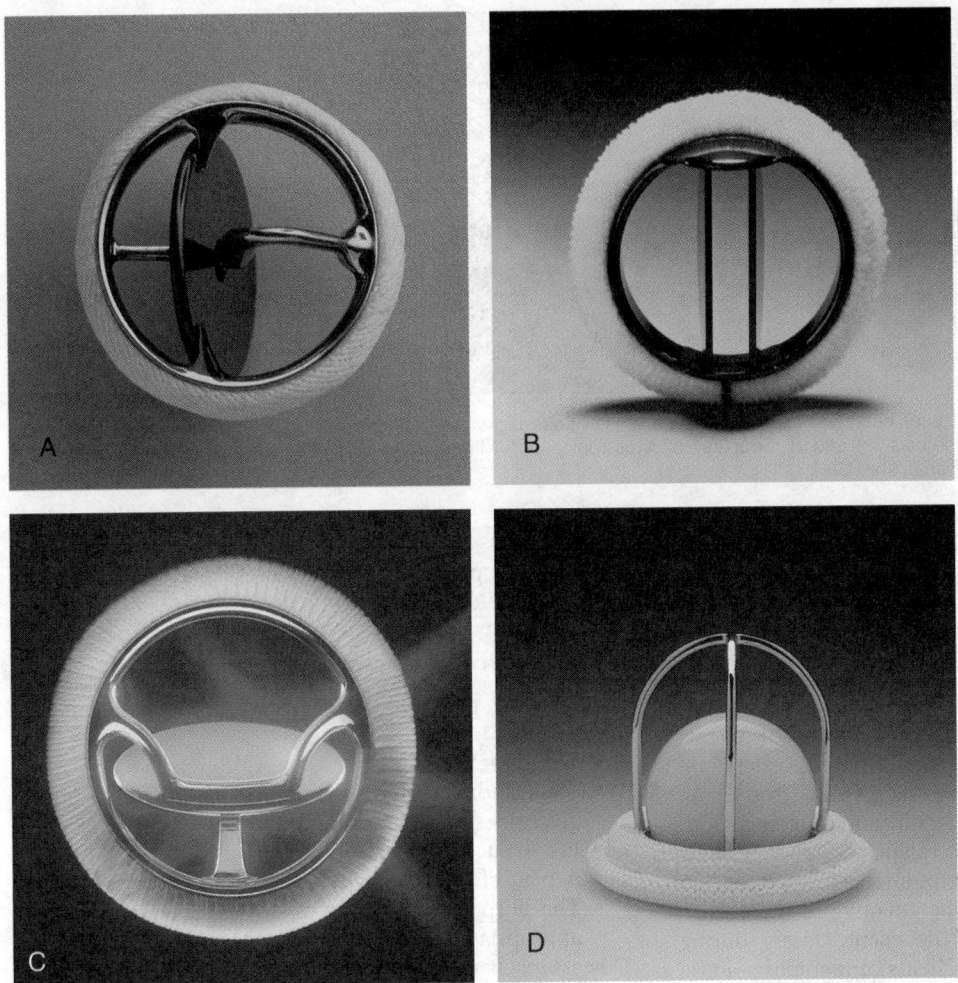

Figure 37–2. Examples of prosthetic (synthetic) heart valves. *A*, Medtronic Hall, a tilting-disk valve. *B*, St. Jude Medical mechanical heart valve. *C*, Monostrat mechanical heart valve. *D*, Starr-Edwards Silastic ball valve. (*A*, Courtesy of Medtronic, Inc., Minneapolis, MN; *B*, Courtesy of St. Jude Medical, Inc. All rights reserved. St. Jude Medical is a registered trademark of St. Jude Medical, Inc.; *C*, Courtesy of Alliance Medical Products, Irvine, CA; *D*, Courtesy of Baxter Healthcare Corporation, Edwards CVS Division, Santa Ana, CA.)

smaller, the physician may suture the leaflets to an annuloplasty ring or take tucks in the client's annulus. Leaflet repair is frequently performed at the same time. Elongated leaflets may be shortened; shortened leaflets may be repaired by lengthening the chordae that bind them in place; and perforated leaflets may be patched with synthetic grafts.

Annuloplasty and leaflet repair result in an annulus of the appropriate size and leaflets that can close completely. Thus, regurgitation is eliminated or markedly reduced.

Replacement Procedures. The development of prosthetic (synthetic) and biological (tissue) valves has improved the surgical therapy and prognosis of valvular heart disease. Prosthetic valves come in a wide variety (Fig. 37–2). Although prosthetic valves are very durable, all clients must receive oral anticoagulation for the rest of their lives because of the possibility of clot formation.

Biological valves may be xenograft (valves from other species), such as a porcine valve (from a pig) (Fig. 37–3) or a bovine valve (from a cow). Because tissue valves are associated with little risk of clot formation, long-term anticoagulation is not indicated. However, xenografts are not as durable as prosthetic valves and usually must be replaced every 7 to 10 years. A xenograft's durability is related to the age of the recipient. Calcium in the blood,

present in larger quantities in younger patients, breaks down the valves. The older the patient, the longer the xenograft will last. Valves donated from human cadavers and pulmonary autographs (the client's own pulmonary valve relocated to the aortic position) are also being used for valve replacement, especially in younger clients.

The mitral valve should be replaced if the leaflets are calcified and immobile. The surgeon excises the valve during cardiopulmonary bypass surgery, and the new valve, either biological or prosthetic, is sutured into place.

An aortic valve is replaced for most symptomatic adults with aortic stenosis and aortic insufficiency. As with mitral valve replacement, the surgeon excises the aortic valve during cardiopulmonary bypass surgery and sutures the new valve into place.

Preoperative Care. Clients undergoing valve surgery have open heart surgery similar to the procedure for clients undergoing a coronary artery bypass graft (CABG) (see Chap. 40). Ideally, surgery is an elective, planned procedure. Therefore, the nurse can assist in preparing the client by instructing the client and family members or a significant other about the management of postoperative pain, incision care, and strategies to prevent respiratory complications (see Chaps. 20 and 22).

The nurse may also introduce the client and the family

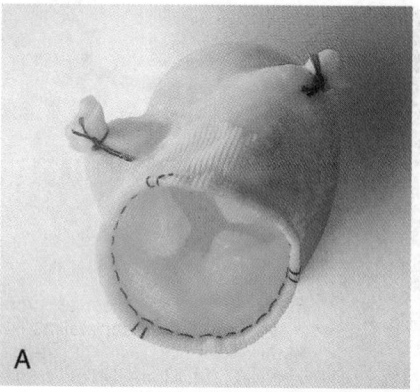 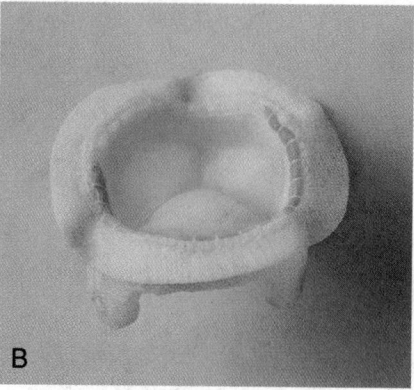 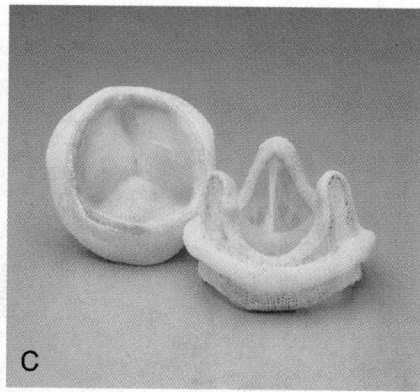

Figure 37–3. Examples of biologic (tissue) heart valves. *A,* Freestyle, a stentless pig valve with no frame. *B,* Hancock II, a stented pig valve. *C,* Carpentier-Edwards bioprosthesis. (*A* and *B,* Courtesy of Medtronic, Inc., Minneapolis, MN; *C,* Courtesy of Baxter Healthcare Corporation, Edwards CVS Division, Santa Ana, CA.)

or the significant other to the staff and the environment of the surgical critical care unit where the client will be transferred after surgery. Clients receiving oral anticoagulants stop taking these medications at least 72 hours before the procedure.

Postoperative Care. Nursing interventions for clients undergoing open heart surgery for valve disorders are similar to those for clients undergoing a CABG (see Chap. 40). However, there are a few significant differences depending in part on the type of valvular surgery. Clients with mitral stenosis often have pulmonary hypertension and stiff lungs. The nurse must be attentive to the client's respiratory status and monitor the client closely during weaning from the ventilator. Clients undergoing aortic valve replacements may be at a higher risk for postoperative hemorrhage, and the nurse is especially vigilant for indications of bleeding.

Clients with valve replacements are also more likely to have significant reductions in cardiac output postoperatively, especially those with aortic stenosis or left ventricular failure from mitral valve disease. The nurse is particularly attentive to monitoring the client's cardiac output and identifying any indications of pump failure. High filling pressures (pulmonary artery wedge pressure greater than 18 mmHg) may be required to maintain an acceptable cardiac output in the immediate postoperative period. The physician may prescribe digoxin (Lanoxin, Novodigoxin✚) for 3 to 6 months postoperatively to maintain cardiac output and to prevent atrial fibrillation. Clients who have had valve replacements with prosthetic valves require lifetime prophylactic anticoagulation therapy to prevent thrombus formation.

➤ Continuing Care

The client with valvular heart disease may be discharged home on medical therapy or postoperatively after valve repair or replacement. Because fatigue is a common problem for clients with valve disorders, the nurse helps the client and family ensure that the home environment is conducive to providing rest. Older clients with aortic stenosis may reside in long-term care.

➤ *Health Teaching*

The teaching plan for the client with valvular heart disease includes
- The disease process
- Medications, including diuretics, vasodilators, cardiac glycosides, antibiotics, and anticoagulants
- Prophylactic use of antibiotics
- A plan of work, activity, and rest to conserve energy
- The purpose and nature of surgical intervention, if appropriate

Because clients with defective or repaired valves are at risk for infective endocarditis, the nurse teaches them to adhere to the precautions described for the client with endocarditis. The nurse instructs clients to inform all health care providers of the valvular heart disease history; the clients are also told that they require antibiotic administration before all invasive procedures and tests. Instructions for the client are described in (Chart 37–9.)

Chart 37–9

Education Guide: Valvular Heart Disease

- Notify all of your health care providers that you have a defective heart valve.
- Remind the health care provider of your valvular problem when you have any dental work (cleaning, filling, or extraction), any examination by instrument (cystoscopy, endoscopy, or sigmoidoscopy), or any other invasive procedure (arteriogram, surgery).
- Request antibiotic prophylaxis before and after these procedures if the health care provider does not offer it.
- Clean all wounds and apply antibiotic ointment to prevent infection.
- Notify your health care provider immediately if you experience fever, petechiae (pinpoint red dots on your skin), or shortness of breath.

The nurse teaches clients taking anticoagulants how to manage their drug therapy successfully and to prevent bleeding. For example, the client should use an electric razor to avoid skin cuts. The client should report any bleeding or excessive bruising to the health care provider. (For more information on anticoagulants, see Chapter 38.)

The nurse teaches clients who have undergone valve surgery how to care for the sternal incision. The nurse instructs clients to watch for and report any fever or drainage or redness at the site. Clients can usually return to normal activity after 6 weeks but should avoid heavy physical labor with their upper extremities for 3 to 6 months to allow healing of the sternotomy incision. Clients who have had valvular surgery should also avoid any dental procedures for 6 months.

Clients with valvular heart disease may have complicated medication schedules as well as long-term antibiotic or anticoagulant therapy. These circumstances may potentially lead to noncompliance. The nurse ensures that the client is an active participant in care decisions. The nurse also provides clear, concise instructions about medication schedules.

The psychological response to valve surgery is similar to that after coronary artery bypass surgery. Clients may experience an altered self-image as a result of the changes required in lifestyle or the visible medial sternotomy incision. In addition, clients with prosthetic valves may have to adjust to a soft but audible clicking sound of the prosthetic valve. The nurse encourages clients to verbalize their feelings about the sternotomy incision and the prosthetic heart valve.

➤ Home Care Management

A home care nurse may be needed to help the client adhere to medication and activity schedules and to detect any problems, particularly with anticoagulant therapy. Clients who have undergone surgery may also require a nurse for assistance with incision care. A home care aide may assist clients with activities of daily living.

➤ Health Care Resources

The American Heart Association is a community resource that provides information to clients about valvular heart disease. A wallet-sized card can be obtained for the client that identifies him or her as needing prophylactic antibiotics. The nurse advises clients receiving anticoagulants to obtain an identification bracelet stating the name of the drug they are taking.

INFLAMMATIONS AND INFECTIONS

Inflammations and infections of the heart frequently follow systemic infections. Recovery from these infections is often prolonged, and clients are at great risk for future heart problems. Inflammation and infection may involve the endocardium (endocarditis), the pericardium (pericarditis), or the entire heart (rheumatic carditis).

Infective Endocarditis
Overview
Pathophysiology

Infective endocarditis (previously called *bacterial endocarditis*) refers to a microbial infection involving the endocardium. The client's own defective valve or a prosthetic valve is most commonly affected, but infection may also occur on apparently healthy endocardium or in septal defects. Current classification of infective endocarditis is by site of involvement, type of pathogen, and definitiveness of diagnosis.

Etiology

Infective endocarditis occurs primarily in clients who are intravenous drug abusers or who have had valve replacements or have structural cardiac defects.

In a client with a cardiac defect, blood may flow rapidly from a high-pressure area to a low-pressure zone, eroding a section of endocardium. Platelets and fibrin adhere to the denuded endocardium, forming a vegetative lesion. During bacteremia, bacteria become trapped in the low-pressure "sinkhole" and are deposited in the vegetation. Additional platelets and fibrin are deposited, causing the vegetative lesion to grow, and the endocardium and valve are destroyed. When the lesion interferes with normal alignment of the valve, valvular insufficiency may result, or, if vegetations become so large that blood flow through the valve is obstructed, the valve appears stenotic.

Possible ports of entry for infecting organisms include

- The oral cavity (especially if dental procedures have been performed)
- Skin rashes, lesions, or abscesses
- Infections (cutaneous, genitourinary, or gastrointestinal)
- Surgery or invasive procedures, including IV line placement

Incidence/Prevalence

The incidence of infective endocarditis is estimated to be 5:100,000 (Matthews, 1994). Men have a higher incidence then women. Mortality rates for infective endocarditis have remained high at 15% to 40% despite antibiotic therapy (Matthews, 1994).

Collaborative Management

 Assessment

Because mortality remains high, early detection of infective endocarditis is essential. Unfortunately, many clients, especially older adults, are misdiagnosed (Matthews, 1994). Clinical manifestations usually occur within 2 weeks of a bacteremia (Chart 37–10).

Assessment usually reveals recurrent fever. Most clients have temperatures from 37.2° to 39.4° C (99° to 103° F). However, many older adults remain afebrile. The severity

> ### Chart 37–10
>
> ## Key Features of Infective Endocarditis
>
> - Fever associated with chills, night sweats, malaise, and fatigue
> - Anorexia and weight loss
> - Cardiac murmur (newly developed or change in existing)
> - Development of heart failure
> - Evidence of systemic embolization
> - Petechiae
> - Splinter hemorrhages
> - Osler's nodes
> - Janeway's lesions

of the symptoms may depend on the virulence of the infecting organism.

➤ Cardiovascular Manifestations

The nurse assesses the client's cardiovascular status. More than 90% of clients with infective endocarditis develop murmurs. The nurse carefully auscultates the precordium, noting and documenting any new murmurs (usually regurgitant in nature) or any changes in the intensity or quality of an old murmur. An S_3 or S_4 heart sound may also be heard.

Heart failure is the most common complication of infective endocarditis. The nurse assesses for right-sided heart failure (as evidenced by peripheral edema, weight gain, and anorexia), as well as left-sided heart failure (as evidenced by fatigue, shortness of breath, and crackles on auscultation of breath sounds).

➤ Embolic Complications

Arterial embolization is a major complication in up to 50% of clients with infective endocarditis. Fragments of vegetation break loose and travel randomly through the circulation. When the left side of the heart is involved, vegetation fragments are carried to the spleen, the kidneys, the gastrointestinal (GI) tract, the brain, and the extremities. When the right side of the heart is involved, emboli enter the pulmonary circulation.

Clients with splenic infarction describe sudden abdominal pain with radiation to the left shoulder. When performing an abdominal assessment, the nurse notes rebound tenderness on palpation. The classic pain described by the client with renal infarction is flank pain with radiation to the groin, accompanied by hematuria or pyuria.

Emboli to the central nervous system cause either transient ischemic attacks (TIAs) or a cerebrovascular accident (CVA). The client may appear confused, have reduced concentration and aphasia, or have dysphagia. Pleuritic chest pain, dyspnea, and cough are often described by the client who is experiencing pulmonary infarction related to embolization.

➤ Peripheral Manifestations

Petechiae (pinpoint red spots) occur in up to 40% of clients with endocarditis. The nurse examines the mucous membranes, the palate, the conjunctivae, and the skin above the clavicles for small red, flat lesions. The nurse also examines the distal third of the nail bed for the black longitudinal lines or small red streaks called *splinter hemorrhages* (Fig. 37–4).

Osler's nodes and Janeway's lesions are also considered classic manifestations of endocarditis, although they may occur with other conditions. The nurse inspects the pads of the fingers, hands, and toes for Osler's nodes, which are reddish tender lesions with a white center. Janeway's lesions (Fig. 37–5) are nontender hemorrhagic lesions found on the fingers, toes, nose, or earlobes. Splenomegaly and clubbing of the fingers may occur in clients who have had infective endocarditis for longer than 6 weeks.

➤ Diagnostic Assessment

A positive blood culture is of prime diagnostic and therapeutic importance. Both aerobic and anaerobic specimens are obtained for culture. Some slow-growing organisms may take 3 weeks and require a specialized medium to isolate. So, cultures should be monitored by the lab for 3 to 4 weeks. Low hemoglobin and hematocrit levels may also be found.

Echocardiography has improved the ability to accurately diagnose infective endocarditis. Transesophageal echocardiography (TEE) allows visualization of cardiac structures that are difficult to see with transthoracic echocardiography (TTE). TEE provides good resolution and is very sensitive for discovering valvular abnormalities, ena-

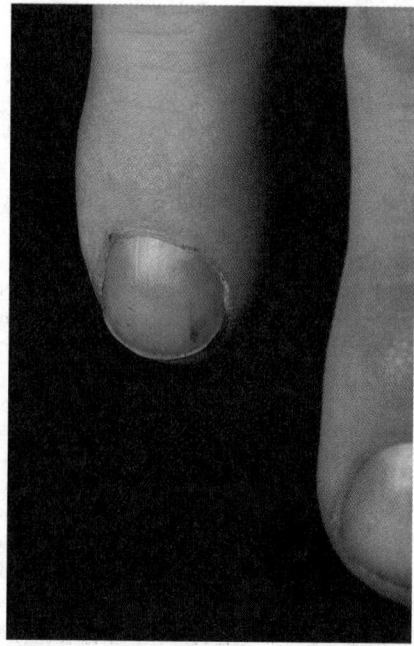

Figure 37–4. Splinter hemorrhage lesions in endocarditis. (From Callen, J. P., et al. [1993]. *Color atlas of dermatology.* Philadelphia: W. B. Saunders.)

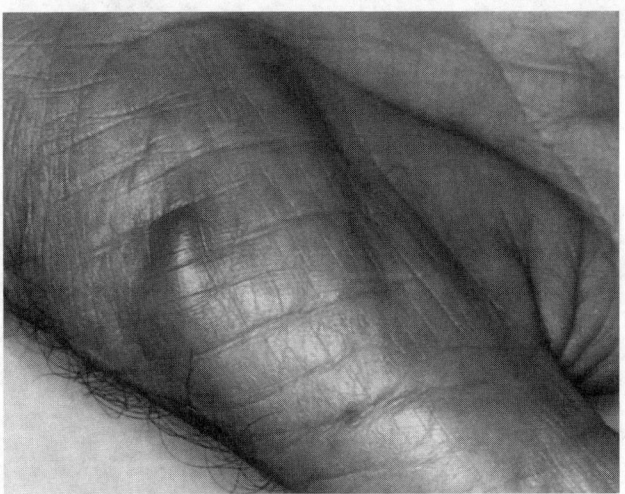

Figure 37–5. Janeway's lesions on the palm. (From Braverman, I. M. [1998]. *Skin signs of systemic disease* [3rd ed.]. Philadelphia: W. B. Saunders.)

bling the clinician to diagnose infective endocarditis more accurately (see Chap. 35).

The most reliable criteria for diagnosing endocarditis include positive blood cultures, a new regurgitant murmur, and evidence of endocardial involvement by echocardiography (Durack, 1995).

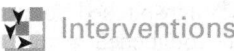 Interventions

Care of the client with endocarditis usually includes antibiotics, rest, and supportive therapy for heart failure. If these interventions are successful, then surgery is usually not required.

➤ *Nonsurgical Management*

The major component of treatment for endocarditis is drug therapy. Other interventions help to prevent the life-threatening complications.

Drug Therapy. Antibiotics are the mainstay of treatment, with the choice of antibiotics depending on the specific organism involved. Because vegetations surround and protect the bacteria, an appropriate antibiotic must be given in a sufficiently high dose to ensure a bactericidal effect. Antibiotics are most often given intravenously, with the course of treatment lasting 4 to 6 weeks. In most cases, the ideal antibiotic is one of the penicillins.

Until recently, clients with endocarditis were hospitalized for up to 6 weeks for intravenous (IV) antibiotic therapy. Now clients are hospitalized for 5 to 7 days to institute IV therapy and then are discharged for continued IV therapy at home. During hospitalization, the nurse assesses the client's response to therapy. Clients are responding to antimicrobial therapy and may be considered for home therapy when they are afebrile, have negative blood cultures, and have no signs of heart failure or embolization.

Anticoagulants are of no value in preventing emboliza-

tion from vegetations. They are avoided unless they are required to retard thrombus formation on a prosthetic valve because they may result in bleeding.

Other Interventions. Complete bed rest need not be enforced unless clients have fever or signs of heart failure. However, the nurse carefully monitors activities to allow adequate rest. The nurse explains proper oral and general body hygiene and consistently uses appropriate aseptic technique when caring for the client to protect the client from contact with potentially infective organisms. Nursing assessment for signs of heart failure (including rapid pulse, fatigue, cough, and dyspnea; new heart murmurs; and early signs of embolization) continues throughout the client's antibiotic regimen.

➤ *Surgical Management*

The cardiac surgeon may be consulted if antibiotic therapy is ineffective in sterilizing a valve, refractory heart failure develops secondary to a defective valve, large valvular vegetations are present, or multiple embolic events occur. Current surgical interventions for infective endocarditis include
- Removing the infected valve (either biological or prosthetic)
- Removing congenital shunts
- Repairing injured valves and chordae tendineae
- Draining abscesses in the heart or elsewhere

Preoperative and postoperative care of clients having surgery involving the valves is similar to that described earlier for clients undergoing a valve replacement.

 Continuing Care

Continuing care for clients with infective endocarditis is essential to resolve the problem and avoid complications. Clients and families involved in the treatment need to be motivated and have the knowledge, physical ability, and resources to administer IV antibiotics at home. The home health nurse may be contacted to complete teaching started in the acute care institution and to monitor client compliance and health status.

The home care nurse and pharmacist arrange for appropriate supplies to be available to the client at home. Supplies include the prepared antibiotic, IV tubing, alcohol wipes, IV access device, normal saline solution, and heparin or saline lock flush solution drawn up in syringes. A heparin or saline lock or central catheter is positioned at a new venous site that is easily accessible to the client or a family member.

The nurse teaches the client, family members, or a significant other how to administer the antibiotic and care for the infusion site while maintaining aseptic technique. The client or a family member demonstrates this technique before the client is discharged from the hospital. The nurse emphasizes the importance of maintaining a blood level of the antibiotic by administering the antibiotics as scheduled.

The nurse encourages the client to maintain proper hygiene, particularly oral hygiene. Clients are advised to use a soft toothbrush, to brush their teeth at least twice a day, and to rinse the mouth with water after brushing. Clients should not use irrigation devices or floss the teeth because bacteremia may result. The nurse instructs clients to wash lacerations well and apply an antibiotic ointment.

Clients must remind health care providers, including their dentists, of their endocarditis and request prophylactic antibiotic coverage for every invasive procedure, including dental care (Table 37–3). This is essential because studies have documented low compliance with prophylaxis regimens by health care providers (Guzzetta, 1992).

The nurse teaches the client self-monitoring for the manifestations of endocarditis, including the complications of heart failure and embolic phenomena. The client is instructed to monitor his or her temperature daily and record it for up to 6 weeks. Clients are also taught to report fever, chills, malaise, weight loss, increase in fatigue, or dyspnea to their primary care provider.

Pericarditis

Overview

Pericarditis is an inflammation or alteration of the pericardium, the membranous sac that encloses the heart. There are two general types of pericarditis: acute pericarditis and chronic constrictive pericarditis.

Acute pericarditis may be fibrous, serous, hemorrhagic, purulent, or neoplastic. Acute pericarditis is most commonly associated with

- Malignant neoplasms
- Idiopathic causes
- Infective organisms (bacteria, viruses, or fungi)
- Post–myocardial infarction (MI) syndrome (Dressler's syndrome)
- Postpericardiotomy syndrome
- Systemic connective tissue disease

The cause of the pericarditis determines its presentation. Acute viral pericarditis commonly follows a respiratory infection and is more common in men aged 20 to 50 years. Dressler's syndrome occurs in 5% to 15% of clients who experience an MI from 1 to 12 weeks after infarction. Postpericardotomy syndrome occurs in 10% to 40% of clients after cardiac surgery.

Chronic constrictive pericarditis occurs when chronic pericardial inflammation causes a fibrous thickening of the pericardium. It is caused by tuberculosis, radiation therapy, trauma, renal failure, or metastatic cancer. In chronic constrictive pericarditis, the pericardium becomes rigid, preventing adequate filling of the ventricles and eventually resulting in cardiac failure.

Collaborative Management

 Assessment

Assessment findings include substernal precordial pain that radiates to the left side of the neck, the shoulder, or the back. Pain is classically grating and oppressive and is aggravated by breathing (mainly on inspiration), coughing, and swallowing. The pain is worse when the client is in the supine position and may be relieved by the client's sitting up and leaning forward. The nurse asks all of the questions to evaluate chest discomfort (see Chap. 35) because it is important that the pain of pericarditis be differentiated from that of acute myocardial infarction.

The nurse may hear a pericardial friction rub with the diaphragm of the stethoscope positioned at the left lower sternal border. This is a scratchy, high-pitched sound; it is produced when the inflamed, roughened pericardial layers create friction as their surfaces rub together.

Clients with acute pericarditis may have an elevated white blood cell count and ECG changes consisting of ST-T wave elevation in all leads, with a T-wave inversion occurring after ST segments return to baseline. Clients with infectious pericarditis usually have fever. Blood specimens for culture may be obtained to assess for possible

TABLE 37–3

Antibiotic Prophylaxis* for Clients Susceptible to Infective Endocarditis		
Procedure	**Standard Regimen**	**For Clients Allergic to Penicillin**
Dental, oral, upper respiratory tract, or esophageal procedures and surgery	One of the following: Amoxicillin 2 g PO Ampicillin 2 g IM or IV	One of the following: Clindamycin (Cleocin) 600 mg PO or IV Cephalexin (Keflex) 2 g PO Azithromycin (Zithromax) 500 mg PO Clarithromycin (Biaxin) 500 mg PO Cefazolin (Ancef) 1 g IM or IV
Genitourinary tract and gastrointestinal tract surgery or instrumentation	One of the following: Ampicillin (2 g IM or IV) plus gentamicin (1.5 mg/kg—not to exceed 120 mg—IM or IV) 30 min before the procedure. Then, ampicillin 1 g IM/IV or amoxicillin 1 g PO 6 hr later. Ampicillin 2 g IM or IV Amoxicillin 2 g PO	One of the following: Vancomycin 1 g IV given over 1–2 hr plus gentamicin (1.5 mg/kg—not to exceed 120 mg—IM or IV) Vancomycin (as above) without the gentamicin)

*PO doses are given 1 hr prior to the procedure; IM or IV doses are given or completed 30 min prior to the procedure.

bacterial infection. Echocardiograms may demonstrate a pleural effusion.

Clients with chronic constrictive pericarditis show signs of right-sided heart failure, elevated systemic venous pressure with jugular distention, hepatic engorgement, and dependent edema. The client usually complains of exertional fatigue and dyspnea. These clients may have thickening of the pericardium on echocardiography or computed tomography (CT) scan. ECG changes include inverted or flat T waves. Atrial fibrillation is common.

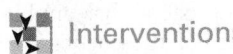 Interventions

➤ Medical Therapy

The client with acute pericarditis may be hospitalized for diagnostic evaluation, observation for complications, and symptom relief. The health care provider usually prescribes nonsteroidal anti-inflammatory drugs for the relief of pain. Clients who do not obtain pain relief within 24 to 48 hours and who do not have bacterial pericarditis may receive corticosteroid therapy. The nurse assesses for pain relief and assists the client to assume positions of comfort, usually sitting upright and leaning slightly forward. If the pain is not relieved within 24 to 48 hours, the nurse notifies the primary care provider.

The various causes of pericarditis require specific therapies. For example, bacterial pericarditis (acute) usually requires antibiotics and pericardial drainage. The usual clinical course of acute pericarditis is short term, from 2 to 6 weeks; however, episodes may recur. Chronic pericarditis caused by malignant disease may be treated with radiation or chemotherapy, while uremic pericarditis is treated by hemodialysis.

The definitive treatment for chronic constrictive pericarditis is surgical excision of the pericardium (pericardiectomy).

➤ Monitoring for Complications of Pericarditis

A significant complication of pericarditis is pericardial effusion, which occurs when the space between the parietal and visceral layers of the pericardium fills with fluid. Pericardial effusion puts the client at risk for cardiac tamponade, excessive fluid within the pericardial cavity. Tamponade restricts diastolic ventricular filling, and cardiac output drops. Findings of cardiac tamponade include
- Jugular venous distention
- Paradoxical pulse, a systolic blood pressure 10 mmHg higher or more on expiration than on inspiration (Chart 37–11)
- Decreased cardiac output
- Muffled heart sounds

➤ Management of Acute Cardiac Tamponade

Acute tamponade may occur when small volumes (20 to 50 mL) of fluid accumulate in the pericardium. The nurse reports any suspicion of this complication to the physician immediately. The physician may initially manage the decreased cardiac output with increased fluid volume administration while awaiting a chest x-ray or echocardiogram to confirm the diagnosis. Unfortunately, these tests

---

Chart 37–11

Nursing Care Highlight: Care of the Client with Pericarditis

- Assess the nature of the client's chest discomfort. (Pericardial pain is typically substernal; it is worse on inspiration and decreases when the client leans forward.)
- Auscultate for a pericardial friction rub.
- Assist the client to a position of comfort.
- Provide anti-inflammatory agents as prescribed.
- Explain that anti-inflammatory agents usually decrease the pain within 48 hr.
- Avoid the administration of aspirin and anticoagulants because these may increase the possibility of tamponade.
- Auscultate the blood pressure carefully to detect paradoxical blood pressure (pulsus paradoxus), a sign of tamponade:
  - Palpate the blood pressure and inflate the cuff above the systolic pressure.
  - Deflate the cuff gradually, and note when sounds are first audible on expiration.
  - Identify when sounds are also audible on inspiration.
  - Subtract the inspiratory pressure from the expiratory pressure to determine the amount of pulsus paradoxus (>10 mmHg is an indication of tamponade).
- Inspect for other indications of tamponade, including jugular venous distention with clear lungs, muffled heart sounds, and decreased cardiac output.
- Notify the physician if tamponade is suspected.

---

are not always helpful because the fluid volume around the heart may be too small to visualize. Hemodynamic monitoring in a specialized critical care unit usually demonstrates compression of the heart, with all pressures (right atrial, pulmonary artery, and wedge) being similar and elevated (plateau pressures).

The physician may elect to perform a pericardiocentesis to relieve the pressure on the heart. Under echocardiographic or fluoroscopic and hemodynamic monitoring, the cardiologist inserts an 8-inch (20.3-cm) long 16- or 18-gauge pericardial needle into the pericardial space. The physician and the nurse monitor the needle's position, recognizing that ST- and T-wave changes indicate myocardial injury, and the needle must be withdrawn slightly. When the needle is properly positioned, a catheter is inserted, and all available pericardial fluid is withdrawn. The nurse monitors the pulmonary artery, wedge, and right atrial pressures during the procedure. The pressures should return to normal as the fluid compressing the heart is removed.

After the pericardiocentesis, the nurse closely monitors the client for the recurrence of tamponade. Often, pericardiocentesis alone does not resolve acute tamponade. The nurse should be prepared to provide adequate fluid volumes to increase cardiac output and to prepare the client for emergency sternotomy if tamponade recurs.

If the client experiences a recurrence of tamponade or recurrent effusions or adhesions from chronic pericarditis, a portion or all of the pericardium may need to be removed to allow adequate ventricular filling and contraction. The surgeon may perform a pericardial window, the removal of a portion of the pericardium permitting the excessive pericardial fluid to drain into the pleural space. In more severe cases, pericardiectomy, removal of the toughened encasing pericardium, may be necessary.

Rheumatic Carditis

Overview

Rheumatic carditis occurs in about 40% of clients with rheumatic fever and affects more than 1 million Americans. It is a sensitivity response that develops after an upper respiratory tract infection with group A beta-hemolytic streptococci. The precise mechanism by which the infection causes inflammatory lesions in the heart is not established. However, inflammation is evident in all layers of the heart. The inflammation results in impaired contractile function of the myocardium, thickening of the pericardium, and valvular damage.

Rheumatic myocarditis is characterized by the formation of Aschoff's bodies, small nodules in the myocardium that are replaced by scar tissue. A diffuse cellular infiltrate also develops and appears to be responsible for the heart failure. The pericardium becomes thickened and covered with exudate, and a serosanguineous pleural effusion may develop. However, the most serious damage occurs to the endocardium, with inflammation of the valve leaflets developing. Hemorrhagic and fibrous lesions form along the inflamed surfaces of the valves, resulting in stenosis or regurgitation primarily of the mitral and aortic valves.

Rheumatic fever may be a complication of 3% of group A beta-hemolytic throat infections. Although the primary attacks occur most often in childhood, rheumatic fever may occur in adulthood. The incidence of rheumatic carditis had been decreasing consistently until the mid-1980s. At that time, a resurgence of rheumatic fever began in both the United States and Europe.

Collaborative Management

Rheumatic carditis is one of the major indicators of rheumatic fever. Common clinical manifestations are
- Tachycardia
- Cardiomegaly
- Development of a new murmur or a change in an existing murmur
- A pericardial friction rub
- Precordial pain
- Changes in the ECG (prolonged PR interval)
- Indications of heart failure
- Evidence of an existing streptococcal infection

Primary prevention is extremely important. The nurse teaches all clients to consult their health care providers and receive appropriate antibiotic therapy if they develop the following indications of streptococcal pharyngitis: moderate to high fever, abrupt onset of a sore throat, a reddened throat with exudate, and enlarged tender lymph nodes. Penicillin is the antibiotic of choice for treatment. Erythromycin (ERYC, Erythromid✦) is the alternative for penicillin-sensitive clients.

The signs of rheumatic carditis must be recognized promptly, and antibiotic therapy must be instituted immediately for secondary prevention. The client is urged to continue the antibiotic administration for the full 10 days to prevent reinfection. The nurse suggests ways to manage the fever, such as maintaining hydration and administering antipyretics. The nurse encourages the client to obtain adequate rest.

The nurse emphasizes tertiary prevention in client education, explaining that a recurrence of rheumatic carditis is probable with reinfection by a streptococcal organism. Thus, antibiotic therapy is essential for streptococcal infection. The nurse also informs the client that antibiotic prophylaxis is necessary for the rest of the client's life to prevent infective endocarditis (see earlier).

Cardiomyopathy

Overview

Cardiomyopathy is a subacute or chronic disorder of cardiac muscle. It is not common, occurring in only 10 to 20 per 100,000 population. The cause is usually unknown.

Treatment is usually palliative, not curative; approximately 50% of clients die within 2 years of symptom onset. Clients have to deal with a shortened life span along with numerous changes in lifestyle.

Cardiomyopathies are classified into three categories on the basis of abnormalities in structure and function: dilated cardiomyopathy, hypertrophic cardiomyopathy, and restrictive cardiomyopathy (Table 37-4).

Dilated Cardiomyopathy

In 87% of cardiomyopathy, dilated cardiomyopathy (DCM) is the structural abnormality. In DCM, there is extensive damage to the myofibrils and interference with myocardial metabolism. There is normal ventricular wall thickness but dilation of both ventricles and impairment of systolic function. Decreased cardiac output from the inadequate pumping of the heart causes the client to experience dyspnea on exertion, decreased exercise capacity, fatigue, and palpitations. DCM is twice as common in men as in women and occurs most often in middle age.

Hypertrophic Cardiomyopathy

The cardinal features of hypertrophic cardiomyopathy (HCM), are asymmetric ventricular hypertrophy of the left ventricle and disarray of the myocardial fibers. The left ventricular hypertrophy leads to a hypercontractile left ventricle with rigid ventricular walls. Obstruction in the left ventricular outflow tract is seen in 75% to 80% of clients with HCM. The abnormal stiffness of the ventricle in HCM results in diastolic filling abnormalities. In approximately 50% of clients, HCM is transmitted as a single-gene autosomal dominant trait.

Restrictive Cardiomyopathy

Restrictive cardiomyopathy, the rarest of the three cardiomyopathies, results in restriction of filling of the ventricles. It is caused by endocardial and/or myocardial disease

TABLE 37–4

Pathophysiology, Signs and Symptoms, and Treatment of Cardiomyopathies

Dilated Cardiomyopathy	Hypertrophic Cardiomyopathy		Restrictive Cardiomyopathy
	Nonobstructed	Obstructed	
Pathophysiology			
Fibrosis of myocardium and endocardium Dilated chambers Mural wall thrombi prevalent	Hypertrophy of all walls Hypertrophied septum Relatively small chamber size	Same as for nonobstructed except for obstruction of left ventricular outflow tract associated with the hypertrophied septum and mitral valve incompetence	Mimics constrictive pericarditis Fibrosed walls cannot expand or contract Chambers narrowed; emboli common

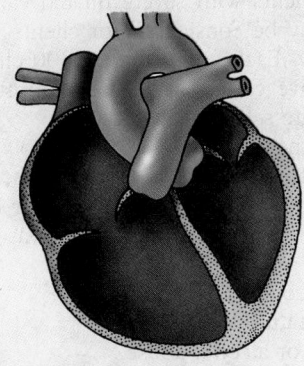 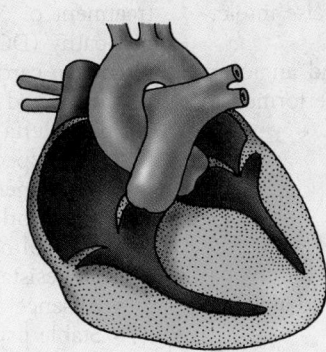

Signs and Symptoms			
Fatigue and weakness Heart failure (left side) Dysrhythmias or heart block Systemic or pulmonary emboli S_3 and S_4 gallops Moderate to severe cardiomegaly	Dyspnea Angina Fatigue, syncope, palpitations Mild cardiomegaly S_4 gallop Ventricular dysrhythmias Sudden death common Heart failure	Same as for nonobstructed except with mitral regurgitation murmur Atrial fibrillation	Dyspnea and fatigue Heart failure (right-sided) Mild to moderate cardiomegaly S_3 and S_4 gallops Heart block Emboli
Treatment			

Symptomatic treatment of heart failure
Vasodilators
Control of dysrhythmias
Surgery: heart transplant
	For both:
	  Symptomatic treatment
	  Beta-blockers
	  Conversion of atrial fibrillation
	  Surgery: ventriculomyotomy or muscle resection with mitral valve replacement
	Digitalis, nitrates, and other vasodilators **contraindicated** with the obstructed form
			Supportive treatment of symptoms
			Treatment of hypertension
			Conversion from dysrhythmias
			Exercise restrictions
			Emergency treatment of acute pulmonary edema

Data from Wynne, J., & Braunwald, E. (1992). The cardiomyopathies and myocarditis. In E. Braunwald (Ed.), *Heart disease: A textbook of cardiovascular medicine* (3rd ed.). Philadelphia: W. B. Saunders.

and produces a clinical picture similar to that of constrictive pericarditis.

Collaborative Management

 Assessment

Findings in cardiomyopathy depend on the structural and functional abnormalities. Left ventricular or biventricular failure is characteristic of *dilated* cardiomyopathy (DCM). Some clients with DCM are asymptomatic for months to years and have left ventricular dilation identified on x-ray. Other clients experience sudden, pronounced symptoms of left ventricular failure such as progressive dyspnea on exertion, orthopnea, palpitations, and activity intolerance. Right-sided heart failure develops late in the disease and is associated with a poor prognosis. Atrial fibrillation occurs in 25% of clients and is associated with embolism.

The clinical picture of *hypertrophic* cardiomyopathy

(HCM) results from the hypertrophied septum, which in 80% of cases causes a mechanical obstruction and thereby reduces stroke volume and cardiac output. Most clients are asymptomatic until late adolescence or early adulthood. The primary symptoms of HCM are exertional dyspnea (90% of clients), angina (75% of clients), and syncope. The chest pain is atypical in that it usually occurs at rest, is prolonged, has no relation to exertion, and is not relieved by the administration of nitrates. A high incidence of ventricular dysrhythmias is associated with HCM. Sudden death occurs and may be the first manifestation of the disease.

The earliest clinical finding in *restrictive* cardiomyopathy is exertional dyspnea. Cardiac output cannot increase during periods of exertion because of the fixed ventricular volume. The client also reports weakness, exercise intolerance, palpitations, and syncope.

Echocardiography, radionuclide imaging, and angiocardiography during cardiac catheterization are performed to diagnose and to differentiate cardiomyopathies.

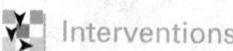 Interventions

The treatment of choice for the client with cardiomyopathy varies with the type of cardiomyopathy and may include both medical and surgical interventions.

➤ *Nonsurgical Management*

The care of clients with dilated or restrictive cardiomyopathy is initially the same as for clients with heart failure. Drug therapy includes the use of diuretics, vasodilating agents, and cardiac glycosides to increase cardiac output. Because clients are at risk for sudden death, the nurse urges them to report any palpitations, dizziness, or fainting, which might indicate a dysrhythmia. Antidysrhythmic drugs or implantable cardiac defibrillators may be used to control life-threatening dysrhythmias. Beta-blockers (e.g., metoprolol) are used experimentally for clients with excessive sympathetic stimulation and resting tachycardia. If cardiomyopathy has developed in response to a toxin, clients are instructed to avoid further exposure. The nurse teaches all clients with cardiomyopathy to abstain from alcohol ingestion because of its cardiac depressant effects.

Management of obstructive hypertrophic cardiomyopathy (HCM) includes administration of negative inotropic agents such as beta-adrenergic blocking agents and calcium antagonists. They decrease the outflow obstruction that accompanies exercise and decrease heart rate, resulting in less angina, dyspnea, and syncope. Vasodilators and cardiac glycosides are contraindicated in clients with obstructive HCM because vasodilating and positive inotropic effects may augment the obstruction.

➤ *Surgical Management*

The type of surgery performed depends on the type of cardiomyopathy.

Excision of Hypertrophied Septum. When clients with obstructive HCM do not respond to medical therapy, surgery may be considered. The most commonly used surgical treatment (ventriculomyomectomy) includes ex-

cising a portion of the hypertrophied ventricular septum resulting in a widened outflow tract. Surgery results in long-term improvement in exercise tolerance in most clients with HCM.

Cardiomyoplasty. Cardiomyoplasty is used for some clients with DCM who cannot undergo cardiac transplantation and are asymptomatic at rest. The latissimus dorsum muscle is dissected free of its distal insertion and wrapped around the heart. For the next 2 months, the muscle is stimulated with increasing frequency until it can contract in synchrony with each heartbeat. Six months after surgery, the client should begin to feel the effects of an enhanced cardiac output.

Heart Transplantation. Heart transplantation is the treatment of choice for clients with severe dilated cardiomyopathy (DCM) and may be considered for clients with restrictive cardiomyopathy. Each year, about 2,300 clients in the United States receive cardiac transplants, most for DCM. Criteria for candidate selection include

- Life expectancy less than 1 year
- Age generally less than 65 years
- New York Heart Association (NYHA) class III or IV
- Normal or only slightly increased pulmonary vascular resistance
- Absence of active infection
- Stable psychosocial status
- No evidence of drug or alcohol abuse

The surgeon transplants a heart from a donor with a comparable body weight and ABO compatibility into a recipient less than 6 hours after procurement. In the most common procedure *(orthotopic transplantation)*, the surgeon removes the diseased heart, leaving the posterior walls of the client's atria. The remnant atria serve as the anchor for the donor heart; anastomoses are made between the recipient and donor atria, aorta, and pulmonary arteries (Fig. 37–6). Because the remaining remnant of the recipient's atria contains the sinoatrial node, two unrelated P waves are visible on ECG.

The postoperative care of the heart transplant recipient is similar to that of the conventional cardiac surgery client (UNOS, 1996). However, the nurse must be especially vigilant to identify occult bleeding into the pericardial sac with the potential for tamponade. The recipient's pericardium has usually stretched considerably to accommodate the diseased, hypertrophied heart. This predisposes the client to concealed postoperative bleeding (UNOS, 1996).

The transplanted heart is denervated, unresponsive to vagal stimulation. The client's heart rate approximates 100 beats per minute, responding slowly with increases in heart rate, contractility, and cardiac output to exercise, stress, or position change. In the early postoperative phase, the nurse may titrate isoproterenol (Isuprel) to support the heart rate and maintain cardiac output. Atropine, digitalis, and carotid sinus pressure are not used because they do not have their usual effects on the heart because of denervation. Denervation of the heart may cause pronounced orthostatic hypotension in the immediate postoperative phase, and the nurse cautions the client to change position slowly.

To suppress natural defense mechanisms and prevent transplant rejection, clients require immunosuppressant

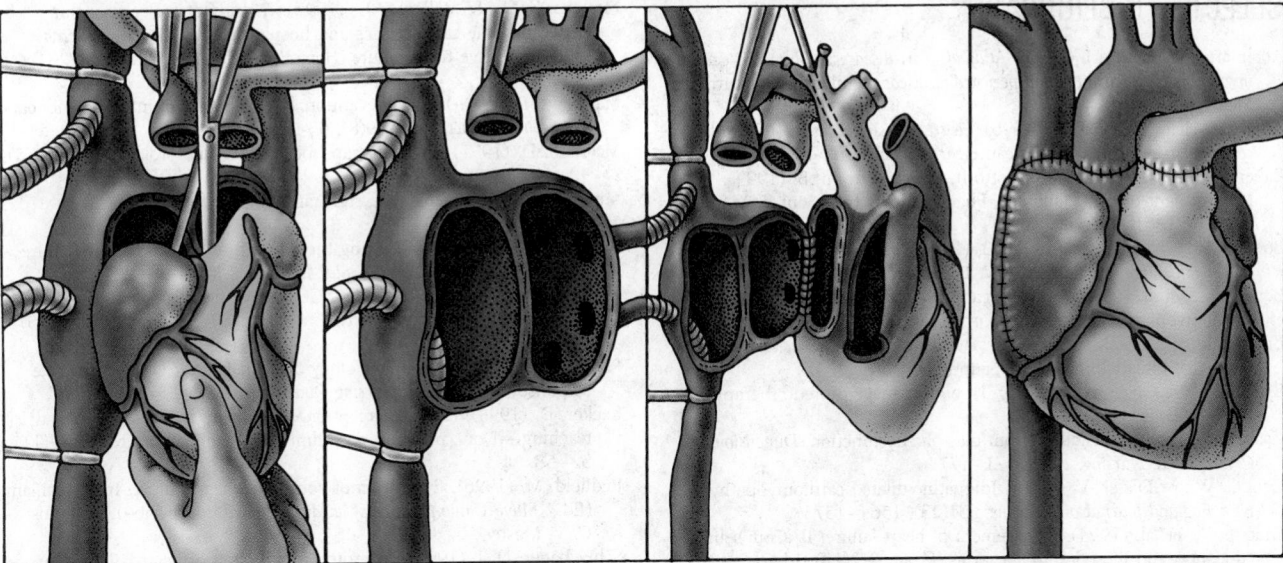

1. After the recipient is placed on cardiopulmonary bypass, the heart is removed.

2. The posterior walls of the recipient's left and right atria are left intact.

3. The left atrium of the donor heart is anastomosed to the recipient's residual posterior atrial walls, and the other atrial walls, the atrial septum, and the great vessels are joined.

POSTOPERATIVE RESULT

Figure 37–6. Heart transplantation.

therapy for the rest of their lives. Most commonly, the physician prescribes therapy with cyclosporine (Sandimmune) and azathioprine (Imuran). Nurses must be vigilant about handwashng and aseptic technique because clients are immunosuppressed and infection is the major cause of death, usually developing in the immediate post-transplant period or during treatment for acute rejection.

Most clients experience their initial episode of acute rejection of the transplanted heart in the first 3 months after transplantation. Symptoms of rejection of the heart are nonspecific, occurring late in the rejection process. They include cardiac dysrhythmias (especially atrial dysrhythmias), hypotension, weakness, fatigue, and dizziness. To detect rejection, the surgeon performs right endomyocardial biopsies at regularly scheduled intervals and whenever symptoms occur.

Approximately 75% of clients survive 3 years after transplantation; most return to NYHA class I or II status (UNOS, 1996). Five years after transplantation, many of the surviving clients (20% to 40%) have evidence of coronary artery disease (CAD) presenting as diffuse plaque in the arteries of the donor heart. Because the heart is denervated, clients do not usually experience angina and regularly scheduled exercise tolerance tests and angiography are required to identify CAD.

To delay the development of CAD, clients are encouraged to follow a prudent lifestyle similar to the client with CAD (see Chap. 40). The physician may prescribe a calcium channel blocker such as diltiazem (Cardizem) to decrease the rate of coronary artery narrowing. The nurse stresses the importance of compliance with dietary modifications and medication regimens. The client is encour-

aged to participate in a regular exercise program but cautioned to allow at least 10 minutes of warm up and cool down for the denervated heart to adjust to changes in activity level.

CASE STUDY for the Client with Heart Failure

■ An 85-year-old woman is one of your nursing home residents. She has a long history of heart failure, myocardial infarction, pulmonary emphysema, hypertension, and degenerative joint disease. Her medications include Lasix 20 mg qd, Vasotec 5 mg qd, digoxin 0.125 mg qd, KCl 40 mEq qd, and Motrin 200 mg qd.

Today the resident complains that she "just doesn't feel right." The nursing assistant reports that her pulse is weak and irregular at 116 bpm, and her skin feels cooler than usual. You go to her room for further assessment.

QUESTIONS:

1. When taking a history from this client, what important questions would you ask?
2. What physical assessments techniques would you perform?
3. During the assessment, you find that she is dyspneic at rest, has a respiratory rate of 32, a blood pressure of 180/95, is very anxious, and has crackles in the bases of her lungs. What should you do first?

SELECTED BIBLIOGRAPHY

Abelmann, W. H. (Ed.). (1995). *Atlas of heart diseases: Volume II. Cardiomyopathies, myocarditis, and pericardial disease.* Philadelphia: Current Medicine.

American Heart Association. (1996). *Heart and stroke facts: 1996 statistical supplement.* Dallas: American Heart Association.

Baker, D. W., Konstam, M. A., Bottorff, M., & Bertram, B. (1994). Management of heart failure: I. Pharmacologic treatment. *JAMA, 272*(17), 1361–1365.

Booker, M. F., & Ignatavicius, D. D. (1996). *Infusion therapy: Techniques and medications.* Philadelphia: W. B. Saunders.

Bove, L. A., et al. (1995). Nursing care of patients undergoing dynamic cardiomyoplasty. *Critical Care Nurse, 15*(3), 96–104.

Braunwald, E. (1997). *Heart disease: A textbook of cardiovascular medicine* (5th ed.). Philadelphia: W. B. Saunders.

Byers, J. F., & Goshorn, J. (1995). How to manage diuretic therapy. *AJN, 95*(2), 38–43.

Cash, A. (1996). Heart failure from diastolic dysfunction. *Dimensions of Critical Care Nursing, 15*(4), 171–177.

Dec, G. W., & Fuster, V. (1994). Idiopathic dilated cardiomyopathy. *New England Journal of Medicine, 331*(23), 1564–1573.

Dracup, K., et. al. (1994). Management of heart failure: II. Counseling, education and lifestyle modifications. *JAMA, 272*(18), 1442–1445.

Dracup, K., Dunbar, S., & Baker, D. W. (1995). Rethinking heart failure. *AJN, 95*(7), 23–27.

Durack, D. T. (1995) Prevention of infective endocarditis. *New England Journal of Medicine, 332*(1), 38–44.

Fowler, N. (1995). Pericardial disease. In W. H. Abelmann (Ed.), *Atlas of heart disease: Volume II. Cardiomyopathies, myocarditis, and pericardial disease* (pp. 13.1–13.15). St. Louis: C. V. Mosby.

Funk, M., & Krumholtz, H. M. (1996). Epidemiologic and economic impact of advanced heart failure. *Journal of Cardiovascular Nursing, 10*(2), 11–28.

*Guzzetta, C. (1992). Infective endocarditis. In B. Dossey (Ed.), *Critical care nursing: Body-mind-spirit* (3rd ed., p. 523). Philadelphia: J. B. Lippincott.

Hawthorne, M. H., & Hixon, M. E. (1994). Functional status, quality of life and mood disturbance in patients with heart failure. *Progress in Cardiovascular Nursing, 9*(1), 22–32.

Hixon, M. E. (1994). Aging and heart failure. *Progress in Cardiovascular Nursing, 9*(1), 4–12.

Jaarsma, T., Dracup, K., Walden, J., et al. (1996). Sexual function in patients with advanced heart failure. *Heart and Lung, 25*(4), 262–270.

Jensen, G. A., & Miller, D. S. (1995). The heart of aging: Special challenges of cardiac ischemic disease and failure in the elderly. *AACN Clinical Issues, 6*(3), 471–481.

Kayser, S. R. (1994). Management of chronic congestive heart failure: Part II—Selection of treatment. *Progress in Cardiovascular Nursing, 9*(2), 30–37.

Konick-McMahon, J. (1997). Discharged with dobutamine. *RN, 60*(4), 24–28.

Konstam, M., Dracup, K., Baker, D., et al. (1994). *Heart failure: Evaluation and treatment of patients with left ventricular systolic dysfunction.* Clinical practice guideline No. 11. Rockville, MD: U.S. Department of Health and Human Services, Public Health Service, Agency for Health Care Policy and Research. AHCPR Pub. No. 94-0612.

Korzeniowski, O., & Kaye, D. (1992). Infective endocarditis. In E. Braunwald (Ed.), *Heart disease: A textbook of cardiovascular medicine* (4th ed., pp. 1078–1105). Philadelphia: W. B. Saunders.

Martens, K. H., & Mellor, S. D. (1997). A study of the relationship between home care services and hospital readmission of patients with congestive heart failure. *Home Healthcare Nurse, 15*(2), 123–129.

Matthews, D. (1994). The prevention and diagnosis of infective endocarditis. *Nurse Practitioner, 19*(8), 53–59.

McGrath, D. (1997). Clinical snapshot: Mitral valve prolapse. *AJN, 97*(5), 40–41.

Miner, P. D. (1994). Infective endocarditis. *Nursing Clinics of North America, 29*(2), 269–283.

Moser, D. K. (1996). Maximizing therapy in the advanced heart failure patient. *Journal of Cardiovascular Nursing, 10*(2), 29–46.

Newkirk, T., & Leeper, B. (1996). Congestive heart failure: Mapping the way to quality outcomes. *AJN: Critical Care Issues Supplement, 96*(5), 25–28.

Pratt, N. G. (1995). Pathophysiology of heart failure: Neuroendocrine response. *Critical Care Nursing Quarterly, 18*(1), 22–31.

Recker, D. (1994). Patient perception of preoperative cardiac surgical teaching—Done pre- and postadmission. *Critical Care Nurse, 14*(1), 52–58.

Redfield, M. (1996). Evaluation of congestive heart failure. In E. Guiliani (Ed.), *Mayo Clinic practice of cardiology* (3rd ed., p. 569). St. Louis: C. V. Mosby.

Schwabauer, N. J. (1996). Retarding progression of heart failure: Nursing actions. *Dimensions of Critical Care Nursing, 15*(6), 307–317.

Shine, L., & Howland-Gradman, J. (1996). Aortic stenosis in elderly: Valvuolplasty versus surgery. *AJN: Critical Care Issues Supplement.* May, pp. 7–11.

Sullivan, M. J. (1994). New trends in cardiac rehabilitation in patients with chronic heart failure. *Progress in Cardiovascular Nursing, 9*(1), 13–21.

Swearubgen, P. L., & Keen, J. H. (Eds.). (1995). *Manual of critical care* (3rd ed.). St. Louis: Mosby–Year Book.

UNOS. (1996). *Donation and transplantation: Nursing curriculum.* UNOS.

U.S. Department of Health and Human Services, Agency for Health Care Policy and Research. (1994). *Heart failure: Evaluation and care of patients with left-ventricular systolic dysfunction.* Rockville, MD: U.S. Department of Health and Human Services.

SUGGESTED READINGS

Cash, A. (1996). Heart failure from diastolic dysfunction. *Dimensions of Critical Care Nursing. 15*(4), 171–177.

This article presents a detailed explanation of the pathophysiology of diastolic heart failure. It describes tests to differentiate diastolic from systolic heart failure and describes possible management strategies for diastolic heart failure.

Konick-McMahon, J. (1997). Discharged with dobutamine. *RN, 60*(4), 24–28.

This article describes clients who might benefit from home dobutamine therapy for heart failure, and discusses the cost of therapy and insurance criteria for coverage. Finally, it describes education essential for the client and caregiver for the home dobutamine therapy to be effective.

Schwabauer, N. J. (1996). Retarding progression of heart failure: Nursing actions. *Dimensions of Critical Care Nursing. 15*(6), 307–317.

This article describes tests that evaluate myocardial performance, monitor neurohormonal activity, and assess functional status of the patient with heart failure. Nursing actions to enhance myocardial performance and functional status are described.

Chapter 38

INTERVENTIONS FOR CLIENTS WITH VASCULAR PROBLEMS

Disorders of the vascular (blood vessel) system cause many problems and may lead to complete shutdown of all body organs or eventually death. Each year, vascular disorders result in disability or death, and the financial impact is overwhelming.

Although vascular disease can affect any portion of the human body, such as the heart, brain, and kidneys, the peripheral vascular system and its associated diseases are described here.

Arteriosclerosis and Atherosclerosis

Overview

Arteriosclerosis is a thickening, or hardening, of the arterial wall. Atherosclerosis, a type of arteriosclerosis, involves the formation of plaque within the arterial wall. Atherosclerosis is the most common cause of arterial obstruction. The process of atherosclerosis can lead to cardiovascular diseases, such as coronary artery disease (CAD), cerebrovascular disease, and peripheral vascular disease (PVD). Cardiovascular disease is the primary cause of death in the United States. Over 1 million people die of heart and blood vessel disease each year (American Heart Association, 1995).

Pathophysiology

The exact pathophysiology of atherosclerosis is not known, but it is thought to occur in the following way (Fig. 38–1). A fatty streak appears on the intimal surface (inner lining) of the artery. At this stage, the fatty streak may appear flattened or elevated, but it generally does not affect the integrity of the arterial wall.

Next, a fibrous plaque develops. This plaque is described as a white, glistening, fibrous elevation that covers a lipid core. At this stage, the plaque is elevated enough to partially or completely occlude the blood flow of an artery.

In the final stage, the fibrous lesions become calcified, hemorrhagic, ulcerated, or thrombosed. The rate of progression of this process may be influenced by genetic factors; certain chronic diseases, such as diabetes mellitus; and lifestyle habits, including smoking, eating habits, and level of exercise.

Etiology

Theories

The exact etiology of atherosclerosis is unknown, but several theories attempt to explain its cause. It is believed

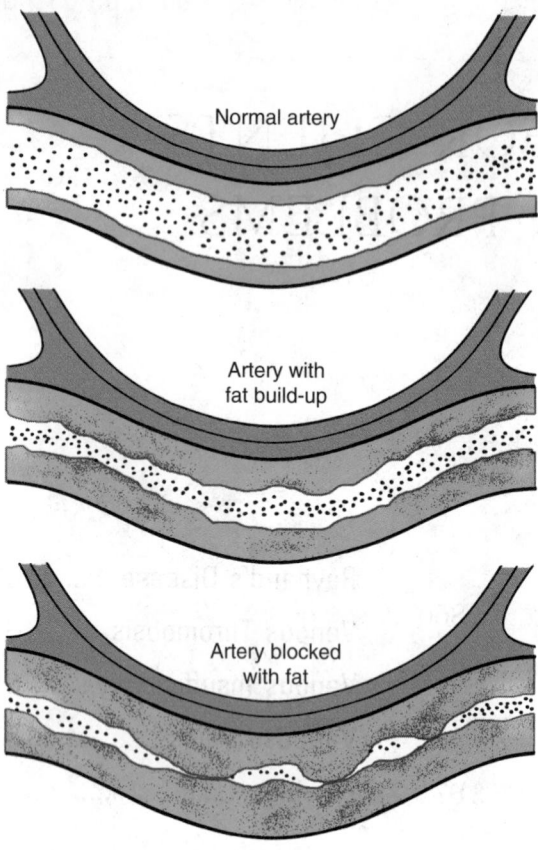

Figure 38–1. Pathophysiology of atherosclerosis.

that an injury to the intimal layer of the artery may initiate the development of atherosclerosis. One popular theory (*platelet aggregation*) is that, after the intimal injury has occurred, platelets form a cluster at the arterial wall and produce a peptide that stimulates the proliferation of the smooth muscle cells of the intima. Eventually, this proliferation can narrow the artery enough to compromise the flow of blood or completely occlude arterial blood flow.

Another theory, the *lipid hypothesis,* assumes that, after an intimal injury, a group of blood lipids (fats) accumulate. Again, this accumulation can partially or completely occlude arterial blood flow. The principal lipids involved are cholesterol and triglyceride.

Many theorists believe that a combination of these two events is the most appropriate view of the atherosclerotic process and that this can occur in any arterial wall of the body. Usually, the disease affects the larger arteries, such as the coronary arterial beds, the major branches of the aorta, the visceral branches of the aorta, the terminal abdominal aorta, the carotid and vertebral arteries, or any combination of these.

Factors Causing Arterial Injury

Intimal injury of the major arteries of the body can be attributed to many factors. Hypertension can cause a mechanical injury, whereas elevated levels of low-density lipoproteins (LDLs) and decreased levels of high-density lip-

oproteins (HDLs) can cause chemical injuries to the intimal wall. Chemical injury can also be caused by elevated levels of toxins in the bloodstream, which may occur with renal failure, or by circulating carbon monoxide in the bloodstream from cigarette smoking. The intimal wall can be weakened by the natural process of aging or by physiologic disorders, such as diabetes.

Genetic predisposition and diabetes have a fairly direct effect on the development of atherosclerosis. Some families demonstrate inherited hyperlipidemia, an elevation in levels of blood lipids. In these people, the liver makes excessive cholesterol, which accounts for the development of atherosclerosis. In some people with hereditary atherosclerosis, however, the blood cholesterol level is normal. The reason for the development and progression of plaque in these people is not understood.

People with severe diabetes mellitus frequently have premature and severe atherosclerosis, often involving the microvasculature. This occurs because diabetes promotes an increase in LDL in plasma. In addition, intimal arterial damage may result from the effect of hyperglycemia.

Factors indirectly related to atherosclerosis include obesity, a sedentary lifestyle, and stress. Clients who are obese are at greater risk, most often because of concomitant elevations in cholesterol levels. Long-term physical activity is important in maintaining ideal body weight; it is also thought to help in maintaining optimal blood pressure and cholesterol levels and improved glucose tolerance. The effect of stress may be due to its effect on the sympathetic and parasympathetic release of catecholamines and an acute rise in blood pressure.

Incidence/Prevalence

It is not known exactly how many people have atherosclerosis, but small plaques are almost always present in the arteries of young adults. The incidence can be better quantified by assessing diseases that result from this process.

WOMEN'S HEALTH CONSIDERATIONS

Although the process of atherosclerosis does not appear to differ between men and women, coronary artery disease (CAD) is much less common in premenopausal women than in age-matched men because of the lipid-lowering effect of estrogen. Postmenopausal women have similar rates of CAD as men in the same age group. People in the United States have a higher incidence of CAD related to atherosclerosis than in other industrialized nations (American Heart Association, 1995).

Collaborative Management

 Assessment

➤ *Vital Signs*

Because of the high incidence of hypertension in clients with atherosclerosis, the nurse assesses the blood pressure in both arms. The heart is also thoroughly assessed because concomitant cardiac disease is often present.

The nurse palpates pulses at all of the major sites on

the body and notes any differences. Carotid arteries are palpated separately because of the risk of inadequate cerebral perfusion. The nurse also palpates for temperature differences in the lower extremities and checks capillary filling. Prolonged capillary filling (>3 seconds in young to middle-aged adults; >5 seconds in older adults) generally indicates poor circulation. An extremity with significant atherosclerotic disease may be cool or cold, with a diminished or absent pulse.

➤ Assessment for Bruits

After palpating the pulses, the nurse auscultates each large artery from the carotid to the dorsalis pedis with a stethoscope or a Doppler probe. Many clients with vascular disease have a bruit in the larger arteries. A bruit is described as a turbulent, swishing sound, which can be soft or loud in pitch. The mere existence of a bruit is considered abnormal, but the role it plays in indicating the severity of vascular disease is not understood. The nurse should document the location of bruits. They often occur in the carotid, aortic, femoral, and popliteal arteries and usually indicate some degree of narrowing of the arterial wall. The rate and intensity of the pulse in each artery during auscultation is also noted. A decrease in intensity and audibility or a complete loss of a pulse may indicate an arterial occlusion. The nurse records at which point the pulse intensity changes and reports these findings immediately to the health care provider.

➤ Laboratory Assessment

Serum cholesterol levels are often elevated in clients with atherosclerosis. It is recommended that clients keep their cholesterol levels below 200 mg/dL. The National Cholesterol Education Program has recommended screening guidelines based on three classifications of cholesterol levels (Table 38–1).

Elevated cholesterol levels must be validated by low-density lipoprotein (LDL) and high-density lipoprotein (HDL) determinations. Elevated LDL levels indicate that a person is at an increased risk for atherosclerosis. Low or normal levels of HDL also indicate an increased risk. A desirable LDL cholesterol level is one below 130 mg/dL, whereas a desirable HDL cholesterol level is 35 mg/dL or above. In some people, particularly women, an elevated cholesterol level may be due to an elevated HDL level, which is not considered a risk.

Triglyceride levels may also be elevated with atherosclerosis. A level of 200 mg/dL or above indicates hypertriglyceridemia. Elevated triglyceride levels may not cause atherosclerosis, but an elevated triglyceride level is often associated with the condition.

Interventions

Atherosclerosis progresses for years before clinical manifestations are evident. Clients with or at risk for atherosclerosis can often be identified by cholesterol screening. Because of the high incidence of atherosclerosis in the United States, all people 20 years of age and older are advised to have their serum cholesterol level evaluated.

Diet Therapy. Clients with LDL values of 130–159 mg/dL are advised to follow a fat-modified diet. In collaboration with the dietitian, the nurse instructs clients with LDLs of 160 mg/dL or greater to follow a more structured diet aimed at decreasing saturated fat and cholesterol and, if appropriate, promoting weight loss. A decrease in fat, particularly saturated fat, is considered more important than simply decreasing the cholesterol number because saturated fat is one of the main determinants of cholesterol synthesis in the body.

In the United States, 37% of the total caloric intake in the diets of many people is made up of fat, and this over consumption of fat and cholesterol leads to hypercholesterolemia—an elevated total blood cholesterol level (Whitney et al., 1994). Elevated cholesterol levels, however, can often be decreased if fat in the diet is limited to no more than 30% of the caloric intake.

TABLE 38–1

Classification of Serum Cholesterol Levels

Serum Cholesterol Level (mg/dL)	Classification	Intervention
<200	• Optimal level	• Provide dietary information • Determine cholesterol levels again within 5 years
200–239 with *no* CAD or risks for CAD	• Borderline high blood cholesterol	• Provide dietary information • Determine cholesterol level again within 1 year
200–239 *with* CAD or risks for CAD 240 or higher, with or without CAD or risks for CAD	• High blood cholesterol	• Obtain serum LDL and HDL cholesterol levels • If LDL is 130–159, advise client to follow fat-modified diet, and repeat LDL annually • If LDL is 160 or higher, provide dietary therapy and frequent monitoring

CAD, coronary artery disease; LDL, low-density lipoprotein; HDL, high-density lipoprotein.

To assess what 30% of the caloric intake is, clients first need to determine their ideal daily caloric intake. They can then calculate their fat limit in grams (see Table 38–2). In addition to tracking fat in grams, people need to assess the fatty acid content of foods.

Step One Diet. The Step One American Heart Association diet, which is often recommended to decrease serum cholesterol level, calls for a total fat intake of less than 30%, with less than 10% of total caloric intake coming from saturated fat, up to 10% of total calories coming from polyunsaturated fat, and 10% to 15% coming from monounsaturated fat. Cholesterol intake with this diet is limited to less than 300 mg daily.

In collaboration with the dietitian, the nurse educates the client about the fat content of foods in terms of the total degree of fat (Table 38–2) and saturation. Meats and eggs contain mostly saturated fats. Because canola (rapeseed) oil is rich in monounsaturated fat and safflower and sunflower oil are rich in polyunsaturated oils, they are recommended over highly saturated oils, such as palm or coconut oil. Cholesterol is found only in animal sources, such as meat and eggs, which are also high in saturated fats.

Step Two Diet. The client's serum cholesterol levels are retested 6 and 12 weeks after the initial dietary intervention. If the cholesterol level has not significantly decreased, the client may be referred to a registered dietitian for instruction on a more restricted diet, such as the Step Two Diet. The Step Two Diet limits saturated fat to less than 7% of total calories and cholesterol to less than 200 mg/day.

In addition to elevated LDLs, other variations of hyperlipidemias put clients at risk for atherosclerosis. A low-fat, low-cholesterol diet, however, can play a significant role in improving a lipid profile, regardless of the lipid alteration.

Smoking Cessation. Cigarette smoking lowers levels of HDL cholesterol and dramatically increases the rate of progression of atherosclerosis.

The nurse advises all clients who smoke to stop smoking and all clients to avoid secondhand smoke. The nurse describes the relationship of smoking to atherosclerosis and assesses the client's willingness to change this behavior. Nurses and other health care providers can refer to the Agency on Health Care Policy and Research's Practice Guidelines on Smoking Cessation. This reference provides

TABLE 38–2

Fat Content of Selected Foods

Food	Fat (g)	Calories	Food	Fat (g)	Calories
Beef (3 oz with removable fat trimmed)			**Poultry** *Continued*		
Corned beef	16	213	Chicken drumstick, meat only, 1 average	2	76
Eye of round (roasted)	5	151	Turkey, light meat with skin	7	168
London broil, braised (choice)	12	208	Turkey, light meat only	3	133
T-bone steak, broiled (choice)	9	182	Turkey, dark meat with skin	10	188
Luncheon Meats (1 slice)			Turkey, dark meat only	6	160
Louis Rich 96% fat-free turkey pastrami	0	25	**Eggs**		
Oscar Mayer bologna	4	50	1 large	5	75
Weaver Chicken Frank with cheese	12	140	Fleischmann's Egg Beaters, ¼ c	0	60
			Morningstar Scramblers, ¼ c	3	60
Seafood (3 oz cooked unless otherwise indicated)			**Milk and Other Dairy Products**		
			Milk (1 c)		
Haddock	1	95	Whole	8	150
Lobster	1	83	2% fat	5	120
Swordfish	4	132	1% fat	3	100
Tuna, canned in oil and drained	7	158	Skim	0	90
Tuna, canned in water and drained	0	111	**Cream (1 tbsp)**		
Shrimp	1	84	Half and half	2	20
Shrimp, breaded and fried	10	206	Heavy whipping cream	6	52
Poultry (3 oz roasted unless otherwise indicated)			Sour cream	3	27
			Cheese		
Chicken breast, meat with skin	7	165	American, 1 oz	9	106
Chicken breast, meat only	3	142	Cheddar, 1 oz	9	114
Chicken drumstick, meat with skin, batter dipped and fried, 1 average	11	193	Cottage cheese, creamed, 1 c	9	217
			Cottage cheese, 1% fat, 1 c	2	164
			Cream cheese, 1 oz	10	99
			Ricotta, ½ c	16	216
			Ricotta, part-skim, ¼ c	10	171
			Swiss, 1 oz	8	107

strategies to assist clients to quit smoking. A smoking cessation group, such as the American Cancer Society's "Fresh Start," may help the client with this difficult process. Most formal programs encourage people to stop smoking "cold turkey."

Johns Hopkins Hospital has developed a "stage of readiness" model that classifies clients into one of six stages (Stillman, 1995). The nurse can assess the client's readiness to stop smoking using this model (Table 38–3).

Clients may also consider using the nicotine patch (Nicoderm, Habitrol, ProStep), which helps relieve nicotine withdrawal symptoms. The patch is about 50% effective in helping clients to stop smoking and is available over the counter. The dose is determined by the client's weight and the extent to which he or she smokes. Clients are urged to stop smoking completely when the nicotine patch is initiated. The nurse informs clients that if they continue to smoke while using the patch, their risks for adverse effects are increased because the peak levels of nicotine are higher than those experienced from smoking alone. Serious cardiovascular effects, such as angina and dysrhythmias, may result from the patch, although the most common side effect is skin irritation. Patches cost approximately $100 a month, or a total of $300 over 3 months. Many health insurance programs will not cover the costs associated with nicotine patches unless the client is enrolled in a smoking cessation program.

Nicotine gum (Nicorette) is necessary if a client feels the need to smoke. Clients should not chew more than 30 pieces of gum per day (Schlafer, 1993).

TRANSCULTURAL CONSIDERATIONS

African-Americans have a higher prevalence of smoking than other ethnic groups. African-American women are less likely to stop smoking than Caucasian women. The reason for this difference is not known (Allen & Phillips, 1997).

Exercise. Regular exercise is recommended to promote optimal lipid levels, and it can actually prevent atherosclerosis. Exercise can also lead to regression of atherosclerotic plaque and the building of collateral circulation in people with atherosclerosis. The level of exercise required to provide protection from atherosclerotic dis-

TABLE 38–2

Fat Content of Selected Foods *Continued*

Food	Fat (g)	Calories	Food	Fat (g)	Calories
Milk and Other Dairy Products *Continued*			**Spreads and Oils** *Continued*		
Weight Watchers American Pasteurized Process Cheese Product, 1 slice	2	45	Margarine, 1 tsp	4	34
			Diet margarine, 1 tsp	2	17
Yogurt			Vegetable oil (corn, safflower, olive, peanut, soybean, sunflower, and sesame), 1 tbsp	14	120
Colombo, plain, 8 oz	7	150	Vegetable oil, spray, 2.5-sec spray	1	6
Colombo, plain, nonfat lite, 8 oz	0	110	**Salad Dressings**		
Breads			Blue cheese, 1 tbsp	8	77
Bagel, 1	1	163	French, 1 tbsp	6	67
English muffin, 1	1	135	Italian, 1 tbsp	7	69
Whole-wheat bread, 1 slice	1	61	Russian, 1 tbsp	8	76
Other Grains			Thousand Island, 1 tbsp	6	59
Pasta, 1 c cooked	1	159	**Sweets**		
White rice, 1 c cooked	1	223	Apple pie, ⅛	12	282
Pancakes, 4-in plain	2	62	Cheesecake, ⅛	13	278
Waffles, 7-in plain	8	206	Chocolate pudding, 1 c	12	385
French toast, 1 slice	7	153	Chocolate syrup, 2 tbsp	1	92
Fruits and Vegetables			Fudge topping, 2 tbsp	5	124
Apple, 1 medium	1	81	Ice cream, Sealtest, vanilla, chocolate, or strawberry, ½ c	6	140
Banana, 1 medium	1	105	Orange sherbet, ½ c	3	92
Orange, 1 medium	1	65	Popsicle ice pop	0	50
Raisins, ⅓ c	1	150	**Snack Foods**		
Avocado, ½ medium	15	153	Lay's Bar-B-Q Flavored Potato Chips, 1 oz	9	150
Broccoli, ½ c cooked	0	23	Orville Redenbacher's Natural Microwave Popping Corn, 4 c popped	7	110
Carrot, raw, 1 medium	0	31			
Corn, canned, ½ c	1	66			
Green beans, ½ c cooked	0	22	Popcorn, air-popped, 1 c	0	23
Peas, ½ c cooked	0	67	Pringle's Light Potato Chips, 1 oz	8	150
Spreads and Oils					
Butter, 1 tsp	4	36			

TABLE 38–3

Stage-of-Readiness Model for Smoking Cessation		
Stage	**Description of Stage**	**Nursing Strategies**
Precontemplation	Clients have no desire to quit smoking	Teach negative effects of smoking; reassure client that feelings are part of addiction process; deliver a "fear" message related to poor health consequences
Contemplation	Clients have thought about smoking cessation but have taken no action	Provide specific examples of how smoking is affecting the client; stress health benefits if client quits smoking
Preparation	Client has taken some steps to quit smoking	Provide behavioral reinforcement; help the client identify cues that lead to smoking, such as after eating; help the client identify coping strategies
Action	Client quits smoking	Provide positive reinforcement to prevent relapse
Maintenance	Client has not smoked for 6 months	Continue with positive reinforcement

Information from Stillman, F. A. (1995). Smoking cessation for the hospitalized cardiac patient: Rationale for and report of a model program. *Journal of Cardiovascular Nursing, 9,* 25–36.

ease has not been established. The nurse instructs clients at risk for or with atherosclerosis—when it results from hyperlipidemia, hypertension, or diabetes—to undergo an exercise tolerance (treadmill or stress) test before undertaking an exercise program, such as aerobics, walking, or running.

Drug Therapy. Clients with elevated total and LDL cholesterol levels that do not respond adequately to dietary intervention are started on lipid-lowering agents (Chart 38–1). Drug choice is dependent on the triglyceride levels. Because most of these drugs can produce major side effects, they are generally given only when nonpharmacologic management has been unsuccessful. Bile acid-binding resins, such as cholestyramine (Questran) or colestipol (Colestid), may be recommended initially because of their low toxicity. Medications such as lovastatin (Mevacor), simvastatin (Zocor), and fluvastatin (Lescol) lower both LDL and triglyceride levels. These statins are contraindicated in active liver disease and pregnancy as they can cause muscle myopathies and marked increases in liver functions. Nicotinic acid lowers LDL and VLDL cholesterol levels and increases HDL cholesterol level. It is used as a single agent or in combination with an acid-binding

Chart 38–1

Drug Therapy for Hyperlipidemia

Drug	Usual Dosage	Nursing Interventions	Rationale
Bile acid sequestrants, e.g., cholestyramine Questran Colestipol (Colestid)	• 12–24 g/day • 30 g/day	• Encourage clients to increase fluid intake and consider stool softeners/psyllium if needed	• Chloestyramine is constipating
Nicotinic acid (Nicobid, Nicolar, Nia-Bid [niacin])	• 1.5–3 g/day • Maximum dose 6 g/day	• Encourage clients to take with meals • Increase dose gradually	• Flushing of skin and pruritus are common side effects, which can be minimized when drug is taken with meals
Fibric acid, usually derivatives, e.g., gemfibrozil (Lopid)	• 600 mg bid • 1–2 mg	• Instruct clients to take with meals if nausea or gastrointestinal discomfort occurs	• Although well tolerated, nausea and gastrointestinal discomfort may occur and can be prevented if taken with meals
HMG-CoA reductase inhibitors, e.g., Lovastatin (Mevacor) Simvastatin (Zocor) Fluvastatin (Lescol)	• Starting dose 20 mg; increased to 40–80 mg • 10–40 mg/day • 20–40 mg/day	• Instruct clients to report muscle tenderness	• Although rare, myopathy has occured as a side effect

resin drug or a statin. Low doses (1.0–1.5 g/day) are generally well tolerated, but higher doses can result in an elevation of hepatic enzymes and various other side effects. Gemfibrozil (Lopid) raises HDL and lowers triglyceride and VLDL cholesterol levels, but is not as effective in lowering LDL.

Hypertension

Overview

Hypertension is generally defined as a systolic blood pressure greater than or equal to 130 mmHg and/or a diastolic blood pressure greater than or equal to 85 mmHg (Joint National Committee, 1993). Generally, hypertension is determined by three separate readings unless the systolic pressure is 210 mmHg or higher and the diastolic pressure is 120 mmHg or more.

Hypertension has been classified into four stages (Table 38–4). The significance of this disease is that it is a major risk factor for coronary, cerebral, renal, and peripheral vascular disease. However, control of hypertension has resulted in significant decreases in cardiovascular morbidity and mortality.

Although mortality rates have declined over the last 20 years, hypertension costs over $500 million per year and accounts for the largest number of health care provider visits per year, as well as the largest consumption of prescription drugs (Eaton et al., 1996). To achieve the Healthy People 2000 objective of increased blood pressure control among clients with hypertension, nurses must be able to assess and intervene appropriately in the care of these clients.

Pathophysiology

The systemic arterial pressure is a product of the cardiac output and the total peripheral resistance (Fig. 38–2). Cardiac output is determined by stroke volume and heart rate. Control of peripheral resistance is maintained by the autonomic nervous system and circulating hormones, such as norepinephrine and epinephrine. Consequently, any factor producing an alteration in peripheral resistance, heart rate, or stroke volume affects the systemic arterial pressure.

TABLE 38–4

Stages of Hypertension		
Stage 1	Systolic, 140–159 mmHg Diastolic, 90–99 mmHg	
Stage 2	Systolic, 160–179 mmHg Diastolic, 100–109 mmHg	
Stage 3	Systolic, 180–209 mmHg Diastolic, 110–119 mmHg	
Stage 4	Systolic, ≥210 mmHg Diastolic, ≥120 mmHg	

From U.S. Department of Health and Human Services. (1993). *The Fifth Report of the Joint National Committee on Detection, Evaluation, and Treatment of High Blood Pressure* (NIH Publication). Washington, DC: U.S. Government Printing Office.

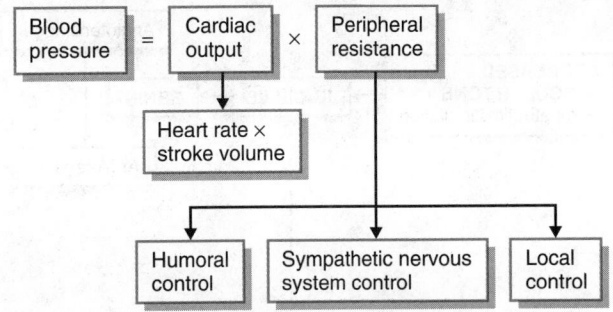

Figure 38–2. The components of blood pressure.

Regulation of Blood Pressure

Stabilizing mechanisms exist in the body to exert an overall regulation of systemic arterial pressure and to prevent circulatory collapse. Four control systems play a major role in maintaining blood pressure: the arterial baroreceptor system, regulation of body fluid volume, the renin-angiotensin-aldosterone system, and vascular autoregulation.

Arterial Baroreceptors

The arterial baroreceptors are found primarily in the carotid sinus but also in the aorta and the wall of the left ventricle. These baroreceptors monitor the level of arterial pressure. The baroreceptor system counteracts a rise in arterial pressure through vagally mediated cardiac slowing and vasodilation with decreased sympathetic tone. Therefore, reflex control of circulation elevates the systemic arterial pressure when it falls and lowers it when it rises. Why this control fails in hypertension is unknown. There is evidence for upward resetting of baroreceptor sensitivity so that pressure rises are inadequately sensed even though pressure decreases are not.

Regulation of Body Fluid Volume

Changes in fluid volume also affect the systemic arterial pressure. If there is an excess of salt and water in a person's body, the blood pressure rises through complex physiologic mechanisms that change the venous return to the heart, producing a rise in cardiac output. If the kidneys are functioning adequately, a rise in systemic arterial pressure produces diuresis and a fall in pressure. Pathologic conditions that change the pressure threshold at which the kidneys excrete salt and water alter the systemic arterial pressure.

Renin-Angiotensin-Aldosterone System

Renin, angiotensin, and aldosterone also regulate blood pressure (Fig. 38–3) (see also Chap. 14). The kidney produces renin, an enzyme that acts on a plasma protein substrate to split off angiotensin I, which is removed by a converting enzyme in the lung to form angiotensin II, then angiotensin III. Angiotensins II and III have strong vasoconstrictor action on blood vessels and are the controlling mechanism for aldosterone release. The signifi-

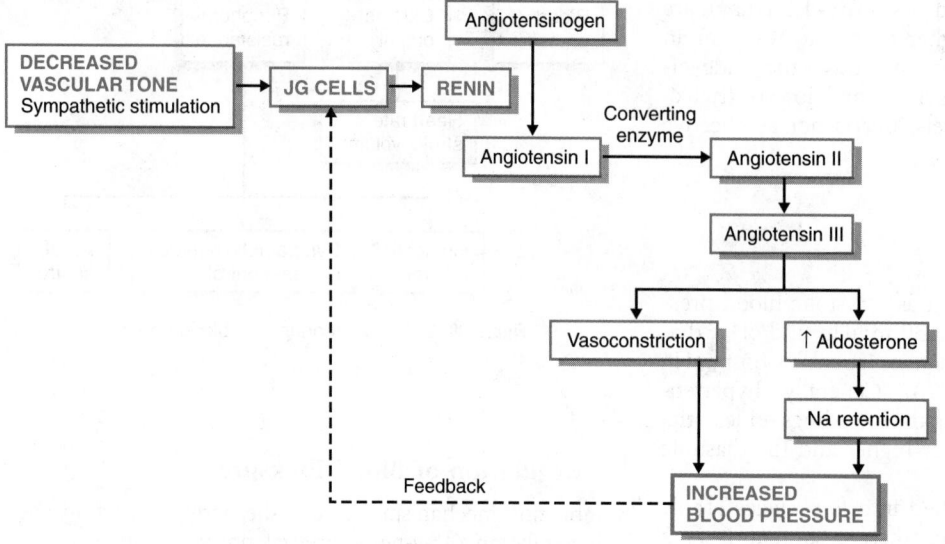

Figure 38–3. The effect of the renin-angiotensin system on blood pressure control. (From Copstead, L. E. C. [1995]. *Perspectives on Pathophysiology.* Philadelphia, W. B. Saunders.)

cance of aldosterone in hypertension is most evident in primary aldosteronism. By increasing the activity of the sympathetic nervous system, angiotensins II and III also appear to inhibit sodium excretion, resulting in an elevation in blood pressure.

Inappropriate secretion of renin may cause increased peripheral vascular resistance in essential (primary) hypertension. In high blood pressure, renin levels should be expected to fall because the increased renal arteriolar pressure should inhibit renin secretion. In most people with essential hypertension, however, renin levels are normal.

Vascular Autoregulation

The process of vascular autoregulation, which keeps perfusion of tissues in the body relatively constant, appears to be important in causing hypertension accompanying salt and water overload. This mechanism is poorly understood.

Complications of Hypertension

Sustained blood pressure elevation in clients with essential (primary) hypertension results in damage to blood vessels in vital organs. Essential hypertension produces medial hyperplasia (thickening) of the arterioles. As the blood vessels thicken and perfusion decreases, body organs are damaged; these changes can result in myocardial infarctions, cerebrovascular accidents, peripheral vascular disease, or renal failure.

Malignant hypertension is a severe type of elevated blood pressure that is rapidly progressive. A person with malignant hypertension usually has symptoms such as morning headaches, blurred vision, and dyspnea and/or symptoms of uremia (accumulation in the blood of substances ordinarily eliminated in the urine). Clients are often in their 30s, 40s, or 50s. The diastolic blood pressure is greater than 110 mmHg and frequently much higher, ranging from 130 to 170 mmHg. Unless interven-

tion occurs promptly, a client with malignant hypertension may experience renal failure, left ventricular failure, or stroke.

Etiology

Hypertension can be essential (primary) or secondary (Table 38–5). Essential hypertension accounts for 95% of all cases (Massie, 1995).

TABLE 38–5

Etiology of Hypertension

Essential (Primary)
- No known cause
- Associated risk factors
  - Family history of hypertension
  - High sodium intake
  - Excessive calorie consumption
  - Physical inactivity
  - Excessive alcohol intake
  - Low potassium intake

Secondary
- Renal vascular and renal parenchymal disease
- Primary aldosteronism
- Pheochromocytoma
- Cushing's disease
- Coarctation of the aorta
- Brain tumors
- Encephalitis
- Psychiatric disturbances
- Pregnancy
- Medications
  - Estrogen (e.g., oral contraceptives)
  - Glucocorticoids
  - Mineralocorticoids
  - Sympathomimetics

Essential Hypertension

Although there is no known cause for essential hypertension, several associated risk factors have been discovered on the basis of common characteristics of people with this disease:

- A family history of hypertension
- High sodium intake
- Excessive calorie consumption
- Physical inactivity
- Excessive alcohol intake
- Low potassium intake

A family history of hypertension is a major risk factor. In families with hypertension, there may be a defect in renal secretion of sodium or a heightened sympathetic nervous response to stress.

Secondary Hypertension

Specific disease states and medications can increase a person's susceptibility to hypertension; a person with this type of elevation in blood pressure has secondary hypertension.

Diseases

Renal vascular and renal parenchymal diseases are two of the most common causes of secondary hypertension. Hypertension can develop when there is any sudden damage to the kidneys. Renovascular hypertension is associated with narrowing of one or more of the main arteries carrying blood directly to the kidneys. Renal parenchymal diseases are related to infection, inflammation, and changes in kidney structure and function.

Dysfunction of the adrenal medulla or the adrenal cortex can cause secondary hypertension. Adrenal-mediated hypertension is due to primary excesses of aldosterone, cortisol, and catecholamines. In *primary aldosteronism,* excessive aldosterone causes hypertension and hypokalemia (low potassium levels). Primary aldosteronism usually arises from benign adenomas of the adrenal cortex. *Pheochromocytomas* originate most commonly in the adrenal medulla and result in excessive secretion of catecholamines. In *Cushing's syndrome,* excessive glucocorticoids are excreted from the adrenal cortex. The cause of Cushing's syndrome may be either adrenocortical hyperplasia or adrenocortical adenoma (see Chap. 66).

Coarctation of the aorta is a congenital narrowing of the aorta that may cause hypertension. Occurring at any level of the thoracic or abdominal aorta, the narrowing restricts blood flow through the aortic arch, resulting in an elevated blood pressure above the constriction. After surgical repair, the elevation in blood pressure eventually subsides.

Secondary hypertension is also associated with other neurogenic disturbances, such as brain tumors, encephalitis, and psychiatric disturbances.

Medications

Medications that can cause secondary hypertension include estrogen, glucocorticoids, mineralocorticoids, sympathomimetics, cyclosporine, and erythropoietin. The use of estrogen-containing oral contraceptives is probably the most common cause of secondary hypertension in women. Discontinuation of medications capable of causing hypertension often reverses this problem.

Incidence/Prevalence

It is estimated that 50 million Americans, or 1 in every 4 adults, have high blood pressure or are currently being treated for hypertension.

ELDERLY CONSIDERATIONS

As adults age they are more likely to develop hypertension (Massie, 1995). In fact, the most prevalent cardiovascular disease in the elderly is hypertension, which is a significant risk factor for death in that population (Matteson et al., 1997).

TRANSCULTURAL CONSIDERATIONS

In the United States, the incidence of hypertension among African-Americans is two times greater than that for Caucasians. Hypertension is more prevalent in African-Americans and Caucasians living in the southeastern United States than in African-Americans and Caucasians living in other parts of the country.

WOMEN'S HEALTH CONSIDERATIONS

African-American women have a higher incidence of hypertension than Caucasian women, Hispanic, women, Caucasian men, and African-American men. Studies are beginning to show that hypertension is being found in African-American teenage girls, especially those who are obese (Allen & Phillips, 1997).

Collaborative Management

 Assessment

➤ History

When obtaining the history, the nurse considers a client's risk factors for hypertension. The nurse ascertains the client's age; ethnic origin or race; family history of hypertension; average dietary intake of calories, sodium- and potassium-containing foods, and alcohol; and exercise habits. Past and present history of renal or cardiovascular disease and current use of medications are also assessed.

➤ Physical Assessment/Clinical Manifestations

When a diagnosis of hypertension is made, most clients have no symptoms; however, they may experience headaches, dizziness, or fainting as a result of the elevated blood pressure. The nurse obtains blood pressure readings in both of the client's arms. Two or more readings are taken at each visit, with the average reading obtained used as the value for the visit. To detect postural (orthostatic) changes, the nurse should also take readings with the client in the supine (lying) or sitting position and at least 2 minutes later with the client standing.

Funduscopic examination of the eyes is done by a skilled practitioner to observe vascular changes in the retina. The appearance of the retina can be a reliable index of the severity and prognosis of hypertension. The Keith-Wagener (KW) classification of retinal changes in hypertension is commonly used to stage changes:

- Stage I is characterized by minimal arteriolar narrowing.
- Stage II involves more marked narrowing of arterioles and arteriovenous nicking (changes at the arteriovenous crossings).
- Stage III shows circular or flame-shaped hemorrhages, fluffy "cotton wool" exudates.
- Stage IV, the most severe, is the same as stage III but with the addition of papilledema (malignant hypertension is always associated with papilledema).

Physical assessment is helpful in diagnosing several conditions that produce secondary hypertension. The presence of abdominal bruits is typical of clients with renovascular disease. Tachycardia, sweating, and pallor suggest pheochromocytoma or adrenal medulla tumor. Coarctation of the aorta is often characterized by elevation of blood pressure in the arms, with normal or low blood pressure in the lower extremities. Femoral pulses are also delayed or absent.

➤ Psychosocial Assessment

The nurse assesses for psychosocial stressors that can worsen the client's hypertension and that may affect the client's ability to collaborate in a treatment. Job-related, economic, and other life stressors are evaluated, as well as the client's response to these stressors.

Some clients may have difficulty coping with the lifestyle changes needed to control hypertension. The nurse assesses the coping strategies that the client has used in the past (see Chap. 8).

➤ Laboratory Assessment

Although no laboratory tests are diagnostic of essential hypertension, several laboratory tests can assess possible causes of secondary hypertension. The presence of protein, red blood cells, pus cells, and casts in the urine; elevated levels of blood urea nitrogen (BUN); and elevated serum creatinine levels indicate renal disease. In clients with a pheochromocytoma, a urinary test for the presence of catecholamines is positive. An elevation in levels of serum corticoids and 17-ketosteroids in the urine is diagnostic of Cushing's disease.

➤ Radiographic Assessment

No specific x-rays can diagnose hypertension. Routine chest radiography may be of assistance in recognizing left ventricular hypertrophy that results from hypertension.

Intravenous pyelography (IVP) is performed when clinical findings suggest renovascular hypertension. Renal arteriography is undertaken to establish the exact location and the extent of any lesions, the degree of obstruction, and the basic pathologic change in the renal arteries.

➤ Other Diagnostic Assessment

An electrocardiogram (ECG) is of value in determining the degree of cardiac involvement. Left atrial abnormality

is the first electrocardiographic sign of cardiac involvement resulting from hypertension.

 Analysis

➤ Common Nursing Diagnoses and Collaborative Problems

Common nursing diagnoses for a client with hypertension include

1. Knowledge Deficit related to information misinterpretation or unfamiliarity with information resources
2. Risk for Ineffective Management of Therapeutic Regime

➤ Additional Nursing Diagnoses and Collaborative Problems

The client may also have one or more of the following diagnoses:

- Altered Tissue Perfusion (renal, cerebral, cardiopulmonary, and peripheral) related to decreased blood flow
- Altered Nutrition: Risk for More than Body Requirements related to learned eating behaviors, ethnic and cultural values, lack of social support for weight loss, and/or imbalance between activity level and caloric intake
- Fatigue related to altered body chemistry (medications)
- Altered Sexuality Patterns related to effects of medical treatment (drugs)
- Ineffective Individual Coping related to effects of chronic illness and major changes in lifestyle
- Risk of Noncompliance with treatment regimen

The following collaborative problems may also occur in some clients with hypertension:

- Potential for Cerebrovascular Hemorrhage
- Potential for Retinal Hemorrhage

 Planning and Implementation

➤ Knowledge Deficit

Planning: Expected Outcomes. The client is expected to verbalize an understanding of the management of hypertension.

Interventions. For the client with essential hypertension, the nurse initially recommends the following lifestyle modifications:

- Sodium restriction
- Weight reduction
- Moderation of alcohol intake
- Exercise
- Relaxation techniques
- Tobacco avoidance

These modifications are considered the foundation of hypertension control. If these modifications are unsuccessful, the health care provider considers the use of antihypertensive drugs.

There is no surgical treatment for essential hypertension. However, surgery may be indicated for certain causes of secondary hypertension, such as renal vascular disease, coarctation of the aorta, and pheochromocytoma.

Sodium Restriction. In collaboration and consultation with the dietitian, the nurse advises all clients with hypertension to decrease their sodium chloride intake from the average of 150 mmol/L (150 mEq/L) to less than 100 mmol/L (100 mEq/L) each day (less than 2.3 g of sodium). To accomplish this goal, clients should avoid adding salt at the table, avoid cooking with salt, avoid adding seasonings that contain sodium, and limit eating canned, frozen, or other processed foods.

The dietitian reviews a 3-day dietary recall with the client to identify whether sodium intake has been excessive. In collaboration with the dietitian, the nurse suggests spices, herbs, fruits, and other non-salt-containing substances, such as powdered garlic and onion, to enhance the flavor of meat, chicken, seafood, and snacks. The nurse and dietitian instruct clients to read the labels on processed foods and to avoid those that are high in sodium. Salt substitutes are an alternative to salt, but the client needs a physician's order to use them. This order is necessary because salt substitutes are high in potassium, and the client may have hyperkalemia (high potassium levels) associated with a concomitant problem, such as renal impairment. Although hyperkalemia is unusual, it can also occur in clients who are taking potassium-sparing diuretics.

While salt is restricted, the client should include recommended daily allowances of potassium, calcium, and magnesium in the diet. Studies are not conclusive, but data suggest that low levels of these electrolytes are associated with high blood pressure.

Weight Reduction. If a client's weight is more than 10% above ideal, the nurse encourages the client to lose weight. The nurse discusses the rationale for reducing or maintaining weight and plans a weight-reducing diet with the dietitian and client. The nurse may then refer the client to a group or organization for weight reduction.

Because of the relationship of saturated fat and cholesterol to weight, a weight-reduction plan is formulated with the following limits:

- Total fat, less than 30% of daily caloric intake
- Saturated fat, less than 10%
- Cholesterol, less than 300 mg/day

Table 38–6 describes how to calculate grams of fat.

Moderation of Alcohol Intake. The nurse instructs clients to limit alcohol intake to no more than 1 oz of ethanol (2 oz of liquor, 8 oz of wine, 24 oz of beer) daily. The client is taught that alcohol consumption may elevate arterial blood pressure and can add "empty" calories.

Exercise. With the physician's approval and in collaboration with the physical therapist, the nurse can help the client develop a regular exercise program. The therapist usually recommends that the client perform regular aerobic exercise, such as brisk walking, running, cycling, swimming, or stair climbing, 30–45 minutes three to five times a week. The client should initiate exercise gradually and should stop and notify the physician if severe short-

TABLE 38–6

How to Determine Dietary Fat Limits

Procedure	Example
1. Begin with the number of calories consumed in a day	• 1800 kcal
2. Multiply the number of calories by 0.3 (30% of total calories) to determine the maximal number of calories that should be obtained from fat	• 1800 × 0.30 = 540 kcal/day from fat
3. Divide by 9 (1 g of fat contains 9 kcal) to determine the maximal number of grams of fat in the diet per day	• 540 ÷ 9 = 60 g/day of fat. To limit fat intake to no more than 30% of calories, the client must take in no more than 60 g of fat daily

ness of breath, fainting, or chest pain occurs. Clients should avoid muscle-building isometric exercise (weight lifting, wrestling, rowing) because it may raise blood pressure to dangerous levels.

Tobacco Avoidance. Although cigarette smoking is unrelated to hypertension, it is a major risk factor for cardiovascular disease. Therefore, the client who smokes is strongly urged to stop. With input from the nurse and physician, the client plans a smoking cessation program that best fits into his or her lifestyle. The nurse explains the nicotine patch and smoking cessation programs and implements follow-up to assess the client's plans for quitting (see earlier discussion of smoking cessation under Arteriosclerosis and Atherosclerosis).

Drug Therapy. Drug therapy is individualized for each client, with consideration given to the client's culture, age, concomitant illness, severity of blood pressure elevation, and cost of drugs and follow-up. Therapy may not be instituted for clients with diastolic readings between 90 and 94 mmHg because there is controversy about the advantage of treatment in this group.

Treatment of hypertension generally begins with a single drug. Once-a-day drug therapy is best, because the more doses required each day, the higher the risk that a client will not follow the treatment regimen. Several classifications of medications are available to control hypertension. Examples of commonly used drugs are listed in Chart 38–2.

Diuretics. Three basic types of diuretics are used to decrease blood volume and lower blood pressure:

- Thiazide diuretics, such as hydrochlorothiazide (HydroDIURIL, Urozide✦), prevent sodium and water reabsorption in the distal tubules while promoting potassium excretion.
- Loop (high-ceiling) diuretics, such as furosemide (Lasix, Furoside✦), depress sodium reabsorption in the ascending loop of Henle and promote potassium excretion

Chart 38–2

Drug Therapy for Hypertension

Drug	Usual Dosage	Nursing Interventions	Rationale
Diuretics			
Thiazides			
Chlorothiazide (Diuril)	• 125–500 mg/day	• Monitor potassium levels and watch for muscle weakness or irregular pulse.	• Hypokalemia is a common occurrence.
Hydrochlorothiazide (Esidrix, HydroDIURIL)	• 12.5–50 mg/day	• Encourage intake of foods high in potassium (e.g., bananas and orange juice).	• Depleted potassium needs to be replaced.
Loop Diuretics			
Furosemide (Lasix, Furoside✶)	• 20–40 mg/day	• Same as for thiazide diuretics.	• Same as for chlorothiazide.
Ethacrynic acid (Edecrin)	• 25–100 mg/day		
Potassium-Sparing Diuretics			
Spironolactone (Aldactone)	• 25–100 mg/day	• Monitor potassium levels and watch for muscle weakness or irregular pulse.	• Hypokalemia or hyperkalemia may occur.
Triamterone (Dyrenium)	• 50–100 mg/day		
Beta-Blocking Agents			
Propranolol (Inderal, Apo-Propranolol✶)	• 40–240 mg/day	• Monitor pulse rate.	• A drop in pulse is expected, and bradycardia may occur.
Atenolol (Tenormin)	• 25–100 mg once a day		
Nadolol (Cogard)	• 20–240 mg/day	• Watch for shortness of breath or cough.	• Bronchospasm caused by blockage of beta-receptors in the lungs may occur.
Metoprolol (Lopressor)	• 50–200 mg/day		
		• Instruct client to report any difficulty in sexual function, fatigue, weakness, or depression.	• Although these are common side effects, newer beta-blocking agents may be more "selective" in terms of side effects.
		• Instruct clients with diabetes to monitor blood glucose levels.	• Hypoglycemic symptoms may be blocked in clients taking beta-blocking agents.
Calcium Channel Blockers			
Nifedipine (Procardia, Adalat)	• 10–30 mg tid	• Monitor blood pressure.	• A drop in blood pressure occurs within 30 min after oral administration.
		• Assess for dizziness.	
		• Assess lower extremities.	• Pedal edema can occur as a result of peripheral vasodilation.

■ Potassium-sparing diuretics, such as spironolactone (Aldactone, Norospiroton✶), act on the distal tubule to inhibit reabsorption of sodium ions in exchange for potassium, thereby retaining potassium.

Diuretics are the drugs of choice for clients who have asthma, chronic airway limitation, and chronic renal disease and for selected clients with congestive heart failure. They are particularly effective for African-American clients.

Diuretics are relatively inexpensive, and adherence to the medication regimen is enhanced because the drug can usually be prescribed on a once-a-day or, at most, a twice-a-day schedule. However, the frequent voiding that occurs after a person takes a diuretic may interfere with one's daily activities. The most frequent side effect associated with diuretics is hypokalemia (low potassium levels). The nurse monitors the client's serum potassium level and assesses for signs and symptoms of irregular pulse and muscle weakness, which may indicate hypokalemia. The nurse advises clients receiving potassium-depleting diuretics to eat foods high in potassium, such as bananas and orange juice. However, the client may need a potas-

Chart 38–2. Drug Therapy for Hypertension   Continued

Drug	Usual Dosage	Nursing Interventions	Rationale
Verapamil (Calan, Isoptin)	• 40–80 mg q8h, 240 mg SR once a day	• Monitor blood pressure and pulse. • Encourage intake of foods high in fiber.	• Hypotension and decreased heart rate may occur. • Constipation is a common side effect.
Diltiazem hydrochloride (Cardizem)	• 30–60 mg q8h	• Monitor blood pressure and pulse.	• Hypotension and decreased heart rate may occur.
Angiotension-Converting-Enzyme Inhibitors			
Captopril (Capoten)	• 6.25 mg tid initially, increased to 50 mg tid	• Instruct client to stay in bed for 3 hr after the first dose.	• Severe hypotension may follow the first dose.
Enalapril (Vasotec)	• 2.5 mg/d initially, increased to 10–40 mg/day	• Monitor blood pressure.	• Hypotension needs to be detected promptly.
Lisinopril/Zestil (Prinvil)	• 5 mg/d initially, increased to 10–40 mg/day	• Monitor renal function tests.	
Central Alpha Agonists			
Clonidine hydrochloride (Catapres)	• 0.1–1.2 mg h.s. or 0.1–0.3 mg once a week transdermally	• Administer at bedtime. • Instruct client to report rash associated with transdermal route.	• Sedation is a common side effect. • Bothersome skin rashes occur in about 25% of clients using transdermal patch.
Methyldopa (Aldomet)	• 250–500 mg qid	• Instruct client to sit on the side of the bed for several minutes before arising and to avoid changing position suddenly. • Warn clients that sedation can occur when drug is initiated and dose is increased. • Instruct male clients to report any difficulty in sexual functions.	• Postural hypotension is a common complication. • This information can assist clients in planning activity and rest periods. • Impotence is a common side effect.
Vasodilators			
Hydralazine (Apresoline)	• 10–50 mg qid	• Monitor pulse rate.	• Tachycardia may occur as a result of reflex increase in sympathetic activity.
Alpha$_1$-receptor blockers Doxazosin (Cardura)	• 1.0–16 mg/day	• Monitor blood pressure.	• A drop in blood pressure can occur between 2 and 6 h after initial dose or dose increases.
Terazosin (Hytrin)	• 1.0–20 mg/day	• Assess for dizziness.	• Give first dose at bedtime to avoid postural hypotension.

sium supplement to maintain adequate serum potassium levels (see Chap. 16). The nurse assesses clients taking potassium-sparing diuretics for hypokalemia and hyperkalemia. Both of these electrolyte disturbances are characterized by weakness and irregular pulse.

Beta-Adrenergic Blocking Agents. Beta-blockers lower blood pressure by blocking beta-receptors in the heart and peripheral vessels, reducing cardiac rate and output. By blocking beta-adrenergic receptors in the heart, beta-blockers cause a decrease in heart rate and decreased contractility. Bradycardia (slow heart rate) and heart fail-

ure may result. Beta-blockers can also prohibit bronchodilation by blocking beta-receptors in the lungs. Therefore, clients with a history of asthma or bronchospasm are generally not given these drugs, and all clients taking these drugs must be monitored for shortness of breath and wheezing.

Common side effects of beta-blockers include fatigue, weakness, depression, and sexual dysfunction, although the potential for side effects depends on the "selective" blocking effects of the drug. A variety of beta-blockers are available, and they differ from each other in terms of their cardioselectivity (primarily beta$_1$ effects, with less beta$_2$ effects), lipid solubility, and sympathomimetic activity throughout the body.

Diabetic clients who take beta-blockers may not have the usual signs and symptoms of hypoglycemia because the sympathetic nervous system is blocked. Counterregulatory responses to hypoglycemia, such as gluconeogenesis, may also be inhibited by certain beta-blockers.

Calcium Channel-Blocking Agents. Calcium channel blockers, such as verapamil hydrochloride (Calan), nifedipine (Procardia, Adalat), and diltiazem (Cardizem), lower blood pressure by interfering with the transmembrane flux of calcium ions, resulting in reduced vasoconstriction.

TRANSCULTURAL CONSIDERATIONS

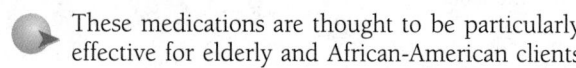

These medications are thought to be particularly effective for elderly and African-American clients.

Verapamil and diltiazem can affect atrial-ventricular conduction and often lower the heart rate. Oral nifedipine can reduce blood pressure quickly, often decreasing blood pressure by 25% within 30 minutes. Sublingual administration of nifedipine, given by puncturing the capsule and placing the liquid contents under the tongue, acts within 10–15 minutes.

Angiotensin-Converting Enzyme Inhibitors. Angiotensin-converting enzyme (ACE) inhibitors are also used as single or combination agents in the treatment of hypertension. The angiotensin-converting enzyme converts angiotensin I to angiotensin II, one of the most powerful vasoconstrictors in the body. ACE inhibitors include captopril (Capoten), enalapril (Vasotec), and lisinopril (Prinivil).

The client receiving an ACE inhibitor for the first time is instructed to stay in bed for 3–4 hours to avoid the severe hypotensive effect that can occur with initial use. The nurse monitors the client's blood pressure every 15 minutes after this first dose. *Postural (orthostatic) hypotension* may occur with subsequent doses, but it is less severe. The nurse checks for postural hypotension by taking the blood pressure when the client is lying, sitting, and standing. If there is a significant decrease in the systolic blood pressure (<20 mmHg), the nurse notifies the physician.

ELDERLY CONSIDERATIONS

The elderly client is at the greatest risk for postural hypotension because of the cardiovascular changes associated with aging (Chart 38–3).

TRANSCULTURAL CONSIDERATIONS

ACE inhibitors are most effective in young Caucasian adults. They are less effective in African-American clients or older adults.

Central Alpha Agonists. Central alpha agonists act on the central nervous system, preventing reuptake of norepinephrine, resulting in a lowering of peripheral vascular

---

Chart 38–3

Nursing Care Highlights: Assessment and Interventions for Hypertensive Crisis

Assess
- Severe headache
- Extremely high blood pressure
- Dizziness
- Blurred vision
- Disorientation

Intervene
- Place client in a semi-Fowler's position
- Administer oxygen
- Administer IV nitroprusside (Nitropress) or other infusion drug as ordered (for nitroprusside, cover infusion bag to prevent drug breakdown by light)
- Monitor the blood pressure every 5 to 15 minutes until the diastolic pressure is also below 90 and not less than 75; then monitor blood pressure every 30 minutes
- Observe for neurologic or cardiovascular complications, such as seizures; numbness, weakness, or tingling of extremities; dysrhythmias; or chest pain

---

resistance and blood pressure. Common central alpha agonists include clonidine (Catapres) and methyldopa (Aldomet, Apo-Methyldopa✦). Methyldopa can cause unique side effects, such as hemolytic anemia and inflammatory disorders of the liver, although they happen rarely. Because of this potential, clonidine is the more commonly used central alpha agonist. Clonidine can also be given as a transdermal patch, providing control of blood pressure for as long as 7 days. Side effects common to clonidine and methyldopa include sedation, postural hypotension, and impotence.

Vasodilators. Vasodilators lower blood pressure by relaxing vascular smooth muscle tone, thus reducing total peripheral resistance. Vasodilators include minoxidil (Loniten), nitroglycerin (Nitro-Bid), and nitroprusside (Nitropress).

Alpha-Adrenergic Receptor Agonists. Alpha-adrenergic agonists, such as prazosin (Minipress), dilate the arterioles and veins. These drugs can lower blood pressure quickly, but their use is limited because of frequent and bothersome side effects.

The Joint National Committee on Detection, Evaluation, and Treatment of High Blood Pressure (1993) has recommended that initial therapy for hypertension include either a thiazide diuretic or a beta-blocker unless these drugs are contraindicated or ineffective or there are special indications for agents such as calcium antagonists or ACE inhibitors. If after 1–3 months a client's blood pressure does not decrease adequately in response to initial therapy, the health care provider may increase the dose of the drug, substitute a drug from another class of antihypertensives, or add a second drug from another class.

Because of changes in recommendations and the availability of more drug options and more information on drug tolerance, the nurse sees a variety of drug protocols used by the health care provider to meet the individual needs of clients with hypertension.

➤ Risk for Ineffective Management of Therapeutic Regimen

Planning: Expected Outcomes. The client is expected to adhere to the therapeutic regimen, thus minimizing the risk of target organ damage.

Interventions. Clients who require pharmacologic treatment to control essential hypertension usually need to take medication for the rest of their lives. Frequently, though, clients stop taking antihypertensive medications because they have no symptoms. They may also discontinue medication because of cost or side effects.

In collaboration with the pharmacist, the nurse and client discuss the goals of therapy, including potential side effects, to help the client identify potential problems. The nurse then assists the client in tailoring the therapeutic regimen to the client's activities of daily living

Clients who do not comply with antihypertensive treatment are at great risk for target organ damage and hypertensive crisis (malignant hypertension). Clients in hypertensive crisis are admitted to critical care units, where they receive intravenous antihypertensive therapy such as nitroprusside (Nitropress), nitroglycerin (Nitro-Bid, Tridil IV), labetalol (Normodyne), diazoxide (Hyperstat), or sublingual nifedipine (Procardia, Adalat) (Chart 38–4). Hospitalization for complications of hypertension can be financially costly in both medical expenses and lost income.

 Continuing Care

Clients who require pharmacologic treatment to control essential hypertension usually need to take medication for the rest of their lives. Studies have shown that within the first year of therapy, over 50% of clients discontinue their treatment (Eaton et al., 1996). Frequently, clients stop taking antihypertensive medications, assuming that because they have no symptoms the hypertension is under control. Clients may assume that if their blood pressure returns to normal levels with antihypertensives, they no longer need them. Clients may also stop taking antihypertensives because of adverse side effects or cost.

➤ Home Care Management

If possible, the client should obtain a blood pressure monitor for use at home so that the pressure can be checked periodically. The nurse evaluates the client's ability to learn how to check his or her blood pressure. If the client cannot monitor blood pressure, a family member or significant other may be taught how to perform this procedure.

If weight reduction is a goal, the nurse suggests that the client have a scale in the home for weight monitoring.

➤ Health Teaching

The nurse instructs the client about sodium restriction, weight maintenance or reduction, alcohol restriction, stress management, and exercise (see earlier discussion). If necessary, the nurse also explains about the need to stop smoking. The elderly can also benefit from lifestyle modifications (Matteson et al., 1997) (see Chart 38–4).

For clients taking medication for hypertension, the nurse provides oral and written information about the indications, dosage, times of administration, side effects, and drug interactions (see Chart 38–2). The nurse stresses that the medication must be taken as prescribed and that, when all of it has been consumed, the prescription must be renewed on a continual basis. Abrupt discontinuation of medications, such as beta-blockers, can result in angina (chest pain) or myocardial infarction.

The nurse also urges clients to report unpleasant side effects, such as sexual dysfunction. In many instances, an alternative medication can be prescribed to minimize certain side effects.

Hypertension is a chronic illness, and clients may not be prepared to accept this fact. The nurse allows clients to verbalize feelings about this disease and its treatment. Clients are advised that their involvement in the treatment can lead to control of this disease and can prevent complications.

➤ Health Care Resources

A home health nurse may be needed for follow-up to monitor blood pressure. The nurse evaluates the ability of the client or the family to obtain accurate blood pressure measurements and assesses their compliance with treatment. If clients cannot purchase equipment to monitor

---

Chart 38–4

Nursing Focus on the Elderly: Hypertension

- Before initiating drug therapy, obtain blood pressure measurements with the client lying, sitting, and standing to assess for postural changes.
- Monitor the client's standing blood pressure during treatment.
- Instruct the client to avoid caffeine and nicotine for 1 hour before blood pressure measurements to obtain accurate readings.
- Teach the client that dizziness is a symptom of hypotension that should be reported.
- Instruct clients how to avoid orthostatic (postural) hypotension by avoiding sudden changes in position. Clients should arise from bed in three stages: sit in bed for 1 minute; sit on the side of the bed with legs dangling for 1 minute; stand, holding onto a nonmovable object for 1 minute before walking. Clients should also be cautious about heat exposure (hot tub), alcohol intake, and exercise, which can lead to orthostatic hypotension.

blood pressure, the nurse may suggest the American Heart Association, the Red Cross, or a local pharmacy for free blood pressure checks.

 Evaluation

On the basis of the identified nursing diagnoses and collaborative problems, the nurse evaluates the care of the hypertensive client. The expected outcomes are that the client will:

- Explain the rationale for treatment of hypertension
- Maintain blood pressure of less than 130/85 mmHg
- Demonstrate no signs or symptoms of target organ damage, such as renal or heart disease

Peripheral Arterial Disease

Overview

Peripheral vascular disease (PVD) includes disorders that alter the natural flow of blood through the arteries and veins of the peripheral circulation. PVD affects the lower extremities much more frequently than the upper extremities. Generally, a client with a diagnosis of PVD has arterial disease (peripheral arterial disease) rather than venous involvement. Some clients have both arterial and venous disease.

Pathophysiology

Peripheral arterial disease (PAD) is a chronic condition in which partial or total arterial occlusion deprives the lower extremities of oxygen and nutrients. PAD of the lower extremities is sometimes referred to as lower extremity arterial disease (LEAD). Body tissues cannot live without an adequate oxygen and nutrient supply, and tissue eventually dies. Atherosclerosis is the most common cause of chronic altered blood flow. Fatty substances accumulate at the site of vessel wall injury and alter or totally occlude blood flow within the arteries. Tissue damage generally occurs below the arterial obstruction.

Obstructions are classified as inflow or outflow, according to the arteries involved and their relationship to the inguinal ligament (Fig. 38–4). *Inflow* obstructions involve the distal end of the aorta and the common, internal, and external iliac arteries. They are located above the inguinal ligament. *Outflow* obstructions involve infrainguinal arterial segments (the femoral, popliteal, and tibial arteries) and are below the superficial femoral artery (SFA). Gradual inflow occlusions may not cause significant tissue damage; gradual outflow occlusions typically do.

Etiology

Because atherosclerosis is the most common cause of chronic arterial obstruction, the risk factors for atherosclerosis apply to peripheral arterial disease as well. These

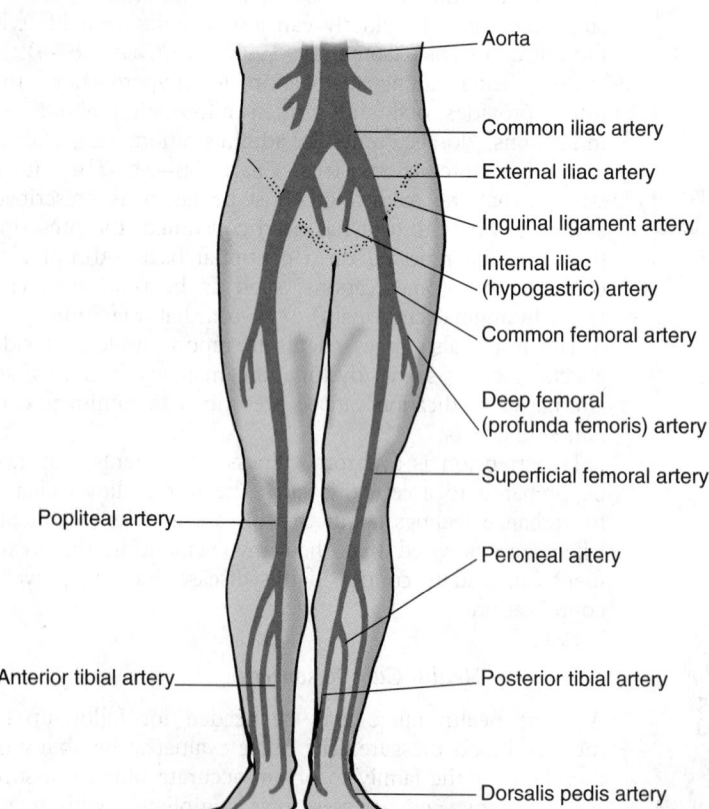

Figure 38–4. Common locations of inflow and outflow lesion.

Labels in figure:
- Aorta
- Common iliac artery
- External iliac artery
- Inguinal ligament artery
- Internal iliac (hypogastric) artery
- Common femoral artery
- Deep femoral (profunda femoris) artery
- Superficial femoral artery
- Popliteal artery
- Peroneal artery
- Anterior tibial artery
- Posterior tibial artery
- Dorsalis pedis artery

include hypertension, hyperlipidemia, diabetes mellitus, cigarette smoking, obesity, and familial predisposition. Advancing age also increases the risk of disease related to atherosclerosis.

Incidence/Prevalence

In the United States, at least 10% of people over age 70 years and 1%–2% of people aged 37–69 years have symptomatic, chronic peripheral arterial disease (American Heart Association, 1995). PAD generally occurs in men older than age 45 years and in postmenopausal women.

Collaborative Management

 Assessment

➤ History

The clinical course of chronic peripheral arterial disease (PAD) can be divided into four stages (Chart 38–5). Clients do not experience symptoms in the early stages of disease.

Pain Assessment. Most clients initially seek treatment for a characteristic leg pain known as *intermittent claudication* (a term derived from a word meaning "to limp"). Usually, clients can walk only a certain distance before a cramping, burning muscle discomfort or pain forces them to stop. The pain subsides after rest. When clients resume walking, they can walk the same distance before the pain returns. The pain is thus considered reproducible. As the disease progresses, clients can walk only shorter and shorter distances before pain recurs. Ultimately, pain may occur even while clients are at rest. The nurse questions the client about the nature and characteristics of leg pain to determine whether the client may be experiencing intermittent claudication.

Rest pain, which may begin while the disease is still primarily in the stage of intermittent claudication, is a numbness or burning, often described as feeling like a toothache, that is severe enough to awaken clients at night. It is usually located in the distal portion of the extremities—in the toes, the foot arches, the forefeet, and the heels—rarely in the calves or ankles. Clients can sometimes achieve pain relief by keeping the limb in a dependent position. Clients with rest pain have advanced disease that may result in limb loss.

Inflow and Outflow Disease. Clients with *inflow* disease experience discomfort in the lower back, buttocks, or thighs. Lower back or buttock discomfort indicates obstruction at or above the common iliac artery or abdominal aorta. Thigh discomfort indicates obstruction at or above the profunda femoris artery.

Clients with *mild* inflow disease experience discomfort after walking about two blocks. This discomfort is not severe but causes the client to stop walking. It is relieved with rest.

Clients with *moderate* inflow disease experience pain in these areas after walking about one or two blocks. The discomfort is described more like pain, but it subsides with rest most of the time.

Severe inflow disease causes the client severe pain after walking less than one block. These clients usually have rest pain.

Clients with *outflow* disease describe burning or cramping in the calves, ankles, feet, and toes. Calf discomfort usually indicates arterial obstruction at or below the superficial femoral or popliteal artery. Instep or foot discomfort indicates an obstruction below the popliteal artery.

The nurse asks specific questions about when the pain occurs and whether it occurs at rest.

Clients with *mild* outflow disease experience discomfort after walking about five blocks. This discomfort is relieved by rest.

Clients with *moderate* outflow disease have pain after walking about two blocks. Intermittent rest pain may be present.

Clients with *severe* outflow disease are usually unable to walk more than one-half block and usually experience rest pain. They may hang their feet off the bed at night for comfort.

Clients with outflow disease complain more frequently of rest pain than do clients with inflow disease.

WOMEN'S HEALTH CONSIDERATIONS

 Women suffer serious problems related to peripheral vascular disease of the lower extremities after

---

Chart 38–5

Key Features of Chronic Peripheral Arterial Disease

Stage I: Asymptomatic
- No claudication is present.
- Bruit or aneurysm may be present.
- Pedal pulses are decreased or absent.

Stage II: Claudication
- Muscle pain, cramping, or burning occurs with exercise and is relieved with rest.
- Symptoms are reproducible with exercise.

Stage III: Rest Pain
- Pain while resting commonly awakens the client at night.
- Pain is described as numbness, burning, toothache-type pain.
- Pain usually occurs in the distal portion of the extremity—toes, arch, forefoot, or heel—rarely in the calf or the ankle.
- Pain is relieved by placing the extremity in a dependent position.

Stage IV: Necrosis/Gangrene
- Ulcers and blackened tissue occur on the toes, the forefoot, and the heel.
- Distinctive gangrenous odor is present.

menopause. In fact, 25% of women aged 55–74 years develop peripheral vascular disease (Gerhard et al., 1995). The major risk factors for women with PVD are cigarette smoking, diabetes mellitus, hypertension, hyperlipidemia, and menopause.

Conservative treatment for women includes exercise training and quitting smoking. Estrogen replacement therapy and cholesterol-lowering drugs may slow the development of arteriosclerosis in the lower extremities in women. Women appear to be at higher risk for amputation than men and should be encouraged to adhere to conservative therapy recommendations to prevent progression of the disease.

➤ Physical Assessment/Clinical Manifestations

Specific findings for peripheral arterial disease (PAD) depend on the severity of the disease. The nurse may observe loss of hair on the lower calf, ankle, and foot; dry, scaly, dusky, pale, or mottled skin; and thickened toenails. With severe arterial disease, the extremity is cold and gray-blue (cyanotic) or darkened. The nurse may also note elevational pallor and dependent rubor. Muscle atrophy can accompany prolonged chronic arterial disease.

The nurse palpates all pulses in both legs. The most sensitive and specific indicator of arterial function is the quality of the posterior tibial pulse. The pedal pulse is not palpable in a small percentage of people. The strength of the pulse should be compared bilaterally. Several scales are available for grading pulse strength. A popular system is presented in Table 38–7.

The nurse may also note early signs of ulcer formation or complete ulcer formation, a complication of peripheral arterial disease. The nurse must differentiate arterial and venous stasis ulcers from diabetic ulcers, which may have a different cause (Chart 38–6).

Initally, *arterial* ulcers are painful and develop on the toes (often the great toe), between the toes, or on the upper aspect of the foot. With prolonged occlusion, the toe(s) can become gangrenous. *Diabetic* ulcers develop on the plantar surface of the foot, over the metatarsal heads, and on the heel—anywhere that pressure is exerted. Diabetic ulcers may not be painful because of diabetic neuropathy. *Venous stasis* ulcers cause minimal pain and occur in the ankle area. The foot is warm, and distal pulses are palpable. The nurse notes discoloration of the lower extremity at the ulcer site. (Skin lesions are discussed in further detail in Chapter 70.)

TRANSCULTURAL CONSIDERATIONS

In clients with dark skin, the soles of the feet and the toenails enable the nurse to detect cyanosis or duskiness in the lower extremities because these areas are less pigmented.

➤ Radiographic Assessment

The most common x-ray for peripheral arterial disease is arteriography of the lower extremities. Because arteriography involves injecting contrast medium into the arterial system, the risks, which include hemorrhage, thrombosis, embolus, and death, are serious. Arteriography is often performed before surgery to pinpoint the exact location of the occlusion. The nurse prepares the client for the procedure and carefully implements follow-up care (see Chap. 35).

➤ Other Diagnostic Assessment

The advent of noninvasive evaluation of arterial disease has become a popular method of diagnosis. Noninvasive testing provides information about the arterial system with minimal risk to the client.

Segmental Systolic Blood Pressure Measurements. Segmental systolic blood pressure measurements of the lower extremities at the thigh, calf, and ankle are a noninvasive method of assessing peripheral arterial disease (PAD). Normally, blood pressure readings in the thigh and calf are higher than those in the upper extremities. With the presence of arterial disease, these pressures are lower than the brachial pressure.

With *inflow* disease, pressures taken at the thigh level indicate the severity of disease. Mild inflow disease may cause a difference of only 10–30 mmHg in pressure on the affected side compared with the brachial pressure. Severe inflow disease can cause a pressure difference of greater than 40–50 mmHg. The ankle pressure is normally equal to or greater than the brachial pressure.

To evaluate *outflow* disease, the nurse compares ankle pressure with the brachial pressure, which provides a ratio known as the *ankle/brachial index* (ABI). This value can be derived by dividing the ankle blood pressure by the brachial blood pressure.

With mild outflow disease, the client has an ankle/brachial index of 0.8–1.0; pressures are decreased by about 10 to 30 mmHg. The client with moderate outflow disease has an ankle/brachial index of 0.5–0.8, with pressure differences of 20–40 mmHg. An ankle/brachial index less than 0.5 indicates severe outflow disease.

Exercise Tolerance Testing. Exercise tolerance testing (by stress test or treadmill) may give valuable information

TABLE 38–7

Pulse Grading Scale	
Value	**Characteristic**
0	No detectable pulse (0/4)
1	Pulse thready, weak, difficult to detect; may fade in and out, easily obliterated by pressure (1/4)
2	Pulse difficult to palpate, hypokinetic, and may be obliterated by pressure; light palpation recommended (2/4)
3	Pulse easily palpable, not easily obliterated by pressure; considered normal in volume (3/4)
4	Pulse strong, bounding, hyperkinetic, easily palpated, not obliterated by pressure; may be pathologic if aortic regurgitation is present (4/4)

Chart 38–6

Key Features of Lower Extremity Ulcers

Feature	Arterial Ulcers	Venous Ulcers	Diabetic Ulcers
History	Client complains of claudication after walking approximately 1–2 blocks Rest pain usually present Pain at ulcer site Two or three risk factors present	Chronic nonhealing ulcer No claudication or rest pain Moderate ulcer discomfort Client complains about ankle or leg swelling	Diabetes Peripheral neuropathy No complaints of claudication
Ulcer location and appearance	End of the toes Between the toes Deep Ulcer bed pale, with even edges Little granulation tissue	Ankle area Brown pigmentation Ulcer bed pink Usually superficial, with uneven edges Granulation tissue present	Plantar area of foot Metatarsal heads Pressure points on feet Deep Pale, with even edges Little granulation tissue
	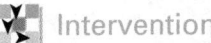		
Other assessment findings	Cool or cold foot Decreased or absent pulses Atrophy of skin Hair loss Pallor with elevation Dependent rubor Possible gangrene When acute, neurologic deficits noted	Ankle discoloration and edema Full veins when leg slightly dependent No neurologic deficit Pulses present May have scarring from previous ulcers	Pulses usually present Cool or warm foot Painless
Treatment	Treat underlying cause (surgical, revascularization) Prevent trauma and infection Client education, stressing foot care	Long-term wound care (Unna boot, damp-to-dry dressings) Elevate extremity Client education Prevent infection	Rule out major arterial disease Control diabetes Client education regarding foot care Prevent infection

Photographs of arterial ulcer and diabetic ulcer from Callen, J. P., Greer, K. E., Hood, A. F., Paller, A. S., & Swinyer, L. J. (1993). *Color atlas of dermatology: Slide set.* Philadelphia: W. B. Saunders.

about clients who are experiencing claudication (muscle pain) without rest pain. The nurse or technician obtains resting pulse volume recordings and has the client walk on a treadmill until the symptoms are reproduced. At the time of symptom onset or after approximately 5 minutes, the nurse or technician obtains another pulse volume recording. Normally, there may be an increased waveform with minimal, if any, drop in the ankle pressures. In clients with arterial disease, the waveforms are decreased (dampened) and there is a decrease in the ankle pressure of the affected limb of 40–60 mmHg for 20–30 seconds. If the return to normal pressure is delayed (longer than 10 minutes), the results suggest abnormal arterial flow in the affected limb.

Plethysmography. Plethysmography can also be performed to evaluate arterial flow in the lower extremities. This measurement provides graph or tracing readings of arterial flow in the limb. If an occlusion is present, the waveforms are dampened to flattened, depending on the degree of occlusion.

Interventions

The nurse first determines whether the altered tissue perfusion is of arterial or venous origin. An accurate assessment often provides this information, but in some people both conditions may exist. In this case, each disease must be considered separately when appropriate interventions are planned.

➤ Nonsurgical Management

The interventions of exercise, position changes, promotion of vasodilation, drug therapy, and invasive nonsurgical procedures are used to increase arterial flow to the affected limb.

Exercise. Exercise may improve arterial blood flow to the affected limb through build up of the *collateral* circulation. (Collateral circulation provides blood to the affected area through smaller vessels that develop and compensate for the occluded vessels.) Exercise is individualized for each client, but people with severe rest pain, venous ulcers, or gangrene should not participate. Other clients with peripheral arterial disease (PAD) can benefit from exercise that is initiated gradually and is slowly increased; an excellent exercise for these clients is walking. The nurse instructs the client to walk until the point of claudication, stop and rest, then walk a little farther. Eventually, clients are able to walk longer distances as collateral circulation develops. The nurse collaborates with the health care provider and physical therapist in determining an appropriate exercise program.

Positioning. Positioning of the client to promote circulation has been somewhat controversial. Some clients have swelling in their extremities. Because swelling prevents arterial flow, these clients should elevate their feet at rest, but the nurse teaches clients to refrain from raising their legs above the heart level. Extreme elevation *slows* arterial blood flow to the feet.

In severe cases, clients with PAD and swelling may sleep with the affected limb hanging from the bed, or they may sit upright in a chair for comfort. The nurse instructs all clients with PAD to avoid crossing their legs, which may interfere with blood flow.

Promoting Vasodilation. Vasodilation can be achieved by providing warmth to the affected extremity and preventing long periods of exposure to cold. The nurse encourages the client to maintain a warm environment at home and to wear socks or insulated shoes at all times. The client is cautioned *never* to apply direct heat to the limb, such as with the use of heating pads or extremely hot water. Sensitivity is decreased in the affected limb, and the client may get burned without feeling it.

The nurse encourages clients to prevent exposure of the affected limb to the cold because cold temperatures cause vasoconstriction (decreasing of the diameter of the blood vessels) and therefore decrease arterial blood flow. Emotional stress, caffeine, and nicotine also can cause vasoconstriction. The nurse emphasizes that complete abstinence from smoking or chewing tobacco is the most effective method of preventing vasoconstriction. The vasoconstrictive effects of each cigarette may last up to 1 hour after the cigarette is smoked.

Drug Therapy. For clients with chronic peripheral arterial disease (PAD), prescribed drugs include hemorrheologic and antiplatelet agents. Pentoxifylline (Trental) is a hemorrheologic agent that increases the flexibility of red blood cells; it decreases blood viscosity by inhibiting platelet aggregation and decreasing fibrinogen and thus increases blood flow in the extremities. Many clients report limited improvement in their daily lives after taking pentoxifylline. Moreover, clients with extremely limited endurance for walking have reported improvement to the point that they can perform some activities (e.g., walk to the mailbox or dining room) that were previously impossible.

Two commonly used drugs for clients with PAD are the antiplatelet agents, such as aspirin (acetylsalicylic acid, Ancasal✚), and dipyridamole (Persantine, Apo-Dipyridamole✚). Aspirin, 325 mg/day, is typically recommended for life for all clients with chronic PAD.

Controlling hypertension can improve tissue perfusion by maintaining pressures that are adequate to perfuse the periphery but not vasoconstrict the vessels. Nurses should make clients aware of the effect of blood pressure on the circulation and should instruct clients in methods of control. For example, clients taking beta-blockers may experience drug-related claudication or an exacerbation of their symptoms. The physician, Nurse Practitioner, and/or nurse closely monitor clients with PAD who are receiving beta-blockers.

Percutaneous Transluminal Angioplasty. Another nonsurgical but invasive method of improving arterial flow is percutaneous transluminal balloon angioplasty (PTBA) (Fig. 38–5). One or more arteries are dilated with a balloon catheter advanced through a cannula, which is inserted into or above an occluded or stenosed artery. When the procedure is successful, it opens the vessel lumen and improves arterial blood flow, creating a smooth inner vessel surface. Clients who are candidates for PTBA must have occlusions or stenoses that are accessible to the catheter. The physician often uses PTA for

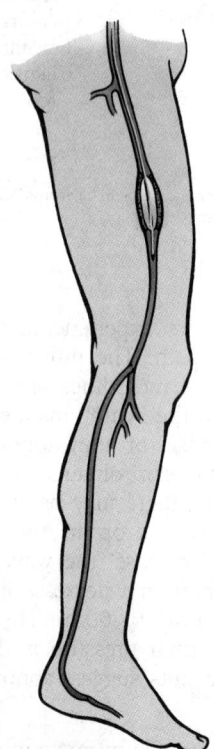

Figure 38–5. Percutaneous transluminal balloon angioplasty.

clients who are poor surgical candidates who cannot withstand general anesthesia or for whom amputation may be inevitable. Clients can experience reocclusion after this procedure, and the procedure may be repeated. Some clients have been occlusion free for up to 3–5 years, whereas others experience reocclusion within a year of PTBA.

During percutaneous transluminal angioplasty, intravascular stents may be placed to ensure adequate blood flow in a stenosed vessel. Candidates for this type of procedure are individuals with stenosis of the common or external iliac arteries. This type of procedure is cost effective and results in shorter hospital stays and earlier recoveries.

Laser-Assisted Angioplasty. Another invasive procedure is laser-assisted angioplasty. A laser probe is advanced through a cannula similar to that used for percutaneous transluminal angioplasty (PTA). Laser-assisted angioplasty is usually reserved for clients with smaller occlusions in the distal superficial femoral, proximal popliteal, and common iliac arteries. Heat from the laser vaporizes the arteriosclerotic plaque to open the occluded or stenosed artery. If significant stenosis remains after the artery is opened, a PTA balloon catheter may be inserted to further dilate the artery.

Preparation of the client for PTA or laser-assisted angioplasty is similar to that for diagnostic angiography. The client must have nothing by mouth (NPO) after midnight. The surgeon may require that the client scrub the groin area with an antiseptic solution.

Post-procedure nursing care involves observing for bleeding at the puncture site. The nurse or assistive nursing personnel closely observes vital signs and frequently checks the distal pulses in both limbs. These clients are typically restricted to bed rest, with the limb straight for approximately 6–8 hours before ambulation. Many of these clients receive anticoagulant therapy, such as heparin (Heplean✦), for approximately 3 days and then dipyridamole (Persantine, Apo-Dipyridamole✦) for 3–6 months at home. Clients usually take aspirin on a permanent basis.

Atherectomy. The technique of mechanical rotational abrasive atherectomy is used to improve blood flow to ischemic limbs in people with peripheral arterial disease. The rotational atherectomy device (Rotablator) is a high-speed rotary, metal bur ranging in size from 1.25 to 4.5 mm in diameter. The distal half of the bur is embedded with fine abrasive bits, which at rotational speeds of 100,000–120,000 rotations per minute result in fine-particle destruction of tissue. The Rotablator is designed to preferentially scrape "hard" surfaces (such as plaque) while minimizing damage to the vessel surface.

► Surgical Management

Clients with severe rest pain or claudication that interferes with the ability to work or threatens loss of a limb become surgical candidates. Arterial revascularization is the surgical procedure most commonly used to increase arterial blood flow in an affected limb.

Surgical procedures are classified as inflow or outflow. Inflow procedures involve bypassing arterial occlusions above the superficial femoral arteries (SFAs). Outflow procedures involve surgical bypassing of arterial occlusions at or below the superficial femoral arteries. For clients who have both inflow and outflow problems, the inflow procedure (for larger arteries) is done before the outflow repair.

Inflow procedures include aortoiliac, aortofemoral, and axillofemoral bypasses. Outflow procedures include femoropopliteal and femorotibial bypasses. Inflow procedures are more successful, with less chance of reocclusion or postoperative ischemia. Outflow procedures are less successful in relieving ischemic pain and are associated with a higher incidence of reocclusion.

Graft materials for the bypasses are selected on an individual basis. For outflow procedures, the preferred graft material is an autogenous saphenous vein. However, these clients can experience systemic vascular disease and may need this vein for coronary artery bypass. When the saphenous vein is not usable, the client's cephalic or basilic arm veins may be used.

Grafts made of synthetic materials, such as polytetrafluoroethylene, Gore-Tex, and Dacron, have also been used when autogenous veins were not available. Although synthetic grafts have achieved adequate patency in arteries above the knee, they have failed to achieve satisfactory results in infrapopliteal outflow vessels. In addition, autogenous veins are often not long enough for use in these vessels. Composite grafts constructed from multiple vein segments offer even better patency to arteries below the knee.

Preoperative Care. Preparing the client for surgery is similar to that described for the client having general or epidural anesthesia (see Chap. 20). Documentation of vital signs and peripheral pulses provides a baseline of information for comparison during the postoperative phase. Depending on the surgical procedure, the client may have an intravenous (IV) line, urinary catheter, central venous catheter, and/or arterial line. To prevent postoperative infection, clients typically receive antibiotic therapy before the procedure.

Operative Procedures. The anesthesiologist or nurse anesthetist places the client under general, epidural, or spinal anesthesia. Epidural or spinal induction is preferred for older adults to decrease the risk of cardiopulmonary complications in this group. If arterial bypass is to be accomplished by autogenous grafts, the surgeon excises the appropriate veins through an incision. The occluded artery is then exposed through an incision, and the conduit veins or synthetic graft material is sutured above and below the occlusion to facilitate blood flow around the occlusion.

For *aortoiliac* and *aortofemoral* bypass surgery, the surgeon makes a midline incision into the abdominal cavity to expose the abdominal aorta, with additional incisions into each groin (Fig. 38–6). Graft material is tunneled from the aorta to the groin incisions, where it is sutured in place.

In an *axillofemoral* bypass (Fig. 38–7), the surgeon makes an incision beneath the clavicle and tunnels graft material subcutaneously with a catheter from the chest to the iliac crest, into a groin incision, where it is sutured in place. Neither the thoracic nor the abdominal cavity is entered. For this reason, the axillofemoral bypass is used for high-risk clients who cannot tolerate a procedure requiring abdominal surgery.

Postoperative Care. Graft occlusion often occurs within the first 24 hours. Therefore, astute nursing care is crucial. The Client Care Plan highlights the most important aspects of postoperative care.

Assessment for Graft Occlusion. The nurse monitors the patency of the graft by checking the extremity every 15 minutes for the first hour, then hourly for changes in color, temperature, and pulse intensity. Warmth, redness, and edema of the affected extremity are often expected outcomes of surgery as a result of increased blood flow. Immediately postoperatively, the operating room or postanesthesia unit (PACU) nurse marks the site where the distal (dorsalis pedis or posterior tibial) pulse is best palpated or heard by Doppler ultrasonography. The nurse communicates this information to the nursing staff on the unit where the client will go.

Pain is frequently the first indicator of postoperative graft occlusion. Many people experience a throbbing pain owing to the increased blood flow to the extremity. This sensation is different from ischemic pain, and the nurse must assess the type of pain that the client is experiencing. If graft occlusion occurs, the client will experience a sharp increase in ischemic pain, described as similar to the pain felt before surgery. The nurse reports severe pain to the surgeon immediately.

Promotion of Graft Patency. To promote graft patency, the nurse monitors the client's blood pressure and notifies the surgeon if the pressure increases or decreases beyond normal limits. Hypotension may indicate hypovolemia, which can increase the risk of clotting. Range of motion of the affected limb is usually limited, with bending of the hip and knee contraindicated. The nurse consults with the surgeon on a case-by-case basis regarding

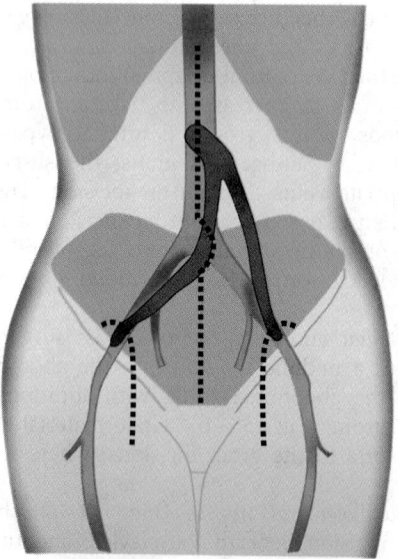

Figure 38–6. In aortoiliac and aortofemoral bypass surgery, a midline incision into the abdominal cavity is required, with an additional incision in each groin.

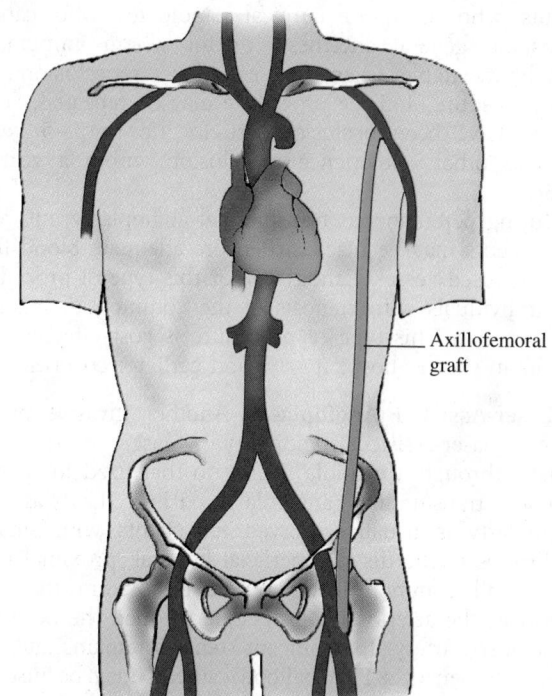

Figure 38–7. An axillofemoral bypass graft.

Axillofemoral graft

limitations of movement, including turning. Clients are restricted to bed rest for at least 24 hours postoperatively.

The nurse instructs all clients to cough and deep breathe every 1–2 hours and to use an incentive spirometer. Clients who have had aortoiliac or aortofemoral bypass are allowed nothing by mouth (NPO) for at least 1 day postoperatively. Clients who have undergone bypass surgery of the lower extremities not involving the aorta or abdominal wall (femoropopliteal or femorotibial bypass) may be on NPO status the night of surgery but are often allowed clear liquids the morning after surgery.

Treatment of Graft Occlusion. If manifestations of graft occlusion occur, the nurse notifies the surgeon immediately. Perfusion through the graft must be resolved promptly to avoid ischemic injury to the limb. Emergency *thrombectomy* (removal of the clot), which the surgeon may perform at the bedside, is the most common treatment for acute graft occlusion. Thrombectomy is associated with excellent results in prosthetic grafts but variable results in autogenous vein grafts, which often necessitate graft revision and even replacement.

Local intra-arterial *thrombolytic therapy* with urokinase (Abbokinase) may be used for acute graft occlusions in selected clients in settings where health providers are experts on its use. The physician considers thrombolytic therapy when the surgical alternative (e.g., thrombectomy with or without graft revision or replacement) carries high morbidity or mortality or when surgery for this type of occlusion has traditionally yielded poor results. When the physician uses urokinase, the nurse closely assesses the client for signs and symptoms of bleeding.

Monitoring for Compartment Syndrome. Compartment syndrome occurs when tissue pressure within a

Client Care Plan

The Client Having Peripheral Arterial Revascularization (Bypass) Surgery

Nursing Diagnosis No. 1: Altered Tissue Perfusion (Peripheral)

Expected Outcomes	Nursing Interventions	Rationale
The client will retain and maintain an increase in arterial blood flow to an extremity previously deprived of arterial blood flow.	■ Assess color, temperature, and pulse intensity of the affected extremity hourly. Notify the surgeon of a significant change.	■ Color, temperature, and pulse intensity immediately postoperatively indicate optimal arterial flow achieved with revascularization. Any increase in pallor or cyanosis or decrease in temperature or pulse intensity indicates postoperative graft occlusion.
	■ Assess the client for pain in the affected extremity, and report, if described, as "severe, similar to the pain before surgery."	■ Severe pain, similar to the pain felt before surgery, is frequently the first indicator of postoperative graft occlusion.
	■ Monitor the client's blood pressure, and report if it is increased or decreased beyond the client's normal limits.	■ Hypotension may indicate hypovolemia, which can increase the risk of clotting. Hypertension may put stress on the graft.
	■ Instruct the client to keep the affected extremity straight, limit movement, and avoid flexion of the knee and hip. Consult with the surgeon about turning the client.	■ Pressure on the graft can facilitate clot formation.
	■ Assess the incision for drainage, edema, and temperature.	■ Edema of the affected extremity is an expected outcome, but excessive edema should be reported.
		■ A small amount of bloody drainage is expected, but excessive bleeding is abnormal.
		■ Warmth, erythema, or a hard, tender area around the incision may indicate infection.

confined body space becomes elevated and restricts blood flow. The resultant ischemia can lead to tissue damage and eventually tissue death. The nurse assesses the client's motor and sensory function of the affected extremity. The extremity should also be assessed for worsening pain, fullness, swelling, and tenseness. These symptoms should be reported to the health care provider immediately. When compartment syndrome is suspected, the nurse continues to assess the extremity and removes or loosens the dressings and places the extremity at the level of the heart.

Assessment of Infection. Graft or wound infections can be life threatening and can endanger the client's limb. The nurse uses sterile technique when in contact with the incision and observes for symptoms of infection at or around the graft and incision sites. If the area over the graft becomes hard, tender, red, or warm, the client may have an infection. The nurse notifies the surgeon if any of these symptoms occurs.

 Continuing Care

➤ Case Management

Peripheral arterial disease is a chronic, long-term problem with frequent complications. PAD may benefit from a case manager who can follow the client across the continuum of care. The goal is to maintain the client in the home environment.

➤ Home Care Management

Managing the client at home often requires an interdisciplinary team approach. Chart 38–7 outlines the assessment highlights for home care clients with peripheral vascular disease. The clinical guide in Figure 38–8 shows how one home care agency documents care for homebound clients with PAD.

➤ Health Teaching

The nurse instructs all clients on methods to promote vasodilation. Clients are taught to avoid raising their legs above the level of the heart unless they also have venous stasis. The nurse provides written and oral instructions on foot care and methods to prevent injury and ulcer development for all clients (Chart 38–8).

The nurse teaches clients receiving pentoxifylline (Trental) to take the drug as prescribed, whether or not they notice improvement, because the drug may take 6–8 weeks to be effective and the effect may not be apparent. Pentoxifylline should be taken with meals to prevent side effects of nausea and vomiting.

Clients receiving dipyridamole (Persantine) are instructed to take the medication 1 hour before meals to promote optimal absorption. The nurse advises clients taking aspirin to take the drug with meals or milk and crackers and to report any nausea or vomiting.

Clients who have had surgery require additional instruction on incision care (see Chap. 22). The nurse encourages all clients to avoid smoking and to limit dietary fat intake to less than 30% of the total daily calories.

The client with chronic arterial obstruction may fear recurrent occlusion or further narrowing of the artery. Clients often fear that they might lose a limb or become debilitated in other ways. Indeed, chronic peripheral arterial disease (PAD) may worsen, especially in clients with diabetes mellitus. The nurse, however, reassures clients that their participation in prescribed exercise, diet, and pharmacologic therapy, along with cessation of smoking, can limit further formation of atherosclerotic plaques.

ELDERLY CONSIDERATIONS

Older clients with peripheral vascular disease may have visual or mobility problems that impede their ability to effectively provide foot care. The nurse can suggest using magnifying mirrors to check the feet and toes for cracks or blisters. Prior to washing the feet with mild soap and warm water, the temperature of the water should be tested with a thermometer or elbow, not the hand. Older adults may be at increased risk for trauma or self-inflicted injury. They should be advised never to go barefoot, to wear cotton socks, and to wear protective shoes. They should be advised to see a podiatrist to trim their toenails and manage corns or calluses.

➤ Health Care Resources

Clients with arterial compromise may need assistance with activities of daily living (ADLs) if activity is limited by pain. The client may need to limit or avoid stair climbing depending on the severity of disease. Clients who have undergone surgery usually need temporary help with activities of daily living.

Clients who must limit activity because of peripheral arterial disease may benefit from the assistance of a home health aide. The client who has undergone surgery may require a home health nurse to assist with incision care. The nurse or case manager arranges for home care resources before the client is discharged.

Acute Peripheral Arterial Occlusion

Overview

Although chronic peripheral arterial disease (PAD) progresses slowly, the onset of acute arterial occlusions may be sudden and dramatic. An embolus is the most common cause of peripheral occlusions, although a local

---

Chart 38–7

Focused Assessment for Home Care: Clients with Peripheral Vascular Disease

- Assess tissue perfusion to affected extremity(ies), including
  - Distal circulation, sensation, and motion
  - Presence of pain, pallor, paresthesias, pulselessness, paralysis, poikilothermia (coolness)
  - Ankle/brachial index
- Assess adherence to therapeutic regime, including
  - Following foot care instructions
  - Quitting smoking
  - Maintaining dietary restrictions
  - Participating in exercise regime
  - Avoiding exposure to cold and constrictive clothing
- Assess ability to manage wound care and prevent further injury, including
  - Use of compression stockings or compression pumps as directed
  - Use of various dressing materials
  - Signs and symptoms to report to nurse
- Assess coping ability of client and family members
- Assess home environment, including
  - Safety hazards, especially related to falls

Multidisciplinary Clinical Guide
Visit Summary

Instructions: Associate Nurse or Practitioner of an Associated Discipline, please complete this visit summary and transmit to the Nursing Case Manager within 24 hours of the completion of each visit.

Date: _____   Name of Patient: _____   and/or Caregiver: _____

Medical Diagnoses: _____

Discipline of Professional Making Visit: _____

Discharge Planning Started: _____

Discipline-Specific Diagnoses Treated at this visit:
_____
_____

Discipline-Specific Goals: (Note any change in goal(s) with reason for change)
_____
_____

Assessment Changes to Be Noted by Case Manager:
_____
_____

Variances from POC Detected: (use key numbers and explain if needed)
_____
_____
_____

Note follow-up care needed or plan for discharge:
_____
_____

Physician Contacted: _____

New Orders: _____

Signature: _____   Date: _____

Variances:

Key _____
1. Psychosocial
2. Environment
3. Physiological
4. Health-related behaviors
5. Other

Figure 38–8. Multidisciplinary clinical guide visit summary. (From Wills, E. M., & Sloan, H. L. [1996]. Assessing peripheral arterial disorders in the home: A multidisciplinary clinical guide. *Home Health Care Nurse, 14*(9), 670–674.)

---

thrombus may be the cause. Occlusion may affect the upper extremities, but it is more common in the lower extremities. Emboli originating from the heart are the most common cause of acute arterial occlusions. Most clients with an embolic occlusion have had an acute myocardial infarction and/or atrial fibrillation within the preceding weeks.

Collaborative Management

 Assessment

Clients with acute arterial occlusion describe severe pain below the level of the occlusion that occurs even at rest.

Criterion		Admission Date:	V	V	V	V	V
KNOWLEDGE	**Assessment Data Key:** 1 = none; 2 = minimal; 3 = basic; 4 = adequate; 5 = superior						
Patient/family	General knowledge about PAD (include smoking)						

Caregiver able to:	1. Inspect daily: blisters, itching, cuts, lesions, redness, pain, swelling, heat, dryness, calluses, corns
	2. Administer hygiene:
	  a. Wash daily with warm water
	  b. Dry carefully between toes
	  c. Change socks, shoes daily						

Selecting footwear	1. Shoes (leather, avoids synthetic)
	  a. Style (wide toe, avoids sandals)
	  b. Inside condition (no foreign objects, nail points, lining intact, no rough areas)
	  c. Wears shoes in- and outdoors
	  d. Correctly breaks in new shoes (wear for 20–30 minutes daily)						

Skin care	1. Corn/callus care
	  a. No chemical products used
	  b. Pumice stone if sensitive
	2. Dry skin care
	  a. Uses superfatted soap
	  b. Water temp 90–105°F
	  c. Emollient to dry areas before drying skin (none between toes)						

Professional care	1. Identifies need for care 2. Reports problems (skin breakdown, edema, ingrown toenails, inability to trim nails safely, shoe problems, rest or night pain) 3. Has routine foot assessment quarterly						
Medications	1. Identifies name and dose 2. Verbalizes reason for use 3. Avoids over-the-counter drugs (interactions with prescriptions)						
Monitors pain and complications	1. Degree and type of pain 2. Identifies one complication (ulcer, gangrene, amputation, functional limitations)						
Exercise/rest	1. Exercise patterns 2. Control of symptoms						
Diet	Knows diet. Type: Activate teaching plan if necessary						

Figure 38–8. *Continued*

The affected extremity is cool or cold, pulseless, and mottled. Minute areas on the toes may be blackened or gangrenous. Clients with acute arterial insufficiency often present with the "six Ps" of ischemia: pain, pallor, pulselessness, paresthesia, paralysis, and poikilothermia (coolness) of the involved extremity.

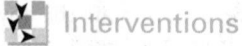 Interventions

The health care provider must initiate treatment promptly to avoid permanent damage or loss of an extremity. Anticoagulant therapy with heparin (Hepalean♣) is usually the first intervention to prevent further clot formation. A bo-

Criterion		Admission Date:	V	V	V	V	V
KNOWLEDGE *(continued)*	**Assessment Data Key:** 1 = none; 2 = minimal; 3 = basic; 4 = adequate; 5 = superior						
Discipline-specific diagnoses and goal dates:	1. Goal date:	Met? (y/n)					
Discipline: Specifiy							
Goal achieved (y/n) Variances: Key 1. Psychosocial 2. Environment 3. Physiological 4. Health-related behaviors 5. Other							
Comments							
BEHAVIOR	**Behavior displayed is appropriate:** Key: 1 = not; 2 = rarely; 3 = inconsistently; 4 = usually; 5 = consistently						
Diet	Type of diet:	Follows diet:					
Smoking	Changes in smoking behavior:						
Medications List:	Medications taken correctly						
Problem solving	Identifies preferences, assists nurse to individualize plan of care (POC)						
Community resources	Needs referrals for: a. Meal preparation d. Healthcare funding b. Transportation e. Support groups c. Personal care f. Shoe fitting, care						
Coping skills	Identifies ways to deal with pain, loss of function						
Beliefs/self-efficacy	a. Identifies beliefs about ability to follow POC b. Beliefs about insensitive feet 1. no pain = no problem 2. no pain means no care is required c. Nurse may have to reinterpret signs and symptoms for client						
Motivation	Client/family motivation to follow POC?						
Diagnoses and goal dates:	1. Goal date:	Met? (y/n)					

Figure 38–8. *Continued*

Criterion		Admission Date:	V	V	V	V	V
BEHAVIOR (continued)	**Behavior displayed is appropriate:** **Key:** 1 = not; 2 = rarely; 3 = inconsistently; 4 = usually; 5 = consistently						
Discipline(s): Specify with diagnosis							
Goal achieved (y/n) Variances: Key 1. Psychosocial 2. Environment 3. Physiological 4. Health-related behaviors 5. Other							
Comments							
STATUS	**Assessment Data Key: Signs & Symptoms:** 1 = extreme; 2 = severe; 3 = moderate; 4 = minimal; 5 = none						
Foot assessment Nails Hygiene Footwear	Inspection: 1. Nails cut straight across or slightly rounded 2. Rate hygiene good, fair, poor 3. Footwear adequate or inadequate a. Socks (materials: cotton, wool, polyester blend) Cautions: nonrestricting fit, no circular garters or constricting clothes, no knee-highs b. Shoes (Check type, fit, condition)						
Skin	1. Color (rubor, pallor, cyanosis, blackened areas) 2. Temperature (check both extremities, note differences) 3. Edema (pitting/nonpitting Grade [1−4]/4)						
Atrophy	Skin (shiny, pale, translucent)						
Changes to foot	1. Toenails (label as thickened, discolored, deformed) 2. Corns/calluses (describe location, size) 3. Deformities (describe in nurse's note; presence of hammer toes, claw toes, bunions)						
Vital signs Post, tibial pulse Blood pressure	Grade pulse (Use 0−4/4 [0 = not palpable, 1 = easily obliterated, 2 = easily palpable, 3 = not easily obliterated, 4 = strong, bounding]) Both arms and do orthostatic if possible						
Ulcerations (location)	Describe completely in nurse's notes and on wound flow sheet						

Figure 38–8. *Continued*

Criterion		Admission Date:	V	V	V	V	V
STATUS *(continued)*	**Assessment Data Key: Signs & Symptoms:** 1 = extreme; 2 = severe; 3 = moderate; 4 = minimal; 5 = none						
Complication potential (Evaluate on admission and every 60 days)	Ulcer, ischemia gangrene, functional limitations						
ABI on admission (Reassess if post-tibial pulse changes)	1. Blood pressure at brachial and ankle locations bilaterally 2. Use Doppler if possible 3. Calculate index from highest readings (A/B = ABI)						
Protective sensation	Measure with Semmes/Weinstein Monofilament. (10 g/0.5). Apply to feet and ankles and random areas (present or not).						
Discipline-specific diagnoses and goal dates:	1. Goal date: Met? (y/n)						
Discipline: Specify							
Goal achieved (y/n) Variances: Key 1. Psychosocial 2. Environment 3. Physiological 4. Health-related behaviors 5. Other							
Comments							

Figure 38–8. *Continued*

Education Guide: Foot Care for the Client with Peripheral Vascular Disease

- Keep your feet clean by washing them with a mild soap in room-temperature water.
- Keep your feet dry, especially between the toes and ankles.
- Avoid injury to your feet and ankles. Wear comfortable, well-fitting shoes. Never go without shoes.
- Keep your toenails clean and filed. Have someone cut them if you cannot see them clearly. Cut your toenails straight across.
- To prevent dry, cracked skin, apply a lubricating lotion to your feet.
- Prevent exposure to extreme heat or cold. Never use a heating pad on your feet.
- Avoid constricting garments.
- If a problem develops, see a podiatrist or physician.
- Avoid extended pressure on your feet or ankles, such as occurs when you lean against something.

lus up to 10,000 U may be ordered. The client may also undergo angiography.

A surgical thrombectomy or embolectomy with local anesthesia may be performed to remove the occlusion. The physician makes an incision, followed by an arteriotomy (a surgical opening into an artery). The physician then inserts a Fogarty catheter into the artery and retrieves the embolus. It may be necessary to close the artery with a patch graft.

Postoperatively, the nurse monitors the affected extremity for improvement in color, temperature, and pulse, as well as other extremities for signs and symptoms of new thrombi or emboli. Pain should significantly diminish after the surgical procedure, although mild incisional pain remains. The nurse watches closely for complications caused by reperfusing the artery after thrombectomy or embolectomy, which include spasms and swelling of the skeletal muscle. Swelling of the skeletal muscles is characterized by edema, pain on passive movement, poor capillary refill, numbness, and muscle tenseness. Fasciotomy (surgical opening into the tissues) may be necessary to prevent further injury and save the limb.

The use of systemic thrombolytic therapy for acute arterial occlusions has been disappointing because bleeding complications have outweighed the benefits obtained. Local intra-arterial thrombolytic therapy with urokinase (Abbokinase) has emerged as an alternative to surgical treatment in selected clients in settings where health providers are familiar with its use and its complications. When urokinase is given, the nurse monitors the client for signs and symptoms of bleeding, bruising, or hematoma. If any of these complications occurs, the nurse notifies the physician immediately.

Aneurysms

Overview

An aneurysm is a permanent localized dilation of an artery, which enlarges the artery to at least two times its normal diameter.

Types of Aneurysms

An aneurysm may be described as *fusiform* (a diffuse dilation affecting the entire circumference of the artery) or *saccular* (an out pouching affecting only a distinct portion of the artery). Aneurysms may also be described as true or false. In true aneurysms the arterial wall is weakened by congenital or acquired problems. False aneurysms occur as the result of vessel injury or trauma to all three layers of the arterial wall.

Dissecting hematomas, traditionally called *dissecting aneurysms,* are more accurately described as *aortic dissections* (see later). Aortic dissections differ from aneurysms in that they are formed when blood accumulates in the wall of an artery.

Aneurysms tend to occur at specific anatomic sites (Fig. 38–9), most commonly in the abdominal aorta. Aneurysms often occur at a point where the artery is not supported by skeletal muscles or on the lines of curves or flexion in the arterial tree.

Pathophysiologic Process

An aneurysm forms when the middle layer (media) of the artery is weakened, producing a stretching effect in the inner layer (intima) and outer layers (adventitia) of the artery. As the artery widens, tension in the wall increases and further widening occurs, thus enlarging the aneurysm. Hypertension (high blood pressure) produces more tension and enlargement within the artery. As the aneurysm grows, the risk of arterial rupture increases.

Abdominal aortic aneurysms account for approximately 75% of all aneurysms. Most of these aneurysms are located between the renal arteries and the aortic bifurcation. Of all abdominal aortic aneurysms greater than 6 cm in diameter, 50% rupture within 1 year; of those aneurysms smaller than 6 cm in diameter, 15%–20% rupture.

Thoracic aneurysms account for approximately 25% of all aneurysms. They commonly develop between the origin of the left subclavian artery and the diaphragm. They are located in the descending, ascending, and transverse sections of the aorta.

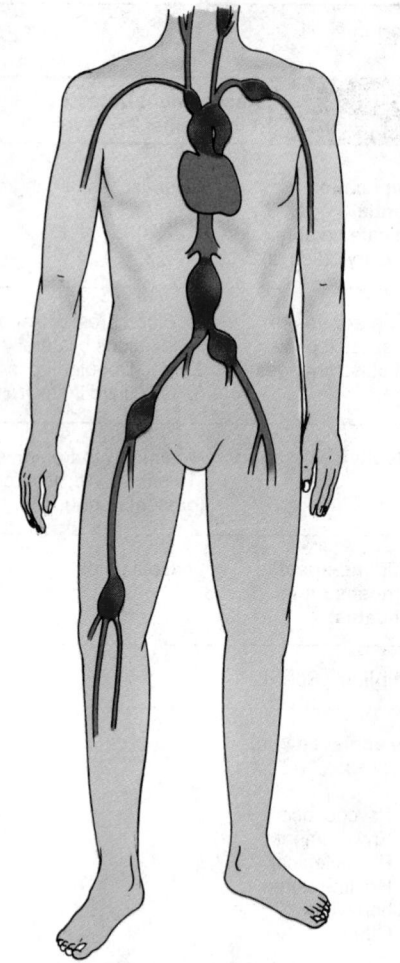

Figure 38–9. Common anatomic sites of arterial aneurysms.

Aneurysms can cause symptoms by exerting pressure on surrounding structures or by rupturing. Rupture of an aneurysm is the most frequent complication and is life threatening because abrupt and massive hemorrhagic shock occurs with the rupture. Thrombi within the wall of an aneurysm can also be the source of emboli in distal arteries below the aneurysm.

Atherosclerosis is the most common cause of all aneurysms, with hypertension and cigarette smoking being contributing factors. Syphilis and Ehlers-Danlos syndrome are other causes of abdominal aortic aneurysms, and there may be a familial risk.

The incidence of abdominal aortic aneurysms, estimated to be between 30 and 66 per 1000 people, is increasing in the Western world. Approximately 15,000 people in the United States die annually from abdominal aneurysms, making it the 13th leading cause of death in the United States. Thoracic aneurysms occur most often in older adults.

Abdominal aortic aneurysms are more common in men than women (with a ratio of 4:1). Approximately 10% of aortic aneurysms are thoracic (Tierney, 1995).

Collaborative Management

 Assessment

Most clients with abdominal aortic or thoracic aneurysms are asymptomatic when their aneurysms are first discovered by routine examination or during radiographic study performed for another reason.

➤ Abdominal Aortic Aneurysms

Because clients may have symptoms, the nurse assesses clients with known or suspected abdominal aortic aneurysm for abdominal, flank, or back pain. Pain related to an abdominal aortic aneurysm is usually steady, with a gnawing quality, unaffected by movement, and may last for hours or days.

The nurse observes for a pulsation in the upper abdomen slightly to the left of the midline between the xiphoid process and the umbilicus. A detectable aneurysm is at least 5 cm in size. The nurse then auscultates for a bruit over the mass but avoids palpating the mass because it may be tender and there is a risk of rupture.

Although some clients have symptoms when the aneurysm is intact, many clients are asymptomatic until the time of rupture. If expansion and impending rupture of an abdominal aortic aneurysm is suspected, the nurse assesses for severe pain of sudden onset in the back or lower abdomen, which may radiate to the groin, buttocks, or legs.

Clients with a rupturing abdominal aortic aneurysm are critically ill in hemorrhagic (hypovolemic) shock. Signs include hypotension, diaphoresis, mental obtundation, oliguria, and dysrhythmias. Retroperitoneal hemorrhage is manifested by hematomas in the flanks. Rupture into the abdominal cavity causes abdominal distention.

➤ Thoracic Aneurysms

When a thoracic aneurysm is suspected, the nurse assesses the client for back pain and manifestations of compression of the aneurysm on adjacent structures. Signs include shortness of breath, hoarseness, and difficulty swallowing.

Thoracic aneurysms are not often detected by physical assessment, but occasionally a mass may be visible above the suprasternal notch.

The client with suspected rupture of a thoracic aneurysm is assessed for sudden and excruciating back or chest pain. Rupture of a thoracic aneurysm is also indicated by hemorrhagic shock (see Chap. 39).

➤ Radiographic Assessment

An abdominal x-ray or lateral film of the spine often shows an abdominal aortic aneurysm. The "eggshell" appearance of the aneurysm is essentially diagnostic.

Computed tomographic (CT) scanning is the standard tool for assessing the size and location of an aortic aneurysm. A thoracic aneurysm can be diagnosed by chest x-ray. A CT scan is used to assess size and location. Aortic arteriography is performed for all clients who are to undergo surgical repair of a thoracic aneurysm.

➤ Other Diagnostic Assessment

Ultrasonography is a noninvasive technique that provides an accurate diagnosis as well as information about the size and location of an abdominal aortic aneurysm.

 Interventions

The size of the aneurysm and the presence of symptoms are the most important parameters in the determination of treatment.

➤ Nonsurgical Management

The goal of nonsurgical management is to maintain the blood pressure at a normal level to decrease the risk of rupture and monitor the growth of the aneurysm.

Because elevated blood pressure can increase the rate of aneurysmal enlargement, hypertension is an important risk factor for rupture. Clients with hypertension are treated with antihypertensives to decrease the rate of enlargement and the risk for early rupture.

For clients with small or asymptomatic aneurysms, frequent CT scans are necessary to monitor the growth of the aneurysm. The nurse emphasizes the importance of following through with scheduled tests to monitor the growth. The nurse also explains the clinical manifestations of aneurysms that need to be promptly reported.

➤ Surgical Management

Surgical management of an aneurysm may be an elective or an emergency procedure. For all clients with either a rupturing abdominal aortic or a thoracic aneurysm, emergency surgery is performed.

Clients with an abdominal aortic aneurysm 6 cm in diameter or wider undergo elective surgery. Some surgeons favor surgical treatment for clients with aneurysms 4–6 cm in diameter if the client is in good health. Clients in good health with aneurysms smaller than 4 cm and clients in poor health with aneurysms 4–6 cm in diameter undergo nonsurgical treatment until the aneurysm reaches 6 cm.

Clients with thoracic aneurysms measuring 7 cm or more in diameter and clients with smaller aneurysms that are producing symptoms are advised to have elective surgery. Clients with aneurysms smaller than 7 cm in diameter that are not causing symptoms are treated nonsurgically until symptoms occur or the aneurysm enlarges to 7 cm.

The most common procedure performed for clients with an abdominal aortic aneurysm is an abdominal aortic aneurysm (AAA) resection or repair (aneurysmectomy). The mortality rate for elective AAA resection is 2%–5%. The mortality rate for emergency surgery for expanding abdominal aortic aneurysms is 5%–15% and 50% for those that have ruptured.

The major surgery for clients with a thoracic aneurysm is a thoracic aneurysm repair. Elective resection of these aneurysms is associated with a 10% mortality rate.

Abdominal Aortic Aneurysm Resection. In an abdominal aortic aneurysm resection, the physician excises the aneurysm from the abdominal aorta to prevent or repair its rupture. The goal is to secure stable aortic integrity and tissue perfusion throughout the body.

Preoperative Care. Interventions are similar to those for clients undergoing surgery with general anesthesia (see Chap. 20). A bowel preparation and emphasis on coughing and deep breathing are very important. Because a significant blood loss often occurs during AAA resection, clients planning elective surgery may be advised to bank their blood for autologous (self) transfusions postoperatively.

The nurse assesses all peripheral pulses to serve as a baseline for comparison postoperatively. The nurse may mark where the pulse is palpated or heard by Doppler ultrasonography to facilitate locating the pulse postoperatively.

Clients with ruptured aneurysms are brought to the operating suite directly from the emergency department. Preoperative care of clients with ruptured aneurysms involves administration of large volumes of intravenous (IV) fluids to maintain tissue perfusion.

Operative Procedure. The surgeon makes a midline abdominal incision from the xiphoid process to the symphysis pubis, or a wide transverse incision from flank to flank, to expose the aneurysm. Clamps are applied just above the aneurysm and below it, the aneurysm is excised, and a preclotted Dacron graft is sutured in an end-to-end fashion (Fig. 38–10).

Postoperative Care. Immediately postoperatively, the client is typically admitted to a critical care unit for 24 to 48 hours, depending on the age and condition of the client. In addition to providing the routine postoperative care discussed in Chapter 22, the nurse assesses for and

assists in the prevention of the postoperative complications that can occur after an AAA repair. These complications include myocardial infarction, graft occlusion or rupture causing hemorrhage, hypovolemia and/or renal failure, respiratory distress, and paralytic ileus.

Myocardial Infarction. During the immediate postoperative period, the client's blood pressure will be monitored with an arterial catheter. Continuous cardiac monitoring will be used to detect any dysrhythmias. Using hemodynamic monitoring, the nurse monitors for low cardiac output and other findings consistent with acute myocardial infarction. The nurse also assesses for other signs of myocardial infarction, including chest pain, shortness of breath, complaints of dyspnea, diaphoresis, anxiety, and restlessness.

Graft Occlusion or Rupture. The nurse or assistive nursing personnel assesses vital signs and circulation every 15 minutes for the first hour, then hourly with assessment of pulses distal to the graft site (including posterior tibial and dorsalis pedis). The nurse reports any signs of graft occlusion or rupture, including

- Changes in pulses
- Cool to cold extremities below the graft
- White or blue extremities or flanks
- Severe pain
- Abdominal distention

The nurse limits elevation of the head of the bed to 45 degrees to avoid flexion of the graft.

Hypovolemia or Renal Failure. Hypovolemia and renal failure occur because there is often a large blood loss during surgery or before if rupture occurred. The nurse assesses urine output via Foley catheter hourly. If urine output is less than 50 mL/hour, the nurse notifies the surgeon. Although advances in surgical technique have decreased the risk of renal failure after clamping during surgery, renal failure may occur. Renal failure caused by acute tubular necrosis is more common after emergency surgery. In addition to monitoring urine output, the nurse and physician monitor serum creatinine and blood urea nitrogen levels daily.

Respiratory Distress. The nurse or assistive nursing personnel assesses the client's respiratory rate and depth every hour and auscultates breath sounds every 4 hours to monitor for respiratory complications. Often, the client is maintained on a ventilator at least overnight to facilitate respiratory exchange. The nurse administers opioids for pain, as ordered, and turns and suctions the client according to protocol. The nurse ensures firm abdominal support of the incision with a pillow or bath blanket, while the client is coughing, to prevent the incision from separating. After the client is extubated, the nurse or assistive nursing personnel assesses that the client turns, coughs, and deep breathes every 1 to 2 hours and increases his or her mobility as ordered.

Paralytic Ileus. Paralytic ileus after AAA repair is expected for 2–3 days. Clients have a nasogastric tube to low suction until bowel sounds return. The nurse listens for bowel sounds every 8 hours and reports their return to the physician. The nurse assesses for prolonged ab-

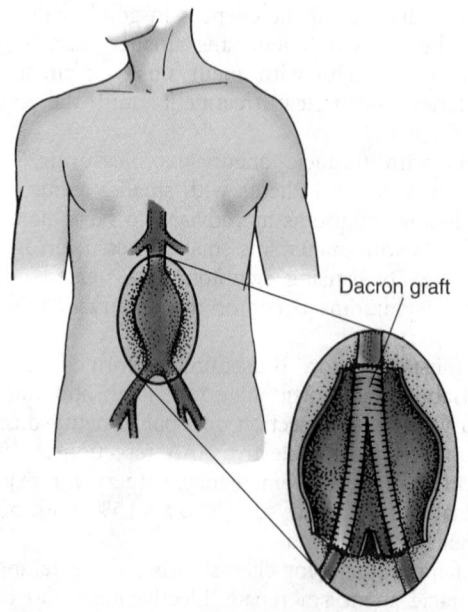

Figure 38–10. Surgical repair of abdominal aortic aneurysm with a woven Dacron graft.

Dacron graft

sence of bowel sounds and distention, which may indicate a prolonged ileus or a bowel infarction.

Thoracic Aneurysm Repair. Repair of thoracic aneurysms is tailored to each client; the procedure depends on the type and location of the aneurysm. Total cardiopulmonary bypass (CPB) is necessary for excision of aneurysms in the ascending aorta, and partial bypass is often used during excision of aneurysms in the descending aorta.

Preoperative Care. The care of the client undergoing thoracic aneurysm resection is similar to that provided for the client having thoracic surgery (see Chap. 34). Clients undergoing cardiopulmonary bypass receive care similar to that described in Chapter 40.

Operative Procedure. The surgeon uses either a thoracotomy or a median sternotomy approach to enter the thoracic cavity. The surgeon exposes the aneurysm and excises it. After excising the aneurysm, the surgeon usually sews a Dacron graft or prosthesis onto the aorta. Saccular aneurysms, which have an out pouching from a distinct portion of the arterial wall, can sometimes be removed without resection of the aorta.

Postoperative Care. The care of a client who has undergone thoracic aneurysm repair is similar to that after other chest surgery. Clients undergoing cardiopulmonary bypass receive care similar to that described in Chapter 40. The nurse assesses for and assists in the prevention of postoperative complications that can occur after a thoracic aneurysm repair. These complications include hemorrhage, ischemic colitis, spinal cord ischemia resulting in paraplegia, respiratory distress, and cardiac dysrhythmias.

Hemorrhage. The nurse assesses vital signs at least hourly, reporting any signs of hemorrhage (a drop in blood pressure, an increase in pulse rate, rapid respirations, diaphoresis) to the physician immediately. The nurse assesses for bleeding or separation at the graft site by noting significant increases in chest drainage from the chest tubes.

Paraplegia. Inadvertent interruption of the blood supply to the spinal cord during thoracic aneurysm repair can result in paraplegia. The nurse assesses the client hourly for sensation and motion in all extremities and reports deficits immediately.

Respiratory Distress. After thoracic aneurysm repair, clients are especially susceptible to respiratory distress from atelectasis or pneumonia. This problem occurs as a result of both cardiopulmonary bypass and incisional discomfort. Both atelectasis and pneumonia may cause shallow breathing and poor cough effort. These clients are often maintained on a ventilator, at least overnight, after surgery. For clients with a median sternotomy, the surgeon firmly splints the incision to prevent separation of the sternum.

Cardiac Dysrhythmias. The nurse assesses all clients recovering from thoracic aneurysm repair for cardiac dysrhythmias. The stress of the thoracic surgery, added to the increased incidence of arteriosclerosis in this group,

may predispose these clients to a myocardial infarction, cardiac dysrhythmias, or heart failure.

 Continuing Care

Most clients after aneurysm repair are discharged home. In rare instances, the postoperative client may be discharged to an extended (long-term) care facility for rehabilitation in the absence of family or other support systems.

➤ *Home Care Management*

If discharged to home, the client must follow the instructions provided by the nurse regarding activity level and incisional care. Because stair climbing may be restricted initially, the client may need a bedside commode if the bathroom is inaccessible.

➤ *Health Teaching*

For clients who have not undergone surgical aneurysm repair, the teaching plan emphasizes the importance of compliance with the schedule of computed tomography (CT) scanning to monitor the size of the aneurysm. The nurse educates the client receiving treatment for hypertension about the importance of continuing to take prescribed medication. The client and family or significant other are instructed about signs and symptoms that they must promptly report to their health care provider:

- Clients with abdominal aortic aneurysms must report abdominal fullness or pain or back pain.
- Clients with thoracic aneurysms must report chest or back pain, shortness of breath, difficulty swallowing, or hoarseness.

The nurse teaches the client who has undergone repair of the aneurysm about activity restrictions, wound care, and pain management. Clients may not engage in activities that involve lifting heavy objects (usually more than 15–20 pounds, or 6.8–9.1 kg) for 6–12 weeks postoperatively. The nurse advises the client to use discretion in activities that involve pulling, pushing, or straining, such as vacuuming, changing bed linens, moving furniture, mopping or sweeping, raking leaves, mowing grass, and chopping wood. Clients should temporarily avoid such hobbies as tennis, swimming, horseback riding, and golf, although putting practice is allowed. Because of postoperative weakness, the client is usually restricted from driving a car for several weeks after discharge.

Clients who have not undergone aneurysm repair may fear rupture and subsequent death. The nurse assesses for the client's and family's perceptions of this potential situation. The nurse reinforces the rationales for CT monitoring of aneurysmal size and for controlling hypertension and encourages clients to verbalize their fears.

➤ *Health Care Resources*

In collaboration with the discharge planner, the nurse assesses the availability of transportation to and from appointments for clients needing CT monitoring. If transportation is a problem, the nurse consults the social worker to assist in arranging this service.

Clients who have undergone surgery may require the services of a home health nurse for assistance with dressing changes. A home health aide may be needed to assist with activities of daily living.

Aneurysms of the Peripheral Arteries

Overview

Although femoral and popliteal aneurysms are relatively uncommon, they are often associated with an aneurysm in another location of the arterial tree. To detect a popliteal aneurysm, the nurse palpates a pulsating mass in the popliteal space. To detect a femoral aneurysm, the nurse palpates a pulsatile mass over the femoral artery. The nurse evaluates both extremities because more than one femoral or popliteal aneurysm may be present.

Collaborative Management

The client may exhibit symptoms of limb ischemia, and the nurse assesses for diminished or absent pulses, cool to cold skin, and pain. Pain may also be present if an adjacent nerve is compressed. The recommended treatment for either type of aneurysm, regardless of the size, is surgery because of the risk of thromboembolic complications associated with their presence.

To treat a femoral aneurysm, the physician excises the aneurysm and restores circulation using a Dacron graft or an autogenous saphenous vein graft. Most surgeons prefer to bypass rather than resect a popliteal aneurysm.

Postoperatively, the nurse monitors for lower limb ischemia. The nurse palpates pulses below the graft to assess graft patency. Often, Doppler ultrasonography is necessary to assess blood flow when pulses are not palpable. Sudden development of pain or discoloration of the extremity is reported immediately to the physician because it may indicate graft occlusion.

Aortic Dissection

Overview

Aortic dissection has traditionally been referred to as a "dissecting aneurysm." However, because this condition is more accurately described as a dissecting hematoma, the term aortic dissection has gained favor.

Aortic dissection is thought to be caused by a sudden tear in the aortic intima, opening the way for blood to enter the aortic wall. Degeneration of the aortic media might be a prerequisite for this condition, with hypertension an important contributing factor.

Aortic dissection is a relatively common event, occurring in at least 2000 people in the United States annually. It is frequently associated with connective tissue disorders such as Marfan's syndrome. It also occurs in older people, peaking in adults in their 50s and 60s and in women in their third trimester of pregnancy.

Because the circulation of any major artery arising from the aorta can be impaired in clients with aortic dissection, this condition is highly lethal and represents an emergency situation.

Dissections are classified in various ways. Debakey's classification contains three groups:

- Type 1: Characterized by an intimal tear in the ascending (proximal) aorta, with extension of the dissection into the descending (distal) aorta
- Type 2: Originates in and is limited to the ascending (proximal) aorta
- Type 3: Arises within the descending (distal) thoracic aorta and often progresses distally

Proximal dissections occur almost twice as often as distal dissections. Although the ascending aorta and descending thoracic aorta are the most common sites, dissection can also occur in the abdominal aorta and other arteries.

Collaborative Management

The most common presenting symptom of aortic aneurysm is pain, with painless dissection occurring rarely. The pain is described as "tearing," "ripping," and "stabbing" and tends to move from its point of origin. Depending on the site of dissection, the client may feel pain in the anterior chest, back, neck, throat, jaw, or teeth.

Diaphoresis, nausea, vomiting, faintness, and apprehension are also common. Blood pressure is usually elevated unless complications, such as cardiac tamponade or rupture, have occurred. A decrease or absence of peripheral pulses is common, as is aortic regurgitation, characterized by a musical murmur heard better along the right sternal border. Neurologic deficits, such as altered level of consciousness, paraparesis, and cerebrovascular accidents, can also occur.

Chest x-ray, Doppler echocardiogram, computed tomography (CT), and aortic angiography are commonly used to confirm the diagnosis.

The goals of emergency treatment include

- The elimination of pain
- A reduction of blood pressure to 100 to 120 mmHg
- A decrease in the velocity of left ventricular ejection

The physician prescribes intravenous (IV) sodium nitroprusside (Nitropress) by continuous drip initially to lower the blood pressure. If this regimen is ineffective, nicardipine hydrochloride (Cardene) may be used. Propranolol (Inderal, Apo-Propranolol✦) is given in increments of 1 mg IV to decrease left ventricular ejection.

Subsequent treatment depends on the location of the dissection. Generally, clients receive continued medical treatment for uncomplicated distal dissections and surgical treatment for proximal dissections.

For clients receiving long-term medical treatment, the systolic blood pressure must be maintained at or below 130–140 mmHg. Beta-blockers (propranolol) and calcium channel antagonists are indicated.

Clients receiving surgical intervention for a proximal dissection always require total cardiopulmonary bypass (see Chap. 40). The surgeon excises the intimal tear and obliterates entry in the false opening by suturing edges of the dissected aorta. Usually, a prosthetic graft is used.

Buerger's Disease

Overview

Buerger's disease (thromboangiitis obliterans) is a relatively uncommon occlusive disease limited to the medium and small arteries and veins. The distal upper and lower limbs are the most frequently affected. Typically, Buerger's disease is identified in young adult males who smoke. Larger arteries, such as the femoral and brachial, become involved in the late stages of the disease. The veins are less commonly involved.

The disease often extends into the perivascular tissues, resulting in fibrosis and scarring that binds the artery, vein, and nerve firmly together. For people who have this disease, cessation of cigarette smoking usually arrests the disease process, but persistence in smoking causes occlusion in the more proximal vessels.

The cause of Buerger's disease is unknown, although there is a strong association with tobacco smoking. A familial or genetic predisposition and autoimmune etiologic factors are also possible.

Collaborative Management

 Assessment

The first clinical manifestation of Buerger's disease is usually claudication (pain in the muscles resulting from an inadequate blood supply) of the arch of the foot. Intermittent claudication may occur in the lower extremities. The pain may be ischemic, occurring in the digits while the client is at rest. Often, there is an aching pain that is more severe at night. Paroxysmal shock-like pain can be the result of ischemic neuropathy. Clients often experience increased sensitivity to cold and complain of coldness and numbness. On physical examination, the nurse notes that the pulses are often diminished in the distal extremities, and the extremities are cool and red or cyanotic in the dependent position.

A diagnosis of Buerger's disease is commonly based on a physical finding of peripheral ischemia, often in association with migratory superficial phlebitis. Ulcerations and gangrene may be seen in the digits. The ulcerations are usually sharply demarcated. The gangrenous lesion can be small or can affect the entire digit.

Arteriograms can be useful in delineating the degree of disease in the arteries. Commonly, arteriography reveals multiple segmental occlusions in the smaller arteries of the forearm, hand, leg, and foot. Plethysmographic studies of the fingers or toes may be diagnostic of the disease in the early stages. These studies can also be useful in following the progression of the disease in more proximal arteries.

Interventions

Nursing interventions are directed at
- Preventing the progression of the disease
- Avoiding vasoconstriction
- Promoting vasodilation
- Relieving pain
- Treating ulceration and gangrene

To prevent progression of Buerger's disease, complete abstinence from tobacco in all forms is essential. The client is instructed to prevent extreme or prolonged exposure to cold to prevent vasoconstriction. The nurse instructs the client about medications that are prescribed for vasodilation, such as nifedipine (Procardia, Adalat). (See Chapter 9 for interventions and nursing management for pain relief.)

The treatment of clients with Buerger's disease is similar to that of clients with peripheral arterial disease (see earlier).

Subclavian Steal
Overview

Subclavian steal occurs in the upper extremities from a subclavian artery occlusion or stenosis. The result is altered blood flow and ischemia in the arm. Subclavian steal can occur in people at any age but is more common in those with risk factors for atherosclerosis. Symptoms include tiredness in the arm with exertion, paresthesias, dizziness, and exercise-induced pain in the forearm when the arms are elevated.

Collaborative Management

Physical examination usually reveals a significant difference in the blood pressures between the arms. A difference greater than 20 mmHg is considered significant. Another important finding is a subclavian bruit, which can occur on the affected side. The subclavian pulse may be decreased on the occluded side compared with the opposite side. The client's arm may also be discolored or cyanotic; however, this finding generally occurs only in severe cases.

Surgery is the recommended intervention when a client has cyanosis or pain. One of three procedures may be used: endarterectomy of the subclavian artery, carotid-subclavian bypass, or dilation of the subclavian artery.

Nursing care encompasses postoperative care of the client and monitoring the arterial flow in the affected arm. The nurse should check brachial and radial pulses frequently and observe for ischemic changes. The nurse also observes the arm for edema, redness, or any other signs.

Thoracic Outlet Syndrome
Overview

Thoracic outlet syndrome is a compression of the subclavian artery at the thoracic outlet by anatomic structures, such as a rib or muscle. The arterial wall may be damaged, producing thrombosis or embolization to distal arteries of the arms. The three common sites of compression in the thoracic outlet are

- The interscalene triangle
- Between the coracoid process of the scapula and the pectoralis minor tendon
- Most commonly, the costoclavicular space

Collaborative Management

Thoracic outlet syndrome is more common in females and in people whose occupations require holding their arms up or leaning over, such as baseball players, golfers, or swimmers. It is also seen in clients who have had trauma such as whiplash or after clavicular fracture. Clients generally complain of neck, shoulder, and arm pain that may be intermittent. The client may also have numbness and moderate edema of the extremity. The pain and numbness are worse when the arm is placed in certain positions, such as over the client's head or out to the side. The client may have overdeveloped neck and shoulder muscles, and the affected arm may appear cyanotic.

Treatment includes physical therapy, exercises, and avoiding aggravating positions, such as elevating the arms. Surgical treatment involves resection of the anatomic structure that is compressing the artery. Surgery is performed only if a client has severe pain, has lost hand function, or is responding poorly to conservative treatment.

Raynaud's Phenomenon

Overview

Raynaud's phenomenon is caused by vasospasm of the arterioles and arteries of the upper and lower extremities, usually unilaterally. *Raynaud's disease* occurs bilaterally. The two terms are sometimes used interchangeably, but, although they are related, there are some differences. Raynaud's phenomenon usually occurs in people older than 30 years; Raynaud's disease can occur between the ages of 17 and 50 years. Raynaud's phenomenon can occur in either sex, but Raynaud's disease is more common in women.

The pathophysiology is the same for both entities. The etiology is unknown. Clients often have an associated systemic connective tissue disease, such as systemic lupus erythematosus or progressive systemic sclerosis (see Chap. 24).

As a result of vasospasm, the cutaneous vessels are constricted and blanching of the extremity occurs, followed by cyanosis. When the vasospasm is relieved, the tissue becomes reddened or hyperemic. The client's extremities are numb and cold, and the client may complain of pain and swelling. Ulcers may also be present. These attacks are intermittent and can be aggravated by cold or stress. In severe cases, the attack lasts longer and gangrene of the digits can occur.

Collaborative Management

Treatment involves relieving or preventing the vasoconstriction by drug therapy. Commonly prescribed drugs are nifedipine (Procardia), cyclandelate (Cyclospasmol), and phenoxybenzamine (Dibenzyline). These vasodilating agents may help to relieve the symptoms, but they can cause uncomfortable side effects, such as facial flushing, headaches, hypotension, and dizziness.

For severe symptoms that cannot be alleviated by drugs, a lumbar sympathectomy can be performed. The physician cuts the sympathetic nerve fibers that cause vasoconstriction of blood vessels in the lower extremities. This method is effective when clients are experiencing foot symptoms. For the upper extremities, a similar procedure—sympathetic ganglionectomy—may provide symptom relief. The long-term effectiveness of these treatments is questionable.

Education of the client is important in prevention of complications. The nurse explains methods to prevent vasoconstriction, such as minimizing exposure to cold and decreasing stress. The client is instructed to wear warm clothes, socks, or gloves when exposed to cool or cold temperatures. Clients should keep their homes at a comfortably warm temperature. The nurse helps the client to identify stressors and provides suggestions for reducing them.

Popliteal Entrapment

Popliteal entrapment causes ischemic symptoms in the affected leg or foot because of anatomic compression of the popliteal artery. Popliteal entrapment occurs in young people, most often in men complaining of intermittent claudication of one or both extremities.

Physical examination may reveal ischemic changes of the affected extremity, with normal function of the unaffected limb. When the client is at rest, the nurse may note diminished distal pulses, although this is a rare finding.

Diagnosis of popliteal entrapment is possible only after an accurate client history, physical examination, and arteriography.

The recommended treatment is surgical repair of the anatomic compression. Reconstruction of the popliteal artery may be necessary to restore arterial blood flow to the limb.

Nursing care involves preventing general postoperative complications and evaluating the patency of the graft or artery postoperatively. The nurse observes for ischemic changes and evaluates distal pulses frequently postoperatively.

Peripheral Venous Disease

To function properly, veins must be patent (unobstructed) with competent valves. Vein function also necessitates the assistance of the surrounding muscle beds to help pump blood toward the heart. If one or more veins are not operating efficiently, they become distended and clinical manifestations occur.

Two distinct phenomena alter the blood flow in veins:

- Thrombus formation (*venous thrombosis*) can lead to pulmonary embolism, a life-threatening complication (see Chap. 34).
- Defective valves lead to *venous insufficiency* and *varicose veins*, which are not life-threatening but are problematic.

Venous Thrombosis

Overview

Thrombus formation constitutes one of health care's greatest challenges. A thrombus (also called a thrombosis) is a blood clot believed to result from an endothelial injury, venous stasis, or hypercoagulability. However, the thrombosis may not be specifically attributable to one element, or it may involve all three elements. Thrombosis is often associated with an inflammatory process. When a thrombus develops, inflammation can occur around the thrombus, thickening the vein wall and consequently leading to embolization (the formation of an embolus).

Thrombophlebitis refers to a thrombus that is associated with inflammation; *phlebothrombosis* is a thrombus without inflammation. Thrombophlebitis can occur in superficial veins; however, it most frequently occurs in the deep veins of the lower extremities.

Deep venous (vein) thrombophlebitis, commonly referred to as *deep venous thrombosis* (DVT), not only is more common but also is more serious than superficial thrombophlebitis because it presents a greater risk for *pulmonary embolism,* in which a dislodged blood clot travels to the pulmonary artery.

Thrombus formation has been associated with stasis of blood flow, endothelial injury, and/or hypercoagulability, known as Virchow's triad. The precise cause of these events remains unknown; however, a few predisposing factors have been identified (see Research Applications for Nursing). Thrombosis has commonly occurred in people undergoing certain surgical procedures. The highest incidence of clot formation occurs in clients who have undergone hip surgery or open prostate surgery. Other conditions that seem to promote thrombus formation are pregnancy, ulcerative colitis, and heart failure.

Immobility can predispose a person to thrombosis. This can occur during prolonged bed rest, such as when a client is confined to bed during the perioperative period. *Phlebitis* (vein inflammation) associated with invasive procedures, such as intravenous therapy, can predispose clients to thrombosis. Severe infections, systemic lupus erythematosus, polycythemia vera, oral contraceptives, and trauma have also been linked to thrombosis.

Collaborative Management

 Assessment

The classic signs and symptoms of deep vein thrombosis (DVT) are calf or groin tenderness and pain, with or without leg swelling. Pain in the calf on dorsiflexion of the foot (Homan's sign) is another possible indicator of DVT, although the reliability of this assessment finding is controversial. The nurse examines the area that the client describes as painful, comparing this site with the contralateral limb. The nurse gently palpates the site, observing for warmth and edema. Signs and symptoms, however, may be absent with thrombophlebitis. Because there are often silent clinical findings, the nurse must have a high index of suspicion for this disorder when caring for clients at high risk.

Localized edema in one extremity may suggest thrombophlebitis. The nurse can measure and compare right and left calf and thigh circumferences for changes over time as an indicator of DVT or venous insufficiency. However, serial leg measurements may not be the most reliable indicator of DVT.

Although diagnostic tests for DVT are available, physical examination findings are often adequate for diagnosis. If a definitive diagnosis is lacking from physical examination alone, other diagnostic tests may be performed, such as venography, Doppler studies, and impedance phlebography.

Venography with contrast medium visualizes clot formation in approximately 95% of people with DVT. However, this study is generally not performed because it may precipitate thrombosis and is very painful.

Duplex ultrasonographic scanning, a noninvasive test, is the preferred diagnostic test for DVT if a definitive diagnosis cannot be made by physical examination. Doppler ultrasonography is also useful in the diagnosis of deep vein thrombosis. Normal venous circulation is characterized by audible signals, whereas thrombosed veins produce little or no flow.

 Interventions

The focus of treatment for thrombophlebitis is to prevent complications, such as pulmonary emboli, and to prevent an increase in size of the thrombus. Deep venous thrombophlebitis (thrombosis) is the most common type of thrombophlebitis. All clients with DVT are hospitalized for treatment.

➤ *Nonsurgical Management*

Deep vein thrombosis (DVT) is most often treated medically, using a combination of rest, drug therapy, and preventive measures.

Rest. Supportive therapy for DVT includes bed rest and elevation of the extremity. Some health care providers order intermittent or continuous warm, moist

▷ Research Applications for Nursing

A Nursing Assessment Tool for Deep Vein Thrombosis Shows Promise

Autar, R. (1996). Nursing assessment of clients at risk for deep vein thrombosis (DVT): The Autar DVT scale. Journal of Advanced Nursing, *23, 763–770.*

This study examined the effectiveness of using the Autar DVT scale to predict the development of deep vein thrombosis (DVT). This scale includes seven risk factors: age, build and body mass index, immobility, special DVT risk, trauma, surgery, and high-risk disease. Studying 21 subjects on two clinical units, the scale was evaluated for reliability, sensitivity, and specificity.

In this study group, the sensitivity of the scale was 100%, and the specificity was 81.2%. The reliability of the scale was reported at 0.98 and had an 83% predicted accuracy.

Critique. The researcher attempted to develop a reliable and valid tool to assess DVT risk. This scale provides a comprehensive nursing assessment to predict individuals at risk for DVT. This study cannot be generalized due to the limited small sample size and to the fact that the subjects were all orthopedic clients. The scale may be helpful in other populations and should be tested in a number of settings and with a number of client groups.

Possible Nursing Implications. This study shows the need to question and validate some of the assessments that nurses have routinely performed without a scientific basis. It clearly raises questions about exploring the various factors that may contribute to the development of DVT.

soaks to the affected area. All clients are evaluated for signs and symptoms of pulmonary embolus (PE), which include shortness of breath and chest pain. Emboli may also travel to the brain or heart, but these complications are not as common as PE (see Chap. 34).

Drug Therapy. Anticoagulants are the drugs of choice for a client with DVT and for clients at risk for DVT. Heparin is used when immediate anticoagulation is indicated, but other agents, such as aspirin or warfarin, may be used for clot prevention.

Heparin Therapy. Most clients with a confirmed diagnosis of an existing blood clot are started on a regimen of intravenous (IV) heparin (Hepalean✲) therapy. Heparin is an anticoagulant agent that, at low doses, interacts with antithrombin III to produce selective inhibition of clotting factor X. At higher doses, heparin inhibits practically all clotting factors. The ultimate result is inhibition of fibrin formation (Pinnell, 1996). Heparin does nothing to the existing clot. The physician prescribes heparin to prevent the formation of other clots, which often develop in the presence of an existing clot, and to prevent enlargement of the existing clot. Over a long period of time, the existing clot is slowly absorbed by the body.

Heparin is initially given by a bolus IV dose of approximately 100 U/kg, followed by constant infusion. The infusion is regulated by a reliable electronic infusion device that protects against accidental free flow of solution. The physician or clinical pharmacist orders concentrations of heparin (in 5% dextrose in water) and the number of units or milliliters per hour to maintain a therapeutic activated partial thromboplastin time (APTT). APTTs are obtained daily, or more frequently, and are reported to the health care provider as soon as the results are available to allow adjustment of heparin dosage. Therapeutic levels of APTTs are usually one to two times normal control levels. The nurse assesses clients for signs and symptoms of bleeding, which include hematuria, frank or occult blood in the stool, ecchymosis, petechiae, an altered level of consciousness, or pain.

Heparin can also decrease platelet counts. Mild reductions are common and are resolved with continued heparin therapy. Severe platelet reductions, although rare, result from the development of antiplatelet bodies between 6 and 14 days into treatment. Platelets aggregate into "white clots" that can cause thrombosis, usually an acute arterial occlusion (Simko & Lockhart, 1996). The provider discontinues heparin administration if severe heparin-induced thrombocytopenia and thrombosis (HITT) ($>100,000$ mm³) occurs. An oral anticoagulant may then be substituted for heparin, if necessary.

The nurse also ensures that protamine sulfate, the antidote for heparin, is available, if needed, for excessive bleeding. Chart 38–9 highlights information important to nursing care and client education associated with anticoagulant therapy.

To prevent DVT, heparin may be given in low doses subcutaneously. The health care provider usually orders a dose of 5000 U every 8–12 hours for high-risk clients, especially after orthopedic surgery. Other pharmacologic agents that may be used for prophylaxis are
■ Low-molecular-weight heparin (e.g., enoxaparin)

Chart 38–9

Nursing Care Highlight: The Client Receiving Anticoagulant Therapy

- Carefully check the dosage of anticoagulant to be administered, even if the pharmacy prepared the medication.
- Monitor the client for signs and symptoms of bleeding, including hematuria, frank or occult blood in the stool, ecchymosis, petechiae, altered mental status (indicating possible cranial bleeding), or pain (especially abdominal pain, which could indicate abdominal bleeding).
- Monitor vital signs frequently for decreased blood pressure and increased pulse (indicating possible internal bleeding).
- Have antidotes available as needed, e.g., protamine sulfate for heparin and vitamin K for warfarin (Coumadin, Warfilone✲).
- Monitor activated partial thromboplastin time (APTT) for clients receiving heparin; monitor prothrombin time (PT) or International Normalized Ratio (INR) for clients receiving warfarin.
- Apply prolonged pressure over venipuncture sites and injection sites.
- When administering *subcutaneous* heparin, apply pressure over the site and do not massage.
- Teach the client going home on an anticoagulant to
  - Use only an electric razor.
  - Take precautions to avoid injury, for example, do not use tools like hammers or saws, where accidents commonly occur.
  - Report signs and symptoms of bleeding, such as blood in the urine or stool, nosebleeds, ecchymosis, or altered mental status.
  - Take the prescribed dosage of medication at the precise time that it was ordered to be given.
  - Not stop taking the medication abruptly; the physician usually tapers the anticoagulant gradually.

- Dextran, an intravenous plasma expander
- Dihydroergotamine (DHE)
- Warfarin (Coumadin, Warfilone✲)
- Aspirin

Warfarin Therapy. After treatment for deep vein thrombosis (DVT) with heparin therapy, and after the signs and symptoms of DVT have greatly resolved, the client is usually started on oral warfarin sodium. Warfarin works in the liver to inhibit synthesis of the four vitamin K–dependent clotting factors. It takes 3–4 days before warfarin can exert therapeutic anticoagulation. For this reason, warfarin administration is started while the intravenous (IV) heparin is being infused. The heparin continues to provide therapeutic anticoagulation until this effect is achieved with warfarin. IV heparin is discontinued at that time.

Therapeutic levels of warfarin are monitored by measuring prothrombin time (PT) and the International Normalized Ratio (INR). Because prothrombin times are often inconsistent and misleading, the INR was developed. Most laboratories report both results. Most clients on warfarin for DVT should have an INR between 2.0 and 3.0 (Coyne, 1997).

The initial dosage of warfarin is usually 10–15 mg daily for 1–2 days. Maintenance therapy generally ranges from 2.5 to 7.5 mg given once a day in the evening. Clients usually receive warfarin for up to 6 months after an episode of DVT.

Nursing assessment for bleeding is similar to that described for clients receiving heparin. The nurse ensures that vitamin K, the antidote for warfarin, is available in case of excessive bleeding (see Chart 38–9).

Thrombolytic Therapy. The use of systemic thrombolytic therapy for deep vein thrombosis (DVT) is effective in dissolving thrombi quickly and completely. The greatest advantage is thought to be the prevention of valvular damage and consequential venous insufficiency, or "postphlebitic syndrome." However, thrombolytic therapy is contraindicated postoperatively, during pregnancy, and after childbirth, trauma, cerebrovascular accidents, or spinal injuries. To be most effective, thrombolytic therapy must be initiated within 5 days after the onset of symptoms.

Tissue plasminogen activator (t-PA) is the thrombolytic that has been studied the most for DVT. It should be used for at least 3 days but not more than 5. The nurse caring for clients receiving t-PA must monitor closely for signs and symptoms of bleeding (see also Chap. 40).

Prevention and Treatment of Peripheral Edema. The client's legs should be elevated when in bed and when in the chair. To help prevent chronic venous insufficiency, clients with active and resolving deep vein thrombosis are often instructed to wear knee or thigh-high compression or elastic stockings.

➤ Surgical Management

A deep venous thrombus is rarely removed surgically unless there is a massive occlusion that does not respond to medical treatment and the thrombus is of recent (1 to 2 days) onset. *Thrombectomy* is the most common surgical procedure for removing the thrombus. Preoperative and postoperative care of clients undergoing thrombectomy are similar to that for clients undergoing arterial surgery (see earlier).

Inferior Vena Caval Interruption. For clients with recurrent deep vein thrombosis or pulmonary emboli that do not respond to medical treatment and for clients who cannot tolerate anticoagulation, inferior vena caval interruption may be indicated to prevent pulmonary emboli.

Preoperative care is similar to that provided for clients receiving local anesthesia (see Chap. 20). If clients have recently been taking anticoagulants, such as warfarin (Coumadin, Warfilone✢) or heparin (Hepalean✢), the nurse consults with the physician about interrupting this therapy in the preoperative period to avoid hemorrhage.

The surgeon inserts a filter device, or "umbrella," percutaneously into the inferior vena cava (Fig. 38–11). The device is meant to trap emboli in the inferior vena cava before they progress to the lungs. Holes in the device allow blood to pass through, thus not significantly interfering with the return of blood to the heart. Popular IVC

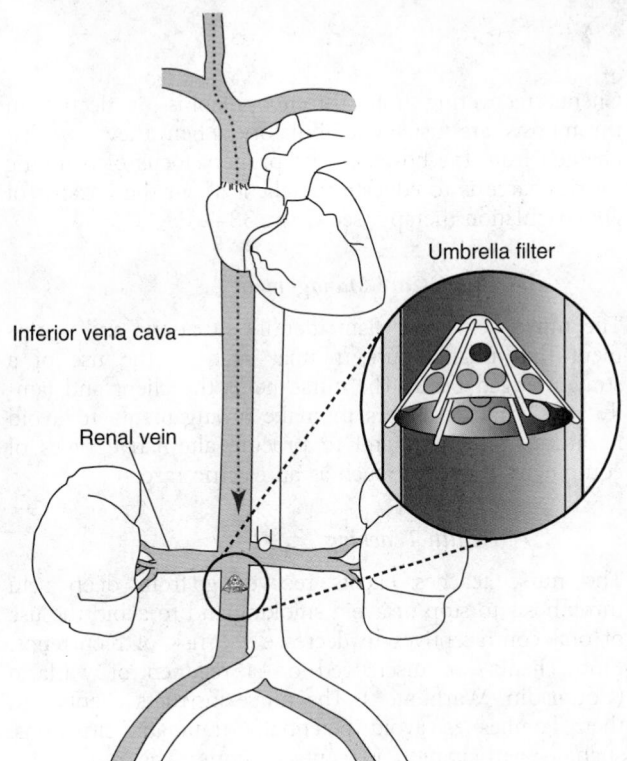

Figure 38–11. An inferior vena caval (IVC) filter.

filters include the bird's-nest filter and the Greenfield filter.

Postoperatively, the nurse inspects the incision on the right side of the chest for bleeding and signs or symptoms of infection. Other postoperative nursing care is similar to that for any client having surgery (see Chap. 22).

Ligation or External Clips. If an inferior vena cava (IVC) filter is not successful in preventing pulmonary emboli or if the filter becomes blocked with thrombi, the surgeon may perform ligation or insert external clips on the inferior vena cava to prevent pulmonary emboli.

Preoperative care for clients undergoing ligation of the vena cava or placement of an external clip is similar to that for clients undergoing abdominal laparotomy. If the client is receiving anticoagulation therapy, the nurse consults with the surgeon about temporary interruption of therapy.

Ligation and insertion of external clips in the inferior vena cava are often performed by means of an abdominal laparotomy. In a ligation, the surgeon ties off the inferior vena cava to block emboli. Application of an external clip, such as the Adams-DeWeese, narrows the inferior vena cava to four serrated transverse slits, 3–5 mm in diameter. If laparotomy is performed, the external clip procedure is preferred because there are fewer hemodynamic and venous complications and a low frequency of recurrent pulmonary emboli associated with its use.

Postoperative care for the client with IVC ligation or external clip placement is similar to that for the client after an abdominal laparotomy.

➤| Continuing Care

Clients recovering from thrombophlebitis or deep vein thrombosis are usually ambulatory when they are discharged from the hospital. The primary focus of planning for discharge is to educate the client about the hazards of anticoagulation therapy (see Chart 38–9).

➤ Home Care Management

The nurse helps the client identify situations and equipment that might cause trauma, such as the use of a straight-edged razor. The nurse helps the client and family or significant others to make arrangements to avoid hazardous situations and to procure alternative types of equipment, if needed, such as an electric razor.

➤ Health Teaching

The nurse teaches clients recovering from deep vein thrombosis to stop or avoid smoking and to avoid the use of oral contraceptives to decrease the risk of recurrence. Most clients are discharged on a regimen of warfarin (Coumadin, Warfilone✦). The nurse instructs clients and their families to avoid potentially traumatic situations, such as participation in contact sports. The nurse provides all clients with written and oral information about the signs and symptoms of bleeding (see earlier). The client must report any of these manifestations to the health care provider immediately.

The anticoagulant effect of warfarin may be reversed by the omission of one or two doses of the drug or by the administration of vitamin K. In case of injury, clients are directed to apply pressure to bleeding wounds and to seek medical assistance immediately. The nurse encourages clients to carry an identification card or wear a medical alert (Medic-Alert) bracelet that states that they are taking warfarin.

The nurse also instructs clients to inform their dentist and other health care providers that they are taking warfarin before receiving treatment or prescriptions. Prothrombin times are affected by many prescription and over-the-counter medications, such as antacids, antihistamines, aspirin, mineral oil, oral contraceptives, and large doses of vitamin C. The action of warfarin is also affected by high-fat and vitamin K–rich foods, such as cabbage, cauliflower, broccoli, asparagus, lettuce, turnips, spinach, kale, fish, liver, and coffee. Clients are therefore instructed to eat a well-balanced diet and to avoid taking additional medications without consulting a health care provider. The nurse arranges for clients to have determinations of prothrombin time 1–2 weeks after discharge.

ELDERLY CONSIDERATIONS

Ⓔ Warfarin is used with caution with older adults or debilitated patients. A reduced dose is often recommended in an effort to prevent spontaneous intracranial bleeding or excessive bleeding related to trauma. Many older adults may have reduced kidney or liver function and a decreased ability to metabolize and excrete the drug. For this reason, it is usually used only when the benefits outweigh the risks. The older adult may have problems adhering to the routine laboratory tests required to monitor the medication's effectiveness.

If the health care provider prescribes antiembolism stockings, the nurse teaches clients how and when to apply them.

Clients who have experienced deep vein thrombosis (DVT) may fear recurrence of a thrombus and may also be concerned about treatment with warfarin and the risk for bleeding. The nurse assures such clients that participation in the prescribed treatment frequently helps in resolving this problem and that ongoing assessment of prothrombin levels and INRs should minimize the risks of bleeding.

➤ Health Care Resources

Clients discharged on warfarin need access to a pharmacy to renew prescriptions and, if feasible, to obtain a Medic-Alert bracelet. Clients also need access to a laboratory for frequent monitoring of prothrombin times and INRs.

Venous Insufficiency
Overview

Venous insufficiency occurs as a result of prolonged venous hypertension, which stretches the veins and damages the valves. This can lead to a back-up of blood and further venous hypertension, resulting in edema. Edema occurs as the by-products of red blood cell break down and infiltrate the surrounding tissues. Because the client cannot eliminate waste products, they accumulate within the tissues. With time, this stasis (stoppage) results in venous stasis ulcers, swelling, and cellulitis.

Venous efficiency is altered when thrombosis occurs or when valves are not functioning correctly. Defective valves can result from prolonged venous hypertension, which stretches the veins and damages valves. This can occur in people who stand or sit in one position for long periods, such as teachers and office personnel. Pregnancy and obesity can also cause chronically distended veins, which lead to damaged valves. Thrombus formation can contribute to valve destruction. Chronic venous insufficiency often occurs in clients who have had thrombophlebitis.

Collaborative Management

 Assessment

Clients with venous insufficiency may have edema in both extremities. There may be *stasis dermatitis* or discoloration along the ankles, extending up to the calf. In people with long-term venous insufficiency or stasis, *ulcers* often form. Ulcer formation can result from the edema or from minor injury to the limb. Venous ulcers typically occur over the malleolus, more often medially than laterally. The ulcer usually has irregular borders. Generally, these ulcers are chronic and difficult to heal (see Chart 38–6). Many clients live with ulcers for years, and recurrence is common. Some clients may lose one or both limbs if ulcers are not controlled.

✦ Interventions

The focus of treating venous insufficiency is to decrease edema and promote venous return from the affected extremity. Clients are not usually hospitalized for venous insufficiency alone unless it is complicated by an ulcer or another disorder is occurring simultaneously.

> ### ➤ *Nonsurgical Management*

Treatment of chronic venous insufficiency is primarily nonsurgical, unless it is complicated by a venous stasis ulcer that requires surgical debridement. The goal of managing venous stasis ulcers is twofold: to heal the ulcer and to prevent stasis with recurrence of ulcer formation.

Treatment of Edema. Clients with chronic venous insufficiency wear elastic or compression stockings, which fit from the middle of the foot to just below the knee or to the thigh. Clients should wear the stockings during the day and evening. The nurse instructs clients to elevate their legs for at least 20 minutes four or five times per day but to avoid long periods of sitting or standing in place. When the client is in bed, the legs should be elevated above the level of the heart (Chart 38–10).

The nurse and physician should also confer about the use of intermittent sequential pneumatic compression of the lower extremities for clients with past or present ve-

---

Chart 38-10

Education Guide: Venous Insufficiency

Elastic Stockings

- Wear elastic stockings as prescribed, usually during the day and evening.
- Put the stockings on upon awakening and before getting out of bed.
- When applying the stockings, do not "bunch up" and apply like socks. Instead, place your hand inside the stocking and pull out the heel. Then place the foot of the stocking over your foot and slide the rest of the stocking up. Be sure that rough seams on the stocking are on the outside, not next to your skin.
- Do not push stockings down for comfort because they may function like a tourniquet and further impair venous return.
- Put on a clean pair of stockings each day. Wash them by hand (not in a washing machine) in a gentle detergent and warm water.
- If the stockings seem to be "stretched out," replace them with a new pair.

Do's and Don'ts

- Elevate your legs for at least 20 minutes four or five times a day. When in bed, elevate your legs above the level of your heart.
- Avoid prolonged sitting or standing.
- Do not cross your legs; crossing at the ankles is acceptable for short periods of time.
- Do not wear tight, restrictive pants; avoid girdles and garters.

---

nous stasis ulcers. If the client is being treated for an open venous ulcer, the device is applied over a dressing such as an Unna boot. The nurse instructs the client to apply the pump as directed during the period of healing. Because of the high incidence of venous ulcer recurrence, clients with chronic venous insufficiency whose ulcers have healed are encouraged to continue compression therapy for life.

Treatment of Venous Stasis Ulcers. Venous stasis ulcers are slightly more manageable than ulcers resulting from arterial disease. They are chronic in nature, with some clients manifesting the same ulcer for years. Ulcers often heal, only to reoccur later in the same area. The client may have simultaneous ulcers for several years.

Dressings. Two types of occlusive dressings are used for venous stasis ulcers: oxygen permeable and oxygen impermeable. Because the role of atmospheric oxygen in wound healing is controversial, opinions vary with regard to which type of dressing is preferred. The oxygen-permeable polyethylene film (e.g., Op Site) and an oxygen-impermeable hydrocolloid dressing (e.g., DuoDerm) are common. Hydrocolloid dressings are left in place for a minimum of 3–5 days for best effect.

Implications for the Elderly. A potential problem is that some occlusive dressings stick to the skin and can cause more damage to friable skin, especially in older clients. Newer dressings have calcium alginate (e.g., Sorbsan), which prevents maceration of healthy tissue.

If the client is ambulatory, an Unna boot may be used. This dressing is constructed of gauze that has been moistened with zinc oxide. The health care provider applies the boot to the affected limb, from the toes to the knee, after the ulcer has been cleaned with normal saline solution. Povidone-iodine (Betadine) and hydrogen peroxide are not used because they destroy granulation tissue. The Unna boot is then covered with an elastic wrap and hardens like a cast; this promotes venous return and prevents stasis. The Unna boot also forms a sterile environment for the ulcer. The physician should change the boot approximately once a week. The nurse instructs the client about what to look for if arterial occlusion should occur from an Unna boot that is too tight.

Drug Therapy. The provider may prescribe topical agents to chemically debride the ulcer, eliminating necrotic tissue and promoting healing. Fibrinolysin and desoxyribonuclease (Elase) are most effective after dry eschar (outer) tissue has been surgically removed. Because these agents can injure healthy tissue, the nurse protects the surrounding skin with an oil-based agent such as petroleum jelly (Vaseline). Injury to healthy tissue can prolong healing time.

If an infection occurs or cellulitis develops, systemic antibiotics are more effective than local ointments. Ointments are not well absorbed in the presence of edema. They may also inhibit the ulcer's healing by occluding the ulcer and prohibiting the needed interactions with air.

Surgical Management. Surgery for chronic venous insufficiency is not usually performed because historically it has not been successful. Attempts at transplanting vein valves have had limited success. Surgical debridement of venous ulcers is similar to that performed for arterial ulcers (see earlier).

 Continuing Care

The goal for the client with chronic venous insufficiency is to manage the client in the home. For clients with frequent acute complications and repeated hospital admissions, case management can help to meet appropriate clinical and cost outcomes.

➤ Home Care Management

The nurse helps clients with chronic venous insufficiency to plan for opportunities and facilities that allow for elevation of the lower extremities in and outside the home. In addition, clients with venous stasis ulcers need to plan for care of the ulcers.

➤ Health Teaching

The nurse instructs clients with chronic venous stasis to
- Avoid standing still if possible
- Elevate their legs when sitting
- Avoid crossing their legs
- Avoid wearing tight girdles, tight pants, and narrow-banded knee-high socks

The physician prescribes support hose or antiembolism stockings. The nurse teaches clients to apply these stockings before they get out of bed in the morning and to remove them just before going to bed at night (see Chart 38–10). The nurse also advises clients that they will probably need to wear these stockings for the rest of their lives.

To improve circulation and aid in weight reduction, the nurse prescribes an exercise program on an individual basis with the health care provider input. The nurse encourages all clients to maintain an optimal weight and may consult with the dietitian to plan a weight-reducing diet. The nurse instructs clients with venous stasis ulcers how to care for the ulcers at home.

Clients with venous stasis disease, especially those with venous stasis ulcers, may require long-term emotional support to assist them in meeting chronic needs. They may also need assistance in coping with necessary lifestyle adjustments, such as changes in occupation.

➤ Health Care Resources

Clients with venous stasis ulcers may need the assistance of a home health nurse to perform dressing changes. Clients with Unna boots will need weekly transportation to their health provider for dressing changes. The nurse will need to arrange for a sequential compression device in the home if the health care provider prescribes one.

Varicose Veins

Overview

Varicose veins are distended, protruding veins that appear darkened and tortuous. They can occur in anyone, but they are common in clients older than 30 years whose occupations require prolonged standing. Varicose veins are also frequently seen in pregnant women, clients with systemic problems, such as heart disease, obese clients, and clients with a family history of varicose veins.

As the vein wall weakens and dilates, venous pressure increases and the valves become incompetent (defective). The incompetent valves enhance the vessel dilation, and the veins become tortuous and distended. The client may complain of pain, especially after standing, and may experience a fullness in the legs. Nursing assessment reveals distended protruding veins.

The Trendelenburg test assists with the diagnosis. The client is placed in a supine position with elevated legs. As the client sits up, the veins would normally fill from the distal end; however, if there are varicosities, the veins fill from the proximal end.

Collaborative Management

Conservative measures are the treatment of choice. These involve wearing elastic stockings and elevating the extremities as much as possible. Clients who continue to have pain or unsightly veins, despite this treatment, may opt for either sclerotherapy or surgical removal of the vein.

Sclerotherapy is performed on small or a limited number of varicosities. The physician injects a solution, such as sodium tetradecyl, directly into the vein. A pressure dressing is applied over the sclerosed vein to keep vessels free of blood for 24–72 hours. The surgeon performs an incision and drainage of trapped blood in the sclerosed vein 14–21 days after injection, followed by application of a second pressure dressing for 12–18 hours.

Varicose veins are surgically removed when they are larger than 4 mm in diameter or are in clusters. The surgeon may use the stab avulsion technique if the saphenous veins are competent. The surgeon exposes varices through 2- to 3-mm stab incisions, grasping the veins with hooks, and dividing and avulsing each vein.

The surgeon may need to strip (remove) affected veins if the saphenous vein is incompetent. The surgeon threads a long wire through an incision above an affected vein, pulling it down through the vein and out through an incision below the vein. After this procedure, the client's legs are bandaged with firm elastic (Ace) bandages.

Postoperatively, the nurse assesses the groin and entire leg for bleeding through the elastic bandage. The nurse instructs the client to keep the legs elevated and to perform range-of-motion exercises of the legs at least hourly. Clients are ambulatory and are often discharged from the hospital by the first postoperative day. At this time, the nurse instructs clients to continue to wear elastic stockings, walk, limit sitting, avoid standing in one place, and elevate their legs when sitting.

Phlebitis

Phlebitis is an inflammation of the superficial veins caused by an irritation, such as intravenous therapy (also see Chap. 17). The client has a reddened, warm area radiating up an extremity, commonly an arm. The client may also experience pain, soreness, and swelling of the extremity.

Treatment involves application of warm, moist soaks, which dilate the vein and promote circulation. Sometimes a heating unit is used to keep the soaks warm. Rarely, ice packs are used. The nurse applies the soaks, making sure that the temperature is not warm enough to burn the client, and assesses for complications, such as tissue necrosis, infection, or pulmonary embolus. After a few days of conservative therapy, the inflammation usually subsides.

Vascular Trauma

Overview

Many types of trauma can result in vascular injury. Injuries to the blood vessels in the upper and lower extremities account for approximately 70% of all vascular injuries to the human body. Vascular injuries to the blood vessels include punctures, lacerations, and transections. Acute blunt or penetrating trauma may result in a false aneurysm or hematoma. Arteriovenous fistulas may be seen after penetrating injuries. The more common causes of penetrating injuries to the blood vessels are gunshot and knife wounds.

Blunt trauma, which is less common, can result from high-speed automobile accidents as a result of the shearing force of rapid deceleration. Vascular trauma can also occur during arterial puncture for arteriographic or hemodynamic studies in which a dissection, hematoma, or occlusive lesion occurs.

Collaborative Management

The history and physical examination aid in establishing the diagnosis in the client with vascular injury. The nurse questions the client or family about the mechanism of injury, the site of injury, the amount of blood loss, and symptoms present after the injury.

The nurse assesses for circulatory, sensory, or motor impairment but is aware that, despite significant trauma, impairment may not be apparent, especially if deep vessels have been injured. Arteriography provides essential information about the vascular injury. Emergency or urgent surgical intervention is warranted for clients with ischemia to maximize successful revascularization.

Management of vascular injuries is often initiated in a hospital emergency department. Careful triage by the nurse is crucial. Snyder and associates (1989) suggest three types of vascular injuries, with variations in the time at which definitive treatment is essential:

■ Category I: These injuries expose clients to immediate threats of survival and must be treated immediately (e.g., tension pneumothorax, cardiac tamponade, exsanguinating hemorrhage).
■ Category II: These injuries are serious but not quite as severe, allowing time for more extensive evaluation before treatment is initiated (e.g., major fractures, abdominal trauma in the presence of stable vital signs, genitourinary trauma).
■ Category III: These injuries permit management of the injury at a more leisurely pace (e.g., lacerations, simple lacerations, contusions).

The most important principles in the management of vascular trauma are establishment of a patent airway, control of bleeding, and restoration of blood flow.

The method of repair varies with the type of vascular injury. Techniques include vein bypass grafting, lateral suture repair, thrombectomy (excision of blood clot), resection with end-to-end anastomosis, and vein patch grafting.

SELECTED BIBLIOGRAPHY

Allen, K. M., & Phillips, J. M. (1997). *Women's health across the lifespan.* Philadelphia: J. B. Lippincott.

Allen, S. L. (1995). Perioperative nursing interventions for intravascular stent placement. *AORN, 61* (4), 689–709.

American Heart Association. (1995). *Heart and stroke facts.* Chicago: American Heart Association.

Autar, R. (1996). Nursing assessment of clients at risk of deep vein thrombosis (DVT): The Autar DVT scale. *Journal of Advanced Nursing, 23,* 763–770.

*Bickerstaff, L. K., Hollier, L. H., Van Peenen, H. J., et al. (1984). Abdominal aortic aneurysm: The changing natural history. *Journal of Vascular Surgery, 1,* 6–12.

Bunt, T. J. (1995). Revascularization versus amputation for elderly patient. *AORN Journal, 62* (3), 433–435.

Cahall, E., & Spence, R. K. (1995). Practical nursing measures for vascular compromise in the lower leg. *Ostomy and Wound Management, 41* (9), 16–32.

Calhoun, D. A., & Oparil, S. (1995). Racial differences in the pathogenisis of hypertension. *American Journal of the Medical Sciences, 310,* 586–590.

Carlson, K. J., & Eisenstat, S. A. (1995). *Primary care of women.* St. Louis: C. V. Mosby.

Clagett, G. P., & Krupski, W. C. (1995). Antithrombotic therapy in peripheral arterial occlusive disease. *Chest, 108* (4), 431S–443S.

Cookingham, A. (1995). Peripheral vascular disease: Education concerns for patients with a chronic disease in the changing health-care environment. *AACN Clinical Issues, 6* (4), 670–676.

Coyne, N. (1997). Current concepts in anticoagulant therapy. *The Journal of Care Management, 3* (4), 28–46, 73.

Dorgan, M. B., Birke, J. A., Moretto, J. A., Patout, C. A., & Rehm, K. B. (1995, November). Performing foot screening for diabetic patients. *American Journal of Nursing, 95,* 32–36.

Dumas, M. A. S. (1995). Intermittent claudication. *American Journal of Nursing, 95* (12), 34.

Eaton, L. E., Buck, E. A., & Catanzaro, J. E. (1996). The nurse's role in facilitating compliance in clients with hypertension. *MEDSURG Nursing, 5,* 339–345, 359.

Fahey, V. A. (1994). *Vascular nursing* (2nd ed.). Philadelphia: W. B. Saunders.

Freis, E. D. (1995). The efficacy and safety of diuretics in treating hypertension. *Annals of Internal Medicine, 122* (3), 223–226.

Gerhard, M., Baum, P., & Raby, K. E. (1995). Peripheral arterial-vascular disease in women: Prevalence, prognosis, and treatment. *Cardiology, 86,* 349–355.

Harris, A. H., Brown-Etris, M., & Troyer-Caudle, J. (1996, January). Managing vascular leg ulcers part I: Assessment. *American Journal of Nursing, 96,* 38–43.

Harris, A. H., Brown-Etris, M., & Troyer-Caudle, J. (1996, February). Managing vascular leg ulcers part II: Treatment. *American Journal of Nursing, 96,* 40–46.

Hatton, D. C., Yue, Q., & McCarron, D. A. (1995). Mechanisms of calcium's effects on blood pressure. *Seminars in Nephrology, 15,* 593–602.

Henderson, L. J., & Kirkland, J. S. (1995). Angioplasty with stent placement in peripheral arterial occlusive disease. *AORN Journal, 61* (4), 671–685.

Hill, E. M. (1995). Perioperative management of patients with vascular disease. *AACN Clinical Issues, 6* (4), 547–561.

Hulley, S. B., & Newman, T. B. (1994). Cholesterol in the elderly. Is it important? *Journal of American Medical Association, 272,* 1372–1373.

*Joint National Committee. (1993). The fifth report of the Joint National Committee on detection, evaluation, and treatment of high blood pressure. *Archives of Internal Medicine, 153,* 154–183.

Kannel, W. B., & Wilson, P. W. (1995). An update of coronary risk factors. *Medical Clinics of North America, 79,* 951–971.

Karch, A. M. (1995). Pain, pills, and possibilities: Drug therapy in peripheral vascular disease. *AACN Clinical Issues, 6* (4), 614–630.

Krenzer, M. E. (1995). Peripheral vascular assessment: Finding your way through arteries and veins. *AACN Clinical Issues, 6* (4), 631–644.

Krikorian, R. K., & Vacek, J. L. (1995). Peripheral arterial disease. *Postgraduate Medicine, 97* (6), 109–119.

Kuncl, N., & Nelson, K. M. (1997). Antihypertensive drugs: Balancing risks and benefits. *Nursing 97, 27* (8), 46–49.

LaPalio, L. R. (1995). Hypertension in the elderly. *American Family Physician, 52,* 1161–1165.

Lewis, C. E. (1996). Characteristics and treatment of hypertension in women: A review of the literature. *American Journal of Medical Sciences, 311,* 193–199.

Littenberg, B. (1995). A practice guideline revisited: Screening for hypertension. *Annals of Internal Medicine, 122,* 937–939.

Lowe, G. D. O., Reid, A. W., & Leiberman, D. P. (1994). Management of thrombosis in peripheral arterial disease. *British Medical Bulletin, 50* (4), 923–935.

Manolio, T. A., Cutler, J. A., Furber, C. D., Psaty, B. M., Whelton, P. K., & Applegate, W. B. (1995). Trends in pharmacologic management of hypertension in the United States. *Archives of Internal Medicine, 15* (5), 829–837.

Massie, B. M. (1995). Systemic hypertension. In L. M. Tierney, S. J. McPhee, & M. A. Papadakis (Eds.), *Current therapy* (pp. 373–390). Norwalk, CT: Appleton & Lange.

Matteson, M. A., McConnell, E. S., & Linton, A. D. (1997). *Gerontological nursing: Concepts and practice* (2nd ed.). Philadelphia: W. B. Saunders.

McKenney, J. M., Proctor, J. D., Harris, S., & Chinchili, V. M. (1994). A comparison of the efficacy and toxic effects of sustained- vs immediate-release niacin in hypercholesterolemic patients. *Journal of American Medical Association, 271,* 672–677.

*National Cholesterol Education Program. (1993). Summary of the second report of the national cholesterol education program. *Journal of American Medical Association, 269,* 3015–3023.

Nunnelee, J. D. (1995, December). Minimize the risk of DVT. *RN,* 28–31.

Pinnell, N. L. (1996). *Nursing pharmacology.* Philadelphia: W. B. Saunders.

Schaefer, E. J., Lamon-Fava, S., Jenner, J. L., McNamara, J. R., Ordovas, J. M., Davis, E., Abolafia, J. M., Lippel, K., & Levey, R. I. (1994). Lipoprotein(a) levels and risk of coronary heart disease in men. *Journal of American Medical Association, 271,* 999–1003.

*Schlafer, M. (1993). *The nurse, pharmacology, and drug therapy: A prototype approach* (2nd ed.). Redwood City, CA: Addison-Wesley.

Schwartz, L. B. (1998). Conventional and alternative therapies for acute deep vein thrombosis. *The Journal of Care Management, 4* (suppl), 9–13.

Simko, L. C., & Lockhart, J. S. (1996). Action stat: Heparin-induced thrombocytopenia and thrombosis. *Nursing 96, 26* (3), 33.

*Snyder, W. H., Thal, E. R., & Perry, M. O. (1989). Vascular injuries of the extremities. In R. B. Rutherford (Ed.), *Vascular surgery* (3rd ed., pp. 613–637). Philadelphia: W. B. Saunders.

Sparks, K. S. (1996). Are you up to date on weight-based heparin dosing? *American Journal of Nursing, 96,* (4) 33–36.

Stillman, F. A. (1995). Smoking cessation for the hospitalized cardiac patient: Rationale for and report of a model program. *Journal of Cardiovascular Nursing, 9,* 25–36.

Tierney, L. M. (1995). Blood vessels and lymphatics. In L. M. Tierney, S. J. McPhee, & M. A. Papadakis (Eds.), *Current therapy* (pp. 391–422). Norwalk, CT: Appleton & Lange.

Warbinek, E., & Wyness, A. (1994). Caring for patients with complications after elective abdominal aortic aneurysm surgery: A case study. *Journal of Vascular Nursing, 12* (3), 73–79.

Wheeler, E. C., & Brenner, Z. R. (1995). Peripheral vascular anatomy, physiology, and pathophysiology. *AACN Clinical Issues, 6* (4), 505–514.

Whitney, E. N., Cataldo, C. B., & Rolfes, S. R. (1994). *Understanding normal and clinical nutrition.* St. Paul: West Publishing Co.

Wills, E. M., & Sloan, H. L. (1996). Assessing peripheral arterial disorders in the home: A multidisciplinary clinical guide. *Home Healthcare Nurse, 14,* 669–682.

Wilson, R. F. (1994). Pre-existing peripheral arterial disease in trauma. *Critical Care Clinics, 10* (3), 567–593.

SUGGESTED READINGS

Cahall, E., & Spence, R. K. (1995). Practical nursing measures for vascular compromise in the lower leg. *Ostomy and Wound Management, 41* (9), 16–32.

This article presents the resources for patient education and treatment for individuals with peripheral vascular disease of the lower extremity. It presents the nursing measures for individuals with chronic venous insufficiency and strategies to improve compliance. Tables that define food label claims, differentiate venous and arterial ulcers, and describe compression devices provide helpful information to nurses.

Kuncl, N., & Nelson, K. M. (1997). Antihypertensive drugs: Balancing risks and benefits. *Nursing 97, 27* (8), 46–49.

This article reviews the major classifications of drugs used for hypertensive clients. The primary focus of the discussion is on health teaching, with an emphasis on how the nurse can teach clients to minimize drug side effects.

Wills, E. M., & Sloan, H. L. (1996). Assessing peripheral arterial disorders in the home: A multidisciplinary clinical guide. *Home Healthcare Nurse, 14,* 669–682.

This article presents a comprehensive approach to care of the client with PAD at home. In addition to the clinical guide presented, the authors discuss the interdisciplinary health problems and interventions that are needed for PAD. A continuing education (CE) test at the end of the article allows the reader to apply for CE credit.

INTERVENTIONS FOR CLIENTS IN SHOCK

The syndrome of shock is a common occurrence in acute care settings, although conditions leading to shock can occur anywhere. Shock is a whole body response to any situation that causes poor oxygenation of tissues and organs. Multisystem organ failure (MOF) and death can result if conditions causing shock are not treated. Nurses can play a vital role in the prevention of shock and its complications by initiating appropriate early interventions. Table 39–1 lists important concepts related to shock.

Overview

Body organs, tissues, and cells need a continuous supply of oxygen for proper metabolism and function. The cardiovascular system delivers oxygen to all tissues and removes cellular wastes. The components of the cardiovascular system are the blood, blood vessels, and heart. When any component of the cardiovascular system does not function properly for any reason, the syndrome of shock can result.

Shock is a pathologic condition rather than a disease state. It is initiated by abnormal cellular metabolism that occurs when insufficient oxygen is delivered to the tissues (Guyton & Hall, 1996). Shock was previously classified as hypovolemic, cardiogenic, vasogenic, or septic, indicating the site of origin of the problem causing shock. The condition, now classified by the specific functional impairment manifested, consists of *hypovolemic shock, cardiogenic shock, distributive shock,* and *obstructive shock* (Effron & Chernow, 1992). Table 39–2 compares the old and new classification systems and common conditions causing each category of shock. Because the functional classification is used by researchers and guides clinicians, it is used in this chapter.

Many clinical manifestations of shock are similar, regardless of the cause or specific impairment. Common findings are due to physiologic compensatory mechanisms. Manifestations unique to any type of shock are due to specific tissue dysfunction. The common clinical features of shock are listed in Chart 39–1.

TABLE 39–1

Key Concepts Related to Shock

- Shock results when too little oxygen reaches cells and tissues.
- Anyone is susceptible to shock.
- Shock progresses in a predictable, orderly fashion.
- Shock is reversible when the compensatory mechanisms are supported and the underlying causes are eliminated.
- Most clinical manifestations of shock are related to the body's compensatory responses to shock and not the cause of shock.
- The nurse always considers the possibility and probability of shock development.
- Subtle changes in heart rate, level of consciousness, and behavior may herald the onset of shock.
- Clients experiencing the early phase of sepsis-induced distributive shock may be warm and pink with a high cardiac output.
- Oxygen administration is an appropriate therapy for any type of shock.
- Changes in systolic blood pressure are not reliable indicators of initial and nonprogressive stages of shock.

Physiology Review

Oxygenation of any organ or tissue depends on how much oxygenated arterial blood perfuses (moves into and through) the organ or tissue. Organ perfusion is related to mean arterial pressure (MAP). Because the cardiovascular system is a closed but continuous circuit, the factors that influence MAP include

- Total blood volume
- Cardiac output
- Size of the vascular bed

Total blood volume and cardiac output are directly related to MAP, so that increases in either total blood volume or cardiac output usually raise MAP. Decreases in either total blood volume or cardiac output eventually lower MAP.

The size of the vascular bed is inversely related to MAP, so that increases in the size of the vascular bed lower MAP and decreases raise MAP (Fig. 39–1). The blood vessels, especially those connected directly to capillaries (arterioles and venules), can increase in size by relaxing the smooth muscle in vessel walls or decrease by

TABLE 39–2

Comparison of New and Old Shock Classification Systems

Classification by Functional Impairment

Hypovolemic	Cardiogenic	Distributive	Obstructive

• Total body fluid decreased (in all fluid compartments)
  • Hemorrhage
  • Dehydration
	• Direct pump failure
	• Fluid volume not affected
	  • Myocardial infarction
	    Valvular problems
	     Stenosis
	     Incompentence
	  • Myopathies
	  • Dysrhythmias
	  • Cardiac arrest
		• Fluid shifted from central vascular space
		• Total body fluid volume normal or increased
		  • Neural-induced loss of vascular tone
		  • Chemical-induced loss of vascular tone
		    Sepsis
		    Anaphylaxis
		    Capillary leak
			• Cardiac function decreased by noncardiac factors
			• Total body fluid volume not affected
			• Central volume decreased
			  • Pulmonary hypertension
			  • Tension pneumothorax
			  • Pericarditis
			  • Thoracic tumor
			  • Tamponade

Classification by Site of Origin

Hypovolemic	Cardiogenic	Vasogenic	Septic

• Central vascular volume decreased
• Total body fluid may or may not be decreased
  • Hemorrhage
  • Dehydration
  • Fluid shifts
    Trauma
    Burns
    Anaphylaxis
	• Direct pump failure
	• Indirect pump failure
	• Decreased cardiac output
	• Total body fluid not decreased
	  • Valvular problems
	    Stenosis
	    Incompetence
	  • Myocardial infarction
	  • Myopathies
	  • Dysrhythmias
	  • Cardiac arrest
	  • Tamponade
	  • Pericarditis
	  • Pulmonary hypertension
	  • Pulmonary emboli
		• Loss of vascular tone
		• Total body fluid not decreased
		  • Neurogenic
		    Head trauma
		    Vasovagal response
		  • Vessel dilation
		    Anaphylaxis
		    Inflammation
			• Loss of vascular tone
			• Eventual reduced cardiac output
			• Seen as a more intense type of vasogenic shock
			  • Infection

Chart 39-1

Key Features of Shock

Cardiovascular

- Decreased cardiac output
- Increased pulse rate
- Thready pulse quality
- Decreased blood pressure
- Narrowed pulse pressure
- Postural hypotension
- Low central venous pressure
- Flat neck and hand veins in dependent positions
- Slow capillary refill in nail beds
- Diminished peripheral pulses

Respiratory

- Increased respiratory rate
- Shallow depth of respirations
- Decreased arterial $PaCO_2$
- Decreased arterial PaO_2
- Cyanosis, especially around lips and nail beds

Neuromuscular

- Early
  - Anxiety
  - Restlessness
- Late
  - Decreased central nervous system activity (lethargy to coma)
  - Generalized muscle weakness
  - Diminished or absent deep tendon reflexes
  - Sluggish pupillary response to light

Renal

- Decreased urinary output
- Increased specific gravity
- Sugar and acetone present in urine

Integumentary

- Cool to cold
- Pale to mottled to cyanotic
- Moist, clammy
- Mouth dry, paste-like coating present

Gastrointestinal

- Decreased motility
- Diminished or absent bowel sounds
- Nausea and vomiting
- Constipation
- Increased thirst

contracting the muscle. When blood vessels dilate but the total blood volume remains the same, blood pressure decreases, and blood flow is slower. When blood vessels constrict but the total blood volume remains the same, blood pressure increases, and blood flow is faster.

Blood vessels contain nerves from the sympathetic division of the autonomic nervous system. Some nerves continuously stimulate vascular smooth muscle, so that the blood vessels are normally partially constricted. This state of variable blood vessel constriction is called *sympathetic tone*. An increase in sympathetic stimulation causes the

vascular smooth muscle to constrict further, raising MAP; a decrease in sympathetic stimulation causes the vascular smooth muscle to dilate, lowering MAP.

Blood flow to body organs varies to adjust to changes in tissue oxygen needs. The body can selectively increase blood flow to some areas while reducing blood flow to others. Some organs, such as the skin and skeletal muscles, can tolerate low levels of oxygen for hours without dying or becoming damaged. Other organs, such as the heart, brain, and liver, tolerate hypoxic conditions (low levels of tissue oxygenation) poorly, and even just a few minutes without adequate oxygen results in serious or permanent damage.

Pathophysiology

The underlying problems common to all types of shock, regardless of cause, are the effects of anaerobic cellular metabolism (metabolism without oxygen), which result from inadequate tissue oxygenation (Shoemaker, 1994). These effects cause adverse changes in tissue function. The body then begins to compensate in an attempt to maintain or restore tissue perfusion and oxygenation even while the triggering events of shock are still present.

When the conditions that cause shock remain uncorrected, shock progresses in a predictable sequence consisting of

1. Initial stage
2. Nonprogressive stage
3. Progressive stage
4. Refractory stage

The stages of shock are identified on the basis of

- How well the client's compensatory mechanisms are working
- The severity of the clinical manifestations
- The reversibility of tissue damage

The main triggering event leading to the recognizable picture of shock is a sustained decrease in mean arterial pressure (MAP) that results from decreased cardiac output, decreased circulating blood volume, or expansion of the vascular bed. A decrease in MAP of 5 to 10 mmHg below the client's baseline value is immediately detected by pressure-sensitive nerve receptors (baroreceptors) located in the aortic arch and the carotid sinus (Guyton & Hall, 1996). This information is transmitted to brain centers, stimulating compensatory mechanisms, which in turn ensure continued blood flow and oxygen delivery to vital organs while limiting blood flow to less vital areas. This moving of blood into selected areas while bypassing others (shunting) leads to the physiologic changes and clinical manifestations of shock.

If the events that caused the initial decrease in MAP are halted at this point, the compensatory mechanisms can return the body to a normal perfused and oxygenated state, even without outside intervention. If the initiating events continue and MAP decreases further, some tissues perform metabolic activities under anaerobic conditions, creating an increase in lactic acid and other harmful me-

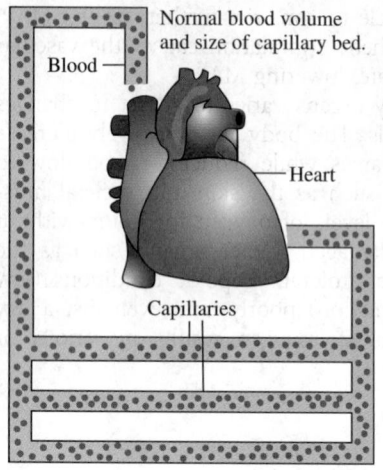

Normal blood volume and size of capillary bed.

Blood

Heart

Capillaries

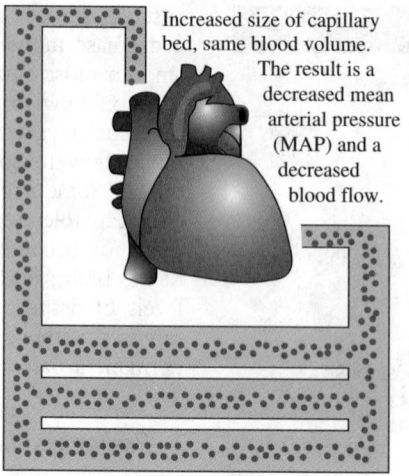

Increased size of capillary bed, same blood volume. The result is a decreased mean arterial pressure (MAP) and a decreased blood flow.

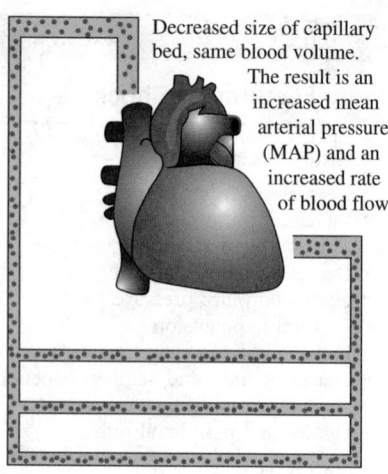

Decreased size of capillary bed, same blood volume. The result is an increased mean arterial pressure (MAP) and an increased rate of blood flow.

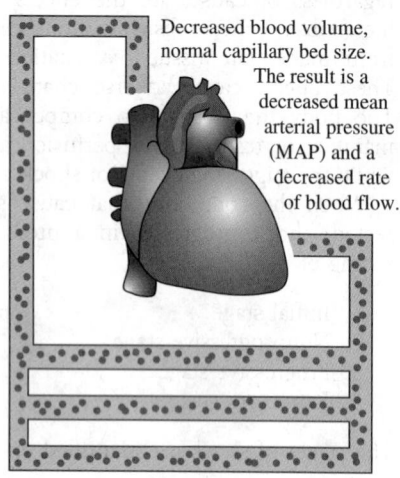

Decreased blood volume, normal capillary bed size. The result is a decreased mean arterial pressure (MAP) and a decreased rate of blood flow.

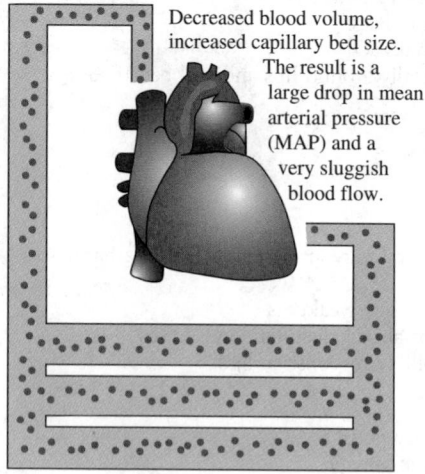

Decreased blood volume, increased capillary bed size. The result is a large drop in mean arterial pressure (MAP) and a very sluggish blood flow.

Figure 39–1. Interaction of blood volume and the size of the capillary bed affecting mean arterial pressure.

tabolites (such as degradative enzymes and oxygen radicals). These substances cause electrolyte and acid-base imbalances that have generalized, tissue-damaging effects and depress cardiac activity. Such effects are temporary and reversible if the cause of shock is corrected within 1 to 2 hours after onset. When conditions causing shock continue for longer periods without interventions, the resulting acid-base imbalance, electrolyte imbalances, and increased levels of toxic metabolites so damage the cells in vital organs that full recovery from shock is no longer possible. Table 39–3 summarizes the progression of shock.

Initial Stage of Shock (Early Shock)

The initial, or early, stage of shock is present when any condition causes MAP to decrease from the client's baseline level by less than 10 mmHg. During this stage, activated compensatory mechanisms are so effective at returning MAP to normal levels that oxygenated blood flow to all vital organs is maintained. Cellular changes in this stage are a decrease in aerobic metabolism and an increase in anaerobic metabolism with production of lactic acid (although overall cellular metabolism is still aerobic).

Compensation, by vascular constriction and heart rate increase, is relatively complete, and both cardiac output and MAP are maintained within the normal range. Because vital organ function is not disrupted, however, the signs and symptoms of shock are subtle and difficult to detect. A heart rate increase from the client's baseline level may be the only manifestation of this early stage of shock.

Nonprogressive Stage of Shock (Compensatory Stage)

The nonprogressive, or compensatory, stage of shock is observed when conditions have caused a 10- to 15-mmHg drop in MAP from baseline level. Renal and chemical compensatory mechanisms are activated because cardiovascular compensation alone is not enough to maintain MAP and to supply needed oxygen to vital organs.

The kidneys and baroreceptors sense a sustained decrease in MAP, resulting in the release of renin, antidiuretic hormone (ADH), aldosterone, and the catecholamines epinephrine and norepinephrine. Renal compensation occurs through the actions of renin, aldosterone, and ADH (see Chap. 14). Renin, secreted by the kidney, starts the reactions that eventually cause de-

TABLE 39–3

Physiologic Events During Shock

Stage of Shock	Physiologic Event

Initial stage	• Decrease in baseline mean arterial pressure (MAP) of 5–10 mmHg
	• Increased sympathetic stimulation
	  • Mild vasoconstriction
	  • Increase in heart rate

Nonprogressive stage	• Decrease in MAP of 10–15 mmHg from the client's baseline value
	• Continued sympathetic stimulation
	  • Moderate vasoconstriction
	  • Increased heart rate
	  • Decreased pulse pressure
	• Chemical compensation
	  • Renin, aldosterone, and antidiuretic hormone secretion
	    • Increased vasoconstriction
	    • Decreased urinary output
	    • Stimulation of the thirst reflex
	• Some anaerobic metabolism in nonvital organs
	  • Mild acidosis
	  • Mild hyperkalemia

Progressive stage	• Decrease in MAP of >20 mmHg from the client's baseline value
	• Anoxia of nonvital organs
	• Hypoxia of vital organs
	• Overall metabolism is anaerobic
	  • Moderate acidosis
	  • Moderate hyperkalemia
	  • Tissue ischemia

Refractory stage	• Severe tissue hypoxia with ischemia and necrosis • Release of myocardial depressant factor from pancreas • Build-up of toxic metabolites

creased urine output, increased reabsorption of sodium, and systemic vasoconstriction (see Chap. 14, Fig. 14–8). ADH is secreted by the posterior pituitary gland. The activity of ADH both increases reabsorption of water in the kidney and causes blood vessel constriction in the skin and other less vital tissue areas. Together, these actions attempt to compensate for shock by maintaining the volume in the central blood vessels (Guyton & Hall, 1996).

Tissue hypoxia is present in nonvital organs and in the kidney but is not great enough to cause severe symptoms or permanent damage. Because some metabolism is anaerobic, acid-base and electrolyte changes occur in response to the build-up of metabolites. Changes include acidosis and hyperkalemia (see Chaps. 16 and 19).

If the client's condition is stable and compensatory mechanisms are supported by medical and nursing interventions, the client can remain in this stage for hours without sustaining permanent damage. Halting the conditions that have caused shock and providing supportive interventions will prevent progression of shock, so that the effects of the nonprogressive stage are reversible.

Progressive Stage of Shock (Intermediate Stage)

The progressive stage of shock, sometimes called the intermediate stage, is characterized by a sustained decrease in MAP of greater than 20 mmHg from baseline level. In this stage, compensatory mechanisms are functioning but no longer able to maintain sufficient oxygen supply, even to vital organs. Compensatory mechanisms require heavy use of oxygen in certain tissues, so that the problem of general inadequate oxygenation becomes even worse. Vital organs develop hypoxia, and less vital organs experience anoxia and ischemia. As a result of inadequate oxygenation and a build-up of toxic metabolites, some tissues develop extensive cell damage and experience cell death.

The progressive stage of shock is a life-threatening emergency. Vital organs can tolerate this situation for only a short time before being permanently damaged. Immediate interventions are required to reverse the effects of this stage of shock. Tolerance of this stage is highly individual and depends greatly on the client's pre-existing health. Usually the client's life can be saved if precipitating conditions are corrected within an hour after the onset of the progressive stage.

Refractory Stage of Shock (Irreversible Stage)

The refractory stage of shock, once called the irreversible stage, is reached when too much cell death and tissue damage have occurred because of too little oxygen getting to the tissues. Vital organs then experience overwhelming changes. This stage is termed refractory because the body is unable to respond effectively to interventions, and the syndrome of shock continues. The remaining cells perform metabolic functions anaerobically. Therapy is ineffective in saving the client's life, even if the underlying cause of shock is corrected and MAP temporarily returns to normal. So much tissue damage has occurred, causing systemic release of toxic metabolites and destructive enzymes, that cellular deterioration of vital organs continues.

This sequence of damage is termed *multisystem organ failure* (MOF), or *multiple organ dysfunction syndrome* (MODS). Once the damage has started, the sequence becomes a vicious cycle as ischemic cells break open and release more harmful metabolites. The metabolites lead to the formation of small clots, disrupting tissue oxygenation, damaging more cells, and thus continuing the devastating cycle. The most profound ongoing change is deterioration of the myocardium. One contributing factor is the release of myocardial depressant factor (MDF) from the ischemic pancreas (Wilson, 1992).

Etiology

Because shock is a manifestation of a pathologic condition rather than a disease state, the causes of shock vary. Specific conditions leading to hypovolemic, cardiogenic, distributive, and obstructive shock are listed in Table 39–4. More than one type of shock can be present at the same time. For example, trauma caused by an automobile accident may trigger both hemorrhage, leading to hypovo-

TABLE 39–4

Types and Causes of Shock

Shock Type	Overall Cause	Specific Cause or Risk Factors

Hypovolemic shock	• Body fluid depletion	• Hemorrhage
		  • Trauma
		  • Gastrointestinal ulcer
		  • Surgery
		  • Inadequate clotting
		    • Hemophilia
		    • Liver disease
		    • Malnutrition
		    • Bone marrow suppression
		    • Cancer
		    • Anticoagulation therapy
		• Dehydration
		  • Vomiting
		  • Diarrhea
		  • Heavy diaphoresis
		  • Diuretic therapy
		  • Nasogastric suction
		  • Diabetes insipidus
		  • Hyperglycemia

Cardiogenic shock	• Direct pump failure	• Myocardial infarction
		• Cardiac arrest
		• Ventricular dysrhythmias
		  • Fibrillation
		  • Tachycardia
		• Cardiac amyloidosis
		• Cardiomyopathies
		  • Viral
		  • Toxic
		• Myocardial degeneration

Distributive shock	• Decreased vascular volume or tone	• Neural-induced
		  • Pain
		  • Anesthesia
		  • Stress
		  • Spinal cord injury
		  • Head trauma
		• Chemical-induced
		  • Anaphylaxis
		  • Sepsis
		  • Capillary leak
		    • Burns
		    • Extensive trauma
		    • Hepatic dysfunction
		    • Hypoproteinemia

Obstructive shock	• Indirect pump failure	• Cardiac tamponade • Arterial stenosis • Pulmonary embolus • Pulmonary hypertension • Constrictive pericarditis • Thoracic tumors • Tension pneumothorax

lemic shock, and a myocardial infarction (MI), leading to cardiogenic shock.

Hypovolemic Shock

Hypovolemic shock occurs when too little circulating (intravascular) fluid volume causes a MAP decrease, so that the body's total need for tissue oxygenation is not met. The most common conditions leading to hypovolemic shock are hemorrhage (external or internal) and dehydration.

Hypovolemic shock caused by external hemorrhage is associated with soft-tissue trauma, wounds, and surgery. Hypovolemic shock caused by internal hemorrhage is associated with blunt trauma, gastrointestinal (GI) ulcers, and poor surgical hemostasis. In addition, external and internal hemorrhage can be caused by any health problem that results in inadequate levels of coagulation factors (see Table 39–4).

Hypovolemia as a result of dehydration can be caused by any condition that decreases fluid intake or increases renal and insensible fluid loss (see Table 39–4).

Cardiogenic Shock

Cardiogenic shock occurs when the actual heart muscle is unhealthy and contractility is directly impaired. Table 39–4 lists common causes of direct pump failure. These conditions decrease cardiac output and afterload, thus reducing MAP. (Chapter 40 provides an in-depth discussion of cardiogenic shock resulting from myocardial infarction.)

Distributive Shock

Distributive shock is characterized by a loss of sympathetic tone, vasodilation, pooling of blood in venous and capillary beds, and increased vascular permeability. All of these factors contribute to decreased mean arterial pressure (MAP) and may be induced either neurogenically or chemically.

Neural-Induced Distributive Shock

Neural-induced loss of MAP occurs when sympathetic stimulation of nerves regulating the vascular smooth muscle is inhibited and the smooth muscles of blood vessels relax, causing vasodilation. Neural-induced vasodilation can be a normal local response to injury, but shock results when the vasodilation is systemic. Common conditions that can cause a systemic loss of sympathetic tone are listed in Table 39–4.

Chemical-Induced Distributive Shock

Chemical-induced distributive shock has three common origins: anaphylaxis, sepsis, and capillary leak syndrome. Chemical-induced distributive shock occurs when certain chemicals or foreign substances within the blood and blood vessels stimulate widespread changes in blood vessel walls. Usually, the chemicals are exogenous (come from outside the body), but this type of shock can be induced by substances normally found in the body.

ANAPHYLAXIS. Anaphylaxis is one result of type I hypersensitivity immune reactions (see Chap. 25). Although it usually begins within seconds to minutes after exposure to a specific allergen, this reaction is termed *delayed* because the person rarely has this type of reaction the first time the allergen is encountered. Rather, anaphylaxis occurs on repeated exposure to the same allergen (Guyton & Hall, 1996). Table 25–8 lists common allergens that can cause anaphylaxis.

Anaphylaxis is due to an antigen-antibody reaction occurring systemically in response to contact with a substance to which the person has a severe hypersensitivity (allergy). The widespread antigen-antibody reaction in-volves the interaction of the allergen, immunoglobulin E (IgE), basophils, and mast cells. The reaction occurs within the walls of blood vessels, myocardial cells, and bronchial epithelium (see Chaps. 23 and 25). Anaphylaxis damages cells and causes the release of large amounts of histamine and other vasoactive amines. These substances are distributed rapidly throughout the circulatory system, causing massive vasodilation and increased capillary permeability, which result in profound hypovolemia and vascular collapse. Decreased cardiac contractility and dysrhythmias occur during anaphylaxis. These symptoms may be direct results of myocardial changes induced by the antigen-antibody reaction, or may be due to the profound hypovolemia. Antigen-antibody reactions in bronchial tissues cause severe edema and pulmonary obstruction, which greatly reduce pulmonary gas exchange. The pulmonary problems, together with inadequate circulation, cause the person to experience extreme hypoxia. Without intervention, this condition results in death.

SEPSIS. Sepsis leading to distributive shock occurs when microorganisms are present in the blood and other normally sterile areas of the body. Often, sepsis is associated with disseminated intravascular coagulation (DIC). Although distributive shock has been reported among clients with viral and yeast sepsis, it is more commonly associated with bacteremia. Organisms often causing sepsis include gram-negative bacteria (*Pseudomonas aeruginosa, Escherichia coli,* and *Klebsiella pneumoniae*) and gram-positive bacteria (*Staphylococcus* and *Streptococcus*) (Beam, 1994; Hazinski, 1994; Lawler, 1994). Table 39–5 lists some of the conditions that predispose clients to sepsis-induced distributive shock.

Sepsis-induced distributive shock results from the large amounts of toxins and endotoxins produced by the bacteria and secreted into the blood, causing a whole body inflammatory reaction. The bacteria-produced toxins and endotoxins react with blood vessels and cell membranes. The resulting reactions, through white blood cell activity, stimulate a variety of inflammatory and immune events known as the *systemic inflammatory response syndrome* (SIRS). These toxin-host interactions stimulate systemic complement activation, altered microcirculation within vascular organs (including selective coagulation and thrombus formation), increased capillary permeability, cell

TABLE 39–5

Conditions That Predispose to Sepsis-Induced Distributive Shock

- Malnutrition
- Immunosuppression
- Large open wounds
- Mucous membrane fissures in prolonged contact with bloody or drainage-soaked packing
- Gastrointestinal ischemia
- Loss of gastrointestinal integrity
- Exposure to invasive procedures
- Malignancy

injury, and increased cellular metabolism (in combination with an inability of some cells to take up necessary oxygen). Metabolism becomes anaerobic because of decreased MAP, clot formation in capillaries, and poor cellular uptake of oxygen. Although bacterial toxins are generally implicated in initiating these events, some evidence indicates that the bacteria in the extracellular fluid, as well as the toxins, can start the SIRS and cause shock.

CAPILLARY LEAK SYNDROME. Capillary leak syndrome leading to distributive shock occurs when there is a shift of fluid from the vascular space to the interstitial space. Such shifts are caused by increased capillary permeability, loss of plasma osmolarity, and increased vascular hydrostatic pressure. Specific conditions associated with fluid shifts include severe burns, bullous skin disease, liver disorders, abdominal ascites, acute peritonitis, paralytic ileus, severe malnutrition, surgical wounds, hyperglycemia, renal disease, hypoproteinemia, and trauma.

Obstructive Shock

Obstructive shock results from conditions that affect the ability of the normal heart muscle to pump effectively. The heart itself is normal, but conditions outside the heart prevent either adequate filling of the heart or adequate contraction of the healthy heart muscle. Some causes of obstructive shock (Effron & Chernow, 1992; Wilson, 1992) are listed in Table 39–4.

Incidence/Prevalence

Because it is a secondary response rather than a separate disease entity, the exact incidence of shock is not known. However, some degree of shock is a common complication among hospitalized clients. Hypovolemic shock is the most common type experienced by clients in emergency departments and after surgery or procedures that involve invasion of a major artery. Cardiogenic shock is the most frequent complication of myocardial infarction, occurring in an estimated 15% of clients who experience damage to 40% or more of the myocardium (Effron & Chernow, 1992). The frequency of distributive shock as a result of sepsis, which ranges in mortality from 40% to 85%, is increasing among clients who are immunocompromised or who have infections (Ackerman, 1994; Clochesy, 1996).

This chapter presents the collaborative management of clients experiencing hypovolemic shock caused by hemorrhage and distributive shock caused by sepsis. Chapter 25 discusses interventions for anaphylaxis, and Chapter 40 discusses care of the client experiencing cardiogenic shock as a result of myocardial infarction.

Collaborative Management

 Assessment

► History

The nurse collects data on risk factors, as well as causative factors, related to hypovolemic shock. Age is impor-

tant because hypovolemic shock associated with trauma is more frequently seen in young adults, whereas sepsis is more common among the elderly. Clients are asked specific questions about recent illness, trauma, procedures, or chronic conditions that may lead to the development of shock. Such conditions include GI ulcers, general surgery, hemophilia, liver disorders, prolonged vomiting, and prolonged diarrhea. The use of such medications as aspirin, diuretics, and antacids may directly cause changes leading to hypovolemic shock or may indicate the presence of a disease or a problem that can contribute to hypovolemic shock.

The nurse inquires about the client's fluid intake and output during the previous 24 hours. Information about urine output is especially critical because the initial and nonprogressive stages of shock are characterized by a reduced urine output, even when fluid intake is normal.

The nurse assesses the client and the immediate environment for obvious signs of factors leading to shock. Areas to examine for signs of hemorrhage include the gums, wounds, and sites of dressings, drains, and vascular access. The nurse observes for any swelling, skin discoloration, or visible manifestations of pain that may indicate internal hemorrhage.

► Physical Assessment/Clinical Manifestations

Most of the observable manifestations of hypovolemic shock result from the physiologic changes that accompany compensatory efforts. Manifestations of shock are first evident as changes in cardiovascular function. As shock progresses, changes in the renal, pulmonary, integumentary, musculoskeletal, and central nervous systems become evident.

Cardiovascular Manifestations

Because shock involves a decrease of mean arterial pressure (MAP) and the resulting early compensatory mechanisms are cardiovascular, the earliest clinical manifestations of hypovolemic shock are also cardiovascular.

Pulse. The nurse or other assistive personnel assesses the central and peripheral pulses for rate and quality. In the initial stage of hypovolemic shock, the pulse rate increases to maintain cardiac output and MAP at normal levels, although the actual stroke volume per beat is usually decreased. Because the cardiac output is decreased, the distal peripheral pulses are more difficult to palpate and are easily blocked with minimal pressure. As hypovolemic shock progresses, superficial peripheral pulses may be absent.

Blood Pressure. Changes in blood pressure are not always present in the initial stage of hypovolemic shock. When assessing the blood pressure of a client at risk for shock, the nurse considers his or her normal baseline blood pressure level. Although a blood pressure measurement of 90/50 may indicate severe shock in one person, it may represent the normal blood pressure value for another healthy, but slightly built adult.

When compensatory efforts include vasoconstriction, the result is an increased diastolic pressure, whereas the systolic pressure remains the same. As a result, the pulse pressure, or the difference between the systolic and diastolic pressure measurements, is smaller. Nursing personnel monitor the client's blood pressure for changes from baseline levels and changes from the previous measurement. For accuracy, the same equipment is used on the same extremity. When the client's condition permits, the nurse measures the blood pressure with the client in the lying, sitting, and standing positions.

As hypovolemic shock progresses and cardiac output changes, the systolic pressure level decreases, reducing the pulse pressure even further. When hypovolemic shock continues and interventions are not adequate, compensation fails, and both the systolic and diastolic pressures decrease. At this stage, blood pressure is difficult to hear. Palpation or a Doppler device may be needed to detect the systolic blood pressure.

Oxygen Saturation. The nurse assesses peripheral oxygen saturation through pulse oximetry. Hemoglobin oxygen saturation values between 90% and 95% are associated with the nonprogressive stage of shock, and values between 75% and 80% are associated with the progressive stage of shock. Any value below 70% is considered a life-threatening emergency and may signal the refractory stage of shock.

Integumentary Manifestations

In hypovolemic shock, the skin is affected by altered perfusion. Because the skin can tolerate low oxygen levels and other vital organs cannot, an early compensatory mechanism for hypovolemic shock is vasoconstriction in the skin and superficial tissues to the extent that perfusion of these tissues is minimal or absent.

The nurse assesses the skin for temperature, color, and degree of moisture. The skin feels cool or cold to the touch, and the color is pale to cyanotic. Color changes are first evident in mucous membranes and in the skin around the mouth. Because pallor or cyanosis may be difficult to observe in many areas in dark-skinned clients, the nurse particularly assesses color changes in oral mucous membranes. As hypovolemic shock progresses, color changes in clients with lighter skin are noted in the extremities and then in the central trunk area. The skin also feels clammy or moist to the touch, not because sweating increases but because the normal fluid lost through the skin does not evaporate quickly on cold skin.

The nurse evaluates capillary refill time by pressing on a fingernail until it blanches and then observing how fast the nail bed resumes color when pressure is released. Normally, the nail bed capillaries resume color as soon as pressure is released. Capillary refill in clients experiencing hypovolemic shock is usually slow and sometimes absent.

Respiratory Manifestations

The nurse assesses the rate, depth, and ease of respiration and also auscultates the lungs for abnormal breath sounds. Respiratory rate increases during hypovolemic shock. This increase is a compensatory mechanism to provide adequate oxygenation to critical tissues. When shock has progressed to the stage at which lactic acidosis is present, the depth of respiration also increases.

Renal/Urinary Manifestations

The renal system compensates for the decreased MAP during hypovolemic shock by conserving body water through decreasing glomerular filtration and increasing the reabsorption of filtrate. The nurse or assistive personnel measures urine output every hour. Urine is assessed for color, specific gravity, and the presence of blood or protein. Urine output is decreased (compared with fluid intake) or even absent in severe shock. Of the four vital organs (heart, brain, liver, and kidney), only the kidney can tolerate hypoxia and anoxia for up to an hour without permanent damage. When hypoxic or anoxic conditions persist beyond this time, clients are at grave risk for acute tubular necrosis and renal failure.

Central Nervous System Manifestations

Clients who have hypovolemic shock are thirsty. This sensation is caused by stimulation of the osmoreceptors in the brain in response to the decreased blood volume (see Chapter 14).

The nurse assesses clients' level of consciousness (LOC) and orientation to person, time, and place. Most causes of hypovolemic shock do not interfere with nerve impulse transmission. Rather, central nervous system manifestations of hypovolemic shock are associated with cerebral hypoxia. In the initial and nonprogressive stages, clients may be restless or agitated and may experience anxiety or a feeling of impending doom that has no obvious cause. As hypoxia progresses, clients become confused and lethargic. Lethargy progresses to somnolence and loss of consciousness as cerebral hypoxia intensifies.

Musculoskeletal Manifestations

Tissue hypoxia, anaerobic metabolism, and lactic acidosis cause skeletal muscle weakness and pain. This weakness is generalized, with no specific pattern of presentation. The accompanying electrolyte disturbances in progressive and refractory stages of shock compound this muscle weakness by interfering with the generation and transmission of action potentials. In this situation, deep tendon reflexes are decreased or absent.

The nurse assesses muscle strength by having the client squeeze the nurse's hand and try to keep the arms flexed while the nurse pulls downward on the lower arms. The nurse assesses deep tendon reflexes by lightly tapping the patellar tendons and Achilles tendons with a reflex hammer and observing the degree of reflexive movement.

▶ Psychosocial Assessment

Changes in mental status and behavior may be early indicators of hypovolemic shock. The nurse observes the client closely and documents behavior. The nurse assesses current mental status by evaluating LOC. The nurse notes whether the client is asleep or awake. If the client is asleep, the nurse attempts to awaken the client and documents the ease with which the client is aroused. If the client is awake, the nurse establishes whether the client is oriented to person, time, and place. The nurse avoids asking questions that can be answered with a "yes" or a "no" response. The nurse documents the manner in

---

Chart 39–2

Laboratory Profile: Hypovolemic Shock

Test	Normal Range for Adults	Significance of Abnormal Findings
pH (arterial)	7.35–7.45	Decreased: insufficient tissue oxygenation causing anaerobic metabolism and acidosis
PaO_2	83–100 mmHg	Decreased: anaerobic metabolism
$PaCO_2$	Females: 32–45 mmHg Males: 35–48 mmHg	Increased: anaerobic metabolism
Lactic acid (venous)	0.9–1.7 mmol/L	Increased: anaerobic metabolism with build-up of metabolites
Hematocrit	Females: 35–47% Males: 39–50%	Increased: fluid shift, dehydration Decreased: hemorrhage
Hemoglobin	Females: 11.7–16 g/dL Males: 13.1–17.2 g/dL	Increased: fluid shift, dehydration Decreased: hemorrhage
Potassium	3.5–4.5 mEq/L or mmol/L	Increased: dehydration, acidosis

PaO_2 = arterial partial pressure of oxygen; $PaCO_2$ = arterial partial pressure of carbon dioxide.
Data from Tietz, N. W. (1995). *Clinical guide to laboratory tests* (3rd ed.). Philadelphia: W. B. Saunders.

---

which the client responds to the questions. The following points are considered during evaluation:

- Is it necessary to repeat questions to obtain a response?
- Does the response answer the question asked?
- Does the client have difficulty with word choices during the responses?
- Is the client irritated or upset by the questions?
- Can the client concentrate on a question long enough to provide an appropriate response, or is attention span limited?

If possible, the nurse questions family members or a significant other to determine whether the behavior and mental status are typical of this client.

➤ Laboratory Assessment

No single laboratory finding confirms or rules out the presence of shock, although changes in laboratory data may support the diagnosis of hypovolemic shock. (Chart 39–2 lists the common laboratory findings associated with hypovolemic shock.) As shock progresses, arterial blood gas values become abnormal. Most commonly, the pH decreases, the arterial partial pressure of oxygen (PaO_2) decreases, and the arterial partial pressure of carbon dioxide ($PaCO_2$) increases. Changes in other laboratory values may be associated with specific causes of hypovolemic shock.

Hematocrit and hemoglobin concentrations decrease with hypovolemic shock caused by hemorrhage. When hypovolemic shock is the result of dehydration or fluid shift, the hematocrit and hemoglobin values are elevated.

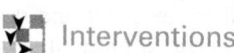 Interventions

Interventions for clients who have hypovolemic shock are focused on reversing the shock, restoring fluid volume, and preventing ischemic complications through support-

ive and drug therapies. Surgery may be necessary to correct the underlying problem leading to hypovolemic shock. Chart 39–3 summarizes nursing care priorities for clients experiencing hypovolemic shock.

➤ Nonsurgical Management

Interventions are aimed at maintaining tissue oxygenation, increasing the body fluid compartment volumes to achieve normal ranges, and supporting the client's operating compensatory mechanisms. Oxygen therapy, intravenous (IV) therapy, fluid replacement therapy, and drug therapies are the management choices for this problem.

Oxygen Therapy

Oxygen therapy is useful whenever shock is present. Oxygen can be administered by mask, hood, nasal cannula, nasopharyngeal tube, endotracheal tube, and tracheostomy tube. Usually, masks and nasal cannulas are used to

---

Chart 39–3

Nursing Care Highlight: The Client in Hypovolemic Shock

- Ensure a patent airway.
- Start an intravenous (IV) catheter or maintain an established catheter.
- Administer oxygen.
- Elevate the client's feet, keeping his or her head flat or elevated to a 30-degree angle.
- Examine the client for overt bleeding.
- If overt bleeding is present, apply direct pressure to the site.
- Take the client's vital signs every 5 minutes until stable.
- Administer medications as ordered.
- Increase the rate of IV fluid delivery.
- Do not leave the client.

provide oxygen to clients in shock. The nurse gives oxygen to the client in liters per minute (for administration via cannula) or concentration by percentage (for administration by mask), as specified by the physician's or nurse practitioner's order.

Intravenous Therapy

The two types of fluids commonly used for volume replacement during hemorrhagic hypovolemia are colloids and crystalloids. Colloids contain large molecules (usually composed of proteins or starches); IV colloid solutions are used to restore plasma volume and colloidal osmotic pressure (see Chap. 14). IV crystalloid solutions are administered for fluid and electrolyte replacement; they contain nonprotein substances, such as minerals, salts, and sugars. A current controversy involves the infusion rate of fluids when hypovolemia is a result of hemorrhage but control of the hemorrhage has not yet been achieved. A consideration is that rapid infusion of IV fluids can increase blood pressure and may increase the rate of blood loss (see Research Application for Nursing).

Colloid Fluid Replacement. Protein-containing colloid fluids are good for restoring vascular osmotic pressure as well as fluid volume. Blood and blood products are frequently used for this purpose and are the treatment of choice when hypovolemia is caused by blood loss. These products include whole blood, packed red blood cells, and plasma.

Whole blood and packed red blood cells increase the hematocrit and hemoglobin concentrations as well as vascular fluid volume. Whole blood is used to replace large volumes of blood loss because it provides increased intravascular volume while improving the oxygen-carrying capacity of the blood. Packed red cells are given for moderate blood loss because they replenish the red cell deficit and improve the oxygen-carrying capacity without adding excessive fluid volume. (Chapter 42 discusses nursing care issues in blood and blood product administration.)

Human plasma, an acellular blood product containing some clotting factors, is given to correct plasma deficits and restore osmotic pressure when the hematocrit and hemoglobin levels are within normal ranges. Plasma protein fractions (such as Plasmanate) and synthetic plasma expanders, such as hetastarch (hydroxyethyl starch, Hespan), increase plasma volume and are frequently used as early treatment for hypovolemic shock before a cause is established.

Crystalloid Fluid Replacement. Crystalloid solutions are given to help establish and maintain an adequate fluid and electrolyte balance. Two common crystalloid solutions are Ringer's lactate and normal saline. Ringer's lactate contains physiologic concentrations of sodium, chloride, calcium, potassium, and lactate in water. This isotonic solution is a good volume expander, and the lactate is a buffer in the presence of acidosis. Normal saline (0.9% sodium chloride in water) is a fluid replacement used to increase the plasma volume when there has been no loss of red blood cells.

Drug Therapy

If the volume deficit is severe and the client does not respond sufficiently to the replacement of fluid volume and blood products, the administration of medications may increase venous return, improve cardiac contractility, or ensure adequate cardiac perfusion through dilation of coronary vessels. Chart 39–4 lists drugs commonly used to treat hypovolemic shock.

Vasoconstricting Agents. A variety of drugs stimulate venous return by causing vasoconstriction and decreasing venous pooling of blood. These actions increase cardiac output and mean arterial pressure (MAP), helping to improve tissue perfusion and oxygenation. Most of these drugs produce serious side effects, and their dosages must be carefully calculated on the basis of the client's size and degree of response (see Chart 39–4).

▶ Research Applications for Nursing

Rapid Infusion of Intravenous Fluids During Hemorrhagic Shock May Increase Bleeding

Matsuoka, T., Hildreth, J., & Wisner, D. (1996). Uncontrolled hemorrhage from parenchymal injury: Is resuscitation helpful? Journal of Trauma, 40(6), 915–922.

A routine intervention for hypovolemic shock is the rapid infusion of crystalloidal and colloidal intravenous fluids in an attempt to increase mean arterial pressure (MAP). The investigators hypothesized that increasing MAP by rapid infusion of intravenous fluid before the cause of hemorrhage is identified and corrected could result in an increased rate of bleeding.

The investigators used an animal model to test this theory. After inflicting a standardized injury to the livers of 120 rats resulting in abdominal hemorrhage, the rats were assigned to one of four interventions groups: no resuscitation, small-volume infusion of isotonic fluid (4 mL/kg), large-volume infusion of isotonic fluid (24 mL/kg), and small-volume infusion of hypertonic saline (HS 4 mL/kg). The variables of blood pressure, intraperitoneal blood volume, and mortality rates were measured. Rats receiving large-volume infusions had higher blood pressures with greater mortality rates and significantly greater intraperitoneal blood volumes than did those receiving small-volume infusions of either fluid. Overall, the best outcomes were seen among the rats receiving small-volume infusions of hypertonic normal saline.

Critique. The study was well controlled and conducted under ideal laboratory conditions; all rat subjects were as similar as possible for most variables. Although animal models have been used successfully to mimic human responses to trauma and interventions for trauma, a major limitation of the study is the size of the animal model. Replication of the study using a larger animal model more comparable to humans is warranted.

Possible Nursing Implications. The results of this study indicate that, although intravenous access and infusion should be a mainstay of intervention for clients with hypovolemic shock, when hemorrhage is suspected, the infusion rate should not be excessive. It is imperative that the health care provider assess all indicators of hemorrhage for response to the infusion therapy.

Chart 39-4

Drug Therapy for Hypovolemic Shock

Drug	Usual Dosage	Nursing Interventions	Rationale
Vasoconstrictors			
Dopamine hydrochloride (Intropin, Revimine*)	• 5–30 μg/kg/min IV (for hypotension) • 2–5 μg/kg/min IV (for renal perfusion)	• Assess the client for chest pain. • Monitor urinary output hourly. • Assess blood pressure every 15 minutes. • Assess the client for headache.	• Dopamine increases myocardial oxygen consumption. • Higher doses decrease renal perfusion and urinary output. • Hypertension is a symptom of overdose. • Headache is an early symptom of drug excess.
Epinephrine (Adrenalin)	• 0.5–1 mg IV initially, followed by 0.5 mg every 5 minutes • May also be given by intracardiac injection	• Monitor the client for dysrhythmias. • Assess the client for chest pain.	• Epinephrine may cause ventricular tachyarrhythmias. • Vasoconstriction may impair cardiac oxygenation.
Norepinephrine (Levophed)	• 0.5–1.0 μg/kg/min continuous IV infusion to maintain blood pressure at 90–100 mmHg	• Assess for extravasation. • Observe the client's extremities for color and perfusion.	• Norepinephrine can cause severe tissue damage and necrosis. • Norepinephrine can cause such vasoconstriction that peripheral ischemia may result.
Phenylephrine (Neo-Synephrine)	• 80–200 μg/min IV	• Assess for chest pain.	• Vasoconstriction may impair cardiac oxygenation.
Agents Enhancing Contractility			
Amrinone (Inocor)	• 0.75–1.5 mg/kg bolus • 5–20 μg/kg/min continuous IV infusion	• Assess blood pressure every 15 minutes. • Do not administer through the same tubing as furosemide.	• Hypertension is a symptom of overdose. • Amrinone and furosemide form a precipitate.
Atropine sulfate	• 0.5–1 mg IV every 5 minutes, up to a total of 2 mg	• Take pulse every 5 minutes. • Monitor urinary output every 30 minutes. • Administer cautiously to clients with glaucoma.	• Atropine sulfate may cause a rebound tachycardia. • Atropine sulfate may cause urinary retention. • Atropine sulfate may precipitate an episode of acute angle-closure glaucoma.
Dobutamine hydrochloride (Dobutrex)	• 2.5–20 μg/kg/min continuous IV infusion	• Assess the client for chest pain. • Assess blood pressure every 15 minutes.	• Dobutamine increases myocardial oxygen consumption. • Hypertension is a symptom of overdose.
Agents Enhancing Myocardial Perfusion			
Sodium nitroprusside (Nitropress, Nipride*)	• 0.5–10 μg/kg/min continuous IV infusion	• Assess blood pressure every 15 minutes.	• Hypotension may result from the systemic dilation of veins and arteries.

Agents Enhancing Myocardial Contractility. Some drugs directly stimulate adrenergic receptor sites on the myocardium (especially beta$_1$-receptors) and increase the contraction of the cardiac muscle cells. Other agents enhance cardiac contractility by slowing the heart rate through altering electrical conduction and allowing the left ventricle a longer filling time. When the filling time is increased, more blood enters the left ventricle and stretches the myocardial fibers. Thus, greater recoil is achieved, and more blood leaves the left ventricle during contraction. Some of these drugs also stimulate the ventricles at the same time. Agents with these types of actions include digoxin (Lanoxin) and dobutamine (Dobutrex).

Agents Enhancing Myocardial Perfusion. The treatment of shock includes giving agents that cause systemic vasoconstriction to help enhance venous return and increase MAP. However, it is important to ensure that the heart is well perfused so that aerobic metabolism is maintained in the cardiac cells and maximum contractility can be achieved. Agents that dilate coronary blood vessels while causing minimal systemic vasodilation are used for this purpose. Care is taken because higher dosages can cause some systemic vasodilation and increase shock.

Monitoring

A major nursing responsibility in caring for the client in hypovolemic shock is monitoring vital signs and level of consciousness (LOC). On the acute nursing unit, the nurse monitors the client's

- Pulse
- Blood pressure
- Pulse pressure
- Central venous pressure
- Respiratory rate
- Skin and mucosal color
- Pulse oximetry values

The nurse performs these assessments at least every 15 minutes until the shock is under control and the client's condition improves. More extensive monitoring of cardiac output (hemodynamic monitoring), including intra-arterial monitoring, mixed venous oxygen saturation (SvO_2), and pulmonary artery wedge pressures, is done in critical care settings.

Clients with shock who require more invasive monitoring, such as central venous pressure (CVP), pulmonary artery pressure (PAP), and pulmonary artery wedge pressure (PAWP), should be transported to a critical care unit. Table 39–6 compares changes seen in hemodynamic patterns with different types of shock.

Insertion of a CVP catheter allows monitoring of the client's right atrial or superior vena cava pressure while providing venous access. Changes in CVP reflect the syndrome of hypovolemic shock. As the circulating volume decreases, the amount of blood returning to the right atrium also decreases, causing the CVP to decrease from baseline levels.

Intra-arterial catheter placement provides a means of monitoring blood pressure continuously and serves as an access for arterial blood sampling. Intra-arterial catheters are inserted into an artery (radial, brachial, femoral, or dorsalis pedis artery). The arterial catheter is attached to pressure tubing and a transducer. The transducer converts the pressure in the artery (mechanical energy) into an electrical signal that is expressed as a visible waveform on an oscilloscope, and a digital numeric value is displayed.

➤ Surgical Management

The nurse monitors the client's fluid loss and uses the nonsurgical interventions described earlier to stabilize the client's hemodynamic status. After a cause has been established, surgical intervention may be necessary to correct the underlying problem. Such interventions include vascular repair or revision, surgical hemostasis of major wounds, oversewing of bleeding ulcers, and chemical scarring (chemosclerosis) of varicosities.

Collaborative Management

 Assessment

Distributive shock caused by sepsis does not resemble other types of shock in that it has two distinctive phases (Figure 39–2). The first phase is relatively long, frequently lasting from hours to a day or longer. The clinical manifestations during this phase are subtle. However, when the client is recognized to be in the first phase of sepsis-induced distributive shock and the appropriate interventions are made, there is a good chance for recovery. The second phase of sepsis-induced distributive shock has a sudden onset and a rapid downhill course. If sepsis-induced distributive shock progresses without intervention to the second phase, chances for the client's recovery are slim. Identification of the first phase of sepsis-induced distributive shock can make the greatest difference in survival among affected clients.

TABLE 39–6

Hemodynamic Pattern Changes Associated with Different Types of Shock				
Type of Shock	Cardiac Output (CO)	Central Venous Pressure (CVP)	Pulmonary Artery Pressure (PAP)	Pulmonary Capillary Wedge Pressure (PCWP)
Hypovolemic	↓	↓	↓	↓
Cardiac	↓	↑	↑	↑
Obstructive	↓	↑	↑	↑
Distributive				
Anaphylactic	↓	↓	↓	↓
Sepsis (early)	↑	Ø	Ø or ↑	Ø or ↑
Sepsis (late)	↓	↓	↓	↓

↑ = increased; ↓ = decreased; Ø = normal or unchanged.
Data from Jones, K. (1996). Shock. In J. Clochesy, C. Breu, S. Cardin, A. Whittaker, & E. Rudy (Eds.), *Critical care nursing* (2nd ed., pp. 1371–1318). Philadelphia: W. B. Saunders.

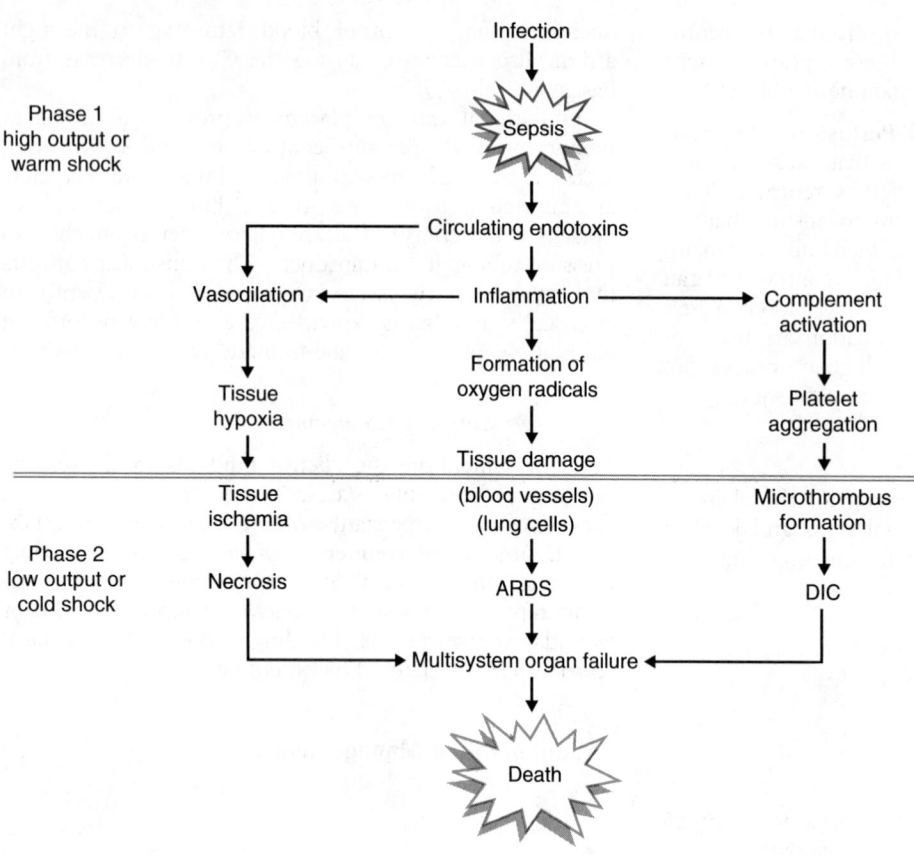

Figure 39–2. The sequence of sepsis-induced distributive shock. (ARDS = adult respiratory distress syndrome; DIC = disseminated intravascular coagulation.)

➤ History

The nurse collects data about risk factors, as well as causative factors, related to sepsis-induced distributive shock. Age is important because sepsis-induced distributive shock can develop more easily among elderly, debilitated people with any degree of immunosuppression. Chart 39–5 lists some of the factors that increase the elderly person's risk for shock. Clients are asked specific questions about recent illness, trauma, or procedures or chronic conditions that may lead to sepsis and distributive shock. The use of some medications may directly cause changes leading to shock. A medication regimen may also indicate a disease or a problem that can contribute to sepsis-induced distributive shock. Such medications include aspirin and aspirin-containing drugs, antibiotics, and chemotherapeutic agents.

➤ Physical Assessment/Clinical Manifestations

Many of the clinical manifestations of the first phase are unique to sepsis-induced distributive shock and, frequently, opposite from those associated with all other types of shock. Chart 39–6 summarizes the clinical manifestations of the first phase of sepsis-induced distributive shock. These findings, affecting the cardiovascular, integumentary, and pulmonary systems, result from the body's reaction to the presence of endotoxins.

Cardiovascular Manifestations

Endotoxins in the client's blood and other extracellular fluids interact with leukocytes as well as blood vessel walls and trigger an inflammatory reaction. In addition, some endotoxins appear to stimulate myocardial tissue directly. As a result, cardiac output is actually increased during the first phase of sepsis-induced distributive shock. This phase also may be called the *high-output* or

---

Chart 39–5

Nursing Focus on the Elderly: Risk Factors for Shock

Type of Shock	Specific Risk Factor
Hypovolemic shock	• Diuretic therapy • Diminished thirst reflex • Immobility
Cardiogenic shock	• Diabetes mellitus • Presence of cardiomyopathies
Distributive shock	• Diminished immune response • Reduced skin integrity • Presence of cancer • Peripheral neuropathy • Cerebrovascular accidents • Institutionalization (hospital or extended care facility) • Malnutrition • Anemia
Obstructive shock	• Pulmonary hypertension • Presence of cancer

---

Chart 39-6

Key Features of Phase 1 Sepsis-Induced Distributive Shock

Assessment	Findings

Assessment

General

Assess the mental status and level of consciousness.

Check the oral temperature.

Cardiovascular System

Check the pulse and blood pressure. Document the pulse pressure with each blood pressure reading.
Check peripheral pulses.
Auscultate heart sounds at four valvular sites, and record the onset of murmur or gallop.

Respiratory System

Observe the rate, rhythm, and effort of breathing. Observe the symmetry of chest expansion.
Percuss and auscultate the lungs. Note the onset of adventitious sounds.
Check blood gas levels.

Integumentary System

Inspect and palpate the skin. Note color, vascularity, moisture, temperature, texture, thickness, mobility, and turgor. Assess the oral mucosa.

Findings

- Irritability, restlessness, lethargy, disorientation, and inappropriate euphoria
- Normal, subnormal, or elevated temperature

- Tachycardia: normal mean arterial blood pressure; widening pulse pressure
- "Bounding" peripheral pulses
- No murmur or gallop

- Tachypnea, hyperventilation

- Crackles and decreased breath sounds

- Respiratory alkalosis

- Warm flushed skin and peripheral edema

---

warm-shock phase. The increased cardiac output is reflected by tachycardia, increased stroke volume, a normal-to-elevated systolic blood pressure, and a normal CVP. The increased cardiac output causes good perfusion of the skin, so that the skin may appear to be normal in color with pink mucous membranes and may feel warm to the touch. This situation is temporary, and eventually the cardiac output greatly diminishes in clients experiencing sepsis-induced distributive shock.

As sepsis-induced distributive shock progresses, disseminated intravascular coagulation (DIC) may accompany it. The presence of the endotoxins and the inflammatory reactions stimulate complement activation (see Chap. 23). These actions cause thousands of small clots to form in the tiny capillaries of vascular organs (e.g., liver, kidney, brain, spleen, and heart). These small clots interfere with the oxygenation in those organs, causing hypoxia and ischemia and making overall metabolism anaerobic. The enormous number of small clots use clotting factors and fibrinogen faster than they can be regenerated by the liver, making clients much more susceptible to hemorrhage. These occurrences mark the beginning of the second phase of sepsis-induced distributive shock. Because some of the blood has already clotted, most of the clotting factors are gone, and blood vessels are dilated; clients are hypovolemic in this phase of distributive shock. The cardiac output now decreases dramatically, as do systolic blood pressure and pulse pressure. This phase is called the *low-output,* or *cold-shock,* phase of sepsis-induced distributive shock, and the clinical manifestations resemble those of the later stages of all forms of shock.

Respiratory Manifestations

In the high-output phase of sepsis-induced distributive shock, respiratory rate and depth are increased. Often, clients experience a respiratory alkalosis.

When sepsis-induced distributive shock progresses to the low-output phase, the possible life-threatening pulmonary complication of adult respiratory distress syndrome (ARDS) may occur. Although this complication has many causes, ARDS in cases of sepsis is thought to be related to the formation of oxygen-free radicals, which damage the pulmonary cells (Wilson, 1992). Oxygen-free radicals can form as a result of oxygen therapy and in response to cellular destruction and subsequent release of oxidizing enzymes. The presence of ARDS in a client who has sepsis-induced distributive shock is an ominous clinical sign associated with a high mortality rate.

Integumentary Manifestations

Often, clients in the early phase of sepsis-induced distributive shock are not recognized as having a problem because the appearance of the skin and mucous membranes leads health care professionals to believe that circulation is unimpaired. Clients feel warm to the touch, and their lips and mucous membranes appear well oxygenated.

When sepsis-induced distributive shock progresses so that circulation is compromised, the skin is cool and clammy with pallor or cyanosis present. In clients with disseminated intravascular coagulation (DIC), petechiae and ecchymoses occur anywhere. Blood may ooze from gums, other mucous membranes, venipuncture sites, and around IV catheters.

➤ *Psychosocial Assessment*

Often, the indicator that all is not well with clients at the beginning of sepsis-induced distributive shock is a change in affect or behavior. The nurse compares their presenting behavior, verbal responses, and general affect with those assessed earlier in the day or the day before and notes changes. Clients may seem just slightly different in their reactions to greetings, comments, or jokes. They may be less patient than usual or act restless or fidgety. Clients may verbalize feelings, such as "I feel as if something is wrong, but I don't know what." If this behavior represents a change from prior assessments, the nurse always considers the possibility of sepsis and shock.

➤ *Laboratory Assessment*

The presence of bacteria in blood and other extracellular fluids supports the diagnosis of sepsis. The nurse obtains specimens of urine, blood, sputum, and any drainage for culture to identify the causative organisms for both diagnostic and therapeutic purposes. Other abnormal laboratory findings associated with sepsis-induced distributive shock include changes in the white blood cell count; the differential leukocyte count may demonstrate a left shift (see Chap. 23). Changes in hematocrit and hemoglobin levels usually are not evident until late in septic shock when the client is hemorrhaging. At that point, the hematocrit and hemoglobin concentrations are low, as are the fibrinogen levels and the platelet count.

 Analysis

A common collaborative problem for clients with sepsis-induced distributive shock is the potential for multisystem organ failure (MOF), also called multiple organ dysfunction syndrome (MODS).

 Planning and Implementation

➤ *Planning: Expected Outcomes*

The client is expected to
- Have normal arterial blood gases
- Maintain a urine output of at least 20 mL/hour
- Have a mean arterial blood pressure within 10 mmHg of baseline

➤ *Interventions*

Interventions for the client experiencing sepsis-induced distributive shock focus on correcting the conditions causing shock and on preventing complications. Chart 39–7 summarizes the nursing care priorities for clients experiencing sepsis-induced distributive shock.

Control of fluid volume deficit associated with sepsis-induced distributive shock is accomplished through supportive and drug therapies. IV therapy is the same as for hypovolemic shock.

Oxygen Therapy. Oxygen therapy is useful whenever inadequate tissue perfusion and inadequate oxygenation

are present, such as during distributive shock. Oxygen therapy for sepsis-induced distributive shock is administered in the same ways as for hypovolemic shock (see p. 390).

Drug Therapy. The same agents used to enhance cardiac output and restore vascular volume in hypovolemic shock are used for sepsis-induced distributive shock. A major focus is the administration of antibiotics to combat sepsis. In addition, agents to counteract disseminated intravascular coagulation (DIC) may be required. Sepsis-induced distributive shock and DIC have two distinctly different phases, and drug therapies for each phase of sepsis-induced distributive shock are different. Drug therapy in the first phase is aimed at preventing coagulation and usually consists of heparin administration. Drug therapy in the second, late phase of sepsis-induced distributive shock is aimed at increasing the blood's ability to clot and usually consists of clotting factor administration.

Antibiotics. Although sepsis and distributive shock can be caused by any microorganism, the most common agents are gram-negative bacteria. When blood cultures have identified specific bacteria, IV antibiotics with known activity against the bacteria are administered. When the causative agent is not known, multiple agents with wide activity are prescribed. A common "triple-antibiotic" regimen includes vancomycin, one of the aminoglycosides, and a systemic penicillin derivative.

Antibodies. Antibodies against the body's mediators for inflammation are being tested for their effectiveness against sepsis-induced distributive shock. Antibodies have been developed against different substances that white blood cells produce to stimulate the inflammatory response. The mediators thought to start the inflammatory

---

Chart 39–7

Nursing Care Highlight: The Client in Sepsis-Induced Distributive Shock

- Ensure a patent airway.
- Start or maintain an established intravenous (IV) catheter.
- Administer oxygen.
- Administer antibiotics.
- Obtain specimens of blood, urine, wound drainage, and sputum for culture.
- Increase the rate of IV fluid delivery.
- Use aseptic technique for any invasive procedure.
- Handle the client gently.
- Examine the client for overt bleeding, especially of gums, injection sites, and IV sites.
- Elevate the client's feet, keeping his or her head flat or elevated to a 30-degree angle.
- Take the client's vital signs every 5 minutes until they are stable.
- Administer medications as ordered:
  - Heparin during phase 1
  - Clotting factors during phase 2
- Do not leave the client.

responses in blood vessels and lead to the cascade of sepsis-induced distributive shock are interleukin-1 (IL-1), interleukin-6 (IL-6), and tumor necrosis factor (TNF). This experimental therapy shows promise in reducing the extensive mortality associated with sepsis-induced distributive shock (Clochesy, 1996; Workman, 1995).

Anticoagulants. When clients are identified as being in the early phase of sepsis-induced distributive shock and are beginning to form numerous small clots, heparin is given to limit unnecessary clotting and to prevent the consumption of clotting factors.

Clotting Factors. When sepsis-induced distributive shock progresses to the point that small clots have formed to such an extent that the client no longer has sufficient clotting factors to prevent hemorrhage, clotting factors are given intravenously. These factors are obtained from pooled human serum. Administration of fresh frozen plasma also helps to replace clotting factors.

Providing a Safe Environment

Primary prevention is possible for some types of shock by identifying clients at risk for conditions and complications leading to sepsis and preventing those complications. Strict adherence to aseptic technique during invasive procedures and during the manipulation of nonintact skin and mucous membranes of clients who are immunocompromised to any degree can help to prevent or limit sepsis and sepsis-induced distributive shock.

Early detection of the clinical manifestations of shock is a major nursing responsibility. Because shock is a common complication of many conditions found among clients in acute care settings, the nurse always considers the possibility of sepsis-induced distributive shock. For early detection, the nurse continuously assesses vital signs for specific changes from normal values or from baseline levels. After distributive shock is recognized, health care providers rapidly take action to halt or change the conditions contributing to shock, to support the client's physiologic compensatory mechanisms, and to prevent life-threatening complications.

> ## Continuing Care

For most clients, shock is a complication of another condition and is resolved before discharge from an emergency department or acute care setting. However, with more clients receiving treatment on an outpatient basis and with earlier discharge from acute care settings, more clients at home are at increased risk for infection and sepsis-induced distributive shock.

➤ Health Teaching

Protecting vulnerable clients from infection and sepsis at home is an important nursing function. The nurse instructs clients about the importance of self-care strategies, such as good hygiene, hand washing, balanced rest and exercise, skin care, and mouth care. If clients or family members do not know how to take a temperature or read

---

Chart 39–8

Education Guide: Infection Precautions

- Avoid crowds and other large gatherings of people, who might be ill.
- Do not share eating utensils or personal toilet articles, such as toothbrushes, toothpaste, washcloths, or deodorant sticks, with others.
- If possible, bathe daily.
- Wash the armpits, groin, genitals, and anal area at least twice a day with an antimicrobial soap.
- Clean your toothbrush daily by either running it through the dishwasher or rinsing it in liquid laundry bleach.
- Wash your hands thoroughly with an antimicrobial soap before you eat or drink, after touching a pet, after shaking hands with anyone, as soon as you come home from any outing, and after using the toilet.
- Wash dishes between use with hot, sudsy water, or use a dishwasher.
- Do not drink water that has been standing for longer than 15 minutes.
- Do not reuse cups and glasses without washing.
- Do not change pet litter boxes.
- Take your temperature at least once a day.
- Refrigerate and prepare food appropriately. Do not eat raw or undercooked meat, fish, poultry, or eggs.
- Report any of the following signs or symptoms of infection to your physician immediately:
  - Temperature greater than 100°F (38°C)
  - Persistent cough (with or without sputum)
  - Pus or foul-smelling drainage from any open skin area or normal body opening
  - Presence of a boil or abscess
  - Urine that is cloudy or foul-smelling or that causes burning on urination
- Do not dig in the garden or work with houseplants.
- Use antibacterial cleansers to clean kitchen and bathroom surfaces at least twice each week. If you clean these areas yourself, wear rubber or vinyl work gloves while cleaning.
- Use a condom when having sex.
- Take all prescribed medications as the physician ordered.

---

a thermometer, the nurse provides instruction and obtains a return demonstration. Clients are instructed to avoid crowds or other people with known illnesses and to notify the health care provider immediately upon experiencing any fever or other sign of infection. Specific recommendations for infection precautions are listed in Chart 39–8.

➤ Home Care Management

The nurse or home health aide evaluates the home environment for safety regarding infection hazards. General cleanliness is noted, and particular attention is paid to the kitchen and bathrooms. Chart 39–9 lists focused client and environmental assessment data to obtain during a home visit.

Chart 39-9

Focused Assessment for Home Care Clients at Risk for Sepsis

- Assess the client for any clinical manifestations of infection including:
  - Temperature, pulse, respiration, and blood pressure
  - Color of skin and mucous membranes
  - The mouth and perianal area for fissures or lesions
  - Any nonintact skin area for the presence of exudates, redness, increased warmth, swelling
  - Any pain, tenderness, or other discomfort anywhere
  - Cough or any other symptoms of a cold or the flu
  - Urine; or ask client whether urine is dark or cloudy; has an odor; or causes pain or burning during urination
- Assess client's and caregiver's compliance with and understanding of infection prevention techniques
- Assess home environment, including
  - General cleanliness
  - Kitchen and bathroom facilities, including refrigeration
  - Availability and type of soap for hand washing
  - Presence of pets, especially cats, rodents, or reptiles

CASE STUDY for the Client with Hypovolemic Shock

■ A 38-year-old woman has returned to the post-anesthesia recovery area 2 hours ago, after having a tubal ligation by colposcopy (through the back wall of the vagina behind the cervix). Her last documented vital signs, taken 30 minutes ago, were as follows: BP, 102/80; pulse, 88; and respirations, 22. You now note that her face is pale, and the skin around her lips has a bluish cast. Her current vital signs are BP, 90/76; pulse, 98; and respirations, 28.

QUESTIONS:

1. What additional assessment techniques would you perform?
2. Where would you look for hemorrhage?
3. What other data would you gather?
4. When you reassess her in 15 minutes, you find her vital signs are now BP, 88/70; pulse, 102; and respirations, 30. She wakens when you shake her arm and complains of back pain and thirst. Given these findings, what are your action priorities?
5. What expected outcomes would be specific to this situation?

SELECTED BIBLIOGRAPHY

Ackerman, M. (1994). The systemic inflammatory response, sepsis and multiple organ dysfunction: New definitions for an old problem. *Critical Care Clinics of North America, 6*(2), 243–250.

Beam, T. (1994). Anti-infective drugs in the prevention and treatment of sepsis syndrome. *Critical Care Clinics of North America, 6*(2), 275–294.

Brown, K. (1994a). Septic shock: How to stop the deadly cascade, part 1. *American Journal of Nursing, 94*(9), 20–27.

Brown, K. (1994b). Septic shock: Critical interventions, part 2. *American Journal of Nursing, 94*(10), 20–26.

Chernow, B. (1996). New advances in the pharmacologic approach to circulatory shock. *Journal of Clinical Anesthesiology, 8*(Suppl. 3), 67s–69s.

Clochesy, J. (1996). Patients with systemic inflammatory response syndrome. In J. Clochesy, C. Breu, S. Cardin, A. Whittaker, & E. Rudy (Eds.), *Critical care nursing* (2nd ed., pp. 1359–1370). Philadelphia: W. B. Saunders.

Cotran, R., Kumar, V., & Robbins, S. (1994). *Robbins pathologic basis of disease* (5th ed.). Philadelphia: W. B. Saunders.

*Effron, M., & Chernow, B. (1992). Shock. In E. Rubenstein & D. Federman (Eds.), *Scientific American: Medicine* (pp. I card III Shock 1-12). New York: Scientific American.

Flavell, C. (1994). Combating hemorrhagic shock. *RN, 57*(12), 26–31.

Grap, M. (1998). Pulse oximetry. *Critical-Care Nurse, 18*(1), 94–99.

Grap, M., Glass, C., & Constatino, S. (1994). Accurate assessment of ventilation and oxygenation. *Medsurg Nursing, 3*(6), 435–443.

Guyton, A., & Hall, J. (1996). *Textbook of medical physiology* (9th ed.). Philadelphia: W. B. Saunders.

Hazinski, M. (1994). Mediator-specific therapies for the systemic inflammatory response syndrome, sepsis, severe sepsis, and septic shock: Present and future approaches. *Critical Care Clinics of North America, 6*(2), 309–319.

Headley, J. (1995). Analyzing normal hemodynamic waveforms. *Nursing95, 25*(3), 32AA–32DD.

Jones, K. (1996). Shock. In J. Clochesy, C. Breu, S. Cardin, A. Whittaker, & E. Rudy (Eds.), *Critical care nursing* (2nd ed., p. 1371). Philadelphia: W. B. Saunders.

Lawler, D. (1994). Hormonal response in sepsis. *Critical Care Clinics of North America, 6*(2), 265–274.

Martin, J. (1995). The Trendelenburg position: A review of current slants about head down tilt. *American Association of Nurse Anesthetists Journal, 63*(1), 29–36.

Matsuoka, T., Hildreth, J., & Wisner, D. (1996). Uncontrolled hemorrhage from parenchymal injury: Is resuscitation helpful? *Journal of Trauma, 40*(6), 915–922.

Mattice, C. (1996). It's not always obvious when a patient's in shock. *RN, 59*(3), 61–62.

Miller, L. (1996). Hemodynamic monitoring. In J. Clochesy, C. Breu, S. Cardin, A. Whittaker, & E. Rudy (Eds.), *Critical care nursing* (2nd ed., pp. 203–234). Philadelphia: W. B. Saunders.

Nawas, Y., & Balk, R. (1994). General approach to shock. *Clinics in Geriatric Medicine, 10*(1), 185–196.

O'Neal, P. (1994). How to spot early signs of cardiogenic shock. *American Journal of Nursing, 94*(5), 36–40.

Price, C. (1994). Acute renal failure: A sequela of sepsis. *Critical Care Clinics of North America, 6*(2), 359–372.

Raimer, F. (1995). Identifying abnormal hemodynamic waveforms. *Nursing95, 25*(4), 32MM–32QQ.

Russell, S. (1994a). Hypovolemic shock: Is your patient at risk? *Nursing94, 24*(4), 34–39.

Russell, S. (1994b). Septic shock: Can you recognize the clues? *Nursing94, 24*(4), 40–48.

Shelton, B. (1994). Disorders of hemostasis in sepsis. *Critical Care Nursing Clinics of North America, 6*(2), 373–387.

Shoemaker, W. (1994). Pathophysiology, monitoring and therapy of acute circulatory problems. *Critical Care Clinics of North America, 6*(2), 295–307.

Stengle, J., & Dries, D. (1994). Sepsis in the elderly. *Critical Care Nursing Clinics of North America, 6*(2), 421–427.

Tangredi, M. (1998). Clinical snapshot: Septic shock. *American Journal of Nursing, 98*(3), 46–47.

Vollman, K. (1994). Adult respiratory distress syndrome. *Critical Care Clinics of North America, 6*(2), 341–358.

*Wilson, R. (1992). *Critical care manual: Applied physiology and principles and therapy* (2nd ed.). Philadelphia: F. A. Davis.

Workman, M. L. (1995). Essential concepts of inflammation and immunity. *Critical Care Clinics of North America, 7*(4), 601–615.

SUGGESTED READINGS

Brown, K. (1994a). Septic shock: How to stop the deadly cascade, part 1. *American Journal of Nursing, 94*(9), 20–27.

Using a case study approach, the author presents the pathophysiology, assessment data, and initial care needs for people with sepsis-induced distributive shock. Self-assessment/CEU questions are included at the end of the article.

Martin, J. (1995). The Trendelenburg position: A review of current slants about head down tilt. *American Association of Nurse Anesthetists Journal, 63*(1), 29–36.
  The author reviews current and historical practice-based research literature about the value of the Trendelenburg position in different clinical situations. The consensus reached for modern techniques is that, although the Trendelenburg position may have some value in specific clinical situations, it is not useful for clients in shock or with head injuries.

Stengle, J., & Dries, D. (1994). Sepsis in the elderly. *Critical Care Nursing Clinics of North America, 6*(2), 421–427.
  This excellent article compares the clinical manifestations of sepsis in elderly people with those considered "classic for the adult population," emphasizing the subtle changes that can be easily overlooked in an elderly client. In addition, the authors describe risk factors, usual clinical course, and treatment.

Chapter 40

INTERVENTIONS FOR CRITICALLY ILL CLIENTS WITH CORONARY ARTERY DISEASE

Since the 1960s, deaths from myocardial infarction (MI) have decreased approximately 30% (American Heart Association [AHA], 1996). This reduction is partly due to improved health promotion, but management of the client with coronary artery disease (CAD) has also changed dramatically.

Most deaths today from MI occur because of dysrhythmias before the client reaches the hospital. During the past 10 years, in-hospital mortality from MI has dropped from 15% to 5%. Advances in cardiac care, especially new strategies for opening and maintaining the patency of obstructed coronary vessels, contributed to this decline.

Overview

Coronary artery disease is the leading cause of death in the United States. This disease affects the arteries that provide blood, oxygen, and nutrients to the myocardium. When blood flow through the coronary arteries is par-

tially or completely blocked, ischemia and infarction (necrosis) of the myocardium may result. Ischemia occurs when insufficient oxygen is supplied to meet the requirements of the myocardium. Infarction occurs when severe ischemia is prolonged and irreversible damage to tissue results.

Pathophysiology

Atherosclerosis is the leading contributor to CAD and death in Western civilizations. Three basic processes occur in atherosclerosis:

- Overgrowth of intimal smooth muscle cells with accumulation of macrophages and T cells
- Formation of a connective tissue matrix in the vessel intima
- Accumulation of lipids, especially cholesterol, in the connective tissue

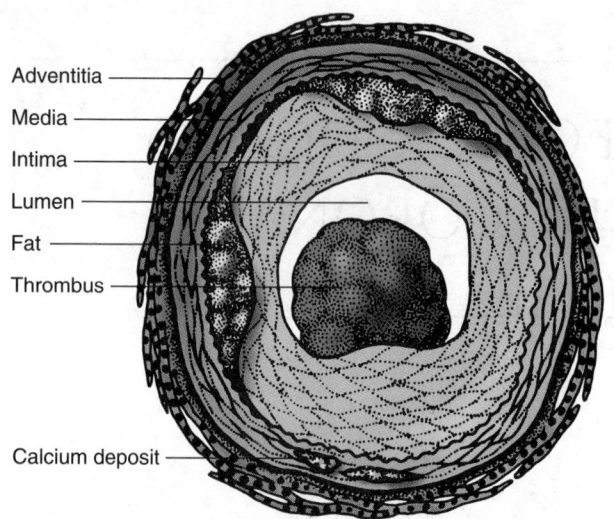

Adventitia
Media
Intima
Lumen
Fat
Thrombus
Calcium deposit

Figure 40–1. A cross-section of an atherosclerotic coronary artery.

These processes narrow the vessel lumen (Fig. 40–1). Blood flow through the restricted lumen may be adequate to perfuse myocardial tissue when the client is at rest.

At rest, the heart extracts a larger amount of oxygen (75%) from its blood flow than does any other major organ in the body. When additional oxygen is needed to meet increased tissue demands, an increase in coronary artery blood flow is required. Once the lumen of a coronary artery is obstructed by more than 70%, blood flow may not be able to increase in response to tissue demands. Increases in myocardial oxygen requirements (e.g., exercise or aortic stenosis) or transient reductions in blood flow (e.g., hypotension or coronary spasm) may result in inadequate oxygen supply to and ischemia of the myocardium. Ischemic myocardium is oxygen-deprived myocardium, and the client typically experiences angina.

Angina Pectoris

Angina pectoris, a name derived from a Latin phrase, means "strangling of the chest." Angina is a temporary imbalance between the coronary arteries' ability to supply oxygen and the cardiac muscle's demand for oxygen. Ischemia that occurs with angina is limited in duration, and it does not cause permanent damage of myocardial tissue.

Angina may be of two predominant types. *Stable angina* is chest discomfort occurring with moderate to prolonged exertion in a pattern that is familiar to the client; frequency, duration, and intensity of symptoms have not increased over the past several months. Stable angina results in only slight limitation of activity. This condition is usually associated with a stable atherosclerotic plaque.

Unstable angina is chest pain or discomfort that occurs at rest or with minimal exertion and causes marked limitation of activity. An increase in the number of attacks and an increase in the intensity of the pain characterize unstable angina. The pain may last longer than 15 minutes or be poorly relieved by rest or nitroglycerin. Unstable angina describes a broad spectrum of disorders, including *new-onset angina, variant (Prinzmetal's) angina, preinfarction angina,* and *crescendo angina.*

The atherosclerotic plaque may rupture in unstable angina, with resultant platelet aggregation, thrombus formation, and vasoconstriction. The incidence of MI (10–30% per year) and death from MI (29% in 5 years) are higher for clients with unstable angina than for those with stable angina (Matrisciano, 1992).

WOMEN'S HEALTH CONSIDERATIONS

Many women experience atypical angina; they may describe angina as a choking sensation that occurs with exertion. Angina is more likely to be the primary presenting symptom of CAD in women (56%) than in men (46%) and is twice as common as MI in women. For 86% of women, compared with 56% of men, angina does not progress to MI.

Myocardial Infarction

Myocardial infarction occurs when myocardial tissue is abruptly and severely deprived of oxygen. When blood flow is acutely reduced by 80%–90%, ischemia develops. Ischemia can lead to necrosis of myocardial tissue if blood flow is not restored. Most MIs are the result of atherosclerosis of a coronary artery, rupture of the plaque, subsequent thrombosis, and occlusion of blood flow. However, other factors may be implicated, such as coronary artery spasm, platelet aggregation, and emboli from mural thrombi (thrombi lining the walls of the cardiac chambers).

Myocardial infarctions often begin with infarction (necrosis) of the subendocardial layer of cardiac muscle. This layer has the longest myofibrils in the heart, the greatest oxygen demand, and the poorest oxygen supply.

Around the initial area of infarction in the subendocardium are two zones: (1) the zone of injury, tissue that is injured but not necrotic; (2) the zone of ischemia, tissue that is oxygen deprived. This pattern is illustrated in Figure 40–2.

Process of Infarction

Infarction is a dynamic process. It does not occur instantly; rather, it evolves over several hours. Hypoxia from ischemia may lead to local vasodilation of blood vessels and acidosis. Imbalances of potassium, calcium, and magnesium as well as acidosis at the cellular level may lead to suppression of normal pacemaker and contractile functions. Automaticity and ectopy are enhanced. Catecholamines released in response to hypoxia and pain may increase the heart's rate and force of contraction. These factors increase oxygen requirements in tissue that is already oxygen deprived. The area of infarction may extend into the zones of injury and ischemia.

The actual extent of the zone of infarction depends on three factors: collateral circulation, anaerobic metabolism, and workload demands on the myocardium.

The infarction may involve only the subendocardium (called a subendocardial MI), or it may spread to the epicardium or to all three layers of cardiac muscle. When all three layers are involved, the MI is termed *transmural.* Subendocardial MIs have less effect on wall motion and cardiac output than transmural infarctions do.

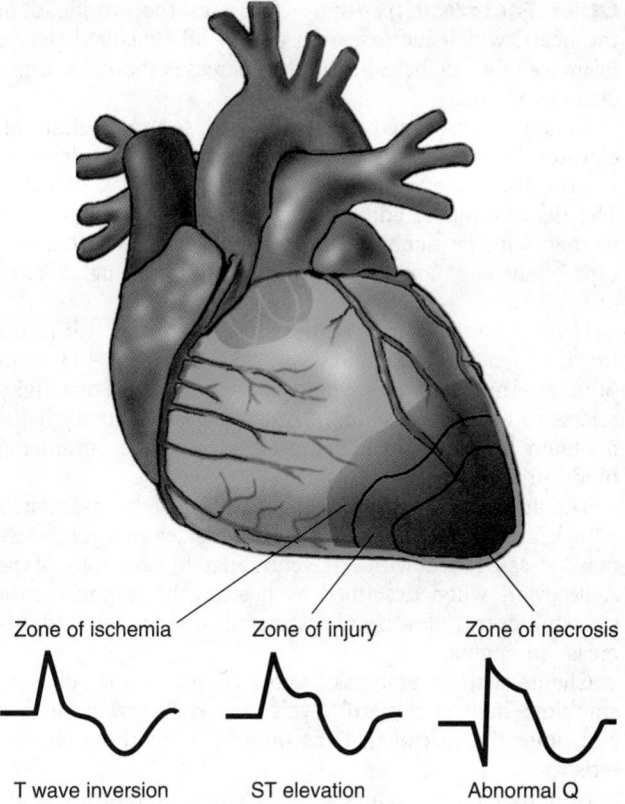

Figure 40-2. Electrocardiogram changes seen in myocardial infarction.

Physiologic Response to the Infarction

Obvious physical changes do not occur in the heart until 6 hours after the infarction, when the infarcted region appears blue and swollen. After 48 hours, the infarct turns gray with yellow streaks as neutrophils invade the tissue and begin to remove the necrotic cells. By 8–10 days after infarction, granulation tissue forms at the edges of the necrotic tissue. Over 2–3 months, the necrotic area eventually develops into a shrunken, thin, firm scar (Pasternak et al., 1992). Scar tissue permanently changes the size and shape of the entire left ventricle (ventricular remodeling). Remodeling may decrease left ventricular function, cause heart failure, and increase morbidity and mortality.

Classification of Myocardial Infarction by Location

The client's response to an MI also depends on which coronary artery or arteries were obstructed and which part of the left ventricle wall was damaged: anterior, lateral, septal, inferior, or posterior. Figure 40–3 details the major coronary arteries, and Table 40–1 describes the structures they perfuse.

Clients with obstruction of the left anterior descending (LAD) artery usually have anterior or septal MIs because the LAD artery perfuses the anterior wall and most of the septal wall of the left ventricle. Anterior wall MIs account for 25% of all MIs and, at 25%, have the highest mortal-ity rate. Clients with anterior MIs are most likely to experience left ventricular heart failure and ventricular dysrhythmias, because a large segment of the left ventricle wall may have been damaged.

The circumflex artery supplies the lateral wall of the left ventricle and possibly portions of the posterior wall or the sinoatrial (SA) and atrioventricular (AV) nodes. Clients with obstruction of the circumflex artery may experience posterior wall MI (2% of MIs) or lateral wall MI (3% of MIs) and sinus dysrhythmias.

In most people, the right coronary artery perfuses the SA and AV nodes as well as the inferior or diaphragmatic portion of the left ventricle. Clients with obstruction of the right coronary artery often have inferior MIs. Inferior wall MIs account for approximately 17% of all MIs and have a mortality rate of about 10%. Clients are most likely to experience bradydysrhythmias or AV conduction defects, especially transient second-degree heart blocks. About one third of clients with inferior MIs have right ventricular MI and right ventricular failure (Braunwald, 1992).

WOMEN'S HEALTH CONSIDERATIONS

Women have higher morbidity and mortality rates after MI than men in part because, when an MI occurs, women are older and sicker and are more likely to have pre-existing diabetes and heart failure. Women also delay longer, an average of 5 hours, before seeking medical assistance for chest pain. These factors often make women ineligible for interventions to reperfuse coronary arteries (Arnstein, Buselli, & Rankin, 1996).

Etiology

Atherosclerosis is the primary factor in the development of coronary artery disease (CAD). Numerous risk factors contribute to atherosclerosis (see Chap. 38). Risk factors are classified as nonmodifiable and modifiable.

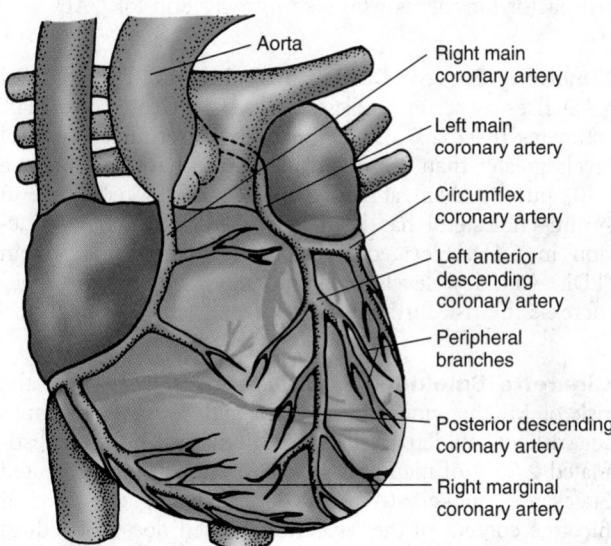

Figure 40-3. Coronary arterial system.

TABLE 40–1

Major Coronary Vessels and the Structures They Perfuse

Left Anterior Descending Coronary Artery
- Most of the left ventricular muscle mass and septum

Left Circumflex Coronary Artery
- Posterior wall of the left ventricle
- SA node in 39% of clients
- AV node in 12% of clients
- Left ventricular muscle in 10% of clients

Right Coronary Artery
- Right ventricle
- Inferior portion of the left ventricle
- SA node in 59% of clients
- AV node in 88% of clients

SA = sinoatrial; AV = atrioventricular.

Nonmodifiable Risk Factors

Nonmodifiable risk factors are personal elements that cannot be altered or controlled. These risk factors, which interact with each other, include age, gender, family history, and ethnic background. The risk of CAD increases with age; 55% of clients who experience an MI are 65 years or older (AHA, 1996).

Premenopausal women have a lower incidence of MI than men do. However, for postmenopausal women in their 70s, the incidence of MI equals that of men. Family history is also a risk factor; people whose parents had CAD are more susceptible.

Modifiable Risk Factors

Modifiable risk factors include elevated serum cholesterol levels, cigarette smoking, hypertension, impaired glucose tolerance, obesity, physical inactivity, and stress. Viagra, a drug to treat impotence, has recently been identified as a risk factor for clients who take nitroglycerin for CAD.

Elevated Serum Cholesterol Levels. The risk of CAD rises as serum cholesterol levels increase. The AHA estimates that 52% of Americans have serum cholesterol levels greater than 200 mg/dL and 20% have levels above 240, putting them at risk for CAD. A 1% reduction in serum cholesterol has been associated with a 2% reduction in CAD. Elevated levels of low-density lipoprotein (LDL) with low levels of high-density lipoprotein (HDL) increase the risk further.

Cigarette Smoking. Cigarette smokers have twice the risk of MI that nonsmokers have and two to four times the risk of sudden cardiac death (AHA, 1996). An estimated 27.5% of men and 22.7% of women in the United States are smokers (AHA, 1996). Reducing the tar and nicotine content of the cigarettes smoked does not reduce the risk of CAD.

Other Factors. *Hypertension* increases the workload of the heart, which increases the risk of MI. *Impaired glucose tolerance* (e.g., diabetes) seriously increases the risks, especially in women.

Obesity is associated with increased serum cholesterol, elevated blood pressure, and abnormal glucose tolerance. It may also have an independent effect on risk of CAD. The distribution of adipose tissue seems to be important; women with fat deposited about the waist rather than the hips often have unfavorable lipid profiles and higher rates of CAD.

Physical inactivity may be the most important risk factor for the general population, because between 40% and 60% of Americans are sedentary, and physical inactivity relates to other risk factors. Regular physical activity helps maintain body weight and muscle mass while optimizing blood pressure and lipid values.

The individual's response to stress may be associated with heart disease. Some evidence indicates that job stress may be associated with left ventricular hypertrophy. *Type A behavior,* when described as hostility in response to a stressful event, has been associated with a twofold increase in angina.

Clients with several risk factors (hypertension, obesity, smoking, high cholesterol levels, and diabetes) have several times the risk of CAD as those without these characteristics.

Although many factors place a client at risk for heart disease, there are well-documented, effective ways of promoting cardiovascular health. Some of these methods are described in Chart 40–1.

TRANSCULTURAL CONSIDERATIONS

Modifiable risk factors vary for people of differing race and ethnic backgrounds. African-Americans do not have significantly higher overall heart disease rates than other groups. However, among African-Americans the incidence of diabetes is 33% higher, and hypertension develops at an earlier age and is more severe at every decade of life. Obesity is significantly more common in African-American women than in the corresponding Caucasian-American populations (U.S. Department of Health and Human Services [DHHS], 1990).

Hispanics have lower death rates from heart disease than non-Hispanics. However, smoking continues in 43% of Hispanic men (higher than in other American populations) (DHHS, 1990). Above-normal weight is more of a problem for Hispanic women, especially Mexican-American women (AHA, 1996) and may be associated with less-than-average physical activity.

Tremendous diversity among the Asian and Pacific Island American populations makes generalizations difficult. However, Filipino-Americans seem to have an increased incidence of hypertension, and more than 60% of native Hawaiians are overweight.

The major modifiable cardiovascular risk factors for Native Americans seem to be obesity and diabetes. The increase in obesity in Native Americans has paralleled the increase in diabetes (DHHS, 1990). In many tribes, more than 20% of the members have diabetes.

Health Promotion Guide: Prevention of Coronary Artery Disease

Smoking
- If you smoke, quit.
- If you don't smoke, don't start.

Diet
- Follow a prudent daily diet:
- Consume sufficient calories for your body: you must obtain
  - 50–55% of your calories from carbohydrates.
  - 30–35% of your calories from complex carbohydrates.
  - 10% of your calories from simple sugars.
  - Less than 30% of your calories from fat.
  - 15% of your calories from monounsaturated fat.
  - 10% of your calories from polyunsaturated fat.
  - The remainder of your calories (5–10%) from saturated fat.
  - 12–20% of your calories from protein.
- Limit your cholesterol intake to less than 300 mg daily.
- Limit your sodium intake to less than 130 mEq daily.

Cholesterol
- Have your cholesterol and low-density lipoprotein (LDL) levels checked regularly.
- If your cholesterol and LDLs are elevated, follow your health care provider's advice.

Physical Activity
- If you are middle aged or older or have a history of medical problems, check with your health care provider before starting an exercise program.
- Appropriate exercise should be enjoyable; burn 400 calories/session, and sustain a heart rate of 120–150 beats per minute, depending on your age.
- Exercise moderately at least three times each week, preferably five.
- Exercise periods should be at least 20–30 minutes long with 10-minute warm-up and 5-minute cool-down periods.
- If you are unable to exercise moderately three to five times each week, walk daily for 30 minutes at a comfortable pace.
- If you are unable to walk 30 minutes daily, walk any distance you can (e.g., park further away from a site than necessary; use the stairs, not the elevator, to go one floor up or two floors down).

Diabetes
- Manage your diabetes with your health care provider.

Blood Pressure
- Have your blood pressure checked regularly.
- If your blood pressure is elevated, follow your health care provider's advice.
- Continue to monitor your blood pressure at regular intervals.

Obesity
- Avoid severely restricted or fad diets.
- Consider a restriction in intake of saturated fats, simple sugars, and cholesterol-rich foods.
- Increase your physical activity.

Incidence/Prevalence

Approximately 1,500,000 MIs occur each year in the United States, and about one third of these people die (AHA, 1996). MI is the single largest cause of death for both men and women. Approximately half of deaths from MI occur in the first hour before reaching the hospital.

Approximately 350,000 people experience angina for the first time each year, and 750,000 people are hospitalized yearly with the diagnosis of unstable angina (Matrisciano, 1992). The AHA estimates that more than 7 million people who have experienced angina or MI are still living (AHA, 1996). The estimated cost of caring for people with CAD is slightly less then $150 billion yearly.

Collaborative Management

 Assessment

➤ History

If chest discomfort is present at the time of the interview, the nurse delays collection of historical data until interventions for pain, vital sign instability, and dysrhythmias are initiated and the discomfort resolves. The nurse obtains information about how the client has managed the current episode of chest discomfort and which medications the client is taking. When the client is *pain-free,* the nurse obtains information about family history and modifiable risk factors, including eating habits, lifestyle, and physical activity levels.

➤ Physical Assessment/Clinical Manifestations

The nurse asks clients to describe the immediate concern. The nurse notes the presence of chest, epigastric, jaw, back, or arm discomfort and asks clients to rate the discomfort on a scale of 0–10, with 10 being the highest level of discomfort. Clients often describe the discomfort as tightness, a burning sensation, pressure, or indigestion. The nurse asks clients what they have already done to try to relieve the pain.

➤ Pain Assessment

The nurse rapidly yet completely assesses the client with ongoing chest pain. Because chest discomfort may occur from a variety of causes (see Table 35–1), it is important to differentiate among the types of chest pain and to identify the source. Both the physician and nurse may question the client to determine the characteristics of the discomfort. Appropriate questions for the nurse to ask concerning the discomfort include onset, location, radiation, intensity, duration, and precipitating and relieving factors.

Chart 40–2 compares and contrasts anginal and infarction pain. Because anginal pain is ischemic pain, it usually improves when the disparity between oxygen supply and demand is resolved. For example, rest reduces tissue demands, and nitroglycerin improves oxygen supply. Discomfort from an MI does not usually resolve with such simple measures. The nurse also notes the presence of any associated symptoms, including nausea, vomiting, di-

---

Chart 40–2

Key Features of Angina and Myocardial Infarction

Angina
Substernal chest discomfort
- Radiating to the left arm
- Precipitated by exertion or stress
- Relieved by nitroglycerin or rest
- Lasting <15 min
- Few associated symptoms

Myocardial Infarction
Substernal chest pressure
- Radiating to the left arm, back, or jaw
- Occurring without cause, primarily early in the morning
- Relieved only by opioids
- Lasting 30 min or more
- Frequent associated symptoms:
  - Nausea
  - Diaphoresis
  - Dyspnea
  - Feelings of fear and anxiety
  - Dysrhythmias

---

aphoresis, dizziness, weakness, palpitations, and shortness of breath.

WOMEN'S HEALTH CONSIDERATIONS

Chest discomfort is often not the initial symptom reported by women experiencing an MI. Women are more likely to have initially atypical symptoms such as heart "flutters" without pain, shortness of breath, fatigue, or depression (Hahn, 1995).

TRANSCULTURAL CONSIDERATIONS

African-Americans have experienced longer delays in seeking treatment for MI and higher mortality rates than Caucasians. One factor thought to contribute to this delay is a greater incidence of dyspnea as an acute symptom of MI among male and female African-Americans rather than the more classic chest discomfort (Lee, 1997).

ELDERLY CONSIDERATIONS

The presence of the associated symptoms without chest discomfort is also significant. In 15%–25% of all clients with MI, primarily older adults and diabetics, chest pain or discomfort may be mild or absent, and clients may complain primarily of the associated symptoms. Twenty-five percent of older adults experiencing MI complain only of shortness of breath (Jensen & Miller, 1995). Clients older then 80 may display disorientation or confusion as a result of poor cardiac output as the major manifestation of MI.

▶ Cardiovascular Assessment

The nurse immediately obtains a blood pressure measurement, determines the heart rate, interprets the cardiac

rhythm, and assesses for dysrhythmias. Sinus tachycardia with premature ventricular contractions (PVC) frequently occurs in the first few hours after MI. If an intravenous (IV) access is available, the nurse ensures that it is patent because the client will most likely receive IV fluids and medications. If an access is not available, the nurse initiates one or contacts the appropriate person to establish an IV route as quickly as possible. The nurse may administer oxygen, titrating the fraction of inspired oxygen (FIO_2) to the client's oxygen (O_2) saturation according to protocols or the physician's order.

Next, the nurse assesses distal peripheral pulses and skin temperature. The skin should be warm, with all pulses palpable. In the client with unstable angina or MI, poor cardiac output may be manifested by cool, diaphoretic skin and diminished or absent pulses.

The nurse auscultates for an S_3 gallop, which often indicates heart failure, a serious and common complication of MI. The nurse also assesses respiratory rate and breath sounds for signs of heart failure. An increased respiratory rate is common because of anxiety and pain, but crackles or wheezes may indicate heart failure. Auscultation of an S_4 heart sound is a common finding in the client who has had a previous MI or hypertension.

The client with MI may experience a temperature elevation for several days after infarction. Temperatures as high as 102° F (38.9° C) may occur in response to myocardial necrosis.

▶ Psychosocial Assessment

Denial is a common early reaction to chest discomfort associated with angina or MI. On average, the client with acute MI waits more than 2 hours before seeking medical attention. Often the client rationalizes that symptoms are due to indigestion or overexertion. In some situations, denial is a normal part of adapting to a stressful event. However, denial that interferes with identification of a symptom, such as chest discomfort, can be harmful to the client. The nurse explains the significance of reporting any discomfort, emphasizing that health care provisions attempt to relieve the discomfort immediately.

Fear, anxiety, and anger are other common reactions of clients and families. Nursing assessment focuses on assisting the client and family members in identifying these feelings. The nurse allows the client and family time to explain their understanding of the event and clarifies any misconceptions.

▶ Laboratory Assessment

Cardiac Enzymes. An MI can be confirmed by abnormally high blood levels of cardiac enzymes and isoenzymes. Of all the cardiac enzymes, creatine kinase (CK) is considered the most sensitive and reliable indicator for diagnosis of MI. Total CK levels rise within 3 hours after the onset of chest pain and peak within 24 hours after damage and death of cardiac tissue. Because total CK also rises with brain or muscle injury, an elevation is not specific for myocardial damage.

When cardiac muscle tissue dies, the CK specific to myocardial cells—CK-MB isoenzyme—enters the bloodstream (serum does not normally contain CK-MB isoenzymes). Peak elevation occurs approximately 12–24 hours after the onset of chest pain; levels return to normal 48–72 hours later. Confirmation of myocardial damage within 2 hours of emergency room admission is possible with the use of stat-CKs and CK subforms. These are gaining popularity as a result of the need to confirm or rule out MI rapidly.

The physician may also use serum measurement of lactate dehydrogenase (LDH) to confirm MI. However, identification of LDH is not as reliable as that of CK-MB. LDH levels start to rise within 12–24 hours after MI, peak between 48 and 72 hours, and fall to normal in 7 days. Thus, they may be useful in diagnosing an MI in a client who has delayed seeking medical help for several days after the onset of chest discomfort. Serum levels of LDH_1 isoenzyme rise higher than serum levels of LDH_2 in the presence of MI. (See Chapter 35 for a more detailed discussion of cardiac enzymes.)

No laboratory test can confirm the diagnosis of angina. Serum enzyme determinations are not useful in assessing the presence of angina. However, serum enzymes remaining within normal limits are an indication that the client has not had an acute MI.

Other Laboratory Tests. The finding of an elevated white blood cell count (10,000–20,000 cells/mm³) helps in the diagnosis of MI. It typically appears on the second day and lasts up to a week.

➤ Radiographic Assessment

Unless there is associated cardiac dysfunction (e.g., valvular disease) or heart failure, the chest x-ray is not diagnostic for angina or MI.

➤ Other Diagnostic Assessment

Electrocardiography. Twelve-lead electrocardiograms (ECG) allow the health care provider to examine the heart from varying perspectives and note both the occurrence and the location of ischemia (angina) or necrosis (infarction).

Ischemic myocardium does not repolarize normally. Thus, 12-lead ECGs obtained during an anginal episode reveal ST depression, T-wave inversion, or both. *Variant angina,* caused by coronary spasm, usually causes elevation of the ST segment during anginal attacks. These ST and T wave changes usually subside when the ischemia is resolved and the pain is relieved. However, the T wave may remain flat or inverted for a period of time. If the client is not experiencing angina at the moment of the test, the ECG for the client with angina is usually normal.

When infarction occurs, three ECG changes are usually observed: ST-segment elevation, T-wave inversion, and an abnormal Q wave (wider than 0.04 seconds or more than one third the height of the QRS complex). Figure 40–2 displays the ECG changes seen in MI.

The Q wave develops because necrotic cells do not conduct electrical stimuli. Hours to days after the MI, the ST- and T-wave changes will return to normal, but the Q wave usually remains permanently. By identifying the lead in which the ECG changes are occurring, the health care provider can identify the extent and location of the infarction.

Stress Test. The health care provider often orders an *exercise tolerance test* (stress test) after the acute stages of an anginal episode or MI to assess for ECG changes consistent with ischemia, evaluate medical therapy, and identify clients who might benefit from referral for invasive therapy.

Scans. *Thallium scans* use radioisotope imaging to assess for ischemia or necrotic muscle tissue related to angina or MI. Areas of decreased or absent perfusion, referred to as cold spots, identify ischemia or infarction. *Multigated acquisition* (MUGA) scans may be used to evaluate left ventricular function.

Cardiac Catheterization. This procedure may be performed to determine the extent and location of obstructions of the coronary arteries. Cardiac catheterization, the "gatekeeper" to invasive management, allows the cardiologist and cardiac surgeon to identify clients who might benefit from percutaneous transluminal angioplasty (PCTA) or coronary artery bypass grafting (CABG). (Chapter 35 describes each of these tests in detail.)

 Analysis

➤ Common Nursing Diagnoses and Collaborative Problems

The client with coronary artery disease (CAD) may have either angina or myocardial infarction (MI). If MI is suspected or cannot be completely ruled out, the client is admitted to a coronary or critical care unit for continuous monitoring. On the basis of the assessment data, the nurse often identifies the following common diagnoses for the client with CAD:

1. Pain related to imbalance between myocardial oxygen supply and demand
2. Altered Tissue Perfusion (cardiopulmonary) related to interruption of blood flow
3. Activity Intolerance related to imbalance between oxygen supply and demand
4. Ineffective Individual Coping related to effects of acute illness, major changes in lifestyle, or loss of control over a body part

For the client experiencing an MI, the most important collaborative problems are

1. Potential for dysrhythmias
2. Potential for heart failure
3. Potential for recurrent chest discomfort and extension of injury

➤ Additional Nursing Diagnoses and Collaborative Problems

Clients with CAD may also experience one or more of the following diagnoses:

■ Fear related to threat of death
■ Altered Sexuality Patterns related to pain and effects of illness
■ Impaired Physical Mobility related to pain or fear of movement

⯈ Planning and Implementation

Pain

Planning: Expected Outcomes. The client is expected to state that chest discomfort is alleviated.

Interventions. The objective of management is to eliminate chest discomfort by providing pain relief, decreasing myocardial oxygen demand, and increasing myocardial oxygen supply. Chart 40–3 summarizes appropriate interventions for the client with chest discomfort.

Drug Therapy. The nurse evaluates the chest pain, obtains the client's vital signs, ensures the patency of an intravenous (IV) access, and notifies the physician of the client's condition. If appropriate, the nurse may administer the prescribed pain medication. One of the initial medications prescribed for chest pain is usually sublingual nitroglycerin (Chart 40–4). Aspirin, 325 mg po (chewed), also may be administered immediately.

Nitroglycerin. Nitroglycerin, a nitrate often referred to as "nitro," increases collateral blood flow, redistributes blood flow toward the subendocardium, and causes dilation of the coronary arteries. The nurse instructs the client to hold the tablet under the tongue and provides 5 mL of water, if necessary, to allow the tablet to dissolve. Pain relief should begin within 1 or 2 minutes and be

---

> **Chart 40–3**
>
> ## Nursing Care Highlight: The Client with Chest Discomfort
>
> - Obtain the client's description of the chest discomfort.
> - Obtain the client's vital signs (blood pressure, pulse, respiration).
> - Assess the client's vascular access.
> - Consult standing orders or notify the physician for specific intervention.
> - Obtain a 12-lead electrocardiogram, if indicated.
> - Provide pain relief medication and ASA as ordered.
> - Administer oxygen therapy as prescribed.
> - Remain calm; stay with the client if possible.
> - Assess the client's vital signs and intensity of pain 5 min after administration of medication.
> - Remedicate (if vital signs remain stable), and check the client every 5 min.
> - Notify the physician if vital signs deteriorate or pain is not relieved after three doses of nitroglycerin.

clearly evident in 3–5 minutes. After 5 minutes, the nurse rechecks the client's pain intensity and vital signs. If the client's blood pressure is less than 100 systolic or 25 mmHg lower than the previous reading, the nurse

---

> **Chart 40–4**
>
> ## Drug Therapy for Coronary Artery Disease

Drug	Usual Dosage	Nursing Interventions	Rationale
Nitrates			
Nitroglycerin (Nitrostat, Tridil)	• 0.3–0.4 mg q5min sublingually, up to three tablets	• Instruct the client to lie down with the head of the bed at a level of comfort when taking the sublingual form.	• Hypotension can be dramatic, immediate, and intensified by the upright position.
		• Monitor blood pressure. Pay attention to orthostatic changes.	• A decrease in blood pressure occurs with vasodilation.
		• Instruct the client to allow the sublingual tablet to dissolve and to avoid swallowing the tablet.	• The sublingual dose is absorbed through the sublingual mucous membranes.
		• Check the expiration date on sublingual tablets. Tablets should be replaced every 3–5 mo.	• The efficacy of the tablets decreases with time.
		• Determine whether pain is relieved.	• Additional medication may be required to relieve pain.
		• Monitor for headache.	• Vasodilation is generalized.
Isosorbide dinitrate (Isordil, Iso-Bid)	• 2.5 mg q4–6h sublingually • 5–30 mg qid PO	• Instruct the client taking sublingual forms to lie down before administration.	• The hypotensive effect can be dramatic and immediate with sublingual administration.
	• 40-mg sustained-release tablet 2–3 times daily	• Monitor blood pressure and assess for dizziness.	• A decrease in blood pressure occurs with vasodilation.

Chart 40–4. Drug Therapy for Coronary Artery Disease Continued

Drug	Usual Dosage	Nursing Interventions	Rationale
Isosorbide mononitrate	• 60 mg extended release tab qd	• Schedule sustained-release form with an 8–12 h dose-free interval.	• Tolerance may develop.
Nitroglycerin patch (Nitro-bid Patch)	• Transdermally started at 5 mg/24 hr (10 cm² system)	• Remove the patch from the client before defibrillation.	• The client may develop a burn.
		• Rotate application sites.	• Rotation prevents skin irritation.
		• Apply the patch to a clean, dry, hairless area.	• The drug is better absorbed when the skin is clean, dry, and hairless.
		• Remove patch for 8–12 hours each day.	• Tolerance will develop.
Beta-Blockers			
Propranolol (Inderal)	• 10–80 mg bid–qid to 240 mg/day PO	• Assess heart rate before administration.	• Beta-blocking effects cause a decrease in heart rate.
	• 1–3 mg at rate not to exceed 1 mg/min IV	• Monitor blood pressure.	• The hypotensive effect is due to a decrease in cardiac output, suppressed renin activity, and beta-blocking effects.
		• Observe for signs of heart failure.	• Heart failure may occur as a result of a decrease in cardiac output.
		• Assess for shortness of breath and wheezing.	• Beta₂-blocking effects in the lungs can cause bronchoconstriction.
Metoprolol (Lopressor, Betaloc❈), a cardioselective beta-adrenergic blocker	• 100–450 mg/day PO	• Assess heart rate before administration; do not administer if heart rate <50.	• Beta-blockers may cause further decreases in heart rate.
	• 5 mg IV over 2 min may be repeated twice for a total of 15 mg	• Monitor BP and hold for systolic <90.	• Decreased blood pressure is an anticipated effect.
		• Assess client for cough, shortness of breath, edema, and weight gain.	• These are indications of heart failure.
Calcium Channel Blockers			
Nifedipine (Procardia, Adalat)	• 10–30 mg tid PO or sublingually	• Monitor blood pressure and assess for dizziness.	• Vasodilation can cause dramatic hypotension, which occurs within minutes, especially after sublingual administration.
		• Assess for headache and edema of the lower extremities.	• These are common side effects.
Verapamil hydrochloride (Calan, Isoptin)	• 40–80 mg qid PO or 120–240 mg sustained-release tablet once a day	• Monitor heart rate.	• This agent slows SA and AV node conduction.
	• 5–10 mg over 2 min IV	• Monitor blood pressure and assess for dizziness.	• Vasodilation decreases blood pressure.
		• Assess for constipation.	• This is a common side effect.
Diltiazem hydrochloride (Cardizem)	• 30–60 mg qid PO or 120–480 mg sustained-release tablet once a day; increase dose slowly	• Monitor blood pressure and assess for dizziness.	• Vasodilation decreases blood pressure.
		• Monitor heart rate.	• This drug slows SA and AV node conduction, but the decrease is not as great as that which occurs with verapamil.

Continued

Chart 40–4. Drug Therapy for Coronary Artery Disease   Continued

Drug	Usual Dosage	Nursing Interventions	Rationale
Antiplatelet Agents			
Aspirin (Empirin, Apoasa✱)	• 80–325 mg PO	• Suggest that the client take the daily dose with food.	• Gastric irritation may occur.
		• Question the client about ringing in the ears.	• Tinnitus may occur with aspirin toxicity.
		• Emphasize to the client that aspirin is an important cardiac medication and should be continued unless the client is told to stop.	• Studies document significantly better survival rates for clients with coronary artery disease receiving aspirin.

SA = sinoatrial; AV = atrioventricular

lowers the head of the client's bed and notifies the physician. If the client is experiencing some but not complete relief and vital signs remain stable, another nitroglycerin tablet may be used. A total of three tablets may be administered in an attempt to relieve anginal pain.

Angina usually responds to nitroglycerin. The client typically states that the pain is relieved or markedly diminished. When simple measures, such as three repeated sublingual nitroglycerin tablets, do not relieve chest discomfort, the client may be experiencing MI. The nurse should inform the physician immediately and prepare the client for transfer to a specialized unit where the client can be closely monitored and appropriately managed.

In a specialized unit, the physician may prescribe IV nitroglycerin for management of the chest pain. The nurse begins the nitroglycerin infusion slowly, checking the client's blood pressure and pain level every 3–5 minutes. The nitroglycerin dose is increased until the pain is relieved, the blood pressure falls excessively, or the maximal prescribed dose is reached. The nurse continues to monitor the blood pressure frequently (Chart 40–5).

Morphine Sulfate. The physician may prescribe morphine sulfate (MS) to relieve chest discomfort that is unresponsive to nitroglycerin. Morphine relieves MI pain, decreases myocardial oxygen demand, and reduces circulating catecholamines. It is usually administered in 2- to 5-mg increments intravenously every 5–15 minutes until the maximal prescribed dose is reached or until the client experiences relief or signs of toxicity. Signs of morphine toxicity include respiratory depression, hypotension, and severe vomiting.

The nurse monitors the client's vital signs and cardiac rhythm every few minutes. These strategies are often enough to relieve the client's pain. If these methods are not adequate, additional interventions, identified later under Altered Tissue Perfusion (Cardiopulmonary), may be attempted.

Other Interventions. Several interventions may assist in relieving chest pain. Supplemental oxygen may increase the amount of oxygen available to myocardial tissue. Therefore, oxygen is often prescribed and administered at 2–4 L/min by nasal cannula titrated to maintain an oxy-gen saturation greater then 92%. If the client's blood pressure is stable, the nurse may assist the client in assuming any position of comfort. Placing the client in semi-Fowler's position often enhances comfort and tissue oxygenation. A quiet, calm environment and explanations of interventions often reduce the client's anxiety and assist in relief of chest pain.

When the pain has subsided and the client is stabilized, the physician may change the client's medication to an oral or topical nitrate. During administration of long-term oral and topical nitrates, a 12-hour nitrate-free period should be maintained to prevent tolerance. The client may complain initially of headache. The physician may prescribe acetaminophen (Tylenol, Exdol) before the nitrate to prevent some of this discomfort.

Altered Tissue Perfusion (Cardiopulmonary)

Planning: Expected Outcomes. The client is expected to exhibit (1) relief of chest discomfort, (2) resolution of ST- and T-wave changes, (3) sinus rhythm (or normal rhythm for the client) rate of approximately 60, and (4) blood pressure within an acceptable range.

Interventions. Because myocardial infarction (MI) is a dynamic process, restoration of perfusion to the injured area often reduces infarct size and improves left ventricular function. Complete, sustained reperfusion of coronary arteries in the first few hours after MI has decreased mortality in MI patients.

Thrombolytic Therapy. Thrombolytic agents are used to dissolve thrombi in the coronary arteries and restore myocardial blood flow. Examples include streptokinase (Kabikinase), tissue plasminogen activator (t-PA, Activase), anisoylated plasminogen-streptokinase activator complex (APSAC), reteplase (Retavase), and urokinase. The physician may order administration of thrombolytics intravenously or by the intracoronary route during cardiac catheterization. Thrombolytic agents are most effective when administered within the first 6 hours of the coronary event. Thrombolytics are underused nationwide in men and women, young and old (Clem, 1995).

Thrombolytic therapy should be given in a unit where the client can be continuously monitored. It is indicated

Chart 40-5

Drug Therapy with Intravenous Vasodilators and Inotropes

Drug	Usual Dosage	Nursing Interventions	Rationale
Nitroprusside sodium (Nipride, Nitropress)	• IV only by infusion device • Begin with 0.2 μg/kg/min • May increase gradually to 10 μg/kg/min	• Monitor BP q2–5 min when initiating therapy. If BP drops excessively, elevate the legs, decrease the dose, and increase fluids per unit policies. • Monitor PAWP, SVR, BP, heart rate, and urine output frequently. • Titrate medication to obtain the desired effect. • Protect from light. • Maintain dose at less than 3 μg/min if possible. • In clients requiring doses >3 μg/min for >24–36 hr, monitor for metabolic acidosis, confusion, or hyperreflexia. Examine blood thiocyanate level.	• This agent is a potent, rapidly reversible vasodilator acting on both peripheral venous and arterial musculature. BP may drop in 2 min. • This agent is light sensitive. • Doses >3 μg/min are associated with thiocyanate or cyanide toxicity. • These are indications of the toxic effects of cyanide.
Nitroglycerin (Tridil)	• IV only by infusion device started at 0.3 μg/min and gradually increased in increments of 3 μg/min until maximum of 20 μg/min	• Monitor BP q1–3 min when initiating therapy. If BP drops excessively, elevate the legs and decrease the dose according to unit policies. • Monitor RAP, PAWP, SVR, BP, heart rate, and urine output frequently. • Titrate medication to obtain the desired effect. • Intermittent administration of IV nitroglycerin should be considered. • Monitor the client for headache.	• This agent dilates coronary arteries. It is a more potent systemic venodilator than an arterial vasodilator. BP may drop in 1 min. • Tolerance may develop rapidly to nitroglycerin administered by continuous IV. • Headache is a frequent side effect of initial nitroglycerin therapy.
Sympathomimetics Dopamine (Intropin)	• IV only by infusion device • Starting dose 2–5 μg/kg/min • Titrate up to 20 μg/kg/min	• Determine the reason for use and the expected result. • Observe the client's heart rate, ECG, BP, PAWP, SVR, CO, and urine output q5min to q1h. • Titrate the dose carefully to maintain the dose range and obtain the desired effect. • Infuse through a central catheter. • Monitor the client for ectopy and angina.	• This agent is a dose-dependent activator of alpha, beta, and dopaminergic receptors. • 2–5 μg/kg/min stimulates dopaminergic receptors, which promotes renal and mesenteric blood flow. • 5 μg/kg/min stimulates beta-receptors. This increases heart rate and contractility. • >10–15 μg/kg/min, alpha effects predominate. This causes peripheral constriction. • Extravasation can cause tissue necrosis and sloughing. • These are adverse effects.

Continued

Chart 40-5. Drug Therapy with Intravenous Vasodilators and Inotropes   Continued

Drug	Usual Dosage	Nursing Interventions	Rationale
Dobutamine (Dobutrex)	• IV only by infusion device, 2–10 μg/kg/min	• Observe the client continuously during administration. • Titrate the drug on the basis of heart rate, ECG findings, BP, PAWP, CO, SVR, and urine output. • Monitor for atrial and ventricular ectopy.	• This agent is a very strong $beta_1$-receptor activator and a moderately strong $beta_2$-activator. • Dysrhythmias are an adverse effect.

PAWP = pulmonary artery wedge pressure; SVR = systemic vascular resistance; BP = blood pressure; RAP = right atrial pressure; ECG = electrocardiogram; CO = cardiac output.

for clients who have chest pain of greater than 30 minutes duration unrelieved by nitroglycerin with indications of transmural ischemia and injury as shown by the ECG. Contraindications include recent abdominal surgery or cerebrovascular accident (CVA), because bleeding may occur when fresh clots are lysed. Table 40–2 lists the current contraindications to thrombolytic therapy.

Before thrombolytic administration, the nurse may need to apply pressure dressings to IV puncture sites or wounds to limit bleeding. Clients who weigh less than 65 kg should have their dose of thrombolytic weight adjusted to lessen the likelihood of bleeding. During administration, the nurse immediately reports any indications of bleeding to the physician. After administration, the nurse observes for signs of bleeding by

- Documenting the client's neurologic status
- Observing all IV sites
- Monitoring clotting studies
- Observing for signs of internal bleeding (watching hemoglobin and hematocrit)
- Testing stools, urine, and emesis for occult blood

Some concerns in thrombolytic administration are associated with the specific thrombolytic. *Streptokinase*, a first-generation thrombolytic agent, is not fibrin specific; thus, it may create systemic bleeding problems. Because it is a bacteria protein, streptokinase can cause a hypersensitivity reaction in the client who has had previous exposure. Therefore, the nurse questions the client about streptococcal infections or doses of streptokinase within the past year. To prevent an allergic reaction, the physician may prescribe steroids or antihistamines before the administration of streptokinase. During administration, the nurse observes the client closely for hives and shivering, the most common responses. The half-life of the drug is 16 minutes.

Second-generation thrombolytics include tissue plasminogen activator (t-PA, Activase), anisoylated plasminogen-streptokinase activator complex (APSAC, Eminase), and reteplase (Retavase). t-PA is fibrin specific, has a short half-life (3–5 minutes), and lacks antigenicity. Because some studies have associated t-PA with a more frequent occurrence of cerebrovascular bleeding, the nurse carefully documents neurologic findings. t-PA is much more expensive than streptokinase.

APSAC is a streptokinase derivative; it has a longer half-life (90–105 minutes) than streptokinase but has the same antigenic properties.

Identification of Coronary Artery Reperfusion. The nurse monitors the client for indications that the clot has been lysed and the artery reperfused. These indications include

- Abrupt cessation of chest pain
- Sudden onset of ventricular dysrhythmias
- Resolution of ST-segment depression
- A peak at 12 hours of CK-MB

After clot lysis with thrombolytics, large amounts of thrombin are released into the system, increasing the risk of vessel re-occlusion. To maintain the patency of the coronary artery after thrombolytic therapy, the physician usually prescribes aspirin and IV heparin. The nurse monitors the activated partial thromboplastin time (aPTT; the usual appropriate range is 1½–2½ times control) and maintains the heparin infusion for 3–5 days, as prescribed.

Drug Therapy. Clients who have had an MI, whether receiving thrombolytics or not, should begin aspirin therapy unless contraindicated. Clients may receive a chewable aspirin immediately and then an enteric-coated aspirin (Ancasal, Ecotrin), 80–325 mg daily or every other day, to prevent platelet aggregation at the site of the obstruction.

TABLE 40-2

Contraindications to Thrombolytic Therapy

Absolute

- Active internal bleeding
- Cerebrovascular processes
  - Recent cerebrovascular accident (within 2 mo)
  - Recent spinal or cerebral surgery
  - Cranial neoplasm
- Prolonged cardiopulmonary resuscitation (CPR)

Relative

- Endocarditis or pericarditis
- Hemostatic defects
- Severe uncontrolled hypertension
- Pregnancy or recent delivery
- Trauma within last 10 days
- Surgery within last 10 days

Beta-adrenergic blocking agents (e.g., metoprolol [Lopressor, Betaloc]) decrease infarction size, ventricular dysrhythmias, and mortality rates in clients with MI. The physician usually prescribes a cardioselective beta-blocking agent within the first 24 hours after MI. Beta-blockers slow the heart rate and decrease the force of cardiac contraction. Thus, these agents prolong the period of diastole and increase myocardial perfusion while reducing the force of myocardial contraction. With beta-blockade, the heart is capable of performing 25% to 30% more work without ischemia. During beta-blocker therapy, the nurse

- Monitors the heart rate (bradycardia is common)
- Checks the BP
- Measures the PR interval
- Checks the client's level of consciousness
- Monitors for any chest discomfort

The nurse assesses the client's lungs for crackles (indicative of heart failure) and wheezes (indicative of bronchospasm). Hypoglycemia, depression, nightmares, and forgetfulness are also problems with beta-blockade, especially in older clients (see Chart 40–4).

Physicians frequently prescribe angiotensin-converting enzyme (ACE) inhibitors within 48 hours of an MI to prevent ventricular remodeling and the development of heart failure. ACE inhibitors have been demonstrated to increase survival after MI (Connors & Lamas, 1995). The nurse monitors the client for hypotension, cough, and changes in serum potassium, creatinine, and blood urea nitrogen. (See Chapter 37 for a more detailed discussion of ACE inhibitors.)

For clients with angina, the health care provider may prescribe calcium channel blockers to enhance vasodilation and myocardial perfusion. Calcium channel blockers are indicated for clients with variant angina or for clients who are hypertensive and continue to have angina despite beta-blocker therapy. They are not indicated for clients after MI. The nurse monitors the client receiving calcium channel blockers for hypotension and headaches, and reviews the frequency of anginal episodes.

Activity Intolerance

Planning: Expected Outcomes. The client is expected to walk at least 200 feet four times a day without chest discomfort or shortness of breath.

Interventions. Activity intolerance is reduced by a planned program of cardiac rehabilitation implemented primarily by the nurse and physical therapist. Cardiac rehabilitation is a process of actively assisting the client with cardiac disease to achieve and maintain a vital and productive life while remaining within the heart's ability to respond to increases in activity and stress. Cardiac rehabilitation can be divided into three phases. *Phase 1* begins with the acute illness and ends up with discharge from the hospital. *Phase 2* begins after discharge and continues through convalescence at home. *Phase 3* refers to long-term conditioning.

In the acute phase (phase 1), the nurse promotes rest and yet ensures some limited mobility. The nurse assists with some activities of daily living (ADL), such as bathing and toileting. Clients progress at their own rate to increasing activity levels, depending on their clinical status, age, and physical capabilities. For example, for the first 24 hours, the client may be maintained on bed rest but allowed to stand to void or to use the bedside commode. The second day, the client may be out of bed sitting in a chair as tolerated, usually for 30 minutes three times a day.

The next step in phase 1 is ambulation of the client in the room and to the bathroom. Finally, the nurse encourages progressive ambulation in the hallway, usually 50, 100, and then 200 feet three times a day. In addition, the client may begin showering for 5 or 10 minutes with warm water; a stool should be available for the client to sit on if necessary.

The nurse assesses the client's heart rate, blood pressure, respiratory rate, and level of fatigue with each level of activity. Decreases in systolic blood pressure greater than 20 mmHg, changes in pulse rate of 20 beats/minute, and complaints of dyspnea or chest pain indicate intolerance of activity. When such signs and symptoms develop, the nurse notifies the physician and does not advance the client to the next level. Older adults with CAD often have needs and concerns different from those of younger adults (Chart 40–6).

Ineffective Individual Coping

Planning: Expected Outcomes. The client is expected to indicate a reduction in anxiety and indicate the beginning of control over life.

Interventions. The nurse assesses the client's level of anxiety while allowing the client to express any anxiety

---

Chart 40–6

Nursing Focus on the Elderly: Coronary Artery Disease

- Recognize that chest pain may not be evident in the older client; associated symptoms, such as dyspnea and confusion, may prevail.
- Although older adults have a greater reduction in mortality from myocardial infarction (MI) with the use of thrombolytics, they also have the most severe side effects. Monitor older clients receiving thrombolytics extremely carefully.
- Dysrhythmia may be a normal age-related change rather than a complication of MI. Determine whether the dysrhythmia is causing significant symptoms, then notify the physician.
- If beta-blockers are used, assess the client carefully for the development of side effects. Exacerbation of the depression already present in older adults is a significant problem with beta-blockade.
- Plan slow, steady increases in activity. Older adults with minimal previous exercise show particular benefit from a gradual increase in activity.
- Older adults should plan longer warm-up and cool-down periods when participating in an exercise program. Their pulse rates may not return to baseline until 30 minutes or longer after exercise.

and attempt to define its origin. Simple, repeated explanations of therapies, expectations, and surroundings may help the client. During the acute phase of illness, the physician may prescribe anxiolytic (antianxiety) medications, such as alprazolam (Xanax). The nurse identifies the client's current coping mechanisms; the most common are denial, anger, and depression.

Denial allows the client to minimize a threat and use problem-focused coping mechanisms. The client may avoid discussing what has happened yet comply with treatment regimens. This type of denial decreases the client's anxiety, and the nurse should not discourage it. However, denial that results in a client's "acting out" and refusing to follow treatment regimens can be harmful. Because this behavior is usually due to extreme anxiety or fear, threats only worsen the behavior. The nurse remains calm and avoids confronting the client but clearly indicates when a behavior is not acceptable and is potentially harmful.

Anger may represent an attempt to regain control of life. The nurse encourages the client to verbalize the source of frustration and provides the client with opportunities for decision-making and control.

Depression may be a client's response to grief and loss of function. The nurse listens as the client verbalizes feelings of loss, being careful not to offer false or general reassurances. The nurse acknowledges that the client is depressed but expects the client to perform activities of daily living (ADL) and other activities within restrictions. The nurse identifies all improvements in the client's condition and shares them with the client. (Chapter 8 describes interventions and positive coping strategies.)

Potential for Dysrhythmias

Planning: Expected Outcomes. The client is expected to resume a normal sinus or normal rhythm for the client and be hemodynamically stable.

Interventions. Dysrhythmias are the cause of death in most clients with myocardial infarction (MI) who die before they can be hospitalized. Even in the early hospitalization period, 70% to 90% of MI clients experience some abnormality of cardiac rhythm. Whenever a dysrhythmia develops in a client with coronary artery disease (CAD), the nurse
- Identifies the dysrhythmia
- Assesses the client's hemodynamic status
- Evaluates the client for chest discomfort

Dysrhythmias are treated when they are causing hemodynamic compromise, are increasing myocardial oxygen requirements, or predispose to lethal ventricular dysrhythmias.

Inferior MI. Typical dysrhythmias for a client with an inferior MI are bradycardias and second-degree AV blocks resulting from ischemia of the AV node. These rhythms tend to be transient. The nurse monitors the client's cardiac rhythm and rate and hemodynamic status. If the client becomes hemodynamically unstable, a temporary pacemaker may be necessary.

Anterior MI. Clients with *anterior* MIs are likely to exhibit ventricular irritability (premature ventricular contractions [PVCs]). Third-degree or bundle branch block is a serious complication in the client with an anterior MI, because it indicates that a large portion of the left ventricle is involved. The physician may insert a pacemaker. The nurse should observe the client closely to detect the development of heart failure. (Appropriate interventions for dysrhythmias are described in Chapter 36.)

Potential for Heart Failure

Planning: Expected Outcomes. The client is expected to regain hemodynamic stability as evidenced by
- Blood pressure and pulse rate within the client's acceptable range
- Adequate urine output
- Mental alertness
- Clear lungs on auscultation
- Palpable peripheral pulses

Interventions. Decreased cardiac output related to heart failure is a relatively common complication after MI. After MI, the client may experience heart failure as a result of left ventricular dysfunction, rupture of the intraventricular septum, papillary muscle rupture with valvular dysfunction, or right ventricular infarction. The most severe form of heart failure, *cardiogenic shock,* accounts for most in-hospital deaths after MI. The type of management used to increase cardiac output depends on the location of the MI and the type of heart failure that resulted from the infarction.

Managing Left Ventricular Failure. When a client with MI experiences damage to the left ventricle, rupture of the intraventricular septum, or tear of a papillary muscle, a reduction occurs in the amount of blood that the heart can eject. This reduction in ejection fraction results in a decreased cardiac output and greater left ventricular residual volumes. Volume and pressure increase first in the left ventricle but eventually in the pulmonary vasculature. When volume and pressure are markedly increased in the pulmonary vasculature, pulmonary complications develop.

Nursing Assessment and Monitoring. The nurse assesses for the development of left ventricular failure and pulmonary edema by auscultating for crackles and identifying their location in the lung fields. Wheezing, tachypnea, and frothy sputum may also occur with pulmonary edema. The nurse auscultates the heart, paying particular attention to the presence of an S_3 heart sound. The nurse monitors for the following signs of poor organ perfusion that may result from decreased cardiac output:
- A change in the client's orientation or mental status
- Urine output less than 30 mL/hr
- Cool, clammy extremities with decreased or absent pulses
- Unusual fatigue
- Recurrent chest pain

In specialized units, hemodynamic monitoring may be instituted to assess the client's preload, afterload, and cardiac output. Hemodynamic monitoring requires the insertion of a pulmonary artery catheter (see Chap. 35). The nurse obtains and records hemodynamic measurements, which include right atrial (RA) pressure, pulmonary artery (PA) systolic and diastolic pressures, pulmonary artery wedge pressure (PAWP) (a measure of preload), systemic vascular resistance (SVR) (a measure of afterload), cardiac output (CO), and cardiac index (CI). Single values of these measurements are less significant than the trend of values combined with the client's clinical manifestations. These measurements help both the nurse and the physician to identify heart failure and guide the administration of fluids and vasoactive drugs.

Classification of Post-myocardial Infarction Heart Failure. Killip categorized heart failure after MI into four classes based on prognosis (Table 40–3).

Class I. Clients with class I heart failure often respond well to reduction in preload with IV diuretics. The nurse monitors the urine output hourly, checks the client's vital signs hourly, continues to assess for signs of heart failure, and reviews the serum potassium level.

Classes II and III. Clients with class II and class III failure may require diuresis and more aggressive medical intervention, such as reduction of afterload or enhancement of contractility. Intravenous nitroprusside or nitroglycerin may be used to decrease both preload and afterload. These drugs are administered as continuous infusions in specialized units where the PAWP and blood pressure can be closely monitored. The client's blood pressure can drop in response to excessive vasodilation (see Chart 40–5).

Positive inotropes, such as dopamine (Intropin), dobutamine (Dobutrex), and amrinone (Inocor), increase the force of cardiac contraction. They are administered by continuous IV infusion. The effects of these drugs on the vasculature and heart rate vary and may be dose dependent. The nurse must understand the anticipated effect of the drug and the desired dosage range. The nurse titrates the infusions to optimize cardiac output. The nurse must use caution when administering these drugs because of the potential risk of increasing myocardial oxygen consumption and further decreasing cardiac output. The nurse continues to assess the client, paying particular attention to the development of chest pain.

TABLE 40–3

The Killip Classification of Heart Failure	
Class	**Description**
I	Absent crackles and S_3
II	Crackles in the lower half of the lung fields and possible S_3
III	Crackles more than halfway up the lung fields and frequent pulmonary edema
IV	Cardiogenic shock

Class IV: Cardiogenic Shock. Killip class IV is cardiogenic shock. In cardiogenic shock, necrosis of more than 40% of the left ventricle has occurred. Most clients have a stuttering pattern of chest pain, resulting in piecemeal extension of the MI. Manifestations of cardiogenic shock include
- Tachycardia
- Hypotension
- Blood pressure less than 90 or 30 mmHg less than the client's baseline
- Urine output less than 30 mL/hr
- Cold, clammy skin with poor peripheral pulses
- Agitation, restlessness, or confusion
- Pulmonary congestion
- Tachypnea
- Continuing chest discomfort

Early detection is essential because established cardiogenic shock has a mortality rate of 65% to 100%.

Medical Management. Medical interventions aim to relieve pain and decrease myocardial oxygen requirements through preload and possibly afterload reduction (see Chart 40–5). The physician orders IV morphine, which is used to decrease pulmonary congestion and relieve pain. Oxygen is administered; intubation and ventilation may be necessary. The nurse uses the information gained from hemodynamic monitoring to titrate drug therapy. Preload reduction may be cautiously attempted with diuretics, nitroglycerin, or nitroprusside, as described with Killip class III clients. Because vasodilation may result in a further decline in blood pressure, the nurse monitors systolic pressure constantly. Vasopressors and positive inotropes may be used to maintain organ perfusion, but such drugs increase myocardial oxygen consumption and can worsen ischemia.

Use of an Intra-aortic Balloon Pump. When clients do not respond to drug therapy with improved tissue perfusion, decreased workload of the heart, and increased cardiac contractility, an intra-aortic balloon pump (IABP) may be inserted. Insertion of an intra-aortic counterpulsation device, such as the IABP, is an invasive intervention that is used to improve myocardial perfusion during an acute MI, reduce afterload, and facilitate left ventricular emptying.

The physician can insert an IABP percutaneously or through surgical cutdown. Inflation of the IABP during diastole increases the client's diastolic pressure and improves coronary perfusion. Deflation of the balloon just before systole reduces afterload at the time of systolic contraction. This facilitates emptying of the left ventricle and improves cardiac output. The balloon catheter is attached to a pump console, which is triggered by an ECG tracing and arterial waveform (Fig. 40–4).

Immediate Reperfusion. Immediate reperfusion is an invasive intervention that shows some promise for clients with cardiogenic shock (Pasternak et al., 1992). The client is taken to the cardiac catheterization laboratory and an emergency left-sided heart catheterization is performed. If the client has a treatable lesion or lesions, the surgeon

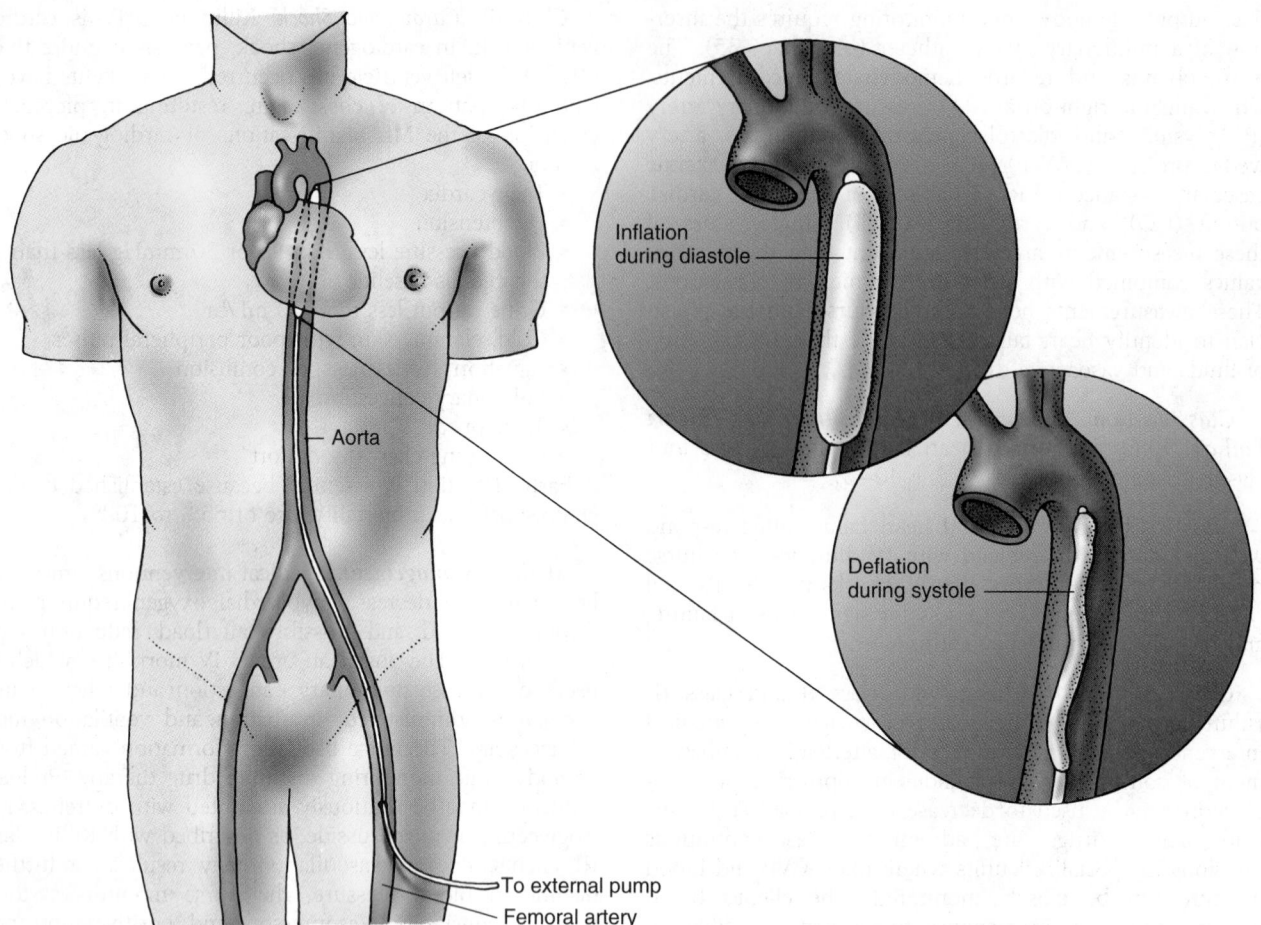

Figure 40–4. Intra-aortic balloon pumping. An intra-aortic balloon catheter is inserted into the femoral artery and advanced into the descending aorta. The polyethylene balloon lies just distal to the left subclavian artery. Immediately after it is inserted, the catheter is connected to the external pump.

performs an immediate percutaneous transluminal coronary angioplasty (PTCA) in the catheterization laboratory, or the client is transferred to the operating suite for coronary artery bypass graft (CABG).

Managing Right Ventricular Failure. Conditions other than left ventricular failure may result in decreased cardiac output after MI. In approximately 30% of clients with inferior MIs, right ventricular infarction and failure develop. In this instance, the right ventricle fails independently of the left. Decreased cardiac output with a paradoxical pulse, clear lungs, and jugular venous distention results when the client is in semi-Fowler's position.

A right ventricular MI may be documented by echocardiography and by an ECG using right-sided precordial leads. The goal of medical management is to improve right ventricular stroke volume by increasing right ventricular fiber stretch or preload. To enhance right ventricular preload, the nurse administers sufficient fluids (as much as 200 mL/hr) to increase right atrial (RA) pressure to 20 mmHg, as ordered. The nurse monitors the pulmonary artery wedge pressure (PAWP) (attempting to maintain it below 15–20 mmHg) and auscultates the lungs to

ensure that left-sided failure is not developing. The nurse monitors the client's cardiac output to ensure that fluid administration is having the desired effect.

Potential for Recurrent Chest Discomfort and Extension of Injury

Planning: Expected Outcomes. The client is expected to experience minimal angina while engaging in ADLs and an exercise program.

Interventions. Recurrent chest discomfort despite medical therapy is one of the major indications for surgical management of coronary artery disease (CAD). Clients who continue to have chest discomfort despite medical therapy may require invasive correction by percutaneous transluminal angioplasty or coronary artery bypass graft (CABG) to resolve angina or prevent MI. Before invasive treatment, a left-sided cardiac catheterization with coronary angiogram (see Chap. 35) is performed to document that the client's lesions are correctable and that left ventricular pump function is adequate.

Percutaneous Transluminal Coronary Angioplasty. Percutaneous transluminal coronary angioplasty (PTCA) is

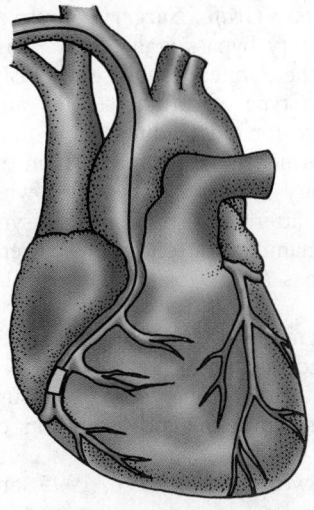 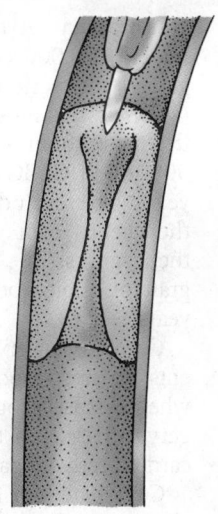 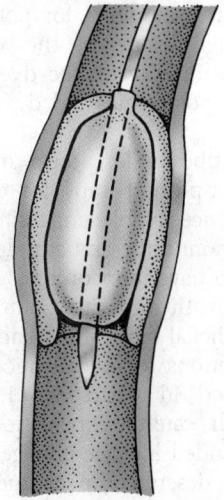 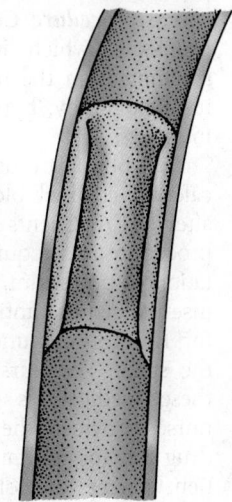

1. The balloon-tipped catheter is positioned in the artery.

2. The uninflated balloon is centered in the obstruction.

3. The balloon is inflated, which flattens plaque against the artery wall.

4. The balloon is removed, and the artery is left unoccluded.

Figure 40–5. Percutaneous transluminal coronary angioplasty.

an invasive but technically nonsurgical technique. It is performed to reduce the frequency and severity of chest discomfort for clients with angina. The risk of complications is not significant.

Indications. Clients who are most likely to benefit from PTCA have single- or double-vessel disease with discrete, proximal, noncalcified lesions. When identifying which lesions are treatable with PTCA, the cardiologist considers the lesion's complexity and location as well as the amount of myocardium at risk. PTCA often will not open complex lesions. Treating lesions located in the left main artery would place a large amount of myocardial tissue at risk should the vessel close acutely; therefore, these lesions are rarely treated with PTCA.

Percutaneous transluminal coronary angioplasty may also be used for the client with an evolving acute MI, either alone or in conjunction with thrombolytic therapy, to reperfuse the damaged myocardium. Approximately 50% of clients needing revascularization are initially treated with PTCA.

Procedure. The physician performs PTCA under fluoroscopic guidance in the cardiac catheterization laboratory. A balloon-tipped catheter is introduced through a guide wire to the occlusion in the coronary vessel. The physician activates a compressor that inflates the balloon at 4–

14 atmospheres of pressure. This process compresses the plaque against the vessel wall and reduces or eliminates the occluding lesion (Fig. 40–5). Balloon inflation may be repeated until angiography indicates decrease of the stenosis (narrowing) to less than 50% of the vessel's diameter.

Intravenous heparin is administered in a continuous infusion to prevent thrombus formation; IV or intracoronary nitroglycerin or sublingual nifedipine is given to prevent coronary spasm. PTCA initially reopens the vessel in more than 90% of appropriately selected clients. However, restenosis occurs in a large number of these clients.

Techniques being used to ensure continued patency of the vessel are laser angioplasty, arthrectomy, and stents. Lasers may be used alone to remove atherosclerotic material from coronary arteries, or they may be used in conjunction with balloon angioplasty to create a smooth lumen about the size of the balloon. Arthrectomy devices can either excise and retrieve plaque or emulsify it. One of the advantages of arthrectomy is that it creates a less bulky vessel with better elastic recoil. Stents are used to maintain the patent lumen obtained by angioplasty or arthrectomy. By providing a supportive scaffold, stents prevent acute closure of the vessel from arterial dissection or vasospasm (Forsha, 1997). Figure 40–6 depicts a stent positioned in a coronary artery.

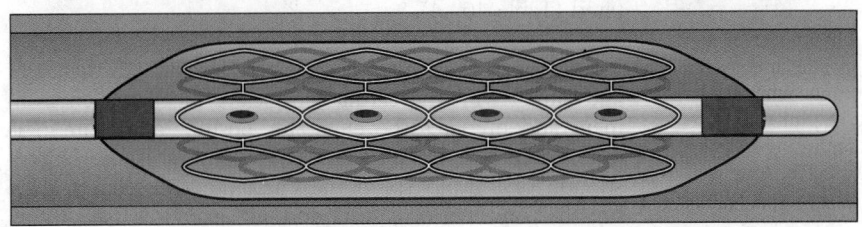

Figure 40–6. A coronary stent open after balloon inflation.

Postprocedure Care. The nurse monitors for potential problems, which include acute closure of the vessel, bleeding from the insertion site, reaction to the dye used in angiography, hypotension, hypokalemia, and dysrhythmias.

The physician usually prescribes a long-term nitrate, calcium channel blocker, and aspirin therapy for clients after PTCA. Clients may experience hypokalemia after the procedure and require careful monitoring and supplementation of potassium. Clients who have intracoronary stents inserted require anticoagulation with warfarin (Coumadin) for 1–3 months until an endothelial covering is laid over the stent. The nursing interventions for clients receiving these medications are described in Chart 40–4. The nurse provides the client with careful explanations of drug therapy and any recommended lifestyle changes. Patient perceptions of PTCA are described in a study by Gulanich and colleagues (1997) (see Research Applications for Nursing).

▶ Research Applications for Nursing

Clients Appreciate Supportive Environment in Angioplasty Laboratory But Experience Postprocedure Discomfort

Gulanich, M., Billey, A., Perino, B., & Keough, V. (1997). Patients' responses to the angioplasty experience: A qualitative study. American Journal of Critical Care, 6(1), 25–32.

This qualitative study examined clients' emotional responses to percutaneous transluminal coronary angioplasty (PTCA). Seven focus group interviews were conducted about the PTCA experience from 45 clients (26 men and 19 women) who had undergone PTCA 3 to 18 months earlier. Most participants described positive experiences during and after PTCA. The most frequent emerging theme was supportive care before, during, and after the procedure. Clients indicated that emotional support and educational preparation for the procedures were very important. However, anger over unmet needs for emotional support and physical comfort was evident. Some clients felt alone during long waits for "tentatively" scheduled procedures. Others complained of back and leg pain from lying flat during and after the procedure. Clients also described discomfort from distended bladders and uncertainty about being allowed to urinate.

Critique. This sample population was drawn from one institution; therefore, generalization to client experiences elsewhere is limited. The interviews were conducted in a group setting. Although investigators encouraged "disagreement" with participants' statements, members of a focus group may be influenced by each other.

Possible Nursing Implications. Because clients move rapidly through health care systems and are awake and aware during PTCA, it is imperative that nurses know what information and interventions clients find most helpful and supportive. This study supports the need for continuing nursing research on comfort measures during and after PTCA as well as on effective methods to educate clients about procedures when time constraints are severe.

Coronary Artery Bypass Graft Surgery. Approximately 490,000 coronary artery bypass graft (CABG) surgeries are performed in the United States each year. CABG is the most common type of cardiac surgery and the most common procedure for older adults; more than 50% of all CABGs are performed on clients older than 65 years. The occluded coronary arteries are bypassed with the client's own venous or arterial blood vessels or synthetic grafts. The internal mammary artery is the current graft of choice because it has a 90% patency rate at 12 years.

Coronary artery bypass grafting is indicated when clients do not respond to medical management of CAD or when disease progression is evident. The decision for surgery is based on the client's symptoms and the results of cardiac catheterization.

Candidates for surgery (Swearingen & Keen, 1995) are clients who have
- Angina with greater than 50% occlusion of the left main coronary artery
- Unstable angina with severe two-vessel or moderate three-vessel disease
- Ischemia with heart failure
- Acute MI
- Signs of ischemia or impending MI after angiography or PTCA

The vessels to be bypassed should have proximal lesions occluding more than 70% of the vessel's diameter but good distal run-off. Bypass of less occluded vessels may result in poor perfusion through the graft and early obstruction. CABG is most effective when good ventricular function remains and the ejection fraction is more than 40%–50%. Clients with lower ejection fractions are poorer risks.

For most clients, the risk is low and the benefits of bypass surgery are clear. Surgical treatment of CAD does not appear to affect the client's life span. Early mortality rates are 1% to 2%. Left ventricular function is the most important long-term indicator of survival. CABG does improve quality of life for most clients; 80%–90% of clients are pain free 1 year after CABG, and 70% remain pain free at 5 years. The percentage of clients experiencing some pain increases sharply after 5 years.

Preoperative Care. CABG surgery may be planned as an elective procedure or performed on an emergency basis. Clients for elective surgery are often admitted the morning of surgery. Preoperative preparations and teaching are completed during prehospitalization interviews. Clients must understand that some medication will need to be adjusted because of the surgery. The nurse ensures that appropriate medications have been discontinued preoperatively and that the necessary ones have been administered (Table 40–4).

Prehospital Preparation. The nurse familiarizes the client and family with the cardiac surgical critical care environment and prepares the client for postoperative care. The nurse demonstrates and has the client return a demonstration of how to splint the chest incision, cough, deep breathe, and perform arm and leg exercises (see Chap. 20). The nurse stresses the following:

TABLE 40-4

Medication Administration Before Coronary Artery Bypass Graft Surgery

Medications Often Discontinued
- Digitalis 12 hr before surgery
- Diuretics 2–3 days before surgery
- Aspirin and anticoagulants 1 week before surgery

Medications Often Administered
- Potassium chloride to maintain potassium between 3.5 and 4.0
- Scheduled beta-blockers
- Scheduled calcium channel blockers
- Scheduled antidysrhythmics
- Scheduled antihypertensives
- Prophylactic antibiotic 20–30 min before surgery

- The client should identify any pain to the nursing staff
- Most of the pain will be in the sternal incision
- Pain medication will be available

The nurse explains that the client should expect to have a sternal incision, possibly a leg incision, one or two chest tubes, a Foley catheter, and several IV fluid catheters postoperatively. An endotracheal tube will be connected to a ventilator for 6–24 hours postoperatively. The client and family must understand that the client will not be able to talk while the endotracheal tube is in place. The client should breathe with the ventilator and not fight it. When describing the postoperative course, the nurse emphasizes that close monitoring and the use of sophisticated equipment are standard treatment.

Psychosocial Preparation. Preoperative anxiety is common. Clients often wait 1–6 weeks for CABG surgery to be scheduled and performed. As the length of the wait increases, anxiety may increase. An appropriate nursing assessment should identify the level of anxiety and the coping methods clients have used successfully in the past. Some clients may find it helpful to define their fears. Common sources of fear include fear of the unknown, fear of bodily harm, and fear of death.

Clients may benefit from detailed information about the surgery, or they may feel overwhelmed by so much material. Some clients need to discuss their feelings in detail or describe the experiences of people they know who have undergone CABG. The nurse assesses clients' anxiety level and helps them to cope. Preoperative anxiety has been positively associated with postpericardiotomy delirium.

Operative Procedure. Coronary artery bypass surgery is performed with the client under general anesthesia and undergoing cardiopulmonary bypass (CPB). The anesthesiologist or nurse anesthetist administers anesthesia and intubates the client. Once the client is anesthetized, one surgical team may begin harvesting the saphenous vein if it is to be used for the graft. The cardiac surgical team begins the procedure with a median sternotomy incision and visualization of the heart and great vessels.

Cardiopulmonary bypass is accomplished by cannulation of the inferior and superior venae cavae. The purpose of CPB is to provide oxygenation, circulation, and hypothermia during induced cardiac arrest. Blood is diverted from the heart to the bypass machine, where it is heparinized, oxygenated, and returned to the circulation through a cannula placed in the ascending aortic arch or femoral artery (Fig. 40-7). During bypass, the client's core temperature is cooled to 82.6°–89.6° F (28–32° C). Cooling decreases the rate of metabolism and demand for oxygen. The heart is perfused with a cardioplegic solution containing potassium, which decreases myocardial oxygen consumption and causes the heart to stop during diastole. This process ensures a still operative field and prevents myocardial ischemia.

Once the heart is arrested, the grafting procedure can begin. The surgeon uses the internal mammary artery (IMA) or a saphenous vein, or both, to bypass lesions in the coronary arteries (Fig. 40-8). The distal end of the IMA is dissected and attached below the lesion on the coronary artery. If the surgeon uses a venous graft, it is anastomosed (sutured) proximally to the aorta and distally to the coronary artery just beyond the occlusion. Thus, myocardial perfusion is improved. After flow rates through the grafts are measured, the heart is rewarmed slowly. The cardioplegic solution is flushed from the heart. The heart regains its rate and rhythm, or it may be defibrillated to return it to a normal rhythm. When the procedure is completed, the client is rewarmed by CPB and weaned from the bypass machine while the grafts are observed for patency and leakage. The surgeon then places atrial and ventricular pacemaker wires and mediastinal chest tubes. Finally, the surgeon closes the sternum with wire sutures.

Postoperative Care. After surgery, the client is transported to a post–open heart surgery unit. There the client undergoes mechanical ventilation for 6–24 hours. The client requires highly skilled nursing care from a nurse qualified to care for clients after cardiac surgery. The nurse connects mediastinal tubes to water seal drainage systems and grounds the epicardial pacer wires and tapes them to the client. The nurse monitors pulmonary artery and arterial pressures and the client's heart rate and rhythm, which are displayed on a monitor. See accompanying clinical pathway for postoperative clients having CABG surgery.

The nurse closely assesses the client for dysrhythmias, such as ventricular ectopic rhythms, bradydysrhythmias, or heart block. The nurse treats symptomatic dysrhythmias according to unit protocols or the physician's order. If the client has symptomatic bradydysrhythmias or heart block, the nurse connects the pacer wires to a pacemaker box and sets the appropriate rate as ordered (see Chap. 36). The nurse also monitors for other complications of CABG surgery, including fluid and electrolyte imbalance, hypotension, hypothermia, hypertension, bleeding, cardiac tamponade, and altered cerebral perfusion. Table 40-5 lists some of the possible postoperative complications of CABG.

Management of Fluid and Electrolyte Imbalance. Assessing fluid and electrolyte balance is a high priority in the

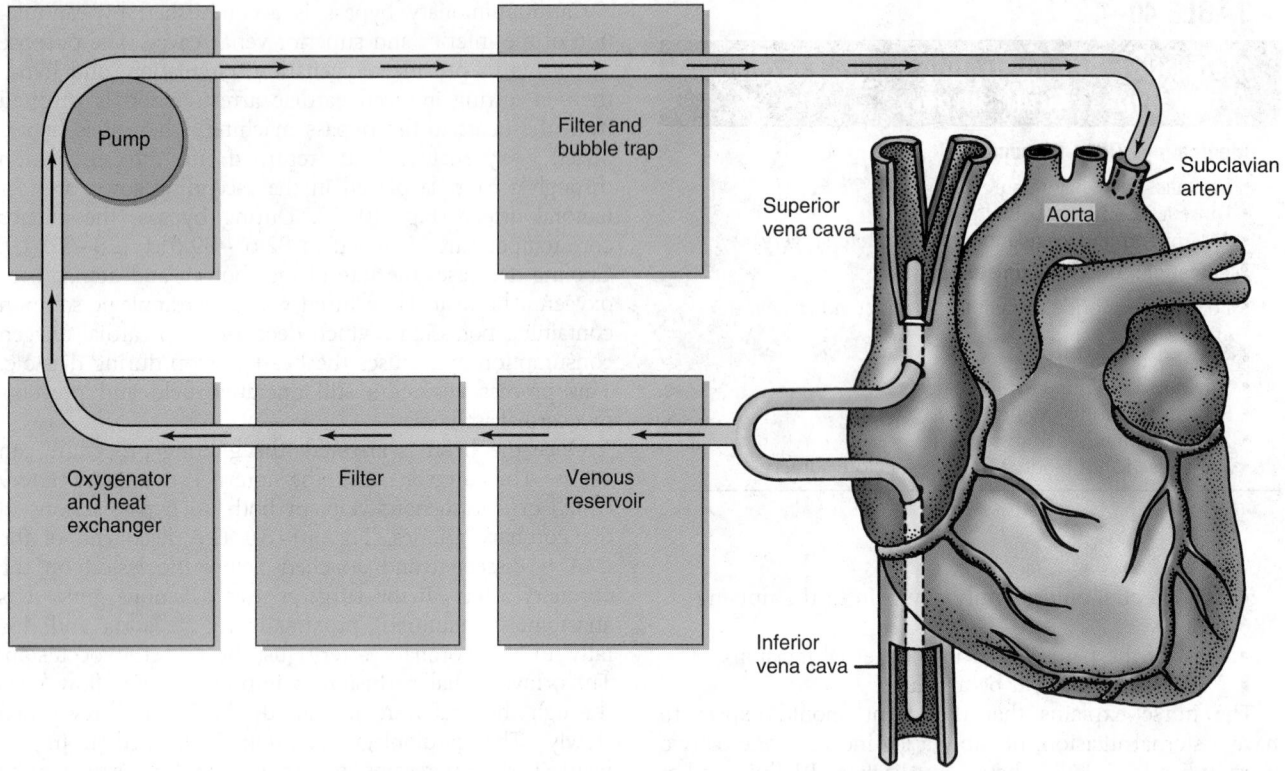

Figure 40–7. Heart-lung bypass circuitry used during cardiopulmonary bypass.

early postoperative period. Clients usually have edema, and fluids may be limited to 1500–2000 mL. However, decisions concerning fluid administration are made on the basis of the client's blood pressure, pulmonary artery wedge pressure (PAWP), right atrial pressure, cardiac output, cardiac index, systemic vascular resistance, and urine output. An experienced nurse interprets assessment findings and adjusts fluid administration on the basis of

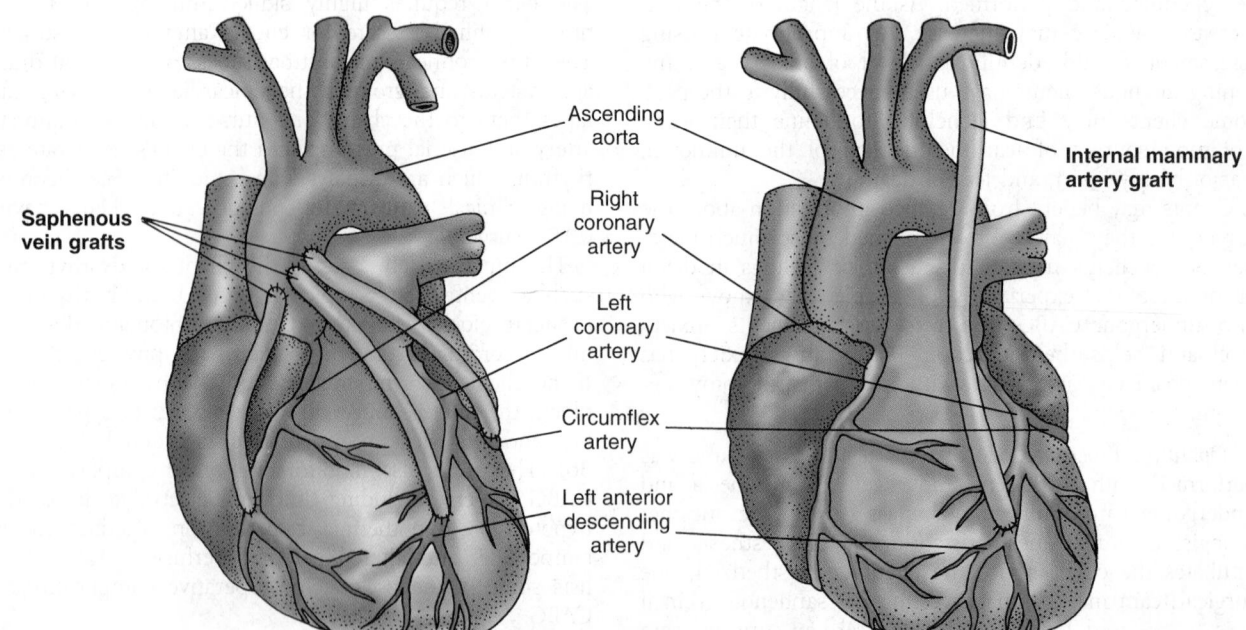

Figure 40–8. Two methods of coronary artery bypass grafting. The procedure used depends on the nature of the coronary artery disease, the condition of the vessels available for grafting, and the client's health status.

TABLE 40-5

Some Possible Postoperative Complications of Coronary Artery Bypass Graft Surgery

Decreased Cardiac Output

- Reduced preload
  - Hypovolemia
  - Hemorrhage
- Increased preload
  - Heart failure
  - Cardiogenic shock
- Increased afterload
  - Hypothermia
  - Increased sympathetic activity
- Dysrhythmias
  - Bradydysrhythmias
  - Conduction defects
  - Tachydysrhythmias
- Myocardial infarction

Pulmonary Dysfunction

- Atelectasis
- Pneumonia
- Pulmonary edema
- Hemothorax/pneumothorax

Neurologic Dysfunction

- Transient neurologic deficits
- Postpericardiotomy delirium
- Cerebrovascular accident

Acute Renal Failure

Gastrointestinal Dysfunction

- Stress ulcer
- Paralytic ileus

Infection

---

standing unit policies or specific orders from the physician.

Serum electrolytes (especially calcium, magnesium, and phosphorus) may be reduced postoperatively and are monitored carefully by both the physician and the nurse. Because the serum potassium level can fluctuate dramatically, electrolyte levels are checked frequently. Potassium depletion is common and may result from hemodilution, diuretic therapy, and nasogastric suction. To prevent dysrhythmias, potassium concentrations are maintained between 4 and 5mEq/L.

If the serum potassium level is depleted, the physician may order IV potassium replacement. The dose of potassium administered exceeds the usual recommended level of no more than 20 mEq of potassium per hour. For a potassium bolus, as much as 40–80 mEq may be mixed in 100 mL of IV solution and given at a rate as high as 40 mEq/hr. The drug must be given through a central catheter and the rate of administration controlled by an infusion pump. The client must be on a cardiac monitor for extremely careful observation.

Management of Hypotension. Hypotension (systolic blood pressure less than 90 mmHg) is a significant problem because it may result in the collapse of a vein graft. The nurse reviews the assessment parameters to identify what might be causing the hypotension. Decreased preload (decreased PAWP) can result from hypovolemia or vasodilation. If the client is hypovolemic, it might be appropriate to increase fluid administration or administer blood. The physician may treat the client with a low PAWP, decreased systemic vascular resistance, and vasodilation with vasopressor therapy to increase the blood pressure. However, if hypotension is the result of left ventricular failure (increased PAWP), IV inotropes might be necessary.

Management of Hypothermia. Although the client is rewarmed to 98.6° F (37° C) before being removed from bypass, it is not uncommon for the temperature to drift downward after the client leaves the surgical suite. The nurse monitors the client's body temperature and institutes rewarming procedures should the temperature drop below 96.8° F (36° C). Rewarming may be accomplished with warm blankets, rewarming lights, or thermal blankets. The danger of rewarming a client too quickly is that the client may begin shivering, resulting in metabolic acidosis and hypoxia. To prevent shivering, rewarming should proceed no faster than 1.8° F (1° C) per hour. The nurse discontinues rewarming when the client's temperature approaches 98.6° F (37° C) and the client's extremities feel warm.

Management of Hypertension. Hypothermia is a significant risk for the client undergoing coronary artery bypass graft (CABG) surgery because it promotes vasoconstriction and hypertension. Other factors contributing to hypertension in the CABG client include CPB, medications, and the client's own sympathetic activity.

When hypertension is defined as a systolic blood pressure greater than 140–150 mmHg, most CABG clients experience hypertension. Hypertension is dangerous because increased pressure promotes leakage from suture lines and may cause bleeding. To return the blood pressure to acceptable limits, the nurse titrates IV nitroprusside or nitroglycerin (see Chart 40–5).

Management of Bleeding. Bleeding occurs to a limited extent postoperatively in all clients. The nurse measures the mediastinal and chest tube drainage at least hourly and reports drainage exceeding 150 mL/hr to the surgeon. Clients with IMA grafts may have more chest drainage. The nurse may autotransfuse the chest drainage to assist with volume management when 500 mL have accumulated or 4 hours have elapsed, depending on the clinical pathway or physician's order. The nurse must maintain the patency of the mediastinal and chest tubes. One effective way of promoting chest tube drainage is to prevent a dependent loop from forming in the tubing.

Management of Cardiac Tamponade. If the client is bleeding and the mediastinal tubes are not kept patent, blood may accumulate around the heart. The myocardium is compressed, and cardiac tamponade results. The fluid accumulating around the heart compresses the atria and ventricles, prevents them from filling adequately, and reduces cardiac output. Hallmarks of cardiac tamponade include

- Sudden cessation of previously heavy mediastinal drainage

Text continued on page 926

University Hospitals
of Cleveland

CARE PATH NAME: CABG/VALVE (SICU)

SICU ELOS: 24 Hours

TOTAL ELOS: 5 Days (Anticipated Discharge on POD 4)

Expected Disposition: Telemetry Unit

Pre-Op Weight: _____ kg.

Collaborative Problem List
1. Home maintenance management
2. Potential for decreased cardiac output
3. Potential for fluid overdrive
4.
5.
6.

Focus	DAY OF SURG.: 1st 15 min.	DAY OF SURG.: 15 min. to 2 hrs.	DAY OF SURG.: 2 hrs to 6 am	POST-OP DAY 1: 6 am to Time of Transfer
Laboratory Tests/ Procedures	• ABG, CBC/diff, Chem 7, Ionized Ca++, Mg++, PT/PTT, surgical isoenzymes Dextrose stick • Pulse oximetry	• EKG, chest x-ray • Dextrose stick as ordered	• Labs q 8 h: CBC (no diff), Chem 7, Ionized Ca++, Mg++, Surg. isoenzymes, ABG after extubation • Others as ordered	• EKG and chest x-ray
Consults	• Respiratory Care Consultant	• Notify Surgical Cardiologist on call		• Order PT Consult on transfer orders for all patients ≥ 75 years old or if in SICU > 48 hours
Physical Assessment	• Complete assessment • Continuous cardiac monitoring • Hemodynamic monitoring q 15 min. & prn • I & O	• Ongoing physical and hemodynamic assessment • Vital signs q 15 min • Wean vent as tolerated and extubate per algorithm.	• Ongoing physical assessment q 4 h • VS/Hemodynamic evaluation q 1-2 h • Weight in AM • Assess bowel sounds • After extubation, O2 at 40-50% VM or nasal cannula and wean O2 as tolerated to Sat. ≥ 92	• VS/Hemodynamic evaluation q 2-4 h
Activity	• Bedrest	• Bedrest: turn q 2 h	• Bedrest: turn q 2 h • Dangle at bedside or sit in cardiac chair 2 h after extubation • In chair at bedside before 5 am	• Sit in chair for breakfast • OOB tid
Diet	• NPO		• Clear liquids after extubation • Assess needs for metoclopramide (Reglan)	• Clear liquids • Advance to low cholesterol diet as tolerated
Medications	• IV: D5 1/4 NS with _____ meq. KCL/L • Antibiotics • MS 2-12 mg IV q 1 h prn • Medications as ordered: Titrate drips according to ordered parameters • Insulin coverage per orders • Other: consider pre-admission meds			• Enteric coated ASA • Dipyridamole (DVH only)

922

Treatments	• Insert NG/OG tube to low continuous suction • Connect to Vent/mode IMV • CT: autotransfusion - 30 cm suction or H2O seal • Document initial CT output • CT/MSCT output q 15 min • Blood replacement: autotransfuse to IL • Blood products as ordered • IAPB/Pacer: stand by • Foley • Warming light or Bair hugger for temp < 35.5° C • Isolate epicardial wires (using 3 cc syringe with syringe cannula)	• D/C NG tube when extubated if bowel sounds present • CT/MSCT output q 1 h. D/C CTs by 6 am • Change epicardial wire dressing when MSCT D/C • Incentive spirometry Q 1 h WA • Encourage C&DB • O2 at 40-50% VM or nasal cannula • Wean as tolerated to keep O2 > 90%	• D/C foley prior to transfer if urine output adequate • D/C Swan Ganz if hemodynamically stable • D/C A-line • D/C Chest tubes • O2 per nasal cannula; Wean as tolerated to keep O2 Sat. > 90%
Discharge Planning		• Assess and document discharge needs when family in to visit to facilitate early D/C planning	• Make referral to Home Care or Social Work if needs are known
Teaching/ Learning		• Discuss "usual post-op" course with family, including anticipated D/C home on POD 4	
Intermediate Outcomes	• Adequate oxygenation/ ventilation • Hemodynamically stable	• Extubate with 4 h post-op • Hemodynamically stable without pharmacological support • CT output ≤ 75 cc/h • Neurologically intact	• Extubate with adequate oxygenation/ventilation • Hemodynamically stable without pharmacological support • Neurologically intact • Swan Ganz and arterial line discontinued • Transferred to telemetry unit on ___/___/___ at _____ hours
Intermediate Outcomes	☐ Met ☐ Not Met (see progress notes)	☐ Met ☐ Not Met (see progress notes)	☐ Met ☐ Not Met (see progress notes)
Date			
RN Signature			

University Hospitals of Cleveland

CARE PATH NAME: CABG/VALVE (TELEMETRY)

ELOS: 4 Days

Expected Disposition: Home

Pre-Op Weight: _____

Collaborative Problem List
1. Home maintenance management
2. Potential for decreased cardiac output
3. Potential for fluid overdrive
4. Potential for activity intolerance
5.
6.

Focus	POST-OP DAY 1: Time of Transfer to 7:00 AM	POST-OP DAY 2	POST-OP DAY 3	POST-OP DAY 4
Laboratory Tests/ Procedures	• Dextrose stick AC and HS (Diabetics) • Pulse ox q shift and prm while on O2 • Telemetry until discontinued	• PT/PTT q d (valve) • EKG • CBC, Chem 7	• Dextrose stick bid (Diabetics) • Pulse ox prn — • CBC, Chem 23 • CXR, EKG	
Consults	• Cardiology consult established in SICU • Respiratory care consult established in SICU • PT evaluation for all patients > 75 years old or with SICU LOS > 48 h and for other patients, if ordered • OT consult and evaluation if ordered • Cardiac rehab. referral • Nutrition Screen (see "Diet") • Home Care Consult if applicable • Social Work Consult today if: • Patient is expected to need short or long term placement • Patient lives alone and/or has inadequate caregiver and is anticipated to have new functional impairment at discharge • Patient currently resides in an extended care facility • Patient has dementia • Patient and family have a confiictual or difficult relationship • Patient has no insurance • Not meeting carepath ambulation criteria		Social Work Consult Today If: • Patient not previously referred and is expected to need short or long term placement • Patient expresses concerns re: obtaining medications at discharge • Patient requires equipment/supplies/home oxygen at discharge • Patient not previously referred and is now expected to require community agency involvement • Patient was being followed by homecare or community agency prior to admission • Other concerns as identified by team	
Physical Assessment	• Nursing assessment q shift • Vital signs q 4 h • Arrhythmia management protocol as needed • I&O q shift, weight qd	• Assess bowel status and medicate as necessary	• Vital signs q shift	
Activity	• OOB tid • Ambulate to bathroom • Ambulate to door (Appx. 20 ft) • Activity participates in ADL • Performs UE and LE exercises on handouts: 5 reps	• OOB to chair for all meals • Ambulate at least 50 ft qid • Independently performs ADLs • 5-10 reps	• Ambulate at least 100 ft tid • Independently performs ADLs • 10-15 reps	• Up ad lib • Ambulate at least 150 ft tid • Climb up/down stairs (Same # as at home) • 20 reps
Diet	• Advance as tolerated to low cholesterol diet • Nutrition Screen: Assess need for diet instruction and consult for nutrition education if indicated • Assess need for metoclopramide (Regan)			

Focus	POST-OP DAY 1: Time of Transfer to 7:00 AM	POST-OP DAY 2	POST-OP DAY 3	POST-OP DAY 4
Treatments	• Check isolated epicardial wires at time of transfer • Temporary pacemaker as ordered • Heparin lock/IVF. D/C IVF when tolerating PO • O2 per NC. Wean as tolerated • D/C O2 when room air pulse ox ≥ 90% • Incentive spirometry q 1 h WA • Encourage C+DB • Arrhythmia management protocol as needed	• Maintain electrical isolation • Evaluate need for temporary pacer. D/C as appropriate • Change CT, graft, epicardial wires, DSGs	• Evaluate possibility of pulling epicardial wires in PM	• D/C epicardial wires; if not already done, apply bandaids • D/C heparin lock
Medications	• Medications as ordered • Beta blocker as ordered • Consider pre-admission meds	• Continue with all medications as ordered • Consider changing IV medications to oral dose		

Discharge Planning/ Teaching	• Orient to Lerner Tower 3 at transfer
	• Assess home care needs
	• Review meds while administering
	• Review activity, incisional care, diet
	• Initiate GRF, if applicable
		• Assess home care needs
		• Review meds while administering
		• Review activity, incisional care, diet
		• Initiate Gold Referral Form (GRF) if applicable
			• Refer to Ambulatory Nutrition Practice or other outpatient nutrition program if further nutrition education identified
			• Review medications, activity, incisional care, diet
			• Update GRF if applicable
			• Initiate D/C folder:
			  Med schedule
			  Med cards
			  PI sheets
			  CTS booklet
			• Cardiac rehab pamphlet
			• Offer videos, PI sheets
				• F/U appts (if known)
				  Final Review:
				• Referral(s) to appropriate agencies
				• Confirm arrangements for equipment
				• Finalize GRF
				• D/C folder
				• Cardiac rehab pamphlet
				• F/U appts

Intermediate Outcomes	• Hemodynamically stable • Pain controlled • Bowel sounds x 4 quads • Ambulates 20 ft with pulse ox ≥ 90% • Home situation assessed and home health services determined • Social Work Consult ordered if indicated by criteria	• Hemodynamically stable • Pain controlled • Ambulates 50 ft and participate in ADLs with pulse ox ≥ 90% • D/C plans discussed with patient/family; plan D/C by 11 AM on Day 4	• Hemodynamically stable • Pain controlled • Ambulates 100 ft and perform ADLs with pulse ox ≥ 90% • No arrhythmias • No signs of hypoxia • Bowel movement x 1 • D/C planning continuing • D/C orders/prescriptions written in evening	• Hemodynamically stable • Pain controlled • Ambulates 150 ft and independently performs ADLs • No arrhythmias • No signs of hypoxia • Bowel movement x 1 • Epicardial wires and graft site sutures D/C'd • D/C plans confirmed • Social Work Consult ordered if indicated by criteria • See discharge outcomes sheet
Intermediate Outcomes	☐ Met ☐ Not Met	☐ Met ☐ Not Met	☐ Met ☐ Not Met	☐ Met ☐ Not Met
Date				
RN Signature				

Discharge Outcomes

Discharge Outcomes	Met	Not Met	Comments	Date/Initials

Patient/family will verbalize understanding of:
a. Medications, Incisional care, Signs/symptoms of infection, Activity progression, Diet, Physician follow-up
b. Epicardial wires removed
c. No signs of bleeding, PT level < 24
d. Arrhythmia free for 24 hours, or controlled arrhythmia
e. Telemetry off
f. No heart failure or treated heart failure
g. Adequate urine output
h. O2 Sat. greater than or equal to 90%
i. CBC, Chem-23, EKG, within normal limits
j. PT/INR within accepted therapeutic range (valve only)
k. Free of uncontrolled infection
l. Adequate bowel movement
  Pain controlled
  Able to ambulate 150 ft. and/or increasing ability to perform ADLs
  Heparin lock out				

University Hospital's carepaths have been developed to assist clinicians in patient management and clinical decision-making. The carepaths are intended to meet the needs of patients in most circumstances. They are not intended to replace a clinician's judgment or establish a protocol for all patients with this diagnosis.

SP-9345 (01/23/97)

Indicate 950001 when ordering new packets.

- Jugular venous distention but clear lung sounds
- Pulsus paradoxus (blood pressure greater than 10 mmHg higher on expiration than on inspiration)
- An equalizing of PAWP and right atrial pressure

Tamponade can be confirmed by echocardiogram or chest x-ray. Pericardiocentesis (see Chap. 37) may not be appropriate for tamponade after CABG because the blood in the pericardium may have clotted. Volume expansion and emergency sternotomy with drainage are then the treatments of choice.

Management of Altered Levels of Consciousness. The client may demonstrate changes in the level of consciousness, which may be permanent or transient. Transient changes related to anesthesia, CPB, or hypothermia occur in as many as 75% of clients. Transient neurologic deficits may include slowness to arouse, memory loss, and confusion.

Clients with transient neurologic deficits usually return to baseline neurologic status over 4–8 hours. Permanent deficits may be associated with a cerebrovascular accident (CVA) during surgery. The client may demonstrate

- Abnormal pupillary response
- Failure to awaken from anesthesia
- Seizures
- Absence of sensory or motor function

The nurse checks the client's neurologic status every 30–60 minutes until the client has awakened from anesthesia; then the nurse checks every 2–4 hours.

Pain Management. The nurse must differentiate between sternotomy pain, which is expected after CABG, and anginal pain, which might indicate graft failure. Typical sternotomy pain is localized, does not radiate, and often becomes worse when the client coughs or breathes deeply. The client may describe the pain as sharp, aching, or burning. Pain may stimulate the client's sympathetic nervous system, which increases the client's heart rate and vascular resistance while decreasing cardiac output. The nurse administers the prescribed medication, in adequate doses, frequently enough to limit pain. However, during the process of weaning the client from mechanical ventilation, it may be necessary to limit pain medication because of the respiratory depressant effects of analgesia.

Transfer from the Special Care Unit. Ventilation is usually provided for 6–24 hours postoperatively, until the client is breathing adequately and is hemodynamically stable. During the first 2 days, the client usually is weaned from the ventilator; has pacer wires, hemodynamic monitoring lines, and mediastinal tubes removed; and is transferred to an intermediate care unit. All CABG clients, but especially those with IMA grafts, are at high risk for atelectasis, so the nurse encourages the client to splint, cough, turn, and deep breathe to raise secretions. The nurse guides the client in a gradual resumption of activity (see clinical pathway). The nurse continues to monitor the client for decreased cardiac output, pain, dysrhythmias, and infection.

Approximately one third of clients with CABG and two thirds of clients with valve replacements experience supraventricular dysrhythmias (especially atrial fibrillation) during the postoperative period, most commonly on the second or third postoperative day. The nurse examines the monitor pattern for atrial fibrillation. When auscultating the heart, the nurse listens for an irregular rhythm. (See Chapter 36 for interventions for atrial fibrillation.)

Sternal wound infections develop between 5 days and several weeks postoperatively in about 2% of clients and represent a significant complication (Hussey & Leeper, 1998). The nurse is alerted to the presence of *mediastinitis* by

- Fever continuing beyond the first 4 days after CABG
- Instability (bogginess or stepping) of the sternum
- Redness or purulent drainage from suture sites
- An increased white blood cell count

The physician may perform a needle biopsy to confirm a sternal infection. Surgical debridement, antibiotic wound irrigation, and IV antibiotics are usually indicated. Four to 6 weeks of IV antibiotics are required if sternal osteomyelitis has developed.

Postpericardiotomy syndrome is a source of chest discomfort in 10% to 40% of postcardiac surgery clients. The syndrome is characterized by pericardial and pleural pain, pericarditis, a friction rub, elevated temperature and white blood cell count, and dysrhythmias. Postpericardiotomy syndrome may occur days to weeks after surgery and seems to be associated with blood remaining in the pericardial sac. The nurse observes the client for the development of pericardial or pleural pain. For most clients, the syndrome is mild and self-limiting. However, the client may require treatment similar to that for pericarditis. The nurse should be prepared to detect pericardial tamponade (see Chap. 37).

Older adults may have different needs and experience slightly different problems after CABG. Nursing concerns related to the older CABG client are detailed in Chart 40–7.

Minimally Invasive Direct Coronary Arterial Bypass. The minimally invasive direct coronary arterial bypass (MIDCAB) may be indicated for clients with a lesion of the left anterior descending artery (LAD). After a 2-inch left thoracotomy incision is made and the fourth rib removed, the left internal mammary artery (IMA) is dissected and attached to the still-beating heart below the level of the lesion in the LAD. Cardiopulmonary bypass (CPB) is not required. Nurses must assess the client postoperatively for chest pain and ECG changes because occlusion of the IMA graft occurs acutely in 10% of clients. Because they have a thoracotomy incision and a chest tube, clients are encouraged to cough and deep breathe. Most clients spend less than 6 hours in a critical care unit and are discharged in 2–3 days.

Transmyocardial Laser Revascularization. Transmyocardial laser revascularization is an experimental procedure for clients with unstable angina and inoperable CAD but areas of reversible myocardial ischemia. After a single-lung intubation, a left anterior thoracotomy is performed and the heart is visualized. A laser is used to create 20–24 long, narrow channels through the left ventricular muscle to the left ventricle. These channels will eventually allow oxygenated blood to flow during diastole from the left ventricle to nourish the muscle. After the surgery, the client is transported to a critical care unit, where the

---

Chart 40-7

Nursing Focus on the Elderly: Coronary Artery Bypass Graft Surgery

- Be aware that perioperative mortality rates are higher for the older client (4%–9%) than for the client younger than 60 years (1%–2%).
- Monitor neurologic and mental status carefully because older adults are more likely to have transient neurologic deficits after coronary artery bypass graft (CABG) surgery than younger adults are.
- Observe for side effects of cardiac drugs because elders are more likely to develop toxic effects from positive inotropes (dobutamine) and potent antihypertensives (nitroglycerin or nitroprusside).
- Monitor the client closely for dysrhythmias because older adults are more likely to have dysrhythmias, such as atrial fibrillation or supraventricular tachycardia, after CABG surgery.
- Be aware that recuperation after CABG surgery is slower for older clients and their average length of hospital stay is longer.
- Teach the client and family that during the first 2 to 5 weeks after discharge, fatigue, chest discomfort, and lack of appetite may be particularly bothersome for older clients.

---

nurse institutes hemodynamic monitoring and monitors for anginal episodes and bleeding disturbances.

 Continuing Care

> ### ➤ Case Management

Case management is most appropriate for clients who meet high-cost, high-volume, and high-risk criteria (Kegel, 1996). Clients with CAD clearly meet all these criteria. Clinical pathways and case management programs for clients who have CAD are in effect in most U.S. hospitals. By focusing on cardiovascular risk reduction and improving the continuity of care, the length and cost of hospital stays have been reduced. Posthospital case management should reduce hospital readmission rates and improve client health.

> ### ➤ Home Care Management

Clients who have experienced myocardial infarction (MI), angina, or coronary artery bypass graft (CABG) surgery are usually discharged to home or to a subacute care setting with pharmacologic therapy and specific activity prescriptions. Hospital stays are approximately 5–7 days for MI and CABG clients and only 2 days for percutaneous transluminal coronary angioplasty (PTCA) clients; therefore, clients are still recovering when they are discharged. Clients may require a home health nurse for assessment and teaching postdischarge and an aide for assistance with ADLs if they are older or weaker (Chart 40–8). Additionally, women, who tend to be older and more frequently living alone when coronary events occur,

may have a greater need for home assistance after CABG surgery (see Research Applications for Nursing). Clients who were residents in long-term care may be returned there after hospitalization for unstable angina, MI, or CABG surgery.

Cardiac rehabilitation is available in many communities for clients after MI or CABG surgery, but only 10% to 30% of clients participate in structured rehabilitation programs. The most frequently cited reasons for nonparticipation are lack of insurance coverage, physicians' directive that it is unnecessary, and client decision that it was not necessary. Clients who participate in structured rehabilitation programs report greater improvement in exercise tolerance and improved ability to control stress. However, there is no difference in clients' return to work.

> ### ➤ Health Teaching

Because hospital stays are short and clients are quite ill during hospitalization, most in-hospital education programs concentrate on survival skills after discharge. As part of home visits or a cardiac rehabilitation program, the nurse identifies the additional educational needs of

---

Chart 40-8

Focused Assessment for Home Health Clients Who Have Had a Myocardial Infarction

- Assess cardiovascular function, including
  - Current vital signs (compare with previous to identify changes)
  - Recurrence of chest discomfort (characteristics, frequency, onset)
  - Indications of heart failure (weight gain, crackles, cough, or dyspnea)
  - Adequacy of tissue perfusion (mentation, skin temperature, peripheral pulses, urine output)
  - Indications of serious dysrhythmia (very irregular pulse, palpitations with fainting or near fainting)
- Assess coping skills, including
  - Is client displaying denial, anger, or fear?
  - Is caregiver providing adequate support?
  - Are client and caregiver having disagreements about treatment?
- Assess functional ability, including
  - Activity tolerance (examine client's activity diary: review distance, duration, frequency, symptoms occurring during client exercise)
  - Activities of daily living (is any assistance needed?)
  - Household chores (who performs them?)
  - Does client plan to return to work? When?
- Assess nutritional status, including
  - Food intake (review client's intake of fats and cholesterol)
- Assess client's understanding of illness and its treatment
  - How to treat chest discomfort
  - Signs and symptoms to report to health care provider
  - Dosage, effects, and side effects of medications
  - How to advance and when to limit activity
  - Modification of risk factors for coronary artery disease

▷ Research Applications for Nursing

Gender Differences in Concerns After Coronary Artery Bypass Graft Surgery

Moore, S. M. (1995). A comparison of women's and men's symptoms during home recovery after coronary artery bypass surgery. Heart & Lung, 24(6), 495–501.

The purpose of this descriptive, comparative study was to determine whether men and women differed in their physical and emotional symptoms during the recovery period after coronary artery bypass graft (CABG) surgery. Secondary analysis was performed on interview data obtained from 40 clients (20 women and 20 men) at three time points within the first 4 weeks after surgery. Questions were asked about specific symptoms experienced as well as recovery concerns, difficulties, and problems. Results showed clear demographic and recovery-specific differences. The women in this study tended to be older, unemployed, and living alone more frequently than the men. Although both men and women reported physical discomfort, men experienced more incisional pain and fatigue and women experienced more physical discomfort associated with their breasts. The most common worry among the men was related to physical recovery. The most common worry among the women was who would assist in their care during home recovery.

Critique. This excellent study points out some gender differences with recovery issues after coronary artery bypass surgery. Although the sample size was small, its composition reflected the national demographics regarding people undergoing CABG.

Possible Nursing Implications. Gender differences are known to exist regarding age at onset, severity of disease, mortality, and time to treatment between men and women experiencing coronary artery disease and myocardial infarction. This is the first study examining possible differences in the postoperative recovery period. The increased age of the women, coupled with the fact that the majority lived alone, has relevance for changes for discharge planning. Additionally, the breast symptoms experienced by the women should be considered for inclusion in home-going information.

the client and family as well as their readiness to learn. The nurse then develops a teaching plan, which usually includes education about the normal anatomy and physiology of the heart, the pathophysiology of angina and MI, risk factor modification, activity and exercise protocols, cardiac medications, and the time to seek medical assistance.

The nurse informs the client about the normal function of the heart and coronary arteries and explains angina and MI. Clients are taught that after MI myocardial healing begins early and is usually complete in 6–8 weeks. Clients who have undergone CABG are told that the sternotomy heals in about 6–8 weeks.

Clients who have undergone CABG require instruction on incisional care for the sternum and the graft site. Clients should inspect the incisions daily for any redness, swelling, or drainage. The leg of a saphenous vein donor site is often edematous. The nurse instructs clients to avoid crossing legs, to wear elastic stockings until the edema subsides, and to elevate the surgical limb when sitting in a chair.

▷ *Risk Factor Modification*

Modification of risk factors is a necessary part of a client's management and involves changing the client's health maintenance patterns. Such modifications may include smoking cessation, altered dietary habits, regular exercise, blood pressure control, and blood glucose control.

Smoking Cessation. For clients who smoke, the nurse explains the detrimental effects on the cardiovascular system of smoking tobacco, especially cigarettes. Many clients spontaneously quit smoking soon after an MI. By encouraging all clients who have smoked to participate in smoking cessation and relapse programs, the nurse ensures that an additional 17%–26% of clients will cease smoking. One effective model uses nurse-managed behavioral intervention with biochemical verification of smoking status (Wenger et al., 1995).

Cholesterol Control. The mainstays of cholesterol control are diet therapy and administration of antihyperlipidemic agents.

Diet Therapy. The nurse collaborates with the dietitian to encourage the client to follow a prudent diet. Less than 30% of the calories in the diet should be from fat, and the fat consumed should be primarily monounsaturated or polyunsaturated. Clients should avoid saturated fats and foods rich in cholesterol. The nurse or dietitian also instructs the client not to add salt at the table. Booklets and cookbooks that can assist the client in learning to cook with reduction of fats, oils, and salt are available from the American Heart Association (AHA).

Weight reduction can normalize plasma lipid and lipoprotein levels in overweight clients. The cardiac rehabilitation nurse collaborates with the dietitian and physical therapist to provide multifactorial rehabilitation, including nutrition education, counseling, behavior modification, and exercise training to assist the overweight client to lose weight permanently (Wenger et al., 1995).

Antihyperlipidemic Agents. Cholesterol reduction with antihyperlipidemic agents, such as pravastatin (Pravacol), has been demonstrated to reduce significantly the risk of further CAD, including recurrent MI, death from CAD, and need for revascularization procedures. Thus, many clients with both normal and high cholesterol levels are encouraged to take these agents after CAD develops.

An area of controversy is the use of antioxidants (such as vitamin E). Some researchers report that the use of such agents counteracts the adverse effects of oxygen free radicals (derived from high cholesterol levels) on blood vessels and protects arteries. Other reports point out that excessive vitamin E increases the risk for liver damage and that the long-term effects of antioxidants are not known.

Physical Activity. The nurse collaborates with the physical therapist to establish an activity and exercise schedule as part of client rehabilitation. The nurse instructs the client to remain near home during the first week after discharge and to continue a walking program. The client may engage in light housework or any activity done sitting that does not precipitate angina. During the second week, the client is encouraged to increase social activities and possibly to return to work part time. By the third week, the client may begin to lift objects as heavy as 15 pounds (such as 2 gallons of milk), but should avoid lifting or pulling heavier objects for the first 6–8 weeks. Chart 40–9 lists suggested instructions for exercise.

The client may begin a simple walking program by walking 400 feet twice a day at the rate of 1 mile/hour the first week after discharge and increasing the distance and rate as tolerated, usually weekly, until the client can walk 2 miles at 3–4 miles/hour. The nurse instructs the client to take a pulse reading before, halfway through, and after exercise. The client should stop exercising if the target pulse rate is exceeded or if dyspnea or angina develops.

After a limited exercise tolerance test, the physical therapist or nurse encourages the client to join a formal exercise program, ideally one that assists the client in monitoring cardiovascular progress. The program should include 5- to 7-minute warm-up and cool-down periods as well as 30 minutes of aerobic exercise. The client should engage in aerobic exercise a minimum of three, but preferably five, times a week.

Complementary Therapies. Complementary therapies can aid in reducing a client's anxiety about progressive activity both in the immediate postoperative period and during the rehabilitation phase. Such techniques as progressive muscle relaxation, guided imagery, and music therapy have been shown to decrease anxiety, reduce depression, and increase client compliance with activity/exercise regimens after CABG (Barnason, Zimmerman, & Nieveen, 1995; Collins & Rice, 1997).

Sexual Activity. Sexual activity is often of great concern to clients and their partners. The nurse informs the client and partner that engaging in their usual sexual activity is unlikely to cause any damage to the client's heart. Clients can resume sexual intercourse on the advice of the physician, usually after exercise tolerance is assessed. The client who can walk one block or climb two flights of stairs without symptoms can usually safely resume sexual activity.

The nurse suggests that initially clients schedule intercourse after a period of rest. Clients might try having intercourse in the morning when they are well rested or wait 1½ hours after exercise or a heavy meal. They may take nitroglycerin before intercourse as a prophylactic measure. The position selected should be comfortable for both the client and his or her partner (e.g., side-lying) so that no undue stress is placed on the heart or suture line.

Blood Pressure Control. The nurse may make arrangements for the client to have blood pressure measured at regular intervals and collaborates with the primary care provider to establish parameters for reporting the blood pressure to the provider. Lifestyle modifications such as weight reduction, physical activity, and reduced sodium diets may assist in the management of hypertension. If the client is taking medication, the nurse assesses the client's compliance with the medication regimen.

Blood Glucose Control. Clients with diabetes mellitus are assessed for their participation in efforts to control hyperglycemia. The nurse reviews the prescribed dosage of insulin or oral hypoglycemic agents with the client and family. The client should demonstrate accurate testing of blood for glucose levels.

Cardiac Medications. The nurse assists the client in understanding the type of cardiac medications prescribed, the benefit of each drug, potential side effects to watch for, and the correct dosage and time of day to take each drug. Medication regimens vary considerably from client to client. However, many clients with angina are discharged taking aspirin, a beta-blocker, a calcium channel blocker, an antihyperlipidemic agent, and a nitrate. Clients who have experienced a myocardial infarction (MI) may require aspirin, a beta-blocker, an antihyperlipidemic agent, and an angiotensin-converting enzyme (ACE) inhibitor. The regimen can be complex. The nurse must determine that the client can comply with the instructions.

Use of sublingual nitroglycerin deserves special attention. The nurse instructs the client to carry nitroglycerin tablets at all times and to keep the tablets in a light-resistant container. Nitroglycerin tablets should be replaced every 3–5 months before they lose their potency and stop tingling when the client places one under the tongue. Chart 40–10 gives instructions for clients about management of chest discomfort at home.

Seeking Medical Assistance. Clients are encouraged to notify their health care provider if they experience
- Heart rate remaining less than 50 after arising
- Wheezing or difficulty breathing
- Weight gain of 3 pounds in 1 week
- Slow persistent increase in nitroglycerin use
- Dizziness, faintness, or shortness of breath with activity

Chart 40–9

Education Guide: Activity for the Client with Coronary Artery Disease

- Begin by walking the same distance at home as in the hospital (usually 400 feet) three times each day.
- Carry nitroglycerin with you.
- Check your pulse before, during, and after the exercise.
- Stop the activity for a pulse increase of more than 20 beats per minute, shortness of breath, angina, or dizziness.
- Exercise outdoors when the weather is good.
- Gradually increase the walking until the distance is ¼ mile twice daily (usually the end of the second week).
- After an exercise tolerance test and with your physician's approval, walk at least three times each week, increasing the distance by ½ mile every other week, until the total distance is 2 miles.
- Avoid straining (lifting, pushups, pull-ups, and straining at bowel movements).

Chart 40–10

Education Guide: Management of Chest Pain at Home

- Keep fresh nitroglycerin available for immediate use.
- At the first indication of chest discomfort, cease activity and sit or lie down.
- Place one nitroglycerin tablet under your tongue and allow it to dissolve.
- Wait 5 minutes for relief.
- If no relief results, repeat the nitroglycerin and wait 5 more minutes.
- If there is no relief, repeat and wait 5 more minutes.
- If there is still no relief, call for transportation to a health care facility.

Clients are encouraged to call for transportation to the hospital if they experience

- Chest discomfort that does not improve after 20 minutes or 3 nitroglycerin tablets
- Extremely severe chest discomfort with weakness, nausea, or fainting.

WOMEN'S HEALTH CONSIDERATIONS

 Women with CAD report requiring more assistance from friends and extended family than men. Male spouses of clients with CAD may be unaccustomed to assuming a caregiving role and the older, widowed or divorced woman may live alone. If a woman is able to develop two or more sources of emotional support, her chance of surviving 5 years is three times higher than if she remains isolated and alone (Arnstein, Buselli, & Rankin, 1996). The cardiac rehabilitation nurse should assess the emotional support available to women with CAD. If there is not adequate support available, the nurse should provide it or arrange for the client to participate in a support group.

Women are less likely to enroll and stay in structured cardiac rehabilitation programs or participate in home walking programs than men. Most cite family and domestic responsibilities for not participating. Although housework is important to the role satisfaction of many older women, it is a poor choice for cardiovascular activity. The home health or cardiac rehabilitation nurse should assess the activity level of the woman with CAD and encourage her to participate in an appropriate exercise program.

➤ Health Care Resources

The American Heart Association (AHA) is an excellent source for booklets, films, video cassettes, cookbooks, and professional service referrals for the client with coronary artery disease (CAD). Many local affiliates have their own cardiac rehabilitation programs for clients to join.

Within the community, cardiac rehabilitation programs may be affiliated with local hospitals, community centers, or other facilities, such as clinics. Many shopping malls open before shopping hours to allow a measured walking program indoors; this is particularly popular with elderly clients and also provides a good support group.

Mended Hearts is a nationwide program with local chapters that provides education and support to CABG clients and their families. Smoking cessation programs and clinics as well as weight reduction programs are found within the community. Many hospitals sponsor health fairs, blood pressure screening, and risk factor modification programs as well.

 Evaluation

The nurse evaluates the client on the basis of the identified nursing diagnoses and collaborative problems. The expected outcomes are that the client will

- State that the chest discomfort is alleviated, appear comfortable, and have resolution of ST- and T-wave changes.
- Remain hemodynamically stable: maintain a normal sinus rhythm or normal rhythm for the client at a rate of approximately 60; maintain blood pressure within an acceptable range, adequate urine output, mental alertness, palpable pedal pulses, and clear lungs on auscultation.
- Walk 200 feet four times a day without chest discomfort or shortness of breath
- Indicate decreased anxiety
- Indicate a sense of having some control over life
- Experience minimal angina while engaging in ADLs or an exercise program.

◗ CASE STUDY for the Client After CABG

■ You are making the first home visit to a 76-year-old man who has been home for 2 days after a 12-day hospitalization for left main coronary artery bypass surgery. His hospital stay was complicated by angina, anxiety, and constipation. He was discharged home taking furosemide (Lasix), 40 mg every day; acetylsalicylic acid (aspirin), 1 tablet every day; metoprolol (Lopressor), 100 mg every day; Metamucil, 1 packet every morning; and allopurinol, 100 mg three times a day. He lives alone in a four-room house; his brother and sister-in-law live next door.

QUESTIONS:

1. What initial information is most important for you to obtain?
2. The client will only answer you in monosyllables. He says he is having trouble sleeping because of shortness of breath and nightmares. What should you do?
3. The client also says his left leg is sore where they removed the saphenous vein. He has been sitting in the chair with his leg dependent all day. What should you do?
4. The client's brother and sister-in-law are extremely worried. They say the client is eating and drinking very little and is leaking liquid stool. The client says he is constipated. What do you think is happening?

SELECTED BIBLIOGRAPHY

American Heart Association. (1996). *1992 Heart and Stroke Facts: 1996 statistical supplement.* Dallas, TX: Author.

Arnstein, P. M., Buselli, E. F., & Rankin, S. H. (1996). Women and heart attacks: Prevention, diagnosis and care. *Nurse Practitioner, 21*(5), 57–69.

Barnason, S., Zimmerman, L., & Nieveen, J. (1995). The effects of music interventions on anxiety in the patient after coronary artery bypass grafting. *Heart & Lung, 24*(2), 124–132.

Beach, E., Smith, A., Luthringer, L., Utz, A., Ahrens, S., & Whitmire, V. (1996). Self-care limitations of persons after acute myocardial infarction. *Applied Nursing Research, 9*(1), 24–28.

Bernat, J. (1997). Smoothing the CABG patient's road to recovery. *American Journal of Nursing, 97*(2), 23–27.

*Braunwald, E. (Ed.). (1992). *Heart disease: A textbook of cardiovascular medicine* (4th ed.). Philadelphia: W. B. Saunders.

Braunwald, E., Mark, D. B., Jones, R. H., et al. (1994). *Diagnosing and managing unstable angina. Quick reference guide for clinicians, #10* (AHCPR Publication No. 94-0603). Rockville, MD: U.S. Department of Health and Human Services.

Bruce, S. L., & Grove, S. K. (1994). The effect of a coronary artery risk evaluation program on serum lipid values and cardiovascular risk levels. *Applied Nursing Research, 7*(2), 67–74.

Carroll, D. (1995). The importance of self-efficacy expectations in elderly patients recovering from coronary artery bypass surgery. *Heart & Lung, 24*(1), 50–59.

Clem, J. R. (1995). Pharmacology of ischemic disease. *AACN Clinical Issues, 6*(3) 404–417.

Collins, J., & Rice, V. (1997). Effects of relaxation intervention in phase II cardiac rehabilitation: Replication and extension. *Heart & Lung, 26*(1), 31–44.

Connors, K. F., & Lamas, G. A. (1995). Postmyocardial infarction patients: Experience from the SAVE trial. *American Journal of Critical Care, 4*(1), 23–28.

Fleury, J., Keller, C., & Murdaugh, C. (1996). Patients with coronary artery disease. In J. Clochesy, C. Breu, S. Cardin, A. Whittaker, & E. Rudy (Eds.), *Critical care nursing* (2nd ed., pp. 336–353). Philadelphia: W. B. Saunders.

Forsha, B. (1997). Scaffolding the coronary arteries: Intracoronary stenting. *Home Healthcare Nurse, 15*(4), 247–255.

Futterman, L. G., Corea, L. F., & Lemberg, L. (1996). Thrombolysis or primary angioplasty? An ongoing controversy in the management of acute myocardial infarction. *American Journal of Critical Care, 5*(2), 160–167.

Futterman, L. G., & Lemberg, L. (1996). Cardiomyoplasty: A potential alternative to cardiac transplantation. *American Journal of Critical Care, 5*(1), 80–86.

Gaw-Ens, B. (1994). Informational support for families immediately after CABG surgery. *Critical Care Nurse, 14*(1), 41–49.

*Gortner, S. R., Dirks, J., & Wolfe, M. M. (1992). The road to recovery for elders after CABG. *American Journal of Nursing, 92*(8), 44–49.

Gulanich, M., Billey, A., Perino, B., & Keough, V. (1997). Patients' responses to the angioplasty experience: A qualitative study. *American Journal of Critical Care, 6*(1), 25–32.

Hahn, M. (1995). Matters of the heart: Women and cardiac disease. *Advance for Nurse Practitioners, 3*(9), 13–19.

Hawthorne, M. H. (1994). Gender differences in recovery after coronary artery surgery. *IMAGE: Journal of Nursing Scholarship, 26*(1), 75–80.

Huerta-Torres, V. (1998). Preparing patients for early discharge after CABG. *American Journal of Nursing, 98*(5), 49–51.

Hussey, L., & Leeper, B. (1998). Sternal wound infection: A case study of a devastating postoperative complication. *Critical Care Nurse, 18*(1), 31–39.

Jarvis, C. (1996). *Physical examination and health assessment* (2nd ed.). Philadelphia: W. B. Saunders.

Jensen, G. A., & Miller, D. S.(1995). The heart of aging: Special challenges of cardiac ischemia and failure in the elderly. *AACN Clinical Issues, 6*(3), 471–481.

Jensen, L., & King, K. (1997). Women and heart disease. *Critical Care Nurse, 17*(2), 45–52.

Kegel, L. M. (1996). Case management, critical pathways, and myocardial infarction. *Critical Care Nurse, 16*(2), 97–111.

Lee, H. O. (1997). Typical and atypical clinical signs and symptoms of myocardial infarction and delayed seeking of professional care among Blacks. *American Journal of Critical Care, 6*(1), 7–13.

Lee, S. (1996). Hospital-home care critical pathways in disease management: Improving case management and patient outcomes in postoperative cardiothoracic surgical patients. *The Journal of Care Management, 2*(3), 42–53.

*Matrisciano, L. (1992). Unstable angina: An overview. *Critical Care Nurse, 12*(8), 30–38.

Meluch, F., & Mitchell, S. (1997). Decreasing intracoronary stent complications. *Dimensions of Critical Care Nursing, 16*(3), 114–121.

Moore, S. M. (1995). A comparison of women's and men's symptoms during home recovery after coronary artery bypass surgery. *Heart & Lung, 24*(6), 495–501.

Moser, D. (1997). Correcting misconceptions about women and heart disease. *American Journal of Nursing, 97*(4), 26–33.

Norris, S. O. (1995). Sternal wound infection. In N. Urban (Ed.), *Guidelines for critical care nursing* (pp. 240–249). St. Louis, MO: C. V. Mosby.

O'Neal, P. V. (1994). How to spot early signs of cardiogenic shock. *American Journal of Nursing, 94*(5), 36–41.

*Pasternak, R., Braunwald, E., & Sobel B. (1992). Acute myocardial infarction. In E. Braunwald (Ed.), *Heart disease: A textbook of cardiovascular medicine* (4th ed., pp. 1200–1291). Philadelphia: W. B. Saunders.

Ray, G. L. (1994) Decisions, decisions: Which thrombolytic is best for your patient? *American Journal of Nursing, 94*(Suppl.), 11–15.

Redeker, N., Mason, D., Wykpisz, E., & Glica, B. (1996). Sleep patterns in women after coronary artery bypass surgery. *Applied Nursing Research, 9*(3), 115–122.

Redeker, N. S., & Sadowski, A. (1995). Update on cardiovascular drugs and elders. *American Journal of Nursing, 95*(9), 34–41.

Riegel, B. (1996). Myocardial infarction. In J. Clochesy, C. Breu, S. Cardin, A. Whittaker, & E. Rudy (Eds.), *Critical care nursing* (2nd ed., pp. 354–379). Philadelphia: W. B. Saunders.

Romeo, K. C. (1995). The female heart: Physiologic aspects of cardiovascular disease in women. *Dimensions of Critical Care, 14*(4), 170–175.

Shuster, P., Wright, C., & Tomish, P. (1995). Gender differences in outcomes of participants in home care programs compared to those in structured cardiac rehabilitation programs. *Rehabilitiation Nursing, 20*(2), 96–100.

Strimike, C. L. (1995). Caring for a patient with an intracoronary stent. *American Journal of Nursing, 95*(1), 40–46.

Swearingen, P. L., & Keen, J. H. (1995). *Manual of critical care: Applying nursing diagnoses to adult critical illness* (2nd ed.). St. Louis, MO: Mosby Year Book.

Tsunoda, D. (1996). Clinical snapshot: Acute myocardial infarction. *American Journal of Nursing, 96*(5), 38–39.

Turner, L., Linden, W., van der Wal, R., & Schamberger, W. (1995). Stress management for patients with heart disease: A pilot study. *Heart and Lung, 24*(2), 145–153.

*U.S. Department of Health and Human Services. (1990). *Healthy people 2000: National health promotion and disease prevention objectives.* Washington, DC: U.S. Government Printing Office.

Valle, B. K., & Lember, L. (1994). Estrogen replacement therapy in women: Prevention and treatment of coronary artery disease. *American Journal of Critical Care, 3*(5), 398–401.

Villaire, M. (1996). Early heart attack care—The critical paradigm shift toward prevention. *Critical Care Nurse, 16*(1), 79–85.

Wenger, N. K., Froelicher, E. S., & Smith, L. K., et al. (1995). *Cardiac rehabilitation as secondary prevention: clinical practice guideline* (quick reference guide for clinicians no. 17, AHCPR publication no. 96-0673). Rockville, MD: U.S. Department of Health and Human Services, Public Health Service, Agency for Health Care Policy and Research and National Heart, Lung, and Blood Institute.

Wright, J. (1995). Pharmacologic management of congestive heart failure. *Critical Care Nursing Quarterly, 18*(1), 32–44.

Workman, M. L. (1994). Anticoagulants and thrombolytics: What's the difference? *AACN Clinical Issues in Critical Care Nursing, 5*(1), 26–34.

SUGGESTED READINGS

Bernat, J. (1997). Smoothing the CABG patient's road to recovery. *American Journal of Nursing, 97*(2), 23–27.
Recent advances in the care of clients undergoing coronary artery bypass graft surgery are identified. The changing client profile

and surgical procedure are described. Risks to vulnerable body systems are detailed specifically.

Hussey, L., & Leeper, B. (1998). Sternal wound infection: A case study of a devastating postoperative complication. *Critical Care Nurse, 18*(1), 31–39.

This excellent article describes the phenomenon of sternal wound infection comprehensively and concisely. The nursing care needs are outlined, and a teaching guide for clients with sternal incisions is included.

Jensen, L., & King, K. (1997). Women and heart disease. *Critical Care Nurse, 17*(2), 45–52.

The influence of gender on cardiovascular anatomy and physiology is discussed. Differences between men's and women's risk factors, diagnoses, and treatment for coronary artery disease are explained. Strategies for prevention, diagnosis, and treatment of CAD in women are detailed.

Meluch, F., & Mitchell, S. (1997). Decreasing intracoronary stent complications. *Dimensions of Critical Care Nursing, 16*(3), 114–121.

The primary focus of this comprehensive article is the nursing management of clients after intracoronary stent implantation. Detailed medication guides are included. Focused assessment techniques are highlighted for the prevention of complications.

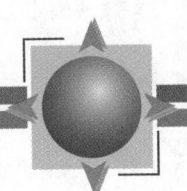

UNIT 8

Management of Clients

with Problems of the

Hematologic System

ASSESSMENT OF THE HEMATOLOGIC SYSTEM

The hematologic system is made up of lymphatic fluid, blood, cellular elements in blood, and blood-forming organs. Blood and lymph circulate through all body tissues and organs, and the functions of the hematologic system influence the health and well-being of all body systems. This chapter and Chapter 23 (Concepts of Inflammation and the Immune Response) review the normal physiology of the hematologic system and the skills necessary to accurately assess the client's hematologic status.

ANATOMY AND PHYSIOLOGY REVIEW
Bone Marrow

Bone marrow is the blood-forming (hematopoietic) organ. It produces most of the cellular elements of the blood, including red blood cells (RBCs), white blood cells (WBCs), and platelets. Bone marrow also is involved in some aspects of the immune response (see Chapter 23).

Each day, the bone marrow in a healthy adult produces and releases about 2.5 billion RBCs, 2.5 billion platelets, and 1 billion granulocytes per kilogram of body weight (Williams et al., 1995).

In the fetus, blood components are formed in the liver

and spleen and, by the last trimester, the bone marrow. At birth, blood-producing marrow is present in every bone. The flat bones (sternum, skull, pelvic and shoulder girdles) contain active blood-producing marrow throughout life. In small, irregularly shaped bones and in the long bones, the amount of functional bone marrow decreases as a person ages, until by age 18, blood production is limited to the ends of the long bones. During adulthood, fatty tissue replaces inactive bone marrow. In elderly people, the proportion of fatty marrow increases to about one half of the marrow found in the sternum and ribs, and only a relatively small portion of the remaining marrow continues active blood production.

The bone marrow produces all blood cells, initially producing stem cells. Bone marrow contains *pluripotent* stem cells, immature and undifferentiated cells capable of maturing into any one of several lines of blood cells—an RBC, WBC, or platelet line, depending on the body's needs (see Fig. 23–3).

The next stage in cell development is the committed stem cell (also called the precursor cell or the unipotent stem cell). A committed stem cell has one specific maturational pathway and matures or differentiates into only one cell type. Committed stem cells are in the active phase of growth but require the presence of a specific

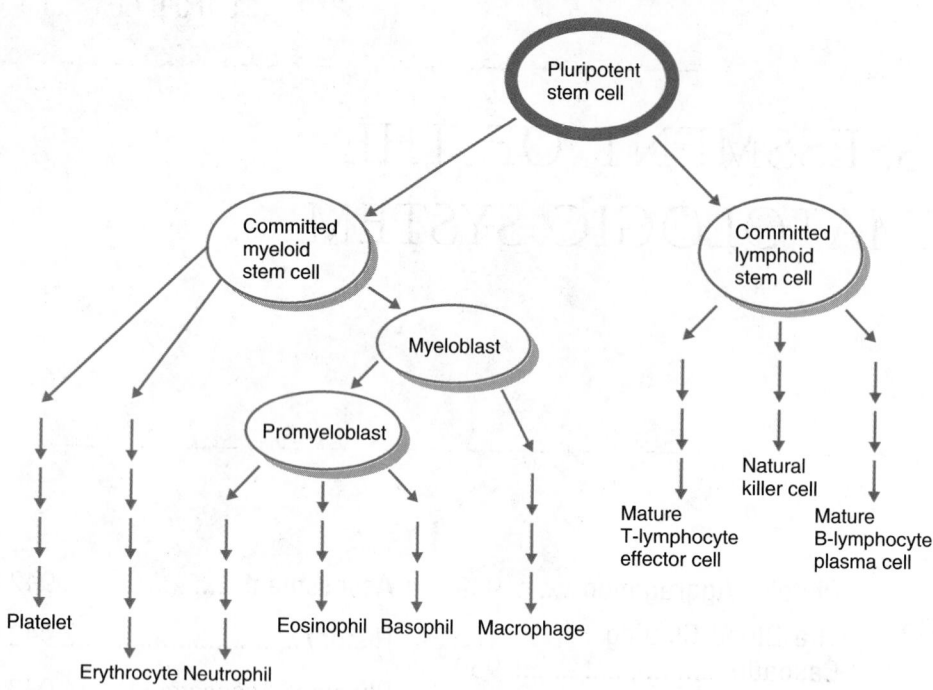

Figure 41–1. Bone marrow cell differentiation and maturational pathways.

growth factor for further development and maturation. For example, erythropoietin is a growth factor made in the kidneys that is specific for the red blood cell line. A variety of other growth factors influence white blood cell and platelet maturation (see Chaps. 23, 27, and 42).

Blood Components

Blood is composed of plasma and cellular elements. Plasma, part of the extracellular fluid of the body, is similar to the interstitial fluid found between tissue cells; however, plasma contains about three to four times more protein than does interstitial fluid. There are three major types of plasma proteins: albumin, globulins, and fibrinogen.

The primary function of albumin is to increase osmotic pressure of the blood, preventing the plasma from leaking into the tissues (see Chap. 14). Globulins perform many functions, such as transporting other substances and protecting the body against infection. Globulins are also the main component of antibodies. Fibrinogen is a protein molecule that can be activated to form a molecule of fibrin. Individual molecules of fibrin assemble to form large structures important in the blood clotting process.

The cellular components of the blood include RBCs, WBCs, and platelets. These blood components differ in structure, site of maturation, and function.

Red Blood Cells (Erythrocytes)

Red blood cells, or erythrocytes, make up the largest proportion of blood cells. Mature RBCs have no nucleus and have a biconcave disk shape. This feature, together with a flexible membrane, allows RBCs to change their shape without breaking as they pass through narrow,

winding capillaries. The number of RBCs a person has varies according to gender, age, and general health, but the normal range is from 4,400,000 to 5,500,000/mm³.

As shown in Figures 41–1 and 41–2, RBCs start out as pluripotent stem cells, enter the myeloid pathway, and progress in stages to the mature RBC, the erythrocyte. Healthy mature RBCs have a life span of approximately 120 days after being released into circulation from the bone marrow. As RBCs age, their membranes become more fragile. These old cells are trapped and destroyed by fixed macrophages in the tissues, the spleen, and the liver. Some intracellular parts of destroyed RBCs, such as iron, are recycled and used in the formation of new RBCs.

Red blood cells are responsible for the formation of hemoglobin (Hgb). Each normal mature RBC contains many thousands of hemoglobin molecules (Guyton & Hall, 1996). The heme portion of each hemoglobin molecule requires a molecule of iron. Only when the heme molecule is complete with iron can it transport up to four molecules of oxygen. Therefore, iron is a critical component of hemoglobin. The globin portion of the hemoglobin molecule carries carbon dioxide. RBCs also serve as a buffer and help maintain acid-base balance.

The most important feature of the hemoglobin molecule is its ability to combine loosely with oxygen. With only a small drop in oxygen tension at the tissue level, a considerable increase in the transfer of oxygen from hemoglobin to tissues occurs. This transfer is also known as *oxygen dissociation*. Some pathologic conditions can alter the speed and quantity of oxygen release to the tissues.

The total number of RBCs a person has is carefully regulated through *erythropoiesis* (selective maturation of stem cells into mature erythrocytes). Regulation ensures

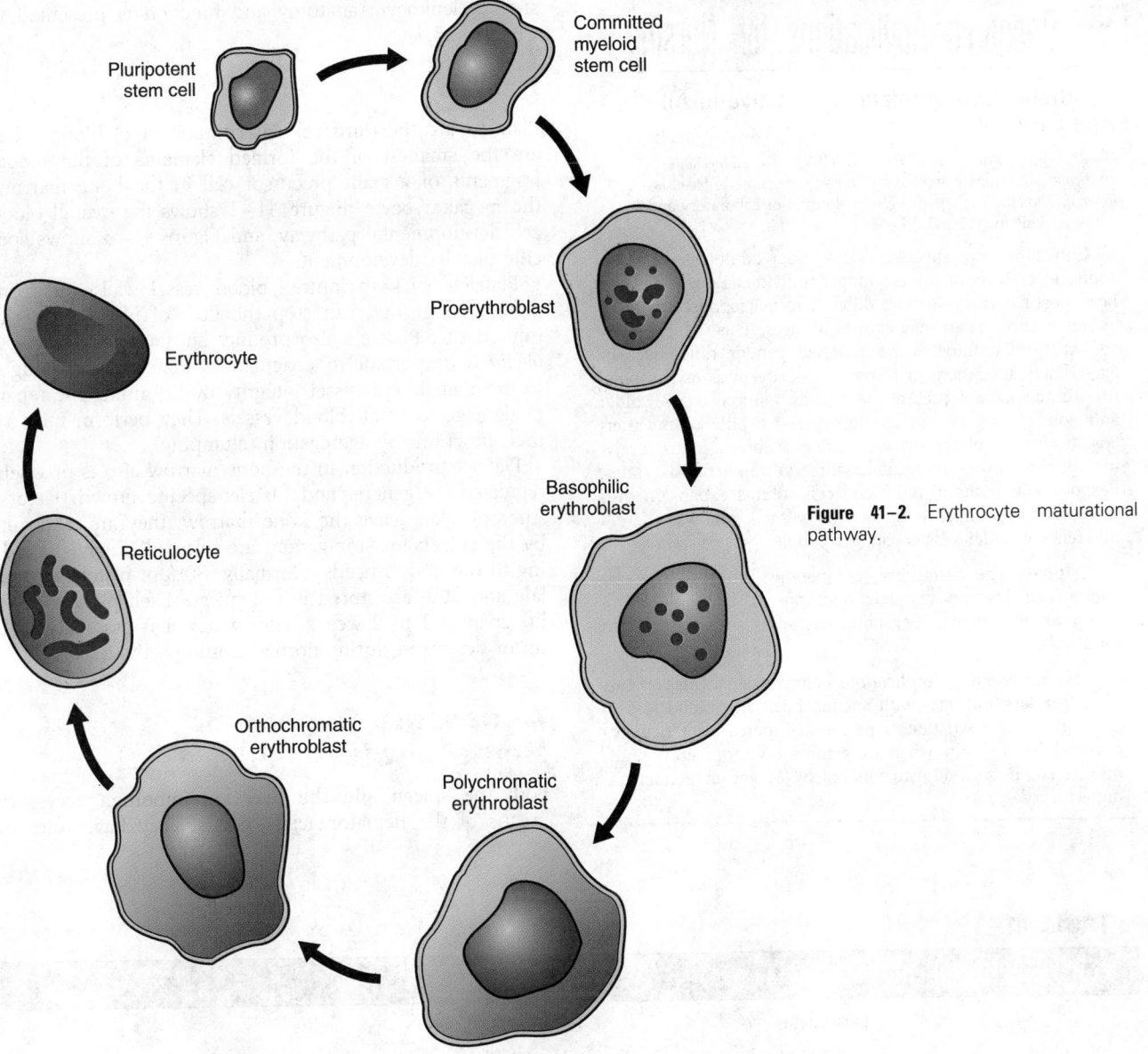

Figure 41-2. Erythrocyte maturational pathway.

that enough RBCs are present for good oxygenation without having an overconcentration, which causes hypercellularity. The trigger for control of erythropoiesis is tissue oxygenation. The kidney produces the RBC growth factor (erythropoietin) at a rate consistent with RBC destruction to maintain a constant normal level of circulating RBCs. When tissue oxygenation is less than normal (*hypoxia*), the kidney increases the production and release of erythropoietin. This growth factor then stimulates the bone marrow to increase RBC production. When tissue oxygenation is excessive, the kidney decreases erythropoietin production, inhibiting RBC production. Synthetic erythropoietin is now available and appears to have the same effect on bone marrow as the naturally occurring erythropoietin in all age groups (see the Research Applications for Nursing box).

Many substances are essential to form hemoglobin and RBCs, including iron, vitamin B_{12}, folic acid, copper, pyridoxine, cobalt, and nickel. A lack of any of these substances can lead to anemia. Anemia is a feature of any of a variety of conditions in which either the function or the number of erythrocytes is insufficient to meet tissue oxygen demands (see Chap. 42).

White Blood Cells (Leukocytes)

White blood cells, or leukocytes, are the second category of blood cells. There are multiple types of leukocytes, each type performing at least one specific function critical to inflammation or immunity (Table 41–1). Most WBCs are formed in the bone marrow and therefore are considered part of the hematopoietic system. However, because leukocytes provide immunity and protect people from the effects of invasion, infection, and injury, a detailed discus-

Research Applications for Nursing

Synthetic Erythropoietin Is Effective in All Age Groups

Goodnough, L., Price, T., & Parvin, C. (1995). The endogenous erythropoietin response and the erythropoietic response to blood loss anemia: The effects of age and gender. Journal of Laboratory and Clinical Medicine, 126(1), 57–64.

Clinicians have speculated that older adults may not respond to erythropoietin as younger individuals do. It has also been postulated that gender differences in responses to exogenous erythropoietin may exist at all ages. This clinical study sought to determine whether actual gender differences or age-related differences in response to exogenous erythropoietin stimulation are present. The study randomized 71 older and younger adults undergoing aggressive phlebotomy therapy to either a placebo group or one of three groups receiving different doses of recombinant erythropoietin six times. Responses in terms of red blood cell volume expansion over time were not different for men or women, nor was there a difference in older versus younger people.

Critique. The descriptive, comparative study design was appropriate for the research questions. Use of a control group to determine endogenous responses adds strength to the results.

Possible Nursing Applications. Nurses can expect clients of all genders and ages with anemia related to blood loss to respond at a known rate of percentage increase for hematocrit and hemoglobin when exogenous erythropoietin is administered. Dosage adjustments solely for age or gender are unnecessary.

sion of leukocyte anatomy and function is presented in Chapter 23.

Platelets

Platelets are the third cellular component of blood. They are the smallest of the formed elements of the blood, fragments of a giant precursor cell in the bone marrow, the megakaryocyte. Figure 41–1 shows the overall blood cell developmental pathway, and Figure 41–3 shows specific platelet development.

Platelets stick to injured blood vessel walls and form platelet plugs that can stop the flow of blood from the injured site. Platelets also produce substances called *phospholipids,* important to coagulation. Platelets are thought to maintain blood vessel integrity by beginning the repair of damage to small blood vessels. They perform most of their functions by aggregation (clumping).

Platelet production in the bone marrow also is precisely regulated by general and platelet-specific growth factors. After platelets leave the bone marrow, they are taken up by the spleen for storage and are released slowly, according to the body's needs. Normally, 80% of platelets circulate and 20% are stored in the spleen. Each platelet has a life span of 1 to 2 weeks, after which it is gradually used up or destroyed during normal clotting activities.

Accessory Organs of Hematopoiesis

Both the spleen and the liver are important accessory organs of the hematopoietic system. They have roles in

TABLE 41–1

Functions of Specific Leukocytes

	Leukocyte	Function
Inflammation	Neutrophil	• Nonspecific ingestion and phagocytosis of microorganisms and foreign protein
	Macrophage	• Nonspecific recognition of foreign proteins and microorganisms; ingestion and phagocytosis
	Monocyte	• Destruction of bacteria and cellular debris; matures into macrophage
	Eosinophil	• Weak phagocytic action; releases vasoactive amines during allergic reactions
	Basophil	• Releases histamine and heparin in areas of tissue damage
Antibody-mediated immunity	B lymphocyte	• Becomes sensitized to foreign cells and proteins
	Plasma cell	• Secretes immunoglobulins in response to the presence of a specific antigen
	Memory cell	• Remains sensitized to a specific antigen and can secrete increased amounts of immunoglobulins specific to the antigen
Cell-mediated immunity	T lymphocyte helper/inducer T cell	• Enhances immune activity through secretion of various factors, cytokines, and lymphokines
	Cytotoxic-cytolytic T cell	• Selectively attacks and destroys non-self cells, including virally infected cells, grafts, and transplanted organs
	Natural killer cell	• Nonselectively attacks non-self cells, especially body cells that have undergone mutation and become malignant; also attacks grafts and transplanted organs

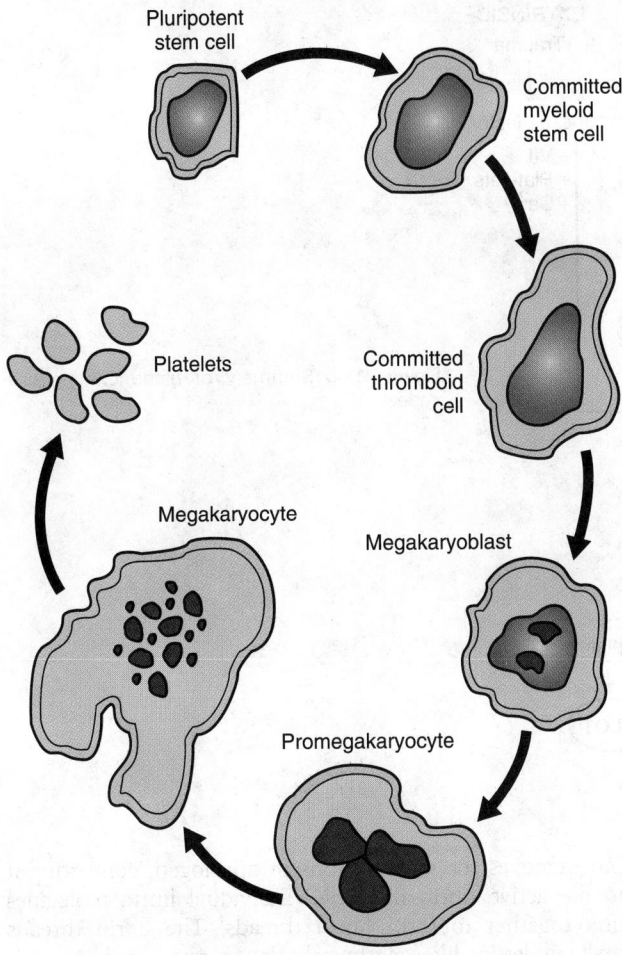

Figure 41–3. Platelet maturational pathway.

the regulation and maturation of blood cells to help maintain hematologic homeostasis.

Spleen

The spleen is located under the diaphragm to the left of the stomach. It contains three types of tissue: white pulp, red pulp, and marginal pulp, which all help balance blood cell production and destruction and assist with immunologic defensive mechanisms. White pulp is filled with lymphocytes and macrophages, filtering the circulating blood and removing unwanted cells (such as bacteria and old RBCs). Red pulp is composed of vascular sinuses that are storage sites for erythrocytes and platelets. Marginal pulp contains the termination sites of many arteries and other blood vessels.

During blood formation, the spleen destroys aged or imperfect RBCs through phagocytosis and mechanical deformation, assists in iron metabolism by breaking down the hemoglobin released from these destroyed cells, stores platelets, and filters antigens. A client who has undergone splenectomy has impairment of some immune functions. As a result, a splenectomized client's body is not efficient at ridding the body of many bloodborne

pathogenic microorganisms and is at a greatly increased risk for infection and sepsis (Workman et al., 1993).

Liver

The liver, important for normal erythropoiesis, is the primary production site for most of the blood clotting factors and prothrombin. In addition, proper liver function, including bile production, is critical to the formation of vitamin K in the intestinal tract. (Vitamin K is essential in the formation of blood clotting factors VII, IX, and X and prothrombin.) Large quantities of whole blood and blood cells can be stored in the liver. The liver also converts bilirubin (one end-product of hemoglobin breakdown) to bile and stores extra iron within a storage protein called ferritin. Small amounts of erythropoietin are synthesized in the liver.

HEMOSTASIS

In hemostasis, selective localized blood clotting occurs in damaged blood vessels while blood circulation to all other areas is maintained. It is a complex process that balances the production of clotting and dissolving factors. Hemostasis begins with the formation of a platelet plug and continues with a series of events that eventually cause the formation of a fibrin clot. Intrinsic and extrinsic factors are involved in fibrin clot formation and blood coagulation.

Platelet Aggregation

Platelets normally circulate as individual cell-like structures. They are not attracted to each other until activated or until the presence of other substances causes platelet membranes to become sticky, allowing aggregation to occur. When platelets become activated and aggregate, they form large, semisolid plugs within the lumens and walls of blood vessels and disrupt blood flow. Some of the substances capable of causing platelets to aggregate include adenosine diphosphate (ADP), calcium, thromboxane A_2, and collagen. Platelets themselves can be stimulated to secrete some of these substances, whereas other substances causing platelet aggregation are exogenous. Formation of a platelet plug can start the cascade reaction that ultimately causes blood coagulation to occur through the formation of a fibrin clot.

The Blood Clotting Cascade

The beginning of the blood clotting cascade is rapidly amplified or enhanced. That is, the final result is much larger than the triggering event. Cascades work like a landslide: A few small pebbles rolling down a steep hillside can dislodge large rocks and pieces of soil, causing a final enormous movement of earth. Just like landslides, cascade reactions are hard to stop once set into motion. Platelet plug formation starting the clotting cascade can result from intrinsic or extrinsic factors.

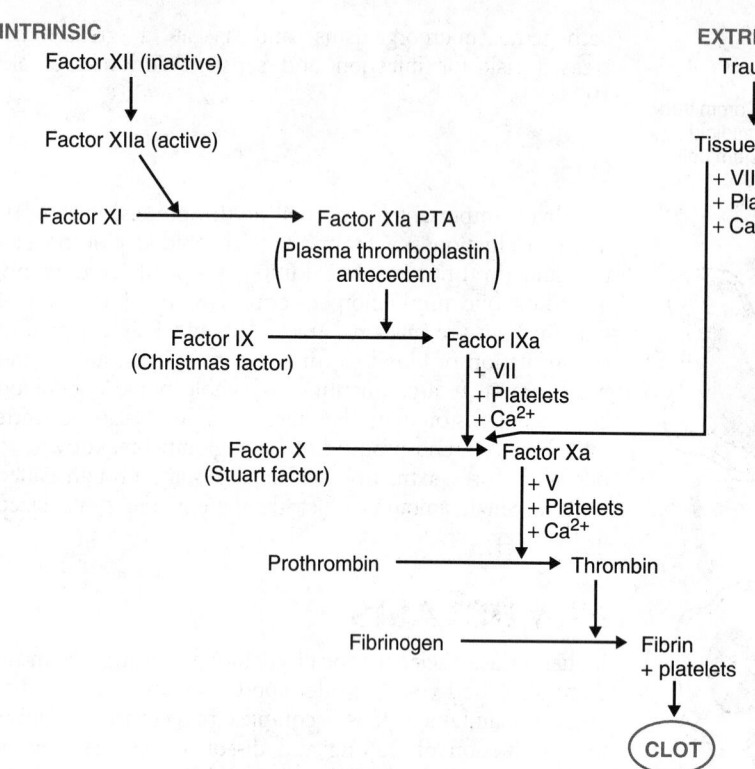

Figure 41–4. Summary of blood clotting cascade.

Intrinsic Factors

Platelet plugs begin to form when changes occur inside blood vessels. Trauma to the blood cells or exposure of the blood to collagen in the linings of blood vessels can cause platelet aggregation, the formation of a platelet plug, and the beginning of the clotting cascade (Fig. 41–4; see also Fig. 42–4). Other intrinsic events stimulating platelet aggregation include antigen-antibody reactions, circulating debris, prolonged venous stasis, and bacterial endotoxins. Having the cascade continue to the point of fibrin clot formation depends on the presence of sufficient amounts of all the various clotting factors and cofactors, presented in Table 41–2.

Extrinsic Factors

Platelet plugs can begin to form due to changes external to the blood vessels. The most common extrinsic events starting the clotting cascade are trauma to tissues and damage to blood vessels. The platelet plug is formed within seconds of the trauma, causing the blood clotting cascade to be started sooner than by the intrinsic pathway, because some of the steps of the intrinsic pathway are bypassed.

Whether initiated by intrinsic or extrinsic factors, the result is the same—the formation of a fibrin clot and coagulation.

Fibrin Clot Formation

Fibrinogen is a large, inactive protein molecule made in the liver and secreted into the blood. An enzyme, throm-

bin, removes the end portions of fibrinogen, converting it to the active fibrin molecule. Individual fibrin molecules link together to form fibrin threads. The fibrin threads make a lattice-like meshwork that forms the base of a blood clot (Fig. 41–5).

After the fibrin mesh is formed, a stabilizing factor (clotting factor XIII) tightens up the mesh, making it more dense. Platelets stick to the threads of the mesh and attract other blood cells and proteins to form an actual blood clot. As this clot retracts, the serum (plasma without the clotting factors) is extruded, and clot formation is complete.

Fibrinolysis

Because blood coagulation occurs through a rapid cascade process, whenever the cascade is set into motion, in theory it keeps forming fibrin clots until all blood throughout the entire body has coagulated. Such widespread coagulation is not compatible with life. Therefore, whenever the blood clotting cascade is started, counterclotting or anticoagulant forces are also started to limit clot formation just to damaged areas, and normal blood flow is maintained everywhere else. When blood clotting and anticlotting actions are appropriately balanced, coagulation occurs only where it is needed and normal circulation is maintained.

The fibrinolytic system dissolves the fibrin clot with special enzymes (Fig. 41–6). The central event of fibrinolysis is the conversion of plasminogen to plasmin. Plasmin, an active enzyme, then digests fibrin, fibrinogen, prothrombin, and factors V, VIII, and XII, thus breaking down the fibrin clot (Colman et al., 1994).

TABLE 41–2

The Coagulation Factors

Factor	Action
I: Fibrinogen	• Factor I is converted to fibrin by the enzyme thrombin. Individual fibrin molecules form fibrin threads, which are the scaffold for clot formation and wound healing.
II: Prothrombin	• Factor II is the inactive precursor of thrombin. Prothrombin is activated to thrombin by coagulation factor X (Stuart-Prower factor). After it is activated, thrombin converts fibrinogen (coagulation factor I) into fibrin and activates factors V and VIII. • Synthesis is vitamin K–dependent.
III: Tissue thromboplastin	• Factor III interacts with factor VII to initiate the extrinsic clotting cascade.
IV: Calcium	• Calcium (Ca^{2+}), a divalent cation, is a cofactor for most of the enzyme-activated processes required in blood coagulation. • Calcium also enhances platelet aggregation and makes red blood cells clump together.
V: Proaccelerin	• Factor V is a cofactor for activated factor X, which is essential for converting prothrombin to thrombin.
VI: Discovered to be an artifact	• No factor VI is involved in blood coagulation.
VII: Proconvertin	• Factor VII activates factors IX and X, which are essential in converting prothrombin to thrombin. • Synthesis is vitamin K–dependent.
VIII: Antihemophilic factor	• Factor VIII together with activated factor IX enzymatically activates factor X. In addition, factor VIII combines with another protein (von Willebrand's factor) to help platelets adhere to capillary walls in areas of tissue injury. • A lack of factor VIII is the basis for classic hemophilia (hemophilia A).
IX: Plasma thromboplastin component (Christmas factor)	• Factor IX, when activated, activates factor X to convert prothrombin to thrombin. • This factor is essential in the common pathway between the intrinsic and extrinsic clotting cascades. • A lack of factor IX is the basis for hemophilia B. • Synthesis is vitamin K–dependent.
X: Stuart-Prower factor	• Factor X, when activated, converts prothrombin into thrombin. • Synthesis is vitamin K–dependent.
XI: Plasma thromboplastin antecedent	• Factor XI, when activated, assists in the activation of factor IX. However, a similar factor must exist in tissues. People who are deficient in factor XI have mild bleeding problems after surgery but do not bleed excessively as a result of trauma.
XII: Hageman factor	• Factor XII is critically important in the intrinsic pathway for the activation of factor XI.
XIII: Fibrin-stabilizing factor	• Factor XIII assists in forming crosslinks among the fibrin threads to form a strong fibrin clot.

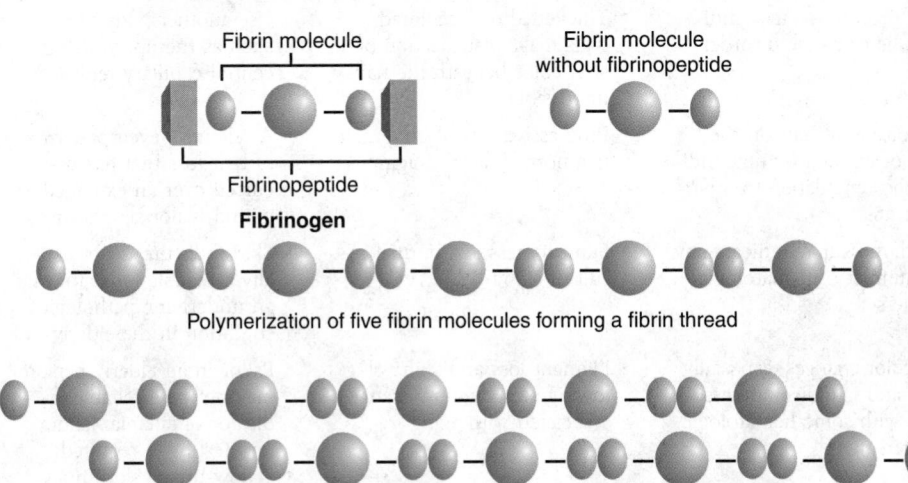

Fibrin molecule

Fibrin molecule without fibrinopeptide

Fibrinopeptide

Fibrinogen

Polymerization of five fibrin molecules forming a fibrin thread

Meshwork of fibrin threads forming scaffold of fibrin clot

Figure 41–5. Activation and polymerization of fibrin to form fibrin clot.

```
                    Plasminogen
                    activators
                         │
Plasminogen ───────────┐ ↓
                       ├──────►  Plasmin          Digestion     Fibrin              Fibrin
                       │        (activated form  ─────────►     clot   ─────────►   degradation
                       ↑        of plasminogen)                                      products
                    Thrombin
```

Figure 41–6. The process of fibrinolysis.

Hematologic Changes Associated with Aging

Aging changes the cellular and plasma components of blood, making accurate assessment of the hematologic system in elderly people more difficult. Chart 41–1 lists assessment tips for this population. Several factors cause a decreased blood volume in elderly people. Total body water is decreased among elderly clients. In addition, elderly people tend to have a lower concentration of plasma proteins and decreased plasma osmotic pressure (possibly related to a decreased dietary intake of proteins), which also causes some loss of blood volume into the interstitial space.

As bone marrow ages, it produces fewer blood cells. Total RBC and WBC counts (especially lymphocyte counts) are lower among elderly people, although platelet counts do not appear to change with age. Lymphocytes become less reactive to antigens and have a loss of immune function. Antibody levels and responses are lower in older adults. The leukocyte count does not rise as high in response to infection in elderly people as in young people (Workman et al., 1993).

Hemoglobin levels also change with age. Hemoglobin levels in men and women fall after middle age. Iron-deficient diets may play a role in this phenomenon.

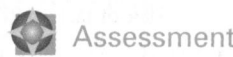 Assessment

➤ *History*

Demographic Data

Age and gender are important variables to obtain in assessments of the client's hematologic status. Bone marrow and immune activity diminish with age.

Chart 41–1

Focus on the Elderly: Hematologic Assessment

Assessment Area	Findings in Hematologic Disorders	Normal Changes in the Elderly	Significance/Alternatives
Nail beds (for capillary refill)	• Pallor or cyanosis may indicate a hematologic disorder	• Thickened or discolored nails make visualization of skin color beneath the nails impossible	• Use another body area, such as the lip, to assess central capillary refill
Hair distribution	• Thin or absent hair on the trunk or extremities may indicate poor circulation to a particular area	• Progressive loss of body hair is a normal facet of aging	• A relatively even pattern of hair loss that has occurred over an extended period is not significant
Skin moisture	• Skin dryness may indicate any of a number of hematologic disorders	• Skin dryness is a normal result of aging	• Skin moisture is not usually a reliable indicator of an underlying pathologic condition in the elderly
Skin color	• Skin color changes, especially pallor and jaundice, are associated with some hematologic disorders	• Pigment loss and skin yellowing are common changes associated with aging	• Pallor in an elderly person may not be a reliable indicator of anemia; laboratory testing is required. • Yellow-tinged skin in an elderly person may not be a reliable indicator of increased serum bilirubin levels; laboratory testing is required

WOMEN'S HEALTH CONSIDERATIONS

W At all ages, women have lower blood cell counts than do men, but this difference is more profound during menstrual years. This gender difference may be related to a dilutional effect of female hormones, which cause an increased volume of vascular fluid, or to differences in bone marrow activity.

It is also important for the nurse to collect information on occupation, hobbies, and the location of housing. This information may indicate exposure to agents or chemicals that affect bone marrow growth and hematologic function.

Personal and Family History

Because many types of bleeding disorders are inherited, the nurse obtains an accurate family history. The nurse asks whether anyone in the family has had hemophilia, frequent nosebleeds, postpartum hemorrhages, excessive bleeding after dental extractions, or continuous heavy bruising in response to relatively mild trauma. Familial information about sickle cell disease or sickle cell trait also is obtained. Although sickle cell disease is seen primarily among African-Americans, anyone may have the trait.

Personal factors to be included in the hematologic assessment are liver function, the presence of known immunologic or hematologic disorders, and current medication use. Because liver function is important in the synthesis of clotting factors, the nurse also asks about jaundice, anemia, and gallstones.

The nurse questions the client about use of blood "thinners" such as sodium warfarin (Coumadin, Warfilone✦) and aspirin. A person who takes aspirin on a daily basis may have bleeding problems, and many over-the-counter medications contain aspirin or other salicylates that disrupt platelet aggregation. The nurse determines all medications that the client is using or has used in the past 3 weeks. Clients are also asked about the use of antibiotics, because prolonged antibiotic therapy can lead to coagulopathies or bone marrow depression. Table 41–3 lists drugs known to alter hematologic function. Previous radiation therapy, especially if marrow-forming bones were in the radiation path, may result in some permanent impairment of hematologic function.

Diet History

Dietary pattern can alter cell quality and blood coagulation. The nurse asks clients to record everything eaten during the previous week. This information is helpful in determining the causes of anemias, as well as deficiencies of proteins, minerals, or vitamins. Diets high in fat and carbohydrates and low in protein, iron, and vitamins can cause many types of anemia as well as a decrease in the functions of all blood cells.

The nurse also asks the client about alcohol consumption. Chronic alcoholism is associated with nutritional deficiencies and liver impairment, both of which can adversely affect the hematologic system.

Some dietary habits can enhance blood clotting. Diets high in vitamin K may increase the rate of blood coagulation. The nurse assesses the amount of raw, leafy green vegetables that the client consumes and whether the client routinely takes supplemental vitamins. The nurse also assesses the amount of calcium consumed within the diet or in supplements.

Socioeconomic Status

The nurse assesses the client's ability to understand and follow instructions related to proper diet, specific procedures and tests, and therapeutic regimens. The nurse also determines the client's personal resources, such as finances and social support. A person with a marginal income may have a diet low in iron and protein. The nurse also notes the client's occupation and asks about potential exposure to chemicals.

Current Health Problem

The nurse determines whether the client has had swelling of lymph nodes or excessive bruising or bleeding and whether the bleeding was spontaneous or induced by trauma. The nurse also inquires about the amount and duration of bleeding after routine dental work. Women are asked about the presence of menorrhagia, or excessive menstrual flow. These clients are asked to estimate the number of pads or tampons used during the most recent menstrual cycle and whether this amount represents a change from the client's usual pattern of menstrual flow. The nurse asks whether clots are present in menstrual blood. The client is asked to estimate clot size using coins or fruit for comparison ("clots are dime-sized" or "clots are the size of lemons").

The nurse determines whether the client experiences dyspnea on exertion, palpitations, frequent infections, fevers, recent weight loss, headaches, or paresthesias. Any or all of these symptoms may accompany hematologic disease.

The single most common symptom of anemia is fatigue. The nurse questions the client about feeling tired, needing more rest, or losing endurance during normal activities. Clients are asked to compare the extent and intensity of their activities during the past month with those of the same month a year ago. The nurse asks about other symptoms associated with anemia, such as vertigo, tinnitus, anorexia, dysphagia, and a sore tongue.

▶ Physical Assessment

The nurse performs a comprehensive physical assessment because hematologic dysfunction affects the whole body. Certain problems are specific for hematologic assessment in elderly clients, as noted in Chart 41–1.

Assessment of the Integumentary System

The nurse inspects the color of the skin for pallor or jaundice and of the mucous membranes and nail beds for pallor or cyanosis. Pallor of the gums, conjunctivae, and palmar creases indicates decreased hemoglobin levels. The

TABLE 41–3

Drugs Impairing the Hematologic System

Generic Name	Common Trade Names
Drugs Causing Bone Marrow Suppression	
Altretamine	Hexalen, Hexastat♣
Amphotericin B	Fungizone
Azathioprine	Imuran
Chemotherapeutic agents*	
Chloramphenicol	Chloromycetin, Novochlorocap♣
Chromic phosphate	Phosphocol
Colchicine	(Generic only)
Didanosine	Videx
Eflornithine	Ornidyl
Foscarnet sodium	Foscavir
Ganciclovir	Cytovene
Interferon alfa	Actimmune, Alferon, Intron-A, Roferon-A, Wellferon-A♣
Pentamidine	Pentam 300, NebuPent, Pentacarinat♣
Sodium iodide	Iodopen
Zalcitabine	Hivid
Zidovudine	AZT, Retrovir, Novo-AZT♣
Drugs Causing Hemolysis	
Acetohydroxamic acid	Lithostat
Chlorpropamide	Diabinese, Glucamide, Novopropamide♣
Doxapram	Dopram
Glyburide	Diabeta, Micronase, Euglucon♣
Mefenamic acid	Ponstel, Ponstan♣
Menadiol diphosphate	Synkayvite
Methyldopa	Aldomet, Dopamet♣
Nitrofurantoin	Macrodantin, Novofuran♣
Amoxicillin	Amoxil, Augmentin, Apo-Amoxi♣
Penicillin G benzathine	Bicillin, Crystapen
Penicillin V	Pen Vee K, Pen Vee, Nu-Pen-VK♣
Primaquine	(Generic only)
Procainamide hydrochloride	Procan-SR, Promide, Pronestyl hydrochloride
Quinidine polygalacturonate	Cardioquin, Quinalan, Novoquinidin♣
Quinine	Legatrin, Quindan
Sulfonamides	Sulfamethoxazole (Gantanol), sulfisoxazole (Gantrisin, Novosoxazole♣)
Tolbutamide	Oramide, Orinase, Apo-Tolbutamide♣, Mobenol♣
Vitamin K	AquaMEPHYTON, Konakion
Drugs Disrupting Platelet Action	
Aspirin	Anacin, Ascriptin, Bufferin, Ecotrin, Entrophen♣, Riphen♣, Triaphen♣
Carbenicillin	Geopen, Pyopen♣
Carindacillin	Geocillin
Dipyridamole	Persantine, Apo-Dipyridamole♣, Novodipiradol♣
Moxalactam	Moxam
Pentoxifylline	Trental
Sulfinpyrazone	Anturane, Antazone♣, Novopyrazone♣
Ticarcillin	Ticar
Ticlopidine	Ticlid
Valproic acid	Dalpro, Depakene, Epvil♣

Data from United States Pharmacopeial Convention, Inc. (1998). *Volume I: Drug information for the health care professional* (18th ed.). Taunton, MA: World Color Book Services.
*General categories of chemotherapeutic agents include alkylating agents, antimitotics, antitumor antibiotics, and antimetabolites.

gums are also assessed for active bleeding in response to light pressure or brushing the teeth with a soft-bristled brush, and any lesions or draining areas are noted. The nurse assesses for signs of bleeding in the form of petechiae and large bruises (ecchymoses). Petechiae are pinpoint hemorrhagic lesions in the skin. Bruises may be confluent or clustered. For hospitalized clients, the nurse determines whether the client is bleeding from sites such as nasogastric tubes, endotracheal tubes, central lines, peripheral intravenous sites, or Foley catheters. The nurse also notes skin turgor and itching, because dry skin or intense itching can indicate hematologic disease.

TRANSCULTURAL CONSIDERATIONS

The nurse may have difficulty assessing people with darker skin for pallor, jaundice, petechiae, and bruising. The oral mucous membranes and the conjunctiva of the eye are areas where pallor and cyanosis are more easily detected, and the roof of the mouth is an area where jaundice can be seen more easily. Petechiae may be visible only on the palms of the hands or the soles of the feet. Bruises can be seen as darker areas of skin and palpated as slight swellings or irregular skin surfaces. The nurse asks the client about pain when skin surfaces are touched lightly or palpated. (Chapter 69 provides additional information on accurate assessment techniques for darker skin.)

Assessment of the Head and Neck

The nurse notes pallor or ulceration of the oral mucosa. The tongue may be completely smooth in pernicious anemia and iron deficiency anemia or smooth and red in nutritional deficiencies. These manifestations may be accompanied by fissures at the corners of the mouth. The nurse also observes for jaundice of the sclera.

All lymph node areas are inspected and palpated. The nurse documents any lymph node enlargement, noting whether palpation of the enlarged node causes pain. In addition, the nurse determines whether the enlarged node moves or remains fixed with palpation.

Assessment of the Respiratory System

The nurse measures the rate and depth of respiration while the client is at rest, and during and after mild physical activity (such as walking 20 steps in 10 seconds). The nurse notes whether the client can complete a ten-word sentence without stopping for a breath. The nurse determines whether the client is fatigued easily, experiences shortness of breath at rest or on exertion, or requires additional pillows to sleep comfortably at night. Many anemias cause these symptoms.

Assessment of the Cardiovascular System

The nurse observes for heaves, distended neck veins, edema, or signs of phlebitis. The nurse auscultates for murmurs, gallops, irregular rhythms, and abnormal blood pressure. In clients with anemia, systolic blood pressure tends to be lower than normal. In conditions of hypercellularity, blood pressure is greater than normal. Severe anemias cause right ventricular hypertrophy and heart disease.

Assessment of the Renal/Urinary System

Because the kidneys are extremely vascular, bleeding problems may manifest as overt or occult hematuria (blood in the urine). The nurse inspects a voided sample of urine for color. Hematuria may be detected by grossly, bloody red or dark brownish-gold urine. Because blood contains significant amounts of proteins, the nurse tests the urine for proteins with a urine test dipstick. The urine sample also is tested for occult blood (Hemoccult test).

Assessment of the Musculoskeletal System

Increased rib or sternal tenderness is an important sign of hematologic malignancy. The nurse examines the superficial surfaces of all bones by applying intermittent firm pressure with the fingertips. The nurse also assesses the client's range of joint motion and notes any swelling or joint pain.

Assessment of the Abdomen

The normal adult spleen is usually not palpable. Enlarged spleens may be detected by percussion, although palpation is more reliable. The spleen lies just beneath the abdominal wall and is identified by its movement during respiration. During palpation, the client lies in a relaxed, supine position while the nurse, standing on the client's right, palpates the left upper quadrant. The nurse palpates gently and cautiously because an enlarged spleen may be tender and easily ruptured.

Palpating the edge of the liver in the right upper quadrant of the abdomen can detect hepatic enlargement. The normal liver may be palpable as much as 4 to 5 cm below the right costal margin but is usually not palpable in the epigastrium. Both the liver and the spleen may be enlarged in hematologic disease.

A common cause of anemia among older adults is a chronically bleeding gastrointestinal lesion. If the lesion is located in the stomach or the small intestine, obvious blood may not be visible in the stool, or such a small amount is passed each day that the client is not aware of it. Therefore, the nurse obtains and tests a stool specimen for occult blood.

Assessment of the Central Nervous System

A thorough examination of cranial nerves and neurologic function is necessary in many clients with hematologic disease. Vitamin B_{12} deficiency impairs cerebral, olfactory, spinal cord, and peripheral nerve function, and severe chronic deficiency may lead to irreversible neurologic degeneration. A variety of neurologic abnormalities may develop in clients who have hematologic malignancies as a consequence of bleeding, infection, or tumor spread. When the client has a known or suspected bleeding disorder and has experienced any head trauma, the nurse expands the physical assessment to include frequent neurologic checks and mental status examinations (see Chap. 43).

Other important signs and symptoms associated with impaired hematologic function include fever, chills, and night sweats.

➤ Psychosocial Assessment

The person with hematologic abnormalities may have a chronic illness, such as hemophilia or cancer, or an acute exacerbation of a chronic disease, such as pernicious anemia. In either instance, each person brings his or her own coping style to the illness. After developing a rapport with the client, the nurse can learn what coping mechanisms the client has used successfully during past illness or crises.

The nurse also asks the client and family members about social support networks, community resources, and financial health. A problem in any of these areas can interfere with the client's compliance with therapy and, ultimately, recovery.

► DIAGNOSTIC ASSESSMENT

Laboratory Tests

In hematologic disease, the most definitive signs are often the laboratory test results. Chart 41–2 lists laboratory data associated with hematologic function.

Tests of Cell Number and Function

Complete Blood Count. A complete blood count (CBC) includes a number of studies: red blood cell (RBC) count, white blood cell (WBC) count, hematocrit, and hemoglobin level. The RBC count measures circulating RBCs in 1 mm^3 of venous blood, and the WBC count measures all leukocytes present in 1 mm^3 of venous blood. To determine the percentages of different kinds of leukocytes circulating in the blood, a WBC count with differential leukocyte count is performed (Chap. 23). The hemoglobin level represents the total amount of he-

---

Chart 41–2

Laboratory Profile: Hematologic Assessment

Test	Reference Range		International Reference Units	Significance of Abnormal Findings
Red blood cell (RBC) count	18–44 yr	F: 3.8–5.1 million/μL M: 4.3–5.7 millon/μL	3.8–5.1 × 10^{12} cells/L 4.3–5.7 × 10^{12} cells/L	• *Decreased levels* indicate possible anemia or hemorrhage • *Increased levels* indicate possible chronic anoxia or polycythemia vera
	45–64 yr	F: 3.8–5.3 millon/μL M: 4.2–5.6 millon/μL	3.8–5.3 × 10^{12} cells/L 4.2–5.6 × 10^{12} cells/L	
	> 64 yr	F: 3.8–5.2 million/μL M: 3.8–5.8 millon/μL	3.8–5.2 × 10^{12} cells/L 3.8–5.8 × 10^{12} cells/L	
Hemoglobin (Hgb)	18–44 yr	F: 11.7–15.5 g/dL M: 13.2–17.3 g/dL	117–155 g/L 132–173 g/L	• Same as for RBC
	45–64 yr	F: 11.7–16.0 g/dL M: 13.1–17.2 g/dL	117–160 g/L 131–172 g/L	
	> 65 yr	F: 11.7–16.1 g/dL M: 12.6–17.4 g/dL	117–161 g/L 126–174 g/L	
Hematocrit	18–44 yr	F: 34–45% M: 39–49%	0.34–0.45 fraction 0.39–0.49 fraction	• Same as for RBC
	45–64 yr	F: 35–47% M: 39–50%	0.35–0.47 fraction 0.39–0.50 fraction	
	> 65 yr	F: 35–47% M: 37–51%	0.35–0.47 fraction 0.37–0.51 fraction	
Mean cell volume (MCV)	80–100 fL (fL = femtoliter)		Same as reference range	• *Increased levels* indicate macrocytic cells, possible anemia • *Decreased levels* indicate microcytic cells, possible iron deficiency anemia
Mean cell hemoglobin (MCH)	26–35 pg/cell (pg = picogram)		Same as reference range	• Same as for MCV
Mean cell hemoglobin concentration (MCHC)	31–37 g/dL cells		310–370 g/L	• *Increased levels* may indicate spherocytosis or anemia • *Decreased levels* may indicate iron deficiency anemia or a hemaglobinopathy
White blood cell count (WBC)	4500–11,000/μL		4.5–11.0 × 10^9 cells/L	• *Increased levels* are associated with infection, inflammation, autoimmune disorders, and leukemia • *Decreased levels* may indicate prolonged infection or bone marrow suppression
Reticulocyte count	0.5%–1.5% of RBCs		0.005–0.015 fraction	• *Increased levels* may indicate chronic blood loss • *Decreased levels* indicate possible inadequate RBC production

Continued

moglobin in peripheral blood. The hematocrit (Hct) is calculated as the percentage of red blood cells in the total blood volume.

Complete blood cell studies can also measure other variables of the circulating cells, including the mean corpuscular volume (MCV), the mean corpuscular hemoglobin (MCH), and the mean corpuscular hemoglobin concentration (MCHC). The MCV measures the average volume or size of a single RBC and is useful for classifying anemias. When the MCV is elevated, the cell is said to be macrocytic, or abnormally large, as seen in megaloblastic anemias. When the MCV is decreased, the cell is abnormally small, or microcytic, as seen in iron deficiency anemia. The MCH is the average amount of hemoglobin in a single RBC. The MCHC measures the average concentration of hemoglobin in a single RBC. When the

CHART 41–2. Laboratory Profile: Hematologic Assessment   Continued

Test	Reference Range	International Reference Units	Significance of Abnormal Findings
Total iron binding capacity (TIBC)	250–425 μg/dL	44.8–76.1 μmol/L	• *Increased levels* indicate iron deficiency • *Decreased levels* may indicate anemia, hemorrhage, hemolysis
Serum haptoglobin	40–240 mg/dL	0.4–2.5 g/L	• *Increased levels* indicate possible inflammatory disease • *Decreased levels* may indicate liver disease or hemolytic disease
Iron (Fe)	F: 50–170 μg/dL M: 65–175 μg/dL	9.0–30.4 μmol/L 11.6–31.3 μmol/L	• *Increased levels* indicate iron excess, hemochromocytosis, liver disorders, megaloblastic anemia • *Decreased levels* indicate possible iron deficiency anemia, hemorrhage
Serum ferritin	F: 10–120 ng/mL M: 20–250 ng/mL	Same as reference range	• Same as for iron
Platelet count	150,000–400,000/μL	150–400 $\times$ 10^9/L	• *Increased levels* may indicate polycythemia vera or malignancy • *Decreased levels* may indicate bone marrow suppression, autoimmune disease, hypersplenism
Hemoglobin electrophoresis	Hgb A$_1$: > 95% Hgb A$_2$: 1.5–3.7% Hgb F: < 2% Hgb S: 0% Hgb C: 0%	> 0.95 fraction 0.015–0.037 fraction < 0.02 fraction 0.0 fraction 0.0 fraction	• *Variations* indicate hemoglobinopathies
Direct Coombs' and indirect Coombs' test	Negative	Negative	• *Positive findings* indicate antibodies to RBCs
Prothrombin time (PT)	11–15 sec	Patient PT/normal/PT (INR) (INR = International Normalized Ratio)	• *Increased time* indicates possible deficiency of clotting factors V and VII • *Decreased time* may indicate vitamin K excess
Bleeding time	2–7 min	Same as reference range	• *Increased time* may indicate inadequate platelet function or number, clotting factor deficiencies
Euglobin lysis time	2–4 hr	Same as reference range	• *Decreased time* may indicate possible fibrinolysis
Fibrin degradation products	< 10 μg/mL	< 10 mg/L	• *Increased levels* may indicate disseminated intravascular coagulation or fibrinolysis

Data from Tietz, N. (1995). *Clinical guide to laboratory tests* (3rd ed.), Philadelphia: W. B. Saunders.
F = female; M = male.

MCHC is decreased, the cell has a hemoglobin deficiency and is hypochromic, as in iron deficiency anemia.

Reticulocyte Count. Another hematologic test helpful in determining bone marrow function is the reticulocyte count. A reticulocyte is an immature RBC, and an elevated reticulocyte count indicates increased RBC production by the bone marrow. Normally, about 2% of circulating RBCs are reticulocytes. An elevated reticulocyte count is desirable in an anemic client or after hemorrhage, when an elevation indicates that the bone marrow is responding appropriately to a decrease in the total RBC mass. An elevated reticulocyte count without a precipitating cause may indicate pathologic conditions, such as polycythemia vera.

Hemoglobin Electrophoresis. Hemoglobin electrophoresis detects abnormal forms of hemoglobin, such as hemoglobin S in sickle cell disease. Hemoglobin A is the major component of hemoglobin in the normal RBC.

Leukocyte Alkaline Phosphatase. Leukocyte alkaline phosphatase (LAP) is an enzyme produced by normal mature neutrophils. Elevated LAP levels occur during episodes of infection or stress. An elevated neutrophil count without an accompanying elevation in LAP level is associated with chronic myelogenous leukemia.

Coombs' Test. The two Coombs' tests (direct and indirect) are used for blood typing. The direct test detects the presence of antibodies (also called antiglobulins) against RBCs that may be attached to a person's RBCs. Although healthy people can make these antibodies, certain diseases, such as systemic lupus erythematosus, mononucleosis, and lymphomas, are associated with the production of antibodies directed against the client's own RBCs. The presence of these antibodies usually causes a hemolytic anemia.

The indirect Coombs' test detects the presence of circulating antiglobulins. The test is used to determine whether the client has serum antibodies to the type of RBCs that he or she is about to receive by blood transfusion.

Serum Ferritin, Transferrin, and Total Iron-Binding Capacity. Serum ferritin, transferrin, and the total iron-binding capacity (TIBC) tests measure iron levels. Abnormal levels of iron and TIBC are characteristic of many diseases, including iron deficiency anemia.

The serum ferritin test measures the quantity of iron present as free iron in the plasma. Because the amount of serum ferritin is proportionally related to the amount of intracellular iron, representing 1% of the total body iron stores, the serum ferritin level provides a means to assess a person's total iron stores. People who have serum ferritin levels within 10 g of the normal range for their gender have adequate iron stores; people with levels 10 g or more lower than the normal range have inadequate iron stores and have difficulty recovering from any hemorrhagic event.

Transferrin is a protein that transports iron from the gastrointestinal tract to the intracellular storage sites. Because the amount of transferrin cannot be easily measured, measuring the amount of iron that can be bound to serum transferrin indirectly determines whether an adequate amount of transferrin is present. This test is the TIBC test. In healthy people, only about 30% of the transferrin is bound to iron in the blood. TIBC is measured by taking a sample of blood and adding measured amounts of iron to it. When the blood no longer binds the iron but allows it to precipitate, the TIBC can be calculated. TIBC increases when a person is deficient in serum iron and stored iron levels. Such a value indicates that an adequate amount of transferrin is present but less than 30% of it is bound to serum iron.

Tests Measuring Bleeding and Coagulation

Capillary Fragility Test. The capillary fragility test, or Rumpel-Leede test, measures vascular hemostatic function by increasing intracapillary pressure in the arm by occluding venous outflow or by applying controlled negative pressure to a skin area. Usually, a blood pressure cuff is inflated to a pressure halfway between the systolic and diastolic pressures and maintained for 5 minutes. The petechiae that appear distal to the cuff are counted. Normally, five to ten petechiae appear. The capillary fragility test can help determine whether excessive bleeding or bruising results from increased capillary fragility or impaired platelet action.

Bleeding Time Test. The bleeding time test evaluates vascular and platelet activity during hemostasis. A small incision (using a special spring-loaded lancet that ensures uniform wound depth) is made in the forearm while a blood pressure cuff remains inflated at 40 mmHg. Blood is blotted from the site at 30-second intervals, and the time required for the bleeding to stop is recorded. Normal bleeding time ranges from 1 to 9 minutes.

Prothrombin Time. The prothrombin time (PT) evaluates the adequacy of the extrinsic coagulation cascade. PT is prolonged when factors II, V, VII, and X are deficient or when liver disease is present. Sodium warfarin (Coumadin, Warfilone✳) therapy is monitored using PT levels. Appropriate warfarin therapy prolongs the PT by one and a half to two times the client's normal PT value. The PT test results are given in seconds, along with a control value. A normal PT is nearly equal to the control value.

Partial Thromboplastin Time. The partial thromboplastin time (PTT) assesses the intrinsic coagulation cascade. It evaluates the presence of factors II, V, VIII, IX, XI, and XII. When any of these factors is deficient, as in hemophilia or disseminated intravascular coagulation (DIC), the PTT is prolonged. Because factors II, IX, and X are vitamin K–dependent and are produced in the liver, liver disease can decrease their concentration and prolong the PTT. Heparin (Calciparin, Liquémin, Hepalean✳) therapy is monitored by PTT. Desired ranges for therapeutic anticoagulation are one and a half to two and a half times normal values.

Platelet Agglutination/Aggregation. Platelet aggregation, or the ability to clump, can be tested by mixing the client's plasma with a substance called ristocetin. The degree of aggregation is noted. Aggregation can be impaired in von Willebrand's disease and during the use of drugs such as aspirin, anti-inflammatory agents, and psychotropic agents.

➤ Radiographic Examinations

Assessment of the client with a suspected hematologic abnormality can include radioisotopic imaging. Isotopes are used to evaluate the bone marrow for sites of active erythropoiesis and sites of iron storage. Radioactive colloids are routinely used to determine organ size and liver and spleen function.

The client is given a radioactive isotope intravenously about 3 hours before the procedure. The client is then taken to the nuclear medicine department for the scan, where he or she must lie still for about an hour. No special client preparation or follow-up care is needed for these tests.

Standard x-rays may be used to diagnose some hematologic disorders. For example, multiple myeloma causes characteristic bone destruction, with a "Swiss cheese" appearance on x-ray.

➤ Bone Marrow Aspiration and Biopsy

Bone marrow aspiration or biopsy is frequently done to evaluate the client's hematologic status when other tests show persistent abnormal findings. Results can provide important information about bone marrow function, including RBC, WBC, and platelet production. Bone marrow aspiration and bone marrow biopsy are similar procedures. In a bone marrow aspiration, cells and fluids are suctioned from the bone marrow. In a bone marrow biopsy, solid tissue and cells are obtained by coring out an area of bone marrow with a large-bore needle.

A physician's order and a signed, informed consent are obtained from the client before a bone marrow aspiration or biopsy is done. Bone marrow aspiration may be performed by a physician, a sanctioned clinical nurse specialist, a nurse practitioner, or a physician assistant, depending on the agency's policy and regional law. The procedure may be performed at the client's bedside, in an examination room, in a laboratory, or in a clinic setting.

On learning what specific tests will be performed on the marrow, the nurse consults the facility's procedure manual and its hematology laboratory to determine how to handle the specimen. Some tests necessitate the addition of heparin or other special solutions to the specimen.

Client Preparation

Most clients experience anxiety or fear before a bone marrow aspiration. Clients who have experienced a bone marrow aspiration may have less or more anxiety, depending on how the previous experience was perceived. The nurse can help reduce anxiety and allay fears by providing accurate information and continuous emotional support. Some clients like to have their hand held during the procedure; other clients may want the nurse to hug or hold their entire upper body.

The nurse explains the procedure to the client and says that he or she will stay with the client during the entire procedure. Occasionally, a friend or family member is permitted to be present to hold the client's hand and provide additional emotional support. If a local anesthetic is to be used, the nurse tells the client that the injection will feel like a stinging or burning sensation. The nurse tells the client to expect a heavy sensation of pressure and pushing while the needle is being inserted. Some clients also can hear a crunching sound or feel a scraping sensation as the needle punctures the bone. The nurse explains that as the marrow is being aspirated by mild suction in the syringe, a brief sensation of painful pulling will be experienced. If a biopsy is performed, the client may feel more pressure and discomfort as the needle is rotated into the bone.

The client is assisted onto an examining table, and the site is exposed, most commonly the iliac crest. If this site is not available or if more marrow is needed, the sternum can be used. If the iliac crest is the site, the client is usually placed in the prone position or, occasionally, in the side-lying position. Depending on the tests to be performed on the specimen, a laboratory technician may also be present to ensure appropriate handling of the specimen.

Procedure

The procedure usually lasts from 5 to 15 minutes. Clients may be uncomfortable and may experience pain. The type and the amount of anesthesia or sedation depend on the physician's preference, the client's preference and previous experience with bone marrow aspiration and biopsy, and the setting.

A local anesthetic solution might be injected into the skin around the site. The client may also receive a mild tranquilizer or a rapid-acting sedative, such as midazolam hydrochloride (Versed) or lorazepam (Ativan, Apo-Lorazepam♣, Novolorazem♣). Some clients do well with guided imagery or autohypnosis.

The procedure for either aspiration or biopsy is invasive, and sterile precautions are observed. The skin over the site is cleaned with a disinfectant solution. For an aspiration, the needle is inserted with a twisting motion and the marrow is aspirated by pulling back on the plunger of the syringe. When sufficient marrow has been aspirated to ensure accurate analysis, the needle is carefully and rapidly withdrawn while the tissues are supported at the site. For a biopsy, a small skin incision is made and the biopsy needle is inserted through the skin opening. Pressure and several twisting motions are performed to ensure coring and loosening of an adequate amount of marrow tissue. External pressure is applied to the site until hemostasis is ensured. A pressure dressing or sandbags may be applied to minimize bleeding at the site.

Follow-Up Care

The site is covered with a dressing after hemostasis is achieved. The site of the aspiration is observed closely for 24 hours for signs of bleeding and infection. A mild analgesic (aspirin-free) is prescribed for discomfort, and ice packs are applied over the aspiration site to limit bruising. The nurse instructs the client to inspect the site every 2 hours for the first 24 hours and to note the presence of active bleeding or bruising. The nurse advises the client not to engage in contact sports or any other activity that might result in trauma to the site for 48 hours.

Information obtained from bone marrow aspiration or biopsy reflects the degree and quality of bone marrow activity present. The counts made on a marrow specimen can indicate whether stem cells, blast cells, committed cells, and more mature cell forms are present in the expected quantities and proportions. In addition, bone marrow aspiration or biopsy can confirm the spread of cancer cells from other tumor sites.

SELECTED BIBLIOGRAPHY

Abboud, C., & Lichtman, M. (1995). Structure of the marrow. In E. Beutler, M. Lichtman, B. Coller, & T. Kipps (Eds.), *William's hematology* (5th ed., pp. 25–38). New York: McGraw-Hill.

Colman, R., Hirsch, J., Marder, V., & Salzman, E. (1994). *Hemostasis and thrombosis: Basic principles and clinical practice* (3rd ed.). Philadelphia: J. B. Lippincott.

Frizzell, J. (1998). Avoiding lab test pitfalls. *American Journal of Nursing, 98*(2), 34–38.

Goodnough, L., Price, T., & Parvin, C. (1995). The endogenous erythropoietin response and the erythropoietic response to blood loss anemia: The effects of age and gender. *Journal of Laboratory and Clinical Medicine, 126*(1), 57–64.

Guyton, A., & Hall, J. (1996). *Textbook of medical physiology* (9th ed.). Philadelphia: W. B. Saunders.

*Hays, K. (1990). Physiology of normal bone marrow. *Seminars in Oncology Nursing, 6*(1), 3–8.

Higgins, C. (1995). Haematology blood testing for anaemia. *British Journal of Nursing, 4*(5), 248–253.

Malaguarnera, M., Bentivegna, P., Giugno, I., DeFazio, I., Motta, M., & Trovato, B. (1996). Erythropoietin in healthy elder subjects. *Archives of Gerontology and Geriatrics, 22*(2), 131–135.

Pitler, L. (1996). Hematopoietic growth factors in clinical practice. *Seminars in Oncology Nursing, 12*(2), 115–129.

Tietz, N. (1995). *Clinical guide to laboratory tests* (3rd ed). Philadelphia: W. B. Saunders.

United States Pharmacopeial Convention, Inc. (1998). *Volume I: Drug information for the health care professional* (18th ed.). Taunton, MA: World Color Book Services.

Williams, W. (1995). Hematology in the aged. In E. Beutler, M. Lichtman, B. Coller, & T. Kipps (Eds.). *Williams hematology* (5th ed., pp. 72–77). New York: McGraw-Hill.

Williams, W., Morris, M., & Nelson, D. (1995). Examination of the blood. In E. Beutler, M. Lichtman, B. Coller, & T. Kipps (Eds.). *Williams hematology* (5th ed., pp. 8–15). New York: McGraw-Hill.

Williams, W., & Nelson, D. (1995). Examination of the marrow. In E. Beutler, M. Lichtman, B. Coller, & T. Kipps (Eds.). *William's hematology* (5th ed., pp. 15–22). New York: McGraw-Hill.

*Workman, M., Ellerhorst-Ryan, J., & Koertge, V. (1993). *Nursing care of the immunocompromised patient.* Philadelphia: W. B. Saunders.

SUGGESTED READINGS

*Hays, K. (1990). Physiology of normal bone marrow. *Seminars in Oncology Nursing, 6*(1), 3–8.

  Although several years old, this excellent article provides useful information on the blood-forming functions of bone marrow. Terms are explained simply and concisely. The reference list contains both informational and research-based sources.

Pitler, L. (1996). Hematopoietic growth factors in clinical practice. *Seminars in Oncology Nursing, 12*(2), 115–129.

  This clinically focused article explains the mechanisms of action and clinical uses of a variety of hematopoietic growth factors. Side effects, precautions, and nursing responsibilities also are addressed.

Chapter 42

INTERVENTIONS FOR CLIENTS WITH HEMATOLOGIC PROBLEMS

Hematologic system disorders can occur in the synthesis, function, or normal destruction of any type of blood cell. The impact of hematologic disorders on the client's well-being depends on the type, degree, and rate of onset of the specific disorder. This chapter discusses hematologic conditions that minimally disrupt activities of daily living (ADLs) as well as potentially life-threatening conditions such as sickle cell disease and leukemia.

RED BLOOD CELL DISORDERS

The major cellular population of the blood is red blood cells (RBCs), or erythrocytes. Physiologic function depends on maintaining the circulating volume of RBCs within the normal range for the person's age and gender and ensuring that the erythrocytes can perform their normal functions. RBC disorders include problems in production, function, and destruction. These problems may result in an insufficient number or function of RBCs (anemia) or an excess of RBCs (polycythemia).

Anemia

Anemia is a reduction in either the number of RBCs, the quantity of hemoglobin, or the hematocrit (the volume of packed RBCs per deciliter of blood). Anemia is a clinical sign, not a diagnosis, because it is a manifestation of a number of abnormal conditions. Anemia can result from dietary deficiency, hereditary disorders, bone marrow disease, and bleeding.

There are many types and causes of anemia. Some anemias arise from a deficiency in one or more of the components needed to make fully functional RBCs. Such anemias can be caused by deficiencies of iron, vitamin B$_{12}$, folic acid, or intrinsic factor. Additional causes include decreased development of the RBC line precursors, decreased rate of erythrocyte production, and increased destruction of RBCs. Table 42–1 lists common causes of various types of anemia. Despite the many causes of anemia, the effects of anemia on the client (Chart 42–1) and the corresponding nursing care are similar for all types of anemia.

Anemias Resulting from Increased Destruction of Red Blood Cells
Sickle Cell Disease
Overview

Sickle cell disease is a condition in which chronic anemia is one of many client problems leading to discomfort,

TABLE 42–1

Common Causes of Anemia

Type of Anemia	Common Causes
Sickle cell disease	• Autosomal recessive inheritance of two defective genes for hemoglobin synthesis
G6PD deficiency anemia	• X-linked recessive inherited deficiency of the enzyme glucose-6-phosphate dehydrogenase.
Autoimmune hemolytic anemia	• Abnormal immune function in which a person's immune reactive cells fail to recognize his or her own red blood cells as self cells

Iron deficiency anemia	• Inadequate iron intake caused by
	  • Iron-deficient diet
	  • Chronic alcoholism
	  • Malabsorption syndromes
	  • Partial gastrectomy
	• Rapid metabolic (anabolic) activity caused by
	  • Pregnancy
	  • Adolescence
	  • Infection

Vitamin B_{12} deficiency anemia	• Dietary deficiency
	• Failure to absorb vitamin B_{12} from intestinal tract as a result of
	  • Partial gastrectomy
	  • Pernicious anemia

Folic acid deficiency anemia	• Dietary deficiency
	• Malabsorption syndromes
	• Drugs
	  • Oral contraceptives
	  • Anticonvulsants
	  • Methotrexate

Aplastic anemia	• Exposure to myelotoxic agents
	  • Radiation
	  • Benzene
	  • Chloromycetin
	  • Alkylating agents
	  • Antimetabolites
	  • Sulfonamides
	  • Insecticides
	• Viral infection (unproven)
	  • Epstein-Barr virus
	  • Hepatitis B
	  • Cytomegalovirus

disability, increased risk for disease, and early death. Once considered a childhood disorder, clients with sickle cell disease who receive appropriate supportive care may live into their 30s and 40s. In addition, there is great individual variation in the severity of the disease and the onset of complications.

Pathophysiology

The primary problem in this hereditary disorder is the formation of abnormal beta chains in the hemoglobin molecule. The hemoglobin molecule of adults is composed of several different substances partially held together by a protein (globin), consisting of two alpha chains and two beta chains of amino acids. This normal adult hemoglobin is called hemoglobin A (HbA). The total hemoglobin of normal healthy adults is usually composed of 98% to 99% HbA with a small percentage of a fetal form of hemoglobin (HbF).

In clients who have sickle cell disease, at least 40% of their total hemoglobin contains an abnormality of the beta chains, hemoglobin S (HbS). HbS is sensitive to changes in the oxygen content of the RBC. When RBCs containing large amounts of HbS are exposed to conditions of decreased oxygen, the abnormal beta chains contract and pile together within the cell, distorting the overall shape of the RBC. These cells assume a sickle shape, become rigid, clump together, and form clusters that obstruct capillary blood flow (Fig. 42–1). Capillary obstruction leads to further tissue hypoxia (reduced oxygen supply) and more sickling, causing blood vessel obstructions and infarctions in the locally affected tissues. Situations that precipitate sickling include hypoxia, dehydration, infections, vascular stasis, low environmental or body temperatures, acidosis, strenuous exercise, and anesthesia.

Usually, sickled cells resume a normal shape when the precipitating condition is removed and proper oxygenation occurs. However, although the outward appearance of the RBCs is normal, at least some of the hemoglobin remains twisted, decreasing cell flexibility. The membranes of the cells become damaged over time, and cells

---

Chart 42–1

Key Features of Anemia

Integumentary Manifestations

• Pallor, especially of the ears, the nail beds, the palmar creases, the conjunctiva, and around the mouth
• Cool to the touch
• Intolerance of cold temperatures
• Nails become brittle and may lose the normal convex shape; over time, nails become concave and fingers assume club-like appearance

Cardiovascular Manifestations

• Tachycardia at basal activity levels, increasing with activity and during and immediately after meals
• Murmurs and gallops heard on auscultation when anemia is severe
• Orthostatic hypotension

Respiratory Manifestations

• Dyspnea on exertion
• Decreased oxygen saturation levels

Neurologic Manifestations

• Increased somnolence and fatigue
• Headache

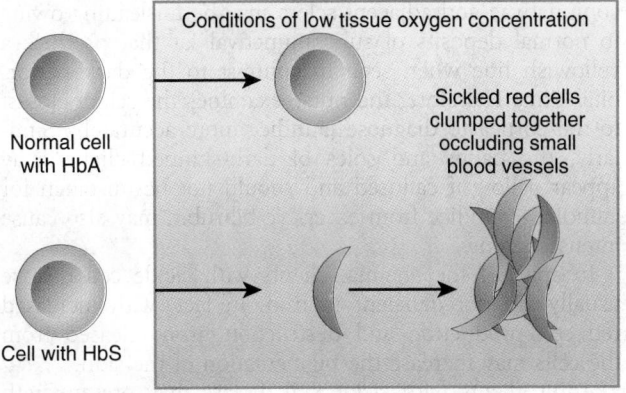

Conditions of low tissue oxygen concentration

Normal cell
with HbA

Cell with HbS

Sickled red cells
clumped together
occluding small
blood vessels

Figure 42–1. Red blood cell actions under conditions of low tissue oxygenation. (HbS = hemoglobin S; HbA = hemoglobin A.)

become irreversibly sickled. Additionally, the altered membranes of cells with HbS make them more fragile and more easily destroyed in the spleen and in other organs that have long, twisted capillary pathways. The average life span of an RBC containing 40% or more of HbS is approximately 20 days, considerably less than the 120-day life span of RBCs containing only HbA. This reduced life span is responsible for hemolytic anemia in clients with sickle cell disease.

The client with sickle cell disease experiences periodic episodes of extensive cellular sickling, or *crises*. The crises have a sudden onset and can occur as frequently as weekly or as seldom as once a year. Many clients are in good health much of the time, with crises occurring sporadically in response to precipitating conditions that stimulate local or systemic hypoxemia (deficient oxygen in the blood).

Repeated occlusions of progressively larger blood vessels have long-term negative effects on tissues and organs (Chart 42–2). Most effects are thought to occur as a result of capillary and blood vessel occlusion leading to tissue hypoxia, anoxia, ischemia, and cell death. Tissues and organs begin to have small infarcted areas that eventually destroy all healthy cells and lead to organ failure. Tissues and organs most commonly affected in this way are the spleen, liver, heart, kidney, brain, bones, and retina.

Etiology

Sickle cell disease is a genetic disorder with an autosomal recessive pattern of inheritance. The formation of the beta chains of the hemoglobin molecule is dependent on a pair of genes. A mutation leads to the formation of HbS instead of HbA. When the client inherits one abnormal gene of this pair, the condition is called *sickle cell trait*. The client can pass the condition on to offspring but has only mild manifestations of the disease under severe precipitating conditions because less than about 30% of the person's hemoglobin is abnormal. When the client inherits two abnormal genes, the condition is called *sickle cell disease* (formerly sickle cell anemia), and the

client has severe manifestations of the disease even under relatively mild precipitating conditions. In addition, if the client has children, each child will inherit one of the two abnormal genes and at least have sickle cell trait.

Incidence/Prevalence

Sickle cell trait and different forms of sickle cell disease occur in people of all races and ethnicities but infrequently among Caucasians.

TRANSCULTURAL CONSIDERATIONS

Sickle cell disease occurs most frequently in African-Americans as well as in African, Mediterranean, Caribbean, Middle Eastern, and Central American populations. Approximately 1 of every 12 African-Americans has the sickle cell trait. One of every 375 African-American infants inherits two abnormal genes (one from each parent) and has overt sickle cell disease (Agency for Health Care Policy and Research, 1993).

Chart 42–2

Key Features of Sickle Cell Disease

Hematologic Manifestations
- Fragile red blood cells that sickle and clump under conditions of low tissue oxygenation, venous stasis, lower environmental or body temperature
  - Anemia
- Tissue hypoxia and ischemia
  - Pain
  - Hardened, enlarged spleen

Respiratory Manifestations
- Pulmonary infarcts
  - Chest pain
  - Pneumonia

Genitourinary Manifestations
- Renal ischemia
  - Decreased urine concentration
- Priapism

Cardiovascular Manifestations
- Cardiac ischemia
  - Myocardial infarctions
  - Chest pain
  - Congestive heart failure
- Cerebrovascular accidents

Musculoskeletal Manifestations
- Necrosis of femur head
- Pain in extremities with moderate physical exercise
- Delayed growth—small stature

Integumentary Manifestations
- Leg ulcers
- Pale, cyanotic skin

Collaborative Management

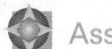 Assessment

➤ History

An adult with sickle cell disease has a long-standing diagnosis of the disorder. However, an adult who has sickle cell trait may have had such mild clinical manifestations that he or she is unaware of the problem until it is diagnosed with an accompanying disorder or when anesthesia is administered.

The nurse asks the client about previous crises, including precipitating events, severity, and usual treatments. Recent activities and situations are explored with the client to determine the probable precipitating condition or event. The nurse also reviews all activities and events during the previous 24 hours, including food and fluid intake, exposure to temperature extremes, types of clothing worn, medications taken, exercise, trauma, stress, and ingestion of alcohol or other recreational drugs. This activity review provides the nurse with important information about fatigue, activity tolerance, and participation in activities of daily living (ADLs).

The nurse also asks about changes in sleep and rest patterns, ability to climb stairs, and any activity that induces shortness of breath. Obtaining a subjective baseline assessment of the individual's perceived energy level using a scale ranging from 1 to 10 (1 = not tired with plenty of energy; 10 = total exhaustion) can be useful in evaluating the degree of fatigue and the effectiveness of later treatments.

➤ Physical Assessment/Clinical Manifestations

Pain is the most common symptom experienced during sickle cell crisis. Jaundice may also be present as a result of increased RBC destruction and release of bilirubin. Other clinical manifestations vary with the site of tissue damage.

Cardiovascular Assessment. The nurse assesses the client's cardiovascular and peripheral vascular status by comparing peripheral pulses, temperature, and capillary refill in all extremities. Extremities distal to blood vessel occlusion are cool to the touch with slow capillary refill and may have diminished or absent pulses. Heart rate may be rapid and blood pressure low to average, with a decreased pulse pressure because lysing of red blood cells (RBCs) leads to anemia.

Integumentary Assessment. The skin may be pale or cyanotic as a result of decreased perfusion and anemia. The nurse examines the lips, tongue, nail beds, conjunctivae, palms, and soles at regular intervals for subtle color changes. With cyanosis, the lips and tongue are gray, and the palms, soles, conjunctivae, and nail beds have a bluish tinge.

Another skin manifestation associated with sickle cell disease is jaundice. Bilirubin, a major component of RBCs, is released when fragile cells are damaged, leading to jaundice. The nurse assesses for jaundice in clients with darker skin by inspecting the oral mucosa, especially the hard palate, for yellow discoloration. Inspection of the conjunctivae and adjacent sclera may be misleading owing to normal deposits of subconjunctival fat that produce a yellowish hue when seen in contrast to the dark periorbital skin. Therefore, the nurse examines the sclera closest to the cornea to diagnose jaundice more accurately. Similarly, the palms and soles of dark-skinned clients may appear yellow if callused and should not be mistaken for jaundice. Jaundice from excessive bilirubin may also cause intense itching.

In spite of the anemia, clients with sickle cell disease usually are not deficient in iron. In fact, with increased red cell production and destruction, iron released from the cells may increase the pigmentation of the skin.

Adult clients with sickle cell disease may present with stasis ulcers or pressure ulcers on the lower extremities. The ulcers usually occur on the lateral or medial aspect of the ankle or on the shin (Blaylock, 1996). The nurse inspects the legs and feet for open lesions or darkened areas that may indicate necrotic tissue.

Abdominal Assessment. Abdominal organs are usually the first to be damaged as a result of multiple episodes of hypoxia and ischemia. The nurse inspects the abdomen for asymmetry or bulging areas, gently palpating it. Affected organs, such as the liver or spleen, may be firm and enlarged with a nodular texture in later stages of the disease.

Musculoskeletal Assessment. Extremities are a common site of vascular occlusion among clients who have sickle cell disease. In addition, joints may be damaged from frequent hypoxic episodes and undergo necrotic degeneration. The nurse inspects the extremities for symmetry and notes any areas of swelling or color difference. Clients are asked to move all joints, and the nurse notes the range of motion and any accompanying pain.

Central Nervous System Assessment. Changes in central nervous system (CNS) function may occur directly or indirectly in clients with sickle cell disease. During crises, clients may have low-grade fever. If the CNS sustains infarcts or repeated episodes of hypoxia, clients may have seizure activity or clinical manifestations of a stroke. Handgrasps are assessed bilaterally. The nurse assesses gait and coordination in those clients who are permitted to walk.

➤ Psychosocial Assessment

Psychosocial assessment is important because behavioral changes may be the first observable clinical manifestations of cerebral hypoxia. The nurse observes the clients and documents presenting behavior. Family members and significant others are questioned to determine whether the presenting behavior and mental status are typical.

Sickle cell disease represents a chronic, painful, life-limiting disorder that can be passed on to one's children. The nurse assesses clients' psychosocial needs in terms of new factors, established support systems, previous and current coping patterns, and disease progression. The nurse also asks clients how they view the disease and what adjustments in lifestyle have been made to accommodate limitations.

➤ Laboratory Assessment

The primary laboratory finding associated with sickle cell disease is the large percentage of HbS present on electrophoresis. A person who has sickle cell trait usually expresses less than 40% HbS, but one with sickle cell disease may express 85% to 95% HbS. This percentage does not change during crises. Another indicator of sickle cell disease is the percentage of RBCs showing irreversible sickling. This value is less than 1% among people who do not have sickle cell disease, is 5% to 50% among people with sickle cell trait, and may exceed 90% among people with sickle cell disease.

A variety of other laboratory tests reflect the problems associated with sickle cell disease, especially during crises. The hematocrit of clients with sickle cell disease is usually low (between 20% and 30%). This value decreases even more dramatically during vascular occlusive crises or aplastic crisis, when the bone marrow temporarily fails to produce cells during physiologically stressful periods (such as infection). The reticulocyte count is elevated, indicating anemia of long duration. Often the mean corpuscular hemoglobin concentration (MCHC) and total bilirubin level are elevated in clients who have sickle cell disease.

The total white blood cell (WBC) count is usually above normal among clients who have sickle cell disease. It is thought that this elevation is related to chronic inflammation resulting from tissue hypoxia and ischemia.

➤ Radiographic Assessment

Bone changes occur as a result of chronically stimulated marrow and hypoxic bone tissue. The skull may show radiographic changes resulting from chronic bone surface resorption and regeneration, giving the skull a "crew cut" appearance. Joint necrosis and degeneration also are obvious on x-ray.

➤ Other Diagnostic Assessment

Electrocardiographic (ECG) changes document cardiac infarcts and tissue damage. Specific ECG changes are related to the area of the myocardium sustaining the damage. Ultrasonography, computed tomography (CT), positron emission tomography (PET), and magnetic resonance imaging (MRI) may reveal soft tissue and organ degenerative changes resulting from inadequate oxygenation and chronic inflammation.

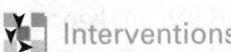 Interventions

The most common health problems for clients with sickle cell disease are pain and the potential complications of sepsis and multiple organ dysfunction. Interventions are aimed at reducing or preventing these problems.

➤ Pain

Pain associated with sickle cell crisis is the result of ischemic tissue injury caused by obstructed blood flow. The pain is often severe enough to require hospitalization and large doses of opioid analgesics (Miller, 1994). Pain is chronic with acute episodes and can occur anywhere in the body, often where circulation is impaired. It is sudden in nature and frequently described as gnawing or throbbing. Subjective reports of pain may be the only evidence, because the chronic nature of the pain may make physiologic changes less obvious.

The subjective nature of the pain, racial prejudice, and concern for addiction often cause these clients to be labeled as difficult (Marchiondo & Thompson, 1996). Health care providers must be aware of their own attitudes when caring for this population, and realize that lack of knowledge and concern for addiction often prevent proper pain management of sickle cell patients. Use of a pain rating scale by all nursing personnel can promote proper pain management. The nurse asks the client to rate pain on a scale ranging from 1 to 10 and evaluates the effectiveness of interventions based on the client's ratings. Use of pain-control contracts can also be useful.

Clients in acute sickle cell crisis often require at least 48 hours of parenteral analgesics. (Chart 42–3 lists specific priorities for nursing care of the client in sickle cell crisis.) Meperidine (Demerol), morphine, and hydromorphone (Dilaudid) are the medications most frequently ordered, administered intravenously (IV) on a routine schedule. Once relief is obtained, the dose can be tapered by 10% to 20% daily (Marchiondo & Thompson, 1996). As needed (PRN) schedules are discouraged because they do not provide adequate relief, and intramuscular (IM) injections are avoided because frequent injections lead to sclerosing of tissue, and absorption may be impaired by poor circulation. Moderate pain may be treated with oral doses of codeine, morphine sulfate, or nonsteroidal anti-inflammatory drugs (NSAIDs). See Chapter 9 for more information on pain management.

➤ Complementary Therapies

Complementary therapies and other nonpharmacologic measures such as keeping the room warm, using distrac-

---

Chart 42–3

Nursing Care Highlight: The Client in Sickle Cell Crisis

- Administer oxygen.
- Administer pain medication as ordered.
- Hydrate the client with normal saline intravenously and with beverages of choice (without caffeine) orally.
- Remove any constrictive clothing.
- Encourage the client to keep extremities extended to promote venous return.
- Do not raise the knee gatch of the bed.
- Elevate the head of the bed no more than 30 degrees.
- Keep room temperature at or above 72° F.
- Avoid taking blood pressure with external cuff.
- Check circulation in extremities every hour.
  - Pulse oximetry of fingers and toes
  - Capillary refill
  - Peripheral pulses
  - Toe temperature

tion and relaxation techniques, proper positioning with support for painful areas, aroma therapy, therapeutic touch, and warm soaks or compresses have all been useful in decreasing pain. However, the nurse must not assume that these methods alone will provide adequate pain relief. Analgesics are required to treat sickle cell pain.

➤ Potential for Sepsis

The client with sickle cell disease is more susceptible to blood-borne infections and infection by encapsulated microorganisms, such as *Streptococcus pneumoniae* and *Haemophilus influenzae*, as a result of decreased spleen function.

Interventions aim at preventing or halting the infection processes, controlling infection, and initiating early, effective treatment regimens for specific infections.

Prevention/Early Detection. A major objective is to protect the client in sickle cell crisis from infection. Frequent, thorough hand washing is of the utmost importance. Any person with an upper respiratory tract infection who must enter the client's room wears a mask. Strict aseptic technique is used for all invasive procedures.

The nurse continually assesses the client for the presence of infection, monitoring daily CBC with differential WBC count. The oral mucosa is inspected during every nursing shift for lesions indicating fungal or viral infection. Lung sounds are auscultated every 8 hours for crackles, wheezes, or diminished breath sounds. Each time the client voids, assistive nursing personnel inspect the urine for odor and cloudiness, and the client is asked about any sensation of urgency, burning, or pain during urination. The client's vital signs are taken at least every 4 hours to assess for fever.

Drug Therapy. Drug therapy is a primary defense against the infections that develop in the client with sickle cell disease. Prophylactic therapy with twice-daily administration of oral penicillin in the penicillin-tolerant client has resulted in dramatic reductions of pneumonia and other streptococcal infections. Drug therapy for an actual infection can control infection and prevent complications associated with sepsis. Agents used depend on the sensitivity of the specific organism causing the infection as well as the extent of the infection.

➤ Potential for Multiple Organ Dysfunction

The threat of multiple organ dysfunction arises from continued vascular occlusions after clumping of sickled cells. Management of sickle cell disease focuses on prevention of vascular occlusion and promotion of adequate oxygenation.

The client in sickle cell crisis is admitted to the acute care hospital. The nurse assesses the client for adequacy of circulation to all body areas. Restrictive clothing is removed, and the client is instructed to avoid keeping the hips or knees in a flexed position.

Dehydration perpetuates cell sickling and must be avoided. Nursing personnel assist the client in maintaining an adequate hydration status. An oral or parenteral intake of at least 200 mL hourly is desired for the client in crisis.

Oxygen is ordered, and the nurse ensures that oxygen therapy is delivered appropriately, including nebulization to prevent dehydration. Transfusion therapy has been used to decrease the incidence of organ dysfunction and stroke (Miller, 1994). RBC transfusions are therapeutic because levels of HbA are sustained while diluting levels of HbS. Transfusions also suppress erythropoiesis, thereby decreasing the production of sickle cells. Transfusions may be administered either in the acute care or clinic setting by a registered nurse. The nurse monitors the client closely for complications of transfusion therapy, discussed later in this chapter.

In some treatment centers, bone marrow transplantation is being performed to correct abnormal hemoglobin permanently. Because bone marrow transplantation is expensive and may result in chronic and life-threatening complications, its risks and benefits need to be seriously considered for each client.

➤ Continuing Care

Sickle cell disease is a progressive disorder with periods of varying degrees of exacerbation. Rarely is there a true remission, although crisis episodes may be infrequent. Care focuses on prevention of complications, an ongoing daily necessity for the client with sickle cell disease. The client with sickle cell disease may be cared for in a variety of settings, including acute care, subacute care, extended or assistive care, and home care.

➤ Health Teaching

Clients are taught to avoid specific activities that lead to hypoxia and hypoxemia. In addition, they are taught to recognize the early signs and symptoms of crisis, so that appropriate treatment can be initiated early to prevent undue pain, complications, and permanent tissue damage. Clients are often given opioid analgesics for self-management of sickle cell crises at home; the nurse teaches clients and families about the correct administration. Additionally, clients are counseled about the hereditary aspects of sickle cell disease, and information concerning prenatal diagnosis, birth control methods, and pregnancy options is offered. ·

WOMEN'S HEALTH CONSIDERATIONS

 Pregnancy in women with sickle cell disease presents special physiologic challenges and may be life threatening. Clients who show evidence of damage to vital organs are advised against becoming pregnant. Usually, barrier methods of contraception (cervical cap, diaphragm, or condoms with or without spermicides) are recommended for women with sickle cell disease. The use of oral contraceptives among these women is controversial, however. Oral contraceptives may increase susceptibility to occlusion by increasing clot formation, especially among smokers. However, the use of oral contraceptives also can reduce menstrual blood loss, thus decreasing the

TABLE 42–2

Indications for Treatment with Blood Components

Component	Volume	Infusion Time	Indications
Packed red blood cells (PRBCs)	• 200–250 mL	• 2–4 hour	• Anemia, hemoglobin <8
Washed red blood cells (WBC-poor PRBCs)	• 200 mL	• 2–4 hour	• History of allergic transfusion reactions • Bone marrow transplant clients
Platelets Pooled	• Approx. 300 mL	• 15–30 minutes	• Thrombocytopenia platelet count <20,000 • Clients who are actively bleeding with a platelet count <80,000
Platelets Single donor	• 200 mL	• 30 minutes	• History of febrile or allergic reactions
Fresh frozen plasma	• 200 mL	• 15–30 minutes	• Deficiency in plasma coagulation factors
Cryoprecipitate	• 10–20 mL/U	• 15–30 minutes	• Hemophilia VIII or von Willebrand's disease
White blood cells (WBCs)	• 400 mL	• 1 hour	• Sepsis, neutropenic infection not responding to antibiotic therapy

degree of anemia. Therefore, the determination of risks versus benefits of oral contraceptives must be individualized.

Glucose-6-Phosphate Dehydrogenase Deficiency Anemia

Overview

Many forms of congenital hemolytic anemia result from defects or deficiencies of one or more enzymes within the red blood cell (RBC). More than 200 such disorders have been identified. Most of these enzymes are needed to complete some critical step in intracellular energy production. The most common type of congenital hemolytic anemia is associated with a deficiency of the enzyme glucose-6-phosphate dehydrogenase (G6PD). This disease is inherited as an X-linked recessive disorder and affects about 10% of all African-Americans (Cotran et al., 1994).

G6PD stimulates critical reactions in the glycolytic pathway. RBCs contain no mitochondria (sites of high-efficiency production of the energy compound adenosine triphosphate [ATP]), so active glycolysis is essential for energy metabolism. Newly produced RBCs from clients with G6PD deficiency have relatively sufficient quantities of G6PD; however, as the cells age, the concentration diminishes drastically. Cells that have reduced amounts of G6PD are more susceptible to hemolysis during exposure to specific drugs (e.g., phenacetin, sulfonamides, aspirin [acetylsalicylic acid], quinine derivatives, thiazide diuretics, and vitamin K derivatives) and toxins.

After exposure to any of these agents, clients experience acute intravascular hemolysis lasting from 7 to 12 days. During this acute phase, anemia and jaundice develop. The hemolytic reaction is self-limited because only older erythrocytes, containing less G6PD, are destroyed.

Collaborative Management

It is imperative that the precipitating drug or the agent responsible for the hemolytic reaction be identified and

totally removed. People should be screened for this deficiency before donating blood, because administration of cells deficient in G6PD can be hazardous for the recipient.

During and immediately after an episode of hemolysis, adequate hydration is essential to prevent precipitation of cellular debris and hemoglobin in the kidney tubules, which can lead to acute tubular necrosis. Osmotic diuretics, such as mannitol (Osmitrol✦), may assist in preventing this complication. Transfusion therapy is indicated when anemia is present and kidney function is normal. Table 42–2 lists indications for transfusion with various types of blood components.

Immunohemolytic Anemia

Overview

Increased RBC destruction through hemolysis can occur in response to many situations, including mechanical trauma, infection (especially malarial infections), and autoimmune reactions. All increase the rate at which RBCs are destroyed by causing lysis (disintegration) of the RBC membrane. The most common types of hemolytic anemias in industrialized countries are the immunohemolytic anemias, also referred to as autoimmune hemolytic anemias (Cotran et al., 1994).

In clients with immunohemolytic anemia, immune system components attack their own RBCs. The exact mechanism that causes immune components to no longer recognize blood cells as self and to initiate destructive processes against RBCs is not known. Some hemolytic anemias are present with other autoimmune disorders (such as systemic lupus erythematosus) or lymphoproliferative disorders. Regardless of the cause, the RBC is viewed as non-self by the immune system and is destroyed.

There are two types of immunohemolytic anemia: warm and cold antibody. The *warm antibody* type is usually associated with immunoglobulin G (IgG) antibody excess. These antibodies are most active at 37° C (98° F) and may be stimulated by drugs, chemicals, or other autoimmune problems. The *cold antibody* type is associated with fixation of complement proteins on immunoglobulin M (IgM), occurs best at 30° C (86° F), and is commonly associated with a Raynaud-like response in which the arteries in the distal extremities constrict profoundly in response to cold temperatures or stress.

Collaborative Management

Treatment depends on clinical severity. Steroid therapy for mild to moderate immunosuppression is the first line of treatment and is temporarily effective in most clients. Splenectomy and more intensive immunosuppressive therapy with cyclophosphamide (Cytoxan, Procytox✱) and azathioprine (Imuran) may be instituted if steroid therapy fails. Plasma exchange therapy to remove attacking antibodies is effective for clients who do not respond to immunosuppressive therapy.

Anemias Resulting from Decreased Production of Red Blood Cells

Anemias associated with decreased RBC production can result from pathologic alterations in any of a variety of physiologic mechanisms. Some anemias arise from failure or inability of the bone marrow to properly synthesize RBCs, others because the body cannot synthesize or absorb a specific component necessary for RBC production.

ELDERLY CONSIDERATIONS

Elderly clients often have restricted diets and may be unable to consume enough meat because of poor dentition or economic reasons, and thus are at risk for iron deficiency anemia (Cotran et al., 1994). The nurse should ask about a family history of anemia. B_{12} deficiency anemia often occurs in individuals 50 to 80 years of age and may be genetically transmitted.

Iron Deficiency Anemia

Overview

The adult body contains between 2 and 6 g of iron, depending on the size of the person and the amount of hemoglobin in the cells. Approximately two thirds of this iron is contained in hemoglobin; the other third is stored in the bone marrow, spleen, liver, and muscle (see Chap. 41). If a person has an iron deficiency, the iron stores are depleted first followed by the hemoglobin stores. As a result, RBCs are small (microcytic), and the client has relatively mild manifestations of anemia, including weakness and pallor. In iron deficiency anemia, serum ferritin values are less than 12 $\mu g/L$.

Iron deficiency anemia is the most common type of anemia and can result from blood loss, increased metabolic energy demands, gastrointestinal malabsorption, and dietary inadequacy. The basic problem of iron deficiency anemia is a decreased supply of iron for the developing RBC. Iron deficiency anemia can occur at any age but is

TABLE 42–3

Common Food Sources of Iron, Vitamin B_{12}, and Folic Acid

Essential Element	Common Food Source
Iron	• Liver (especially pork and lamb) • Red meat • Organ meats • Kidney beans • Whole wheat breads and cereals • Leafy green vegetables • Carrots • Egg yolks • Raisins
Vitamin B_{12}	• Liver • Organ meats • Dried beans • Nuts • Green leafy vegetables • Citrus fruit • Brewer's yeast
Folic acid	• Liver • Organ meats • Eggs • Cabbage • Broccoli • Brussels sprouts

Data from Pennington, J. (1994). *Bowe's and Church's food values of portions commonly used* (16th ed.). Philadelphia: J. B. Lippincott.

more frequent in women, the elderly, and people with poor diets.

Collaborative Management

The primary treatment of clients with iron deficiency anemia is to increase the oral intake of iron, from common food sources, listed in Table 42–3. An adequate diet supplies a person with about 10 to 15 mg of iron per day, of which only 5% to 10% is absorbed (Higgins, 1995). This amount is sufficient to meet the needs of healthy men and healthy women after childbearing age, but is not sufficient to supply the greater needs of menstruating women and adolescents during growth spurts. Fortunately, if iron intake is inadequate or if bleeding or pregnancy occurs, the gastrointestinal (GI) tract is capable of increasing the absorption of iron to about 20% to 30% of the total daily intake (Cotran et al., 1994).

When iron deficiency anemia is severe, iron preparations can be administered intramuscularly. Such preparations are administered using the Z-track method outlined in Chart 42–4.

Vitamin B_{12} Deficiency Anemia

Overview

Proper production of red blood cells (RBCs) depends on adequate deoxyribonucleic acid (DNA) synthesis in the precursor cells, so mitosis and further maturation into

---

Chart 42-4

Nursing Care Highlight: Administering Intramuscular Medications by the Z-Track Method

- Draw medication up into the syringe using aseptic technique.
- Add 0.25 mL of air to the syringe.
- Discard the needle used to draw up the medication.
- Place a new needle (22-gauge, 2–3 inches long) on syringe.
- Make certain that the injection site is in a bright light.
- *Select the dorsal gluteal site only.*
- Identify appropriate landmarks for administration into the upper, outer quadrant.
- Once the site is selected, pull the skin and subcutaneous tissues sideways away from the muscle.
- Clean the site while holding the skin and subcutaneous tissues off to the side.
- Insert the needle deeply into the muscle tissue.
- Aspirate to determine needle placement.
- Iron dextran is black; look very closely to determine whether or not blood is being aspirated into the syringe.
- If blood is aspirated, withdraw needle and begin procedure again from the first step.
- If no blood is aspirated, inject medication slowly, followed by injection of the air-bubble.
- Quickly withdraw the needle.
- Release the skin and subcutaneous tissue.
- *Do not massage the injection site.*

---

functional erythrocytes occur. All DNA synthesis requires adequate amounts of folic acid (folate) to ensure the availability of the nucleotide thymidine, which stimulates DNA synthesis. One function of vitamin B_{12} is to serve as an essential cofactor to activate the enzyme system responsible for transporting folic acid from the extracellular fluid into the cell, where DNA synthesis occurs. Thus, a deficiency of vitamin B_{12} indirectly causes anemia by inhibiting folic acid transportation and limiting DNA synthesis in RBC precursor cells. These precursor cells then undergo improper DNA synthesis and mitosis and increase in size. Only a few are released from the bone marrow. This type of anemia is called *megaloblastic* (macrocytic) because of the large size of these abnormal cells.

Vitamin B_{12} deficiency can result from either inadequate intake (dietary deficiency) or poor absorption from the intestinal tract. Anemia caused by failure to absorb vitamin B_{12} (*pernicious* anemia) results from a deficiency of intrinsic factor (normally secreted by the gastric mucosa) necessary for intestinal absorption of vitamin B_{12}.

Vitamin B_{12} deficiency anemia may be mild or severe, usually develops slowly, and produces few symptoms. Clients usually have severe pallor and slight jaundice. Clients also have glossitis (a smooth, beefy-red tongue), fatigue, and weight loss. Because vitamin B_{12} also is necessary for normal nervous system functioning, especially of the peripheral nerves, clients with pernicious anemia may also have neurologic abnormalities, such as paresthe-sias (abnormal sensations) in the feet and the hands and disturbances of balance and gait (Chart 42–5).

Collaborative Management

When anemia is the result of a dietary deficiency, clients must increase their intake of foods rich in vitamin B_{12} (animal proteins, eggs, dairy products). Vitamin supplements may be prescribed when anemia is severe. For clients who have anemia as a result of a deficiency of intrinsic factor, vitamin B_{12} must be administered parenterally on a regular schedule (usually weekly for initial treatment, then monthly for maintenance).

Folic Acid Deficiency Anemia

Overview

Primary folic acid deficiency can also cause megaloblastic anemia. Clinical manifestations are similar to those of vitamin B_{12} deficiency without the accompanying nervous system manifestations, because folic acid does not appear to affect neuronal function. The absence of neurologic problems is an important diagnostic finding to differentiate folic acid deficiency from vitamin B_{12} deficiency. The disease develops slowly, and symptoms may be attributed to other coexisting diseases.

The three common causes of folic acid deficiency are poor nutrition, malabsorption, and drugs. Poor nutrition, especially a diet lacking green leafy vegetables, liver, yeast, citrus fruits, dried beans, and nuts, is the most common cause. Chronic alcohol abuse and parenteral alimentation without folic acid supplement are other dietary causes. Malabsorption syndromes, such as Crohn's disease, are the second most common cause.

Specific drugs impede the absorption and conversion of folic acid to its active form (tetrahydrofolate) and can also lead to folic acid deficiency and anemia. Such drugs include methotrexate, some anticonvulsants, and oral contraceptives.

Collaborative Management

Folic acid deficiency anemia prevention is aimed at identifying high-risk clients, such as the older, debilitated alcoholic; others prone to malnutrition; and those with increased folic acid requirements. A diet high in folic acid

---

Chart 42-5

Key Features of Vitamin B_{12} Deficiency Anemia

- Severe pallor
- Slight jaundice
- Smooth, beefy-red tongue
- Fatigue
- Weight loss
- Paresthesias of the hands and feet
- Difficulty with gait

and vitamin B_{12} prevents a deficiency (see Table 42–3). By routinely including assessment of dietary habits in a health history, the nurse can determine which clients are at risk for diet-induced anemias and provide appropriate follow-up.

Aplastic Anemia

Overview

Aplastic anemia is a deficiency of circulating erythrocytes resulting from arrested development of RBCs within the bone marrow. It is caused by an injury to the hematopoietic precursor cell, the pluripotent stem cell. Although aplastic anemia sometimes occurs alone, it is usually accompanied by agranulocytopenia (a reduction in leukocytes) and thrombocytopenia (a reduction in platelets). These three problems occur simultaneously because the bone marrow produces not only RBCs but also white blood cells (WBCs) and platelets. Consequently, if the bone marrow is abnormal for any reason or if it has been exposed to a myelotoxin (any substance toxic and damaging to bone marrow), production of erythrocytes, leukocytes, and thrombocytes slows greatly. *Pancytopenia* (a deficiency of all three cell types) is common in aplastic anemia. The onset of aplastic anemia may be insidious or rapid.

The development of aplastic anemia, although relatively rare, is associated with chronic exposure to several myelotoxic agents (see Table 41–3).

In about 50% of cases, the cause of aplastic anemia is unknown. Aplastic anemia may occur as a sequela of viral infection (Cotran et al., 1994), but the mechanism of bone marrow damage is unknown.

Collaborative Management

Blood transfusions are the mainstay of treatment for clients with aplastic anemia. Transfusion is indicated only when the anemia causes real disability or when bleeding is life threatening because of thrombocytopenia. Unnecessary transfusion, however, increases the opportunity for the development of immune reactions to platelets, shortens the life span of the transfused cell, and may increase the rate of rejection of transplanted marrow cells. Transfusions are thus discontinued as soon as the bone marrow begins to produce RBCs.

Because clients with some types of aplastic anemia have a disease course consistent with that of autoimmune problems, immunosuppressive therapy may be helpful. Agents that selectively suppress lymphocyte activity, such as antilymphocyte globulin (ALG), antithymocyte globulin (ATG), and cyclosporine (Sandimmune) have brought about partial or complete remissions. In more severe cases, general immunosuppressive agents, such as prednisone and cyclophosphamide (Cytoxan, Procytox✦), have been effective.

Splenectomy is considered in clients with an enlarged spleen that is either destroying normal RBCs or suppressing their development. Bone marrow transplantation in which defective stem cells are replaced has also resulted in a cure for some clients (Cotran et al., 1994). Cost,

availability, and complications limit this technique for treatment of aplastic anemia, however.

Polycythemia

In polycythemia, the number of RBCs in whole blood is greater than normal. Polycythemia is characterized by hyperviscosity, or increased blood thickness. The problem may be transitory, subsequent to other conditions, or chronic. One type of polycythemia, polycythemia vera (PV), is fatal if left untreated.

Polycythemia Vera

Overview

Polycythemia vera is characterized by a sustained increase in blood hemoglobin concentration to 18 g/dL, a red blood cell (RBC) count of 6 million/mm³, or a hematocrit increase to 55% or greater. PV is an RBC malignancy with three major hallmarks: unrestrained production of massive numbers of RBCs, excessive leukocyte production, and overproduction of thrombocytes. As described in Chart 42–6, extreme hypercellularity of the peripheral blood occurs in people with PV. The skin, especially facial, and mucous membranes have a dark, flushed (plethoric) appearance. These areas may appear purplish or cyanotic because the blood in these tissues is incompletely oxygenated. Most clients experience intense itching related to vasodilation and variation in tissue oxygenation. Blood viscosity is also greatly increased, causing a corresponding increase in vascular friction and peripheral resistance. Superficial veins are visibly distended. Blood moves more slowly through all tissues and thus places increased demands on the pumping action of the heart, resulting in hypertension. In some highly vascular areas, blood flow may become so slow that vascular stasis occurs. Vascular stasis causes thrombosis within the smaller vessels to the extent that the vessels are occluded and the surrounding tissues experience hypoxia, progressing to anoxia and further to infarction and necrosis. Tissues

---

Chart 42–6

Key Features of Polycythemia Vera

- Persistently elevated hematocrit value (>55%)
- Hypertension
- Dark, flushed appearance of the hands and face
- Distention of superficial veins
- Weight loss
- Fatigue
- Intense itching
- Enlarged hemorrhoids
- Swollen, painful joints
- Enlarged, firm spleen
- Infarctions of the heart
  - Chest pain
  - Congestive heart failure
- Cerebrovascular accidents
- Bleeding tendency

most prone to this complication are the heart, spleen, and kidneys, although infarction with loss of tissue and organ function can occur in any organ or tissue.

Because the actual number of cells in the blood is greatly increased and the cells are not completely normal, individual cell life spans are shorter. The shorter life spans, coupled with increased cell production, result in a rapid turnover of peripheral blood cells. This rapid turnover increases the amount of intracellular products (released when cells die) in the blood, adding to the general "sludging" of the blood. These products include uric acid and potassium, which can cause the associated symptoms of gout and hyperkalemia.

Later clinical manifestations of PV are related to abnormal blood cells. Even though the number of circulating erythrocytes is greatly increased, their oxygen-binding capacity is impaired, and clients experience severe generalized hypoxia. In spite of the RBC excess, most clients with PV are susceptible to bleeding problems because of an apparent associated platelet dysfunction (Cotran et al., 1994).

Collaborative Management

Polycythemia vera is a malignant disease that progresses in severity over time. If left untreated, few people with PV live longer than 2 years. Conservative management with repeated phlebotomies (two to five times per week) can prolong life for 5 to 10 years. (Phlebotomy is the routine collection of the client's RBCs to decrease the number of RBCs and diminish blood viscosity.) Maintaining adequate hydration and promoting venous return are essential to prevent thrombus formation. Therapy aims to prevent clot formation and includes the use of anticoagulants. Chart 42–7 lists preventive tips for clients with PV.

As the disease progresses, clients need more intensive therapies that suppress bone marrow activity, including oral alkylating agents and/or irradiation with injections of radioactive phosphorus. Allogeneic bone marrow transplantation, an experimental treatment, is promising, but the results are too limited to determine its application to PV.

WHITE BLOOD CELL DISORDERS

As discussed in Chapter 23, white blood cells (WBCs or leukocytes) provide protection from invading non-self cells and cancer cells in several ways. These protective functions depend on maintaining normal numbers and ratios of many specific mature, circulating leukocytes. When any one type of WBC is present in either abnormally high or low amounts, hematopoietic function and immune function may be altered to some degree, placing clients at risk for specific complications. This section covers the pathologic changes and nursing care requirements for clients with disorders characterized by overgrowth of specific types of WBCs. (See Chapter 25 for the pathologic alterations and care requirements for clients with leukocyte-related problems of immunodeficiency, allergy, and autoimmune disorders.)

Leukemia

Overview

The leukemias are a group of malignant disorders involving abnormal overproduction of a specific WBC type, usually at an immature stage, in the bone marrow. Leukemia may be acute, with a sudden onset and short duration, or chronic, with a slow onset and persistent symptoms over a period of years.

Leukemias are categorized by the specific maturational pathway from which the abnormal cells arose (Devine & Larson, 1994). Leukemias in which the abnormal cells arise from within the committed lymphoid maturational pathways (see Figure 23–3) are lymphocytic or lymphoblastic. Leukemias in which the abnormal cells arise within the committed myeloid maturational pathways are myelocytic or myelogenous. Several subtypes exist for each of these diseases, classified by the degree of maturity of the abnormal cell and the specific cell type involved (Table 42–4).

Pathophysiology

The basic pathologic defect in leukemia is a malignant transformation of the stem cells or early committed precursor leukocyte cells, causing an abnormal proliferation of a specific type of leukocyte. The functionally and structurally abnormal immature leukocytes, produced in excessive quantities in the bone marrow, essentially shut down normal bone marrow production of erythrocytes, platelets, and other functionally mature leukocytes. This situation leads to anemia, thrombocytopenia, and leukopenia of the unaffected WBC types, even though the number of immature, abnormal WBCs in the circulation is greatly elevated. Unless treatment is instituted, clients usually die from infection or hemorrhage. For clients with acute leukemias, these pathologic changes occur rapidly and, without intervention, progress quickly to death. Chronic

---

Chart 42–7
Education Guide: Polycythemia Vera
• Drink at least 3 L of liquids each day.
• Avoid tight or constrictive clothing, especially garters or girdles.
• Wear gloves when outdoors in temperatures lower than 50° F.
• Keep all health care–related appointments.
• Contact your physician at the first sign of infection.
• Take anticoagulants as ordered.
• Wear support hose or stockings while you are awake and up.
• Elevate your feet whenever you are seated.
• Exercise slowly and only on the advice of your physician.
• Stop activity at the first sign of chest pain.
• Use an electric razor, not a manual one.
• Use a soft-bristled toothbrush to brush your teeth.
• Do not floss between your teeth.

TABLE 42–4

Differentiating Characteristics of the Four Types of Leukemia

Leukemia Type	Age at Onset (yr)	Gender Predilection	Racial Predilection	Cell of Origin	Specific Markers	Comments
Acute lymphocytic (ALL)	• <15	• Males	• Caucasian	• B cell	• CALLA+ • Hyperdiploidy • TDT+	• Prognosis poorer for adults than for children • Prognosis better than in AML • Curable in children
Acute myelogenous (AML)	• 15–39	• Equal incidence	• None	• Myeloblast • Myelocyte • Promyelocyte • Myelomonocyte	• TDT− • t(9;22) • t(15;17)	• Prognosis generally poor • Heterogeneous tumor cell populations • Best prognosis with bone marrow transplant
Chronic myelogenous (CML)	• >50	• Males	• None	• Myeloid cell	• Ph^1 chromosome	• Prognosis generally poor; worse if no Ph^1 chromosome • No blockage of maturation of nonmalignant leukocytes • Blastic crisis indicative of more acute disease
Chronic lymphocytic (CLL)	• >50	• Males	• Caucasian	• B cell	• Trisomy 12	• Prognosis poor • Long (4–10 yr) course with rare conversion to acute form • Only leukemia with a possible genetic predisposition

leukemia may be present for many years before overt pathologic changes occur.

Etiology

Epidemiologic studies suggest that many different genetic and environmental factors may be involved in the development of leukemia. Although only a few of these factors have been definitely identified, the basic mechanism appears to involve gene damage of cells, leading to transformation of those cells from a normal to a malignant state. The following constitute possible risk factors: ionizing radiation, chemicals and drugs, marrow hypoplasia, environmental interactions, genetic factors, viral factors, immunologic factors, and the interaction of these factors (Callaghan, 1996).

Ionizing radiation exposure in large quantities appears to be a major risk factor. Exposures ranging from therapeutic irradiation (for such diseases as ankylosing spondylitis and Hodgkin's lymphoma) to environmental irradiation (such as the atomic bomb at Hiroshima or the nuclear accident at Chernobyl) are associated with leukemia.

Chemicals and drugs have been linked to the development of leukemia. Table 41–3 lists many common offenders.

Marrow hypoplasia can increase the risk of leukemia. A reduction or alteration in the production of hematopoietic cells may be responsible. Examples of conditions associated with the later development of leukemia include Fanconi's syndrome, paroxysmal nocturnal hemoglobinuria during its aplastic phase, and myelodysplastic syndromes (Callaghan, 1996).

Genetic factors are suspected as a cause of leukemia because of the increased frequency of leukemia in the following populations: identical twins of clients with leukemia and people with Down syndrome, Bloom syndrome, Fanconi's syndrome, and Klinefelter's syndrome. Chromosomal aberration may be an important factor in these syndromes.

Immunologic factors, especially immune deficiencies, may also favor the development of leukemia. Leukemia among immunodeficient people may be a result of immunosurveillance failure, or the pathologic mechanisms that cause the immune deficiency may also trigger malignant transformation of leukopoietic cells.

Interaction of multiple host and environmental factors may result in leukemia. Because each person tolerates the interaction of these factors differently, it is difficult to determine the origin of any specific leukemia.

Incidence/Prevalence

The leukemias account for 2% of all newly diagnosed cases of cancer and 4% of all cancer deaths (American Cancer Society, 1998). The incidence and frequency of leukemia depend on many factors, including the type of WBC affected, age, gender, race, and geographic locale.

In the United States, an estimated 28,700 new cases of leukemia were projected for 1998 (American Cancer Society, 1998). In this country, leukemia is categorized into any one of four basic types based on the cell type affected and the rate of progression of the leukemia. Characteris-

tics and risk factors associated with these four types of leukemia are presented in Table 42–4.

1. *Acute myelogenous leukemia* (AML) occurs with similar frequency in all ages and is the most common form of leukemia in adults.
2. *Acute lymphocytic leukemia* (ALL) constitutes about 10% of adult leukemias but is most common in children.
3. *Chronic myelogenous leukemia* (CML) constitutes about 20% of adult leukemias, occurring more frequently in people older than 50 years.
4. *Chronic lymphocytic leukemia* (CLL) is the rarest type of leukemia, occurring primarily in people older than 50 years.

Collaborative Management

 Assessment

➤ History

The nurse asks the client about risk factors and causative factors. Age is important because the incidence of adult leukemia increases with age. The client's occupation and hobbies may also reveal specific environmental exposures that increase the risk of leukemia. Previous illnesses and medical history may indicate exposure to ionizing radiation or medications that increase risk as well.

Because of leukemia-related alterations of immune function, the risk for infection is increased in the client with leukemia. The nurse asks the client about the frequency and severity of infectious processes (such as colds, influenza, pneumonia, bronchitis, and unexplained episodes of fever) during the preceding 6 months.

Because platelet function may be diminished in people with leukemia, the nurse questions the client about any overt or hidden excessive bleeding episodes, such as

- A tendency to bruise easily
- Nosebleeds
- Increased menstrual flow
- Bleeding from the gums
- Rectal bleeding
- Hematuria (blood in the urine)
- Prolonged bleeding after minor abrasions or lacerations

If the client has experienced such an episode, the nurse asks whether this type and extent of bleeding constitute the client's usual response to injury or represent a change.

The client with leukemia frequently experiences weakness and fatigue resulting from anemia and increased metabolic and energy demands of the leukemic cells. The nurse asks the client whether he or she has experienced any of the following:

- Headaches
- Behavior changes
- Increased somnolence
- Decreased alertness
- Decreased attention span
- Lethargy, muscle weakness
- Diminished appetite

- Weight loss
- Increased fatigue

Listing activities in the previous 24 hours may disclose additional information about activity intolerance, changes in behavior, and unexplained fatigue. The nurse determines how long the client has had any of these debilitating symptoms.

➤ Physical Assessment/Clinical Manifestations

Because leukemia affects all blood cells, and blood influences the health and functional capacity of all organs and systems, many areas remote from the actual site of origin of malignant cells may be affected (Chart 42–8). The following clinical manifestations are associated with the acute leukemias (Cotran et al., 1994). Some of these findings may also be present in the client with chronic leukemia in the blast phase.

Cardiovascular Manifestations. These are usually related to anemia. The client's heart rate may be increased and blood pressure decreased. Murmurs and bruits may be present. Capillary filling time is increased.

Respiratory Manifestations. These are primarily associated with anemia and infectious complications. The client's respiratory rate increases as the degree of anemia becomes greater. If respiratory tract infections are present, the client may experience signs and symptoms of pneumonia, including cough and shortness of breath. Abnormal breath sounds are present on auscultation.

Integumentary Manifestations. The client's skin and mucous membranes may manifest abnormalities. The skin may be pale and cool to the touch as a result of accompanying anemia. Pallor is especially evident on the face, around the mouth, and in the nail beds. The conjunctiva of the eye also is pale, as are the creases on the palmar surface of the hand (most evident when the skin over the palm of the hand is stretched). Petechiae (raised red spots) may be present on any area of skin surface, especially the lower extremities. The petechiae may be unrelated to any obvious trauma. The nurse carefully inspects for any skin infections or traumatized areas that have failed to heal. The nurse also inspects the client's mouth for evidence of bleeding from the gums and any sore or lesion of the oral cavity indicating infection.

Gastrointestinal Manifestations. Gastrointestinal manifestations may be related to increased bleeding tendency and to fatigue. Weight loss, nausea, and anorexia are common. The nurse examines the rectal area for fissures and tests the stool for occult blood. Many clients with leukemia have diminished bowel sounds and constipation. Enlargement of the liver and spleen and abdominal tenderness also may be present from leukemic infiltration of abdominal viscera.

Central Nervous System Manifestations. Cranial nerve disturbances, headache, and papilledema as a result of leukemic infiltration of the meninges or central nervous system (CNS) and, in advanced cases, seizure activity and coma may occur. Although clients often have fever, this manifestation may be more a response to infection than to malignant changes in the CNS.

Miscellaneous Manifestations. Other manifestations include bone and joint tenderness as a result of marrow involvement and bone resorption. Leukemic cell growth or infiltration may produce enlarged lymph nodes or masses.

➤ Psychosocial Assessment

The client with newly diagnosed leukemia is extremely anxious, because the average layperson equates a diagnosis of any cancer with a death sentence. Current therapies have greatly improved the prognoses of most cancers, yet the public is largely unaware of these advances. The nurse spends time with the client and family to ascertain what the diagnosis means to them and what they expect from the future. Without knowing the client's expectations and feelings, the nurse cannot educate and provide support in an individualized manner or develop a meaningful plan of care.

A diagnosis of leukemia has dramatic implications for a client's lifestyle. Hospitalization for initial treatment often lasts several weeks, and clients become bored, lonely, and isolated. The nurse assesses the client's coping patterns, including activities that the client finds enjoyable and

---

Chart 42–8

Key Features of Acute Leukemia

Integumentary Manifestations
- Ecchymoses
- Petechiae
- Open infected lesions
- Pallor of the conjunctiva, nail beds, and palmar creases and around the mouth

Gastrointestinal Manifestations
- Bleeding gums
- Anorexia
- Weight loss
- Enlarged liver and spleen

Renal Manifestations
- Hematuria

Cardiovascular Manifestations
- Tachycardia at basal activity levels
- Orthostatic hypotension
- Palpitations

Respiratory Manifestations
- Dyspnea on exertion

Neurologic Manifestations
- Fatigue
- Headache
- Fever

Musculoskeletal Manifestations
- Bone pain
- Joint swelling and pain

methods that help the client to relax. A care plan to prevent diversional activity deficit is particularly beneficial for such clients. After initial therapy, the client may be able to resume work, depending on the occupation. However, the client often must make adjustments to accommodate changes in functional status. Repeated hospitalizations may also be necessary.

➤ Laboratory Assessment

The client with acute leukemia usually has decreased hemoglobin and hematocrit levels, a decreased platelet count, and an altered white blood cell (WBC) count. The WBC count may be low, normal, or elevated but usually is quite elevated; counts of 20,000 to 100,000 are common. The client with a higher WBC count on diagnosis has a poorer prognosis (Callaghan, 1996).

The definitive test for leukemia includes various examinations of cells obtained from bone marrow aspiration and biopsy. The bone marrow is full of leukemic blast phase cells. The composition of various cell surface proteins (antigens) on the leukemic cells helps diagnose the type of leukemia (Devine & Larson, 1994). Such markers include the T-11 protein, the enzyme terminal deoxynucleotidyl transferase (TDT), and the common acute lymphoblastic leukemia antigen (CALLA). These markers also indicate prognosis.

Coagulation variables are usually abnormal for the client with acute leukemia. Reduced levels of fibrinogen and other coagulation factors are typical. Whole blood clotting time (Lee-White clotting test) is increased, as is the activated partial thromboplastin time (PTT).

Chromosomal analysis of the malignant bone marrow cells may identify specific marker chromosomes to assist in the diagnosis of leukemia type, predict prognosis, and determine the effectiveness of therapy.

➤ Radiographic Assessment

Specific symptoms determine the feasibility of specific tests. For instance, a client with dyspnea needs chest radiography to determine whether leukemic infiltrates are present in the lung. Skeletal x-rays may help to determine the degree of bone reabsorption present with subperiosteal involvement.

 Analysis

➤ Common Nursing Diagnoses and Collaborative Problems

The following nursing diagnoses are commonly seen in adult clients with acute myelogenous leukemia (AML), the most common type of adult leukemia:

1. Risk for Infection related to decreased immune response
2. Risk for Injury related to thrombocytopenia
3. Fatigue related to decreased tissue oxygenation and increased energy demands

The primary collaborative problem is Potential for Antineoplastic Therapy Adverse Effects.

➤ Additional Nursing Diagnoses and Collaborative Problems

In addition, many clients with AML have one or more of the following nursing diagnoses:

- Impaired Skin Integrity related to prolonged immobility
- Altered Oral Mucous Membrane related to effects of chemotherapy and pancytopenia
- Total Self-Care Deficit related to progressive debilitation and weakness
- Altered Nutrition: Less than Body Requirements related to anorexia, nausea, and vomiting
- Anxiety related to fear of death
- Powerlessness related to an inability to control disease progression
- Altered Family Processes related to acute, life-threatening illness of a family member
- Altered Role Performance related to perceived inability to fulfill parental and other family roles and prolonged hospitalization
- Diversional Activity Deficit related to prolonged hospitalizations.

 Planning and Implementation

Risk for Infection

Planning: Expected Outcomes. After intervention, the client is expected to

- Remain free from cross-contamination–induced infection
- Remain free of autocontamination-induced infection
- Not experience sepsis

Interventions. Infection is a major cause of death in the immunosuppressed client, and septicemia is a common sequela. Infection of the client with leukemia occurs through both *autocontamination* (the client's normal flora overgrows and penetrates the internal environment) and *cross-contamination* (microorganisms from another person or the environment are transmitted to the client). The three most common sites of infection are the skin, respiratory tract, and gastrointestinal tract.

Gram-negative bacteria frequently cause infection, although gram-positive and fungal infections do occur (Dean, Haeuber, & Rivera, 1996). Interventions aim to interrupt or halt the infection processes and control specific infections early. Chart 42–9 emphasizes the importance of thorough assessment for the client at risk for infection. The accompanying client care plan outlines specific interventions for the client with AML.

Drug Therapy for Leukemia. Drug therapy for clients with AML is divided into three distinctive phases: induction, consolidation, and maintenance.

Induction Therapy. This is intensive and consists of combination chemotherapy initiated at the time of diagnosis. This therapy is aimed at achieving a rapid, complete remission of all manifestations of disease (Wujcik, 1996). Institutions and physicians differ in agents used

Chart 42–9

Focused Assessment for Hospitalized or Home Care Clients with Potential or Actual Risk for Infection

General Condition

Age, fatigue, malaise
History of allergies
History of chemotherapy, radiation therapy, or other immunosuppressive therapies such as steroid use
Chronic diseases
History of febrile neutropenia and associated symptoms
Nutritional status
Functional status—problems with immobility
Tobacco use—cigarettes, pipe, cigars, oral
Recreational drug use
Alcohol use
Prescribed and over-the-counter medication use
Baseline and ongoing vital signs—blood pressure, heart rate, respiratory rate, and temperature

Skin and Mucous Membranes

Thorough inspection of all skin surfaces with special attention to axilla, perineum (particularly the anorectal area), and under breasts. Inspect skin for color, vascularity, bleeding, lesions, edema, moist areas, excoriation, irritation, erythema. General condition of hair and nails, pressure areas, swelling, pain, tenderness, biopsy or surgical sites, wounds, enlarged lymph nodes, catheters, or other devices
Inspect the oral cavity, including lips, tongue, mucous membranes, gingiva, teeth, and throat—color, moisture, bleeding, ulcerations, lesions, exudate, mucositis, stomatitis, placque, swelling, pain, tenderness, taste changes, amount and character of saliva, ability to swallow, changes in voice, dental caries, client's oral hygiene routine
History of current skin disorders or problems with the mucous membranes

Head, Eyes, Ears, Nose

Pain, tenderness, exudate, crusting, enlarged lymph nodes

Cardiopulmonary

Respiratory rate and pattern, breath sounds (presence/absence, adventitious sounds), quantity and characteristics of sputum, shortness of breath, use of accessory muscles, dysphagia, diminished gag reflex, tachycardia, blood pressure

Gastrointestinal

Pain, diarrhea, bowel sounds, character and frequency of bowel movements, constipation, rectal bleeding, hemorrhoids, change in bowel habits, sexual practices, erythema, ulceration

Genitourinary

Dysuria, frequency, urgency, hematuria, pruritus, pain, vaginal or penile discharge, vaginal bleeding, burning, lesions, ulcerations, characteristics of urine

Central Nervous System

Cognition, level of consciousness, personality, behavior

Musculoskeletal

Tenderness, pain, loss of function

Modified from Dean, G. E., Haeuber, D., & Rivera, L. M. (1996). Infection. In R. McCorkle, M. Grant, M. Frank-Stromborg, & S. Baird (Eds.), *Cancer nursing: A comprehensive textbook* (2nd ed., p. 975). Philadelphia: W. B. Saunders. Used with permission.

and the treatment schedule, but a typical course of aggressive chemotherapy includes intravenous (IV) administration of cytosine arabinoside (at 100–200 mg/m² of body surface area per day) for 7 days with concomitant administration of daunorubicin (45 mg/m²/per day) for the first 3 days (Devine & Larson, 1994).

A major side effect of these agents is severe bone marrow suppression. As a result, the client becomes even more vulnerable to infection than before the treatment started. Prolonged hospitalizations are common while the client is immunosuppressed. Recovery of hematopoiesis requires at least 2 to 3 weeks, during which time the client must be protected from life-threatening infections. Other adverse reactions include nausea, vomiting, diarrhea, alopecia (hair loss), stomatitis, renal toxicity, hepatic toxicity, and cardiac toxicity. For information on nursing management of adverse reactions to antineoplastic agents, refer to Chapter 27.

Consolidation Therapy. This usually consists of another course of either the same agents used for induction at a different dosage or a different combination of chemotherapeutic agents. This treatment occurs early in remission, and its intent is to cure (Ong & Larson, 1995). At

Text continued on page 971

Client Care Plan

The Client with Acute Myelogenous Leukemia

Nursing Diagnosis No. 1: Risk for Infection related to decreased immune response

Expected Outcomes	Nursing Interventions	Rationale
The client is expected to remain free from cross-contamination–induced infection. ■ Limits close contact with other people ■ Maintains a core body temperature of < 100° F (38° C) ■ Does not have pathogenic organisms in cultures of blood, urine, or wound drainage	■ Initiate protective isolation procedures according to institutional policy (e.g., thorough hand washing between clients, reverse isolation, private room, wear masks). ■ Keep supplies for the client (e.g., paper cups, straws, dressing materials, gloves) separate from supplies for other clients. ■ Limit the number of care personnel entering the client's room. ■ Have the client maintained in a private room. ■ Limit visitors to healthy adults. ■ Reduce exposure to environmental microorganisms by eliminating raw fruits and vegetables in the client's diet and by not having standing water in the client's room (e.g., remove vases, humidifiers, and water games). ■ Clean the client's room at least once per day.	■ These procedures reduce the number of vector-transmissible microorganisms. ■ Separation of these supplies limits the potential for cross-contamination infection. ■ This precaution decreases the client's exposure to non-self microorganisms. ■ Isolation reduces traffic and exposure to non-self microorganisms. ■ This precaution prevents transmission of microorganisms by small children, who may incubate microorganisms and inadvertently transmit them to the client by not adhering to infection control procedures. ■ These measures prevent contact with potentially harmful microorganisms. ■ A clean environment inhibits proliferation of environmental microorganisms.
The client is expected to remain free from auto-contamination–induced infection. ■ Complies with prescribed hygiene measures ■ Maintains a core body temperature of < 100° F (38° C) ■ Does not have pathogenic organisms in cultures of blood, urine, or wound drainage	■ Instruct or assist the client with daily bathing using antimicrobial soap. ■ Touch the client gently to avoid injuring the skin. ■ Instruct and assist the client to perform oral hygiene every 4 hours, including the use of antimicrobial rinses, mouth swabs, and moisturizing rinses. ■ Change IV tubing every 48 hours.	■ Antisepsis reduces microorganisms on skin surfaces. ■ Keeping the skin intact prevents new portals of entry for microorganisms. ■ Proper hygiene reduces the number of oral tract microorganisms. ■ Fresh tubing reduces the risk for contamination.

(Continued)

Client Care Plan

Nursing Diagnosis No. 1: Risk for Infection related to decreased immune response

Expected Outcomes	Nursing Interventions	Rationale
	■ Prevent rectal trauma by initiating a bowel program, including stool softeners and laxatives and sitz baths. ■ Change wound dressings daily, teaching the client or performing central venous catheter site care per institutional protocol. ■ Teach client to identify signs and symptoms of infections and instruct him or her to inform a health care professional should any new symptom occur. ■ Avoid invasive procedures, such as injections, rectal temperatures, and urinary catheterization. ■ Encourage the client to cough and deep breathe; counsel regarding smoking cessation.	■ Preventing constipation reduces intestinal stasis and bacterial overgrowth. ■ Fresh dressings reduce the number of colony-forming microorganisms at the site of a portal of entry and allow inspection of the site for signs and symptoms of infection. ■ Often clients are more in touch with subtle changes that occur to their own person. Involving the client can help with early detection of infection. ■ Invasive procedures and trauma can disrupt mucosal linings and skin, resulting in a portal of entry for infectious organisms. ■ These measures help to prevent respiratory infection.

The client is expected to not experience septicemia.
■ Does not experience a "left shift" in white blood cell (WBC) populations
■ Maintains a core body temperature of <100° F (38° C)
■ Does not have pathogenic organisms in cultures of blood, urine, or wound drainage
■ Maintains a pulse rate and blood pressure (BP) within normal limits
	■ Assess the client for signs and symptoms of infection.
	  ■ Measure oral temperature q4h.
	  ■ Inspect wound areas for redness, swelling, or drainage q8h.
	  ■ Auscultate lungs q8h.
	  ■ Check urine for odor and cloudiness.
	  ■ Monitor pulse and BP q4h.
	■ Monitor the differential WBC, especially the absolute neutrophil count (ANC).
	
	■ If symptoms of infection are present, notify the physician immediately and be prepared to
	  ■ Obtain blood specimens through the venous access device and the peripheral vein before antibiotic therapy is initiated.
		■ These assessments identify the infectious process early so that appropriate interventions can be initiated.
		
		■ These values determine the client's risk for infection and indicate a return of immune function.
		■ Appropriate treatment can be instituted:
		
		  ■ It is important to determine whether microorganisms are present in the blood and whether the venous access device is the source of contamination.

(Continued)

Client Care Plan

Nursing Diagnosis No. 1: Risk for Infection related to decreased immune response

Expected Outcomes	Nursing Interventions	Rationale
	■ Obtain specimens for culture of open lesions, urine, and sputum.	■ It is important to determine the origin of the infection and to identify the infecting organism.
	■ Administer prescribed antibiotic, antifungal, and/or antiviral therapy.	■ These therapeutic measures limit proliferation of microorganisms within the client and prevent progression to sepsis.
The client is expected to not experience injury. ■ Has intact skin and mucous membranes ■ Manifests no bruising or petechiae ■ Does not participate in activities that increase the risk for falls and other injuries	■ Handle the client gently.	■ Gentle handling prevents trauma to sensitive tissues.
	■ Use soft-bristle toothbrush or sponge tooth cleaners. Avoid dental floss.	■ It is important to prevent damage to oral mucous membranes.
	■ Avoid intravenous, intramuscular, and subcutaneous injections.	■ Avoiding injections prevents trauma to the skin and bleeding.
	■ Apply firm but gentle pressure to a needlestick site for at least 10 minutes after removal of the needle.	■ Gentle pressure prevents excessive capillary blood loss.
	■ Offer soft foods cool to warm in temperature.	■ These dietary measures avoid mucous membrane injury.
	■ Permit the client to use only an electric razor for shaving.	■ Electric razors reduce the risk for abrasions or lacerations.
	■ Pad side rails and sharp corners of bed.	■ Padding reduces the risk of contusion injuries.
	■ Remove extra furniture from the client's room.	■ Removing extra furniture increases the client's space and reduces the risk of bumping into environmental objects and becoming injured.
	■ Discourage the client from engaging in activities involving the use of sharp objects (e.g., hand sewing, whittling).	■ Eliminating sharp objects in hobbies reduces the risk of injury.
	■ Use soft cloths, mild soap, and a light touch when bathing the client.	■ These measures prevent abrasion injury.
	■ Avoid dressing the client in clothing that is tight or rubs.	■ Loose clothing reduces risk for abrasion injury.
	■ Avoid taking blood pressures with a standard, external, inflatable cuff.	■ It is important to prevent skin injury from cuff pressure.
	■ Instruct the client to avoid blowing or picking the nose.	■ It is important to minimize the risk of trauma to nasal mucous membranes.
	■ Avoid rectal suppositories, enemas, and rectal thermometers.	■ Rectal mucosa bleeds easily; avoiding these items prevents rectal trauma.

(Continued)

Client Care Plan

Nursing Diagnosis No. 1: Risk for Infection related to decreased immune response

Expected Outcomes	Nursing Interventions	Rationale

The client is expected to not experience significant blood loss.
■ Has normal hematocrit and hemoglobin values
■ Has no manifestation of overt bleeding from wounds or body orifices
	■ Examine the client q4h for signs and symptoms of bleeding, including
	  ■ Increase in abdominal girth
	  ■ Presence of petechiae
	  ■ Oozing from mucous membranes
		■ These measures help determine sites and extent of bleeding.

Nursing Diagnosis No. 2: Risk for Injury related to excessive bleeding secondary to thrombocytopenia

Expected Outcomes	Nursing Interventions	Rationale

■ Maintains pulse rate and BP within normal limits	■ Increase in bruise size
	■ Drainage on dressings and around IV sites
	■ Scleral hemorrhage
	■ Persistent headaches
	■ Vaginal or rectal bleeding
	■ Epistaxis
	■ Examine all body fluids and excrement for the presence of overt or occult blood.
	  ■ Vomitus
	  ■ Urine
	  ■ Stool
	■ Administer ice and topical agents (e.g., Gelfoam, thrombin) to wound sites.
	■ When the client is menstruating, count the number of pads or tampons used and weigh each before and after use.
	
	■ Administer oral medications to stop menses.
	■ Instruct the client in the signs and symptoms of overt and occult hemorrhage.
	
	■ Instruct the client to avoid drug products that contain aspirin and nonsteroidal antiinflammatory drugs (NSAIDs).
	■ Monitor laboratory values (e.g., platelet count, hematocrit, coagulation studies).
	
	■ Administer blood products as ordered.
		■ Ice and topical agents promote blood clotting at the wound site.
		■ Noting the number of pads and tampons used during menstruation can help determine the rate and amount of blood loss.
		■ Interrupting menstruation prevents excessive blood loss.
		■ If clients know the signs and symptoms of overt hemorrhage, they can participate in self-care and accept responsibility in health maintenance.
		■ Aspirin and NSAIDs may trigger bleeding episodes. Limiting their use can prevent excess bleeding.
		■ Laboratory findings can pinpoint potential and actual blood loss and help to determine the need for blood product replacement therapy.
		■ This will provide cells necessary for coagulation and tissue oxygenation.

(Continued)

Client Care Plan

Nursing Diagnosis No. 3: Fatigue related to anemia and increased energy demands

Expected Outcomes	Nursing Interventions	Rationale
The client is expected to be able to participate in some self-care activities without becoming excessively fatigued. ■ Verbalizes symptoms of mild fatigue ■ Performs self-care activities within limitations ■ Identifies alternative means of performing daily activities that require less energy than normal	■ Assist the client in selecting food items high in protein and calories. ■ Provide small meals that require little chewing. ■ Administer blood products as ordered. ■ Assist the client in turning and self-care activities. ■ Allow the client to rest between nursing interventions. ■ Cancel activities not essential to the client's immediate well-being.	■ High-protein and high-calorie foods restore nutritional balance and increase available energy substrates. ■ Small meals prevent the client from becoming fatigued while eating. ■ Blood products replace red blood cells and hemoglobin, ameliorating anemia and decreasing fatigue. ■ These measures conserve the client's energy. ■ Rest conserves the client's energy. ■ Eliminating nonessential activities conserves the client's energy.

some institutions, consolidation therapy is a single course of chemotherapy; at others, it involves regularly scheduled, repeated courses of chemotherapy over 1 to 2 years.

Maintenance Therapy. This may be prescribed for months to years after successful induction and consolidation therapies. The purpose is to maintain the remission achieved through induction and consolidation. Maintenance agents are milder and are often given orally for 2 to 5 years. There are conflicting data regarding the effectiveness of maintenance therapy. Future research will help to determine the benefit of different maintenance protocols on the various types of leukemia (Callaghan, 1996).

WOMEN'S HEALTH CONSIDERATIONS

Pregnancy may increase a woman's risk of developing leukemia, although the current data are inconclusive. The diagnosis of acute leukemia during pregnancy forces a woman to face a difficult ethical dilemma regarding treatment. AML is fatal for the mother if not treated aggressively with chemotherapeutic agents, many of which are harmful and potentially lethal to the fetus. A review of the current literature suggests the following findings regarding chemotherapy treatment for AML during pregnancy:

■ Certain chemotherapeutic and supportive agents may be used judiciously in pregnant women.

■ First-trimester treatment can cause severe fetal malformation or miscarriage.
■ Normal live births to mothers treated after the first trimester are well documented.
■ Infants born to mothers treated during the second and third trimesters did not differ from those born to healthy mothers.
■ Side effects experienced by the mother, such as malnutrition, infection, and death, may harm the fetus.

Nursing care for the pregnant client with leukemia focuses on prevention of infection, bleeding, injury, and premature delivery. The nurse assists the client to maintain adequate nutrition and provides resources to help cope with a diagnosis that can be fatal to both the mother and fetus (Ramirez-Smiley & Ingle, 1995).

Drug Therapy for Infection. Drug therapy is the primary defense against infections that develop in clients undergoing therapy for AML. Agents used depend on the sensitivity of the specific organism causing the infection and the extent of the infection, and are categorized by specificity as antibacterial, antiviral, or antifungal. Figure 42-2 outlines pharmacologic management of the febrile neutropenic client.

Antibiotic and Antibacterial Agents. These agents used for prophylaxis or treatment of infection in clients with AML usually include at least one of the aminoglycosides (amikacin, gentamicin, and tobramycin) and a sys-

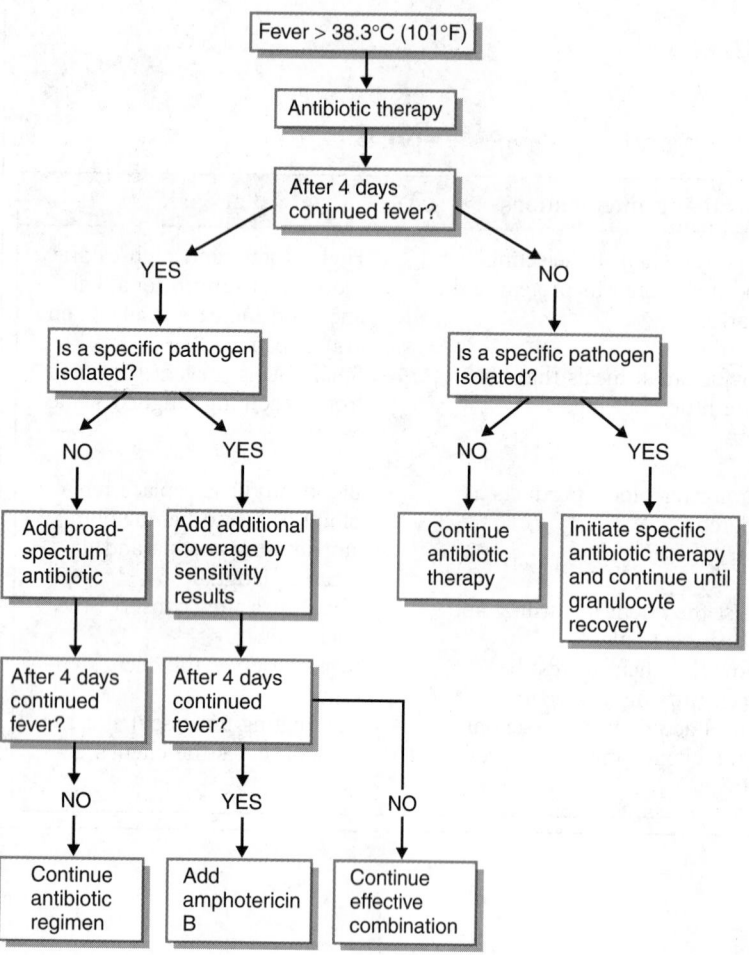

Figure 42–2. Example of antibiotic management for fever in the neutropenic patient.

temic penicillin. Additional, powerful antibiotics used may include vancomycin and drugs from the tetracycline and third-generation cephalosporin classes.

Antifungal Agents. Systemic antifungal agents, used when a fungal infection has been diagnosed or is strongly suggested, include amphotericin B, ketoconazole (Nizoral), and nystatin (Mycostatin, Nadostine✦, Nilstat). In neutropenic clients, antifungal creams such as miconazole nitrate are administered intravaginally to prevent yeast infections.

Antiviral Agents. These are commonly used in clients with leukemia to prevent and treat viral infections. Acyclovir is administered either orally or parenterally before the initiation of antineoplastic agents, especially in clients who are cytomegalovirus positive. If a viral infection is suspected or diagnosed with positive cultures, pharmacologic treatments may include ganciclovir, foscarnet, or steroids (Dean et al., 1996).

The antivirals, although helpful in combating severe infections, are associated with a wide range of serious adverse effects, especially ototoxicity and nephrotoxicity. The nurse carefully monitors the client treated with such drugs for signs of hearing impairment and renal insufficiency.

Infection Control. A major objective in caring for the leukemic client is protection from infection. Nurses and all assistive personnel must use extreme care during all nursing procedures. Frequent, thorough hand washing is of the utmost importance. Anyone with an upper respiratory tract infection who must enter the client's room must wear a mask. Nurses must also observe strict procedures when performing dressing changes or when assisting a physician insert a central venous catheter. The nurse maintains strict aseptic technique in the care of these catheters at all times.

If possible, the nurse ensures that a client is in a private room to minimize cross-contamination. Because infection in the immunosuppressed person is most commonly caused by normal body microorganisms, protective (reverse) isolation has been eliminated from the Centers for Disease Control and Prevention (CDC) guidelines for infection control. However, other environmental precautions are heeded, such as allowing no standing collections of water in vases, denture cups, or humidifiers in the client's room, because they are excellent breeding grounds for microorganisms.

Some institutions prescribe a "minimal bacteria diet" for the client during the neutropenic period. Any uncooked foods, such as raw fruit and vegetables, and pepper are eliminated from the diet because they contain large numbers of microorganisms. Whether clients benefit from this diet is controversial.

In some institutions, the immunosuppressed client is placed in a room with a high-efficiency particulate air (HEPA) filtration or laminar airflow system. These systems decrease the number of airborne pathogens. Again, whether these restrictions benefit clients is debatable.

The nurse continually assesses the client for the presence of infection. This task is difficult because manifestations of infection may not be obvious in the client with leukopenia. The development of fever and the formation of pus (both common indicators of infection) depend on the presence of leukocytes. Therefore, the leukopenic client may have severe infections without pus and with relatively low fevers.

The nurse monitors the client's daily complete blood count (CBC) with differential white blood cell (WBC) count. The nurse inspects the oral mucosa during every nursing shift for lesions indicating fungal or viral infection. The nurse also auscultates the client's lung sounds every 8 hours for crackles, wheezes, or diminished breath sounds. Each time the client voids, the nurse inspects the urine for odor and cloudiness, and then asks the client about any urgency, burning, or pain present on urination.

The nurse takes the client's vital signs at least every 4 hours to assess for fever. A temperature elevation of even 0.5° F or C above baseline is significant for a leukopenic client and indicates infection until proven otherwise.

Many hospital units that specialize in the care of the neutropenic client have specific protocols for antibiotic therapy if infection is suspected. Usually, physicians are notified immediately, and specific specimens are obtained for culture. Blood for bacterial and fungal cultures is obtained from peripheral sites and from the central venous catheter. Urine specimens, sputum specimens, and specimens from open lesions are taken for culture, and chest x-rays taken. After the specimens are obtained, the client begins a regimen of IV antibiotics.

Skin Care. This is important for preventing infection in the leukemic client. The skin may be the client's only intact defense. The nurse teaches the ambulatory client thorough hygiene care and encourages daily bathing. If the client is immobile, turning is necessary every hour and skin lubricants are applied.

Respiratory Care. Respiratory care, including pulmonary hygiene, is performed every 2 to 4 hours. The nurse auscultates the lungs for crackles, wheezes, or diminished breath sounds. The nurse encourages the client to cough and deep breathe or to perform sustained maximal inhalations every hour while awake.

Transplantation. This is now considered a standard treatment for the client with leukemia. This treatment modality began with allogeneic bone marrow transplantation (BMT) (transplantation of human leukocyte antigen [HLA]–identical bone marrow from a sibling) and has advanced to the use of HLA-matched marrow from unrelated donors (Viele, 1996). During the 1980s, autologous BMT was introduced. In this procedure, the donor's own marrow is harvested during a period of remission, frozen, and stored for transplant at a later date. All of these transplant procedures use stem cells harvested from bone marrow.

The newest type of transplantation, peripheral blood stem cell (PBSC) or peripheral blood progenitor cell (PBPC) transplantation, was introduced in the past decade. It involves use of stem cells obtained from the blood rather than the bone marrow (Ford et al., 1996). Multiple pheresis (removal of cells from the plasma) harvests stem cells from the client.

Advances in the field of transplantation have been remarkable. Even as recently as the late 1980s, the client undergoing transplantation would have been seen only in major medical centers. Today, transplant units are becoming commonplace, even in community hospital settings. With long-term survival after transplantation increasing, nurses can expect to be caring for these people if not during the actual transplantation or recovery period, then during the post-transplant period in a variety of health care settings.

Bone marrow transplantation is the treatment of choice for the client with leukemia who has a closely matched donor and who is experiencing temporary remission with induction therapy. Because of BMT success in the client with leukemia, this therapy is now being used for clients with lymphoma, aplastic anemia, inborn errors of metabolism, and many solid tumors (Ford et al., 1996).

For many malignant disorders, the dose-limiting toxicity of treatments is bone marrow suppression. The aim of BMT or PBSC transplantation is to rid the client of all leukemic or other malignant cells through high doses of chemotherapy, often in conjunction with whole body irradiation. These treatments are lethal to the bone marrow and, without replacement of bone marrow function through transplantation of progenitor cells of the hematopoietic system, the client would die of infection or hemorrhage.

The bone marrow is the actual site of production of leukemic cells. Because it can be difficult to ensure that all leukemic cells have been eradicated during induction therapy, the goal is for extremely high doses of chemotherapy to destroy all the affected marrow. The new, healthy marrow then begins the process of hematopoiesis, which results in normal, properly functioning cells and, it is hoped, a permanent cure.

Although marrow donated from a person whose human leukocyte antigens (HLA) match the those of the client is assumed to be disease free, autologous marrow, even if harvested during remission, may contain abnormal cells. In some centers, the harvested autologous marrow is "purged" with chemotherapy or monoclonal antibody treatments to remove any residual leukemia cells. It is not known whether clients who receive purged marrow have better long-term responses than those who receive untreated marrow (Viele, 1996).

Transplantation procedures have five phases: stem cell procurement, conditioning regimen, transplantation, engraftment, and post-transplantation recovery.

Obtaining Stem Cells. Stem cells for transplantation are obtained either by harvest of bone marrow or by pheresis for peripheral blood stem cells. Bone marrow is harvested either from the client directly (autologous marrow) or from an HLA-matched person (allogeneic marrow). For allogeneic marrow, a suitable donor is selected after family members are tested for HLA types. The most preferred transplantations are those between HLA-identical siblings, but transplantation can also be successful between those with closely matched HLA types. The chance of matching with any given sibling is 25%. Several donor registries have been formed that keep records of people willing to donate marrow to provide marrow for clients who do not have a family member HLA match.

After a suitable donor is identified by tissue typing, the donor is taken to the operating room, where sufficient marrow for transplant is harvested through multiple aspirations from the iliac crests. About 500 to 1000 mL of marrow is aspirated, approximately 3% to 5% of the donor's marrow supply (Whedon, 1991). The marrow is then filtered and may be further processed to purge the autologous marrow of any residual cancer cells or to deplete the allogeneic marrow of T cells, which may later cause graft-versus-host disease (GVHD) (described later). Allogeneic marrow is transfused into the recipient immediately; autologous marrow is frozen for later use.

The nurse monitors the donor for signs and symptoms of fluid loss, assesses for complications of anesthesia, and manages postoperative pain. During surgery, donors may lose a significant amount of fluid in addition to the volume of marrow donated. Donors are often hydrated with saline infusions before and immediately after surgery. Occasionally, the donor may require an infusion of packed RBCs.

The nurse assesses the harvest sites to ensure that the dressings are dry and intact and that the donor is not bleeding excessively. Donors often experience pain at the harvest sites (hip), usually managed effectively with oral non–aspirin-containing analgesics. Individual differences do occur, however. Some donors refuse pain medication, but others require opioid analgesics.

There are three phases to obtaining peripheral blood stem cells: mobilization, collection, and reinfusion. During the mobilization phase, chemotherapy or hematopoietic growth factors are administered to the client (Viele, 1996). These agents cause stem cells to circulate in the peripheral blood and the number of WBCs to increase. The stem cells are then collected by pheresis (Ford et al., 1996). Four to seven pheresis procedures, each lasting 2 to 4 hours, are usually required to obtain enough stem cells for PBSC transplantation (Jassak & Riley, 1994). The stem cells are then frozen and stored for reinfusion after the conditioning regimen.

The nurse must monitor the patient closely during pheresis. Common complications include catheter clotting, which may delay pheresis, or hypocalcemia caused by anticoagulants. The client with hypocalcemia may experience chills, paresthesia, abdominal or muscle cramping, or chest pain, and the nurse may need to administer oral calcium supplements to manage these symptoms. The nurse must also monitor vital signs frequently. The client may experience hypotension as a result of fluid volume changes during the procedure.

Conditioning Regimen. Figure 42–3 outlines the timing and steps typically involved in bone marrow transplantation. The day the client receives the bone marrow is considered day T-0. Pretransplantation conditioning days are counted in reverse chronologic order from T-0, just like a rocket countdown. Post-transplantation days are counted in chronologic order from day of transplantation to discharge.

The client must first undergo a conditioning regimen, which varies with the diagnosis and type of transplant to be received. The conditioning regimen serves two purposes: to obliterate, or "wipe out," the client's own bone marrow, thus preparing the client for optimal graft take, and to give higher than normal doses of chemotherapy and/or radiotherapy to obliterate, or wipe out, a malignancy, such as breast cancer. Usually, anywhere from 5 to 10 days is required. The conditioning regimen always includes intensive chemotherapy and sometimes includes radiotherapy, usually total body irradiation (TBI). Each conditioning regimen is individually tailored with the client's specific disease, overall health, and previous treatment taken into account.

A typical conditioning regimen for an adult client receiving an allogenic bone marrow transplant for treatment of acute myelogenous leukemia (AML) is as follows (Workman et al., 1993):

1. Days T-7 through T-5: high-dose chemotherapy to obliterate the client's own bone marrow cells and to eradicate any remaining leukemic cells. Specific agents include busulfan, carmustine, cyclophosphamide, cytosine arabinoside, etoposide, and melphalan. The dosages are many times higher than those used for normal chemotherapy (Ford et al., 1996).

2. Days T-4 through T-2: delivery of fractionated TBI (smaller doses of radiation given over a period of time instead of one larger dose). The typical radia-

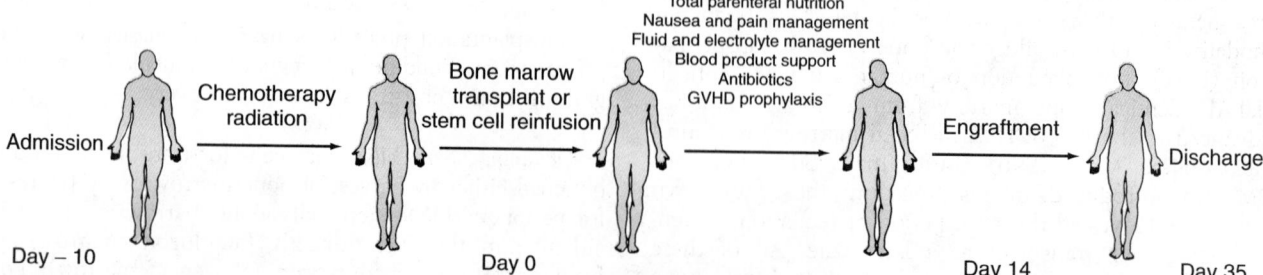

Figure 42–3. Timing and steps of allogeneic bone marrow transplantation. (GVHD = graft-versus-host disease.)

tion dose for TBI is 1200 rad. The client usually receives no cell-killing treatment on day T-1.

During conditioning, bone marrow and normal tissues begin to respond immediately to the chemotherapy and radiotherapy. The client experiences all the expected side effects associated with both therapies. Because the chemotherapy is administered in such high doses, these side effects are much more intense than those seen with either normal chemotherapy or radiation. These side effects include severe nausea and vomiting, mucositis, capillary leak syndrome, diarrhea, and bone marrow suppression.

Late effects from the conditioning regimen are also common, occurring as late as 3 to 10 years after transplantation, and include veno-occlusive disease (VOD), skin toxicities, cataracts, fibrotic pulmonary disease, secondary malignancies, cardiomyopathy, endocrine complications, and neurologic complications.

Transplantation. Day T-0, transplantation day, is separated from the chemotherapy conditioning by at least 2 days to ensure that the chemotherapeutic agent has cleared and will not exert any cytotoxic effects on the transplanted stem cells. The client should have few, if any, circulating WBCs at this point, indicating successful conditioning.

The transplantation itself is very simple. Frozen marrow or PBSCs are thawed in a warm water bath (37°–40° C [99°–102° F]) (Jassak & Riley, 1994). The bone marrow is administered through the client's central catheter like an ordinary blood transfusion but not using blood administration tubing. Usually, the marrow is infused over a 30-minute period, although it may also be administered by IV push directly into the central catheter with syringes.

Side effects of BMT and PBSC transfusion are similar. The client may experience fever and hypertension as a result of a reaction to dimethylsulfoxide (DMSO), the preservative used for storage of stem cells (Ford et al., 1996). To prevent these reactions, the nurse administers acetaminophen, hydrocortisone, and diphenhydramine before the transfusion. Antihypertensives or diuretics may also be required to treat fluid volume changes (Jassak & Riley, 1994). The client may experience red urine secondary to hemolysis of erythrocytes in the infused product.

Engraftment. The transfused PBSCs and marrow cells circulate only briefly in the peripheral blood. Most of the cells, especially the stems cells, find their way to the marrow-forming sites of the recipient's bones and establish residency there. The mechanism by which the donated marrow cells "home in" on the appropriate sites is not yet understood.

Engraftment is the key to the whole transplantation process. In order for the donated marrow or PBSCs to "rescue" the client after large doses of chemotherapy and/or radiotherapy wipe out his or her own bone marrow, the transfused stem cells must survive and grow in the clients' bone marrow sites. When successful, the engraftment process takes 2 to 5 weeks, when the client's WBC, erythrocyte, and platelet counts begin to rise.

Prevention of Complications. The post-transplantation period is difficult. Because the client remains without any natural immunity until the transfused stem cells begin to proliferate and engraftment occurs, infection and severe thrombocytopenia are major problems. The nursing care requirements for this client are virtually identical to those for the client undergoing aggressive induction therapy for AML. Helping the client to maintain hope through this long recovery period is difficult (Larson, 1995). Complications are often severe and life threatening. The nurse should try to encourage the client to maintain a positive attitude and be involved in his or her own recovery (Research Applications for Nursing).

In addition to the problems related to the period of pancytopenia (too few circulating blood cells), other immediate hazards associated with BMT include failure to engraft, development of GVHD, and VOD.

Failure to Engraft. Sometimes the donated marrow or PBSCs fail to engraft. This possibility is discussed in advance with the client and the donor. Failure to engraft occurs more frequently among allogeneic trans-

---

▷ Research Applications for Nursing

What Are the Client's Perceptions of Needs After Bone Marrow Transplantation?

Larson, P. J. (1995). Perceptions of the needs of hospitalized patients undergoing bone marrow transplantation. Cancer Practice, 3(3), 173–179.

This qualitative descriptive study identified patient needs during the first 4 weeks after bone marrow transplant (BMT). A sample of 30 patients were interviewed four times during their hospital stay at approximately 1-week intervals. A constant comparative analysis suggested the following care needs: week 1, team effort of cure; week 2, management of symptoms and side effects; week 3, getting better; week 4, recovery and returning home. Patients perceived that they, as well as physicians, nurses, and family, were responsible for meeting these needs.

Other findings included that patients viewed physicians as in charge of planning and monitoring medical care and verifying that progress was satisfactory. Nurses were perceived as "responsible for carrying out medical orders, managing symptoms, and keeping things in order." The patients wanted family members to be emotionally supportive and to take care of nonmedical needs. Patients perceived their own role as maintaining a positive attitude and participating in their recovery.

Critique. The study was an excellent attempt to capture patients' perceptions of care needs during hospitalization for BMT. The small sample size and the fact that interviews were only conducted at two West Coast BMT centers limited the generalizability of the results. This study further limited its scope to the short-term needs of hospitalized BMT patients. Additional studies are needed to assess patient needs over longer periods of time.

Possible Nursing Implications. Nurses can discuss with patients expectations of their care needs throughout the hospital stay. Helping patients maintain realistic self-expectations and hope is important. Nurses can also monitor emotionally and physically labile periods, which often occur at week 3 or 4, when providing support and managing symptoms is critical.

plant recipients than among autologous marrow or PBSC transplant recipients. The causes may be related to insufficient numbers of cells transplanted, attack or rejection of donor cells by residual immunologically competent recipient cells, infection of transplanted cells, and unknown biological factors. If the transplanted marrow or PBSCs fail to engraft, the client will die unless another transplantation is successful.

Graft-Versus-Host Disease. GVHD is an immunologic event that occurs if the recipient is not immunocompetent and the donor tissue has active leukocytes, especially effector T cells and T-cell precursors. Because the recipient is totally immunosuppressed, the recipient cannot recognize the donated bone marrow cells as foreign or non-self. Instead, the immunocompetent cells of the donated marrow recognize the client's (recipient) cells, tissues, and organs as foreign and mount an immune offense against them. The graft is actually trying to attack the host.

Although all host tissues can be attacked and harmed, the tissues most commonly damaged are the skin, gastrointestinal tract, and liver. Approximately 30% to 70% of all allogeneic BMT recipients experience some degree of GVHD, and more than 15% of the clients who experience GVHD die from its complications (Whedon, 1991). The presence of GVHD indicates that the transplanted cells are competent and have successfully engrafted.

Clients with GVHD are managed with immunosuppressive agents and support of the systems sustaining the heaviest damage. Care is taken to avoid suppressing the new immune system to the extent that either the client becomes more susceptible to infection or the transplanted cells stop engrafting.

Veno-Occlusive Disease. VOD involves occlusion of the hepatic venules by thrombosis and phlebitis. This condition occurs in up to 20% of clients who receive a BMT, and symptoms usually occur within the first 30 days after transplantation. Clients who have received high doses of chemotherapy, especially alkylating agents, are at risk for life-threatening hepatic complications. Clinical signs include jaundice, pain in the right upper quadrant, ascites, weight gain, and liver enlargement.

Because there is no known way of opening the hepatic vessels, treatment is supportive. Early detection enhances the chances of client survival. Fluid management is also crucial. The nurse assesses the client daily for weight gain, fluid accumulation, increases in abdominal girth, and hepatomegaly (Ford et al., 1996).

Risk for Injury

Because normal bone marrow production is severely limited in the client with AML, the number of circulating platelets is severely diminished, creating thrombocytopenia. This condition puts the client with AML at a greatly increased risk for excessive bleeding in response to minimal trauma.

Planning: Expected Outcomes. After intervention, the client is expected to remain free from bleeding.

Interventions. As a result of chemotherapy-induced pancytopenia, the client's platelet count is decreased. During the period of greatest bone marrow suppression (the nadir), the platelet count may be extremely low ($<10,000/mm^3$). The client is at great risk for bleeding once the platelet count falls below $50,000/mm^3$, and spontaneous bleeding frequently occurs when the platelet count is lower than 20,000 (Lin & Beddar, 1996). The nurse's major objectives are to protect the client from situations that could lead to bleeding and to closely monitor any bleeding that does occur.

The nurse assesses the client frequently for evidence of bleeding: oozing, confluent ecchymoses, petechiae, or purpura. All stools, urine, nasogastric drainage, and vomitus are examined visually for blood and tested for occult blood. The nurse measures any blood loss as accurately as possible and measures the client's abdominal girth during every nursing shift. Increases in abdominal girth can indicate internal hemorrhage. Bleeding precautions are instituted (Chart 42–10).

The nurse also monitors laboratory values daily. CBC results are reviewed daily to determine the client's risk for bleeding as well as actual blood loss. The client with a platelet count below $20,000/mm^3$ may need a platelet transfusion. For the client with severe blood loss, packed RBCs may be ordered (see Transfusion Therapy later).

Chart 42–10

Nursing Care Highlight: Bleeding Precautions

- Handle the client gently.
- Use a lift sheet when moving and positioning in bed.
- Avoid intramuscular injections and venipunctures.
- When injections or venipunctures are necessary, use the smallest gauge needle for the task.
- Apply firm pressure to the needlestick site for 10 minutes or until the site no longer oozes blood.
- Apply ice to areas of trauma.
- Test all urine and stool for the presence of occult blood.
- Observe IV sites every 2 hours for bleeding.
- Avoid trauma to rectal tissues:
  - Do not take temperatures rectally.
  - Do not give enemas.
  - Administer well-lubricated suppositories with caution.
  - Advise client not to have anal intercourse.
- Measure abdominal girth daily.
- Teach the client to use an electric razor.
- Teach the client to avoid mouth trauma:
  - Use soft-bristled toothbrush or tooth sponges.
  - Do not floss between teeth.
  - Avoid dental work, especially extractions.
  - Avoid hard foods.
  - Make sure that dentures fit and do not rub.
- Encourage the client not to blow the nose or insert objects into the nose.
- Teach the client to avoid contact sports.
- Teach client to wear shoes with firm soles whenever ambulating.

Fatigue

Because normal bone marrow production is severely limited in clients with AML, the number of circulating erythrocytes is severely diminished, creating a condition of anemia, leading in turn to fatigue. Because leukemic cells tend to have higher rates of metabolism and greater utilization of oxygen, the anemic client with leukemia is at risk for severe fatigue.

Planning: Expected Outcomes. After appropriate intervention, the client is expected to

- Experience no increase in fatigue
- Recognize symptoms of fatigue and alter activity before fatigue becomes excessive

Interventions. These are aimed at decreasing the effects of anemia and conserving the client's energy expenditure.

Diet Therapy. Diet therapy is indirectly related to fatigue and subsequent activity intolerance. The client must ingest enough calories to meet at least basal energy requirements, but increasing dietary intake can be difficult when the client is extremely fatigued. The nurse thus provides small, frequent meals high in protein and carbohydrates. Food items that are liquid or easy to chew also require less effort to eat.

Blood Replacement Therapy. Blood transfusions are sometimes indicated for the client with fatigue. Transfusions increase the blood's oxygen-carrying capacity and replace missing RBCs and some coagulation factors (see Table 42–3). For the leukemic client experiencing fatigue related to anemia, packed RBCs are usually the blood component of choice. (See Transfusion Therapy for a discussion of nursing care during transfusions.)

Drug Therapy. Clients may receive subcutaneous injections of epoetin alfa (Epogen or Procrit) 50 to 100 U/kg three times per week (DeLaPena et al., 1996). This growth factor is naturally secreted by the kidney and boosts the production of RBCs. Epoetin alfa has previously been used in anemia associated with chronic renal failure and human immunodeficiency virus (HIV) clients receiving zidovudine and is now approved for use in anemia associated with chemotherapy (Rieger & Haeuber, 1995).

The nurse administers injections three times a week and assesses for side effects such as hypertension, headaches, fever, myalgia, and rashes (DeLaPena et al., 1996). For more information on hematopoietic growth factors, see Chapter 27.

Conservation of Energy. The nurse examines the hospitalized client's schedule of prescribed and routine activities. Those activities that do not have a direct positive effect on the client's condition are assessed in terms of their usefulness to the client. If the actual or potential benefit of an activity is less than its actual or potential worsening of the client's fatigue, the nurse consults with other members of the health care team about eliminating or postponing it. Candidates for cancellation or postpone-

ment include hair washing, physical therapy, and certain invasive diagnostic tests not required for assessment or treatment of current problems.

 Continuing Care

The leukemic client is discharged after induction chemotherapy or transplantation. Follow-up care is provided on an outpatient basis.

► Home Care Management

Planning for home care for the client with leukemia begins as soon as a client achieves remission. The client will need assistance at home until the condition improves. The nurse assesses the available support mechanisms. Many clients require the services of a visiting nurse to assist with dressing changes for central venous catheters, to assist with hyperalimentation infusions, to transfuse platelets, and to answer questions. Occasionally, the client may require home transfusion therapy for one or more blood components as well (Randolph et al., 1995).

► Health Teaching

The client and the family need to be educated about the importance of continuing therapy and appropriate medical follow-up, despite the unpleasant side effects of therapy. Many clients go home with a central venous catheter in place and require instructions about its care and maintenance. Chart 42–11 lists general guidelines for central venous catheter care at home. These guidelines may be altered depending on the home setting, assistance available, and agency policy.

Protecting the client from infection after discharge from the hospital is just as important as when the client was

---

Chart 42–11

Education Guide: Home Care of the Central Venous Catheter

- To maintain patency, flush the catheter briskly with heparinized saline (10 U/mL) once a day and after completing infusions.
- Change the Luer-lok cap on each catheter lumen weekly.
- Change the dressing every other day:
  - Use clean technique with thorough hand washing.
  - Clean the exit site with alcohol and povidone-iodine (Betadine).
  - Apply antibacterial ointment to the site.
  - Cover the site with dry sterile gauze dressing, taped securely, or with transparent adherent dressing.
- To prevent tension, always tape the catheter to yourself.
- Look for and report any signs of infection (redness, swelling, or drainage at the exit site).
- In case of a break or puncture in the catheter lumen, immediately clamp the catheter between yourself and the opening. *Notify your physician immediately.*

hospitalized. (See Chart 42–9 for focused assessment for the client at risk for infection.) The nurse urges the client to use proper hygiene and avoid crowds or others with infections. Neither the client nor any household member should receive live virus immunization (poliomyelitis, measles, or rubella) for 1 year after transplantation. The client should continue mouth care regimens at home. The nurse emphasizes that the client should immediately notify the physician if he or she experiences any fever or other sign of infection.

Because platelet recovery is usually slower than that of white blood cells (WBCs), many clients return home still at risk for bleeding. The nurse reinforces the safety and bleeding precautions initiated in the hospital, emphasizing that the client follow these precautions until the platelet count is above 50,000. The nurse also instructs the client and family to assess for petechiae, avoid trauma and sharp objects, apply pressure to wounds for 10 minutes, and report any unusual symptoms, including blood in the stool or urine, or headache that does not respond to acetaminophen.

Psychosocial Preparation

The nurse's responsibility in psychosocial preparation of the client before discharge is very important. A diagnosis of leukemia threatens the client's self-esteem and family role (Larson, 1995). The client is confronted with the reality of death, and treatment causes major adjustments in self-image. The client and family also experience changes in the client's body image, level of independence, and lifestyle. Some clients feel threatened by their environment, seeing everything as potentially infectious. The nurse helps the client and family redefine priorities, understand the illness and its treatment, and find hope. The nurse makes referrals to support groups sponsored by organizations such as the American Cancer Society ("I Can Cope" and "Make Today Count"), which can be enormously beneficial to both the client and the family.

➤ Health Care Resources

The client with limited social support may need assistance at home until strength and energy return. A home care aide may suffice for some clients, whereas a visiting nurse may be needed for other clients to reinforce teaching. The client may also need equipment to facilitate ADLs and ambulation. Financial resources are assessed. Treatment of cancer is expensive, and the nurse works closely with the local social services department to ensure that insurance is adequate. If the client is uninsured, other sources, such as drug-company sponsored compassionate aid programs, are explored. The Leukemia Society of America, Inc., offers limited financial assistance for clients with leukemia, sponsors support groups, and provides publications for clients and health care providers.

Prolonged outpatient contact and follow-up will be necessary, and clients will need transportation to the outpatient facility. Many local divisions of the American Cancer Society offer free transportation to clients with cancer, including leukemia.

 Evaluation

The nurse evaluates the care of the client with leukemia based on the identified nursing diagnoses. The expected outcomes include that the client will

- Remain free from cross-contamination–induced infection
- Remain free of autocontamination-induced infection
- Not experience sepsis
- Remain free from episodes of bleeding
- Not experience an increase in fatigue
- Recognize symptoms of fatigue and alter activity before fatigue becomes excessive

Malignant Lymphoma

Malignant lymphomas reflect abnormal proliferation of one type of leukocyte (lymphocytes), but differ from the leukemias in the degree of differentiation of the affected cells and the location of cell production. Lymphomas are malignancies characterized by a proliferation of committed lymphocytes rather than stem cell precursors (as in leukemia). This proliferation occurs not in bone marrow but in other lymphoid tissues scattered throughout the body, especially the lymph nodes and spleen. Lymphomas are actually solid tumors rather than cellular suspensions within the blood and bone marrow, and fall into two major categories among adults: Hodgkin's and non-Hodgkin's.

Hodgkin's Lymphoma

Overview

Hodgkin's lymphoma is a cancer that can affect any age group, although incidence peaks first in people in their mid-to-late 20s and then in people older than 50. Men and women are affected equally in the first group, but the disease is more prevalent in men in the older group (Carson, 1996).

Factors implicated as possible causes of Hodgkin's lymphoma include viral infections and previous exposure to alkylating chemical agents. This cancer usually originates in a single lymph node or a single chain of nodes. The lymphoid tissues within the node undergo malignant transformation, usually initiating some inflammatory processes. These nodes contain a specific transformed cell type, the Reed-Sternberg cell, a characteristic marker of Hodgkin's lymphoma. The disease first metastasizes (spreads) to other adjacent lymphoid structures and eventually invades nonlymphoid tissues.

Collaborative Management

Assessment most often reveals a greatly enlarged but painless lymph node or nodes, usually the earliest manifestation of Hodgkin's lymphoma. The client also often experiences fever, malaise, and night sweats (Table 42–5). More specific clinical manifestations depend on the site (or sites) of malignancy and the extent of disease.

Diagnosis and grade are established when biopsy of a node or mass reveals Reed-Sternberg cells. The client then

TABLE 42–5

Manifestations and Staging Criteria for Hodgkin's Lymphoma

Stage	Manifestations
Stage Ia	• Disease is confined to a single lymph node region or only one extranodal site.
Stage Ib	• Disease is confined to a single lymph node region or only one extranodal site. The client also experiences some or all of the following systemic symptoms: persistent fever, night sweats, and significant weight loss (>10%).
Stage IIa	• Disease is confined to either two or more lymph node regions on the same side of the diaphragm or contiguous extranodal sites on the same side of the diaphragm.
Stage IIb	• Disease is confined to either two or more lymph node regions on the same side of the diaphragm or contiguous extranodal sites on the same side of the diaphragm. Client also experiences some or all of the following systemic symptoms: persistent fever, night sweats, and significant weight loss (>10%).
Stage IIIa	• Disease extends to lymph node regions on both sides of the diaphragm.
Stage IIIb	• Disease extends to lymph node regions on both sides of the diaphragm. The client also experiences some or all of the following systemic symptoms: persistent fever, night sweats, and significant weight loss (>10%).
Stage IIIc	• Disease extends to lymph node regions on both sides of the diaphragm. The client also experiences some or all of the following systemic symptoms: persistent fever, night sweats, and significant weight loss (>10%). The spleen is also involved in disease.
Stage IV	• Disease has widely disseminated foci of involvement, including one or more extranodal tissues and organs.

undergoes extensive staging procedures to determine the exact extent of disease (see Table 42–5). Staging must be detailed and accurate because the treatment regimen is determined by the extent of disease. Staging procedures for Hodgkin's lymphoma include biopsies of distant lymph nodes, lymphangiography, computed tomography (CT) of the thorax and the abdomen, CBC, liver function studies, and bilateral bone marrow biopsies.

Such great progress has been made in treatment regimens that Hodgkin's lymphoma is now one of the most curable types of cancer. Generally, for stage I and II disease without mediastinal node involvement, the treatment of choice is extensive external radiation of involved lymph node regions. With more extensive disease, radiation coupled with an aggressive multiagent chemotherapy

regimen is most effective in achieving a cure. (See Chapter 27 on general care of clients receiving radiation and/or chemotherapy.)

Specific nursing management of the client undergoing treatment for Hodgkin's lymphoma focuses on the side effects of therapy, especially

■ Drug-induced pancytopenia, which results in increased risk for infection, bleeding, and anemia
■ Severe nausea and vomiting
■ Skin irritation and breakdown at the site of radiation
■ Impaired hepatic function either by metastasis to the liver or by the multiagent chemotherapy
■ Permanent sterility for male clients receiving radiation in an inverted-**Y** pattern to the abdominopelvic region along with specific chemotherapeutic agents (client should be informed of this side effect and given the option to store sperm in a sperm bank before treatment)

Non-Hodgkin's Lymphoma

Overview

Non-Hodgkin's lymphoma is the classification for all cancers originating from lymphoid tissues that are not diagnosed as Hodgkin's lymphoma. There are more than 12 subtypes of non-Hodgkin's lymphoma, including low grade, intermediate, and high grade.

The low-grade lymphomas usually arise from B-cell lymphocytes and progress slowly. Although clients with low-grade lymphomas have longer survival rates, the diseases are less responsive to treatment, and consequently, cures are rare.

At the other end of the spectrum are the high-grade lymphomas, which are aggressive tumors of usually mixed cellularity with rapid doubling times. High-grade lymphomas are more responsive to chemotherapy, and the chances for a long-term cure are greater.

Most non-Hodgkin's lymphomas arise from lymph nodes but can originate in virtually any tissue or organ. A low-grade lymphoma also can convert to a higher grade lymphoma. Most non-Hodgkin's lymphomas occur among older adults. Definitive causes are unknown, but viral infection, exposure to ionizing radiation, and exposure to toxic chemicals have all been implicated.

Collaborative Management

Because lymphomas may arise from lymphoid cells in any tissue and because the malignancy can spread to any organ, assessment reveals no specific clinical manifestations other than lymphadenopathy common to all types of lymphoma. Diagnosis is made from the histologic features apparent on biopsy of any suspicious node or mass. Classification of specific lymphoma subtype is based on a complex grading of surface markers, cytogenetic features, cell size, and expression of viral antigens. Staging is similar to that for Hodgkin's lymphoma (see Table 42–5).

Depending on the cell type, prognosis ranges from excellent to poor. Overall, however, clients with non-

Hodgkin's lymphomas have a poorer prognosis than those with Hodgkin's lymphoma. Some types of non-Hodgkin's lymphoma run a protracted course, extending over many years, and are not treated in the early phases. However, for most types of non-Hodgkin's lymphoma, death ensues rapidly if clients are not treated. Treatment consists of radiation therapy and multiagent chemotherapy. Nursing care needs are similar to those for clients with Hodgkin's lymphoma, with additional organ-specific problems taken into account if the disease is widely disseminated.

COAGULATION DISORDERS

Coagulation disorders are synonymous with bleeding disorders, and are characterized by abnormal or increased bleeding resulting from defects in one or more components regulating hemostasis. Bleeding disorders may be spontaneous or traumatic, localized or generalized, lifelong or acquired. They can originate from a defect in the hemostatic processes at the vascular, platelet, or clotting

factor level. Figure 42–4 outlines blood clotting cascades and sites where specific defects and drugs disrupt the hemostatic processes.

Platelet Disorders

Platelets play a vital role in hemostasis. For both the intrinsic and extrinsic pathways, coagulation starts with platelet adhesion and formation of a platelet plug. Any condition that either diminishes the number of platelets or interferes with their ability to adhere (to one another, blood vessel walls, collagen, or fibrin threads) can be manifested as increased bleeding. Platelet disorders can be inherited, acquired, or temporarily induced by the ingestion of substances that limit platelet production or inhibit aggregation.

A drop in the number of platelets below the level needed for normal coagulation is called *thrombocytopenia* (Lapka et al., 1994). Thrombocytopenia may occur as a result of other conditions or treatments that suppress gen-

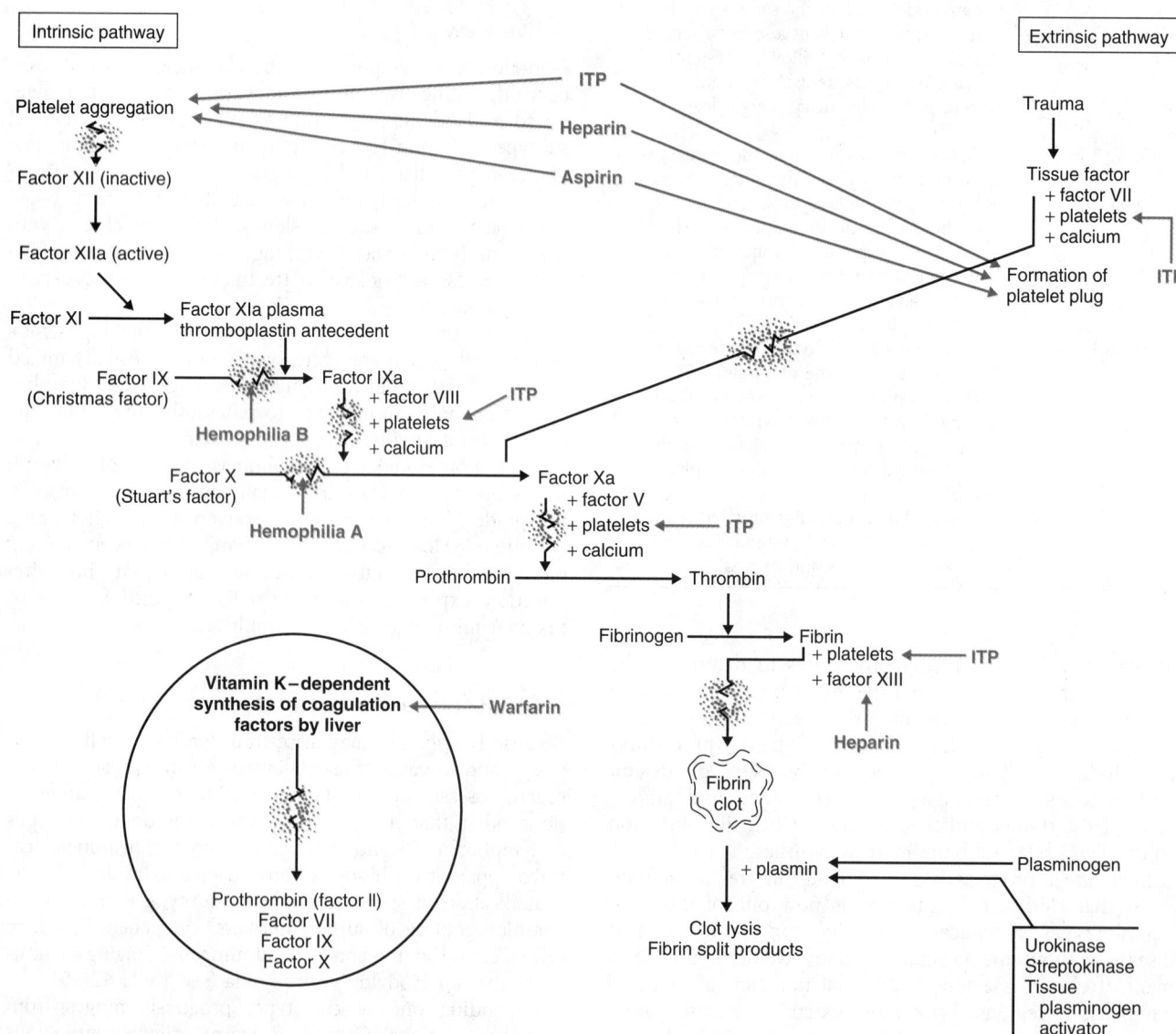

Figure 42–4. Sites of disruption of the coagulation mechanisms by drugs and disease. (ITP = idiopathic thrombocytopenic purpura.)

eral bone marrow activity. It also can occur through processes that specifically limit platelet formation or increase the rate of platelet destruction. The two thrombocytopenic conditions affecting adults are autoimmune thrombocytopenic purpura and thrombotic thrombocytopenic purpura.

Autoimmune Thrombocytopenic Purpura

Overview

Before the underlying cause of autoimmune thrombocytopenic purpura was identified, this condition was known as idiopathic thrombocytopenic purpura (ITP). Although the cause is now thought to be an autoimmune reaction, the condition is still commonly known as ITP. The total number of circulating platelets is greatly diminished in ITP, even though platelet production in the bone marrow is normal.

Clients with idiopathic thrombocytopenic purpura make an antibody directed against the surface of their own platelets (an antiplatelet antibody). This antibody coats the surface of the platelets, making them more susceptible to attraction and destruction by phagocytic leukocytes, especially macrophages (see the discussion of opsonization in Chapter 23). Because the spleen contains a large concentration of fixed macrophages and because the blood vessels of the spleen are long and tortuous, antibody-coated platelets are destroyed primarily in the spleen. When the rate of platelet destruction exceeds that of production, the number of circulating platelets decreases and blood clotting slows.

Although the cause of this disorder appears to be autoimmune, the exact mechanism initiating the production of autoantibodies is unknown. ITP is most common among women between the ages of 20 and 40 and among people with a pre-existing autoimmune condition, such as systemic lupus erythematosus (Cotran et al., 1994).

Collaborative Management

Clinical Manifestations

Clinical manifestations associated with ITP are generally limited to the skin and mucous membranes: large ecchymoses (bruises) on the arms, legs, upper chest, and neck or a petechial rash. Mucosal bleeding occurs easily. If the client has experienced significant blood loss, signs of anemia may also be present.

A rare complication is an intracranial bleeding–induced cerebrovascular accident. The nurse assesses the client for neurologic function and mental status (see Chap. 43). The nurse asks family members or significant others if the client's behavior and responses to the mental status examination are typical or represent a change from usual reactions.

Diagnosis

Idiopathic thrombocytopenic purpura is diagnosed by a decreased platelet count and large numbers of megakaryocytes in the bone marrow. Antiplatelet antibodies may be present in detectable levels in peripheral blood. If the

client experiences any episodes of bleeding, hematocrit and hemoglobin levels also are low.

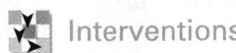 Interventions

➤ Nonsurgical Management

As a result of the decreased platelet count, the client is at great risk for bleeding. Interventions include therapy for the underlying condition as well as protection of the client from trauma-induced bleeding episodes.

Drug Therapy. Agents used to control ITP include drugs that suppress immune function to some degree. The premise for the use of agents such as corticosteroids and azathioprine is to inhibit immune system synthesis of antiplatelet autoantibodies. More aggressive therapy can include low doses of chemotherapeutic agents, such as the antimitotic agents and cyclophosphamide.

Blood Replacement Therapy. For the client with a platelet count of less than 20,000/mm³ who is experiencing an acute life-threatening bleeding episode, a platelet transfusion may be required. Platelet transfusions are not performed routinely because the donated platelets are just as rapidly destroyed by the spleen as the client's own platelets (see Transfusion Therapy later).

Maintaining a Safe Environment. The nurse's major objectives are to protect the client from situations that can lead to bleeding and to closely monitor the amount of bleeding that is occurring. (For nursing care actions, see the earlier nursing diagnosis Risk for Injury under Leukemia.)

➤ Surgical Management

For the client who does not respond to drug therapy, splenectomy may be the treatment of choice. Because the leukocytes in the spleen perform many different immunodefensive functions, the client who has a splenectomy is at increased risk for infection.

Thrombotic Thrombocytopenic Purpura

Overview

Thrombotic thrombocytopenic purpura (TTP) is a rare disorder in which platelets clump together inappropriately in the microcirculation, and insufficient platelets remain in systemic circulation. The client experiences inappropriate clotting; yet the blood fails to coagulate properly when trauma occurs. The clinical picture is similar to that of disseminated intravascular coagulation (DIC) but is not initiated by the same factors. The underlying cause of TTP appears to be an autoimmune reaction in blood vessel cells (endothelial cells) that makes platelets aggregate in the microcirculation.

Collaborative Management

Treatment for the client with TTP focuses on inhibiting the inappropriate platelet aggregation and disrupting the underlying autoimmune process. Immunosuppressive therapy reduces the intensity of this disorder. Interventions to inhibit platelet aggregation include plasma exchange therapy and the administration of platelet aggregation inhibitors, such as aspirin, alprostadil (Prostin), and plicamycin.

Clotting Factor Disorders

Coagulation or bleeding disorders can result from a clotting factor defect, including the inability to produce a specific clotting factor, or production of insufficient quantities, or a less active form of a clotting factor.

Most clotting factor disorders are congenitally transmitted gene abnormalities of one clotting factor. The few acquired clotting factor disorders are related to an inability to synthesize many clotting factors at the same time as a result of liver damage or an insufficiency of clotting cofactors and precursor products. Common congenital disorders that result in defects at the clotting factor level include hemophilias A and B and von Willebrand's disease. DIC may be considered an acquired clotting disorder but is more closely associated with sepsis-induced distributive shock (see Chap. 39).

Hemophilia

Overview

Hemophilia comprises two hereditary bleeding disorders resulting from deficiencies of specific clotting factors. Hemophilia A (classic hemophilia) results from a deficiency of factor VIII and accounts for 80% of hemophilia cases. Hemophilia B (Christmas disease) is a deficiency of factor IX and accounts for 20% of cases.

The incidence of both is 1 in 10,000. Hemophilia is an X-linked recessive trait. Female carriers risk transmitting the gene for hemophilia to half of their daughters (who then are carriers) and half their sons (who will have overt hemophilia). Hemophilia A is, with rare exceptions, a disease affecting males, none of whose sons will have the gene for hemophilia and all of whose daughters will be obligatory carriers. In about 30% of clients with hemophilia, there is no family history, and it is presumed that their disease is the result of a new mutation (Cotran et al., 1994).

The bleeding disorder associated with hemophilia A is so severe that, before blood transfusions were available, hemophiliacs rarely survived past age 3 years. With the availability of blood transfusion and factor VIII therapy, mean survival time has increased so greatly that hemophilia now is commonly seen among adult clients.

The clinical pictures of hemophilia A and B are identical. The client has abnormal bleeding in response to any trauma because of an absence or deficiency of the specific clotting factor. Hemophiliacs form platelet plugs at the bleeding site, but the clotting factor deficiency impairs the hemostatic response and the capacity to form a stable fibrin clot. This produces abnormal bleeding, which may be mild, moderate, or severe, depending on the degree of factor deficiency.

Collaborative Management

Assessment of the client with hemophilia reveals

■ Excessive hemorrhage from minor cuts or abrasions caused by abnormal platelet function
■ Joint and muscle hemorrhages that lead to disabling long-term sequelae
■ A tendency to bruise easily
■ Prolonged and potentially fatal postoperative hemorrhage

The laboratory test results for a true hemophiliac demonstrate a prolonged partial thromboplastin time (PTT), a normal bleeding time, and a normal prothrombin time (PT) (Cotran et al., 1994). The most common health problem associated with hemophilia is degenerating joint function resulting from chronic bleeding into the joints, especially at the hip and knee.

The bleeding problems of hemophilia A can be well managed by either regularly scheduled IV administration of factor VIII cryoprecipitate or intermittent administration as needed, depending on activity level and injury probability (see Transfusion Therapy). However, the cost of cryoprecipitate is prohibitive for many people with hemophilia. In addition, because the precipitated clotting factors are derived from pooled human serum, a risk of viral contamination remains (even with the use of heat-inactivated serum). Major complications of hemophilia therapy during the 1980s were infection with hepatitis B virus, cytomegalovirus, and human immunodeficiency virus (HIV). Although heat-inactivated serum and the elimination of HIV-positive donors have reduced these risks, they have not yet been eliminated. New techniques for producing synthetic factor VIII will lead to uncontaminated and less expensive sources of this vital substance.

TRANSFUSION THERAPY

Any blood component may be removed from a donor and transfused to benefit a recipient. Components may be transfused individually or collectively, with varying degrees of benefit to the recipient.

Pretransfusion Responsibilities

Nursing actions during transfusions aim largely at prevention or early recognition of adverse transfusion reactions. Preparation of the client for transfusion therapy is imperative, and institutional blood product administration procedures should be carefully followed. Before administering any blood product to a client, the nurse reviews the agency's policies and procedures (Chart 42–12 presents a general guideline).

Legally, a physician's order is needed to administer blood or its components. The order specifies the type of component to be delivered, the volume to be transfused, and any special conditions the physician judges to be important. The nurse verifies the order for accuracy and completeness. The nurse also evaluates the need for transfusion, considering both the client's clinical condition and the laboratory values. In many hospitals, a separate con-

Nursing Care Highlight: Guidelines for Transfusion Therapy

Nursing Actions	Rationale
Before Infusion	
1. Assess laboratory values.	• Many institutions have specific guidelines for blood product transfusions (i.e., platelet count <20,000 or hemoglobin <8.0).
2. Verify the medical order.	• Legally, a physician's order is required for transfusions. The order should state the type of product, dose, and transfusion time.
3. Assess the client's vital signs, urine output, skin color, and history of transfusion reactions.	• Determine whether the client can tolerate infusion. Baseline information may be needed to help identify transfusion reactions.
4. Obtain venous access. Use a central catheter or 19-gauge needle, if possible.	• The larger bore needle allows cells to flow more easily without occluding the lumen of the catheter.
5. Obtain blood products from a blood bank. Transfuse immediately.	• Once a blood product has been released from the blood bank, the product should be transfused as soon as possible (e.g., red blood cell transfusions should be completed within 4 hours of removal from refrigeration).
6. With another registered nurse, verify the client by name and number, check blood compatibility, and note expiration time.	• Human error is the most common cause of ABO incompatibility reactions.
7. Administer the blood product using the appropriate filtered tubing.	• Filters are needed to remove aggregates and possible contaminants.
8. If the blood product needs to be diluted, use *only* normal saline solution.	• Hemolysis occurs if any other intravenous solution is used.
9. Remain with the client during the first 15–30 minutes of the infusion.	• Hemolytic reactions occur most often within the first 50 mL of the infusion.
10. Infuse the blood product at the ordered rate.	• Fluid overload is a potential complication of rapid infusion.
11. Monitor vital signs.	• Vital sign changes often indicate transfusion reactions.
12. When the transfusion is completed, discontinue infusion and dispose of the bag and tubing properly.	• Bloodborne pathogens may be spread inadvertently through improper disposal.
13. Document.	• The client record should indicate type of product infused, product number, volume infused, time of infusion, and any adverse reactions.

sent form must be obtained for the administration of blood products before a transfusion is performed.

A blood specimen is obtained for cross-matching (the testing of the donor's blood and the recipient's blood for compatibility). The procedure and responsibility for obtaining this specimen are specified by hospital policy. In most hospitals, a new cross-matching specimen is required at least every 48 hours.

Because of the viscosity of blood components, a 19-gauge needle or larger is used, whenever possible, for venous access. Both Y tubes and straight tubing sets are available for blood component administration. A blood filter (approximately 170 μ) to remove aggregates from the stored blood products is included with component administration equipment and must be used to transfuse all blood products. In massive transfusion, a microaggregate filter (20–40 μ) may be used (Kefer et al., 1996).

Normal saline is the solution of choice for administration. Ringer's lactate and dextrose in water are contraindicated for administration with blood or blood products because they cause clotting or hemolysis of blood cells

(Bradbury & Cruickshank, 1995). *Medications are never added to blood products.*

Before the transfusion is initiated, it is essential to determine that the blood component delivered is correct. Two registered nurses simultaneously check the physician's order, the client's identity, and whether the hospital identification band name and number are identical to those on the blood component tag. The blood bag label, the attached tag, and the requisition slip are examined to ensure that the ABO and Rh types are compatible. The expiration date is also checked, and the product is inspected for discoloration, gas bubbles, or cloudiness, indicators of bacterial growth or hemolysis (Huston, 1996).

Transfusion Responsibilities

The nurse takes the client's vital signs, including temperature, immediately before initiating the transfusion. Infusion begins slowly. A nurse remains with the client for the first 15 to 30 minutes. Any severe reaction usually occurs with administration of the first 50 mL of blood. The nurse assesses vital signs 15 minutes after initiation of the transfusion to detect signs of a reaction. If there are none, the infusion rate can be increased to transfuse 1 unit in about 2 hours (depending on the client's cardiovascular status). The nurse takes the client's vital signs every hour throughout the transfusion or as specified by agency policy.

Blood components without large amounts of RBCs can be infused more quickly. The identification checks are the same as for RBC transfusions. Physiologic changes in elderly clients may necessitate that blood products be transfused at a slower rate. See Chart 42-13 for other nursing care needs of older clients undergoing transfusion therapy.

Types of Transfusions
Red Blood Cell Transfusions

Red blood cells are administered to replace erythrocytes lost as a result of trauma or surgical interventions. Clients with clinical conditions that result in the destruction or abnormal maturation of RBCs may also benefit from RBC transfusions. Packed RBCs, supplied in 250-mL bags, are a concentrated source of RBCs and are the most common component administered to RBC-deficient clients.

Blood transfusions are actually transplantations of tissue from one person to another. The donor and recipient blood must thus be carefully checked for compatibility to prevent potentially lethal reactions (Table 42-6). Com-

patibility is determined by two different types of antigen systems (cell surface proteins): the ABO system antigens and the Rh antigen, present on the membrane surface of RBCs.

Red blood cell antigens are inherited. For the ABO antigen system, a person inherits one of the following:

- A antigen (type A blood)
- B antigen (type B blood)
- Both A and B antigens (type AB blood)
- No antigens (type O blood)

Within the first few years of a child's life, circulating antibodies develop against the blood type antigens that were not inherited. For example, a child with type A blood will form antigens against type B blood. A child with type O blood has not inherited either A or B antigens and will form antibodies against RBCs that contain either A or B antigens. If erythrocytes that contain a foreign antigen are infused into a recipient, the donated tissue can be recognized by the immune system of the recipient as non-self, and the client may have a reaction to the transfused products (Kefer et al., 1996).

The mechanism of the Rh antigen system is slightly different. An Rh-negative person is born without the antigen and does not form antibodies unless he or she is specifically sensitized to the it. Sensitization can occur with RBC transfusions from an Rh-positive person or from exposure during pregnancy and birth. Once an Rh-negative person has been sensitized and antibody development has occurred, any exposure to Rh-positive blood can cause a transfusion reaction. Antibody development can be prevented by administration of Rh-immune globulin as soon as exposure to the Rh antigen is suspected. People who have Rh-positive blood can receive an RBC transfusion from an Rh-negative donor, but Rh-negative people must never receive Rh-positive blood (Bradbury & Cruickshank, 1995).

Platelet Transfusions

Platelets are administered to clients with platelet counts below 20,000 mm^3 and to thrombocytopenic clients who are actively bleeding or scheduled for an invasive procedure (Kefer et al., 1996). Platelet transfusions are usually pooled from as many as 10 donors, and do not have to be of the same blood type as the client. For clients who are candidates for bone marrow transplant (BMT) or who

TABLE 42-6

Compatibility Chart for Red Blood Cell Transfusions				
	Recipient			
Donor	**A**	**B**	**AB**	**O**
A	X		X	
B		X	X	
AB			X	
O	X	X	X	X

require multiple platelet transfusions, single-donor platelets may be ordered. Single-donor platelets are obtained from one person and decrease the amount of antigen exposure to the recipient, helping prevent the formation of platelet antibodies. The chances of allergic transfusion reactions to future platelet transfusions are thus reduced.

Platelet infusion bags usually contain 300 mL for pooled platelets and 200 mL for single-donor platelets. Because the platelet is a fragile cell, platelet transfusions are administered rapidly after being brought to the client's room, usually over 15 to 30 minutes. A special transfusion set with a smaller filter and shorter tubing is used.

Standard transfusion sets are not used with platelets because the filter traps the platelets, and the longer tubing increases platelet adherence to the lumen. Additional platelet filters help remove WBCs in the platelet concentrate. These filters are connected directly to the platelet transfusion set and are used for clients who have a history of febrile reactions or who will require multiple platelet transfusions.

The nurse takes the client's vital signs before the infusion, 15 minutes after infusion is initiated, and at its completion. The client may be premedicated with meperidine or hydrocortisone to minimize the chances of a reaction. The client can become febrile and experience rigors (severe chills) during transfusion, but these symptoms are not considered a true transfusion reaction. IV administration of amphotericin B, an antifungal agent given to many leukemic clients, is discontinued during platelet transfusion and not resumed for at least 1 hour after transfusion. Amphotericin B can cause severe allergic reactions that are difficult to distinguish from transfusion reactions.

Plasma Transfusions

Historically, plasma infusions have been administered to replace blood volume, and they are occasionally still used for this purpose. It is more common for plasma to be immediately frozen after donation. Freezing preserves the clotting factors, and the plasma can then be used for clients with clotting disorders. Fresh frozen plasma (FFP) is infused immediately after thawing while the clotting factors are still viable.

ABO compatibility is required for transfusion of plasma products. The volume of the infusion bag is approximately 200 mL. The infusion takes place as rapidly as the client can tolerate, generally over 30 to 60 minutes, through a regular Y-set or straight-filtered tubing.

Cryoprecipitate

Cryoprecipitate is a product derived from plasma. Clotting factors VIII and XIII, von Willebrand's factor, fibronectin, and fibrinogen are precipitated from pooled plasma to produce cryoprecipitate. This highly concentrated blood product is administered to clients with clotting factor disorders at a volume of 10 to 15 mL/unit. Although cryoprecipitate can be infused, it usually is given by IV push within 3 minutes. Dosages are individualized, and it is best if the cryoprecipitate is ABO compatible.

Granulocyte Transfusions

At some centers, neutropenic clients with infections receive granulocyte transfusions for WBC replacement. However, this practice is highly controversial because the potential benefit to the client must be weighed against the potential severe reactions that often accompany granulocyte transfusions (Kefer et al., 1996). The surface of granulocytes contains numerous antigens that can cause severe antibody-antigen reactions when infused into a recipient whose immune system recognizes these antigens as nonself. In addition, transfused granulocytes have a very short life span and are probably of minimal benefit to the client (see Chap. 23). There is some evidence that treatment with antibiotics alone results in better survival rates.

Granulocytes are suspended in 400 mL of plasma and should be transfused over 45 to 60 minutes (Kefer et al., 1996). Institutional policies often require more stringent monitoring of clients receiving granulocytes. A physician may need to be present on the hospital unit and vital signs taken every 15 minutes throughout the transfusion. Administration of amphotericin B and granulocyte transfusions should be separated by 4 to 6 hours (Kefer et al., 1996).

TRANSCULTURAL CONSIDERATIONS

Although transfusion with blood products is relatively common in acute care settings, the nurse remains sensitive to those clients who view receiving blood or blood products of others as repugnant, even sinful. Approximately 800,000 Jehovah's Witnesses live in the United States (Marelli, 1994). The tenets of this religion include that receiving human or animal blood is the same as "consuming" blood, an act specifically prohibited in the Old Testament. Devout Jehovah's Witnesses believe that to receive blood condemns them to eternal damnation. When possible, transfusion therapy with human blood products is avoided for this group. When clients are transfused with blood products against their will, the nurse shows respect for the client's distress and religious beliefs.

Some of the newer therapies for clients with anemia or hypovolemia may reduce the need for transfusion of human or animal blood products. One such therapy is the increasing use of hemoglobin substitutes, also known as "artificial blood." These agents increase the oxygen-carrying and oxygen-releasing power of the client's own blood.

Transfusion Reactions

Clients can experience any of the following transfusion reactions: hemolytic, allergic, febrile, bacterial, circulatory overload, and transfusion-associated graft-versus-host disease. The nurse is vigilant to prevent serious complications through early detection and initiation of appropriate treatment.

Hemolytic Transfusion Reactions

Hemolytic transfusion reactions are caused by blood type or Rh incompatibility. When blood containing antibodies against the recipient's blood is infused, antigen-antibody complexes are formed and released into the circulation. These complexes can destroy the transfused cells and initiate inflammatory responses in the recipient's blood vessel walls and organs (Huston, 1996). The ensuing reaction may be mild, with fever and chills, or severe, with disseminated intravascular coagulation (DIC) and circulatory collapse. Other clinical signs include

- Apprehension
- Headache
- Chest pain
- Low back pain
- Tachycardia
- Tachypnea
- Hypotension
- Hemoglobinuria
- A sense of impending doom

The onset of this type of reaction may be immediate or may not occur until subsequent units have been transfused.

Allergic Transfusion Reactions

Allergic transfusion reactions are most often seen in the client with a history of allergy. The client may have urticaria, itching, bronchospasm, or occasionally anaphylaxis. Onset of this type of reaction usually occurs during or up to 24 hours after the transfusion. The client with a history of allergy can be given buffy coat–poor or washed RBCs in which the WBCs and plasma are removed. This procedure minimizes the possibility of an allergic reaction.

Febrile Transfusion Reactions

Febrile transfusion reactions occur most commonly in the client with anti-WBC antibodies, a situation seen after multiple transfusions (Bradbury & Cruickshank, 1995). The recipient experiences

- Sensations of cold
- Tachycardia
- Fever
- Hypotension
- Tachypnea

Again, the physician can order buffy coat–poor RBCs or single-donor HLA-matched platelets. Leukocyte filters may also be used to trap WBCs and prevent their transfusion into the client.

Bacterial Transfusion Reactions

Bacterial transfusion reactions are seen after transfusion of contaminated blood products. Usually, a gram-negative organism is the source because these bacteria grow rapidly in blood stored under refrigeration. Symptoms include

- Tachycardia
- Hypotension
- Fever

- Chills
- Shock

Onset is rapid. (See Chapter 39 for care of the client experiencing sepsis-induced distributive shock.)

Circulatory Overload

Circulatory overload can occur when a blood product is administered too quickly. This complication is most common with whole blood transfusions or when the client requires multiple transfusions. The elderly are most at risk for this condition. See Chart 42–13. Symptoms include

- Hypertension
- Bounding pulse
- Distended jugular veins
- Dyspnea
- Restlessness
- Confusion

The nurse can both manage and prevent this complication by monitoring intake and output, transfusing blood products more slowly, and administering diuretics. See Chapter 15 for management of clients with fluid overload.

Transfusion-Associated Graft-Versus-Host Disease

Transfusion-associated graft-versus-host disease (TA-GVHD) is an infrequent but life-threatening complication that can occur in both immunosuppressed and immunocompetent clients. Its cause in immunosuppressed clients is similar to that of GVHD associated with allogeneic BMT, discussed earlier in this chapter, in which donor T-cell lymphocytes attack host tissues.

The cause of TA-GVHD in immunocompetent hosts is uncertain. Reactions are more common when the host and donor share similar human leukocyte antigens (HLAs), such as in first-degree relatives or individuals with similar ethnic background (Spector, 1995). Symptoms typically occur within 1 to 2 weeks and include thrombocytopenia, anorexia, nausea, vomiting, chronic hepatitis, weight loss, and recurrent infection.

Transfusion-associated GVHD has a 90% mortality rate, but can be prevented by transfusing irradiated blood products, thus preventing TA-GVHD by destroying T cells and their cytokine products (Spector, 1995).

Autologous Blood Transfusion

Autologous blood transfusions involve collection and transfusion of the client's own blood. Advantages of this type of transfusion are guaranteed compatibility and elimination of the risk of transmitting diseases such as hepatitis or HIV (Smith et al., 1995). The four types of autologous blood transfusions are preoperative autologous blood donation, acute normovolemic hemodilution, intraoperative autologous transfusion, and postoperative blood salvage.

Preoperative autologous blood donation, the most common type of autologous blood transfusion, involves collection of whole blood from the client, division into components, and then storage for later use (such as after a scheduled surgical procedure). As long as hematocrit and hemoglobin levels are within a safe range, client-donors donate blood on a weekly basis until the prescribed amount of blood is obtained. Fresh packed RBCs may be stored for 42 days. For individuals with rare blood types, blood may be frozen for up to 10 years. Platelets and plasma may be collected via pheresis (Gerber, 1994). Some cardiovascular problems and bacteremia are contraindications for autologous blood donation.

Acute normovolemic hemodilution involves withdrawal of a client's RBCs and volume replacement just before a surgical procedure. The goal is to decrease RBC loss during surgery. The blood is stored at room temperature for up to 6 hours and reinfused after surgery. This type of autologous transfusion is appropriate for healthy clients, but is contraindicated for individuals who are anemic or who have poor renal function (Gerber, 1994).

Intraoperative autologous transfusion and *postoperative blood salvage* involve the recovery and reinfusion of a client's own blood, collected either from an operative field or postoperatively from a wound. Several commercial products are available that collect, filter, and drain the blood into a transfusion bag (Smith et al., 1995). This autologous blood is often used for trauma or surgical clients with severe blood loss and must be reinfused within 6 hours.

The nurse transfuses autologous blood products using the guidelines previously mentioned. Although the client receiving autologous blood is not at risk for most types of transfusion reactions, the nurse must still assess for circulatory overload or bacterial transfusion reactions that can occur as a result of contamination.

CASE STUDY for the Client with Hematologic Complications

■ A 25-year-old woman is hospitalized on your unit for acute myelogenous leukemia. She completed induction chemotherapy 4 days ago, and today her major complaint is feeling tired and weak. Last night she reports waking up with epistaxis after an episode of coughing. Today's CBC with differential indicates an absolute neutrophil count of 180, a platelet count of 8000, and a hematocrit of 19.4.

QUESTIONS:

1. Given the treatment and laboratory values, what other type of symptoms might you expect?
2. What type of transfusions might be ordered?
3. What nursing interventions would help protect this client from infection?

SELECTED BIBLIOGRAPHY

*Agency for Health Care Policy and Research. (1993). *Sickle cell disease: Screening, diagnosis, management, and counseling in newborns and infants.* Rockville, MD: Author.

American Cancer Society. (1998). *Cancer facts and figures 1998.* 98-300M–No. 5008.98. Atlanta, GA: Author.

Blaylock, B. (1996). Sickle cell ulcers. *MedSurg Nursing, 5*(1), 41–43.

Bradbury, M., & Cruickshank, J. P. (1995). Blood and blood transfusion reactions: 2. *British Journal of Nursing, 4*(15), 861–868.

Callaghan, M. (1996). Leukemia. In R. McCorkle, M. Grant, M. Frank-Stromborg, & S. Baird (Eds.), *Cancer nursing: A comprehensive textbook* (2nd ed., pp. 752–772). Philadelphia: W. B. Saunders.

Carson, C.(1996). Hodgkin's disease and non-Hodgkin's lymphoma. In R. McCorkle, M. Grant, M. Frank-Stromborg, & S. Baird (Eds.), *Cancer nursing: A comprehensive textbook* (2nd ed., pp. 729–751). Philadelphia: W. B. Saunders.

Chernow, B., Jackson, E., Miller, J., & Wiese, J. (1996). Blood conservation in acute care and critical care. *AACN Clinical Issues: Advanced Practice in Acute and Critical Care, 7*(2), 191–197.

Cotran, R., Kumar, V., & Robbins, S. (1994). *Robbins pathologic basis of disease* (5th ed.). Philadelphia: W. B. Saunders.

D'Andrea, B., Belliveau, D., Birmingham, J., & Cooper, D. (1997). High-dose chemotherapy followed by stem cell transplant: The clinical/home care experience. *Journal of Care Management, 3*(2), 46–58, 80–85.

Dean, G. E., Haeuber, D., & Rivera, L. M. (1996). Infection. In R. McCorkle, M. Grant, M. Frank-Stromborg, & S. Baird (Eds.), *Cancer nursing: A comprehensive textbook* (2nd ed., pp. 963–978). Philadelphia: W. B. Saunders.

DeLaPena, L., Woolery-Antill, M., Tomaszewiski, J. G., Gantz, S., Bernato, D. L., DiLorenzo, K., Molenda, C., & Kryk, J. A. (1996). Hematopoietic growth factors. *Cancer Nursing, 19*(2), 135–150.

Devine, S. M., & Larson, R. A. (1994). Acute leukemia in adults: Recent developments in diagnosis and treatment. *CA: A Cancer Journal for Clinicians, 44,* 326–352.

Eisenberg, D. (1997). Advising patients who seek alternative medical therapies. *Annals of Internal Medicine, 127*(1), 61–69.

*Ford, R. (1991). Bone marrow transplantation. In S. Baird, R. McCorkle, & M. Grant (Eds.), *Cancer nursing: A comprehensive textbook* (pp. 385–406). Philadelphia: W. B. Saunders.

Ford, R., McDonald, J., Mitchell-Supplee, K. J., & Jagels, B. A. (1996). Marrow transplant and peripheral blood stem cell transplantation. In R. McCorkle, M. Grant, M. Frank-Stromborg, & S. Baird (Eds.), *Cancer nursing: A comprehensive textbook* (2nd ed., pp. 505–530). Philadelphia: W. B. Saunders.

Gerber, L. (1994). Autologous blood transfusion: Why and how. *Journal of Intravenous Nursing, 17*(2), 65–69.

Higgins, C. (1995). Haematology blood testing for anaemia. *British Journal of Nursing, 4*(5), 248–253.

Hurley, C. (1997). Ambulatory care after bone marrow or peripheral blood stem cell transplantation. *Clinical Journal of Oncology Nursing, 1*(1), 19–21.

Huston, C. J. (1996). Hemolytic transfusion reaction. *American Journal of Nursing, 96*(3), 47.

Jacobs, L. A., & Piper, B. F. (1996). The phenomenon of fatigue and the cancer patient. In R. McCorkle, M. Grant, M. Frank-Stromborg, & S. Baird (Eds.), *Cancer nursing: A comprehensive textbook* (2nd ed., pp. 1193–1210). Philadelphia: W. B. Saunders.

Jassak, P. F., & Riley, M. B. (1994). Autologous stem cell transplant: An overview. *Cancer Practice, 2*(2), 141–145.

Kefer, C. A., Godwin, J., & Jassak, P. F. (1996). Blood component therapy. In R. McCorkle, M. Grant, M. Frank-Stromborg, & S. Baird (Eds.), *Cancer nursing: A comprehensive textbook* (2nd ed., pp. 485–503). Philadelphia: W. B. Saunders.

Lapka, D. M. V., Wild, L. D., & Barbour, L. A. (1994). Heparin-induced thrombocytopenia and thrombosis: A case study and clinical overview. *Oncology Nursing Forum, 21*(5), 871–876.

Larson, P. J. (1995). Perceptions of the needs of hospitalized patients undergoing bone marrow transplantation. *Cancer Practice, 3*(3), 173–179.

Lin, E. M., & Beddar, S. M. (1996). Abnormalities in hemostasis and hemorrhage. In R. McCorkle, M. Grant, M. Frank-Stromborg, & S. Baird (Eds.), *Cancer nursing: A comprehensive textbook* (2nd ed., pp. 979–1008). Philadelphia: W. B. Saunders.

Marchiondo, K., & Thompson, A. (1996). Pain management in sickle cell disease. *MedSurg Nursing, 5*(1), 29–33.

Marelli, T. (1994). Use of a hemoglobin substitute in the anemic Jehovah's Witness patient. *Critical Care Nurse, 14*(1), 31–38.

McBrien, N. (1997). Thrombotic thrombocytopenic purpura. *American Journal of Nursing, 97*(2), 28–29.

Miller, C. (1994). The role of transfusion therapy in treatment of sickle cell disease. *Journal of Intravenous Nursing, 17*(2), 70–73.

Morrison, V. A. (1994). Chronic leukemias. *CA: A Cancer Journal for Clinicians, 44,* 353–377.

Ong, S. T., & Larson, R. A. (1995). Current management of acute lymphoblastic leukemia in adults. *Oncology, 9*(5), 433–442.

Poliquin, C. (1997). Overview of bone marrow and peripheral blood stem cell transplantation. *Clinical Journal of Oncology Nursing, 1*(1), 11–17.

Ramirez-Smiley, M., & Ingle, B. (1995). Leukemia during pregnancy. *Oncology Nursing Forum, 22*(9), 1363–1367.

Randolph, S. R., Kelley, C. H., & McBride, L. H. (1995). Discharge planning for bone marrow recipients. *Journal of Care Management, 1*(4), 13, 14, 29–33.

Richardson, A., Ream, E., Wilson-Barnett, J. (1998). Fatigue in patients receiving chemotherapy: Patterns of change. *Cancer Nursing, 21*(1), 17–30.

Rieger, P. T., & Haeuber, D. (1995). A new approach to managing chemotherapy-related anemia: Nursing implications of epoetin alpha. *Oncology Nursing Forum, 22*(1), 71–81.

Smith, R. N., Fallentine, J., Kessel, S., & Maloney, M. (1995). Autotransfusion. *Nursing95, 25*(3), 52–55.

Spector, D. (1995). Transfusion-associated graft-versus-host disease: An overview and two case reports. *Oncology Nursing Forum, 22*(8), 97–101.

Vernon, S., & Pfeifer, G. (1997). Are you ready for bloodless surgery? *American Journal of Nursing, 97*(9), 40–46.

Viele, C. S. (1996). Chronic myelogenous leukemia and acute promyelocytic leukemia: New bone marrow transplantation options. *Oncology Nursing Forum, 23*(3), 488–502.

Walker, F., Roethke, S. K., & Martin, G. (1994). An overview of the rationale, process, and nursing implications of peripheral blood stem cell transplantation. *Cancer Nursing, 17*(2), 141–148.

*Whedon, M. B. (1991). *Bone marrow transplantation principles, practice and nursing insights.* Boston: Jones and Bartlett.

*Workman, M. L., Ellerhorst-Ryan, J., & Koertge, V. (1993). *Nursing care of the immunocompromised patient.* Philadelphia: W. B. Saunders.

Wujcik, D. (1996). Update on the diagnosis of and therapy for acute promyelocytic leukemia and chronic myelogenous leukemia. *Oncology Nursing Forum, 23*(3), 478–486.

SUGGESTED READINGS

Bradbury, M., & Cruickshank, J. P. (1995). Blood and blood transfusion reactions: 2. *British Journal of Nursing, 4*(15), 861–868.

This article describes different types of transfusion reactions, their etiology, and presenting symptoms. Detailed guidelines for nursing management of hemolytic, febrile, urticarial, septic, and anaphylactic transfusion reactions are provided in a tabular format.

Gerber, L. (1994). Autologous blood transfusion: Why and how. *Journal of Intravenous Nursing, 17*(2), 65–69.

The author describes the four different types of autologous blood transfusions: preoperative blood donation, acute normovolemic hemodilution, intraoperative blood recovery, and postoperative blood salvage. Patient eligibility, indications, and contraindications for each modality are also explained.

Jassak, P. F., & Riley, M. B. (1994). Autologous stem cell transplant: An overview. *Cancer Practice, 2*(2), 141–145.

This informational article helps the reader understand the rationale for bone marrow transplantation, with a complete description of the transplantation process. The authors highlight supportive care issues, particularly those required after the client goes home.

Marelli, T. (1994). Use of a hemoglobin substitute in the anemic Jehovah's Witness patient. *Critical Care Nurse, 14*(1), 31–38.

The author uses a case report approach to present the clinical applications and limitations of Fluosol DA, a hemoglobin substitute used to treat anemia. Jehovah's Witness views on blood transfusion are presented, with historic and physiologic information about Fluosol DA. Specific nursing needs for clients receiving hemoglobin substitutes are addressed.

Wujcik, D. (1996). Update on the diagnosis of and therapy for acute promyelocytic leukemia and chronic myelogenous leukemia. *Oncology Nursing Forum, 23*(3), 478–486.

The diagnosis and treatment of these leukemias are the focus of this article, with pathophysiology, diagnostic parameters, and common treatments discussed in detail. This is a valuable article for students who have clinical experience caring for clients with leukemia or who are considering this setting for employment.

UNIT 9

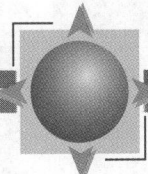

Problems of Mobility,

Sensation, and Cognition:

Management of Clients

with Problems of the

Nervous System

ASSESSMENT OF THE NERVOUS SYSTEM

The nervous system is the basis for all human function. It is the center of thinking, memory, judgment, sensation, movement, cognition, communication, behavior, and personality. In addition to its direct control over many processes, the nervous system innervates many other body systems and thus indirectly influences their functions. For example, damage to the spinal nerves that innervate the diaphragm may result in respiratory arrest.

The nurse may encounter clients with neurologic dysfunction throughout the health care system in various settings, including the acute care hospital, the ambulatory care center, the rehabilitation facility, and the home. Disorders of the nervous system can range from acute life-threatening emergencies to chronic, long-term conditions resulting in significant impairments, disability, or handicap.

ANATOMY AND PHYSIOLOGY REVIEW

The major divisions of the nervous system are the central nervous system (CNS) and the peripheral nervous system (PNS)

The brain and spinal cord are the major components of the CNS. The PNS is composed of 12 pairs of cranial nerves, 31 pairs of spinal nerves, and the autonomic ner-

vous system. The autonomic nervous system is further subdivided into the sympathetic and parasympathetic fibers.

The nervous system contains two types of cells: neurons, which transmit or conduct nerve impulses, and glial cells, which have an interdependent role with the neuron.

Nervous System Cells

Neurons

Structure

The basic unit of the nervous system, the neuron, functions to transmit impulses. Some neurons are motor (facilitating movement), and some are sensory (facilitating sensation); some process information, and some retain information. When a neuron receives an impulse from another neuron, the effect may be excitation or inhibition as well as conduction of the impulse. Each neuron (Fig. 43–1) has a cell body, or soma; short, branching processes called a dendrite; and a single axon.

Dendrites may have many branches or few. Each dendrite synapses with another cell body, axon, or dendrite and brings information to the cell body from other neurons. The dendritic process is described as an afferent pathway. Although only one axon extends from each neu-

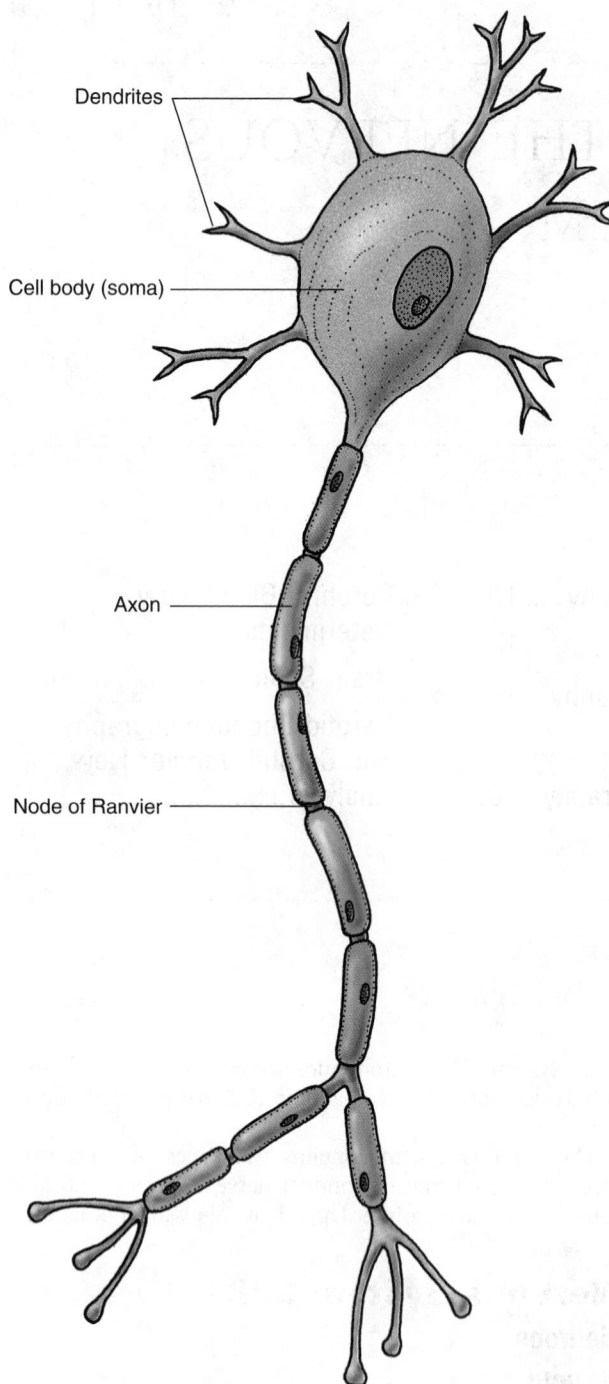

Dendrites

Cell body (soma)

Axon

Node of Ranvier

Figure 43–1. The structure of a typical neuron.

major role in impulse conduction, as shown in Figure 43–1. The enlarged, distal end of each axon is called the synaptic, or terminal, knob. Within the synaptic knobs are the mechanisms for manufacturing, storing, and releasing a transmitter substance. Each neuron produces a specific transmitter substance (such as acetylcholine or serotonin) capable of either enhancing or inhibiting the impulse, but not both.

Mechanism for Nerve Impulse Conduction

Sodium (Na^+) and chloride (Cl^-) ions are heavily concentrated in the area outside of the cell, the interstitial space. Within the cell, in the intracellular space, potassium ions (K^+) and other organic material are present. The inside of the cell is negatively charged compared with the interstitial space. Because of the different concentration of Na^+ and K^+, a neuron, even at rest, is constantly charged.

With a strong enough stimulus, the permeability of the cell membrane to Na^+ and K^+ is changed, and depolarization begins. Certain proteins within the membrane function as gates, or channels, that open for either sodium or potassium, but not both. With depolarization, sodium diffuses through the membrane first. It is believed that calcium plays a part in controlling the amount of sodium that diffuses through the membrane by controlling the gates. After sodium has entered the cell, potassium begins to leave the cell. Sodium is actively pumped out of the cell, and repolarization occurs. In nerve membrane, as an action potential or impulse occurs at one point on the membrane, the impulse excites adjacent cells so that the impulse is conducted all along the nerve fiber membrane. If the impulse is not of sufficient strength, there will be no action potential.

Synapses

Impulses are transmitted to their eventual destination through synapses. There are two distinct types of synapses: *neuron to neuron* and *neuron to muscle* (or gland). Between the terminal knob and the next cell is a small space called the synaptic cleft. The knob, the cleft, and the portion of the cell to which the impulse is being transmitted constitute the synapse.

Factors Affecting Transmission

Several factors affect the transmission of an impulse. Distance is one of the established factors. Synapses on or near the body of the cell have greater influence than those farther along the dendrite. The strength of the stimulus can also be influenced by other mechanisms, such as inhibition by another neuron, inadequate supply of transmitter substance, and extracellular fluid (ECF) changes. Lack of oxygen or the effects of hypnotics and anesthetics can quickly depress nerve cell activity.

Changes in ECF pH also affect neuron transmission. For example, acidosis depresses nerve cell activity. Alkalosis, on the other hand, excites nerve cells. Increased nerve cell activity occurs with the use of some drugs, such as caffeine (in coffee), theophylline (in tea and asthma drugs), theobromine (in cocoa), and strychnine.

ron, it may have few or many branches. The axonal process, called the efferent pathway, transmits impulses from its cell body to other neurons.

Many but not all axons are covered by a myelin sheath, or a white lipid covering. The myelinated axons appear whitish and are therefore also called white matter. The nonmyelinated axons have a grayish cast and are called gray matter. Myelinated axons have gaps in the myelin called nodes of Ranvier. The nodes of Ranvier play a

Transmitters

Transmitters are chemical substances that enhance or inhibit nerve impulses. These include

- Acetylcholine
- Serotonin
- Dopamine
- Norepinephrine
- Gamma-amino butyric acid (GABA)
- Substance P
- The endorphins and enkephalins

Other substances, although not specifically identified as transmitters, are considered probable transmitters. Table 43–1 summarizes what is currently known about them.

Glial Cells

Glial cells, which vary in size and shape, are divided into two main classes. Microglia cells play a scavenger role by responding to infection or trauma to the central nervous system. Macroglia cells are further divided into four subsets:

- *Astroglia* (star-shaped) cells provide the physical support for the neurons, regulate the chemical environment, and nourish the neurons.
- *Oligodendrocyte* and *Schwann* cells form the myelin sheath around axons.
- *Ependymal* cells form the lining of ventricles and the central canal of the spinal cord. They are also part of

TABLE 43–1

Sites, Functions, and Actions of Transmitters, Probable Transmitters, and Neuromodulators

Transmitter Substance	Site	Function/Comments	Action
Amines			
Acetylcholine	• Brain, brain stem, basal ganglia, autonomic nervous system	• Nerve and muscle transmission • Parasympathetic and preganglionic sympathetic system	• Excitatory, but some inhibitory
Gamma-aminobutyric acid (GABA)	• Brain, brain stem, basal ganglia, spinal cord, cerebellum	• Nerve and muscle transmission • Possibly one-third of brain neurons	• Inhibitory
Histamine	• Brain, spinal cord, PNS	• Not many data	• Questionable
Serotonin	• Medial brain stem, hypothalamus, dorsal horn of spinal cord	• Possible onset of sleep, mood control; pain pathway inhibitor in spinal cord	• Inhibitory
Catecholamines			
Dopamine	• Substantia nigra to basal ganglia	• Complex movements, emotional response regulation, attention	• Usually inhibitory
Norepinephrine (epinephrine parallels)	• Hypothalamus, brain stem, reticular formation, cerebellum, sympathetic nervous system	• Maintenance of arousal, reward system, dreaming sleep, mood regulation	• Mainly excitatory
Amino Acids			
Aspartic acid	• Brain, spinal cord interneurons	• Sensation	• Excitatory
Glutamic acid	• Sensory pathways	• Sensation	• Excitatory
Glycine	• Spinal cord interneurons	• Muscle control	• Inhibitory
Polypeptides*			
Substance P	• Brain, neurons in spinal cord	• Pain transmission	• Excitatory
Endorphins, enkephalins	• Thalamus, hypothalamus, spinal cord, pituitary	• Pleasure sensation, reward system, analgesia (inhibits release of substance P), released with ACTH (corticotropin) during stress	• Probably excitatory

*Other polypeptides under investigation as probable transmitters are vasopressin (ADH), gastrin, cholecystokinin, glucagon, insulin, somatostatin, angiotensin, melanocyte-stimulating hormone (MSH), luteinizing hormone–releasing hormone (LH-RH), and thyrotropin-releasing hormone (TRH). Prostaglandins, also under investigation, are thought to be modulators.

the blood-brain barrier and help regulate the composition of cerebrospinal fluid (CSF).

Central Nervous System

The central nervous system (CNS) is composed of the brain, which directs the regulation and function of the nervous system as well as all other systems of the body, and the spinal cord, which initiates reflex activity and transmits impulses to and from the brain.

Bone

The brain and spinal cord are encased, respectively, in the cranium and the vertebral column. For the most part, they are well protected. However, there are some areas of vulnerability, such as the nasal sinuses, the palate of the throat, the ears, and the cervical spine. The upright position of humans creates additional strain on the vertebrae and musculature. There are 7 cervical, 12 thoracic, 5 lumbar, 5 fused sacral, and 4 fused coccygeal vertebrae. Although there are some differences in structure, all of the vertebrae protect the spinal cord and give structure to the body.

Brain

Meninges

The meninges form the immediate protective covering of the brain and the spinal cord.

- The pia mater, a thin, delicate, and vascular membrane, adheres to the brain and the spinal cord.
- The arachnoid, the next layer, is thin and delicate but also fibrous. CSF fills the web-like tissue.
- The dura mater, the outer layer, is heavy, fibrous, and nonelastic. There are actually two layers of dura. The outer layer adheres to the cranium and becomes the periosteum. The inner layer covers the brain.

Situated between the arachnoid and pia mater is the subarachnoid space, where CSF circulates. The subdural space is located between the inner dura and the arachnoid. A potential space, referred to as the epidural space, is located between the skull and the outer layer of the dura.

Between the two layers of dura are the venous sinuses. The inner layer of dura dips down between the two hemispheres and is called the falx. The dura also lies between the cortex and the cerebellum and is called the tentorium. The falx and the tentorium decrease or prevent the transmission of force from one hemisphere to another and protect the lower brain stem. Clinical references may be made to a lesion (e.g., a tumor) as being *supratentorial* or, if it is in the cerebellum, *infratentorial*.

Cerebrum

The right and left hemispheres of the cerebral cortex are joined by the corpus callosum. The dominant hemisphere in most people is the *left* hemisphere (even for many left-handed people). Within the deeper structures of the cerebrum are the right and left lateral ventricles. At the base

TABLE 43–2

Brain Lobe Functions	
Frontal Lobe	• The primary motor area (also known as the motor "strip") • Broca's speech center on the dominant side • An eye field • Access to current sensory data • Access to past information or experience • Affective response to a situation • Regulates behavior based on judgment and foresight • Judgment prevents distraction • Ability to develop long-term goals • Ability to weigh the pros and cons of a situation or action
Parietal Lobe	• Understand sensation, texture, size, shape, and spatial relationships • Three-dimensional (spatial) perception • Important for singing, playing musical instruments, and processing nonverbal visual experiences • Perception of body parts and body position awareness • Taste impulses for interpretation
Temporal Lobe	• Auditory center for sound interpretation • Complicated memory patterns • Wernicke's area for speech
Occipital Lobe	• Primary visual center
Limbic Lobe	• Emotional and visceral patterns connected with survival • Learning and memory

of the cerebrum near the ventricles is a group of neurons called the basal ganglia. Composed of the caudate nucleus, putamen, and globus pallidus, the basal ganglia regulate movement and body tone.

The cerebral cortex is divided into lobes by sulci (fissures) and are named the same as the overlying bone, with the exception of the limbic lobe. The name and function of each lobe can be found in Table 43–2.

Since the early 1900s, attempts have been made to classify neurons by their cellular structure and then to relate that to function. Brodmann's map represents one means to classify neurons by their cellular structure and then to relate that to function. (Fig. 43–2).

Two important speech areas of the cerebrum are *Broca's* and *Wernicke's area*. Broca's area is composed of neurons responsible for the formation of words, or speech. This requires respiratory activation of the vocal cords, which must occur at the same time as tongue and mouth movements. This association area (Wernicke's area) plays a significant role in higher-level brain function. It enables processing of words into coherent thought and recognizing the idea behind written or printed words (language).

The general interpretive area enables a person to process complex thoughts, remember the notes of music,

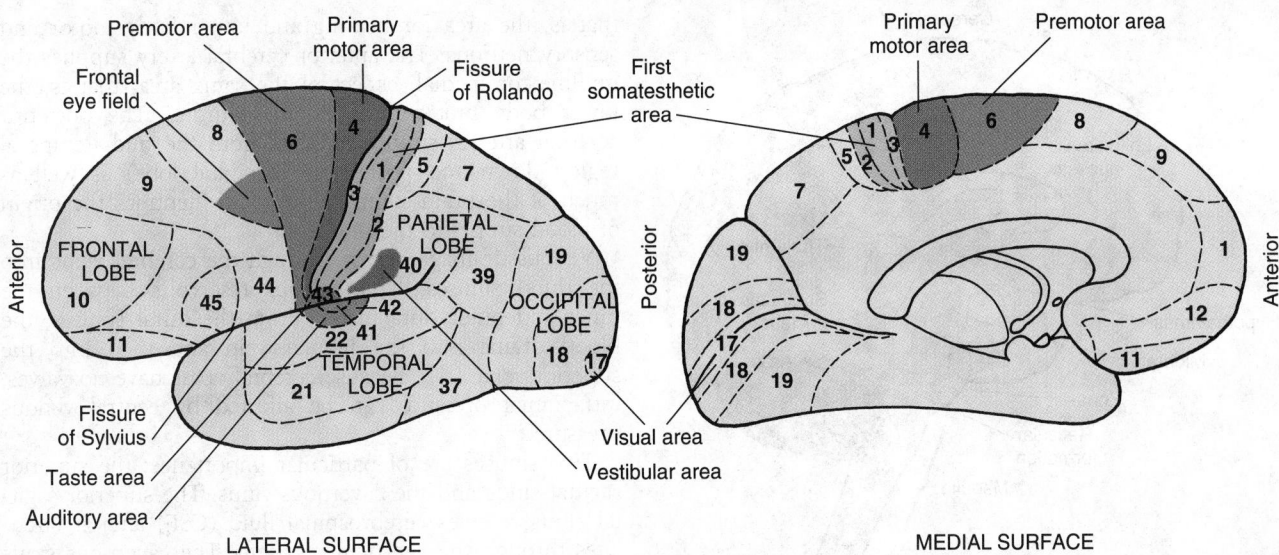

Figure 43-2. The functions of the brain according to Brodmann's map. *1–3*, Primary somatic sensory area (overlap with *4*). *4*, Primary motor area. *5*, Somatesthetic association cortex. *6*, Premotor area. *7*, Somatesthetic association cortex. *8*, Frontal eye field. *9–14*, Prefrontal or orbitofrontal association cortex (judgment, foresight, behavior), autonomic centers (respiratory, circulatory, renal, gastrointestinal; *11* and *12* have no clearly assigned function). *17*, Visual area. *18* and *19*, Visual association cortex. *21* and *22*, Ideation, sensory, language, also *37* (posterior part: auditory association cortex [Wernicke's area]). *37*, See *21* and *22*. *39* and *40*, Ideation, sensory, language, angular gyrus. *41*, Auditory area. *42*, May also function as auditory area. *43*, Taste area. *44* and *45*, Dominant hemisphere (motor speech centers and related functions), lips, and tongue (Broca's center). *47*, No clearly assigned function. (Modified from Barr, M. L., & Kiernan, J. A. [1988]. *The human nervous system: An anatomical viewpoint* [5th ed.]. Philadelphia: J. B. Lippincott.)

recite a speech heard or read long ago, recall childhood experiences, and so forth. Damage to this area on the dominant side after the age of 5 years is catastrophic.

Diencephalon

The diencephalon, which lies below the cerebrum (see Fig. 43–3), includes the thalamus, the hypothalamus, and the epithalamus.

The thalamus is the major "relay station," or "central switchboard," for the central nervous system. The hypothalamus is an integral part of the autonomic nervous system control and plays an essential role in intellectual function. The epithalamus contains the roof of the third ventricle and the pineal gland. See Table 43–3 for additional information concerning the diencephalon.

Hypophysis (Pituitary Gland)

The hypophysis is situated in the sella turcica of the ethmoid bone and is connected to the hypothalamus by tissue called the hypophyseal stalk. The hypophysis has two lobes, each releasing specific hormones into the circulation under the regulation of the hypothalamus.

Brain Stem

The brain stem (Fig. 43–3), includes the midbrain, pons, and medulla. The functions of these structures are presented in Table 43–4.

Throughout the brain stem are special cells that constitute reticular formation tissue, which controls awareness and alertness. For example, this tissue awakens a person from sleep when an arm or leg has become ischemic ("gone to sleep"), when there is abdominal pain, or be-

cause it is time to rise. Many sensory fibers branch and terminate here. The reticular formation area has abundant connections with the cerebrum, the rest of the brain stem, and the cerebellum. This is referred to as the *reticular activating system* (RAS). Within the reticular formation

TABLE 43-3

Diencephalon Functions	
Thalamus	• All sensation except smell • Sensation perceived at the thalamic level is crude and cannot be localized or quantified
Hypothalamus	• Regulates water metabolism, appetite, sleep-wake cycle, temperature control, and thirst • Hormonal activity • Posterior pituitary hormones, such as vasopressin and oxytocin • Anterior pituitary hormone excretion • Growth, thyrotropin, and follicle-stimulating hormones, prolactin, and corticotropin • Emotions and drives basic to self-preservation
Epithalamus	• By young adulthood often calcified and is radiopaque • Used as a point of reference on an x-ray or a computed tomography scan
Subthalamus	• Contains sensory tracts • Connections to basal ganglia

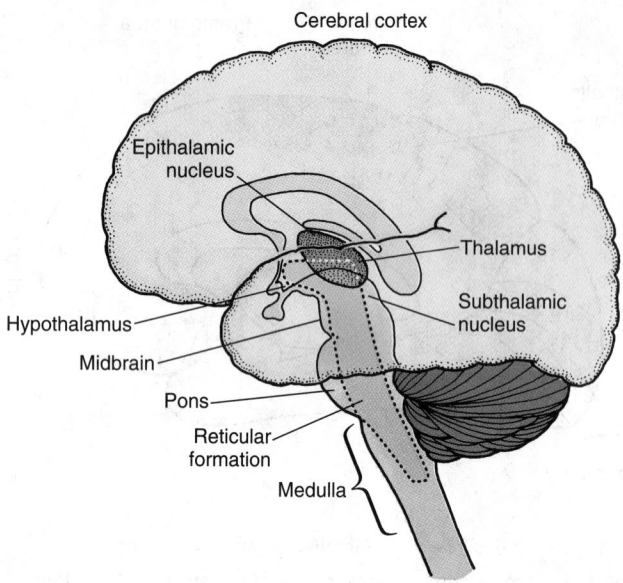

Figure 43–3. The structures of the brain stem and the diencephalon.

tissue, groups of specific neurons have functions other than control of alertness. These neurons are referred to as brain stem nuclei.

Cerebellum

The cerebellum receives instantaneous and continuous information about the condition of muscles, joints, and tendons. Cerebellar function enables a person to

- Keep a moving part from overshooting the intended destination
- Move from one skilled movement to another in an orderly sequence
- Predict distance or gauge the speed with which one is approaching an object
- Control voluntary movement
- Maintain equilibrium

Cerebellar control of the body is *ipsilateral* (situated on the same side). The right side of the cerebellum controls the right side of the body, and the left cerebellum controls the left side of the body.

Cerebral Circulation

The circulation in the brain originates from the carotid and vertebral arteries (Fig. 43–4). The internal carotid arteries branch into the anterior and middle cerebral arteries. The two posterior vertebral arteries become the basilar artery, which then divides into two posterior cerebral arteries. The anterior, middle, and posterior cerebral arteries are joined together by small communicating arteries to form a ring, the circle of Willis.

The circle of Willis is about the level of the pons or the level of the upper nose or lower border of the eye. The middle cerebral artery supplies the lateral surface of the cerebrum from about the mid–temporal lobe upward;

that is, the area for hearing and upper body motor and sensory neurons. The anterior cerebral artery supplies the midline, or medial, aspect of the same area; that is, the lower body motor and sensory neurons. The posterior cerebral arteries supply the area from the mid–temporal region down and posteriorly (occipital lobe) as well as much of the brain stem. Table 43–5 identifies the origin of blood supply to the brain.

Venous drainage occurs through the cerebral veins into the dural sinuses, large venous reservoirs between the inner and outer dura mater. From the dural sinuses, the blood drains into the jugular vein and then into the superior vena cava. Because cerebral veins have no valves, intracranial pressure can be affected by central venous pressure.

Two sinuses are of particular importance: the superior sagittal sinus and the cavernous sinus. The superior sagittal sinus receives cerebrospinal fluid (CSF) after it circulates through the ventricular system. The cavernous sinus is located near the eye and receives venous blood from the eye. In addition, the carotid artery passes through the cavernous sinus (the only place in the body where an artery passes through a vein); thus, the potential exists for development of a fistula between an artery and a vein (usually from trauma).

Blood-Brain Barrier

The blood-brain barrier seems to exist because the endothelial cells of the cerebral capillaries, along with ependymal cells, are joined tightly together. This keeps some substances in the plasma out of the cerebrospinal circulation and out of brain tissue. Substances that can pass through the blood-brain barrier include oxygen, carbon dioxide, alcohol, anesthetics, and water.

TABLE 43–4

Brain-Stem Structure Functions	
Medulla	• Cardiac-slowing center • Respiratory center • Cranial nerves IX (glossopharyngeal), X (vagus), XI (spinal accessory), and XII (hypoglossal) emerge from the medulla, as do portions of cranial nerves VII (facial) and VIII (acoustic)
Pons	• Cardiac acceleration and vasoconstriction centers • Pneumotaxic center helps control respiratory pattern and rate • Four cranial nerves originate from the pons: V (trigeminal), VI (abducens), VII (facial), and VIII (acoustic)
Midbrain	• Contains the cerebral aqueduct or aqueduct of Sylvius • Location of periaqueductal gray, which, when stimulated, may abolish pain • Cranial nerve nuclei III (oculomotor) and IV (trochlear) located here

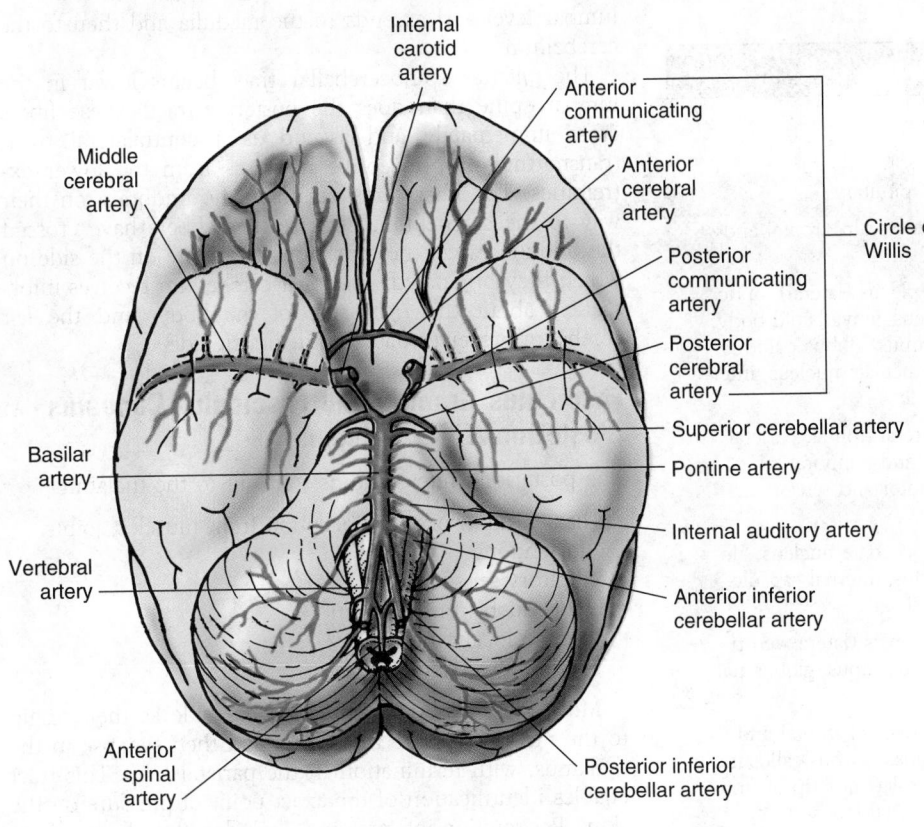

Internal
carotid
artery

Anterior
communicating
artery

Anterior
cerebral
artery

Middle
cerebral
artery

Posterior
communicating
artery

Circle of
Willis

Posterior
cerebral
artery

Superior cerebellar artery

Figure 43–4. Cerebral circulation and the circle of Willis at the base of the brain.

Basilar
artery

Pontine artery

Internal auditory artery

Vertebral
artery

Anterior inferior
cerebellar artery

Anterior
spinal
artery

Posterior inferior
cerebellar artery

Cerebrospinal Fluid Circulation

Cerebrospinal fluid (CSF) surrounds and cushions the brain and spinal cord. While circulating through the subarachnoid space, the fluid is continuously reabsorbed by the arachnoid villi and then channeled into the superior sagittal sinus (Fig. 43–5). Expanded areas of subarachnoid space, where there are large amounts of CSF, are called *cisterns*. The largest cistern is the lumbar cistern, the site of lumbar puncture (L2–S2).

Spinal Cord

The spinal cord controls body movement; regulates visceral function; processes sensory information from the extremities, trunk, and many internal organs, and transmits information to and from the brain. It contains gray matter (neuron cell bodies) that is H-shaped and surrounded by white matter (myelinated axons). The white matter is divided into posterior, lateral, and anterior columns. Groups of cells in the white matter (ascending and descending tracts) have been fairly well identified (Fig. 43–6). The gray matter divisions are posterior, intermediolateral, and anterior.

Ascending Tracts

As a general rule, ascending tracts begin in the spinal cord and end in the brain. Three ascending tracts are important for understanding the client with neurologic

problems: spinothalamic tracts, spinocerebellar tracts, and fasciculi gracilis and cuneatus (posterior white columns).

SPINOTHALAMIC TRACTS. As the name indicates, spinothalamic tracts begin in the spinal cord and end primarily in the thalamus. The spinothalamic tracts carry sensations of pain, temperature, light touch, and pressure. The axon fibers from the cells decussate (cross) the anterior white and gray commissures to the opposite side and become the contralateral (situated on the opposite side) spinothalamic tract. These fibers continue up to the thalamus. Some branches terminate in the reticular formation of the medulla and pons.

A pain or temperature impulse enters the posterior horn on the same side on which the sensation occurs. It is transmitted to other cells in several laminae, is further propelled to the opposite spinothalamic tract, and continues up to its ultimate destinations—the thalamus and the parietal lobe (Fig. 43–7).

POSTERIOR AND ANTERIOR SPINOCEREBELLAR TRACTS. Spinocerebellar tracts begin in the spinal cord and end in the cerebellum. The *posterior* spinocerebellar tract transmits impulses of proprioception (awareness of position and movements of body parts), or kinesthesia, mostly from the lower extremities. The impulses enter the posterior gray horn and synapse with tract cells in lamina VII. Spinocerebellar axons then form the tract on the *same,* or ipsilateral, side. This tract begins at the second

TABLE 43–5

Blood Distribution to the Brain

Artery	Distribution
Internal Carotid Artery Branches	
Hypophyseal	• Posterior pituitary
Ophthalmic	• Eye, frontal scalp, frontal and ethmoid sinuses
Anterior choroidal	• Choroid plexus (lateral), optic tract, uncus, amygdaloid body, hippocampus, globus pallidus, lateral geniculate nucleus, internal capsule
Middle cerebral	• Insula; lateral frontal, parietal, occipital, and temporal lobes (major motor and sensory areas)
Lenticulostriate	• Putamen, caudate nucleus, globus pallidus, internal capsule, corona radiata
Other	• Choroid plexus (lateral ventricles), hippocampus, globus pallidus
Anterior cerebral	• Medial surface of frontal and parietal lobes, corpus callosum, superior or lateral strip of frontal and parietal lobes
Vertebral Artery Branches	
Posterior cerebellar	• Medulla • Posterior cerebellum, inferior vermis, cerebellar nuclei, choroid plexus (fourth ventricle), posterolateral medulla
Basilar Artery Branches	
Anterior inferior cerebellar	• Cortex and inferior surface cerebellum, cerebellar nuclei, upper medulla, lower pons
Internal auditory	• Inner ear
Pontine	• Pons
Superior cerebellar	• Cortex, white matter and nuclei of cerebellum, pons, superior cerebellar peduncle, inferior peduncle, inferior colliculus
Posterior Cerebral Artery Branches	
	• Medial, inferior temporal, and occipital lobes
Calcarine	• Visual cortex
Other	• Posterior and lateral thalamus, subthalamus, pituitary, mammillary bodies, and midbrain; choroid plexus of lateral and third ventricle, dorsal thalamus
Circle of Willis	• Hypothalamus, caudate nucleus, putamen, globus pallidus, internal capsule, external capsule, thalamus, subthalamus, cerebral peduncles

lumbar level and ascends to the medulla and then to the cerebellum.

The *anterior* spinocerebellar tract begins lower in the lumbar spine than does the posterior tract. These fibers cross immediately and ascend as a contralateral tract, transmitting proprioceptive impulses from the lower extremities. The fibers cross again in the midbrain on their way to the cerebellum. Because these fibers have crossed the midline twice, the sensations terminate on the side on which they originated. The *right* cerebellum receives information about the *right* side of the body, and the *left* cerebellum receives data about the *left* side.

Fasciculus Gracilis and Fasciculus Cuneatus (Posterior White Columns)

The posterior white columns transmit to the thalamus

- The sensation of proprioception from muscles, joints, and tendons
- Vibratory sense
- Light touch from the skin
- Discrete localization
- Two-point discrimination

Most of the fibers ascend the *same* side as their origin to the medulla, where they cross and then synapse in the thalamus, with termination in the parietal lobe. This tract enables identification of the exact point of pressure on the skin. Recognition of pressure includes the shape of an object (with eyes closed), movement across the skin (a number being written or a fly crawling), and acknowledgment of two points of touch close together.

Descending Tracts

Descending tracts *begin* in the brain and *end* in the spinal cord. The major descending tract of importance for understanding neurologic problems is the lateral corticospinal, or pyramidal, tract. The corticospinal tract originates in the motor cortex of the frontal lobe and portions of the parietal lobe. At the level of the medulla, the lateral tract fibers cross to the opposite side. After crossing, the fibers descend to a predetermined level and synapse with interneurons of the gray matter. A few fibers connect directly with lower motor neurons. The cervical area has a high concentration of fibers synapsing with interneurons, which possibly reflects the complexity of hand and finger movements.

The motor neurons of the other descending tracts and the basal ganglia used to be referred to as an extrapyramidal system. It was thought that pyramidal neurons initiated voluntary muscle activity and extrapyramidal neurons initiated automatic or nonvoluntary muscle action. The descending tracts and the basal ganglia are necessary for the smooth function of all motor activity. The term *extrapyramidal* is still often used clinically to connote the origin of abnormal spontaneous movement.

Spinal Cord Circulation

The blood supply for the cord comes from three main arteries. The anterior spinal artery originates from a branch of the vertebral arteries. The two posterior spinal

Arachnoid villi or granulations
Superior sagittal sinus
Interventricular foramen
Lateral ventricle
Subarachnoid space
Straight sinus
Dura mater
Skull
Third ventricle
Choroid plexus of third ventricle
Cerebral aqueduct
Foramen of Luschka
Choroid plexus of fourth ventricle
Central canal
Foramen of Magendie

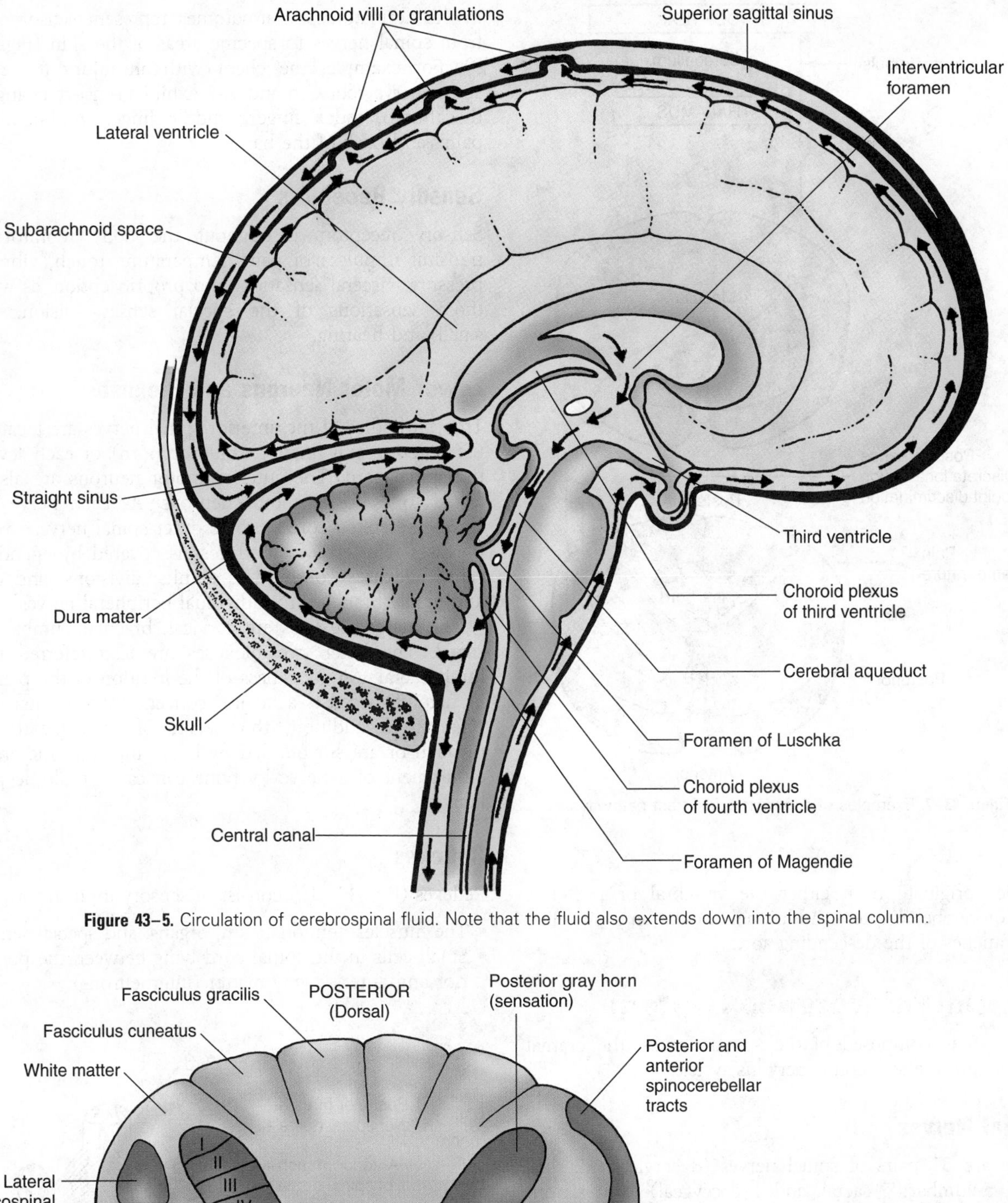

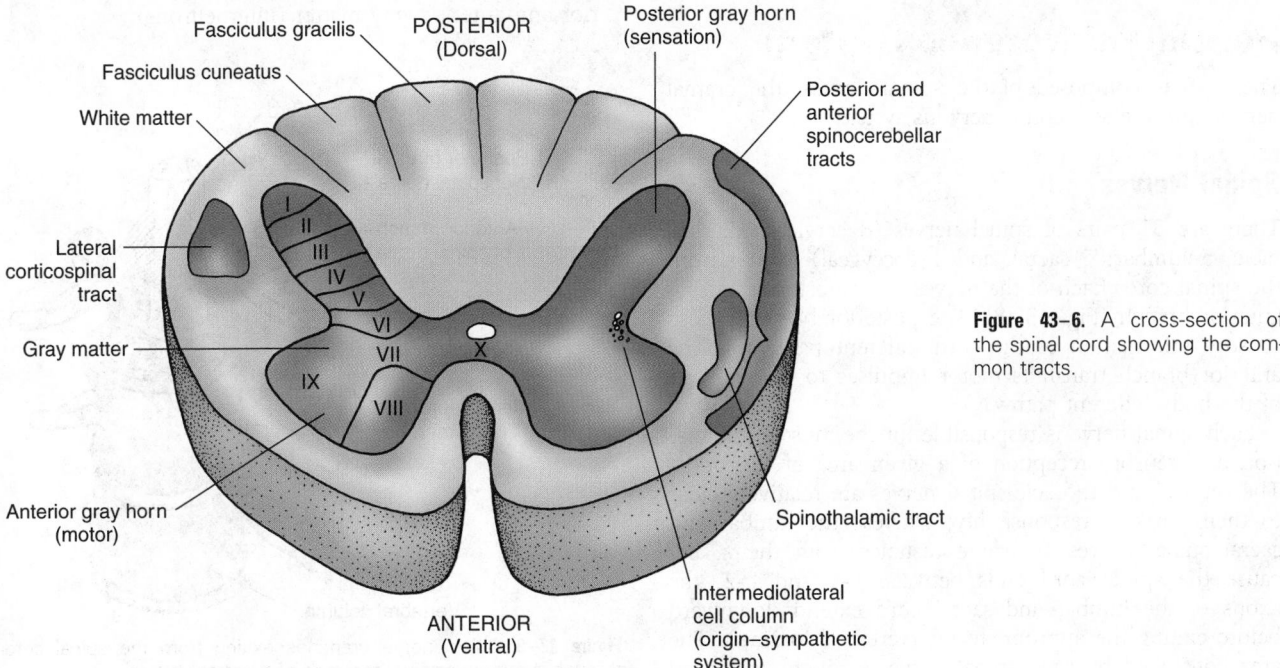

Figure 43–5. Circulation of cerebrospinal fluid. Note that the fluid also extends down into the spinal column.

Fasciculus gracilis
POSTERIOR (Dorsal)
Posterior gray horn (sensation)
Fasciculus cuneatus
White matter
Posterior and anterior spinocerebellar tracts
Lateral corticospinal tract
I
II
III
IV
V
VI
VII
VIII
IX
X
Gray matter
Anterior gray horn (motor)
Spinothalamic tract
Intermediolateral cell column (origin–sympathetic system)
ANTERIOR (Ventral)

Figure 43–6. A cross-section of the spinal cord showing the common tracts.

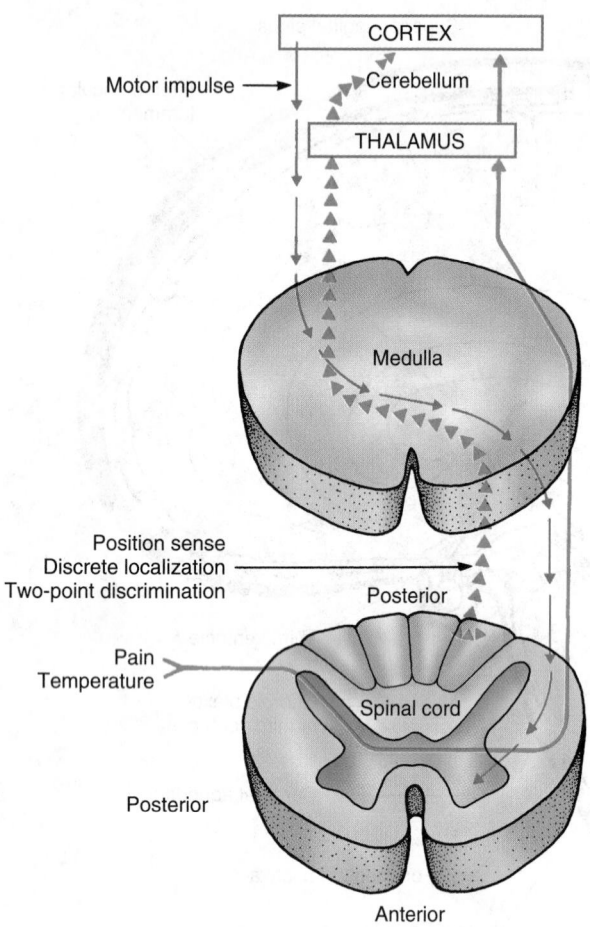

Figure 43–7. Examples of common spinal tract pathways.

arteries originate from either the vertebral or posterior inferior cerebellar artery. Additional circulation is supplied by branches of the descending aorta.

Peripheral Nervous System

The PNS is composed of the spinal nerves, the cranial nerves, and the autonomic nervous system.

Spinal Nerves

There are 31 pairs of spinal nerves (8 cervical, 12 thoracic, 5 lumbar, 5 sacral, and 1 coccygeal) exiting from the spinal cord. Each of the nerves has a posterior and an anterior branch (Fig. 43–8). The posterior branch carries sensory information to the cord (afferent pathway). The anterior branch transmits motor impulses to the muscles of the body (efferent pathway).

Each spinal nerve is responsible for the muscle innervation and sensory reception of a given area of the body. The cervical and thoracic spinal nerves are relatively close to their areas of responsibility, whereas the lumbar and sacral spinal nerves are some distance from theirs. Because the spinal cord ends between L-1 and L-2, the axons of the lumbar and sacral cord extend downward before exiting the appropriate intervertebral foramen. The area controlled by each spinal nerve is roughly reflected

in the dermatomes. Dermatomes represent sensory input from spinal nerves to specific areas of the skin (Fig. 43–9). For example, the client with an injury to cervical spinal nerve root C-6 and C-7 exhibits sensory changes in the thumb, index finger, middle finger, middle of the palm, and back of the hand.

Sensory Receptors

Sensory receptors throughout the body monitor and transmit impulses of pain, temperature, touch, vibration, pressure, visceral sensation, and proprioception, as well as those sensations of the special senses—vision, taste, smell, and hearing.

Lower Motor Neurons and Plexuses

The cell bodies of the anterior spinal nerves are located in the anterior gray matter (anterior horn) of each level in the spinal cord. The anterior motor neurons are also referred to as lower motor neurons. As each nerve axon leaves the spinal cord, it joins other spinal nerves to form plexuses (clusters of blood vessels covered by ependymal cells). Plexuses continue as trunks, divisions, and cords and finally branch into individual peripheral nerves.

The major plexuses are cervical, brachial, lumbar, and sacral. The latter two plexuses are also referred to as lumbosacral. An awareness of the location of the plexuses is helpful because a major concentration of nerves is present. In addition, the nerves of each plexus pass through or are surrounded by bone. Injury to the area or entrapment of a nerve by bone can cause multiple problems.

Reflexes

Reflexes (Fig. 43–10) consist of sensory input from

- The muscles, tendons, skin, organs, and special senses
- Small cells in the spinal cord lying between the posterior and anterior gray matter (interneurons)

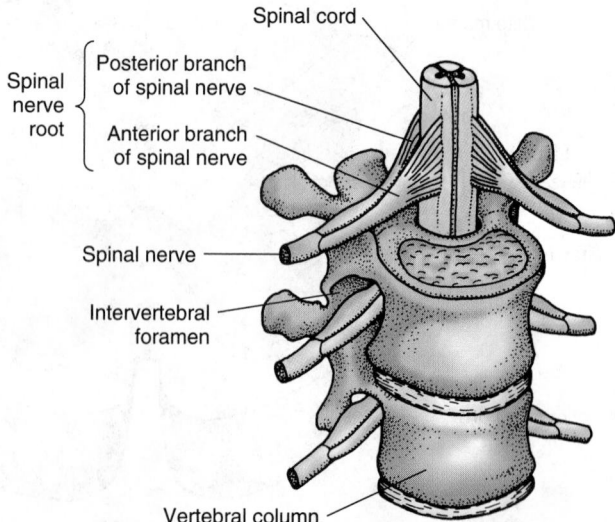

Figure 43–8. Spinal nerve branches exiting from the spinal cord through the intervertebral foramen of a vertebra.

C-2
C-3
C-4
C-5
T-2
T-3
T-4
T-5
T-6
T-7
T-8
T-9
T-10
T-11
T-12
C-6
T-1
L-1
S-3
S-4
S-5
C-8
C-7
L-2
L-3
L-4
L-5
S-1
S-2
Coccyx

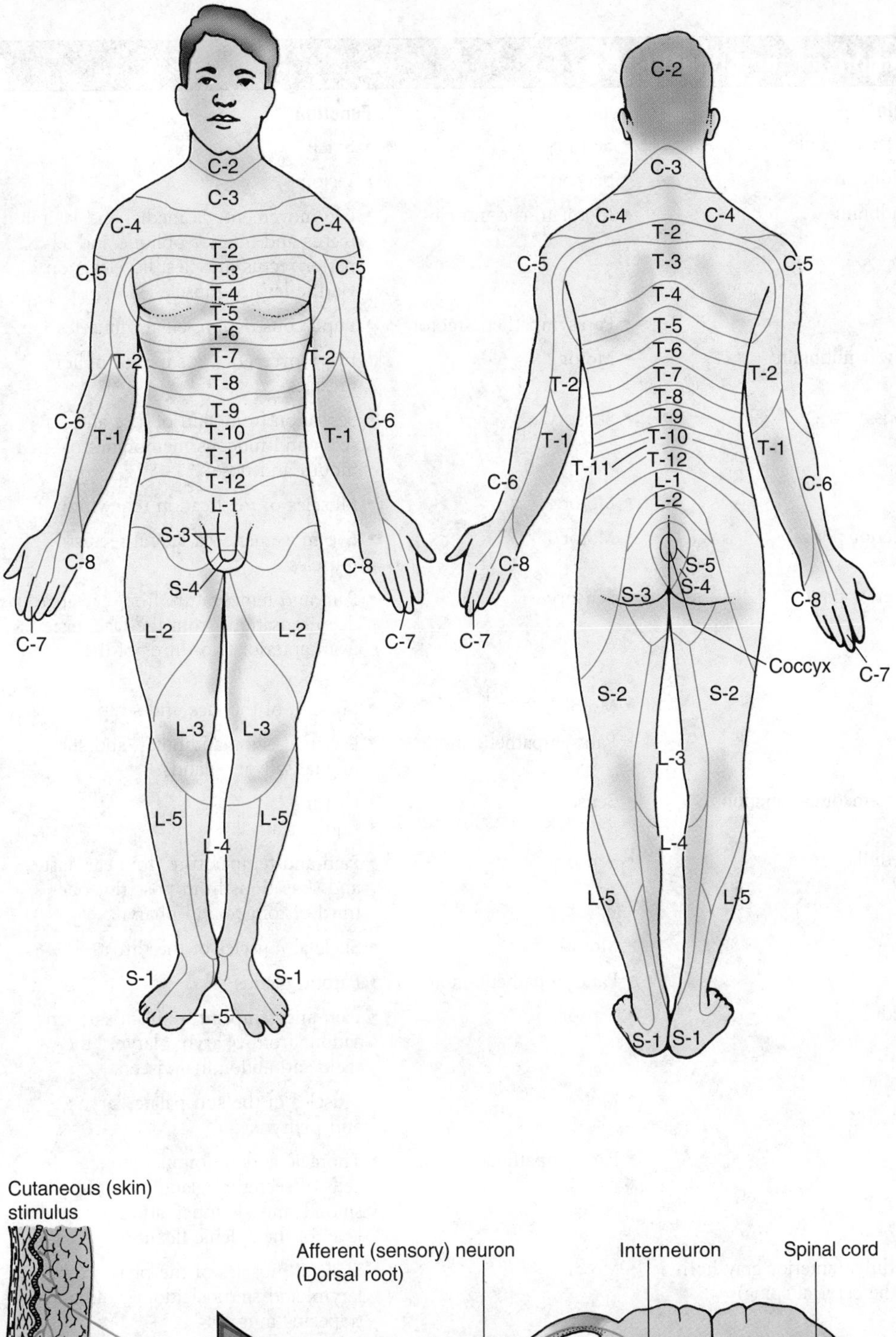

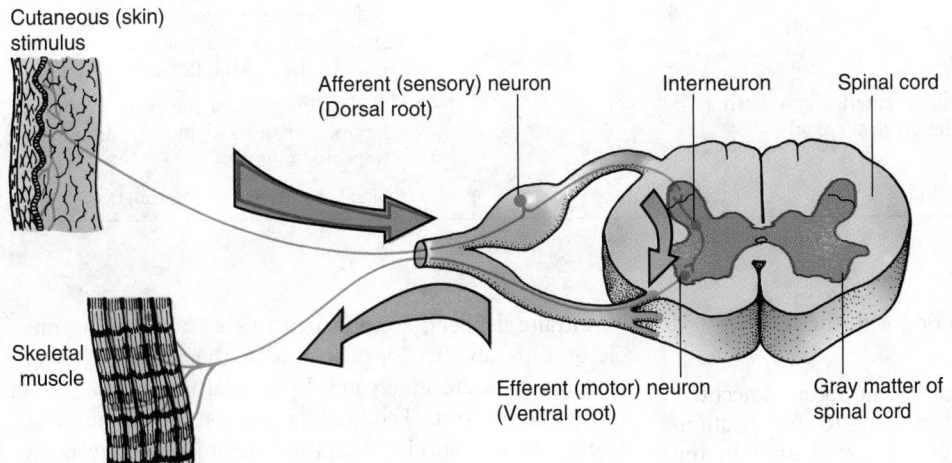

Figure 43–9. Dermatomes (cutaneous innervation of spinal nerves).

Cutaneous (skin) stimulus
Afferent (sensory) neuron (Dorsal root)
Interneuron
Spinal cord
Skeletal muscle
Efferent (motor) neuron (Ventral root)
Gray matter of spinal cord
Motor end plate response (contraction)

Figure 43–10. An example of reflex activity. Stimulation of skin results in involuntary muscle contraction (reflex arc).

TABLE 43–6

Origins, Types, and Functions of the Cranial Nerves

Cranial Nerve	Origin	Type	Function
I: Olfactory	• Olfactory bulb	• Sensory	• Smell
II: Optic	• Midbrain	• Sensory	• Vision
III: Oculomotor	• Midbrain	• Motor to eye muscles	• Eye movement via medial and lateral rectus and inferior oblique and superior rectus muscles; lid elevation via the levator muscle
		• Parasympathetic-motor	• Pupil constriction; ciliary muscles
IV: Trochlear	• Lower midbrain	• Motor	• Eye movement via superior oblique muscles
V: Trigeminal	• Pons	• Sensory	• Sensation from skin of face and scalp and mucous membranes of mouth and nose
		• Motor	• Muscles of mastication (chewing)
VI: Abducens	• Inferior pons	• Motor	• Eye movement via lateral rectus muscles
VII: Facial	• Inferior pons	• Sensory	• Pain and temperature from ear area; deep sensations from the face; taste from anterior two-thirds of the tongue
		• Motor	• Muscles of the face and scalp
		• Parasympathetic-motor	• Lacrimal, submandibular, and sublingual salivary glands
VIII: Vestibulocochlear	• Pons-medulla junction	• Sensory	• Hearing • Equilibrium
IX: Glossopharyngeal	• Medulla	• Sensory	• Pain and temperature from ear; taste and sensations from posterior one-third of tongue and pharynx
		• Motor	• Skeletal muscles of the throat
		• Parasympathetic-motor	• Parotid glands
X: Vagus	• Medulla	• Sensory	• Pain and temperature from ear; sensations from pharynx, larynx, thoracic and abdominal viscera
		• Motor	• Muscles of the soft palate, larynx, and pharynx
		• Parasympathetic-motor	• Thoracic and abdominal viscera; cells of secretory glands; cardiac and smooth muscle innervation to the level of the splenic flexure
XI: Spinal accessory	• Medulla (anterior gray horn of the cervical spine)	• Motor	• Skeletal muscles of the pharnyx and larynx and sternocleidomastoid and trapezius muscles
XII: Hypoglossal	• Medulla	• Motor	• Skeletal muscles of the tongue

■ The anterior motor neurons, along with the muscles they innervate

Sensory data from a specific peripheral location account for a change in the motor impulses going to that location. This closed circuit, which requires no mediation in the cerebral cortex, is called the reflex arc.

Muscle tone is achieved by special fibers in the middle of the muscle. These special fibers, called muscle spindle or intrafusal fibers, are attached to the surrounding muscle and are able to contract only at their ends. The contractible ends are innervated by special motor fibers from the anterior horn. The middle portion of the intrafusal fibers contains special receptors that measure the degree of stretch of the muscle. These receptors identify a change in length of the muscle as well as measure the rate of change in length.

Cranial Nerves

There are 12 cranial nerves. The name, number, origin, type, and function of the cranial nerves are summarized in Table 43–6.

Autonomic Nervous System

The autonomic nervous system (ANS) is composed of two parts: the sympathetic nervous system (SNS) and the parasympathetic (PAS) nervous system. Through the use of biofeedback and other mechanisms, some ANS functions can be brought under conscious control.

Sympathetic Nervous System

The cells of origin for the sympathetic nervous system are located in the gray matter of the spinal cord from T-1 through L-2 or L-3. Therefore, this part of the ANS is considered *thoracolumbar* because of its anatomic location.

STRUCTURE. Lying beside the spinal cord on either side is a chain of ganglia extending the length of the cord. This chain of ganglia is called the sympathetic chain. Sympathetic axons leave the spinal nerve immediately and enter the sympathetic chain. Some fibers synapse within the sympathetic chain, and others do not.

FUNCTION. If almost any portion of the sympathetic nervous system is stimulated, the whole system responds (the fight-or-flight response). During periods of excessive sympathetic stimulation

- Skeletal muscle vessels dilate.
- The heart pumps faster.
- The liver releases extra glucose.
- The thyroid is stimulated.
- Sweating increases.
- Kidney vessels constrict.

During true emergencies, this is a helpful mechanism; with false emergencies (such as being unduly anxious), this mechanism wastes resources.

Parasympathetic Nervous System

The cells of origin for the parasympathetic (PAS) nervous system are located in the gray matter of the spinal cord from S-2 to S-4 (sacral area of the spinal cord) plus portions of cranial nerves III, VII, IX, and X. The PAS nervous system conserves the body's resources.

Parasympathetic fibers to the viscera have some sensory ability in addition to motor function. Sensations of irritation, stretching of an organ, or decrease in tissue oxygen are transmitted to the thalamus through pathways not yet fully understood. Because pain from internal organs is often felt below the body wall innervated by the spinal nerve, it is presumed that there are connections between the viscera and body structure that relay pain sensations. Table 43–7 compares the action of sympathetic and parasympathetic systems in the body.

TABLE 43–7

Effects of the Autonomic Nervous System on Various Organs of the Body

Organ	Effect of Sympathetic Stimulation	Effect of Parasympathetic Stimulation
Eye		
Pupil	• Dilated	• Constricted
Ciliary muscle	• Slight relaxation	• Constricted
Glands		
Nasal	• Vasoconstriction and slight secretion	• Stimulation of copious (except pancreas) secretion (containing many enzymes for enzyme-secreting glands)
Lacrimal		
Parotid		
Submandibular		
Gastric		
Pancreatic		
Sweat glands	• Copious sweating (cholinergic)	• Sweating of the palms of the hands
Apocrine glands	• Thick, odoriferous secretion	• None
Heart		
Muscle	• Increased rate • Increased force of contraction	• Slowed rate • Decreased force of contraction
Coronary arteries	• Dilated (beta$_2$); constricted (alpha)	• Dilated
Lungs		
Bronchi	• Dilated	• Constricted
Blood vessels	• Mildly constricted	• ? Dilated
Gut		
Lumen	• Decreased peristalsis and tone	• Increased peristalsis and tone
Sphincter	• Increased tone (most times)	• Relaxed (most times)

Table continued on following page

TABLE 43–7

Effects of the Autonomic Nervous System on Various Organs of the Body *Continued*		
Organ	**Effect of Sympathetic Stimulation**	**Effect of Parasympathetic Stimulation**
Liver	• Glucose released	• Slight glycogen synthesis
Gallbaldder and bile ducts	• Relaxed	• Contracted
Kidney	• Decreased output and renin secretion	• None
Bladder		
Detrusor	• Relaxed (slight)	• Excited
Trigone	• Contracted	• Relaxed
Penis	• Ejaculation	• Erection
Systemic arterioles		
Abdominal	• Constricted	• None
Muscle	• Constricted (alpha-adrenergic) • Dilated (beta$_2$-adrenergic) • Dilated (cholinergic)	• None
Skin	• Constricted	• None
Blood		
Coagulation	• Increased	• None
Glucose	• Increased	• None
Lipids	• Increased	• None
Basal metabolism	• Increased up to 100%	• None
Adrenal medullary secretion	• Increased	• None
Mental activity	• Increased	• None
Piloerector muscles	• Contracted	• None
Skeletal muscle	• Increased glycogenolysis • Increased strength	• None
Fat cells	• Lipolysis	• None

From Guyton, A. C. (1991). *Textbook of medical physiology* (8th ed.). Philadelphia: W. B. Saunders.

Neurologic Changes Associated with Aging

Motor/Sensory Ability

Motor changes in the elderly are interrelated with sensory function and musculoskeletal status (Chart 43–1). Any problems affecting nerves, bones, muscles, or joints affect motor ability. The elderly person may have tremors without rigidity, and deep tendon reflexes may be hypoactive. Balance and coordination may be impaired as a result.

Sensory changes in older people can affect their daily activities. Pupils decrease in size, which restricts the amount of light entering the eye. The pupils also adapt more slowly. Touch sensation decreases, which may precipitate falls because the elderly person may not feel pebbles or small objects underfoot. Vibration sense may be lost in the ankles and feet. Hearing also decreases, especially for high-pitched sounds (presbycusis).

Mental Status

Intellect does not decline as a result of aging; however, a person may experience decrease in intellectual level caused by insufficient oxygen supply to the brain or drug interactions. Some older adults may need more time than does a younger person to process questions, learn new information, solve problems, or complete analogies.

Subtle memory changes are typical for many elderly people. Long-term memory seems better than recall (recent) or immediate (registration) memory. The elderly may need more time to retrieve information. These changes may be partly due to the loss of cerebral neurons, which is associated with the aging process.

Insomnia, anxiety, and depression among the elderly may cause some changes in mental status. Circadian rhythm disorders may lead to wakefulness until later at night, with extended sleeping in the morning (a pattern opposite to most health care facility routines). Many elderly people require less sleep than do their younger counterparts.

HISTORY

The neurologic history and assessment begin the moment the nurse firsts meets the client. During the introduction, the nurse notes the client's appearance and assesses his or her speech, affect, and motor function. The nurse provides privacy and makes the client as comfortable as possible. If the client appears to have cognitive deficits or has

---

Chart 43–1

Nursing Focus on the Elderly: Changes in the Nervous System Related to Aging

Physiologic Changes	Nursing Implications	Rationale
Recent memory loss	• Reinforce teaching by repetition and written teaching aids.	• Intellect is not impaired but the learning process is slowed. Repetition helps the client learn new information and recall it when needed.
Decreased touch sensation	• Remind the client to look where his or her feet are placed when walking. • Instruct the client to wear shoes that provide good support when walking. • If the client is unable, change the client's position frequently (every hour) while he or she is in bed or the chair.	• Decreased sensation may cause the client to fall.
Change in perception of pain	• Ask the client to describe the nature and specific characteristics of pain. • Monitor additional assessment variables to detect possible health problems.	• Accurate and complete nursing assessment ensures that the interventions will be appropriate for the elderly person in pain.
Change in sleep patterns	• Ascertain sleep patterns and preferences. • Adjust the client's daily schedule to his or her sleep pattern and preference as much as possible (e.g., evening versus morning bath).	• Most elderly clients require less sleep than younger clients do. However, frequent rest periods are needed.
Altered balance or coordination	• Instruct the client to move slowly when changing positions. • If needed, advise the client to hold on to hand rails when ambulating. • Assess the need for an ambulatory aid, such as a cane.	• The client may fall if moving too quickly. • Assistive and adaptive aids provide support and prevent falls.

---

trouble speaking or hearing, the nurse asks a family member or significant other to stay with the client during the history-taking to help secure accurate information. Chart 43–2 elaborates on the information the nurse obtains from the client or the family as part of the history.

Personal and Family History

Questions about the client's past medical history as well as the family and dietary history are necessary for any bearing they might have on the present problem. Ethnic and cultural background may be an influence, depending on the degree of socialization to the health care system.

Questions about the client's level of activities of daily living (ADL) may highlight subtle changes in neurologic function. Knowing the level of daily activity also helps the nurse establish a baseline for later comparison with changes resulting from improving or worsening neurologic function. The nurse asks whether the client is right- or left-handed. This information is important for several reasons:

- The client may be somewhat stronger on the dominant side, and this is expected.
- The client has a greater degree of independence if the dominant hand and arm can be free of tubing and tape.
- The effects of cerebral injury or disease are more pronounced if the dominant hemisphere is involved.

Current Health Problem and Social History

The nurse obtains information from the client as outlined in Chart 43–2.

PHYSICAL ASSESSMENT

The nurse may not perform the initial physical examination but must be knowledgeable about those components within the scope of nursing practice. There are times when the nurse is the first person to see the client and performs a neurologic examination as a part of the complete physical assessment. Establishment of baseline data for the client is most important. Nurses must constantly make comparisons with each assessment (e.g., to findings 5 minutes or an hour earlier, to the client's baseline, between the right and left sides, and to the expected progression for the client). Much of the neurologic assessment can be done with the client sitting or lying down.

Assessment of Mental Status

While collecting the history data, the nurse makes observations about the client's mental status, speech, and behavior:

Chart 43-2

Nursing Care Highlight: Personal and Family History Data for a Neurologic Assessment

Demographic Data
- Age
- Sex

Past Medical History
- Client's past medical history
- Family's past medical history
- Previous injuries or congenital problems
- Chronic diseases
  - Hypertension
  - Diabetes mellitus
  - Lung disease
- Previous neurologic problems
  - Headaches
  - Seizures
  - Head or spine trauma
  - Eye problems

Current History
- Current symptoms
  - Blurred vision
  - Headache
  - Speech or swallowing difficulty
  - Numbness, tingling
  - Weakness, clumsiness
  - Bowel or bladder difficulties
  - Nausea or vomiting
  - Personality seizures
- Allergies
  - Food
  - Medications
  - Environmental
- Pain tolerance
  - Medications taken for pain
  - Behaviors to reduce pain
- Medications
  - Prescribed
  - Illicit
  - Over-the-counter
- Activities of daily living

Social History
- Usual recreational activities
- Level of physical activity each day
- Hobbies
- Alcohol consumption and use of recreational drugs
- Smoking, use of any tobacco products
- Sleep habits
  - Changes in pattern, duration, or intensity
- Work history
  - Exposure to toxic agents
- Ethnic and cultural background
- Handedness (right or left)
- Educational background

- Are the client's answers appropriate?
- Is the client's behavior appropriate?
- Is the speech pattern of normal tone, rate, rhythm, and volume?

- Are the answers complete?
- Is the client's appearance neat or untidy?
- Is the client cooperative, hostile, or anxious?

Although the mental status examination is often left until last, it may be better to complete it as part of the initial physical assessment, especially if neurologic problems have been noted.

ELDERLY CONSIDERATIONS

Normal mental status in the elderly varies, but the nurse should be aware of some general considerations during the mental status assessment. Elderly clients may take longer to process and answer questions, particularly if they do not understand the relevancy. Their attention span may be short, and they may be guided by internal rather than external motivation. Depending on age, previous occupation, and retirement activities, a client may find some of the cognitive tests difficult or impossible to perform. The nurse should then change the questions to focus on the client's immediate life. If the client's behavior seems appropriate, the mental status assessment can be shortened. If the behavior is not appropriate, the nurse performs an in-depth mental status assessment; a tool, such as the Mini-Mental State Exam (MMSE) described in Chapter 44, is used for this assessment. The MMSE is an organized way to assess memory, attention, speech, language, and cognition, described in more detail in the next section.

Level of Consciousness and Orientation

The nurse determines level of consciousness (LOC) by observing the client's level of responsiveness to the environment. A change in the LOC is the first indication that central neurologic function has declined. The client who is alert is awake and responsive. Clients who are less than alert are labeled lethargic (sleepy but arousable), stuporous (arousable with difficulty), or comatose (not arousable). (Assessment of the client who is less than alert because of trauma or surgery, for example, is discussed in Chapters 44 and 47.)

To better identify the client's level of cognitive function or exact state of consciousness, the nurse describes the client's behavior in response to stimulation. The client is asked questions that indicate orientation to *person, place,* and *time*. During the history-taking, responses that indicate orientation to person, place, and time include

- The client's ability to relate the onset of symptoms
- The name of his or her physician
- The year and month
- His or her address
- The name of the referring physician or health care agency

Advanced age, time of day, medications, and the need for sleep affect a client's responses.

Memory

Memory is one of the most important criteria for neurologic assessment. If the client cannot remember, most of the verbal assessment tests are either not feasible or at best unreliable. Loss of memory, especially recent memory, tends to be an *early* sign of neurologic problems. Three facets of memory are tested: long-term (remote) memory, recall (recent) memory, and immediate memory. Some elderly clients may not be as capable with recall or immediate memory, and this may be acceptable for that person.

The nurse can test *remote,* or long-term, memory by asking clients about their birth date, schools attended, the city of birth, or anything from the past. The nurse must be able to verify the answers. Nurses often ask the maiden name of the client's mother; this is sometimes listed on the admission form and can be checked.

The nurse can test *recall* (recent) memory fairly well during the history-taking by assessing

- The accuracy of the medical history
- Dates of clinic or physician appointments
- The time of admission
- Health care providers seen within the past few days
- Mode of transportation to the hospital or clinic

The nurse tests *immediate* (new) memory by giving the client two or three unrelated words, such as "apple," "street," and "chair," and asking him or her to repeat the words to make sure they were heard. After about 5 minutes, while continuing with the examination, the nurse asks the client to repeat the words. A person normally should be able to do this correctly.

Attention

The nurse asks the client to repeat three numbers, such as 4, 7, and 3. The series is increased by one number with each successful repetition until seven or eight digits are achieved. If the client has difficulty at any level (cannot repeat the series), the nurse repeats the numbers. If the client cannot repeat, the nurse stops the procedure. Next, the nurse asks the client to repeat the numbers backward, starting again with three digits and increasing by one each time. Normally, a person should be able to repeat five to eight digits forward and four to six backward. Education, occupation, interest, culture, anxiety, and depression affect mental status, and what is considered normal may not be so for a particular client.

The nurse can also use the serial seven test to test attention. The client is asked to count backward from 100 by 7 (the examiner stops when the client reaches 65 successfully). Depending on education and other factors, it may be better to ask the person to subtract by three or to add forward by five. The nurse must use judgment in deciding which of these tests to use.

Language and Copying

The nurse can assess most language and copying skills during the initial interview. The client demonstrates language comprehension by following the nurse's directions on admission (e.g., getting undressed and providing a urine specimen). Was there any hesitancy in speech, indi-

cating that the client groped for words? If so, the nurse points to items and asks the client to name them, such as a drinking glass, the door, or the bed.

The nurse tests reading comprehension by writing a simple command and giving it to the client (e.g., "close your eyes"). Writing can be tested by asking the client to write a sentence. The nurse must remember that some clients are not able to read or write and modify the examination accordingly. The nurse usually tests copying ability by having the client copy something the nurse has drawn. The figures used most frequently are a cross, a circle, a diamond, and a square. The figures drawn by the client should look similar to those drawn by the nurse.

Cognition

The nurse assesses higher intellectual function by asking about favorite hobbies, current events, the names of the last few presidents, or the meaning of a statement. The nurse can evaluate abstract reasoning by asking the meaning of proverbs (e.g., "A stitch in time saves nine." or "A rolling stone gathers no moss."). Nurses can also assess the client's judgment, at least partially, during the interview. Did the client make rational decisions in dealing with his or her symptoms? The nurse can evaluate judgment by asking such questions as "What would you do if stopped for speeding?" and "What would you do if there was a fire in the wastepaper basket?" Remember, testing of cognition (general knowledge, abstraction, and judgment) is influenced by culture.

Assessment of Cranial Nerves

Cranial nerves are typically not tested unless the client has a suspected problem affecting one or more nerves.

Cranial Nerve I: Olfactory

With the client's eyes closed, the nurse tests one of the client's nostrils at a time; the client occludes the other with a finger. The nurse asks the client to identify familiar odors, such as coffee, tobacco, mint, or soap. Alcohol sponges and ammonia are not used because they stimulate the trigeminal nerve rather than the olfactory nerve. Lack of or decreased smell sensation may not be significant. However, it may affect the client's appetite, so adequate nutrition may be a problem. Decreased sensation occurs with age, smoking, colds, and allergies. It is more significant if the client reports that smell was suddenly lost without a predisposing factor or that odors are distorted.

Cranial Nerve II: Optic

Each eye is tested individually, with the other eye covered but open. The nurse tests *central vision,* or visual acuity, using the Snellen chart. If the client is literate, he or she reads out loud from a pocket reader card, a magazine, or a newspaper. Clients are tested with and without their glasses if glasses are used for far or near vision.

The nurse can assess the client's visual fields or peripheral vision by asking the client to focus his or her eye on the nurse's nose. The nurse wiggles one finger of each hand in the superior visual field, asking the client to indicate where the movement is. The client should see movement on both sides. The nurse then repeats the test in the inferior visual field. For testing the second eye, the nurse wiggles the finger of only one hand to prevent the client from repeating the previous answers. The nurse then tests the superior and inferior fields using a finger of each hand. If the client cannot see the fingers in one or more of the fields, further testing is required. The fundus, or optic disk, is inspected with the ophthalmoscope to check for vascular problems, retinal disease, papilledema, or optic atrophy. Nurses require special training to use the ophthalmoscope.

Cranial Nerve III: Oculomotor

Pupil constriction is tested with the room darkened, if possible. The nurse brings the penlight in from the side or from above or below the client's head and shines the light in the client's eye. The pupil should constrict, and it should stay constricted (*direct* response). The nurse also watches for *consensual* response in the eye not being tested (consensual response is less than direct response). Pupils should be *equal* in size, *round*, *regular*, and react to *light* and *accommodation* (PERRLA). Using a millimeter ruler or other measuring device, the nurse estimates the size of both pupils. Clients who have had eye surgery for cataracts or glaucoma often have irregularly shaped pupils. Clients using eye drops for either cataracts or glaucoma may have unequal pupils if only one eye is treated.

The nurse assesses accommodation by bringing an object from far to near the client's eyes. The pupils should constrict and the eyes converge (turn in to focus on the object). Accommodation need not be tested if constriction to light is normal. Some medications may affect constriction and dilation.

As a person ages, the pupils become less regular and round and adaptation from dark to light is longer. The pupils should react to light with the same rate of speed and to the same degree. Glaucoma, cataract surgery, and iridectomy may influence the shape and size of the pupil as well as its reaction to light. With the light stimulus still present, a pupil may dilate slightly after constricting (hippus); this reaction may be normal. In a few people, one pupil may be larger than the other (anisocoria); this may also be normal if there are no other eye symptoms. The client is usually aware of the size difference. The client with Adie's pupil has one pupil that is larger than the other; in addition to the size difference, the pupil is slow to react to light.

The nurse assesses lid elevation. The upper eyelid should rest approximately at the top or slightly below the top of the pupil. The strength and closure of the lid are a function of cranial nerve VII (see later) but can be tested with the eye examination.

The nurse evaluates eye movement (upward, downward, and medial) by assessing cranial nerve VI.

Cranial Nerve IV: Trochlear

Eye movement (inferior and medial) is tested with assessment of cranial nerve VI.

Cranial Nerve V: Trigeminal

The client's eyes are closed for the sensory portion of trigeminal nerve testing. The nurse asks the client to indicate when touch is felt by saying "now." By stroking a piece of cotton over the client's face (light touch), the nurse tests all three branches of the trigeminal nerve (ophthalmic branch—forehead; maxillary branch—cheek; mandibular branch—jaw). The nurse alternates sides for comparison. Next, by using an object that has sharp and dull components, such as a safety pin, the nurse asks the client to indicate whether the sensation is sharp or dull and then repeats the process. The motor aspect can be tested with the client's eyes open. The nurse palpates the temporal and masseter (jaw) muscles (with one hand on each side) for strength and equality (Fig. 43–11).

The corneal reflex has traditionally been tested by using a wisp of cotton and touching the edge of the cornea, which normally causes blinking. However, this procedure can cause abrasion to the cornea. In a routine examination, the examiner will see blinking and need not test the corneal reflex. If there is concern that the corneal reflex is absent, there are two safer tests. One is to bring a hand quickly toward the client's face in a threatening motion. If the client has vision, this will cause blinking. Alternatively, the nurse can use a syringe full of air and, while holding it 4–6 inches away from the client's eyes, expel the air gently toward the eyes. Another alternative is to place one or two drops of sterile saline into each eye. The client will blink if the reflex is intact.

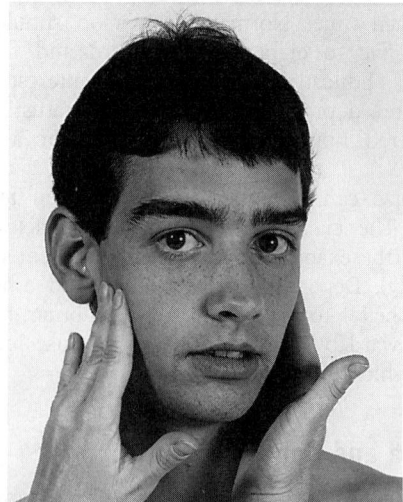

Figure 43–11. Assessment of cranial nerve V function. (From Jarvis, C. [1996]. *Physical examination and health assessment* [2nd ed.]. Philadelphia: W. B. Saunders.)

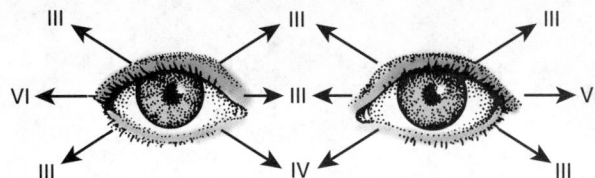

Figure 43–12. Checking extraocular movements in the six cardinal positions indicates the functioning of cranial nerves III, IV, and VI.

Cranial Nerve VI: Abducens

Cranial nerve VI controls lateral eye movement. Together with cranial nerves III and IV, cranial nerve VI is tested by checking the six cardinal positions of gaze. The nurse asks the client to follow the nurse's finger or a held object while keeping the head still. The nurse starts at the 1 o'clock position and moves clockwise through the six positions shown in Figure 43–12. The nurse pauses in the horizontal and vertical positions to check for nystagmus (involuntary oscillation of the eyes) or deviation. Some nystagmus in the extreme lateral position is normal. Severe lateral nystagmus or nystagmus in any other position is abnormal. If there is weakness or paralysis of a particular muscle, the eye will not turn in that direction.

Cranial Nerve VII: Facial

Only the motor portion of the facial nerve is tested. Taste on the anterior portion of the tongue is tested with cranial nerve IX. While looking for symmetry of both sides, the nurse asks the client to frown, smile, wrinkle the forehead, and puff out the cheeks. The nurse tests eyelid closure and strength by asking the client to close the eyes tightly and keep them closed while the nurse tries to pry them open.

Cranial Nerve VIII: Vestibulocochlear (Acoustic)

Hearing is tested initially with the client's eyes closed. The nurse rubs a thumb and finger together next to the client's ear and asks where sound is heard. The nurse then repeats this maneuver for the other ear. A watch can also be used, or the nurse can whisper close to each ear. (Quartz and electronic watches do not tick.)

The nurse may use the Weber and Rinne tests (with the client's eyes open) to check for conductive or sensorineural hearing loss. Conductive hearing loss is caused by external-ear and middle-ear problems, such as excessive cerumen, the presence of pus, ossicle fusion, or a damaged eardrum. Sensorineural hearing loss is due to cochlear or nerve damage.

In the *Weber* test, a vibrating tuning fork is placed on top of the client's head or forehead. The client should hear sound equally in both ears. (Touching the fork tines will stop the vibration; therefore, the fork must be held by the handle only.) With conductive loss, the sound is

heard louder in the ear with the deficit because the sound bypasses the obstruction. With sensorineural loss, the sound is louder in the better ear. The *Rinne* test measures the difference between bone and air conduction. A vibrating tuning fork is placed on the mastoid bone until sound is no longer heard and then moved near the external ear canal. With a normal or *positive* test result, the client hears the sound about twice as long by air conduction as by bone. In conductive hearing loss, the client hears the sound longer through bone (*negative* Rinne test result). The sound is heard longer by air than by bone (positive test result) in sensorineural loss (see Chap. 50).

Equilibrium, although regulated by cranial nerve VIII, is generally tested with the cerebellum at the end of the examination to avoid having the client stand and sit excessively.

Cranial Nerve IX: Glossopharyngeal

The motor portion is tested with cranial nerve X assessment. Taste (the posterior third of the tongue) is often not tested unless the client reports loss of taste. When testing taste, remember that the tongue must be rinsed between the sweet, sour, bitter, and salty samples. Taste occurs only when the substance is in solution, so the tongue must be moist for a true test result. As a normal process of aging, taste for sweets and salt may be decreased.

Cranial Nerve X: Vagus

To test the motor portion, the nurse asks the client to say "Ah" when looking into the throat. The uvula and palate should rise bilaterally and equally. Stimulating the gag reflex with a tongue blade reflects sensitivity to a stimulus. The ability to swallow and normal phonation and articulation also imply intact nerves IX and X.

Cranial Nerve XI: Spinal Accessory

The nurse assesses the strength of the client's sternocleidomastoid and trapezius muscles by having the client turn the head against resistance (provided by the nurse's hand on the side of the face toward the turn). The test is then repeated in the other direction. In the second test, the client shrugs the shoulders upward against the resistance of the nurse's hands placed on the client's shoulders (Fig. 43–13).

Cranial Nerve XII: Hypoglossal

The nurse tests motor innervation to the tongue by asking the client to stick out the tongue. The nurse checks for deviation to one side or the other. The tongue deviates toward the same side where the lesion has occurred in the brain. The nurse can test the strength of the tongue by asking the client to push against a tongue blade held at one side of the tongue. The test is then repeated on the other side.

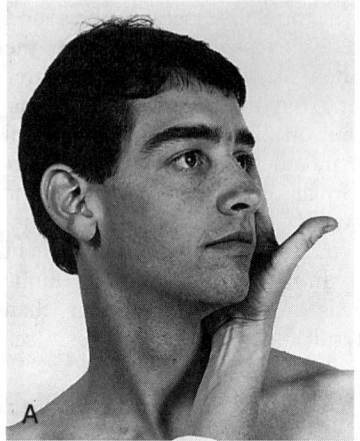 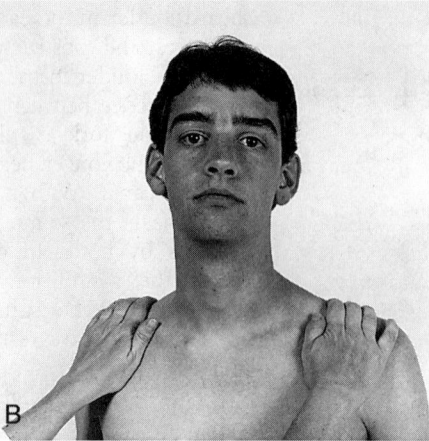

Figure 43–13. Assessment of cranial nerve XI function. (From Jarvis, C. [1996]. *Physical examination and health assessment* [2nd ed.]. Philadelphia: W. B. Saunders.)

Assessment of Sensory Function

The sensory examination is done in a manner as expedient as possible. The entire procedure soon causes fatigue to the client and makes test results questionable. An accurate assessment can be achieved from a few tests for the client who has not complained of any sensory loss. Sensory testing of the face is completed with testing of the trigeminal nerve.

Pain and Temperature

Pain and temperature sensations are transmitted by the same nerve endings. Therefore, if one sensation is tested and found to be intact, it can safely be assumed that the other is intact. The testing of temperature sensation is usually not accurate because it is difficult to keep vials of water at the appropriate temperatures (hot and cold). Testing of pain sensation is relatively easy and more reliable.

The nurse assesses for pain sensation with any object perceived as being sharp or dull. A safety pin or paper clip (dispose in the sharps' receptacle after each client use) has a sharp and a dull end. The nurse instructs the client to keep the eyes closed and to indicate whether the touch is sharp or dull. It may be necessary first to demonstrate what will be done with the client's eyes open. The sharp and dull stimuli should be interchanged at random so the client does not anticipate the type of the next stimulus. Not all areas need to be tested unless the client has suffered a spinal cord injury. Testing at one site on the upper arm, the lower arm, the hand, the thigh, the lower leg, and the foot suffices. If testing is begun on the hands and feet, there is no need to test the more proximal parts of the extremities because the tracts transmitting pain and temperature sensations are intact. The nurse compares reactions on each side. A sensation reported as dull when the stimulus was actually sharp necessitates more finite testing. A client with sensory loss is generally aware of the loss and points it out to the nurse.

Light Touch

The nurse assesses for light touch by taking a piece of cotton or a cotton swab and lightly stroking the client's skin over some of the dermatomes. While the client's eyes are closed, the nurse asks the client to say "now" when touched. Testing once on each hand or wrist and each ankle or foot should be sufficient. Light touch discrimination is likely to be normal if pain and temperature sensations are intact.

Touch Discrimination and Two-Point Discrimination

With the client's eyes closed, the nurse touches the client with a finger and asks that he or she point to the area touched. This procedure is repeated on each extremity at various points randomly picked rather than in sequence. Next, the nurse touches the client on each side of the body on corresponding sites at the same time. The client should be able to point to both sites. An inability to sense touch on one side is called the extinction phenomenon (a subtle test for sensory loss).

With two objects, such as cotton-tipped applicators, the nurse then touches the client in two places on the same extremity. A person can normally identify two points fairly close together, depending on where the stimuli are. The more nerve innervation an area has, the closer is two-point discrimination. For instance, two points around the mouth, on the fingers and the feet, or around the eyes can be identified at closer range than can two points the same distance apart on the leg or the back. These tests are not done unless response to light touch is abnormal or a posterior column problem is suspected.

Proprioception: Position Sense and Vibration Sense

Position sense is tested with the client's eyes closed. The nurse grasps the great toe on either side between thumb and index finger and moves the toe up or down, asking the client to indicate the direction of movement. The nurse should not grasp the toe by the anterior and posterior aspects because the pressure of the fingers will indicate the direction of movement. The same test is done on the fingers if upper-extremity problems are apparent.

Vibration sense is tested with the use of the tuning fork. After the client closes his or her eyes, the nurse places a vibrating tuning fork on the bony part of the ankle or the wrist. The client indicates the onset and cessation of vibration. The length of time the client feels the vibration can be compared with a normal response by using the nurse as a control.

ELDERLY CONSIDERATIONS

Posterior column function decreases with age. In the elderly, duration of vibration sensation may be normally decreased.

Graphesthesia and Stereognosis

The nurse assesses for *graphesthesia* (the ability to recognize numbers or letters when traced or written on the skin) by using an object, such as a capped pen, to write a number or a letter on the palm of the client's hand. The client can normally identify letters or numbers correctly. *Stereognosis* is the recognition by feel alone of an object placed in the hand. A key, a coin, and a pen are ordinary objects that should be recognized. With both tests, the client's eyes are closed.

Abnormal Sensory Findings

Abnormal sensory findings may have a peripheral nervous system (PNS) or a central nervous system (CNS) cause. The neuropathies of diabetes, malnutrition, and vascular problems are attributable to a PNS cause and generally involve the whole extremity or both extremities. Damage to a specific spinal nerve may not result in significant sensory loss because the spinal nerves overlap. Injury to several adjacent spinal nerves is manifested as decreased or absent sensation in the dermatomes of those nerves.

CNS problems can occur within the spinal cord, the brain stem, the cerebellum, and the cerebral cortex. Sensory deficits attributable to spinal cord damage vary with the location of the damage. Involvement of only the posterior column leads to lost proprioception below the level of the damage on the same side or on both sides (if both right and left posterior columns are involved). A lesion involving only the right spinothalamic tract results in loss of pain and temperature sensation below the lesion on the *left* side. Problems in the brain stem, the thalamus, and the cortex generally result in loss of sensation on the *contralateral* (opposite) side of the body. Cerebellar lesions affect sensation on the *same* side of the body as the lesion.

Assessment of Motor Function

Throughout the physical assessment, the nurse observes the client for involuntary tremors or movements. These movements, if present, need to be characterized as accu-

rately as possible; for example, "pill rolling with the thumbs and fingers at rest" or "intention tremors of both hands" (tremors occurring when the person tries to do something).

Muscle Strength

The nurse can test motor function best by putting each joint and extremity through a range of motion with and without resistance. The head and neck muscles are tested during the examination of the cranial nerves. The nurse measures hand strength by asking the client to grasp and squeeze two fingers of each of the nurse's hands. The nurse then compares the grasps for equality of strength. After comparison, the nurse tries to withdraw the fingers from the client's grasp and compares the ease or difficulty as another means of evaluating strength. The client should release the grasps on command, which is another assessment of consciousness and the ability to follow commands.

The nurse usually tests the client's strength against resistance by asking the client to resist the nurse's bending or straightening of the client's arm, hand, leg, or foot being tested (Fig. 43–14). A five-point rating scale is commonly used (see Chap. 52, Table 52–1). The results of testing are sometimes recorded as 5/5, 3/5, and so forth, indicating the criteria that were used and the status of the client at that testing. The nurse must evaluate and compare strength on each side. Later testing results are compared with these and other previous results to indicate progress or regression.

Cerebral/Brain-Stem Integrity

Cerebral or brain-stem integrity is assessed in the following procedure. The nurse asks the client to close the eyes and hold the arms perpendicular to the body with palms

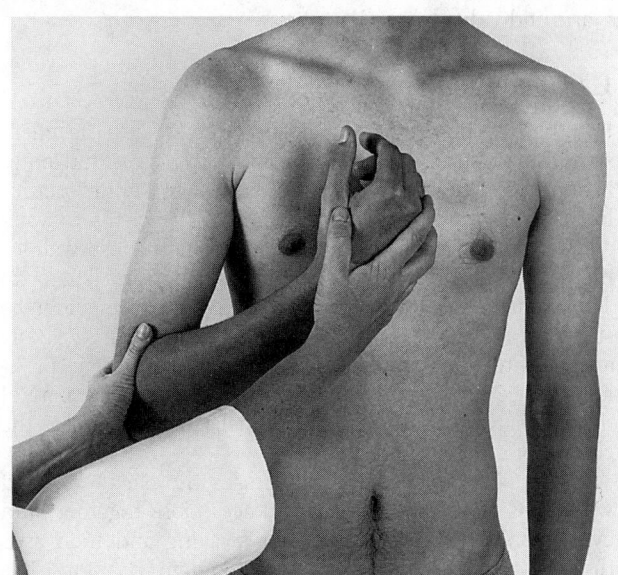

Figure 43–14. Testing for strength against resistance. (From Jarvis, C. [1996]. *Physical examination and health assessment.* [2nd ed.]. Philadelphia: W. B. Saunders.)

up for 15–30 seconds. If there is a cerebral or brain-stem reason for muscle weakness, the arm on the weak side will start to fall, or "drift," with the palm pronating (turning inward). The same can be done for the lower extremities, with the client lying on his or her stomach with the legs bent upward at the knees. However, it is easier for most clients to sit on the side of the bed and extend the legs outward.

Abnormal Motor Findings

Peripheral motor problems are caused by injury, neuropathies, vascular problems, or a localized lesion in the opposite motor cortex. Tremors, unintentional movements (clonus), and changes in gait or posture represent problems in the basal ganglia or specialized nuclei of the brain stem or cerebellum. Motor cortex lesions, such as cerebrovascular accidents (stroke), cause weakness or paralysis on the contralateral side of the body.

Assessment of Cerebellar Function
Coordination

Most of the assessment of cerebellar function can be done with the client sitting on the side of the bed or examining table. Fine coordination of muscle activity is tested. With the client's eyes closed, the nurse asks the client to perform the following:

- Run the heel of one foot down the shin of the other leg and repeat with the other leg (the client should be able to do this smoothly and keep the heel on the shin).
- Place the hands palm-up and then palm-down on each thigh, repeating as fast as possible (this can normally be done rapidly).
- With arms out at the side, touch finger to nose two or three times, with eyes open and then with eyes closed (this can be done with alternating arms or with each arm individually).

Gait and Equilibrium

For the last part of the cerebellar assessment, the client stands for testing of gait and equilibrium. Gait and equilibrium are usually tested at the end of the entire neurologic assessment. First, the nurse asks the client to walk across the room and return. The client is observed for inequality in steps, difficulty maneuvering, and so forth. To evaluate balance, the nurse then asks the client to stand on one foot and then on the other. Tiptoe walking and heel-to-toe walking can also demonstrate gait problems. Knee bends and one-leg squats are used as part of the testing, but these may be normally impossible for the elderly or nonathletic clients.

To test equilibrium, the nurse asks the client to stand with arms at the sides, feet and knees close together, and eyes open. The nurse checks for swaying and then asks the client to close the eyes and maintain position. The nurse should be close enough to prevent falling if the client cannot stay erect. If the client sways with the eyes closed but not when the eyes are open (the Romberg sign), the problem is probably *proprioceptive*. If the client sways with eyes open and closed, the neurologic disturbance is probably *cerebellar* in origin.

If the client is not able to perform any of these activities smoothly, the problem is manifested on the same side as the cerebellar lesion. If both lobes of the cerebellum are involved, the incoordination is bilateral.

Assessment of Reflex Activity
Procedure

The nurse assesses deep tendon reflexes (DTRs) and superficial (cutaneous) reflexes (Table 43–8). The *deep tendon reflexes* of the biceps, triceps, brachioradialis, and quadriceps muscles and of the Achilles tendon are tested in a routine neurologic assessment. Striking the tendon with the hammer should cause contraction of the muscle (Fig. 43–15). The appropriate muscle contraction indicates an intact reflex arc. The nurse taps each tendon quickly but not with too much force.

The *cutaneous* (superficial) reflexes usually tested are the plantar reflexes and sometimes the abdominal reflexes. The plantar reflex is tested by a pointed but not sharp object, such as the handle end of the reflex hammer or the rounded end of bandage scissors. The sole of the client's foot is stroked from the heel up the lateral side and then across the ball of the foot to the medial side. The normal response is plantar flexion of all toes. Dorsiflexion of the great toe and fanning of the other toes (Babinski's sign) is abnormal in anyone older than 2 years and represents the presence of central nervous system disease. (Positive Babinski's sign, meaning an abnormal response, and negative Babinski's sign, meaning a normal response, are clinically used terms but are not correct. Babinski's sign is present if the reaction is abnormal.) Babinski's sign can occur with drug and alcohol intoxication or after a seizure.

To test the abdominal reflex, the nurse strokes the client's abdomen in all four quadrants diagonally toward the umbilicus. The umbilicus should deviate toward the

TABLE 43–8

Deep Tendon and Superficial Reflexes

Deep Tendon Reflexes

- Jaw closure
- Biceps
- Triceps
- Brachioradialis
- Patellar
- Achilles

Superficial Reflexes

- Corneal
- Palatal
- Pharyngeal
- Abdominal (upper and lower)
- Cremasteric
- Gluteal
- Plantar

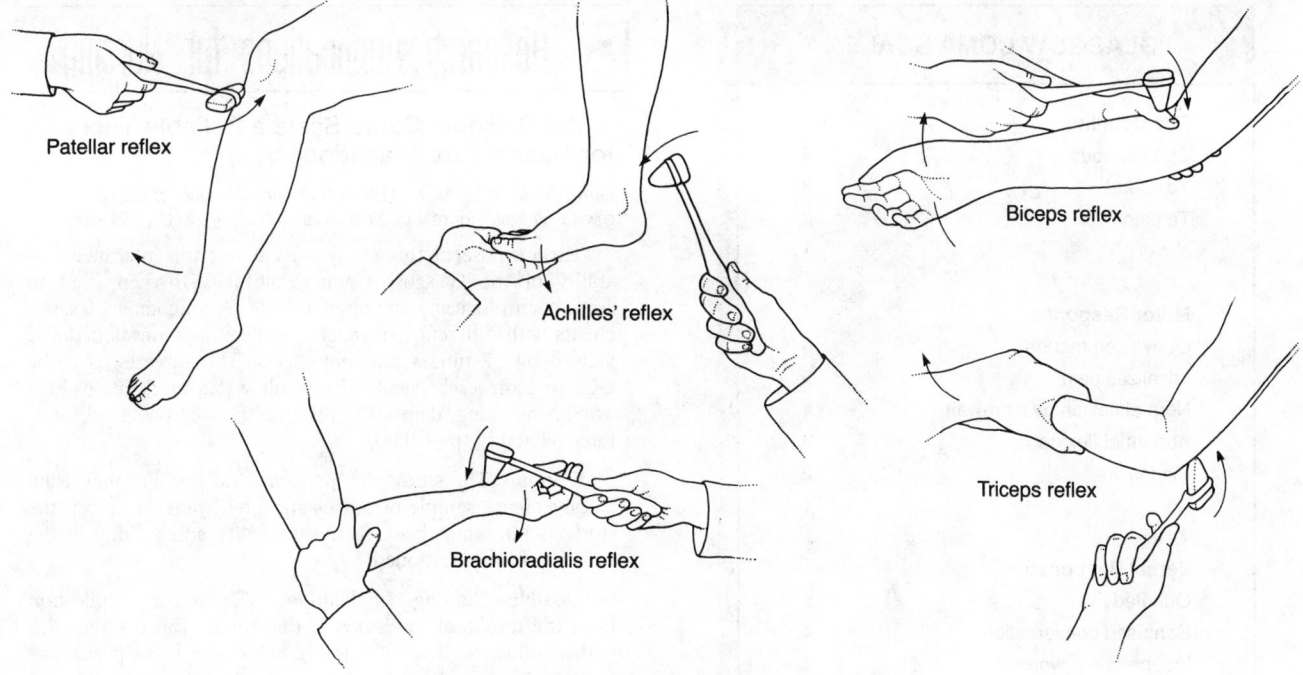

Figure 43-15. Procedures for testing deep tendon reflexes.

stimulus, but obesity may mask the reflex. The abdominal reflex can be absent in both upper and lower motor neuron disease.

Abnormal Reflex Findings

Hyperactive reflexes indicate possible upper motor neuron disease, tetanus, or hypocalcemia. Hypoactive reflexes may result from lower motor neuron disease (damage to the spinal cord); disease of the neuromuscular junction; muscle disease; or metabolic diseases, such as diabetes mellitus, hypothyroidism, or hypokalemia.

Although people can display hyperactive, hypoactive, or even absent reflexes, *asymmetry* is an important finding because it probably indicates a disease process. The results of reflex testing are recorded by use of a stick figure and a scale of 0-4 (Fig. 43-16). A score of 2 (++) is considered normal, although scores of 1 (hypoactive) or 3 (stronger than normal) may be normal for a particular client.

Rapid Neurologic Assessment

The nurse performs a complete neurologic assessment when the client is admitted to a health care facility or is seen for the first time by a physician or a nurse practitioner. As part of the client's routine or ongoing neurologic ("neuro") assessment or in the event of a sudden change in the client's neurologic status, the nurse may perform a rapid "neuro" assessment.

In many health care agencies, a form of the Glasgow Coma Scale (GCS) (Fig. 43-17) is used. Some agencies have expanded the GCS to be more comprehensive. The GCS establishes baseline data in each of the following areas: eye opening, motor response, and verbal response.

The client is assessed and assigned a numerical score for each of these areas. A score of 15 represents normal neurologic functioning. The tool has been shown to be reliable as one measure of neurologic assessment (see Research Applications for Nursing).

The nurse must use the most appropriate stimulus for eliciting the client's response. If the client is not awake and responding to commands, it may be necessary to use painful stimuli to obtain the best response. The client's response to central pain (brain response) is assessed first.

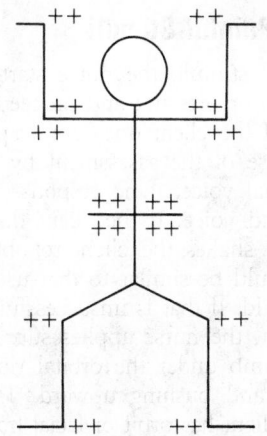

0	Absent, no response
1 (+)	Weaker than normal, hypoactive
2 (++)	Normal
3 (+++)	Stronger or more brisk than normal
4 (++++)	Hyperactive
	(Note: 1 and 3 may be normal for some individuals)

Figure 43-16. A stick figure and scale for recording reflex activity.

GLASGOW COMA SCALE*

Eye Opening	
Spontaneous	4
To sound	3
To pain	2
Never	1
Motor Response	
Obeys commands	6
Localizes pain	5
Normal flexion (withdrawal)	4
Abnormal flexion	3
Extension	2
Nil	1
Verbal Response	
Oriented	5
Confused conversation	4
Inappropriate words	3
Incomprehensible sounds	2
None	1

* The highest possible score is 15

Figure 43–17. The Glasgow Coma Scale. The highest possible score is 15.

Research Applications for Nursing

Is the Glasgow Coma Scale a Reliable Tool for Health Care Practitioners?

Juarez, V. J., & Lyons, M. (1995). Interrater reliability of the Glasgow Coma Scale. Journal of Neuroscience Nursing, 27(5), 283–286.

The purpose of this study was to test the interrater reliability of the Glasgow Coma Scale (GCS) when used to assess neurologically impaired clients. A videotape of seven clients with different neurologic problems was developed and viewed by 57 nurses and physicians. The subjects used the GCS to score each client. The result was a moderate-to-high agreement rating, demonstrating that the tool has good interrater reliability ($p = 0.00$).

Critique. The study was performed at one hospital using a convenience sample of nurses and physicians. However, the study is important because the reliability and validity of the GCS has been questioned.

Possible Nursing Implications. The major implication from the results of this study is that nurses can use the GCS with confidence. The GCS is a reliable tool to help evaluate clients with neurologic impairments.

in the value of the information gained from frequent or prolonged sternal rubs.

The client may respond to painful stimuli in several ways. Although the client's initial response to pain may be abnormal flexion or extension, continued application of pain for no more than 20–30 seconds may demonstrate that the client can localize or withdraw. If the client does not respond after 20–30 seconds, it is not necessary to continue to apply the painful stimulus.

If the client responds by moving, but not all extremities move, the nurse assesses the client's peripheral response to pain. The nurse places a pen or pencil on top of the client's nail bed at the base of the cuticle and applies pressure. This maneuver is done only on the extremity that did not move.

Level of Consciousness

In addition to using the Glasgow Coma Scale, the nurse assesses the client's level of consciousness (LOC). This area of the assessment must be meticulously recorded and described as a change in LOC. Even a subtle change is the first indicator of a deterioration in the client's neurologic status. These changes include complaints of headache; restlessness, irritability, or being unusually quiet; slurred speech; and a change in the level of orientation.

Decerebrate or decorticate posturing (Fig. 43–18) as well as pinpoint or dilated nonreactive pupils is a late sign of deterioration. The physician should be notified immediately. Decortication (Fig. 43–18A) is abnormal posturing seen in the client with lesions that interrupt the corticospinal pathways. The client's arms, wrists, and fingers are flexed with internal rotation and plantar flexion of the legs. Decerebration (Fig. 43–18B) is abnormal posturing and rigidity characterized by extension of the cli-

On the basis of the client's response, peripheral pain may be assessed. Failure to apply painful stimuli appropriately may lead the nurse to make an erroneous conclusion about the client's neurologic status.

Response to Painful Stimuli

To apply painful stimuli, the nurse starts with the least noxious irritation or pressure and proceeds to more painful stimulation if the client does not respond. The nurse begins each phase of the assessment by speaking to the client in a normal voice; if no response is obtained, the nurse uses a loud voice. If the client does not respond, the nurse gently shakes the client to obtain a response. The shaking should be similar to that used in attempting to wake up a child. If that is unsuccessful, painful stimuli are applied. First, the nurse applies supraorbital pressure by placing a thumb under the orbital rim in the middle of the eyebrow and pushing upward. This technique is not used if the client has orbit or facial fractures.

A second technique to elicit pain is to pinch the trapezius muscle located at the angle of the shoulder and neck muscle. If the client remains unresponsive, the nurse rubs the sternum. The nurse makes a fist and rubs the knuckles of the hand against the client's sternum in a twisting motion. The tissue in this area is tender, and bruising is not unusual. Therefore, the nurse must exercise judgment

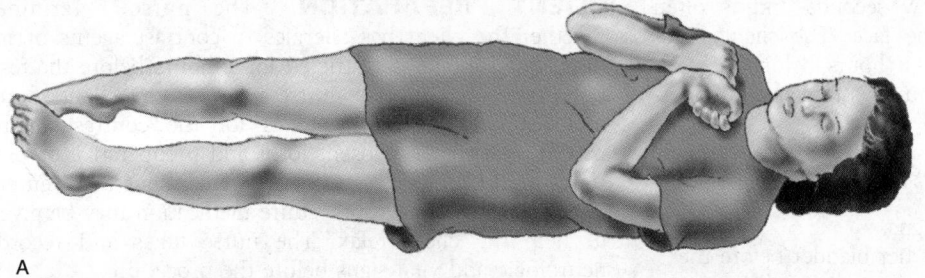

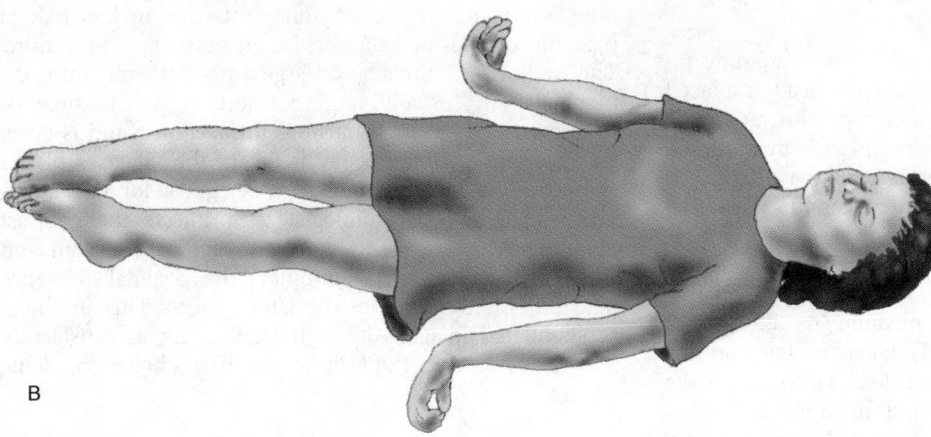

Figure 43–18. Posturing. *A,* Decorticate posturing. *B,* Decerebrate posturing.

ent's arms and legs, pronation of the arms, plantar flexion, and opisthotonos. It is usually associated with dysfunction in the brain-stem area.

DIAGNOSTIC ASSESSMENT
Laboratory Tests

For clients with a neurologic problem resulting from or concomitant with systemic infection, blood cultures are necessary to identify the causative agent of the infection. Although any client must have the cause of infection determined, this is especially true for clients with CNS disease. The blood-brain barrier is often not intact in neurologic disease, and the client is more susceptible to infection of the nervous system (meningitis or encephalitis).

Radiographic Examinations
X-Rays of the Skull and Spine

Plain x-rays of the skull and spine are used to determine bony fractures, curvatures, bone erosion, bone dislocation, and possible calcification of soft tissue, which can damage the nervous system.

Several views are taken—anteroposterior, lateral, oblique—and, when necessary, special views of the facial bones. In head trauma and multiple injuries, cervical fracture must be ruled out by radiography as one of the first priorities.

The nurse explains that the x-ray procedure for the skull and spine is similar to that for a chest x-ray, that the client will have to remain still during the procedure,

and that the exposure to radiation is minimal. If the client is in traction, the nurse may need to accompany the client to assist with positioning if a portable x-ray unit is not available. Any client who cannot walk from a wheelchair to the x-ray table should go to the radiology department on a stretcher. The client is positioned for each of the views desired and is asked not to move just before each x-ray. Follow-up care is not required.

Cerebral Angiography

Cerebral angiography (arteriography) illuminates the cerebral circulation. Contrast medium is injected into an artery (usually the femoral), and x-rays are taken sequentially as the contrast medium flows with the blood for visualizing carotid, vertebral, and cerebral circulation. The test is used for diagnosis of vascular aneurysms, malformations, displacements, and occluded or leaking blood vessels.

Contrast Media Method

CLIENT PREPARATION. The nurse ascertains that the client has no allergies to contrast agents or iodine. The procedure is initially explained to the client by the person obtaining the written consent, usually the radiologist. The nurse can clarify the explanation by answering questions and reinforcing the following important points:

- The necessity for not moving during the procedure
- The necessity for immobilization of the head
- The expectation of burning or heat sensation from the contrast medium as it is injected

The sensation lasts just a few seconds and is often noted behind the eyes or in the face. The client is allowed nothing by mouth for 6–8 hours before the test. Most hospitals require that the nurse complete a preoperative checklist. The nurse

- Removes the client's hairpins, jewelry, hearing aids, and/or dentures
- Records neurologic and vital signs
- Asks the client to empty his or her bladder before the procedure
- Administers the preangiography hypnotic, sedative, or analgesic as ordered by the physician

PROCEDURE. The client is placed on an examining table and secured with straps. The client's head is placed within a headrest device or immobilized with tape. The radiologist locates the artery to be used either by cutdown or palpation and threads a catheter into the artery. Although the carotid or vertebral artery can be used, the femoral or brachial artery is preferred because complications are fewer. Patency of the catheter is maintained with intravenous (IV) fluid.

The radiologist injects contrast medium (usually 40–50 mL), and x-rays are automatically taken as the contrast material moves through the circulation. The major risks are allergic response to the contrast medium and vasospasm, either of which may end the test. Vasospasm may be severe enough to cause occlusion and subsequent ischemia or infarction. The resultant tissue ischemia can cause hemiparesis, paralysis, or speech difficulties, depending on the artery in spasm. This risk is about 0.5% to 1%. After the catheter is removed, pressure is maintained over the puncture site for 5 minutes or more to prevent arterial bleeding.

FOLLOW-UP CARE. The nurse takes the client's vital signs and neuro signs according to hospital policy. The client is usually restricted to bed rest for 6 hours. The extremity into which the contrast medium was injected is kept straight and immobilized for approximately the length of the bed rest. The nurse checks the extremity for adequate circulation, which is demonstrated by

- Skin color and temperature
- Pulses distal to the injection site
- Capillary refill

The nurse inspects the injection site frequently for evidence of bleeding. A pressure dressing, sandbag, ice bag, or combination of the three may be maintained over the site for 6–12 hours to prevent bleeding, swelling, or hematoma formation. The nurse checks neurologic and vital signs frequently (every 15–20 minutes) for the first hour or two and compares them with the preangiography signs. Oral or IV fluid intake is increased (if fluids are not contraindicated) to help the client excrete the contrast material, which takes approximately 24 hours.

Digital Subtraction Angiography

Digital subtraction angiography (DSA) is used to evaluate the carotid and other cerebral arteries.

CLIENT PREPARATION. The nurse determines whether the client has allergies to contrast agents or iodine. Food intake is restricted for 2 hours before the test, but fluids are not. The nurse instructs the client to remain still during the test (as for the contrast media method). A signed consent form and preoperative or preprocedural checklist is necessary. The client must empty his or her bladder. Preprocedure medication may be given to help the client relax. The nurse takes and records neurologic and vital signs before the procedure.

PROCEDURE. Because DSA is done through the intravenous route, it has the advantage of causing less risk of bleeding or spasm. DSA can be an outpatient procedure. The radiologist threads a large angiocatheter into the brachial vein (usually) and positions it in the superior vena cava near the right atrium. Intravenous fluid is given via catheter. An initial x-ray is taken; the image is placed in a computer, to be used as a reference for the subsequent images. The radiologist then injects the contrast medium. As subsequent images appear on a screen and are transferred to the computer, the original reference image is subtracted from the later images. This produces a heightened image. Although DSA is not as satisfactory as the contrast method, it is the best choice for some clients.

FOLLOW-UP CARE. The client's vital signs and neuro signs are checked frequently. The nurse checks the extremity into which the contrast medium was injected for adequate circulation (as outlined for the contrast media method). The nurse checks the IV injection site for any bloody drainage because of the large size of the catheter. Unless increased fluid intake is contraindicated, the nurse encourages the client to increase fluid intake for 24 hours after the procedure to help excretion of the contrast medium. There are no activity restrictions.

Myelography

To perform myelography, a contrast medium or dye is inserted into the subarachnoid space of the spine. A lumbar puncture is the usual insertion site. Myelography enables the vertebral column, intervertebral disks, spinal nerve roots, and blood vessels to be visualized.

After the procedure, the client is usually managed in the same manner as the client who had a lumbar puncture (described later). Although this test is still performed, it is becoming less popular as computed tomography (CT) and magnetic resonance imaging (MRI) replace such invasive diagnostic techniques. This procedure is usually done as an ambulatory procedure.

Computed Tomography

Computed tomography (CT) scanning has been a significant tool in advancing neurologic diagnoses. With the aid of a computer, pictures are taken at many horizontal levels, or slices, of the brain or spinal cord. A contrast medium may be used to enhance the image. CT scans distinguish bone and soft tissue, such as the brain, the vascular system, and the ventricular system. Tumors, infarctions, hemorrhage, hydrocephalus, and bone malformations can be identified.

CLIENT PREPARATION. The nurse explains the procedure and ascertains whether the client has allergies to iodine. The nurse instructs the client to remove hairpins, hairpieces, or wigs. If contrast medium is used, food is withheld for 4–6 hours before the test. Fluids are generally not withheld. The nurse alerts the physician if the client seems unduly anxious, fearful, or unable to cooperate. Preprocedure sedation may be ordered, although it is not usually necessary. A consent form is obtained by the health care provider.

PROCEDURE. The client is placed on a movable table. The client's head is positioned in a holding device, which is then secured. The angles for the desired pictures are determined by the x-ray technician. The client must be completely still during the test, which may be difficult. The table is then positioned within the machine, a large cylinder-type structure. Some clients are fearful of the machine or of being confined in a small space. A noncontrast series of pictures is taken first. Contrast media enhance the visualization of the vascular system and are frequently used. Except for the intravenous injection of contrast media, the procedure is noninvasive. The entire procedure takes 10 minutes or less with the newer machines and 40 minutes with older machines or the use of contrast media.

FOLLOW-UP CARE. The nurse checks for a delayed allergic response to the contrast medium, if it was used. If a contrast medium was used, the resultant diuresis may require the administration of replacement fluids.

Positron Emission Tomography/Single-Photon Emission Computed Tomography

Positron emission tomography (PET) scanning is a new diagnostic tool available only in larger medical centers at present. Its benefit over a computed tomography (CT) scan or magnetic resonance imaging (MRI) is that it provides information about the *function* of the brain. Current CT scanners and MRI provide information about the *structure* of the central nervous system.

The physician injects the client with the molecule deoxyglucose, which is tagged to an isotope. The isotope emits activity in the form of positrons, which are scanned and converted into an image by computer. The image is displayed in color. The more active a given part of the brain, the greater the glucose uptake. This test is being used extensively for diagnosis of and research on Alzheimer's disease and other dementias, epilepsy, and movement disorders. The level of radiation is equivalent to that of five or six x-rays but much less than exposure during CT. Because the radioisotopes have such a short life, there must be a cyclotron on the premises to prepare them. This limits the number of medical centers able to offer the test.

This limitation of PET may be overcome through the use of single-photon emission computed tomography (SPECT). Radionuclides that emit gamma rays are administered by intravenous injection or inhalation for SPECT. Gamma-emitting radionuclides have longer half-lives; thus, the need for a cyclotron near the scanner is eliminated. Although SPECT is less expensive than PET, the resolution of the images is limited. SPECT is particularly useful in studying cerebral blood flow and cerebral blood volume, among other things.

CLIENT PREPARATION. The nurse explains the test and withholds caffeine, alcohol, and tobacco for 24 hours before the test, according to agency policy. The client should eat a meal 3–4 hours before the procedure (if the client is diabetic, no insulin is given before the test). The nurse withholds any other drugs that alter glucose metabolism.

PROCEDURE. The client sits on a reclining chair in front of the scanner. An intravenous line is started in each hand or arm—one to inject the isotope and the other to obtain blood samples. The arm used for blood samples is warmed to get arterial (shunted) and venous blood. The client may be blindfolded and have earplugs inserted for all or part of the test and must be still for 1 to 1½ hours. The client is asked to perform certain mental functions, which activate different areas of the brain.

FOLLOW-UP CARE. The radioisotope is eliminated in the urine, which requires no special precautions. Follow-up care is not required.

Other Diagnostic Tests
Lumbar Puncture

Lumbar puncture (spinal tap) is the insertion of a spinal needle into the subarachnoid space between the third and fourth and sometimes the fourth and fifth lumbar vertebrae. Lumbar puncture is used to

- Obtain pressure readings with a manometer
- Obtain cerebrospinal fluid (CSF) for analysis
- Check for spinal blockage attributable to a spinal cord lesion
- Inject contrast medium or air for diagnostic study
- Inject spinal anesthetic (see Chap. 21)
- Inject certain medications
- Reduce mild to moderate increased intracranial pressure in certain conditions

The procedure is contraindicated in clients with symptoms suggestive of increased intracranial pressure, except under extreme conditions (the procedure is then different from the one described here), because of the danger of sudden release of CSF pressure. The sudden release of CSF pressure causes a sudden shift of cranial tissue known as *uncal herniation,* which results in more brain damage. The procedure is also contraindicated in clients with skin infections at or near the puncture site because of the danger of introducing infective organisms into the CSF.

CLIENT PREPARATION. An informed consent form is signed by the client. The nurse explains the procedure to the client, noting that some discomfort may be felt when the local anesthetic is injected. Some clients experience pain in the leg when the spinal needle is inserted. The nurse asks the client to empty his or her bladder as a comfort measure. The nurse then positions the client on whichever side he or she is most comfortable, with the client's back close to the edge of the bed or examining table. When the physician is ready, the nurse asks the client to bring the knees up as close as possible to the trunk and to assume a "fetal" position (using the arms to hold the knees in place) with head bent forward. Some clients need help in achieving and maintaining this position. To help the client maintain the position, the nurse grasps the client behind the knees and the back of the lower neck. A pillow under the head and between the knees aids body alignment.

PROCEDURE. The physician cleans the skin site thoroughly. The injection site is determined, and the physician injects a local anesthetic. A few minutes after the anesthetic is injected, the physician inserts a spinal needle with stylet between the third and fourth lumbar verte-

brae. The nurse instructs the client to inform the physician if there is shooting pain or a tingling sensation. After determining proper placement in the subarachnoid space by removing the stylet and seeing CSF, the physician instructs the client to relax a little so the pressure reading will be more accurate. Opening and closing pressure readings are taken and recorded. Usually three to five test tubes of CSF are collected and numbered sequentially. After the specimens are collected, the needle is withdrawn; slight pressure is applied; and an adhesive bandage strip is placed over the insertion site. The nurse may or may not be able to help with the collection and numbering of the specimens, depending on the client's ability to remain quiet. If the client is restless or unable to cooperate, the procedure may need two people assisting instead of one. The nurse considers this possibility before beginning the procedure.

Examination of CSF has been a useful diagnostic tool for some time, and recent technical advances are increasing the number of analyses that can be done on CSF. The normal characteristics of CSF and some of the more common abnormalities are given in Table 43–9. Gram stain

TABLE 43–9

Significance of Cerebrospinal Fluid Findings

Findings	Significance
Pressure	
70–180 mmH$_2$O (5–13 mmHg)	• Normal range
68–195 mmH$_2$O (4–15 mmHg)	• Upper limits of normal
Color/Appearance	
Clear, colorless	• Normal
Pink-red to orange	• Red blood cells present
Yellow	• Bilirubin present owing to hemolysis of red blood cells; possible causes include subarachnoid hemorrhage, jaundice, increased CSF protein, hypercarotenemia, or hemoglobinemia
Brown	• Methemoglobin present, indicating previous meningeal hemorrhage
Unclear or hazy	• Cell count greater than 200/mL
Cells	
0–5 small lymphocytes/mm^3	• Normal
More than 5 lymphocytes/mm^3	• Reaction to infection, tumor, chemical substance, or blood
Proteins	
Total	
15–45 mg/100 mL (or less than 1% of serum levels)	• Normal
45–100 mg/100 mL	• Paraventricular tumor
50–200 mg/100 mL	• Viral infection
More than 500 mg/100 mL	• Bacterial infection, Guillain-Barré syndrome
Less than 15 mg/100 mL	• Meningismus, pseudotumor cerebri, hyperthyroidism, normal finding after lumbar puncture
Immune Gamma Globulin (IgG, the most important protein)	
3%–12% of *total* protein	• Normal
More than 3%–12% of total protein	• Multiple sclerosis, neurosyphilis, or viral infection

Table continued on following page

smears test for particular types of meningitis, such as tubercular meningitis. CSF can be cultured, and sensitivity studies determine the best choice of antibiotic if an infection is diagnosed. A specific test for neurosyphilis is the fluorescent treponemal antibody–absorption (FTA-ABS) test. Cytologic studies of CSF can identify tumor cells.

FOLLOW-UP CARE. After lumbar puncture, the client is restricted to bed rest in a flat position for 4–8 hours, as prescribed by the physician or determined by hospital policy, to prevent CSF leakage from the puncture site. The nurse instructs the client to increase fluid intake (to 3000 mL if possible) for 24–48 hours to facilitate CSF production. A decrease in CSF may cause a severe, throbbing headache (also called a spinal headache). The nurse administers analgesics as ordered for headache if it occurs. If the lumbar puncture was done to reduce intracranial pressure, neurologic signs, especially level of consciousness, are assessed more frequently until stability is ensured. Complications of lumbar puncture, although uncommon, include infection, CSF leakage, and hematoma formation.

Magnetic Resonance Imaging

Magnetic resonance imaging (MRI) is one of the newest diagnostic tools for detecting neurologic problems. Through the use of a large magnetic field and the introduction of a specific radio frequency, protons of the body absorb and emit energy. This energy is then converted to a picture or an image on a screen or magnetic tape. The images are clear for all densities of tissue. MRI is particularly useful as a diagnostic tool for multiple sclerosis. It surpasses computed tomography (CT) in clarity for many types of tissue and lesions, such as meningiomas and acoustic neuromas as well as arteriovenous malformations and other cerebral anomalies. MRI does not involve exposure to radiation and is noninvasive (see Chap. 52).

Client preparation is similar to that for a CT scan. A

TABLE 43–9

Significance of Cerebrospinal Fluid Findings *Continued*	
Findings	**Significance**
Albumin/Globulin Ratio	
8:1	• Normal
Glucose	
45–80 mg/100 mL (dL)	• Normal
Less than 45 mg/100 mL (usually accompanied by the presence of pathologic organisms)	• Bacterial, fungal, or viral meningitis; CNS leukemia; or cancer
Electrolyes and Minerals	
Sodium	
144–154 mEq/L	• Normal (abnormal values are not disease-specific)
Potassium	
2.4–3.1 mEq/L	• Normal (abnormal values are not disease-specific)
Chloride	
118–132 mEq/L	• Normal (abnormal values are not disease-specific)
Calcium	
2.1–2.7 mEq/L	• Normal (abnormal values are not disease-specific)
Other Characteristics	
Lactic Acid	
10–20 mg/100 mL	• Normal
More than 10–25 mg/100 mL	• Systemic acidosis or increased CSF glucose metabolism
Urea	
10–15 mg/100 mL	• Normal
More than 10–15 mg/100 mL	• Uremia, meningitis, or urea administration
Glutamine	
Less than 20 mg/100 mL	• Normal
More than 20 mg/100 mL	• Hepatic coma or cirrhosis of liver
Lactate Dehydrogenase	
10% of serum level	• Normal
More than 10% of serum level	• Bacterial meningitis, inflammatory diseases of CNS

signed consent form is obtained. The client is asked to remove anything metal such as watches, rings, earrings, necklaces, credit cards, and so on. Importantly, the client is questioned concerning any implanted devices, such as metal clips in the brain, metal prosthesis, or other metal implanted devices such as a pacemaker.

The procedure is similar to that of a CT scan. Many of the devices are more open, lessening the possibility that the client will feel claustrophobic. No special follow-up care is needed other than monitoring routine vital and neurologic signs.

Electroencephalography

Electroencephalography (EEG) records the electrical activity of the cerebral hemispheres. Each graphic recording represents the voltage changes in various areas of the brain (determined by recording the difference between two electrodes). The test is performed to

- Determine the general activity of the cerebral hemispheres
- Determine the origin of seizure activity (epilepsy)
- Determine cerebral function in pathologic conditions other than epilepsy, such as tumors, abscesses, cerebrovascular disease, hematomas, injury, metabolic diseases, degenerative brain disease, and drug intoxication
- Differentiate between organic and hysterical or feigned blindness or deafness
- Monitor cerebral activity during surgical anesthesia
- Diagnose sleep disorders (all-night EEG)
- Determine brain death

CLIENT PREPARATION. The test is done on an ambulatory (outpatient) basis. Chart 43–3 lists instructions for the client preparing to have an EEG.

The nurse explains the purpose and procedure for the test. If the EEG is ordered with the client "sleep-de-

prived," the client should be kept awake from about 2 to 3 AM through the rest of the night. CNS depressants and stimulants are usually not administered for 24 hours before the test. The physician indicates whether anticonvulsants are to be withheld. If anticonvulsants are withheld, the nurse monitors the client for signs of seizure activity. The nurse withholds coffee, tea, and other stimulants, but food and other fluids are given because hypoglycemia affects brain activity. The nurse checks to make sure the hair is clean and free from hairpins, sprays, or oils.

PROCEDURE. The client is placed on a reclining chair or bed. Usually, 16–24 electrodes are attached to the scalp with a jelly-like substance, according to an internationally accepted procedure, and connected to the machine. The physician or EEG technician places a glue over the electrodes to prevent slippage. The client must lie still with eyes closed during the initial recording. The rest of the test engages the client in certain activities: hyperventilation, photic stimulation, and sleep.

Hyperventilation produces cerebral vasoconstriction and alkalosis, which increases the likelihood of seizure activity. The client is asked to breathe deeply 20 to 30 times for 3 minutes.

In *photic stimulation,* a strobe light (a bright light) is placed in front of the client. Frequencies of 1–20 flashes per second are used with the client's eyes open and then closed. The EEG shows waves corresponding to each flash of light or waves indicating seizure activity if the client's seizures are photosensitive in origin.

Sleep is either natural or induced by an oral or IV sedative. EEG waves indicative of temporal lobe epilepsy can be demonstrated best during sleep.

Throughout the test, which takes 40–60 minutes, the technician watches the client closely and records any movement. These movements alter the record and must be labeled as artifacts. Examples of artifacts are tongue movement, eye blinking, muscle tenseness, and nervousness.

FOLLOW-UP CARE. The nurse removes the jelly-like substance and glue from the scalp and hair, if this is not done in the EEG laboratory, with acetone and then shampoo. Any medications that were withheld are reinstituted. Provision for a nap is made if the client was deprived of sleep before the test.

Electromyography

Electromyography (EMG) records the electrical activity of peripheral nerves by testing muscle activity (see Chap. 52 for a description of client preparation, procedure, and follow-up care).

Caloric Test and Electronystagmography

Caloric stimulation and electronystagmography (ENG) test vestibular function. In *caloric testing,* the examiner instills cold water into the ear canals to elicit nystagmus. For the ENG test, electrodes placed near the eyes transmit eye

---

Chart 43–3

Nursing Care Highlight: The Client Having an Electroencephalogram

- Thoroughly explain the procedure to the client.
- If the order is for the client to be "sleep-deprived," tell the client to awaken about 2 to 3 AM and stay awake for the rest of the night.
- Instruct the client to avoid central nervous system depressants or stimulants; withhold anticonvulsants only if instructed by the physician.
- Tell the client not to drink caffeine-containing fluids, such as coffee or tea, on the day of the test.
- Reassure the client that the test is not dangerous or uncomfortable.
- Ask the client to wash his or her hair on the morning of the test and remove all hairpins, sprays, or oils.
- Inform the client that after the test, the hair will need to be washed again to remove the electrode glue.

movements, which are recorded on graph paper. The two tests can be done separately or together.

CLIENT PREPARATION. The nurse explains the test and withholds food and fluids for 6–8 hours before the caloric test to lessen vomiting. (There are no restrictions for the ENG test.) As a comfort measure, the nurse asks the client to empty the bladder. For the caloric test, the tympanic membranes must be intact (with no perforations). The physician performing the test checks the tympanic membranes. For the ENG test, the nurse asks the client to remove any make-up around the eyes.

PROCEDURE. The client is positioned on a chair (usually in a diagnostic laboratory), with the head tilted forward 30 degrees. The client is instructed to maintain eye contact with a certain object, which enables the examiner to observe eye movement during the test.

For the *caloric test,* the examiner irrigates one ear with cold water for 30 seconds. The normal result is *slow* movement of the eyes *toward* the side of irrigation, followed by *fast* movement to the *opposite* side. After 5 minutes, the examiner irrigates the ear with warm water. The normal result is nystagmus to the irrigated side. The other ear is then tested in the same way. The instillation of fluid usually produces nausea, vertigo and, occasionally, vomiting. The client may be placed in another position or asked to perform some cerebellar assessments (finger-to-nose touch or the Romberg test). Abnormal findings of no nystagmus or nystagmus in directions other than normal are elicited in Meniere's disease, coma, certain brain tumors, and pathologic states of the brain stem.

For *ENG,* the client is recumbent. Electrodes are secured to the skin near the eyes and then attached to a machine that records the eye movements graphically. The client must keep the eyes closed during the entire test and may be asked to change positions at various intervals. The examiner may instill a small amount of cold or warm water (0.2 mL) into the ear canal as a stimulus.

FOLLOW-UP CARE. For the caloric test, the client is restricted to bed rest until abatement of any nausea, vomiting, or vertigo. ENG requires no follow-up care unless a caloric stimulus was used.

Oculoplethysmography

Oculoplethysmography studies carotid artery blood flow by monitoring one of the carotid artery's branches, the ophthalmic artery. The systolic pressure of each ophthalmic artery is measured by raising the intraocular pressure above systolic ophthalmic arterial pressure. The examiner instills anesthetic eyedrops, places suction cups that resemble contact lenses on the cornea, and applies pressure. The pressure is then released. The reappearance of pulsation is measured as the systolic pressure of the ophthalmic artery. The eyes are compared for circulatory assessment. Other than explaining the test and checking for

corneal abrasion after the procedure, the nurse need offer no follow-up care.

Cerebral Blood Flow Determination

Cerebral blood flow can be determined for many areas of the brain with use of radioactive substances. The nurse explains the test and withholds CNS depressants and stimulants, if drugs have previously been ordered, for 24 hours before the test. The nurse checks to make sure the client's hair is clean and hairpins are removed.

The client must be able to relax mentally and physically during the procedure. The technician attaches sensors or probes connected to a computer to the scalp. The radioactive isotope (usually xenon) is injected intravenously, or the client inhales the radioactive gas (xenon) through a mouthpiece (with the nostrils occluded) or a mask for 1 minute. The client receives various stimuli during the test. Increases in local blood flow can be seen with any neuronal activity, such as reading, hand movement, seizures, and temperature elevation (up to 42° C [107.6° F]). Local blood flow decreases with degenerative disease, comas of metabolic origin, increased intracranial pressure, or subarachnoid hemorrhage. Follow-up care for this test is not required.

Brain Scan

The brain scan is a radionuclide imaging study. A radioactive substance is injected to detect certain pathologic conditions. The test is especially useful in evaluating vascular abnormalities, such as aneurysms, and locating tumors, hematomas, and abscesses. As technological advances in diagnostic testing continue, this test is being performed less frequently.

The nurse explains the test and asks the client to empty the bladder as a comfort measure. A signed consent form may be necessary, depending on agency policy.

During the procedure, the physician injects the client with a radioactive isotope, usually technetium (Tc 99m). There is a delay in the test of up to 2 hours while the isotope is absorbed by the brain. The client is placed on a table and must remain still with hands at the sides for the duration of the test. The test takes 1–2 hours, depending on the number of scannings used.

For follow-up care, the nurse provides fluid to promote elimination of the isotope (urine does not need special handling).

Carotid Phonoangiography and Carotid Doppler Flow Analysis

Carotid phonoangiography and carotid Doppler flow analysis tests determine narrowing or occlusion of the carotid arteries. The lumen size of the carotid artery can be measured through the use of amplified sound, which is then converted to a graphic picture. An electronic microphone is placed over the client's carotid arteries for phonoangiography; a directional Doppler probe is used in the flow analysis. The nurse explains the tests. There is no client preparation or follow-up care.

SELECTED BIBLIOGRAPHY

Bentson, J. R. (1996). Magnetic Resonance Imaging. In J. R. Youmans (Ed.) *Neurological surgery* (4th ed. Vol. 1). Philadelphia: W. B. Saunders.

Buzea, C. E. (1995). Understanding computerized EEG monitoring in the intensive care unit. *Journal of Neuroscience Nursing, 27*(5), 292–297.

Cason, C. L., & Sample, J. C. (1995). Preparatory information for myelogram. *Journal of Neuroscience Nursing, 27*(3), 182–187.

Darovic, G. (1997). Assessing pupillary responses. *Nursing97, 27*(2), 49.

Geary, S. M. (1995). Nursing management of cranial nerve dysfunction. *Journal of Neuroscience Nursing, 27*(2), 102–108.

Hickey, J. (1996). *The clinical practice of neurological and neurosurgical nursing.* Philadelphia: J. B. Lippincott.

Jarvis, C. (1996). *Physical examination and health assessment.* (2nd ed.). Philadelphia: W. B. Saunders.

Juarez, V. J., & Lyons, M. (1995). Interrater reliability of the Glasgow Coma Scale. *Journal of Neuroscience Nursing, 27*(5), 283–286.

Martin, H. H. (1996). *Neuroanatomy text and atlas.* Philadelphia: W. B. Saunders.

Monti, E. J., Kerr, M. E., & Bender, C. (1995). Monitoring neuromuscular function. *Journal of Neuroscience Nursing, 27*(4): 252–256.

Pressman, E. K., Zeidman, S. M., & Summers, L. (1995). Primary care for women: Comprehensive assessment of the neurological system. *Journal of Nurse Midwifery, 40*(2), 163–171.

Quisling, R. Q., & Peters, K. R. (1996). Computed tomography. In J. R. Youmans (Ed.), *Neurological surgery* (4th ed., Vol. 1) Philadelphia: W. B. Saunders.

Raila, F. A. (1996). Radiology of the skull. In J. R. Youmans (Ed.), *Neurological surgery* (4th ed., Vol. 1) Philadelphia: W. B. Saunders.

Shpritz, D. W. (1995). Understanding neurologic assessment. *Journal of Postanesthesia Nursing, 10*(4), 216–222.

Stewart, N. (1996). Neurological observation. *Professional Nurse, 11*(6), 377–378.

Weisberg, L. A., Garcia, C., & Strub, R. (1996). *Essentials of clinical neurology.* St. Louis: C. V. Mosby.

Wooten, C. (1996). The top ten ways to detect deteriorating central neurological status. *Journal of Trauma Nursing, 3*(1), 25–27.

Youmans, J. R. (1996). *Neurological surgery* (4th ed., Vol. 1). Philadelphia: W. B. Saunders.

SUGGESTED READINGS

Geary, S. M. (1995). Nursing management of cranial nerve dysfunction. *Journal of Neuroscience Nursing, 27*(2), 102–108.

The strength of this article is that it provides the reader with the understanding of how to manage the patient with cranial nerve dysfunction. The focus is on specific nursing interventions directed toward minimizing complications and ensuring a better outcome for the patient. The author stresses the role of the interdisciplinary team and the importance of patient and family education and support.

Shpritz, D. W. (1995). Understanding neurological assessment. *Journal of Postanesthesia Nursing, 10* (4), 216–222.

The author describes the most critical elements in a rapid neurologic assessment. Most importantly, the relationship of assessment parameters, its corresponding anatomical correlate, and patient response are presented in a concise and useful format.

Chapter 44

INTERVENTIONS FOR CLIENTS WITH PROBLEMS OF THE CENTRAL NERVOUS SYSTEM: BRAIN

Dysfunction of the central nervous system (CNS) may be a mild disorder that a person can learn to live with, a devastating disorder that drastically affects the client and the family, or a degree between the two extremes. With newer diagnostic tools and treatment methods, the rate and the quality of recovery and rehabilitation are improving steadily. Neurologic impairment tends to involve many aspects of the person's life: the neurologic problem itself, family life alteration or disruption, occupational changes, body image and self-worth conflicts, and, frequently, the realization of a continuous need for numerous resources.

HEADACHES

Probably few people have not experienced a headache. Headaches account for 18.3 million, or 43.2 per 1000, outpatient visits per year (Barrett, 1996). Headaches occur when pain-sensitive areas of the head have been stimulated, although much of the brain is not pain sensitive (Table 44–1). A useful acronym to assess headache pain is PQRST: *p*ain, *p*rovocation, *q*uality, *r*egion, strength and *t*ime course (Ryan, 1996). In addition to the neurologic assessment, psychosocial issues should be addressed, because depression can manifest as chronic headache. Clients with headaches are managed in the outpatient setting by the physician, nurse practitioner, or physician assistant.

Migraine Headache

Overview

A migraine headache is an episodic vascular disorder manifested by pain in the head, often accompanied by anorexia, photophobia, and nausea with or without vomiting. Clients tend to have the same clinical manifestations each time they have a migraine and may have to refrain from regular activities for several days if they cannot control or relieve the headache in its early stage.

Migraine attacks begin in early childhood or near puberty, affect primarily females, and continue periodically, with diminishing severity, until middle age. Menopause may cause an exacerbation. People may continue to have migraine headaches into old age, although this is not typical. Classic migraine episodes tend to increase in frequency during pregnancy, although the usual migraine incidence decreases in most pregnant women.

TABLE 44–1

Pain-Sensitive and Non–Pain-Sensitive Areas of the Head

Pain-Sensitive Areas

- Skin, subcutaneous tissue, muscles, and periosteum of the skull
- Extracranial and intracranial vessels
- Eye, ear, nasal cavity, and sinuses
- Dura mater at the base of the brain
- Cranial nerves V, IX, and X
- First three cervical nerves

Non–Pain-Sensitive Areas

- Skull bone
- Most of pia, arachnoid, and dura mater
- Brain parenchyma
- Ependyma and choroid plexus

Collaborative Management

 Assessment

Migraine with aura, or "classic migraine," usually occurs in three phases. The migraine without aura, previously referred to as the common migraine, begins without an aura before the onset of the headache, or, if present, the aura may be unrecognized as such. The signs and symptoms of both types of migraines are found in Chart 44–1.

 Interventions

The priority for care of the client experiencing a migraine is pain management, which may be achieved by drug therapy and nondrug measures initiated by the health care provider or nurse.

Drug Therapy. The health care provider may prescribe drug therapy to prevent and treat migraine headaches.

Preventive Therapy. Unless otherwise contraindicated, the health care provider may initially prescribe a beta-adrenergic blocker, such as propranolol (Inderal, Apo-Propranolol✦), nadolol (Corgard), atenolol (Tenormin), or timolol (Blocadren, Apo-Timol✦) or an ergot derivative, such as methysergide (Sansert), which blocks serotonin to prevent attacks. Antidepressants, such as amitriptyline (Elavil, Levate✦) and nortriptyline (Pamelor), are not used in the elderly but may be prescribed for younger age groups. These drugs are not without risk, and the client must be under close medical supervision while taking them. The nurse reviews the dosage, side effects, and importance of notifying the physician if side effects, such as orthostatic hypotension and drowsiness, occur.

Calcium channel blockers, such as verapamil (Calan), nifedipine (Procardia, Apo-Nifed✦), and diltiazem (Cardizem), and monoamine oxidase inhibitors (phenelzine [Nardil]) have all been used with success to prevent mi-

graine headaches. Many neurologists recommend prophylactic therapy with one aspirin daily unless this is contraindicated.

Treatment of Headaches. The drug aimed at alleviating pain after the headache has started is typically ergotamine tartrate (Cafergot), although nonsteroidal antiinflammatory drugs, such as indomethacin (Indocin, Indocid✦) or naproxen (Naprosyn, Novonaprox✦), have been used with some success to relieve pain. The health care provider may order antiemetics, such as prochlorperazine (Compazine), to help control nausea and vomiting.

Sumatriptan succinate (Imitrex) is given or self-administered for intractable migraines when other drugs do not work. It is available in 25-mg tablets or as a subcutaneous injection. Sumatriptan specifically stimulates 5-HT1 (serotonin) receptors, causing cranial vasoconstriction. For many clients, this drug is highly effective for pain, nausea, vomiting, and light and sound sensitivity with few side effects. The drug is contraindicated in clients with actual or suspected ischemic heart disease or in those with Prinzmetal's angina because of the potential of coronary vasospasm. Chart 44–2 summarizes commonly used medications for migraine headaches. This chart is not inclusive; new medications are introduced on the market regularly.

Complementary Therapies. At the beginning of a migraine attack, clients may be able to alleviate pain if they lie down and darken the room. They may want their eyes covered as well and should be allowed to sleep undisturbed until awakening.

The nurse explores the possibility of using behavior therapy in conjunction with drug therapy. Behavior therapy includes biofeedback, exercise classes, and relaxation techniques, which are generally offered in a center such as a specialized headache clinic (also see Chapter 4 on complementary therapies). Often a combination of these alternative methods is recommended for best results. These resources are becoming more available and paid for by managed-care companies; they can provide clients with active participation in their program of pain control. An additional positive factor is that these programs usually allow the clients to interact with others with the same or similar problems. Knowing that they are not alone helps relieve fear and allows clients an opportunity to exchange ideas with others.

Modification of Potential Triggering Factors. The nurse collaborates with the client and other health care providers to determine which factors, if any, may trigger the development of a headache. For example, foods containing monosodium glutamate, mature cheese, sausage, sauerkraut, dark chocolate, citrus fruit, and red wine may trigger headache. Many clients are sensitive to odors from cigarette or cigar smoke, paint or gasoline fumes, perfumes, or aftershave lotion.

The nurse assures clients that minor lifestyle changes may be necessary, but that a complete change is usually not necessary. For example, clients may need to avoid red wine if it triggers a migraine attack but may substitute white wine.

Clients may also need to modify their lifestyle to decrease stress if stress is a contributing factor to migraine attacks.

Cluster Headache

Overview

The cluster headache, also referred to as histamine cephalalgia, is less common than migraine headache. It occurs more frequently in men than in women and generally begins in the third or fourth decade of life.

The pain of these unilateral (one-sided), oculotemporal or oculofrontal headaches is often described as excruciating, boring, and nonthrobbing. The headaches occur every 8 to 12 hours and up to 24 hours daily at the same time for about 6 to 8 weeks (hence the term cluster), followed by a period of remission for 9 months to a year.

This episodic form is the most common, although there is a chronic form in which there may not be a remission for more than a year. The average duration of each headache is 10 to 45 minutes.

The headache is accompanied by ipsilateral (same side) tearing of the eye, rhinorrhea or congestion, ptosis, and miosis. There may be bradycardia, flushing or pallor of the face, increased intraocular pressure, and increased skin temperature.

The pain may radiate to the forehead, temple, or cheek. The temporal artery may be prominent and tender. Physical activity during the attack consists of pacing, walking, or sitting and rocking. This is the only headache type in which this behavior occurs. During periods of remission, alcohol does not induce a headache (as it does during the headache period). The onset of the headaches is associated with relaxation, napping, or rapid eye movement (REM) sleep.

The cause of cluster headaches is unknown. There is no genetic or family link, diet has no effect, and the disorder is unrelated to personality type.

Collaborative Management

The nurse asks the client about prescribed and nonprescribed drugs for both the prevention and alleviation of the headache as well as over-the-counter drugs the client may be taking. Interventions used by the client may include relaxation techniques, meditation, acupuncture, or massage therapies. The client is asked to recall a typical week's activities and any recent changes in lifestyle and to identify specifically bedtimes and waking times, which helps the nurse assess changes in activity or lack of continuity in the sleep-wake cycle.

Pain control may be accomplished by drug and nondrug measures initiated by the nurse. The client's understanding of the preventive measures is important in the management of cluster headaches.

Drug Therapy. The health care provider typically prescribes dihydroergotamine, 1 mg, at bedtime. If the headache occurs more than one time per day, dihydroergotamine 0.5 mg TID may be required. Lidocaine 4% solution (intranasal) has been found to decrease the pain associated with a cluster headache. Prophylactic drug therapy starts immediately at onset of headache for 2 weeks and is gradually discontinued. Chart 44–2 outlines the nursing implications for clients receiving drug therapy. Because an informed person is better able to comply with the therapeutic plan, the nurse instructs the client in all aspects of the drugs being taken.

Other Pain Relief Measures. During the periods of attack, the nurse instructs the client to wear sunglasses and to sit facing away from the window, which helps to decrease exposure to light and glare. If the health care provider orders oxygen, the nurse or assistive nursing personnel gives 100% oxygen via mask at 5 L/minute with the client in a sitting position. The oxygen is administered for no longer than 15 minutes and is discontinued when the headache is relieved. Oxygen reduces cerebral blood flow and inhibits activity of the carotid bodies, which are sensitive to oxygen levels in the body. To

Chart 44-2

Drug Therapy for the Prevention and Treatment of Migraine Headaches in the Adult Client

Drug	Usual Dosage	Interventions	Rationale
Agents that Decrease Platelet Aggregation			
Acetylsalicylic acid (aspirin)	• 600 mg daily PO	• Assess for prior salicylate intolerance. • Check for petechiae.	• Drug can cause hearing impairment, tinnitus, gastric bleeding or irritation, and depressed plasma ascorbic acid level. • Drug prolongs bleeding time.
Dipyridamole (Persantine, Apo-Dipyramidole✦)	• 50 mg tid PO	• Give with a glassful of water. • Observe for signs of gastric distress.	• Water aids absorption and decreases gastric distress. • Drug may need to be taken with meals.
Agents used for Prevention of Attacks			
Propranolol (Inderal, Detensol✦, Apo-Propranolol✦) Atenolol (Tenormin) Calcium channel blockers (nimodipine)	• 60 mg in divided doses initially and increased gradually to 240 mg in divided doses orally	• Administer the last dose of the day at bedtime. • Check for petechiae. • Teach the client to take pulse. • Teach slow position changes. • Assess other drug use. • Assess overall health status. • Ensure gradual withdrawal.	• Bedtime administration prevents early morning vasodilation. • Drug decreases platelet aggregation. • Drug causes bradycardia. Notify the physician if pulse is slower than baseline or irregular. Pulse may not rise in response to stress, such as fever and exercise. • Drug lowers blood pressure, and the client may become hypotensive, especially when changing position. • Propranolol is contraindicated if the client is taking MAO inhibitors. • Propranolol is contraindicated if the client has asthma or acute congestive heart failure. • Gradual withdrawal prevents severe symptoms.
Methysergide (Sansert)	• 2–6 mg in divided doses PO	• Administer with meals. • Assess for fibrotic, cardiovascular, and CNS complications. • Teach slow position changes. • Withdraw gradually	• Food helps prevent gastrointestinal (GI) disturbances. • There is a high incidence of side effects: *fibrotic*—retroperitoneal fibrosis (oliguria, dysuria, urinary obstruction, and increased blood urea nitrogen) and pleuropulmonary fibrosis (dyspnea, chest pain, pleural friction rubs, and effusion) (drug should be stopped every 3 months for at least 2 weeks to prevent fibrosis); *cardiovascular*—peripheral edema, phlebitis, claudication, postural hypotension, and heart murmurs; *CNS*—insomnia, vertigo, confusion, euphoria, feelings of depersonalization, distortion of body image, anxiety, depression, hallucinations, nightmares, ataxia, and parethesia. • Drug can cause orthostatic hypotension. • Gradual withdrawal prevents rebound headache.

Continued

Chart 44-2 Drug Therapy for the Prevention and Treatment of Migraine Headaches in the Adult Client
Continued

Drug	Usual Dosage	Interventions	Rationale
Cyproheptadine (Periactin)	• 2 mg tid PO	• Give with food or milk. • Assess other drug use. • Assess overall health status.	• Food or milk prevents gastric distress. • Drug may increase and prolong effects of alcohol, barbiturates, narcotic analgesics, tranquilizers, and other CNS depressants. Contraindicated if the client is taking MAO inhibitors. • Drug is contraindicated if the client has asthma or glaucoma.
Phenelzine (Nardil) or tricyclic antidepressant, such as imipramine hydrochloride (Tofranil, Impril❈)	• 30–60 mg daily in divided doses	• Teach avoidance of foods and liquids containing tyramine. • Teach slow position changes. • Assess for appearance of GI, renal, muscular, or neural symptoms.	• MAO inhibitor increases norepinephrine in tissues. Tyramine forms pressor amines in body. • Drugs have some paradoxic hypotensive effects. • Side effects can be often eliminated by adjusting the dosage.
Amitriptyline (Elavil) (use with caution in the elderly)		• Assess for headache or palpitation. • Withdraw slowly.	• Drugs are discontinued if prodromal signs of hypertensive crisis occur. • Gradual withdrawal prevents rebound headache.
Belladonna, phenobarbitol, and ergotamine tartrate (Bellergal-S)			

Agents Used for Early Alleviation of Attacks

Drug	Usual Dosage	Interventions	Rationale
Caffeine (ergotamine tartrate combination) (Cafergot)	• 100 mg, caffeine, 1.0 mg ergotamine: 2 tablets at start of attack, then 1 tablet every 30 min PO	• Watch timing of administration. • Assess overall health status.	• Dose late in the day may prevent sleep. • Drug is contraindicated in peripheral vascular and coronary artery disease, hypertension, and renal or hepatic disease. Dosage should not exceed 6 tablets per attack.
Indomethacin (Indocin, Indocid❈)	• 150–200 mg in divided doses PO	• Give with meals or milk.	• Food or milk decreases gastric irritation.
Isometheptene, dichloralphenazone, and acetaminophen (Midrin)	• Two capsules; can repeat once	• Take last dose at bedtime.	• Bedtime administration reduces the incidence of frontal morning headache. If frontal headache persists, the dosage may be reduced or the drug stopped.
Lidocaine	• Intranasal	• Monitor for side effects such as numbness in throat and nose, irritated nasal passages.	• Client may experience a bitter aftertaste. • Lidocaine is suggested as an alternative to Imitrex because of lower cost, less serious side effects.
Naproxen sodium (Anaprox)	• 275-mg tablets: 3 tablets, then 2 more in 1 hr if no results	• Assess overall health status.	• This drug is contraindicated if the client is sensitive to aspirin or has renal or hepatic disease.
Naproxen (Naprosyn)	• 250-mg tablets: 3 tablets, then 1 more in 1 hr if no results	• Monitor weight. • Assess for possible infections.	• In cardiovascular disease, water and sodium retention occur. • Drug may mask signs and symptoms of latent infections.

Continued

Chart 44–2 Drug Therapy for the Prevention and Treatment of Migraine Headaches in the Adult Client
Continued

Drug	Usual Dosage	Interventions	Rationale
Agents Used for Control of Nausea or Vomiting			
Metoclopramide (Reglan, Maxeran❤)	• 10–20 mg PO	• Give at onset of attack and 30 min before other migraine drugs. • Assess overall health status. • Assess for CNS symptoms (extrapyramidal).	• Drug helps regain peristalsis and aids absorption of other drugs. • Drug is contraindicated in those with epilepsy or history of breast cancer. • These are most likely to occur in younger adults: restlessness, involuntary movements, facial grimacing, rigidity, and tremors.
Promethazine hydrochloride (Phenergan, Histanil❤)	• 50 mg PO once (or IM)	• Give with food, milk, or glassful of water. • Teach slow position changes. • Assess overall health status. • Encourage frequent oral hygiene. • Assess other medications being taken.	• Food, milk, or water minimizes GI distress. • Drug has a hypotensive effect. • Drug is contraindicated in angle-closure glaucoma, epilepsy, and urinary retention. • Mouth dryness may be a problem. • Over-the-counter medications should not be taken without physician approval, nor should CNS depressants, including alcohol.
Agents Used for Intractable Headache			
Ketorolac	• 60 mg IM	• Assess for pain relief. • Assess for allergies to aspirin and non-steroidal anti-inflammatory agents. • Give immediately at onset of headache.	• This drug is contraindicated in clients with renal or hepatic disease and with concurrent cardiac or antihypertensive medication therapy.
Sumatriptan succinate (Imitrex)	• Give only for severe headache: 6 mg SC (may repeat × 1) or 25 mg PO up to 4 times per day	• Assess for pain relief. • Monitor for chest pain, dizziness; monitor liver enzyme levels when drug used for long term.	• Drug usually works quickly to relieve pain and other symptoms. • Drug can cause coronary vasospasm; long-term use can cause liver toxicity.

MAO = monoamine oxidase inhibitors; CNS = central nervous system; GI = gastrointestinal; PO = orally; IM = intramuscularly; SC = subcutaneously.

prevent future attacks brought on by precipitating factors, the nurse discusses the relationship among such factors (bursts of anger, prolonged anticipation, excessive physical activity, and excitement), the postactivity period, and the onset of cluster headaches. The nurse also explains the necessity and importance of a consistent sleep-wake cycle.

Other Types of Headache

Headaches occur from many other causes (Table 44–2). (For a discussion of headaches caused by common non-neurologic problems, see elsewhere in the text.)

EPILEPSY

Overview

Epilepsy is a chronic disorder characterized by recurrent, unprovoked seizure activity and may be inherited. It is the result of brain or central nervous system (CNS) irritation. A seizure is an abnormal, sudden, excessive discharge of electrical activity within the brain.

Primary or idiopathic epilepsy is not associated with any identifiable brain lesion. Secondary epilepsy results from an underlying brain lesion, most commonly a tumor or trauma. Seizures may also be caused by metabolic

TABLE 44–2

Differential Features of Common Headache Types

Type	Pathophysiology, Signs, and Symptoms	Treatment Approaches	Comments
Ophthalmoplegic migraine	• Headache with paralysis of cranial nerve III (usually) persists for days or weeks. Ptosis occurs. Pupils usually not affected.	• Carotid aneurysm and tumors must be ruled out.	• Paralysis may become permanent.
Basilar artery migraine	• Brain stem symptoms of tinnitus, vertigo, ataxia, dysarthria, blurring of vision, diploplia, and loss of consciousness are present. May have transient global amnesia. More commonly occurs in young girls and women. Lasts 10–30 minutes and is followed by occipital headache.	• Tumors must be ruled out.	
Tension headache	• Pathophysiology is unknown. Usually bilateral in occipitalnuchal, temporal, or frontal region. May be diffuse over top of the head. Pain is dull and aching. Descriptions include feeling of fullness, tightness, or vise or band around head. Gradual onset, but lasts days, weeks, months, or years. More common in women than in men, and occurrence almost as great as that for migraine. Most likely to begin in middle age or when anxiety and depression are present.	• Massage, relaxation. Antianxiety drugs include diazepam (Valium, Apo-Diazepam✦) and alprazolam (Xanax, Apo-Alpraz✦). One of the above plus amitriptyline (Elavil, Levate✦) in presence of depression.	• Aspirin and psychotherapy do not help.
Traumatic headache from head injury	• Often occurs from subdural hematoma. Pain is deep seated and steady. Unilateral or generalized and accompanied by drowsiness, confusion, stupor, coma, or hemiparesis.	• Identification and correction of possible focus.	• See text.
Meningeal irritation headache from infection or hemorrhage	• Dilation and congestion of inflamed vessels. Irritation of nerve endings in meninges from serotonin, plasma kinins, or possibly increased intracranial pressure. Acute onset of pain, which is severe, generalized, deep seated, and constant with nuchal rigidity.	• Rest, time, and antibiotics if infection is cause.	• See text.

Table continued on following page

TABLE 44–2

Type	Pathophysiology, Signs, and Symptoms	Treatment Approaches	Comments
Post–lumbar puncture (LP) headache	• No satisfactory pathophysiologic explanation at present. Possible reasons—leakage of CSF through needle tract or low CSF pressure causes brain to exert painful traction on vessels or dural attachments. Pain is occipital, frontal, and nuchal. Steady pain is evident after LP on arising.	• Time, fluids to aid CSF production.	• If severe neck and head pain continues, bacteria introduced by needle must be considered. See Chap. 43.
Headaches from disease of ligaments, joints, or muscles of upper spine from arthritis or whiplash.	• Pain referred to occiput and nape of neck. Steady ache and often more painful after immobility.	• Massage, heat.	• See Chap. 24.
Ocular—hypermetropia (hyperopia) or astigmatism	• Sustained contraction of frontotemporal muscles during prolonged close use. Steady ache.	• Correction of visual defect.	• See Chap. 49.
Cranial arteritis			• See Chap. 24.
Sinus headache from infection or blockage	• Pressure and irritation of sinus walls.		• See Chap. 31.
Headaches occurring during sexual activity	• Pathophysiology unknown. Resembles pain of ruptured aneurysm, except there are no other symptoms. Severe, throbbing, explosive type at time of orgasm. Persists for several minutes to hours.	• None.	• Hypertensive hemorrhage, rupture of aneurysm, or AVM does occur during sexual activity.
Headaches related to medical problems: Hypertension Fever Carbon monoxide exposure Chronic pulmonary disease with hypercapnia Hypothyroidism Cushing's disease Corticosteroid withdrawal Chronic ergotamine ingestion Chronic exposure to nitrites Adrenal insufficiency Aldosterone-producing adrenal tumors Pheochromocytoma Acute anemia with hemoglobin below 10 g/dL Constipation Birth control hormones		• Treat cause or underlying medical condition	

CSF = cerebrospinal fluid; LP = lumbar puncture; AVM = arteriovenous malformation.

disorders, acute alcohol withdrawal, electrolyte disturbances (e.g., hyperkalemia, water intoxication, hypoglycemia), and heart disease. Seizures resulting from these problems are not considered as epilepsy (McNew et al., 1997).

In spite of intense public education programs, social barriers and discriminatory practices against people who have seizures continue to exist.

Types of Seizures

The International Classification of Epileptic Seizures recognizes three broad categories of seizure disorders (Table 44–3).

Generalized Seizures

Four types of generalized seizures may occur and involve both cerebral hemispheres. The *tonic-clonic* seizure (formerly called a *grand mal* seizure), lasting 2 to 5 minutes, begins with a tonic phase that is characterized by stiffening or rigidity of the muscles, particularly of the arms and legs, and immediate loss of consciousness. It is followed by clonic or rhythmic jerking of all extremities. The client may bite his or her tongue and may become incontinent of urine or feces. Occasionally, only tonic or clonic movement may occur. Fatigue, confusion, and lethargy may last up to an hour after the seizure.

The *absence seizure*, previously referred to as a *petit mal* seizure, is more common in children. It consists of brief (often just seconds) periods of loss of consciousness and blank staring, as though the person is daydreaming. The client returns to baseline immediately after the seizure.

The *myoclonic* seizure is characterized by a brief jerking or stiffening of the extremities, which may occur singly or in groups. Lasting for just a few seconds, the contractions may be symmetric or asymmetric.

The *atonic* (akinetic) seizure (formerly known as drop attacks), is characterized by a sudden loss of muscle tone, lasting for seconds. In most cases, these seizures cause the client to fall.

Partial Seizures

Partial seizures, also called *focal* seizures, begin in a part of one cerebral hemisphere. They are further subdivided into two main classes: complex partial seizures and simple partial seizures.

Complex partial seizures cause the client to lose consciousness, or black out, for 1 to 3 minutes. Characteristic behavior known as automatisms (the client is not aware of the behavior) may occur, such as lip smacking, patting, picking at clothes, and so forth. In the period after the seizure, the client may experience amnesia. Because the area of the brain most often involved in this type of epilepsy is the temporal lobe, complex partial seizures are often called *psychomotor* seizures or *temporal lobe* seizures.

The client with a simple partial seizure remains conscious throughout the episode. The client often reports an aura (unusual sensation) before the seizure takes place. This may consist of a déjà vu phenomenon, perception of an offensive smell, or sudden onset of pain. During the seizure, the client may have unilateral movement of an extremity, experience unusual sensations, or have autonomic or psychic symptoms. Autonomic changes include a change in heart rate, skin flushing, and epigastric discomfort.

Unclassified Seizures

Unclassified, or idiopathic, seizures account for about half of all seizure activity. They occur for no known reason and do not fit into the generalized or partial classifications.

Risk Factors

Certain risk factors can trigger a seizure, such as increased physical activity, emotional stress, excessive fatigue, alcohol or caffeine consumption, or certain foods or chemicals.

Collaborative Management

 Assessment

A complete description of the type of seizure activity that occurs and events surrounding the seizure assists in determining the best treatment plan. The nurse or other health care provider obtains information from the client and family or significant other regarding the presence of an aura before the seizure (preictal phase).

 Interventions

Secondary epilepsy and seizures that are not considered as epileptic are managed by removing or treating the underlying condition or cause of the seizure. In most cases, primary epilepsy is managed through drug therapy.

Nonsurgical Management. Most seizures can be completely or almost completely controlled through the administration of antiepileptic drugs (AEDs), sometimes referred to as anticonvulsants, for specific types of seizures. The nurse plays an important role in drug therapy and seizure management.

TABLE 44–3

Classification of Seizure Disorders
Generalized Seizures
• Generalized absence (petit mal)
• Generalized tonic-clonic (grand mal)
• Myoclonic
• Atonic
Partial Seizures (Focal Seizures)
• Simple partial
• Complex partial
Unclassified Seizures*

* Incomplete data.

Drug Therapy. Drug therapy is the major component of management (Chart 44–3). Generally, the health care provider introduces one drug at a time to achieve seizure control. If the chosen drug is not effective, the dosage may be increased or another drug introduced. At times, seizure control is achieved only through a combination of medications. The dosage of medications is adjusted to achieve therapeutic blood levels without causing major side effects.

The nurse administers the medications on time to maintain therapeutic blood levels and maximal effectiveness. The client is instructed to avoid drugs and foods that might interfere with the absorption or metabolism of the AED. For instance, warfarin (Coumadin, Warfilone♣) should not be given with phenytoin (Dilantin). In addition, the nurse observes for side and adverse effects of the prescribed medications.

Promising new drugs are being investigated for the treatment of epilepsy. Divalproex sodium is used as first-line treatment of partial-onset seizures and simple and

---

Chart 44–3

Drug Therapy: Commonly Used Antiepileptic Drugs

Drug	Indication for Use	Nursing Implications
Carbamazepine (Tegretol, Tegretol XR, Mazepine♣)	All types except absence, myoclonic, and atonic seizures	• Give with meals. • Monitor for diplopia or blurred vision, N/V, and leukopenia.
Clonazepam (Klonopin, Rivotril♣)	Absence, myoclonic, atonic seizures	• Monitor CBC. • Monitor for lethargy, diplopia, ataxia, slurred speech, and thrombocytopenia.
Diazepam (Valium, Apo-Diazepam♣); lorazepam (Ativan)	Status epilepticus	• Monitor for respiratory distress if given IV. • Monitor VS carefully.
Divalproex (Depakote); valproic acid (Depakene)	All types of seizures	• Monitor for hair loss, tremor, increased liver enzymes, bruising, and N/V. • Monitor CBC, PT/PTT, and AST.
Ethosuximide (Zarontin)	Absence seizures	• Watch for N/V, skin rash, lethargy, and anorexia. • Monitor CBC and liver function tests.
Felbamate (Felbatol)	Refractory partial seizures	• Monitor CBC carefully because drug can cause aplastic anemia. • Monitor liver function tests. • Watch for anorexia and weight loss.
Gabapentin (Neurontin)	Partial seizures	• Watch for increased appetite and weight gain. • Monitor for ataxia, irritability, dizziness, fatigue.
Lamotrigine (Lamictal)	Partial seizures	• Watch for diplopia, drowsiness, ataxia, N/V, and life-threatening rash when given with valproic acid.
Phenobarbital (Barbita, Luminal♣)	Partial seizures, generalized tonic-clonic seizures	• Monitor for drowsiness, sleep disturbances, cogitive impairment, and depression.
Phenytoin (Dilantin); fosphenytoin (Cerebyx)	All types, except absence, myoclonic, and atonic seizures; for status epilepticus	• Monitor for gastric distress, gingival hyperplasia, anemia, ataxia, and nystagmus. • Check CBC and calcium levels. • For IV phenytoin, flush catheter with saline before and after administration. • For fosphenytoin, use phenytoin equivalent for dosing.
Primidone (Mysoline, Sertan♣)	Refractory partial or generalized tonic-clonic seizures	• Monitor for vertigo and lethargy. • Watch for drug interactions with phenobarbital and isoniazid.
Topiramate	Partial seizures	• Monitor for ataxia, confusion, dizziness, and fatigue.

N/V = nausea and vomiting; CBC = complete blood cell count; IV = intravenously; PT = prothrombin time; PTT = partial thromboplastin time; AST = aspartate aminotransferase.

complex partial seizures. It has also been used as an adjunctive therapy to treat multiple seizure types (Beydoun et al., 1997).

ELDERLY CONSIDERATIONS

Epilepsy is especially likely to affect the elderly secondary to cerebrovascular disease, metabolic changes, and head trauma. It is especially important to monitor their medication closely because of changes in metabolism and elimination of epileptic drugs associated with aging. The elderly are at risk for adverse drug reactions from the epilepsy medication itself or other medications prescribed to treat concurrent medical problems.

Seizure Precautions. In the hospital setting, when a client has a history of seizures, the nurse takes precautions to prevent the client from injury if a seizure occurs. Seizure precautions vary, depending on health care agency policy. In most agencies, it is recommended that oxygen and suctioning equipment with airway be readily available. It is also appropriate to insert a saline lock in clients who do not have an intravenous (IV) access and are at significant risk for generalized tonic-clonic seizures. The saline lock provides ready access if IV medication must be given to stop the seizure.

The use of padded side rails is controversial, but it is usually inappropriate. Although the side rails are rarely the source of significant injury, they should be in the "up" position at all times. More importantly, padded side rails may embarrass the client and the family. The bed is kept in the lowest position in case the client falls out of bed.

Padded tongue blades do not belong at the bedside and should never be inserted into the client's mouth after a seizure begins, because the jaw may clench down as soon as the seizure begins. Forcing a tongue blade or airway into the mouth is more likely to chip the client's teeth and increase the risk of aspiration of tooth fragments than to prevent the client from biting the tongue. Further, improper placement of a padded tongue blade can obstruct the client's airway.

Seizure Management. The actions taken by the nurse should be appropriate for the type of seizure experienced by the client. For example, for a simple partial seizure, the nurse may only have to observe, document, and time the length of the seizure. The client engaged in activities that may cause harm is directed away from the activity. The client who loses consciousness during a seizure, usually during a generalized tonic-clonic or complex partial seizure, should be turned on the side (Chart 44–4). If possible, the nurse turns the client's head to the side to prevent aspiration and allow secretions to drain. The nurse removes any objects that might injure the client.

It is not unusual for the client to become cyanotic during a generalized tonic-clonic seizure. The cyanosis is generally self-limiting, and no treatment is needed. Some health care providers prefer to give the high-risk client (e.g., elderly, critically ill, or debilitated) oxygen by nasal cannula or face mask during the postictal period. The client is not restrained because this may cause injury and may exacerbate (worsen) the situation, causing more sei-

---

Chart 44–4

Nursing Care Highlight: Care of the Client During a Tonic-Clonic or Complete Partial Seizure

- Protect the client from injury.
- Do not force anything into the client's mouth.
- Turn the client to the side.
- Loosen any restrictive clothing the client is wearing.
- Maintain the client's airway and suction as needed.
- Do not restrain the client; guide the client's movements if necessary.
- At the completion of the seizure
  - Take the client's vital signs.
  - Perform neurologic checks.
  - Keep the client on his or her side.
  - Allow the client to rest.
  - Document the seizure (see Chart 44–5).

---

zure activity. The client with atonic seizures, however, may benefit from a protective vest when sitting in a chair to keep from falling. For any type of seizure, the nurse carefully observes the seizure and documents assessment findings (Chart 44–5).

Chart 44–5

Nursing Observations and Documentation of a Seizure

- How often the seizures occur
  - Date, time, and duration of the seizure
- A description of each seizure
  - Tonic, clonic
  - Staring spells, blinking
  - Automatism
- Whether more than one type of seizure occurs
- The sequence of seizure progression
  - Where the seizure began
  - Body part first involved
- Observations during the seizure
  - Changes in pupil size and any eye deviation
  - Level of consciousness
  - Presence of apnea, cyanosis, and salivation
  - Incontinent of bowel or bladder during the seizure
  - Eye fluttering
  - Movement and progression of motor activity
  - Lip smacking or other automatism
  - Tongue or lip biting
- How long the seizures last
- When the last seizure took place
- Whether the seizures are preceded by an aura
  - Dizziness, numbness, or visual
  - Gustatory or auditory disturbances
- What the client does after the seizure
  - Feels drowsy or weak
  - May resume normal behavior
  - May be unaware that the seizure took place
- How long it takes for the client to return to preseizure status

Status Epilepticus Management. Status epilepticus is seizure activity that lasts longer than 30 minutes or a series of seizures that occur in rapid succession. It is a potential complication of all types of seizures. The usual causes of status epilepticus include

- Sudden withdrawal from anticonvulsant medication
- Infections
- Acute alcohol withdrawal
- Head trauma
- Cerebral edema
- Metabolic disturbances

Convulsive status epilepticus is a neurologic emergency in the client with generalized tonic-clonic seizures and must be treated promptly to prevent irreversible brain damage and possibly death from hypoxia, cardiac dysrhythmias, lactic acidosis, or brain damage. The nurse notifies the physician immediately if this condition occurs and establishes an adequate airway promptly. (Intubation by an anesthesiologist or nurse anesthetist may be necessary.) Oxygen is given as indicated by the client's condition. If not already in place, intravenous (IV) access is established and the client should receive 0.9% sodium chloride (Chart 44–6).

Medications that the physician uses to treat status epilepticus include IV diazepam (Valium, Rival✦) or lorazepam (Ativan, Apo-Lorazepam✦) to stop motor movement, followed by phenytoin (Dilantin) or fosphenytoin (Cerebyx) to prevent recurrence (McNew et al., 1997). A fairly new drug, fosphenytoin can be administered intramuscularly as well as IV and is compatible with most IV solutions. After administration, fosphenytoin converts to phenytoin in the body. Therefore, the U.S. Food and Drug Administration requires the dosage to be written as a phenytoin equivalent (PE); 150 mg of fosphenytoin equals 100 mg of phenytoin. Fosphenytoin should never be given faster than 50 mg/minute, because rapid administration may lead to cardiac dysrhythmias. General anesthesia may be used as a treatment of last resort to stop the seizure activity.

The nurse, physician, or clinical pharmacist monitors serum drug levels closely for the first 3 days after the start of the anticonvulsant medication and thereafter as indicated. Other nursing interventions are found in Chart 44–6.

Surgical Management. A small percentage of clients with epilepsy cannot be fully controlled with medications. When all other treatment options are exhausted, surgery may be indicated to improve the quality of the client's life.

Care of the client is similar to that described for clients undergoing a craniotomy (see Chap. 47). Preoperative diagnostic tests include magnetic resonance imaging (MRI), or single-photon emission computed tomography (SPECT)/positron emission tomography (PET) scan as described in Chapter 43. An intracarotid amobarbital test (Wada) and neuropsychological testing is also done. The Wada test assesses hemispheric lateralization of language and memory after intracarotid injection of amobarbital, a short-acting anesthetic. This procedure establishes the safety of surgery in terms of language preservation and memory. Neuropsychological testing evaluates memory, visuospatial function, language function, and intelligence quotient to identify deficiencies in a restricted brain region that might correspond to areas believed to be the epileptogenic region. It is also used to compare the client's preoperative and postoperative cognitive functioning.

Conventional Surgical Procedures. The client with seizures that do not respond to medication may benefit from surgical excision of the seizure area of the brain. The procedure involves continuous recording of the client's electroencephalogram (EEG), close observation, and, in many hospitals, video monitoring of the client at all times, except during personal care activities. After the seizure area is identified, electrodes are surgically implanted into the brain tissue to identify the extent of the focal area. This step is followed by additional continuous EEG and video monitoring of the client at all times (except during personal care) as well as close observation by the nursing staff. The area is excised if it can be safely removed without affecting vital areas of brain function.

Anterior temporal lobe resection is the safest and most effective procedure for the client with complex partial seizures of temporal origin. Multiple suboccipital transection done over all areas of seizure foci as well as over other stereotactic volumetric radiofrequency lesions of the intracranial structures may be performed.

The more traditional surgical approach, the corpuscallosotomy, is used to treat tonic-clonic or atonic seizures in clients who are not candidates for other surgical procedures. The surgeon sections the anterior two thirds of the corpus callosum, preventing neuronal discharges from passing between the two hemispheres of the brain. This surgery usually reduces the number and severity of the seizures, making them more amenable to more conventional drug therapy.

Vagal Nerve Stimulation. Clients with multifocal or bihemisphere seizure foci may not be candidates for surgical excision because this may result in severe neurologic deficits. Several centers in the United States are participating in a study that involves placing a vagal nerve stimulating device to control partial seizures. The stimulating device is surgically implanted below the left clavicle in

---

Chart 44–6

Care for the Client in Status Epilepticus

- Support the ABCs (*a*irway, *b*reathing, and *c*irculation).
  - Prepare for possible intubation.
  - Protect the client from injury.
- Do not force an airway into the client's mouth; provide oxygen via nasal cannula or face mask.
- Establish intravenous access if not already available and begin infusion of 0.9% saline.
  - Administer drugs as ordered and observe the client for side effects or signs of toxicity from the medications.
  - Monitor vital signs and cardiac rhythm.

the sternocleidomastoid muscle. The vagus nerve is dissected free between the carotid artery and the jugular vein, and an electrode is placed. Each month the amplitude, frequency, and stimulation time of the device are adjusted. Preliminary results with a few clients have demonstrated a decrease in seizure frequency (Ben-Menachem, 1994).

Alternative Therapies. Several alternative therapies are being tried with success in some client groups. For example, the ketogenic diet seems to help children who have myoclonic, atonic, or generalized seizures. The diet mimics starvation by converting fats into energy instead of carbohydrates (McNew et al., 1997).

Client and Family Education. The nurse provides an educational program for the client, family, or significant other in a manner that can be easily understood (Chart 44-7). The nurse ascertains what they understand about the disorder, corrects any misinformation, and presents new information as the client and family are able to understand it.

The nurse emphasizes that the drug must not be stopped, even if the seizures have stopped. Discontinuing the drug can lead to the recurrence of seizures or the life-threatening complication of status epilepticus. Some clients may stop taking the medication simply because they do not have the money to purchase their medications. The nurse refers limited-income clients to the social services department for financial assistance or to a case manager to locate other resources.

All states prohibit discrimination against people who have epilepsy. Clients who work in occupations in which a seizure might cause serious harm to themselves or others (e.g., construction workers, operators of dangerous equipment, pilots, railroad engineers) may need to find alternative employment. They may need to curtail or modify strenuous or potentially dangerous physical activity to avoid harm, although this varies with each client.

INFECTIONS
Meningitis
Overview

Meningitis is an inflammation of the arachnoid and pia mater of the brain and the spinal cord. Bacterial and viral organisms are most often responsible for meningitis, although fungal and protozoal meningitis also occur. Bacterial meningitis occurs most frequently; early detection and treatment are associated with a more favorable outcome. Viral meningitis is usually self-limiting, and the client has a complete recovery.

The organisms responsible for meningitis enter the central nervous system (CNS) via the bloodstream at the blood-brain barrier. Direct routes of entry occur as a result of penetrating trauma, surgical procedures, or a ruptured cerebral abscess. Otorrhea (ear discharge) or rhinorrhea (nasal discharge), which may be caused by a basilar skull fracture, may lead to meningitis owing to the direct communication of cerebrospinal fluid (CSF) with the environment. The invading organisms migrate throughout the CNS via the subarachnoid space. The presence of the organism in the subarachnoid space produces an inflammatory response in the pia mater, the arachnoid, the cerebrospinal fluid (CSF), and the ventricles. The exudate formed may spread to both cranial and spinal nerves, causing further neurologic deterioration.

Bacterial Meningitis

Bacterial meningitis is seen most often in fall and winter, when upper respiratory tract infections commonly occur. The most frequently involved organisms responsible for bacterial meningitis include *Streptococcus pneumoniae and Neisseria meningitidis* (Table 44-4). Meningococcal meningitis is the only type of bacterial meningitis that occurs in outbreaks and is most likely to occur in areas of high population density, such as college dormitories, military barracks, crowded living areas, and prisons.

Most often, the client has a predisposing condition, such as otitis media, pneumonia, acute sinusitis, or sickle cell anemia, that increases the likelihood of meningitis. A fractured skull or brain or spinal surgery may contribute to the development of meningitis. Meningitis is also common in people with compromised immune systems, such

TABLE 44-4

Common Bacteria that Cause Meningitis
- *Haemophilus influenzae*
- *Neisseria meningitidis* (meningococcal)
- *Diplococcus pneumoniae* (pneumococcal)
- Streptococci, group A
- *Staphylococcus aureus*
- *Escherichia coli*
- *Klebsiella*
- *Proteus*
- *Pseudomonas*

as those with acquired immunodeficiency syndrome (AIDS) and acquired or congenital immunoglobulin deficiency.

Viral Meningitis

Viral meningitis is sometimes referred to as aseptic meningitis. It often occurs as a sequela to a variety of viral illnesses, including measles, mumps, herpes simplex, and herpes zoster. The formation of exudate that is common in bacterial meningitis does not occur, and no organisms are obtained for culture from the CSF. Inflammation occurs over the cerebral cortex, the white matter, and the meninges. The susceptibility of the brain tissue to the virus varies, depending on which type of cell is involved. The herpes simplex virus alters cellular metabolism, which quickly results in necrosis of the cells. Other viruses cause an alteration in the production of enzymes or neurotransmitters, which results in dysfunction of the cells and possible neurologic defects.

Fungal Meningitis

Cryptococcal meningitis is the most commonly seen fungal infection that affects the central nervous system of clients with AIDS. The clinical manifestations vary among people because of their compromised immune system, which affects the inflammatory response. For example, some clients have fever and others do not. Almost all clients have headache, nausea, and vomiting and show a decline in mental status.

Collaborative Management

 Assessment

The nurse performs a complete neurologic assessment to detect changes associated with a diagnosis of meningitis or suspected meningitis as outlined in Chart 44–8.

Meningeal Irritation. Meningeal irritation is indicated by nuchal rigidity and a positive Kernig's sign and Brudzinski's sign. Nuchal rigidity is manifested by a stiff neck and soreness, particularly when the client's neck is flexed. The nurse may elect to test for both Kernig's and Brudzinski's signs. A positive response occurs in the presence of bacterial meningitis but is absent in viral meningitis. The client lies supine in bed for both tests.

To elicit Kernig's sign, the nurse flexes the client's leg at the hip, brings the knee to a 90-degree angle (Fig. 44–1), and then attempts to extend the knee. If meningitis is present, the client will experience pain and spasm of the hamstring muscle when the leg is straightened. Pain occurs secondary to meningeal irritation and spinal nerve root inflammation (from exudate around the roots).

To test the Brudzinski reflex, the nurse gently flexes the client's head and neck onto the chest. A positive response is indicated by flexion of the hips and knees.

Increased Intracranial Pressure. The nurse also assesses the client for complications that may occur, including increased intracranial pressure (ICP) resulting from the presence of exudate, which can lead to hydrocephalus

---

> **Chart 44–8**
>
> ### Nursing Care Highlight: Focused Assessment for Meningitis
>
> Level of consciousness
> Orientation to person, place, and year
> Pupil reaction and eye movements
> - Photophobia
> - Nystagmus
> - Abnormal eye movements
>
> Motor response
> - Normal early in disease process
> - Hemiparesis, hemiplegia, and decreased muscle tone may occur later.
> - Cranial nerve dysfunction
>   - Cranial nerves III, IV, VI, VII, VIII
> - Memory changes
> - Attention span (usually short)
> - Personality and behavior changes
>   - Bewilderment
> - Severe, unrelenting headaches
> - Generalized muscle aches and pain
> - Nausea and vomiting
> - Fever and chills
> - Tachycardia
> - Red macular rash (meningococcal meningitis)

---

and cerebral edema. Left untreated, increased ICP can lead to herniation of the brain and death (see Chap. 47).

Seizure activity may be caused by irritation of the cerebral cortex. Because of abnormal stimulation of the hypothalamic area, excessive amounts of antidiuretic hormone (ADH) (vasopressin) are produced. This results in water retention and dilution of serum sodium attributable to increased excretion of sodium by the kidneys. This syndrome of inappropriate antidiuretic hormone (SIADH) production may lead to further increases in ICP (see Chap. 66).

Vascular Dysfunction. To assess the client's vascular status, the nurse

- Observes the color and temperature of the extremities
- Determines the presence of peripheral pulses
- Identifies any indicators of abnormal bleeding

Septic emboli in the blood may block circulation in the small vessels of the hands and feet, leading to gangrene. Excessive fibrinolysis that occurs in bacteremia and infections from viruses, fungi, or protozoa may lead to disseminated intravascular coagulation (DIC). Vascular involvement of the cerebral arteries, veins, and venous sinuses may lead to seizures and hemiparesis.

Laboratory Assessment. The most significant laboratory test used in the diagnosis of meningitis is the analysis of the client's cerebrospinal fluid (CSF). A lumbar puncture is usually not done in the presence of increased ICP. The CSF is analyzed for cell count and protein. Glucose concentrations are determined, and culture, sensitivity, and Gram's stain studies are performed.

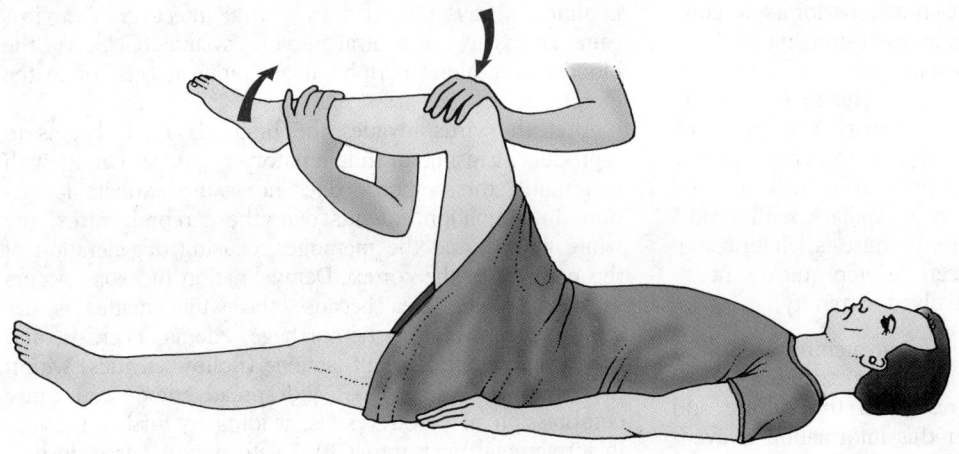

Figure 44–1. Kernig's sign, which indicates meningitis. Flexion of the hip and knee causes pain.

Counterimmunoelectrophoresis (CIE) may be performed to determine the presence of viruses or protozoa in the CSF. CIE is also indicated if the client has received antibiotics before the CSF was obtained. To identify a possible bacterial source of infection, specimens for culture are obtained and Gram's stains of the blood, urine, throat, and nose are performed. Table 44–5 compares CSF findings in those with bacterial and viral meningitis.

A complete blood count (CBC) is performed, with attention to the white blood cell (WBC) count, which is generally elevated well above the normal value. Serum electrolyte values are also assessed with attention to sodium count. Hyponatremia may occur secondary to SIADH, a complication of bacterial meningitis.

Other Diagnostic Studies. X-rays of the chest, air sinuses, and mastoids are taken to determine the presence of infection. A computed tomographic (CT) scan may be performed to identify increased ICP, presence of a brain abscess, or developing hydrocephalus.

Interventions

The most important nursing intervention for clients with meningitis is the accurate monitoring and recording of their neurologic status, vital signs, and vascular assess-ment. Other areas of nursing care are found in Chart 44–9.

Neurologic Assessments. The client's neurologic status and vital signs are assessed at least every 4 hours or more often if clinically indicated. The nurse assesses for neurologic changes indicative of cerebral complications, especially increased intracranial pressure (ICP). The health care team provides intervention for the client with increased ICP as discussed in Chapter 47. The client is at risk for seizure activity, and care should be provided as discussed in the section on epilepsy.

The nurse includes complete cranial nerve testing as part of the routine neurologic assessment because of possible cranial nerve involvement. Particular attention is given to cranial nerves III, IV, VI, VII, and VIII, as discussed earlier. A sixth cranial nerve defect (inability to move the eyes laterally) may indicate the development of hydrocephalus. Other indicators of hydrocephalus include the usual signs of increased ICP and the presence of urinary incontinence in the previously continent client. Urinary incontinence occurs secondary to the client's decreasing level of consciousness (LOC).

TABLE 44–5

Cerebrospinal Fluid (CSF) Findings in Meningitis		
Finding	**Bacterial Meningitis**	**Viral Meningitis**
Appearance	• Cloudy, turbid	• Clear
White blood cells	• Increased	• Increased
Protein	• Increased	• Increased, slightly elevated
Glucose	• Increased	• Normal
CSF pressure	• Elevated	• Varies

Chart 44–9

Nursing Care Highlight: The Client with Meningitis

- Take vital signs and perform neurologic checks every 2 to 4 hours, as ordered.
- Perform nerve assessments, with particular attention to cranial nerves III, IV, VI, VII, and VIII, and monitor for changes.
- Manage pain through drug and nondrug methods.
- Provide interventions to treat or prevent increased intracranial pressure.
- Perform vascular assessment and monitor for changes.
- Give medications as ordered, and document the client's response.
- Protect the client from injury; use seizure precautions.
- Maintain isolation precautions per hospital policy.

Vascular Assessments. The nurse performs a complete vascular assessment during each nursing shift or more often, if indicated, to prevent and detect early vascular compromise from septic emboli. This severe complication is most frequently seen in circulation to the hand. The nurse assesses the client's temperature, color, pulses, and capillary refill (by applying pressure to nail bed and looking for blood return). Normal capillary refill occurs within 3 seconds. If vascular compromise is left unrecognized and untreated, gangrene can develop quickly, possibly leading to the loss of the involved extremity.

Drug Therapy. To avoid life-threatening complications, the health care provider usually prescribes a broad-spectrum antibiotic until the results of the culture and Gram's stain are available. After this information is available, the specific antibiotic to treat the client's type of meningitis is given. Table 44–6 lists some of antibiotics commonly used. In administering these drugs, the nurse begins the medication within 1 to 2 hours after it is ordered and monitors and documents the client's response to the medication.

The client with bacterial meningitis may experience increased ICP, and seizure activity may occur. Medications used by the physician to treat these complications include hyperosmolar agents, steroids, and anticonvulsants.

People who have been in close contact with a client who has meningococcal meningitis must have prophylaxis treatment with rifampin.

Monitoring for Complications. The health care team monitors the client for other complications, including shock, coagulation disorders, septic complications (bacterial endocarditis), and prolonged fever.

Encephalitis
Overview

Encephalitis is an inflammation of the brain parenchyma (brain tissue) and often the meninges. It affects the cerebrum, the brain stem, and the cerebellum. Encephalitis is most often caused by a viral agent, although bacteria, fungi, or parasites may also be involved. Viral encephalitis

is almost always preceded by a viral infection. The virus gains access to the central nervous system (CNS) via the bloodstream, along peripheral or cranial nerves, or in the meninges.

After the virus invades the brain tissue, it begins to reproduce, causing an inflammatory response. Unlike with meningitis, this response does not cause exudate formation. Inflammation extends over the cerebral cortex, the white matter, and the meninges, causing degeneration of the neurons of the cortex. Demyelination of axons occurs in the involved area because the white matter is destroyed. This leads to hemorrhage, edema, necrosis, and the development of small lacunae (hollow cavities) within the cerebral hemispheres. Widespread edema can cause compression of blood vessels, leading to further increase in intracranial pressure (ICP). Death may occur from herniation and increased ICP.

Arboviruses

Arboviruses can be transmitted to humans through the bite of an infected mosquito or tick. The most common types of encephalitis seen are eastern and western equine, St. Louis, and California. Clients who have an insect bite that is large and reddened or becomes infected should be monitored for symptoms of encephalitis.

Encephalitis associated with tick bites tends to occur more frequently in the spring; encephalitis associated with mosquitoes occurs in middle to late summer. The incubation period for both types is 5 to 15 days. Summer is also the peak time for encephalitis caused by the enteroviruses, except the mumps virus, which is more prevalent in early winter. The incubation period varies, depending on the virus involved. Because clients are often unaware of tick bites, the nurse asks about outdoor activities.

Enteroviruses

Echovirus, coxsackievirus, poliovirus, herpes zoster, and viruses that cause mumps and chickenpox are the common enteroviruses associated with encephalitis.

Herpes Simplex Type 1

Herpes simplex virus type 1 (HSV1) causes the third type of viral encephalitis, the most frequently occurring nonepidemic encephalitis in North America. Clients with herpes encephalitis often have a history of cold sores. Mortality rates for HSV1 encephalitis can be as high as 40% to 50%, whereas mortality for the other types is much lower (Hickey, 1996).

Amebae

Amebic meningoencephalitis is caused by the amebae *Naegleria* and *Acanthamoeba*. Both are found in warm freshwater areas and can enter the nasal mucosa of people swimming in ponds or lakes. The amebae may also be found in soil and decaying vegetation. Although this infection has not been seen frequently in the past, the incidence in North America is increasing, perhaps because the ponds and lakes are becoming more polluted.

TABLE 44–6

Common Antibiotics Specific to Organisms Causing Meningitis	
Antibiotic	**Organisms**
Penicillin G	• Pneumococci • Meningococci • Streptococci
Gentamicin	• *Klebsiella* • *Pseudomonas* • *Proteus*
Chloramphenicol	• *Haemophilus influenzae*
Cephalosporin	• *Neisseria meningitidis*
Cefotaxime	• *Streptococcus pneumoniae*

Collaborative Management

 Assessment

The typical client with encephalitis has a fever and complains of nausea, vomiting, and a stiff neck. Other signs and symptoms include

- Changes in level of consciousness and mental status
- Motor dysfunction
- Focal neurologic deficits
- Symptoms of increased intracranial pressure ICP

The nurse assesses the client's level of consciousness (LOC) using the Glasgow Coma Scale (see Chap. 43). The client may be lethargic, stuporous, or comatose. Mental status changes include acute confusion, delirium, irritability, and personality and behavior changes (especially noted in the presence of herpes simplex). The nurse examines the client for signs of meningeal irritation by assessing for the presence of nuchal rigidity and Kernig's or Brudzinski's sign (described earlier under Meningitis). Motor changes exhibited by the client may vary from a mild weakness to hemiplegia. The client may have muscle tremors, spasticity, an ataxic gait (postencephalitic parkinsonism), myoclonic jerks, and increased deep tendon reflexes. Seizure activity is not uncommon. The client often experiences fever, nausea, vomiting, headache, and vertigo.

Cranial nerve involvement is exhibited by ocular palsies, facial weakness, and nystagmus. The herpes zoster lesion affects cranial and spinal nerve root ganglia, which is clinically manifested by a rash, severe pain, itching, burning, or tingling in the areas innervated by these nerves.

In severe cases of encephalitis, the client may exhibit increased ICP resulting from cerebral edema, hemorrhage, and necrosis of brain tissue. The nurse observes the client's vital signs for indications of a widened pulse pressure, bradycardia, and irregular respirations. The client's pupils become increasingly dilated and less responsive to light. Left untreated, increased ICP leads to herniation of the brain tissue and possibly death.

Interventions

Nursing interventions for the client with encephalitis are similar to those for the client with meningitis, with the exception of drug therapy. Supportive nursing care and prompt recognition and treatment of increased intracranial pressure (ICP) are essential components of management. The nurse also maintains a patent airway to prevent the development of atelectasis or pneumonia, which can lead to further brain hypoxia from inadequate amounts of oxygen in the circulating blood.

The nurse or assistive nursing personnel encourages and assists the client to turn, cough, and deep breathe at least every 2 hours. Deep tracheal suctioning may be performed, even in the presence of increased ICP, if the findings of the respiratory assessment indicate that the client's respiratory status is compromised, possibly causing cerebral hypoxia.

The nurse also checks the client's vital signs and neurologic signs every 2 hours or more frequently if clinically indicated. The head of the bed is elevated 30 to 45 degrees unless this is contraindicated (e.g., after lumbar puncture or in the client with severe hypotension).

Acyclovir (Zovirax) is the drug of choice for the treatment of herpes encephalitis and is associated with a significantly lower mortality rate than vidarabine (Vira-A) or adenine arabinoside (ara-A). Drug therapy is most effective if used early, before the client becomes stuporous or comatose. This usually occurs within 4 to 6 days after the appearance of the initial neurologic symptoms. No specific drug therapy is available for infection by arboviruses or enteroviruses.

If there are permanent neurologic disabilities, the client with encephalitis is usually discharged to a rehabilitation setting or a long-term care facility. The client with minimal neurologic problems is discharged to the home setting.

Botulism

Overview

Botulism is a neurotoxic disorder caused by the bacterium *Clostridium botulinum*. Most cases of botulism are caused by eating improperly canned foods. Symptoms usually appear 12 to 36 hours after ingestion of affected food. Less often, the bacterium can enter the body through a wound and produces the toxin in the traumatized area.

The bacterium impairs the release of acetylcholine (ACh) at the motor nerve synapse. This causes a motor paralysis that affects both voluntary and involuntary motor activity.

Collaborative Management

Clients with botulism have the following signs: extraocular and facial muscle paralysis, bulbar palsies, strabismus, blurred vision, diplopia, dysarthria, flaccid paralysis, dysphagia, vertigo, deafness, nausea, and vomiting.

Paralysis of the respiratory muscles is not uncommon. The diagnosis is based on history, clinical presentation, and isolation of the *C. botulinum* organism in the stool. Anaerobic blood cultures may also isolate the organism.

Treatment consists of the rapid administration of trivalent botulism antitoxin. Clients with secondary bacterial infections are treated with antibiotics. Supplemental care is given to prevent respiratory complications and complications of immobility as well as to provide nutritional support.

Tetanus

Overview

Tetanus, also known as lockjaw, is caused by *Clostridium tetani* and is easily prevented through immunization. Tetanus infection is frequently transmitted through a wound contaminated with the bacterium, which is commonly found in soil.

On entering the wound, the bacterium multiplies rapidly and produces the toxin *tetanospasmin*. The toxin enters the central nervous system and spinal motor ganglia through the bloodstream. The toxin interferes with the normal activity of the inhibitory postsynaptic potentials. This causes the anterior horn cells to become overstimulated and transmit excessive stimuli to the muscles. The result is opisthotonos (spasm causing head and feet to bend backward and the body bowed forward), muscle rigidity, cramps, muscle spasms, stiffness, and headache. The incubation period is 1 to 3 days.

Diagnosis is made on the basis of history and clinical findings almost exclusively, and there are no definitive tests for tetanus.

Collaborative Management

Treatment includes the prompt (within 72 hours) intramuscular (IM) administration of the antitoxin human tetanus immune globulin or hyperimmune equine or bovine serum. Antibiotics may be prescribed to treat superimposed infections. The physician may order sedatives, antianxiety agents, and muscle relaxants to decrease muscle spasms and increase the client's comfort. If necessary, propranolol (Inderal) is given to treat cardiac irregularities. Aggressive respiratory support and intervention are ordered as needed. Other interventions are directed toward preventing the complications of immobility. The mortality rate for untreated tetanus is high.

PARKINSON'S DISEASE

Overview

Parkinson's disease, also referred to as paralysis agitans, is a debilitating, neurologic disease affecting motor ability. It is characterized by muscle rigidity, bradykinesia, slow movement, and tremor. Although the exact cause of Parkinson's disease is not known, evidence suggests it might be related to a genetic defect of chromosome 4 (Youdim & Riederer, 1997). It occurs most often in people older than 50 years. Parkinson's syndrome may be seen in those younger than 40 years, secondary to certain medications, or as result of trauma or ischemia to the substantia nigra.

For motor activity to occur, the actions of the cerebral cortex, basal ganglia, and cerebellum must be integrated. The basal ganglia are a group of neurons located deep within the cerebrum at the base of the brain near the lateral ventricles. When basal ganglia are stimulated, muscle tone in the body is inhibited and voluntary movements are refined. This process is accomplished by the secretion of two neurotransmitters: dopamine (DP) and acetylcholine (ACh).

Dopamine is produced in the substantia nigra as well as in the adrenal glands, and it is transmitted to the basal ganglia along a connecting neural pathway for secretion when needed. Acetylcholine is produced and secreted by the basal ganglia as well as in the nerve endings in the periphery of the body. ACh-producing neurons transmit excitatory messages throughout the basal ganglia. Dopamine inhibits the function of these neurons, allowing control over voluntary movement. This system of checks and balances allows for refined, coordinated movement, such as picking up a pencil and writing.

Parkinson's disease results from widespread degeneration of the substantia nigra, leading to a decrease in the amount of dopamine. Dopamine produced in the adrenal glands is not available because it is quickly metabolized in the body. When DP levels are decreased, a person loses the ability to refine voluntary movement. The large number of excitatory ACh-secreting neurons remains active, creating an imbalance between excitatory and inhibitory neuronal activity. The resulting excessive excitation of neurons prevents a person from controlling or initiating voluntary movement.

In addition to changes in voluntary movement, some clients experience autonomic nervous system symptoms, such as excessive perspiration and orthostatic hypotension; however, the cause of these symptoms is unclear. Some clients also experience dementia.

Parkinson's disease is separated into stages according to the symptoms and degree of disability (Table 44-7). Stage 1 is mild disease with unilateral limb involvement. Bilateral limb involvement occurs in stage 2. In stage 3, the client exhibits significant gait disturbances and moderate generalized disability. Stage 4 is characterized by severe disability, akinesia (no initiation of movement), and muscle rigidity. The client with stage 5 disease is completely dependent in all activities of daily living (ADLs). Other classifications refer simply to mild, moderate, and severe disease,

Collaborative Management

 Assessment

The nurse collects data related to the time and progression of symptoms noticed by the client or the family. Early signs and symptoms, such as fatigue, slight tremor, and problems with manual dexterity, may be ignored, especially by the elderly client, who may assume that these behaviors are normal changes associated with aging.

TABLE 44-7

Stages of Parkinson's Disease
Stage 1: Initial Stage
• Unilateral limb involvement
• Minimal weakness
• Hand and arm trembling
Stage 2: Mild Stage
• Bilateral limb involvement
• Mask-like facies
• Slow, shuffling gait
Stage 3: Moderate Disease
• Gait disturbances increase
Stage 4: Severe Disability
• Akinesia
• Rigidity
Stage 5: Complete Dependence

Chart 44–10

Key Features of Parkinson's Disease

Posture
- Stooped posture
- Flexed trunk
- Fingers abducted and flexed at the metacarpophalangeal joint
- Wrist slightly dorsiflexed

Gait
- Slow and shuffling
- Short, hesitant steps
- Propulsive gait
- Difficulty stopping quickly

Motor
- Bradykinesia
- Akinesia
- Tremors
- "Pill-rolling" movement
- Mask-like facies
- Difficulties chewing and swallowing
- Uncontrolled drooling, especially at night
- Fatigue
- Difficulty getting in and out of bed
- Little arm swinging when walking
- Change in handwriting (gets smaller)

Speech
- Soft, low-pitched voice
- Dysarthric
- Echolalia (automatic repetition of what another person says) and repetition of sentences
- Change in voice volume, phonation, or articulation

Autonomic Dysfunction
- Orthostatic hypotension
- Excessive perspiration
- Oily skin
- Seborrhea
- Flushing
- Changes in skin texture
- Blepharospasm

Psychosocial Assessment
- Emotionally labile
- Depression
- Paranoia
- Easily upset
- Rapid mood swings
- Cognitive impairments (i.e., dementia)
- Delayed reaction time
- Sleep disturbances

Other signs and symptoms are found in Chart 44–10, which summarizes the clinical manifestations of Parkinson's disease.

The nurse begins the assessment by checking for evidence of rigidity, or resistance to passive movement of the extremities. Rigidity is evaluated as the nurse performs passive range of motion (ROM) of the extremities. Rigidity is classified as

- Cogwheel, manifested by a rhythmic interruption of the muscle movement
- Plastic, defined as mildly restrictive movement
- Lead pipe, or total resistance to movement

Rigidity is present early in the disease process and progresses over time. The nurse further observes the client's ability to relax a muscle or move a selected muscle group.

Changes in facial expression or a mask-like facies with wide-open, fixed, staring eyes is caused by rigidity of the facial muscles (Fig. 44–2). This rigidity can lead to difficulties in chewing and swallowing, particularly if the pharyngeal muscles are involved. Uncontrolled drooling may occur.

A diagnosis of Parkinson's disease is made on the basis of the clinical findings. There are no specific diagnostic tests. Analysis of cerebrospinal fluid (CSF) may show a decrease in dopamine levels, although the results of other studies are usually normal.

Interventions

Drug therapy, physical or occupational therapy, and, as a last resort, palliative surgery may be performed to assist the client in remaining mobile for as long as possible. Chart 44–11 provides an overview of nursing management of the client with Parkinson's disease.

➤ Nonsurgical Management

Drug Therapy. A variety of medications are used to control tremor and rigidity. Medication administration is closely monitored, and the physician adjusts the dosage or changes the medication as the client's condition war-

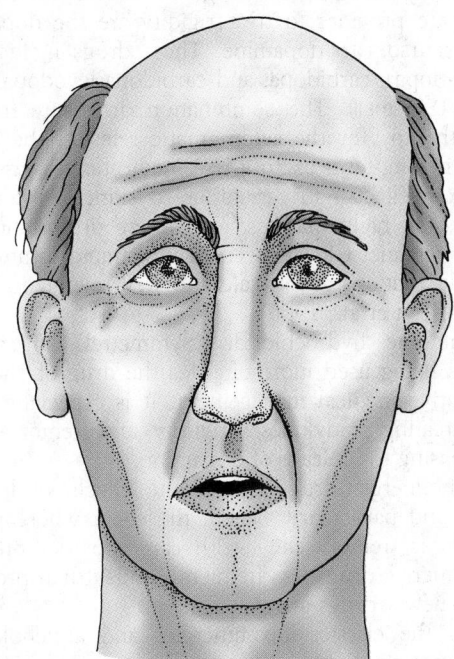

Figure 44–2. The mask-like facial expression typical of clients with Parkinson's disease.

Nursing Care Highlight: The Client with Parkinson's Disease

- Administer medications promptly on schedule to maintain continuous therapeutic drug levels.
- Monitor for side effects of medications, especially orthostatic hypotension, hallucinations, and acute confusional state.
- Collaborate with physical and occupational therapists to keep the client as mobile and as independent in activities of daily living as possible.
- Allow the client time to perform activities of daily living and mobility skills.
- Implement interventions to prevent complications of immobility, such as constipation, pressure ulcers, and contractures.
- Schedule appointments and activities late in the morning to prevent rushing the client, or schedule them at the time of the client's optimal level of functioning
- Teach the client to speak slowly and clearly; use alternative communication methods such as a communication board.
- Monitor the client's ability to eat and swallow; monitor actual food and fluid intake.
- Provide high-protein, high-calorie foods or supplements to maintain weight.
- Recognize that Parkinson's disease affects the client's body image; focus on the client's strengths.
- Assess for depression and anxiety.

rants. The nurse ensures that the drug is given at the prescribed times to keep the client's serum level of the drug constant.

Types of Drugs. The drugs of choice used by the health care provider to treat rigidity are the dopaminergics, precursors to dopamine. These drugs include levodopa (L-dopa), carbidopa, and carbidopa-levodopa combinations (Sinemet). The combination drugs are the most potent therapy for the symptomatic relief of the disease. However, long-term use of these medications is associated with side effects, for example, dyskinesias (abnormal movements), hallucinations, and severe orthostatic hypotension. Sinemet CR has been demonstrated to ameliorate motor fluctuations and is safe and well tolerated (Wolters and Msarleen et al., 1996).

Amantadine hydrochloride (Symmetrel), an antiviral agent, is being used more often as the drug of choice for conservative medical management. It is especially beneficial in treating bradykinesia, rigidity, and tremor and acts by increasing the release of dopamine.

Anticholinergic drugs extend the effects of levodopa therapy and particularly benefit the client whose primary symptom is tremor. The health care provider prescribes anticholinergic drugs less frequently today than previously because newer drugs are available.

When the classic dopaminergics and anticholinergics fail or are no longer effective, bromocriptine mesylate (Parlodel) may be prescribed to activate the release of dopamine. It may be used alone or in combination with Sinemet. Some providers may prescribe bromocriptine mesylate early in the course of treatment of the client with Parkinson's disease. It is especially useful in the client who has experienced such side effects as dyskinesias or orthostatic hypotension while receiving levodopa.

Additional therapeutic strategies used for Parkinson's disease include the administration of monoamine oxidase (MAO) inhibitors to reduce the metabolic breakdown of dopamine and catechol O-methyltransferase inhibitors to retard the breakdown of levodopa. Dextromethorphan glial-derived neurotrophic factor administered directly into the brain is undergoing clinical trials (Hickey, 1996).

Drug Toxicity. For the client on long-term drug therapy regimens, drug tolerance or drug toxicity often develops. Drug toxicity is evidenced by delirium, cognitive impairments, decreased effectiveness of the drug, or hallucinations. Delirium may be difficult to assess in the client who is already suffering from chronic dementia from Parkinson's disease or another disease. If possible, the nurse compares the client's current cognitive and behavioral status with his or her baseline before drug therapy began.

When drug tolerance is reached, the client finds that the drug's effects do not last as long as previously. The treatment of drug toxicity or tolerance includes
- A reduction of medication dosage
- A change of medications or frequency of administration
- A drug holiday (particularly with levodopa therapy)

During a drug holiday, which typically lasts up to 10 days, the client receives no medications. The client must be carefully monitored during this time.

Exercise/Ambulation. In collaboration with the physical therapist, the nurse plans and implements an active and passive range-of-motion (ROM), muscle-stretching, and activity program. The prescribed program includes exercises for the muscles of the face and tongue to facilitate swallowing and speech. A speech and language pathologist may also be consulted.

Because of the potential for respiratory problems, the nurse or respiratory therapist teaches the client how to perform breathing exercises, including diaphragmatic and abdominal exercises. The nurse instructs the client with orthostatic hypotension to wear elastic stockings and change positions slowly, especially when moving from a sitting to a standing position, to allow for adequate cerebral blood flow.

Self-Care. The nurse and the health care team encourage the client to participate as much as possible in the performance of self-care or ADL skills. The nurse and rehabilitation specialists make the environment conducive to independence in activity and as stress-free and safe as possible. Consultations with occupational and physical therapists are obtained for training in ADLs and the use of adaptive devices, if needed, to facilitate independence.

Nutrition. If intake is not sufficient, the client is weighed weekly. Food intake is recorded daily or as needed based on the client's needs. The nurse consults the dietitian for calorie calculation and diet planning. Supplemental feedings with high-protein, high-calorie liquids or puddings may be given several times a day to maintain weight. (Chapter 64 covers additional interventions for clients with undernutrition.) The nurse and dietitian carefully monitor the client's swallowing and chewing abilities as well as the ability to feed independently. The client who attempts self-feeding may drop a large portion of the food on the lap instead of getting the food into the mouth. The nurse carefully monitors actual food intake. Usually, a soft diet or thick, cold fluids, such as milk shakes, are more easily tolerated. Smaller, more frequent meals or a commercial powder, such as Thick-It, added to liquids may assist the client who has difficulty swallowing. The client is positioned properly with the head elevated to facilitate swallowing and prevent aspiration.

When possible, the nurse schedules medications so that peak action occurs during mealtime, facilitating independence in feeding.

Communication. The nurse instructs the client to speak slowly and clearly and to pause and take deep breaths at appropriate intervals during each sentence. Unnecessary environmental noise should be eliminated, if possible, to maximize the listener's ability to hear and understand the client. The nurse and the family ask the client to repeat words they do not understand, and they watch the client's lips and nonverbal expressions for cues as to the meaning of conversation. The nurse instructs the client to organize thoughts before speaking and encourages the client to use facial expression and gestures, if possible, to assist with communication. In addition, the client should exaggerate words to increase the listener's ability to understand.

If the client cannot communicate verbally, he or she must use alternative methods of communication, such as a communication board, mechanical voice synthesizer, computer, or electric typewriter. The client's ability to use these devices must be assessed before a decision is made about the method to use.

Psychosocial Support. About 40% of clients with Parkinson's disease are classified as demented. Clients experience changes in gait and tremors that are uncontrollable. In the late stages of the disease, they cannot move without assistance, have difficulty with articulation, have minimal facial expression, and may drool. Clients often state that they are embarrassed, and they tend to avoid social events or groups of people. Clients should not be forced into situations in which they feel ashamed of their appearance. They should be encouraged to undertake activities that do not require small muscle dexterity, such as light, modified aerobic exercises.

The nurse emphasizes the client's abilities or strengths and provides positive reinforcement when the client has met daily goals. The client, the family or significant others, and the nurse mutually set realistic goals that can be achieved. Assisting the client with grooming and hygiene is also important in maintaining a positive body image (see also Chap. 10).

► *Surgical Management*

Several options are available if surgery for the client with Parkinson's disease is needed. Surgery is a last resort when drugs are ineffective in symptom management.

Stereotactic Pallidotomy. This is a very effective treatment for Parkinson's disease. First, the target area within the pallidum via a CT or MRI scan is identified. Next, the stereotactic head frame is placed on the client. IV sedation is given and a bur hole is made into the cranium; an electrode or cylindrical rod is inserted into the target area. The target area receives a mild electrical stimulation, and the client's reaction is assessed for reduction of tremor and rigidity. If this result does not occur or if unexpected visual, motor, or sensory symptoms appear, the probe is repositioned. When the probe is in the ideal location, a temporary lesion is made. If this is successful, the permanent lesion is made. The client is monitored in the postanesthesia care unit (PACU) for about 1 hour and then returns to the inpatient unit for continuing postoperative care.

Analogous Tissue Transplant. An experimental surgical procedure is now being conducted at several medical centers throughout the United States for clients with Parkinson's disease. Small pieces of the client's own adrenal gland are transplanted into the basal ganglia of the brain. A right adrenalectomy is performed followed by a right frontal craniotomy. The surgeon removes a small area from the caudate nucleus of the basal ganglia and implants the adrenal medullary graft directly into the area. Wire clips hold the implant in place, and a subdural catheter is inserted for intracranial monitoring. A collection reservoir is also implanted during the procedure so that the surgeon can easily obtain cerebrospinal fluid (CSF) for postoperative analysis of dopamine content.

The client selected for brain graft surgery must meet strict criteria (Table 44–8). Postoperatively, the client is transferred to the critical care unit, where the nurses must plan care for the client with a craniotomy, adrenalectomy, and Parkinson's disease. After a stay in the primary critical care unit for about 1 week, the client is then transferred to a step-down unit for further care for another 3 to 5 days. Although the transplantation is considered palliative rather than curative, case reports have been very encouraging that the procedure may control symptoms and reverse the client's disability.

TABLE 44–8

Criteria for Brain Graft Surgery

- Younger than 65 years
- No dementia
- No history of end-stage cardiac, pulmonary, or renal disease
- Confirmation of two adrenal glands by computed tomography (CT) scan
- Informed consent, including understanding the procedure, risks, and potential effects
- Parkinson's disease with muscle rigidity and bradykinesia as the major clinical manifestations
- History of some response to medication, but with inadequate relief of symptoms and severe side effects

Modified from Bradbury, K. M., & Bauer, M. (1991). Brain graft surgery: A new treatment for Parkinson's disease. *Critical Care Nurse, 10*(8), 22. Used with permission.

Fetal Tissue Transplant. Fetal tissue transplantation is an experimental and highly controversial procedure. Fetal substantia nigra tissue is transplanted into the caudate nucleus of the brain. Preliminary reports suggest that clients show substantial clinical improvement after receiving the transplanted tissue (Iacono, 1995).

ALZHEIMER'S DISEASE

Overview

Alzheimer's disease, also known as dementia, Alzheimer's type (DAT), is a chronic, progressive, degenerative disease that accounts for 60% of the dementias occurring in people older than 65 years. It may also be seen less commonly in people in their 40s and 50s, which is referred to as early dementia, Alzheimer's type, or presenile dementia, Alzheimer's type. It is characterized by loss of memory, judgment, and visuospatial perception and a change in personality. Over time, the client becomes increasingly cognitively impaired; severe physical deterioration takes place and death occurs.

Pathophysiology

Structural Changes in the Brain

The brain of the older adult weighs less and occupies less space in the cranial vault than does the brain of a younger person. Other changes in the brain that occur with aging include widening of the cerebral sulci, narrowing of the gyri, and enlargement of the ventricles. In the presence of Alzheimer's disease, these normal changes are greatly accelerated. Brain weight is reduced further, and there is marked cerebral atrophy. The cerebral sulci and fissures as well as the ventricles are enlarged more than those of persons of the same age without Alzheimer's disease. Areas of the brain particularly affected are

- The precentral gyrus of the frontal lobe
- The superior temporal gyrus
- The hippocampus
- The substantia nigra

Microscopic changes of the brain found in people with Alzheimer's disease include neurofibrillary tangles, senile or neuritic plaques, and granulovascular degeneration.

Neurofibrillary tangles are a classic finding at autopsy in the brains of clients with Alzheimer's disease. They consist of tangled masses of fibrous elements throughout the neurons. The same tangles and chemical changes are found in people with Down syndrome.

Senile plaques are composed of degenerating nerve terminals and are found particularly in the hippocampus, an important part of the limbic system. Deposited within the plaques are increased amounts of an abnormal protein called *amyloid*. When amyloid infiltrates body tissue, it causes the tissue to decrease or lose function.

Although vascular degeneration occurs in the normally aging brain, its presence is significantly increased in clients with Alzheimer's disease. It accounts for at least partial loss of the ability of nerve cells to function properly. This pathologic change contributes to the mortality associated with this disorder.

Chemical Changes in the Brain

In addition to the structural changes in the brain associated with Alzheimer's disease, abnormalities in the neurotransmitters (acetylcholine [ACh], norepinephrine, dopamine [DP], serotonin) may occur. ACh in the brain is reduced as much as 75% and leads to a decrease in the amount of acetyltransferase in the hippocampus. This loss is significant because the decrease in acetyltransferase interferes with cholinergic innervation to the cerebral cortex. This results in dysfunction of cognition, recent memory, and the ability to acquire new memories. The exact role of the reduction of neurotransmitters in the development of Alzheimer's disease is not well understood.

Etiology

The exact cause of Alzheimer's disease is unknown. Several theories and risk factors have been proposed: genetics, chemical imbalances, environmental agents, and immunologic changes.

There is little doubt that for many clients with Alzheimer's disease there is a genetic predisposition to the development of the disease. Studies of families are ongoing to determine the exact genetic pathway that is responsible. Twin studies suggest that a defect may occur on chromosome 14. Chromosomes 1 and 19 have been implicated in some forms of familial Alzheimer's disease. However, less than 10% of the cases are inherited by an autosomal dominant mechanism (Hier, 1997). Amyloid beta-protein encoded on chromosome 21 has been detected in non-neuronal tissues and blood vessels of clients with Alzheimer's disease. People with Down syndrome often develop dementia with characteristic features of DAT.

Chemical changes in the brain, particularly the role of acetylcholine and amyloid, are also being studied. Clients with Alzheimer's disease may have a shortage of the neurotransmitter acetylcholine and an abnormal build-up of amyloid (Hickey, 1996). The abnormal build-up of amyloid appears to be directly related to the lack of ACh.

Environmental agents, especially certain viruses such as herpes zoster and herpes simplex, and aluminum toxicity have been suggested as environmental causes. Clients who have experienced a head injury may be more at risk for Alzheimer's disease and at an earlier age than others.

Research concerning immunologic causes of Alzheimer's disease has been inconclusive, and further studies are needed.

Incidence/Prevalence

Alzheimer's disease may affect anyone older than 40 years, although it occurs more often in those older than 65 years.

WOMEN'S HEALTH CONSIDERATIONS

When Alzheimer's disease occurs in old age, it tends to affect women slightly more frequently than men. Worldwide, Alzheimer's disease occurs in more than 20 million people; some 5 million people in the United States older than 65 years have the disease. It is the fourth leading cause of death, after heart attacks, cancer, and strokes. The cost to care for those with the disease is estimated at more than $90 billion annually (Hickey, 1996).

Collaborative Management

 Assessment

The client with Alzheimer's disease often presents with cognitive impairment, although many other disorders, drugs, and environmental factors can cause changes in cognition. A thorough history and physical examination is necessary to differentiate Alzheimer's disease from other possibly reversible causes (Table 44–9). The nurse obtains information from the client, family members, and significant others, because the client may be unaware of the problems, denying their existence or covering them up.

The most important information to be obtained concerns the onset, duration, progression, and course of the client's symptoms obtained. The nurse questions the client and the family about changes in memory or increasing forgetfulness and the ability to perform activities of daily living (ADLs). Further information obtained includes current employment status, work history, and ability to fulfill household responsibilities, including cleaning, grocery shopping, and preparing meals. The nurse elicits a history concerning changes in driving ability, ability to handle routine financial transactions, and language and communication skills. In addition, any changes in personality and behavior are recorded.

The history taking concludes with a review of the client's medical history. The nurse asks about a history of head trauma, viral illness, and exposure to metal or toxic waste and a family history of Alzheimer's disease.

➤ Physical Assessment/Clinical Manifestations

Stages of Alzheimer's Disease. The clinical manifestations associated with Alzheimer's disease can be grouped into three broad stages on the basis of the progress of the disease (Chart 44–12). The client does not necessarily progress from one stage to the next in an orderly fashion. A stage may be bypassed, or the client may exhibit symptoms of one or several stages. Every client exhibits different disease stages and clinical manifestations. Consequently, some authorities now use more broad terms such as early (mild), moderate, and severe.

The primary focus of the nurse's neurologic assessment of clients with Alzheimer's disease is to identify abnormalities in cognition, including language, personality, and behavior. Physical manifestations of neurologic impairment (seizures, tremors, or ataxia) tend to occur late in the disease process.

Changes in Cognition. Cognition refers to the ability of the brain to process, store, retrieve, and manipulate information. Therefore, the nurse assesses the client for deficits in the following abilities:

- Attention and concentration
- Judgment and perception

TABLE 44–9

Causes of Cognitive Impairment in the Elderly

Neurologic Causes
- Vascular insufficiency
- Infections
- Trauma
- Tumors
- Normal pressure hydrocephalus

Cardiovascular Causes
- Myocardial infarction
- Dysrhythmias
- Congestive heart failure
- Cardiogenic shock
- Endocarditis

Pulmonary Causes
- Infection
- Pneumonia
- Hypoventilation

Metabolic Causes
- Electrolyte imbalance
- Acidosis/alkalosis
- Hypoglycemia/hyperglycemia
- Acute and chronic renal failure
- Fluid volume deficit
- Hepatic failure
- Porphyria

Drug Intoxication
- Misuse of prescribed medications
- Side effects of medications
- Incorrect use of over-the-counter medications
- Ingestion of heavy metals

Nutritional Deficiencies
- B vitamins
- Vitamin C
- Hypoproteinemia

Environmental Causes
- Hypothermia/hyperthermia
- Unfamiliar environment
- Sensory deprivation/overload

Psychological Causes
- Depression
- Anxiety
- Pain
- Fatigue
- Grief
- Paranoia

- Learning and memory
- Communication and language
- Speed of information processing

Typical symptoms experienced by the client include memory impairment, as well as new memory, and defects in information retrieval resulting from dysfunction in the hippocampal, frontal, or parietal region. Alterations in communication abilities, such as apraxia (inability to use objects appropriately), aphasia (inability to speak or understand), anomia (inability to find words), and agnosia

Key Features of Alzheimer's Disease

Early, or Stage I

- Forgets names; misplaces household items
- Mild memory loss
- Short attention span
- Subtle changes in personality and behavior
- No social or employment problems
- Cognitive impairment, problems with judgment
- Decreased performance, especially when stressed
- Unable to travel alone to new destinations
- Decreased knowledge of current events
- Loss of judgment

Moderate, or Stage II

- Severe impairment of all cognitive functions
- Gross intellectual impairments
- Complete disorientation to time, place, and event
- Possible depression, agitated
- Physical impairment
- Loss of ability to care for self
- Visuospacial deficits
- Speech and language deficits

Severe, or Stage III

- Completely incapacitated
- Totally dependent in activities of daily living
- Motor and verbal skills lost
- General and focal neurologic deficits

(loss of sensory comprehension), are due to dysfunction of the temporal and parietal lobes. Frontal lobe impairment produces difficulties with judgment, inability to make decisions, decreased attention span, and diminished ability to concentrate. As the disease progresses, the client loses all cognitive abilities, is totally unable to communicate, and becomes less aware of the environment.

To assess the presence of cognitive impairment, the nurse can use one of several assessment tools. One of the most popular tools is Folstein's Mini-Mental State Examination (MMSE), also known as the "mini-mental" (Folstein et al., 1975) (Fig. 44–3). The client performs certain cognitive tasks that are scored and added for a total score of 0 to 30. The lower the score, the greater is the severity of the dementia. It is not unusual for a client with advanced Alzheimer's disease to score below 5.

Although the MMSE is used very frequently, the client must be able to read. For the client who cannot read or for a quicker screening test, the nurse can use a SET test, which is useful for the elderly client. The nurse asks the client to name 10 items in each of four categories: fruits, animals, colors, and towns (FACT). Other categories can be used, if necessary. The client receives 1 point for each item, for a possible maximum score of 40. Clients who score above 25 do not have dementia. Although this assessment is more comprehensive and easy to administer, it should not be used for clients with hearing impairments or aphasia. Other tests used to measure cognitive

impairments include the Dementia Rating Scale and the Blessed Scale for Activities of Daily Living.

Changes in Behavior and Personality. One of the most difficult aspects of Alzheimer's disease that families, significant others, and health care professionals cope with are the behavioral changes that can occur in advanced disease. The nurse assesses for

- Aggressiveness, especially verbal and physical abusive tendencies
- Rapid mood swings
- Increased confusion at night ("sundowning") or in excessively fatigued clients

If the client is not too ill to ambulate, he or she may also wander and become lost or may go into other rooms to rummage through another's belongings. Hoarding objects like washcloths is also common.

For some clients with dementia, emotional and psychiatric problems accompany the primary disease. Some clients experience paranoia, illusions, hallucinations, and depression. The nurse assesses clients for these behaviors and documents their occurrence. (See a psychiatric nursing textbook for a complete discussion of these disorders.)

Although drug therapy is not effective in treating dementia, certain drugs may help to control the emotional and psychiatric manifestations such as depression, anxiety, paranoia, and aggression, associated with the primary disease.

Changes in Self-Care Skills. Changes in the client's self-care skills observed by the family, significant others, or nurse include

- Decreased interest in personal appearance
- Selection of clothing that is inappropriate for the weather or event
- Loss of bowel and bladder control
- Decreased appetite or ability to eat

Over time, the client becomes less mobile and muscle contractures develop; the client eventually becomes totally immobile, requiring total physical care.

► *Psychosocial Assessment*

In people with Alzheimer's disease, the cognitive changes as well as biochemical and structural dysfunctions affect personality and behavior. In the early stage, clients often recognize that they are experiencing memory or cognitive changes and may attempt to hide the problems, deny them, or become depressed over the changes. Older clients typically attribute the changes to "old age."

As the disease progresses, clients begin to display major changes in emotional and behavioral affect. Of particular importance is the need for the nurse to assess clients' reactions to changes in routine or environment. For example, a hospital admission is very traumatic for most clients with dementia. It is not unusual for clients to exhibit a catastrophic response or overreact to any change by becoming excessively aggressive or abusive.

As clients become unaware of their behavior, the focus of the psychosocial assessment shifts to the family and significant others. The nurse assesses their ability to cope

Maximum Score	Score	
		Client _____ Examiner _____ Date _____

Orientation

| 5 | ( ) | What is the (year) (season) (date) (day) (month)? |
| 5 | ( ) | Where are we (state) (country) (town) (hospital) (floor)? |

Registration

| 3 | ( ) | Name 3 objects: 1 second to say each. Then ask the client all 3 after you have said them. Give 1 point for each correct answer. Then repeat them until he/she learns all 3. Count trials and record. |

Trials _____

Attention and Calculation

| 5 | ( ) | Serial 7's. 1 point for each correct answer. Stop after 5 answers. Alternatively spell "world" backward. |

Recall

| 3 | ( ) | Ask for the 3 objects repeated above. Give 1 point for each correct answer. |

Language

2	( )	Name a pencil and a watch. (2 points)
1	( )	Repeat the following: "No ifs, ands, or buts." (1 point)
3	( )	Follow a 3-stage command: "Take a paper in your hand, fold it in half, and put it on the floor." (3 points)
1	( )	Read and obey the following: CLOSE YOUR EYES. (1 point)
1	( )	Write a sentence. (1 point)
1	( )	Copy a design. (1 point)
_____		Total Score

Figure 44–3. The Mini-Mental State Examination. (Reprinted with permission from Folstein, M. E., Folstein, S. E. [1975]. Mini-Mental State: A practical method for grading the cognitive state of patients for the clinician. *Journal of Psychiatric Research,* *12.* Copyright 1975, Pergamon Press plc.)

with the chronicity and progression of the disease and identifies possible support systems.

➤ *Laboratory Assessment*

No laboratory tests exist to confirm the diagnosis of Alzheimer's disease; diagnosis is made on the basis of brain tissue examination at autopsy, which confirms the presence of neurofibrillary tangles and neuritic plaques. Because of the seriousness of the procedure and the potential complications, a brain biopsy is rarely performed to obtain a definitive diagnosis.

Several studies indicate that measurement of protein in the cerebrospinal fluid (CSF), together with clinical observation, is a useful screening tool to diagnosis Alzheimer's disease (Trojanowski, 1995).

Genetic testing, specifically for apolipoprotein E (Apo E), may be helpful as an ancillary test (not a predictive test) for the differential diagnosis of Alzheimer's disease. Four genes have been found to be associated with Alzheimer's disease. Three are associated with early onset (before age 65) and one gene, *Apo E,* is associated primarily with late onset.

A variety of laboratory tests may be performed to rule out other treatable causes of dementia or delirium, including

- A complete blood count
- Determination of serum electrolyte levels, blood urea nitrogen, glucose
- Determination of vitamin B_{12} levels
- Determination of folate levels
- Thyroid and liver function tests
- A serologic test for syphilis
- Drug toxicity screening tests (over-the-counter and illegal drugs)
- Alcohol screening tests

➤ *Radiographic Assessment*

Computed tomography (CT) and positron emission tomography (PET) may be performed to rule out other causes of neurologic diseases. The CT scan typically shows cerebral atrophy and ventricular enlargement, wide sulci, and shrunken gyri in the later stages of the disease. The PET scan, which measures glucose in living cells, shows a significant decrease in metabolic activity in the brains of people with Alzheimer's disease.

➤ *Other Diagnostic Assessment*

Magnetic resonance imaging (MRI) can also rule out other causes of neurologic disease. The electroencephalogram (EEG) shows slow-wave delta activity indicative of dementia in the second and third stages of Alzheimer's disease.

In an effort to identify clearly the nature and extent of the client's cognitive dysfunction, several neuropsychological tests are administered by the physician, usually a neurologist. The tests used depend on physician preference and the ability of the client to participate in testing. All of the tests focus on the client's cognitive ability and may be repeated over time to measure changes.

 Analysis

> ### *Common Nursing Diagnoses and Collaborative Problems*

The common nursing diagnoses pertinent to the client with Alzheimer's disease are
1. Altered Thought Processes and Self-Care Deficit related to limited attention span, loss of memory, depression, and/or exposure to unfamiliar environment
2. Risk for Injury related to memory loss, wandering, behavior changes, and/or seizure activity
3. Ineffective Family Coping: Compromised related to the client's deteriorating condition and constant care demands
4. Sleep Pattern Disturbance related to unfamiliar environment, overstimulation, and/or confusion

> ### *Additional Nursing Diagnoses and Collaborative Problems*

In addition to the common diagnoses, the client may exhibit one or more of the following nursing diagnoses:
- Impaired Verbal Communication related to aphasia, anomia, agnosia, and apraxia
- Altered Nutrition: Less than Body Requirements related to self-care deficit and anorexia
- Total (Urinary) Incontinence and Bowel Incontinence related to cognitive and self-care deficits
- Social Isolation related to personality and behavior changes
- Impaired Physical Mobility related to contractures and other effects of debilitating disease
- Risk for Impaired Skin Integrity related to immobility or impaired nutritional status
- Self-Care Deficit (Total) related to cognitive deficit
- Risk for Violence related to behavior changes
- Hopelessness related to inability to control the progression of disease

 Planning and Implementation

Altered Thought Processes

Planning: Expected Outcomes. The outcomes are that the client is expected to (1) be oriented to person, place, or time, in early DAT, if possible, and (2) have no or decreased episodes of agitation.

Interventions. The client with memory problems benefits from a structured and consistent environment. Many

TABLE 44–10

Factors that Can Worsen Alzheimer's Disease

- Stroke
- Subdural hematoma
- Space-occupying lesion
- Decrease in blood supply to the brain
- Myocardial infarction
- Dysrhythmias
- Hypoglycemia
- Impaired renal function
- Impaired hepatic function
- Infection
- Impaired vision and hearing
- Sudden changes in surroundings
- Pain and discomfort
- Drugs
- Physical restraint

variables, including physical illness and environmental factors, can worsen or exacerbate the clinical manifestations of Alzheimer's disease (Table 44–10). The nurse assesses for the presence of these factors so that they can be addressed if present.

Structuring the Environment. The health care team collaborates to identify conditions in the environment that can be modified to increase the client's ability to function. The two most important actions that are necessary for the client with Alzheimer's disease are preventing overstimulation and providing a structured and orderly environment.

Preventing Overstimulation. When a client is admitted to a new setting or environment (hospital, assisted living, or long-term care facility), the staff works with the admitting department to select a room that is in the quietest area of the unit and away from obvious exits, if possible. A private room may be needed if the client has a history of agitation or wandering. The television should remain off unless the client turns it on or requests that it be turned on.

Nursing research on sound has studied noise levels within both acute and long-term care settings. In addition to disturbed sleep, other negative effects of high noise levels included decreased nutritional intake, changes in blood pressure and pulse rates, and feelings of increased stress and anxiety. The client with Alzheimer's disease is especially susceptible to these changes and needs to have as much undisturbed sleep at night as possible. Fatigue increases the client's confusion and behavioral manifestations, such as agitation and aggressiveness.

The nurse also assesses the client's assigned room for pictures on the wall that could be misinterpreted as people or animals that could harm the client. An abstract painting or wallpaper might look like a fire or an explosion and might scare the client. The nurse checks all areas of the room for adequate nonglare lighting and potentially frightening shadows.

Providing Consistency. The nurse plans ways to provide consistency for the client. For example, objects such as furniture, a hairbrush, and eyeglasses should be kept in the same place. A daily routine is established, posted in view of the client, and followed as much as possible. In some settings, each room has a communication board on which scheduled activities and other data to promote orientation are listed such as day of the week, month, and year. Pictures of people familiar to the client can be placed on this board.

Orientation and Validation Therapy. The nurse explains changes in routine before the occurrence and again immediately before they take place. Clocks and single-date calendars also help the client maintain day-to-day orientation to the environment in the early stages of the disease process. For the client with early disease, reality orientation is usually appropriate. Family members and health care professionals should frequently reorient the client to the environment.

For the client in the later stages of Alzheimer's disease, reality orientation is usually ineffective and often increases agitation. The health care team uses validation therapy for the client with moderate or severe Alzheimer's disease. Using validation therapy, the staff member recognizes and acknowledges the client's feelings and concerns. For example, rather than argue with the client who insists that he or she has not had breakfast (even though the nurse saw the client eat it), the nurse obtains juice, toast, or other food item for the client.

Promoting Independence in Activities of Daily Living. Altered thought processes affect the client's ability to perform activities of daily living (ADLs). The nurse allows the client to perform as much self-care as possible. The nurse also teaches the family or significant other that every effort should be made to allow the client to maintain independence in daily living skills as long as possible. For example, in the home setting, complete clothing outfits that can be easily removed and put on (e.g., shirt, slacks, underwear, and socks) can be placed on a single hanger and the client selects from these groupings. When possible, the client should participate in meal preparation, grocery shopping, and other household routines.

The nurse may need to consult with the occupational therapist for a complete evaluation and assistance in helping the client become more independent. Adaptive devices, such as grab bars in the bathtub or shower area, elevated commode, and adapted eating utensils, may enable the client to maintain independence in grooming, toileting, and feeding.

Promoting Bowel and Bladder Continence. The client may remain continent of bowel and bladder for long periods if taken to the bathroom or given a bedpan or urinal every 2 hours or more often during the day and possibly less frequently at night. The staff encourages the client to drink adequate fluids to promote optimum voiding. A client may refuse to drink enough fluids because of a fear of incontinence. The staff assures the client that he or she will be toileted on a regular schedule to prevent incontinent episodes.

When clients with Alzheimer's disease are in the hospital or other unfamiliar place, they may get out of bed unassisted during the night and fall while trying to locate

the bathroom. In some institutions, the side rails on beds are required to be up for all clients older than 60 or 65. If the client climbs over the side rail and falls, the injury is likely to be worse than if the bed had been left in the lowest position and the side rail left down (preferably the lower rail in a split rail system). The nurse maintains an unobstructed path between the bed and bathroom at all times. For clients who are too weak to walk to the bathroom, a bedside commode may be used.

Some clients may void in inappropriate places, such as the sink or wastepaper basket. As a reminder of where they should toilet, the nurse may place a picture of the commode on the bathroom door. Depending on written signs for identification is useless because most clients lose their ability to read as the disease progresses.

Assisting with Facial Recognition. As the disease progresses, the client may experience prosopagnosia (an inability to recognize oneself and other familiar faces). The nurse encourages the family to provide the client with pictures of family members and close friends that are labeled with the person's name on the picture. Additionally, the nurse advises the family to reminisce with the client about pleasant experiences from the past. The nurse may also conduct reminiscence therapy while assisting the client with ADLs or performing a treatment or assessment. Referring the client to a personal item in the room may help the client begin to talk about its meaning in the present and in the past.

It is not unusual for the client to talk to his or her image in the mirror. This behavior should be allowed as long as it is not harmful. If the client becomes frightened by the mirror image, the nurse covers the mirror. In some health care settings, a picture of the client is placed on the room door to help with facial recognition and to help the client locate his or her room. Having a picture of the client also helps the staff locate the client in case of elopement (running away).

Promoting Communication. The nurse assists the client with communication problems and nonlistening behaviors by attracting the client's attention before conversing with the intervention known as *redirection.* The environment should be as free of distractions as possible. The nurse speaks directly to the client in a slow and distinct manner. Sentences should be clear and short. The client is asked to perform one task at a time, and sufficient time must be allowed for completion. It may be necessary to break each task down into many small steps.

As the client's disease progresses, the client is unable to perform tasks when asked. The nurse shows the client what needs to be done or provides the cues to remind the client how to perform the task. For example, if the nurse wishes to clean the client's dentures but the client refuses to remove them from the mouth, the nurse leaves a denture cup, which may trigger the client's memory about the need to remove and clean dentures. When possible, the nurse explains and demonstrates the task that the client is asked to perform.

Drug Therapy. A variety of drugs are being used or are under investigation to improve the client's cognitive abilities in mild disease. To date most have limited effectiveness, and few have shown any long-term improvement in the client's cognitive or functional abilities. Ergoloid mesylate (Hydergine) may be used in the early stages of the disease. Although cognitive abilities, ability to perform ADLs, and mood usually improve for a short period of time, side effects, such as orthostatic hypotension and dizziness, frequently occur.

Several cholinergic drugs are under investigation in the hope that they might improve the client's memory. To date, no improvement has been seen in clients receiving acetylcholine (ACh) precursors. Tetrahydroaminoacridine (THA) (tacrine), doneprezil hydrochloride (Aricept), and physostigmine salicylate (Antilirium) are ACh esterase inhibitors that have improved cognitive function in some clients for short periods of time. Tacrine (Cognex) and Aricept are used in clients with early- to middle-stage Alzheimer's disease. The use of tacrine may be limited because of side effects, especially liver damage, when given for long periods. Liver function studies are frequently performed. Clients may also experience gastrointestinal (GI) disturbances and, sometimes, worsening confusion. Aricept has fewer side effects and seems to be as effective as tacrine. When these drugs are effective, clients may experience an improved cognitive function and self-care ability for variable periods of time.

Some clients with Alzheimer's disease experience depression, and they may be treated with fluvoxamine (Lurox), sertraline (Zoloft), desipramine (Norpramin), maprotiline (Ludiomil), or trazodone (Desyrel). Antidepressants such as amitriptyline (Elavil, Levate♣) should not be used because of their anticholinergic effect. The nurse observes for the therapeutic effects of these medications and reports side effects, such as increased delirium, drowsiness, orthostatic hypotension, and urinary retention, to the health care provider as soon as possible.

Psychotropic drugs, also called antipsychotic and neuroleptic drugs, should be reserved for clients with emotional and psychiatric disorders that sometimes accompany dementia, such as hallucinations and delusions. In clinical practice, however, the nurse may find that these drugs are sometimes inappropriately used for agitation, combativeness, or restlessness.

Psychotropic drugs are considered chemical restraints because they decrease mobility and clients' ability to care for themselves. Therefore, most geriatricians recommend that these medications be used as a last resort and with caution for a specific emotional or psychiatric behavior in low doses, because most clients with dementia are elderly (see Chap. 6). The specific drug prescribed depends on side effects, the condition of the client, and anticipated outcomes. For example, some geriatricians favor thioridazine (Mellaril, Novoridazine♣) over haloperidol (Haldol, Peridol♣), a commonly prescribed medication for the elderly, because of haloperidol's potency and tendency to be overprescribed. The nurse observes for drug side effects, including increased confusion and extrapyramidal symptoms (e.g., rigidity, tremors), drooling, constipation, and urinary retention, and promptly reports these to the physician.

Complementary Therapies. A number of alternative or complementary therapies are being researched that may prevent Alzheimer's disease, retard its occurrence, or slow its progression in the elderly. Examples of these therapies include vitamin E, ibuprofen, and nicotine patches.

Risk for Injury

Planning: Expected Outcomes. The outcomes are that the client is expected to remain free from physical harm and not injure anyone else.

Interventions. Many clients with Alzheimer's disease tend to wander and may easily become lost. In later stages of the disease, some clients may become severely agitated and physically or verbally abusive to others.

Coping with Restlessness and Wandering. The nurse teaches the home caregiver that the client should always wear an identification badge or bracelet. The nurse checks the client frequently and places the client in a room that can be monitored easily. The room may need to be close to the nurse's station (if the noise level in the nurses' station can be managed) and away from exits and stairs. Some health care agencies place large stop signs or red tape on the floor in front of exits. Others have installed alarm systems to indicate when a client is opening the door.

Restlessness may be decreased if the client is taken for frequent walks. If the client begins to wander, the nurse redirects the client and tries to determine where the client is trying to go. For example, if the client insists on going shopping for clothes, the nurse or other caregiver might redirect the client to his or her closet to select clothing that will not be recognized as his or her own. This type of activity can be repeated a number of times because the client has lost short-term memory.

In any setting, clients should be kept busy with structured activities. In a health care agency, an activity or recreational therapist may work with clients as a group or individually to determine the type of activity that is appropriate for the stage of the disease. Puzzles, board games, and art activities are often appropriate. Music and art therapy are becoming very popular in acute and long-term care for clients with dementia (see Research Applications for Nursing).

Physical restraints, such as protective vests and geri-chairs with lap boards, should be used only as a last resort because they often increase the restlessness and cause agitation. Federal regulations in long-term care facilities in the United States mandate that all residents have the right to be free of both physical and chemical restraints.

Ensuring Safety. Clients with Alzheimer's disease may become injured because they cannot recognize objects or situations as harmful. All potentially dangerous objects (e.g., knives, needles, and cleaning solutions) are removed or secured. Clients are often unaware that their driving ability is impaired and usually want to continue this activity even if their driver's license is suspended secondary to the disease. Automobile keys must be secured and the client appropriately informed.

Late in the disease process, the client may experience seizure activity. The nurse institutes seizure precautions

➤ Research Applications for Nursing

Does Music Help Decrease Agitation in Elderly Clients with Dementia?

Ragneskog, H., Kihlgren, M., Karlsson, I., & Norberg, A. (1996). Dinner music for demented patients: Analysis of video-recorded observations. Clinical Nursing Research, 5(3), 262–277.

In a nursing home, demented clients were exposed to selections of dinner music during three periods of 2 weeks. The reactions of five clients were recorded on video and analyzed. All of the clients ate their meals more quietly and calmly. At least one client fed herself more than usual, and all clients spent more time enjoying their meal when music was played.

Critique. This pilot study was an attempt to show that distraction and calming music can decrease restlessness and agitation in clients experiencing dementia. The convenience sample was extremely small, and the study needs to be replicated.

Possible Nursing Implications. Music is a simple, yet effective nursing intervention for clients who are restless and agitated. Clients who are less agitated tend to eat better, thus improving nutritional status. This type of intervention is preferred over drug therapy, which is typically used for agitated clients.

and takes appropriate action during a seizure episode (see prior discussion of Epilepsy).

Minimizing Agitation. In the event of agitated behavior, the nurse talks calmly and softly and attempts to redirect the client to a more positive behavior or activity. If the client remains agitated, the nurse ensures the client's safety and leaves the room after explaining that he or she will return later. Frequent visual checks must be done during this time.

If the client is connected to any type of tubing or other device, he or she may try to disconnect it or pull it out. These devices should be used sparingly in the client with dementia. If intravenous (IV) access, for example, is needed, the nurse places the catheter or cannula in an area that the client cannot easily see. Some health care agencies recommend covering the site with an elastic bandage, although this prevents quick visual inspection of the IV site.

Another way to manage this problem is to provide a diversion. For example, if the client is doing an activity or holding an item such as a stuffed animal or doll, he or she might be less likely to pay attention to medical devices. The nurse asks the family or significant other to provide the client's favorite keepsake, which may help to divert the client's attention. Some nursing units include items used for this purpose.

Ineffective Family Coping

Planning: Expected Outcomes. The desired outcome is that the family is expected to obtain appropriate support services to enable them to adjust and cope with the client's physical and mental problems.

Interventions. The client with Alzheimer's disease requires continual, 24-hour supervision. Severe cognitive changes leave the client unable to manage finances, property, and personal care. The nurse advises the family to seek legal counsel regarding the client's competency and the need to obtain guardianship or durable medical power of attorney. The family can be referred to the local Alzheimer's disease support group for literature and information concerning the disease and related problems. The nurse establishes a supportive environment for family members and encourages them to express their feelings to other family members. Family members are encouraged to maintain their own social network and obtain respite from care of the client. The nurse can help the family and significant others to cope with the long-term nature of this disease by providing a list of resources readily available in the community.

Sleep Pattern Disturbance

Planning: Expected Outcomes. The expected outcome is that the client will sleep through the night.

Interventions. The client with Alzheimer's disease often has difficulty sleeping at night but tends to nap frequently during the day. One way to establish the usual day-night pattern is to keep the client very active during the day. A daily routine that consists of a balance between passive activities and those requiring more strenuous exercise, such as walking or stretching activities, usually facilitates sleep at night. The client may want to take a nap in the late afternoon, but this should be discouraged if possible. In the last stage of the disease, the client may sleep often during the day and night.

To facilitate sleep, a pre-bedtime ritual is established. The routine usually consists of personal hygiene activities (e.g., bathing, toileting, brushing teeth) and environmental control measures to reduce noise and eliminate distractions. A back rub or small snack may help the client prepare for sleep.

The nurse adjusts the client's treatment and medication schedule to provide for uninterrupted sleep. If more conventional measures fail to induce sleep, the physician may prescribe a low dose of medication, such as chloral hydrate (Novochlorhydrate).

➤ Continuing Care

➤ Home Care Management

Alzheimer's disease is a chronic progressive condition that eventually leaves the client completely disoriented and totally dependent on others for all aspects of care. In the early stages, the client may be cared for at home with little need for outside interventions. Whenever possible, the client and family should be assigned to a case manager, who can assess their needs for health care resources and facilitate appropriate placement throughout the continuum of care.

The client usually begins to withdraw from friends and social events as memory impairments and personality and

Chart 44–13

Education Guide: Reducing Caregiver Stress

Maintain realistic expectations for the person with Alzheimer's disease.

- Take each day one at a time.
- Try to find the positive aspects of each incident or situation.
- Use humor with the person who has Alzheimer's disease.
- Set aside time each day for rest or recreation away from the client, if possible.
- Seek respite care periodically for longer periods of time.
- Use the resources of the Alzheimer's Association, including attending local support group meetings.
- Explore alternative care settings early in the disease process for possible use later.
- Establish advance directives with the Alzheimer's client early in the disease process.

behavior changes become more apparent. This increases the family's responsibilities to minimize the impact of social isolation and decreased activity. The family may begin to decrease their own social activities as the demands of the client's care take more of their time. The nurse should emphasize to the family the importance of maintaining their own social contacts and leisure activities. Many family members experience caregiver stress, which affects their physical, mental, and emotional health. Chart 44–13 lists strategies for reducing caregiver stress. (Chapter 8 also describes interventions for stress management and coping that the nurse can teach the family.)

It is now possible in most areas of the United States for the family to arrange respite care. The client may be placed in a respite facility for the weekend or for several weeks to give the family a rest from the constant care demands of the client. The family may also be able to obtain respite care in the home through a home care agency or the Alzheimer's Association. The nurse stresses that respite care is for a short period of time; it is not a permanent placement. Some health care agencies have opened adult day care centers or specialty units for clients with Alzheimer's disease. In the day care center, clients spend all or part of the day at the facility and participate in activities as their condition permits. Although these centers are usually open only on weekdays, this arrangement allows the caregiver to work or participate in other activities.

The nurse teaches the family to be prepared in the event that the client becomes restless, agitated, abusive, or combative. In addition, the family can learn how to use reality orientation or validation therapy, depending on the stage of the disease.

▶ Health Teaching

Usually the client with Alzheimer's disease is cared for in the home until late in the disease process. Because health insurance coverage in the United States and family finances are usually insufficient to cover the services of a private duty nurse or home care aide, the care is typically provided by family members. The client care plan developed by the nurse or case manager, in conjunction with the family, must be reasonable and realistic for the family to implement.

The nurse teaches the family how to assist the client with bathing, dressing, toileting, and other self-care activities. The nurse and the occupational therapist collaborate to teach the family and the client how to use adaptive equipment, such as a brace, a sling, a cane, or modified eating utensils. The client may have difficulty chewing, swallowing, or tasting foods and may not be able to eat without assistance. The nurse, the family, and the dietitian should develop a diet plan to maximize the client's nutritional intake. In the late stage of Alzheimer's disease, the client's intake often decreases and the client loses weight. (Chapter 64 discusses the interventions for preventing or managing undernutrition.)

The nurse also teaches the family what to do in the event of a seizure and how to protect the client from injury. The family is instructed to notify the physician if the seizure is prolonged or if the client's seizure pattern changes.

Drug Therapy

The nurse explains the name, time, and route of administration; the dosage; and the side effects of all medications to the family or other caregiver. The family is instructed to check with the client's physician before using any over-the-counter medications because they may interact with prescribed medication.

The nurse emphasizes the need for the client to have an established exercise program to maintain mobility as long as possible as well as to prevent complications of immobility. The nurse collaborates with the family and the physical therapist (PT) to develop an individualized exercise program. The PT may continue to work with the client at home until goals are achieved.

Safety

The nurse instructs the family or other caregiver to take special precautions to maintain the client safely at home. The environment must be uncluttered, consistent, and structured. All hazardous items (e.g., cleaning fluids, power tools, insect spray) are removed or secured. All electrical sockets not in use should be covered with safety plugs. Hand rails and grab bars should be installed in the bathroom; hand rails should be along all stairways and a guardrail placed around porches or open stairwells. Because the client may have a tendency to wander, especially at night, the family may want to install alarms to all outside doors, basement, and the client's bedroom. All outside and basement doors should have dead-bolt locks to prevent the client from going outside un-supervised. The temperature of the water heater should be adjusted to prevent accidental burns. Night-lights should be used in the client's bedroom, hallway, and bathroom.

 Health Care Resources

When the client can no longer be cared for at home, referral to a long-term care (LTC) facility may be needed. Early in the course of the disease, the nurse should advise the family that placement may be needed in the late stages of the disease. This allows the family to begin the search process for an appropriate facility before a crisis develops and immediate placement is needed. A number of LTC facilities specialize in the care of clients with Alzheimer's disease and other dementias. These units generally have a high staff-client ratio and are architecturally designed to meet the special needs of this type of client. The national office of the Alzheimer's Association in the United States has a publication that outlines criteria for a dementia unit.

All families should be referred to their local chapter of the Alzheimer's Disease and Related Disorders Association (often called the Alzheimer's Association). This organization provides information and support services to clients and their families, including seminars, audiovisual aids, and publications.

 Evaluation

On the basis of the identified nursing diagnoses and collaborative problems, the nurse evaluates the care of client with Alzheimer's disease. Outcomes include that the client is expected to

- Remain at home for as long as possible
- Maintain independence in activities of daily living (ADLs) and self-care skills as long as possible
- Remain free of injury from falls, seizure activity, and environmental hazards

HUNTINGTON'S DISEASE

Overview

Huntington's disease (HD), also called Huntington's chorea, is a hereditary disorder transmitted as an autosomal dominant trait at the time of conception. The causative gene is located on chromosome number 4. The offspring of a parent with the disease has a 50% chance of eventually manifesting the disease. In the United States, it is estimated that 25,000 people have the disease, and another 20,000 to 50,000 are thought to carry the gene (Hickey, 1996). Men and women are equally affected, and symptoms begin between 30 and 50 years of age. The clinical onset of HD is gradual. The two main symptoms of the disease are progressive mental status changes, lead-ing to dementia, and choreiform movements (rapid, jerky movements) in the limbs, trunk, and facial muscles. Dementia is related to the destruction of neurons within the cerebral cortex; it may also be associated with excessive amounts of dopamine found within the cerebral cortex and limbic systems of those affected.

Two structures within the basal ganglia are involved in the development of HD: the caudate nucleus and the putamen. Both structures have close connections to the cerebral cortex and are closely associated with neurotransmitters. Neurotransmitters are secreted at the synapse, or junction, of one neuron with another, and it is through their specific excitation or inhibition of neurons that fine, controlled, integrated motor activity occurs.

In the presence of HD, there is a decrease in the amount of γ-aminobutyric acid (GABA) and acetylcholine, both excitatory neurotransmitters. Dopamine is not affected. This shift in balance between dopamine, an inhibitory neurotransmitter, and GABA at the synapse leads to uninhibited motor activity. The result is brisk, jerky, purposeless movements, particularly of the hands, face, tongue, and legs, which the client is unable to stop.

The diagnosis of HD is made on the basis of a family history of the disease, clinical assessment, and laboratory findings. Clinical manifestations include chorea, poor balance, hesitant or explosive speech, dysphagia, impaired respiration, and bowel and bladder incontinence. Mental status changes include decreased attention span, poor judgment, memory loss, personality changes, and dementia (later in the disease process).

TRANSCULTURAL CONSIDERATIONS

Huntington's disease is most prevalent in people of western European ancestry (Paulus-Thomas et al., 1997).

Collaborative Management

There is no known cure or treatment of clients with HD. The only way to prevent transmission of the gene is for those affected to refrain from having children. Genetic counseling is important for children of clients with the disease. It is now possible to test people at risk for the disease to determine whether or not the gene is present on chromosome 4. However, the test is still under investigation, and large-scale studies have not been completed. Therefore, the results of testing may be subject to error, although this risk has been greatly reduced. Before the testing procedure is undertaken, counseling is necessary to ensure that the client has voluntarily decided in favor of testing and is not being pressured by family or friends. In addition, counseling helps to determine whether the benefits of knowing the results outweigh the risks of a positive result (e.g., depression or suicide).

Management is symptomatic. Some symptoms can be managed with medications, but there is no cure. The client's status deteriorates, and death occurs from complications of immobility, such as pneumonia, sepsis, or heart disease, within 15 years of the onset of symptoms.

CASE STUDY for the Client with Central Nervous System Disorders

■ An elderly client was recently discharged from the hospital for evaluation of seizure activity. His history reveals that he has late-stage Alzheimer's disease, Parkinson's disease, hypertension, and type II diabetes mellitus, which is controlled by diet. He lives at home, where his wife and daughter take care of him. His discharge medications include phenytoin (Dilantin), 100 mg BID; hydrochlorothiazide (Hydro-DIURIL), 50 mg QD; Sinemet, 25/100 TID; and haloperidol (Haldol), 1 mg QN. The client has been referred for home care nursing follow-up.

QUESTIONS:

1. On the initial home visit by the nurse, what assessments should be done?
2. The wife and daughter need teaching about his antiepileptic medication. What teaching should be included?
3. During the initial home visit, the client experienced a generalized seizure. What action should the nurse take?

SELECTED BIBLIOGRAPHY

Abudi, S., Bar-Tal, Y., Ziv, L., & Fish, M. (1997). Parkinson's disease symptoms—Patient's perspective. *Journal of Advanced Nursing, 25*(1), 54–59.

Barrett, E. (1996). Primary care for women. Assessment and management of headache. *Journal of Nurse Midwifery, 41*(2), 117–124.

Barrett, J. J. (1997). Knowledge about Alzheimer's disease among primary care physicians, psychologists, nurses and social workers. *Alzheimer's Disease Association, 11*(2), 99–106.

Becker, W. J., Riess, C. M., & Hoag, J. (1996). Effectiveness of subcutaneous dihydroergotamine by home injection for migraine. *Headache, 36*(3), 144–148.

Ben-Menachem, R. (1994). Vagus nerve stimulation and treatment of partial seizures: A controlled study of the effects on seizures. *Epilepsia, 35*(3), 637–643.

Beydoun, A., Sacellares, J. C., & Shu, V. (1997). Safety and efficacy of divalproex sodium monotherapy in epilepsy. *Neurology, 48*(1), 182–189.

Blacker, D., et al. (1997). Apo E-4 and the age of onset of Alzheimer's disease. *Neurology, 48*(1), 139–141.

Callanan, M. (1996) Sexual assessment and intervention for people with epilepsy. *Clinical Nursing Practice in Epilepsy, 3*(1), 7–9.

Chiocca, E. M. (1995). Meningococcal meningitis. *American Journal of Nursing, 95*(5), 25.

Cleeland, E. A., & Davis, L. L. (1997). Depression in elders with dementia: Implications for home healthcare practice. *Home Healthcare Nurse, 15*(11), 780–787.

Comair, Y. C. (1995). Functional hemispherectomy. *Journal of Neurosurgery, 1*, 52–57.

Crawford, P., et al. (1996). Generic prescribing for epilepsy. Is it safe? *Seizure, 5*(1), 1–5.

Cysyk, B. J. (1996). A deep vein thrombosis prevention program for patients undergoing long term invasive epilepsy monitoring. *Journal of Neuroscience Nursing, 28*(5), 298–304.

Dewar, S., Passano, E., Itzhak, F., & Engel J. (1996). Intracranial electrode monitoring for seizure localization: Indications, methods and prevention of complications. *Journal of Neuroscience Nursing, 28*(5), 280–292.

Dorton, D. M. (1995). The care of the patient with Parkinson's disease. *Journal of Post Anesthesia Nursing, 10*(2), 102–106.

Fisher, J. H., Turnbull, T., Ulman, B., et al. (1995). Safety, tolerance, and pharmacokinetics of fosphenytoin (Cerebyx) versus Dilantin. *Neurology, 45*(Suppl. 4), A202.

*Folstein, M., Folstein, S., & McHugh, P. (1975). Mini-Mental State: A practical method for grading the cognitive state of patients for the clinician. *Journal of Psychiatric Research, 12*, 189–198.

Gilbert, M., Counsell, C. M., & Snively, C. (1996). Pallidotomy: A surgical intervention for control of Parkinson's disease. *Journal of Neuroscience Nursing, 28*(4), 215–221.

Goldensohn, E. S., Rausch, R., Cloyd, J. C., et al. (1996). *Epilepsy in the elderly: Distinctive considerations in diagnosis and treatment.* Advisory Board of the Epilepsy Foundation of America.

Hier, D. B. (1997). Alzheimer's disease. *Surgical Neurology, 47*(1), 84–85.

Heyman, A., Peterson, B., Fillenbaum, G., & Pieper, C. (1996). The Consortium to Establish a Registry for Alzheimer's Disease: Part XIV. Demographic and clinical predictors of survival in patients with Alzheimer's disease. *Neurology, 46*(3), 656–660.

Hickey, J. V. (1996). *The clinical practice of neurological and neurological nursing* (2nd ed.). Philadelphia: Lippincott-Raven.

Hollister, L., & Gruber, N. (1996). Drug treatment of Alzheimer's disease. Effects on caregiver burden and patient quality of life. *Drugs and Aging, 8*(1), 47–55.

Hyde, R. S. (1996). Home healthcare nurses knowledge of Alzheimer's disease. *Home Healthcare Nurse, 14*(5), 391–397.

Iacono, R. P. (1995). The results, indications, and physiology of posteroventral pallidotomy for patients with Parkinson's disease. *Neurosurgery, 36*(6), 1118–1125.

Jaffe, W. (1995). Homelessness and epilepsy: Overcoming the barriers to healthcare. *Clinical Nursing Practice in Epilepsy, 2*(2), 12–13.

Kennedy, D., & Barter, R. (1995). Client assessment tools: A means to enhance nurse-client-physician collaboration. *Journal of Neuroscience Nursing, 27*(5), 312–318.

Khachaturian, Z. S., & Radebaugh, T. S. (1996). *Alzheimer's disease cause(s), diagnosis, treatment and care.* New York: CPC Press.

Kovach, C. R. (1997). Preventing agitated behavior during bath time. *Geriatric Nurse, 18*(3), 112–114.

Long, L. (1996). Epilepsy: A review of seizure types, etiologies, diagnosis, treatment, and nursing implications. *Critical Care Nurse, 16*(4), 83–92.

Lovecchio, F., & Jacobson, S. (1997). Approach to generalized weakness and peripheral neuromuscular disease. *Emergency Medical Clinical North America, 8*(3), 605–623.

Marshall, J., Edwards, C., & Lambert, M. (1997). Administration of medicines by emergency nurse practitioners according to protocols in emergency departments. *Journal of Accident Emergency Medicine, 7*(4), 233–237.

McKurth, A., et al. (1997). Tolcapone improves motor function and reduces levodopa requirements in patient with Parkinson's disease experiencing motor fluctuations. *Neurology, 48*(1), 81–87.

McNew, C. D., Hunt, S., & Warner, L. S. (1997). How to help your patient with epilepsy. *Nursing97, 27*(9), 57–63.

Mitchell, S. L., Kiely, D. K., Kiel, D. P., & Lipsitz, L. A. (1996). The epidemiology, clinical characteristics and natural history of older nursing home residents with a diagnosis of Parkinson's disease. *Journal of American Geriatric Society, 44*(4), 294–399.

Montagna, P., et al. (1997). Male preponderance: Similar pathway to migraine. *Neurology, 48*(1), 113–118.

Neal, L. J. (1996a). The home care client with Alzheimer's disease: Part 1. Assessment tool for activities of daily living. *Home Healthcare Nurse, 14*(3), 175–178.

Neal, L. J. (1996b). The home care client with Alzheimer's disease: Part II. Interventions. *Home Healthcare Nurse, 14*(4), 265–267.

Nussbaum, E. (1996). Migraines. *American Journal of Nursing, 96*(10), 36–37.

Patil, A. A., Andrews, R., & Torkelson, R. (1995). Stereotactic volumetric radiofrequency lesions of intracranial structures for control of intractable seizures. *Stereotactic Functional Neurosurgery, 64*(5), 123–133.

Patil, A. A., Andrews, R., & Torkelson, R. (1997). Surgical treatment of intractable seizures with multilobar or bi-hemispheric seizure focus. *Surgical Neurology, 41*(1), 72–78.

Paulus-Thomas, J., Gross, M. E., & Thull, D. L. (1997). Huntington disease: The long and the short of it. *Genetics in Practice, 4*(1), 1–3.

Perry, J. A., & Olshansky, E. F. (1996). A family's coming to terms with Alzheimer's disease. *Western Journal of Nursing Research, 18*(1), 12–28.

Ragneskog, H., Kihlgren, M., Karlsson, I., & Norberg, A. (1996). Dinner music for demented patients: Analysis of video-recorded observations. *Clinical Nursing Research, 5*(3), 262–277.

Ryan, C. W. (1996). Evaluation of patients with chronic headache. *American Family Physician, 54*(3), 1051–1057.

Sacks, H. S. (1997). The botulism hazard. *Annals of Internal Medicine, 26*(11), 918–919.

Sanders, P. T. (1996). Safety in long term EEG/video monitoring. *Journal of Neuroscience Nursing, 28*(5), 305–313.

Scholtz, M. J. (1997). A new treatment option for trigeminal neuralgia. *RN, 60*(8), 70.

Shua-Haim, J. R. (1996). Alzheimer's syndrome not Alzheimer's disease. *Journal of the American Geriatric Society, 44*(1), 96–97.

Sierzant, T. (1996a). Dealing with memory impairments: A practical approach. *Clinical Nursing Practice in Epilepsy, 3*(4), 11–13.

Sierzant, T. (1996b). Surgical options for individuals with epilepsy: Opportunities for nursing interventions. *Clinical Nursing Practice in Epilepsy, 3*(2), 4–7.

Sloane, P. D., & Barrick, A. L. (1996). Improving long term care for persons with Alzheimer's disease. *Journal of American Geriatric Society, 44*(1), 91–92.

Tackenberg, J. N. (1996). Anatomic correlates of psychological events related to temporolimbic epilepsy. *Journal of Neuroscience Nursing, 28*(2), 73–81.

Toth, T., Papp, C., Nemeti, M., & Papp, Z. (1997). Questions and problems in direct predictive testing for Huntington's disease. *American Journal Medical Genetics, 71*(2), 238–239.

Trojanowski, J. et al. (1995). Relationship between plaques, tangles, and dystrophic process in Alzheimer's disease. *Neurobiology of Aging, 16*(3), 335–340.

Wallhagen, M. I., & Brod, M. (1997). Perceived control and well-being in Parkinson's disease. *Western Journal of Nursing Research, 19*(11), 11–31.

Wolters, E. C., & Msarleen, H. J. (1996). International double blind study of Sinemet CR and standard Sinemet in 170 patients with fluctuating Parkinson's disease. *Journal of Neurology, 243*, 235–240.

Yen, P. K. (1997). Weight loss resulting from Alzheimer's disease. *Geriatric Nurse, 18*(3), 132–133.

Youdim, B. H., & Riederer, P. (1997). Understanding Parkinson's disease. *Scientific American Medicine, 39*(1), 52–59.

U.S. Newswire. (1997, July 17). Epilepsy Foundation welcomes approval of new therapy device, p. 24.

SUGGESTED READINGS

Cleeland, E. A., & Davis, L. L. (1997). Depression in elders with dementia: Implications for home healthcare practice. *Home Healthcare Nurse, 15*(11), 780–787.

This excellent article provides practice tips on how to assess depression in the elderly, including a comparison of five tools commonly used to measure depressive symptoms. Home care nursing interventions are described using a case study approach. A care plan for the case and general guidelines for counseling caregivers of elders with dementia and depression are delineated.

Khachaturian, Z. S., & Radebaugh, T. S. (1996). *Alzheimer's disease cause(s), diagnosis, treatment and care.* New York: CPC Press.

This book is an excellent resource for professionals who care for clients with Alzheimer's disease. The authors have included comprehensive coverage using an interdisciplinary approach to care.

McNew, C. D., Hunt, S., & Warner, L. S. (1997). How to help your patient with epilepsy. *Nursing97, 27*(9), 57–63.

This article presents a comprehensive overview of seizures, including assessment and documentation of seizure activity, drug therapy for epilepsy, and interventions for status epilepticus. A continuing education quiz is offered at the end of the article.

INTERVENTIONS FOR CLIENTS WITH PROBLEMS OF THE CENTRAL NERVOUS SYSTEM: THE SPINAL CORD

Problems of the spinal cord range may be acute or chronic, short term or long term. Some problems require surgery, whereas others require extensive rehabilitation. The spinal cord neurons do not regenerate, and damage to neuronal fibers is permanent.

BACK PAIN

Overview

Back pain is one of the most common reasons for visiting a health care provider. Back problems are costly in terms of time lost from work and medical treatment and are the most frequent cause of disability for persons younger than 45 years. About 1% of the U.S. population is chronically disabled at any given time as a result of back problems. The cervical (upper back) vertebrae and lumbosacral (lower back) vertebrae are most commonly affected. It is estimated that the annual societal cost of back problems ranges from $20 to $50 billion (Bigos et al., 1994a,b).

Pathophysiology

Cervical Back Pain

Cervical involvement usually results from a herniation of the nucleus pulposus in an intervertebral disk (also spelled disc). As seen in Figure 45–1, the herniation occurs laterally where the annulus fibrosus is weakest and the posterior longitudinal ligament is thinned. The result is spinal nerve root compression, with subsequent motor and sensory manifestations, typically in the neck and down the affected arm. The disk between the fifth and sixth cervical vertebrae (C5–6) is affected most often.

If the disk does not rupture, nerve compression may be caused by osteophyte (bony outgrowth) formation from degenerative joint disease. The osteophyte presses on the intervertebral foramen, which results in a narrowing of the disk. A client with nerve compression may experience either continuous or intermittent chronic pain.

Cervical pain—acute or chronic—may also occur from muscle strain or ligament sprain. If these injuries occur in

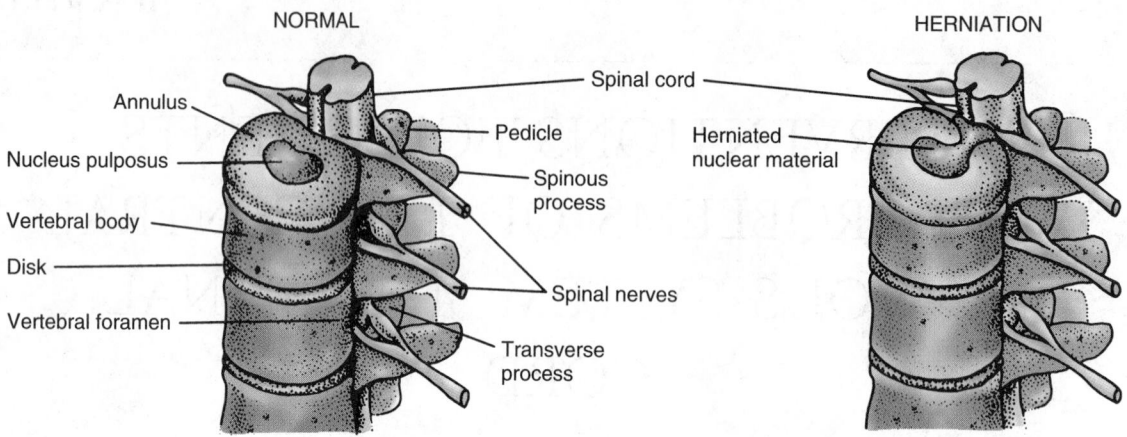

Figure 45-1. Herniation of the nucleus pulposus.

the workplace, the client may be eligible for workers' compensation benefits.

Lumbosacral Back Pain

Lumbosacral back pain, more often referred to as low back pain (LBP), is more common than cervical pain. Acute pain is caused by muscle strain or spasm, ligament sprain, disk injury from hyperflexion or degeneration, or herniation of the nucleus pulposus from the center of the disk. Herniated disks occur most often between the fourth and fifth lumbar vertebrae (L4-L5) but may occur at other levels. A herniated nucleus pulposus in the lumbosacral area can press on the adjacent spinal nerve (usually the sciatic nerve), causing severe, burning, or stabbing pain down into the leg or foot. The specific area of pain depends on the level of herniation.

Muscle spasms of the affected leg may also occur. The pain is usually aggravated by sneezing, coughing, or straining. If LBP continues for 3 months or if repeated episodes of pain occur, the client has chronic back pain.

Etiology

Acute back pain usually results from trauma. The client typically hyperflexes or twists the back during a vehicular accident, or the injury occurs when the client lifts a heavy object. Obesity places increased stress on back muscles and typically contributes to the occurrence or the severity of back pain. Congenital spinal conditions and scoliosis can also lead to back discomfort.

ELDERLY CONSIDERATIONS

For elderly clients, the cause of back pain is usually degenerative joint disease, a type of arthritis that is seen with aging. Cervical pain is common in clients with advanced rheumatoid arthritis who experience cervical disk subluxation (dislocation), most often at the C1-C2 level. Other factors contributing to back pain in the elderly are presented in Chart 45-1.

WOMEN'S HEALTH CONSIDERATIONS

Chronic back pain in women may result from having poor posture or from wearing high-heeled shoes. Excessively high heels cause the body to compensate to maintain balance; the lower back becomes more lordotic, which strains the back muscles.

Many of the problems related to acute back pain can be prevented by recognition of the causes of back pain (see earlier) and appropriate action. For example, good posture, proper lifting techniques, and exercise can significantly decrease the incidence of low back pain. Chart 45-2 summarizes information on the prevention of low back pain.

Collaborative Management

 Assessment

➤ *Physical Assessment/Clinical Manifestations*

The nurse assesses the client's posture and gait. Some clients have so much pain that they walk in a stiff, flexed state, or they may be unable to bend at all. If a client has low back pain, the nurse may note a limp, which may indicate sciatic nerve impairment. Walking on heels or toes often causes severe pain in the affected leg, the back, or both.

The nurse inspects the back for vertebral alignment and swelling caused by muscle spasm. Local muscle spasms are common in clients with back pain, and muscle spasms in the affected extremity are not uncommon. It is thought that a compressed nerve becomes inflamed and irritates adjacent muscle tissue. Clients complain of stabbing, continuous pain in the muscle close to the affected disk. In clients with cervical injury, pain radiates down one arm; in clients with lumbosacral involvement, pain radiates down the posterior leg. The pain usually does not extend the entire length of the limb; clients with low back pain report sharp, burning posterior thigh or calf pain. They may also report the same type of pain in the middle of one buttock.

Chart 45-1

Focus on the Elderly: Factors Contributing to Low Back Pain

- Changes in support structures
  - Spinal stenosis
  - Hypertrophy of the intraspinal ligaments
  - Arthritis
- Changes in vertebral support
  - Vertebral malalignment
    - Scoliosis
    - Lordosis
- Vascular changes
  - Diminished blood supply to the spinal cord or cauda equina caused by arteriosclerosis
  - Blood dyscrasias
- Intervertebral disk degeneration

The nurse palpates the back and the involved extremity for tenderness, which is frequently present. The nurse assesses for sensory changes by asking whether there is paresthesia or numbness in the involved limb. Both extremities should be checked for sensation by using a pin or paper clip and a cotton ball for comparison of light and deep touch. The client may feel sensations in both limbs but may experience a stronger sensation in the unaffected side. The client with a severe case may lose both bowel and bladder control from sacral nerve involvement.

If the sciatic nerve is compressed, the client reports severe pain when raising a straight leg. To complete the neurologic assessment, the nurse evaluates muscle tone and strength. In severe, chronic conditions, muscles in the extremity or in the back atrophy. The client has difficulty with movement, and certain movements elicit more pain than others. The client with cervical pain may lose handgrip strength and may be unable to carry as much weight as before the injury.

► Diagnostic Assessment

The client's evaluation begins with flat plate x-rays with anterior, posterior, and lateral views. The health care provider frequently orders computed tomography (CT) or magnetic resonance imaging (MRI), done with or without contrast media enhancement, to visualize the herniated disk. Less often, the caregiver may order a myelogram, which is an invasive procedure that may or may not detect the problem.

Electrodiagnostic studies such as electromyography (EMG), nerve conduction studies, somatosensory evoked potentials (SSEP), and motor evoked potentials (MEP) may help differentiate motor neuron diseases, peripheral neuropathies, peripheral nerve entrapment, and radiculopathies. These are especially useful in chronic diseases because it takes at least 3 weeks for pathologic changes to produce symptoms. Chapter 43 describes these tests in more detail.

 Interventions

Management of clients with back pain varies with the severity and the chronicity of the problem. Most clients with acute LBP need only a short-term treatment regimen. The client, family members, and the nurse can become frustrated if treatment measures are ineffective. The health care provider initially implements conservative measures, but if these are unsuccessful, surgery may be indicated.

Nonsurgical Management. Nonsurgical management of back pain may include rest and proper positioning, exercise, anti-inflammatory analgesics, heat or ice therapy, and other pain relief measures and preventive measures in the work setting.

Rest and Positioning. The basic treatment of acute low back pain is typically 1 to 2 days of rest. The Agency for Health Care Policy and Research (AHCPR) Guidelines (Bigos et al., 1994a,b) recommend no longer than 4 days of bed rest, because the side effects of prolonged bed rest may be worse that a gradual return to usual activity. The Williams position is typically more comfortable and therapeutic for the client with low back pain. In this position, the client lies in the semi-Fowler's position and flexes the knees to relax the muscles of the lower back and to relieve pressure on the spinal nerve root.

A firm mattress or a back board placed under a soft mattress, provides back support. A flat position is particularly helpful for the client with a muscle injury. For a client with a herniated disk causing spinal nerve root compression in the lumbar spine, a flat position may aggravate the pain. The client usually gains pain relief from reclining or sleeping in the Williams position (just described).

Exercise. Exercises are used to strengthen the back, relieve pressure on compressed nerves, and protect the

Chart 45-2

Health Promotion Guide: Prevention of Low Back Pain

- Use proper body mechanics, with specific attention to bending, lifting, and sitting.
- Assess the need for assistance with your household chores or other activities.
- Participate in a regular exercise program, especially one that promotes back strengthening, such as swimming and walking.
- Do not wear high-heeled shoes.
- Use good posture when sitting, standing, or walking.
- Avoid prolonged sitting or standing. Use a foot stool to lessen back strain.
- Keep weight within 10% of ideal body weight. Ensure adequate calcium intake.
- Stop smoking. If you are not able to stop, cut down on the number of cigarettes or decrease the use of other forms of tobacco.

back from reinjury. A variety of exercise programs are available to treat low back pain. Isometric exercises are generally the most effective (Barker, 1994).

The nurse collaborates with the physical therapist (PT) to develop an individualized exercise program. The type of exercises prescribed depends on the location and nature of the injury and the type of pain. The client does not begin exercises until acute pain is reduced by other means. Several specific exercises for low back pain are provided in Chart 45–3.

Drug Therapy. The health care provider often prescribes muscle relaxants, such as cyclobenzaprine hydrochloride (Flexeril), and nonsteroidal anti-inflammatory drugs, such as aspirin and ibuprofen (Motrin, Amersol✦). Opioid analgesics are no more effective than the nonsteroidal analgesics and should be avoided if at all possible. If they must be used, the course of therapy should be short (Bigos et al., 1994a,b). An epidural or local steroid injection may also be helpful. (Chapter 9 describes drug therapy and nursing implications for the care of clients in acute or chronic pain in detail.)

Heat and Ice Therapy. Some clients with back pain experience temporary relief from the application of heat. Heat increases blood flow to the affected area and promotes healing of injured nerves. The nurse or therapist recommends moist heat in the form of heat packs or hot towels for 20 to 30 minutes at least four times a day. Hot showers or baths are also often beneficial. The physical therapist may administer deep heat therapy, such as ultrasound treatments and diathermy. The therapist and nurse monitor the effects of heat treatment by assessing the client's skin condition and the relief of pain.

Some clients prefer ice instead of heat to relieve pain. Ice therapy using ice packs or ice massage may be applied over the affected area for 10 to 15 minutes every 1 to 2 hours. For some clients, a course of alternating ice and heat applications may be effective.

Diet Therapy. Weight control frequently helps to reduce chronic back pain by decreasing the work on the vertebrae necessitated by excess weight. If the client's weight exceeds the ideal by more than 10%, caloric restriction is necessary.

Therefore, health care providers must be sensitive when reinforcing the need for clients to lose weight to prevent or to lessen chronic back pain. The nurse collaborates with the dietitian to plan and implement an appropriate calorie-restricted diet plan. Positive reinforcement and self-esteem building are integral to the diet plan.

Other Pain Relief Measures. Other measures to reduce pain include distraction, imagery, and music therapy. Physical therapy with manipulation of the low back during the first month of symptoms may be beneficial (Bigos et al., 1994a,b). Shoe insoles may also help decrease pain when standing for prolonged periods of time. Preventive measures for the occupational setting may include a corset and supportive back belts. A structured educational program about low back problems in the work setting has also been found helpful in decreasing both injuries and time lost from work.

Chart 45–3

Education Guide: Typical Exercises for Chronic or Postoperative Low Back Pain

Exercise	Instructions
Extension Exercises	
Stomach lying	• Lie face down with a pillow under your chest.
Upper trunk extension	• Lie face down with your arms at your sides and lift your head and neck.
Prone pushups	• Lie face down on a mat and, keeping your body stiff, push up to extend your arms.
Flexion Exercises	
Pelvic tilt	• Lying on your back with your knees bent, tighten your abdominal muscles to push your lower back against the mat.
Semi–sit-ups	• Lying on your back with your knees bent, raise your upper body at a 45-degree angle and hold this position for 5–10 sec.
Knee to chest	• Lying on your back with your knees bent, tighten your abdominal muscles to push your lower back against the mat. Now bring one or both knees to your chest and hold this position for 5–10 sec.

Surgical Management. When conservative measures fail to relieve back pain after 1 month or neurologic deficits progress, the surgeon usually performs surgery.

Common Operative Procedures. The most common operative procedures are diskectomy, laminectomy, and spinal fusion. These open surgical procedures can cause major complications, including nerve injuries, diskitis, and dural tears.

In a conventional diskectomy, the spinal nerve is usually lifted to remove the offending portion of the disk. A laminectomy is the removal of one or more vertebral laminae plus osteophytes, if present, and the herniated nucleus pulposus. Both procedures are performed through a 3- to 4-inch (7.5 to 10 cm) longitudinal incision. The standard hospital stay is 2 to 3 days, but may be shorter or longer depending on the client's condition and the reimbursement source. A sample client version clinical pathway for a lumbar laminectomy is included in this chapter.

When repeated laminectomies are performed or the spine is unstable, the surgeon may perform a spinal fusion to stabilize the affected area. Chips of bone are removed, typically from the client's iliac crest, and are grafted between the vertebrae for support and to strengthen the back.

For clients who may be difficult to fuse, implantable direct current stimulation (DCS) may be used to promote bone fusion. Studies show that DCS has a success rate of 90% or more (Kahanovitz & Pashos, 1996).

Alternative Operative Procedures. Three alternatives to a laminectomy that have varying degrees of popularity are percutaneous lumbar diskectomy, microdiskectomy, and laser-assisted laparoscopic lumbar diskectomy. The primary advantage of these surgical procedures is a shortened hospital stay and the possibility of the procedure being done on an outpatient basis. Spinal cord complications are also less likely.

Percutaneous Lumbar Diskectomy. Using local anesthesia for this procedure, the surgeon inserts a metal cannula, or endoscope, adjacent to the affected disk under fluoroscopy. A special cutting tool is threaded through the cannula for removal of pieces of the disk that are compressing the nerve root.

Microdiskectomy. A microdiskectomy involves microscopic surgery through a 1-inch incision. This procedure allows for easier identification of anatomic structures, improved precision in removing small fragments, and decreased tissue trauma and pain.

Laser-Assisted Laparoscopic Lumbar Diskectomy. This procedure combines a laser with modified standard disk instruments inserted periumbilically through the laparoscopic cannula. It may be used to treat herniated disks that, although bulging, have not encroached the vertebral canal. The primary risks of this surgery are infection and nerve root injury. The client is typically discharged in 24 to 48 hours.

Preoperative Care. Because lumbar back surgery is performed more often than cervical back surgery, preoperative and postoperative care for lumbar procedures is described here. Preoperative care of the client preparing for a laminectomy is similar to that for any client undergoing surgery (see Chap. 20). The nurse and physical therapist teach the client what to expect postoperatively and how to move in bed. The client should be warned that various sensations, such as numbness and tingling, may be experienced in the affected leg or both legs, because of the manipulation of nerves and muscles during surgery.

The client with a fusion is usually braced postoperatively. The brace is fitted by the physical therapist and made before surgery. The nurse in the surgeon's office or the clinic teaches the client about the importance of wearing the brace, as instructed during the healing process.

The surgeon explains where the bone for grafting will be obtained from. Whenever possible, the client's own bone is used, but supplemental bone from a bone bank may be needed. The surgeon provides verbal and written information about the type and the source of bone for surgery. The client signs an informed consent form preoperatively.

Postoperative Care. Early postoperative nursing care focuses on preventing and assessing complications that might occur in the first 24 to 48 hours (Chart 45–4). As for any client undergoing surgery, the nurse or assistive nursing personnel measures vital signs at least every 4 hours during the first 24 hours to assess for fever and for hypotension, which could indicate bleeding or severe pain. The nurse performs a complete neurologic assessment every 4 hours as well. Of particular importance is the client's ability to feel sensation in the extremities and to move them.

The nurse carefully checks the client's ability to void. Pain and a flat position in bed make voiding difficult, especially for men. Inability to void may indicate damage to the sacral spinal nerves, which control the detrusor muscle in the bladder. The client with a diskectomy or a laminectomy typically gets out of bed with assistance on the evening of surgery, which may facilitate voiding.

Pain control may be achieved with intramuscular opioid analgesia or patient-controlled analgesia (PCA). Either morphine or meperidine hydrochloride (Demerol) may be used during the first 24 hours, depending on the client's age and mental status. The physician typically prescribes oral opioids after the parenteral drug administration is discontinued. The nurse assures the client that pain will decrease as the incision area heals.

The nurse inspects the surgical dressing for blood or any other type of drainage. Clear drainage may mean cerebrospinal fluid (CSF) leakage, and the nurse must report such a finding to the surgeon immediately. Bulging at the incision site may be due to a CSF leak or a hematoma, both of which are also reported to the surgeon.

The nurse or assistive nursing personnel also empties and measures the drainage from the surgical drain, usually a Jackson-Pratt or Hemovac drain. Because the drainage is usually minimal, the surgeon usually removes the drain in 24 to 36 hours.

Correct turning of the client in bed is especially important. The nurse or assistive nursing personnel logrolls the client every 2 hours from side to back and vice versa. In logrolling, the client is turned all at once while the client's back is kept as straight as possible. For large clients, a turning sheet may be used. Either turning method may require additional assistance, depending on how much the client can assist. When the nurse or assistive nursing personnel helps the client in getting out of bed, the client's back is kept straight and the client is placed in a straight-backed chair, with the feet resting comfortably on the floor.

As for any client postoperatively, the nurse instructs the client to deep breathe every 2 hours to prevent atelectasis and pneumonia. Until the client can ambulate independently, the client wears graduated compression stockings, sequential compression devices (SCDs), or

Patient Daily Guidelines Following Lumbar Laminectomy©

Arrow symbol means "*continue what you are doing*" →

	Day of Surgery	Day One	Day Two	Day Three (Probable Day of Discharge)
Vital Signs	Your nurse closely monitors: Your responsiveness to stimulation, speech, movement of your arms and legs, dressing and vital signs.	Your nurse will continue to monitor you closely.	→	→
I & O	**Intake and output (I & O)** Nursing staff records all fluids and solids taken in and put out. If you eat, drink or go to the bathroom without assistance, tell the staff.	Staff continues to record *I & O*.	*I & O* record discontinued.	
Hemovac	**Hemovac fluids** The hemovac collects drainage from the incision, it is measured and recorded.	Drainage from hemovac measured and recorded.	Dressing changed or removed. Hemovac may be discontinued.	
IV Fluids	**IV Fluids** - are given through an intravenous device (allowing access to a vein) and recorded.	IV fluids may be discontinued. IV device remains in place.	After completion of antibiotics, IV device may be discontinued.	
Triflow	Breathing exercise - Use the Triflow breather 10 times every hour while awake.	Continue using Triflow.	→	→
TEDS	You may wear sequential and/or thigh high TED hose. Once, each shift the nurse removes and reapplies them.	Continue wearing TEDS. Removed and reapplied once each shift.	Ask your doctor if you need to wear TEDS at home.	→
Pain Control	Ask your nurse for pain medication every three to four hours. The goal is for you to remain comfortable. After surgery you may be given injections. At some point this changes to pills.	Continue to ask for pain medication as you need it.	→	→
Diet	Clear liquid diet. Water, juices and tea as desired.	Return to presurgery diet. Your bowels should return to presurgery activity.	If you haven't had a bowel movement, tell a nurse.	→
Bathing	Nursing staff helps you bathe.	Nursing staff, if needed, can assist you to bathe.	After the dressing is removed, you may shower.	→
Activity	Progress, with assistance, from walk to standing to walking. Walk often, as tolerated. **Logroll every two hours.** The nursing staff assists you to roll from side to side. **Pillow** - When lying on your back, or either side, place pillow beneath knees. You are taught and encouraged to maintain correct body alignment and mechanics.	Progress with assistance, from standing to walking. The staff assists you to logroll. **Body mechanics:** Keep back straight. Bend with knees. Don't sit a long time. **Ask doctor for guidelines.**	Assistance is available when walking in the halls. Walk often, as long as you feel comfortable. Change position every two hours when in bed. Logroll to turn to side. **Patient Survey:** You will be given a *Patient Questionnaire.* Please complete and give it to your nurse prior to leaving the hospital.	**Discharge Teaching:** You'll receive information about caring for yourself at home. Make sure all questions are asked and answered. Any medications taken at home will be discussed. Written prescriptions given.

This tool is intended as a guideline only. Each person is an individual and responses may vary. If you have any questions please talk to your doctor.

P 8414   **May - 92**

Clinical Pathway Lumbar laminectomy. Client version. (Patricia Barnes, RN, BSN, ONC; Ann Beaver, RN, BSN; Pamela Cronk, RN, BSN; Cynthia Economou, RN; Andrea Kidd, RN, BSN; Cynthia Mosher, RN, BSN, CNS; Susan Stockton, RN, BSN, ONC; courtesy of William Beaumont Hospital, Royal Oak, MI.)

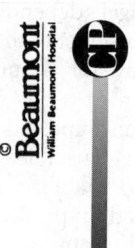

Beaumont
William Beaumont Hospital

Nursing Care Highlight: The Client with Major Complications of Lumbar Spinal Surgery

Complication	Assessment/Interventions
Cerebrospinal fluid (CSF) leakage	• Observe for clear fluid on or around the dressing. • If CSF is present, test for glucose. (The test result is positive if glucose is present.) • Report CSF leakage immediately to the surgeon. (The client is usually kept on flat bed rest for 7–10 days while the dural tear heals.)
Fluid volume deficit	• Monitor vital signs carefully for hypotension and tachycardia. • Monitor intake and output; monitor drain output, which should not be more than 250 mL in 8 hr during the first 24 hr. Drainage should taper within 12 hr after surgery. (The surgeon removes the drain in 24–36 hr.)
Acute urinary retention	• Assist the client to the bathroom or a bedside commode as soon as possible postoperatively. • Assist male clients to stand at the bedside as soon as possible postoperatively. • Give bethanechol (Urecholine) chloride as ordered to stimulate the detrusor muscle of the bladder.
Paralytic ileus	• Monitor for the return of bowel sounds. • Assess for abdominal distention, nausea, and vomiting.
Fat embolism syndrome (FES) (more common in people with spinal fusion)	• Observe for and report chest pain, dyspnea, anxiety, and mental status changes (particularly common in the elderly). • Note petechiae around the neck, upper chest, buccal membrane, and conjunctiva. • Monitor arterial blood gas values for decreased PaO_2.
Persistent or progressive lumbar radiculopathy (nerve root pain)	• Report pain not responsive to opioids. • Document the location and nature of pain. • Administer analgesics as ordered.
Infection (e.g., wound diskitis, hematoma)	• Monitor the client's temperature carefully (a slight elevation is normal). Increased temperature elevation or a spike after the second postoperative day is possibly indicative of infection. • Report increased pain at the wound site or in the legs. • Give antibiotics as ordered. • Use sterile technique for dressing changes.

PaO_2 = partial pressure of arterial oxygen.

pneumatic compression boots (PCBs) to prevent deep venous thrombosis (DVT) and possible pulmonary emboli. Elderly clients are especially susceptible to these complications of immobility.

When a spinal fusion is performed in addition to a laminectomy, more care is taken with mobility and positioning. The client usually stays in bed for 24 hours, and the nurse or assistive nursing personnel logrolls the client every 2 hours. The nurse inspects both the iliac and spinal incision areas for problems, as previously described.

A brace or other type of thoracolumbar support is worn when the client is out of bed. The nurse discourages prolonged sitting or standing.

➤ Continuing Care

The client with back pain who does not have surgery is typically managed at home. If back surgery is performed, the client is usually discharged to home with support from family or significant others.

➤ Home Care Management

The nurse informs the client and family members or a significant other that the client should have a firm mattress to provide support for the entire vertebral column. A bed board or large piece of plywood placed under a soft mattress may suffice. After back surgery, the client may not be allowed to climb stairs for several weeks. It is essential that facilities to meet personal needs be on one level in the home. The client can usually return to work in 2 to 6 weeks, depending on the nature of the job and the extent of and type of surgery. Weight that may be lifted is initially limited to 5 pounds. The amount is gradually increased as healing occurs.

➤ Health Teaching

In collaboration with the dietitian and physical therapist, the nurse instructs the client to do the following:
- Continue with a weight-reduction diet, if needed
- Use moist heat as needed
- Perform strengthening exercises, as initiated in the hospital setting

---

Chart 45-5

Health Promotion Guide: Use of Proper Body Mechanics to Prevent Back Injury

- Size up the load to determine the number of persons needed to perform task.
- When lifting an object, keep your back straight, do not bend at the waist; lift with your large thigh muscles.
- Push objects rather than pull them.
- Do not twist your back.
- Avoid prolonged sitting or standing. Use a foot stool to lessen back strain.
- Sit in chairs with good support; sleep on a firm mattress.
- Avoid shoulder stooping—use proper posture.
- Do not walk or stand in high-heeled shoes for prolonged periods (for women).

The physical therapist reviews and demonstrates the principles of body mechanics and muscle-strengthening exercises. The client is then asked to demonstrate these principles (Chart 45-5).

The health care provider may want the client to continue taking medications such as anti-inflammatory drugs and muscle relaxants. The nurse reminds the client and the family about the possible side effects of drugs and what to do if they occur. If the client has a spinal fusion, he or she may need to wear a brace or a thoracolumbar support for 3 to 6 months while the fusion heals completely. The client may not be able to return to full functioning for 6 to 12 months after a spinal fusion.

The client with an acute episode of back pain typically returns to usual activities but may fear a recurrence. The nurse reminds the client that if caution is used, the client may never have another episode. For the client with chronic pain, however, the continuous or repeated pain can be frustrating and tiring. If pain is unremitting, surgery is indicated. The nurse encourages the client and family members to set short-term goals and to take steps toward recovering slowly.

In a few clients, back surgery may not be successful. This situation, referred to as failed back surgery syndrome (FBSS), is a complex combination of organic, psychological, and socioeconomic factors. Repeated surgical procedures often discourage these clients, who must continue nonsurgical management of pain after multiple operations. Nerve blocks and other pain management modalities may be needed on a long-term basis (see Chap. 9).

➤ Health Care Resources

The nurse identifies support systems (e.g., family, church groups, and clubs) for the client after back surgery or with FBSS. For example, a spouse may help the client with exercises or may perform the exercises with the client. Members of a church group may help run errands and do household chores.

The client with back pain may continue physical therapy on an ambulatory basis after discharge. For unresolved pain, the client may be referred to pain specialists or clinics, which are usually found in large metropolitan hospitals. A case manager may be assigned to the client to help with resource management and utilization.

SPINAL CORD INJURY
Overview

Spinal cord injury (SCI) has received increased public attention and research as a result of Christopher Reeve's spinal cord trauma. Loss of motor function, sensation, reflex activity, and bowel and bladder control often result from SCI. In addition, the client may experience significant behavior and emotional problems as a result of changes in body image, role performance, and self-concept.

Spinal cord injuries are classified as complete or incomplete. A complete injury is one in which the spinal cord has been severed or damaged in a way that eliminates all innervation below the level of the injury. Injuries that allow some function or movement below the level of the injury are described as incomplete.

Pathophysiology
Autonomic Nervous System Syndromes

Specific syndromes seen after spinal cord injury (SCI) and damage to the autonomic nervous system (ANS) are spinal shock and autonomic dysreflexia.

Spinal shock occurs immediately after injury as a result of disruption in the communication pathways between upper motor neurons and lower motor neurons. Also known as neurogenic shock, it is characterized by

- Flaccid paralysis
- Loss of reflex activity below the level of the lesion
- Bradycardia
- Paralytic ileus (occasionally)
- Hypotension

It may last from a few days to several months.

Autonomic dysreflexia, or hyper-reflexia, is usually seen in injuries above the level of the sixth thoracic vertebra. It generally occurs after the period of spinal shock is completed. This syndrome results from uninhibited sympathetic discharge; that is, the sympathetic nervous system (SNS) is no longer controlled by higher centers in the cerebral cortex, owing to disruption in impulse transmission. Chart 45-6 summarizes the key features of this life-threatening complication.

Chart 45-6

Key Features of Autonomic Dysreflexia

- Severe, rapidly occurring hypertension
- Bradycardia
- Flushing above level of lesion
- Severe, throbbing headache
- Nasal stuffiness
- Sweating
- Nausea
- Blurred vision

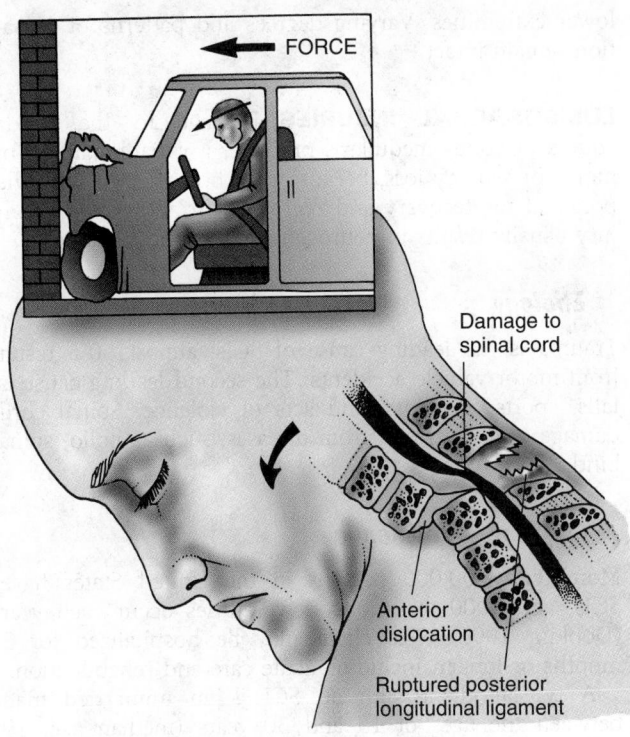

Figure 45-2. Hyperflexion injury of the cervical spine.

Mechanisms of Injury

When sufficient force is applied to the spinal cord, damage results in neurologic deficits. Sources of force include injury to the vertebral column (fracture, dislocation, and subluxation) or penetrating trauma (gunshot or knife wounds). Although in some cases the cord itself may remain intact, at other times the cord undergoes a destructive process caused by a contusion, a compression, or a concussion.

Four mechanisms may result in SCI: hyperflexion; hyperextension; axial loading, or vertical compression; and excessive rotation. Penetrating injuries to the cord may also occur.

A hyperflexion injury (Fig. 45-2) occurs when the head is suddenly and forcefully accelerated forward, causing extreme flexion of the neck. This type of injury often occurs in head-on collisions and diving accidents. Flexion injury to the lower thoracic and lumbar spine may occur when the trunk is suddenly flexed on itself, as occurs in a fall on the buttocks. The posterior ligaments can be stretched or torn, or the vertebrae may fracture or dislocate. Either process may disrupt the integrity of the spinal cord, causing hemorrhage, edema, and necrosis.

Hyperextension injuries (Fig. 45-3) occur most often in automobile accidents in which the client's vehicle is struck from behind or during falls when the client's chin is struck. The head is suddenly accelerated and then decelerated. This stretches or tears the anterior longitudinal ligament, fractures or subluxates the vertebrae, and perhaps ruptures an intervertebral disk. As with flexion injuries, the spinal cord may easily be damaged.

Diving accidents, falls on the buttocks, or a jump in which a person lands on the feet can cause many of the injuries attributable to axial loading (vertical compression) (Fig. 45-4). The blow to the top of the head causes the vertebrae to shatter. Pieces of bone enter the spinal canal and damage the cord.

Rotation injuries are caused by turning the head beyond the normal range.

Penetrating injuries to the spinal cord are classified by the velocity of the vehicle (e.g., knife or bullet) causing the injury. Low-velocity, or low-impact, injuries cause damage directly at the site or localized damage to the spinal cord or the spinal nerves. In contrast, high-velocity injuries that occur from gunshot wounds cause both direct and indirect damage.

As mentioned earlier, the spinal cord may be contused, lacerated, or compressed as a result of injury. Petechial hemorrhage into the central gray matter, and later into white matter, can be caused by contusion and laceration of the spinal cord. Together with compression of the cord from hemorrhage of a lacerated blood vessel or bony fragments, spinal cord edema develops. Necrosis of the spinal cord occurs from compromised capillary circulation and venous return.

Extent of Injury

Incomplete SCIs are more common than complete lesions. A client experiencing an incomplete lesion typically has preservation of a mixed pattern of motor, sensory, and reflex function. Specific syndromes result from incomplete

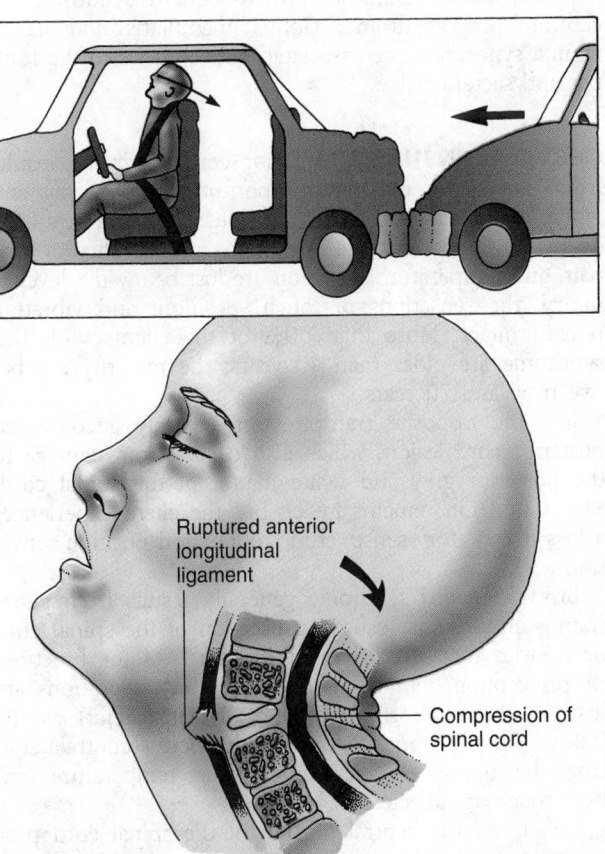

Figure 45-3. Hyperextension injury of the cervical spine.

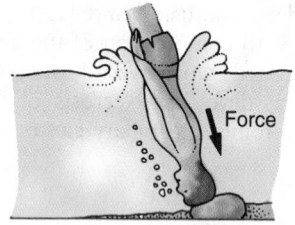
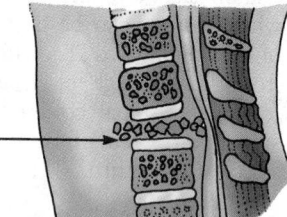

Figure 45–4. Axial loading (vertical compression) injury of the cervical spine and the lumbar spine.

lesions (Fig. 45–5). A "pure" syndrome may not be seen. Cervical injuries may produce anterior cord syndrome, posterior cord syndrome, Brown-Séquard syndrome, or central cord syndrome. Conus medullaris and cauda equina syndromes are associated with injuries to the lumbar and sacral cord.

CERVICAL INJURIES. Anterior cord syndrome results from damage to the anterior portion of both gray and white matter of the spinal cord, usually as a result of decreased blood supply. Although motor function and pain and temperature sensation are lost below the level of injury, the sensations of touch, position, and vibration remain intact. More than 50% of the clients with this syndrome are older than 40 years; the majority are between 50 and 70 years.

Just the opposite transpires in a rarely encountered posterior cord lesion, which also occurs from damage to the posterior gray and white matter of the spinal cord. Motor function remains intact, but the client experiences a loss of vibratory sense, crude touch, and position sensation.

Brown-Séquard syndrome generally results from penetrating injuries that cause hemisection of the spinal cord or injuries that affect half of the cord. Motor function, proprioception, vibration, and deep touch sensations are lost on the same side of the body (ipsilateral) as the lesion. On the opposite side of the body (contralateral) from the injury, the sensations of pain, temperature, and light touch are affected.

Lesions of the central portion of the spinal cord produce a central cord syndrome. Loss of motor function is more pronounced in the upper extremities than in the

lower extremities. Varying degrees and patterns of sensation remain intact.

LUMBOSACRAL INJURIES. Damage to the cauda equina or conus medullaris produces a variable pattern of motor or sensory loss, because peripheral nerves have the potential for recovery and regrowth. In addition, this injury usually results in neurogenic bowel and bladder.

Etiology

Trauma is the leading cause of SCIs; almost 50% result from motor vehicle accidents. The second leading cause is falls, sports accidents, and acts of violence. Spinal cord damage can also result from diseases, such as polio, spina bifida, and tumors.

Incidence/Prevalence

More than 200,000 persons in the United States have SCIs, and 8000 to 10,000 new injuries occur each year (Dobkin, 1996). The client may be hospitalized for 3 months or longer, including acute care and rehabilitation.

A typical client with an SCI is an unmarried man between the ages of 15 and 30 years (median age, 19 years). Peak incidence of injury occurs in the summer or warmer months.

Collaborative Management

Assessment

➤ History

When obtaining a history from a client with an SCI, the nurse gathers as much data as possible about how the accident occurred and the probable mechanism of injury. The nurse specifically asks about the position of the client immediately after the injury, the symptoms that occurred after the injury, and the changes that have occurred since the initial appearance of signs and symptoms. In addition, if possible, prehospital rescue personnel are questioned about the type of immobilization devices used and whether any problems occurred during stabilization and transport of the client to the hospital. The nurse asks about the medical treatment given at the scene of injury or in the emergency room (e.g., medications and intravenous [IV] fluids).

The nurse also determines the client's medical history, including a history of arthritis of the spine, congenital deformities, osteoporosis or osteomyelitis, cancer, and previous injury or surgery of the neck or the back. These health problems may cause or contribute to an SCI. If the client has experienced a cervical SCI, the nurse documents a detailed history of any respiratory problems.

➤ Physical Assessment/Clinical Manifestations

Initial Assessment. The first priority for the client with an SCI is to assess the client's respiratory pattern and ensure an adequate airway. The client with a cervical SCI is at high risk for respiratory compromise because the

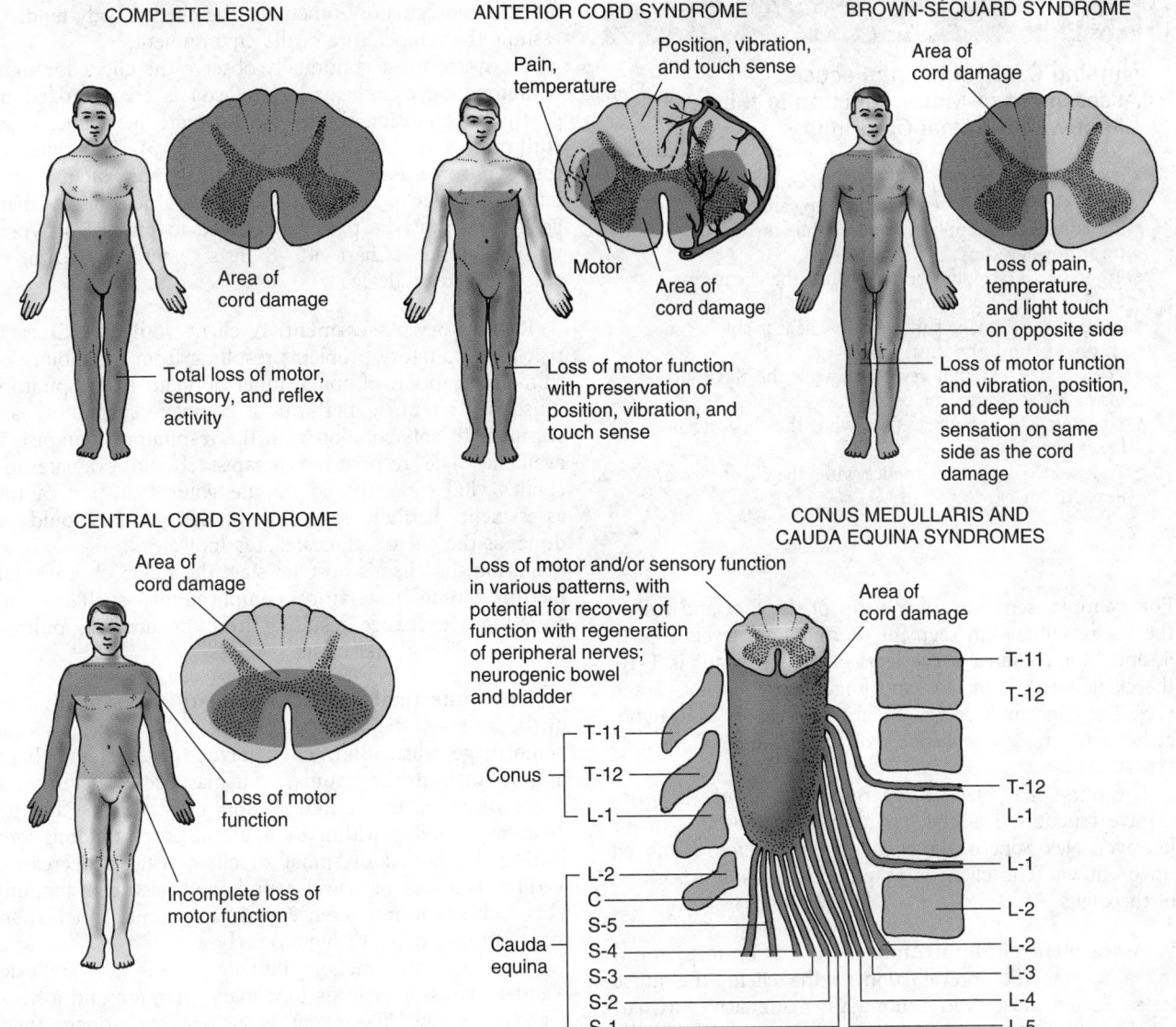

COMPLETE LESION

Area of cord damage

Total loss of motor, sensory, and reflex activity

ANTERIOR CORD SYNDROME

Position, vibration, and touch sense

Pain, temperature

Motor

Area of cord damage

Loss of motor function with preservation of position, vibration, and touch sense

BROWN-SÉQUARD SYNDROME

Area of cord damage

Loss of pain, temperature, and light touch on opposite side

Loss of motor function and vibration, position, and deep touch sensation on same side as the cord damage

CENTRAL CORD SYNDROME

Area of cord damage

Loss of motor function

Incomplete loss of motor function

CONUS MEDULLARIS AND CAUDA EQUINA SYNDROMES

Loss of motor and/or sensory function in various patterns, with potential for recovery of function with regeneration of peripheral nerves; neurogenic bowel and bladder

Area of cord damage

T-11
T-12

Conus — T-11
T-12
L-1

T-12
L-1

L-1

Cauda equina
L-2
C
S-5
S-4
S-3
S-2
S-1

L-2
L-2
L-3
L-4
L-5

Figure 45–5. Common spinal cord syndromes.

cervical spinal nerves (C-3 through C-5) innervate the phrenic nerve, which controls the diaphragm. Endotracheal intubation may be necessary to prevent respiratory arrest.

The nurse also assesses the client for indications of hemorrhage or bleeding around fracture sites or intra-abdominal hemorrhage. Other indicators of hemorrhage include hypotension and tachycardia with a weak and thready pulse.

The client's neurologic status is usually assessed by the Glasgow Coma Scale (see Chapter 43 for description of tool). Cognitive impairment as a result of an associated traumatic brain injury (TBI) or substance abuse is seen in up to 50% of traumatic SCIs (Dobkin, 1996). The nurse performs a detailed assessment of the client's motor and sensory status to assist in determining the level of injury and to serve as baseline data for future comparison. The level of injury is the lowest neurologic segment with intact or normal motor and sensory function. Quadriplegia (also called tetraplegia) (paralysis) or quadriparesis (weakness) involves all four extremities, as seen with cervical cord injury. Paraplegia (paralysis) or paraparesis (weakness) involves only the lower extremities, as seen in lower thoracic and lumbosacral injuries or lesions.

Assessment of Sensation. Sensation is carried from the peripheral nerves to the spinal cord and up to the cerebral cortex via a variety of sensation-specific tracts. Injury to the spinal cord may prohibit sensory impulses from reaching the brain. To test sensory abilities, the nurse first asks the client to close his or her eyes. Next, the nurse touches the skin with a clean safety pin or cotton-tipped applicator and asks the client whether he or she can feel the pinprick or light touch. Bilateral responses are compared. The nurse follows the sensory distribution of the skin dermatomes (see Chap. 43, Fig. 43–3), beginning the examination in the area of reported loss of sensation and ending where sensation becomes normal.

Chart 45–7

Nursing Care Highlight: Focused Assessment of Motor Function in the Client with a Spinal Cord Injury

- To assess C4–5, apply downward pressure while the client shrugs his or her shoulders upward.
- To assess C5–6, apply resistance while the client pulls up his or her arms.
- To assess C-7, apply resistance while the client straightens his or her flexed arms.
- To assess C-8, make sure that the client is able to grasp an object and form a fist.
- To assess L2–4, apply resistance while the client lifts his or her legs from the bed.
- To assess L-5, apply resistance while the client dorsiflexes his or her feet.
- To assess S-1, apply resistance while the client plantar flexes his or her feet.

For example, sensation of the top of the foot and calf of the leg is spinal skin segment (dermatome) levels L-3, L-4, and L-5. The area at the level of the umbilicus is T-10, the clavicle is C-3 or C-4, and finger sensation is C-7 and C-8. The client may report a complete sensory loss, hypoesthesia (decreased sensation), or hyperesthesia (increased sensation).

The nurse may elect to determine the client's proprioceptive function. The client is again asked to close his or her eyes. Next, one of the client's fingers or toes is moved up or down. The client is asked to identify the position of the digits.

Assessment of Motor Ability. In addition to performing a routine motor evaluation of the client, the nurse tests selected muscles in a more systematic fashion (Chart 45–7). The nurse asks the client to flex and extend the elbows, elevate both arms off the bed, and flex and extend the wrists and fingers. The client with spinal injuries at the fifth or sixth cervical vertebra are often able to flex, but not extend, their arms. Next, the nurse observes the client's ability to move the lower extremities. The client is requested to wiggle the toes, flex and extend the feet and knees, and move one or both hips.

The nurse or health care provider may also test deep tendon reflexes (DTRs), including the biceps (C-5), triceps (C-7), patellar (L-3), and ankle (S-1). It is not unusual for these reflexes, as well as all motor function or sensation, to be absent immediately after the injury owing to spinal shock. After spinal shock has resolved, the reflexes may return if the lesion is incomplete or involves upper motor neurons.

Cardiovascular Assessment. Cardiovascular dysfunction is usually the result of disruption of the autonomic nervous system, especially if the injury is above the sixth thoracic vertebra. Bradycardia, hypotension, and hypothermia result from loss of sympathetic input and may lead to cardiac dysrhythmias. In addition, the lack of sympathetic or hypothalamic control causes the client to

lose thermoregulatory functions; the client's body tends to assume the temperature of the environment.

The nurse must continually observe the client for signs of autonomic dysreflexia. Dysreflexia is characterized by severe hypertension, bradycardia, severe headache, nasal stuffiness, and flushing (see Chart 45–6). The cause of this syndrome is a noxious stimulus, most often a distended bladder or constipation. This is a neurologic emergency and must be promptly treated to prevent a hypertensive stroke. Chart 45–8 lists emergency care of autonomic dysreflexia.

Respiratory Assessment. A client with an SCI is at risk for respiratory problems resulting from immobility or from interruption of spinal innervation to the respiratory muscles. The nurse performs a complete respiratory assessment in collaboration with the respiratory therapist, if available. The respiratory therapist should evaluate the client's vital capacity and minute volume as part of the assessment. Periodic repetition of these tests should be done, as the client's clinical status indicates.

During the client's hospital stay, the nurse observes for life-threatening respiratory complications, such as impaired gas exchange resulting from pneumonia, pulmonary emboli, and atelectasis.

Gastrointestinal and Genitourinary Assessment. The nurse assesses the client's abdomen for indications of hemorrhage, distention, or paralytic ileus. Hemorrhage may result from the trauma, or it may occur later from a stress ulcer or the administration of steroids. Paralytic ileus may develop within 72 hours of hospital admission. During the period of spinal shock, peristalsis decreases, leading to a loss of bowel sounds and gastric distention. This lack of or interference with autonomic innervation may lead to a reflex or hypotonic bowel.

Autonomic dysfunction initially causes an areflexic bladder, which later leads to urinary retention and a neurogenic bladder. The client is at risk for urinary tract

Chart 45–8

Nursing Care Highlight: Emergency Care of the Client Experiencing Autonomic Dysreflexia

- Raise the head of the bed to a high Fowler position.
- Call the physician and notify him or her of the emergency.
- Loosen tight clothing on the client.
- Check the Foley catheter tubing (if present) for kinks or obstruction.
- If a Foley catheter is not present, check for bladder distention and catherize immediately.
- Check the client for fecal impaction; if present, disimpact immediately using anesthetic ointment.
- Check the room temperature to ensure that it is not too cool or drafty.
- Monitor blood pressures every 10–15 min.
- Give nitrates or hydralazine (Apresoline, Novo-Hylazin✦) as ordered.

infection from an indwelling urinary catheter, from intermittent catheterizations, or from bladder distention, stasis, and overflow.

Musculoskeletal Assessment. The nurse assesses the client's muscle tone and size. Muscle wasting results from long-term flaccid paralysis seen in clients with lower motor neuron (LMN) lesions. Incomplete lesions or upper motor neuron (UMN) lesions may cause muscle spasticity, which can lead to contractures after spinal shock has resolved.

The nurse assesses the condition of the client's skin, especially over pressure points, at least twice daily. Any reddened area is carefully assessed and monitored for change. It may be necessary to use an air mattress, special beds, or other techniques to prevent skin breakdown.

Another complication of prolonged immobility is heterotopic ossification (bony overgrowth, often into muscle). It is evidenced by swelling, redness, warmth, and decreased range of motion (ROM) of the involved extremity. Changes in the bony structure are not evident until several weeks after the initial symptoms appear.

➤ Psychosocial Assessment

If possible, the nurse assesses the client's preinjury psychosocial status by obtaining information about the client's usual methods of coping with illness, difficult situations, and disappointments. The nurse determines the client's level of independence or dependence and his or her comfort level in discussing feelings and emotions with family members or close friends. Clients who are emotionally secure, with a positive self-image, a supportive family, and financial and job security, often adapt to their injury. Information about the client's religious beliefs or cultural background also assists the nurse in developing the plan of care. The client with an SCI must cope with changes in body image, self-esteem, independence, role relationships, and sexuality (also see Chaps. 10 and 11).

In addition, the nurse assesses family members or significant others to determine how well they are coping with the client's injury and changes in their roles. The client and significant others must be prepared for extensive rehabilitation and changes in lifestyle. Financial constraints may pose additional stress.

➤ Laboratory Assessment

The health care provider orders routine laboratory studies for the client with an SCI to establish baseline data or to prepare for surgery. A urinalysis is used to check for the presence of blood in the urine after trauma. Arterial blood gas analysis is used to monitor the respiratory status of a client at risk for respiratory insufficiency. The findings should be within normal limits unless the client has a history of heavy smoking or preinjury pulmonary disease or is experiencing respiratory failure, as indicated by decreased oxygen levels, increased carbon dioxide levels, and respiratory acidosis.

➤ Diagnostic Assessment

The physician orders a complete spine radiographic series to identify vertebral fractures, subluxation, or dislocation.

Computed tomography (CT) or magnetic resonance imaging (MRI) may be performed to determine the degree and extent of damage to the spinal cord and to detect the presence of blood and bone within the spinal column. Electromyography (EMG), somatosensory evoked potentials (SSEP), and motor evoked potentials (MEP) may also help distinguish levels of injury.

 Analysis

➤ Common Nursing Diagnoses and Collaborative Problems

The most common nursing diagnoses related to the care of a client with an SCI are
1. Altered (Spinal Cord) Tissue Perfusion related to compression, contusion, and/or edema
2. Ineffective Airway Clearance, Ineffective Breathing Pattern, and Impaired Gas Exchange related to decreased innervation to muscles of respiration or immobility
3. Impaired Physical Mobility and/or Self-Care Deficit (the level depends on the extent and level of the injury) related to quadriplegia, quadriparesis, paraplegia, or paraparesis
4. Altered Urinary Elimination and Constipation related to neurogenic bowel and bladder
5. Impaired Adjustment related to depression, fear, a change in body image, or altered role performance

➤ Additional Nursing Diagnoses and Collaborative Problems

Some clients may have one or more of the following:
- Risk for Impaired Skin Integrity related to immobility
- Altered Sexuality Patterns and Sexual Dysfunction related to decreased or absent innervation of the reproductive system
- Pain related to trauma, spasticity, and/or immobility
- Risk for Injury related to immobility and decreased sensation

Additional collaborative problems include
- Potential for Deep Venous Thrombosis (DVT)
- Potential for Sepsis
- Potential for Hypoxemia
- Potential for Atelectasis, Pneumonia

 Planning and Implementation

➤ Altered (Spinal Cord) Tissue Perfusion

Planning: Expected Outcomes. The client is expected to demonstrate adequate spinal cord tissue perfusion and exhibit no further deterioration in neurologic status.

Interventions. If the client has experienced fractured vertebrae, the primary concern of the physician is to reduce and immobilize the fracture to prevent further damage to the spinal cord from bone fragments. The health care provider typically utilizes nonsurgical techniques using traction or external fixation, but surgery may be necessary to stabilize the spine and prevent further spinal cord damage.

Nonsurgical Management. The nurse assesses the client's vital signs and neurologic status, especially respiratory function and motor and sensory changes in the extremities, every 4 hours or more often if clinically indicated. In the first 24 hours after injury, the client is at risk for neurogenic shock, which is manifested by hypotension and bradycardia. Caused by loss of autonomic function, neurogenic shock is most often associated with cervical spinal injuries.

The client with a cervical spine injury is usually placed in fixed skeletal traction to realign the vertebrae, facilitate bone healing and prevent further injury.

Immobilization: Cervical Injuries. The most commonly used devices for immobilization are the halo fixation device and cervical tongs (Gardner-Wells, Barton, or Crutchfield tongs), which may be used in conjunction with a Stryker frame or kinetic treatment table. Either device is inserted by the physician into the outer aspect of the client's skull and may be used with a Stryker frame or kinetic treatment table to maintain spinal alignment and allow frequent turning. The addition of traction to the cervical tongs assists in reducing the fracture. Traction may or may not be used with the halo fixator. Traction weights may be ordered by the physician.

The halo fixator is a static traction device. Four pins (or screws) are inserted into the client's skull. The metal halo ring may be attached to a plastic vest or cast when the spine is stable, allowing increased client mobility. The client should never be moved or turned by holding or pulling on the halo device. The nurse checks the client's skin frequently to ensure that the jacket or the cast is not causing pressure. The nurse should be able to insert one finger easily under the jacket or the cast.

The nurse monitors the client's neurologic status for changes in movement or decreased strength. The weights of the traction should hang freely at all times. Releasing the traction could cause further neurologic damage. The nurse maintains the client in alignment and ensures that the ropes for the traction remain within the pulley. The insertion sites of the tongs or halo device are monitored for signs of infection. The nurse follows the hospital's policy for pin site care, which may specify the use of solutions such as hydrogen peroxide and saline (Fig. 45–6).

Immobilization: Thoracic and Lumbar/Sacral Injuries. The client with a thoracic injury is placed on bed rest; immobilization with a Fiberglas or plastic body cast may be done (see also Chap. 54). For lumbar and sacral injuries, immobilization of the spine is typically accomplished with a brace or a corset worn when the client is out of bed. Newer lightweight, custom-fit thoracic lumbar sacral orthoses (TLSOs) are preferred over heavier braces or splints, such as the Taylor splint.

Drug Therapy. Methylprednisolone (Solu-Medrol) in high dosages within 8 hours of injury is now the widely recognized first course of treatment. Clients receiving this medication show significant improvement in motor and sensory function (Marciano et al., 1995). Dextran, a plasma expander, may be used to increase capillary blood flow within the spinal cord and to prevent or treat hypotension. Atropine sulfate is used to treat bradycardia if the pulse rate falls below 50 to 60 beats per minute. Hypotension, if severe, is treated with inotropic and sympathomimetic agents such as dopamine hydrochloride (Intropin) and isoproterenol.

Research continues to explore interventions in pharmacologic and surgical management of SCIs. Naloxone and thyrotropin-releasing hormone (TRH) have shown promise in improving spinal cord blood flow. Sygen is being researched for use in acute SCI, but may also be studied for chronic SCI. Another drug, 4-AP, remains in clinical trials for clients whose SCI is older than 18 months (Tompkins, 1997).

For clients with severe muscle spasticity (usually UMN injuries), medications to help control spasticity include

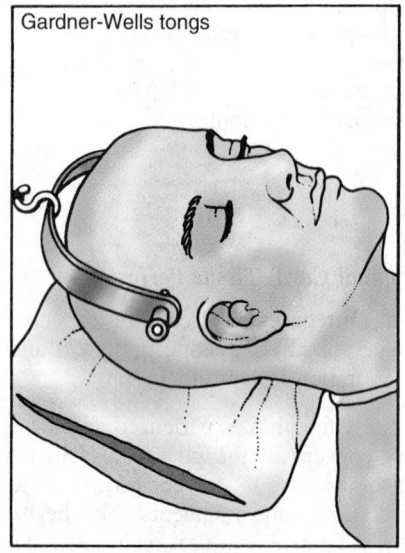
Gardner-Wells tongs

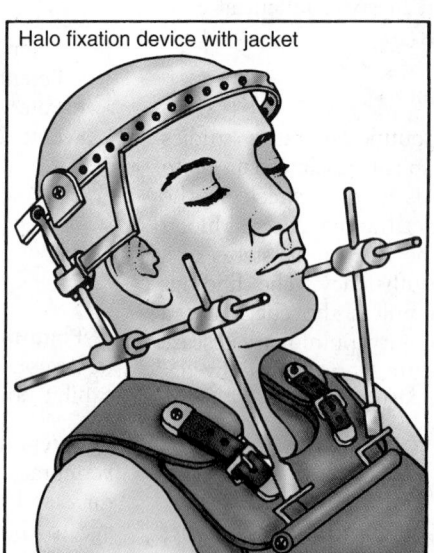
Halo fixation device with jacket

Figure 45–6. Types of cervical spine traction.

dantrolene (Dantrium) and baclofen (Lioresal). Other drugs to prevent or to treat complications of immobility may be needed later during the rehabilitative phase. For example, etidronate disodium (Didronel) may be ordered for the client with heterotopic ossification.

Surgical Management. Emergency surgery may be indicated if there is evidence of spinal cord compression. The procedure is usually necessary to remove bone fragments from a vertebral fracture, evacuate a hematoma, or remove penetrating objects, such as a bullet. A decompressive laminectomy (removal of one or more laminae) allows for cord expansion from edema if other more conventional measures fail to prevent neurologic deterioration. (Postoperative care is discussed earlier.)

Additional surgical procedures to stabilize and support the spine may be performed at the discretion of the physician, depending on the client's condition and the extent of the injury. Typical procedures include a spinal fusion and the insertion of metal or steel rods, such as Harrington rods, to stabilize thoracic spinal injuries. Postoperatively, the client usually wears a brace, a corset, or lumbosacral support (TLSO) to keep the operative area immobilized during recovery. (See also Chapter 53 under Collaborative Management of Scoliosis.)

Postoperatively, the nurse assesses the client's neurologic status and vital signs at least every hour for the first 4 to 6 hours after surgery and then, if the client is stable, every 4 hours. Complications of surgery, such as hematoma and edema, are manifested by a deterioration in neurologic status.

The client is also at risk for cardiovascular instability because of loss of sympathetic innervation. The client is logrolled when being moved to maintain skeletal alignment or placed on a special bed such as a Roto-Rest bed. (A complete discussion of postoperative nursing care is found in Chapter 22.)

➤ Ineffective Airway Clearance; Ineffective Breathing Pattern; Impaired Gas Exchange

Planning: Expected Outcomes. The client is expected to maintain a patent airway and not experience respiratory complications, such as pneumonia, atelectasis, and aspiration.

Interventions. Clients with injuries at and above the sixth thoracic vertebra are especially at risk for respiratory complications as a result of impaired functioning of the intercostal muscles. Depending on the level of injury, intubation or tracheotomy with mechanical ventilation may be needed. The nurse or assistive nursing personnel turns the client at least every 2 hours and instructs the client to breathe as deeply as possible. The nurse can assist quadriplegic clients to cough by placing his or her hands on either side of the rib cage or upper abdomen below the diaphragm. This technique is sometimes called "assisted coughing," "quad cough," or "cough assist." As the client inhales, the nurse pushes upward to help the client expand the lungs and cough.

The nurse also encourages the client to use an incentive spirometer. The nurse or respiratory therapist performs a respiratory assessment every 8 hours to determine the effectiveness of these strategies. In some cases, it may be necessary to perform oral or nasal suctioning if the client cannot clear the airway of secretions effectively.

➤ Impaired Physical Mobility; Self-Care Deficit

Planning: Expected Outcomes. The client is expected to be free from complications of immobility and learn to perform activities of daily living (ADLs) as independently as possible.

Interventions. The client with an SCI is especially at risk for pressure ulcers, contractures, and deep venous thrombosis or pulmonary emboli.

Preventing Complications of Immobility. To decrease the high risk of pressure sores, the nurse or assistive nursing personnel turns and repositions the client, while in bed, at least every 2 hours. When sitting in a chair, the client is repositioned or taught to reposition himself or herself more often than every 2 hours, because most of the client's weight is placed on one area, the ischial tuberosities. Special pressure relief devices, such as gel pads, may be used in the wheelchair or the bed, but these do not eliminate the need for regular turning and repositioning.

The nurse inspects, as well as teaches the client to inspect, the skin frequently to determine the client's tolerance for sitting and to detect reddened areas. The nurse attempts to blanch the reddened areas over the ischial tuberosities by pressing on the areas and looking for blanching to occur. If blanching does not occur, the area is vulnerable to skin breakdown.

To decrease the risk of contractures as a result of immobility, the nurse or assistive nursing personnel performs ROM exercises at least once every 8 hours. The nurse collaborates with the physical therapist and the occupational therapist:
- To determine the most appropriate positioning and exercise techniques
- To assess the need for hand and wrist splints
- To develop a plan to prevent foot drop (usually clients wear high-topped tennis shoes for prevention)

The nurse assesses the client's lower extremities for indications of deep venous thrombosis (DVT). Signs and symptoms include leg or calf pain, localized tenderness, swelling, and redness. Some clients may be totally asymptomatic. Graduated compression stockings (GCS) or pneumatic compression boots (PCBs) are typically ordered. Sodium heparin, 5000 units every 12 hours subcutaneously, or sodium warfarin (Coumadin, Warfilone✱) in therapeutic dosages may be ordered to prevent DVT or embolus formation. Low-molecular-weight (LMW) heparin is a more recent treatment. It provides the same level of antithrombotic activity as heparin but may decrease hemorrhage risk. (For further discussion of measures to prevent complications of immobility, see Chapter 13.)

Preventing Orthostatic Hypotension. Clients with cervical cord injuries are especially at high risk for orthostatic (postural) hypotension, although any client who is immobilized may have this problem. If the client moves from a lying position to a sitting or standing position too quickly, he or she may experience hypotension, which could result in dizziness and falls. Because of interrupted autonomic innervation, the blood vessels do not constrict quickly enough to push blood up into the brain, which causes the dizziness or lightheadedness often experienced by these clients.

The nurse observes the client carefully for indications of orthostatic hypotension when the head of the bed is raised and when the client is permitted to dangle the legs over the side of the bed or get up in a chair. Blood pressure is measured in each position.

To help prevent orthostatic hypotension, the nurse teaches the client to change position slowly. Some clients wear elastic corsets around the trunk to help facilitate blood flow. Thigh-high antiembolism stockings or elastic (Ace) wraps around both legs may also be used. Chart 45–9 summarizes the most important aspects of care of clients with an SCI.

Promoting Self-Care. The most important part of promoting self-care is setting realistic goals on the basis of the client's potential functional level. Even clients with a cervical SCI may be able to learn how to perform most ADLs independently. The nurse collaborates with the physical therapist and the occupational therapist to evaluate how the client can best transfer from a bed to the wheelchair and feed, dress, and bathe. Various assistive/adaptive devices are available to help clients regain their independence.

Many clients with SCI can no longer ambulate. These clients become wheelchair dependent and must learn new skills. The physical therapist carefully measures the client and orders a custom-made wheelchair for each client. If the client is unable to self-propel the chair manually, electronic devices are available so that the client can use the mouth, the neck, or the upper arm to ambulate in the chair.

➤ *Altered Urinary Elimination; Constipation*

Planning: Expected Outcomes. The client is expected to achieve continence of stool and urine.

Interventions. Clients with SCIs have reflex or neurogenic loss of bowel and bladder control. Many of these clients can become continent if they rigorously adhere to an established program. The type of program depends on the client's usual elimination pattern and whether the injury involved upper motor neurons (UMNs) or lower motor neurons (LMNs). Urologic evaluation may be needed to identify bladder type.

Establishing a Bladder Retraining Program. As soon as the client is medically stable, the indwelling Foley catheter is removed. Initially, the physician may prescribe an intermittent catheterization program. The nurse typically catheterizes the client every 4 hours as ordered and more frequently if the urinary output is greater than 500 mL. Over time, the intervals between catheterizations are increased and adjusted to the client's fluid intake and sleep times.

After the acute care phase has passed, the client may be able to initiate voiding by using specific techniques.

> **Chart 45–9**
>
> ### Nursing Care Highlight: The Client with a Spinal Cord Injury
>
> - Assess the client's respiratory status; monitor for atelectasis, pneumonia, and pulmonary embolus.
> - Take vital signs q4h or more often if clinically indicated; monitor for orthostatic hypotension.
> - Perform neurologic status checks q4h or more often if clinically indicated.
>   - Notify the physician immediately of a deterioration in motor status.
>   - Watch for and immediately treat autonomic dysreflexia.
> - Give pain medication as ordered; document the client's response.
> - Prevent immobility complications.
>   - Have the client TCDB q2h.
>   - Use pneumatic compression boots or graduated compression stockings.
>   - Check the skin and bony prominences for redness and breakdown.
> - Assess bladder function.
>   - Palpate the abdomen for distention.
>   - Begin a bladder retraining program as appropriate.
>   - Assess intake and output.
> - Assess bowel function.
>   - Auscultate bowel sounds.
>   - Palpate for distention.
>   - Chart stool frequency.
>   - Begin a bowel program as appropriate.
> - Monitor the nutritional status, including a calorie count, and collaborate with the dietitian to identify an appropriate diet.
> - Assess psychological status.
>   - Communicate with the client.
>   - Answer questions honestly; refer questions that you cannot answer to someone who can.
>   - Assess for signs of depression or anger.

TCDB = turn, cough, and deep breathe.

Clients with UMN (spastic) bladder problems (injury above the sacrum) may be able to stimulate voiding by
- Stroking the inner thigh
- Pulling on pubic hair and hair of the upper thigh
- Pouring warm water over the perineum
- Tapping the bladder area to stimulate the detrusor muscle

Some health care providers prescribe a drug to stimulate voiding, such as bethanechol (Urecholine) chloride. Bethanechol is a cholinergic agent that facilitates contraction of the detrusor muscle and is usually given twice to four times daily about 1 hour before attempts to void.

Clients with injuries to the lumbosacral area usually have an LMN (flaccid) bladder. Clients with flaccid bladders may achieve emptying of the bladder by performing a Valsalva maneuver or tightening the abdominal muscles. These techniques are not successful for all LMN injuries. To ascertain the effectiveness of these maneuvers, the nurse catheterizes the client for residual urine after voiding. Some clients rely solely on catheterization twice or three times daily to empty the bladder. All clients are encouraged to drink 2000 to 2500 mL of fluid each day to prevent urinary tract infection and calculus formation. Clients with an LMN injury may decrease fluid intake after 6 or 7 PM each evening to prevent catheterization in the middle of the night.

The client with any SCI is at risk for pyelonephritis, hydronephrosis, renal failure, and kidney stones (see Chaps. 74 and 75).

Establishing a Bowel Retraining Program. The essential elements of a bowel program are
- A consistent time for bowel elimination
- A high fluid intake (at least 2000 mL/day) unless fluid intake is restricted
- A high-fiber diet
- Rectal stimulation with or without suppositories
- If needed, stool softener medications such as docusate sodium (Colace) and docusate sodium and cas-anthranol (Peri-Colace)

If the client has sustained an LMN injury, the resulting flaccid large bowel may require the client to perform or to have manual disimpaction. Additional stimuli used to facilitate a bowel movement include scheduling toileting 30 minutes to 1 hour after meals to optimize the gastro-colic reflex and teaching the client to perform a Valsalva maneuver. Massaging the abdomen from right to left along the outline of the large intestine may also be helpful. (Additional information about bladder and bowel retraining is provided in Chapter 13.)

➤ Impaired Adjustment

Planning: Expected Outcomes. The client is expected to demonstrate the ability to cope with the changes caused by the injury and verbalize his or her feelings about the injury and changes in lifestyle.

Interventions. The nurse uses the information obtained from the psychosocial assessment to identify strategies to help the client adjust to the disability. The client is invited to ask questions, which the nurse should answer openly and honestly. The nurse should refer questions about prognosis and potential for complete recovery to the health care provider because the timing and extent of recovery vary for each client. The nurse encourages the client to discuss his or her perceptions of the situation and the coping strategies that can be used. The client should feel free to express personal feelings and emotions in an acceptable manner. The client may behave in a socially unacceptable manner (excessive anger, verbal abuse, use of illegal drugs), and the nurse attempts to redirect this behavior. In addition, the nurse begins a client education program to clarify misconceptions as well as to provide health teaching. Referrals to clergy, rabbis, or other spiritual leaders or to a psychologist or a psychiatric liaison nurse may be needed to help clients adjust to their unexpected life change. Support groups are available for clients and families.

Clients with SCIs should be referred to a social worker or a financial counselor for review of their insurance and financial status and to appropriate social service agencies

as necessary. Coverage of rehabilitation is not provided in many insurance policies.

 Continuing Care

Case managers are ideal care coordinators to act as SCI client advocates. In some settings, case managers begin working with clients in the emergency department to establish a positive image of SCI rehabilitation (Hesslegrave, 1997). Rehabilitation begins in the critical care unit when clients are hemodynamically stable and spinal shock has subsided. Clients are usually transferred from the acute care setting to a rehabilitation setting, where they learn more about self-care, mobility skills, and bladder and bowel retraining. The length of stay in the rehabilitation hospital or unit is typically 1 to 3 months, depending on medical complications that may occur, such as infections.

➤ Home Care Management

If the client is discharged home or returns home for a weekend visit from the rehabilitation setting, the environment must be assessed to ensure that it is free from hazards and can accommodate the client's special needs (e.g., a wheelchair). The occupational or physical therapist, in collaboration with rehabilitation and home health nurse, usually assesses the home environment where the client will be staying on a temporary or permanent basis. Ease of accessibility is particularly important at the entrance of the home as well as the bathroom, the kitchen, and the bedroom. The height of the client's bed may need to be adjusted to facilitate smooth transfer into or out of the bed.

All adaptive devices that the client will use at home should be ordered and delivered to the rehabilitation facility. This enables the nurse and other therapists to ensure that the items fit correctly and that the client and family know how to use them correctly.

➤ Health Teaching

The teaching plan for the client with an SCI includes
- Physical mobility and activity skills
- Activities of daily living (ADLs) skills
- Bowel and bladder retraining program
- Skin care
- Medication regimen
- Sexuality education

This information should be reinforced with written handouts or other client education material that the client, family members, or significant others can use after the client is discharged to the home.

Learning mobility skills is important so that the client can negotiate movement on sidewalks and carpeting and other flooring surfaces. The client must also be able to negotiate sidewalk curbs while walking independently with crutches or a cane or while in a wheelchair.

Some clients are discharged home or to a rehabilitation setting with a halo vest. A halo vest has a significant physical and psychological impact on clients. Physically, clients find it difficult to perform mobility skills and ADLs independently, especially dressing, bathing, and

---

Chart 45–10

Education Guide: Use of a Halo Device*

- Be aware that the weight of the halo device alters balance. Be careful when leaning forward or backward.
- Wear loose clothing, preferably with hook and loop (Velcro) fasteners or large openings for head and arms.
- Bathe in the bathtub or sponge bathe. (Some physicians allow showers.*)
- Wash under the lamb's wool liner of the vest to prevent rashes or sores; use powders or lotions sparingly under the vest.
- Have someone change the liner if it becomes odorous.
- Support the head with a small pillow when sleeping to prevent unnecessary pressure and discomfort.
- Try to resume usual activities to the extent possible; keep as active as possible. (The weight of the device may cause fatigue or weakness.) Avoid contact sports or swimming, however.
- Do not drive, because vision is impaired with the device.
- Keep straws available for drinking fluids.
- Cut meats and other food in small pieces to facilitate chewing and swallowing.
- If going outside in cold temperatures, wrap the pins with cloth to prevent the metal from getting cold.
- Have someone clean the pin sites as recommended by physician or hospital protocol.
- Observe the pin sites daily for redness or drainage; report changes to the physician.
- Increase fluids and fiber in the diet to prevent constipation.
- Use a position of comfort during sexual activity.

*Home care instructions may vary depending on hospital or physician preference.

---

feeding. From a psychological perspective, clients perceive an altered body image. The nurse teaches the client going home or to a rehabilitation setting how to care for and adjust to the halo device (Chart 45–10).

Activities of daily living training for the client with SCI includes a structured exercise program to promote strength and endurance. The occupational therapist instructs the client in the correct use of all adaptive equipment. The nurse, in collaboration with the therapists, instructs family members or the caregiver in transfer skills, feeding, bathing, dressing, positioning, and skin care as appropriate. The nurse collaborates with the dietitian to help the client maintain an ideal body weight and to promote bowel and bladder elimination. The nurse also reinforces the need to follow the client's individualized bowel and bladder program. The client is instructed in the procedures to follow if problems develop.

The nurse teaches the client about the name, purpose, dosage and timing of administration, and side effects of all medications. The client should understand the possible interaction of prescribed medication with over-the-counter medication or illegal drugs and alcohol.

The goal of sexuality education is to answer the client's questions and to correct any misinformation. Unless the nurse has specific training or experience in sexuality counseling of people with SCIs, detailed questions should be directed to a sexuality counselor.

➤ *Psychosocial Preparation*

Psychosocial adaptation is one of the critical factors in determining the success of rehabilitation. The case manager or acute care nurse can help the client prepare for discharge or transfer to a rehabilitation hospital. The nurse assists the client to verbalize feelings and fears about body image, self-concept, role performance, and self-esteem. The nurse should prepare the client for the reactions of those outside the security of the hospital environment. In the acute care setting, the nurse, family members, or friends can take the client to the hospital lobby or, if permitted, to the cafeteria or outside on the hospital grounds. The nurse should tactfully and non-judgmentally let the client know when behavior is unacceptable for the time and place where it occurs as well as encouraging more positive behaviors. The use of role-playing or anticipating responses to potential problems is helpful. For example, the client can practice answering questions from children about why he or she is in a wheelchair or cannot move parts of the body.

➤ *Health Care Resources*

The nurse or case manager refers the client and family or significant others to the local, state or province, and national organizations for those with SCIs. These include the National Spinal Cord Injury Association and the Spinal Cord Injury Hotline. Many consumer-oriented books, journals, and films are also available. Support groups may also be helpful to help the client and family adjust to a changed lifestyle and to provide solutions to commonly encountered problems.

If the quadriplegic client returns home, a full-time caretaker or personal assistant is usually required. The caretaker may be a family member or a nursing assistant employed to help provide care and companionship. The paraplegic client is often able to function without assistance after an appropriate rehabilitation program.

 Evaluation

The nurse evaluates the care provided by determining whether the client

- Exhibits no deterioration in neurologic status
- Maintains a patent airway and experiences no respiratory complications
- Is free from complications of immobility
- Performs ADLs as independently as possible with or without the use of assistive or adaptive devices
- Achieves continence of stool and urine
- Demonstrates the ability to cope with the change caused by the injury

SPINAL CORD TUMORS

Overview

Spinal cord tumors occur most frequently in the thoracic area, followed by an almost equal distribution in the lumbar and cervical region. Signs and symptoms depend on the location of the tumor and its speed of growth.

Pathologic effects of a spinal cord tumor are more often related to compression of the cord than to invasion of the spinal cord itself. As the tumor expands within the vertebral column, it compresses the cord or the spinal nerve roots. Further growth leads to displacement of the cord. Additionally, a large tumor may disrupt the vascular supply to the cord by compression or obstruct the normal flow of cerebrospinal fluid (CSF). Venous occlusion by the tumor may lead to spinal cord congestion and infarction.

The appearance of neurologic signs and symptoms is related to the rate of tumor growth. The spinal cord can often accommodate a slowly growing lesion. With time, the cord may become significantly misshapen and displaced, but the client has surprisingly few symptoms. On the other hand, a rapidly growing tumor quickly leads to spinal cord compression and edema and the development of neurologic symptoms, such as numbness and paralysis.

Primary spinal cord tumors arise from the epidural vessels, spinal meninges, or glial cells of the cord. Their cause is unknown. Approximately 20% to 30% of spinal cord tumors develop as a consequence of metastatic tumors from the lungs, the breasts, the kidney, and the gastrointestinal tract.

Anatomically, spinal cord tumors may be extramedullary or intramedullary. Intramedullary tumors originate within the spinal cord itself, in the central gray matter and the anterior commissure. Extramedullary tumors are found within the spinal dura but outside the cord; they are further defined anatomically as extradural and intradural tumors. Extradural or epidural tumors occur between the vertebrae and the spinal dura. These tumors develop in the surrounding bone and cause destruction of the vertebral bodies. Intradural tumors are located within the dura and originate from the pia-arachnoid, the spinal roots, or the denticulate ligaments.

Spinal cord tumors account for only about 1% of all tumors in adults. Thoracic tumors account for 50% of all spinal cord tumors; cervical tumors occur 20% of the time, followed by lumbosacral tumors (30%). The majority of tumors are benign. They occur equally in both men and women and manifest in chests between 20 and 60 years of age. Spinal cord tumors are rarely seen in advanced elderly clients (American Association of Neuroscience Nurses [AANN], 1993).

Collaborative Management

 Assessment

➤ *Physical Assessment/Clinical Manifestations*

Clinical manifestations depend on the location of the tumor (Chart 45–11) and its rate of growth.

The most frequent complaint of the client with a spinal cord tumor is pain. Pain results from spinal cord compression, infiltration of the spinal tracts, or irritation of the spinal roots. The nurse assesses the quality, severity, and intensity of the pain. In addition, the nurse asks the client to describe factors that exacerbate and relieve the

---

Chart 45–11

Key Features of Spinal Cord Tumors

General
- Pain
- Sensory loss or impairment
- Motor loss or impairment
- Sphincter disturbance (bladder before bowel)

Cervical
- High cervical
  - Respiratory distress
  - Diaphragm paralysis
  - Occipital headache
  - Quadriparesis
  - Stiff neck
  - Nystagmus
  - Cranial nerve dysfunction
- Low cervical
  - Pain in the arms and the shoulders
  - Weakness
  - Paresthesia
  - Motor loss
  - Horner's syndrome
  - Increased reflexes

Thoracic
- Sensory loss
- Spastic paralysis
- Positive Babinski's sign
- Bladder and bowel dysfunction
- Pain in the chest and the back
- Muscle atrophy
- Muscle weakness in the legs
- Foot drop

Lumbosacral
- Low back pain
- Paresis
- Spastic paralysis
- Sensory loss
- Bladder and bowel dysfunction
- Sexual dysfunction
- Decreased-to-absent ankle and knee reflexes

---

pain. Radicular (nerve root) pain is described as stabbing or dull, with intermittent episodes of sharp, piercing pain. The pain may be increased when the client coughs, strains, or sneezes. Lying flat may increase pain as a consequence of stretching involved spinal nerve roots.

Involvement of the pyramidal (corticospinal) tract may lead to motor deficits. The nurse assesses for weakness, clumsiness, spasticity, and hyperactive reflexes and compares the responses on both sides of the body. Other presenting signs include ataxia, hypotonia, and a positive Babinski's sign. Spastic paralysis is seen most often, although a flaccid paralysis may be seen with tumors affecting the spinal roots, an intramedullary tumor in the enlargements of the cervical or lumbar area, or an extramedullary tumor complicated by spinal shock. A flaccid paralysis may also be noted in the presence of a cauda equina lesion.

The nurse also assesses for sensory loss on each side of the body and compares the responses. Early symptoms of sensory loss include a slowly progressive numbness or tingling, pain, and temperature loss. The sensory deficit is further marked by a decreased appreciation of touch, inability to sense vibration, and loss of position sense. The client often reports a tight, band-like feeling around the trunk. Brown-Séquard syndrome or central cord syndrome may be manifested (see earlier).

Loss of bladder control frequently precedes loss of bowel control in the client with a spinal cord tumor. Typically, bladder dysfunction is manifested by hesitancy, dribbling, incontinence, urgency, or acute retention. Bowel dysfunction is manifested by constipation. The nurse must remember that the client is often embarrassed to admit to bladder or bowel dysfunction.

A lesion in the sacral area may cause a decrease in genital sensation and thus impair the client's sexual function and enjoyment. Men may be unable to have an erection or to ejaculate.

➤ Diagnostic Assessment

A lumbar puncture (LP) is usually performed by the physician to obtain cerebrospinal fluid (CSF) for analysis. The LP is generally not performed until after a myelogram or computed tomography (CT) scan or magnetic resonance imaging (MRI) is done. The fluid obtained is generally xanthochromic; protein count is elevated and tumor cells may be present.

Routine x-rays or tomographic scans of the spine are obtained to detect a narrowing of the spinal canal, destruction of the vertebrae, or the presence of calcification. A myelogram, useful when a block is incomplete, indicates the level, extent, and boundaries of a tumor.

An MRI scan with and without enhancement provides more detail of the pathologic condition of the spinal cord than either a CT scan or myelography. Electromyography may help make a differential diagnosis to rule out multiple sclerosis or amyotrophic lateral sclerosis (ALS).

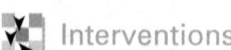 Interventions

Nursing care of the client with a spinal cord tumor includes obtaining vital signs and checking neurologic status at least every 4 hours and more often as clinically indicated. As for any client with a spinal cord problem, the nurse must pay meticulous attention to the client's motor and sensory status. The nurse reports any changes immediately to the physician.

➤ Surgical Management

The primary management modality is surgery. The goal of surgical intervention is to remove as much of the tumor as possible. Often this is not feasible and other treatment is indicated, such as radiation therapy. Emergency surgery is indicated if the client experiences a rapid loss of motor and sensory function as well as loss of bladder and bowel control. Table 45–1 summarizes the treatment of spinal cord tumors of various types and locations.

General preoperative care is performed (see Chap. 20). The nurse devotes particular attention to detailed documentation of the client's motor and sensory status.

The neurosurgeon, often in collaboration with an orthopedic surgeon, performs a laminectomy and surgical decompression and total or partial resection of the tumor. Depending on the extent of the tumor, a spinal fusion may be necessary. Occasionally, a cordotomy, or palliative sectioning of sensory roots, is done to control intractable pain. Laminectomies are discussed earlier in this chapter.

General postoperative care is provided, as discussed in Chapter 22. After surgery, the nurse assesses the client's vital signs and neurologic status every 1 to 2 hours until they are stable and then every 4 hours. The client is logrolled and repositioned every 2 hours. The nurse inspects the incision site for drainage and signs of infection. The client with a cervical cord tumor must also be carefully monitored for respiratory compromise. Postoperative nursing care for a client undergoing a laminectomy was discussed earlier in this chapter.

➤ Nonsurgical Management

Radiation Therapy. Radiation therapy may be necessary, depending on the tumor type. The spinal cord cannot tolerate high doses of radiation. Overexposure to radiation may lead to radiation myelopathy, which develops during 6 to 12 months. It is manifested by progressive spinal cord degeneration and neurologic deficits such as Brown-Séquard syndrome. With time, the client experiences spastic paralysis, loss of sensation, and bowel and bladder dysfunction; death may occur. (Care of the client undergoing radiation therapy is described in detail in Chapter 27.)

Pain Control. Pain control may be accomplished by pharmacologic and nonpharmacologic measures. Patient-controlled analgesia (PCA) with morphine or meperidine hydrochloride (Demerol) is frequently used to provide pain relief immediately postoperatively. The client is gradually switched to oral analgesics before discharge. The nurse assesses the client's level of pain, provides appropriate pain relief medication, and documents the client's response to the medication. If the drug therapy does not provide pain relief, the nurse collaborates with the health care provider to identify a more effective medication.

Turning and proper positioning of the client often enhance pain relief. The nurse or assistive nursing personnel provides range-of-motion (ROM) exercises to prevent atrophy and contractures, which can increase pain. Hypnosis, music therapy, and imagery techniques are other methods of pain relief that the client may use (see Chaps. 4 and 9).

Prevention of Complications of Immobility. The client who is immobilized from a spinal cord tumor or has spinal surgery is especially at risk for pressure sores and deep venous thrombosis (DVT) or pulmonary emboli. The nurse or assistive nursing personnel turns the client, while in bed, at least every 2 hours. When the client is sitting in a chair, the nurse repositions the client every 30 to 60 minutes. (Pressure relief measures are discussed more completely in Chapter 13.)

The nurse inspects the client's skin frequently to deter-

TABLE 45–1

Location and Treatment of Spinal Cord Tumors

Type	Location	Symptoms	Treatment
Extramedullary Tumors			
Vertebral hemangioma	• Thoracic or lumbar spine (more common in women; this type of tumor is essentially an atrioventricular shunt fed by the intercostal and lumbar arteries)	• Back pain • Paraparesis • Radicular pain	• Embolization of the mass followed by surgical excision
Meningioma	• Cervical or thoracic area (more common in women)	• Vague sensory loss • Midline back pain	• Resection of tumor • Radiation therapy
Chordoma	• Cervical or sacrococcygeal area	• Slow growing; locally invasive • Low back pain • Bowel or bladder dysfunction	• Resection of tumor • Unresponsive to radiation therapy
Schwannoma or neurofibroma	• Thoracic or cervical area	• Radicular pain • Motor weakness	• Surgical resection • Unresponsive to radiation therapy
Hemangioblastoma	• Thoracic area	• Progressive neurologic dysfunction • Motor weakness • Sensory dysfunction	• Surgical excision (prognosis is good)
Intramedullary Tumors			
Astrocytoma type I or II	• Cervical or thoracic area (slightly more common in men)	• Slowly progressive • May mimic multiple sclerosis • Back or neck pain • Paresthesia • Paresis	• Surgical excision and drainage of the cyst • Radiation therapy
Malignant astrocytoma		• Rapid neurologic deterioration • Pain • Paralysis • Sensory impairment	• Surgical excision • Radiation therapy • Chemotherapy (prognosis is poor)
Ependymoma	• Cauda equina or cervical area (more common in men)	• Slowly progressive; gradual onset • Back pain, worse at night • Radicular pain • Motor weakness • Sensory dysfunction	• Surgical excision • Radiation therapy (prognosis is good with total excision of the tumor)
Spinal Cysts			
Dermoid and epidermoid	• Conus medullaris or thoracic area (slightly more common in men)	• Back pain • Saddle anesthesia • Leg weakness • Sphincter dysfunction	• Surgical excision • May reoccur
Teratoma	• Lumbar area	• Progresive spastic paralysis	• Surgical excision
Lipoma	• Cervical and thoracic areas	• Sensory dysfunction	• Surgical excision

mine tolerance for sitting and to detect the presence of reddened areas. The reddened areas over the ischial tuberosities are blanched. If unable to blanch, the area is prone to breakdown. The nurse collaborates with physical and occupational therapists to determine the most appropriate positioning and exercise techniques and to assess the need for assistive devices. It may be necessary for the

client to be placed on a water bed or air bed to prevent or treat pressure ulcers.

The nurse assesses the client's lower extremities for indications of DVT. Sequential compression devices may be used in place of or as an adjunct to graduated compression stockings. The health care provider may order sodium heparin, 5000 units every 12 hours subcutaneously, or sodium warfarin (Coumadin, Warfilone✦) in therapeutic dosages to help prevent DVT or embolus formation.

Bowel and Bladder Program. The nurse asks the client about his or her normal defecation pattern. On the basis of the information from the client, the nurse establishes a bowel program. The essential elements of this program are

- A consistent time for bowel elimination
- A high fluid intake (2000 mL/day) unless fluid intake is restricted
- A high-fiber diet
- Rectal stimulation with or without suppositories
- If needed, stool softener medications, such as docusate sodium (Colace) and docusate sodium and casanthranol (Peri-Colace)

Manual disimpaction may be necessary if the client has lower motor neuron (LMN) symptoms.

The client's bladder program is determined by the specific dysfunction, usually urinary retention. The nurse or assistive nursing personnel monitors the client's voiding pattern and strictly measures and records intake and output. The nurse assesses the client for suprapubic distention and other indications of retention, such as overflow and dribbling. The client is encouraged to empty the bladder every 2 hours.

 ## Continuing Care

➤ *Home Care Management*

The nurse collaborates with the client and family members or significant others to identify and suggest corrections for potential hazards in the home. If necessary, referral is made to a home care nurse, social worker, or case manager to assess the need for structural alterations to the home. Structural alterations may be needed to accommodate ambulatory aids, such as a walker, and to enable the client to perform ADLs.

Some clients may be discharged from the acute care hospital to a rehabilitation setting, where they can learn to function as independently as possible. (Chapter 13 describes rehabilitation in detail.)

➤ *Health Teaching*

The teaching plan for the client with a spinal cord tumor depends on the level of dysfunction present. With decompression of the tumor, the severity of the client's symptoms often lessens. Deficits that may remain include mobility and sensory loss. Learning mobility skills can enable the client to negotiate movement on sidewalks and carpeting and other flooring surfaces. The client must also be able to negotiate sidewalk curbs independently. The physical or occupational therapist instructs the client in the correct use of all adaptive equipment. The nurse reinforces the individualized bowel and bladder program.

The goal of sexuality education in the acute care setting is to answer the client's questions and correct any misinformation. Unless the nurse has had specific training or experience in sexuality counseling of people with spinal cord tumors or injuries, more detailed questions should

be directed to a sexuality counselor. (Chapter 11 presents specific nursing interventions for clients needing sexuality counseling.)

➤ *Psychosocial Preparation*

The prognosis for the client with malignant tumors or secondary tumors is poor. The nurse determines what the physician and family members have told the client about diagnosis and prognosis. The nurse observes the client and listens for and records evidence that indicates the client needs information. The nurse can help the client prepare for discharge or transfer to a rehabilitation hospital by assisting the client to verbalize feelings and fears about prognosis, body image, self-concept, role performance, and self-esteem.

➤ *Health Care Resources*

Clients and family members or significant others should be referred to local, state or province, and national organizations for people with spinal cord injuries, which are applicable to spinal cord tumors. These groups often have information available for clients with spinal cord tumors. For clients with a malignancy, the nurse refers them to the American Cancer Society. Referral to support groups may also assist clients and family with adaptation to lifestyle changes.

MULTIPLE SCLEROSIS

Overview

Multiple sclerosis (MS) is a progressive degenerative disease that affects the myelin sheath and conduction pathway of the central nervous system (CNS). It is one of the leading causes of neurologic disability in persons 20 to 40 years of age. This chronic disease is characterized by periods of remission and exacerbation (flare). As the severity and the duration of the disease progress, the periods of exacerbation become more frequent.

Pathophysiology

Nerve impulses are transmitted from one nerve cell to another along unmyelinated fibers or via the nodes of Ranvier in myelinated axon fibers. In the presence of MS, the myelin sheath is damaged, causing an inflammatory response. The inflammation reduces the thickness of the myelin sheath. Impulses are still transmitted, but they are not as effective as before. The damaged myelin is then removed by astrocytes (scavenger cells). These cells form scar tissue, known as plaque, that interferes with normal pulse transmission.

The white fiber tracts that connect the neurons in the brain and spinal cord are generally involved. Especially affected areas include optic nerves, pyramidal tracts, posterior columns, brain stem nuclei, and the periventricular region of the brain. Although the myelin surrounding the axon is involved, the axon itself is relatively spared until late in the disease process, when scarring occurs. Initially, however, recovery of the myelin occurs with remission of symptoms. Eventually, with repeated exacerbations of the disease, damage becomes permanent.

Four types of MS are seen (Kelley, 1996):

- Benign or stable
- Relapsing-remitting
- Relapsing-progressive
- Chronic-progressive

Of clients with MS, 20% have the benign type and demonstrate no active disease or clinical deterioration in the preceding year. Those with benign MS present with a few episodes of mild attacks; there is minimal or no disability.

The classic picture of the relapsing-remitting type occurs in 25% of the cases of MS and is characterized by increasingly frequent attacks. The course of the disease may be mild or moderate, depending on the degree of disability. Relapses develop over 1 to 2 weeks, resolve over 4 to 8 months, and then return the client to baseline.

Relapsing-progressive MS occurs most frequently and is similar to the relapsing-remitting MS. It is characterized by the absence of periods of remission, and the client's condition does not return to baseline. Progressive, cumulative symptoms and deterioration occur during several years. This type of MS can convert to the chronic progressive type over time.

Chronic progressive MS is similar to relapsing-progressive MS, but its initial presentation is more insidious with spinal cord and cerebellar symptoms. At some point, it converts to a progressive course without periods of remission.

Etiology

The exact cause of MS remains unknown. Research continues on viral, immunologic, and genetic etiologic factors. The viral theory suggests that MS is caused by a slow virus that has been dormant for many years.

The immune theory suggests that an unidentified factor (probably a virus) triggers an autoimmune response in the CNS. Both humoral and cell-mediated immune system dysfunction have been implicated. This theory is supported by research data that immunoglobulin G (IgG) and oligoclonal bands in the CSF of clients with MS are elevated.

Although no genetic pattern of transmission has been found, genetic markers HLA-DR2 (on chromosome 6) and immunoglobulin Gm (on chromosome 14) are more frequently found in MS clients. The risk is greater if an identical twin has MS (Barker, 1994).

Incidence/Prevalence

Multiple sclerosis usually occurs in people between the ages of 20 and 40 years, although cases may occur in those younger than 15 years and older than 50 years. Approximately 350,000 people in the United States are currently affected. Women are affected slightly more often than men (Barker, 1994). MS is seen more often in the colder climates of the northeastern, Great Lakes, and Pacific northwestern states. Studies have indicated that if one relocates after the age of 15 years from an area of high incidence to one of a lower incidence, the risk factor

of the higher area is carried. For people younger than 15 years, the risk factor is not carried. These studies suggest that the risk factor for MS occurs about the age of 15 years. Life expectancy for those with MS is about 85% of that of the general population, or about 35 years after the onset of symptoms.

TRANSCULTURAL CONSIDERATIONS

 There is a greater prevalence of MS in Caucasians, and the disease is more common in higher socioeconomic groups than urban residents (AANN, 1993).

Collaborative Management

Assessment

➤ History

Multiple sclerosis often mimics other neurologic diseases. Therefore, obtaining a thorough history is essential for accurate diagnosis. The nurse begins by asking the client for a history of changes in vision, motor skills, and sensations, all early indicators of MS. The symptoms are often vague and nonspecific in the early stages of the disease. Of significance is the client's report that symptoms were first noticed several years earlier, but because they disappeared, medical attention was not sought. The nurse questions the client about the progression of symptoms, with particular attention to determining whether the symptoms are intermittent or whether they are becoming progressively worse. The nurse should find out the date (month and year) when the client first noticed the clinical manifestations.

Next, the nurse questions the client about factors that aggravate the symptoms, such as fatigue, stress, overexertion, temperature extremes, or a hot shower or bath. The client and the family are questioned about any personality or behavioral changes that have occurred (e.g., euphoria, poor judgment, inattentiveness). In addition, they are questioned about a family history of MS.

➤ Physical Assessment/Clinical Manifestations

Multiple sclerosis produces a wide variety of signs and symptoms. Any myelinated fibers of the brain and spinal cord may be affected. To determine a client's specific manifestations, the nurse performs a complete neurologic assessment.

Motor Assessment. First, the nurse assesses the client's motor status. The client often reports increased fatigue and stiffness of the extremities, particularly of the legs. Flexor spasms at night may awaken the client from sleep. Further examination of the client reveals increased, or hyperactive, deep tendon reflexes; clonus; positive Babinski's reflex; and absent abdominal reflexes. The client's gait may be unsteady owing to weakness of the legs and spasticity.

Significant cerebellar findings exhibited include intention tremor (tremor when performing an activity), dysmetria (inability to direct or limit movement), and dysdiadochokinesia (inability to stop one motor impulse and substitute another). Motor movements are often clumsy; the client may lose balance easily and may exhibit signs of poor coordination.

During examination of the cranial nerves and brain stem function, the client may report tinnitus, vertigo, and hearing loss. The client may show indications of facial weakness and have dysphagia. Speech problems include dysarthria, ataxia, and slow, scanning speech.

Typical clinical findings from assessment of the client's visual acuity, visual fields, and pupils include

- Blurred vision
- Diplopia
- Decreased visual acuity
- Scotomas (changes in peripheral vision)
- Nystagmus (involuntary, rapid eye movements)

Sensory Assessment. The sensory findings include hypalgesia (diminished sensitivity to pain), paresthesia, facial pain, and decreased temperature perception. The client may report numbness, tingling, burning, or crawling sensations.

If demyelination of the spinal cord has occurred, the client may experience bowel and bladder dysfunctions as well as alterations in sexuality. The client may have an areflexic bladder or experience frequency, urgency, or nocturia. Bowel problems include altered rectal tone and constipation as well as incontinence. Problems with sexuality include impotence, difficulty in sustaining an erection, and decreased vaginal secretion.

Cognitive Assessment. Finally, the nurse examines the client for mental status changes. Cognitive changes are usually seen late in the course of the disease and include decreased short-term memory, decreased concentration, decreased ability to perform calculations, inattentiveness, and impaired judgment. Chart 45–12 summarizes the common clinical manifestations of MS.

➤ Psychosocial Assessment

After the initial diagnosis of MS, the client is often anxious. Apathy, emotional lability, and depression are fairly common. The client may be euphoric or giddy, either as a result of the disease itself or because of the medications used to treat the disease. The nurse assesses the client's previously used coping and stress management skills in preparing the client for a chronic, usually debilitating disease. (Chapter 8 discusses stress and adaptation.)

➤ Laboratory Assessment

No one specific procedure is definitively diagnostic for MS. However, the collective results of a variety of tests are usually conclusive. During an acute attack, changes may be evident. Abnormal cerebrospinal fluid (CSF) findings include an elevated protein level and a slight increase in the white blood cell count. CSF electrophoresis reveals an increase in the myelin basic protein and the presence of oligoclonal bands (IgG). IgG bands are seen in most clients with MS.

➤ Other Diagnostic Assessment

The health care provider usually orders a computed tomography (CT) scan, which may show an increased den-

---

Chart 45–12

Key Features of Multiple Sclerosis

- Muscle weakness and spasticity
- Fatigue
- Intention tremors
- Dysmetria
- Numbness or tingling sensations (paresthesia)
- Hypalgesia
- Ataxia
- Dysarthria
- Dysphagia
- Diplopia
- Nystagmus
- Scotomas
- Decreased visual and hearing acuity
- Tinnitus, vertigo
- Bowel and bladder dysfunction
- Alterations in sexual function, such as impotence
- Cognitive changes, such as memory loss, impaired judgment, and decreased ability to solve problems or perform calculations

---

sity in the white matter and MS plaques. Magnetic resonance imaging (MRI) demonstrates the presence of plaques and is considered diagnostic for MS. However, a complete diagnostic evaluation is necessary to exclude other pathology.

Results of visual, auditory, and brain stem evoked potential studies are often abnormal. In people with advanced disease, the electromyogram findings may be grossly abnormal.

The diagnosis of MS is based on the presence of neurologic dysfunction in more than one area of the CNS and occurring over time combined with laboratory and neuroimaging assessment.

 Interventions

The client with MS is often weak and easily fatigued. The nurse teaches the client the importance of planning activities and allowing sufficient time to complete activities. For example, the client should check that all items needed for work are gathered before leaving the house. Items used on a daily basis should be easily accessible.

Exercise Program. In collaboration with physical and occupational therapists, an exercise program including range-of-motion (ROM) exercises and stretching and strengthening exercises is developed. The nurse encourages the client to ambulate as tolerated, using assistive ambulation devices as needed, including a cane, walker, wheelchair, or electric cart (Amigo). Additional assistive/adaptive devices may be needed to enable the client with tremor, spasticity, and weakness to remain independent in activities of daily living (ADLs). (Chapter 13 describes additional interventions to increase physical mobility and promote ADL independence.)

The nurse emphasizes the importance of avoiding rigorous activities that cause an increase in body temperature. Increased temperature may lead to increased fatigue as well as diminished motor ability and decreased visual acuity resulting from changes in the conduction abilities of the injured axons.

Drug Therapy. A variety of medications are used to treat and control the disease and attempt to slow its progression.

Steroid Therapy. The health care provider uses methylprednisolone (Solu-Medrol) to reduce edema and the inflammatory response. One gram is administered intravenously daily for 3, 5, or 7 days depending on the provider and the extent of the client's symptoms. These medications often decrease the length of time the client's symptoms are exacerbated and often improve the degree of recovery.

Common nursing interventions while the client is receiving these medications include

- Carefully monitoring fluid and electrolyte levels
- Testing the client's serum glucose concentration
- Providing dietary or supplemental potassium
- Observing for indications of gastrointestinal (GI) bleeding, such as gastric pain or blood in the stool
- Documenting any changes in personality (e.g., euphoria and insomnia)
- Minimizing the client's exposure to people with communicable or infectious diseases

Immunosuppressive Therapy. Immunosuppressive therapy with a combination of cyclophosphamide (Cytoxan) and methylprednisolone is used for the treatment of chronic progressive MS to stabilize the disease process. Research has shown interferon beta-1b (Betaseron) to decrease the frequency and severity of exacerbations. Interferon beta-1a (Avonex) has received Food and Drug Administration (FDA) approval for the treatment of relapsing forms of MS to slow the accumulation of physical disability and decrease frequency of exacerbations.

Adjunctive Drug Therapy. The health care provider may prescribe baclofen (Lioresal), diazepam (Valium, Apo-Diazepam✦), or dantrolene sodium (Dantrium) to lessen muscle spasticity. Severe spasticity may be treated with intrathecal baclofen administered through a surgically implanted pump. A surgical tendon release may also be performed by the physician if spasms prevent the client from learning mobility and ADL skills.

Paresthesia may be treated with carbamazepine (Tegretol) or tricyclic antidepressants (amitriptyline). Propranolol hydrochloride (Inderal) and clonazepam (Klonopin) have been used to treat cerebellar ataxia. If fatigue cannot be controlled through the use of nondrug measures, amantadine hydrochloride (Symmetrel) may be prescribed.

Complementary Therapies. A number of complementary therapies have been reported by clients with MS to be successful in minimizing their symptoms, including bee stings and nutritional supplements. These modalities are being researched for their efficacy.

Interventions for Visual Disturbances. An eyepatch that is alternated from eye to eye every few hours usually relieves diplopia. If the client has peripheral visual deficits, the nurse teaches scanning techniques by having the client move his or her head from side to side. Changes in visual acuity may be assisted by corrective lenses.

The nurse or assistive nursing personnel orients the client to the environment and keeps it free from clutter. The environment should be as standardized as possible to enable the client to memorize or to anticipate the placement of objects.

 Continuing Care

➤ Home Care Management

To help the client maintain maximum strength, function, and independence, continuity of care through an interdisciplinary team in both the rehabilitation and home setting is necessary. Admission to a rehabilitation center is brief but usually provides a program to improve functional ability. In collaboration with the discharge planner and the occupational therapist, the nurse or case manager assesses the client's home for any hazards before discharge. Any items that might interfere with mobility, such as scatter rugs, are removed. In addition, care must be taken to prevent injury resulting from visual problems. The home environment should remain as structured and free from clutter as possible. Later, as the disease progresses, the home may need to be adapted for wheelchair accessibility. Any assistive or adaptive device needed by the client should be available before discharge from the hospital.

➤ Health Teaching

The health care provider explains to the client and family the development of MS and those factors that may exacerbate the symptoms. The importance of avoiding overexertion, stress, extremes of temperatures, high humidity, and people with upper respiratory tract infections is emphasized. The nurse explains all medications to be taken on discharge, including time and route of administration, dosage, purpose, and side effects. The client is taught how to differentiate expected side effects from adverse or allergic reactions and is given the name of a resource person to call if questions arise. Written instructions are provided as a resource to the client and caregivers at home.

The physical therapist develops an exercise program appropriate for the client's tolerance level. The client is instructed in techniques for self-care, daily living skills, and the use of required adaptive equipment. The nurse should also include information on the following programs: bowel and bladder management, skin care, nutrition, and positioning techniques. (Chapter 13 describes these aspects of chronic illness and rehabilitation in detail.)

The client is taught to obtain adequate rest and to avoid undue stress. It is equally important for the client to engage in regular social diversional activities. Often the client is anxious about discharge from the hospital and worries about how long the remission will last or when the disease will progress further.

Because personality changes are not unusual, the nurse teaches the family or significant others strategies that enable them to cope with these changes. For example, the family may develop a nonverbal signal to alert the client of potentially inappropriate behavior (e.g., a talkative person may be reminded to be quiet if a family member displays a prearranged signal). This action avoids embarrassment for the client.

➤ Health Care Resources

The client with MS is able to live independently in the early stages of the disease. As the client's condition deteriorates, the assistance of a home care nurse or a family member may be required (see Research Applications for Nursing). Another alternative may be placement in a long-term care facility.

The nurse or case manager refers the client and family members or significant others to the local and national MS societies. Other community resources available include meal delivery services (e.g., Meals on Wheels),

transportation services for the disabled, and homemaker services.

AMYOTROPHIC LATERAL SCLEROSIS

Overview

Amyotrophic lateral sclerosis (ALS), also known as Lou Gehrig's disease, is a progressive degenerative disease involving the motor system. It is characterized by atrophy of the hands, forearms, and legs. The disease results in paralysis and death. There is no known cause, no cure, no specific treatment, no standard pattern of progression, and no method of prevention (Shpritz, 1996). Unlike the case with many other neural degenerative diseases, the sensory and autonomic nervous systems are not involved. Mental status changes do not result from the disease.

Amyotrophic lateral sclerosis may occur at any age. The incidence in the United States is 1.5 per 100,000. The usual age of onset is between 40 and 70 years. ALS is more prevalent in men than women. Death typically occurs within 3 to 5 years after the onset of symptoms and is attributable to respiratory failure.

The cause of the disease is unknown. Researchers are exploring many theories, including viral, bacterial, genetic, metabolic, neurotoxins, minerals, hormones, and defects in the immune system. Findings suggest that the metabolism of a potential toxic amino acid, glutamate, is abnormal in ALS clients. Genetic research has found that the genes that normally destroy toxic free radicals may be defective in ALS clients.

Collaborative Management

 Assessment

The clinical manifestations of ALS include fatigue, muscle atrophy, and weakness. Early symptoms include
- Fatigue while talking
- Tongue atrophy
- Dysphagia
- Weakness of the hands and arms
- Fasciculations of the face
- Nasal quality of speech
- Dysarthria

As the disease progresses, muscle atrophy, particularly of the trapezius and sternocleidomastoid muscles, develops. Muscle weakness and atrophy extend until a flaccid quadriplegia develops. Eventually, the respiratory muscles become involved, leading to respiratory compromise, pneumonia, and death.

Diagnosis is based on clinical and diagnostic test findings and by ruling out other causes of the motor changes. There is no specific test to diagnose ALS. The electromyogram demonstrates fibrillations and fasciculations of the muscles. A muscle biopsy specimen typically demonstrates small, angulated, atrophic fibers. Other diagnostic studies reveal motor strength deficits in serial muscle testing; abnormal pulmonary function test results, such as a decreased vital capacity (less than 2 L); and dysphagia.

▷ Research Applications for Nursing

Caregivers Use Coping Strategies in Meeting Needs of Persons with MS

Gullick, E. E. (1995). Coping among spouses or significant others of persons with multiple sclerosis. Nursing Research, 4(4), 220–225.

Meeting the dependency needs of persons with MS in managing everyday activities is frequently reported by caregivers to be overwhelming, yet little is known about how spouses or significant others cope with this responsibility. The purposes of this study were to identify the coping strategies used by caregivers of persons with MS and to determine whether differences existed among the coping strategies with respect to frequency used, dependency status of the person with MS, presence or absence of illness in the caregiver, and the person's gender and relationship to the person with MS.

Results indicate that spouses and significant others differed in the types of coping strategies used. The dependence of the person with MS on the caregiver and the health status of the caregiver influenced the frequency and type of coping strategies used.

Critique. Although the study used a convenience sample, Dr. Gullick explored an issue that has a great impact on the well-being of both the client and the caregivers.

Possible Nursing Implications. The impact of MS on spouses and significant others cannot be underestimated. The need for factual information to assist with problem solving is great. Counseling and health teaching the caregivers as to the total impact that the illness can have on family dynamics is essential.

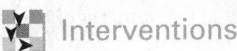 Interventions

There is no known cure for ALS, and treatment is symptomatic. Riluzole (Rilutek) was approved by the FDA as the only drug for use with ALS clients. It is not a cure, but it does extend survival time. Nursing interventions are directed toward preventing complications of immobility and promoting comfort. In addition, the nurse provides ongoing support and counseling to the client and the family as they begin to cope with the impact of this terminal disease.

POLIOMYELITIS

Overview

Poliomyelitis (polio) is an acute viral disease characterized by destruction of the motor cells of the anterior horn of the spinal cord, the brain stem, and the motor strip in the frontal lobe. This communicable disease may be relatively asymptomatic or may lead to paralysis or death. The incubation period is 7 to 10 days.

The virus is transmitted either through droplet infection or via the fecal or oral route and the gastrointestinal (GI) tract. After the virus enters the body, it settles in the lymph nodes of the throat and the ileum and multiplies. The virus then invades the CNS, causing inflammation, scarring, and shrinking of the cell body of the involved motor cell. If the disease progresses, necrosis of the neuron occurs and results in permanent neurologic dysfunction.

Poliomyelitis, although rare in North America today, is seen most often in the summer and fall months. It affects males more often than females; male clients are more at risk for paralysis. The disease can be prevented by immunization with Salk's or Sabin's vaccine. The importance of immunization against this disease cannot be underestimated. Outbreaks of poliomyelitis continue to occur throughout the world; with the ease of travel in today's world, poliomyelitis can easily be introduced back into North America.

Collaborative Management

The clinical manifestations of poliomyelitis include
- Fever
- Chills
- Excessive perspiration
- Severe muscle aches and weakness, especially of the legs, neck, and back
- Drowsiness
- Irritability
- Increased deep tendon reflexes
- Abdominal tenderness
- Nausea
- Vomiting
- Dysphagia
- Headache

Diagnosis is made on the basis of the clinical presentation and positive throat or stool cultures for the poliovirus.

Treatment is symptomatic. Analgesics are prescribed to relieve pain. Antibiotics may be indicated to prevent secondary infections. Nursing interventions are directed at providing supportive care and preventing the complications of immobility. The client's respiratory status is carefully monitored to prevent respiratory arrest resulting from paralysis of the muscles of respiration.

Postpolio Syndrome

A syndrome known as postpolio syndrome or postpolio sequelae (PPS) has been identified in people who have recovered from poliomyelitis. It refers to the new onset of weakness, pain, and fatigue in polio survivors, 10 to 40 years after the initial episode of the disease. The exact cause is not known. Decompensation, exhaustion, and loss of overworked motor neurons may contribute to PPS. Temporary or permanent disability can result from PPS.

The client suspected of having or being predisposed to PPS should have a complete physical examination and diagnostic tests for muscular, neurologic, and pulmonary function. If test results are abnormal, the interdisciplinary health care team teaches the client how to make lifestyle modifications to preserve energy and physiologic function. Swimming in warm water is widely recommended to promote comfort and flexibility. Adaptive and orthotic devices may be needed to prevent high energy consumption and maintain muscle function.

Having PPS is a frightening experience. The client who survived the initial disease has to face the chronic, potentially debilitating sequelae. Support groups are becoming readily available around the United States, and information is available through the Polio Network News.

CASE STUDY with Critical Thinking Exercises

▪ John Oswald is a 35-year-old construction worker who was admitted to your unit after an on-the-job accident. He was diagnosed with a herniated nucleus pulposus at L4–5 and had a lumbar diskectomy. This is Mr. Oswald's first hospitalization. He is married and has a 4-year-old daughter. His wife, Connie, is a school teacher. He has just returned from the PACU.

QUESTIONS:

1. What is a herniated nucleus pulposus? How would you explain it to John and his wife?
2. What are your priorities in planning your nursing interventions for John?
3. How would you get John out of bed safely?
4. What referrals do you feel are essential for Mr. Oswald in planning his return home?

SELECTED BIBLIOGRAPHY

Abel, N. A., & Smith, R. A. (1994). Intrathecal baclofen for treatment of intractable spinal spasticity. *Archives of Physical Medicine & Rehabilitation, 75*(1), 54–58.

Adsit, P. A., & Bishop, C. (1995). Autonomic dysreflexia—Don't let it be a surprise. *Orthopaedic Nursing, 14*(3), 17–20.

*American Association of Neuroscience Nurses. (1993). *Core curriculum for neuroscience nursing.* Chicago: Author.

Arbour, R. (1994). Laser and ultrasound technology in aggressive management of central nervous system tumors. *Journal of Neuroscience Nursing, 26*(1), 30–35.

Azouvi, P., Mane, M., et al. (1996). Intrathecal baclofen administration for control of severe spinal spasticity: Functional improvement and long-term follow-up. *Archives of Physical Medicine & Rehabilitation, 77*(1), 35–39.

Barker, E. (1994). *Neuroscience nursing.* St. Louis: C. V. Mosby.

Bartfeld, H., & Mo, D. (1996). Recognizing post-polio syndrome. *Hospital Practice,* May 15, 95–116.

Bensimon, G., Lacomblez, L., & Meininger, V. (1994). A controlled trial of riluzole in amyotrophic lateral sclerosis. ALS/riluzole study group. *New England Journal of Medicine, 330*(9), 585–591.

Bigos, S., Bowyer, Q., Braen, G., et al. (1994a). *Acute low back problems in adults: Clinical practice guideline No. 14* (AHCPR Publication No. 95-0642). Rockville, MD: Agency for Health Care Policy and Research, Public Health Service, U.S. Department of Health and Human Services.

Bigos, S., Bowyer, Q., Braen, G., et al. (1994b). *Acute low back problems in adults: Clinical practice guideline, quick reference guide No. 14* (AHCPR Publication No. 95-0643). Rockville, MD: Agency for Health Care Policy and Research, Public Health Service, U.S. Department of Health and Human Services.

Canobbio, M. M. (1996). *Mosby's handbook of patient teaching.* St. Louis: C. V. Mosby.

Day, L. (1995). Gene therapy for ALS. *Journal of Neuroscience Nursing, 27*(4), 260.

Dobkin, B. H. (1996). *Neurologic rehabilitation.* Philadelphia: FA Davis.

Fowler, S. B. (1995). Deep vein thrombosis and pulmonary emboli in neuroscience patients. *Journal of Neuroscience Nursing, 27*(1), 224–228.

Gilbert, M., & Counsell, C. M. (1995). Coordinated care for the SCI patient. *SCINursing, 12*(3), 87–89.

Good, D. M., Bower, D. A., & Einsporn, R. L. (1995). Social support: Gender differences in MS spousal caregivers. *Journal of Neuroscience Nursing, 27*(5), 305–311.

Greene, D., Chen, D., et al. (1994). Prevention of thromboembolism in spinal cord injury: Role of low molecular weight heparin. *Archives of Physical Medicine & Rehabilitation, 75*(3), 290–292.

Gullick, E. E. (1995). Coping among spouses or significant others of persons with multiple sclerosis. *Nursing Research, 44*(4), 220–225.

Halstead, L. S., & Grimby, G. (1995). *Post-polio syndrome.* St. Louis: C. V. Mosby.

Hesslegrave, B. (1997). Case management and spinal cord management. *The Case Manager, 8*(3), 89–94.

Hodge, A. L. (1995). Addressing issues of sexuality with spinal cord injured persons. *Orthopaedic Nursing, 14*(3), 21–24.

IFNB Multiple Sclerosis Study Group and the University of British Columbia MS/MRI Analysis Group. (1995). Interferon beta 1-b in the treatment of multiple sclerosis. *Neurology, 45*(7), 1277–1285.

Kahanovitz, N., & Pashos, C. L. (1996). The role of implantable direct current stimulation in the critical pathway for lumbar spinal fusion. *The Journal of Care Management, 2*(6), 46–48, 53–54, 56, 58.

Kelley, C. L. (1996). The role of interferon in the treatment of MS. *Journal of Neuroscience Nursing, 28*(2), 114–120.

Kelley, C. L., & Smeltzer, S. C. (1994). Betaseron: The new MS treatment. *Journal of Neuroscience Nursing, 26*(1), 52–56.

Kuehn, A. F., & Winters, R. K. (1994). A study of symptom distress, health locus of control, and coping resources of aging post-polio survivors. *Image—The Journal of Nursing Scholarship, 26*(4), 325–331.

Malmivaara, M. D., et al. (1995). The treatment of low back pain—Bedrest, exercise, or ordinary activity? *New England Journal of Medicine, 332*(6), 351–355.

Marciano, F. F., Greene, K. A., Aposolides, P. J., Dickman, C. A., & Sonntag, V. K. H. (1995). Pharmacological management of spinal cord injuries: Review of the literature. *BNI Quarterly, 11*(2), 2–11.

Schultz, D. L. (1995). The role of the neuroscience nurse in lumbar fusion. *Journal of Neuroscience Nursing, 27*(2), 90–95.

Segatore, M. (1995). The skeleton after spinal cord injury. Part 1. Theoretical aspects. *SCINursing, 12*(3), 82–86.

Shaddinger, D. E. (1995). An acute spinal cord injury: My family's experience. *Journal of Neuroscience Nursing, 27*(4), 236–239.

Shpritz, D. W. (1996). *Delmar's rapid nursing intervention—Neurologic.* Albany, NY: Delmar Publishers.

Spoltone, T. A., & O'Brien, A. M. (1995). Rehabilitation of the spinal cord injured patient. *Orthopaedic Nursing, 14*(3), 7–16.

Stice, K. A., & Cunningham, C. A. (1995). Pulmonary rehabilitation with respiratory complications of post-polio syndrome. *Rehabilitation Nursing, 20*(1), 37–42.

Stone, L. A., Frank, J. A., Albert, P. S., et al. (1995). The effect of interferon-B on blood-brain barrier disruptions demonstrated by contract-enhanced magnetic resonance imaging in relapsing-remitting multiple sclerosis. *Annals of Neurology, 37*(5), 611–619.

Tompkins, J. A. (1997). High and low tech case management for the spinal cord injured patient. *The Case Manager, 8*(3), 83–88.

Werner, P. (1997). New medications for brain and spinal cord injury: Minimizing the second injury. *The Journal of Care Management, 3*(1), 46–56.

SUGGESTED READINGS

Shaddinger, D. E. (1995). An acute spinal cord injury: My family's experience. *Journal of Neuroscience Nursing, 27*(4), 236–239.

In this article, the author shares a personal experience of an acute spinal cord injury, which resulted in paraplegia for her brother after an accident 12 years ago. Through the use of a journal, Ms. Shaddinger kept track of what the experience was like for her and her family. The support and love of family, flexibility of visiting hours, and being kept informed of her brother's progress were most important to the family's coping with this devastating event.

Hesslegrave, B. (1997). Case managers and spinal cord management. *The Case Manager, 8*(3), 89–94.

This article describes the role of the case manager in the care of the client with spinal cord injury (SCI). Resources for SCI rehabilitation are provided as is a CEU quiz at the end of the article.

INTERVENTIONS FOR CLIENTS WITH PROBLEMS OF THE PERIPHERAL NERVOUS SYSTEM

Peripheral nervous system (PNS) disorders range in severity from life-threatening conditions, such as Guillain-Barré syndrome and myasthenia gravis (which may require intensive nursing care), to relatively benign conditions, such as polyneuritis, peripheral nerve trauma, and cranial nerve disorders (e.g., trigeminal neuralgia and Bell's palsy). Although hospitalization is rarely required for these less serious dysfunctions, the nurse may encounter them as secondary disorders in hospitalized clients as well as in clients in outpatient (ambulatory) or community settings. These conditions may be extremely painful, and disfigurement may result.

Guillain-Barré Syndrome

Overview

Guillain-Barré syndrome (GBS) is an acute inflammatory process characterized by varying degrees of motor weakness and paralysis. It may be referred to by a variety of other names such as *acute idiopathic polyneuritis* and *polyradiculoneuropathy*.

In this condition, the client's life and ultimate potential for rehabilitation depend almost entirely on the effectiveness of nursing care. The nurse's expertise in providing care, monitoring for and preventing complications, and offering emotional support to the client and significant others is essential. With skilled care, the mortality rate can be very low. Mortality generally results from complications of respiratory compromise, such as pulmonary emboli or respiratory arrest.

Pathophysiology

In Guillain-Barré syndrome, the immune system starts to destroy the myelin sheath that surrounds the axons. Segmental demyelination, the destruction of myelin between the nodes of Ranvier, is the major pathologic finding in GBS. Saltatory conduction, the leaping of impulses from node to node of Ranvier, is thus affected. The result is dispersion of impulses, slow conduction velocities, or conduction block in the late stages of the disease. Although the heavily myelinated cranial and motor nerves are affected more frequently than are the thinly myelinated pain, touch, and temperature nerve fibers, sensory function is often affected. Additionally, the brain may receive inappropriate sensory signals, resulting in tingling, "crawling skin," or pain.

On microscopic examination, aggregates of lymphocytes are seen at the points of myelin breakdown, yet the axons usually remain intact. In some instances, there may be secondary damage to the cell body, the neurilemma, or the axon; this can delay recovery or result in permanent deficits.

Three stages make up the *acute* course of GBS:

- The *initial period* (1–3 weeks), which begins with the onset of the first definitive symptoms and ends when no further deterioration is noted
- The *plateau period* (several days to 2 weeks)
- The *recovery phase* (4–6 months), which is thought to coincide with remyelination and axonal regeneration

Chronic inflammatory demyelinating polyneuropathy (CIDP) is a type of GBS that progresses over a longer period; complete recovery rarely occurs. The condition in which relapsing attacks of GBS occur, called chronic relapsing polyneuropathy, is treated with prednisone, 100 mg every day, tapering slowly to 10–20 mg every day, based on clinical improvement.

Etiology

The cause of GBS remains obscure. Most of the evidence implicates a cell-mediated immunologic reaction. Research suggests that the humoral immune system is involved as well. Defects of T lymphocytes (T cells) and B lymphocytes (B cells) of the lymphatic system may be the basis of the syndrome. T cells are responsible for cell-mediated immunity and the phagocytosis of bacteria. B lymphocytes produce and secrete immunoglobulin, which form the humoral arm of the immune system. Normally, these antibodies combine with antigens, such as viruses, and prevent the organisms from having a harmful effect. This antigen-antibody combination also induces an inflammatory reaction by attracting T cells.

The client with GBS often relates a history of acute illness, trauma, surgery, or immunization 1 to 8 weeks before the onset of neurologic signs and symptoms. Other risk factors identified in epidemiologic studies include an upper respiratory tract infection or gastrointestinal (GI) illness in 50% of cases and positive antibodies to cytomegalovirus or Epstein-Barr virus. It is believed that the prodromal (earlier) event causes a limited malfunction of the immune system, which sensitizes the T cells to the client's myelin. In response to several antigens, some clients apparently form a demyelinating antibody that has a direct toxic effect on nerves or attracts a cellular immune response; this ultimately destroys myelin (Hickey, 1996).

Incidence/Prevalence

The annual incidence of GBS is approximately 1.9 cases per 100,000 population in the United States. It generally affects people between the ages of 30 and 50 years; men and women are equally affected. The mortality rate in the elderly is 5% higher than in the general population. GBS is seen more frequently in clients with Hodgkin's disease, systemic lupus erythematosus, and human immunodeficiency virus infection.

In 3%–10% of cases, a chronic or recurrent GBS develops. The chronic syndrome has been linked to the

use of immunosuppressive agents, such as corticosteroid (e.g., prednisone [Deltasone, Winpred✦]) or cyclophosphamide (Cytoxan), for the treatment of this disorder.

TRANSCULTURAL CONSIDERATIONS

 Guillain-Barré syndrome (GBS) has worldwide distribution, is not seasonal, and affects people of all races and ages. Higher rates, however, have been noted in people 45 years of age or older. The incidence of the disease is 50%–60% higher in Caucasians than in African-Americans (Giger & Davidhizar, 1995).

Collaborative Management

Assessment

➤ History

In addition to biographical data, such as age, sex, and cultural background, the nurse collects a complete medical and surgical history. Any antecedent illness (infection or other illness) 1–8 weeks before the onset of GBS is explored. The nurse asks the client to describe the symptoms in chronologic order, if possible.

➤ Physical Assessment/Clinical Manifestations

Manifestations of GBS depend on the degree of weakness and progression of symptoms.

Common Clinical Manifestations. Although features may vary (Chart 46–1), most people with GBS relate an abrupt onset. Typically, GBS does not affect

---

Chart 46–1

Key Features of Guillain-Barré Syndrome

Motor Manifestations

Ascending symmetric muscle weakness → flaccid paralysis without muscle atrophy
Decreased or absent deep tendon reflexes (DTRs)
Respiratory compromise (dyspnea, diminished breath sounds, decreased tidal volume and vital capacity) and failure
Loss of bowel and bladder control (less common)

Sensory Manifestations

Paresthesias
Pain (cramping)

Cranial Nerve Manifestations

Facial weakness
Dysphagia
Diplopia
Difficulty speaking

Autonomic Manifestations

Labile blood pressure
Cardiac dysrhythmias
Tachycardia

the client's level of consciousness, cerebral function, or pupillary signs.

Clinical Variations. The clinical variations of GBS reflect the areas of earliest or most severe involvement. *Ascending* GBS is the most common clinical pattern. Weakness and paresthesia begin in the lower extremities and progress upward to include the trunk and arms or affect the cranial nerves. The client may exhibit symptoms of an ascending flaccidity or weakness, evolving over a period of hours to several days (1–10 days). The extent of the motor deficit ranges from mild paresis to total quadriplegia. In about half of these cases, the client experiences some degree of respiratory compromise. Although they may be diminished during the initial assessment, deep tendon reflexes are absent in limbs that become paralyzed. *Pure motor* GBS is identical to the ascending variant, except sensory signs and symptoms are absent.

In clients with *descending* GBS, the nurse initially observes weakness of the face or bulbar muscles of the jaw, the sternocleidomastoid muscles (head rotators), and the muscles of the tongue, pharynx, and larynx. Weakness progresses downward to involve the limbs. This type may quickly affect the client's respiratory function. The nurse carefully monitors the client for breathlessness during speech, shallow respirations, dyspnea, and decreased tidal volume.

This variation often includes ophthalmoplegia (paralysis or weakness of the eye muscles), causing diplopia, or, if the pupillary response to light is affected, functional blindness may result. Thus, the nurse assesses visual function while providing information, explanation, and support to the client experiencing visual disturbances. In this variation, numbness is more common in the hands than in the feet. Deep tendon reflexes are decreased or absent.

The *Miller-Fisher variant* consists of a triad of ophthalmoplegia (paralysis of ocular [eye] muscles), areflexia (no reflexes), and severe ataxia (defective muscle coordination). The client's motor strength and sensory function are normal. The client's pupillary response to light is occasionally affected by the ophthalmoplegia, which results in functional blindness. Although respiratory complications are rare in clients with this variant, respiratory function is monitored frequently.

With any of the variants, *cranial nerve* involvement most often affects the facial nerve (cranial nerve VII). Involvement of the facial nerve results in the inability to smile, frown, whistle, or drink from a straw. In addition to monitoring these functions of cranial nerve VII, the nurse assesses the client for dysphagia and paralysis of the larynx. Less frequently affected cranial nerves include the glossopharyngeal (IX), vagus (X), spinal accessory (XI), and hypoglossal (XII). The client's inability to cough, gag, or swallow results from involvement of cranial nerves IX and X. The nurse monitors the client closely for varying blood pressure (hypertensive and hypotensive episodes or postural hypotension) and tachycardia. These symptoms are characteristic of *autonomic dysfunction,* which is linked to vagus nerve (X) deficit. The nurse assesses cranial nerve XI (spinal accessory) by asking the client to perform shoulder shrugs. Hypoglossal nerve (XII)

deficit is evidenced by deviation or paralysis of the tongue.

➤ Psychosocial Assessment

In addition to determining the client's usual roles and responsibilities, occupation, motivation, and available support systems, the nurse assesses the client's ability to cope with this devastating illness and the accompanying fear and anxiety. Generally, the disease is self-limiting and the paralysis is temporatry in nature.

➤ Laboratory Assessment

Although no single clinical or laboratory finding confirms the diagnosis of Guillain-Barré syndrome (GBS), the physician performs a lumbar puncture to evaluate cerebrospinal fluid (CSF). Albuminocytologic dissociation, an increase in CSF protein level without an increase (or only a slight to moderate increase) in the cell count, is a distinguishing feature of GBS. However, high protein levels may not be noted until after 1–2 weeks of illness, reaching a peak in 4–6 weeks. The CSF lymphocyte count is normal.

Peripheral blood tests may show a moderate leukocytosis early in the illness. The number of leukocytes rapidly returns to normal in the absence of complications or concurrent illness. The erythrocyte sedimentation rate (ESR) is typically within normal limits.

➤ Other Diagnostic Assessment

Electrophysiologic studies demonstrate demyelinating neuropathy. The degree of abnormality found on testing does not always correlate with the clinical severity. Within 3 weeks of symptoms, nerve conduction velocities are depressed. Denervated potentials (fibrillations) develop in some cases later in the illness. Electromyographic (EMG) findings, which reflect peripheral nerve function, are normal early in the illness. Electrophysiologic changes appear only after denervation of muscle has been present for 4 weeks or longer.

Respiratory function is frequently compromised in clients with GBS. Vital capacity may be decreased, and arterial blood gas values may be abnormal (decreased PaO_2, increased $PaCO_2$, or increased pH).

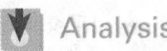 Analysis

➤ Common Nursing Diagnoses and Collaborative Problems

The common nursing diagnoses pertinent to clients with GBS are

1. Ineffective Breathing Pattern, Ineffective Airway Clearance, and Impaired Gas Exchange related to respiratory muscle weakness or paralysis, inability to cough and deep breathe effectively, and immobility
2. Impaired Physical Mobility related to weakness, paralysis, and ataxia

3. Pain related to paresthesia
4. Impaired Verbal Communication related to intubation or paralysis of the muscles required for speech
5. Powerlessness related to the inability to perform activities of daily living (ADL) and usual role responsibilities
6. Anxiety related to powerlessness, uncertain prognosis, and fear of the unknown
7. Anticipatory Grieving related to loss of function and inability to perform usual roles and responsibilities
8. Self Care Deficit (level depends on extent and stage of disease) related to weakness or paralysis

➤ Additional Nursing Diagnoses and Collaborative Problems

In addition to the common nursing diagnoses, the client may also have one or more of the following nursing diagnoses:

- Impaired Home Maintenance Management related to lack of knowledge or inadequate support systems
- Sensory/Perceptual Alterations (Tactile, Kinesthetic, and Visual) related to paresthesia and diplopia
- Risk for Impaired Skin Integrity related to altered sensation, altered nutrition, or immobility
- Body Image Disturbance and Self Esteem Disturbance related to loss of body function, physical changes, and dependency
- Altered Nutrition: Less than Body Requirements related to difficulty chewing, dysphagia, paralysis of extremities, anxiety, or depression
- Risk for Fluid Volume Deficit related to cranial nerve paralysis, dysphagia, and paralysis of the extremities
- Constipation, Diarrhea, or Bowel Incontinence related to inadequate oral intake, immobility, and impaired communication
- Decreased Cardiac Output related to autonomic dysfunction

A possible collaborative problem is Potential for Respiratory Paralysis which results in death if the disorder is not managed.

 Planning and Implementation

➤ Ineffective Breathing Pattern, Ineffective Airway Clearance, Impaired Gas Exchange

Planning: Expected Outcomes. The desired outcomes are that the client is expected to have an effective air exchange, have a vital capacity within acceptable limits, and have arterial blood gas levels within normal limits.

Interventions. In the acute (initial) phase, the nurse monitors the client closely, generally in a critical care unit, for signs of respiratory distress, such as dyspnea, air hunger, confusion (resulting from hypoxia), and cyanosis. In addition, the nurse monitors respiratory rate, rhythm, and depth every 1–4 hours; checks the client's vital capacity every 2–4 hours; and auscultates the lungs at 4-hour intervals.

Arterial blood gas values are monitored for acid-base abnormalities and decreasing oxygen saturation. Deterioration of vital capacity to less than 15–20 mL/kg and the inability to clear secretions may be indications for elective intubation. Equipment for performing an endotracheal intubation and a ventilator are kept available in case of respiratory emergency.

The nurse maintains (or assists the client to maintain) a patent airway by correct positioning, suctioning, and adjusting endotracheal or nasotracheal airways. For prevention of infection, sterile technique is maintained in suctioning the client. The nurse or assistant nursing personnel assesses and documents the color, consistency, and amount of secretions. Chest physiotherapy and frequent position changes are combined with breathing exercises (coughing and deep breathing) to prevent pneumonia and atelectasis. Oxygen may be administered by nasal cannula at a flow rate prescribed by the health care provider.

➤ Impaired Physical Mobility

Planning: Expected Outcomes. The outcomes are that the client is expected to participate, actively or passively, in mobilization and not experience complications related to immobility.

Interventions. During the initial period, when symptoms may be developing rapidly, the nurse assesses motor (muscle) function every 2–4 hours. A reproducible method that is readily understood by all members of the health care team is used for this assessment, such as Lovett's scale for determining muscle strength (see Table 52–1). Nursing interventions to provide for mobility and prevent complications depend on the degree of motor deficit. To ensure the client's safety, the nurse assists with ambulation, transfers from bed to chair, position changes, and maintenance of proper body alignment. The nurse always encourages maximal independence. Range-of-motion (ROM) exercises are performed actively or passively every 2–4 hours. The nurse instructs family members in these techniques.

Because pulmonary emboli are frequent complications of immobility, the health care provider may prescribe subcutaneous heparin injections every 12 hours. Antiembolism stockings are used to promote venous return. The nurse or assistant nursing personnel removes the stockings at least once every 24 hours for 15–30 minutes and observes the client's skin condition and circulation. Other prevention measures are determined by agency policy or health care provider preference.

Drug Therapy. The treatment of GBS depends on ventilatory assistance and supportive nursing care. In most cases, the disease is self-limiting and recovery is complete. Adrenocorticotropic hormone (ACTH), 25–40 units three times a day intramuscularly or subcutaneously, shortens the syndrome's duration, although further investigation is needed to determine its therapeutic usefulness. Treatment with immunoglobins has shown promising success to the point that it may replace the need for plasmapheresis. Immunoglobin therapy side effects include such minor annoyances as mild fever, myalgia, and headache, to major complications such as aseptic meningitis, retinal necrosis, and acute renal failure.

Plasmapheresis. In the method of plasmapheresis, plasma is selectively separated from whole blood. The blood cells are returned to the client without the plasma. Plasma ususally replaces itself or the client is transfused with normal plasma or a colloidal substitute. Plasmapheresis removes the circulating antibodies thought responsible for the disease. Immune human serum globulin (gamma globulin) may be given to restore serum antibodies removed during the treatment. The use of this measure has resulted in reductions in

- Length of hospitalization
- Period of ventilatory dependency
- Amount of time required by the client to resume walking

If the procedure is instituted 2 weeks or longer after the onset of illness, however, it seems to be of little value. In clients with chronic, recurrent GBS, beneficial responses, although temporary, can be maintained with repeated plasmapheresis or with the addition of immunosuppressive therapy.

Before the procedure, the physician obtains vascular access either through a shunt, similar to the type used for hemodialysis, or with a dual-lumen catheter, such as the Quinton catheter. The arterial inlet or port is used for blood flow to a machine called a blood cell separator, in which the antibodies are separated from the plasma. Blood is returned to the client through the venous return port. The usual protocol is an exchange of 200–250 mL/kg of plasma, 1–2 days apart, for a total of three to four exchanges over a course of 8–10 days.

Nursing responsibilities for the client undergoing plasmapheresis include providing information and reassurance to the client, weighing the client before and after the procedure, and administering proper care to the shunt. Proper shunt care includes maintaining shunt patency, checking for bruits every 2–4 hours, keeping double bulldog clamps at the bedside, and observing the puncture site for bleeding or ecchymosis.

The nurse monitors the client's vital signs and observes for signs of complications throughout the procedure (Chart 46–2).

> ➤ *Pain*

Planning: Expected Outcomes. The primary outcome is that the client is expected to have adequate pain relief as evidenced by client report of pain relief.

Interventions. The nurse assesses the severity and nature of the client's pain, which is often worse at night. The typical pain experienced by the client is often not relieved by medication other than opiates, which can be administered via a patient-controlled analgesia (PCA) pump or continuous intravenous drip. The nurse documents the client's response to the pain medication and notifies the physician if the client does not receive sufficient pain relief.

Other pain relief measures include repositioning the client frequently, relaxation techniques, guided imagery, and distractions, such as music or visitors. (Chapter 8 discusses these pain relief measures in detail.)

> ➤ *Impaired Verbal Communication*

Planning: Expected Outcomes. The desired outcome is that the client is expected to communicate effectively with the staff, family, and/or significant others.

Chart 46–2

Nursing Care Highlight: Interventions for Complications of Plasmapheresis

Complication	*Nursing Interventions*
Trauma or infection at vascular access site	Keep the site clean and dry. Monitor the site for redness, swelling, drainage of other signs of infection.
Hypovolemia with resultant hypotension, tachycardia, dizziness, and diaphoresis	Monitor fluid and electrolyte status and vital signs. Administer fluids as prescribed. Provide an explanation of side effects and reassure the client.
Hypokalemia and hypocalcemia	Monitor fluid and electrolyte balance. Administer replacement electrolytes, as ordered. Observe for cardiac dysrhythmias.
Temporary circumoral and distal extremity paresthesias, muscle twitching, nausea, and vomiting related to administration of citrated plasma	Add calcium gluconate or calcium chloride to exchange fluids, as prescribed. Provide explanations, comfort measures, and reassurance.

Interventions. The client may have difficulty communicating because the muscles required for the production of speech are weak, or the client may be on a mechanical ventilator because the respiratory muscles are paralyzed. In either case, in collaboration with the speech and language pathologist, the nurse assists the client in developing a communication system. A simple technique involves eye blinking or moving a finger to indicate yes and no. A communications board can be developed with the letters of the alphabet or a list of common requests, such as the need to be repositioned or the need for pain medication. Both the staff and the client's visitors must know how the client's communication system operates.

➤ *Powerlessness*

Planning: Expected Outcomes. The outcomes are that the client is expected to (1) increase the ability to identify factors that are under independent control, (2) make decisions regarding care, treatment options, and the future, when possible, and (3) participate in care within the limitations of the illness.

Interventions. The nurse assesses feelings of powerlessness by encouraging the client to verbalize feelings about the illness and its effects. Previous decision-making patterns, roles, and responsibilities are examined. By asking the client and the family to describe their usual lifestyles and situations when they coped both effectively and ineffectively, the nurse may identify factors that influence coping ability. The nurse is then better able to identify interventions that facilitate a greater sense of control for the client and the family.

The nurse provides information about the pathophysiology and natural progression of the syndrome and describes tests, procedures, and routines to increase the client's knowledge and sense of control. The client is encouraged to make choices and to participate in care as much as possible. The nurse gives positive feedback for doing so.

The client's own cosmetics, personal hygiene items, and clothing are used, when feasible, to provide a sense of the familiar and control. The nurse ensures environmental control by keeping the call light, television control, telephone, and other necessary items within the client's reach. Alternative communication methods, such as chalk and a blackboard, may be needed if the client cannot verbally express needs.

➤ *Anxiety; Anticipatory Grieving*

Planning: Expected Outcomes. The outcomes are that the client is expected to cope effectively, adapting to the changes in roles and responsibilities associated with the disease process, and verbalize feelings related to anxiety, fear, and grief.

Interventions. The nurse assesses the client and family or significant others for verbal and nonverbal behaviors that indicate anxiety, fear, and grieving. Sadness, depression, anger, guilt, crying or the inability to cry, denial, and withdrawal may be noted. The nurse helps establish a trusting, therapeutic nurse/client relationship. The client and the family or significant other are encouraged to discuss fears and concerns. The client's usual coping strategies and remaining strengths are identified and capitalized on. The family is encouraged to spend time with the client and to assist with care, providing range-of-motion (ROM) exercises, massages, and other comfort measures. The nurse provides as much information as is needed and, if indicated, initiates referrals to the social services department, the hospital chaplain or appropriate spiritual resource, and local support groups.

➤ *Self Care Deficit*

Planning: Expected Outcomes. The outcomes are that the client is expected to adapt to his or her deficits and plan for optimal ability to perform daily living skills.

Interventions. The nurse assesses the client's ability to perform activities of daily living (ADL). While monitoring the client's emotional and mental status, the nurse determines the client's level of acceptance of the disability. Assistance is offered as necessary, but the client is encouraged to perform ADL independently, if possible. The nurse or assistive nursing personnel monitor the client's response to or tolerance of activity and provide adequate rest periods between activities and therapy sessions. Activities are coordinated with the interventions of other health care team members (occupational, speech, and physical therapists). Assistive devices and instructions for their use are provided for the client. The nurse freely gives positive feedback for any gains noted in the client's self-care activities. The family or significant other is encouraged to become involved in all aspects of the rehabilitation process.

 Continuing Care

The severity and course of Guillain-Barré syndrome (GBS) are extremely variable, which makes it difficult to predict prognosis. By the time the client is discharged from the hospital, major problems, such as respiratory paralysis, are resolved. The most likely residual effects at discharge are related to mobility, self-care, and perhaps sensory alteration and disturbed self-concept. For clients who experience total quadriparesis or respiratory paralysis, the course of the rehabilitation phase is even more variable and may require weeks to years.

Planning for the client's discharge begins on admission. The client may be discharged to home. The nurse, discharge planner, or case manager makes appropriate referrals to a home care agency and community agencies for assistance in the home setting after the client is discharged. Clients who require more intensive physical and occupational therapy may be discharged to a skilled nursing facility or rehabilitation setting before returning home.

➤ Health Teaching

The nurse or case manager provides oral and written information and reinforces the teaching provided by the interdisciplinary health care team. A family member or significant other is included in the education process throughout the client's hospitalization.

The client and family are given both oral and written instructions in techniques to facilitate mobility and prevent skin breakdown. If mobility remains markedly impaired, the nurse and physical therapist emphasizes the need for ROM exercises, positioning and frequent turning techniques, and prevention of skin breakdown.

The nurse and rehabilitation team ensure that the client and the family understand how to use assistive devices safely and properly, providing written instructions and diagrams as necessary. If paresthesia persists, the nurse instructs the client and the family to visually examine the affected limbs several times daily. After discharge from the hospital, the client must be monitored for recurrent disease by the physician.

The psychosocial adjustment needed may be minimal to dramatic, depending on the client's residual deficit, age, sex, usual roles and responsibilities, usual coping strategies, available support systems, and occupation. As the client begins to function in familiar surroundings, it is likely that self-concept will improve. Residual deficits rarely require permanent changes in lifestyles or roles. To provide the necessary support, the nurse encourages the client and the family to discuss their feelings with one another. The nurse helps the client identify other support systems, such as church members, social club members, or spiritual resources.

➤ Home Care Management

If the client is discharged to home while still dependent on assistive devices, the interdisciplinary health care team makes certain that the necessary equipment has been delivered after evaluation of the home setting. These activities may be coordinated by the case manager. The occupational therapist checks to see that grab bars for bathtub and toilet transfers, if needed, are properly installed. Any modifications to the home need to be completed before the client's arrival. Throw rugs are removed if they pose a hazard. Ramps are installed, doorways are widened, and commodes are provided if the client remains wheelchair dependent.

➤ Health Care Resources

Self-help groups for clients with chronic illness are common. The nurse consults with the client and the physician and seeks referrals to these groups if indicated. The Guillain-Barré Foundation provides information about local resources and information for clients and their families.

 Evaluation

On the basis of the identified nursing diagnoses and collaborative problems, the nurse evaluates the care of the client with GBS. Outcomes include that the client is expected to

- Have an effective respiratory rate, cough effectively, and have adequate gas exchange in the lungs
- Participate in mobilization to the greatest extent possible to prevent complications of immobility
- Verbalize relief from pain and be able to use relaxation and imaging techniques to reduce pain
- Perform ADL as independently as possible
- Verbalize feelings relative to emotional status and coping abilities, using family members, the nurse, and other sources for support (with the family or significant others)
- Develop appropriate coping strategies on the basis of personal strengths and previous experiences (with the family or significant others)

Myasthenia Gravis

Overview

Myasthenia gravis (MG) means "grave muscle weakness" or weakness of the voluntary or striated muscles. It may take many forms, from mild disturbances of the ocular muscles to rapidly developing generalized weakness that may lead to death from respiratory failure. It is characterized by remissions and exacerbations (worsening). MG is a chronic, neuromuscular, autoimmune disease that involves a decrease in the number and effectiveness of acetylcholine (ACh) receptors at the neuromuscular junction.

Pathophysiology

The major pathologic defect in MG is that nerve impulses are not transmitted to the skeletal muscle at the neuromuscular junction. Clients with MG develop specific antibodies to one or more ACh receptor sites, possibly because of autoimmune injury. The antibodies accelerate the degeneration of ACh receptors.

There is no evidence of central or peripheral nervous system disease in MG. The muscle appears normal macroscopically, and there is usually no evidence of atrophy. On microscopic examination, lymphocytic infiltrates may be seen within muscles and other organs, yet these findings have been inconsistent.

The thymus gland is often abnormal. Thymoma (encapsulated thymus gland tumor) occurs in approximately 15% of cases, and 70% of the remaining cases show hyperplasia of the thymus. There is also a very strong association between MG and hyperthyroidism. Genetic factors may play a role in the development of MG (Weisberg et al., 1996).

Etiology

Although the precipitating event remains unclear, research strongly suggests that MG is caused by antibodies to ACh receptors. Evidence also suggests a relationship between MG and hyperplasia of the thymus gland.

Incidence/Prevalence

The incidence of MG is estimated at 0.4/100,000 in the United States. Although it may begin at any age, onset of MG before 10 years or after 60 years of age is rare. The peak age at onset is between 20 and 30 years. Before age 40 years, women are affected two to three times more often than are men (Hickey, 1996).

ELDERLY CONSIDERATIONS

 In later life, the incidence in the sexes is about equal. Men predominate among myasthenic clients with thymoma, and these men tend to be 50–60 years old.

Collaborative Management

Assessment

In addition to the standard biographical data and nursing history, the nurse assesses the client with MG for the rapid onset of fatigue. Subjective complaints of muscle weakness that increases on exertion or as the day wears on and improves with rest are noted. The nurse asks the client to describe symptoms, specifically noting the affected muscle groups and any limitation or inability of the client in performing activities of daily living (ADL). Additional areas of inquiry include any history of ptosis (drooping eyelids) or diplopia (double vision), difficulty chewing or swallowing, and the type of diet best tolerated. Signs and symptoms of respiratory difficulty, choking, or weakness of the voice are also elicited. The client is asked about any difficulty holding up the head, brushing the teeth, combing the hair, or shaving. The nurse inquires about the presence of paresthesia or aching in weakened muscles. Last, any history of thymus gland tumor is elicited.

Although the onset of MG is usually insidious, some instances of fairly rapid development have been preceded by infection, emotional upset, pregnancy, or anesthesia. Thus, the nurse inquires about any history of these events. A temporary increase in weakness may be noted after vaccination, menstruation, and exposure to extremes in environmental temperature.

➤ Physical Assessment/Clinical Manifestations

If the client can cooperate fully, the diagnosis of MG may be established by the demonstration of *progressive* paresis of affected muscle groups that is resolved, at least in part, by rest (Chart 46–3). The most common symptoms (exhibited by more than 90% of clients) are related to involvement of the levator palpebrae or extraocular muscles. The nurse assesses the client for ocular palsies, ptosis, diplopia, and weak or incomplete eye closure.

These symptoms may last only a few days at the onset, then resolve, only to return weeks or months later. Normal pupillary responses to light and accommodation are present.

For most clients, the muscles of facial expression, chewing, and speech are affected. The nurse notes the client's smile, which may be transformed into a snarl; the jaw may hang so that the client must prop it up with the hand. Difficulty in chewing and swallowing, choking, and regurgitation of fluids through the nose may lead to considerable weight loss. The nurse inquires about the client's nutritional status and any recent loss of weight. It may be more difficult for the client to eat after talking. After extended conversations, the voice may become weaker or exhibit a nasal twang. In some clients, the tongue shows one central and two lateral longitudinal fissures.

Less often involved are the muscles of the shoulders, the flexors of the neck, and the hip flexors. Because limb weakness is more often *proximal,* the client may have difficulty climbing stairs, lifting heavy objects, or raising the arms overhead. Neck weakness may be mild or severe enough to cause difficulty holding the head erect. Among the trunk muscles, the erector spinae are most frequently affected: This results in difficulty sustaining a sitting or walking posture.

In the most advanced cases, all muscles are weakened, including those associated with respiratory function and the control of bladder and bowel function. Thus, in severe cases, the nurse inquires about bowel and bladder function. Respiratory function is assessed regularly.

Atrophy of muscles, although rarely marked in degree, occurs in a small percentage of clients with myasthenia gravis (MG). The client's tendon reflexes should be assessed, but they are not often affected. The nurse assesses for pain, which is seldom a major complaint. However, many clients report some aching of the weakened muscles. Paresthesia affecting the muscles of the face, the hands, and the thighs is not associated with any loss of sensation. Lost or decreased sensations of smell and taste have been reported. There is no alteration of consciousness.

Chart 46–3

Key Features of Myasthenia Gravis

Motor Manifestations

Progressive muscle weakness (proximal) that usually improves with rest
Poor posture
Ocular palsies
Ptosis
Weak or incomplete eye closure
Diplopia
Respiratory compromise
Loss of bowel and bladder control
Fatigue

Sensory Manifestations

Muscle achiness
Paresthesias
Decreased smell and taste

In *Eaton-Lambert syndrome,* a special form of myasthenia often observed in combination with small cell carcinoma of the lung, the muscles of the trunk and the pelvic and shoulder girdles are the most frequently affected. Although weakness increases after exertion, there may be a temporary increase in muscle strength during the first few contractions, followed by rapid decrements. Diagnosis is confirmed by electromyography. Treatment includes removing the tumor, managing the cancer, and administering medications to release acetylcholine (ACh). Additional therapies may include plasmapheresis and immunosuppressive therapy.

Osserman (1958) introduced a clinical staging classification for MG still in use at many medical centers (Table 46–1).

► Laboratory Assessment

In virtually all cases, the diagnosis of MG is obvious from the history and physical examination findings. MG may be immediately confirmed by the client's response to cholinergic drugs. A standard series of laboratory studies is usually performed for clients with known or suspected MG. Thyroid function should be tested. Serum protein electrophoresis evaluates the client for immunologic disorders. Thyrotoxicosis (excessive thyroid hormone) is present in approximately 5% of myasthenic clients. Rheumatoid arthritis, systemic lupus erythematosus, and polymyositis are associated with the disease as well.

TABLE 46–1

Osserman's Clinical Staging of Myasthenia Gravis

Class I: Ocular Myasthenia

Ptosis and diplopia
Mild; no mortality

Class IIA: Mild Generalized Myasthenia with Slow Progression

No crises
Drug responsive
Low mortality

Class IIB: Moderate Generalized Myasthenia

Severe skeletal and bulbar involvement
No crises
Drug response less than satisfactory
Low mortality

Class III: Acute Fulminating Myasthenia

Rapid progression with respiratory crises
Poor drug response
High incidence of thymoma
High mortality

Class IV: Late Severe Myasthenia

Progression during 2 years from class I to class II
Poor response to medication
High mortality

Adapted with permission from Adams, R. D., & Victor, M. (1985). *Principles of neurology* (3rd ed.). New York: McGraw-Hill.

Testing for acetylcholine receptor antibodies (AChRab) has become an important diagnostic criterion: 85%–95% of clients with MG have AChRab, and there are virtually no false-positive results. Thus, a positive antibody test result confirms the diagnosis, but a negative finding does not exclude the disease (Weisburg et al., 1996).

► Radiographic Assessment

Because some clients with MG have thymoma, the client is assessed for this condition. The thymus, an H-shaped gland located in the upper mediastinum beneath the sternum, is one organ in which ACh receptor antibodies are formed. Although thymoma can often be seen on routine frontal and lateral chest x-rays, special studies should be done of any area suggestive of thymoma in the anterior mediastinum. The nurse prepares the client for these tests or for computed tomography (CT) scan by explaining the equipment and what the client may expect during the tests.

► Other Diagnostic Assessment

Tensilon Testing. Pharmacologic tests with the cholinesterase inhibitors edrophonium chloride (Tensilon) and neostigmine bromide (Prostigmin) have been in use since the 1950s. Tensilon is used more often because of its rapid onset and brief duration of action. This drug inhibits the breakdown of ACh at the postsynaptic membrane, which increases the availability of ACh for excitation of postsynaptic receptors. To perform the test, the physician first estimates the strength of certain cranial muscles. Initially, 2 mg (0.2 mL) is injected intravenously; if this is tolerated, an additional 8 mg (0.8 mL) is injected after 30 seconds. Within 30–60 seconds of the first dose, most myasthenic clients show a marked improvement in muscle tone that lasts 4–5 minutes. False-positive test results may be caused by increased muscle effort by the client. False-negative findings may be seen if the tested muscle is extremely weak or refractory to the drug.

This test may also be used to help determine whether increasing weakness in the previously diagnosed myasthenic client is due to *cholinergic crisis* (overmedication with anticholinesterase drugs) or to *myasthenic crisis* (under medication with cholinesterase inhibitors). In cholinergic crisis, muscle tone does not improve after the administration of Tensilon. Instead, weakness may actually increase, and fasciculations (muscle twitching) may be noted around the eyes and face. The Tensilon test poses a danger of ventricular fibrillation and cardiac arrest, although these rarely occur. Atropine sulfate is the antidote for Tensilon and must be available for these complications.

Electromyography. A common diagnostic test performed by the physician or technician is electromyography (EMG). Although electrical testing of the normal neuromuscular junction produces no change in the amplitude of muscle contraction, the amplitude of the muscle's response diminishes with progressive stimulation. A decrease in amplitude of more than 10% between the first and fifth responses generally indicates defective neuromuscular transmission characteristic of, although not unique to, MG. Testing of several muscles may be done to increase the likelihood of detecting an abnormality. Testing may be performed after exercise or exposure of the muscle to curare or to ischemia.

Single-fiber EMG is even more sensitive in detecting defects of neuromuscular transmission. This test compares the stability of the firing of one muscle fiber with that of another fiber innervated by the same motor neuron. The time interval between the two firings normally shows a minor degree of variability, called jitter. Defective transmission increases jitter or actually blocks successive discharges.

Interventions

The hallmark of MG is muscle weakness that increases when the client is fatigued and limits the client's mobility and ability to participate in activities. Treatment efforts for this disease fall into two categories:

- Treatment that affects the symptoms of MG without influencing the actual course of the disease (anticholinesterases or cholinergic drugs)
- Therapeutic efforts for inducing remission, such as the administration of immunosuppressive drugs or corticosteroids, plasmapheresis, and thymectomy (removal of the thymus gland)

➤ Nonsurgical Management

The nurse assesses the client's motor strength before and after periods of activity. Assistance is provided as necessary to prevent the client from becoming fatigued. The nurse teaches the client to participate in activities early in the day or during the energy peaks that follow the administration of medications. The nurse also helps the client to plan the periods of rest necessary for avoiding excess fatigue.

Providing Assistance with Activities. During periods of maximal weakness, the nurse or assistive nursing personnel may need to provide assistance with ambulation, transfers from bed to chair or toilet or commode, position changes, and maintenance of body alignment.

Active or passive range-of-motion (ROM) exercises are performed every 2–4 hours. The nurse assesses skin integrity and instructs family members or significant others in these techniques. The client is repositioned and bony prominences are assessed at least every 2 hours for skin breakdown and contractures. The nurse also uses heel and elbow protectors, eggcrate or alternating-pressure mattresses, and other devices for preventing pressure ulcers. The nurse collaborates with the physical and occupational therapy departments for assistance with mobility, self-care, and energy conservation techniques.

Drug Therapy. Three groups of drugs are typically prescribed for the treatment of myasthenia gravis (MG)—

anticholinesterases, corticosteroids, and immunosuppressants. The nurse is responsible for administering these medications *on time* to maintain blood levels and thus facilitate increased muscle strength. The nurse also monitors and documents the client's responses. The nurse instructs the client and the family about the indications for, effectiveness of, and side effects of the drugs used in treatment of MG.

Anticholinesterase Drugs. Anticholinesterase drugs, sometimes referred to as antimyasthenics, increase the response of muscles to nerve impulses. Thus, muscle strength is improved. The anticholinesterase drugs of choice are neostigmine (Prostigmin), pyridostigmine (Mestinon, Regonol), and ambenonium (Mytelase). The nurse may expect day-to-day variations in dosage, depending on the client's fluctuating symptoms.

A potential side effect of these medications is cholinergic crisis. This is generally treated with atropine sulfate. The nurse must administer these medications on time for consistent blood levels to be maintained. The nurse administers the medications with a small amount of food to help alleviate gastrointestinal side effects and instructs the client to eat meals 45 minutes to 1 hour after taking these medications. This is very important if the client has bulbar involvement to avoid aspiration. Drugs containing magnesium, morphine or its derivatives, curare, quinine, quinidine, procainamide, and hypnotics or sedatives should be avoided because these substances may increase the client's weakness. Antibiotics, such as neomycin, kanamycin, polymyxin B, and certain tetracyclines, impair transmitter release and increase myasthenic symptoms as well.

Sudden increases in weakness and the inability to clear secretions, swallow, or breathe adequately indicate that the client is experiencing crisis. There are two types of crises:

- Myasthenic crisis, an exacerbation of the myasthenic symptoms caused by undermedication with anticholinesterase drugs
- Cholinergic crisis, an acute exacerbation of muscle weakness caused by overmedication with cholinergic (anticholinesterase) drugs

Myasthenic crisis is often preceded by some type of infection. In either crisis, an adequate airway and artificial respiration must be maintained. Because myasthenic and cholinergic crises have many common characteristics, the type of crisis the client is experiencing must be identified for effective treatment to be provided (Table 46–2). In many clients, increasing myasthenic symptoms leads to an overdose of anticholinesterase drugs. As a result, the client may experience a *mixed* crisis. The Tensilon test (described earlier), although not always conclusive, is an important procedure for differentiation. Tensilon produces a temporary improvement in myasthenic crisis but no improvement or worsening of symptoms in cholinergic crisis.

Nursing management of the client in myasthenic crisis is directed at early detection and maintenance of adequate respiratory function. The acutely ill client may need intensive nursing care for monitoring and maintenance of

TABLE 46–2

Characteristics of Myasthenic and Cholinergic Crises

Myasthenic Crisis	Cholinergic Crisis	Mixed Crisis
Increased pulse and respiration	Nausea	Apprehension
Rise in blood pressure	Vomiting	Restlessness
Anoxia	Diarrhea	Dyspnea
Cyanosis	Abdominal cramps	Dysphagia
Bowel and bladder incontinence	Blurred vision	Dysarthria
	Pallor	Increased lacrimation
Decreased urinary output	Facial muscle twitching	Increased salivation
Absence of cough and swallow reflex	Pupillary miosis	Diaphoresis
	Hypotension	Generalized weakness

body functions. The client may require mechanical ventilation. Anticholinesterase drugs are withheld because they increase respiratory secretions and are usually ineffective in the first few days after the crisis begins. Medications are reinstituted gradually and at lower dosages.

In *cholinergic* crisis, anticholinergic drugs are withheld while the client is maintained on a ventilator. Atropine (1 mg intravenously) may be given and repeated, if necessary. When atropine is ordered, the nurse must observe the client carefully; secretions are thickened by the drug, which causes more difficulty with airway clearance and possibly the development of mucous plugs. Unless such complications as pneumonia or aspiration develop, the client in crisis improves rapidly after the appropriate drugs have been given. The nurse continues to provide assistance as necessary because the client tires easily after minimal exertion.

Corticosteroids. Corticosteroids, such as prednisone (Deltasone, Winpred✸), may be used with anticholinesterase drugs in the treatment of MG. Worsening of symptoms during the first 7–10 days of prednisone therapy should be expected. The client is usually kept on prednisone for 6 months; then the dosage is gradually decreased over 12–16 months. Moderate- to low-dose corticosteroid therapy is particularly useful to reduce the diploplia and frequency of deterioration to generalized disease in ocular MG.

Immunosuppressants. Immunosuppression with azathioprine (Imuran), methotrexate (Mexate), and cyclophosphamide (Cytoxan, Procytox✸) has resulted in some clinical improvement and reduction in acetylcholine receptor antibody (AChRab) levels.

Plasmapheresis. Plasmapheresis is a method by which offending autoantibodies are removed from the plasma. The physician prescribes immunosuppressive drugs, which are administered concurrently to decrease the formation of additional antibodies. Complications and nursing management of the client undergoing plasmapheresis

are presented in the earlier discussion of Guillain-Barré syndrome and in Chart 46–2.

Respiratory Support. Although not all clients with MG have respiratory compromise, the nurse must provide ongoing assessment and maintenance of respiratory function. Both myasthenic crisis (undermedication) and cholinergic crisis (overmedication) increase muscle weakness and the client's risk for respiratory compromise. The diaphragm and the respiratory and intercostal muscles may be affected, inhibiting the client's ability to maintain adequate ventilation, breathe deeply, and cough effectively. In addition, dysphagia may result in the aspiration of foods, fluids, or saliva, which compounds the respiratory problems. Because of their respiratory muscle involvement, many of these clients have an increased risk of pulmonary infections.

The client who cannot cough effectively may require oropharyngeal or nasopharyngeal suctioning. The nurse may need to teach assisted cough technique, similar to that used by quadriplegics (see Chap. 45). Chest physiotherapy consisting of postural drainage, percussion, and vibration mobilizes secretions and helps prevent pneumonia and atelectasis. The nurse keeps an Ambu bag, equipment for oxygen administration, and endotracheal intubation equipment at the bedside in case of respiratory distress.

Because breathing difficulty or the inability to breathe easily is frightening, the nurse should be aware of the client's mental and emotional status during periods of respiratory compromise. Finally, while monitoring and documenting the client's response, the nurse administers the medications prescribed for muscle weakness, bronchodilation, and pulmonary congestion.

Self-Care. Generalized weakness and fatigue affect the myasthenic client's ability to participate in activities of daily living (ADL). Impaired fine motor control and shoulder weakness, which result in difficulty raising the arms, often compound the problem. Self-care deficits may be complete or partial, depending on the severity of the illness, the client's response to drugs, and the client's ability to tolerate activity without excessive fatigue.

To establish abilities and limitations, the nurse assesses the client's ability to perform ADL. Although the nurse encourages the client to perform activities as independently as possible, he or she provides whatever assistance is necessary to avoid undue frustration and fatigue. For maximizing independence and making attempts at self-care successful, activities are planned to follow the administration of medication. The nurse monitors and documents the client's response or tolerance to activity, providing alternating periods of activity and rest. Rest is critical because increased fatigue can precipitate a crisis. In addition, occupational and physical therapists evaluate the client for assistive-adaptive devices. In collaboration with the nurse, they teach the client and the family energy conservation techniques and ideas for making work and self-care easier after discharge from the hospital.

Assistance with Communication. Weakness of speech and facial muscles often results in dysarthric and nasal speech. Thus, it may be difficult for myasthenic clients to make their speech understood by others.

The nurse assesses the functions of cranial nerves V, VII, IX, X, and XII (see Chap. 43) to determine the client's ability to communicate. The client is instructed to speak slowly while the nurse attempts to lip-read. The nurse repeats the information to verify that it is correct. Questions that can be answered with yes or no or by gestures may be used along with alternative communication systems, such as eye blinking; flash cards; magic slates; notebook and pencil; and picture, letter, or word boards. The nurse collaborates with the speech and language pathologist for suggestions and support.

Nutritional Support. The client with myasthenia gravis (MG) may have difficulty maintaining an adequate intake of food and fluid because the muscles needed for chewing and swallowing become weakened and tire easily. In collaboration with the dietitian, occupational therapist, and speech and language pathologist, the client's nutritional status and his or her ability to receive adequate oral nutrition are evaluated. Small, frequent meals and high-calorie snacks are often well tolerated. The nurse monitors the effectiveness of the nutrition program by recording calorie counts, intake and output, serum albumin levels, and daily weights (Chart 46-4). If the client is not able to swallow, a feeding tube may be used.

Eye Protection. The client's inability to completely close the eyes may lead to corneal abrasions and further compromise vision and comfort. During the day, the nurse or family member applies artificial tears to keep the corneas moist and free from abrasion. A lubricant gel and shield may be applied to the eye at bedtime to provide more extensive coverage. To help relieve diplopia, the eyes should be alternately covered with a patch for 2–3 hours at a time.

Chart 46–4

Nursing Care Highlight: Improving Nutrition in Clients with Myasthenia Gravis

Assess the client's gag reflex and ability to chew and swallow.

Provide frequent oral hygiene as needed.

Collaborate with the dietitian, speech and language pathologist, and occupational therapist to plan and implement meals that the client can eat and enjoy.

Offer small, frequent meals.

Cut food into small bites and encourage the client to eat slowly.

Observe client for choking, nasal regurgitation, and aspiration.

Provide high-calorie snacks or supplements such as puddings.

Keep the head of the bed elevated during meals and for 30–60 minutes after the client eats.

Avoid liquids because they can easily cause choking and aspiration; provide a soft diet.

Monitor food intake carefully.

Weigh the client daily.

Monitor serum transferrin and albumin levels.

Administer anticholinesterase drugs, as ordered: 30–60 minutes before meals.

➤ Surgical Management

For clients with MG, thymectomy is an alternative method of treatment. The procedure is not always immediately effective, and it may take several years for remission to occur, if at all. Clients who have the surgery within 2 years of the onset of myasthenic symptoms show the most improvement.

Preoperative Care. The nurse teaches the client coughing and deep-breathing exercises and the use of incentive spirometry. The nurse demonstrates airway suctioning and discusses wound care, intravenous infusions, and the critical care unit environment (if indicated). Because there is no way to predict whether remission or improvement will occur, it is important to avoid making promises, although optimism is warranted.

Immediately before surgery, the nurse may administer pyridostigmine (Mestinon), as ordered, with a small amount of water to keep the client stable during and after surgery. If steroids have been used, they are also given before surgery and are tapered during the postoperative period. The nurse also administers antibiotics immediately before and for several days after surgery. Plasmapheresis may be used preoperatively and postoperatively to decrease circulative antibodies more quickly.

Operative Procedure. One of two surgical approaches may be used: the transcervical incision or the sternal split. Advocates of the transcervical approach claim a lower morbidity rate and more rapid recovery with less postoperative discomfort. The client often requires only a small dressing and an intravenous line. The sternal split, however, allows the surgeon to directly visualize the mediastinum. Thus, because more precise and complete removal of all thymic tissue is ensured, this may be the approach of choice.

When thymoma is present, all contiguous involved structures such as the pericardium, the innominate vein, a portion of the superior vena cava, and a portion of the lung, are removed. A single chest tube is placed in the anterior mediastinum. The client may be admitted to the critical care unit postoperatively.

Postoperative Care. Although clients with adequate respiratory function may be extubated immediately after the procedure, most clients require a gradual weaning from the ventilator. Prolonged ventilatory assistance is rare, however. After the client is extubated, the nurse pays conscientious attention to pulmonary hygiene. The nurse provides suctioning as necessary and encourages the client to turn, cough, and breathe deeply and to use incentive spirometry every 2 hours. In addition to observing respiratory function and providing bronchial hygiene, the nurse observes the client for signs of pneumothorax or hemothorax, such as

- Chest pain
- Sudden shortness of breath
- Diminished or delayed chest wall expansion
- Diminished or absent breath sounds
- Restlessness or a change in vital signs (decreasing blood pressure or a weak, rapid pulse)

For the sternal surgical technique, the nurse provides chest tube care. Both surgical approaches require meticulous wound care. The nurse also remains alert for signs of infection, such as increasing or purulent drainage; redness, warmth, or swelling around the wound; and elevated temperature. Finally, the nurse provides appropriate client and family teaching in preparation for discharge from the hospital.

 Continuing Care

The client with myasthenia gravis (MG) may be cared for in a variety of settings, including the home, subacute unit, rehabilitation setting, or long term care facility.

The client discharged from the hospital may be weak and may require the assistance of a family member, home care nurse, physical therapist, occupational therapist, and/or home care aide.

➤ Health Teaching

The more that the client and family know about the disease and the drugs used for treatment, the less likely it is that complications will develop.

Disease Process. The client and the family are encouraged to ask questions. Concerning the disease process, the nurse discusses its episodic nature (exacerbations and remissions) and factors that predispose the client to exacerbation, such as infection, stress, surgery, hard phys-

TABLE 46–3

Factors Precipitating or Worsening Myasthenia Gravis

Various medications, including
    Antidysrhythmics
    Beta-blocking agents
    Antibiotics
    Antirheumatic drugs
    Antispasmodics
    Antihistamines
    Opioids
    Phenytoin (Dilantin)
    Antidepressants (tricyclics)
Rheumatoid arthritis
Alcohol
Hormonal changes
Stress
Infection
Seasonal temperature changes
Heat
Surgery

ical exercise, sedatives, and enemas or strong cathartics (Table 46–3). The client is instructed to collaborate with the health care provider to monitor muscle strength, ability to perform activities of daily living (ADL), and need to adjust medications.

Lifestyle Changes. The nurse stresses the importance of making such lifestyle adaptations as avoiding heat (e.g., sauna, hot tubs, and sunbathing), crowds, overeating, erratic changes in sleep habits, or emotional extremes. The nurse describes the signs of exacerbation, such as increased weakness, increased diplopia, ptosis, and problems with chewing or swallowing. The client is instructed to plan activities to allow for rest periods.

Drug Therapy. The medication regimen is provided in a written format that includes the drugs' names, purposes, dosages, times scheduled, administrative routes, and side effects. The nurse explains that the drugs are normally taken before such activities as eating, participating in sports, or engaging in work. The nurse stresses the importance of maintaining therapeutic blood levels by taking the medications on time as prescribed and not missing or postponing doses. In addition, the nurse informs the client of the side effects of anticholinesterase drugs. Additional health teaching regarding medications is found in Chart 46–5.

Finally, the nurse advises the client to avoid such medications as morphine, curare, quinine, quinidine, procainamide, mycin-type antibiotics, and drugs containing magnesium. These agents markedly increase muscle weakness.

In preparing the client for discharge, the nurse also explains the signs and symptoms of myasthenic and cholinergic crises and the need to contact the physician or other health care professional whenever either type of

---

Chart 46–5

Education Guide: Helpful Hints for Medication Teaching of Clients with Myasthenia Gravis

Keep medication and a glass of water at your bedside if you are weak in the morning.

Wear a watch with alarm function (or beeper) to remind you to take medications.

Post your medication schedule so others know it.

Plan strenuous activities, when possible, when medication peaks.

Keep extra supply of medications in your car or at work. Be sure they are secured.

Do not take any over-the-counter medications without checking with your health care provider.

---

crisis is suspected. Because respiratory compromise often occurs in myasthenic clients, family members are encouraged to gain skills in resuscitation procedures. An Ambu bag, suctioning equipment, and oxygen should be available in the home for clients susceptible to crisis. Family members should be instructed in their proper use.

Psychosocial Preparation. The episodic nature of MG, the potential or actual loss of independence, and body image changes (e.g., the inability to smile) affect the client's adjustment. During discharge planning, the case manager (CM) considers such factors as age, sex, usual roles and responsibilities, available support systems, occupation, and financial status. Because the client's and the family's need for psychosocial adjustment may range from minimal to dramatic, the CM remains sensitive to their needs and provides information and support. The CM encourages family members or significant others to discuss their feelings with one another.

➤ Home Care Management

Clients with MG are usually managed at home. Hospitalization is restricted to the diagnostic and evaluation processes, myasthenic or cholinergic crisis resulting in respiratory failure, or periods of exacerbation when respiratory function is threatened.

Unless the client requires assistive devices, little preparation of the home setting is required. In consultation with physical and occupational therapists, the CM makes certain that needed equipment has been delivered and properly installed. In addition, the CM makes sure that the client and family members can use the equipment safely. If the client is wheelchair dependent, the discharge planner or CM ensures that any necessary modifications to the home (such as the installation of ramps or widening of doorways) have been completed before the client's discharge from the hospital.

➤ Health Care Resources

In consultation with the health care provider, the client, and the family, the staff nurse or CM may initiate refer-

rals to home health agencies and to local self-help groups for people who have chronic illnesses and their families. The Myasthenia Gravis Foundation, headquartered in New York City, has education and research programs and provides assistance with financial aid and community resources. The CM encourages the client to obtain and wear a medical alert (MedicAlert) bracelet or necklace and to carry identification at all times.

Polyneuritis and Polyneuropathy

Overview

Systemic diseases, infections, trauma, vascular or metabolic disturbances, and such exogenous substances as alcohol, medications, industrial agents, and heavy metals may damage cranial and peripheral nerves. Although the term *polyneuritis* implies an inflammatory process, it may denote noninflammatory lesions as well. Thus, the terms *polyneuritis, polyneuropathy,* and *peripheral neuropathy* may describe syndromes whose clinical hallmarks are muscle weakness with or without atrophy, pains and paresthesia or loss of sensation, impaired reflexes, and autonomic manifestations, or combinations of these symptoms.

The most common type of neuropathy is a symmetric polyneuropathy in which the client experiences decreased sensation along with the feeling that an extremity is asleep. Tingling, burning, tightness, or aching sensations generally start in the feet and progress to the level of the knee before being noted in the hands (glove and stocking neuropathy). Other clients may complain of unsteadiness, clumsiness, the inability to recognize objects by feel, and injury without pain. Diabetic neuropathy is a common example, as are the neuropathies resulting from renal or hepatic failure, alcoholism, acquired immunodeficiency syndrome (AIDS), and drug or toxic exposures. Common factors associated with polyneuropathy are presented in Table 46–4.

Collaborative Management

 Assessment

Although peripheral neuropathy rarely necessitates hospitalization, the nurse is likely to encounter clients with this condition in a variety of settings, particularly among the elderly or in clients with a related illness. Nursing assessment includes a detailed medical history and examination of the client's sensory and motor abilities. The client can often outline a specific area of sensory deficit. Because the client may be unaware of decreased sensation, the nurse assesses the distal extremities for light touch using cotton balls or cotton-tipped applicators and for pain using a safety pin. The nurse assesses position sense, or kinesthetic sensation, by gently grasping the involved digit or extremity on its sides. With the client's eyes closed, the nurse changes the position of the digit or extremity. The client is asked to describe how the position was changed. The client should be able to acknowledge even slight movements. A tuning fork may be placed on bone promi-

TABLE 46–4

Factors Associated with Polyneuropathy

Diseases

Amyloidosis
Alcoholism
Carcinomas
Diabetes mellitus
Diphtheria
Hepatic failure
Malabsorption or malnutrition
Porphyria
Renal failure (uremia)
Trauma
Vascular disease

Vitamin Deficiencies

Vitamin B_1 (thiamine)
Vitamin B_6 (pyridoxine)
Vitamin B_2 (riboflavin)
Vitamin B_c (folic acid)
Vitamin B_{12}
Niacin

Drug Use

Nitrofurantoin
Vincristine
Isoniazid
Phenytoin
Amitriptyline
Hydralazine

Environmental Exposures

Heavy metals
Industrial solvents

nences to test for sensitivity to vibration. The examination is started at distal sites. More proximal areas are tested only if the client fails to perceive the duration of the vibration at the distal site.

The nurse examines the extremities for any signs of injury of which the client may be unaware. The nurse also assesses the client for

- Orthostatic hypotension
- Abnormal sweating
- Miosis (abnormal constriction of the pupil)
- Sphincter disturbances, such as loss of bowel and bladder control
- Other autonomic dysfunctions that may accompany the neuropathy

All abnormal findings are documented and brought to the health care provider's attention.

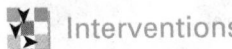 Interventions

Medical management of clients with peripheral neuropathy consists of removal or treatment of the underlying cause and symptomatic therapy, including supportive care and physiotherapy. The diet is generally supplemented with vitamins, especially if vitamin deficiency is an underlying cause. However, there is no evidence that vitamins in excess of those contained in a well-balanced diet have

any effect on forms of polyneuropathy unrelated to vitamin deficiency.

With removal of the toxic agent or correction of the metabolic defects, recovery may be rapid if the continuity of the nerves has not been interrupted. If there has been axonal destruction, recovery may require several months. After severe degeneration, there may be permanent weakness, atrophy, decreased reflexes, and sensory deficits.

The nurse is responsible for extensive client teaching. For clients with decreased sensation in their feet and legs, the nurse explains the importance of proper foot care (Chart 46–6). In addition, the nurse assists the client who has decreased sensation to recognize potential hazards, such as

- Exposure to extremes of environmental temperature (e.g., frostbite)
- Bathwater or dishwater that may be too hot
- Contact of the feet with heat sources (such as heating pads or radiators) while sleeping
- Burns associated with cooking

The nurse discourages smoking because the resultant vasoconstriction may worsen the neuropathy. The importance of maintaining adequate nutrition is emphasized. Clients with postural hypotension are taught to arise slowly and wear support or elastic stockings to minimize pooling of blood in the legs.

Many clients, especially those with the acute forms of polyneuropathy associated with drugs or exposure to toxic substances, experience anxiety, impaired coping, and changes in such family processes as role responsibilities and sexual functioning. Thus, it is vital for the nurse to establish a trusting nurse/client relationship and to provide psychosocial support. In consultation with the physician, social worker, chaplain or religious leader, and physical and occupational therapists, the nurse focuses on

Chart 46–6

Education Guide: Peripheral Neuropathy of the Lower Extremities

Wash your feet and legs with mild soap each day; rinse and dry well.
Apply lanolin or lubricating lotion to your feet and legs once or twice daily.
Inspect your feet and legs daily; report skin changes or open areas to your physician or other health care provider.
Wear white or colorfast stockings or socks, and change them daily.
Check the temperature of bathwater with a thermometer before putting your feet into the water.
Do not use heating pads or other heat sources on your feet.
Do not use sharp devices to remove corns or calluses (use a pumice stone) or to cut nails. Seek professional podiatry care on a regular basis.
Wear support or elastic stockings if you have orthostatic hypotension or dependent edema.
Wear well-fitted shoes; avoid going barefoot.

the client's abilities and strengths and helps identify new ways of coping, meeting needs, and restructuring activities.

Peripheral Nerve Trauma

Overview

The peripheral nerves are subject to injuries associated with mechanical or vehicular accidents, certain sports, injection of particular drugs, military conflicts or wars, and acts of violence (e.g., knife or gunshot wounds). Specific mechanisms of injury include

- Partial or complete severance of a nerve or nerves
- Contusion, stretching, constriction, or compression of a nerve or nerves
- Ischemia
- Electrical, thermal, or radiation injury

Most commonly affected are the median, ulnar, and radial nerves of the arms and the peroneal, femoral, and sciatic nerves of the legs (Fig. 46-1).

After a nerve is transected, the nerve distal to the injury degenerates and retracts within 24 hours. Motor and sensory dysfunction distal to the lesion coincide with the loss of electrical excitability as the nerve fibers degenerate. Recovery occurs as Schwann cells of the neurilemma proliferate from both the proximal and distal stumps. Dividing mitotically, these cells form neurilemmal cords, which act as guidelines for the regenerating axon. Tiny unmyelinated sprouts are generated at the proximal axon and grow 1–4 mm each day. Some can cross the transected gap through guidance by the neurilemma to find their way to the distal stump. The better aligned the union, the more normal the functional return (Fig. 46–2).

Successfully realigned nerves remyelinate, grow to their former size, and eventually claim conduction velocities of 80% of their former capacity (Hickey, 1996). Successful reinnervation is adversely affected by loss of anatomic continuity of the nerve, infection, and increasing age. With disorganization of the nerve or mismatched realignments, functional weakness or unintentional muscle movements as well as poor sensory discrimination and localization of stimuli may result.

Some sensory function may return before the regeneration process can occur. This is because nerves proximal to the injured neurons are stimulated to produce collat-

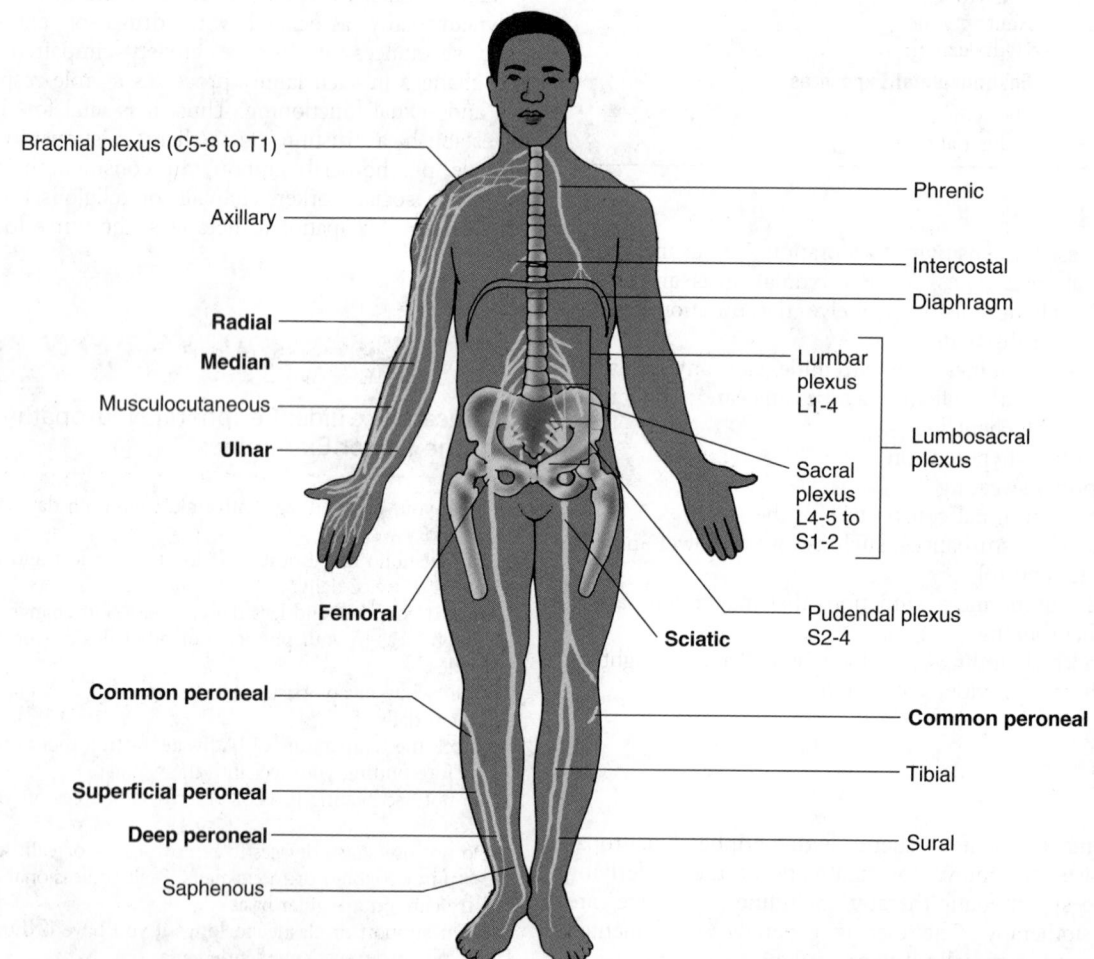

Figure 46–1. Distribution of selected peripheral nerves in the body. The nerves most commonly affected by trauma are highlighted in **bold** type.

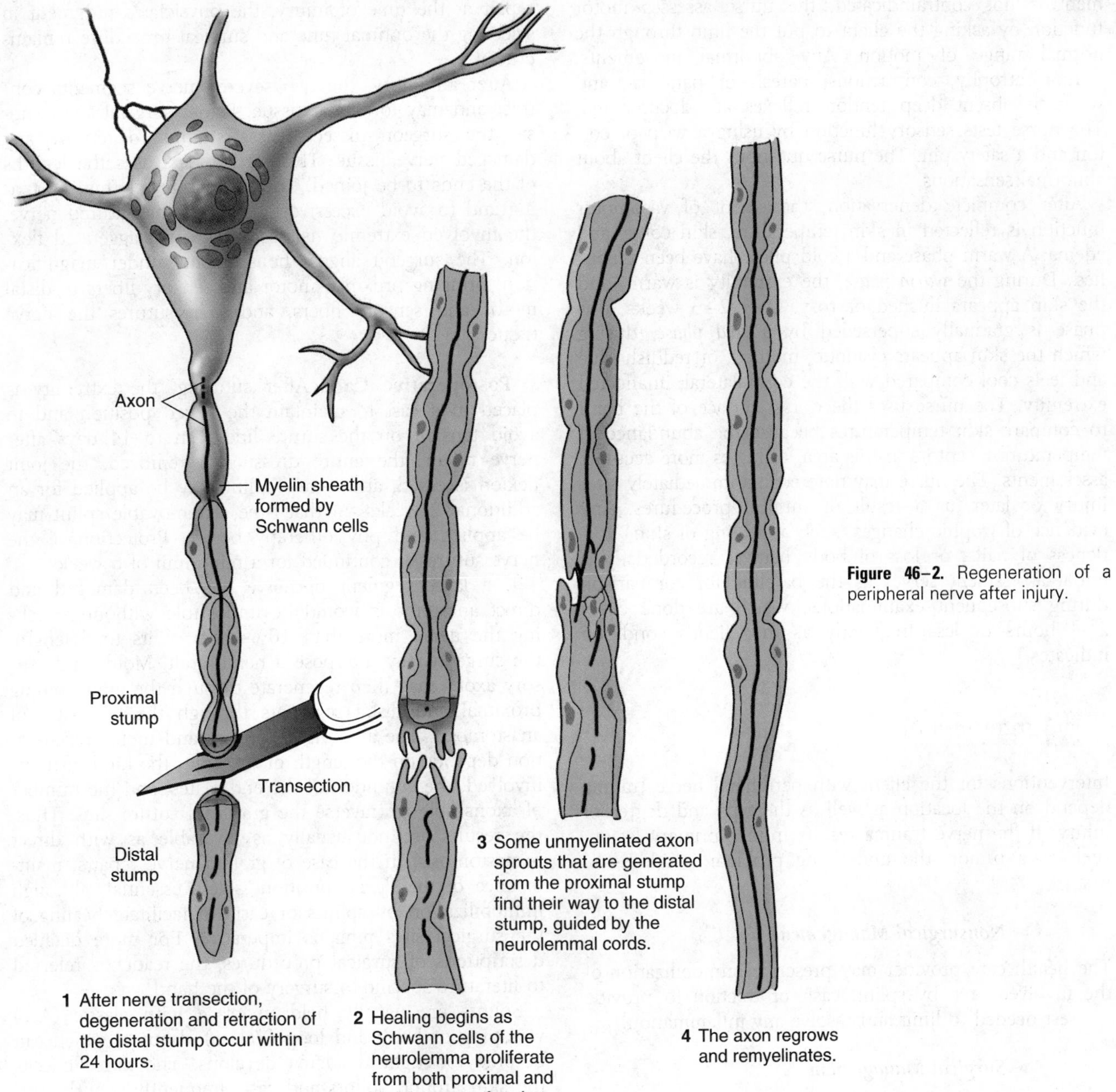

Axon

Myelin sheath
formed by
Schwann cells

Proximal
stump

Transection

Distal
stump

3 Some unmyelinated axon
sprouts that are generated
from the proximal stump
find their way to the distal
stump, guided by the
neurolemmal cords.

Figure 46–2. Regeneration of a
peripheral nerve after injury.

1 After nerve transection,
degeneration and retraction of
the distal stump occur within
24 hours.

2 Healing begins as
Schwann cells of the
neurolemma proliferate
from both proximal and
distal stumps, forming
neurolemmal cords
that will guide the
regenerating axon.

4 The axon regrows
and remyelinates.

eral innervation to the affected areas. These collaterals provide some innervation before the axon itself has regenerated sufficiently.

Collaborative Management

Assessment

The primary nursing considerations for the client with peripheral nerve trauma are assessment of function, maintenance of function, and rehabilitation.

The client may relate a history of extremity or pelvic trauma, penetrating injury, recent surgery, use of crutches, or pain after medication injections. In addition to weakness or flaccid paralysis, the client may complain of burning sensations distal to the trauma or pain that increases on tactile or environmental stimulation. Skin and nail changes of the affected extremities may be noted by the client as well.

The nurse performs a physical assessment to determine which neurologic functions are intact. In acute trauma, the injury should first be evaluated by the physician to determine whether movement is contraindicated. If movement is not contraindicated, the nurse assesses motor function by asking the client to put the limb through the normal range of motion. Any abnormal movements, tremor, atrophy, contractions, paresis or paralysis, and weak or absent deep tendon reflexes are documented. The nurse tests sensory function by using a wisp of cotton and a safety pin. The nurse questions the client about abnormal sensations.

After complete denervation, the extent of vasomotor function is reflected in skin temperature, skin color, and edema. A warm phase and a cold phase have been identified. During the *warm phase,* the extremity is warm, and the skin appears flushed or rosy. Over 2–3 weeks, this phase is gradually superseded by a *cold phase,* during which the skin appears cyanotic, mottled, or reddish blue and feels cool compared with the contralateral, unaffected extremity. The nurse uses the dorsal surface of the hand to compare skin temperatures because the abundance of temperature receptors in this area facilitates more accurate assessments. The nurse may note edema immediately after injury or later, as a result of surgical procedures. Any evidence of trophic changes, such as scaling of skin, brittleness of nails, or loss of body hair, is recorded. This initial assessment serves as the baseline for comparison during subsequent examinations, which are done every 2–4 hours or less frequently as the client's condition indicates.

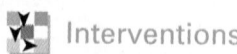 Interventions

Interventions for the client with peripheral nerve trauma depend on the location as well as the type and degree of injury. If the nerve trauma results from a primary lesion, such as a tumor, the underlying problem is addressed first.

➤ Nonsurgical Management

The health care provider may prescribe immobilization of the involved area by splint, cast, or traction to provide the rest needed to limit and resolve any inflammation.

➤ Surgical Management

The purpose of surgical management is to restore function of the damaged nerve(s).

Preoperative Care. There are usually no special preoperative interventions for the client undergoing peripheral nerve repair. (Chapter 20 describes the general care of the client before surgery.)

Operative Procedures. If the nerve is lacerated or transected, surgery may be indicated. Restorative procedures include resecting and suturing to reapproximate the severed nerve ends, nerve grafts, and nerve and tendon transplants.

Since surgeons first began to repair injured nerves, the timing of these procedures has been controversial. In the past, with delay of repair for 3–8 weeks after injury, associated injuries could heal and the surgeon could better assess the extent of nerve damage. Although microsurgery and the use of lasers now allow primary nerve repair at the time of injury, the physician's judgment in selecting the optimal time and surgical procedure remains crucial.

After an injury, the two severed nerve segments contract and may form scar tissue. Before surgical anastomosis, the surgeon dissects these stumps to remove any damaged nerve tissue. This further decreases the lengths of the ends to be joined. To compensate for this shortening and to avoid excessive tension on the sutured nerve, the involved extremity is positioned in exaggerated flexion. The surgeon aligns the segments under magnification, bringing proximal motor and sensory fibers to distal motor and sensory fibers, and then sutures the nerve tissue.

Postoperative Care. After suturing, the extremity is placed in a cast to maintain the flexed position and to avoid tension on the suture line. Ten to 14 days after nerve repair, the entire dressing is removed, the joint flexion is eased, and a new splint may be applied for an additional 2 weeks. At that time, a removable splint may be applied and physiotherapy begun. Protection of the nerve sutures is continued for a minimum of 6 weeks.

If a large segment of nerve has been damaged and direct anastomosis would be impossible without stretching the nerve more than 10%–15% of its total length, the surgeon may interpose a nerve graft. Motor and sensory axons may then regenerate through the graft, joining proximal and distal segments through the two sites of anastomosis. The amount of sensory and motor regeneration depends on the length of the graft, the kind of nerve involved, the condition of the end plates, and the number of axons able to traverse the graft and suture sites. Thus, the results are not usually as favorable as with direct reanastomosis. In the case of grafted nerve repairs, maintenance of the flexed position is less essential, although immobilization by splints or casts to facilitate healing of the surgical sites remains imperative. For more detailed descriptions of surgical procedures, the reader is referred to literature specific to surgery of the hand.

Splints are usually held in place with elastic (Ace) wrapping or hook and loop (Velcro) closures, which can become too tight if edema develops. The nurse checks the skin around splints and casts frequently (hourly, initially) for tightness, warmth, and color. If the client complains of discomfort, tingling, or coolness or if the color is blanched, the cast or splint may be too tight; the nurse promptly informs the physician. The nurse immediately reports any indication of drainage under a splint or cast.

Skin care is essential. Atrophy of the epidermis and underlying tissue causes the skin to become more fragile and more susceptible to injury and breakdown. The decreased skin nutrition and decreased vascularity associated with denervation cause delayed healing, which further compounds the problem. The nurse thoroughly examines the skin for evidence of irritation or injury and assists or instructs the client to wash and dry the involved areas carefully. If the skin is dry, lanolin or cocoa butter may be used as a lubricant. Because sensation may be absent or inhibited, the nurse instructs the client to protect involved areas from extremes in temperature or other sources of potential trauma.

➤ Rehabilitation

Physiotherapy is the major approach for rehabilitation after surgical repair. The nurse reinforces and helps the client perform exercises learned in these sessions. Because the regeneration of nerves and subsequent return of sensory and motor function may be extremely slow and pain producing, the client may become discouraged and depressed. If the disability is permanent, the client needs encouragement and assistance to cope with the changes in body image, self-esteem, and lifestyle.

Restless Legs Syndrome

Overview

Restless legs syndrome (RLS) affects between 5% and 15% of the U.S. population, but most health care providers do not know what it is. The incidence may be higher in nursing home and home care clients, who often have diabetes and renal failure, two conditions that are correlated with RLS (Boucher, 1997).

The client complains of intense "crawling-type" sensations in the limbs and subsequently feels the need to move the limbs repeatedly. These symptoms are worse at night and when the client is still for a period of time. For that reason, clients with RLS often refer to themselves as "night walkers."

Collaborative Management

Diagnosis is made on the history and there is no known etiology. Potential contributing factors include vitamin and mineral deficiencies, anemias, polyneuropathies, diabetes mellitus, renal failure, and substances such as caffeine, alcohol, tricyclics, and beta-blockers.

The management of RLS is symptomatic and involves treating the underlying cause or contributing factor, if known. The nurse recommends measures for promoting sleep. For some clients, the health care provider orders antiembolism stockings or medications that have proven to be effective for some clients, e.g., clonidine hydrochloride (Catapres, Dixarit✦), carbamazepine (Tegretol, Mazepine✦), and clonazepam (Clonidine, Rivotril✦) (Boucher, 1997). The Restless Legs Foundation is an excellent resource for information and client and family support.

Diseases of the Cranial Nerves

The nurse may encounter clients with cranial nerve disease in various practice settings. The cranial nerves may be affected in association with other disorders of the nervous system or as a result of trauma. The most common disorders, those affecting cranial nerves V (trigeminal) and VII (facial), are discussed here.

Trigeminal Neuralgia

Overview

ELDERLY CONSIDERATIONS

 Trigeminal neuralgia, or *tic douloureux*, usually appears in people older than 50 years. The elderly are affected at a frequency of 15 cases per 100,000, with a female to male ratio of 2:1 (Weisberg, et al., 1996). This disorder

- Entails a specific type of facial pain, which occurs in abrupt, intense paroxysms
- Is usually provoked by minimal stimulation of a trigger zone
- Is unilateral and confined to the area innervated by the trigeminal nerve, most often the second and third branches (Fig. 46–3)

Clients younger than 30 years with pain in more than one branch of the trigeminal nerve may be further evaluated to rule out the possibility of a tumor or multiple sclerosis.

When describing the pain, clients use terms such as "excruciating," "sharp," "shooting," "piercing," "burning," and "jabbing." Between bursts of pain, which last from seconds to minutes, there is usually no pain. The nurse usually finds no sensory or motor deficits on examination, although the condition can be agonizing for the client. The fear of precipitating attacks often causes clients to avoid talking, smiling, eating, or attending to such hygienic needs as shaving, washing the face, and brushing the teeth.

The cause of trigeminal neuralgia is thought to be related to impaired inhibitory mechanisms in the brain stem caused by excessive firing of irritated fibers in the trigeminal nerve. In addition, trauma and infection of the teeth, jaw, or ear may be contributing factors.

The course of trigeminal neuralgia is characterized by bouts of pain for several weeks or months followed by spontaneous remissions. The length of these remissions may vary from days to years, but attack-free periods tend to become shorter as the client grows older. Symptoms rarely disappear permanently.

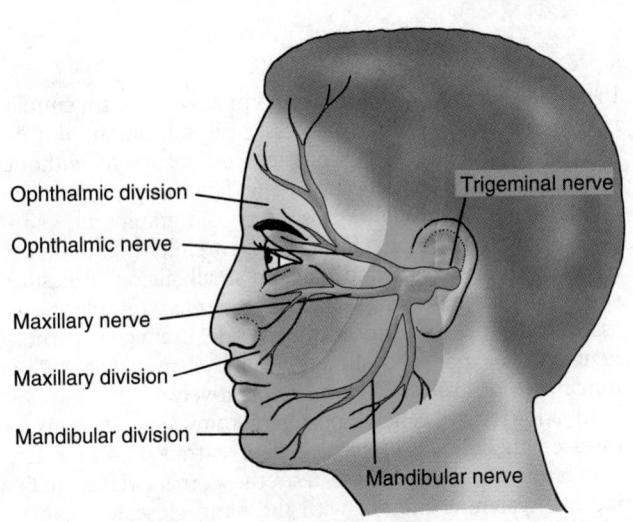

Figure 46–3. Distribution of the trigeminal nerve and its three divisions: ophthalmic, maxillary, and mandibular.

Collaborative Management

Management of the client with trigeminal neuralgia is determined by the amount of pain the client is experiencing. Conservative measures are usually tried first.

Nonsurgical Management. Medical management is accomplished with the use of drugs, such as carbamazepine (Tegretol, Apo-Carbamazepine, Mazepine♣), phenytoin (Dilantin), baclofen (Lioresal), and occasionally amitriptyline (Elavil, Meravil♣) or diazepam (Valium, E-Pam♣). Initial therapy should always be nonsurgical, and drugs may be used singly or in combination. Surgical management may be considered if the client and the physician agree that the pain or the toxic effects of drug therapy are worse than the risk of surgery.

Approximately 70% of clients respond to carbamazepine, 20–1200 mg daily, alone or in combination with phenytoin in average daily doses of 200–400 mg. Fosphenytoin may also be given intravenously to abort an acute attack. Phenytoin and fosphenytoin are anticonvulsants believed to decrease the paroxysmal afferent impulses in much the same way as when these drugs are used in the treatment of seizure disorders.

Injection of alcohol into the affected branch of the trigeminal nerve may relieve pain for periods of up to 16 months. Injection into the gasserian ganglion, where sensory root fibers arise, may provide permanent pain control but with greater risk of extraocular palsies, keratitis, blindness, or masticatory paralysis. In both blocking procedures, complete anesthesia to the portion of the face innervated by the injected branch results.

Surgical Management. The purpose of surgery is to relieve the client's pain.

➤ Preoperative Care

In addition to the general preoperative care provided to all clients (see Chap. 20), the surgeon thoroughly explains the surgical benefits and any expected neurologic deficits. The nurse reinforces the information provided by the surgeon.

➤ Operative Procedures

In some clients, a small artery compresses the trigeminal nerve as it enters the pons. Surgical relocation of this artery may relieve the pain of trigeminal neuralgia without compromising facial sensation. The *Jannetta procedure* accomplishes this through a posterior fossa craniotomy. Under microscopic vision, the surgeon carefully lifts the loop of artery off the nerve and places a small silicone (Silastic) sponge between the vessel and the nerve. Complications associated with this procedure include headache, permanent cranial nerve dysfunction, and hemorrhage. The nurse provides routine care postoperatively.

In addition to general postcraniotomy care, the nurse assesses the client's corneal reflex, extraocular muscles, and facial nerve. The nurse tests the corneal reflex, making a threatening motion with the hand close to the eye. The client will blink if the reflex is intact. The nurse

assesses extraocular muscles by asking the client to follow a finger through the six cardinal positions (see Chap. 43) while observing for conjugate eye movements. For assessing the facial nerve, the nurse asks the client to wrinkle the forehead, frown, wink, squeeze the eyes closed, whistle, and blow air out of the cheeks. Last, the nurse evaluates the client for abnormal sensations and pain as well as ability to chew. The nurse documents any abnormal findings and reports them to the physician. In a similar microvascular procedure, one or all branches of the trigeminal nerve are visualized and dissected.

Radiofrequency rhizotomy may provide lasting relief of pain without compromising touch or motor function. During this procedure, the client is sedated with small doses of diazepam, midazolam hydrochloride (Versed), or fentanyl (Sublimaze) but is alert and able to respond verbally to questions. The physician inserts a needle electrode and advances it under radiographic control to the appropriate area, where a heat lesion is made. After each needle insertion, the corneal and ciliary reflexes, as well as sensation in the face, are checked. The advantages of this procedure include

- Long-term pain relief
- Relatively short hospital stays
- Tolerance by the elderly
- Absence of facial paralysis
- Preservation of the sensation of touch

The possibility of puncturing the internal carotid artery and the occurrence of anesthesia dolorosa are disadvantages (Hickey, 1996). The affected side is permanently insensitive to pain.

➤ Postoperative Care

The nurse applies an ice pack to the operative site on the jaw for 4 hours. A soft diet is prescribed, and the client is discouraged from chewing on the affected side until the paresthesia is abated. The nurse instructs the client to avoid rubbing the eye on the affected side because the protective mechanism of pain will no longer warn of injury (Chart 46–7). The nurse teaches the client to inspect the eye daily for redness or irritation and to report this or blurred vision to the physician. The client may also develop herpes simplex around the lips. The nurse encourages the client to schedule regular dental examinations because the absence of pain may not warn the client of potential problems.

Chart 46–7

Education Guide: Trigeminal Nerve Rhizotomy

Avoid rubbing your eye on the affected side.
Inspect your eye daily for redness and irritation.
See your dentist regularly for examinations.
When possible, chew your food on the unaffected side.

Psychosocial considerations for the client with trigeminal neuralgia include disappointment with ineffective drug protocols or surgical procedures as well as fear that the pain may recur with any activity. The client may fail to move the face in an attempt to prevent pain. This behavior may be misinterpreted by others as withdrawal, antisociability, or depression. The nurse's goal is to help the client cope with the condition and to develop strategies for dealing with identified problems.

Facial Paralysis

Overview

Facial paralysis, or *Bell's palsy* (acute paralysis of cranial nerve VII) was first described by Sir Charles Bell of England in 1821. The incidence is 23 per 100,000; men and women are equally affected (Hickey, 1996). Although the incidence may be slightly higher among diabetics, the condition occurs in all ages and at all times of the year.

The onset is acute. Maximal paralysis is attained within 48 hours in about half the clients and within 5 days in almost all clients. Pain behind the ear or on the face may precede paralysis by a few hours or days. The disorder is characterized by a drawing sensation and paralysis of all facial muscles on the affected side. The client cannot close the eye, wrinkle the forehead, smile, whistle, or grimace. The face appears mask-like and sags. Taste is usually impaired to some degree, but this seldom persists beyond the second week of paralysis.

Although the cause of Bell's palsy remains obscure, it may be the result of an inflammatory process. Although clients with Bell's palsy are rarely hospitalized, the nurse may encounter them in outpatient settings, such as clinics or physicians' offices or emergency departments.

Collaborative Management

Medical management consists of the administration of prednisone (Deltasone, Winpred✦), 30–60 mg daily, during the first week after the onset of symptoms. Analgesics may help relieve the pain. Nursing care is directed toward managing the major neurologic deficits and providing psychosocial support. Because the eye does not close, the cornea must be protected from drying and subsequent ulceration or abrasion. The nurse instructs the client to manually close the eyelid at intervals and to instill artificial tears four times daily. The eye may be patched or taped closed at bedtime.

The client may be unable to chew, sip fluids through a straw, or control drooling on the affected side. Thus, mealtime may become a problem. The nurse encourages the client to eat and drink using the unaffected side of the mouth. The nurse may be needed to provide emotional support and suggestions for coping and adapting. Frequent, small meals may be better tolerated, and clients may require a soft diet. The nurse explains simple techniques of massage; application of warm, moist heat; and facial exercises.

A facial sling may prevent drooping of the affected side. As muscle tone improves, the nurse instructs the client to grimace, wrinkle the brow, force the eyes closed, whistle, and blow air out of the cheeks three or four times daily for 5 minutes in front of a mirror.

Although 80% of clients recover fully within a few weeks or months, approximately 15%–20% have some residual weakness; a few have permanent neurologic deficits (Hickey, 1996). These clients require a great deal of support because body image and self-esteem are drastically affected. The nurse is a valuable source of both information and psychosocial support.

📍 CASE STUDY for the Client with Guillain-Barré Syndrome

■ An anxious female client presents in the Emergency Department (ED) of a community hospital with complaints of leg cramps, lower extremity muscle weakness, and facial weakness. When taking her history, the nurse finds that these symptoms began earlier in the day and have worsened. The client states that she is a physical therapist and is concerned that she may have Guillain-Barré syndrome (GBS). The ED physician confirms this diagnosis and admits the client to the general medical-surgical unit.

Q U E S T I O N S :

1. What is the nurse's priority in the care of the client at this time?
2. What is a possible cause of the client's GBS?
3. What should the nurse teach her about the disorder?

SELECTED BIBLIOGRAPHY

Barker, F. G., Jannetta, D. J., Larkins, N. V., & Jho, H. D. (1996). Long term outcomes after microvascular decompression for trigeminal neuralgia. *New England Journal of Medicine, 334*(5), 1077–1083.

Boucher, M. A. (1997). Restless legs syndrome in home healthcare. *Home Healthcare Nurse, 15*(8), 550–556.

Froelich, J., & Eagle, C. J. (1996). Anaesthetic management of the patient with myasthenia gravis and trachial stenosis. *Canadian Journal of Anaesthesia, 43*(1), 84–89.

Giger, J. N. & Davidhizar, R. E. (1995). *Transcultural nursing: Assessment and intervention* (2nd ed.). St. Louis: Mosby–Year Book.

Hardy, E. M. (1994). Myasthenia gravis: An overview. *Orthopaedic Nursing, 13*(6), 37–42.

Hickey, J. V. (1996). *The clinical practice of neurological and neurosurgical nursing.* Philadelphia: J. B. Lippincott.

Kernich, C. A. (1996). Myths and facts about myasthenia gravis. *Nursing96, 26*(7), 21.

Kernich A., & Kaminski, H. J. (1995) Myasthenia gravis: Pathophysiology diagnosis and collaborative care. *Journal of Neuroscience Nursing, 27*(4), 207–218.

Kupersmith, M. J., et al. (1996). Beneficial effects of corticosteroids on ocular myasthenia gravis. *Archives of Neurology, 53*(8), 802–804.

McMahon-Parkes, K. (1997). Guillain-Barré syndrome: Biological basis, treatment, and care. *Intensive Critical Care Nurse, 13*(1), 42–48.

Midroni, G. (1996). Chronic inflammatory polyradicular demyelinating neuropathy, usual clinical features and therapeutic response. *Neurology, 46*(5), 1206–1212.

O'Donnell, L. (1995). Caring for patients with myasthenia gravis. *Nursing95, 25*(3), 60–61.

*Osserman, H. M. (1958). *Myasthenia gravis.* New York: Grune and Stratton.

Putman, M. T. (1996). Myasthenia gravis and upper airway obstruction. *Chest, 209*(2), 400–404.

Rees, J. (1995). Guillain-Barré syndrome. Clinical manifestations and directions for treatment. *Drugs, 49*(6), 912–920.

Scrivani, S., Mathews, E. W., Keith, D., & Slawk, E. (1995). Percutaneous differential radiofrequency thermal rhizotomy for treatment of trigeminal neuralgia. *Journal of Orofacial Pain, 9*(1), 36–41.

Taha, J. M., & Tew, J. M. (1996). Comparison of surgical treatments for trigeminal neuralgia: Reevaluation of radiofrequency rhizotomy. *Neurosurgery, 38*(5), 865–871.

Weisberg, L. A., Garcia, C., & Strub, R. (1996). *Essentials of clinical neurology.* St. Louis: Mosby–Year Book.

Yang, J., et al. (1996). Trigeminal neuralgia versus atypical facial pain: A review of the literature and case report. *Oral Surgery, Medicine, Pathology, Radiology, and Endodontics, 81*(4), 424–432.

SUGGESTED READINGS

O'Donnell, L. (1996). An elusive weakness: Myasthenia gravis. *MED-SURG Nursing, 5*(1), 44–49

The article provides an excellent description of the variety of signs and symptoms that the client with myasthenia gravis may experience and why it is often difficult to diagnose. It includes an excellent overview of pathophysiology, diagnosis, and clinical management of the client. The nursing care section provides practical and useful information for the nurse caring for the client with a potentially life-threatening condition.

McConaghy, D. J. (1994). Trigeminal neuralgia: A personal review and nursing implications. *Journal of Neuroscience Nursing, 26*(2), 85–90.

The author discusses the medical, surgical, and pharmacologic treatment of trigeminal neuralgia. The nursing interventions suggested are especially noteworthy, as the author has personal experience with trigeminal neuralgia.

Chapter 47

INTERVENTIONS FOR CRITICALLY ILL CLIENTS WITH NEUROLOGIC PROBLEMS

CHAPTER

HIGHLIGHTS

Some neurologic problems, such as cerebrovascular accident (CVA), head injury, brain tumor, and brain abscess, can cause increased intracranial pressure (ICP), a life-threatening complication. Through prompt recognition and aggressive management of this complication, permanent neurologic dysfunction or death may be prevented.

CEREBROVASCULAR ACCIDENT

Overview

A cerebrovascular accident (or cerebral vascular accident [CVA]), commonly referred to as a *stroke,* is a disruption in the normal blood supply to the brain. It often occurs suddenly and produces focal neurologic deficits. Although the number of stroke deaths has decreased during the past several years, CVA remains the third most common cause of death in the United States and the primary cause of adult disability. The direct and indirect cost of stroke is $30 billion annually.

The National Stroke Association now uses the term "brain attack" to describe stroke. Stroke is a medical emergency that strikes suddenly and should be treated immediately to prevent neurologic deficit and permanent disability.

Pathophysiology

Pathophysiologic Changes in the Brain

The brain must receive a constant flow of blood for normal function, because it is unable to store oxygen or glucose. In addition, blood flow is important for the removal of metabolic waste, carbon dioxide, and lactic acid. If deprived of its blood flow, the brain can be permanently damaged within a few minutes.

Through the processes of cerebral autoregulation, blood flow is maintained at a fairly constant rate of 1000 mL/min. In response to blood pressure changes or changes in carbon dioxide tension, the cerebral arteries dilate or constrict.

In the event of a CVA, ischemia occurs in the brain tissue supplied by the affected artery, and brain dysfunction results. Ischemia leads to hypoxia or anoxia and hypoglycemia. These processes then cause infarction or death of the neurons, the glia, and the involved area of the brain. In addition, brain metabolism after stroke is affected in the involved area as well as in the contralateral (opposite side) hemisphere.

Small lacunar infarcts may also occur. Lacunae are small, deep cavities within the brain that result from occlusion of a small vessel. This occlusion leads to infarct and necrosis of the area of the brain supplied by the affected vessel. Lacunar infarcts occur almost exclusively

TABLE 47–1

Differential Features of the Types of Stroke			

Feature	Ischemic		Hemorrhagic
	Thrombotic	**Embolic**	
Evolution	• Intermittent or stepwise improvement between episodes of worsening • Completed stroke	• Abrupt development of completed stroke • Steady progression	• Usually abrupt onset
Onset	• Daytime (10 AM–12 PM) • Gradual (minutes to hours)	• Daytime • Sudden	• Daytime • Sudden, may be gradual if caused by hypertension
Level of consciousness	• Preserved (client is awake)	• Preserved (client is awake)	• Deepening stupor or coma
Contributing associated factors	• Hypertension • Atherosclerosis	• Cardiac disease	• Hypertension • Vessel disorders
Prodromal symptoms	• Transient ischemic attack		
Neurologic deficits	• Deficits during the first few weeks • Slight headache • Speech deficits • Visual problems • Confusion	• Maximal deficit at onset • Paralysis • Expressive aphasia	• Focal deficits • Severe, frequent
Cerebrospinal fluid	• Normal, possibly presence of protein	• Normal	• Bloody
Seizures	• No	• No	• Usually
Duration	• Improvements during weeks to months • Possibly permanent deficits	• Rapid improvements	• Variable, possibly permanent neurologic deficits

in the internal capsule, the basal ganglia, and the thalamus. They produce either a pure motor deficit (internal capsule) or a pure sensory deficit (thalamus). A lacunar infarct is generally regarded as a type of ischemic stroke (see later).

Types of Cerebrovascular Accidents

CVAs are generally classified as ischemic (occlusive) or hemorrhagic. Ischemic strokes are further divided into thrombotic strokes and embolic strokes (Table 47–1).

ISCHEMIC STROKE. An ischemic stroke is caused by occlusion of a cerebral artery by either a thrombus or an embolus (Fig. 47–1). A stroke that is caused by a thrombus is referred to as a thrombotic stroke, whereas a stroke caused by an embolus is referred to as an embolic stroke.

Thrombotic Stroke. Thrombotic strokes account for over half of all strokes and are commonly associated with the development of atherosclerosis of the blood vessel wall (see Fig. 47–1). Arteriosclerosis is a noninflammatory degenerative disease affecting almost any cerebral blood vessel. As a result of plaques or atheromatous deposits that gradually build up on the interior of the vessel wall, the artery loses its elasticity and becomes hardened. The thrombus extends along the interior of the artery, gradually occluding the lumen of the artery. This process may occur during many years, and often collateral circu-

lation to the involved area develops. As the artery becomes completely occluded, blood flow to the area is markedly diminished. Decreased blood flow causes transient ischemia, which progresses to complete ischemia and infarction of the brain tissue. Within 72 hours, the area is edematous and necrotic, and cavities develop. The bifurcations (divisions) of the common carotid artery and the vertebral arteries at their junction with the basilar artery are the most common sites involved. Because of the gradual occlusion of the arteries, thrombotic strokes tend to have a slow onset.

A lacunar stroke is another type of thrombotic stroke. A lacunar stroke causes a soft area or cavity to develop in the white matter or the deep gray matter of the brain. This type of stroke may result in significant neurologic dysfunction if it damages a critical area in the brain.

Embolic Stroke. An embolic stroke is caused by an embolus or a group of emboli that break off from one area of the body and travel to the cerebral arteries via the carotid artery (see Fig. 47–1). The usual sources of emboli are cardiac. Emboli can occur in clients with nonvalvular atrial fibrillation, ischemic heart disease, rheumatic heart disease, and mural thrombi following an MI or a prosthetic heart valve. Another source of emboli may be plaque that breaks off from the carotid sinus or the internal carotid artery. Emboli tend to become lodged in the smaller cerebral blood vessels at their point of bifurcation

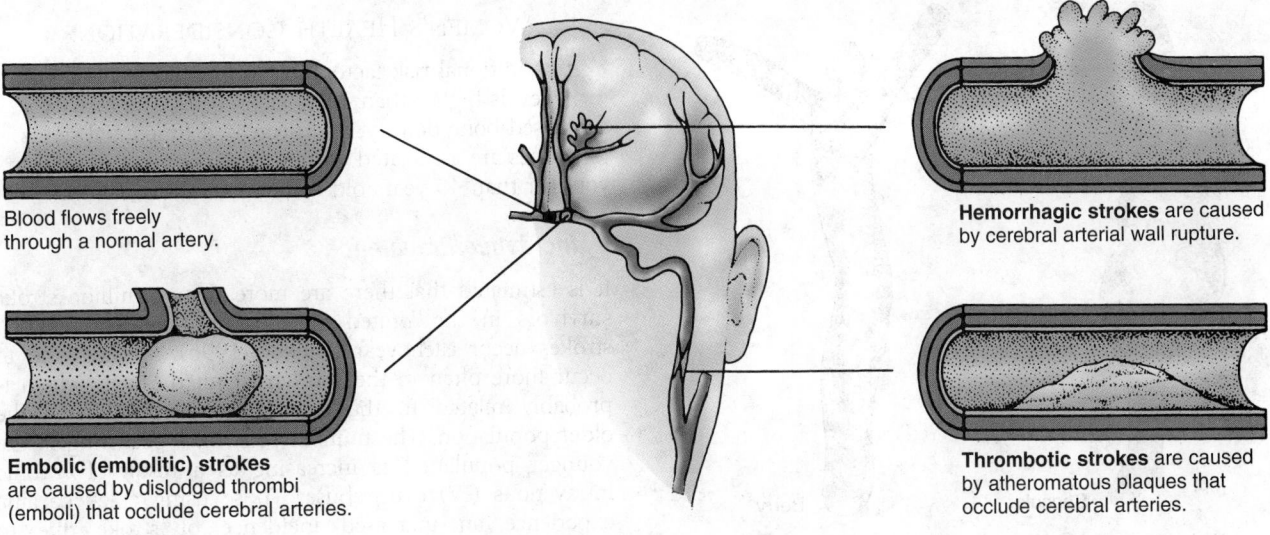

Blood flows freely
through a normal artery.

Embolic (embolitic) strokes
are caused by dislodged thrombi
(emboli) that occlude cerebral arteries.

Hemorrhagic strokes are caused
by cerebral arterial wall rupture.

Thrombotic strokes are caused
by atheromatous plaques that
occlude cerebral arteries.

Figure 47–1. The types of stroke.

or where the lumen narrows. Embolic strokes account for about a third of all strokes.

The middle cerebral artery (MCA) is most frequently involved. As the emboli occlude the vessel, ischemia develops, and the client experiences the clinical manifestations of the stroke. Often, however, the occlusion is temporary, and the embolus breaks into smaller fragments, enters smaller blood vessels, and is absorbed. For these reasons, embolic strokes are characterized by the sudden development and rapid occurrence of focal neurologic deficits, followed by clearing of the symptoms during several hours or a few days. However, a cerebral hemorrhage may result if significant damage to the wall of the involved vessel has occurred.

Transient Ischemic Attack and Reversible Ischemic Neurologic Deficit. Ischemic strokes are frequently preceded by warning signs, such as a transient ischemic attack (TIA)—also called "silent" strokes—(Chart 47–1) or a reversible ischemic neurologic deficit (RIND). Both cause transient focal neurologic dysfunction attributable to a brief interruption in cerebral blood flow, possibly owing to cerebral vasospasm or transient systemic arterial hypertension. The difference between a TIA and an RIND is the length of time that the client is symptomatic. A TIA lasts a few minutes to less than 24 hours, whereas symptoms of an RIND last longer than 24 hours but less than a week. Both TIAs and RINDs damage the brain tissue, which is evidenced by magnetic resonance imaging (MRI) or computed tomography (CT). Multiple TIAs increase the risk of major stroke.

Hemorrhagic Stroke

The second major classification of stroke is hemorrhagic stroke (see Fig. 47–1). In this type of stroke, the integrity of the vessel is interrupted, and bleeding occurs into the brain tissue or the spaces surrounding the brain (ventricular, subdural, subarachnoid). Hemorrhage into the brain tissue generally results from a ruptured saccular (berry)

aneurysm, rupture of an arteriovenous malformation (AVM) or, more commonly, hypertension. Although the exact mechanisms involved are unknown, it is hypothesized that elevated systolic and diastolic pressures cause changes within the arterial wall that leave it susceptible to rupture. An intracerebral hemorrhage occurs when the vessel ruptures.

A ruptured cerebral aneurysm is another cause of hemorrhagic stroke. An *aneurysm* is an abnormal ballooning or blister on the involved artery (Fig. 47–2). Aneurysms may be congenital or traumatic. A congenital aneurysm is a developmental defect in the media and elastica of the vessel wall. Both etiologies weaken the vessel wall. Continued force on the weakened vessel wall from elevated blood pressure causes the vessel wall to become stretched and thinned. Although rupture may occur at any time, it usually happens during activity. Aneurysms are often

---

Chart 47–1

Key Features of Transient Ischemic Attack

Visual Deficits
- Blurred vision
- Diplopia (double vision)
- Blindness in one eye
- Tunnel vision

Motor Deficits
- Transient weakness (arm, hand, or leg)
- Gait disturbance (ataxic)

Sensory Deficits
- Transient numbness (face, arm, or hand)
- Vertigo

Speech Deficits
- Aphasia
- Dysarthria (slurred speech)

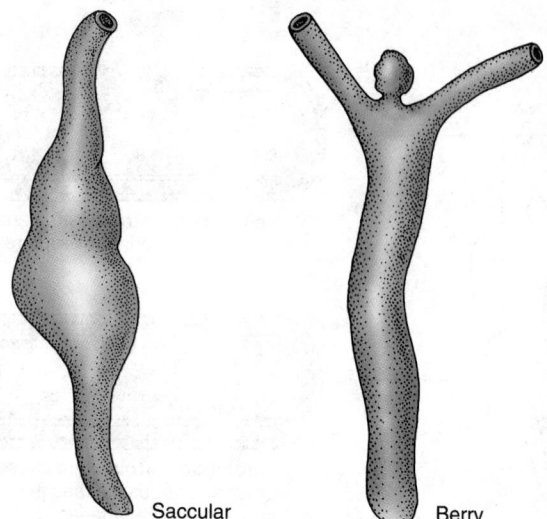

Figure 47–2. Two common types of cerebral aneurysms.

found at branchings of major cerebral arteries (Fig. 47–3). Rupture of the aneurysm causes bleeding into the subarachnoid space or directly into the ventricles or the development of an intracerebral hematoma. Vasospasm, a sudden and transient constriction of a cerebral artery, often occurs after a cerebral hemorrhage. Blood flow to distal areas of the brain supplied by the artery is markedly diminished, leading to cerebral ischemia and infarction and further neurologic dysfunction.

An *arteriovenous malformation* is a developmental abnormality that occurs during embryonic development. It is a tangled or spaghetti-like mass of malformed, thin-walled, dilated vessels (Fig. 47–4). The congenital absence of a capillary network in these vessels forms an abnormal communication between the arterial and venous systems. The vessels may eventually rupture, causing bleeding into the subarachnoid space or into the intracerebral tissue.

Etiology

Strokes are caused by an occlusion in an artery from a thrombus or an embolus; they are also due to hemorrhage resulting from hypertension, a ruptured aneurysm, or an AVM. Certain major risk factors have been identified that increase the likelihood of cerebrovascular disease, especially hypertension, diabetes mellitus, heart disease, and nonvalvular atrial fibrillation.

Other risk factors include

- Smoking
- Substance abuse (particularly cocaine)
- Obesity
- A sedentary lifestyle
- High stress levels
- Elevated serum cholesterol, lipoprotein, and triglyceride levels
- Previous CVA or TIA
- Heavy alcohol use
- Sudden discontinuation of antihypertensive medications (causes hemorrhagic stroke)

WOMEN'S HEALTH CONSIDERATIONS

Additional risk factors for women are hemoglobin levels higher than 14 g, lack of physical activity, decreased bone density, and decreased functional status. Migraines are associated with ischemic strokes in women younger than 45 years old (Allen & Phillips, 1997).

Incidence/Prevalence

It is estimated that there are more than 3 million stroke survivors in the United States. Approximately 550,000 strokes occur each year (Hickey, 1996). Strokes tend to occur more often in the southern United States, which is probably related to the geographic distribution of the older population. The number of strokes occurring in the younger population is increasing as a result of chronic intravenous (IV) drug abuse. Those using crack cocaine experience an increased incidence of stroke due to changes in the clotting mechanism caused by the drugs or the sudden increase in systolic blood pressure (BP).

ELDERLY CONSIDERATIONS

Stroke may occur at any age; however, it usually occurs in people older than 45 years, with an increased frequency in people older than 65 years. Males have a higher rate of stroke than females by a 3:1 ratio. There are 150,000 deaths that occur per year as a result of strokes (Hickey, 1996).

TRANSCULTURAL CONSIDERATIONS

African-Americans are affected more frequently than other groups, possibly as a result of the high fre-

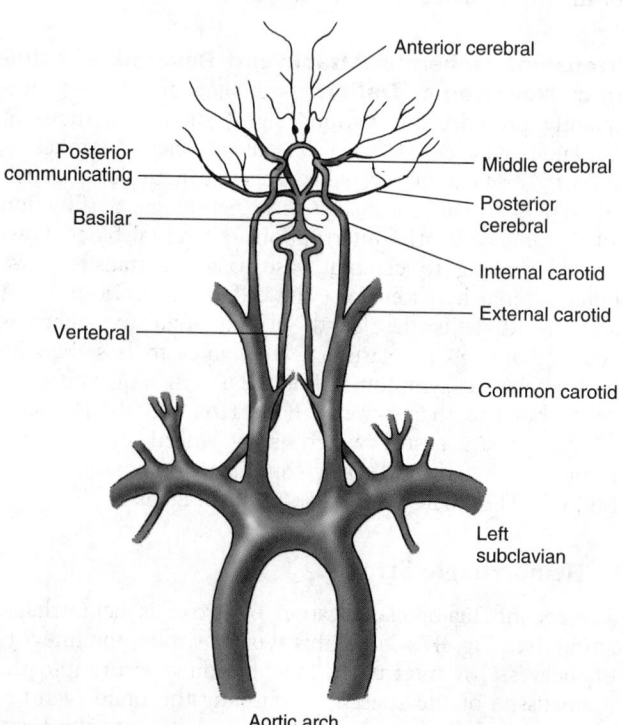

Figure 47–3. Common locations for cerebral aneurysms.

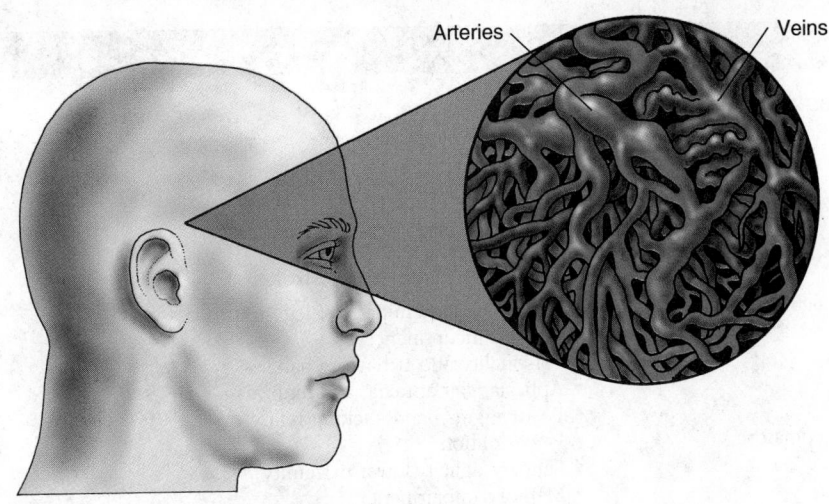

Figure 47-4. Appearance of an arteriovenous malformation. Note dilated, entangled blood vessels.

quency of hypertension and diabetes in this group. A study of 660,000 medical records of clients 15–44 years old found that ischemic strokes were twice as common in African-Americans as in Caucasians; hemorrhagic strokes were three times more common among African-Americans (Allen & Phillips, 1997).

Collaborative Management

 Assessment

➤ History

An accurate history is important in the diagnosis of a stroke. The information obtained assists in the identification of the area of the brain involved as well as the cause of the stroke. The nurse obtains a history of the client's activity when the stroke began. Ischemic strokes frequently occur during sleep, whereas hemorrhagic strokes tend to occur during activity. Next, the nurse asks the client or a family member how the symptoms progressed. The nurse also elicits a history of the onset of the stroke. Symptoms of an embolic or hemorrhagic stroke tend to occur abruptly, whereas thrombotic strokes generally have a more gradual progression. The nurse must also determine the severity of the symptoms; for example, whether they got worse after the initial onset (hemorrhagic stroke) or began to improve (embolic stroke). It is important to determine whether the symptoms come and go, possibly indicating a TIA or an RIND.

During the interview, the nurse observes the client's level of consciousness (LOC) and assesses for indications of intellectual or memory impairments or difficulties with speech or hearing. The client or family member is questioned about the presence of any sensory or motor changes, visual problems, problems with balance or gait, and changes in reading or writing abilities.

In addition, the nurse asks about past medical history, with specific attention directed toward a history of head trauma, diabetes, hypertension, heart disease, anemia, obesity, and headache. A list of any medications the client currently takes is obtained, including prescribed, over-the-counter, and recreational (illicit) drugs. Medications that could contribute to stroke include anticoagulants, aspirin, vasodilators, and illegal drugs. To complete the history-taking, the nurse obtains data about the client's social history, including education, employment, travel, leisure activities, and personal habits (e.g., smoking, diet, exercise pattern, and drug and alcohol use).

➤ Physical Assessment/Clinical Manifestations

Neurologic Assessment. The nurse performs a complete neurologic examination of the client. Specific neurologic and other signs and symptoms exhibited by the client depend on the extent and location of the insult and the arteries involved (Chart 47–2).

Cognitive Changes. The client may exhibit a variety of cognitive problems in addition to changes in the level of consciousness. Level of consciousness may vary, depending on the extent of increased intracranial pressure caused by the CVA. The nurse assesses the client for indications of denial of the illness; neglect syndrome or hemiparesis; spatial and proprioceptive (awareness of body position in space) dysfunction; impairment of memory, judgment, or problem-solving and decision-making abilities; and decreased ability to concentrate and attend to tasks. The client's dysfunction in one or more of these areas may be more pronounced, depending on the hemisphere involved (Chart 47–3).

The right cerebral hemisphere is more involved with visual and spatial awareness and proprioception. A person who has a stroke involving the right cerebral hemisphere is often unaware of any deficits and may be disoriented to time and place (see Research Applications for Nursing). Personality changes include impulsivity and poor judgment. The left cerebral hemisphere, the dominant hemisphere in all but about 15%–20% of the population, is the center for language, mathematic skills, and analytic thinking. Therefore, a left hemisphere cerebrovascular accident (CVA) results in aphasia (inability to use or comprehend language), alexia (reading problems), and agraphia (difficulty with writing). Persons with left-hemisphere CVAs tend to be slow and cautious.

Chart 47–2

Key Features of Stroke Syndromes

Middle Cerebral Artery Strokes

- Contralateral hemiparesis: arm > leg
- Contralateral sensory deficit
- Homonymous hemianopsia
- Unilateral neglect or inattention
- Aphasia, anomia, alexia, agraphia, and acalculia
- Impaired vertical sensation
- Spatial deficit
- Perceptual deficit
- Visual field deficit
- Altered level of consciousness: drowsy to comatose

Posterior Cerebral Artery Strokes

- Perseveration
- Aphasia, amnesia, alexia, agraphia, visual agnosia, and ataxia
- Loss of deep sensation
- Decreased touch sensation
- Possible choreoathetoid movements
- Stupor; coma

Internal Carotid Artery Strokes

- Contralateral hemiparesis
- Sensory deficit
- Hemianopsia, blurred vision, blindness
- Aphasia (dominant side)

Internal Carotid Artery Strokes

- Headache
- Bruit

Anterior Cerebral Artery Strokes

- Contralateral hemiparesis: leg > arm
- Bladder incontinence
- Personality and behavior changes
- Aphasia, gait apraxia, and amnesia
- Positive grasp and sucking reflex
- Perseveration
- Sensory deficit (lower extremity)
- Memory impairment
- Apraxic gait

Vertebrobasilar Artery Strokes

- Headache and vertigo
- Coma
- Memory loss and confusion
- Flaccid paralysis
- Areflexia, ataxia, and vertigo
- Cranial nerve dysfunction
- Dysconjugate gaze
- Visual deficits (uniorbital) and homonymous hemianopsia
- Sensory loss: numbness

Motor Changes. The motor examination provides information about which cerebral hemisphere is involved. A right hemiplegia (paralysis on one side of the body) or hemiparesis (weakness) indicates a stroke involving the left cerebral hemisphere, because the motor nerve fibers cross in the medulla before entering the spinal cord and periphery. Conversely, a left hemiplegia or weakness indicates a right cerebral hemisphere CVA.

In addition to assessing motor strength, the nurse gauges the client's muscle tone. The client with hypo-

Chart 47–3

Key Features of Left and Right Hemisphere Cerebrovascular Accidents

Feature	Left Hemisphere*	Right Hemisphere
Language	• Aphasia • Agraphia • Alexia	• Impaired sense of humor
Memory	• Deficit may be present	• Disoriented to time, place, and person • Cannot recognize faces
Vision	• Unable to discriminate words and letters • Reading problems • Deficits in the right visual field	• Visual spatial deficits • Neglect of the left visual field • Loss of depth perception
Behavior	• Slow • Cautious • Anxious when attempting a new task • Depression or a catastrophic response to illness • Sense of guilt • Feeling of worthlessness • Worries over future • Quick anger and frustration	• Impulsive • Unaware of neurologic deficits • Confabulates • Euphoric • Constantly smiles • Denies illness • Poor judgment • Overestimates abilities (risk for injury)
Hearing	• No deficit	• Loses ability to hear tonal variations

*Location for speech in all but 15% to 20% of people.

Research Applications for Nursing

Mental Status Exam Helps Predict Outcomes in Right Hemispheric Stroke

Sisson, R.A. (1995). Cognitive status as a predictor of right hemisphere stroke outcomes. Journal of Neuroscience Nursing, 27(3), 152–156.

The purpose of this study was to examine the relationship between emotional, behavioral, and cognitive status and functional activity status of stroke survivors. This research is significant in that it focuses on clients with right hemispheric stroke; the majority of stroke research has targeted those who have experienced a left-sided stroke. Somatic concerns, memory deficit, depressive mood, and mental fatigue were the most frequently occurring mental status changes seen 6 months post stroke. There was a correlation between cognitive ability and functional ability as measured on the Barthel Functional Index and the Neurobehavioral Rating Scale (NRS).

Critique. This research was a pilot study to examine clients with right hemisphere strokes. Although the sample was small (n = 15), it showed a need for further research in the area.

Possible Implications for Nursing. While conducting a neurologic assessment is routine, more attention to the mental status examination and the incorporation of the results in planning care is needed. The mental status assessment can assist in determining readiness for rehabilitation and for planning realistic goals. Teaching and counseling the caregivers about the sequelae of stroke as reflected in the mental status examination can help the caregiver cope more effectively with the outcome of a right hemispheric stroke.

---

tonia, or flaccidity, is unable to overcome the forces of gravity, and the extremities tend to fall to the side. The extremities feel heavy, and muscle tone is inadequate for balance, equilibrium, or protective mechanisms. Hypertonia (spastic paralysis) tends to cause fixed positions or contractures of the involved extremities. Range of motion (ROM) of the joints is restricted, and shoulder subluxation may easily occur from either spasticity or flaccidity. The nurse also assesses proprioception (position sense), head and trunk control, balance, coordination, and gait.

Loss of inhibitory nervous control from the cerebral cortex results in a spastic (upper motor neuron), uninhibited bladder. Bowel function may also be affected.

Sensory Changes. The sensory examination conducted by the nurse evaluates the client's response to touch and painful stimuli. In addition, the nurse determines the client's ability to distinguish between two tactile stimuli presented simultaneously. Finally, the nurse assesses the client's ability to respond to stimuli that require proprioceptive and tactile processing together with cortical integration. The client who has had a stroke may be unable to write, comprehend reading material, use an object correctly (agnosia), or carry out a purposeful motor activity (apraxia).

The nurse also evaluates the client for indications of neglect syndrome, which is particularly evident with right cerebral hemisphere strokes. In this syndrome, the client is unaware of the existence of his or her left or paralyzed side. The typical picture is that of the client sitting in a wheelchair, leaning to the left with the arm caught in the wheelchair wheel. When questioned, the client often states that everything is fine and believes that he or she is sitting up straight in the chair. Another typical example of neglect syndrome is the client who washes or dresses only one side of the body.

Another important part of the nursing assessment focuses on the client's visual ability. Infarction or ischemia involving the carotid artery may cause pupillary abnormalities, ptosis, visual field deficits, or pallor and petechiae of the conjunctiva. Amaurosis fugax, a brief episode of blindness in one eye, results from retinal ischemia caused by ophthalmic or carotid artery insufficiency. Hemianopsia, or blindness in half of the visual field, results when there is damage to the optic tract or the occipital lobe. Most often this deficit occurs as homonymous hemianopsia, in which there is blindness in the same side of both eyes (Fig. 47–5). The client with this condition must turn his or her head to scan the complete range of vision. Otherwise, the client does not see half of the visual field. For example, the client eats only half of a meal because that is the only portion seen.

Cranial Nerve Intactness. The nurse conducts a review of each cranial nerve, with particular attention to abnormalities of cranial nerves V, VII, IX, X, and XII. Damage to these cranial nerves may cause difficulties with chewing (V), facial paralysis or paresis (VII), dysphagia (inability to swallow) (IX and X), an absent gag reflex (IX), or impaired tongue movement (XII). The client may have a great deal of difficulty with chewing or swallowing foods and liquids and is at risk for aspiration pneumonia. In addition, the client may become constipated from inadequate fluid intake.

Cardiovascular Assessment. At the completion of the neurologic assessment, the nurse performs a complete physical assessment. Of particular importance is the assessment of the client's cardiovascular system. Clients with embolic strokes often have heart murmur, dysrhythmias, or hypertension. It is not unusual for the client to be admitted to the hospital with a blood pressure value greater than 180–200/110–120. Although a somewhat higher blood pressure (150/100) is needed to maintain cerebral perfusion after a stroke, pressures above this limit may lead to another stroke.

➤ Psychosocial Assessment

A typical client with a stroke is older than 60 years of age, is hypertensive, and has varying degrees of motor weakness and level of consciousness. Language and cognitive deficits may also occur, and the client may experience behavior and memory problems.

The nurse determines the client's reaction to illness, especially in relation to changes in body image, self-concept, and ability to perform activities of daily living (ADL). In collaboration with the client's family and friends, the nurse identifies any difficulties in coping mechanisms or personality changes. (See also Chapter 8 on stress and coping.)

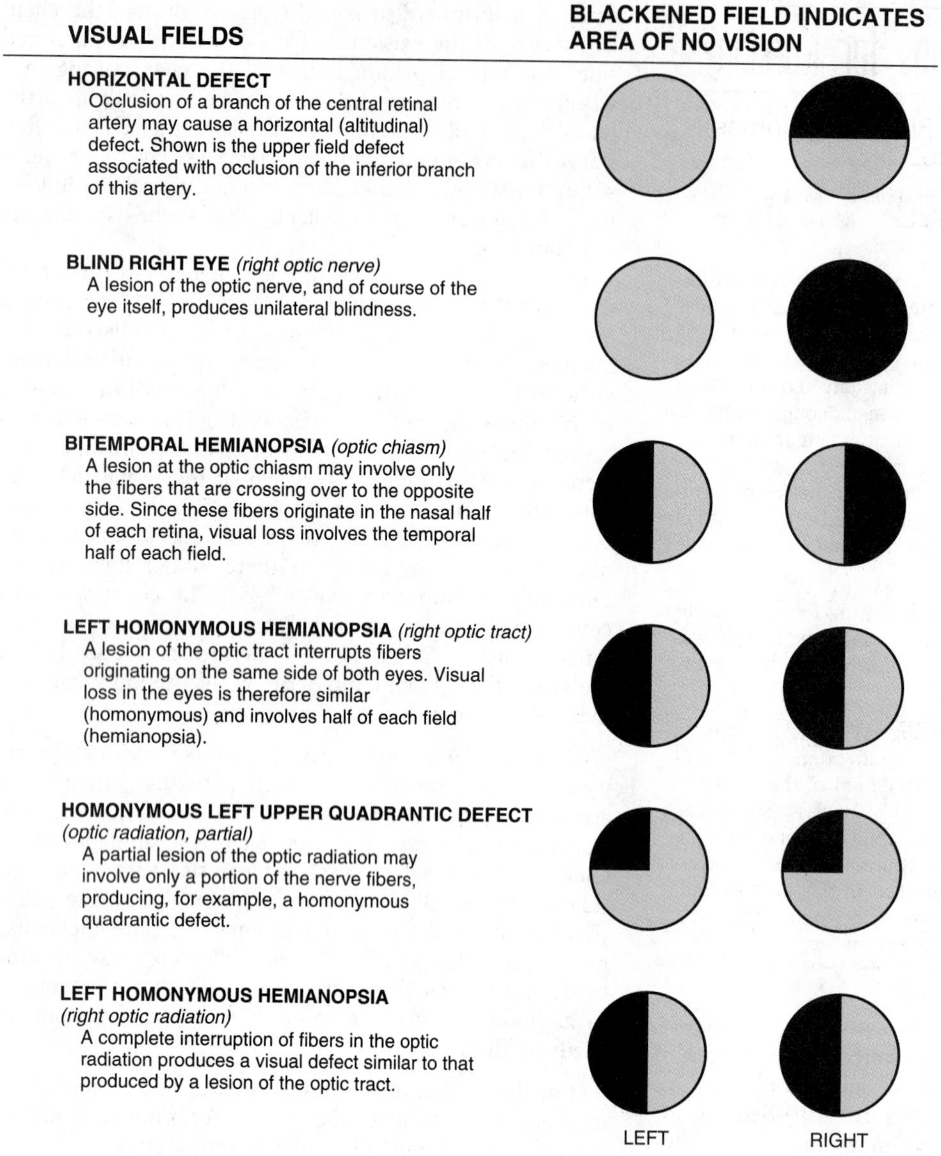

VISUAL FIELDS

BLACKENED FIELD INDICATES AREA OF NO VISION

HORIZONTAL DEFECT
Occlusion of a branch of the central retinal artery may cause a horizontal (altitudinal) defect. Shown is the upper field defect associated with occlusion of the inferior branch of this artery.

BLIND RIGHT EYE *(right optic nerve)*
A lesion of the optic nerve, and of course of the eye itself, produces unilateral blindness.

BITEMPORAL HEMIANOPSIA *(optic chiasm)*
A lesion at the optic chiasm may involve only the fibers that are crossing over to the opposite side. Since these fibers originate in the nasal half of each retina, visual loss involves the temporal half of each field.

LEFT HOMONYMOUS HEMIANOPSIA *(right optic tract)*
A lesion of the optic tract interrupts fibers originating on the same side of both eyes. Visual loss in the eyes is therefore similar (homonymous) and involves half of each field (hemianopsia).

HOMONYMOUS LEFT UPPER QUADRANTIC DEFECT
(optic radiation, partial)
A partial lesion of the optic radiation may involve only a portion of the nerve fibers, producing, for example, a homonymous quadrantic defect.

LEFT HOMONYMOUS HEMIANOPSIA
(right optic radiation)
A complete interruption of fibers in the optic radiation produces a visual defect similar to that produced by a lesion of the optic tract.

LEFT   RIGHT

Figure 47–5. Visual field defects produced by selected lesions in the visual pathways. (Modified from Bates, B. [1991]. *A guide to physical examination and history taking* [5th ed.]. Philadelphia: J. B. Lippincott.)

The nurse also assesses the client's financial status and occupation, because these aspects of the client's life may be altered by the residual neurologic deficits from the CVA. Clients who do not have disability or health insurance may worry about how their family will cope financially with the disruption in their lives.

The nurse assesses for emotional lability, especially if the frontal lobe of the brain has been affected. In such cases, the client laughs and then cries unexpectedly for no apparent reason. It is important that the nurse explain these uncontrollable emotions to the family or significant others so that they do not feel responsible for the client's reactions.

➤ Laboratory Assessment

Clinical history and presentation often are sufficient to diagnose a stroke. No definitive laboratory tests confirm the diagnosis of a stroke. Elevated hematocrit and hemoglobin levels are associated with a severe or major stroke.

An elevated white blood cell count may indicate the presence of an infection, possibly subacute bacterial endocarditis or a response to physiologic stress. Generally, the health care provider orders a prothrombin time (PT) or international normalized ratio (INR), and partial thromboplastin time (PTT) to establish baseline coagulation information in case anticoagulation therapy is initiated. These diagnostic tests may also provide supportive evidence that a hemorrhagic stroke has occurred. If there is no indication of increased intracranial pressure (ICP), a lumbar puncture may be performed to obtain cerebrospinal fluid (CSF) for analysis. Blood in the spinal fluid or a high CSF red blood cell count is indicative of a subarachnoid hemorrhage.

➤ Radiographic Assessment

Computed tomography (CT) or MRI assists in the differential diagnosis of a stroke. The primary purpose of the initial scan is to identify the presence of hemorrhage or a cerebral aneurysm. This diagnostic test shows the presence of ischemia and is invaluable in establishing baseline information for future comparison in case the client's condition deteriorates. In addition, the scans enable the physician to identify pathologic changes that may mimic a stroke, such as a brain tumor or a hematoma, both of which are unrelated to cerebrovascular disease. As the stroke progresses, later CT scans or MRI may show the presence of edema and tissue necrosis not evident on the initial scan.

Information about the status of the cerebral vessels is obtained by angiography, digital subtraction angiography, or magnetic resonance angiography (MRA). These studies reveal abnormal vessel structures or identify the area of vessel wall rupture and vasospasm. Skull radiography is generally not performed, although it may detect the presence of abnormal calcification of a vessel or a pineal shift, both of which may indicate the presence of cerebral hemorrhage.

➤ Other Diagnostic Assessment

Noninvasive blood flow studies such as carotid artery ultrasound or carotid Doppler sonography provide additional information about the cerebral vasculature. An electroencephalogram (EEG) is rarely of any diagnostic value.

To assist in the determination of a cardiac cause of a stroke, the health care provider may order an electrocardiogram (ECG), a Holter monitor test, cardiac enzymes evaluation, and an echocardiogram. As with other neurologic diseases, it is not unusual to find the following changes on the ECG: inverted T wave, ST depression, and QT elevation and prolongation.

 Analysis

➤ Common Nursing Diagnoses and Collaborative Problems

The most common nursing diagnoses pertinent to the care of the client with a cerebrovascular accident (CVA) are

1. Altered (Cerebral) Tissue Perfusion related to interruption of arterial blood flow and a possible increase in ICP
2. Impaired Physical Mobility and Self Care Deficit related to hemiparesis or hemiplegia, decreased level of consciousness, or cognitive dysfunction
3. Sensory/Perceptual Alterations related to decreased sensation, neglect, or visual impairment
4. Unilateral Neglect related to right cerebral hemisphere dysfunction or hemianopsia
5. Impaired Verbal Communication related to decreased circulation in the brain
6. Impaired Swallowing related to weakness of the muscles necessary for swallowing and a decreased gag reflex
7. Total (Urinary) Incontinence and Bowel Incontinence related to neurologic dysfunction, decreased sensation, cognitive dysfunction, immobility, or expressive aphasia

➤ Additional Nursing Diagnoses and Collaborative Problems

Additional Nursing Diagnoses

In addition to the common nursing diagnoses, some clients with stroke have one or more of the following nursing diagnoses:

- Risk for Aspiration related to impaired swallowing
- Body Image Disturbance related to physical or cognitive disability
- Altered Role Performance related to change in physical capacity to perform role
- Risk for Injury related to neglect syndrome, visual disturbances, and paralysis or weakness
- Sexual Dysfunction related to altered body function
- Colonic Constipation related to lack of adequate fluid intake, immobility, or lack of physical activity

Additional collaborative problems include

- Potential for Deep Vein Thrombosis
- Potential for Increased Intracranial Pressure
- Potential for Seizures
- Potential for Hypoxemia
- Potential for Atelectasis and Pneumonia

 Planning and Implementation

Altered (Cerebral) Tissue Perfusion

Planning: Expected Outcomes. The client is expected to maintain adequate cerebral tissue perfusion, maintain or improve level of consciousness, and not experience additional neurologic problems.

Interventions. Interventions are primarily determined by the type of stroke and the extent of the stroke. Strokes are now being called "brain attacks" to parallel medical response to "heart attack." For selected clients with ischemic strokes, early intervention with thrombolytic therapy to dissolve the clot can prevent neurologic deficit.

Unless major medical complications occur, the health care provider manages the client conservatively with drug therapy and aggressive rehabilitation to promote an optimal level of well-being and function. The clinical pathway in this chapter outlines the care for a client with a CVA. In some cases, the physician may need to intervene surgically to prevent further neurologic dysfunction.

Nonsurgical Management. Nursing interventions are initially aimed at monitoring for neurologic changes or complications associated with a CVA. The client is at risk for continued progression of the stroke or increased intracranial pressure (ICP). The nurse performs a comprehensive neurologic assessment when the client is admitted to the hospital and at the beginning of each nursing shift. The nurse performs neurologic checks using the Glasgow Coma Scale (see Chap. 43) or other neurologic assessment tools at least every 4 hours or more often as indicated by the client's condition.

Monitoring for Increased Intracranial Pressure. The client is at most risk for increased intracranial pressure (ICP) resulting from edema during the first 72 hours after the onset of the stroke. The nurse must be alert for symp-

Text continued on page 1120

University Hospitals of Cleveland

Stroke Collaborative Carepath: Inpatient

Priority 2: ELOS 5-7 Days

Significant sensory/motor deficits with rehab potential

Expected Disposition: Rehab Facility

Care Coordinator _____

Collaborative Problem List:

1. Potential altered mobility 2° stroke.
2. Safety related to altered mobility
3. Potential inability to perform ADL's 2° weakness
4. Need for education re: signs and symptoms of stroke

Stamp Patient Name and Number in Space Above

Focus	1 - 12 Hours Post ED Admit Date	13 - 24 Hours Post ED Admit Date	Day 2 Post Stroke Day___ Date	Day 3 Post Stroke Day___ Date	Day 4 Post Stroke Day___ Date	Day 5 Post Stroke Day___ Date	Day 6 Post Stroke Day___ Date

Tests, Labs, Procedures	☐ Head CT if not completed in ED
	☐ CXR if not completed in ED
	☐ 12 Lead EKG if not completed in ED
	☐ **LABS (if not completed in ED)**
	☐ CBC ☐ Chem-7
	☐ CXR ☐ Coag-file
	☐ Fibrinogen level
	☐ U/A and C&S
	
	Fibrinogen Levels
	IV: 1 hr _____
	    3 hrs _____
	    5 hrs _____
	IA: 1 hr _____
	    2 hrs _____
		☐ Angio completed
		☐ Serial angio's performed
		☐ 12 Lead EKG at 24° post thrombolytic
		
		☐ Fibrinogen levels q12° x 3
		☐ PT/PTT q12° x 3
			☐ MD: Following tests ordered:
			☐ MRA
			☐ MRI
			☐ EEG
			☐ Carotid Ultrasound
			☐ Trans-Esophageal ECHO
			☐ Trans-Thoracic Doppler
			☐ Trans-Cranial Doppler
				☐ PT, PTT if needed
				
				☐ Check ECHO results with 24° of test
						☐ PT, PTT if needed	

Consults	☐ MD: PT, OT, ST evaluation ordered	☐ RN: Assess swallowing ☐ ST: Cognitive-linguistic evaluation and swallow test if needed	☐ Cardiology consult if needed ☐ PT and/or ☐ OT and/or ☐ ST evaluation completed with recommended plan of care in chart	☐ Other consults as needed ☐ PT, ☐ OT, ☐ ST session(s) as scheduled	☐ PT, ☐ OT, ☐ ST session(s) as scheduled	☐ PT, ☐ OT, ☐ ST session(s) as scheduled	☐ PT, ☐ OT, ☐ ST session(s) as scheduled

sh/astrptwo.doc 11/30/94
University Hospitals' carepaths have been developed to assist clinicians in patient management and clinical decision-making. The carepaths are intended to meet the needs of patients in most circumstances. They are not intended to either replace a clinician's judgment or to establish a protocol for all patients with this diagnosis.

Page 1 of 4

Priority Two

1116

Focus	1 - 12 Hours Post ED Admit Date	13 - 24 Hours Post ED Admit Date	Day 2 Post Stroke Day___ Date	Day 3 Post Stroke Day___ Date	Day 4 Post Stroke Day___ Date	Day 5 Post Stroke Day___ Date	Day 6 Post Stroke Day___ Date
Physical Assessment	☐RN:Admission assessment completed ☐RN:Skin integrity assessed ☐RN:Complete vascular checks per routine if femoral sheath placed ☐RN:Vital signs completed q___ ☐RN:Neuro checks completed q___ ☐RN:Obtain FIM at pt/family interview ☐Continuous EKG monitoring ☐NIH Stroke Scale completed: 30mins___ 1Hour___ 2Hours___	☐RN: Continue neuro checks q hour ☐RN: Assess need for Dobhoff ☐MD:remove sheath ☐RN:Assess femoral site for hematoma/bleed ☐RN:Vital sign q___ ☐NIH Stroke Scale completed: 24 hours___	☐RN: Neuro checks q shift ☐Assess need for longterm PEG tube ☐Vital signs q shift ☐NIH Stroke Scale completed: 48 hours___	☐Vital signs q shift ☐Perform FIM if not already done ☐NIH Stroke Scale completed within 24° of discharge___	☐Vital signs q shift ☐RN: Obtain post-stroke FIM within 24° of discharge ☐NIH Stroke Scale completed within 24° of discharge___	☐Vital signs q shift ☐RN: Obtain post-stroke FIM within 24° of discharge ☐NIH Stroke Scale completed within 24° of discharge___	☐Vital signs q shift ☐RN: Obtain post-stroke FIM within 24° of discharge ☐NIH Stroke Scale completed within 24° of discharge___
Activity	☐Bedrest with head of bed flat to 30°	☐Bedrest with HOB flat to 30°	☐Bedrest with HOB flat to 30°	☐OOB with assist ☐Document on transfer	☐OOB with assist ☐Document gait	☐OOB with assist	☐OOB with assist
Treatments	☐Admit to NSU ☐IVF as ordered ☐Embolism precautions as ordered: ☐TED hose ☐SCD's ☐Safety precautions	☐Foley to CD ☐RN: IVF's if ordered ☐Embolism precautions as ordered: ☐TED hose ☐SCD's ☐Safety precautions	☐Transfer to Tow 4 ☐RN: IVF's if ordered ☐Embolism precautions as ordered: ☐TED hose ☐SCD's ☐Safety precautions	☐RN: DC IVF's if not already done ☐Place heplock ☐Continue SCD's if indicated ☐PT☐OT as scheduled	☐Maintain heplock ☐D/C SCD's if ambulatory ☐PT☐OT as scheduled	☐PT☐OT as scheduled	☐PT☐OT as scheduled
Diet	☐NPO upon admission ☐RN: assess pt. swallowing ability	☐Diet as ordered: ☐NPO ☐Regular ☐Soft ☐Pureed ☐Other___ or ☐Dobhoff tube feeds	☐Assess pt.'s ability to tolerate regular diet or ☐Assess pt.'s Dobhoff tube feeds	☐Maintain diet as ordered	☐Maintain diet as ordered ☐Note PEG feedings ☐Teach pt. and family PEG tube care	☐Maintain diet as ordered	☐Maintain diet as ordered

sh/a:strpftwo.doc 11/30/94

University Hospitals' carepaths have been developed to assist clinicians in patient management and clinical decision-making. The carepaths are intended to meet the needs of patients in most circumstances. They are not intended to either replace a clinician's judgment or to establish a protocol for all patients with this diagnosis.

Priority Two

University Hospitals of Cleveland

Stroke Collaborative Carepath: Inpatient
Priority Two

Care Coordinator_____

Stamp Patient Name and Number in Space Above

Focus	1 - 12 Hours Post ED Admit Date	13 - 24 Hours Post ED Admit Date	Day 2 Post Stroke Day ___ Date	Day 3 Post Stroke Day ___ Date	Day 4 Post Stroke Day ___ Date	Day 5 Post Stroke Day ___ Date	Day 6 Post Stroke Day ___ Date
Medications	☐ Urokinase protocol IV/IA ☐ Heparinization protocol ☐ Hydration	☐ Continue anticoagulation if ordered ☐ Check PT/PTT	☐ Continue anticoagulation if ordered ☐ Check PT/PTT	☐ Continue anticoagulation if ordered ☐ Check PT/PTT	☐ Continue anticoagulation if ordered ☐ Check PT/PTT	☐ Continue anticoagulation if ordered ☐ Check PT/PTT	☐ Heparin IV DC'd if not done already ☐ Pt. instruction re: po anticoagulation if indicated
Discharge Planning		☐ RN: Give stroke information to patient and family ☐ RN: Consult SW for rehab placement planning	☐ RN, ☐ MD, ☐ OT, ☐ PT, ☐ SW, ☐ ST: Start Gold Form and F/U on MD disposition orders ☐ MD: Discuss rehab placement with pt./family ☐ SW: Explore rehab insurance coverage ☐ SW: Discuss facilities with pt. and family after MD discussion and encourage family to tour facilities ☐ SW: Contact facilities if already identified by pt. and family	☐ RN, ☐ MD, ☐ OT, ☐ PT, ☐ SW, ☐ ST: Complete Gold Form ☐ SW: Discuss preferences and insurance issues with pt. and family ☐ SW: Fax Gold Form and chart to facilities ☐ SW: Contact facilities if not already done ☐ Facilities: Review Gold Form or come to UHC to assess pt.	☐ Facilities: Review Gold Form or come to UHC to assess pt. ☐ RN, ☐ MD, ☐ OT, ☐ PT, ☐ SW, ☐ ST: Update Gold Form ☐ SW: Obtain pt./fam decision on facility ☐ SW: Coordinate pt. accept by preferred facility or negotiate next preference and comm. outcome with team, pt. family ☐ MD: Write D/C orders and scripts and sign ambulance form ☐ SW: Arrange transportation, request chart copying, coordinate D/C time ☐ MD/RN: If pt. on coumadin, schedule F/U coag study or ☐ MD/RN: If pt. on Ticlid, schedule F/U WBC studies	☐ Prepare pt. for discharge to: ☐ Home ☐ Traditional Rehab ☐ Skilled Nursing ☐ Secretary: Copy chart ☐ RN: Ensure that chart, updated Gold Form, signed ambulance form, and "Day of Discharge Summary" accompany pt. at D/C	

sh/a:strprtwo.doc 11/30/94
University Hospitals' carepaths have been developed to assist clinicians in patient management and clinical decision-making. The carepaths are intended to meet the needs of patients in most circumstances. They are not intended to either replace a clinician's judgment or to establish a protocol for all patients with this diagnosis.

Priority Two

Focus	1 - 12 Hours Post ED Admit Date	13 - 24 Hours Post ED Admit Date	Day 2 Post Stroke Day ___ Date	Day 3 Post Stroke Day ___ Date	Day 4 Post Stroke Day ___ Date	Day 5 Post Stroke Day ___ Date	Day 6 Post Stroke Day ___ Date
Caregiver Signatures	Day ___ Eve ___ Night ___	Day ___ Eve ___ Night ___	Day ___ Eve ___ Night ___	Day ___ Eve ___ Night ___	Day ___ Eve ___ Night ___	Day ___ Eve ___ Night ___	Day ___ Eve ___ Night ___

MD: ___ SW: ___ PT: ___ OT: ___ ST: ___

Stroke Collaborative Carepath: Priority Two Outcomes

Intermediate Outcomes	Met	Not Met	N/A	Comments	Date/Signature
1. Pt. placed on Brain Attack Protocol within three hours of symptoms.					
2. Stroke carepath documentation initiated in the ED at the time of diagnosis.					
3. Pt. prioritized on day of admission.					
4. ECHO results available within 24° of ECHO.					
5. Anti-coagulant or anti-platelet agent determined by Day 2.					
6. PT/OT evaluation with recommended plan of care in chart by Day 3.					
7. Pre-admission FIM completed by Day 3.					
8. Discharge disposition determined by Day 3.					
9. NIH Stroke Scale completed at scheduled intervals.					
10.					

Discharge Outcomes	Met	Not Met	N/A	Comments	Date/Signature
1. Pt. participates in ADL's with assistance.					
2. Pt. tolerates therapy 3-4 hours/day.					
3. PT. can tolerate OOB and sit in chair 2 consecutive hrs.					
4. ECHO results available within 24° of test.					
5. Pt./family understand and support rehab plan/goals.					
6. Pt./family know facility to which pt. will go, appx. LOS, and plan for Home Care upon D/C.					
7. Pt. maintains adequate nutritional intake.					
8. Pt. states risk factors for CVA					
9. Pt. describes stroke and TIA signs/sx, and what action to take should signs/sx occur.					
10. FIM completed within 248 of discharge.					
11. Pt. has follow-up appt. scheduled at time of discharge.					
12.					

sh/a:strprtwo.doc 11/30/94
University Hospitals' carepaths have been developed to assist clinicians in patient management and clinical decision-making. The carepaths are intended to meet the needs of patients in most circumstances. They are not intended to either replace a clinician's judgment or to establish a protocol for all patients with this diagnosis.

Page 4 of 4

Priority Two

1119

toms of increased ICP (Chart 47–4) and report any deterioration in the client's neurologic status to the health care provider.

The nurse elevates the head of the client's bed to 30–45 degrees and maintains the client's head in a midline, neutral position to facilitate venous drainage from the brain. In collaboration with the health care team, the nurse plans the client's care to avoid activities and procedures that may increase ICP, particularly if the client has focal neurologic deficits and indications of cerebral edema. Extreme hip and neck flexion should be avoided. Extreme hip flexion may increase the intrathoracic pressure, whereas extreme neck flexion prohibits venous drainage from the brain.

Additional management measures include avoiding the clustering of nursing procedures (e.g., giving a bath followed immediately by changing the bed linen) and hyperoxygenating the client before suctioning (if needed). The nurse should fully assess the need for suctioning because it may cause increased ICP. A quiet environment is particularly important for the client experiencing a headache, which frequently occurs in the presence of an aneurysm or increased ICP attributable to blood in the subarachnoid space or pressure within the cranial vault. The client may have photophobia; therefore, the nurse or assistive nursing personnel keep the lights in the client's room lowered.

The client's vital signs are monitored closely, at least every 4 hours. The nurse notifies the health care provider if the client's blood pressure exceeds acceptable levels. Generally, the health care provider allows the client to be slightly hypertensive (blood pressure of 150/100) to facilitate adequate cerebral tissue perfusion. A higher blood pressure could lead to a hemorrhagic stroke or rebleeding of an aneurysm (if present).

Clients admitted to a critical care unit are connected to a cardiac monitor and observed for dysrhythmias. The nurse performs a cardiac assessment, with particular attention directed toward auscultation of heart sounds to identify the presence of cardiac murmurs. Murmurs may place the client at increased risk for emboli. Hemodynamic monitoring may be needed to monitor and evaluate physiologic stability and response to therapy.

Drug Therapy. The type of drugs prescribed by the health care provider for the client with a stroke depends on the type of stroke and the neurologic dysfunction that resulted from the stroke. In general, the goals of drug therapy are to prevent further thrombotic episodes (anticoagulation), augment blood flow, and protect the neurons (Barker, 1994).

Thrombolytics. In 1996, the American Heart Association issued new guidelines for the use of tissue plasminogen activator (tPA), a thromolytic drug, to treat acute ischemic strokes. The stroke should be verified by CT imaging and given within 3 hours of the onset of symptoms. Clients who have bleeding complications or are on anticoagulants are not candidates for this therapy (Adams et al., 1996).

Another thrombolytic drug—streptokinase—has been used for the same purpose. Some researchers have shown no differences in clients who received the drug and those who did not (Donnan et al., 1996). Therefore, the use of thrombolytic therapy to treat early acute ischemic strokes is controversial.

Anticoagulants. The use of anticoagulants and antiplatelet agents to treat the client with a stroke is also controversial and depends on the health care provider's preference. The principle drugs used are aspirin, heparin, low molecular weight heparinoids, and Coumadin. If the client received a thrombolytic, an intravenous anticoagulant is usually ordered as a follow-up treatment.

The provider typically orders sodium heparin (Hepalean✦) subcutaneously or via a continuous IV infusion to prevent progression of TIAs or evolving strokes. Baseline prothrombin time (PT) and partial thromboplastin time (PTT) values are usually obtained before the initiation of heparin therapy, 6–8 hours after the start of the infusion, and every morning while the client is receiving heparin therapy. The therapeutic goal is to achieve 1½ to 2 times the client's normal baseline PT and PTT values. The PT is used to monitor oral anticoagulant therapy, whereas the PTT is used to monitor heparin therapy. The World Health Organization now advocates the use of the international normalized ratio (INR) to monitor warfarin therapy. Target INR value for most clients with strokes is 2.0–3.0; for strokes of cardiac origin, the goal is 3.0–4.5.

Sodium heparin and other anticoagulants, such as sodium warfarin (Coumadin, Warfilone✦), may cause bleeding. The nurse observes for signs of blood in the client's urine or stool, epistaxis, bleeding gums, and easy bruising. Anticoagulant therapy is contraindicated in clients who have ulcers, uremia, or hepatic failure.

Enteric-coated or other forms of aspirin (Ancasal✦) have proved useful primarily in the prevention of recurrent stroke or TIA. Aspirin has been shown to reduce the risk of stroke by 30% and subsequent TIAs by 20% to 22% (Barker, 1994). These drugs prevent clotting of the blood by reducing platelet adhesiveness. Anticoagulants

---

Chart 47–4

Key Features of Increased Intracranial Pressure

- Decreased level of consciousness (lethargy to coma)
- Behavior changes: restless, irritable, and confused
- Headache
- Nausea and vomiting
- Change in speech pattern
- Aphasia
- Slurred speech
- Change in sensorimotor status
- Pupillary changes: dilated and nonreactive or constricted and nonreactive pupils
- Cranial nerve dysfunction
- Ataxia
- Seizures
- Cushing's triad
- Abnormal posturing
  - Decerebrate ⎫
  - Decorticate ⎭ latest stage

and antiplatelet medications are contraindicated in the presence of hemorrhagic stroke because they may cause further bleeding. Ticlopidine hydrochloride (Ticlid) is a newer antiplatelet drug used in the treatment of TIAs.

Other Drugs. The health care provider may prescribe anticonvulsants, such as phenytoin (Dilantin), to treat seizures if they occur.

Calcium channel blockers (e.g., nimodipine [Nimotop]) to treat cerebral vasospasm, which usually occurs between 4 and 14 days after the stroke, inhibits blood flow to the area and worsening ischemia. These drugs work by relaxing the smooth muscles of the vessel wall and reducing the incidence and severity of the spasm, thus improving neurologic functioning. Calcium channel blockers possibly also dilate collateral vessels to ischemic areas of the brain. Cerebral vasospasm is responsible for almost 40% of the deaths that occur after rupture of a cerebral aneurysm. Stool softeners, analgesics for pain, and antianxiety drugs may also be ordered.

Monitoring for Other Complications. The client with an aneurysm or AVM must be monitored for the presence of hydrocephalus and vasospasm. Hydrocephalus may occur as a consequence of blood in the cerebrospinal fluid, which prevents it from being reabsorbed properly by the arachnoid villi. Eventually, the ventricles become enlarged and, if hydrocephalus is left untreated, increased intracranial pressure occurs. The nurse observes for clinical manifestations of hydrocephalus, which include a change in level of consciousness (drowsy to coma), gait disturbances, and behavior changes.

Vasospasm, or a narrowing of the cerebral vessels, leads to cerebral ischemia and infarction. It is characterized by a decreased level of consciousness, motor and reflex changes, and increased neurologic deficits, such as cranial nerve dysfunction and aphasia. The symptoms may fluctuate with the occurrence of vasospasm.

Rebleeding or rupture is a frequent complication for the client with an aneurysm or AVM. It tends to occur within 24 hours of the initial bleed or rupture and 7–10 days later. It is manifested by severe headache, nausea and vomiting, decreased level of consciousness, and additional neurologic deficits.

Surgical Management. The surgical procedure depends on the cause of the stroke.

Endarterectomy. Carotid endarterectomy is the most widely used surgical procedure to prevent progressing stroke with symptomatic clients with recurrent TIAs and in clients with carotid stenosis who are symptomatic (Barker, 1994). The purpose of an endarterectomy is to remove atherosclerotic plaque from the inner lining of the artery, usually the carotid artery. It is hoped that this will open the artery enough to re-establish blood flow.

Extracranial-Intracranial Bypass. In this surgical procedure, the surgeon performs a craniotomy and bypasses the blocked artery by making a graft or a bypass from the first artery to the second artery. The procedure establishes blood flow around the blocked artery and re-establishes blood flow to the involved areas. Clinical trials have shown little or no differences in the effectiveness and

benefit of these procedures in preventing stroke. Despite this finding, these procedures continue to be performed. The two most common techniques are the superficial middle temporal artery to middle cerebral artery (STA-MCA) graft and the occipital to posterior inferior cerebellar artery (PICA) bypass. The procedures are used in only selected clients in whom it is believed that more conservative therapy would not be beneficial.

Management of Arteriovenous Malformations. The usual treatment of an AVM is interventional therapy to occlude abnormal arteries or veins. The same procedure may be performed to occlude the vessels surrounding an aneurysm. The physician inserts a microcatheter into the carotid artery, or more often into the femoral artery, and threads it to the vessel to be embolized. The physician then injects an embolic agent, such as platinum coils, detachable silicone balloons, liquid acrylic, or polyvinyl alcohol, to embolize the involved arteries (Fig. 47-6). If the AVM is large, the physician may elect to occlude the artery gradually to allow a gradual change in the blood supply to the surrounding brain. In this case, the embolization procedure is carried out during 1–2 weeks. Whenever possible, the involved vessels are totally removed surgically. The surgeon ligates the vessels and removes the defect. Gamma radiation delivered through the Gamma knife produces sloughing of the endothelial lining of the vessels to prevent further vessel enlargement. Improved microsurgical techniques have significantly reduced morbidity and mortality rates, and these proce-

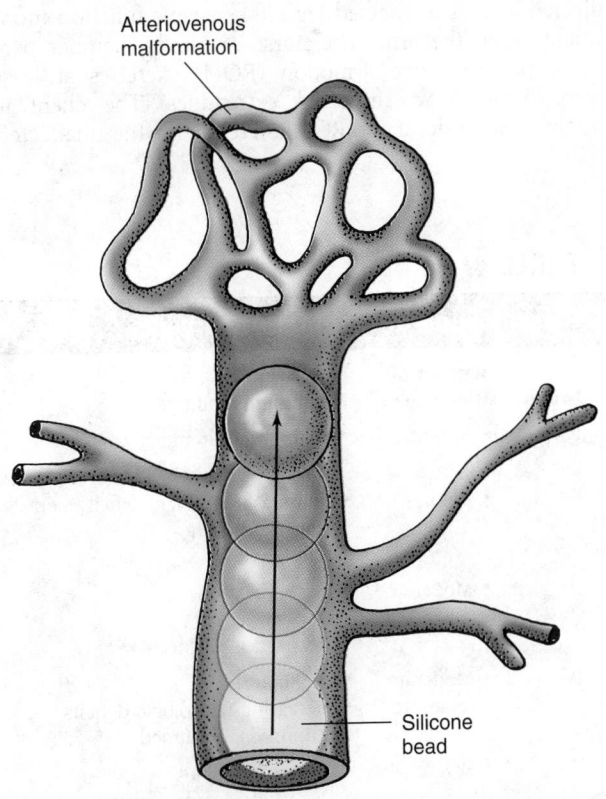

Figure 47-6. Embolization procedure to treat an AVM. The embolic agent travels to the area to cause vessel thrombosis.

dures are becoming the treatment of choice in many medical centers.

Management of Cerebral Aneurysms. Cerebral aneurysms are repaired via craniotomy as soon as the client's condition is stabilized. Surgery may be postponed for clients with a grade IV or V aneurysm (Table 47–2) because their condition makes them high-risk surgical candidates. During surgery, the aneurysm is clipped or a clamp is placed at the base, or neck, of the aneurysm, which prevents blood from entering the area. If the aneurysm does not have a neck, it may be wrapped with muscle, muslin, or a plastic coating to reinforce the wall to prevent rebleeding. Timing of surgery and specific interventions are usually determined by individual physician preferences. Visitors may be limited, and measures to decrease the client's stress and increase comfort are usually ordered.

Management of Intracranial Bleeding. For some clients who have hemorrhagic strokes, blood clots may be removed via craniotomy to relieve intracranial pressure. Craniotomies are discussed later in this chapter in the section on Head Injury.

Impaired Physical Mobility; Self Care Deficit

Planning: Expected Outcomes. The client is expected to increase tolerance and endurance for therapies, not experience complications of immobility, and become independent in activities of daily living (ADL).

Interventions. Clients who have experienced a stroke may exhibit flaccid or spastic paralysis. It is not unusual for the client to have a spastic arm and flaccid leg on the affected side. The affected leg often regains function more quickly than the arm. The nurse or family member performs passive range-of-motion (ROM) exercises at least every 6 hours for involved extremities. The client is taught how to do active ROM exercises for the unaffected

TABLE 47–2

Classification of Cerebral Aneurysms		
Grade	Amount of Bleeding	Neurologic Findings
I	• Minimal	• Neurologically intact • Slight headache
II	• Mild	• Minimal neurologic deficit, alert • Severe headache • Stiff neck
III	• Moderate	• Facial deficits • Drowsy, sleepy • Headache, stiff neck
IV	• Moderate to severe	• Hemiparesis • Increasing neurologic deficits • Stuporous, obtunded
V	• Severe	• Comatose • Decorticate or decerebrate posturing

side. When able, the client may perform passive exercises on the affected side.

Careful positioning is necessary to maintain proper alignment of the body and to decrease spasticity or increase muscle tone in flaccid extremities. The affected hand or lower leg may need splinting to prevent contractures. The nurse collaborates with the physical and occupational therapists to determine the most appropriate splinting technique and positions for the client when the client is lying, sitting, and transferring from the bed to a chair.

A major complication of immobility is the development of deep vein (venous) thrombosis (DVT). The nurse provides care to prevent this complication by the application of sequential compression stockings or pneumatic compression boots, frequent positioning changes, and mobilization of the client. The nurse reports any indications of DVT to the health care provider and documents the finding in the client's chart. (Chapter 38 describes DVT in detail.)

Sensory/Perceptual Alterations

Planning: Expected Outcomes. The major concern of clients with sensory or perceptual changes is learning to adapt to the deficits. Therefore, the client is expected to adapt to sensory or perceptual changes in vision and proprioception and sensation and to be free from injury.

Interventions. Clients who have right hemisphere brain damage typically have difficulty with visual-perceptual or spatial-perceptual tasks. They have problems with depth and distance perception and with discrimination of right from left or up from down. Because of these problems, they have difficulty performing routine activities of daily living (ADL). The nurse and significant others help the client adapt to these disabilities by using frequent verbal and tactile cues and by breaking down tasks into discrete steps. The nurse and assistive nursing personnel approach the client from the unaffected side; the client's unaffected side should face the door of the room.

The client who has experienced a stroke may have difficulties with ambulating and may lack depth perception and may have altered proprioception (position sense). The nurse teaches the client who has visual field deficits to turn his or her head from side to side and to scan with the eyes to compensate for the disability. Objects should be placed within the client's field of vision; a mirror may be helpful to assist the client to visualize more of the environment. If the client has diplopia (double vision), a patch may be placed over the affected eye. The nurse and assistive nursing personnel ensure a safe environment by removing clutter from the room.

The client who has a left hemisphere lesion generally experiences memory deficits and may show significant changes in the ability to carry out simple tasks. To assist the client with memory problems, the nurse reorients the client to the month, year, day of the week, and circumstances surrounding admission to the hospital. The nurse establishes a routine or schedule for the client that is as structured, repetitious, and consistent as possible. Information is presented in a simple, concise manner. A step-by-step approach is often most effective because the client can master one step before moving to the next. When possible, the family or significant other should bring in pictures and other objects that are familiar to the client.

The client may be unable to plan and to execute tasks in an organized manner. Apraxia, or the inability to perform previously learned motor skills or commands, may be present. Typically, the client with apraxia exhibits a slow, cautious, and hesitant behavior style.

Unilateral Neglect

Planning: Expected Outcomes. The client is expected to learn and use techniques to compensate for the one-sided neglect.

Interventions. Unilateral neglect, or neglect syndrome, occurs most commonly in clients who have a right cerebral stroke. However, it can occur in any client who experiences hemianopsia, in which the vision of one or both eyes is affected. This problem places the client at additional risk for injury owing to an inability to recognize his or her physical impairment or to a lack of proprioception.

The primary role of the nurse is to teach the client to touch and use both sides of the body. For example, the nurse and assistive nursing personnel encourage the client to wash both the affected and unaffected sides of the body. When dressing, the nurse reminds the client to dress the affected side first. If hemianopsia is present, the nurse also teaches the client to turn his or her head from side to side to expand the visual field. This scanning technique is also useful when the client is eating or ambulating (see earlier in this chapter).

Impaired Verbal Communication

Planning: Expected Outcomes. The client is expected to develop strategies for alternative methods of communication.

Interventions. Language or speech problems are usually the result of a stroke involving the dominant hemisphere. In all but 15% to 20% of the population, the left cerebral hemisphere is the speech center. Speech and language problems may be the result of aphasia or dysarthria. Although aphasia is caused by cerebral hemisphere damage, dysarthria is due to loss of motor function to the tongue or the muscles of speech, causing slurred speech.

Aphasia can be classified in a number of ways. Most commonly, aphasia is classified as expressive, receptive, or global (mixed) (Table 47–3). Expressive (Broca's, or motor) aphasia is the result of damage in Broca's area of the frontal lobe. It is a motor speech problem—the client generally understands what is said but is unable to communicate verbally. The client also has difficulty with writing. Rote speech and automatic speech, such as responses to greeting, are often intact. The client is aware of the deficit and may become frustrated and angry.

Receptive (Wernicke's, or sensory) aphasia is due to injury involving Wernicke's area in the temporoparietal area. The client is unable to understand the spoken and often the written word. Although the client may be able to talk, the language is often meaningless. Neologisms (made-up words) are common parts of speech.

TABLE 47–3

Types of Aphasia

Expressive
- Referred to as Broca's, or motor, aphasia
- Difficulty speaking
- Difficulty writing

Receptive
- Referred to as Wernicke's, or sensory, aphasia
- Difficulty understanding spoken words
- Difficulty understanding written words
- Speech often meaningless
- Neologisms

Global (Mixed)
- Combination of difficulty understanding words and speech
- Difficulty with reading and writing

More often, the client exhibits language dysfunction in both the areas of expression and reception; this is known as a global, or mixed, aphasia. Reading and writing ability are equally affected. Few clients exhibit either expressive *or* receptive aphasia. In most cases, one type is dominant, but two or more types are present.

The nurse collaborates with the speech-language pathologist (SLP) in working with the client who has aphasia or dysarthria. The aphasic client requires repetitive directions to understand or to complete a task. Each task should be broken down into component parts and given to the client one step at a time. The nurse faces the client and speaks slowly and clearly. The client should be given sufficient time to understand and process the information and to respond. The nurse encourages the client to communicate and reinforces this behavior positively. Family members or significant others and staff repeat the names of objects used on a routine basis. For example, the nurse states "This is the toothbrush" when assisting the client to brush his or her teeth. If necessary, a picture board or communication board should be developed by the SLP for the client who has Broca's aphasia. It consists of a picture of an activity (e.g., someone eating) and the printed description below. The client can point to the activity or object desired.

It is difficult to understand the client who is dysarthric. The same techniques used by the nurse for the client with aphasia can be used for the person with dysarthria. Facial muscle exercises may be performed to strengthen the muscles used for speech. Many clients who are dysarthric are also aphasic.

Impaired Swallowing

Planning: Expected Outcomes. The client is expected to eat and drink fluids without aspiration and to maintain or attain ideal or usual body weight.

Interventions. The nurse assesses the client's ability to swallow before feeding. The nurse observes the client for facial drooping, drooling, and a weak, hoarse voice. To assess the swallowing reflex, the nurse places the thumb and the index finger on either side of the client's Adam's apple, or laryngeal protuberance, and asks the client to swallow. The nurse should be able to feel the client's larynx elevate. Next, the nurse checks the client's gag and cough reflex. The nurse collaborates with the speech-language pathologist, who specializes in swallowing evaluations, to determine the extent of the client's swallowing problem. In some cases, the health care provider may order a barium swallow to detect the specific cause of the swallowing problem.

Positioning the client to facilitate the swallowing process is extremely important. The client should eat all meals sitting in a chair or sitting straight up in bed. The client's head and neck are positioned slightly forward and flexed. Generally, clients with swallowing problems are able to tolerate or swallow soft or semisoft foods and fluids (mechanically soft or dental diet, junior baby foods, custards, scrambled eggs) better than thin liquids (water, juice, or milk) or a regular meal. Powdered thickener (Thick-It) may be added to thicken foods to a more manageable consistency. The nurse collaborates with the dietitian to find an appropriate diet for the client with dysphagia. The nurse monitors the client's weight at least twice a week to ensure that the client is receiving adequate nutrition. Supplements such as milk shakes and Ensure may be needed to meet caloric and protein requirements. Calorie counts may be necessary to evaluate nutritional intake fully.

Foods that stimulate saliva production and thus facilitate swallowing include beef broth and foods that are sweet, sour, or salty. The nurse instructs the client to place food in the back of the mouth on the unaffected side to prevent trapping of food in the affected cheek.

Some clients are able to swallow without difficulty, but because they are easily distracted and impulsive, they are at risk for aspiration. These clients require a distraction-free environment with minimal disruption from television, visitors, or environmental noise. The nurse observes the client for indications of fatigue because this can significantly interfere with the desire and ability to eat.

Total (Urinary) Incontinence; Bowel Incontinence

Planning: Expected Outcomes. The client is expected to become continent of urine and stool.

Interventions. The client may be incontinent of urine and stool because of an altered level of consciousness, impaired innervation, or an inability to communicate the need to urinate or defecate. Before beginning an education program to correct these problems, the nurse must first establish the causes. Typically, the client who has had a stroke can relearn both bowel and bladder control. To begin a bladder training program, the nurse places the client on the bedpan or the commode or offers the urinal every 2 hours. The nurse encourages the client to have a total fluid intake of 2000 mL or more per day unless contraindicated. Catheterizations to check for residual urine after voiding (postvoiding residuals) may be done in the early part of the bladder retraining program to ensure that the client is emptying the bladder. Retained urine can lead to a urinary tract infection.

Before establishing a bowel training program, the nurse determines the client's normal time for bowel elimination and any routine that helps to ensure an acceptable evacuation. If possible, this routine is followed, and the client is placed on the bedpan or the commode at the same time as the previous schedule at home. The nurse collaborates with the dietitian to provide a diet high in bulk and fiber. The nurse encourages the client to drink apple or prune juice to help promote bowel elimination. A stool softener (Colace) may be ordered. Suppositories or digital stimulation may also assist in reestablishing a bowel routine. (A complete discussion of bowel and bladder training programs is in Chapter 13.)

 Continuing Care

The client with a cerebrovascular accident (CVA) may be discharged to home, a rehabilitation center, or a long-term care facility, depending on the extent of the disability and the availability of family or caregiver support. Some clients experience no significant neurologic dysfunction as a result of their stroke and are able to return home and live independently or with minimal support. Other clients are able to return home but require ongoing assistance with activities of daily living, as well as supervision to prevent accidents or injury. Speech, physical, or occupational therapy is conducted in the home or on an outpatient (ambulatory) basis. Clients admitted to a rehabilitation or long-term care facility require continued or more complex nursing care as well as extensive physical, occupational, recreational, and speech-language, or cognitive, therapy. The goal of rehabilitation is to maximize the client's abilities in all aspects of life.

➤ Health Teaching

The teaching plan for the client with a stroke includes the medication schedule, mobility transfer skills, communication skills, safety precautions, dietary management, activity levels, and self-care skills. Health teaching should focus on tasks that must be performed by the client and the family after discharge. The nurse should provide both written and verbal instruction. Return demonstrations assist the nurse in evaluating the family members' competency in tasks required for the client's care.

The client must take the prescribed medication to prevent another stroke and to keep hypertension under control. The nurse teaches the client and the family the name of the drug, the dosage, the timing of administration and how to take it, and possible side effects. In collaboration with the physical and occupational therapists, the nurse teaches the client how to climb stairs safely, if able; transfer from bed to chair; get into and out of a car; and use any aids to mobility. Finally, the client and family members are taught how to use any equipment needed to increase independence in self-care skills. The most important information the nurse provides the client is what to do in an emergency and whom to call for nonemergency questions.

It is not unusual for clients to become depressed within 6 months after discharge from the hospital, particularly elderly Caucasian men. Generally, this is self-limiting, although the client may require the administration of antidepressants, such as amitriptyline hydrochloride (Elavil, Levate✦), for a short time. Emotional lability is also common. The family is advised to avoid being over-protective and is assisted to establish realistic and achievable goals.

Families may feel overwhelmed by the continuing demands placed on them by the client. Depending on the location of the lesion, the client may be anxious, slow, cautious, hesitant, and lack initiative (left hemisphere lesions), or impulsive and seemingly unaware of any deficit. The family members or other caregivers need to spend time away from the client on a routine basis to continue to provide full-time care without sacrificing their own physical and emotional health. The nurse may refer the family to a social worker for further support and counseling.

➤ Home Care Management

Collaboration with the case manager is needed if the client is discharged to the home setting. Needs for assistive or adaptive and safety equipment must be identified. The extent of this assessment depends on the disabilities experienced by the client. The home of the client with hemiparesis should be free from scatter rugs or other obstacles in the walking pathways. The bathtub and the toilet should be equipped with grab bars. Antiskid patches or strips should be placed in the bathtub to prevent the client from slipping. The physical or occupational therapist works with the client and the family or significant others to obtain all needed assistive devices *before* discharge from the hospital, the rehabilitation setting, or the long-term care facility. Appointments for outpatient speech, physical, and occupational therapy must also be arranged before discharge.

➤ Health Care Resources

Resources available to the client include a variety of publications from the American Heart Association, including *Stroke: A Guide for Families* and *Stroke: Why Do They Behave That Way?* The National Stroke Association also provides publications and videotapes for caregivers and patients. *Recovering After a Stroke: A Patient and Family Guide* is available from the Agency for Health Care Policy and Research. The nurse refers the client and family members or significant others to local stroke support groups.

 Evaluation

The nurse evaluates the care provided by determining whether the client
- Maintains adequate cerebral tissue perfusion
- Maintains or improves his or her level of consciousness
- Experiences no additional neurologic problems
- Adapts to sensory or perceptual changes in vision, proprioception, and sensation
- Increases tolerance and endurance for therapies

- Uses assistive or adaptive devices as needed
- Exhibits no complications of immobility
- Is free from injury
- Becomes independent in activities of daily living (ADL)
- Develops strategies for alternative methods of communication
- Eats and drinks fluids without aspiration
- Maintains or attains ideal or usual body weight
- Is continent of urine and stool

HEAD INJURY
Overview

Craniocerebral trauma, commonly referred to as head trauma, is a traumatic insult to the brain caused by an external physical force that may produce a diminished or altered state of consciousness. It may result in impairment of cognitive abilities or physical functioning as well as disturbance of behavior or emotional functioning. These impairments may be either temporary or permanent and cause partial or total functional disability or psychosocial maladjustment. In the United States, head injury has taken more lives of people 18–34 years of age than all other causes combined for that age group. Taking into account both inflationary and real changes, the total cost of head injury in 1992 in the United States was estimated at $10 billion. This includes direct costs (hospitalization and rehabilitation) and indirect costs (lost wages and productivity).

Pathophysiology

Various terms are used to describe brain injuries that are produced when a mechanical force is applied either directly or indirectly to the brain. A force produced by a blow to the head is a direct injury, whereas a force applied to another body part with a rebound effect to the brain is an indirect injury. The brain responds to these forces by forward movement within the rigid cranial vault. The brain may also rebound or rotate on the brain stem, causing diffuse axonal injury (shearing injuries). This moving brain may be contused or lacerated as it moves over the inner surfaces of the cranium, which is irregularly shaped and sharp. Damage most frequently occurs to the frontal and temporal lobes of the brain, especially the raised surfaces of the summits of the gyri.

Primary Brain Injury

Primary brain damage results from the physical stress (force) within the brain tissue caused by open or closed trauma. An open head injury occurs when there is a fracture of the skull or the skull is pierced by a penetrating object. The integrity of the brain and the dura is violated, and there is exposure to outside, or environmental, contaminants. Damage may occur to the underlying vessels, the dural sinus, the brain, and the cranial nerves. A closed head injury is the result of blunt trauma; the integrity of the skull is not violated. It is the more serious of the two types of injury, and the damage to the brain tissue depends on the degree and mechanisms of injury.

Open Head Injury

The types of fractures associated with an open head injury are linear, depressed, open, and comminuted.

A *linear* fracture is a simple, clean break in which the impacted area of bone bends inward, whereas the area around it bends outward; linear fractures account for about 80% of all skull fractures. In a *depressed* fracture, the bone is pressed inward into the brain tissue to at least the thickness of the skull. In an *open* fracture, the scalp is lacerated, creating a direct opening to the brain tissue. The *comminuted* fracture involves fragmentation of the bone, with depression of the bone into the brain tissue.

A unique fracture is a basilar skull fracture. It occurs at the base of the skull, usually extending into the anterior, middle, or posterior fossa, and results in cerebrospinal fluid (CSF) leakage from the nose or ears. Of significance with this fracture is the potential development of hemorrhage caused by damage to the internal carotid artery; damage to cranial nerves I, II, VII, and VIII; and infection.

The majority of penetrating injuries to the skull are caused by gunshot wounds and knife injuries. The degree of injury to the brain tissue depends on the velocity, mass, shape, and direction of impact. High-velocity injuries produce the greatest damage to brain tissue. As with any open head injury, the client with a penetrating injury is at high risk for infection from the object that pierces the skull as well as from other environmental contaminants.

Closed Head Injury

Close head injuries, caused by blunt trauma, lead to concussions, contusions, and lacerations of the brain.

The damage to the brain may be mild, as occurs in a concussive injury, or it may be more severe, causing diffuse axonal injury or widespread injury to the white matter of the brain. A *concussion* is characterized by a brief loss of consciousness. Damage occurs to the gray matter of the cerebral cortex or possibly to the diencephalon or the brain stem. The damage to the axons is functional, not structural, which is why permanent neurologic dysfunction is generally not seen. (However, some authorities believe that both functional and structural damage are involved.) A *contusion* is a bruising of the brain tissue and is most frequently found at the site of impact (coup injury) or in a line opposite the site of impact (contrecoup injury) (Fig. 47–7). The base of the frontal and temporal lobes is most often involved. A *laceration* causes actual tearing of the cortical surface vessels, which may lead to secondary hemorrhage, and is therefore more serious than a contusion.

Types of Force

Other factors that must be considered in the dynamics of head injury are the type of force and the mechanisms of injury involved (Fig. 47–8). An acceleration injury is caused by the head in motion. A deceleration injury occurs when the head is suddenly stopped or hits a stationary object. These forces may be sufficient to cause the cerebrum to rotate about the brain stem, resulting in

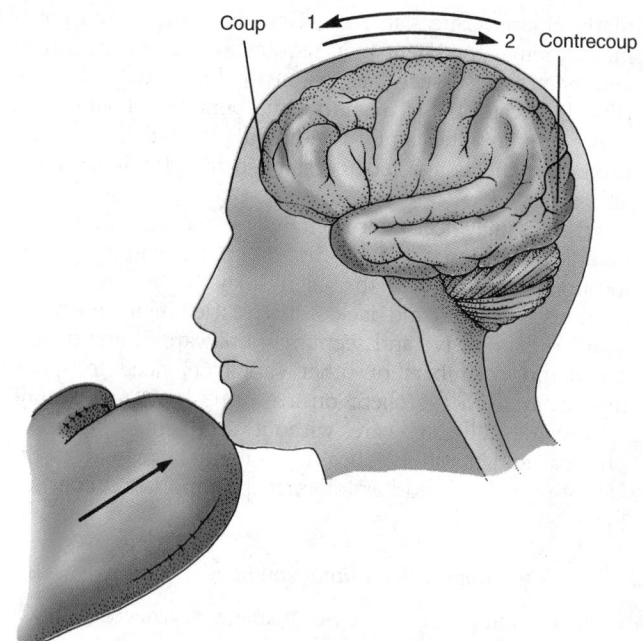

Figure 47–7. Coup (site of impact) injury to frontal area of brain, and contrecoup injury to frontal and temporal areas of the brain.

shearing, straining, and distortion of the brain tissue, particularly of the axons in the brain stem and cerebellum. Small areas of hemorrhage may develop around the blood vessels that sustain the impact of these forces (stress), with destruction of adjacent brain tissue. Particularly affected are the basal nuclei and the hypothalamus.

Secondary Responses and Insults

Secondary responses to brain injury include any neurologic damage that occurs after the initial injury. Secondary injuries or responses increase the morbidity and mortality after head trauma. The most frequently occurring response is the development of increased intracranial pressure (ICP) attributable to edema, hemorrhage, hematoma development, impaired cerebral autoregulation, or hydrocephalus. Hypoxemia, hypercapnia, or systemic hypotension may precipitate increased ICP. Damage to the brain tissue occurs primarily because the delivery of oxygen and glucose to the brain is interrupted.

INCREASED INTRACRANIAL PRESSURE. The brain is composed of brain tissue, blood, and cerebrospinal fluid (CSF). It is encased in the relatively rigid skull. Within this space, there is little room for any of the components to expand or increase in volume. Through the processes of accommodation and compliance, the ICP is maintained at its normal level of 10–15 mmHg despite transient increases in pressure that occur with straining during defecation, coughing, or sneezing. According to the Monro-Kellie hypothesis, any increase in the volume of one component must be compensated for by a decrease in the volume of one of the other components.

As a first response to an increase in the volume of any

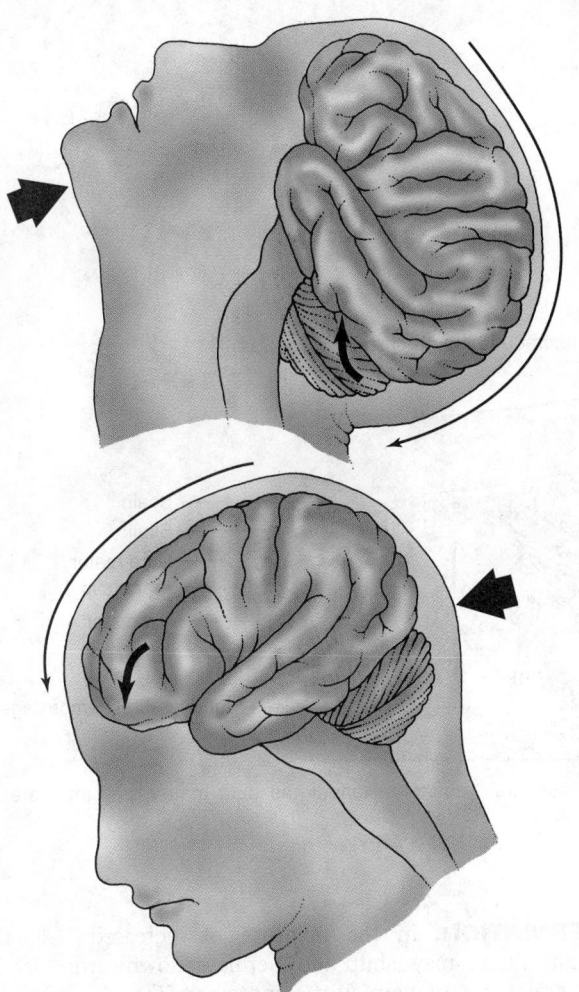

Figure 47–8. Head movement during acceleration-deceleration injury typically seen in motor vehicle accidents.

of these components, the CSF is shunted or displaced from the cranial compartment to the spinal subarachnoid space, or the rate of CSF absorption is increased. An additional response, if needed, is a decrease in cerebral blood volume by the displacement of cerebral venous blood into the sinuses. As long as the brain is able to compensate for the increase in volume and to remain compliant, there are minimal increases in ICP.

Increased ICP is the leading cause of death from head trauma in clients who reach the hospital alive. It occurs when compliance no longer takes place and the brain cannot accommodate further volume changes. As the ICP increases, cerebral blood flow decreases, leading to tissue hypoxia, a decrease in serum pH level, and an increase in carbon dioxide level. This process causes cerebral vasodilation, edema, and a further increase in the ICP, and the cycle continues. If the condition is untreated, the brain herniates downward toward the brain stem, causing irreversible brain damage and possibly death (uncal herniation).

Two types of edema may cause increased ICP: vasogenic and cytotoxic. A third type (interstitial edema) occurs in the presence of acute brain swelling.

Vasogenic edema is seen most often as a cause of increased ICP in the adult. It is characterized by an increase in brain tissue volume caused by an abnormal permeability of the walls of the cerebral vessels, which allows protein-rich plasma infiltrate to leak into the extracellular space of the brain. The fluid collects primarily in the white matter.

Cytotoxic, or cellular, edema may occur as a result of a hypoxic insult, which causes a disturbance in cellular metabolism, the sodium pump, and active ion transport. The brain is quickly depleted of available oxygen, glucose, and glycogen and converts to anaerobic metabolism. The sodium pump fails, and sodium enters the cells and pulls water from the extracellular space. A concomitant decrease in serum sodium level to less than 120 mEq/L occurs. As a result, there is an abnormal accumulation of fluid in the brain cells and a decrease in the extracellular fluid space. Cytotoxic edema may lead to vasogenic edema and further increase in ICP.

Interstitial edema occurs in the presence of acute brain swelling and is associated with elevated blood pressure or increased CSF pressure. Edema develops rapidly in the perivascular and periventricular white space and can be controlled through measures to reduce the client's blood pressure, decrease the cerebrospinal fluid (CSF) pressures, or increase the cerebral perfusion pressure. Cerebral perfusion pressure (CPP) is the amount of pressure needed to deliver oxygen and nutrients to brain tissue. CPP is influenced by oxygenation, cerebral blood volume, blood pressure, cerebral edema, and intracranial pressure. Maintenance of a CPP above 60 mmHg provides adequate metabolic needs.

HEMORRHAGE. Hemorrhages, which cause hematomas (clots), are classified as secondary injury and are caused by vascular damage from the shearing force of the trauma. All hematomas are potentially life-threatening because they act as space-occupying lesions and are surrounded by edema. Three types of hemorrhages include epidural hematoma, subdural hematoma, and intracerebral hemorrhage.

Epidural Hematoma. An epidural hematoma (Fig. 47–9) results from arterial bleeding into the space between the dura and the inner table of the skull. It is frequently caused by a fracture of the temporal bone, which houses the middle meningeal artery. Epidural hematomas are characterized by the presence of a "lucid interval" lasting for minutes, during which time the client is awake and talking. This follows momentary unconsciousness that occurred within minutes of the injury. The client then becomes increasingly symptomatic and may progress to coma.

Subdural Hematoma. A subdural hematoma (SDH) (see Fig. 47–9) results from venous bleeding into the space beneath the dura and above the arachnoid. It results most frequently from tearing of the bridging veins within the cerebral hemispheres or from laceration of the brain tissue. Bleeding from this injury occurs more slowly than from the epidural injury. Subdural hematomas are subdivided into acute, subacute, and chronic. An acute SDH presents within 48 hours after impact; the subacute

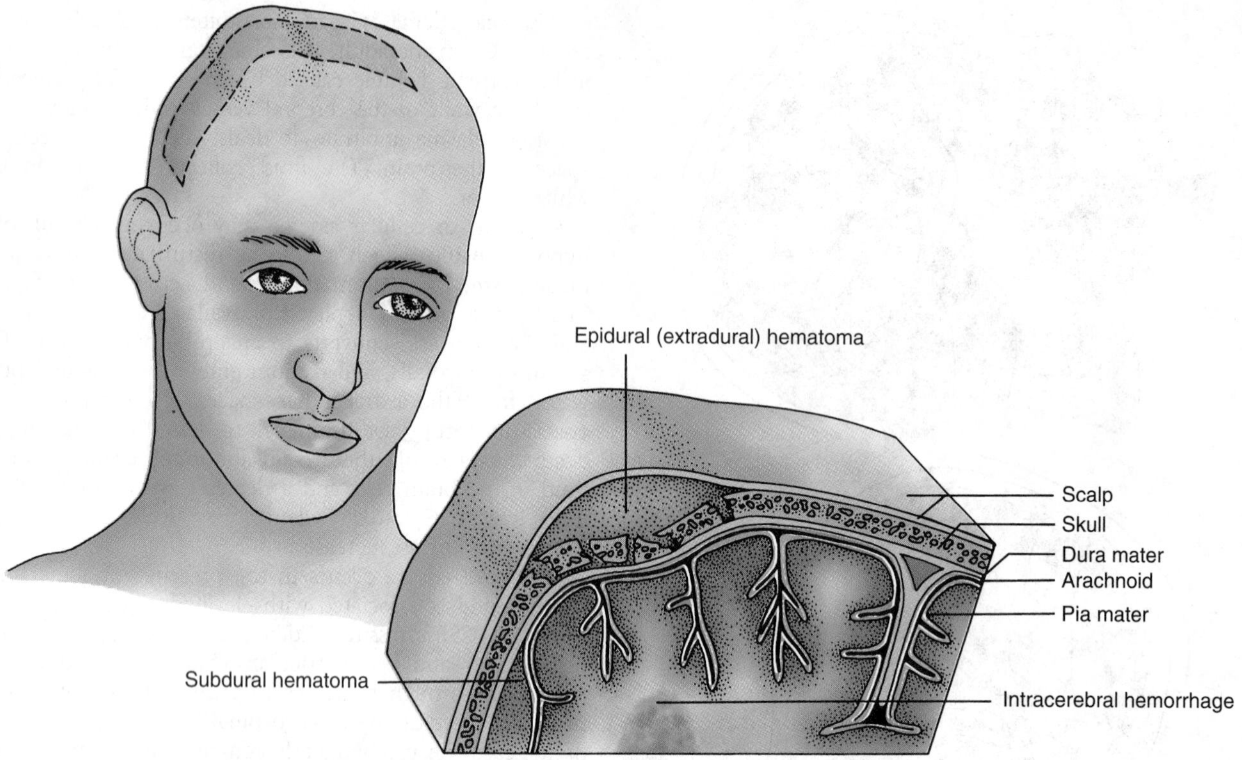

Figure 47–9. Epidural hematoma (outside the dura mater of the brain), subdural hematoma (under the dura mater), and intracerebral hemorrhage (within the brain tissue).

SDH between 48 hours and 2 weeks; the chronic SDH from 2 weeks to several months following injury. Subdural hematomas have the highest mortality rate.

Intracerebral Hemorrhage. An intracerebral hemorrhage (see Fig. 47–9) is the accumulation of blood within the brain tissue caused by the tearing of small arteries and veins in the subcortical white matter. Brain stem hemorrhage occurs as a result of direct trauma, fractures, or torsion injuries to the brain stem.

LOSS OF AUTOREGULATION. Through the process of cerebral autoregulation, the blood flow to the brain remains relatively constant, despite variations in systemic blood pressure. Loss of autoregulation causes the cerebral blood flow to fluctuate passively with the systemic blood pressure. Systemic hypertension may cause an increase in intracranial pressure (ICP) (from an increase in cerebral blood flow) and the potential for vasogenic edema. Hypoxemia and hypercapnia cause marked cerebral vasodilation and therefore an increase in cerebral blood flow, which contributes to increased ICP.

HYDROCEPHALUS. Hydrocephalus is an abnormal increase in the cerebrospinal fluid (CSF) volume. It is caused by dilation of the cerebral ventricles, resulting either from the impairment of CSF absorption in the arachnoid villi or from obstruction of the CSF circulation pathway. This increase in the CSF volume may lead to increased ICP.

HERNIATION. In the presence of increased ICP, the brain tissue may shift and herniate downward. Of the several types of herniation syndromes (Fig. 47–10), uncal, or transtentorial, herniation is the most clinically significant because it is life-threatening. It is caused by a shift of one or both areas of the temporal lobe, known as the uncus. This shift creates pressure on the third cranial nerve and results in dilated and nonreactive pupils, ptosis, and a rapidly deteriorating level of consciousness. Central herniation is caused by a downward shift of the brain stem and the diencephalon from a supratentorial lesion. It is clinically manifested by Cheyne-Stokes respirations and pinpoint nonreactive pupils.

A shift of the cingulate gyrus below the falx cerebri is known as cingulate herniation. A type of infratentorial herniation—cerebellar tonsillar herniation—occurs when the cerebellar tonsils shift and compress the medulla. This may lead to respiratory and cardiovascular compromise or arrest. All herniation syndromes are potentially life-threatening, and the physician must be notified immediately when they are suspected.

Etiology

The most common cause of head injury in the United States is accidents involving motor vehicles, which include both automobiles and motorcycles. All too often, alcohol and drugs are contributing factors to the accident. Falls, acts of violence, and sports-related injuries are the next most common causes.

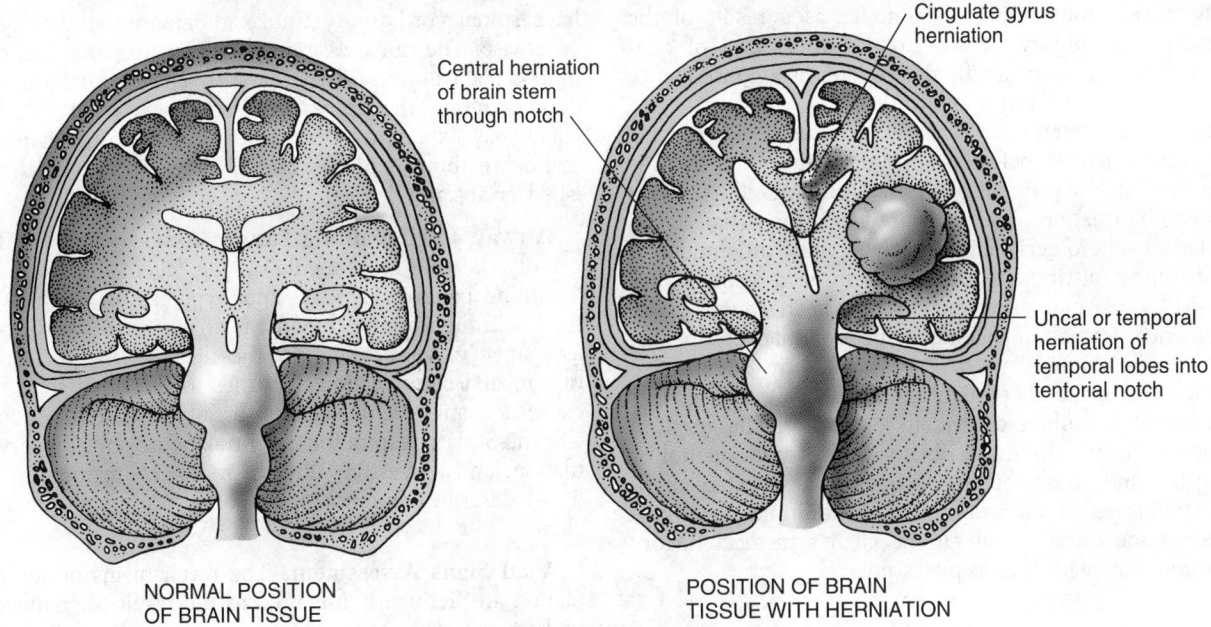

Figure 47–10. Herniation syndromes.

(Labels in figure:)
Central herniation of brain stem through notch

Cingulate gyrus herniation

Uncal or temporal herniation of temporal lobes into tentorial notch

NORMAL POSITION OF BRAIN TISSUE

POSITION OF BRAIN TISSUE WITH HERNIATION

Incidence/Prevalence

Approximately 300,000 clients are admitted to the hospital yearly with head injuries. The mortality rate is 19.3% (56,000 deaths annually). One third of all trauma-related deaths in the United States each year is the result of head injuries. Of these people with head injuries, some 100,000 are left with permanent neurologic dysfunction. Studies indicate that the summer and spring months, evenings, nights, and weekends are associated with a high number of injuries.

Head injuries occur three times more often in male than in female clients. More than 70% occur in people between the ages of 10 and 39 years, with a peak incidence between 15 and 24 years of age.

ELDERLY CONSIDERATIONS

 Clients older than 60 years of age have a higher mortality rate as they are at higher risk for developing secondary injury related to the initial traumatic brain injury (Chart 47–5).

Collaborative Management

Assessment

➤ History

Obtaining an accurate history from a client who has sustained craniocerebral trauma may be difficult because of either the seriousness of the injury or the presence of amnesia. It is not unusual for the client to experience retrograde or anterograde amnesia: loss of memory for the events before or after the injury, respectively. The client with a serious head injury is often admitted to the hospital unconscious or in a confused and combative state. If the client is unable to provide information, the history can be obtained from rescue workers or witnesses to the injury. The nurse should ask when, where, and how the injury occurred. Did the client lose consciousness? If so, for how long was the client unconscious, and has there been a change in the level of consciousness?

The nurse obtains information about the events immediately after the injury. Clients with a severe injury may have several different reactions. The client may be completely unresponsive after the injury; alternatively, the client may initially be responsive and, within a few minutes to several hours, the client's condition may deteriorate rapidly. In another typical presentation, the client is ini-

---

Chart 47–5

Nursing Focus on the Elderly: Head Injury

- Is the fifth leading cause of death
- 65–75–year-old age group has second highest incidence of head injury of all age groups
- Falls and motor vehicle accidents are most common cause
- The following factors contribute to high mortality:
  - Falls causing subdural hematomas (closed head injuries)—especially chronic subdural hematoma
  - Poorly tolerated systemic stress, increased by admission to a high-stimuli environment
  - Medical complications, such as hypotension, hypertension, and cardiac problems
  - Decreased protective mechanisms, which make clients susceptible to infections (especially pneumonia)
  - Decreased immunologic competence, further diminished by head injury

tially unconscious for a few minutes as a result of the primary brain injury, returns to a normal level of consciousness, and then rapidly deteriorates as a consequence of secondary insult to the brain.

The nurse determines whether the client experienced any seizure activity before or after the injury or if there is a history of a seizure disorder. It is important to obtain precise information about the circumstances of falls, particularly in the older client. The nurse must differentiate a head injury attributable to a fall from a head injury caused by a stroke, an aneurysm, or a heart attack. Other pertinent information includes hand dominance, any diseases of or injuries to the eyes, and any allergies to medications or food, particularly seafood. People allergic to seafood are often allergic to contrast media used in diagnostic tests. The nurse obtains a history of alcohol or drug use and abuse, because drugs or alcohol may mask the symptoms of increased ICP. In addition, the nurse asks routine questions about the client's medical history in accordance with the hospital's policies.

➤ Physical Assessment/Clinical Manifestations

No two injuries are alike—the client with a head injury may have a variety of signs and symptoms depending on the severity of injury and the resulting increase in intracranial pressure (ICP) (see Chart 47–4). The goals of the nursing assessment are the establishment of baseline data and the early detection of and prevention of increased ICP, systemic hypotension, hypoxia, or hypercapnia (increased blood levels of carbon dioxide). The early detection of subtle changes in the client's neurologic status enables the health care team to prevent or to treat potentially life-threatening complications.

Because it is estimated that 5% to 20% of clients with head trauma have associated cervical spinal cord injuries, all clients with head trauma are treated as though they have spinal cord injury until radiographic studies prove otherwise. The nurse assesses for indicators of spinal cord injury, such as loss of motor and sensory function, tenderness along the spine, and abnormal head tilt. The client may experience respiratory problems and diaphragmatic breathing, and his or her reflexes may be diminished or absent.

Airway and Breathing Pattern Assessment. The first priority is the assessment of the client's airway and breathing pattern. Hypoxia and hypercapnia are best detected through arterial blood gas analysis, but the nursing assessment is vital to identify the client at risk for respiration-related complications. Injuries to the brain stem may cause a change in the client's breathing pattern, such as Cheyne-Stokes respirations; central neurogenic hyperventilation; and apneustic, cluster, or ataxic breathing. Table 47–4 describes common respiratory patterns of comatose clients.

Vital Signs Assessment. The mechanisms of autoregulation are frequently impaired as the result of craniocerebral trauma. The more serious the injury, the more severe the impact on autoregulation. The nurse or assistive nursing personnel monitor the client's blood pressure and pulse to detect possible changes in cerebral blood flow caused by impaired autoregulation as a result of hypotension or hypertension. The Cushing reflex, a classic, yet late sign of increased intracranial pressure (ICP), is manifested by severe hypertension with a widened pulse pressure and bradycardia. As the ICP increases, the pulse becomes thready, irregular, and rapid. Cerebral blood flow increases in response to hypertension, and vasogenic edema may occur, further increasing the ICP. In contrast, hypotension and tachycardia are symptomatic of hypovolemic shock. This decrease in blood volume may lead to decreased cerebral perfusion pressure and eventually to ischemia and infarct of the brain tissue.

TABLE 47–4

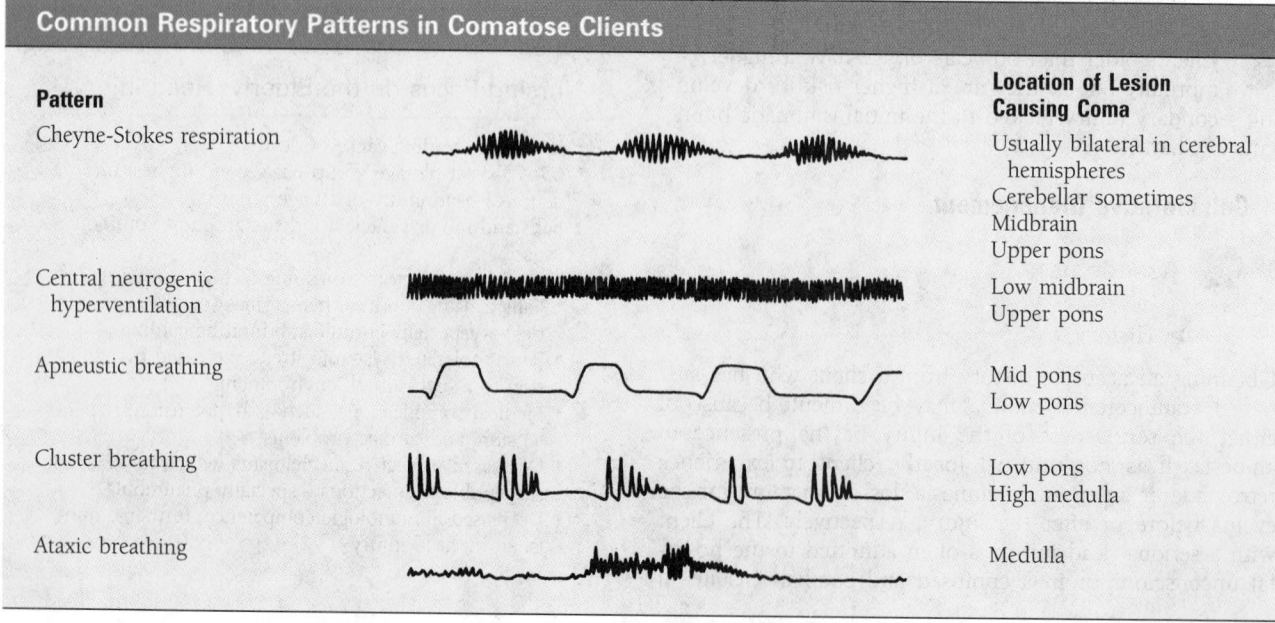

Common Respiratory Patterns in Comatose Clients		
Pattern		**Location of Lesion Causing Coma**
Cheyne-Stokes respiration		Usually bilateral in cerebral hemispheres Cerebellar sometimes Midbrain Upper pons
Central neurogenic hyperventilation		Low midbrain Upper pons
Apneustic breathing		Mid pons Low pons
Cluster breathing		Low pons High medulla
Ataxic breathing		Medulla

Hypovolemic shock is usually due to intra-abdominal bleeding or bleeding into the soft tissue around major fractures, not to intracranial bleeding. Cardiac dysrhythmias may result from chest trauma, bruising of the heart, or interference with the autonomic nervous system.

Neurologic Assessment. Many hospitals use the Glasgow Coma Scale to assess the client's neurologic status (see Chap. 43). The most important variable to assess is the level of consciousness. A decrease or change in the level of consciousness is typically the first sign of a deterioration in the client's neurologic status. Changes in the content of consciousness or orientation are due to injury to the cerebral cortex. A decrease in arousal or increased sleepiness and coma are caused by injury in the reticular activating system within the brain stem. Early indicators of a change in the level of consciousness include behavior changes, such as restlessness or irritability, and are often subtle in nature.

Eye Assessment. The nurse elicits a history of previous eye injury or medications that affect pupillary dilation and constriction such as anticholinergics and adrenergics. The nurse also checks the client's pupils for size and reaction to light. Any changes in pupil size, shape, and reactivity must be reported to the health care provider immediately as these changes indicate an increase in ICP. Depending on which areas of the brain are damaged, the pupillary changes or eye signs will differ. Pinpoint and nonresponsive pupils are indicative of brain-stem dysfunction at the level of the pons. Of particular importance is the ovoid pupil, which is regarded as the midstage between a normal-sized pupil and a dilated pupil. This finding indicates the development of increased ICP.

The nurse checks gross vision, if the client's condition permits. The nurse can have the client read any printed material, such as the nurse's name tag, or count the number of fingers that the nurse holds within the client's visual field. Loss of vision is usually caused by injury to the occipital lobe, which produces temporary cortical blindness.

If the client is able to cooperate, the nurse tests cranial nerves III, IV, and VI. Extraocular movements may be diminished owing to the presence of increased ICP and hydrocephalus. Damage to the optic chiasm, the optic tract, or the optic radii may cause visual field deficits or diplopia. In the unconscious client, the oculocephalic and oculovestibular tests are performed to test the integrity of the brain stem and the integrity of cranial nerves III, VI, and VII. Chapter 43 describes these techniques in detail.

Motor Assessment. The nurse also assesses for bilateral motor responses to avoid missing lateralizing signs. The client's motor loss or dysfunction usually appears contralateral to the site of the lesion. For example, a left-sided hemiparesis is indicative of an injury to the right cerebral hemisphere. A deterioration in motor function or the development of abnormal posturing (decerebrate or decorticate posturing) or flaccidity is another indicator of increased ICP. These changes are attributable to dysfunction within the pyramidal system or cerebral peduncles. Brain stem or cerebellar injury may cause ataxia, decreased or increased muscle tone, and weakness.

Additional Neurologic Assessment. If the client is able to cooperate, a full neurologic assessment is completed as outlined in Chapter 43. Particular attention is paid to cranial nerves I, V, VII, IX, and X. The first cranial nerve is frequently damaged where the frontal lobe passes over the irregularly shaped bones of the anterior and middle fossa; this results in the loss of smell (anosmia). Cranial nerves V, VII, IX, and X are important for chewing and swallowing abilities and phonation. The client's ability to speak must be assessed, with particular attention directed toward differentiating aphasias (caused by injury to the cerebral cortex) from communication impairments (caused by damage to the cranial nerves and cerebellum). Damage to the cranial nerves occurs from disruption of the nerve trunk, either intracranially or along its extracranial course in the skull or face. Cranial nerve damage may be the result of direct trauma or compression associated with pressure or hemorrhage.

The nurse assesses for other signs of increased intracranial pressure (ICP) (see Chart 47–4). These include severe headache, nausea, vomiting, seizures, and papilledema (seen by ophthalmoscopic examination). Papilledema, also known as a choked disk, is edema and hyperemia of the optic disk. It is always a sign of increased ICP. Headache and seizures are a response to the injury and may or may not be associated with increased ICP. In general, a single neurologic finding is not indicative of increased ICP. The nurse must keep in mind, however, that the client can have a marked increase in ICP yet be relatively asymptomatic.

The nurse carefully assesses the client's ears and nose for any signs of cerebrospinal fluid (CSF) leaks that result from a basilar skull fracture. CSF placed on a white absorbent background can be distinguished from other fluids by the "halo" sign, a yellowish stain surrounded by bloody drainage. In addition, CSF tests positively for glucose when a strip testing method (Dipstix) is used. If there is a CSF leak, the client should be assessed for any signs of nuchal rigidity (stiff neck), which may indicate infection or blood in the CSF. Nuchal rigidity is not checked until a spinal cord injury has been ruled out.

The client's head is palpated to detect the presence of fractures or hematomas. The nurse looks for areas of ecchymosis, tender areas of the scalp, and lacerations.

Clients with a *minor* head injury should be assessed for signs and symptoms of post-traumatic sequelae. The symptoms include a wide array of physical and cognitive problems, ranging from persistent headache, weakness, and dizziness to personality and behavior changes, loss of memory, and problems with perception, reasoning abilities, and concept formation. The symptoms may persist for a few days or weeks to several months after the injury. For some clients, severe physical and cognitive problems remain, despite a relatively benign initial clinical presentation and normal diagnostic test findings.

▶ Psychosocial Assessment

The person who has had a *major* head injury is never the same as before the injury. Most often, the client with a major head injury has personality changes manifested by temper outbursts, depression, risk-taking behavior, and denial of disability. The client may become talkative and develop a very outgoing personality. Memory, especially recent or short-term memory, is affected, which should not be confused with problems of aphasia. The client's ability to learn new information and concentration may be affected. Finally, the client may exhibit problems with insight and planning. All of these problems may lead to difficulties within the family structure and with social and work-related interactions. Coping strategies that have been used in the past must be assessed to determine the client's ability to adapt to the changes in physical and cognitive abilities. Clients with a mild head injury, while having no focal signs, may still have disability symptoms 1 year after injury.

The nurse assesses family dynamics, particularly if the client is discharged to the family's care directly from the acute care hospital. The family or significant others must also cope with the changes in the client's physical appearance and cognitive abilities. Many families are angry at the client for being injured, especially when the client's behavior or their own behavior resulted in an injury that could have been prevented. They may feel guilty that they did not or were not able to prevent the injury. The family or significant others may feel overwhelmed by the complexity of care the client requires and the long recovery period. Both the family and the client need to develop coping strategies to deal with the potential role reversals and role changes caused by the injury.

➤ Laboratory Assessment

There are no laboratory tests to diagnose primary brain injury; however, several laboratory tests are used to diagnose or indicate measures to prevent secondary brain insult. Arterial blood gases are analyzed, with particular attention paid to oxygen and carbon dioxide levels. The health care provider also orders a complete blood count and determination of serum glucose and electrolyte levels and osmolality. These tests are performed to monitor the client's hemodynamic status or to identify electrolyte imbalance or the presence of infection.

➤ Radiographic Assessment

The health care provider orders computed tomography scanning to identify the extent and scope of injury to the brain. This diagnostic test can identify the presence of a lesion that requires surgical intervention, such as an epidural or subdural hematoma. Radiography of the cervical spine and the skull is done to rule out fractures and dislocations. A chest x-ray is taken to identify fractured ribs or other chest injuries. A flat-plate of the abdomen may be obtained to assist in the diagnosis of abdominal bleeding or bowel laceration.

➤ Other Diagnostic Assessment

Magnetic resonance imaging is particularly useful in the diagnosis of diffuse axonal injury but not recommended for clients with ICP monitoring devices or other invasive monitoring devices. As the client's condition stabilizes, the

physician may order other diagnostic tests to identify the extent of the injury to the brain. For example, the integrity of the cerebral vessels is measured through the use of Doppler flow studies or an arteriogram; cerebral perfusion is measured by cerebral blood flow studies. Evoked potentials provide information on the functioning sensory pathways and may be useful in predicting outcome.

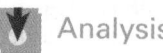 Analysis

➤ Common Nursing Diagnoses and Collaborative Problems

The common nursing diagnoses when caring for a client with craniocerebral trauma are
1. Altered (Cerebral) Tissue Perfusion related to impaired circulation and increased intracranial pressure (ICP)
2. Sensory/Perceptual Alterations related to decreased level of consciousness, damage to the parietal lobe, or injury to the olfactory nerve
3. Impaired Gas Exchange related to pooling of secretions, poor cough reflex, and altered breathing pattern
4. Risk for Injury related to seizures, agitation, restlessness, and confusion
5. Impaired Physical Mobility and Self Care Deficit (the level depends on the extent of injury) related to neurologic dysfunction or fatigue
6. Altered Nutrition: Less than Body Requirements related to an inability to chew or swallow or cognitive dysfunction
7. Body Image Disturbance and Altered Role Performance related to cognitive dysfunction and physical disabilities

➤ Additional Nursing Diagnoses and Collaborative Problems

In addition to the common nursing diagnoses, some clients experience one or more of the following:
- Altered Thought Processes related to brain damage from injury and hypoxia
- Impaired Verbal Communication related to aphasia
- Post-Trauma Response related to sudden and unexpected injury
- Pain related to the injury
- Powerlessness related to cognitive and physical disabilities
- Ineffective Family Coping: Compromises related to changes in the client's role and physical and cognitive disabilities

Some clients with major head injury are at risk for complications. These include
- Potential for Hypoxemia
- Potential for Increased Intracranial Pressure (ICP)
- Potential for Atelectasis and Pneumonia
- Potential for Seizures
- Potential for Deep Vein Thrombosis
- Potential for Sepsis

Planning and Implementation

Altered (Cerebral) Tissue Perfusion

Planning: Expected Outcomes. The client is expected to maintain a normal ICP, maintain appropriate vital signs and arterial blood gas values, and achieve improvement in level of consciousness.

Interventions. The client with a *severe* head injury is admitted to the critical care unit or a trauma center. Clients with *minor* head injuries are either admitted to the general nursing unit, where they are closely observed for at least 24 hours, or sent home from the emergency department with instructions (Chart 47–6).

The health care provider treats the client with medication and supportive measures to prevent increased ICP. If these measures fail, surgery may be indicated to remove necrotic brain tissue, the tips of the temporal lobe, or part of the frontal lobe. These procedures are used only if more conservative measures to treat increased ICP or cerebral edema fail. Evacuation of hematomas may be needed to reduce or prevent increased ICP.

Nonsurgical Management. Nursing interventions for all clients with a head injury are directed toward preventing or detecting increased ICP, promoting fluid and electrolyte balance, and monitoring the effects of treatments and medications.

Chart 47–6

Education Guide: Minor Head Injury

- If the person is sleeping, wake him or her every 3–4 hr for the first 2 days, asking name, where the client is, and identification of caregiver.
- Expect the person to complain of headache, nausea, or dizziness for at least 24 hr. If these symptoms are severe or do not improve, contact the physician immediately or take the person back to the emergency department.
- For a headache, give acetaminophen (Tylenol) every 4 hr as needed.
- Avoid giving the person sedatives, sleeping pills, or alcoholic beverages for at least 24 hr unless the physician instructs otherwise.
- Do not allow the person to engage in strenuous activity for at least 48 hr.
- Do not allow nose blowing or ear cleaning for 48 hr.
- If any of the following symptoms occur, take the person back to the emergency department immediately:
  - Blurred vision
  - Drainage from the ear or nose
  - Weakness
  - Slurred speech
  - Progressive sleepiness
  - Vomiting
  - Worsening headache
  - Unequal pupil size
- Keep follow-up health care provider appointments.

Assessment of Vital Signs. The nurse or assistive nursing personnel take and record the client's vital signs every 1–2 hours. The physician may order medications to prevent severe hypertension or hypotension. The client in the critical care unit is connected to a cardiac monitor to detect any cardiac dysrhythmias. Nonspecific ST-segment or T-wave changes may occur, possibly in response to stimulation of the autonomic nervous system or an increase in the level of circulating catecholamines. The nurse documents and reports cardiac irregularities to the health care provider.

The client with a head injury is often admitted with a fever, which is a defense mechanism in the presence of trauma. Fever as a consequence of infection may develop later in the course of the disease. A third type of fever is a central fever caused by hypothalamic damage. It is manifested by an absence of sweating and no diurnal (daily) variation; the fever is high and lasts several days to weeks. In addition, this type of fever responds better to cooling (hypothermia blanket, sponge bath) than to the administration of antipyretic drugs, such as acetaminophen (Tylenol, Ace-Tabs♦).

Positioning. The nurse positions the client to avoid extreme flexion or extension of the neck and to maintain the head in the midline, neutral position. The nurse logrolls the client during turning to avoid extreme hip flexion and keeps the head of the bed elevated 30–45 degrees. All of these measures enhance venous drainage, which helps prevent increased ICP.

Hyperventilation. Prophylactic hyperventilation during the first 20 hours after injury is usually avoided as it may produce ischemia by causing cerebral vasoconstriction with a resulting decrease in cerebral blood volume and ICP. However, in acute neurologic deterioration, hyperventilation may be used for brief periods. Intracranial hypertension that does not respond to standard treatment may also require hyperventilation for longer periods of time (AANS, 1997).

The client who requires mechanical ventilation is hyperventilated to maintain an arterial carbon dioxide pressure ($PaCO_2$) of 27–35 mmHg. Carbon dioxide is a very potent vasodilator that can contribute to increases in ICP. The $PaCO_2$ must not be allowed to fall to less than 20 mmHg, which may result in hypoxia caused by *severe* vasoconstriction. Arterial oxygen levels (PaO_2) are maintained between 80 and 100 mmHg to prevent cerebral vasodilation resulting from hypoxemia. Arterial blood gas values are monitored at least twice per day and after each change in the ventilator setting.

Induction of Barbiturate Coma. For clients whose ICP cannot be controlled by other means, the health care provider may place the client in a barbiturate coma using pentobarbital sodium (Nembutal, Novopentobarb♦) to decrease elevated ICP. This drug works by decreasing the metabolic demands of the brain and cerebral blood flow, stabilizing cell membranes, decreasing formation of vasogenic edema, and producing a more uniform blood supply. The provider adjusts the dosage to maintain complete unresponsiveness. As a consequence, it is difficult for the nurse to recognize subtle or unsubtle neurologic changes. The client requires mechanical ventilation, sophisticated hemodynamic monitoring, and ICP monitoring. Complications of barbiturate coma include cardiac dysrhythmias, hypotension, and fluid and electrolyte disturbances.

Drug Therapy. Glucocorticoids (dexamethasone [Decadron, Dexasone♣] and methylprednisolone sodium succinate [Solu-Medrol, Medrol♣]) have no demonstrated benefit in the management of increased ICP as a result of head injury or cerebral infarction. Mannitol (Osmitrol♣), an osmotic diuretic, is used to treat cerebral edema by pulling water out of the extracellular space of the edematous brain tissue but not cross the blood-brain barrier. It is most effective when given in boluses rather than a continuous infusion. Furosemide (Lasix), a loop diuretic, is often used as adjunctive therapy to reduce the incidence of rebound from mannitol and also enhances its therapeutic action. Furosemide also reduces edema and blood volume, decreases sodium uptake by the brain, and decreases production of CSF at the choroid plexus.

The nurse gives mannitol through a filter in the IV tubing or, if given by IV push, drawn up through a filtered needle to eliminate microscopic crystals. The nurse strictly monitors the client receiving either osmotic or loop diuretics for intake and output and observes for severe dehydration and indications of acute renal failure, weakness, edema, and changes in urinary output. A Foley catheter must be inserted to maintain strict measurement of output. The client's serum and urine osmolality are checked daily.

Codeine or fentanyl (Sublimaze) may be used with ventilated clients to decrease agitation and control restlessness. These agents can be easily reversed with naloxone (Narcan). Neuromuscular blocking agents (NMBA), such as pancuronium bromide (Pavulon), have no analgesic effect but when used with sedation help decrease cerebral metabolic rate associated with agitation. Neuromuscular muscular blocking agents *must never be used without sedation.*

Anticonvulsants, such as phenytoin (Dilantin), are given to prevent seizures. Acetaminophen (Tylenol, Ace-Tabs♣) and aspirin (Ancasal♣) are given to clients who are febrile (temperature greater than 39° C [101° F]) to reduce fever.

Fluids and Electrolytes. The client with craniocerebral trauma is at risk for diabetes insipidus and the syndrome of inappropriate antidiuretic hormone (SIADH) because the pituitary gland may be injured or compressed from cerebral edema (see later discussion).

Fluid overload can occur in the client with multiple trauma from the rapid administration of IV fluids, plasma expanders, or corticosteroids. Fluids may be restricted to 2 L/day initially to decrease increased ICP and swelling. The amount of fluid restriction is also influenced by response to diuretic therapy and evaluation of laboratory values. Serum osmolality should be maintained below 310 mOsm. Urine specific gravity is checked every 1–4 hours. Serum and urine osmolality and electrolytes are monitored frequently.

Surgical Management. The physician may elect to insert an intracranial pressure (ICP) monitoring device to evaluate the client's pressure more closely. All devices are inserted through a bur hole that is placed in the skull using a twist drill. Each device is connected to a transducer that is connected to a monitor. The monitor is able to record the pressure waves and to provide a digital readout of the pressure.

Intracranial Pressure Monitoring. Various types of devices for monitoring ICP are used (Fig 47–11). An *intraventricular catheter* (IVC) is a small tube that is inserted into the anterior horn of the lateral ventricle of the nondominant cerebral hemisphere. The advantage of this system is that cerebrospinal fluid (CSF) can be drained to decrease ICP, and specimens can be obtained for laboratory analysis. The *subarachnoid screw* or *bolt* is a hollow device that is placed into the subarachnoid space for direct pressure measurement. A disadvantage of the system is that CSF cannot be drained to treat increased ICP; however, it is less invasive, thus lowering the risk of infection (Table 47–5).

An *epidural catheter* or *sensor* is a transducer that is placed between the skull and the dura, leaving the dura intact. A similar device is the *subdural catheter,* placed under the dura mater. Its major advantage is the decreased risk of infection from an open dural space. The *fiberoptic transducer tipped pressure sensor* is a newer device for ICP monitoring. It is easily transported and can be placed in the subdural or subarachnoid space, in the ventricle, or directly into brain tissue.

The nurse follows the agency's protocols for the management of these devices. The waveform should be observed for signs of damping, which indicates that the device is not functioning and the pressure that is displayed may not be accurate. If this problem occurs, the nurse checks that the transducer is at the level of the ventricle. The transducer is recalibrated and rebalanced, and the tubing is checked for air bubbles. If the waveform remains damped, the nurse should notify the physician.

Craniotomy. In extreme cases, if the client's ICP cannot be controlled, the physician may elect to perform a craniotomy to remove ischemic tissue or the tips of the temporal lobes. The removal of nonvital brain tissue allows expansion of brain tissue without further compromise of the ICP. A craniotomy may also be performed to remove epidural or subdural hematomas. (Care of the client with a craniotomy is discussed in the section on Brain Tumor later in this chapter.)

Sensory/Perceptual Alterations

Planning: Expected Outcomes. The major concern of the client with sensory or perceptual changes is to develop strategies to adapt to the changes. Therefore, the client is expected to adapt to the residual neurologic dysfunction.

Interventions. The client with a *major* head injury may exhibit changes in the following areas: sense of smell; ability to taste, swallow, or feel the presence of food within the oral cavity; and vision, pain, and temperature sensation. As a result, the client is at risk for nutritional deficits, which may interfere with the healing proc-

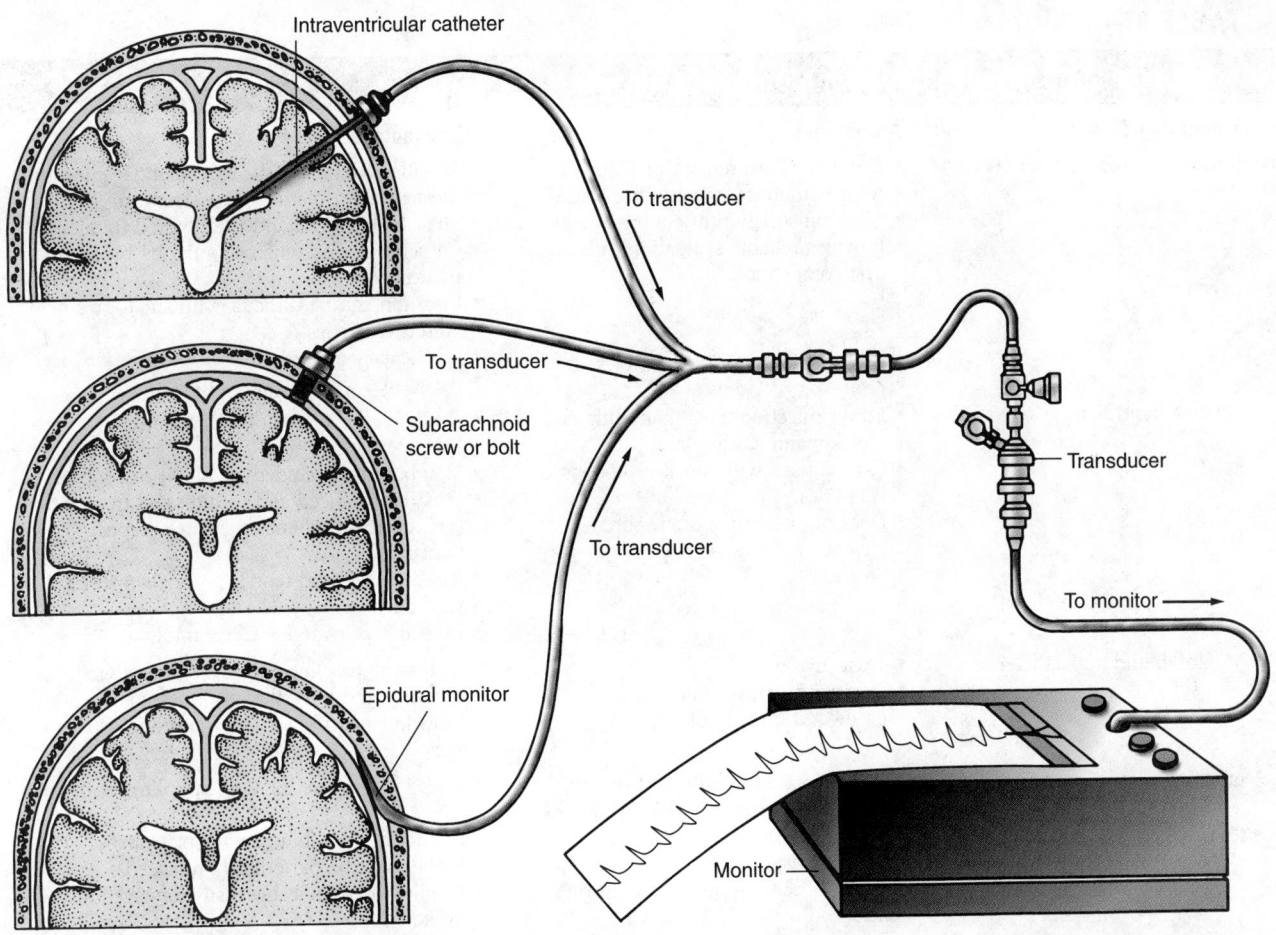

Figure 47–11. Common types of intracranial pressure (ICP) monitoring devices: intraventricular catheter, subarachnoid screw or bolt, and epidural monitor.

ess. The client may be injured from falling over objects outside the field of vision, or burn injuries could occur because of the inability to perceive variations in water temperatures.

The nurse ensures that mealtime and the surrounding environment is a pleasant experience and positions the client to maximize swallowing ability. In collaboration with the speech-language pathologist, the nurse identifies strategies to prevent food from accumulating in the cheek of the affected side. Generally, clients who have swallowing problems are able to tolerate or swallow soft or semi-soft foods and liquids (mechanical soft or dental diet, junior baby foods, custards, scrambled eggs) better than thin liquids (water, juice, or milk). Powdered thickener (Thick-It) may be added to thicken foods to a more manageable consistency. The nurse collaborates with the dietitian to find a diet appropriate for the client with dysphagia.

If there is a large lesion of the parietal lobe, the client may experience loss of sensation for pain, temperature, touch, and proprioception, preventing the client from responding appropriately to environmental stimuli. A hazard-free environment is necessary to prevent injury (e.g., from burns, if the client's coffee is too hot, or falls, if the side rails on the bed are not kept up). A sensory stimula-

tion program should be integrated into the comatose or stuporous client's routine care activities. Sensory stimulation is done to facilitate a client's meaningful response to the environment. The nurse presents visual, auditory, or tactile stimuli one at a time and explains the purpose and the type of stimulus presented. For example, the nurse shows a picture of the client's mother and says to the client, "This is a picture of your mother." The picture is shown to the client several times, and the same words are used to describe the picture. If auditory tapes are used, they should not be longer than 10–15 minutes. If the stimulus is presented for a longer period, it simply becomes "white" noise, or meaningless background noise.

The client may be disoriented and experience a short-term memory loss. The nurse always introduces himself or herself to the client before any interaction. The nurse's explanations of procedures and activities are short and simple and are given immediately before and throughout the procedure. A sleep-wake cycle must be maintained, with scheduled rest periods. The nurse orients the client to time (day, month, and year) and place and explains the reason for the client's hospitalization. The nurse reassures the client that the client's family knows where the client is and that the client is safe. The nurse should ask the family to bring in familiar objects, such as pictures.

TABLE 47-5

Advantages and Disadvantages of Monitoring Devices

Monitoring Device	Advantages	Disadvantages
Intraventricular catheter (IVC)	• Accurate measurement of ICP. • Allows drainage or sampling of CSF. • Allows instillation of contrast media. • Provides reliable evaluation of cerebral compliance.	• Provides additional site for potential infection. • Most invasive method for monitoring ICP. • Must be balanced and recalibrated frequently. • Catheter can become occluded by blood or tissue. • Insertion can be difficult with small or collapsed ventricles. • CSF leakage can occur around insertion site. • Associated with increased infection rate.
Subarachnoid bolt or screw	• Lower infection rates than with IVC. • Quickly and easily placed. • Can be used with small or collapsed ventricles. • Does not penetrate brain parenchyma.	• Tendency for dampened waveform. • Less accurate at high ICP. • May become occluded by blood or tissue. • Must be balanced and recalibrated frequently (i.e., q4h and whenever client is repositioned). • Baseline drift and tendency for dampened waveform. • Does not provide for CSF sampling.
Subdural/epidural catheter or sensor	• Least invasive. • Decreased risk for infection. • Easily and quickly placed.	• Increasing baseline drift over time; therefore, accuracy and reliability are questionable. • Does not provide for CSF sampling or drainage.
Fiberoptic transducer tipped catheter	• Can be placed in subdural or subarachnoid space, in ventricle, or into brain tissue. • Easily transported. • Requires zeroing only once (during insertion). • Baseline drift to 1 mmHg/day. • Decreased risk of infection. • Less waveform artifact. • No need to adjust transducer to the client's position. • Easy to insert.	• Does not provide for CSF sampling or drainage. • Cannot be recalibrated after placement. • Probe must be periodically replaced. • Fragile fiberoptic cable easily damaged and broken.

Orientation cues within the environment, such as a large clock with numbers or a single-date calendar, should be provided.

Impaired Gas Exchange

Planning: Expected Outcomes. The client is expected to be free from respiratory infection and atelectasis and have adequate arterial blood gas values.

Interventions. Pulmonary secretions tend to pool as a result of a decreased level of consciousness, ineffective cough, or an altered breathing pattern. The secretions may be thick because of the fluid intake restriction used to prevent cerebral edema. Chest physiotherapy and frequent turning may be needed as indicated by the results of the respiratory assessment.

The client with increased intracranial pressure (ICP) should be carefully observed when suctioned. If the client is intubated, he or she should be manually hyperventilated (preoxygenated) with 100% oxygen for 60 seconds between each pass of the catheter. The client should be allowed a rest period of a few minutes after suctioning to prevent increased ICP. Lidocaine given intravenously or endotracheally may be used to suppress the cough reflex, which would increase ICP.

Risk for Injury

Planning: Expected Outcomes. The client is expected to be free of injuries that result from seizure activity, restlessness, agitation, or confusion.

Interventions. The client is at risk for seizure activity, and actions are taken as outlined in the discussion of epilepsy (see Chap. 44). The nurse and assistive nursing personnel keep the bed in a low position with the side rails up. If the client pulls out the intravenous (IV) line or nasogastric tube, hand mittens may be applied. The client's extremities should be restrained *only* if absolutely necessary, and the use of restraints should begin with single-limb or opposite restraints. Restraining any extremity increases the client's agitation and fear. The nurse always obtains a physician's order for the use of restraints of any kind for no more than 24 hours. The mitten is removed, the restrained hand is exercised, and the mitten is reapplied. The client's behavior is observed and documented at least every hour. Most agencies have a special restraint documentation form that is used for this purpose.

The nurse or assistive nursing personnel orient the client to the surroundings as needed and provides a quiet environment. The nurse closely monitors the client's response to television programs or the radio. Often, the client is unable to differentiate these situations or programs from what is happening within his or her own environment.

Impaired Physical Mobility; Self Care Deficit

Planning: Expected Outcomes. The client is expected to be free from complications of immobility and to be able to ambulate and perform activities of daily living (ADL) independently with or without adaptive or assistive devices.

Interventions. Chapter 13 discusses mobility and ADL skills in detail as well as ways to prevent the complications of immobility. Several additional interventions are provided here.

It is especially important to prevent pulmonary complications in the client with head injury because they may further compromise neurologic status. The nurse or assistive nursing personnel turn the client at least every 2 hours. Chest physiotherapy may be performed if attention is directed toward preventing increased ICP. It may be necessary to sedate the client before the procedure or to avoid placing the client in Trendelenburg's position. The client should wear pneumatic compression boots or sequential compression stockings until fully mobile to prevent venous stasis that could lead to either a pulmonary embolus or deep vein (venous) thrombosis. Administration of prophylactic anticoagulants such as heparin, aspirin, or low-molecular-weight heparinoids may be ordered.

In collaboration with the physical therapist and occupational therapist, a program of exercises to maintain function, prevent complications of immobility, and accomplish ADLs is implemented. The nurse, assistive nursing personnel, or significant other provides passive or active-assistive range-of-motion exercises at least once every 8 hours, with particular attention given to the joints of the fingers and the wrist. Splints for the affected limbs should be custom-fitted by physical or occupational therapists. The client whose feet are flaccid may wear high-topped tennis shoes to prevent foot drop. Such shoes may be used for the client who is spastic, only after consultation with the occupational or physical therapist. The nurse or assistive nursing personnel remove splints and supportive shoes and inspect the skin for signs of irritation several times each day.

Altered Nutrition: Less Than Body Requirements

Planning: Expected Outcomes. The client is expected to maintain body weight within 10% of the ideal body weight or at the usual body weight and maintain adequate hydration.

Interventions. The client who is moderately to severely injured usually has a decreased level of consciousness, at least temporarily. As a result, the client is unable to chew or swallow and must receive nutrition and fluids by an alternative method. The client initially receives IV fluids until stabilized. If there is no improvement in the client's level of consciousness, long-term nutritional support via enteral feeding is usually instituted. A small-lumen nasogastric or nasoduodenal tube or percutaneous endoscopic gastrostomy (PEG) tube is used for continuous or intermittent feeding. Small bore tubes decrease the risk for aspiration in a client who is at high risk. (Care of the client receiving enteral feeding is described in Chapter 64.)

With the use of either type of tube, the nurse weighs the client daily, collaborates with the dietitian to determine if caloric needs are being met, and monitors the serum albumin level to ensure adequate protein intake. The client is assessed daily for signs of dehydration, such as dry mucous membranes and poor skin turgor. Supplements such as milk shakes and Ensure may be needed to meet caloric and protein requirements.

Body Image Disturbance; Altered Role Performance

Planning: Expected Outcomes. The client is expected to develop confidence in his or her abilities and begin to adapt to changes in physical appearance and abilities.

Interventions. To assist the client in developing a positive self-concept, the nurse must first establish a trusting relationship with the client. The nurse can help establish trust by having a nonjudgmental attitude and providing open and honest communication. The client is encouraged to ask questions about his or her care and to verbalize his or her thoughts, fears, and anxieties. The nurse should answer any questions honestly and correct any misinformation. The client should participate as much as possible in all decision-making about treatment. The nurse emphasizes the client's abilities while assisting him or her to adapt to disabilities. The nurse allows the client privacy; however, the client should be encouraged to balance a need for privacy with appropriate social interaction.

 Continuing Care

The client with a *major* head injury requires ongoing rehabilitation following hospitalization. Information on the selection of a head injury rehabilitation facility can be obtained from the National Head Injury Foundation (NHIF). Other preparation includes the development of a detailed client care plan to be given to the rehabilitation facility. This enables the provision of consistent care and decreases the initial anxiety related to the changes that the client may experience. The nursing discharge summary states medications, including the dosage, possible reactions, and special preparation; the current client care plan; techniques used to motivate or calm the client; and strategies to assist the family to adapt to the situation.

The goal of rehabilitation after head injury is to maximize the client's ability to return to his or her highest level of functioning. Rehabilitation activities such as occupational therapy (OT), physical therapy (PT), and speech therapy may continue in the home after discharge from the rehabilitation facility. Adaptation of the home environment to safely accommodate the client may be needed. The family may require assistance in obtaining adaptive devices needed for ADLs and ambulation.

➤ Health Teaching

The staff nurse or case manager provides the client and family with both written and verbal instructions. The teaching plan for the client with craniocerebral trauma includes strategies to adapt to sensory dysfunction and to cope with the personality or behavior problems that may arise and a review of seizure precautions. The nurse explains the purpose, dosage, schedule, and route of administration of any medications. The client is encouraged to participate in activities as tolerated. Demonstrations and return demonstrations of care activities may facilitate competence of family members in skill performance. The nurse stresses the importance of regular follow-up visits with therapists and health care providers.

With the family and the client, the nurse reinforces the same strategies used in the hospital to treat sensory or perceptual changes. In addition, the family or significant others are taught about the importance of not moving furniture or other objects in the home to a different place because this can lead to an injury in the client with visual problems or might confuse the client with cognitive impairments.

Clients with personality and behavior problems respond best to an environment that is structured and consistent. The nurse instructs the family to develop a home routine that provides structure, repetition, and consistency. The family must also be instructed on the importance of reinforcing positive behaviors and not reinforcing negative behaviors.

The nurse teaches the client who has sustained a *minor* head injury (e.g., a concussion) that post-trauma syndrome may occur. This syndrome is a group of clinical manifestations including but not limited to

- Personality changes
- Irritability
- Headaches
- Dizziness
- Restlessness
- Nervousness
- Insomnia
- Memory loss

Many clients with head injuries experience some of these manifestations during recovery. However, some clients have these problems for weeks, months, or even years to the extent that they interfere with daily activities, such as employment. The prolonged pattern is classified as post-trauma syndrome. The exact cause of the phenomenon is not known, but physiologic and psychological theories have been espoused. Support groups and professional counseling are the most effective interventions.

Most clients who had moderate-to-severe craniocerebral trauma are discharged with physical as well as cognitive

disabilities. Changes in personality and behavior are not unusual. The family must learn to cope with the client's increased fatigue, irritability, temper outbursts, depression, and memory problems. Frequently, these clients require constant supervision at home, and eventually the families feel socially isolated. The nurse instructs the family to plan for regular respite care, either in a structured day-care respite program or through relief provided by a friend or a neighbor. The family members, particularly the primary caretaker, may become depressed, with feelings of loneliness. Family members may experience isolation, increased responsibilities, and role reversals. In addition, the family may feel angry at the client because of the additional responsibilities (financial or emotional) that his or her care has placed on them. To help the family cope with these problems, the nurse suggests that they join and actively participate in a local head injury support group.

The client needs assistance in identifying realistic expectations for discharge. Because of cognitive deficits, it may not be possible for the client to return to previous employment or educational pursuits. The client may experience a sense of isolation and loneliness, because personality and behavior changes make it difficult to resume or maintain preinjury social contacts.

➤ Home Care Management

Little home care preparation is needed for the client with a concussion unless he or she is experiencing symptoms of post-traumatic sequelae. The nurse and the discharge planner assess the client's home for potential hazards before discharge from the hospital. There must be functioning smoke and fire alarms, because the client with a head injury often loses the sense of smell. This information can be obtained from the admission data or by a home visit. Home adaptations and referrals to outside agencies should be completed before the client is discharged from the hospital.

➤ Health Care Resources

The nurse or case manager refers families and significant others and clients to the National Head Injury Foundation (NHIF), as well as to the local or state group, for information and support. The NHIF and its state chapters maintain lists of rehabilitation facilities for clients with head injuries. The NHIF will send family members and other interested persons guidelines for selecting a rehabilitation facility. Families should inquire about the facility's experience in caring for the person with a head injury, how many admissions the facility has had in the previous 2–3 years, and the results or outcome statistics on those clients (e.g., how many went home and at what functional recovery level—poor, fair, or good).

Other helpful groups include the National Easter Seal Society and National Institute of Handicapped Research.

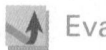 Evaluation

The nurse evaluates the care provided by determining whether the client

- Maintains a normal ICP
- Maintains appropriate vital signs and arterial blood gas values
- Achieves improvement in the level of consciousness
- Develops strategies to adapt to residual neurologic dysfunction
- Is free from respiratory infections and atelectasis
- Has adequate ABG values
- Does not experience injury
- Does not experience complications of immobility
- Is able to ambulate and perform ADLs independently with or without adaptive or assistive devices
- Maintains body weight within 10% of the ideal body weight or at the usual body weight
- Maintains adequate hydration
- Develops confidence in his or her abilities
- Begins to adapt to changes in physical appearance and abilities

BRAIN TUMORS

Overview

Brain tumors can arise anywhere within the brain structures and are named according to the cell or tissue from which they originate. Primary tumors originate within the central nervous system (CNS) and rarely metastasize outside this area. Secondary brain tumors result from metastasis from other areas of the body, such as the lungs, the breast, the kidney, and the gastrointestinal tract.

Pathophysiology

Primary brain tumors occur as a rapid proliferation or abnormal growth of cells normally found within the CNS. Secondary brain tumors occur as malignant cells from other tumors outside the CNS that metastasize to the brain. Regardless of the origin, the tumor expands in an irregular fashion and invades, infiltrates, or compresses normal brain tissue. This leads to

- Cerebral edema
- Increased intracranial pressure (ICP)
- Focal neurologic deficits
- Obstruction of the flow of cerebrospinal fluid (CSF)
- Pituitary dysfunction

Complications of Tumors

Cerebral edema, or more specifically vasogenic edema, results from changes in capillary endothelial tissue permeability, which allows plasma to seep into the extracellular spaces. This leads to increased ICP, and herniation of the brain tissue may occur. A variety of focal neurologic deficits result from edema, infiltration, and compression of surrounding brain tissue. The cerebral blood vessels may become compressed because of edema and increased ICP. This compression leads to ischemia of the area supplied by the vessel. In addition, the tumor may infiltrate the walls of the vessel, causing it to rupture and hemorrhage into the tumor bed or adjacent brain tissue. Approximately 33% of clients who have brain tumors experience seizure activity attributable to interference with the brain's normal conduction pathways.

Increased ICP may also result from obstruction of the flow of CSF or displacement of the lateral ventricles by the expanding lesion. Typically, a tumor obstructs the aqueduct of Sylvius or one of the ventricles or encroaches on the subarachnoid space. Posterior fossa tumors may obstruct the flow of CSF from the fourth ventricle to the foramen of Luschka or Magendie. With any brain tumor, the obstruction of normal CSF flow causes hydrocephalus and eventually leads to increased ICP.

Pituitary dysfunction may occur as the tumor compresses the pituitary gland and causes the syndrome of inappropriate antidiuretic hormone or diabetes insipidus. These disorders result in severe fluid and electrolyte imbalances and can be life-threatening (see Chapter 66 for a complete description).

Classification of Tumors

Brain tumors are generally classified as malignant or benign (Table 47–6). Although benign tumors are generally associated with a favorable outcome, this is often not the case with malignant tumors. However, benign tumors may be malignant by virtue of their location. If the tumor cannot be completely removed or treated, it continues to grow. As it invades other brain tissue, cerebral edema, focal neurologic deficits, and increased ICP occur. Herniation of the brain tissue eventually leads to death. Benign tumors may undergo histologic changes and become malignant.

A second classification system is based on location. Supratentorial tumors, which occur most often in the adult, are located in the area above the tentorium, the tent-like fold of dura that surrounds the cerebellar hemisphere and supports the occipital lobe. In other words, supratentorial tumors are located within the cerebral hemispheres. Located beneath the tentorium is the infratento-

---

Chart 47–7

Key Features of Common Brain Tumors

Cerebral Tumors
- Headache (most common feature)
- Vomiting unrelated to food intake
- Changes in visual acuity and visual fields; diplopia (visual changes caused by papilledema)
- Hemiparesis or hemiplegia
- Hypokinesia
- Hyperesthesia, paresthesia, decreased tactile discrimination
- Seizures
- Aphasia
- Changes in personality and/or behavior

Brain Stem Tumors
- Hearing loss (acoustic neuroma)
- Facial pain and weakness
- Dysphagia, decreased gag reflex
- Nystagmus
- Hoarseness
- Ataxia and dysarthria (cerebellar tumors)

TABLE 47–6

Classification of Brain Tumors

Benign
- Acoustic neuroma
- Meningioma
- Pituitary adenoma
- Astrocytoma
  - Grade 1 (may undergo changes and become malignant)
- Chondroma
- Craniopharyngioma
- Hemangioblastoma

Malignant
- Astrocytoma
  - Grade 2
  - Grade 3
  - Grade 4 (also known as glioblastoma multiforme)
- Oligodendroglioma
- Ependymoma
- Medulloblastoma
- Chondrosarcoma
- Glioma
- Lymphoma

rial area, the area of the brain stem structures and cerebellum.

A third classification system is according to the cellular, histologic, or anatomic origin of the tumor. The nervous system is composed of two types of cells: neurons, which are responsible for nerve impulse conduction, and neuroglial cells, which provide support, nourishment, and protection for neurons. Four specific types of cells are neuroglial cells: astrocytes, oligodendroglia, ependymal cells, and microglia.

When classifying tumors according to this system, tumors are named by their cell type. For example, an astrocytoma is a tumor of astrocytes.

Gliomas. Gliomas are malignant tumors; they account for 45%–60% of all brain tumors in adults and arise from the neuroglial cells of the brain and the brain stem. Malignant gliomas have a peak incidence in people 40–60 years of age. They infiltrate and invade surrounding brain tissue. The most common type of glioma is the astrocytoma, which may be found anywhere within the cerebral hemispheres. It is usually treated by surgery, followed by radiation and chemotherapy. Oligodendrogliomas, another type of glioma, are generally located within the frontal lobes of the brain. These are slow-growing tumors and usually are calcified. Surgical removal is possible, and the long-term prognosis for the client is good. A glioblastoma is a highly malignant, rapidly growing, invasive astrocytoma. Although improved surgical techniques and advanced treatment have improved the outlook and quality of life for a client with this type of tumor, less than 15% of affected clients survive 18 months after diagnosis. Ependymomas arise from the lining of the ventricles and are difficult to treat surgically because of their location. Radiation and shunting

procedures to control hydrocephalus caused by the tumor's blocking normal CSF flow are the treatment of choice. Chemotherapy may also be used for these tumors.

Gliomas are graded according to their cellular differentiation or how closely the tumor cells resemble normal cells. Grade I tumors are well differentiated; grade II tumors are moderately differentiated; grade III tumors are poorly differentiated and may rapidly change to grade IV tumors, which are poorly differentiated. A grade III or IV astrocytoma is referred to as glioblastoma multiforme and is associated with a poor outcome. Grade I and II tumors frequently undergo cellular changes and become grade III or IV.

Meningiomas. Meningiomas arise from the coverings of the brain (the meninges). They are the most common benign tumor, with a peak incidence at age 45 years. Females are affected more than males by a 2:1 ratio. This tumor is encapsulated, globular, and well-demarcated and causes compression and displacement of surrounding brain tissue. Although complete removal of the tumor is possible, it tends to recur. It tends to occur in areas where the meninges predominate.

Pituitary Tumors. Pituitary tumors that occur in the anterior lobe account for 10%–25% of brain tumors and may cause endocrine dysfunction. The most common type of pituitary tumor is the adenoma, subdivided into the chromophobe, secretory, and nonsecretory adenomas. The tumors are benign and frequently occur in young and middle-aged adults. Often the presenting symptoms are visual disturbances, and they produce hypopituitary signs (loss of body hair, diabetes insipidus, sterility, visual field defects, and headaches).

Acoustic Neuromas. Acoustic neuromas arise from the sheath of Schwann cells in the peripheral portion of cranial nerve VIII. They are also referred to as cerebellar pontine angle (CPA) tumors to describe their anatomic location. Acoustic neuromas compress brain tissue and tend to surround adjacent cranial nerves (cranial nerves VII, V, IX, X), making surgical removal difficult without causing permanent cranial nerve dysfunction. Females are twice as likely to have acoustic neuromas as males. Common symptoms include hearing loss, ringing in the ears, and dizziness.

Metastatic, or secondary tumors, account for nearly 30% of brain tumors. Metastatic cells from the lungs, the breast, the colon, the pancreas, and the kidney can travel to the brain via the blood and the lymphatic system. Multiple metastatic lesions are not uncommon.

Etiology

The exact cause of brain tumors is unknown. Several areas under investigation include genetic changes, heredity, errors in fetal development, ionizing radiation, electromagnetic fields, environmental hazards, diet, viruses, and injury.

Incidence/Prevalence

Brain tumors account for 2.4% of all cancer deaths. Each year in the United States, 36,000 new cases of primary brain tumors are diagnosed; 18,000 secondary tumors are found.

Brain tumors in the adult population are seen primarily in clients 40–60 years of age.

ELDERLY CONSIDERATIONS

 Meningiomas are seen more frequently in middle-aged and elderly women, whereas gliomas are seen slightly more often in men. The incidence rate is higher in men, greater in Caucasians, and increases with age (Barker, 1994).

Collaborative Management

Assessment

The clinical manifestations of brain tumors vary with the site of the tumor. In general, symptoms of a brain tumor include

- Headaches—usually more severe upon awakening in the morning
- Nausea and vomiting
- Visual symptoms
- Seizures
- Changes in mentation or personality
- Papilledema (swelling of the optic disk)

Neurologic deficits result from the destruction, distortion, or compression of brain tissue. Supratentorial tumors usually result in paralysis, seizures, memory loss, cognitive impairment, language impairment, or vision problems. Infratentorial tumors produce ataxia, autonomic nervous system dysfunction, vomiting, drooling, hearing loss, and vision impairment. As the tumor grows, intracranial pressure increases, and the symptoms become progressively more severe.

Diagnosis is based on history, neurologic assessment, clinical examination, and results of neurodiagnostic testing. Noninvasive diagnostic studies—computed tomography (CT), magnetic resonance imaging (MRI), and skull films—are conducted first. The CT and MRI identify the size, location, and extent of the tumor. Whereas the MRI may be used for initial diagnostic evaluation, the CT is often used for follow-up during the hospital course. Cerebral angiography is usually not indicated to diagnose a brain tumor but may be used to provide additional information about the vascular supply to the tummor. Electro-encephalography (EEG), lumbar puncture (LP), myelogram, brain scan, and positron emission tomography (PET) may be indicated to provide further information about the tumor's size, location, and characteristics. Laboratory tests may also be ordered to evaluate endocrine function, renal status, and electrolyte balance.

Interventions

When possible, the nurse obtains a history from the client as well as from the family, including current signs and symptoms. A complete neurologic assessment is needed to establish baseline data and to determine the nature and extent of neurologic deficits.

Nonsurgical Management. The goal of treatment of brain tumors is to decrease the tumor size, improve the quality of life, and improve survival time. The type of treatment selected depends on the tumor size and location, client symptoms and general condition, and whether the tumor is recurrent. Treatment of brain tumors may include radiation, chemotherapy, and surgery. A number of experimental treatment modalities are being investigated, including blood brain barrier disruption, recombinant DNA, monoclonal antibodies, new antineoplastic drugs, immunotherapy, and hyperthermia. Gliadel wafers have recently been approved by the U.S. Food and Drug Administration for use as adjunct therapy in clients with recurrent glioblastoma multiforme. The wafers are placed in the resection cavity of the tumor (Rhone-Poulenc, 1996).

Drug Therapy. The health care provider may prescribe a variety of medications to treat the client's symptoms and to prevent complications. Analgesics, such as codeine and acetaminophen (Tylenol, Ace-Tabs), are given for headache. Dexamethasone (Decadron) is usually given to control cerebral edema. Research supports the efficacy of administration of glucocorticoids for the treatment of edema resulting from brain tumors. Phenytoin (Dilantin) is used to prevent seizure activity. Histamine blockers such as ranitidine hydrochloride (Zantac) or Axid are given to decrease gastric acid secretion and prevent the development of stress ulcers. Prochlorperazine dimaleate (Compazine) and other antiemetics are used to treat nausea and vomiting.

Radiation Therapy and Chemotherapy. Radiation therapy may be used alone, after surgery, or in combination with chemotherapy and surgery. (Chapter 27 discusses radiation treatment for cancer in detail.) Chemotherapy is used primarily as an adjunct to surgery. It may be given alone or in combination with radiation and surgery. There is no known "curative regimen" (Barker, 1994). Chemotherapy usually involves more than one agent and may be given intravenously, intra-arterially, or intrathecally through an Ommaya reservoir (Fig. 47–12).

Radiosurgical Procedures. Radiosurgical procedures are an alternative to surgery. These techniques include the modified linear accelerator using accelerated x-rays, particle accelerator using beams of protons (cyclotron), isotope seeds implanted in the tumor (brachytherapy), and the gamma knife.

The gamma knife is a type of stereotactic radiosurgical procedure that uses a single high dose of ionized radiation that focuses 201 beams of cobalt-60 radiation to selectively destroy intracranial lesions without damaging surrounding healthy tissue. Combining neurodiagnostic imaging tools, including the MRI, CT, magnetic resonance angioigraphy (MRA), and angiography, with the gamma knife allows for precise localization of deep-seated or anatomically difficult lesions and delivery of a customized dose of cobalt-60 radiation to the desired area only. Treatment usually takes less than an hour and clients require only overnight hospitalization. Advantages of this technique include its noninvasive nature; less risk than the traditional craniotomy, surgical precision; and de-

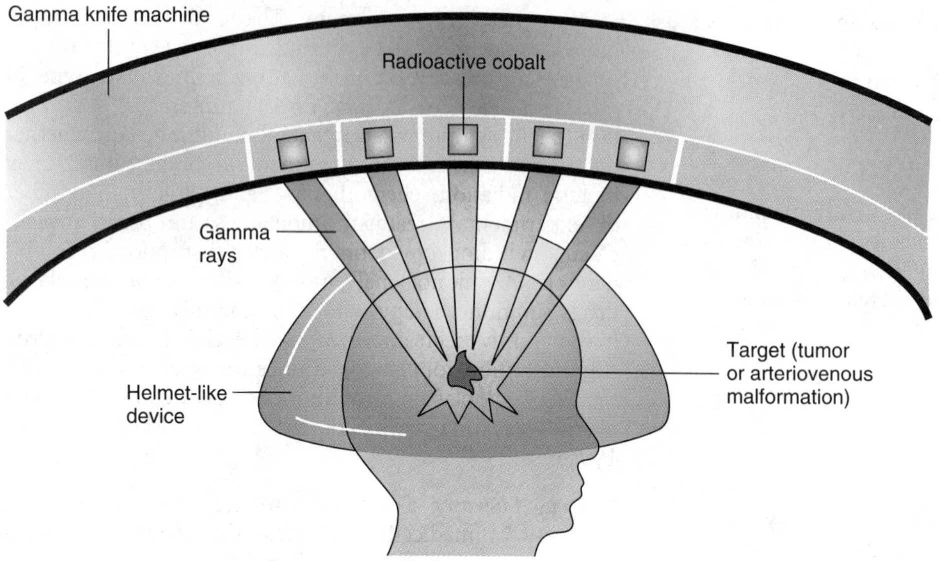

Figure 47–12. A gamma knife treatment. The radiation beams are widely dispersed over the surface of the head to prevent damage to healthy brain tissue. The beams are intense only at the point of the target.

creased cost, morbidity, length of hospital stay, and recovery time.

The gamma knife is used primarily for brain tumors or arteriovenous malformations (AVM) that are in an inaccessible location that makes them unresectable by craniotomy. Tumors typically treated are acoustic neuromas, meningiomas, and metastatic tumors. The gamma knife may also be used with clients who refuse conventional surgery, for clients whose age and physical condition precludes general anesthesia, as an adjunct to radiation therapy, and for recurrent or residual AVM or tumors after embolization or craniotomy.

Surgical Management. The most important modality in the treatment of brain tumors is a craniotomy, but the challenge for the surgeon is to remove the tumor as completely as possible without damaging normal tissue. Postoperatively, the client is usually admitted to the critical care unit.

Postoperative Assessment. The accompanying Client Care Plan highlights the major aspects of postoperative nursing care. The focus of postoperative care is to monitor the client to detect changes in status and to prevent or minimize complications, especially increased ICP. The nurse assesses the client's neurologic and vital signs every 30 minutes for the first 4–6 hours after surgery and then every hour. If the client is stable for 24 hours, the frequency of these checks may be decreased to every 2–4 hours, depending on the agency's policy. Potential neurologic deficits include decreased level of consciousness, motor weakness or paralysis, aphasia, visual changes, and personality changes. Periorbital edema and ecchymosis of one or both eyes is not unusual and is treated with cold compresses to decrease swelling. The nurse irrigates the affected eye with warm saline solution or artificial tears to improve the client's comfort.

The client in the critical care unit is routinely connected to the cardiac monitor. Dysrhythmias may occur after posterior fossa surgery or be due to fluid and electrolyte imbalance. Other nursing interventions include

strict recording of the client's intake and output and a fluid restriction to 1500 mL/day. Range-of-motion exercises to all extremities are performed at least once per nursing shift. The nurse or assistive nursing personnel assist the client to turn, cough, and breath deeply every 2 hours. Sequential compression stockings or pneumatic compression boots are kept in place until the client is ambulating to prevent the development of deep vein thrombosis.

Positioning. Clients who have had supratentorial surgery should have the head of the bed elevated 30–45 degrees to promote venous drainage from the head. The nurse positions the client to avoid extreme hip or neck flexion and maintains the client's head in a midline, neutral position. The client may be turned side-to-side or remain supine. However, if a large tumor has been removed, it is recommended that the client be placed on the nonoperative side to prevent displacement of the cranial contents by gravity. The client with an infratentorial craniotomy should be kept flat and positioned on either side for 24–48 hours. This prevents pressure on the neck-area incision site. It also prevents pressure on the internal tumor excision site from higher cerebral structures. The client should be NPO status for 24 hours, because edema of the cranial nerve controlling swallowing and the gag reflex may place the client at risk for aspiration.

Monitoring the Dressing. The nurse checks the head dressing every 1–2 hours for signs of drainage. The area of drainage is marked once during each shift for baseline comparison. A small or moderate amount of drainage is expected. Some clients may have a Hemovac, Jackson-Pratt, or other surgical drain in place for 24 hours after surgery. The nurse measures the drainage every 8 hours and then records the amount and color; a typical amount of drainage is 30–50 mL per shift (8 hours). The nurse follows the manufacturer's and the physician's instructions to maintain suction within the drain. Excessive amounts of drainage (a saturated head dressing or greater than

Client Care Plan

The Client Requiring a Craniotomy

Nursing Diagnosis No. 1: Knowledge Deficit related to the surgical procedure.

Expected Outcomes	Nursing Interventions	Rationale
The client will verbalize preoperative and postoperative routines.	Provide preoperative teaching: ■ Answer questions. ■ Reinforce information provided by the surgeon.	An informed client is less anxious and fearful.
The client will be free of postoperative complications.	■ Explain preoperative preparation such as laboratory work, chest x-rays, electrocardiogram. ■ Explain anesthesia procedures. ■ Explain the procedure for preparing the client's head for surgery. Tell the client and the family how long the procedure will take and where the client will go after surgery (perianesthesia care unit or critical care unit). Discuss how the client will look after surgery. Tell the family where to wait while the client is in surgery. Ensure that all permits are signed. If possible, arrange a visit to the critical care unit for the client and the family to meet the staff. Explain routine postoperative care—head dressing, urinary catheter, endotracheal tube, IVs, incentive spirometry, pain management.	The client's hair is shaved in the surgical site. The client will have a head dressing, may have periorbital edema and bruising, and may be intubated and on a ventilator.

(Continued)

50 mL/8 hr) should be reported immediately to the physician.

Monitoring Laboratory Values. Laboratory studies that are monitored postoperatively include complete blood count, serum electrolyte levels and osmolality, coagulation studies, and arterial blood gas measurements.

The client's hematocrit and hemoglobin concentration may be abnormally low from blood loss during surgery or perhaps elevated if the blood was replaced. Hyponatremia may occur as a result of fluid volume overload, syndrome of inappropriate antidiuretic hormone (SIADH), or steroid administration. Hypokalemia may cause cardiac irritability. Weakness, a change in the level of consciousness, and confusion are symptoms of hyponatremia and hypokalemia. Hypernatremia may be caused by meningitis, dehydration, or diabetes insipidus (DI). It is manifested by muscle weakness, restlessness, extreme thirst, and dry mouth. Untreated hypernatremia may lead to seizure activity. Arterial blood gas values are monitored to ensure adequate cerebral oxygenation.

Ventilating the Client. Often the client is electively mechanically ventilated and hyperventilated for the first 24–

Client Care Plan

Nursing Diagnosis No. 2: Risk for Altered (Cerebral) Tissue Perfusion related to the surgical procedure.

Expected Outcomes	Nursing Interventions	Rationale
The client's level of consciousness and neurologic status will improve or remain the same.	Check vital signs and neurologic signs every hour postoperatively or more often as clinically indicated. Report changes to the physician. Monitor for signs of increased ICP. Implement nursing measures to prevent increased ICP: ■ Elevate the head of the bed 30–45 degrees. ■ Position the client in bed to avoid extreme hip and neck flexion. ■ Maintain the client's head in a midline, neutral position. ■ Avoid clustering nursing activities. ■ Avoid talking about the client at the bedside. ■ Provide a quiet environment.	The client is at risk for increased intracranial pressure (ICP).
	Record strict measurement of intake and output. Monitor serum electrolyte levels, serum and urine osmolality, and urine specific gravity. Administer medications as ordered if ICP increases.	Fluid intake is generally restricted postoperatively. The client is at risk for dehydration and fluid and electrolyte imbalance.
	Check the head dressing for drainage: ■ Circle and date the area if drainage. ■ Notify the physician of a significant increase in drainage. ■ Notify physician of cerebrospinal fluid (CSF) drainage immediately.	A small amount of bloody drainage is not unusual; CSF drainage is not normal.

48 hours after surgery to prevent increased ICP. The goal of hyperventilation is to maintain the client's arterial carbon dioxide level at 27–35 mmHg, with normal arterial oxygen levels. This produces cerebral vasoconstriction, which decreases ICP. If the client is awake or attempting to breathe at a rate other than that set on the ventilator, medications such as fentanyl citrate (Sublimaze) are given. The client who is intubated is suctioned if indicated by the findings of frequent respiratory assessments. The nurse remembers to hyperoxygenate the client before suctioning.

Drug Therapy. Medications routinely given postoperatively include anticonvulsants, histamine blockers, and corticosteroids. Analgesics such as codeine are given for pain, and acetaminophen is given for fever or mild pain. Some physicians may elect to administer prophylactic antibiotics to prevent infection.

Preventing Postoperative Complications. Postoperative complications are listed in Table 47–7.

Increased Intracranial Pressure. The major postoperative complication is increased ICP from cerebral edema, hem-

Client Care Plan

Nursing Diagnosis No. 3: Pain related to the surgical procedure.

Expected Outcomes	Nursing Interventions	Rationale
The client's pain will be alleviated or reduced.	Assess level and extent of pain. Give pain medication as ordered; document the client's response. Assess the effectiveness of pain relief and collaborate with the physician for an effective pain management protocol. Use nonpharmaceutical pain relief measures such as imagery, relaxation, distraction, or music, as needed. Organize a plan of care to allow the client uninterrupted periods of rest. Apply an ice pack to the eyes as needed. Provide comfort measures: ■ Back rub. ■ Cool compress to forehead. Provide frequent mouth care: ■ Apply moisturizer to the lips. ■ Provide ice chips.	Pain management enables the client to participate fully in the plan of care. The client may have periorbital edema. The client's mouth may be dry because of the fluid restriction.

orrhage, or obstruction of the normal flow of cerebrospinal fluid (CSF). Symptoms of increased ICP include severe headache, deteriorating level of consciousness, restlessness, irritability, and dilated or pinpoint pupils that are slow to react or nonreactive to light.

Treatment of increased ICP includes placing the client supine with the head of the bed elevated 30–45 degrees unless contraindicated. The client's head should be maintained in a midline, neutral position to facilitate venous drainage from the brain. Osmotic diuretics such as mannitol (Osmitrol), glucocorticoids, or loop diuretics may be given to decrease cerebral edema. After computed tomography or other diagnostic tests to determine the exact cause of increased ICP, the client may be connected to a ventilator and hyperventilated. An ICP monitoring device may be inserted to measure ICP more accurately. Surgery may be needed to correct the problem (e.g., hematoma) or to relieve pressure. (Treatment of increased ICP is discussed more fully earlier in this chapter.)

Cerebral edema is frequently present before surgery and may be further increased by tissue manipulation during the surgical procedure. Edema usually reaches a peak within 72 hours after surgery and, if no further complications occur, gradually subsides during the next few weeks. Cerebral edema is manifested by a change in the

level of consciousness and other symptoms of increased ICP.

Hematomas. Subdural and epidural hematomas and intracranial hemorrhage are manifested by severe headache, a change in the level of consciousness, progressive neurologic deficits, and herniation syndromes. Bleeding into the posterior fossa may lead to sudden cardiovascular and respiratory arrest. Treatment of a hematoma necessitates surgical removal, whereas an intracranial hemorrhage is treated with aggressive medical management (e.g., osmotic diuretics and ICP monitoring).

Hydrocephalus. Hydrocephalus is caused by obstruction of the normal CSF pathway from edema, an expanding lesion such as a hematoma, or blood in the subarachnoid space. Rapidly progressive hydrocephalus produces the classic symptoms of increased ICP. Slowly progressive hydrocephalus is manifested by headache, decreased level of consciousness, irritability, blurred vision, and urinary incontinence. Often, this is self-limiting and resolves without any treatment or with daily lumbar punctures to remove CSF. If treatment is required, a surgical shunt is inserted to drain CSF to another area of the body. Usually, a ventriculoperitoneal or, less often, a ventriculoatrial or lumbar peritoneal shunt procedure is performed. A

TABLE 47–7

Postoperative Complications of Craniotomy

- Increased ICP
- Hematomas
  - Subdural hematoma
  - Epidural hematoma
  - Subarachnoid hemorrhage
- Hypovolemic shock
- Hydrocephalus
- Respiratory complications
  - Atelectasis
  - Hypoxia
  - Pneumonia
  - Neurogenic pulmonary edema
- Wound infection
- Meningitis
- Fluid and electrolyte imbalances
  - Dehydration
  - Hyponatremia
  - Hypernatremia
- Seizures
- CSF leak
- Cerebral edema

major complication of a shunting procedure is a subdural hematoma from tearing of bridging veins. An external lumbar drain may also be used temporarily. Additional information about shunts may be found in neuroscience nursing texts.

Respiratory Problems. Respiratory complications include atelectasis, pneumonia, and neurogenic pulmonary edema. Atelectasis and pneumonia can be prevented by providing appropriate pulmonary hygiene, turning the client frequently, and encouraging the client to take several deep breaths to expand the lungs each hour. The provision of humidified air and incentive spirometry are useful techniques to prevent these complications. Other treatment modalities include endotracheal or oral tracheal suctioning and chest physiotherapy. These measures may cause an increase in the client's ICP. However, close monitoring of the client's status and ICP waveforms allows the client to receive the benefits of aggressive pulmonary hygiene despite potential risk.

Neurogenic pulmonary edema is a life-threatening complication of neurosurgical procedures, but it is infrequent. Its symptoms are the same as those of acute pulmonary edema; however, there are no associated cardiac problems. In spite of aggressive treatment, most clients with neurogenic pulmonary edema do not survive the insult.

Wound Infection. Wound infections occur more often in older and debilitated clients and clients with a history of diabetes, long-term steroid use, obesity, and previous infections. The client may contribute to the problem by rubbing or scratching the wound. If infection is present, the wound appears reddened and puffy. It may begin to separate and is sensitive to touch and feels warm. The client may or may not be febrile. Treatment is based on

the degree and extent of the infection. The nurse may treat a localized infection by simply cleaning with alcohol or by applying local antibiotics. For more severe infections, systemic antibiotic administration may be required. If the underlying bone is involved, it may need to be removed.

Meningitis. Meningitis is an inflammation of the meninges and may occur as a result of wound infection, a cerebrospinal fluid (CSF) leak, or contamination during surgery. (The reader is referred to the discussion of meningitis in Chapter 44 for a more complete explanation of this complication.)

Fluid and Electrolyte Imbalances. Complications related to fluid and electrolyte imbalance include diabetes insipidus and syndrome of inappropriate antidiuretic hormone (SIADH). Diabetes insipidus is seen most often after supratentorial surgery, especially procedures involving the pituitary gland or hypothalamus. Failure of the posterior pituitary gland to secrete antidiuretic hormone (ADH) leads to failure of the renal tubules to reabsorb water. The client's urinary output increases dramatically (it may be up to 10 L/day), and the urine specific gravity drops to below 1.005. Urine osmolality decreases, whereas serum osmolality increases. The client may become dehydrated, and if this condition is left untreated, hypovolemic shock develops. Fluid replacement to replace urinary losses and prevent dehydration may be accomplished by having the client who can do so increase oral intake or use IV fluids. Hormonal replacement may also be necessary, especially if fluid loss is greater than 6 L/24 hr.

Aqueous vasopressin is short-acting, lasting only 6–8 hours. For long-term replacement therapy, desmopressin acetate (DDAVP) administered as a nasal spray is the drug of choice.

SIADH occurs when the posterior pituitary gland secretes too much ADH, causing water retention. The client becomes anuric, with a urinary output of less than 20 mL/hr. Sodium concentration in the urine is normal or elevated, whereas the serum sodium level falls. Other indications of SIADH are loss of thirst, irritability, muscle weakness, and decreased level of consciousness. SIADH is treated by fluid restriction, which is usually sufficient to correct the hyponatremia. Slow IV infusion of 3% hypertonic sodium may be needed for severe hyponatremia (<118 mEq/L).

Clients with complications related to fluid and electrolyte imbalance have strict measurement of their intake and output. An accurate daily weight measurement is an essential aspect of nursing care. The nurse assesses the client carefully for indications of fluid overload or dehydration during treatment. Serum electrolyte levels and osmolality are measured daily or more often if clinically indicated.

➤ Continuing Care

The client with a brain tumor is managed at home if possible. The nurse or case manager mobilizes health resources to support the client and family at home.

➤ Health Teaching

It is important that the client and the family fully understand the importance of any recommended follow-up health care appointments. The nurse writes the date, time, and place on a card and gives it to the client or family member, significant other, or other caregiver. The nursing discharge summary should state the name of the person who has given follow-up information.

Information given to the client and the family or significant others includes the name of the medications, the dosage, the timing of administration, and number of days to take the medication, and any side effects. The nurse tells the client what to do or whom to call if any adverse reactions occur. The client is taught to refrain from taking any over-the-counter medications unless authorized by the health care provider.

The nurse instructs the client to maintain a program of regular physical exercise within the limits of any disabilities. Referral to the dietitian may be necessary to ensure adequate caloric intake for the client receiving radiation or chemotherapy.

Seizures are a potential complication that can occur at any time for as long as 1 year or more postoperatively. The nurse provides the client and the family with information about seizure precautions and what to do if a seizure occurs.

If long-term changes or disability is expected, the client needs to be prepared for major lifestyle changes. Chapter 13 discusses coping with disability in more detail.

➤ Home Care Management

Unless the client has a permanent disability, no special home care preparation is needed. Clients with hemiparesis need assistance to ensure that their home is accessible, depending on their method of mobility (e.g., cane, walker, or wheelchair). The environment should be made safe to prevent falls. For example, scatter rugs should be removed and grab bars placed in the bathroom.

Information about the selection of rehabilitation or chronic care facility, if needed, can be obtained from the social worker or the discharge planner. The facility selected should have experience in providing care for neurologically impaired clients. A psychologist should be available to provide input in the evaluation of the cognitive disabilities often exhibited by the client.

➤ Health Care Resources

The nurse refers the client and the family or significant others to the American Brain Tumor Association or the National Brain Tumor Foundation. The American Cancer Society is also an appropriate community resource for clients with malignant tumors. Home care agencies are available to provide both the physical and rehabilitative care that the client may need at home. Hospice services may be needed for the terminally ill client.

BRAIN ABSCESS

Overview

A brain abscess is a purulent infection of the brain in which pus forms in the extradural, subdural, or intracerebral area of the brain. The causative organisms are most often bacteria, which invade the brain directly or indirectly.

Organisms from the ear, the sinus, or the mastoid area generally enter the brain by traveling along the wall of the cerebral veins and therefore may spread to any area of the brain. At times, the organisms (especially those from the ear) erode the bone, form a tract, and enter the brain directly. Septic emboli from the heart, the lungs, or a dental or peritonsillar abscess may break off and enter the systemic circulation. These organisms may become lodged in a cerebral vessel and produce a localized infection. Penetrating trauma, open head injuries, and neurosurgical procedures provide a potential means for the direct entry of an organism into the brain. In the past 15 years, the number of clients with a brain abscess as a consequence of immunosuppression, organ transplantation, and acquired immunodeficiency syndrome (AIDS) has increased rapidly.

The organisms cause a local infection. Acute inflammation surrounds the involved area. Within a few days, necrosis of the tissue takes place, and pus formation and liquefaction of the tissue occur. This is followed by the development of cerebral edema owing to localized vascular congestion in response to inflammation. During the subsequent 2 weeks, the area becomes encapsulated, first by fibrous granulation tissue and later by collagenous connective tissue. The abscess usually occurs deep within the cerebral hemisphere and involves the white matter of the brain. Occassionally, the abscess does not become encapsulated; instead, it spreads through the brain tissue to the subarachnoid space and ventricular system.

The organisms most often involved in the formation of brain abscesses are bacteria, such as *Streptococcus, Staphylococcus,* and *Streptococcus pneumoniae.* Enterobacteriaceae, *Proteus, Escherichia,* and *Psuedomonas* account for 24% of all abscesses. Yeast and fungi are now implicated in 9% to 17% of cases of cerebral abscess formation, particularly in the client who is immunosuppressed. *Toxoplasma gondii* is the most frequently seen CNS opportunistic infection in the AIDS population.

Most brain abscesses occur in the frontal and temporal lobes. It is estimated that 5%–20% of affected clients have more than one abscess. Mortality rates vary from 30%–60%; abscesses that occur in the immunosuppressed client are associated with a higher mortality rate.

Collaborative Management

 Assessment

➤ Physical Assessment/Clinical Manifestations

The clinical manifestations of a brain abscess are insidious. The client may present with headache, fever, and focal neurologic deficits or nonspecific signs and symptoms (Chart 47–8). The nurse begins the examination by performing a complete neurologic assessment. The client is usually mildly lethargic and somewhat confused. The pupillary response to light is normal in the early stages. As increased ICP progresses, the pupils dilate and become nonresponsive. Examination of the client's visual fields

Chart 47–8

Key Features of Brain Abscess

Early Manifestations
- Headache
- Fever
- Focal neurologic deficits
- Lethargy

Late Manifestations
- Confusion
- Increased intracranial pressure (ICP)
- Dilated and nonresponsive pupils
- Visual field deficits
- Cushing's triad

often reveals a temporal field blindness (decrease in peripheral vision). If the abscess affects the cerebral hemispheres, nystagmus and a dysconjugate gaze may be noted. Motor examination reveals a generalized weakness. More significant motor problems, such as hemiplegia, may be apparent in the presence of a frontal lobe abscess. An ataxic gait is seen with cerebellar abscess. Sensory impairment varies, although the client often exhibits no sensory deficits. The client may have varying degrees of aphasia in the presence of a frontal or temporal lobe abscess. Seizure activity may occur owing to irritation of the cortical tissue. Late in the disease process, more severe symptoms of increased ICP occur, including severe headache, coma, a widened pulse pressure, bradycardia, and irregular respirations. The client with AIDS often presents with systemic infection, central nervous system involvement, and lymphoma.

➤ Diagnostic Tests

A complete blood count and erythrocyte sedimentation rate (ESR) are typically performed. The white blood cell count and ESR are usually elevated, indicating the presence of infection. If the abscess is encapsulated, the white blood cell count may be normal. The nurse obtains specimens for aerobic and anaerobic (when possible) cultures of the blood, ear, nose, and throat to determine the primary source of infection.

The health care provider orders a computed tomography scan to determine the presence of cerebritis, hydrocephalus, or a midline shift. Magnetic resonance imaging is also useful in detecting the presence of an abscess early in the course of the disease. An electroencephalogram can localize the lesion in most cases and shows high-voltage slow-wave activity; electrical silence may be noted in the area of the abscess. Radiography of the sinuses and the mastoid is often indicated. A lumbar puncture is not usually performed because of the risks of cerebral herniation.

The nurse assesses the client, using the Glasgow Coma Scale (see Chap. 43) at least every 2 hours or more often if clinically indicated. Included in this assessment are the

client's vital signs. The client is at risk for increased ICP, which may initially be manifested by a change in the level of consciousness. Late signs of increased ICP include seizures, pupillary changes, and a widened pulse pressure and bradycardia. The nurse elevates the head of the client's bed 30–45 degrees to promote venous drainage from the head. Other interventions for the treatment of increased ICP are discussed earlier in the chapter in the section on Head Injury.

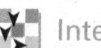 Interventions

The nurse gives the medications ordered by the physician to treat the abscess (Table 47–8). Typically used antibiotics include penicillin G benzathine (Bicillin) and nafcillin sodium (Nafcil, Unipen). Metronidazole (Flagyl, Novonidazol✲) may be used if an anaerobic organism is the causative agent. These agents are particularly useful in the early stages (cerebritis) of abscess formation. A combination of antibiotics is used, particularly if the abscess resulted from septic emboli. Anticonvulsants, such as phenytoin (Dilantin), may be used prophylactically to prevent seizures. The nurse strictly adheres to the medication schedule to maintain therapeutic blood levels. Analgesics may be ordered to treat the client's headache.

The physician may surgically drain an encapsulated abscess via a bur hole to reduce the mass effect of the lesion. The physician may elect to perform a craniotomy to remove the abscess in certain cases. The decision to perform surgery is based on the client's general condition, the stage of abscess development, and the site of the abscess. The nurse provides routine preoperative and postoperative care for the client undergoing a craniotomy, as discussed earlier in the section on Brain Tumors.

The client with a brain abscess is discharged to home if few or no neurologic deficits are present. Those clients with severe dysfunction are usually transferred to long-term care or a rehabilitation facility.

TABLE 47–8

Antibiotics Used to Treat Brain Abscess

Organism	Treatment
Streptococcus	• Penicillin • Chloramphenicol
Anaerobes Staphylococcus	• Metronidazole • Nafcillin • Methicillin • Vancomycin
Enterobacteriaceae Toxoplasma	• Cefotaxime • Pyrimethamine • Sulfonamides • Trimethoprim-sulfamethoxazole • Clindamycin • Fluconazole

CASE STUDY with Critical Thinking Exercises

■ Ann Townsend is a 20-year-old female who fell from a third-story balcony during a fraternity party. Upon arrival, paramedics assessed the following: unresponsive to verbal or painful stimuli, Glasgow Coma Score 3, BP 70/30, HR 40 and irregular, R-6 shallow and irregular, pupils unequal with the right larger than the left and sluggishly responsive, and corneal, cough, and gag reflexes intact. The paramedics resuscitated her in the field and transported her to a regional trauma center on a back board with a cervical collar in place. She has been intubated and has had an orogastric tube and a large-bore IV inserted.

In addition to the neurologic injury, Ann has a fractured lower left leg and an occipital laceration. She has no significant medical history, but her blood alcohol level is .17.

In the emergency room her status has not changed significantly. Complete laboratory studies, including typing and matching for four units of blood, were done. Extensive x-rays and a CT scan were obtained. The CT scan showed a large left frontoparietal lobe hematoma with a midline shift. Ann is taken to the operating room, and a left frontoparietal craniotomy is performed. The epidural hematoma is evacuated, the leg fracture is treated through an open reduction and internal fixation (ORIF), and an intraventricular catheter is placed. Ann is transferred to the ICU.

In the ICU, Ann is placed on mechanical ventilation and hyperventilated via an endotracheal tube. She has a urinary catheter, an arterial line, a triple lumen catheter, EKG monitoring, and ICP monitoring via an IVC. She requires frequent suctioning, turning, and assessment.

Within 3 hours postoperatively, Ann is responding appropriately and is able to follow simple commands. Her BP and HR fluctuate but can be controlled with medication. Her ICP ranges 13–25 mmHg, with the increases noted with nursing activities, and requires mannitol occasionally for control.

Ann's parents have been in to visit and are very upset about the fact that Ann appears to have been drinking at the fraternity party.

QUESTIONS:

1. What medications can the nurse anticipate the physician ordering for Ann?
2. When planning your care for Ann you are aware that many interventions can cause an increase in ICP. How would you plan your nursing care to avoid precipitating an increase in Ann's ICP?
3. What referrals do you feel are essential for both Ann and her parents in planning for Ann's eventual discharge from the hospital?
4. How would you explain Ann's neurologic injury to her parents?

SELECTED BIBLIOGRAPHY

Acorn, S. A. (1995). Assisting families of head injured survivors through a family support programme. *Journal of Advanced Nursing, 21*(5), 872–877.

Adams, H. P., Brott, T. G., Furlan, A. J., et al. (1996). Guidelines for thrombolytic therapy for acute stroke: A supplement to the guidelines for the management of patients with acute ischemic stroke. *Circulation, 94*(1), 167–171, 174.

Alexander, M. P. (1995). Mild traumatic brain injury: Pathophysiology, natural history and client management. *Neurology, 45*, 1253–1260.

Allen, K. M., & Phillips, J. M. (1997). *Women's health across the lifespan: A comprehensive perspective*. Philadelphia: J. B. Lippincott.

American Association of Neurological Surgeons. (1997). *Guidelines for the management of severe head injuries*. Chicago: Author.

American Association of Neuroscience Nurses (AANN). (1997). *Clinical guidelines series: Intracranial pressure monitoring*. Chicago: Author.

American Brain Tumor Association. (1996). *A primer of brain tumors*. Des Plaines, IL: American Brain Tumor Association.

Armstrong, S. L. (1994). Cerebral vasospasm: Early detection and intervention. *Critical Care Nurse 14*(4), 33–37.

Barker, E. (1994). *Neuroscience nursing*. St. Louis: Mosby.

Blank-Reid, C. (1996). How to have a stroke at an early age: The effects of crack, cocaine, and other illicit drugs. *Journal of Neuroscience Nursing, 28*(1), 19–27.

Brem, S., Rozental, J. M., & Moskal, J. R. (1995). What is the etiology of human brain tumors? A report on the first Lebow Conference. *Cancer, 76*(4), 709–713.

Canobbio, M. M. (1996). *Mosby's handbook of patient teaching*. St. Louis: Mosby.

Choi, S. C., Barnes, T. Y., Bullock, R., Germanson, T. A., Marmarou, A., & Young, H. F. (1994). Temporal profile of outcomes in severe head injury. *Journal of Neurosurgery, 81*(2), 169–173.

Chudley, S. (1994). The effects of nursing activities on ICP. *British Journal of Nursing, 3*(9), 454–459.

Counsell, C., Gilbert, M., Snively, C. (1995). Nimodipine: A drug therapy for treatment of vasospasm. *Journal of Neuroscience Nursing, 27*(1), 53–56.

Dobkin, B. H. (1996). *Neurologic rehabilitation*. Philadelphia: F. A. Davis.

Donnan, G. A., Davis, S. M., Chambers, B. R., et al. (1996). Streptokinase for acute ischemic stroke with relationship to time of administration. *JAMA, 276*(12), 961–966.

Eisenhart, K. (1994). New perspectives in the management of adults with severe head injury. *Critical Care Nursing Quarterly, 17*(2), 1–12.

Evans, R. W. (1996). *Neurology and trauma*. Philadelphia: W. B. Saunders.

Fowler, S. B. (1995). Deep vein thrombosis and pulmonary emboli in neuroscience patients. *Journal of Neuroscience Nursing, 27*(4), 224–228.

German, K. (1994). Intracranial pressure monitoring in the 1990's. *Critical Care Nursing Quarterly, 17*(1), 21–32.

Gershman, G. E., Duncam, P. W., Stason, W. B., et al. *Post stroke rehabilitation: Assessment, referral and patient management. Clinical practice guidelines and quick reference guide for clinicians, No. 16*. Rockville, MD. U.S. Department of Health & Human Services Public Health Service, Agency for Health Care Policy and Research. AHCPR Publication No. 95-0663. May 1995.

Gershman, G. E., Duncam, P. W., Stason, W. B., et al. *Post stroke rehabilitation: Clinical practice guidelines, No. 16*. Rockville, MD. U.S. Department of Health & Human Services Public Health Service, Agency for Health Care Policy and Research. AHCPR Publication No. 95-0662. May 1995.

Gersin, K., Grindlinger, G. A., Lee, V., Dennis, R. C., Wedel, S. K., & Cachecho, R. (1994). The efficacy of sequential compression devices in multiple trauma patients with severe head injury. *Journal of Trauma, 37*(2), 205–208.

Hickey, J. V. (1996). *The clinical practice of neurological and neurosurgical nursing*. Philadelphia: J. B. Lippincott.

*Laws, E. R., & Thapar, K. (1993). Brain tumors. *CA: A Cancer Journal for Clinicians, 43*(5), 263–271.

Macabasco, A., & Hickmam. J. (1995). Thrombolytic therapy for brain attack. *Journal of Neuroscience Nursing, 27*(3), 138–151.

Martin, K. M. (1994). Loss without death: A dilemma for the head-injured patient's family. *Journal of Neuroscience Nursing, 26*(3), 134–139.

Mock, C. N., Maier, R. V., Boyle, E., Pilcher, S., & Rivara, F. P. (1995). Injury prevention strategies to promote helmet use decrease severe head injuries at a level I trauma center. *Journal of Trauma, 39*(1), 29–35.

Monti, E. J. (1995). Monitoring neuromuscular function. *Journal of Neuroscience Nursing, 27*(4), 252–257.

Rhone-Polenc Rorer Pharmaceuticals. (1996). Gliadel package insert.

Rusy, K. L. (1996). Rebleeding and vasospasm after subarachnoid hemorrhage: A critical care challenge. *Critical Care Nurse, 16*(1), 41–48.

Shepherd, T. J., & Fox, S. W. (1996). Assessment and management of hypertension in the acute ischemic stroke patient. *Journal of Neuroscience Nursing, 28*(1), 5–12.

Shpritz, D. W. (1996). *Delmar's rapid nursing interventions—neurologic.* Albany, NY: Delmar Publishers.

Slazinski, T., & Johnson, M. C. (1994). Severe diffuse axonal injury in adults and children. *Journal of Neuroscience Nursing, 26* (3), 151–154.

Sosnowski, C., & Ustik, M. (1994). Early intervention: Coma stimulation in the ICU. *Journal of Neuroscience Nursing, 26*(6), 336–341.

Sosin, D. M., Sniezek, J. E., & Waxmeiler, R. J. (1995). Trends in deaths associated with traumatic brain injury, 1979 through 1992. *JAMA, 273*(22), 1778–1780.

Stass, D. T. (1995). A sensible approach to mild traumatic brain injury. *Neurology, 45,* 1251–1252.

Stewart-Amidei, C. (1995). Quality of life in the neuro-oncology patient. *Journal of Neuroscience Nursing, 27*(4), 219–223.

Stewart-Amidei, C. (1996). Brain attack: Abstracts from the 1995 Neuroscience Nursing Clinical Symposium. *Journal of Neuroscience Nursing, 28*(1), 44–55.

Van de Kelft, E., Segnarbieux, F., Candon, F., Couchet, P., Frerebeau, P., & Daures, J. P. (1994). Clinical recovery of consciousness after traumatic coma. *Critical Care Medicine, 22*(7), 1108–1113.

Whitney, F. (1994). Drug therapy for acute stroke. *Journal of Neuroscience Nursing, 26*(2), 111–117.

Winkelman, C. (1994). Advances in managing increased cranial pressure: A decade of selected research. *AACN Clinical Issues, 5*(1), 9–14.

SUGGESTED READINGS

Winkelman, C. (1994). Advances in managing increased cranial pressure: A decade of selected research. *AACN Clinical Issues, 5*(1), 9–14.

Among the eight clinical topics identified by the American Association of Critical Care Nurses as priorities for nursing research is the examination of the effect of nursing activities, environmental stimuli, and human interactions on intracranial pressure (ICP). This article is an excellent review of the pathophysiology and treatment of intracranial hypertension. Recent research focusing on the causes and treatment of increased ICP is highlighted. Investigational therapies are also described.

German, K. (1994). Intracranial pressure monitoring in the 1990's. *Critical Care Nursing Quarterly, 17*(1), 21–32.

This article is an excellent overview of the concept of ICP monitoring, including the types of monitoring systems and interpretation and utilization of the data obtained from ICP monitors. Ethical considerations related to the use of ICP monitoring in the changing health care environment are discussed.

Blank-Reid, C. (1996). How to have a stroke at an early age: The effects of crack, cocaine, and other illicit drugs. *Journal of Neuroscience Nursing, 28*(1), 19–27.

There has been an increase in the number of stroke deaths in the 14–24– and the 45–54–year-old age groups. One of the most significant factors is the increased use of illicit drugs such as crack, cocaine, heroin, amphetamines, and PCP. This article is an excellent in-depth discussion of the commonly used drugs that contribute to stroke. The classification, characteristics, overdose, interventions, and withdrawal symptoms of the drugs are presented. Nursing considerations include sample questions to use in taking a history of illicit drug use and common findings seen in substance-abusing clients.

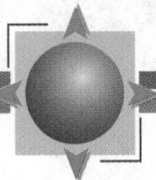

Problems of Sensation:

Management of Clients

with Problems of the

Sensory System

Chapter 48

ASSESSMENT OF THE EYE AND VISION

CHAPTER

HIGHLIGHTS

Vision is most people's key to the world. The eye is the sensory organ responsible for vision. Many conditions can affect the eye and vision. Assessment of the eye and vision provides the nurse with important data regarding clients' general health status and the degree to which they can participate in their own health care.

ANATOMY AND PHYSIOLOGY REVIEW
Structure

The eyeball, a spherical organ about 2.5 cm in length and 2.3 cm in diameter, is located in the anterior portion of the *orbit*. The orbit, the bony structure of the skull that surrounds the eye, protects the eye as well as the associated muscles, nerves, vessels, and most of the lacrimal apparatus.

Layers of the Eyeball

The eye has three layers, or coats (Fig. 48–1). The external layer consists of the sclera (the opaque tissue making up the "whites" of the eye) and the transparent cornea, on the front of the eye.

The middle layer, or *uvea*, is heavily pigmented. This layer consists of the choroid, the ciliary body, and the iris. The *choroid*, a dark brown membrane between the sclera and the retina, lines most of the sclera. The choroid contains many blood vessels that supply nutrients to the retina.

The *ciliary body* connects the choroid with the iris and secretes aqueous humor. The *iris* is the colored portion of the external eye; its central circular opening is the *pupil*. The muscles of the iris contract and relax to regulate pupil size and the amount of light entering the eye.

The innermost layer is the *retina*, a thin, delicate structure through which the sensory fibers that transmit impulses to the optic nerve are distributed. The retina contains blood vessels and two classes of photoreceptors called *rods* and *cones*. The rods function at low levels of light and provide peripheral vision. The cones function at bright levels of light and provide color and central vision.

The *optic fundus* is viewed at the back of the eye with an ophthalmoscope. This area contains the *optic disk*, a creamy pink to white depressed area in the retina (Fig. 48–2). The *optic nerve* enters the eyeball at this point. The optic disk is sometimes referred to as the *blind spot* because it contains only nerve fibers and no photoreceptor cells. To one side of the optic disk is a small, yellowish-pink area called the *macula lutea*. The central area of the macula is the *fovea centralis*, where vision is the most acute.

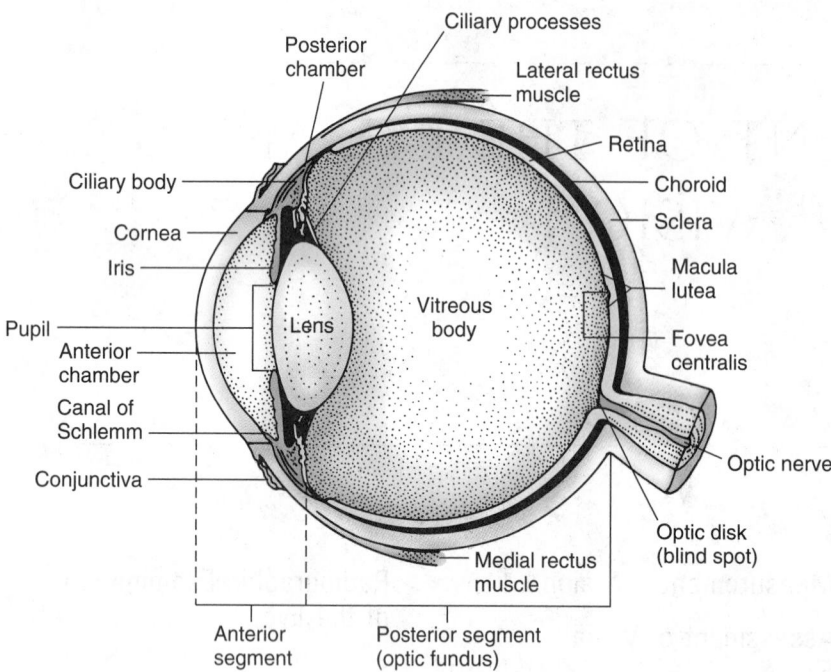

Figure 48–1. Anatomic features of the eye.

Refractive Media

Light waves pass through the following structures of varying densities on the way to the retina: cornea, aqueous humor, lens, and vitreous humor. Each of these structures causes the light waves to bend, or *refract,* to some degree and focus images on the retina. These structures constitute the *refracting media* of the eye.

The *cornea* is the transparent layer that forms the external coat of the anterior portion of the eye (see Fig. 48–1). The *aqueous humor* is a clear, watery fluid that

Optic disk

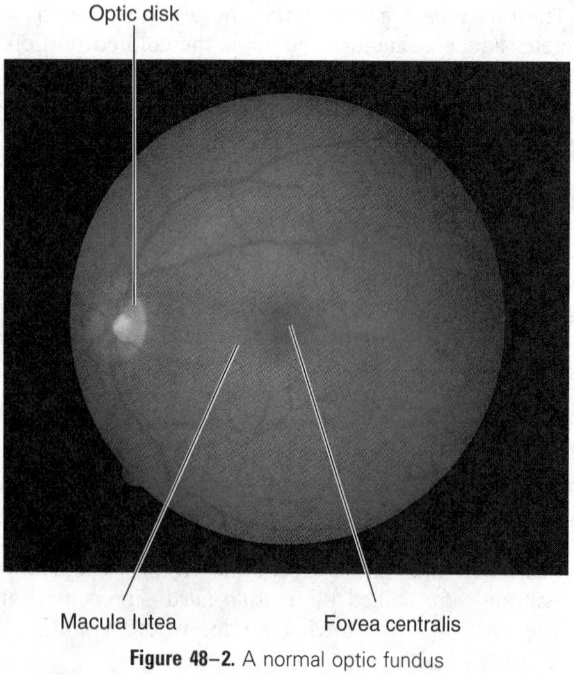

Figure 48–2. A normal optic fundus

Macula lutea   Fovea centralis

fills the anterior and posterior chambers of the eye. Aqueous humor is continually produced by the ciliary processes and passes from the posterior chamber through the pupil into the anterior chamber. This fluid drains through the *canal of Schlemm* into the systemic circulation to maintain a balanced intraocular pressure (IOP, or the pressure within the eye).

The *lens* is a circular, biconvex structure that lies behind the iris and in front of the vitreous body. It is normally transparent. The lens bends rays of light entering through the pupil so that they focus on the retina. The curvature of the lens enables a person to focus on near or distant objects.

The *vitreous body* consists of a gelatinous substance that occupies the vitreous chamber, the space between the lens and the retina. This gelatinous body transmits light and gives shape to the posterior eye.

External Structures

The *eyelids* are thin, movable folds of skin that protect the eyes from entry of a foreign body, shut out light during sleep, and keep the cornea moist. The upper eyelid is larger than the lower one. The place at which the two eyelids meet at the corner of the eye is called the *canthus.*

The *conjunctivae* are mucous membranes of the eye. The *palpebral* conjunctiva is a thick, vascular membrane that lines the posterior surface of each eyelid. Located over the sclera is the thin, transparent *bulbar* conjunctiva.

Tears are produced by a small *lacrimal gland,* located in the upper outer part of each orbit (Fig. 48–3). Tears flow across the eye and corneal surface toward the nose and into the lower inner canthus. They drain out through the *punctum,* found at each of the innermost lid margins,

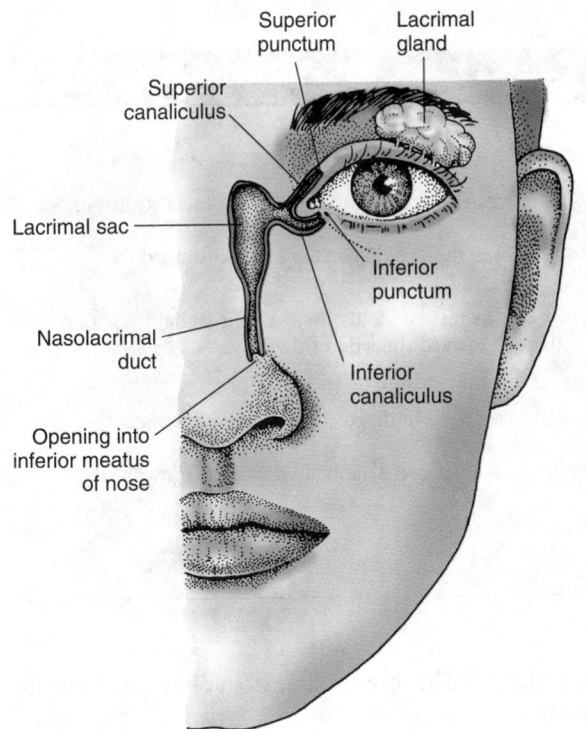

Figure 48–3. Anterior view of the eye and adjacent structures.

into the *lacrimal duct* and *sac,* and then into the nose through the nasolacrimal duct.

Muscles

There are seven voluntary muscles of the orbit; six rotate the eye and coordinate eye movements (Fig. 48–4; Table 48–1 summarizes their functions.) Coordinated eye movements ensure that the retina of each eye receives an image at the same time, so only a single image is perceived.

Nerves

The extraocular muscles are innervated by the following cranial nerves: oculomotor (cranial nerve III), trochlear (cranial nerve IV), and the abducens (cranial nerve VI). The *optic nerve* (cranial nerve II) is the nerve of sight, connecting the optic disk to the brain. The ophthalmic division of the trigeminal nerve (cranial nerve V) innervates the sensory portion of the blink reflex, stimulated when the cornea is touched. The facial nerve (cranial nerve VII) innervates the lacrimal glands and musculature involved in lid closure. (Assessment of these nerves is discussed in Chapter 43.)

Blood Vessels

The *ophthalmic artery* supplies blood to the structures in the orbit. The central artery of the retina branches off the ophthalmic artery and supplies blood to the retina. The ciliary arteries supply the sclera, choroid, ciliary body, and iris. Venous drainage is through the two *ophthalmic veins.*

Function

Three functions of the eye provide clear images of near and far objects. These functions are refraction, pupillary constriction, and accommodation.

Refraction

The different curved surfaces and refractive media of the eye allow light to pass through to the retina. Each surface and media refract light differently. Refraction is the process of bending the light rays to focus an image on the retina. *Emmetropia* is the ideal refraction of the eye: with the lens at rest (unaccommodated), light rays from a distant source (6 m or more) are focused into a sharp image on the retina. Figure 48–5 shows the normal refraction of light within the eye. Images fall on the retina inverted and reversed left to right. For example, an object in the lower nasal visual field strikes the upper outer area of the retina.

Errors of refraction are common. *Hyperopia* (also called hypermetropia or far-sightedness) is a condition in which the eye does not refract light enough and images converge behind the retina (see Fig. 48–5). Vision beyond 20 feet is normal, but near vision is poor. Hyperopia is corrected with a convex lens.

Myopia (near-sightedness) is a condition in which the eye overrefracts or overbends the light, so images are focused in front of the retina (see Fig. 48–5). Near vision is normal, but distance vision is poor. Myopia is corrected with a biconcave lens.

Astigmatism is a refractive error caused by unevenly curved surfaces in the eye, creating visual distortion. Usually astigmatism is associated with uneven corneal surfaces.

Pupillary Constriction

The pupil regulates the amount of light that enters the eye. If the level of light to one or both eyes is increased, both pupils constrict. The amount of constriction depends on how much light is available and how well the retina

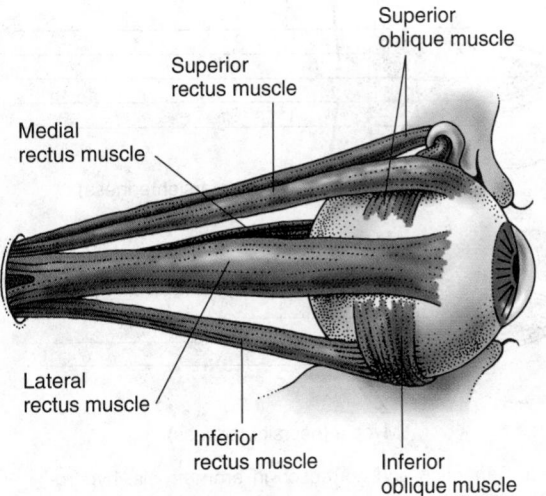

Figure 48–4. The extraocular muscles.

TABLE 48–1

Functions of Ocular Muscles	
Muscle	**Movement on Contraction**
Levator palpebrae	• This muscle lifts the upper eyelid.
Superior rectus	• Together with the lateral rectus, this muscle moves the eye diagonally upward toward the side of the head. • Together with the medial rectus, this muscle moves the eye diagonally upward toward the middle of the head.
Lateral rectus	• Together with the medial rectus, contraction of this muscle holds the eye in a straight position. • Contracting alone, the lateral rectus turns the eye toward the side of the head.
Medial rectus	• Contracting alone, the medial rectus turns the eye toward the nose.
Inferior rectus	• Together with the lateral rectus, this muscle moves the eye diagonally downward toward the side of the head. • Together with the medial rectus, this muscle moves the eye diagonally downward toward the middle of the head.
Superior oblique	• Contraction pulls the eye downward.
Inferior oblique	• Contraction pulls the eye upward.

can adapt to light changes. Pupillary constriction is called *miosis,* and pupillary dilation is called *mydriasis.* Medications can alter pupillary constriction.

Accommodation

The healthy eye can focus sharp images on the retina whether the image is close to the eye or more distant. The process of maintaining a clear visual image when gaze is shifted from a distant to a near object is known as *accommodation.* The eye is able to adjust its focus by changing the curve of the lens.

Eye Changes Associated with Aging

Visual acuity is reduced with age. Age-related changes within the eye, the nervous system, and in the structures supporting the eye affect visual function (Chart 48–1).

Age-Associated Structural Changes

In the elderly, decreased eye muscle tone impairs the ability to maintain an upward gaze and to sustain convergence. The lower eyelid may relax and fall away from the eye (ectropion), exposing more of the eye and leading to dry eye symptoms.

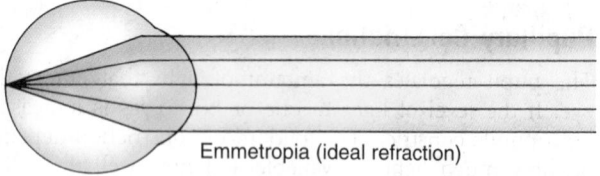

Emmetropia (ideal refraction)

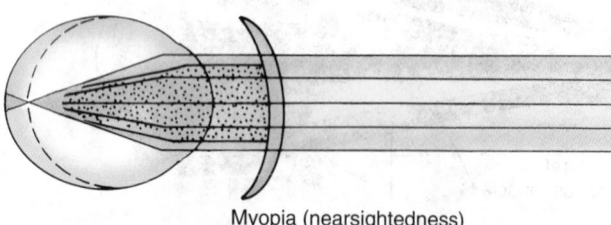

Hyperopia (hypermetropia, or farsightedness)

Myopia (nearsightedness)

Figure 48–5. Refraction and correction in emmetropia, hyperopia, and myopia.

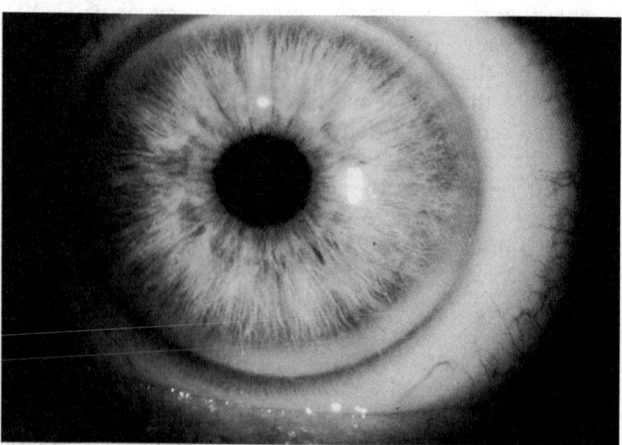

Figure 48–6. Arcus senilis of the iris.

Chart 48–1

Nursing Focus on the Elderly: Changes in the Eye Related to Aging

Structure/Function	Change
Appearance	• Eyes appear to be sunken • Arcus senilis forms • Sclera yellows
Cornea	• Cornea flattens, which causes astigmatism and blurring of vision
Ocular muscles	• Muscle strength is reduced, which results in a diminished capacity to maintain an upward gaze and to sustain convergence
Lens	• Elasticity is lost, which increases the near point of vision • Lens hardens and becomes compact • Cataracts form
Iris	• Decrease in ability to dilate results in small pupil size and poor adaptation to darkness
Pupil	• Pupil size smaller • Aperture size takes longer to change, which reduces ability to see in dim light
Color vision	• Discrimination among colors of short wavelength (green, blue, violet) decreases
Tears	• Diminished tear production results in dry eyes

Arcus senilis, an opaque ring formed within the circumference of the cornea, results from deposition of fatty globules (Fig. 48–6). Although it is a common finding, not all elderly people have arcus senilis. This change does not affect vision.

The transparency and shape of the cornea change with age. After age 65, the cornea flattens and the curvature of its surface is irregular. This change produces or worsens astigmatism. As a result, images are distorted and blurred.

Degenerative changes occur in the sclera; fatty deposits cause the sclera to develop a yellowish tinge. As the sclera thins, a bluish color may be noted. With increasing age, the iris has less ability to dilate and clients have difficulty adapting to a darker environment. Older adults may need additional light for reading.

Age-Associated Functional Changes

With aging, the lens yellows, affecting the eye's ability to transmit and focus light. The aging lens hardens, shrinks, and loses elasticity. As the lens loses elasticity, the eye's ability to accommodate is gradually lost. The *near point* of vision, the closest distance at which the eye can see an object clearly, increases. Near objects (especially reading material) must be placed farther from the eye to be seen clearly. This age-related change is termed *presbyopia.* The *far point,* or the farthest point at which an object can be distinguished, decreases. Thus, the elderly person has a narrower visual field.

As a person ages, color sensitivity across the entire light spectrum is lost, as is discrimination among colors of short wavelengths (such as green, blue, and violet). More light is needed to stimulate the visual receptors. Intraocular pressure (IOP) is slightly higher in older than in younger adults.

HISTORY
Demographic Data

The client's age is an important factor to consider when assessing the visual processes and eye structure. The incidence of glaucoma and cataract formation increases with aging. Presbyopia commonly begins in the 40s.

The client's gender also may be significant. For example, retinal detachments are more common in men, and dry eye symptoms are more common in women.

Personal and Family History

The nurse asks the client about a family history of eye problems, because some conditions, such as a refractive error, show a familial tendency. The nurse also asks about any systemic medical conditions that could have ocular involvement or cause complications (Table 48–2).

The client is asked about past accidents, injuries, surgeries, or blows to the head that may have led to the present findings. The nurse asks specifically about previous laser surgeries, because clients often do not classify laser treatment as surgery. The nurse asks about the types of sports the client plays, because some injuries are more common to specific sports.

The client is questioned about medications used, particularly decongestants and antihistamines. The ocular effects associated with these drugs are well documented. Many clients do not consider over-the-counter eyedrops to be medication. The nurse notes the name, strength, dose, and schedule of administration for all ophthalmic medications. Many systemic drugs can cause ocular disturbances (see Table 48–2). Clinical manifestations of ocular drug effects include pruritus (itching), foreign body

TABLE 48–2

Extraocular Conditions Affecting the Eye and Vision	
Category	**Condition/Factor**
Systemic disorders	Diabetes mellitus
	Hypertension
	Lupus erythematosus
	Sarcoidosis
	Thyroid dysfunction
	Acquired immunodeficiency syndrome
	Cardiac disease
	Multiple sclerosis
Drugs	Antihistamines
	Decongestants
	Antibiotics
	Opioids
	Anticholinergics
	Cholinergic agonists
	Sympathomimetics
	Oral contraceptives
	Antineoplastic agents
	Corticosteroids
	Carbonic anhydrase inhibitors
	Beta-blockers

sensation, redness, tearing, photophobia (sensitivity to light), and the development of cataract or glaucoma.

Diet History

Because some ocular problems are associated with vitamin deficiencies, the nurse asks questions about the client's food choices. For example, vitamin A deficiency can cause conjunctival xerosis (dryness), keratomalacia, and blindness.

Socioeconomic Status

The nurse asks the client about his or her work and specifically how the eyes are used. In some occupations, such as computer programming, constant exposure to monitor screens may lead to eyestrain and the need for eyeglasses. Machine operators are at risk for eye injury because of the high speeds at which particles can be thrown at the eye. The nurse asks clients who work in industrial settings about the use of protective eyewear, such as goggles. Chronic exposure to infrared or ultraviolet light may cause photophobia and cataract formation.

Current Health Problem

The nurse asks the client about the onset of visual changes. Has the change occurred rapidly or slowly? A client with a sudden or persistent loss of vision within the past 48 hours should be seen immediately by an ophthalmologist, as should the client experiencing trauma, a foreign body in the eye, sudden ocular pain, or redness. The nurse asks the client whether the same symptoms are present to the same degree in both eyes.

The nurse asks the following questions if ocular injury or eye trauma is involved:

- How long ago did the injury occur?
- What was the client doing when it happened?
- If a foreign body might be involved, what was its source?
- Was any first aid administered at the scene? If so, what actions were taken?

PHYSICAL ASSESSMENT
Inspection

The nurse looks for head tilting, squinting, or other noticeable postural characteristics that offer clues to compensatory stances for attaining clear vision. For example, clients with double vision may cock the head to the side in an attempt to focus the two images into one.

The nurse observes for symmetry in the appearance of the eyes. The nurse checks that the eyes are an equal distance from each other, the same size, and of the same degree of prominence. The eyes also are assessed for their placement in the orbits and for symmetry of movement. *Exophthalmos* (proptosis) is a condition in which the eyes protrude; in *enophthalmos*, the eyeballs are sunken.

The nurse assesses the eyebrows and eyelashes for distribution of hair growth. The direction of the eyelashes is determined. Eyelashes normally extend outward and away from the eyelid. The nurse looks at the eyelid to assess *ptosis* (drooping), redness, lesions, or swelling. The lids normally close completely, with the upper and lower lid edges touching. When the eyes are open, the upper lid covers a small portion of the iris. The edge of the lower lid lies below the line between the cornea and sclera. No sclera should be visible between the eyelid and the iris.

Scleral and Corneal Assessment

The sclera is examined for color; it is usually white. A yellow color may indicate jaundice or systemic problems. In dark-skinned people, however, the normal sclera may appear yellow, and small, pigmented dots may be visible (Jarvis, 1996).

The nurse can best observe the cornea by directing a light at it obliquely from several angles. The cornea should be transparent, smooth, shiny, and bright. Any cloudy areas or specks may be the result of accidents or injuries.

The nurse assesses the blink reflex by bringing a fist quickly toward the client's face; clients who have vision blink. Alternatively, the nurse can expel a syringe full of air toward the eyes. The client blinks if the reflex is intact.

Pupillary Assessment

The pupils are usually round and of equal size. Approximately 5% of people normally have a slight but noticeable difference in the size of the pupils, termed *anisocoria*. The size of pupils varies in people exposed to the same amount of light. Pupils are smaller in older adults. People with myopia have larger pupils; people with hyperopia have smaller pupils. The normal pupil diameter is between 3 and 5 mm.

The nurse observes the pupils for response to light: increasing light causes pupillary constriction, whereas decreasing light causes dilation. Constriction of both pupils is the normal response to direct light. Pupils also constrict in response to accommodation. The nurse assesses pupillary reaction to light by asking the client to look straight ahead while quickly bringing the beam of a flashlight in from the side and directing it at the right (oculus dexter, or OD) pupil (see Chap. 43). The constriction of the OD pupil is a direct response to shining the flashlight into that eye. Constriction of the left (oculus sinister, or OS) pupil from shining of the light at the OD pupil is known as a *consensual response*. Direct and consensual responses are assessed for each eye.

Each pupil is evaluated for speed of reaction. The pupil should immediately constrict when a light is directed at it. This rapid response is termed *brisk*. If the pupil takes more than 1 second to constrict, the response is termed *sluggish*. Pupils that fail to react are termed *nonreactive* or *fixed*. Reactivity speed of OD and OS pupils is compared and any discrepancy noted.

In assessing for accommodation, the nurse holds the index finger about 18 cm from the client's nose and moves it toward the nose. The client's eyes normally converge during this movement, and the pupils constrict equally. When accommodation stops, the pupils begin to enlarge and return to their normal size.

Measurement of Vision

Vision is measured by various tests. Each eye is tested separately, and then both eyes are tested together. Clients who routinely wear corrective lenses are tested both without and with their corrective lenses.

Acuity

Visual acuity tests measure both distance and near vision. The Snellen chart, or "eye chart," is a simple tool to measure distance vision. The chart has letters, numbers, pictures, or a single letter presented in various positions (Fig. 48–7). The client stands 20 feet from the chart, covers one eye, and uses the other eye to read the line that appears most clear. If the client can do this accurately, the nurse asks the client to read the next lower line. This sequence is repeated to the last line on which the client can correctly identify most characters. The procedure is then repeated for the other eye. Findings are recorded as a comparison between what the client can read at 20 feet, and the distance at which a person with normal vision can read the same line. For example, 20/50 means that the client is able to see at 20 feet from the chart what a "healthy eye" can see at 50 feet.

For clients in a confined space that does not permit a 20-foot distance to the eye chart or who cannot see the 20/400 character, the nurse assesses visual acuity by holding fingers in front of the client's eyes and asking the client to count them (Fig. 48–8). This procedure is repeated five times. Acuity is recorded as "count fingers

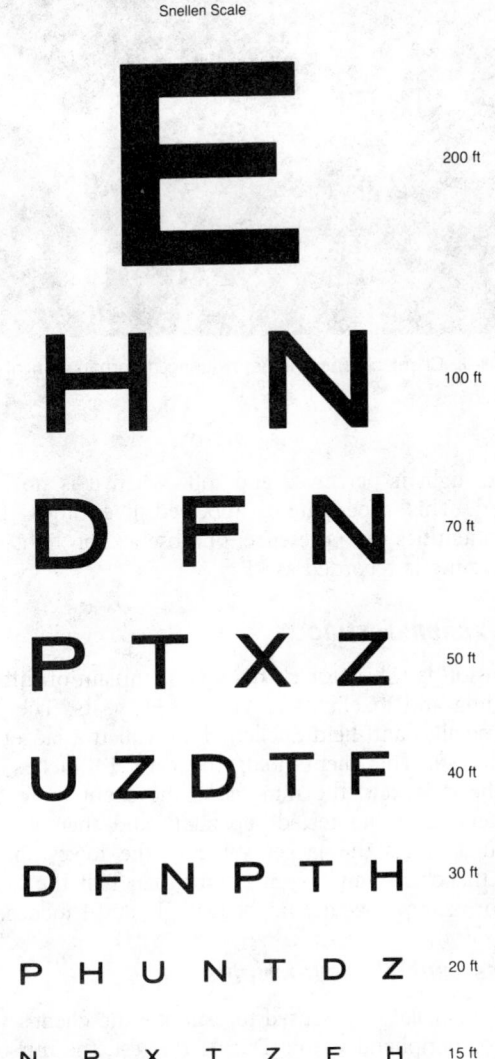

LETTER CHART FOR 20 FEET
Snellen Scale

Figure 48–7. A typical Snellen chart. (Courtesy of the National Society to Prevent Blindness.)

vision at 5 feet" or the farthest distance at which the client can count the fingers correctly.

Clients who cannot count fingers are tested for *hand motion (HM) acuity*. The nurse stands about 2 to 3 feet in front of the client. The eye not being tested is covered. A light is directed onto the hand from behind the client. The nurse demonstrates the three possible directions in which the hand can move during the test (stationary, left-right, or up-down). The nurse moves the hand slowly (1 second per motion) and asks the client, "What is my hand doing now?" This procedure is repeated at least five times. Visual acuity is recorded as HM at the farthest distance the client correctly identifies most of the hand motions.

If the client cannot detect hand movement, the nurse tests acuity by measuring *light perception* (LP). The nurse first asks the client to cover the left eye (OS). In a darkened room, from a distance of 2 to 3 feet, the nurse directs the beam of a penlight at the right eye (OD) for 1 to 2 seconds. Clients are instructed to say "on" when the

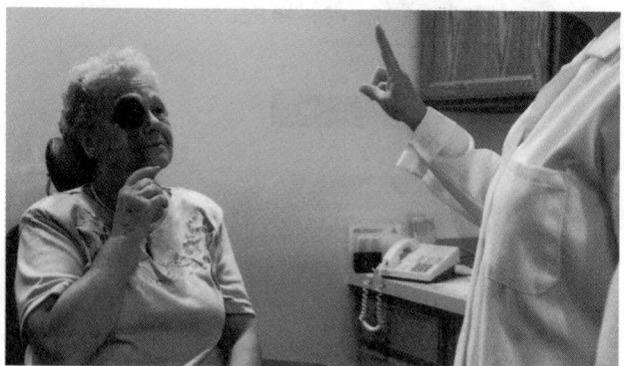

Figure 48–8. Client counting fingers during determination of visual acuity.

beam of light is perceived and "off" when it is no longer detected. This procedure is repeated five times. If the client identifies the presence or absence of light three times, acuity is recorded as LP.

Near-Vision Testing

Near vision is tested for clients who complain of difficulty in reading and in clients older than 40 years. The nurse uses a small, hand-held Snellen chart, called a Jaeger card (Fig. 48–9). The client holds the card 14 inches away from the eyes, and the nurse asks the client to read the characters. Eyes are tested separately and then together. The nurse notes the Jaeger value of the lowest line on which the client can identify more than half the characters. For example, acuity might read "J2 at 14 inches."

Assessment of Visual Fields

A *confrontational* test is used to examine the client's visual fields, or peripheral vision. During the test, the nurse and the client sit facing each other, looking directly into each other's eyes throughout the test. The nurse covers his or her right eye (OD) and the client covers the left eye (OS), so that both have approximately the same visual field. The nurse moves a finger or an object from a nonvisible area into the client's line of vision.

This test provides only a crude estimate of the client's visual fields but can reveal large-field defects, such as hemianopia (blindness in one half of the field of vision), quadrantanopia (blindness in one fourth of the field of vision), or large scotomas (blind spots in the visual field).

Assessment of Extraocular Muscle Function

Assessment of extraocular muscle function includes three components: the corneal light reflex, the six cardinal positions of gaze, and the cover–uncover test. The nurse also observes for parallelism of the eyes and smoothness of ocular movements.

The corneal light reflex determines alignment of the two eyes. After asking the client to stare straight ahead, the nurse shines a penlight at both corneas from a distance of 12 to 15 inches. The bright dot of light reflected from the shiny surface of the cornea should be in a symmetric position (e.g., at the 1 o'clock position in the

right eye and at the 11 o'clock position in the left eye). An asymmetric reflex indicates a deviating eye and possible muscle imbalance.

The six cardinal positions of gaze (see Chap. 43) are used to assess muscle function, because the eye will not turn to a particular position if the muscle is weak or if the controlling nerve is affected. The nurse asks the client to hold his or her head still and to move the eyes to follow a small object, such as a pen. The nurse moves the object to the following positions:

To the client's right (lateral)
Upward and right (temporal)
Down and right
To the client's left (lateral)
Upward and left (temporal)
Down and left

ROSENBAUM POCKET VISION SCREENER

		distance equivalent
95		20/800
874	Point · Jaeger	20/400
2843	26 16	20/200
638 ЕШЭ XOO	14 10	20/100
8745 ЭМШ OXO	10 7	20/70
63925 МЕЭ XOX	8 5	20/50
428365 ШЕМ oxo	6 3	20/40
374258 ЭШЭ x x o	5 2	20/30
937826 шmE x o o	4 1	20/25
428739 Ewm o o x	3 1+	20/20

Card is held in good light 14 inches from eye. Record vision for each eye separately with and without glasses. Presbyopic patients should read thru bifocal segment. Check myopes with glasses only.

DESIGN COURTESY J. G. ROSENBAUM, M.D., CLEVELAND, OHIO

PUPIL GAUGE (mm.)

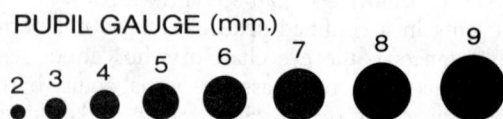

2 3 4 5 6 7 8 9

Figure 48–9. A typical Jaeger card. (Courtesy of SMP Division, Cooper Laboratories [P.R.], Inc., San German, Puerto Rico.)

While the client moves the eyes to these positions, the nurse observes for eye parallel movements and any deviation of movement. *Nystagmus,* an involuntary rhythmic, rapid twitching of the eyeball, is a normal finding for the far lateral gaze. It may also be caused by abnormal innervation or prolonged reduced vision.

A different method of assessing muscle function is the cover–uncover test. The nurse asks the client to use both eyes to look at a specific fixed point, such as the nurse's nose. One of the client's eyes then is covered with a card. The nurse observes the uncovered eye to see whether it moves to fix on the object; if the eye moves, it was not straight before the other eye was covered. The nurse then removes the cover and observes for any movement in the eye just uncovered. The nurse records the presence and direction of any deviations of eye movement.

Assessment of Color Vision

Several methods are available for testing color vision. The most frequently used tool is the *Ishihara chart,* which consists of numbers composed of colored dots within a circle of colored dots (Fig. 48–10). Testing each eye separately, the nurse asks the client what numbers he or she sees on the chart. The ability to read the numbers depends on the normal functioning of the client's color vision.

PSYCHOSOCIAL ASSESSMENT

Clients undergoing changes in visual perception may express anxiety and fear related to a loss of vision. Clients with severe visual defects may be unable to perform normal activities of daily living and may need to change leisure activities (see Research Applications for Nursing). The sense of dependency resulting from diminished vision

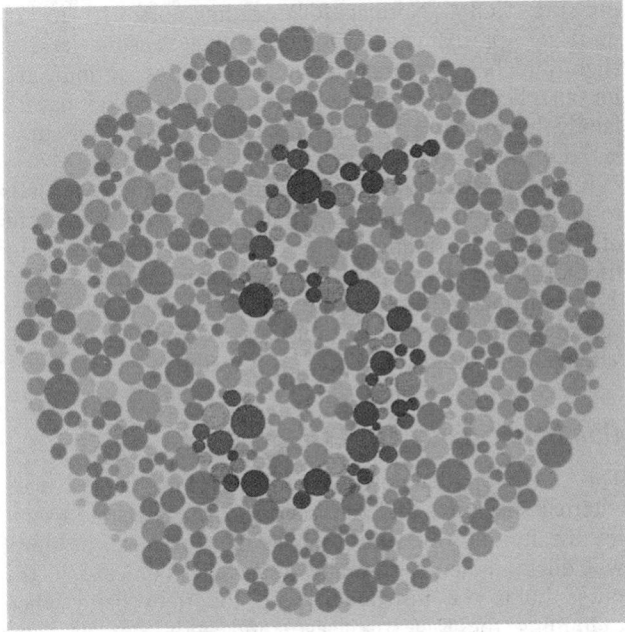

Figure 48–10. An Ishihara chart for testing color vision.

► Research Applications for Nursing

How Can the Visually Impaired Elderly Maintain Social Interaction?

Kelly, M. (1995). Consequences of visual impairment on leisure activities of the elderly. Geriatric Nursing, 16(6), 273–275.

The purposes of this prospective descriptive study were to assess the visual impairments experienced by a group of 88 indigent, community-dwelling elders and to identify the impact of decreased vision on their daily lives. The research methods used were interviews, assessment of visual acuity, and administration of the Inventory of Functional Visual Status questionnaire. Ninety-six percent wore eyeglasses; 39% of subjects had reduced vision not correctable by glasses (cataracts and macular degeneration). Only 12 clients indicated that they had difficulties participating in leisure activities to the degree they would like because of their vision problems. Most participants were not aware of the availability of resources and inexpensive assistive devices for visual impairment.

Critique. The investigator concluded that the amount of functional ability does not always correlate with the degree of visual impairment. The article did not provide data regarding how long the participants had experienced vision problems, what changes they had made in activities of daily living or leisure activities, or what coping methods were used. Nor did the article report the degree of satisfaction that elders with visual problems had in leisure activities compared with elders with minimal visual problems. Incorporation of qualitative methods into research regarding the impact of diminishing vision on functional status may have strengthened this study.

Possible Nursing Implications. Much of the isolation experienced by older clients may be related to reduced vision. Relatively simple changes in lighting and the use of inexpensive assistive devices can maximize limited sight. When caring for an older client, the nurse needs to consider the possibility of some degree of visual impairment, make appropriate adjustments in the immediate environment, and be a source of information regarding local resources for the visually impaired.

can affect a person's self-esteem. The nurse investigates the client's feelings about the visual disturbances and assesses the effectiveness of the client's coping techniques. The nurse also discusses the client's concerns with family members or significant others to establish the availability of support for the client. The nurse determines the client's current knowledge and use of available services for the visually impaired.

DIAGNOSTIC ASSESSMENT
Laboratory Tests

Cultures and smears of corneal or conjunctival swabs and scrapings aid in the diagnosis of infections. A sample of the exudate is obtained for culture before antibiotics or topical anesthetics are instilled. Swabs are taken from the conjunctivae and any ulcerated or inflamed areas.

Radiographic Examinations

Computed Tomography

Computed tomography (CT) is a radiographic diagnostic method in which a cross-sectional image is formed using computers. It is valuable in visualizing the globes, extraocular muscles, and optic nerves. It is a sensitive method for detecting tumors in the orbital space. Data are obtained by scanning the skull and orbits with beams of low-intensity x-rays. Because contrast material is not usually administered, no special client preparation or follow-up care is required. The nurse informs the client that there is no pain with this test. However, the client must be positioned in a confined space and keep the head still during the procedure.

Radioisotopic Scanning

Radioisotopes are used to locate tumors and lesions in various body organs. Isotope studies differentiate intraocular tumor and hemorrhage, especially in the choroid layer.

CLIENT PREPARATION. After the informed consent process, the client receives a tracer dose of the radioactive isotope, either orally or by injection.

PROCEDURE. The client is asked to lie still and breathe normally. The scanner measures the radioactivity emitted by the radioactive atoms concentrated in the area being studied for tumor. Clients who are restless, anxious, or agitated may require sedation.

FOLLOW-UP CARE. The nurse assures the client that the amount of radioisotope used as a tracer is extremely small and that the client is not radioactive. No other special follow-up care is required.

Other Diagnostic Tests

A variety of techniques are used to examine specific ocular structures. Such techniques are not necessary in the routine visual assessment of all people, but may be indicated for those clients with special risks, symptoms, or exposures. Such techniques require special skill and are used only by physicians, optometrists, or advanced-practice nurses.

Slit-Lamp Examination

The slit lamp (Fig. 48–11) permits examination of anterior ocular structures under microscopic magnification. The client leans on a chin rest to stabilize the head. A narrow beam (slit) of light is aimed so that it brightly illuminates only a narrow segment of the eye. This technique allows the examiner to locate accurately the position of any abnormality in the cornea, lens, or anterior vitreous humor. The slit beam also may help identify abnormal presence of cells in the aqueous humor.

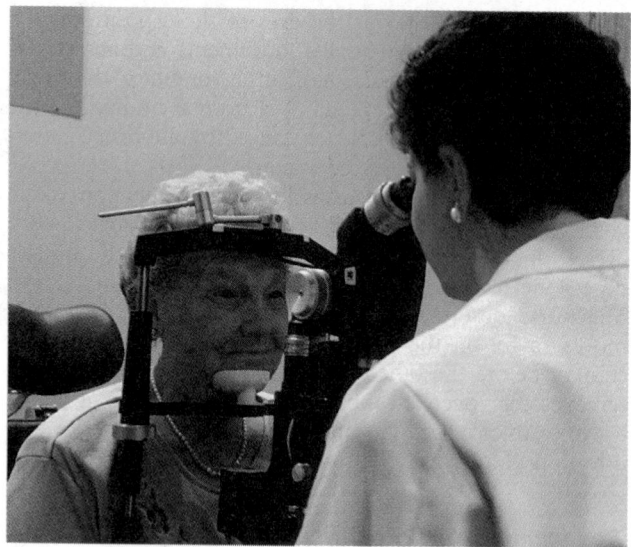

Figure 48–11. Slit-lamp ocular examination.

Corneal Staining

Corneal staining consists of the instillation of fluorescein or other topical dye into the conjunctival sac. The dye outlines irregularities of the corneal surface that are not easily visible. Corneal staining is indicated in cases of corneal trauma, pathologic conditions caused by a contact lens, the presence of foreign bodies, corneal abrasions or ulcers, or other corneal disorders.

The procedure is noninvasive and is performed under aseptic conditions. The dye is applied topically to the eye, and the eye is then viewed through a blue filter. Nonintact areas of the cornea stain a bright green color.

Tonometry

A tonometer is an instrument for measuring intraocular pressure (IOP). Normal IOP readings are 10 to 21 mmHg. Approximately 5% of normal clients have a slightly higher pressure. Tonometer readings are indicated for all clients older than 40 years. Adults who have a family history of glaucoma should have their IOP measured once or twice a year.

Intraocular pressure varies throughout the day. It tends to be highest in the morning, but it may peak at any time of the day, depending on the individual. Therefore, the time of IOP measurement is always documented.

Several methods and instruments are available to measure IOP (Fig. 48–12). Table 48–3 compares the advantages and disadvantages of each method.

Ophthalmoscopy

The direct ophthalmoscope allows viewing of the eye's external structures and the interior. It is easiest to examine the fundus when the room is dark because the pupil will dilate. When performing direct ophthalmoscopy, the nurse holds the instrument with the right hand when examining the OD (right eye) and with the left hand

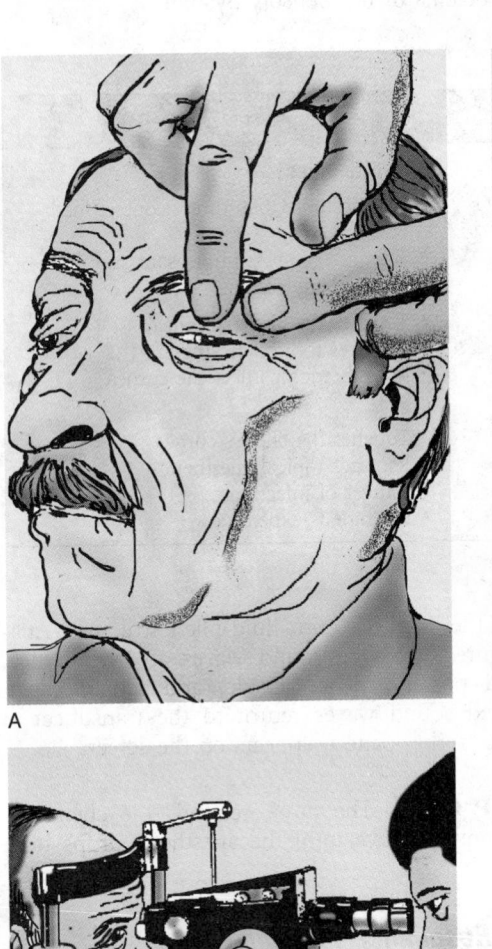

A

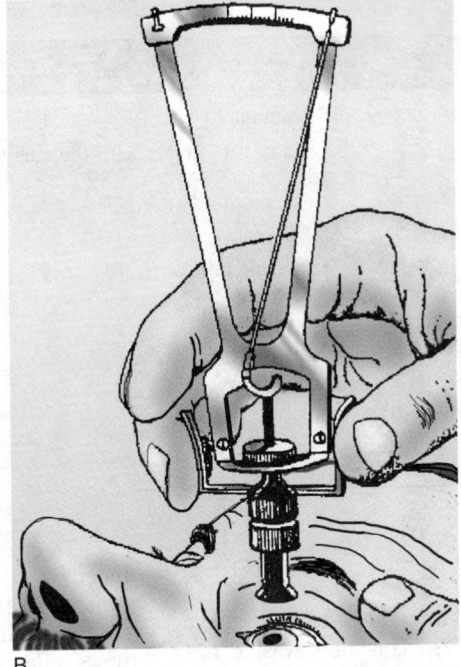

B

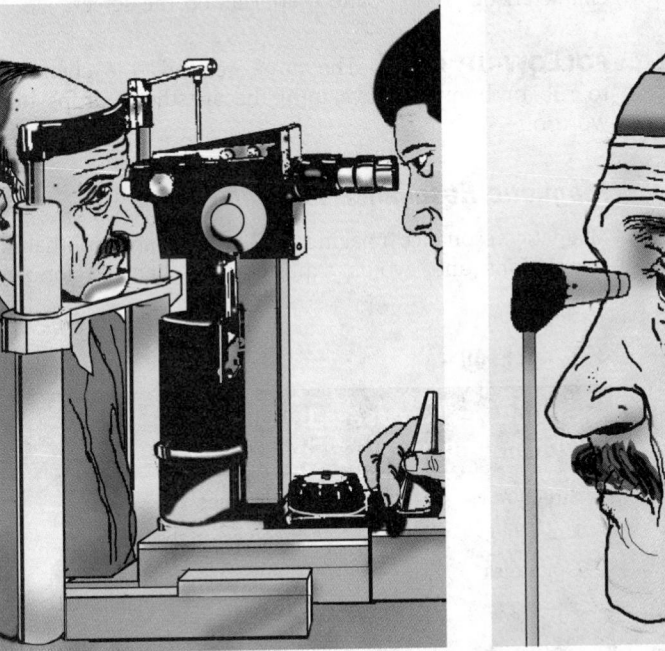

C

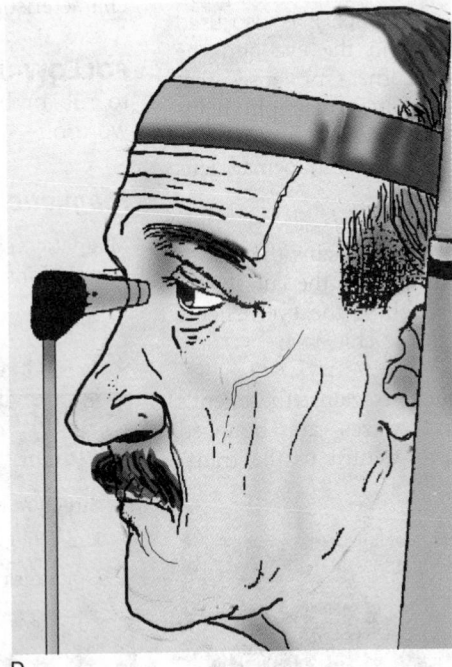

D

Figure 48–12. Methods of intraocular pressure estimation. *A,* Finger palpation is useful only when a large difference exists between the intraocular pressure of the two eyes, as in unilateral angle-closure glaucoma. *B,* Schiøtz tonometry can be learned readily. Because the tonometer is relatively inexpensive, it can be used in every physician's office to screen for chronic simple glaucoma. *C,* The air-puff tonometer can be used for screening large numbers of patients but is far more expensive than Schiøtz's tonometer. *D,* Goldman's applanation tonometer, used with a slit-lamp, is the standard instrument for glaucoma diagnosis and management for most ophthalmologists. It is expensive and requires considerable skill.

when examining the OS (left eye). The nurse stands on the same side as the eye being examined. The client is instructed to look straight ahead at an object on the wall behind the nurse. A thumb can be placed on the client's eyebrow to assist the examiner in knowing the distance from the ophthalmoscope to the client. The ophthalmoscope is held firmly against the nurse's face and is aligned so that the examiner's eye sees through the sight hole (Fig. 48–13).

When using the ophthalmoscope, the nurse approaches the client's eye from about 12 to 15 inches away and approximately 15 degrees lateral to the client's line of vision. As the ophthalmoscope is directed at the pupil, a red glare (the *red reflex*) is seen in the pupil. The red reflex is a reflection of the light on the vascular retina. Absence of the red reflex may indicate an opacity in the lens. With both of the nurse's eyes open and blinking normally, the nurse moves toward the pupil while following the red reflex. The retina should then be visible through the ophthalmoscope. Structures examined through the ophthalmoscope include the optic disk, optic vessels, fundus, and macula. Table 48–4 lists the features that should be observed in each structure.

TABLE 48-3

Types of Tonometry

Type of Tonometry	Advantages	Disadvantages
Noncontact (air-puff) tonometer A puff of air indents the cornea	• No direct contact with the client's cornea • No anesthesia needed • Very rapid	• Less accurate than direct contact methods • The puff of air is unpleasant and may startle the client
Schiøtz tonometer A small pressure gauge is placed on the cornea, and a weighted plunger is depressed	• Reliable readings • Portable • Low cost	• Touches the client's cornea • Requires topical anesthetic • May abrade or infect the cornea
Goldman's applanation tonometer The machine exerts a force against the cornea	• Highly accurate • Rapid	• Touches the client's cornea • Requires topical anesthetic • Danger of infection • Machine is expensive

Ultrasonography

Ultrasonography is used to examine the orbit and eye with high-frequency sound waves. This noninvasive test aids in the diagnosis of trauma, intraorbital tumors, proptosis, and choroidal or retinal detachments. It is also used to determine gross outline changes in the eye and the orbit of clients who have cloudy corneas or lenses that prevent examination of the fundus. Ultrasonography helps calculate the length of the eye, one of the measurements used to determine the strength of an intraocular lens implant needed after cataract surgery.

CLIENT PREPARATION. The nurse explains the test to the client and instills anesthetic drops into the cul-de-sac. The client is cautioned to avoid rubbing the eye. Clients are seated upright with the chin in the chin rest.

PROCEDURE. The probe is touched against the client's anesthetized cornea, and sound waves are bounced through the eye. The sound waves return to the trans-

ducer when they strike a non–fluid-filled structure. Anatomic structures reflecting sound waves are the cornea, anterior and posterior lens capsule, and retina. When these reflected sound waves return to the transducer, a characteristic "spike" pattern appears on the screen.

FOLLOW-UP CARE. The nurse reminds the client not to rub or bump the eye until the anesthetic drops have worn off.

Magnetic Resonance Imaging

Magnetic resonance imaging (MRI) has many ophthalmic applications and avoids exposing the client to ionizing

TABLE 48-4

Structures to Assess by Direct Ophthalmoscopy

Structure	Observations
Red reflex	• Presence or absence
Optic disk	• Color • Margins (sharp or blurred) • Cup size • Presence of rings or crescents
Optic blood vessels	• Size • Color • Kinks or tangles • Light reflection • Narrowing • Nicking at arteriovenous crossings
Fundus	• Color • Tears or holes • Lesions • Bleeding
Macula	• Presence of blood vessels • Color • Lesions • Bleeding

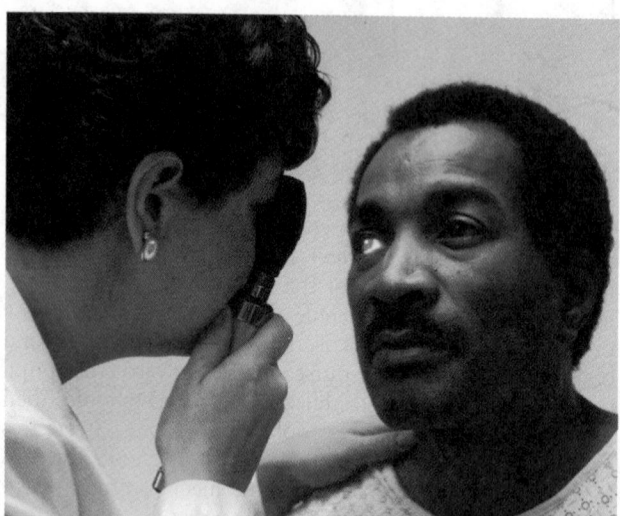

Figure 48-13. Proper technique for direct ophthalmoscopic visualization of the retina.

radiation. It is contraindicated with an actual or suspected metallic foreign body, because the magnetic pull can move the metal fragment and damage the eye.

The nurse explains to the client that the MRI study is performed in an enclosed space (although MRI units with open sides are becoming more available). Sedation may be necessary. If the client needs to be sedated, pulse oximetry is performed during the procedure because direct visualization for assessment of the client's respiratory status is not possible. The nurse ensures that all metallic jewelry is removed from the client until the procedure is completed.

Fluorescein Angiography

Fluorescein angiography provides a detailed image and permanent record of the ocular circulation. Photographs are taken in rapid succession after the intravenous administration of dye. This test is useful for the diagnosis of conditions affecting the circulation of the retina, such as diabetic retinopathy and macular degeneration, or for the diagnosis of intraocular tumors.

CLIENT PREPARATION. The nurse explains the procedure to the client, asks about allergies and previous reactions to dyes, and instills mydriatic (a drug causing pupil dilation) eyedrops about an hour before the test. Chart 48-2 lists the steps for correct instillation of eyedrops. The nurse makes sure that informed consent is obtained from the client or responsible person. The nurse warns the client that the dye may cause the skin to appear yellow for several hours after the test. The stain is gradually eliminated through the urine, which causes a change in urine color.

PROCEDURE. Venous access must be obtained. After the examiner validates that the catheter is in the vein, 5 mL of a 10% solution of fluorescein is injected into the client's peripheral vein. A camera is set up with ophthalmologic equipment to photograph retinal and choroidal blood vessels as the dye passes through these vessels. The procedure takes only minutes because the vessels fill quickly.

FOLLOW-UP CARE. After the test, the client may feel weak and nauseated. After the nausea resolves, clients are encouraged to drink fluids to remove the dye from their systems. The nurse encourages the client to rest and emphasizes that any yellow staining of the skin will disappear in a few hours. After the test, urine will be bright green until the dye is excreted. The nurse instructs the client to avoid direct sunlight after the test until pupil dilation returns to normal.

Electroretinography

Electroretinography is the process of graphing the retina's response to light stimulation. An electroretinogram is obtained by placing a contact lens electrode on a client's anesthetized cornea. Lights at varying speeds and intensities are flashed, and the neural response is graphed. The measurement from the cornea is identical to the response

---

> ### Chart 48-2
>
> ### Nursing Care Highlight: Instillation of Ophthalmic Drops
>
> - Wash your gloves.
> - Don gloves if secretions are present.
> - Explain the procedure to the client.
> - Check the name, strength, and expiration date of the solution.
> - Stand behind the client.
> - Instruct the client to tilt the head backward, open the eyes, and look up.
> - Have the client's head rest against your body.
> - Pull the lower lid downward against the cheekbone.
> - Hold the medication bottle like a pencil, with the tip down.
> - Rest the wrist holding the bottle on the client's cheek.
> - Without touching the tip of the bottle to the client's conjunctiva, squeeze the bottle gently and release the correct number of drops into the conjunctival pocket.
> - Gently release the lower eyelid.
> - Instruct the client to close the eyes gently, without squeezing the lids together.

that would be obtained if electrodes were placed directly on the retina.

Preparation includes instillation of an anesthetic into the eye. Afterward, the client is reminded to avoid rubbing the eye until the effects of the anesthetic have disappeared.

This procedure is especially helpful in detecting and evaluating retinal vascular changes such as diabetic or hypertensive retinopathy; traumatic alterations to the retinal blood supply, such as with a retinal detachment; toxic changes from the use of drugs; and systemic disorders, such as vitamin A deficiency.

SELECTED BIBLIOGRAPHY

Carter, T. (1994). Age-related vision changes: A primary care guide. *Geriatrics, 49*(9), 37–45.

Cleary, B. (1997). Age-related changes in the special senses. In M. Matteson, E. McConnell, & A. Linton (Eds.), *Gerontological nursing: Concepts and practice* (2nd ed., pp. 384–405). Philadelphia: W. B. Saunders.

Cleary, M. (1995). Helping the person who is visually impaired: Concerns, questions, remedies, & sources. *Journal of Ophthalmic Nursing and Technology, 14*(5), 205–211.

Cotran, R., Kumar, V., & Robbins, S. (1994). *Robbins pathologic basis of disease* (5th ed.). Philadelphia: W. B. Saunders.

Jarvis, C. (1996). *Physical examination and health assessment* (2nd ed). Philadelphia: W. B. Saunders.

Kavanaugh, K., & Tate, B. (1996). Recognizing and helping older persons with vision impairments. *Geriatric Nursing, 17*(2), 68–71.

Jubeck, M. (1994). Teaching the elderly: A common sense approach. *Nursing94, 24*(5), 70–71.

Kelly, M. (1995). Consequences of visual impairment on leisure activities of the elderly. *Geriatric Nursing, 16*(6), 273–275.

Kelly, M. (1996). Medications and the visually impaired elderly. *Geriatric Nursing, 17*(2), 60–62.

*Ruehl, C., & Schremp, P. (1992). Nursing care of the cataract patient: Today's outpatient approach. *Nursing Clinics of North America, 3*, 727–743.

Sandler, R. (1995). Clinical snapshot: Glaucoma. *American Journal of Nursing, 95*(3), 34–35.

Shoemaker, J. (1997). Adult vision screening by nonphysicians. *Journal of Ophthalmic Nursing & Technology, 16*(5), 244–250.

*Sullivan, N. (1983). Vision in the elderly. *Journal of Gerontological Nursing, 9*(4), 228–235.

*Vader, L. (1992). Vision and vision loss. *Nursing Clinics of North America, 27*(3), 705–714.

Vaughan, D., Asbury, T., & Riordan-Eva, P. (Eds.). (1995). *General ophthalmology* (14th ed.). Norwalk, CT: Appleton & Lange.

SUGGESTED READINGS

Cleary, B. (1997). Age-related changes in the special senses. In M. Matteson, E. McConnell, & A. Linton (Eds.), *Gerontological nursing: Concepts and practice* (2nd ed., pp 384–405). Philadelphia: W. B. Saunders.

This chapter provides excellent information for age-related changes in all special sensory areas. For vision, the authors first describe normal eye structure and function, and then discuss all expected age-related changes. Suggestions to assist clients in maintaining activities while vision diminishes are presented.

Kavanaugh, K., & Tate, B. (1996). Recognizing and helping older persons with vision impairments. *Geriatric Nursing, 17*(2), 68–71.

This article provides the reader with practical suggestions to assist older adults with a variety of visual problems. A useful item included in the text is a quality assurance check list for assessing "low-vision friendly environments."

*Sullivan, N. (1983). Vision in the elderly. *Journal of Gerontological Nursing, 9*(4), 228–235.

Although written more than a decade ago, this article remains a classic in its presentation of visual assessment and interventions for elderly clients with visual impairments. When each physiologic change is discussed, multiple suggestions are made for helping the older client to maintain independence, physical function, and social interaction in spite of the visual impairment.

*Vader, L. (1992). Vision and vision loss. *Nursing Clinics of North America, 27*(3), 705–714.

This unique article presents the concept of vision in terms of its personal and historical meaning. The role of eyes and vision in mysticism, religion, sexuality, and art is explored. Attitudes toward blindness are addressed from a historical and contemporary viewpoint.

Chapter 49

INTERVENTIONS FOR CLIENTS WITH EYE AND VISION PROBLEMS

Many conditions can adversely affect vision. Some conditions occur gradually, such as cataract, and others can result from an acute insult or illness. Visual changes affect each client in a unique manner, and the nurse uses a holistic approach to guide client care.

EXTERNAL EYE DISORDERS
Eyelid Disorders

The eyelid is composed of small muscles and thin skin. The eyelid protects the external eye surface and is responsible for the distribution of tears. Disorders can be related to changes in the structure, function, or position of the eyelid. Lid structure may also be altered by age (Figs. 49-1 and 49-2).

Blepharitis
Overview

Blepharitis, a common inflammation of the eyelid margins, is seen most frequently in the elderly and is often associated with *dry eye syndrome* (see later). The lack of a tear film accompanying this disorder may lead to bacterial

invasion of the eye structures, because tears are bacteriostatic.

Collaborative Management

Clients usually have itchy, red, and burning eyes. Seborrhea of the eyebrows and eyelids is often present. Upon slit-lamp examination, greasy scales and mattering may be seen on the eyelid-eyelash margin.

Blepharitis is best controlled by a regimen of eyelid care using warm moist compresses followed by gentle scrubbing with dilute baby shampoo. The nurse instructs the client not to rub the eyes because this action can spread the infection to other eye structures.

Entropion
Overview

An entropion is an inversion of the eyelid that results in eyelashes rubbing against the conjunctiva. It may be a congenital condition or may develop later in life, usually after age 40 years. Entropion can be caused by spasms of the muscle of the eyelid or by scarring and deformity of the eyelid itself as a result of trauma, chemical or thermal

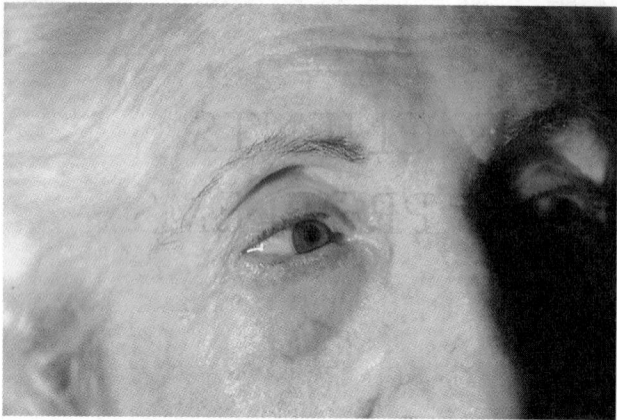

Figure 49–1. Eyelid eversion (ectropion).

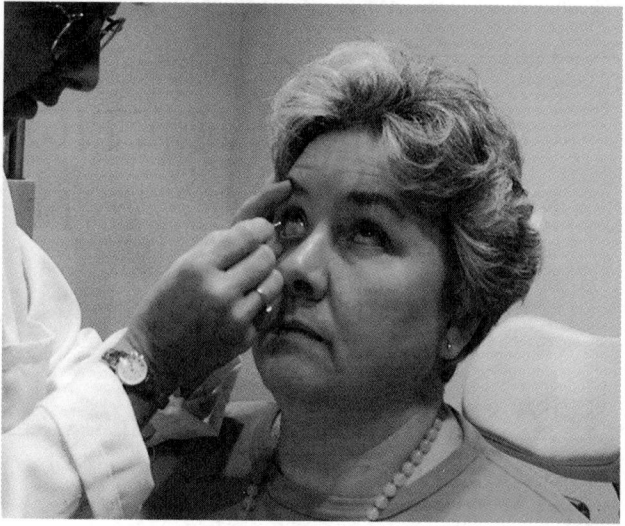

Figure 49–3. Application of ophthalmic ointment.

burns, atonia, or inflammation. Elderly clients are susceptible to entropion because of a loss of tissue support with aging.

Collaborative Management

The client usually reports "feeling something in my eye." Pain and tearing may also be present. On inspection, the eyelid is turned inward, and the conjunctiva may appear inflamed. Corneal abrasion may be present as a result of irritation from the eyelashes.

Surgery may correct the position of the eyelid by either tightening the orbicular muscle (thus moving the eyelid to a normal position) or directly preventing inward rotation of the eyelid margin. After surgery, the eye is usually covered with a patch, and the client is discharged a few hours later.

The nurse demonstrates instillation of eyedrops and evaluates the client's ability to instill the drops. The nurse instructs the client to leave the patch in place until he or she is seen by the ophthalmologist and to inform the ophthalmologist of any pain or drainage under the patch. If the client is to care for sutures, the nurse demonstrates how to clean the suture line with a cotton swab and the prescribed solution. A small amount of antibiotic oint-

ment may be applied (Fig. 49–3). Chart 49–1 describes the correct technique for applying ophthalmic ointment; Chart 49–2 summarizes important information on ophthalmic drugs.

Ectropion

Overview

An ectropion is the outward sagging and eversion of the eyelid (see Fig. 49–1). It may be congenital but is more often associated with aging. Ectropion is caused by relaxation of the orbicular muscle associated with aging, injury

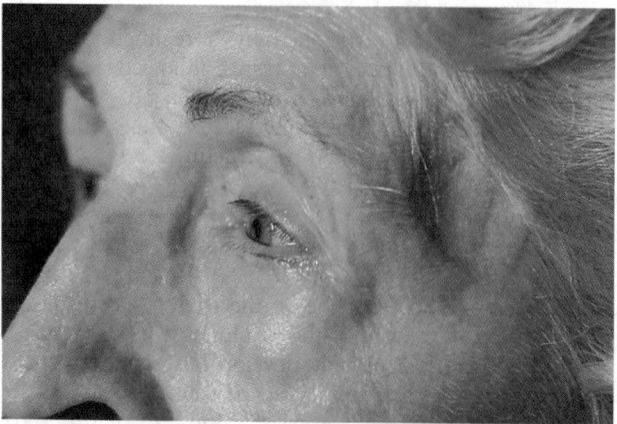

Figure 49–2. "Bags" under the eyes.

Chart 49–1

Nursing Care Highlight: Instillation of Ophthalmic Ointment

- Wash your hands.
- Wear gloves.
- Explain the procedure to the client.
- Check the name, strength, and expiration date of the medication.
- Instruct the client to tilt the head backward, open the eyes, and look up.
- Pull the client's lower lid downward, toward the cheekbone, creating a "pocket" in the lower lid.
- Hold the tube like a pencil, with the tip downward.
- Rest the wrist holding the tube on the client's cheek.
- Do not touch the tip of the tube to the conjunctiva.
- Squeeze the tube gently until a small amount of ointment is in the pocket.
- Release the lower eyelid.
- Instruct the client to close the eye gently.
- Tell the client that vision may be blurred by the ointment.
- Instruct the client to remove the ointment before driving or operating equipment.

Chart 49–2

Drug Therapy for Eye Problems

Drug	Nursing Interventions	Rationale
Topical Anesthetics Proparacaine HCl, or proxymetacine (AK-Taine, Alcaine, Ocu-Caine, Ophthetic) Tetracaine HCl, cocaine HCl (Pontocaine)	• Use nasal punctal occlusion. • Remind the client not to rub or touch the eye while it is anesthetized. • Patch the eye if the client leaves facility before the anesthetic wears off. • Do not use discolored solution. • Store the bottle tightly closed.	• This technique decreases systemic absorption and side effects. • Touching may injure the eye. • The use of a patch prevents injury, such as corneal abrasion. • Discoloration is a sign of altered drug composition. • Air may cause drug contamination and oxidation.
Topical Steroids Prednisolone acetate (Ocu-Pred, Ophtho-Tate✦) Prednisolone phosphate (Inflamase) Dexamethasone (Dexair, DexOtic, Maxidex✦) Betamethasone (Betnesol) Fluorometholone (Fluor-Op, Liquifilm)	• Shake vigorously before use. • Monitor the client for signs of corneal ulceration. • Advise the client not to share eyedrops with others.	• Medication is a suspension; shaking is required to distribute the medication evenly in the solution. • Steroid use predisposes the client to local infection. • Disease transmission is possible when sharing eyedrops.
Anti-infective Agents Gentamicin (Alcomicin✦, Garamycin, Genoptic) Tobramycin (Tobrex) Ciprofloxacin (Ciloxan) Erythromycin (Ilotycin) Chlortetracycline (Aureomycin) Sulfisoxazole (Gantrisin)	• Be sure to obtain a specimen for culture before use. • Clean exudate from the eyes before administering drops. • Reinforce the importance of completing the prescribed medication regimen.	• Use of an antibiotic before a culture specimen is obtained may alter culture results. • Cleansing decreases the risk of contaminating the medication and increases contact of the conjunctiva with the medication. • Compliance is critical to maintain a therapeutic level of medication.
Antibiotic-Steroid Combinations Tobramycin with dexamethasone (TobraDex) Neomycin sulfate with polymyxin B sulfate and dexamethasone (Maxitrol)	• This is the same as for each component alone.	• This is the same as for each component alone.
Topical Antiviral Agents Idoxuridine (Herplex, Stoxil) Trifluridine (Viroptic) Vidarabine (Vira-A)	• Refrigerate and protect from light. • Monitor the client for itching lids and burning eyes.	• Cool temperatures and absence of light ensures medication stability. • Sensitivity to this drug is common.
Adrenergics Dipivefrin HCl (Propine)	• Instruct the client to use nasal punctal occlusion during administration. • Monitor the client's heart rate and blood pressure.	• Nasal punctal occlusion decreases systemic absorption and side effects. • Systemic absorption increases the heart rate and blood pressure.
Beta-Blockers Betaxolol HCl (Betoptic) Carteolol (Ocupress) Levobunolol (Betagan) Metipranolol (OptiPranolol)	• Instruct the client to use nasal punctal occlusion during administration. • Monitor the client's heart rate and blood pressure.	• Nasal punctal occlusion decreases systemic absorption and side effects. • Systemic absorption slows the heart rate and may decrease blood pressure, causing orthostatic hypotension.

Continued

CHART 49–2. Drug Therapy for Eye Problems Continued

Miotics		
Carbachol (Isopto Carbachol, Miostat) Pilocarpine HCl (Isopto Carpine, Miocarpine✦, Pilocar, Spersacarpine✦)	• Warn the client that visual acuity is decreased in low-light environments. • Use with caution in clients who have urinary tract obstruction.	• This drug causes severe pupillary constriction. • This drug mimics parasympathetic system and can cause urinary retention.
Mydriatics and Cycloplegics		
Atropine (Atropair, Minims Atropine✦, Ocu-Tropine) Cyclopentolate (Cyclogyl, Minims Cyclopentate✦) Phenylephrine (Minims Phenylephrine, Neo-Synephrine, Ocu-Phrin, Spersaphrine✦) Tropicamide (Minims Tropicamide✦, Mydriacyl, Tropicacyl)	• Instruct the client to wear sunglasses until the drug wears off. • Instruct the client to avoid driving or operating hazardous machinery until the drug wears off. • Instruct the client to use nasal punctal occlusion during administration.	• The drug causes photophobia. • The drug causes blurred vision. • This technique decreases systemic absorption and side effects.

or paralysis of the seventh cranial nerve, or scarring caused by trauma, burns, or ulcers. This lid position does not permit tears to wash adequately over the eye anterior surface. Corneal drying and ulceration also result from an inability to keep the cornea moist.

Collaborative Management

Clients frequently complain of constant tearing. Outward deviation of the eyelid is noted on close observation.

Surgery is required to restore proper lid alignment. After surgery, the eye is covered with a patch and the client is discharged. Nursing interventions are the same as those for the client with an entropion.

Ptosis

Overview

Ptosis is the drooping of, or inability to use, the upper eyelid. This disorder can be congenital or can result from muscle dysfunction, excessive weight of the eyelids from edema, inflammation, tumors, or any injury to the third cranial nerve.

Collaborative Management

If the ptosis is slight and does not alter appearance or visual function, no intervention is needed. Outpatient surgery is performed to improve elevation of the eyelid if visual acuity or appearance is adversely affected.

The nurse assesses the eye and eyelid for redness or purulent drainage and reports any evidence of infection to the ophthalmologist. Cool compresses are applied after surgery to decrease edema formation.

Nursing interventions include instilling an ophthalmic antibiotic or an antibiotic-steroid combination ointment, such as tobramycin plus dexamethasone (TobraDex), and teaching the client how to instill it. The nurse instructs the client to keep the eye as clean as possible and to avoid rubbing the eyelid.

Hordeolum

Overview

A hordeolum, or *stye*, can be external or internal. An external hordeolum is an infection of the sweat glands in the eyelid, occurring near the exit of the eyelashes from the eyelid, called the *eyelid-eyelash margin*. A localized, red, swollen, tender area is noted on the skin surface side of the margin. An internal hordeolum is caused by an infection of the eyelid sebaceous glands. The most common causative organisms are *Staphylococcus aureus, Staphylococcus epidermidis,* and *Streptococcus.* The hordeolum and its localized redness usually affect only one eyelid at a time. Vision is not affected.

Chart 49–3

Education Guide: Application of an Ocular Compress

1. Wash your hands.
2. Fold a clean washcloth into fourths.
3. Soak the washcloth with running tap water that is warm to your inner wrist. (If cool compresses are needed, follow the same steps using cold running tap water.)
4. Place the cloth over your *closed* eye.
5. Keep the cloth in place with minimal pressure until the cloth cools.
6. Refold the washcloth so that a different "fourth" will be held against the eye.
7. Resoak the cloth with running tap water.
8. Repeat applications three times for as many times each day as are ordered by your physician.

Chart 49–4

Nursing Care Highlight: Application of an Eyepatch

Nonpressure Eyepatch

1. Assemble the equipment:
   - Eyepatch
   - Skin preparation
   - Nonallergenic paper tape
2. Explain the procedure to the client.
3. Wash your hands.
4. Apply a skin preparation to the client's forehead and cheek.
5. Instruct the client to close both eyes gently.
6. Place a patch over the closed eyelid.

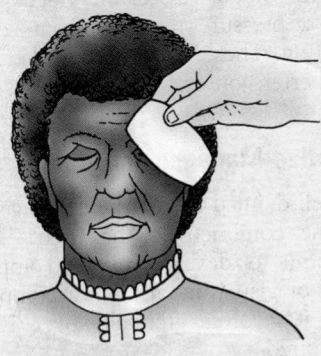

7. Apply tape from the cheek to the middle of the forehead in a diagonal line.

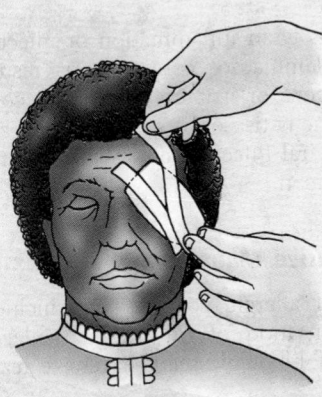

8. Cover the patch with overlapping pieces of tape.

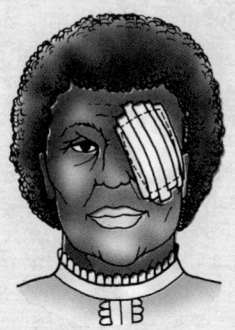

Pressure Eyepatch

1. Assemble the equipment:
   - Two eyepatches for each eye requiring treatment
   - Skin preparation pad
   - Nonallergenic paper tape
2–5. Follow corresponding steps under Nonpressure Eyepatch.
6. Fold one eyepatch in half, place it over the closed eyelid, and apply a second eyepatch (unfolded) over the folded one.

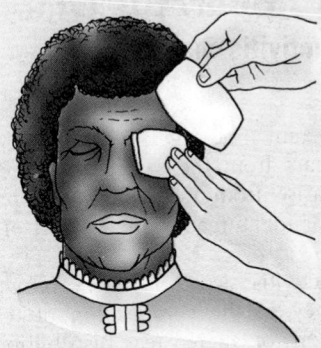

7, 8. Follow corresponding steps under Nonpressure Eyepatch.

Collaborative Management

Small, beady, edematous areas may be noted on the skin side of the eyelid or on the conjunctival side of the eyelid-eyelash margin. As the hordeolum forms, it fills with purulent material, which causes pain.

Treatment includes use of warm compresses four times a day and an antibacterial ointment. When the lesion opens, either spontaneously or after use of warm compresses, the purulent material drains and pain subsides.

Nursing interventions include applying a clean washcloth compress and instructing the client in this application. Chart 49–3 describes the proper technique for applying ocular compresses.

After the compresses have been applied for the prescribed time, the nurse instills antibiotic ointment. The client is advised that ointments may cause blurred vision and is taught to remove the ointment from the eyes before driving or operating machinery. To remove the ointment, the client closes the eye and gently wipes the closed eyelid from the inner canthus outward.

Chalazion

Overview

A chalazion is a sterile, granulomatous inflammation of a sebaceous gland in the eyelid. It begins with inflammation and tenderness, similar to the hordeolum, and is characterized by a gradual painless swelling at the gland. In its fully developed state, no inflammatory signs are present.

Collaborative Management

Most chalazia point on the conjunctival side of the eyelid. The client has eye fatigue, sensitivity to light, and possibly epiphora (excessive tearing).

Treatment includes the use of warm compresses for 15 minutes four times a day, followed by instillation of ophthalmic ointment. The physician excises the chalazion if it is large enough to affect vision, is cosmetically unsatisfactory to the client, or recurs frequently.

After excision, antibiotic ointment is instilled and the eye is covered with a patch. Steps for proper application of a nonpressure eyepatch are described in Chart 49–4.

The client is instructed to leave the eyepatch intact for 4–6 hours, and then remove the patch and begin applying warm, moist compresses. Antibiotic eyedrops are instilled after the use of the compresses. The nurse instructs the client to report any evidence of infection, increasing redness, purulent drainage, or reduced vision to the ophthalmologist immediately.

Lacrimal Apparatus Disorders

Keratoconjunctivitis Sicca

Overview

The lacrimal system moistens the external eye with tears and removes tears from the external surface of the eye. Problems can arise from insufficient tear production or from infection or inflammation in any part of the lacrimal system.

Keratoconjunctivitis sicca, or *dry eye syndrome*, results from a deficiency in the composition of tears, lacrimal gland malfunction, or altered tear distribution. Decreased tear production can also occur during antihistamine, beta-adrenergic blocking agent, or anticholinergic drug therapy. Diseases associated with decreased tear production include rheumatoid arthritis, leukemia, sarcoidosis, multiple sclerosis, mumps, and lymphoma. Radiation or chemical burns can also decrease lacrimal system function. Injury to the facial nerve (cranial nerve VII) can inhibit tearing.

Collaborative Management

The client has a foreign body sensation, burning and itching eyes, and photophobia (increased sensitivity to light). The corneal light reflex is dulled or distorted. The tear film may contain strands of mucus.

Treatment depends on the severity of the symptoms. Artificial tears (HypoTears, Refresh) are prescribed for daytime use to reduce dryness, and can be used as often as necessary. At night, a lubricating ointment (Lacri-Lube S.O.P., Refresh P.M.) is used. If the dry eye syndrome is caused by an abnormal eyelid position or function, surgery may be required.

Conjunctival Disorders

The conjunctiva is a thin mucous membrane that acts as a protective coating for the eye. Because of its location, the conjunctiva is subject to trauma and exposure to noxious gases and is susceptible to infection.

Subconjunctival Hemorrhage

Overview

Subconjunctival blood vessels are fragile and can break after increased pressure resulting from sneezing, coughing, or vomiting. These hemorrhages also may be associated with hypertension or blood dyscrasias.

Collaborative Management

The small, well-defined area of hemorrhage appears bright red under the conjunctiva. The client is usually quite concerned about its development and appearance. However, no pain or visual impairment accompanies the hemorrhage, and it resolves gradually over 10–14 days; no treatment required.

Conjunctivitis

Overview

Conjunctivitis is an inflammation or infection of the conjunctiva. Inflammatory conjunctivitis results from exposure to allergens or irritants and is not contagious. Infectious conjunctivitis occurs frequently as a result of bacterial or viral infection and is readily transmitted from person to person.

Collaborative Management

Symptoms of allergic conjunctivitis include conjunctival edema, a sensation of burning, vascular injection (engorgement of blood vessels), excessive tearing, and itching.

Treatment includes the instillation of vasoconstrictors and corticosteroid eyedrops. The client is instructed to refrain from using make-up until all symptoms of conjunctivitis subside.

Bacterial conjunctivitis, or "pink eye," is caused by S. aureus, Haemophilus influenzae, or Pseudomonas aeruginosa. Symptoms include blood vessel dilation, mild conjunctival edema, tearing, and discharge. The discharge is watery at first and then gradually becomes thicker, with shreds of mucus.

The causative microorganism of bacterial conjunctivitis is identified by obtaining specimens of the discharge for culture. Treatment is aimed at controlling the infection. A broad-spectrum topical antibiotic is administered until specific sensitivities of the microorganism are determined.

Nursing interventions are focused on preventing the spread of the disease. For example, cross-contamination may cause involvement of the other eye. The amount, color, and type of drainage are noted. The nurse reviews hygienic principles with the client, including hand washing after touching the eye and before instilling eyedrops. The client is warned not to touch the unaffected eye without first washing the hands and to avoid sharing washcloths and towels with others.

Trachoma

Overview

Trachoma is a chronic, bilateral scarring form of conjunctivitis caused by *Chlamydia trachomatis*. Trachoma infection is the chief cause of blindness in the world. Incidence is highest in warm, moist climates where hygienic practices are substandard.

Collaborative Management

The incubation period is 5–14 days. Initially, trachoma resembles bacterial conjunctivitis. Symptoms include tearing, photophobia, edema of the eyelids, and conjunctival edema. Follicles form on the upper eyelid conjunctiva. As the disease progresses, the eyelid scars and turns inward, causing the eyelashes to abrade the cornea.

Specimens are obtained for culture to identify the causative organism. A 4-week course of oral tetracycline (Achromycin, Apo-Tetra✦) or erythromycin (Apo-Erythro✦, E-Mycin, E.E.S.) is given. These drugs may be applied topically if the systemic forms are unavailable.

Nursing interventions focus on infection control. The client is instructed to wash the hands before and after touching the eyes. The nurse advises the client to keep his or her washcloths separate from those of unaffected people and to launder them separately. The nurse also emphasizes the importance of completing the prescribed course of antibiotics.

Corneal Disorders

Overview

For a sharp image to be produced on the retinal receptors, the cornea must be transparent and intact. Corneal problems are the leading cause of visual impairment in the United States and Canada. Corneal disorders may be caused by degeneration of the cornea (keratoconus; Fig. 49–4); deposition of substances in the cornea, altering its refracting power (dystrophies); inflammation from either irritation or infection (keratitis); or ulceration of the corneal surface. Table 49–1 lists common causes of corneal disorders.

Collaborative Management

► Physical Assessment/Clinical Manifestations

The client with a corneal disorder usually has pain or reduced vision, photophobia, and eye secretions are also

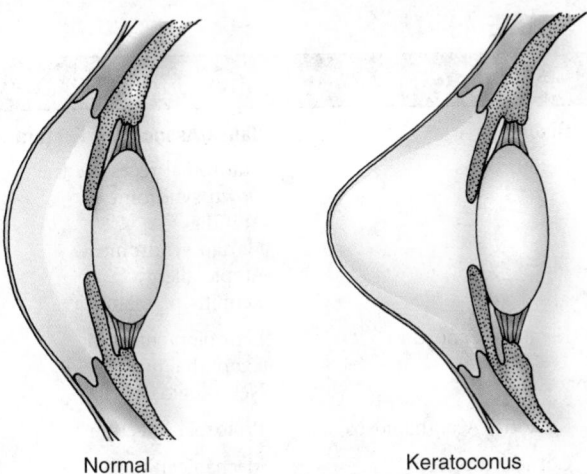

Normal   **Keratoconus**

Figure 49–4. Profiles of a normal eyeball and one with keratoconus.

common. The nurse notes cloudy or purulent fluid on the eyelids or eyelashes. The nurse always wears gloves during the examination when secretions are noted.

The cornea may look hazy or cloudy. An altered corneal light reflex may be noted. The cornea may no longer be intact, and patchy areas may be visible on examination. When fluorescein is used, these areas appear green.

No definitive tests exist to confirm corneal disease. However, several tests, including microbial culture and corneal scrapings, can help determine which organism is causing a corneal ulcer. For microbial culture, swabs from the ulcer and its margins are obtained and sent to the laboratory to identify microorganisms. For corneal scrapings, the cornea is anesthetized with a topical agent, and a sterile spatula is used to remove samples from the center and edge of the ulcer.

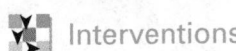 Interventions

► Nonsurgical Management

Treatment for the client with a corneal disorder is aimed at reducing symptoms, restoring corneal clarity, and enhancing the client's ability to use his or her remaining vision.

Drug Therapy. Antibiotics, antifungals, and antivirals are prescribed to reduce the number of microorganisms. Clients are first started on a broad-spectrum antibiotic regimen after the culture. This antibiotic may be changed when the results of the culture are known. Steroids may be used in selected cases of ocular herpes to reduce the inflammatory response in the eye. Drugs can be administered topically as eyedrops, injected subconjunctivally, or administered intravenously. Chart 49–5 lists the principles of eyedrop administration.

Vision Enhancement. The nurse assists clients in using their functional vision, suggesting sunglasses and indirect lighting if glare creates difficulties. The nurse also informs them about assistive devices, such as magnifiers and special light fixtures.

TABLE 49-1

Common Causes of Corneal Disorders	
Disorder	**Cause/Associated Factors**
Keratoconus	Autosomal recessive trait
	Down syndrome
	Aniridia
	Marfan syndrome
	Atopic allergy
	Retinitis pigmentosa
Keratitis (exposure)	Ectropion/entropion
	Exophthalmos
	Neurologic deficits
Keratitis (Acanthamoeba)	Protozoal infection
Corneal ulcers	Mechanical injury
	Chemical injury
	Drying
	Infection

Chart 49-5

Nursing Care Highlight: Eyedrop Administration

- Administer drugs at frequent, precise intervals. *The timing of administration is critical.* Clients with eye problems are often given several broad-spectrum antibiotics. If each drug is administered every hour, create separate dosage schedules. For example, give antibiotic A at 7:00, 8:00, 9:00, and 10:00. Then give antibiotic B at 7:30, 8:30, 9:30, and 10:30.
- If two medications must be administered *at the same time, separate instillation by 5 minutes.* For example, a client with glaucoma and a bacterial ulcer receives timolol (Apo-Timop✽, Timoptic) at 7:00 and tobramycin (Tobrex) at 7:05.
- If the same medication is required for both eyes and one eye is infected, use *separate* bottles of medication.
- Clearly label each bottle for the appropriate eye (OS for the left eye, OD for the right eye).
- Wear gloves when ocular drainage is present.
- Wash your hands before and after administering eyedrops.

➤ Surgical Management

Keratoplasty, or corneal transplant, is the surgical removal of diseased corneal tissue and replacement with tissue from a human donor cornea. Transplantation restores vision by removing corneal opacities or scars created by injury or infection or by correcting a corneal dystrophy.

There are two approaches: lamellar and penetrating. In the lamellar approach (partial-thickness keratoplasty), the superficial cornea is removed and replaced with donor tissue. In penetrating keratoplasty, the full thickness of the client's cornea is removed and replaced with donor tissue. The penetrating approach is used most often because it produces optimal visual clarity.

Preoperative Care. Corneal transplantation is performed as a scheduled surgical procedure or when donor tissue becomes available. Usually, the client is quite anxious. The nurse's calm approach is helpful during discussions with the client. The nurse assesses the client's knowledge of the surgery and of preoperative and postoperative routines, providing information as needed.

The nurse examines the client's eyes for signs of infection and immediately reports any redness, watery or purulent drainage, or edema around the eye to the ophthal-

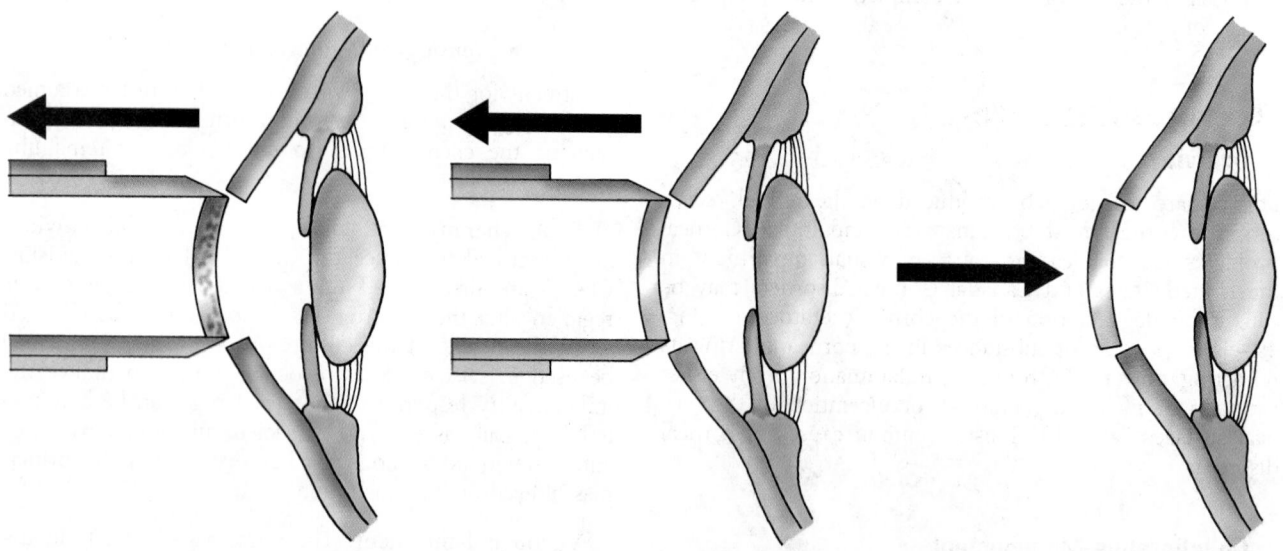

The diseased cornea is removed with a trephine.

A button, or graft, of donor cornea is removed with the same trephine so that the cuts are identical.

The donor cornea is placed on the eye and stitched into place with suture material that is finer than a human hair.

Figure 49-5. The steps involved in corneal transplantation (penetrating keratoplasty).

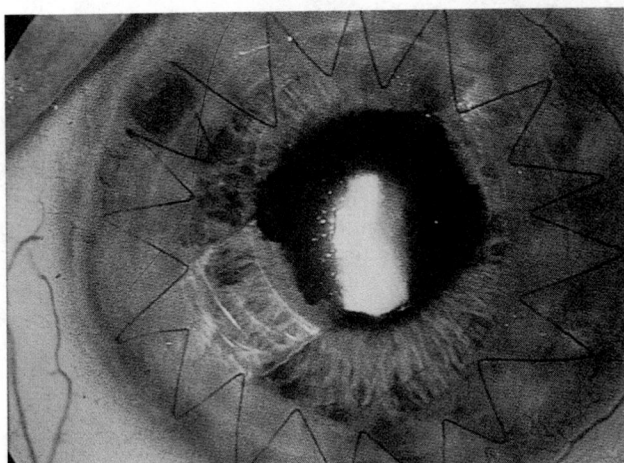

Figure 49-6. The appearance of the eye with sutures in place after corneal transplantation. (Courtesy of John A. Costin, MD.)

mologist. Antibiotic drops are instilled into the eye to reduce the number of microorganisms present. An intravenous catheter is inserted to administer fluids and medication.

Operative Procedure. The surgeon removes the center 7 to 8 mm of the diseased cornea (Fig. 49-5) with a trephine, a circular knife that operates much like a cookie cutter. The same trephine is used to cut a button of tissue from the donor cornea. The donor corneal button, also called the graft, is positioned on the eye and sutured into place with a running suture. Figure 49-6 shows sutures in place in the eye after corneal transplantation.

During a keratoplasty, the client is usually under regional anesthesia. The nerves around and behind the eye are numbed so that the client cannot move or see out of the eye.

Postoperative Care. After the procedure is completed, a subconjunctival antibiotic injection is given and an antibiotic ointment instilled. The eye is covered with a pressure patch and a protective metal or plastic shield. This initial dressing is left in place until the next day. The nurse does not remove or change the dressing without a specific order from the ophthalmologist.

The nurse notifies the ophthalmologist of any significant changes in vital signs or of drainage on the dressing. The client is instructed to lie on the nonoperative side to reduce intraocular pressure (IOP). During the immediate postoperative period, the client cannot see out of the affected eye because of the eyepatch and shield.

If the client is to maintain the patches after discharge, the nurse shows the client how to apply a patch and obtains a return demonstration from the client. The client is instructed to wear the shield at night for 1 month and whenever around small children or pets.

Complications after corneal transplant surgery include bleeding, wound leakage, infection, and graft rejection. Bleeding from the eye or suture line may be caused by inadequate hemostasis or IOP. Wound leakage is caused by incomplete wound closure.

Although the cornea has no blood supply, graft rejection is still possible. The inflammatory process starts in the donor cornea near the graft margin and moves centrally. Vision is reduced, and the cornea becomes cloudy. The client is treated with frequent applications of topical corticosteroids. If the rejection process continues, the cornea becomes opaque, and blood vessels may begin to branch into the opaque tissue.

Eye Donation. Tissue for a keratoplasty is obtained from a local eye or tissue bank. An eye bank obtains its supply of corneal tissue from volunteer donors. These donors must be free from infectious disease or cancer at the time of death.

If a deceased client is a potential eye donor, the nurse
- Raises the head of the bed 30 degrees
- Instills antibiotic eyedrops, such as Neosporin or tobramycin
- Closes the eyes and applies a small ice pack to the closed eyes
- Contacts the family and physician to discuss eye donation (see Research Applications for Nursing)

▷ Research Applications for Nursing

Continuing the Nursing Care for a Deceased Client Leaves a Positive Impression on Relatives

Doerling, J. (1996). Families' experiences in consenting to eye donation of a recently deceased relative. Heart & Lung, 25(1), 72-78.

The purpose of this descriptive study was to explore the experiences of families consenting to eye donation of a recently deceased relative. Relatives from 16 donors were randomly selected and interviewed within 3 to 12 months after the death. All interviews were conducted in person in the participant's home. Among the 16 donors, 12 donations were solicited by health care personnel, most frequently a nurse, and 4 donations were initiated by relatives. Most participants were comfortable with their decision, even when the eyes were used for research rather than for transplantation. Participants generally stated that they believed the person who solicited the donation was a caring individual but also that they wanted more explanations from physicians about the causes of death. In addition, they stated that an insufficient amount of debriefing time with a health care professional had been allotted to them. The follow-up letter from the eye bank was viewed positively by the participants.

Critique. This study supported the results of other studies: people making the decision to donate organs of dying relatives believe it is the "right thing to do," especially if the donor had previously signed an organ donor card. Additional study exploring the perceptions of relatives approached for organ donation but who refuse to consent might provide greater insight into how best to interact with them.

Possible Nursing Implications. The results of this study imply that the perception of caring on the part of the health care professional approaching family members for organ donation was a determining factor in giving consent. Nurses should keep this factor in mind when approaching a family and not maintain a "professional distance."

Scleral Disorders

Episcleritis

Overview

Episcleritis is a localized inflammation of the episclera, usually close to the corneal margin. Its cause is unknown, but hypersensitivity reactions are suspected. It is a common finding in clients with rheumatoid arthritis, syphilis, herpes zoster, and tuberculosis. Episcleritis is usually unilateral and affects men and women equally.

Collaborative Management

The eyeball appears pink or purple, with edema of the episclera and hyperemia of the episcleral vessels. Signs and symptoms include ocular redness, pain, lacrimation, and photophobia. Diagnosis is made on the basis of the clinical symptoms and ocular examination.

Episcleritis is usually self-limiting and disappears in 1 to 2 weeks. Topical corticosteroids may be used to reduce inflammation. Because corticosteroids may predispose the client to corneal ulcers, the nurse instructs the client to report any ocular injury to the ophthalmologist.

INTRAOCULAR DISORDERS
Lens Disorders

Cataract

Overview

The lens is a biconvex, transparent, refractive elastic structure suspended behind the iris. A cataract is an opacity of the lens that distorts the image projected onto the retina (Fig. 49–7). The degree of disability created by the cataract is determined by the location and density of the opacification as well as the client's age, occupation, and living arrangements. Intervention is indicated when visual acuity has been reduced to a level that the client finds unacceptable or that adversely affects lifestyle.

Pathophysiology

With aging, the lens gradually loses water and increases in density. This increased density results from the com-

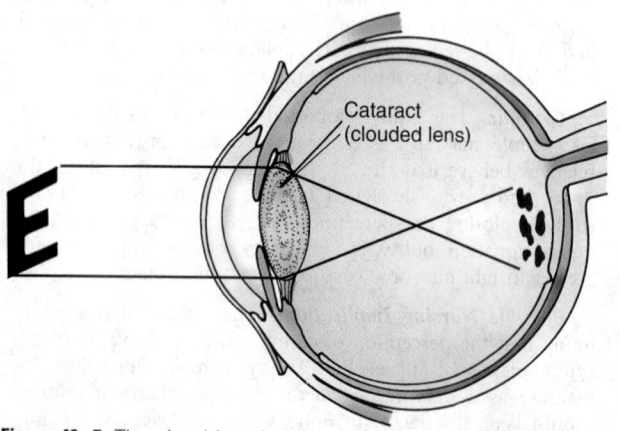

Figure 49–7. The visual impairment produced by the presence of a cataract.

TABLE 49–2

Common Causes of Cataracts	
Cataract Type	**Cause/Associated Factors**
Age-related	Lens water loss and fiber compaction
Traumatic	Blunt injury to eye or head Penetrating eye injury Intraocular foreign bodies Radiation exposure, therapy
Toxic	Corticosteroids Phenothiazine derivatives Miotic agents
Associated	Diabetes mellitus Hypoparathyroidism Down syndrome Chronic sunlight exposure
Complicated	Retinitis pigmentosa Glaucoma Retinal detachment

pression of older lens fibers and the production of new fibers in the outer layers. Opacities can develop in any part of the lens or capsule. A cataract forms as compaction of fibers reduces lens water content and causes lens proteins to precipitate. Over time, a progressive, painless, and bilateral loss of lens transparency occurs; however, the rate of progression in each eye is seldom similar.

Etiology

Cataracts are classified by nature or by onset. They may be present at birth or develop at any time. Cataracts may be age-related or result from trauma or exposure to toxic substances. Cataract formation also is associated with specific diseases and other ocular disorders (see Table 49–2).

Incidence/Prevalence

Cataracts develop in approximately 5 to 10 million people worldwide every year. The age-related cataract is the most common. Some degree of cataract formation is expected in all people older than 70 years (Vaughan et al., 1995).

Collaborative Management

 Assessment

> *History*

When taking a history from a client with known or suspected cataracts, the nurse notes the client's age, because cataracts are most prevalent in the elderly. The nurse asks about other predisposing factors, including

- Recent or past trauma to the eye
- Exposure to radioactive materials or x-rays
- Systemic disease (such as diabetes mellitus, hypoparathyroidism, Down syndrome, and atopic dermatitis)

- Use of medications (such as corticosteroids, chlorpromazine, or miotic drugs)
- Intraocular disease (such as recurrent uveitis)

The nurse asks the client to describe his or her vision. For example, the nurse might say, "Tell me what you can see well and what you have difficulty seeing." This technique helps the nurse determine the impact of visual deficits on the client.

➤ Physical Assessment/Clinical Manifestations

Early manifestations of cataract development include slightly blurred vision and decreased color perception (Chart 49–6). As lens opacification continues, the client may complain of a decrease in vision that adversely affects daily activities. Central lens opacities may divide the visual axis, creating the optical defect of seeing two blurred images. This visual deterioration can progress to blindness if no surgical intervention is performed. *No pain or eye redness is associated with age-related cataract formation.*

Visual acuity is significantly reduced. Vision can be tested using a Snellen chart and brightness acuity testing (see Chap. 48). The nurse evaluates the client's acuity under various lighting conditions, which can help determine the exact location of the cataract in the lens and the degree of visual disability.

The nurse examines the lens with the direct ophthalmoscope and describes any observed densities by size, shape, and location. As the cataract matures, the opacification makes visualization of the retina increasingly difficult. Eventually, fundus reflection is absent, with no red reflex. When this occurs, the pupil is white (Fig. 49–8), the most easily detected symptom of a cataract.

➤ Psychosocial Assessment

Loss of eyesight is usually gradual, and the client may not be aware of the change until such activities as reading, meal preparation, and driving are affected. Fear of losing one's eyesight can be overwhelming, and the client may exhibit great anxiety during an ocular evaluation. When questioning the client about eyesight, the nurse uses a calm approach and empathizes with the client's fears.

Chart 49–6

Key Features of Cataracts

Early
- Blurred vision
- Decreased color perception

Late
- Diplopia
- Reduced visual acuity progressing to blindness
- Absence of red reflex
- Presence of white pupil

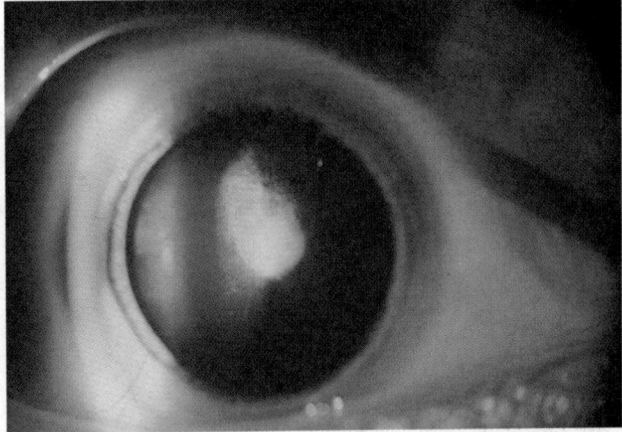

Figure 49–8. The appearance of an eye with a mature cataract. (Courtesy of John A. Costin, MD.)

 Analysis

➤ Common Nursing Diagnoses and Collaborative Problems

The most common diagnosis for the client with a cataract is Sensory/Perceptual Alterations (Visual) related to ocular lens opacity.

➤ Additional Nursing Diagnoses and Collaborative Problems

The client also may present with one or more of the following diagnoses:
- Fear related to loss of eyesight, scheduled surgery, or inability to regain eyesight
- Risk for Injury related to decreased vision, age, or presence in an unfamiliar environment
- Social Isolation related to reduced visual acuity, fear of injury, decreased ability to navigate in the community, or fear of embarrassment
- Self-Care Deficit related to visual impairment
- Knowledge Deficit (cataract pathophysiology and treatment) related to lack of information or misinterpretation of previously acquired information
- Impaired Home Maintenance Management related to age, limited vision, or activity restrictions imposed by surgery

 Planning and Implementation

➤ Sensory/Perceptual Alterations (Visual)

Planning: Expected Outcomes. The desired outcome is that the client's vision improves.

Interventions. Surgery and a variety of nursing interventions facilitate the client's recovery of vision.

Preoperative Care. The nurse provides clients with accurate information so that she or he can make informed decisions about treatment. The nurse teaches the client

EXTRACAPSULAR
CATARACT EXTRACTION

INTRACAPSULAR
CATARACT EXTRACTION

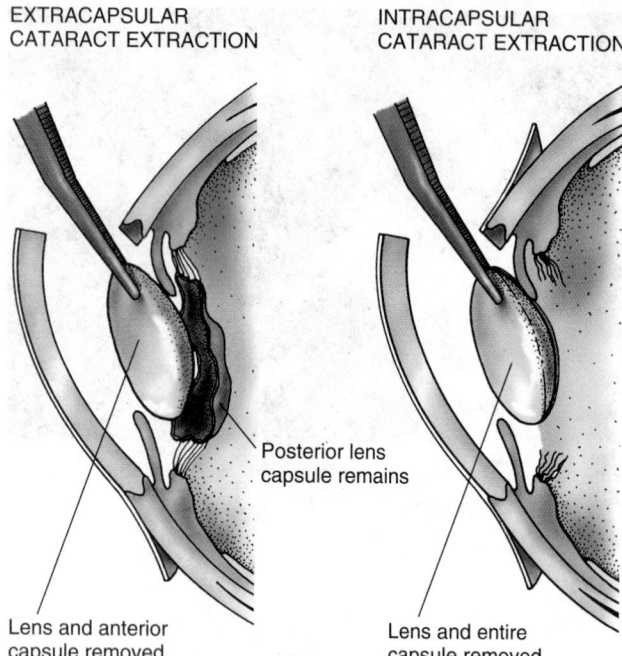

Posterior lens
capsule remains

Lens and anterior
capsule removed

Lens and entire
capsule removed

Figure 49–9. Surgical approaches to lens removal for cataracts.

about the nature of cataracts, their progression, and their treatment.

Because cataract surgery is usually an outpatient procedure and most clients are elderly, adequate preoperative teaching is problematic. The nurse assesses how well the client's vision allows participation in the daily living skills of dressing, eating, and ambulating.

The nurse reviews presurgical events. An intravenous infusion may be started in the client's room or in the operating room. A sedative is given preoperatively, and oral acetazolamide (Acetazolam✦, Diamox) may be given on the morning of surgery to reduce intraocular pressure (IOP). The nurse instills a series of sympathomimetic drugs preoperatively, such as phenylephrine (Neo-Synephrine, Spersaphrine✦), to achieve mydriasis and vasoconstriction. The nurse also administers parasympatholytic drops, such as tropicamide (Minims Tropicamide✦, Mydriacyl) or cyclopentolate hydrochloride (Cyclogyl, Minims Cyclopentolate✦), to induce paralysis and render the ciliary muscles unable to move the lens.

After the client is in the surgical area, a local anesthetic is administered into the muscle cone behind the eye to achieve anesthesia and ensure eye paralysis. The client may receive an intravenous injection of midazolam (Versed) to create a few minutes of light anesthesia during the administration of local anesthesia.

Operative Procedure. Extraction of the cataractous lens can be extracapsular or intracapsular (see Fig. 49–9). The most common procedure is extracapsular cataract extraction (ECCE). The anterior portion of the capsule is ruptured and removed. The ophthalmologist then expresses, or removes, the lens cortex and nucleus. Any remaining lens material is carefully removed from the eye. The posterior lens capsule is left inside the eye.

In intracapsular cataract extraction, the ophthalmologist removes the lens and capsule completely. The advantage of this approach is the ease with which the procedure is performed. The major disadvantage is that the protective posterior capsule is removed, placing the eye at greater risk for retinal detachment and resulting in the loss of a supportive structure for the intraocular lens (IOL) implant.

Postoperative Care. Immediately after surgery, the nurse administers an antibiotic subconjunctivally and instills an antibiotic plus steroid ointment. The closed eye is covered with a patch and a protective shield. The client is positioned in semi-Fowler position or on the nonoperative side. The nurse observes the dressing for evidence of drainage and reports any drainage to the surgeon.

The ophthalmologist usually performs the first dressing change and examines the eye with a slit-lamp microscope the next day. Steroid-antibiotic eyedrops, such as tobramycin and dexamethasone (TobraDex), are instilled.

Mild itching caused by the small stitches used to close the incision is normal. Cool compresses are usually beneficial. Discomfort at the site is usually controlled by a mild analgesic, such as acetaminophen (Abenol✦, Tylenol) or acetaminophen with oxycodone (Endocet✦, Percocet, Tylox). Aspirin is avoided because of its effects on blood coagulation.

Pain may indicate a serious complication, such as increased IOP or hemorrhage. The nurse instructs the client to contact the ophthalmologist if pain accompanied by nausea or vomiting is present.

After the dressing is removed, eye protection must be worn at all times to guard against injury. During the day, the client may wear glasses or the protective shield; at night, the protective shield alone is sufficient.

To minimize intraocular pressure (IOP) increases, the major complication during the postoperative period, the nurse enforces activity restrictions and teaches these to the client and family. Activities that can cause a sudden rise in IOP are listed in Table 49–3.

Another major complication is infection. The client is instructed to observe for increasing redness of the eye, a change in visual acuity, tearing, and photophobia. Creamy white, dry, crusty drainage on the eyelids and lashes is normal. Yellow or green drainage must be reported, however.

Bleeding into the anterior chamber of the eye also may occur, usually several days after surgery. Blood may come from the incision, iris, or ciliary body. The client is in-

TABLE 49–3

Activities That Increase Intraocular Pressure
• Bending from the waist
• Sneezing, coughing
• Blowing the nose
• Straining to have a bowel movement
• Vomiting
• Sexual intercourse
• Keeping the head in a dependent position
• Wearing tight shirt collars

structed to report any change in vision immediately to the ophthalmologist.

Rehabilitation Options. After surgery, the eye has no accommodative power and has lost most of its refractive ability (aphakia). A replacement lens is required to focus light rays in the retina. Aphakia is corrected by the use of eyeglasses, contact lenses, or an intraocular lens (IOL) implant to attain clear, functional vision.

Eyeglasses. Aphakic spectacles must be worn during waking hours for the rest of the client's life if this option is selected. This method of visual rehabilitation is the least expensive but is seldom selected because of cosmetic and functional drawbacks. Images are slightly distorted, and peripheral vision is limited.

Contact Lenses. Contact lenses are an alternative corrective method for aphakia. The chief advantage of contact lenses over eyeglasses is that image size with a contact lens is only 7% larger than normal, so images from both eyes can be fused into one. With contact lenses, the visual field is neither distorted nor constricted. Unfortunately, the manual dexterity required to insert and remove contact lenses limits the number of clients who can manage them without assistance. Disposable, extended-wear contact lenses, which are worn for a 2-week period and then discarded, may help solve this problem.

Intraocular Lens Implant. At the time of surgery or at a later date, a small, clear, high-density plastic lens can be implanted. The major advantages of an IOL implant include minimal (1–3%) distortion of the image produced and an immediate return to binocular vision. Disadvantages include higher cost, slightly increased rate of complications, and risk of lens rejection.

 Continuing Care

The client undergoing cataract surgery is usually discharged on the day of surgery. Because of early discharge, the nurse is essential in helping the client and family with plans for the return to home, assisted living, or extended care.

► *Health Teaching*

The nurse reviews signs and symptoms of complications after cataract surgery with the client and family before the client's discharge, including

- Sharp, sudden pain
- Bleeding or increased discharge
- Lid swelling
- Decreased vision
- Flashes of light or floating shapes

The nurse instructs the client to wear a shield over the operative eye at night to prevent accidental injury during sleep. The procedure for instilling eyedrops is reviewed with the client or caretaker. If the client is concerned that the drops may not be correctly instilled, the nurse may advise the client to refrigerate the eyedrops. Then, when the eyedrop falls into the conjunctival sac, the client will experience a cool feeling.

The nurse also tells the client to avoid activities that might increase IOP (see Table 49–3). If an IOL implantation has not been performed, the nurse explains the proper use of cataract eyeglasses. The client is instructed to look through the center of the corrective lenses and to turn the head, rather than only the eyes, when looking to the side.

The client may wash his or her hair a day or two after surgery, but only with the head tilted back, such as in a beauty salon or barber shop. For the immediate postoperative period, the client is advised to stand in the shower with the face held away from the shower head. Washing hair or standing in the shower in the usual manner allows soap and water too close to the eye, which can cause irritation and predispose to infection.

Cooking and light housekeeping are permitted, but vacuuming should be avoided for several weeks because of the forward flexion involved and the rapid, jerky movements required. The client is also advised to refrain from driving, operating machinery, and participating in certain sports, such as golf, until given specific permission from the ophthalmologist.

► *Home Care Management*

Meals can be prepared ahead and frozen, and groceries purchased in sufficient amounts to preclude frequent trips to the store. Articles in low kitchen cupboards can be moved to the countertops. If the client has difficulty instilling eyedrops, a supportive neighbor, friend, or family member can be taught the procedure. Adaptive equipment that positions the bottle of eyedrops directly over the eye can also be purchased.

Safety is a primary concern on the client's return home. The client wears an eye shield at night on the operative eye for several weeks after surgery. If the client also has a cataract in the opposite eye, vision may be severely reduced. Chart 49–7 lists items to cover in the focused assessment of a client in the home environment after cataract surgery.

► *Health Care Resources*

If the client lives alone and has no family or significant others, the nurse arranges for a home care nurse to assess the client and the home situation. The client must be able to instill eyedrops, but may be unable to perform this task independently. A friend, neighbor, or family member can be taught this technique.

 Evaluation

The nurse evaluates care of the client with cataracts on the basis of the nursing diagnoses identified. The desired outcomes may include that the client is expected to

- Demonstrate improved vision
- Recognize signs and symptoms of complications after cataract removal
- Instill eyedrops correctly
- State activities that might increase IOP
- Remain free from injury after cataract removal
- Use cataract eyeglasses as prescribed

Chart 49-7

Focused Assessment for Home Care Clients After Cataract Surgery

- Assess the eye and vision, including
  - Visual acuity in both eyes using a Jaeger card
  - Visual fields of both eyes
  - Compare operative eye to nonoperative eye for presence or absence of
    Redness
    Tearing
    Drainage
- Ask the client about
  - Pain in or around the operative eye
  - Any change in visual acuity (decreased or improved) in the operative eye
  - Whether any of the following has been noticed in the operative eye:
    Dark spots
    Increase in the number of floaters
    Bright flashes of light
- Assess the home environment for
  - Safety hazards (especially tripping and falling hazards)
  - Kitchen hazards
  - Level of room lighting
- Assess client compliance with and understanding of treatment and limitations, including
  - Signs and symptoms to report
  - Medication regimen
  - Activity restrictions
- Assess function ability
  - Activities of daily living
  - Compliance with medication regimen

Glaucoma

Overview

Glaucoma comprises a group of ocular diseases characterized by increased IOP. When IOP is greater than the tissues can tolerate, the cells of the retina and the optic nerve are damaged. If the condition progresses, blindness results. In most common forms of glaucoma, vision is lost gradually and painlessly, without the person's awareness.

Pathophysiology

Intraocular pressure is a measure of fluid (aqueous humor) pressure. A normal IOP of 10 to 21 mmHg is maintained as balance between production and outflow of aqueous humor. IOP can be raised by an abnormally high resistance to outflow of aqueous fluid through the anterior chamber or by excess production of aqueous humor. In people with glaucoma, aqueous humor builds up inside the eye, and the increased pressure compromises blood flow to the optic nerve and retina. The sensitive nerve tissue becomes ischemic and dies. Tissue damage usually starts in the periphery and moves inward toward the fovea centralis. Left untreated, glaucoma can result in blindness.

There are several causes and types of glaucoma (Table 49-4). Glaucoma is classified as primary, secondary, or associated. In primary glaucoma, the most common form, the structures involved in circulation and reabsorption of the aqueous humor undergo direct pathologic change.

Primary open-angle glaucoma (POAG), the most common form of primary glaucoma, is usually bilateral and asymptomatic in the early stages. There is a resistance to the outflow of aqueous humor through the chamber angle. Because the fluid cannot leave the eye at the same rate at which it is produced, IOP gradually builds.

Angle-closure glaucoma (also called closed-angle glaucoma, narrow-angle glaucoma, and acute glaucoma) is much less common, has a sudden onset, and is treated as an emergency. The basic problems are a narrowed angle and an anteriorly displaced iris. Displacement of the iris against the cornea narrows or closes the chamber angle, which obstructs the outflow of aqueous humor. This can happen suddenly and without warning.

Secondary glaucoma results from ocular diseases that cause a narrowed angle or an increased volume of fluid within the eye. These diseases or conditions indirectly disrupt the activity of the structures involved in circulation and reabsorption of aqueous humor. This can happen suddenly and without warning.

Incidence/Prevalence

Glaucoma is a common cause of blindness in industrialized countries. Incidence is age-related, affecting as many as 10% of people older than 80 years (Vaughan et al., 1995).

Collaborative Management

Primary open-angle glaucoma develops slowly, usually without symptoms. The gradual losses of visual fields associated with this disease remain undetected because central vision remains unaffected. At times, the client may note foggy vision, diminished accommodation, mild aching in the eyes, or headaches, and may require frequent

TABLE 49-4

Common Causes of Glaucoma	
Glaucoma Type	**Cause/Associated Factors**
Primary	Aging
	Heredity
	Central retinal vein occlusion
Secondary	Uveitis
	Iritis
	Neovascular disorders
	Trauma
	Ocular tumors
	Degenerative disease
	Eye surgery
Associated	Diabetes mellitus
	Hypertension
	Severe myopia
	Retinal detachment

Chart 49–8

Key Features of Glaucoma

Early
- Increased intraocular pressure
- Diminished accommodation

Late
- Diminished visual fields (loss of peripheral vision)
- Decreased visual acuity not correctable with glasses
- Halos around lights
- Headache or eye pain (acute closed-angle glaucoma)
- Increased cup-to-disk ratio
- Pale optic disk

changes in eyeglass prescriptions. Late symptoms of glaucoma that occur after irreversible damage to optic nerve function include visual field losses, decreased visual acuity not correctable with eyeglasses, and the appearance of halos around lights. Chart 49–8 lists common clinical manifestations of glaucoma.

 Assessment

➤ Physical Assessment/Clinical Manifestations

Examination of the client with glaucoma with an ophthalmoscope reveals cupping and atrophy of the optic disk. The disk becomes wider and deeper and turns a white or gray color (Fig. 49–10).

To determine the extent of peripheral field losses, visual fields are measured. A visual field examination maps the areas seen by the eye while it fixates on a central point. The test searches for *scotomas* (blind spots). In chronic open-angle glaucoma, the visual fields initially show a small crescent-shaped defect that gradually progresses to a nasal and superior field defect. In acute angle-closure glaucoma, the visual fields can quickly become significantly decreased.

The clinical manifestations of acute angle-closure glaucoma differ from those of open-angle glaucoma. The onset of symptoms is acute, and the client complains of sudden, excruciating pain around the eyes that radiates over the sensory distribution of the fifth cranial nerve. Headache or brow ache, nausea, vomiting, and abdominal discomfort also may occur. Other symptoms may include seeing colored halos around lights and sudden blurred vision with decreased light perception.

On examination, the sclera may appear reddened and the cornea foggy. Ophthalmoscopic examination reveals a shallow anterior chamber, cloudy aqueous humor, and a moderately dilated nonreactive pupil.

➤ Other Diagnostic Assessment

Tonometry. Intraocular pressure, as measured by tonometry, is elevated in glaucoma. If an elevated reading is found, the nurse takes several readings over a period of

time at various times of the day to determine a pattern, because IOP varies during the day. In open-angle glaucoma, the tonometry reading is between 22 and 32 mmHg (normal is 10–21 mmHg). In angle-closure glaucoma, the tonometry reading may be 30 mmHg or higher.

Tonography. This combines the use of an electronic indentation tonometer with a recording device. The ease of outflow of aqueous humor from the eye is measured while a weight rests on the globe. The slope of the graph is significant. A flat tracing indicates interference with the rate of outflow, as in glaucoma. A steep downhill tracing indicates adequate drainage.

Gonioscopy. A special lens that eliminates the corneal curve facilitates the view of the drainage angle in the anterior chamber of the eye. The entire 360-degree circumference of the iridocorneal angle is examined to provide vital diagnostic information. The presence of adhesions, aberrant blood vessels, sites of previously undiagnosed trauma, and other data are noted as possible causes of secondary glaucoma.

 Interventions

➤ Nonsurgical Management

Blindness from glaucoma can often be prevented by early detection, lifelong treatment, and a commitment to close monitoring and follow-up care. Usually some degree of vision loss is experienced. Chart 49–9 provides information that the nurse can use to assist the elderly client with low vision to remain as independent as possible.

Drug Therapy. Drug therapy for glaucoma focuses on reducing IOP through two mechanisms:
- Physically constricting the pupil so that the ciliary muscle is contracted, which allows better circulation of the aqueous humor to the site of absorption
- Inhibiting the production of aqueous humor

Pupillary Constriction. Drugs that constrict the pupil and contract the ciliary muscle (miotics) such as pilocar-

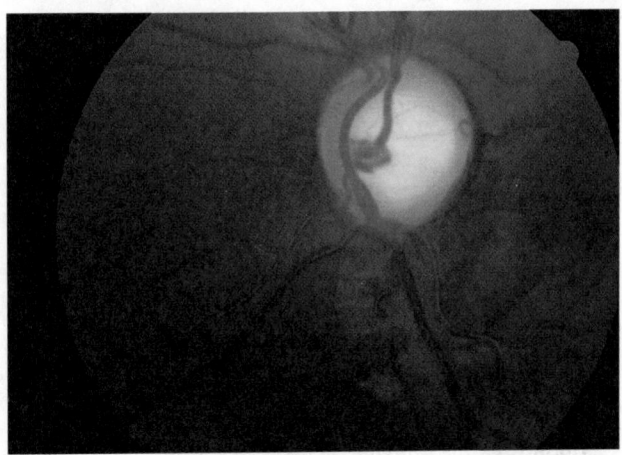

Figure 49–10. The optic fundus of a client with glaucoma.

Chart 49–9

Nursing Focus on the Elderly: Promote Independent Living in Clients with Low Vision

Medications

- Having a neighbor, relative, friend, or visiting nurse visit once a week to measure the proper medications for each day may be helpful.
  - If the client is to make medications more than once each day, it is helpful to use a container of a different shape (with a lid) each time. For example, if the client is to take medication at 9:00 AM, 1:00 PM, and 9:00 PM, the 9:00 AM medications would be placed in a round container, the 1:00 PM medications in a square container, and the 9:00 PM medications in a triangular container.
  - It is helpful to place each day's medication containers in a separate box with raised letters on the side of the box spelling out the day.
- "Talking clocks" are available to the client with low vision.

Communication

- Telephones with large, raised block numbers may be helpful. The best models are those with black numbers on a white phone or white numbers on a black phone.
- Telephones that have a programmable, automatic dialing feature are very helpful. Programmed numbers should include those for the fire department, police, relatives, friends, neighbors, and 911.

Safety

- It is best to leave furniture the way the client wants it and not move it.
- Throw rugs are best eliminated.
- Appliance cords should be short and kept out of walkways.
- Lounge-style chairs with built-in footrests are preferable to footstools.
- Nonbreakable dishes, cups, and glasses are preferable to breakable ones.
- Cleansers and other toxic agents should be labelled with large, raised letters.
- Hook-and-loop (Velcro) strips at hand level may help to mark the locations of switches and electrical outlets.

Food Preparation

- Meals on Wheels is a service that many elderly people find helpful. This service brings meals at mealtime, cooked and ready to eat. The cost of this service varies, depending on the client's ability to pay.

- Many grocery stores offer a "shop by telephone" service. The client can either complete a computer booklet indicating types, amounts, and brands of items desired, or the store will complete this booklet over the telephone by asking the client specific information. The store then delivers groceries to the client's door (many stores also offer a "put away" service) and charges the client's bank card.
- A microwave oven is a safer means of cooking than a standard stove, although many elderly clients are afraid of microwave ovens. If the client has and will use a microwave oven, others can prepare meals ahead of time, label them, and freeze them for later use. Also, many complete, microwavable frozen dinners that comply with a variety of dietary restrictions are available.
- Friends or relatives may be able to help with food preparation. Often, relatives do not know what to give an elderly person for birthdays or other gift-giving occasions. One suggestion is a homemade prepackaged frozen dinner that the client enjoys.

Personal Care

- Handgrips should be installed in bathrooms.
- The tub floor should have a nonskid surface.
- Male clients should use an electric shaver rather than a razor.
- Choosing a hairstyle that is becoming but easy to care for (avoiding parts) will help in independent living.
- Home hair care services may be available.

Diversional Activity

- Some clients are able to use large-print books, newspapers, and magazines (available through local libraries and vision services).
- Books, magazines, and some newspapers are available on audiotape.
- Clients experienced in knitting or crocheting may be able to create items fashioned from straight pieces, such as afghans.
- Card games, dominoes, and some board games available in large, high-contrast print may be helpful for clients with low vision.

---

pine hydrochloride (Isopto Carpine, Pilocar, Spersacarpine♦) are commonly used to treat glaucoma. In acute angle-closure glaucoma, constriction of pupil size is also desired, because it stretches the iridocorneal angle and enhances aqueous outflow. Carbachol (Isopto Carbachol, Miostat) may be used in conjunction with or in place of pilocarpine. Echothiophate iodide (Phospholine Iodide) produces miosis and increases outflow. The nurse reminds the client that miotics may cause blurred vision for 1 to 2 hours after use and that adaptation to dark environments is difficult because of the pupillary constriction.

Inhibition of Aqueous Humor. Beta-blockers such as

timolol (Apo-Timoptic♦, Timoptic) and levobunolol (Betagan) are the drug of choice for decreasing IOP. When used as eyedrops, beta-blockers reduce aqueous humor production without causing pupil constriction.

Carbonic anhydrase inhibitors, such as acetazolamide (Acetazolam♦, Diamox) and methazolamide (Neptazane), reduce aqueous humor production to help maintain a lowered IOP. Epinephrine, 0.5%–2%, and dipivefrin hydrochloride (Propine) also reduce aqueous humor production. Epinephrine-containing agents are not used in angle-closure glaucoma because of the pupillary dilation caused by their sympathomimetic action.

Osmotic agents may be administered systemically for a client with angle-closure glaucoma as part of emergency treatment to rapidly reduce IOP. Such agents include oral glycerin (Osmoglyn) and mannitol (Osmitrol♦).

> ➤ *Surgical Management*

Laser Surgery. When a medical regimen for the open-angle glaucoma client has been ineffective at controlling IOP, laser surgery is indicated.

Preoperative Care. Nursing interventions include informing the client about laser technology, expected sights and sounds commonly heard during this procedure, and expected outcomes.

Operative Procedure. A laser trabeculoplasty burns the trabecular meshwork, scarring it and causing the meshwork fibers to tighten. This tightening of the fibers allows increased outflow of aqueous humor and thus a reduction in IOP. Topical or local anesthesia is used. Clients commonly experience a temporary increase in IOP immediately after this procedure.

Laser surgery is also indicated for the client with angle-closure glaucoma. The laser creates a hole in the periphery of the iris, which allows aqueous humor to flow from the posterior chamber to the anterior chamber and then into the trabecular meshwork.

Postoperative Care. The client is instructed to arrange for transportation home; driving is prohibited after the surgery. Because laser procedures can sometimes increase IOP, the pressure should be reevaluated 1 hour after surgery and before discharge. The ophthalmologist may prescribe an ocular steroid, such as prednisolone acetate (Ocu-Pred, Ophtho-Tate♦).

Standard Surgical Therapy. In open-angle glaucoma that fails to respond to pharmacologic and laser therapy and in selected cases of angle-closure glaucoma, surgical intervention is required. This surgery either creates a new drainage channel for aqueous humor or destroys the structures responsible for its production.

Glaucoma surgery is performed either in a hospital or on an outpatient basis. The usual length of stay is several hours to several days.

After surgery, the ophthalmologist administers an antibiotic subconjunctivally. The eye is covered with a patch after an antibiotic-steroid ointment is inserted, and a protective shield is applied over it. The client is instructed to avoid taking aspirin, to not lie on the operative side, and to report any brow pain, severe eye pain, or nausea.

The most serious complication of hypotonia after glaucoma surgery is choroidal hemorrhage. If IOP is too low to maintain normal pressure, fluid may enter the suprachoroid space and cause a choroidal detachment. The accumulation of fluid in this space may strain the many blood vessels located there. Symptoms of choroidal hemorrhage include

- Acute pain deep in the eye
- Decreased vision
- Vital sign changes

Ocular Chamber Disorders: Vitreous Hemorrhage
Overview

The vitreous is the avascular gelatinous body that makes up the posterior two thirds of the eye and provides the eye's shape. Vitreous hemorrhage, bleeding into the vitreous cavity, may result from aging, systemic diseases, or trauma or may occur spontaneously. With aging, the vitreous may spontaneously detach from the retina. If blood vessels are torn, bleeding into the vitreous results. Diseases that disrupt the retinal blood vessels, such as hypertensive retinopathy and proliferative diabetic retinopathy, also may cause blood leakage into the vitreous.

Collaborative Management

Symptoms of vitreous hemorrhage include reduced visual acuity; the degree of reduction varies with the severity of the hemorrhage. A mild hemorrhage may cause the client to see a red haze or series of vitreous "floaters." The client experiencing a moderate hemorrhage may graphically describe seeing "black streaks" or "tiny black dots." Severe hemorrhage may cause the client's visual acuity to be reduced to hand motion. Eye examination reveals a noticeably reduced red reflex because light rays have difficulty reaching the retina. Ultrasonography is used to determine the location and extent of the hemorrhage.

A vitreous hemorrhage may be absorbed slowly with no treatment. If the hemorrhage is still present several weeks to months later, a *vitrectomy* (surgical removal of the vitreous) is indicated.

Uveal Tract Disorders: Uveitis
Overview

The uveal tract is composed of three separate but interrelated parts: the iris, the ciliary body, and the choroid. The most common problem associated with these structures is inflammation, or uveitis. Uveitis may occur in the anterior or posterior portion of the eye.

Anterior uveitis can include inflammation of the iris, inflammation of the ciliary body, or both. The cause of anterior uveitis is unknown but is associated with exposure to allergens, infectious agents, trauma, or systemic disease (rheumatoid arthritis, ankylosing spondylitis, herpes simplex, herpes zoster). Symptoms include periorbital aching; tearing; blurred vision; photophobia; a small, irregular, nonreactive pupil; and engorgement of scleral vessels.

Posterior uveitis is the common term for *retinitis*, inflammation of the retina, and *chorioretinitis*, inflammation of both the choroid and the retina. Posterior uveitis is associated with tuberculosis, syphilis, and toxoplasmosis.

The onset of symptoms is slow and insidious. Visual impairment in the affected eye, the primary symptom, results from protein-rich fluid, fibrin, and cells leaking into the vitreous cavity. The pupil is small, nonreactive, and irregularly shaped. Black dots are visible against the red background of the fundus. Chorioretinal lesions appear as grayish-yellow patches on the retinal surface.

Collaborative Management

Treatment of the client with anterior or posterior uveitis is symptomatic. The treatment plan includes resting the ciliary body with a cycloplegic agent. The pupil is dilated to prevent adhesions between the iris and the lens. Steroid drops are administered every hour to decrease the inflammatory response of the eye and to prevent adhesions of the iris to the cornea and lens. Subconjunctival injections of steroids may be used in posterior uveitis or when topical steroids have been ineffective. Analgesics that contain neither aspirin nor opioids are ordered for pain. Antibiotics may be initiated for the client with posterior uveitis or when infection is present with anterior uveitis.

Cool or warm compresses are applied for ocular pain. Darkening the room and wearing sunglasses reduce the discomfort of photophobia. Because the client's vision is blurred from the cycloplegic drops, the nurse instructs the client not to drive or operate machinery. The nurse reviews the signs and symptoms of bacterial and fungal ulcers and the indications of increased IOP.

Retinal Disorders
Hypertensive Retinopathy
Overview

Many Americans have hypertension. In people with hypertensive disease, vascular changes occur in the eyes that lead to retinal damage and decreased visual acuity.

Hypertensive retinopathy is classified by grades. With each increasing grade, progressive changes are noted in the retina. A direct relationship exists between arteriole narrowing and elevation of the diastolic blood pressure.

Collaborative Management

As blood pressure increases, retinal arterioles narrow and take on a characteristic "copper wire" appearance (Fig. 49–11). Nicking, or narrowing, of the vessel at arteriovenous crossings is apparent. If blood pressure remains elevated, areas of localized ischemia, known as soft exudates, or "cotton wool" spots, develop as a result of occlusion of the arteriole. Small hemorrhages may be noted. The client may also complain of headaches and vertigo. Left untreated, hypertensive retinopathy can produce serous retinal detachments.

Treatment focuses primarily on management of the systemic hypertension (see Chap. 38) and controlling IOP.

Diabetic Retinopathy
Overview

Diabetic retinopathy refers to the vascular complications of diabetes in the retina. The longer the person has diabetes, the greater is the incidence and severity of retinop-

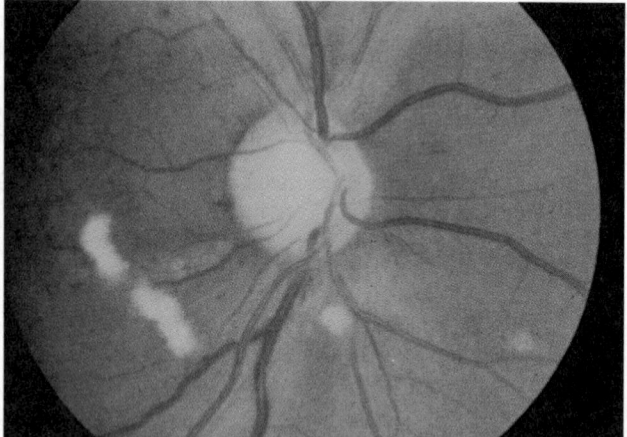

Figure 49–11. The optic fundus of a client with hypertension.

athy (Cotran et al., 1994). Another factor influencing the severity of retinopathy is blood glucose control. Good control is believed to lessen the severity of the disease. There are two types of diabetic retinopathy: background and proliferative.

In background diabetic retinopathy, the supporting cells of the retinal vessels die, and the capillary walls of the retina thicken and allow fluid to leak. As this fluid is absorbed, thick yellow-white deposits, or hard exudates, are formed. The retinal capillaries become diseased and lose their ability to transport needed oxygen and nutrients via red blood cells. Outpouches in the walls of capillaries (microaneurysms) are formed. These fragile capillaries bleed easily and cause intraretinal hemorrhages in the nerve fiber layer of the retina (Fig. 49–12). Visual acuity is diminished by reduction of the capillary blood supply to the retina or by macular edema.

In clients with proliferative diabetic retinopathy, a network of fragile new blood vessels develops, leaking blood and protein into the surrounding tissue. Development of these blood vessels is stimulated by the hypoxic state of the retina that results from poor capillary perfusion of retinal tissues. New blood vessels grow in the retina, encroach onto the iris, and grow into the posterior face of the vitreous. The vitreous contracts and pulls away from the retina, causing blood vessels to break and bleed into the vitreous.

Collaborative Management

Treatment of the client with diabetic retinopathy depends on the degree of retinal involvement. Laser therapy can be used to seal microaneurysms, resulting in decreased bleeding. The light scattering of laser burns across the retina can also decrease the retina's need for oxygen and control the growth of new blood vessels.

A vitrectomy is performed if frequent bleeding occurs into the vitreous and the body is unable to reabsorb it or if fibrin bands threaten to detach the retina. Fibrin bands within the vitreous are severed with a cutter and

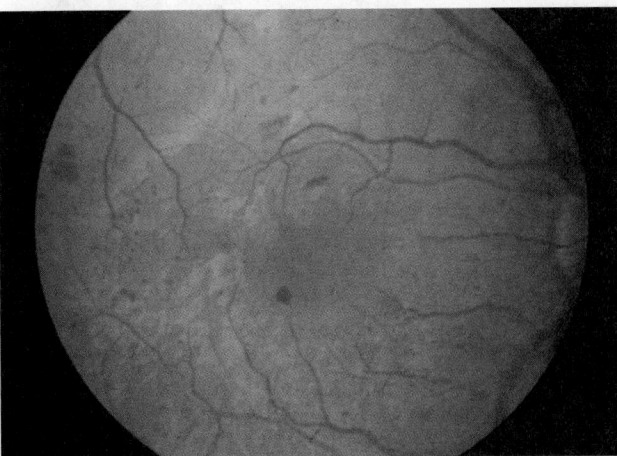

Figure 49–12. The optic fundus of a client with diabetes.

then flushed away. An endolaser may be used in the eye during surgery to seal leaking or bleeding blood vessels.

Macular Degeneration

Overview

Macular degeneration (deterioration of the macula) can be atrophic (age related, or *dry*) or exudative (*wet*). Atrophic degeneration is characterized by sclerosing of retinal capillaries, causing macular cells to become ischemic and necrotic. Rod and cone photoreceptors die. Central vision declines, and clients describe "mild blurring and distortion."

Clients with exudative degeneration experience a sudden decrease in vision after a serous detachment of pigment epithelium in the macula. Blood vessels invade this injured area and cause fluid and blood to accumulate under the macula (like a blister), resulting in scar formation and progressive distortion of vision.

Collaborative Management

Treatment of atrophic macular degeneration aims to help the client maximize remaining vision. The associated loss of central vision may interfere with the client's ability to read, write, recognize safety hazards, and drive. The nurse suggests alternative strategies (such as large-print books and public transportation) and referrals to community organizations that provide a wide range of adaptive equipment.

Management of clients with exudative macular degeneration is geared toward halting the initiating process and identifying further changes in visual perception. Fluid and blood may resorb in a small percentage of clients with exudative degeneration. Laser therapy to seal the leaking blood vessels in or near the macula may also limit the extent of the damage.

Retinal Holes, Tears, and Detachments

Overview

A retinal hole is a break in the integrity of the peripheral sensory retina. Frequently, a retinal hole is associated with trauma, or it can occur with aging.

A retinal tear is a more jagged and irregularly shaped break in the retina. It can result from traction on the retina.

A retinal detachment is the separation of the sensory retina from the pigmented epithelium. Retinal detachments are classified by the nature of their development.

Rhegmatogenous detachments occur following a hole or tear in the retina caused by mechanical force, creating an opening for the vitreous to filter into the subretinal space. When sufficient fluid collects in this space, the retina detaches.

Traction detachments are created when the retina is pulled away from the epithelium by bands of fibrous tissue in the vitreous.

Exudative detachments are caused by fluid accumulation in the subretinal space, association with a systemic disease, and ocular tumors. No retinal break occurs.

Collaborative Management

The onset of a retinal detachment is usually sudden and painless because no pain fibers are located in the retina. Clients may suddenly see bright flashes of light (photopsia) or floating dark spots in the affected eye. During the initial phase of the detachment or if the detachment is partial, the client may describe a sensation of a curtain being pulled over part of the visual field. The visual field loss corresponds to the area of detachment.

 Assessment

On ophthalmoscopic examination, detachments appear as gray bulges or folds in the retina that quiver with movement. This appearance is in marked contrast to the flat pink-orange color of the choroid as it shows through the transparent retina. Depending on the cause of the detachment, a hole or tear also may be seen at the edge of the detachment.

 Interventions

If a retinal hole or tear is discovered before it causes a detachment, the ophthalmologist may elect to close or seal the break. Closure prevents the accumulation of fluid under the retina, reducing the likelihood of a detachment. Treatment aims to create an inflammatory response that will bind the retina and choroid together around the break. This inflammatory response can be created through external application of cryotherapy (a freezing probe), photocoagulation (laser), or diathermy (high-frequency current).

Spontaneous reattachment of the retina is rare. Surgical repair is required to place the retina in contact with the underlying structures. One such repair procedure is scleral buckling.

Preoperative Care. Clients requiring retinal surgery are noticeably anxious and fearful about a possible permanent loss of vision. The nurse provides accurate information and calm reassurance to allay such fears.

Depending on the location and size of the retinal break, activity restrictions may be necessary immediately to prevent further tearing or detachment and to promote drainage of any subretinal fluid.

The nurse places an eyepatch over the client's affected eye to reduce eye movement. Topical medications to inhibit accommodation and constriction of the pupil are administered before surgery.

Operative Procedure. The surgery is performed under general anesthesia. In scleral buckling, the ophthalmologist repairs wrinkles or folds in the retina so the retina can assume its normal smooth position, and the sclera flattens against the retina. To promote reattachment, a small piece of silicone is placed against the sclera and held in place by an encircling band (Fig. 49–13). These devices keep the retina in contact with the choroid and sclera to promote scar tissue formation and attachment. Any subretinal fluid present is drained.

To further encourage retinal reattachment, a gas such as sulfahexafluoride (SF6) or silicone oil can be used. These agents have a specific gravity less than that of the vitreous humor or air, and they float up against the retina to hold it in place until healing occurs.

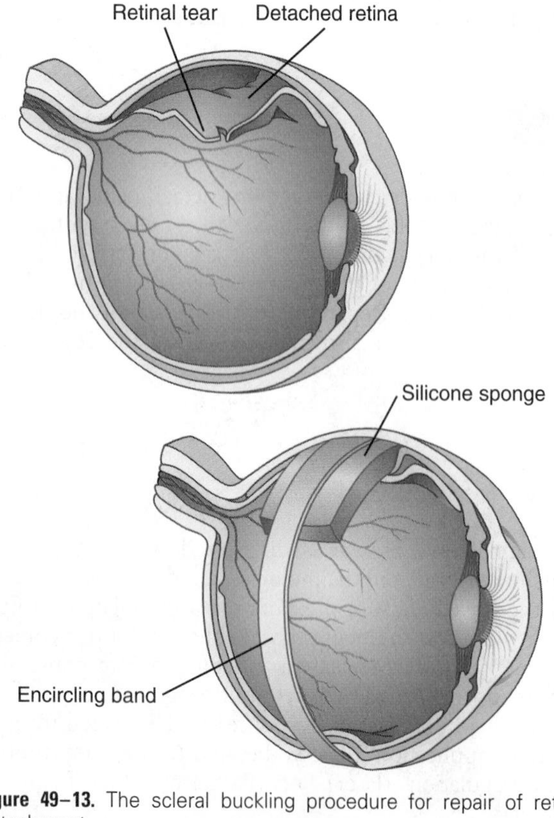

Postoperative Care. After retinal reattachment surgery, an eyepatch and shield are applied. The nurse monitors the client's vital signs and evaluates the eyepatch and shield for any drainage.

Activity status varies. If gas or oil has been used, the nurse positions the client on his or her abdomen to allow the gas to float against the retina. The client's head is turned to the operative eye, lying with the unaffected eye down, for several days until the gas has been absorbed. As an alternative, the client can sit on the side of the bed and place the head on an over-the-bed table. Bathroom privileges are allowed once the client is fully awake.

The client may experience nausea and pain postoperatively. The nurse administers analgesics and antiemetics as prescribed. The nurse reports any complaint of a sudden increase in pain or pain accompanied by nausea to the ophthalmologist, because these symptoms may indicate the development of complications. The nurse also instructs the client to avoid activities that increase IOP (see Table 49–3).

In the first week after retinal detachment surgery, the client should avoid reading, writing, and close work, such as needlepoint, because these activities cause rapid eye movements. The nurse teaches the client about the signs and symptoms associated with infection and detachment. The client is instructed to notify the nurse or physician if any signs or symptoms occur.

Retinitis Pigmentosa

Overview

Several types of bilateral retinal disorders are characterized by progressive degeneration of the retina and a loss of visual receptors, leading to blindness. Retinitis pigmentosa is a condition in which retinal cells degenerate and the pigmented cells of the retina grow and move into the sensory areas of the retina, causing further retinal degeneration. Different forms of this disorder can be inherited as an autosomal dominant trait, an autosomal recessive trait, or an X-linked recessive trait (Cotran et al., 1994).

Collaborative Management

The most common early clinical manifestation experienced by a person with retinitis pigmentosa is night blindness. Over time, decreased visual acuity progresses to total blindness. Ophthalmoscopic examination of the retina shows excessive pigmentation in a lattice-like pattern. Cataracts may accompany this disorder.

No current therapy has proved effective in preventing or slowing the degenerative process. Because some retinal destruction resembles that seen with vitamin A deficiency, a regimen of vitamin A, along with decreased exposure of the retina to bright light, is being tried.

REFRACTIVE ERRORS

Overview

The ability of the eye to focus images on the retina depends on the anteroposterior diameter of the eye and

Retinal tear   Detached retina

Silicone sponge

Encircling band

Figure 49–13. The scleral buckling procedure for repair of retinal detachment.

the refractive power of the lens system. *Refraction* is the bending of light rays. Problems in either area can result in refractive errors.

Myopia

In myopia, or *near-sightedness,* the refractive ability of the eye is too strong for the eye length. Images are bent so that they fall in front of, not on, the retina.

Hyperopia

In hyperopia, *hypermetropia* or *far-sightedness,* the refractive ability of the eye is too weak, causing images to be focused behind the retina. A shorter anteroposterior diameter of the eye may contribute to the development of hyperopia.

Presbyopia

As people age, the crystalline lens loses its elasticity and is less able to alter its shape to focus the eye for close work. As a result, images fall behind the retina. Presbyopia usually occurs in people in their 30s and 40s.

Astigmatism

Astigmatism occurs when the curve of the cornea is uneven. Because light rays are not refracted equally in all directions, a focus point on the retina is not achieved.

Collaborative Management

 Assessment

Refractive errors are diagnosed through a process known as refraction. The client is asked to view an eye chart while lenses of different strengths are systematically placed in front of the eye, and then asked whether the lenses sharpen or worsen vision. The power or strength of the lens necessary to permit focusing of the image on the retina is expressed in measurements called diopters.

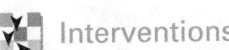 Interventions

➤ Nonsurgical Management

Errors of refraction must be corrected through the use of a lens to permit light rays to focused on the retina (see Fig. 48–5). Myopic vision is corrected to bring the image forward onto the retina with a concave lens. Hyperopic vision is corrected with convex lenses to move the focused image back to the retina.

Eyeglasses. These commonly correct errors of refraction. Advantages of eyeglasses, when compared with other refractive error corrections, include ease of use, durability, availability, and low cost. Disadvantages include an alteration in physical appearance, weight of the frame on the nose, and reduced peripheral vision (vision is corrected only when the client looks through the center of the lens).

Contact Lenses. These can also correct refractive errors. Round plastic disks rest against the cornea and fit under the eyelid.

Hard Lenses. Hard contact lenses correct refractive errors by changing the shape of the cornea, which increases its refracting ability, and by placing the specific refractive power and shape needed in front of the eye so that light rays can be correctly focused onto the retina.

Complications of hard contact lens wear include corneal edema, which occurs when the lenses are worn for an extended period. Corneal abrasions can result from overwear, which dries the epithelium and causes minute breaks, or from the irritation of the contact lens against the cornea.

Soft Lenses. Soft contact lenses are larger but better tolerated than hard contact lenses. They resemble the thickness of plastic wrap and can be worn for longer periods because the lenses' hydrophilic character allows greater corneal access to moisture and oxygen. Most soft lens wear problems are related to lens deterioration, deposits in the lens, and lack of compliance with lens care practices.

There are two types of soft contact lenses: daily-wear lenses (worn during waking hours) and extended-wear contact lenses. Extended-wear lenses can be worn continuously for several days to several weeks, depending on the client's environment, activities, and tolerance of the lenses.

➤ Surgical Management

Surgery is becoming a popular alternative for the treatment of refractive errors.

Radial Keratotomy. Radial keratotomy (RK) is an outpatient surgical procedure for the treatment of mild to moderate myopia. Eight to 16 diagonal incisions are made through 90% of the peripheral cornea. Because the central cornea is not incised, vision is not diminished. These incisions flatten the cornea, which decreases the length of the eye and allows the image to be focused closer to the retina.

Slight overcorrection or undercorrection of the refractive error is possible, so the client still must wear some form of visual correction after the surgery. Other complications include corneal scarring.

Epikeratophakia. In this procedure, donor corneal tissue is surgically grafted onto the client's own cornea to alter its refractive ability. The donor corneal tissue is frozen and reshaped to the specific strength and size needed.

Photorefractive Keratectomy. Photorefractive keratectomy (PRK) is a new alternative for people with mild to moderate stable myopia and low astigmatism. PRK is not a laser version of radial keratotomy but a completely different procedure. An excimer laser pulses a brief but powerful beam of ultraviolet light on the central cornea. This beam removes small portions of the tissue surface, reshaping the cornea to properly focus an image on the retina.

Photorefractive keratectomy is performed under local

anesthesia as an outpatient procedure. One eye is treated at a time, usually at least 3 months apart. The eye is patched after surgery. Complete healing to the best vision may take up to 6 months.

Most people do not need corrective lenses for distance vision after PRK but may still need reading glasses. Expected side effects of PRK in the postoperative period include pain, hazy vision, light sensitivity, tearing, and pupillary enlargement. Possible complications include night vision difficulty, corneal clouding, undercorrection, far-sightedness, increased intraocular pressure (IOP), and glare.

TRAUMATIC DISORDERS

Trauma to the eye or periorbital area can result from almost any activity. Care varies depending on the area of the eye affected and whether the globe has been penetrated.

Hyphema

Overview

A hyphema is blood in the anterior chamber. It is produced when a force is applied to the eye and is sufficient to break the integrity of the blood vessels in the eye.

Collaborative Management

If the hyphema is large, it may obstruct the pupil and reduce visual acuity, possibly causing pain and photophobia. Hemolysis of the blood occurs, and the blood is filtered out of the eye through the trabecular meshwork. If the hemolyzed blood obstructs the trabecular meshwork, an increased IOP results.

The client with a hyphema is treated by bed rest in a semi-Fowler position to aid gravity in keeping the hyphema away from the optical center of the cornea. Minimal or no sudden eye movements are permitted for 3 to 5 days to decrease the likelihood of rebleeding. Cycloplegic eyedrops may be ordered to place the eye at rest, and the eye is protected by a shield and covered with a patch. Television and reading are restricted. Hyphema usually resolves in 5 to 7 days.

Contusion

Overview

A contusion of the eyeball and surrounding tissue is produced by traumatic contact with a blunt object. The force of the contact pushes the eye back in the orbit. The globe is compressed and stretching of the ocular soft tissues occurs, which can produce damage and possible rupture of the globe.

Results of the injury may not be seen immediately. These results include edema of the eyelids, subconjunctival hemorrhage, corneal edema, and hyphema.

Collaborative Management

Periorbital ecchymosis, or "black eye," a common contusion injury, is usually caused by blunt trauma. Bleeding into the soft tissue occurs, creating the characteristic purple bruise. The color fades gradually and disappears in approximately 10 days. Visual acuity is usually not affected. Other symptoms include orbital pain, photophobia, eyelid edema, and diplopia.

Treatment begins at the time of injury. Ice is applied immediately. The client should receive a thorough eye examination to rule out any other eye injuries.

Foreign Bodies

Overview

Eyelashes, dust, fingernails, dirt, and airborne particles can come in contact with the conjunctiva or cornea and produce a mechanical irritation or abrasion. If nothing is seen on the cornea or conjunctiva, the eyelids are everted to examine the palpebral and bulbar conjunctivae.

Collaborative Management

The client complains of "feeling something in my eye" or of blurry vision. Pain is a common symptom if the corneal epithelium is injured. Tearing and photophobia may be noted.

Evaluation of vision precedes treatment. The nurse examines the eye of any client with a suspected or known corneal abrasion with fluorescein, followed by ocular irrigation with normal saline (0.9%) to gently remove the particles. Ophthalmologic irrigation is described in Chart 49–10.

After the foreign body is removed and the eyepatch applied, the nurse tells the client how long the patch must be left in place, usually overnight. The client is reminded to seek follow-up care to have the patch removed and the eye examined.

Lacerations

Overview

Lacerations are caused by sharp objects and projectiles. Lacerations can occur to any part of the eye, but the most common areas of involvement are the eyelids and the cornea.

Collaborative Management

Initially, the eye is closed and a small ice pack is applied to decrease bleeding. The client receives medical attention as soon as possible.

If the client can open the eye, the nurse checks visual acuity and cleans the eyelids. Minor lacerations of the eyelid can be sutured in an emergency department, an urgent care center, or an ophthalmologist's office. A microscope is necessary in the operating room if the client has a laceration that involves the eyelid margin, affects the lacrimal system, involves a large area, or has jagged edges.

Corneal lacerations are considered an ocular emergency because ocular contents may prolapse through the laceration. Symptoms include severe eye pain, photophobia, tearing, decreased visual acuity, and inability to open the

Nursing Care Highlight: Ocular Irrigation

1. Assemble equipment:
   - Normal saline IV (1000-mL bag)
   - Macrodrip IV tubing
   - IV pole
   - Eyelid speculum
   - Topical anesthetic (proparacaine hydrochloride)
   - Gloves
   - Collection receptacle (emesis basin works well)
   - Towels
   - pH paper
2. Quickly obtain a history from the client while flushing the tubing with normal saline:
   - Nature and time of the injury
   - Type of irritant or chemical (if known)
   - Type of first aid administered at the scene
   - Any allergies to the "caine" family of medications
3. Evaluate the client's visual acuity *before* treatment:
   - Ask the client to read your name tag with the affected eye while covering the good eye.
   - Ask the client to "count fingers" with the affected eye while covering the good eye.
4. Put on gloves.
5. Place a strip of pH paper in the cul-de-sac of the client's affected eye.
6. Instill proparacaine hydrochloride eyedrops as ordered.
7. Place the client in a supine position with the head turned slightly toward the affected eye.
8. Have the client hold the affected eye open, or position an eyelid speculum.
9. Direct the flow of normal saline across the affected eye from the nasal corner of the eye toward the outer corner of the eye.
10. Assess the client's comfort during the procedure.
11. If both eyes are affected, irrigate them simultaneously using separate personnel and equipment.

eyelid. If the laceration is the result of a penetrating injury, an object may be noted protruding from the eye. *This object must never be removed except by the ophthalmologist, because it may be holding ocular structures in place.*

Antibiotics are initiated to reduce the likelihood of an infection. Depending on the depth of the laceration, scarring may develop. If the scar alters vision, a corneal transplant may be needed later. If the ocular contents have prolapsed through the laceration or if the injury is severe, enucleation (surgical eye removal) may be indicated.

Penetrating Injuries

Overview

Clients with penetrating ocular injuries have the poorest visual prognosis. Glass, high-speed metallic or wood particles, BB pellets, and bullets are common causes of penetrating injuries. The particles can enter the eye through the eyelid, sclera, or cornea and can lodge in or behind the eyeball.

Collaborative Management

The client usually complains of some eye pain and relates a history of "suddenly feeling hit in the eye." An entrance wound may be visible. Depending on the location of the entrance and the resting place of the projectile, vision may be affected.

X-rays and computed tomography (CT) scans of the orbit are obtained. Ultrasonography of the globe and orbit may also be performed.

Usually, surgery is performed to remove the foreign object. In some cases, foreign bodies need to be removed by a vitrectomy. Intravenous antibiotics are started before surgery to reduce the chance of an infection or endophthalmitis. A tetanus booster is administered if necessary.

Visual acuity is assessed and documented. If the client cannot see print, the nurse must note whether the client can count fingers or see directional movement of the nurse's hand. If the client cannot see movement, the nurse assesses the client's ability to see light.

OCULAR MELANOMA

Overview

Melanoma is the most common intraocular malignant tumor in adults. This unilateral tumor occurs most often in the uveal tract among people in their 30s and 40s.

Because of its rich blood supply and vascular channels, an ocular melanoma can spread easily. Common pathways for metastatic spread are direct, through the sclera, or indirect, through invasion of other intraocular structures.

Collaborative Management

Symptoms of malignant melanoma may not be readily apparent; the lesion may be discovered during a routine examination. Blurring of vision may be evident if the macular area is invaded. Visual acuity is reduced if the tumor grows inward toward the center of the eye from the choroid, thus altering the visual pathway. Increased intraocular pressure (IOP) can result if the tumor invades the canal of Schlemm and obstructs outflow of aqueous humor. A change in iris color may occur if the tumor infiltrates the iris. Sudden loss of a portion of the visual field may result from tumor invasion of the subretinal space, producing retinal detachment.

Diagnostic tests for a malignant melanoma lesion depend on lesion size and growth rate. Ultrasonography is performed to determine lesion location and size.

Treatment also depends on lesion size and growth rate and the condition of the other eye. Small lesions of the iris not affecting the iris root are not excised but are monitored until growth is observed. Lesions of the choroid can be treated by surgical enucleation or by radiation therapy with a radioactive cobalt plaque.

Chart 49–11

Nursing Care Highlight: Insertion and Removal of an Ocular Prosthesis

Insertion

1. Assemble equipment:
   - Prosthesis
   - Gloves
   - Towel
2. Explain the procedure to the client.
3. Wash your hands.
4. Cover the work area with a cloth or towel.
5. Don gloves
6. Remove the prosthesis from its container and rinse it with tepid water.
7. Lift the client's upper lid using your nondominant hand.

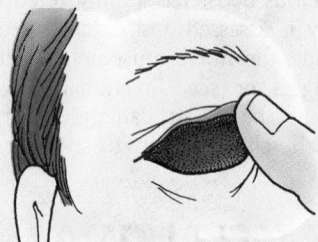

8. Place the prosthesis between the thumb and forefinger of your dominant hand. The notched end of the prosthesis should be closest to the client's nose.

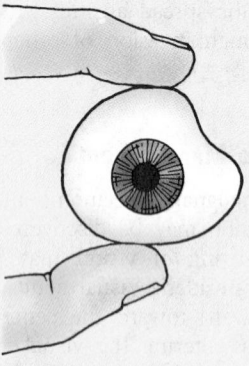

9. Insert the prosthesis with the top edge slipping under the upper lid. Continue until most of the iris is covered by the upper lid.

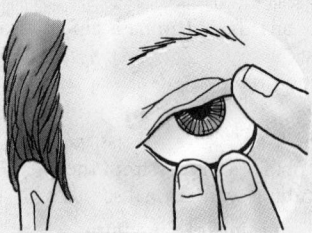

10. Gently release the upper eyelid.
11. Retract the lower lid slightly until the bottom edge of the prosthesis slips behind it.

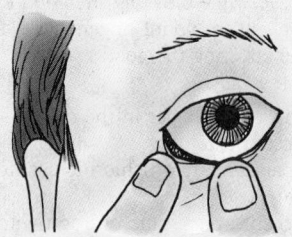

12. Release your hands slowly.

Removal

1. Assemble equipment:
   - Normal saline-filled labeled container
   - Gloves
2. Explain the procedure to the client.
3. Wash your hands.
4. Don gloves.
5. Instruct the client to sit up and tilt the head slightly downward.
6. Place your hand against the client's cheek, palm side up.
7. Pull the lower lid slightly down and laterally.
8. Allow the prosthesis to slide out onto your hand, or pull gently if necessary.
9. Place the prosthesis in a container filled with normal saline labeled with the client's name. Cover the container.

Surgery

Enucleation (surgical removal of the entire eyeball) is performed with the client under general anesthesia. After the eye is removed, a ball implant is inserted to provide a firm base for the socket prosthesis and to facilitate the best cosmetic result.

The implant is covered with surrounding tissue, mus-cles, and conjunctiva. A plastic conformer is placed over the conjunctiva to maintain the shape of the eyelids until a prosthesis can be fitted. After the dressing is removed, a pressure patch is placed over the eye for 24 hours.

Until the prosthesis is fitted, usually 1 month after surgery, an antibiotic-steroid ointment is inserted into the cul-de-sac once a day. Steps for the insertion and removal of the prosthesis are given in Chart 49–11.

Radiation Therapy

Cobalt plaque therapy can reduce the size and thickness of malignant melanomas. The plaque, a round, flat disk about the size of a dime containing a radioactive material, such as cobalt 60 or iodine 125, is sutured to the sclera overlying the tumor site. The length of time the plaque remains sutured to the sclera depends on the size of the tumor and the dose of radiation to be delivered.

Complications of radiation therapy include tumor vasculopathy, retinopathy, glaucoma, necrosis of the sclera, and cataract formation. Vitreous hemorrhage may develop as the tumor becomes smaller.

While the plaque is in place, the eye may or may not be covered with a patch. Cycloplegic eyedrops and an antibiotic-steroid combination are administered. The nurse teaches the client how to instill eyedrops.

OCULAR MANIFESTATIONS OF HUMAN IMMUNODEFICIENCY VIRUS INFECTION

Human immunodeficiency virus (HIV) infection affects many ocular structures and can significantly impair vision. The ocular effects of this disease are seen in 75% of clients diagnosed with acquired immunodeficiency syndrome (AIDS). (Chapter 25 discusses care of clients with HIV disease.) Ocular manifestations of HIV disease can be infectious or noninfectious.

Noninfectious Manifestations

Kaposi's Sarcoma

Overview

Kaposi's sarcoma (KS) is the most common lesion noted in the anterior segment of the eye in AIDS clients. It is present in approximately 30% of clients diagnosed with AIDS.

Collaborative Management

The most common sign of KS is a nontender, reddish-purple discoloration or nodule in the lower fornix or on the eyelid. If the lesion impairs eyelid closure, signs of exposure keratitis may be noted. Pain is the most common symptom of ocular KS.

Treatment goals for clients with ocular KS are to remove the sarcoma with the smallest degree of structural alteration possible and to preserve visual function. KS lesions are not removed unless they impair the structure or function of the eye or are cosmetically unacceptable to the client. Treatment options are chemotherapy, radiation, and excision.

AIDS Retinopathy

Overview

Noninfectious AIDS retinopathy presents itself most commonly as cotton wool spots, retinal hemorrhages, or reti-

nitis. Cotton wool spots are fluffy white opacities that indicate focal retinal ischemia. The retinal ischemia involves the nerve fiber layer and is caused by the occlusion of retinal arterial and venous vessels, contributing to development of capillary nonperfusion.

Collaborative Management

Cotton wool spots are usually seen in the peripapillary area of the retina. Because of their fluffy appearance, they are sometimes mistaken for cytomegalovirus (CMV) retinitis; however, these spots appear to regress and fade over time. Retinal hemorrhages are seen in both the superficial and the deep layers of the retina. Roth's spots, areas of hemorrhage with a white central area, have also been observed.

Cotton wool spots are not treated but monitored as indicators of microvascular perfusion. Treatment of retinal hemorrhage and retinitis for clients with AIDS is the same as that for other clients with these retinal disorders.

Infectious Manifestations

Cytomegaloretinitis

Overview

The second most common ocular manifestation of HIV and a common opportunistic infection in clients with AIDS is cytomegalovirus (CMV) retinitis. Direct viral invasion of retinal cells causes damage and necrosis. The initial occurrence of CMV retinitis is usually unilateral. Involvement of the opposite eye often follows as a result of the viremia.

Collaborative Management

Clients with CMV retinitis have granular white dots on the retina that somewhat resemble cotton wool spots. However, these dots are deep and have an increased density. The lesions tend to occur close to major blood vessels and form patches of opacification. Left untreated, these patches expand and occlude retinal blood vessels. Atrophy and papilledema of the optic nerve also can occur. Hemorrhages are present and vision can be affected, depending on the location of the retinitis. Untreated CMV retinitis progresses to acute retinal necrosis.

CMV retinitis is diagnosed on the basis of client history and ocular findings. Clients with HIV disease may be asymptomatic, presenting for treatment of another ocular problem. Rapid detection of CMV retinitis is critical because of its fast progression. Because the goal of treatment is to arrest the disease quickly to maintain as much functional vision as possible, the nurse alerts clients with HIV infection to the signs and symptoms of CMV retinitis. These symptoms include any change in vision and the appearance of flashes of light or floaters.

Treatment of the client with CMV retinitis involves use of ganciclovir or trisodium phosphonoformate (Foscarnet). These drugs slow the proliferative nature of the disease but do not kill the virus. Recurrence is common.

BLINDNESS
Overview

Varied forms of blindness exist and may affect any or all dimensions of vision, including color, light, image, movement, and acuity. Clients are classified as legally blind if their best visual acuity with corrective lenses in the better eye is 20/200 or less or if the widest diameter of the visual field in that eye is no greater than 20 degrees.

Blindness can occur in one or both eyes. When one eye is affected, the horizontal field of vision is narrowed and depth perception is impaired.

Central vision can be impaired by diseases involving the macula, such as macular edema or macular degeneration. The loss of side vision affects the client's ability to drive and his or her awareness of hazards in the periphery. Loss of peripheral vision is associated with glaucoma.

Collaborative Management

The nurse teaches the client several techniques to better use existing vision. Moving the head slightly up and down can enhance a three-dimensional effect. When shaking hands or pouring water, the client can line up the object and move toward it. The client should choose a position that favors the good eye; for example, people with vision in the right eye should position people and items on their right.

Nursing interventions for the client with reduced sight fall into four areas: orientation, ambulation, self-care, and support.

Orientation

Most clients seen in health care settings have varied degrees of sight. Most clients categorized as "blind" had sight at some time and thus have a background knowledge of size and shape on which the nurse can rely when providing information. When talking with a client who has limited sight or is blind, the nurse always uses a normal tone of voice.

The nurse first orients the client to the immediate environment and communicates the approximate size of the room. One object in the room, such as an examination chair or hospital bed, serves as the focal point during the nurse's description. The nurse guides the client to the focal point and orients him or her to the environment from that point. For example, the nurse might say, "To the left of the bed is a chair." The nurse then describes all other objects in relation to the focal point. The nurse accompanies the client to other important areas, such as the bathroom, so that the client can learn their locations. The nurse highlights the location of the toilet, sink, and toilet paper holder. The client with limited sight is never left in the center of an unfamiliar room.

Clients with limited sight prefer to establish the location of important objects, such as the call bell, water pitcher, and clock. Once their location has been fixed, these items are not moved without the client's consent. The location of movable items, such as chairs, stools, and wastebaskets, are not disturbed without consulting the client.

At mealtime, the nurse or assistive nursing personnel sets up food on the tray using clock placement. For example, "There is sliced ham at 6 o'clock; peas are located at 3 o'clock; to the right of the plate is coffee; salt and pepper are next to the coffee."

Ambulation

When assisting a client with limited sight to ambulate, the nurse allows the client to grasp the nurse's arm at the elbow. The arm is kept close to the nurse's body so that the client can detect the direction of movement. When obstacles are noted in the path ahead, the nurse alerts the client.

Clients may use a cane to detect obstacles, such as furniture, walls, or curbs. The cane is held in the dominant hand several inches off the floor and sweeps the ground where the client's foot will be placed next. The laser cane sends out signals to help a blind client detect obstacles.

Self-Care

The ability to control the environment is important to the client with a visual impairment. The nurse knocks on the door before entering the client's hospital room or any other environment of a client with limited sight. The nurse states his or her name and reason for visiting when entering the room.

Support

Clients' reaction to the loss of sight is similar to the reaction to loss of a body part. Newly blind clients may experience a brief period of physical or psychological immobility. A period of grieving is needed for the "dead" (nonseeing) eye. Clients often experience hopelessness

> ### CASE STUDY for the Client with Acute Angle-Closure Glaucoma
>
> ■ One of your assistive nursing personnel, a 45-year-old woman, comes to you complaining of sudden, excruciating pain around the left eye and left cheek, accompanied by nausea. She asks to lie down for a while.
>
> While talking to her, you notice that her left pupil is dilated more than the right and does not react when you move her from a dimly lighted room to one that is brighter. You also notice that the sclera of the left eye is red with enlarged blood vessels radiating outward from the iris. She is anxious and crying.
>
> Q U E S T I O N S :
> 1. What assessment techniques should you perform?
> 2. What questions should you ask?
> 3. Given these findings, what should be your plan of action?
> 4. What are the expected outcomes for this situation?

and denial. With time, anger usually gives way to acceptance. The ability to cope may begin within days, but some clients may need months to mourn.

Clients benefit from the honest, empathetic support that nurses can provide. They need to hear that it is normal to mourn, to cry, and to feel the loss. Nurses help clients move toward acceptance by encouraging the mastery of one task at a time and by providing positive reinforcement for each success.

SELECTED BIBLIOGRAPHY

Bass, S., & Giovinazzo, V. (1996). Laser treatment of macular disease. *Optometry Clinics, 5*(1), 161–173.

Birt, L. (1995). Making sense of photorefractive keratectomy. *Nursing Times, 91*(44), 30–31.

Brady, B. (1995). Macular degeneration: Helping your patient cope. *Nursing95, 25*(6), 62–64.

Carter, T. (1994). Age-related vision changes: A primary care guide. *Geriatrics, 49*(9), 37–45.

Cleary, M. (1995). Helping the person who is visually impaired: Concerns, questions, remedies, & sources. *Journal of Ophthalmic Nursing and Technology, 14*(5), 205–211.

Cooper, J. (1996). Improving compliance with glaucoma eye-drop treatment. *Nursing Times, 92*(32), 36–37.

Cotran, R., Kumar, V., & Robbins, S. (1994). *Robbins pathologic basis of disease* (5th ed.). Philadelphia: W. B. Saunders.

Doerling, J. (1996). Families' experiences in consenting to eye donation of a recently deceased relative. *Heart & Lung, 25*(1), 72–78.

Eichenbaum, J. (1996). Vitamins for cataracts and macular degeneration. *Journal of Ophthalmic Nursing and Technology, 15*(2), 65–67.

Jubeck, M. (1994). Teaching the elderly: A commonsense approach. *Nursing94, 24*(5), 70–71.

Kearney, K. (1997). Retinal detachment. *American Journal of Nursing, 97*(8), 50.

Kelly, M. (1996). Medications and the visually impaired elderly. *Geriatric Nursing, 17*(2), 60–62.

LaRussa, F., & Holsted, D. (1995). Photorefractive and phototherapeutic procedures. *Optometry Clinics, 4*(4), 51–67.

Long, K., & Long, R. (1994). Treating open-angle glaucoma. *Nurse Practitioner Forum, 5*(4), 205–206.

Oshinskie, L. (1996). Age-related macular degeneration. *Optometry Clinics, 5*(1), 25–53.

*Plona, B., & Schremp P. (1992). Nursing care of patients with ocular manifestations of human immunodeficiency virus infection. *Nursing Clinics of North America, 27*(3), 793–805.

*Ruehl, C., & Schremp, P. (1992). Nursing care of the cataract patient: Today's outpatient approach. *Nursing Clinics of North America, 27*(3), 737–743.

Sandler, R. (1995). Clinical snapshot: Glaucoma. *American Journal of Nursing, 95*(3), 34–35.

Servodidio, C.(1995). Nursing care of the choroidal melanoma patient. *Seminars in Perioperative Nursing, 4*(4), 211–219.

Sivalingam, E. (1996). Glaucoma: An overview. *Journal of Ophthalmic Nursing and Technology, 15*(1), 15–18.

*Smith, S. (1992). Diabetic retinopathy. *Nursing Clinics of North America, 27*(3), 745–759.

Vaughan D., Asbury, T., & Riordan-Eva, P. (1995). *General ophthalmology* (14th ed.). Norwalk, CT: Appleton & Lange.

*Woods, S. (1992). Macular degeneration. *Nursing Clinics of North America, 27*(3), 761–775.

SUGGESTED READINGS

Eichenbaum, J. (1996). Vitamins for cataracts and macular degeneration. *Journal of Ophthalmic Nursing and Technology, 15*(2), 65–67.
   This article explores the potential role of antioxidants in the prevention and treatment of several visual disorders. The reader is advised to help clients understand the difference between early studies indicating how these agents might work and long-term studies that establish effectiveness and potential toxicities.

Kelly, M. (1996). Medications and the visually impaired elderly. *Geriatric Nursing, 17*(2), 60–62.
   A case presentation approach is used to highlight the problems visually impaired older clients encounter in taking prescribed medications. Suggestions for increasing accuracy are presented. The author stresses the difference between visual acuity and functional safety with visual impaired clients.

*Woods, S. (1992). Macular degeneration. *Nursing Clinics of North America, 27*(3), 761–775.
   This article provides an in-depth discussion of the pathophysiology, clinical manifestations, and nursing care needs of people with macular degeneration. High-quality photographs of macular changes in the retina are included. The nursing interventions cited are specific and appropriate.

Chapter 50

ASSESSMENT OF
THE EAR AND HEARING

CHAPTER
HIGHLIGHTS

Health assessment of the ear and a client's hearing ability are especially important for nurses. Many ear and hearing difficulties have insidious onsets and may be affected by several medications. An understanding of the anatomy and physiology of the ear is essential. Table 50–1 defines terms commonly used in assessing the ear and hearing.

ANATOMY AND PHYSIOLOGY REVIEW
Structure

The ear consists of three structural parts: external, middle, and inner; each is integral to the hearing process.

External Ear

The external ear develops in the embryo at the same time as the kidneys and urinary tract. Therefore, any person with a defect of the external ear must also be examined for possible malformations of the renal and urinary systems.

The external ear is embedded in the temporal bone bilaterally at the level of the eyes, attached to the head by skin and cartilage at approximately a 10-degree angle. The external ear extends from the pinna through the external canal to the tympanic membrane, or eardrum (Fig. 50–1). The external ear canal is slightly S-shaped and lined with *cerumen* (wax)-producing glands, sebaceous glands, and hair follicles. The hair follicles and cerumen protect the tympanic membrane and the middle ear. In the adult, the distance from the opening of the external canal to the tympanic membrane is approximately 2.5–3.75 cm (1–1½ inches). The external ear includes the *mastoid process,* the bony ridge located over the temporal bone behind the pinna.

Middle Ear

The middle ear begins at the medial side of the tympanic membrane. It consists of the *epitympanum,* a compartment containing the three bony *ossicles* (Fig. 50–2): the malleus, the incus, and the stapes. The proximal end of the eustachian tube also opens in the middle ear.

The *tympanic membrane* is a thick, transparent sheet of tissue providing a barrier between the external ear and middle ear. The landmarks on the tympanic membrane include (Fig. 50–3) the annulus, pars flaccida, and pars tensa. The tympanic membrane is attached to the first

TABLE 50–1

Terminology Commonly Used in Ear and Hearing Assessment	
Term	**Definition**
Cerumen	• Wax-like secretion of the external ear canal
Conductive hearing loss	• Hearing loss resulting from a physical disruption in the transmission of sound waves
Decibel	• A unit of sound for expressing loudness
Masking	• The process of hiding a specific sound from one ear while the other ear is tested for its ability to hear that sound
Meniere's disease	• An intermittent but progressive deterioration of hearing and balance
Otitis media	• Inflammation/infection of the middle ear
Otosclerosis	• Formation of spongy bone around structures of the middle and inner ear, leading to low-tone hearing impairment
Ototoxic	• Damaging to the structures important for hearing
Presbycusis	• Age-related degenerative changes in the ear, leading to decreased hearing acuity
Sensorineural	• Hearing loss resulting from neural defects
Spondee	• Words of two syllables on which equal stress is placed during pronunciation
Vestibular hearing loss	• Relating to the functions of the ear for the sense of balance and position

round and the oval windows. The eustachian tube originates from the floor of the middle ear at the proximal end and opens at the distal end in the nasopharynx. The distal opening in the nasopharynx is surrounded by adenoid lymphatic tissue (Fig. 50–4). The eustachian tube allows equalization of pressure on both sides of the tympanic membrane. Secretions from the middle ear drain through it.

Inner Ear

The inner ear, lying on the other side of the oval window, contains the semicircular canals, the cochlea, and the distal end of the eighth cranial nerve (see Fig. 50–2). The *semicircular canals* contain fluid and hair cells connected to the sensory nerve fibers of the vestibular portion of the eighth cranial nerve, which help to maintain the sense of balance.

The *cochlea* is the spiral organ of hearing, divided into the scala tympani and the scala vestibuli. Reissner's membrane stretches across the scala vestibuli and forms the duct of the cochlea, or the scala media. The scala media is filled with *endolymph,* a fluid similar to intracellular fluid. The scala tympani and scala vestibuli are filled with *perilymph.* Endolymph and perilymph protect the cochlea and the semicircular canals, which literally float in the fluids, cushioning them against abrupt movements of the head.

The *organ of Corti* is the receptor end-organ of hearing located on the basilar membrane of the cochlea. The cochlea contains hair cells that detect vibration from sound and stimulate the eighth cranial nerve.

Function

The ear's main function is hearing, accomplished when sound is delivered through the air to the external ear canal and the temporal bone covering the mastoid air cells. The sound waves strike the mastoid and the movable tympanic membrane, which is connected to the first bony ossicle, the malleus. The sound wave vibrations are transferred from the tympanic membrane to the malleus,

bony ossicle, the *malleus,* at the *umbo* (see Fig. 50–3). The bony ossicles behind the tympanic membrane are joined, although not rigidly, allowing vibratory movement.

The pars flaccida and pars tensa are parts of the tympanic membrane. The pars flaccida is that portion of the tympanic membrane above the short process of the malleus; the pars tensa is that portion surrounding the long process of the malleus. It is usually transparent, opaque, or pearly gray and mobile when air is injected into the external canal. The umbo is seen through the tympanic membrane as a white dot at the end of the long process of the malleus. The short process of the malleus, the long process of the malleus, and the umbo are structures seen through the transparent tympanic membrane.

The middle ear is separated from the inner ear by the

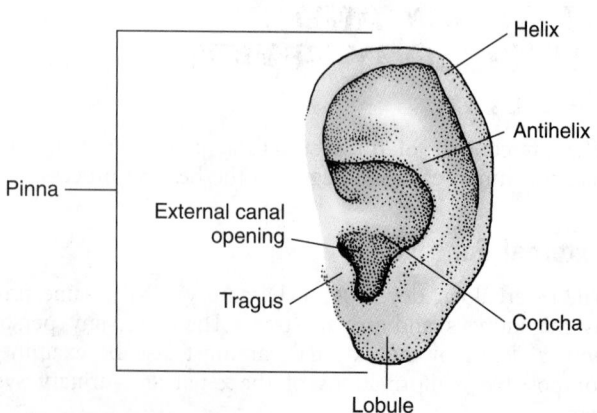

Figure 50–1. Anatomic features of the external ear.

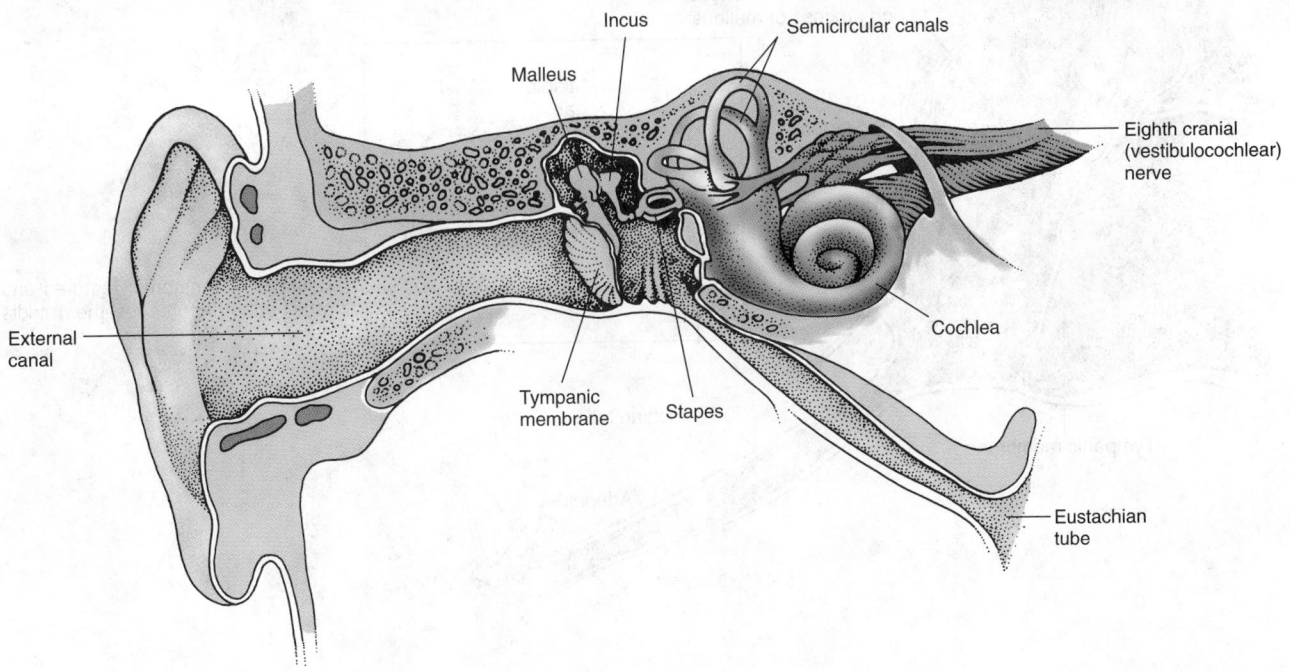

Figure 50–2. Anatomic features of the internal ear.

the incus, and the stapes. From the stapes, the vibrations are transmitted to the cochlea. Receptors there transduce (change) the vibrations into action potentials, conducted to the brain as neural impulses by the cochlear portion of the eighth cranial (or auditory) nerve. Sound is processed and interpreted by the brain.

Ear and Hearing Changes Associated with Aging

Ear and hearing changes related to aging are summarized in Chart 50–1. Some of these changes are harmless (see Research Applications for Nursing); others pose serious threats to the hearing ability of older clients and call for nursing interventions.

HISTORY

The nurse obtains a thorough history from the client. Informal hearing assessment begins as the nurse observes the client listening to and answering questions. The client's posture and appropriateness of responses provide additional information about the client's hearing acuity.

During the interview, the nurse sits in adequate light, facing the client, which allows the client to see the nurse speaking. The nurse is careful to use ordinary language. The nurse also assesses demographic data, personal and family history, socioeconomic status, and the current health problem.

Demographic Data

The gender of the client is important. Some auditory disorders, such as otosclerosis, are more common in

women; others, such as Meniere's disease, are more common in men. Age is also a significant factor in hearing loss.

Personal and Family History

Personal history includes information on past or current signs and symptoms of ear pain, ear discharge, vertigo,

RIGHT TYMPANIC MEMBRANE

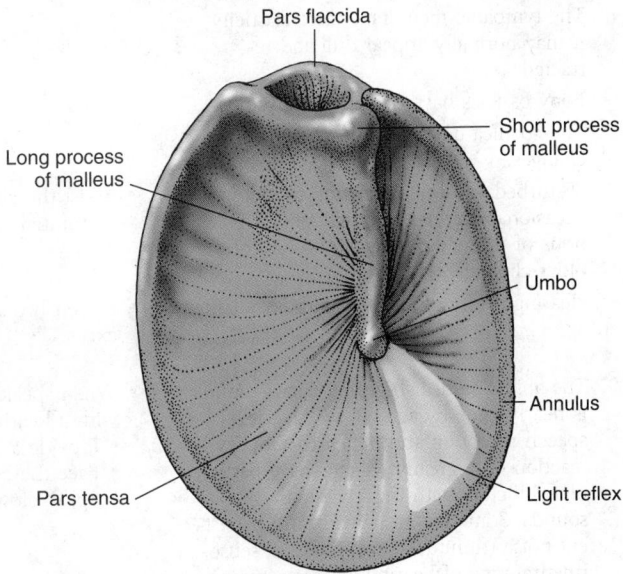

Figure 50–3. Landmarks on the tympanic membrane.

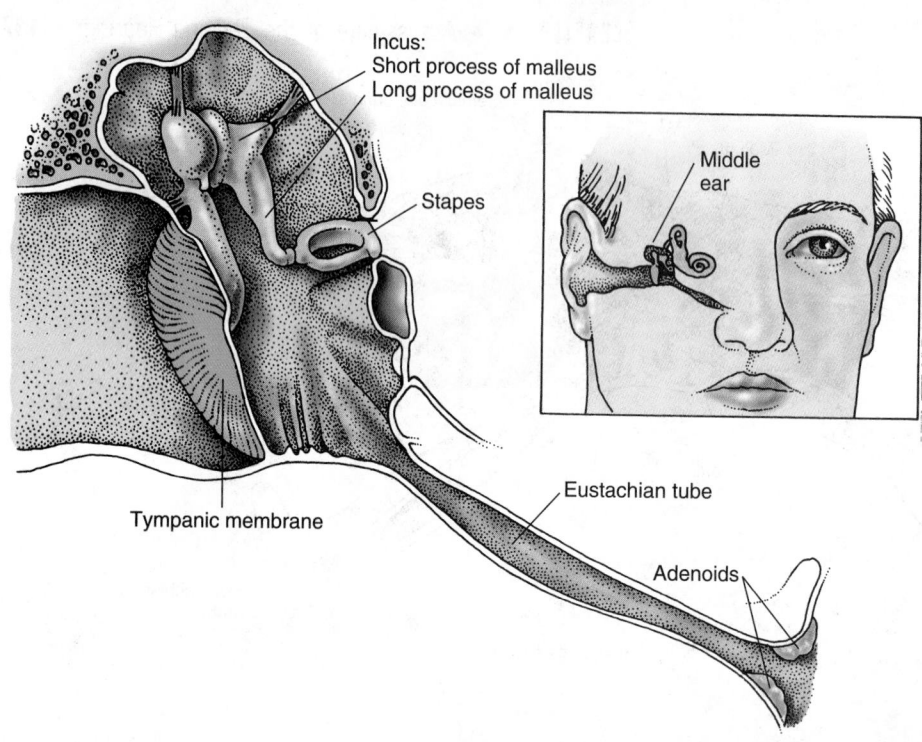

Incus:
Short process of malleus
Long process of malleus

Stapes

Middle
ear

Figure 50–4. Anatomic features and attached structures of the middle ear.

Tympanic membrane

Eustachian tube

Adenoids

Chart 50–1

Nursing Focus on the Elderly: The Ear and Hearing

Physiologic Change	Nursing Implications	Rationale
The pinna becomes elongated because of normal loss of subcutaneous tissue and decreased tissue elasticity.		
Hair becomes coarser and longer, especially in men.		
Cerumen-producing glands decrease in number and function.	• Irrigate ear canal weekly.	• Irrigation removes excess cerumen, preventing impaction and enhancing transmission of sound waves.
Cerumen tends to be drier in older clients; it becomes impacted, which causes hearing loss.	• Place 1–2 drops of oil into ear canal 8 hr before irrigation.	• Oil softens impacted cerumen, facilitating removal.
The tympanic membrane loses elasticity; it may normally appear dull and retracted.		
Bony ossicles have decreased movement.		
The cochlea undergoes degenerative changes.		
Disturbed vestibular function results in occasional dizziness, vertigo, and sensations of unsteadiness in 50%–60% of older clients.	• Assist the client with standing and initial ambulation.	• The nurse provides a stable point of reference. Assistance decreases the risk of falling as a result of vestibular disorientation.
Hearing acuity diminishes with advancing age.	• Establish that a hearing deficiency exists.	• Determine whether interventions are needed. Not all elderly clients have diminished hearing acuity.
The ability to hear high-frequency sounds is nearly gone by age 60, which affects speech reception and increases auditory reaction time greatly. Clients have particular difficulty with the *f, s, sh,* and *pa* sounds. Some older clients hear a persistent noise (tinnitus). Presbycusis (a sensorineural type of hearing loss) is common in the aged.	• When speaking to an older client with a hearing deficiency: • Provide a quiet environment. • Face the client. • Speak slowly in a deeper voice.	• This makes it easier for the client to hear and communicate. • Extraneous noise may interfere with the client's auditory perception. • The client can benefit by being able to see lip movement. • The client may be able to discern lower frequencies more easily.

Research Applications for Nursing

Aging Causes Ear Size Changes

Heathcote, J. A. (1995). Why do old men have big ears? British Medical Journal, 311(7021), 1668.

This study examined the external ear size of males as they aged. External ear length was measured in 206 men ranging in age from 53 to 75 years. It was found that, on average, the external ear increased in size on average 0.22 mm/year.

Critique. External ear length has long been thought to increase with age, yet no empirical data supported this. This study only examined men, and no explanation was offered for why the male external ear increases in size.

Possible Nursing Implications. Older male patients can be reassured that increasing external ear length is common.

tinnitus, decreased hearing, and difficulty understanding people when they talk or difficulty hearing environmental noises. The nurse asks the client about any history of

- Ear trauma
- Ear surgery
- Past infections
- Excessive cerumen
- Ear itch
- Any invasive instruments routinely used to clean the ear
- Type and pattern of ear hygiene
- Exposure to loud noise or music
- Air travel (especially in unpressurized aircraft)
- Swimming habits and the use of protective ear devices for swimming

If the client uses a hearing aid, the nurse determines how well it works, the date of the last hearing test, the type of test given, and the results. The nurse asks the client about other conditions that may impair hearing, such as allergies, upper respiratory tract infection, hypothyroidism, arteriosclerosis, head trauma, and recent head, facial, or dental surgery.

A thorough medication history is crucial because many drugs are ototoxic (Table 50–2).

The nurse asks about occupation and hobbies involving exposure to excessive environmental noise or music. The nurse also investigates the use of protective ear devices or any devices inserted into the ear, such as telephone operator headsets or stethoscopes. Information about hearing loss among family members is important because some types of hearing loss are hereditary or have a genetic component.

Socioeconomic Status

The nurse assesses the client's socioeconomic status to determine the availability of health care. Clients of lower socioeconomic status often do not seek health care for ear-related problems until hearing damage is extensive.

However, clients at any socioeconomic level might hesitate to have their hearing loss diagnosed because of the fear of wearing a hearing amplification device.

Current Health Problems

The nurse assesses current ear-related health problems, asking whether the client has noticed any "trouble with" his or her ears, ear pain, or discharge, including any earwax. The nurse asks the client about any change in hearing or associated problems, like ringing in the ears. If a change in hearing is reported, the nurse asks whether one or both ears are involved and whether the change

TABLE 50–2

Impact of Ototoxic Substances on Auditory Function

Drug	Auditory Effects
Antibiotics	
Amikacin (Amikin)	++
Chloramphenicol (Chloromycetin, Novochlorocap✦)	+ to ++
Erythromycin (Apo-Erythro✦, E.E.S., E-Mycin, Novorythro✦)	+ to ++
Gentamicin (Cidomycin✦, Garamycin)	++
Kanamycin (Kantrex)	++
Neomycin	++
Streptomycin	++
Tobramycin (Nebcin)	++
Vancomycin (Lyphocin, Vancocin)	++
Diuretics	
Acetazolamide (Apo-Acetazolamide✦, Diamox)	++
Furosemide (Apo-Furosemide✦, Lasix, Furoside✦)	++
Ethacrynic acid (Edecrin)	++
Nonsteroidal Antiinflammatory Agents	
Salicylates (Apo-Asa✦, Ascriptin, Bufferin, Enthrofen✦)	++
Ibuprofen (Advil, Amersol✦, Motrin, Novoprofen✦)	+
Naproxen (Anaprox, Apo-Napro-Na✦, Naprosyn, Novonaprox✦)	+
Indomethacin (Indocid✦, Indocin)	+
Miscellaneous	
Cisplatin (Abiplatin✦, Platinol)	++
Mechlorethamine (Mustargen)	+
Quinine (Legatrin, Novoquinine✦, Quinamm)	+
Quinidine (Apo-Quinidine✦, Cardioquin, Quinidex)	+

+ = slight impact; ++ = significant impact.

was sudden or gradual. The nurse also questions the client about any problems with dizziness or balance.

PHYSICAL ASSESSMENT

Inspection and palpation are the only examination techniques used to assess the ear. The nurse begins the examination by placing the client in either a sitting or a supine position. Uncooperative clients are carefully restrained to prevent injury to the external canal. Any hearing aids should be removed during the examination. After the otoscopic examination, the nurse inspects the hearing aid for cracks, debris, and a proper fit. Ear examination is divided into external ear and mastoid assessment, otoscopic assessment, and auditory assessment.

External Ear and Mastoid Assessment

The mastoid process is inspected for redness and swelling, which indicate inflammation. To assess for tenderness, the nurse gently taps with one finger over the mastoid process, compresses the tragus with one finger, and gently manipulates the pinna forward and backward. Any tenderness suggests an inflammatory process in either the external ear or the mastoid.

The entire external ear is inspected for configuration, location of attachment to the head, and condition of the visible external canal. The normal pinna is uniformly shaped without additional skin tags or deformity. The pinna should be attached vertically to the side of the head at a posterior angle of no greater than 10 degrees. It should fall within or touch the eye-occiput line, an imaginary line drawn from the greatest protuberance on the occiput to the lateral canthus of the eye. The nurse notes variations from the normal ear shape and attachment.

Abnormalities of the pinna include swelling, nodules, and lesions. In chronic gout, accumulations of uric acid crystals result in hard, irregular, painless nodules called tophi on the helix and antihelix portions of the pinna. Other painless nodules on the pinna might be due to basal cell carcinoma or rheumatoid arthritis. Small, crusted, ulcerated, or indurated lesions on the pinna that fail to heal could be squamous cell carcinoma.

The normal external canal is free from lesions, dry, clean, and not reddened. The nurse assesses for abnormalities, including

- Furuncles
- Large accumulations of cerumen
- Scaliness
- Redness
- Swelling of or drainage from the ear associated with a foreign object, trauma, or infection

The nurse also notes any drainage (blood, cerebrospinal fluid, pus, or serous fluid) and its character.

Otoscopic Assessment

An instrument called an otoscope is used to examine the ear. Many types are available. An otoscope (Fig. 50–5)

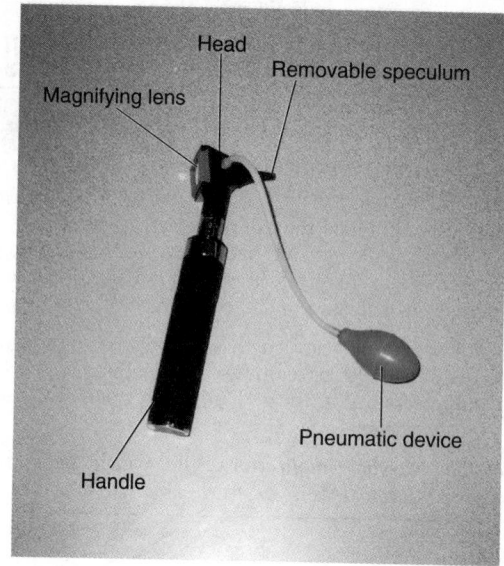

Figure 50–5. Functional components of an otoscope.

consists of a light, handle, magnifying lens, and a pneumatic attachment for injecting air into the external canal to test mobility of the tympanic membrane.

Specula of various diameters attach to the head of the otoscope; the largest that most comfortably fits the client's external canal is selected for the examination. The nurse never blindly introduces the speculum into the external canal because of the risk of perforating the tympanic membrane.

If the client experiences any pain during external ear examination, the nurse attempts a cautious otoscopic examination. (The speculum will cause extreme pain if it comes in contact with inflamed tissue in the external canal.) The nurse must become familiar with and memorize all the structures of the tympanic membrane and middle ear before attempting to visualize them with an otoscope.

When performing an otoscopic examination, the nurse tilts the client's head slightly away and holds the otoscope upside down, like a large pen (Fig. 50–6). This position permits the nurse's hand to lie against the client's head for support. If the client moves, both the nurse's hand and the otoscope move as well, preventing damage to the external canal or tympanic membrane. The nurse holds the otoscope in the dominant hand and gently pulls the pinna up and back with the nondominant hand. The nurse visualizes the external canal while slowly inserting the speculum. The nurse uses caution and avoids jamming the speculum into the walls of the external canal, which causes pain.

After the pinna is correctly displaced and the otoscope is comfortably introduced in the external canal, the nurse observes the tympanic membrane for color, intactness, and shape. The nurse further assesses for lesions and amount and consistency of cerumen and hair. The normal external canal is skin-colored, intact, without lesions, and with various amounts of soft cerumen and small, fine hairs.

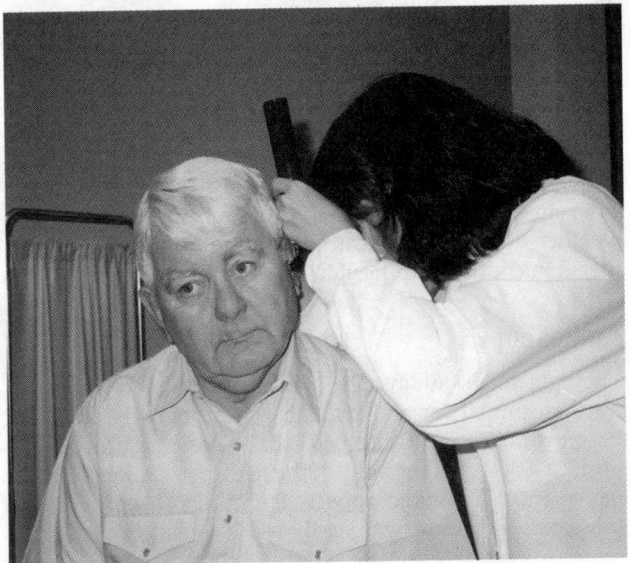

Figure 50–6. Proper technique for an otoscopic examination.

Next, the nurse assesses the tympanic membranes for intactness, normal structures seen through the tympanic membrane (the long and short processes of the malleus and the umbo), portions of the tympanic membrane itself (light reflex, pars flaccida, and pars tensa), and the color, shape, lesions, and mobility of the membrane. Figure 50–7 shows an otoscopic view of a normal tympanic membrane. The normal tympanic membrane is always intact. The long process of the malleus is seen through the tympanic membrane as a whitish streak extending from the short process of the malleus to the umbo. A normal variation in some people with allergies is vascularity over the long process, although this might be an early indication of otitis media.

The short process of the malleus is seen through the tympanic membrane as a white structure, which seems more three-dimensional (projecting out toward the otoscope) than the other structures on the tympanic membrane. The umbo appears as a round, white dot.

The long and short processes of the malleus, in addition to the umbo, are always easily identified in the normal ear. Abnormal variations are caused by serous otitis and otitis media, among other disorders.

Reflection of the otoscope's light off the tympanic membrane reveals the *light reflex,* a clearly demarcated triangle of light in the normal ear. The base of the triangle is on the annulus, and the point of the triangle on the umbo. When the light reflex is spotty or multiple because of changed tympanic membrane shape from either retraction or bulging, the light reflex is termed *diffuse.*

The tympanic membrane is normally shiny and transparent, opaque, or pearly gray. Abnormal variations include red (as seen in otitis media) and dull or retracted (as seen in serous otitis).

The normal tympanic membrane is slightly concave, allowing the pars tensa portion to move gently on testing with a puff of air from the pneumatic device on the otoscope.

The normal tympanic membrane is free from lesions. The most common lesion is scarring caused by previous ear infection and perforation. A scar thickens the tympanic membrane, which makes it difficult or impossible to see through the membrane at the point of the scar, and reduces the mobility of the tympanic membrane.

The nurse tests the mobility of the tympanic membrane by gently injecting a small puff of air through the pneumatic device into the external canal and watching the pars tensa portion for movement. The normal tympanic membrane moves gently. Decreased or absent mobility results from scarring, retraction, bulging, presence of fluid in the middle ear, and decreased mobility of the ossicles associated with aging.

TRANSCULTURAL CONSIDERATIONS

Cerumen is generally moist and tan or brown in Caucasian and African-American clients. It is dry and light brown to gray in Asians and Native Americans. The color of the lining of the external ear canal varies with the client's skin tone.

Auditory Assessment

After completing bilateral external ear and otoscopic examinations, the nurse assesses the client's hearing acuity. Sound is transmitted by air conduction and bone conduction. Air conduction of sound is normally more sensitive than bone conduction. If hearing acuity is decreased, the hearing loss is categorized as

- Conductive hearing loss, resulting from any physical obstruction of sound wave transmission (such as a foreign body in the external canal, a retracted or bulging tympanic membrane, or fused bony ossicles)

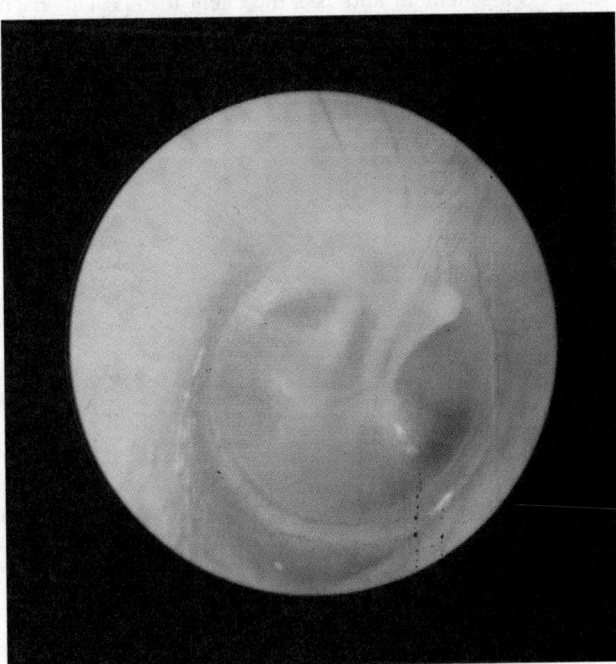

Figure 50–7. Otoscopic view of a normal tympanic membrane.

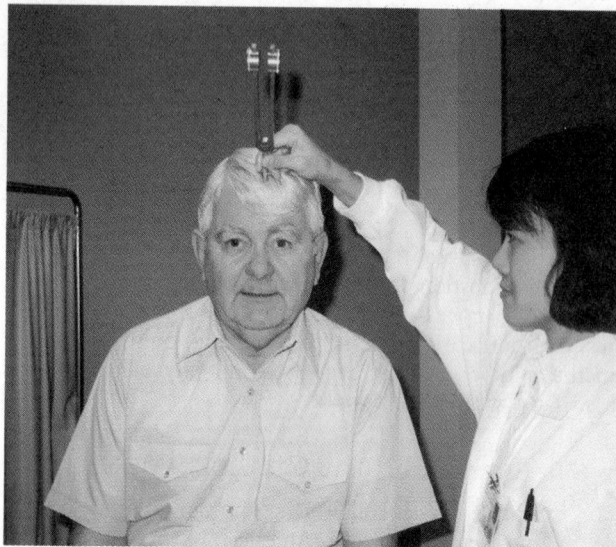

Figure 50–8. Correct placement of the tuning fork for the Weber test.

- Sensorineural hearing loss, resulting from a defect in the cochlea, the eighth cranial nerve, or the brain itself
- Mixed conductive and sensorineural hearing loss, a profound hearing loss

Each of the auditory function tests determines the degree of hearing loss and differentiates the type of loss.

Voice Test

The nurse can conduct a simple hearing acuity test by asking the client to block one external ear canal while standing 30 to 60 cm (1–2 feet) away. The nurse quietly whispers a statement and asks the client to repeat it. Each ear is tested separately. If the client does not respond correctly, a louder whisper is used. If the nurse suspects that the client is lip reading, the nurse's hand can be used to block the client's view of the nurse's mouth.

Watch Test

A ticking watch is used to test hearing acuity for high-frequency sounds. The nurse holds a ticking watch about 12.7 cm (5 inches) from each of the client's ears and asks whether the ticking is heard. The client with normal hearing should be able to hear it.

Audioscopy

The lightweight audioscope allows the examiner to visualize the external ear and tympanic membrane. Hearing can be measured at a 40-decibel (dB) intensity at frequencies of 500, 1000, 2000, and 4000 cycles per second (cps) or hertz (Hz). The audioscope is larger than a conventional otoscope, and nurses can easily use it to assess hearing.

Tuning Fork Tests

Hearing acuity can be tested by the Weber and Rinne tuning fork tests. Tuning fork tests are useful, although limited, in differentiating between conductive and sensorineural hearing losses. The frequency range of the tuning fork used for these tests corresponds to that of normal speech: 512 or 1024 Hz. To perform this assessment, the nurse stands in front of the sitting client.

Weber Tuning Fork Test

To perform the Weber tuning fork test, the nurse places the vibrating tuning fork in the middle of the client's head, at the midline of the forehead, or above the upper lip over the teeth. Many clients object to the vibration over the upper lip, so the preferred site is the midline of the skull (Fig. 50–8). The nurse takes care to hold the vibrating tuning fork by the stem only, not by the vibrating forks. The nurse asks the client in which ear the sound is louder. The normal test result is sound heard

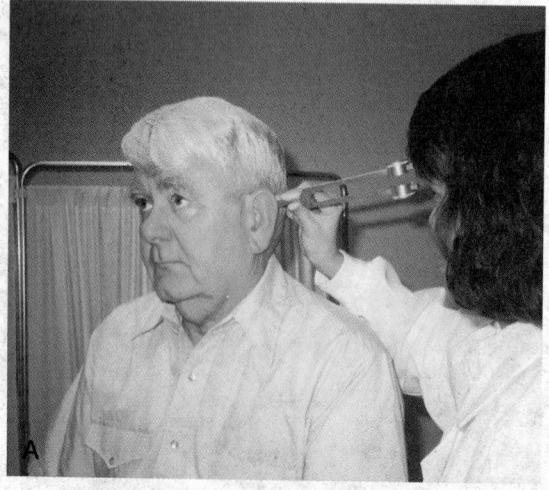

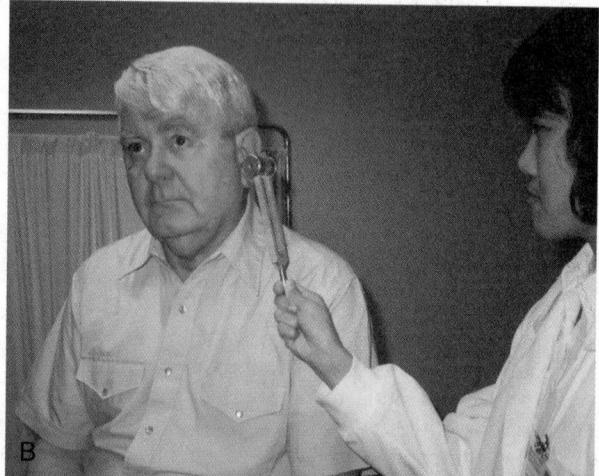

Figure 50–9. (A, B) Correct placement of the tuning fork for the Rinne test.

equally in both ears. If the client hears the sound louder in one ear, the term *lateralization* describes the side hearing the loudest.

Rinne Tuning Fork Test

The Rinne tuning fork test compares the client's hearing by air and bone conduction. Sound is normally heard two to three times longer by air than by bone conduction. The nurse performs the Rinne tuning fork test by placing the vibrating tuning fork stem on the client's mastoid process. The client indicates when he or she no longer hears the sound and the nurse quickly brings the tuning fork in front of the pinna without touching the client, asking whether he or she still hears the sound (Fig. 50–9). The nurse records the duration of both phases, bone conduction followed by air conduction, and compares the times. The client normally continues to hear the sound two times longer in front of the pinna after not hearing it with the tuning fork touching the mastoid process.

PSYCHOSOCIAL ASSESSMENT

The client may become irritable, frustrated, and depressed by an inability to hear and respond appropriately. The inability to hear results in frustrating experiences and often isolates the client from the world. Depression may result from the sensory isolation of hearing loss. The nurse is sensitive to the client and conducts the interview at a pace appropriate to that client.

The nurse investigates the client's social and work relationships to determine whether the client experiences isolation because of hearing problems. In addition, the nurse encourages the client to express feelings related to hearing loss and discuss changes in daily living activities for coping. The nurse also obtains information from family members, especially if the client denies having a hearing problem. Throughout the assessment, the nurse remains patient and empathic.

DIAGNOSTIC ASSESSMENT
Laboratory Tests

Laboratory tests are not of value in determining hearing acuity. For an external ear infection, microbial culture and antibiotic sensitivity tests can determine the causative organism and the most appropriate antibiotic.

Radiographic Examinations
Tomography

Tomography is an x-ray that blurs the tissues above and below a single layer or plane of tissue to provide exacting detail. It can be used to assess pathologic conditions of the mastoid, middle ear, and inner ear structures. This highly sophisticated test helps diagnose both conductive and sensorineural hearing losses.

To prepare the client for tomography, the nurse

- Carefully explains the procedure and its purpose
- Informs the client that approximately 45 minutes are required for the procedure

- Asks women whether they are pregnant; clients in the first trimester of pregnancy should delay tomography
- Ensures that all jewelry is removed before the procedure begins

Women in the latter phases of pregnancy are protected with a lead apron over the abdomen and pelvis. Lead eye shields cover the corneas to diminish the radiation dose to the eyes. Clients must remain still, in a supine position, during the procedure.

No special follow-up care is needed.

Polytome X-Ray Studies

Polytome x-rays are a modification of standard tomography to achieve a multidimensional picture. This study, with or without contrast enhancement, is helpful in diagnosing lesions of the temporal bone.

Computed Tomography

Computed tomography (CT), with or without contrast enhancement, reveals the structures of the ear in great detail by multiple x-rays of the head, which are then averaged by a computer. CT is especially helpful in diagnosing acoustic tumors.

Arteriography and Venography

When polytome x-rays suggest a tumor, arteriography may be done. The physician inserts a catheter into the carotid artery and injects dye to radiographically determine the tumor's vascularity and origin of blood supply. Venography is usually done if polytome x-rays do not clearly show involvement of the jugular bulb of the carotid canal; x-rays are taken after a catheter is threaded into the jugular vein or the femoral vein and dye is injected.

Other Diagnostic Assessment
Magnetic Resonance Imaging

Magnetic resonance imaging (MRI) is a noninvasive, nonradioactive diagnostic tool that uses a computer to generate images. Because of its superior contrast resolution, no bony artifacts can obscure tissue. Therefore, MRI has great sensitivity to soft-tissue changes. Clients with internal metal vascular clips cannot have MRI.

Audiometry

Audiometry is the measurement of hearing acuity. To understand audiometry, the nurse must first understand audiometric testing terminology.

Frequency is the highness or lowness of tones (expressed in hertz). The greater the number of vibrations per second, the higher the frequency (pitch) of the sound; the fewer vibrations per second, the lower the pitch.

Intensity of sound is expressed in decibels. The lowest intensity at which a young, normal ear can detect sound (about 50% of the time) is 0 dB. Sound at 110 dB is so intense (loud) that it is painful for most people with normal hearing. Conversational speech is generally around

TABLE 50-3

Decibel Intensity and Safe Exposure Time for Common Sounds		
Sound	Decibel Intensity (dB)	Safe Exposure Time*
Threshold of hearing	0	
Whispering	20	
Average residence or office	40	
Conversational speech	60	
Car traffic	70	>8 hr
Motorcycle	90	8 hr
Chain saw	100	2 hr
Rock concert, front row	120	3 min
Jet engine	140	Immediate danger
Rocket launching pad	180	Immediate danger

* For every 5-dB increase in intensity, the safe exposure time is cut in half.

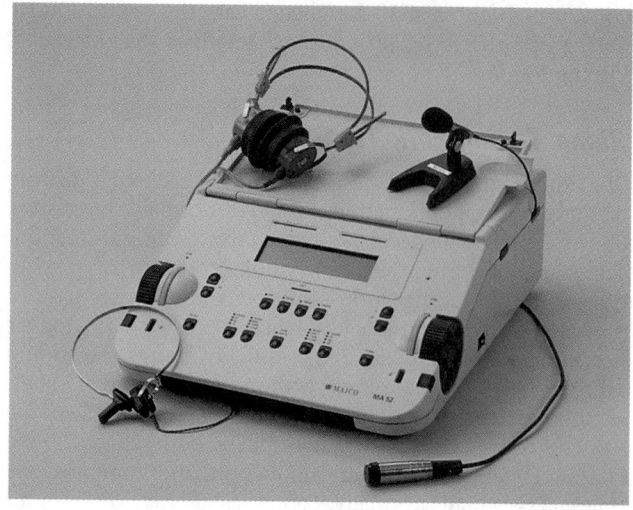

Figure 50–10. A pure tone audiometer. (Courtesy of Maico, Inc., Minneapolis, MN.)

60 dB, and a soft whisper is around 20 dB (Table 50–3). A hearing loss of 45–50 dB renders the person unable to hear speech without a hearing aid. A person with a hearing loss of 90 dB may not be able to hear speech even with a hearing aid.

Threshold is the lowest level of intensity at which pure tones and speech are heard by a client (about 50% of the time). *Pure tones* are generated by an *audiometer* (Fig. 50–10) to determine hearing acuity. There are two types of audiometry: pure tone and speech.

Pure Tone Audiometry

Tones generated by an audiometer are presented to the client at frequencies for hearing speech, music, and other common sounds. Pure tone audiometry is performed by air conduction testing or bone conduction testing. The results of pure tone audiometry are plotted on an *audiogram* (Fig. 50–11). For some clients, the hearing of one ear is "masked" while the hearing of the other ear is tested.

AIR CONDUCTION TEST. Pure tone air conduction testing determines whether a client hears normally or has a hearing loss. It is designed to test air conduction hearing sensitivity (through earphones) at frequencies of 125, 250, 500, 750, 1000, 1500, 2000, 3000, 4000, 6000, and 8000 Hz, but thresholds are usually confined to the frequencies of 250, 500, 1000, 2000, 4000, and 8000 Hz.

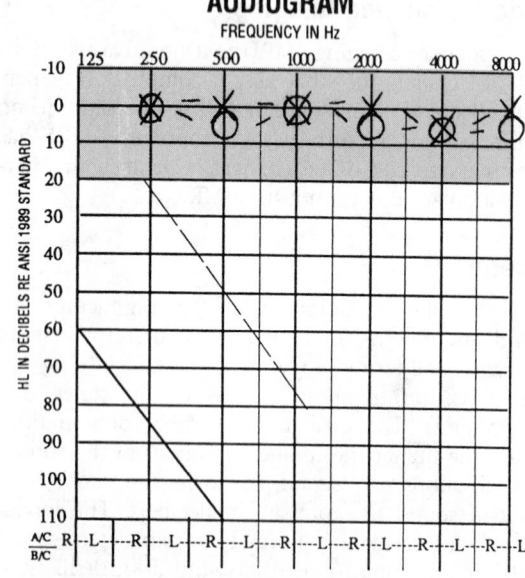

Audiogram Key	Left	Right		Left	Right
AC Unmasked	x	o	AC Masked	☐	Δ
BC Unmasked	>	<	BC Masked	]	[
No Response	↓	↙	SF		S

Figure 50–11. Audiogram pattern depicting normal hearing. (Courtesy of the Cleveland Hearing and Speech Center, Cleveland, OH.)

The intensities for the pure tones generally range from 10 to 110 dB.

CLIENT PREPARATION. The client is placed in a sound-isolated room in which ambient noise does not exceed American National Standards Institute noise standards. The nurse sits facing the client because the client's facial expressions are frequently helpful in evaluating responses. Hearing-impaired clients may benefit from lip reading the nurse's instructions. The nurse instructs the client as follows:

"I am going to test your hearing. The object of the test is to find the point at which you can just barely hear the tones. The tones will sound like soft bells or tuning forks. Every time you hear one, no matter how soft, signal by raising your hand (or pushing the button) on the side you hear the tone."

(If the client cannot raise a hand or push a button because of physical or motor disabilities, a yes-no verbal response is appropriate.)

"When you no longer hear the tone, lower your hand (or release the button). This lets me know when you hear the tone and when it goes away."

PROCEDURE. The ear with the better hearing is tested first. Before beginning the test, the nurse adjusts the audiometric equipment by

1. Setting the frequency control at 1000 Hz and the hearing level control at 40 dB
2. Putting on the earphones and listening to the tone while switching from one ear to the other
3. In each earphone, listening to the tone while gradually turning the hearing level control toward 0 dB
4. Testing the signal cord and light to make sure they are working

The nurse follows the steps in Chart 50–2 to obtain a profile of a client's hearing for pure tones across the frequencies tested, from low to high frequencies. No special follow-up care is needed.

Bone Conduction Test

Pure tone bone conduction testing determines whether the hearing loss detected by air conduction testing is due to conductive or sensorineural factors, or a combination. It is used only when the results of air conduction testing are abnormal. There are restrictions on both the frequency and intensity of the sound produced by the device. The frequencies are usually restricted to those between 250 and 4000 Hz. Because a bone conduction oscillator requires great power to vibrate the skull, maximal outputs for bone conduction are also lower.

CLIENT PREPARATION. The nurse explains that hearing sensitivity for bone conduction is going to be checked. The sounds and how the client should respond are the same as for the air conduction test.

PROCEDURE. The ear with greater acuity is tested first.

If neither ear is "better," it makes no difference which is tested first.

The bone conduction vibrator is placed behind the pinna, firmly on the mastoid process. The nurse then follows steps 4–9 of Chart 50–2. Remember that restrictions are placed on both the intensity and the frequency

---

Chart 50–2

Nursing Care Highlight: Pure Tone Air Conduction Audiometry

1. After explaining the procedure to the client, place the earphones on the client. Make sure that the side marked *left* is on the left ear and the side marked *right* is on the right ear. The earphones must cover the ears.
2. If the client reports a hearing difference between the two ears, test the ear with better hearing first.
3. Begin the testing at 1000 Hz. This frequency is near the middle of the ear's sensitivity spectrum, and it has been demonstrated to have good test-retest reliability.
4. Adjust the audiometer so that the tone is inaudible unless the interrupter switch is depressed. Start with the hearing level control at its minimal reading, either 0 or −10 dB. Depress the interrupter switch and gradually increase the intensity of the tone until the client signals that the tone is heard. Increase the intensity of the tone beyond this point by about 20 dB to give the client an opportunity to hear it well.
5. Now reduce the intensity of the tone in 5-dB steps until the client indicates that the tone is no longer heard. Note the last intensity level, in the 5-dB decrement steps, at which the client signaled. The last point at which the client indicated that the tone was still heard should be his or her threshold for hearing for that frequency. The threshold can be tested for reliability by increasing the tone by 20 dB once again and then descending in 5-dB steps until once again the lowest point in intensity is reached.
6. If you have succeeded in obtaining a consistent threshold at 1000 Hz, change the frequency control to 500 Hz and start again. The preferred method is to test the lower frequencies first (500 and 250 Hz) and then to move higher, usually 2000, 4000, and 8000 Hz. At each frequency, the procedure is the same as that for 1000 Hz.
7. After you have completed the threshold measurements on the first ear, switch the output selector to the opposite earphone. Proceed in the same manner to obtain thresholds for the other ear, also beginning at 1000 Hz.
8. If the thresholds of the second ear seem to differ by 40 dB or more from those of the first ear, masking of the better hearing ear is indicated to rule out its participation in the test.
9. In operating the interrupter switch, make sure that you do not fall into rhythmic patterns that the client can follow. The pattern of tonal presentations should be irregular so that the client cannot predict when the tone will be presented.

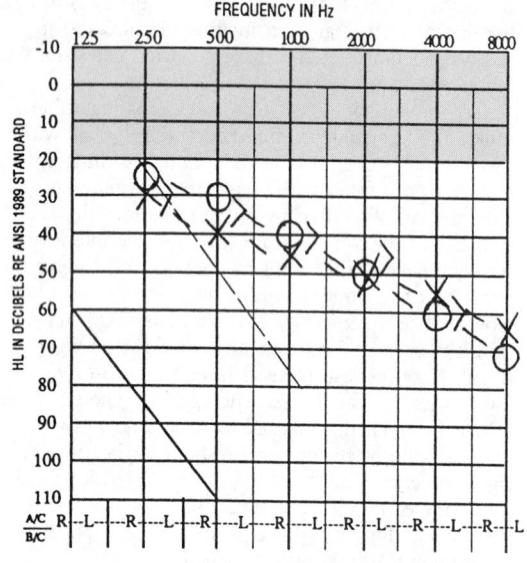

AUDIOGRAM

Pattern Depicting
Conductive Hearing Loss

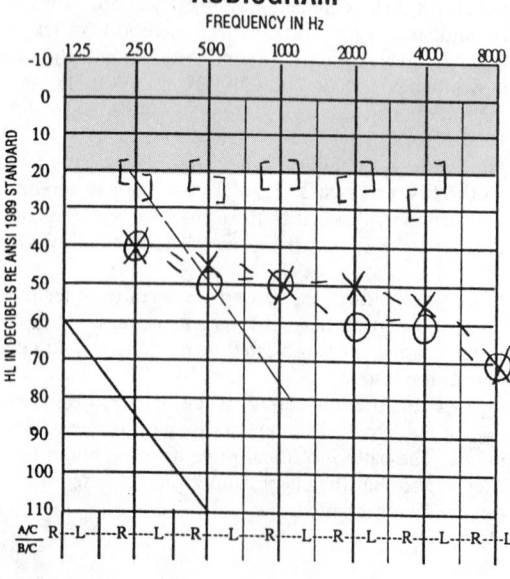

AUDIOGRAM

Pattern Depicting
Sensorineural Hearing Loss

AUDIOGRAM

Pattern Depicting Conductive and
Sensorineural Hearing Loss

Audiogram Key	Left	Right		Left	Right
AC Unmasked	x	o	AC Masked	□	△
BC Unmasked	>	<	BC Masked	]	[
No Response	↘	↙	SF		S

Figure 50–12. Audiogram patterns depicting various types of hearing loss. (Courtesy of the Cleveland Hearing and Speech Center, Cleveland, OH.)

used in bone conduction testing. Restrictions are usually described on the face of the audiometer.

No special follow-up care is needed.

INTERPRETATION OF RESULTS. Audiometric evaluation determines whether the client's hearing is within normal limits or, with a hearing impairment, whether the hearing loss is conductive, sensorineural, or mixed. The type of loss can be determined by the configuration of the audiogram after completion of pure tone air and bone conduction audiometry.

In the hands of an experienced clinician, the audiometer is a useful tool for evaluating the extent and type of hearing loss. For interpreting the results of a hearing test, the expertise of the person who performed the test and the reliability of the client's responses must be considered. In reality, the audiogram is the best estimate by the diagnostician of the client's hearing, based on observations of the client's auditory behavior in the testing situation.

Figure 50–11 is an audiogram showing normal results of air and bone conduction tests. Hearing is generally considered normal when the pure tone thresholds are at 10 dB or better. The line at 0 dB on the audiogram represents the hearing thresholds of a young person with normal hearing. Figure 50–12 depicts audiogram representations of various types of hearing loss.

Speech Audiometry

In speech audiometry, the client's ability to hear spoken words is measured through a microphone connected to an audiometer. The two components of speech audiometry are the speech reception threshold and speech discrimination.

SPEECH RECEPTION THRESHOLD. This is the level of intensity at which a client can repeat simple words. In testing this threshold, the nurse tries to determine how intense (or loud) a simple speech stimulus must be before the client can hear it well enough to repeat it correctly. In one common test, lists of two-syllable words called *spondee* are used (i.e., words in which there is generally equal stress on each syllable, such as airplane, railroad, and cowboy).

The speech reception threshold measured by the audiometer is the hearing level at which the client can repeat simple words correctly 50% of the time. The test is administered essentially the same as for the pure tone tests, but the microphone is activated through the audiometer. The intensity dial on the audiometer regulates word level intensity.

SPEECH DISCRIMINATION. Speech discrimination testing establishes the client's ability to discriminate among similar sounds or among words that contain similar sounds. The ability to understand speech is considered the most important measurable aspect of human auditory function. Speech discrimination testing assesses the client's understanding of speech. A hearing loss may not only decrease sensitivity to sound but also impair understanding of what is being said.

A standard format contains lists of 25 or 50 monosyllabic (one-syllable) words, such as carve, day, toe, and ran, phonemically balanced (designed to include the phonemes of American English in the proper proportion), and with equal word difficulty between lists. The lists are presented to the client through earphones at a selected loudness level, generally about 30–40 dB above the speech reception threshold, or at the client's most comfortable listening level. A percentage score is derived from the number of words repeated correctly.

Tympanometry

Tympanometry assesses compliance (mobility) of the tympanic membrane and structures of the middle ear as a function of systematically varied air pressure in the external auditory canal. The progression or resolution of serous otitis and otitis media can be accurately monitored with this procedure.

Tympanometry is helpful in distinguishing middle-ear pathologic conditions, such as otosclerosis, ossicular disarticulation, otitis media, and perforation of the tympanic membrane. It is also valuable for assessing patency of the eustachian tube and for observing postsurgical recovery of middle-ear function.

SELECTED BIBLIOGRAPHY

Benjamin, B., Bingham, B., Hawke, M., & Stammberger, H. (1995). *A color atlas of otorhinolaryngology*. Philadelphia: Lippincott-Raven.

Bess, F. H., & Humes, L. E. (1995). *Audiology: The fundamentals*. Baltimore: Williams & Wilkins.

Ginsberg, I. A., & White, T. P. (1994). Otologic disorders and examination. In J. Katz, (Ed.), *Handbook of clinical audiology* (4th ed., pp. 6–24). Baltimore: Williams & Wilkins.

Guyton, A. C. (1995). *Textbook of medical physiology* (9th ed.). Philadelphia: W. B. Saunders.

Heathcote, J. A. (1995). Why do old men have big ears? *British Medical Journal, 311*(7021), 1668.

Hull, R. H. (1995). *Hearing in aging*. San Diego: Singular Publishing Group.

Hull, R. H. (1996). *Aural rehabilitation: Serving children and adults*. San Diego: Singular Publishing Group.

Jarvis, C. (1996). *Physical examination and health assessment* (2nd ed.). Philadelphia: W. B. Saunders.

Jubeck, M. (1994). Teaching the elderly: A commonsense approach. *Nursing94, 24*(5), 70–71.

Lipscomb, D. L. (1996). The external and middle ear. In J. Northern (Ed.), *Hearing disorders* (3rd ed., pp. 1–13). Boston: Allyn and Bacon.

Martin, F. N. (1994). The human ear and tests of hearing. In F. Martin (Ed.), *Introduction to audiology* (5th ed., pp. 3–15). Englewood Cliffs, NJ: Prentice-Hall.

Meador, J. A. (1995). Cerumen impaction in the elderly. *Journal of Gerontological Nursing, 21*(12), 43–45.

Mitchell, I. C. (1994). An approach to ear, nose and throat assessment. *Australian Family Physician, 23*(11), 2087–2093.

Russell, J. (1995). Ear screening. *Community Nurse, 1*(4), 14, 16.

Ryan, A. R., & Dallos, P. (1996). The physiology of the cochlea. In J. Northern (Ed.), *Hearing disorders* (3rd ed., pp. 15–31). Boston: Allyn and Bacon.

Seidel, H. M., Ball, J. W., Dains, J. E., & Benedict, G. W. (1994). *Mosby's guide to physical examination* (3rd ed.). St. Louis: C. V. Mosby.

Yantis, P. A. (1994). Puretone air-conduction thresholds testing. In J. Katz (Ed.), *Handbook of clinical audiology* (4th ed., pp. 97–108). Baltimore: Williams & Wilkins.

SUGGESTED READINGS

Benjamin, B., Bingham, B., Hawke, M., & Stammberger, H. (1995). *A color atlas of otorhinolaryngology*. Philadelphia: Lippincott-Raven.
   This book has beautiful color photographs of many external and middle-ear conditions. The book also briefly covers the anatomy and physiology of the ear.

Meador, J. A. (1995). Cerumen impaction in the elderly. *Journal of Gerontological Nursing, 21*(12), 43–45.
   This excellent article summaries the problems faced by older clients with cerumen impaction and clearly discusses four methods for cerumen removal. Patient education information is also included.

Chapter 51

INTERVENTIONS FOR CLIENTS WITH EAR AND HEARING PROBLEMS

Accurate hearing enhances all aspects of communication between a person and his or her environment. Hearing problems can be caused by disorders of the different structures involved in processing sound, as the result of non–hearing-related disorders, or as the result of treatment for other conditions. Early recognition and intervention may minimize hearing loss and help the client to maintain her or his maximal level of communication.

CONDITIONS AFFECTING THE EXTERNAL EAR

Many conditions affect the structures of the external ear, including congenital malformation, trauma, and infectious or noninfectious lesions of the pinna, the auricle, and the auditory canal. Congenital anomalies range from a crumpling or falling forward of the pinna to absence (atresia) of the auditory canal. Congenital disorders of the external ear do not necessarily mean that middle-ear and inner-ear structures are affected, because each structure develops differently. Additionally, trauma can damage or destroy the auricle and external canal. Surgical reconstruction, done in phases, can reform the pinna with skin grafts and plastic prostheses. Trauma to the auricle resulting in hematoma necessitates the removal of blood via needle aspiration to prevent calcification and hardening, a cauliflower (boxer's) ear.

Benign cysts or polyps of the auricle or the external canal are surgically removed if they grow large enough to block the canal and affect hearing. Malignant cells, most commonly basal cell carcinoma, can also be found on the pinna. In general, treatment consists of simple excision. As the lesion becomes larger, its proximity to the skull and facial nerve makes treatment more difficult.

External Otitis
Overview

External otitis is an infective, inflammatory, or allergic response of the external auditory canal or auricle. When irritating or infective agents come into contact with the skin of the external ear, either an allergic response or inflammation with or without infection results. The skin becomes red, swollen, and tender to touch or movement.

TABLE 51–1

Differential Features of External Otitis and Otitis Media			
Problem	**Etiology**	**Clinical Manifestations**	**Treatment**
External otitis	• Allergic reaction • Bacterial or viral infection • Swimming • Local trauma	• Pain • Itching • Hearing loss • Plugged feeling in ear • Redness and edema • Exudate	• Topical antibiotics • Corticosteroids • Oral analgesics • Local heat
Otitis media	• Bacterial or viral infection • Sterile accumulation of fluid	• Pain • Pressure in ear • Hearing loss • Tinnitus • Fever • Malaise • Nausea or vomiting • Bulging tympanic membrane • Fluid behind tympanic membrane	• Systemic antibiotics • Analgesics • Local heat • Antipyretics • Antihistamines • Decongestants • Myringotomy

Swelling of the auditory canal can lead to hearing loss because of obstruction of the canal. Allergic external otitis is commonly caused by contact with cosmetics, hair sprays, earphones, earrings, and hearing aids. The most common infectious organisms, usually bacterial or fungal, are *Pseudomonas aeruginosa, Streptococcus, Staphylococcus,* and *Aspergillus.* Table 51–1 compares external otitis and otitis media.

External otitis occurs more often in hot, humid environments, especially in the summer, and is commonly referred to as *swimmer's ear* because of the high incidence in people involved in water sports. Additionally, clients who have traumatized and opened lesions in their external auditory canal with sharp objects such as hairpins, with cotton-tipped applicators, or through headphones are more susceptible to external otitis.

Necrotizing or malignant external otitis is the most virulent form of external otitis; the organism spreads beyond the external auditory canal into the adjacent structures of the ear and skull. The high mortality rate seen with malignant external otitis results from complicating disorders such as meningitis, brain abscess, and destruction of certain cranial nerves, especially the facial nerve (cranial nerve VII).

Collaborative Management

 Assessment

Clinical manifestations of external otitis include a variety of complaints, ranging from mild itching to pain with movement of the pinna or tragus. Clients have pain with physical manipulation of the pinna and tragus or when upward pressure is applied to the external canal. Clients report that they feel as though the ear is plugged and their hearing reduced.

The nurse uses extreme caution during otoscopic examination to avoid exerting pressure on the walls of the external canal, which causes excessive pain. Drainage from the ear, when present, is often greenish white. The nurse is careful to dispose of the otoscope tip and wash his or her hands thoroughly between examining opposite ears to prevent cross-contamination. Hearing loss can be severe on the affected side when inflammation causes obstruction of the tympanic membrane.

 Interventions

Treatment of external otitis focuses on reducing local inflammation, edema, and pain. The nurse or assistive nursing personnel applies heat locally for 20 minutes three times a day, using towels warmed with water and then wrapped in a plastic bag, or heating pads placed on a low setting. Bed rest is often helpful in limiting head movements, thereby reducing pain.

Topical antibiotic and steroid therapies are the most effective means of decreasing inflammation and pain. The nurse reviews with the client the proper way to instill eardrops, as shown in Chart 51–1. The nurse observes the client to make sure that he or she uses proper technique. If edema has caused an obstruction of the external canal, an earwick is inserted past the blockage, with medicated drops applied to the outside end (Fig. 51–1). A long piece of gauze dressing serves as an earwick, which the physician or nurse practitioner inserts using forceps to push carefully through the blocked external auditory canal to the tympanic membrane. The earwick may be removed when medication can flow freely into the canal. Thorough hand washing is strictly enforced. Systemic oral or intravenous antibiotics are used in severe cases, especially when cellulitis is present or the auricular lymph nodes are enlarged.

Analgesics, including opioids, may be necessary for pain relief during the initial days of therapy. Acetylsalicylic acid (aspirin, Enthrophen♣) or acetaminophen (Tylenol, Abenol♣) can be given to relieve less severe pain.

After the inflammation has subsided, diluted alcohol may be dropped into the ear to keep it clean and dry and prevent recurrence. The nurse teaches the client not to use cotton-tipped applicators to dry the ears, because their use could lead to trauma to the canal and increase the risk of infection or inflammation. The use of ear plugs when engaging in water sports is recommended for clients with recurrent episodes of external otitis after swimming.

Furuncle
Overview

Often called localized external otitis, a furuncle is caused by bacterial infection, usually *Staphylococcus*, of a hair follicle. A furuncle is located on the outer half of the external canal.

Collaborative Management

The clinical manifestations of a furuncle include intense local pain to light touch. The area is swollen and pink, with tight skin covering the area, possibly with a purulent head. No drainage is noted unless the furuncle has ruptured. Hearing is impaired if the lesion occludes the canal.

Treatment is consistent with that of other types of external otitis: local and systemic antibiotic administration and localized heat application. An earwick may be used

with one-half strength Burow's solution to relieve pain. The furuncle might need to be incised and drained if it does not resolve with the use of antibiotics.

Cerumen or Foreign Bodies
Overview

Many objects can enter or be placed in the external auditory canal. Cerumen, or wax, is the most common cause of an impacted canal. Vegetables, beads, pencil erasers, and insects are other common items that may also enter the ear, with or without the client's help. Although uncomfortable, these are rarely true emergencies, and the nurse takes care when removing cerumen or foreign bodies.

Collaborative Management

 Assessment

Clients have a sensation of fullness in the ear, with or without associated hearing loss, and ear pain, itching, and bleeding from the ear.

 Interventions

When the occluding material is cerumen, the nurse irrigates the canal with a mixture of water and hydrogen peroxide at body temperature (Fig. 51-2), following guidelines for proper irrigation (Chart 51-2). Removal of wax by irrigation is a slow process and may take more than one sitting; however, when cerumen obstruction is the cause of hearing loss, its removal results in increased hearing. Between 50 and 70 mL of solution is the maxi-

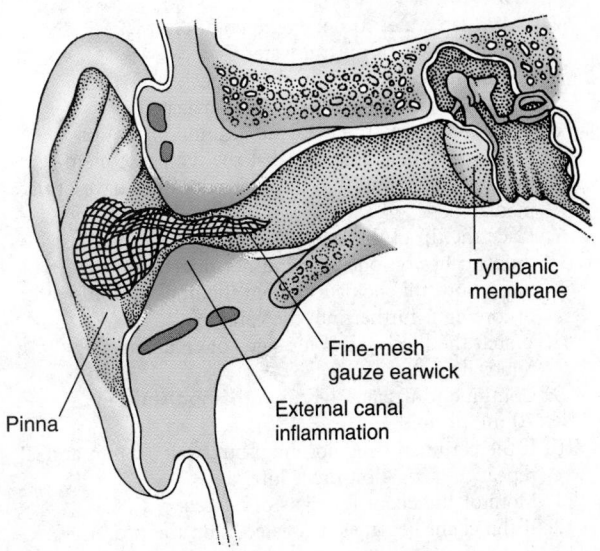

Figure 51-1. Earwick for instillation of antibiotics into the external canal. When edema occludes the external auditory canal, it is difficult for antibiotic solutions to enter the canal adequately. An earwick is placed through the meatus. Solutions placed on the external portion of the earwick are absorbed through the canal.

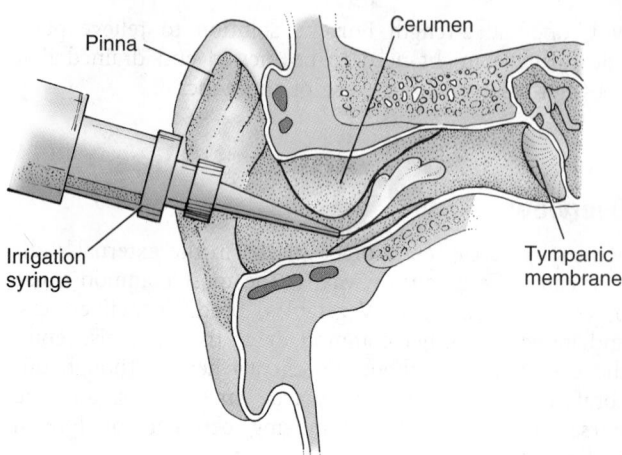

Figure 51–2. Irrigation of the external canal. Cerumen and debris can be removed from the ear by irrigation with warm water. The stream of water is aimed above or below the impaction to allow back-pressure to push it out rather than further down the canal.

mal amount that the client can tolerate at one sitting. Irrigation is contraindicated in clients who have tympanic membrane perforation or otitis media.

If the cerumen is thick and dry or cannot be removed easily, the health care provider may prescribe a ceruminolytic product such as Cerumenex to soften the wax before trying to remove it. Another way to soften cerumen is to add three drops of glycerin to the ear at

---

Chart 51–2

Nursing Care Highlight: Ear Irrigation

1. Gather the proper equipment: basin, syringe, otoscope, towel.
2. Warm tap water to body temperature.
3. Fill a syringe with warm water.
4. Place a towel around the client's neck.
5. Place a basin under the ear to be irrigated.
6. Use an otoscope to check the location of the impacted cerumen; ascertain that the tympanic membrane is intact and that the client does not have otitis media.
7. Place the tip of the syringe at an angle so that the fluid pushes on one side and not directly on the impaction (this helps to loosen the impaction instead of forcing it further into the canal).
8. Watch the fluid return for signs of cerumen plug removal.
9. Continue to irrigate the ear with approximately 70 mL of fluid.
10. If the cerumen does not drain out, wait 10 min and repeat the irrigation procedure.
11. Monitor the client for signs of nausea.
12. If the client becomes nauseated, stop the procedure.
13. If the cerumen cannot be removed by irrigation, the client may place mineral oil into the ear three times/day for 2 days to soften dry, impacted cerumen, after which irrigation may be repeated.

Chart 51–3

Nursing Focus on the Elderly: Cerumen Impaction

- Assess the hearing of all elderly clients using simple voice tests (see Chap. 50).
- Perform a gentle otoscopic inspection of the external canal and tympanic membrane of any elderly client who has a problem with hearing acuity, especially the client who wears a hearing aid.
- Use ear irrigation to remove any impacted cerumen.
- Make certain that the irrigating fluid is 37° C (approx. 98° F) to reduce the chance of stimulating the vestibular sense.
- Use no more than 5–10 mL of irrigating fluid at a time.
- If nausea, vomiting, or dizziness develop, stop the irrigation immediately.
- Teach the client how to irrigate his or her own ears.
- Obtain a return demonstration of ear irrigation from the client, observing for specific areas in which the client may need assistance.
- Encourage the client to wash the external ears daily using a soapy, wet washcloth over the index finger (best done in the shower or while washing the hair).

---

bedtime and three drops of hydrogen peroxide twice a day. After several days of this treatment, the cerumen is more easily removed through irrigation. In some cases, a small curette or cerumen spoon may be used to scoop out the wax. *Only trained health care professionals should use this method, because damage to the canal or the tympanic membrane is likely with improper technique.* Refer to Chart 51–3 for special nursing care considerations of elderly clients with cerumen impaction.

When the foreign object is vegetable matter, irrigation is *not* used because this material expands with hydration, worsening the impaction.

Insects are killed before removal unless they can be coaxed out by a flashlight or a humming noise. Mineral oil or diluted alcohol is instilled into the ear to suffocate the insect, which is then removed with ear forceps.

If the client has local irritation, an antibiotic or steroid ointment may be applied to prevent infection and reduce local irritation. Hearing acuity is tested by the nurse if hearing loss is not resolved by removal of the object.

In rare cases, surgical removal of the foreign object is necessary. The object is removed through the transcanal route using a wire bent at a 90-degree angle. The wire is looped around and the object pulled out. Because this procedure is painful, general anesthesia is necessary.

CONDITIONS AFFECTING THE MIDDLE EAR
Otitis Media
Overview

The three most common forms of otitis media are acute, chronic, and serous otitis media. Each affects the middle-ear structures but has slightly different causes, incidences, and pathologic changes. If otitis progresses or remains untreated, permanent conductive hearing loss may occur.

Acute otitis media and chronic otitis media, also known as suppurant or purulent otitis media, are similar in pathophysiology. An infecting agent introduced into the middle ear causes an inflammation within the mucosa, leading to swelling and irritation of the ossicles within the middle ear. This process is followed by a purulent inflammatory exudate. Onset is sudden in acute disease, with a relatively short duration of 3 weeks or less. Chronic otitis media usually follows repeated acute episodes, has a longer duration, and can be associated with greater morbidity or injury to the middle ear.

The eustachian tube and mastoid, connected to the middle ear by a continuation of cells, are also affected by the infection. If the tympanic membrane perforates and infective materials spill into the external ear, external otitis also develops, which untreated thickens and scars the middle ear. Necrosis of the ossicles leads to destruction of the middle-ear structures.

Collaborative Management

 Assessment

The chief complaint of the client with acute or chronic otitis media is ear pain with or without manipulation of the external ear structures. Chronic otitis media pain is much less severe than that associated with acute otitis media. As the pressure in the middle ear increases, there is a greater sensation of fullness in the ear, and hearing is diminished and distorted. The client may notice a sticking or cracking sound in the ear on yawning or swallowing or tinnitus as a low hum or a low-pitched sound. Conductive hearing loss may occur as a result of physical obstruction in sound wave transmission. Headaches are common, and systemic symptoms such as malaise, fever, nausea, and vomiting can occur. As the pressure on the middle ear impinges on the inner ear, the client may have slight dizziness or vertigo.

Otoscopic examination findings vary, depending on the

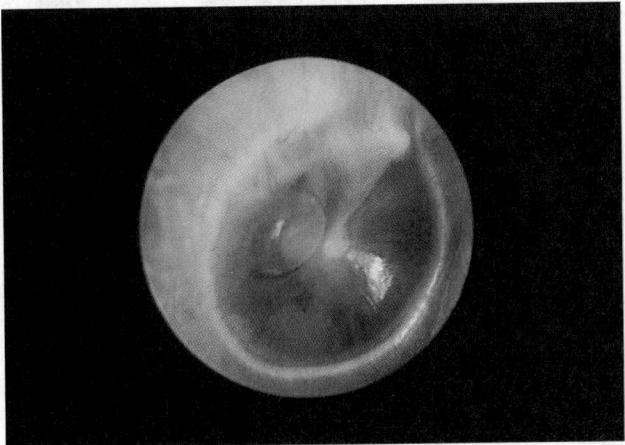

Figure 51–3. Otoscopic view of otitis media.

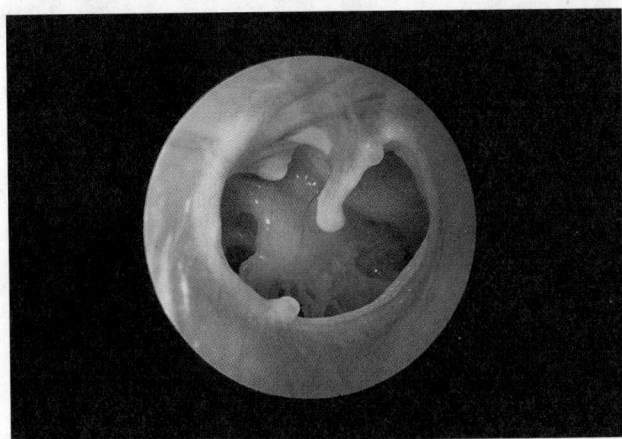

Figure 51–4. Otoscopic view of a perforated tympanic membrane.

stage of the disease. The tympanic membrane is initially retracted, which allows clear visualization of the ear landmarks. At this early stage, the client has only vague ear discomfort; however, as the disease progresses, the tympanic membrane's blood vessels dilate and appear red (Fig. 51–3). In the third stage, the tympanic membrane becomes red, thickened, and bulging, with loss of landmarks. Decreased membrane mobility is evident on inspection with a pneumatic otoscope. Exudate behind the membrane may be visible.

If the disease progresses, the tympanic membrane spontaneously perforates and pus or blood drains from the ear (Fig. 51–4). This discharge may be pulsating when viewed through the otoscope. When the membrane ruptures, the client notices a marked decrease in pain as the pressure on middle-ear structures is relieved (Fig. 51–5). Tympanic perforations from any cause may heal if the underlying problem is controlled. The membrane covering appears thinner over the healed perforation. A simple central perforation does not interfere with hearing unless the ossicles of the middle ear are damaged or the perforation is large. However, repeated perforations with extensive scarring can cause hearing loss.

Drainage cultures after a perforation from uncontrolled otitis media may reveal the infecting agent. Cultures are usually not taken unless previous treatment has been ineffective. When the tympanic membrane is not perforated, a needle aspiration or myringotomy draws fluid for culture.

 Interventions

Nonsurgical Management. Treatment can be as simple as leaving the client in a quiet environment without distractions. Bed rest limits head movements that intensify the pain. Localized heat may be applied by using a heating pad adjusted to a low setting. Application of cold may occasionally relieve pain.

Systemic antibiotic therapy can decrease pain by reducing inflammation. Analgesics such as acetylsalicylic acid (aspirin, Enthrophen✤) and acetaminophen (Tylenol, Abenol✤) aid in pain relief, and their antipyretic effects

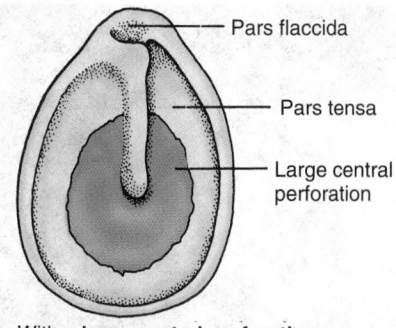

With a large central perforation,
clients complain of significant hearing loss.

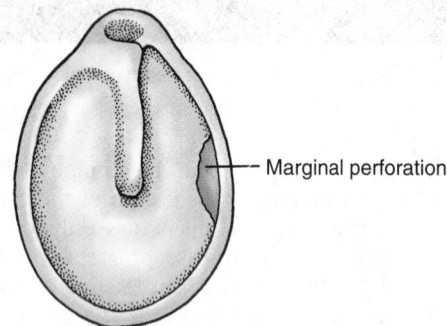

With a marginal perforation,
clients might complain of significant hearing loss.

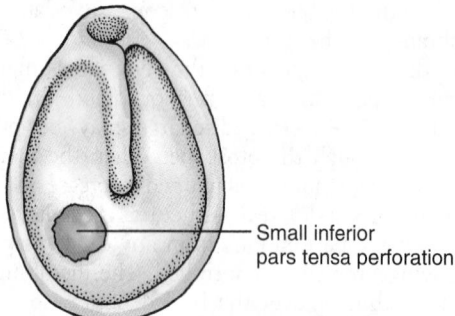

With a small inferior pars tensa perforation,
clients do not complain of much interference with hearing.

Figure 51–5. Perforations of the tympanic membrane. Central perforations heal more quickly than marginal perforations. Marginal perforations that do not heal allow cholesteatoma formation.

helps the client feel better by relieving an elevated temperature. When the client has severe pain, opioid analgesics such as codeine and meperidine hydrochloride (Demerol) also may be used.

Oral and nasal antihistamines and decongestants are prescribed to decrease mucus production in the nasopharynx and to decrease fluid in the middle ear. The body then can reabsorb the fluid, reducing pressure and pain.

Surgical Management. If the pain persists after initial antibiotic therapy and the tympanic membrane continues to bulge, a myringotomy, a surgical perforation of the pars tensa of the tympanic membrane, is performed. Myringotomies drain middle-ear fluids and almost immediately relieve pain.

Preoperative Care. The nurse reassures the client that the myringotomy will relieve pain and is usually per-

formed without anesthesia. Many people are apprehensive about a perforation and its effect on hearing. To relieve some of this anxiety, the nurse discusses the reasons for the procedure with the client and encourages relaxation techniques such as deep breathing before and during the procedure. Systemic antibiotic therapy continues before and after this procedure. The nurse cleans the external canal with a bacteriostatic solution such as povidone-iodine (Betadine) before the myringotomy.

Operative Procedure. The small surgical incision can be performed in an office or clinic setting and heals rapidly. An alternative is the removal of fluid from the middle ear via needle aspiration. For relief of pressure caused by serous otitis media, a small grommet (polyethylene tube) may be surgically placed through the tympanic membrane to allow continuous drainage of middle-ear fluids (Fig. 51–6).

Postoperative Care. Care must be taken to keep the external ear and canal free from other substances while the incision is healing. The nurse instructs the client to keep his or her head dry by not washing the hair or showering for several days. Other postoperative instructions are given in Chart 51–4.

Mastoiditis
Overview

The epithelial lining of the middle ear is continuous with the epithelial lining of the mastoid air cells, embedded in the temporal bone. Mastoiditis is a secondary disorder resulting from untreated or inadequately treated otitis media and can be acute or chronic. Before antibiotic therapy,

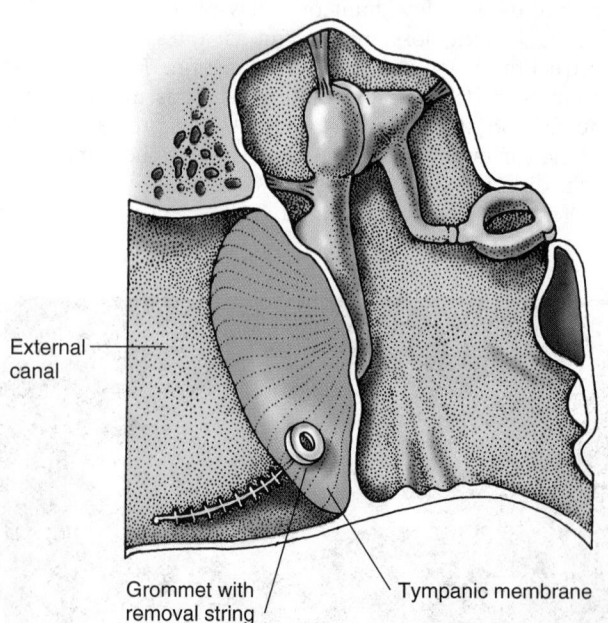

Figure 51–6. Grommet through the tympanic membrane. A small grommet is placed through the tympanic membrane away from the margins, which allows prolonged drainage of fluids from the middle ear. The grommet can be removed later and the tympanic membrane allowed to heal naturally or patched with a small piece of homogenous tissue.

Chart 51–4

Education Guide: Recovery from Ear Surgery

- Avoid straining when you have a bowel movement.
- Do not drink through a straw for 2–3 wk.
- Avoid air travel for 2–3 wk.
- Avoid coughing excessively for 2–3 wk.
- Stay away from people with colds.
- If you need to blow your nose, blow gently, one side at a time with your mouth open.
- Avoid getting your head wet, washing your hair, and showering for 1 wk.
- Keep your ear dry for 6 wk by placing a ball of cotton coated with petroleum jelly (such as Vaseline) in your ear. Change the cotton ball daily.
- Avoid rapidly moving the head, bouncing, and bending over for 3 wk.
- Change your ear dressing every 24 hr as directed.
- Report excessive drainage immediately to your physician.

mastoiditis was a leading cause of death in children and of hearing loss in adults. Today, antibiotic therapy is aimed at treating the middle-ear infection before it progresses to mastoiditis.

Collaborative Management

 ### Assessment

The clinical manifestations of mastoiditis include swelling behind the ear and pain with minimal movement of the tragus, the pinna, or the head. Pain is not relieved by myringotomy. Cellulitis develops on the skin or external scalp over the mastoid process. Otoscopic examination reveals a red, dull, thick, immobile tympanic membrane with or without perforation. Postauricular lymph nodes are tender and enlarged. Clients with mastoiditis also have low-grade fever, malaise, and anorexia.

 ### Interventions

Nonsurgical Management. Antibiotic therapy aims at preventing the continued spread of infection from the otitis media or mastoiditis, but it has limited use in actual mastoiditis treatment because of the difficulty of achieving effective antibiotic levels within the bony structure of the mastoid. Cultures from the ear drainage or by myringotomy determine the sensitivities of infecting organisms to specific antibiotics.

Surgical Management. Surgical removal of the infected tissue is necessary if the client does not respond to antibiotic administration within a few days. A simple or modified radical mastoidectomy with tympanoplasty is the most common treatment. All infected tissue must be removed so that the infection does not spread to other

structures, and a tympanoplasty is performed to reconstruct the ossicles and the tympanic membrane to restore hearing. Client preparation, operative procedure, and follow-up care for tympanoplasty are discussed later under Hearing Loss.

Complications arise when infective material has not been removed completely or when other structures outside the mastoid and middle ear are contaminated. Complications of mastoiditis include damage to the abducens and facial cranial nerves (cranial nerves VI and VII), decreasing the client's ability to look laterally (cranial nerve VI) and causing a drooping of the mouth on the affected side (cranial nerve VII). Other complications include vertigo, meningitis, brain abscess, chronic purulent otitis media, and wound infection.

Trauma
Overview

Trauma and damage may occur to the tympanic membrane and ossicles by infection, by direct damage to the structures, or through rapid changes in the middle-ear cavity pressure. Foreign objects placed in the external canal may exert pressure on the tympanic membrane and cause perforation. If the objects continue through the canal, the bony structure of the stapes, incus, and malleus may be damaged. Blunt injury to the basal skull and ears can also damage middle-ear structures through fractures extending to the middle ear. Rapid slapping of the external ear increases the pressure in the external auditory canal, tearing the eardrum when the pressure is great enough. The tympanic membrane has a limited stretching ability and gives way under high pressure. Excessive nose blowing and rapid changes of pressure that occur with nonpressurized air flight (barotrauma) can cause a pressure increase within the middle ear. High pressure damages the ossicles and can cause outward perforation of the eardrum.

Collaborative Management

Tympanic membrane perforations usually heal within 24 hours. Repeated perforations, especially from chronic otitis media, heal slower, with tympanic scarring. Depending on the amount of damage to the ossicles, hearing may or may not return. Hearing aids can improve hearing in this type of hearing loss. Surgical reconstruction of the ossicles and tympanic membrane through a tympanoplasty or a myringoplasty may also improve hearing (see later discussion of nursing care after tympanoplasty).

Preventive measures should be taken to avoid trauma. The nurse instructs clients to avoid inserting objects into the external canal. Ear protectors can be used when blunt trauma is likely, especially in such sports as boxing.

Neoplasms
Overview

Tumors of the middle ear are rare. The most common type of tumor is the glomus jugulare, a highly vascular benign lesion arising from the jugular vein. Extremely rare malignant tumors include primary adenocarcinoma, adenoid cystic carcinoma, and mucoepidermoid carcinoma. The growth of any lesion within the middle-ear fossa disrupts conductive hearing, erodes the ossicles, and has the potential to involve the inner ear and adjacent cranial nerves.

Collaborative Management

Clients experience progressive hearing loss and tinnitus. Infection and pain are rarely associated with glomus jugulare tumors. A physical examination reveals bulging of the tympanic membrane or a mass extending to the external auditory canal. The highly vascular nature of the glomus jugulare tumor gives it a reddish color and a visible pulsation when seen through the eardrum.

Diagnosis is made by physical examination, tomography, and angiography. Neoplasms are removed by surgery, which generally sacrifices hearing in the affected ear. If all the margins of the tumor can be seen clearly through the tympanic membrane, a transcanal approach is used to remove the lesion. When the tumor margins extend past the tympanic membrane, further diagnostic tests are necessary to determine the extent of growth and vascular involvement. Radiation therapy is used to decrease the vascularity of the glomus jugulare tumor but is not the preferred method of treatment. Benign lesions are removed because, with continued growth of the neoplasm, cranial structures other than the middle ear can be affected, further damaging the facial or trigeminal nerve. When possible, reconstructive surgery of the middle-ear structures is performed later to restore conductive hearing.

CONDITIONS AFFECTING THE INNER EAR
Tinnitus
Overview

Tinnitus is one of the most common complaints of clients with ear or hearing disorders.

Collaborative Management

Symptoms of tinnitus range from mild ringing, which can go unnoticed during the day, to a loud roaring in the ear, which can interfere with thinking and attention span. When clients report tinnitus, the nurse is alert to the wide variety of pathologic disorders and other factors that cause tinnitus: presbycusis, otosclerosis (irregular bone growth around ossicles), Meniere's disease, certain drugs, exposure to loud noise, and other inner-ear abnormalities.

The exact pathophysiology and treatment of tinnitus vary with the underlying cause. When no underlying cause can be found or the disorder is untreatable, therapy focuses on ways to mask the tinnitus with background sound, noisemakers, and music during sleeping hours. Ear mold hearing aids can amplify sounds to drown out the tinnitus during the day. The American Tinnitus Association assists clients in coping with tinnitus when other therapy is unsuccessful.

Vertigo and Dizziness
Overview

Vertigo and dizziness are common clinical manifestations of many ear disorders. Dizziness is a disturbed sense of a person's proper relationship to space. Clients vary greatly in defining dizziness. Vertigo is often used interchangeably with dizziness, but the definition, as well as the cause, is somewhat different. True vertigo is a real sense of whirling or turning in space.

The visual system, the vestibular system (cochlea, semicircular canals), and the proprioceptive system (muscles and nerve endings) combine to give input to the cerebellum about balance. Dysfunction in any of these areas leads to a disturbed sense of balance or motion. Common factors affecting the ear that cause vertigo include Meniere's disease, labyrinthitis, acoustic neuromas, benign paroxysmal vertigo, trauma, motion sickness, and drug or alcohol ingestion.

Collaborative Management

Associated symptoms of vertigo include nausea, vomiting, falling, nystagmus, hearing loss, and tinnitus. Until the underlying cause of the vertigo can be treated, each clinical manifestation is treated. Clients are advised to

- Restrict head motions and move more slowly
- Maintain adequate hydration, especially after vomiting
- Take medications with antivertiginous effects, such as dimenhydrinate (Dramamine, Gravol✦), diazepam (Valium, Apo-Diazepam✦), and scopolamine (Transderm Scōp, Transderm-V✦).

Many clients are dissatisfied with treatment because side effects of the medications, especially drowsiness, can be worse than the vertigo. The nurse cautions clients to maintain a safe, uncluttered environment to prevent accidents during periods of vertigo and to use a cane or walker to maintain balance. The nurse further instructs clients not to drive or operate machinery when taking antivertiginous drugs.

Labyrinthitis
Overview

Labyrinthitis is an infection of the labyrinth, which occasionally occurs as a complication of acute or chronic otitis media. Infection results from an erosion of the bony capsule, allowing infective materials to invade the inner ear. Labyrinthitis often results from the growth of a cholesteatoma (benign overgrowth of squamous cell epithelium) from the middle ear into the lateral semicircular canal. Labyrinthitis may follow middle-ear or inner-ear surgery when infection is present. When the infecting organism is viral, the labyrinthitis may be part of a systemic viral infection such as an upper respiratory tract infection or infectious mononucleosis.

Collaborative Management

Clinical manifestations include hearing loss, tinnitus, spontaneous nystagmus to the affected side, and vertigo with associated nausea and vomiting. Meningitis is the most common complication of labyrinthitis.

Treatment of labyrinthitis includes the use of systemic antibiotics such as ampicillin (Omnipen, Apo-Ampi♦). Clients are advised to stay in bed in a darkened room until clinical manifestations have diminished. Antiemetics, such as chlorpromazine hydrochloride (Thorazine, Novo-Chlorpromazine♦), and antivertiginous medications, such as dimenhydrinate (Dramamine, Gravol♦), relieve symptoms.

The client also needs psychosocial support. Hearing loss may be permanent on the affected side, although vertigo subsides as the inflammation resolves. Persistent balance problems may improve with gait training and physical therapy.

Meniere's Disease
Overview

Meniere's disease is characterized by the triad of tinnitus, unilateral sensorineural hearing loss, and vertigo occurring in attacks that can last for several days. Clients are almost totally incapacitated during an attack, and several days are needed for full recovery. The pathologic changes of Meniere's disease are either overproduction or decreased reabsorption of endolymphatic fluid, causing a distortion of the entire inner-canal system. This distortion leads to decreased hearing from dilation of the cochlear duct, vertigo because of damage to the vestibular system, and tinnitus from unknown cause. Involvement is generally unilateral. The initial hearing loss is reversible, but repeated damage to the cochlea, caused by increased fluid pressure, leads to permanent hearing loss.

The cause of Meniere's disease is unknown but is associated with viral or bacterial infections, allergic reactions, and biochemical disturbances that increase fluid imbalances. Mild long-term stress also seems to be associated with Meniere's disease.

Collaborative Management

 Assessment

The onset of Meniere's disease symptoms usually occurs in people between the ages of 20 and 50 years, with a greater prevalence in men and Caucasians. Times of severe, debilitating attacks alternate with almost symptom-free periods. Clients often have certain clinical manifestations before an attack of vertigo, such as headaches, increasing tinnitus, and a feeling of fullness in the affected ear. Clinical manifestations are unilateral in 60% to 70% of the cases.

Clients describe the tinnitus as a continuous, low-pitched roar or a humming sound, which worsens just before and during a severe attack. Hearing loss is initially of the low-frequency tones but worsens to include all levels after repeated episodes. Hearing loss is worse during an attack. In the early stages of Meniere's disease, periods of remission are marked by normal or nearly normal hearing, but permanent hearing loss develops as the attacks increase.

When questioned, clients describe the vertigo as periods of whirling, which might even cause them to fall. The vertigo is so intense that even while lying down clients hold the bed or ground to prevent the whirling. The severe vertigo usually lasts 3 to 4 hours, but clients continue to feel dizzy long after the attack. Nausea and vomiting are common. Other clinical manifestations include nystagmus, rapid eye movements, and severe headaches.

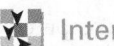 Interventions

Nonsurgical Management. The nurse instructs clients to make slow head movements to prevent worsening of the vertigo. Dietary and lifestyle changes, such as salt and fluid restrictions that reduce the amount of endolymphatic fluid, are recommended. Clients are advised to stop smoking because of its vasoconstrictive effects.

Drug therapy aims to control the vertigo and vomiting and restore normal balance. Mild diuretics are prescribed to decrease endolymph volume. Nicotinic acid has been found to be useful because of its vasodilatory effect. Antihistamines such as diphenhydramine hydrochloride (Benadryl, Allerdryl♦) and dimenhydrinate (Dramamine, Gravol♦) help reduce the severity of or stop an acute attack. Antiemetics such as chlorpromazine hydrochloride (Thorazine, Novo-Chlorpromazine♦), droperidol (Inapsine), and trimethobenzamide hydrochloride (Arrestin, Tigan) help control the nausea and vomiting. Diazepam (Valium, Apo-Diazepam♦) calms the anxious client; controls vertigo, nausea, and vomiting; and allows the client to rest quietly during an attack.

Surgical Management. Surgical treatment of Meniere's disease remains controversial because the hearing in the affected ear is often sacrificed. When medical therapy is ineffective and the client's functional hearing level has decreased significantly, surgery is performed. The most radical procedure involves resection of the vestibular nerve or total removal of the labyrinth (*labyrinthectomy*), performed via the transcanal route. The footplate of the stapes is moved aside, and the labyrinth removed through the oval window with fine forceps.

Another procedure performed early in the course of the disease is *endolymphatic decompression* with drainage and shunt. The endolymphatic sac is drained, and a small tube is inserted to enhance fluid drainage. Some clients report relief of vertigo and preservation of their hearing.

If an endolymphatic decompression has been performed, manipulation of the vestibular structures of the inner ear causes postoperative vertigo. The nurse reassures the client that the vertigo is temporary as a result of the surgical procedure, not the disease.

Acoustic Neuroma
Overview

An acoustic neuroma is a benign tumor of the vestibular, or acoustic, nerve. However, its location makes it destructive, because it frequently involves the cerebellum. Depending on the size and exact location of the tumor, damage to hearing, facial movements, and sensation can occur. Other neurologic-pathologic disorders associated with a lesion occupying intracranial space may also result.

Collaborative Management

Clinical manifestations begin with tinnitus and progress to gradual sensorineural hearing loss in more than 90% of clients. Later, clients experience constant mild vertigo. As the tumor enlarges, adjacent cranial nerves are damaged.

Acoustic neuromas are diagnosed with computed tomography (CT) scanning and magnetic resonance imaging (MRI). Audiograms diagnose sensorineural hearing loss. Cerebrospinal fluid assays show increased pressure and positive results for protein.

Surgical removal via a craniotomy is necessary, and the remaining hearing is sacrificed. Extreme care is taken to preserve the function of the facial nerve (cranial nerve VII). (Routine postcraniotomy care is discussed in Chapter 47). Acoustic neuromas rarely recur after surgical removal.

HEARING LOSS

Pathophysiology

Hearing loss is one of the most common physical handicaps in North America. Hearing loss may be conductive, sensorineural, or a combination (Fig. 51–7). Conduc-tion hearing loss occurs when sound waves are blocked from contact with inner-ear nerve fibers because of external-ear or middle-ear disorders. If the inner-ear or sensory fibers that lead to the cerebral cortex are damaged, the hearing loss is termed sensorineural. Combination hearing loss is known as mixed conductive-sensorineural.

The differences in conductive and sensorineural hearing loss are summarized in Table 51–2. Disorders that lead to a conductive hearing loss can often be corrected with no or minimal permanent damage. Sensorineural hearing loss is often permanent, and measures must be taken to reduce further damage or to amplify sounds as a means to improve hearing.

Etiology

Common Causes of Conductive Hearing Loss

Any inflammatory process or obstruction of the external or middle ear by cerumen or foreign objects leads to a conductive hearing loss. Changes in the tympanic membrane such as bulges, retractions, and perforations may indicate damage to middle-ear structures, which leads to conductive hearing loss. Tumors, scar tissue build-up, and overgrowth of soft bony tissue (otosclerosis) on the ossicles from previous middle-ear surgery also lead to conductive hearing loss.

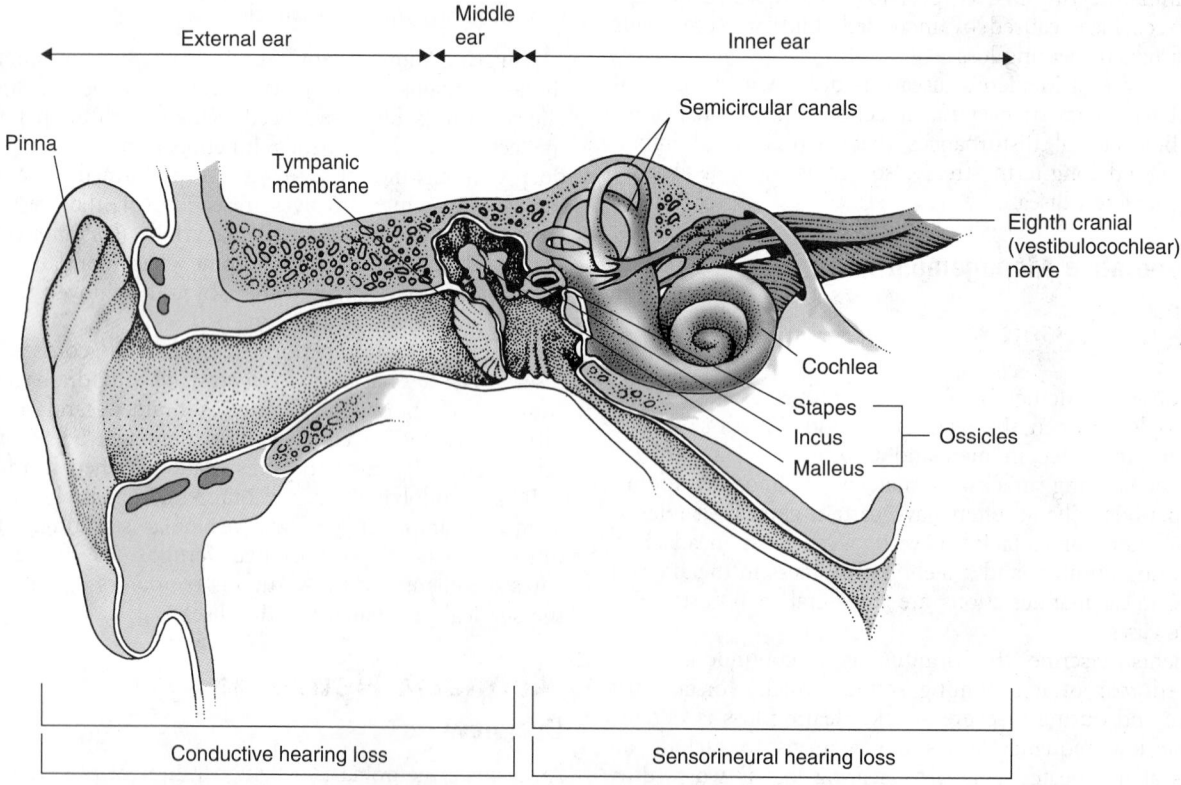

Figure 51–7. Anatomy of hearing loss. Hearing loss can be divided into three types: (1) conductive (difficulty in the external or the middle ear), (2) sensorineural (difficulty in the inner ear or the acoustic nerve), and (3) mixed conductive-sensorineural (a combination of the two).

TABLE 51–2

Differential Features of Conductive and Sensorineural Hearing Loss

Feature	Conductive Hearing Loss	Sensorineural Hearing Loss
Causes	• Cerumen • Foreign body • Perforation of the tympanic membrane • Edema • Infection of the external or middle ear • Tumors • Otosclerosis	• Prolonged exposure to noise • Presbycusis • Ototoxic substances • Meniere's disease • Acoustic neuroma • Diabetes mellitus • Labyrinthitis • Infection • Myxedema
Assessment findings	• Evidence of obstruction with otoscope • Abnormality in tympanic membrane • Speaking softly • Hearing best in a noisy environment • Rinne's test: air conduction greater than bone conduction • Weber's test: lateralization to affected ear	• Normal appearance of external canal and tympanic membrane • Tinnitus common • Occasional dizziness • Speaking loudly • Hearing poorly in loud environment • Rinne's test: air conduction less than bone conduction • Weber's test: lateralization to unaffected ear

Common Causes of Sensorineural Hearing Loss

When the inner ear or auditory nerve (cranial nerve VIII) is damaged, sensorineural hearing loss develops. Prolonged exposure to loud noise can damage the hair cells of the cochlea. Many drugs are toxic (ototoxic) to the inner-ear structures, and their effects on hearing can be transient or permanent, unilateral or bilateral, dose related or non-dose related. When ototoxic drugs (such as those listed in Table 50–2) are given to clients with reduced renal function, increased ototoxicity can result because elimination of these drugs takes longer. Older clients are especially susceptible to ototoxicity because of a decline in renal function.

Presbycusis is a common cause of sensorineural hearing loss associated with the catabolic processes of aging. This hearing loss is commonly caused by degeneration or atrophy of the ganglion cells in the cochlea, loss of elasticity of the basilar membrane, or a decreased vascular supply to the inner ear. Other causes of sensorineural hearing loss include inherited disorders, metabolic and circulatory disorders (such as arteriosclerosis and hypertension), bacterial or viral infections, prolonged fever, Meniere's disease, diabetes mellitus, and ear surgery. Each is thought to accelerate degenerative changes of the cochlea. Trauma to the ear or the head also contributes to sensorineural hearing loss.

Incidence/Prevalence

Because hearing loss may be gradual and affect only some aspects of hearing, many adults are unaware their hearing is impaired. The actual incidence of hearing loss is not known, although it is estimated that approximately 30% of adults older than 60 years have some degree of hearing loss (Palumbo, 1990). The prevalence sharply increases to 90% among elderly institutionalized clients.

Collaborative Management

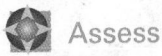 Assessment

➤ History

The nurse asks clients how long they have noticed a difference in their hearing and whether the changes occurred suddenly or gradually. Age is an important factor because some ear and hearing changes occur with advanced age and chronic otitis media is diagnosed more often in the older adult. The nurse notes occupational exposure to loud or continuous noises as well as current or previous use of ototoxic drugs. Clients are also asked about histories of external-ear and middle-ear infections and whether tympanic membrane perforation accompanied the infection. The nurse questions clients about any history of direct trauma to the ears. Because some types of hearing loss have a genetic predisposition, the nurse asks whether any family members are hearing impaired.

When pain accompanies acute-onset hearing loss, the nurse asks clients whether they have had a recent upper respiratory tract infection and about any allergies affecting the upper respiratory system.

➤ Physical Assessment/Clinical Manifestations

Chart 51–5 presents focused assessment techniques for clients with suspected hearing loss. Hearing loss may be sudden or gradual and is often bilateral. The ability to hear high-frequency soft discriminating consonants is lost first, especially "s," "sh," "f," "th," and "ch" sounds. Clients often state that they have no problem with hearing

---

Chart 51–5

Focused Assessment for the Client with Suspected Hearing Loss

- Assess whether the client has any of the following ear complaints:
  - Pain
  - Feeling of fullness or congestion
  - Dizziness or vertigo
  - Tinnitus
  - Difficulty understanding conversations, especially in a noisy room
  - Difficulty hearing sounds
  - Needing to strain to hear
  - Needing to turn head to favor one ear or needing to lean forward to hear
- Assess visible ear structures, particularly external canal and tympanic membrane:
  - Position and size of pinna
  - Patency of the external canal; presence of cerumen or foreign bodies, edema, and inflammation
  - Condition of tympanic membrane; intact, edema, fluid, inflammation
- Assess functional ability, including
  - Frequency of asking people to repeat statements
  - Withdrawal from social interactions or large groups
  - Shouting in conversation
  - Failing to respond when not looking in the direction of the sound
  - Answering questions incorrectly

---

but cannot understand specific words. They might think that the speaker is mumbling. Clients often experience high-pitched, continuous bilateral tinnitus. Vertigo may be present, depending on the extent of inner-ear involvement.

Tuning Fork Tests. Tuning fork tests help diagnose hearing loss (see Chap. 50). With Weber's test, the client can usually hear sounds well in the ear with a suspected conductive hearing loss because of the preserved bone conduction. With Rinne's test, the client reports that sound transmitted by bone conduction is louder and more sustained than that transmitted by air conduction.

Otoscopic Examination. The nurse performs an otoscopic examination to assess the external auditory canal, the tympanic membrane, and structures of the middle ear visible through the tympanic membrane (see Chap. 50). Physical findings from examination vary, depending on the cause of the hearing loss.

Obstruction of the external auditory canal can result in hearing loss. The nurse inspects the canal and notes the following:

- Whether the canal is open
- The amount and character of cerumen present
- The integrity of the skin lining the canal

Special note is also made of redness, exudates, lesions, and the presence of foreign objects.

Middle-ear infections can also diminish hearing. In infection or inflammation, the tympanic membrane appears red, thickened, and bulging, with a loss of landmarks. Loss of mobility of the membrane is evident when inspected with a pneumatic otoscope. The nurse notes the presence of any scars or perforations on the tympanic membrane. With close observation, the nurse may be able to see an exudate behind the membrane.

▶ Psychosocial Assessment

For the person with a hearing loss, communication can become a struggle, and he or she may isolate themselves because of the difficulty in talking and listening. Social isolation can lead to depression, fear, and despair. The nurse is sensitive to emotional changes that may be related to reduced hearing and a decline in conversational skills.

▶ Laboratory Assessment

No laboratory tests can definitively diagnose hearing loss. However, some laboratory findings can indicate pathologic problems that might affect hearing.

White blood cell counts are elevated in the client with acute or chronic otitis media. Microbial culture and antibiotic sensitivity tests can determine the causative organism and the most appropriate antibiotic therapy when infection causes hearing loss.

The client with hearing loss associated with peripheral neuropathy may have other systemic diseases, including poorly controlled diabetes mellitus. The fasting blood glucose level may be elevated and the blood, even when diluted, positive for serum acetone.

▶ Radiographic Assessment

Radiographic assessment can determine nonauditory problems affecting hearing ability. Some auditory problems can be diagnosed using radiographic techniques: skull x-rays, to determine bony involvement in otitis media and the location of otosclerotic lesions; CT and MRI to determine soft-tissue involvement and the presence and location of tumors.

▶ Other Diagnostic Assessment

Audiometry can make a differential diagnosis and determine the extent and type of hearing loss. An audiogram shows whether hearing loss is only conductive or whether it has a sensorineural component. This is important to determine a possible cause of the hearing loss and to plan appropriate interventions.

 Analysis

▶ Common Nursing Diagnoses and Collaborative Problems

Two nursing diagnoses are common in clients with any degree of hearing impairment:

1. Sensory/Perceptual Alterations (Auditory) related to obstruction, infection, damage to the middle ear, or damage to the auditory nerve
2. Anxiety related to an inability to communicate

➤ Additional Nursing Diagnoses and Collaborative Problems

The client with hearing loss or impairment also may have one or more of the following diagnoses:

- Knowledge Deficit related to treatment and prevention
- Activity Intolerance related to pain
- Social Isolation related to pain and decreased hearing
- High Risk for Injury related to altered auditory perception and infection
- Pain related to an inflammatory process and fluid in the middle ear
- Impaired Physical Mobility related to vertigo

 Planning and Implementation

➤ Sensory/Perceptual Alterations (Auditory)

Planning: Expected Outcomes. The client is expected to either

- Experience an increase in auditory sensory perception to a functional level or
- Maintain existing levels of hearing

Interventions. Interventions aim at identifying the problem, halting the pathologic processes, and improving auditory sensory perception.

Nonsurgical Management. Nonsurgical interventions include early detection of hearing impairment, use of drug therapy and comfort measures, and use of assistive devices to amplify or augment the client's auditory perception.

Early Detection. Early detection helps correct the problem causing the hearing loss. When hearing loss is gradual, the client can compensate. The nurse assesses for indications of hearing loss, as listed in Chart 51-5.

Drug Therapy. Drug therapy is aimed at either correcting the underlying pathologic change or reducing the side effects of the various disorders associated with hearing loss. Local (topical) antibiotics are administered to clients with external otitis. Systemic antibiotics are necessary when clients have other auditory infections. By treating the infection, local edema is resolved and hearing improved. When pain accompanies hearing disorders, local or systemic analgesics are often used, depending on the type and location of the pain. Many ear disorders disturb equilibrium, causing vertigo and dizziness with nausea and vomiting. Antiemetic, antihistamine, antivertiginous, and benzodiazepine drugs can help correct nausea, vertigo, and dizziness.

Assistive Devices. Many devices are useful for clients with permanent progressive hearing loss. Telephone amplifiers increase telephone volume, allowing the caller to speak in a normal voice. Flashing lights activated by the ringing telephone or doorbell alert clients visually. In some cases, clients may be referred for the use of a specially trained dog to help them be aware of sounds (ringing telephones or doorbells, cries of other people, and potential dangers), like a seeing eye dog assists a blind person.

Small portable audio amplifiers can assist the nurse in communicating with clients experiencing hearing loss but who have chosen to not use a hearing aid. Use of audio amplifiers or allowing clients to use a stethoscope helps nurses to communicate with elders and other clients who need additional volume to hear speech (see Research Applications for Nursing).

Hearing Aids. A hearing aid is a miniature electronic amplifier, usually used for clients with a conductive hearing loss. Hearing aids are less effective for sensorineural hearing loss and may make functional hearing worse by amplifying background noise. The amplifier can be worn in one or both ears. Local agencies offer special aural

---

➤ Research Applications for Nursing

Amplification Enhances Communication with the Hearing Impaired

Erber, N. (1994). *Communicating with Elders: Effects of amplification.* Journal of Gerontological Nursing, 20(10), 6–10.

This comparative descriptive study evaluated whether mechanical amplification affected communication ability in 68 elders living in a residential care facility. All participants exhibited some form of acquired hearing loss, and although 43 owned hearing aids, only 25 wore them on a regular basis. The investigators chose to use a small portable audio amplifier to augment conversational sounds mechanically. Each participant had two short conversations with one investigator while another investigator observed the interactions. One conversation was with amplification, the other without. Both interviewer and observer rated the participants' conversational fluency on a scale ranging from 1 (*very poor*) to 5 (*very good*) for each conversation. As might be expected, conversational fluency was mostly higher using the amplifier. Several participants did not demonstrate any change in performance, but none was rated lower while using the amplification device. Fourteen participants scored the maximum rating without amplification; thus, no improvement with amplification was possible.

Critique. The investigators were careful to control for various potential extraneous factors, including differences among different voices, environmental distractions associated with miscommunication, and unfamiliar subject matter. Reasons why more than half of the hearing-impaired participants either did not possess or did not wear hearing aids is not adequately addressed.

Possible Nursing Implications. Many elderly clients have diminished hearing. Teaching and general conversation can be facilitated by using an amplification device. The nurse should also explore why certain hearing-impaired elderly do not own or do not choose to use a hearing aid. A short-term amplification device may be easier for the client to use and can be effective in transferring information from nurse to client.

Chart 51–6

Education Guide: Hearing Aid Care

- Keep the hearing aid dry.
- Clean the ear mold with mild soap and water while avoiding excessive wetting.
- Clean debris from the hole in the middle of the part that goes into your ear with a toothpick or a pipe cleaner.
- Turn off the hearing aid and remove the battery when not in use.
- Check and replace the battery frequently.
- Keep extra batteries on hand.
- Keep the hearing aid in a safe place.
- Avoid dropping the hearing aid or exposing it to temperature extremes.
- Adjust the volume to the minimal hearing level to prevent feedback squeaking.
- Avoid using hair spray, cosmetics, oils, or other hair and face products that might come into contact with the receiver.
- If the hearing aid does not work:
  - Change the battery.
  - Check the connection between the ear mold and the receiver.
  - Check the on/off switch.
  - Clean the sound hole.
  - Adjust the volume.
  - Take the hearing aid to an authorized service center for repair.

ing to television and radio and reading aloud can help the client get used to new sounds. The tone or volume of the hearing aid can be adjusted. The most important and difficult aspect of a hearing aid is the amplification of background noise as well as voices. The client must learn to concentrate and filter out background noises.

The client must also learn to care for the hearing aid (Chart 51–6). Hearing aids are delicate electronic devices that should be handled only by people who know how to care for them properly. The cost of the aids varies greatly, but represents a significant investment.

Cochlear Implants. Cochlear implantation may help clients with sensorineural hearing loss. A small computer converts sound waves into electronic impulses. Electrodes are placed by the internal ear, with the computer attached to the external ear. The electronic impulses then directly stimulate nerve fibers. Some clients have a 50% return of their hearing with this method.

Surgical Management. Many surgical interventions are available for clients with specific disorders leading to hearing loss.

Tympanoplasty. This is reconstruction of the middle ear to improve hearing caused by conductive hearing loss. The surgical procedures vary from simple reconstruction of the tympanic membrane (myringoplasty) to replacement of the ossicles within the middle ear. A type I tympanoplasty is used for a myringoplasty and a type II for greater damage and to provide more extensive reconstruction (Figure 51–8).

Preoperative Care. The nurse gives specific instructions to the client scheduled for a tympanoplasty. Antibiotic drops eliminate any remaining infecting organism. Before surgery, a solution of equal parts of vinegar and sterile water irrigates the ear to restore its normal pH. The client follows other measures to decrease the chances of postoperative infection, such as avoiding people with upper res-

rehabilitation classes for the hearing impaired, helping the wearer obtain the most benefit from this device.

Here are some special tips to help the client adjust to the hearing aid. Hearing with a hearing aid can be different from natural hearing. The client is encouraged to start using the hearing aid slowly, initially wearing the hearing aid only at home and only during part of the day. Listen-

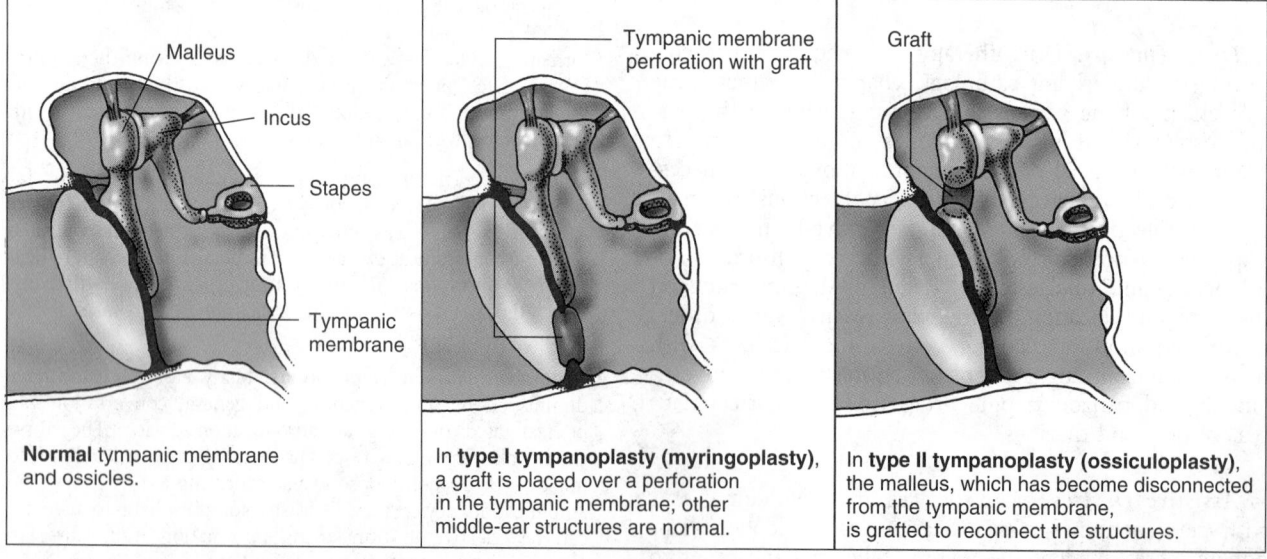

Figure 51–8. A normal tympanic membrane and two types of tympanoplasties.

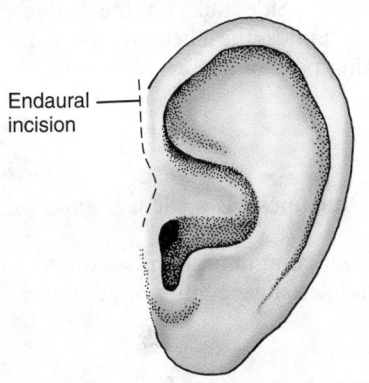

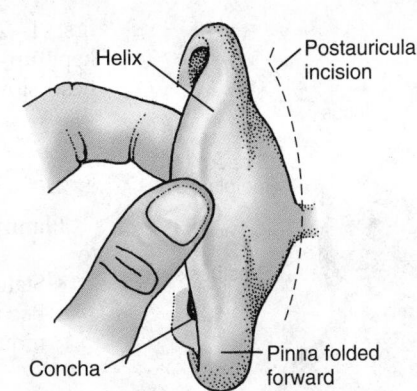

Figure 51–9. Surgical approaches for the ear. The endaural approach is used when the external canal is too small to use for a transcanal approach (not shown because no external incision is used). The postauricular approach is used for more extensive repair of the middle-ear and inner-ear structures.

piratory tract infections, getting adequate rest, eating a balanced diet, and maintaining an adequate fluid intake.

The nurse assures the client that initial hearing loss after surgery is normal because of the packing in the canal but that it will improve on removal. The nurse explains the importance of deep breathing and coughing postoperatively but emphasizes that forceful coughing increases pressure in the middle ear and must be avoided.

Operative Procedure. Surgical treatment is initiated only if the middle ear is free from infection and if the condition of the eustachian tube does not promote continued infection. If an infection is present, the graft is more likely to become infected and not heal properly. Surgery of the tympanic membrane and ossicles necessitates the use of a microscope and is considered a delicate procedure. Local anesthesia can be used, although general anesthesia is often chosen to prevent the client from moving.

The surgeon can repair the tympanic membrane with a variety of materials, including temporal muscle fascia, a split-thickness skin graft, and venous tissue. If the ossicles are damaged, more extensive measures must be taken to repair or replace them. The surgeon reaches the ossicles via transcanal approach, an endaural incision, or the postauricular route with a mastoidectomy (Figure 51–9).

The surgeon then removes diseased tissue and cleans the middle-ear cavity. The ossicles are closely assessed for damage and the extent to which repair or replacement is necessary. The surgeon uses autogenous cartilage or bone, cadaver ossicles, stainless steel wire, or polytetrafluoroethylene (Teflon) to repair or replace the ossicles.

Postoperative Care. An antiseptic-soaked gauze, such as iodoform gauze (Nu-Gauze), is packed in the auditory canal. If the postauricular or endaural incision is used, an external dressing is placed over the operative site. Dressings are kept clean and dry, and the nurse uses sterile technique when changing them. The client is kept flat with the operative ear up for at least 12 hours postoperatively. Prophylactic antibiotic therapy is used to prevent infections from recurring.

Clients generally report hearing improvement after the canal packing is removed. Until that time, the nurse communicates as with a hearing-impaired client, directing conversation to the unaffected ear. The nurse also instructs the client in postoperative care and activity restrictions (see Chart 51–4).

Stapedectomy. A partial or complete stapedectomy with prosthesis effectively corrects hearing loss. This procedure is most effective for clients with hearing loss related to otosclerosis.

Preoperative Care. To prevent the introduction of infective material to the middle-ear structures, no signs or symptoms of external otitis can be present at surgery. The nurse instructs the client to follow measures that prevent middle-ear or external-ear infections (Chart 51–7).

The nurse reviews the expected outcomes and possible complications of the surgery. Hearing is initially worse after a stapedectomy. The success rate of this procedure is high; however, as with all ear procedures, it carries a risk of failure that might lead to total deafness on the affected side or damage to the cranial nerves. Other possible complications include prolonged vertigo, infection, and facial nerve damage. A decision to proceed with surgery should

---

Chart 51–7

Health Promotion Guide: Prevention of Ear Infection or Trauma

- Do not use small objects such as cotton-tipped applicators, matches, toothpicks, and hairpins to clean your external ear canal.
- Wash your external ear and canal daily in the shower or while washing your hair.
- Blow your nose gently.
- Do not occlude one nostril while blowing your nose.
- Sneeze with your mouth open.
- Wear sound protection around loud or continuous noises.
- Avoid activities with high risk for head or ear trauma, such as wrestling, boxing, motorcycle riding, and skateboarding.
- Wear head and ear protection when engaging in these activities.
- Keep the volume on head receivers at the lowest setting that allows you to hear.
- Frequently clean objects that come into contact with your ear (headphones, telephone receivers, and so on).
- Avoid environmental conditions with rapid changes in air pressure.

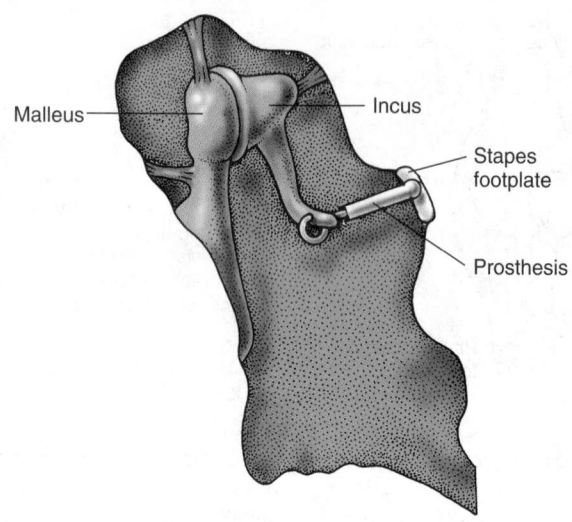

Figure 51–10. Prosthesis used with stapedectomy. The stapes is removed, leaving the footplate. After a hole is drilled in the footplate, a metal or plastic prosthesis is connected to the incus and inserted through the hole to act as a vibration device, much as the stapes worked before the development of otosclerosis.

be made with the client's full knowledge and understanding of these complications.

Operative Procedure. A stapedectomy is usually performed through the external auditory canal under local anesthesia. The head and neck of the stapes and, less often, the footplate are removed. After removal of the immobile bone, a small hole is drilled in the footplate; a metal or plastic prosthesis in the shape of a piston is connected between the incus and footplate (Figure 51–10). Sounds cause the prosthesis to vibrate as the stapes did. After stapedectomy, up to 90% of clients experience restoration of practical hearing.

Postoperative Care. The nurse informs the client that noticeable improvement in hearing may not occur until 6 weeks after surgery. Initially, the ear packing interferes with hearing. Postoperative swelling in the ear continues to affect hearing until the edema has resolved. Medications for pain assist the client in maintaining comfort, and antibiotics such as neomycin (Myciguent) are given prophylactically to reduce the risk of infection at the surgical site. The nurse instructs the client to follow the postoperative procedures in Chart 51–4.

The surgical procedure is performed in an area where cranial nerves VII, VIII, and X might be damaged by direct trauma or by postoperative swelling. The nurse observes for complications of surgery by assessing for facial nerve damage or muscle weakness and changes in tactile sensation or taste. Vertigo, nausea, and vomiting are common complaints because of the proximity to inner-ear structures.

Antivertiginous drugs, such as meclizine hydrochloride (Antivert, Bonamine✱), and antiemetic medications, such as droperidol (Inapsine), are given. Care is taken to prevent injury, especially during times of increased vertigo. The nurse assists the client with ambulating during the

first 1–2 days after surgery. Side rails on the bed are kept up, and the nurse reminds the client to move the head slowly when changing positions to avoid vertigo.

➤ *Anxiety*

Planning: Expected Outcomes. The client is expected to
- State that anxiety about communication is reduced
- Become proficient in alternative communication techniques

Interventions. Interventions focus on facilitating communication and reducing anxiety.

Facilitating Communication. The nurse uses the techniques listed in Chart 51–8 to communicate with a hearing-impaired client. Shouting to the client is of little benefit, because the sound may be projected at a higher frequency and the client less able to understand. The most obvious means of communicating with such a client is by the written word (if the client is able to see, read, and write) or with pictures of familiar phrases and objects. Some television programming is now closed captioned (subtitled) for the hearing impaired.

Assistive Devices. Assistive devices, described earlier under Sensory/Perceptual Alterations, can greatly increase communication for the client with a hearing impairment.

Lip Reading. Lip reading and sign language can also enhance communication. In a formal lip-reading class, clients are taught the special cues to look for when lip reading and how to understand body language. However,

---

Chart 51–8

Nursing Care Highlight: Communicating with a Hearing-Impaired Client

- Position yourself directly in front of the client.
- Make sure that the room is well lighted.
- Get the client's attention before you begin to speak.
- Move closer to the better hearing ear.
- Speak clearly and slowly.
- Do not shout (shouting raises the frequency of the sound and often makes understanding more difficult).
- Keep hands and other objects away from your mouth when talking to the client.
- Attempt to have conversations in a quiet room with minimal distractions.
- Have the client repeat your statements rather than just indicating assent.
- Rephrase sentences and repeat information to aid in understanding.
- Use appropriate hand motions.
- Write messages on paper if the client is able to read.

the best lip reader still misses more than 50% of what is being said. Because hearing is assisted by even minimal lip reading, clients are encouraged to wear their eyeglasses when talking with someone to see subtle movements of the lips.

Sign Language. For clients with more severe hearing loss, special languages have been developed, including American Sign Language (ASL). Such languages combine speech with hand movements that signify letters, words, and phrases. These languages take time and effort to learn, and many people are unable to learn language, just as many people cannot learn foreign languages. However, as hearing-impaired persons become less able to function, they may be better motivated to learn.

Managing Anxiety. A major source of anxiety is the possibility of permanent hearing loss. The nurse provides honest and accurate information about the likelihood of hearing returning. When hearing impairment is likely to be permanent or become more profound, the nurse reassures clients that communication and social interaction can be maintained.

To reduce anxiety and prevent social isolation, clients use remaining resources to make social contact satisfying. The most obvious way to decrease social isolation is by improving communication (as previously described). The nurse asks about past or present diversional activities to identify clients' most satisfying activities and social interactions and determine the amount of effort necessary to continue them. Activities can be altered to maximize clients' satisfaction. Someone accustomed to large gatherings might choose smaller groups instead. A quiet evening meal at home with friends might substitute for dinner in a noisy restaurant.

Continuing Care. Lengthy hospitalization is rare for most clients with ear and hearing disorders. If surgical repair is necessary and the procedure is completed without complications, the hospital stay is usually only 1 to 3 days.

➤ Health Teaching

The nurse gives clients written instructions about how to take medications and when to return for follow-up care. If the client cannot read, the nurse gives these instructions to a family member who may assist with care. The nurse teaches clients how to instill eardrops (see Chart 51–1) and irrigate the ears (see Chart 51–2), and asks for a return demonstration.

To promote health and prevent late postoperative infections, clients are instructed to follow the suggestions in Chart 51–7. For clients who use a hearing aid, the nurse teaches them how to use it effectively.

➤ Home Care Management

Clients who experience persistent vertigo either associated with the disorder or as a side effect of surgery remain in danger of falling. The home must, therefore, be assessed for potential hazards and to determine whether family members or significant others are available to assist the client with meal preparation and other activities of daily living. Home care nurses and nonprofessionals contacted ahead of time can help greatly.

➤ Health Care Resources

If clients do not have family or friends to help during the postoperative period, a referral to a home care agency is necessary. Assistance with meal preparation, cleaning, and personal hygiene can be contracted with the hospital discharge planners.

Follow-up hearing tests are scheduled for clients when the lesions are well healed, in about 6 to 8 weeks. Pre- and posttreatment audiograms are compared, and evaluation for further intervention to improve hearing begins. A complication of an unsuccessful surgery is continued disability or complete loss of hearing in the affected ear. Surgery is performed on the ear with the greatest hearing loss. If the surgery does not improve the hearing, clients must decide either to attempt surgical correction of the other ear or to continue to use an amplification device. When the underlying disorder causing the hearing impairment is progressive, this decision is difficult. The nurse supports clients by listening to their concerns and giving additional information when needed.

Information and support can come from several organizations, such as the American Speech-Language-Hearing Association, which publishes informative articles to help clients reduce hearing loss. Many public and private institutions offer hearing evaluations. The National Association of Hearing and Speech Agencies and Self-Help for Hard-of-Hearing People (Shhh) both supply information and counseling for clients with hearing disorders.

 Evaluation/Outcomes

On the basis of the identified diagnoses, the nurse evaluates the care given to the client. Desired outcomes for the client with hearing loss may include the following: the client is expected to

- State that the hearing loss has been at least partially relieved
- State that anxiety is reduced
- Demonstrate proper technique for using assistive devices
- Identify potential postoperative hazards
- State the importance of follow-up hearing assessments
- Be able to communicate effectively with family, friends, coworkers, and health care professionals
- Maintain satisfactory social contacts
- State that the pain is reduced or alleviated
- Describe the proper use of antibiotic therapy
- Demonstrate proper techniques when using eardrops, ointments, powders, or irrigation liquids
- Identify and avoid potential causes of otitis media
- Seek assistance with activities of daily living until vertigo and dizziness have subsided

CASE STUDY for the Client with External Otitis

■ B.B., a 38-year-old woman, comes to your outpatient clinic with complaints of left ear pain for the past 3 days and new onset of purulent green-yellow ear drainage. B.B. describes aching pain and a feeling of fullness in her left ear as well. She denies fever, anorexia, fatigue, and malaise. She states she has a history of recurrent external ear infections.

QUESTIONS:

1. What else should you ask the client?
2. What physical signs might you expect in a client with external otitis?
3. What teaching would you reinforce to prevent the recurrence of external otitis?
4. What expected outcomes are specific to this situation?

SELECTED BIBLIOGRAPHY

*Barnes, L., & Peel, R. (1992). *Head and neck pathology: A text/atlas of differential diagnosis.* New York: Igaku-Shoin.

Becker, W. (1994). *Ear, nose and throat diseases: A pocket reference* (2nd ed.). New York: Thieme Medical.

Benjamin, B., & Hawke, M. (1995). *A color atlas of otorhinolaryngology.* Philadelphia: Lippincott-Raven.

*Callaway, T., & Tucker, C. M. (1986). Rehabilitation of deaf black individuals: Problems and intervention strategies. *Journal of Rehabilitation, 52*(4), 53–56.

Chmiel, R., & Jerger, J. (1996). Hearing aid use, central auditory disorder, and hearing handicap in elderly persons. *Journal of the American Academy of Audiology, 7*(3), 190–202.

Clinical guidelines. Adult screening for hearing. (1996). *Nurse Practitioner: American Journal of Primary Health Care, 21*(6), 106, 108, 115.

*Colman, B. (1992). *Hall & Colman's diseases of the nose, throat, and ear* (14th ed.). Edinburgh: Churchill Livingstone.

Davidson, T., & Neuman, T. (1994). Managing ear trauma. *Physician & Sports Medicine, 22*(7), 27–32.

Ebert, D., & Heckerling, P. (1995). Communications with deaf patients: Knowledge, beliefs, and practices of physicians. *Journal of the American Medical Association, 273*(3), 227–229.

Erber, N. (1994). Communicating with elders: Effects of amplification. *Journal of Gerontological Nursing, 20*(10), 6–10.

*Facione, N. (1990). Otitis media: An overview of acute and chronic disease. *Nurse Practitioner, 15*(10), 11–20.

*Glasscock, M., & Shambaugh, G. (Eds.). (1990). *Surgery of the ear.* Philadelphia: W. B. Saunders.

Hardingham, M. (1995). Adenoma of the middle ear. *Archives of Otolaryngology: Head & Neck Surgery, 121*(3), 342–344.

*Hayback, P. (1993). Tuning in to ototoxicity: The inside story. *Nursing93, 23*(6), 34–41.

Heath, I. (1994). Tinnitus and health anxiety. *British Journal of Nursing, 3*(10), 502–505.

Lindblade, D., & McDonald, M. (1995). Removing communication barriers for the hearing-impaired elderly. *MedSurg Nursing, 4*(5), 379–385.

Luey, H., Glass, L., & Elliot, H. (1995). Hard-of-hearing or deaf: Issues of ears, language, culture, and identity. *Social Work: Journal of the National Association of Social Workers, 40*(2), 177–82.

*Mahoney, D. (1993). Cerumen impaction: Prevalence and detection in nursing homes. *Journal of Gerontological Nursing, 19*(6), 23–28.

Martin, R. (1994). How to care for the external ear. *Hearing Journal, 47*(2), 43–44.

McAllen, P. (1996). Hospital extra. Managing Meniere's disease. *American Journal of Nursing, 96*(6, Nurse Practice Extra Suppl.), 16E–F, 16H.

Meador, J. (1995). Clinical outlook. Cerumen impaction in the elderly. *Journal of Gerontological Nursing, 21*(12), 43–45.

Medical diagnosis and treatment (36th ed.). (1997). Los Altos, AC: Lang Medical.

Newland, J. (1994). Adult otitis media. *American Journal of Nursing, 94*(4, Nurse Practice Extra Suppl.), 16F.

*O'Rourke, C., Britten, F., Gatschet, C., & Krien, T. (1993). Effectiveness of hearing screening protocol for the elderly. *Geriatric Nursing, 14*(2), 66–69.

*Palumbo, M. (1990). Hearing access 2000: Increasing awareness of the hearing impaired. *Journal of Gerontological Nursing, 16*(9), 26–31.

Parker, W. (1995). Meniere's disease: Etiologic considerations. *Archives of Otolaryngology: Head and Neck Surgery, 121*(4), 377–382.

Put Prevention into practice: Screening for hearing loss. (1994). *Journal of the American Academy of Nurse Practitioners, 6*(9), 439–443.

Roberts, A. (1994). Systems of life: The ear and hearing 1. *Nursing Times, 89*(45), 33–36.

Roberts, A. (1994). Systems of life: The ear and hearing 2. *Nursing Times, 89*(49), 41–44.

Roberts, A. (1994). Systems of life: The ear and hearing 3. *Nursing Times, 90*(2), 45–48.

Rosenhall, U., & Pedersen, K. (1995). Presbycusis and occupational hearing loss. *Occupational Medicine: State of the Art Reviews, 10*(3), 593–607.

*Ross, V., Echevarria, K., & Robinson, B. (1991). Geriatric tinnitus: Causes, clinical treatment, and prevention. *Journal of Gerontological Nursing, 17*(10), 6–11.

*Ruddy, J., & Bickerton, R. (1992). Optimum management of the discharging ear. *Drugs, 43*(2), 219–235.

Schuller, D. (1994). *DeWeese and Saunders' Otolaryngology—head and neck surgery* (8th ed.). St. Louis: C. V. Mosby.

Selesnick, S. (1996). Diseases of the external auditory canal. *Otolaryngology Clinics of North America, 29*(5).

Sorensen, V., & Bonding, P. (1995). Can ear irrigation cause rupture of the normal tympanic membrane? *Journal of Laryngology and Otology, 109*(11), 1039–1040.

Stephens, D., France, L., & Lormore, K. (1995). Effects of hearing impairment on the patient's family and friends. *Acta Oto-Laryngologica, 115*(2), 165–167.

*Taylor, K. (1993). Geriatric hearing loss: Management strategies for nurses. *Geriatric Nursing, 14*(2), 74–78.

Thurgood, K., & Thurgood, G. (1995). Ear syringing: A clinical skill. *British Journal of Nursing, 4*(12), 682–687.

*Tolson, D. (1991). Making sense of...hearing aids. *Nursing Times, 87*(18), 36–38.

Winslow, E. H. (1994). Hearing loss? Check for impacted cerumen. *American Journal of Nursing, 94*(10), 55.

SUGGESTED READINGS

Lindblade, D., & McDonald, M. (1995). Removing communication barriers for the hearing-impaired elderly. *MedSurg Nursing, 4*(5), 379–385.

This very detailed article reviews causes and consequences of hearing loss as well as advantages and disadvantages of different communication methods available for the deaf and hearing impaired. The article describes how the nurse and community can support the hearing-impaired older person. Finally, a protocol is outlined to assess and manage the older person with hearing loss to assist the nurse organize care strategies.

Meador, J. (1995). Clinical outlook. Cerumen impaction in the elderly. *Journal of Gerontological Nursing, 21*(12), 43–45.

This short article concisely describes key points to consider when treating the client with cerumen impaction. The author describes general information about the production and normal elimination of cerumen and various ways to remove cerumen mechanically. A discussion of possible complications of cerumen impaction and removal is included.

Thurgood, K., & Thurgood, G. (1995). Ear syringing: A clinical skill. *British Journal of Nursing, 4*(12), 682–687.

Although the major purpose of this article is to describe the clinical skill of ear irrigation, information about the anatomy and physiology of the ear and hearing is included as well. The authors provide a thorough protocol for ear irrigation, along with a discussion of the potential problems the nurse will face when performing routine irrigations. Client education information is also included to assist the nurse in health maintenance teaching.

UNIT 11

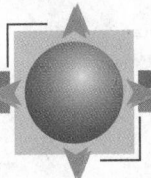

Problems of Mobility:

Management of Clients

with Problems of the

Musculoskeletal System

ASSESSMENT OF THE MUSCULOSKELETAL SYSTEM

Accounting for as much as 75% of the body's weight, the musculoskeletal system is one of the largest body systems. It includes bones, joints, and skeletal muscles and their supporting structures. Disease and trauma frequently affect any part of the system, and yet its assessment is often overlooked by nurses.

ANATOMY AND PHYSIOLOGY REVIEW
Skeletal System

The skeletal system consists of 206 bones and multiple joints. The growth and development of these structures occur during childhood and adolescence and are not discussed in this text.

Bones
Types

Bones may be classified by their shape. *Long bones,* such as the femur, are cylindric with rounded ends; they often bear weight. *Short bones*—for example, the phalanges—are small and bear little or no weight. *Flat bones,* such as the sternum, protect vital organs and often contain blood-forming cells. Bones that have unique shapes are known as *irregular bones:* for example, the carpal bones in the wrist. The *sesamoid bone* is the least common type and develops within a tendon; the patella is a typical example.

Structure

As shown in Figure 52–1, the outer layer of bone, or cortex, is composed of dense, compact bone tissue. The inner layer, in the medulla, contains spongy, cancellous tissue. Almost every bone has both tissue types but in varying quantities. The long bone typically has a shaft, or diaphysis, and two knob-like ends, or epiphyses.

The structural unit of the cortical, compact bone is the haversian system, as detailed in Figure 52–1. The haversian system is a complex canal network containing microscopic blood vessels, which supply nutrients and oxygen to bone, and lacunae, which are small cavities that house osteocytes (bone cells). The canals run longitudinally within the hard, cortical bone tissue.

The softer, cancellous tissue contains large spaces, or trabeculae, filled with red and yellow marrow. Hematopoiesis (production of blood cells) occurs in the red marrow. The yellow marrow contains fat cells, which can be dislodged and enter the bloodstream to cause fat embo-

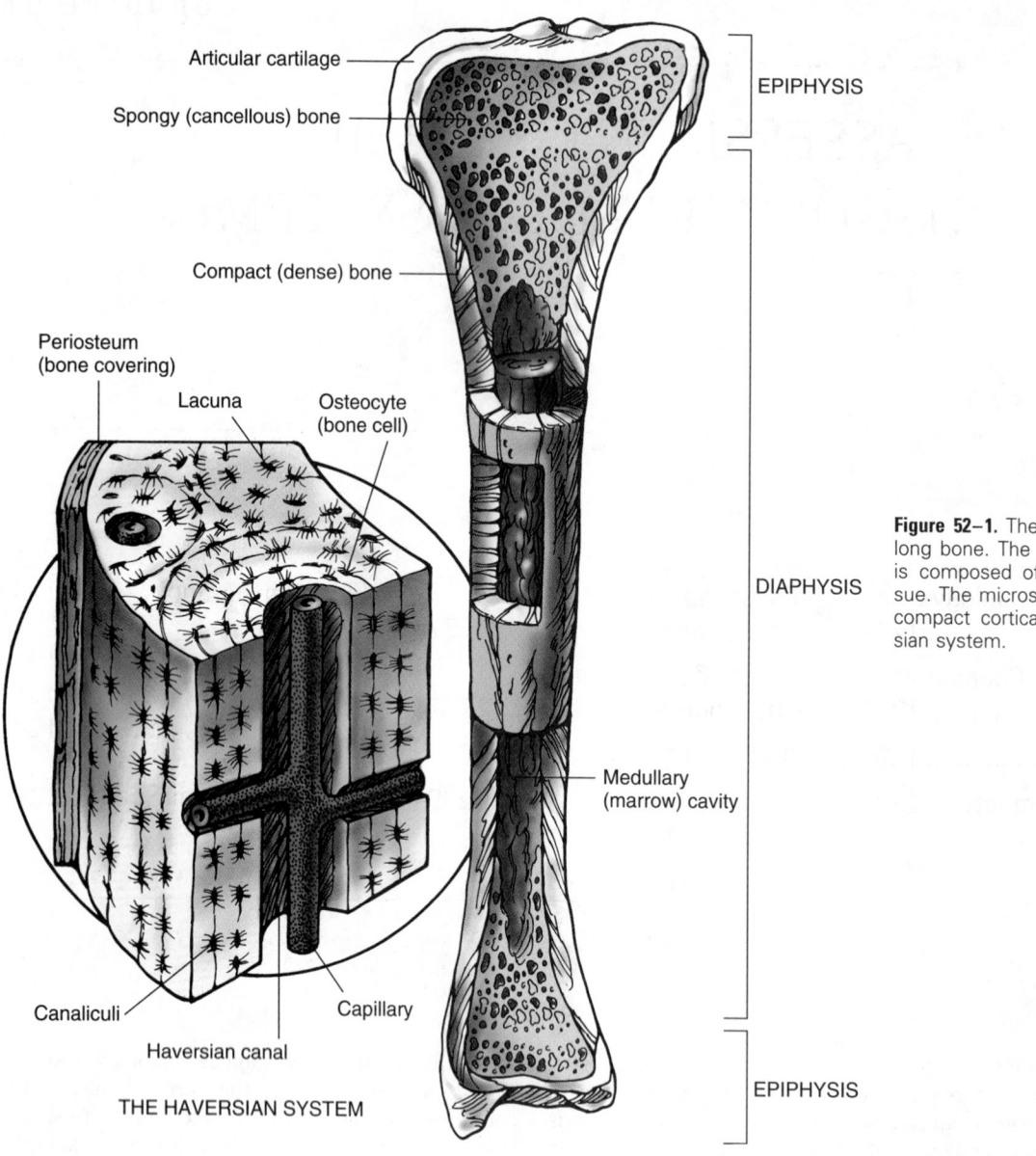

Articular cartilage

Spongy (cancellous) bone

Compact (dense) bone

Periosteum
(bone covering)

Lacuna

Osteocyte
(bone cell)

EPIPHYSIS

DIAPHYSIS

Medullary
(marrow) cavity

Canaliculi

Capillary

Haversian canal

THE HAVERSIAN SYSTEM

EPIPHYSIS

Figure 52–1. The structure of a typical long bone. The cortex, or outer layer, is composed of dense, compact tissue. The microscopic structure of this compact cortical tissue is the haversian system.

lism syndrome (FES), a life-threatening complication. Volkmann's canals connect bone marrow vessels with the haversian system and periosteum, the outermost covering of the bone. Osteogenic cells, which later differentiate into *osteoblasts* (bone-forming cells) and *osteoclasts* (bone-destroying cells), are found in the deepest layer of the periosteum.

Bone also contains a matrix (also called *osteoid*) consisting chiefly of collagen, mucopolysaccharides, and lipids. Deposits of inorganic calcium salts (carbonate and phosphate) in the matrix provide the hardness of bone.

Bone is a very vascular tissue; its estimated total blood flow is between 200 and 400 mL/minute. Each bone has a principal nutrient artery, which enters near the middle of the shaft and branches into ascending and descending vessels. These vessels supply the cortex, the marrow, and the haversian system. Sympathetic and afferent (sensory) fibers constitute the sparse nerve supply to bone. Dilation of blood vessels is controlled by the sympathetic nerves.

The afferent fibers transmit the pain experienced by clients who have primary lesions of the bone.

Growth and Metabolism

After puberty, bone reaches its maturity and maximal growth. Bone is a dynamic tissue, however, undergoing a continuous process of formation and resorption, or destruction, at equal rates until the age of 35 years. In later years, bone resorption accelerates, decreasing bone mass and predisposing clients to injury. (See Chapter 53 for a discussion of the effects of aging on bone metabolism.)

Bone growth and metabolism are affected by numerous minerals and hormones, including

- Calcium
- Phosphorus
- Calcitonin
- Vitamin D
- Parathyroid hormone (PTH)

- Growth hormone
- Glucocorticoids
- Sex hormones

CALCIUM AND PHOSPHORUS. Bone accounts for approximately 99% of the calcium in the body and 90% of the phosphorus. The serum concentrations of calcium and phosphorus maintain an inverse relationship; for example, when calcium levels rise, phosphorus levels decrease. When serum levels of calcium and phosphorus are altered, calcitonin and PTH work to maintain equilibrium. If the calcium level of the blood is decreased, for example, the bone (which stores calcium) releases calcium into the vascular system in response to PTH stimulation.

CALCITONIN. Calcitonin is produced by the thyroid gland and *decreases* the serum calcium concentration if it is increased above its normal level. Calcitonin inhibits bone resorption and increases renal excretion of calcium and phosphorus as needed.

VITAMIN D. Vitamin D and its metabolites are produced in the body and transported in the blood to promote the absorption of calcium and phosphorus from the small intestine. They also seem to enhance PTH activity in the release of calcium from the bone. A decrease in the body's vitamin D level can result in osteomalacia in the adult. An external source of vitamin D may be given to clients at risk for or diagnosed with osteomalacia. (Vitamin D metabolism and osteomalacia are detailed in Chapter 53.)

PARATHYROID HORMONE. When serum calcium levels are lowered, parathyroid hormone (PTH, or parathormone) secretion increases and stimulates bone to promote osteoclastic activity and *donate* calcium to the blood. PTH reduces the renal excretion of calcium and facilitates its absorption from the intestine. Conversely, when serum calcium levels increase, PTH secretion diminishes to preserve the bone calcium supply; this is an example of the feedback loop system of the endocrine system.

GROWTH HORMONE. Growth hormone—secreted by the anterior lobe of the pituitary gland—is responsible for increasing bone length and determining the amount of bone matrix formed before puberty. During childhood, an increased secretion results in gigantism, and a decreased secretion results in dwarfism. In the adult, an increase causes acromegaly, which is characterized by bone and soft-tissue deformities (see Chap. 66).

GLUCOCORTICOIDS. Adrenal glucocorticoids regulate protein metabolism, either increasing or decreasing catabolism to reduce or intensify the organic matrix of bone. They also aid in regulating intestinal calcium and phosphorus absorption.

SEX HORMONES. Estrogens stimulate osteoblastic activity and inhibit PTH. When estrogen levels decline at menopause, women are susceptible to low serum calcium levels with subsequent bone loss (osteoporosis). Androgens, such as testosterone, promote anabolism and in-

crease bone mass. External sources of estrogen and testosterone may be prescribed for clients at risk for or diagnosed with osteoporosis.

Function

The skeletal system

- Provides a framework for the body
- Supports the surrounding tissues (e.g., muscle and tendons)
- Assists in movement through muscle attachment and joint formation
- Protects vital organs, such as the heart and lungs
- Manufactures blood cells in red bone marrow
- Provides storage for mineral salts (e.g., calcium and phosphorus)

Joints

A joint is a space in which two or more bones come together. The primary function of a joint is to provide movement and flexibility in the body.

Types

The three types of joints in the body are

- Synarthrodial, or completely immovable (e.g., in the cranium)
- Amphiarthrodial, or slightly movable (e.g., in the pelvis)
- Diarthrodial (synovial), or freely movable (e.g., the elbow and knee)

Although any of these joints can be affected by disease or injury, the diarthrodial joints are most commonly involved.

Structure and Function

The diarthrodial, or synovial, joint is the most common type of joint in the body. Synovial joints are so named because they are the only type lined with synovium, a membrane that secretes synovial fluid for lubrication and shock absorption. As illustrated in Figure 52–2, the synovium lines the internal portion of the joint capsule but does not normally extend onto the surface of the cartilage at the spongy bone ends. Articular cartilage consists of a collagen fiber matrix impregnated with a complex ground substance. Bursae, small sacs located at joints to prevent friction, are also lined with synovial membrane.

Synovial joints are subtyped by their anatomic structures. *Ball-and-socket* joints (shoulder, hip) permit movement in any direction. *Hinge* joints (elbow) allow motion in one plane, flexion, and extension. The knee is often classified as a hinge joint, but it rotates slightly as well as flexes and extends. It is best described as a *condylar* type of synovial joint. The gliding movement of the wrist is characteristic of the *biaxial* joint. *Pivot* joints permit rotation only, as in the radioulnar area.

Muscular System

There are three types of muscle in the body: smooth, cardiac, and skeletal. Smooth, or nonstriated, involuntary

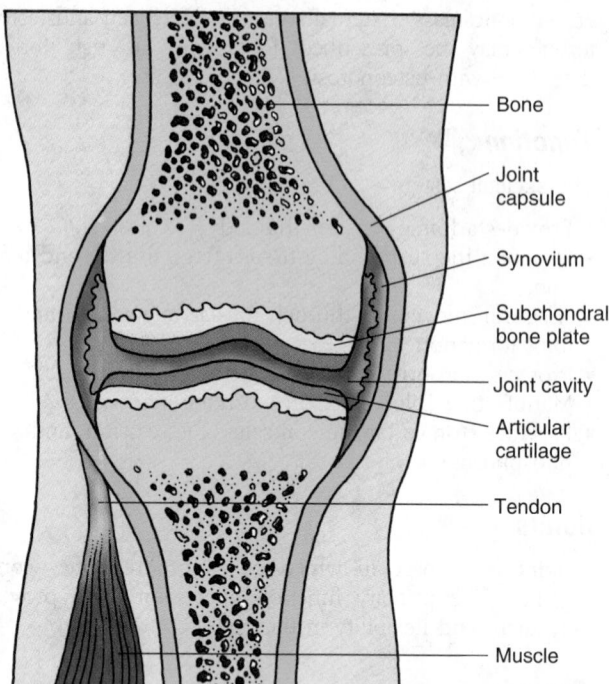

Bone
Joint capsule
Synovium
Subchondral bone plate
Joint cavity
Articular cartilage
Tendon
Muscle

Figure 52–2. The structure of a diarthrodial joint. Synovium lines the joint capsule but does not extend into the articular cartilage.

muscle is responsible for contractions of organs and blood vessels and is controlled by the autonomic nervous system. Cardiac muscle, or the myocardium, is also controlled by the autonomic nervous system. The smooth and cardiac muscles are discussed with the body systems to which they belong in the assessment chapters.

Structure

In contrast to smooth and cardiac muscle, skeletal muscle is voluntarily controlled by the central and peripheral nervous systems. The junction of a peripheral motor nerve and the muscle cells that it supplies is sometimes referred to as a motor end plate. Muscle fibers are held in place by connective tissue in bundles, or fasciculi. The entire muscle is surrounded by dense, fibrous tissue (fascia) containing the muscle's blood, lymph, and nerve supply.

Function

The primary function of skeletal muscle is movement of the body and its parts. When bones, joints, and supporting structures are adversely affected by injury or disease, the adjacent muscle tissue is often involved, limiting mobility. During the aging process, muscle fibers decrease in size and number, even in well-conditioned people. This senile atrophy is compounded when muscles are not regularly exercised, and they deteriorate from disuse.

Supporting Structures

In addition to the articular cartilage of joints, several types of cartilage occur in other areas. *Costal* cartilage connects the sternum to the rib cage. *Hyaline* cartilage is

in the septum of the nose, larynx, and trachea. The external ear and epiglottis contain *yellow* cartilage. In all areas, the tissue is flexible and elastic and can withstand enormous tension.

Other important supporting structures that are susceptible to injury include *tendons,* bands of tough, fibrous tissue that attach muscles to bones, and *ligaments,* which attach bones to other bones at joints.

Musculoskeletal Changes Associated with Aging

As one ages, bone density decreases, causing postural changes and predisposing a person to fractures. Synovial joint cartilage degenerates owing to the repeated use of joints, especially weight-bearing joints such as the hips and the knees. The result is often degenerative joint disease. Muscle tissue atrophy occurs, but its rate may be slowed by increased activity and exercise. Collectively, these changes cause decreased coordination, gait changes, and predisposition to falls with injury. Chart 52–1 lists the major anatomic and physiologic changes and the associated nursing interventions.

HISTORY

In assessment of a client with an actual or potential musculoskeletal problem, a detailed history aids the nurse in identifying diagnoses and subsequent interventions.

Demographic Data

Young men are at the greatest risk for trauma related to motor vehicle accidents.

WOMEN'S HEALTH CONSIDERATIONS

The age and sex of the client are important indicators in musculoskeletal disorders. Elderly women, for example, are most likely to have metabolic bone disease, such as osteoporosis. Women of any age are at the highest risk for most types of arthritis.

Personal and Family History

Accidents, illnesses, and medications may relate to a client's current problem. When taking a personal health history, the nurse questions the client about all traumatic incidents, regardless of date of occurrence. An injury to the lumbar spine 30 years previously may contribute to a client's current complaint of low back pain. An automobile accident that resulted in no apparent personal injury can be the cause of arthritis years after the event.

Previous or concurrent diseases may also affect musculoskeletal status. For example, a diabetic client treated for a foot ulcer is at high risk for acute or chronic osteomyelitis (bone infection). In addition, diabetes slows the healing process. Certain disorders have a familial or genetic tendency. Osteoporosis (age-related bone loss), for instance, often occurs in several generations of a family; bone cancer tends to be genetically linked. It is also

---

Chart 52–1

Nursing Focus on the Elderly: Changes in the Musculoskeletal System Related to Aging

Physiologic Change	Nursing Implications	Rationale
Decreased bone density	• Teach safety tips to prevent falls.	• Porous bones are more likely to fracture.
Increased bone prominence	• Prevent pressure on bone prominences.	• There is less soft tissue to prevent skin breakdown.
Kyphotic posture: widened gait, shift in the center of gravity	• Teach proper body mechanics; instruct the client to sit in supportive chairs with arms.	• Correction of posture problems prevents further deformity; the client should have support for bony structures.
Cartilage degeneration	• Provide moist heat, such as a shower.	• Moist heat increases blood flow to the area.
Decreased ROM	• Assess the client's ability to perform ADL and mobility.	• The client may need assistance with self-care skills.
Muscle atrophy, decreased strength	• Teach exercises.	• Exercises increase muscle strength.
Slowed movement	• Do not rush the client; be patient.	• The client may become frustrated if hurried.

---

important for the nurse to determine a history of previous hospitalizations and illnesses or complications.

The nurse also asks about previous and current use of medications. Some drugs, such as steroids, can affect calcium metabolism. Other drugs may be taken to relieve musculoskeletal pain.

Diet History

An evaluation of the client's diet history helps determine the cause of a musculoskeletal problem and anticipate complications of inadequate nutrition.

ELDERLY CONSIDERATIONS

An inadequate intake of calcium or protein foods or insufficient exposure to sunlight predisposes the elderly person to loss of bone and muscle tone. Homebound or institutionalized elderly clients are particularly at risk if they are not exposed to sunlight.

Inadequate protein or insufficient vitamin C in the diet inhibits healing of bone and tissue. Obesity places excess stress and strain on bones and joints, with resultant fractures and cartilage degeneration. In addition, obesity inhibits mobility in clients with musculoskeletal problems, which predisposes them to complications, such as respiratory and circulatory problems.

Socioeconomic Status

When assessing a client with a possible musculoskeletal alteration, the nurse inquires about lifestyle. A person's occupation can cause or contribute to an injury. For instance, fractures are not uncommon in clients whose jobs require manual labor, such as carpenters and mechanics. Certain factory or clerical jobs may predispose a person to carpal tunnel syndrome (entrapment of the median

nerve in the wrist). Construction workers may experience back injury from prolonged standing and excessive lifting. Amateur and professional athletes frequently experience acute musculoskeletal injuries, such as joint dislocations and fractures, or chronic disorders, such as degenerative joint disease.

Socioeconomic status may be related to the client's occupation and, therefore, affect the likelihood of musculoskeletal problems. For example, an executive working in an office is less likely to sustain a musculoskeletal injury than is a painter or roofer engaged in manual labor and such activities as climbing ladders.

TRANSCULTURAL CONSIDERATIONS

The body proportions of African-Americans differ from those of Caucasians, Asian-Americans, and Native Americans. African-Americans have shorter trunks and longer legs than other groups do. Their long bones are significantly longer and narrower than those of Caucasians. All bones are denser, and African-American men have denser bones than do African-American women. Caucasian women have the least amount of bone density of any group, which makes them the most susceptible to osteoporosis and fracture (Giger & Davidhizar, 1995).

Many African-Americans also have a lactose intolerance: that is, an inability to convert lactose to glucose and galactose. Because milk and dairy products are good sources of calcium for bone building but are rich in lactose, African-Americans may need to obtain their calcium from other food sources, such as dark green, leafy vegetables. Inuits also have a low tolerance for milk, and the adult diet is low in calcium (Giger & Davidhizar, 1995).

Ethnic and cultural background may also be helpful in ascertaining a client's tolerance to pain. There may be differences in reactions to pain among cultural populations, as discussed in Chapter 9. The nurse uses this information to aid in pain assessment.

Current Health Problem

The nurse gathers data pertinent to the client's presenting complaint as follows:

- Date and time of onset
- Factors that cause or exacerbate (worsen) the problem
- Course of the problem (e.g., intermittent or continuous)
- Clinical manifestations (as expressed by the client) and the pattern of their occurrence
- Measures that improve clinical manifestations (e.g., heat)

The most common complaint of people with musculoskeletal problems is pain. The pain may be acute or chronic, depending on its onset and duration. The nurse may use the P-Q-R-S-T model to elicit a complete assessment of the client's pain:

P Provoking incident? (Was there a certain incident or event that precipitated the pain or caused an exacerbation of the pain?)

Q Quality of pain? (What does the pain feel like in descriptive terms? Is it burning, throbbing, stabbing?)

R Region, radiation, and relief? (Exactly where is the pain located? Does the pain travel or radiate? Does anything help relieve the pain?)

S Severity of the pain? (How severe is the pain? The client may use a pain scale [see Chap. 9] or describe how the pain has interfered with his or her ability to function.)

T Time? (How long does the pain last? When does it occur? Is it worse at night or during the day? If the pain awakens a person at night, the source of the pain is most likely inflammatory, not degenerative.)

With any pain assessment, it is always best if the client describes the pain in his or her own words and points to its location, if possible.

PHYSICAL ASSESSMENT

Although bones, joints, and muscles are usually assessed simultaneously in a head-to-toe approach, each subsystem is described separately for emphasis and understanding. For physical assessment of the musculoskeletal system, the nurse incorporates inspection, palpation, active range of motion, and special techniques for specific problems. A general assessment is described in this chapter. More specific assessment techniques are discussed in the interventions chapters that follow for each musculoskeletal problem.

Assessment of the Skeletal System

General Inspection

The nurse observes the client's posture, gait, and mobility for gross deformities and impairment.

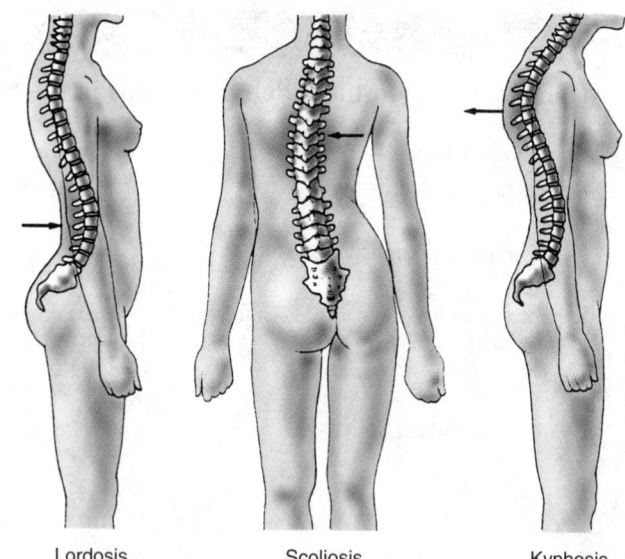

Lordosis   Scoliosis   Kyphosis

Figure 52–3. Common spinal deformities.

Posture

Posture includes the person's body build and alignment when standing and walking. The nurse observes the curvature of the spine and the length, shape, and symmetry of extremities. Figure 52–3 illustrates some common spinal deformities. Muscle mass is also inspected for size and symmetry.

Gait

Most clients with musculoskeletal problems eventually have a problem with gait. The two phases of normal, automatic gait (Fig. 52–4) are the stance phase and the swing phase.

The nurse or therapist evaluates the client's balance, steadiness, and ease and length of stride; a limp or other asymmetric leg movement or deformity is noted. An abnormality in the stance phase of gait is called an *antalgic* gait. When part of one leg is painful, the person shortens the stance phase on the affected side. An abnormality in the swing phase is called a *lurch*. This abnormal gait occurs when the muscles in the buttocks and/or leg are too weak to allow the person to change weight from one foot to another. In this case, the shoulders are moved either side to side or front to back for help in shifting the weight from one leg to another. Some clients, such as those with chronic hip pain and muscle atrophy from degenerative joint disease, have a combination of the antalgic gait and lurch.

Mobility

In collaboration with the physical or occupational therapist, the nurse observes the client's need for or use of ambulatory devices, such as canes and walkers, during transfer from bed to chair and while walking and climbing stairs. The nurse also assesses mobility by asking the client to perform simple activities of daily living (ADL),

STANCE PHASE

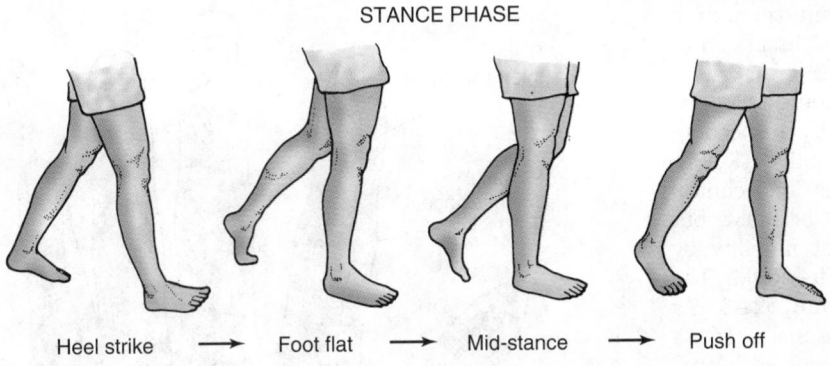

Heel strike → Foot flat → Mid-stance → Push off

Figure 52–4. The phases of gait.

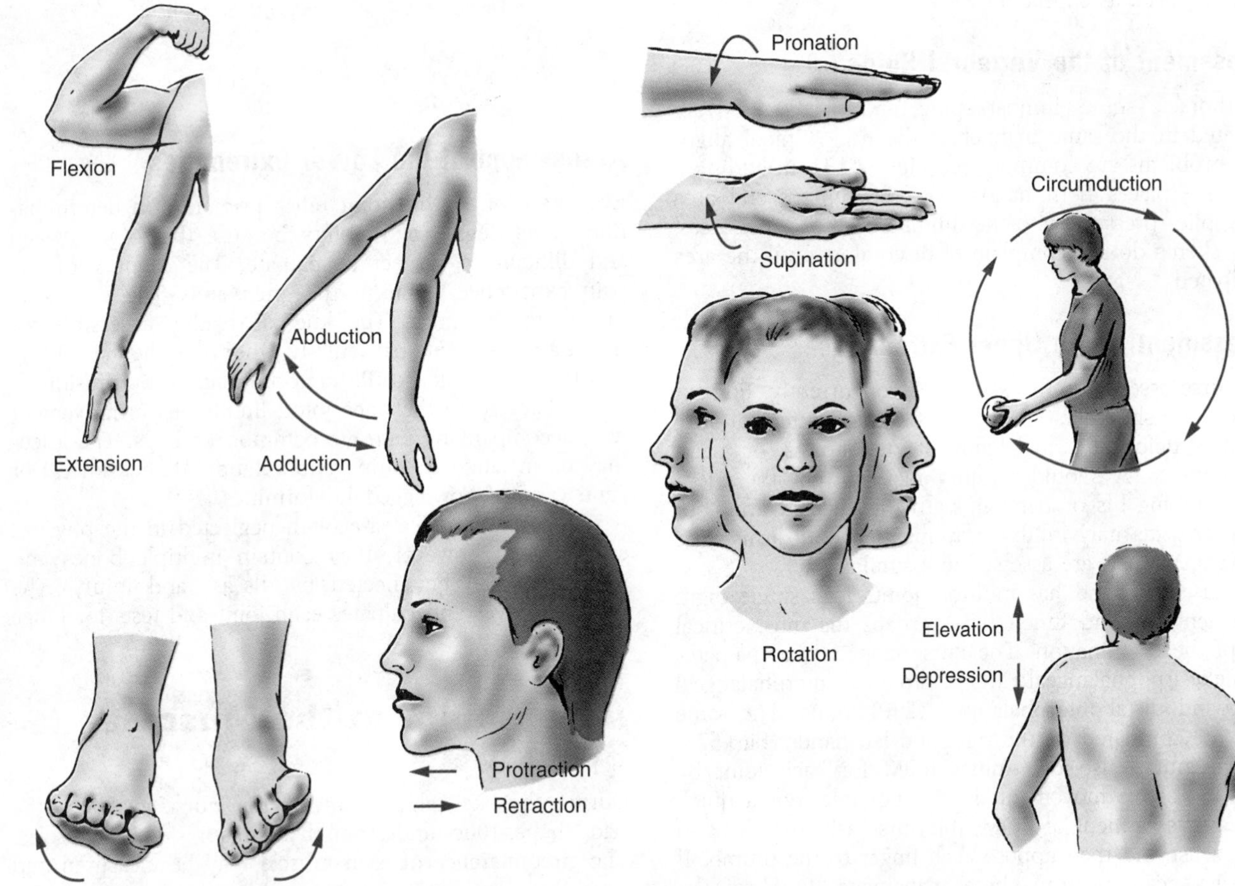

SWING PHASE

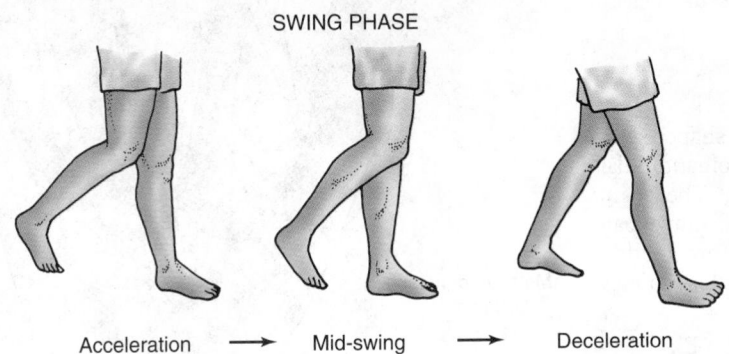

Acceleration → Mid-swing → Deceleration

Flexion

Extension

Abduction

Adduction

Pronation

Supination

Rotation

Circumduction

Elevation ↑

Depression ↓

Protraction

Retraction

Eversion   Inversion

Figure 52–5. Movements of the skeletal muscles. (Modified from Jarvis, C. [1996]. *Physical examination and health assessment* [2nd ed.]. Philadelphia: W. B. Saunders.)

such as putting on shoes. Pain and deformity may limit physical mobility and function. (A complete discussion of functional assessment is found in Chapter 13.)

After performing a functional assessment, the nurse assesses major bones, joints, and muscles by inspection, palpation, and determination of range of motion (ROM). A goniometer (used by physical therapists and clinical specialists) provides an exact measurement of ROM, but the nurse can estimate the degree of joint mobility by having the client put each joint through its ROM. The nurse uses the movements shown in Figure 52–5. As long as the client can function to meet personal needs, a limitation in ROM may not be significant. For each anatomic location, the nurse observes the skin for color, elasticity, and lesions that may relate to musculoskeletal dysfunction.

Assessment of the Head and Neck

The nurse inspects and palpates the skull for shape, symmetry, tenderness, and masses. The temporomandibular joints (TMJs) are best evaluated by palpation. The client is asked to open his or her mouth while the nurse palpates the TMJs. Common abnormal findings are tenderness or pain, crepitus (a grating sound), and a spongy swelling caused by excess synovium and fluid.

The nurse then inspects and palpates each vertebra of the spine in the neck. Clinical findings may include malalignment; tenderness; or inability to flex, extend, and rotate the neck as expected.

Assessment of the Vertebral Spine

The thoracic spine, lumbar spine, and sacral spine are evaluated in the same manner as the neck. Spinal alignment problems are common (see Fig. 52–3). In addition, the nurse places both hands over the lumbosacral area and applies pressure with the thumbs to elicit tenderness. Many clients do not complain of discomfort until the area is palpated.

Assessment of the Upper Extremities

The nurse assesses both extremities concurrently. For example, both shoulders are inspected and palpated for size, swelling, deformity, malalignment, tenderness or pain, and mobility. A shoulder injury may prevent the client from combing his or her hair with the affected arm, but severe arthritis may inhibit movement in both arms. The elbows and wrists are assessed in a similar way.

Because the hand has multiple joints in a single digit, assessment of hand function is perhaps the most critical part of the examination. The nurse inspects and palpates the metacarpophalangeal (MCP), proximal interphalangeal (PIP), and distal interphalangeal (DIP) joints. The same digits are compared on the right and left hands (Fig. 52–6). The nurse also determines ROM for each joint by observing active movement, if it is possible. For a quick and easy assessment of ROM, the nurse asks the client to make a fist and then appose each finger to the thumb. If the client can perform these maneuvers, ROM of the hand is not seriously restricted.

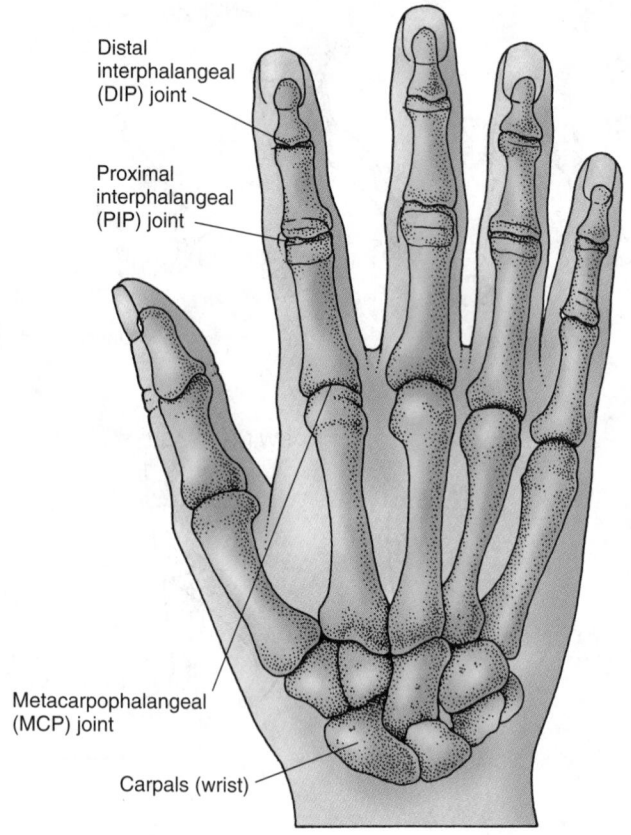

Figure 52–6. The small joints of the hand.

Assessment of the Lower Extremities

Evaluation of the hip joint relies primarily on determination of its degree of mobility because the joint is deep and difficult to inspect or palpate. The client with hip pain experiences pain in the *groin* area. The pain may radiate to the knee. The knee is readily accessible for nursing assessment, particularly when the client is sitting and the knee is flexed. Fluid accumulation, or effusion, is easily detected in the knee joint; limitations in movement with accompanying pain are common findings. The knees may be malaligned, as in genu valgum ("knock-knee") or genu varum ("bowlegged") deformities.

The ankles and feet are often neglected in the physical examination; however, they contain multiple bones and joints that can be affected by disease and injury. The nurse observes and palpates each joint and tests for range of motion.

Assessment of the Muscular System

During the skeletal assessment, the nurse evaluates the size, shape, tone, and strength of major skeletal muscles. The circumference of each muscle may be measured and compared symmetrically for an estimation of muscle mass.

TABLE 52–1

Lovett's Scale for Determining Muscle Strength	
Rating	**Description**
5	• Normal: ROM unimpaired against gravity with full resistance
4	• Good: can complete ROM against gravity with some resistance
3	• Fair: can complete ROM against gravity
2	• Poor: can complete ROM with gravity eliminated
1	• Trace: no joint motion and slight evidence of muscle contractility
0	• Zero: no evidence of muscle contractility

ROM, range of motion

In addition to inspecting and palpating the skeletal muscles, the nurse asks the client to demonstrate muscle strength. For instance, to determine grip strength, the nurse asks the client to squeeze a sphygmomanometer bulb and records the level of pressure achieved. This method provides a precise measurement that can be used to observe improvement or deterioration of muscle ability. In another method, the nurse applies resistance by holding the extremity and asking the client to move it. Although movement against resistance is not easily quantified, several scales are available for grading the client's strength. A commonly used scale is delineated in Table 52–1.

PSYCHOSOCIAL ASSESSMENT

The data from the history and physical examination provide clues for the nurse in anticipating psychosocial problems. For instance, the client with multiple fractures who requires extensive immobilization and therapy is at high risk for sensory deprivation. Prolonged absence from employment or permanent disability may cause the client to lose his or her job or occupation. Further stress may be experienced if chronic pain ensues and the client cannot cope with numerous stressors simultaneously. Deformities resulting from musculoskeletal disease or injury can affect a person's body image and self-concept.

DIAGNOSTIC ASSESSMENT
Laboratory Tests

Chart 52–2 lists the major laboratory tests used in assessing clients with musculoskeletal disorders. There is no special client preparation or follow-up care for any of these tests. The nurse teaches the client the purpose of the test and the procedure that can be expected. (Tests performed for clients with connective tissue diseases, such as rheumatoid arthritis, are described in Chapter 24.)

Serum Calcium and Phosphorus

The concentrations of calcium and phosphorus, or phosphate (inorganic phosphorus), have an inverse relationship. In a healthy state, when the calcium level decreases, the phosphorus level increases, and vice versa. Disorders of bone and the parathyroid gland are often reflected in an alteration of the serum calcium or phosphorus level.

Alkaline Phosphatase

Alkaline phosphatase (ALP) is an enzyme normally present in blood. The concentration of ALP increases with bone or liver damage. In metabolic bone disease and bone cancer, the enzyme concentration rises in proportion to the osteoblastic activity, which indicates bone formation. The level of ALP is normally slightly increased in the elderly.

Serum Muscle Enzymes

The major muscle enzymes affected in skeletal muscle disease or injury are

- Creatine kinase (CK), formerly called creatine phosphokinase (CPK)
- Aspartate aminotransferase (AST), formerly called serum glutamic-oxaloacetic transaminase (SGOT)
- Aldolase (ALD)
- Lactate dehydrogenase (LDH)

As a result of damage, the muscle tissue releases additional amounts of these enzymes, which increases serum levels.

The serum CK level begins to rise 2 to 4 hours after muscle injury and is elevated early in muscle disease, such as muscular dystrophy. The CK molecule has two subunits: M (muscle) and B (brain). Three isoenzymes have been identified. Skeletal muscle CK (CK-MM, or CK_3) is the only isoenzyme that rises in concentration with damage to skeletal muscle.

AST is moderately elevated (three to five times normal) in certain muscle diseases, such as muscular dystrophy and dermatomyositis. The levels of the isoenzymes aldolase A (ALD-A) and LDH_5 also increase in clients with these disorders.

Radiographic Examinations
Standard Radiography

The skeleton and its supporting structures are readily visible on standard x-rays. Anteroposterior projections are the initial screening views. Other approaches, such as lateral or oblique, depend on the part of the skeleton to be evaluated.

Observations of bone density, alignment, swelling, and intactness are made. The conditions of joints can be determined, including the size of the joint space, the smoothness of articular cartilage, and synovial swelling. Soft-tissue involvement may also be evident but not clearly differentiated.

The nurse informs the client that the x-ray table is

Chart 52-2

Laboratory Profile: Musculoskeletal Assessment

Test	Normal Range for Adults	Significance of Abnormal Findings

Serum calcium	• 8.6–10.0 mg/dL (2.15–2.50 mmol/L)
	• **>60 y:** Slightly lower
	• **>90 y:** 8.2–9.6 mg/dL
		• *Hypercalcemia* (increased calcium)
		  • Metastatic cancers of the bone
		  • Paget's disease
		  • Bone fractures in healing stage
		• *Hypocalcemia* (decreased calcium)
		  • Osteoporosis
		  • Osteomalacia

Serum phosphorus	• 2.7–4.5 mg/dL (0.87–1.45 mmol/L)
	• **>60 y:** 2.3–3.7 mg/dL (M)
	  2.8–4.1 mg/dL (F)
		• *Hyperphosphatemia* (increased phosphorus)
		  • Bone fractures in healing stage
		  • Bone tumors
		  • Acromegaly
		• *Hypophosphatemia* (decreased phosphorus)
		  • Osteomalacia

Alkaline phosphatase (ALP)	• 25–100 U/L	• *Elevations* may indicate
		  • Metastatic cancers of the bone
		  • Paget's disease
		  • Osteomalacia

Serum muscle enzymes
  Creatine kinase (CK₃)
	• Total CK:
	  • Men: 38–174 U/L (M)
	  • Women: 26–140 U/L (F)
	• **>90 y:** 21–203 (M)
	  22–99 (F)
		• *Elevations* may indicate
		  • Muscle trauma
		  • Progressive muscular dystrophy
		  • Effects of electromyography

Lactate dehydrogenase (LDH)	• Total LDH: 140–280 U/L
	• **60–90 y:** 110–210 U/L
	• **>90 y:** 99–284 U/L
	• LDH₅: 0%–5%
		• *Elevations* may indicate
		  • Skeletal muscle necrosis
		  • Extensive cancer
		  • Progressive muscular dystrophy

Aspartate aminotransferase (AST)	• 8–10 U/L (slightly lower in women)
	• **>60 y:** 11–26 U/L (M)
	  10–20 U/L (F)
		• *Elevations* may indicate
		  • Skeletal muscle trauma
		  • Progressive muscular dystrophy

Aldolase (ALD)	• 1.0–7.5 U/L	• *Elevations* may indicate
		  • Polymyositis and dermatomyositis
		  • Muscular dystrophy

M, males; F, females.

hard and cold and instructs the client to remain still during the filming process.

Tomography and Xeroradiography

Whereas standard x-rays superimpose one structure on another, tomography produces planes, or slices, for focus and blurs the images of other structures. This procedure is helpful in detailing the musculoskeletal system because the many close structures make visualization difficult.

Xeroradiography highlights the contrast between structures. Margins and edges can be clearly seen (edge enhancement). Disadvantages of xeroradiography are the higher radiation dose to the client and its inability to determine tissue densities.

Myelography

Myelography involves the injection of contrast medium, or dye, into the subarachnoid space of the spine, usually by lumbar puncture. The vertebral column, intervertebral

disks, spinal nerve roots, and blood vessels can be visualized. Although this test is still performed, it is becoming less popular as computed tomography (CT) and magnetic resonance imaging (MRI) replace such invasive diagnostic techniques (see Chap. 43).

Arthrography

An arthrogram is an x-ray of a joint after contrast medium (air or solution) has been injected to enhance its visualization. Double-contrast arthrography, which uses both air and solution, may be performed when a traumatic injury is suspected. The physician can often determine bone chips, torn ligaments, or other loose bodies within the joint.

CLIENT PREPARATION. The most common joints studied are the knee and the shoulder. The nurse questions the client about allergy to seafood or iodine.

The nurse informs the client that the test may be uncomfortable because of pressure at the needle insertion site. The joint may be swollen for several days after the test, and strenuous physical activity should be avoided for 12 to 24 hours. The joint may be wrapped, and ice may be applied at intervals for the first few hours after the test to decrease swelling.

PROCEDURE. If the knee is examined, the client is placed in a sitting position to flex the joint. After a local anesthetic is applied, the physician injects an iodine-based contrast medium directly into the joint through a medial or lateral approach. The client feels pressure but should not experience pain. X-rays are then taken of the joint, which may be put through range of motion (ROM) during the test.

FOLLOW-UP CARE. Because the contrast medium mixes with synovial fluid, it is not withdrawn after the procedure. As a result, the client's joint is enlarged and slightly uncomfortable. Some clients state that they feel the solution moving in the joint and hear "clicking" noises for several days until the solution is absorbed by the body.

The nurse instructs the client to resume usual activities but to avoid strenuous exercise, such as participating in contact sports, for at least 12 hours after the test. An elastic bandage may be worn around the joint for several days. The application of ice may reduce some of the swelling.

Computed Tomography

Computed tomography (CT) has gained wide acceptance for the detection of musculoskeletal problems, particularly those of the vertebral column. It may be used with or without a contrast medium, which is given orally or intravenously. If the administration of a contrast agent is planned, the nurse checks that the client has been allowed nothing by mouth (NPO) for at least 4 hours and is not allergic to iodine.

As a noninvasive procedure, the CT scan requires minimal nursing intervention except for client education. During the procedure, the client must remain still for 30 to 60 minutes on a hard table while encased in the machine. Complaints of claustrophobia and annoyance from the clicking sounds made by the scanner on rotation are common, but the nurse reassures the client that there is no danger from the machine.

Other Diagnostic Tests
Bone Biopsy

In a bone biopsy, the physician extracts a specimen of bone for microscopic examination. This invasive test may confirm the presence of infection or neoplasm. Two techniques may be used to retrieve the specimen: needle (closed) or incisional (open) biopsy.

CLIENT PREPARATION. The nurse teaches the client about the procedure and post-test care. The open technique is more invasive and requires more care.

PROCEDURE. The physician may perform bone biopsy in the client's room, in a special procedures room in the radiology department, or in the operating room with use of local or general anesthesia. If the client is not given general anesthesia, this procedure is quite painful. After anesthesia is induced, the physician inserts a long needle into the bone cortex or makes a small incision to reveal the bone tissue. A sterile dressing is applied after extraction of the osseous tissue. If an incision is made, the physician uses a pressure dressing.

FOLLOW-UP CARE. The post-care nurse inspects the biopsy site for bleeding, swelling, and hematoma formation, the most common complications of bone biopsy during the first 24 hours after the procedure. Because the pressure dressing inhibits observation, the nurse monitors the client's level of pain. If internal bleeding or marked swelling occurs, the client complains of severe pain instead of the mild to moderate discomfort usually associated with the procedure. For decreasing the likelihood of bleeding, the client is taught to immobilize the affected extremity for 12 to 24 hours. If bone infection occurs as a complication of bone biopsy, the client's temperature may be elevated 1 to 3 days after the procedure.

A mild analgesic often relieves the discomfort resulting from the procedure. After an open biopsy, the nurse teaches the client to reapply the dressing daily over the incision site while inspecting the wound for signs of inflammation or infection, such as redness, warmth, and tissue swelling.

Muscle Biopsy

Muscle biopsy is done for the diagnosis of atrophy (as in muscular dystrophy) and inflammation (as in polymyositis). The procedure and care for clients undergoing muscle biopsy are the same as those for clients undergoing bone biopsy.

Electromyography

Electromyography (EMG) is usually accompanied by nerve conduction studies for determining the electrical potential generated in an individual muscle. EMG helps in the diagnosis of neuromuscular, lower motor neuron, and peripheral nerve disorders. Figure 52–7 shows an electromyograph, the instrument used to perform EMG.

CLIENT PREPARATION. The nurse informs the client that EMG may cause temporary discomfort, especially when the client is subjected to episodes of electrical current. For selected clients, mild sedation is ordered. The physician may also order a temporary discontinuation of skeletal muscle relaxants several days before the procedure to prevent medication from having effects on the test results.

PROCEDURE. The test may be performed at the bedside or in an EMG laboratory. When both EMG and nerve conduction studies are done, nerve conduction is usually tested first. Flat electrodes are placed along the nerve to be evaluated, and low electrical currents are

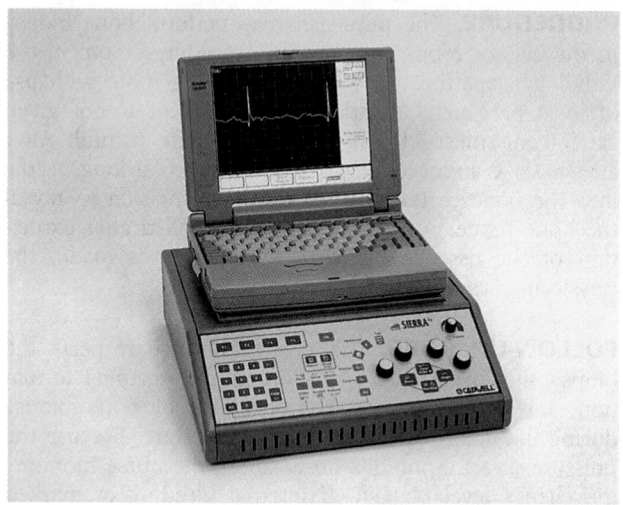

Figure 52–7. An electromyograph. (Courtesy of Cadwell Laboratories, Kennewick, WA.)

passed through the electrodes to the nerve and muscle innervated. If nerve conduction is accomplished, the muscle contracts.

For testing muscle potential, multiple needle electrodes varying from ½ to 3 inches (1.3 to 7.5 cm) are inserted. The client may be asked to perform activities for measurement of muscle potential during minimal and maximal contraction. The degree of nerve and muscle activity is recorded on an oscilloscope, which provides a graphic readout for later interpretation.

FOLLOW-UP CARE. A few medical complications are associated with EMG. The nurse provides comfort measures and inspects the needle sites for hematoma formation. The nurse can apply ice to prevent this complication. The client may complain of increased pain and anxiety after the test.

Arthroscopy

An arthroscope is a tubular device inserted into a joint for direct visualization; the knee and shoulder are most commonly evaluated. In addition, synovial biopsy and surgical procedures to repair traumatic injury can be accomplished with the arthroscope.

CLIENT PREPARATION. Because the knee is most commonly "scoped," the care described for the client undergoing arthroscopy relates to that joint. Arthroscopy is performed on an ambulatory basis or as same-day surgery. Clients who cannot flex their knees at least 40 degrees or who have infected knees are not candidates for the procedure. The client must be able to flex the knee, and joint infection may worsen from the mechanical trauma of arthroscope insertion.

If possible, the client should have a physical therapy consultation before arthroscopy to learn the leg exercises that are necessary after the test, especially if the procedure will be surgical. Straight-leg raises (SLRs) and quad-

riceps setting exercises (isometrics with the leg extended) are practiced in sets of ten each. Range-of-motion (ROM) exercises are also taught but may not be allowed immediately after arthroscopic surgery. The nurse in the surgeon's office or at the surgical center can teach these exercises or reinforce the information provided by the physical therapist. The nurse also explains the procedure and post-test care.

PROCEDURE. The client is usually given local, light general, or epidural anesthesia, depending on the purpose of the procedure. In some settings, a large pneumatic tourniquet is used around the thigh to minimize bleeding during the procedure. Medications promoting vasoconstriction for control of bleeding may be used alone or in conjunction with the tourniquet.

The knee is flexed to at least 40 degrees, and saline or Ringer's lactate is used to irrigate the knee. As shown in Figure 52–8, the arthroscope is inserted through a small incision less than ¼ inch (0.6 cm) long. Multiple incisions may be required to allow inspection at a variety of angles. After the procedure, a bulky pressure dressing and an elastic bandage may be applied, depending on the amount of manipulation during the test or surgery.

FOLLOW-UP CARE. The nurse evaluates the neurovascular status of the client's affected leg frequently, in accordance with nursing standards of care. Initially, the typical protocol is every hour. The technique for this assessment is described in Chapter 54.

The nurse encourages the client to perform exercises as taught before the examination. For the mild discomfort experienced after the diagnostic arthroscopy, the physician prescribes a mild analgesic, such as acetaminophen (Tylenol, Ace-Tabs✦). The client seldom has activity restrictions and often returns to normal daily activities immediately. When arthroscopic surgery is performed, the physician usually prescribes an opioid-analgesic combination, such as oxycodone and acetaminophen (Percocet).

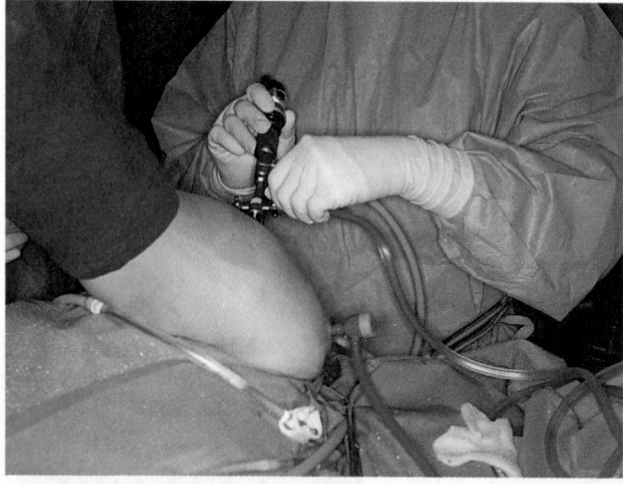

Figure 52–8. An arthroscope is used in the diagnosis of pathologic changes in the joints. This client is undergoing arthroscopy of the shoulder.

Although complications are not common, the nurse monitors and teaches the client to monitor for

- Hypothermia (decreased body temperature) resulting from the use of the tourniquet during the procedure
- Increased joint pain attributable to mechanical injury
- Thrombophlebitis
- Infection

Severe joint or leg pain after discharge may indicate a possible complication and warrants that the client contact the physician immediately. The physician may see the client about 1 week after the test to check for complications.

Bone Scan

The bone scan is a radionuclide test in which radioactive material is injected for visualization of the entire skeleton. It is used primarily to detect tumors, arthritis, osteomyelitis, osteoporosis, vertebral compression fractures, and unexplained bone pain.

CLIENT PREPARATION. A nuclear medicine physician or technician injects the client intravenously with the radioactive isotope of technetium (Tc 99m) several hours before the scanning procedure. As a bone-seeking substance, the isotope migrates to bone. The nurse assures the client that the dose is minimal and that no complications will result from receipt of the material. The client is asked to void immediately before the scan to prevent an obliterated view of the pelvis.

PROCEDURE. The client is taken to the nuclear medicine department and placed on the scanning table. For an accurate image, the client must be able to lie still for 30 to 60 minutes during scanning. Clients who are elderly, restless, or in pain may find this test uncomfortable and may need mild sedation. The examiner looks for areas of bone in which there is increased uptake, or concentration, of the isotope. These hot lesions indicate abnormal bone metabolism, a sign of bone disease. Cold lesions, in which there is decreased uptake, indicate poor blood flow to bone, as in severe arteriosclerosis.

FOLLOW-UP CARE. The amount of radioactivity in the isotope is minimal and presents no hazard to the client or the nurse. The substance is excreted in urine and stool. Because the substance rapidly deteriorates in the body, no special precautions are required for handling excreta. The nurse encourages the client to push fluids to facilitate urinary excretion. Repeated scans may be taken, but no additional injection of the radioisotope is required.

Gallium/Thallium Scans

The gallium or thallium scan is similar to the bone scan but is more specific and sensitive in detecting bone problems. Gallium citrate (Ga 67) is the radioisotope most commonly used. This substance also migrates to brain, liver, and breast tissue and therefore is used in examination of these structures when disease is suspected.

For clients with osteosarcoma, thallium (Tl 201) is bet-

ter than gallium or technetium for diagnosing the extent of the disease. Thallium has traditionally been used for the diagnosis of myocardial infarctions but is now also used for evaluation of cancers of the bone.

CLIENT PREPARATION. Because bone takes up gallium slowly, the nuclear medicine physician or technician administers the isotope 1 to 2 days before scanning. Other tests that require contrast media or other isotopes cannot be given during this time.

The nurse instructs the client that the radioactive material poses no threat to the client because it readily deteriorates in the body. Because gallium is excreted through the intestinal tract, it tends to collect in feces before the scanning procedure.

PROCEDURE. Depending on the tissue to be examined, the client is taken to the nuclear medicine department 1 to 2 days after injection. The procedure takes 30 to 60 minutes, during which time the client must lie still for accurate test results to be achieved. Mild sedation may be necessary to facilitate relaxation and cooperation during the procedure for confused elderly clients or those in severe pain.

FOLLOW-UP CARE. No special care is required after the test. The radioisotope is excreted in stool and urine, but no precautions are taken in handling the excreta. The nurse encourages the client to push fluids to facilitate urinary excretion.

Magnetic Resonance Imaging

Magnetic resonance imaging (MRI), with or without the use of contrast media, can be used to diagnose musculoskeletal disorders. Its use is expanding and replacing some of the more traditional tests, such as bone scans. The MRI is more accurate than CT and myelography for many spinal disorders (Patel & Lauerman, 1997).

The image is produced through the interaction of magnetic fields, radio waves, and atomic nuclei showing hydrogen density. Simply put, the radiowaves "bounce" off the body tissues being examined. Because each tissue has its own density, the computer image clearly distinguishes normal and abnormal tissues. For some tissues, the cross-sectional image is better than that produced by radiography or computed tomography. The lack of hydrogen ions in cortical bone makes it easily distinguishable from soft tissues. The test is particularly useful in identifying problems with muscle, tendons, and ligaments.

The nurse ensures that the client removes all metal objects and checks for clothing zippers and metal fasteners. Although joint implants that are titanium- or stainless steel–based are safe, pacemakers and surgical clips are not. Chart 52–3 lists questions that the nurse must consider in preparing the client for MRI. Open MRIs prevent the claustrophobia that occurs with the older, encased machines.

Gadolinium-DTPA (diethylenetetramine-pentaacetic acid) is the only contrast agent approved for MRI. It is most commonly used to diagnose degenerative vertebral disease and recurrent disc herniation, sometimes referred to as

---

Chart 52–3

Nursing Care Highlight: The Client Preparing for Magnetic Resonance Imaging

- Is the client pregnant?
- Does the client have magnetic metal fragments or implants, such as an aneurysm clip?
- If the client has an IV catheter, can it be converted to a heparin lock temporarily?
- Does the client have a pacemaker or electronic implant?
- Can the client be without supplemental oxygen for an hour?
- Can the client tolerate the supine position for 20–30 minutes?
- Can the client lie still for 20–30 minutes?
- Does the client need life-support equipment?
- Can the client communicate clearly and understand verbal communication?

---

the failed back surgery syndrome (Patel & Lauerman, 1997).

Ultrasonography

Sound waves produce an image of the tissue in ultrasonography. An ultrasound procedure may be used to visualize

- Soft-tissue disorders, such as masses and fluid accumulation
- Traumatic joint injuries
- Osteomyelitis
- Surgical hardware placement

A jelly-like substance applied to the skin over the site to be examined promotes the movement of a metal probe. No special preparation or post-test care is necessary.

SELECTED BIBLIOGRAPHY

Bates, B. (1995). *A guide to physical examination and history taking.* Philadelphia: J. B. Lippincott.

Binkley, N. (1995). Assessment and management of the patient with osteoporosis. *Topics in Geriatric Rehabilitation, 10*(4), 64–74.

Burke, M. M., & Walsh, M. B. (1997). *Gerontologic nursing: Wholistic care of the older adult.* St. Louis: Mosby–Year Book.

Eliopoulos, C. (1995). *Gerontological nursing.* Philadelphia: J. B. Lippincott.

Giger, J. N., & Davidhizar, R. E. (1995). *Transcultural nursing: Assessment and intervention* (2nd ed.). St. Louis: Mosby–Year Book.

Guyton, A. C. (1995). *Textbook of medical physiology.* Philadelphia: W. B. Saunders.

Jarvis, C. (1996). *Physical examination and health assessment* (2nd ed.). Philadelphia: W. B. Saunders.

Matteson, M. A., McConnell, E. S., & Linton, A. D. (1997). *Gerontological nursing: Concepts and practice* (2nd ed.). Philadelphia: W. B. Saunders.

Neal, L. (1997). Basic musculoskeletal assessment: Tips for the home health nurse. *Home Healthcare Nurse, 15*(4), 227–235.

Patel, P. R., & Lauerman, W. C. (1997). The use of magnetic resonance imaging in the diagnosis of lumbar disc disease. *Orthopaedic Nursing, 16*(1), 59–65.

Scura, K. W., & Whipple, B. (1997). How to provide better care for the postmenopausal woman. *American Journal of Nursing, 97*(4), 36–44.

Tietz, N. W. (1995). *Clinical guide to laboratory tests* (3rd ed.). Philadelphia: W. B. Saunders.

SUGGESTED READINGS

Neal, L. (1997). Basic musculoskeletal assessment: Tips for the home health nurse. *Home Healthcare Nurse, 15*(4), 227–235.

This article reviews the fundamentals of musculoskeletal assessment, including history taking, observation, examination, and documentation. A documentation form for the assessment is included, as well as a continuing education test to obtain CEUs.

Patel, P. R., & Lauerman, W. C. (1997). The use of magnetic resonance imaging in the diagnosis of lumbar disk disease. *Orthopaedic Nursing, 16*(1), 59–65.

This article reviews the use of magnetic resonance imaging (MRI) in the diagnosis of spinal disorders, especially degenerative disk disease and for primary or recurrent herniated disks. The advantages of MRI over other diagnostic modalities is clearly explained. A contrast agent may be needed to help visualize the pathologic process.

Chapter 53

INTERVENTIONS FOR CLIENTS WITH MUSCULOSKELETAL PROBLEMS

Musculoskeletal problems are very common among all age groups. This chapter focuses on selected disorders not covered in Chapter 24 on connective tissue diseases. Musculoskeletal disorders include metabolic bone diseases, bone tumors, and a variety of deformities and syndromes. The elderly client is at the greatest risk for the development of many of these disorders, particularly metabolic bone diseases. Osteoporosis, osteomalacia, and Paget's disease can cause severe deformity and disability.

The incidence of bone cancer is also increasing in both the young and the elderly population. As technological advances occur and clients survive longer with primary lesions, metastatic cancer becomes more prevalent.

METABOLIC BONE DISEASES
Osteoporosis
Overview

Osteoporosis is a metabolic disease in which bone demineralization results in decreased density and subsequent fractures. The wrist, hip, and vertebral column are most frequently affected. Osteoporosis is a major health problem in many countries. The estimated cost for osteoporosis-related health care in the United States is more than $10 billion each year (National Osteoporosis Foundation, 1995).

Pathophysiology

Bone is a dynamic tissue. Throughout a person's life span, new bone is formed by osteoblastic activity, whereas old bone is resorbed through osteoclastic activity, a process known as bone modeling. Bone mass, or density, peaks between 30 and 35 years of age. After the peak years, bone resorption activity exceeds bone-building activity, and bone mass density decreases. Trabecular, or cancellous (spongy), bone is lost first, followed by a loss of cortical (compact) bone. As a result of decreased bone density, more than 1.5 million fractures per year occur in people older than 45 years. Hip fractures account for 250,000 of cases.

Bone mass decreases rapidly in postmenopausal women as serum estrogen levels diminish. Approximately 40% to 45% of a woman's bone mass is lost during her life span. It is estimated that 50% of all women older than 65 have symptomatic osteoporosis.

1243

Classification of Osteoporosis

Osteoporosis is an irreversible osteopenia (bone mass loss). There are two major types: primary and secondary.

Primary osteoporosis is the most common and is not associated with an underlying pathologic condition. Secondary osteoporosis results from an associated medical condition, such as hyperparathyroidism, long-term drug therapy, such as with corticosteroids, and prolonged immobility, such as that seen with spinal cord injury (Table 53–1). Treatment of the secondary type is directed toward the cause of the osteoporosis when possible.

Primary osteoporosis can be divided into two subtypes. *Type I* (postmenopausal) osteoporosis occurs in women between the ages of 55 and 65 years. Estrogen presumably prevents or decreases the rate of bone resorption in women and is, therefore, unavailable in sufficient quantities after menopause. Vertebral and wrist fractures are common in this group because the predominant bone type in these areas is cancellous.

Type II (senile) osteoporosis occurs in those older than 65 years and affects women twice as often as men. Hip and vertebral fractures are frequently seen in clients with type II disease.

Theories of Osteoporosis Development

The exact pathophysiology of osteoporosis remains a mystery. Two theories of disease development have been advocated. First, osteoporosis may result from decreased osteoblastic activity. The osteoblasts, or bone-forming cells, may have a shortened life span or may be less efficient in the osteoporotic client. The second, and more popular, theory suggests an increase in osteoclastic (bone resorption) activity. The latter theory has gained increased recognition over the past few years, and has resulted in treatment directed toward measures to prevent rapid bone resorption.

Etiology

The exact cause of osteoporosis is unknown; however, numerous risk factors have been identified. Osteoporosis most frequently occurs in women after menopause as a result of decreased estrogen levels. Women lose approximately 2% of their bone mass every year in the first 5 years after menopause (Segatore, 1995).

In addition, body build seems to predict the occurrence of the disease. Osteoporosis occurs more frequently in thin, lean-built women, particularly those who do not exercise regularly. Obese women can store estrogen in their tissues for use as necessary to maintain a normal level of serum calcium. Exercise decreases bone resorption and stimulates bone formation. Immobilization, such as prolonged bed rest, produces rapid bone loss.

Studies by Chappard and colleagues (1995) showed that immobilization secondary to spinal cord injury (SCI) causes rapid loss of trabecular bone tissue, similar to the rate of bone loss after menopause. Clients in the study had an average of 33% bone loss 6 months after the SCI.

The relationship of osteoporosis to dietary factors is not as well established. A diet deficient in calcium and vita-

TABLE 53–1

Causes of Secondary Osteoporosis

Diseases/Conditions

- Diabetes mellitus
- Hyperthyroidism
- Hyperparathyroidism
- Cushing's syndrome
- Growth hormone deficiency
- Metabolic acidosis
- Female hypogonadism
- Paget's disease
- Osteogenesis imperfecta
- Rheumatoid arthritis
- Prolonged immobilization
- Marfan's syndrome
- Bone cancer
- Cirrhosis
- Chronic airway limitation

Drugs (Chronic Use)

- Corticosteroids
- Heparin
- Anticonvulsants
- Ethanol

min D stimulates the parathyroid gland to produce parathyroid hormone (PTH). PTH triggers the release of calcium from the bony matrix. Malabsorption, caused by disease or drugs, also contributes to low serum calcium levels. Institutionalized or homebound people who are not exposed to sunlight may be at risk because they do not receive adequate vitamin D for the metabolism of calcium.

Protein deficiency may also contribute to the incidence of bone demineralization, although this theory is controversial. Because 50% of serum calcium is protein bound, protein is needed for calcium utilization; however, excessive protein intake may increase calcium loss in the urine.

Alcohol consumption and cigarette smoking have also been cited as possible risk factors. Although the exact mechanisms are not known, these substances may promote acidosis, which in turn increases bone loss. Excessive caffeine intake, for example, from coffee and tea, can increase calcium loss in the urine.

Certain drugs can cause bone loss, especially corticosteroids, phenytoin (Dilantin), heparin, and furosemide (Lasix) (Ashworth, 1997).

Hereditary factors may play a role, but this hypothesis has not been confirmed. Several of the suspected risk factors, such as body build, are determined in part by heredity; however, heredity or a genetic influence alone probably is not predictive for osteoporosis.

ELDERLY CONSIDERATIONS

Ɛ   Aging is a major risk for osteoporosis. As aging occurs, serum concentrations of 1,25-dihydroxycholecalciferol, a vitamin D metabolite, decrease. In addition, osteoporosis is often accompanied by low levels of serum calcitonin, a hormone secreted by the thyroid gland that helps maintain a normal serum calcium level.

Incidence/Prevalence

Between 25 and 35 million Americans, 80% of them women, have osteoporosis (Department of Health and Human Services, 1990). The incidence of the disease is greater in women than in men (at least 5:1) because men usually have larger bones.

Osteoporosis results in 1.3 million fractures each year, 250,000 of which are hip fractures. In people older than 90 years, one third of women and one fifth of men experience at least one hip fracture. The mortality for elderly clients with hip fractures is between 20% and 50%, and the debilitating effects can be devastating (Ashworth, 1997).

TRANSCULTURAL CONSIDERATIONS

Caucasian women are affected more often than African-American women. It is well documented that African-American women have 10% more bone mass than Caucasian women. Northern European and Asian American women are at a higher risk than Caucasian women (Segatore, 1995). Postmenopausal women are at the highest risk, regardless of cultural background or race (Matteson et al., 1997).

Collaborative Management

 Assessment

Typically, a diagnosis of osteoporosis is made after the client sustains a vertebral, wrist, or hip fracture. The client may be asymptomatic before admission with one or more bone fractures.

➤ *Physical Assessment/Clinical Manifestations*

When performing a musculoskeletal assessment, the nurse inspects and palpates the vertebral column. The classic "dowager's hump," or kyphosis of the dorsal spine, is usually present (Fig. 53–1). The client often states that height has been shortened, perhaps as much as 2–3 inches (5–7 cm) within the previous 20 years. Studies have shown that people with the greatest loss in height have the highest rate of bone loss (see Research Applications for Nursing).

Accompanying the spinal deformity is the complaint of back pain, which frequently occurs after lifting, bending, or stooping. The pain may be sharp and acute in onset. Pain is worse with activity and is relieved by rest. Palpation of the vertebrae, particularly the lower thoracic and lumbar vertebrae, usually increases the client's discomfort. Therefore, palpation should be gentle.

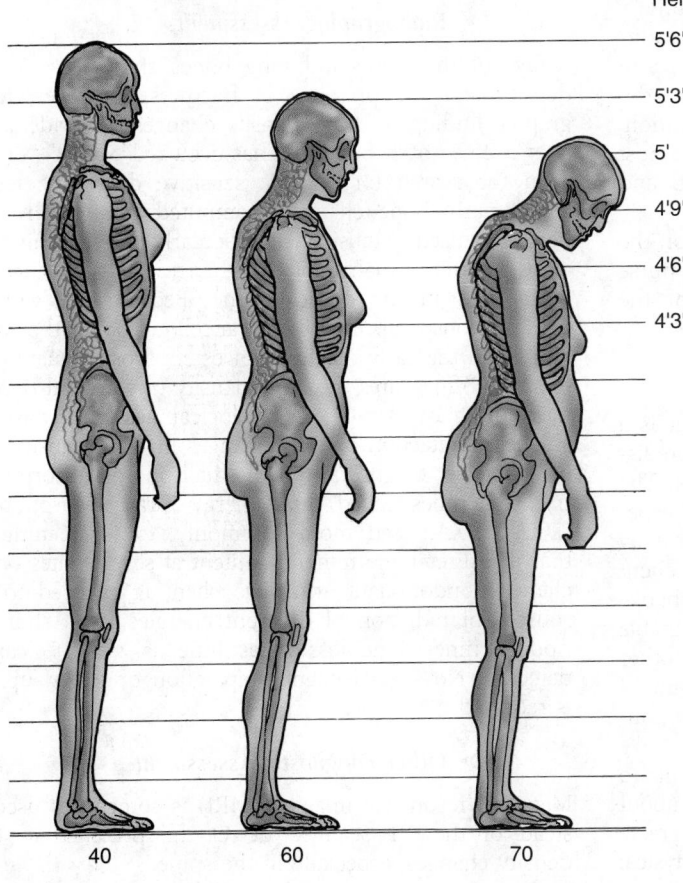

Figure 53–1. A normal spine at age 40 years and the osteoporotic changes at ages 60 and 70 years. These changes can cause a loss of as much as 6 inches in height and can result in the so-called dowager's hump *(far right)* in the upper thoracic vertebrae.

▶ Research Applications for Nursing

People Who Lose Inches from Their Height Lose Bone Mass, Too!

Hunt, A. H. (1996). The relationship between height change and bone mineral density. Orthopaedic Nursing, 15(3), 57–71.

This exploratory study investigated the relationship between height loss and low bone density as a possible screening tool for osteoporosis. The convenience sample of 76 women (mean age, 60.4 years) were clients in a bone health clinic; 61 had a diagnosis of osteoporosis. Heights and bone density measurements were taken on all participants. Recalled height was subtracted from measured height to determine height loss. There was strong evidence that those with the lowest bone mass had the greatest height loss.

Critique. The individuals comprising the convenience sample were Caucasian and ranged in age from 25 to 88 years. There were no controls for these variables. The study should be replicated using a greater cross-sampling.

Possible Nursing Implications. Although a limited convenience sample was used, the researchers point out that nurses should assess height loss as a screening tool for high-risk clients for osteoporosis. These data could then be used for referrals so that the clients could receive more extensive testing and work-up for the disease.

Back pain accompanied by tenderness and voluntary restriction of spinal movement suggests one or more compression vertebral fractures, the most common type of osteoporotic fracture. Movement restriction and spinal deformity may result in constipation, abdominal distention, and respiratory compromise in severe cases. The most likely area for fracture occurrence is between T-8 and L-3.

Fractures are also common in the distal end of the radius and the upper third of the femur (hip). The nurse directs special attention to these areas as part of the physical assessment.

▶ Psychosocial Assessment

The typical clinical picture of the osteoporotic client is a postmenopausal woman with back pain who is predisposed to multiple bone fractures from trivial trauma. The nurse assesses the client's concept of body image, especially if the client is severely kyphotic. The client may have difficulty finding clothes that fit properly. The client may have curtailed social interactions because of a change in appearance or the physical limitations of being unable to sit in chairs in restaurants, movie theaters, and other places. Alterations in sexuality may occur as a result of poor self-esteem or the discomfort imposed by positioning during intercourse.

Because osteoporosis readily predisposes a client to fractures, the client must be extremely cautious about activities. As a result, the threat of fracture can create anxiety and fear and a limitation of social or physical activities. The nurse assesses for the presence of these feelings because they may affect the client's response to health care. For instance, the client may be anxious to the point that he or she will not exercise as prescribed for fear that a fracture will occur.

▶ Laboratory Assessment

There are no definitive laboratory tests that confirm a diagnosis of primary osteoporosis; however, a number of biochemical markers can provide information about bone modeling. A battery of tests can be performed to rule out secondary osteoporosis or other metabolic bone diseases, such as osteomalacia and Paget's disease. These include determination of serum calcium, vitamin D, phosphorus, and alkaline phosphatase levels.

Urinary calcium levels are also assessed. Serum protein measurements and thyroid function tests are performed to exclude hyperthyroidism.

A simple, more specific and sensitive test to evaluate bone resorption is being used with SCI clients and other at-risk clients. The Upyr Crosslinks assay measures urinary concentrations of pyridinium (Upyr), a collagen substance found in bone and cartilage. An increase in urinary levels indicates increased bone resorption (loss). The advantage of this test is its ability to detect bone loss early. Additionally, there is no special client preparation for the test. The disadvantage of the test is its cost, because it is relatively new. However, Upyr and other biochemical markers of bone modeling may be used in the future as a routine screening test (Hunt et al., 1995).

▶ Radiographic Assessment

X-rays of the spine and long bones show loss of bone density and the presence of fractures. However, radiographic findings of bone density changes are evident only after a 25%–40% bone loss has occurred.

In the search for a more sensitive diagnostic test to detect early bone changes, computed tomography (CT) has been used extensively, particularly for the spine. CT allows better visualization of changes in the cancellous bone than in the cortical bone. Because the vertebral column consists primarily of cancellous bone, the test is helpful in the early diagnosis of osteoporosis. Quantitative CT (QCT) measures the bone density of vertebral bone.

In the past decade, technological advances have enabled the detection of early changes in bone density. One of the newer diagnostic tools is dual-photon absorptiometry, sometimes called dual energy x-ray absorptiometry (DXA). DXA, used more commonly, is a screening test that measures bone mineral content at several sites on the client's nondominant arm. The client is exposed to two sources of radiation of different energies for a short period of time. Bone loss of as little as 1%–3% can be detected. No special client preparation or follow-up care is required.

▶ Other Diagnostic Assessment

Magnetic resonance imaging (MRI) is sometimes used instead of the CT scan to detect the presence of bone density changes, especially in the spine.

Interventions

Because the client is predisposed to fractures, drugs and diet therapy are used to retard bone resorption and form new bony tissue. These measures help to reduce the chance of fracture and subsequent complications (see Client Care Plan).

Drug Therapy. The health care provider may prescribe estrogen, calcium supplements, vitamin D, alendronate (Fosamax), or a combination of several drugs to treat osteoporosis as well as to prevent it (Chart 53–1). Other agents have been given, but with limited success.

Estrogen. Estrogen replacement is effective in preventing bone loss. Studies have shown a remarkable reduction of fractures in women undergoing estrogen therapy (Matteson et al., 1997). It is recommended, however, that the drug be initiated within 3–5 years after menopause; later induction may not be beneficial.

The health care provider may prescribe low doses of conjugated estrogens, such as 0.625 mg of Premarin (C.S.D.✦), because the side effects of the drug, such as cervical cancer, are potentially serious. Some providers do not use the drug for preventive purposes. Others believe that the benefit of estrogen in preventing potentially debilitating and life-threatening fractures outweighs its risks. The health care provider often prescribes progesterone with the estrogen to minimize cancer occurrence. For middle-aged women, especially those in their 40s (sometimes referred to as the "transition years"), birth control pills may be used to provide these supplements.

A newer form of estrogen, the estrogen patch (Estraderm, Estrace, Femogex✦), delivers an even, continuous amount of estrogen when applied several times each week. These patches are available in several doses, from 4 mg/10 cm (0.05 mg/24 hours) to 8 mg/10 cm (0.1 mg/24 hours).

Calcium. If a person cannot ingest sufficient quantities of calcium in the diet, calcium supplements are used. Natural calcium sources, such as oyster shells, are preferable. Supplements should be started in the high-risk population as early as age 40 years, because bone resorption accelerates after age 35 years. Calcium carbonate, found in over-the-counter (OTC) drugs such as Tums, is probably the most efficacious. Forty percent of calcium carbonate is elemental calcium that can be used by the body. For example, a 600-mg tablet contains about 240 mg of elemental calcium.

The client should take calcium supplements under the supervision of a health care provider. As shown in Chart 53–1, hypercalcemia (excess serum calcium) can cause serious damage to the urinary system. The amount of calcium prescribed is affected by the addition of estrogen therapy and the presence of risk factors for osteoporosis.

In the United States, the typical daily intake of dietary calcium is between 450 and 550 mg. The recommended daily allowance (RDA) of calcium is 800 mg. Many clinicians and researchers believe that the RDA is insufficient to meet the calcium requirements of postmenopausal women. The premenopausal woman may need at least 1000 mg/day, and postmenopausal women may require as much as 1500 mg or more daily to prevent osteoporosis. An increased calcium intake may prevent bone loss in men as well. Foods rich in calcium include milk and dairy products and dark-green, leafy vegetables (see Chapter 14 for a list of foods high in calcium).

Vitamin D. Vitamin D supplementation may be necessary for the institutionalized or homebound client. An adequate level of vitamin D is needed for optimal calcium absorption in the intestines. The prescribed dosage is usually 400 to 800 IU/day. Higher doses can produce toxic effects, such as hypercalcemia and hyperphosphatemia.

Alendronate. Alendronate (Fosamax) is a newer but widely used drug, classified as a bone resorption inhibitor. It is used for the prevention of osteoporosis in postmenopausal women and for the treatment of hypercalcemia in clients with Paget's disease or hypercalcemia resulting from cancer. The usual oral dosage is 5 mg/day (Hodgson et al., 1997).

Although side effects are not common, when they do occur they tend to be serious. Esophagitis and esophageal ulcers have been reported with the use of Fosamax, especially when the pill is not completely swallowed. The nurse teaches clients taking this drug to take it early in the morning with 8 ounces of water. They should not lie down until after breakfast. If chest pain occurs, a symptom of esophageal irritation, they should discontinue the drug and contact their health care provider.

Other Drugs. Other drugs that may be used include sodium fluoride, androgens, calcitonin, and metabolites of vitamin D.

Sodium Fluoride. In combination with estrogen and calcium, sodium fluoride stimulates the formation of new bone and may inhibit bone loss. The side effects of the drug, however, must be considered in relation to its benefits. The drug is currently reserved for investigative settings or is used with extreme caution by the clinician.

Androgens. Androgens, such as testosterone propionate (Testex, Malogen✦), have been successful in decreasing bone resorption. When given to postmenopausal women, however, androgens cause masculine traits and may lead to liver disease. Androgens may decrease bone resorption in men, particularly the elderly.

Calcitonin. Calcitonin inhibits bone loss, but it is expensive and is administered by injection. These disadvantages prohibit its use in most settings over a long period of time. Another naturally occurring hormone, parathyroid hormone (PTH), is being tested for its ability to strengthen bone by its bone formation capability.

Vitamin D Metabolites. Metabolites of vitamin D, such as 1,25-dihydroxyvitamin D (calcitriol), can help to inhibit bone resorption, but they remain experimental. There is little clinical evidence to support this hypothesis.

Selective Estrogen Receptor Modulators (SERMs). A new class of drugs is being studied and may soon obtain Food and Drug Administration (FDA) approval in the United States. Early studies suggest that raloxifene, one of the

Text continued on page 1252

Client Care Plan

The Client with Osteoporosis

Nursing Diagnosis No. 1: Risk for Injury (Fracture) related to trivial accidents or falls

Expected Outcomes	Nursing Interventions	Rationale

The client will not experience falls and fracture resulting from falls.	▪ Create a hazard-free environment for the client while he or she is in the hospital or other setting.
	  ▪ Get the client out of bed with bed height in lowest position.
	  ▪ Teach the client to wear nonskid slippers.
	  ▪ Inspect the floor for spills and the room for equipment that may cause tripping or stumbling.
	  ▪ Provide additional lighting for an elderly client.
	  ▪ Place necessary items close to bed within easy reach (e.g., water pitcher and call bell).
	  ▪ Keep two side rails up, especially for elderly clients who are confused.
	  ▪ Teach the importance and use of hand rails in the bathroom.
		▪ Creating a hazard-free environment reduces the risk of falls and subsequent fracture.

	▪ Provide ambulatory support as needed.
	  ▪ Assess the need for a cane or a walker.
	  ▪ Consult with a physical therapist.
	  ▪ Teach the client to call for assistance.
	  ▪ Teach the client to take his/her time when getting out of bed and walking.
		▪ Ambulatory aids provide additional support when walking and help prevent rushing, which contributes to falls. Elderly clients often hurry to the bathroom to prevent incontinence.

	▪ When helping with activities of daily living (ADLs), prevent the client from accidentally hitting side rails, door frames, and so on.	▪ Striking hard surfaces can cause bone fracture, as bones are porous from calcium loss.
	▪ Teach the client to bend or stoop slowly and not to lift or move heavy objects such as hospital furniture.	▪ Quick body movements can easily lead to vertebral compression fractures in the osteoporotic client.

(Continued)

Client Care Plan

Expected Outcomes	Nursing Interventions	Rationale
	■ Monitor side effects for any drugs the client may be taking for concurrent medical conditions.	■ Diuretics, phenothiazines, and tranquilizers can cause dizziness, drowsiness, and weakness, predisposing the client to falls.

	■ Teach the important of diet in preventing further osteoporosis.
	  ■ Refer to dietary consultation.
	  ■ Teach the client which foods are high in calcium content.
	  ■ Teach the need to decrease caffeine and alcohol intake.
		■ Dietary calcium is needed to maintain serum level, thus preventing additional loss from bone. Caffeine excess can increase calcium loss in urine; alcohol excess can promote acidosis, which increases bone resorption.

	■ Teach the effect of cigarette smoking on bone remodeling (if the client is a smoker).	■ Cigarette smoking can promote acidosis.

Nursing Diagnosis No. 2: Impaired Physical Mobility related to decreased muscle tone, dysfunction secondary to previous fractures, or pain secondary to recent fractures

Expected Outcomes	Nursing Interventions	Rationale

The client will increase mobility to the level of ADL independence.	■ Consult with the physical therapist regarding an exercise program to include strengthening and weight-bearing exercises.
	  ■ Assist the client as necessary with exercises.
	  ■ Teach the client that ADLs do not replace prescribed exercises.
	  ■ Teach the importance of exercises.
		■ Strengthening exercises increase joint movement, increase muscle tone, and stimulate blood circulation to bone and muscle tissue. Weight-bearing exercises decrease the rate of bone loss and increase bone formation.

	■ Assist with ADLs as necessary, allowing the client to be as independent as possible.	■ Pain and poor muscle tone may limit the client's ability to be independent, especially after a fracture.
	■ Assess the need for assistive and adaptive devices to perform ADLs; consult with the occupational therapist to obtain appropriate equipment.	■ Devices may be needed for the client to be ADL independent. Overuse and reliance, however, should be discouraged.

(Continued)

Client Care Plan

Nursing Diagnosis No. 3: Pain related to effects of vertebral fracture

Expected Outcomes	Nursing Interventions	Rationale
The client will experience alleviation or reduction of pain so that client can be independent in care.	■ Assess the need for pain medication: opioid or nonopioid analgesics, muscle relaxants, or anti-inflammatory drugs.	■ Clients usually receive pain medication on a prn schedule. Elderly clients often do not request pain medication even if needed; therefore, the nurse must anticipate this need.

	■ Maintain orthotic devices for vertebral fracture.
	  ■ Check that the brace or corset fits properly.
	  ■ Inspect the skin where the device causes pressure.
	  ■ Apply the device for use when the client gets out of bed.
		■ Orthotic devices maintain spine alignment and provide spinal column support.

	■ Apply moist heat to back (heat packs or hot compresses) as needed to reduce pain. (The physical therapist may do this.) (Also see Chap. 9.)	■ Heat increases blood circulation to affected areas, thus relieving muscle spasms, which cause pain.

Chart 53–1

Drug Therapy for Osteoporosis

Drug	Usual Dosage	Nursing Interventions	Rationale
Calcium, preferably calcium carbonate (e.g., Os-Cal, Tums, Caltrate-600, and Ca-Plus)	• 1.0–1.5 g in divided doses PO	• Give 1 hr before meals	• Calcium may cause gastrointestinal irritation if taken on empty stomach; free hydrochloric acid is needed for calcium absorption.
		• Give a third of daily dose at bedtime. Push fluids.	• Calcium is most readily utilized by the body when the client is fasting and immobile. Increased fluid intake aids in preventing the formation of calcium-based urinary stones.
		• Assess for a history of urinary stones.	• Calcium supplements are not given to clients who are susceptible to urinary stone formation.
		• Monitor serum calcium level.	• Hypercalcemia, or calcium excess, is a side effect of calcium supplementation.

Chart 53–1. Drug Therapy for Osteoporosis   Continued

Drug	Usual Dosage	Nursing Interventions	Rationale
		• Monitor urinary calcium level (no more than 4 mg/kg in 24 hr).	• The kidneys attempt to excrete excess calcium.
		• Observe for signs of hypercalcemia.	• Hypercalcemia can result in urinary stones, cardiac arrhythmias, and an increase or decrease in skeletal muscle tone.
Conjugated estrogen (e.g., Premarin, Estinyl, and Estrace C.D.S.♣, Transderm) may be given with progesterone on d 16–25	• 0.425–1.25 mg PO for 25 d/mo • 0.05 mg/24 hr or 0.1 mg/24 hr transdermally	• Assess for history of tumors, hypertension, thromboembolytic disease, or liver or gallbladder disease.	• Estrogen therapy is withheld from clients with susceptibility to an exacerbation of one or more of these problems.
		• Teach the importance of gynecologic exams every 6 months.	• Endometrial and breast cancer can result from estrogen therapy.
		• Teach breast self-examination.	• Clients can detect potentially malignant lesions early so that treatment can begin immediately.
		• Observe for vaginal bleeding.	• Vaginal bleeding is a side effect of estrogen therapy and a sign of possible endometrial cancer.
		• Monitor blood pressure.	• Hypertension and other cardiovascular complications may result from combined estrogen-progesterone therapy.
		• Observe for thrombus formation.	• Deep vein thrombosis is a complication of combined estrogen-progesterone therapy.
		• Monitor serum liver enzyme and cholesterol levels.	• An elevation of liver enzyme levels may be indicative of liver involvement resulting from estrogen. An elevated cholesterol level can result in hypertension and thrombus formation.
Vitamin D (e.g., ergocalciferol, calcitriol, and calcifediol)	• 7000–8000 IU PO	• Observe for signs of hypercalcemia and hyperphosphatemia.	• Calcium and phosphate excess can result from excessive vitamin D therapy.
		• Monitor renal status.	• Excessive serum calcium levels can result in urinary stone formation.
Alendronate (Fosamax)	• 5 mg/d PO	• Take early in AM with 8 oz water; do not lie down until after breakfast.	• Although not common, esophagitis or esophageal ulcers may result from alendronate therapy.
Sodium fluoride	• 40–90 mg in divided doses	• Give 15 min before meals or with meals.	• Gastric irritation may result if sodium fluoride is given when the stomach is empty.
		• Observe for synovitis or joint inflammation.	• Synovitis is a side effect of sodium fluoride therapy.

new SERMs, increases bone mass 2%–3% a year. SERMs are designed to mimic estrogen in some parts of the body while blocking its effects elsewhere. It may not replace estrogen, however.

Diet Therapy. The dietary considerations for the treatment of a client with a diagnosis of osteoporosis are the same as those for preventing the disease. Calcium and vitamin D intake is increased, and alcohol and caffeine consumption is discouraged. For the client who has sustained a fracture, intake of protein, vitamin C, and iron is increased to promote bone healing.

Prevention of Falls. The client must be careful to prevent falls and other activities that can cause a fracture. A hazard-free environment is necessary to meet this goal, and the nurse must teach the client about its importance.

Many hospitals and long-term care facilities have risk management programs in which clients are assessed for their risk for falls. For clients at high risk, programs such as the Falling Star protocol have reduced falls by making the staff aware of the client's high risk. In this program, a star is placed at the head of the client's bed to designate the person at high risk. (Chapter 6 discusses fall prevention in health care agencies and at home in more detail.)

Exercises. In collaboration with the health care provider, the physical therapist (PT) prescribes exercises for strengthening the abdominal and back muscles. These exercises improve posture and provide an improved support for the spine. Abdominal isometrics, deep breathing, and pectoral stretching are stressed to increase pulmonary capacity. Exercises for the extremity muscles include isometric, resistive, and range of motion (ROM). The nurse encourages active ROM exercises, which improve joint mobility and increase muscle tone.

In addition to the muscle-strengthening component, a general weight-bearing exercise program is implemented. Walking, both slow and fast, and bicycling are recommended daily activities. The nurse teaches the client that certain jarring recreational activities, such as bowling and horseback riding, may cause vertebral compression and should be avoided.

Pain Management. The pain management program depends on the intensity and duration of the pain. With treatment, pain from spinal fractures often resolves 6 to 8 weeks after injury; treatment usually includes drug therapy and orthotic devices. The health care provider prescribes analgesics, opioid and nonopioid, during the acute phase of the pain (i.e., from the time of injury to as long as several weeks). Muscle relaxants, which ease the discomfort associated with muscle spasms, are frequently used for spinal fractures. Nonsteroidal anti-inflammatory drugs (NSAIDs) are beneficial for pain relief and for decreasing spinal nerve root inflammation from crushed vertebrae. The nurse monitors the need for medication as well as the side effects that can contribute to injury. The nurse is especially alert to the problems associated with NSAIDs, particularly in the elderly, such as gastrointestinal bleeding and congestive heart failure.

Orthotic Devices. Known as dorsolumbar orthoses, orthotic devices immobilize the spine during the acute

pain phase and provide spinal column support (Fig. 53–2). The physical therapist or orthotist custom-fits the client for this lightweight device. The client is taught to inspect the skin for irritation and report tolerance to the device.

➤ Continuing Care

Clients with osteoporosis are usually managed at home. However, some clients experience fractures that may require hospitalization.

The osteoporotic client who has one or more fractures can be discharged to the home setting. In some instances, the client is discharged to a long-term care facility for rehabilitation or permanent residence when support systems are not available.

➤ Home Care Management

If the client is discharged to a home setting, the nurse must assess the environment for potential hazards before discharge. The nurse uses the data base completed at time of admission by the nurse or occupational therapist to ascertain whether alterations in the home environment are necessary. For example, if scatter rugs are used in the home, the client is advised to have these removed to reduce the chance of falling.

A two-story house or apartment may be a problem if physical mobility is limited or if adequate support railing is not available to assist with stair climbing. The social worker, discharge planner, or case manager, in conjunction with the nurse, helps the client identify adaptations

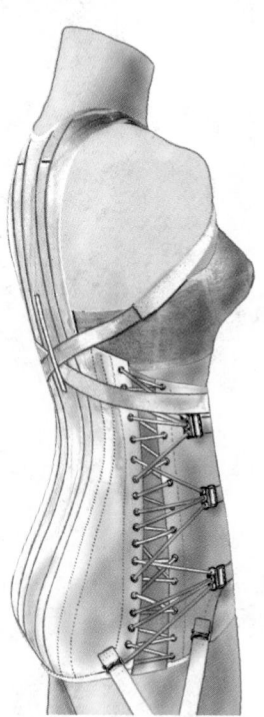

Figure 53–2. A dorsolumbar orthosis. (Courtesy of Truform Orthotics and Prosthetics, Cincinnati, OH.)

that may have to be made to create as hazard free an environment as possible.

Assistive or adaptive devices for personal use may also be needed at home, if only for a short time. Devices to assist with activities of daily living (ADLs), such as a dressing stick to put on pants, are helpful in maintaining the client's independence. The occupational therapist works with the nurse to determine the need for assistive devices. (Chapter 13 describes the promotion of ADL independence in detail.)

The nurse and physical therapist assess the need for ambulatory aids in the home. A walker or cane may provide the additional support necessary to prevent falls.

➤ Health Teaching

The teaching plan for the client with osteoporosis includes prevention of falls, exercise, diet therapy, and drug therapy. Psychosocial support is also important to help the client maintain the highest quality of life possible.

Prevention of Falls. Clients must be extremely careful to prevent falls. Ambulatory aids should be used for additional support, although some clients refuse to be seen in public with a cane or walker. Similarly, clients may not want to wear orthotic devices because of embarrassment or discomfort. The nurse and physical therapist (PT) provide a thorough explanation of the necessity and the proper method for using these devices.

Exercise. The PT prescribes a structured exercise program, which the nurse reinforces. Strengthening, ROM, and weight-bearing exercises are taught. Follow-up physical therapy visits ensure that clients have learned the exercises and are compliant.

Diet Therapy. The nurse emphasizes the importance of a diet rich in calcium-containing foods. A diet consultation before discharge can help clients select foods they like and that are high in the essential nutrients. If a fracture has occurred, the nurse encourages clients to eat foods rich in vitamin C, protein, and iron. The nurse also instructs them to decrease caffeine and alcohol consumption and to stop smoking.

Drug Therapy. For clients who will be homebound or institutionalized, sunlight exposure should be promoted as an essential source of vitamin D. The importance of sunlight should be stressed to the long-term care facility where clients may be transferred.

Psychosocial Support. Because clients are often afraid they will sustain a fracture, it is extremely important to allay their fears to the extent possible. The degree of osteoporosis determines the likelihood of injury. The more severe the osteoporosis, the more limited the activities should be. For example, a severely osteoporotic woman may sustain vertebral compression fractures from stooping or bending. For most clients, an aggressive treatment plan prevents fractures from trivial trauma.

Explaining the importance of orthotic and ambulatory aids in the prevention of injury increases compliance and decreases reluctance to use the devices. A supportive spouse, family member, or significant other can encourage clients to adhere to the treatment plan.

ELDERLY CONSIDERATIONS

Because most osteoporotic clients are elderly, they may not comply with the diet. Often the elderly client is used to eating less than the required daily nutrients. Consumption of milk and dairy products is usually minimal. As a result, the health care provider prescribes calcium supplements for long-term maintenance. The nurse instructs clients to take only the prescribed amount; too much calcium can lead to hypercalcemia.

If placed on estrogen therapy, clients need to have frequent gynecologic checkups to detect early signs of cervical cancer. The nurse teaches clients how to monitor for side effects. Follow-up visits to the internist or orthopedist are scheduled frequently to monitor calcium blood levels and determine further progression of osteoporosis.

➤ Health Care Resources

If the client cannot return home after a fracture, placement in a nursing may be necessary, at least for a short time. The hospital nurse or case manager documents the client's needs on the transfer chart and communicates the special considerations required.

If returning to a home environment, the client may need equipment for activities of daily living (ADLs) and ambulation. Financial resources are assessed before equipment is obtained. If insurance or other third-party payer will not reimburse the client, other sources are explored. Religious and support organizations are possible resources for free materials. Items are often donated to these groups for use as needed in the community. Rental of equipment is also an option. The hospital or local medical supplier can provide estimates of renting versus purchasing the needed equipment. The equipment should be accessible before the client returns home.

A home care nurse may be needed for follow-up in the home environment. The nurse in this setting can be contacted to assist in the discharge planning for the client, to assess potential environmental hazards, and to obtain equipment and supplies. The home health nurse determines the need for physical or occupational therapy, social work, and homemaking personnel in the home.

In addition to home care resources, the Osteoporosis Foundation provides information to clients and health care professionals regarding the disease and its treatment. Large metropolitan hospitals often have osteoporosis specialty clinics and support groups for osteoporotic clients.

Osteomalacia

Overview

Osteomalacia is a reversible metabolic disease in which there is a defect in the mineralization of bone. Unlike in osteoporotic tissue, in osteomalacia the amount and quality of bone matrix (osteoid) are normal but mineralization is delayed or inadequate (Table 53–2).

Pathophysiology

Osteomalacia is the adult equivalent of rickets, or vitamin D deficiency, in children. In its natural form, vitamin D is obtained from the ultraviolet radiation of the sun and

TABLE 53–2

Differential Features of Osteoporosis and Osteomalacia		
Characteristic	Osteoporosis	Osteomalacia
Definition	• Decreased bone mass	• Demineralized bone
Pathophysiology	• Lack of calcium	• Lack of vitamin D
Radiographic findings	• Osteopenia, fractures	• Pseudofractures, Looser's zones, fractures
Calcium level	• Normal	• Low or normal
Phosphate level	• Normal	• Low or normal
Parathyroid hormone	• Normal	• High or normal
Alkaline phosphatase	• Normal	• High

from certain foods. In combination with calcium and phosphorus, the vitamin is necessary for bone formation.

Vitamin D is actually a group of vitamins, including vitamins D_2 and D_3. The naturally occurring substance is D_3 (cholecalciferol), which is manufactured by photochemical activation in the skin when triggered by the sun's ultraviolet light. As illustrated in Figure 53–3, the D_3 from either the skin or food is carried to the liver bound to an alpha-globulin as transcalciferin. There, part of the substance is converted to 25-hydroxycholecalciferol, or calcidiol.

Calcidiol is then transported to the kidney for transformation into the major active vitamin D metabolite, 1,25-dihydroxycholecalciferol, or calcitriol. The amount of calcitriol produced is regulated by parathyroid hormone (PTH) and the blood level of phosphate, the inorganic form of phosphorus. Calcitriol production increases when there is an increase in PTH or a decrease in serum phosphate levels.

Calcitriol is needed for optimal intestinal absorption of calcium and works in combination with PTH for the release of calcium from bone to assist in serum calcium regulation. Consequently, calcitriol or vitamin D deficiency results in decreased calcium absorption from the gut, which in turn leads to PTH stimulation and a decrease in both serum phosphate and calcium levels.

In osteomalacia, a primary or secondary vitamin D deficiency causes insufficient bone mineralization. Nonmineralized or poorly mineralized osteoid accumulates over the surfaces of both cortical and cancellous bone.

Etiology

In addition to primary vitamin D deficiency related to lack of sunlight exposure or dietary intake, vitamin D deficiency attributable to various pathologic conditions may result in osteomalacia (Table 53–3). Malabsorption of the vitamin from the small bowel is a common post-surgical complication of partial or total gastrectomy and bypass or resection surgery of the small intestine. Small-bowel disease, such as Crohn's disease, may cause decreased vitamin absorption.

Liver and pancreatic disorders interrupt vitamin D metabolism and decrease the production of usable substance. Renal failure or disease interferes with the synthesis of calcitriol, the most active vitamin metabolite.

Conditions that contribute to phosphate depletion (hypophosphatemia) lead to osteomalacia. Osteomalacia is also a complication of the intake of certain drugs, particularly anticonvulsants, barbiturates, and fluoride. The exact mechanism for the drug effects is not known.

Incidence/Prevalence

Until recently, osteomalacia was considered nonexistent in Western countries.

ELDERLY CONSIDERATIONS

Although the disease is not thought to be common, researchers and clinicians are exploring its incidence in the elderly. In the geriatric population, significant

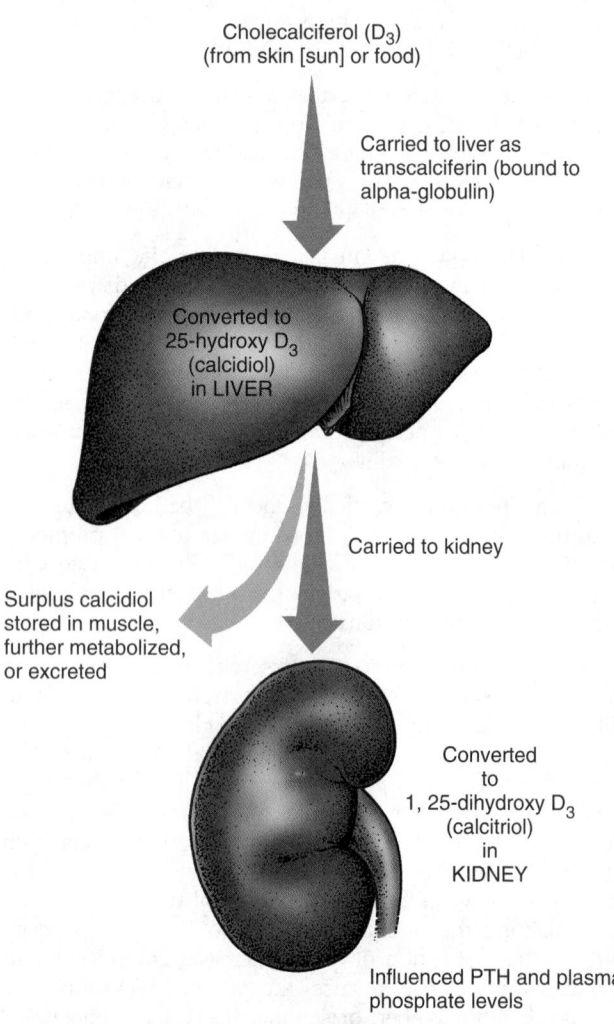

Cholecalciferol (D_3)
(from skin [sun] or food)

Carried to liver as transcalciferin (bound to alpha-globulin)

Converted to 25-hydroxy D_3 (calcidiol) in LIVER

Surplus calcidiol stored in muscle, further metabolized, or excreted

Carried to kidney

Converted to 1, 25-dihydroxy D_3 (calcitriol) in KIDNEY

Influenced PTH and plasma phosphate levels

Figure 53–3. Process of vitamin D metabolism in the body.

TABLE 53-3

Causes of Osteomalacia

Vitamin D Disturbance
- Inadequate production
- Lack of sunlight exposure
- Dietary deficiency
- Abnormal metabolism
- Drug therapy
  - Phenytoin (Dilantin)
  - Fluoride
  - Barbiturates
- Liver disease
- Renal disease
- Inadequate absorption
  - Postgastrectomy
  - Malabsorption syndrome
- Inflammatory bowel disease

Kidney Disease
- Chronic renal failure
- Renal tubular disorders
  - Acidosis
  - Hypophosphatemia

Familial Metabolic Error
- Hypophosphatemia

numbers of people are deprived of sun exposure, maintain poor diets, or both. Although there are no statistical data to indicate the incidence of osteomalacia in the United States, health care professionals are continuing to study its occurrence in nursing homes and other residences for the elderly. As a result, osteomalacia is recognized as a health problem for the elderly population.

Collaborative Management

 Assessment

The important data for the nurse to obtain for a client with osteomalacia or suspected osteomalacia include age, exposure to sunlight, and skin pigmentation. The elderly person who has been homebound or chronically institutionalized is at greatest risk. People who have dark skin and consume minimal protein are more at risk than light-skinned people with the same dietary habits. The nurse also takes a thorough diet history to determine the intake of foods containing vitamin D and calcium.

➤ Physical Assessment/Clinical Manifestations

Osteomalacia is easily confused with osteoporosis; many of the clinical manifestations are similar, and both disorders may occur at the same time.

In the early stages of osteomalacia, the manifestations are nonspecific. Muscle weakness and bone pain are often misdiagnosed as arthritis or rheumatism. In some cases, proximal muscle weakness in the shoulder and pelvic girdle areas is the only complaint.

Muscle weakness in the lower extremities may cause a waddling and unsteady gait, which contributes to falls and subsequent fractures. Hypophosphatemia leads to an inadequate production of muscle cell adenosine triphosphate, thus resulting in a decrease in muscle cell energy. If hypocalcemia is present, muscle cramping may accompany the weakness.

The nurse assesses muscle strength and observes the client's gait. The nurse records complaints of muscle cramps and bone pain. The skeletal discomfort is often vague and generalized. The spine, ribs, pelvis, and lower extremities are most often affected. The client usually describes the pain as aggravated by activity and worse at night.

In addition to the client's subjective complaint of pain, the nurse palpates the bones affected for tenderness. Bone tenderness can be elicited by pressure on the tibia or rib cage. The nurse observes skeletal malalignment as long bone bowing or spinal deformity, similar to that seen in osteoporosis. In extreme cases, the pelvis narrows such that vaginal childbirth is difficult.

If osteomalacia is untreated, vertebral, rib, and long bone fractures may occur. The client may be misdiagnosed as having bone cancer or osteoporosis.

➤ Diagnostic Assessment

Table 53-3 shows the changes in laboratory values that help to support the diagnosis of osteomalacia. X-rays of bone tissue with osteomalacia show a decrease in the trabeculae of cancellous bone and lack of osteoid sharpness. The classic diagnostic finding specific to the disease, however, is the presence of radiolucent bands (Looser's lines or zones). Looser's zones are pseudofractures; they represent stress fractures that have not mineralized. They often appear symmetrically in the inner femora, ribs, and inferior pubic rami and may progress to complete fractures with minimal trauma.

 Interventions

Because the nursing diagnoses for osteomalacia are the same as those for osteoporosis, the client goals are also similar. An increase in vitamin D through dietary intake, sun exposure, and drug supplementation is promoted. The nurse teaches the client about foods high in vitamin D and the importance of frequent sun exposure for the manufacture of the vitamin.

The RDA of vitamin D is 10 μg, or 400 IU. Because the elderly are at risk for bone demineralization from aging as well as for osteomalacia, a safe and adequate daily requirement may be as high as 15 to 20 μg, or 600 to 800 IU. Chart 53-2 lists interventions for helping elderly clients meet the daily requirement of vitamin D.

Paget's Disease

Overview

Paget's disease, or osteitis deformans, is a metabolic disorder of bone remodeling, or turnover, in which increased resorption or loss results in bone deposits that are weak, enlarged, and disorganized. First described in 1876 by Sir James Paget, an English surgeon, the disease was thought

---

Chart 53–2

Nursing Focus on the Elderly: Meeting the Daily Requirement for Vitamin D

- Advise clients to get sun exposure for at least 5 minutes weekly, even in the summer and winter.
- Recommend that clients eat food high in calcium to promote vitamin D absorption and utilization in the small intestines.
- Suggest that clients eat natural and fortified foods containing vitamin D, including milk and dairy products, such as ice cream (or ice milk), yogurt, and cheese.
- Recommend that clients exercise on a regular basis (at least three times a week for 20 to 30 minutes) to prevent bone loss.

---

to be an inflammatory process, infectious in origin. Until the 1960s, Paget's disease was considered a medical curiosity and given little attention. With the growing number of elderly people in Western countries, interest in the disease has increased and treatment has improved.

Three pathophysiologic phases of the disorder have been described: active, mixed, and inactive.

In the first phase (the active phase), a prolific increase in osteoclasts (cells that break down bone) causes massive bone destruction and deformity. The osteoclasts of pagetic bone are large and multinuclear, unlike the osteoclasts of normal bone tissue.

In the mixed phase, the osteoblasts (bone-forming cells) react in a compensatory manner to form new bone. The result is bone that is disorganized and chaotic in structure. The new trabecular bone has a mosaic pattern with a volume twice that of normal bone.

When the osteoblastic activity exceeds the osteoclastic activity, the inactive phase occurs. The newly formed bone becomes sclerotic and ivory hard. The number of osteoclasts begins to return toward normal.

As a result of the metabolic bone process, the vascularity of the newly formed bone tissue is increased. The arterial capillaries of pagetic bone become hypertrophied, causing marrow sinus and venous system distention. Paget's disease occurs in one bone or in multiple sites. The most common areas of involvement are the vertebrae, the femur, the skull, the sternum, and the pelvis.

The exact cause of Paget's disease is unknown, but it may be the result of a latent viral infection contracted in young adulthood and manifesting as a disease 20 to 40 years later. Bone biopsy specimens have revealed an antigen from a respiratory virus and measles. Because the disorder is present in monozygotic twins, a familial autosomal dominant pattern has been suggested. The disease has been noted in up to 30% of people with a positive family history for Paget's disease.

ELDERLY CONSIDERATIONS

Paget's disease is primarily a disease of the older age group. It occurs in a very small percentage of people younger than 40 years.

TRANSCULTURAL CONSIDERATIONS

Because Paget's disease occurs more frequently in Europe and less often in Asia and Scandinavia, there may be a possible link between the disease and ethnic origin.

Collaborative Management

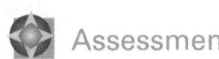 Assessment

➤ Physical Assessment/Clinical Manifestations

Of clients with Paget's disease, 80% are asymptomatic. The disease may be confined to one bone. The disease is often accidentally discovered during a routine laboratory or radiographic examination. In more severe disease, the manifestations are diverse and potentially fatal (Chart 53–3).

Musculoskeletal Assessment. Bone pain causes the client to seek medical attention. The pain is aching, poorly described, deep, and worsened by pressure and weight bearing. It is most noticeable at night or when the client is resting, and the pain is typically mild to moderate. Back pain and headache are common complaints.

The pain associated with the disorder may result from metabolic bone activity, secondary arthritis, impending fracture, or nerve impingement. Arthritis occurs at the joints of the affected bones, but its relationship to Paget's disease is unclear. Nerve impingement is particularly common in the lumbosacral area of the vertebral column, presenting as back pain that radiates along one or both lower extremities.

The nurse assesses the location and extent of the client's pain to determine the bone areas involved. The

---

Chart 53–3

Key Features of Paget's Disease of the Bone

Musculoskeletal Manifestations

- Bone and joint pain (may be in a single bone) that is aching, poorly described, and aggravated by walking
- Low back and sciatic nerve pain
- Bowing of long bones
- Loss of normal spinal curvature
- Enlarged, thick skull
- Pathologic fractures
- Osteogenic sarcoma

Skin Manifestations

- Flushed, warm skin

Other Manifestations

- Apathy, lethargy, fatigue
- Hyperparathyroidism
- Gout
- Urinary or renal stones
- Heart failure from fluid overload

nurse also observes the client's posture, stance, and gait to identify gross bony deformities that exist in Paget's disease. Because of the enlargement of the vertebrae, loss of normal spinal curvature, and lower-extremity malalignment, the client is usually short. Long bone bowing in the arms and legs with subsequent varus deformity of the elbows and knees is often symmetric. Flexion contractures of the hips are often present.

When performing a musculoskeletal assessment in a client with Paget's disease, the nurse pays particular attention to the size and shape of the skull, which is soft, thick, and enlarged. Involvement of the temporal bone may lead to deafness and vertigo, whereas basilar complications can compress any of the cranial nerves and result in neurologic compromise. Platybasia, or basilar invagination, causes brain stem manifestations that threaten life. In some cases, the bony enlargement of the skull blocks cerebrospinal fluid (CSF), resulting in hydrocephalus.

Pathologic fractures may be the presenting clinical manifestation of the disorder. As many as 30% of clients with Paget's disease sustain at least one incomplete or complete fracture. The femur and the tibia are most often affected, and fracture of these bones can result from minimal trauma. The fracture line is usually perpendicular to the long axis of the bone, and healing is unpredictable in view of abnormal metabolic activity within the bone.

The most dreaded complication of Paget's disease is neoplasm, most commonly osteogenic sarcoma (see later discussion of bone cancer). Sarcomas occur in about 1% of clients with pagetic bone. They appear primarily in the pelvis, the femur, and the humerus and carry a grave prognosis owing to early metastasis to the lung or extensive local invasion. Frequently, they are multifocal, and they occur more often in men. When severe bone pain is present in a client with Paget's disease, neoplasm is suspected.

Skin Assessment. The nurse assesses the client's skin for its color and temperature. In people with Paget's disease, the skin is flushed and warm because of increased vascularity. In addition, the nurse assesses the client's energy level. The client usually complains of apathy, lethargy, and fatigue.

Other Manifestations. Other less common manifestations of Paget's disease include hyperparathyroidism and gout. Secondary hyperparathyroidism leads to an increase in serum and urinary calcium levels. In severe cases, calcium excess results from prolonged immobilization. Calcium deposits occur in joint spaces or as stones in the urinary tract. Hyperuricemia (serum uric acid excess) and gout occur because the increased metabolic activity of bone creates an increase in nucleic acid catabolism.

In a few cases, increased vascularity causes an increase in cardiac output, resulting in congestive heart failure. Cardiac complications tend to occur only when more than a third of the skeleton is involved.

➤ Laboratory Assessment

Increases in serum alkaline phosphatase (ALP) and urinary hydroxyproline levels are the primary laboratory findings indicating the probability of Paget's disease.

Overactive osteoblasts cause the alteration in ALP level. An evaluation of the 24-hour urinary hydroxyproline level reflects an increase in bone collagen turnover and indicates the degree of the disease process. The higher the value of hydroxyproline, the greater is the severity of Paget's disease.

The calcium levels in blood and urine are normal or elevated. The immobilized client is more likely to have an increase in calcium levels as a result of calcium moving from bone into the blood.

Paget's disease often causes an elevation of uric acid because nucleic acid from overactive bone metabolism increases. This finding may be misinterpreted as primary gout.

➤ Radiographic Assessment

X-rays of pagetic bone reveal radiolucent, or punched-out, areas indicative of increased bone resorption. Depending on the phase of the disease, the overall bone mass is enlarged and the cortices are thickened. Malalignment deformities, fractures, and secondary arthritic changes may be present.

Computed tomography (CT) is useful in the detection of sarcomas, changes in the skull, and spinal cord or nerve compression.

➤ Other Diagnostic Assessment

Bone scans using radioactive isotopes are only slightly more sensitive than routine x-rays in delineating the bone changes of Paget's disease. When the diagnosis is difficult, the physician may perform a bone biopsy. Magnetic resonance imaging (MRI) may also be used for the same purpose as the CT scan.

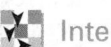 **Interventions**

Nonsurgical or surgical management may be necessary to reduce the client's pain. Nonsurgical interventions are used initially.

Nonsurgical Management. Drug therapy is the primary intervention used for pain relief. Not only can drugs relieve pain but they may cause the disease to go into remission for a period of time. Other pain relief measures are also used.

Drug Therapy. The purpose of drug therapy in Paget's disease is to relieve pain and to decrease bone resorption. Mild to moderate pain may be alleviated by aspirin or nonsteroidal anti-inflammatory drugs (NSAIDs), such as ibuprofen (Motrin, Apo-Ibuprofen✦). When the calcium level is more than twice the normal value and multisystem disease is present, the physician usually prescribes more potent drugs, such as calcitonin, etidronate disodium (EHDP), mithramycin, or alendronate (Fosamax).

Calcitonin. Calcitonin (calcitonin-salmon [Calcimar]) is a thyroid hormone that is 75% effective in initiating a remission of Paget's disease. It seems to retard bone resorption and, subsequently, relieve pain. The drug often causes a dramatic decrease in the alkaline phosphatase level in a few weeks. Given subcutaneously in doses of 50 to 100 μg three times a week, calcitonin is a fairly safe medication but has side effects, including nausea, flushing, and rash. Most of these effects occur within 1 hour of drug administration. The usual duration of therapy is 6 months, followed by a 6-month course of etidronate disodium (EHDP).

Etidronate Disodium. Etidronate disodium (EHDP) (Didronel) is prescribed orally in a dosage range of 5–20 mg/kg per day and tends to have a longer lasting effect on Paget's disease compared with calcitonin. The dosage is kept to a minimum because high dosages may cause osteomalacia or vitamin D deficiency. Its major disadvantage is that the drug is poorly absorbed from the small intestine. Therefore, EHDP should be taken on an empty stomach 1–2 hours after breakfast or at bedtime with water or juice. Milk or milk products inhibit the drug's absorption as well. Diarrhea may occur in a few clients, but this problem is treated with an antidiarrheal medication.

Calcitonin and EHDP are often the first drugs prescribed and are often used in combination. If repeated courses of these drugs are not effective, mithramycin may be added to the drug regimen. A newer drug, alendronate, may be used instead of mithramycin.

Mithramycin. Mithramycin (plicamycin, Mithracin) is a potent antineoplastic and antibiotic with many side effects. It is reserved for clients with marked hypercalcemia or severe disease with neurologic compromise. By suppressing both osteoblast and osteoclast activity, the drug can relieve bone pain in 4–5 days. The usual dosage range is 10–25 μg/kg per day intravenously, with 15 μg/kg the most commonly administered dosage. The nurse observes for signs of toxicity to the liver, gastrointestinal tract, and kidneys. Liver and kidney function test results and intake and output are monitored daily. Because mithramycin also suppresses platelets, daily platelet counts and bleeding precautions are taken. When liver enzyme levels become extremely high, drug therapy is interrupted temporarily.

Alendronate. Alendronate, better known by its trade name Fosamax, is a bone resorption inhibitor and calcium regulator. It corrects hypercalcemia and decreases the occurrence of fractures. For Paget's disease, the typical intravenous (IV) dosing is 10 mg per day for 5 days, infused over 1 hour. Side effects from IV use are not common.

Other Pain Relief Interventions. In addition to administering medication, the nurse uses physical measures to reduce pain. These measures may include application of heat, massage, and institution of an exercise program, and they are performed in conjunction with a physical therapist. The client may be fitted for an orthotic device to immobilize and provide support for the vertebrae or long bones. (Additional interventions for pain relief, such as relaxation techniques, are discussed in Chapter 9.)

The nurse provides the client with the address for the Paget's Disease Foundation and the local chapter of the Arthritis Foundation. These resources provide information and support for the client and family or significant others.

Surgical Management. When a client with Paget's disease has secondary arthritis and pain relief is not achieved, the client may undergo a partial or total joint replacement (see Chap. 24).

OSTEOMYELITIS

Overview

Osteomyelitis is the term used to describe any infection of the bone. Even with current antibiotic treatment options, osteomyelitis continues to be a common problem and a difficult challenge for the health care team.

Pathophysiology

Osteomyelitis is divided into two major types: acute and chronic. An infection lasting less than 4 weeks is acute; an infection lasting longer than that time is chronic.

Regardless of the type of osteomyelitis, the pathophysiologic process is the same. On invasion by one or more pathogenic microorganisms, the bone, and often the surrounding soft tissues, becomes inflamed. The resulting increased vascularity promotes edema. Within several days, vessel thromboses develop, causing ischemia (decreased blood flow) to the involved bone, which consequently dies. The presence of necrotic bone (sequestrum) retards bone healing and causes superimposed infection, often in the form of bone abscess. As shown in Figure 53–4, the cycle repeats itself as the superimposed infection leads to further inflammation, vessel thromboses, and necrosis. Increased attention has been given to the mechanisms by which pathogens invade bone tissue: hematogenous spread, direct inoculation, or contiguous spread.

Acute Osteomyelitis

Acute hematogenous osteomyelitis occurs more often in children, but it is becoming increasingly common in adults, particularly the elderly. An infection occurring in another part of the body moves to and invades bone tissue, particularly the long bones (such as the femur)

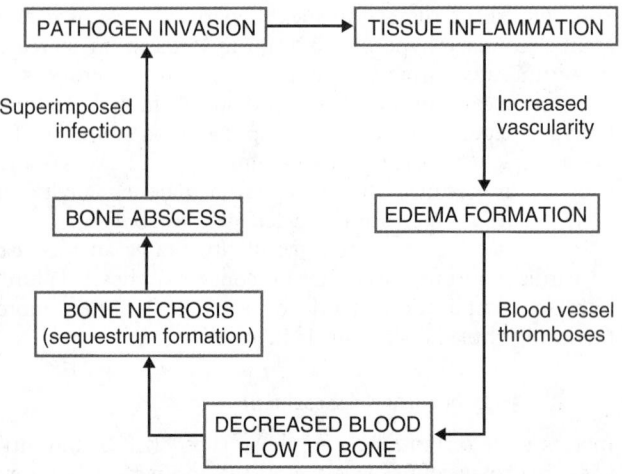

Figure 53-4. Infection cycle of osteomyelitis.

and the vertebrae. Pathogenic microbes favor bone that has a rich vascular supply and a marrow cavity.

Osteomyelitis resulting from direct inoculation frequently occurs in adults. The client experiences penetrating trauma, which allows the offending organism direct access to bone tissue. The microbe may originate from the client's skin or from a penetrating object, such as a nail.

Contiguous spread of microorganisms occurs when surrounding soft tissue becomes infected. This mechanism is common in adults who have vascular compromise, as in those with diabetes or peripheral vascular disease. The client with vascular insufficiency is typically older than 50 years and has soft-tissue infections of the small bones in the feet or hands. Many different types of microbes invade the adjacent bone simultaneously.

Chronic Osteomyelitis

Chronic osteomyelitis may result from any of the acute types. The adult with a compromised vascular supply is at greatest risk for chronic infection. Advanced age and concurrent disease may prolong the course of the infection for as long as a year or more.

Etiology

Each type of bone infection has its own causative factors. Acute hematogenous spread results from bacteremia, underlying disease, or nonpenetrating trauma. Urinary tract infections, particularly in older men, tend to spread to the lower vertebrae. Long-term intravenous (IV) catheters, such as Hickman catheters, are primary sources of infection. Clients undergoing long-term hemodialysis and IV drug abusers are also at risk for osteomyelitis. *Salmonella* infections of the gastrointestinal tract may spread to bone. Clients with sickle cell anemia and other hemoglobinopathies frequently experience multiple episodes of salmonellosis, which can cause bone infection.

Minimal trauma of the nonpenetrating type can cause hemorrhages or small-vessel occlusions, leading to bone necrosis. Regardless of the source of infection, many infections are caused by *Staphylococcus aureus*.

In contrast, penetrating trauma leads to acute osteomyelitis by direct inoculation. A concurrent soft-tissue infection may be present as well. Animal bites, puncture wounds, and bone surgery can result in bone infection. The most common offending organism is *Pseudomonas aeruginosa,* but other gram-negative bacteria may be found.

Contiguous spread occurs when adjacent soft tissues are infected. Poor dental hygiene and radiation therapy can predispose the mandible to infection.

ELDERLY CONSIDERATIONS

Malignant external otitis media involving the base of the skull and mastoid bones is seen in elderly diabetic clients. The most common case of contiguous spread is found in the client with diabetes or peripheral vascular disease who has a slow-healing foot ulcer. Multiple organisms are responsible for the subsequent osteomyelitis.

If bone infection is misdiagnosed or inadequately treated, chronic osteomyelitis occurs. Inadequate treatment results when the treatment period is too short or when the treatment is delayed or inappropriate. Gram-negative bacteria alone or mixed with gram-positive organisms account for nearly 50% of all chronic bone infections.

Collaborative Management

 Assessment

The client with acute osteomyelitis manifests fever, usually above 38° C (101° F). The area around the infected bone swells and is tender when palpated. Erythema (redness) and heat may also be present.

When vascular insufficiency is suspected, the nurse assesses circulation in the distal extremities. Draining ulcers may be present on the feet or hands, indicating inadequate healing ability as a result of poor circulation.

Bone pain, with or without other manifestations, is a common complaint of clients with bone infection. The pain is described as a constant, localized, pulsating sensation that intensifies with movement. When there is severe vascular compromise, clients may not feel discomfort because of nerve damage from lack of blood supply.

Fever, swelling, and erythema are less common in those with chronic osteomyelitis. Ulceration resulting in sinus tract formation, localized pain, and drainage are more characteristic of chronic infection (Chart 53–4).

The client with osteomyelitis usually has an elevated white blood cell (leukocyte) count, often double the normal value. In chronic infection, normal or slight elevations are not uncommon.

The erythrocyte sedimentation rate (ESR) may be normal early in the course of the disease but rises as the condition progresses. The rate may remain elevated for as long as 3 months after drug therapy is discontinued.

If bacteremia is present, a blood culture identifies the

Chart 53–4

Key Features of Acute and Chronic Osteomyelitis

Acute Osteomyelitis
- Fever, temperature usually above 38° C (101° F)
- Swelling around the affected area
- Erythema of the affected area
- Tenderness of the affected area
- Bone pain that is constant, localized, and pulsating; intensifies with movement

Chronic Osteomyelitis
- Ulceration of the skin
- Sinus tract formation
- Localized pain
- Drainage from the affected area

offending organisms to determine which antibiotics should be used in treatment. Approximately 50% of clients with acute hematogenous infection have positive blood cultures.

Although bone changes cannot be detected early with standard x-rays, changes in blood flow can be seen early in the course of the disease by radionuclide scanning. A bone scan, using technetium or gallium, is extremely helpful in the diagnosis of osteomyelitis and identifies most cases.

In some cases, magnetic resonance imaging (MRI) may be more sensitive in the diagnosis of osteomyelitis than traditional bone scanning.

The definitive diagnosis of osteomyelitis may be made by bone biopsy. A culture of soft tissue or sinus tract may not identify the offending microbes invading the bone. Often the organisms affecting soft tissue and bone are different, and each must be treated.

▶ Interventions

The specific treatment protocol depends on the type and number of microbes present in the infected tissue. If other measures fail to resolve the infectious process, surgical management may be needed.

Nonsurgical Management. To reverse osteomyelitis, the health care provider initiates antibiotic therapy as soon as possible. Contact precautions prevent the spread of the offending organism to other clients and health personnel (see Chapter 28 for a discussion of contact precautions).

Drug Therapy. Intravenous (IV) antibiotic therapy is usually prescribed for several weeks for acute osteomyelitis. More than one antibiotic may be needed to combat the presence of multiple types of organisms. The hospital or home care nurse gives the drugs at specifically ordered times so that therapeutic serum levels are achieved. The nurse must become familiar with the drugs' actions, side effects, toxicity, interactions, and precautions for administration. Family members in the home setting are taught how to administer the antibiotics.

The optimal drug regimen for clients with chronic osteomyelitis is not well established. Prolonged therapy for more than 3 months may be needed to eliminate the infection. Because of the cost of lengthy hospital stays, clients are typically discharged to the home setting with central IV catheters, such as the Hickman catheter, for medication administration. After discontinuation of IV drugs, oral antibiotic therapy may be needed for weeks or months. A cost-saving alternative to IV drug therapy is the use of newer and more potent oral antibiotics, such as fleroxacin (Megalone).

In addition to parenteral or oral drug administration, the wound may be irrigated, either continuously or intermittently, with one or more antibiotic solutions. The nurse is responsible for drug administration and uses sterile technique at all times. A technique in which beads are impregnated with an antibiotic and packed into the wound provides direct contact of the antibiotic with the offending organism.

Infection Control. If an open wound or ulcer is present in the hospital setting, the client's treatment usually includes standard precautions for limited infections in which the wound is covered, but this practice varies according to health care agency policy. Contact precautions are reserved for more severe infections, particularly when the purulent material cannot be adequately contained by a dressing. The open area is covered, and strict aseptic technique is used when dressings are changed to prevent further contamination.

Wounds may be managed through the window of a cast, which must remain dry during dressing or irrigation procedures.

Hyperbaric Oxygen Therapy. One fairly new treatment to increase tissue perfusion for clients with chronic, unremitting osteomyelitis is the use of the hyperbaric chamber or portable device to administer hyperbaric oxygen (HBO) therapy. These devices are usually available in large teaching hospitals and may not be accessible to all clients who may benefit from them. With HBO therapy, the affected area is exposed to a high concentration of oxygen that diffuses into the tissues to promote healing. In conjunction with high-dose antibiotic therapy and surgical debridement, HBO has proved very useful in treating a number of anaerobic infections.

Surgical Management. Antibiotic therapy alone may not be sufficient to meet the goals of treatment. Surgical techniques are used to minimize the disfigurement that heretofore has been a devastating result of severe osteomyelitis. Most often, surgery is reserved for clients with chronic osteomyelitis.

Sequestrectomy. Because bone cannot heal in the presence of necrotic tissue, a sequestrectomy is performed to debride the infected bone and allow revascularization of tissue.

Bone Grafts. The excision of devitalized and infected bone often results in a sizable cavity, or bone defect. The use of cancellous bone grafts to obliterate bone defects began in the 1940s and is still used widely today. One of the most popular surgical techniques is the Papineau procedure, or open cancellous bone graft, used primarily with large bone and soft-tissue defects.

As a three-step procedure, the surgeon excises necrotic bone, grafts the bone, and covers the skin, if necessary (Fig. 53–5). The donor bone is most often taken from the client's posterior ileum. The surgeon tightly packs small chips of bone into the cavity and applies a pressure dressing. In 4 or 5 days, the first postoperative dressing is done in the operating room under sterile conditions. Daily sterile dressings are applied until about 2 weeks later, when the graft stabilizes. If needed, the surgeon performs a skin graft, usually a simple split-thickness graft, between 8 and 16 weeks after the bone graft.

Bone Segment Transfers. When infected bone is extensively resected, reconstruction with microvascular bone

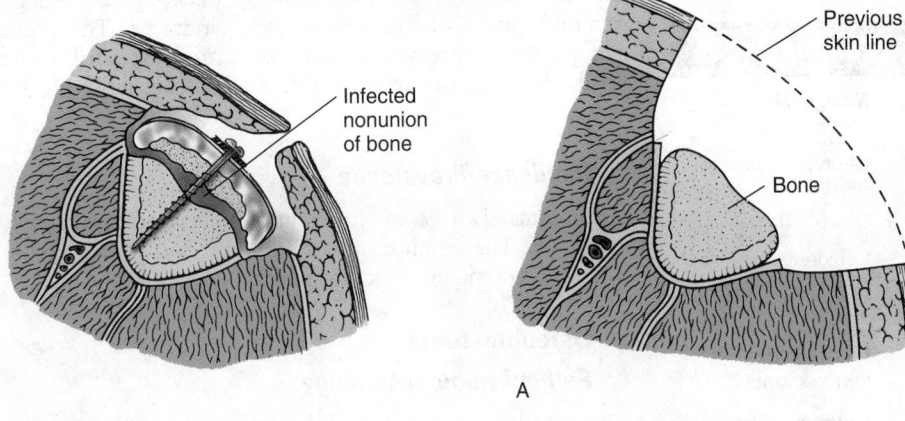

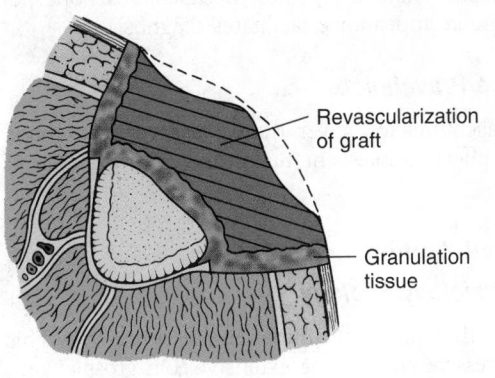

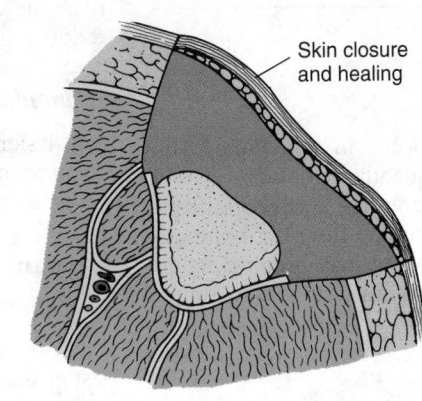

Figure 53–5. Three stages of the Papineau procedure: *A*, stage I: excision and stabilization, allowing tissue to granulate. *B*, stage II: open cancellous bone graft showing vascularization. *C*, stage III: skin coverage if not spontaneous.

transfers may be useful. In general, a bone transfer is reserved for larger skeletal defects.

The most common donor sites are the client's fibula and iliac crest. The bone graft may have an attached muscle or skin flap, if necessary. The steps of the procedure are similar to those of cancellous grafting in that debridement precedes bone transfer.

Muscle Flaps. If the bony defect is relatively small, a muscle flap may be the only surgery required. Local muscle flaps are used in the treatment of chronic osteomyelitis when soft tissue does not obliterate the dead space, or cavity, resulting from bone debridement. The flap provides wound coverage and enhances blood flow to promote healing. A split-thickness skin graft is often applied several days after the muscle flap.

Amputation. When the previously described surgical procedures are not appropriate or successful, the affected limb may need to be amputated. (The physical and psychological care for a client who has undergone an amputation is discussed in Chapter 54.)

For all of the surgical procedures and their recovery phases, long-term antibiotic treatment is necessary. The preoperative and postoperative nursing care is similar to that for repair of musculoskeletal trauma.

BONE TUMORS
Benign Bone Tumors
Overview

Benign bone tumors are often asymptomatic and may be discovered on routine x-ray examination or as the cause of pathologic fractures. The cause of benign bone tumors is not known.

Tumors may arise from several types of tissue. The major classifications (Table 53–4) include chondrogenic (from cartilage), osteogenic (from bone), and fibrogenic (from fibrous tissue and found most often in children). The cause of bone tumors, like other neoplasms, is unknown. Although many specific benign tumors have been identified, only the common ones are described here.

Chondrogenic Tumors
Osteochondroma
Pathophysiology/Etiology

The most common benign bone tumor is osteochondroma. Although its onset is usually in childhood, the tumor grows until skeletal maturity and may not be diagnosed until adulthood. The tumor may be a single growth

TABLE 53-4

Classification of Primary Bone Tumors	
Benign	**Malignant**
Chondrogenic	
Osteochondroma	Chondrosarcoma
Chondroma	
Osteogenic	
Osteoid osteoma	Osteosarcoma
Osteoblastoma	
Giant cell tumor	
	Fibrogenic
	Fibrosarcoma
	Unknown Origin
	Ewing's sarcoma

or multiple growths and can occur in any bone. The femur and the tibia are most frequently involved.

On gross appearance, the tumor has a large cartilaginous cap with a bony stalk protruding from the bone. As the cap grows, the tumor ossifies and may become malignant. About 10% of osteochondromas change into sarcomas.

Incidence/Prevalence

Osteochondromas account for about 40% of all benign bone tumors and typically affect males more often than females.

Chondroma

Pathophysiology/Etiology

The chondroma, or endochondroma, is closely related to the osteochondroma in histologic (cellular) presentation. Unlike the osteochondroma, however, the chondroma is a lesion of mature hyaline cartilage affecting primarily the hands and the feet. The ribs, the sternum, the spine, and the long bones may also be involved. Chondromas are slow growing and frequently cause pathologic fractures after trivial injury.

Incidence/Prevalence

Chondromas are found in people of all ages, occur in both males and females, and can affect any bone.

Osteogenic Tumors

Osteoid Osteoma

Pathophysiology/Etiology

The osteoid osteoma is distinguished by its pinkish, granular appearance, resulting from the proliferation of osteoblasts. Unlike other tumors, a single lesion is usually less than 0.4 inch (1 cm) in diameter. Any bone can be affected, but the femur and the tibia are most often involved. When the osteoid osteoma occurs in the spinal

column and sacrum, the client's clinical manifestations resemble those of the lumbar disk syndrome. The client complains of unremitting bone pain, probably attributable to the increase in prostaglandin levels associated with the tumor.

Incidence/Prevalence

Approximately 10% of all benign bone tumors are osteoid osteomas. The lesion occurs in children and young adults, with a predominance among males.

Osteoblastoma

Pathophysiology/Etiology

Often called the *giant osteoid osteoma,* the osteoblastoma affects the vertebrae and long bones. The tumor is larger than the osteoid osteoma and lies in cancellous bone. Its reddish, granular appearance facilitates diagnosis.

Incidence/Prevalence

The lesion accounts for fewer than 1% of primary bone tumors and affects adolescent males and young adults of both sexes.

Giant Cell Tumor

Pathophysiology/Etiology

The origin of the giant cell tumor remains uncertain. This lesion is aggressive and can be extensive. On gross examination, the lesions are gray to reddish-brown and may involve surrounding soft tissue. Although classified as benign, giant cell tumors can metastasize to the lung.

Incidence/Prevalence

Unlike most other benign bone tumors, giant cell tumors affect women older than 20 years; the peak incidence occurs in clients in their 30s. Approximately 18% of all benign bone tumors are giant cell.

Collaborative Management

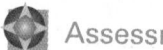 Assessment

➤ *Physical Assessment/Clinical Manifestations*

If a client experiences clinical manifestations of a benign bone tumor, pain is the most frequent complaint. The pain can range from mild to moderate, as seen with chondromas, to unremitting and intense, typical with osteoid osteomas. Pain can be caused by direct tumor invasion into soft tissue, compressing peripheral nerves, or by a resulting pathologic fracture.

In addition to collecting information regarding the nature of the client's pain, the nurse observes and palpates the suspected involved area. When the tumor affects the lower extremities or the small bones of the hands and feet, local swelling may be detected as the neoplasm enlarges. In some cases, muscle atrophy or muscle spasm may be present. The nurse palpates the bone and muscle to detect these changes and elicit tenderness.

► *Diagnostic Assessment*

Routine radiography and conventional tomography are extremely beneficial in localizing and visualizing neoplasms of the bone. Benign tumors are characterized by sharp margins, intact cortices, and smooth, uniform periosteal bone.

Computed tomography (CT) is less useful, except in complex anatomic areas, such as the spinal column and sacrum. The test is helpful in evaluating the extent of soft-tissue involvement.

When the diagnosis of a benign tumor is uncertain, an open or needle biopsy of the bone is performed. The open, surgical method is preferred to obtain a sufficient amount of tissue.

A bone scan is not specific in distinguishing a benign from a malignant tumor, but it allows the extent of the lesions to be better visualized compared with most radiographic examinations.

Magnetic resonance imaging (MRI) may be helpful in viewing problems of the spinal column.

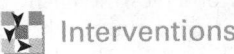 Interventions

Nonsurgical Management. The physician uses drug therapy and surgery in combination when possible. Non-drug pain relief measures are also used. Depending on the client's preference and tolerance, measures such as application of heat or cold may be helpful to relieve pain.

In addition to ordering analgesics to reduce pain, the health care provider usually prescribes one or more nonsteroidal anti-inflammatory drugs (NSAIDs) to inhibit prostaglandin synthesis and thus relieve pain in the client with osteoid osteoma. The nurse observes for drug actions and side effects, administering the drug after meals or with milk and crackers.

Surgical Management. The most common surgical procedure used for clients with benign bone tumors is curettage, or simple excision of the tumor tissue. If the tumor is small, surgery may not be indicated. When the lesion is extremely extensive, as in giant cell tumor, the neoplasm is removed with care to restore or maintain the function of the adjacent joint, most often the knee. In some cases, the knee is replaced with a prosthetic device or is fused (arthrodesis). Bone grafting may be needed. (The nursing care for clients having these surgical procedures is discussed in Chapter 24.)

Malignant Bone Tumors
Overview

Malignant bone tumors may be primary (those that originate in bone; see Table 53–4) or secondary (those that originate in other tissues and metastasize to bone). Primary tumors occur most frequently in people between 10 and 30 years and make up a small percentage of bone cancers. As for other forms of cancer, the exact cause of bone cancer is unknown. Metastatic lesions most often occur in the older age group and account for most bone cancers.

Primary Tumors
Osteosarcoma
Pathophysiology/Etiology

Osteosarcoma, or osteogenic sarcoma, is the most common type of primary malignant bone tumor. More than 50% occur in the distal femur, followed, in decreasing order of occurrence, by the proximal tibia and humerus. Flat bone and long bone incidence is about equal in people older than 25 years.

Osteosarcoma is a relatively large lesion, causing pain and swelling of short duration. The involved area is usually warm as the vascularity to the site increases. The central portion of the mass is sclerotic from increased osteoblastic activity; the periphery is soft, extending through the bone cortex in the classic sunburst appearance associated with the neoplasm. An inward expansion into the medullary canal is also common.

Osteosarcoma may be osteoblastic, chondroblastic, or fibroblastic, depending on the tissue of origin. Regardless of source, the lesion typically metastasizes to the periphery of the lung within 2 years of treatment; metastasis usually results in death.

Incidence/Prevalence

Osteosarcoma occurs more often in males than in females (2:1), between ages 10 and 30 years, and in older clients with Paget's disease. Clients who have received radiation for other forms of cancer or who have benign lesions are also at a high risk.

Ewing's Sarcoma
Pathophysiology/Etiology

Although Ewing's sarcoma is not as common as other tumors, it is the most malignant. Like other primary tumors, it causes pain and swelling. In addition, systemic manifestations, particularly low-grade fever, leukocytosis, and anemia, characterize the lesions. The pelvis and the lower extremity are most often affected. Pelvic involvement is a poor prognostic sign.

On a cellular level, the tumor is similar to bone lymphoma. On x-ray, the characteristic mottled destructive pattern and "onion skin" appearance of the bone surface distinguish the neoplasm as Ewing's sarcoma. Like other malignant tumors, it is not encapsulated and often extends into soft tissue. Death results from metastasis to the lungs and other bones.

Incidence/Prevalence

Five percent of all malignant bone tumors are Ewing's sarcoma. Although the tumor can be seen in clients of any age, it usually occurs in children and young adults in their 20s. Men are affected more often than women.

Chondrosarcoma
Pathophysiology/Etiology

In contrast to the client with osteosarcoma, the client with chondrosarcoma experiences dull pain and swelling for a long period. The tumor typically affects the pelvis and proximal femur near the diaphysis. Arising from cartilaginous tissue, the lesion destroys bone and often calcifies. The client with chondrosarcoma has a better prognosis than the client with osteogenic sarcoma.

Incidence/Prevalence

Chondrosarcoma occurs in middle-aged and older people, with a slight predominance in men, and accounts for fewer than 10% of all malignant bone tumors.

Fibrosarcoma
Pathophysiology/Etiology

Arising from fibrous tissue, fibrosarcomas can be divided into subtypes. The most malignant subgroup is the malignant fibrous histiocytoma (MFH). Most often, its clinical presentation is slow and insidious, without specific manifestations. Local tenderness, with or without a palpable mass, occurs in the long bones of the lower extremity. Like other bone cancers, the lesion can metastasize to the lungs.

Incidence/Prevalence

Although MFH affects people of all ages, it typically occurs in middle-aged men. Fortunately, the lesion is not common.

Metastatic Bone Disease
Pathophysiology/Etiology

Primary tumors of the prostate, breast, kidney, thyroid, and lung are called *bone-seeking* cancers; they metastasize to the bone more often than other primary tumors. The vertebrae, pelvis, femur, and ribs are the bone sites commonly affected. Simply stated, primary tumor cells, or seeds, are carried to bone through the bloodstream. Almost all metastatic lesions are of epithelial origin and begin in the bone marrow.

Pathologic fractures, which occur in 10%–15% of cases, are a major concern in management. The most commonly affected areas for fracture are the acetabulum and the proximal femur.

Incidence/Prevalence

Metastatic bone tumors greatly outnumber primary malignant neoplasms. Metastatic bone disease primarily affects people older than 40 years. In clients with a history of cancer and local pain, metastasis is suspected. The incidence of bone metastasis ranges from 20% to 70%, depending on the statistical reporting source. It is suspected that the reported incidence of metastasis is grossly understated.

Collaborative Management

 Assessment

➤ History

The data collected for the client suspected of having a malignant tumor are similar to those required for the client with a benign growth. In addition, the nurse asks whether the client has had previous radiation therapy for cancer and elicits information about the client's general health state.

➤ Physical Assessment/Clinical Manifestations

The clinical manifestations seen in the client with malignant tumor or metastatic disease vary, depending on the specific type of lesion. Most often, the client has a group of nonspecific complaints, including pain, local swelling, and a tender, palpable mass. Marked disability may be present in advanced metastatic bone disease.

In a client with Ewing's sarcoma, a low-grade fever may occur because of the systemic features of the neoplasm. For this reason, Ewing's sarcoma is often confused with osteomyelitis. Fatigue and pallor resulting from anemia are also common.

In performing a musculoskeletal assessment, the nurse inspects the involved area and palpates the mass for size characteristics and tenderness. The nurse also determines the client's ability to perform mobility tasks and activities of daily living (ADLs). The nurse observes the client performing mobility skills and may record the results on a functional assessment tool (see Chap. 13). The degree of disability can then be determined for comparison with later measurements after medical and nursing intervention.

➤ Psychosocial Assessment

Often clients with a malignant bone tumor are young adults whose socially productive life is just beginning. They needs support systems to help cope with the diagnosis and its treatment. Family, significant others, and health care professionals are major components of the needed support. The nurse assesses the systems available to clients.

Clients frequently experience a loss of control over their lives when a diagnosis of malignancy is made. As a result, they become anxious and fearful about the outcome of their illness. Coping with the diagnosis becomes a challenge. They go through the grieving process; initially, there is denial. The nurse identifies the anxiety level and assesses the stage or stages of the grieving process. The nurse also identifies any maladaptive behavior, indicating ineffective coping mechanisms. (Chapter 27 further elaborates on the psychosocial assessment for clients with malignancy.)

➤ Laboratory Assessment

The client with a malignant or metastatic bone tumor typically shows elevated serum alkaline phosphatase (ALP) levels, indicating the body's attempt to form new bone by increasing osteoblastic activity.

The client with Ewing's sarcoma or metastatic bone lesions frequently has a normocytic anemia. In addition, leukocytosis is common with Ewing's sarcoma.

In some clients with bone metastasis from the breast, kidney, and lung, the serum calcium level is elevated. Massive bone destruction stimulates release of the mineral into the bloodstream.

In clients with Ewing's sarcoma and bone metastasis,

often the erythrocyte sedimentation rate (ESR) is elevated, probably attributable to secondary tissue inflammation.

➤ Radiographic Assessment

As for benign bone tumors, routine x-rays and computed tomography (CT) allow for adequate visualization of malignant lesions. Although each tumor type has its own characteristic radiographic pattern, certain findings are common to all. Malignant tumors typically show poor margination, bone destruction, irregular periosteal new bone, and cortical breakthrough.

Metastatic lesions may increase or decrease bone density, depending on the amount of osteoblastic and osteoclastic activity. CT is helpful in determining the extent of soft-tissue damage.

➤ Other Diagnostic Assessment

Bone Biopsy. A bone biopsy may be performed to diagnose tumor type. A needle biopsy is usually done when metastasis to the bone is suspected. An open method, through surgical incision, is preferred for primary lesions. The surgeon keeps the incision as small as possible. The biopsy scar is removed during bone cancer surgery to eliminate a possible source of tumor seeds.

After biopsy, the cancer is staged according to the grade of the tumor. One popular method is the TNM staging system, which uses determinations of **t**umor size, **n**odal involvement, and evidence of **m**etastasis.

Another surgical staging method is to correlate the tumor grade (high or low), tumor site (intracompartmental or extracompartmental), and presence of metastatic disease (positive or negative). Staging guides the health care team in their decision regarding treatment.

Bone Scan. Although a bone scan is not helpful in determining the type of tumor, it allows the extent of the cancer to be visualized. A scan is almost always ordered when bone metastasis is suspected.

 Analysis

➤ Common Nursing Diagnoses and Collaborative Problems

The following nursing diagnoses are common to clients with malignant bone lesions:
1. Pain and Chronic Pain related to direct tumor invasion into soft tissue
2. Anticipatory Grieving related to change in body image or impending death
3. Body Image Disturbance related to effects of chemotherapy, radiation therapy, or surgery

The common collaborative problem is the potential for fractures.

➤ Additional Nursing Diagnoses and Collaborative Problems

In addition to the common diagnoses seen in most clients, one or more of the following diagnoses may be applicable on the basis of the assessment findings:

- Fear and Anxiety related to medical diagnosis, possible disfiguring surgery, or impending death
- Ineffective Individual Coping related to nonacceptance of medical diagnosis
- Ineffective Family Coping: Compromised related to nonacceptance of medical diagnosis
- Dysfunctional Grieving related to inability to cope with medical diagnosis
- Impaired Physical Mobility related to size and extent of tumor, weakness, and/or effects of terminal metastatic disease
- Altered Nutrition: Less than Body Requirements related to increased metabolic process secondary to cancer
- Sleep Pattern Disturbance related to pain
- Total Self-Care Deficit related to impaired physical mobility and weakness
- Altered Role Performance related to temporary or permanent inability to maintain role in family or community
- Spiritual Distress related to fear of death

 Planning and Implementation

Pain and Chronic Pain

Planning: Expected Outcomes. The desired outcome is that the client is expected to experience a reduction or alleviation of pain associated with the bone lesion.

Interventions. Because the pain is often due to direct tumor invasion, treatment is aimed at reducing the size of or removing the tumor. A combination of nonsurgical and surgical management is often used to promote client comfort and eliminate the complications of bone cancer.

Nonsurgical Management. In addition to analgesics for local pain relief, chemotherapeutic agents and radiation therapy are often administered in an attempt to cause tumor regression. In clients with vertebral metastatic disease, bracing and immobilization with cervical traction reduce back pain.

Drug Therapy. The physician may prescribe chemotherapy to be given alone or in combination with radiation or surgery. Certain proliferating tumors, such as Ewing's sarcoma, are sensitive to cytotoxic medications. Others, such as chondrosarcomas, are often totally drug resistant. Chemotherapy seems to work best for small, metastatic lesions and may be administered before or after surgery. For most tumors, the physician orders a combination of agents. At present, there is no universally accepted protocol of chemotherapeutic agents. The drugs selected are determined in part by the primary source of the cancer in metastatic disease. For example, when metastasis occurs from breast cancer, estrogens and progesterones may be used.

The nurse observes the client carefully for side and toxic effects and monitors laboratory tests diligently. (Chapter 27 discusses the nursing care associated with the administration of cytotoxic agents.)

Radiation Therapy. Radiation is used for selected types of malignant tumors. For clients with Ewing's sarcoma and early osteosarcoma, radiation may be the treatment of choice in reducing tumor size and thus pain.

For clients with metastatic disease, radiation is given primarily for palliation. The therapy is directed toward the painful sites in an attempt to provide a more comfortable life span. One or more treatments are given, depending on the extent of disease. With precise planning, radiation therapy can be used with minimal complications. (The nursing care for clients receiving radiation therapy is described in Chapter 27.)

Surgical Management. The treatment of primary bone tumors is surgery, often combined with radiation or chemotherapy.

Preoperative Care. Preoperatively, the nurse thoroughly evaluates the client to assist the physician in the selection of the surgical procedure to be performed. In addition to the nature, progression, and extent of the tumor, the client's age and general health state are taken into consideration. Chemotherapy may be administered preoperatively.

As for any client preparing for cancer surgery, the client with bone cancer needs psychological support from the nurse and other members of the health care team. The nurse assesses the level of understanding of the client and the family or significant others. As a client advocate, the nurse encourages the expression of concerns and questions and provides information regarding hospital routines and procedures. Spiritual support is important to some clients, who may prefer to contact their own clergy, rabbi, or spiritual leader or talk with the clergy affiliated with the hospital. The nurse helps to arrange for spiritual assistance if needed.

Postoperative needs are anticipated and planned for as much as possible before the client undergoes surgery. The nurse informs the client what to expect postoperatively and how to help ensure adequate recovery.

Operative Procedures. Wide or radical resection procedures are commonly performed for clients with bone sarcomas. Wide excision is the removal of the lesion surrounded by an intact cuff of normal tissue and leads to cure of low-grade tumors only. A radical resection includes the removal of the lesion, the entire muscle, bone, and other tissues directly involved. It is the only procedure adequate for high-grade tumors of the bone.

In the past, limb amputation was commonly performed for bone tumors, with or without disarticulation (joint removal). Today, advances in reconstructive surgery allow for the resection of the tumor and repair of the resulting bony defect to salvage the limb. Bone defects are corrected by

- Total joint replacements with prosthetic implants, either whole or partial
- Custom metallic implants
- Allografts from the iliac crest, rib, or fibula

In a few cases, arthrodesis (joint fusion) may be the procedure of choice. (Total joint replacements are discussed in Chapter 24.)

As an alternative to total replacement, an allograft may be implanted with internal fixation for those clients who do not have metastases. This is a common procedure for sarcomas of the proximal femur. Allografts for the knee are also performed, particularly in young adults. Preoperative chemotherapy is given to enhance the likelihood of success. Allografts with adjacent tendons and ligaments are harvested from cadavers and can be frozen or freeze-dried for a prolonged period. The graft is fixed with a series of bolts, screws, or plates. The nurse observes for signs of hemorrhage, infection, and fracture.

For clients with metastatic disease, intractable pain is surgically treated with percutaneous cordotomy (cutting of the spinal nerve roots). Cryosurgery (cold application) may reduce pain and tumor size.

Postoperative Care. The surgical incision for a limb salvage procedure is often extensive. A pressure dressing with wound suction is typically maintained for up to 5 days.

The client who has undergone a limb salvage procedure has resulting impaired physical mobility and a self-care deficit. The nature and extent of the alterations depend on the location and extent of the surgery.

Promotion of Physical Mobility. Usually, muscle strengthening and range-of-motion (ROM) exercises begin immediately postoperatively and continue for at least a year. After upper-extremity surgery, the client can engage in active-assistive exercises by using the opposite hand to help achieve motions such as forward flexion and abduction of the shoulder. Continuous passive motion (CPM) using a CPM machine may be initiated as early as the first postoperative day for either upper-extremity or lower-extremity procedures.

After lower-extremity surgery, the emphasis is on the strengthening of the quadriceps muscles by using passive and active motion when possible. Maintaining muscle tone is an important prerequisite to weight-bearing, which progresses from toe touch or partial weight-bearing to full weight-bearing by 3 months postoperatively.

The client who has had a bone graft has a plaster cast that remains in place for several months. Weight-bearing is prohibited until there is evidence that the graft is incorporated into the adjacent bone tissue.

During the recovery phase, the client also needs assistance with activities of daily living (ADLs), particularly if the surgery involves the upper extremity. The nurse assists if needed, but at the same time tries to encourage the client to do as much as possible unaided.

Neurovascular Assessment. Surrounding tissues, including nerves and blood vessels, may be sacrificed during surgery. Vascular grafting is common, but the lost nerve is usually not replaced. The nurse assesses the neurovascular status of the affected extremity and its digits thoroughly and frequently. Splinting or casting of the limb may also cause neurovascular compromise and needs to be checked for proper placement.

Pelvic lesions, although not commonly seen, are also excised. Reconstruction generally entails bone fusion with muscle and nerve preservation. A hip spica cast or brace may be necessary until graft incorporation has occurred. The client may need a cane for ambulation.

The major complications peculiar to reconstructive surgery for which the nurse should observe are superficial and deep wound infection, dislocation or loosening of the implants, and rapid neurovascular compromise.

An increase in pain or temperature or a rapid deterioration in circulatory status alerts the nurse to notify the physician promptly.

Psychological Support. In addition to needing psychological help in coping with physical disabilities, the client may need help coping with the surgery and its effects postoperatively. Having identified the available support systems preoperatively, the nurse helps to mobilize them for use after surgery.

As a result of most of the surgical procedures, the client experiences an alteration in body image. The nurse can suggest ways to minimize cosmetic changes. For example, a shoulder droop can be covered by a custom-made pad worn under clothing. The client can cover lower-extremity defects with pants.

Anticipatory Grieving

Planning: Expected Outcomes. The desired outcomes are that the client is expected to work through the grieving process and accept the prognosis. In some cases, the cure for cancer may be as devastating as the cancer itself, as when amputation is needed.

Interventions. The nurse's most important role is to be an active listener and to allow the client and family or significant others to verbalize their feelings. Counselors and members of the clergy or spiritual leaders may provide additional assistance in promoting acceptance of the diagnosis, treatment, or, possibly, impending death. (Chapter 12 provides information about death and dying.)

The nurse acts as an advocate for the client and the family and often promotes the physician-client relationship. For instance, the client may not completely understand the medical or surgical treatment plan but may be hesitant to question the physician. The nurse's intervention increases communication, which is essential in successful management of the client with cancer.

Body Image Disturbance

Planning: Expected Outcomes. The desired outcomes are that the client is expected to experience an improvement in feelings about the alteration in body image and accept the resulting physical changes.

Interventions. The client's self-perception of body image is closely associated with the ability to accept the illness. The nurse recognizes and accepts the client's view about the body image alteration. A trusting nurse-client relationship allows the client freedom to verbalize negative feelings. The client's strengths and remaining capabilities are emphasized. Realistic mutual goals regarding lifestyle are established. (Chapter 10 provides a discussion about altered body image.)

Potential for Fractures

Planning: Expected Outcomes. As with other bone diseases in which pathologic fracture is a possible complication (e.g., osteoporosis), the outcome is that the client is expected to avoid falls and minimize trauma to prevent fractures. In people with metastatic bone disease, fractures more readily occur and are not as preventable because of resulting destructive bone changes. A more realistic outcome for people with metastatic disease, then, may be that the client's pain will be minimized through treatment of the fracture.

Interventions. Radiation or surgery may be required to reinforce or replace the diseased bone to prevent fracture. In recent years, surgical techniques have also been improved for fracture fixation.

Nonsurgical Management. Newer techniques in radiation therapy have improved the incidence of bone healing for actual and impending pathologic fractures. To improve muscle tone and, consequently, to reduce the risk for fracture, the client performs strengthening exercises. Physical therapy on an ambulatory basis is commonly prescribed.

Surgical Management. The principles of surgery for metastatic fractures include
- Replacing as much defective bone as possible
- Being thorough in technique to avoid a second procedure
- Aiming to return the client to a functional state with a minimum of hospitalization and immobilization

Fractures of the proximal femur are very common. Prosthetic replacement reinforced with polymethyl methacrylate is preferred over open reduction and internal fixation (ORIF) when feasible. The surgeon uses intramedullary rods (IMs) and compression screws for more distal fractures. Prophylactic fixation may be indicated for microscopic fractures that cause chronic pain. (Chapter 54 discusses the nursing management for clients with fractured hip repair.)

 Continuing Care

After medical treatment for a primary malignant tumor, the client is usually managed at home with follow-up care. The client with metastatic disease may remain in the home or, when home support is not available, may be admitted to a long-term care facility for extended or hospice care. The client's care may be managed by a case manager.

► Health Teaching

For the client receiving intermittent chemotherapy on an ambulatory basis, the nurse emphasizes the importance of keeping appointments. The nurse reviews the side effects and toxic effects of the medications. The client is taught how to treat minor side effects and when to alert the health care provider. If the drugs are administered at home via long-term IV catheter, the nurse explains the care involved with daily dressing changes and potential catheter complications. (Chapter 17 describes the health teaching required for a client receiving infusion therapy at home.)

The client receiving radiation therapy is also taught the importance of keeping appointments and recognizing the complications of treatment. The nurse reviews interventions that can be used at home for minor complications.

If the client has surgery, the client has a wound and limited mobility. The nurse teaches the client how to care for the wound and perform ADLs and mobility activities independently. Physical and occupational therapists assist in ADL teaching and provide or recommend assistive and adaptive devices if necessary. The physical therapist also teaches the proper use of ambulatory aids, such as crutches, and exercises.

Pain management can be a major problem, particularly in the client with metastatic bone disease. The nurse reviews nondrug pain relief measures, including relaxation and music therapy. The nurse emphasizes those techniques that worked during hospitalization.

The client with bone cancer typically fears that the malignancy will return. The nurse acknowledges this possibility but reinforces confidence in the health care team and medical treatment chosen.

Realistic goals regarding return to work, recreational activities, and so forth are mutually established. The nurse encourages the client to resume a functional lifestyle but cautions that it should be gradual. Certain activities, such as participating in sports, may be prohibited.

The client with advanced metastatic bone disease needs to prepare for death. The nurse and other support personnel assist the client through the stages of death and dying and identify resources that can help the client write a will, visit with distant family members, or do whatever he or she thinks is needed to die in peace.

➤ Home Care Management

In collaboration with the occupational therapist, the nurse evaluates the client's home environment for structural barriers that may hinder mobility. The client may be discharged with a cast, crutches, or a wheelchair.

Accessibility to eating and toileting facilities is essential to promote independence. Because the client with metastatic disease is susceptible to pathologic fractures, potential hazards that may contribute to falls or injury should be removed.

➤ Health Care Resources

In addition to family and significant others, cancer support groups available to anyone with cancer are helpful to the client with bone cancer. Organizations such as I Can Cope provide information and emotional support; others such as CanSurmount are geared more toward client and family education. The appendix provides a complete listing of resources.

The hospital staff nurse, discharge planner, or case manager also ensures that follow-up care, including nursing care and physical or occupational therapy, is

available in the home. The client with terminal cancer may choose to become part of a hospice program (see Chap. 12).

 Evaluation

On the basis of the identified nursing diagnoses and collaborative problems, the nurse evaluates the care provided for the client with primary or metastatic bone cancer. The expected outcomes may include that the client will

- State that pain is reduced or alleviated
- Perform ADLs and ambulation activities independently
- Seek health care resources as needed, including cancer support groups
- State that body image perception is improved
- Return to a functional lifestyle (or accept impending death in the case of advanced metastasis)
- State that anxiety regarding medical diagnosis and treatment is decreased

DISORDERS OF THE HAND
Carpal Tunnel Syndrome
Overview

Carpal tunnel syndrome (CTS) is a common condition in which the median nerve in the wrist becomes compressed, causing pain and numbness. The carpal tunnel is a rigid canal lying between the carpal bones and a fibrous tissue sheet called the flexor retinaculum. As seen in Figure 53–6, a group of nine tendons enveloped by synovium share space with the median nerve in the carpal tunnel. When the synovium becomes swollen or thickened, the nerve is compressed.

The median nerve supplies the motor, sensory, and autonomic function for the first three digits of the hand and the palmar aspect of the fourth. Because of the median nerve's proximity to other structures, wrist flexion

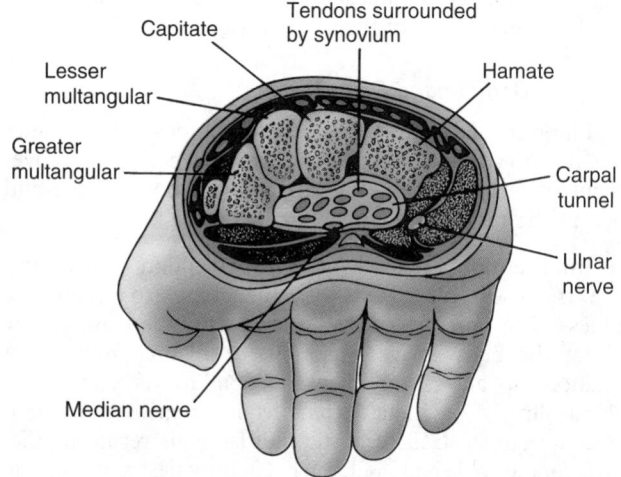

Figure 53–6. Anatomy of the carpal tunnel.

causes nerve impingement against the flexor retinaculum; extension causes increased pressure in the distal portion of the carpal tunnel.

Carpal tunnel syndrome (CTS) usually manifests as a chronic problem; acute cases are rare. Excessive hand exercise, edema or hemorrhage into the carpal tunnel, or thrombosis of the median artery can lead to acute CTS. Clients with a Colles' fracture of the wrist or hand burns are particularly at risk for rapid CTS development.

In most cases, however, the causative factors may not result in neurologic deficit for years. CTS is a common complication of certain metabolic and connective tissue diseases. For example, synovitis (inflammation of the synovium) occurs in clients with rheumatoid arthritis. The hypertrophied synovium compresses the median nerve. In other chronic disorders such as diabetes mellitus, inadequate blood supply can cause median nerve neuropathy, or dysfunction, resulting in CTS.

Carpal tunnel syndrome is also a potential occupational hazard. People whose jobs require repetitive hand activities involving pinch or grasp during wrist flexion, such as factory workers, computer operators, and jackhammer operators, are predisposed to CTS. CTS can also result from overuse in sports activities such as golf, tennis, and racquetball.

In a few cases, CTS may be a familial or congenital problem, manifesting in adulthood. Space-occupying lesions, such as ganglia, tophi, and lipomas, can also result in nerve compression.

Carpal tunnel syndrome occurs in adults of all ages but peaks between 30 and 60 years. Women are five times more likely to experience the problem than men. Most often CTS affects the dominant hand, but it can occur in both hands simultaneously. Children and adolescents are beginning to experience CTS as a result of the increased use of computers in everyday life.

Collaborative Management

 Assessment

On the basis of client history and complaint of hand pain and numbness, a medical diagnosis is often made without further assessment. The nurse questions clients regarding the nature, intensity, and location of the pain. Clients often state that the pain is worse at night as a result of flexion or direct pressure during sleep. The pain may radiate to the arm, the shoulder and neck, or the chest.

In addition to the complaint of numbness, clients with CTS may also experience paresthesia (painful tingling). Sensory changes usually precede motor manifestations by weeks or months.

➤ *Physical Assessment/Clinical Manifestations*

The nurse performs several tests to elicit abnormal sensory findings. Phalen's wrist test, sometimes called *Phalen's maneuver,* produces paresthesia in the median nerve distribution within 60 seconds. The client is asked to relax the wrist into flexion or place the backs of the hands together and flex both wrists simultaneously (Fig.

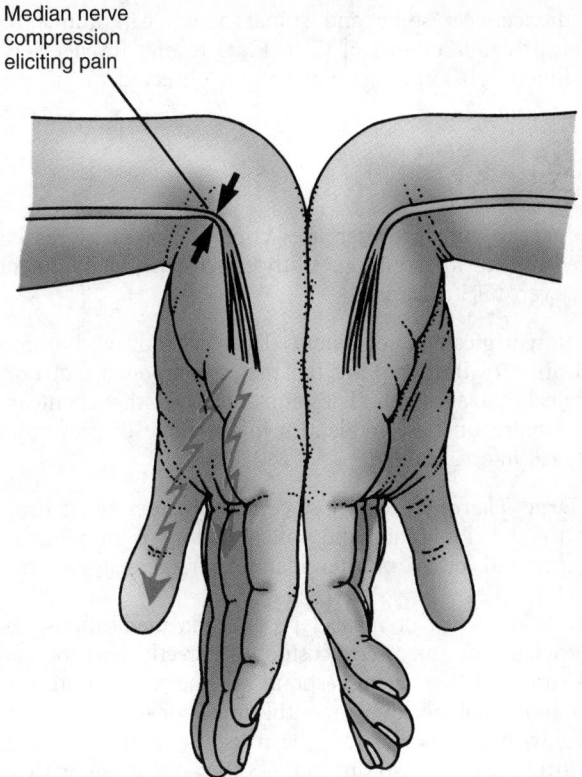

Median nerve compression eliciting pain

Figure 53–7. Phalen's maneuver for detection of carpal tunnel syndrome.

53–7). Of clients with CTS, 80% have a positive Phalen's test result.

The same sensation can be elicited by tapping lightly over the area of the median nerve in the wrist (*Tinel's sign*). If the test is unsuccessful, a blood pressure cuff can be placed on the upper arm and inflated to the client's systolic pressure. The result is frequently pain and tingling.

Motor changes begin with a weak pinch, clumsiness, and difficulty with fine movements, and then progress to muscle weakness and wasting. The nurse tests for pinching ability and asks the client to perform a fine-movement task, such as threading a needle. Strenuous hand activity worsens the subjective complaints.

In addition to inspecting for muscle atrophy and task performance, the nurse observes the wrist for swelling attributable to edema or lesions. The area is palpated, and characteristics are described.

Autonomic changes may be evidenced by skin discoloration; nail changes, such as brittleness; and increased or decreased palmar sweating.

➤ *Diagnostic Assessment*

Routine x-rays are ordered to visualize bone changes, space-occupying lesions, and synovitis. If these causative factors are not suspected, a client with CTS may not need x-rays.

The health care provider may order electromyography (EMG) when a definitive diagnosis is uncertain. Problems of the cervical spine and spinal nerves can mimic the clinical manifestations of CTS. EMG testing reveals nerve dysfunction before muscle atrophy is observed.

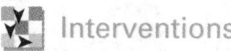 Interventions

The health care provider uses conservative measures before surgical intervention. With either type of treatment, however, CTS can recur.

Nonsurgical Management. Drug therapy and immobilization of the wrist are the major components of nonsurgical management. The nurse teaches the client the importance of these modalities in the hope of preventing surgical intervention.

Drug Therapy. The most commonly prescribed drugs for the relief of pain and inflammation, if present, are aspirin and other nonsteroidal anti-inflammatory drugs (NSAIDs).

In addition to or instead of systemic medications, the physician may inject corticosteroids directly into the carpal tunnel. If the client responds to the medication, several additional weekly or monthly injections are given.

As with any medication, the nurse monitors the effects of drug therapy. Aspirin and NSAIDs are given with or after meals to reduce gastric irritation.

Immobilization. A splint may be used to immobilize the wrist during the day, during the night, or both. Many clients experience temporary relief with splinting. The occupational therapist places the client's wrist in the neutral or slight extension position. Even when a splint is not used, the nurse instructs the client to minimize hand activities, at least temporarily.

Surgical Management. Surgery is necessary in about half of clients with CTS. Surgery can relieve the pressure on the median nerve by providing nerve decompression.

Preoperative Care. The nurse in the physician's office or same-day surgical center reinforces the teaching provided by the surgeon regarding the nature of the surgery. Postoperative care is reviewed so that the client knows what to expect.

Operative Procedures. When CTS is a complication of rheumatoid arthritis, a synovectomy (removal of excess synovium via incision) may resolve the problem. Removal of a space-occupying lesion, if present, also decompresses the nerve. Whatever the cause of nerve compression, the physician removes it either by cutting or by the newer laser technique. In some cases, CTS recurs months to years after surgery.

An alternative to the traditional inner wrist incision is an endoscopic procedure. The surgeon makes a very small incision (less than ½ inch [1.2 cm]) through which the endoscope is inserted. The surgeon then uses special instruments, which may include laser, to free the trapped median nerve.

Postoperative Care. In addition to vital sign monitoring, the nurse checks the client's pressure dressing carefully for drainage and tightness. If the endoscopic procedure has been performed, the dressing is very small. The surgeon may require the client's hand and arm to be elevated above heart level for 1 or 2 days to reduce swelling from surgery. The nurse checks the neurovascular status of the digits every hour during the postoperative period, encouraging the client to move all fingers of the affected hand frequently. The nurse offers pain medication and assures the client that he or she will be given a prescription for analgesics for use at home during recovery.

After surgery, the client's wrist is placed in a splint that allows thumb and finger movements. The splint is usually applied after the sutures have been removed and is used for at least 2 weeks.

Hand movements, including lifting heavy objects, may be restricted for 4–6 weeks. The client can expect weakness and discomfort for weeks or perhaps months. The nurse teaches the client how to assess for neurovascular status.

The client must realize that the surgical procedure might not be a cure. For instance, synovitis may recur in the client with rheumatoid arthritis and may recompress the median nerve. Multiple operations and other treatments are not uncommon for the client with carpal tunnel syndrome.

The client may need assistance with routine daily tasks or even self-care activities during recovery. The nurse ensures that assistance in the home is available, usually provided by the family or significant others.

Dupuytren's Contracture

Dupuytren's contracture, or deformity, is a slowly progressive contracture of the palmar fascia resulting in flexion of the fourth or fifth digit of the hand. The third digit is occasionally affected. Although Dupuytren's contracture is a fairly common problem, the cause is unknown. It usually occurs in older men, tends to be familial, and can be bilateral.

When function becomes impaired, surgical release is required. A partial or selective fasciectomy (removal of fascia) is performed. After removal of the dressing and drain, a splint may be used. Nursing care is similar to that for the client with carpal tunnel repair.

Ganglion

A ganglion is a round, cyst-like lesion often overlying a wrist joint or tendon. The synovium surrounding the tendon degenerates, allowing the tendon sheath tissue to become weak and distended. Ganglia are painless on palpation, but they can cause joint discomfort after prolonged joint use or minor trauma, such as a strain. The lesion can disappear and then recur. Ganglia are most likely to develop in people from 15 to 50 years of age.

Although the fluid within the lesion can be aspirated, total excision is preferred. The postoperative care is the same as that for the client undergoing other hand surgery.

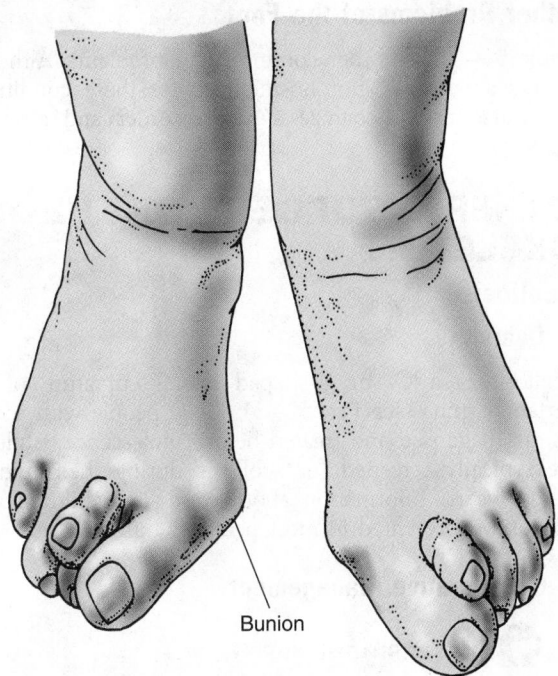

Figure 53–8. Appearance of hallux valgus with a bunion.

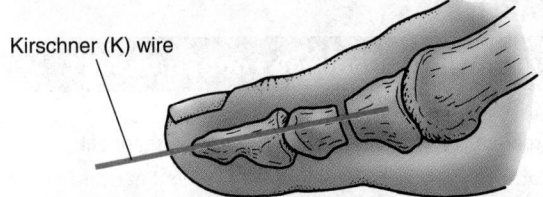

Figure 53–9. Use of Kirschner wires to repair hallux valgus and other toe deformities.

DISORDERS OF THE FOOT

Hallux Valgus

The hallux valgus deformity, sometimes referred to as a bunion, is a common foot problem. The great toe deviates laterally at the metatarsophalangeal (MTP) joint (Fig. 53–8). Although hallux valgus is often congenital, it can occur as a result of arthritis or poorly fitted shoes. As the deviation worsens, the bony prominence enlarges and causes pain, particularly when shoes are worn. Women are affected more frequently than men.

The surgical procedure, a simple bunionectomy, involves removal of the bony overgrowth and bursa. When other toe deformities accompany the condition or if the bony overgrowth is large, several osteotomies, or bone resections, may be performed. In this case, Kirschner wires are inserted vertically through the toes until healing occurs (Fig. 53–9). If both feet are affected, one foot is treated at a time.

Hammertoe

Often clients have hammertoes and hallux valgus deformities simultaneously. As shown in Figure 53–10, a hammertoe is the dorsiflexion of any metatarsophalangeal (MTP) joint with plantar flexion of the adjacent proximal interphalangeal (PIP) joint. The second toe is most often affected. As the deformity worsens, corns may develop on the dorsal side of the toe and calluses may appear on the plantar surface. Clients are uncomfortable when wearing shoes and walking.

Hammertoe is treated by surgical correction of the deformity with osteotomies and the insertion of Kirschner wires for fixation (see Figure 53–9). The postoperative course is similar to that for the client with hallux valgus repair. The client uses crutches until full weight-bearing is allowed 3 to 4 weeks postoperatively.

Morton's Neuroma

In the client with Morton's neuroma, or plantar digital neuritis, a small tumor grows in a digital nerve of the foot. The client usually describes the pain as an acute, burning sensation in the web space. The pain involves the entire surface of the third and fourth toes.

Treatment involves surgical removal of the neuroma and application of a pressure dressing. Ambulation is usually permitted immediately after surgery.

Tarsal Tunnel Syndrome

Tarsal tunnel syndrome is the ankle version of the carpal tunnel syndrome. The posterior tibial nerve in the ankle becomes compressed, resulting in loss of sensation and pain in a portion of the foot. Typically, the median and lateral plantar branches, which supply the sole of the foot and the distal phalanges, are affected by the nerve compression.

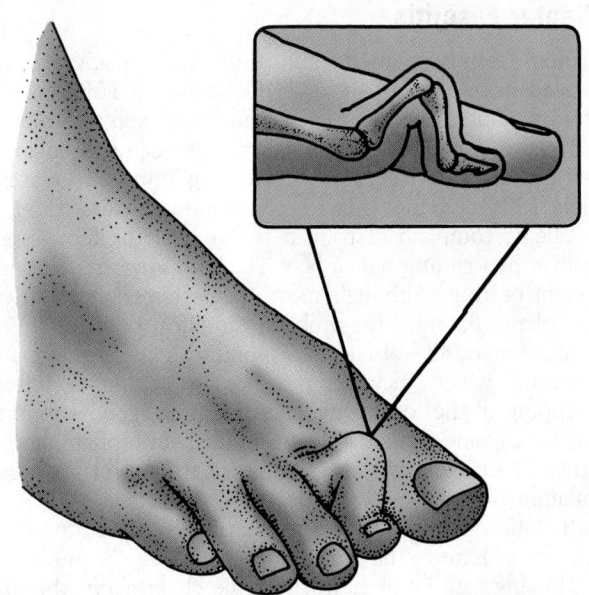

Figure 53–10. Hammertoe of the second metatarsophalangeal (MTP) joint.

TABLE 53–5

Treatment of Common Foot Problems

Problem	Description/ Cause	Treatment
Corn	• Induration and thickening of the skin caused by friction and pressure, painful conical mass	• Surgical removal by podiatrist
Callus	• Flat, poorly defined mass on the sole over a bony prominence caused by pressure	• Padding and lanolin cremes, overall good skin hygiene
Ingrown nail	• Nail sliver penetration of the skin, causing inflammation	• Removal of sliver by podiatrist, warm soaks, antibiotic ointment
Hypertrophic ungual labium	• Chronic hypertrophy of nail lip caused by improper nail trimming; results from untreated ingrown nail	• Surgical removal of necrotic nail and skin, treatment of secondary infection

Diagnosis and treatment are similar to those for carpal tunnel syndrome.

Plantar Fasciitis

Plantar fasciitis is an inflammation of the plantar fascia located in the area of the arch of the foot. It is frequently seen in middle-aged and elderly adults as well as athletes, especially runners. In ambulatory care settings, plantar fasciitis accounts for 10% of running injuries (Quaschnick, 1996). Obesity is also a contributing factor.

Clients complain of pain in the arch of the foot, especially when getting out of bed. The pain is worsened with weight-bearing. Although most clients experience unilateral plantar fasciitis, the problem can affect both feet.

More than 90% of clients respond to conservative management, which includes rest, ice, stretching exercises, strapping of the foot to maintain the arch, good supporting shoes, and orthotics. Nonsteroidal anti-inflammatory drugs or steroids may also be needed to control pain and inflammation.

If conservative measures are unsuccessful, endoscopic surgery to remove the inflamed tissue may be required.

Nursing care involves teaching the client about the importance of complying with the treatment plan and coordinating care with the physical therapist for instruction in exercise.

Other Problems of the Foot

Table 53–5 cites other common foot problems. Although clients are usually not hospitalized for these conditions, the nurse may recognize a foot disorder and alert the physician.

OTHER DISORDERS OF THE SKELETON

Scoliosis

Overview

Scoliosis is a C- or S-shaped lateral curvature of the vertebral spine (see Fig. 52–3). Many people with scoliosis are diagnosed and treated before adolescence. Children are typically screened for scoliosis during their middle-school years. Information about caring for children with scoliosis is presented in most pediatric nursing texts.

Collaborative Management

 Assessment

In the adult with scoliosis, the impairment is usually cosmetic, although severe deviations of more than 50 degrees can compromise cardiopulmonary function. The abnormal curvature can cause low back pain, for which treatment is initiated. Women are affected more frequently than men.

Methods of treating adult scoliosis differ from those used for children. The adult spinal column is less flexible and, therefore, less likely to respond to exercises, weight reduction, bracing, and casting for correction of the deformity. In the adult, the disorder is progressive and can result in an additional 1 degree of deviation each year.

Clients who had undergone scoliosis surgery 20–25 years ago are returning with progressive, debilitating back pain from degenerative disk disease below the fusion and with "flat back" syndrome, a loss of lumbar curvature. In some of these clients, fusion was not accomplished with instrumentation, and surgery may be necessary to resolve the pain.

 Interventions

Surgical intervention is the most common treatment for the adult. The procedure consists of surgical fusion and insertion of instrumentation. The surgeon performs one or more spinal fusions by packing cancellous bone chips, usually from the iliac crest, between the affected vertebrae for support and stabilization. Both an anterior and a posterior approach may be needed. In this case, the surgeon may perform them during the same operative day or may stage them 7–10 days apart.

The metal instrumentation straightens the spine and immobilizes the fused area during healing (Figure 53–11). The earlier instrumentation systems include those by Harrington, Dwyer, and Luque. In the 1980s, Cotrel-Dubousset (CD) implants became popular and are still commonly used today. Other systems similar to the CD im-

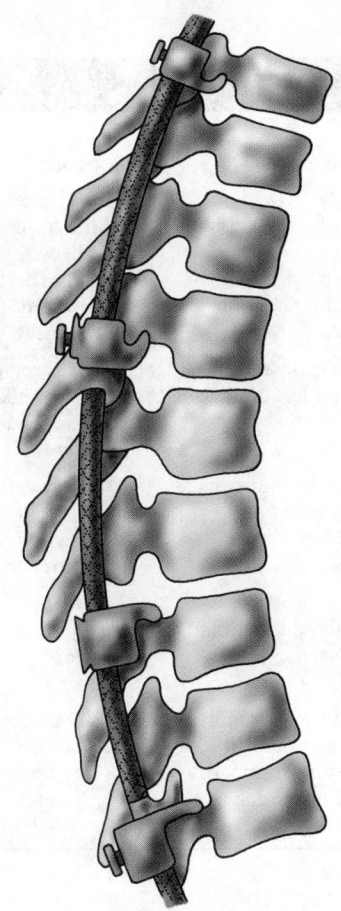

Figure 53–11. Correction of the lateral spine contour with Cotrel-Dubousset instrumentation and spinal fusion.

plant include the Texas Scottish Rite Hospital system (TSRH) and the ISOLA system.

The nursing care of the client undergoing corrective surgery for scoliosis is similar to that for the client undergoing a laminectomy or spinal fusion (see Chap. 45). The major difference is the length of postoperative immobilization, which can be several days in bed with Harrington or Dwyer procedures. Luque and CD instrumentation allow the client to be out of bed the same evening or day after surgery. A thoracolumbosacral (dorsolumbar) orthosis (TLSO) is typically used to support the vertebral column (see Fig. 53–2).

With the newer surgical techniques, the client may return to work in about 3 weeks and can resume activities such as swimming and bicycling. Recreational sports, such as tennis, are usually resumed in 6 weeks with CD implant surgery, but other surgery may prevent the client from performing these activities until 3–6 months postoperatively. Many clients are allowed to return to contact sports within a year or less.

Osteogenesis Imperfecta

Although there are several types of osteogenesis imperfecta (OI), the milder tarda form with autosomal inheritance is more prevalent in adults. In this rare hereditary disease, a defect of connective tissue formation results in fragile and deformed bones. In addition to multiple fractures and poor skeletal development, the client may have blue sclera; soft, brownish teeth; and presenile deafness.

The treatment is palliative, and the client's life span is frequently shortened.

The physician prescribes steroids, calcium, vitamin C, and sodium fluoride. Physical therapy, casting or bracing, and intramedullary rodding are used to maintain mobility and promote ambulation if possible. The nurse refers the client to the Osteogenesis Foundation (in the United States) or the "Brittle Bones" society in other countries for information and support.

MUSCULAR DISEASES
Progressive Muscular Dystrophies
Overview

At least nine types of muscular dystrophy (MD) have been clinically identified. They can be broadly categorized as slowly progressive or rapidly progressive. The slowly progressive types are most commonly seen in adults.

Five forms of MD are often seen in adults. Each type has its own distinct characteristics and causes, but all are progressive (Table 53–6).

The exact pathophysiologic mechanisms are unknown, but three theories have been advocated.

The vascular theory suggests that a lack of blood flow causes the typical degeneration of muscle tissue seen in muscular dystrophy. Microscopic necrotic areas in dystrophied muscle tissue support this hypothesis, although this finding does not explain the marked degree of degeneration frequently seen in the disease.

The neurogenic theory proposes a disturbance in nerve-muscle interaction. Research has failed, however, to locate the nature of the disturbance.

The most popular belief is the membrane theory. This theory suggests that cell membranes are genetically altered, causing a compromise in cell integrity. An increase in the activity of muscle proteolytic enzymes may accompany the membrane alteration, leaving the muscle cell vulnerable to degeneration. Increased enzyme activity has been documented in the client with dystrophied muscles.

The cause of MD is unknown, but there may be a genetic influence for most of the major types. Some forms of MD are transmitted as autosomal dominant or recessive traits, whereas others are sex linked.

The most commonly occurring type of MD is the severe X-linked recessive variety initially described by Guillaume Duchenne in 1868. Each year, 20–33 cases are reported per 100,000 live male births. In an X-linked recessive disorder, one half of the male children of an unaffected mother, or carrier, manifest the disease. Becker's dystrophy is also inherited in an X-linked recessive manner, but it is less common than Duchenne's dystrophy. The other types of MD seen in adults can occur in either sex.

Collaborative Management

Diagnosis of MD is often difficult because the clinical manifestations are similar to those of other muscular dis-

TABLE 53–6

Differential Features of Common Muscular Dystrophies

Dystrophy	Onset	Genetics	Clinical Manifestations	Progression
Duchenne (severe X-linked)	• 18 mo–4 yr	• Sex-linked recessive, expression in males	• Symmetric pelvic and shoulder girdle muscle weakness, waddling gait, cardiac involvement common, mental retardation in one third	• Severely progressive, leading to inability to walk between 7 and 11 yr of age, death from cardiac or respiratory failure in 20s or 30s
Becker (benign X-linked)	• 5–25 yr	• Sex-linked recessive, expression in males	• Wasting of pelvic and shoulder muscles, normal cardiac and mental function	• Gradual progression, inability to walk 25 yr after onset, usually normal life span
Limb-girdle	• Usually 20s or 30s	• Usually autosomal dominant, expression in either sex	• Upper-extremity and neck muscles and lower-extremity and hip muscle weakness	• Extremely variable, severe disability within 10–20 yr after onset, life span shortened by 10–20 yr
Facioscapulohumeral (Landouzy-Dejerine)	• Usually in 20s	• Autosomal dominant, expression in either sex	• Facial and shoulder girdle muscle involvement	• Usually benign, normal life span
Myotonic (Steinert)	• Birth to 40s	• Autosomal dominant, expression in either sex	• Muscle atrophy with multiple organ involvement (e.g., heart, lungs, smooth muscle, and endocrine system)	• Usually gradual if onset in adulthood

orders. Muscle biopsy frequently confirms the diagnosis. Muscle weakness and trophic changes are characteristic of all types of MD. Serum muscle enzyme values may be elevated, and electromyographic (EMG) findings are frequently abnormal.

Management of the client with MD is supportive and involves the entire health care team. Physical and occupational therapy helps the client maintain as much function and independence as possible. Major organ or body system involvement is medically managed, but the client's life span is often shortened from these manifestations of the disease. No drug has been found to slow the progression of the disorder, although steroids and immunosuppressive agents have been tried.

An experimental treatment called myoblast transfer therapy (MTT) is being studied and supported by the FDA. MTT involves injections of healthy muscle cells (myoblasts) taken from a donor and multiplied in a laboratory. The cells are then given to the client with MD where they theoretically fuse with each other and the recipient's unhealthy muscle cells.

Nursing interventions focus on making the client as comfortable as possible and reinforcing techniques and exercises taught in the physical therapy program. The nurse's role in caring for a client with cardiac or other organ involvement is the same as for any client with dysfunction of these areas.

Other Muscular Disorders

Most muscle diseases are classified as neuromuscular disorders, such as myasthenia gravis, or connective tissue diseases, such as polymyositis. Therefore, these disorders are discussed in Chapters 46 and 24, respectively.

 CASE STUDY **for the Client with Acute Osteomyelitis**

■ A 58-year-old man with a history of diabetes mellitus, coronary artery disease, hypertension, and pulmonary emphysema sees his nurse practitioner with a foot wound. He states that he attempted to cut out an ingrown toenail last week, but his "little knife" slipped and entered the soft tissue around the nail. On inspection, the area is red, warm, and slightly tender. He has a temperature of 39° C (101.8°).

Q U E S T I O N S :

1. What other physical assessment should be performed at this time?
2. What laboratory tests will the nurse practitioner most likely order?
3. What treatments may the client have based on his probable diagnosis?

SELECTED BIBLIOGRAPHY

Ashworth, L. (1997). Can alendronate help my osteoporosis? *Home Care Provider, 2*(1), 37–39.

Chappard, D., Minaire, P., Privat, C., et al. (1995). Effects of tiludronate on bone loss in paraplegic patients. *Journal of Bone and Mineral Research, 10,* 112–118.

Dawe, D., & Curran-Smith, J. (1994). Going through the motions. *The Canadian Nurse, 90*(1), 31–33.

*Department of Health and Human Services. (1990). *Healthy people 2000.* Rockville, MD: Author.

*Ficner, H. B. (1993). Revision surgery in adult scoliosis patients. *Orthopaedic Nursing, 12*(2), 23–33.

Fraser, D. R. (1995). Vitamin D. *Lancet, 345,* 104–107.

Hodgson, B. B., Kizior, R. J., & Kingdon, R. T. (1997). *Nurse's drug handbook 1997.* Philadelphia: W. B. Saunders.

Hunt, A. H. (1996). The relationship between height change and bone mineral density. *Orthopaedic Nursing, 15*(3), 57–71.

Hunt, A. H., Civitelli, R., & Halstead, L. (1995). Evaluation of bone resorption: A common problem during impaired mobility. *SCINursing, 12*(3), 90–94.

Kessenich, C. R., & Rosen, C. J. (1996). Vitamin D and bone status in elderly women. *Orthopaedic Nursing, 15*(3), 67–71.

LeBoff, M. S. (1997). Metabolic bone disease. In W. N. Kelley, E. D. Harris, S. Ruddy, & C. B. Sledge (Eds.), *Textbook of rheumatology,* (5th ed., pp. 1563–1580). Philadelphia: W. B. Saunders.

Maher, A. B., Salmond, S. W., & Pellino, T. A. (1994). *Orthopaedic nursing.* Philadelphia: W. B. Saunders.

Marchigiano, G. (1997). Osteoporosis: Primary prevention and intervention strategies for women at risk. *Home Care Provider, 2*(2), 76–82.

Matteson, M. A., McConnell, E. S., & Linton, A. D. (1997). *Gerontological nursing: Concepts and practice* (2nd ed.). Philadelphia: W. B. Saunders.

National Osteoporosis Foundation. (1995). *Position paper: Current perspective on diagnosis, prevention, and treatment of osteoporosis.* Washington, DC: Author.

Piasecki, P. A. (1996). Nursing care of the patient with metastatic bone disease. *Orthopaedic Nursing, 15*(4), 25–33.

Quaschnick, M. S. (1996). The diagnosis and management of plantar fasciitis. *Nurse Practitioner, 21*(4), 50–63.

Segatore, M. (1995). The skeleton after spinal cord injury. Part 1. Theoretical aspects. *SCINursing, 12*(3), 82–86.

Tietz, N. W. (1995). *Clinical guide to laboratory tests.* Philadelphia: W. B. Saunders.

Torgerson, D. J., & Kanis, J. A. (1995). Cost-effectiveness of preventing hip fractures in the elderly population using vitamin D and calcium. *Quarterly Journal of Medicine, 88,* 135–139.

SUGGESTED READINGS

Kessenich, C. R., & Rosen, C. J. (1996). Vitamin D and bone status in elderly women. *Orthopaedic Nursing, 15*(3), 67–71.

This study demonstrated a correlation between lack of vitamin D intake and decreased bone density in elderly women living in northern New England. Vitamin D supplementation, especially during the fall and winter months, may help prevent bone loss.

Piasecki, P. A. (1996). Nursing care of the patient with metastatic bone disease. *Orthopaedic Nursing, 15*(4), 25–33.

This article describes the nursing care of the client with metastatic bone disease, a common consequence of cancer. Nursing management includes assessment, psychological support, and client education. Pain management is a primary concern to clients.

Chapter 54

INTERVENTIONS FOR CLIENTS WITH MUSCULOSKELETAL TRAUMA

Musculoskeletal injury is one of the primary causes of disability in the United States. Trauma to the musculoskeletal system ranges from simple muscle strain to multiple bone fractures with severe soft tissue damage. With advancing age, a person is more likely to develop decreased bone mass (osteoporosis), which causes fractures. Hip, wrist, vertebral, and pelvic fractures are common in late adulthood.

FRACTURES

Overview

A fracture is a break or disruption in the continuity of a bone. Fractures can occur anywhere in the body and at any age. All fractures have the same basic pathophysiologic mechanism and nursing management, regardless of fracture type or location.

Pathophysiology

Classification of Fractures

A fracture is classified by the extent of the break as

- Complete—the break is across the entire width of the bone in such a way that the bone is divided into two distinct sections

- Incomplete—the fracture does not divide the bone into two portions because the break is through only part of the bone

A fracture is described by the extent of associated soft-tissue damage as open (or compound) or closed (or simple). The skin surface over the broken bone is disrupted in a compound fracture, which causes an external wound. These fractures are often graded in order to define the extent of tissue damage. Grade I is the least severe injury, and skin damage is minimal. In grade II, an open fracture is accompanied by skin and muscle contusions. The most severe injury is grade III, in which there is damage to skin, muscle, nerve tissue, and blood vessels; the wound is more than 6–8 cm (2.4–3.2 inches) in diameter (Maher et al., 1994).

A closed (simple) fracture does not extend through the skin. Therefore, there is no visible wound.

Figure 54–1 illustrates common types of fractures. The nurse needs to be familiar with the differences in these types because they often dictate the specific nursing care required for the client.

In addition to being identified by type, fractures are characterized by their cause. A pathologic (spontaneous) fracture occurs after minimal trauma to a bone that has been weakened by disease. For example, a client with bone cancer or osteoporosis can easily sustain a patho-

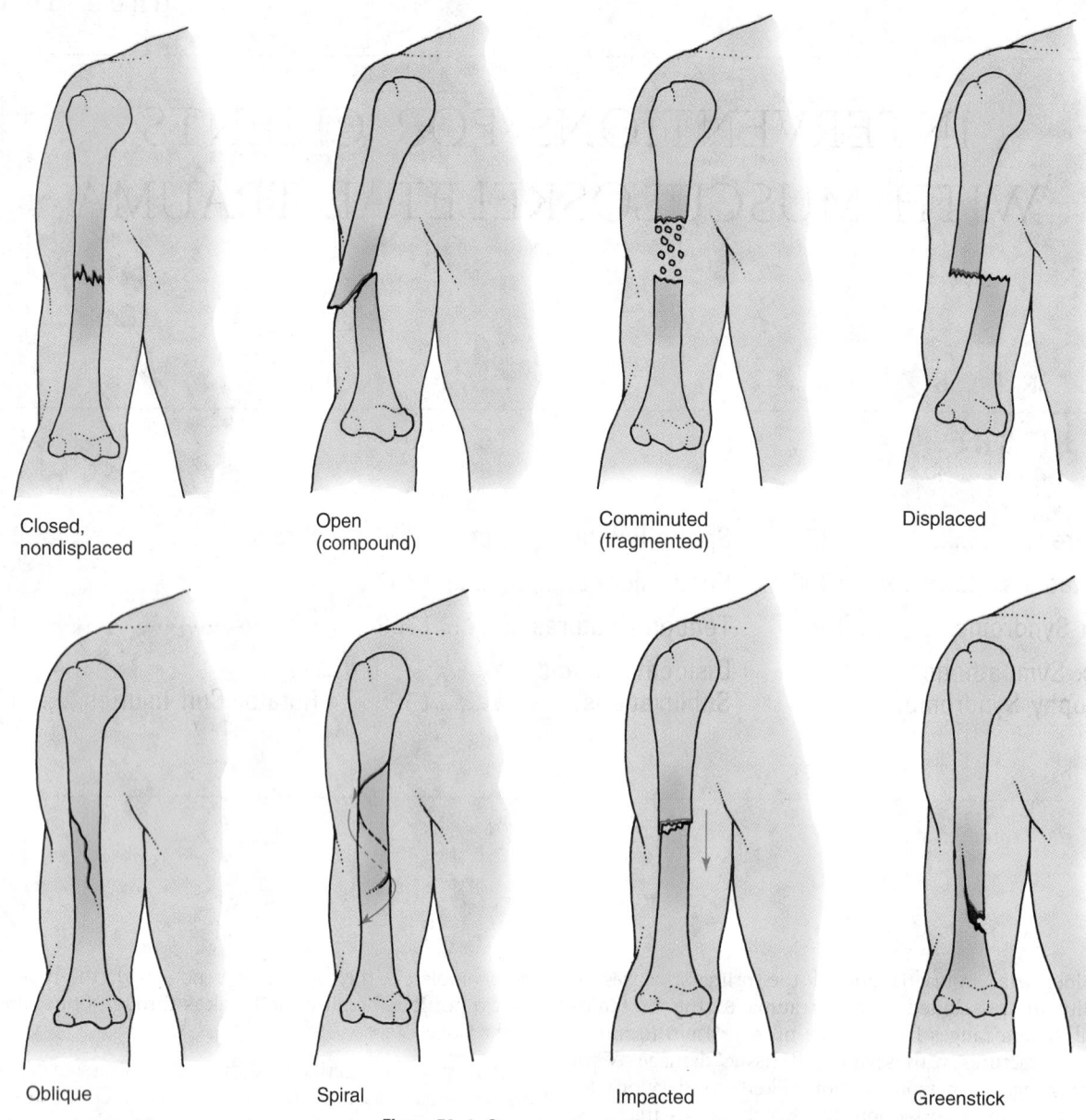

Closed,
nondisplaced

Open
(compound)

Comminuted
(fragmented)

Displaced

Oblique

Spiral

Impacted

Greenstick

Figure 54–1. Common types of fractures.

logic fracture. A fatigue or stress fracture results from excessive strain and stress on the bone.

Stages of Bone Healing

When a bone is broken, the body immediately begins the healing process to repair the injury and restore the body's equilibrium. Within 48–72 hours after the injury, a hematoma forms at the site of the fracture because bone is extremely vascular. Blood supply to and within the bone usually diminishes, which causes an area of bone necrosis. Fibroblasts and osteoblasts migrate to the area to begin the granulation stage of healing.

As a result of vascular and cellular proliferation, the fracture site is surrounded by new vascular tissue known as a callus. Callus formation is the beginning of a nonbony union. As healing continues, the callus is trans-

formed from a loose, fibrous tissue into bone. Osteoclasts and phagocytes remove the debris, and necrotic bone is resorbed. This process is often referred to as bone *remodeling*.

Figure 54–2 summarizes the stages of bone healing. In young, healthy adult bone, healing takes about 6 weeks. In the elderly person who has reduced bone mass, healing time is lengthened; complete healing frequently takes 3–6 months.

ELDERLY CONSIDERATIONS

Healing can be affected by a number of factors in addition to the aging process. Bone formation and strength rely on adequate nutrition. Calcium, phosphorus, vitamin D, and protein are necessary for production of new bone (see Chap. 53). For women, the loss of estro-

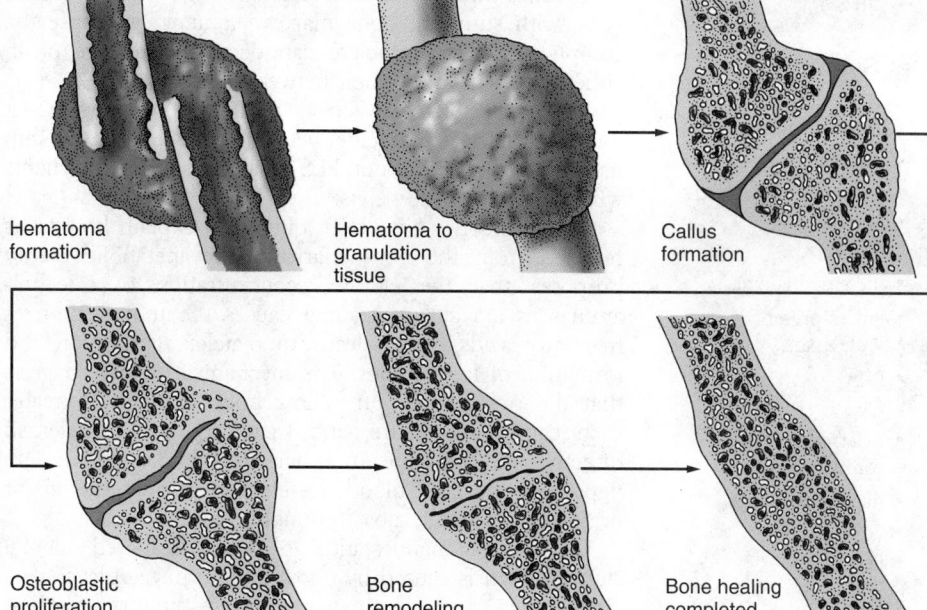

Hematoma formation

Hematoma to granulation tissue

Callus formation

Osteoblastic proliferation

Bone remodeling

Bone healing completed

Figure 54–2. The stages of bone healing.

gen after menopause is detrimental to the body's ability to form new bone tissue. Concurrent diseases can also affect the rate at which bone heals. For instance, peripheral vascular diseases, such as arteriosclerosis, reduce arterial circulation to bone; thus the bone receives less oxygen and nutrients needed for repair.

Complications of Fractures

Regardless of the type or location of the fracture, several life-threatening complications can result from the injury. The nurse must be able to recognize the clinical manifestations of impending complications so that treatment can be started immediately. In some cases, careful monitoring and assessment can prevent these complications.

ACUTE COMPARTMENT SYNDROME. Compartments are sheaths of inelastic fascia that support and partition muscles, blood vessels, and nerves in the body. Acute compartment syndrome (ACS) is a serious condition in which increased pressure within one or more compartments causes massive compromise of circulation to the area. The most common sites for ACS are the compartments in the lower leg and the dorsal and volar compartments of the forearm.

The pressure to the compartment can be from an external or internal source. Tight, bulky dressings and casts are examples of external pressure. Blood or fluid accumulation is a common source of internal pressure. ACS is not limited to clients with musculoskeletal problems; clients with severe burns, extensive insect bites, or massive infiltration of intravenous fluids are also susceptible to compartment syndrome. In these situations, edema increases pressure in one or more compartments.

Pathophysiologic Changes. The primary pathophysiologic changes of increased compartment pressure are

sometimes referred to as the ischemia-edema cycle. Capillaries within the viable muscle dilate, which raises capillary pressure. Capillaries become more permeable because of the release of histamine by the ischemic muscle tissue. As a result, plasma proteins leak into the interstitial fluid space, and edema occurs. Edema causes pressure on nerve endings and subsequent pain. Blood flow to the area is reduced, and further ischemia results. The color of the tissue pales, and pulses begin to weaken; the affected area is usually palpably tense. If the condition is not treated, cyanosis, tingling, numbness, paresis, and severe pain occur. Chart 54-1 summarizes the sequence of pathophysiologic events in compartment syndrome and the associated clinical assessment findings.

Acute compartment syndrome is not common, but it creates an emergency situation when it does occur. Within 4–6 hours after the onset of compartment syndrome, neuromuscular damage is irreversible. The limb can become useless in 24–48 hours.

Possible Results of Compartment Syndrome. Specific problems resulting from compartment syndrome include infection, persistent motor weakness in the affected extremity, contracture, and myoglobinuric renal failure. In extreme cases, amputation may be necessary.

Infection from the necrotic tissue may become severe enough that amputation of the limb is warranted. *Motor weakness* from injured nerves is not reversible, and the client may require braces or other orthotic devices for assistance in movement. Volkmann's *contractures*, which can begin within 12 hours of the pressure increase, result from shortening of the ischemic muscle and nerve involvement.

Myoglobulinuric renal failure is a potentially fatal complication of compartment syndrome. It commonly occurs when large or multiple compartments are involved. Injured muscle tissues release myoglobulin (muscle protein)

Chart 54–1

Key Features of Compartment Syndrome

Physiologic Change	Clinical Findings
• Increased compartment pressure	• No change
• Increased capillary permeability	• Edema
• Release of histamine	• Increased edema
• Increased blood flow to area	• Pulses present • Pink tissue
• Pressure on nerve endings	• Pain
• Increased tissue pressure	• Referred pain to compartment
• Decreased tissue perfusion	• Increased edema
• Decreased oxygen to tissues	• Pallor
• Increased production of lactic acid	• Unequal pulses • Flexed posture
• Anaerobic metabolism	• Cyanosis
• Vasodilation	• Increased edema
• Increased blood flow	• Tense muscle swelling
• Increased tissue pressure	• Tingling • Numbness
• Increased edema	• Paresthesia
• Muscle ischemia	• Severe pain
• Tissue necrosis	• Paresis

---

into the circulation, and the protein is then filtered by the kidneys. Although the exact pathophysiologic mechanisms are unknown, it is suspected that myoglobulin causes renal vasoconstriction or has a direct toxic effect on the kidney. The release of myoglobulin also causes metabolic acidosis, hyperkalemia, and sepsis. In severe cases, it may necessitate amputation of the affected limb.

SHOCK. Bone is quite vascular; therefore, there is a risk of bleeding with bone injury. In addition, trauma can sever adjacent arteries and cause hemorrhage; consequently, hypovolemic shock can develop rapidly. (The pathophysiology of hypovolemic shock is described in Chapter 39.)

FAT EMBOLISM SYNDROME. Fat embolism syndrome (FES) is a serious complication, usually resulting from a fracture, in which fat globules are released from the yellow bone marrow into the bloodstream. FES may also occur, although less often, with pancreatitis, diabetic coma, osteomyelitis, and sickle cell anemia. Factors that increase a client's risk for fat emboli include elevated serum glucose or cholesterol level, increased capillary fragility, and inability to cope with physiologic stress.

The release of fat emboli is most likely with fractures of

long bones or multiple fractures, although a break in any bone with sufficient bone marrow content can cause the complication. The problem can occur at any age or in either sex, but young men between ages 20 and 40 years and older persons between ages 70 and 80 years are at the greatest risk. The elderly client with a fractured hip has the highest risk, but FES is also common in clients with fractures of the pelvis.

Several theories have been offered to explain how fat is released from the bone marrow. The metabolic theory proposes that the elevated concentration of catecholamines as a result of trauma causes the mobilization of free fatty acids, which leads to platelet aggregation and formation of fat globules. The mechanical theory suggests that the pressure within yellow bone marrow is greater than capillary pressure, and therefore fats are released directly from the bone. In either case, the fat globules are deposited in small blood vessels that supply the major organs of the body, most commonly the lungs.

The *earliest* manifestation of FES is altered mental status, which is caused by a low arterial oxygen level. The client then typically experiences respiratory distress, tachycardia, hypertension, tachypnea, fever, and petechiae, a macular, measles-like rash over the neck, upper arms, and/or chest and abdomen. Petechiae are characteristic of fat emboli, but the physiologic basis for their development is not known.

Laboratory findings in FES include

- Increased erythrocyte sedimentation rate
- Decreased serum albumin and calcium levels
- Decreased red blood cell and platelet counts
- Increased serum lipase level

These changes in blood values are poorly understood, but they aid in diagnosis of the condition.

Fat embolism usually occurs within 48 hours of the fracture and can result in respiratory failure or death, often from pulmonary edema. When the lungs are affected, the complication may be misdiagnosed as a pulmonary embolism from a blood clot (Chart 54–2).

THROMBOEMBOLITIC COMPLICATIONS. Deep venous thrombosis (DVT) frequently develops in people who are immobile because of trauma, surgery, or disability. It is the most common complication of lower-extremity surgery or trauma and the most frequently fatal complication of musculoskeletal surgery. A person who smokes, is obese, has heart disease, or has a history of thromboembolitic complications is at an increased risk for DVT. The incidence of life-threatening embolic conditions is highest in elderly clients, particularly during the first 2–3 days after musculoskeletal surgery.

Certain fracture sites are more often associated with life-threatening thrombi. For example, DVT that leads to pulmonary embolism is more likely to develop in clients with fractures of the lower extremities and pelvis. Local venous stasis or trauma increases the chance of DVT in clients with musculoskeletal trauma. (A further discussion of DVT is found in Chapter 38.)

INFECTION. Any time there is trauma to tissues, the body's defense system is disrupted. Wound infections are

Chart 54-2

Key Features of Pulmonary Emboli: Fat Embolism Versus Blood Clot Embolism

Characteristic	Fat Embolism	Blood Clot Embolism
Definition	• Obstruction of the pulmonary vascular bed by fat globules	• Obstruction of the pulmonary artery by a blood clot or clots
Origin	• 95% from fractures of the long bones; occurs usually within 48 hr	• 85% from deep venous thrombosis in the legs or pelvis; can occur anytime
Assessment findings	• Altered mental status (earliest sign) • Increased respirations, pulse, temperature • Chest pain • Dyspnea • Decreased level of consciousness • Petechiae (50%–60%) • Retinal hemorrhage (not common) • Mild thrombocytopenia	• Same as for fat embolism, except no petechiae
Treatment	• Bed rest • Gentle handling • Oxygen • Hydration (intravenous fluids) • Possibly steroid therapy	• Preventive measures (e.g., leg exercises, antiembolism stockings) • Bed rest • Oxygen • Possibly mechanical ventilation • Heparin therapy • Thrombolytics • Possible surgery: ligation of vena cava, vena cava umbrella

the most common type of infection resulting from orthopedic trauma; they range from superficial skin infections to deep wound abscesses. Infection can also be caused by indwelling hardware used to repair a fracture surgically, such as pins, plates, and rods. Clostridial infections can result in gas gangrene or tetanus and can prevent the bone from healing properly.

Bone infection, or osteomyelitis, is most common with open fractures in which skin integrity is lost and after surgical repair of a fracture (see Chap. 53). For clients experiencing this type of trauma, the risk of hospital-acquired (nosocomial) infections is increased.

AVASCULAR NECROSIS. Avascular necrosis (AVN) is sometimes referred to as aseptic or ischemic necrosis or osteonecrosis. Blood supply to the bone is disrupted, which results in the death of bone tissue. AVN is most frequently a complication of hip fractures or any fracture in which there is displacement of bone. Surgical repair of fractures can also lead to AVN because the hardware can interfere with circulation.

DELAYED UNION, NONUNION, AND MAL-UNION. Delayed union describes a fracture that has not healed within 6 months of injury. Some fractures never achieve union; that is, they never completely heal (nonunion); others heal incorrectly (malunion). These problems are most common in clients with tibial fractures, fractures for which a number of different treatment techniques have been used (e.g., cast, traction), and pathologic fractures. Union may also be delayed or not

achieved in the elderly client. If bone does not heal, the client typically experiences pain and immobility from deformity.

Etiology

The primary cause of a fracture is trauma from a motor vehicle accident (MVA) or fall. The trauma experienced may be a direct blow to the bone or an indirect force from muscle contractions or pulling forces on the bone. Sports, vigorous exercise, and malnutrition are contributing factors. Bone diseases, such as osteoporosis, increase the risk of a fracture in the elderly.

Incidence/Prevalence

The incidence of fractures depends on the location of the injury. Rib fractures are the most common type in the adult population. Femoral shaft fractures occur most often in young and middle-aged adults. The incidence of proximal femur (hip) fractures is highest in the elderly population. Humeral fractures are common in adults; the older the person, usually the more proximal the fracture. Wrist (Colles') fractures are typically seen in the middle-aged and elderly population.

WOMEN'S HEALTH CONSIDERATIONS

It is estimated that more than 1 million fractures occur annually in the United States result from osteoporosis, and most occur in middle-aged and elderly women (Maher et al., 1994).

TRANSCULTURAL CONSIDERATIONS

 Hip fractures occur less often in African Americans and in men of any race than in Caucasian women because the incidence of osteoporosis is lower in these groups (Giger & Davidhizar, 1995).

Collaborative Management

Assessment

➤ History

The nurse collects data to determine the cause of the fracture, which helps in developing an individualized plan of care for the client.

Preceding Events. The nurse asks the client to recall the specific events up to the time of the injury. Some type of force, such as incision, crush, acceleration or deceleration, shearing, and friction, leads to most musculoskeletal injuries (Maher et al., 1994). As a result, several body systems are frequently affected.

Incisional (as from a knife wound) and crush injuries cause hemorrhage and disrupt blood flow to major organs. Acceleration or deceleration injuries cause direct trauma to the spleen, brain, and kidneys when these organs are moved from their fixed locations in the body. Shearing and friction damage the skin and cause a high level of wound contamination.

By asking about the events leading to the injury, the nurse can determine which forces have been experienced and therefore which body systems or parts of the body to assess. For example, a forward fall often results in Colles' fracture of the wrist because the person tries to catch himself or herself with an outstretched hand. Knowing the mechanism of injury also helps the nurse determine whether other types of injury, such as head and spinal cord injury, may be present.

Other History. A medication history, including substance abuse (recreational drug use), is important regardless of age. For example, a young adult may have had an excessive amount of alcohol, which contributed to a motor vehicle accident or to a fall at the work site. Many elderly persons also consume alcohol and an assortment of prescribed and over-the-counter drugs, which can cause dizziness and loss of balance.

A medical history elicits possible causes of the fracture and gives clues as to how long it will take for the bone to heal. Certain diseases, such as bone cancer and Paget's disease, cause pathologic fractures that often do not achieve union.

The nurse asks about the client's occupation and recreational activities. Some occupations are more hazardous than others; for instance, construction work is potentially more physically dangerous than is office work. Certain hobbies and recreational activities are also extremely hazardous (e.g., skiing and bungee jumping). Contact sports, such as football and ice hockey, often result in musculoskeletal injuries, including fractures. Other activities do not have such an obvious potential for injury but can

cause fractures nonetheless. For instance, daily jogging and frequent marching in a band can lead to fatigue fractures.

Because inadequate nutrition contributes to fractures and can inhibit bone healing, the nurse takes a complete nutritional history. Health promotion counseling is a major focus for comprehensive health care today (Scura & Whipple, 1997).

ELDERLY CONSIDERATIONS

This history is especially important for the elderly. For example, some elderly clients eat poorly because of loss of companionship and poor finances. They may be unable to prepare meals and thus rely on others for proper nutrition.

➤ Physical Assessment/Clinical Manifestations

Body System Assessment. The client with a fracture often sustains trauma to other body systems. Consequently, the nurse assesses all major body systems *first* for life-threatening complications, including head, thoracic, and abdominal injuries. The assessment of these areas is described elsewhere in this text.

Musculoskeletal Assessment. When inspecting the site of a possible fracture, the nurse observes for a change in bone alignment. The bone may appear deformed, or a limb may be internally or externally rotated. Accompanying these deviations may be an alteration in the length of the extremity (usually a shortening) or a change in bone shape. The nurse asks the client to move the involved body part. If pain is elicited, the movement is stopped immediately. Range of motion (ROM) is typically decreased. When the affected part is moved, the nurse may hear crepitation, a continuous grating sound created by bone fragments.

The nurse also observes the skin for integrity. If the skin is intact (closed fracture), the area over the fracture may be ecchymotic (bruised) from bleeding into the underlying soft tissues. Subcutaneous emphysema, the appearance of bubbles under the skin because of air trapping, is not uncommon but is seen later.

Swelling at the fracture site is rapid and can result in marked neurovascular compromise. Therefore, the nurse performs a thorough neurovascular assessment and compares the injured area with its symmetric counterpart. Skin color and temperature, sensation, mobility, pain, and pulses are assessed distal to the fracture site. If the fracture involves an extremity, the nurse checks the nails for capillary refill by applying pressure to the nail and observing for the speed of blood return. If nails are brittle or thick, the skin adjacent to the nail is assessed. Chart 54–3 describes the procedure for a neurovascular assessment, which is sometimes called a circulation check ("circ. check") or CMS (circulation, movement, sensation) assessment.

For an open fracture, the nurse determines the degree of soft-tissue damage and the amount of overt bleeding. The area may be lightly palpated for tenderness, but a sterile glove is worn if the skin is disrupted.

Chart 54–3

Nursing Care Highlight: Assessment of Neurovascular Status in Clients with Musculoskeletal Injury

Characteristic	Assessment Technique	Normal Findings
Skin color	• Inspect the area distal to the injury.	• No change in pigmentation compared with other parts of the body.
Skin temperature	• Palpate the area distal to the injury (the dorsum of the hands is most sensitive to temperature).	• The skin is warm.
Movement	• Ask the client to move the affected area or the area distal to the injury (active motion). • Move the area distal to the injury (passive motion).	• The client can move without discomfort. • No difference in comfort compared with active movement.
Sensation	• Ask the client if numbness or tingling is present (paresthesia). • Palpate with a safety pin or paper clip (especially the web space between the first and second toes or the web space between the thumb and forefinger).	• No numbness or tingling. • No difference in sensation in the affected and unaffected extremities. • Loss of sensation in these areas indicates perineal nerve or median nerve damage.
Pulses	• Palpate the pulses distal to the injury.	• Pulses are strong and easily palpated; no difference in the affected and unaffected extremities.
Capillary refill	• Press the nail beds distal to the injury until blanching occurs (or the skin near the nail if nails are thick and brittle).	• Blood returns (return to usual color) within 3 seconds (5 seconds for elderly clients).
Pain	• Ask the client about the location, nature, and frequency of the pain.	• Pain is usually localized and is often described as stabbing or throbbing.

Clients often complain of moderate to severe pain at the site of the fracture or in an adjacent or distal area. For example, clients with a fractured hip may have groin pain or pain referred to the back of the knee. Pain is usually due to muscle spasm and edema, which result from the fracture. In clients with one or more fractured ribs, severe pain occurs when deep breaths are taken. The nurse assesses the client's respiratory status, which may be severely compromised from pain or pneumothorax (air in the pleural cavity).

Special Assessment Considerations. For fractures of the shoulder and upper arm, the physical assessment is best done with the client in a sitting or standing position, if possible, so that shoulder drooping or other abnormal positioning can be seen. The nurse supports the affected arm and flexes the elbow to promote comfort during the assessment. For more distal areas of the arm, the assessment is done with the client in a supine position so that the extremity can be elevated to reduce swelling.

The nurse places the client in a supine position for assessment of the lower extremities and pelvis. A client with an impacted hip fracture may be able to walk for a short time after injury, although this is not recommended. The client with any type of hip fracture has pain and decreased range of motion in the hip.

Some fractures can cause internal organ damage, resulting in hemorrhage. When a pelvic fracture is suspected, the nurse assesses the client's vital signs, skin color, and level of consciousness for indications of possible hypovolemic shock. The urine is checked for blood, which indicates damage to the urinary system, often the bladder.

➤ Psychosocial Assessment

The psychosocial status of a client with a fracture depends on the extent of the injury and other complications. Hospitalization is usually not required for a single, uncomplicated fracture, and the client may return to usual daily activities within a few days. Healing is usually complete in a young adult in 4–6 weeks.

In contrast, a client suffering multiple trauma can be hospitalized for weeks and may undergo many surgical procedures and other treatments. For these clients, disruptions in lifestyle can create a high level of stress.

The stresses that result from a chronic condition affect relationships between the client and family members or significant others. The nurse assesses the client's feeling about himself or herself as a person and asks about how the client coped with previously experienced stressful events. The client's body image and sexuality may be altered by deformity, treatment modalities for fracture repair, and/or long-term immobilization.

➤ Laboratory Assessment

No special laboratory tests are available for clients who have fractures. The client's hemoglobin level and hematocrit are often low because of bleeding caused by the injury. If extensive soft-tissue damage accompanies the fracture, the erythrocyte sedimentation rate (ESR) may be elevated, which indicates the expected inflammatory response. If the ESR increases during fracture healing, the client may have a bone infection. During the healing stages, serum calcium and phosphorus levels are often increased as the bone releases these elements into the blood.

➤ Radiographic Assessment

The health care provider orders standard x-rays and tomograms to confirm a diagnosis of fracture. These reveal the bone disruption, malalignment, or deformity. If the x-ray does not show a fracture but the client is symptomatic, the x-ray is usually repeated with additional views.

The computed tomography (CT) scan is useful in detecting fractures of complex structures, such as the hip and pelvis. It also identifies compression fractures of the spine.

➤ Other Diagnostic Assessment

The health care provider may order a bone scan (with technetium or gallium) for help in detecting certain types of fractures, particularly pathologic and fatigue fractures. It is impossible for fractures of small bones or occult fractures to be visualized by conventional x-rays as early as by a bone scan. In addition, the bone scan can better determine fracture complications, such as delayed bone healing, nonunion, infection, and avascular necrosis.

Magnetic resonance imaging (MRI) is useful in determining the amount of soft-tissue damage that may have occurred with the fracture. It is also helpful in visualizing vertebral and skull fractures.

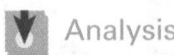 Analysis

➤ Common Nursing Diagnoses and Collaborative Problems

The common nursing diagnoses for clients with fractures include
  1. Risk for Peripheral Neurovascular Dysfunction related to bone and soft-tissue trauma and immobility
  2. Pain related to bone disruption, soft-tissue damage, muscle spasm, and edema
  3. Risk for Infection related to bone trauma and soft-tissue damage
  4. Impaired Physical Mobility related to pain
  5. Altered Nutrition: Less than Body Requirements related to additional metabolic need for healing of bone and soft tissues

➤ Additional Nursing Diagnoses and Collaborative Problems

In addition to the common nursing diagnoses, a client with a fracture may have one or more of the following diagnoses:
- Activity Intolerance related to pain and impaired mobility
- Constipation related to prolonged immobility (particularly in the elderly)
- Ineffective Individual Coping related to prolonged immobility, hospitalization, and/or lifestyle changes
- Ineffective Family Coping: Compromised related to the client's prolonged hospitalization and/or lifestyle changes
- Diversional Activity Deficit related to prolonged hospitalization and rehabilitation
- Anticipatory Grieving related to altered lifestyle
- Self Care Deficit related to pain and immobility
- Body Image Disturbance related to deformity and/or treatment modality
- Sexual Dysfunction related to pain and immobility
- Sleep Pattern Disturbance related to chronic pain and prolonged hospitalization
- Fear related to possible nursing home placement and/or death (particularly in the elderly)
- Impaired Skin Integrity and Impaired Tissue Integrity related to bone injury

Collaborative problems that may be appropriate for a client with a severe fracture include
- Potential for acute compartment syndrome
- Potential for hypovolemic shock
- Potential for fat embolism syndrome
- Potential for thromboembolitic complications
- Potential for avascular necrosis
- Potential for delayed healing, malunion, or nonunion

 Planning and Implementation

Risk for Peripheral Neurovascular Dysfunction

Planning: Expected Outcomes. The client is expected to have sufficient blood flow for adequate oxygen and nutrients to be provided to tissues, especially distal to the fracture site.

Interventions. A fracture can occur anywhere. The nurse provides emergency interventions until medical treatment in a hospital is available.

Emergency Care. A fracture may be accompanied by multiple injuries to vital organs. Therefore, the nurse *first* assesses the client for respiratory distress, bleeding, and head injury. If any of these is present, the nurse provides lifesaving care before being concerned about the fracture.

The fracture injury is then assessed (Chart 54–4). If the person is clothed, the nurse or another person trained in first aid cuts away clothing from the fracture site for best visualization. Bleeding is controlled by direct pressure on the area and digital pressure over the proximal artery nearest the fracture. At the same time, to prevent

Nursing Care Highlight: Emergency Care of the Client with an Extremity Fracture

1. Remove the client's clothing (cut, if necessary) to inspect the affected area.
2. Apply direct pressure on the area if there is bleeding and pressure over the proximal artery nearest the fracture.
3. Keep the client warm and in a supine position.
4. Check the neurovascular status of the area distal to the extremity: temperature, color, sensation, movement, and capillary refill. Compare affected and unaffected limbs.
5. Immobilize the extremity by splinting; include joints above and below the fracture site.
6. Cover the affected area with a clean cloth (e.g., a handkerchief).

shock, the nurse checks vital signs, places the client in a supine position, and keeps the client warm with coverings.

The nurse also

- Inspects the fracture site for intactness of skin, swelling, and deformity (e.g., shortening and rotation)
- Palpates the area *lightly* to determine temperature (coolness), decreased sensation, and blanching
- Assesses distal pulses by comparing affected and unaffected extremities, if applicable
- Assesses for motor function by asking the client to move an area distal to the fracture. For example, if a femoral fracture is suspected, the client is asked to move the ankle and foot on the affected side. The upper portion of the leg remains immobilized.

To prevent further damage, reduce pain, and increase circulation, the nurse immobilizes the area of the fracture by splinting. Any object or device that extends to the joints above and below the fracture can be used as a splint. At the scene of an accident, the nurse may need to improvise by using available materials, such as a tree limb or a board. If the skin is broken, the nurse applies a clean (preferably sterile) cloth loosely to prevent further contamination of the wound.

In the emergency department, physician's office, or clinic, fracture management begins with reduction and immobilization of the fracture.

- Reduction, or realignment of the bone ends for proper healing, is accomplished by a closed method (e.g., traction) or an open (surgical) procedure.
- Immobilization is achieved by the use of bandages, casts, traction, internal fixation, or external fixation.

The health care provider selects the treatment method on the basis of the fracture's type, location, and extent. These interventions prevent further injury and reduce discomfort. The nurse is responsible for maintaining these devices and for assessing, preventing, and intervening for complications that can result from their use.

Nonsurgical Management. Nonsurgical management typically involves closed reduction and immobilization

with a bandage, splint, cast, or traction. For each modality, the nurse's primary concern is assessment and prevention of neurovascular dysfunction or compromise.

Neurovascular Monitoring. The nurse performs a neurovascular assessment (see Chart 54-3) at frequent intervals if the client is admitted to the hospital, depending on the severity and extent of the fracture and agency policy. The nurse pays particular attention to *early* signs and symptoms of acute compartment syndrome (ACS) by doing a thorough pain assessment. The client with early ACS typically complains of severe, diffuse pain that is not relieved by analgesics; pain during passive motion is greater than pain during active motion. If the client presents with this complaint, the nurse notifies the health care provider *immediately*.

In some cases, clients at especially high risk for ACS are monitored by an invasive procedure. The method involves placement of a device (needle, wick, or slit catheter) into a compartment to measure its pressure. Critical pressures depend on which technique is used. The pressure reading is digitally displayed and should be within 10-30 mmHg of the client's diastolic blood pressure.

If ACS is verified, the surgeon may perform a fasciotomy by making an incision through the skin and subcutaneous tissues into the fascia of the affected compartment. This procedure relieves the pressure to restore circulation to the affected area. After fasciotomy, the nurse packs and dresses the open wound on a regular basis until secondary closure occurs, usually in 4-5 days. At that time, the surgeon usually debrides the wound and may apply a skin graft to promote healing.

Closed Reduction. Closed reduction is the most common nonsurgical method for managing a simple fracture. While applying a manual pull, or traction, on the bone, the health care provider manipulates the bone ends so that they realign. Anesthesia or analgesia may be used during this procedure to minimize pain. An x-ray verifies that the bone ends are approximated before the bone is immobilized.

Bandages and Splints. For certain areas of the body, such as the scapula and clavicle, an elastic or muslin bandage may be used to immobilize the bone during healing. Because upper-extremity bones do not bear weight, splints may be sufficient to keep bone fragments in place. Figure 54-3 illustrates the use of a wrist splint for fracture immobilization. A durable, flexible material

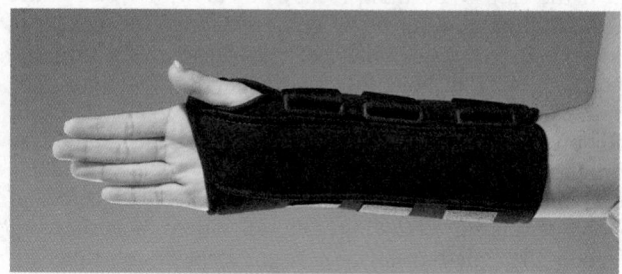

Figure 54-3. A universal wrist and forearm splint used for immobilization. (Courtesy of Smith & Nephew, Inc., Bracing and Support Systems.)

for splinting, Thermoplast, allows custom fitting to the client's body part.

The nurse's primary responsibility is to assess the area distal to the bandage or splint for neurovascular compromise. The client usually complains of increased discomfort that is not relieved by analgesics if the splint or bandage is too tight. The nurse teaches the client how to assess for circulatory changes. The nurse reminds the client to keep the device as dry and clean as possible for preventing skin breakdown and infection.

Casts. For more extensive fractures or fractures of the lower extremity, the physician or orthopedic technician applies a cast to hold bone fragments in place after reduction. A cast is a rigid device that immobilizes the affected body part while allowing other body parts to move. A cast also allows early mobility and reduces pain. Although its most common use is for fractures, a cast may be applied for correction of deformities (such as a rotated ankle) or for prevention of deformities (such as those seen in some clients with rheumatoid arthritis).

Cast Materials. Several types of materials are used to make the cast. The traditional plaster of Paris (anhydrous calcium sulfate) cast requires application of a well-fitted stockinette under the material. If the stockinette is too tight, it may impair circulation; if it is too loose, wrinkles can lead to the development of pressure ulcers and subsequent skin breakdown. Web padding is applied over the stockinette, followed by wet plaster rolls wrapped around the extremity or other body part. The cast feels hot because an immediate chemical reaction occurs, but it soon becomes damp and cool. This type of cast takes 24–72 hours to dry, depending on the size and location of the cast. A wet cast feels cold, smells musty, and is grayish. The cast is dry when it feels hard and firm, is odorless, and has a shiny white appearance.

On occasion, the plaster cast may have rough edges, which can crumble and cause skin irritation. To resolve this problem, the nurse petals the cast if the underlying stockinette does not cover the edges of the cast. Small strips of tape are placed over the rough edges to protect the skin. If the skin under the cast was disrupted, the physician, orthopedic technician, or specially trained nurse cuts a window into the cast so that the wound can be observed and cared for. A window is also an access for taking pulses, removing wound drains, or relieving abdominal distention when the client is in a body or spica cast.

If the cast is too tight, it may be cut with a cast cutter to relieve pressure or allow tissue swelling. The physician may choose to bivalve the cast (cut it lengthwise into two equal pieces) if bone healing is almost complete. The nurse can remove either half of the cast for inspection or for provision of care. The two pieces are then reunited by an elastic bandage wrap.

Synthetic materials for casts include fiberglass and polyester-cotton knit (Fig. 54–4). These materials are lighter than plaster and require minimal drying time. Fiberglass casts are dry in 10–15 minutes and can bear weight 30 minutes after application. Polyester-cotton casts take 7 minutes to dry and can withstand weight-bearing in approximately 20 minutes. Some health care providers

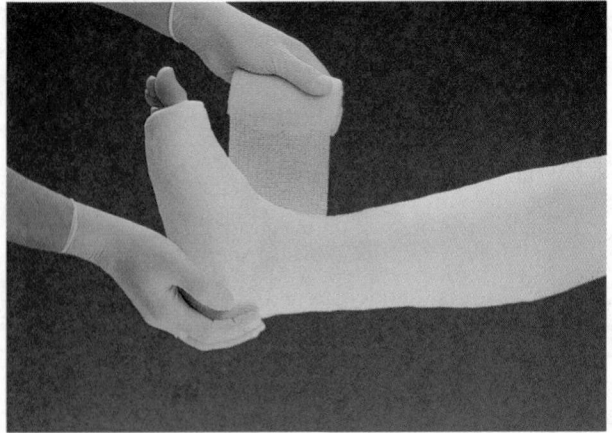

Figure 54–4. Application of a fiberglass synthetic cast. (Courtesy of Smith & Nephew Casting, Memphis, TN.)

use plaster of Paris casts for lower extremities and synthetic casts for upper extremities because plaster casts can bear more weight for a longer time.

Types of Casts. Casts can be generally divided into four main groups: arm casts, leg casts, cast braces, and body or spica casts. Table 54–1 describes specific casts that are used for various parts of the body.

When a client is in bed with an *arm cast,* the nurse uses a sling to elevate the arm above the client's heart to reduce swelling. The hand should be higher than the elbow. Ice may be ordered for the first 24–48 hours. When the client is out of bed, the nurse supports the arm with a sling placed around the neck to alleviate fatigue caused by the weight of the cast. The sling should distribute the weight over a large area of the client's shoulders and trunk, not just the neck.

A *leg cast* permits mobility and requires the client to use ambulatory aids, such as crutches. A cast shoe, sandal, or boot that attaches to the foot or a rubber walking pad attached to the sole of the cast assists the client in ambulation and helps prevent falls or damage to the cast (see Fig. 54–4). The nurse elevates the affected leg on several pillows to reduce swelling and applies ice for the first 24 hours or as ordered.

A *cast brace* enables the client to bend unaffected joints while the fracture is healing. The fracture must show signs of healing and minimal tissue edema before application of this cast. Two cylindric casts are made and connected by a hinge to allow joint movement. As healing occurs, the casts may be removed and replaced with a soft brace.

A *body cast* encircles the trunk of the body; a *spica cast* encases a portion of the trunk and one or two extremities. A client with either of these casts presents a special challenge for nursing care. Potential complications related to severe impairment in mobility include

- Skin breakdown
- Respiratory dysfunction, such as pneumonia and atelectasis
- Constipation
- Joint contractures

TABLE 54–1

Types of Casts Used for Musculoskeletal Trauma

Type and Characteristics of Cast	Use
Upper-Extremity Casts	
Short-arm cast (SAC) (extends from below the elbow to and including part of the hand)	• Stable fractures of the wrist (metacarpals, carpals, or distal radius)
Long-arm cast (LAC) (includes the upper arm to and including part of the hand)	• Unstable fractures of the wrist, distal humerus, radius, and ulna
Hanging-arm cast (same as LAC but heavier, with added loop at the mid-forearm)	• Fractures of the humerus that cannot be aligned by LAC • Light traction is possible while the client is in bed or by an attached strap that extends around the neck
Thumb spica (gauntlet) cast (similar to SAC with the thumb casted in abduction)	• Fractures of the thumb
Shoulder spica cast (the shoulder is casted in abduction with the elbow flexed)	• Unstable fractures of the shoulder girdle or humerus; dislocations of the shoulder
Lower-Extremity Casts	
Short-leg cast (SLC) (from below the knee to the base of the toes)	• Fractures of the ankle, metatarsals, and foot
Long-leg cast (LLC) (from the mid-upper thigh to the base of the toes)	• Unstable fractures of the tibia, fibula, and ankle
Walking cast (a walking device on the bottom of SLC or LLC)	• Same as for SLC or LLC
Leg cylinder (similar to SLC, but the ankle and foot are not casted)	• Stable fractures of the tibia, fibula, and knee
Long-leg cylinder (similar to LLC, but the ankle and foot are not casted)	• Stable fractures of the distal femur, proximal tibia, and knee
Cast Braces (or Brace Casts)	
Patellar weight-bearing cast (similar to SLC or leg cylinder)	• Midshaft or distal shaft fractures of the femur
External polycentric knee hinge cast (a hinge connects the lower and upper leg and allows 90 degrees of knee flexion)	• Same as for the patellar weight-bearing cast
Body Casts	
Hip spica (extends from below the nipple line down the affected leg [single], down the leg and half of the unaffected leg [1½], or down both legs [double])	• Dislocation of the hip • Pelvic and hip injuries
Risser's cast (the body jacket extends from the shoulders to beyond the iliac crests and hips, with a large opening over the anterior chest)	• Scoliosis • Thoracic spinal fractures
Halo cast (the body jacket contains a halo brace)	• Fractures of the cervical spine

In addition to physical limitations, the client in a body cast may experience *cast syndrome,* which is similar to a claustrophobic reaction. The client exhibits behaviors of acute anxiety, such as hyperventilation, diaphoresis, hypertension, and increased heart rate. Other physiologic manifestations are due to decreased gastrointestinal motility, which results in nausea, vomiting, and abdominal distention from paralytic ileus (cessation of peristalsis). Paralytic ileus is thought to be related to traction on the superior mesenteric artery, which reduces blood flow to the bowel. The management of ileus for this client is the same as for any client with the complication.

Cast Care. Before the cast is applied, the nurse explains the purpose of the cast and the procedure for its application to the client. For a plaster cast, it is particularly important for the nurse to warn the client about the heat that will be felt immediately after the wet cast is applied. The new cast, sometimes called a green cast, is not covered; this facilitates air-drying.

When a client with a wet plaster cast is moved and turned, the nurse handles the cast with the palms of the hands to prevent indentations and resultant areas of pressure on the client's skin. The client is turned every 1–2 hours to allow air to circulate and dry all parts of the cast. If the client is hospitalized, the nurse or assistive nursing personnel places a sign at the head of the client's bed as a reminder that the cast is wet and requires special handling. The client may be placed on a firm mattress, fracture bed, Roto-Rest bed, or other special bed to keep the cast aligned during the drying period. If the health care provider orders that the cast be elevated to reduce swelling, a cloth-covered pillow is used instead of one encased in plastic, which could cause the cast to retain heat and prevent drying. Elevation of the casted extremity reduces edema but may impair arterial circulation to the affected limb.

For preventing contamination by urine or feces, the perineal area of a dry long-leg or body cast is encased in a plastic, protective covering. Fracture pans are preferred to traditional bedpans because they are smaller and more comfortable for the client. Care is taken to prevent spillage onto the cast.

The nurse checks to ensure that the cast is not too tight and frequently monitors the client's neurovascular status, usually every hour for the first 24 hours after application (see Chart 54–3 for a description of the procedure and normal findings). The nurse should be able to insert a finger between the cast and the skin.

Once the plaster cast is dry, it is inspected at least once every 8 hours for drainage, cracking, crumbling, alignment, and fit. Areas of drainage on the cast are circled, dated, and monitored for change. It is not unusual, however, for bloody drainage to seep through the cast from an open fracture site. The nurse immediately reports sudden increases in the amount of drainage or a change in the integrity of the cast to the health care provider. After swelling decreases, it is not uncommon for the cast to become too loose and need replacement. If the client is not admitted to the hospital, he or she is given instructions regarding cast care, as discussed later in the Continuing Care section.

Cast Complications. During hospitalization, the nurse assesses for other complications resulting from casting that can be serious and life-threatening, such as infection, circulation impairment, and peripheral nerve damage. If the client returns home after cast application, the client and family are taught how to monitor for these complications and when to notify the health care provider.

Infection most often results from breakdown of skin under the cast (pressure necrosis). If pressure necrosis occurs, the client typically complains of a very painful "hot spot" under the cast, and the cast may feel warmer in the affected area. The nurse smells the area for mustiness or an unpleasant odor that would indicate infected material. If the infection progresses, a fever may develop.

Circulation impairment and peripheral nerve damage can result from constriction of the cast. The nurse performs frequent neurovascular assessments, as described in Chart 54–3. A client with a new cast may require hourly assessments. A client with a cast that is 3 or 4 days old usually requires assessments every 4–8 hours.

The client with a cast may be immobilized for a prolonged period, depending on the extent of the fracture and the type of cast. The nurse assesses for complications of immobility (see Chap. 13), such as skin breakdown, pneumonia, atelectasis, thromboembolism, and constipation.

Before the cast is removed, the nurse informs the client that the cast cutter will not injure the skin but that heat may be felt during the procedure. Specific nursing interventions required for a client with a cast are delineated in Chart 54–5.

Because of prolonged immobilization, a joint may become contracted, usually in a fixed state of flexion, or degenerative arthritis may develop from lack of weight-bearing, which is necessary for cartilage viability. Muscle can also atrophy from lack of exercise during prolonged immobilization of the affected body part, usually an extremity.

Traction. Traction is the application of a pulling force to a part of the body to provide reduction, alignment, and rest. Traction can also decrease muscle spasm (thus relieving pain) and prevent or correct deformity and tis-

---

Chart 54–5

Nursing Care Highlight: The Client with a Cast

- Monitor the neurovascular status of the casted extremity every 1–2 hr for the first 24 hr and every 4 hr thereafter:
  - Perform a circulation check as described in Chart 54–3.
  - Ask the client if the cast feels too tight.
  - Have the cast cutter available.
- Maintain cast integrity:
  - Turn the client every 1–2 hr.
  - Use the palms when handling a wet cast.
  - Do not turn the client by holding on to the abductor bar (e.g., hip spica).
  - Do not cover a wet cast or place it on a plastic-coated pillow.
  - Protect other parts from irritation caused by the rough surface of a synthetic cast.
  - Keep set plaster cast dry during bathing by covering it completely with plastic (also, tuck plastic into the ends to prevent water seepage under the cast).
  - Immerse a synthetic cast in water during bathing, if permitted.
  - Clean a soiled plaster cast with mild detergent and a damp cloth as necessary.
  - Inspect the cast when performing circulation checks for crumbling and cracking.
- Maintain skin integrity:
  - Examine the skin around the cast edges for redness and irritation.
  - Trim its edges to prevent roughness.
  - Petal the edge with 1- to 2-inch adhesive strips if stockinette edging is not used.
  - Do not use skin lotions or powder around the cast.
  - Teach the client not to place foreign objects inside the cast (e.g., wire hanger to scratch under the cast).
  - Smell the cast for foul odor and palpate for hot areas every shift.
  - Inspect the cast for an increase in drainage every shift.

---

sue damage. A client in traction is usually hospitalized longer but can generally move and exercise more readily without the weight and limitations of a cast.

Mechanical traction can be

- Continuous, as in fracture treatment
- Intermittent, for relief of muscle spasm in other types of musculoskeletal/neurologic trauma, such as low back pain (LBP)

Traction may also be classified as running traction or balanced suspension. In running traction, the pulling force is in one direction and the client's body acts as countertraction. Moving the body or bed position can alter the countertraction force. Balanced suspension provides the countertraction so that the pulling force of the traction is not altered when the bed or client is moved.

Types of Traction. Traction is typically referred to one of five types: skin, skeletal, plaster, brace, and circumferential.

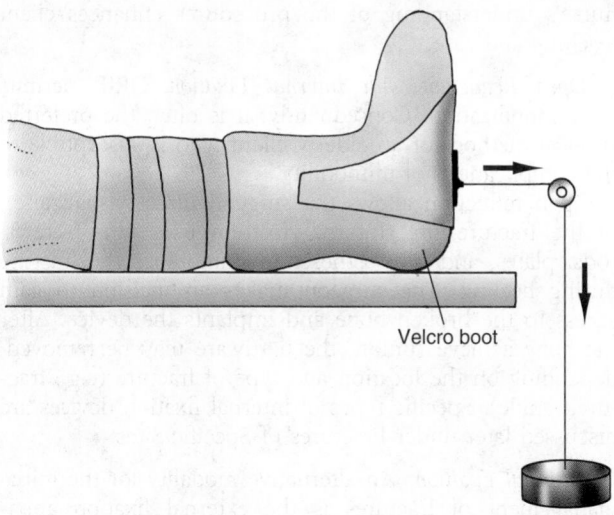

Figure 54–5. Buck's traction with a hook-and-loop fastener (Velcro) boot, commonly used for hip fractures.

Velcro boot

Skin traction involves the use of a Velcro boot (Buck's traction) (Fig. 54–5), belt, or halter, which is secured around a body part. The primary purpose of skin traction is to decrease painful muscle spasms that accompany fractures. The weight used as a pulling force is limited (5–10 pounds [2.3–4.5 kg]) to prevent injury to the skin.

In skeletal traction, pins (e.g., Steinmann), wires (e.g.,

Kirschner), tongs (e.g., Crutchfield), or screws are surgically inserted directly into bone. These allow the use of longer traction time and heavier weights (usually 15–30 pounds [6.8–13.6 kg]). Skeletal traction aids in bone re-alignment.

Plaster traction combines skeletal traction and a plaster cast. A brace traction device exerts a pull for correction of alignment deformities.

Circumferential traction uses a belt around the body, such as pelvic traction for low back problems.

Table 54–2 describes commonly used types of traction for various parts of the body.

Traction Care. The nurse may set up or assist in the set-up of traction. In larger or specialty hospitals or units, orthopedic technicians may set up traction. Once traction is applied, the nurse is responsible for maintaining the correct balance between traction pull and countertraction force. Weights are not usually removed without a physician's order; they are not usually lifted manually or allowed to sit on the floor. Weights should be freely hanging at all times. The nurse teaches this important point to staff members on the unit and to other personnel, such as in the radiology department.

The nurse inspects the skin at least every 8 hours for signs of irritation and inflammation. When possible, the nurse removes the belt or boot that is used for skin traction every 8 hours to inspect under the device.

TABLE 54–2

Types of Traction Used for Musculoskeletal Trauma	
Type and Characteristics of Traction	**Use**
Upper-Extremity Traction	
Sidearm skin or skeletal traction (the forearm is flexed and extended 90 degrees from the upper part of the body)	• Fractures of the humerus with or without involvement of the shoulder and clavicle
Overhead or 90–90 traction, skin or skeletal (the elbow is flexed and the arm is at a right angle to the body over the upper chest)	• Same as above (depends on the physician's preference)
Plaster traction (pins inserted through the bone are fixed in the cast)	• Fractures of the wrist
Lower-Extremity Traction	
Buck's extension traction (skin) (the affected leg is in extension)	• Fractures of the hip or femur preoperatively • Prevention of hip flexion contractures; reduction of low back muscle spasms (bilateral Buck's) • Hip dislocation
Russell's traction (similar to Buck's, but a sling under the knee suspends the leg)	• Fracture of the end of the tibia
Balanced skin or skeletal traction (the limb is usually elevated in a Thomas splint with Pearson's attachment, or a Böhler-Braun splint is used)	• Fractures of the femur and pelvis
Spinal Column and Pelvic Traction	
Cervical halter (a strap under the chin)	• Cervical muscle spasms, strain/sprain, or arthritis
Cervical skeletal (e.g., halo brace, Crutchfield tongs)	• Cervical fractures of the spine • Muscle spasms
Pelvic belt (a strap around the hips at the iliac crests is attached to weights at the foot of the bed)	• Pain, strain, sprain, or muscle spasms, in the lower back
Pelvic sling (a wide strap around the hips is attached to an overhead bar to keep the pelvis off the bed)	• Pelvic fractures and other pelvic injuries

When skeletal traction is used, the nurse pays particular attention to the points of entry of pins, wires, or screws for signs of inflammation or infection. A small amount of clear fluid drainage ("weeping") is expected. Most health care providers prefer that the nurse perform pin care every day. No standardized method or protocol for pin care throughout the United States has been established. Some health care providers and nurse specialists believe that cleaning the pins disrupts the skin's natural barrier to infection and advise against this care. In any case, the nurse observes pin sites at least every 8 hours for drainage, color, odor, and severe redness, which indicate inflammation and possible infection. Infection of the pin tract may result in osteomyelitis.

The nurse is responsible for checking traction equipment to ensure its proper functioning. All ropes, knots, and pulleys are inspected at least every 8 hours for loosening, fraying, and positioning. The nurse checks the weight for consistency with the health care provider's order. At times, the health care provider or qualified technician changes the weight without notifying the nurse or modifying the written order; the nurse contacts the person responsible for a new order for confirmation of the change. Sometimes one of the weights is accidentally displaced by a staff member or visitor who bumps into it. The nurse replaces the weights if they are not correct and notifies the health care provider or orthopedic technician.

If the client complains of severe pain from muscle spasm, the weights may be too heavy, or the client may need realignment. The nurse reports the pain to the health care provider if body realignment fails to reduce the discomfort. The nurse also assesses the neurovascular status of the affected body part to detect changes of circulatory compromise and subsequent tissue damage. As for clients with casts, circulation is usually monitored every hour for the first 24 hours after traction is applied and every 4 hours thereafter (see Chart 54–3).

ELDERLY CONSIDERATIONS

Elderly clients often have peripheral vascular disease, connective tissue disease, and/or diabetes. Therefore, they are at high risk for problems caused by skin or skeletal traction because of inadequate circulation and sensation. Traction of any type is not the ideal treatment for the elderly client because it necessitates a prolonged period of immobilization; serious complications can result, such as pneumonia and pulmonary emboli. Abrasions, ulcers, and other skin problems should be reported to the health care provider. Care must be taken to avoid pressure on the bony prominences and superficial nerves. Pressure on the peroneal nerve at the point where it passes around the neck of the fibulas must also be avoided, or footdrop could occur (Styrcula, 1994).

Surgical Management. For some types of fractures, casts and traction are not appropriate or sufficient treatment techniques. Open reduction with internal fixation (ORIF) is a common method of reducing and immobilizing a fracture. When this method is not feasible, external fixation with closed reduction is used. Although the nurse does not decide which surgical technique is used, the nurse's understanding of the procedures enhances client teaching and care.

Open Reduction with Internal Fixation. ORIF permits early mobilization. Consequently, it is often the preferred surgical method for an elderly client who is susceptible to the complications of immobility.

Open reduction allows the surgeon direct visualization of the fracture site. Internal fixation uses pins, screws, rods, plates, and/or prostheses to immobilize the fracture during healing. The surgeon makes an incision to gain access to the broken bone and implants the device. After the bone achieves union, the hardware may be removed, depending on the location and type of fracture (e.g., fractured ankle). Specific types of internal fixation devices are discussed later under Fractures of Specific Sites.

External Fixation. An alternative modality for the initial management of fractures is the external fixation apparatus, as shown in Figure 54–6. After fracture reduction, the physician makes small percutaneous incisions so that pins may be implanted into the bone. Several small holes are drilled into the bone, and metal pins are inserted through or into the bone. The pins are held in place by a large, external metal frame to prevent bone movement.

Advantages and Disadvantages. External fixation has several advantages over other immobilization techniques:
- There is minimal blood loss, in comparison with internal fixation.
- The device allows early ambulation and exercise of the affected body part while relieving pain.

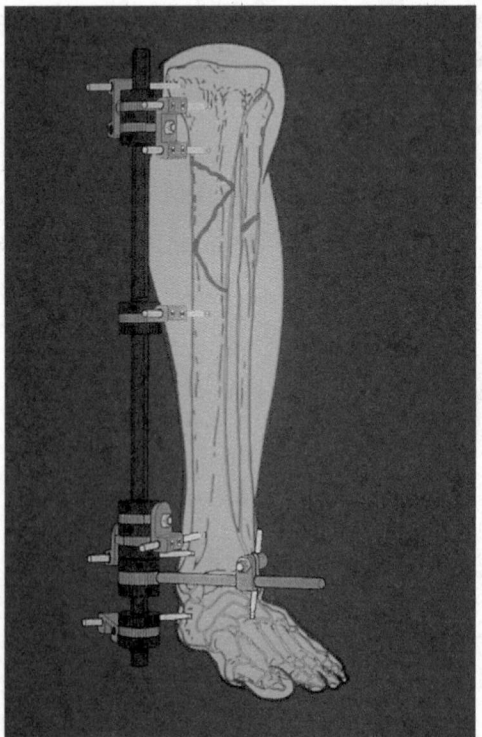

Figure 54–6. The Hex-Fix external fixation system for tibial fractures. (Courtesy of Smith & Nephew, Inc., Orthopaedic Division, Memphis, TN.)

- In open fractures, in which skin and tissue trauma accompanies the fracture, the device permits easy access to the wound and promotes healing. This method is often preferred to the use of a window in a cast for wound care.

A major disadvantage of external fixation is pin tract infection. Pin tract infections can lead to osteomyelitis, which is serious and difficult to treat (see Chapter 53 for discussion of osteomyelitis). For prevention of these infections, some agencies have a pin care procedure that is performed several times a day. The procedure is similar to that described earlier for skeletal traction pins (see Traction Care). As with skeletal traction, the need for special cleaning of the pins and the area around the pins is controversial. Regardless of whether pin care is done, the nurse inspects the pin sites at least daily for severe redness, swelling, and purulent drainage.

Care of the Client with an External Fixator. As with any fracture treatment, the nurse assesses the neurovascular status of the extremity distal to the fracture. External fixators may be used for an extremity or for fractures of the pelvis. External fixation is not long-term treatment for fractures. After a fixator is removed, the client may be placed in a cast until healing is complete.

The client with an external fixator may experience a body image disturbance. The frame is large and bulky, and the affected area may have massive tissue damage with dressings. The nurse is sensitive to this possibility in planning care.

Ilizarov Procedure. A relatively new external fixation procedure in the United States is sometimes used for malunion or nonunion fractures: the Ilizarov technique. The procedure originated in Russia more than 50 years ago.

A circular external fixation device stimulates bone growth. Unlike the traditional fixator, the Ilizarov external fixator promotes rotation, angulation, shortening, lengthening, and/or widening of bone while allowing healing of the soft-tissue defect. It is most commonly used in adults for congenital anomalies (especially dwarfism), joint contractures, segmental bone defects, and deformities from malunion or nonunion fractures. The nursing care of the client with this device is similar to the care of the client with other external fixation systems. Screening and teaching are particularly important because the client adjusts and cares for the apparatus for a prolonged time.

Preoperative Care. For stabilizing the fracture, the client may be placed in traction for several days before surgery. This procedure is typical of the management of a fractured hip, in which Buck's traction is often used preoperatively (see Fig. 54–5). The nurse teaches the client and family or significant others what to expect during and after the surgery. The preoperative care for a client undergoing musculoskeletal surgery is similar to that for any client preparing for surgery with general or epidural anesthesia. (See Chapter 20 for a thorough discussion of preoperative nursing care.)

Postoperative Care. The postoperative care for a client having ORIF or external fixator application is similar to

that provided for any client undergoing surgery (see Chapter 22 for discussion of postoperative care). However, because bone is a vascular, dynamic body tissue, the client is at risk for certain complications specific to fractures and musculoskeletal surgery. These problems (e.g., fat embolism and deep venous thrombosis) are discussed in the earlier section on pathophysiology.

Procedures for Nonunion. Some surgical repairs are not successful because the bone does not heal. Several additional options are available to the surgeon to promote bone union, such as electrical bone stimulation, bone grafting, and the newest therapy, ultrasound fracture treatment.

For selected clients, electrical bone stimulation may be successful. This procedure is based on research showing that bone has inherent electrical properties that are used in healing. The exact mechanism of action is unknown. Table 54–3 provides important information about the types of stimulators that may be used.

Another method of treating nonunion is bone grafting. A bone graft may also replace diseased bone or increase bone tissue for joint replacement. In most cases, chips of bone are taken from the client's iliac crest or other site and are packed or wired between the bone ends to facilitate union. Allografts from cadavers may also be used. These grafts are frozen or freeze-dried and stored under sterile conditions in a bone bank, usually in a hospital.

Bone banking from living donors is increasingly popular. If qualified, clients undergoing total hip replacement may donate their femoral heads to the bank for later use in bone grafting procedures for other clients. Careful screening ensures that the bone is healthy and that the donor client has no communicable disease. The bone cannot be donated without the client's written consent.

The newest advance in fracture healing modalities is low intensity pulsed ultrasound (also called Exogen therapy). Used for slow-healing fractures or for fresh fractures as an alternative to surgery, ultrasound treatment has yielded excellent results. The client applies the treatment for about 20 minutes each day. It has no contraindications or adverse effects. The outcomes of ultrasound fracture treatment have been so effective that health insurers are covering the cost of treatment in many cases.

➤ Pain

Planning: Expected Outcomes. The client is expected to experience a reduction or alleviation of pain after appropriate interventions.

Interventions. The nonsurgical or surgical management of fractures through reduction and immobilization helps reduce pain and prevents neurovascular injury. The client often requires drug therapy and other pain relief measures to meet the goal.

Drug Therapy. Musculoskeletal pain related to soft-tissue damage, bone disruption, and muscle spasm is one of the most severe types of pain that can be experienced. The client often has the pain for a prolonged time, which makes pain management difficult. The health care pro-

TABLE 54–3

Features of Electrical Bone Stimulation

Technique	Description	Duration of Treatment	Risk	Client Responsibilities
Noninvasive electromagnetic coils system	• Uses external coils on the skin or a cast to induce weak electrical currents in bones called pulsing electromagnetic fields	• 5–6 mo	• None known because the current is weak • The system is not used on the arms if the client has a pacemaker	• Use 10–12 hr/day, preferably at night without interruption • Avoid weight-bearing until consent is given by the health care provider • Notify the health care provider if the alarm signals, which indicates equipment malfunction
Semi-invasive percutaneous stimulator	• One or more electrodes are placed at the fracture site, with one or more placed on the skin (the number depends on the type, severity, and treatment of the fracture)	• 3 mo	• Local skin irritation from electrodes (anode or cathode); breakage of cathode pins	• Avoid weight-bearing • Change the anode pad every 48 hr to avoid skin irritation
Fully implantable, direct current stimulator	• The entire system is placed at the fracture site under the skin; no external apparatus	• 5–6 mo	• Usual risk of complications with bone surgery	• Follow the health care provider's advice for weight-bearing and activity; can often begin immediately after surgery

vider commonly prescribes opioid analgesics, anti-inflammatory drugs, and muscle relaxants.

For clients with chronic, severe pain, opioid and non-opioid drugs are alternated or given together for prevention of drug dependence. The nurse and client mutually decide on the best times for the strong pain relievers to be administered (e.g., before a complex dressing change and at bedtime). The nurse observes the client carefully for the effectiveness of the medication and its side effects. An early sign of acute compartment syndrome is often the sudden inability of pain medication to relieve pain. (Chapter 9 discusses the various methods of pain management, including epidural analgesia and patient-controlled analgesia.)

Complementary Therapies. With chronic, severe pain, the client cannot depend solely on drugs for relief. The nurse uses temporary pain relief measures, such as ice or heat, depending on the cause of the pain. If swelling causes pressure on the affected area, ice and elevation of the affected body part may be appropriate. Muscle spasms are best relieved by application of heat and massage. Other physical measures include a warm, soothing bath, a back rub, and the use of therapeutic touch.

If these measures are not effective in reducing pain, the nurse uses distraction, imagery, or music therapy as alternatives. The nurse teaches the client relaxation techniques, such as deep breathing, for use during periods of

severe pain. (Chapter 9 discusses these techniques in detail.)

➤ Risk for Infection

Planning: Expected Outcomes. The client is expected to be free of a wound or bone infection.

Interventions. When caring for a client with a fracture, particularly an open fracture, the nurse uses strict aseptic technique for dressing changes and wound irrigations. Signs and symptoms of local inflammation with purulent drainage are reported immediately to the physician. Other infections, such as pneumonia and urinary tract infection, may also occur days after the fracture. The nurse or assistive nursing personnel monitors the client's vital signs every 4–8 hours; increases in temperature and pulse often indicate systemic infection.

For most clients with an open fracture, the health care provider prescribes one or more broad-spectrum antibiotics prophylactically. This treatment is especially important in clients with fractures requiring surgical repair.

➤ Impaired Physical Mobility

Planning: Expected Outcomes. The client is expected to be free of complications of impaired mobility and independent in ambulation and mobility, such as transferring from bed to chair.

Interventions. The interventions necessary for this diagnosis can be grouped into two types: those that help prevent complications of impaired mobility, and those that help increase the client's mobility.

Prevention of Complications. The nurse plays a vital role in preventing and assessing complications in immobilized clients with fractures. Additional information about nursing care for preventing problems associated with immobility is found in Chapter 13 and in the discussion of specific complications in the earlier section on pathophysiology.

ELDERLY CONSIDERATIONS

The risk of each complication is dramatically increased if surgery is performed. The elderly client is at the greatest risk; physiologic changes and prolonged immobility predispose the elderly to these complications.

Promotion of Mobility. The use of crutches or a walker increases mobility and assists in ambulation. The client may progress to use of a cane.

Crutches. Crutches are the most commonly used ambulatory aid for many types of musculoskeletal trauma (e.g., fractures, sprains, and amputations). In most agencies, the physical therapist fits the client for crutches and teaches the client how to ambulate with them on flat surfaces and stairs. The nurse's role may be to reinforce the instructions and evaluate whether the client is using the crutches correctly.

Walking with crutches requires strong upper extremities, balance, and coordination. For this reason, crutches are not used as often for elderly clients. To prepare for using crutches, the client practices upper-extremity-strengthening exercises. The unaffected extremity and gluteal muscles are also strengthened because they carry the weight that is usually supported by the affected extremity.

Recommended leg exercises include quadriceps setting ("quad sets"), gluteal sets, and straight-leg raises (SLR). There are several ways of performing each of these exercises. For quad sets, the supine client flattens the knee by pushing it against the bed. This position is held for 5 to 10 seconds as the quadriceps muscle of the thigh tenses. This procedure is alternated five times for each leg. For gluteal sets, the supine client bends the knees, tightens the buttocks, and raises the buttocks slightly off the bed. This procedure is repeated 5–10 times, depending on the client's tolerance.

The therapist pads the tips and axillary bars of the crutches; padding prevents the tips from slipping and the bars from damaging the axillae. For preventing pressure on the axillary nerve, there should be two to three finger-breadths between the axilla and the top of the crutch when the crutch tip is at least 6 inches (15 cm) diagonally in front of the foot. The crutch is adjusted by the therapist so that the elbow is flexed no more than 30 degrees when the palm is on the handle (Fig. 54–7).

There are several types of gaits for walking with crutches. The most common one for musculoskeletal injury is the three-point gait, which allows minimal weight-bearing on the affected leg. The physical therapist initially teaches the use of crutches. The nurse may review this

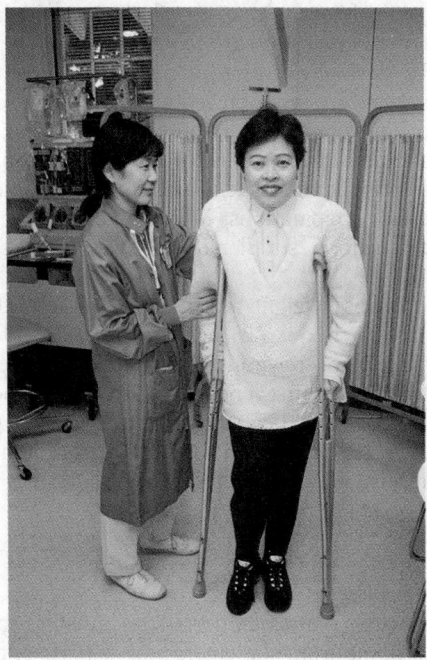

Figure 54–7. Assisting the client with crutch-walking. Note how the therapist guards the client and how the client's elbows are at no more than 30 degrees of flexion.

information and observe the client for correct use of these aids.

Walker. A walker is most often used by the elderly client who needs additional support for balance. The physical therapist assesses the strength of the upper extremities and the unaffected leg. Strength is improved with exercise as needed.

Cane. A cane is sometimes used if the client needs only minimal support for an affected leg. The straight cane offers the least support. A hemi-cane or quad-cane provides a broader base for the cane and therefore more support for the client. The cane is placed on the *unaffected* side and should create no more than 30 degrees of flexion of the elbow. The top of the cane should be parallel to the greater trochanter of the femur.

➤ *Altered Nutrition: Less than Body Requirements*

Planning: Expected Outcomes. The client is expected to maintain an adequate dietary intake to promote healing and prevent complications.

Interventions. Nursing interventions focus on meeting the client's nutritional needs. The nurse assesses the client's food likes and dislikes and collaborates with the dietitian to plan meals that are both appealing and nutritional. For promotion of bone and tissue healing, the client needs a high-protein, high-calorie diet. Supplements of vitamins B and C are also required for tissue nutrition. Many clients with fractures are immobilized for extended periods; thus they are predisposed to hypocalcemia, which results in loss of calcium from bone and in subsequent bone fragility. The nurse teaches the client to increase intake of foods high in calcium, particularly milk and milk products if they are tolerated.

In 7–10 days after injury, a negative nitrogen balance can develop in an immobilized client because of an increase in catabolism without compensatory protein intake. The nurse offers frequent small feedings and supplements of high-protein liquids, such as Ensure or Carnation Instant Breakfast preparations. Milk shakes are an excellent protein and calorie supplement as well as a source of calcium.

Because of less weight-bearing, the immobilized client with a fracture frequently becomes anemic. Blood loss from the injury or reparative surgery contributes to the anemic state. The nurse encourages intake of foods high in iron content. The health care provider may prescribe an oral iron supplement. It is not uncommon for the client to receive a daily multivitamin with iron.

 Continuing Care

The client with an uncomplicated fracture is usually discharged to home from the emergency department. Elderly clients with hip or other fractures or clients with multiple trauma are hospitalized and then often transferred to a rehabilitation setting or to a long-term care facility for rehabilitation or permanent residence. To ensure continuity of care, the case manager or the discharge planner in the hospital communicates the client's plan of care to the health care agency receiving the client.

➤ **Health Teaching**

The client with a fracture may be discharged from the hospital, emergency department, office, or clinic with a bandage, splint, cast, or external fixator. The nurse gives verbal and written instructions to the client on the care of these devices. (Chart 54–6) describes care of the affected extremity after removal of the cast.

The client may also need to continue wound care at home. The nurse teaches the client and caregiver how to assess and dress the wound to promote healing and prevent infection. The client is taught how to recognize complications (discussed earlier in this chapter) and when and where to contact professional health care should complications occur.

Chart 54–6

Education Guide: Care of the Extremity After Cast Removal

- Remove scaly, dead skin carefully by soaking—do not scrub.
- Move the extremity carefully. Expect discomfort, weakness, and decreased range of motion.
- Support the extremity with pillows or your orthotic device until strength and movement return.
- Exercise slowly as instructed by your physical therapist.
- Wear support stockings or elastic bandages to prevent swelling (for lower extremity).

Additional educational needs depend on the type of fracture and fracture repair. Care of external fixators and casts is discussed earlier in this chapter.

➤ **Home Care Management**

If the client is discharged to home, the nurse or case manager assesses the home environment for structural barriers to mobility, such as stairs.

ELDERLY CONSIDERATIONS

A home assessment is particularly important for elderly clients. A cast is bulky and requires room for maneuvering and ambulating. In collaboration with the therapy team, the nurse instructs the client and family or significant others to remove scatter rugs and other items that can contribute to falls. The rooms should not be cluttered with furniture, so that the client can maneuver with crutches, a walker, or a cane. An elevated toilet seat or shower chair may be needed to promote independence in toileting.

➤ **Health Care Resources**

The nurse identifies potential or actual problems in the hospital and arranges for follow-up care at home. For example, professional counseling for depression may need to continue after the client's discharge from the hospital. A social worker may need to help the client apply for funds to pay medical bills. If there is severe bone and tissue damage, the nurse must be realistic and help the client understand the long-term nature of the recovery period—particularly if the client experiences a major complication, such as infection, while in the hospital. Multiple treatment techniques and surgical procedures required for complications can be mentally and emotionally draining for the client and family. A vocational counselor may be needed to help the client seek a different type of job, depending on the nature of the fracture.

The client with a severe injury and multiple treatment modalities may need follow-up care in the home by a home health nurse. An elderly or incapacitated client may need assistance with activities of daily living, which is provided by home health aides. The nurse in the hospital anticipates the client's needs and arranges for these services, usually with the assistance of the social worker.

It is extremely important for the hospital nurse to communicate the client's needs to the nurse or aide who will care for the client at home. A physical therapist may come to the home, or the client may go to a clinic, hospital, or private office for follow-up physical therapy after discharge from the hospital. An occupational therapist assists with retraining in the home environment for activities of daily living; adaptations in the home enable the client to be independent.

 Evaluation

On the basis of the identified nursing diagnoses and collaborative problems, the nurse evaluates the care provided to the client with a fracture. Expected outcomes include that the client

- Maintains adequate tissue perfusion, as evidenced by bone and soft-tissue healing
- States that pain is reduced or alleviated
- Does not acquire an infection of the bone or soft tissues
- Independently ambulates with or without ambulatory aids and provides self-care
- Does not experience complications of immobility
- Maintains an adequate nutritional intake, as evidenced by bone and soft-tissue healing

Fractures of Specific Sites

Upper Extremity Fractures

Fractures of the Clavicle

Fractures of the clavicle typically result from a fall on an outstretched hand, a fall on the shoulder, or a direct injury. Most clavicular fractures are self-healing; a splint or bandage is used for immobilization. Complicated fractures, although uncommon, may require open reduction with internal fixation (ORIF) by pins, wires, or screws.

Fractures of the Scapula

Scapular fractures are not common and are usually caused by direct impact to the area. Serious internal trauma can accompany these fractures, including pneumothorax, pulmonary contusion, and fractured ribs.

The shoulder is immobilized with a sling and swathe or a shoulder immobilizer until the fracture heals, usually in 2–4 weeks. Intra-articular neck and glenoid fractures may require surgical intervention with plate and screw fixation.

Fractures of the Humerus

Fractures of the proximal humerus, particularly impacted or displaced fractures, are common in the elderly. An impacted injury is usually treated conservatively, with a sling for immobilization. A displaced fracture often requires ORIF with pins or a prosthetic device.

Humeral shaft fractures are generally corrected by closed reduction and the application of a hanging arm cast or splint. If necessary, the fracture is repaired surgically (with an intramedullary rod or metal plate and screws) or with external fixation. Nonunion of the bone and radial nerve palsy are frequent complications of this fracture. Bone grafting facilitates union; prolonged splinting is necessary while the radial nerve regenerates.

A direct blow to the condyles of the distal humerus can cause either or both condyles to fracture, usually in a T- or Y-shaped configuration. The most serious complication is damage to the brachial or median nerve. Condylar fracture is usually treated by ORIF with a series of screws, although skeletal traction and casting can be used.

Fractures of the Olecranon

Fractures of the olecranon are relatively common in adults and typically result from a fall on the elbow. Many are successfully treated by closed reduction and the application of a cast. The healing process usually takes more than 2 months, and several additional months may be needed before full use of the elbow is achieved. ORIF is performed for displaced fractures, and a splint is worn during the healing phase.

Fractures of the Radius and Ulna

Forearm fractures of the ulna without accompanying injury to the radius are rare. As with other fractures of long bones, closed reduction with casting may be the appropriate treatment. If the fracture is displaced, ORIF with intramedullary (IM) rods or plates and screws is required.

WOMEN'S HEALTH CONSIDERATIONS

Colles' fracture, or distal radius fracture, is common in the elderly (particularly women); it results most often from a fall on an open hand. The distal radius has a large percentage of cancellous bone, the type that is initially affected by osteoporosis. (Chapter 53 describes osteoporosis, or loss of bone mass, in detail.) The options for reduction and immobilization include splinting, casting, plaster-and-pin fixation, or external fixation with a frame (if soft-tissue damage is present).

Fractures of the Wrist and Hand

One or more of the bones in the wrist and hand can break, but the most common fracture is of the carpal scaphoid bone in young adult men. This is also one of the most misdiagnosed fractures because it is poorly visualized on an x-ray. Closed reduction and casting for 6–12 weeks is the treatment of choice. If the bone does not heal, open reduction and bone grafting are performed.

Fractures of the metacarpals and phalanges are usually not displaced, which makes their treatment less difficult than that of other fractures. Metacarpal fractures are immobilized for 3–4 weeks. Phalangeal fractures are immobilized in finger splints for 10–14 days.

Lower Extremity Fractures

Fractures of the Hip

Hip fractures include those involving the upper third of the femur and are classified as intracapsular (within the joint capsule) or extracapsular (outside the joint capsule). These types are further divided according to fracture location (Fig. 54–8).

ELDERLY CONSIDERATIONS

Hip fractures occur most frequently in elderly persons, particularly women who have osteoporosis. Repair of hip fracture is rapidly becoming the most common surgical procedure for people older than 85 years. As many as 50% of elderly clients who sustain a hip fracture die within 1 year of injury from medical complications caused by the fracture or by immobility that occurs after the fracture.

Falls cause most hip fractures; impaction or displacement, especially of the femoral neck, often results. If the degree of osteoporosis is so severe that it prevents surgi-

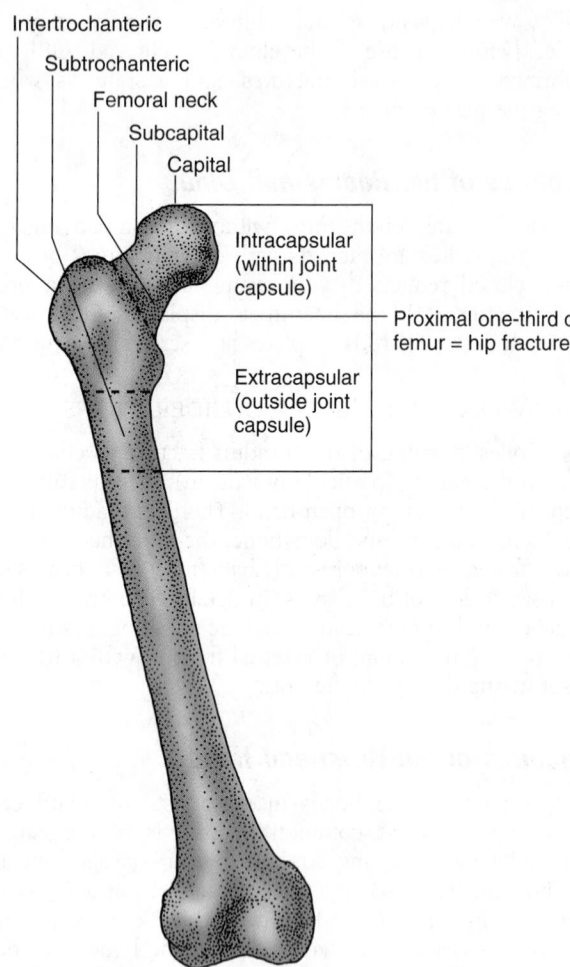

Figure 54–8. The types of hip fractures.

cal intervention, the client may be incapacitated for the remainder of his or her life.

The treatment of choice is surgical repair, when possible, to allow the elderly client to get out of bed. Depending on the exact location of the fracture, open reduction with internal fixation (ORIF) may include an intramedullary rod, pins, a prosthesis, or a fixed sliding plate (such as a compression screw). The client with a compression screw can usually ambulate a few days after surgery and has a decreased chance of infection and nonunion, in comparison with clients for whom other procedures are used. If the femoral neck or head is fractured, a prosthetic device is implanted. Figures 54–9 and 54–10 illustrate examples of these devices used for ORIF of the hip. Nonsurgical options are Buck's traction and skeletal traction, followed by use of a cast brace.

Hip fractures are common. Nurses in all health care settings need to know how to care for the special needs of the elderly client with hip fracture (Client Care Plan). The care is similar to that needed by elderly clients having a total hip replacement (see Chap. 24).

Elderly clients having a fractured hip repair are cared for at home by family or other lay caregivers or are admitted for rehabilitation in a nursing home or other type facility. Williams et al. (1996) studied the effects of

caregiving on family members as they provided care for female clients recovering from hip fractures. The researchers found that caregivers need information and support in their role. Nurses should be more aware of the burden of caregiving in the home and assist in meeting the needs of the family or other lay caregivers (See Research Applications for Nursing).

Fractures of the Femur

Fractures of the lower two thirds of the femur usually result from trauma, often a motor vehicle accident. A femoral fracture is seldom immobilized by casting because the powerful muscles of the thigh become spastic, which causes displacement of bone ends. Extensive hemorrhage is associated with femoral fracture.

Skeletal traction, followed by a cast brace or hip spica cast, is the typical nonsurgical treatment. Surgical treatment is ORIF with nails, rods, or a compression screw. In a few cases, external fixation may be employed. Healing time for a femoral fracture may be 6 months or longer.

Fractures of the Patella

Like most other fractures, patellar fractures result from direct impact. The surgeon typically repairs the fracture by closed reduction and casting or internal fixation with screws.

Fractures of the Tibia and Fibula

Trauma to the lower leg most often causes fractures of both the tibia and the fibula, particularly the lower third ("tib-fib" fractures).

The three basic treatment techniques are closed reduction with casting, internal fixation, and external fixation. If closed reduction is used, the client wears a cast for at least 8–10 weeks. Delayed union is not unusual with this

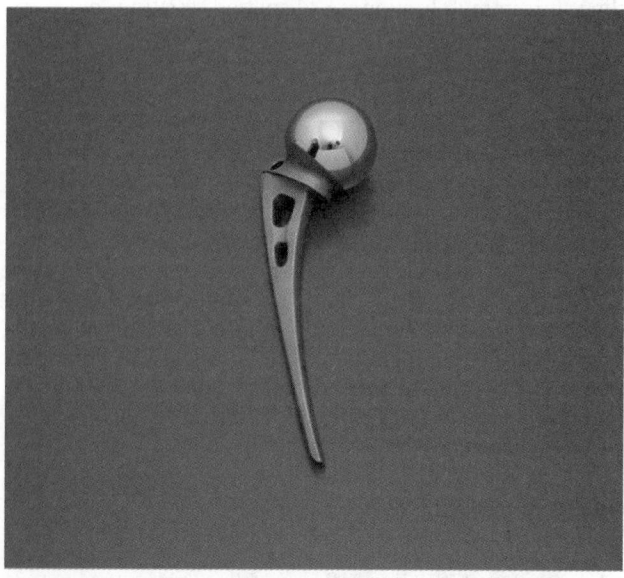

Figure 54–9. The Moore prosthesis, which is used for hip fractures. (Courtesy of the Orthopaedic Division of Smith & Nephew, Inc., Memphis, TN.)

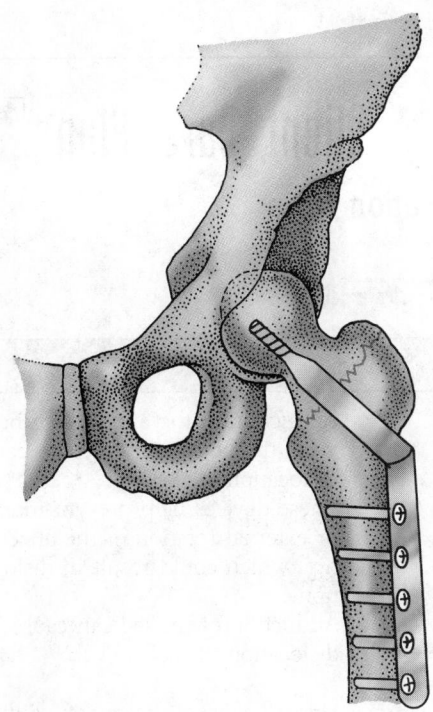

Figure 54–10. A compression hip screw used for open reduction internal fixation (ORIF) of the hip.

type of fracture. Internal fixation with nails or a plate and screws, followed by a long leg cast for 4–6 weeks, is another option. When the fractures cause extensive skin and soft-tissue damage, the initial treatment may be external fixation, often for 6–10 weeks.

Fractures of the Ankle and Foot

Ankle fractures are described by their anatomic place of injury. For example, a bimalleolar (Pott's) fracture involves the medial malleolus of the tibia and the lateral malleolus of the fibula. Because of the instability of the ankle joint, the fracture can result from supination and eversion, pronation and abduction, or pronation and eversion. These forces generally create spiral, transverse, or oblique breaks, which are often difficult to treat and present problems in healing. A combination of closed and open techniques may be used, depending on the severity and extent of the fracture. An arthrodesis (fusion) may be needed if the bone does not heal.

Treatment of fractures of the foot or phalanges is similar to that of other fractures, with either closed or open reduction. Phalangeal fractures are more painful than but not as serious as most other types of fractures.

Fractures of the Ribs and Sternum

Chest trauma may cause fractures of the ribs or sternum; the most commonly fractured ribs are numbers 4 through 8. The major concern with rib and sternal fractures is the potential for puncture of the lungs, heart, or arteries by bone fragments or ends. Fractures of the lower ribs may damage underlying organs, such as the liver, spleen, or kidneys.

Fractures of the Pelvis

Because the pelvis is close to major organs and blood vessels, associated internal damage is the chief concern in fracture management. After head injuries, pelvic fractures are the second most common cause of death from trauma. In young adults, pelvic fractures typically result from motor vehicle accidents or falls from buildings; falls are the most common cause in the elderly. The major concern related to pelvic injury is venous oozing or arterial bleeding. Loss of blood volume leads to hypovolemic shock.

Internal abdominal trauma is assessed by checking for the presence of blood in the urine and stool and by watching the abdomen for the development of rigidity or swelling. The trauma team may use peritoneal lavage for assessment of hemorrhage.

Fractures of the pelvis are divided into two broad categories: non–weight-bearing and weight-bearing fractures.

When a non–weight-bearing part of the pelvis is fractured, such as one of the pubic rami or the iliac crest, treatment can be as minimal as bed rest on a firm mattress or bed board. This type of fracture can be quite painful, and the client may need stool softeners to facilitate defecation. Well-stabilized fractures usually heal in 2 months.

A weight-bearing fracture, such as a fractured sacrum or acetabulum, may necessitate the use of skeletal traction, double-hip spica cast, open reduction with internal fixation, or external fixator. Clients are kept non–weight-

---

▷ Research Applications for Nursing

Are Caregiver Expectations of Hip Fracture Recovery Realistic?

Williams, M. A., Oberst, M. T., Bjorklund, B. C., & Hughes, S. H. (1996). Family caregiving in cases of hip fracture. Rehabilitation Nursing, 21(3), 124–131, 138.

In this prospective study, 57 family caregivers were provided with information before the client's hospital discharge and again 2, 8, and 14 weeks after discharge. The caregivers were then asked about caregiving demands and problems, their mood, expectations about recovery, and advice to future caregivers. All clients receiving care were women who had lived at home before the fracture.

Nonspouses reported the most demands and problems, and their distress did not improve. These caregivers seemed to have unrealistic expectations about the length of the recovery period. By 14 weeks, 35% felt that the client's mobility was worse than they had expected. The most frequent advice to future caregivers was to be patient.

Critique. This study is one of the few that have examined the effects of caregiving on families. The impact of education and support was measured as perceived by the caregivers, not judgments made by the researchers or others.

Possible Nursing Implications. As the population ages and more care is provided in the home setting, support and education for caregivers become increasingly crucial. The nurse plays a major role in providing information and emotional support to both client and family members.

Client Care Plan

The Client with an Open Reduction and Internal Fixation for a Fractured Hip

Nursing Diagnosis No. 1: Risk for Injury related to subluxation or dislocation

Expected Outcomes	Nursing Interventions	Rationale
The client will not experience subluxation or dislocation of the operative hip during the hospital stay.	▪ Place an abduction pillow, a splint, or bed pillow between the client's legs in bed. ▪ Use a leg cradle or similar device to align the affected leg.	▪ Adduction of the affected leg beyond the body's midline can cause dislocation of the hip. ▪ These devices help prevent internal or external rotation of the affected hip, which could result in dislocation.

	▪ Turn the client carefully toward either side to prevent adduction (check the physician's order).
	▪ Do not flex the operative hip beyond 90 degrees.
	  ▪ Use an elevated toilet seat.
	  ▪ Have the client sit in a supporting chair with straight back and seat.
	▪ Teach the client not to cross the legs.
		▪ Adduction of the leg can cause dislocation of the hip.
		
		▪ Hyperflexion of the operative hip can cause dislocation.
		
		▪ Crossing the legs causes adduction.

Nursing Diagnosis No. 2: Pain related to surgical incision

Expected Outcomes	Nursing Interventions	Rationale
The client will experience alleviation or reduction of surgical pain.	▪ Give pain medication as needed; anticipate the client's need if the client cannot verbalize (epidural or patient-controlled analgesia may be used). ▪ Give pain medication after the physical therapy session or other periods of increased activity. ▪ Use a fracture pan instead of a traditional bedpan. ▪ Assess the appropriateness of using a transcutaneous electrical nerve stimulation (TENS) unit (consult the physician). ▪ Use nondrug pain relief measures, such as distraction, music, and relaxation exercises as needed.	▪ Relieving the client's pain helps the client to participate more fully in the plan of care. ▪ A fracture pan does not require as much lifting by the client; lifting increases pain. ▪ Nondrug pain relief measures may reduce the use of opioid analgesia.

Client Care Plan

Nursing Diagnosis No. 3: Risk for Infection related to impaired skin integrity

Expected Outcomes	Nursing Interventions	Rationale
The client will not experience surgical wound infection.	■ Inspect the surgical dressing for drainage and document the type and amount. ■ Monitor and measure the drainage collected in a surgical drain, such as Hemovac (keep the suction device compressed to prevent hematoma formation, which increases the risk of infection). ■ After removal of the surgical dressing, inspect the incision for redness, swelling, and warmth. ■ If a dressing is used, change the dressing by using sterile technique. ■ Monitor vital signs every 4 hr for 1–3 days.	■ Purulent drainage indicates wound infection. ■ Drains allow the removal of exudate, which can be a medium for bacterial growth. ■ Signs of inflammation may indicate an infectious process. ■ Sterile conditions reduce the chance of infection. ■ Elevated pulse and temperature may indicate wound infection.

Nursing Diagnosis No. 4: Impaired Physical Mobility related to hip precautions and surgical pain

Expected Outcomes	Nursing Interventions	Rationale

The client will experience increased physical mobility.	■ Reinforce transfer and ambulation techniques (walker or crutches) as taught by the physical therapist.
	  ■ Have the trapeze and overhead frame on the bed before surgery and teach the client to use the device.
	  ■ Teach the client to bear weight to tolerance (or to bear weight partially for at least 6 wk postoperatively).
	■ Assess the client's need for assistive-adaptive devices to perform activities of daily living (ADL) independently; consult with an occupational therapist.
	■ Assess for and prevent complications of prolonged immobility, such as deep venous thrombosis, skin breakdown, or hypostatic pneumonia. (See Chap. 13 and earlier portions of this chapter for nursing assessment and prevention of complications.)
		■ Increasing mobility promotes the client's independence and return to society as a functional member.
		
		■ Complications of immobility cause the client discomfort and prolonged hospitalization.

bearing (NWB) or partial weight-bearing (PWB) for 6–8 weeks and progress to full weight-bearing by about 12 weeks.

Fractures at Other Sites

Because the skull and vertebral column protect the brain and spinal cord, these fractures are described in Chapter 47. The nurse must be aware of the special care required for these clients because of possible neurologic damage resulting from these fractures. Fractures of the mandible or nose and other facial trauma are discussed elsewhere in the text.

Amputations
Overview

An amputation is the removal of a part of the body. The nurse recognizes that the psychosocial ramifications of the procedure are often more devastating than the physical impairment that results. The loss experienced by the client is complete and permanent and causes a change in body image and often in self-esteem. As with other types of loss, the client can be expected to progress through phases of the grieving process.

Pathophysiology
Surgical Amputation

Amputations range from removal of part of a digit to removal of nearly half the entire body. The surgeon performs an amputation by one of two methods: open (or guillotine) method or closed (or flap) method.

The open method is used for clients who have or are likely to develop an infection. The wound remains open, and drains allow exudate to escape from the site until the infection clears. The surgeon may suture the skin flaps over the wound at a later time.

In the closed technique, the surgeon pulls the skin flaps over the bone end and sutures them in place as part of the amputation procedure. One or more drains are typically inserted.

In either the closed or open method, the surgeon attempts to preserve as much of the part as possible and to keep major joints intact for maximal postoperative mobility.

Traumatic Amputation

Not all amputations are surgically planned. Some, classified as traumatic amputations, occur when a body part is severed unexpectedly (e.g., by a chain saw). Because the amputated part in these clients is usually healthy, attempts to replant it may be made.

One of the most likely replantations involves one or more digits. The current recommendation for pre-hospital care is that the severed digit be wrapped in a cool, dry cloth and moistened with normal saline, if possible. The digit should then be placed in a sealed plastic bag. The bag is placed in ice water. Contact between the digit and the water is avoided to prevent tissue damage. Any semi-detached parts of the digit should not be removed.

Levels of Amputation

LOWER EXTREMITY. Lower-extremity amputations are performed much more frequently than upper-extremity amputations are. Five types of lower-extremity (LE) amputations may be performed (Fig. 54–11).

The loss of any or all of the small toes presents a minor disability. Loss of the great toe is significant because it affects balance, gait, and "push off" ability during walking. Midfoot amputations, such as the Lisfranc and Chopart, and the Syme amputation are common procedures for peripheral vascular disease. In the Syme amputation, most of the foot is removed but the ankle remains. The advantage of this surgery over traditional amputations below the knee is that weight-bearing can be accomplished without use of a prosthesis and without pain.

There is intense effort to preserve knee joints with below-knee amputation (BKA) rather than above-knee amputation (AKA). When the cause for the amputation extends beyond the knee, however, above-knee or higher amputations are performed. Hip disarticulation, or removal of the hip joint, and hemipelvectomy procedures are more common in younger clients than in elderly clients, who cannot easily handle the cumbersome prostheses required for ambulation. The higher the level of amputation, the more energy is required for ambulation. These higher level procedures are typically done for cancer of the bone, osteomyelitis, or trauma. Hemicorporectomy (hemipelvectomy and translumbar amputation) is a rare radical procedure performed as a last resort for cancer.

UPPER EXTREMITY. Fewer than 10% of all amputations are upper-extremity amputations. An amputation of

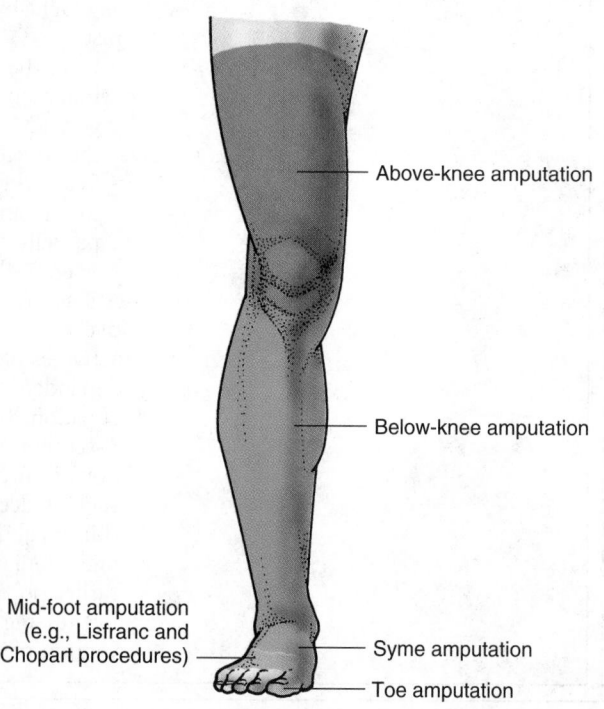

Figure 54–11. Common levels of lower-extremity amputation.

any part of the upper extremity is generally more incapacitating than one of the leg. The arms and hands are necessary for activities of daily living, such as feeding, bathing, dressing, and driving a car. As much length as possible is saved to maintain function. Early replacement with a prosthetic device is vital for the client with this type of amputation.

Complications of Amputations

Common complications of elective or traumatic amputations include

- Hemorrhage
- Infection
- Phantom limb pain
- Problems associated with immobility
- Neuroma
- Flexion contractures

HEMORRHAGE. When a person loses part or all of an extremity either by surgery or by trauma, major blood vessels are severed, which causes bleeding. If the bleeding is uncontrolled, the client is at risk for hypovolemic shock and possibly death.

INFECTION. As with any surgical procedure or trauma, infection can occur in the wound or the bone (osteomyelitis). The elderly client who is debilitated and confused is at the greatest risk because excreta may soil the wound, or the client may remove the dressing and pick at the incision.

PHANTOM LIMB PAIN. Phantom limb pain (PLP) is a frequent complication of amputation. As many as 80% of all amputees experience residual limb (sometimes referred to as "stump") pain or PLP at intervals throughout the first postoperative year (Yetzer, 1996). PLP is rare in clients who experience traumatic amputations.

No one theory explains or predicts PLP. Three theories are being researched:

- The peripheral nervous system theory
- The central nervous system theory
- The psychological theory

The peripheral nervous system theory implies that sensations remain as a result of severing peripheral nerves during the amputation. The central nervous system theory is actually a group of theories. One of the most popular is that the normal sympathetic reflex causing vasoconstriction during surgery does not shut off. As a result, decreased circulation to the residual limb causes pain. Neither of these physiologic theories completely explains PLP. Most likely, a psychological component helps predict and explain this phenomenon. Stress, anxiety, and depression often worsen or trigger an episode of PLP but are not likely to be the causative factors.

When experiencing PLP, the client complains of pain in the removed body part, most often shortly after surgery. The pain is often described either as an intense burning or crushing sensation or as cramping. Some clients say they feel as if the removed part is in a distorted, uncomfortable position; they experience numbness and tingling as well as pain, sometimes called phantom limb sensation.

Some clients report that the most distal area of the removed part feels as if it is retracted into the residual limb end. For most clients, the pain is triggered by touching the residual limb, by temperature and barometric pressure changes, by concurrent illness, by fatigue, and by emotional stress. Routine activities, such as urination, can trigger the pain in other clients. If the pain is long-standing, especially before the amputation, any stimulus can cause the pain, including touching any part of the body.

PROBLEMS ASSOCIATED WITH IMMOBILITY. Because the client experiences reduced mobility as a result of surgery, the complications of atelectasis, pneumonia, thromboembolism, and skin breakdown can readily occur. These problems are discussed in the section on pathophysiology of fractures earlier in this chapter.

NEUROMA. Neuroma—a sensitive tumor consisting of nerve cells found at severed nerve endings—forms most often in amputations of the upper extremity but can occur anywhere.

FLEXION CONTRACTURES. Flexion contractures of the hip or knee are seen in clients with amputations of the lower extremity. This complication must be avoided so that the client can ambulate with a prosthesis.

Etiology

Most knowledge about amputations was obtained during World War II when trauma necessitated a loss of one or more body parts. Today, with highly sophisticated microsurgery for revascularization of tissues to save limbs, amputations related to trauma are less likely to be needed. Amputations are also performed less often for

- Thermal injuries, such as frostbite and burns
- Tumors
- Infections
- Metabolic disorders, such as Paget's disease
- Congenital anomalies

Limb salvage procedures, such as those described in Chapter 53 (under Interventions in the section on bone cancer), have reduced the need for amputation.

Traumatic amputations most often result from accidents. A person may be cleaning lawn mower blades or a snow blower without disconnecting the machine. A motor vehicle or industrial machine accident may also cause an amputation.

ELDERLY CONSIDERATIONS

The primary indication for surgical amputation is *ischemia* from peripheral vascular disease in the elderly client (see Chapter 38 for discussion of this disease). The rate of lower-extremity amputation, for example, is much greater among diabetic clients than among nondiabetic clients because of peripheral neuropathy and peripheral vascular disease. In addition, these elderly diabetic clients have visual, cardiac, and kidney problems. A client with an amputation of one leg because of poor circulation will often have an amputation of the other leg within 3–5 years (Yetzer, 1996).

Incidence/Prevalence

Surgical amputations are not as common as they were before 1980, although more than 60,000 are performed each year in the United States (Yetzer, 1996).

The typical client undergoing the procedure is a middle-aged or elderly diabetic man with a lengthy history of smoking. The client most likely has failed to care for his feet properly, which has resulted in a nonhealing, infected foot ulcer and possibly gangrene.

The second largest group having amputations consists of young men who experience motorcycle or other vehicular accidents or who are injured at work by industrial equipment. These men may either experience a traumatic amputation or have a surgical amputation because of a severe crushing injury and massive soft-tissue damage.

TRANSCULTURAL CONSIDERATIONS

 The incidence of lower-extremity amputations is greater in the African-American population because the incidence of major diseases leading to amputation, such as diabetes and arteriosclerosis, is greater in this population (Giger & Davidhizar, 1995).

Collaborative Management

Assessment

➤ Physical Assessment/Clinical Manifestations

The nurse's primary concern preoperatively is to assess circulation in other parts of the body when the client has peripheral vascular disease. The nurse assesses skin color, temperature, sensation, and pulses in both affected and unaffected extremities. Capillary refill is evaluated by applying pressure to the nail bed and waiting for the brisk return of normal color. In the elderly client, however, this test may be difficult to do because the nails may be thick and opaque. In this situation, the skin near the nail bed can be assessed (see Chart 54–3).

➤ Psychosocial Assessment

People react differently to the loss of a body part. The nurse needs to be aware that an amputation of a portion of one finger can be traumatic to the client, and therefore the loss must not be underestimated. The client undergoing an amputation faces a complete, permanent loss. The nurse assesses the client's psychological preparation for a planned amputation and expects the client to experience the grieving process. Adjustment to a traumatic, unexpected amputation is often more difficult than accepting a planned one. The young client may be bitter, hostile, and uncooperative. In addition to loss of a body part, the client may lose a job, the ability to participate in favorite recreational activities, or a social relationship if the other person cannot accept the body change. (Chapter 12 discusses the nursing assessment for a client experiencing loss.)

The client is faced with an altered self-concept. The physical alteration that results from an amputation affects body image and self-esteem. For example, a client may think that an intimate relationship with a mate is no longer possible. An elderly client may feel a loss of independence. The nurse assesses the client's feelings about himself or herself to identify areas in which the client needs emotional support. (See Chapter 10 for a complete discussion of body image and assessment tools.)

The nurse tries to determine the client's willingness and motivation to withstand prolonged rehabilitation after the amputation. Asking questions about how the client has dealt with previous life crises can provide clues. The client's willingness to change careers or other activities is also determined. Adjustment to the amputation and rehabilitation is less difficult if the client is willing to make necessary changes.

In addition to assessing the client's psychosocial status, the nurse assesses the family's or significant others' reaction to the surgery. The family's response usually correlates directly with the client's progress during recovery and rehabilitation. The family can be expected to grieve for the loss and must be allowed to adjust to the change in the client.

The nurse also assesses the client's coping abilities and helps the client identify personal strengths and weaknesses. The nurse ascertains the client's religious or spiritual beliefs because certain groups require that the amputated body part be stored for later burial with the rest of the body.

➤ Diagnostic Assessment

Routine preoperative x-rays, such as a chest x-ray, are done as appropriate for any client having surgery. The surgeon determines which tests are performed to assess for viability of the limb. A large number of noninvasive techniques are available to assist the physician in this evaluation. For complete accuracy, the physician does not rely on any single test.

One procedure is measurement of segmental limb blood pressures, which can also be used by the nurse at the bedside. In this test, an ankle/brachial index (ABI) is calculated by dividing ankle systolic pressure by brachial systolic pressure. A normal ABI is greater than or equal to 1.00.

Blood flow in an extremity can also be assessed by many other noninvasive tests, including Doppler ultrasonography and transcutaneous oxygen pressure ($TcPO_2$). The ultrasonography measures the velocity of blood flow in the limb. The $TcPO_2$ measures oxygen pressure to indicate blood flow in the limb.

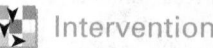 Interventions

Clients undergoing amputation today are not confined to a wheelchair. Advancements in the design of prosthetics have enabled clients to become independent in ambulation. Therefore, complications from extended bed rest are not common, even for the elderly client.

Assessment of Tissue Perfusion. The nurse's primary focus is to monitor for signs indicating that there is sufficient tissue perfusion but no hemorrhage. The skin flap at the end of the residual limb should be pink in a light-skinned person and not discolored (lighter or darker than other skin pigmentation) in a dark-skinned client. The area should be warm but not hot. The nurse assesses the closest proximal pulse for strength and compares it with that in the other extremity. If the client has bilateral vascular disease, however, comparison of limbs is not an accurate way of measuring blood flow.

Management of Pain. Pain management for the client with an amputation is not unlike that for any client in pain (see Chap. 9). If the client complains of phantom limb pain (PLP), the nurse recognizes that the pain is real. It is not therapeutic for the nurse to remind the client that the limb cannot be hurting because it is missing. To prevent increased pain, the nurse handles the residual limb carefully when assessing the site or changing the dressing.

Drug Therapy. Some studies have shown that opioids are not as effective for PLP as for residual limb pain. The health care provider prescribes medication on the basis of the type of PLP the client experiences. For instance, beta-blocking agents such as propranolol (Inderal, Apo-Propranolol♣, Detensol♣) are used for constant, dull burning. Anticonvulsant therapy may be used for knife-like pain; antispasmodics may be prescribed for muscle spasms or cramping.

Complementary Therapies. Over 50 treatments for PLP have been used worldwide. Transcutaneous electrical nerve stimulation (TENS) has had the most consistent pain relief rates. Other treatment measures include
- Ultrasound therapy
- Massage
- Exercises
- Biofeedback
- Distraction therapy
- Hypnosis
- Psychotherapy

Prevention of Infection. The surgeon typically prescribes broad-spectrum prophylactic antibiotics for several days postoperatively. The initial pressure dressing and drains are usually removed by the surgeon 48–72 hours after surgery. The nurse
- Inspects the wound site for signs of inflammation (e.g., redness and swelling)
- Monitors the healing process
- Records the characteristics of drainage, if present
- Changes the soft dressing every day until the sutures are removed

The below-the-knee limb may be casted in the operating suite for protection, prevention of edema, and prevention of knee contractures. On the third postoperative day, a window is opened in the distal end of the cast to inspect the suture line (Yetzer, 1996).

Promotion of Ambulation. The nurse or physician consults with a physical therapist to initiate exercises as soon as possible after surgery. If the amputation is a planned one, the therapist often works with the client before surgery to start muscle-strengthening exercises and to evaluate the need for aids, such as crutches. If the client can be instructed preoperatively in the use of these devices, learning how to ambulate after surgery is facilitated.

Exercise. For clients with above-knee amputations (AKA) or below-knee amputations (BKA), the nurse teaches range-of-motion exercises for prevention of flexion contractures, particularly of the hip and knee. A trapeze and an overhead frame, as shown in Figure 54–12, aid in strengthening the upper extremities and allow the client to move independently in bed.

A firm mattress is essential for preventing contracture with a lower-extremity amputation. The nurse assists the client into a prone position every 3–4 hours for 20- to 30-minute periods. This position may be uncomfortable for the client initially, but it is necessary to prevent hip flexion contractures. The nurse instructs the prone client to pull the residual limb close to the other leg and contract the gluteal muscles of the buttocks. For below-knee amputations, the nurse also teaches the client to push the residual limb down toward the bed while supporting it on a pillow. After the sutures are removed, the physical therapist may begin resistive exercises with a "sling-and-spring" apparatus which can also be used at home.

Elevation of a lower-leg residual limb on a pillow while the client is in a supine position is controversial. Some practitioners advocate avoiding this procedure at all times because it promotes hip or knee flexion contracture. Others allow elevation for the first 24 hours to reduce swelling and subsequent discomfort. The nurse inspects the residual limb daily to ensure that it lies completely flat on the bed.

Prostheses. For an elective amputation, the nurse arranges for the client to see a certified prosthetist-orthotist (CPO) so that planning can begin for the client's postoperative needs. Arrangements for replacing an upper extremity are especially important so that the client can provide self-care. Clients are sometimes fitted with a temporary prosthesis at the time of surgery. Other clients,

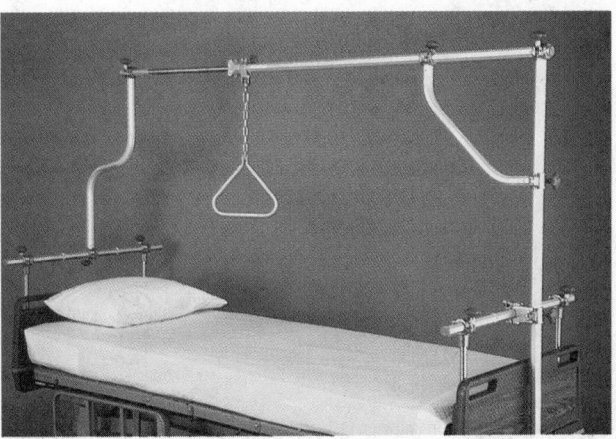

Figure 54–12. The placement of an overhead frame and trapeze on a bed.

particularly the elderly client with vascular disease, are fitted after the residual limb has healed.

When the client is fitted with a lower extremity prosthesis, he or she should bring a sturdy pair of shoes. The prosthesis will be adjusted to that heel height (Yetzer et al., 1994).

Preprosthetic Care. Several devices help shape and shrink the residual limb in preparation for the prosthesis. Rigid removable dressings are preferred because they decrease edema, protect and shape the limb, and allow easy access to the wound for inspection. The Jobst air splint, a plastic inflatable device, is sometimes used for this purpose. This device is usually inflated to 20 mmHg for 22 of 24 hours a day. One of its disadvantages is air leakage.

Wrapping with elastic bandages can be effective in reducing edema, shrinking the limb, and holding the wound dressing in place. Most surgeons prefer elastic bandages over a shrinker sock, although it is easier for the client to apply a sock than to wrap elastic bandages.

For wrapping to be effective, the nurse reapplies the bandages every 4–6 hours or more often if they become loose. Figure-eight wrapping prevents restriction of blood flow. The nurse decreases the tightness of the bandages while wrapping in a distal-to-proximal direction. After wrapping, the nurse anchors the bandages to the most proximal joint, such as above the knee for below-knee amputations (Fig. 54–13).

Prosthesis Application. The design of and materials for prostheses have improved dramatically over the years. Computer-assisted design and manufacturing (CAD-CAM) is now available for a custom fit.

One of the biggest developments in lower-extremity prosthetics is the ankle-foot prosthesis. The Flex-foot is used by more active amputees.

Promotion of Body Image. The client often experiences feelings of inadequacy as a result of losing a body part, especially the elderly person who was in poor health before surgery. If it is possible, the nurse arranges for the client to meet with a rehabilitated amputee. If the client is elderly, an elderly amputee is the ideal person with whom the client should interact.

Use of the word *stump* for referring to the remaining portion of the limb is controversial. Clients have reported feeling as if they were part of a tree when the term was used. However, some rehabilitation specialists who routinely work with amputees believe the term is appropriate because it forces the client to realize what has happened

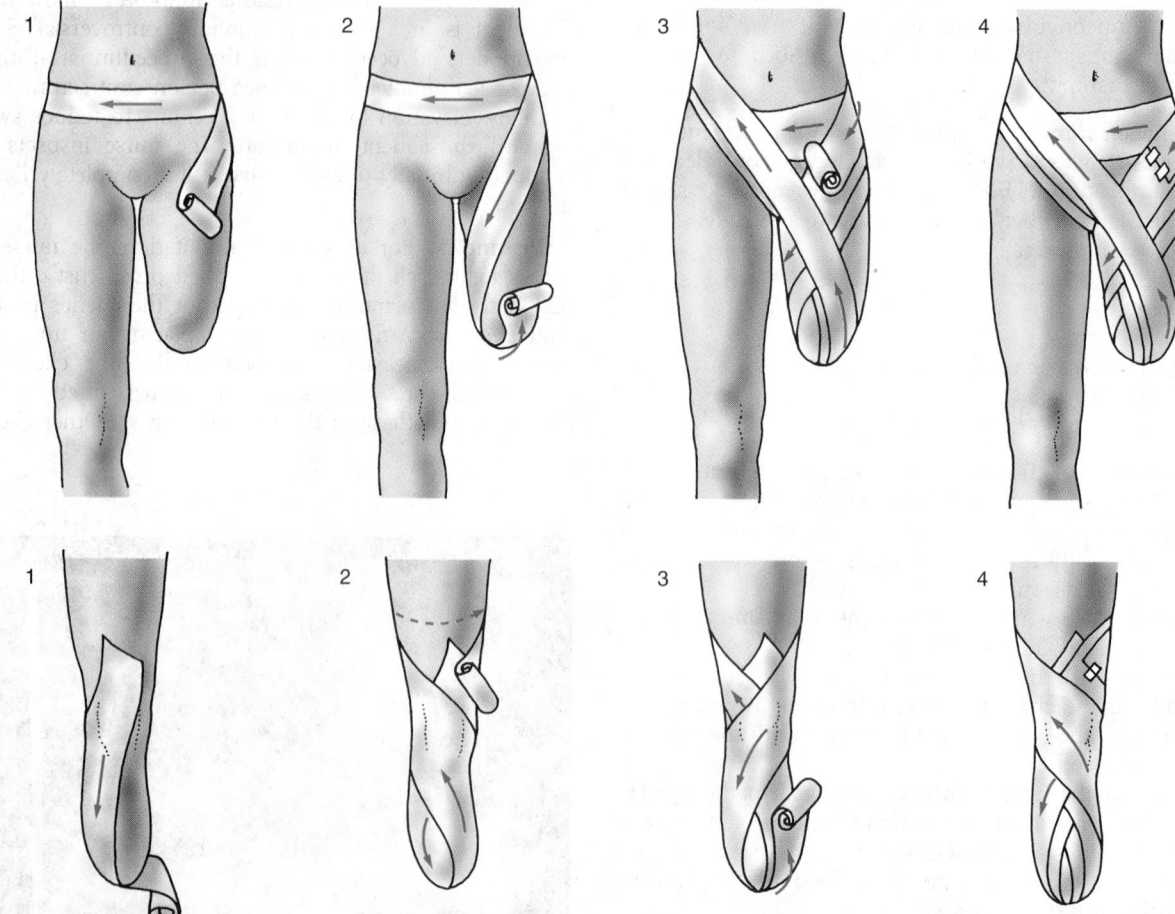

Figure 54–13. A common method of wrapping an amputation stump. *Top,* wrapping for above-knee amputation. *Bottom,* wrapping for below-knee amputation.

and enhances adjustment to the amputation. This discussion uses *residual limb* instead.

The nurse assesses the client's verbal and nonverbal references to the affected area. Some clients behave euphorically and seem to have accepted the loss. The nurse should not jump to the conclusion that acceptance has occurred. The nurse asks the client to describe his or her feelings about changes in body image and self-esteem. The client may verbalize acceptance but refuse to look at the area during a dressing change. This inconsistent behavior is not unusual and should be noted by the nurse. (See Chapter 10 for further nursing interventions for the client with an altered body image.)

Promotion of Lifestyle Adaptations. The client may believe that it will be impossible to return to a previous lifestyle, including intimate relationships, job, and recreational activities. With advancements in prostheses, many clients can return to their jobs and other activities. Professional athletes who use prostheses are quite successful in sports. Clients with amputations ski, hike, bowl, and participate in other physically demanding activities. Over 20,000 amputees in the United States currently participate actively in sports; about a fourth of them are engaged in organized competition.

If a job or career change is necessary, the nurse consults with a social worker for evaluation of the client's other skills that can be used in another capacity. A supportive family or significant other is important for the client's adjustment to this change. The client may also think that an intimate relationship is no longer possible because of physical changes. The nurse works with the sexual partner to help in the client's adjustment to the amputation. Professional assistance from a sex counselor or psychologist may be needed.

For any client with an amputation, the nurse helps the client to set realistic goals, to take one day at a time. The nurse helps the client recognize personal strengths, which are emphasized and taken into account in setting goals. If the client is not realistic, frustration and disappointment may dampen the client's motivation during rehabilitation. (Basic principles of rehabilitation are discussed in Chapter 13.)

 Continuing Care

The client is discharged directly to home or to a rehabilitation facility, depending on the extent of the amputation. In the few cases in which rehabilitation is not feasible (e.g., for a debilitated, confused elderly client), the client may be discharged to a long-term care facility.

> ### ➤ *Health Teaching*

After the sutures are removed (several weeks after surgery), the client begins residual limb care. The home care nurse teaches the client how to care for the residual limb and the prosthesis, if it is available. The limb should be rewrapped three times a day with an elastic bandage applied in a figure-eight manner (see Fig. 54–13) by the client or family member. After the residual limb is healed,

---

> ## Chart 54–7
>
> ### Education Guide: Prosthesis Care
>
> - Have a wooden prosthesis refinished at least every 6 months.
> - Clean the prosthesis socket with mild soap and water, and dry it completely.
> - Replace worn inserts and liners when they become too soiled to clean adequately.
> - Check all mechanical parts, such as bolts, periodically for unusual sounds or movements.
> - Grease the mechanical parts as instructed by your prosthetist.
> - Use garters to keep socks or stockings in place.
> - Replace your shoes, when they wear out, with new ones of the same height and type.

it is cleaned each day with the rest of the body during bathing with soap and water, and it is inspected for signs of inflammation or skin breakdown.

Prostheses require special care for ensuring their reliability and proper function. (Chart 54–7) summarizes discharge teaching for the amputee with a prosthesis.

A client who seemed to adjust to the amputation during hospitalization may realize that it is difficult to cope with the loss after discharge from the hospital. The nurse in the hospital setting should tell the client that this can happen. During the hospital stay, the nurse helps the client to identify strong support systems on which the client can rely after discharge. The home care or rehabilitation nurse reinforces this supporting information.

> ### ➤ *Home Care Management*

The client with amputation of a lower extremity needs to have enough room at home to maneuver a wheelchair if the leg prosthesis is not yet available. The client must be able to use toileting facilities and have access to areas necessary for self-care, such as the kitchen. Structural changes may be required before the client goes home.

> ### ➤ *Health Care Resources*

For the elderly client or for the client with an extensive amputation, such as a hemipelvectomy, the hospital nurse arranges for follow-up care in the home by a home care nurse (Chart 54–8). Physical therapy may continue in the home or on an outpatient basis.

The client with an upper-extremity amputation may need occupational therapy to relearn activities of daily living. The nurse also makes arrangements for vocational or family counseling, as needed. Some clients are discharged to a rehabilitation facility for 2–3 weeks for these services. (Chapter 13 describes the rehabilitation phase of health care in detail.) The nurse teaches the client to explore amputee support groups that may be available in the client's community.

CRUSH SYNDROME

When multiple compartments in the leg or arm are injured, crush syndrome (CS) can occur. CS is a potentially life-threatening, systemic complication after a severe crush injury. Its pathophysiologic mechanism is similar to that of acute compartment syndrome (see earlier Complications of Fractures section).

Specific causes of CS include

- Prolonged use of a pneumatic antishock garment (PASG) or military antishock trousers (MAST) (For this reason, these devices are seldom used today.)
- Wringer-type injuries
- Natural disasters, such as earthquakes
- Work-related injuries, such as being trapped under heavy equipment or material
- Drug/alcohol overdose, when one or more limbs may be compressed by body weight for a prolonged time

Regardless of the cause, CS is characterized by

- Acute compartment syndrome
- Hypovolemia
- Rhabdomyolysis (myoglobulin release from skeletal muscle into the bloodstream)
- Acute tubular necrosis (ATN) resulting from hypovolemia and rhabdomyolysis

REFLEX SYMPATHETIC DYSTROPHY SYNDROME

Reflex sympathetic dystrophy syndrome (RSDS) is a poorly understood complex disorder that includes pain, trophic changes, and vasomotor instability probably caused by an abnormally hyperactive sympathetic nervous system. It most often results from traumatic injury and commonly occurs in the feet and hands.

Millions of people worldwide suffer from RSDS, and all age groups are affected (Greipp & Thomas, 1994). The syndrome tends to progress through three classic stages. In stage 1, which lasts 1–3 months, the client complains of locally severe, burning pain; edema; vasospasm;

and muscle spasm. Over the next 3 months, clients in stage 2 have more severe, diffuse pain and edema, muscle atrophy, and spotty osteoporosis, as shown on x-ray. In the final stage, Stage 3, the client presents with marked muscle atrophy, intractable (unrelenting) pain, severely limited mobility of the affected area, contractures, and marked, diffuse osteoporosis (Greipp & Thomas, 1994).

The first priority of management is pain relief. Nurses play an important role in pain management, which includes drug therapy as well as an array of nonpharmacolgic modalities. Chapter 9 discusses pain management in detail.

In collaboration with the physical and occupational therapist, the nurse also assists in maintaining adequate range of motion. The skin of a client with RSDS tends to alternate between warm, swollen, and red to cool, clammy, and bluish. Skin care needs to be gentle, with minimal stimulation.

The nurse helps the client in coping with RSDS. Psychotherapy may be indicated. The RSDS Association is available to help clients organize or locate support groups and other resources for clients with this syndrome.

SPORTS-RELATED INJURIES

In addition to the bone and muscle problems already discussed, trauma can cause cartilage, ligament, and tendon injury. Many musculoskeletal injuries are the result of participation in sports or other strenuous physical activities. These injuries have become so common that large metropolitan hospitals have clinics and physicians for the specialty of sports medicine.

Although the specific types of injury are numerous, this chapter includes only the most common ones seen by the nurse in a hospital setting. The principles of injury to one part of the body are analogous to those of similar injuries in other parts. For example, a tendon rupture in a knee is cared for in the same manner as a tendon rupture in the wrist. Because the knee is most frequently injured, it is discussed as a typical example of other areas of the body. (Chart 54–9) lists general emergency measures for sports-related injuries.

Knee Injuries

Trauma to the knee results in internal derangement, a broad term for disturbances of an injured knee joint. When surgery is required to resolve the problem, most surgeons prefer to perform the procedure through an arthroscope when possible. (A general description of arthroscopy is presented in Chapter 52.)

Meniscus Injuries

Overview

There are two semilunar cartilages, or menisci, in the knee joint: medial and lateral. These pads act as shock absorbers, but they can tear. Tearing is usually a result of twisting the leg when the knee is flexed and the foot is placed firmly on the ground. The medial meniscus is much more likely to tear than is the lateral meniscus because it is less mobile. Internal rotation causes a tear in the medial meniscus; external rotation causes a tear in the lateral meniscus.

Tears can be anterior or posterior, longitudinal or transverse. In the medial meniscus, a longitudinal tear, or "bucket-handle" injury, often causes the knee to lock; that is, the torn cartilage jams between the femur and tibia and prevents extension of the knee. Surgery is frequently required for this type of injury. In transverse tears, the knee does not lock, and surgery may not be required.

Collaborative Management

The client with a torn meniscus typically has pain, swelling, and tenderness in the knee. A clicking or snapping sound can often be heard when the knee is moved.

A common diagnostic technique is the McMurray test. The examiner flexes and rotates the knee and then presses on the medial aspect while slowly extending the leg. The test result is positive if clicking is palpated or heard. A negative finding, however, does not rule out a tear.

For a locked knee, the treatment may be manipulation followed by casting for 3–6 weeks. If the problem recurs, a partial or total meniscectomy is performed. An open meniscectomy requires a surgical incision for removal of all or part of the meniscus and is rarely performed. Most surgeons prefer to remove only the affected portion, which can be accomplished through an arthroscope during a closed meniscectomy as a same-day surgical procedure. As described in Chapter 52, an arthroscope is a metal tubular instrument used for examination or surgery of joints. One or more small incisions (less than 1/4 inch [0.6 cm] long) are made in the knee for insertion of the arthroscope. The surgeon threads a cutting device through the arthroscope for removal of the torn cartilage while the knee is irrigated with saline or Ringer's lactate solution, depending on the type of equipment used. The surgeon may use a laser during the procedure, depending on the type and severity of the injury. A bulky pressure dressing is applied after the procedure, and the affected leg is wrapped in elastic bandages.

As for any postoperative client, the nurse checks the surgical dressing for bleeding and monitors the client's vital signs after the client is readmitted to the unit. The nurse performs circulation checks, as outlined in Chart 54–3, usually every hour for the first few hours and then every 4 hours.

The client begins leg exercises immediately after surgery to strengthen the leg, prevent thrombophlebitis, and reduce swelling. Quadriceps setting, in which the client straightens the leg while pushing the knee against the bed, is done in sets of 10 or more. Straight-leg raises are also performed as soon as the client awakens from anesthesia. Range-of-motion exercises are usually not started for several days.

To prevent the client from bending the affected knee, the physician may order a knee immobilizer, such as the one shown in (Fig. 54–14). The nurse elevates the leg on one or two pillows per the physician's preference and applies ice to reduce postoperative swelling. Full weight-bearing is restricted for several weeks, depending on the amount of cartilage removed. The client is usually discharged from the hospital with crutches in less than 23 hours.

Ligament Injuries

Overview

The cruciate and collateral ligaments in the knee are predisposed to injury, often from sports or vehicular accidents. The anterior cruciate ligament (ACL) is the most frequently torn ligament in the knee. The combination of ACL, medial meniscus, and medial cruciate ligament injuries simultaneously is called O'Donoghue's unhappy triad. Athletes often experience ACL injuries during skiing or gymnastics.

When the ACL is torn, the person feels a snap; the

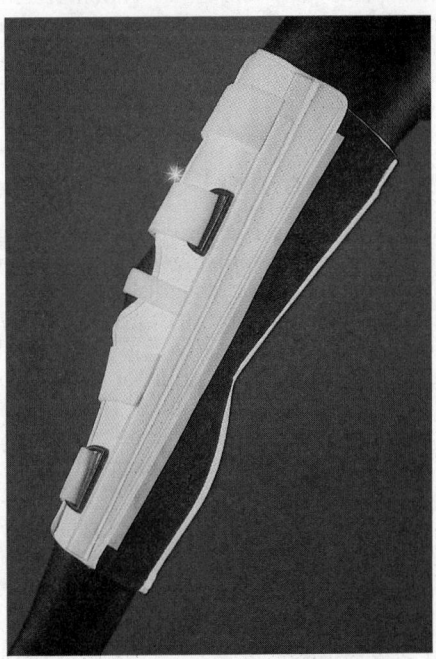

Figure 54–14. A knee immobilizer. (Courtesy of Zimmer, Inc., Warsaw, IN.)

knee gives way because of ACL laxity. Within hours, the knee is swollen, stiff, and painful.

Collaborative Management

The diagnosis of ACL deficiency is made by x-rays, magnetic resonance imaging (MRI), or an arthrometer (an instrument for measuring the amount of tibial displacement).

Treatment may be nonsurgical or surgical, depending on the severity of the injury and the anticipated activity of the client. Exercises, bracing, and limits on activities may be sufficient while the ligament heals. If medical management is not effective, surgery may be needed.

The surgeon repairs the tear by reattaching the torn portions of the ligaments, and the leg is placed in a cast. If the ligament cannot be repaired, reconstructive surgery may be performed with use of autologous grafts. Since the early 1980s, the U.S. Food and Drug Administration has approved several artificial knee ligaments. The Gore-Tex ligament is a permanent implant. The ligament augmentation device is used temporarily while an autograft heals. Both of these materials can be implanted through an arthroscope.

Complete healing of knee ligaments after surgery can take 6–9 months or longer. Nursing management is similar to the care of any client in a cast, which is described earlier in this chapter.

Tendon Ruptures

Rupture of the patellar tendon is common in young adults who participate in strenuous sports. In the elderly client, quadriceps tendon rupture may occur from a fall down several steps. As for severe ligament damage, the tendon is surgically repaired; the leg is immobilized in a cast for 6–8 weeks. If the tendon is beyond repair, a tendon transplant (also known as tendon reconstruction) is performed. A tendon is removed from one part of the body and transplanted to the affected area. The nursing care for these clients is similar to that discussed earlier for a client with a cast.

Dislocations and Subluxations

Dislocation of a joint occurs when the articulating surfaces are no longer in proximity. If dislocation is not complete, the joint is partially dislocated, or subluxed. Dislocation can occur in any diarthrodial (synovial) joint but is common in the shoulder, hip, knee, and fingers. This injury is most often the result of trauma but can be congenital or pathologic (resulting from joint disease, such as arthritis).

The typical manifestations of dislocation are

- Pain
- Immobility
- Alteration in contour of the joint
- Deviation in length of the extremity
- Rotation of the extremity

The health care provider performs a closed manipulation, or reduction, of the joint and forces it back into its original position while the client is anesthetized. The joint is immobilized by a cast or bandage until healing occurs.

Recurrent dislocations are common in the knee and shoulder. For this problem, the joint is fixed with wires to prevent further displacement; a cast, splint, or traction is applied for 3–6 weeks.

Strains

A strain is an excessive stretching of a muscle or tendon when it is weak or unstable. Strains are sometimes referred to as muscle pulls. Falls, lifting heavy items, and exercise often cause this injury.

Strains are classified according to their severity:

- A first-degree (mild) strain causes mild inflammation but little bleeding. Swelling, ecchymosis, and tenderness are usually present.
- A second-degree (moderate) strain involves tearing of the muscle or tendon fibers without complete disruption. Muscle function may be impaired.
- A third-degree (severe) strain involves a ruptured muscle or tendon with separation of muscle from muscle, tendon from muscle, or tendon from bone. Severe pain and disability result from severe strains.

Management usually involves cold and heat applications, exercise, and activity limitations. The health care provider may prescribe anti-inflammatory drugs to decrease inflammation and pain. Muscle relaxants may also be used. In third-degree strains, surgical repair of the ruptured muscle or tendon may be necessary.

Sprains

A sprain is excessive stretching of a ligament. Twisting motions from a fall or sports activity typically precipitate the injury. Sprains are classified according to severity:

- A first-degree (mild) sprain involves tearing of a few fibers of a ligament. Function of the joint is not impaired.
- In a second-degree (moderate) sprain, more fibers are torn, but stability of the joint remains intact.
- A third-degree (severe) sprain causes marked instability of the joint.

Pain and swelling characterize ligament injuries.
The treatment for mild (first-degree) sprains is minimal:

- Rest
- The use of ice
- A compression bandage, which is applied for a few days to reduce swelling and provide joint support

Second-degree sprains require casting for 4 to 6 weeks while the tear heals. For severe ligament damage (third-degree sprain), surgery is the treatment of choice, as discussed earlier for ligament injuries of the knee.

Rotator Cuff Injuries

The musculotendinous or rotator cuff of the shoulder functions to stabilize the head of the humerus in the glenoid cavity during shoulder abduction. The rotator cuff typically undergoes degenerative changes as one gets older. Young adults usually sustain a tear of the cuff by substantial trauma, including a fall, throwing a ball, or heavy lifting. Older adults tend to have small tears related to aging, repetitive motions, or falls.

Clients with a torn rotator cuff have shoulder pain and cannot initiate or maintain abduction of the arm at the shoulder. When the arm is abducted, the client usually drops the arm because abduction cannot be maintained (drop arm test).

The health care provider usually treats the client conservatively with nonsteroidal anti-inflammatory drugs, physical therapy, sling support, and ice/heat applications while the tear heals.

For clients who do not respond to conservative treatment or for those who have a complete tear, the surgeon repairs the cuff. After surgery, the client's affected arm is usually immobilized for several weeks in a sling. Pendulum exercises are started on the third or fourth postoperative day and progress to active exercises in about 2 weeks. If the surgery is extensive, the client's arm may be immobilized for a longer time before exercises begin.

 CASE STUDY for Client with Fractured Hip

■ An elderly resident in a nursing home falls during a dance activity in the day room. When you check her, you find that she is grimacing and complains of severe left knee pain. Her left leg is slightly externally rotated and you suspect a fractured hip. She cries and tells you that she is afraid that she has a fractured hip and will die, as her best friend did last year.

QUESTIONS:

1. What other assessments should you conduct at this time?
2. What should you tell the resident to allay her fears?
3. What will the most likely treatment be for the resident after she is admitted to the hospital?

SELECTED BIBLIOGRAPHY

Bomar, K. S., & Calandruccio, J. H. (1996). Crush injuries to the hand and forearm. *Orthopaedic Nursing, 15*(6), 56–65.

Bradley, C. F., & Kozak, C. (1995). Nursing care and management of the elderly hip fractured patient. *Journal of Gerontological Nursing, 21*(8), 15–22.

Brown, C., Henderson, S., & Moore, S. (1996). Surgical treatment of patients with open tibial fractures. *AORN Journal, 63*(5), 875–881, 885–896.

Davis, A. E. (1995). Hip fractures in the elderly: Surveillance methods and injury control. *Journal of Trauma Nursing, 2*(1), 15–21.

*Dykes, P. C. (1993). Minding the 5Ps of neurovascular assessment. *American Journal of Nursing, 93*(6), 38–39.

Giger, J. N., & Davidhizar, R. E. (1995). *Transcultural nursing: Assessment and intervention* (2nd ed.). St. Louis: Mosby–Year Book.

Greipp, M. E., & Thomas, A. F. (1994). Reflex sympathetic dystrophy syndrome: A longitudinal study. *MEDSURG Nursing, 3*(5), 378–384.

Hart, K. (1994). Using the Ilizarov External Fixator in bone transport. *Orthopaedic Nursing, 13*(1), 35–40.

Houldin, A. D., & Hogan–Quigley, B. (1995). Psychological interventions for older hip fracture patients. *Journal of Gerontological Nursing, 21*(12), 20–26.

Jarvis, C. (1996). *Physical examination and health assessment* (2nd ed.). Philadelphia: W. B. Saunders.

Lamb, K. V., Waszkiewicz, M., & Davis–Kipnis, N. (1996). Dual disabilities: When a stroke patient fractures a hip. *Orthopaedic Nursing, 15*(5), 13–20.

Maher, A. B., Salmond, S. W., & Pellino, T. A. (1994). *Orthopaedic nursing.* Philadelphia: W. B. Saunders.

Paier, G. S. (1996). Specter of the crone: The experience of vertebral fracture. *Advances in Nursing Science, 18*(3), 27–35.

Pellino, T. A. (1994). How to manage hip fractures. *American Journal of Nursing, 94*(4), 46–50.

Santy, J. (1994). Hip fractures: Can nursing make a difference? *British Journal of Nursing, 3*(7), 335–339.

Scura, K. W., & Whipple, B. (1997). How to provide better care for postmenopausal women. *American Journal of Nursing, 97*(4), 36–44.

Stamatos, C. A., Sorenson, P. A., & Telfer, K. M. (1996). Meeting the challenge of the older trauma patient. *American Journal of Nursing, 96*(5), 40–48.

Styrcula, L. (1994). Traction basics: Part IV—Traction for lower extremities. *Orthopaedic Nursing, 13*(5), 59–68.

Tingle, J. (1995). Care of the elderly with hip fractures: Legal and clinical risk management implications. *British Journal of Nursing, 4*(22), 1298–1299.

Williams, M. A., Oberst, M. T., Bjorklund, B. C., & Hughes, S. H. (1996). Family caregiving in cases of hip fracture. *Rehabilitation Nursing, 21*(3), 124–131, 138.

Yetzer, E. A. (1996). Helping the patient through the experience of an amputation. *Orthopaedic Nursing, 15*(6), 45–49.

Yetzer, E., Kauffman, G., & Sopp, F. (1994). Development of a patient education program for new amputees. *Rehabilitation Nursing, 14*(3), 355–358.

Zavotsky, K. E., & Banavage, A. (1996). Management of the patient with complex orthopaedic fractures. *Orthopaedic Nursing, 14*(5), 53–54, 56–57.

SUGGESTED READINGS

Lamb, K. V., Waszkiewicz, M., & Davis–Kipnis, N. (1996). Dual disabilities: When a stroke patient fractures a hip. *Orthopaedic Nursing, 15*(5), 13–20.

   Both hip fracture and stroke incidence increases with age. This article discusses incidence of these disabilities, describes the pathophysiology of stroke, and uses a case study to outline specific nursing interventions for the client with these concurrent health problems. A quiz at the end of the article may be taken for continuing education credit.

Yetzer, E. A. (1996). Helping the patient through the experience of an amputation. *Orthopaedic Nursing, 15*(6), 45–49.

   This article discusses the information needed by both the amputee and his or her family about preoperative and postoperative care. The nurse plays a major role in providing education and emotional support.

Zavotsky, K. E., & Banavage, A. (1995). Management of the patient with complex orthopaedic fractures. *Orthopaedic Nursing, 14*(5), 53–54, 56–57.

   Clients who sustain complex fractures as a result of trauma can develop devastating complications, such as wound and systemic infections, and fracture nonunion. This article describes the management of open complex fractures through a case study approach.

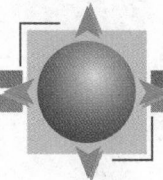

Problems of Digestion,

Nutrition, and

Elimination: Management

of Clients with Problems

of the Gastrointestinal

System

ASSESSMENT OF THE GASTROINTESTINAL SYSTEM

The gastrointestinal (GI) tract is a tube that extends from the mouth to the anus (Fig. 55–1). Its main function is to digest food, with the aid of other organs such as the pancreas and the liver. Nutritional assessment is discussed in Chapter 64.

Problems of the GI tract range from minor discomforts such as an oral ulceration to severe, potentially debilitating diseases such as cancer.

ANATOMY AND PHYSIOLOGY REVIEW
Overview of the Gastrointestinal Tract

Structure

The GI tract has generally the same structure throughout its 25-to 30-foot length. The hollow part of the tube, the lumen, is surrounded by a layer of surface and epithelial cells called the mucosa. The mucosa also includes a thin layer of smooth muscle and some exocrine gland cells, which secrete digestive and protective juices. This layer is surrounded by the submucosa, which is made up of connective tissue and additional exocrine gland cells. The outermost layer is composed of both circular and longitu-

dinal smooth muscles, which work to keep contents moving through the tract.

Function

The GI tract has three major functions: transportation, digestion, and absorption. *Transportation* of water and food through the GI tract is the first function. After food is ingested, it is swallowed, propelled along the lumen, and eliminated as waste products of digestion. *Digestion,* the second function of the GI tract, is a mechanical and chemical process whereby complex foodstuffs are broken down into simpler forms that can be used by the body. During digestion, the GI tract secretes many hormones and enzymes that aid in food breakdown. After the digestive process is complete, the tract absorbs the nutrients. This third function, *absorption,* is carried out as nutrients pass through the intestinal walls into the body's circulatory system for uptake by individual cells (Fig. 55–2).

Nerve Supply

Innervation of the GI tract occurs in two ways. First, intrinsic contractile stimulation is provided by two internal nerve plexuses: the *myenteric* plexus, an outer plexus found in the longitudinal and circular smooth muscle,

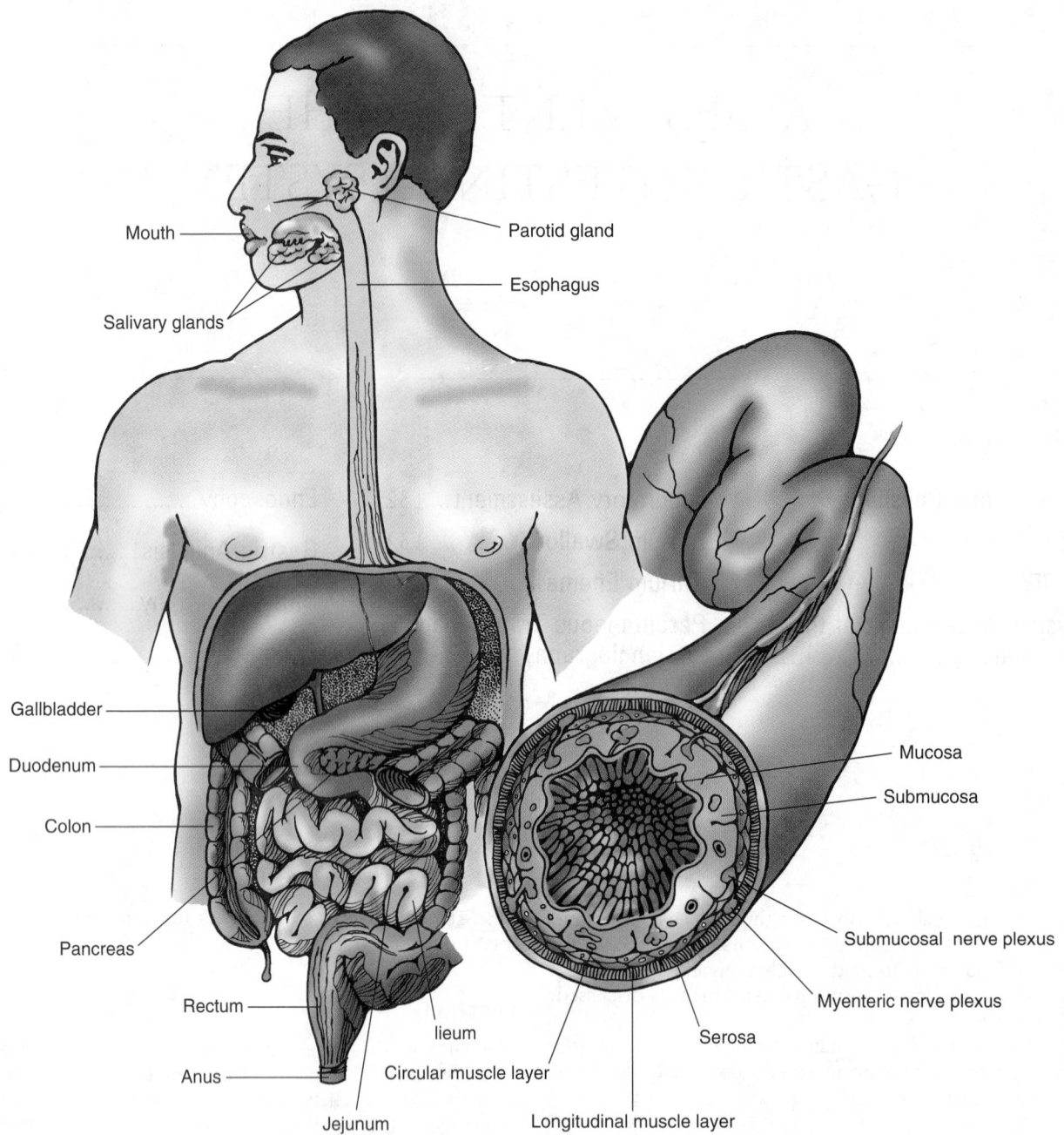

Figure 55–1. The gastrointestinal system (GI tract) can be thought of as a tube (with accessory structures) extending from the mouth to the anus for a 25-foot length. The structure of this tube (shown enlarged) is basically the same throughout its length.

and the *submucosal* plexus, an inner nerve plexus in the submucosa. These nerve plexuses connect with each other along the entire length of the GI tract to maintain the tone of the smooth muscle and to stimulate movements.

The second type of innervation is provided by the autonomic nervous system, which connects with nerve fibers from the intrinsic nerve plexuses. Parasympathetic stimulation is provided mainly by the vagus nerve (cranial nerve X), which innervates the esophagus, the stomach, and, to a lesser extent, the small intestine, the gallbladder, and part of the large intestine. This stimulation causes increased motor and secretory activity and relaxation of sphincters. Sympathetic stimulation via the thoracic and

lumbar splanchnic nerves is provided to all parts of the GI tract; it slows movement, inhibits secretions, and contracts sphincters.

Blood Supply

The blood supply to the GI tract originates from the aorta and branches to the many arteries throughout the length of the tract: celiac, gastric, splenic, common hepatic, internal and external iliac, and superior and inferior mesenteric arteries. The venous system that carries absorbed nutrients away from the lumen of the GI tract consists of the gastric vein, the splenic vein, and other veins that

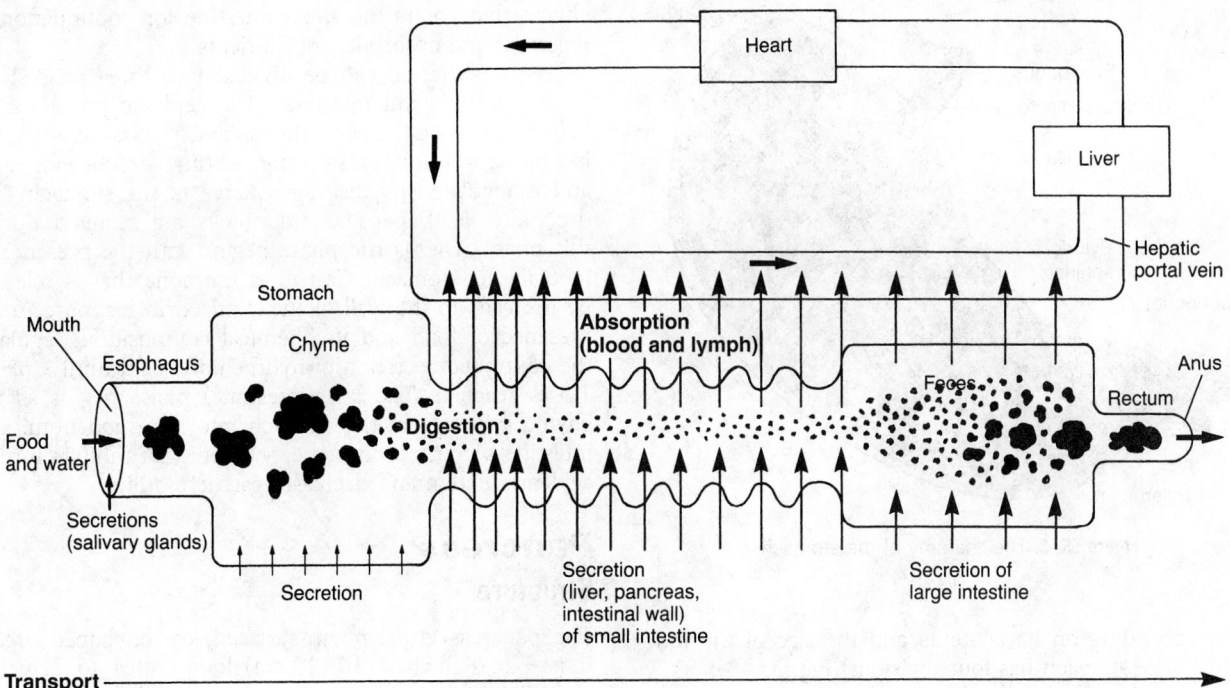

Figure 55–2. A conceptual view of the gastrointestinal system. (From Vander, A. J., Sherman, J. H., & Luciano, D. S. Human physiology [5th ed.]. Copyright 1990 by McGraw-Hill, Inc. Used by permission of McGraw-Hill Book Company.)

drain into the portal vein of the liver. This blood circulates through the liver to the hepatic vein and returns to the heart via the inferior vena cava.

Mouth and Pharynx

Structure

The mouth is lined with mucous membranes and contains the teeth, the gums, and three pairs of salivary glands: the parotid, the submaxillary, and the sublingual glands.

The pharynx (throat) extends from the soft palate to the esophagus. It is lined with mucous membranes and contains three pairs of organs: the adenoids, the lingual tonsils (at the base of the tongue), and the palatine tonsils (often simply referred to as the tonsils).

Function

Swallowing, or deglutition, begins after food is taken into the mouth and chewed. Saliva is secreted in response to the presence of food in the mouth and begins to soften the food. Saliva contains mucin and an enzyme, salivary amylase (also known as ptyalin), which begins the breakdown of carbohydrates.

The three phases of swallowing are voluntary, pharyngeal, and esophageal. As the food softens, the tongue forces the bolus of food to the rear of the mouth toward the pharynx. This process is the voluntary phase. The pharyngeal phase is under reflex control and is thus no longer a voluntary act. As the bolus is forced into the pharynx, the soft palate elevates, which seals the nasal cavity. At this time, the swallowing reflex also inhibits

respirations and allows the opening of the esophagus so that the food can enter. The esophageal phase begins as a peristaltic wave and passes the food down the esophagus to the stomach, which takes about 9 seconds.

Esophagus

Structure

The esophagus is approximately 10 inches (25 cm) long; it is a tube that extends from the pharynx to the stomach and passes through the hiatus in the center of the diaphragm. It lies posterior to the trachea. The esophagus is lined with skeletal muscle in the upper one third and smooth muscle in the lower two thirds, and it contains mucus-secreting glands. The esophagus is innervated by both sympathetic and parasympathetic fibers.

Function

The esophagus receives the bolus of food from the pharynx. The esophageal walls secrete mucus to lubricate the food and to aid in the transport of the bolus to the stomach. As peristalsis pushes the bolus along the esophagus, the cardiac sphincter relaxes to allow the bolus to enter the stomach.

Stomach

Structure

The stomach is located in the midline and left upper quadrant of the abdomen. It is approximately 10 inches (25 cm) long and 4 inches (10 cm) wide but varies in

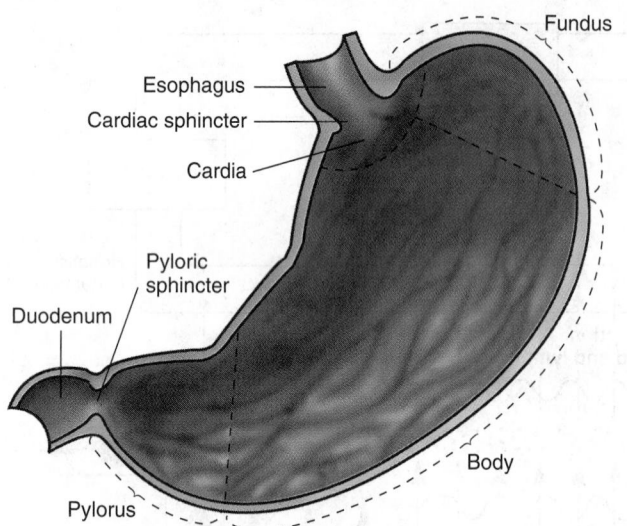

Figure 55–3. The anatomy of the stomach.

size, depending on its contents and the size of the individual. The stomach has four divisions (Fig. 55–3):

- The cardia, the area where the esophagus joins the stomach
- The fundus, the enlarged left area above the esophageal opening
- The body, the main area of the stomach
- The pylorus, the lower area that meets the duodenum

Both ends of the stomach are guarded by sphincters (cardiac and pyloric), which aid in the transport of food through the gastrointestinal (GI) tract and also prevent backflow.

Function

The stomach is a temporary reservoir for food. It secretes 2 to 3L of gastric juice per day, which contains hydrochloric acid, water, mucus, the enzymes pepsin and lipase, and intrinsic factors that begin the digestive process (Table 55–1). The stomach also mixes or churns the food, breaking apart the large food molecules and mixing them with gastric secretions to form chyme, which has a thick consistency. The pylorus regulates the amount of

chyme that enters the small intestine for continuation of digestion and absorption of nutrients.

Gastric secretion can be divided into three phases: cephalic, gastric, and intestinal. The cephalic phase occurs before the food reaches the stomach. Gastric secretion begins as a result of smelling, tasting, or chewing food and is regulated by the vagus nerve to the stomach. Hydrochloric acid, pepsin, and mucus are secreted during this phase. The gastric phase begins with the presence of food in the stomach. Gastrin, a hormone that is released by the cells in the wall of the stomach in response to the presence of food and its chemical composition, regulates the continued secretion of hydrochloric acid until a pH of 1.5 is reached. The last (intestinal) phase begins as the chyme passes from the stomach into the duodenum. The intestine secretes a hormone, secretin, that inhibits further acid production and decreases gastric motility.

Pancreas
Structure

The pancreas is a smooth-surfaced, carrot-shaped organ. It is 4 to 8 inches (10–20 cm) long and 1 to 2 inches (2.5–5 cm) wide. It lies retroperitoneally in the upper abdominal cavity behind the stomach and extends horizontally from the duodenal C loop to the spleen.

The pancreas has two major ducts (Fig. 55–4). The duct of Wirsung, more commonly referred to as the pancreatic duct, runs through the pancreas from left to right, with other ducts emptying into it at right angles. It comes close to the common bile duct, with both ducts passing into the wall of the duodenum to form the ampulla of Vater. The second duct, the accessory duct of Santorini, drains the lower part of the head of the pancreas and enters the duodenum about 0.8 inches (2 cm) above the duct of Wirsung, through the sphincter of Oddi. This duct is not present in all people.

Function

Two major cellular bodies within the pancreas have separate functions: exocrine and endocrine. The *exocrine* pancreas consists of acinar cells, which secrete the enzymes that are necessary for the digestion of carbohydrates, fats, and proteins: trypsin, chymotrypsin, amylase, and lipase (Table 55–2). The *endocrine* pancreas is made up of the

TABLE 55–1

Gastrointestinal Hormones		
Hormone	**Source**	**Effect**
Gastrin	• Secreted by the gastric mucosa in the presence of peptides	• Stimulates gastric motility and secretion of hydrochloric acid
Secretin	• Secreted by the duodenum in the presence of hydrochloric acid	• Stimulates the secretion of pancreatic juice and bile from the liver
Pancreozymin	• Secreted by the duodenum in the presence of hydrochloric acid and peptides	• Stimulates the secretion of pancreatic juice
Cholecystokinin	• Secreted by the duodenum in the presence of amino acids and fatty acids	• Stimulates the secretion of pancreatic enzymes and bile from the gallbladder

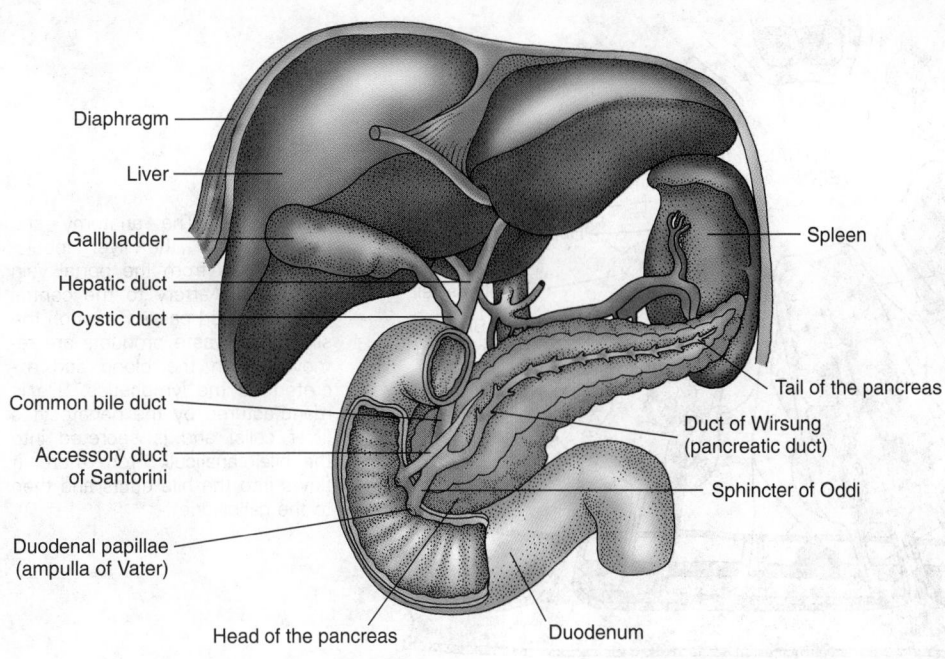

Figure 55–4. The anatomy of the pancreas, the liver, and the gallbladder.

Labels (clockwise): Diaphragm, Liver, Gallbladder, Hepatic duct, Cystic duct, Common bile duct, Accessory duct of Santorini, Duodenal papillae (ampulla of Vater), Head of the pancreas, Duodenum, Sphincter of Oddi, Duct of Wirsung (pancreatic duct), Tail of the pancreas, Spleen

islets of Langerhans, with alpha cells producing glucagon and beta cells producing insulin. Chapter 65 describes the endocrine function of the pancreas.

Liver and Gallbladder
Structure
Liver

The liver is the largest organ in the body and is mainly located in the right upper quadrant of the abdomen.

It has two major lobes, a larger right lobe and a smaller left lobe. The lobes are divided by the falciform ligament, which attaches the liver to the diaphragm. The liver is made up of functioning units called lobules (Fig. 55–5). It has a connective tissue covering, called the Glisson capsule, which protects the organ. Hepatocytes, or liver cells, are arranged into cellular plates, which radiate from a central vein. Small bile channels fit between the plates and empty into terminal bile ducts. The right and left hepatic ducts transport bile from the liver.

TABLE 55–2

Major Digestive Enzymes and Bile			
Substance	**Source**	**Substrate**	**End-Product**
Salivary amylase (ptyalin)	• Salivary glands	• Starch	• Dextrins, maltose
Gastric pepsin (protease)	• Stomach	• Proteins	• Polypeptides
Gastric lipase	• Stomach	• Emulsified fats	• Fatty acids* and glycerol*
Bile (contains no enzymes)	• Liver; stored and released from the gallbladder	• Unemulsified fats	• Emulsified fats
Trypsin	• Pancreas	• Proteins and polypeptides	• Polypeptides and amino acids*
Chymotrypsin	• Pancreas	• Proteins and polypeptides	• Polypeptides and amino acids*
Carboxypeptidase	• Pancreas	• Polypeptides	• Smaller polypeptides
Amylase	• Pancreas	• Starch	• Maltose, lactose, and sucrose
Lipase	• Pancreas	• Bile and emulsified fats	• Glycerol* and fatty acids*
Enterokinase	• Duodenal mucosa	• Trypsinogen	• Trypsin
Peptidases	• Intestine	• Peptides	• Amino acids*
Lactase	• Intestine	• Lactose (milk sugar)	• Glucose* and galactose*
Maltase	• Intestine	• Maltose (malt sugar)	• Glucose*
Sucrase	• Intestine	• Sucrose (cane sugar)	• Glucose* and fructose*

*End-product ready for digestion.

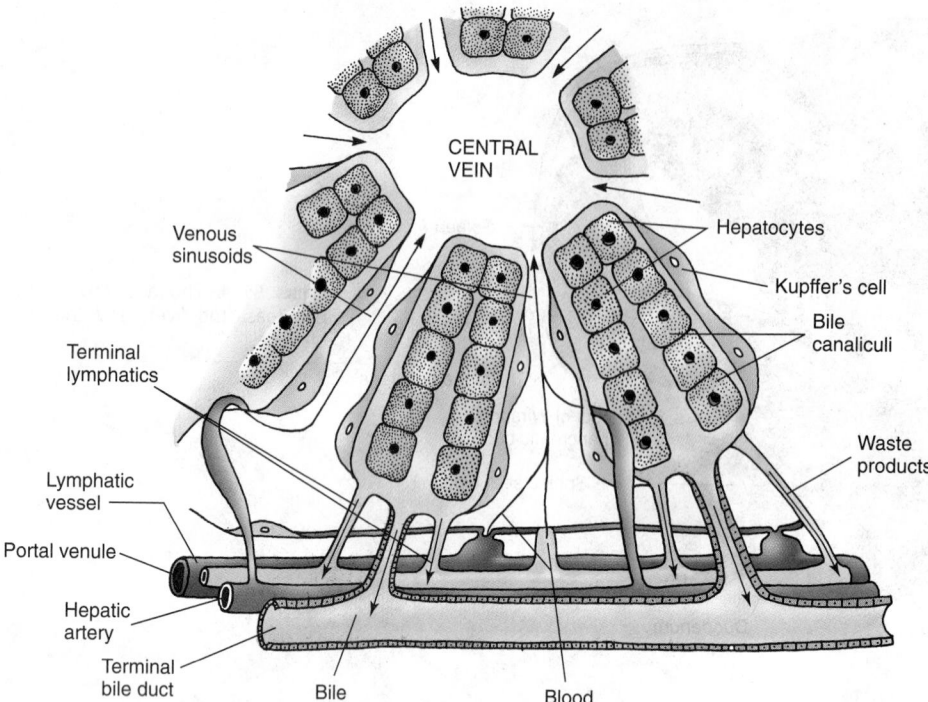

Figure 55–5. The anatomy and physiology of the liver lobule. Blood flows from the portal vein and hepatic artery to the central vein. As blood passes through the sinusoids, waste products are removed from the blood and excreted via the lymphatics. Bile is manufactured by the hepatocytes (liver cells) and is secreted into the bile canaliculi. From there, it flows into the bile ducts and then to the gallbladder.

Gallbladder

The gallbladder is a pear-shaped bulbous sac that is about 3 to 4 inches (8–10 cm) long. It is located beneath and attached to the liver. The gall bladder has three portions: the neck, which is continuous with the cystic duct; the body, or main portion; and the fundus, the lower bulbous section. The cystic duct connects it to the common bile duct.

Function

Liver

The liver performs more than 400 functions in three major categories: storage, protection, and metabolism. The liver stores several minerals and vitamins: copper, iron, magnesium, vitamin B_{12}, folic acid, vitamin B_6, niacin, and the fat-soluble vitamins A, D, E, and K.

The protective function of the liver involves phagocytic Kupffer's cells, which are part of the body's reticuloendothelial system. They engulf harmful bacteria and anemic red blood cells. The liver also detoxifies potentially harmful compounds such as drugs, chemicals, and alcohol that are ingested.

The liver functions in the metabolism of proteins that are vital for human survival. It breaks down amino acids to remove ammonia (NH_3), which is then converted to urea and is excreted via the kidneys. In addition, the liver synthesizes several plasma proteins, such as albumin, prothrombin, and fibrinogen. The liver's role in carbohydrate metabolism involves storing and releasing glycogen as the body's energy requirements change. The liver synthesizes, breaks down, and temporarily stores fatty acids and triglycerides.

The liver forms and continually secretes bile. Bile is

essential for the emulsification of fat. The constituents of bile are bile salts, cholesterol, phospholipids (lecithin), water, electrolytes, and bile pigments (bilirubin). The secretion of bile increases in response to gastrin, secretin, and cholecystokinin. Bile is secreted into small ducts that empty into the common bile duct and into the duodenum at the sphincter of Oddi. However, if the sphincter is closed, the bile goes to the gallbladder for storage.

Gallbladder

The gallbladder concentrates and stores the bile that has come from the liver. It releases the bile into the duodenum via the common bile duct when fat is present.

Small Intestine

Structure

The small intestine is a 1-inch (2.5-cm) round tube that consists of three divisions: the duodenum, jejunum, and ileum. The duodenum is the first 10 inches (25 cm) of the small intestine and is attached to the distal end of the pylorus. It is C-shaped, curving left around the head of the pancreas and bending behind the transverse portion of the large intestine. After bending forward and downward, the small intestine is termed the jejunum for the next 4 to 6 feet. The last 8 to 12 feet of the small intestine is called the ileum.

The inner surface of the small intestine has circular folds of mucosa and submucosa called plicae circulares, which project into the lumen to increase the surface area for digestion and absorption. Villi, which are microscopic finger-like projections, cover the plicae circulares to increase further the absorptive surface of the small intestine.

Function

The small intestine has three main functions:

- Movement (mixing and peristalsis)
- Digestion
- Absorption

The small intestine mixes and transports the chyme by movements called segmental contractions. The contents are moved back and forth over short distances, thereby allowing the chyme to mix with many digestive enzymes. It takes an average of 3 to 10 hours for the contents to be propelled by peristalsis through the small intestine. The ileocecal valve, between the small and large intestines, opens only to allow the passage of chyme.

The small intestine finishes the digestion of the chyme. Many digestive hormones and enzymes aid in this process, each having a specific function (see Tables 55-1 and 55-2). Carbohydrates, fats, proteins, vitamins, water, and electrolytes are absorbed by both diffusion and active transport (see Chap. 14).

Large Intestine

Structure

The large intestine is a tube, 2.5 inches (6 cm) in diameter, that is the last 5 to 6 feet of the gastrointestinal (GI) tract. It begins at the cecum, a pouch that extends below the junction with the ileum. The appendix is an outgrowth of the cecum. The colon consists of four divisions: the ascending, transverse, descending, and sigmoid colons. The sigmoid colon empties into the rectum. The large intestine is made up of smooth muscle and secretes only mucus to protect the bowel wall against the fecal contents.

Function

The large intestine's functions are movement, absorption, and elimination. Movement in the large intestine consists of mainly segmental contractions, like those in the small intestine, to allow enough time for the absorption of water. In addition, three or four strong peristaltic contractions per day are triggered by colonic distention in the proximal large intestine to propel the contents toward the rectum. Here, the material is stored until the urge to defecate occurs.

Absorption of water and some electrolytes occurs in the large intestine to reduce the fluid volume of the chyme, which creates a more solid material, the feces, for elimination.

Gastrointestinal Changes Associated with Aging

Physiologic changes of the GI system occur with aging. In some cases, specific age-related changes have not been validated by research. For example, dryness of the mouth has typically been considered an age-related change. However, some sources have questioned whether dry mouth is actually a normal physiologic change or if other factors, such as hydration and medication, affect the amount of saliva secreted. GI changes associated with aging are summarized in Chart 55-1.

HISTORY
Demographic Data

The nurse or assistive nursing personnel collects demographic data about the client, such as age, sex, culture, and occupation. This information can provide hints to the nurse about predispositions to particular GI tract disorders. For example, many cancers of the GI tract are familial and are seen more frequently in male than in female clients (e.g., colon cancer).

Gastrointestinal ulcers also correlate with certain demographic data. They are seen more frequently in people with high-stress occupations and in men more often than in women. Duodenal ulcers are seen more frequently in young adults, whereas gastric ulcers are more common in older adults.

ELDERLY CONSIDERATIONS

Many GI tract cancers are also correlated with age; the elderly are generally at higher risk for GI cancers. In addition, the incidence of hiatal hernia increases with each decade of life. Diverticulosis and gallstones are also seen increasingly in people older than 40 years of age.

TRANSCULTURAL CONSIDERATIONS

Ulcerative colitis is more prevalent among people of Jewish descent, and lactose intolerance is more common in African-Americans (Huether, 1996). The incidence of GI cancers also varies among ethnic groups. For example, stomach cancer is prevalent among the Japanese, as a consequence of their high intake of raw fish (Giger & Davidhizar, 1995). Chinese people are known to be at high risk for esophageal, stomach, and liver cancer. The intake of certain foods, such as fermented and moldy foods, and the nitrosamines that are found in pickled vegetables and certain grains, is thought to be a possible contributing factor to these cancers. The Chinese are at low risk for colon and rectal cancer, but these cancers are increasing among Chinese-Americans who eat the typical high-fat American diet (King & Locke, 1988).

Personal and Family History

A review of the client's overall health status is an important part of every history. The nurse questions the client about previous gastrointestinal (GI) disorders or abdominal surgery. The client's history of diabetes mellitus, liver disease, pancreatic disease, heart disease, cancer, jaundice, hemorrhoids, bleeding disorders, hernia, ulcers, colitis, gallbladder disease, abdominal aneurysm, or alcoholism is noted. The family's health status is also assessed.

The nurse asks the client about prescription medications being taken, how much and when the drugs are administered, and why they have been prescribed. The nurse also explores whether the client takes over-the-counter medications, which the client may buy and use

---

Chart 55–1

Nursing Focus on the Elderly: Changes in the Gastrointestinal System Related to Aging

Structure	Physiologic Change	Disorders Related to Change	Nursing Implications	Rationale
Stomach	• Atrophy of the gastric mucosa is characterized by a decrease in the ratio of gastrin-secreting cells to somatostatin-secreting cells. This change leads to decreased hydrochloric acid levels (hypochlorhydria).	• Decreased hydrochloric acid levels lead to decreased absorption of iron and vitamin B_{12} and to proliferation of bacteria. Atrophic gastritis occurs as a consequence of bacterial overgrowth.	• Encourage frequent feedings of bland foods high in vitamins and iron. • Assess for epigastric pain.	• Frequent feedings help prevent gastritis. • Assessment helps detect gastritis.
Large intestine	• Peristalsis decreases and nerve impulses are dulled.	• Decreased sensation to defecate can result in postponement of bowel movements, which leads to constipation and impaction.	• Encourage a high-fiber diet and 1500 mL of fluid intake daily (if not contraindicated). • Encourage as much activity as tolerated.	• These interventions increase the sensation of needing to defecate.
Pancreas	• Distention and dilation of pancreatic ducts change. Calcification of pancreatic vessels occurs with a decrease in lipase production.	• Decreased lipase level results in decreased fat absorption and digestion. Steatorrhea, or excess fat in the feces, occurs because of decreased fat digestion.	• Encourage small frequent feedings. • Assess for diarrhea.	• Small, frequent feedings help prevent steatorrhea. • Diarrhea may be steatorrhea.
Liver	• A decrease in the number and size of hepatic cells leads to decreased liver weight and mass. This change and an increase in fibrous tissue lead to decreased protein synthesis and changes in liver enzymes. Enzyme activity and cholesterol synthesis are diminished.	• Decreased enzyme activity depresses drug metabolism, which leads to accumulation of drugs—possibly to toxic levels.	• Assess all clients for adverse effects of all drugs, even those administered in normal doses.	• Assessment detects drug toxicity.

---

independently. Many clients do not consider drugs that they can buy on their own to be important. In particular, the nurse asks whether aspirin, nonsteroidal anti-inflammatory drugs (NSAIDs) (such as ibuprofen), vitamin supplements, laxatives, antacids, or enemas are taken. Large amounts of aspirin or NSAIDs can predispose the client to GI ulcer disease and GI bleeding. Similarly, long-term use of laxatives or enemas can cause dependence on such stimulation and result in constipation.

Finally, the nurse investigates the client's travel history. The nurse asks the client whether he or she has traveled out of the country recently. This information may give some clue about a possible cause of a GI symptom, especially diarrhea.

Diet History

A diet history is important when assessing GI tract function. The nurse determines whether the client is eating a special diet. The client is asked to describe the usual foods that are eaten daily and the times of the meals. The nurse thus gains information about the client's knowledge of the food pyramid and the importance of a balanced diet (see Chap. 64).

The nurse explores with the client any changes that have occurred in eating habits as a result of illness. The client's diet, usual and current appetite, and any recent changes in eating habits are also assessed. The nurse determines the occurrence of nausea, vomiting, and dyspepsia (indigestion, or heartburn), along with a description of each symptom in terms of frequency, duration, and association with meals. The nurse also asks about changes in taste and any difficulty or pain with swallowing (dysphagia). The nurse asks the client whether any foods are avoided and, if so, why they are avoided. It is also important to assess alcohol and caffeine consumption, because both substances are associated with many GI disorders, such as gastritis and peptic ulcer disease. (A complete diet history is described in Chapter 64.)

TRANSCULTURAL CONSIDERATIONS

Cultural and religious patterns are important to a GI tract diet history. The nurse determines which foods pose a problem for the client. For example, the spices or hot pepper used in cooking in many cultures can aggravate or precipitate GI tract complaints, such as indigestion. The nurse should also note religious patterns such as fasting or abstinence.

Some people may not be able to tolerate certain foods or chemicals. For instance, lactose intolerance is a well-documented condition in African-Americans. About 75% of African-Americans have this problem (Giger & Davidhizar, 1995). Lactose intolerance causes GI symptoms of bloating, cramping, and diarrhea as a result of lack of the enzyme lactase. Lactase is needed to convert lactose in milk and other dairy products to glucose and galactose.

Socioeconomic Status

Knowledge of the client's socioeconomic status can give the nurse valuable clues for determining the client's ability to obtain food, medications, and medical care. People who have limited budgets, such as the elderly or the unemployed, may not be able to obtain a balanced diet. They may also substitute less expensive over-the-counter medications, which may not have the same effects or protective coatings, for prescription medications.

Current Health Problem

Gastrointestinal tract clinical manifestations are often vague and difficult for the client to describe. The nurse explores each complaint in detail, assessing the exact location of the problem, what precipitates or alleviates it, when it worsens, and how long it lasts (Chart 55–2). The following examples are topics to explore with clients about specific GI tract symptoms.

A change in bowel habits is a significant complaint. The nurse explores with the client:

- The frequency of bowel movements
- The color and consistency of the feces
- The occurrence of diarrhea or constipation
- Effective action taken to relieve diarrhea or constipation

> ### Chart 55–2
>
> ### Nursing Care Highlight: Questions to Include in a Gastrointestinal Assessment
>
> - Have you noticed changes in your bowel habits? If so, what are they?
> - Have you experienced any sudden weight gain or loss?
> - Do you or have you ever smoked? If so, how much?
> - Have you had or do you currently have pain? If so, where is the pain and what, if anything, makes it better?
> - Have you had nausea or vomiting? If vomiting occurred, describe the vomitus.
> - Have you noticed any skin changes, such as jaundice or rashes?
> - Has your appetite change? Has it increased? Decreased?
> - Do you have any problem with swallowing?
> - Have you had indigestion or feelings of bloating or fullness? If so, when and how often did the feelings occur?

- The meaning of diarrhea and constipation to the client
- The presence of abdominal distention or gas

An unexplained weight gain or weight loss is often an early warning sign to the client that something is wrong. The nurse assesses the client for his or her

- Normal weight
- Weight gain or loss
- Period of time for weight change
- Change in appetite or oral intake

Smoking predisposes the client to several types of cancer, especially oral cancer, because nicotine is a gastrointestinal (GI) irritant. The nurse asks whether the client has ever smoked. If the client smokes, the nurse obtains a smoking history from the client, including the number of packs of cigarettes smoked per day for how many years. The nurse also asks about a history or current use of cigars, pipe tobacco, or chewing tobacco. If the client has stopped smoking or is using tobacco in another form, the nurse asks when and why this was done.

Pain is a common complaint in clients with GI tract disorders. The nurse asks the client about

- The presence of pain
- The location of the pain
- Radiation to another site
- Factors that make the pain better or worse
- The time of day when the pain is worst

The nurse also asks about the relationship of food intake to the onset or worsening of pain. For example, a high-fat meal frequently triggers gallbladder pain.

Changes in the skin can result from several GI tract disorders, such as liver and biliary system obstruction. The nurse asks the client about

- Skin discolorations or rashes
- Itching

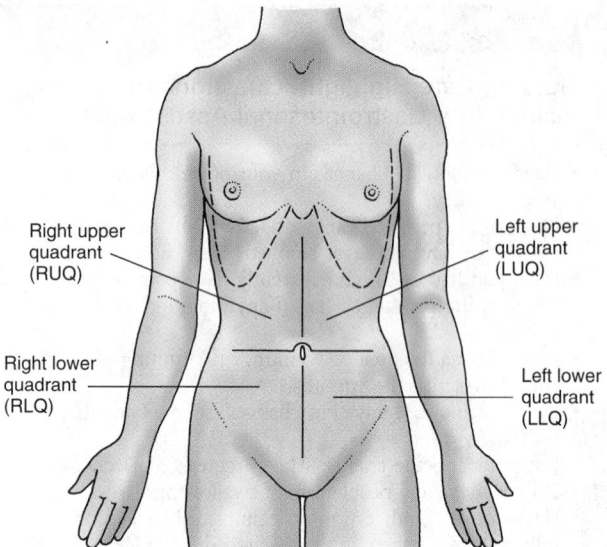

Figure 55–6. A topographic division of the abdomen into quadrants.

- Jaundice
- Increased susceptibility to bruising
- Increased tendency to bleed

PHYSICAL ASSESSMENT

Physical assessment of the GI system involves a comprehensive examination of the client's nutritional status, the mouth and pharynx, the abdomen, and the extremities. (Nutritional assessment is discussed in detail in Chapter 64.)

Mouth and Pharynx

Assessment of the mouth involves inspection and palpation. To begin the examination of the mouth, the nurse puts on gloves, faces the client, and inspects the lips for color, symmetry, and any abnormalities, such as ulcers. The nurse asks the client to open and close the mouth and notes the client's ability to perform this movement and its symmetry. To continue, the nurse needs a penlight and a tongue depressor. The nurse inspects the inner surfaces of the lips and the oral mucosa, starting on the client's left side and moving in a clockwise fashion. The nurse notes the color and condition of the membranes. To view the tongue, the nurse asks the client to stick the tongue out of the mouth. The tongue is inspected for color, coating, ulcers, and variations in size and shape.

The nurse inspects the teeth and gums for

- Gross evidence of dental caries
- The absence of teeth
- Inflammation
- Signs of bleeding

The gums should be pink, moist, and smooth. If the client wears dentures, they are removed. The nurse can recommend that the client seek follow-up dental care if the nurse detects any problems. Throughout this examination, the nurse is alert to any significant mouth odors

that suggest disease. For instance, a fruity smell may indicate uncontrolled diabetes mellitus.

For further examination of the oral cavity, the nurse asks the client to open his or her mouth wide to inspect the pharynx. The nurse observes the color and any signs inflammation. The presence of the tonsils and exudate, ulcerations, or swellings is noted. The nurse asks the client to say "ah" and observes the normal retraction of the uvula with an intact vagus nerve (cranial nerve X).

Abdomen

During the abdominal examination, the nurse usually begins at the client's right side and proceeds in a systematic fashion (Fig. 55–6):

- Right upper quadrant (RUQ)
- Left upper quadrant (LUQ)
- Left lower quadrant (LLQ)
- Right lower quadrant (RLQ)

Table 55–3 lists the organs that lie in each of these topographic areas.

The nurse determines from the history whether there is pain or tenderness and examines the area of pain last. This sequence should prevent the client from tensing abdominal muscles because of the pain, which would make

TABLE 55–3

Location of Body Structures in Each Abdominal Quadrant

Right Upper Quadrant (RUQ)
- Most of the liver
- Gallbladder
- Duodenum
- Head of the pancreas
- Hepatic flexure of the colon
- Part of the ascending and transverse colon

Left Upper Quadrant (LUQ)
- Left lobe of the liver
- Stomach
- Spleen
- Body and tail of the pancreas
- Splenic flexure of the colon
- Part of the transverse and descending colon

Left Lower Quadrant (LLQ)
- Part of the descending colon
- Sigmoid colon
- Left ureter
- Left ovary and fallopian tube
- Left spermatic cord

Right Lower Quadrant (RLQ)
- Cecum
- Appendix
- Right ureter
- Right ovary and fallopian tube
- Right spermatic cord

Midline
- Abdominal aorta
- Uterus (if enlarged)
- Bladder (if distended)

the examination difficult. The nurse examines any area of tenderness cautiously and instructs the client to state whether it is too painful. The nurse also observes the client's face for signs of distress or pain.

The nurse assesses the client's abdomen by using the four techniques of examination, but in a sequence different from that used for other body systems:

- Inspection
- Auscultation
- Percussion
- Palpation

This sequence is preferred so that palpation and percussion do not increase intestinal activity and hence increase bowel sounds. Palpation is not performed if the client has suspected appendicitis or an abdominal aneurysm.

Before the abdominal assessment, the nurse instructs the client to empty his or her bladder, then to lie in a supine position with the knees bent, keeping the arms at the sides to prevent inadvertent tensing of the abdominal muscles.

Inspection

The nurse inspects the skin and notes the following:

- Overall color of the abdomen
- Hair distribution
- The presence of discolorations (rashes, lesions, striae, petechiae, scars, distended superficial veins, jaundice, and any other pigmentation changes)
- Abdominal distention
- Bulging flanks
- Taut, glistening skin

The nurse assesses the architecture of the client's abdomen by observing its contour and symmetry. The contour of the abdomen is the client's abdominal profile and is either rounded, flat, concave, or distended. Contour is best seen if one stands at the side of the bed. The nurse notes whether the contour is symmetric or asymmetric. An asymmetric abdomen, best seen from the foot of the bed, could be the result of a hernia, tumor, or previous abdominal surgery. The nurse inspects the shape and position of the umbilicus for any deviations.

Finally, the nurse inspects the client's abdominal movements, including the normal rising and falling with inspiration and expiration, and notes any distress during movement. Occasionally, pulsations may be visible, particularly in the area of the abdominal aorta. Peristaltic movements are rarely seen on inspection unless the client is thin and has markedly increased peristalsis. If such movements are observed, the nurse notes the quadrant of origin and the direction of peristaltic flow. This finding is reported to the physician because it might indicate an intestinal obstruction.

Auscultation

The nurse performs auscultation of the abdomen with the diaphragm of the stethoscope. The nurse places the stethoscope lightly on the abdominal wall and listens for bowel sounds in all four quadrants. If the client is obese,

the nurse may need to apply more pressure with the stethoscope.

Bowel sounds are created as air and fluid move through the gastrointestinal (GI) tract. They are normally heard as soft clicks and gurgles every 5 to 15 seconds, with a normal frequency range of 5 to 30 per minute. The nurse listens for the character and frequency of the sounds. Bowel sounds may be irregular, so the nurse must listen for at least one full minute in each quadrant to confirm the absence of bowel sounds. Bowel sounds are diminished or absent after abdominal surgery or in the client with peritonitis or paralytic ileus. Increased bowel sounds, especially loud gurgling sounds, result from hypermotility of the bowel. These sounds are usually heard in the client with diarrhea or gastroenteritis or above a complete intestinal obstruction.

The nurse also auscultates the abdomen for circulatory sounds, especially bruits. The nurse places the bell of the stethoscope lightly on the abdomen and listens for a blowing or "swooshing" sound. The nurse can listen over the abdominal aorta, the renal arteries, and the iliac arteries. A bruit heard over the aorta usually indicates the presence of an aneurysm. If this sound is heard the nurse discontinues the examination and notifies the physician immediately.

The nurse can auscultate for two other abnormal circulatory sounds—friction rubs and venous hums. A friction rub, which sounds like two pieces of leather rubbing together, can be heard over the spleen or the liver and indicates the presence of a splenic infarct or a hepatic tumor. A continuous venous hum is heard in the periumbilical region in the presence of engorged liver circulation, as in hepatic cirrhosis.

Percussion

Percussion is used during the abdominal assessment to determine the size of solid organs and to detect the presence of masses, fluid, and air. The nurse elicits percussion notes by placing the middle finger of one hand over the abdominal area to be percussed. The nurse strikes his or her finger lightly several times and systematically assesses each quadrant by comparing sounds over different areas. The percussion notes normally heard in the abdomen are termed tympanic (the high-pitched, loud, musical sound of an air-filled intestine) or dull (the medium-pitched, softer, thud-like sound over a solid organ such as the liver).

To percuss the size of the liver span, the nurse begins from below the right nipple in the mid-clavicular line and is careful to percuss between ribs. The percussion note should change from resonance of the lung tissue to dullness of the liver when the upper liver border is reached. The nurse marks the area where percussion tones change. Then the nurse percusses up from the iliac crest in the mid-clavicular line until the percussion note changes from tympany of the bowel to dullness of the liver at the lower border. Again, the nurse marks this area. The distance between the two marks is the approximate liver span, which is normally 2 to 4 inches (5–10 cm).

The nurse may use percussion techniques to determine the size and position of the spleen at the tenth intercostal space in the left mid-axillary line. Percussion can also be used to detect a distended bladder. The percussion notes that are elicited over the spleen or a distended bladder are dull because these are solid organs.

Palpation

Palpation of the abdomen consists of two types—light palpation and deep palpation. Only highly skilled nurses, such as clinical nurse specialists and nurse practitioners, should perform deep palpation.

LIGHT PALPATION. The technique of light palpation is used to detect large masses and areas of tenderness and to help the client achieve muscular relaxation. The nurse places the palm and fingers of the hand lightly on the abdomen and proceeds smoothly and systematically from quadrant to quadrant; the nurse depresses to a depth of 0.5 to 1 inch (1.25–2.5 cm). Any areas of tenderness or guarding are noted, because these areas are examined last and cautiously during deep palpation. While performing light palpation, the nurse is alert to signs of rigidity or muscle spasticity. If the nurse thinks that the client is relaxed, which is best determined while palpating abdominal muscles on expiration, rigidity is probably involuntary. This rigidity could indicate the presence of peritoneal inflammation.

DEEP PALPATION. Deep palpation is used to further determine the size and shape of abdominal organs and masses. The nurse uses the palm and fingers of one or both hands and proceeds deliberately around the abdominal wall to a maximal depth. If both hands are used (bimanual palpation), one hand is placed on top of the other for palpation of a deep organ.

Two techniques are used for palpating the liver (Fig. 55–7). For the first technique, the nurse stands at the client's right side and places the left hand under the client's back at the lower part of the rib cage. Then the nurse places the right hand on the client's abdomen below the lower border of the liver toward the client's head. As the client takes a breath, the nurse presses the hand in and up under the rib cage until a maximal depth is

reached. The client is instructed to take a deep abdominal breath while the nurse tries to feel the lower edge of the liver as it descends. The liver may or may not be palpable.

The second technique for palpating the liver is the hooking technique (see Fig. 55–7). The nurse stands at the client's right side behind the shoulder and places both hands, next to one another, below the lower border of the liver. The client is instructed to take a deep breath while the nurse presses in with the fingers of both hands at the costal margin. The nurse attempts to feel the lower border of the liver as it descends.

Palpation is also used to detect an enlarged spleen; however, the spleen must be three times its original size before it is palpable. The same two techniques for palpating the liver are used for the spleen, but on the left side. The pancreas, the gallbladder, and the left kidney are not usually palpable in most healthy adults.

MEASUREMENT OF ABDOMINAL GIRTH. To complete the abdominal examination, the nurse may need to measure the client's abdominal girth (circumference) if ascites or distention was noted earlier. The nurse uses a tape measure to measure around the fullest part of the abdomen, usually at the umbilicus. The nurse places a small pen mark on the abdomen to show where the measurement was taken to ensure that future measurements are taken at the same place for comparison.

Other Findings

The nurse inspects the skin of the neck, shoulders, and chest for the presence of spider telangiectases, typically indicative of liver cirrhosis. The nurse also assesses the lower extremities for edema. If edema is present, the nurse checks circulation to the tissue by evaluating the quality of the dorsalis pedis and posterior tibial pulse.

A clinical finding known as asterixis, also called "liver flap," is assessed. The nurse asks the client to put both arms on a flat surface and extend the hands upward. The nurse notes whether the client's fingers flap while in this position, which indicates hepatic encephalopathy. Aste-

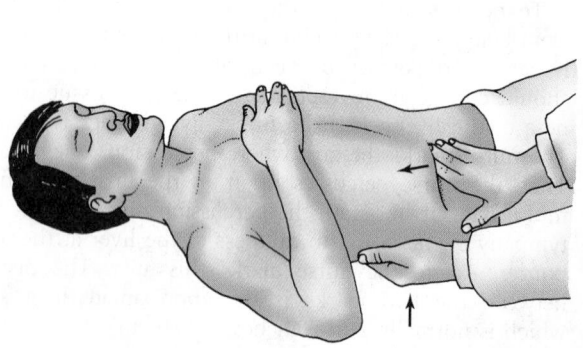
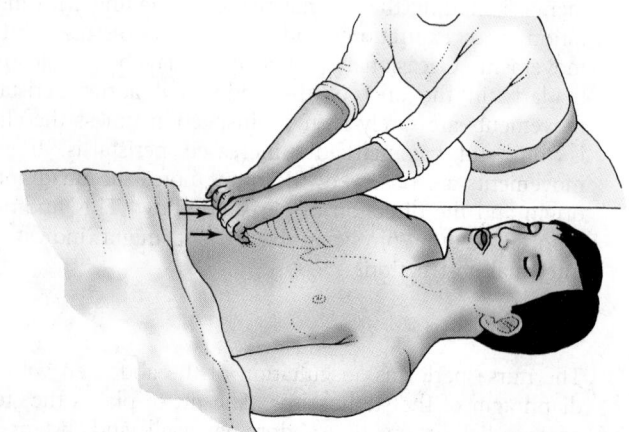

Figure 55–7. Two techniques for palpation of the liver.

rixis can also be assessed initially by noting changes in the client's handwriting.

PSYCHOSOCIAL ASSESSMENT

Psychosocial assessment focuses on how the current complaint affects the client's lifestyle. The nurse asks the client whether there has been any interruption of or disturbance to usual activities, including employment. For example, has the client been able to work or has he or she had to stay away from work because of illness? The nurse questions the client about the stress level of the job or any other recent emotional stresses experienced. Stress in one's life is associated with the development of certain gastrointestinal (GI) tract disorders.

The nurse also asks about the client's current financial status. Financial problems can be a source of stress and may precipitate GI disorders. In addition, poor finances, especially in elderly, unemployed, or uninsured clients, may prevent the client from obtaining appropriate medical care or a proper diet.

DIAGNOSTIC ASSESSMENT
Laboratory Assessment

To make an accurate assessment of the many possible causes of gastrointestinal (GI) tract abnormalities, blood, urine, and stool specimen tests can be performed.

Blood Tests

Chart 55–3 lists blood tests commonly used by the physician in diagnosis of GI disorders. A complete blood count (CBC) aids in the diagnosis of anemia and detects changes in the blood's formed elements. The prothrombin time measures coagulation factors produced in the liver. This test is useful in evaluating the levels of these clotting factors, which are abnormally increased in diseases of the liver. Serum protein electrophoresis is also useful for eval-

uation of GI tract disorders. It is a test to measure the serum protein fractions in the blood, which are important for the maintenance of oncotic and capillary pressures.

Many electrolytes are altered in GI tract dysfunction. For example, calcium is absorbed in the GI tract. It is measured to detect blood clotting deficiencies, GI tract malabsorption, and renal and endocrine disorders.

Many blood studies are important in the evaluation of liver function. Aspartate aminotransferase (AST), formerly referred to as serum glutamic-oxaloacetic transaminase (SGOT), and alanine aminotransferase (ALT), formerly referred to as serum glutamic-pyruvic transaminase (SGPT), are two enzymes found in the liver and other organs. These enzymes are released into circulation when the liver is damaged. The enzyme lactate dehydrogenase (LDH) is necessary for the conversion of lactic acid to pyruvic acid. One form of LDH is found in the liver. Serum levels of alkaline phosphatase, which is an enzyme that is found in the liver and intestines, are elevated in clients with biliary obstruction or liver disease.

Bilirubin is the primary pigment in bile, which is normally conjugated and excreted by the liver and biliary system. Bilirubin is measured as total serum bilirubin, conjugated (direct) bilirubin, and unconjugated (indirect) bilirubin. These measurements are important in the evaluation of jaundice and of liver and biliary tract functioning.

The serum level of ammonia is also measured to evaluate hepatic function. Ammonia is normally used to rebuild amino acids or is converted to urea for excretion. Elevated ammonia levels are seen in cirrhosis of the liver.

Serum amylase and serum lipase levels are evaluated to identify acute pancreatic dysfunction. Amylase is formed by the pancreas for digestion of starches, and lipase is necessary for the digestion of fats.

Two oncofetal antigens, CA19-9 and CEA, are evaluated to monitor the success of cancer therapy and to assess for the recurrence of cancer in the gastrointestinal tract. These antigens may also be increased in benign GI conditions.

Chart 55–3

Laboratory Profile: Gastrointestinal Assessment

Test	Normal Range for Adults	Significance of Abnormal Findings

Calcium (total)	18–60 y: 8.6–10.0 mg/dL or 2.15–2.50 mmol/L
	60–90 y: 8.8–10.2 mg/dL or 2.20–2.55 mmol/L
	>90 y: 8.2–9.6 mg/dL or 2.15–2.40 mmol/L
		Decreased values indicate possible
		  Malabsorption
		  Renal failure
		  Acute pancreatitis

Potassium	Male: 3.5–4.5 mEq/L or 3.5–4.5 mmol/L
	Female: 3.4–4.4 mEq/L or 3.4–4.4 mmol/L
		Decreased values indicate possible
		  Vomiting
		  Gastric suctioning
		  Diarrhea
		  Drainage from intestinal fistulas

Continued

Chart 55–3. Laboratory Profile: Gastrointestinal Assessment Continued

Albumin	3.9–5.1 g/dL 18–60 y: 3.4–4.8 g/dL	*Decreased* values indicate possible hepatic disease
Alanine aminotransferase (ALT)	18–60 y, male: 10–40 units/L 　　　female: 7–35 units/L 60–90 y, male: 13–40 units/L 　　　female:10–28 units/L >90 y, male: 6–38 units/L 　　　female: 5–24 units/L	*Increased* values indicate possible 　Liver disease 　Hepatitis 　Cirrhosis
Aspartate aminotransferase (AST)	18–60 y, 8–20 units/L >60 y, male: 11–26 units/L 　　　female: 10–20 units/L	*Increased* values indicate possible 　Liver disease 　Hepatitis 　Cirrhosis
Lactate dehydrogenase (LDH)	140–280 units/L	*Increased* values indicate possible damaged liver caused by hepatitis and other hepatocellular disorders
Alkaline phosphatase	25–100 U/L or 0.43–1.70 μKat/L	*Increased* values indicate possible 　Hepatic disease 　Biliary obstruction
Bilirubin 　Total serum	18–60 y: 0.3–1.2 mg/dL or 5–21 μmol/L 60–90 y: 0.2–1.1 mg/dL or 3–19 μmol/L >90 y: 0.2–0.9 mg/dL or 3–15 μmol/L	*Increased* values indicate possible 　Hemolysis 　Biliary obstruction 　Hepatic damage
Conjugated (direct)	<0.2 mg/dL or <3.4 μmol/L	*Increased* values indicated possible biliary obstruction
Unconjugated (indirect)	<1.1 mg/dL or <19 μmol/L	*Increased* values indicate possible 　Hemolysis 　Hepatic damage
Ammonia	19–60 μg/dL or 11–35 μmol/L	*Increased* values indicate possible hepatic disease such as cirrhosis
Xylose absorption	5-g dose in 2 hr: >20 mg/dL or >1.3 mmol/L 25-g dose in 2 hr: >25 mg/dL or >1.7 mmol/L	*Decreased* values in blood and urine indicate possible malabsorption in the small intestine
Serum amylase	18–60 y: 27–131 IU/L or 0.46–2.23 μKat/L 60–90 y: 24–151 IU/L or 0.41–2.57 μKat/L	*Increased* values indicate possible acute pancreatitis
Serum lipase	13–141 units/L or 0.22–2.40 μKat/L >60 y: 0–302 units/L or 0.0–5.13 μKat/L	*Increased* values indicate possible acute pancreatitis
Cholesterol	<200 mg/dL or <5.18 mmol/L	*Increased* values indicate possible 　Pancreatitis 　Biliary obstruction *Decreased* values indicate possible liver cell damage
Carbohydrate antigen 19-9 (CA19-9)	<37 AU/mL	*Increased* values indicate possible 　Cancer of the pancreas, stomach, colon 　Acute pancreatitis 　Inflammatory bowel disease
Carcinoembryonic antigen (CEA)	Nonsmoker: <2.5 ng/mL Smoker: up to 5 ng/mL	*Increased* values indicate possible 　Colorectal, stomach, pancreatic cancer 　Ulcerative colitis 　Crohn's disease 　Hepatitis 　Cirrhosis

Urine Tests

The level of amylase in urine is also measured for the evaluation of acute or chronic pancreatitis. After an attack of acute pancreatitis, levels of amylase remain high in the urine after serum levels have returned to normal.

Urine urobilinogen is a form of bilirubin that is converted by the intestinal flora and excreted in the urine. Its measurement is useful in the evaluation of hepatic and biliary obstruction (Chart 55–4).

Stool Tests

Several stool examinations are used in the evaluation of GI tract dysfunction (see Chart 55–4). Stool testing for occult blood is called the fecal occult blood test (FOBT). The FOBT measures the presence of blood in the stool from GI bleeding, a common finding associated with colorectal cancer.

WOMEN'S HEALTH CONSIDERATIONS

Compared with women of lower socioeconomic status, women of higher socioeconomic status are more likely to have regular physical examinations that include an annual FOBT and a proctosigmoidoscopy every 3 to 5 years after the age of 50. Annual fecal occult blood testing reduces mortality from colorectal cancer in women (Allen & Phillips, 1997).

Stool samples for ova and parasites are collected to aid in the diagnosis of parasitic infection. Stool samples tested for fecal fats are evaluated for steatorrhea and malabsorption. Fat is normally absorbed in the small intestine in the presence of biliary and pancreatic secretions. In malabsorption, fat is abnormally excreted in the stool.

Radiographic Examinations
Flat Plate of the Abdomen

A flat plate x-ray visualizes organs in the abdomen. This simple film has the ability to reveal abnormalities such as masses, tumors, and strictures or obstructions to normal movement. This x-ray is generally the first one that the physician orders when diagnosing a gastrointestinal (GI) problem. There is no required client preparation, except that the client should wear a hospital gown and remove any jewelry or belts, which may interfere with the film.

Barium Swallow

A barium swallow examination is a test of the pharynx and esophagus done to detect tumors, strictures, ulcers, or other motility disorders. The test is often indicated for a client with a complaint of indigestion or dysphagia.

Client Preparation

The client is permitted nothing by mouth (NPO) after midnight the evening before the test. The nurse instructs the client about the barium preparation, including its consistency and chalk-like taste.

Procedure

The barium swallow examination is performed with the client in an upright position. During the test, the client

Chart 55–4

Laboratory Profile: Common Urine and Stool Tests Used in Gastrointestinal Assessment

Test	Normal Range for Adults	Significance of Abnormal Findings
Urine bilirubin	Negative	*Increased* values indicate possible Biliary obstruction Cirrhosis Hepatitis
Urobilinogen	Urine: 0.1–1.0 Ehrlich unit/mL	*Increased* values indicate possible Hepatitis Cirrhosis *Absence* indicates possible obstructive jaundice
Urine amylase	Various levels, depending on unit of measure	*Increased* values indicate possible Acute pancreatitis Pancreatic obstruction
Stool for occult blood	Negative	*Presence* indicates possible Carcinoma Peptic ulcer Ulcerative colitis
Ova and parasites	Negative	*Presence* is diagnostic of infection
Fecal fat	<7 g/24 hr with normal diet	*Increased* values indicate possible Crohn's disease Malabsorption syndrome Pancreatic disease

swallows a barium sulfate mixture while fluoroscopy is used to follow the passage of the barium down the esophagus. The client may be placed in other positions, lying flat or moving from side to side. This test is usually done *after* a barium enema or gallbladder radiographic series to prevent the mixture used in the barium swallow from interfering with the other examinations.

Follow-Up Care

After the test, the nurse or the radiologic technician instructs the client to drink plenty of fluids to eliminate the barium from the colon. Barium retention could result in an intestinal obstruction. An elderly client or a client who is susceptible to constipation may need a mild laxative or stool softener to facilitate barium elimination. The nurse or the technician cautions the client that stools will be chalky white or lighter in color for approximately 1 to 3 days. When all barium is expelled, stools return to a normal brown color.

Abdominal distention and decreased or absent bowel sounds associated with constipation or obstipation may suggest barium impaction. The nurse instructs the client to report these signs and symptoms to the physician immediately.

Upper Gastrointestinal Series and Small-Bowel Series

An upper GI (UGI) radiographic series is an x-ray visualization of the esophagus, stomach, and duodenum. The small-bowel radiographic series, also known as a small-bowel follow-through (SBFT), continues the tracing of the barium through the small intestines up to and including the ileocecal junction. These tests are typically performed for a client with complaints of indigestion, abdominal pain, nausea, vomiting, or weight loss.

Client Preparation

The client is NPO after midnight the evening before the test. The nurse instructs the client about the barium preparation and its consistency and that he or she will have to drink about 16 ounces of the barium. The nurse also tells the client about the rotating x-ray table and the many positions that are required for this test.

Procedure

The client drinks a mixture of barium sulfate, and fluoroscopy is used to trace the barium through the esophagus and stomach. The client stands against the x-ray table for this part of the test. The table then moves the client to a lying position for more views of the stomach and duodenum. Lying in a prone position, the client drinks more barium as quickly as possible while x-rays are taken. The technician or the radiology nurse is aware that this position is uncomfortable for elderly people. A pillow for comfort and a sheet to prevent chilling are supplied for these clients whenever possible.

If a small-bowel radiographic series is included, the client drinks additional barium, and more x-rays are taken at intervals. This series can take several hours, de-pending on how long it takes the barium to reach the cecum.

Follow-Up Care

After either of these series, the nurse teaches the client to drink plenty of fluids to help eliminate the barium. For some clients, especially elderly clients, a mild laxative or stool softener may be necessary. The nurse or the radiologic technician instructs the client that stools may be chalky white for 24 to 72 hours as barium is excreted. As with the barium swallow, the nurse teaches the client that when all barium is passed, brown stools return. If the client is at home, the nurse instructs him or her to report abdominal fullness, pain, or a delay in return to brown stools.

Barium Enema

A barium enema (BE) examination, also known as a lower GI radiographic series, is an x-ray visualization of the large intestine. This test is usually ordered for a client with a complaint of blood or mucus in the stool or a change in bowel pattern, such as diarrhea or constipation.

Client Preparation

Adequate client preparation for a barium enema study is very important. Whenever possible, the client is placed on a low-residue diet 2 days before the test. The client consumes clear liquids the evening before the examination and is NPO after midnight until the test is completed. In addition, the physician usually orders a potent laxative, such as magnesium citrate, and an oral liquid preparation for cleaning the bowel the evening before the examination. In some cases, a cleansing enema is needed or required by the agency's procedure.

The preparation for a barium enema study can be stressful for the client. In a classic study, Pieper (1992) found that clients scheduled for a barium enema study slept poorly the night before the procedure and experienced fatigue and anxiety (see Research Applications for Nursing box).

Procedure

During the barium enema examination, a rectal catheter is inserted. The barium mixture is instilled by gravity slowly, and the client is instructed to hold the barium while films are taken. The client may have abdominal cramps and the urge to defecate as the barium enema is given. This procedure can be extremely uncomfortable, especially for elderly clients. The client is instructed to take slow, deep breaths and to hold the anal sphincter as tightly closed as possible. The test takes about 45 minutes to 1 hour.

Follow-Up Care

The nurse or the radiologic technician teaches the client to drink plenty of fluids to eliminate the barium. A mild laxative or cleansing enema may be needed for those who are susceptible to constipation, especially elderly clients.

▷ Research Applications for Nursing

Clients Have Increased Anxiety, Fatigue, and Insomnia When Scheduled for Certain Gastrointestinal Diagnostic Tests

Pieper, B. (1992). A study of persons undergoing outpatient gastrointestinal radiography. Journal of Enterostomal Therapy, 19, 54–58.

This study examines the effects of the preparation and procedure on 36 people having a barium enema study and 31 people having an upper gastrointestinal (GI) radiographic series. Thirty-six additional people who had x-rays that did *not* require preparation were used as a control group. The variables were blood pressure, heart rate, fatigue, anxiety, quality of sleep before the test, and perceived energy expenditure during the test. All variables were measured before and after the test. Perceptions of fatigue and anxiety were reported to the researcher by telephone 24 hours after the procedure.

Research participants who had a barium enema study reported that they slept poorly the night before the test and rated a greater energy expenditure during the examination than did the subjects in the other two groups. Barium enema study subjects also had clinically small (but statistically significant) increases in blood pressure after the test. Participants in the barium enema group and participants in the control group reported less anxiety over time.

Critique. The use of a control group was an appropriate design for this research study. All groups were similar in demographic data. Because blood pressure was measured in a sitting position, potential orthostatic changes were not detected. Previous studies found that orthostatic blood pressure changes accompany certain GI tests.

Possible Nursing Implications. The researcher suggests that individuals scheduled for a barium enema should arrange transportation to and from the radiology facility, because this is a potentially exhausting procedure. The nurse should perform client education prior to any scheduled diagnostic procedure to help decrease client anxiety.

The nurse informs the client that the stools will be chalky white for about 24 to 72 hours.

Percutaneous Transhepatic Cholangiography

Percutaneous transhepatic cholangiography is an x-ray of the biliary duct system with an iodine dye. This procedure is usually performed when a client has jaundice or persistent upper abdominal pain even after cholecystectomy. It can also be performed during surgery.

A laxative is usually given to the client the evening before the procedure. The client is given nothing by mouth (NPO) for 12 hours before the test, and the nurse asks about allergies to iodine or seafood. If the client has either of these allergies, the nurse informs the physician.

During the test, the client is instructed to hold his or her breath on expiration while a needle is inserted into the liver under x-ray visualization. The dye is injected slowly until the biliary tree is filled. X-rays are taken as the dye reaches the biliary duct system. The procedure usually takes 30 minutes to 1 hour.

After a percutaneous transhepatic cholangiography, the client is confined to bed for 6 hours, and the nurse inspects the injection site for bleeding or swelling. The nurse checks vital signs frequently, as ordered, and observes the client for abdominal distention or tenderness.

Gallbladder Series

A gallbladder (GB) radiographic series, or oral cholecystography, is an x-ray visualization of the gallbladder after oral ingestion of radiopaque dye. Although not commonly done, the test may be performed to identify causes of obstruction, such as stones. A gallbladder radiographic series should be done before any barium studies.

Before the gallbladder radiographic series, the nurse checks with the client about any allergies to iodine or seafood. On the day before the test, the client eats a fat-free or low-fat diet and takes six radiopaque iodine tablets (iopanoic acid [Telepaque]) approximately 2 hours after the evening meal. One tablet is taken with water every 5 minutes until all six tablets are consumed. The nurse instructs the client that the tablets can cause diarrhea. The client is NPO from midnight before the test until after the test is completed.

The client is usually in the x-ray department for about 60 minutes while several views of the gallbladder are taken.

There is no follow-up care after a gallbladder radiographic series.

Intravenous Cholangiography

Intravenous cholangiography (IVC) is an x-ray of the gallbladder and biliary ducts. This test is performed if the gallbladder is not visualized by a gallbladder radiographic series, or if biliary symptoms occur in a client who has had a cholecystectomy. It may also be done during surgery.

Before the test, the nurse checks with the client about any allergies to iodine or seafood and reports allergies to the physician.

The client may be in the x-ray department for 2 to 4 hours for IVC. The client is given an intravenous injection of a contrast material, and x-rays are taken at 20-minute intervals for 1 hour, or until the biliary ducts are visualized. The gallbladder should be visualized in 1 to 2 hours.

No follow-up care is needed after IVC.

Computed Tomography

Computed tomography (CT), also referred to as a CT scan, is a cross-sectional x-ray visualization that can detect tissue densities and abnormalities in the abdomen, liver, pancreas, spleen, and the biliary tract. CT may be performed with or without contrast media, depending on the physician's preference.

Client preparation involves education about the procedure. If the use of contrast media is scheduled, the nurse asks the client about allergies to seafood and iodine. There may be food and fluid restrictions.

The radiologic technician instructs the client to lie still and to hold his or her breath when asked. The client is placed on the examining table, and a series of x-rays are taken. Contrast media may be given by intravenous injection for a second set of x-rays to enhance the images. The test takes approximately 1 to 2 hours to complete.

No follow-up care is needed after a CT scan.

Other Diagnostic Tests

Endoscopy

Endoscopy is direct visualization of the gastrointestinal (GI) tract by means of a flexible fiberoptic endoscope. Endoscopes of various sizes are used for different areas of the GI tract. Visualization of the esophagus, the stomach, the biliary system, and the bowel is possible. Endoscopy is usually ordered to evaluate bleeding, ulceration, inflammation, masses, tumors, and cancerous lesions. Obtaining specimens for biopsy and cytologic studies is also possible through the endoscope. There are several types of endoscopic examinations.

Esophagogastroduodenoscopy

Esophagogastroduodenoscopy (EGD) is a visual examination of the esophagus, stomach, and duodenum. An examination of only the esophagus is called an esophagoscopy; an examination of the stomach is a gastroscopy.

Client Preparation

The client preparing for the upper GI endoscopic examination usually is NPO after midnight the evening before the test, or 8 to 12 hours before the procedure. The nurse explains that during the test a flexible tube is passed down the esophagus. The physician usually orders medication, such as midazolam hydrochloride (Versed) or diazepam (Valium, E-Pam✦), to relax the client. Atropine may be administered to dry secretions. In addition, a local anesthetic is sprayed to anesthetize the client's throat and facilitate passage of the tube. The nurse explains that this anesthetic will calm the gag reflex and that swallowing will be difficult. If the client has dentures, they are removed.

Procedure

After the medications are administered, the client is usually placed on his or her side with a towel or basin at the mouth for secretions. The physician passes the tube through the mouth and into the esophagus (Fig. 55–8). The client is asked to swallow to facilitate tube passage.

Follow-Up Care

After endoscopy, the nurse checks the client's vital signs frequently, as ordered, usually every 30 minutes until the sedation wears off. The nurse keeps the bed side rails raised during this time. The client remains on NPO status until the gag reflex returns. The nurse monitors the client for signs of perforation, such as pain, bleeding, and fever.

Endoscopic Retrograde Cholangiopancreatography

Endoscopic retrograde cholangiopancreatography (ERCP) includes visual and radiographic examination of the liver, gallbladder, and pancreas. The physician may perform a papillotomy, a small incision in the sphincter around the ampulla of Vater, to remove gallstones.

Client Preparation

For an ERCP, the client is prepared in the same manner as for EGD, including having nothing by mouth (NPO) after midnight before the test. The nurse asks the client about prior exposure to x-ray dye and any sensitivities or allergies.

Procedure

The endoscopic portion of an ERCP is similar to EGD, except that the endoscope is advanced farther, to the duodenum and into the biliary tract. The radiologist or the radiologic technician injects contrast medium, and x-ray films are taken to evaluate the biliary tract. An ERCP lasts from 30 minutes to 2 hours.

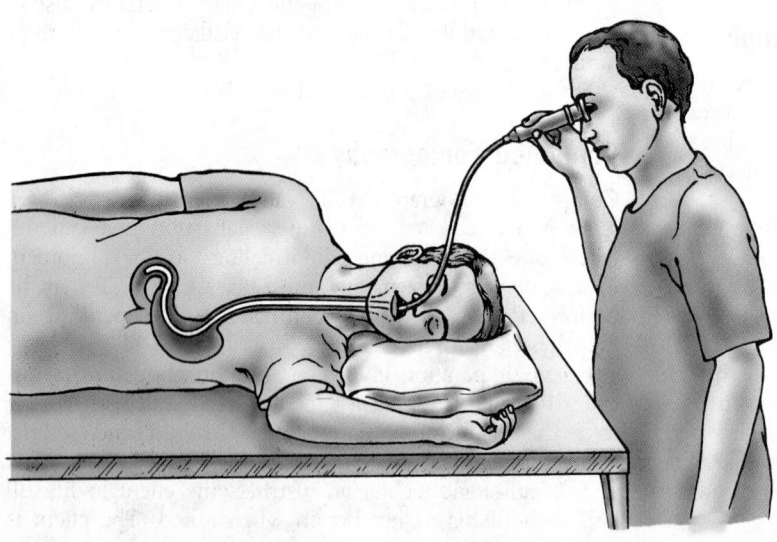

Figure 55–8. Esophagogastroduodenoscopy (EGD) allows visualization of the esophagus, the stomach, and the duodenum. If the esophagus is the focus of the examination, the procedure is called esophagoscopy. If the stomach is the focus, the term gastroscopy is used.

Follow-Up Care

After an ERCP, the nurse assesses the client's vital signs based on the agency's protocol for the frequency of vital sign monitoring. The client remains on NPO status until the gag reflex returns.

The nurse assesses the client for several postprocedure complications, including cholangitis, perforation, sepsis, and pancreatitis. These problems do not occur immediately after the procedure but may take several hours to 2 days to develop (Malarkey & McMorrow, 1996).

Colonoscopy

Colonoscopy is an endoscopic examination of the entire large bowel. The physician may also obtain tissue biopsy specimens or perform polyp removal through the colonoscope.

Client Preparation

The client should have a liquid diet for at least 24 hours before a colonoscopy and is usually NPO after midnight the evening before the procedure. An oral liquid preparation for cleaning the bowel (e.g., polyethylene glycol–electrolyte solution [GoLYTELEY]) is given to the client the evening before the examination.

The nurse chills the solution to make it more palatable. Even though it has a salty taste, the nurse should not dilute the solution or add ice. The nurse instructs the client to drink the preparation quickly—8 ounces (240 mL) every 10 minutes until all 4 L are consumed. This solution produces a watery diarrhea that begins in approximately 1 hour. The bowel clears in 4 to 5 hours. In some cases, the client may require laxatives, suppositories (e.g., bisacodyl [Dulcolax]), or one or more cleaning enemas.

Procedure

The physician orders medication to aid in relaxation, usually midazolam hydrochloride (Versed). Initially, the client is placed on the left side with the knees drawn up while the endoscope is passed into the rectum or colostomy up into the bowel. He or she may be asked to change positions later during the procedure.

To decrease peristaltic activity, the physician may administer intravenous glucagon or atropine. Because vasovagal reflex can occur during the procedure causing bradycardia, atropine should be available (Malarkey & McMorrow, 1996). The entire procedure lasts from 20 to 60 minutes.

Follow-Up Care

The nurse checks the client's vital signs per agency protocol or physician order. Side rails are kept up until sedation wears off. The nurse observes the client for signs of perforation and hemorrhage. The nurse instructs the client that a feeling of fullness and cramping and passage of flatus are expected for several hours after the test.

If a polypectomy or tissue biopsy has been performed, the client may see a small amount of blood in the first stool after the colonoscopy. Excessive bleeding should be reported immediately to the health care provider (Chart 55–5).

Proctosigmoidoscopy

Proctosigmoidoscopy is an endoscopic examination of the rectum and sigmoid colon using a flexible or rigid scope.

The client should have a liquid diet for at least 24 hours before a sigmoidoscopy; usually, a cleansing enema or sodium biphosphate (Fleet's) enema is given the morning of the procedure. A laxative may also be ordered the evening before the test.

For a proctosigmoidoscopy, the client is placed on the left side in the knee-chest position or on a special table in the proctoscopic position. The examination usually lasts about 30 minutes.

After the procedure, the care is similar to that after a colonoscopy (described earlier).

Gastric Analysis

The stomach's secretion of hydrochloric acid and pepsin is measured for evaluation of gastric and duodenal disorders. There are two tests in gastric analysis: basal gastric secretion and gastric acid stimulation. Basal gastric secretion measures the secretion of hydrochloric acid between meals. Gastric acid stimulation is a follow-up test to basal gastric secretion if only small amounts of secretion are collected.

Client Preparation

The client is NPO for at least 12 hours before the test. The nurse inserts a nasogastric (NG) tube and removes and discards the residual contents of the stomach.

Procedure

The nurse attaches the NG tube to suctioning equipment and collects the contents at 15-minute intervals for 1

Chart 55–5

Nursing Care Highlight: Care of the Client After a Colonoscopy

- Do not allow the client to take anything by mouth until sedation wears off and the client is alert.
- Take vital signs every 15 to 30 minutes until the client is alert.
- Keep the bed rails up until the client is alert.
- Assess for rectal bleeding or blood clots.
- Remind the client that fullness and mild abdominal cramping are expected for several hours.
- Assess for manifestations of bowel perforation, including *severe* abdominal pain and guarding. Fever may occur later.
- Assess for manifestations of hypovolemic shock, including dizziness, lightheadedness, decreased blood pressure, tachycardia, pallor, and altered mental status (may be the first sign).

hour. The nurse collects each sample and labels the time and volume of each specimen.

For the gastric acid stimulation test, the NG tube is left in place, and a drug that stimulates gastric acid secretion (e.g., pentagastrin or betazole dihydrochloride [Histalog]) is given to the client. Fifteen minutes after the injection of the drug, specimens are again collected at 15-minute intervals for 1 hour. The nurse collects, labels, and measures the specimens.

Depressed levels of gastric secretion suggest the presence of gastric carcinoma. Increased levels of gastric secretion indicate Zollinger-Ellison syndrome and duodenal ulcers (see Chap. 58).

Follow-Up Care

After the test is completed, the NG tube is removed unless it is needed for another purpose. No other follow-up is necessary.

Ultrasonography

Ultrasonography is a technique in which high-frequency, inaudible vibratory sound waves are passed through the body. Echoes of the sound waves that are created vary with tissue density changes. It is commonly used to image soft tissues, such as the liver, the spleen, the pancreas, the gallbladder, and the biliary system.

The client is usually allowed nothing by mouth (NPO) for 8 to 12 hours before ultrasonography of the abdomen. The nurse informs the client that it will be necessary to lie still during the study. Clients must have a full bladder for accurate visualization.

The client is placed in a prone or a supine position. The technician applies insulating gel to the end of the transducer and on the area of the abdomen under study. This gel allows airtight contact of the transducer with the client's skin. The technician moves the transducer back and forth over the skin until the desired images are obtained. The study takes about 15 to 30 minutes. No follow-up care is necessary after ultrasonography.

Endoscopic Ultrasonography

Endoscopic ultrasonography (EUS) provides images of the gastrointestinal (GI) wall and high-resolution images of the digestive organs. The ultrasonography is performed through the endoscope. This procedure is useful in diagnosing the presence of lymph node tumors, mucosal tumors, and tumors of the pancreas, stomach, and rectum. The client preparation and follow-up care are similar to those for both endoscopy and ultrasonography.

Liver Scan

A liver scan is a nuclear medicine technique. It is more correctly called a liver-spleen scan, because an intravenous injection of a radioactive colloid is given that is taken up primarily by the liver and secondarily by the spleen. The scan evaluates the liver and the spleen for tumors or abscesses, organ size and location, and vascularity.

The nurse instructs the client about the need to lie still during the scanning. The client is assured that the colloid injection has only small amounts of radioactivity and is not dangerous.

The technician or the physician gives the radioactive injection through an intravenous line, and a wait of about 15 minutes is necessary for uptake. The technician places the client in many different positions while the scanning takes place. No follow-up care is necessary after a liver scan.

SELECTED BIBLIOGRAPHY

Allen, K. M., & Phillips, J. M. (1997). *Women's health across the lifespan.* Philadelphia: Lippincott-Raven.

Dammel, T. (1997). Fecal occult blood testing: Looking for hidden danger. *Nursing97, 27*(7), 44–45.

Ferrucci, J. (1997). Colonoscopy and barium enema: Radiologist's response. *Gastroenterology, 112*(1), 294–297.

Fischbach, F. (1996). *A manual of laboratory and diagnostic tests* (5th ed.). Philadelphia: Lippincott-Raven.

Giger, J. N., & Davidhizar (1995). *Transcultural nursing: Assessment and interventions* (2nd ed.). St. Louis: Mosby-Year Book.

Huether, S. E., (1996). Structure and function of the digestive system. In S. E. Huether & K. L. McCance (Eds.), *Understanding pathophysiology* (pp. 917–943). St. Louis: Mosby-Year Book.

Jarvis, C. (1996). *Physical examination and health assessment* (2nd ed.). Philadelphia: W. B. Saunders.

Joffrion, L. P., & Leuszler, L. B. (1995). The gastrointestinal system and its problems in the elderly with nutritional considerations. In M. Stanley & P. G. Beare (Eds.), *Gerontological nursing* (pp. 241–254). Philadelphia: F. A. Davis.

*King, H., & Locke, F. B. (1988). The national mortality survey of China: Implications for cancer control and prevention. *Cancer Detection and Prevention, 13,* 157–166.

Linton, A. D. (1997). Age-related changes in the gastrointestinal system. In M. A. Matteson, E. S. McConnell, & A. D. Linton (Eds.), *Gerontological nursing: Concepts and practice* (2nd ed.; pp. 317–335). Philadelphia: W. B. Saunders.

Malarkey, L. M., & McMorrow, M. E. (1996). *Nurse's manual of laboratory tests and diagnostic procedures.* Philadelphia: W. B. Saunders.

Nowazek, V., & Neeley, M. (1996). Health assessment of the older patient. *Critical Care Nursing Quarterly, 19*(2), 1–6.

*Pieper, B. (1992). A study of persons undergoing outpatient gastrointestinal radiography. *Journal of Enterostomal Therapy, 19,* 54–58.

Porth, C. M., (1994). *Pathophysiology concepts of altered health states* (4th ed.). Philadelphia: J. B. Lippincott.

*Renkes, J. (1993). GI endoscopy: Managing the full scope of care. *Nursing93, 23*(6), 50–55.

Siconolfi, L. A. (1995). Clarifying the complexity of liver function tests. *Nursing95, 25*(5), 39–46.

Tilkian, S. M., Conover, M. B., & Tilkian, A. G. (1995). *Clinical and nursing implications of laboratory tests.* St. Louis: Mosby-Year Book.

Watson, J., & Jaffe, M. S. (1995). *Nurse's manual of laboratory and diagnostic tests* (2nd ed.). Philadelphia: F. A. Davis.

Wellman, N. (1997) A case manager's guide to nutrition screening and intervention. *The Journal of Care Management, 3*(2), 12–27.

SUGGESTED READINGS

Dammel, T. (1997). Fecal occult blood testing: Looking for hidden danger. *Nursing97, 27*(7), 44–45.

This brief article describes the fecal occult blood test (FOBT) and how to use the Hemoccult SENSA slide method. The author also lists dos and don'ts to help ensure accuracy of the test results. Color photos illustrate each step of the FOBT procedure.

Siconolfi, L. A. (1995). Clarifying the complexity of liver function tests. *Nursing95, 25*(5), 39–46.

This article summarizes the major functions of the liver and presents a chart on specific tests and their significance. The author also includes a section on what to watch for in the client who has liver dysfunction. A quiz for continuing education credit completes the article.

Chapter 56

INTERVENTIONS FOR CLIENTS WITH ORAL CAVITY PROBLEMS

CHAPTER HIGHLIGHTS

Basic functions, such as eating, breathing, and speaking, can be severely impaired by problems of the oral cavity. Although problems of the oral cavity are limited to a small anatomic area, the effects can be widespread and have an impact on the person's lifestyle and general health.

Prevention and management of dental disease, such as dental caries and gingivitis, are not discussed in this chapter. Most basic nursing textbooks include this information. Chart 56–1 lists ways for maintaining a healthy oral cavity.

STOMATITIS

Stomatitis is an inflammation of the oral cavity, or mouth, which is located from the lips to the first tonsillar arch. Stomatitis is different from pharyngitis, inflammation of the pharynx, because pharyngitis occurs within the pharyngeal boundaries of the first tonsillar arch (including the arch, the tonsils, and the soft palate) to the posterior pharyngeal wall. (Chapter 31 discusses pharyngitis in detail.)

Overview

Stomatitis is classified by the cause of the inflammation. *Primary* stomatitis includes aphthous stomatitis, herpes simplex stomatitis, Vincent's stomatitis, and traumatic ulcers. *Secondary* stomatitis generally results from infection by opportunistic viruses or bacteria when the client's resistance is lowered by a local or systemic disorder.

The oral mucosa is often the first site to show a systemic disease. The etiologic factors implicated in stomatitis are bone marrow disorders, allergies, systemic diseases, drugs, nutritional disorders, and emotional disturbances.

Stomatitis is also a common side effect of radiation therapy to the head and neck and of some chemotherapeutic agents. (See Chapter 27 for nursing care of the client undergoing radiation and chemotherapy.)

Primary Stomatitis
Aphthous Stomatitis
Pathophysiology/Etiology

Aphthous stomatitis, also known as aphthous ulcers or canker sores, is a common self-limiting condition with an unclear pathogenesis. An immunologic response to oral cavity antigens appears to play a role in the development of this type of stomatitis; however, contributing factors include psychological stress, a genetic predisposition, vitamin B_{12}, iron, and folate deficiencies. Viruses, allergies, and trauma are possible causes as well.

Aphthous stomatitis develops in four phases. The first phase is the premonitory phase, characterized by tingling, burning, or a hyperesthetic sensation that lasts as long as 24 hours. The second phase is the preulcerative phase and is characterized by painful erythematous macules or papules with erythematous halos that last from 18 hours to 3 days. The third phase is the ulcerative phase that last 1 to 16 days. During this phase, discrete ulcers appear singly or in groups and measure 2 to 10 mm with a dusky erythematous halo around a gray-yellow membrane-covered ulcer. During the last phase, healing occurs usually without scarring and takes about 2 weeks. Aphthous stomatitis is localized only to the oral cavity.

Incidence/Prevalence

Aphthous stomatitis is very common, with about 20% of the population affected at some time (Goroll & May, 1995). In approximately one third of those affected with aphthous stomatitis, the lesions are recurrent and can continue for 40 years. Some women experience recurrences premenstrually.

Herpes Simplex Stomatitis

Pathophysiology/Etiology

Stomatitis caused by the herpes simplex virus (HSV) occurs as a primary or secondary (or recurrent) infection; secondary infections are more common. Two types of HSV have been identified: HSV type 2, which causes genital lesions (discussed in Chapter 80), and HSV type 1, which is responsible for nongenital lesions.

The initial exposure to the virus results in a primary HSV infection, also called acute herpetic stomatitis. The uniformly sized vesicles occur most frequently on the tongue, the palate, and the buccal and labial mucosae. The vesicles rupture soon after appearing, leaving painful ulcerated areas surrounded by erythematous margins (Fig. 56–1). The lesions at this stage are similar to aphthous ulcers. The ulcerated areas heal in 10 to 14 days.

The mucosal vesicles are generally accompanied by acute inflammation of the gingiva, occasionally with herpetic lesions. The tongue has a characteristic white coating, and the client complains of a foul odor to the breath. Primary HSV infections are characterized by symptoms of generalized infection, including malaise, fever, and lymphadenopathy.

Incidence/Prevalence

Herpes simplex virus infection is extremely common. Primary herpetic stomatitis is usually contracted in childhood but may be seen in adults.

Vincent's Stomatitis

Pathophysiology/Etiology

Vincent's stomatitis, or necrotizing stomatitis, is an acute bacterial infection of the gingiva. The disease has a sudden onset and is related to a decreased resistance of tissues to normal oral bacterial flora. Systemic etiologic factors that decrease tissue resistance include poor nutrition, leukemia, and severe infections such as pyelonephritis. Poor oral hygiene and extreme emotional stress have been suggested as contributing factors.

The disease is characterized by erythema, ulceration, and necrosis of the gingival margins; the slough of skin that is left is easily scraped off. The gingival papillae between the teeth appear worn away and raw (Fig. 56–2). Clients complain of severe pain, foul breath, thick ropy secretions, and increased salivation. The gingivae often bleed spontaneously or from mild irritation, such as chewing. Systemic clinical manifestations can include malaise, poor appetite, and, occasionally, enlargement of cervical (neck) lymph nodes.

Incidence/Prevalence

Necrotizing gingivitis occurs frequently in adults, and the incidence seems to increase with aging. Older adults have

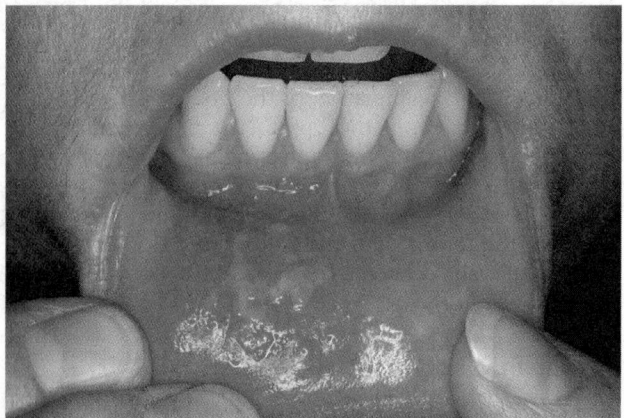

Figure 56–1. Herpes simplex stomatitis. (From Callen, J. P., Greer, K. E., Hood, A. F, et al. [1993]. *Color atlas of dermatology.* Philadelphia: W. B. Saunders Co.)

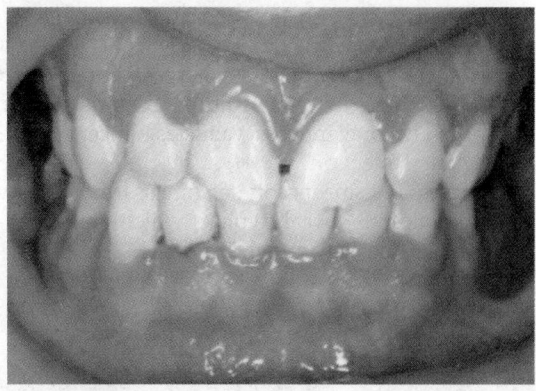

Figure 56-2. Acute necrotizing ulcerative gingivitis. (From Carranza, F. A., Jr., & Newman, M. G. [1996]. *Clinical periodontology* [8th ed.]. Philadelphia: W. B. Saunders Co.)

an increased susceptibility to infections because of decreased immunocompetence.

Traumatic Ulcers

Pathophysiology/Etiology

Traumatic ulcers can be differentiated from aphthous ulcers on the basis of history and clinical manifestations. The client is usually able to recall a physical (such as cheek biting) or thermal (such as a pizza burn) injury. Traumatic oral lesions are similar to aphthous ulcers but are less sharply defined and are generally not as painful.

Incidence/Prevalence

Traumatic ulcers are commonly found in clients with malocclusion, ill-fitting dentures, or broken teeth and in those who habitually bite their oral mucosa.

Secondary Stomatitis

Lichen Planus

Pathophysiology/Etiology

Lichen planus is a chronic dermatosis involving both the skin and the oral mucous membrane. Oral lesions are present in many cases of lichen planus, and they are often the first manifestation of the disease. Symmetric, white oral lesions of various patterns (linear, interlacing lines, spots, or plaques) are most common in the pharynx (Fig. 56-3) but are also found on the tongue and the buccal or labial mucosa. The lesions tend to be domed and shiny, although those on the tongue are often flat and dull. These oral lesions rarely ulcerate and are generally asymptomatic. Clients occasionally complain of a burning feeling, especially from lesions on the tongue. Most people have a spontaneous remission in 6 months to 2 years after the onset of the disease.

The etiology is unknown, but psychosomatic, genetic, allergic, and infectious processes have been proposed. Prognosis for cure is poor. Spontaneous flares and remissions are hallmarks of the disease.

Incidence/Prevalence

Lichen planus occurs with equal frequency in men and women and is usually a disease of middle-aged Caucasians.

Candidiasis (Moniliasis)

Pathophysiology/Etiology

Candida albicans is part of the normal flora of the oral cavity. It is the yeast-like fungus that causes candidiasis (or thrush), which is sometimes referred to as a yeast infection. With recurrent candidiasis, as with all secondary stomatitis, a causative systemic disorder should be sought. Because antibiotic therapy destroys the normal flora that usually prevent fungal infections, candidiasis can occur in clients receiving long-term antibiotic therapy. Chemotherapy diminishes the ability of the immune system to prevent infection, so clients receiving chemotherapy often develop candidiasis.

Candidiasis appears as white patches (often described as milk curds) on the tongue, the palate, and the buccal mucosa (Fig. 56-4). When these patches are wiped away, the underlying surface appears red and sore. Clients rarely complain of actual pain but describe the lesions as dry or hot.

Incidence/Prevalence

Candidiasis of the oral cavity is common in clients undergoing immunosuppressive therapy (chemotherapy, radiation to the head, steroid therapy, or antirejection medication) and clients with immunodeficiency disease, such as human immunodeficiency virus (HIV) infection.

ELDERLY CONSIDERATIONS

Elderly clients are especially at high risk for candidiasis because aging causes a decrease in immune function. Clients who are diabetic, malnourished, or under emotional stress are also at high risk.

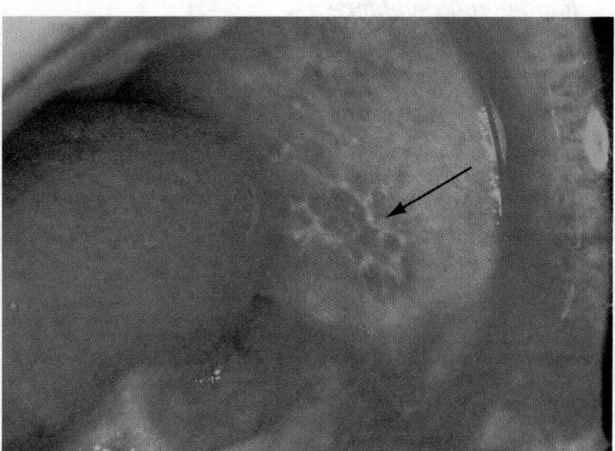

Figure 56-3. Oral lichen planus *(arrow).* (Courtesy of Dr. Andrew Martof, Charlottesville, VA.)

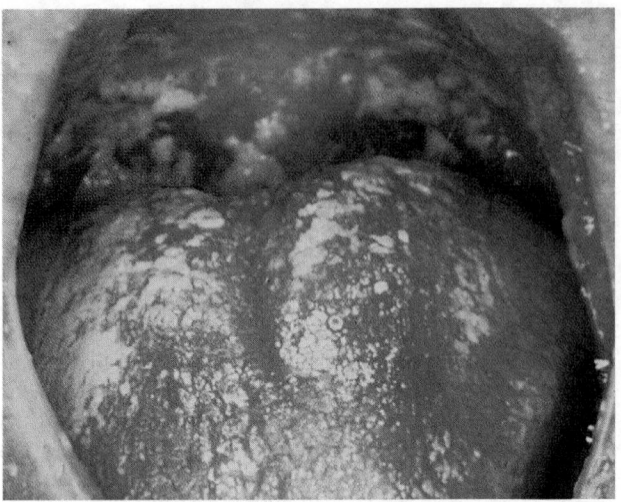

Figure 56-4. Oral candidiasis. (From Radford, J., & Thatcher, N. [1988]. The toxicity of cancer chemotherapy in adults. *Cancer Care, 5*:4-7.)

Herpes Simplex Stomatitis

Pathophysiology/Etiology

The lesion of secondary herpes simplex stomatitis is the typical cold sore or fever blister. This is caused by a recurrent herpes simplex virus (HSV) type 1 infection. The current theory is that the virus lies dormant after primary exposure (which is often subclinical; that is, not resulting in generalized symptoms of stomatitis). HSV is then reactivated by an upper respiratory infection, a febrile episode, exposure to actinic radiation (sunlight), trauma, emotional stress, menstruation, or immunologic compromise.

These lesions usually appear on the lip at the edge of the labial mucosa; they can also occur in other areas of the lip or around the mouth. There may be one or several vesicular lesions. The vesicles erupt soon after appearing, crust over, and heal in 7 to 10 days.

Incidence/Prevalence

Secondary herpes simplex stomatitis is a common disorder seen frequently in immunocompromised clients, such as those receiving chemotherapy for cancer, those on anti-rejection medication, and those with HIV infection.

Collaborative Management

 Assessment

As in any examination of the oral cavity, the nurse wears nonsterile gloves for protection against infection. Adequate lighting, including a flashlight or penlight, and a tongue blade facilitate the examination.

Using clean gloves, the nurse assesses the oral cavity of the client with stomatitis for lesions, coating, cracking, and fissures. Characteristics of the lesions are described in terms of location, size, shape, color, and drainage. Odors are also described.

Fluid from herpetic vesicles in herpes simplex stomatitis may be obtained for viral culture. Bacterial culture of exudate from the oral mucosa validates Vincent's stomatitis or secondary infection.

Gram stains or smears of scrapings from the white lesions of candidiasis reveal hyphae, which are thread-like processes associated with fungi.

 Interventions

Interventions for the client with stomatitis focus on proper oral hygiene, drug therapy, and diet therapy.

Oral Hygiene. The nurse assesses the client's current regimen of oral hygiene. Modifications may be needed when oral discomfort occurs. For example, the nurse suggests the use of gauze sponges to replace brushing during painful episodes of stomatitis.

The client with lesions of the oral cavity generally tolerates gentle mouth care with lukewarm, soothing solutions. Most commercial mouthwashes are contraindicated because they have a high alcohol content, which causes a burning sensation in irritated or ulcerated oral mucosa. Mouth rinses with normal saline, baking soda (1 tsp in 8 ounces of water [5 mL in 240 mL of water]), or half-strength hydrogen peroxide are tolerated better than commercial products and soothe inflamed tissues. Clients who experience difficulty in swallowing because of increased or tenacious secretions can use oral suction equipment with a dental tip or a tonsil tip (Yankar catheter) to clear saliva.

Frequent gentle mouth care enhances debridement of ulcerated lesions and can prevent superinfections. Frequent oral care also promotes a general feeling of well-being. Chart 56-2 lists appropriate activities for special oral care.

Drug Therapy. Anti-infectives and analgesics, opioid and nonopioid, are often required for the client with stomatitis.

Anti-Infectives. The health care provider prescribes systemic antibiotics for clients with Vincent's stomatitis. When inflammation and edema threaten the airway, the client is hospitalized for observation and treated with systemic steroids as well as intravenous (IV) antibiotics.

Antibiotics are of little value in viral or fungal stomatitis unless a secondary infection is present. Systemic antibiotics are ineffective for lichen planus and are not recommended.

A regimen of IV acyclovir (Zovirax) is usually prescribed for immunocompromised clients who contract herpes simplex stomatitis. Acyclovir is typically administered to clients with normal renal function at a dose of 5 mg/kg, infused at a constant rate over 1 hour every 8 hours for 7 days. Clients with competent immune systems may be given acyclovir in oral or topical form.

For clients with oral *Candida* infection, an antifungal agent is prescribed, such as nystatin (Mycostatin, Nadostine✱) oral suspension 600,000 units four times daily for 7 to 10 days. The nurse teaches the client to swish the solution around in the mouth before swallowing. Oral troches (lozenges) may also be effective. Systemic steroids can be of benefit in long-standing lichen planus.

Analgesics. The nurse assesses the need for analgesics. On the basis of the client's subjective report of pain relief and objective symptoms of pain, the nurse evaluates the effect of the chosen regimen.

Topically applied agents or oral analgesics temporarily relieve severe oral pain (Table 56–1). Coating agents, such as kaolin and magnesium hydroxide (milk of magnesia), relieve the severe oral pain of aphthous ulcers; they provide a soothing feeling as well as protect the

TABLE 56–1

Drugs Commonly Used for Oral Pain Relief

Oral Agents
- Lidocaine 2%, viscous
- Diphenhydramine (Benadryl) elixir
- Antacid suspension of choice
- Diphenhydramine elixir
- Kaopectate
- Acetaminophen with codeine elixir (codeine phosphate 12 mg, acetaminophen 120 mg/5 mL)

Topical Agents
- Dyclonine (Dyclone) 0.5%
- Butyl aminobenzoate 2%
- Tetracaine 2%
- Benzalkonium chloride 0.5%
- Cetyldimethylethylammonium bromide (Cetacaine) 0.005%

lesions from further irritation. Gentian violet, 0.5% to 1% aqueous solution painted on *Candida* lesions every other day for 1 week, decreases local irritation. Topical swishes are available, such as 50/50 diphenhydramine hydrochloride (Benadryl) and kaolin with pectin, lidocaine (Xylocaine) viscous solution, and dyclonine hydrochloride (Dyclone). These medications provide topical analgesia as well as local anti-inflammatory effects.

The health care provider often prescribes topical swishes for herpes simplex virus (HSV) stomatitis and lichen planus. These suspensions can be offered to the client in frozen form; the numbing effects of the cold provide longer analgesia. Topical corticosteroids are indicated for aphthous ulcers, lichen planus, and primary HSV lesions. Triamcinolone cream is frequently applied with the finger or a cotton-tipped applicator, or the corticosteroid can be injected directly into the lesion.

Diet Therapy. Liquid, soft, or blenderized foods cause less discomfort with painful oral lesions and help maintain adequate nutrition. A change in the consistency of food often eliminates irritation. Citrus juices or spicy or hot foods can cause oral irritation and should be avoided. Cold, icy drinks are usually well tolerated. The nurse assesses the client's ability to maintain adequate fluid intake and nutrition by mouth. In severe cases of stomatitis, nutrition may have to be supplemented by milkshakes or commercial liquid nutritional supplements, such as Ensure or Boost. In some cases, short-term nasogastric feeding may be necessary.

TUMORS
Overview

Tumors of the oral cavity, whether benign or malignant, can change many aspects of the client's daily routine. Swallowing or chewing may be altered, speech may be affected, and/or pain may limit the client's ability to perform activities of daily living.

Tumors of the oral cavity often have a profound effect on the client's body image as well. The nurse must be aware of the many implications of tumors of the oral cavity in assisting the client to decide on a treatment regimen. The nurse helps the client maintain independence and control during treatment.

Tumors of the oral cavity can be classified as premalignant, malignant, or benign. Most benign lesions in the oral cavity arise from the many minor salivary glands in the oral mucous membrane. (See Neoplasms of the Salivary Glands.)

Premalignant Lesions
Leukoplakia
Pathophysiology/Etiology

Leukoplakia is a white spot or patch on the oral mucous membrane that is not a result of other processes, such as lichen planus or candidiasis. The lesion can occur in any area of the mucous membrane but is most common on the buccal mucosa; however, lingular lesions have the greatest risk of malignant transformation. Leukoplakia is usually asymptomatic, but clients may complain of slight burning or itching in the area of the lesion.

Leukoplakia is potentially premalignant. In 10% of cases, leukoplakia represents premalignant changes that show dysplasia on biopsy (Kelly, 1995).

The major etiologic factors in the development of oral leukoplakia are mechanical factors, such as poorly fitting dentures, broken or poorly repaired teeth, chronic cheek nibbling, and problems with malocclusion that result in long-term irritation of the oral mucous membrane.

The dryness, heat, and tobacco products associated with smoking are also implicated, as is excessive heat from food and beverages. Leukoplakia is sometimes referred to as the smoker's patch.

Heredity may also place the client at risk for these lesions. By lowering the resistance of the mucous membrane, poor nutrition can enhance susceptibility to leukoplakia.

Incidence/Prevalence

Leukoplakia of the oral mucous membrane is a relatively common disorder, usually seen in people in their 40s. Men are twice as likely as women to have leukoplakia; however, the incidence of leukoplakia in women is rising because more women are smoking.

Erythroplakia

Erythroplakia is a red, velvety patch on the oral mucosa. It is generally asymptomatic, is not raised or indurated, and is often discovered on routine oral examinations. Erythroplakia is highly suggestive of an early carcinoma (Kelly, 1995). The incidence of erythroplakia is similar to that of leukoplakia.

Malignant Tumors
Squamous Cell Carcinoma
Pathophysiology/Etiology

Oral cancers are most often squamous cell carcinomas that arise from tiny flat cells lining various parts of the oral cavity. Because these tumors usually grow slowly, the lesion may be large before the onset of symptoms unless ulceration is present. Half of all oral cancers metastasize or become invasive before they are diagnosed. Symptoms of a squamous cell tumor include

- A sore or lesion in the oral cavity or in the neck (cervical metastasis)
- Trouble with wearing dentures
- Mild irritation of the tongue
- Sore throat
- Loose teeth
- Pain in the tongue or ear

The American Joint Committee on Cancer has devised the TNM classification system for tumors of the lip and oral cavity (Table 56–2). Each lesion is defined by

T—the size or degree of penetration of the tumor
N—the presence, size, number, and location of involved cervical lymph nodes
M—the presence of distant metastasis (spread)

Use of tobacco in all of its forms (cigarettes, cigars, smokeless tobacco, and snuff) is an independent risk factor for the development of oral cancer (Bundgaard et al., 1996). Heavy alcohol consumption appears to increase the risk of oral cancer as well, but the mechanism is not well understood. These two factors combined seem to be especially destructive to the oral mucosa.

As with leukoplakia, poor nutritional status accompanies many cases of oral cancer. Family history often reveals a trend in cancer incidence, which might indicate an inherited trait. Poor oral hygiene is also associated with oral cancer. Deficient oral hygiene might render the mucous membrane less resistant to infection and trauma. Other possible etiologic factors include previous low-dose ionizing radiation to the head or neck, occupational exposure to carcinogens, and pollution.

Incidence/Prevalence

Oral cancers represent 4% of all cancers in men and 2% of all cancers in Women in the United States; squamous cell carcinoma accounts for more than 90% of them. The peak incidence of oral cancer for women is in the sixth decade. For men, the incidence is equally frequent after the age of 50 years (Kelly, 1995).

TRANSCULTURAL CONSIDERATIONS

The relative 5-year survival rate for Caucasians with oral cavity and pharynx cancer is 55%, compared with a relative 5-year survival rate of 33% for African-Americans with oral cavity cancer (American Cancer Society, 1996).

ELDERLY CONSIDERATIONS

Approximately half of all oral cancers and most deaths associated with oral cancers occur in people over 65 (American Cancer Society, 1996).

Basal Cell Carcinoma
Pathophysiology/Etiology

Basal cell carcinoma of the oral cavity occurs primarily on the lips. The lesion is asymptomatic and resembles a raised scab. With time, the lesion evolves into a characteristic ulcer with a raised pearly border. Basal cell carcinomas do not metastasize but can aggressively involve the skin of the face. The major etiologic factor in basal cell carcinoma is exposure to sunlight.

Incidence/Prevalence

Basal cell carcinoma is the second most common type of oral cancer but is much less frequent than squamous cell carcinoma.

TABLE 56–2

TNM Classification for Tumors of the Lip and Oral Cavity

Primary Tumor (T)

- TX Primary tumor cannot be assessed
- T0 No evidence of primary tumor
- Tis Carcinoma in situ
- T1 Tumor 2 cm or less in greatest dimension
- T2 Tumor more than 2 cm but not more than 4 cm in greatest dimension
- T3 Tumor more than 4 cm in greatest dimension
- T4 (Lip) Tumor invades adjacent structures (e.g., through the cortical bone, the tongue, and the skin of the neck)
- T4 (Oral cavity) Tumor invades adjacent structures (e.g., through the cortical bone, into the deep [extrinsic] muscle of the tongue, the maxillary sinus, and the skin)

Lymph Node (N)

- NX Regional lymph nodes cannot be assessed
- N0 No regional lymph node metastasis
- N1 Metastasis in a single ipsilateral lymph node, 3 cm or less in greatest dimension
- N2 Metastasis in a single ipsilateral lymph node, more than 3 cm but not more than 6 cm in greatest dimension; or multiple ipsilateral lymph nodes, none more than 6 cm in greatest dimension; or bilateral or contralateral lymph nodes, none more than 6 cm in greatest dimension
  - N2a Metastasis in a single ipsilateral lymph node more than 3 cm but not more than 6 cm in greatest dimension
  - N2b Metastasis in multiple ipsilateral lymph nodes, none more than 6 cm in greatest dimension
  - N2c Metastasis in bilateral or contralateral lymph nodes, none more than 6 cm in greatest dimension
- N3 Metastasis in a lymph node more than 6 cm in greatest dimension

Distant Metastasis (M)

- MX The presence of distant metastasis cannot be assessed
- M0 No distant metastasis
- M1 Distant metastasis

Stage Grouping

0	Tis	N0	M0
I	T1	N0	M0
II	T2	N0	M0
III	T3	N0	M0
	T1	N1	M0
	T2	N1	M0
	T3	N1	M0
IV	T4	N0	M0
	T4	N1	M0
	Any T	N2	M0
	Any T	N3	M0
	Any T	Any N	M1

From American Joint Committee on Cancer. (1988). O. H. Beahrs, D. E. Hanson, R. V. Hatter, & M. H. Myers (Eds.), *Manual for staging of cancer* (3rd ed.). Philadelphia: J. B. Lippincott.

TRANSCULTURAL CONSIDERATIONS

Clients who work outdoors or who sunbathe excessively are more likely to have basal cell carcinomas, especially Caucasians with fair skin.

Kaposi's Sarcoma

Kaposi's sarcoma appears as painless red-purple oral plaques, which later change to nodular form. It is most often associated with acquired immunodeficiency syndrome (AIDS). (See Chapter 25 for a complete discussion.)

Collaborative Management

 Assessment

➤ *History*

The nurse begins assessment of the client with a tumor of the oral cavity by obtaining a history of the current problem. The nurse asks about occupation and exposure to known oral carcinogens or irritants, such as sunlight or other source of ultraviolet radiation, mechanical irritation, chronic exposure to heat (from foods or tobacco products), or use of alcohol and/or tobacco products.

The nurse identifies areas in which client education is needed for altering behaviors that are potentially harmful to the oral mucosa. A family history of cancer and a history of previous oral cancer alert health care providers to be especially vigilant for the appearance of neoplastic disease.

The nurse assesses the client's routine oral hygiene regimen and use of dentures or oral appliances, which might add to discomfort or mechanically irritate the mucosa. The nurse questions the client about hemoptysis, which might indicate an ulcerative lesion. The oral hygiene regimen may need to be modified if the current routine is inadequate or the client experiences discomfort when performing oral care.

The nurse determines the status of the client's past and current appetite and nutritional state, including difficulty with chewing or swallowing. A continuing trend of weight loss may be related to metastasis, heavy alcohol intake, difficulty in eating or chewing, or an underlying disorder.

➤ Physical Assessment/Clinical Manifestations

The nurse thoroughly assesses the oral cavity for any lesions, evidence of pain, or restriction of movement. The nurse notes any alteration in speech attributable to tongue restriction.

Because cervical metastasis is frequently associated with lesions of the buccal mucosa and the tongue, the nurse completes the physical assessment by palpating the cervical lymph nodes (Fig. 56–5). The nurse uses enough pressure to palpate structures under the skin, rather than rubbing the fingers over the tissues.

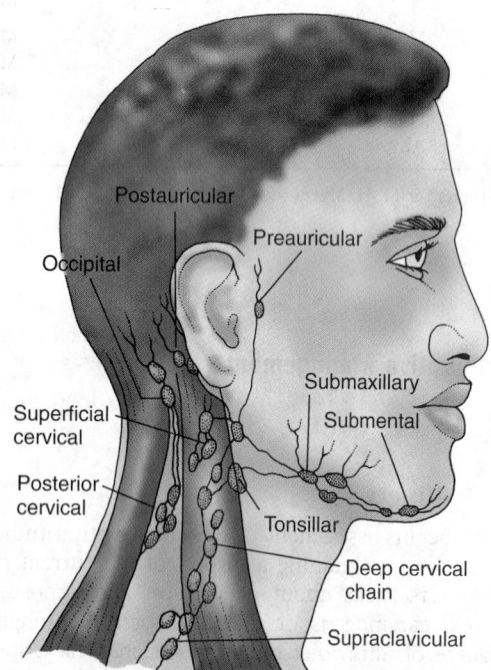

Figure 56–5. The lymph nodes of the cervical region.

Postauricular
Preauricular
Occipital
Submaxillary
Superficial cervical
Submental
Posterior cervical
Tonsillar
Deep cervical chain
Supraclavicular

➤ Psychosocial Assessment

Fear of cancer is probably the most important factor in the client's failure to seek professional assessment when oral lesions are noted. The nurse explores the client's fears and anxieties, providing information as needed about diagnosis and treatment.

The nurse assesses the meaning of cancer to the client, because this often varies. Some clients fear death; others fear pain or loss of family roles. The nurse evaluates the client's support system and past mechanisms of coping. This may help identify available supports during the current crisis of diagnosis of oral cancer.

Because the functioning and the appearance of the oral cavity are strongly linked with body image and sexuality, the nurse assesses the impact of oral lesions on the client's self-concept. In addition, the nurse assesses the client for any educational or cultural limitations to instruction or therapy.

➤ Radiographic Assessment

The health care provider may order an x-ray of the skull and/or computed tomography (CT) to determine whether the cancer has spread into other adjacent structures.

➤ Other Diagnostic Assessment

Biopsy is the definitive method for diagnosis of oral cancer; therefore, the physician obtains a biopsy specimen of the oral tissue to assess for malignant or premalignant changes. Biopsies can be performed with local anesthesia or with the client under general anesthesia. When general anesthesia is used, biopsy is usually combined with endoscopy (bronchoscopy, esophagoscopy, laryngoscopy, or a combination of these procedures).

 Analysis

➤ Common Nursing Diagnoses

The priority for nursing diagnoses in caring for the client with an oral tumor are:
1. Risk for Ineffective Breathing Pattern, related to obstruction by the tumor, edema, or secretions
2. Altered Oral Mucous Membrane, related to effects of the tumor

➤ Additional Nursing Diagnoses

In addition, the client may have one or more of the following nursing diagnoses:
- Impaired Verbal Communication, related to tumor or surgery
- Body Image Disturbance, related to altered oral mucous membrane, surgery, chemotherapy, or radiation therapy
- Pain, related to altered oral mucous membrane
- High Risk for Infection, related to altered oral mucous membrane

- Altered Nutrition: Less than Body Requirements, related to pain and/or edema

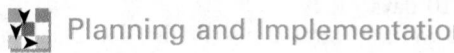

Planning and Implementation

Risk for Ineffective Breathing Pattern

Planning: Expected Outcomes. The most important outcome is that the client is expected to maintain a patent airway.

Interventions. Nursing measures for maintaining airway patency center on decreasing the tenacity of oral secretions, enabling the client to expectorate oral secretions, and decreasing edema in the head and neck area.

In some cases, the physician may perform a tracheotomy to maintain airway patency.

Nonsurgical Management. The nurse assesses the client's current regimen of oral hygiene. Modifications might be needed because of oral discomfort, bleeding, or edema. Gauze sponges, vigorous rinsing, and a water pick are appropriate alternatives to brushing.

Clients with ulcerative or bleeding lesions may not be able to use commercial mouth rinses. Many commercial mouth rinses have a high alcohol content, which can cause a burning sensation in the area of the lesion. The nurse or assistive nursing personnel modifies the rinse solution according to whether the secretions need to be vigorously evacuated or merely thinned and rinsed out. A solution of 1 tsp baking soda in 8 ounces of water is soothing and well tolerated by many clients. The nurse may elect a solution of half hydrogen peroxide and half normal saline. (See also Chart 56–2.)

Measures to Decrease Oral Secretions. If the oral cavity requires more vigorous cleaning, the nurse uses oral suction equipment with a dental tip or a tonsil tip (Yankar catheter) to aid the client in expectorating oral secretions. The suction equipment is available for the client to use as needed.

The nurse also assesses the client's fluid balance and hydration. Increasing fluid intake and improving general hydration thin the oral secretions and thereby facilitate their removal.

Measures to Decrease Edema. Clients at risk because of edema often receive steroids for reducing inflammation. Antibiotics may be ordered to reduce the risk of infection, which can increase the inflammation and edema in the lesion.

The nurse elevates the head of the bed to at least 30 degrees; this aids in decreasing edema by gravity. A cool mist by face tent may assist with oxygen transport and control of edema.

Surgical Management. The client with an oral lesion is occasionally not able to sustain a normal breathing pattern preoperatively. This may be caused by the tumor, secretions, edema, or a combination. A tracheotomy re-establishes a patent airway and can be performed by the physician under local or general anesthesia.

The tracheostomy tube is usually left in place until edema resolves and the airway is patent. If the tumor is the major cause of the oral airway blockage, however, the tracheostomy may be maintained through the perioperative period until the tumor has been excised and oral healing begins. After postoperative edema resolves, the client is decannulated (the tracheostomy tube is removed). (Refer to Chapter 30 for nursing care of the client with a tracheostomy.)

Altered Oral Mucous Membrane

Planning: Expected Outcomes. The desired outcome is that the client is expected to maintain or re-establish oral mucosal integrity.

Interventions. The health care provider evaluates the client's cancer and its extent as part of the decision-making process for treatment. The client may elect nonsurgical treatment, surgery, or a combination.

Nonsurgical Management. The two standard nonsurgical treatments of cancer of the oral cavity are radiation therapy and chemotherapy. The two modalities can be administered separately but are often combined for an additive effect.

Radiation Therapy. Radiation therapy for oral cancers can be given by external beam. External radiation passes through the skin or mucous membrane to the tumor site. Another option is the implantation of radioactive substances directly into the tumor area (interstitial radiation therapy). The physician chooses the type of radiation therapy on the basis of tumor site and staging.

Interstitial radiation is used for smaller lesions that do not infiltrate surrounding tissues. The radioactive materials can be

- Seeds, which are permanently implanted into the tissue
- Needles or wires, which are extracted at the end of therapy
- Radiation catheters or holders, which are later loaded with radioactive materials
- A "mold" of radioactive material placed directly over the lesion for a specific time

Interstitial therapy delivers the radiation close to the tumor and rarely involves adjacent tissues. The dose is often difficult to calculate, however, and the client must remain hospitalized. Radiation isolation precautions must be instituted while the materials are active or in place. A tracheostomy may be required with interstitial implants because of edema and increased oral secretions. (See Chapter 27 for nursing care of clients undergoing radiation therapy.)

Chemotherapy. The client may receive one or more chemotherapeutic agents (Table 56–3). The advantages of chemotherapy instead of surgery or radiation for cancer of the oral cavity continue to be eveluated.

The nurse instructs the client undergoing chemotherapy about the anticipated side effects of the medication, which vary with each agent. The nurse administers antiemetic medications as prescribed and provides other comfort measures as needed.

TABLE 56–3

Common Chemotherapeutic Drugs Used in Clients with Squamous Cell Carcinoma of the Head and Neck

- Methotrexate
- Bleomycin
- Cisplatin (*cis*-platinum)
- Cyclophosphamide
- Doxorubicin
- Vincristine
- 5-Fluorouracil
- Hydroxyurea

- The need for vital signs to be taken frequently postoperatively
- The need to take nothing by mouth (remain NPO) for 7 to 10 days
- The need to have intravenous (IV) lines in place for 2 to 3 days
- Postoperative medications and activity (out of bed on the first postoperative day)
- Any drains involved (Hemovac drain or Foley catheter)

The nurse also assesses the client's ability to read and write. The client and the nurse select the method of communication the client will use postoperatively with staff and family members (e.g., magic slate, picture board, or pad and pencil).

For oral care for the client receiving chemotherapy or radiation therapy, foam brushes instead of standard toothbrushes are often used. Ransier et al. (1995) found that foam brushes soaked in chlorhexide were effective in reducing bacteria and controlling candidiasis (see Research Applications for Nursing box). A topical solution containing diphenhydramine, 2% viscous lidocaine, kaolin with pectin, and nystatin decreases pain and helps prevent secondary stomatitis (Aubertin, 1997).

Surgical Management. The physician can often excise small, noninvasive lesions of the oral cavity in an ambulatory setting with local anesthesia. The surgical defect is usually small enough to be closed by sutures. These smaller lesions are also responsive to *carbon dioxide laser therapy* or *cryotherapy* (extreme cold application), which can be performed as an outpatient procedure in a surgicenter but may require general anesthesia.

Small oral cancers are equally responsive to radiation therapy and to surgery. Excision is often more appealing to the client. However, ambulatory surgery or, at most, a 1- to 2-day hospital stay is preferred to commuting daily for weeks to undergo external beam radiation.

More invasive lesions require more extensive surgical excision, usually in combination with radiation therapy. Not all lesions can be excised by the peroral (through the mouth) approach (Fig. 56–6).

Preoperative Care. Before excision of a lesion of the oral cavity, the nurse assesses and documents the client's level of understanding of the disease process, the rationale for the surgery, and the planned intervention. Information is reinforced as needed. The nurse identifies family members and support people and includes them in all teaching.

The nurse reviews the type of anesthesia, any preoperative medications, and any postoperative limitations. For small local excisions, postoperative restrictions include a liquid diet for a day, then soft foods. There are no activity limitations. Analgesics are prescribed for the client.

The nurse instructs the client undergoing composite tissue resection about

- The likelihood of tracheostomy and its concomitant nursing care (oxygen therapy and suctioning)
- The temporary loss of speech because of the tracheostomy

▷ Research Applications for Nursing

Are Better Methods for Oral Hygiene Available for Clients Undergoing Radiation or Chemotherapy?

Ransier, A., Epstein, J., Lunn, R., & Spinelli, J. (1995). A combined analysis of a toothbrush, foam brush, and a chlorhexidine-soaked foam brush in maintaining oral hygiene. Cancer Nursing, 18(5), 393–396.

Because during chemotherapy and/or radiation therapy clients often develop mucositis and ulcerations, gentle forms of oral hygiene are often sought. Foam brushes are often used during this time rather than a standard toothbrush. Oral hygiene is important in reducing the oral bacteria that can possibly lead to systemic infections in the immunocompromised person. The purpose of this study was to demonstrate that foam brushes alone are ineffective in reducing bacterial plaque levels. The researchers showed that a foam brush soaked in chlorhexidine was effective in reducing plaque gram-positive aerobes and controlling candidiasis.

Critique. The sample of 56 healthy individuals was recruited. The criteria for selection were not discussed, nor was the consent rate reported. The study was conducted in two parts. In the first part, the subjects were randomly assigned to a group that brushed with a regular brush for a week and a foam brush for the second week, and a group was assigned the procedure in the reverse order. The subjects were evaluated by a dental hygienist after the first week and after the second week for plaque and gingival health. The second phase of the study was the same, except that the subjects were directed to soak the foam brush in 0.2% aqueous chlorhexidine. They also were evaluated by a dental hygienist at the end of weeks one and two. It is difficult to generalize these findings to a larger population because the study was done on healthy adults rather than immunosuppressed individuals.

Possible Nursing Implications. Because oral hygiene is an important part of nursing care for clients undergoing chemotherapy and/or radiation therapy, it is essential to note that foam brushes alone are not as effective as regular toothbrushes. Nurses caring for these clients should consider a change in oral hygiene procedures and include an antibacterial solution when foam brushes are indicated for mouth care.

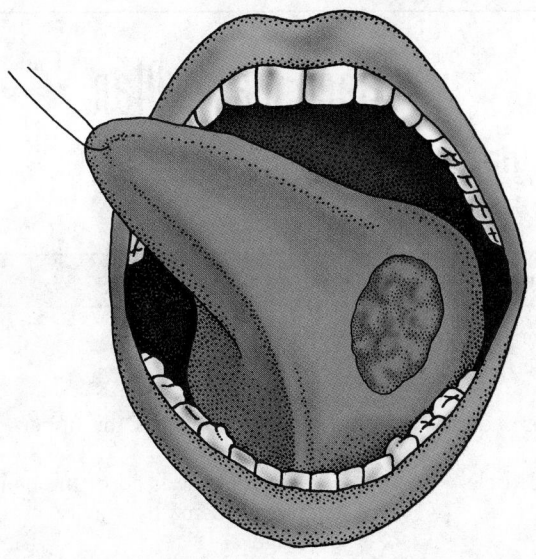

Figure 56–6. A peroral incision for surgery of the oral cavity.

Operative Procedures. An external approach is often necessary. The surgeon may approach the oral cavity from under the mandible or may split the lower lip and retract the lips and cheek for exposure. The mandible is occasionally split as well and pushed aside for oral access; it is wired at the end of the operation.

The most extensive oral operations are composite resections, which combine partial or total glossectomy (tongue removal) and partial mandibulectomy. In the *commando* (co-mandible) *procedure,* the surgeon excises a segment of the mandible with the oral lesion, usually in conjunction with a radical neck dissection (see Chapter 31).

Postoperative Care. After local excision of an oral lesion, the nurse instructs the client in gentle oral hygiene. The nurse advises the client to avoid extremely hot foods and beverages, spicy foods, hard or crisp foods, and alcohol until the area is fully healed.

Maintaining Airway Patency. After extensive excision or composite resection, the most important nursing intervention is maintaining airway patency (see Client Care Plan). The client may not recall on awakening from anesthesia that a tracheostomy tube is in place. The client may initially panic because of the inability to speak. The nurse reminds the client why he or she cannot speak and reassures the client that the vocal cords are intact. The nurse provides the client with the predetermined method of communication.

After oral edema has decreased and the tracheostomy tube has been changed to a noncuffed type, the client can speak by plugging the stoma with the fingertip. The nurse and physician determine the appropriateness of instructing the client in this technique.

Clients who have undergone extensive resection may have slurred speech or difficulty in phonating. The nurse assesses the need for consultation with a speech/language pathologist.

Protecting the Operative Area. The nurse protects the oral suture line from trauma by prohibiting any oral hy-giene, oral suctioning, and oral temperature checks until the physician approves these measures. After healing has begun, the nurse provides the client with gentle mouth care for cleaning away tenacious secretions and stimulating flow of saliva. The nurse elevates the head of the bed to at least 30 degrees to assist in decreasing edema by gravity. The nurse and assistive nursing personnel encourage the client to be out of bed after the first postoperative day. If skin grafting was done, the nurse inspects the donor site (generally on the anterior thigh) during every nursing shift for bleeding or manifestations of infection. (For specific nursing care for the client with a radical neck dissection, refer to Chapter 31.)

Relieving Pain. The nurse relies on subjective and objective data to assess the client's need for analgesics and the effectiveness of the medications given.

The client who has undergone a split-thickness skin graft often perceives the greatest amount of pain at the donor site. Comfort measures related to a painful donor site include providing a mechanism for keeping bed linens off the site and consulting the physician about using a heat lamp on the site several times a day.

Promoting Nutrition. Clients who have undergone extensive resections of the oral cavity remain NPO for 5 to 7 days or longer. This allows healing in the oral cavity before food contacts the incision. Nasogastric feeding or total parenteral nutrition is needed during this time. The tubes are usually inserted in the operating room.

When oral fluid intake is begun, the nurse assesses for and documents difficulty in swallowing, aspiration, or leakage of saliva or fluids from the suture line.

A speech and language pathologist is often consulted to assist the client with swallowing techniques. A swallowing impairment may be a problem, but it is usually temporary. The client is encouraged to practice swallowing.

 Continuing Care

Continuing care for the client with an oral tumor depends on the severity of the tumor, the treatment for the tumor, and available support systems for the client. Most clients are maintained at home during follow-up care.

➤ Health Teaching

The nurse instructs the client and family about medications, diet or feedings, any treatments (such as tracheostomy care, suture line care, and dressing changes), and early symptoms of infection.

The dietitian discusses food preparation and eating schedules with the client and the family food preparer before discharge from the hospital. In collaboration with the dietitian, the nurse instructs the client and the family how to assess the nutritional intake of the client who is just beginning to eat. In case of decreased nutritional intake, the nurse provides guidelines about whom to notify.

To increase retention of the information, the client and the family demonstrate all skills they are taught. The nurse documents their understanding of the treatments.

(*Text continued on page 1348*)

Client Care Plan

The Client Undergoing Excision of a Tumor of the Oral Cavity

Nursing Diagnosis No. 1: Ineffective Airway Clearance related to edema

Expected Outcomes	Nursing Interventions	Rationale
The client is expected to maintain a patent airway.	■ Provide nursing care for the client with a tracheostomy (see Chapter 30).	■ See Chapter 30.
	■ Use methods to decrease edema as instructed.	■ Edema can obstruct the upper airway.
	■ Keep the head of the bed elevated to at least 30 degrees.	■ Elevation of the head of the bed decreases edema by gravity drainage.
	■ Monitor and record intake and output, including output from drains, during each nursing shift.	■ Monitoring can indicate fluid overload or retention and the patency of drains.
	■ Ensure patency of surgical drains. Document and report any significant change in the color or character of drainage and any obstructing clots.	■ Surgical drains are a major means of removing serous drainage and blood after surgery. Continuous suction provided by surgical drains is necessary for the viability of flaps after surgery.
	■ Notify the physician if leaks or whistling is noted from the surgical drain. Apply antibacterial ointment over the leak to attempt to seal the site.	■ Leaks or whistling can indicate malfunction of the surgical system.
	■ Avoid pressure on flaps. If the client has a tracheostomy, check to see that ties are not constricting the flap. Prevent kinking of the flap by head position.	■ Pressure on the flap impedes gravity drainage of edema. Pressure also impedes blood flow to the flap and can compromise flap viability.

Nursing Diagnosis No. 2: Impaired Verbal Communication related to tracheostomy

Expected Outcomes	Nursing Interventions	Rationale
The client is expected to demonstrate the ability to communicate with family and staff members postoperatively.	■ Use methods to provide the client with a means of communication.	■ Communication assistance provides a means for the client to express feelings and needs to health care professionals and family.
	■ Assess and document the client's ability to hear and understand the spoken voice preoperatively.	■ This establishes a baseline of communication abilities.
	■ Assess and document the literacy level preoperatively. Have the client demonstrate the ability to write.	■ Assessment provides a baseline for determining choices of nonverbal communication.

(Continued)

Client Care Plan

Expected Outcomes	Nursing Interventions	Rationale
	■ Discuss and agree on an alternative system of communication, such as pad and pen, magic slate, or picture board. Document the system agreed on. ■ Consult with a speech therapist postoperatively as appropriate. ■ Remind the client postoperatively of the temporary nature of lack of speech as appropriate (e.g., because of tracheostomy or edema).	■ Documentation of a prearranged system of communication will inform other health care workers and provide continuity of communication between the client and the family. ■ Speech/language pathologists can assist the client in determining alternative communication methods. The client has a sense of input and control over his or her environment. ■ Speech loss or difficulties due to surgery for oral tumors are often temporary and can be restored by plugging the tracheostomy to speak or waiting until edema has decreased.

Nursing Diagnosis No. 3: Risk for Infection related to altered mucous membranes

Expected Outcomes	Nursing Interventions	Rationale
The client is expected to experience no signs or symptoms of infection or trauma at the surgical site.	■ Prevent trauma to the surgical site. ■ Do not reposition or replace the nasogastric tube in a client with pharyngeal anastomoses. ■ Do not start oral care until it is cleared by the physician. ■ Do not suction the oral cavity without a physician's order. ■ Avoid pressure on the donor site if skin grafting was done (the site is usually on the thigh; prevent bed linens and the like from rubbing the site). ■ Do not obtain oral temperatures for the client undergoing oral surgery. ■ Monitor the surgical site for early detection of infection or complications. ■ Assess the cutaneous suture line for redness, drainage, and other signs of infection. ■ Clean sutures during each nursing shift with half-strength hydrogen peroxide; dry the area and apply a small amount of antibacterial ointment.	■ Trauma could puncture or irritate the intraoral incision, the donor site, or cutaneous sutures; trauma could open a potential route of infection. ■ Monitoring can detect complications and early signs of infection as soon as possible. ■ Redness, drainage, and tenderness can be early signs of infection. ■ Crusts and secretions are ideal media for bacterial growth.

(Continued)

Client Care Plan

Expected Outcomes	Nursing Interventions	Rationale
	■ Assess the donor site during each nursing shift. Document and report signs of bleeding or infection.	■ Frequent assessments can lead to early detection of complications.
	■ Apply the heat lamp to the donor site per the physician's order three times a day for 10 minutes.	■ The heat lamp promotes drying of the donor area if a skin graft was done, prevents bacterial infection by preventing the formation of a warm, wet medium, and is soothing to the client.
	■ After drains are removed, clean sites with half-strength hydrogen peroxide; dry the area and apply a small amount of antibacterial ointment. Assess drain sites while performing care for early signs of infection.	■ Crusts and secretions provide good media for bacterial growth.
	■ Monitor vital signs per the physician's orders. Document and report any significant changes.	■ Increased pulse and temperature can be early indications of infection. Discreet bleeding can be indicated by increased pulse and decreased blood pressure.
	■ Assess potentially compromised skin flaps.	■ Continual assessment and documentation monitor flap progress.

Nursing Diagnosis No. 4: Altered Nutrition: Less than Body Requirements related to NPO status

Expected Outcomes	Nursing Interventions	Rationale
The client is expected to maintain adequate nutritional intake by nasogastric tube until oral feedings are begun.	■ Use methods to provide nutritional support while the client can take nothing by mouth (NPO).	■ Nutrients are provided and tissue growth is promoted while the client is NPO.
	■ Remind the client of NPO status when he or she is alert.	■ Elderly clients may demonstrate memory deficit; clients are often NPO until the intraoral incision has healed.
	■ Monitor intravenous hydration while the client is NPO and before tube feedings are begun; monitor and record intake and output during every nursing shift.	■ Evaluation of hydration status can alert the nurse to fluid overload or retention; the elderly are often susceptible to overload of fluids.
	■ Assess and document bowel sounds during every nursing shift until tube feedings are well tolerated.	■ A baseline for bowel sounds is established; the return of bowel sounds postoperatively is often an indication to begin tube feedings.
	■ Measure and record weight daily.	■ Weight changes indicate fluid status.

(Continued)

Client Care Plan

Expected Outcomes	Nursing Interventions	Rationale
	■ Maintain proper functioning of the nasogastric tube: While the client is attached to suction, measure and record drainage during every nursing shift. When tube feedings are begun, flush the tube carefully with water after each feeding or medication administration.	■ Patency of the tube is noted by continued drainage and by flushing of the tube.
The client will demonstrate ability to assist with tube feedings.	■ Provide the client with written and oral instructions about tube feedings.	■ Written instructions provide the client with resources when the nurse is not available. Because of memory deficits, elderly clients often benefit from being able to review procedures several times.
	■ Include the family in all teaching.	■ Including the family ensures support for the client in performing the procedures.
	■ Have the client perform a return demonstration of the procedure.	■ Return demonstration aids in retention of the learned procedure and provides a means of evaluation for the nurse.
The client will maintain adequate oral nutritional intake with minimal dysphagia or aspiration.	■ When oral fluids are begun, assess and document difficulty in swallowing, aspiration, or leakage.	■ Clients occasionally have difficulty with oral feeding after oral excisions; assessment provides documentation or real or perceived difficulty.
	■ If the client is experiencing difficulty in swallowing, check with the physician about a consultation with a speech therapist for assessment of or assistance with swallowing.	■ Speech therapists are often expert at evaluating swallowing disorders; providing the client with techniques of head positioning and breath holding or oral exercises can help overcome minor swallowing difficulties.
	■ Offer encouragement to continue to practice eating. Assure the client that this impairment is often temporary.	■ Clients often become discouraged at the inability to perform a previously reflexive maneuver. Providing the client with encouragement and hope often increases motivation and dedication to practice.
	■ Consult with the dietitian as appropriate.	■ Often a change in food consistency eases swallowing difficulties. Liquids are often poorly tolerated at first; semisolids are tolerated best.
	■ When oral feedings are begun, check with the physician about starting oral care measures.	■ Providing the client with oral hygiene can aid in cleaning the oral cavity of tenacious secretions, which often hinder swallowing efforts, and also provides the client with a sense of oral normalcy and well-being.

ELDERLY CONSIDERATIONS

For the elderly client with metastatic or invasive oral cancer, skilled home care nursing services are required for pain management, nutrition maintenance, and emotional support. Elderly clients often take subtherapeutic doses of analgesics for fear of becoming addicted. The home care nurse teaches the client about the need to promote comfort to improve nutrition and prevent depression. (See Chapter 9 for further information on pain management in the elderly).

Nutrition is one of the most difficult challenges. Pain and mucositis from treatment may decrease appetite and limit intake. The home care nurse encourages fluids to prevent dehydration and suggests that clients eat foods they enjoy.

Loss of appetite and weight may also be a sign of depression. Feelings of helplessness, fear, and anxiety are common among elderly clients with metastatic cancers. Chart 56–3 summarizes the focused nursing assessment for the client with oral cancer being cared for at home.

➤ Home Care Management

Minimal home care preparation is required for the client undergoing biopsy or minor excision of a lesion of the oral cavity. Home care needs for the client who has undergone extensive excision depend on the condition of the client at the time of discharge.

The client who has been decannulated is often taking a soft diet by mouth before discharge. Occasionally, however, clients are discharged from the hospital while still requiring tracheostomy suction, oral suction, and nasogastric feedings. Suction equipment, nutritional supplies, and nursing care can be provided by home care companies. (See Chapter 64 for home care preparation for the client receiving home parenteral nutrition and Chapter 30 for home care preparation for the client with a tracheostomy.)

➤ Health Care Resources

The nurse accepts the feelings the client displays and encourages the client to verbalize fears and concerns. A social worker or other health care professional may be needed for client and family counseling.

Chart 56–3

Focused Assessment of the Elderly Client with Oral Cancer

- Assess the mouth and surrounding tissues for candiadiasis, mucositis, pain, and loss of appetite and taste.
- Monitor the client's weight.
- Monitor nutritional and fluid intake.
- Assess for difficulty in eating or speech.
- Assess pain status and measures used to control pain.
- Monitor the client's response to medications.
- Identify psychosocial problems, such as depression, anxiety, and fear.

Clients who undergo composite resection often experience depression related to a change in body image. Excision of a portion of the mandible can leave the client with a facial defect that may be difficult to hide. Speech is often affected as well. Clients who undergo a total glossectomy may be able to speak with special training and the use of an intraoral prosthesis fashioned by a maxillofacial prosthodontist. The prosthesis is similar to dentures, with augmentation to approximate the oral articulating surfaces.

The nurse consults the social worker or case manager for assistance in obtaining special equipment or nutritional resources required by the client at home. The case manager assesses the financial needs of the client and makes referrals to government, community, and religious organizations as needed.

 Evaluation

The nurse considers the common nursing diagnoses to evaluate the care of the client with a tumor of the oral cavity. The expected outcomes include that the client

- Maintains a patent oral airway by handling oral secretions
- Maintains nutritional status by eating a balanced diet
- Communicates thoughts and feelings to family members, friends, and health care personnel
- Maintains the integrity of the oral mucous membrane

DISORDERS OF THE SALIVARY GLANDS

Acute Sialadenitis

Overview

Acute sialadenitis, the inflammation of a salivary gland, can be of bacterial, viral, or allergic origin. The most common causative organisms are *Staphylococcus aureus, Staphylococcus pyogenes, Streptococcus pneumoniae,* and *Escherichia coli.* This disorder most commonly affects the parotid or submandibular gland in adults.

A decrease in production of saliva usually precipitates acute sialadenitis, as in dehydrated or debilitated clients or in clients who take nothing by mouth (NPO) postoperatively for an extended time. The bacteria or viruses enter the gland through the ductal opening in the oral cavity. Systemic medications, such as phenothiazines, chloramphenicol, and oxytetracycline, can also precipitate an episode of acute sialadenitis. Untreated infections of the salivary glands can evolve into abscesses, which can rupture and spread infection into the tissues of the neck and the mediastinum.

Collaborative Management

Assessment findings include pain and swelling of the face over the affected gland. These symptoms increase with meals. Fever and general malaise also occur, and purulent drainage can often be massaged from the affected duct in the oral cavity (Chart 56–4).

Treatment includes the administration of intravenous (IV) and measures to increase the flow of saliva, such as

- Hydration
- Application of warm compresses
- Massage of the gland
- Use of sialagogues (substances that stimulate flow of saliva)

Sialagogues include lemon slices and fruit-or citrus-flavored candy. Massage is accomplished by milking the edematous gland with the fingertips toward the ductal opening. Elevation of the head of the bed promotes gravity drainage of the edematous gland.

Acute sialadenitis is best prevented by adherence to routine oral hygiene. This practice prohibits infections from ascending to the salivary glands from the oral cavity.

Postirradiation Sialadenitis

The salivary glands are sensitive to ionizing radiation, such as from radiation therapy or radioactive iodine treatment of thyroid cancers. Exposure of the glands to radiation produces xerostomia (very dry mouth caused by severe reduction in flow of saliva) within 24 hours. Radiation to the salivary glands can also produce pain and edema, which generally abate after several days.

Xerostomia may be temporary or permanent, depending on the dose of radiation and the percentage of total salivary gland tissue irradiated. Little can be done to relieve the client's dry mouth during the course of radiation therapy. Frequent sips of water and frequent mouth care, especially before meals, are the most effective interventions. After the course of radiation therapy has been completed, saliva substitutes may provide moisture for 2 to 4 hours at a time. Over-the-counter solutions are available, or solutions may be mixed with methylcellulose (Cologel), glycerin, and saline.

Calculi

Salivary calculi, or stones, can occur within the gland itself or in the gland's ductal system. In general, calculi within the gland produce few symptoms unless they become infected. Salivary calculi within the ducts, however, often obstruct the flow of saliva unless they are naturally expelled.

Symptoms of obstruction by salivary calculi include sudden pain and swelling of the affected gland, most commonly when the client is eating. The physician at-

tempts to dilate the duct and the duct opening with increasingly larger sizes of bougies (dilators) and milks the gland to help the calculus pass spontaneously. If dilation and massage fail to remove an obstructing calculus, surgery may be necessary.

Neoplasms of the Salivary Glands

Overview

Tumors of the salivary glands are relatively rare; they constitute only 3% of all oral tumors. The parotid gland is the salivary gland most commonly affected by neoplastic disease.

The most common benign tumor of the salivary gland is the mixed tumor. A mixed tumor usually occurs as a small, slow-growing mass. The client is usually asymptomatic.

Malignant tumors of the salivary glands are most commonly classified as mucoepidermoid, epidermoid, and adenoid cystic carcinomas. Malignant neoplasms are characterized by more rapid growth than that of benign tumors and are generally associated with pain. Involvement of the facial nerve, more common with malignant tumors, results in facial weakness or paralysis (partial or total) on the affected side.

Biopsy of a salivary gland tumor that is suspected of being malignant is contraindicated. Rupture of the capsule (tumor covering) of the mass can spread tumor cells into unaffected tissues.

Collaborative Management

The treatment of choice for both benign and malignant tumors of the salivary glands is surgical excision. However, radiation therapy is frequently used for salivary gland cancers that are large, have recurred, show evidence of residual disease after excision, or are highly malignant.

Clients who have undergone parotidectomy (surgical removal of the parotid glands) or submandibular gland surgery are at risk for weakness or loss of function of the facial nerve because the nerve courses directly through the gland. The nurse assesses the client's ability to

- Wrinkle the brow
- Raise the eyebrows
- Squeeze the eyes shut
- Wrinkle the nose
- Pucker the lips
- Puff out the cheeks
- Grimace or smile

Acute Malocclusion

Overview

Malocclusion is an altered position of the teeth or an altered position of the mandible or maxilla to which the teeth are attached. Fractures of the teeth or mandible most often cause the acute onset of malocclusion (as opposed to the chronic malocclusion of congenital facial deformity or malpositioned teeth). Malocclusion often causes temporomandibular joint (TMJ) dysfunction.

Fractures of the mandible create malocclusion when the fractured bone fragment is displaced. Fractures of the mandible are rarely fatal but require treatment for prevention of further malocclusion or deformity due to improper healing.

Fractures of the teeth cause malocclusion by changing the fit of the maxillary teeth (upper teeth) against the mandibular teeth (lower teeth). Malocclusion caused by tooth fractures also requires professional treatment for preventing infection of the pulp of the tooth as well as correcting the malocclusion.

Tooth fractures and mandibular fractures result from trauma. Many occur from motor vehicle accidents, work accidents, sports, and assault. The facial bones absorb the impact of the trauma and protect the spinal cord and the brain from injury.

Fractures of the mandible are also caused by falls in the elderly, who are more susceptible to osteoporosis. Mandibular fractures are common because of the prominence and rigidity of the mandible.

Teeth can also be fractured by biting down on hard objects (e.g., a bone or foreign object). Teeth become more susceptible to fracture as a result of decay or poor nutrition, which can soften the teeth.

Incidence figures vary, but fractures of the teeth are fairly common, especially in the elderly and those with devitalized teeth. Fractures of the mandible are more frequent than other facial fractures (with the exception of nasal fractures), in part because of the mandible's prominent position.

Collaborative Management

 Assessment

The nurse observes the client while obtaining the history of the facial deformity. It is helpful to observe the client carefully when the facial muscles are at rest as well as in motion, such as during talking or eating. As the client opens and closes the jaw, the nurse gently palpates over the area of the teeth and mandible, including the TMJ. During palpation, the nurse assesses for pain, abnormality or restriction of movement, crepitance (grinding sensation and sound caused by bone fragments), and change in sensation.

The interior of the oral cavity is inspected. The nurse notes the presence of broken teeth, the status of the dentition, and the intactness of the oral mucous membrane.

For eliciting tenderness, teeth can be tapped with a tongue blade. The nurse palpates the mandibular rim in the oral cavity and assesses for abnormal movement, pain, and crepitance.

Edentulous (without teeth) clients who do not wear dentures may be unaware of a mandibular fracture because symptoms of malocclusion are lacking. Clinical manifestations of mandibular fracture include pain on motion, lack of sensation from damage to cranial nerve V, drooling (pain often overstimulates the salivary glands), disfigurement, and disability in opening the mouth.

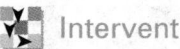 Interventions

Clients with acute malocclusion require surgical intervention in most cases. However, other therapies and interventions are also used.

➤ Nonsurgical Management

Nonsurgical management of acute malocclusion resulting from tooth or mandibular fracture includes drug therapy, comfort measures, oral hygiene, and diet therapy.

Drug Therapy

The health care provider usually prescribes prophylactic antibiotics because of the possibility of wound contamination from foreign objects or normal oral flora. Opioid and nonopioid analgesics are often required; fractures of the teeth or mandible can be painful, especially during eating. The efficient use of analgesics can enhance clients' compliance with the treatment regimen.

Comfort Measures

Much of the discomfort of tooth or mandibular fracture is related to pressure from edema. The nurse instructs the client to keep the head of the bed elevated or to sleep on several pillows; these measures encourage gravity drainage of edema. The nurse also cautions the client to avoid sleeping on the injured side for preventing further discomfort.

The nurse recommends the application of ice packs to the affected area during the first 24 hours after the fracture. The ice decreases swelling and often provides an analgesic effect as well.

Oral Hygiene

Oral hygiene measures often must be altered when malocclusive fractures occur; vigorous brushing or commercial rinses may increase discomfort.

The nurse advises the client to maintain adequate oral hygiene by using lukewarm saline or sodium bicarbonate rinses and brushing with a soft brush (when appropriate). The use of a water pick on a gentle setting can be effective. By instructing the client to maintain oral hygiene, the nurse assists the client in preventing infection as well as promoting oral well-being.

The nurse assesses and evaluates the method of oral hygiene. The nurse alters the regimen as needed to eliminate uncomfortable elements, thereby increasing compliance. (See also Chart 56–2.)

Diet Therapy

The nurse counsels the client and the family food preparer about diet changes for lessening discomfort. Soft foods that require little or no chewing or blenderized foods are recommended if the client has pain caused by pressure from chewing. Hot and cold foods and beverages are avoided; thermal extremes can stimulate exposed tooth pulp or nerves.

In collaboration with the dietitian, the nurse provides the client and the family with guidelines for maintaining a proper balance of nutritional elements while the client requires soft foods or other changes in food consistency.

➤ Surgical Management

Surgical management of malocclusion from tooth fracture or mandibular fracture involves tooth extraction, pulpectomy, crown repair, and reduction of the mandibular fracture.

Preoperative Care

Clients who do not require open reduction of mandibular fractures are often treated with topical anesthetics while the wires are placed. With these clients, the nurse discusses

- The need for a liquid diet while in intermaxillary fixation (IMF)
- The need for continued oral hygiene while in occlusion
- The presence of pain and available analgesics

The nurse instructs clients undergoing open reduction to expect the following postoperatively:

- IV fluids until a liquid diet can be taken without nausea
- Nasogastric suction for 24 hours (if the teeth are placed in occlusion during the surgery)
- The presence of pain and the availability of analgesics
- The need to get out of bed the first postoperative day
- The application of dressings over the incision if the reduction is not done through an intraoral incision

Operative Procedures

In performing a *pulpectomy,* the oral surgeon removes the entire pulp of the tooth and aseptically fills and seals the cavity to eliminate further infection. Even without living pulp, the tooth usually remains well rooted in the gingiva and can be of use to the client. The pulpectomy procedure generally takes 1 to 2 hours and is usually performed with local anesthesia.

For a *crown repair,* the dentist restores the contours of the tooth with gold, porcelain, or a blend of these materials. The client may or may not require a pulpectomy before crown placement.

Reduction of the mandibular fracture involves placing the mandible in proper alignment and maintaining reduction until the fracture is healed, usually for 6 weeks. The surgeon often places clients with nondisplaced fractures in IMF (the mandibular teeth are occluded to the maxillary teeth and wired or banded without requiring further reduction) (Fig. 56–7).

Displaced fractures often require open reduction. A surgical incision exposes the mandible, and the fracture is reduced during surgery. The client is placed in IMF postoperatively. An external acrylic splint may be required for severely comminuted (splintered) fractures when open reduction cannot provide adequate support.

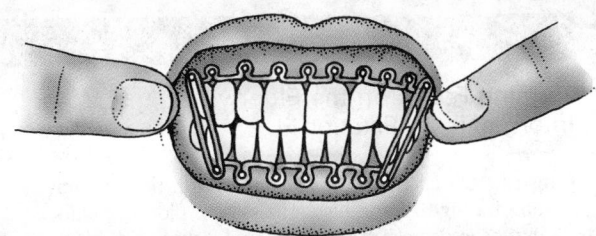

Figure 56–7. Teeth wired in intermaxillary fixation.

Postoperative Care

The most important nursing intervention in caring for a client who has been placed in IMF is maintaining a patent airway.

Immediate Postoperative Care The nurse monitors the airway closely as the client wakes from general anesthesia in IMF. The elderly client may be disoriented or agitated from the anesthesia (Chart 56–5).

Vomitus and oral secretions are extremely difficult to clear from the airway when the teeth are wired or banded in occlusion. The nurse takes care to visualize the positioning of the bands or wires that will require cutting should the client experience airway difficulty. Prevention of vomiting is a major nursing goal.

Often, bands or wires are not placed until the client is fully awake from anesthesia; this circumvents the problem of vomiting after general anesthesia. If the client is placed in IMF in the operating suite, a nasogastric tube may suction and empty the stomach of gastric contents until the client is fully awake.

Continuing Postoperative Care. After the client in IMF is fully alert and begins to take a liquid diet, the nurse instructs the client and the family to notify the nursing staff of symptoms of nausea. The physician prescribes antiemetics to help the client overcome the nausea. If the client begins to vomit, the nurse cuts the wires with wire cutters kept at the bedside or cuts the bands with scissors to clear the client's oral airway. Suction equipment is kept at the bedside for help in clearing the oral airway in emergencies. Bands or wires are also cut for other respiratory emergencies, such as respiratory arrest and the need for cardiopulmonary resuscitation.

The nurse inspects the incision for signs of infection or bleeding. Depending on agency policy or the physician's preference, the nurse cleans cutaneous suture lines two to four times a day with half-strength hydrogen peroxide (half hydrogen peroxide, half normal saline). A small amount of antibacterial ointment may be applied to prevent infection, prevent crusting, and decrease scarring.

The nurse instructs the client in oral care for maintaining dental health as well as preventing infection if there is an intraoral incision. With the teeth wired in occlusion, brushing of the lingual aspects of the teeth is impossible. The nurse checks with the physician about the advisability of using a soft brush to clean the outer aspects of the

---

Chart 56-5

Nursing Focus on the Elderly: Intermaxillary Fixation

- Instruct the client and home caregiver in the preparation of a high-calorie blenderized diet. Elderly clients often have decreased appetites, and liquid diets fill them up quickly.
- Encourage the client to seek dental care once intermaxillary fixation (IMF) is removed. Elderly clients often have poor dentition or ill-fitting dentures; weight loss and the inability to clean the oral cavity properly with IMF can compound their dental problems.
- Instruct the client to cough and deep breathe every 2 hours postoperatively for prevention of atelectasis and pneumonia.
- Investigate whether the client is at risk for falls, which could have contributed to the fracture; determine the need for assistance or a change in living arrangements.
- Give written instructions to reinforce verbal teaching; recent memory may be impaired in the elderly client.
- Assess upper arm mobility for the ability to cut bands in an emergency. Determine the need for assistance as needed.
- Encourage the client to get out of bed as soon as possible postoperatively to permit full lung expansion. Assist the client out of bed; be alert for orthostatic hypotension.
- Be alert for signs of pain and anticipate the need for pain medication.

---

teeth. Oral rinses are the most effective methods of oral cleaning to date for the client in intermaxillary fixation (IMF). Rinses applied under pressure, such as with a water pick or bulb syringe, provide debridement. The nurse also supplies the client with a lip emollient to prevent cracked lips because clients in IMF cannot lick their lips.

For comfort measures and to decrease edema and the risk of aspiration, the nurse raises the head of the bed to at least 30 degrees after the client is fully awake from general anesthesia. To determine the need for analgesics and the effectiveness of the analgesic regimen, the nurse assesses the client's subjective sensation of discomfort and objective signs. The nurse carefully assesses the level of analgesia achieved to prevent oversedation and a decrease in important reflexes, especially the gag reflex. If the gag reflex is diminished, the client may aspirate.

Wires used to place the client in IMF often press against the gingivae and lips. This can be painful, especially if oral edema is placing the wires in direct contact with oral structures. The nurse assesses the need for topical anesthetics. Bone wax, beeswax, or dental wax can be rubbed over protruding wires to soften sharp edges and prevent further trauma. Assisting the client to be more comfortable in IMF often increases the client's compliance with measures needed during IMF and encourages the client not to tamper with the bands and wires.

Clients in IMF cannot chew and must take all nutrition in liquid or blenderized form through a straw. The nurse

collaborates with a dietitian to instruct the client and the family in preparing a nutritionally balanced liquid diet. The food preparer must often be creative to provide enough variation in a potentially monotonous diet. Clients in IMF often lose 10 to 20 pounds (4.5–9 kg) in 6 weeks. Special care must be taken to assess the client's nutritional status and prevent excessive weight loss. The nurse also monitors the client's bowel elimination pattern because fiber may be inadequate in a liquid diet.

 Continuing Care

Little home care preparation is needed for the client who has undergone repair or extraction of a fractured tooth. For clients who have had repair of a fractured mandible, the nurse assesses the client's need for a blender for food preparation and a water pick for oral care.

The nurse instructs the family and the client about treatments (such as suture line care and dressing changes), oral care, medications, diet, and early detection of infection. The client in IMF is counseled about safety precautions while the teeth are wired in occlusion. The nurse cautions that scissors or wire cutters should be with the client at all times; the nurse teaches the client which wires to cut in an emergency. Swimming and water activities are contraindicated with IMF because water entering the oral cavity is difficult to clear quickly.

The nurse instructs the client to avoid carbonated beverages because the fizzing in the oral cavity can often cause sensations of choking. Inhaled air from the use of straws and excessive carbonation can cause abdominal distention. Alcoholic beverages are contraindicated while the client is maintained in IMF; not only is there a potential for vomiting after excessive alcohol intake but also the effect of alcohol decreases the gag reflex. The nurse also advises the client to avoid contact sports or any activities that could reinjure the fracture area.

The nurse instructs the client to seek professional dental assistance after the wires are removed. The minimal hygiene measures during the 6-week period of IMF often result in numerous dental caries, which require attention.

As with clients who have other disorders of the oral cavity, clients who have undergone tooth repair or extraction because of fracture or who are in IMF for mandibular fracture often experience a disturbance in body image. The appearance of oral disorders is often difficult to hide. In addition, the client in IMF experiences changes in speech patterns and eating. If the nurse anticipates that the client may experience a disturbance in body image, the topic is introduced to the client and the family before discharge from the hospital. The nurse encourages the client to verbalize these feelings and assures the client that such feelings are common and to be expected.

The nurse may need to collaborate with a speech/language pathologist for alternative communication ideas. A communication board is typically used, but other methods are available.

The nurse collaborates with the discharge planner or social worker to

- Assist the client with financial needs
- Obtain equipment

- Supply special dietary needs at home
- Assist in counseling the client who is experiencing difficulty returning to social roles

Home health nurses

- Assess the home situation
- Ascertain the ability of the client and the family to perform the treatment or supply the diet at home
- Provide ongoing evaluation of the client at home (e.g., assess nutritional status and pain control)
- Provide emotional support to the client and the family
- Determine the need for other health care workers at home

CASE STUDY for the Client with Oral Cavity Cancer

■ A 56-year-old man is seen in the clinic with a sore he has had in his mouth for 3 months that he claims "isn't healing." He tells you that he is a heavy smoker but is only a social drinker. He is diagnosed with squamous cell carcinoma. You are meeting with him to review his plan of care.

QUESTIONS:

1. What lifestyle concerns need to be addressed to plan care?
2. What additional information would be helpful to plan care with this client?
3. This client chooses to have surgical treatment, and a composite tissue resection is scheduled. What instructions should you provide for this client before surgery?

SELECTED BIBLIOGRAPHY

American Cancer Society. (1996). *Cancer facts & figures—1996*. Atlanta: American Cancer Society, Inc. 96-300M-No. 5008.96.

Aubertin, M. A. (1997). Home care of the elderly oral cancer patient. *Home Healthcare Nurse, 15*(6), 381–390.

Barnes, L., MacMillan, C., Ferlito, A., Rinaldo, A., Altavilla, G., & Doglioni, C. (1996). Basaloid squamous cell carcinoma of the head and neck: Clinicopathological features and differential diagnosis. *Annals of Otology Rhinology and Laryngology, 105,* 75–82.

Bartkiw, T., & Pynn, B. (1994). Burning mouth syndrome: An overlooked condition in the geriatric population. *Geriatric Nursing, 15*(5), 241–245.

Berger, A., Henderson, M., Nadoolman, W., Duffy, V., Cooper, D., Saberski, L., & Bartoshuk, L. (1995). Oral capsaicin provides temporary relief for oral mucositis pain secondary to chemotherapy/radiation therapy. *Journal of Pain & Symptom Management, 10*(3), 243–248.

Bundgaard, T., Bentzen, S., Wildt, J., Sorensen, F., Sogaard, H., & Nielsen, J. (1996). Histopathologic, serologic, epidemiologic, and clinical parameters in the prognostic evaluation of squamous cell carcinoma of the oral cavity. *Head & Neck, March/April,* 142–152.

Coleman, S. (1995). An overview of the oral complications of adult patients with malignant haematological conditions who have undergone radiotherapy or chemotherapy. *Journal of Advanced Nursing, 22,* 1085–1091.

Dollar, B., & Lawson, G. (1994). Protocol for nursing assessment and management of stomatitis. *Home Healthcare Nurse, 12*(2), 25–27.

Dose, A. (1995). The symptom experience of mucositis, stomatitis, and xerostomia. *Seminars in Oncology Nursing, 11*(4), 248–255.

Friedman, M., Venikatesan, T., & Caldarelli, D. (1996). Intralesional vinblastine for treating AIDS-associated Kaposi's sarcoma of the oropharynx and larynx. *Annals of Otology Rhinology and Laryngology, 105,* 272–274.

Ganley, B. (1995). Effective mouth care for head and neck radiation therapy patients. *MEDSURG Nursing, 4*(2), 133–141.

Goroll, A., & May, L. (1995). Management of aphthous stomatitis. In A. Goroll, L. May, & A. Mulley (Eds.), *Primary care medicine: Office evaluation and management of the adult patient* (3rd ed.). Philadelphia: J. B. Lippincott.

Kelly, J. (1995). Screening for oral cancer. In A. Goroll, L. May, & A. Mulley (Eds.), *Primary care medicine: Office evaluation and management of the adult patient* (3rd ed., pp. 983–985). Philadelphia: J. B. Lippincott.

Lawson, W. (1994). Erythematous oral lesions: Which are benign, which are more worrisome? *Consultant, 34*(10), 1446–1448.

Ransier, A., Epstein, J., Lunn, R., & Spinelli, J. (1995). A combined analysis of a toothbrush, foam brush, and a chlorhexidine-soaked foam brush in maintaining oral hygiene. *Cancer Nursing, 18*(5), 393–396.

Rhodus, N., Moller, K., Colby, S., & Bereuter, J. (1995). Dysphagia in patients with three different etiologies of salivary dysfunction. *ENT Journal, 74*(1), 39–48.

SUGGESTED READINGS

Aubertin, M. A. (1997). Home care of the elderly oral cancer patient. *Home Healthcare Nurse, 15*(6), 381–390.
This excellent, comprehensive article describes the special needs of elderly home care clients experiencing oral cancers. The author discusses the home care nurse's role in prevention, early detection, and treatment. A quiz for continuing education credit follows the article.

Dollar, B., & Lawson, G. (1994). Protocol for nursing assessment and management of stomatitis. *Home Healthcare Nurse, 12*(2), 25–27.
This article provides a quick comprehensive nursing assessment of stomatitis and possible causative agents. Nursing interventions are outlined as they relate to specific nursing diagnoses.

Dose, A. (1995). The symptom experience of mucositis, stomatitis, and xerostomia. *Seminars in Oncology Nursing, 11*(4), 248–255.
Mucositis, stomatitis, and xerostomia are common problems for people undergoing chemotherapy and/or radiation therapy. This article provides an overview of these problems, the symptoms related to each, and the current therapy. Nursing interventions and implications for practice, education, and research are concisely presented.

Chapter 57

INTERVENTIONS FOR CLIENTS WITH ESOPHAGEAL PROBLEMS

The esophagus is a distensible muscular tube located behind the trachea that acts primarily as a conduit for food from the mouth to the stomach. It passes through the diaphragm at the esophageal hiatus and extends to the gastroesophageal junction (see Fig. 55–1). Despite its structural simplicity, the esophagus is susceptible to a variety of inflammatory, structural, motor, and neoplastic disorders, which range in severity from mild and annoying to life-threatening. Because many of the treatment strategies involve diet and lifestyle modifications rather than definitive medical or surgical therapy, nurses have significant influence in the successful management of esophageal disorders.

Gastroesophageal Reflux Disease

Overview

Esophageal reflux is the backward flow of gastrointestinal contents into the esophagus without associated retching and vomiting. It is a very common disorder with potentially serious clinical consequences.

Gastroesophageal reflux disease (GERD) is multifactorial and describes a syndrome that results from esophageal reflux. Reflux produces its characteristic symptoms by exposing the esophageal mucosa to the irritating effects of gastric and/or duodenal contents. These contents gradually break down the mucous barrier of the esophagus. A person with acute symptoms of inflammation is often

described as having *reflux esophagitis,* but this term is not as descriptive or inclusive as *GERD.*

Pathophysiology

The reflux of gastric contents into the esophagus is normally prevented by the presence of two high-pressure areas that remain relatively contracted in the resting phase. A 3-cm segment at the proximal end of the esophagus is called the upper esophageal sphincter (UES), and another 2- to 4-cm portion just proximal to the gastroesophageal junction is referred to as the lower esophageal sphincter (LES). These areas are under muscular, hormonal, and neural control. The function of the LES is supported by its anatomic placement in the abdomen, where the surrounding pressure is significantly higher than in the low-pressure thorax. Sphincter function is also augmented by the acute angle (angle of His) that is formed as the normal esophagus enters the stomach.

Esophageal reflux can occur when gastric volume or intra-abdominal pressure is elevated, when the sphincter tone of the LES is decreased, or when the LES undergoes inappropriate relaxation.

Virtually everyone experiences reflux occasionally. People may even experience frequent episodes of reflux and be asymptomatic. However, the esophagus has only a limited resistance to the damaging effects of acidic gastrointestinal (GI) contents. GERD develops when the esophageal mucosal barrier breaks down and an inflammatory response is initiated. The degree of esophageal inflammation appears to be primarily related to the extent and duration of acid exposure, the number of reflux episodes, and the acidity of the refluxed material.

Refluxed material is returned to the stomach by a combination of gravity, saliva, and peristalsis. The effectiveness of the clearance mechanism is very important. An inflamed esophagus cannot eliminate the refluxed material as quickly or efficiently as a healthy one, and the duration of exposure is therefore increased with each reflux episode.

Hyperemia (increased blood flow) and erosion occur in the esophagus in response to the chronic inflammation. Gastric acid and pepsin are responsible for most of the injury. Minor capillary bleeding frequently accompanies the erosion, although frank hemorrhage is rare. During the process of healing, the body may substitute a columnar epithelium (Barrett's epithelium) for the normal squamous cell epithelium of the lower esophagus. This new tissue is more resistant to acid and therefore supports esophageal healing; however, this is premalignant tissue and is associated with an increased risk of adenocarcinoma (cancer). The fibrosis and scarring that also accompany the healing process can produce esophageal stricture. The stricture leads to progressive difficulty in swallowing. Uncontrolled esophageal reflux also creates a risk for other serious complications, such as esophageal ulceration, hemorrhage, and aspiration pneumonia. GERD has been implicated as one of the causes of adult-onset asthma, laryngitis, and dental deterioration.

Etiology

The inappropriate relaxation of the lower esophageal sphincter LES in response to an unknown stimulus is believed to be the primary cause of GERD. However, many symptomatic clients have resting LES pressures that are within normal limits, and most clients with GERD produce normal amounts of acid.

Nighttime reflux is most important because the swallowing rate decreases by two thirds during sleep, and the recumbent position significantly interferes with the ability of the esophagus to clear the refluxed material. Therefore, the duration of exposure to this acid material is significantly increased at night.

For many years, it was assumed that the presence of a sliding hiatal hernia (see later), which displaced the LES into the thorax, was the primary etiologic factor in GERD. Hiatal hernia is much more common in the general population than was previously estimated. Although most clients with hiatal hernias experience reflux, not all clients who experience reflux have hiatal hernias. The two conditions are now considered to be related but separate. The symptoms of GERD correlate better with incompetency of the LES than they do with the presence of a hiatal hernia. Any condition that delays gastric emptying and thereby maintains a high gastric volume and pressure can also contribute to reflux. Physiologic changes in the elderly put this population at high risk for GERD. Clients who are obese are also at high risk for GERD.

A number of environmental and physical factors have been identified that influence the tone and contractility of

TABLE 57-1

Factors Contributing to Decreased Lower Esophageal Sphincter Pressure

- Fatty foods
- Caffeinated beverages, such as coffee, tea, and cola
- Chocolate
- Nicotine in cigarette smoke
- Beta-adrenergic blocking drugs
- Calcium channel blockers
- Nitrates
- Theophylline
- Diazepam (Valium, E-Pam)
- Peppermint, spearmint
- Alcohol
- Anticholinergic drugs
- High levels of estrogen and progesterone

the LES. As presented in Table 57–1, LES pressure is *lowered* by entities such as fatty foods, nicotine in cigarette smoke, and chocolate. LES tone can be *increased* by gastrin release, protein ingestion, antacids, metoclopramide (Reglan, Maxeran♣), and cholinergic agents, such as bethanechol (Urecholine).

Other conditions besides GERD can produce esophagitis, although GERD is by far the most common. Herpes and monilial infections of the esophagus can produce acute inflammation. Ingestion of corrosive substances produces severe esophagitis and can cause irreversible esophageal damage. Radiation to the lung, esophagus, or mediastinum frequently produces an acute esophagitis that is directly dose related.

Clients who have a nasogastric tube often experience esophagitis. The tube keeps the cardiac sphincter open and allows acidic contents from the stomach to enter the esophagus.

Incidence/Prevalence

Gastroesophageal reflux disease (GERD) can occur at any age, but it is more common in people older than 50 years of age. The incidence of GERD is probably significantly underestimated because many people with mild disease simply accept it as a normal condition and relate the symptoms to episodes of stress or dietary indiscretion. GERD probably produces daily symptoms in as much as 7% of the population and at least monthly symptoms in 36% to 45% (Robinson, 1994).

Collaborative Management

 Assessment

> ### Physical Assessment/Clinical Manifestations

The clinical manifestations of reflux may vary substantially in severity (Chart 57–1). Diagnosis of GERD is made principally by a history of dyspepsia, also called pyrosis or heartburn, which is the characteristic symptom. Clients often describe this pain as being a substernal or

---

Chart 57–1

Key Features of Gastroesophageal Reflux Disease

- Heartburn (pyrosis) (pain may radiate upward or to back)
- Regurgitation (may lead to aspiration or bronchitis)
- Coughing, hoarseness, or wheezing at night
- Water brash
- Dysphagia
- Odynophagia (painful swallowing)
- Chest pain
- Belching
- Flatulence
- Nausea and vomiting (rare)
- Unexplained weight loss (rare)

---

retrosternal burning sensation that tends to radiate upward. If severe, the pain may radiate to the neck or jaw or may be referred to the back. The pain is typically worsened when a person bends over, strains, or is in a recumbent position. With severe GERD, the pain occurs after each meal and persists for 20 minutes to 2 hours. Clients usually experience prompt relief with the ingestion of fluids or antacids. Some clients experience *atypical chest pain,* which mimics angina and needs to be carefully differentiated from cardiac disease.

Regurgitation, which is not associated with either belching or nausea, is another common symptom. The client reports the occurrence of warm fluid traveling up the throat. If the fluid reaches the level of the pharynx, the client notes a sour or bitter taste in the mouth. This effortless regurgitation frequently occurs when the client is in the upright position. If regurgitation occurs when the client is recumbent, the danger of aspiration is increased.

If the client experiences regurgitation, the nurse carefully auscultates the chest for any evidence of aspiration. The nurse assesses for coughing, hoarseness, or wheezing at night, which may be related to recumbent regurgitation. Clients who have had long-term regurgitation may have bronchitis.

Water brash is a less common symptom. A reflex salivary hypersecretion occurs in response to reflux. Water brash must be carefully distinguished from regurgitation. The client reports a sensation of fluid in the throat; however, because the fluid is saliva, it does not have a sour or bitter taste.

Chronic GERD can involve dysphagia (difficulty in swallowing). In 33% of clients with GERD, dysphagia may be the presenting symptom. This symptom is usually fairly mild; it is not progressive and occurs with the first swallow of each meal. Dysphagia does not interfere with oral nutrition or produce weight loss. If a client reports progressive or persistent dysphagia, careful assessment is required, because it usually indicates the development of a stricture or adenocarcinoma. The nurse assesses the following:

- The degree of dysphagia
- Whether it occurs with ingestion of solids, liquids, or both
- Whether it is intermittent or occurs with each swallowing effort

Odynophagia (painful swallowing) is a possible symptom, although it is relatively rare in people with uncomplicated reflux disease. Severe and long-lasting chest pain may be present if spasms occur in the esophagus that cause the muscle to contract with excess force. The pain can be agonizing and last for hours.

Eructation, flatulence, or bloating after eating are other common complaints. Nausea and vomiting occur infrequently, and unplanned weight loss is rare.

➤ Radiographic Assessment

The most accurate method of diagnosis of gastroesophageal reflux disease (GERD) is through 24-hour pH monitoring; this involves placing pH probes 2 inches (5 cm) above the lower esophageal sphincter (LES). Then, a barium swallow with fluoroscopy outlines the structure of the esophagus and its peristaltic patterns. Twenty-four–hour ambulatory pH monitoring is used widely but is helpful only in evaluating acid reflux.

➤ Other Diagnostic Assessment

The health care provider orders esophageal manometry, or motility testing, when the diagnosis is unclear. Water-filled catheters are inserted via the client's nose or mouth and are connected to transducers that record pressures from various sites in the esophagus as the catheters are withdrawn. Manometry quantifies the resting pressure of the lower esophageal sphincter and helps to evaluate sphincter competence.

In Bernstein's test, an acidic solution is infused via a tube into the distal esophagus. Clients with normal esophageal mucosa experience no symptoms when acid is infused, but clients with esophagitis experience immediate heartburn.

Scintigraphy involves preloading the stomach via the mouth or tube with a liquid radioisotope. Scintillation counts are then taken over the lower esophagus and compared with counts obtained over the stomach. If a client is experiencing frequent reflux, the radioisotope will be refluxed back into the esophagus, which significantly elevates the scintillation counts over the lower esophageal region. Scintigraphy may be used in conjunction with pH monitoring.

Although endoscopic examination through esophagoscopy is rarely necessary to establish the diagnosis of GERD, physicians perform it routinely to rule out malignancy, to take tissue specimens for biopsy, and to evaluate complications.

⬛ Interventions

Interventions begin with thorough teaching about GERD as a chronic condition that warrants ongoing management. This knowledge base is essential for the client's understanding of and adherence to the prescribed regimen of drugs, diet therapy, and lifestyle modifications.

Nonsurgical Management. In most cases, GERD can be controlled by diet therapy, education, lifestyle changes, and drug therapy.

Diet Therapy. In clients with relatively mild GERD, diet therapy alone may relieve symptoms. In collaboration with the dietitian, the nurse explores the client's basic meal patterns, likes, and dislikes. The nurse and dietitian then work with both the client and the family or significant other to discover modifications that may decrease reflux symptoms. It is essential that the family members who do the shopping and cooking be included in this discussion if adherence at home is to be successful.

Because fatty foods, coffee, tea, cola, chocolate, and alcohol all decrease lower esophageal sphincter (LES) pressure, the nurse counsels the client to limit or eliminate these substances in the daily diet. The client should also restrict spicy foods and acidic foods, such as orange juice, until esophageal healing can occur because these foods irritate the inflamed tissue and cause heartburn.

Because large meals increase the volume pressure in the stomach and delay gastric emptying, the nurse instructs the client to eat four to six small meals each day rather than three large ones. Carbonated beverages should also be avoided because they increase the pressure in the stomach. Clients are encouraged to avoid evening snacks and to eat no food for at least 3 hours before going to bed, as reflux episodes are most damaging at night. This restriction may be the most difficult one for the client. The nurse also advises the client to eat slowly and chew thoroughly to facilitate digestion and prevent eructation (belching). The nurse encourages the client to investigate which particular diet changes best reduce the frequency and severity of the symptoms. In some cases, avoiding caffeine relieves symptoms.

Client Education. One of the most sensitive areas involves teaching the client about the importance of not smoking. Smoking causes a prompt and significant drop in LES pressure and optimally should be stopped.

The nurse explains about proper positioning to decrease pain. Teaching the client to elevate the head of the bed by 8–12 inches (3.2–4.8 cm) for sleep is the single most important aspect of educating the client about GERD. Nighttime reflux is extremely common, and infrequent swallowing, in combination with a recumbent position, significantly impairs esophageal clearance. Although wooden blocks have traditionally been recommended to elevate the head of the bed, the use of foam wedges may also achieve satisfactory results. The client or the client's spouse or partner may find elevation of the bed unacceptable at first. The nurse emphasizes the importance of this intervention and investigates all possible approaches for achieving compliance (Chart 57–2).

Lifestyle Changes. If the client is obese, the nurse collaborates with the dietitian to examine approaches to weight reduction. Decreasing intra-abdominal pressure reduces reflux symptoms in many clients. Other lifestyle factors also cause increased abdominal pressure, and the nurse explores these with the client. Constrictive clothing,

---

> ### Chart 57–2
>
> ## Education Guide: Lifestyle Modifications to Control Reflux
>
> * Eat four to six small meals a day.
> * Limit or eliminate fatty foods, coffee, tea, cola, and chocolate.
> * Reduce or eliminate from your diet any food or spice that causes pain.
> * Limit or eliminate alcohol and tobacco.
> * Do not snack in the evening, and take no food for 2–3 hours before you go to bed.
> * Eat slowly, and chew your food thoroughly to reduce belching.
> * Remain upright for 1–2 hours after meals if possible.
> * Elevate the head of your bed 8–12 inches on wooden blocks, or with a foam wedge. Never sleep flat in bed.
> * If you are overweight, lose weight.
> * Do not wear constrictive clothing.
> * Avoid heavy lifting, straining, and working in a bent-over position.

---

lifting heavy objects or straining, and working in a bent-over or stooped position should all be avoided. The nurse emphasizes that these general adaptations are an essential and effective component of disease management and can produce prompt results in uncomplicated cases.

Drug Therapy. Drug therapy is usually initiated by the client with antacid self-medication or the over-the-counter histamine receptor antagonists such as cimetidine (Tagamet) and ranitidine (Zantac). If these measures are not effective, the client then typically seeks medical care.

Antacids. In uncomplicated cases of GERD, antacids are effective for occasional episodes of heartburn. Antacids have an acid-neutralizing effect and usually produce prompt symptomatic relief. They are inadequate, however, for the control of frequent symptoms, because their duration of action is too short and their nighttime effectiveness is minimal.

Either aluminum hydroxide or magnesium hydroxide may be used. Maalox and Mylanta consist of a combination of these two agents, and clients frequently tolerate them better because the side effects, such as constipation and diarrhea, are less. The nurse instructs the client to take the antacid 1 hour before and 2–3 hours after each meal. Some antacids are prepared as double-strength (DS) suspensions or tablets. The advantage of DS preparations is that the client can take a smaller amount of the drug. For example, 30 mL of regular Mylanta equals 15 mL of Mylanta-II (DS preparation).

Gaviscon, a combination of aluminum hydroxide and magnesium carbonate, is a commonly used and very effective medication for GERD. It forms a viscous foam that floats on top of the gastric contents and theoretically decreases the incidence of reflux. If reflux occurs, the foam enters the esophagus first and buffers the acid in the refluxed material. The nurse reminds the client to take this drug when food is in the stomach.

Histamine Receptor Antagonists. With histamine receptor antagonists available over the counter (OTC) and widely advertised for heartburn, many clients will self-medicate with these agents before seeking medical attention. When clients present with uncontrolled symptoms, the health care provider usually prescribes a *higher* dose of a histamine receptor antagonist that is not available OTC, such as ranitidine (Zantac), famotidine (Pepcid), or nizatidine (Axid). Cimetidine (Tagamet, Apo-Cimetidine, Novocimetidine♦) is not used as often as the longer-acting preparations. Ranitidine and the other preparations are longer acting, and less frequent dosing is necessary. They also appear to produce fewer side effects and are safe for long-term administration. Although these drugs do not affect the occurrence of reflux directly, they do reduce gastric acid secretion, provide symptomatic improvement, and support healing of the inflamed esophageal tissue.

Other Drugs. The health care provider may add bethanechol (Urecholine) or metoclopramide (Reglan, Maxeran♦) to the drug regimen for clients who experience severe and ongoing symptoms of reflux. Bethanechol increases lower esophageal sphincter (LES) pressure and significantly increases the rate of esophageal clearance. Because bethanechol is a cholinergic drug, it increases the secretion of gastric acid and usually requires the simultaneous administration of a histamine receptor antagonist and antacids. Bethanecol is usually prescribed in 25-mg doses four times a day. The nurse teaches the client to take bethanechol 30–60 minutes before meals and warns the client about typical side effects, which include abdominal cramping, diarrhea, increased salivation, and urinary urgency.

The primary action of metoclopramide is to increase the rate of gastric emptying. It does not affect gastric acid secretion or directly heal esophageal tissue. Its use is also associated with a high incidence of neurologic and psychotropic side effects, such as fatigue, anxiety, ataxia, and hallucinations. Long-term use is not recommended.

The proton pump inhibitors are typically reserved for the treatment of clients with severe GERD. These potent drugs can reduce gastric acid secretion by about 90% over a 24-hour period and can be given in a single daily dose. Photon pump inhibitors promote rapid tissue healing, but recurrence is common when the drug is stopped. Safety for long-term use has not been established. Omeprazole (Prilosec) is usually prescribed in a 20-mg oral dose once a day for 4–8 weeks.

As part of teaching about drug therapy, the nurse asks about other drugs that the client uses routinely or intermittently. Anticholinergics, calcium channel blockers, theophylline, and diazepam (Valium, Meval♦) all decrease LES pressure or delay gastric emptying and should be avoided if possible.

Cisapride (Propulsid) is a gastrointestinal prokinetic agent (a drug that improves GI motility) that has been approved for the symptomatic treatment of clients with nocturnal heartburn caused by GERD. Treatment is usually started with a dose of 10 mg four times a day before meals and at bedtime, and the dose is increased if necessary. (Chart 57–3) summarizes information about drugs often used in the treatment of GERD.

Surgical Management. Antireflux surgery is usually indicated for otherwise healthy clients who have not responded positively to aggressive medical management. Various surgical procedures may be used. Three major surgical procedures include Nissen fundoplication, Hill's repair, and Belsey's repair. Laparoscopic fundoplication is being tested in sites around the country and will undoubtedly become a common procedure as the technique is perfected (Soper and Jones, 1994; Tucker et al., 1996). (For a more complete description of the three major procedures, see Surgical Management in the discussion of hiatal hernia later in this chapter.)

The Nissen fundoplication (Fig. 57–1) is used most frequently. In each of these procedures, the surgeon wraps and sutures the gastric fundus around the esopha-

---

Chart 57–3

Drug Therapy for Gastroesophageal Reflux Disease (GERD)

Drug	Usual Dosage	Nursing Interventions	Rationale
Antacids, either aluminum or magnesium salts	• 30 mL PO between meals and as needed (PRN) throughout the day and at bedtime	• Give 1 hr before meals, 2–3 hr after meals, and at bedtime. • Give PRN as instructed by physician. • Observe the client for constipation of diarrhea. • Suggest use of combination mixtures or alternating use of aluminum and magnesium products.	• Antacids neutralize acid and produce prompt relief of heartburn. • Aluminum products produce constipation, and magnesium products induce diarrhea. • Balancing their effects is important for client adherence.

Continued

Chart 57–3. Drug Therapy for Gastroesophageal Reflux Disease (GERD)   Continued

Drug	Usual Dosage	Nursing Interventions	Rationale
Gaviscon, antacid plus alginic acid	• 1 tablet or 10–20 mL PO throughout the day and at bedtime	• Give after meals and at bedtime.	• Alginic acid forms a viscous foam that floats on top of the gastric contents, impeding reflux or buffering its effects when it occurs.
Histamine receptor antagonists:		• Instruct the client to take the drug with meals.	• These drugs dramatically suppress gastric acid secretion and promote healing.
Cimetidine (Tagamet, Apo-Cimitine✤, Novocimetidine✤)	• 300 mg qid (four times a day) PO or 900–1200 mg PO at bedtime	• Observe the client for side effects; fatigue, headache, and diarrhea are common.	
Ranitidine (Zantac)	• 150 mg bid (twice a day) PO		• Ranitidine and famotidine are more potent, longer-acting drugs, yet they produce fewer side effects.
Famotidine (Pepcid)	• 40 mg PO at bedtime or 20 mg PO bid		
Bethanechol (Urecholine)	• 25 mg qid PO	• Instruct the client to take the drug 30–60 minutes before meals. • Continue with antacids and histamine receptor antagonists as ordered. • Observe the client for typical side effects: abdominal cramping, diarrhea, urinary urgency, and increased salivation. • Counsel the client about control of side effects.	• This drug increases lower esophageal sphincter (LES) pressure and increases the rate of esophageal clearance. • Bethanecol has cholinergic effects and increases the secretion of gastric acid. • Typical associated cholinergic effects occur with the use of bethanechol.
Metoclopramide (Reglan)	• 10 mg tid (three times a day) or qid PO	• Instruct the client to take the drug before meals. • Teach the client to report any neurologic or psychotropic side effects, such as restlessness, anxiety, ataxia, or hallucinations.	• This drug increases the rate of gastric emptying. • Long-term drug use produces adverse effects in up to one third of clients.
Omeprazole (Prilosec, Losec✤)	• 20–30 mg PO daily	• Instruct the client to take the drug before meals. • Observe the client for typical side effects: abdominal cramping, diarrhea, headache.	• Gastric acid suppression is greater than 90%. Action is prolonged but GI effects are severe in some clients.
Cisapride (Propulsid)	• 10–20 mg PO qid before meals and bedtime	• Do not give to clients with GI hemorrhage, mechanical obstruction, or gastric/abdominal perforation.	• The drug worsens these conditions because it increases GI motility.

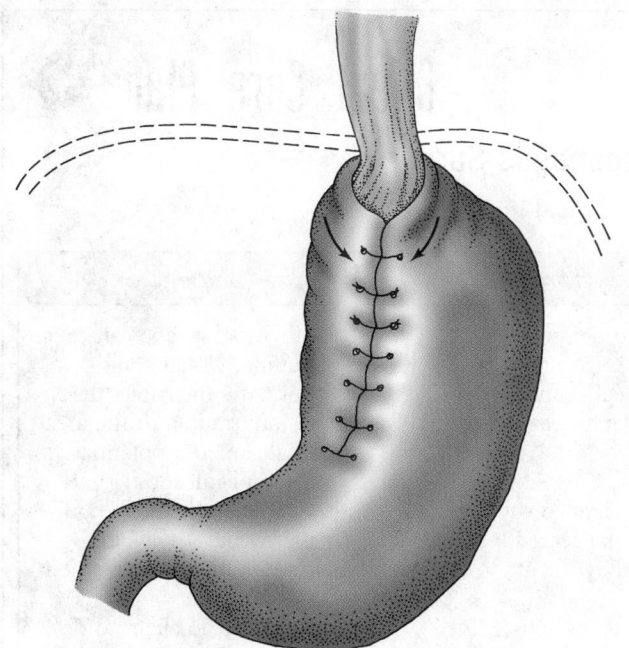

Figure 57–1. Nissen fundoplication for gastroesophageal reflux disease or hiatal hernia repair.

gus, which anchors the LES area below the diaphragm and reinforces the high-pressure area. The Client Care Plan outlines nursing care of clients undergoing esophageal surgery. Clients who have surgery are encouraged to continue to follow the basic antireflux regimen of antacids and diet therapy, because the rate of recurrence is significant.

Placement of the synthetic Angelchik prosthesis also is used for clients with severe reflux. This surgical procedure is an alternative and is associated with fewer long-term problems with achalasia (failure of the lower esophageal muscles and sphincter to relax properly). The surgeon performs a laparotomy and ties a C-shaped silicone prosthesis filled with gel around the distal esophagus (Fig. 57–2). The prosthesis anchors the LES in the abdomen and reinforces sphincter pressure. Dysphagia is the primary complication. Other problems may develop from the presence of a foreign body.

Hiatal Hernia
Overview

The esophageal hiatus is the opening in the diaphragm through which the esophagus passes from the thorax to the abdomen. Hiatal hernias, also called diaphragmatic hernias, occur when the lower portion of the esophagus, a portion of the stomach, or both, move into the thorax through the hiatus. Clients with hiatal hernias may be completely asymptomatic, or they may experience daily symptoms that are similar to those of clients with gastroesophageal reflux disease (GERD).

Pathophysiology

The two major types of hiatal hernias are sliding and paraesophageal (rolling).

Sliding Hernia

Sliding hernias are the most common type and account for 90% of the total number of hiatal hernias. The esophagogastric junction and a portion of the fundus of the stomach slide upward through the esophageal hiatus into the thorax (Fig. 57–3). The hernia generally moves freely and slides into and out of the thorax when changes in position or intra-abdominal pressure occurs. Although volvulus (twisting) and obstruction do occur rarely, the major concern in a client with a sliding hernia is the development of esophageal reflux and its complications. The development of reflux appears to be related to the chronic exposure of the lower esophageal sphincter (LES) to the low pressure of the thorax, which significantly reduces its effectiveness. The hernia itself seems to cause few, if any, problems.

Rolling Hernia

In a client with a paraesophageal hernia, the gastroesophageal junction remains below the diaphragm, but the fundus and possibly portions of the stomach's greater curvature roll into the thorax beside the esophagus (see Fig. 57–3). The herniated portion of the stomach may be small or quite large, and in rare cases, the stomach completely inverts into the thorax. Reflux is rarely a concern because the LES remains anchored below the diaphragm; however, the risks of volvulus, obstruction, and strangulation are high. The development of iron deficiency anemia is common, resulting from slow bleeding because venous obstruction causes the gastric mucosa to become engorged and ooze. Significant bleeding or hemorrhage is rare.

Etiology

Sliding hiatal hernias are believed to develop from muscle weakening in the esophageal hiatus, which loosens the esophageal supports and permits the lower portion of the esophagus to rise into the thorax. The sliding hiatal hernia is a straightforward type of muscle weakness that seems to be consistent with the aging process, although congenital weaknesses, trauma, obesity, or surgery may play a significant role. The development of the hernia is the result of the combined effects of weakened support structures and prolonged increases in abdominal pressure.

Muscle weakening does not appear to cause paraesophageal hernias. Instead, it is theorized that the stomach is not properly anchored below the diaphragm and the hernia results from an anatomic defect rather than a structural weakness.

Incidence/Prevalence

Hiatal hernia is one of the more common disorders that affect the upper gastrointestinal tract, and it affects women more often than men.

Client Care Plan

The Client Undergoing Traditional Open Esophagus Surgery

Nursing Diagnosis No. 1: Risk for Infection related to surgical incision

Expected Outcomes	Nursing Interventions	Rationale
The client will manifest no signs or symptoms of infection.	■ Do not reposition or replace the nasogastric tube. Do not perform endotracheal suctioning on a client with esophageal anastomosis or repair.	■ Moving the tube can cause trauma, which could puncture or irritate the incision; trauma to the area might open a potential route of infection.
	■ Encourage the client to suction or expectorate oral secretions rather than swallow them.	■ Clients are kept on nothing by mouth (NPO) status to avoid active peristalsis.
	■ Assess the cutaneous suture line for redness, drainage, and other signs of infection. Observe the dressing for bleeding; document and report any findings to the physician.	■ Monitor the client to detect complications and early signs of infection as soon as possible.
	■ Clean sutures once each shift with half-strength peroxide; dry the area and apply a small amount of antibacterial ointment.	■ Cleaning removes crusts and secretions, which could be ideal media for bacterial growth.
	■ Monitor vital signs per the physician's orders. Document and report any significant changes to the physician.	■ Monitoring provides early detection of and intervention for hemorrhage or infection.

Nursing Diagnosis No. 2: Risk for Altered Nutrition: Less than Body Requirements related to NPO status and surgical disruption of the esophagus

Expected Outcomes	Nursing Interventions	Rationale
The client will maintain adequate nutritional intake by nasogastric tube until oral feedings are begun.	■ Remind the client of NPO status when the client is alert.	■ Elderly clients may demonstrate memory deficit; clients are often NPO until the intraoral incision is healed.
	■ Monitor IV hydration while the client is NPO and before tube feedings are begun; monitor and record intake and output every shift.	■ Monitor hydration status for overload or retention; elderly clients are often susceptible to overload of fluids.
	■ Assess and document bowel sounds every shift until tube feedings are well tolerated.	■ Establish a baseline for bowel sounds; return of bowel sounds postoperatively is often an indication to begin tube feedings.

Client Care Plan

Expected Outcomes	Nursing Interventions	Rationale
	■ Measure and record the client's weight daily.	■ Weight gives information on fluid status.
	■ Maintain proper functioning of the nasogastric tube; while it is attached to suction, measure and record drainage every shift. When tube feedings are begun, flush the tube carefully with water after each feeding or medication administration.	■ Monitor and maintain patency to permit drainage and to allow a route for the administration of medications and nutrition.
	■ Elevate the head of the bed 30 degrees at rest and 90 degrees for feeding and for 1/2 hr after feeding.	■ Raising the head helps prevent reflux; the incidence of reflux is greatest during and 1/2 hr after tube feedings.
	■ Provide the client with written and oral instructions regarding tube feedings.	■ Written as well as oral instructions provide the client with resources when the nurse is not available.
	■ Include the family/significant other in all teaching.	■ Including loved ones ensures support for the client to perform the procedures.
	■ Have the client give a return demonstration of the procedure.	■ A return demonstration aids in retention of the learned procedure and provides a means of evaluation for the nurse.
	■ When oral fluids are begun, assess and document difficulty in swallowing, aspiration, or leakage, including signs of increased pulse rate, increased temperature, increased respiratory rate, subcutaneous emphysema, or change in chest tube drainage indicating contamination from the GI tract.	■ Clients occasionally have difficulty in swallowing after esophageal surgery; assessment provides documentation of real or perceived difficulty. The nurse observes carefully for signs of leakage from the esophageal anastomosis site or from a perforation.
	■ If the client is experiencing difficulty in swallowing, consult a speech-language pathologist for assessment or assistance in swallowing.	■ Speech-language pathologists are often expert at evaluating swallowing disorders; providing the client with techniques of head positioning, breath holding, or oral exercises can help overcome minor swallowing difficulties.
	■ Collaborate with the dietitian as appropriate.	■ Often a change in food consistency eases swallowing difficulties.

(Continued)

Client Care Plan

Expected Outcomes	Nursing Interventions	Rationale
	■ Observe the client for any epigastric burning, retrosternal or back pain, or pain radiating to the chin or shoulder indicative of esophageal reflux; document any findings.	■ Esophageal reflux, once documented, can be treated by positioning the client or dietary changes; analgesics may be required before mealtimes.

Nursing Diagnosis No. 3: Pain related to incision or reflux

Expected Outcomes	Nursing Interventions	Rationale
The client will verbalize control of pain, facilitating adequate nutritional intake and participation in activities of daily living.	■ Assess and document the level of pain, relying on subjective and objective symptoms of pain and pain relief. Assess and document relief obtained from the analgesic regimen.	■ Clients are often unwilling to demonstrate evidence of pain and are often unwilling to use analgesics, particularly opioids, as often as prescribed.
	■ Assess the client for pain related to esophageal reflux or perforation: epigastric burning; pain radiating to shoulder, chin, or back; change in vital signs; change in character of chest tube drainage (if present); subcutaneous emphysema. Document and report all findings to the physician.	■ Early detection of esophageal perforation is imperative to begin effective treatment; documentation of reflux communicates need to prevent reflux aspiration to other health care workers.
	■ Instruct client to keep the head of the bed raised 30 degrees at all times and 90 degrees at meals and for 1/2 hr after meals.	■ Raising the head of the bed not only reduces edema by facilitating gravity drainage, but also facilitates food passage and prevents esophageal reflux.
	■ Explore dietary modifications with the client to alleviate discomfort related to reflux.	■ Smaller, more frequent meals with a change in food consistency can reduce discomfort associated with reflux.
	■ Explore various positioning changes to facilitate food passage and alleviate symptoms of reflux.	■ Varying positions assumed while eating and after eating can reduce discomfort associated with reflux or dysphagia.
	■ Instruct the client to use analgesic medication 1/2 hr before meals, chest physiotherapy, and other treatments as needed.	■ Assuring a peak analgesic effect during activities that the client reports as being most uncomfortable can increase compliance with those activities and efforts to obtain adequate nutritional intake.

Client Care Plan

Expected Outcomes	Nursing Interventions	Rationale
	■ Instruct the client and family/significant other about medications prescribed: timing, side effects, and restrictions; provide written as well as oral instructions.	■ Written and oral instructions are given because the client may have memory loss.
	■ Instruct the client to monitor his or her own comfort.	■ The client gains a feeling of control concerning discomfort.

ELDERLY CONSIDERATIONS

The incidence of sliding hiatal hernias increases for both sexes with age and reaches a prevalence of approximately 60% in the sixth decade of life. As many as 80% of clients with hiatal hernias are asymptomatic or experience only mild transient symptoms associated with reflux.

Collaborative Management

Assessment

The nurse assesses the client's general physical appearance and nutritional status and helps the client identify the location of any pain. Because the primary symptoms of sliding hiatal hernias are associated with reflux, the nurse carefully assesses for heartburn, regurgitation, pain, dysphagia, and belching (Chart 57–4). The nurse also auscultates the thorax and lungs, as pulmonary symptoms similar to asthma may be triggered by episodes of aspiration, particularly at night.

Clients with paraesophageal (rolling) hernias rarely experience reflux symptoms. The nurse assesses for symptoms that are related to the stretching or displacement of thoracic contents by the hernia. Clients may report a feeling of fullness after eating and may even experience breathlessness or a feeling of suffocation if the hernia interferes with breathing. Some clients experience chest pain that mimics angina. Symptoms are typically worse when the client is in a recumbent position.

The barium swallow study with fluoroscopy is the most specific diagnostic test for identifying hiatal hernia. Paraesophageal hernias are usually clearly visible, and sliding hernias can often be observed as the client is moved through a series of positions that increase intra-abdominal pressure.

Clients with sliding hernias usually experience the symptoms of reflux. Therefore, any or all of the diagnostic tests that are used for gastroesophageal reflux disease (GERD) may be used to fully evaluate the extent of reflux and the degree of esophageal damage (see earlier under Other Diagnostic Assessment for GERD).

Interventions

Clients with hiatal hernias may be managed either medically or surgically. The health care provider's choice of management is based on the severity of the client's symptoms and the risk of serious complications. Sliding hiatal hernias are most frequently treated medically, whereas large paraesophageal hernias are treated surgically because of the high rate of complications.

Nonsurgical Management. Basic interventions for the client with hiatal hernia closely follow the regimen out-

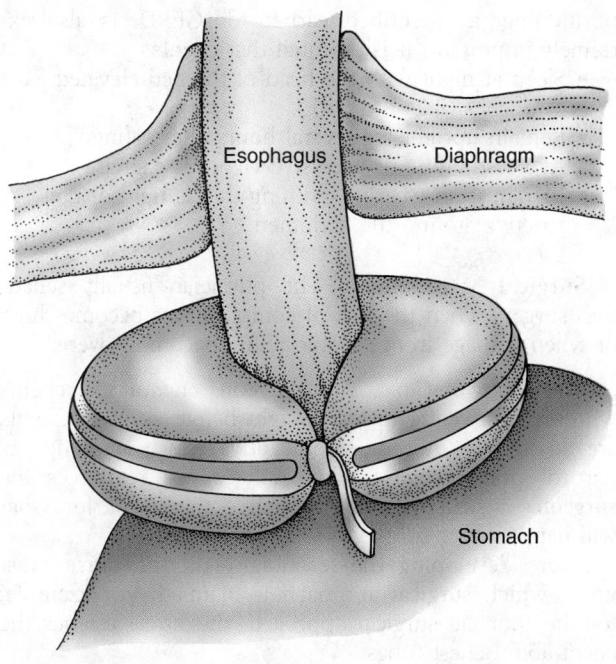

Figure 57–2. Placement of the Angelchik antireflux prosthesis.

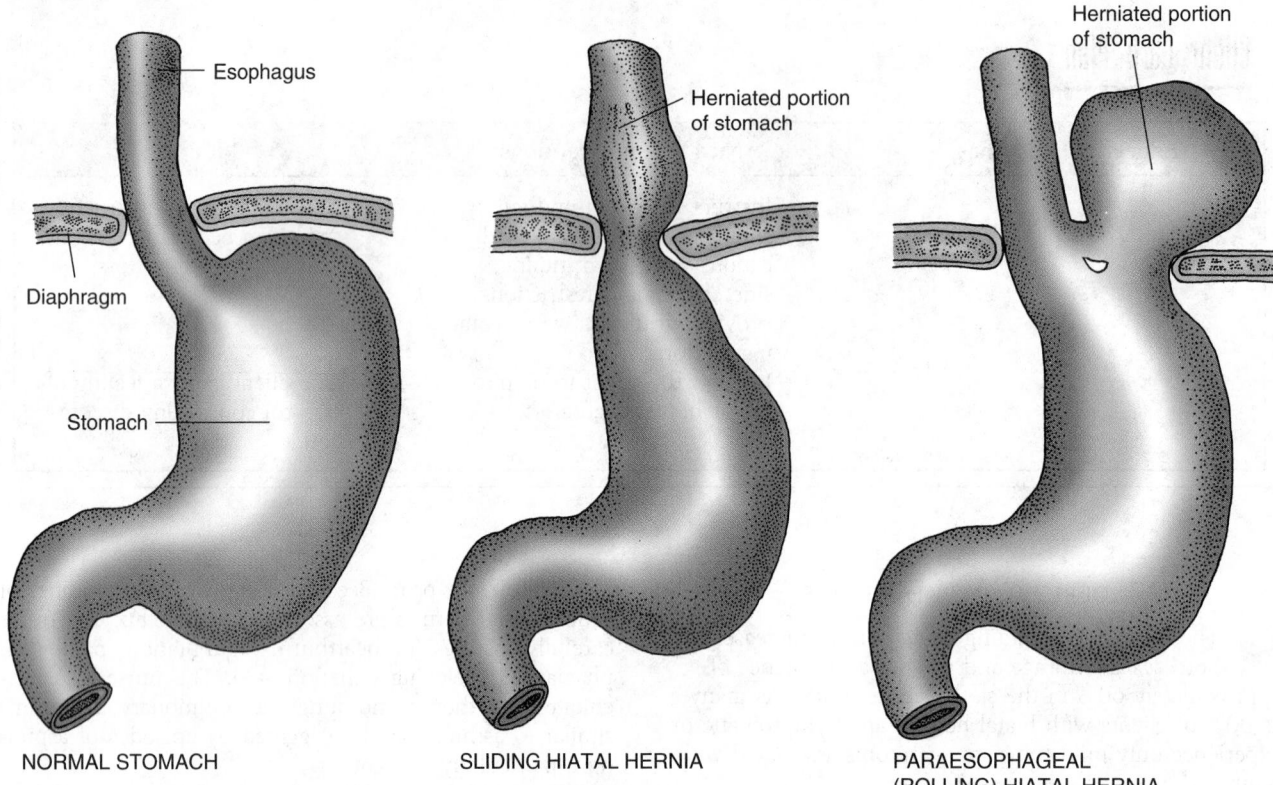

Figure 57–3. A comparison of the normal stomach and sliding and paraesophageal (rolling) hiatal hernias.

lined for those with GERD and include drug therapy, diet therapy, lifestyle modifications, and client education.

The health care provider typically prescribes antacids and histamine receptor antagonists, such as ranitidine (Zantac), in an attempt to control reflux and its symptoms.

Diet therapy is also an integral part of the conservative management of hiatal hernia and follows the guidelines discussed earlier for GERD. The client is reminded not to snack before bed. In collaboration with the dietitian, the nurse works with the client to modify the diet to reduce body weight, if appropriate, because obesity increases intra-abdominal pressure and worsens both the hernia and the symptoms of reflux.

The nurse carefully explains the underlying condition to increase the client's understanding of the disorder and adherence with the treatment regimen. Teaching about positioning, as described earlier for GERD, is also extremely important. It is essential that clients

- Sleep at night with the head of the bed elevated 8–12 inches (3.2–4.8 cm)
- Remain upright for several hours after eating
- Avoid straining or excessive vigorous exercise
- Refrain from wearing clothing that is tight or constrictive around the abdomen

Surgical Management. The physician usually schedules surgery when the risk of complications becomes high or when damage from chronic reflux becomes severe.

Preoperative Care. The surgeon encourages clients who are overweight to lose weight before surgery. Clients are advised to quit or significantly reduce smoking. As part of preoperative teaching, the nurse reinforces the surgeon's instructions and prepares the client for what will happen after surgery.

Before developing the teaching plan, the nurse must know which surgical approach is planned. For example, for the thoracic surgical approach, the nurse teaches the client about chest tubes.

The nurse informs the client that a nasogastric tube

Chart 57–4

Key Features of Hernias

Sliding Hiatal Hernias

- Heartburn
- Regurgitation
- Chest pain
- Dysphagia
- Belching

Paraesophageal Hernias

- Feeling of fullness after eating
- Breathlessness after eating
- Feeling of suffocation
- Chest pain that mimics angina
- Worsening of manifestations in a recumbent position

will be inserted during surgery and will remain in place for several days. Oral intake is started gradually with clear liquids after peristalsis is re-established or to stimulate peristalsis. The nurse also instructs the client in techniques for effective deep breathing and use of the incentive spirometer. Because the surgery involves the diaphragm, these measures are essential to prevent postoperative respiratory complications. The high incision makes deep breathing extremely painful for the client. Teaching and reassurance about adequate postoperative analgesia help promote client cooperation and compliance.

Operative Procedures. The repair of *paraesophageal* hernias is similar to other hernia procedures, in that straightforward anatomic repair is the primary focus. There is no need to alter or modify lower esophageal sphincter (LES) function. Simple repair of the defect in the diaphragm, however, does not successfully control the reflux problems associated with *sliding* hiatal hernias. All of the current surgical approaches for sliding hernias also involve reinforcement of the LES to restore sphincter competence and prevent reflux. Eventual recurrence can be a problem for a client with either type of hernia.

Although several hiatal hernia repair procedures are in use, each involves LES reinforcement through some degree of fundoplication. The surgeon wraps a portion of the stomach fundus around the distal esophagus to anchor it and reinforce the LES.

The Nissen repair, shown in Figure 57–1, is the procedure most commonly used. An abdominal approach is usually chosen. The surgeon wraps the fundus a full 360 degrees around the lower esophagus. The sphincter reinforcement is tight and usually controls reflux effectively.

In the Hill repair, an abdominal approach is also used, but the fundoplication is 180 degrees around the esophagus. The angle of His is restructured to accentuate the angle at which the esophagus enters the stomach.

The Belsey repair usually involves a 280-degree esophageal wrap and a thoracic approach. Surgeons do not agree about which surgical repair is most appropriate or effective, because each procedure has unique advantages and disadvantages.

Postoperative Care. Postoperative care after hiatal hernia repair closely follows that required after any esophageal surgery (see Client Care Plan). The nurse carefully assesses for complications of fundoplication surgery and reports their occurrence to the physician (Chart 57–5).

Respiratory Care. Prevention of respiratory complications is the primary focus of postoperative care. The nurse or assistive nursing personnel elevate the head of the client's bed at least 30 degrees to lower the diaphragm and facilitate lung expansion. The nurse or assistive nursing personnel help the client get out of bed and ambulate as soon as possible. The incision must be supported during coughing to reduce pain and to prevent excessive strain on the suture line, especially with obese clients.

Incentive spirometry and deep breathing are routinely used after surgery to maintain patency of the airways. Adequate analgesia is essential for client compliance and should be administered as needed. Clients with a smoking history or chronic airway limitation require more aggressive respiratory management by the respiratory therapist to prevent atelectasis and pneumonia. Clients with large hiatal hernias have a high risk for developing respiratory complications (see Research Applications for Nursing).

Nasogastric Tube Management. Another important part of postoperative management is care of the nasogastric (NG) tube. The large-diameter NG tube inserted during surgery prevents the fundoplication wrap from becoming too tight around the esophagus. The NG drainage is initially dark brown with old blood, but it should become normal yellowish-green within the first 8 hours after surgery. The nurse checks for proper placement of the tube in the stomach every 4–8 hours. The nurse also ensures that the NG tube is properly anchored and that it cannot be displaced, because it cannot be safely reinserted without risking perforation of the incision.

Regular assessment of the patency of the tube is essential to keep the stomach decompressed, thus preventing retching or vomiting, which can strain or rupture the stomach sutures. Because the tube is irritating, the nurse or assistive personnel provide frequent oral hygiene. The nurse also assesses the client's hydration status regularly, including accurate measures of intake and output. Adequate fluid replacement helps to keep respiratory secretions thin.

Chart 57–5

Nursing Care Highlight: Assessment of Postoperative Complications of Fundoplication Procedures

Complication	Indicators of Complication
Temporary dysphagia	• The client has difficulty swallowing when oral feeding begins.
Gas bloat syndrome	• The client has difficulty belching to relieve distention.
Atelectasis, pneumonia	• The client experiences dyspnea, chest pain, and/or fever.
Obstructed nasogastric tube	• The client has nausea, vomiting, and/or abdominal distention. The nasogastric tube does not drain.

Research Applications for Nursing

Do People with Hiatal Hernias Have Weaker Lower Esophageal Sphincters and More Severe Gastroesophageal Reflux Disease?

Patti, M., Goldberg, H., Arcerito, M., Bortolasi, L., Tong, J., & Way, L. (1996). Hiatal hernia size affects lower esophageal sphincter function, esophageal acid exposure, and the degree of mucosal injury. The American Journal of Surgery, 171, 182–186.

The role of hiatal hernia in the pathophysiology of gastroesophageal reflux disease (GERD) has been debated for several decades; therefore, the purpose of this study was to determine the relationship among the presence and size of a hiatal hernia and the dysfunction of the lower esophageal sphincter (LES), efficacy of esophageal acid clearance, the amount of gastroesophageal reflux, and the degree of mucosal injury. The researchers found that people with large hiatal hernias had more abnormal acid clearance, more refluxed acid, and more profound LES dysfunction than people with small or no hiatal hernia. These factors correlated to the degree of mucosal damage.

Critique. The sample of 95 was selected from a group of clients who were referred to the Swallowing Center of the University of California, San Francisco. The methods the investigators used to determine the extent of GERD (symptom evaluation, endoscopy, esophageal manometry, 24-hour esophageal pH monitoring, and upper gastrointestinal series) are the accepted standard of practice. The selection criteria for the sample were not discussed, nor was the consent rate reported. It is difficult to generalize these findings to a larger population without this information; however, these findings support other reports in the literature related to the presence and size of hiatal hernias and the degree of reflux involved.

Possible Nursing Implications. Because 83% of the clients with large hiatal hernias had respiratory symptoms (coughing or wheezing), nurses caring for these people should perform careful respiratory assessments to monitor for the possible development of pneumonia. Because the degree of esophageal injury increased with the size of the hiatal hernia, nurses should prepare focused teaching plans to emphasize ways to minimize acid reflux through lifestyle and diet alterations.

Nutrition. The client may begin oral intake with clear fluids after peristalsis is re-established or in an effort to stimulate peristalsis. Some surgeons create a temporary gastrostomy for feeding to allow for undisturbed healing of the repair. The client gradually progresses to a near-normal diet during the first 6 weeks. A few foods, such as caffeinated or carbonated beverages and alcohol, are either restricted or eliminated. The food storage area of the stomach is reduced by the surgery, and meals need to be both smaller and more frequent.

The nurse carefully supervises the first oral feedings, because temporary dysphagia is common. Persistent dysphagia usually indicates that the fundoplication is too tight, and dilation may be required.

Another common complication of fundoplication surgery is the gas bloat syndrome, in which clients are unable to voluntarily eructate (belch). The syndrome is usually temporary but may persist. The nurse teaches the

client to avoid drinking carbonated beverages; eating gas-producing foods, especially high-fat foods; chewing gum; and drinking with a straw.

Many clients acquire the habit of aerophagia (air swallowing) from attempting to reverse or clear acid reflux. The nurse teaches these clients to consciously relax before and after meals, eat and drink slowly, and chew all food thoroughly.

Air in the stomach that cannot be removed by belching can be extremely uncomfortable for the client. Frequent position changes and ambulation are effective interventions for eliminating air from the gastrointestinal tract.

▶ Continuing Care

For clients having one of the three major surgical repairs, activity is restricted during the standard 4- to 6-week postsurgical recovery period. For laparoscopic surgery, activity is typically restricted for a shorter time, and the client can return to his or her usual lifestyle more quickly. The nurse instructs the client to avoid straining and prevent constipation. For long-term management, the nurse teaches the client, family, or significant other about appropriate diet modifications, but the use of stool softeners or bulk laxatives is recommended for the first postoperative weeks until healing is complete.

The nurse instructs the client to inspect the healing incision daily and to notify the physician or health care provider if swelling, redness, tenderness, discharge, or fever occurs.

The nurse advises the client to avoid contact with people with respiratory infections and to contact the physician if symptoms of a cold or influenza develop. Persistent coughing can cause the incision or the fundoplication to dehisce. If possible, the client should not smoke.

The nurse and dietitian educate the entire family or significant other about diet. Full support is essential for the client to successfully modify the size and timing of meals. Relatively few ongoing diet restrictions are needed, but eating too much or eating the wrong kinds of foods can produce discomfort if the client cannot belch. The client is the best judge of what foods produce discomfort, and the nurse encourages cautious experimentation with new foods. The nurse instructs the client to report the recurrence of reflux symptoms to the physician.

Although most clients experience a sense of relief when the chronic symptoms of reflux are surgically relieved, unrealistic expectations can be a problem. Although severe surgical complications are relatively rare, conditions such as gas bloat syndrome and dysphagia are common and may persist. The nurse helps the client prepare for these problems, as well as for the potential that reflux may not be completely controlled or may occur again. Although surgery controls the condition, a cure is rare and lifestyle modifications need to be ongoing.

Achalasia

Overview

Achalasia is a condition in which the lower esophageal muscles and sphincter fail to relax appropriately in response to swallowing. It is characterized by chronic and progressive dysphagia. Regurgitation of ingested food may also occur.

The pathophysiology and etiology of achalasia remain unclear. The disorder may result from a neuromuscular defect localized to the inner circular muscle layer of the esophagus. Degeneration of ganglion cells appears to cause a loss of nerves that innervate the smooth muscle of the lower esophagus. Over time, peristaltic failure plus spasm can produce a massively dilated esophagus, which further slows food passage. Achalasia is an uncommon disorder that affects people of all ages and both sexes equally.

Collaborative Management

 Assessment

The nurse assesses for the primary symptoms of achalasia when obtaining a history from the client with this disorder. Symptoms includes dysphagia, chest pain, and regurgitation. This assessment may be more difficult in the elderly client because chest pain may not be the primary presenting symptom. In addition, the onset and/or duration of symptoms should be determined.

Achalasia is often a chronic condition; however, the symptoms get worse over time, which makes the client more aware of the problems. The nurse questions the client about factors that aggravate the symptoms (such as body position or diet changes) as well as medications or home treatments that relieve the symptoms. The nurse asks the client about a history of previous esophageal surgery or trauma, which can add to the progressive dysphagia. Respiratory history and current respiratory difficulties are particularly important with regard to their direct relationship to reflux, regurgitation, and aspiration.

To determine the effect of the esophageal symptoms, the nurse takes a nutritional history, including dietary habits, food tolerances, and weight loss.

The nurse also notes the presence of halitosis (foul mouth odor), which can be caused by regurgitation of previously ingested food. The nurse assesses the client's weight and compares it with the client's report of past weight.

A barium swallow study frequently shows a narrow "bird's beak" junction at the esophageal hiatus and esophageal dilation, with possible retained food and fluid. Esophageal manometry is used to evaluate peristalsis and sphincter pressure. Expected findings from manometry are elevated resting pressures at the lower esophageal sphincter (LES) with slow low-amplitude or absent peristalsis. The sphincter frequently fails to relax when the client swallows.

Interventions

Drug and Diet Therapy. Various categories of medications have been investigated to lower esophageal pressures and to relax the LES. Anticholinergic drugs, nitrates, gastrointestinal hormones, and calcium channel blockers have all been used, but none has proved to be consistently effective. Nonopioid and opioid analgesics may occasionally be administered. Drug therapy is basically symptom driven and is not recommended as an alternative to more definitive therapy.

The nurse advises the client to experiment with changes in diet, because they can often ease the pressure and reflux associated with achalasia. The nurse discusses with the client any food habits that he or she has noted that aggravate or relieve the symptoms. Semisoft foods are often better tolerated, as are warm foods and liquids. Eating several smaller meals rather than three larger meals during the day facilitates the passage of food. The nurse collaborates with the dietitian for additional suggestions about diet changes and nutritional balance.

Nocturnal reflux of foods and liquids from the dilated esophagus into the hypopharynx and oral cavity often can be prevented if the client sleeps with the head of the bed elevated or in a semisitting position. The nurse also advises the client to experiment with various changes in position while eating, because these changes can reduce pressure sensations during meals. Some clients benefit from arching the back while swallowing. The nurse cautions the client to avoid wearing restrictive clothing, which can increase esophageal pressure and regurgitation.

Esophageal Dilation. Several methods can be used for dilation of the esophagus. The traditional treatment is the passage of progressively larger sizes of esophageal bougies (dilators). Another method, balloon dilation (polyurethane balloons on a catheter) of the esophagus, is the most effective treatment for achalasia. Typically, pneumatic dilators are positioned across the esophageal junction with fluoroscopy and local anesthesia. The balloon, which is filled with air or water, is inflated to a predetermined level for 30–60 seconds (Fig. 57–4). The basal LES pressure is lowered by this method by tearing of the esophageal sphincter muscle fibers.

The procedure is performed on an outpatient (ambulatory) basis. The nurse monitors the client for bleeding and signs of perforation, such as chest and shoulder pain, elevated temperature, subcutaneous emphysema (air under the skin), or hemoptysis (coughing up blood).

The nurse teaches the client to expectorate rather than swallow secretions. The client is allowed nothing by mouth (NPO) for about an hour and is instructed to swallow only liquids for 24 hours. The procedure may be repeated in 2–3 months if needed. Most clients report improvement in swallowing.

Esophagomyotomy. Surgical procedures for clients with achalasia are aimed at facilitating the passage of food. Esophagomyotomy, in which the LES is incised, has been used successfully for decades. Both thoracic and abdominal approaches are used according to the surgeon's preference and experience. An antireflux wrap (fundoplication) may or may not be part of the procedure.

Esophagomyotomy is a more complex surgical treatment for achalasia than is dilation. General anesthesia is required, and the client is hospitalized for several days. A thoracotomy approach permits exposure of the esophagus. The surgeon cuts muscle fibers around the LES to open

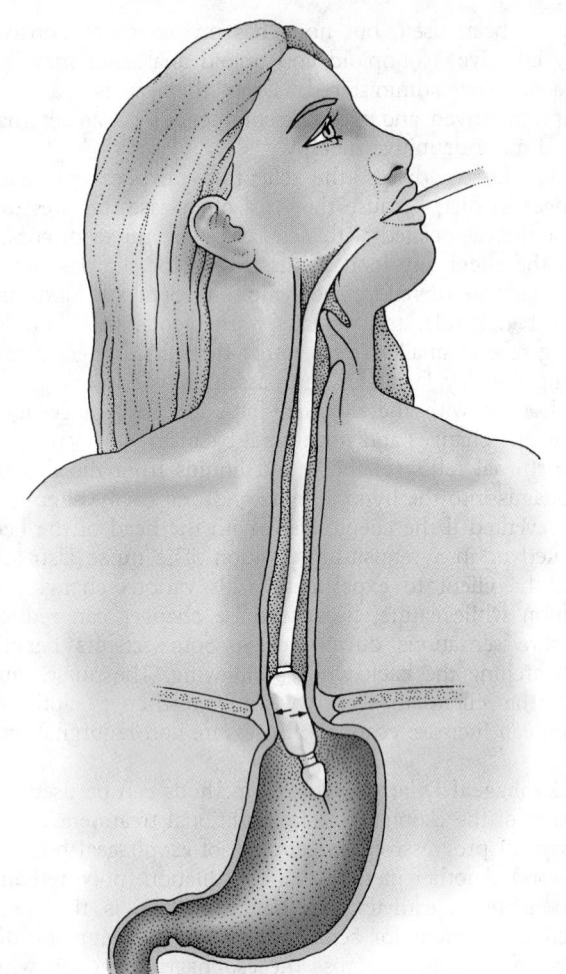

Figure 57–4. Balloon (pneumatic) dilation of the lower esophagus.

the sphincter and thereby provide less obstruction to food passage.

For long-term refractory achalasia, the surgeon may attempt excision of the affected portion of the esophagus, with or without replacement by a segment of colon or jejunum (partial esophagectomy).

Postoperative care for clients undergoing esophagomyotomy or esophagectomy includes managing chest tubes and drains, assessing healing of the thoracotomy or abdominal incision, pain control, and managing nasogastric feedings. (See Chapter 22 for general postoperative care and Chapter 34 for care of the client with a thoracotomy.)

Esophageal Tumors

Overview

Both benign and malignant tumors may occur in the esophagus. Benign tumors, usually in the form of leiomyomas, are extremely uncommon and are usually asymptomatic. No specific treatment is required unless they produce symptoms, and then they are generally excised. Cancer of the esophagus is uncommon in the United State; however, it is almost always fatal. The tumor is almost never diagnosed early enough to allow for effective intervention.

Pathophysiology

Cancer may develop at any point within the esophagus. Approximately 85% of esophageal cancers are squamous epidermoid tumors, half of which develop in the middle third of the esophagus, 35% in the lower third, and 15% in the upper third. The remainder of the tumors are adenocarcinomas, which develop in the lower third and may result from chronic reflux. Esophageal tumors of all types evolve as part of a slow process that begins with tissue changes that are at first benign.

Esophageal tumors exhibit rapid local growth because there is no serosal layer to limit their extension, and because the esophageal mucosa is richly supplied with lymphatics, there is early spread of tumors to lymph nodes. The tumors themselves are typically intraluminal ulcerating lesions with a tendency to encircle the wall of the esophagus and to extend up and down its length.

Cancer of the esophagus is a progressive disease, and complications are expected. Most clients experience pulmonary complications related to fistula formation and aspiration, and these are a frequent cause of death. The close anatomic relationships of the various structures in the neck and chest also contribute to the early symptoms associated with obstruction and compression within other structures. Total esophageal obstruction is inevitable if therapy is not successful. Invasion of the tumor into major vessels can produce life-threatening hemorrhage.

Etiology

Geographic and environmental factors may affect the development of esophageal cancer. Chronic trauma and the long-term effects of other esophageal problems (e.g., achalasia, stricture, hiatal hernia) also influence the incidence statistics but in only a minor way. In the United States, the long-term heavy consumption of alcohol and use of tobacco are believed to account for 80% to 90% of the cases of esophageal cancer. In other parts of the world where esophageal cancer is common, the incidence appears to be linked to high levels of nitrosamines, smoked opiates, and contaminants in the soil and foodstuffs. Diets that are chronically deficient in fresh fruits and vegetables, vitamins, and proteins are also implicated.

Incidence/Prevalence

In the United States, cancer of the esophagus accounts for fewer than 1% of all newly diagnosed cancers and 4% of all tumors involving the gastrointestinal tract. Esophageal cancer is extremely virulent and has a 5-year survival rate of less than 5%.

TRANSCULTURAL CONSIDERATIONS

Over the past several decades, there have been statistically significant annual increases in the incidence of cancer of the esophagus in the United States, particularly in African-Americans. Esophageal cancer mortality rates for this group are now second only to cancer of the lung.

In areas of northwest China, around the Caspian Sea in Russia and Iran, and in the Transkei region of southern Africa, the incidence is extremely high. Residents of some provinces in China have a 30%–40% probability of dying of esophageal cancer. The causes of these extreme variations are being researched but have not been satisfactorily explained.

In North America, cancer of the esophagus typically affects men between the ages of 50 and 80 years. Men are affected more than women, African-Americans are affected more than Caucasians, and Asian-American men are affected more than the general population (Giger & Davidhizar, 1995).

Collaborative Management

 Assessment

➤ History

The nurse assesses the client's race, cultural background, age, sex, and any pertinent history of alcohol consumption, tobacco use, dietary habits, and other esophageal problems, such as stricture or reflux.

Cancer of the esophagus is a silent tumor in its early stages, with few, if any, signs to identify on assessment. By the time the tumor causes symptoms, it usually has spread rather extensively. Clients commonly experience a weight loss of as much as 40–50 pounds (18.2–22.7 kg) over a 2- to 3-month period. The weight loss is a nonspecific assessment feature, which may be related to anorexia, dysphagia, or the discomfort produced by the tumor's presence. The nurse carefully assesses the client's diet pattern and any modifications that have been made in response to the symptoms.

➤ Physical Assessment/Clinical Manifestations

The nurse assesses the client's general physical appearance and nutritional status and asks about recent weight loss.

Because the most important diagnostic feature of esophageal cancer is dysphagia, the nurse carefully assesses its severity and extent. Clients usually report a sensation that food is sticking in the throat or the substernal area. Tumor-induced dysphagia is both persistent and progressive. It is initially associated with swallowing solids, particularly meat, and then progresses rapidly over a period of weeks or months to difficulty in swallowing soft foods and liquids. Late in the disease, even saliva can induce choking. Careful assessment of the dysphagia is an important part of the diagnosis because the dysphagia that is associated with other esophageal disorders is not usually continuous. Dysphagia does not usually appear until at least 60% of the esophageal diameter is narrowed by the tumor.

Odynophagia (painful swallowing) is present in most clients and is reported as a steady, dull, substernal pain that may radiate. The presence of pain that is severe or persistent often indicates tumor invasion of mediastinal structures. The nurse also assesses for the occurrence of regurgitation, vomiting, foul breath, and chronic hiccups, which often accompany advanced disease. In most clients,

pulmonary complications develop at some point, and the nurse assesses for the presence of chronic cough, increased secretions, and a history of recent infections.

Tumors in the upper esophagus may involve the larynx and thus cause hoarseness. Chart 57–6 summarizes the clinical manifestations of esophageal tumors.

➤ Psychosocial Assessment

The symptoms and diagnosis of esophageal cancer can affect a client in profound ways. The disease produces significant daily symptoms, requires major modifications in basic eating patterns, and is terminal. The fear of choking can transform normal mealtimes into frightening experiences that the client may wish to avoid. The nurse carefully assesses the client's response to the diagnosis and prognosis and explores the client's coping strengths and resources. The nurse thoroughly assesses the impact of the disease on the client's usual pattern of activities. The client's home situation is assessed, including family members and friends who can provide support or direct assistance with care. The nurse also assesses the potential financial impact of the disease and its treatment.

➤ Laboratory Assessment

Slow occult bleeding from the tumor may produce decreased hemoglobin and hematocrit values, but laboratory tests are not definitive for esophageal cancer.

➤ Radiographic Assessment

To arrive at a diagnosis of esophageal cancer, the physician first uses a barium swallow study with fluoroscopy. The tumor margins of large masses can often be outlined during the test. A negative result does not rule out cancer, however, and further diagnostic evaluation is usually indicated.

➤ Other Diagnostic Assessment

The physician performs an endoscopic examination to inspect the esophagus and to obtain specimens for cytologic studies, biopsy, and staging. Multiple tissue samples may be required when the suspected tumor is in the distal esophagus, because clear tissue samples are difficult to obtain.

If surgery is planned, the physician may also use computed tomography, gallium scans, and bronchoscopy to

---

Chart 57–6

Key Features of Esophageal Tumors

- Persistent and progressive dysphagia (most diagnostic feature)
- Feeling of food sticking in the throat
- Odynophagia (painful swallowing)
- Severe, persistent chest pain
- Regurgitation
- Chronic cough with increasing secretions
- Hoarseness

help determine the extent of the disease. (These tests are described elsewhere in this text.)

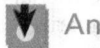

Analysis

➤ Common Nursing Diagnoses and Collaborative Problems

The most common nursing diagnosis associated with cancer of the esophagus is Altered Nutrition: Less than Body Requirements, related to impaired swallowing.

➤ Additional Nursing Diagnoses and Collaborative Problems

In addition, one or more of the following nursing diagnoses may be appropriate:

- Pain, related to the pressure of the tumor mass in the esophagus or mediastinum
- Impaired Swallowing, related to obstruction by tumor or effects of radiation
- Ineffective Individual Coping and Ineffective Family Coping: Compromised, related to disease effects and terminal prognosis
- Anticipatory Grieving, related to declining physical status and terminal prognosis
- Spiritual Distress, related to impending death

The client with esophageal tumors also has the potential for airway obstruction or aspiration.

Planning and Implementation

➤ Altered Nutrition: Less than Body Requirements

Planning: Expected Outcomes. The outcome is that the client is expected to ingest sufficient balanced nutrients to meet the body's needs and to maintain a stable weight.

Interventions. Treatment options for cancer of the esophagus include

- Radiation therapy
- Dilation of strictures
- Prosthesis insertion
- Chemotherapy
- Nutritional support
- Radical surgery

None of the available approaches has significantly improved either the 5-year survival rates or the terminal prognosis. Therefore, there is little agreement about how aggressive treatment should be for each client. Clients with cancer of the esophagus almost always suffer greatly, and relieving symptoms becomes an essential consideration.

Nonsurgical Management. Treatment decisions are based on location and size of the tumor, the presence of metastasis, the client's concurrent health status, and the client's ability to withstand radical surgery.

Nonsurgical interventions are usually directed at the palliation of symptoms. The physician selects nonsurgical

management when a client is either unable or unwilling to undergo extensive surgery.

Radiation Therapy. Radiation therapy is the treatment of choice for palliation. Radiation reduces the tumor's size and offers clients consistent short-term relief. High doses of radiation, however, can result in esophageal stricture or stenosis, which may require dilation. Normal esophageal tissue is very sensitive to the effects of radiation. The treatment is typically administered during a 6- to 8-week period in an attempt to minimize these negative effects. Radiation therapy is a successful palliative measure that improves the client's quality of life, but it also consumes a significant portion of the client's remaining time.

In the first weeks of treatment, radiation produces edema and epithelial desquamation, which often create acute esophagitis and odynophagia (painful swallowing). Profound anorexia, nausea, and vomiting may also result. Symptoms persist until treatment is completed. The nurse assesses the client frequently to determine the incidence and severity of symptoms. Systemic analgesics are often required to control discomfort, and the nurse administers oral lidocaine (Xylocaine Viscous) before each attempt at oral feeding.

The nurse works with the client to modify the diet to meet nutritional needs and maintain comfort. Small, frequent, soft or semiliquid meals are offered. Sweet, light foods are often tolerated best, and protein powder may be used to supplement the nutritional content of the diet. The nurse maintains accurate records of calorie counts, intake and output, and daily weights and assesses skin turgor and mucous membranes regularly. In collaboration with the physician and dietitian, the nurse assesses the need for enteral nutrition if oral intake is insufficient.

For clients receiving radiation therapy, frequent gentle mouth care is important. Clients are at risk for monilial esophagitis, and the nurse is alert to any abrupt worsening of the client's symptoms. (Chapter 27 describes additional nursing interventions for the client undergoing radiation therapy.)

Esophageal Dilation. Esophageal dilation may be performed as necessary throughout the course of the disease to achieve temporary symptomatic relief of dysphagia. The physician uses dilation to reduce the tumor obstruction and to treat the strictures that frequently follow radiation therapy. In the hands of a skilled physician, malignant tumors may be dilated safely. The treatment is repeated as often as needed to preserve the client's ability to swallow (see the earlier text on achalasia).

Prosthesis Insertion. The physician may insert a semirigid prosthesis to bypass disabling dysphagia and to prevent aspiration in clients with advanced disease or with tracheoesophageal (TE) or esophagobronchial (EB) fistulas. Insertion of a prosthesis can maintain an open esophagus and preserve the client's ability to take oral nourishment. The procedure is not without risk: The prosthesis can become dislodged, can migrate, or can perforate the esophagus as tumor bulk increases.

The nurse's primary care emphasis is the prevention of aspiration because the tube interrupts the function of the lower esophageal sphincter (LES) and permits free reflux of gastric contents. The nurse supervises the client closely, offers small oral feedings, and ensures that the client does not lie flat in bed.

Drug Therapy. In recent years, chemotherapy combining several antineoplastic drugs has been used more frequently as part of the primary treatment of esophageal cancer. Chemotherapy appears to be most effective when given in combination with radiation, surgery, or both. Most drug regimens include cisplatin (Platinol). Other drugs include antacids and analgesics to relieve the symptoms of heartburn and odynophagia.

Diet Therapy. Maintaining adequate nutrition is essential for clients with esophageal cancer. Interventions often take different forms as the disease progresses. The nurse collaborates with the dietitian to modify the diet when dysphagia develops. The nurse teaches the client to select soft or semiliquid foods and to enrich these meals with milk powder or commercial protein supplements. Most clients tolerate small, frequent feedings better than large meals. Attempts are made to prepare and serve meals as attractively as possible, and the client's personal likes and dislikes are carefully considered.

Ongoing efforts are made to preserve the client's ability to swallow, but feeding tubes may be needed temporarily when dysphagia is severe. In clients with complete obstruction or life-threatening fistula formation, it may be necessary to create a gastrostomy or jejunostomy. Because these measures radically disrupt normal eating and do not enable clients to swallow even saliva, they are considered to be the least desirable option. When tube feedings are used, blenderized regular foods with liberal additional water are preferable to commercial products because they are less likely to induce diarrhea. Short-term parenteral nutrition is also used to improve a client's nutritional status quickly, particularly before surgery (see Chap. 64). The nurse carefully monitors daily weights, calorie counts, and intake and output to evaluate the client's response to the interventions.

Positioning. Careful positioning is essential for clients who are experiencing frequent regurgitation or who have prosthetic tubes to keep the esophagus patent. The nurse teaches the client to remain upright for several hours after meals and to avoid lying completely flat. The head of the bed is always elevated 30 degrees or more to prevent reflux.

Surgical Management. Radical surgery represents the only definitive treatment for esophageal cancer and is the preferred treatment for otherwise healthy clients. The procedures are extensive, however, and are associated with a high mortality rate, especially for elderly clients with concurrent health problems. Survival rates after surgery remain low.

Preoperative Care. Adequate client preparation for surgery may require anywhere from 5 days to 2–3 weeks of nutritional support. Ideally, this supplementation is given orally; however, most clients usually require tube feeding or parenteral nutrition. The nurse carefully monitors the client's weight, intake and output, and fluid and electrolyte balance. Meticulous oral care is performed four times daily to decrease the risk of postoperative infection. Some clients may also receive radiation therapy before surgery.

The remainder of preoperative nursing care focuses on teaching and psychologic support. The client may feel ambivalent about signing permission for this radical surgery. The nurse ensures that the client is knowledgeable about the surgery and its outcomes. The physician's instructions are clarified and reinforced as needed. The nurse explains the following:

■ The number and sites of all incisions
■ Wound drainage tubes
■ Chest tubes
■ The nasogastric tube
■ Intravenous lines

The client visits the critical care unit, if possible, and initiates contacts with unit staff.

The nurse instructs the client about routines for turning, coughing, deep breathing, and chest physiotherapy. The crucial nature of postoperative respiratory care is emphasized. The nurse addresses the probable need for ventilator support because respiratory management is a major focus of postoperative care. If colon interposition is planned, the client also undergoes a complete bowel preparation with laxatives and enemas before surgery.

The client faces extensive surgery with a high surgical mortality rate. It is natural for the client to be extremely anxious and ambivalent. The nurse encourages the client to talk about personal feelings and fears and involves the family or significant others in all preoperative teaching and discussions. A primary nurse or case manager can be extremely helpful in providing continuity of care and support to the entire family.

Operative Procedures. Subtotal or total *esophagectomy* is usually required because tumors are frequently quite large and involve distant lymph nodes. Several procedures have been used, but the preferred surgical procedure is an *esophagogastrostomy.* The diseased portion of the esophagus is removed, and the cervical portion is anastomosed (connected) to the stomach. The cervical portion of the stomach is then brought up into the thorax through the esophageal hiatus (Fig. 57–5). This procedure is the simplest, yet it involves both laparotomy and thoracotomy incisions.

For a client with tumors in the upper esophagus, radical neck dissection and laryngectomy may also be required because of spread of the disease to the larynx. When the tumor involves the stomach or the stomach is otherwise unsuitable for anastomosis, the surgeon may instead perform a colon interposition. A section of right or left colon is removed and brought up into the thorax to substitute for the esophagus (see Fig. 57–5).

In addition to the usual surgical risks of hemorrhage, shock, and infection, these radical operations create a serious risk of leakage at the anastomosis site. This situation is especially true with colon interpositions because several anastomosis sites are vulnerable to the effects of tension, poor blood supply, and delayed healing. If the client successfully recovers from surgery, he or she is still at risk for aspiration from regurgitation because the

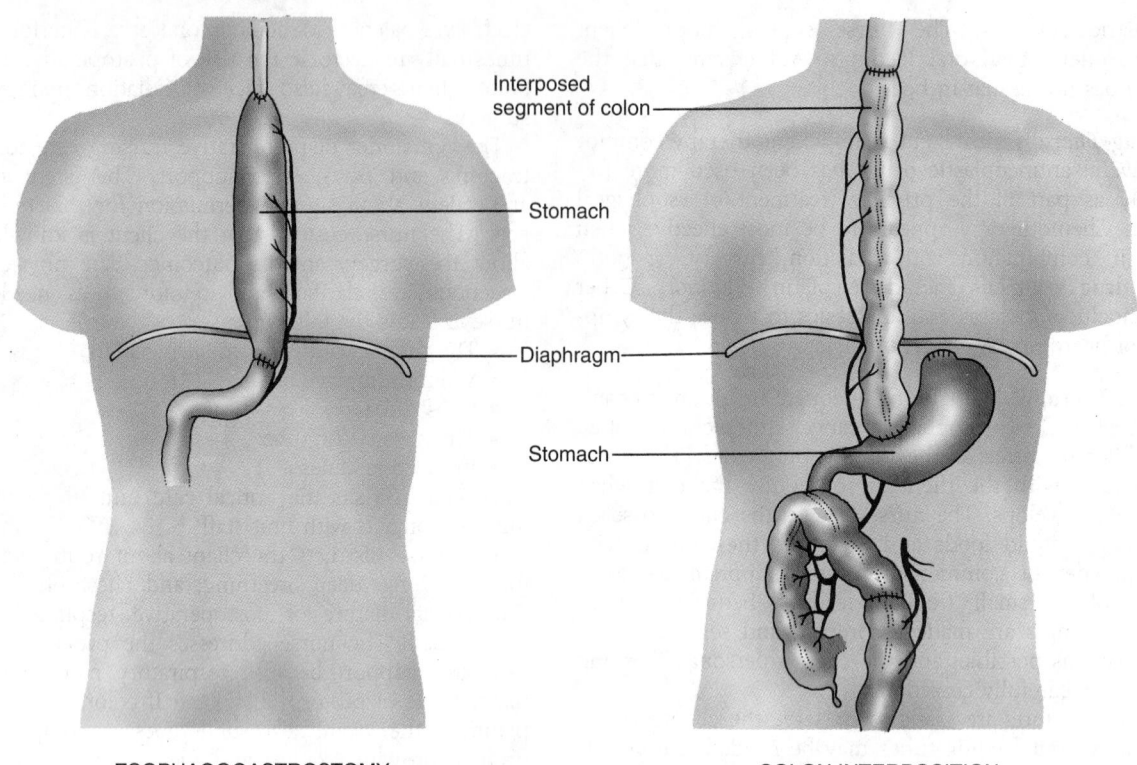

ESOPHAGOGASTROSTOMY   COLON INTERPOSITION

Figure 57–5. Surgical approaches to the treatment of esophageal cancer.

sphincter effect of the lower esophagus has been eliminated.

Postoperative Care. The client requires meticulous postoperative care and is at risk for multiple serious complications. The Client Care Plan outlines client interventions for esophageal surgery.

Respiratory Care. Respiratory care is the *highest* postoperative priority, and the client is usually intubated for at least the first 24 hours. The nurse assesses the client's respiratory status every 1–2 hours and begins turning and coughing routines. Chest physiotherapy is initiated as ordered, usually every 2–4 hours. Incisional support and adequate analgesia are essential for effective coughing and should be administered regularly if the client's vital signs remain stable. The nurse keeps the client in a semi-Fowler's or high Fowler's position to support ventilation and to prevent reflux. The physician prescribes prophylactic antibiotics and supplemental oxygen; blood gases are ordered regularly. The nurse ensures the patency of the water seal drainage system for chest tubes.

Wound Management. Wound management is another significant postoperative concern because the client has multiple incisions and drains. The nurse provides incisional support during turning and coughing to prevent dehiscence. Anastomosis leakage is a dreaded complication, which may appear about 5–7 days after surgery.

The nurse carefully assesses for fever, fluid accumulation, general signs of inflammation, and symptoms of early shock, such as tachycardia and tachypnea.

The nurse reports any findings to the physician immediately.

Nasogastric Tube Management. The nurse monitors the nasogastric (NG) tube for patency and carefully secures the tube to prevent dislodgment, which can disrupt the sutures at the anastomosis. The nurse *does not* independently irrigate or reposition the NG tube in clients who have had esophageal surgery. The initial NG drainage is bloody but should change to a greenish-yellow color by the end of the first postoperative day. The continued presence of blood may indicate bleeding at the suture line. The nurse provides oral hygiene every 2–4 hours while the tube is in place. After initial stabilization, the client is given 3–5 mL of water every 15–30 minutes. If this fluid is satisfactorily tolerated, the quantity is increased to an ounce (30 mL) at a time. The nurse supervises the client during all initial swallowing efforts and ensures that the client is in an upright position. To keep the gastrointestinal tract decompressed, the nurse leaves the NG tube in place while feedings are initiated. The nurse continues to assess for signs of leakage (Chart 57–7).

Unless another time interval is specified, the client is allowed nothing by mouth (NPO) for 4–5 days until intestinal motility is well established. The client receives intravenous fluids or parenteral nutrition but is kept slightly dehydrated to avoid circulatory overload.

If leaks do not appear, the client slowly adds blenderized and semisolid foods. The nurse helps the client establish the quantity of food that can be swallowed safely

Chart 57-7

Nursing Care Highlight: The Client with a Nasogastric Tube in Place After Esophageal Surgery

- Check for tube placement every 4 to 8 hours.
- Ensure that the tube is patent (open) and draining; drainage should turn from bloody to yellowish-green by the end of the first postoperative day.
- Secure the tube well to prevent dislodgment.
- Do not irrigate or reposition the tube without a physician's order.
- Provide meticulous oral and nasal hygiene every 2 to 4 hours.
- Keep the head of the bed elevated to at least 30 degrees.
- When the client is permitted to have a small amount of water, place the client in an upright position and observe for dysphagia (difficulty swallowing).
- Observe for leakage from anastomosis site, as indicated by fever, fluid accumulation, and manifestations of early shock (tachycardia, tachypnea, altered mental status).

and comfortably and reviews the importance of eating small meals and maintaining an upright position. The food storage area of the stomach has been radically decreased, and gravity is the client's only real defense against reflux.

 Continuing Care

Most clients require a lot of assistance at home after discharge, particularly if they live alone or with an elderly spouse. Treatment of esophageal cancer is radical. Even if major postoperative complications do not occur, the client is likely to have ongoing concerns about respiratory care, incisional healing, and nutritional support. The nurse gathers accurate and detailed data about the client's social situation and assists the physician in making decisions about home care needs.

➤ *Health Teaching*

Wound healing is also an ongoing concern. The nurse teaches the client and family to inspect the incisions daily for redness, tenderness, swelling, and discharge.

The nurse prepares written instructions about the signs of anastomosis leakage and the importance of reporting them to the physician or other health care provider immediately.

Nutritional support remains a concern. The nurse encourages the client to continue increasing oral feedings as tolerated. The client is reminded to eat a high-calorie, high-protein diet that contains soft and easily swallowed foods. Meals should be small and frequent, and nutritionally empty foods are avoided. Eggnogs and milk shakes

may be easily prepared and enriched to supplement meals. If sufficient oral intake is not possible, the family may need instruction about tube feedings or parenteral nutrition at home.

The nurse emphasizes the importance of keeping the client upright after meals and elevating the head of the bed on blocks. Families are counseled that dysphagia or odynophagia may recur because of stricture or tumor regrowth. These symptoms should be promptly reported to the health care provider.

Despite radical surgery, the client with cancer of the esophagus still has a terminal illness and a relatively short life expectancy. Emphasis is placed on the improved quality of life that surgery provides. As the client's condition eventually worsens, realistic planning is important, and the client and family are assisted to plan together for the future. The nurse assists family members in exploring and accepting formal and informal sources of support. The nurse helps the family or significant others arrange for hospice care.

➤ *Home Care Management*

The care given in the hospital is continued to some degree after discharge. Both the client and family or significant others must be well informed about the care needed. Ongoing respiratory care is a priority, and family members are instructed to assist with ambulation, splinting incisions, and chest physiotherapy. The nurse teaches the family to protect the client from infection and to contact the physician immediately if signs of respiratory infection develop. The client is encouraged to be as active as possible and to avoid excessive bed rest and its complications at all costs.

➤ *Health Care Resources*

The nurse initiates referrals to community or home care organizations to assist the family in providing the needed home care. In addition, the nurse informs the family about the services available through the American Cancer Society. The nurse may also acquaint the family with area hospice services for future planning.

 Evaluation

Evaluation is based on each client's specific nursing diagnoses and stated outcomes. It also reflects the understanding that the client's disease is ultimately fatal. Desired outcomes may include that the client will

- Take in sufficient balanced nutrients to meet the body's needs
- Maintain a stable weight
- Swallow without discomfort
- Maintain a patent airway and be free from respiratory infection
- Adapt to the stresses of the diagnosis and receive meaningful support from family or significant others
- Discuss the prognosis and make realistic plans for the future with the family and significant others

Diverticula

Overview

Diverticula in the esophagus are outpouchings that result in a blind pouch in which ingested foods and liquids are trapped, often to be regurgitated later. Clients complain of symptoms similar to those of achalasia (discussed earlier), such as regurgitation, nocturnal cough, halitosis, sour taste in the mouth, dysphagia, and feelings of pressure or fullness.

Diverticula may develop anywhere along the length of the esophagus. The most common form is *Zenker's diverticulum,* commonly located near the hypopharynx. It occurs most often in older adults. Clients with esophageal diverticula can be at risk for esophageal perforation because the mucosa is without the protection of the normal esophageal muscle layer. Diverticula may result from congenital weakness of the esophageal wall, esophageal trauma, or development of fibrotic scar tissue in response to chronic inflammation or erosion. The incidence of all forms is rare.

Collaborative Management

 Assessment

Typical symptoms of diverticula include dysphagia, regurgitation, halitosis (bad breath), and feelings of fullness or pressure.

Variations occur as a result of food choices, mealtimes, activity, and positioning. The presence of respiratory symptoms indicates the possibility of regurgitation and aspiration. The barium swallow study is indicated to observe for filling of the diverticula. Endoscopy is rarely performed because of the risk of accidental perforation.

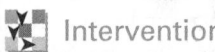 Interventions

Diet therapy and positioning are the major interventions for controlling symptoms related to diverticula. In collaboration with the dietitian, the nurse assists the client in exploring variations in the size and frequency of meals and in food texture and consistency. Semisoft foods and smaller meals are often best tolerated and may reduce or relieve the symptoms of pressure and reflux. The nurse explores individual food tolerances and intolerances with the client.

As with other forms of reflux, nocturnal problems associated with diverticula are best managed by sleeping with the head of the bed elevated and avoiding the recumbent position for at least 2 hours after eating. The client is also counseled to avoid vigorous exercise after meals. The nurse advises the client to avoid restrictive clothing and frequent stooping or bending.

Surgical management is aimed at excision of the diverticula and reapproximating the mucosa. Most physicians use the cervical surgical approach, above the clavicle. The client takes nothing by mouth for several days to promote healing and receives intravenous fluids for hydration, tube feedings, and then oral fluid and food. The nurse assists in pain relief and monitors for complications such as bleeding or perforation. A nasogastric (NG) tube is placed during surgery for decompression and is *not* irrigated or repositioned unless specifically ordered by the surgeon. Later this tube may be used for feeding.

Continuing care includes teaching the client and family about

- Tube feeding and resuming an oral diet
- Positioning guidelines to prevent reflux
- Warning signs of complications

Community resources are usually not needed for uncomplicated cases.

Trauma

Overview

Trauma to the esophagus (Table 57–2) can result from blunt injuries, chemical burns, surgery or endoscopy, or the stress of protracted severe vomiting.

Trauma may affect the esophagus directly, impairing swallowing and nutrition, or it may create problems and complications in related structures, such as the lungs or mediastinum. The incidence of most forms of esophageal trauma is low in adults.

When excessive force is exerted on the esophageal mucosa, it may perforate or rupture, allowing the caustic acid secretions to enter the mediastinal cavity. These tears are associated with a high mortality rate related to shock, respiratory impairment, or sepsis.

Chemical injury is usually a result of accidental or intentional ingestion of caustic substances. The oral cavity is also usually damaged. The damage is rapid and severe. Acid burns tend to affect the superficial layers of the esophagus; alkaline substances cause deeper penetrating injuries. Strong alkalis can cause full perforation of the esophagus within a minute. Additional problems may include aspiration pneumonia and hemorrhage. Strictures may develop as scar tissue forms. Table 57–3 lists caustic substances frequently found in the home.

Collaborative Management

 Assessment

Most clients with esophageal trauma are initially evaluated and treated in the emergency room. Assessment focuses

TABLE 57–2

Causes of Esophageal Perforation
• Straining
• Seizures
• Trauma
• Foreign objects
• Instruments or tubes
• Chemical injury
• Complications of esophageal surgery
• Ulcers

TABLE 57–3

Active Ingredients of Common Household Corrosives

Type	Corrosive	Active Ingredient
Acids	• Mister Plumber	• Sulfuric acid 8.5%
Liquid	• Lysol Toilet Bowl Cleaner	• Hydrochloric acid
	• Sno-Bol Toilet Bowl Cleaner	• Hydrochloric acid 15%
Granular	• ZUD Rust and Stain Remover	• Oxalic acid
	• Sani-Flush Toilet Bowl Cleaner	• Sodium bisulfite 75%
	• Vanish Toilet Bowl Cleaner	• Sodium acid sulfate 62%
Alkalis	• Liquid Drāno	• Sodium hydroxide 9.5%
	• Crystal Drāno	• Sodium hydroxide 80%
	• Liquid Plumr	• Sodium hypochlorite and hydroxide 8%
	• Easy-Off Liquid Oven Cleaner	• Sodium hydroxide
	• Mr. Muscle Oven Cleaner	• Sodium hydroxide
	• Industrial/Professional Drano	• Sodium hydroxide 32%
	• Ammonia	• Ammonium hydroxide
Bleaches	• Clorox	
	• Peroxide	
Thermal agents	• Dry ice	
	• Hot water	
	• Clinitest tablets	
Detergents	• Cascade (dish)	• Sodium tripolyphosphate
	• Amway (dish)	• Sodium tripolyphosphate

on the nature of the injury and the circumstances surrounding it. The nurse assesses for the presence of pain, dysphagia, vomiting, and bleeding.

If the risk of extending the damage is not excessive, the physician may order an x-ray or endoscopic study to evaluate tears or perforation.

 Interventions

After the injury, the client is allowed nothing by mouth to prevent further leakage of esophageal secretions. A nasogastric or gastrostomy tube is used for drainage and to rest the esophagus. Esophageal rest is maintained for at least 10 days after injury to allow for initial healing of the mucosa. The physician orders total parenteral nutrition (TPN) to provide calories and protein for wound healing while the client is not eating.

To prevent sepsis, the physician prescribes broad-spectrum antibiotics. High-dose corticosteroids may be administered to suppress inflammation and prevent strictures. The physician may prescribe opioid and nonopioid analgesics for pain management. When caustic burns involve the oral cavity, topical agents, such as 50/50 diphenhydramine hydrochloride (Benadryl) and kaolin with pectin (Kaopectate) or topical lidocaine (Xylocaine Viscous), may be used for topical analgesia and local anti-inflammatory action.

If nonsurgical management is not effective in healing traumatized esophageal tissue, the client may need surgery to remove the damaged tissue. The client with severe injuries may require resection of part of the esophagus with a gastric pull-through and repositioning or replacement by a bowel segment. (See Surgical Management in the discussion of esophageal tumors.)

 CASE STUDY for the Client with Gastroesophageal Reflux Disease

■ A 59-year-old woman presents in the physician's office with a diagnosis of possible gastroesophageal reflux disease (GERD). She has a history of arthritis, for which she takes Motrin 200 mg qid.

Q U E S T I O N S :

1. What questions should you ask when taking a history from this woman?
2. What information should you include when doing a teaching plan for this client?

SELECTED BIBLIOGRAPHY

Benini, L., Sembenini, C., Castellani, G., Bardelli, E., Brentegani, M., Giorgetti, P., & Vantini, I. (1996). Pathological esophageal acidification and pneumatic dilatation in achalasia patients. *Digestive Diseases and Sciences, 41*(2), 365–371.

Devault, K., & Castell, D. (1995). Guidelines for the diagnosis and treatment of gastroesophageal reflux disease. *Archives of Internal Medicine, 155*, 2165–2173.

Galmiche, J., & Janssens, J. (1995). The pathophysiology of gastro-oesophageal reflux disease: An overview. *Scandinavian Journal of Gastroenterology, Suppl 211*, 7–18.

Giger, J. N., Davidhizar, R. E. (1995). *Transcultural nursing: Assessment and intervention* (2nd ed.) St. Louis: Mosby.

Killen, J. (1996). Understanding dysphagia: Interventions for care. *MEDSURG Nursing, 5*(2), 99–105.

Meshkinpour, H., Haghighat, P., & Meshkinpour, A. (1996). Quality of life among patients treated for achalasia. *Digestive Diseases and Sciences, 41*(2), 352–356.

Miller, C. (1994). Alleviating the discomfort of gastroesophageal reflux disease. *Geriatric Nursing, 15*(3), 171–172.

Molina, E., Stollman, N., Grauer, L., Reiner, D., & Barkin, J. (1995). Conservative management of esophageal nontransmural tears after pneumatic dilation for achalasia. *American Journal of Gastroenterology, 91*(1), 15–18.

Patti, M., Goldberg, H., Arcerito, M., Bortolasi, L., Tong, J., & Way, L. (1996). Hiatal hernia size affects lower esophageal sphincter function, esophageal acid exposure, and the degree of mucosal injury. *American Journal of Surgery, 171,* 182–186.

Robinson, M. (1994). Gastroesophageal reflux disease: Selecting optimal therapy. *Postgraduate Medicine, 95*(2), 88–102.

Sackier, J. (1996). New applications of laparoscopy in gastrointestinal surgery. *American Family Physician, 53*(1), 237–242.

Shoenut, P., Yamashiro, Y., Orr, W., Kerr, P., Micflikier, A., & Kryger, M. (1996). Effect of severe gastroesophageal reflux on sleep stage in patients with aperistaltic esophagus. *Digestive Diseases and Sciences, 41*(2), 372–376.

Soper, J., & Jones, D. (1994). Laparoscopic Nissen fundoplication. *Surgical Rounds, 10,* 573–581.

Triadafilopoulos, G., Kaczynska, M., & Iwane, M. (1996). Esophageal mucosal eicosanoids in gastroesophageal reflux disease and Barrett's esophagus. *American Journal of Gastroenterology, 91*(1), 65–74.

Tucker, J., Ramshaw, B., Newman, C., Sims, M., Mason, E., Duncan, T., & Lucas, G. (1996). Laparoscopic fundoplication in the treatment of severe gastroesophageal reflux disease: Preliminary results of a prospective trial. *Southern Medical Journal, 89*(1), 60–64.

SUGGESTED READINGS

DeVault, K., & Castell, D. (1995). Guidelines for the diagnosis and treatment of gastroesophageal reflux disease. *Archives of Internal Medicine, 155,* 2165–2173.

These guidelines were prepared for the Practice Parameters Committee of the American College of Gastroenterology as the preferable approach to gastroesophageal reflux disease (GERD). The guidelines were developed by reviewing the world literature including all the current research published on GERD. General concepts in diagnosis and treatment of reflux are discussed.

Killen, J. (1996). Understanding dysphagia: Interventions for care. *MED-SURG Nursing, 5*(2), 99–105.

This article provides an excellent overview of the mechanics of swallowing and assessment and evaluation of dysphagia. Specific nursing interventions, as well as the physiology and rationale for each intervention, are delineated.

Chapter 58

INTERVENTIONS FOR CLIENTS WITH STOMACH DISORDERS

Gastritis and peptic ulcer disease are the two most common stomach disorders. Gastric cancer is less frequently seen but is a serious health problem with an often poor prognosis.

GASTRITIS

Overview

The term gastritis implies inflammation of the gastric mucosa. It refers to any diffuse lesion in the gastric mucosa that is histologically identified as inflammation. Gastritis may be classified as acute or chronic. The categories refer to the pattern of inflammation rather than to a specific time course.

Exact incidence figures for gastritis have not been reported. Acute gastritis is frequently associated with upper gastrointestinal (GI) bleeding. The incidence of gastritis is higher in men than in women, is highest in people in their 40s and 50s, and is greater in heavy smokers and in alcoholics.

Pathophysiology

The mucosal barrier normally protects the stomach from digesting itself by a process called acid autodigestion. Prostaglandins provide this protection.

When the mucosal barrier fails, gastritis results. After the barrier is broken, mucosal injury occurs and is worsened by histamine release and cholinergic nerve stimulation. Hydrochloric acid can then diffuse back into the mucosa and injure small vessels. This back-diffusion results in edema, hemorrhage, and erosion of the stomach's lining. Alcohol, aspirin, and reflux of duodenal contents can also alter the diffusion barrier.

The pathologic changes of gastritis include vascular congestion, edema, acute inflammatory cell infiltration, and degenerative changes in the superficial epithelium.

The early pathologic manifestation of gastritis is a thickened, reddened mucous membrane with prominent rugae, or folds. As the disease progresses, the walls and lining of the stomach thin and atrophy. With progressive gastric atrophy from chronic mucosal injury, the function of the chief and parietal cells deteriorates. When the function of the acid-secreting cells deteriorates, the source of intrinsic factor is lost.

The intrinsic factor is critical for absorption of vitamin B_{12}. When body stores of vitamin B_{12} are eventually depleted, pernicious anemia results. Degeneration may be observed in the chief and parietal cells. Stomach secretions gradually decrease in amount and concentration of acid until they consist of only mucus and water.

Chronic gastritis is associated with an increased risk of gastric cancer. Hemorrhage may occur after an episode of acute gastritis or with ulceration caused by chronic gastritis.

Acute Gastritis

Inflammation of the gastric mucosa or submucosa after exposure to local irritants is called acute gastritis. Various degrees of mucosal necrosis and inflammatory reaction occur in acute disease. The diagnosis cannot be based solely on clinical symptoms without histologic confirmation. Complete regeneration and healing usually occur within a few days. If the muscularis is not involved, complete recovery usually ensues with no residual evidence of gastric inflammatory reaction.

Chronic Gastritis

Diffuse inflammation of the mucosal lining of the stomach is defined as chronic gastritis. Chronic gastritis usually heals without scarring, but it can progress to hemorrhage and the formation of an ulcer.

Chronic gastritis may be divided into three categories: type A, type B, and atrophic. Type A chronic gastritis involves the body and fundus of the stomach, is autoimmune in cause, and accompanies pernicious anemia. Type B chronic gastritis usually affects the antrum but may involve the entire stomach. *Helicobacter pylori,* a gram-negative organism, has been associated with this condition.

Chronic atrophic gastritis affects all layers of the stomach; the number of fundal, parietal, and chief cells is decreased. It is associated with both gastric ulcer and gastric cancer. The muscularis is thickened, and inflammation is present. Visceral afferent nerve stimulation causes the symptoms, which are not related to the actual extent of the inflammation. Chronic atrophic gastritis is characterized by total loss of fundal glands, minimal inflammation, thinning of the gastric mucosa, and intestinal metaplasia (abnormal tissue development).

Etiology

Acute Gastritis

Acute gastritis is caused by local irritation from

- Radiation
- Drugs, including alcohol, analgesics (especially anti-inflammatory agents) in large doses, cytotoxic agents, caffeine, corticosteroids, antimetabolites, and indomethacin (Indocin, Novomethacin✦)
- Bacterial endotoxins from staphylococci, *Escherichia coli,* or salmonella
- Accidental or intentional ingestion of corrosive substances, including acids or alkalis (such as lye, Mister Plumber, or Drano)

In the client with burns or trauma, or the postoperative client who is allowed nothing by mouth (NPO), gastritis may result from lack of stimulation of normal secretions. The temperature of foods and the use of spices have *not* been documented as a cause of acute gastritis.

Chronic Gastritis

Chronic gastritis is associated with atrophy of the gastric glands and may be caused by any condition that allows reflux of bile and bile acids into the stomach. Fifty per-

cent of clients who have gastric ulcers have associated chronic gastritis. Gastrojejunostomy may also result in chronic gastritis.

Chronic local irritation by alcohol, drugs, smoking, radiation, infectious agents (e.g., *H. pylori*), and environmental agents may cause the disorder. Advanced age, genetic factors (e.g., pernicious anemia), illness (e.g., diabetes or renal disease), and autoimmune disorders are endogenous factors associated with chronic gastritis.

Drugs contributing to chronic gastritis include nonsteroidal anti-inflammatory drugs (NSAIDs), aspirin, and steroids. Cigarette smokers may be vulnerable because of the reduced bicarbonate content of pancreatic secretions, and a decreased pyloric sphincter pressure allows reflux from the duodenum into the stomach.

Chronic Atrophic Gastritis

Atrophic gastritis is a type of chronic gastritis. It is seen most frequently in the elderly. It occurs after exposure to toxic substances in the workplace (e.g., benzene, lead, and nickel) and is associated with infection, sepsis, brain lesions, and renal failure.

Although atrophic gastritis is often present in people with gastric cancer, it is not always considered a precancerous lesion. Gastric carcinoma develops in fewer than 10% of clients who have atrophic gastritis.

Chart 58–1 lists guidelines for preventing gastritis.

Collaborative Management

 Assessment

▶ *Physical Assessment/Clinical Manifestations*

The physical assessment does not yield significant findings in uncomplicated gastritis but does in acute and chronic gastritis.

Acute Gastritis. In clients with acute gastritis or after exposure to an etiologic agent, there is a rapid onset of epigastric discomfort, anorexia, cramping, nausea, vomiting, and gastric hemorrhage (Chart 58–2). The sympto-

---

Chart 58–1

Health Promotion Guide: Gastritis Prevention

- Avoid drinking excessive amounts of alcoholic beverages.
- Use caution in taking large doses of aspirin, nonsteroidal anti-inflammatory drugs (such as ibuprofen and indomethacin), and corticosteroids. Prolonged use of small doses of corticosteroids may cause gastritis.
- Avoid excessive intake of caffeine-containing beverages.
- Avoid eating contaminated foods or drinking contaminated water.
- Stop smoking
- Protect yourself against exposure to toxic substances in the workplace, such as lead and nickel.

Chart 58-2

Key Features of Gastritis

Acute Gastritis

- Rapid onset of epigastric pain
- Anorexia
- Abdominal cramping
- Gastric hemorrhage
- Dyspepsia (heartburn)

Chronic Gastritis

- Vague complaint of epigastric pain that is relieved or worsened by food
- Anorexia
- Vomiting
- Intolerance of fatty and spicy foods
- Weight loss
- Pernicious anemia

matic state is limited to a few hours or days and varies with the cause. Aspirin-related gastritis may result in dyspepsia (heartburn). Gastritis from alcohol abuse may cause vomiting and hematemesis. Gastritis or food poisoning caused by endotoxins, such as staphylococcal endotoxin, is abrupt in onset; severe nausea and vomiting often occur within 5 hours of ingestion of the contaminated food.

Chronic Gastritis. Chronic gastritis often produces vague complaints. Periodic epigastric pain may simulate ulcer-like distress, which is relieved on ingestion of food. The pain, however, is most often less radiating (see Chart 58-2). Some clients have anorexia and pain exacerbated by eating and vomiting. Spicy or fatty foods may not be tolerated.

The discomfort from *atrophic* gastritis is not relieved by antacid therapy, nor do clients experience pain at night. Weight loss may mimic that in gastric cancer, but bleeding is uncommon. Pernicious anemia may result from depletion of intrinsic factor, which is required for the absorption of vitamin B_{12} and is normally secreted from the gastric mucosa.

➤ Diagnostic Assessment

The health care provider may order a barium swallow examination to rule out other gastric diseases. Esophago-gastroduodenoscopy (EGD) via an endoscope with biopsy is the most effective tool for diagnosing gastritis. The superficial mucosal changes of gastritis may not be seen. The health care provider uses biopsy to establish a definitive diagnosis of the type of gastritis or the presence of gastric cancer. A cytologic examination of the biopsy specimen rules out gastric cancer.

Interventions

Clients with gastritis are not often seen in the acute care setting unless they have an exacerbation of acute or chronic gastritis resulting in fluid and electrolyte imbalance or bleeding. Management is directed toward supportive care for relieving the symptoms and removing the cause of discomfort.

Acute gastritis is treated symptomatically and supportively because the healing process is spontaneous, usually occurring within a few days. If the cause is removed, pain and discomfort usually subside. If hemorrhage is severe, a blood transfusion may be necessary; fluid replacement is indicated in clients with severe fluid loss. Surgery, such as partial gastrectomy, pyloroplasty, and/or vagotomy, may be indicated for clients with major bleeding or ulceration.

Nonsurgical Management. The client frequently experiences gastritis from noxious agents. Identification and elimination of the causative factors can often relieve the pain. Drugs and diet therapy are used for clients with gastritis. In the acute phase, when discomfort is present, physical rest is recommended.

Drug Therapy. In the acute phase, the nurse directs actions toward relief of pain and discomfort. The health care provider may order medications that block and buffer gastric acid secretions to relieve pain.

H_2-receptor antagonists are commonly used to block gastric secretions. These agents include ranitidine (Zantac), cimetidine (Tagamet, Apo-Cimetidine✶, Novo-cimetidine✶), famotidine (Pepcid), and nizatidine (Axid). Sucralfate (Carafate, Sulcrate✶), a mucosal barrier fortifier, may also be prescribed. Antacids used as buffering agents include aluminum hydroxide with magnesium hydroxide (Maalox) and aluminum hydroxide with simethicone and magnesium hydroxide (Mylanta) (Chart 58-3). The nurse monitors for symptom relief and side effects of these medications and notifies the health care provider of any untoward effects or worsening of gastric distress.

Clients with chronic gastritis may require vitamin B_{12} for prevention or treatment of pernicious anemia. If *H. pylori* is found in biopsy specimens, the health care provider may initiate treatment to eradicate the infection and reverse or prevent impairment of mucosal defenses. A common drug regimen for *H. pylori* infection is bismuth subsalicylates (e.g., Pepto-Bismol), metronidazole (Flagyl, Novonidazol✶), and tetracycline or ampicillin (Amcill, Ampicin✶).

In collaboration, the nurse, health care provider, and pharmacist instruct clients about the medications associated with gastric irritation. These medications include chemotherapeutic agents, aspirin, corticosteroids, erythromycin (E-Mycin, Erythromid✶), and nonsteroidal anti-inflammatory agents, such as indomethacin (Indocin, Novemethacin✶) and ibuprofen (Motrin, Advil, Amersol✶, Novoprofen✶).

The health care provider may change the dose, frequency, or type of medication if symptoms of gastric irritation appear or persist. The nurse instructs clients to avoid stomach-irritating over-the-counter (OTC) medications, such as aspirin and ibuprofen.

Diet Therapy. The nurse and dietitian instruct the client with gastric disease to limit intake of any foods and spices that cause distress. Tea, coffee, cola, chocolate,

Chart 58-3

Drug Therapy for Peptic Ulcer Disease

Drug	Usual Dosage	Nursing Interventions	Rationale
Antacids			
Magnesium hydroxide with aluminum hydroxide (Maalox, Mylanta)	• 50–80 mEq 1 hr + 3 hr pc (after meals) + hs (at bedtime	• Give 1 hr and 3 hr after meals and at bedtime • Use liquid rather than tablets • Do not give other drugs within 1–2 hr of antacids. • Assess the client for a history of renal disease. • Assess the client for a history of congestive heart failure. • Observe the client for the side effect of diarrhea.	• Hydrogen ion load is high after ingestion of foods. • Suspensions are more effective than chewable tablets. • Antacids interfere with absorption of other drugs. • Hypermagnesemia may result. • These antacids have a high sodium content. • Magnesium often causes diarrhea.
Aluminum hydroxide (Amphojel)	• 50–80 mEq 1 hr + 3 hr pc + hs	• Give 1 hr after meals and at bedtime • Use liquid rather than tablets if palatable. • Do not give other drugs within 1–2 hr of antacids. • Observe the client for the side effect of constipation. If constipation occurs, consider alternating with magnesium antacid. • Use for clients with renal failure	• Hydrogen ion load is high after ingestion of food. • Suspensions are more effective than chewable tablets. • Antacids interfere with absorption of other drugs. • Aluminum causes constipation, and magnesium has a laxative effect. • Aluminum binds with phosphates in the GI tract.
H₂ Antagonists			
Ranitidine (Zantac)	• 150 mg (2/d) bid PO or 300 mg hs; 50 mg q/6h IV or 8 mg/hr IV (continuous)	• Give single dose at bedtime.	• Bedtime administration suppresses nocturnal acid production.
Famotidine (Pepcid)	• 40 mg once a day or in two divided doses; 20 mg IV q12h	• Give single dose at bedtime.	• Bedtime administration suppresses nocturnal acid production. Compliance may improve with less frequent administration.
Nizatidine (Axid)	• 150 mg bid or 300 mg hs	• Give single dose at bedtime.	• Bedtime administration suppresses nocturnal acid production. Compliance may improve with less frequent administration.
Cimetidine (Tagamet, Apo-Cimetidine✴, Novocimetidine✴)	• 400 mg bid or 800 mg PO at bedtime; 50 mg/hr IV (continuous) or 300 mg IV q6h	• Give clients 60 yr and older reduced dose. • Give single dose at bedtime. • IV administration requires slow infusion. • Give 1 hr before or after antacids. • Closely watch clients with impaired renal or hepatic function for side effects.	• Side effect of confusion occurs most often in elderly clients. • Bedtime administration suppresses nocturnal acid production. • Bradycardia or cardiac arrest may occur with rapid administration. • Antacids interfere with absorption. • Metabolism by the liver and elimination by the kidneys will increase drug level.

Continued

Chart 58-3. Drug Therapy for Peptic Ulcer Disease Continued

Drug	Usual Dosage	Nursing Interventions	Rationale
Mucosal Barrier Fortifiers			
Sucralfate (Carafate, Sulcrate✦)	• 1 g qid (4/d) or 2 g bid	• Give 1 hr before and 2 hr after meals, and at bedtime. • Do not give within 30 min of giving antacids or other drugs.	• Food may interfere with drug's adherence to mucosa. • Antacids may interfere with effect.
Antisecretory Agents			
Omeprazole (Prilosec, Losec✦)	• 20 mg bid or 40 mg hs	• Have the client take capsule whole • Give single dose at bedtime for ulcer disease.	• Delayed-release capsules allow absorption after granules leave the stomach. • Bedtime administration suppresses nocturnal acid production.
Lansoprazole (Prevacid)	• 15 or 30 mg hs		

mustard, paprika, cloves, pepper, and hot spices may increase the client's discomfort. Alcohol and tobacco should be avoided.

After the client has an acute episode of gastritis, the nurse helps the client to identify foods that aggravate discomfort. New foods should be introduced one at a time. Avoidance of substances that cause symptoms is important. Most clients seem to progress better with a soft, bland diet, and smaller, more frequent meals.

Stress Reduction. The nurse assesses factors that decrease the client's tolerance of pain or discomfort (e.g., lack of knowledge, anxiety, and fatigue), and explains the effects of fatigue and anxiety on discomfort. The nurse may further assist the client with various techniques that reduce stress and discomfort, such as progressive relaxation, cutaneous stimulation, guided imagery, and distraction (see Chap. 4).

Surgical Management. Partial gastrectomy, pyloroplasty, vagotomy, or even total gastrectomy may be indicated for clients who have major bleeding from severe erosive gastritis. Such surgery is necessary only if more conservative measures have not controlled the bleeding. Surgical interventions are discussed later with surgical management of peptic ulcer disease.

Peptic Ulcer Disease

Overview

Peptic ulcers occur in the stomach, proximal duodenum, and, rarely, in the lower esophagus. Approximately 4–8 million people in the United States have symptoms related to active ulcer disease.

Peptic ulcer disease (PUD) is a break in the continuity of the mucosa. PUD may occur in any part of the gastrointestinal (GI) tract that comes in contact with hydrochloric acid and pepsin. Because of anatomic and physiologic differences of the various types, the term *peptic* does not precisely describe these ulcers. In this chapter, PUD, a chronic disorder, refers to gastric and duodenal ulcers (Fig. 58–1).

Pathophysiology

Types of Ulcers

GASTRIC ULCERS. Gastric ulcers are usually found at the junction of the fundus and the pylorus, but smaller ulcers may also occur in the antrum. Most gastric ulcers occur on the lesser curvature of the stomach near the pylorus (Fig. 58–2).

A gastric ulcer is a break in the gastric mucosal barrier that extends into the muscularis mucosae. This barrier overlies the gastric epithelium and differs from the glycoprotein mucus that covers the epithelium. The secretion of mucus and bicarbonate provides a first line of defense in maintaining a near-normal pH on the gastric epithelium and protects the barrier against acid. Gastromucosal prostaglandins increase resistance of the gastric mucosa to ulceration. The integrity of the mucosal barrier is enhanced by the rich blood supply of the mucosa of the stomach and duodenum.

When a mucosal break occurs, hydrochloric acid injures the epithelium. Gastric ulcers may then result from back-diffusion of acid or dysfunction of the pyloric sphincter (see Fig. 58–1). The pyloric sphincter may not function normally or may not respond to secretin and cholecystokinin (hormones that increase the pressure and prevent reflux). Without normal functioning and competence of the pyloric sphincter, bile refluxes into the stomach. This reflux of bile acids may break the integrity of the mucosal barrier and produce hydrogen ion back-diffusion, which leads to mucosal inflammation. Toxic agents and bile then destroy the lipid plasma membrane of the gastric mucosa. Antral motility near the ulcer is often decreased with gastric ulcers. A decreased blood flow to the gastric mucosa may also alter the defense barrier and thereby allow ulceration to occur.

Agents that break the mucosal barrier (such as acetylsalicylic acid [aspirin], alcohol, and nonsteroidal anti-inflammatory drugs [NSAIDs]), disrupt the mucosal protection, and hydrochloric acid flows back into the mucosa. Release of histamine results in greater acid production, vasodilation, and increased capillary permeability.

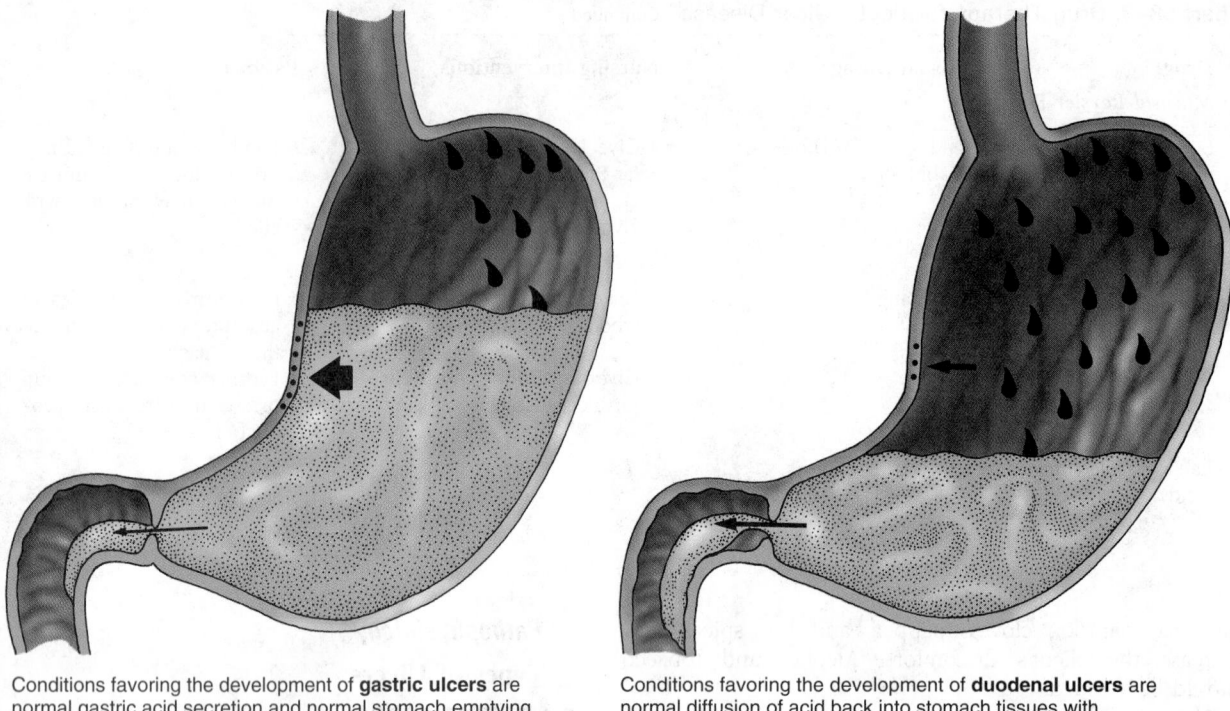

Conditions favoring the development of **gastric ulcers** are normal gastric acid secretion and normal stomach emptying with *increased diffusion of gastric acid back into the stomach tissues.*

Conditions favoring the development of **duodenal ulcers** are normal diffusion of acid back into stomach tissues with *increased secretion of gastric acid* and *increased stomach emptying.*

Figure 58–1. The pathophysiology of peptic ulcer.

When ulceration is rapid, bleeding may occur as vessel walls are eroded. With slower-forming ulcers, the inflammatory and thrombotic processes result in ulcer symptoms, and bleeding is less likely. Ulcers heal slowly because of a poor blood supply to the area. Gastric ulcers tend to heal less quickly than doduodenal ulcers, and more complications tend to occur in the elderly.

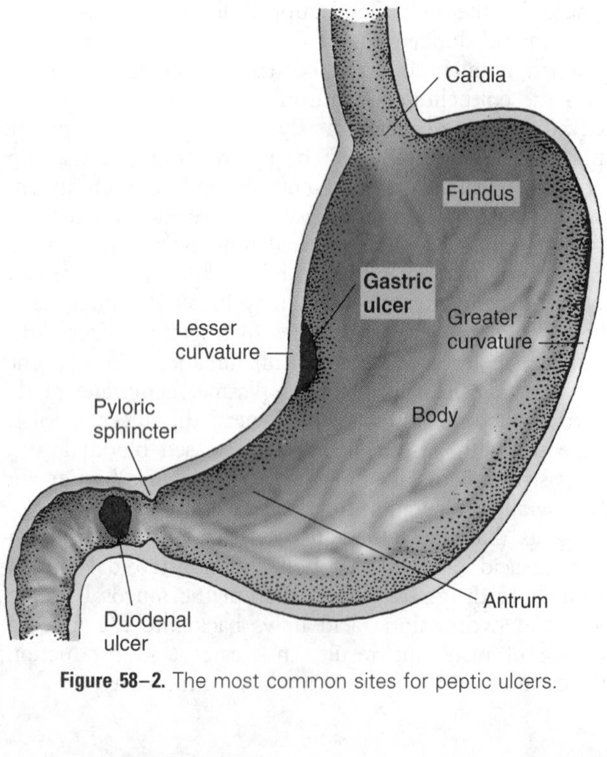

DUODENAL ULCERS. A duodenal ulcer is a chronic break in the duodenal mucosa extending through the muscularis mucosae; it leaves a scar with healing. Duodenal ulcers occur in the duodenum, are the most common type of peptic ulcer, and are almost never malignant. Increased acid secretion due to greater parietal cell mass or vagal activity is associated with duodenal ulcers. With vagal stimulation, the parietal cells and G cells release gastrin; gastrin stimulates the production of pepsin and hydrochloric acid.

Gastric activity affects the regulation of secretions. Gastrin is stimulated by the presence of protein or by distention of the antrum. Sensitivity to gastrin increases secretion of gastric hydrochloric acid in clients with a duodenal ulcer. The client with a duodenal ulcer secretes a larger amount of gastric juices, and normal mechanisms may not control gastrin release. A pH of 2.5–3 inhibits the secretion of gastrin and limits the amount of hydrochloric acid secreted. Acid chyme from the stomach also inhibits gastric secretions. Cholecystokinin, secretin, gastric inhibitory peptides, and fat inhibit the effects of gastrin. Secretin stimulates the pancreas to secrete bicarbonates to neutralize duodenal acid.

The characteristic feature of duodenal ulcer is high gastric acid secretion, although a wide range of secretory levels is found. In clients with duodenal ulcers, pH levels are low in the duodenum for long periods. Acid secretion is stimulated by protein-rich meals, calcium, and vagal

Figure 58–2. The most common sites for peptic ulcers.

excitation. Combined with hypersecretion, a rapid empty-ing of food from the stomach reduces the buffering effect of food and delivers a large acid bolus to the duodenum (see Fig. 58–1). Inhibitory secretory mechanisms and pancreatic secretion may be insufficient to control the acid load.

Up to 90% of clients with duodenal ulcer disease test positive for *H. pylori* infection (Davis, 1996). This infection is most prevalent in developing countries where sanitation and housing are poor. Experts agree that peptic ulcer disease is an infectious illness and treat it as such. If this spiral gram-negative organism is found in gastric mucosal biopsy specimens, treatment with antibiotics and antisecretory medications is indicated.

STRESS ULCERS. A stress ulcer occurs after an acute medical crisis or trauma, such as head injury, burn, respiratory failure, shock, or septic state. Bleeding caused by gastric erosion is the principal manifestation of acute stress ulcers.

Lesions are multiple and occur in the proximal portion of the stomach. They begin as focal areas of ischemia and evolve into erosions and sometimes ulcerations that may progress to massive hemorrhage. Little is known about the cause of stress ulcers, but ischemia is probably a contributing factor. In the presence of elevated hydrochloric acid, ischemia can progress to erosive gastritis and subsequent ulcerations. Increased hydrogen ion back-diffusion and mucosal ischemia may result.

Complications of Ulcers

The most common complications of peptic ulcer disease are hemorrhage, perforation, pyloric obstruction, and intractable disease.

HEMORRHAGE. Minimal bleeding from ulcers is manifested by occult blood in a tarry stool (melena). With massive bleeding, the client vomits bright red or coffee-ground blood (hematemesis) (Fig. 58–3). Bleeding is the most serious complication of peptic ulcer.

Hemorrhage tends to occur more often in clients with gastric ulcers and in the elderly. Hematemesis usually indicates bleeding at or above the duodenojejunal junction (upper GI bleeding). Melena may occur in clients with gastric ulcers but is more common in those with duodenal ulcers. Gastric acid digestion of blood typically results in a granular dark vomitus; the digestion of blood within the duodenum and small intestine may result in a black stool.

PERFORATION. In clients with perforation, the gastroduodenal contents (acid peptic juice, bile, and pancreatic juice) empty through the anterior wall of the stomach or duodenum into the peritoneal cavity. Sudden, sharp pain begins in the mid–epigastric region and spreads over the entire abdomen. The amount of pain depends on the amount and type of GI contents spilled. The characteristic pain causes the client to be apprehensive; the abdomen is tender, rigid, and board-like. The client assumes the knee-chest position in an attempt to decrease the tension on the abdominal muscles.

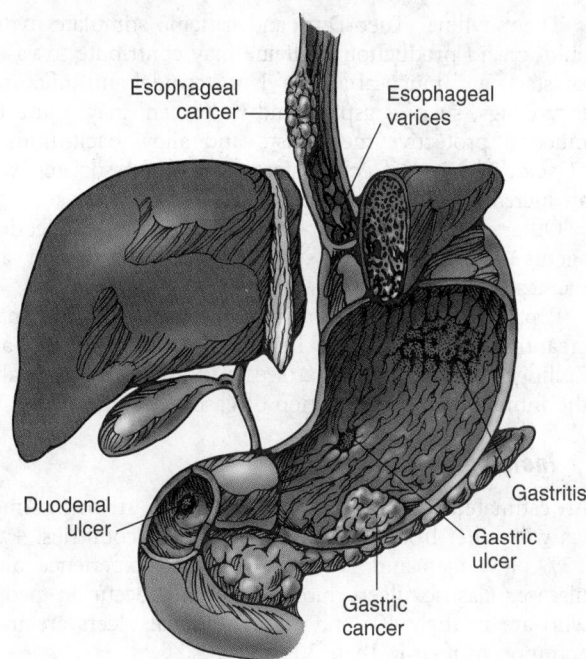

Figure 58–3. Common causes of upper gastrointestinal bleeding.

The client may become desperately ill within hours. Chemical peritonitis soon occurs; bacterial septicemia and hypovolemic shock follow. Peristalsis diminishes, and paralytic ileus develops. Perforation is a surgical emergency.

PYLORIC OBSTRUCTION. Pyloric obstruction is manifested by vomiting caused by stasis and gastric dilation. Obstruction occurs at the pylorus (the gastric outlet) and is caused by scarring, edema, inflammation, or a combination of these factors.

When vomiting persists, the client may experience hypochloremic (metabolic) alkalosis from loss of large quantities of acid gastric juice (hydrogen and chloride ions) in the vomitus. Hypokalemia may also result from the vomiting or metabolic alkalosis. The health care provider typically hospitalizes the client so that the client may receive intravenous (IV) fluid and electrolyte replacement.

INTRACTABLE DISEASE. One third of all clients with ulcers have a single episode with no recurrence. Intractability may develop from other complications of ulcers, excessive stressors in the client's life, and the client's inability to make necessary lifestyle changes. The client no longer responds to conservative management, or recurrences of symptoms interfere with activities of daily living (ADL). In general, the client continues to have recurrent pain and discomfort despite treatment.

Etiology

Certain drugs may contribute to gastroduodenal ulceration by altering gastric secretion, producing localized damage to mucosa, and interfering with the healing process.

Theophylline (Theo-Dur) and caffeine stimulate hydrochloric acid production. Caffeine may contribute to vascular stasis and mucosal anoxia. Nonsteroidal anti-inflammatory drugs, such as aspirin and ibuprofen, may injure the mucosal protective mechanism and allow back-diffusion of acid. The use of corticosteroids is also associated with an increased incidence of peptic ulceration.

Other factors contributing to PUD include infectious agents, such as *H. pylori;* smoking; alcohol; radiation, and increased stress.

Peptic ulceration is also seen in clients who have pancreatitis, Crohn's disease, hepatic or biliary disease, and Zollinger-Ellison syndrome (see later); these diseases alter the inhibition and stimulation of gastric secretion.

Incidence/Prevalence

An estimated 5%–10% of the population in North America will suffer from PUD. In industrialized countries, 4%–15% of women and 10%–15% of men experience ulcer disease. Gastric ulcers most commonly occur in people who are in their 40s and 50s. Duodenal ulcers are most common in men in their 30s and 40s.

Collaborative Management

 Assessment

➤ History

The nurse collects data related to the causes of and risk factors for ulcer disease. The nurse records the client's age, sex, and occupation. The client's overall lifestyle is evaluated, and actual or perceived daily stressors are identified. The client is questioned about

- Diet factors, such as caffeine and alcohol intake
- Intake of irritants
- Overall eating patterns
- Use of tobacco

A history of current or past medical conditions focuses on gastrointestinal (GI) tract problems. The nurse determines whether the client has taken or is taking any over-the-counter or prescription drugs, such as corticosteroids, aspirin, and other nonsteroidal anti-inflammatory drugs (NSAIDs). The nurse also asks whether the client has ever undergone radiation treatments.

The nurse obtains a history of GI upset, pain and its relationship to eating and sleep, and actions taken to relieve symptoms. Classic symptoms have a definite relationship to eating. With a duodenal ulcer, discomfort is relieved by eating food or taking antacids; with a gastric ulcer, discomfort increases with eating, especially after drinking warm liquids (Table 58–1). With a duodenal ulcer, pain often wakes the person from sleep. After relieving the pain with food or antacid, the person returns to sleep and awakens in the morning without pain. Pain may also be exacerbated by certain foods (such as tomatoes, hot spices, fried foods, onions, alcohol, or caffeine drinks) and certain medications (such as aspirin, NSAIDs, or corticosteroids).

➤ *Physical Assessment/Clinical Manifestations*

The client typically describes discomfort, pain, or heartburn (the chief symptoms) as circumscribed in an area about 2.5–12.5 cm (1–5 in) between the xiphoid cartilage and umbilicus in the epigastrium or just to the right of the midline. *Gastric* ulcer pain often occurs in the upper epigastrium, with localization to the left of the midline; *duodenal* ulcer pain is in the right epigastrium

TABLE 58–1

Differential Features of Gastric and Duodenal Ulcers		
Feature	**Gastric Ulcer**	**Duodenal Ulcer**
Age	• Usually 50 yr and older	• Usually 40–50 yr
Gender	• Male/female ratio of 1.1:1	• Male/female ratio of 2.2:1
Blood group	• No differentiation	• Most frequently O
General nourishment	• May be malnourished	• Usually well nourished
Stomach acid production	• Normal secretion or hyposecretion	• Hypersecretion
Occurrence	• Mucosa exposed to acid-pepsin secretion	• Mucosa exposed to acid-pepsin secretion
Clinical course	• Healing and recurrence	• Healing and recurrence
Pain	• Occurs ½-1 hr after a meal; at night: rarely	• Occurs 2–3 hr after a meal; at night: often awakens client between 1 and 2 AM
	• Not helped by ingestion of food, sometimes even increased	• Relieved by ingestion of food
Response to treatment	• Healing with H_2 receptor antagonists	• Healing with H_2 receptor antagonists
Hemorrhage	• Hematemesis more common than melena	• Melena more common than hematemesis
Malignant change	• Perhaps in less than 10%	• Rare
Recurrence	• Less likely after surgery	• Occurs after modest resection
Surrounding mucosa	• Atrophic gastritis	• No gastritis

(Table 58–1). Steady pain near the midline of the back between the sixth and tenth thoracic vertebrae may indicate a perforated posterior wall caused by a duodenal ulcer. The nurse then assesses for a feeling of fullness or hunger. Distention of the duodenal bulb produces epigastric pain, which may radiate to the back and thorax. Pain is less frequently the initial complaint in the elderly client; melena is a more frequent presenting sign of ulcer disease in this group.

Vomiting may be a symptom with ulcer disease, most commonly with pyloric sphincter dysfunction. Vomiting results from gastric stasis associated with pyloric obstruction. Appetite is generally maintained in clients with peptic ulcer unless pyloric obstruction is present.

To assess for fluid volume deficit, possibly secondary to bleeding, the nurse takes orthostatic vital signs of all clients suspected of peptic ulcer disease (PUD). Orthostatic changes are characterized by a decrease of more than 20 mmHg in systolic blood pressure, 10 mmHg in diastolic blood pressure, and/or an increase in pulse when the client rises from a lying to an erect (sitting or, if possible, standing) position. The nurse also assesses the client for dizziness, especially when the client is upright. Dizziness is another symptom of fluid volume deficit.

➤ *Psychosocial Assessment*

The nurse assesses
- The impact of ulcer disease on the client's lifestyle, occupation, family, and social and leisure activities
- The client's ability and willingness to alter the work environment and daily schedule to reduce occupational stressors or to integrate therapeutic plans
- Family and individual stressors
- Usual patterns of coping and problem-solving

The nurse evaluates the impact that lifestyle changes will have on the client. Questions about lifestyle, occupation, and leisure can yield important information. This assessment determines the client's ability to comply with the prescribed treatment regimen and to obtain the needed social support to alter lifestyle.

➤ *Laboratory Assessment*

Hemoglobin and hematocrit values may be low, indicating bleeding. The stool specimen may be positive for occult blood if bleeding is present.

➤ *Radiographic Assessment*

An upper GI series (barium swallow) may show evidence of PUD. This is often the initial test for a client who does not have severe symptoms. If perforation is suspected, the health care provider usually orders a flat plate of the abdomen first to identify the presence of free air.

➤ *Other Diagnostic Assessment*

The major diagnostic test for PUD is esophagogastroduodenoscopy (EGD). The procedure may be done at the bedside on an emergent basis if bleeding is suspected. Visualization of the ulcer crater by EGD allows the health care provider to take specimens for *H. pylori* testing and for biopsy and cytologic studies for ruling out gastric

cancer. EGD may be repeated at 4- to 6-week intervals while the health care provider evaluates the progress of healing in response to therapy.

Recently, the Food and Drug Administration approved a breath test to detect *H. pylori*. The client drinks a carbon-enriched urea solution. If *H. pylori* is present, the bacteria break down the solution and release carbon dioxide, which the client inhales in a collection container for analysis. In addition to its noninvasive nature, this test assesses the entire stomach and may prove especially helpful after the client has been treated to determine if treatment was successful (Heslin, 1997).

 Analysis

➤ *Common Nursing Diagnoses and Collaborative Problems*

The common nursing diagnosis for clients with peptic ulcer disease (PUD) is Pain (acute or chronic) related to gastric and duodenal mucosal injury.

The most common collaborative problem is Potential for Hemorrhage, Perforation, or Obstruction.

➤ *Additional Nursing Diagnoses and Collaborative Problems*

In addition to the common diagnoses and collaborative problems, the client may present with one or more additional nursing diagnoses, including
- Ineffective management of therapeutic regime related to unfamiliarity with resources related to medications, diet, and signs and symptoms to report
- Ineffective Individual Coping related to intractable progressive disease requiring significant lifestyle alterations
- Altered Nutrition: Less than Body Requirements related to anorexia, nausea, or diet constraints
- Sleep Pattern Disturbance related to discomfort
- Risk for Injury related to orthostatic hypotension

 Planning and Implementation

➤ *Pain*

Planning: Expected Outcome. The client is expected to experience a reduction or alleviation of pain after treatment.

Interventions. The health care provider generally manages pain with specific ulcer therapy. The nurse monitors the client for worsening pain and reports it to the health care provider. In the ambulatory care setting, the nurse case manager may monitor the costs and efficacy of various treatment protocols and monitor the recurrence rate.

Drugs and diet therapy promote the comfort of clients with PUD. The nurse assists the client to understand the meaning of discomfort. For relief of signs and symptoms, the nurse stresses the importance of following the treatment plan to decrease gastric stimulation.

Clients with indigestion are usually treated symptomatically on an ambulatory basis for 6–8 weeks. If symptoms do not disappear after this period, if there is no relief within 10 days, or if complications occur, the health care provider typically orders further diagnostic evaluation. Repeated upper gastrointestinal (GI) x-rays are taken to document healing. If healing has not occurred, EGD and biopsy treatment may be repeated. Ulcer disease can be a chronic disease; treatment programs used to heal the ulcer may not prevent recurrence.

ELDERLY CONSIDERATIONS

Older adults may not seek medical care when they experience dyspepsia or ulcer disease. They may also use over-the-counter remedies, often delaying appropriate treatment for ulcer disease. Symptoms of peptic ulcer disease may not be typical, and thus the clinical presentation may be confusing. Older adults often suffer from one or more chronic illnesses, such as arthritis, that require the use of nonsteroidal anti-inflammatory medications, which place them at increased risk for ulcer disease.

In the elderly, hypoglycemic agents and smoking may affect ulcer symptoms, whereas cardiovascular medications and diseases, esophagitis, and NSAIDs may influence ulcer healing. Persistence of ulcer symptoms in older adults suggests persistent ulcer disease (DiMario et al., 1996).

Older adults who suffer acute strokes may be an increased risk for gastrointestinal hemorrhage (Davenport, Dennis, & Warlow, 1996). There is evidence that older adults may be at increased risk for complications and death following acute peptic ulcer bleeding (Hudson et al., 1995).

Drug Therapy. The primary objective of drug therapy in the treatment of peptic ulcers is eradication of *H. pylori* infections and to provide rest for the stomach (see Chart 58–3). Currently, the use of an antisecretory medication combined with azithromycin and amoxicillin is the first line of therapy for individuals with ulcer disease. The rationale for drug therapy involves different mechanisms:

- The treatment of *Helicobacter* infections (bismuth preparations)
- The reduction of secretions (hyposecretory drugs)
- The neutralization or buffering of acid (antacids)
- The protection of the mucous barrier (mucosal barrier fortifiers) by decreasing the activity of pepsin and hydrochloric acid

Special considerations for administering ulcer medications to the elderly client are listed in Chart 58–4.

Hyposecretory Drugs. Hyposecretory drugs, which cause a reduction in acid secretions, include antisecretory agents, H₂ receptor antagonists, and prostaglandin analogs.

Antisecretory Agents. Both omeprazole (Prilosec, Losec♣) and Prevacid (lansoprazole) suppress the H⁺K⁺-ATPase enzyme system of gastric acid production. The main use of these drugs is in gastroesophageal reflux disease, but they are now being used in selected clients

---

Chart 58–4

Nursing Focus on the Elderly: Giving Ulcer Medications Safely

- Check the drug dose carefully. Drug absorption may be delayed and drug metabolism slowed in the elderly client; thus, a smaller dose is required.
- Check the client's weight and nutrition status. Distribution may be altered, especially if the client is malnourished.
- Assess the client's complete drug regimen. Elderly clients may be more susceptible to side effects from multiple drugs.
- Monitor the client carefully for signs of overdose or adverse effects.
- Monitor the client receiving cimetidine (Tagamet) carefully for confusion and other central nervous system reactions.
- Keep dosage schedules simple when a client is at home.
- Assess the client's understanding of instructions related to medications. Provide a written list and instructions.

---

with duodenal ulcer disease. Capsules must be taken whole. In ulcer disease, the usual dose is 20 mg at bedtime for 2–4 weeks. Some health care providers use these drugs on a long-term basis.

H₂-Receptor Antagonists. Drugs that block histamine-stimulated gastric secretions are effective in the management of ulcer disease. In lower-dose forms, available over the counter, these medications may be used for indigestion and heartburn. H₂-receptor antagonists block the action of the H₂ receptors of the parietal cells. The most common drugs are ranitidine (Zantac), famotidine (Pepcid), and nizatidine (Axid). These drugs inhibit gastric acid secretion in response to all stimuli. When given orally for ulcer disease, these drugs are generally administered in a single dose at bedtime.

Prostaglandin Analogs. Prostaglandins are naturally abundant in the GI tract. They are thought to inhibit acid secretion and contribute to the gastric mucosal barrier by increasing bicarbonate and mucus production. Misoprostol (Cytotec), the most commonly used drug in this category, *prevents* NSAID-induced ulcers. Some NSAIDs are being manufactured that are in combination with misoprostol. A significant adverse effect of this drug is that it can cause miscarriage; thus, it is contraindicated for pregnant women.

Antacids. The ideal antacid is one that decreases acidity, is effective for a prolonged period, is pleasant to take orally, is not constipating or cathartic in effect, and is not absorbed to cause systemic side effects.

Antacids buffer gastric acid and prevent the formation of pepsin. Clients need to understand that antacids do not influence healing or prevent recurrence but that they do seem to decrease pain and discomfort. Liquid suspensions are the most therapeutic form, but tablets may be more convenient and enhance compliance.

The nurse instructs the client that for therapeutic effect, sufficient antacid must be ingested to neutralize the hourly production of acid. For optimal effect, antacids are given about 2 hours after meals to reduce the hydrogen ion load in the duodenum. Antacids may be effective 30 minutes up to 3 hours after ingestion. A common antacid dosage schedule for active ulcer disease is 1 and 3 hours after each meal and at bedtime. Antacids taken with an empty stomach are quickly evacuated; thus, the neutralizing effect is reduced.

Calcium carbonate (Tums) is a potent antacid but may cause constipation. It triggers gastrin release, which causes a rebound acid secretion. Magnesium carbonate and magnesium oxide are also potent antacids but are laxatives. Aluminum hydroxide, aluminum phosphate, and aluminum carbonate are not as effective as other types of antacids because they only partially neutralize the acid and are constipating. Magnesium-based products are often given alternately with aluminum-based products to balance the constipating effects. Combined magnesium and aluminum preparations, such as Mylanta and Gelusil, are more palatable to the client and are designed to minimize the constipating and diarrheal effects of each other. Although sodium bicarbonate (baking soda) is a potent antacid, its effects are brief; it is also absorbed systemically, which may result in metabolic alkalosis. The nurse ensures that the client understands the negative effects of sodium bicarbonate, such as gastric distention, pulmonary edema, and electrolyte imbalances.

Antacids can interact with certain drugs, such as phenytoin, tetracyclines, and ketoconazole, and interfere with their effectiveness. The nurse determines what other drugs the client is using before recommending a specific antacid. Medications are administered 1–2 hours before or after the antacid. The nurse informs the client that flavored antacids, especially wintergreen, should be avoided. The flavoring increases the emptying time of the stomach; thus, the desired effect of the antacid is negated.

The nurse teaches the client with past or present heart failure to avoid antacids with a high sodium content, such as some aluminum hydroxide, magnesium hydroxide, sodium bicarbonate, and simethicone combination products (Gelusil and Mylanta). Magaldrate (Riopan) has the lowest sodium concentration. Aluminum hydroxide (ALternaGEL) and some combination products (Maalox Plus tablets, Mylanta II tablets, and Gelusil tablets) have a high sugar content. The aluminum and magnesium hydroxide combination products (Maalox and Mylanta II) neutralize well at small doses. Combination therapy with H_2-receptor antagonists and antacids is common and seems to be effective.

Aluminum- and magnesium-based products must also be administered cautiously to elderly clients and to those with renal impairment. These substances cannot be eliminated adequately by the kidneys and are consequently retained in excessive amounts in the body.

Mucosal Barrier Fortifiers. Sucralfate (Carafate) is sulfonated disaccharide that forms complexes with proteins at the base of a peptic ulcer. This protective coat prevents further digestive action of both acid and pepsin.

Sucralfate does not inhibit acid secretion and has minimal acid-neutralizing ability, but it is effective in the treatment of ulcers. It may be used in conjunction with H_2 receptor antagonists and antacids but should not be administered within 1 hour of the antacid. It is given on an empty stomach 1 hour before each meal and at bedtime. Constipation is the main side effect.

Diet Therapy. The value of diet in the management of ulcer disease is highly controversial. There is no evidence that restriction of diet promotes or accelerates healing. Food itself acts as an antacid by neutralizing gastric acid for 30–60 minutes. An increased rate of gastric acid secretion, called rebound, may follow. If diet therapy is used, it may be directed toward neutralizing acid and reducing hypermotility, which may alleviate symptoms.

The nurse instructs the client to avoid substances that increase acid secretion, including caffeine-containing beverages (coffee, tea, and cola). Decaffeinated coffee may be allowed if it is tolerated, but both caffeinated and decaffeinated coffees contain peptides that stimulate gastrin release.

In collaboration, the nurse and dietitian teach the client to exclude any foods that cause discomfort. During the acute symptomatic phase, the diet is often bland and nonirritating. The nurse encourages the client to avoid foods that reproduce any symptoms of gastric distress. Bedtime snacks are avoided because they may stimulate gastric acid secretion. For some clients, six daily meals may help, but this regimen is no longer a regular part of therapy. Milk may be taken in small amounts but is a poor neutralizer and may cause rebound acid secretion. Clients should avoid alcohol and tobacco because of their stimulatory effects.

Rest and Decreased Activity. The nurse teaches the client with PUD to avoid intense physical activity because it reduces motor activity, which stimulates gastric secretions. Physical *and* mental rest are important. The number and intensity of environmental stimuli are decreased in order to prevent increased gastric acid stimulation.

When ulcer symptoms appear, the nurse assists the client in altering a stressful work routine and implementing plan that enables rest. The nurse teaches coping and relaxation techniques specific to the client's stress (see Chap. 8).

► *Potential for Hemorrhage, Perforation, and Obstruction*

Planning: Expected Outcomes. The client is expected to experience no complications of peptic ulcer disease (PUD), such as hemorrhage, perforation, or obstruction. If complications do occur, they must be treated promptly.

Interventions. Monitoring and early recognition of complications are critical to the successful management of PUD. In some cases, the health care provider must treat the complications surgically.

Nonsurgical Management. Nonsurgical treatments depend on the type of complication. The nurse monitors the client carefully and immediately reports changes to the health care provider.

Management of Hemorrhage. The nurse observes the symptoms to determine the severity of the hemorrhage. The health care provider or nurse inserts a nasogastric (NG) tube to

- Ascertain the presence or absence of blood in the stomach
- Assess the rate of bleeding
- Prevent gastric dilation
- Administer saline lavage

A Salem sump or Levin tube is typically used. The nurse irrigates the NG tube to maintain patency and prevent obstruction with clotted blood.

In a person with mild bleeding (less than 500 mL), only slight weakness and perspiration may be present. Blood loss of more than 1 L/24 hr may cause signs and symptoms of shock, such as hypotension; weak, thready pulse; chills; palpitations; and diaphoresis.

In severe bleeding, the nurse keeps an accurate and up-to-date record of the client's hemoglobin and hematocrit values, which may indicate significant blood loss. Any client in whom active bleeding is suspected must be admitted to the hospital and monitored carefully for signs of hemorrhage. Some clients are admitted directly to the critical care unit.

The nurse carefully describes and documents bleeding, including the occurrence of hematemesis and melena; the color, amount, and consistency of blood; the frequency of bleeding, and vital signs.

Bright red blood signifies new bleeding; dark red blood indicates old bleeding. The nurse immediately notifies the health care provider of major episodes of hemorrhage.

Therapy for massive bleeding is aimed at

- Treating hypovolemic shock
- Preventing dehydration and electrolyte imbalance
- Stopping the bleeding
- Providing rest

The health care provider uses early endoscopy (esophagogastroduodenoscopy [EGD]) in conjunction with laser coagulation to control bleeding or determine the need for surgery. Clients are confined to bed, allowed nothing by mouth (NPO), and given IV fluids until the bleeding subsides.

Saline Lavage. Saline lavage is traditionally accomplished with insertion of a large-bore nasogastric tube. Iced saline in volumes of 50–200 mL may be instilled manually. The saline and blood are repeatedly withdrawn until returns are clear or light pink, without clots.

For protection against exposure to blood, practitioners may use a closed system for irrigation and suction. A Y-connector is attached to the nasogastric tube. A bag of normal saline is attached to tubing at one end of the Y-connector. Wall suction is attached to tubing at the other end of the connector. After the stomach is initially drained by suctioning, the tubing attached to suction is clamped off, and up to 200 mL of normal saline is allowed to drain into the client through the NG tube. After the saline is instilled, the tube connecting the saline to the NG tube is clamped off, and the clamp to suction is released. The nurse instructs the client to lie on the left side during this procedure to limit the flow of saline out of the stomach and prevent aspiration.

There is considerable controversy about the value of iced saline for lavage. Iced saline controls bleeding through its vasoconstrictive effect. The concern about using iced saline is that it might cause a decrease in perfusion to the gastric mucosa, thus leading to more mucosal damage. It can also stimulate a vagal response, which decreases systemic perfusion. Because of these effects, saline at room temperature is preferred. The saline solution is cooler than body temperature, yet not as cold as an iced solution.

Vasopressin Therapy. Intra-arterial administration of vasopressin (via infusion pump) has successfully controlled acute hemorrhage. The health care provider typically orders a rate of 0.2–0.4 units/min. The nurse is alert for complications from the pharmacologic effect of vasopressin, which include

- Pain at the injection site or local necrosis
- Gangrene
- Chest pain (angina; pain related to myocardial infarction)
- Difficulty in urinating
- Nausea and vomiting
- Abdominal or stomach cramps
- Belching
- Diarrhea
- Water intoxication (evidenced by drowsiness, listlessness, headache, confusion, and weight gain)

This procedure is contraindicated for clients with cardiac problems.

Other Treatment Measures. The health care provider may perform EGD to visualize the esophagus and stomach directly and identify bleeding sites. Injection therapy, laser photocoagulation, heater probe therapy, and electrocoagulation through the endoscope may then be used to control the hemorrhage. The treatment of active upper gastrointestinal bleeding with endoscopic electrocoagulation has decreased the length of hospital stays, the need for transfusions, and the number of surgical procedures.

Absolute bed rest to keep the client's blood pressure down and to decrease intestinal motility is essential for several days after bleeding has subsided. When bleeding stops, the health care provider usually permits bathroom privileges (BRP). Opioids, if ordered, are administered with caution. Morphine sulfate can cause nausea and vomiting, but it may be used for the client who is extremely restless or apprehensive.

During the first few days after hemorrhage, gastric pH should be increased to between 5.5 and 7.0 and maintained at that level to control secretory activity. To accomplish this, the health care provider may prescribe ranitidine (Zantac) or cimetidine (Tagamet) every 4–6 hours or as a continuous intravenous drip for a few days. The use of antacids complements the effectiveness of H_2 antagonists for maintaining the pH level of gastric secretions. Anticholinergics are not recommended for clients with gastric hemorrhage because decreased gastric motility may delay gastric emptying.

Management of Perforation. For preventing peritonitis from the gastrointestinal (GI) contents that have entered the peritoneum, perforation is managed by the immediate replacement of fluid, blood, and electrolytes and the administration of antibiotics. The nurse maintains nasogastric suction to drain gastric secretions and, thus, prevent further peritoneal spillage. The client remains NPO, and the nurse carefully monitors intake and output. The nurse or assistive nursing personnel check the client's vital signs at least hourly and monitors the client for clinical manifestations of septic shock, such as fever, pain, tachycardia, lethargy, anxiety, and prostration.

Management of Pyloric Obstruction. Pyloric obstruction is caused by edema, spasm, or scar tissue. Symptoms of obstruction related to difficulty in emptying the stomach include feelings of fullness, distention, or nausea after eating and vomiting of copious amounts of undigested food.

Treatment of obstruction is directed toward restoration of fluid and electrolyte balance and decompression of the dilated stomach. If necessary, surgical intervention is used.

Obstruction related to edema and spasm generally responds to medical therapy. First, the stomach must be decompressed with nasogastric suction. Metabolic alkalosis and dehydration are then treated. The nasogastric tube is clamped after about 72 hours, and the client is checked for retention of gastric contents. If the amount retained is not more than 350 mL in 30 minutes, the health care provider may allow oral fluids.

Surgical Management. Surgery of the stomach is used to

- Reduce the acid-secreting ability of the stomach
- Treat a surgical emergency that develops as a complication of peptic ulcer disease (PUD)
- Treat clients who do not respond to medical therapy or in whom complications develop

Most chronic, recurring ulcers are eventually treated surgically. When an ulcer does not respond to intensive medical therapy or when a definitive diagnosis cannot be made by x-ray and esophagogastroduodenoscopy, the health care provider performs surgery. Clients with duodenal ulcer may require surgery for hemorrhage, perforation, obstruction, or intractability.

Preoperative Care. Before surgery, a nasogastric (NG) tube is inserted (if this has not already been done) and connected to suction to remove secretions and empty the stomach. This allows surgery to take place without contamination of the peritoneal cavity by gastric secretions.

Chart 58–5 describes the procedure for inserting the NG tube and nursing care associated with NG tube maintenance. The NG tube remains in place postoperatively to prevent the accumulation of secretions, which may lead to vomiting or gastrointestinal (GI) distention and pressure on the suture line.

Other preoperative nursing measures for the client undergoing gastric surgery are the same as those for any client having abdominal surgery and general anesthesia (see Chap. 20).

Operative Procedures. If perforation occurs, the surgeon closes the perforation after the escaped gastric contents have been evacuated. If the perforation is small and closes immediately by adhering to the adjacent tissues, the loss of gastric contents is small. In this instance, the client may recover without surgery. Penetration into the pancreas results in serious, continuous pain and requires surgery.

Vagotomy. Vagotomy eliminates the acid-secreting stimulus to gastric cells and decreases the responsiveness of parietal cells. In a vagotomy, each branch of the vagus nerve may be

- Completely cut (truncal vagotomy)
- Partially cut to preserve the hepatic and celiac branches (selective vagotomy)
- Partially cut to denervate only the parietal cell mass, thus preserving innervation of both the antrum and the pyloric sphincter (superselective vagotomy)

Selective vagotomy avoids the problems of impaired emptying and diarrhea that follow the truncal vagotomy. Vagotomy also eliminates the need for a drainage anastomosis to offset the gastric stasis, yet it reduces acid secretion and preserves the function of the antrum. In the proximal (parietal cell) vagotomy, the surgeon severs only the gastric portion of vagal nerves that innervate the upper two thirds of the stomach (Fig. 58–4).

Pyloroplasty. The surgeon often performs pyloroplasty with a vagotomy to widen the exit of the pylorus. This facilitates emptying of stomach contents. The most common procedure is the Heineke-Mikulicz pyloroplasty (Fig. 58–5). In this procedure, the surgeon enlarges the pyloric stricture by incising the pylorus longitudinally and sutures the incision transversely.

Gastroenterostomy. A simple gastroenterostomy permits neutralization of gastric acid by regurgitation of alkaline duodenal contents into the stomach. The surgeon creates

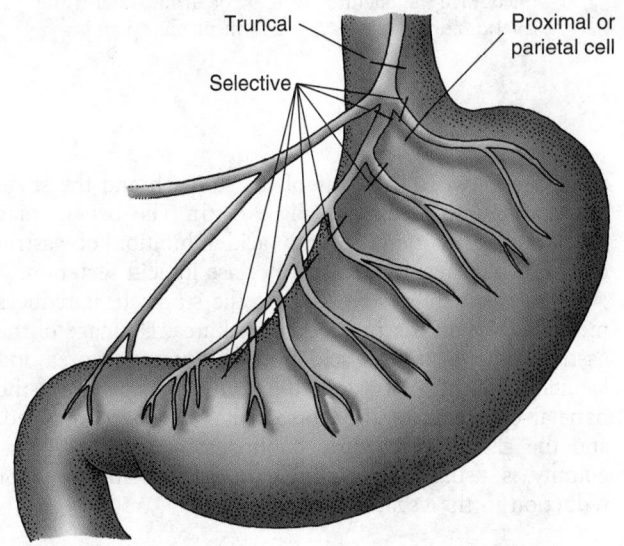

Figure 58–4. The types of vagotomies.

Chart 58–5

Nursing Care Highlight: Nasogastric Tubes

1. Inform the client about the procedure and its potential discomfort.
2. Seat the client with pillows behind the shoulders.
3. Lubricate the tube with a water-soluble lubricant.
4. Measure the length of the tube to be passed.
   a. Measure from the bridge of the nose to the ear lobe to the xiphoid process.
   b. Indicate this length with a piece of tape on the tube.

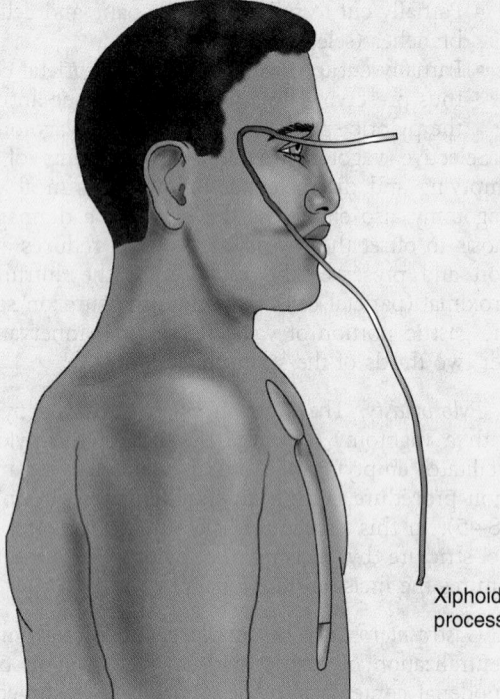

Xiphoid process

5. Determine which nostril is more patent.
6. Encourage the client to swallow or drink water if the level of consciousness and treatment plan permit.

7. Insert the tube.
   a. Pass the tube gently into the nasopharynx. Ask the client to swallow repeatedly while the tube is advanced.
   b. If resistance is met, rotate the tube slowly, aiming downward and toward the closer ear.
   c. In the intubated or semiconscious client, flex the client's head toward the chest while passing the tube.
8. Withdraw the tube immediately if any change is noted in the client's respiratory status.
9. Test for tube placement by using one or more of the following techniques.
   a. Obtain a sample of the gastric contents by aspirating with a 50-mL catheter-tipped syringe.
   b. Test the pH of the gastric contents (should be between 1 and 3.5).
   c. Obtain an order for an x-ray to confirm placement.
10. Connect the tube to suction at low pressure.
    a. The Levin tube is connected to intermittent low suction.
    b. The Salem sump or Anderson tube is connected to continuous low suction.
11. Secure the tube to the client's nose with adhesive tape and to the client's gown.
    a. Tie a slipknot around the tube with a rubber band.
    b. Pin a rubber band to the client's gown.
12. Check the client's intake and output every 4 hr or more often, as indicated.
13. Observe the client for nausea, vomiting, abdominal fullness, or distention.
14. If irrigation is indicated, use only a normal saline solution.
15. Observe the client for alterations in fluid and electrolyte balance.
16. If indicated, instruct the client about movement that will not dislodge the tube and cause nasal irritation.
17. Remove the adhesive tape securing the tube to the nose daily and PRN to clean skin; reapply tape.

---

a passage between the body of the stomach and the small bowel, often the jejunum (Fig. 58–6). The benefit may be offset by interference with acid inhibition of gastrin release, which results in a net increase in acid secretion.

If the gastroenterostomy drains the stomach, it reduces motor activity in the pyloroduodenal area. Drainage of the gastric contents diverts acid from the ulcerated area and facilitates healing. However, the secretory capacity of the parietal cell mass of the stomach has not been reduced, and the gastrin mechanism continues to function. A vagotomy is usually combined with gastroenterostomy for reduction in the vagal influences.

Antrectomy. The surgeon performs antrectomy (removal of the antrum) to reduce acid-secreting portions of the stomach. A *subtotal gastrectomy,* sometimes referred to

as a partial gastrectomy, is accomplished by either a Billroth I or a Billroth II procedure.

Billroth I. A Billroth I procedure removes part of the distal portion of the stomach, including the antrum; the remainder is anastomosed to the duodenum. This operation is more properly called a *gastroduodenostomy* (Fig. 58–7). The surgeon removes the gastrin source in the antrum of some of the acid-pepsin–secreting parietal cells. This helps to decrease the incidence of the dumping syndrome, which often occurs after this operation.

Billroth II. In a Billroth II resection, or *gastrojejunostomy,* the surgeon anastomoses the proximal remnant of the stomach to the proximal jejunum. It is the procedure most often used for gastric ulcer. The Billroth II technique is also preferred for the treatment of duodenal ulcer

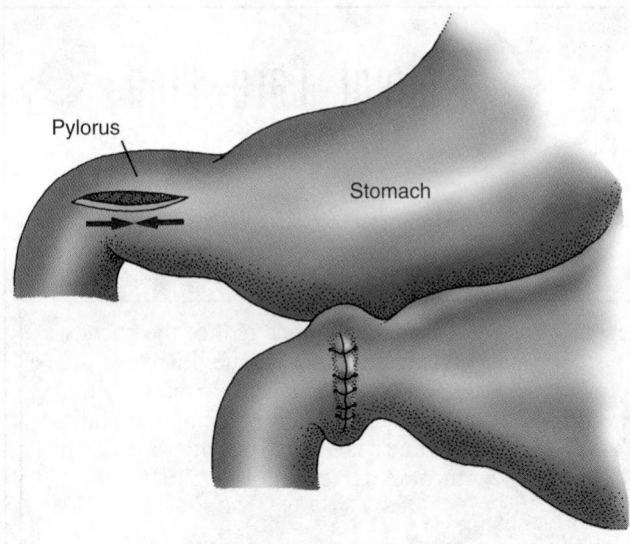

Figure 58–5. The Heineke-Mikulicz pyloroplasty.

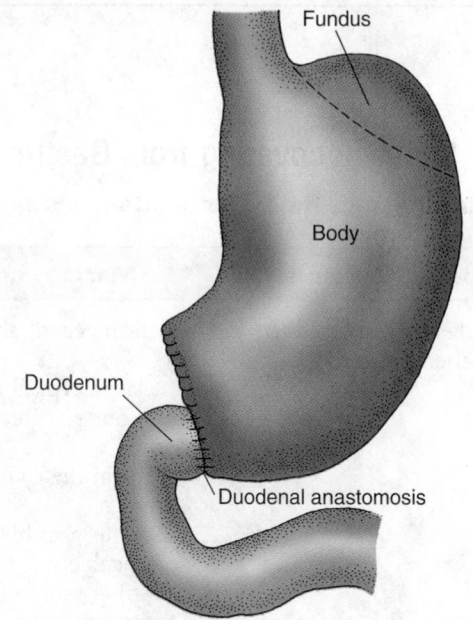

Figure 58–7. The Billroth I procedure (gastroduodenostomy). The distal portion of the stomach is removed, and the remainder is anastomosed to the duodenum. The shading shows the portion removed.

because the ulcer recurs less frequently. The duodenal stump is preserved to permit bile flow to the jejunum, as shown in Figure 58–8.

Postoperative Care. The postoperative care for all of the surgical procedures is similar (Client Care Plan). The nurse provides the usual postoperative care for clients receiving general anesthesia (see Chap. 22).

Care of the Nasogastric Tube. Patency of the nasogastric (NG) tube in the client who has had gastric surgery is critical for preventing the retention of gastric secretions. The nurse assesses that no more than a scant amount of blood drains from the tube and that the client does not

develop abdominal distention. If these problems occur, the nurse reports them immediately to the surgeon. The nurse must never irrigate or reposition the nasogastric tube after gastric surgery unless specifically ordered by the surgeon (see Research Applications for Nursing).

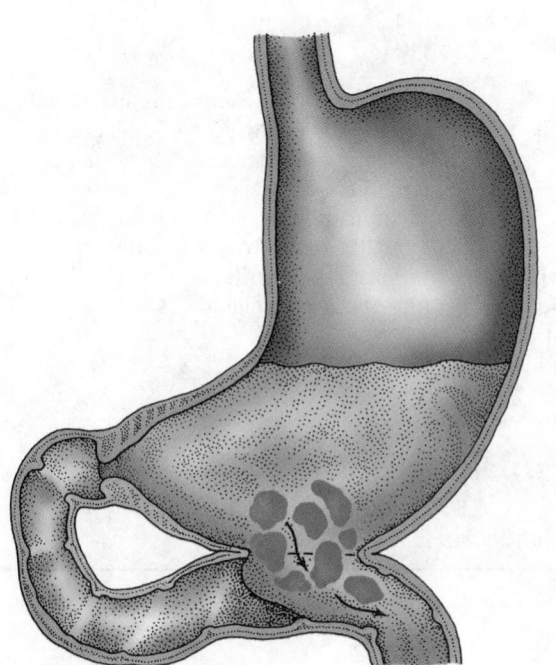

Figure 58–6. Gastroenterostomy, which is the creation of a passage between the body of the stomach and the jejunum.

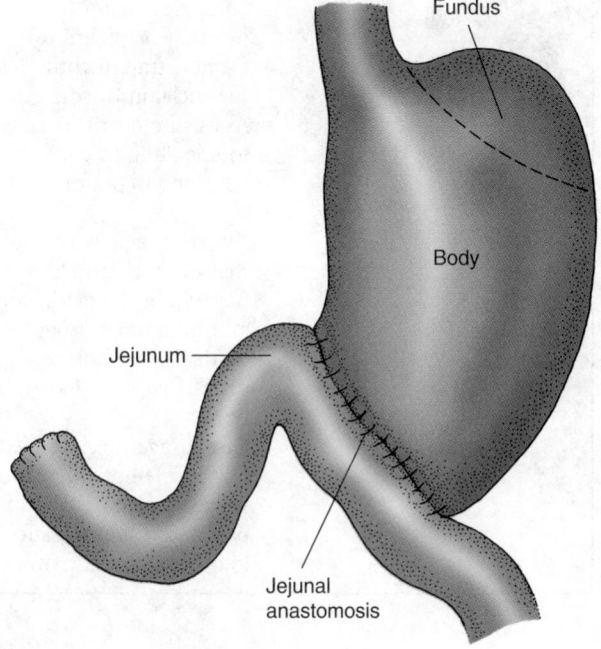

Figure 58–8. The Billroth II procedure (gastrojejunostomy). The lower portion of the stomach is removed, and the remainder is anastomosed to the jejunum. The shading shows the portion removed. A remaining duodenal stump is closed.

Client Care Plan

The Client Recovering from Gastric Surgery

Nursing Diagnosis No. 1: Pain related to surgery

Expected Outcomes	Nursing Interventions	Rationale

The client is expected to experience reduced pain.	▪ Teach the client about pain experiences
	  ▪ Relate a typical disease process or course with realistic expectations.
	  ▪ Explain the cause of pain, if known.
	  ▪ Explain possible effects of fatigue and anxiety.
	  ▪ Instill a sense of control of the situation in relation to the temporary nature of the problem.
	  ▪ Assess the client's sleep patterns and influence of pain on sleep.
	  ▪ Encourage rest and provide an opportunity for rest during the day.
		▪ These interventions reduce the client's anxiety level and fatigue. Increased anxiety and fatigue ultimately intensify the pain experience by reducing the body's or mind's adaptive capacity to deal with uncomfortable stimuli or situations.

	▪ Assess pain relief measures commonly used by the caregiver and encourage the use of mutually acceptable methods. ▪ Teach techniques commonly used, such as relaxation, cutaneous stimulation, and massage. ▪ Encourage positioning to improve chest expansion (i.e., semi-Fowler's position or reclining). ▪ Demonstrate techniques to splint the incision during coughing.	▪ Pain relief measures enable the client and family to manage pain and discomfort. Thus, a sense of control is promoted, and the use of invasive methods avoided.
	▪ Assist the client in assessing for factors leading to exacerbations of pain or discomfort.	▪ Identification of factors eliminates individualized pain triggers. Some are known gastric irritants, yet not all factors affect each client.
	▪ Avoid, or use with caution, drugs that decrease mucosal resistance (acetylsalicylic acid, nonsteroidal anti-inflammatory agents, adrenocorticotropic hormone, steroids) or drugs that alter gastric acid production. ▪ Discourage the use of stimulants (e.g., caffeine and nicotine) or spices (e.g., mustard, paprika, pepper, and Tabasco sauce) that are known to cause pain or discomfort.	▪ Identification of factors eliminates individualized pain triggers. Some are known gastric irritants, yet not all factors affect each client.

(Continued)

Client Care Plan

Expected Outcomes	Nursing Interventions	Rationale
	■ Eliminate the use of alcohol. Avoid the concurrent use of alcohol and aspirin.	■ Alcohol irritates the mucosal lining and may provoke gastritis. Alcohol and aspirin together greatly irritate the mucosal lining.
	■ Encourage an adequate diet for meeting nutritional needs. Emphasize the inclusion of nonirritating foods.	

	■ Administer medications as ordered to:
	  ■ Block histamine-stimulated gastric secretions (H_2 receptor antagonists)
	  ■ Neutralize or buffer gastric acids (antacids)
	  ■ Protect the mucous barrier (mucosal barrier fortifiers)
		■ The use of medications provides the stomach an opportunity to rest. This rest leads to decreased gastric acid secretion and promotes tissue healing and, ultimately, a reduction in pain and discomfort.

	■ Assess the client's response to the medication.
	  ■ Return in ½ hr to determine effect.
	  ■ Rate the severity of pain and the amount of relief.
	  ■ Identify when the pain begins to increase.	

	■ Consult the primary-care provider if a dosage or interval change is required.	
	■ Reduce or eliminate common medication side effects.	
	■ Gradually increase food until the client is able to eat three to six meals a day.	■ Return of function of the stomach and intestines is evaluated.
	■ If discomfort recurs, decrease the size of meals and the amount of fluids.	
	■ Instruct the client to report signs of complications, a feeling of fullness, weakness, and hematemesis.	

Nursing Diagnosis No. 2: Risk for Fluid Volume Deficit related to nausea, vomiting, and possible hemorrhage or perforation

Expected Outcomes	Nursing Interventions	Rationale
The client is expected to maintain vascular, cellular, and intracellular perfusion as evidenced by: ■ Intact mental status ■ Stable blood pressure ■ Warm, dry skin ■ Urinary output of at least 30 mL/hr	■ Assess for nausea, vomiting, black or bloody stools, occult blood in stools, thirst, diaphoresis, pain, increased pulse, and decreased blood pressure; also assess urinary output and hemoglobin and hematocrit values.	■ Assessment detects fluid volume deficit and evaluates its severity. If fluid volume deficit occurs, these same interventions assess the effectiveness of treatment.

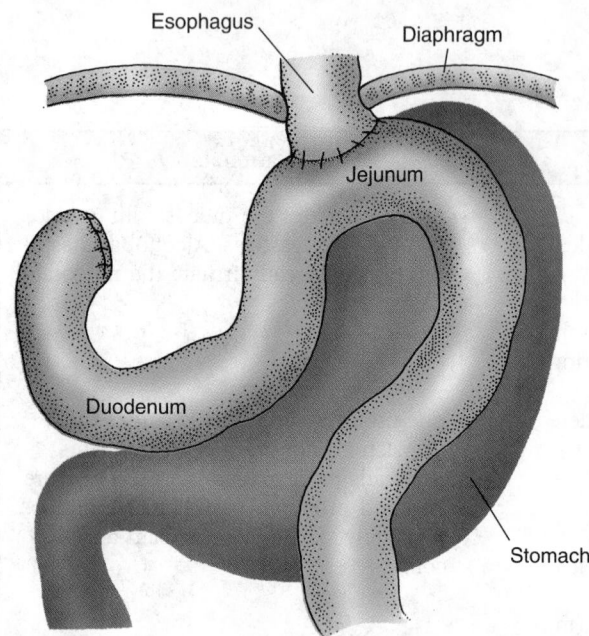

Figure 58–9. Total gastrectomy, with anastomosis of the esophagus to the jejunum (esophagojejunostomy), is the principal medical intervention for extensive gastric cancer.

Monitoring for Postoperative Complications. The nurse observes the client carefully for possible complications and reports them immediately to the health care provider. In the immediate postoperative period, many complications may occur. Table 58–2 summarizes surgical procedures and potential complications.

Acute *gastric dilation* is manifested by epigastric pain and a feeling of fullness, hiccups, tachycardia, and hypotension. This problem generally improves rapidly after the health care provider clears a plugged NG tube or inserts a new one.

The *dumping syndrome* results from gastric resection in which the pylorus is bypassed. It is most likely after a Billroth II procedure, occurs soon after surgery, and subsides in 6 months to 1 year. Dumping syndrome is a postprandial problem associated with the rapid entry of ingested food into the jejunum without proper mixing and without the normal digestive processes of the duodenum having been accomplished.

The nurse observes for *early* manifestations of this syndrome, which typically occur 5–30 minutes after eating. Symptoms include vertigo, tachycardia, syncope, sweating, pallor, palpitations, and the desire to lie down.

The early manifestations may be due to the rapid movement of extracellular fluids into the bowel to convert the hypertonic bolus into an isotonic mixture. This rapid fluid shift decreases the circulating blood volume, which causes the symptoms.

The *late* manifestations of dumping syndrome, which occur 2–3 hours after eating, are caused by a release of an excessive amount of insulin. The insulin release follows a rapid rise in the blood glucose level resulting from the rapid entry of high-carbohydrate food into the jejunum. The nurse observes for intestinal manifestations, which include epigastric fullness, distention, diarrhea, abdominal cramping, nausea with only occasional vomiting, and borborygmi (very loud gurgling bowel sounds).

Some clients experience a strong desire to defecate. Severe pain is usually not a part of this syndrome. Intestinal manifestations are caused by the distention of the jejunum, which increases intestinal peristalsis and motility.

The health care provider manages the dumping syndrome by advising the client to decrease the amount of food taken at one time and prescribing a high-protein, high-fat, low-carbohydrate diet (Table 58–3). Pectin administered in the form of a dry powder may *prevent* the syndrome. The client can delay gastric emptying by not taking fluids with meals, by eating in a recumbent or semirecumbent position, or by lying down after meals. The health care provider may order sedatives and antispasmodics to delay gastric emptying.

Alkaline *reflux gastritis* is a complication of gastric surgery in which the pylorus is bypassed or removed, such as pyloroplasty, gastric resection with gastroduodenostomy (Billroth I procedure), and gastrojejunostomy (Billroth II procedure). The reflux of duodenal contents with bile acids results in reflux gastritis. Injury to the gastric

► Research Applications for Nursing

Is Medication as Effective When Administered Through a Nasogastric Tube?

Elfant, A. B., Levine, S. M., Peikin, S. R., Cencora, B., Mendez, L., Pello, M. J., Atabek, U. M., Alexander, J. B., Spence, R. K., & Camishion, R. C. (1995). Bioavailability of medication delivered via nasogastric tube is decreased in the immediate postoperative period. American Journal of Surgery, 169(4), 430–432.

The researchers determined the bioavailability of acetaminophen delivered via nasogastric (NG) tubes in hospitalized clients following abdominal surgery. A standard dose of acetaminophen was administered orally prior to surgery and 3 hours postoperatively via the tube. NG tubes were clamped for a period of 30 minutes following the administration of the medication. Serum levels of acetaminophen were measured at the time of administration and 40 and 90 minutes after each dose. The researchers reported significantly lower serum levels when the medication was give via the NG tube following surgery.

Critique. This is one of few studies that have examined the effectiveness the medications when administered through an NG tube. More research needs to be conducted that might support the need for different dosing when NG administration is needed.

Nursing Implications. This study supports the premise that the bioavailability of acetaminophen is decreased when it is administered via an NG tube when compared with oral administration. Nasogastric and feeding tubes are commonly used for the administration of medications in a variety of clinical situations. Health care providers and nurses must be aware that the bioavailability of acetaminophen as well as other medications may be reduced when administered via a tube. Nurses must observe clients receiving medications via an NG tube and not assume that the client is receiving the full therapeutic benefit of the administered medication(s).

TABLE 58-2

Surgical Management of Peptic Ulcer Disease and Potential Complications of Peptic Ulcer Disease

Surgery	Description	Possible Adverse Effects
Vagotomy Truncal (total abdominal vagotomy)	• Cuts the vagus nerve at the esophageal level; severs both anterior and posterior trunks; destroys vagal and abdominal innervation; destroys gastrointestinal motility	• Gastric emptying is inhibited; pyloroplasty or antrectomy must be performed to prevent gastric stasis • Some clients experience a feeling of fullness after eating (33%), dumping syndrome (10%), or diarrhea (10%)
Selective	• Cuts the vagus nerve to the stomach, but other abdominal innervation remains; acid production stops	• Gastric emptying is inhibited; pyloroplasty or antrectomy must be performed to prevent gastric stasis
Proxima, or parietal cell (can be done without pyloroplasty or antrectomy)	• Cuts the parietal branches of the vagus nerve; alters innervation to acid-producing cells but does not alter gastric motility	• Few negative consequences because innervation of the antrum and the pyloric sphincter remains
Vagotomy with antrectomy	• Cuts the vagus nerve and removes the antrum (lower half) of the stomach; removes the source of gastrin secretion	• Some clients may have a feeling of fullness after eating, dumping syndrome, diarrhea, anemia, or malabsorption
Pyloroplasty	• Enlarges the pylorus by surgically enlarging the pyloric sphincter	• The stomach may empty too rapidly
Vagotomy and pyloroplasty	• Cuts the right and left branches of the vagus nerve; widens the existing pyloric sphincter to prevent stasis and to enhance emptying of the stomach	• The stomach may empty too rapidly
Subtotal gastrectomy Billroth I (gastroduodenostomy after resection) hemigastrectomy	• Removes the distal one third to one half of the stomach and anastomoses with the duodenum; removes the antral portion of the stomach and the pylorus	• Dumping syndrome, anemia, malabsorption, weight loss, or bile reflux may occur
Billroth II (gastrojejunostomy after resection)	• Removes the distal segment of the stomach and antrum and anastomoses with the jejunum; retains the duodenum; secretions of the liver and pancreas flow to the jejunum; preferred procedure	• Infection in the duodenum, malabsorption-related weight loss, vitamin B_{12} deficiency, or dumping syndrome may occur
Total gastrectomy (esophagojejunostomy)	• Removes the stomach from the level of the lower esophageal sphincter to the duodenum and anastomoses the duodenum to the esophagus	• Gastric function is altered • Dumping syndrome and anemia may occur

mucosal barrier by the bile acids may allow back-diffusion of hydrogen ions. Symptoms include persistent pain and nausea and vomiting that are accentuated after meals. Epigastric burning is only partially relieved by vomiting.

Delayed gastric emptying is often present after gastric surgery and usually resolves within 1 week. Edema at the anastomosis or adhesions obstructing the distal loop may be mechanical causes. Metabolic causes (such as hypokalemia, hypoproteinemia, or hyponatremia) should be considered. The edema is resolved with nasogastric suction, maintenance of fluid and electrolyte balance, and proper nutrition.

Gastrojejunocolic fistula is a postoperative complication associated with recurrent peptic ulcer disease. The fistula arises from perforation of a recurrent ulceration at the gastrojejunal anastomosis site. The clinical manifestations are caused by bacterial overgrowth in the small intestine.

The nurse assesses for fecal vomiting, diarrhea, weight loss, and anorexia. Belching of fecal-smelling gas may occur. Surgery may be necessary to correct the fistula.

Afferent loop syndrome may occur when the duodenal loop is partially obstructed after a Billroth II resection. Pancreatic and biliary secretions fill the intestinal loop, which becomes distended. Painful contractions attempt to propel these secretions from the loop. When secretions finally enter the jejunum, the excessive pressure forces them back into the stomach, and vomiting occurs. The nurse reports these symptoms if they occur. Treatment usually consists of nasogastric suction until operative edema subsides.

Monitoring Nutritional Status. Several problems of nutrition develop from partial removal of the stomach, including

TABLE 58-3

Diet for Dumping Syndrome

Food Group	Foods Allowed or Encouraged	Foods to Use with Caution	Foods That Must Be Excluded
Soups		• Fluids 1 hr before and after meals	• Spicy soups
Meat and meat substitutes	• 8 oz or more per day: fish poultry, beef, pork, veal, lamb, eggs, cheese, and peanut butter		• Spicy meats or meat substitutes
Potato and substitutes	• Potato, rice, pasta, starchy vegetables	• Foods made with milk	• Highly spiced potatoes or substitutes
Bread and cereal	• White bread, rolls, muffins, crackers, and cereals	• Whole-grain bread, rolls, crackers, and cereals	• Breads with frosting or jelly, sweet rolls, and coffee cake
Vegetables	• Two or more cooked vegetables	• Gas-producing vegetables, such as cabbage, onions, broccoli, or raw vegetables	
Fruits	• Limit three per day: unsweetened cooked/canned fruits	• Unsweetened juice or fruit drinks 30–45 minutes after meals; fresh fruit	• Sweetened fruit or juice
Beverages	• Dietetic drinks	• Limit to 1 hr after meals; caffeine-containing beverages, such as coffee, tea, and cola; if tolerated, diet carbonated beverages	• Milk shakes, malts, and other sweet drinks; regular carbonated beverages and alcohol
Fats	• Margarine, oils, shortening, butter, bacon, and salad dressings	• Mayonnaise	• Any fats with milk products
Desserts	• Fruit (see Fruits)	• Sugar-free gelatin, pudding, and custard	• All sweets, cakes, pies, cookies, candy, ice cream, and sherbet
Seasonings and miscellaneous	• Diet jelly, diet syrups, sugar substitutes	• Excessive amounts of salt	• Excessive amounts of spices, sugar, jelly, honey, syrup, or molasses

General Principles
• Five to six small meals daily
• Relatively high fat and protein content
• Low roughage
• Relatively low carbohydrate content
• No milk, sweets, or sugars
• Liquid between meals *only*

■ Deficiency of vitamin B_{12}, folic acid, and iron
■ Impaired calcium metabolism
■ Reduced absorption of calcium and vitamin D

These problems are caused by a shortage of intrinsic factor, which results from the resection and inadequate absorption because of rapid entry of food into the bowel. In the absence of intrinsic factor, clinical manifestations of pernicious anemia occur. These manifestations are corrected by the administration of vitamin B_{12}. The health care provider may also prescribe folic acid or iron preparations.

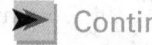 Continuing Care

➤ Home Care Management

Clients are discharged to the home setting to continue recuperation. Clients who have undergone surgery or have had complications, such as hemorrhage, may require assistance with activities of daily living. The primary focus of home care preparation is teaching individual risk factors for preventing recurrence of the ulcer.

➤ Health Teaching

The nurse instructs the client and family or significant others about factors related to the development of an ulcer. A risk assessment assists the client in identifying gastric irritants and lifestyle stressors. Strategies for lifestyle changes are developed with the client.

The nurse teaches the client about symptoms that should be brought to the attention of the health care provider after discharge from the hospital, such as abdominal pain; nausea and vomiting; black, tarry stools; and weakness or dizziness.

The client describes the symptoms to the nurse in return to demonstrate understanding. The nurse also teaches the client about diets to be used for avoiding postprandial distention or the dumping syndrome (see earlier).

For postsurgical clients, especially those who have had partial stomach removal, a smaller meal may be required. In collaboration with the dietitian, the nurse instructs the client to

- Have small and more frequent meals
- Avoid drinking liquids with meals
- Refrain from skipping meals or going a long time without eating
- Abstain from hot, spicy foods
- Eliminate caffeine and alcohol consumption
- If a smoker, quit smoking

The client is also taught to avoid any over-the-counter product containing aspirin or ibuprofen. The nurse schedules a follow-up visit to the health care provider. The importance of keeping all follow-up appointments is emphasized.

The nurse assists the client in

- Identifying how stress affects the client's life
- Identifying situations that are stressful
- Describing feelings during stressful situations
- Developing an awareness of patterns of coping with stressors

The nurse encourages the client to learn and use relaxation techniques, such as exercise, yoga, biofeedback, humor, and imagery (see Chap. 8). Psychotherapy may be indicated to help some clients cope with stress. Ulcer disease may recur, so it is essential for the client and family to understand how modified living, working, and eating habits minimize the risks of ulcer recurrence.

➤ Health Care Resources

No special equipment is needed. On occasion, clients may require dressings after surgical intervention. Referral to home care agencies may be indicated if clients and family members or significant others require instruction on any dimension of follow-up care, such as dressing changes, IV therapy, monitoring of potential complications, and continued nutritional problems (Chart 58–6).

Family members may need help to modify eating habits and patterns.

 Evaluation

On the basis of the identified nursing diagnoses and collaborative problems, the nurse evaluates the care for the client with ulcer disease. The expected outcomes may include that the client will

- State that pain is reduced or alleviated and that comfort is achieved
- Identify potential causes of and risks for recurrence of disease
- Follow a nutritious diet that includes essential nutrients
- State and report early symptoms of recurrence or complications
- Adhere to a plan for follow-up care and return to the previous level of function in 6–8 weeks

---

Chart 58–6

Focused Assessment for Ambulatory Care with Ulcer Disease

- Assess gastrointestinal and cardiovascular status, including:
  - Vital signs, including orthostatic vital signs
  - Skin color
  - Presence of abdominal pain (location, severity, character, duration, precipitating factors, and relief measures)
  - Character, color, and consistency of stools
  - Changes in bowel elimination pattern
  - Hemoglobin and hematocrit
  - Bowel sounds; palpate for areas of tenderness
- Assess nutritional status, including:
  - Dietary patterns and habits
  - Intake of caffeine and alcohol
  - Relationship of food to symptoms
- Assess medication history
  - Use of steroids
  - Use of NSAIDs
  - Use of over-the-counter medications
- Assess client's coping style
  - Recent stressors
  - Past coping style
- Assess client's understanding of illness and ability to comply with therapeutic regime
  - Symptoms to report to health care provider
  - Expected and side effects of medications
  - Food and drug interactions

Zollinger-Ellison Syndrome

Zollinger-Ellison syndrome is a hormonally induced peptic ulcer. It is associated with autonomous secretion of gastrin by a rare islet cell tumor in the pancreas (gastrinoma). The characteristic features are hypersecretion of acid (with a high ratio of basal acid output to maximal acid output) and hypergastrinemia (increased secretion of gastrin).

In addition to the peptic ulcer associated with gastrinoma, diarrhea may be a manifestation of this disorder. The diarrhea may be associated with fat maldigestion from a low level of duodenal-inactivating pancreatic lipase or with malabsorption related to acid-induced injury of the villi.

Clinical manifestations are largely related to gastric acid hypersecretion. In part, this situation is due to hyperplasia of the gastric mucosa induced by the trophic effect of gastrin.

The aim of therapy is to suppress acid secretion. Control of the hypersecretion controls the client's symptoms. For most clients, the health care provider prescribes large doses of H_2 receptor antagonists, such as ranitidine (Zantac). Anticholinergic drugs supplement their use.

The health care provider uses 2-hour gastric aspirations or 24-hour pH monitoring to evaluate symptom control. Endoscopy is also indicated to evaluate clinical response. If medical therapy fails, the health care provider may choose to perform a vagotomy and pyloroplasty to supplement the use of H_2 receptor antagonists for controlling hypersecretion. A total gastrectomy is the surgical approach of choice for this disorder if vagotomy, pyloroplasty, and medical therapy are inadequate.

Gastric Carcinoma

Overview

Gastric carcinoma refers to malignant neoplasms in the stomach. Adenocarcinomas are the most common type of cancer; malignant lymphoma is the second most common.

Although the incidence of gastric cancer is decreasing in the United States, it is the sixth most common cause of cancer-related death. The onset is insidious, and the disease is often advanced when detected.

Pathophysiology

Gastric adenocarcinoma develops from the mucous membrane within the stomach. Early gastric cancer is defined in pathologic terms (disease involving only the mucosa or submucosa), but it is seldom symptomatic. On microscopic examination, the cells resemble intestinal metaplasia (abnormal tissue development). Most gastric cancers develop in the pyloric and antral regions.

Gastric cancers have several methods of extension, including

- Spread within the gastric wall and into regional lymphatics
- Direct invasion of adjacent organs (e.g., liver, pancreas, and transverse colon)
- Hematogenous spread via the portal vein to the liver and via the systemic circulation to the lungs and bones (the most common mode of metastasis)
- Peritoneal seeding into the involved gastric serosa to the omentum, peritoneum, ovary, and pelvic cul-de-sac

Peritoneal seeding may produce a firm mass (referred to as a rectal shelf, or Blumer's shelf), which is an indicator of advanced cancer. The intramural lymphatics readily allow horizontal spread within the gastric wall. Extramural lymphatics carry tumor deposits to lymph nodes in more than 50% of operable cases.

In people with advanced gastric cancer, there is invasion of the muscularis or beyond. These lesions are not amenable to curative resection. Overall, results of treatment have not significantly improved during the past 40 years.

Most clients in the United States have stage III or stage IV disease (late stages) when the cancer is diagnosed. Clients with lesions at the cardia or fundus have a poor prognosis because the lesions are usually advanced when detected. The prognosis and treatment depend on the stage of disease and the general health status of the client.

Etiology

No etiologic factor has been proven conclusively to cause gastric cancer. Pernicious anemia, gastric polyps, chronic atrophic gastritis, and achlorhydria (absence of secretion of hydrochloric acid) seem to be associated with an increased risk for gastric cancer. Because of changes in the gastric mucosa, carcinogens may be absorbed more when gastritis has been present.

Gastric cancer seems to be positively correlated with the ingestion of starch, pickled foods, salted fish, salted meat, and nitrates from processed foods and with a high salt consumption. It is negatively correlated with the ingestion of whole milk, fresh vegetables, and vitamin C. Cigarette smoking is associated with gastric carcinoma, and genetic factors may play a role because there is an increased incidence in direct relatives of clients with gastric cancer.

Gastric surgery, especially a Billroth II procedure for benign conditions, seems to increase the risk for gastric cancer, probably because of the development of atrophic gastritis. Bile reflux may also result in mucosal changes. Most cancers occur 20 years after the original surgical procedure.

Incidence/Prevalence

In the United States and other Western countries, the incidence of gastric carcinoma has steadily decreased over the past 50 years. However, 24,000 new cases are diagnosed each year, causing an estimated 14,000 deaths. The decline in the death rate is believed to be due primarily to the decreasing incidence of the disease rather than to improvements in treatment.

TRANSCULTURAL CONSIDERATIONS

Gastric cancer occurs more frequently in men than in women. The incidence and mortality rates increase with age, in African Americans and Japanese Americans, and in lower socioeconomic groups. The highest incidence of gastric cancer is in men older than 70 years. In the United States, the incidence of gastric cancer is higher in the North Central and Northeast regions (Giger & Davidhizar, 1995).

Collaborative Management

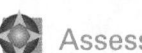 Assessment

➤ Physical Assessment/Clinical Manifestations

Although clients with *early* gastric cancer may have no symptoms, indigestion (heartburn) and abdominal discomfort are the *most* common symptoms (Chart 58–7). These symptoms are often ignored, however, or a change in diet or use of antacids relieves them. As the tumor grows, these symptoms become more severe and do not respond to diet changes or antacids. The second most frequent symptom is loss of appetite accompanied by a bloated feeling, weight loss, and fatigue. As the disease becomes more advanced, vomiting represents pronounced dilation, thickening of the stomach wall, or pyloric obstruction. Obstructive symptoms appear earlier with tumors located near the pylorus than with fundic lesions. There are no physical findings specifically associated with early gastric cancer. Clients with advanced disease may present with occult blood in the stools and may have iron-deficiency anemia, causing pallor.

Chart 58–7

Key Features of Early Versus Advanced Gastric Cancer

Early Gastric Cancer

- Indigestion
- Abdominal discomfort relieved with antacids
- Loss of appetite
- Bloated feeling
- Weight loss
- Fatigue

(*Note:* Many clients with early gastric cancer have no clinical manifestations.)

Advanced Gastric Cancer

- Vomiting
- Occult blood in the stool
- Iron deficiency anemia
- Palpable epigastric mass
- Enlarged lymph nodes
- Pallor
- Cachexia
- Other distant manifestations:
  - Virchow's nodes
  - Blumer's shelf
  - Krukenberg's tumor

In *advanced* gastric carcinoma, physical assessment findings may be absent, or a palpable epigastric mass may suggest hepatomegaly from metastatic disease or ascites. Hard, enlarged lymph nodes in the left supraclavicular chain, left axilla, or umbilicus may be the result of metastasis from gastric cancer. Masses on the right suggest metastasis in the perigastric lymph nodes or liver. Signs of distant metastasis include

- Virchow's (sentinel or signal) nodes (enlarged supraclavicular lymph nodes, especially on the left)
- Blumer's shelf (resulting from peritoneal seeding)
- Infiltration of the umbilicus
- Krukenberg's tumor (metastatic ovarian tumor)

Acanthosis nigricans, a dermatosis with roughness and pigmentation found in the axilla, is associated with cancer of the stomach. Recurrent episodes of thrombophlebitis unexplained by local findings in the extremities should alert the health care provider of the possibility of an intra-abdominal (especially gastric and pancreatic) cancer.

➤ Diagnostic Assessment

In clients with advanced disease, anemia is evidenced by low hematocrit and hemoglobin values. Clients may have macrocytic or microcytic anemia associated with decreased iron or vitamin B_{12} absorption. The stool may be positive for occult blood.

Hypoalbuminemia and abnormal results of liver tests (such as bilirubin and alkaline phosphatase) occur with advanced disease and with hepatic metastasis. The level of carcinoembryonic antigen (CEA) is elevated in *advanced* cancer of the stomach.

➤ Radiographic Assessment

An upper gastrointestinal (GI) series is usually the first diagnostic test. A polypoid mass, ulcer crater, or thickened fibrotic gastric wall may suggest gastric cancer.

➤ Other Diagnostic Assessment

The health care provider uses esophagogastroduodenoscopy (EGD) for definitive diagnosis of gastric cancer. The lesion can be viewed directly in this study. Benign and malignant lesions can be delineated. Cytologic brushing or gavage and biopsy treatment may determine the presence of cancer cells.

 Interventions

Management of gastric cancer includes drug therapy, radiation, and/or surgery.

Nonsurgical Management. Although surgery is the only potentially curative treatment, radiation may be used as an adjuvant therapy. Adjuvant chemotherapy is not routinely used for curative treatment. Radiation and chemotherapy commonly prolong survival of clients with advanced gastric disease.

Drug Therapy. Fluorouracil (5-FU) is the most common chemotherapeutic agent for gastric cancer. The FAM protocol, which combines 5-FU, doxorubicin (Adriamycin), and mitomycin C, has also been used for treatment of advanced gastric cancer. (Chapter 27 discusses chemotherapy in detail.)

Radiation Therapy. When used as adjuvant therapy with surgery, radiation may be given before surgery to shrink a tumor or postoperatively to kill residual tumor cells. Intraoperative radiotherapy is being studied.

The most common side effects experienced by clients undergoing radiation include impaired skin integrity, fatigue, and anorexia. Nausea, vomiting, and diarrhea may occur approximately 1 week after treatment is initiated and continue but diminish for a month or more after treatment (see Chap. 27).

Surgical Management. In early gastric cancer, surgery is usually curative. Curative resection can be offered to only 40%–60% of clients, however, because the remainder has advanced disease. Most clients with advanced disease are candidates for palliative surgical treatment. Metastasis in the supraclavicular lymph nodes (Virchow's nodes), inguinal lymph nodes, liver, umbilicus, or perirectal wall indicates that the opportunity for cure by resection has been lost. Palliative resection may significantly improve the quality of life for a client suffering from obstruction, hemorrhage, or pain.

Preoperative Care. The health care provider gives the client and the family an explanation of the disease and the available treatment options (potentially curative or palliative). The nurse reinforces and clarifies the information given. Preoperative care is similar to that provided for the client undergoing general anesthesia and abdominal surgery (see Chap. 20).

Operative Procedures. When the tumor is located in the distal (lower) two thirds of the stomach, a subtotal gastrectomy typically is performed. The surgeon uses a Billroth I or Billroth II procedure (see surgical management of peptic ulcer disease). The omentum, spleen, and relevant nodes are also removed.

For the client with a growth in the upper third of the stomach, a total gastrectomy is required. Because the disability after total gastrectomy is so severe, this procedure is not performed routinely or palliatively. In this procedure, the surgeon removes the entire stomach, with en bloc removal of the spleen and omentum. The surgeon sutures the esophagus to the duodenum or jejunum to reestablish continuity of the GI tract.

Clients with tumors at the gastric outlet who are not candidates for subtotal or total gastrectomy may undergo gastroenterostomy for palliation. The surgeon creates a passage between the body of the stomach and the small bowel, often the duodenum (see Fig. 58–7).

Postoperative Care. Clients require the standard postoperative care that is given to clients who receive general anesthesia (see Chap. 22). Complications after gastric surgery may include

- Duodenal stump leakage
- Hemorrhage
- Obstruction
- Gastric dilation resulting in reflux gastritis
- Delayed gastric emptying
- Anemia
- Nutritional deficiency
- Dumping syndrome

These complications are discussed earlier in the peptic ulcer disease section.

Nutritional therapy is a vital aspect of preoperative and postoperative management of the client with gastric cancer. Severe tissue wasting is a major clinical complication in clients with advanced disease. Early satiety, abdominal distention, and pain may contribute to inadequate intake of nutrients. Clients may lose up to 10% of total body weight. Steatorrhea related to malabsorption may contribute to this problem if a total or partial gastrectomy has been performed.

Pain medication may relieve discomfort and thus allow the client to eat or drink more comfortably. Medications for relief of nausea, such as prochlorperazine (Compazine) and thiethylperazine (Torecan), may also improve the client's appetite.

To correct malnutrition before surgery, the health care provider may prescribe supplements to the diet and/or total parenteral nutrition (TPN). Vitamins with minerals, iron, and protein supplements are essential for correction of nutritional deficits. To improve calorie intake, the nurse works with the client and family or significant others to determine the client's food preferences, cultural norms, and usual eating habits. Clients tend to do better when they eat frequent small meals and avoid spicy foods. In collaboration with the dietitian, the nurse guides the client and family in providing the most nutrients and calories. Counseling about methods of preparation and types of food that increase calorie and protein intake is essential. The nurse maintains intake, output, and calorie counts on a daily basis and records weights at least weekly (see Chap. 64).

TPN may also be used postoperatively to provide necessary nutrients and prevent further deficiencies until oral intake is adequate. Oral intake should begin with fluids and progress to solids as tolerated by the client. For clients who had esophageal or stomach surgery, regurgitation may result from eating too much or too fast. After oral feedings are restarted, the nurse observes the client for signs and symptoms of the dumping syndrome. The nurse teaches the client the manifestations of the syndrome and how to avert it by frequent meals (six daily feedings) and a diet of high-protein, high-fat, low-carbohydrate foods (see Table 58–3). This diet is intended for clients who have recovered sufficiently from gastric surgery to eat regular foods but who are experiencing, or are likely to experience, the dumping (or jejunal) syndrome caused by the formation of a concentrated hyperosmolar solution.

The basic principles of the diet are the same as those for the postgastrectomy diet, except that regular foods are used in place of bland foods. Liquids should not be taken with meals. Milk and dairy products are usually eliminated because many clients are lactose-intolerant and have symptoms after the ingestion of milk-containing products.

If adequate nutrition cannot be attained with diet management after 2–3 months, TPN may be necessary, either alone or to supplement oral intake. Weight loss of 10% or more of usual body weight necessitates consideration of TPN. The nurse informs the client that an IV line will be placed to allow this therapy. Home TPN is available (see Chapter 64 for discussion of care needed with TPN). Malabsorption of iron, vitamin B_{12}, and calcium may necessitate replacement therapy.

 Continuing Care

Clients who have undergone total gastrectomy and those who are debilitated with advanced gastric cancer are discharged to home with maximal assistance or to a subacute unit. Clients who have undergone subtotal gastrectomy but who are not debilitated may be discharged to home with partial assistance for activities of daily living. Many clients experience recurrence of the cancer and need regular follow-up examinations and radiographic assessments.

The client and family need a list of medications to be taken and when they should be given. The nurse demonstrates home treatments, such as dressing changes; the client and family members responsible for care demonstrate these procedures in return.

➤ *Home Care Management*

The nurse or discharge planner assesses for ease of reaching the bathroom, bedroom, and kitchen facilities, enabling the client to have mobility and care. It is important to know who will help care for the client at home and who will provide the family caregiver with relief or assistance.

> ## Health Teaching

The nurse instructs the client and family or significant others about recommended nutritional therapy, pain management, and medications. If clients are discharged with dressings, the nurse teaches about clean dressing changes. The nurse identifies the signs and symptoms of incisional infection (such as fever, redness, and drainage) that are to be reported. Clients who will be receiving radiation therapy or chemotherapy require instructions related to the side effects of these treatments. See Chapter 27 for education for clients receiving chemotherapy or radiation therapy.

Clients may fear returning home because of their inability to care for themselves adequately and to control or minimize pain. Enlisting family and health care resources for the client may ease some of this anxiety. The family needs adequate information and support systems to make the transition to home care easier for the client. If family members or significant others are still trying to cope with the diagnosis and poor prognosis of the client, their coping abilities will be impaired. If prognosis is poor, the client and the family need continued professional support to cope with death and dying. (Chapter 27 discusses the psychosocial aspects of cancer, and Chapter 12 describes nursing interventions for the dying client.)

Clients and families need continued support and an empathic approach from the nurse. It is essential that clients for whom cure is not possible, those in whom relapse has occurred, and those who do not respond to treatment do not feel abandoned. Clients and families must be included in making all decisions about further care. Many clients with gastric cancer must make a trade-off between quality of life and possible survival. The psychosocial dimensions of care are as important a consideration as are the diagnostic and therapeutic dimensions.

> ## Health Care Resources

A home health referral provides ongoing assessment, assistance, and encouragement to the client and family or significant others at home. A home health nurse can help with physical care procedures and can provide valuable psychological support as well. This combination of resources helps minimize anxiety.

Other referrals that might be necessary are to a dietitian, professional counselor, and clergy or religious or spiritual leader. Referral to a hospice team is a critical component of home care. So that comprehensive care is ensured, the coordinator or case manager of the client's care should be the person to arrange the referrals. Appropriate support groups, such as I Can Cope provided by the American Cancer Society, can be a major resource (see Chap. 27).

CASE STUDY for the Client with Ulcer Disease

■ A 48-year-old woman comes to the employee health office complaining of heartburn, indigestion, and pain during the middle of the night. She is a computer technician who has recently served as the project coordinator at work for a computer and software upgrade.

She is in generally good health and has no history of health problems or concerns. She does report taking some over-the-counter ibuprofen and antacids as needed, and she typically drinks six cups of coffee a day. You ask her to go into the examination room for a further assessment.

QUESTIONS:

1. When taking a history from this client, what important questions should you ask?
2. Which components of physical assessment should you perform?
3. She tells you her stools are dark and appear black. Given this statement, what should you do first?

SELECTED BIBLIOGRAPHY

Ben-Menachem, T., McCarthy, B. D., Fogel, R., Schiffman, R. M., Patel, R. V., Zarowitz, B. J., Nerenz, D. R., & Bresalier, R. S. (1996). Prophylaxis for stress-related gastrointestinal hemorrhage: A cost effectiveness analysis. *Critical Care Medicine, 24*(2), 338–345.

Bertoni, G., Sassatelli, R., Nigrisoli, E., Tansini, P., Bianchi, G., Casa, G. D., Bagni, A., & Bedogni, G. (1996). Triple therapy with Azithromycin, Omeprazole, and Amoxicillin is highly effective in the eradication of *Helicobacter pylori*: A controlled trial versus Omeprazole plus Amoxicillin. *The American Journal of Gastroenterology 91*(2), 258–263.

Cello, J. P. (1995). *Helicobacter pylori* and peptic ulcer disease. *American Roentgen Review, 164,* 283–286.

Ching, C. K., & Lam, S. K. (1995). Drug therapy of peptic ulcer disease. *British Journal of Hospital Medicine, 54,* 101–106.

Cook, D. J., Reeve, B. K., Guyatt, G. H., Heyland, D. K., Griffith, L. E., Buckingham, L., & Tryba, M. (1996). Stress ulcer prophylaxis in critically ill patients: Resolving discordant metal-analyses. *Journal of American Medical Association, 275*(4), 308–314.

Cromwell, D. M., & Pasricha, P. J. (1996). Endoscopy or empirical treatment for peptic ulcer disease: Decision, decisions *Gastroenterology, 110*(4), 1314–1316.

Cryer, B., & Feldman, M. (1994). Peptic ulcer disease in the elderly. *Seminars in Gastrointestinal Disease, 5*(4), 166–178.

Davenport, R. J., Dennis, M. S., & Warlow, C. P. (1996). Gastrointestinal hemorrhage after acute stroke. *Stroke, 27*(3), 421–424.

Davis, S. (1996). Triple therapy and *Helicobacter pylori. Australian Family Physician, 25*(1), 53–59.

DiMario, F., Leandro, G., Battaglia, G., Pitotto, A., DelSanto, P., Vianello, F., Franceschi, M., Ferrana, M., Dal Bianco, T., & Vigneri, S. (1996). Do concomitant diseases and therapies affect the persistence of ulcer symptoms in the elderly? *Digestive Diseases and Science, 41*(1), 17–21.

Elfant, A. B., Levine, S. M., Peikin, S. R., Cencora, B., Mendez, L., Pello, M. J., Atabek, U. M., Alexander, J. B., Spence, R. K., & Camishion, R. C. (1995). Bioavailability of medication delivered via nasogastric tube is decreased in the immediate postoperative period. *American Journal of Surgery, 169*(4), 430–432.

Fuchs, C. S., & Mayer, R. J. (1995). Gastric carcinoma. *The New England Journal of Medicine, 333*(1), 32–41.

Giger, J. N. & Davidhizar, R. E. (1995). *Transcultural nursing: Assessment and Intervention,* (2nd ed.). St. Louis: Mosby.

Greenberg, P. D., Koch, J., & Cello, J. P. (1996). Clinical utility and cost effectiveness of *Helicobacter pylori* testing for patients with duodenal and gastric ulcer. *The Amercian Journal Gastroenterology, 91*(2), 228–232.

Heslin, J. M. (1997). Peptic ulcer disease. *Nursing97, 27*(1), 34–40.

Heximer, B. (1996, July). Spontaneous balloon rupture. *RN,* 22–25.

Hudson, N., Faulkner, G., Smith, S. J., et al. (1995). Late mortality in elderly patients surviving acute peptic ulcer bleeding. *Gut, 37*(2), 177–181.

Jaspersen, D. (1995). *Helicobacter pylori* eradication: the best long-term prophylaxis for ulcer bleeding recurrence? *Endoscopy, 27*(8), 622–625.

Lanza, L. L., Walker, A. M., Bortnichak, E. A., & Dreyer, N. A. (1995). Peptic ulcer and gastrointestinal hemorrhage associated with nonsteroidal anti-inflammatory drug use in patients younger than 65 years: A large health maintenance organization cohort study. *Archives of Internal Medicine, 155*(13), 1371–1377.

Levine, M. S., & Rubesin, S. E. (1995). The *Helicobacter pylori* revolution: Radiologic perspective. *Radiology, 195,* 593–596.

McConnell, E. A. (1994). Managing a nasoenteric-decompression tube. *Nursing, 24,* 18.

Meko, J. B., & Norton, J. A. (1995). Management of patients with Zollinger-Ellison syndrome. *Annual Review of Medicine, 46,* 395–411.

Navab, F., & Steingrub, J. (1995). Stress ulcer: Is routine prophylaxis necessary? *The American Journal of Gastroenterology, 90*(5), 708–712.

Olbe, L., Hamlet, A., Dalenback, J., & Fandriks, L. (1996). A mechanism by which *Helicobacter pylori* infection of the antrum contributes to the development of duodenal ulcer. *Gastroenterology, 110*(5), 1386–1394.

Perri, F., Ghoos, Y. F., Maes, B. D., Geypens, B. J., Ectors, N., Geboes, K., Hiele, M. I., & Rutgeerts, P. J. (1996). Gastric emptying and *Helicobacter pylori* infection in duodenal ulcer disease. *Digestive Disease and Science, 41*(3), 462–468.

Pound, S. E., & Heading, R. C. (1995). Diagnosis and treatment of dyspepsia in the elderly. *Drugs and Aging, 7*(5), 347–354.

Raskin, J. B., White, R. H., Jaszewski, R., Korsten, M. A., Shubert, T. T., & Fort, J. G. (1996). Misoprostol and ranitidine in the prevention of NSAID-induced ulcers: A prospective, double-blind, multicenter study. *The American Journal of Gastroenterology, 91*(2), 223–227.

Rauws, E. A. & van der Hulst, R. W. (1995).Current guidelines for the eradication of *Helicobacter pylori* in peptic ulcer disease. *Drugs, 50*(6), 984–990.

Rauws, E. A. J., & Tytgat, G. N. J. (1995). *Helicobacter pylori* in duodenal and gastric ulcer. *Bailliere's Clinical Gastroenterology, 9*(3)529–547.

Roth, S. H. (1995). From peptic ulcer to NSAID gastropathy's: An evolving nosology. *Drugs and Aging, 6*(5), 358–367.

Sawyers, J. (1995). Gastric carcinoma. *Currrent Problems in Medicine, 32*(2), 106–178.

Talley, N. J. (1996). Modern management of dyspepsia. *Australian Family Physician, 25*(1), 47–52.

Thijs, J. C., Kuipers, E. J., van Zwet, A. A., Pena, A. S., & deGraff, J. (1995). Treatment of *Helicobacter pylori* infections. *Quality Journal of Medicine, 88,* 369–389.

Weber, H. C., Orbuch, M., & Jensen, R. T. (1995). Diagnosis and management of Zollinger-Ellison syndrome. *Seminars in Gastrointestinal Disease, 6*(2), 79–89.

SUGGESTED READINGS

Heslin, J.M. (1997). Peptic ulcer disease. *Nursing97, 27*(l), 34–40.

This article describes peptic ulcer disease (PUD) and its effect on the esophagus (only 5% occurs here), stomach, and duodenum. A chart outlining the major groups of drugs used in PUD includes special considerations for nursing practice. A CEU quiz can be found at the end of the article.

Heximer, B. (1996, July). Spontaneous balloon rupture. *RN* 22–25.

This article describes nursing interventions to prevent and detect rupture of the balloon of gastrostomy tube. These types of tubes may be used for decompression and, eventually, feeding purposes following gastric surgery. The author provides a helpful discussion of commonly occurring problems, such as migration of the gastrostomy tube, overinflation or deterioration of the balloon, and increased intra-abdominal pressure. A number of helpful suggestions are provided regarding monitoring and caring for these devices.

Sawyers, J. (1995). Gastric carcinoma. *Current Problems in Medicine, 32*(2) 106–178.

This paper serves as a complete review about gastric cancer, including its history. It discusses precancerous lesions as well as the factors associated with the development of malignant changes. This monograph also gives a complete description of the diagnostic evaluation and the staging and classification of this disease. Surgery, radiation, chemotherapy, and new approaches to treatment are explained and discussed thoroughly.

Chapter 59

INTERVENTIONS FOR CLIENTS WITH INTESTINAL DISORDERS

Intestinal disorders can be classified as inflammatory or noninflammatory. This chapter reviews noninflammatory intestinal disorders. Noninflammatory intestinal disorders include obstructions, malignant neoplasms, malabsorption, and trauma.

Many intestinal disorders are clinically manifested by changes in stool pattern, abdominal pain, and rectal bleeding (Fig. 59–1). These symptoms can be vague and insidious in onset or abrupt with significant insult to the client. Identification of the specific disorder is often difficult because of common symptoms among people with various intestinal diseases.

IRRITABLE BOWEL SYNDROME

Overview

Irritable bowel syndrome (IBS), also called spastic bowel, nonulcerative colitis, and mucous colitis, is the most common digestive disorder in the United States. IBS is not a true colitis in that there is no inflammation. It primarily entails a change in bowel habits with crampy, abdominal pain; there is no organic disease.

The diagnosis of IBS is made through the exclusion of other diseases that mimic its symptoms. Diagnostic studies strongly suggest that IBS is a disorder of intestinal motility. This change in motility may result from anxiety, stress, depression, fear, food, drugs, toxins, and colonic distention.

Because of motility changes, the bowel elimination pattern changes to one of diarrhea, constipation, or alternating diarrhea and constipation. Clients may report an onset of IBS in adolescence or later in life. Bowel function changes progressively and eventually forms a characteristic pattern. The most common pattern is diarrhea alternating with constipation. The course of the illness is generally specific to the client, and most clients can identify factors that precipitate exacerbations, such as diet, stress, or anxiety. There are no changes in the bowel mucosa and, therefore, no serious health consequences. However, the irregular bowel patterns and associated cramps often wreak havoc on the person's lifestyle.

The exact cause of IBS is unknown, and it is considered a functional disorder. Physical factors, such as diverticular disease, ingestion of coffee or other gastric stimulants, or lactose intolerance, may contribute to IBS. IBS follows a pattern of intermittent remissions and exacerbations.

Reliable data for the incidence of IBS are not available. IBS is estimated to affect up to 20% of the general population in Western countries (McQuaid, 1995).

TRANSCULTURAL CONSIDERATIONS

More than two thirds of the population with IBS are women. The incidence is higher among Caucasians and people of Jewish descent. Most people report symptoms before the age of 35 (McQuaid, 1995).

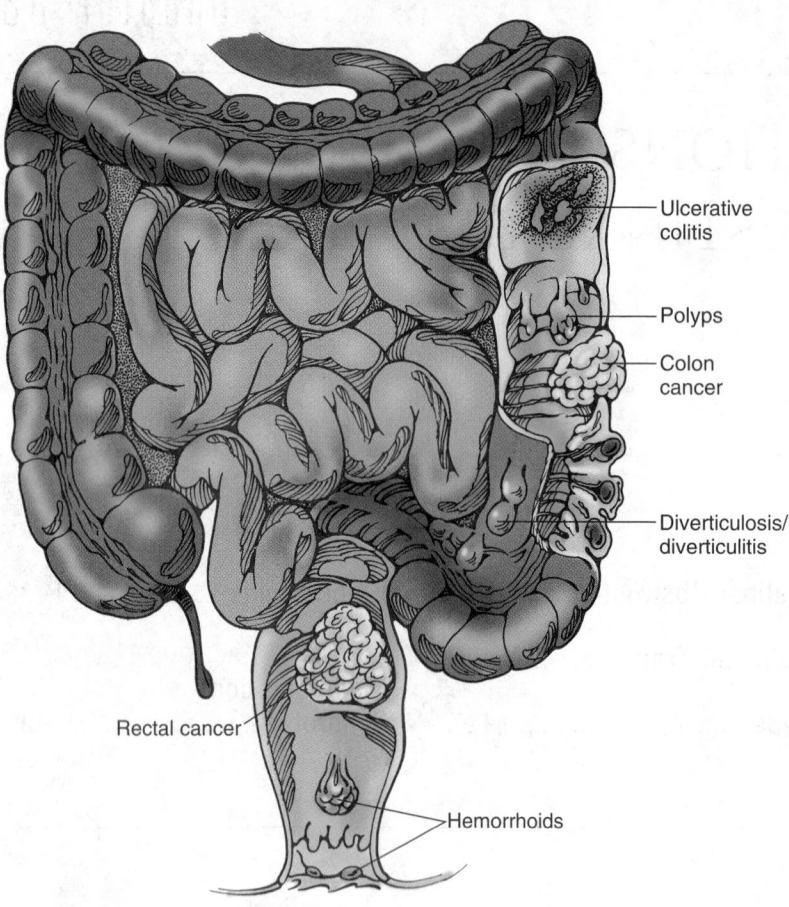

Ulcerative colitis

Polyps

Colon cancer

Diverticulosis/ diverticulitis

Rectal cancer

Hemorrhoids

Figure 59–1. Common causes of lower gastrointestinal bleeding.

Collaborative Management

 Assessment

Irritable bowel syndrome is typically diagnosed after many episodes of diarrhea or constipation. A flare consisting of worsening cramps, abdominal pain, and diarrhea or constipation usually brings the client to the health care provider. The most common symptom of IBS is pain in the left lower quadrant of the abdomen. The client reports increased pain after eating and relief after a bowel movement. Nausea may be associated with mealtime and defecation. The crampy abdominal patterns are accompanied by constipation or diarrhea. The constipated stools are small and hard, generally followed by several softer stools. The diarrheal stools are soft and watery, and mucus is frequently present in the stools.

Clients with IBS frequently complain of belching, gas, anorexia, and bloating. Some clients may also experience fatigue, anxiety, headaches, and difficulty concentrating.

The nurse inspects and auscultates the abdomen. Bowel sounds are generally within normal range and may be somewhat quiet with constipation. When percussing the abdomen, tympanic sounds may be heard over loops of filled bowel. On palpation, there may be diffuse tenderness, which is generally worse if the sigmoid colon is palpable. The rectal examination may reveal hard or soft stool.

The client generally looks well but perhaps fatigued.

Weight is stable, and nutritional and fluid levels are within normal ranges.

An IBS client may appear tense and anxious and may have recently undergone stress or emotional tension. The client is often unaware of any correlation between stressors and changes in bowel patterns. The nurse can assist the client to correlate pertinent life events to bowel patterns (e.g., by a time line of life events).

Routine laboratory work (including a complete blood count, serologic tests, serum albumin, erythrocyte sedimentation rate, and stools for occult blood) is normal in IBS. The health care provider routinely orders a barium enema examination for clients suspected of having IBS. Colonic spasm is often noted during the procedure; however, this finding is not diagnostic. In the absence of other diagnostic findings, colonic spasm supports the diagnosis (Fig. 59–2).

The evaluation of IBS is not complete without flexible sigmoidoscopy in adults younger than 40 years and colonoscopy in adults older than 40 years. This examination often demonstrates intense spastic contractions, which frequently stimulate painful sensations. Otherwise, the bowel mucosa appears continuous, smooth, and pink.

Interventions

The client with IBS is most often cared for on an ambulatory basis. Interventions are directed at the relief and

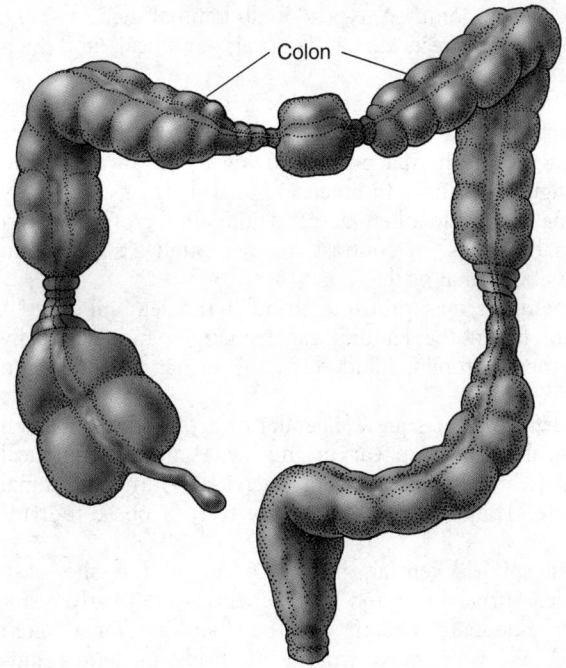

Figure 59–2. Spastic contractions of the colon, as they occur with irritable bowel syndrome.

management of symptoms. The health care provider may use a number of treatment modalities, including drug therapy, diet therapy, stress management, exercise, and modification of daily routines.

Drug Therapy. The health care provider typically prescribes bulk-forming laxatives, antidiarrheal agents, and anticholinergic agents. The use of one or a combination of products can help in managing unpleasant symptoms.

The bulk-forming laxatives, such as psyllium hydrophilic mucilloid (Metamucil) or calcium polycarbophil (Mitrolan), are generally taken at mealtimes with a glassful of water. The hydrophilic properties of these medications help prevent dry, hard, or liquid stools.

Antidiarrheal agents, such as diphenoxylate hydrochloride with atropine sulfate (Lomotil), loperamide (Imodium), or camphorated tincture of opium (paregoric), help decrease cramping and frequent stools (Chart 59–1). Long-term therapy with these drugs, however, is not recommended because these agents carry a certain risk of dependency.

Anticholinergics or antispasmodics, such as dicyclomine hydrochloride (Bentyl, Bentylol✤) and propantheline bromide (Pro-Banthine, Popanthel✤), help relieve abdominal cramping and intestinal spasm. If clients experience postprandial (after eating) discomfort, the client should take these medications 30–45 minutes before mealtime.

Diet Therapy. Dietary fiber and bulk help produce bulky, soft stools and establish regular bowel habits. The client should ingest approximately 30–40 g of fiber each day. Eating regular meals, drinking 8–10 cups of liquid each day, and chewing food slowly promote normal bowel function. The nurse may need to collaborate with the dietitian to help the client and family or significant others with meal planning.

The nurse assists the client to identify and eliminate offending or upsetting foods. Regular mealtimes are emphasized. The client is advised to avoid alcohol, excess caffeine, and other gastric irritants. Milk and milk products are to be avoided if the client has a documented lactose intolerance or if the client can specify milk as an aggravating factor.

Chart 59–1

Drug Therapy for the Treatment of Diarrhea

Drug	Usual Dosage	Nursing Interventions	Rationale
Diphenoxylate hydrochloride and atropine sulfate (Lomotil)	• 1 tablet 6 times/day; no more than 6 tablets in 24 hr	• Assess for abdominal distention, pain, and fever.	• These symptoms may indicate a bacterial organism in the gastrointestinal (GI) tract. Diarrhea should not be suppressed in the presence of GI infection.
		• Assess for sedation, dry mouth, urinary retention, and rash.	• These are common side effects.
Loperamide (Imodium)	• 2 mg after each loose stool; maximum of 16 mg/day	• Assess for abdominal distention, pain, and fever.	• These symptoms may indicate a bacterial organism in the GI tract. Diarrhea should not be suppressed if GI infection is present.
		• Assess for drowsiness, fatigue, and dry mouth.	• These are common side effects.
Camphorated tincture of opium (paregoric)	• 0.6 mL qid PO; no more than 6 mL/day	• Assess for abdominal distention, pain, and fever.	• These symptoms may represent a bacterial infection.
		• Assess for nausea and vomiting.	• These are side effects.

Stress Management. Stress management is based on the client's current and ongoing stressors and available resources. After the nurse completes a detailed psychosocial assessment, the nurse and the client set expected outcomes and plan appropriate interventions. Relaxation techniques can help the client learn skills for managing the illness. Understanding the illness empowers the client to take certain actions (e.g., diet modification and exercise) that can significantly affect the course of the illness.

If the client is in a stressful work or family situation, personal counseling may be helpful. The nurse assists the client in making appointments or makes appropriate referrals. The opportunity to discuss problems and attempt creative problem solving is often helpful. (Chapter 8 describes additional nursing interventions for assisting the client to cope.)

Exercise and Modification of Daily Routines. The nurse teaches the client that regular exercise is important for managing stress and promoting regular bowel elimination. The client must be alert to the urge to defecate and evacuate promptly to avoid straining. The client should plan to allow time and privacy in the bathroom. The nurse assists the client in maintaining a stool count and determining the consistency, color, and character of the stools.

HERNIATION

Overview

A hernia is a weakness in the abdominal muscle wall through which a segment of the bowel or other abdominal structure protrudes. Hernias can also penetrate through any other defect in the abdominal wall, through the diaphragm, or through other structures in the abdominal cavity.

Hernias generally result from a defect in the integrity of the muscle wall and increased intra-abdominal pressure. Defects in the muscle wall result from weakened collagen or widened spaces at the inguinal ligament. These muscle weaknesses can be inherited or acquired as part of the aging process. Increases in intra-abdominal pressure as a result of pregnancy, obesity, abdominal distention, ascites, heavy lifting, or coughing can also contribute to their occurrence.

The most common types of abdominal hernias (Fig. 59–3) are indirect, direct, femoral, umbilical, and incisional.

An *indirect* inguinal hernia is a sac formed from the peritoneum that contains a portion of the intestine or omentum. The hernia pushes downward at an angle into the inguinal canal. Indirect inguinal hernias frequently become large and often descend into the scrotum. *Direct* inguinal hernias, in contrast, pass through a weak point in the abdominal wall.

Femoral hernias protrude through the femoral ring. A plug of fat in the femoral canal enlarges and eventually pulls the peritoneum and often the urinary bladder into the sac.

Umbilical hernias are congenital or acquired. Congenital umbilical hernias appear in infancy. Acquired umbilical hernias directly result from increased intra-abdominal pressure. They are most frequently seen in obese individuals.

Incisional, or ventral, hernias occur at the site of a previous surgical incision. These hernias frequently result from inadequate healing of the incision, most often caused by postoperative wound infections, inadequate nutrition, and obesity.

Hernias may also be classified as reducible, irreducible (incarcerated), or strangulated.

A hernia is *reducible* when the contents of the hernial sac can be replaced into the abdominal cavity by gentle pressure. An *irreducible* (incarcerated) hernia cannot be reduced or placed back into the abdominal cavity. A hernia is *strangulated* when the blood supply to the herniated segment of the bowel is cut off by pressure from the hernial ring (the band of muscle around the hernia). If a hernia is strangulated, there is ischemia and obstruction of the bowel loop. This can lead to necrosis of the bowel and possibly bowel perforation. Signs of strangulation are abdominal distention, nausea, vomiting, pain, fever, and tachycardia.

ELDERLY CONSIDERATIONS

The elderly client with a strangulated hernia may not complain of pain but usually has nausea and vomiting. A change in mental status may also occur.

Any of these symptoms require immediate medical and

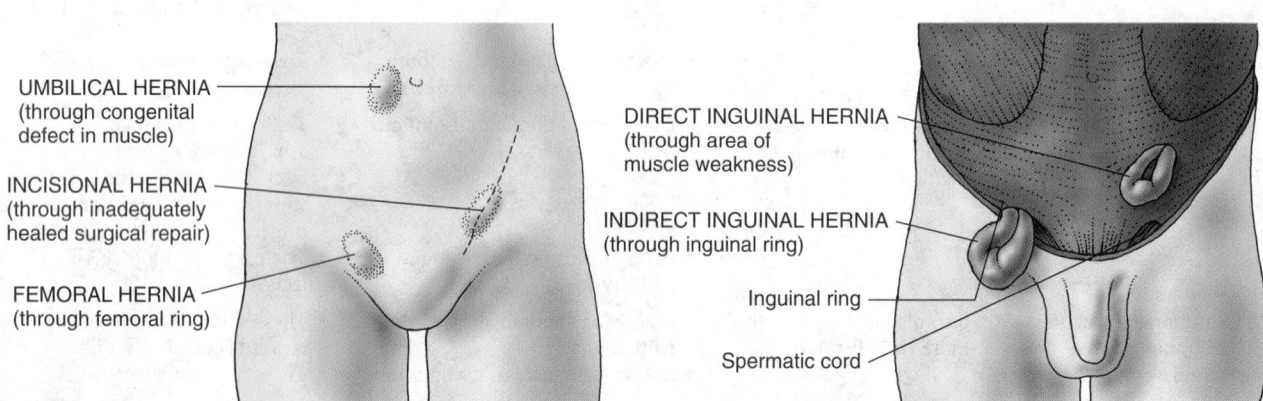

Figure 59–3. The types of abdominal hernia.

eventually surgical intervention. Any hernia that is not reducible requires immediate surgical evaluation.

The most important elements in the development of a hernia are congenital or acquired muscle weakness and increased intra-abdominal pressure. The most significant factors contributing to increased intra-abdominal pressure are obesity, pregnancy, and lifting of heavy objects.

Hernias can occur at any age, but specific incidence statistics are not available. Any condition that contributes to an increase in intra-abdominal pressure can lead to development of a hernia, especially if there is a pre-existing weakness in the abdominal wall.

Indirect inguinal hernias, the most common type, are most frequent in men because they follow the tract that develops when the testes descend into the scrotum before birth. Direct hernias occur more often in the elderly. Femoral and adult umbilical hernias are most common in obese or pregnant women. Incisional hernias occur in people who have abdominal surgery.

Collaborative Management

 Assessment

The client with a hernia typically comes to the health care provider's office or the emergency department with a complaint of a "bunch" or "lump" felt on the abdomen. The client frequently describes an incident of straining or lifting when "something popped."

To perform an abdominal assessment, the nurse inspects the abdomen when the client is lying and standing. If the hernia is reducible, it may disappear when the client is lying flat. The nurse asks the client to strain or perform the Valsalva maneuver and observes for bulging.

The nurse auscultates the abdomen for active bowel sounds. Absent bowel sounds may indicate obstruction and strangulation.

To palpate the hernia, the health care provider gently examines the ring and its contents by inserting a finger in the ring and noting any changes when the client coughs. The nurse never forces the hernia to reduce; this maneuver can cause strangulated intestine to rupture.

If a male client suspects a hernia in his groin, the health care provider has him stand for the examination. Using the right hand for the client's right side and the left hand for the client's left side, the health care provider invaginates the loose scrotal skin with the index finger, following the spermatic cord upward to the external inguinal cord. At this point, the client is asked to cough, and the health care provider notes any palpable herniation.

Interventions

The nurse advises the client to contact the physician if any symptoms of incarceration or strangulation occur.

Nonsurgical Management. The nurse teaches the client that no attempt should be made to reduce an incarcerated hernia. The health care provider may prescribe a truss for elderly or debilitated clients who are poor surgical risks. A truss is a pad made with firm material; it is held in place over the hernia with a belt to help keep the abdominal contents from protruding into the hernial sac. If a truss is used, it is applied only after the physician has reduced the hernia. The client usually applies the truss before arising. The nurse teaches the client to assess the skin under the truss daily and to protect it with a light layer of powder.

Surgical Management. Surgical repair of a hernia is generally the treatment of choice. Surgery is often performed on an outpatient basis for adult clients who have no pre-existing health conditions that would complicate the operative course. In same-day surgery centers, anesthesia may be local, regional, or general, and the surgery may be laparoscopic. More extensive surgery, such as a bowel resection or temporary colostomy, may be necessary if strangulation results in a gangrenous section of bowel. Clients having extensive surgery are hospitalized.

Herniorrhaphy is the surgery of choice for hernia repair. Hernioplasty is performed less frequently but can be performed in conjunction with a herniorrhaphy.

Preoperative Care. The nurse prepares the client for surgery (see Chap. 20). The client may be instructed to have one or two enemas the night before or the morning of surgery, depending on the surgeon's preference. If outpatient surgery is planned, the nurse assists the client to make appropriate arrangements for travel to home and home care.

Operative Procedure. During a herniorrhaphy, the surgeon makes an abdominal incision and replaces the contents of the hernial sac into the abdominal cavity before closing the opening. When a hernioplasty is performed, the surgeon reinforces the weakened muscle wall with mesh, fascia, or wire. The surgeon may opt to perform the surgery through a laparoscope instead of using the open surgical method.

Postoperative Care. Postoperative care of the client is the same as that described in Chapter 22, except that clients who undergo surgery for hernias are told to avoid coughing. To promote lung expansion, the nurse encourages deep breathing and frequent turning. With repair of an indirect inguinal hernia, the physician often orders a scrotal support and ice bags applied to the scrotum to prevent swelling, which often contributes to pain. Elevation of the scrotum with a soft pillow and bed rest also help prevent and control swelling. The nurse encourages early ambulation on the day of surgery if it is not contraindicated by scrotal swelling or pre-existing conditions. Ambulation helps promote comfort and a feeling of well-being and decreases the risk of postoperative complications.

In the immediate postoperative period, the client may experience difficulty voiding. The nurse allows the male client to stand to allow a more natural position for gravity to facilitate voiding and bladder emptying. Techniques to stimulate voiding, such as allowing water to run, may also be used. Careful monitoring of intake and output alerts the nurse to voiding problems early. The nurse carefully palpates the abdomen for distention. A fluid intake of at least 1500–2500 mL/day prevents dehydration and maintains urinary function. Most surgeons order catheterization every 6–8 hours if the client cannot void. The interval between catheterizations should not be prolonged; a distended bladder can stress the incision and increase discomfort.

Most clients have uneventful recoveries after hernia repairs. After surgery, surgeons generally allow clients to return to their usual activities, with avoidance of straining and lifting for 2 weeks. Depending on the site and the extent of repair and the client's general physical condition, this period may be extended to 6 weeks.

The nurse provides oral instructions and a written list of symptoms to be reported, including fever, chills, wound drainage, redness or separation of the incision, and increasing incisional pain.

The client is also instructed to keep the wound dry and clean and to replace the sterile dressing daily if indicated. If the surgeon allows, showering is permitted.

COLORECTAL CANCER

Overview

Cancer of the small intestine is rare and is not discussed in this text. Cancer of the colon and rectum, however, is the fourth most common cancer in American men and women when grouped separately and the second most common when men and women are combined. Cancer of the colon is second only to lung cancer as a cause of all deaths attributed to cancer in the United States (Parker, Tong, Bolden, & Wingo, 1997). Although the death rate from large-bowel cancer may be decreasing slightly, this disease is lethal in a significant number of cases because it is often not detected until an advanced stage, when metastasis has occurred.

WOMEN'S HEALTH CONSIDERATIONS

Colorectal cancer is the third most common type of cancer in women in America, occurring in 6% (1 in 17) of women from birth to death (Parker, Tong, Bolden, & Wingo, 1997). Women with histories of breast, endometrial, or ovarian cancer should be advised of their increased risk of the disease and monitored closely by health care providers.

A diet high in animal fat and low in fiber has been associated with colon cancer in women. For this reason, it is recommended that women reduce their dietary intake of fat and increase their intake of fruits, vegetables, and whole grains. Maintaining normal body weight may also be a helpful strategy in reducing the risks of developing cancer.

Pathophysiology

Pathologic Changes

Tumors occur in different areas of the colon. The percentages in Figure 59–4 represent an increased incidence of cancer in the proximal sections of the large intestine in the last 20 years (Schroy, 1996).

Most colorectal carcinomas are thought to develop from an adenomatous polyp. Tumors usually grow undetected

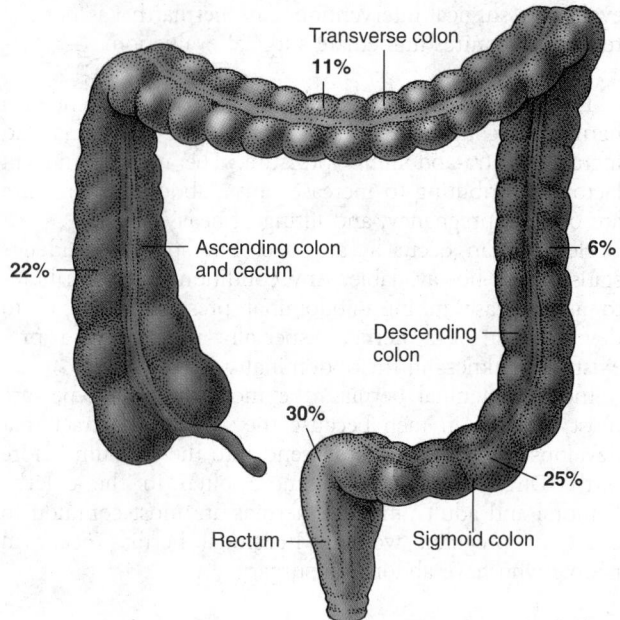

Figure 59–4. The incidence of cancer in relation to colorectal anatomy.

until symptoms slowly and insidiously appear. The disease can spread by several methods. The tumor may spread locally into deeper layers of the bowel wall, reaching the serosa and the mesenteric fat. The tumor may then begin to attach to other neighboring organs. It may enlarge into the lumen of the bowel or spread through the lymphatics or the circulatory system. The circulatory system is entered directly from the primary tumor through blood vessels in the bowel or via the lymphatics. After tumor cells enter the circulatory system, the cells most commonly travel to the liver.

Colon tumors can also spread by peritoneal seeding during surgical resection of the tumor. Seeding occurs when a tumor is excised and cancer cells break off from the tumor into the peritoneal cavity. The liver and peritoneal cavity are common sites of metastasis and relapse. Other sites include the pelvis, the retroperitoneum, and the lungs. If metastasis occurs, it is usually multifocal (several sites at one time), but some clients will have isolated or local recurrence of disease.

Complications

Complications related to the increasing growth of the tumor locally or through metastatic spread include bowel perforation with resultant peritonitis, abscess formation, and fistula formation to the urinary bladder or the vagina.

The tumor may invade neighboring blood vessels and cause frank bleeding. A tumor growing into the bowel lumen can gradually obstruct the intestine and eventually block it completely. Tumor extending beyond the bowel wall may place pressure on neighboring organs (uterus, urinary bladder, and ureters) and cause symptoms that mask those of the cancer.

Twenty percent of clients diagnosed with colorectal cancer are diagnosed at the time of an emergency hospitalization for bowel obstruction or other life-threatening complication (Hardcastle, 1997).

Etiology

The exact cause of colorectal cancer is unknown. Risk factors include personal history of adenomatous polyps, history of two or more first-degree relatives with bowel cancer, familial polyposis syndromes, inflammatory bowel disease, and personal history of breast, ovarian, or endometrial cancer.

It is theorized that decreased bowel transit time and certain foods containing chemical mutagens may place individuals at risk for colorectal cancer (Table 59–1). These foods also aid in decreasing bowel transit time, which would increase the time that the bowel is exposed to carcinogens. A high-fat diet, particularly animal fat from red meats, increases bile acid secretion and anaerobic bacteria, which are thought to be carcinogenic within the bowel. Fried and broiled meats and fish are also thought to contain chemical mutagens that are carcinogenic. Diets with large amounts of refined carbohydrates that lack fiber decrease bowel transit time.

Because almost all colorectal tumors develop from an adenoma, the *primary* risk factor for colorectal cancer is the presence of an adenoma. There are three types of colorectal adenoma: tubular, villous, and tubulovillous (see later discussion of polyps). Even though almost all colorectal cancers originate from adenomas, only 2% to 5% of all colorectal adenomas become malignant. Villous adenomas have the highest potential for malignant change (Markowitz & Winawer, 1997).

The factor that initiates the change from a benign adenoma to a malignant tumor is unknown. Familial polyposis is a hereditary disorder transmitted as an autosomal dominant trait; it is characterized by an early onset of multiple adenomatous polyps of the colon and rectum. The risk for cancer in cases of familial polyposis approaches 100% from age 40–50 years of life. Screening for cancer in individuals with familial polyposis begins at age 10–20, and a prophylactic colectomy is generally performed before age 50 years. People who have had

ulcerative colitis are also at risk for colorectal cancer. The risk increases with younger age at onset and larger extent of colon involvement. After 8–10 years, those who have ulcerative colitis extending proximal to the rectum are recommended to have annual colonoscopies with biopsies.

Incidence/Prevalence

Approximately 131,200 people in the United States were diagnosed with colorectal cancer in 1997, with an estimated 54,900 deaths (Jessup, Menck, Fremgen, & Winchester, 1997). Most clients with colorectal cancer are older than 50 years; only 2% to 6% are younger than 40. The peak incidence occurs in clients in their 70s and 80s. Colorectal cancer occurs with slightly greater frequency in men, and cancer of the rectum is more common in men. Cancer of the right colon is more common in women.

TRANSCULTURAL CONSIDERATIONS

 Both male and female African-Americans have an increased frequency of colorectal cancer in advanced stages at time of diagnosis, and consequently an increase in colorectal death rates, as opposed to Caucasian American males and females (Jessup et al., 1997). Hispanics are also slightly more likely to be diagnosed with advanced colorectal cancer than non-Hispanic Caucasians. Asian-Americans have a pattern of diagnosis similar to that of non-Hispanic Caucasians.

Collaborative Management

Assessment

➤ History

In taking a history from a client with colorectal cancer, the nurse obtains the client's diet history and questions the client about major risk factors, such as personal history of breast, ovarian, or endometrial cancer; ulcerative colitis; Crohn's disease; familial polyposis; adenomas; or a family history of colorectal cancer. The nurse also assesses client's participation in age-specific screening guidelines for colorectal cancer (see Chap. 27).

The nurse also asks about changes in bowel habits, such as diarrhea or constipation, with or without blood in the stool. The client may also report fatigue (related to anemias), abdominal fullness, pain, or weight loss, which unfortunately are signs of advanced disease.

➤ Physical Assessment/Clinical Manifestations

The signs of colorectal cancer depend on the location of the tumor. However, the most common signs are rectal bleeding, anemia, and change in stool.

Blood may be manifested microscopically in stools for occult blood or more vividly as mahogany or bright-red stools. Gross blood is not usually detected with tumors of the right colon but is common (but not massive) with tumors of the left colon and rectum.

The first noted manifestations of colorectal cancer may be a palpable mass, partial or complete obstruction of the colon, or perforation of the colon characterized by ab-

TABLE 59–1

Foods that Affect a Person's Risk for Colorectal Cancer

Foods to Avoid
- Red meat
- Animal fat
- Fatty foods
- Fried or broiled meats and fish
- Refined carbohydrates (e.g., concentrated sweets)

Foods to Consume
- Fruits and vegetables, especially cruciferous vegetables from the cabbage family (e.g., broccoli, cabbage, cauliflower, brussels sprouts)
- Whole-grain products
- Adequate fluids, especially water

dominal distention and pain. These findings as well as cachexia indicate advanced disease.

➤ Psychosocial Assessment

People often delay seeking health care because of the fear of a cancer diagnosis. Cancer is commonly equated with pain and death. Many people are not aware of the advances in treatment and the increased survival rates. Early detection is critical to the control of colorectal cancer, and the delay in seeking health care can dramatically reduce the chance for survival.

People who live healthy lifestyles and follow health guidelines may experience anger when clinical manifestations appear. These clients may feel a sudden loss of control, helplessness, and shock. The diagnostic process is generally extensive and can be tiresome and anxiety provoking for the client and the family. The nurse enables the client to ventilate his or her feelings during this process.

➤ Laboratory Assessment

Hemoglobin and hematocrit values are usually decreased, which indicates anemia. A positive test result for occult blood in the stool confirms bleeding in the gastrointestinal (GI) tract. The client *avoids* meat, peroxidase-containing foods (horseradish and beets), aspirin, and vitamin C for 48 hours before giving a stool specimen. The nurse assesses whether the client is taking nonsteroidal anti-inflammatory drugs (such as ibuprofen, corticosteroids, or salicylates). The nurse then consults the physician about prescribing other medications in place of these or at least taking their ingestion into account in the guaiac test results. These foods and medications may stimulate bleeding when no true bleeding exists and lead to false-positive results. Two separate stool samples are tested on 3 consecutive days. Negative results do not completely rule out the possibility of colon cancer.

Carcinoembryonic antigen (CEA) may be elevated in 70% of people with colorectal cancer. There is no relationship between the CEA level and the stage of colon cancer. CEA is not specifically associated with the colorectal cancer, and it may be elevated in the presence of other benign or malignant diseases. CEA is often used to monitor the effectiveness of treatment and identify disease recurrence.

➤ Radiographic Assessment

A barium enema examination may confirm the presence of tumor and identify its location. This test may demonstrate an occlusion in the bowel where the tumor is decreasing the size of the lumen. Small lesions may not be identified by this test. Barium enemas are generally performed after sigmoidoscopy and colonoscopy.

Computed tomography (CT) helps confirm the existence of a mass and the extent of disease. Chest x-ray and liver scan may locate distant sites of metastasis.

➤ Other Diagnostic Assessment

The physician commonly performs a colonoscopy to identify tumors. Biopsy of the mass can also be done during this procedure.

 Analysis

➤ Common Nursing Diagnoses and Collaborative Problems

The client with cancer of the colon typically has the nursing diagnosis of grieving related to disturbance in self-concept and potentially terminal illness.

The most common collaborative problem is potential for metastasis.

➤ Additional Nursing Diagnoses and Collaborative Problems

In addition, the client with colorectal cancer may have one or more of the following nursing diagnoses:
- Pain related to tumor obstruction of the intestine, with possible pressure on other organs
- Risk for Ineffective Management of Therapeutic Regimen related to unfamiliarity with the disease process, the diagnostic work-up, treatment options, and the treatment plan
- Ineffective Family Coping: Compromised related to alteration in roles, lifestyle changes, and fear of the client's death
- Altered Nutrition: Less than Body Requirements related to the diagnostic work-up
- Fear related to the disease process
- Powerlessness related to the presence of life-threatening illness and its treatment

Some clients are also at risk for the following collaborative problems for which the nurse assesses:
- Potential for Paralytic Ileus
- Potential for Hypovolemia/Shock

 Planning and Implementation

Grieving

Planning: Expected Outcomes. The client is expected to identify, develop, and use effective coping methods in dealing with the perceived changes and losses experienced.

Interventions. The client and the family are faced with the issues of the disease cancer, the possible loss of body functions, and altered body functions.

The nurse observes and identifies
- The client's and family's current methods of coping
- Effective sources of support used in past crises
- The client's and family's present perceptions of the health problem

The nurse encourages the client to verbalize feelings about the colostomy, if one has been performed (see Operative Procedure under Surgical Management later). The nurse acknowledges that sadness, anger, feelings of loss, and depression are normal responses to this change in body function.

It may help to discuss the colostomy as one aspect of the client's care rather than making it the focus of care, just as defecation is only one aspect of the client's physiologic functioning. The nurse encourages the client to look at and touch the stoma. When the client is physically able, the nurse encourages the client's participation in colostomy care. The nurse assists the client and the family in formulating questions and verbalizing needs. The nurse observes whether the client has processed the necessary information and has learned the psychomotor skills for colostomy care. Participation helps to restore the client's sense of control over lifestyle and thus facilitates improved self-esteem.

Potential for Metastasis

Planning: Expected Outcomes. The client is expected to experience cure or prolonged survival, an enhanced quality of life, and no complications of cancer, including metastasis.

Interventions. Surgery is usually the primary treatment for tumors in the colon or rectum. Radiation therapy and chemotherapy may be used as adjuncts for controlling symptoms or preventing cancer recurrence.

Nonsurgical Management. The physician assesses each client with cancer to determine the best treatment plan. Age, concurrent illness, and quality of life are considered.

Radiation Therapy. Preoperative radiation may be administered to the client who has a large colorectal tumor, although this is not routinely done. This therapy aids in creating more definite tumor margins, which facilitates resection of the tumor during surgery.

Radiation can be used postoperatively in clients with high risk of recurrence because of tumor involvement in margins of tissue removed during surgery or, less frequently, after local excision for early-stage colorectal tumors. As a palliative measure, radiation therapy reduces pain, hemorrhage, bowel obstruction, or metastasis to the lung in advanced disease.

The nurse explains the radiation therapy procedure to the client and the family and monitors for possible side effects (e.g., diarrhea and fatigue). The nurse implements interventions to reduce side effects of the therapy. (See Chapter 27 for care of clients undergoing radiation therapy.)

Chemotherapy. Adjuvant chemotherapy after primary surgery is recommended for clients with stage II and stage III disease (cancer invades at least into the muscle) to improve survival (National Institutes of Health Consensus Conference, 1990). The drug of choice is intravenous (IV) 5-fluorouracil (5-FU) with or without levamisole or leucovorin. In 1997, Camptosar (irinotecan) was approved as second-line treatment for metastatic disease if disease has recurred or progressed after treatment with 5-FU (Pharmacia & Upjohn Co.). Intrahepatic arterial chemotherapy, often with 5-FU, may be administered to clients with liver metastasis.

Surgical Management. Size of the tumor, location, extent of metastasis, condition of bowel integrity, and condition of the client determine which surgical procedure is performed for colorectal cancer (Table 59-2). Because the majority of colorectal cancers are diagnosed when the cancer has extended beyond the tumor, the three most common surgeries performed are *radical colon resection*

TABLE 59-2

Surgical Procedures for Colorectal Cancers in Various Locations

Tumor Location	Procedures
Right-sided colon tumors	• Right hemicolectomy for smaller lesions • Right ascending colostomy or ileostomy for large, widespread lesions • Cecostomy (opening into the cecum with intubation to decompress the bowel)
Left-sided colon tumors	• Left hemicolectomy for smaller lesions • Left descending colostomy for larger lesions (e.g., the Hartmann procedure)
Sigmoid colon tumors	• Sigmoid colectomy for smaller lesions • Sigmoid colostomy for larger lesions (e.g., the Hartmann procedure) • Abdominoperineal resection for large, low sigmoid tumors (near the anus) with colostomy (the rectum and the anus are completely removed, leaving a perineal wound)
Rectal tumors	• Resection with anastomosis or pull-through procedure (preserves anal sphincter and normal elimination pattern) • Colon resection with permanent colostomy • Abdominoperineal resection with colostomy

(resection of tumor and regional lymph nodes) with reanastomosis; *radical colon resection* with *colostomy (temporary or permanent),* and *abdominal-perineal (AP) resection.*

Small tumors indicate an early stage of cancer, are well differentiated without evidence of vascular or lymphatic invasion, can be removed with clean margins, and may be treated with local excision, postoperative radiation, and close follow-up. A transanal approach without an abdominal incision is the technique most commonly used, which decreases the risk for postoperative complications and shortens the hospital stay. Only 5% of clients with colorectal cancer, however, meet the criteria of early-stage cancer, as just outlined.

Colon Resection (Radical). A colon resection involves excision of that part of the colon with tumor and leaves an area of clean margins. If the integrity of the intestine is optimal (e.g., without inflammation as in bowel obstruction or perforation), and the rectal sphincter can be left intact, reanastomosis can usually be accomplished, and an ostomy can be avoided. If healing of a reanastomosed bowel is thought to be in jeopardy, a temporary or permanent colostomy will be performed.

Preoperative Care. The nurse assists the client to prepare for colon resection by reinforcing the physician's explanation of the planned surgical procedure. The client is told as accurately as possible what anatomic and physiologic changes will occur with surgery. Before evaluating the tumor and colon in surgery, the physician might not be able to determine whether a colostomy will be necessary. If this is the case, the physician informs the client that a colostomy is a possibility. If the surgeon informs the client that a colostomy is inevitable, the nurse consults an enterostomal therapist (ET) to advise on optimal placement of the ostomy and instructs the client about the rationale and general principles of ostomies. An ET is a registered nurse who has completed specialized training and is certified in ostomy nursing care.

The client who requires low rectal surgery is faced with the risk of postoperative sexual dysfunction and urinary incontinence as a result of nerve damage during surgery. The physician discusses the risk for these problems with the client before surgery, and the nurse allows the client to verbalize concerns and questions related to this risk. The nurse prepares the client for abdominal surgery with general anesthesia (see Chap. 20).

If the bowel is not obstructed or perforated, elective surgery is planned. The client receives a thorough cleaning of the bowel, or "bowel prep," to minimize bacterial growth and prevent complications. For a bowel prep, the client is usually instructed to restrict the diet to clear liquids for 1–2 days before surgery. Mechanical cleaning is accomplished with laxatives and enemas or with "whole gut lavage." For whole gut lavage, the client ingests large quantities of a sodium sulfate and polyethylene glycol solution (e.g., GoLYTELY). This solution overwhelms the absorptive capacity of the small bowel and clears feces from the colon. To reduce the risk of infection, the surgeon may prescribe oral or intravenous (IV) antibiotics to be given the day before surgery.

Operative Procedure. The surgeon makes an incision in the abdomen and explores the abdominal cavity to determine resectability of the tumor. The portion of the colon with tumor is excised, and the two open ends of the bowel are irrigated before anastomosis of the colon. If an anastomosis is not feasible because of the location of the tumor or the condition of the bowel (e.g., inflammation), a colostomy is created.

A colostomy may be created in the ascending, transverse, descending, or sigmoid colon (Fig. 59–5). One of three basic techniques is used to construct a colostomy. A loop stoma is made by bringing a loop of colon to the skin surface, severing and everting the anterior wall, and suturing it to the abdomen wall. Loop colostomies are usually performed in the transverse colon and are usually temporary (Bradley & Pupiales, 1997). An external rod is used to support the loop until the intestinal tissue adheres to the abdominal wall. Care must be taken to avoid displacing the rod, especially during appliance changes.

An end stoma is often constructed when a colostomy is

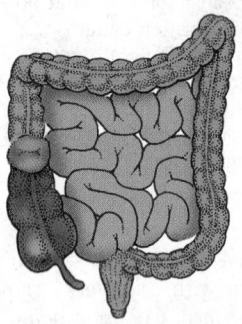

The **ascending colostomy** is done for right-sided tumors.

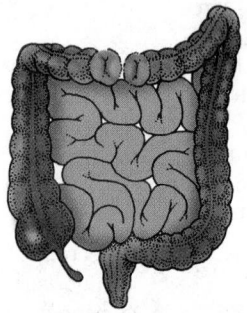

The **transverse (double-barreled) colostomy** is often used in such emergencies as intestinal obstruction or perforation because it can be created quickly. There are two stomas. The proximal one, closest to the small intestine, drains feces. The distal stoma drains mucus.

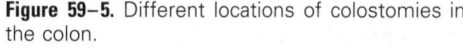

Figure 59–5. Different locations of colostomies in the colon.

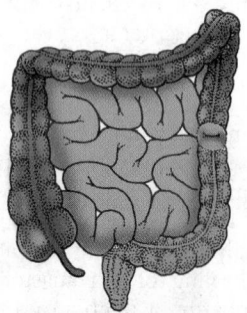

Descending colostomy

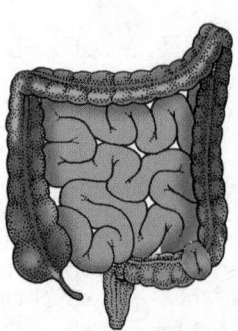

Sigmoid colostomy

intended to be permanent and is most often located in the descending or sigmoid colon. However, it may also be done in conjunction with a Hartmann procedure, when the surgeon oversews the distal stump of the colon and places it in the abdominal cavity, preserving it for future reattachment. An end stoma is constructed by severing the end of the proximal portion of the bowel and bringing it out through the abdominal wall.

The least common colostomy is the double-barrel stoma, which is created by dividing the bowel and bringing both the proximal and distal portions to the abdominal surface to create two stomas. The proximal end (closest to the client's head) is the functioning stoma, which eliminates stool; the distal (farthest from the head) stoma is considered nonfunctioning, although it may secrete some mucus. The distal stoma is sometimes referred to as a mucous fistula.

Postoperative Care. Clients who have had colon resection without colostomy receive care similar to that of clients undergoing any abdominal surgery (see Chap. 22).

The client who has a colostomy may return from surgery with an ostomy pouch system in place. If there is no pouch system in place, the nurse places a petrolatum gauze dressing over the stoma to keep it moist and covers the gauze with a dry, sterile dressing. In collaboration with the enterostomal therapist (ET), the nurse places a pouch system as soon as possible. The colostomy pouch system allows more convenient and acceptable collection of stool than a dressing does.

The nurse assesses the color and integrity of the stoma. A healthy stoma should be reddish-pink and moist and will protrude about 2 cm from the abdominal wall. A small amount of bleeding at the stoma is common, but any appreciable bleeding is reported to the surgeon.

The nurse observes and reports if the stoma has

- Signs of ischemia and necrosis (dark red, purplish, or black color; dry, firm, or flaccid)
- Unusual bleeding
- Mucocutaneous separation (breakdown of suture line securing stoma to abdominal wall)

The nurse also assesses the condition of the periostomal skin and frequently checks the pouch system for proper fit and signs of leakage. The periostomal skin should be intact, smooth, and nonreddened.

The colostomy should start functioning 2–4 days postoperatively. When the colostomy begins to function, the pouch may need to be emptied frequently for excess gas collection. It should be emptied when it is one third to one half full of stool. Stool is liquid immediately postoperatively but becomes more solid, depending on where in the colon the stoma was placed. For example, the stool from a colostomy in the ascending colon is liquid, the stool from a colostomy in the transverse colon is pasty, and the stool from a colostomy in the descending colon is more solid (similar to usual stool expelled from the rectum).

Abdominal-Perineal Resection. When rectal tumors are present, the rectum and rectal support structure may need to be removed. An abdominoperineal resection usually requires a permanent colostomy for evacuation. However, with improvements in surgical techniques, more cli-

ents can undergo colon resection with the rectal sphincter left intact; thus, the need for a colostomy is avoided.

Preoperative Care. The preoperative care for the client undergoing abdominal perineal resection is similar to that provided for the client undergoing colon resection (see earlier).

Operative Procedure. The surgeon removes the distal sigmoid colon, the rectosigmoid colon, the rectum, and the anus through combined abdominal and perineal incisions. A permanent end sigmoid colostomy is created.

Postoperative Care. Postoperative care after an abdominoperineal resection is similar to that given after a colon resection with the creation of a sigmoid colostomy. The nurse collaborates with the ET to provide colostomy care and client and family education.

The perineal wound is generally surgically closed, and two bulb suction drains, such as Jackson-Pratt drains, are placed in the wound or through stab wounds near the wound. The drains help prevent drainage from collecting within the wound and are usually left in place for several days, depending on the character and amount of drainage.

Monitoring drainage from the perineal wound and cavity is important because of the possibility of infection and abscess formation. Serosanguineous drainage from the perineal wound may be observed for 1–2 months after surgery. Complete healing of the perineal wound may take 6 to 8 months. This wound can be a greater source of discomfort than the abdominal incision and ostomy, and more care may be required. The client may experience phantom rectal sensations because sympathetic innervation for rectal control has not been interrupted. Pain and itching may occasionally occur after healing. There is no physiologic explanation for these sensations. Interventions may include use of antipruritic medications, such as benzocaine, and sitz baths. The nurse

- Explains the physiology of perineal sensations to the client
- Continually assesses for signs of infection, abscess, or other complications
- Implements methods for promoting wound drainage and comfort (Chart 59–2)

 Continuing Care

After hospitalization for surgery, the client with colorectal cancer is usually managed at home. Radiation therapy or chemotherapy is typically done on an ambulatory (outpatient) basis. Hospitalization may be required at another time if signs or symptoms of recurrent tumor or metastasis occur. For the client with advanced cancer, hospice care is an option (see Chapter 12 for discussion of hospice care).

▶ *Home Care Management*

The nurse assesses all clients for their ability to perform incision care and activities of daily living (ADL) within limitations. For the client who has undergone colostomy, the nurse or case manager reviews the home situation to

Chart 59-2

Nursing Care Highlight: Perineal Wound Care

Wound Care
- Place an absorbent dressing (Kerlix or abdominal pad) over the wound.
- Instruct the client that he or she may
  - Use a feminine napkin as a dressing
  - Wear jockey-type shorts rather than boxers

Comfort Measures
- If ordered, soak the wound area in a sitz bath for 10–20 min 3 or 4 times/day.
- Administer pain medication as ordered and assess its effectiveness.
- Instruct the client about permissible activities. The client should
  - Assume a side-lying position in bed; avoid sitting for long periods
  - Use foam pads or a soft pillow to sit on whenever in a sitting position.
  - Avoid the use of air rings or rubber doughnut devices.

Prevention of Complications
- Maintain fluid and electrolyte balance by monitoring intake and output and by monitoring output from the perineal wound.
- Observe suture line integrity and monitor wound drains; watch for erythema, edema, bleeding, purulent drainage, unusual odor, and excessive or constant pain.

aid the client in arranging for care. So that the ostomy products will function properly, the client and the family must keep supplies in an area (preferably the bathroom) where the temperature is neither hot nor cold (skin barriers may become stiff or melt in extreme temperatures). The enterostomal therapist (ET) may serve as the case manager for the client with a colostomy when discharged home to ensure continuity of care.

No changes are needed in sleeping accommodations. Some clients move into a separate room or into twin beds. This can lead to physical and emotional distancing from their spouse and significant others. A rubber covering may initially be placed over the bed mattress if clients feel insecure about the pouch system.

➤ Health Teaching

Clients who have undergone a colon resection without colostomy receive instruction for specific needs, similar to that given to clients who have undergone abdominal surgery. In addition to this information, the nurse teaches all clients with colon resections to watch for and report clinical manifestations of intestinal obstruction and perforation (e.g., cramping, abdominal pain, nausea, and vomiting).

Rehabilitation after ostomy surgery requires that clients and family members learn the principles of colostomy

care and the psychomotor skills to facilitate this care. Providing information is important, but the nurse must also allow adequate opportunity for clients to learn the psychomotor skills involved in ostomy care before discharge. Sufficient practice time is planned for clients and family or significant others so that they can handle, assemble, and apply all ostomy equipment. The nurse teaches clients and family (Table 59–3)
- About the stoma
- Measurement of stoma
- Choice, use, care, and application of the pouch system
- Skin protection
- Dietary control
- Control of gas and odor
- Potential problems and solutions
- Tips on how to resume normal activities, including work, travel, and sexual intercourse

The appropriate pouch system must be selected and fitted to the stoma. Clients with flat, firm abdomens may use either flexible (bordered with paper tape) or nonflexible (full skin barrier wafer) pouch systems. A firm abdomen with lateral creases or folds needs a flexible system. Clients with deep creases, flabby abdomens, a retracted stoma, or a stoma that is flush or concave to the abdominal surface would benefit from a convex appliance with a stoma belt (Bradley & Pupiales, 1997). This type of system presses into the skin around the stoma, causing the stoma to protrude. This protrusion helps tighten the skin and prevents leaks around the stoma opening onto the periostomal skin.

Measurement of the stoma is necessary to determine the size of the stomal opening on the appliance. The opening should be wide and long enough to not only cover the periostomal skin but also to avoid stomal trauma. The stoma will shrink within 6–8 weeks of surgery; therefore, it will need to be measured at least once weekly during this time and as needed if the client gains or loses weight. The client and family caregiver should be taught to trace the pattern of the stomal area on the wafer portion of the appliance and to cut an opening about 1/16 inch larger than the stomal pattern (Wound Ostomy and Continence Nurses Society, 1992) to ensure that stomal tissue will not be constricted.

Skin preparation may include clipping periostomal hair or shaving the area to achieve a smooth surface, prevent unnecessary discomfort when the wafer is removed, and minimize risk of infected hair follicles. The client is advised to avoid using moisturizing soaps to clean the area because the lubricants can interfere in adhesion of the appliance. The client and family caregiver are taught to apply a skin sealant and allow it to dry before application of the appliance to facilitate less painful removal of tape or adhesive. If periostomal skin becomes raw, the client or caregiver checks to see whether the sealant contains alcohol, and reconsiders using it to avoid burning to the skin. Stoma powder or paste, or a combination, may also be used for erythematous periostomal skin.

Control of gas and odor from the colostomy is often a significant goal for new ostomates. Although a leaking or inadequately closed pouch is the usual cause, flatus can

TABLE 59–3

Solutions to Special Problems in Ostomy Use

Problems	Solutions
Odor	
Foods	
Dairy products (boiled milk, eggs, and some cheese), fish, onion, garlic, coffee, alcohol, nuts, prunes, beans, cabbage, cucumber, asparagus, radish, broccoli, turnips, peas, highly seasoned foods	• Spinach, cranberry juice, yogurt, buttermilk, dark green vegetables (parsley is particularly helpful), increased vitamin C in food or vitamin preparations
Drugs	*Oral Medications*
Antibiotics, vitamins, iron	• Chlorophyll tablets (Derifil) for fecal odors (absorb gas) • Charcoal tablets • Bismuth bicarbonate (0.6 g tid with meals) • Bismuth subgallate (Devrom or Biscaps) 1 or 2 tablets with meals and 1 tablet hs
	Pouch Preparations
	• Odor-proof pouch or pouch with odor-control mechanism • Manufactured preparations (place small amounts in pouch): Banish II or Superbanish (United), Odor-Guard (Marlan), Ostobon (Pettibone Labs), activated charcoal, ostomy deodorant (Sween), Nilodor, Devko tablets (Parthenon Co.), D-Odor, M-9 (Mason Lab) • Sodium bicarbonate solution (soaked cotton balls in pouch) • Vanilla, peppermint, lemon, or almond extracts (put 10 drops into pouch or soak cotton balls) • Favorite spice, cloves, or cinnamon (place ¼ tsp in pouch) • Mouthwash (e.g., Cēpacol, Listerine) (several drops in pouch or soaked cotton balls in pouch)
	Cleaning Reusable Pouches
	• Wisk and water (1:1 solution) • Baking soda and water (1:1 solution) • Household white vinegar and water (1:1 solution) • Manufactured products: Uri-Kleen, Uni-Wash (United), PeriWash (Sween), Skin Care cleaner (Bard) • Baking soda (after drying the pouch, powder inside with baking soda)
Flatulence	
Activities	
Eating fast and talking at same time, gum chewing, smoking, snoring, skipping meals, emotional upset	• Avoid these activities; eat solids before taking liquids
Foods	*Pouch Adaptation*
Mushrooms, onions, beans, cabbage, brussels sprouts, spinach, cheese, eggs, beer, carbonated beverages, fish, highly seasoned foods, some fruit drinks, corn, pork, peas, coffee, high-fat foods	• Use pouches with gas or odor filters

Table continued on following page

also contribute to the odor. The nurse teaches the client and family caregiver that there are generally no forbidden foods for ostomates, but that certain foods and habits can effect flatus or contribute to odor when the pouch is open. Broccoli, brussels sprouts, cabbage, cauliflower, cucumber, mushrooms, and peas often cause flatus, as does chewing gum, smoking, beer drinking, and skipping meals. Crackers, toast, and yogurt can help prevent gas. Asparagus, broccoli, cabbage, turnips, eggs, fish, and gar-

lic contribute to odor when the pouch is open. Buttermilk, cranberry juice, parsley, and yogurt will help prevent odor; charcoal filters, pouch deodorizers, or placement of a breath mint in the pouch will eliminate odors. The client should be cautioned not to put aspirin tablets in the pouch because they may cause ulceration of the stoma.

The client with a sigmoid colostomy may benefit from colostomy irrigation to regulate elimination. The nurse

TABLE 59-3

Solutions to Special Problems in Ostomy Use *Continued*

Problems	Solutions
Skin Irritation	
Allergy	
Erythema, erosion, edema, weeping, bleeding, itching, burning, stinging, irritation the same shape as the allergic material	• Creams: Sween cream, Unicare cream, or Hollister Skin Conditioning Cream (use small amount and rub in; tapes will adhere when dry)
Chemical Exposure	• Powders (karaya gum, Stomahesive, cornstarch) used with skin gel (Skin Prep, Skin Gel)
Stool, urine, glues, solvents, soaps, detergents, proteolytic digestive enzymes	• Antacids: aluminum hydroxide (Amphojel, Maalox) used with skin sealant (Skin Prep, Skin Gel)
Epidermal Hyperplasia	• Skin sealant alone (for slightly reddened skin)
Increased formation of epidermal cells causing a generalized thickening of the outer layer of the skin	• Skin barriers: one application left on for 24 hr or longer may clear irritations quickly
Mechanical Trauma	• Pastes (Hollister Premium, Stomahesive) used to fill in creases and spaces
Pressure, friction, or stripping of the skin (e.g., adhesives, tape, belts)	• Hair dryer on cool setting to decrease moisture
	• Do not patch or tape leaks; correct the leakage problem immediately
Skin Irritation	
Infection	
Candida albicans infection indicated by pustular, reddened, weepy, white spots	**For Candidiasis**
Radiation Therapy	• Use nystatin (Mycostatin) powder, cover with skin sealant (Skin Prep or Skin Gel)
	• Use drying agent (e.g., acroflavin)
	• Place skin barrier (Stomahesive) over site

discusses this technique with the client and the family to determine its feasibility and perceived worth. If this method is chosen, the nurse teaches the client and the family how to perform colostomy irrigation (Chart 59–3). A variety of teaching tools may be used. Written instructions are helpful because the client can take these home for future reference. Repetition is necessary in teaching the client these new skills. Anxiety, fear, discomfort, and other distractions alter the client's and family's ability to learn and retain information.

In addition to instructing the client about the clinical manifestations of obstruction and perforation, the nurse also advises the client with a colostomy to report any fever or sudden onset of pain or swelling around the stoma (Chart 59–4).

The diagnosis of cancer can be emotionally immobilizing for the client and family or significant others, but treatment may be welcomed because it may provide hope for control of the disease. The nurse explores the client's reactions to the illness and perceptions of planned interventions.

The client's reaction to ostomy surgery, which may include disfigurement, may involve

- Feelings of being offensive to others
- Feelings of feeling dirty, with a reduced sense of value
- Fear of rejection

The nurse allows the client to verbalize these feelings (see Chapter 10 on body image). By teaching the client how to physically manage the ostomy, the nurse assists the client in restoring self-esteem and improving body image, which leads to solid relations with others. Inclusion of family and significant others in the rehabilitation process also helps maintain relationships and raise the client's self-esteem.

➤ Health Care Resources

Several resources are available to complement nursing care, maintain continuity of care in the home environment, and provide for client needs that the nurse is not able to meet.

The nurse makes a referral to the case manager or social worker, who can

- Provide further emotional counseling to the client and family or significant others
- Aid in managing the financial concerns that the client and family may have
- Arrange home care or extended care (e.g., in a nursing home, group home, or hospice) as needed

The nurse makes a referral to the enterostomal therapist (ET) to

- Aid in preoperative stoma teaching
- Evaluate and mark the stoma site
- Help with postoperative care and teaching
- Provide consultation for problems in care
- Provide assistance with the discharge process

The enterostomal therapist may also conduct an outpatient clinic for ongoing client needs.

Chart 59-3

Education Guide: Colostomy Irrigation

Irrigation Procedure

1. Assemble the necessary equipment:
   • An irrigating kit with a sleeve
   • Tubing with a clamp
   • A cone
   • A container for the irrigation solution
   • Skin care items
   • A new pouch system ready for application
2. Remove the old pouch and dispose of it.
3. Clean the stoma and the skin.
4. Apply the irrigating sleeve, and place the end of the sleeve into the toilet.
5. Fill the irrigation container with 500 to 1000 mL of lukewarm water. Initial irrigations are usually performed with 500 mL of fluid or less to prevent over-distention and cramping.
6. Suspend the irrigating container with the bottom of the container at shoulder level.
7. Allow the solution to flow through the tubing to remove air from the tubing.
8. Lubricate the cone tip and gently insert the cone tip into the stoma. Do not force it. Hold tip securely in place to prevent backflow. Open clamp and allow solution to flow in steadily over 5 to 10 minutes.
9. When the desired amount of solution has entered or the client senses colonic distention, close the clamp and remove the cone.
10. Wait approximately 30 to 45 minutes for returns. When initial returns are complete (usually 10–15 minutes), the client may close the bottom of the sleeve and move around.
11. When evacuation of the stool is complete, remove the irrigation sleeve, clean the stoma, and apply a new pouch system.
12. Clean the irrigating equipment, then dry and store it.

Special Tips

1. You may wish to wear a small stomal covering instead of a pouch system between irrigations.

2. If cramping occurs while you are irrigating, stop irrigation and wait. After cramping subsides and you are ready to resume the procedure, try the following: slow down the flow of solution, lower the container, or warm the water.
3. Make sure that air is out of the tubing before putting it into the stoma.
4. If water does not flow easily, try changing the position of the cone, checking the tubing for kinks and the level of the container, and relaxing with several deep breaths.
5. If no returns occur, try gently massaging the abdomen or drinking warm liquids.

Approaches to Common Problems

1. If spillage occurs between irrigations, try:
   • Decreasing the rate of infusion
   • Decreasing the amount of irrigant used
   • Limiting how far the catheter is inserted into the bowel
   • Allowing a longer time for evacuation
2. If your bowel retains the solution after irrigation, try
   • Changing position
   • Walking around
   • Massaging your abdomen gently
   • Drinking something hot
3. If returns are less than usual, you may need to wear a pouch.
4. If returns after irrigation are clear, decrease the frequency of irrigation.
5. If you feel weak or faint during irrigation, stop the procedure and lie down. When weakness subsides, change your position to facilitate evacuation.
6. Call your physician if weakness does not resolve.
7. If you have had weakness during irrigation that resolved quickly, use warmer water at a slower rate and try inserting the cone or catheter less deeply in the stoma when you irrigate the next time.
8. If weakness or faintness is a recurrent problem, notify your physician.

The nurse provides information about the United Ostomy Association, a self-help group of people who have ostomies. Literature, such as the organization's publication (*Ostomy Quarterly*), and information about a local chapter are given to the client. This organization conducts a visitor program that sends specially trained visitors (who have an ostomy) to talk with clients. After obtaining the client's consent, the nurse makes a referral to the visitor program so that the visitor can see the client preoperatively as well as postoperatively. A physician's consent for visitation is generally necessary.

The local division or unit of the American Cancer Society (ACS) can provide necessary medical equipment and supplies, home health services, travel accommodations, and other resources for the client who is undergoing cancer treatment or ostomy surgery. The nurse informs the client and family of the programs available through the local division or unit.

Because of short hospital stays, clients with new ostomies receive most of their instruction on colostomy care from nurses working for home care agencies. This resource also facilitates client needs for physical care, medication management, and emotional support for clients with or without colostomies. If the client has advanced colorectal cancer, a referral for hospice services in the home, nursing home, or other long-term care setting may be appropriate.

The nurse informs the client and the family what ostomy supplies are needed and where they can be purchased. Price and location are considered before recommendations are made to the client. (See Suggested Reading for resources on ostomy product suppliers.)

Chart 59-4

Focused Assessment for the Home Care Client with a Colostomy

- Assess gastrointestinal status, including
  - Dietary and fluid intake and habits
  - Presence or absence of nausea and vomiting
  - Weight gain or loss
  - Bowel elimination pattern and characteristics and amount of effluent (stool)
  - Bowel sounds
- Assess condition of stoma, including
  - Location, size, protrusion, color, and integrity
  - Signs of ischemia such as dull coloring or dark or purplish bruising
- Assess periostomal skin for
  - Presence or absence of excoriated skin, leakage underneath drainage system
  - Fit of appliance and effectiveness of skin barrier and appliance
- Assess client and family coping skills, including
  - Self-care abilities in the home
  - Acknowledgment of changes in body image and function
  - Sense of loss

 Evaluation

The nurse evaluates the care provided for the client with colorectal cancer. The expected outcomes may include that the client will

- Recover from surgery by a return of gastrointestinal (GI) function with stable respiratory, cardiovascular, and renal systems
- Demonstrate appropriate incision care and, if applicable, appropriate colostomy care with minimal assistance
- Acquire or maintain effective coping patterns by verbalizing the diagnosis of cancer and its treatment

INTESTINAL OBSTRUCTION

Overview

Intestinal obstruction is a common and serious disorder caused by a variety of conditions. The obstruction can be partial or complete. It can occur anywhere in the intestinal tract, although the ileum in the small intestine (the narrowest part of the intestinal tract) is the most common site. Because obstruction is very common and is linked to many other disorders, the nurse assesses for clinical manifestations of obstruction in all clients with gastrointestinal (GI) disorders.

Pathophysiology

Types of Obstruction

Partial and total obstructions can be either mechanical or nonmechanical. Mechanical obstruction can be caused by disorders outside the intestine (e.g., adhesions and hernias) or blockages in the lumen of the intestine (e.g., tumor, inflammation, stricture, or fecal impaction).

Nonmechanical obstruction (also known as paralytic ileus or adynamic ileus because it is a result of neuromuscular disturbance) does not involve a physical obstruction in or outside the intestine. Instead, muscle activity of the intestine is decreased, which results in a slowing of the movement of intestinal contents.

In both mechanical and nonmechanical obstruction, the intestinal contents accumulate at the area of obstruction and above it. The intestinal contents are composed of ingested fluid and saliva; gastric, pancreatic, and biliary secretions; and swallowed air.

Intestinal distention results from the intestine's inability to absorb these contents and mobilize them down the intestinal tract. Peristalsis increases in an effort to move the intestinal contents forward. The increase in peristalsis stimulates more secretions, which leads to additional distention; this causes edema of the bowel with increased capillary permeability. Plasma leaking into the peritoneal cavity and fluid trapped in the intestinal lumen markedly decrease the absorption of fluid and electrolytes into the vascular space. Reduced circulatory blood volume and electrolyte imbalances typically occur. Hypovolemia ranges from mild to extreme (hypovolemic shock).

Specific fluid and electrolyte problems depend on the part of the intestine that is blocked:

- An obstruction high in the small intestine causes a loss of gastric hydrochloride, which can lead to metabolic alkalosis.
- An obstruction below the duodenum but above the large bowel results in loss of both acids and bases so that acid-base imbalance need not be significant.
- Obstruction at the end of the small intestine and lower in the intestinal tract causes loss of alkaline fluids, which can lead to metabolic acidosis.

Complications of Obstruction

Renal insufficiency or even death can be a consequence of severe hypovolemia. Peritonitis with or without actual perforation is another major complication.

Bacteria in the intestinal contents lie stagnant in the obstructed intestine. This is not a problem unless the blood flow to the intestine is compromised. However, with so-called closed-loop obstruction (blockage in two different areas) or a strangulated obstruction (obstruction with compromised blood flow), the risk for peritonitis is great. Bacteria without blood supply can form an endotoxin, and release of the endotoxin into the peritoneal or systemic circulation can cause septic shock. With strangulated obstruction, there can also be a major blood loss into the intestine and the peritoneum.

The mortality rates vary from about 10% for small-bowel obstruction to 30% for large-bowel obstruction. Strangulated small-bowel obstruction has a mortality ranging from 20%–75%; strangulated large-bowel obstruction has a 60% mortality rate.

Etiology

Mechanical obstruction can result from any of the following:

- Adhesions
- Tumors
- Hernias
- Foreign bodies, such as gallstones and fecal impactions
- Strictures from Crohn's disease and radiation or congenital strictures
- Intussusception (telescoping of a segment of the intestine within itself)
- Volvulus (twisting of the intestine) (Fig. 59–6)
- Fibrosis from such disorders as endometriosis
- Vascular disorders, such as emboli and arteriosclerotic narrowing of mesenteric vessels

Adhesions are the most common cause of mechanical obstruction in the small intestine. Adhesions are bands of granulation and scar tissue that develop many years after abdominal surgery, encircling the intestine and constricting its lumen. Other common causes of colon obstruction are tumors, followed by diverticulitis and volvulus.

Paralytic (or adynamic) ileus is a nonmechanical obstruction, the most common of all intestinal obstructions. It is caused by physiologic, neurogenic, or chemical imbalances associated with decreased peristalsis from trauma or the effect of a toxin on autonomic intestinal control, as in

- Abdominal surgery and trauma
- Hypokalemia
- Myocardial infarction
- Pneumonia
- Spinal injuries

- Peritonitis
- Vascular insufficiency

Vascular insufficiency results when arterial or venous thrombosis or an embolus decreases blood flow to the mesenteric blood vessels surrounding the intestines. Vascular insufficiency to the bowel, also referred to as intestinal ischemia, can also occur when blood flow is reduced as a result of congestive heart failure or severe shock. Severe insufficiency of blood supply can result in infarction of surrounding organs (e.g., bowel infarction).

Paralytic ileus can be caused by handling of the intestines during abdominal surgery. It occurs to some degree after any abdominal surgical procedure; intestinal function is lost for a few hours to several days.

Incidence/Prevalence

Obstruction of the intestines occurs in approximately 20% of all clients who are seen for acute abdominal pain. It is the most common reason for surgery of the small intestine. Because bowel obstruction is a result of other disorders, statistics on the incidence of bowel obstruction are not readily available.

Obstruction of the intestines occurs in all age groups, but the incidence differs with age. In adults, 75% of all obstructions occur in the small intestine and 15% in the large intestine. In order of occurrence, adhesions, hernias, and tumors are the most common causes of small-bowel obstruction; cancer of the colon, diverticulitis, and volvulus cause most large-bowel obstruction in adults.

ELDERLY CONSIDERATIONS

 The physiologic changes associated with aging, such as decreased peristalsis and decreased mobility, contribute to fecal impactions in older adults. Fecal impactions can lead to partial or complete bowel obstruction.

Collaborative Management

Assessment

➤ *History*

To obtain the history of a client with a suspected or known intestinal obstruction, the nurse gears questions to factors that place the client at risk for obstruction. The nurse elicits the medical history (always identifying the time of diagnosis and treatment), specifically obtaining information about abdominal surgery, radiation therapy, inflammatory bowel disease, gallstones, hernias, and tumors. A diet history is also obtained. The nurse asks about the recent occurrence of nausea or vomiting and the time of the last bowel movement.

The nurse assesses for a family history of colorectal cancer and asks the client about blood in the stool or a change in bowel pattern. This information is important because these symptoms might indicate a colon tumor, and tumors are the most common cause of mechanical obstruction of the colon.

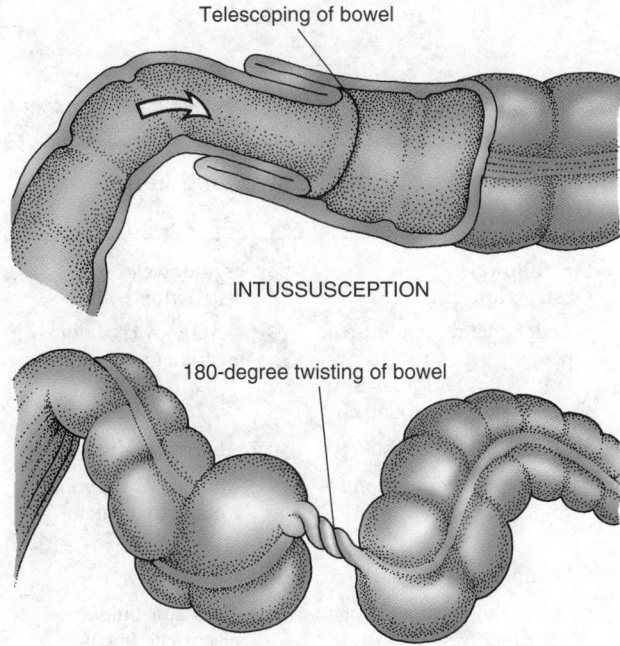

Telescoping of bowel

INTUSSUSCEPTION

180-degree twisting of bowel

VOLVULUS

Figure 59–6. Two types of mechanical obstruction.

➤ *Physical Assessment/Clinical Manifestations*

Mechanical Obstruction. The client with mechanical obstruction in the proximal (high) small intestine often has upper abdominal "discomfort." Obstruction of the mid or distal small intestine often causes episodic periumbilical cramping. Lower abdominal cramping pain is characteristic of large-bowel obstruction. The client describes cramping in the mid-abdominal region that comes and goes but is usually relatively comfortable between episodes. The client with an ischemic bowel, however, may describe severe pain, which is disproportional to physical findings.

On examination of the abdomen, the nurse may observe peristaltic waves. The nurse auscultates for proximal high-pitched bowel sounds (borborygmi) associated with the cramping early in the obstructive process as the intestine tries to push the mechanical obstruction forward. In later stages of mechanical obstruction, the bowel sounds are absent, especially distal to the obstruction. Abdominal distention is the hallmark of intestinal obstruction. It can vary from relatively none to severe, with taut, shiny skin; the umbilicus rises higher in the abdomen as the distention increases.

Nausea and vomiting are common with mechanical obstruction; vomitus varies in consistency, depending on the location of the obstruction. An obstruction above the ileum causes early and profuse vomiting, which initially contains partially digested food and chyme. As the intestine empties with vomiting, the contents become more watery, with bile and mucus. An obstruction below the ileum may not cause vomiting; if it does, the vomiting occurs in a different pattern and with different contents.

The ileocecal valve in the large intestine tries to prevent regurgitation of intestinal contents below it. However, if the valve cannot contain the intestinal contents, vomiting occurs. The vomitus from a mechanical obstruction in the large intestine is orange-brown and has a foul odor. The foul odor results from bacterial overgrowth in intestinal contents proximal to the obstruction, or it may actually be due to fecal contamination. Late stages of mechanical obstruction in the small intestine can also feature this type of vomitus from bacterial overgrowth or fecal contents. Bacterial overgrowth can also cause the client to have fecal breath.

Obstipation is a characteristic manifestation of complete mechanical obstruction of the small and large intestines, although feces distal to the obstruction may empty after symptoms begin.

Nonmechanical Obstruction. In most types of nonmechanical obstruction (paralytic, or adynamic, ileus), the pain is described as a constant, diffuse discomfort. Colicky cramping is not characteristic of this type of obstruction. Pain associated with obstruction attributable to vascular insufficiency or infarction is usually severe and constant. On auscultation of the abdomen, the nurse notes decreased bowel sounds in early obstruction and absent bowel sounds in later stages. Vomiting of gastric contents and bile is frequent, but the vomitus rarely has a foul odor and is rarely profuse. Obstipation may or may not be present. Singultus (hiccups) is common with all types of intestinal obstruction.

Temperature with obstruction is rarely higher than 37.8° C (100° F). Temperature higher than this, with or without guarding and tenderness, and a sustained elevation in pulse indicate strangulated obstruction or peritonitis. Chart 59–5 compares small-bowel and large-bowel obstruction.

➤ *Laboratory Assessment*

No laboratory test confirms a diagnosis of mechanical or nonmechanical obstruction. White blood cell (WBC) counts may be normal unless there is a strangulated obstruction, in which case there may be leukocytosis. Hemoglobin, hematocrit, creatinine, and blood urea nitrogen (BUN) values are often elevated, indicating dehydration. Serum sodium, chloride, and potassium concentrations are reduced because of loss of fluid and electrolytes.

High obstruction in the small intestine is likely to show elevated serum venous carbon dioxide concentration and other values indicative of metabolic alkalosis. Obstruction in the large intestine is likely to show low serum venous carbon dioxide concentration and other values suggestive of metabolic acidosis.

➤ *Radiographic Assessment*

The health care provider obtains flat-plate and upright abdominal x-rays as soon as an obstruction is suspected. Distention of loops of intestine with fluid and gas in the small intestine, with the absence of gas in the colon, indicates an obstruction in the small intestine. However, x-rays are often normal when a strangulated obstruction actually exists in the small intestine. Therefore, obstruction cannot be ruled out on the basis of x-ray findings.

Obstruction of the large intestine often shows gas distention of the colon on abdominal x-rays. Free air under the diaphragm on an abdominal x-ray indicates a perforated intestine.

Chart 59–5

Key Features of Small-Bowel and Large-Bowel Obstruction

Small-Bowel Obstruction	Large-Bowel Obstruction
• Abdominal discomfort/pain, possibly accompanied by visible peristaltic waves in upper and mid abdomen	• Severe lower abdominal cramping
• Abdominal distention	• Abdominal distention
• Nausea and early, profuse vomiting	• Minimal or no vomiting (may contain fecal material)
• Obstipation	• Obstipation
• Severe fluid and electrolyte imbalances	• No major fluid and electrolyte imbalances
• Metabolic alkalosis	• Metabolic acidosis

➤ *Other Diagnostic Assessment*

The physician may perform endoscopy (sigmoidoscopy or colonoscopy) or a barium enema study to determine the cause of the obstruction if the risk of perforation is not great. The examination chosen depends on the suspected location of the obstruction.

🔷 Interventions

If the obstruction is partial and there is no evidence of strangulation, nonsurgical management is the treatment of choice. Decompression of the intestinal tract is commonly implemented at the same time that fluid and electrolyte balance is being restored.

Nonsurgical Management. In addition to being allowed nothing by mouth (NPO), clients with intestinal obstruction typically have a nasogastric (NG) tube or a nasointestinal (NI) tube inserted. These tubes decompresses the bowel by draining fluid and air and are attached to suction; the type of suction depends on the type of tube inserted.

Nasointestinal Tubes. The physician occasionally inserts intestinal tubes (such as the Miller-Abbott, Cantor, and Harris tubes) for obstruction of the small intestine. These longer tubes extend into the small intestine; mercury-filled balloons at the end of a lumen act as a bolus of food, stimulating peristalsis and advancing down the intestinal tract (Fig. 59–7). The Cantor and Harris tubes are single-lumen tubes with mercury-filled balloons at the tips and suction ports within the same lumen, proximal to the tip. The Miller-Abbott tube has two separate lumens for mercury and drainage.

The nurse assists with progression of the tube by helping the client change position every 2 hours and, if ordered, by advancing the tube 3–4 inches at specified times. These tubes are never taped to the nose until they reach a specified position in the intestine. As the tube is being inserted and advanced, it drains by gravity. The nurse monitors the drainage; if drainage stops, the nurse obtains a physician's order to inject 10 mL of air. The nurse does not irrigate the NI tube with fluid unless ordered by the physician. If ordered, the nurse attaches low intermittent suction to the suction lumen when the tube has stopped advancing. Chart 59–6 summarizes the nurse's role in caring for clients with NI tubes.

Many physicians avoid the use of NI tubes because insertion of the mercury-filled lumen is often difficult; the time it takes to insert the tube also delays treatment. Insertion of this tube can be uncomfortable for clients. However, most clients with an obstruction have at least an NG tube in place, unless the obstruction is mild.

Nasogastric Tubes. Salem sumps and Anderson tubes are commonly used NG tubes that sit distally in the stomach and are attached to *low continuous* suction. Levin tubes are connected to *low intermittent* suction.

At least every 4 hours, the nurse assesses the client with an NG tube for proper placement of the tube, tube patency, and output (Research Applications for Nursing). The nurse also assesses for

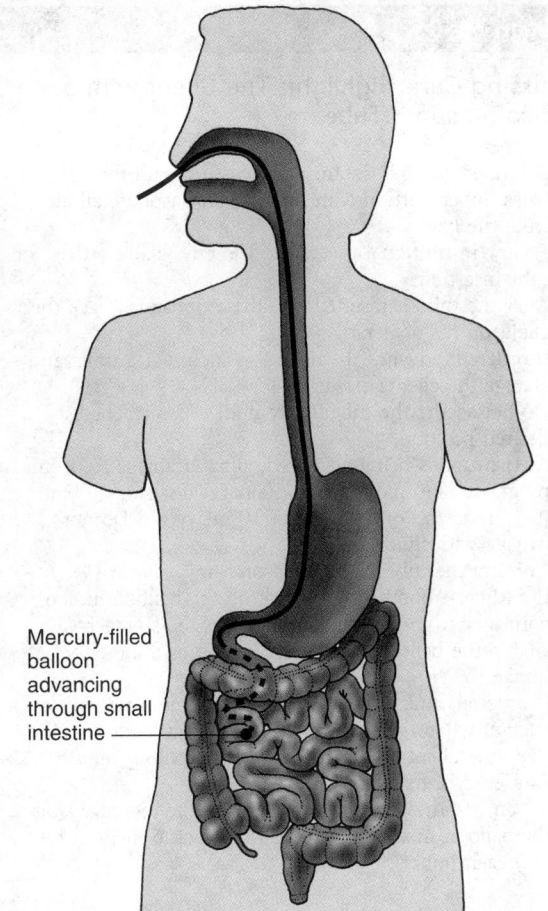

Mercury-filled balloon advancing through small intestine —

Figure 59–7. A nasointestinal tube is passed down the intestinal tract. The mercury-filled balloon at the end of the lumen stimulates peristalsis.

- Skin integrity at the point of insertion at least daily
- Peristalsis by auscultating for bowel sounds with the suction disconnected (suction will mask peristaltic sounds)

The nurse evaluates for flatus or bowel movements and measures the abdominal girth at the same point each day. The client is also assessed for nausea and asked to report this manifestation.

If problems are noted with NG tubes, the effect of nonfunctioning tubes is immediately determined. For example, some tubes move out of optimal drainage position or become plugged. In this case, the nurse notes a decrease in gastric output or stasis of the tube's contents. The nurse assesses the client for nausea, vomiting, increased abdominal distention, and placement of the tube.

After appropriate placement is established, the contents are aspirated, and the tube is irrigated with 30 mL of normal saline every 4 hours or as needed to maintain patency.

Other Nonsurgical Techniques. Most types of nonmechanical obstruction respond to NG decompression along with medical treatment of the primary disorder. Incomplete mechanical obstruction can sometimes be successfully treated without surgery. Obstruction caused by fecal

---

Chart 59–6

Nursing Care Highlight: The Client with a Nasointestinal Tube

- Before inserting a Cantor or Harris tube, fill the balloon bag's upper portion with mercury and aspirate all air from the bag.
- Follow institutional policy and the physician's orders for tube insertion.
- After the tube is inserted into the esophagus, place the client on his or her right side.
- If ordered, advance the tube 2–4 inches at a time, and change the client's position.
- Do not secure the tube firmly until it has reached its desired position.
- As the tube is being advanced, allow drainage to occur by gravity and monitor the drainage. If it stops, obtain the physician's order to inject 10 mL of air. Do not irrigate with fluid.
- Confirm the tube's placement on x-ray.
- If a Miller-Abbott tube is used, fill the balloon lumen with mercury when the tube reaches the stomach.
- Clamp the balloon lumen and label it as a mercury lumen.
- If ordered, attach the suction lumen to intermittent low suction when the tube reaches the specified destination.
- Keep the client NPO and provide scrupulous mouth care every 2 hr and PRN.
- When withdrawing the tube, remove the mercury from the balloon first, and pull the tube back 6 inches (2.4 cm) each hour.

---

impaction usually resolves after disimpaction and enema administration. Intussusception may respond to hydrostatic pressure changes during a barium enema.

Fluid and Electrolyte Replacement. Intravenous (IV) fluid replacement and maintenance are indicated for all clients with intestinal obstruction because of some degree of vascular fluid loss. On the basis of electrolyte, BUN, and serum creatinine levels as well as the client's overall condition, the surgeon orders normal saline or a balanced salt solution with potassium. Blood replacement may be indicated in strangulated obstruction because of blood loss into the bowel or the peritoneal cavity.

The nurse or assistive nursing personnel monitors the client's vital signs and other measures of fluid status (e.g., urinary output, skin turgor, and mucous membranes). The nurse also assesses for edema from third spacing because fluid is lost mostly from the vascular space into surrounding spaces (e.g., peritoneal cavity). In collaboration with the dietitian, the physician may order total parenteral nutrition (TPN) to improve the nutritional status of the client, especially if the client has had chronic nutritional problems and has been NPO for an extended period. (Chapter 64 covers the nursing care of clients receiving TPN.)

Because of fluid losses, the client with intestinal obstruction is characteristically thirsty. The nurse provides frequent mouth care to help maintain moist mucous

membranes. Lemon-glycerin swabs are avoided because they can increase mouth dryness. A small amount of ice chips may be allowed if the client is not having surgery; however, a physician's order should be obtained. Ice chips can provide more free water than electrolytes; thus, potassium and hydrochloric acid are washed out of the NG tube. The nurse monitors the client carefully for intake and output to avoid electrolyte imbalance and false interpretation of gastric output measurements.

Pain Management. The abdominal distention commonly noted with intestinal obstruction can cause a great deal of discomfort, especially when distention is severe. The colicky, crampy pain that comes and goes with mechanical obstruction and the nausea, vomiting, dry mucous membranes, and thirst contribute to the client's discomfort. The nurse must continually assess the character and location of the pain. The nurse immediately reports any pain that significantly increases or changes from a colicky, intermittent type to a constant discomfort. Such changes can indicate perforation of the intestine or peritonitis.

Opioid analgesics are normally withheld in the diagnostic period so that clinical manifestations of perforation or peritonitis are not masked. The nurse explains to the client and the family the rationale for not giving analge-

---

▷ Research Applications for Nursing

An Effective Means of Securing NG Tubes Is Essential

Comparison of nasogastric tube securing methods and tube types in medical intensive care patients. American Journal of Critical Care, 4(3), 198–203.

This study examines the most effective and safest method to secure nasogastric (NG) tubes in medical intensive care clients. Pink tape, clear tape, or a butterfly was used in 264 taping episodes of 103 clients. The pink tape stayed in place for an average of 100 hours, whereas the clear tape stayed in place an average of 56 hours. The butterfly device was least effective and stayed in place on the average of 30 hours. The researchers also found that duodenal tubes stayed secure longer than sump tubes.

Critique. This is an important topic for clinical nursing research. The researchers used a convenience sample, but randomly assigned subjects to treatment groups, which enhanced the internal validity of the study. The researchers also considered variables such as level of alertness, confusion, sedation, mobility, and use of restraints. This study was conducted with clients in medical intensive care units; therefore, the results cannot be generalized. The study should be replicated in a variety of clinical settings and include other materials and devices used to secure these types of tubes.

Possible Nursing Implications. Nurses need to be aware that traditional approaches to care may or may not be the most effective and should be researched carefully. Displacement of NG tubes leads to problems such as aspiration and additional costs in terms of supplies, nursing time, and discomfort for clients. Identifying and using the most effective strategy to secure these tubes is essential to nursing practice.

sics. If an analgesic is ordered, it is most likely meperidine hydrochloride (Demerol); morphine causes decreased intestinal motility, which may lead to nausea and vomiting. However, meperidine can also cause nausea and vomiting. The nurse must be alert to this side effect, because nausea and vomiting are also signs of NG obstruction or worsening bowel obstruction.

The nurse helps the client obtain a position of comfort with frequent position changes to promote increased peristalsis. A semi-Fowler's position helps alleviate the pressure of abdominal distention on the chest; not only is this a good comfort technique, but it also facilitates adequate thoracic excursion and normal breathing patterns.

Discomfort is generally less with nonmechanical obstruction than with mechanical obstruction. With both types of obstruction, discomfort is aggravated by ingestion of food or fluids.

Surgical Management. In all cases of complete mechanical obstruction and in many cases of incomplete mechanical obstruction, surgical intervention is necessary to relieve the obstruction. Strangulated obstruction is always complete, and surgical intervention is, therefore, always required. An exploratory laparotomy is initially performed for most clients with obstruction. More specific surgical procedures depend on the cause of the obstruction.

Exploratory laparotomy is a surgical opening of the abdominal cavity to explore for abnormalities (in this case, the cause of the intestinal obstruction).

Preoperative Care. The nurse provides preoperative teaching as discussed in Chapter 20. If time permits, all clients who require surgery for obstruction have NG or intestinal intubation and suction before surgery.

Operative Procedure. The surgeon enters the abdominal cavity and explores for obstruction. If adhesions are found to be the cause of the obstruction, the adhesions are lysed (released). Obstruction caused by tumor or diverticulitis requires colon resection with primary anastomosis or temporary or permanent colostomy. If obstruction is caused by intestinal infarction, embolectomy, thrombectomy, or colon resection (partial removal) may be necessary, particularly if the intestine is gangrenous.

Postoperative Care. Postoperative care for the client undergoing exploratory laparotomy with lysis of adhesions, colon resection, thrombectomy, or embolectomy is similar to that described in Chapter 22 and earlier in this chapter. All clients have an NG tube in place until peristalsis (as characterized by return of bowel sounds) resumes. The client may be weaned off the NG tube by slowly discontinuing suction and then clamping the tube for a scheduled time. Residual drainage is checked at each stage to assess peristalsis without decompression before removing the NG tube.

➤ Continuing Care

All clients with intestinal obstruction are hospitalized. The length of stay depends on the cause of the obstruction and the treatment necessary to relieve it. If surgery is performed, 1 week of hospitalization is often required. Clients who have complicated obstruction, such as strangulation or incarceration, are at greater risk for peritonitis, sepsis, and shock. The hospital stay may be several weeks, depending on the severity of complications.

Clients with nonmechanical (adynamic) intestinal obstruction are less likely to require a lengthy hospitalization because of the obstruction alone. Adynamic obstruction generally responds to NG intubation and suction within a few days.

➤ Home Care Management

For the client who has had an intestinal obstruction, home care preparation depends on the cause of the obstruction and the treatment required. Clients who have resolution of obstruction without surgical intervention are assessed for their knowledge of strategies to avoid recurrent obstruction. For example, if fecal impaction was the cause of the obstruction, the nurse assesses the client's ability to carry out a bowel regimen independently. For clients who have undergone surgery, the nurse evaluates their ability to function at home with the added tasks of incision care and possibly colostomy care.

➤ Health Teaching

The nurse instructs the client to report any abdominal pain or distention, nausea, or vomiting, with or without constipation, which might indicate recurrent obstruction. The client, however, should be reassured that recurrent paralytic ileus is not usually a problem. The client who has had mechanical obstruction from fecal impaction (often the elderly client) needs to have a structured bowel regimen to prevent recurrence (Chart 59–7). The nurse instructs this client to adhere to high-fiber diets, to exercise, and to drink at least 24 ounces of water daily,

---

Chart 59–7

Nursing Focus on the Elderly: Fecal Impaction

- Teach the client to eat high-fiber foods, including plenty of raw fruits and vegetables and whole-grain products.
- Encourage the client to drink adequate amounts of fluids, especially water.
- Do not routinely administer a laxative; teach the client that laxative abuse decreases abdominal muscle tone and contributes to an atonic colon.
- Encourage the client to exercise regularly, if possible. Walking every day is an excellent exercise for promoting intestinal motility.
- Use natural foods to stimulate peristalsis, such as warm beverages and prune juice.
- Take bulk-forming products, such as Metamucil, to provide fiber.
- Check the client's stool for amount and frequency; oozing of soft or diarrheal stool often indicates a fecal impaction.
- Have the client sit on a toilet or bedside commode, rather than on a bedpan, for elimination.

unless contraindicated. The physician may also order bulk-forming laxatives to help the client maintain a consistent elimination pattern.

The nurse teaches the client who has had surgery about incision care, drug therapy, and activity limitations. Drug therapy consists of an oral opioid analgesic, such as oxycodone hydrochloride with acetaminophen (Tylox, Percocet, Endocet✦), to be taken as needed for incisional discomfort.

With resolution of obstruction, the client focuses on the cause and necessary treatment. Psychosocial preparation depends on these two factors. The client who had curative treatment of the underlying cause most likely requires less support than the client who underwent treatment of obstruction related to a serious disease that will require further treatment.

The nurse allows the client to express fears and concerns about the future. The nurse assesses the client's understanding and needs with regard to treatment plans.

> ### ➤ *Health Care Resources*

The need for follow-up appointments depends on the cause of and the treatment required for the obstruction. If the client is at risk for fecal impaction, the nurse can arrange for a home health nurse to assess the gastrointestinal (GI) function and dietary habits of the client on an ongoing basis. A home health nurse should also be arranged if the client needs help with incision or colostomy care.

ABDOMINAL TRAUMA

Overview

Abdominal trauma is defined as injury to the structures located between the diaphragm and the pelvis, which occurs when the abdomen is subjected to blunt or penetrating forces. Organs injured may include the large or small bowel, spleen, duodenum, pancreas, kidneys, and urinary bladder.

At least one half of all blunt abdominal trauma occurs from motor vehicle accidents (MVA) (Sommers & Johnson, 1997). Other causes of blunt trauma include falls, aggravated assaults, and contact sports. *Penetrating abdominal trauma* is caused by gunshot, stabbing, or impalement with an object. The liver is the most commonly injured organ in blunt and penetrating trauma. The spleen is the most commonly injured organ in blunt abdominal trauma. The small intestine is the third most commonly injured organ in abdominal trauma; 80% of injuries are caused by gunshot wounds (GSW).

TRANSCULTURAL CONSIDERATIONS

Motor vehicle accidents are three times more common in males than females in the 15- to 24-year age group. European-Americans have a death rate 40% higher from MVAs than do African-Americans in the 15- to 34-year age group (Sommers & Johnson, 1997). Penetrating injuries from GSWs and stab wounds are more common in preteen and young adults than in older adults and are more common in African-Americans than European-Americans.

Collaborative Management

 Assessment

In the emergency phase of treatment, health care providers focus on the risks of hemorrhage, shock, and peritonitis. Mental status and skin perfusion are *priority* nursing assessments. Skin perfusion is the most reliable clinical guide in assessing hypovolemic shock:

- In a person with mild shock, the skin is pale, cool, and moist.
- With moderate shock, diaphoresis is more marked and urinary output ceases.
- With severe shock, changes in mental status are manifested by agitation, disorientation, and recent memory loss.

The nurse assesses for abdominal trauma by asking the client about the presence, location, and quality of pain. The abdomen, flanks, back, genitalia, and rectum are inspected for contusions, abrasions, lacerations, ecchymosis, penetrating injuries, and symmetry. All of the client's clothes must be removed. If pneumatic garments such as antishock trousers are in place, they are usually not removed unless aggressive fluid replacement has been given to the client, a surgical team is immediately available to intervene, and the attending physician orders it to be done. After pneumatic garments are removed, uncontrolled hemorrhage can occur. Antishock trousers have a constrictive effect on hemorrhage in the trunk and facilitate circulatory return to the heart. However, they can cause compartment syndrome to the lower extremities and, consequently, are not used routinely.

To perform an adequate inspection, the nurse turns the client while maintaining spinal immobilization. Ecchymosis may signify internal bleeding. Ecchymosis around the umbilicus is known as *Cullen's sign* and may indicate retroperitoneal bleeding into the abdominal wall. Ecchymosis in either flank, known as *Turner's sign,* also indicates retroperitoneal bleeding.

The nurse auscultates the abdomen for bowel sounds. Absent or diminished bowel sounds may be caused by the presence of blood, bacteria, or a chemical irritant in the abdominal cavity. The nurse also auscultates for bruits in the abdomen, which indicate renal artery injury.

The nurse percusses the abdomen next. An abnormal sign associated with abdominal trauma is resonance over the right flank with the client lying on the left side. This is known as *Ballance's sign,* which is found with a ruptured spleen. Resonance over the liver, which is normally dull, is due to free air, which is pathologic. Dullness over hollow organs that normally contain gas, such as the stomach and the large and small intestines, may indicate blood or fluid. Light abdominal palpation identifies areas of tenderness, rebound tenderness, guarding, rigidity, and spasm. If the nurse palpates a mass, it may be blood or a fluid collection.

The client without obvious significant bleeding or definite signs of peritoneal irritation undergoes abdominal radiography, diagnostic peritoneal lavage, and computed tomography (CT). For peritoneal lavage, the physician inserts a large-bore catheter into the abdomen and allows fluid to enter the abdominal cavity. If the return drainage from the abdomen is pink or grossly bloody, the health care team prepares the client for surgery.

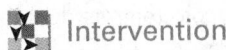 Interventions

Nonsurgical Management. Nursing interventions include placement of at least two large-bore intravenous (IV) catheters in the upper extremities. IV catheters in the lower extremities are not used; if the vasculature has been injured, fluid can pool in the abdomen. The physician may insert a central venous catheter to assist with rapid fluid volume infusion. IV fluid consists of a balanced saline solution, crystalloids, and possibly blood.

The physician typically orders
- Arterial blood gas analysis
- Complete blood count
- Serum electrolyte, glucose and amylase, and blood urea nitrogen (BUN) determinations
- Liver function tests
- Clotting studies

Hemoglobin and hematocrit do not initially reflect true blood loss; values appear higher than they actually are because of hemoconcentration from volume loss. Serial hemoglobin and hematocrit measurements identify true blood loss. An elevated white blood cell (WBC) count may indicate a ruptured spleen. Elevation of serum amylase activity may signal injury to the pancreas or the bowel. All laboratory work is compiled so that values can be compared and subtle changes noted.

The client is attached to a cardiac monitor in the emergency department. The nurse inserts an indwelling urinary catheter (Foley), unless there is blood at the urinary meatus. Initially and hourly thereafter, the nurse evaluates urinary outputs for bleeding and specific gravity. The nurse checks for blood and protein in the urine. If there is an open abdominal wound or evisceration, the nurse covers it with a sterile dry dressing unless the physician orders otherwise. Unless it is contraindicated, as in the case of a concomitant skull fracture, the physician or nurse inserts a nasogastric (NG) tube, which is kept in place to identify bleeding and to minimize the risk of vomiting and aspiration. The nurse administers antibiotics as ordered to reduce the risk of peritonitis.

If the client with known abdominal trauma has no definite clinical manifestations of active bleeding or abdominal injury, the client is admitted to the hospital for observation. Blunt trauma can cause active, but often not obvious, damage. The nurse assesses for abdominal or referred pain and nausea. Every 15–30 minutes in the early postinjury period and then hourly, the nurse evaluates
- Mental status
- Vital signs
- Clinical findings, such as vomiting, guarding, rigidity, and rebound tenderness
- Skin temperature
- Bowel sounds
- Urinary output

The nurse reports any change immediately to the physician.

It is more important for the nurse to recognize the high risk of an active abdominal injury and assess for general signs of abdominal injury (e.g., hemorrhage and peritonitis) than to identify the exact nature of the abdominal injury. Analgesics for pain are not prescribed at this time so that clinical manifestations are not masked or overlooked. The nurse explains the rationale for withholding analgesics to the client and family or significant others.

Surgical Management. For the client with severe abdominal trauma, the surgeon performs an exploratory laparotomy and repair of abdominal injuries immediately if there are definite signs of peritoneal irritation. These signs include
- Rebound tenderness
- Significant bleeding from an NG tube or the rectum
- Active blood loss that cannot be associated with an injury outside the abdomen
- Evisceration
- A gunshot wound (GSW) with possible peritoneal involvement

Most stab wounds require exploratory laparotomy, but as many as 25% are superficial and do not involve the peritoneum. Using local anesthesia, the surgeon explores and cleans superficial stab wounds; the client does not require an exploratory laparotomy.

Before discharge from the hospital, the client who has experienced abdominal trauma is taught the signs and symptoms of abdominal bleeding whether or not surgery has been performed. The nurse instructs the client to report abdominal pain, nausea, vomiting, bloody or black stools, fever, weakness, and dizziness.

Hemorrhage can occasionally occur weeks after blunt abdominal trauma, despite medical evaluation. For the client who undergoes surgery or exploration of wounds, the nurse provides instructions on wound care before discharge from the hospital.

POLYPS

Overview

Polyps in the intestinal tract are small growths covered with mucosa and attached to the surface of the intestine. Although most are benign, polyps are significant in that some have the potential to become malignant.

Polyps are identified by their tissue type. The presence of adenomas always necessitates medical consultation because of their malignant potential. Although only 2%–5% of adenomas progress to cancer, almost all colorectal cancers develop from an adenoma (Markowitz & Winawer, 1997). Adenomas are further classified as villous or tubular. Of these, villous adenomas pose a greater cancer risk.

Familial polyposis and Gardner's syndrome are inherited syndromes characterized by progressive development of hundreds to thousands of colorectal adenomas. Unless these syndromes are treated, colorectal cancer inevitably occurs by the fourth to fifth decade of life (Markowitz & Winawer, 1997).

Other types include hyperplastic and hamartomatous polyps. Hyperplastic polyps, which include mucosal and

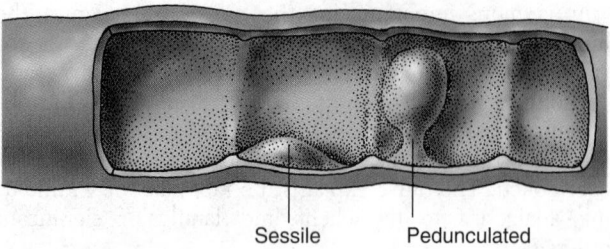

Figure 59–8. Pedunculated and sessile polyps. Pedunculated polyps, such as tubular adenomas, are stalk-like. Sessile polyps, such as villous adenomas, are broad-based.

inflammatory varieties, are entirely benign with no malignant potential. Hamartomatous polyps include juvenile and Peutz-Jeghers syndrome polyps. Although both are generally benign, rare reports of malignant changes have been reported in juvenile polyps.

In addition to being classified by their tissue type, polyps are described according to their appearance (Fig. 59–8). Pedunculated polyps are stalk like; a thin stem attaches them to the intestinal wall. They become elongated as peristalsis pulls them into the lumen of the intestine. Polyps attached to the intestinal walls by a broad base are described as sessile. A malignant polyp may be pedunculated or sessile.

Collaborative Management

Polyps are usually asymptomatic and are discovered during routine diagnostic testing or tests for blood in the stool. However, they can cause gross rectal bleeding, intestinal obstruction, or intussusception. Diagnostic studies involve a barium enema examination and proctosigmoidoscopy or colonoscopy for ruling out cancer. Biopsy specimens of polyps can be obtained, or the entire polyp can be removed (polypectomy) with use of an electrocautery snare that fits through the sigmoidoscope or colonoscope. This often eliminates the need for abdominal surgery to remove a suspicious or definitely malignant polyp. The client with familial polyposis or Gardner's syndrome most often requires a total colectomy (colon removal) to prevent the development of cancer.

Nursing care focuses on client education. The nurse instructs the client about

- The significance of polyps
- What clinical manifestations to watch for and report
- The need for ongoing monitoring by the health care team

The client with a known benign polyp that does not need to be removed has frequent sigmoidoscopic or colonoscopic examinations to monitor for any growth or change in the polyp or an increase in the number of polyps. If the client has had a polypectomy, follow-up sigmoidoscopic or colonoscopic examinations are needed, because there is an increased risk of multiple polyps in the client who has had at least one polyp.

Nursing care of the client after polypectomy of the colorectal area includes monitoring for abdominal disten-

tion and pain, rectal bleeding, mucopurulent rectal drainage, and fever.

A small amount of blood might appear in the stool after a polypectomy, but this should be temporary. (Care for the client who has had a total colectomy is described in Chapter 60, under Crohn's disease.)

HEMORRHOIDS

Overview

Hemorrhoids are unnaturally swollen or distended veins in the anorectal region. They are common and not significant unless they cause pain or bleeding. These distended veins begin as part of the normal structure in the anal region. With limited distention, the veins function as a valve overlying the anal sphincter that assists in continence. Increased intra-abdominal pressure causes elevated systemic and portal venous pressure, which is transmitted to the anorectal veins. Arterioles in the anorectal region shunt blood directly to the distended anorectal veins, which increases the pressure. With repeated elevations in pressure from increased intra-abdominal pressure and engorgement from arteriolar shunting of blood, the distended veins eventually separate from the smooth muscle surrounding them. The result is prolapse of the hemorrhoidal vessels.

Hemorrhoids are internal or external (Fig. 59–9). Internal hemorrhoids, which cannot be seen on inspection of the perineal area, lie above the anal sphincter. External hemorrhoids lie below the anal sphincter and can be seen on inspection of the anal region. Prolapsed hemorrhoids can become thrombosed or inflamed, or they can bleed.

The most common causes of repeated increased abdominal pressure resulting in hemorrhoids are straining at stool, pregnancy, portal hypertension, and colorectal cancer.

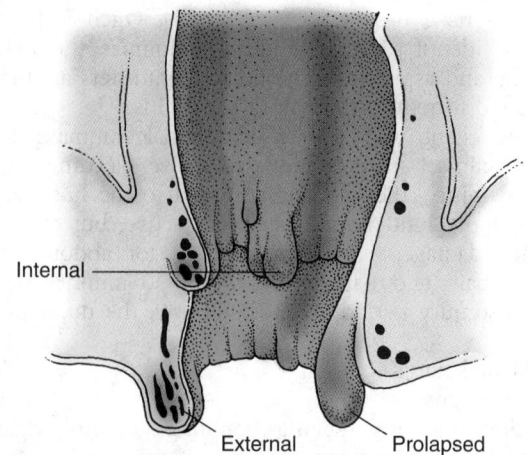

Figure 59–9. Internal, external, and prolapsed hemorrhoids. Internal hemorrhoids lie above the anal sphincter and cannot be seen on inspection of the anal area. External hemorrhoids lie below the anal sphincter and can be seen on inspection of the anal region. Hemorrhoids that enlarge, fall down, and protrude through the anus are called prolapsed hemorrhoids.

Collaborative Management

 Assessment

The most common symptoms of hemorrhoids are bleeding and prolapse. Blood is characteristically bright red and is found on toilet tissue or outside the stool. Pain is a common symptom and is often associated with thrombosis, especially if thrombosis occurs suddenly. Other symptoms include itching and mucous discharge. Diagnosis is made by inspection, digital examination, proctoscopy, or proctoscopic ultrasonography.

 Interventions

Nonsurgical Management. Treatment is conservative and is aimed at reducing symptoms with a minimum of discomfort, cost, and time lost from usual activities. Local treatment and diet therapy are initiated when symptoms begin. Application of cold packs to the anorectal region for 3–4 hours at the onset of pain, followed by hot sitz baths three or four times a day, is often enough to relieve discomfort, even if the hemorrhoids are thrombosed.

Witch hazel soaks (e.g., Tucks) are also effective. Topical anesthetics, such as lidocaine (Xylocaine), are useful for severe pain. Dibucaine (Nupercainal) ointment, an over-the-counter remedy, may be applied for mild to moderate pain. This ointment should be used only temporarily, however, because it can mask worsening symptoms and delay diagnosis of a severe disorder. If itching or inflammation is present, the health care provider prescribes a steroid preparation, such as hydrocortisone.

Diets high in fiber and fluids are recommended to promote regular bowel movements without straining. Stool softeners, such as docusate sodium (Colace), can be used temporarily. Irritating laxatives are avoided. The health care provider may prescribe oral analgesics for pain if the hemorrhoids are thrombosed.

Conservative treatment should alleviate symptoms in 3–5 days. If symptoms continue or recur frequently, the client may require surgical intervention.

Surgical Management. The surgeon can perform several procedures for symptomatic hemorrhoids. The type of surgery depends on the degree of prolapse, whether there is thrombosis, and the overall condition of the client. Surgical methods include sclerotherapy, elastic band ligation, cryosurgery, and hemorrhoidectomy.

In *sclerotherapy,* the surgeon injects a sclerosing agent into the tissues around the hemorrhoids to obliterate the vessels. Sclerotherapy can be done on an outpatient basis without long-term pain. However, it can be done only for low-grade hemorrhoids.

Elastic band ligation is considered a better method because of its success rate. One or two rubber bands are put on at one outpatient visit, and repeated visits may be needed for ligation of all hemorrhoids. Local pain after ligation does occur, and hemorrhage may also occur.

Cryosurgery, which can be done on an outpatient basis, involves freezing the hemorrhoid with a probe to cause necrosis. Because of its many disadvantages (e.g., profuse and foul drainage lasting up to 6 weeks, hemorrhage, large painful skin tags, and incomplete destruction), cryosurgery is no longer a widely accepted method.

Hemorrhoidectomy, the standard treatment, can now be performed in an outpatient setting. Approximately 10% of clients with symptomatic hemorrhoids undergo hemorrhoidectomies. The most common problem after hemorrhoidectomy is pain, which is severe for 1–2 days after surgery. Urinary retention can also occur because of rectal spasms and anorectal tenderness. Hemorrhage, which may be internal and not visible or external, is a rare but potential complication.

The nurse teaches clients with hemorrhoids about the need for adhering to high-fiber, high-fluid diets to promote regular bowel patterns and for local treatments. The nurse advises clients to avoid stimulant laxatives, which are habit forming.

For clients who undergo any type of surgical intervention, the nurse monitors for hemorrhage and pain postoperatively. These clients, in particular, require ongoing interventions for pain because of its severity. Appropriate nursing interventions include

- Assisting clients to a side-lying position
- Keeping fresh ice packs over the dressing until the packing is removed (if ordered by the physician)
- Using moist heat (as in sitz baths) three or four times a day after the first 12 hours postoperatively

Vasodilation from the sitz bath redirects blood to the rectal area, which might cause the client to feel faint. The nurse may place an ice bag on the client's head during the sitz bath to prevent feelings of faintness. A flotation pad can be used under the buttocks for sitting.

The client's first postoperative bowel movement may be very painful. The physician usually prescribes stool softeners, such as docusate sodium, to begin on the first postoperative day. Opioid analgesics are administered before the client attempts to defecate, and the caregiver should stay near the client during the first defecation. All clients who have undergone hemorrhoidectomy are monitored for urinary retention. Measures to facilitate voiding are provided as needed, such as

- Administration of analgesics
- Provision of privacy
- Stimulation by running water
- Spirits of peppermint in the commode

MALABSORPTION SYNDROME

Overview

Malabsorption is a syndrome associated with a variety of disorders and intestinal surgical procedures. One or multiple nutrients are not digested or absorbed as a result of a generalized flattening of the mucosa of the small intestine.

With various disorders, physiologic mechanisms limit absorption of nutrients because of one or more of the following abnormalities:

- Bile salt deficiencies
- Enzyme deficiencies
- Bacteria

- Disruption of the mucosal lining of the small intestine
- Alteration in lymphatic and vascular circulation
- Decrease in gastric or intestinal surface area

The nutrient that is malabsorbed depends on which abnormality exists and the specific location of the abnormality in the intestinal tract.

Deficiencies of bile salts can lead to malabsorption of fats and fat-soluble vitamins. Bile salt deficiencies can result from decreased synthesis of bile in the liver, bile obstruction, or alteration of bile salt absorption in the small intestine.

Enzymes normally found in the intestine split disaccharides (complex sugars) to monosaccharides (simple sugars). Examples of these enzymes are lactase, sucrase, maltase, and isomaltase. Lactase deficiency is the most common disaccharide enzyme deficiency. Without sufficient amounts of this enzyme, the body is not able to break down lactose. Lactase deficiency can be due to genetic transmission, injury to intestinal mucosa from viral hepatitis, bacterial proliferation in the intestine, and sprue. Deficiencies of the other disaccharide enzymes are rare.

Pancreatic enzymes are also necessary for absorption of vitamin B_{12}. With destruction or obstruction of the pancreas or insufficient pancreatic stimulation, these nutrients are malabsorbed. Chronic pancreatitis, pancreatic carcinoma, resection of the pancreas, and cystic fibrosis can cause these malabsorption problems.

Loops of bowel can accumulate intestinal contents when there is a decrease in peristalsis, which can result in bacterial overgrowth. Bacteria at these sites break down bile salts, and fewer salts are available for fat absorption. These bacteria can also ingest vitamin B_{12}, which contributes to vitamin B_{12} deficiency. This phenomenon can occur after a gastrectomy or with progressive systemic sclerosis and diabetic enteropathy.

Disruption of the mucosal lining of the intestine is responsible for the malabsorption that occurs with celiac (nontropical) sprue, tropical sprue, Crohn's disease, and ulcerative colitis.

In *celiac (nontropical) sprue,* the absorptive surface area in the intestine is lost; there is malabsorption of most nutrients. Celiac sprue is thought to be due to a genetic immune hypersensitivity response to gluten or its breakdown products or to result from the accumulation of gluten in the diet with peptidase deficiency.

Tropical sprue is caused by an infectious agent that has not been identified but is thought to be bacterial. Mucosal changes occur in a more widespread manner than in celiac sprue. However, the changes are not as severe as in celiac sprue. Tropical sprue results in malabsorption of fat, folic acid, and vitamin B_{12} in later stages of the disease.

The inflammation in Crohn's disease interferes with the surface of cells absorbing bile salts and, therefore, leads to fat malabsorption. In ulcerative colitis, protein loss may occur.

Obstruction to lymphatic flow in the intestine can lead to loss of plasma proteins along with minerals (such as iron, copper, and calcium), vitamin B_{12}, folic acid, and lipids. Lymphatic obstruction can be caused by

- Tumors
- Inflammation
- Radiation enteritis
- Crohn's disease
- Lymphoma
- Whipple's disease
- Congestive heart failure
- Constrictive pericarditis

Interference with blood flow to the intestinal mucosa, which occurs in celiac and superior mesenteric artery disease, results in malabsorption.

With intestinal surgery, there is loss of surface area to facilitate absorption. Resection of the ileum results in vitamin B_{12}, bile salt, and other nutrient deficiencies. Gastric surgery is one of the most common causes of malabsorption and maldigestion. Other conditions associated with maldigestion and malabsorption include small-bowel ischemia and radiation enteritis.

Collaborative Management

 Assessment

Clinical manifestations of malabsorption vary, but steatorrhea (greater than normal amounts of fat in the feces) is a common sign. Steatorrhea is a result of bile salt deconjugation, nonabsorbed fats, or bacteria in the intestine. Other clinical manifestations include

- Weight loss
- Fatigue
- Decreased libido
- Easy bruising
- Anemia (with iron and folic acid or vitamin B_{12} deficiency)
- Bone pain (with calcium and vitamin D deficiency)
- Edema (caused by hypoproteinemia)

Laboratory studies reveal a decrease in mean corpuscular volume (MCV), mean corpuscular hemoglobin (MCH), and mean corpuscular hemoglobin concentration (MCHC); these decreases indicate hypochromic microcytic anemia resulting from iron deficiency. Increased MCV and variable MCH and MCHC indicate macrocytic anemia resulting from vitamin B_{12} and folic acid deficiencies. Serum iron levels are low in protein malabsorption because of insufficient gastric acid for use of iron. Serum cholesterol levels may be low from decreased absorption and digestion of fat. Low serum calcium levels may indicate malabsorption of vitamin D and amino acids. Low levels of serum vitamin A (retinol) and carotene, its precursor, indicate a bile salt deficiency and malabsorption of fat. Serum albumin and total protein levels are low if protein loss occurs. A quantitative fecal fat analysis is elevated in either malabsorption or maldigestion.

A lactose tolerance test result that shows less than a 20% rise in the blood glucose level over the fasting blood glucose level indicates lactose intolerance. A monosaccharide test validates or rules out lactase deficiency. The xylose absorption test can reveal low urine and serum D-xylose levels if malabsorption in the small intestine is present, a common finding in celiac sprue.

The Schilling test measures urinary excretion of vitamin

B_{12} for diagnosis of pernicious anemia and a variety of other malabsorption syndromes. The bile acid breath test assesses the absorption of bile salt.

Biopsy of the small intestine is performed via an oral endoscopic procedure for diagnosis of tropical sprue or celiac sprue. Ultrasonography is used to diagnose pancreatic tumors and tumors in the small intestine that are causing malabsorption. X-rays of the gastrointestinal (GI) tract reveal pancreatic calcifications, tumors, or other abnormalities that cause malabsorption. Barium enema examination shows mucosal changes representative of celiac sprue or other abnormalities.

 Interventions

Interventions for most malabsorption syndromes focus on avoidance of dietary substances that aggravate malabsorption and supplementation of nutrients. Surgical or nonsurgical management of the primary disease may be indicated. Drug therapy may also improve or resolve malabsorption.

Dietary management includes a low-fat diet for clients who have gallbladder disease, severe steatorrhea, cystic fibrosis, and progressive systemic sclerosis.

A low-fat diet may or may not be indicated for pancreatic insufficiency because this disorder improves with enzyme replacement. Some clinicians believe that limitation of fat intake is not necessary with enzyme replacement. Dietary intake of fat is actually beneficial to the client because it has a high amount of calories. After a total gastrectomy, a high-protein, high-calorie diet and small, frequent meals are recommended. Lactose-free or restricted diets are available for clients with lactase deficiency, and gluten-free diets are available for clients with celiac sprue.

The physician orders nutritional supplements according to the specific deficiency. Common supplements include

- Water-soluble vitamins, such as folic acid, vitamin B_{12}, and vitamin B complex
- Fat-soluble vitamins, such as vitamin A, vitamin D, and vitamin K
- Minerals, such as calcium, iron, and magnesium
- Pancreatic enzymes, such as pancrelipase (Pancrease, Viokase)

Antibiotics are used to treat tropical sprue, Whipple's disease, and other disorders involving bacterial overgrowth. Tropical sprue is treated with trimethoprim and sulfamethoxazole (Bactrim, Septra). Bacterial overgrowth can be caused by a variety of disorders but is often treated with tetracycline and metronidazole (Flagyl, Novonidazol✦). Steroids are sometimes given in celiac disease to decrease inflammation.

Drug therapy controls the clinical manifestations of the malabsorption disorder. Antidiarrheal agents, such as diphenoxylate hydrochloride and atropine sulfate (Lomotil), camphorated tincture of opium (paregoric), or kaolin with pectin (Kaopectate, Kao-Con✦), are often used to control diarrhea and steatorrhea (see Chart 59–1). Anticholinergics, such as dicyclomine hydrochloride (Bentyl, Bentylol✦), are often given before meals to inhibit gastric

---

Chart 59–8

Nursing Care Highlight: Special Skin Care for Clients with Chronic Diarrhea

- Use medicated wipes or premoistened disposable wipes rather than toilet tissue to clean the perineal area.
- Clean the perineal area well with mild soap and warm water after each stool; rinse soap from the area well.
- If the physician allows, provide a sitz bath several times a day.
- Apply a thin coat of vitamin A & D ointment or other medicated protective covering, such as aloe products, after each stool.
- Keep the client off the affected buttock area.
- For open areas, cover with thin DuoDerm or Tegaderm occlusive dressing to promote rapid healing.
- Observe for fungal or yeast infections, which appear as dark red rashes. Obtain an order for medication if this problem occurs.

---

motility. IV fluids may be necessary to replenish fluid losses associated with diarrhea.

The nurse provides special measures to protect the client's skin when diarrhea occurs (Chart 59–8). The nurse conducts an ongoing assessment for clinical manifestations of malabsorption and relates these to activities and dietary intake. For example, clients with steatorrhea are monitored for fluid and electrolyte imbalances and are encouraged to ingest electrolyte-rich liquids liberally. The nurse teaches clients the rationale for dietary, drug, and surgical management of nutritional deficiencies and evaluates interventions on the basis of changes in or resolution of clinical manifestations.

CASE STUDY for the Client with a Bowel Obstruction

■ You are making a home visit to a 69-year-old man with a history of a stroke at age 59. He is wheelchair dependent and has chronic constipation, angina, and social isolation. His only surgical history was a cholecystectomy and appendectomy at 45 years of age. His only medications are milk of magnesia and nitroglycerin taken as needed. At the start of the home visit, he tells you "My bowels have not moved in 1 week; my magnesia is not working."

QUESTIONS:

1. In this situation, what questions should you ask?
2. Which components of the physical examination should you perform?
3. What health problems may the client be experiencing?
4. Which conditions place him at risk for a bowel obstruction?
5. During the health assessment, you cannot hear any bowel sounds. The client's abdomen is distended and tender to the touch. On the basis of these assessment findings, what is the most appropriate action?

SELECTED BIBLIOGRAPHY

American Cancer Society. (1997). Colorectal cancer. *CA: Cancer Journal for Clinicians, 47*(2).

American Dietetic Association and The Canadian Dietetic Association. (1995). Women's health and nutrition. *Journal of the American Dietetic Association, 95*(3), 362–366.

Banerjee, A. K., Jehle, E. C., Shorthouse, A. J., & Buess, G. (1995). Local excision of rectal tumours. *British Journal of Surgery, 82*, 1165–1173.

Bassotti, G., & Whitehead, W. E. (1994). Biofeedback as a treatment approach to gastrointestinal tract disorders. *The American Journal of Gastroenterology, 89*(2), 158–164.

Bradley, M., & Pupiales, M. (1997). Essential elements of ostomy care. *American Journal of Nursing, 97*(7), 38–46.

Brandt, B. T., DeAntonio, P., Dezort, M. A., & Eyman, L. M. (1996). Hepatic cryosurgery for metastatic colorectal carcinoma. *Oncology Nursing Forum, 23*(1), 29–36.

Burns, S. M., Martin, M., Robbins, V., et al. (1995). Comparison of nasogastric tube securing methods and tube types in medical intensive care patients. *American Journal of Critical Care, 4*(3), 198–203.

Cheek, C. M., Williams, M. H., & Farndon, J. R. (1995). Trusses in the management of hernia today. *British Journal of Surgery, 82*(12), 1611–1613.

Clouse, R. E. (1994). Antidepressants for functional gastrointestinal syndromes. *Digestive Diseases and Sciences, 39*(11), 2352–2363.

Cumbie, B. (1996). Action stat: Bowel obstruction. *Nursing96, 26*(1), 33.

Drossman, D. A. (1994). Irritable bowel syndrome. *The Gastroenterologist, 2*, 315–326.

Fong, Y., Blumgart, L. H., & Cohen, A. (1995). Surgical treatment of colorectal metastases to the liver. *CA: A Cancer Journal for Clinicians, 45*(1), 50–62.

Forgacs, I. (1995). Clinical gastroenterology. *British Medical Journal, 310*, 114–116.

Gorard, D. A., & Farthing, M. J. G. (1994). Intestinal motor function in irritable bowel syndrome. *Digestive Diseases, 12*, 72–74.

*Hampston, B. G., & Bryant, R. A. (1992). *Ostomies and continent diversions: Nursing management.* St. Louis, MO: Mosby Year Book.

Hardcastle, J. D. (1997). Colorectal cancer. *CA: A Cancer Journal for Clinicians, 47*, 66–68.

Jacob, D. R., Slavin, J., & Marquart, L. (1995). Whole grain intake and cancer: A review of the literature. *Nutrition and Cancer, 24*(3), 221–229.

Jenks, J. M., Morin, K. H., & Tomaselli, N. (1997). The influence of ostomy surgery on body image in patients with cancer. *Applied Nursing Research, 10*(4), 174–180.

Jessup, J. M., Menck, H. R., Fremgen, A., & Winchester, D. P. (1997). Diagnosing colorectal carcinoma: Clinical and molecular approaches. *CA: A Cancer Journal for Clinicians, 47*, 70–92.

Longstreth, G. F. (1994). Irritable bowel syndrome and chronic pelvic pain. *Obstetrical and Gynecological Survey, 49*(7), 505–507.

Macho, J. R., Lewis, F. R., & Krupski, W. C. (1994). Management of the injured patient. In L. W. Way (Ed.), *Current surgical diagnosis and treatment* (10th ed., pp. 213–233). Norwalk, CT: Appleton & Lange.

Markowitz, A. J., & Winawer, S. J. (1997). Management of colorectal polyps. *CA: A Cancer Journal for Clinicians, 47*, 93–112.

McQuaid, K. R. (1995). Alimentary tract. In L. M. Tierney, S. J. McPhee, & M. A. Papdakis (Eds.), *Current medical diagnosis and treatment* (pp. 476–554). Norwalk, CT: Appleton & Lange.

*National Institutes of Health Consensus Conference. (1990). Adjuvant therapy for patients with colon and rectal cancer. *Journal of the American Medical Association, 284*, 1444–1450.

Nelson, R. L. (1996). Screening of average-risk individuals for colorectal cancer and postoperative evaluation of patients with colorectal cancer. *Surgical Clinics of North America, 76*(1), 35–45.

Nixon, D. W. (1995). Diet and chemoprevention of colon polyps and colorectal cancer. *Seminars in Surgical Oncology, 11*, 411–415.

Parker, S. L., Tong, T., Bolden, S., & Wingo, P. A. (1997). Cancer statistics 1997. *CA: A Cancer Journal for Clinicians, 47*, 5–27.

Pharmacia & Upjohn Co. (1997). Data on file. Kalamazoo, MI: Author.

Ross, S. C., & Srivastava, S. (1996). National cancer institute workshop on genetic screening for colorectal cancer. *Journal of the National Cancer Institute, 88*(6), 331–339.

Saunderlin, G. (1994). Celiac disease: A review. *Gastroenterology Nursing, 17*(3), 100–105.

Schroy, P. C. (1996). Gastrointestinal and liver tumors. In J. Noble (Ed.), *Textbook of primary care medicine* (2nd ed., pp. 634–650). St. Louis, MO: C. V. Mosby.

Schumpelick, V., Treutner, K. H., & Arlt, G. (1994). Inguinal hernia repair in adults. *Lancet, 344*(8919), 375–379.

Seaman, S. (1996). Basic ostomy management. *Home Healthcare Nurse, 14*(5), 335–343.

Sommers, M. S., & Johnson, S. A. (1997). *Davis's manual of nursing therapeutics for diseases and disorders.* Philadelphia: F. A. Davis.

Spiller, R. C. (1994). Irritable bowel or irritable mind? *British Medical Journal, 309*(17), 1646–1647.

Thompson, W. G. (1994). Irritable bowel syndrome. *Canadian Family Physician, 40*, 307–316.

Toribara, N. W., & Sleisenger, M. H. (1995). Screening for colorectal cancer. *New England Journal of Medicine, 332*(13), 861–867.

Town, J. (1997). Bringing acute abdomen into focus. *Nursing97, 27*(5), 52–57.

*U.S. Department of Health and Human Services. (1990). *Healthy people 2000: National health promotion and disease prevention objectives.* Washington, DC: Author.

Van Dam, J., Bond, J. H., & Sivak, M. V. (1995). Fecal occult blood screening for colorectal cancer. *Archives of Internal Medicine, 155*, 2389–2402.

*Wound Ostomy and Continence Nurses Society. (1992). *Standards of care: Patient with ileostomy, patient with colostomy, patient with urinary diversion.* Costa Mesa, CA: Author.

Zalcberg, J. R., Friedlander, M. L., Collopy, B. T., Barton, M., & Gray, B. (1996). Treatment principles in advanced colorectal cancer. *Australian and New Zealand Journal of Surgery, 66*, 202–205.

Zimbalist, E. H., & Plumer, A. R. (1995). Genetic and environmental factors in colorectal carcinogenesis. *Digestive Disease, 13*, 365–378.

SUGGESTED READINGS

American Cancer Society. (1997). Colorectal cancer. *CA: A Cancer Journal for Clinicians, 47*(2).

This entire issue provides an up-to-date review of detection and management issues related to colorectal cancer. The guest editorial is particularly helpful in that it provides concise information on controversial issues (e.g., benefits of Hemoccult testing as a screening tool, and need to thoroughly assess symptomatic clients, even if younger than age 40) that have relevance to the health care needs of all Americans.

Bradley, M., & Pupiales, M. (1997). Essential elements of ostomy care. *American Journal of Nursing, 97*(7), 38–46.

This article provides a concise, up-to-date overview of ostomy surgeries, types of stomas and their characteristics, complications of ostomies, and tips for choosing and applying appliances and providing skin care to promote wound healing and prevent skin breakdown. Dietary considerations, sexual concerns, and information on sources of support and ostomy supplies are provided for nurses to share with ostomates.

Jenks, J. M., Morin, K. H., & Tomaselli, N. (1997). The influence of ostomy surgery on body image in patients with cancer. *Applied Nursing Research, 10*(4), 174–180.

This nursing study used a variety of tools to measure changes in body image in 45 clients treated with an ostomy for either bowel or bladder cancer. Surprisingly, body image scores did not change significantly between the preoperative period and the postoperative period when clients had their new ostomies.

Chapter 60

INTERVENTIONS FOR CLIENTS WITH INFLAMMATORY INTESTINAL DISORDERS

Because of common symptoms among people with various types of intestinal diseases, inflammatory and infectious intestinal disorders are often difficult to differentiate. Some disorders are acute and easily treated; others are chronic and may be life threatening. The nurse's involvement in assessing and managing intestinal disorders is essential to early diagnosis and successful treatment.

ACUTE INFLAMMATORY BOWEL DISORDERS

Appendicitis, peritonitis, and gastroenteritis are the most common acute inflammatory bowel problems. If not treated early, major systemic complications can result.

Appendicitis

Overview

Appendicitis is acute inflammation of the vermiform appendix, the small, finger-like pouch attached to the cecum of the colon. The appendix is about the thickness of a pencil, from 2 to 6 inches (0.8–2.4 cm) long. Its usual location is the right iliac region, just below the ileocecal valve; however, it can be positioned in another area of the abdomen. Acute appendicitis is the most common cause of acute inflammation in the right lower quadrant. Consequently, it is one of the most common indications for emergency abdominal surgery.

The appendix has no known function. As part of the cecum, it fills with food and empties on a regular basis. Inflammation of the appendix can occur when the lumen of the appendix is obstructed. Inflammation leads to infection as bacteria invade the wall of the appendix.

When the lumen is obstructed, the mucosa continues to secrete fluid until the pressure within the lumen exceeds venous pressure. Blood flow to the appendix is restricted, and infection causes more swelling, which further impedes blood flow. Gangrene from hypoxia or perforation can occur in 24–36 hours. If this process occurs slowly, adjacent organs may wall off the appendiceal area, and a localized abscess develops. If the infectious process occurs rapidly, peritonitis may result. All complications of peritonitis are serious (see Peritonitis later).

It is thought that chronic infection of the appendix can occur, but this is not usually the cause of abdominal pain that lasts for weeks or months. Recurrent acute appendicitis does occur, often with complete remission of inflammation between acute attacks.

In most clients with appendicitis, there is no identifiable cause of obstruction of the appendiceal lumen. However, it has been suggested that calculi composed of fecal material (fecaliths), calcium-phosphate–rich mucus, and inorganic salts may be the most common cause of the initial obstruction. Other causes of obstruction include tumors, viral infections, or worms.

Although appendicitis affects a person at any age, the peak incidence is between the ages of 20 and 30 years. Appendicitis occurs slightly more often in females.

ELDERLY CONSIDERATIONS

 Appendicitis is relatively rare at extremes in age; however, perforation is more common in the elderly, who show a higher mortality rate. Because the diagnosis of appendicitis is difficult to establish in elderly people, this may account for the higher rates of perforation, infectious complication, and mortality. Older people may have a decreased response to the usual pain signals and vague or mild symptoms.

Collaborative Management

 Assessment

The nurse asks the client about symptoms, paying specific attention to the location and sequence of pain in relation to other symptoms. With *classic* appendicitis, abdominal pain in the epigastric or periumbilical area is the initial symptom. Within a few hours after the initial onset, it then shifts to the right lower quadrant. Pain may not be localized, however, and it can exist anywhere in the abdomen or flanks. Abdominal pain that increases with cough or movement and is relieved by flexion of the right hip or knees suggests a perforated appendix with peritonitis. Anorexia and nausea with or without vomiting are common, but they occur *after* the initial symptom of pain.

Abdominal tenderness on palpation is the most common, important, and reliable symptom. In later stages of inflammation, tenderness becomes more localized and is noted with palpation of the right lower quadrant. This area is referred to as McBurney's point; it is located midway between the anterior iliac crest and the umbilicus in the right lower quadrant (Fig. 60–1). The nurse may feel tenseness of the muscles (muscle rigidity) over the tender area. Rigidity over the whole abdomen, accompanied by tense positioning and guarding, indicates a perforated appendix with peritonitis. "Rebound tenderness" describes a sensation of severe pain that occurs after deep pressure is applied and released. This maneuver, which involves pressing a finger into the abdomen at a point away from the pain, is performed only by the physician.

The client's temperature is usually normal or slightly elevated at 99° to 100.5° F (37.2°–38° C). A temperature of 101° F (38.2° C) or higher suggests the presence of peritonitis. If the client has fever, tachycardia is present.

Because the clinical manifestations associated with

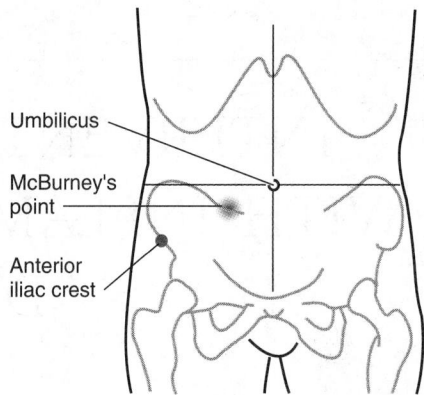

Figure 60–1. McBurney's point is located midway between the anterior illiac crest and the umbilicus in the right lower quadrant. This is the classic area for localized tenderness during the later stages of appendicitis.

many other medical conditions are similar to those of acute appendicitis, arriving at a diagnosis is often difficult. It is important for the nurse to determine the sequence of symptoms. For example, nausea and vomiting that precede abdominal pain often indicate gastroenteritis.

Clinical manifestations that do not follow the classic pattern can also occur, due to variations in the anatomic location of the appendix. The appendix can be located deep in the pelvis, in the right upper quadrant, or even in the left lower quadrant.

Laboratory findings do not establish the diagnosis, but there is often a moderate elevation of the white blood cell (WBC) count (leukocytosis) to 10,000–18,000/mm^3 with a "shift to the left" (an increased number of immature WBCs). A WBC count elevation to greater than 20,000/mm^3 may indicate a perforated appendix.

Interventions

All clients with suspected or confirmed appendicitis are hospitalized and examined by a surgeon. If the diagnosis is questionable, the health care team observes the client before surgical exploration.

Nonsurgical Management. After admission to the hospital, the physician keeps the client with suspected or known appendicitis on nothing by mouth (NPO) status to prepare for the possibility of emergency surgery and to avoid aggravating the inflammatory process. The nurse administers intravenous fluids, as ordered, to prevent fluid and electrolyte imbalance and to replenish fluid volume. If the semi-Fowler's position can be tolerated, the nurse advises the client to maintain this position so that abdominal drainage, if any, can be contained in the lower abdomen.

Once the diagnosis of appendicitis is confirmed, the surgeon schedules surgery. The nurse may administer opioid analgesics, as ordered, while the client is being prepared for surgery. The client with suspected appendicitis should not receive laxatives or enemas, which can cause perforation of the appendix. Heat should never be applied to the client's abdomen because this may increase circulation to the appendix and result in increased inflammation and perforation.

Surgical Management. Surgery is required as soon as possible. If the diagnosis is not definitive but the client is at high risk for complications from suspected appendicitis, the surgeon may perform an exploratory laparotomy to rule out appendicitis.

Preoperative Care. Preoperative teaching is often limited because the client is in pain or may be transferred to the operating suite for emergency surgery. The nurse prepares the client for general anesthesia and surgery (see Chap. 20).

Operative Procedures. Appendectomy, as the name implies, is the removal of the inflamed appendix. In a *traditional,* uncomplicated appendectomy, the surgeon removes the appendix through an incision approximately 3 inches (7.5 cm) long in the right lower quadrant. The incision is larger if the appendix is in an atypical position or if peritonitis is present.

An appendectomy may also be done via *laparoscopy.* The surgical procedure is similar to that for a cholecystectomy via laparoscopy (see Chap. 62). The surgeon makes several small incisions through which an endoscope is inserted. A cutting instrument is threaded through the endoscope, and the appendix is removed.

Postoperative Care. Postoperative care of the client who has undergone an appendectomy includes the care required for any client who has received general anesthesia (see Chap. 22). For clients who have undergone a traditional appendectomy, the incision is located over Mc-Burney's point if the appendix was in the typical location. The incision may be as long as the length of the abdomen, depending on the area explored in surgery and the location of the appendix. Drains may protrude from the incision site if an abscess was present or if the appendix perforated. The drains are left in place for several days. If peritonitis occurred, a nasogastric (NG) tube is placed to decompress the stomach and prevent abdominal distention. If an abscess or peritonitis was present, the nurse administers antibiotics as ordered by the physician. Opioid analgesics are administered for pain as needed. The client is typically out of bed on the evening after surgery or the first postoperative day.

The client who has had an uncomplicated appendectomy via laparoscopy may stay overnight or may be discharged on the day of surgery. In this case, no NG tubes or drains are needed.

The client who has undergone an uncomplicated appendectomy usually recovers rapidly. After a traditional surgical procedure, the client is usually discharged on the third postoperative day and can resume normal activity in 2–4 weeks. If surgery has been complicated by perforation or peritonitis, the client is hospitalized for 7 days or longer.

If the client is discharged to a home setting, the nurse assesses the client's ability to function with the added tasks of incision care, drug therapy, and some activity restrictions. The nurse assesses the client's home environment and the need for support to meet physical needs.

Peritonitis

Overview

Peritonitis is an acute inflammation of the peritoneum (the lining of the abdominal cavity). It can be primary or secondary, localized or generalized. Peritonitis is a life-threatening illness and is associated with several abdominal disorders.

Pathophysiology

Pathologic Changes. When the peritoneal cavity is contaminated, the body initially produces an inflammatory reaction that walls off a localized area to fight the infection. This local reaction involves vascular dilation and increased capillary permeability, allowing for transport of leukocytes and subsequent phagocytosis of the offending organisms. This walling-off process can result in abscess formation or fibrous adhesions, which may or may not cause further pathologic change. If the peritonitis is contained, generalized peritonitis need not occur. If the offending stimulus is too massive to be contained, diffuse peritonitis occurs, leading to serious systemic complications.

Complications. Vascular dilation continues along with hyperemia and a fluid shift. The body responds to the infectious process by shunting extra blood to the area of inflammation. Fluid is shifted from the extracellular fluid (ECF) compartment into the peritoneal cavity, connective tissues, and the gastrointestinal (GI) tract ("third spacing"). This shift of fluid out of the vascular space can result in a significant decrease in circulatory volume. The rate of decreasing circulatory volume is proportional to the degree of peritoneal involvement. Decreased circulatory volume can result in insufficient perfusion of kidneys, leading to renal failure with electrolyte imbalance.

Peristalsis slows or stops in response to severe peritoneal infection, and the lumen of the bowel becomes distended with gas and fluid. Fluid that normally flows to the small bowel and the colon for reabsorption accumulates in the intestine in volumes of 7–8 L daily. The toxins or bacteria responsible for the peritonitis can also enter the bloodstream from the peritoneal area, leading to bacteremia, or septicemia (bacterial invasion of the blood).

Respiratory problems can occur due to increased abdominal pressure against the diaphragm from intestinal distention and fluid shifts to the peritoneal cavity. Pain can interfere with ventilatory efforts when the client has an increased oxygen demand because of the infectious process.

Types of Peritonitis. Peritonitis can be primary or secondary. Primary peritonitis is an acute bacterial infection that is not associated with a perforated viscus or organ. Bacterial infection is the usual cause and may be associated with an infection by the same organism somewhere else in the body, which reaches the peritoneum via the vascular system. Tuberculous peritonitis, which originates from tuberculosis elsewhere in the body, is a type of primary peritonitis. Clients with alcoholic cirrhosis and ascites, in the absence of a perforated organ, often manifest peritonitis, which may be due to leakage of bacteria through the wall of the intestine.

Secondary peritonitis is usually caused by bacterial invasion as a result of perforation or of rupture of an abdominal viscus. It can also result from severe chemical reactions to pancreatic enzymes, digestive juices, or bile released into the peritoneal cavity.

Etiology

Peritonitis is caused by contamination of the peritoneal cavity by bacteria or chemicals. The most common etiologic feature of bacterial invasion within the peritoneal cavity is perforation, associated with

- Appendicitis
- Peptic ulcer
- Diverticulitis
- Gangrenous gallbladder
- Gangrenous obstruction of the small bowel
- Strangulated hernia
- Volvulus
- A spleen or liver condition
- Ectopic pregnancy

Other causes of peritonitis include

- Perforating tumors
- Ulcerative colitis
- Foreign bodies (from trauma)
- Leakage or contamination during a surgical procedure
- Contamination of trochar, catheter, or solution used for peritoneal dialysis
- Administration of intraperitoneal chemotherapy

Bacterial invasion can occur from an ascending infection through the reproductive tract, as in salpingitis or a septic abortion. Bacteria responsible for peritonitis include *Escherichia coli, Streptococcus, Staphylococcus, Pneumococcus,* and *Gonococcus.*

Incidence/Prevalence

Primary peritonitis accounts for only a small percentage of the cases of peritonitis. The incidence of secondary peritonitis is difficult to determine because data usually relate to the underlying cause, such as appendicitis or peptic ulcer.

Collaborative Management

 Assessment

➤ Physical Assessment/Clinical Manifestations

Physical findings of peritonitis (Chart 60–1) depend on whether it is early or late in the disease course, the body has been able to localize the process, and the inflammation has progressed to generalized peritonitis.

The client appears acutely ill, lying still, possibly with knees flexed. Movement is guarded, and the client may report and show signs of pain (e.g., facial grimacing) with

---

> **Chart 60–1**
>
> ## Key Features of Peritonitis
>
> - Abdominal pain (localized, poorly localized, or referred to the shoulder or thorax)
> - Rigid, "board-like" abdomen
> - Distended abdomen
> - Nausea, anorexia, vomiting
> - Diminishing bowel sounds
> - Inability to pass flatus or feces
> - Rebound tenderness in the abdomen
> - High fever
> - Tachycardia
> - Dehydration from high fever (poor skin turgor)
> - Decreased urinary output
> - Hiccups
> - Possible compromise in respiratory status

---

cough or movement of any type. Pain may be sharp and localized in the abdomen, poorly localized in the abdomen, or referred to either the shoulder or the thoracic area. The abdomen may be rigid (sometimes referred to as "board-like"), distended, or both. The nurse may auscultate bowel sounds, but these usually disappear with progression of the inflammation.

In the client with localized peritonitis, the abdomen is tender on palpation in a well-defined area of the abdomen, with rebound tenderness in this area. With generalized peritonitis, tenderness is widespread. The client may have a high fever because of the infectious process, with tachycardia occurring in response to the fever. The nurse assesses whether the client has dry mucous membranes with poor tissue turgor and a low urinary output. Low urinary output occurs because fluid accumulates in the peritoneal cavity, the GI tract, and connective tissues, resulting in a fluid deficit in the vascular space. Hiccups may occur as a result of diaphragmatic irritation. Depending on the severity of peritonitis, the nurse may find that the client has a compromised respiratory status.

➤ Diagnostic Assessment

White blood cell (WBC) counts are commonly elevated to 20,000/mm^3 with a high neutrophil count. The physician usually orders a series of blood culture studies to determine whether septicemia has occurred and to identify the causative organism to enable appropriate therapy.

The health care provider orders laboratory tests to assess fluid and electrolyte balance and renal status, including electrolytes, blood urea nitrogen (BUN), creatinine, hemoglobin, and hematocrit. Arterial blood gas values are obtained to assess respiratory function and acid-base balance.

Abdominal x-rays are obtained to assess for free air or fluid in the abdominal cavity, which indicates perforation. The x-ray may also show dilation, edema, and inflammation of the small and large intestines.

The physician performs diagnostic peritoneal lavage by instilling 1 L of fluid through a peritoneal dialysis catheter. A positive lavage fluid is characterized by the following:

- More than 500 WBCs per cubic milliliter of fluid
- More than 50,000 red blood cells (RBCs) per milliliter
- Bacteria on Gram stain

Bile-stained green fluid may indicate a ruptured gallbladder or perforated intestine, which can lead to chemical peritonitis.

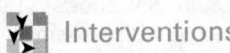 Interventions

All clients with peritonitis are hospitalized because of the critical nature of the illness. If complications are extensive, the client may be in a critical care unit. The most important nursing intervention is thorough assessment of all body systems to identify complications early.

Nonsurgical Management. The physician prescribes intravenous (IV) fluids and broad-spectrum antibiotics immediately after establishing the diagnosis of peritonitis. A nasogastric (NG) tube is inserted to decompress the stomach and the intestine, and the client is allowed nothing by mouth (NPO). The nurse administers oxygen, as ordered, according to the client's respiratory status.

Surgical Management. Abdominal surgery is the optimal treatment for identifying and repairing the cause of the peritonitis. If the client is so critically ill that surgery would be life threatening, it may be delayed. Surgery focuses on controlling the contamination, removing foreign material from the peritoneal cavity, and draining collected fluid.

The surgeon performs an *exploratory laparotomy* ("exploratory lap") to remove or repair the inflamed or perforated organ. The abdominal cavity is opened surgically and explored for inflamed and perforated organs or other abnormalities.

Preoperative Care. The preoperative care for the client undergoing exploratory laparotomy is similar to that described in Chapter 20 for the client receiving general anesthesia.

Operative Procedures. For an exploratory laparotomy, the surgeon makes an incision through the abdominal wall and explores the abdominal cavity. Part or all of a perforated or inflamed organ may be removed, depending on that organ's function. For example, an appendectomy is performed for an inflamed appendix; a colon resection, with or without colostomy, is indicated for a perforated diverticulum or perforated colon secondary to a tumor. Before the abdominal cavity is closed, the surgeon irrigates the peritoneum with antibiotic solutions. Two to four catheters may also be inserted to drain the cavity and provide a route for irrigation postoperatively.

Postoperative Care. Postoperative care is similar to that for other clients undergoing surgery (see Chap. 22). Because clients with peritonitis may have actual or potential multisystem complications, the nurse initially monitors the client's level of consciousness, vital signs, respiratory status (respiratory rate and breath sounds), and fluid and electrolyte status (I&O and laboratory values) at least hourly.

Positioning. The nurse maintains the client in a semi-Fowler's position to promote drainage of peritoneal contents in the inferior region of the abdominal cavity. This position also facilitates adequate respiratory excursion in that the diaphragm and abdominal contents are impinging on respiratory muscles.

Wound Care. The client is likely to have multiple incisions and drains. Because contamination at the time of surgery impedes healing of an incision with edges well approximated (by first intention), incisions are allowed to heal by second or third intention. These incisions necessitate meticulous care involving manual irrigation or packing, as ordered by the surgeon. If the surgeon orders peritoneal irrigation through a drain, the nurse maintains sterile technique during manual irrigation, usually by using a catheter-tipped syringe. The nurse determines that the client is not retaining irrigant by ensuring the absence of abdominal distention or pain and by monitoring irrigant intake and output.

As a result of the loss of fluids from the extracellular space to the peritoneal cavity, intravenous (IV) fluid replacement and maintenance are indicated for all clients with peritonitis. Fluid volume deficit also occurs due to nasogastric suctioning and the client's NPO status. Normal saline or a balanced salt intravenous infusion with potassium is administered according to electrolyte, blood urea nitrogen, and serum creatinine values. To assess fluid volume, the nurse monitors the client's vital signs, urinary output, skin turgor, integrity of mucous membranes, and, most importantly, weight. The nurse also assesses for edema from third spacing.

ELDERLY CONSIDERATIONS

 The elderly client often does not have characteristic signs and symptoms of dehydration. A change in mental status may be an early sign of fluid deficit. The nurse assesses skin turgor on an elderly client using the skin over the forehead or sternum.

The younger client with peritonitis is characteristically thirsty because of fluid losses. The nurse provides frequent mouth care to help maintain moist mucous membranes. The use of lemon-glycerin swabs is avoided because they can increase dryness.

▶ Continuing Care

The client with peritonitis is hospitalized for 5–10 days. The length of hospitalization depends on how localized the infectious process is and how severe the systemic reaction becomes. Clients who have a localized abscess drained and respond to antibiotics and IV fluids—without respiratory, renal, or cardiac complications—are discharged in 1–2 weeks. Clients who experience complications of peritonitis, along with sepsis or shock, may require mechanical ventilation or hemodialysis, with hospital stays lasting for weeks to months. Discharge planning varies with the degree of involvement of all body systems.

If the client is being discharged home, the nurse assesses the client's ability to function at home with the added task of incision care and a diminished activity tolerance.

The nurse provides the client with written and oral instructions to report

- Drainage
- Swelling
- Bleeding
- Redness
- Warmth
- Odor from the wound
- Temperature higher than 101° F (38.2° C)
- Abdominal pain

The nurse also instructs the client in proper handwashing and dressing change techniques, which includes directions to dress wounds separately to avoid cross-contamination.

The physician prescribes an oral opioid analgesic and, possibly, an antibiotic. The nurse reviews information about these medications with the client and caregiver.

The nurse also explains diet and activity limitations. Diet depends on the type of surgery performed and the client's specific food tolerances at the time of discharge. All clients are told to refrain from any lifting for *at least* 6 weeks. Other activity limitations are made on an individual basis with the physician's recommendation.

Peritonitis is a life-threatening and, consequently, a frightening illness. Incisional care can be demanding, and activity intolerance can be overwhelming. If complications have resolved, the nurse reassures clients that they can realistically expect to resume their previous lifestyle. Convalescence is often longer than that required for other types of surgery, however, because of the multisystemic involvement.

Clients with incisions healing by second or third intention may require dressings, solution, and catheter-tipped syringes to irrigate the wound. The nurse may arrange for a home health nurse to assess, irrigate, or pack a wound and change a dressing as needed. If a client needs assistance with activities of daily living, a home health aide or temporary placement in a skilled care facility may be indicated.

Gastroenteritis

Overview

Gastroenteritis (GE) is an inflammation of the mucous membranes of the stomach and intestinal tract. It primarily affects the small bowel and can be of either viral or bacterial origin. Both the viral and bacterial forms have similar manifestations and are considered self-limiting in their course unless complications occur. All organisms that are implicated in gastroenteritis cause diarrhea; however, these organisms have distinguishing characteristics.

Authors disagree on classification of the infectious diseases described as gastroenteritis. Some investigators include shigellosis when discussing gastroenteritis; others consider shigellosis separately as a dysentery. Dysenteries affect the *large* bowel; gastroenteritis affects the *small* bowel. Other authors classify infectious disease of the intestine as bacterial, viral, and parasitic, without using the term *gastroenteritis*.

Food poisoning is sometimes described in conjunction with gastroenteritis, with specific reference to the organism causing the food poisoning. Gastroenteritis, however, differs from food poisoning with regard to transmission in the body, incubation time, and effect on immunity.

The following discussion of gastroenteritis includes the viral forms (epidemic viral, rotavirus), the bacterial forms (*Campylobacter, Escherichia coli*), and shigellosis (Table 60–1). (Organisms associated with food poisoning and parasitic infections are discussed later.)

Pathophysiology/Etiology
Pathologic Changes

Both viral and bacterial organisms entering the intestinal tract cause an inflammatory response and the resulting symptoms of gastroenteritis in one of the following ways:

- The organism releases enterotoxin, which acts on the small intestine, causing local inflammation, which results in diarrhea (e.g., some *Shigella* forms and enterotoxigenic *E. coli*).
- The organism penetrates the intestine, causing cellular destruction, necrosis, and a potential for ulceration. Diarrhea occurs, often with white blood cells (WBCs) or red blood cells (RBCs) (e.g., *Shigella* and *Campylobacter*).
- The organism attaches to mucosal epithelium but does not penetrate it. Cells of the intestinal villi are destroyed, and malabsorption results (e.g., rotavirus).

All of these situations result in *increased* gastrointestinal (GI) motility, with fluids and electrolytes being secreted into the intestine at fast rates. Invading organisms have increased capabilities of attaching to the intestinal mucosa if the normal intestinal flora is altered. This can occur in clients who are receiving antibiotics, who are malnourished, and who are debilitated.

Types of Gastroenteritis

Viral Gastroenteritis. Viral gastroenteritis can be an epidemic viral type or a rotavirus type.

Epidemic viral gastroenteritis can be caused by many types of parvovirus-like organisms. The reservoir of these viruses is humans, and the viruses are transmitted via the fecal-oral route in food and water. The incubation period ranges from 10 to 51 hours. The organism is transmissible during the acute stage of the illness.

Many types of rotaviruses cause *rotavirus* gastroenteritis. The reservoir of these viruses is in humans. The viruses are transmitted via the fecal-oral route and, possibly, via the respiratory tract. Incubation is 48 hours. The period of communicability is during the acute stage and shortly after. Rotavirus infection is generally limited to infants and young children; by age 2 years, most children have acquired antibodies against most types of these viruses.

Bacterial Gastroenteritis. There are three general types of bacterial gastroenteritis:

TABLE 60–1

Common Types of Gastroenteritis and their Characteristics	
Type	**Characteristics**
Viral gastroenteritis	
Epidemic viral	• Caused by many parvovirus-type organisms • Transmitted by the fecal-oral route in food and water • Incubation period 10–51 hr • Communicable during acute illness
Rotavirus	• Transmitted by the fecal-oral and, possibly, the respiratory routes • Incubation in 48 hr • Most common in infants and young children
Bacterial gastroenteritis	
Campylobacter enteritis	• Transmitted by the fecal-oral route or by contact with infected animals or infants • Incubation period 1–10 days • Communicable for 2–7 weeks
Escherichia coli diarrhea	• Transmitted by fecally contaminated food, water, or fomites
Shigellosis	• Transmitted by direct and indirect fecal-oral routes • Incubation period 1–7 days • Communicable during the acute illness to 4 weeks after the illness • Humans possibly carriers for months

- *Campylobacter* enteritis ("traveler's diarrhea")
- *E. coli* diarrhea (also referred to as "traveler's diarrhea")
- Shigellosis (bacillary dysentery)

The etiologic feature of *Campylobacter* enteritis is the bacterium *Campylobacter jejuni*. Its reservoirs are domestic or wild animals and birds. *C. jejuni* is transmitted by

- Ingestion of water or food contaminated with feces
- Contact with infected animals or infants
- The fecal-oral route

Incubation ranges 1–10 days. The organism is communicable for several days to weeks throughout the course of the infection (usually 2–7 weeks). Carriers of the bacteria are rare.

The reservoirs of *E. coli* are humans, who are often asymptomatic. The organism is transmitted through fecally contaminated food, water, or fomites.

Shigellosis is caused by different groups of *Shigella* bacteria, which have many strains. The reservoirs of these bacteria are humans. Direct or indirect fecal-oral transmission can occur from an infected person or carrier. Incubation is 1–7 days. The illness can be communicated during the acute phase to 4 weeks after the onset of the illness. A person may be a carrier of this illness for months after the acute illness.

Incidence/Prevalence

Epidemic viral gastroenteritis occurs throughout the world and is very common. As its name suggests, this disease often occurs in epidemic outbreaks among groups of people. *Campylobacter* enteritis occurs worldwide, commonly in epidemic outbreaks. Its incidence is highest during warm months.

Diarrhea caused by *E. coli* also occurs worldwide, commonly in epidemics. The highest incidence is in areas of poor sanitation during warm months.

Shigellosis occurs worldwide in every age group but is most frequent in children under the age of 10 years. Children and the elderly are more susceptible to *Shigella* because of their immature or depressed immune systems. Outbreaks of shigellosis are common in areas with crowded living conditions.

Collaborative Management

 Assessment

Nausea and vomiting can occur with all types of gastroenteritis but are usually limited to the first 1 or 2 days of the illness. All clients with gastroenteritis classically have diarrhea. The consistency and amount vary with the causative organism.

Diarrhea associated with epidemic viral gastroenteritis is typically limited to 24–48 hours. Rotavirus gastroenteritis causes watery diarrhea, lasting up to 8 days; rectal bleeding can occur. *Campylobacter* enteritis causes foul-smelling stools with blood, which can number 20–30 per day for up to 7 days. *E. coli* gastroenteritis may or may not cause blood or mucus in the stool; diarrhea can last for up to 10 days. *Shigella* causes stools with blood and mucus, which can continue for up to 5 days.

The client who has gastroenteritis usually appears ill. Temperature can be normal or elevated from 101° to 103° F (38.2°–39.2° C).

In clients with *Campylobacter* enteritis or shigellosis, the temperature may be as high as 105° F (40° C). Abdominal pain is typically present.

In clients with epidemic viral gastroenteritis, myalgia (muscle aches), headache, and malaise are often reported. The nurse notes slight abdominal distention. The nurse auscultates hyperactive bowel sounds and finds diffuse tenderness on palpation. However, there should be *no* rebound tenderness, which might indicate peritonitis. Depending on the amount of fluids lost through diarrhea and vomiting, the client may have varying degrees of dehydration manifested by poor skin turgor, dry mucous membranes, orthostatic blood pressure changes, hypotension, and oliguria.

Dehydration may be severe, and shock may occur if diarrhea is prolonged. Dehydration occurs rapidly in elderly clients.

As part of the laboratory assessment, Gram stain of stool is usually done before culture. Many white blood cells (WBCs) on Gram stain suggest shigellosis. The presence of WBCs and RBCs in stool indicates *Campylobacter* gastroenteritis.

A stool culture that is positive for enterotoxigenic *E. coli* is diagnostic of *E. coli* diarrhea. Culture of stool that is positive for *Shigella* when there are pus cells or WBCs present on examination of stool is diagnostic of shigellosis.

Sophisticated electron microscopy and immunoassay procedures can identify epidemic viral gastroenteritis or rotavirus gastroenteritis; however, such examinations are rarely done because they are expensive and tedious to perform.

Interventions

For clients with most types of gastroenteritis, treatment is supportive. Therapy is focused on fluid replacement, and the amount and route of fluid administration are determined by the client's fluid status.

Fluid Replacement. For cases of mild gastroenteritis, the client is treated on an outpatient basis. If fluid volume is severely depleted, the client is admitted to the hospital for administration of intravenous (IV) fluids. For elderly clients at home or in a long-term care setting, oral rehydration therapy (ORT) with commercially prepared products, such as Resol, may prevent hospitalization.

The nurse obtains weight, orthostatic blood pressure readings, and other vital signs at the time of admission. Hypotonic IV fluids, such as half-strength normal saline (0.45% sodium chloride), are infused as ordered. The nurse monitors the client's vital signs, intake and output, and weight. A rapid gain or loss of 1 kg (2.2 lbs) of body weight is equivalent to the gain or loss of 1 L of fluid. Standard precautions are consistently observed when handling vomitus and stool.

The physician may order a potassium supplement to be added to IV fluids if the client's serum potassium level is low. To help assess renal function and prevent hyperkalemia, the nurse verifies that the client is voiding before and during potassium replacement. The client is advised to rest in bed, especially during periods of nausea or vomiting, and to avoid quick movements, which can make nausea more severe.

Depending on the type of gastroenteritis, the local health department may need to be notified. It is mandatory that every case of shigellosis be reported. In some endemic areas, *Campylobacter* enteritis needs to be reported on a case-by-case basis. Other types of gastroenteritis must be reported only if they occur in epidemic proportion. The nurse checks with state and local health department guidelines for reporting requirements.

Diet Therapy. Diet therapy is the same for the client who remains at home and the client in the hospital. If the client is not actively vomiting, the nurse recommends small volumes of clear liquids with electrolytes (such as Gatorade) for 24 hours. The frequency and amount of oral intake can be increased if nausea and vomiting are *not* present. If nausea and vomiting continue, the nurse withholds food and fluids until these symptoms subside. The nurse advises the client *not* to drink water because it does not contain any electrolytes to replace those lost. After 24 hours, the diet for all clients can be advanced to include saltine crackers, toast, and jelly. When the client can tolerate this, bland foods, such as nonfatty soup, custard, yogurt, cottage cheese, mashed or baked potatoes, and cooked vegetables, may be added. The client may progress to a regular diet as tolerated.

Drug Therapy. Drugs that suppress intestinal motility, such as anticholinergics and antiemetics, are *not* routinely given for bacterial or viral gastroenteritis. Use of these drugs can be dangerous; the infecting organisms need to be eliminated from the body, and these agents may interfere with the evacuation of the organisms.

If the gastroenteritis is due to shigellosis, anti-infective agents, such as sulfamethoxazole with trimethoprim (Septra, Bactrim), are administered.

For relatively short-term diarrhea—24 to 48 hours— the diagnosis is based primarily on the client's history and clinical manifestations without validation by a stool examination. When diarrhea is severe or persists for long periods, the stool is examined in an effort to determine the causative organism and to begin specific treatment. It should be determined whether the diarrhea is caused by *Salmonella* or parasites because these organisms respond to specific medications (see later). Diarrhea that continues longer than 10 days is probably *not* due to gastroenteritis, and a thorough investigation for the cause is warranted.

Skin Care. Frequent stools that are rich in electrolytes and enzymes, and frequent wiping and washing of the anal region, can irritate the skin. The nurse teaches the client to avoid toilet paper, washcloths, towels, and harsh soaps. Ideally, the client can gently clean the area with warm water or absorbent cotton, followed by thorough drying with absorbent cotton. If stool sticks to excoriated skin, the client can apply a cream, oil, or gel on a damp, warm washcloth to facilitate removal of stool. Hydrocortisone cream or protective barrier cream should be applied to the skin between stools. Witch hazel compresses (e.g., Tucks) and sitz baths for 10 minutes, two to three times daily, can also relieve discomfort. If seepage of stool is a problem, the client can put absorbent cotton next to the anal orifice and keep it in place with snug underwear.

For clients who are incontinent, the nurse keeps the

Health Promotion Guide: Measures to Prevent the Transmission of Gastroenteritis

- Wash your hands meticulously with an antibacterial soap, especially after having a bowel movement.
- Do not share your dishes, glasses, or toothpaste.
- Keep the commode clean to prevent exposure to your stool.
- Do not prepare or handle food that will be consumed by others.

perineal and buttock areas clean and dry. The use of incontinent pads instead of briefs allows air to circulate to the skin and prevents irritation.

Health Teaching. The nurse teaches the client and the family about the importance of minimizing the risk of transmission of gastroenteritis. Clients are advised to

- Wash their hands meticulously with an antibacterial soap, especially after bowel movements
- Restrict the use of glasses, dishes, eating utensils, and tubes of toothpaste to themselves only
- Maintain clean bathroom facilities to avoid exposure to stool
- Maintain good personal hygiene

Clients adhere to these precautions for up to 7 weeks after the illness or up to several months if *Shigella* was the offending organism. If the client is employed as a food handler, the public health department should be consulted for recommendations about the return to work (Chart 60–2).

CHRONIC INFLAMMATORY BOWEL DISEASES

The term *chronic inflammatory bowel disease* describes several disorders for which the clinical manifestations and

treatment are similar. About 25,000 new cases are diagnosed each year in the United States. Ulcerative colitis and Crohn's disease (regional enteritis) are the most common chronic disorders in this category of inflammatory bowel problems (Table 60–2).

Ulcerative Colitis
Overview

Ulcerative colitis is a chronic inflammatory process of the large bowel (colon) or rectum that can result in poor absorption of vital nutrients. Over time, the client experiences episodes of physical discomfort and disruption of lifestyle. The affected client may have only minor periodic health problems, necessitating only ambulatory care, or serious problems, such as malnutrition and physical debilitation, requiring multiple hospitalizations.

Pathophysiology
Pathologic Changes

Ulcerative colitis is characterized by diffuse inflammation of the intestinal mucosa; the result is a loss of surface epithelium with ulceration and, possibly, abscess formation. Generally, the disease begins in the rectum and proceeds in a uniform, continuous manner proximally toward the cecum. Ulcerative colitis is characterized by periods of remission and exacerbation.

Clients with *acute* ulcerative colitis (during an exacerbation or "attack" of the disease) may have vascular congestion, hemorrhage, edema, and ulceration of the bowel mucosa. As the disease course progresses, *chronic* changes occur, such as muscle hypertrophy, deposition of fat and fibrous tissue, and a narrower and shorter large bowel.

Complications

Complications of ulcerative colitis include

- Hemorrhage
- Abscess formation
- Toxic megacolon
- Malabsorption
- Bowel obstruction

TABLE 60–2

Differential Features of Ulcerative Colitis and Crohn's Disease		
Feature	**Ulcerative Colitis**	**Crohn's Disease**
Location	• Begins in the rectum and proceeds in a continuous manner toward the cecum	• Most often in the terminal ileum, with patchy involvement through all layers of the bowel
Etiology	• Unknown	• Unknown
Peak incidence at age	• 15–35 yr	• 15–35 yr
Stools	• 10–20 liquid, bloody stools per day	• 5–6 soft, loose stools per day, rarely bloody
Complications	• Hemorrhage • Perforation • Fistulas • Nutritional deficiencies	• Fistulas • Nutritional deficiencies

- Bowel perforation with resultant peritonitis and fistula formation
- Increased risk of colon cancer
- Extraintestinal clinical manifestations, such as arthritis

Table 60–3 describes common complications.

Etiology

The cause of ulcerative colitis is unknown. Many theories have been formulated, including infectious agents (bacterial, fungal, or viral) and allergies. There appears to be a genetic predisposition, as indicated by familial clustering of the disease. Immunologic theories, including autoimmune dysfunction, have been explored because of the extraintestinal manifestations of the disease. Psychological factors, such as stress and hostile feelings, have also been implicated; however, some researchers speculate that these are either a result of inflammatory bowel disease or a contributing factors to the severity of the attack, not the direct cause.

Incidence/Prevalence

The annual incidence of ulcerative colitis is approximately two to seven new cases per 100,000 persons. The preva-lence is 40–100 cases per 100,000 people in the United States.

Peak incidence is between the ages of 15 and 40 years, and another peak occurs between ages 55 and 60 years. Females are more often affected than men. Jewish Caucasians are at highest risk compared with other Caucasian groups.

TRANSCULTURAL CONSIDERATIONS

 Ulcerative colitis is four to five times more common among people of Jewish origin and commonly affects Caucasians in developed Western society. It is seen more frequently in Ashkenazi Jews than in non-Jews or any other Jewish group (Giger & Davidhizar, 1995).

Collaborative Management

Assessment

➤ History

The nurse collects data on family history of inflammatory bowel disease and previous and current therapy for illness, including dates and types of surgery. Obtaining a diet history is essential. The history should include the client's usual dietary patterns and the relationship of elimination patterns to intolerance of milk and milk products and greasy, fried, spicy, or hot foods. The nurse asks about the symptoms of acute ulcerative colitis, which often include 10–20 liquid, bloody stools per day, anorexia, and fatigue.

➤ Physical Assessment/Clinical Manifestations

The client with ulcerative colitis may have symptoms that vary with the acuteness of onset and with complications of the disease process. The nurse assesses for bowel sounds. Palpation may reveal areas of increased or localized tenderness. Rebound tenderness may suggest peritonitis. The nurse may note localized areas of abdominal pain or cramping over areas of diseased bowel.

The nurse assesses the bowel elimination pattern, noting the color, consistency, and character of stool and the presence or absence of blood in all stools. The nurse notes the relationship between the occurrence of diarrhea and the timing of meals, pain, emotional distress, and activity. The client may be febrile and tachycardic, indicating possible complications, such as peritonitis, dehydration, and bowel perforation.

➤ Psychosocial Assessment

The nurse evaluates the client's understanding of the illness and its impact on his or her lifestyle. The client is encouraged and supported while the following are explored:

- The relationship of life events to disease exacerbations
- Job-related stress factors that produce symptoms
- Effects of smoking and alcohol on the frequency of stool
- The occurrence of crampy pain

TABLE 60–3

Complications of Ulcerative Colitis and Crohn's Disease

Complication	Description
Hemorrhage/perforation	• Lower gastrointestinal bleeding results from erosion of the bowel wall.
Abscess formation	• Localized pockets of infection develop in the ulcerated bowel lining.
Toxic megacolon	• Paralysis of the colon causes dilation and subsequent bowel obstruction.
Malabsorption	• Essential nutrients cannot be absorbed through the diseased intestinal wall, causing anemia and malnutrition (most common in Crohn's disease).
Bowel obstruction	• Obstruction results from toxic megacolon or cancer.
Fistulas	• Fistulas can occur anywhere, but usually track between the bowel and bladder. Pyuria and fecaluria result.
Colorectal cancer	• Clients with ulcerative colitis for 7–10 years or longer have a high risk for colorectal cancer. This complication accounts for about one third of all deaths related to ulcerative colitis.
Extraintestinal complications	• Complications include arthritis, hepatic and biliary disease (especially cholelithiasis), oral and skin lesions, and ocular disorders, such as iritis. The cause is unknown.

- The effect of pain and diarrhea on sleep habits
- Family and social support systems

Many clients are very apprehensive regarding the frequency of stools and the presence of blood. The uncontrollability of the disease symptoms, particularly diarrhea, can be disruptive and stress-producing.

More severe illness can limit the client's activities outside the home. As a result of the excessive diarrhea, the client may become dependent on the proximity of a bathroom. Eating may be associated with pain and cramping, as well as an increased frequency of stools. Mealtimes may become unpleasant experiences for clients.

► Laboratory Assessment

As a result of chronic blood loss, hematocrit and hemoglobin levels may be low. An increased white blood cell (WBC) count and elevated erythrocyte sedimentation rate are consistent with inflammatory disease. Sodium, potassium, and chloride concentrations may be depleted by the frequent diarrheal stools and the malabsorption that results from the diseased bowel.

Viral and bacterial dysenteries can cause symptoms similar to those of ulcerative colitis. Before an invasive diagnostic work-up, the stools are examined for occult blood, ova (eggs), and parasites, and specimens for culture are obtained. Other problems must be ruled out before a definitive diagnosis of ulcerative colitis is made.

► Radiographic Assessment

Barium enemas with air contrast demonstrate differences between Crohn's disease and ulcerative colitis and identify complications, mucosal patterns, and the distribution and depth of disease involvement.

► Other Diagnostic Assessment

The sigmoidoscopic examination is probably the most definitive diagnostic procedure for ulcerative colitis. The physician can directly visualize the sigmoid and transverse colon. Common findings include an edematous, friable bowel mucosa with a loss of vascular pattern and frequent ulcerations.

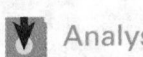 Analysis

► Common Nursing Diagnoses and Collaborative Problems

The following nursing diagnoses are common in clients with ulcerative colitis:

- Diarrhea related to inflammation of the bowel mucosa
- Acute and Chronic Pain related to inflammation of the bowel mucosa

The most common collaborative problem is Potential for Gastrointestinal Bleeding.

► Additional Nursing Diagnoses and Collaborative Problems

Clients may have one or more of the following nursing diagnoses:

- Altered Nutrition: Less than Body Requirements related to diarrhea and malabsorption
- Body Image Disturbance related to change in body function
- Activity Intolerance related to generalized weakness
- Altered Health Maintenance related to knowledge deficit about the disease process
- Ineffective Individual Coping related to physical illness and hospitalization

Some clients may have additional collaborative problems, including

- Potential for fluid and electrolyte imbalances
- Potential for anemia
- Potential for abscesses, fissures, and/or fistulas

 Planning and Implementation

► Diarrhea

Planning: Expected Outcomes. The client is expected to experience decreased diarrhea through control of the inflammation of the intestinal lining.

Interventions. Many measures are used to relieve symptoms and to reduce intestinal motility, decrease inflammation, and promote intestinal healing. Medical management of ulcerative colitis is the preferred and initial treatment option.

Nonsurgical Management. Nonsurgical management includes drug and diet therapy. Physical and emotional rest are also very important.

Drug Therapy. The health care provider uses a combination of drugs to meet the treatment goals, including salicylate compounds, corticosteroids, immunosuppressants, and antidiarrheals.

Salicylate Compounds. Oral mesalamine (Asacol; Pentasa) is used for its anti-inflammatory effect in the acute phase of the illness. The recommended dose of Asacol is 800 mg three times a day or Pentasa 4 g daily in divided doses. Olsalazine (Dipentum) 1 g daily is a salicylate used for maintenance therapy. Side effects of oral mesalamine include occasional flare-ups of colitis.

Clients with mild to moderate colitis of the distal bowel may be treated with mesalamine suppositories, given two or three times daily, or retention enemas (Rowasa enema) given once daily at hour of sleep.

Corticosteroids. Corticosteroid therapy, used orally or intravenously, may be prescribed during exacerbations of the disease. Prednisone (Deltasone, Winpred✱) 40–100 mg daily can be given orally; prednisolone (Delta-Cortef) 100 mg daily may be given intravenously. For clients with rectal symptoms, topical steroids in the form of small-retention enemas may be prescribed. Hydrocortisone rectal foam (Cortifoam) is ordered one to two times daily for 2–3 weeks, then every other day. Hydrocortisone enemas (Cortenema) are given at hour of sleep for 21 days, then tapered and discontinued.

Immunosuppressive Drugs. If inflammation of the intestinal wall is so severe that it does not respond to steroids, oral mercaptopurine (Purinethol) may be given at a dose of 1.5 to 2.5 mg/kg daily. Side effects of this medication include thrombocytopenia, leukopenia, anemia, renal failure, infection, headache, gastrointestinal ulceration, stomatitis, and hepatotoxity.

Antidiarrheal Drugs. To provide symptomatic management of diarrhea, antidiarrheal drugs may be ordered. Common antidiarrheal drugs include diphenoxylate hydrochloride and atropine sulfate (Lomotil), loperamide (Imodium), and camphorated tincture of opium (paregoric) (see Chart 59–1). Codeine sulfate and morphine sulfate can also be effective. These drugs decrease the

frequency of stools, usually by reducing the volume of liquid in the stools.

Diet Therapy. The severity of the client's ulcerative colitis determines the type of diet required. Clients with severe symptoms are kept on nothing by mouth (NPO) status to ensure bowel rest. The physician orders total parenteral nutrition (TPN) for these clients (see Chap. 64). Clients with slightly less severe symptoms may be given elemental formulas such as Vivonex or Ensure, which are absorbed in the upper bowel, thus minimizing bowel stimulation. Clients with significant but less severe symptoms may be restricted to a low-fiber (low-residue)

TABLE 60–4

Guidelines for a Low-Fiber Diet

Foods Allowed	Foods Not Allowed
Beverages	
Only 2 glasses of milk, if allowed, boiled or evaporated; strained fruit juices, coffee, tea, and carbonated beverages	Alcohol
Eggs	
Prepared in any manner, except fried	Fried
Cheese	
Cottage, cream, milk, American, and Tillamook (use in small amounts)	Highly flavored
Meats or Poultry	
Roasted, baked, or broiled tender beef, lamb, liver, veal, fish, chicken, or turkey	Tough meats, pork; fried or highly spiced meats
Soups	
Bouillon, broth, and strained cream soups from foods allowed	Any others
Fats	
Butter, margarine, oils, 30 mL (1 oz) of cream daily	None
Vegetables	
Canned or cooked vegetables, such as asparagus, beets, carrots, peas, potatoes, pumpkin, squash, spinach, and young string beans; tomato juice	Raw or whole cooked vegetables (e.g., potato with skin)
Fruits	
Strained fruit juices; cooked or canned apples, apricots, Royal Ann cherries, peaches, pears, dried fruit purée, and ripe banana and avocado; all of the above *without skins or seeds*	All other raw or cooked fruits
Bread and Crackers	
Refined bread, toast, rolls, and crackers	Pancakes, waffles, and whole-grain bread or rolls
Cereals	
Cooked cereal, such as Cream of Wheat, Malt-O Meal, strained oatmeal, cornmeal, cornflakes, puffed rice, Rice Krispies, and puffed wheat	Whole-grain cereals; other prepared cereals
Potatoes/Rice/Pasta	
White rice, macaroni, noodles, and spaghetti	Fried potato, potato chips, and brown rice
Desserts	
Gelatin desserts, tapioca, angel food or sponge cake, plain custards, water ice or ice cream without fruit or nuts, and rennet or simple puddings	Rich pastries, pies, and anything with nuts or dried fruit
Sweets	
Sugar, jelly, honey, syrups, gumdrops, hard candy, plain creams, milk chocolate	Other candy; jam, marmalade
Miscellaneous Foods	
Cream sauce and plain gravy	Nuts, olives, popcorn, rich gravies, pepper, spices, and vinegar

Modified from Williams, S. R. (1989). *Nutrition and diet therapy* (6th ed.). St. Louis: Times Mirror/Mosby College Publishing.

diet. However, because the role of diet in IBD is not well defined, and because individual tolerance to foods vary, clients with controlled symptoms may only need to limit or omit those foods that cause them discomfort or diarrhea. All clients should be cautioned that caffeinated beverages, pepper, alcohol, and smoking are common gastrointestinal (GI) stimulates that could cause discomfort.

Clients following a low-fiber diet should avoid foods such as whole-wheat grains, nuts, and fresh fruits or fresh vegetables (Table 60–4). Clients may begin with one form of diet therapy and progress to a more advanced diet as symptoms diminish, with the goal of preventing hyperactive bowel activity.

Rest. At the onset of treatment, the client's activity is generally restricted because the required rest can reduce intestinal activity, provide comfort, and promote healing. The nurse ensures that the client has easy access to a bedpan, commode, or bathroom in case of urgency or tenesmus.

Surgical Management. When clients experience severe complications of ulcerative colitis, surgery may be indicated. Indications for surgery include bowel perforation, toxic megacolon, hemorrhage, colon cancer, and conventional treatment failure. The surgeon may choose one of several surgical procedures to alleviate these problems.

Total Proctocolectomy with Permanent Ileostomy. Total proctocolectomy (or colectomy) with permanent ileostomy has traditionally been the surgery of choice (Research Applications for Nursing).

Preoperative Care. When an ileostomy is indicated, the nurse provides extensive explanations to the client and family or significant other. Preoperative teaching includes aspects that relate to abdominal surgery (see Chap. 20) and those that relate to ileostomy. The surgeon consults with the enterostomal therapist (a nurse specializing and certified in skin and ostomy care) preoperatively for recommendations on the location of the ostomy (stoma). A visit from an ostomate (a client with an ostomy) may be appropriate before surgery if the client agrees to this. The surgeon orders oral or parenteral antibiotics, such as neomycin sulfate (Mycifradin, Neo-fradin), to clean the bowel. Mechanical cleansing of the bowel with enemas or laxatives may also be required.

Operative Procedure. During a total proctocolectomy with traditional permanent ileostomy, the colon, rectum, and anus are removed, followed by closure of the anus. The surgeon brings the end of the terminal ileum out through the abdominal wall and forms a stoma, or ostomy. The stoma is usually placed in the right lower quadrant of the abdomen, below the belt line (Fig. 60–2). The surgeon makes a perineal incision to remove the rectum and supporting tissues.

Postoperative Care. Initially after surgery, the output from the ileostomy is loose, dark-green liquid and may contain some blood. Over time, a process called ileostomy adaptation occurs. The small intestine begins to absorb increased amounts of sodium and water, a former function of the large intestine, which was removed by surgery. Stool volume decreases and becomes thicker (paste-like)

▷ Research Applications for Nursing

Clients Facing Colectomy Benefit from Assistance with Decision-Making

Kelly, M. P. (1994). Patients' decision making in major surgery: The case of total colectomy. Journal of Advanced Nursing, 19(6), 1168–1177.

This qualitative study examined clients' decision-making processes when faced with total colectomy and ileostomy. A convenience sample of 45 individuals who had a colectomy or were about to have surgery for ulcerative colitis were interviewed. When first faced with surgery, subjects reported being surprised and not fully understanding the seriousness of their illness. Strategies that assisted in the decision-making process included seeking and obtaining information, caregiver and counselor support, and processing the physician's recommendations. Subjects consistently reported that they were involved in the decisions leading to surgery.

Critique. This was a retrospective study and was conducted with a convenience sample. Therefore, the results cannot be generalized to other populations. However, it is an important exploratory study about the decision-making process regarding surgery for ulcerative colitis. The results of this study support the premise that decision-making can be a complex process that integrates education and information with social and psychological factors.

Possible Nursing Implications. The process by which clients make decisions about colectomy for ulcerative colitis remains unclear. This study suggests that there are a number of strategies that may support the decision-making process. These include education, information, counseling, and an opportunity to grieve. Nurses should remember that each client's response to ulcerative colitis and possible surgery is highly individual. However, nurses can provide emotional support and education to help clients in the decision-making process. Further research should be conducted to examine this decision-making process in a concurrent fashion with various populations.

and turns yellow-green or yellow-brown. The effluent (fluid material) usually has little odor or a sweet odor. Any foul or unpleasant odor may be a symptom of some underlying problem (e.g., blockage or infection).

Depending on the frequency and irritation of stool drainage, the client must wear a pouch system at all times. Disposable systems are most often used.

Prevention of skin problems (irritation, excoriation, ulceration) is critical for the client with an ileostomy. Output from the small intestine is rich in proteolytic enzymes and bile salts, which can quickly irritate and injure the skin. A pouch system that has some type of skin barrier (gelatin or pectin) provides sufficient protection for most clients. Other products are also available.

Most clients undergoing surgical intervention for ulcerative colitis have lived with chronic illness for some time. Clients may welcome surgery, for it provides a sense of relief from the multiple problems that have been occurring. Initially, however, the client may not perceive life with an ileostomy as a positive alternative. Nursing research has begun to examine the quality of life after an ileostomy. Interventions that may enhance quality of life

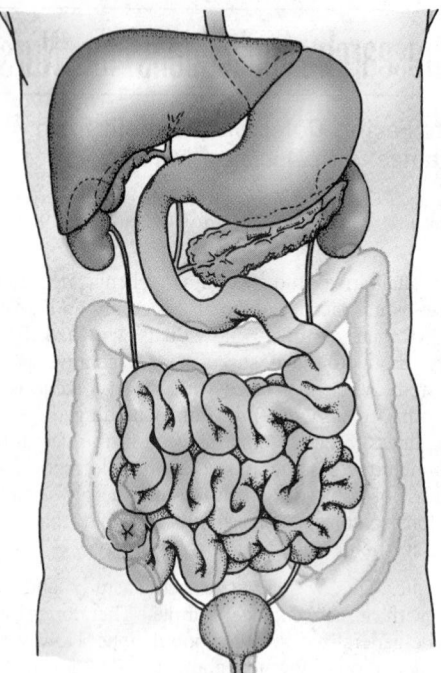

Figure 60–2. Total proctocolectomy with a permanent ileostomy. This involves removal of the colon, the rectum, and the anus with closure of the anus. Note the missing colon, rectum, and anus with the resultant stoma in the right lower quadrant.

include providing the opportunity to discuss feelings regarding the effect of the illness and the perceived effects of surgical interventions.

Surgery results in the loss of a body organ and the partial or total loss of a body function. The physical appearance of the body also changes. Client goals include

- Becoming able to provide self-care
- Adapting one's lifestyle to include care of an ostomy
- Resuming pre-surgery activities

If the client's lifestyle was limited before surgery because of the illness, the goal is a more positive and productive lifestyle after surgery.

Total Colectomy with Continent Ileostomy. As an alternative to the traditional ileostomy with an external pouch, the surgeon may create an internal system—Kock's ileostomy, or ileal reservoir. This procedure is sometimes referred to as a "continent" ileostomy. The surgeon constructs an intra-abdominal pouch or reservoir from the terminal ileum (Fig. 60–3), where stool can be stored in the pouch until it is drained by the client. The care of a Kock's ileostomy involves the connection of the pouch to the stoma, which is constructed with a nipple-like valve made from an intussuscepted portion of the ileum. The stoma is flush with the skin.

The nursing care for a client with a Kock's ileostomy is similar to the care of the client with a proctocolectomy and ileostomy (see earlier). Immediately postoperatively, an indwelling Foley catheter is placed in the pouch, which is connected to low intermittent suction and irrigated as ordered.

The nurse monitors the character and quality of effluent (drainage). Approximately 2 weeks after surgery, the nurse teaches the client to drain the stoma. Initially, the pouch holds only 50–75 mL; over time, the pouch capacity reaches 500–700 mL. The client drains the pouch several times a day. When the pouch needs to be emptied, the client experiences a sensation of fullness. The client drains the pouch by inserting a urinary catheter. The client wears a small dressing over the stoma to keep it moist and to protect clothing from the moist stoma. Advantages to this procedure include

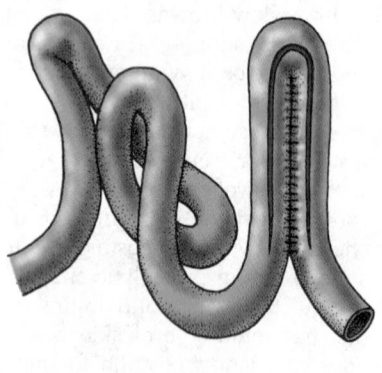

1. A reservoir, in which the client will retain stool until draining it, is constructed from a loop of ileum folded and sutured together, then cut.

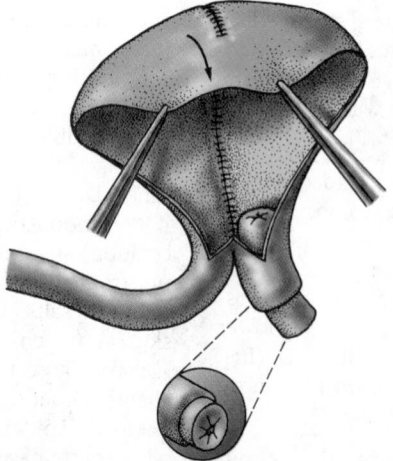

2. A portion of the ileum is intussuscepted to form a nipple valve, and the upper part of the stitched and cut ileum is pulled down and sutured to form a pouch.

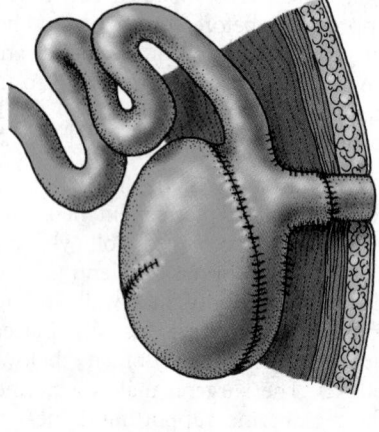

3. The nipple valve, which shuts tight against pressure from a filled pouch, is pulled through the stoma and sutured flush with the abdomen.

Figure 60–3. The creation of a Kock (continent) ileostomy.

- The client does not need to wear an external pouch for collection of stool
- The client experiences minimal skin problems
- There is no leakage of flatus or stool

Unfortunately, between 20% and 40% of Kock's ileostomies malfunction, usually because the nipple-like valve does not work properly.

In clients who undergo Kock's ileostomy, a gastrostomy tube is inserted through the abdominal wall directly into the stomach. This tube, which is connected to suction, is more effective than a nasogastric (NG) tube in preventing discomfort and complications.

Total Colectomy with Ileoanal Anastomosis. During this procedure, the surgeon removes the colon and the rectum and sutures the ileum into the anal canal. This surgery may be performed in two stages. A temporary colostomy is formed first, and, when the anastomosis is healed, the colostomy is reversed. Care of the client undergoing this procedure is similar to patients undergoing a colectomy. With an ileoanal anastomosis, perineal irritation is a common occurrence as a result of frequent, loose stools. The nurse should provide careful perineal care.

Ileoanal Reservoir. This technique has become popular for clients with ulcerative colitis because it spares the rectal sphincter and eliminates the need for an ostomy. During this procedure, the surgeon removes the colon and sutures the ileum into the rectal stump to form a reservoir.

Preoperative Care. The preoperative care for a client undergoing an ileoanal anastomosis is similar to that for a client undergoing an ileostomy. However, clients do not require a visit from an enterostomal therapist or ostomate.

Operative Procedure. Ileoanal anastomosis occurs in two stages (Fig. 60–4). In the first stage, the surgeon excises the rectal mucosa, performs an abdominal colectomy, constructs the reservoir or pouch to the anal canal, and creates a temporary loop ileostomy. The loop ileostomy is necessary to allow adequate healing of the internal pouch and all anastomosis sites and to allow for an increase in the capacity of the internal reservoir through fluid instillations. After 3–4 months, the client returns to have the loop ileostomy closed. Stool formation resembles that in clients who have had a traditional ileostomy.

Postoperative Care. The nurse provides the usual postoperative interventions as for clients who have undergone other types of abdominal surgery. All clients requiring surgical intervention for ulcerative colitis have an abdominal incision. Initially, most clients are maintained on NPO status, and a nasogastric (NG) tube is used for suction. (See Chapter 58 for care of the client with an NG tube.)

► Acute and Chronic Pain

Planning: Expected Outcomes. The client is expected to experience relief from painful abdominal cramping that occurs with ulcerative colitis.

Interventions. Pain control may be accomplished by drug and nondrug measures. The client's symptoms can cause physical discomfort, which can also contribute to emotional discomfort. The use of a variety of symptom-

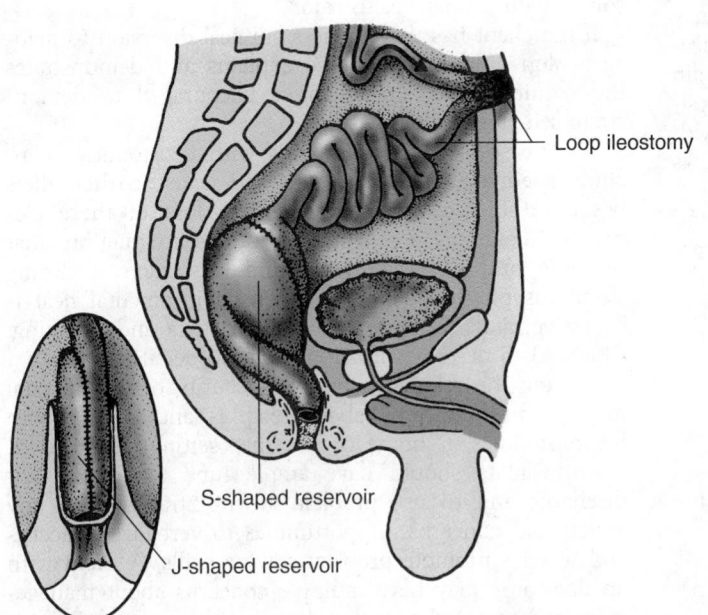

Stage 1.
After removal of the colon, a temporary loop ileostomy is created and an ileoanal reservoir is formed. The reservoir is created in an S-shaped reservoir (using three loops of ileum) or a J-shaped reservoir (suturing a portion of ileum to the rectal cuff, with an upward loop).

Loop ileostomy

S-shaped reservoir

J-shaped reservoir

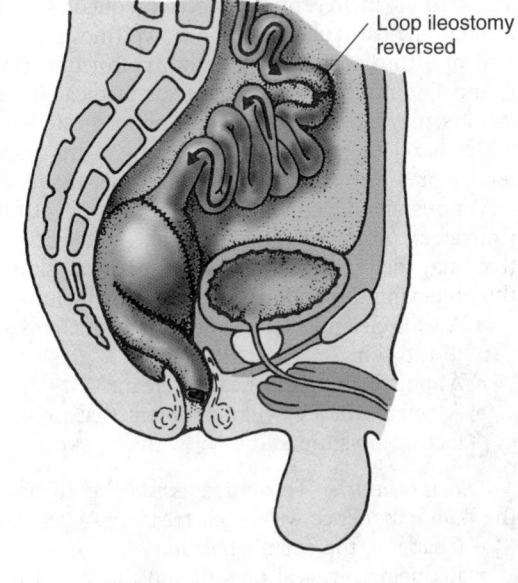

Loop ileostomy reversed

Stage 2.
After the reservoir has had time to heal—usually several months—the temporary loop ileostomy is reversed, and stool is allowed to drain into the reservoir.

Figure 60–4. The creation of an ileoanal reservoir.

reducing interventions and supportive measures can provide increased comfort.

Drug Therapy. Antidiarrheal medications are used to control the diarrhea and thereby reduce the resulting discomfort (see Chart 56–1). The physician may prescribe anticholinergics, such as propantheline bromide (Pro-Banthine), before meals to provide relief from the pain and cramping that may occur with diarrhea. Opioids are used sparingly and cautiously. These drugs can mask symptoms of life-threatening complications.

Pain Monitoring. The nurse assesses for pain and pays particular attention to any changes in the client's complaints of and responses to pain. Changes in the pain experience may suggest disease complications, such as increased inflammation, obstruction, hemorrhage, or peritonitis.

Pain assessment includes the following:

- Character and intensity of pain (use rating scale)
- Pattern of occurrence (e.g., before or after meals, during the night, before or after bowel movements)
- Duration of the pain

Diet Therapy. Dietary measures, discussed earlier under Diarrhea, help to control symptoms and thereby promote relief from discomfort. The nurse evaluates the effects of implemented dietary measures on an ongoing basis.

Perineal Skin Care. Perineal skin can be irritated by the frequent contact of the diarrheal stool and frequent cleaning. This irritation can be a major contributor to the client's discomfort. The nurse explains special measures for skin care. For example, cleaning the perineal area with mild soap and warm water after each bowel movement keeps the skin free of any stool. Frequent sitz baths may be helpful, particularly after a bowel movement. Application of a thin coat of mineral oil, petroleum jelly, vitamin A and D ointment, aloe creams, or medicated foam applications may provide relief. Use of medicated wipes with witch hazel (e.g., Tucks) is soothing if the rectal area is tender or sensitive from the use of toilet tissue.

Various manufacturers of ostomies (e.g., Hollister and Convatec) produce a three-product system for skin care that may help prevent and heal perineal skin irritation, thus relieving discomfort. Such systems include

- A skin-cleaning solution that is gentle and soothing to the skin
- A moisturizing and healing cream
- A petroleum jelly–like ointment that prevents contact of moisture and stool with the skin

Other Measures. The nurse assists the client in altering the pain experience with such measures as

- Changing the client's position
- Reducing physical pressure on the site of pain
- Applying heat
- Encouraging participation in diversional activities
- Emphasizing adequate rest and activity
- Involving the client in plans of care
- Providing information and explanations
- Allowing opportunities for the client to voice feelings and concerns

Such measures contribute to a therapeutic environment

and assist the client in acquiring the ability to deal with pain.

➤ *Potential for Gastrointestinal Bleeding*

Planning: Expected Outcomes. The client is expected to experience no GI bleeding. If bleeding does occur, the goal is to stop it using the appropriate treatment options.

Interventions. The nurse's primary responsibility is to monitor the client closely for signs and symptoms of internal bleeding. All stools are checked for blood, using both gross and occult examination. Other manifestations include hypotension, tachycardia, restlessness, and a change in mental status, especially among the elderly. If any of these signs and symptoms are present, the nurse notifies the health care provider immediately. Chapter 58 describes the management of GI bleeding in detail.

 ## Continuing Care

➤ *Case Management*

The client with ulcerative colitis is managed at home, but may require hospitalization during exacerbations. Clients with uncontrolled or severe colitis may be assigned a case manager to facilitate quality care in a cost effective way.

➤ *Health Teaching*

The nurse educates the client about the nature of ulcerative colitis with regard to its acute episodes, remissions, and symptom management. The nurse emphasizes that even though the cause is unknown, relapses can be resolved with proper health care.

If the client has undergone a surgical diversion to manage colon effluent, the nurse explains and demonstrates the required care. The client is encouraged to demonstrate self-care of the ileostomy.

The nurse also teaches clients with ileostomies to include adequate amounts of salt and water in their diets because the ileostomy promotes the loss of these elements. Clients are taught to be cautious in situations that promote profuse sweating or fluid loss, such as during strenuous physical activities, when environmental heat is excessive, and during episodes of diarrhea and vomiting. Chart 60–3 describes ileostomy care in detail.

Leaving the relative safety and security of the hospital may prompt concerns about relapses and coping with responsibilities at home or in other settings, such as at work. Clients should have ample time to prepare for discharge and to use problem-solving strategies for any anticipated concerns. Opportunities to verbalize concerns and worries promote problem-solving skills. A client with an ileostomy may have multiple concerns about management at home and sexual and social adjustments. Considering possible sexual issues helps the client identify and discuss these concerns with the sexual partner. Social situations may precipitate some anxieties related to decreased self-esteem and a disturbance in the client's body image. The nurse helps the client explore possible concerns in addressing and resolving these potentially stressful events (see also Chapter 10 on body image).

Chart 60–3

Education Guide: Ileostomy

Pouch Care

- Empty your pouch when it is ⅓ to ½ full.
- Change the pouch during inactive times, such as before meals, before retiring at night, on waking in the morning, and 2–4 hr after eating.
- Change the entire pouch system every 3–7 days.

Skin Protection

- Use a pectin-based skin barrier (not karaya gum) to protect your skin from contact with contents from the ostomy.
- Use skin care products, such as skin sealants and ostomy skin creams, if your skin continues to come into contact with ostomy contents.
- Watch your skin for any irritation or redness.

Diet

- Chew food thoroughly.
- Be cautious of high-fiber and high-cellulose foods. You may need to eliminate these from the diet if they cause severe problems (diarrhea, constipation, or blockage). Examples include popcorn, peanuts, coconut, Chinese vegetables, string beans, tough fiber meats, shrimp and lobster, rice, bran, and skinned vegetables (tomatoes, corn, and peas).

Medications

- Avoid taking enteric-coated and capsule medications.
- Inform any health care provider who is prescribing medications for you that you have an ostomy. Before having prescriptions filled, inform your pharmacist that you have an ostomy.
- Do not take any laxatives or enemas. You should usually have loose stool and should contact a physician if no stool has passed in 6–12 hr.

Symptoms to Watch for

- Report any drastic increase or decrease in drainage to your health care provider.
- If stomal swelling, crampy abdominal pain, or distention occurs or ileostomy contents stop draining, do the following:
  - Remove the pouch with faceplate.
  - Lie down, assuming a knee-chest position.
  - Begin abdominal massage.
  - Apply moist towels to the abdomen.
  - Drink hot tea.
  - If none of these maneuvers is effective in resuming ileostomy flow, or if abdominal pain is severe, call your health care provider right away.

► Home Care Management

The nurse assesses the client's ability to obtain prescribed medications, to obtain rest, and to follow dietary restrictions after discharge. Clients who have undergone surgery are also assessed for their ability to provide incision and, possibly, ostomy (or Kock's pouch) care.

► Health Care Resources

If a client requires assistance with activities of daily living, the nurse may help to arrange the services of a home care aide. If the client is discharged from the hospital with an ileostomy, the nurse makes a referral to a home health agency. A home care nurse can provide assessment and guidance in integrating ostomy care into the client's lifestyle and possibly provide wound care, including the monitoring of wound healing (Chart 60–4). The client needs to know where to purchase ostomy supplies along with the name, size, and manufacturer's order number. The nurse contacts local and regional supply companies for prices and availability of supplies (Seaman, 1996).

The nurse can identify the local stoma support group by contacting the United Ostomy Association. A local support group and the Crohn's & Colitis Foundation of America may be of assistance in obtaining supplies. The nurse also informs the client and family or significant others of available ostomy outpatient clinics and enterostomal therapists. If the client agrees, a visit from an ostomate can be initiated or continued on an outpatient basis.

 Evaluation

On the basis of the identified nursing diagnoses and collaborative problems, the nurse evaluates the care of the

Chart 60–4

Focused Assessment for Home Care: Clients with Inflammatory Bowel Disease

- Assess gastrointestinal function and nutritional status, including
  - Abdominal cramping or pain
  - Bowel elimination pattern; specifically frequency, characteristics and amount of stools, presence or absence of blood in stools
  - Dietary and fluid intake and habits (include relationship of specific foods to cramping and stools)
  - Weight gain or loss
  - Signs and symptoms of dehydration
  - Presence or absence of fever, rectal tenesmus, or urgency
  - Bowel sounds
  - Condition of perianal skin, including presence or absence of perianal fistula or abscess
- Assess client and family coping skills, including
  - Current and ongoing stress level and coping style
  - Availability of support system
- Assess home environment, including
  - Adequacy and availability of bathroom facilities
  - Opportunity for rest and relaxation
- Assess ability to manage therapeutic regime, including
  - Knowledge of medications
  - Signs and symptoms to report
  - Dietary management
  - Availability of community resources
  - Importance of follow-up care

client with ulcerative colitis. Expected outcomes may include that the client will

- Be free of diarrhea, rectal bleeding, and cramping
- Maintain adequate hydration
- Have an awareness of factors that influence active disease and use this knowledge to adapt his or her lifestyle for better control of exacerbations
- Maintain ideal body weight
- Be aware of and adhere to the prescribed drug regimen

Additionally, the client with an ileostomy can be expected to

- Perform his or her own pouch care
- Maintain peristomal skin integrity
- Verbalize dietary restrictions
- Demonstrate behaviors that integrate the ostomy into his or her lifestyle
- Verbalize signs and symptoms of stoma complications

Crohn's Disease

Overview

Crohn's disease, also known as *regional enteritis* or *granulomatous colitis,* is an inflammatory bowel disease that can affect any part of the gastrointestinal tract, from the mouth to the anus. Crohn's disease is similar to ulcerative colitis in that the cause is unknown, and its clinical manifestations and treatment are similar. It may be related to an infectious, immune, or psychological factor, such as excessive stress.

In people with Crohn's disease, the terminal ileum is most frequently involved. The lesions are patchy and often extend through all bowel layers, at which point bowel fistulas can develop. The result is severe diarrhea and malabsorption of vital nutrients. Like ulcerative colitis, Crohn's disease is characterized by periods of remission and exacerbation.

Chronic pathologic changes include thickening of the bowel wall, thus narrowing of the bowel lumen and strictures. In advanced disease, the bowel mucosa demonstrates nodular swelling (granulomas) intermingled with deep ulcerations.

The complications associated with Crohn's disease are similar to those from ulcerative colitis. As shown in Table 60–3, hemorrhage is more common in ulcerative colitis, but severe small intestinal malabsorption is more common in Crohn's colitis. Bowel cancer may develop in the client with Crohn's disease, but usually after the disease has been present for 15–20 years.

Fistulas are common. Those that extend through the serosa and into nearby loops of bowel or between two portions of the intestine are called *enteroenteric* fistulas. Fistulous tracts that form from diseased segments of the bowel to the skin, umbilicus, and perineum are called *enterocutaneous* fistulas (Fig. 60–5). Fistulas can also extend from the bowel to other organs and body cavities, such as the bladder or vagina.

In the United States, the annual incidence of Crohn's disease is approximately 2 per 100,000 people. The peak incidence is between 20 and 40 years of age. There is a higher incidence among twins and siblings, suggesting a genetic connection.

TRANSCULTURAL CONSIDERATIONS

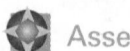 Crohn's disease is more common among people of Jewish descent, Caucasians, and those of middle European origin. Studies indicate that Jewish males are affected most often (Giger & Davidhizar, 1995).

Collaborative Management

Assessment

➤ *Physical Assessment/Clinical Manifestations*

The clinical presentation of Crohn's disease can vary greatly from client to client. When performing an abdominal assessment, the nurse often notes findings that are consistent with those in acute appendicitis, for example, tenderness, guarded movement, and a palpable mass in the right lower quadrant.

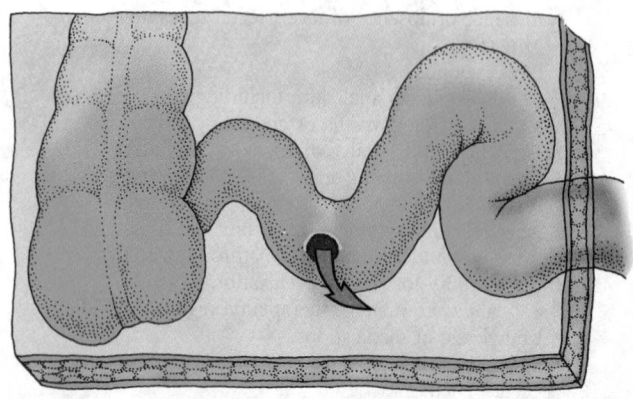

External enterocutaneous

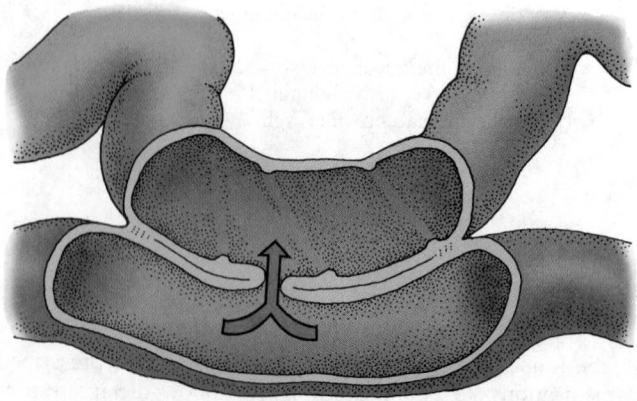

Enteroenteric

Figure 60–5. The types of fistulas that are complications of Crohn's disease.

Depending on the parts of the bowel involved, the nurse can identify several clinical manifestations. Most clients report diarrhea, abdominal pain, and low-grade fever. If the disease occurs only in the ileum, diarrhea occurs five or six times per day, often with a soft loose stool. Steatorrhea (fatty diarrheal stools) is common. The stool may contain bright-red blood, but this is a rare finding.

Abdominal pain from the inflammatory process is usually constant and is located in the right lower quadrant. Clients also experience periumbilical pain before and after bowel movements. If the lower colon is diseased, pain is often experienced in both lower abdominal quadrants. Fever is commonly present with complications such as fistulas and severe inflammation.

Weight loss may indicate serious nutritional deficiencies. Clients often experience nutritional problems as a result of anorexia, self-imposed dietary restrictions, decreased absorption of multiple vital nutrients, and fluid and electrolyte loss.

The marked inflammatory bowel changes decrease the small bowel's ability to absorb nutrients. These problems may be worsened by surgery and fistulas. The nurse is acutely aware of how important it is to detect clinical manifestations of peritonitis, bowel obstruction, and nutritional and fluid imbalances. The early detection of a change in the client's status helps to minimize these life-threatening complications.

➤ Psychosocial Assessment

The client experiencing Crohn's disease needs a complete psychosocial assessment. The chronicity of the problem and the troublesome complications can greatly affect clients and their families. The assessment should be ongoing and should continuously reflect the client's status as well as the family's.

➤ Diagnostic Assessment

The health care provider may order a number of laboratory studies for clients with Crohn's disease; however, no disease-specific tests are available to confirm the diagnosis. The diagnosis is made by ruling out disorders with similar clinical manifestations. Typical findings include

- Negative stool cultures
- Occult blood in the stool
- Low serum albumin levels, resulting from protein loss due to poor absorption

Serum levels of folic acid and cobalamin (vitamin B_{12} group) are generally low because of malabsorption. The nurse may note decreased hemoglobin and hematocrit values as a result of slow blood loss. An elevated erythrocyte sedimentation rate is consistent with the presence of inflammation. White blood cells in the urine may indicate infection (pyuria), which may be caused by ureteral obstruction or enterovesical (bowel to bladder) fistula.

The results of the contrast barium enema and upper gastrointestinal (GI) series often provide more specific diagnostic information. X-rays show narrowing, ulcerations, strictures, and fistulas consistent with Crohn's disease. In the acute illness, these tests are often deferred until the risk of perforation lessens.

Depending on which areas of the bowel are diseased, the sigmoidoscopic examination may not be diagnostic. If the rectosigmoid colon is involved, the physician may see ulcerations and inflamed mucosa, areas of fissure, fistula, and abscess formation of the perianal and perirectal areas.

Colonoscopy is used when other tests, especially the barium enema examination, have not led to a specific diagnosis.

 Interventions

Treatment of Crohn's disease is similar to that described earlier under nonsurgical management of ulcerative colitis. Specific interventions will vary, depending on which complications have occurred. Fistulas can occur with acute exacerbations of Crohn's disease. Clients with fistulas often experience complications, such as systemic infections, skin problems, malnutrition, and fluid and electrolyte imbalances.

The degree of associated problems depends on

- The site of the fistula
- The client's general health status
- The character and amount of discharge from the fistula

Nonsurgical Management. Treatment of the client with a fistula is multidimensional and includes nutrition and electrolyte therapy, skin care, and prevention of infection.

Nutrition and Electrolyte Therapy. Establishing adequate nutrition and fluid and electrolyte balance takes priority in the care of the client with a fistula. GI secretions are high in volume, electrolytes, and enzymes. The client is at high risk for malnutrition, dehydration, and hypokalemia. The nurse assesses the client for these complications (see Chaps. 15, 16, and 64).

The physician orders fluids and electrolyte replacement by oral liquids and nutrients as well as intravenous (IV) fluids. An antidiarrheal agent, such as diphenoxylate hydrochloride or atropine sulfate (Lomotil), may be prescribed to decrease fluid loss from diarrhea.

When a fistula begins to develop, the client's nutritional status is usually compromised. After the fistula has developed, nutritional status worsens. The client requires at least 3000 kcal/day to promote healing of the fistula. If the client cannot take adequate oral fluids and nutrients, the physician may order total parenteral nutrition (TPN). In collaboration with the dietitian, the nurse

- Carefully monitors the client's tolerance to diet
- Assists the client in selecting high-calorie, high-protein, high-vitamin, low-fiber meals
- Offers enteral supplements, such as Ensure and Vivonex
- Records food intake for accurate calorie counts

Skin Care. Proteolytic enzymes and bile contribute to the problem of skin irritation and excoriation. Skin irritation needs to be prevented; this is usually accomplished through the use of skin barriers, application of pouches, and insertion of drains (Fig. 60–6). By applying a pouch to the draining fistula, the nurse prevents skin irritation and can measure the effluent (drainage).

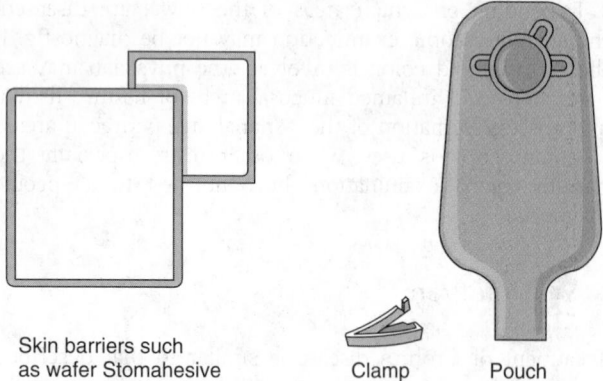

Skin barriers such
as wafer Stomahesive   Clamp   Pouch

Figure 60–6. Skin barriers, such as wafers, are cut to fit ⅛ inch around the fistula. A drainable pouch is applied over the wafer. Effluent should drain into the bag and not contact the skin.

In one approach to drainage management, the nurse covers the area surrounding the fistula with barriers, such as Stomahesive or DuoDerm, and then applies a wound drainage system over the fistula, securing it to the protective dressing. The skin adjacent to the fistula is cleaned with normal saline solution and gently patted dry.

The nurse collaborates with the enterostomal therapist (ET) to provide wound management. Wound drainage must *never* be allowed to be in direct contact with skin without prompt cleaning because intestinal fluid enzymes are caustic.

Prevention of Infection. Clients with fistulas are at extremely high risk for intra-abdominal abscesses and sepsis. Intra-abdominal fistulas are treated with careful nursing interventions, containment of wound drainage, and antibiotic therapy. The nurse observes for subtle signs of infection or sepsis, such as fever, abdominal pain, or change in mental status.

Surgical Management. Surgery to remove diseased portions of intestine is controversial for clients with Crohn's disease because risk for recurrence is considerable. However, those who continue to have symptoms after long-term medical treatment, and those with complications such as fistulas, may undergo small-bowel resection and anastomosis with or without colon resection. Strictureplasty may be performed for bowel strictures related to Crohn's disease. This procedure, which involves incising along the length of the stricture and suturing the incised area on the horizontal plane, allows for an increase in the bowel diameter. Preoperative and postoperative care for each of these surgical procedures is similar to care for clients undergoing other types of abdominal surgery.

➤ Continuing Care

The discharge care plan for the client with Crohn's disease is similar to that for the client with ulcerative colitis (described earlier). If the client has a draining fistula, the nurse helps the client plan for care of the fistula at home.

➤ *Health Teaching*

Before the client is discharged, the nurse explains and demonstrates fistula care. The client needs opportunities to practice the care in the hospital. Ideally, the client should be independent in fistula care before leaving the hospital, but, because of the perirectal or vaginal location of the fistula or an obese abdomen, the client may need assistance in this care. If this is the case, a family member or a caregiver must learn and practice the care, or the nurse can arrange for home health care services.

The remainder of the teaching plan for the client with Crohn's disease is similar to that for the client with ulcerative colitis. Like the client with ulcerative colitis, the client with Crohn's disease must identify stressors and methods to eliminate or reduce their impact. The nurse provides an atmosphere of trust and caring and encourages the client to verbalize concerns. Interventions should build self-esteem and promote independence.

➤ *Home Care Management*

The client's home should be arranged so that the client has easy access to the bathroom as well as privacy to perform fistula care and to rest. To ensure adequate nutrition, the client should have easy access to a well-supplied kitchen of readily prepared foods.

➤ *Health Care Resources*

The client with Crohn's disease benefits from the same health care resources as the client with ulcerative colitis. If the client needs equipment for fistula care, such as skin barriers and wound drainage bags, the nurse or case manager contacts medical supply companies or local pharmacies to ascertain their availability and price.

The nurse assesses the client's and the family's ability to monitor the progress of fistula healing and to watch for signs and symptoms of infection and sepsis. The assistance of a home health nurse may be considered for these tasks.

A home health aide might be considered for clients who cannot meet their nutritional needs, who need help with meal preparation, and who need help in purchasing groceries.

Diverticular Disease
Overview

The term diverticular disease describes the illnesses that traditionally have been identified as "diverticulosis" and "diverticulitis." Diverticulosis is the presence of several abnormal outpouchings or herniations (diverticula) in the wall of the intestine. Diverticulitis is the inflammation of one or more diverticula.

Pathophysiology/Etiology

Diverticula can occur in any part of the small or large intestine, but they occur most frequently in the sigmoid colon (Fig. 60–7), where high pressures are generated to push stool into the rectum. In and of themselves, diverticula cause few problems. If undigested food or bacteria

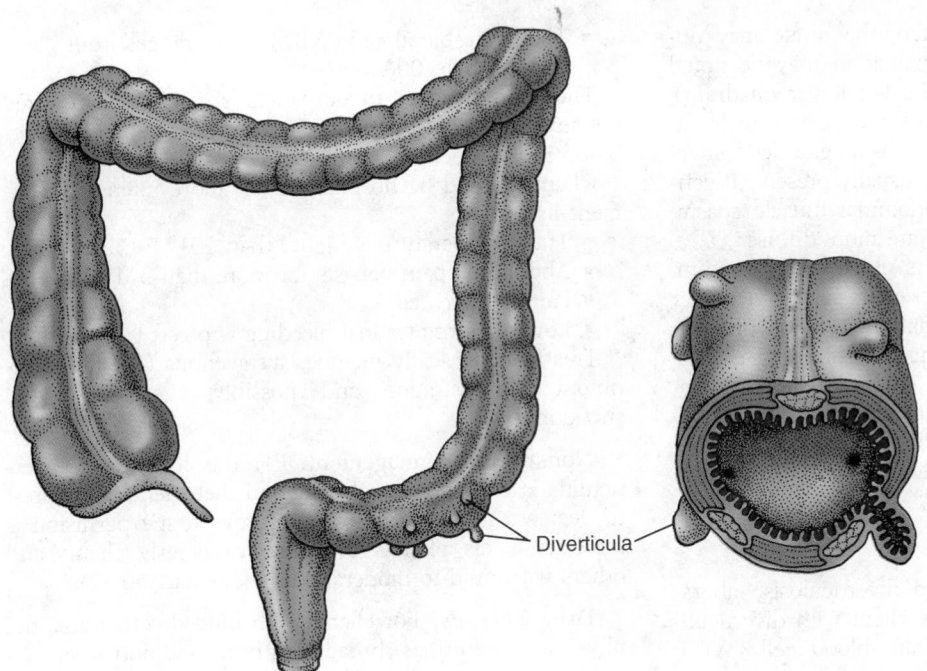

Figure 60-7. Several abnormal out-pouchings, or herniations, in the wall of the intestine, which are diverticula. These can occur anywhere in the small or large intestine but are found most often in the sigmoid as shown in this figure. Diverticulitis is the inflammation of a diverticulum that occurs when undigested food or bacteria become trapped in a diverticulum. Clinical Pathway: Peritonitis. (Courtesy of Harbor Hospital Center, Baltimore, MD.)

Diverticula

become trapped in a diverticulum, however, blood supply to that area diminishes and bacteria invade the diverticulum. Diverticulitis results when the diverticulum perforates and a local abscess forms. The perforated diverticulum can also progress to an intra-abdominal perforation with generalized peritonitis.

Bleeding from diverticula can range from minor, localized bleeding to massive hemorrhage. Minor bleeding is often due to localized inflammation in areas of vascular granulation tissue at the base of the diverticulum. Hemorrhage can result when a blood vessel is eroded within a diverticulum. Inflammation secondary to recurrent diverticulitis can lead to narrowing of the bowel lumen, which may result in obstruction. Inflammation can also result in fistulas to other organs, such as the bladder and the vagina.

ELDERLY CONSIDERATIONS

 A diverticulum results when significantly high pressure in the intestinal lumen pushes the intestine out, creating a herniation. Diverticula seem to occur at points of weakness in the intestinal wall, often at areas where blood vessels interrupt muscular continuity. The muscle weakness develops as part of the aging process.

Diets with small amounts of fiber have been implicated in the development of diverticula in that they cause less bulky stool and possibly constipation. For diverticulosis and diverticulitis to occur, there must be an increase in intraluminal pressure and muscle contractions to move fecal material through the colon.

The etiologic factor in diverticulitis may be retained undigested food in diverticula, which compromises the blood supply to that area and facilitates bacterial invasion of the sac.

Incidence/Prevalence

The incidence of diverticulosis is difficult to determine, but it is estimated that millions of people are affected. Diverticular disease affects one third of adults over age 60 years. Although diverticulosis is common, only one of five people with this disease have symptoms. Diverticular disease seems to occur equally in men and women.

Collaborative Management

◆ Assessment

The diagnosis of diverticulosis is usually made incidentally when a client has x-rays of the gastrointestinal (GI) tract to rule out other illnesses. Occasionally, diverticulosis causes symptoms. For clients with uncomplicated diverticulosis, the nurse asks about a history of intermittent pain in the left lower quadrant and a history of constipation.

➤ Physical Assessment/Clinical Manifestations

When assessing the client with diverticulosis, the nurse may find no clinical manifestations specific to this disorder. Occasionally, the nurse may elicit tenderness on abdominal palpation.

The client with diverticulitis has abdominal pain, most often localized to the left lower quadrant. The pain may be intermittent at first but becomes progressively steady. Occasionally, pain may be suprapubic or may occur on one side. Abdominal pain is generalized if peritonitis has occurred. The client's temperature is elevated, ranging from a low-grade fever to 101° F (38.2° C) with chills. Tachycardia results from fever, and nausea and vomiting are frequently present.

On examination of the abdomen, the nurse may observe distention. Tenderness on palpation may be noted over the area involved (usually the left lower quadrant). The colon may be palpable. If localized peritoneal irritation is present, localized muscle spasm, guarded movement, and rebound tenderness are usually present. If generalized peritonitis is present, abdominal muscle spasm, guarding, and rebound tenderness are more diffuse.

If the perforated diverticulum is close to the rectum, the physician or nurse practitioner may palpate a tender mass during the rectal examination. Blood pressure checks may show orthostatic changes. If bleeding is massive (rare with diverticulitis), the client may have hypotension and dehydration that result in shock. If generalized peritonitis has occurred, sepsis and manifestations of hypotension and septic or hypovolemic shock can occur.

➤ Diagnostic Assessment

For the client with uncomplicated diverticulosis, laboratory studies are not indicated. The client with diverticulitis, however, has an elevated white blood cell (WBC) count. In stool tests for occult blood, results are positive in 20% of clients (also called a positive guaiac). Urinalysis may show a few red blood cells if the left ureter is in proximity to a perforated diverticulum.

X-rays of the intestinal tract with barium contrast show diverticula. An upper gastrointestinal (GI) series shows diverticula of the small intestine, and barium enema examination shows diverticula of the large intestine. X-rays are not indicated in clients with uncomplicated diverticulosis because symptoms are usually minimal or nonexistent.

The client with diverticulitis usually does *not* undergo invasive x-ray studies (e.g., barium enema) in the acute phase of the illness because of the risk of perforating a local abscess. A barium enema examination may be completed after the client has been treated with antibiotics and the inflammation has resolved. A flat plate of the abdomen may reveal free air and fluid in the left lower quadrant, suggesting an abscess or free air under the diaphragm, indicating perforation. The health care provider may also order a computed tomography (CT) scan to diagnose an abscess or thickening of the bowel related to diverticulitis.

Ultrasonography, a noninvasive test, may reveal bowel thickening or an abscess. The physician may perform a sigmoidoscopy or colonoscopy *after the acute phase* of the illness, usually to rule out the presence of a tumor in the large intestine, particularly if the client has rectal bleeding. If the sigmoidoscope or colonoscope enters a diverticulum, however, the chances of perforating the diverticulum are high.

◈▸ Interventions

Clients may be treated on an ambulatory basis when
- Symptoms are mild
- Their temperature is lower than 101° F (38.2° C)

- The white blood cell (WBC) count ranges from 13,000 to 15,000/mm³

The client who is an outpatient should be monitored for any prolonged or increased fever, abdominal pain, or blood in the stool.

Clients should be hospitalized for more intensive treatment if
- Their temperature is higher than 101° F (38.2° C)
- Abdominal pain persists for more than 3 days
- Pain is increased
- Lower gastrointestinal bleeding is present

Treatment typically includes intravenous (IV) fluid, antibiotic administration, and, possibly, nasogastric (NG) suctioning.

Nonsurgical Management. For the client with diverticulitis, a combination of drug and diet therapy with rest to decrease inflammation and improve tissue perfusion is indicated. This plan is preferred for elderly clients and others with mild to moderate disease (Chart 60–5).

Drug Therapy. For clients with mild diverticulitis, the physician prescribes broad-spectrum antibiotics and a mild analgesic for pain. The physician admits clients with more severe pain to the hospital and orders intravenous (IV) antibiotics. Anticholinergics, such as propantheline bromide (Pro-Banthine), may reduce intestinal hypermotility.

For clients with severe diverticulitis, an opioid analgesic, such as meperidine hydrochloride (Demerol) or morphine sulfate, can alleviate pain.

Laxatives are avoided because they increase intestinal motility. Enemas are avoided because they increase intraluminal pressure. The nurse assesses the client for clinical

---

Chart 60–5

Nursing Focus on the Elderly: Diverticulitis

- Provide antibiotics, analgesics, and anticholinergics as ordered. Observe elderly clients carefully for side effects of these drugs, especially confusion (or increased confusion), urinary retention or failure, and orthostatic hypotension.
- Do not give laxatives or enemas. Teach the client and the family about the importance of avoiding these measures.
- Encourage the client to rest and to avoid activities that may increase intra-abdominal pressure, such as straining and bending.
- While diverticulitis is active, provide a *low*-fiber diet (see Table 60–4). When the inflammation resolves, provide a *high*-fiber diet. Teach the client and family about these diets and when they are appropriate.
- Because elderly clients do not always experience the typical pain or fever expected, observe carefully for signs of active disease.
- Perform frequent abdominal assessments to determine distention and tenderness on palpation.
- Check stools for occult or frank bleeding.

manifestations of fluid and electrolyte imbalance on an ongoing basis.

Rest. The nurse instructs the client to remain in bed during the acute phase of illness. The nurse advises the client to refrain from lifting, straining, coughing, or bending to avoid an increase in intra-abdominal pressure, which can result in perforation of the diverticulum.

Diet Therapy. During the acute phase of the illness, the client's diet is restricted to clear liquids. Clients who have more severe symptoms are admitted to the hospital and are kept on NPO status. A nasogastric tube is inserted if nausea, vomiting, or abdominal distention is severe. The nurse administers IV fluids, as ordered, for hydration. In collaboration with the dietitian, the client increases dietary intake slowly as symptoms subside. When inflammation has resolved and bowel function returns to normal, a fiber-containing diet is introduced gradually. If active diverticulitis recurs, fiber intake is stopped for the acute phase of the illness.

Surgical Management. The client with diverticulitis may need to undergo surgery if one of the following occurs:

- Rupture of diverticulum with subsequent peritonitis
- Pelvic abscess
- Bowel obstruction
- Fistula
- Presence of a mass or suspected tumor
- Persistent fever or pain after 4 days of medical treatment
- Uncontrolled bleeding

The surgeon performs emergency surgery if peritonitis, bowel obstruction, or pelvic abscess is present. Colon resection, with or without colostomy, is the most common surgical procedure for clients with diverticular disease.

Preoperative Care. Preparation of the client for surgery depends on the circumstances. The surgery might be performed on an emergency basis, with just a few hours' or days' notice (after unsuccessful medical treatment), or it might be done with a few weeks' notice (as when resection is performed for recurrent diverticulitis). The surgeon informs the client whether a temporary or permanent colostomy might be required.

If the client is *not* in the acute stage of diverticulitis, a thorough bowel preparation *may* be given, consisting of enemas and laxatives daily for 2–3 days before surgery. Because of the risk of perforation, however, the surgeon may forgo an aggressive bowel preparation. If a client has an acutely inflamed diverticulum or persistent fever and abdominal pain, the bowel preparation is most likely withheld.

The client who is to undergo emergency surgery or who has not responded to medical intervention is maintained on NPO status with a nasogastric tube in place. These clients receive IV fluids with appropriate electrolyte replacements.

For clients without acute inflammation, a well-structured preoperative diet is ordered. The client usually has a low-fiber diet for 4–5 days, followed by a full-liquid diet for 2 days, then a clear-liquid diet the evening before surgery.

Preoperative teaching about colostomies depends on the surgeon's plan and how certain the need for colostomy is. If a colostomy is a possible outcome, the enterostomal therapist (ET) or staff nurse describes its function and purpose. The nurse need not discuss colostomy care in detail unless the client wants this information.

Operative Procedures. In a resection of the colon, the surgeon excises the portion that is inflamed or diseased, and, if possible, creates an anastomosis of the colon to restore patency. Inflammation and infection, however, may preclude the feasibility of an anastomosis. If this is the case, the surgeon may perform a colostomy. Select clients may be candidates for colostomy closure and anastomosis, after the bowel has been allowed to rest 3 to 6 months.

Postoperative Care. The immediate physical care for clients undergoing colon resection for diverticulitis is the same as for clients undergoing abdominal surgery.

Wound Care. The client has a drain in place at the abdominal incision site for 2–3 days. If a colostomy has been performed, it may be covered with a dressing because it does not drain for approximately 2 days, or a colostomy bag may be placed over the stoma. If the stoma is visible, the nurse monitors its color and integrity. The stoma should be pinkish to cherry red without retraction or prolapse into the abdomen.

Diet Therapy. The client is kept on NPO status after a colon resection with or without a colostomy, with a nasogastric (NG) tube in place for 2–3 days. When peristalsis returns, the nurse removes the NG tube, according to the physician's order, and introduces clear liquids *slowly.* *Gradually,* the client's diet is advanced to solids, depending on the return of peristalsis and bowel function.

If the client has had a colostomy, it should start functioning in 2–4 days. Most clients who undergo surgery and colostomy formation for diverticulitis have a sigmoid colostomy because the sigmoid colon is the most common site of diverticulitis. Drainage from a sigmoid colostomy initially is loose stool, but eventually it becomes formed. A tight seal around the stoma is essential to avoid contact of feces with the skin. (Colostomy care is detailed in Chapter 59.)

Emotional Support. If a colostomy has been performed, the nurse gives the client opportunity to express feelings about the ostomy. The nurse discusses these feelings with the client, acknowledging that anger and depression are normal responses. When the client is physically able, the nurse encourages him or her to look at the stoma and touch the apparatus.

▶ Continuing Care

The length of hospitalization for a client with diverticulitis ranges from 4–10 days, depending on the response to medical treatment and the need for surgery. Discharge plans vary with the treatment.

➤ *Health Teaching*

Diet Therapy. All clients with diverticular disease need instructions on proper diet and rationale for the diet. The nurse and dietitian encourage the client with diverticulosis to eat a diet high in cellulose and hemicellulose types of fiber. These substances can be found in wheat bran, whole-grain breads, and cereals. The client should ingest at least 15 g of bran daily. This requirement can be derived from four slices of 100% whole-wheat bread and a 3-oz serving of all-bran cereal. The nurse also teaches the client to eat fruits and vegetables with a high-fiber content to add bulk to stools.

The client who is not accustomed to eating high-fiber foods should add them to the diet gradually to avoid flatulence and abdominal cramping. If the client cannot tolerate the recommended fiber requirement, a bulk-forming laxative, such as psyllium hydrophilic mucilloid (Metamucil), can be taken to increase fecal size and consistency. Clients should *avoid all fiber* when they have symptoms of *diverticulitis* because high-fiber foods are irritating.

The nurse explains that hot or cold foods and liquids cause gas, and these should be avoided. The client should also avoid alcohol because it irritates the bowel.

In collaboration with the dietitian, the nurse teaches the overweight client to begin a weight-reduction program because excessive weight worsens the symptoms of diverticular disease. The nurse suggests several techniques for helping the client lose weight, such as

- Establishing goals for weight loss
- Implementing a 24-hour recall of diet to identify problem areas
- Counting calories
- Using sample diets and menus
- Attending support groups

The nurse provides the same information to the client with active diverticulitis but emphasizes that the client should *not* add the recommended fiber until fever and abdominal pain have totally resolved. The client who has undergone surgery is usually taking solid food by the time of discharge from the hospital.

Surgical Follow-Up. Clients who have had abdominal surgery need oral and written instructions on incision care and the signs and symptoms to watch for and report. These are similar to the instructions given to clients after other types of abdominal surgery. The nurse provides instructions on colostomy care for clients who have a temporary or permanent colostomy.

Acute Diverticulitis. The nurse instructs clients *with any type of diverticular disease*, orally and in writing, about signs and symptoms of acute diverticulitis, including fever; abdominal pain; and bloody, mahogany, or tarry stools.

The nurse advises all clients to avoid the use of laxatives (other than bulk-forming types) and enemas. All clients can also benefit from avoiding the activities that increase intra-abdominal pressure, such as straining at stool, bending, or lifting heavy objects.

The nurse reassures clients with diverticulosis that this disorder need not cause problems if a proper diet is followed. The nurse informs clients with diverticulitis that this illness does not commonly recur and that, with proper diet and elimination patterns, recurring episodes and potential complications can be avoided.

The client with a colostomy has special needs with regard to the alteration in body image and loss of body function. The nurse encourages the client to verbalize concerns about body image (see Chap. 10).

Clients who have undergone surgery may need assistance with incision and colostomy care. The nurse arranges for a home health nurse to assess wound healing and proper functioning of the ostomy and the appliance. If the client is interested, the nurse can arrange for a visit from an ostomy volunteer or an enterostomal therapist. For information about other ostomy resources, the nurse or the client can contact the United Ostomy Association.

➤ *Home Care Management*

For the client with diverticulitis who has responded to medical treatment, home care focuses on proper diet. The nurse assesses the client's ability to obtain and prepare the recommended high-fiber foods.

The client who has required surgical intervention has the added responsibilities of incision care and, possibly, colostomy care, with some temporary limitations placed on activities.

Anorectal Abscess

Overview

Anorectal abscesses most often result from obstruction of the ducts of glands in the anorectal region by feces, foreign bodies, or trauma. Stasis of obstructing contents occurs and causes infection that spreads into adjacent tissue. Most abscesses begin as cryptitis (a pocket of infection in an anal crypt).

Rectal pain is the first symptom. There may be no clinical manifestations at the time of the first physical assessment, but local swelling, erythema, and tenderness on palpation are apparent within a few days after onset of pain. The client may report a history of diarrhea before the occurrence of rectal pain. If the abscess is a chronic condition, discharge, bleeding, and pruritus (itching) may exist. Fever occurs if larger abscesses are present.

Collaborative Management

Anorectal abscesses are managed by surgical incision and drainage. The physician can often incise simple perianal and ischiorectal abscesses using a local anesthetic. For clients with more extensive abscesses, a regional or general anesthetic may be needed. Systemic antibiotics are given only for clients who

- Are immunocompromised
- Are diabetic
- Have valvular disease or a prosthesis
- Have extensive cellulitis

Incision and drainage (I&D) in these clients is performed after antibiotic therapy.

Nursing interventions are focused on assisting the client to maintain comfort and optimal perineal hygiene (Chart 60–6). The nurse encourages the use of sitz baths, anal-

---

Chart 60–6

Nursing Care Highlight: Promoting Perineal Comfort

- Keep the perineal area clean with mild soap.
- Pat the perineal area dry instead of rubbing it.
- Provide warm sitz baths or warm compresses to the area.
- If the area is acutely inflamed, apply cold packs.
- Provide a chair cushion or a soft, inflatable ring for the seated client. For the elderly or debilitated client, monitor the skin carefully to prevent pressure sores.
- Use absorbent pads for drainage, if any, and change them often.
- Use premoistened wipes for cleaning the perineal area after a bowel movement.
- Use witch hazel wipes (e.g., Tucks) to relieve pain.
- Give bulk-forming agents, such as psyllium mucilloid (Metamucil), as ordered, to reduce pain associated with defecation.
- Apply a topical anesthetic cream to the perineal area, as ordered.
- Give oral analgesics, as prescribed, for pain relief.
- Do not administer enemas or give potent laxatives.

---

gesics, bulk-producing agents, and stool softeners during the perioperative period until healing occurs. The nurse also emphasizes the importance of ongoing perineal hygiene after all bowel movements and the maintenance of a regular bowel pattern with a high-fiber diet.

Anal Fissure

Overview

An anal fissure (a "fissure in ano") is an elongated ulcerated laceration between the anal canal and the perianal skin. Fissures can be primary or secondary, acute or chronic.

Primary fissures are idiopathic with no known cause. *Secondary* fissures are associated with another disorder (e.g., Crohn's disease, tuberculosis, or leukemia) or with trauma (e.g., from a foreign body, childbirth, or perirectal surgery). Constipated stool, diarrhea, or spasm of the anal sphincter is another possible cause.

Collaborative Management

An acute anal fissure is superficial and resolves spontaneously or with conservative treatment. Chronic fissures recur, and surgical treatment may be needed. Pain during and after defecation is the most common symptom. Bleeding noted outside of the stool or on toilet tissue is the next most common symptom. Other symptoms associated with chronic fissures are pruritus, urinary frequency or retention, dysuria, and dyspareunia (painful intercourse).

The health care provider makes the diagnosis by inspecting and stretching the perianal skin. If the client is having pain at the time of the examination, diagnostic testing is usually limited to inspection. If the client is not

in severe pain, a digital examination and possibly a sigmoidoscopy are performed. When painless or multiple fissures are present, the physician may perform a barium enema and sigmoidoscopy to rule out an associated inflammatory bowel disorder.

Management of an acute fissure is nonsurgical, with interventions aimed at local, symptomatic pain relief and softening of stool to reduce trauma to the area. Warm sitz baths and analgesia are recommended along with the use of bulk-producing agents, such as psyllium hydrophilic mucilloid (Metamucil), which help minimize pain associated with defecation. If fissures do not respond to medical management within several days to weeks, surgical excision of the fissure with a local anesthestic may be necessary.

The nurse explains the appropriate pain control measures to the client. When nonsurgical management is initiated, the nurse instructs clients to notify the health care provider if pain is not relieved within a few days. The nurse instructs the client who undergoes surgery to continue with the same pain management and bowel regimen, including sitz baths, analgesics, and bulk-forming agents. The client is reminded to report any drainage or bleeding from the rectum to the health care provider.

Anal Fistula

Overview

An anal fistula (a "fistula in ano") is an abnormal tract-like communication between the anal canal and the skin outside the anus. Most anal fistulas result from anorectal abscesses, which are caused by obstruction of anal glands (see Anorectal Abscess, earlier). Fistulas can also be associated with tuberculosis, Crohn's disease, or cancer.

Collaborative Management

The client with an anal fistula has pruritus (itching), purulent discharge, and tenderness or pain that is worsened by bowel movements. The physician uses a proctoscope to identify the source of symptoms and to locate the fistula. Because fistulas do not heal spontaneously, surgery is necessary. To perform a fistulotomy, the surgeon incises the tissue overlying the tract and performs curettage (scraping) of the base. The incision site heals by secondary intention. In a client with a high fistula, a special surgical technique is necessary because important sphincters are often affected. Postoperatively, the nurse instructs the client about sitz baths, analgesics, and the use of bulk-producing agents or stool softeners to minimize pain.

Parasitic Infection

Overview

Parasites can enter and invade the gastrointestinal (GI) tract and cause infections leading to varying degrees of illness. Parasites commonly enter through the mouth by means of fecal-oral transmission, for example,

- From contaminated food or water
- During sexual oral-anal practices
- From contact with feces from a contaminated person

Common parasites that cause infection in humans are *Entamoeba histolytica,* which causes amebiasis (amebic dysentery), and *Giardia lamblia,* which causes giardiasis (Table 60–5).

Infection with Entamoeba histolytica

Humans are the only known hosts for *E. histolytica.* This organism occurs in cysts and trophozoites (sporozoan parasites). Trophozoites die rapidly after they leave the body in stool. Cysts, however, can remain viable in the right type of environment for weeks or months. Humans who eliminate cysts are infectious. Flies have been found to be vectors for transmission of the cysts, and transmission is increased in areas that use human excrement for fertilizer.

Amebiasis occurs worldwide, but it is most prevalent and severest in tropical areas. Prevalence rates are as high as 40% in areas with poor sanitation, crowding, and poor nutrition. Amebiasis causes 40,000–100,000 deaths annually worldwide. The disease causes less severe symptoms and often goes undiagnosed in temperate climates. The organism may occur in 2% to 5% of some populations in the United States (Goldsmith, 1994a).

E. histolytica either feeds on bacteria in the intestine or invades and ulcerates the mucosa of the large intestine. The parasite can be limited to the GI tract (intestinal amebiasis), or it can extend outside the intestines (extraintestinal amebiasis). People can have intestinal amebiasis without having any symptoms, or symptoms can range from mild to severe.

Infection with Giardia lamblia

G. lamblia is a protozoal parasite that causes superficial invasion, destruction, and inflammation of the mucosa in the small intestine. Like *E. histolytica,* *G. lamblia* also has a trophozoite and cyst form, and cysts can transmit the organism. Humans are hosts to this organism, but beavers and dogs may be reservoirs for infection. Giardiasis is also a well-recognized problem in travelers, campers, male homosexuals, and immunosuppressed people.

Modes of transmission are similar to those for amebiasis; in the United States, however, giardiasis is much more prevalent and is the most common parasitic infection. Giardiasis affects only the intestinal system, causing acute diarrhea, chronic diarrhea, or malabsorption syndrome. The acute phase usually is self-limiting, lasting days or weeks. The chronic phase can last for years. Diarrhea is usually mild in both forms, but it can be severe. As stools increase in frequency, they become more watery, greasy, frothy, and malodorous with mucus. Weight loss and weakness are also common. Malabsorption can occur with diarrhea that continues for longer than 3 weeks. Manifestations result from malabsorption of fat, protein, vitamin B_{12}, and lactase deficiency.

Infection with Cryptosporidium

Cryptosporidium is another parasitic infestation manifested by diarrhea that commonly occurs in immunosuppressed clients, particularly those with human immunodeficiency virus (HIV) (see Chapter 25 under HIV infection).

Collaborative Management

 Assessment

Mild to moderate *Entamoeba histolytica* infestation causes clinical manifestations, including
- The passage of a few strongly odoriferous stools daily, possibly with mucus but without blood
- Abdominal cramping
- Flatulence
- Fatigue
- Weight loss

Clients experience characteristic remissions and recurrences. Severe amebic dysentery is manifested by frequent, more liquid, and odoriferous stools, with mucus *and* blood. Fever up to 105° F (40° C), tenesmus (ineffectual and painful straining to defecate), generalized abdominal tenderness, and vomiting can also occur. The ulcerations characteristic of invading amebiasis that occur in the colon can cause pain, bleeding, and obstruction. Ulcerations can also be localized in the rectum, resulting in formed stool with blood. Complications are rare but include appendicitis and bowel perforation.

Extraintestinal amebiasis can occur without symptoms of intestinal infection. The most common form is amebic liver abscess, which causes symptoms of fever, pain, and an enlarged liver. The abscess can rupture, and death can result if the infection is not treated and complications occur.

The diagnosis of amebiasis is made by examination of stool for parasites. Because *E. histolytica* organisms are difficult to detect, serial examinations of stool are needed if the disease is suspected. The use of sigmoidoscopy may detect ulcerations in the rectum or colon. Exudate obtained during sigmoidoscopic examination is studied for the parasite. The white blood cell count can be as high as 20,000/mm³ when severe dysentery is present.

The diagnosis of giardiasis is also confirmed by stool examination for parasites. Because organisms may not be detected for at least 1 week after symptoms appear, multiple stool samples should be examined. Duodenal aspirate can also be examined for the parasite.

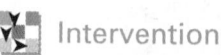 Interventions

Interventions for Amebiasis. Treatment for all types of amebiasis mandate the use of amebicide drugs. The physician commonly prescribes metronidazole (Flagyl,

TABLE 60–5

Parasites that Commonly Cause Diarrhea	
Parasite	**Infection**
Entamoeba histolytica	• Ambiasis (amebic dysentery)
Giardia lamblia	• Giardiasis
Cryptosporidium	• Cryptosporidiosis

Novonidanzol✦) and diloxanide furoate (Entamide) or diloxanide furoate and tetracycline hydrochloride (Sumycin) followed by chloroquine. Clients with severe dysentery require intravenous fluids for replacement and maintenance of fluid volume and possibly opiates, such as diphenoxylate hydrochloride and atropine sulfate (Lomotil), to control bowel motility. Clients with extraintestinal amebiasis or severe dehydration are hospitalized. Clients with asymptomatic, mild, or moderate disease are treated as outpatients with drug therapy. For all clients, at least three stools are examined for parasites at 2- to 3-day intervals, starting 2–4 weeks after drug therapy has been completed.

Interventions for Giardiasis. Treatment for giardiasis is drug therapy. Tinidazole (Fasigyn) is the drug of choice, and metronidazole is the alternative. Stools are examined 2 weeks after treatment is begun to assess for eradication.

The nurse explains modes of transmission and ways to avoid the spread of infection and recurrent contact with parasitic organisms. Clients are taught that they can transmit the infection to others until amebicides effectively kill the parasites. The nurse instructs clients to

- Avoid contact with stool
- Keep toilet areas clean
- Wash their hands meticulously with an antimicrobial soap after bowel movements
- Maintain personal hygiene
- Avoid stool from dogs and beavers

The client is also advised to avoid sexual practices that allow rectal contact until drug therapy is completed. The nurse informs the client that all household and sexual contacts should undergo stool examinations for parasites. If the water supply is suspected as the source, a sample is obtained and sent for analysis. Multiple infections are common in households, often as a result of contaminated water supplies. Well water and water from areas with inadequate or no filtration equipment can be sources of contamination.

Helminthic Infestation

Helminths are worm-like animals; they are often parasitic and capable of causing infectious disease in humans. There are many species of helminths and, for purposes of classification, are divided into three general categories:

- Roundworms (nematodes)
- Flukes (trematodes)
- Tapeworms (cestodes)

Helminths can cause various degrees of GI symptoms in humans. Most often, they enter the human body through the skin or via the oral route with ingestion of food, water, or other substances contaminated with worms. Some helminths gain access to the human body via insects, such as flies and mosquitoes. Helminths that are typically transmitted via insects are limited to tropical areas, however, and are not discussed here. Flukes (trematodes), which are passed to humans via snail-contaminated water, are also limited to tropical and subtropical areas outside the United States and are not discussed here.

Roundworms

Roundworms are commonly the cause of helminthic infections in the United States and worldwide. These infections include enterobiasis, trichinosis, and hookworm.

Enterobiasis

Enterobiasis ("pinworm infection") is caused by *Enterobius vermicularis* and is the most common helminthic infection in the United States. It is transmitted by oral ingestion of contaminated food, drink, or fomites. The most common clinical manifestations of infection include nocturnal perianal pruritus, vaginitis, insomnia, and restlessness.

The client may have vague gastrointestinal (GI) symptoms, such as abdominal pain, nausea, vomiting, and diarrhea. However, many infected clients have no symptoms. Diagnosis is made when eggs of the helminth are found on perianal skin or on cellulose tape that has been applied to perianal skin.

Treatment of enterobiasis includes meticulous hand-washing techniques after defecation and before meals to prevent spread of the worms to others. Drug therapy is indicated for all clients with symptoms and in some clients who are infected but are not symptomatic. Household cohabitants of an infected client may be treated with drug therapy even if they are asymptomatic. Pyrantel pamoate (Antiminth, Combantrin✦) or mebendazole (Vermox, Nemasole✦) is given orally in one dose, which is repeated at 2 and 4 weeks.

Infection with pinworms is curable and is not usually associated with complications; however, recurrences are common.

Trichinosis

Trichinosis is another helminthic disease caused by roundworms. The incidence in the United States has decreased to fewer than 100 cases annually, but many mild or asymptomatic cases are not diagnosed (Goldsmith, 1994b). *Trichinella spiralis,* which lives in the intestine of humans, pigs, bears, and rats, causes trichinosis. The organism is usually transmitted to people who ingest undercooked pork or pork products. Ingestion of other meats, such as ground beef, can also promote transmission if a meat grinder has been used for both beef and pork. Incubation is 12 hours to 28 days after ingestion. Clinical manifestations range from none to severe; death rarely results.

There are three stages of illness:

- The intestinal stage
- The stage of muscular invasion
- The stage of convalescence

The intestinal stage is often characterized by diarrhea, cramps, and malaise. During the stage of muscular invasion, the client experiences

- Fever
- Muscle pain
- Periorbital and facial edema
- Photophobia
- Conjunctivitis

- Pain on swallowing
- Dyspnea
- Coughing
- Hoarseness

Vague muscle pain and malaise characterize the convalescence phase, which can last for several months.

A diagnosis of trichinosis is conformed by a history of ingestion of raw or undercooked meat. White blood cell (WBC) and eosinophil counts are elevated for 2 weeks after meat is ingested. Biopsy of skeletal muscle shows larvae of the *Trichinella* organism. Worms are rarely seen in feces.

During the intestinal stage, the client is treated with oral mebendazole. During the stage of muscle invasion, the client must be hospitalized to receive high doses of corticosteroids.

Hookworms

Hookworms are also roundworms. They differ from pinworms and *Trichinella* in that they initially enter the human body through the skin. Hookworm disease is caused by either *Ancylostoma duodenale* or *Necator americanus*.

Hookworms infect a quarter of the world's population, but the disease is rare in areas outside the tropics or in areas with little rain (Goldsmith, 1994b). Worms are infective outside the body in warm, moist soil for up to 1 week. Transmission occurs when larvae penetrate through the skin. The organism can migrate to pulmonary capillaries via the bloodstream and enter alveoli. Cilia carry the organisms up the respiratory tree to the pharynx and the mouth, where they are swallowed and enter the gastrointestinal (GI) tract. Hookworms probably also enter the GI tract when a person ingests contaminated food.

Early symptoms of hookworm disease include a pruritic, erythematous, raised vesicular inflammation of the skin. Infection in the GI tract may produce no symptoms, or it may cause anorexia, diarrhea, or mild abdominal and epigastric discomfort. Bleeding and anemia may occur when worms suck blood at sites of attachment in the GI tract. If blood loss is severe, the client may have symptoms of iron deficiency anemia, such as pallor, hair thinning, deformed nails, pica, and shortness of breath.

Diagnosis of hookworm infection is based on the presence of ova (eggs) in the feces. Occult blood is often present in stool. There may be a low hemoglobin concentration and hematocrit values or low serum iron level and high iron-binding capacity, indicating hypochromic microcytic anemia. The WBC counts and eosinophil counts are elevated.

All clients with symptoms receive iron therapy and a diet high in protein and vitamins for at least 3 months after anemia is corrected. Pyrantel pamoate (Antiminth) or mebendazole (Vermox) is given for a complete recovery.

Tapeworms

Five types of tapeworms (cestodes) may infect humans: cattle, fish, dog, pig, and rodent. Tapeworm infections generally cause either no symptoms or only occasional gastrointestinal upset, such as nausea, diarrhea, or abdominal pain.

Transmission of tapeworms occurs when a person ingests undercooked beef, raw fish, and other contaminated food or water or accidentally swallows infected lice or fleas from dogs. People can also accidentally ingest arthropods, such as cockroaches, in stored foods or cereals.

The diagnosis of tapeworm infestation is made by laboratory examination of eggs found in stool (test of stool for ova and parasites). Clients are treated with medications for this type of infection.

When caring for clients with helminths, the nurse follows standard precautions or body substance precautions when in contact with any stool. All clients are taught to wash their hands after defecating and before eating. Clients should avoid ingesting undercooked beef, fish, and pork and drinking water that may be contaminated. After petting dogs, clients should take care to keep their mouth closed and wash their hands. All stored foods should be kept tightly closed to avoid contamination by cockroaches and other insects.

Food Poisoning

Food poisoning results when a person ingests infectious organisms in food. Unlike gastroenteritis, food poisoning is not directly communicable from person to person, and incubation periods are shorter. Like gastroenteritis, it causes diarrhea, nausea, and vomiting. The nurse can differentiate food poisoning from gastroenteritis by obtaining a thorough history of common food intake in clients who have common symptoms of acute diarrhea, nausea, and vomiting.

Three common types of food poisoning are caused by bacterial toxins:

- Staphylococcal infection
- *Escherichia coli* infection
- Botulism (Table 60–6)

Salmonellosis is also sometimes classified as a type of food poisoning. All cases of botulism and salmonellosis need to be reported to the local health department. Cases of staphylococcal and *E. coli* food poisoning are reported if epidemic outbreaks occur.

Staphylococcal Infection

Staphylococcus is found in meats and dairy products and can be transmitted by people, who are carriers of the organism. For staphylococcal food poisoning to occur, there must be contamination of food and a period of time (hours) during which the organisms multiply. This can take place during the slow cooling of food after it is cooked.

Symptoms of staphylococcal food poisoning include an abrupt onset of vomiting, abdominal cramping, and diarrhea. The person usually has symptoms 2–4 hours after ingesting the contaminated food. There is no fever, but the client is weak.

A diagnosis can be made when stool culture yields 100,000 enterotoxin-producing staphylococci; however, symptoms rarely last more than 24 hours, and people do not always seek medical attention. Antimicrobial drug therapy is not usually indicated, unless an agent produces

TABLE 60-6

Common Types of Food Poisoning

Type	Characteristics
Staphylococcal infection	• Caused by contaminated meats and dairy products • Can be transmitted by human carriers • Causes abrupt onset of vomiting and diarrhea without fever
Escherichia coli infection	• Caused by meat contaminated with animal feces • Causes abrupt vomiting, diarrhea, abdominal cramping, and fever
Botulism	• Commonly associated with improperly canned foods, especially fruits and vegetables • Nausea, vomiting, diarrhea, and weakness progressing to paralysis • Diplopia, dysphagia, and dysarthria
Salmonellosis	• Caused by contaminated food or drink but can be transmitted by the fecal-oral route • Fever, nausea, vomiting, abdominal cramping, and diarrhea lasting for 3–5 days

progressive systemic involvement. Parenteral fluids may be necessary if fluid volume is grossly depleted.

Escherichia coli *Infection*

Escherichia coli (E. coli) is not usually associated with food poisoning. In late 1992, however, more than 500 cases of E. coli food poisoning occurred in the United States when people ate contaminated meat in a fast-food restaurant. Many children were hospitalized with vomiting, diarrhea, abdominal cramping, and fever, and some subsequently died. The investigation of this outbreak showed that the hamburger meat used in the restaurant had been contaminated with fecal material during preparation in the slaughterhouses where the beef was initially cut and ground. E. coli is found in feces. Treatment of the client with E. coli food poisoning includes intravenous fluids and antibiotic therapy.

Botulism

Botulism is a type of food poisoning that occurs after a person ingests a toxin in food contaminated with *Clostridium botulinum*. Botulism is most frequently associated with home-canned foods, particularly vegetables, fruits, condiments, and, less commonly, meat and fish. It can be associated with commercially prepared products and with products not adequately heated to destroy toxins before they are eaten.

Incubation is usually 18–36 hours. After this time, symptoms occur causing a mild illness or a severe illness with paralysis, respiratory failure, and death. Initial symptoms include diplopia, dysphagia, and dysarthria.

Weakness can progress rapidly from the neck to arms, thorax, and legs. Paralytic ileus, severe constipation, and urinary retention can also occur. Nausea, vomiting, and abdominal pain may occur before or after the onset of paralysis.

The diagnosis is made on the basis of the client's history and a stool culture of *C. botulinum*. The serum may be positive for toxins.

Treatment with trivalent botulism antitoxin (ABE) is given as soon as the diagnosis is made if the client is not hypersensitive to it. The physician may lavage the client's stomach to stop absorption of toxin. All clients are hospitalized to observe for and treat respiratory paralysis. Nothing is given orally until swallowing and respiratory difficulties pass. The physician orders intravenous fluids as needed. If respiratory paralysis occurs, tracheostomy and mechanical ventilation are implemented. If ventilation can be maintained, the client can survive with no neurologic deficits after the illness.

To prevent botulism, the nurse teaches clients the importance of discarding cans of food that are punctured or swollen or that have defective seals. Containers for foods that are home-canned must be sterilized by boiling for 20 minutes to destroy *C. botulinum* spores before canning.

Salmonellosis

Salmonellosis is a bacterial infection caused by the *Salmonella* organism. Some consider this infection to be a food poisoning and others a gastroenteritis. It occurs after a person ingests contaminated food or drink, which characterizes it as food poisoning. However, salmonellosis can also be transmitted from person to person via the fecal-oral route.

Incubation is 8–48 hours after the person has ingested the contaminated food or liquid. Symptoms usually last for 3–5 days and include fever with or without chills, nausea, vomiting, cramping abdominal pain, and diarrhea, which may be bloody.

Salmonellosis is usually self-limiting, but bacteremia with localization in joints or bone may occur. The definitive diagnosis is made by stool culture.

Treatment is symptomatic, and drug therapy is not usually indicated unless bacteremia occurs; in that case, the physician prescribes antibiotics.

Clients may be carriers of the bacterium up to 1 year. The nurse instructs all clients with *Salmonella* infection and their contacts to wash their hands before meals and after defecating to avoid transmission of the organism.

CASE STUDY for the Client with Inflammatory Bowel Disease

■ Ms. Irene Bender is a 68-year-old woman admitted to the hospital for a colectomy and ileostomy for ulcerative colitis. Her surgeon describes her as extremely anxious. Ms. Bender's mother died unexpectedly following surgery about 5 years ago. Her other health problems include hyperthyroidism and anemia. She has had a 30-lb weight loss since the onset of her illness 18 months ago. She has lived

Continued on following page

CASE STUDY *Continued*

alone since her mother's death. She has few friends, and her sisters and brothers visit her infrequently.

Her nasogastric tube is removed 3 days following surgery. The physician has ordered sips of fluids orally. Ms. Bender calls you to her room and tells you that her stomach is "going to explode." She appears very restless and is twisting her hands. You begin a further assessment.

QUESTIONS:

1. Should your assessment initially focus on her physical complaints or on her mood and behavior?
2. What further questions should you ask?
3. What are the priority areas of assessment?
4. During the abdominal assessment, you find that her abdomen is distended and there are no bowel sounds. Given these assessment findings, what should you do first?

SELECTED BIBLIOGRAPHY

Belmonte, C., Klas, J. V., Perez, J. J., Wong, W. D., Rothenberger, D. Z., Goldberg, S. M., & Madoff, R. D. (1996). The Hartmann procedure. First choice or last resort in diverticular disease. *Archives of Surgery, 131*(6), 612–615.

Bennett, W. G., & Cerda, J. J. (1996). Benefits of dietary fiber. Myth or medicine. *Postgraduate Medicine, 99*(3), 153–156, 166–168.

Brydolf, M., & Segesten, K. (1994). Physical health status in young subjects after colectomy: An application of the Roy model. *Journal of Advanced Nursing, 20*(3), 500–508.

Calder, J. D., & Gajraj, H. (1995). Recent advances in the diagnosis and treatment of acute appendicitis. *British Journal of Hospital Medicine, 54*(4), 129–133.

Cox, J. (1995). Inflammatory bowel disease: Implications for the medical-surgical nurse. *MEDSURG Nursing, 4*(6), 427–434.

Doherty, D. B. (1994). What you need to know about inflammatory bowel disease. *American Journal of Nursing, 94*(7), 24–31.

Franz, M. G., Norman, J., & Fabri, P. J. (1995). Increased morbidity of appendicitis with advancing age. *American Surgeon, 61*(1), 40–44.

Giese, L. A., & Terrell, L. (1996). Sexual health issues in inflammatory bowel disease. *Gastroenterology Nursing, 19*(1), 12–17.

Giger, J. N., Davidhizar, R. E. (1995). *Transcultural nursing: Assessment and intervention* (2nd ed.). St. Louis: C. V. Mosby.

Godet, P. G., May, G. R., & Sutherland, L. R. (1995). Meta-analysis of the role of oral contraceptive agents in inflammatory bowel disease. *Gut, 37*(5), 668–673.

Goldsmith, R. S. (1994a). Infectious diseases: Protozoal. In L. M. Tierney, S. J. McPhee, and M. A. Papadakis (Eds.), *Current medical diagnosis and treatment 1994* (pp. 1215–1245). Norwalk, CT: Appleton & Lange.

Goldsmith, R. S. (1994b). Infectious diseases: Helminthic. In L. M. Tierney, S. J. McPhee, and M.A. Papadakis (Eds.), *Current medical diagnosis and treatment 1994* (pp. 1246–1275). Norwalk, CT: Appleton & Lange.

Jacobs, D. R., Slavin, J., & Marquart, L. (1995). Whole grain intake and cancer: A review of the literature. *Nutrition and Cancer, 24*(3), 221–229.

Kelly, M. P. (1994). Patients' decision making in major surgery: The case of total colectomy. *Journal of Advanced Nursing, 19*(6), 1168–1177.

Lo, C. Y., & Chu, K. W. (1996). Acute diverticulitis of the right colon. *American Journal of Surgery, 171*(2), 244–246.

Lucarotti, M. E., Freeman, B. J., Warren, B. F., & Durdey, P. (1995). Synchronous proctocolectomy and ileoanal pouch formation and the risk of Crohn's disease. *British Journal of Surgery, 82*(6), 755–756.

Macho, J. R., Lewis, F. R., & Krupski, W. C. (1994). Management of the injured patient. In L. W. Way (Ed.), *Current surgical diagnosis and treatment* (10th ed. pp. 213–233). Norwalk, CT: Appleton & Lange.

Mader, T. J. (1994). Acute diverticulitis in young adults. *Journal of Emergency Medicine, 12*(6), 779–782.

O'Dell, K. (1995). Infection control. Personal contacts. *Nursing Times, 91*(46), 58–60.

Ollinger-Snyder, P., & Matthews, M. E. (1996). Food safety: Review and implications for dieticians and dietetic technicians. *Journal of the American Dietetic Association, 96*(2), 163–168, 171.

Pacelli, F., Doglietto, G. B., Alfieri, S., Piccioni, E., Sgadari, A., Gui, D., & Crucitti, F. (1996). Prognosis in intraabdominal infections. Multivariate analysis on 604 patients. *Archives of Surgery, 131*(6), 641–645.

Phillips, S. (1995). Gut reaction. *Nursing Times, 91*(1), 44–45.

Phillips, S., & Warren, J. (1995). Supporting the patient with inflammatory bowel disease. *Nursing Times, 91*(27), 38–39.

Seaman, S. (1996). Basic ostomy management: Assessment and pouching. *Home Healthcare Nurse, 14*(5), 334–345.

Shuler, F. W., Newman, C. N., Angood, P. B., Tucker, J. G., & Lucas, G. W. (1996). Nonoperative management for intra-abdominal abscesses. *American Surgeon, 62*(3), 218–222.

Takacs, L. F., & Kollman, C. E. (1994). An inflammatory bowel disease support group for teens and their parents. *Gastroenterology Nursing, 17*, 11–13.

Willis, J. (1995). Stoma care: Principles and product type. *Nursing Times, 91*(4), 43–45.

Zurita, V. F., Rawls, D. E., & Dyck, W. P. (1995). Nutritional support in inflammatory bowel disease. *Digestive Diseases, 13*(2), 92–107.

SUGGESTED READINGS

Doherty, D. B. (1994). What you need to know about inflammatory bowel disease. *American Journal of Nursing, 94*(7), 24–30.

This author presents information regarding the types of inflammatory bowel diseases, their manifestations, and treatment approaches. There is a complete discussion of the lifestyle changes that occur with these disease processes and strategies to assist clients to cope effectively. Using a case study approach, the author clearly presents nursing care in a number of clinical situations.

Ollinger-Snyder, P., & Matthews, M. E. (1996). Food safety: Review and implications for dietician and dietetic technicians. *Journal of the American Dietetic Association, 96*(2), 163–168, 171.

This article discusses the six pathogens transmitted via food by infected food handlers. The authors present the factors that contribute to foodborne illnesses and strategies to prevent and control these illnesses. Strategies to limit the incidence of foodborne illnesses are reviewed.

Seaman, S. (1996). Basic ostomy management: Assessment and pouching. *Home Healthcare Nurse, 14*(5), 334–345.

This excellent article, written by an enterostomal therapist, describes how to assess a stoma, where to locate ostomy supplies, and how to trouble shoot problems. A chart outlining common peristomal skin complications and a list of national ostomy suppliers are included. A CEU quiz is found at the end of the article.

Chapter 61

INTERVENTIONS FOR CLIENTS WITH LIVER PROBLEMS

The liver is the largest and one of the most vital internal organs, performing more than 400 functions and affecting every system in the body. When the liver cannot perform its complex activities, hepatic failure results. Liver diseases range in severity from mild hepatic inflammation to chronic end-stage cirrhosis.

Cirrhosis

Overview

Cirrhosis is a chronic, progressive liver condition. It usually develops insidiously and has a prolonged, destructive course. As an end-stage process, it is essentially an irreversible reaction to hepatic inflammation and necrosis.

Pathophysiology

Cirrhosis is characterized by diffuse fibrotic bands of connective tissue, which distort the liver's normal architecture. Extensive degeneration and destruction of hepatocytes (hepatic, or liver, cells) occur. In attempts to regenerate with new nodule formation, a disorganized lobular pattern develops. Flow alterations in the vascular system and lymphatic bile duct channels result from compression caused by the proliferation of fibrous tissue.

Types of Cirrhosis

There are four major types of cirrhosis (Table 61–1):

- Laënnec's, or alcoholic
- Postnecrotic
- Biliary
- Cardiac

LAËNNEC'S CIRRHOSIS. Laënnec's cirrhosis, or alcoholic cirrhosis, may also be called nutritional, or portal, cirrhosis. Alcohol has a direct toxic effect on liver cells (hepatocytes), causing liver inflammation (alcoholic hepatitis), which usually precedes the onset of alcoholic cirrhosis. Metabolic changes in the liver that are induced by alcohol lead to fatty infiltration of the hepatocytes and scarring between the lobules. The liver becomes enlarged, with cellular degeneration and infiltration by fat, leukocytes, and lymphocytes (white blood cells). As the inflammatory process decreases, the destructive phase increases. Early scar formation is caused by fibroblast infiltration and collagen formation. Damage to the hepatic parenchyma progresses as a result of malnutrition and repeated exposure to the hepatotoxin (alcohol). If alcohol is withheld, the fatty infiltration is reversible. If alcohol abuse continues, widespread scar tissue formation and fibrosis infiltrate the liver as a result of cellular necrosis.

1463

TABLE 61–1

Major Types of Cirrhosis of the Liver

Type	Description
Laënnec's cirrhosis (most common type)	• Caused by long-term use of alcohol. • The liver becomes enlarged, firm, and hard in early disease; smaller and nodular in end-stage disease.
Postnecrotic cirrhosis	• Caused by massive hepatic cell necrosis, usually from acute viral hepatitis or exposure to certain hepatotoxins, such as industrial chemicals.
Biliary cirrhosis	• Caused by chronic biliary obstruction, bile stasis, and inflammation. • The liver becomes fibrotic; hepatic cells are destroyed.
Cardiac cirrhosis	• Caused by severe or chronic heart failure (also called vascular cirrhosis). • The liver becomes enlarged and congested with venous blood, resulting in cell necrosis from anoxia.

In people with early cirrhosis, the liver capsule is enlarged, firm, and hard. The regenerated nodules give the capsule a hobnailed, or bumpy, appearance. As the pathologic process of cirrhosis progresses, the liver shrinks in size. The capsule is covered by fine nodules surrounded by gray connective tissue.

POSTNECROTIC CIRRHOSIS. Postnecrotic cirrhosis occurs after massive liver cell necrosis. Broad bands of scar tissue cause destruction of liver lobules and entire lobes. First the liver enlarges; then it becomes shrunken with large nodules, representing macronodular structural changes throughout the organ. Postnecrotic cirrhosis occurs as a complication of acute viral hepatitis or after exposure to industrial or chemical hepatotoxins, such as carbon tetrachloride. This type of cirrhosis is suspected in clients who exhibit signs of chronic liver disease and do not have a history of excessive alcohol intake.

BILIARY CIRRHOSIS. Biliary cirrhosis develops as a result of chronic biliary obstruction, bile stasis, inflammation, or diffuse hepatic fibrosis. *Primary* biliary cirrhosis results from intrahepatic bile stasis. *Secondary* biliary cirrhosis is caused by obstruction of the hepatic or common bile ducts, which produces bile stasis in the liver. The accumulation of excessive hepatic bile leads to progressive fibrosis, hepatocellular destruction, and regenerated nodules. Severe obstructive jaundice is a key clinical manifestation in both types of biliary cirrhosis.

CARDIAC CIRRHOSIS. Cardiac cirrhosis, or vascular cirrhosis, is associated with severe right-sided heart failure. It develops in clients with long-standing heart failure after cor pulmonale, constrictive pericarditis, and valvular insufficiency (see Chap. 37). The liver becomes enlarged, is congested with venous blood, and appears edematous and dark in color. The liver serves as a reservoir for large amounts of venous blood that the failing heart cannot pump back into the systemic circulation. The increase in hepatic volume and pressure causes severe venous congestion. The liver becomes anoxic, which results in hepatic cell necrosis and fibrosis.

Complications of Cirrhosis

Common problems and complications associated with hepatic cirrhosis depend on the amount of damage sustained by the liver. The loss of hepatic function contributes to the development of metabolic abnormalities. Hepatic cell degeneration may lead to

- Portal hypertension
- Ascites (accumulation of abdominal fluid)
- Bleeding esophageal varices
- Coagulation defects
- Jaundice
- Portal-systemic encephalopathy (PSE) with hepatic coma
- Hepatorenal syndrome

PORTAL HYPERTENSION. Portal hypertension is a major complication of cirrhosis. It is a persistent increase in pressure within the portal vein. Portal hypertension results from increased resistance or obstruction to the flow of blood through the portal vein and its tributaries. The blood meets resistance to flow and seeks collateral venous channels around the high-pressure area.

Blood flow backs into the spleen, causing splenomegaly. Veins in the esophagus, stomach, intestines, abdomen, and rectum become dilated. Portal hypertension can result in ascites, esophageal varices, prominent abdominal veins (caput medusae), and hemorrhoids.

ASCITES. Ascites is the accumulation of free fluid containing almost pure plasma within the peritoneal cavity. Increased hydrostatic pressure from portal hypertension causes plasma to leak into the peritoneal cavity. The accumulation of plasma protein, primarily albumin, in the peritoneal fluid reduces the amount of circulating plasma protein in the blood. When this decrease is combined with the liver's inability to synthesize albumin because of impaired hepatocyte functioning, the effective serum colloid osmotic pressure is decreased in the circulatory system.

Increased hepatic lymph formation also contributes to ascites formation. The lymphatic system is unable to channel the increased amounts of lymph, and the resultant weeping of liver plasma ("liver sweat") occurs. The decrease of effective intravascular circulation from massive ascites may cause renal vasoconstriction, triggering the renin-angiotensin system. This results in sodium and water retention, which increases hydrostatic pressure and lymph formation, and the vicious circle of ascites formation continues.

BLEEDING ESOPHAGEAL VARICES. As the blood backs up away from the liver, it enters the esophageal and gastric vessels that carry it into the systemic circulation. Bleeding esophageal varices occur when these fragile, thin-walled esophageal veins are distended or irritated and rupture. Variceal bleeding may be caused by

- Any chemical irritant, such as alcohol, medications, and refluxed gastric acid
- Mechanical trauma from abrasions by poorly chewed food, vomiting, or nasogastric (NG) tube insertion
- Increased pressure in the esophagus, caused by vigorous physical exercise, coughing, or retching and vomiting

Varices occur most frequently in the distal end of the esophagus but are also noted in the proximal esophagus and stomach. Gastric ulceration or erosion also puts the client at risk for hemorrhage from the stomach. Endoscopy, if possible, can differentiate between gastric and esophageal bleeding.

The client loses large volumes of blood from hematemesis and may go into shock from hypovolemia. Bleeding esophageal varices are a medical emergency and necessitate immediate medical intervention (described later under Planning and Implementation).

COAGULATION DEFECTS. In people with cirrhosis, there is a decrease in the synthesis of bile fats in the liver, preventing the absorption of fat-soluble vitamins (such as vitamin K). Without vitamin K, clotting factors II, VII, IX, and X are not produced in sufficient quantities, and the client is susceptible to bleeding and easy bruising. Therefore, when a client has bleeding esophageal varices, the blood does not clot and hemorrhage occurs.

JAUNDICE. Jaundice found in clients with hepatic cirrhosis is caused by one of two mechanisms (Table 61–2): hepatocellular disease or intrahepatic obstruction. Hepatocellular jaundice develops because the liver cannot metabolize bilirubin. The liver's normal uptake of bilirubin from the blood is impaired; decreased excretion results in excessive circulating bilirubin levels. Intrahepatic obstructive jaundice results from edema, fibrosis, or scarring of the hepatic bile channels and bile ducts, interfering with normal bile and bilirubin excretion.

PORTAL SYSTEMIC ENCEPHALOPATHY (PSE). PSE is also known as *hepatic encephalopathy* and *hepatic coma* in the later stages. It is a clinical disorder seen in end-stage hepatic failure and cirrhosis. PSE is manifested by neurologic symptoms. It is characterized by an altered level of consciousness, impaired thinking processes, and neuromuscular disturbances.

PSE may develop insidiously in clients with chronic liver disease and go undetected until the late stages. In acute liver dysfunction, the symptoms develop rapidly. Four stages of development (prodromal, impending, stuporous, comatose) have been identified (Table 61–3). The client's symptoms may gradually progress to coma or fluctuate among the four stages.

The exact mechanisms of PSE have not been identified. The most probable cause is impaired ammonia metabolism. Most of the ammonia in the body is found in the gastrointestinal (GI) tract. Protein provided by the diet is transported to the liver by the portal vein. The liver breaks down protein, resulting in the formation of ammonia. The liver further converts ammonia to glutamine, which is stored, and then to urea for excretion. Urea diffuses into the body fluids and is eventually excreted in the urine by the kidneys.

Some ammonia is normally formed in the GI tract by the action of intestinal bacteria on protein products. Gastric juices are also a source of ammonia, and peripheral tissue metabolism produces some ammonia. In addition, the kidney may be a source of endogenous ammonia if hypokalemia is present.

When the liver is incapable of adequate protein degradation and cannot convert ammonia to urea, an excessive amount of circulating ammonia develops. The elevated ammonia levels are toxic to central nervous system tissue (glial and nerve cells), interfering with normal cerebral metabolism and function.

Factors that may precipitate PSE include

- High-protein diet
- Infections
- Hypovolemia
- Hypokalemia
- Constipation
- GI bleeding (which causes a large protein load in the intestines)

TABLE 61–2

Laboratory Diagnostic Differentiation of Jaundice			
Test	**Hepatocellular Jaundice**	**Obstructive Jaundice**	**Hemolytic Jaundice**
Serum bilirubin			
Indirect (unconjugated)	• Increased	• Slightly increased	• Increased
Direct (conjugated)	• Increased	• Moderately increased	• Normal
Urine bilirubin	• Increased	• Increased	• None
Urobilinogen			
Stool	• Normal to decreased	• None	• Increased
Urine	• Normal to increased	• None	• Increased

TABLE 61–3

Stages of Portal-Systemic Encephalopathy

Stage I: Prodromal

- Subtle manifestations that may not immediately be recognized
- Personality changes
- Behavior changes (agitation, belligerence)
- Emotional lability (euphoria, depression)
- Impaired thinking
- Inability to concentrate
- Fatigue, drowsiness
- Slurred or slowed speech
- Sleep pattern disturbances

Stage II: Impending

- Continuing mental changes
- Mental confusion
- Disorientation to time, place, or person
- Asterixis (see Fig. 61–3)

Stage III: Stuporous

- Progressive deterioration
- Marked mental confusion
- Stuporous, drowsy, but arousable
- Abnormal electroencephalogram tracing
- Muscle twitching
- Hyperreflexia
- Asterixis

Stage IV: Comatose

- Unresponsiveness, leading to death in 85% of clients progressing to this stage
- Unarousable, obtunded
- Response to painful stimulus
- No asterixis
- Positive Babinski's sign
- Muscle rigidity
- Fetor hepaticus (characteristic liver breath—musty, sweet odor)
- Seizures

- Drugs, such as hypnotics, opioids, sedatives, analgesics, and diuretics

PSE may also occur after paracentesis or shunting procedures. The prognosis for a client with PSE depends on the severity of the underlying cause, the precipitating factors, and the degree of liver dysfunction.

HEPATORENAL SYNDROME. The development of hepatorenal syndrome indicates a poor prognosis for the client with hepatic failure. It is one of the primary causes of death in end-stage cirrhosis. Progressive oliguric renal failure associated with hepatic failure results in function impairment of kidneys with normal anatomic and morphologic features. This syndrome is manifested by

- A sudden decrease in urinary flow
- Elevated blood urea nitrogen and creatinine levels, with abnormally decreased urine sodium excretion
- Increased urine osmolarity

Hepatorenal syndrome often occurs after clinical deterioration from GI bleeding or the onset of PSE. Drugs such as indomethacin (Indocin) and possibly acetaminophen (Tylenol, Exdol♣) and aspirin (acetylsalicylic acid [ASA]) may precipitate renal failure when administered to the client with cirrhosis. Hepatorenal syndrome is generally accompanied by elevated serum ammonia levels with an increase in jaundice and serum bilirubin levels. The kidneys cannot excrete these products in the urine. Hepatorenal syndrome may also complicate other liver diseases, including acute hepatitis and hepatic malignancy.

Etiology

The exact factors contributing to cirrhosis have not been clearly defined. There is a genetic component, with a familial tendency to develop cirrhosis, as well as a familial hypersensitivity to alcohol in some people. Many alcoholics do not experience cirrhosis, whereas others have cirrhosis even when adequate nutrition is maintained.

The cause varies with the type of cirrhosis. Laënnec's (alcoholic) cirrhosis results from alcohol's hepatotoxic effect. Poor nutritional intake compounds the problem of a malnourished liver in most adults. Postnecrotic cirrhosis usually occurs after acute viral hepatitis, which may result from blood transfusions. It is seen after exposure to industrial or chemical hepatotoxins (e.g., carbon tetrachloride, arsenic, and phosphorus). Biliary cirrhosis results from chronic biliary obstruction and inflammation. Cardiac cirrhosis is associated with prolonged hepatic venous congestion. Cirrhosis often develops as an idiopathic process.

Incidence/Prevalence

Cirrhosis may develop at any age. Cirrhosis and chronic liver disease was the tenth leading cause of death in 1994, accounting for more than 25,500 deaths (Singh et al., 1995). Of all cases of cirrhosis, 10% to 30% are postnecrotic and 5% to 10% are primary biliary (Porth, 1994). More than 65% of all cases of cirrhosis are alcohol-related, but cirrhosis occurs in only approximately 25% of alcoholics (Huether et al., 1996). Laënnec's (alcoholic) cirrhosis is the most common form of cirrhosis in industrialized countries. Laënnec's cirrhosis is more common in men than in women.

TRANSCULTURAL CONSIDERATIONS

 Mortality from cirrhosis in the United States is higher in non-Caucasians (Huether et al., 1996). The cause is unknown.

Collaborative Management

■ Assessment

➤ *History*

The nurse obtains historical data from clients with suspected cirrhosis, including age, sex, race, and employment history, especially exposure to harmful chemical toxins. The nurse determines whether there is a history of alcoholism in the family. The client is asked to describe his or her alcohol intake, including the amount consumed during what period of time. The nurse also asks the client about previous medical conditions, such as acute viral hepatitis, biliary tract disorders, viral infections, recent blood transfusions, and a history of heart failure or respiratory disorders.

➤ Physical Assessment/Clinical Manifestations

Because cirrhosis has an insidious onset, many of the early signs and symptoms are vague and nonspecific. The client may report

- Generalized weakness
- Weight loss
- Gastrointestinal symptoms (loss of appetite, early morning nausea and vomiting, dyspepsia, flatulence, and changes in bowel habits, with constipation and bouts of diarrhea)

The client may also report abdominal pain and liver tenderness, but these symptoms are often ignored by the client.

Hepatic function abnormalities are often detected when a physical examination or laboratory tests are completed for an unrelated illness or problem. The development of late signs of advanced cirrhosis may impel the client to seek medical treatment. GI bleeding, jaundice, ascites, and spontaneous bruising indicate deteriorating hepatic function and represent complications of cirrhosis.

The nurse thoroughly assesses the client with liver dysfunction or hepatic failure, because these disease processes affect every body system (Fig. 61–1). The clinical picture and course vary from client to client, depending on the severity of hepatic failure. When the nurse begins the assessment, an inspection may reveal

- Obvious yellowing of the skin (jaundice) and of the sclerae (icterus)
- Dry skin
- Rashes
- Purpuric lesions, such as petechiae (manifested as round, pinpoint red-purple lesions) or ecchymosis (large purple, blue, or yellow bruises)

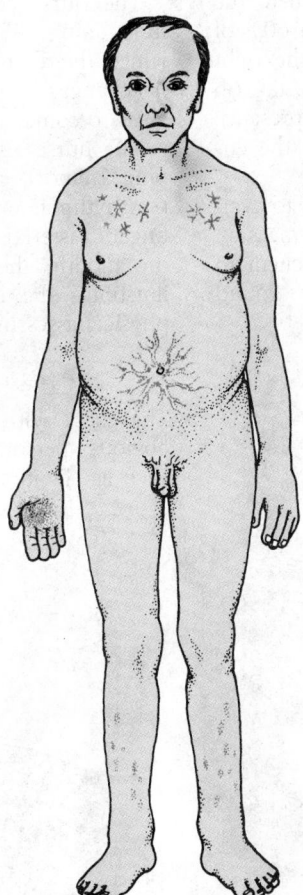

NEUROLOGIC FINDINGS
Asterixis
Paresthesias of feet
Peripheral nerve degeneration
Portal-systemic encephalopathy
Reversal of sleep-wake pattern
Sensory disturbances

GASTROINTESTINAL (GI) FINDINGS
Abdominal pain
Anorexia
Ascites
Clay-colored stools
Diarrhea
Esophageal varices
Fetor hepaticus
Gallstones
Gastritis
GI bleeding
Hemorrhoidal varices
Hepatomegaly
Hiatal hernia
Hypersplenism
Malnutrition
Nausea
Small nodular liver
Vomiting

RENAL FINDINGS
Hepatorenal syndrome
Increased urine bilirubin

ENDOCRINE FINDINGS
Increased aldosterone
Increased antidiuretic hormone
Increased circulating estrogens
Increased glucocorticoids
Gynecomastia

IMMUNE SYSTEM DISTURBANCES
Increased susceptibility to infection
Leukopenia

CARDIOVASCULAR FINDINGS
Cardiac arrhythmias
Development of collateral circulation
Fatigue
Hyperkinetic circulation
Peripheral edema
Portal hypertension
Spider angiomas

PULMONARY FINDINGS
Dyspnea
Hydrothorax
Hyperventilation
Hypoxemia

HEMATOLOGIC FINDINGS
Anemia
Disseminated intravascular coagulation
Impaired coagulation
Splenomegaly
Thrombocytopenia

DERMATOLOGIC FINDINGS
Axillary and pubic hair changes
Caput medusae
Ecchymosis
Increased skin pigmentation
Jaundice
Palmar erythema
Pruritus
Spider angiomas

FLUID AND ELECTROLYTE DISTURBANCES
Ascites
Decreased effective blood volume
Dilutional hyponatremia or hypernatremia
Hypocalcemia
Hypokalemia
Peripheral edema
Water retention

Figure 61–1. The clinical picture of a client with liver dysfunction. Signs and symptoms vary according to the progression of the disease. Early signs and symptoms are noted in color.

- Warm and bright-red palms of the hands (palmar erythema)
- Vascular lesions with a red center and radiating branches, known as "spider angiomas" (telangiectasias, spider nevi, or vascular spiders), occurring on the nose, the cheeks, the upper thorax, and the shoulders

The nurse also inspects the extremities and the sacrum for peripheral, dependent edema.

Abdominal Assessment. The nurse may readily detect *massive* ascites as a distended abdomen with bulging flanks. The umbilicus may protrude, and dilated abdominal veins, or caput medusae, may radiate from the umbilicus. Ascites can cause physical problems; for example, orthopnea and dyspnea from increased abdominal distention can interfere with lung expansion. The client may have difficulty maintaining an erect body posture, and problems with balance may affect walking. The nurse inspects and palpates for the presence of inguinal or umbilical hernias, which are likely to develop in clients with ascites because of increased intra-abdominal pressure.

Minimal ascites is often more difficult to detect. Advanced assessment techniques, such as the percussion test for shifting dullness and the presence of a fluid wave, may be performed.

When performing an assessment of the abdomen, the nurse keeps in mind that hepatomegaly occurs in 60% of all cases of early cirrhosis. The nurse palpates the right upper quadrant for an enlarged liver below the costal (rib cage) border. The nurse may also ascertain the presence of hepatomegaly by percussing for dullness over the enlarged liver.

The nurse takes abdominal girth measurements to evaluate the progression of ascites (Fig. 61–2). To measure the client's abdominal girth, the nurse asks the client to lie flat, and then the nurse pulls a tape measure around the largest diameter of the client's abdomen. The girth is measured at the end of exhalation. The nurse marks the client's abdominal skin and flanks to ensure that the tape measure placement is the same on subsequent readings.

Other Physical Assessment. The nurse assesses nasogastric (NG) tube drainage (if present), vomitus, and stool for the presence of blood. This may be indicated by frank blood in the excrement or by a positive result of an *o*-toluidine test for occult blood content (guaiac, Hema-Check). Gastritis, stomach ulceration, or oozing esophageal varices may be responsible for the presence of blood (melena).

The nurse may note fetor hepaticus, the distinctive breath odor of chronic liver disease and portal-systemic encephalopathy (PSE). It is characterized by a fruity or musty odor. Fetor hepaticus results from the damaged liver's inability to metabolize and detoxify mercaptan, which is produced by bacterial degradation of methionine, a sulfurous amino acid.

Amenorrhea may occur in women, and men may exhibit testicular atrophy, gynecomastia (enlarged breasts), and impotence as a result of inactive hormones. Clients with problems of the hematologic system caused by hepatic failure may have bruising, petechiae, and an enlarged spleen.

The nurse continually assesses the clients' neurologic functioning. PSE is manifested by neurologic changes, which the alert nurse should recognize. These often subtle changes in mentation and personality frequently progress to coma, a late complication of PSE.

The nurse also assesses for asterixis (liver flap or flapping tremor), a coarse tremor characterized by rapid, nonrhythmic extensions and flexions in the wrists and fingers. Asterixis also appears in the ankles, the corners of the mouth, the eyelids, and the tongue. Figure 61–3 illustrates the technique used to elicit asterixis during physical assessment.

➤ Psychosocial Assessment

The client with hepatic cirrhosis may undergo subtle or obvious personality, cognitive, and behavior changes, such as agitation and belligerence. He or she may exhibit

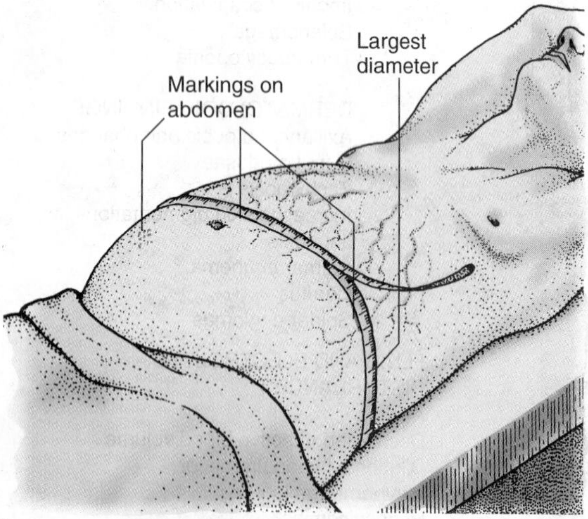

Figure 61–2. How to measure abdominal girth. With the client supine, the nurse brings the tape measure around the client and takes a measurement at the level of the umbilicus. Before removing the tape, the nurse marks the client's abdomen along the sides of the tape on the client's flanks (sides) and midline to ensure that later measurements are taken in the same place.

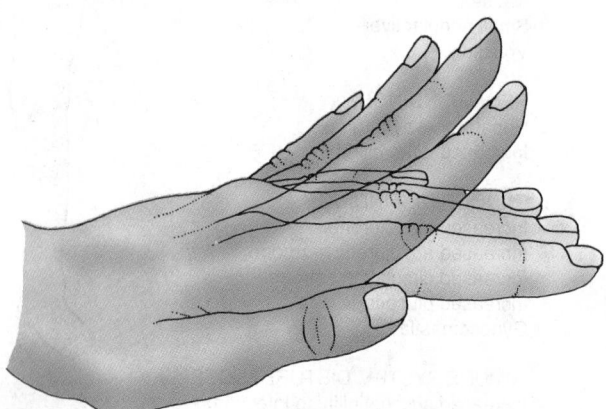

Figure 61–3. To elicit asterixis (flapping tremor), have the client extend the arm, dorsiflex the wrist, and extend the fingers. Observe for rapid, nonrhythmic extensions and flexions.

signs of emotional lability, euphoria, or depression, or he or she may experience sleep pattern disturbances. The nurse performs a psychosocial assessment to identify needs and help guide client care.

For clients with alcohol-induced cirrhosis who do not adhere to treatment plans, repeated hospitalizations are common. The nurse assesses the impact of the hospitalizations on the client's lifestyle and self-esteem. The nurse asks the client about financial capabilities to help determine whether referrals are needed for assistance.

➤ *Laboratory Assessment*

Characteristic abnormalities are common in laboratory studies of clients with liver disease (Table 61–4).

Liver enzyme levels are elevated. Serum levels of aspartate aminotransferase (AST), previously called serum glutamic-oxaloacetic transaminase (SGOT); alanine aminotransferase (ALT), previously called serum glutamic-pyruvic transaminase (SGPT); and lactate dehydrogenase (LDH) are elevated because these substances are released into the blood with the destruction of hepatic cells. Alkaline phosphatase levels are sensitive to mild extrahepatic or intrahepatic biliary obstruction and are therefore increased in clients with cirrhosis.

Total serum bilirubin levels also rise. Indirect bilirubin levels rise in clients with cirrhosis because of the failing liver's inability to conjugate bilirubin. Therefore, bilirubin is present in the urine (urobilinogen) in increased amounts. Fecal urobilinogen concentration is decreased in clients with biliary tract obstruction, which occurs in biliary cirrhosis.

Total serum protein and albumin levels are decreased in clients with severe or chronic liver disease as a result of decreased synthesis by the liver. Serum levels of globulins (alpha, beta, and gamma) are elevated because of the liver's increased synthesis of globulins by the reticuloendothelial system, indicating an immune response to hepatic disease.

Prothrombin time (PT) is prolonged because the liver has decreased synthesis of prothrombin, reflecting hepatocellular or obstructive biliary tract disease. Anemia may be reflected by altered complete blood count (CBC), with decreased hemoglobin and hematocrit values. The white blood cell (WBC) count may also be decreased. Increased toxins in the blood lead to premature cell death. Ammonia levels are elevated in the presence of advanced liver disease and PSE because conversion of ammonia to urea for excretion is decreased.

➤ *Radiographic Assessment*

Abdominal x-rays may reveal an enlarged liver, gas or cysts within the liver and the biliary tract, calcification of the liver, and massive ascites.

The upper gastrointestinal (GI) radiographic series is an examination of the esophagus, the stomach, and the small bowel. It may show the presence of esophageal varices or gastric or duodenal ulceration, all of which complicate the care of a client with cirrhosis.

The physician may order angiographic studies to identify actual arterial bleeding sites within the stomach. Computed tomography (CT) is helpful in detecting mini-

TABLE 61–4

Assessment of Abnormal Laboratory Findings in Liver Disease	
Abnormal Finding	**Significance**
Serum Enzymes	
Elevated serum aspartate aminotransferase (AST)*	• Hepatic cell destruction, hepatitis (most specific indicator)
Elevated serum alanine aminotransferase (ALT)**	• Hepatic cell destruction, hepatitis
Elevated lactate dehydrogenase (LDH)	• Hepatic cell destruction
Elevated serum alkaline phosphatase	• Obstructive jaundice, hepatic metastasis
Bilirubin	
Elevated serum total bilirubin	• Hepatic cell disease
Elevated serum direct conjugated bilirubin	• Hepatitis, liver metastasis
Elevated serum indirect unconjugated bilirubin	• Cirrhosis
Elevated urine bilirubin	• Hepatocellular obstruction, viral or toxic liver disease
Elevated urine urobilinogen	• Hepatic dysfunction
Decreased fecal urobilinogen	• Obstructive liver disease
Serum Proteins	
Increased serum total protein	• Acute liver disease
Decreased serum total protein	• Chronic liver disease
Decreased serum albumin	• Severe liver disease
Elevated serum globulin	• Immune response to liver disease
Other Tests	
Elevated serum ammonia	• Advanced liver disease or portal-systemic encephalopathy (PSE)
Prolonged prothrombin time (PT) or INR†	• Hepatic cell damage and synthesis of prothrombin

*Formerly serum glutamic-oxaloacetic transaminase (SGOT).
**Formerly serum glutamic-pyruvic transaminase (SGPT).
†INR, International Normalized Ratio.

mal ascites and provides information about the volume and character of fluid collections.

➤ *Other Diagnostic Assessment*

The physician may perform an esophagogastroduodenoscopy (EGD) to directly visualize the upper GI tract and to detect the presence of bleeding or oozing esophageal varices, stomach irritation and ulceration, or duodenal ulceration and bleeding. Injection sclerotherapy may be done during the endoscopic procedure to halt variceal bleeding as a palliative measure (see later under Planning and Implementation).

Radioisotope liver scans show abnormal hepatic thickening and identify liver masses. The physician uses liver biopsy as the definitive test for cirrhosis. Hepatic tissue biopsy reveals destruction and fibrosis of hepatic cells, indicative of cirrhosis.

 Analysis

> ➤ *Common Nursing Diagnoses and Collaborative Problems*

The most common nursing diagnosis for the client with cirrhosis is Fluid Volume Excess related to portal hypertension (causing ascites) and decreased serum colloid osmotic pressure.

The primary collaborative problems are

1. Potential for Hemorrhage
2. Potential for Portal Systemic Encephalopathy (PSE)

> ➤ *Additional Nursing Diagnoses and Collaborative Problems*

The client with cirrhosis may also exhibit one or more of the following nursing diagnoses:

■ Altered Nutrition: Less than Body Requirements related to anorexia; nausea; and faulty absorption, metabolism, and storage of nutrients and vitamins
■ Ineffective Breathing Pattern related to ascites and decreased diaphragmatic excursion and pressure on diaphragm from ascites
■ Pain related to abdominal pressure
■ Risk for Infection related to a decreased number of white blood cells
■ Risk for Impaired Skin Integrity related to pruritus secondary to jaundice, edema, and ascites
■ Ineffective Individual Coping related to chronic and potentially fatal disease process
■ Sexual Dysfunction related to altered hormonal function and decreased libido

Additional collaborative problems include

■ Potential for Drug Toxicity
■ Potential for Hypokalemia

 Planning and Implementation

Fluid Volume Excess

Planning: Expected Outcomes. The client is expected to experience a decrease in extravascular and intra-abdominal fluid.

Interventions. During the early stages of ascites, when fluid accumulations are minimal, interventions are aimed at preventing the accumulation of additional fluid and mobilizing the existing fluid collection. Nonsurgical treatment measures usually control ascites. If respiratory or abdominal functioning is compromised, however, surgical measures may be necessary.

Nonsurgical Management. Supportive measures to control abdominal ascites include diet therapy, drugs, paracentesis, and comfort measures. The nurse determines whether the client is adhering to the treatment plan.

Diet Therapy. The health care provider usually places the client with abdominal ascites on a low sodium diet as an initial means of controlling fluid accumulation in the abdominal cavity. The amount of daily sodium intake restriction typically varies from 500 mg to 2 g. In collaboration with the dietitian, the nurse explains the purpose of the diet and advises the client to eliminate table salt, salty foods (such as potato chips, pretzels, and snack foods), canned and frozen vegetables, and salted butter or margarine. (See Chapter 16 for a list of high sodium foods.) The absence of salt in low sodium diets is distasteful to most people, so the nurse suggests alternative flavoring additives, such as lemon, vinegar, parsley, oregano, and pepper. The nurse consults with the dietitian about additional flavoring substitutes and low sodium products and diet instructions.

The health care provider may limit the client's fluid intake if serum sodium levels fall. The kidneys retain sodium, and dilutional hyponatremia results, primarily from excessive fluid volume. Fluids, both intravenous (IV) and oral, are restricted to 1000 to 1500 mL/day in an effort to reverse the fluid overload and raise the serum sodium level. The nurse calculates the permitted amount of oral fluids on the basis of the ordered IV intake.

In general, clients with cirrhosis are malnourished and have multiple dietary deficiencies. Vitamin supplements, such as thiamine, folate, and multivitamin preparations, are added to the IV fluids because of the liver's inability to store vitamins. When IV fluid administration is discontinued, oral vitamins are given.

Drug Therapy. The health care provider usually orders a diuretic, such as spironolactone (Aldactone), to help reduce ascites. More potent diuretics are sometimes needed. The primary goal of diuretic therapy is to reduce fluid accumulation and to prevent cardiac and respiratory impairment.

The nurse monitors diuretic therapy by assessing intake and output, weighing the client daily, measuring the client's abdominal girth, and monitoring electrolyte levels. Serious electrolyte imbalances may accompany diuretic therapy. Hypokalemia and hyponatremia may occur as a result of treatment. (See Chapter 16 for discussion of electrolyte imbalances.) Depending on the diuretic selected, the physician may order an oral or IV potassium supplement.

Clients with cirrhosis often require antacid therapy for gastrointestinal symptoms. Because most antacids are high in sodium, the physician prescribes a low sodium antacid such as magaldrate (Riopan).

Paracentesis. If dietary restrictions and the administration of drugs fail to control ascites, abdominal paracentesis may be indicated (Chart 61–1). The procedure is performed at the bedside. The physician inserts a trocar catheter into the abdomen to remove and drain ascitic fluid in the client's peritoneal cavity.

Once a primary treatment modality for ascites, paracentesis is more commonly used as a diagnostic tool to examine the ascitic fluid. It is also used as a palliative

Nursing Care Highlight: Paracentesis

- Explain the procedure and answer the client's questions.
- Obtain vital signs, measure the client's abdominal girth, and weigh the client.
- Ask the client to void completely or drain the Foley catheter.
- Position the client. Assist him or her to sit in an upright position at the side of the bed with the feet propped on a stool. Support the client to maintain this position during the procedure.
- Monitor vital signs every 15 minutes during the procedure.
- Measure the drainage and record on the intake and output record.
- Describe the collected fluid (e.g., clear, straw-colored, hazy, or cloudy). Send specimens for laboratory analysis.
- After the physician removes the trocar catheter, apply a dressing to the puncture site. Assess for fluid leakage.
- Position the client in bed and maintain bed rest until vital signs are stable and return to baseline.

measure to relieve abdominal pressure, inasmuch as ascites may cause severe respiratory and abdominal distress. To relieve acute symptoms, the physician slowly drains the ascitic fluid (usually 1–3 L). The potential for hypovolemia with fluid volume deficit may occur with rapid fluid removal because these clients have adjusted to the excessive fluid volume in the abdomen. Rapid, drastic removal of the ascitic fluid leads to decreased abdominal pressure, which may contribute to vasodilation and shock. The nurse observes for impending signs of shock from fluid shifting during and immediately after the procedure.

Repeated paracentesis procedures are contraindicated because of the increased incidence of protein depletion, hypovolemia, and electrolyte imbalances (hypokalemic alkalosis), which can contribute to the development of portal-systemic encephalopathy in the client with cirrhosis.

Comfort Measures. Excessive ascitic fluid volume in the abdomen may cause the client to experience respiratory difficulty. Dyspnea may develop as a result of increased intra-abdominal pressure, which limits thoracic expansion and diaphragmatic excursion. The nurse or assistive nursing personnel elevates the head of the bed to at least 30 degrees or as high as the client wishes in an effort to minimize shortness of breath. The nurse or assistive nursing personnel can also encourage the client to sit in a chair. This upright position, with the client's feet elevated to discourage dependent ankle edema, often relieves dyspnea.

The nurse or assistive nursing personnel uses a standard upright bedside scale to weigh the client if the client can stand. Weighing the client on a bed scale necessitates that the client lies flat; this supine position can cause the client to feel increasingly short of breath and can increase anxiety.

Surgical Management. When medical management fails to control ascites, the physician may choose surgical intervention to divert ascites into the venous system by creating a shunt. This surgical bypass shunting procedure is associated with high mortality among clients with severe liver dysfunction. Therefore, it has limited use as an effective treatment for ascites. Clients with ascites are poor surgical risks because of their susceptibility to infection, as evidenced by

- A decreased WBC count
- Disseminated intravascular coagulation (DIC)
- Bleeding esophageal varices
- Anesthesia reactions

Preoperative Care. Because the client with cirrhosis has many underlying medical problems, an optimal physical state is desired before surgery is performed. Electrolyte imbalances are corrected, and abnormal coagulation is treated with the administration of fresh frozen plasma and vitamin K. Packed red blood cells are made available for transfusion because these clients have bleeding tendencies.

Operative Procedures. One of several types of shunts may be created.

Peritoneovenous Shunt. A peritoneovenous shunt, also known as a peritoneojugular or LeVeen shunt (Fig. 61–4), drains ascites through a one-way valve into a silicone rubber tube that terminates in the superior vena cava. A pressure gradient develops between the peritoneal cavity and the vena cava, facilitating the flow of ascitic fluid through the valve into the venous system. During inspiration, the diaphragm descends, increasing peritoneal fluid (ascites) pressure, and the pressure in the superior vena cava increases, creating the needed gradient. A pressure difference of greater than 3 cm H_2O is necessary to open the valve. The valve closes when the pressure is decreased.

After the shunt has been inserted, the client is expected to lose weight, show a decrease in abdominal girth, have increased urinary output, and exhibit an increased renal excretion of sodium. These clinical improvements result from restored adequate peripheral circulation.

Denver Shunt. The Denver shunt has a subcutaneous pump that can be manually compressed. It is often preferred for clients whose ascites contains large particles (common in neoplastic ascites). These particles can cause flow to become sluggish and result in a clotted shunt. Compressing the Denver shunt's pump helps irrigate the tubing to maintain patency.

Postoperative Care. The nurse provides the usual postoperative care for a client undergoing abdominal surgery (see Chap. 22). The nurse remains aware that the ascitic fluid is routed into the venous system. This excessive fluid results in vascular volume expansion and hemodilution. The nurse monitors the client's vital signs carefully; an increase in blood pressure reflects an increase in volume. If the client has a central venous or pulmonary artery catheter in place, the nurse determines whether pressure is elevated. Breath sounds are auscultated for the presence of crackles, indicating excessive lung fluid. The

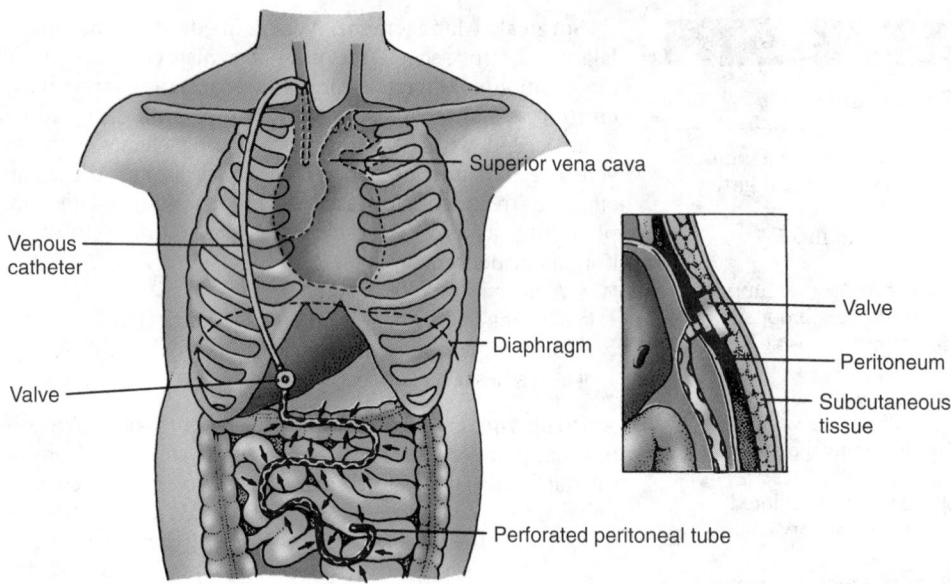

Superior vena cava

Venous catheter

Valve

Diaphragm

Valve

Peritoneum

Subcutaneous tissue

Perforated peritoneal tube

Figure 61-4. Peritoneovenous (LeVeen) shunting for treatment of ascites.

nurse administers a diuretic, such as furosemide, as ordered to rid the body of excessive fluid.

The nurse reports abnormal results of coagulation studies (prothrombin time [PT] and partial thromboplastin time [PTT]) to the physician. Reabsorption of clotting factors in ascitic fluid may further inhibit an already altered clotting mechanism and lead to disseminated intravascular coagulation and bleeding abnormalities.

The nurse or assistive nursing personnel measures the client's weight, abdominal girth, and urinary output each shift to determine the effectiveness of the shunting procedure.

Potential for Hemorrhage

Planning: Expected Outcomes. The client is expected not to hemorrhage.

Interventions. During the acute phase of bleeding, early interventions are based on identifying the source of bleeding and initiating treatment to halt it. Because massive esophageal bleeding can cause rapid blood loss, emergency interventions are initiated. If the client is a known alcoholic with a history of variceal bleeding, measures to treat the esophageal varices are initiated and valuable time is not wasted looking for another source of bleeding.

Nonsurgical Management. The health care team intervenes quickly to control bleeding by providing gastric intubation, balloon tamponade, drug therapy, replacement of blood products, injection sclerotherapy, or transjugular intrahepatic portal-systemic shunt (TIPS). The client is managed in the critical care unit. After the acute bleeding episode has been controlled, the client may require surgical intervention to decrease portal hypertension, thereby decreasing the risk of further variceal bleeding.

Gastric Intubation. Early in the hospitalization, the client's reports of hematemesis should be investigated. The physician usually inserts an 18-gauge Salem sump tube and lavages the stomach until the fluid returned is clear.

The introduction of saline or water lavage may be used to achieve vasoconstriction of the bleeding gastric ulceration or varices. The physician may add norepinephrine (Levophed) to the solution to produce further constriction.

If the bleeding site has been identified by endoscopy as a gastric ulcer, the physician initiates medical treatment with drug therapy (antacids and histamine receptor antagonists) and blood product replacement. If bleeding continues from the ulcer, surgical intervention is necessary.

Esophagogastric Balloon Tamponade. If the physician suspects that hematemesis has occurred because of bleeding esophageal varices, he or she inserts an esophagogastric tamponade tube. Bleeding varices are a medical emergency necessitating immediate intervention. The primary nursing intervention is maintenance of a patent airway. Vomiting and the accumulation of blood in the oropharynx may result in aspiration, occlusion of the airway, and respiratory compromise. The nurse attempts to keep the client's oropharynx clear by suctioning secretions, turning the client's head, and keeping the head of the bed elevated during vomiting episodes to prevent aspiration.

Types of Esophagogastric Tubes. The classic method of treating bleeding esophageal varices is by compressing the bleeding vessels with a Sengstaken-Blakemore tube (Blakemore tube). This tube has two balloons (Fig. 61-5). When inflated, the large esophageal balloon compresses the esophagus. The smaller gastric balloon helps anchor the tube and exerts pressure against bleeding varices in the distal esophagus and the cardia of the stomach. A third lumen terminates in the stomach and is connected to suction, allowing aspiration of gastric contents and blood. A Salem sump tube is used in conjunction with the Sengstaken-Blakemore tube and is placed in the proximal esophagus to enable clearing of collected esophageal secretions, saliva, and blood.

Another esophagogastric balloon tube often used is the Minnesota tube (see Fig. 61-5). Like the Sengstaken-Blakemore tube, the Minnesota tube has an additional

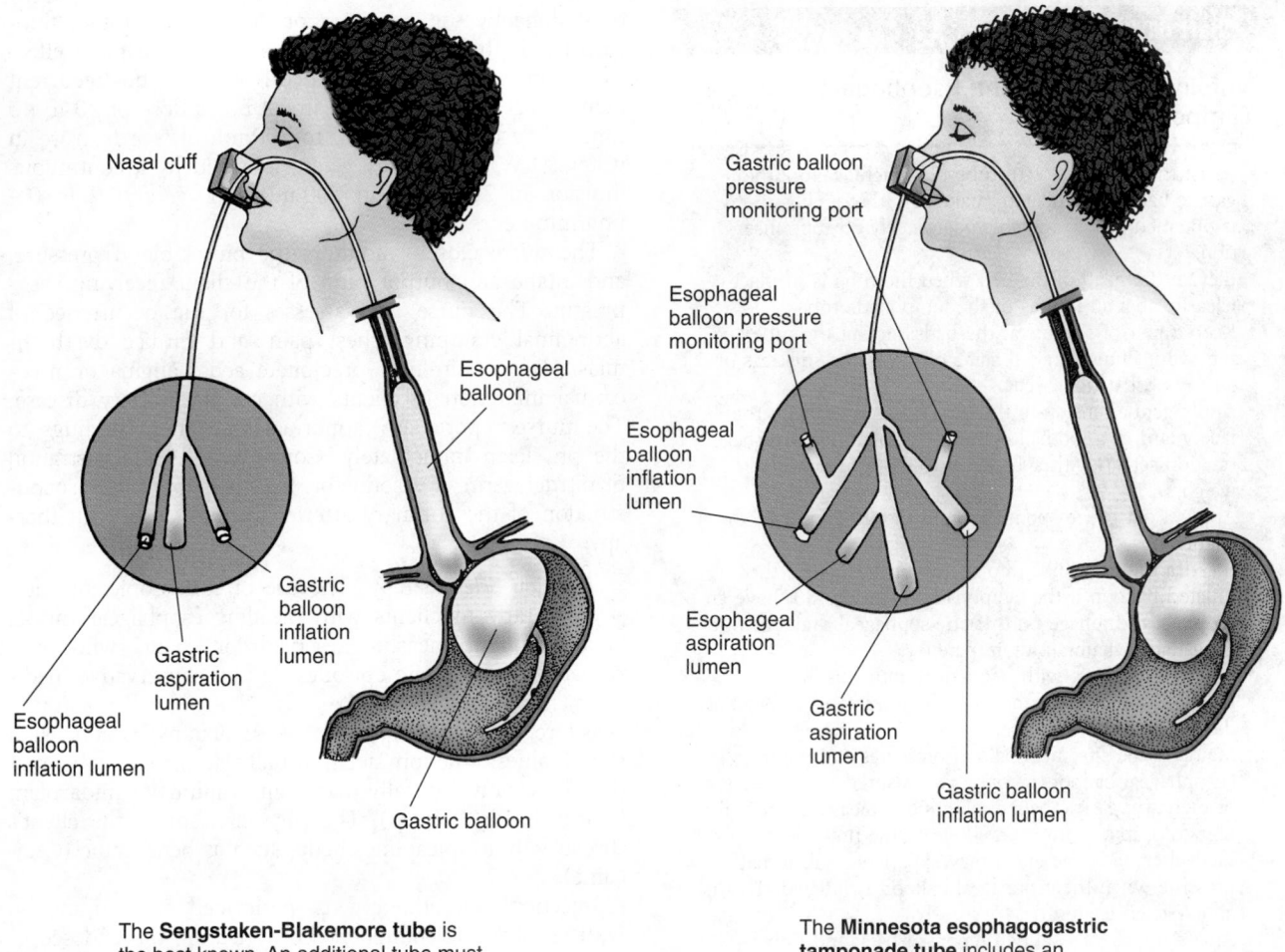

The **Sengstaken-Blakemore tube** is the best known. An additional tube must be placed in the proximal esophagus.

The **Minnesota esophagogastric tamponade tube** includes an esophageal aspiration lumen.

Figure 61–5. A comparison of esophageal tamponade tubes.

lumen (port), which is above the esophageal balloon to suction esophageal secretions. This eliminates the necessity for an additional tube, such as the Salem sump tube.

Insertion of an Esophagogastric Tube. Before the physician inserts the tamponade tube, the nurse inspects it and inflates and deflates the balloons to check for integrity and leaks. Each lumen is identified and labeled to prevent errors in adding or removing pressure and air volume.

The physician usually anesthetizes the client's nose and oropharynx, introduces the tube through the nares, and gently inserts it into the stomach. After the tube placement is verified, the stomach is aspirated and irrigated. The gastric balloon is inflated with up to 300 mL of air. The nurse assists the physician in securing the tube and applying traction, which provides additional tamponading pressure. This is accomplished by taping the tube to the face guard of a football helmet or by securing it to an overbed traction apparatus and applying a 1-pound (0.45-kg) traction weight.

Care of the Client with an Esophagogastric Tube. Inflation of the esophageal balloon is measured with a sphygmomanometer. Pressure should be maintained between 20 and 25 mmHg. The nurse periodically checks the bal-

loon pressures and volumes to prevent loss of pressure (with further bleeding or erosion) or rupture of the esophagus caused by overinflation (Chart 61–2). The esophagogastric balloon is usually removed after 48 hours. The nurse attaches the esophageal and gastric drainage lumina to low intermittent suction and monitors the amount and type of drainage.

Placement of the tamponade tube should halt variceal bleeding. After bleeding is controlled, the traction is released and the esophageal pressure is gradually decreased. The gastric balloon is deflated, and the tube is removed. Another tube should be kept at the bedside for potential reinsertion if bleeding recurs.

The nurse and assistive nursing personnel should be alert for sudden respiratory compromise with acute distress caused by airway obstruction from upward displacement of the esophageal balloon. A pair of scissors is *always* kept at the bedside. If the tube becomes dislodged, the nurse cuts both balloon ports to rapidly deflate the balloon and quickly removes the tube.

Blood Transfusions. Massive hemorrhage necessitates replacement by blood products. Blood is drawn to identify the client's blood type. Until the blood is available, the

---

Chart 61–2

Nursing Care Highlight: Esophageal Tamponade Tubes

- Assist the physician with tube placement. Before the gastric balloon is inflated, make sure that a chest x-ray is obtained and is available *immediately* on tube insertion.
- Elevate the head of the bed when the tube is in place.
- Clearly label all lumina of the tamponade tube.
- Keep a pair of scissors at the bedside. Cut the tube and remove it immediately if signs of respiratory distress or airway obstruction occur.
- Apply gentle tension to the tube by securing it to the face guard of a football helmet or applying an overhead traction set-up with a 1-pound (0.45-kg) traction weight.
- Apply a cut gauze sponge around the tube under the client's nose.
- Insert a drainage tube into the esophagus above the inflated balloon if the tamponade tube does not have an esophageal drainage port. If an esophageal drainage port is available, maintain drain patency.
- Provide the client with frequent mouth care.
- Restrain the client's hands loosely *if necessary* to prevent dislodgement of the tube.
- Maintain the specified balloon pressures and volumes. (Esophageal balloon pressure is measured in millimeters of mercury; gastric balloon volume is measured in milliliters or cubic centimeters.) Release the pressure at specified intervals. (The client may experience substernal pressure when the esophageal balloon is inflated. This is an expected feeling.)
- Assess the client's sudden report of back and upper abdominal pain. Monitor vital signs for a drop in blood pressure and an increase in the heart rate. Report these signs immediately.

---

nurse administers large crystalloid (IV fluids) or colloid (plasma) volumes, as ordered, into large-bore IV access routes to maintain blood pressure.

The nurse administers packed red blood cells and fresh frozen plasma (per physician order and agency policy) to replace blood volume and clotting factors. The physician and the nurse monitor trends in hemoglobin and hematocrit levels, and additional blood products are transfused as indicated.

Drug Therapy. The physician may use a vasoconstrictor, such as vasopressin (Pitressin), to temporarily control hemorrhage by lowering pressure within the portal blood flow system. This drug causes contraction of smooth muscle in the vascular bed. By constricting preportal splanchnic arterioles, blood flow is decreased to the abdominal organs, which reduces portal pressure and portal blood flow.

Vasopressin is administered by infusion pump intravenously or through a catheter placed in the superior mesenteric artery. The IV route is indicated initially because it allows easy, rapid access. The insertion of a superior mesenteric artery catheter is an invasive proce-

dure done by the physician or radiologist through fluoroscopy. Both infusion methods have demonstrated effective short-term control of variceal bleeding, but recurrent hemorrhage is common. An initial bolus dose of 20 to 40 units of vasopressin in 100 to 200 mL of 5% dextrose in water (D_5W) is typically given, followed by a continuous infusion of 200 units in 500 mL of D_5W at 0.2 to 0.4 unit/minute.

The nurse closely monitors the pulse, blood pressure, and intake and output ratio of the client receiving vasopressin. The nurse also assesses for the occurrence of abdominal cramping, chest pain, and cardiac dysrhythmias. Vasopressin may precipitate acute angina or myocardial infarction in clients with coronary artery disease. The nurse reports any abnormal assessment findings to the physician immediately. Concurrent IV administration of nitroglycerin, a vasodilator, may help prevent vasoconstriction of the coronary arteries during vasopressin therapy.

Injection Sclerotherapy. The use of endoscopic injection sclerotherapy in clients with bleeding esophageal varices is a treatment measure reserved for clients who have repeated hemorrhagic episodes despite conservative medical management.

Before the endoscopy, the nurse obtains baseline vital signs values. The physician usually administers the first dose of sedative, usually diazepam (Valium) or midazolam hydrochloride (Versed). The physician sprays the client's throat with a topical anesthetic, such as benzocaine (Cetacaine).

Injection sclerotherapy is performed in conjunction with esophagogastroduodenoscopy. During the endoscopic examination, the physician introduces a sclerosing agent, or sclerosant (such as morrhuate sodium, sodium tetradecyl sulfate, and ethanolamine oleate), through a flexible injector (Fig. 61–6).

Bleeding from the varices should stop within 2 to 5 minutes. If it continues, the physician makes a second injection attempt below the bleeding site. Prophylactic injection sclerotherapy may be done on other distended, nonbleeding varices. Because the procedure is usually done during an acute bleeding episode, the nurse or assistive nursing personnel closely monitors the client's vital signs during this hour-long procedure, which is done at the bedside or in an endoscopy clinic.

The client may report noncardiac chest discomfort, which is relieved by analgesia, for 24 to 72 hours after the injection. The nurse assesses the complaint of chest pain and administers pain medication. Esophageal perforation and ulceration are other complications of the treatment, and these cause severe chest pain. The nurse immediately reports acute changes to the physician.

Because aspiration may also occur and cause pneumonia and pleural effusion, the nurse assesses lung sounds for decreased aeration and adventitious sounds. After injection sclerotherapy, caution is necessary when nasogastric (NG) tubes are used and inserted. Some physicians prefer not to reinsert NG tubes, to decrease the risk of injury to the sclerosed esophagus.

Endoscopic Ligation. A fairly new method used to treat bleeding esophageal varices is endoscopic variceal ligation.

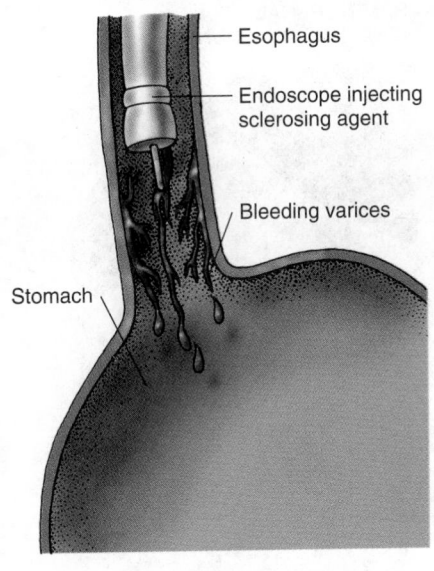

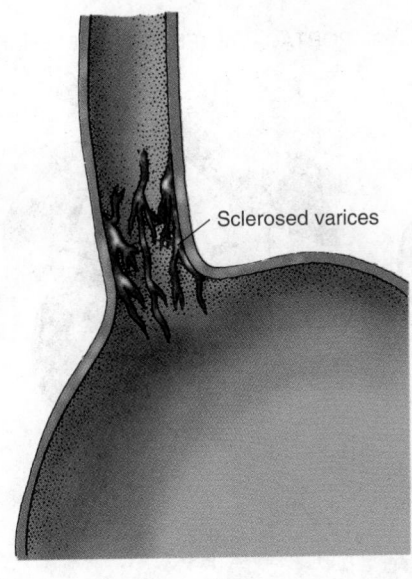

Figure 61-6. Injection sclerotherapy.

Before

After

This procedure uses bands to ligate the bleeding varices and is now considered the treatment of choice by many physicians (Laine et al., 1996; Saeed, 1996).

Transjugular Intrahepatic Portal-Systemic Shunt. Insertion of a transjugular intrahepatic portal-systemic shunt (TIPS) is a nonsurgical procedure that is performed in the radiology department in a special procedures room or an interventional radiology suite. This procedure is usually reserved for clients who have not responded to any other nonsurgical management. With the client under IV conscious sedation, the physician implants a shunt, passed through a catheter, between the portal vein and the hepatic vein. This technique reduces portal venous pressures and therefore controls bleeding.

Before the procedure, the physician obtains informed consent from the client. The client should know that the procedure is painful, even though droperidol (Inapsine), meperidine hydrochloride (Demerol), or midazolam hydrochloride (Versed) is given in high doses for IV conscious sedation.

Despite the potential for complications, such as stenosis and thrombosis, TIPS is an alternative for clients awaiting liver transplantation or for those who are unable to have surgery (Becker et al., 1996). After TIPS, the client can usually go home within 2 to 4 days instead of the 10 to 14 days after a surgical procedure.

Surgical Management. Portal-systemic shunts are considered a last-resort intervention for clients with portal hypertension and esophageal varices. The high mortality rate associated with shunting procedures occurs because clients with end-stage liver disease have coagulation abnormalities, are susceptible to infection, tolerate anesthesia poorly, and have ascites. In recent years, liver transplantation has also been commonly performed for end-stage cirrhosis (see discussion of transplantation later in chapter).

Surgical bypass shunting procedures decrease portal hypertension by diverting a portion of the portal vein blood flow from the liver. The goal is to decrease the incidence of variceal bleeding while maintaining sufficient blood flow to the liver, preserving hepatocellular function.

Preoperative Care. The client with hepatic cirrhosis has multiple underlying problems. The client with esophageal bleeding must be transfused before surgery with packed red blood cells and fresh frozen plasma to correct clotting deficiencies.

Operative Procedures. The shunting procedures most commonly used are the portacaval and splenorenal shunts (Fig. 61-7).

The portacaval shunt diverts the portal venous blood flow into the inferior vena cava to decrease portal pressure. The portal vein is anastomosed to the inferior vena cava. Splenorenal shunting involves splenectomy with the anastomosis of the splenic vein and the left renal vein. There are several variations of these procedures. With the *mesocaval* shunt, the superior mesenteric vein is anastomosed to the inferior vena cava.

Portal-systemic decompression shunting procedures are not performed as frequently as they once were because of the occurrence of complications such as bleeding, portal-systemic encephalopathy (PSE), shunt thrombosis, and infection. A shunt may decrease the occurrence of variceal bleeding, but the survival time of the client is usually not prolonged.

Postoperative Care. The client is usually admitted to the critical care unit immediately after surgery. The extent of care needed depends on the client's preoperative health status, extent of hepatic disease, and magnitude of the procedure.

The nurse provides constant observation and careful monitoring, including frequent assessment of vital signs, central venous pressure, and pulmonary artery pressure (if indicated) and hourly intake and urinary output measurements. These clients are usually maintained on me-

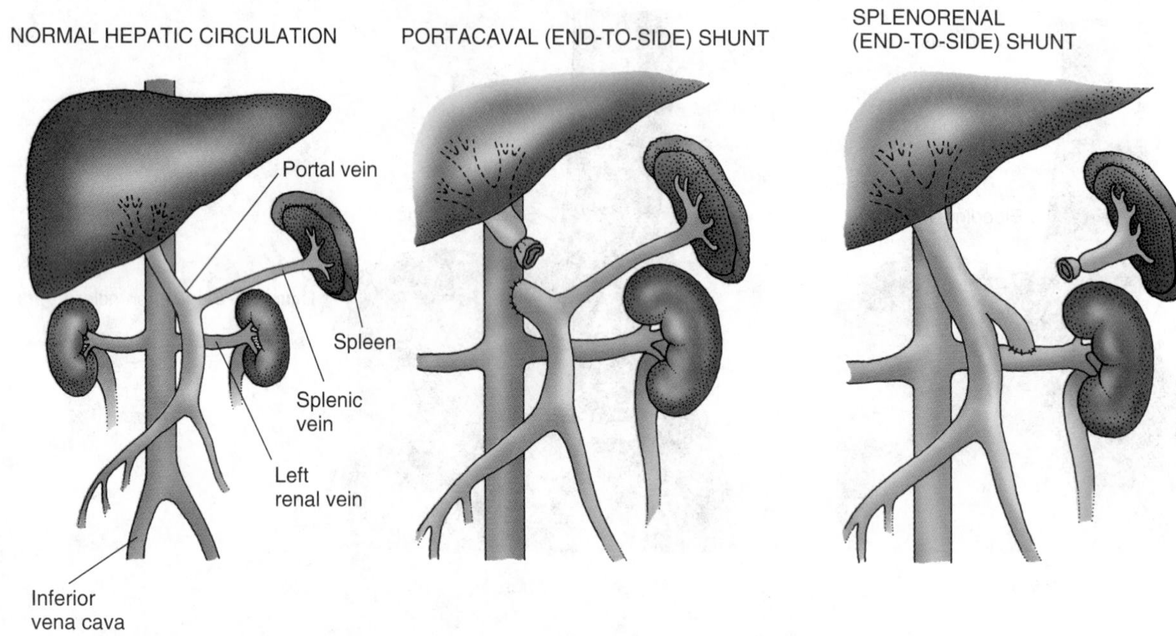

NORMAL HEPATIC CIRCULATION   PORTACAVAL (END-TO-SIDE) SHUNT   SPLENORENAL (END-TO-SIDE) SHUNT

Figure 61–7. Surgical shunting diverts portal venous blood flow from the liver to decrease portal and esophageal pressure.

chanical ventilation for several days. The nurse, in collaboration with the physician and the respiratory therapist, monitors respiratory status, protects the client's artificial airway (endotracheal tube), and checks the ventilator for correct settings. The usual postoperative care measures to prevent atelectasis and pneumonia are instituted.

During the postoperative period, the nurse exercises discretion in providing opioid analgesia for pain relief and sedation, although the intubated client has an increased need for sedatives. These drugs are contraindicated in clients with chronic hepatic failure, because most drugs are metabolized in the liver.

After these shunting procedures, clients are susceptible to oliguria. They are often hypovolemic as a result of
- Uncompensated blood loss
- Excessive fluid loss from prolonged exposure of the peritoneal space during surgery, resulting in fluid evaporation
- The recurrence of ascites
- Preoperative fluid restriction
- Diuretic therapy

The nurse administers the ordered fluid volume and assesses the effects of the volume by monitoring for increased blood pressure, decreased heart rate, and increased urinary output. The nurse reports excessive increases in the central venous pressure or pulmonary artery pressure after fluid challenge. Volume replacement may be given as fresh frozen plasma (to correct postoperative coagulopathy), IV solution boluses, and packed red blood cells.

Recurrent esophageal variceal bleeding after a portal-systemic shunt is not uncommon and may indicate the return of elevated portal pressures caused by a thrombosed (clotted) shunt. A rapid reaccumulation of abdominal fluid may also suggest a failed shunt or excessive sodium administration. The physician may need to rein-

stitute diuretic therapy. The nurse continues to measure the client's abdominal girth and reports sudden girth increases to the physician.

The nurse should be alert for the development of post-shunt encephalopathy, because it occurs commonly in these clients (see care measures for portal systemic encephalopathy [PSE]).

These clients have increased nutritional requirements and are often given total parenteral nutrition (TPN) to provide the needed calories, vitamins, and minerals. The nurse also administers albumin intravenously several times per day to replace the albumin lost in ascites. (See Chapter 64 for care associated with TPN administration.)

Potential for Portal Systemic Encephalopathy

Planning: Expected Outcomes. The client is expected not to experience portal systemic encephalopathy.

Interventions. During the early stages of PSE in clients with hepatic cirrhosis, interventions are focused on decreasing ammonia formation in an effort to decrease progressive cerebral dysfunction. The diseased liver cannot convert ammonia to a less toxic form, and ammonia is carried by the circulatory system to the brain, in which high levels are toxic to normal cerebral function. The aim of PSE management is to halt this process.

Because ammonia is formed in the gastrointestinal (GI) tract by the action of bacteria on protein, nonsurgical treatment measures to decrease ammonia production include dietary limitations and drug therapy to reduce the bacterial breakdown. The nurse collaborates with the dietitian and the physician to plan and implement these treatment measures.

Diet Therapy. The client with cirrhosis has increased

nutritional requirements. The client needs high-carbohydrate, moderate-fat, and high-protein foods. When the client has elevated serum ammonia levels and exhibits the signs of PSE, however, the diet is often modified. The client's intake of dietary protein is typically limited in an effort to reduce the excessive breakdown of protein into ammonia by intestinal bacteria.

The client's diet usually includes low-protein foods as well as simple carbohydrates, such as fruit juice. As the client's mental status deteriorates, proteins may be totally eliminated from the diet. When PSE fluctuates among the four stages, the nurse avoids giving the client foods high in protein content, such as meat, fish, poultry, eggs, and dairy products.

Clients with cirrhosis often experience GI bleeding, resulting in the formation of increased amounts of ammonia as intestinal bacteria attempt to metabolize the blood cells. GI bleeding may precipitate hepatic coma (stage IV of PSE). These clients are maintained on nothing by mouth (NPO) status with a nasogastric tube or an esophageal tamponade tube, depending on the source of the bleeding. Nutritional maintenance with IV total parenteral nutrition is often necessary.

Drug Therapy. Several types of drugs can eliminate or reduce ammonia levels in the body.

Lactulose. The physician orders the administration of lactulose (Cephulac) to promote the excretion of ammonia in the stool. Lactulose, a disaccharide with high molecular weight, is a viscous, sticky, sweet-tasting liquid that the nurse administers either orally or by nasogastric tube. When giving the drug orally, the nurse dilutes the lactulose with fruit juice to help the client tolerate the sweet taste. Lactulose retention enemas are often necessary when the client cannot tolerate oral administration or when liquids are contraindicated in the upper GI tract.

Lactulose creates an acid environment in the bowel by keeping ammonia in its ionized state, resulting in a fall of the colon's pH from 7 to 5. This causes ammonia to leave the circulatory system and move into the colon, which reverses the normal passage of ammonia from the colon to the bloodstream. The acid environment also discourages the growth of bacteria. Lactulose draws water into the bowel because of its high osmotic gradient, producing a laxative effect and facilitating evacuation of ammonia from the bowel.

The desired effect of lactulose is two to three soft stools per day with an acid fecal pH. During the acute phase of PSE, lactulose is administered in a dosage of 20 to 30 g at 4-hour intervals until stools are achieved and then decreased to three or four times per day. As a retention enema, lactulose is given in a dosage of 200 g diluted in 1000 mL of water at 4- to 6-hour intervals.

The nurse or assistive nursing personnel closely observes for watery diarrheal stools, which may signify excessive lactulose administration. The client may complain of intestinal bloating and cramping. The nurse also monitors daily for decreasing ammonia levels, which would reflect a positive effect of drug therapy, and for hypokalemia and dehydration, which can result from numerous stools.

Neomycin Sulfate. Neomycin sulfate (Mycifradin Sulfate), a broad-spectrum antibiotic, is given to act as an intestinal antiseptic. It destroys the normal flora in the bowel, diminishing protein breakdown and decreasing the rate of ammonia production. Maintenance doses of neomycin are given orally, but it may also be administered as a retention enema.

Because constipation may lead to increased bacterial action on retained stool, with a resulting increase in ammonia levels, stool softeners should be included in the long-term treatment plan. The administration of medications that are potentially toxic to the liver, such as opioid analgesics, sedatives, and barbiturates, must be restricted.

Other Drugs. Because the client with portal systemic encephalopathy (PSE) exhibits progressive neurologic changes and is often confused, combative, uncooperative, or belligerent, the nurse may need to give sedatives to prevent the client from self-harm or harm of others. In such cases, the judicious use of drugs such as oxazepam (Serax) is warranted.

Levodopa (Dopar, Larodopa) has been used with some success in the treatment of chronic PSE. The use of levodopa (a precursor of dopamine and norepinephrine) is based on the theory that there are defective neurotransmitters in encephalopathy. Deficient dopamine and norepinephrine are replaced by false transmitters, the amine products from the breakdown of dietary protein. The pathway for normal transmission is provided by synthetic levodopa.

Neurologic Assessment. The nurse or assistive nursing personnel continually assesses the client for changes in level of consciousness and orientation. An individualized neurologic assessment is developed for each client; it includes the assessment of simple tasks, such as name writing, bilateral handgrasping, and performing serial subtractions and additions.

The nurse also continually assesses for the presence of asterixis (liver flap) and fetor hepaticus (liver breath). These signs suggest worsening encephalopathy.

 Continuing Care

If the client with hepatic cirrhosis survives life-threatening complications, he or she is usually discharged from the hospital after treatment measures have combated the acute medical problems. The client may be discharged to the home or to a long-term care facility. If the client is discharged to the home, a home health referral may be needed. These chronically ill clients are frequently readmitted, and continuing care is aimed at preventing rehospitalization. The client may benefit from hospice care. A case manager to coordinate interdisciplinary care is often utilized.

► Health Teaching

The client is discharged to the home setting with an individualized teaching plan (Chart 61-3) covering diet therapy, drug therapy, and alcohol abstinence.

Chart 61–3

Education Guide: Cirrhosis

Diet Therapy

- Consume a diet high in calories, protein, and vitamins, unless your health care provider has told you to avoid high-protein foods.
- If you have excessive fluid in the abdomen, follow the low-sodium diet prescribed for you.
- Eat small, frequent meals that are nutritionally well balanced.
- Include in your diet daily supplemental liquids, such as Ensure or Ensure Plus, and a multivitamin. Low-protein supplements are available if needed.

Drug Therapy

- Take the diuretics prescribed for you. If you experience weakness or cardiac irregularities, report these symptoms to your health care provider.
- Take the H_2-receptor antagonist prescribed for you to prevent gastrointestinal bleeding.
- Do *not* take any other medication unless specifically ordered by your health care provider.

Alcohol Abstinence

- Do not consume any alcohol.
- Seek support services for help.

Diet Therapy. In collaboration with the dietitian, the nurse provides strict dietary instructions. Most clients need a diet high in calories, protein, and vitamins. The dietitian plans meals and menus with the client's favorite foods and provides lists of foods high in caloric, protein, and vitamin content.

For some clients, certain food items need to be restricted. The client with ascites requires a diet low in sodium. The nurse advises the client to eat nutritious, well-balanced meals but to limit the amount of or totally eliminate sodium in the diet. The nurse prepares a list of foods high in sodium content, which should be eliminated in the diet. These foods include table salt, snack foods (potato chips, pretzels), canned and frozen vegetables, and salted margarine and butter. The client and family members are instructed to read food labels and to avoid purchasing foods with a high sodium content.

The client with portal-systemic encephalopathy must avoid high-protein foods at home in an effort to decrease the incidence of progressive neurologic dysfunction. The nurse and the dietitian instruct the client and the family or significant other to modify the diet by limiting the ingestion of high-protein foods, such as meat, fish, poultry, eggs, and dairy products. If the client's nutritional intake is decreased after discharge, multivitamin supplements and supplemental liquid feedings, such as Ensure, are usually needed.

Drug Therapy. The client is often discharged while receiving diuretics. The nurse provides written instruction and the health care provider's prescription for the di-

uretic. The nurse also supplies written information about signs and symptoms of potential electrolyte imbalances, such as hypokalemia, which may result from diuretic therapy. The client may need to take a potassium supplement.

If the client has had problems with bleeding from gastric ulcers, the physician prescribes antacids or an H_2-receptor antagonist agent, such as ranitidine hydrochloride (Zantac). The nurse provides written guidelines and administration schedules for all medications to be taken at home.

The nurse advises the client to avoid all over-the-counter medications and to consult the physician for follow-up medical care. The client is instructed to notify the physician immediately if any gastrointestinal bleeding is noted, so that reevaluation can be initiated quickly.

Alcohol Abstinence. One of the most important aspects of continuing care for the nurse to stress is the need for alcohol abstinence. Avoiding alcohol can

- Prevent further fibrosis of the liver from scarring
- Allow the liver to regenerate
- Prevent gastric and esophageal irritation
- Reduce the incidence of bleeding
- Prevent other life-threatening complications

➤ Home Care Management

The nurse, the client, and the family or significant other identify any physical adaptations needed to prepare the client's home for convalescence. The client's rest area should be close to a bathroom because diuretic therapy increases the frequency of urination. If the client has difficulty reaching the toilet, additional equipment, such as urinals, bedpans, and bedside commodes, are necessary. If the client has an altered mental status and has urinary incontinence, special adult-sized incontinence pads or briefs may be helpful.

For the client who has undergone surgical intervention, initial home activity may be limited. The client may be confined to one floor. It may be necessary to obtain a hospital bed for the client who has chronic hepatic failure as a result of long-term problems. If the client experiences shortness of breath from massive ascites, elevating the head of the bed and maintaining the client in a semi- to high-Fowler's position may help alleviate respiratory distress. Alternatively, a reclining chair with a foot elevator may be used.

➤ Health Care Resources

The client with chronic cirrhosis may require a home care nurse to assess the client's tolerance of dietary restrictions. The home care nurse can also monitor the effectiveness of drug therapy or the surgical shunt in controlling ascites. Individual and group therapy sessions may be arranged to assist the client in dealing with abstinence from alcohol. The nurse may refer the client and family to self-help groups, such as Alcoholics Anonymous and Al-Anon. The client may also desire spiritual support. Other possible resources include hospice and long-term care in a nursing home.

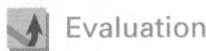 Evaluation

On the basis of the identified nursing diagnoses and collaborative problems, the nurse evaluates the care of the client with cirrhosis. Outcomes include that the client will

- Experience a decrease in extravascular and intra-abdominal fluid
- Not experience hemorrhage
- Not experience PSE
- Have quality of life

Hepatitis
Overview

Hepatitis is the widespread inflammation of liver cells. *Viral* hepatitis is the most prevalent type and can be acute or chronic. Viral hepatitis results from an infection caused by one of five major categories of viruses:

- Hepatitis A virus (HAV)
- Hepatitis B virus (HBV)
- Hepatitis C virus (non-A, non-B, or HCV)
- Hepatitis D virus (hepatitis delta virus, or HDV)
- Hepatitis E virus (HEV)

Hepatitis F and G have also been identified but are uncommon.

Liver injury with inflammation can also develop after exposure to a number of pharmacologic and chemical agents by inhalation, ingestion, or parenteral (IV) administration. *Toxic* and *drug-induced* hepatitis can result from exposure to hepatotoxins, such as industrial toxins, alcohol, and medications. Hepatitis may also occur as a secondary infection during the course of infections with other viruses, such as Epstein-Barr, herpes simplex, varicella-zoster, and cytomegalovirus.

Clients usually recover from hepatitis but may have residual liver damage. Mortality from hepatitis is relatively low, but severe hepatitis may be fatal.

Pathophysiology

After the liver has been exposed to causative agents, such as a virus, it becomes enlarged and congested with inflammatory cells, lymphocytes, and fluid, resulting in right upper quadrant pain and discomfort. As the disease process continues and progresses, the liver's normal lobular pattern becomes distorted, owing to widespread inflammation, necrosis, and hepatocellular regeneration. Pressure within the portal circulation increases because of the distortion, interfering with the blood flow into the hepatic lobules. Edema of the liver's bile channels results in intrahepatic obstructive jaundice.

Specific data on the pathogenesis of hepatitis A, C, D, and E are limited. Investigational evidence suggests that clinical manifestations of acute HBV inflammation are determined by an immunologic response of the host (client). Immune complex–mediated tissue damage may contribute to the extrahepatic manifestations of acute hepatitis B. Clinical responses include an urticarial rash (hives) and arthritic joint pain.

The recovery phase of hepatitis is marked by active phagocytosis and enzyme activity; damaged hepatic cells are removed, allowing for regeneration of the cells. Unless serious complications develop, most clients recover normal hepatic function after a viral hepatic insult. Regeneration usually occurs within 2 to 4 months.

Classification of Hepatitis
Viral Hepatitis

The five types of acute viral hepatitis vary by mode of transmission, manner of onset, and incubation periods (Table 61–5). These viruses are classified as enteral or parenteral, in reference to the mechanism of transmission.

Enteral forms, hepatitis A and E, are transmitted by the fecal-oral route. Parenteral forms, hepatitis B, C, and D, are transmitted via venous blood transfer or through intimate sexual contact. Vaccines to prevent hepatitis A and B are currently available.

HEPATITIS A. The causative agent of hepatitis A (HAV), formerly known as *infectious* hepatitis, is probably a ribonucleic acid (RNA) virus of the enterovirus family. HAV is characterized by a mild course similar to that of a typical viral syndrome and often goes unrecognized. It is spread by the fecal-oral route by the oral ingestion of fecal contaminants. Sources of infection include contaminated water, shellfish caught in contaminated water, and food contaminated by food handlers infected with HAV. The virus may also be spread by oral-anal sexual activity. The incubation period of hepatitis A is usually 15 to 50 days, with an average of 4 weeks (Benenson, 1995; Jackson & Rymer, 1994). The disease is usually not life-threatening.

HEPATITIS B. Hepatitis B (HBV), formerly known as *serum* hepatitis, is caused by a double-shelled particle containing deoxyribonucleic acid (DNA) composed of a core antigen (HBcAg), a surface antigen (HBsAg), and an independent protein (HBeAg) that circulates in the blood.

The primary mode of transmission of HBV is via the percutaneous and permucosal route by contamination with blood and serous fluid. Lower concentrations of HBV are also found in semen, vaginal fluid, and saliva. Although transmission can occur through bites, there are no documented cases of transmission through kissing. Hepatitis B may be spread through the following modes of transmission:

- Sexual contact (heterosexual and homosexual)
- Sharing needles
- Accidental needlesticks or injuries from sharp instruments (in health care personnel)
- Blood transfusion
- Hemodialysis
- Acupuncture, tattooing, ear or body piercing
- Perinatal (maternal-fetal)

The clinical course of hepatitis B may be varied. It may have an insidious onset with mild signs and symptoms, or it may result in serious complications such as fulminant hepatitis, chronic hepatitis, cirrhosis, and hepatocellular carcinoma. The incubation period is generally 45 to

TABLE 61–5

Differential Features of the Five Types of Viral Hepatitis*

Feature	Hepatitis A	Hepatitis B	Hepatitis C (Non-A, Non-B Hepatitis)	Delta Hepatitis	Hepatitis E
Synonyms	• Infectious hepatitis	• Serum hepatitis	• Post-transfusion		• Epidemic non-A, non-B hepatitis or enterically transmitted hepatitis
Diagnosis of acute disease	• Anti-HAV IgM in serum	• HBsAg in serum	• Anti-HCV	• Anti-HDV titer increase	• Anti-HEV
Incubation period	• 15–50 days	• 48–180 days	• 14–180 days	• 14–56 days	• 15–64 days
High-risk groups	• More common in young children and institutional settings	• All age groups affected, especially drug addicts, clients undergoing long-term hemodialysis, and heath care personnel	• All ages drug users; hemophilia patients	• Drug addicts	• Persons living in under-developed countries
Season	• Fall and early winter	• All year	• All year	• All year	• All year
Transmission	• Usually by oral-fecal route among persons living in close contact; ingestion of contaminated water or contaminated shellfish	• Usually by transfusion of blood and blood products or some other form of inoculation, especially parenteral drug abuse; sexual contact	• Primarily blood	• Coinfects with hepatitis B; nonpercutaneous, close personal contact	• Oral-fecal route; transmitted principally by contaminated water
Clinical findings	• Majority of type A infections mild and anicteric; symptoms similar to those of influenza • Fatigue, anorexia, low-grade fever, abdominal discomfort, arthralgias, rashes, enlarged tender liver, light stools, dark urine, jaundice	• Changes similar to those of hepatitis A • Tends to have more severe symptoms; sometimes necessitates hospitalization for extended periods	• Changes similar to those of hepatitis A	• Changes similar to those of hepatitis A, but symptoms often more severe than those in hepatitis A and hepatitis B	• Resembles hepatitis A

	Hepatitis A (HAV)	Hepatitis B (HBV)	Hepatitis C (HCV)	Hepatitis D (HDV)	Hepatitis E (HEV)
Elevated serum AST and ALT levels (early), hyperbilirubinemia, abnormal liver function test results	Yes				
Virus in feces	Yes	Not infectious	Not identified	Not identified	Possible
Virus in serum	During acute phase and incubation period—rare	HBsAg is in serum throughout the clinical course	Yes	Present during entire phase of hepatitis B	Yes
Nosocomial problem	No	Yes	Yes	Yes	No
Mortality	Less frequent	More frequent	Unknown	Increased	Unknown
Incidence of chronic active hepatitis as a complication	Low	Somewhat higher	Yes	Yes	No
Associated with post-transfusion hepatitis	No	Rarely (causes 5%–8% of cases)	Yes	No	No
Immune globulin (IG) (prophylaxis)	IG	HBIG or IG	No	None; recommended IG	None identified
Serologic test (specific antigen)	HA Ag	HBsAg, HB Ag	Not identified	HD Ag	None identified
Vaccine	Yes	Yes	No	Prevention of hepatitis B with vaccine prevents hepatitis D	No
Antibody	Anti-HAV	Anti-HB$_3$m, anti-HBc, anti-HBe	Anti-HCV	Anti-HD	Anti-HEV

*Anti-HAV, antibody to HAV; IgM, immunoglobulin M; HBsAg, hepatitis B surface antigen; anti-HCV, antibodies to HCV; anti-HDV, antibodies to HDV; anti-HEV, antibodies to HEV; AST, aspartate aminotransferase; ALT, alanine aminotransferase; HBIG, hepatitis B immune globulin; HA Ag, hepatitis A antigen; HB Ag, hepatitis B antigen; HD Ag, hepatitis D antigen; anti-HB$_3$m; anti-HBc; anti-HBe.

180 days, but hepatitis B commonly develops 60 to 90 days after exposure. Chronic HBV infection develops in about 1% to 10% of adult clients with acute HBV infection (Benenson, 1995; Hepatitis Branch, 1997).

HEPATITIS C. The causative virus of hepatitis C (HCV) is an enveloped, single-stranded RNA virus. It is transmitted through percutaneous exposure to blood and plasma. The highest incidence (70% to 90%) occurs in drug users (injecting) and in individuals with hemophilia. The incubation period is 14 to 180 days, with the average incubation period being 42 to 63 days. (Benenson, 1995; Jackson & Rymer, 1994) More than 50% of infected individuals develop chronic hepatitis (Kowdley, 1996).

HEPATITIS D. Hepatitis D (delta hepatitis, or HDV) is caused by a defective RNA virus that needs the helper function of HBV. HDV coinfects with HBV and needs its presence for viral replication. Hepatitis D can coinfect a client with HBV or can occur as a superinfection in a client with chronic HBV. Superinfection usually develops into chronic HDV. The incubation period is approximately 14 to 56 days. The disease is transmitted primarily by parenteral routes, like HBV (Benenson, 1995; Hepatitis Branch, 1997).

TRANSCULTURAL CONSIDERATIONS

In the United States, Canada, and northern Europe, hepatitis D (delta infection) is most prevalent in people exposed to blood and blood products (e.g., drug addicts and hemophiliacs).

The prevalence of hepatitis D usually corresponds to the prevalence of hepatitis B. Southern Italy, Africa, South America, and parts of Russia and Romania have a high prevalence, whereas northern Italy, Spain, Turkey, and Egypt have a moderate prevalence (Benenson, 1995; Hepatitis Branch, 1997).

HEPATITIS E. The hepatitis E virus (HEV) was originally identified by its association with water-borne epidemics of hepatitis in the Indian subcontinent and has since occurred in epidemics in Asia, Africa, and Mexico. In the United States, hepatitis E has been found only in travelers returning from these endemic areas. The nonenveloped, single-stranded RNA virus is transmitted via the fecal-oral route, and the clinical course resembles that of hepatitis A. HEV has an incubation period of 15 to 64 days. There is no evidence of a chronic form of HEV (Benenson, 1995).

TRANSCULTURAL CONSIDERATIONS

Hepatitis E occurs most frequently in developing countries such as India, parts of Africa, and Mexico (Porth, 1994). The attack rate is highest in young adults (Benenson, 1995).

Toxic and Drug-Induced (Chemical Hepatitis)

Two major types of toxic hepatitis have been recognized.

DIRECT TOXIC HEPATITIS. Direct toxic hepatitis (DTH) results in necrosis and fatty infiltration of the liver. Agents causing toxic hepatitis are generally systemic poisons or are converted in the liver to toxic metabolites. People with repeated, regular exposure to an offending agent, such as alcohol (alcoholic hepatitis), or with a dose-related toxicity range can have direct toxic hepatitis. For example, acetaminophen (Tylenol), a commonly used over-the-counter (OTC) analgesic, can cause severe hepatic necrosis when taken in large amounts, as in suicide attempts or accidental ingestion by children.

Industrial toxins, such as carbon tetrachloride, trichloroethylene, and yellow phosphorus, also have a direct toxic effect on the liver.

IDIOSYNCRATIC TOXIC HEPATITIS. Idiosyncratic toxic hepatitis (ITH) results in morphologic changes to the liver that are similar to those found in viral hepatitis. In idiosyncratic drug reactions, the occurrence of hepatitis is unpredictable and infrequent. It may occur at any time during or shortly after exposure to the drug. Agents that result in idiosyncratic toxic hepatitis include

- Halothane, an anesthetic agent
- Methyldopa (Aldomet, Dopamet♣), an antihypertensive drug
- Isoniazid (INH, Isotomine♣), an antituberculosis drug
- Phenytoin (Dilantin), an anticonvulsant

Treatment of toxic and drug-induced hepatitis is supportive. Withdrawal of the suspected agent is indicated at the first sign of a reaction. Chemical exposure of the liver to drugs and toxins has resulted in the development of chronic active hepatitis and cirrhosis.

Complications of Hepatitis

Failure of the liver cells to regenerate, with progression of the necrotic process, results in a severe, frequently fatal form of hepatitis known as *fulminant* hepatitis. This form of massive hepatic necrosis is rare.

When liver inflammation continues for longer than several months (usually defined as 6 months), the hepatitis is considered to be chronic. *Chronic* hepatitis usually occurs as a result of hepatitis B or hepatitis C. Superimposed infection with delta hepatitis agent (HDV) in clients with chronic HBV may also result in chronic hepatitis.

In a person with *chronic active* hepatitis (CAH), liver damage is progressive and is characterized by hepatic necrosis, acute inflammation, and progressive fibrosis. The client may be asymptomatic for long periods of the hepatic disease process, or the continued fibrosis may lead to liver failure, cirrhosis, and death. Chronic active hepatitis may be manifested by

- Persistent clinical symptoms and hepatomegaly
- The continual presence of HBsAg (hepatitis B surface antigen)
- Elevated, fluctuating serum levels of aspartate aminotransferase (AST), bilirubin, and alkaline phosphatase for 6 months or longer after the acute hepatitis episode

Liver biopsy is necessary to establish the diagnosis of chronic hepatitis.

In people with *chronic persistent* hepatitis and *chronic lobar* hepatitis, liver damage does not progress after the initial insult. These types of hepatitis result from infections with hepatitis B and C viruses. In these nonprogressive disorders, the development of cirrhosis is rare and the recovery prognosis is good.

Most clients with chronic persistent hepatitis are asymptomatic, and physical findings are normal. Laboratory data may reveal a mild elevation of serum AST and alkaline phosphatase levels that may persist for up to 1 year.

Etiology

Causes of hepatitis include

- Viral infections
- Drugs, chemicals, and toxins
- Blood transfusion reactions from exposure to the hepatitis virus
- Hyperthyroidism
- Ingestion of ethyl alcohol, resulting in alcoholic hepatitis

Viral inflammation of the liver is the most common form of hepatitis. The viruses are described in the Classification of Hepatitis section.

Routine screening of blood donors and the elimination of commercial blood sources have markedly decreased the incidence of hepatitis B caused by blood transfusion. However, the risk of viral hepatitis after a transfusion remains a significant problem and is dependent on the method by which blood products are processed. Multiple pooled donor products carry the greatest risk. Clients undergoing hemodialysis are also at a high risk for hepatitis B.

Case reporting to local health departments for all types of *viral* hepatitis is mandatory. Measures to prevent viral hepatitis are listed in Charts 61–4 and 61–5.

Incidence/Prevalence

During the time period of 1982 to 1993 in the United States, the types of acute viral hepatitis cases were as follows: hepatitis A, 47%; hepatitis B, 34%; hepatitis C, 16%. Hepatitis A is most common among school-age children and young adults. There were 26,796 cases reported in 1994.

Hepatitis B occurs primarily in young adults between the ages of 20 and 39 years. The incidence of hepatitis B decreased during the first half of the 1990s. The widespread use of the hepatitis B vaccine is a likely contributing factor. In 1994, 12,517 cases were reported. The number one mode of transmission is sexual contact.

The prevalence of hepatitis C is highest in individuals with hemophilia and injecting drug users. In 1994, 4470 cases were reported (Benensen, 1995; Centers for Disease Control and Prevention, 1995; Hepatitis Branch, 1997).

Collaborative Management

 Assessment

➤ History

If viral hepatitis is suspected, the nurse asks the client whether he or she has had known exposure to a person with hepatitis A or B. The nurse determines whether the client has had recent blood transfusions or undergoes hemodialysis for renal failure. The client should be asked about

- Sexual activities
- Social activities
- Injectable drug use
- Recent ear or body piercing and/or tattooing
- Close living accommodations, such as military barracks, correctional institutions, overcrowded apartments, long-term care facilities

The client's employment history is obtained. The nurse specifically questions the client about employment as a health care worker. The nurse also asks the client about recent travel to a foreign country or to an area with inadequate environmental sanitation. The client is questioned about the ingestion of water from a possibly contaminated source or the recent ingestion of shellfish.

➤ Physical Assessment/Clinical Manifestations

Viral Hepatitis. The courses and clinical manifestations of all five types of viral hepatitis are similar (see Table 61–5). The nurse assesses the client's general subjective complaints, determining whether symptoms occurred acutely (hepatitis A and E) or insidiously (hepatitis B and C).

The client may verbalize feelings of fatigue and loss of appetite. The nurse explores further to assess whether the client is experiencing

- Abdominal pain
- Arthralgia (joint pain)
- Myalgia (muscle pain)
- Diarrhea/constipation
- Fever
- Irritability
- Lethargy
- Malaise
- Nausea/vomiting

The nurse palpates the right upper abdominal quadrant to assess for liver tenderness. The client may report right upper quadrant pain with jarring movements. The skin, sclerae, and mucous membranes are inspected for the presence of jaundice. The client may present for medical treatment only after jaundice appears, believing that other vague symptoms are related to an influenza-like syndrome.

Jaundice in hepatitis results from intrahepatic obstruction and is caused by edema of the liver's bile channels. Dark urine and clay-colored stools are often reported by the client as well. The nurse obtains a urine and stool specimen for visual inspection and laboratory analysis. The nurse also inspects the skin for the presence of rashes in clients with suspected hepatitis B and hepatitis C. Irregular patches of erythema, redness, or urticaria (hives) may occur. The client often reports pruritus (itching) and may have skin abrasions from scratching.

The client with hepatitis A usually has a fever; temperature may range from 100° to 104° F (38° to 40° C). Fever may be low-grade or absent with hepatitis B and hepatitis C.

Toxic and Drug-Induced Hepatitis. The clinical picture in toxic and drug-induced hepatitis depends on the causative agent. Idiosyncratic reactions may result in clinical manifestations that are indistinguishable from those of viral hepatitis or may simulate extrahepatic bile duct obstruction symptoms, such as severe jaundice, rash, arthralgia, and fever.

➤ Psychosocial Assessment

Viral hepatitis usually occurs as an acute illness. Its symptoms may be mild and abate rapidly or go undetected. The clinical manifestations of hepatitis B can persist for up to 6 months. Emotional problems for affected clients often center on their anger about being sick and being fatigued. General malaise, inactivity, and vague complaints contribute to depression and despondency. These clients worry about the long-term effects and complications.

Clients with viral hepatitis often feel guilty about having exposed others to the virus. Infectious diseases such as hepatitis continue to have a social stigma. The client may feel embarrassed by the isolation and hygiene precautions that are imposed in the hospital and that continue to be necessary at home. This embarrassment may cause the client to limit social interactions. Self-imposed visitor restrictions may be instituted by the client out of fear of spreading the virus to family and friends.

Family members are sometimes afraid of contracting the disease and may distance themselves from the client. The nurse allows the client and the family to verbalize these feelings and explores the reasons for these fears. Precautionary isolation measures evoke anxiety for the client and the family.

If transmission of hepatitis B is caused by generally unacceptable social behavior, such as illicit drug use and homosexual activity, the client may feel guilty and ashamed. Clients are unable to return to work until the results of blood tests for serologic markers are negative. The loss of wages and the cost of hospitalization for a client without insurance coverage may produce great anxiety and financial burden for the client and the family.

➤ Laboratory Assessment

The presence of hepatitis A and B is indicated by acute elevations in levels of liver enzymes, indicating liver cellular damage, and by specific serologic markers.

Serum Liver Enzymes. Levels of alanine aminotransferase (ALT) may be elevated to more than 1000 mU/mL and may rise to as high as 4000 mU/mL in severe cases of viral hepatitis. The aspartate aminotransferase (AST) levels may rise to 1000 to 2000 mU/mL. Alkaline phosphatase levels may be normal (30 to 90 IU/L) or mildly elevated. Serum total bilirubin levels are elevated to greater than 2.5 mg/dL and are consistent with the clinical appearance of jaundice. Elevated levels of bilirubin are also present in the urine.

Serologic Markers. The presence of hepatitis A is established when hepatitis A virus (HAV) antibodies (anti-HAV) are identified in the blood. Ongoing inflammation of the liver by HAV is evidenced by the presence of immunoglobulin M (IgM) antibodies, which persist in the blood for 4 to 6 weeks. Previous infection is indicated by the presence of immunoglobulin G (IgG) antibodies. These antibodies persist in the serum and provide permanent immunity to HAV.

The presence of the hepatitis B virus (HBV) is established if serologic testing confirms the presence of hepatitis B antigen-antibody systems in the blood. HBV is a double-shelled DNA virus consisting of an inner core and an outer shell. Antigens located on the surface, or shell, of the virus (HBsAg) are the most significant serologic marker, and their presence establishes the diagnosis of hepatitis B. As long as HBsAg is present in the blood, the client is considered infectious. Persistence of this serologic marker after 6 months or longer indicates a carrier state or chronic hepatitis. Normally, the HBsAg levels decline and disappear after the acute hepatitis B episode. The presence of antibodies to HBsAg (anti-HBs) in the blood indicates recovery and immunity to hepatitis B.

Hepatitis B early antigen (HBeAg) is detected in the serum about 1 week after the appearance of HBsAg. Its presence determines the infective state of the client. Clients who test positively for both HBsAg and HBeAg are more contagious than those who are HBsAg-positive and HBeAg-negative.

The presence of delta hepatitis can be confirmed by the identification of intrahepatic delta antigen or, more often, a rise in the hepatitis D virus antibodies (anti-HD) titer. Circulating hepatitis D antigen (HD Ag) is diagnostic of acute disease but is detected only briefly in the serum.

There have been advances in the development of serologic tests for hepatitis C. The first-generation enzyme immunoassay (EIA) detects antibody to hepatitis C virus (anti-HCV). This assay does not distinguish between IgM and IgG. At present, a second-generation EIA with the ability to detect antibody to additional antigen is in use. At this time, there is no acceptable reliable serologic screening test to identify hepatitis C. There is an increased number of false-positive results with the current screening test. In some instances, seroconversion with hepatitis C may be delayed for up to a year. Although the improved immunoassays increase specificity and sensitivity for anti-HCV testing, definitive diagnosis still relies on a combination of clinical, biochemical, and serologic features.

There are no known serologic markers for hepatitis E.

➤ Other Diagnostic Assessment

Chronic hepatitis is diagnosed by percutaneous liver biopsy. The biopsy distinguishes between chronic active and chronic persistent hepatitis.

The finding of fatty infiltrates in liver biopsy specimens and inflammation with neutrophils is consistent with Laennec's (alcohol-induced) hepatitis.

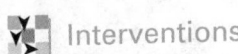 Interventions

The client with viral hepatitis can be mildly or acutely ill, depending on the severity of the inflammation. Some clients are not hospitalized. There is no specific treatment for viral hepatitis, except for hepatitis C. Hepatitis C has been treated with interferon-alpha, which boosts the body's immune system, with some success. The plan of care for all clients with viral hepatitis is based on measures to rest the liver, promote cellular regeneration, and prevent complications (see Client Care Plan).

Nonsurgical Management. During the acute stage of viral hepatitis, interventions are aimed at resting the inflamed liver to promote hepatic cell regeneration. Rest is an essential intervention to reduce the liver's metabolic demands and increase its blood supply. Treatment is generally supportive.

Physical Rest. The nurse and assistive nursing personnel assess the client's response to activity and rest periods. Strict bed rest may be indicated during the early icteric phase of hepatitis. The client is usually tired and expresses feelings of general malaise. Most often, complete bed rest is not required, but rest periods alternating with periods of activity are indicated and are frequently sufficient to promote hepatic healing.

The nurse individualizes the client's plan of care and changes it as needed to reflect the severity of symptoms, fatigue, and the results of liver function tests and enzyme determinations. Scheduled rest periods should be adhered to by the client and the nursing staff. Activities such as providing self-care and ambulating are gradually added to the activity schedule as tolerated.

Psychological Rest. Emotional and psychological rest is essential for the client. Because bed rest and inactivity can be anxiety-producing, the nurse includes diversional activities in the plan of care. If the client is interested, the nurse asks the client's family to bring in small crafts projects; reading materials, such as magazines, books, and newspapers; or a portable radio. The hospital usually provides a television and a telephone in each room. The nurse also encourages staff and family members to spend time in the client's room.

Diet Therapy. A special diet is usually not required. The diet may be high in carbohydrates and calories with moderate amounts of fat and protein. Small, frequent meals are often preferable to three standard meals. The nurse asks the client about food preferences because favorite foods are tolerated better than randomly selected foods. The nurse or assistive nursing personnel encourages the client to prepare the dietary menu, selecting foods that are appealing. The nurse consults with the dietitian about providing high-calorie snacks.

The health care provider typically orders supplemental vitamins. If caloric intake is low, the nurse may need to provide supplemental commercial feedings, such as Ensure. If the client cannot tolerate these feedings orally, the provider may order a feeding tube.

The nurse asks the client's family to prepare favorite foods from home and bring them to the hospital if possible. Fried and fatty foods should be avoided. The nurse encourages the family to prepare meals high in carbohydrates and proteins.

Drug Therapy. An antiemetic to relieve nausea, such as trimethobenzamide hydrochloride (Tigan) and dimenhydrinate (Dramamine), may be prescribed. Prochlorperazine maleate (Compazine), a phenothiazine, is avoided because of its potential hepatotoxic effects.

Comfort Measures. Some foods and smells may stimulate nausea. The nurse or assistive nursing personnel removes the stimulus causing the nausea, if possible. In an effort to stimulate appetite, the nurse or assistive nursing personnel provides mouth care or instructs the client to perform mouth care before meals. The meal may be more

Client Care Plan

The Client with Viral Hepatitis

Nursing Diagnosis No. 1: Activity Intolerance related to general malaise

Expected Outcomes	Nursing Interventions	Rationale
The client will gradually increase activity to the level experienced before hepatitis occurred.	▪ Provide several periods of rest during the day. ▪ Organize care so that the client is not fatigued. ▪ Reinforce the need for bed rest in the immediate recovery period. ▪ Gradually add activities to the client's daily schedule. For example, self-care activities are allowed before ambulation. ▪ Provide or encourage diversional activities on the basis of the client's interests, such as reading, watching television, or doing small crafts. ▪ Encourage family members and significant others to visit the client for short periods.	▪ Rest promotes healing of the liver; inflammation of hepatic cells decreases. ▪ Diversions such as visits and independent activities decrease anxiety, which can prevent rest. The nurse needs to caution against excessive visitation, as the client may become more fatigued.

Nursing Diagnosis No. 2. Altered Nutrition: Less than Body Requirements related to anorexia, nausea, and vomiting

Expected Outcomes	Nursing Interventions	Rationale
The client will achieve an optimal intake of nutrients and calories to promote liver tissue healing.	▪ Provide a diet high in carbohydrates and calories; provide moderate amounts of fat and protein, in collaboration with the dietitian. ▪ Provide small, frequent meals that are attractively presented. ▪ Provide foods that the client likes; allow the client to select meals from the menu. ▪ Offer high-calorie, high-protein snacks such as milk shakes. ▪ Provide supplemental vitamins and liquid feedings, such as Ensure or Ensure Plus, as ordered. ▪ Avoid fried and fatty foods, which can increase nausea. ▪ Administer antiemetic medication, such as trimethobenzamide hydrochloride (Tigan), as ordered. ▪ Remove noxious odors or move unpleasant objects or substances away from the client.	▪ A diet high in carbohydrates and calories provides energy. Protein is needed for hepatic cell regeneration. ▪ The appearance of a large meal can cause anorexia. ▪ Eating a large quantity of food can cause abdominal distention and nausea or vomiting. ▪ Antiemetics diminish nausea and vomiting, allowing the client to consume adequate oral nutrition. ▪ Noxious odors or substances, such as a full bedside commode, can contribute to nausea.

palatable when the client is sitting up in a chair. The nurse empties bedpans, urinals, and bedside commodes promptly and provides an air freshener for the room if it is tolerated by the client.

Surgical Management. Liver transplantation may be performed for clients with chronic hepatitis (see later discussion of liver transplantation).

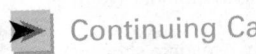

➤ Health Teaching

The nurse teaches the client and the family to observe measures to prevent infection transmission. In addition, the nurse instructs the client with viral hepatitis to avoid alcohol and any nonprescription, over-the-counter medications, particularly acetaminophen (Tylenol, Exdol✚) and sedatives, for 3 to 12 months. These drugs are hepatotoxic.

The client must determine patterns for rest on the basis of physical tolerance of increased activity. The nurse encourages the client to increase activity gradually to prevent fatigue. The client should eat small, frequent meals of high-carbohydrate and low-fat foods. In collaboration with the dietitian, the nurse provides diet teaching and menu planning.

The nurse teaches the client to follow precautionary measures and avoid sexual activity until hepatitis B surface antigen (HBsAg) testing results are negative (Chart 61–6).

➤ Home Care Management

Home care management varies according to the type of hepatitis. A primary focus is preventing the spread of the infection. For hepatitis transmitted by the fecal-oral route, careful hand washing and sanitary disposal of feces are important. Standard precautions are used for hepatitis transmitted percutaneously and permucosally. Therefore, education is very important.

➤ Health Care Resources

Clients with viral hepatitis and their families may contact the local health department for further information on infection control and prevention. Clients discharged home with limited activity tolerance or minimal family support may need the assistance of a home care aide in performing activities of daily living, particularly meal preparation.

Fatty Liver

A fatty liver is caused by the accumulation of triglycerides and other fats in the hepatic cells. In severe cases, fat may constitute as much as 40% of the liver's weight and cause changes in liver function. Minimal, temporary fatty changes are usually reversible by eliminating the cause. The most common cause of fatty liver is chronic alcoholism. Other causes include

- Malnutrition
- Diabetes mellitus
- Obesity
- Pregnancy
- Prolonged total parenteral nutrition (TPN)
- Exposure to large doses of drugs toxic to the liver

Fatty infiltration of the liver may result from faulty fat metabolism in the liver and mobilization of fatty acids from adipose tissue.

Many clients with a fatty liver are asymptomatic. The most common, typical finding is hepatomegaly. Other symptoms include

- Right upper abdominal pain
- Ascites
- Edema
- Jaundice
- Fever
- Signs of late cirrhosis, depending on the severity of the fat infiltration and the longevity of the occurrence

A liver biopsy confirms excessive fat in the liver. Interventions are aimed at removing the underlying cause of the infiltration and providing dietary restrictions.

Hepatic Abscess
Overview

Although hepatic abscesses are uncommon, they carry a high mortality rate. Liver abscesses occur when the liver is invaded by bacteria or protozoa. These organisms destroy the liver tissue, producing a necrotic cavity filled with infective agents, liquefied liver cells and tissue, and leukocytes. The infectious necrotic tissue walls off the abscess from the healthy liver.

A *pyogenic* liver abscess occurs when bacteria invade the liver. Infecting organisms include *Escherichia coli* and *Klebsiella, Enterobacter, Salmonella, Staphylococcus,* and *Enterococcus* species. Pyogenic abscesses are generally multiple. The usual cause is acute cholangitis, occurring as a complication of cholelithiasis. Pyogenic liver abscesses may also result from liver trauma, abdominal peritonitis, and sepsis, or an abscess can extend to the liver after pneumonia or bacterial endocarditis.

The protozoan *Entamoeba histolytica* causes an *amebic* hepatic abscess, which may occur after amebic dysentery. These abscesses usually occur in the form of a single abscess in the right hepatic lobe.

Chart 61–6

Education Guide: Viral Hepatitis

- Avoid all medications, including over-the-counter drugs, such as acetaminophen (Tylenol, Exdol✚), unless prescribed by your physician.
- Avoid all alcohol.
- Rest frequently throughout the day and get adequate sleep at night.
- Eat small, frequent meals with a high-carbohydrate, low-fat content.
- Avoid sex until antibody testing results are negative.
- Follow the guidelines for prevention of transmission of the disease [see Chart 61–5].

Collaborative Management

Clients with hepatic abscesses are generally ill. On occasion, an abscess is not diagnosed until autopsy. In clients with a pyogenic liver abscess, the onset of symptoms is usually sudden. Amebic abscesses cause a more insidious onset of symptoms. Common complaints include

- Right upper abdominal pain with a palpable, tender liver
- Anorexia
- Weight loss
- Nausea and vomiting
- Fever and chills
- Shoulder pain
- Dyspnea
- Pleural pain if the diaphragm is involved

A hepatic abscess is usually diagnosed by liver scan. Hepatic arteriography differentiates an abscess from a malignancy. Blood cultures assist in identifying the causative organism in pyogenic abscesses, and stool cultures may identify *E. histolytica*. With ultrasonographic guidance, a liver abscess may be aspirated percutaneously. Surgical drainage is indicated only for a single pyogenic abscess or for an amebic abscess that fails to respond to long-term antibiotic treatment.

Liver Trauma

Overview

The liver is the most common organ to be injured in clients with penetrating trauma of the abdomen (such as gunshot wounds, stab wounds, and rib fractures) and the second most commonly injured organ in clients who have blunt abdominal trauma. Liver damage or injury should be suspected whenever any upper abdominal or lower chest trauma is sustained. The liver is frequently injured by steering wheels in vehicular accidents. Common injuries to the liver include simple lacerations, multiple lacerations, avulsions (tears), and crush injuries.

The liver is a highly vascular organ, receiving approximately 29% of the body's cardiac output. When hepatic trauma occurs, blood loss can be massive. The client may exhibit signs of hemorrhagic shock, such as

- Hypotension
- Tachycardia
- Tachypnea
- Pallor
- Diaphoresis
- Cool, clammy skin
- Confusion

A decreased hematocrit may confirm suspected blood loss. Clinical manifestations include right upper quadrant pain with abdominal tenderness, distention, guarding, and rigidity. Abdominal pain exaggerated by deep breathing and referred to the right shoulder (Kehr's sign) may indicate diaphragmatic irritation (Chart 61–7).

Collaborative Management

When hepatic and other abdominal organ trauma is suspected, the physician performs an emergency peritoneal

---

Chart 61–7

Key Features of Liver Trauma

- Right upper quadrant pain with abdominal tenderness
- Abdominal distention and rigidity
- Guarding of the abdomen
- Increased abdominal pain exaggerated by deep breathing and referred to the right shoulder (Kehr's sign)
- Indicators of hemorrhage and hypvolemic shock:
  - Tachycardia
  - Tachypnea
  - Pallor
  - Diaphoresis
  - Cool, clammy skin
  - Confusion or other change in mental state

---

lavage to confirm injury. If trauma is present, the lavage reveals gross blood or a high red blood cell count.

The physician then performs an exploratory laparotomy to identify and control the source and type of bleeding. Often, minor surgical interventions, such as suture placement, wound packing, decompression, or a combination of these procedures, are performed to halt bleeding. In some extensive liver injuries, liver lobe resection is required.

Clients with hepatic trauma require administration of multiple blood products, packed red blood cells, and fresh frozen plasma, as well as massive volume infusion to maintain adequate hydration. Postoperatively, the client with hepatic trauma is admitted to a critical care unit. The nurse monitors the client for persistent bleeding. Complete blood count and coagulation studies must be closely monitored for trends in changes.

Carcinoma of the Liver

Overview

Carcinoma of the liver usually develops as a metastatic process. Because of the increased vascularity of the liver, the organ is a common site for metastasis from (1) primary cancers of the esophagus, the stomach, the colon, the rectum, the breasts, and the lungs or (2) a malignant melanoma. Liver cancer accounts for about 2% of cancers in North America and occurs most often in men over 60 (Meissner, 1996).

TRANSCULTURAL CONSIDERATIONS

Primary hepatic carcinoma (cancer originating within the liver) is rare in the United States. In other parts of the world, such as Africa, however, it is one of the most common malignancies. The geographic variation probably reflects the prevalence of chronic hepatitis B infection in other countries. Hepatitis B virus is thought to be the primary carcinogen in as many as 80% of clients with primary hepatic cancer worldwide. Between 30% and 70% of clients with primary hepatic cancer also have cirrhosis, and the risk of hepatic cancer is 40 times greater in clients who have cirrhosis.

Primary hepatic cancer has also been associated with viral hepatitis, trauma, nutritional deficiencies, and exposure to carcinogens and hepatotoxins, such as aflatoxin, thorium dioxide, *Senecio* alkaloids, and the fungus *Aspergillus*.

The most common form of primary hepatic cancer is hepatoma. Clinical manifestations of hepatoma include jaundice, ascites, bleeding, and encephalopathy.

Clients with liver metastasis initially complain of epigastric or right upper quadrant abdominal pain, fatigue, anorexia, and weight loss. Later they typically experience the same manifestations of hepatoma. A nuclear radioisotope liver scan detects metastasis in many cases; however, ultrasonography with needle biopsy may be required to confirm the metastasis.

Collaborative Management

Liver cancer is usually fatal within 6 months of diagnosis (Meissner, 1996). Surgical management may be indicated for clients with a single metastatic lesion confined to one liver lobe. Liver lobe resection for surgical excision of metastasis has been successful in achieving survival rates of up to 5 years.

Unfortunately, 75% of clients are not candidates for surgical excision because their tumors are unresectable. A newer procedure, cryosurgical ablation of the liver, has produced remissions that offer hope for long-term survival (Leininger, 1997).

In this procedure, the surgeon makes a subcostal or midline abdominal incision and selects which tumors are appropriate for either resection or cryoablation. The cryotherapy probes circulate liquid nitrogen and freeze the tumors.

Postoperatively, the client is admitted to the critical care unit for monitoring of complications, including hypothermia, renal failure, and bleeding. Chart 61–8 highlights the nursing care needed during the immediate postoperative period.

Other standard treatments for liver cancer include high-dose chemotherapy and hepatic artery ligation to deprive the metastatic lesion of oxygen. Both treatments can be accomplished without systemic effect because of the unique portal vein circulation in the liver. Hepatic chemotherapy is administered by a surgically implanted infusion pump, which enables controlled infusion for up to 14 days at a time. (See Chapter 27 for discussion of intra-arterial chemotherapy.)

Liver Transplantation

Overview

The first liver transplantation was performed in 1963, and in 1983 it was decided that liver transplantation no longer be considered experimental (Kahn & Starzl, 1995). One-year survival rates improved from approximately 30% in the 1970s to approximately 85% to 90% by the end of the 1980s. The 5-year survival rate is approaching 60%. During 1994, 3650 liver transplant operations were performed in the United States (Dienstag, 1994; Roberts, 1996).

> **Chart 61–8**
>
> ### Nursing Care Highlight: Immediate Postoperative Care of the Client Having Cryosurgical Ablation of the Liver
>
> - Monitor vital signs frequently.
> - Check urine pH every 4 to 6 hours (indicates whether myoglobin has been released from destroyed tissue that can cause acute renal failure).
> - Monitor intake and output every 1 to 2 hours.
> - Maintain Salem sump nasogastric tube at low continuous suction.
> - Maintain warming blanket at >37° C.
> - Observe for bleeding
> - Empty Jackson-Pratt drains every 8 hours.
> - Provide pain medication as ordered via patient-controlled analgesic (PCA) pump.
> - Monitor IV fluids with KCl and sodium bicarbonate as ordered.
> - Administer anti-ulcer medication as ordered.
> - Maintain NPO and bed rest.
> - Monitor laboratory results, especially SMA-13, arterial blood gases, and urine myoglobin.

The client with end-stage liver disease who has not responded to conventional medical or surgical intervention is a potential candidate for liver transplantation. In the adult, diseases treated by liver transplantation include

- Primary or secondary biliary cirrhosis and chronic active hepatitis with cirrhosis
- Hepatic metabolic diseases, such as protoporphyria and Wilson's disease
- Budd-Chiari syndrome (hepatic vein thrombosis)
- Primary sclerosing cholangitis

Liver transplantation is not commonly performed for clients with malignant neoplasms. Because the tumor is likely to recur in immunosuppressed clients, the procedure remains controversial.

The client for potential transplantation undergoes extensive physiologic and psychological assessment and evaluation by physicians and nurses to identify contraindications to the procedure.

Clients who are not considered candidates for transplantation are those with severe end-stage liver disease with life-threatening complications, such as

- Hepatorenal syndrome
- Repeated episodes of esophageal variceal bleeding
- Sepsis
- Severe cardiovascular instability with advanced cardiac disease
- Acquired immunodeficiency syndrome (AIDS)
- Diabetes mellitus
- Severe respiratory disease

Additional identified risk factors include the existence of

- Portal vein thrombosis
- Advanced catabolic state
- Active alcoholism

- Age older than 60 years
- Primary and metastatic malignant disease
- A lack of knowledge and understanding of the procedure and necessary postoperative care measures
- A poor psychosocial support system
- Psychological instability

Liver transplantation has become the most effective treatment of clients with an increasing number of acute and chronic liver diseases, although they are more common in children than adults (see Research Applications for Nursing). Indications and contraindications continue to vary among transplantation centers and are continually revised (Kahn & Starzl, 1995).

Donor livers are obtained primarily from head trauma victims and in the United States are distributed through a nationwide program, United Network of Organ Sharing. This system distributes donor livers on the basis of regional considerations and recipient acuity. Recipients with the highest level of acuity receive highest priority (Dienstag, 1994).

Acute Graft Rejection

The success of all transplantations has greatly improved since the introduction in 1980 of cyclosporine (cyclo-

sporin A), an immunosuppressant drug (see Chap. 25). Cyclosporine has been the primary agent to prevent rejection of the donor organ graft, but azathioprine (Imuran) and prednisone (Deltasone) are also used. Most recipients receive a combination of cyclosporine, steroids, and azathioprine (Kahn & Starzl, 1995).

A new immunosuppressant agent discovered in 1984, FK506, is more potent than cyclosporine. FK506 has been shown to be effective as a form of rescue therapy for a client who continues to reject the liver graft. Other immunosuppressive drugs currently being tested include brequinar sodium, dyspergaulin, and RS61443 (Kirsch, Robson, & Trey, 1995).

The rejection response after liver transplantation still occurs in a majority of clients, starting 1 to 2 weeks after surgery. Clinical manifestations of acute rejection include tachycardia, fever, right upper quadrant or flank pain, decreased bile pigment and volume, and increasing jaundice. Laboratory findings include elevated serum bilirubin, alkaline phosphatase levels, and increased prothrombin time and aminotransferase levels.

Transplant rejection is treated with intravenous doses of methylprednisolone (Solu-Medrol). If this drug is not effective, antibodies to lymphocytes such as OKT3 may also be used (Dienstag, 1994). OKT3 is T cell–specific and more potent; however, it increases the client's risk of infection. If none of these drugs is effective, a rapid deterioration of liver function occurs. Multisystem organ failure, including respiratory and renal involvement, develops, along with diffuse coagulopathies and portal-systemic encephalopathy. The only alternative for treatment is emergency transplantation.

▷ Research Applications for Nursing

What Is the Impact of Liver Transplantation on Quality of Life?

LoBiondo-Wood, G., Williams, L., Wood, R. P., & Shaw, B. W. (1997). Impact of liver transplantation of quality of life: A longitudinal perspective. Applied Nursing Research, 10 (1), 27–32.

The primary purpose of this longitudinal study was to explore the impact of liver transplantation on the quality of life (QOL) of adult liver transplant recipients. The researchers also examined whether demographic or condition-related variables influenced QOL.

The QOL Index—Liver Transplant Version was completed by 41 subjects before transplantation and then again 3, 6, 12, and 18 months after transplantation. Data collection occurred over 3 years.

Data analysis showed a significant increase in overall QOL between pre- and post-tranplantation times. Of the demographic variables, only age and income correlated significantly with overall QOL.

Critique. Previous studies examining QOL have used one or two variables to measure QOL, had a small sample size, and collected data on post-transplant clients on only one occasion. This study improved on previous methodology by measuring multiple variables, having a larger sample size, and following clients over a longer period of time after transplantation.

Possible Implications for Nursing. Nurses should be closely involved with transplant recipients and their families to initiate discussion and answer questions about changes in QOL. Longitudinal studies of family perceptions about QOL are needed to help nurses better support families during the transplantation process.

Infection

Infection is another potential threat to the transplanted graft and the client's survival. Immunosuppressant therapy, which must be used to prevent and treat organ rejection, significantly increases the client's susceptibility to and risk of infection. Other risk factors include the presence of multiple tubes and intravascular lines, immobility, and prolonged anesthesia.

According to Roberts (1996), the average client acquires at least one bacterial infection and has a 40% to 50% chance of developing a viral or fungal infection. In the early post-transplantation period, common infections include pneumonia, wound infections, and urinary tract infections. Opportunistic infections usually develop after the first postoperative month and include cytomegalovirus, mycobacterial infections, and parasitic infections (Dienstag, 1994). In addition, latent infections such as tuberculosis and herpes simplex are frequently reactivated.

The physician prescribes broad-spectrum antibiotics for prophylaxis during and after surgery. The nurse obtains culture specimens from all lines and tubes and collects specimens for culture at predetermined time intervals dictated by the agency's policy. If an infection is detected, the physician prescribes organism-specific anti-infective agents.

Other Complications

The biliary anastomosis is susceptible to breakdown, obstruction, and infection. If leakage occurs or if the site becomes necrotic or obstructed, an abscess can form, or peritonitis, bacteremia, and cirrhosis may develop. Other potential complications include

- Hemorrhage
- Hepatic artery thrombosis
- Fluid and electrolyte imbalances
- Pulmonary atelectasis
- Acute renal failure
- Chronic graft rejection
- Psychological maladjustment

Collaborative Management

Care of the client undergoing liver transplantation requires an interdisciplinary team approach. Case managers are an important part of the team. After the client is identified as a candidate and a donor organ is procured, the actual liver transplantation surgical procedure usually takes 8 hours; the range is 6 to 18 hours (Dienstag, 1994). The procedure involves five anastomoses between

recipient and donor organs, including the following vascular anastomosis sites:

- Suprahepatic inferior vena cava
- Infrahepatic vena cava
- Portal vein
- Hepatic artery
- Biliary tract

The biliary anastomosis site varies, depending on the client's extrahepatic biliary tract. Two common sites are end-to-end anastomosis between the donor and the recipient common bile duct and anastomosis between the donor common bile duct and the recipient jejunum.

In the immediate postoperative period, the client who has undergone liver transplantation is managed in the critical care unit and requires aggressive monitoring and care. The nurse assesses for signs and symptoms of complications of surgery and immediately reports their occurrence to the physician (Table 61–6).

The nurse monitors the client's temperature and reports temperatures greater than 38° C (100° F) and increased abdominal pain, distention, and rigidity, which are indicators of peritonitis. Nursing assessment also includes monitoring for a change in neurologic status that could indi-

TABLE 61–6

Assessment and Prevention of Common Postoperative Complications Associated with Liver Transplantation

Complication	Assessment	Prevention
Acute graft rejection	• Occurs from the 4th to 10th postoperative day • Manifested by tachycardia, fever, right upper quadrant (RUQ) or flank pain, diminished bile drainage or change in bile color, or increased jaundice • Laboratory changes include increased levels of serum bilirubin, transaminases, and alkaline phosphatase and prolonged prothrombin time.	• Prophylaxis with immunosuppressant agents, such as cyclosporine • Early diagnosis to treat with more potent antirejection drugs, such as OKT3
Infection	• Can occur at any time during recovery • Frequent cultures of tubes, lines, and drainage • Manifested by fever or excessive, foul-smelling drainage (urine, wound, or bile); other indicators depend on the location and the type of infection.	• Antibiotic prophylaxis • Early diagnosis and treatment with organism-specific anti-infective agents
Hepatic complications (bile leakage, abscess formation, hepatic thrombosis)	• Manifested by decreased bile drainage, increased RUQ abdominal pain with distention and guarding, nausea or vomiting, increased jaundice, and clay-colored stools • Laboratory changes include increased levels of serum bilirubin and transaminases.	• Keep the T tube in a dependent position; empty frequently, recording the quality and quantity of drainage. • Report manifestations to the physician immediately. • May necessitate surgical intervention
Acute renal failure	• Caused by hypotension, antibiotics, cyclosporine, acute liver failure, or hypothermia • Indicators of hypothermia include shivering, hyperventilation, increased cardiac output, vasoconstriction, and alkalemia. • Early indicators of renal failure include changes in urinary output, increased BUN and creatinine levels, and electrolyte imbalance.	• Keep the client warm. • Observe for early signs of renal failure and report them immediately to the physician.

*BUN, blood urea nitrogen

cate encephalopathy from a nonfunctioning liver. Signs of coagulopathy (e.g., continuous bloody oozing from a catheter, a drain, and incision sites; petechiae; or ecchymosis) are reported to the physician immediately, because they can indicate impaired function of the transplanted liver.

CASE STUDY for the Client with Cirrhosis

■ You are a staff nurse on a busy medical unit. One of the nursing assistants tells you that Mr. Biddix may be confused. You know that Mr. Biddix, age 50, was admitted last evening with a medical diagnosis of alcoholic cirrhosis. When you question the nursing assistant about why she feels that Mr. Biddix is confused, she responds that he is talking about needing to catch the next bus that goes by his door.

Q U E S T I O N S :

1. According to the medical diagnosis, what complication may be occurring in Mr. Biddix?
2. What assessment and laboratory data do you need to obtain immediately?
3. What is the usual medical treatment for this complication? Why is this treatment used?

SELECTED BIBLIOGRAPHY

Anti-Otong, D. (1995). Helping the alcoholic patient recover. *American Journal of Nursing, 95*(8), 22–29.

Becker, Y. T., Reed, G., Lind, C. D., & Richards, W. O. (1996). The role of elective operation in the treatment of portal hypertension. *The American Surgeon, 62,* 171–177.

Benenson, A. (1995). *Control of communicable diseases manual* (16th ed.). Washington, DC: American Public Health Association.

Busuttil, R. W., Shaked, A., Millis, J. M., et al. (1994). One thousand liver transplants. The lessons learned. *Annals of Surgery, 219*(5), 490–497.

Butler, R. W. (1994). Managing the complications of cirrhosis. *American Journal of Nursing, 94*(3), 46–49.

Carveth, J. A. (1995). Perceived patient deviance and avoidance by nurses. *Nursing Research, 44*(3), 173–177.

Centers for Disease Control and Prevention. (1995). Summary of notifiable diseases, United States, 1994. *MMWR, 43*(53), 6.

Cirolia, B. (1996). Understanding edema. *Nursing, 26*(2), 66A–70.

Colquhoun, S. D. (1996). Hepatitis C: A clinical update. *Archives of Surgery, 131,* 18–23.

Dienstag, C. (1994). Liver transplantation. In K. J. Isselbacher, E. Braunwald, J. D. Wilson, et al. (Eds.), *Harrison's principles of internal medicine* (13th ed., pp. 1501–1504). New York: McGraw-Hill.

Hepatitis Branch, Centers for Disease Control and Prevention. (1997, April 28). Epidemiology and prevention of viral hepatitis A to E: An overview. http://www.cdc.gov/ncidod/diseases/hepatitis/slideset/httoc.htm.

Huether, S. E., McCance, K. L., & Danek, G. D. (1996). Alterations of digestive function. In S. E. Huether & K. L. McCance (Eds.), *Understanding pathophysiology* (pp. 944–990). St. Louis: Mosby–Year Book.

Jackson, M. M., & Rymer, T. E. (1994). Viral hepatitis—Anatomy of a diagnosis. *American Journal of Nursing, 94*(1), 43–48.

Kahn, D., & Starzl, T. (1995). Liver transplantation. In R. Kirsch, S. Robson, & C. Trey (Eds.), *Diagnosis and management of liver disease* (pp. 281–285). London: Chapman & Hall Medical.

Kowdley, K. (1996). Update on therapy for hepatobiliary diseases. *Nurse Practitioner, 21*(7), 78–88.

Laine, L., Stein, C., & Sharma, V. (1996). Randomized comparison of ligation plus sclerotherapy in patients with bleeding esophageal varices. *Gastroenterology, 110,* 529–533.

Leininger, S. M. (1997). Managing patients with cryosurgical ablation of the prostate and liver. *MEDSURG Nursing, 6*(6), 359–363, 386.

LoBiondo-Wood, G., Williams, L., Wood, R., & Shaw, B. (1997). Impact of liver transplantation on quality of life: A longitudinal perspective. *Applied Nursing Research, 10*(1), 27–32.

Meissner, J. E. (1996). Caring for the patient with liver cancer. *Nursing96, 26*(1), 52–53.

O'Hanlon-Nichols, T. (1995). Portal hypertension. *American Journal of Nursing, 95*(11), 38.

Payne, J. L., McCarty, K. R., Drougas, J. G., et al. (1996). Outcomes analysis for 50 liver transplant recipients: The Vanderbilt experience. *The American Surgeon, 62,* 320–325.

Porth, C. M. (1994). *Pathophysiology concepts of altered health states* (4th ed.). Philadelphia: J. B. Lippincott.

Roberts, J. P. (1996). Liver transplantation. In J. C. Bennett & F. Plum (Eds.), *Cecil textbook of medicine* (20th ed., pp. 800–802). Philadelphia: W. B. Saunders.

Runyon, B. A. (1994). Care of patients with ascites. *New England Journal of Medicine, 330*(5), 337–342.

Saeed, Z. A. (1996). Endoscopic therapy of bleeding esophageal varices: Ligation is still the best. *Gastroenterology, 110,* 635–638.

Siconolfi, L. A. (1995). Clarifying the complexity of liver function tests. *Nursing95, 25*(5), 39–44.

Singh, G. K., Mathews, T. J., Clarke, S. C., et al. (1995). Annual summary of births, marriages, divorces, and deaths: United States, 1994. *Monthly Vital Statistics Report, 43*(13).

Starzl, T., Marchioro, T., Von Kaulla, K., et al. (1997). Liver transplantation. *Gastroenterology, 112*(1), 288–291.

SUGGESTED READINGS

Butler, R. W. (1994). Managing the complications of cirrhosis. *American Journal of Nursing, 94*(3), 46–49.

This author discusses the pathophysiology, complications, and management of clients with cirrhosis. The focus is on prevention and early detection of life-threatening problems for the client with late-stage cirrhosis.

Jackson, M. M., & Rymer, T. E. (1994). Viral hepatitis—Anatomy of a diagnosis. *American Journal of Nursing, 94*(1), 43–48.

This case study examines the "detective work" required to diagnose viral hepatitis. Also included is a guide to the five major types of viral hepatitis.

Siconolfi, L. A. (1995). Clarifying the complexity of liver function tests. *Nursing95, 25*(5), 39–44.

This author provides a comprehensive discussion of liver function tests, including interpretation. Also included is a brief review of liver functions and problems.

Chapter 62

INTERVENTIONS FOR CLIENTS WITH PROBLEMS OF THE GALLBLADDER AND PANCREAS

Disorders of the gallbladder and the pancreas initially occur as single-organ processes. If the primary disorder is untreated, however, the inflammatory response may extend to other organs. The anatomic proximity of the liver, the gallbladder, and the pancreas and the possibility of impeded flow of bile from the liver through the biliary (gallbladder) ductal system contribute to potential complications and multiorgan involvement in disease processes. Obstruction of bile flow by gallstones, edema, stricture, and tumors can cause inflammation of the gallbladder, the liver, or the pancreas, depending on the location of the obstruction in the biliary system. For example, gallstone impaction of the cystic duct causes cholecystitis, whereas gallstones lodged in the ampulla of Vater impede the flow of bile and pancreatic secretions, which can result in pancreatitis.

BILIARY DISORDERS

Cholecystitis

Overview

Gallbladder disease is a common health care problem in the United States. Cholecystitis may occur as an acute or chronic inflammation of the gallbladder wall (Table 62–1). Chronic inflammation may be complicated by an acute attack if an obstruction is present.

Pathophysiology

Acute Cholecystitis

Acute cholecystitis (inflammation of the gallbladder) usually develops in association with cholelithiasis (gallstones), although it can occur without the presence of gallstones. Cholelithiasis is discussed in detail later in this chapter.

Cholecystitis occurring in the absence of gallstones (acalculous cholecystitis) is believed to be due to bacterial invasion via the lymphatic or vascular route. *Escherichia coli* is the most common causative bacterium found. *Streptococcus* and *Salmonella* are also present.

When the gallbladder is inflamed, trapped bile is reabsorbed and acts as a chemical irritant to the gallbladder wall, having a toxic effect. The presence of bile, in combination with impaired circulation, edema, and distention of the gallbladder, causes ischemia of the gallbladder wall, resulting in tissue sloughing with necrosis and gangrene. Perforation of the gallbladder wall may occur. If the perforation is small and localized, an abscess may form. If the perforation is large, peritonitis may result.

TABLE 62–1

Comparison of Acute and Chronic Cholecystitis	
Acute Cholecystitis	**Chronic Cholecystitis**
• Inflammation present	• Inflammation followed by fibrosis
• Most commonly occurs as a result of cholelithiasis (gallstones) but can occur from bacterial invasion or biliary spasm	• Most commonly occurs as a result of cholelithiasis
• Bile obstruction *not* common	• Bile obstruction common; may result in cholangitis and pancreatitis
• Jaundice *not* common	• Jaundice very common

In some cases, painful episodes of cholecystitis may be the result of organ or bile duct spasticity. The spasticity temporarily prevents the release of an adequate amount of bile for fat digestion.

Chronic Cholecystitis

Chronic cholecystitis results when inefficient emptying of bile by the gallbladder and gallbladder muscle wall disease persist. It may be caused by or lead to the formation of gallstones. In chronic cholecystitis, the gallbladder becomes fibrotic and contracted, which results in decreased motility and deficient absorption.

Pancreatitis and cholangitis (inflammation of the common bile duct) can occur as complications of cholecystitis. Pancreatitis and cholangitis result from the backup of bile throughout the biliary tract. Bile obstruction leads to jaundice.

Jaundice (the yellow discoloration of skin and mucous membranes) and icterus (yellow discoloration of the sclera) can occur in clients with acute cholecystitis but is most commonly seen in clients with chronic gallbladder inflammation. Impeded or obstructed bile flow caused by edema of the ducts or gallstones contributes to *extrahepatic obstructive* jaundice. Jaundice in cholecystitis may also be caused by direct liver involvement. The inflammation of the liver's bile channels or bile ducts may cause *intrahepatic* obstructive jaundice, resulting in an increase in circulating levels of bilirubin, the principal pigment of bile.

When the concentration of bilirubin in the blood increases to greater than 2 mg/dL, jaundice occurs (Malarkey & McMorrow, 1996). Excessive bile salts accumulate in the skin, causing pruritus (itching) or a burning sensation.

In a person with obstructive jaundice, the normal flow of bile into the duodenum is blocked. Bilirubin is unable to reach the large intestine, where it is converted to urobilinogen. Because urobilinogen accounts for the normal brown color of feces, clay-colored stools result. Water-soluble bilirubin is normally excreted by the kidneys in the urine. When an excess in circulating bilirubin occurs, the urine becomes dark and foamy because of the kidneys' effort to clear the bilirubin.

Etiology

The exact etiology of cholecystitis is unknown. Other than the formation of gallbladder calculi, causes of acute cholecystitis include

- Trauma
- Inadequate blood supply
- Prolonged anesthesia/surgery
- Adhesions
- Edema
- Neoplasms
- Long-term fasting
- Prolonged dehydration
- Gallbladder trauma
- Prolonged immobility
- Excessive opioid use

Any condition that affects the regular filling or emptying of the gallbladder or causes "gallbladder shock" (a decrease in blood flow to the gallbladder) can result in acute cholecystitis. Cholecystitis has also been attributed to anatomic problems, such as twisting or kinking of the gallbladder neck or cystic duct, and pancreatic enzyme reflux into the gallbladder.

Incidence/Prevalence

A high incidence of biliary tract disease and cholecystitis occurs in people with a sedentary lifestyle, a familial tendency to biliary disease, obesity, and diabetes mellitus.

WOMEN'S HEALTH CONSIDERATIONS

 The incidence of gallbladder disease is higher in women, especially European American women. By age 60 years, nearly one-third of obese women develop biliary disease (Allen & Phillips, 1997).

Collaborative Management

Assessment

➤ *Physical Assessment/Clinical Manifestations*

There is no typical presentation for clients with acute cholecystitis. Clinical manifestations vary in intensity and frequency (Chart 62–1).

Key Features of Cholecystitis

- Episodic or vague abdominal pain or discomfort that can radiate to the right shoulder.
- Pain triggered by a high-fat or high-volume meal
- Anorexia
- Nausea or vomiting
- Dyspepsia
- Eructation
- Flatulence
- Feeling of abdominal fullness
- Rebound tenderness (Blumberg's sign)
- Fever
- Jaundice, clay-colored stools, dark urine, steatorrhea (most common with chronic cholecystitis)

The nurse or assistive nursing personnel obtains the client's height and weight and determines the client's sex, age, race, and ethnic group. The nurse questions the client about food preferences and determines whether excessive fat and cholesterol are included in the diet. The client is asked whether any foods are not tolerated. The nurse asks whether any of the following gastrointestinal (GI) symptoms occur in relation to the intake of fatty food: flatulence, dyspepsia (indigestion), eructation (belching), anorexia, nausea, vomiting, and abdominal pain or discomfort.

The nurse asks the client to describe the pain, including its intensity and duration, precipitating factors, and measures that relieve the pain, if any. The pain may be described as indigestion of varying intensity, ranging from a mild, persistent ache to a steady, constant pain in the right upper abdominal quadrant. The pain may radiate to the right shoulder or scapula. The abdominal pain of chronic cholecystitis may be vague and nonspecific. The usual pattern of more acute pain is episodic. Clients often refer to these episodes as "gallbladder attacks."

The nurse also asks the client to describe his or her daily activity or exercise routines to determine whether the client's lifestyle is sedentary. The client is asked whether there is a family history of gallbladder disease, because a familial tendency exists for biliary tract diseases.

It is difficult to use abdominal palpation and percussion in assessment of the client with acute cholecystitis. The gallbladder may be tender on palpation. With right subcostal palpation, pain increases with deep inspiration (Murphy's sign). Guarding and rigidity as well as rebound tenderness (Blumberg's sign) are reliable indicators of peritoneal irritation.

Assessment for rebound tenderness and deep palpation is reserved for clinical nurse specialists or Nurse Practitioners. To elicit rebound tenderness, the nurse pushes his or her fingers deeply and steadily into the client's abdomen, then quickly releases the pressure. Pain that results from the rebound of the palpated tissue indicates peritoneal inflammation. Deep palpation below the liver border in the right upper quadrant may reveal a sausage-shaped mass, representing the distended, inflamed gall-

bladder. Percussion over the posterior rib cage intensifies localized abdominal pain.

In *chronic* cholecystitis, clients may have insidious symptoms and may not seek medical treatment until late symptoms such as jaundice, clay-colored stools, and dark urine result from an obstructive process. Steatorrhea (fatty stools) occurs because fat absorption is decreased owing to the lack of bile. Bile is needed for the absorption of fats and fat-soluble vitamins in the intestine. As with any inflammatory process, the client may have an elevated temperature of 37°–39° C (99°–102° F), tachycardia, and dehydration from fever and vomiting.

➤ Diagnostic Assessment

There are no laboratory tests specific for gallbladder disease. Serum levels of alkaline phosphatase, aspartate aminotransferase (AST), and lactate dehydrogenase (LDH) may be elevated, indicating abnormalities in liver function. The direct (conjugated) and indirect (unconjugated) serum bilirubin levels are elevated if an obstructive process is present. An increased white blood cell (WBC) count indicates inflammation. If there is pancreatic involvement, serum and urine amylase levels are elevated.

If cholecystitis is suspected, the health care provider may order an oral cholecystogram (OCG) or gallbladder (GB) radiographic series to confirm the presence of biliary tract disease in clients seen as outpatients. Additional radiographic studies are done when cholelithiasis is suspected. If the gallbladder is not visualized during cholecystography or when only faint opacification occurs, inflammatory disease such as cholecystitis is suspected. The provider may also order an upper GI radiographic series to rule out other causes of abdominal pain, such as gastritis and peptic ulcer disease.

Technetium-labeled acetanilido iminodiacetic acid (^{99m}Tc HIDA) is also used to detect abnormal hepatobiliary function. The HIDA scan may have faster diagnostic capabilities than oral cholecystography because the pretest fasting period necessary for the HIDA scan is 4–6 hours. Additionally, cholecystography is not performed if the serum total bilirubin level is greater than 1.8 mg/dL.

Ultrasonography of the gallbladder has largely replaced the oral cholecystogram for diagnosing gallbladder disease. Gallbladder ultrasound is noninvasive and highly accurate (Porth, 1994; Malarkey & McMorrow, 1996).

 Interventions

During the acute phase of cholecystitis, treatment measures are directed at resting the inflamed gallbladder in an effort to reduce the inflammatory process and relieve the pain. Nonsurgical interventions are implemented, but if these are unsuccessful, the client requires surgery.

Nonsurgical Management. Nonsurgical measures to relieve pain include diet and drug therapy. The physician, the nurse, and the dietitian often collaborate when implementing these interventions.

Diet Therapy. For clients with acute cholecystitis, the health care provider may recommend withholding food and fluids or modifying the diet by avoiding high-fat or high-volume meals. These dietary measures decrease stimulation of the gallbladder and help prevent pain, nausea, and vomiting. For clients with severe nausea and vomiting, decompression of the stomach may be necessary. A nasogastric tube is inserted to empty the stomach contents. (The nurse's role in caring for a client with a nasogastric tube is described in Chapter 58.)

The nurse encourages the client with chronic cholecystitis to consume a low-fat diet to decrease stimulation of the gallbladder. Smaller, more frequent meals assist some clients in tolerating food better.

Drug Therapy. For clients in severe pain, the physician may order opioid analgesics, such as meperidine hydrochloride (Demerol), to relieve abdominal pain and spasm. Morphine is not given because it can cause spasms of the sphincter of Oddi and increase pain. Antispasmodic agents, such as anticholinergics (e.g., dicyclomine hydrochloride [Bentyl, Lomine✦]), may be used to relax the smooth muscles, preventing biliary contraction. Decreased muscle contraction minimizes secretions and assists in the reduction of pain. The health care provider usually prescribes antiemetics, such as trimethobenzamide hydrochloride (Tigan), to relieve nausea and vomiting.

Surgical Management. The usual surgical treatment of clients with acute and chronic cholecystitis is cholecystectomy, the removal of the gallbladder. Two operative procedures are available to the surgeon for performing a cholecystectomy: the traditional approach and laparoscopic laser cholecystectomy.

Traditional Cholecystectomy. The use of the traditional surgical approach has markedly declined during the past decade. The client undergoing this surgery is usually hospitalized.

Preoperative Care. The nurse provides the usual preoperative care in the operating suite on the day of surgery (see Chap. 20). The nurse reinforces teaching of aggressive measures to prevent respiratory complications. To minimize abdominal/incisional jarring during coughing, deep breathing, and turning, the nurse demonstrates splinting methods such as use of a pillow or folded blanket. These clients are also susceptible to postoperative atelectasis, especially the elderly and smokers. The nurse instructs the client in the use of sustained maximal inspiration (SMI) devices, such as an incentive spirometer.

The importance of early mobilization in preventing complications is also emphasized. The nurse informs the client to expect to get out of bed the evening of surgery.

Operative Procedure. The surgeon not only removes the gallbladder through a right subcostal incision but also often explores the biliary ducts for the presence of stones. If the common bile duct (CBD) is explored, the surgeon typically inserts a T-tube drain to ensure patency of the duct (Fig. 62–1). Trauma to the common bile duct stimulates inflammation, which can impede bile flow and contribute to bile stasis. In addition, the surgeon usually inserts a drainage tube, such as a Penrose or Jackson-Pratt drain. The drainage tube is positioned in the gallbladder bed to prevent fluid accumulation. The drainage is usually serosanguineous (serous fluid mixed with blood) and is bile-stained in the first 24 hours postoperatively.

Postoperative Care. Postoperative incisional pain relief after traditional cholecystectomy is usually achieved with

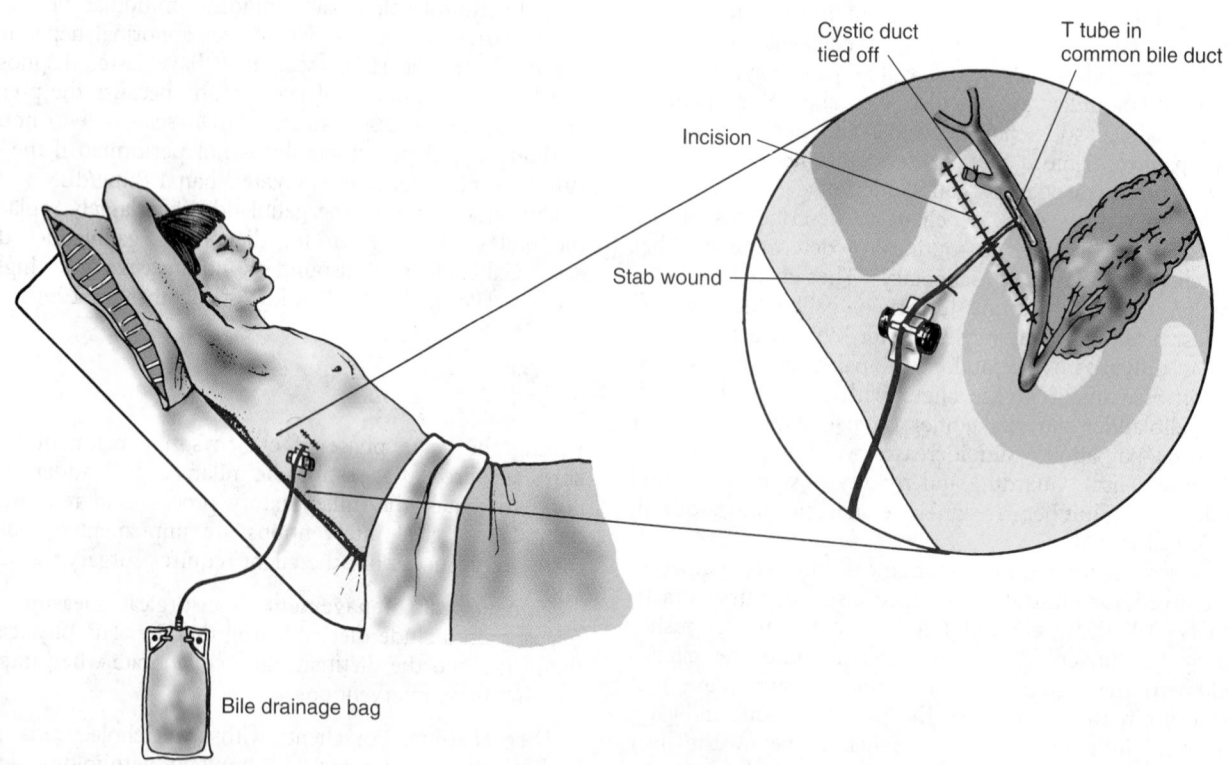

Cystic duct
tied off

T tube in
common bile duct

Incision

Stab wound

Bile drainage bag

Figure 62–1. Placement of a T tube.

meperidine hydrochloride (Demerol) using a patient-controlled analgesia (PCA) pump. Morphine is generally not given because it can constrict the sphincter of Oddi and cause biliary ductal spasm. The client participates in coughing and deep breathing exercises more readily when pain is minimized. Therefore, the nurse plans the coughing and deep breathing exercises when pain relief is optimal.

Antiemetics may be necessary for clients with episodes of postoperative nausea and vomiting. The nurse administers the antiemetic early, as ordered, to prevent retching associated with vomiting to decrease the incidence of pain related to muscle straining.

The nurse cares for the incision, the surgical drain, and the T tube. The surgeon typically removes the surgical dressing and drain within 24–48 hours after surgery. The T tube, however, may remain in place for 6 weeks or longer. Chart 62–2 highlights the important nursing care activities associated with the T-tube system.

The client usually receives nothing by mouth (NPO) for about 8–24 hours postoperatively. If gallbladder disease is severe, a nasogastric (NG) tube provides stomach decompression during this period. When peristalsis returns, the nurse removes the NG tube as ordered. The physician places the client on a clear liquid diet. The nurse gradually advances the diet from clear liquids to solid foods as tolerated by the client. Within a day or two, the client resumes the ingestion of solid foods and is discharged to home.

The amount of fat allowed in the client's diet after cholecystectomy depends on the client's tolerance of fat. In the early postoperative period, if bile flow is reduced, a low-fat diet may reduce discomfort and prevent nausea. For most clients, a special diet is not required. The nurse advises the client to eat nutritious meals and avoid excessive intake of fat. If the client is obese, the nurse recommends a weight-reduction program. The nurse collaborates with the physician and the dietitian in planning the appropriate diet.

Laparoscopic Cholecystectomy. Laparoscopic cholecystectomy, introduced in 1989, has quickly gained in popularity (see accompanying clinical pathway). It is now considered the treatment of choice by many surgeons and is performed more often than the traditional, open cholecystectomy.

Preoperative Care. The laparoscopic procedure is commonly done on an outpatient (ambulatory) basis in a same-day surgery suite. The surgeon explains the procedure; the nurse answers questions and reinforces the physician's instructions. There is no special preoperative preparation for the client. However, the physician typically orders the usual preoperative laboratory tests and requires the client to be on NPO status before the surgery. (Chapter 20 describes general preoperative care for the client undergoing anesthesia.)

Operative Procedure. The surgeon makes a 10-mm midline puncture at the umbilicus. The abdominal cavity is insufflated with 3–4 L carbon dioxide. A trocar catheter is inserted, through which a laparoscope is introduced. The laparoscope is attached to a video camera,

---

> ### Chart 62–2
>
> ### Nursing Care Highlight: The Client with a T Tube
>
> - Assess the amount, color, consistency, and odor of drainage at least q4h, then q8h. In the initial postoperative period, expect bloody drainage, which changes to green-brown bile. Bile output is 400 mL/day with a gradual decrease in amount. Report bile drainage amounts in excess of 1000 mL/day.
> - Collect and administer excess bile output to the client by the nasogastric tube or give synthetic bile salts, such as dehydrocholic acid (Decholin).
> - Report sudden increases in bile output after a normally decreasing output pattern is established (9–10 days postoperatively).
> - Assess for foul odor and purulent drainage, which indicate infection or extensive inflammation. Report changes in drainage to the physician.
> - Inspect the skin around the T tube insertion site for signs of inflammation, including redness, swelling, and erythema, and observe for frank bile leakage. Keep the dressing dry. (Use the hospital's procedure and provide drain care and dressing change per protocol. The site is usually cleaned and the dressing changed daily.)
> - Keep the drainage system below the level of the gallbladder. Maintain the client in the semi-Fowler's position.
> - *Never* irrigate, aspirate, or clamp a T tube without a physician's order.
> - Assess the drainage system for pulling, kinking, or tangling of tubing, especially when the client is positioned toward the right side. Assist the client with early turning and ambulation.
> - When ordered by the physician, raise the drainage bag to the level of the abdomen (usually on the fourth or fifth postoperative day). Then, assess the client for feelings of fullness, nausea, or pain.
> - Clamp the T tube for 1–2 hr per physician's orders before and after meals. Assess the client's response for tolerance of food.
> - Observe stools for return of brown color 7–10 days postoperatively.

---

and the abdominal organs are viewed on a monitor. The surgeon makes three small punctures through which to introduce laparoscopic forceps to manipulate the gallbladder. A laser is used to dissect the gallbladder away from the liver bed and to close off the cystic artery and the duct. The surgeon mobilizes the gallbladder and then extracts it through the midline puncture site.

Postoperative Care. Removing the gallbladder with the laproscopic technique reduces the risk of wound complications. Some clients have a problem with "free air pain" from carbon dioxide retention in the abdomen. The nurse teaches the client the importance of early ambulation to promote absorption of the carbon dioxide. Far less opioid analgesia is necessary after the laparoscopic procedure.

Following laparoscopic surgery, the client can return to usual activities, including work, much sooner than if an

Clinical Pathway for Laparoscopic Cholecystectomy

Aspect of Care	Preadmission/ Preoperative	Preoperative/DOS	Postoperative
Assessment	Physician assessment	Preoperative check, nursing assessment, psychosocial assessment	Vital signs, intake and output; assess: abdomen, bowel sounds, pain, breath sounds, incisions
Teaching	Education by physician; review clinical pathway with client and family	Teach/demonstrate turn, cough, and deep breathe	Review discharge information: pain control, activity, wound care, complications
Consults	Anesthesia if indicated; social workers, dietitian, spiritual guide		
Laboratory Tests and Diagnostic Tests	CBC, EKG if age >40 years; liver/pancreas screen		If indicated: CBC, H&H
Medications	Assess allergies; identify home medications	Preoperative medications—taken at home; IVF antibiotic per hospital protocol	Analgesic, antiemetic
Treatments/Interventions	NPO after midnight		Elevate head of bed; Band-Aids, turn, cough, and deep breathe; emotional support Encourage fluids, solid food per client choice
Activity	Activity ad lib		Progressive ambulation
Discharge Planning	Determine needs: transportation, financial, home health		Arrangements made based on preoperative assessment needs; follow-up appointment with MD

Adapted from *Clinical path: Outpatient laparoscopic cholecystectomy*, 1995, Saint Joseph's Hospital, Asheville, NC; and Ignatavicius, D. D., & Hausman, K. A. (1995). *Clinical pathways for collaborative practice.* Philadelphia: W. B. Saunders.

open cholecystectomy had been done. Most clients are able to resume usual activities within 1–3 weeks (see Research Applications for Nursing).

 Continuing Care

➤ *Health Teaching*

For the client having a cholecystectomy, discharge teaching for the client and the family may include
- Pain management
- Diet therapy
- Wound, drain, and incision care
- Activity restrictions
- Complication recognition
- The need for health care follow-up

In postoperative teaching and discharge planning, the nurse should include a supportive spouse, family member, or significant other to provide reinforcement of information and to assist the client in adhering to the treatment plan.

Diet therapy for the client who has had a cholecystectomy is based on the client's tolerance of fats. A special diet may not be needed. In this case, the nurse advises the client to eat nutritious, well-balanced meals. If the client has a poor tolerance of fats, the nurse recommends a low-fat diet and provides the client and the family or significant other with a list of foods to avoid (Table 62–2). The dietitian may provide printed menu-planning guidelines. Some clients need to maintain a low-fat diet for 6 months or longer. They are advised to add fatty foods to the diet slowly and as tolerated.

Research Applications for Nursing

Clients Recovering From Laparoscopic Cholecystectomy Need Accurate Information on What to Expect Postoperatively

Carson, C., Seidel, S., & Bushmiaer, M. (1996). Recovery from laparoscopic cholecystectomy procedures. AORN Journal, 63(6), 1099–1113.

Laparoscopic cholecystectomy client education materials usually portray recovery occurring within 3 to 5 days after surgery with relatively little pain and minimal disruption of daily activities. The focus of this study was to examine the postoperative experience of 53 adults who had routine, uncomplicated laparoscopic cholecystectomy procedures. Using a Likert-type scale, clients rated their pain, nausea, vomiting, and fatigue. Data were also gathered on appetite and activity. The data were collected preoperatively, before discharge, and after discharge on days 1, 2, 3, 4, and 7. Compared with previous studies, clients in this study reported more intense pain and nausea. Regular eating patterns were slower to return, taking 7 days before the majority of participants (92%) had resumed their regular diet. Moreover, by the seventh day after surgery, only 51% of the study participants had resumed their usual activities.

Critique. The study needs to be replicated with extended parameters such as larger sample size, extended postoperative data gathering period, expanded client diversity, and the effectiveness of preoperative client education.

Possible Nursing Implications. It is important that preoperative client education in regard to what the client can expect postoperatively be as accurate as possible. In view of the results of this study, preoperative instruction for a client scheduled for a laparoscopic cholecystectomy should include the following about postoperative expectations: Pain is common for at least the first 2 days after surgery and may persist for 7 or more days; although the majority of the pain is incisional/abdominal in nature, discomfort may also occur in the shoulder, rib cage, or back; and it may take 7 or more days before the resumption of usual activity occurs. It is also important to stress that these criteria are given as examples only.

If the client has problems tolerating three large meals a day, the nurse advises the client to try smaller, more frequent meals. A weight-reduction diet for obese clients is recommended, and appropriate dietary teaching is tailored to provide dietary guidelines and recommendations.

After traditional cholecystectomy, clients are leaving the hospital sooner after surgery than in the past. Some clients are sent home with T-tube drainage systems intact. The nurse instructs the client and one or more family members to inspect the incision wound and the T-tube drainage site for signs and symptoms of inflammation. These signs and symptoms include redness, swelling, warmth, extreme tenderness, excessive drainage, and increased incisional pain. Any of these findings should be reported to the physician or the Nurse Practitioner. The nurse provides the client with oral and written instructions for drainage tube care (Chart 62–3).

The client with cholecystitis who either refuses or postpones surgery must be instructed on the signs of potential complications of chronic cholecystitis, including fever, recurrent abdominal pain, and jaundice. If these signs occur, the client should notify the health care provider for prompt medical care.

► Home Care Management

After traditional cholecystectomy, clients usually need short-term assistance with procuring foods, preparing meals, performing dressing changes, and caring for the T tube. Clients who have undergone traditional gallbladder surgery may also need transportation to follow-up appointments with the health care provider. The surgeon typically allows these clients to return to their usual activities 4–6 weeks after surgery

► Health Care Resources

For clients at home with a T tube or for advanced elderly clients who cannot manage self-care, a home care nurse may be needed to provide support and follow-up nursing care and teaching. The home care nurse assesses the client's adaptation to the treatment plan and evaluates wound healing and the integrity of the T-tube drainage system. The home care nurse also determines the need for further wound and skin care interventions and implements these interventions as needed.

Cholelithiasis

Overview

Cholelithiasis, the presence of one or more gallstones, is the most common disorder of the biliary tract. In more than 90% of clients with cholecystitis, the cause of inflammation is bile stasis resulting from impaction of the cystic duct by gallstones. Chronic cholecystitis occurs when repeated episodes of cystic duct obstruction result in chronic inflammation.

TABLE 62–2

Foods for Clients with Cholecystitis or Cholelithiasis To Avoid

Foods High in Cholesterol	Gas-Forming Vegetables
Dairy Products	• Cabbage
• Whole milk	• Onions
• Ice cream	• Broccoli
• Butter	• Cauliflower
• Cream	• Sauerkraut
• Cheese	• Radishes
Other Foods	• Cucumbers
• Fried, fatty foods	• Beans
• Rich pastries	
• Gravies	
• Nuts	
• Chocolate	
• Egg yolks	
• Avocado	

Chart 62–3

Education Guide: Home Care for the Client with a T Tube

- Wear loose-fitting clothes.
- Wear older clothes to prevent ruining good-quality clothes.
- If staining occurs, soak the garment in a solution of detergent, baking soda, and bleach.
- Take showers instead of baths.
- Avoid heavy lifting and strenuous activity.
- Remove the dressing around the T tube every day. Hold the tube in place and use an alcohol wipe to clean the skin around the tube. Apply a pre-cut dressing around the catheter, and tape it in place.
- Empty the drainage bag at the same time each day. Allow the bile to flow from the bag's spout; do not disconnect the system.
- Watch the amount, color, and odor of the drainage, and report any change in drainage, abdominal pain, nausea, or vomiting to your physician.
- Coil the drainage tubing and secure it to your abdomen by taping or using a belt with hook and loop fasteners (Velcro). Keep the drainage bag below the level of the T tube.
- Inspect the wound for signs of infection, including redness, swelling, warmth, abdominal firmness, pain, and purulent drainage at the tube site. Take your temperature and report a temperature of 100° F (37° C) or greater to your physician.
- Return to the hospital as scheduled for a cholangiogram.

Pathophysiology

Pathologic Changes

The exact pathophysiology of gallstone formation is not clearly understood. Contributing factors may include

- Supersaturation of bile with cholesterol
- Excessive bile salt losses
- Decreased gallbladder-emptying rates
- Changes in bile concentration or bile stasis within the gallbladder

Gallstones may lie dormant within the gallbladder or may move to other areas of the biliary tree as the gallbladder empties and refills with bile. Stones may migrate and lodge within the gallbladder neck, the cystic duct, or the common bile duct, causing obstruction (Fig. 62–2). Gallstones interfere with or totally obstruct normal bile flow from the gallbladder to the duodenum, causing vascular congestion as a result of impeded venous return. Edema and congestion occur and contribute to the initial inflammatory process. When bile cannot flow from the gallbladder, the stasis of bile and local irritation from the gallstones lead to cholecystitis (described earlier).

Cholangitis, usually associated with choledocholithiasis (common bile duct stones), involves infection of the bile ducts. *Ascending* cholangitis, inflammation of the biliary tree, occurs after bacterial invasion of the ducts. Bacterial invasion can lead to life-threatening *suppurative* cholangitis when symptoms are not recognized quickly and pus accumulates in the ductal system.

Types of Gallstones

The gallbladder provides an excellent environment for the production of gallstones. In particular, the gallbladder only occasionally mixes its normally abundant mucus and a highly viscous, concentrated bile. The constant temperature within the gallbladder also contributes to stone formation by delaying bile emptying, causing biliary stasis.

Gallstones are composed of substances normally found in bile, such as cholesterol, bilirubin, bile salts, calcium, and various proteins. Stones are classified as either cholesterol stones or pigment stones.

Cholesterol stones form as a result of metabolic imbalances of cholesterol and bile salts. They are the most common type found in people in the United States.

Pigment stones are small, are brown or black, and usually occur in clusters as a result of metabolic imbalances of unconjugated bilirubin. Black pigment stones are composed primarily of calcium bilirubinate and are the most often found pigment stones in clients in the United States.

Etiology

There appears to be a familial tendency in the development of cholelithiasis, but this may be related to familial dietary habits (excessive dietary cholesterol intake) and sedentary lifestyles in some families. Gallstones are seen more frequently in obese clients, probably as a result of impaired fat metabolism. People ingesting low-calorie or liquid protein diets are also susceptible to gallstones.

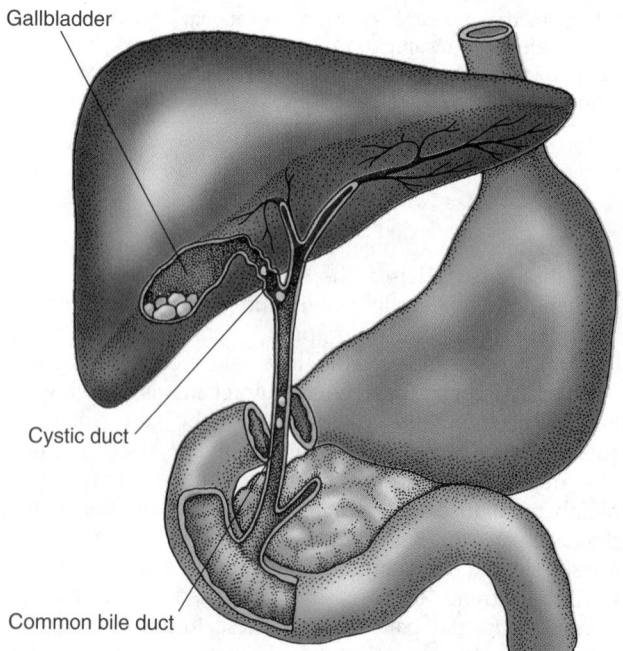

Figure 62–2. Gallstones within the gallbladder and obstructing the common bile and cystic ducts.

These diets cause the liberation of cholesterol from tissues; the cholesterol is excreted as crystals in bile.

WOMEN'S HEALTH CONSIDERATIONS

 Pregnancy tends to worsen gallstone formation. Pregnancy and drugs, such as estrogen and birth control pills, alter hormone levels and delay muscular contraction of the gallbladder, causing a decreased rate of bile emptying. The incidence of gallstones is higher in women who have had multiple pregnancies. Combinations of causative factors increase the incidence of stone formation, especially in women. For example, an obese pregnant woman or an obese woman taking birth control pills may be at higher risk.

Cholelithiasis is seen with hemolytic blood disorders, with bowel disease such as Crohn's disease, and after jejunoileal bypass surgery as a treatment of morbid obesity. Stone formation and cholecystitis are also common in clients with type 1 diabetes.

Incidence/Prevalence

Cholelithiasis is prevalent in developed countries, with an incidence of 10%–20%. The incidence is higher in women than in men. Male clients who have cholelithiasis are usually 50 years of age or older. Cholelithiasis has been diagnosed in more than 20 million people in the United States, and 1 million new cases are reported yearly. Two-thirds of people with gallstones also experience chronic cholecystitis (Greenberger & Isselbacher, 1994; Huether et al., 1996).

TRANSCULTURAL CONSIDERATIONS

Caucasians and Native Americans, particularly members of the Navajo and Pima tribes, have a higher incidence of gallstones, although the disorder is also prevalent in Asian-Americans and African-Americans (Giger & Davidhizar, 1995).

Collaborative Management

Assessment

The same historical data base may be obtained for clients with cholecystitis and cholelithiasis (see Cholecystitis earlier).

➤ *Physical Assessment/Clinical Manifestations*

The severity of pain and presentation of symptoms in the client with cholelithiasis depend on
- Whether the stone is stationary or mobile
- The size and location of the stone
- The degree of obstruction
- The presence and extent of inflammation

Initially, the pain of cholelithiasis is usually a steady, mild ache located in the mid–epigastric area. It may increase in intensity and duration and may radiate to the right shoulder or back.

The severe pain of *biliary colic* is produced by obstruction of the cystic duct of the gallbladder. When a stone is moving through or is lodged within the duct, tissue spasm occurs in an effort to mobilize the stone through the small duct. This intense pain may be so severe that it is accompanied by tachycardia, pallor, diaphoresis, and prostration (extreme exhaustion).

Any of the clinical manifestations seen in acute or chronic cholecystitis may occur in cholelithiasis (see Chart 62–1). Clients with chronic cholecystitis and acute ductal obstruction may experience the excruciating pain of biliary colic as well. On inspection, the nurse may observe jaundice of the skin, the sclera, the upper palate, and the oral mucous membranes. If gallstones occlude the common bile duct, prolonged severe inflammation and hepatic damage may also occur.

➤ *Laboratory Assessment*

There are no specific laboratory tests for cholelithiasis. As in cholecystitis, the serum alkaline phosphatase, lactate dehydrogenase, aspartate aminotransferase, and direct and indirect bilirubin levels may be elevated. Examination of a random stool specimen reveals absent or low levels of urobilinogen in the feces, indicating an obstructive process. If pancreatic involvement accompanies gallstone impaction, serum and urine amylase levels are elevated.

➤ *Radiographic Assessment*

Calcified gallstones are easily visualized on abdominal x-ray examination. An oral cholecystogram is diagnostic when the stones are radiopaque. The physician may order intravenous (IV) cholecystography (or cholangiography) for clients who are unable to absorb oral contrast agents. An ultrasound may be ordered as a screening test. The gallbladder and ductal systems are outlined, and the stones present are visualized.

Percutaneous transhepatic cholangiography is a fluoroscopic examination of the biliary ducts and may be used to diagnose obstructive jaundice and visualize stones located in the ducts.

➤ *Other Diagnostic Assessment*

Ultrasonography of the gallbladder is now considered the test of choice to confirm the diagnosis of cholelithiasis and distinguish between obstructive and nonobstructive jaundice. Ultrasound of the gallbladder is reported to be 95% accurate in detecting gallstones.

Interventions

The health care provider may institute supportive medical treatment for clients with cholelithiasis as an alternative for or before surgical removal of the gallbladder and gallstones.

Nonsurgical Management. Some gallstones do not produce problems or cause pain. Acute pain occurs when the gallstones move into the duct or partially or totally obstruct the duct. Measures aimed at resting the inflamed gallbladder are the same as those discussed earlier for cholecystitis.

Diet Therapy. In general, the client must adhere to a low-fat diet to prevent further pain of biliary colic. If gallstones are causing an obstruction of bile flow, the health care provider orders replacement of fat-soluble vitamins, such as vitamins A, D, E, and K, and the administration of bile salts to facilitate digestion and vitamin absorption. Food and fluids are withheld if nausea and vomiting occur.

Drug Therapy. Pain caused by acute obstruction with gallstones necessitates opioid analgesia with meperidine hydrochloride (Demerol). Morphine is not used because it can cause biliary spasm and constrict the sphincter of Oddi. Antispasmodic or anticholinergic drugs, such as dicyclomine hydrochloride (Bentyl, Lomine✦), may be given to relax smooth muscles and decrease ductal tone and spasm. The provider orders antiemetics to control nausea and vomiting.

Bile acid therapy has been effective in dissolving gallstones, depending on the type of stones. Chenodeoxycholic acid (CDCA; chenodiol; Chenix) reduces cholesterol stones by maintaining a normal amount of cholesterol solubility in bile. Chenodiol may be effective in dissolving small stones (less than 5 mm), but large stones (larger than 2 cm) usually cannot be dissolved (Kowdley, 1996). This treatment is generally reserved for elderly clients who have mild or asymptomatic gallstone disease and those who are poor surgical risks. Unfortunately, it may take up to 2 years to dissolve gallstones. These drugs are expensive, and stones can recur if the client is not maintained on low drug dosages for prolonged periods. The nurse observes for and reports diarrhea, the common side effect of chenodiol therapy.

Ursodiol (Actigall) has been approved in the United States as an anticholelithic agent since 1988. This drug dissolves small (less than 20 mm) cholesterol gallstones. As is the case for chenodiol, ursodiol may take 4 months to 2 years to dissolve the stone or stones. Moreover, in up to 50% of treated clients, the stones recur within 5 years. Therefore, this treatment is best for clients who have mild or infrequent clinical manifestations, those who refuse surgery, or those clients who are poor surgical risks, such as the "frail" elderly.

Obstructive jaundice in cholelithiasis is caused by impeded bile flow through the common bile duct as a result of gallstone obstruction. It may lead to excessive accumulation of bile salts in the skin. As a result, severe pruritus may occur. Cholestyramine resin (Questran) binds with bile acids in the intestine, forming an insoluble compound that is excreted in the feces, removing excessive bile salts and decreasing itching. The nurse mixes the powder form of the drug with fruit juices or milk. It is given before meals and at bedtime.

Extracorporeal Shock Wave Lithotripsy. Extracorporeal shock wave lithotripsy is a noninvasive procedure that is being used as an ambulatory treatment of clients with gallstones in some settings. A machine, a lithotriptor, generates powerful shock waves to shatter the gallstones (Fig. 62–3). Clients who are eligible for this procedure must have three or fewer cholesterol stones (measuring between 5 and 30 mm), have a functioning gallbladder, and have no history of liver or pancreatic disease. Clients who have pacemakers or who are pregnant are not candidates for lithotripsy.

During the hour-long procedure, up to 1500 shocks are repeated until the gallstone is completely fragmented. The minute particles are then able to travel through the biliary ductal system to be excreted via the intestines. Because some clients experience mild pain as gallbladder spasms occur in an effort to expel the tiny stone fragments, the physician may use intravenous (IV) conscious sedation with fentanyl citrate (Alfenta, Sublimaze) or midazolam hydrochloride (Versed).

Eating and drinking are permitted almost immediately after the procedure. The nurse informs the client that right upper quadrant pain after the procedure is not uncommon and usually resolves in 2 days. Acetaminophen (Tylenol, Exdol✦) often provides enough analgesia to relieve this pain.

Percutaneous Transhepatic Biliary Catheter Insertion. The physician may insert a percutaneous transhepatic biliary catheter under fluoroscopic guidance. This procedure decompresses obstructed extrahepatic ducts so that bile can flow (Fig. 62–4). It is primarily used for

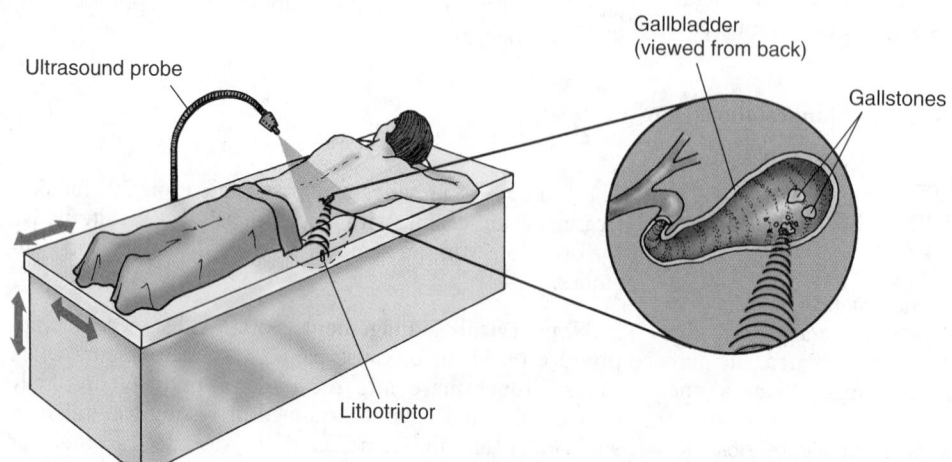

Ultrasound probe

Gallbladder (viewed from back)

Gallstones

Lithotriptor

Figure 62–3. Biliary lithotripsy. With the assistance of a computer and an ultrasound monitor, the physician positions the client over a shock wave generator (lithotriptor) by means of a table that moves upward and downward, forward and backward, and side to side. When the client is positioned properly, the physician fires the lithotriptor. Particles slough off the gallstones until they are completely fragmented, and the fragments pass through the biliary ductal systems.

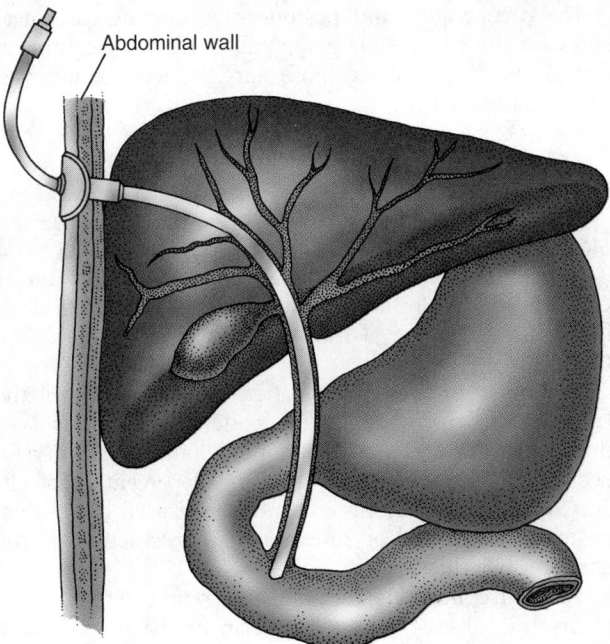

Figure 62–4. Transhepatic biliary catheterization.

Abdominal wall

Chart 62–4

Nursing Care Highlight: The Client with a Transhepatic Biliary Catheter

- Change the catheter insertion site dressing daily, according to the hospital's policy. Recommended care includes cleaning the skin with hydrogen peroxide and applying antibiotic ointment and a small sterile dressing to the site.
- During the first several days after catheter insertion, unclamp the catheter and allow it to drain into an external drainage system (per physician order).
- Using a three-way stopcock system located between the catheter and the drainage bag, irrigate the catheter twice daily with 5–20 mL of bacteriostatic (preservative-free) saline. Check the physician's orders for the amount of solution and the frequency of irrigation. Flush to the client and to the bag to ensure that the tubing is patent. (Occlude the stopcock with a sterile cap when the irrigation procedure is complete.)
- Instruct the client that he or she may experience discomfort during irrigation. Observe for abdominal cramping or excessive pain, and notify the physician if any occurs.
- If pain is severe and abdominal rigidity develops, notify the physician immediately.
- Assess the client for decreasing jaundice. Stools should change from clay-colored to normal brown and urine from dark to straw-colored. Monitor serum bilirubin test results for decreasing levels.
- Assess the client for fever, chills, and hypotension, and report these findings to the physician.
- Inspect the catheter for the presence of blood, and notify the physician immediately if any occurs.
- Inspect the catheter for patency.
- Drainage bag should remain in dependent position. Do not place on bed or above level of client.
- Affix bag to client's gown (not to the bed).
- Provide discharge instructions to the client or a family member, including
  - Dressing care
  - Signs of catheter malfunction, infection, and dislodgment
  - Outpatient and cholangiography appointments

---

inoperable hepatic, pancreatic, or bile duct carcinoma. It may be a nonsurgical alternative for the treatment of biliary obstruction caused by gallstones and hepatic dysfunction associated with obstructive jaundice and biliary sepsis in the high-risk candidate. Nursing care associated with this treatment is outlined in Chart 62–4.

Surgical Management. One of several procedures may be indicated in the surgical treatment of cholelithiasis (Table 62–3). *Cholecystotomy* (an opening into the gallbladder) can be an emergency procedure to remove gallstones. This procedure is often performed for elderly clients or critically ill clients with life-threatening multisystem problems who may not withstand a prolonged surgical procedure. If the stones are located in the common bile duct, a *choledocholithotomy* (an incision into the common bile duct to remove stones) is necessary. If the

TABLE 62–3

Common Gallbladder Surgical Procedures

Surgical Procedure	Description
Traditional cholecystectomy	• Removal of the gallbladder through a high (subcostal) abdominal incision
Laparoscopic laser cholecystectomy	• Removal of the gallbladder by laser through a laparoscope
Cholecystotomy	• Opening into gallbladder to remove gallstones
Choledochotomy	• Incision into the common bile duct
Choledocholithotomy	• Incision into the common bile duct to remove gallstones

common bile duct is explored, the surgeon inserts a T-tube drain into the duct to ensure patency until edema subsides and to allow collection of excessive bile drainage.

A simple, traditional *cholecystectomy* or laparoscopic cholecystectomy is performed when stones are confined to the gallbladder. The common bile duct and adjacent ducts are explored for the presence of additional stones or stone fragments and crystals in the traditional surgical procedure (see Cholecystitis earlier).

After cholecystectomy with T-tube placement, the surgeon may prescribe drugs to stimulate bile production and bile flow from the liver. Bile flow promotes the digestion and absorption of the fats, fat-soluble vitamins, and cholesterol in the duodenum. Hydrocholeretic drugs, such as dehydrocholic acid (Decholin, Cholan-HMB), which are synthetic bile salts, increase the solubility of cholesterol. Increased solubility prevents the accumulation of cholesterol in bile, thereby decreasing the recurrence of biliary calculi and promoting drainage of (potentially infected) bile through the T-tube drainage system.

A postoperative T-tube cholangiogram can identify retained stones. Direct visualization of the biliary tract with an endoscope (*choledochoscopy*) enables the removal of calculi retained in the common bile duct. Choledochoscopy is performed through a T tube or an incision into the common bile duct. An instrument with a small basket-like attachment is used to snare the stone (Fig. 62–5). If this method fails, a fiberoptic endoscope is introduced into the duodenum. An incision into the papillae (papillotomy) allows the stone to pass into the duodenum.

The preoperative and postoperative nursing care measures for the client undergoing gallbladder surgical procedures are the same as those for cholecystectomy (see Cholecystitis earlier).

 Continuing Care

Most often, the client with cholelithiasis has surgery and is discharged home postoperatively (see earlier under Cholecystitis). More frequently than in the past, the client is discharged with a T-tube drainage system intact (see Chart 62–3).

The nurse provides information to the client and the family about the potential for postcholecystectomy syndrome. The clinical manifestations of biliary tract disease occur after cholecystectomy in a small percentage of clients. Postcholecystectomy syndrome is caused by residual or recurring calculi or inflammation or stricture of the common bile duct.

The nurse instructs the client to report symptoms of biliary tract disease to the physician or the nurse practitioner, including jaundice of the skin or sclera, darkened urine, light-colored stools, pain, fever, or chills.

Cancer of the Gallbladder

Overview

Primary cancer of the gallbladder is rare. Adenocarcinoma and squamous cell carcinoma of the gallbladder account for the majority of gallbladder cancers. They typically

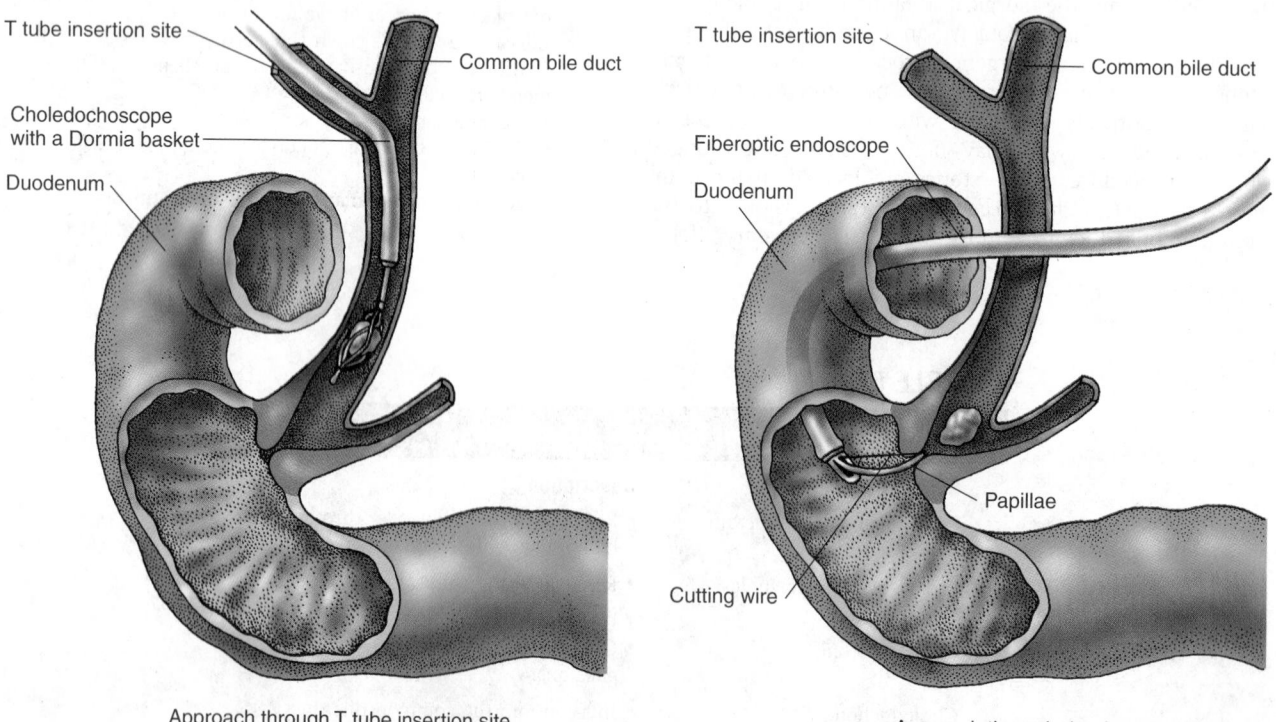

Approach through T tube insertion site

Approach through duodenum

Figure 62–5. Cholendoscopic removal of gallstones.

infiltrate the liver and ducts, as well as the gallbladder. These rare gallbladder carcinomas appear more frequently in clients with pre-existing chronic cholecystitis and cholelithiasis.

The diagnosis of gallbladder cancer is difficult. Early symptoms are insidious in onset and similar to those of chronic cholecystitis and cholelithiasis. Characteristic signs and symptoms include

- Anorexia
- Weight loss
- Nausea
- Vomiting
- General malaise
- Jaundice
- Hepatosplenomegaly
- Chronic, progressively severe epigastric or right upper quadrant pain

A moderately tender, irregularly shaped mass may be palpated. Often, gallbladder carcinoma is discovered during oral cholecystography for diagnosis of suspected cholecystitis or during cholecystectomy.

Collaborative Management

The prognosis for the client with cancer of the gallbladder is poor. Surgical intervention is usually performed and may be extensive. A bile drainage tube (transhepatic biliary catheter) may be inserted to relieve symptoms such as jaundice and itching (see Chart 62–4).

PANCREATIC DISORDERS

Acute Pancreatitis

Overview

Acute pancreatitis is a serious and, at times, life-threatening inflammatory process of the pancreas, resulting in autodigestion of the organ by its own enzymes. The pathologic changes occur in variable degrees. The severity of pancreatitis depends on the extent of inflammation and tissue destruction, ranging from mild involvement evidenced by edema and inflammation to necrotizing hemorrhagic pancreatitis. This severe form of pancreatitis is characterized by diffusely bleeding pancreatic tissue with fibrosis and tissue death.

Pathophysiology

The activation of an inflammatory process of the pancreas may occur after any insult or injury that causes obstruction of the pancreatic duct. Direct toxic injury to the pancreatic cells and the production and release of pancreatic enzymes (trypsin, elastase, phospholipase A, lipase, and kallikrein) result from the obstructive damage. After pancreatic duct obstruction, increased pressure within the pancreas and the pancreatic ducts may contribute to ductal rupture, allowing spillage of trypsin and other enzymes into the pancreatic parenchymal tissue.

In acute pancreatitis, four major pathophysiologic processes occur: lipolysis, proteolysis, necrosis of blood vessels, and inflammation.

Lipolysis

The hallmark of pancreatic necrosis is enzymatic fat necrosis of the endocrine and exocrine cells of the pancreas by the enzyme lipase. Fatty acids are released during this lipolytic process and combine with ionized calcium to form a soap-like product. The initial rapid lowering of serum calcium levels is not readily compensated for by the parathyroid gland. Because the body needs ionized calcium and cannot use bound calcium, hypocalcemia occurs.

Proteolysis

The pathogenesis of pancreatitis involves autodigestion of the pancreatic parenchyma organ by the enzymes normally produced by the pancreas (Fig. 62–6). Trypsin activates the major proteolytic enzymes involved in autodigestion. The agent that triggers the premature activation of these enzymes has not been identified and is being investigated. Proteolysis involves the splitting of proteins by hydrolysis of the peptide bonds, with the formation of smaller polypeptides. Proteolytic activity may lead to thrombosis and gangrene of the pancreas. Pancreatic destruction may be localized and confined to one area or may involve the entire organ.

Necrosis of Blood Vessels

Elastase is activated by trypsin, causing the dissolving of elastic fibers of the blood vessels and ducts. The necrosis of blood vessels results in bleeding, ranging from minor bleeding to massive hemorrhage of pancreatic tissue. Another pancreatic enzyme, kallikrein, causes the release of vasoactive peptides, bradykinin, and a plasma kinin known as kallidin. These substances contribute to vasodilation and increased vascular permeability, further compounding the hemorrhagic process. This massive destruction of blood vessels by necrosis may lead to generalized hemorrhage, with blood escaping into the retroperitoneal tissues. The client with hemorrhagic pancreatitis is critically ill, and extensive pancreatic destruction and shock may lead to death. The majority of deaths in clients with acute pancreatitis result from irreversible shock.

Inflammation

The inflammatory stage occurs when leukocytes cluster around the hemorrhagic and necrotic areas of the pancreas. A secondary bacterial process may lead to suppuration of the pancreatic parenchyma or formation of an abscess (see later discussion of pancreatic abscess). Mild infected lesions may be absorbed. When these infected lesions are severe, calcification and fibrosis occur. If the infected fluid becomes walled off by fibrous tissue, a pancreatic pseudocyst is formed (discussed later in this chapter).

Theories of Enzyme Activation

Several theories explain the triggering mechanisms leading to enzyme activation in acute pancreatitis. The bile reflux ("common channel") theory proposes that an obstruction

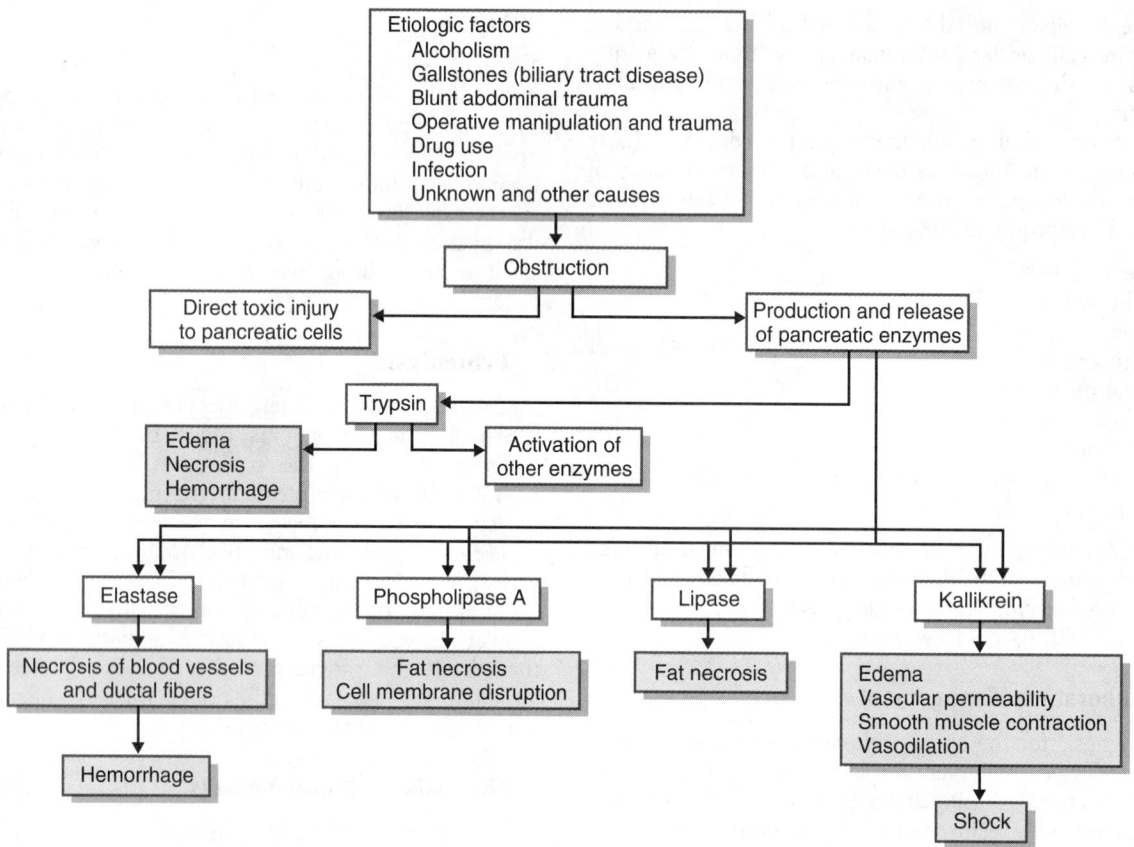

Figure 62–6. The process of autodigestion in acute pancreatitis.

of the common channel (the common bile duct and the main pancreatic duct channel) causes reflux of the bile into the pancreatic tissue, resulting in activation of the enzymes. Not all biliary tracts have this common channel. If the common channel is absent, the common bile and pancreatic ducts merge into the duodenum separately.

According to the hypersecretion-obstruction theory, rupture of the pancreatic duct occurs, with disruption or tearing of the cell membrane, allowing pancreatic secretions and enzymes to leak back into the parenchymal tissue.

The exact mechanism of alcohol-induced changes in pancreatitis is unclear. Alcohol appears to have a direct metabolic effect on the pancreas by stimulating hydrochloric acid and secretin production, which in turn stimulates exocrine functions of the pancreas. Alcohol also causes edema of the duodenum and the ampulla of Vater, obstructing the flow of pancreatic secretions. Alcohol may decrease the tone of the sphincter of Oddi and cause sphincter spasm with duodenal reflux.

According to the fourth theory, reflux of duodenal contents can occur from biliary tract disease, gallstones in the bile duct (causing the sphincter of Oddi to dilate), or generalized loss of tone caused by alcohol ingestion. Duodenal contents can enter the pancreatic duct through the weakened sphincter, activating the pancreatic enzymes.

The generalized abdominal pain of acute pancreatitis is related to peritoneal irritation. Ductal release of digested proteins and lipids into the peripancreatic tissues, along

with stretching of the pancreatic tissue, causes the seepage of these substances into the mesentery. The resultant peritonitis stimulates the sensory nerves, contributing to intense pain in the back and flanks.

Complications of Acute Pancreatitis

Acute pancreatitis may result in severe, life-threatening complications. Jaundice occurs from swelling of the head of the pancreas, which impedes bile flow through the common bile duct. The bile duct may also be compressed by calculi or a pancreatic pseudocyst, with total bile flow obstruction, resulting in severe jaundice. Transient hyperglycemia from the release of glucagon and the decreased release of insulin results from damage to the pancreatic islet cells.

Left lung pleural effusions frequently develop in the client with acute pancreatitis. Amylase effusions probably occur when exudate containing pancreatic enzymes passes from the peritoneal cavity into the pleural cavity via the transdiaphragmatic lymph channels. Atelectasis and pneumonia may also occur, especially in elderly clients.

Multisystem organ failure occurs as a sequela to necrotizing hemorrhagic pancreatitis. The client is at risk for adult respiratory distress syndrome (ARDS). This severe form of pulmonary edema is caused by disruption of the alveolar-capillary membrane and is a serious complication of acute pancreatitis. (see Chapter 34 for a discussion of ARDS). In acute pancreatitis, pulmonary failure accounts for more than half of all deaths that occur in the first 7 days of the disease.

Coagulation defects are another major potential complication and may result in death. Complex physiologic changes in the pancreas cause release of necrotic tissue and enzymes into the bloodstream, resulting in altered coagulation. Disseminated intravascular coagulation (DIC) involves hypercoagulation of the blood, with consumption of clotting factors and the development of microthrombi.

Shock in acute pancreatitis results from peripheral vasodilation from the released vasoactive substances and the retroperitoneal loss of protein-rich fluid from proteolytic digestion. Hypovolemia may result in decreased renal perfusion and acute renal failure (Ambrose & Dreher, 1996). Paralytic ileus results from peritoneal irritation and seepage of pancreatic enzymes into the abdominal cavity.

Etiology

The cause of pancreatitis is not known. Many factors can produce injury to the pancreas. Most commonly cited are alcoholism and biliary tract disease with gallstones. Iatrogenic acute pancreatitis may occur as a result of trauma from surgical manipulation after biliary tract, pancreatic, gastric, and duodenal procedures, such as cholecystectomy, the Whipple procedure, and partial gastrectomy.

Other etiologic factors include

- Pancreatic tumors, cysts, and abscesses
- Abnormal organ structure
- Penetrating gastric or duodenal ulcers, resulting in peritonitis
- Viral infections, such as with coxsackievirus B
- Toxicities of drugs, including opiates, sulfonamides, thiazides, steroids, and oral contraceptives

The exact mechanism by which these and other drugs cause pancreatitis is unknown.

Blunt abdominal trauma, as well as metabolic disturbances (e.g., hyperparathyroidism and hyperlipidemia), has caused episodes of pancreatitis. Pancreatic inflammation has been reported after renal failure, fasciculitis (inflammation of fascia), renal transplantation, and endoscopic retrograde cholangiopancreatography (ERCP), a diagnostic procedure.

Heredity has been cited as a predisposing factor; in some cases, neurogenic or emotional factors have been involved. In many cases, the cause is never identified (i.e., idiopathic acute pancreatitis).

Incidence/Prevalence

Alcoholism is the most frequent cause of acute pancreatitis in the middle-aged male population. Episodes of pancreatitis usually occur after excessive alcohol consumption. These attacks are especially common during holidays and vacations. Steady, heavy alcohol intake for 5–10 years is likely to produce pancreatitis. Women are affected most often after cholelithiasis and biliary tract disturbances.

Of clients with acute pancreatitis, death results in approximately 10%. With early diagnosis and treatment, mortality can be reduced. Death occurs at a higher rate in the elderly population and in clients with postoperative pancreatitis. The prognosis for recovery is favorable for pancreatitis associated with biliary tract disease and poor if pancreatitis accompanies alcoholism. Mortality rises as high as 60% when necrosis and hemorrhage occur.

Collaborative Management

 Assessment

➤ History

The nurse asks the client with acute pancreatitis to state the reason for seeking medical treatment. Most often, the primary reason is relief of abdominal pain. The nurse asks the client whether abdominal pain is related to alcohol ingestion or eating a high-fat meal. The nurse asks the client about alcohol intake, including the amount of alcohol consumed during what period of time. The client is questioned about a family history of alcoholism, pancreatitis, or biliary tract disease. The client is asked whether any biliary tract problems, such as gallstones, have been experienced. The nurse determines whether any abdominal surgical interventions, such as cholecystectomy, or diagnostic procedures, such as ERCP, have been performed recently.

The nurse assesses for the presence of other medical problems known to cause pancreatitis, including peptic ulcer disease, renal failure, vascular disorders, hyperparathyroidism, and hyperlipidemia.

The client is asked whether any recent viral infections have been experienced and to list all prescription and over-the-counter (OTC) drugs taken recently.

➤ Physical Assessment/Clinical Manifestations

Clinical manifestations of acute pancreatitis vary widely and depend on the severity of the inflammation. Typically, a client is diagnosed after presenting with abdominal pain, the most frequent symptom. The nurse obtains in-depth data about the pain. The client often states that the pain had a sudden onset and is located in the mid–epigastric area or the left upper quadrant, with radiation to the back, left flank, or left shoulder. The pain is described as intense and continuous. The client may admit that the pain has been aggravated by eating a fatty meal, ingesting alcohol, or lying in a recumbent position. The nurse determines whether the pain is relieved by positioning. Often, the client finds relief by assuming the fetal position (with the knees drawn up to the chest and the spine flexed) or when sitting upright and bending forward.

The client may report weight loss with nausea and vomiting. When performing an abdominal assessment, the nurse may find the following on inspection:
- Generalized jaundice
- Gray-blue discoloration of the abdomen and periumbilical area (Cullen's sign)
- Gray-blue discoloration of the flanks (Turner's sign), caused by pancreatic enzyme leakage to cutaneous tissue from the peritoneal cavity

The nurse listens for bowel sounds; absent or decreased

bowel sounds usually indicate paralytic (adynamic) ileus. On light palpation, the nurse notes abdominal tenderness, rigidity, and guarding from peritonitis. A palpable mass may be found if a pancreatic pseudocyst is present. Pancreatic ascites creates a dull sound on percussion.

The nurse or assistive nursing personnel takes and records vital signs frequently to assess for elevated temperature, tachycardia, and decreased blood pressure. The nurse uses these data to determine whether complications are occurring. Respiratory complications, such as left lung pleural effusions, atelectasis, and pneumonia, are common in clients with acute pancreatitis. The nurse performs a respiratory assessment, auscultating the lung fields for adventitious sounds or decreased aeration, and observes respirations for dyspnea or orthopnea.

The nurse assesses changes in vital signs, which may indicate the life-threatening complication of shock. Hypotension and tachycardia may result from pancreatic hemorrhage, excessive fluid volume shifting, or the toxic effects of abdominal sepsis from enzyme damage. The nurse also observes the client for changes in behavior and sensorium that may be related to alcohol withdrawal or indicate hypoxia or impending sepsis with shock.

➤ Psychosocial Assessment

Excessive alcohol intake, particularly in men, is the most frequent cause of acute pancreatitis. Thus, the nurse tactfully explores the client's alcohol intake history. The nurse and the client discuss the intake of alcohol and the reasons for overindulging. The nurse asks the client when increased drinking episodes occur. In particular, the nurse asks whether binges occur during holidays, vacations, or weekends or revolve around particular activities, such as card playing or television viewing. The nurse also questions whether the client has recently experienced any traumatic event, such as the death of a family member or a job loss, that may have contributed to increased alcohol consumption.

➤ Laboratory Assessment

Diagnostic laboratory abnormalities are found in clients with acute pancreatitis (Table 62–4). Elevated serum amylase and lipase levels provide the most reliable and direct evidence of pancreatitis and are considered the cardinal diagnostic signs of pancreatitis. Serum amylase levels usually increase in 12–24 hours and remain elevated for 3–4 days. Lipase is considered more specific in the diagnosis of acute pancreatitis, and serum levels remain elevated for up to 2 weeks. Amylase levels in 2-hour urine collections are also elevated owing to the inflammatory process and remain elevated for up to 2 weeks. If pancreatitis is accompanied by biliary dysfunction, serum bilirubin and alkaline phosphatase levels are elevated. Elevated white blood cell count and serum glucose levels are also common in acute pancreatitis (Ambrose & Dreher, 1996).

Decreased serum calcium and magnesium levels are seen with fat necrosis. Calcium levels may fall and remain decreased for 7–10 days. Calcium levels that consistently remain below 8 mg/dL are associated with a poor prognosis.

➤ Radiographic Assessment

Computed tomography (CT) provides a reliable diagnosis of acute pancreatitis. This noninvasive technique may be used to rule out pancreatic pseudocyst or ductal calculi. A chest x-ray may reveal hemidiaphragm elevation on the left side or pleural effusion.

➤ Other Diagnostic Assessment

In the client with severe pancreatitis, ultrasonography and magnetic resonance imaging (MRI) of the pancreas help confirm an initial clinical impression, assess for the degree of inflammatory resolution, and reveal common bile duct dilation from obstruction or gallstones.

A bentiromide test may also be performed to assess pancreatic functioning. A pancreas-specific medication

TABLE 62–4

Causes of Laboratory Diagnostic Abnormalities in Acute Pancreatitis

Abnormal Finding	Cause
Cardinal Diagnostic Tests	
Increased *serum* amylase	• Pancreatic cell injury
Elevated *serum* lipase	• Pancreatic cell injury
Elevated *urine* amylase	• Pancreatic cell injury
Other Diagnostic Tests	
Elevated serum glucose	• Pancreatic beta-cell injury, resulting in impaired carbohydrate metabolism
Decreased serum calcium	• Fatty acids combined with calcium; seen in fat necrosis
Elevated bilirubin	• Hepatobiliary obstructive process
Elevated alkaline phosphatase	• Hepatobiliary involvement
Elevated white blood cell count	• Inflammatory response

(bentiromide) is given to the client who has had nothing by mouth after midnight. The medication is broken down by the pancreas in a manner similar to that in which the normal pancreas assists in food digestion. A 6-hour urine specimen is obtained because part of the drug is secreted in the urine. Pancreatic function is determined by the amount of drug found in the urine specimen.

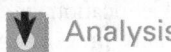 Analysis

➤ Common Nursing Diagnoses and Collaborative Problems

The following priority diagnoses occur commonly in clients with acute pancreatitis:
1. Pain related to the effects of pancreatic inflammation and enzyme leakage
2. Altered Nutrition: Less than Body Requirements related to the effects of pancreatic dysfunction, nausea, vomiting, and anorexia

➤ Additional Nursing Diagnoses and Collaborative Problems

The client may also have one or more of the following nursing diagnoses:
- Fluid Volume Deficit related to pancreatic hemorrhage, fluid loss into the abdominal cavity, and vomiting
- Ineffective Breathing Pattern related to the complications of pleural effusion or adult respiratory distress syndrome
- Risk for Activity Intolerance related to debilitation
- Anxiety related to severe illness and possible chronic condition
- Sleep Pattern Disturbance related to pain
- Altered Health Maintenance related to a knowledge deficit about the illness, its causative factors, and the treatment plan

The client with pancreatitis is also likely to have a Potential for Hyperglycemia.

 Planning and Implementation

➤ Pain

Planning: Expected Outcomes. The client is expected to experience relief of abdominal pain.

Interventions. Abdominal pain is the prominent symptom of pancreatitis. The main focus of nursing care is aimed at reducing discomfort and pain by the use of measures that decrease gastrointestinal (GI) tract activity, thus decreasing pancreatic stimulation.

Nonsurgical Management. The health care team initially attempts to achieve pain relief with nonsurgical interventions. These interventions include fasting, drug therapy, and comfort measures.

Fasting. In an effort to rest the pancreas and reduce pancreatic enzyme secretion, food and fluids are withheld in the acute period. The health care provider orders IV

fluid administration to maintain hydration. IV replacement of calcium and magnesium may also be needed.

Nasogastric (NG) drainage and suction may be necessary to decrease gastric distention and to suppress pancreatic secretion. Gastric decompression prevents gastric digestive juices from flowing into the duodenum. Because paralytic (adynamic) ileus is a common complication of acute pancreatitis, prolonged nasogastric intubation may be necessary. The nurse assesses for the presence of bowel sounds before the NG tube is removed.

Drug Therapy. Meperidine hydrochloride (Demerol) is the drug of choice for relieving abdominal pain associated with acute pancreatitis. Meperidine hydrochloride causes less incidence of spasm of the smooth musculature of the pancreatic ducts and the sphincter of Oddi than do opiate drugs, such as morphine. In mild pancreatitis, the pain usually subsides in 3–4 days; however, with severe, acute pancreatitis, the abdominal pain and tenderness may persist for up to 2 weeks. The nurse individualizes dosages and intervals of medication administration, as ordered, according to the severity of the disease and the symptoms.

Pancreatic stimulation is reduced by decreasing the release of secretin. Secretin is an intestinal hormone that stimulates the release of enzymes and bicarbonate from the pancreas when acidic chyme is present in the duodenum. Antacids administered orally or via an NG tube that is clamped for 20 minutes neutralize gastric secretions. The health care provider orders histamine receptor antagonists, such as ranitidine hydrochloride (Zantac), to decrease hydrochloric acid production so that pancreatic enzymes are not activated by an acid pH. These interventions also are useful in reducing the occurrence of GI erosion and bleeding. Anticholinergics, such as dicyclomine hydrochloride (Bentyl, Lomine✢), are indicated to decrease vagal stimulation, decrease GI motility, and inhibit pancreatic enzyme and bicarbonate volume and concentration.

Comfort Measures. Helping the client to assume the fetal position (with the legs drawn up to the chest) may decrease the abdominal pain of pancreatitis.

If the client has an NG tube in place, the nurse provides frequent oral hygiene measures to keep mucous membranes moist and free from inflammation or crusting. Because of the drying effect of anticholinergic drugs and the absence of oral fluids, the mouth and oral cavity may be extremely dry and parched, causing considerable discomfort for the client.

Pain may also be substantially reduced by lowering the client's anxiety level. The nurse provides thorough explanations of procedures. The client is encouraged to express the emotions and responses he or she is experiencing. The nurse also provides reassurance and diversional activities, such as television, music, and reading material, and encourages visitors to direct attention away from pain.

Surgical Management. Surgical intervention for acute pancreatitis is usually not indicated. However, complications of pancreatitis, such as pancreatic pseudocyst and abscess, may necessitate surgical drainage. If pancreatitis is caused by biliary tract obstruction, the physician may perform a laparotomy (abdominal exploration) for common bile duct exploration and the release of obstruction.

Preoperative Care. In addition to general preoperative care measures, the client usually has a nasogastric tube inserted and begins IV fluids. The nurse teaches the client to expect a pancreatic drainage tube and explains its care during the postoperative period.

Operative Procedure. When an abscess or pseudocyst is incised and drained under general anesthesia, drainage tubes are inserted, sutured in place, and connected to low suction (80 mmHg or less) to prevent further tissue erosion.

Postoperative Care. Postoperatively, the nurse monitors drainage tubes for patency by assessing for kinks in the tubes and maintaining the ordered drain suction pressure and system integrity. The nurse records the output amount from the drain and describes the character of the drainage. A sump-type drain is usually inserted. The nurse ascertains that the drain is functioning, indicated by a hissing noise from the sump lumen.

The nurse provides meticulous skin care and dressing changes. The nurse monitors for the first signs of redness or skin irritation because pancreatic enzyme drainage is particularly excoriating to the skin. Skin barriers, such as a Stomahesive wafer around the drainage tube and aluminum paste, are applied to repel drainage from the skin. The nurse continually assesses for further deterioration of the tissue. The nurse also collaborates with an enterostomal therapist (ET) for measures to promote skin integrity, such as the use of individualized ostomy appliances and the application of topical ointments.

➤ Altered Nutrition: Less Than Body Requirements

Planning: Expected Outcomes. The client is expected to have sufficient nutritional intake to maintain body weight and a decrease in pancreatic stimulation.

Interventions. The client is maintained on nothing-by-mouth status in the early stages of pancreatitis. If the client is severely nutritionally depleted, total parenteral nutrition (TPN) is indicated (see Chap. 64). If TPN is used for nutritional support, the nurse assesses for glucose intolerance by monitoring for elevated blood glucose levels. This is extremely important in clients with pancreatitis because pancreatic dysfunction affects the release of insulin. Some clients require insulin administration during an acute episode of the disease.

When food is tolerated during the recovery phase, the physician usually orders small, frequent, moderate- to high-carbohydrate, high-protein, low-fat meals. Foods should be bland with little spice; caffeine-containing foods, such as tea, coffee, and cola, as well as alcohol should be avoided.

To boost caloric intake, commercial liquid preparations, such as Ensure and Isocal, supplement the diet. If caloric intake is less than desired, a nasogastric tube may be required for enteral feedings. The health care provider may also prescribe fat-soluble and other vitamin and mineral replacement supplements.

 Continuing Care

➤ *Health Teaching*

Education needs to be started early in the hospitalization period but after acute episodes of pain have subsided. The nurse assesses the client's and family members' or significant others' knowledge of the disease.

The goals of discharge planning and education are to avoid further episodes of pancreatitis and prevent progression to a chronic disease. The nurse instructs the client to abstain from alcohol to prevent further pain attacks and extension of inflammation and pancreatic insufficiency. The nurse tells the client that, if alcohol is consumed, pain will be experienced, and further autodigestion of the pancreas will lead to chronic pancreatitis and chronic pain.

The nurse also teaches the client to notify the physician after discharge to home if acute abdominal pain or biliary tract disease (as evidenced by jaundice, clay-colored stools, or darkened urine) occurs. These signs and symptoms are possible indicators of complications or disease progression.

➤ *Home Care Management*

Little special preparation is needed at the client's home, but home care measures must be individualized for each client's circumstances. Some clients with acute pancreatitis may be severely weakened from their acute illness and need to confine activity to one floor, limiting stair climbing and other strenuous activities until they regain their strength.

➤ *Health Care Resources*

Clients with acute pancreatitis require visits by a home health nurse if the hospital course was complicated. In these cases, home health care may be needed for wound care and assistance with activities of daily living (ADL). The client requires medical follow-up with the primary care physician or nurse practitioner for monitoring of the disease process. For clients with alcoholism, the nurse provides information about community assistance resources, such as Alcoholics Anonymous (AA). Family members may attend support groups such as Al-Anon and Al-Ateen.

 Evaluation

On the basis of the identified nursing diagnoses and collaborative problems, the nurse evaluates the care of the client with acute pancreatitis. Expected outcomes include that the client will

- Experience an alleviation of or reduction in abdominal pain
- Maintain adequate nutritional intake with a decrease in pancreatic stimulation
- Not experience a recurrence of pancreatitis

Chronic Pancreatitis

Overview

Chronic pancreatitis is a progressive, destructive disease of the pancreas, characterized by remissions and exacerbations (recurrence). Inflammation and fibrosis of the tissue contribute to pancreatic insufficiency and diminished function of the organ. Chronic pancreatitis usually develops after repeated episodes of alcohol-induced acute pancreatitis. It may also be associated with chronic obstruction of the common bile duct. Chronic pancreatitis may develop in the absence of a known acute disorder.

Pathophysiology

Types of Chronic Pancreatitis

Alcohol-induced chronic pancreatitis is also known as *chronic calcifying pancreatitis* (CCP). It is characterized by protein precipitates that plug the ducts and lead to ductal obstruction, atrophy, and dilation. As the protein plugging becomes diffuse, the epithelium of the ducts undergoes histologic changes, resulting in metaplasia (cell replacement) and ulceration. This inflammatory process causes fibrosis of the pancreatic tissue. Intraductal calcification and marked pancreatic parenchymal destruction develop in the late stages of chronic pancreatitis. Cystic sacs containing pancreatic secretions and enzymes form on the pancreas. The organ becomes hard and firm as a result of acinar cell atrophy and pancreatic insufficiency.

Chronic obstructive pancreatitis develops from inflammation, spasm, and obstruction of the sphincter of Oddi. Inflammatory and sclerotic lesions occur in the head of the pancreas and around the ducts, causing an obstruction and backflow of pancreatic secretions (see the earlier discussion of acute pancreatitis and its complications).

Pathophysiologic Changes

Pancreatic insufficiency in chronic pancreatitis is characterized by the loss of exocrine function. Pancreatic exocrine secretion is divided into two components: aqueous bicarbonate and enzymes.

The aqueous component neutralizes the duodenal contents and pancreatic enzymes that are essential to normal digestion and absorption. Most clients with chronic pancreatitis have a decreased output of pancreatic secretion and bicarbonate. Pancreatic enzyme secretion must be reduced by more than 80% to produce steatorrhea resulting from severe malabsorption of fats. These characteristic stools are pale, bulky, and frothy and have an offensive odor. The action of colonic bacteria on unabsorbed lipids and proteins is responsible for the foul odor. On inspection of the stools, the fat content is visible. In severe chronic pancreatitis, stool fat output may exceed 40 g/day.

Fat malabsorption also contributes to weight loss and muscle wasting, or a decrease in muscle mass, and leads to general debilitation of the client. Protein malabsorption results in a "starvation" edema of the feet, legs, and hands caused by decreased levels of circulating albumin.

The loss of pancreatic endocrine function is responsible for the development of frank diabetes mellitus in clients with chronic pancreatic insufficiency (see Chapter 68 for a complete discussion of diabetes mellitus).

The client with chronic pancreatitis may have pulmonary complications, such as pleuritic pain, pleural effusions, and pulmonary infiltrates. Pancreatic ascites may impede diaphragmatic excursion and decrease lung expansion, resulting in impaired ventilation. In the ill client with chronic pancreatitis, adult respiratory distress syndrome may develop.

Etiology

The cause of chronic calcifying pancreatitis is persistent excessive alcohol intake that results in repeated episodes of acute pancreatitis. The most common cause of chronic obstructive pancreatitis is cholelithiasis and biliary tract disease, which results in persistent inflammation. Other etiologic factors include pancreatic pseudocyst, postoperative ductal scarring, and cancer of the pancreas or duodenum. All of these factors can produce obstruction of the pancreatic duct. Prolonged starvation and prolonged use of parenteral feedings for nutritional support can result in pancreatic atrophy, causing pancreatic insufficiency.

Incidence/Prevalence

Alcohol-induced pancreatitis is predominantly found in men, but the incidence in women is increasing. In women, it occurs more frequently among those with biliary tract disease (cholecystitis and cholelithiasis). The age at occurrence of chronic pancreatitis is variable but is usually between 45 and 60 years.

Collaborative Management

 Assessment

Clinical manifestations of chronic pancreatitis differ from those of an acute inflammation. Abdominal pain is the major clinical manifestation (Chart 62–5). The client with

---

Chart 62–5

Key Features of Chronic Pancreatitis

- Intense abdominal pain (major clinical manifestation) that is continuous and burning or gnawing
- Abdominal tenderness
- Ascites
- Possible left upper quadrant mass (if pseudocyst or abscess is present)
- Respiratory compromise manifested by adventitious or diminished breath sounds, dyspnea, or orthopnea
- Steatorrhea; clay-colored stools
- Weight loss
- Jaundice
- Dark urine
- Polyuria, polydipsia, polyphagia (diabetes mellitus)

chronic pancreatitis typically describes the pain as a continuous burning or gnawing dullness with periods of acute exacerbation. The pain is intense and relentless. The frequency of acute exacerbations may increase as the pancreatic fibrosis develops.

The nurse performs the same abdominal assessment as for clients with acute pancreatitis, but the findings may not be as significant. Abdominal tenderness is less intense. A mass may be palpated in the left upper quadrant, indicative of a pancreatic pseudocyst or abscess (see later). Massive pancreatic ascites may be present, producing dullness on abdominal percussion.

Because respiratory complications can accompany the condition, the nurse performs a respiratory assessment, auscultating the lung fields for adventitious sounds or decreased aeration. The nurse observes respirations for dyspnea or orthopnea.

The client is asked to collect a random stool specimen, if able, or asked to describe the stools. The nurse inspects the specimen for the presence of steatorrhea. These foul-smelling fatty stools may increase in volume as pancreatic insufficiency progresses and lipase production decreases. The nurse observes the client's anal area for excoriation resulting from frequent defecation.

The client may also experience weight loss, muscle wasting, jaundice, dark urine, and the signs and symptoms of diabetes mellitus, such as polyuria, polydipsia, and polyphagia.

In chronic pancreatitis, significant laboratory findings include elevated serum bilirubin, alkaline phosphatase, and amylase levels. Transient serum glucose elevations are common. Stool specimens may be examined for elevated levels of fat and trypsin.

The only definitive diagnostic test for chronic pancreatitis is the identification of calcification of pancreatic tissue in a biopsy specimen. The physician may order a secretin test to assess pancreatic exocrine function. Secretin is a hormone that stimulates hepatic and pancreatic secretion. In this test, the client swallows a double-lumen gastrointestinal (GI) tube. The tip should reach the duodenum, with the proximal lumen port located in the stomach. Gastric and duodenal contents are aspirated before and after IV administration of secretin. Abnormally low volumes of enzymes and bicarbonate in the GI contents may indicate chronic pancreatitis.

Abdominal ultrasonography is also a helpful diagnostic tool, especially to reveal pseudocysts. Endoscopic retrograde cholangiopancreatography may reveal ductal system abnormalities, such as calcification and strictures, or it may delineate the presence of pancreatic pseudocyst.

Interventions

The focus of caring for the client with chronic pancreatitis is to manage pain and assist the client in maintaining a sufficient nutritional intake.

Nonsurgical Management. Nonsurgical interventions primarily include drug and diet therapy.

Drug Therapy. The major intervention for the pain of chronic pancreatitis is drug therapy. In addition, the nurse teaches the client to avoid ingesting irritating substances that can precipitate pain.

Analgesia. The nurse medicates the client, as ordered, according to the assessment of the level and intensity of pain, and evaluates the effectiveness of the drug intervention. Opioid analgesia with meperidine hydrochloride (Demerol) is most frequently used, but opioid dependency may become a problem. Nonopioid analgesics may be tried to relieve pain (see Chapter 9 for other interventions for chronic pain).

If drug dependency becomes a problem, behavior modification programs and drug and alcohol counseling are necessary. The health care provider may need to admit these clients to drug and alcohol dependency programs.

Enzyme Replacement. Pancreatic enzymes are essential dietary supplements (Chart 62–6). These are generally given with meals or snacks to aid in digestion and absorption of fat and protein. Drugs such as pancreatin (Dizymes tablets) and pancrelipase (Cotazym, Viokase, or Pancrease) are prescribed in capsule, tablet, or powder form and contain amylase, lipase, and protease. Cotazym also contains calcium carbonate to increase depleted calcium levels. The nurse mixes the powder form in applesauce or a fruit juice to make it more palatable. Enzyme preparations should not be mixed with foods containing proteins because the enzymatic action dissolves the food into a watery substance. The nurse advises the client to wipe his or her lips with a wet towel to prevent the skin irritation and breakdown that residual enzymes can cause.

The dosage of pancreatic enzymes depends on the severity of malabsorption and maldigestion. The nurse records the number of stools per day and the stool consistency to monitor the effectiveness of enzyme therapy. If pancreatic enzyme treatment is effective, the stools should become less frequent and less fatty.

Insulin Therapy. If the client has diabetes, the health care provider prescribes insulin or oral hypoglycemic agents for glucose control. Clients maintained on TPN are particularly susceptible to labile glucose levels and may require regular insulin additives to the solution. The nurse closely monitors blood glucose levels so that hyper-

---

Chart 62–6

Nursing Care Highlight: Enzyme Replacement for the Client with Chronic Pancreatitis

- Give pancreatic enzymes before or with meals.
- Tell the client to swallow the tablets without chewing to minimize oral irritation.
- Mix the powder form in applesauce or fruit juice.
- Do not mix enzyme preparations in protein-containing foods.
- Have the client wipe his or her lips after taking enzymes to avoid skin irritation.
- Do not crush enteric-coated preparations.
- Monitor serum uric acid levels (pancrelipase can cause an increase in uric acid levels).

glycemia is controlled and insulin or diabetic shock is prevented. The use of glucose monitoring meters allows frequent assessment of glucose levels during the critical insulin dosage adjustment period. The nurse, laboratory technician, or assistive nursing personnel checks glucose levels every 2–4 hours.

Other Drugs. The health care provider may also prescribe histamine receptor antagonists, such as ranitidine hydrochloride (Zantac), to decrease gastric acid. Gastric acid destroys the lipase needed to break down fats.

Diet Therapy. Protein and fat malabsorption results in significant weight loss and decreased muscle mass in the client with chronic pancreatitis. Therefore, the nutritional interventions for the client with acute pancreatitis are also relevant for clients in the chronic phase of pancreatitis. The client often limits food intake to avoid the recurrent pain, which is exacerbated by eating. For this reason, nutrition maintenance is often difficult to achieve, and clients are provided with TPN, including vitamin and mineral replacement.

For long-term dietary management, the client needs increased calories, up to 4000–6000 kcal/day, to maintain weight. Foods high in carbohydrates and protein also assist in the healing process. Foods high in fat are avoided because they cause or increase diarrhea.

Surgical Management. Surgery is not a primary intervention for the treatment of chronic pancreatitis. It may be indicated for intractable abdominal pain, incapacitating relapses of pain, or complications, such as abscesses and pseudocysts.

The underlying pathologic changes determine the procedure indicated. The surgeon incises and drains an abscess or pseudocyst. Cholecystectomy or choledochotomy (incision of the common bile duct) is indicated if biliary tract disease is an underlying cause of pancreatitis. If the pancreatic duct sphincter is fibrotic, the surgeon performs a sphincterotomy (incision of the sphincter) to enlarge it.

In pancreaticojejunostomy, the pancreatic duct is opened and anastomosed to the jejunum to relieve obstruction. This procedure relieves pain and preserves pancreatic tissue and function. The preoperative and postoperative care are similar to those for clients undergoing the Whipple procedure (see Pancreatic Carcinoma later). A partial pancreatectomy (resection of the pancreas) may be performed for clients with advanced pancreatitis or disabling pain. Vagotomy with gastric antrectomy is done to alter nerve stimulation and decrease pancreatic secretion (see Chapter 58 for a discussion of nursing care).

In a few cases, a pancreas transplantation may be done. However, this procedure is performed most often for clients with severe, uncontrolled diabetes. (Chapter 68 discusses pancreas transplantation.)

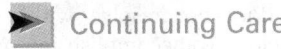 Continuing Care

➤ *Health Teaching*

Because there is no known cure for chronic pancreatitis, client and family education is aimed at preventing further acute exacerbations of this chronic disease, providing long-term care, and promoting health maintenance (Chart 62–7).

Diet Therapy. The nurse instructs the client to avoid known precipitating factors, such as the ingestion of caffeinated beverages and alcohol. The nurse elicits the participation of the family or significant other in diet planning and food preparation. Diet instructions focus on eating bland, low-fat, frequent meals and avoiding rich, fatty foods. The nurse and dietitian stress the importance of dietary compliance and the need for increased nutritional intake to prevent acute exacerbations of this chronic illness. Written instructions on diet and pancreatic enzyme replacement therapy are essential.

The nurse instructs the client and significant other or family members on the importance of adhering to the pancreatic enzyme replacement treatment. The client must take the prescribed enzymes with meals and snacks to aid in the digestion of food and promote the absorption of fats and proteins. The nurse teaches the client to take the enzymes at the beginning of the meal and to report to the health care provider any increase in the occurrence of foul-smelling, frothy, fatty stools; abdominal distention; and cramping so that pancreatic enzyme replacement may be increased as needed. The nurse also instructs the client to report any skin excoriation or breakdown so that therapeutic interventions to promote skin integrity can be instituted.

Skin Care. The frequency of continent or incontinent defecation poses challenging skin care problems. The nurse instructs the client to keep his or her skin dry and free from the abrasive fatty stools that are excoriating to the skin. The skin should be cleaned thoroughly after each stool and a soothing emollient, such as Sween, applied. To prevent breakdown and maintain skin integrity, a skin barrier may be needed. Many products on the market, such as zinc oxide cream, actively repel stool from the skin.

Drug Therapy. The client and family members must be able to state the desired effect of the prescribed drugs, the schedule for drug administration, and potential side effects. The nurse provides written guidelines as reinforcement.

Chart 62–7

Education Guide: Prevention of Exacerbations of Chronic Pancreatitis

- Avoid things that make your symptoms worse, such as drinking caffeinated beverages.
- Avoid alcohol ingestion.
- Eat bland, low-fat meals; avoid gastric stimulants such as spices.
- Eat small meals and snacks high in calories.
- Take the pancreatic enzymes that have been prescribed for you with or before a meal.
- Rest frequently; restrict your activity to one floor until you regain your strength.

If the client develops diabetes mellitus as a result of chronic pancreatitis from endocrine dysfunction, management of elevated glucose levels after discharge from the hospital may necessitate oral hypoglycemic agents or insulin injections. If this is the case, the client and the family require in-depth teaching concerning diabetes, its signs and symptoms, medical management, insulin administration, dietary management, urine and blood glucose monitoring, and general care information. (See Chapter 68 for a discussion of diabetes.)

➤ Home Care Management

The client with chronic pancreatitis is usually discharged to home, but some clients may require care in a long-term care setting.

If the client is discharged to home, the activity area should be limited to one floor until the client regains strength and can increase activity. Toilet facilities must be easily accessible because of chronic steatorrhea and frequent defecation. If toilet facilities are not available in the immediate rest area, a bedpan or bedside commode is obtained for the home.

➤ Health Care Resources

Chronic illnesses are devastating for families. The high costs of medical insurance, medical treatment, and drug therapy cause serious financial problems. Often, the client with chronic pancreatitis is unable or unwilling to work. Case management to coordinate care and manage resources should be instituted during hospitalization.

The client may require home visits by nurses and a dietitian, depending on the severity of the chronic health problems and home maintenance and support needs. The home care nurse assesses the client for pain management, compliance with dietary guidelines and alcohol abstinence, the effectiveness of pancreatic enzyme therapy, and the psychosocial adaptation to a chronic illness.

The nurse or case manager refers the client to a counselor or a self-help group, such as Alcoholics Anonymous, if appropriate.

Pancreatic Abscess

Overview

Pancreatic abscesses are the most serious complication of pancreatitis. If untreated, they are always fatal. After surgery, the recurrence rate is higher than 30%. The abscesses form from collections of purulent liquefaction of the necrotic pancreas.

Pancreatic abscesses occur after severe acute pancreatitis, exacerbations of chronic pancreatitis, and biliary tract surgery. The development of a single abscess or multiple abscesses results from extensive inflammatory necrosis of the pancreas that is readily invaded by infectious organisms, such as *Escherichia coli, Klebsiella, Bacteroides, Staphylococcus,* and *Proteus.* They can erode through the retroperitoneum into the bowel mesentery, the mediastinum, the pleural space, or the pelvis.

Collaborative Management

Clients with pancreatic abscesses often appear more seriously ill than clients with pseudocysts. Clinical manifestations are similar; however, the temperature in clients with abscesses may spike to as high as 104° F (40° C). Blood cultures are helpful in revealing the infective organism. Pleural effusions commonly accompany these abscesses. Ultrasonography and computed tomography cannot differentiate between pancreatic pseudocysts and abscesses.

Pancreatic abscesses that are not surgically drained carry a 100% mortality. Drainage should be performed as soon as possible to prevent sepsis. Antibiotic treatment alone does not resolve the abscess. Mortality remains as high as 60%, even after surgical drainage. Many clients require multiple drainage procedures for recurrent abscesses.

Pancreatic Pseudocyst

Overview

Pancreatic pseudocysts develop as a complication of acute or chronic pancreatitis. Pseudocysts occur in pancreatitis caused by alcoholism, biliary tract disease, or abdominal and surgical trauma. Pseudocysts develop in 10% to 20% of all people with pancreatitis, and mortality is reported at approximately 10%.

Pancreatic pseudocysts, or false cysts, are so named because, unlike true cysts, they do not have an epithelial lining. Pseudocysts are encapsulated sac-like structures that form on or surround the pancreas. The pseudocyst wall is inflamed, vascular, and fibrotic. It may contain up to several liters of straw-colored or dark-brown viscous fluid, the enzymatic exudate of the pancreas.

Collaborative Management

A pseudocyst can be palpated as an epigastric mass in approximately 50% of cases. The primary presenting symptom is epigastric pain radiating to the back. Other common clinical manifestations include abdominal fullness, nausea, vomiting, and jaundice.

Pseudocysts are diagnosed, and their growth and resolution monitored, by serial abdominal ultrasonographic examination or computed tomography.

Complications of pseudocyst formation include
- Hemorrhage
- Infection
- Obstruction of the bowel, biliary tract, or splenic vein
- Abscess
- Fistula formation
- Pancreatic ascites

Pseudocysts may spontaneously resolve, or they may rupture and produce hemorrhage. Surgical intervention is necessary if the pseudocyst does not resolve within 6 weeks or if complications develop. To accomplish internal drainage, the surgeon creates an opening (ostomy) between the pseudocyst and the stomach (cystogastrostomy), the jejunum (cystojejunostomy), or the duodenum (cystoduodenostomy). To provide external drainage, the surgeon inserts a sump drainage tube to remove pancreatic secretions and exudate. Pseudocysts recur in almost 10% of cases. Pancreatic fistulas are common after surgery, and skin breakdown from corrosive pancreatic enzymes presents a major nursing care challenge (see the text on acute pancreatitis earlier).

Pancreatic Carcinoma

Overview

Cancer of the pancreas is one of the most deadly neoplasms. The median survival rate after diagnosis is 4.1 months (Ahlgren, 1996).

Pathophysiology

Pancreatic tumors usually originate from epithelial cells of the pancreatic ductal system. If the tumor is discovered in the early stages, the tumor cells may be localized within the glandular organ; however, this is highly unlikely. Most often, the tumor is discovered in the late stages of development and may be a well-defined mass or be diffusely spread throughout the pancreas.

The tumor may be a primary cancer, or it may result from metastasis from cancers of the lung, breast, thyroid, or kidney or from skin melanoma. Primary pancreatic tumors are generally adenocarcinomas and grow in well-differentiated glandular patterns. Pancreatic adenocarcinoma grows rapidly and spreads to surrounding organs (stomach, duodenum, gallbladder, and intestine) by direct extension and invasion of lymphatic and vascular systems. This highly metastatic lesion may eventually invade the lung, peritoneum, liver, spleen, and lymph nodes.

Clinical manifestations depend on the site of origin or metastasis. The head of the pancreas is the most common site of pancreatic carcinoma. Pancreatic tumors are usually small lesions with poorly defined margins. Jaundice results from tumor compression and obstruction of the common bile duct and gallbladder dilation, causing the organ to enlarge.

Carcinomas of the body and tail of the pancreas are usually large and invade the entire tail and body. These tumors may be palpable abdominal masses, especially in the thin client. Through metastatic spread via the splenic vein, metastasis to the liver may cause hepatomegaly (enlargement of the liver up to two to three times its normal size). Carcinomas of the body and tail spread more extensively than do pancreatic head carcinomas, with invasion of the retroperitoneum, vertebral column, spleen, adrenals, colon, or stomach.

Regardless of where it originates, pancreatic cancer spreads rapidly through the lymphatic and venous systems to other organs.

Thrombophlebitis is a common complication of pancreatic carcinoma. It is attributed to an increase in the levels of thromboplastic factors in the blood. Necrotic products of the pancreatic tumor are believed to have thromboplastic properties, resulting in the blood's hypercoagulable state. Thrombophlebitis is due to the client's confinement to bed and extensive surgical manipulation.

Etiology

The exact cause of pancreatic carcinoma is unknown. Research shows a strong relationship with certain risk factors such as cigarette smoking; a diet high in protein and fat; food additives, especially nitrates and nitrites; and a family history of pancreatic cancer (McEwen et al., 1996).

Incidence/Prevalence

Pancreatic carcinoma comprises only 3% to 4% of all cancers in North America, but ranks fourth as a cause of cancer death. It is second among gastrointestinal sites for both cancer incidence and mortality (Ahlgren, 1996).

In 1994, approximately 27,000 new cases occurred in the United States, and there were 25,000 deaths (American Cancer Society, 1994). Only 2.3% to 5.2% of clients with pancreatic cancer are alive 5 years after diagnosis.

ELDERLY CONSIDERATIONS

Cancer of the pancreas has its highest rates of incidence in people between 65 and 79 years old (Porth, 1994; Tierney et al., 1996). The incidence rate is higher in men.

TRANSCULTURAL CONSIDERATIONS

Cancer of the pancreas occurs in developed countries. The highest incidence is among African-Americans, especially men between the ages of 35 and 70 (Ahlgren, 1996; McEwen et al., 1996).

Collaborative Management

 Assessment

The client's first clue to the presence of pancreatic carcinoma may be the appearance of jaundice, which is a late sign (Chart 62–8). Jaundice appears as the initial sign in two-thirds of all cases because the gallbladder and liver

---

Chart 62–8

Key Features of Pancreatic Carcinoma

- Jaundice (initial but late sign)
- Clay-colored stools
- Dark urine
- Abdominal pain, usually vague, dull, or nonspecific
- Leg or calf pain (from thrombophlebitis)
- Weight loss
- Anorexia
- Nausea or vomiting
- Flatulence
- Gastrointestinal bleeding
- Ascites

are commonly involved. As the tumor spreads, the green-gold skin color associated with obstructive jaundice progressively worsens. On noting the jaundice, the nurse asks the client whether the color of the stool and urine has changed. As a result of the obstructive process, the stool is clay colored and the urine is dark and frothy. The nurse inspects the skin for dryness and scratch marks, indicating pruritus from jaundice.

By the time jaundice appears, the pancreatic carcinoma is usually in an advanced stage. The nurse may be able to palpate the enlarged gallbladder and liver. In advanced cases, the pancreatic tumor may be palpated as a firm, fixed mass in the left upper abdominal quadrant or epigastric region.

The nurse questions the client about abdominal pain, which may be described as a vague, constant dullness in the upper abdomen and nonspecific in nature. Pain is a common early complaint in clients with pancreatic carcinoma. It is also present in the advanced stages of the disease. Pain may be related to eating or activity.

In addition, the nurse asks the client whether he or she is experiencing pain in other areas of the body. Referred back pain may be caused by pressure on the nerve plexus, and some clients have leg or calf pain with swelling and redness as a result of thrombophlebitis, a complication of pancreatic carcinoma.

The nurse or assistive nursing personnel weighs the client and determines the extent of weight loss and whether it has occurred rapidly. The client is questioned about food intake and intolerances. Anorexia accompanied by early satiety, nausea, flatulence, and vomiting are common. Gastrointestinal bleeding may develop from esophageal or gastric varices caused by the tumor pressing on the portal vein.

The nurse performs a general abdominal assessment. In particular, the nurse percusses the abdomen for dullness, which may indicate the presence of ascites. Pancreatic ascites occurs in the advanced stages of the disease process.

There are no specific blood tests to diagnose pancreatic carcinoma. Serum amylase and lipase levels, as well as alkaline phosphatase and bilirubin levels, are elevated. The degree of elevation depends on the acuteness or chronicity of the pancreatic and biliary damage. Elevated carcinoembryonic antigen (CEA) levels occur in 80% to 90% of clients with pancreatic carcinoma. This test may provide early information about the presence of tumor cells.

Computed tomography can confirm the presence of a tumor and can differentiate the tumor from a cyst.

Biopsy of pancreatic tissue by needle aspiration reveals malignant cells. Ultrasonographic examinations do not distinguish pancreatic carcinoma from other pancreatic disorders. Endoscopic retrograde cholangiopancreatography (ERCP) visualization and cytologic study of aspirate provide the most definitive diagnostic data. Aspiration of pancreatic ascitic fluid by abdominal paracentesis may reveal malignant cells and elevated amylase levels. When the secretin test is performed, duodenal or gastric aspirate may reveal a malignant cytologic finding (see Chronic Pancreatitis).

 Interventions

Management of the client with pancreatic carcinoma is geared toward preventing tumor spread and decreasing pain. These measures are not curative, only palliative. The cancers are often multifocal and recur despite treatment.

Nonsurgical Management. As for other types of cancer, chemotherapy or radiation is used to relieve pain. (See Chapter 27 for nursing interventions associated with these treatment modalities.)

Drug Therapy. The nurse medicates the client with opioid analgesics, usually morphine, and provides comfort measures before the pain escalates and reaches a peak in an effort to keep the pain under control. Because of the poor prognosis, drug dependency is not a consideration. High doses of opioid analgesics may be needed for the intense abdominal and back pain in the late stages of the disease.

Chemotherapeutic interventions for pancreatic carcinoma have had limited success. Combining agents such as fluorouracil (5-fluorouracil [5-FU]) and carmustine (BCNU) has been more successful than single-agent chemotherapy. 5-FU is an antimetabolite that interferes with deoxyribonucleic acid (DNA) synthesis in rapidly dividing cells. Two other drugs prescribed are mitomycin C (Mutamycin), an antitumor antibiotic that inhibits synthesis of ribonucleic acid (RNA), and streptozocin (Zanosar), a nitrosourea that interferes with the replication of DNA. The nurse provides the client with symptomatic relief and comfort measures for the toxic side effects of chemotherapeutic agents.

Radiation Therapy. Intensive external beam radiation therapy to the pancreas may offer pain relief by shrinking tumor cells, alleviating obstruction, and improving food absorption; it does not improve survival rates. Implantation of radioactive (I-125) seeds, in combination with systemic or intra-arterial administration of floxuridine (FUDR), have been used. The client may experience discomfort during and after the radiation treatments. Supportive nursing interventions for the relief of symptoms are indicated.

Surgical Management. The most effective management of pancreatic carcinoma is surgical intervention. Clients with tumors confined to the head of the pancreas are candidates for curative resection. Clients with tumors of the body and tail generally are not candidates for surgery because, in most cases, their tumors have spread to other organs. The surgeon may perform either a total pancreatectomy or the Whipple procedure.

Preoperative Care. The client with pancreatic carcinoma is a poor surgical risk because of malnutrition and debilitation. A nasogastric (NG) tube for decompression is inserted, and the administration of IV fluids or total parenteral nutrition is started before surgery.

The client experiences anorexia with early satiety and, frequently, nausea and vomiting, making the oral intake of nutrition difficult to maintain. Management is geared toward providing optimal nutrition preoperatively and postoperatively.

Tube Feedings. As long as intestinal function is adequate, the client may be maintained nutritionally with enteral tube feedings. After tube feedings are tolerated, a small-lumen silicone feeding tube, such as a Dobbhoff tube, is inserted to avoid the complications of larger lumen tubes, such as sinusitis and nasal irritation. Specific nutrients are provided by commercially prepared products chosen by the health care provider or dietitian. Feedings are given by bolus or continuous infusion, depending on the client's tolerance and residual volumes.

Often, in the late stages of pancreatic carcinoma or during the Whipple procedure, the physician inserts a small catheter into the jejunum (jejunostomy) so that enteral feedings may be given. This feeding method is preferred to prevent reflux and to facilitate absorption. Feedings are initiated in low concentrations and volumes and are gradually increased as tolerated. The nurse delivers feedings by a tube feeding pump to maintain a constant volume and assesses for diarrhea frequency as a means to measure tolerance (see Chap. 64).

Total Parenteral Nutrition. For optimal nutrition, hyperalimentation by TPN may be necessary in addition to tube feedings or as a single measure to provide nutrition. When central venous access is required, a Hickman catheter or other type of catheter may be necessary. Meticulous IV line care is an important nursing management measure to prevent catheter sepsis. Sterile dressing changes every 48–72 hours and site observation are extremely important. The nurse performs fingersticks to obtain blood for glucose measurements. These measurements help to monitor the client's tolerance of dextrose in the solution and pancreatic function. (Additional nursing care measures for the client receiving TPN are given in Chapter 64.)

Operative Procedure. The classic surgery, the Whipple procedure (radical pancreaticoduodenectomy), involves extensive surgical manipulation and is used to treat cancer of the head of the pancreas. The procedure entails resection of the proximal head of the pancreas, the duodenum, a portion of the jejunum, the stomach (partial or total gastrectomy), and the gallbladder with anastomosis of the pancreatic duct (pancreaticojejunostomy), the common bile duct (choledochojejunostomy), and the stomach (gastrojejunostomy) to the jejunum (Fig. 62–7). In addition, the surgeon may remove the spleen (splenectomy).

As a palliative measure to relieve biliary obstruction in the likelihood of extensive tumor invasion, a simple surgical intervention, such as cholecystojejunostomy, may be done as a bypass procedure.

Postoperative Care. In addition to routine postoperative care measures, the client undergoing a radical pancreaticoduodenectomy requires intensive nursing care and is usually admitted to a surgical critical care unit. The nurse assesses for potential complications of the Whipple procedure (Table 62–5).

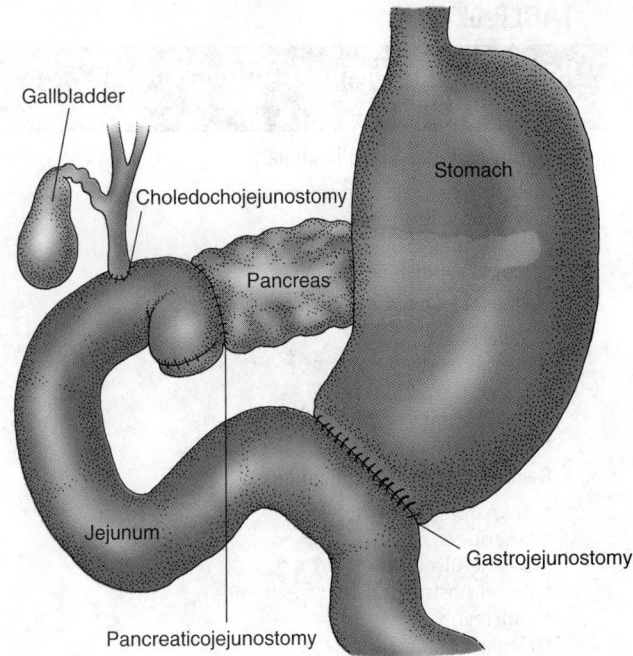

Figure 62–7. The three anastomoses that constitute the Whipple procedure: choledochojejunostomy, pancreaticojejunostomy, and gastrojejunostomy.

Gastrointestinal Drainage Monitoring. The monitoring of gastrointestinal drainage and NG tube patency is an important aspect of postoperative nursing care. Drainage tubes are strategically placed during surgery to remove drainage and secretions from the area and to prevent stress on the anastomosis sites. The nurse assesses the tubes and drainage devices for undue stress or kinking and maintains the drainage tubes in a dependent position. The nurse frequently checks suction gauge pressure to keep the desired suction level. Most often, Salem sump tubes are used and connected to low continuous suction (80 mmHg or less) to maintain drain patency.

The nurse monitors the drainage for color, consistency, and amount. The drainage should be serosanguineous; the appearance of clear, colorless, bile-tinged drainage or frank blood with an increase in output may indicate disruption or leakage of an anastomosis site.

If the NG tube is obstructed, the nurse instills air first. If this method does not keep the drainage lumen open, irrigation with 10–20 mL of normal saline is gently performed.

The development of a fistula (an abnormal passageway) is the most common and most serious postoperative complication. Biliary, pancreatic, or gastric fistulas result from partial or total breakdown of an anastomosis site. The secretions that drain from the fistula contain bile, pancreatic enzymes, or gastric secretions, depending on which anastomosis site is ruptured. These secretions, particularly pancreatic fluid, are corrosive and irritating to the skin, and internal leakage causes a chemical peritonitis. Peritonitis necessitates treatment with multiple antibiotics.

TABLE 62–5

Potential Complications of the Whipple Procedure

Cardiovascular Complications

- Hemorrhage at anastomosis sites with hypovolemia
- Myocardial infarction
- Heart failure
- Thrombophlebitis

Pulmonary Complications

- Atelectasis
- Pneumonia
- Pulmonary embolism
- Adult respiratory distress syndrome
- Pulmonary edema

Gastrointestinal Complications

- Adynamic (paralytic) ileus
- Gastric retention
- Gastric ulceration
- Bowel obstruction from peritonitis
- Pancreatitis
- Hepatic failure
- Thrombosis to mesentery

Wound Complications

- Infection
- Dehiscence
- Fistulas—pancreatic, gastric, and biliary

Metabolic Complications

- Unstable diabetes mellitus
- Renal failure

Positioning. The nurse places the client in the semi-Fowler's position to reduce stress on the suture line and anastomosis, as well as to optimize lung expansion. Stress on the gastric suture line can be minimized by maintaining NG tube drainage at a low suction level to keep the remaining stomach (if a partial gastrectomy is done) or the jejunum (if a total gastrectomy is done) free from excessive fluid build-up and pressure. The NG tube is also used to reduce stimulation of the remaining pancreatic tissue.

Assessment of Fluids and Electrolytes. Because the Whipple procedure is extensive and can take 6–10 hours to complete, maintaining fluid and electrolyte balance can be difficult. The clients tend to experience significant intraoperative blood loss and a tendency to bleed postoperatively. The intestine is exposed to air for long periods, and evaporation of fluid occurs. Significant losses of fluid and electrolytes occur from nasogastric and other drainage tubes. Additionally, these clients are usually malnourished and have low serum levels of protein and albumin, which maintain colloid osmotic pressure within the circulating system. Reduction in the serum osmotic pressure makes the client susceptible to third spacing of body fluids, with fluid moving from the intravascular to the interstitial space.

For these reasons, the nurse closely monitors vital signs for decreased blood pressure and increased heart rate,

decreased vascular pressures with a central venous line or pulmonary artery catheter (Swan-Ganz catheter), and decreased urinary output to detect early signs of hypovolemia and prevent shock. The nurse is also alert for pitting edema of the extremities, dependent edema in the sacrum and back, and an intake that far exceeds output. Nutritional repletion via hyperalimentation and the administration of albumin promote the shift of fluid from the interstitial space back into the intravascular space.

Maintenance of ordered IV fluid volume replacement is important. The nurse monitors hemoglobin levels and hematocrit results to assess for blood loss and the need for blood transfusions. The nurse monitors electrolyte results for decreased serum levels of sodium, potassium, chloride, and calcium. IV fluid concentrations must be altered to correct these electrolyte imbalances. The physician orders replacement of electrolytes as needed.

Glucose Monitoring. Immediately after the Whipple procedure, the client may have transient hyperglycemia or hypoglycemia as a result of stress and surgical manipulation of the pancreas. Most of the endocrine cells (islets of Langerhans, responsible for insulin and glucose secretion) are located in the body and tail of the pancreas. In most clients, up to half of the gland remains, and diabetes does not develop; however, a large number of clients are diabetic before surgery. The nurse monitors glucose levels frequently during the early postoperative period and administers insulin injections, as prescribed.

 Continuing Care

➤ Health Teaching

When the client is sent home, many of the care measures are palliative and aimed at providing relief of symptoms such as pain. Care measures and teaching information are similar to those for clients with chronic pancreatitis.

In many cases, the diagnosis of pancreatic cancer is made a few months before death occurs. The client needs time to adjust to the diagnosis, which is usually made too late for cure or prolonged survival. The nurse helps the client identify what needs to be done to prepare for death. For example, the client may want to write a will or see family members and friends whom he or she has not seen recently. The client needs to make specific requests for the funeral or memorial service known to family members or significant others. These actions help the client prepare for death in a dignified manner. (Chapter 12 discusses anticipatory grieving and preparation for death in detail.)

➤ Home Care Management

The stage of progression of pancreatic carcinoma and available home care resources dictate whether the client can be sent home or whether additional institutional care is needed in a nursing home or hospice setting. Special home care preparations depend on the client's physical and activity limitations and should be tailored for each client's needs.

The nurse provides emotional support for the client and the family to deal with issues related to this illness.

The nurse assists family members to ascertain realistically and objectively the amount of physical care required for the client. The family members must be told that their own physical and emotional health is at risk during this stressful period and that supportive counseling is indicated. If the family does not have a religious affiliation or a spiritual leader (e.g., a minister or a rabbi) to provide support, the nurse suggests alternative counseling options. It is appropriate for the nurse to make the initial contact or appointment based on client or family desire.

▶ Health Care Resources

Regular home care nursing and assistive nursing personnel visits are scheduled to assist the client and family by providing physical, psychological, and supportive care. The nurse supplies information about local hospice care and cancer support groups (see Chapter 12 for information on hospice care).

CASE STUDY for the Client with Acute Pancreatitis

■ You are a charge nurse on a medical unit of a large teaching hospital. The Emergency Department (ED) is sending you a new admission, Ms. Putnam, age 48, with a medical diagnosis of acute pancreatitis. Upon her arrival on your unit, you fully assess Ms. Putnam. Included in your assessment findings are the following data:

1. VS: T = 100.2° F; P = 104; R = 22; BP = 100/60
2. Sharp pain in the mid-epigastric area radiating to the back, rated as 8 (scale 0 to 10)
3. Vomited twice in ED; reports that she is still nauseated
4. Bowel sounds hypoactive at 2 per minute

QUESTIONS:

1. Why is it important to monitor vital signs of the client with acute pancreatitis?
2. What position may help to decrease the client's pain?
3. What medication will probably be ordered for the client's pain and why?
4. What does the nausea, vomiting, and hypoactive bowel sounds indicate?

SELECTED BIBLIOGRAPHY

Ahlgren, J. (1996). Epidemiology and risk factors in pancreatic cancer. *Seminars in Oncology, 23*(2), 241–250.

Allen, K. M., & Phillips, J. M. (1997). *Women's health across the lifespan: A comprehensive perspective.* Philadelphia: J. B. Lippincott.

Ambrose, M. S., & Dreher, H. M. (1996). Pancreatitis: Managing a flare-up. *Nursing96, 26*(4), 33–39.

American Cancer Society. (1994). *Cancer facts and figures 1994.* Atlanta: American Cancer Society.

*Bagg, A. (1988). Whipple's procedure: Nursing guidelines. *Critical Care Nurse 8*(5), 34–45.

Carson, C., Seidel, S., & Bushmiaer, M. (1996). Recovery from laparoscopic cholecystectomy procedures. *AORN Journal, 63*(6), 1099–1113.

Conner, M., & Deane, D. (1995). Patterns of patient controlled analgesia and intramuscular analgesia. *Applied Nursing Research, 8*(2), 67–72.

*Fain, J. A., & Amato-Vealey, E. (1988). Acute pancreatitis: A gastrointestinal emergency. *Critical Care Nurse, 8*(6), 47–63.

Giger, J. N., & Davidhizar, R. E. (1995). *Transcultural nursing: Assessment and Intervention* (2nd ed.). St. Louis: C. V. Mosby.

Greenberger, N. J., & Isselbacher, K. J. (1994). Diseases of the gallbladder and bile ducts. In K. J. Isselbacher, E. Braunwald, J. D. Wilson, J. B. Martin, A. S. Fauci, & D. L. Kesper (Eds.), *Harrison's principles of internal medicine* (13th ed., p. 1504). New York: McGraw Hill.

* Holland, P., & Hussain, I. (1989). Biliary lithotripsy: Nonsurgical treatment of gallstones. *Society of Gastrointestinal Assistants Journal, 3,* 158–162.

Huether, S. E., McCance, K. L., & Danek, G. D. (1996). Alterations of digestive function. In S. E. Huether & K. L. McCance (Eds.), *Understanding pathophysiology* (pp. 944–990). St. Louis: C. V. Mosby.

*Jeffres, C. (1989). Complications of acute pancreatitis. *Critical Care Nurse, 4*(9), 38–46.

Katz, J. (1997). Back to basics: Providing effective patient teaching. *AJN, 97*(5), 33–36.

Kowdley, K. (1996). Update on therapy for hepatobiliary diseases. *Nurse Practitioner, 21*(7), 78–88.

*Mathews, J. S., Maher, K. A., & Cattau, E. L. (1989). The role of endoscopic retrograde cholangiopancreatography injection training sessions for the gastroenterology nurse and associate. *Gastroenterology Nursing, 12*(2), 106–108.

Malarkey, L. M., & McMorrow, M. E. (1996). *Nurse's manual of laboratory tests and diagnostic procedures* (pp. 508–594). Philadelphia: W. B. Saunders.

McEwen, D., Sanchez, M., Rosario, A., & Allen, W. (1996). Managing patients with pancreatic cancer. *AORN Journal, 64*(5), 716–734.

McGrath, P., Sloan, D., & Kenady, D. (1996). Surgical management of pancreatic carcinoma. *Seminars in Oncology, 23*(2), 200–212.

Noone, J. (1995). Acute pancreatitis: An Orem approach to nursing assessment and care. *Critical Care Nurse, 15*(4), 27–35.

Nowazek, V. (1996). Nursing management of the patient with acute pancreatitis. In S. D. Ruppert, J. G. Kernicki, & J. T. Dolan (Eds.), *Dolan's critical care nursing* (2nd ed., pp. 832–847). Philadelphia: F. A. Davis.

Peterson, A. (1997). Analgesics. *RN, 60*(4), 45–50.

Pinto, K. (1996). Acalculous cholecystitis: A case report. *Nurse Practitioner, 21*(10), 120–122.

Porth, C. M. (1994). *Pathophysiology concepts of altered health states* (4th ed., pp. 843–871). Philadelphia: J. B. Lippincott.

Ransohoff, D. F., & McSherry, C. K. (1995). Why are cholecystectomy rates increasing? *JAMA, 273*(20), 1621–1622.

Steer, M. L., Waxman, I., & Freedman, S. (1995). Chronic pancreatitis. *New England Journal of Medicine, 332*(22), 1482–1490.

Tierney, L. M., McPhee, S. J., & Papadakis, M. A. (1996). *Current medical diagnosis and treatment* (35th ed.). Stamford: Appleton & Lange.

SUGGESTED READINGS

Ambrose, M. S., & Dreher, H. M. (1996). Pancreatitis: Managing a flare-up. *Nursing96, 26*(4), 33–39.
  The authors discuss the pathophysiology, etiology, and clinical manifestations of the client with acute pancreatitis. Nursing assessment and interventions to manage the complex problems of clients with pancreatitis are described.

Kowdley, K. (1996). Update on therapy for hepatobiliary diseases. *Nurse Practitioner, 21*(7), 78–88.
  This article provides an excellent, comprehensive update on viral hepatitis, gallstones, and liver transplants. The main focus is on recent developments in diagnosis and medical treatment.

McEwen, D., Sanchez, M., Rosario, A., & Allen, W. (1996). Managing patients with pancreatic cancer. *AORN Journal, 64*(5), 716–734.
  This article provides a comprehensive review of cancer of the pancreas. Areas discussed include etiology, treatment options, and nursing care.

Chapter 63

INTERVENTIONS FOR CLIENTS WITH ANOREXIA NERVOSA AND BULIMIA NERVOSA

Anorexia nervosa is frequently misdiagnosed as a physical illness. Bulimia nervosa is often a hidden disorder. The medical-surgical nurse must be familiar with these syndromes because early diagnosis and intervention can eliminate years of suffering for the anorexic or bulimic person.

ANOREXIA NERVOSA

Overview

Anorexia nervosa is a sometimes life-threatening illness that takes the form of indirect self-destructive behavior. It occurs primarily in females, with onset most often during adolescence. It is a clinical syndrome of self-induced starvation. The anorexic refuses to eat because of an intense fear of losing control of eating and thus becoming fat. Anorexics suffer from a disturbed body image and continue to feel fat even when they are emaciated.

Pathophysiology

The term *anorexia nervosa* is a misnomer. Anorexics do not experience a true loss of appetite until late in starva-

tion; clients experience the feeling of hunger but ignore it. As the illness progresses, anorexics continue to refuse food and are preoccupied with thoughts of food. It is not unusual for anorexics to be well educated in the area of nutrition. They may become gourmet cooks or "health food" advocates and insist that their families eat well while they continue to avoid food and lose weight.

The anorexic who controls weight by limiting nutritional intake has the *restricting* type of anorexia nervosa. Some anorexics limit intake and also use laxatives and/or diuretics as purgatives to further decrease the effect of ingested calories. Anorexics may indulge in binge-eating and purge by vomiting. These people have the *binge-eating/purging* type of anorexia nervosa.

Although the anorexic and family frequently search for a physical cause for the weight loss experienced, anorexia nervosa is a psychiatric rather than a physical illness. The anorexic often experiences medical complications from the effects of starvation and unhealthy behaviors such as purging (vomiting, laxative abuse, and diuretic abuse). It is crucial, however, to recognize that the medical problems are the *results,* not the cause, of the illness.

Criteria for Diagnosis

For many years, Russell's criteria (1970) have guided health care practitioners in diagnosing anorexia nervosa:

- Self-induced starvation
- A morbid fear of fatness
- An abnormality in reproductive hormone functioning that leads to amenorrhea in females and decreased sexual interest and function in males

The presence of these hallmarks of the disorder alerts the nurse to the possibility that the client may be suffering a psychiatric, not a medical, condition. The American Psychiatric Association has outlined the features of anorexia nervosa in the *Diagnostic and Statistical Manual of Mental Disorders, Fourth Edition, Revised* (DSM-IV) (1994). The criteria listed in Chart 63–1 describe the hallmark features of the disease. *DSM-IV* defines two types of anorexia nervosa: the restricting type and the binge-eating/purging type. Diagnosis is made on the basis of these standardized criteria, not from the results of extensive testing designed to eliminate all possible physical conditions.

The Body's Response to Anorexia Nervosa

Certain clinical manifestations are indications of the body's efforts to protect itself and to function on its limited food intake, including lowered body temperature, bradycardia, and amenorrhea. To maintain vital functioning, the body attempts to decrease fuel requirements by lowering the core body temperature and decreasing the basal metabolic rate. The reduced core body temperature causes a decrease in enzyme production.

The circulating norepinephrine level decreases, resulting in a reduced heart rate. A decrease in blood pressure, as well as cold hands and feet with occasional cyanosis, may occur because of reduced blood flow. In some anorexics,

---

TABLE 63–1

Factors Contributing to Anorexia Nervosa

- Societal pressure to be thin
- Family dynamics
- Developmental issues
- Personality characteristics
- Triggering events in vulnerable person (including sexual abuse)
- Biological predisposition

---

the skin has a covering of fine, downy lanugo hair, but why it develops is not clear. Bone marrow function decreases, resulting in anemia that is usually microcytic or normocytic. The gastrointestinal tract becomes more efficient and absorbs whatever it receives. There is evidence that gastric emptying time is decreased in anorexics, although the full significance of this alteration is not clear.

Changes in the endocrine system protect the body by stopping menses to preserve energy. Cessation of menses (amenorrhea) prevents pregnancy, which would require thousands of stored calories to maintain. Changes in thyroid hormone levels account for the decreased metabolic rate mentioned earlier.

A chronic state of anorexia nervosa can produce such changes as atrophy of the heart muscle, decreased liver function, impaired renal function, chronic anemia, and osteoporosis.

Etiology

The cause of anorexia nervosa is not fully understood. Many hypotheses have been generated and discussed over the past century as anorexia nervosa has been studied and treated (Bemporad, 1996). The disorder appears to be the result of the interaction of many factors in a vulnerable person. The multifactorial concept of the illness blends many of the hypotheses proposed. Contributing etiologic factors of anorexia nervosa are listed in Table 63–1. Because everyone is unique, the degree of importance of each factor varies from person to person. Some factors may not be present at all, whereas others contribute to and perpetuate the illness. Chart 63–2 suggests ways in which parents can help prevent eating disorders.

Cultural Influences

One possible contributing factor to the development of anorexia relates to societal values and a cultural obsession with thinness. Western media advertising suggests that "thin is beautiful." A person may feel societal, family, and peer pressure to maintain a thin body. This often occurs when an adolescent is struggling with issues of identity, individuation, and fears about impending sexuality. These concerns may be present before coping skills have been fully developed. The adolescent may have body image disturbances (Thompson, 1996). A poor self-image and certain personality characteristics, such as perfectionism or compulsiveness, may increase a person's vulnerability. Many experts suggest that familial patterns of behavior,

---

Chart 63–1

Key Features of Anorexia Nervosa (DMS-IV Diagnostic Criteria)

1. Refusal to maintain body weight at or above a minimally normal weight for age and height (e.g., weight loss leading to maintenance of body weight less than 85% of expected; or failure to gain weight during period of growth, leading to body weight less than 85% of expected)
2. Intense fear of gaining weight or becoming fat, even though underweight
3. Disturbance in the way body weight or shape is experienced, undue influence of body weight or shape on self-evaluation, or denial of the seriousness of the current low body weight
4. In postmenarcheal females, amenorrhea, i.e., the absence of at least three consecutive menstrual cycles

Modified from American Psychiatric Association (1994). *Diagnostic and statistical manual of mental disorders* (4th ed., revised). Washington, DC: American Psychiatric Association.

Health Promotion Guide: How Parents Can Prevent Eating Disorders

- Teach your children to eat in moderation from all food groups and avoid excess fats and sweets.
- Be a role model for your children. Show them healthy eating and dieting behaviors.
- Foster self-esteem in your children based on the importance of who they are and the skills they have, not on their physical characteristics.
- Seek family counseling during times of conflict or significant change.
- Early intervention is important. Young adolescents struggling with identity concerns and who show abnormal eating behaviors are at risk.
- Eating disorders are often secretive. Get them out in the open, and get help.

marital disharmony, and the adolescent's attempts to become independent play a role. Clients may associate the onset of illness with a triggering event, such as pressure to pass exams, a break-up with a boyfriend, dieting, or changes in the family caused by divorce or death.

Biological Factors

Some researchers have suggested that anorexia nervosa is the result of a hormonal or hypothalamic dysfunction that predisposes a person to the disorder. Others have identified a higher than expected incidence of affective illness, that is, depression and bipolar illness, in families of anorexics. Further support of a genetic link is evidenced by the high incidence of anorexia nervosa in twins and triplets.

Biopsychosocial Model

The biopsychosocial model for anorexia nervosa, illustrated in Figure 63-1, shows the interrelationship of the factors and the resulting cycle of illness and consequences

of illness-related behaviors. Dieting may begin as a response to social influences and expectations or as an intrapsychic avoidance of sexual feelings and a defense against anxiety. The dieting results in severe weight loss accompanied by physiologic and mental changes.

Incidence/Prevalence

Since at least 1950, experts in the United States and around the world have shared concern over the increased incidence and prevalence of anorexia nervosa. For many years the literature has reported a much higher incidence of anorexia nervosa in women than in men. Women outnumber men by approximately 9 to 1. The prevalence rate of anorexia nervosa is 0.5% to 1% for women (Thompson, 1996).

In a study of 50-year trends in the incidence of anorexia nervosa, Lucas et al. (1991) found the disease to be more common than previously recognized. These researchers report increased incidence among 15- to 24-year-old females but not among older women or males. The overall prevalence rate per 100,000 was 14.6 (0.15%) for females and 1.8 (0.02%) for males. Some experts believe the prevalence data on eating disorders are understated.

Although the illness is usually diagnosed in adolescent girls, Lucas et al. (1991) identified it in both women and men, with the age of onset ranging from 10 to 57 years. Males make up 5% to 10% of the population with anorexia nervosa. The incidence in the male population may be underestimated because of the reluctance of some men to acknowledge that they have an illness that is primarily associated with females.

An anorexia nervosa–like syndrome has also been reported in older people. However, more research is needed before comparisons can be made between younger and older people with abnormal eating attitudes and behaviors and altered body image.

Incidence in Selected Populations

People who participate in sports or belong to professions that demand low weight are at an increased risk for development of anorexia nervosa. Ballet dancers, models,

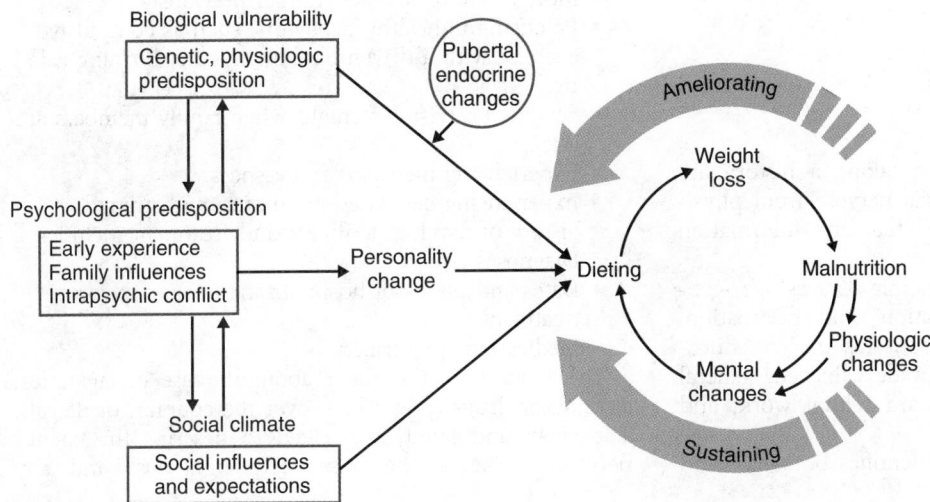

Figure 63–1. Biopsychosocial model for anorexia nervosa. (From Lucas, A. R. [1981]. Toward the understanding of anorexia nervosa as a disease entity. *Mayo Clinic Proceedings, 56,* 258.)

jockeys, gymnasts, wrestlers, and actresses are examples. An increased incidence among dietitians may reflect the interest of the anorexic in food and nutrition when choosing a profession rather than participation in the profession being a risk factor in and of itself.

Mortality Rate

A meta-analysis revealing a mortality rate of 5.9% was reported by Neumarker (1997). This analysis indicated that when the duration of illness is 4 to 5 years, the mortality rate is 5%. This rate increases to 15% to 20% when the duration of illness is 20 to 30 years. Neumarker (1997) pointed out that variability exists not only in the method of determining mortality rate but also in data and evaluations related to causes of death in anorexia nervosa. Causes ranged from suicide to sudden death.

A new 12-year follow-up study by Herzog et al. (1997) show that some of the laboratory data obtained at the initial evaluation may predict a fatal or chonic course. In their study

- Serum albumin levels less than 3.6 g/L and body weight less than 60% of average weight at initial examination best predicted a lethal course
- High serum creatinine and uric acid levels predicted a chronic course

Transcultural Considerations

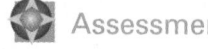

Anorexia nervosa is most commonly diagnosed in females from the middle and upper classes in Western cultures.

A review of the literature on eating disorders in minority groups by Crago et al. (1996) revealed very few studies. However, the available studies reported that eating disorders occur less frequently in African-American and Asian-American females than in Caucasian females. Eating disorders are equally common among Hispanic females as Caucasian females and more frequent in Native American females. Risk factors identified among minority females include being younger, heavier (being overweight versus perceiving oneself as overweight), well educated, and more often identified with white middle-class values.

Collaborative Management

Assessment

➤ History

Data collected by the nurse when taking a history are invaluable in differentiating anorexia nervosa from physical illness. The client is reassured that any information volunteered is confidential.

The nurse obtains such demographic data as age, gender, socioeconomic status, education, and occupation. The nurse also asks the client about his or her educational history, including highest grade achieved, general level of performance, attitude toward school work, and career plans.

A history of medical problems identifies both past and current diagnoses with information about each problem and how the diagnosis was made. The nurse gathers specific information about gastrointestinal symptoms (nausea, vomiting, esophagitis, irritable bowel syndrome, constipation). The client is asked to describe any difficulties or concerns about his or her physical functioning, such as weakness, fatigue, intolerance to cold, change in sleep habits, swelling in any body part, and seizures.

The nurse pays special attention to the client's weight history and gathers data on current weight, height, and body build. The client is asked to describe the onset of weight loss by giving information about

- Age and weight at the time of onset
- Reason for the weight loss such as dieting, divorce of parents, break-up with boyfriend or girlfriend, or a physical illness
- Highest and lowest weights
- Fluctuations in weight
- Changes in appetite

In taking the sexual history from a female client, the nurse asks about

- Age at breast development
- Age, weight, and height at menarche
- Menstrual history
- Details about amenorrhea, if present

Both male and female clients are questioned about their preparation for puberty and how they acquired sexual information. Keeping in mind that the anorexic client is often sexually inactive, the nurse tactfully explores the client's attitude toward sexual development and sexuality. A matter-of-fact, nonjudgmental approach by the nurse helps to put the anorexic at ease with what might be a difficult topic. It may be necessary to postpone some of the questions about sexual orientation and experiences until the client has established trust in the nurse.

The nurse obtains specific information about the client's attitudes and behavior related to food and weight (Chart 63–3). By asking such questions as "Do you like the way you look?" and "Are you happy with the size of all your body parts?" the nurse can obtain information that helps to identify the presence of a perceptual distortion in body image (see Chap. 10).

The history of the client's activity levels can uncover changes; for example, the client may be

- More active or less active than previously
- Practicing unhealthy behaviors, such as compulsive exercise with a driven quality aimed at burning calories
- Secretly exercising at night when family members are asleep
- Experiencing increased restlessness
- Experiencing decreased endurance and strength

A history of psychiatric illness and treatment includes

- Diagnoses
- Dates and places of hospitalizations or outpatient treatment
- Medications prescribed

The nurse asks the client about the use of cigarettes, alcohol, or drugs (prescribed, over the counter, or illegal). The client and family are asked to describe the client's personality before the onset of weight loss and any

Chart 63–3

Nursing Care Highlight: The Client with Possible Anorexia Nervosa

- Ask the client about changes in appetite and about the use of appetite-suppressing drugs. Be alert to denial.
- Ask when the client eats, what and in what quantity, and which foods the client avoids.
- Ask whether the client has any unusual thoughts about food, hoards food, or feels compelled to cook for others.
- Ask about vomiting and use of laxatives, diuretics, and syrup of ipecac.
- Ask about any unusual food-related behaviors, such as chewing then spitting food out, hiding food or throwing it away, cutting food into small pieces, and practicing unusual mealtime rituals.
- Ask how frequently the client weighs self, and assess the client's opinion of her or his ideal body weight. Does the client desire to lose more weight? Does she or he take unusual pride in losing weight? Is there any body image disturbance?
- Ask whether the client is fearful of becoming fat. Does the client fear that certain ingested foods will go directly to certain body parts? That foods touching the body will be absorbed as calories? Does the client feel guilty or depressed after eating?

changes perceived since that time. The nurse pays special attention to reports of a tendency toward

- Perfectionism
- Self-criticism
- Compulsiveness
- Low mood or fluctuations
- Anxiety
- Phobias

This information helps the nurse document the client's ability to describe mood and feelings to uncover the presence of alexithymia (the inability to identify inner feelings), a major feature of anorexia nervosa.

The nurse questions the client about the family history, such as

- Parents' ages, education, careers, general health, and relationship with the client (e.g., very close to mother but cannot relate to father, or vice versa)
- Ages and sex of siblings and their relationships with the client
- Family functioning and conflict
- Family history of psychiatric illness, such as eating disorders, alcoholism, depression, or bipolar illness
- Family members' attitudes about food and weight

The nurse might ask, "Is anyone or has anyone been overweight or underweight? Is anyone constantly dieting? Is anyone being teased about weight?"

The family's reaction to the client's illness is very important, for example:

- Denying a serious problem
- Looking for a medical reason for the weight loss

- Blaming oneself or each other for the client's illness
- Anger at or disgust with the client

➤ *Physical Assessment/Clinical Manifestations*

Most clients with anorexia nervosa come to medical attention when weight loss is readily apparent. Amenorrhea may occur before excessive weight loss is noticed. As profound weight loss occurs—15% or more of total body weight—physical assessment reveals signs of hypothermia (decreased core body temperature to 35° C [95° F] or lower). Other vital signs are also lowered. Blood pressure may be as low as 60/40 mmHg, or there may be orthostatic blood pressure changes (a drop in pressure when the client changes from lying to sitting or sitting to standing positions). The client's heart rate may range from 40 to 60 beats per minute, and the respiratory rate may be slow. The nurse questions the client to determine whether the weight loss has been slow and gradual. If so, the accompanying decrease in vital signs is probably not cause for alarm because the body has adjusted to the changes. The client may complain of intolerance to cold temperatures, dizziness, and weakness but is usually not in acute distress. Table 63–2 summarizes the physical consequences of anorexia nervosa.

General Physical Appearance. The client's extremities are cool and sometimes cyanotic on examination. Al-

TABLE 63–2

Physical Consequences of Eating Disorder Behaviors

Restricting	Purging/Binge-Eating
Metabolic acidosis	Seizures
Bradycardia	Cardiac dysrhythmias
Atrophy of heart muscle	Gastrointestinal symptoms
Orthostatic hypotension	Gastric dilation/rupture
Anemia	Hypokalemic alkalosis
Hypoalbuminemia	Loss of bowel reactivity
Hypocalcemia	Irritable bowel syndrome
Hypophosphatemia	Prolapsed rectum
Hypercholesterolemia	Steatorrhea
Decreased triiodothyronine	Enlarged parotid glands
Increased growth hormone	Enamel erosion of teeth
Amenorrhea or irregular menses	Esophagitis
Decreased sexual drive	Abnormal liver function
Decreased muscle mass/ weakness	Dehydration
Decreased subcutaneous fat	Urinary tract infection
Lowered core temperature	Renal complications
Acrocyanosis/sensitivity to cold	Muscle weakness
Pedal edema	Peripheral parathesias
Lanugo hair	Finger clubbing/swelling
Delayed gastric emptying	Calluses on abdomen
Constipation	Scars on dorsum of hand
Malnutrition	Death
Osteoporosis	
Death	

though many anorexics do not purge by vomiting, the nurse observes for evidence of scars on the knuckles of the hands and calluses from digital pressure on the abdomen that indicate self-induced vomiting. An absence of such signs, however, should *not* be interpreted as the absence of self-induced vomiting. The emaciated anorexic loses muscle mass and subcutaneous fat, and a prominent bone structure is revealed. Severe emaciation, which creates the appearance of a skeleton covered with skin (e.g., a weight of 60 pounds for a 5-foot, 5-inch female), may be shocking to the nurse. The nurse takes special care not to transmit this reaction to the client. The client's body may also be covered with fine lanugo hair, which may be especially evident on the extremities, shoulders, and face.

During the physical assessment, the nurse may also note the presence of *edema* anywhere on the body. The cause of this edema is not clear; it is usually *not* related to kidney or liver failure but probably to mild protein deficiency and a reduced plasma albumin level. This symptom may become more prominent during refeeding but resolves as the client approaches normal weight.

Parotid gland tenderness and swelling alert the nurse that the client probably practices self-induced vomiting. Other indicators are discolored tooth enamel and excessive numbers of caries ("cavities"), which result from frequent exposure to gastric acids during vomiting.

Complications of Anorexia Nervosa. The physical complications that accompany anorexia nervosa vary with the degree of starvation and the method of weight control that the client uses. Anorexics who are food restrictors usually have fewer complications than anorexics who also use vomiting, laxatives, and diuretics to maintain low weight. Such behaviors lower potassium levels and may result in a state of hypokalemic metabolic alkalosis, which can cause seizures and cardiac dysrhythmias. A decreased potassium level can result from starvation as well as from purging, but in this case it is not as severe. The nurse is more likely to see metabolic acidosis with food restriction and starvation related to the conversion of fat to fatty acids and ketones. (See Chapter 19 for a discussion of acid-base imbalances.)

The nurse observes for tetany (intermittent tonic muscular contractions), which may result from hypocalcemia. Hypophosphatemia (low phosphate levels), when severe, may induce the clinical manifestations of paresthesia (abnormal tingling or prickling sensations), convulsions, coma, or death.

Some practices of anorexics seem to protect them, to some extent, from the severe effects of starvation. Many anorexics take multiple vitamins, which counteract the effects of a vitamin-deficient diet and may protect against peripheral neuropathies and paresthesias. Anorexics seem to fear intake of protein somewhat less than the intake of fatty and high-carbohydrate foods. This ingestion of small amounts of protein may help them avoid the features of malnutrition seen in those with marasmus or kwashiorkor (severe protein depletion). Some anorexics, but not all, who engage in high levels of regular exercise may be affected less by the loss of bone mass of osteoporosis associated with estrogen deficiency and low calcium in-

take than those anorexics who do not exercise. Return to normal weight is essential in reversing the clinical manifestations outlined above.

➤ *Psychosocial Assessment*

There is evidence that anorexia nervosa affects clients of both sexes, ranging in age from very young to old, as well as clients from diverse cultural backgrounds. Most often, however, anorexics are Caucasian, adolescent or young adult females from middle-class to upper-class families; they are high achievers academically and exhibit a high level of motivation and compliance. Parents frequently describe their anorexic adolescent as having been a "perfect" child. Before the onset of illness, the adolescent was popular with peers and involved in social activities, frequently excelling in athletics. Although seemingly successful in facing the challenges of adolescence, the anorexic suffers from a sense of ineffectiveness and low self-esteem.

Along with the physical symptom of weight loss, the client has a severe distortion in body image. The anorexic's attitude toward the weight loss is significant to the diagnosis in that the client seems to enjoy losing weight and takes pride in extreme thinness. Anorexics do not see a thin, emaciated body in the mirror. Instead, they see "fat thighs" or a "protruding stomach." Along with this distorted body image, the nurse may find that the client does not correctly perceive stimuli within the body, that is, fails to recognize feelings of hunger.

The onset of anorexia nervosa seems to occur when the client is struggling with the identity issues of adolescence. The illness may be triggered by an emotionally stressful situation, such as a change in family structure or a move to a new city. Peer pressure may influence the onset of the illness, as when a group of adolescents begins to diet and one person continues to diet to extreme thinness. There is reason to believe, however, that adult clients with certain vulnerabilities are at risk for becoming anorexic. Although the average age of onset is 17 years (Smolak & Levine, 1996), clinicians have noted its occurrence after age 25, including several case reports of eating disorders that began after age 55.

Assessment of the Family. Family dynamics are often a major contributing factor to the development of anorexia nervosa. Questions are asked by the nurse about
- A tendency toward rigidity in the parents and strong parental control
- Parental overinvolvement with one or all children
- Poor conflict resolution and communication problems
- Domination of one parent over the other
- Tendency for the client to be emotionally very close to one parent but somewhat distanced from the other

The anorexic desires parental approval and strives for perfection. Anorexics attempt to attain a sense of independence, achievement, and control over life while combating an unrealistic fear of failure. Maintaining thinness may be one way in which adolescents try to maintain self-confidence. Regulating food intake and exercising strict self-discipline become a way of exerting control and of proving that there is one thing that the person can do extremely well. In the interview with the client and family, the nurse observes the interaction process, noting areas of tension or conflict, overprotectiveness, or family members' answering questions for others—especially parents speaking for the adolescent.

Assessment of Mental Status. A mental status examination is part of the psychosocial assessment. During this examination, the nurse identifies an alteration in the state of consciousness that may accompany starvation and an alteration in mood state, such as depression. The nurse asks the client about feelings of self-worth and hopelessness, the ability to enjoy life, and suicidal thoughts. Depression reported by anorexics at their low weight, however, often resolves when weight returns to normal. The nurse also inquires about obsessions, compulsions, phobias, and any unusual ideas about food.

The anorexic may have peculiar ideas about what food does inside the body and sometimes outside the body. For example, the client may fear that food will produce fat, which will be deposited on the thighs, or that crumbs falling on oneself will cause absorption of calories and weight gain. When assessing for the presence of ritualistic behavior, the nurse may find that the client always goes through a certain fixed routine at mealtimes, such as sitting a certain way in a chair, using only certain utensils, or arranging food items in a certain way on the plate. The anorexic may have a self-imposed requirement of a set number of repetitions of a certain exercise for each calorie ingested. Standing or moving about constantly to burn more calories, rather than sitting, is another common behavior in anorexics.

Assessment of Sexual Adjustment. Some clients have a history of childhood sexual abuse. Both male and female anorexics exhibit poor sexual adjustment. Delayed sexual development is common in adolescent anorexics, and there is a decreased interest in sex among adult anorexics. The quality and number of social relationships tend to decline as the anorexic's preoccupation with food and body increases. The client and family are asked to describe changes in behavior, such as decreased involvement with peers and family and changes in participation in school activities. The nurse might ask whether the client does things with the family, for example, go on family outings, watch television together, eat with other family members. Questions such as "Do you enjoy going to school dances or sports events?" and "Do you have a special boyfriend or girlfriend?" may illuminate a change in behavior.

The nurse also assesses the client's strengths. The nurse may identify positive coping skills in both client and family. The client's high motivation and desire for success are positive when they are used to regain health rather than maintain a lower weight. Effective communication skills assist the anorexic in exploring issues with health care professionals. (Chapter 8 provides invaluable information on planning nursing care that emphasizes and encourages positive coping behaviors.)

➤ *Laboratory Assessment*

Hematology and Blood Chemistries. Blood abnormalities, such as profound anemia, are demonstrated by a complete blood count with differential. The SMA-7 (7/60) and SMA-12 provide useful information.

Hypoalbuminemia indicates protracted undernutrition. Serum transferrin values may reflect a protein deficiency. Possible fluid and electrolyte abnormalities that can cause cardiac dysrhythmias and renal failure include hypokalemia, hypochloremia, hypomagnesemia, and hypocalcemia.

Hypoglycemia may be severe in restrictors who fast for extended periods. An elevated blood urea nitrogen (BUN) level indicates dehydration. Purging through vomiting, laxative abuse, or diuretic abuse can cause dehydration and hypokalemia along with severe renal problems. A nephropathy related to low potassium levels can cause interstitial fibrosis and impaired renal function.

Serum amylase levels are elevated in anorexics who purge by vomiting. The nurse makes it a priority to obtain a baseline level and uses amylase tracking to determine whether the client is engaging in vomiting behavior. The level rises about 2 hours after the client has purged by vomiting. Once the client ceases the vomiting behavior, it takes about a week for these high levels to return to normal.

Endocrine Studies. In female anorexics, endocrine studies identify low levels of luteinizing hormone, follicle-stimulating hormone, and estrogen; in male anorexics, the studies identify decreased testosterone levels. Thyroid studies, such as thyroxine (T_4), triiodothyronine resin uptake (T_3RU), plasma triiodothyronine (T_3), and thyroid-stimulating hormone (TSH) determinations, often reveal low-normal T_4 and subclinical T_3 values with normal TSH concentrations.

Table 63–3 summarizes the abnormal laboratory

TABLE 63–3

Laboratory Findings in Clients with Anorexia Nervosa

- Anemia
- Hypoalbuminemia
- Hypokalemia
- Hypochloremia
- Hypomagnesemia
- Hypocalcemia
- Metabolic alkalosis
- Hypoglycemia
- Elevated blood urea nitrogen (BUN)
- Elevated serum amylase
- Decreased luteinizing hormone
- Decreased testosterone
- Low normal thyroxine (T_4)
- Slightly elevated liver enzymes (aspartate aminotransferase [AST], alanine aminotransferase [ALT])
- Elevated serum cholesterol

test values commonly seen in clients with anorexia nervosa.

➤ Other Diagnostic Assessment

The hospital's consulting psychiatrist and/or psychiatric consultation-liaison nurse should be asked to evaluate the client as part of the process of establishing a diagnosis. These consultants may also assist in arranging for appropriate psychological testing to be done by a psychologist. Such tests include
- The Minnesota Multiphasic Personality Inventory (MMPI)
- An intelligence quotient test (Wechsler's Adult Intelligence Scale [WAIS])
- A perceptual distortion test
- A depression scale
- An eating disorder scale (the Eating Attitudes Test [EAT]), developed by Garner and Garfinkel
- The Eating Disorder Inventory (EDI), developed by Garner et al. (Fig. 63–2)

(For additional information on the purpose, methods, and meaning of results of psychiatric tests, consult a psychology or psychiatric nursing textbook.)

 Analysis

➤ Common Nursing Diagnoses and Collaborative Problems

The priority nursing diagnoses for the client with anorexia nervosa are
1. Altered Nutrition: Less than Body Requirements related to inadequate food intake
2. Pain (abdominal) related to reintroduction of certain foods
3. Fluid Volume Deficit related to self-imposed fluid restriction or purging behaviors
4. Risk for Fluid Volume Excess related to fluid retention during refeeding

---

INSTRUCTIONS

This is a scale that measures a variety of attitudes, feelings, and behaviors. Some of the items relate to food and eating. Others ask you about your feelings about yourself. THERE ARE NO RIGHT OR WRONG ANSWERS SO TRY VERY HARD TO BE COMPLETELY HONEST IN YOUR ANSWERS. RESULTS ARE COMPLETELY CONFIDENTIAL. Read each question and fill in the circle under the column which applies best to you. Please answer each question *very* carefully. Thank you.

	ALWAYS	USUALLY	OFTEN	SOMETIMES	RARELY	NEVER
1. I eat sweets and carbohydrates without feeling nervous	O	O	O	O	O	O
2. I think that my stomach is too big	O	O	O	O	O	O
3. I wish that I could return to the security of childhood	O	O	O	O	O	O
4. I eat when I am upset	O	O	O	O	O	O
5. I stuff myself with food	O	O	O	O	O	O
6. I wish that I could be younger	O	O	O	O	O	O
7. I think about dieting	O	O	O	O	O	O
8. I get frightened when my feelings are too strong	O	O	O	O	O	O
9. I think that my thighs are too large	O	O	O	O	O	O
10. I feel ineffective as a person	O	O	O	O	O	O
11. I feel extremely guilty after overeating	O	O	O	O	O	O
12. I think that my stomach is just the right size	O	O	O	O	O	O
13. Only outstanding performance is good enough in my family	O	O	O	O	O	O
14. The happiest time in life is when you are a child	O	O	O	O	O	O
15. I am open about my feelings	O	O	O	O	O	O
16. I am terrified of gaining weight	O	O	O	O	O	O
17. I trust others	O	O	O	O	O	O
18. I feel alone in the world	O	O	O	O	O	O
19. I feel satisfied with the shape of my body	O	O	O	O	O	O
20. I feel generally in control of things in my life	O	O	O	O	O	O

Figure 63–2. A portion of the Eating Disorder Inventory. (Adapted and reproduced by special permission of Psychological Assessment Resources, Inc., Lutz, FL 33549, from Garner D., Olmstead M. P., & Polivy J., *The eating disorder inventory*. Copyright, 1984, 1991 by Psychological Assessment Resources, Inc. Further reproduction is prohibited without permission from PAR, Inc.)

5. Constipation related to decreased intake and/or laxative abuse
6. Anxiety related to increased food intake and consequent weight gain
7. Body Image Disturbance related to misperception of body size
8. Ineffective Individual Coping related to fears of loss of self-control and fatness
9. Noncompliance with therapeutic recommendations related to food refusal, vomiting, laxative abuse, overexercising, or decision to leave hospital against medical advice
10. Altered Family Processes related to difficulty in coping with client's illness and hospitalization

➤ Additional Nursing Diagnoses and Collaborative Problems

Anorexia nervosa is a complex disorder, and the client may have one or more of the following nursing diagnoses:

- Decreased Cardiac Output related to alterations in rhythm caused by hypokalemia (this can be a life-threatening problem; it is not common in the restricting type but may be seen in the binge-eating/purging type of anorexia nervosa. See Planning and Implementation under Bulimia Nervosa.)
- Hypothermia related to low weight
- Risk for Injury (fracture) related to low-estrogen condition and calcium deficiency with decreased bone mass
- Activity Intolerance related to starved state and muscle weakness
- Sleep Pattern Disturbance related to hyperactivity and nocturnal exercise habits
- Altered Growth and Development related to inadequate food intake
- Sexual Dysfunction related to altered body function and psychosocial vulnerabilities
- Sensory/Perceptual Alterations related to inability to recognize physical and emotional states of hunger and safety or to identify emotions
- Self-Esteem Disturbance related to issues of personal identity and issues of role performance
- Social Isolation related to preoccupation with illness behaviors and thoughts of food
- Ineffective Family Coping: Compromised or disabling related to changes in family dynamics brought about by illness
- Altered Health Maintenance related to recurrent episodes of illness and/or knowledge deficit

 Planning and Implementation

➤ Altered Nutrition: Less Than Body Requirements

Planning: Expected Outcomes. The expected outcomes are that the client will establish an eating pattern that meets daily nutritional needs and maintain a healthy weight.

Interventions. The nurse can determine a healthy weight for the client by using the Metropolitan Height and Weight Tables (see Chap. 64). The data developed by Frisch and McArthur (1974) (Table 63–4) are also used to calculate the minimal weight needed for the onset or restoration of menses. Initial interventions are aimed at saving the client from death by starvation. Later interventions stress the return to a healthy weight and normal body functioning, for example, establishment of a regular menstrual cycle.

Diet Therapy. The physician usually orders an initial diet of 1200 to 1600 kcal/day. The nurse accepts the challenge of helping the anorexic eat "normally" by mouth. The number of calories is increased gradually to ensure a steady weight gain of 2 to 4 pounds (0.9 to 1.8 kg) per week. This gradual increase in calories may also help to decrease the anxiety the client experiences at the beginning of treatment (Salisbury et al., 1995). Persistent refusal of food and fluid for 24 hours by a severely starved client necessitates the use of intravenous (IV) fluids. Liquid feedings via nasogastric tube or total parenteral nutrition may also be necessary, depending on the extent of food refusal. Transfer to a psychiatric facility specializing in the treatment of eating disorders is considered when the client's refusal of food continues unabated or when purging behaviors persist after food is consumed.

The nurse collaborates with the dietitian and client in selecting an appropriate diet. The client may experience anxiety when asked to select foods from a menu. The nurse assists the client in making decisions and sets firm limits regarding the selection of items from each category on the menu. The nurse does not give the client a choice about the amount and type of food to be eaten. When the client is extremely distressed by the process of food selection, the nurse makes all selections. Ultimately, the nurse assists the client in viewing diet as one way of regaining control. Selection and intake of a healthy diet provide a positive means for the client to eat, gain weight, and gain control over activities and behavior.

Prevention of Complications. Introducing a diet of 1200 to 1600 kcal/day, given in three meals and one or two snacks, can prevent painful abdominal distention and the dangerous complication of gastric dilation. In a person with gastric dilation, motility is lost and the stomach fills with food that does not pass through to the duodenum. The stomach contents must be evacuated to avoid rupture. IV fluids are given temporarily until motility is restored.

➤ Pain

Planning: Expected Outcomes. The client is expected to experience minimal abdominal discomfort during refeeding related to the reintroduction of certain foods.

Interventions. Abdominal pain usually results from gastric distention, cramping from lactose intolerance, and difficulty with the digestion of fats. Interventions, therefore, are directed at assisting the client's body to adjust by introducing small amounts of food initially (1200 to 1600 kcal/day) and by gradually including lactose and fats over the first few weeks of refeeding. The daily number of

TABLE 63-4

Minimal Weight Necessary for the Onset or Restoration of Menstrual Cycles, by Height

Height		Menarche or Primary Amenorrhea			Secondary Amenorrhea		
		Minimal* Weight (10th Percentile)		Average Weight (50th Percentile)	Minimal† Weight (10th Percentile)		Average Weight (50th Percentile)
in	cm	lb	kg	kg	lb	kg	kg
53.1	135	66.7	30.3	34.9	74.6	33.9	38.9
53.9	137	68.6	31.2	36.0	76.8	34.9	40.1
54.7	139	70.6	32.1	37.0	79.0	35.9	41.2
55.5	141	72.6	33.0	38.0	81.2	36.9	42.4
56.3	143	74.4	33.8	39.0	83.4	37.9	43.5
57.1	145	76.3	34.7	40.1	85.6	38.9	44.7
57.9	147	78.3	35.6	41.1	87.8	39.9	45.8
58.7	149	80.3	36.5	42.1	90.0	40.9	47.0
59.4	151	82.3	37.4	43.1	92.2	41.9	48.1
60.2	153	84.3	38.3	44.2	94.4	42.9	49.3
61.0	155	86.2	39.2	45.2	96.6	43.9	50.4
61.8	157	88.2	40.1	46.2	98.8	44.9	51.5
62.6	159	90.2	41.0	47.2	101.0	45.9	52.7
63.4	161	92.2	41.9	48.3	103.2	46.9	53.8
64.2	163	93.9	42.7	49.3	105.4	47.9	55.0
65.0	165	95.9	43.6	50.3	107.6	48.9	56.1
65.7	167	97.9	44.5	51.4	109.8	49.9	57.3
66.5	169	99.9	45.4	52.4	112.0	50.9	58.4
67.3	171	101.9	46.3	53.4	114.0	51.8	59.6
68.1	173	103.8	47.2	54.4	116.2	52.8	60.7
68.9	175	105.8	48.1	55.5	118.4	53.8	61.8
69.7	177	107.8	49.0	56.5	120.6	54.8	63.0
70.5	179	109.6	49.8	57.5	122.8	55.8	64.1
71.3	181	111.8	50.8	58.5	125.2	56.9	65.3

Data from Frisch, R. E. & McArthur, J. W. (1974). *Science, 185,* 949–951. From Frisch, R. E. (1977). Food intake, fatness and reproductive ability. In R. A. Vigersky (Ed.), *Anorexia nervosa* (pp. 149–161). New York: Raven Press.
*Equivalent to 17% fat/body weight.
†Equivalent to 22% fat/body weight.

calories can be increased gradually because more calories will be needed at the end of treatment to gain weight.

The health care provider prescribes a low-lactose, low-lipid diet. Milk products and fats are introduced slowly during the second or third week of refeeding. If cramping is severe, they are withdrawn and reintroduced later.

Opioid pain medications are never indicated because they contribute to the danger of decreased stomach and bowel motility. Acetaminophen (Tylenol, Ace-Tabs✦, Exdol✦) relieves minor abdominal discomfort. Antacids may provide some relief from indigestion. The nurse encourages the client to tolerate symptoms without medications as much as possible because proper diet management minimizes distress in a few days.

> ## ➤ Fluid Volume Deficit

Planning: Expected Outcomes. The client is expected to experience a correction of fluid volume deficit and maintain an adequate fluid volume during the treatment period.

Interventions. Clients who have severely restricted their food and fluid intake before hospitalization are as-

sessed for fluid volume deficit. The nurse assesses blood pressure, urinary output and concentration, and the condition of the skin and mucous membranes. The client with a fluid volume deficit typically has

- Low blood pressure
- Small volumes of very concentrated urine (specific gravity of 1.020 to 1.025)
- Tenting of the skin
- Dry membranes

The nurse offers fluids such as water, juice, soda, coffee, and tea; milk products are avoided. Because the anorexic's body has made a gradual adjustment to a state of severely limited food and fluid intake, fluids are carefully introduced at a rate and in quantities that will not compromise the cardiovascular system and create a fluid volume overload.

Fluids are offered hourly. The nurse maintains a strict record of intake and output. If the client is experiencing symptoms of impending shock, the physician immediately orders IV fluids, such as normal saline, to replenish volume. IV fluids are also indicated if the client refuses fluids orally for 24 hours.

To increase the likelihood of the client's cooperation

and to prevent the complications of volume deficit, the nurse explains the consequences of inadequate fluid intake.

➤ Risk for Fluid Volume Excess

Planning: Expected Outcomes. The client is expected to experience minimal refeeding edema.

Interventions. Refeeding edema is common in the early days of nutritional rehabilitation and can cause discomfort. The client may complain of swelling in ankles, knees, fingers, and face. The edema is usually most severe in the lower extremities. The condition is annoying, but it does not appear to have a serious cause (such as kidney or liver failure). Interventions that prevent edema and provide increased comfort for the client are indicated.

Diuretics are not recommended and are avoided unless the client begins to experience serious complications, such as heart failure.

Refeeding edema responds well to a low-salt diet. Fluid restriction, limited to 1000 to 1500 mL/day, is helpful for clients with severe edema. The caloric intake is also held constant for several days.

The client's most frequent complaint is discomfort. The nurse provides a comfortable chair and foot rest and encourages the client to keep the feet elevated for several hours a day. The client is advised to remove rings from the fingers and to avoid restrictive clothing and shoes. Older anorexics who have been chronically ill for several years seem to be most troubled by refeeding edema and may experience it for an extended time, sometimes for weeks. The nurse teaches the client how to manage prolonged edema.

➤ Constipation

Planning: Expected Outcomes. The client is expected to establish a regular bowel elimination pattern without the use of laxatives.

Interventions. Normal physiologic bowel action is preferable to the use of bowel action stimulated by cathartics. The nurse teaches chronic laxative abusers to find noncathartic ways to enhance elimination. However, anxiety related to weight gain may prompt even the non–laxative-abusing anorexic to request laxatives or enemas and to exaggerate the extent of the problem. The nurse seeks interventions that encourage physiologic bowel action and prevent such complications as fecal impaction.

Drug Therapy. A bowel regimen that includes a bulk laxative (hydrophilic colloid), such as psyllium (Metamucil), and a stool softener, such as docusate (Colace), given twice daily assists in the development of a regular bowel elimination pattern. Persistent constipation lasting longer than 3 or 4 days may be treated with a cathartic suppository, such as bisacodyl (Dulcolax, Bisacolax♣). If this measure is ineffective, a sodium phosphate (Fleet) enema is suggested.

When the regular bowel regimen, suppositories, or enemas do not adequately relieve constipation, the nurse suspects a fecal impaction. Digital disimpaction may be necessary.

Diet Therapy. The nurse collaborates with the dietitian to provide the starved anorexic with a diet that has an adequate fiber content (3 to 6 g daily). For clients with bowel elimination problems, the fiber content may be gradually increased until it includes 12 to 18 g of fiber. An adequate fluid intake (at least 1500 mL/day) is essential. The dietitian also includes foods that enhance elimination, such as wheat bran, fresh fruits, fresh vegetables, and prunes or prune juice (Chart 63–4).

Other Interventions. Physical activity enhances regular bowel elimination. Although the starved anorexic is restricted from rigorous exercise, walking around the unit is usually permitted. Warm fluids, such as coffee, tea, or hot water, stimulate the gastrocolic reflex and may be helpful.

➤ Anxiety

Planning: Expected Outcomes. The client is expected to state that anxiety is decreased.

Interventions. The nurse is instrumental in assisting the anorexic to overcome anxiety so that it does not interfere with establishing a healthy eating pattern and consistent weight gain. The client needs emotional support and encouragement during mealtimes or when snacks are eaten. A member of the nursing staff is present while the client eats and interrupts statements on the client's part related to the number of calories being consumed or potential weight gain. The nursing staff member guides the client through the meal with reminders to continue eating or to try an untouched food on the plate. The staff member encourages social conversation unless the client uses talking as a means to avoid eating. In this case, the staff member discourages conversation during the meal. Although supportive measures are emphasized, the introduction of antianxiety agents before meals may be necessary in the early stages of nutritional rehabilitation.

The nursing staff member does not bargain with the client to exchange foods or to eliminate any of the offered foods. The staff member reminds the client that food is

---

Chart 63–4

Nursing Care Highlight: Anorexia Nervosa

- Help the client select an appropriate diet within the calorie limits allowed.
- Avoid milk products and fatty foods initially; introduce them slowly later, if permitted, to prevent abdominal cramping.
- Offer fluids to prevent constipation and prevent hunger, but stay within the prescribed fluid restriction for clients with severe edema.
- Provide foods high in fiber, such as bran, fresh fruits and vegetables, prunes, or prune juice, to prevent or treat constipation.
- Collaborate with the dietitian in planning the client's diet.

the "medicine" that will save her or his life and, therefore, holds firm in the expectation that all food presented will be eaten.

The period after meals or snacks is often one during which the anorexic feels anxious about the number of calories consumed. A member of the nursing staff provides emotional support and shows acceptance of the client's feelings.

Drug Therapy. Extremely anxious clients who do not begin to eat despite supportive nursing interventions may require an antianxiety agent before meals are presented. The physician may prescribe a short-acting anxiolytic agent such as lorazepam (Ativan, Novolorazem✣), 0.5 mg 1 hour before meals, to decrease anxiety so that the client can decide to eat.

Other Interventions. Allowing the client to control some decisions may decrease anxiety. The nurse determines which decisions are negotiable and which are not. For example, after the menu is planned, it is not renegotiated, but the time or place of the meal may be. The nurse might ask, "Do you want to have breakfast at 7 AM or 8 AM today?" or "Do you want to eat in your room or in the lounge this morning?" Allowing the client input into other non–food-related decisions may also decrease anxiety and increase cooperation. The use of deep breathing exercises and relaxation techniques may give the client an increased sense of control.

➤ Body Image Disturbance

Planning: Expected Outcomes. The client is expected to develop a realistic perception of body size.

Interventions. The anorexic client often has disturbances in self-concept related to personal identity, self-esteem, and role performance. The most common disturbance, however, is in the area of body image, which manifests itself as an inability to perceive body size and needs accurately. The nurse encourages the client who overestimates the size of her or his own body or who believes that one part or all of the body is too large, even though emaciated, to express feelings about body size and function as well as feelings about self. The nurse points out misperceptions but does not argue with the client. For example, if the client states that his or her stomach is too large, the nurse can respond by acknowledging that the client's body is once more becoming stronger and healthier and is functioning more normally.

The nurse is supportive and makes affirmative statements when the client expresses an accurate perception of body size and function. For example, the nurse can give positive feedback if the client states a feeling of hunger before a meal. The nurse assists the client, on an ongoing basis, in accepting the changes that are taking place in body size and function. The nurse also provides an opportunity for the client to communicate concerns and to identify strengths.

➤ Ineffective Individual Coping

Planning: Expected Outcomes. The client is expected to demonstrate behaviors and verbalize statements that indicate self-control and coping.

Interventions. The nurse concentrates efforts on assisting the client to use previously developed healthy coping measures and to learn new methods of coping. The nurse collaborates with the hospital's consulting psychiatrist and/or psychiatric consultation-liaison nurse to provide care related to the diagnosis. Individual therapy with one of these health professionals during the period of hospitalization enhances the supportive therapy provided by the nurse. Group therapy is not commonly available in the acute hospital setting.

Together with the client, the nurse explores new ways of coping with the problems of everyday living. Unless a diagnosis of depression is made for which antidepressant therapy is indicated, the client is not given medication.

The client may begin individual therapy with a psychiatrist, a psychologist, or the psychiatric consultation-liaison nurse in the health care facility. It is essential that provisions be made for psychotherapy to continue after discharge.

Groups organized by recovering anorexics and/or families may be available after discharge. These groups help clients and families to become better educated about anorexia nervosa and provide a support system during periods of extreme stress. These are not psychotherapy groups and are not usually led by health professionals.

Other support groups may be offered in the health care facility or community setting and are led by a health care professional, often a nurse.

In many facilities, occupational therapy departments provide services for medical clients. If such services are unavailable, the nurse can arrange with the inpatient psychiatric service to include the client in groups that provide

- Assertiveness training
- Relaxation techniques
- Creative expressions
- Art therapy
- Dance therapy

The group setting provides a vehicle for interaction and socialization with others who can give feedback about the client's behaviors.

➤ Noncompliance

Planning: Expected Outcomes. The client is expected to comply with the treatment plan and continue to participate in a treatment program as recommended by the interdisciplinary team.

Interventions. Anorexics have developed behaviors over time that, although unhealthy, help them cope with the problems of adolescence and life. The fear of fatness that is part of the illness contributes significantly to the maintenance of these unhealthy behaviors and makes the likelihood of noncompliance predictable. Interventions that increase the likelihood of compliance are those discussed for the preceding nursing diagnoses.

There is no magic formula for solving the problem of noncompliance. Monitoring behavior and providing support are key nursing interventions that, when combined with motivation on the client's part to move away from illness and toward health, can deeply influence successful completion of a treatment program. The psychiatric consultation-liaison nurse is an important resource for planning care with the nurse.

Noncompliance with treatment for anorexia nervosa can be life-threatening. The nurse teaches the client and family specifics related to the illness and treatment plan and emphasizes the consequences of noncompliance (see Table 63–2). The nurse, often with assistance from a case manager, helps to locate an inpatient psychiatric program, when indicated, or arranges outpatient psychiatric treatment.

During a crisis, anorexic clients may be treated on a medical unit where ongoing treatment is not an option. The client and family may not understand that anorexia nervosa is a psychiatric illness and that many specialized programs are available. Such teaching and assistance, with referral by the nurse, may prevent serious complications and years of suffering for the client and family.

The parents of a minor with anorexia nervosa that has reached a life-threatening stage may need information about placing their child in a psychiatric facility. This placement can be done even when the child does not want treatment. An adult whose illness has reached the life-threatening stage may also be committed for care to a psychiatric facility by two physicians who conclude that the client is a danger to herself or himself. Laws for such commitment vary from state to state, and the institution's legal department can provide the treatment team with such information. Eating disorder clients who are not in a life-threatening state are now treated in intensive outpatient day programs.

➤ Altered Family Processes

Planning: Expected Outcomes. The family is expected to demonstrate an understanding of the client's illness and support the client by following the recommendations of the interdisciplinary health care team.

Interventions. Families are usually frightened for their anorexic loved one. They may be frustrated and angry about behaviors that they do not understand. They may feel guilty that perhaps they contributed to the illness or that they cannot seem to stop it. The nurse helps the family to understand the illness and the method of treatment being implemented by the team. The nurse explains the details of the emotional and physical manifestations of anorexia nervosa to help the family understand the treatment approach and rationale for specific interventions.

The nurse helps families who are in considerable distress to contact the social worker responsible for the client's case. The social worker assesses the family dynamics and provides therapy as needed. If the social worker cannot provide family therapy, an outside referral may be necessary.

➤ Continuing Care

The client with anorexia nervosa who has established a regular pattern of weight gain and whose behavior indicates a motivation to change behaviors may be discharged to the home and receive psychiatric treatment in an outpatient program (Chart 63–5). Clients whose behavior indicates a life-threatening situation are transferred to a psychiatric facility for inpatient treatment. The ideal

---

Chart 63–5

Focused Assessment for Clients with Anorexia Nervosa Being Managed in the Community

* Assess nutritional status, including
  * Current weight; any gain or loss
  * Food and fluid intake
  * Tenting of skin
* Assess cardiovascular and gastroenterologic status, including
  * Vital signs
  * Muscle weakness
  * Edema
  * Gastrointestinal complaints
  * Evidence of vomiting
  * Evidence of diarrhea
* Assess functional ability, including
  * Mobility and ambulation
  * Activity intolerance
  * Evidence of overexercising
* Assess psychological state, including
  * Fear of fatness
  * Denial of seriousness of low body weight
  * Body image disturbance
  * Perfectionistic traits
  * Ritualistic behavior, especially food-related behavior
  * Changes in self-esteem
  * History of recent stressors
  * Preoccupation with food, calories, weight
  * Evidence of depression
  * Evidence of anxiety
  * Evidence of poor sexual adjustment
* Assess family dynamics, including
  * Conflict
  * Strong parental control
  * Parental over-involvement
  * Evidence that one parent is emotionally distant
  * Family attitudes about food, weight, and dieting
  * History of eating disorders in other family members
  * History of other psychiatric illness in family members
* Assess client's and family's understanding of illness and its treatment, including
  * Importance of eating together in relaxed atmosphere
  * Signs and symptoms to report to nurse
  * Need for client and family psychiatric intervention

---

placement is a facility specializing in the treatment of eating disorders.

➤ Health Teaching

During the client's hospital stay, the nurse instructs the client and family in how to recognize and understand the physical, behavioral, and emotional characteristics of anorexia nervosa. The teaching plan is individualized to identify the problems specific to the client, for example, food restriction, laxative abuse, hypothermia, hypokalemia, or distorted body image (Chart 63–6). The nurse emphasizes the importance of viewing anorexia nervosa as a psychiatric illness that is treated most effectively by mental health professionals through individual, group, and

---

Chart 63–6

Education Guide: Anorexia Nervosa

- Use the food patterns and exchanges that your dietitian has provided to plan your meals.
- Drink about 1500 mL of fluid per day to prevent fluid overload, but drink enough fluids to avoid constipation.
- Avoid laxatives to promote bowel elimination.
- Do not discuss conflicts or try to solve problems at mealtimes.
- Exercise regularly each day for 20 to 30 minutes.
- Participate in local support groups for encouragement.
- Report any signs of electrolyte imbalance, such as muscle weakness from hypokalemia, to your doctor.

---

family therapy. The primary focus is to help the client differentiate emotional hunger from physical hunger.

In collaboration with the dietitian, the nurse explains how to use food patterns and food exchanges. For the family whose anorexic member is returning home, the nurse stresses the importance of eating together as a family. The client is encouraged to normalize both eating and family relationships. The nurse cautions the family not to use mealtimes to resolve conflicts and to avoid centering on the anorexic and commenting on eating behavior.

The nurse also discusses the type and amount of exercise suggested for the client. This is very important if the anorexic has a history of overexercising.

➤ *Psychosocial Preparation*

Whether the client is discharged home with outpatient treatment or to an inpatient psychiatric setting, the client and family need much education and support. It is often difficult for clients and families to accept a psychiatric diagnosis because of the fear that they will be stigmatized and perhaps labeled "crazy." The nurse encourages them to discuss their fears and concerns to correct misconceptions about the illness and its treatment. The nurse emphasizes the availability of health care professionals and lay support groups. The nurse acknowledges that the illness is very serious and that patience and hard work are necessary on the part of each family member. The nurse encourages families to explore family dynamics and to confront existing problems, such as marital conflict.

➤ *Home Care Management*

It is absolutely essential for the client to have either inpatient or outpatient therapy arranged before being discharged from the medical unit. The client is usually under treatment for 2 to 3 years.

➤ *Health Care Resources*

If the client cannot return home for outpatient treatment, arrangements are made for appropriate inpatient treatment. The psychiatrist, case manager, and/or psychiatric consultation-liaison nurse provide information about inpatient facilities and assist the family in obtaining such treatment.

In some communities, anorexia nervosa organizations offer support groups for clients and families. Hospitals with treatment programs may also provide support. Support groups do not take the place of individual or group psychotherapy for the client, and they do not replace family therapy for the client and family. They do provide the opportunity for interaction with other people who have firsthand knowledge of the effects of anorexia nervosa and who can empathize and offer information about dealing with the illness. If such resources are unavailable, the nurse may recommend videotapes containing interviews with clients recovering from eating disorders.

The client and family may seek appropriate resource information from The National Anorexic Aid Society and two other organizations—Anorexia Nervosa and Related Eating Disorders and Anorexia Nervosa and Associated Disorders.

 Evaluation

The nurse examines the effectiveness of the interventions described in the plan of care to resolve each nursing diagnosis identified. The client is expected to
- Establish an eating pattern that meets daily nutritional needs
- Maintain a healthy weight
- Experience minimal abdominal discomfort during the refeeding period related to the reintroduction of certain foods into the diet
- Experience a correction of fluid volume deficit
- Maintain an adequate fluid volume during the treatment period
- Establish a regular bowel elimination pattern without the use of laxatives
- State that anxiety is decreased
- Develop a realistic perception of body size
- Demonstrate behaviors and verbalize statements that indicate self-control and coping
- Comply with the treatment plan
- Continue to participate in a treatment program as recommended by the treatment team

The family is expected to
- Demonstrate an understanding of the client's illness
- Support the client by following the recommendations of the interdisciplinary health care team

BULIMIA NERVOSA

Overview

Bulimia nervosa is an eating disorder that is characterized by episodes of binge-eating that recur, are uncontrolled, and involve the ingestion of a large amount of food in a short time. This binge-eating is usually followed by some form of purging behavior, such as vomiting and the excessive use of laxatives or diuretics.

Like the anorexic, the bulimic has an intense fear of fatness. This intense fear distinguishes the bulimic from people who binge-eat for pleasure or to reduce stress.

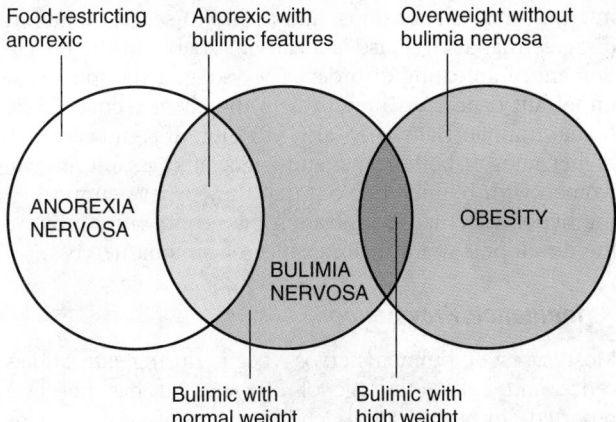

Figure 63–3. Schematic representation of the overlapping relationship between eating disorders and obesity. (Adapted from Fairburn, C. [1982]. Binge-eating and bulimia nervosa. *SK&F Publications, 1,* 15.)

Some controversy exists about whether bulimia nervosa is a separate syndrome from anorexia nervosa because the clinical manifestations of bulimia—binge-eating and purging—occur in people at varied body weights, ranging from starved to overweight.

Figure 63–3 illustrates the overlapping nature of eating disorders and obesity; some clients with anorexia nervosa maintain low weight by food restriction alone, but others use purging behaviors to rid themselves of unwanted calories and at times indulge in an eating binge.

Normal-weight bulimics who experience the binge-purge cycle frequently have a 10-pound (4.5-kg) weight fluctuation. The high-weight bulimic experiences the binge-purge cycle and overlaps with the obese client who may binge-eat but purge or have a morbid fear of fatness.

Pathophysiology

The bulimic secretly eats enormous quantities of food—often concentrated sweets or fats—very rapidly, without appreciating the taste. The onset of a binge may be precipitated by a variety of factors, such as hunger, boredom, anger, anxiety, and depression.

Eating binges may also be triggered by physical causes that are not yet understood. Bouts of overeating may be provoked or facilitated by hypothalamic reactions to starvation. Bulimics spend much of their day in a starved state and may actually suffer from chronic malnutrition with resulting metabolic and endocrine symptoms of starvation.

Binge-eating behavior usually results in feelings of depression and self-deprecating thoughts. Approximately half of bulimics binge-eat daily or more often. During a binge most bulimics consume far more calories than would be eaten in a normal meal. Binge-purge episodes are interspersed with periods of minimal food intake, and many bulimics do not eat normal meals.

Purging behavior is an attempt to regain a sense of control and to eliminate the calories ingested. Most bulimics report that vomiting is their preferred method of purging.

The diagnostic criteria for bulimia nervosa of the American Psychiatric Association are identified in Chart 63–7. The DSM-IV criteria guide decisions regarding diagnosis and treatment. DSM-IV describes two types of bulimia nervosa: (1) purging type and (2) nonpurging type.

Etiology

It is possible to describe typical bulimic behavior, but it is much more difficult to identify the cause. Many bulimics experience the onset of symptoms after undertaking a rigid diet to lose weight. Studies designed to identify factors that precipitate the binge-purge syndrome involve self-reporting by bulimic clients. Factors identified are

- Depression
- Loneliness
- Boredom
- Anger
- Interpersonal conflicts related to job or relationships
- Issues of individuation and identity

The illness often starts in the late teens and coincides with loss of or separation from family and friends. The social pressure to be thin that is experienced by both sexes, but particularly women, is a major factor contributing to the development of bulimia nervosa.

The appetite regulation center in the hypothalamus is the focus of most biological models, which suggest a dysregulation of neurotransmitters, especially serotonin, and hormones (Cochrane, 1995). Biological risk factors include a history of being at least slightly overweight and a vulnerability to fluctuation in mood state.

People with diabetes mellitus may have an increased risk for developing bulimia nervosa. Mannucci et al.

Chart 63–7

Key Features of Bulimia Nervosa (DSM-IV Diagnostic Criteria)

1. Recurrent episodes of binge-eating characterized by both
   - Eating, within any 2-hour period, an amount of food definitely larger than most people would eat during a similar period of time under similar circumstances
   - A sense of lack of control over eating during the episode
2. Recurrent, inappropriate compensatory behavior to prevent weight gain, such as self-induced vomiting; misuse of laxatives, diuretics, enemas, or other medications; fasting; or excessive exercise
3. Binge eating and inappropriate compensatory behaviors that both occur, on average, at least twice a week for 3 months
4. Self-evaluation is unduly influenced by body shape and weight
5. The disturbance does not occur exclusively during episodes of anorexia nervosa

Modified from American Psychiatric Association (1994). *Diagnostic and statistical manual of mental disorders* (4th ed., revised). Washington, DC: American Psychiatric Association.

(1997) report that binge eating may start as a response to hypoglycemic reactions. Clients with type I diabetes who overeat do not usually gain weight unless insulin dosage is increased, but they experience glycosuria and impaired metabolic control. The combination of diabetes mellitus and bulimia nervosa creates a serious and often life-threatening health problem.

People at risk frequently have disturbed familial relationships. In addition, clients with bulimia nervosa often have personality traits that reflect problems with self-esteem, impulse control, and self-discipline. Casper and Lyubomirsky (1997) found that components of individual psychopathology most directly associated with bulimia nervosa were depressive symptoms, suicidality, and impulsive behavior.

Figure 63–4 illustrates the relationship between etiologic factors and pathways that end in a binge-purge cycle.

WOMEN'S HEALTH CONSIDERATIONS

Although being a woman immediately places a person at risk for developing an eating disorder, there is now question about the relationship of childhood sexual abuse and the development of an eating disorder. Vanderlinden and Vandereycken (1996) cite many reports of serious traumatic experiences, especially physical and sexual abuse, in clients with eating disorders. They report that sexual abuse is more often reported in bulimic rather than restricting clients. Their review of the reports in the literature revealed prevalence data of sexual abuse during childhood in eating disorder clients that ranged from 28% to 70%. Their own studies showed the highest prevalence of sexual abuse in clients who had purging behaviors and significant co-morbidity such as depression, alcohol abuse, stealing, promiscuity, and self-mutilation. They further suggest that sexual abuse is a risk factor for eating disorders even though a linear causal link does not exist. Kearney-Cooke and Striegel-Moore (1996) agree that sexual abuse has a lasting effect on body image, identity,

interpersonal relationships, and ability to self-regulate but disagree that such abuse is a causal variable in the development of an eating disorder. They suggest the most important concern is how to help the client recover from sexual trauma. Dansky et. al (1997) found significantly higher rates of both sexual and aggravated assault among women with bulimia nervosa that they believe support the hypothesis that victimization may contribute to both the development and maintenance of bulimia nervosa.

Incidence/Prevalence

Most cases of bulimia nervosa begin during late adolescence and before the age of 25 years. It has not been reported in prepubertal children (Smolak & Levine, 1996). A prevalence ratio of 1.0% to 3.0% has been identified (Thompson, 1996).

TRANSCULTURAL CONSIDERATIONS

A review of recent studies of bulimia nervosa and recurrent binge-eating comparing behaviors of Caucasian women and African-American women by Striegel-Moore and Smolak (1996) suggested that symptoms of eating disorders are more common in African-American women than was previously recognized. Furthermore, they may be more likely to develop a binge-eating disorder. Reports also indicate that African-American women favor the use of laxatives over vomiting as a method of purging.

Collaborative Management

 Assessment

The nurse gathers data from the client and family. The history gathered from the bulimic client is similar to that gathered from the anorexic (see earlier). Changes in the emphasis of questions are suggested. When gathering data about medical problems and clinical manifestations, the

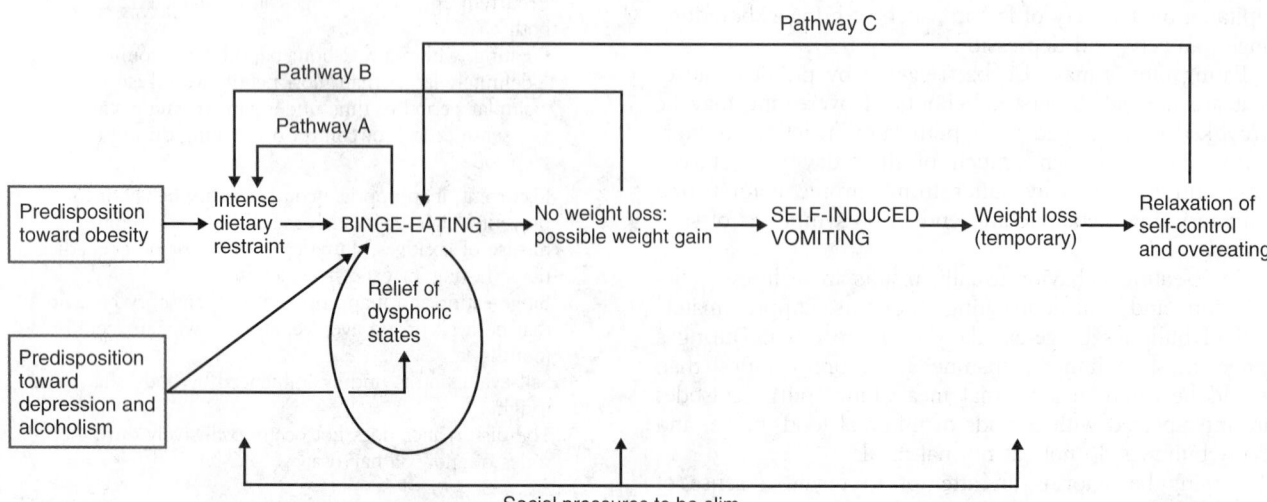

Figure 63–4. Etiologic factors and their relationship to the binge-purge cycle. (Adapted from Fairburn, C. [1982]. Binge-eating and bulimia nervosa. *SK&F Publications, 1,* 13.)

nurse emphasizes questions related to the episodes of vomiting and laxative abuse.

➤ *Physical Assessment/Clinical Manifestations*

Although the client with bulimia nervosa has what looks like a normal, healthy body, bulimic practices create a high risk for serious physical complications. The bulimic may be only slightly underweight, of normal weight, or overweight. Table 63–4 lists physical consequences of eating disorders; those associated with purging behaviors are particularly applicable to the bulimic client.

General Physical Appearance. During the physical assessment by the nurse, the client may reveal complaints of weakness, tiredness, constipation, and depression. Such complaints, coupled with an irregular pulse, alert the nurse to a possible electrolyte imbalance resulting from practices of vomiting or from laxative or diuretic abuse. Ipecac syrup abuse can cause cardiotoxicity. Purging behaviors can lead to serious abnormalities in electrolyte levels, such as hypokalemia and cardiac dysrhythmias, which can result in cardiac arrest and sudden death.

The chronic hypokalemia that results from frequent vomiting, laxative abuse, and diuretic abuse can also cause kidney disturbances or damage. The nurse assesses for current evidence of pain or signs of urinary tract infection because these are often evident in bulimic clients who experience dehydration and ketonuria. The nurse considers other serious complications of electrolyte imbalance, such as seizures and peripheral paresthesias (pricking or tingling sensations on the skin).

The frequent practice of purging by vomiting causes dry mouth and swelling of the parotid glands with some tenderness but usually not pain. The nurse assesses the teeth for signs of frequent exposure to gastric acid from vomiting, for example:

- Loss of tooth enamel
- A color change to brown or gray
- Caries (tooth decay)
- Periodontal disease

Complications of Bulimia Nervosa. Gastrointestinal tract disturbances range from esophagitis (inflammation of the esophagus) to the serious complication of gastric dilation (extreme expansion of the stomach caused by binge-eating). Gastric dilation has caused stomach rupture and even death. The nurse assesses the client for abdominal distention, listens for bowel sounds, and questions the client about abdominal pain. Abdominal distention with pain in the absence of bowel sounds signifies an emergency situation. Chronic laxative abuse can lead to permanent loss of bowel reactivity and prolapse of the rectum. Other signs of laxative abuse include

- Recurrent abdominal pain
- Steatorrhea (fatty stools)
- Finger swelling or clubbing

Dieting and purging cause fluctuations in fluid balance; episodes of dehydration alternate with rebound water retention. The nurse often detects an immediate weight gain and edema in the hands and feet related to rebound fluid retention after cessation of purging behavior. Proper fluid balance gradually returns after the client completely stops

purging behaviors. The presence of edema in clients who purge is sometimes called *pseudo-Bartter syndrome*. The persistent release of renin from the kidneys results in increased angiotensin in the blood. The angiotensin acts on the adrenal glands and causes release of aldosterone, which conserves sodium. Saving sodium causes water to be retained, and, because the blood vessels cannot hold all the water, it leaks out and collects in dependent areas.

Frequent fluctuations in weight may also interfere with the regularity of the menstrual cycle. Even at normal weight, the bulimic may have irregular menses or amenorrhea.

The nurse assesses skin integrity by observing for tenting, which may be present if dehydration is severe. Scars on the knuckles and calluses on the abdomen may indicate self-purging behaviors. Scars from cuts or burns may indicate self-mutilating behaviors or suicide attempts.

➤ *Psychosocial Assessment*

Although researchers agree that the typical bulimic in Western society is young, female, and Caucasian, there is less agreement about other risk factors. Some of these include low self-esteem, personality characteristics, depression, body image disturbance, chronic dieting, socioeconomic status, family history of eating disorders, obesity, or other psychiatric disorders. When compared with the client with anorexia nervosa, the client with bulimia nervosa has a greater awareness of inner states—both physiologic, such as hunger, and psychological, such as depression. The bulimic's decreased ability to control urges and impulses can lead to difficulties in several areas besides food and weight. The bulimic has a poorly defined self-image and low self-esteem and is frequently sensitive to criticism while experiencing an excessive need for approval.

Bulimics are usually aware that eating relieves emotional distress but also starts the cycle that leads to feelings of low self-esteem and depression. The bulimic feels the discomfort related to the eating disorder, is aware of personal mood state, and can describe feeling depressed, demoralized, and hopeless. These feelings may lead to thoughts of suicide or to actual attempts, which initiate the client's first contact with health care providers.

The nurse asks about such prior or current treatment for depression and its effectiveness. If the client reveals any suicide attempts, the nurse assesses the lethality of the attempt by asking about the method used, the number of attempts, and what happened to prevent completion of the attempt. If the client has resorted to nonlethal cutting or burning, the nurse assesses for evidence of a pattern of self-mutilating behavior that the client may be using to relieve tension and decrease anxiety.

The nurse assesses family dynamics initially and on an ongoing basis to identify the extent of the client's support system as well as any conflictual relationships among family members.

The nurse gathers information about the family's knowledge of the client's illness behaviors and their attitudes about them. The nurse determines what efforts have been made to help the client and by which family members. Intensely close or distant relationships are identified.

The nurse observes family interaction and notes whether family members speak for each other. By asking how family members resolve conflicts and angry feelings, the nurse may gain useful information about the relationship of bulimic episodes to a lack of conflict resolution. The nurse assesses how the family presents itself, for instance, as perfect, overprotective, or chaotic.

▶ Laboratory Assessment

The health care provider orders an SMA-7 (7/60) and SMA-12 (12/60), which yield valuable data about the client's electrolyte and fluid balance and kidney function. An elevated blood urea nitrogen (BUN) level indicates dehydration. Dehydration associated with hypokalemia can predispose the client to serious renal problems.

A complete blood count with differential reveals blood abnormalities such as anemia or a bleeding tendency. Monitoring the magnesium level is important because low levels can result in dysrhythmias, weakness, bowel dysfunction, and cognitive problems.

The nurse monitors the client's serum amylase level on admission and routinely because *high* levels suggest that the client is practicing vomiting behavior. The serum amylase level rises within about 2 hours after vomiting and takes about 1 week to return to normal after vomiting behavior ceases.

In female bulimics who are amenorrheic or who have irregular menses, luteinizing hormone, follicle-stimulating hormone, and estrogen levels may be low. Male bulimics who report a loss of interest in sex may have low testosterone levels.

Thyroid studies show normal levels of thyroxine (T_4) and triiodothyronine (T_3) resin uptake, but lower on average than normal plasma T_3 in most bulimics. These determinations may be useful in the differential diagnosis, such as hyperthyroidism or Addison's disease.

▶ Other Diagnostic Assessment

An electrocardiogram (ECG) is essential in the physical assessment of the bulimic client. The ECG screens for dysrhythmias that may be life threatening. Dysrhythmias are the result of hypokalemia (deficient potassium levels) or toxicity from ipecac (an agent that induces vomiting).

The physician includes a routine chest x-ray. Upper and lower gastrointestinal (GI) tract studies may be necessary if the client has seriously damaged the GI tract. The GI tract may have been injured from vomiting, which exposes the esophageal mucosa to acidic gastric contents, or from laxative abuse, which produces the clinical manifestations of irritable bowel syndrome.

Psychological testing is indicated and is facilitated by collaboration with the hospital's consulting psychiatrist and/or psychiatric consultation-liaison nurse. The tests ordered for a bulimic client are similar to those suggested for the anorexic. The tests are usually performed by a clinical psychologist (see Other Diagnostic Assessment in the earlier discussion of anorexia nervosa). It is crucial that the nurse involve psychiatric specialists if the bulimic client is admitted to the hospital as a result of a suicide attempt or if the client has expressed depression or suicidal thoughts.

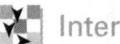 Interventions

Clients who purge by vomiting or by using laxatives and diuretics are at risk for depleting potassium chloride levels and creating a state of hypokalemic metabolic alkalosis. The depletion of this electrolyte results in low potassium levels and shrinkage of the effective arterial blood volume. Cardiac dysrhythmias and sudden cardiac arrest can result. (See Chapter 16 for more information on fluid and electrolyte imbalances.)

The bulimic who habitually uses ipecac syrup to induce vomiting is also at risk because of its potential for causing cardiotoxicity. When a bulimic client is admitted to the hospital, the nurse is especially alert for signs of an irregular pulse and blood volume depletion, such as orthostatic blood pressure changes and tachycardia when the client stands. The nurse or assistive nursing personnel take the client's vital signs on admission and frequently thereafter, usually every 3 to 4 hours.

▶ Drug Therapy

The physician may treat mild potassium depletion (3.0 to 3.4 mEq/L) in an otherwise asymptomatic client with oral supplements. In clients with more serious electrolyte imbalance, intravenous sodium chloride solution with potassium is administered.

Some experts in the treatment of bulimia nervosa advocate the use of a monoamine oxidase (MAO) inhibitor, such as tranylcypromine sulfate (Parnate) or phenelzine sulfate (Nardil). Because some clinical findings suggest that decreased brain serotonin level may be involved in bulimia nervosa, some experts treat with drugs that facilitate serotonergic neurotransmission, such as

- Fluoxetine (Prozac)
- Sertraline hydrochloride (Zoloft)
- Paroxetine (Paxil)
- Nefazodone (Serzone)
- Venlafaxine (Effexor)

It is thought that these agents decrease the client's urge to binge. Another drug has been used by Geretsegger et al. (1995), who report a significant reduction in binges after a 4-week trial of isapirone, a partial 5HT(1A) agonist. Other clinicians prefer a supportive, behavioral approach without drugs to break the binge-purge cycle.

The bulimic client may also experience relief from depression as well as help in controlling binge-eating by treatment with tricyclic antidepressants, such as nortriptyline hydrochloride (Aventyl) and desipramine hydrochloride (Norpramin). These older drugs are used cautiously, however, because of their side effects and the risk of overdose by suicidal clients.

▶ Diet Therapy

The nurse teaches the client to eat adequate amounts of food from the food pyramid. Nursing supervision provides emotional support and prevents binging behavior during the stressful period when the client is breaking the binge-purge cycle. The dietitian determines the client's daily nutritional needs according to the basal metabolic rate and suggests the appropriate daily food pattern and number of calories to be consumed. These requirements are relatively low for the bulimic, for instance, 1000 to 1200 kcal/day. The bulimic may feel deprived with the small amount of food allowed and may be tempted to binge and purge.

The nurse teaches the client to select the correct portion sizes and to think in terms of food patterns rather than calorie counting. Bulimics are encouraged to eat slowly and to avoid bolting down their food without really tasting it. Most clients with eating disorders are not permitted to use diet foods and drinks during treatment. The exception is the bulimic who gains weight easily and can eat only a small number of calories (e.g., 1000) to maintain a constant weight; these clients may use artificial sweeteners and diet foods and drinks.

The nurse collaborates with the dietitian in selecting a low-sodium diet (2 g/day) to minimize fluid retention. The amount of fluid intake is limited to about 1000 mL daily while edema is severe.

The nurse explains the wide swings in fluid balance that result when a person uses vomiting and purgatives to control weight. The nurse tells clients to expect edema, especially in the fingers, ankles, and face, and an initial weight gain when they discontinue purging behaviors. Because the weight gain may be significant, for instance, 5 to 10 pounds (2.3 to 4.5 kg), the nurse supports the client emotionally to prevent resumption of purging behaviors out of fear of fatness. The nurse reassures the client that the client's body will readjust its fluid balance and that the edema will resolve.

➤ Exercise

The nurse explains the importance of increasing the activity level and establishing a regular exercise routine. Bulimic clients who gain weight on few calories find exercise to be particularly important because it allows for increased caloric intake. The nurse cautions the client to avoid extremes, such as overexercising or underexercising.

➤ Psychotherapy

Regular psychotherapy sessions with a mental health professional provide an opportunity for the client

- To further develop and maintain control over eating habits
- To experience decreased anxiety
- To learn strategies for dealing with intense feelings and stress

The goal of increasing the client's sense of effectiveness—and thus increasing self-esteem and improving self-concept—may seem out of reach for the client. The nurse helps the client realize that this is a long-term goal that is achieved by accomplishing a series of small successes. The nurse emphasizes that the process is enhanced by the development of a trusting therapeutic relationship with a mental health professional.

The nurse helps to arrange the client's follow-up treatment for ongoing physical problems before discharge. The decision about specific psychiatric treatment is also made before discharge from the medical unit.

The nurse may give the client and family information about local resources for people with eating disorders and

▷ Research Applications for Nursing

Response to Intensive Treatment of Bulimia Nervosa

Olmsted, M. P., Kaplan, Q. S., Rockut, W., & Jacobsen, M. (1996). Rapid responders to intensive treatment of bulimia nervosa. International Journal of Eating Disorders, 19, 279–285.

This article is a report of research completed in a day-treatment program that included a nurse-therapist as a research associate (M.J.). The purpose of the study was to examine patterns of response to treatment of bulimia nervosa. Another desired outcome was to determine the benefit of being able to differentiate rapid from slow responders to treatment.

The study subjects included 166 women who met criteria for bulimia nervosa and were vomiting at least eight times a month. Treatment was provided in a day-hospital program that ran 8 hours a day, 5 days a week, and had an intensive group therapy focus. The treatment duration was individually determined and averaged 10.4 weeks. Symptom frequencies were assessed at the beginning and end of treatment using the Eating Disorder Inventory, Beck Depression Inventory, Hamilton Rating Scale for Depression, Social Adjustment Scale Self Report, and Eating Disorder Examination.

Forty-one percent of the participants were identified as rapid responders, with decreased symptoms during the first 4 weeks of treatment. Of the 166 participants, 31% were considered slow responders, who had symptom frequencies of three or less over the last 4 weeks of treatment. In addition, 18% of the participants were partial responders and 10% nonresponders. Two-year follow up data suggested a more favorable prognosis for rapid responders, that is, the rate of relapse was 15.8% for rapid responders, 57% for slow responders, and 66.7% for partial responders.

The researchers found that a significant subgroup of their study population of severely ill bulimia nervosa clients had a rapid and enduring response to treatment. However, they were unable to identify the likely rapid responders before treatment.

Critique. This study had a respectable sample size and used a variety of standardized instruments for measurement. However, the exact nature of the method of treatment was not specified. It is unclear whether other variables might account for the results of the study. Methods for deciding on the use of medication as part of the treatment were not identified. An important follow-up study identified by the researchers would examine the number of weeks of treatment most beneficial to rapid and slow responders.

Possible Nursing Implications. The article describes a day-treatment program that successfully treats clients with severe bulimia nervosa. It supports the current trend toward outpatient treatment and identifies the nurse-therapist as a key member of the interdisciplinary team.

their families. The nurse can obtain such information from the state department of mental health and hygiene. Further information is available from the American Anorexia/Bulimia Association, Inc. These resources provide general information about the illness and specific information about local treatment programs and support groups. Clients and families may benefit from attending groups established and maintained by people who are struggling with similar issues and problems. The family is encouraged to participate in family therapy provided in a day-hospital program or other outpatient treatment program (see Research Applications for Nursing). Woodside et al. (1995) reported a significant improvement in family functioning after such treatment.

CASE STUDY for the Client with Anorexia Nervosa

■ A 40-year-old married mother of two with a history of anorexia nervosa with bulimic features since her early teens is one of your clients. She has had at least three psychiatric hospitalizations in the past for this disorder. She has admitted to taking up to 100 laxatives a day in the past and says she now takes five a day. She has been treated for major depression with antidepressant therapy for the past 5 years and has been admitted to your surgical floor ten times in the last 3 years. She has history of hypertension, stomach ulcers, and prolapsed rectum. Surgeries include cholecystectomy, Bilroth I with bilateral truncal vagotomy, hernia repair, exploratory laparotomy for partial duodenal obstruction, partial removal of bezoar, and feeding jejunostomy tube placement. She has been admitted today to rule out another bezoar. She has had the jejunostomy tube for several months and verbalizes her understanding that she can eat nothing by mouth. She admits to drinking diet soda but denies eating any food, and she states she has no idea how a bezoar might have formed. You know from past hospitalizations that she was frequently observed buying candy in the hospital gift shop, and staff found empty candy wrappers in her room. Staff suspected she was vomiting regularly, but it was not directly observed and she denied it. She tells you today that she has continued to see her therapist regularly and is still taking Zoloft for depression. The client admits to hoarding food at home but denies eating by mouth or vomiting while at home. Her weight is under 100 pounds despite her report that she is using her jejunoscopy tube to administer her liquid nutritional feedings. She has been seen by the psychiatric consultation-liaison nurse and the consultation-liaison psychiatrist during past hospitalizations. You are interested in helping her to use healthy coping strategies during this hospital stay.

Q U E S T I O N S :

1. What specific questions will you ask the client related to her eating disorder?
2. What resource personnel would you use to assist in developing a plan of care for this patient?
3. What suggestions do you have for the plan of care?

SELECTED BIBLIOGRAPHY

American Psychiatric Association (1994). *Diagnostic and statistical manual of mental disorders* (4th ed., revised). Washington, DC: American Psychiatric Association.

*Andersen, A. E. (1985). *Practical comprehensive treatment of anorexia nervosa and bulimia.* Baltimore: The Johns Hopkins University Press.

Bemporad, J. R. (1996). Starvation through the ages. *International Journal of Eating Disorders, 19,* 217–237.

Casper, R. C., & Lyubomirsky, S. (1997). Individual psychopathology relative to reports of unwanted sexual experiences as predictor of a bulimic eating pattern. *International Journal of Eating Disorders, 21,* 229–236.

Cochrane, C. E. (1995). Eating regulation responses and eating disorders. In G. W. Stuart & S. J. Sundeen (Eds.), *Principles and practice of psychiatric nursing* (5th ed., pp. 607–632). St. Louis: C. V. Mosby.

Crago, M., Shisslak, C., & Estes, L. (1996). Eating disorders among American minority groups: A review. *International Journal of Eating Disorders, 19,* 239–248.

Crow, S. J., Salisbury, J. J., Crosby, R. D., & Mitchell, J. E. (1997). Serum electrolytes as markers of vomiting in bulimia nervosa. *International Journal of Eating Disorders, 21,* 95–98.

Dansky, B. S., Brewerton, T. D., Kilpatrick, D. G., & O'Neil, P. M. (1997). The national women's study: Relationship of victimization and posttraumatic stress disorder to bulimia nervosa. *International Journal of Eating Disorders, 21,* 213–228.

Davis, W. N. (1998). Eating disorders and case management. *The Case Manager, 9*(1), 35–39.

*Frisch, R. E., & McArthur, J. W. (1974). Menstrual cycles: Fatness as a determinant of minimum weight for height necessary for their maintenance or onset. *Science, 185,* 949–951.

Geretsegger, C., Greimel, K., Roed, I., & Hesselink, J. (1995). Isapirone in the treatment of bulimia nervosa: An open pilot study. *International Journal of Eating Disorders, 17,* 359–363.

Herzog, W., Deter, H.-C., Fiehn, W., & Petzold, E. (1997). Medical findings and predictors of long-term physical outcome in anorexia nervosa: A prospective 12-year follow-up study. *Psychological Medicine, 27,* 269–279.

Kearney-Cooke, A., & Striegel-Moore, R. (1996). Treatment of childhood sexual abuse in anorexia nervosa and bulimia nervosa: A feminist psychodynamic approach. In M. F. Schwartz & L. Cohn (Eds.), *Sexual abuse and eating disorders* (pp. 155–178). New York: Brunner/Mazel.

*Lasegue, C. (1985). On hysterical anorexia. In A. E. Andersen (Ed.), *Practical comprehensive treatment of anorexia nervosa and bulimia* (pp. 19–27). Baltimore: The Johns Hopkins University Press. (Reprinted from *Archives of General Medicine,* 1873, 2, 367.)

*Lucas, A. R., Beard, C. M., O'Fallon, W. M., & Kurland, L. T. (1991). 50-Year trends in the incidence of anorexia nervosa in Rochester, Minn.: A population-based study. *American Journal of Psychiatry, 148,* 917–922.

Mannucci, E., Ricca, V., & Rotella, C. (1997). Clinical features of binge eating disorder in type I diabetes: A case report. *International Journal of Eating Disorders, 21,* 99–102.

Neumarker, K.-J. (1997). Mortality and sudden death in anorexia nervosa. *International Journal of Eating Disorders, 21,* 205–212.

Olmsted, M. P., Kaplan, Q. S., Rockut, W., & Jacobsoen, M. (1996). Rapid responders to intensive treatment of bulimia nervosa. *International Journal of Eating Disorders, 19,* 279–285.

*Russell, G. F. M. (1970). Anorexia nervosa: Its identity as an illness and its treatment. In J. H. Price (Ed.), *Modern trends in psychological medicine* (Vol. 2, pp. 131–164). London: Butterworths.

Salisbury, J. J., Levine, A. S., Crow, S. J., & Mitchell, J. E. (1995). Refeeding, metabolic rate, and weight gain in anorexia nervosa: A review. *International Journal of Eating Disorders, 17,* 337–345.

Smolak, L., & Levine, M. P. (1996). Adolescent transitions and the development of eating problems. In L. Smolak, M. P. Levine, & R. Striegel-Moore (Eds.), *The developmental psychopathology of eating disorders: Implications for research, prevention, and treatment* (pp. 207–234). Mahway, NJ: Lawrence Erlbaum Associates.

Striegel-Moore, R., & Smolak, L. (1996). The role of race in the development of eating disorders. In L. Smolak, M. P. Levine, & R. Striegel-Moore (Eds.), *The developmental psychopathology of eating disorders: Implications for research, prevention, and treatment* (pp. 259–284). Mahway, NJ: Lawrence Erlbaum Associates.

*Theander, S. (1985). Outcome and prognosis in anorexia nervosa and bulimia: Some results of previous investigations, compared with those of a Swedish long-term study. *Journal of Psychiatric Research, 19,* 493–508.

Thompson, J. K. (1996). *Body image, eating disorders, and obesity: An integrative guide for assessment and treatment.* Washington, DC: American Psychological Association.

Vanderlinden, J., & Vandereycken, W. (1996). Is sexual abuse a risk factor for developing an eating disorder? In M. F. Schwartz & L. Cohn (Eds.), *Sexual abuse and eating disorders* (pp. 17–22). New York: Brunner/Mazel.

Woodside, D. B., Shekter-Wolfson, L., Garfinkel, P. E., Olmsted, M. P., Kaplan, A. S., & Maddocks, S. E. (1995). Family interactions in bulimia nervosa I: Study design, comparisons to established population norms, and changes over the course of an intensive day hospital treatment program. *International Journal of Eating Disorders, 17,* 105–115.

SUGGESTED READINGS

Bemporad, J. R. (1996). Starvation through the ages. *International Journal of Eating Disorders, 19,* 217–237.

This is an excellent review of the history of eating disorders. The purpose of the review was to identify factors that foster or inhibit the development of eating disorders.

Cochrane, C. E. (1995). Eating regulation responses and eating disorders. In G. W. Stuart & S. J. Sundeen (Eds.), *Principles and practice of psychiatric nursing* (5th ed., pp. 607–632). St. Louis: C. V. Mosby.

This book chapter provides an in-depth description of the treatment of anorexia nervosa, bulimia nervosa, and binge-eating disorder. It is written by a doctorally prepared nurse psychotherapist who cares for clients in both the inpatient and outpatient setting.

Waller, D., Fairburn, C., McPherson, A., Kay, R., Lee, A., & Nowell, T. (1996). Treating bulimia nervosa in primary care: A pilot study. *International Journal of Eating Disorders, 19,* 99–103.

These British clinicians report on a pilot study that used cognitive behavioral treatment for bulimia nervosa. The unusual aspect of this study was that the treatment was administered by general practice physicians or nurses in the primary care setting. The authors concluded that the results of this study indicate that this form of treatment can benefit a significant proportion of the clients with bulimia nervosa seen in the primary care setting.

Chapter 64

INTERVENTIONS FOR CLIENTS WITH MALNUTRITION AND OBESITY

Nutrition plays a major role in promoting and maintaining health. The client in good nutritional health has a decreased risk of having a catastrophic event, such as a myocardial infarction, and can regain optimal function more quickly if such an event occurs.

Nutritional health not only contributes to positive care outcomes but also saves health care dollars. For example, the cost of treating malnourished clients is more than twice that of treating clients in good nutritional health (Wellman, 1997).

As part of a comprehensive health assessment, the nurse should include nutritional screening to identify clients who have nutritional deficits or are at risk for developing nutritional deficits. Nurses may also conduct a complete nutritional assessment (Grindel & Costello, 1996).

NUTRITION STANDARDS
Dietary Planning

Several national standards are available for planning and evaluating nutrition. The standard most widely accepted in the United States is the Recommended Dietary Allowances (RDA), established by the Food and Nutrition Board (FNB) of the National Research Council/National Academy of Sciences. These standards were originally published in 1943. The most current revision in 1989 establishes recommendations for energy intake, protein,

vitamins, and minerals for a healthy population. Healthy adults require approximately 1800 calories a day and 0.8 g of protein per kilogram of body weight to meet basal energy needs.

The RDA can be used to estimate the adequacy of nutrient intake over time. However, if a client does not meet 100% of the RDA, it is incorrect to assume that the client is nutritionally deficient. The risk of inadequate intake for any nutrient is not presumed to be increased until less than 70% of the RDA is consumed. It is also incorrect to assume that all clients in a specific population who meet 100% of the RDA are not at risk for malnutrition.

The FNB, with the involvement of Health Canada, has recommended Dietary Reference Intakes (DRI) replace the RDA. The first DRI released recommended intake of nutrients related to bone health (Food and Nutrition Board, 1997).

The established standard of Canada, the Recommended Nutrient Intakes (RNI), is similar to that of the United States.

Disease Prevention and Health Promotion

The role of diet and nutrition in disease has been a subject of interest for many years. The current focus is on the prevention of disease and health promotion. In 1995,

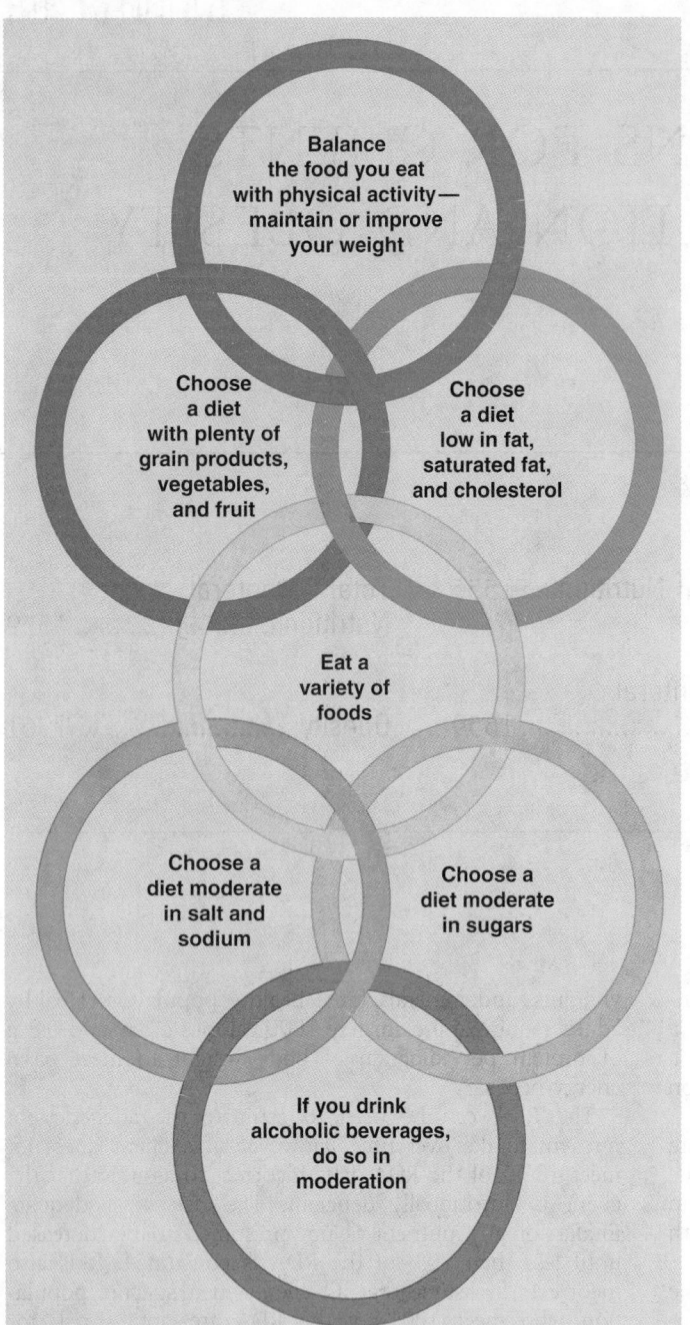

Figure 64–1. Dietary guidelines developed by the U. S. Departments of Agriculture and Health and Human Services.

the Dietary Guidelines for Americans were revised by the U.S. Departments of Agriculture (USDA) and Health and Human Services (HHS). These seven guidelines emphasize the importance of selecting foods to maintain a healthful diet with balance, moderation, and variety (Fig. 64–1). One of the most noticeable changes from previous editions occurs in the weight guideline. For the first time, diet and physical activity are emphasized in the second guideline with the goal of maintaining or improving body weight (Kennedy et al., 1996).

The Nutrition Recommendations for Canadians (Table 64–1) are similar to the Dietary Guidelines for Ameri-

cans. In addition, they recommend limiting the caffeine content of the diet to no more than the equivalent of four cups of coffee per day and adding fluoride to community water supplies to a level of 1 mg/L.

The USDA developed the Food Guide Pyramid (Fig. 64–2) in 1992 to translate food recommendations into a practical graphic format. A pyramid format was chosen to communicate three key dietary principles—variety, moderation, and proportionality. The pyramid design emphasizes building the diet on a base of grains, fruits, and vegetables. Moderate quantities of lean meats, protein sources, and dairy products are added while intake of fats

TABLE 64-1

Nutrition Recommendations for Canadians

- The sodium content of the Canadian diet should be reduced.
- The Canadian diet should include no more than 5% of total energy as alcohol, or two drinks daily, whichever is less.
- The Canadian diet should contain no more caffeine than the equivalent of four cups of regular coffee per day.
- Community water supplies containing less than 1 mg/L of fluoride should be fluoridated to that level.
- The Canadian diet should provide energy consistent with the maintenance of body weight within the recommended range.
- The Canadian diet should include essential nutrients in amounts specified in the Recommended Nutrient Intakes.
- The Canadian diet should include no more than 30% of energy as fat (33 g/1000 kcal or 39 g/5000 kJ) and no more than 10% as saturated fat (11 g/1000 kcal or 13 g/5000 kJ).
- The Canadian diet should provide 55% of energy as carbohydrates (138 g/1000 kcal or 165 g/5000 kJ) from a variety of sources.

From Communications/Implementation Committee, Minister of National Health and Walfare. (1990). *Action towards healthy eating. Canada's guidelines for healthy eating and recommended strategies for implementation* (Cat. No. H39-166/1990E). Ottawa: Branch Publications Unit.

and sweets is limited. This guide to daily food choices has replaced the basic four food groups as the standard for evaluating the nutritional adequacy of dietary intake. Table 64–2 suggests daily servings of each food group

and clarifies what a serving is. Adherence to this pattern will result in a nutritionally adequate intake if a variety of foods is chosen.

A variety of vegetarian diet patterns are being adopted by increasing numbers of people for health, environmental, and moral reasons. The lacto-vegetarian eats milk, cheese, and dairy foods but avoids meat, fish, poultry, and eggs. The lacto-ovo-vegetarian includes eggs also. The vegan eats only foods of plant origin. Vegans can develop megaloblastic anemia as a result of vitamin B_{12} deficiency. Vegans should include a daily source of vitamin B_{12} in their diets, such as a fortified breakfast cereal, fortified soy beverage, or meat analog (American Dietetic Association, 1997). All vegetarians should ensure that they get adequate calcium, iron, zinc, and vitamins D and B_{12}. Well-planned vegetarian diets can provide adequate nutrition. The Vegetarian Food Pyramid (Fig. 64–3), endorsed by the Vegetarian Resource Group, can assist vegetarians with daily food choices.

NUTRITIONAL ASSESSMENT

Malnutrition and obesity are common nutrition problems that occur as progressive changes within the client. When nutritional deficiencies or excesses develop, the body adapts through the use of homeostatic mechanisms. As the intake moves farther away from the accepted range, however, the body accommodates by reducing functional levels or changing the status or size of the affected body compartments. The nutritional status of a client can be determined by the presence or absence of these adaptations.

Nutritional status reflects the balance between nutrient

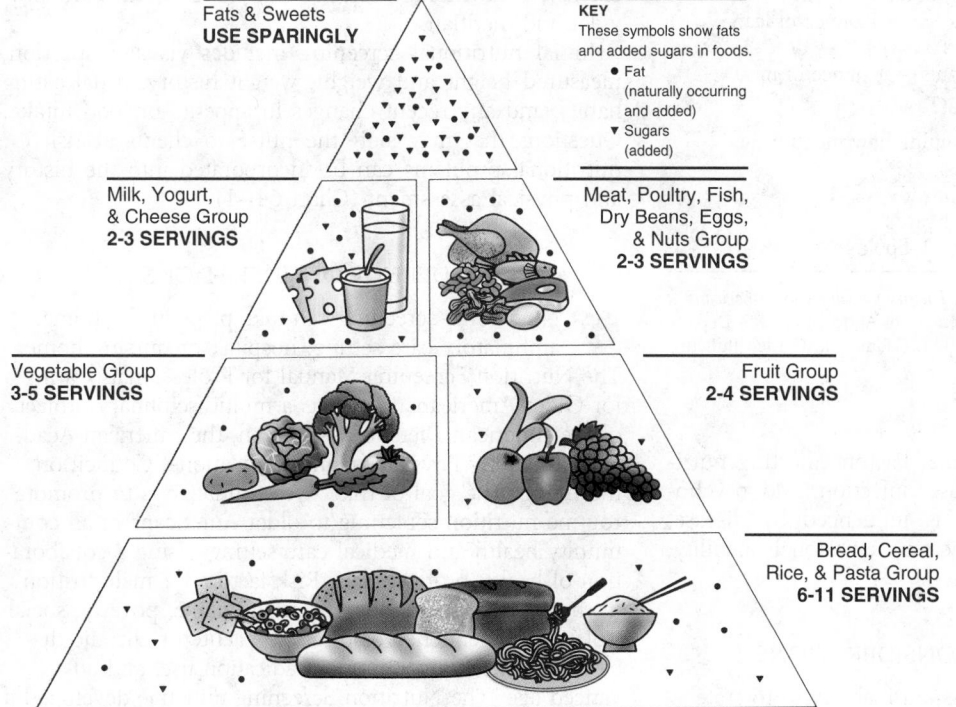

Figure 64–2. The U. S. Department of Agriculture (USDA) Food Guide Pyramid.

TABLE 64-2

Serving Sizes for Each Food Group

With the Food Guide Pyramid, what counts as a "serving" may not always be a typical "helping" of what you eat. Here are some examples of servings.

Bread, Cereal, Rice, and Pasta

6 to 11 servings recommended
Examples of one serving:

- 1 slice of bread
- 1 ounce ready-to-eat cereal
- ½ cup cooked cereal, rice, or pasta

Vegetables

3 to 5 servings recommended
Examples of one serving:

- 1 cup raw leafy vegetables
- ½ cup other vegetables, cooked or chopped raw
- ¾ cup vegetable juice

Fruits

2 to 4 servings recommended
Examples of one serving:

- 1 medium apple, banana, or orange
- ½ cup chopped, cooked, or canned fruit
- ¾ cup fruit juice

Milk, Yogurt, and Cheese

2 to 3 servings recommended
Examples of one serving:

- 1 cup milk or yogurt
- 1½ ounces natural cheese
- 2 ounces process cheese

Meat, Poultry, Fish, Dry Beans, Eggs, and Nuts

2 to 3 servings recommended
Examples of one serving:

- 2–3 ounces cooked lean meat, poultry, or fish
- ½ cup cooked dry beans or 1 egg = 1 ounce of lean meat
- 2 tbsp peanut butter or ⅓ c nuts = 1 ounce of meat

How Much Is an Ounce of Meat?

Here's a handy guide for determining how much meat, chicken, fish, or cheese weighs:
1 ounce = the size of a match box
3 ounces = the size of a deck of cards
8 ounces = the size of a paperback book

Adapted from *Nutrition and your health: Dietary guidelines for Americans* (4th ed.). Washington, DC: U.S. Department of Agriculture, U.S. Department of Health and Human Services, 1995) (Home and Garden Bulletin No. 232).

requirements and nutrient intake. Factors affecting nutrient requirements include disease, infection, and psychological stress. Nutrient intake is influenced by disease, eating behavior, economic factors, emotional stability, medication, and cultural factors.

TRANSCULTURAL CONSIDERATIONS

 Lactose intolerance, that is, an inability to tolerate milk and milk products, is a relatively common condition that occurs in a number of ethnic groups. It is found in over 66% of Mexican-Americans and 79% of African-Americans, as well as in some Native American tribes, Asian-Americans, and Ashkenazic Jews (Giger & Davidhizar, 1995). The cause of lactose intolerance is an insufficient amount of the lactase enzyme that converts lactose into absorbable glucose.

Optimal nutritional care is a major nursing goal for clients with malnutrition and obesity. Evaluation of nutritional status is an important part of total client assessment. A thorough assessment of nutritional status includes

- Review of the diet history
- Food and fluid intake record
- Laboratory data
- Food-medication interactions
- Physical examination and health history
- Anthropometric measurements
- Psychosocial assessment

Monitoring the nutritional care of a client is as important as the initial assessment. The health care provider, nurse, and dietitian collaborate to identify clients at risk for nutritional problems.

Initial Nutritional Screening

Not every client needs a complete nutritional assessment, but it is important to identify clients at risk for nutritional problems through screening. Initial nutritional screening of the client provides the nurse with an inexpensive, quick way of determining which clients will need more extensive nutritional assessment by the health care provider and dietitian.

Initial nutritional screening includes visual inspection, measured height and weight, weight history, usual eating habits, and any recent changes in appetite or food intake. Questions that may alert the nurse to clients at risk for nutritional problems can be incorporated into the history and physical assessment (Chart 64–1).

ELDERLY CONSIDERATIONS

Nutritional screening can take place in the home, ambulatory care setting, hospital, or nursing home. The Nutrition Screening Manual for Professionals Caring for Older Americans (1991) is a multidisciplinary project of the American Dietetic Association, the American Academy of Family Physicians, and the National Council on the Aging. The goal of this 5-year initiative is to promote routine nutrition screening to older Americans in all community health and medical care settings using a collaboration of health professionals. Risk factors for malnutrition in the elderly include inappropriate intake, poverty, social isolation, dependency or disability, acute or chronic diseases or conditions, chronic medication use, and advanced age. The Nutrition Screening initiative developed a three-tiered approach to nutrition screening:

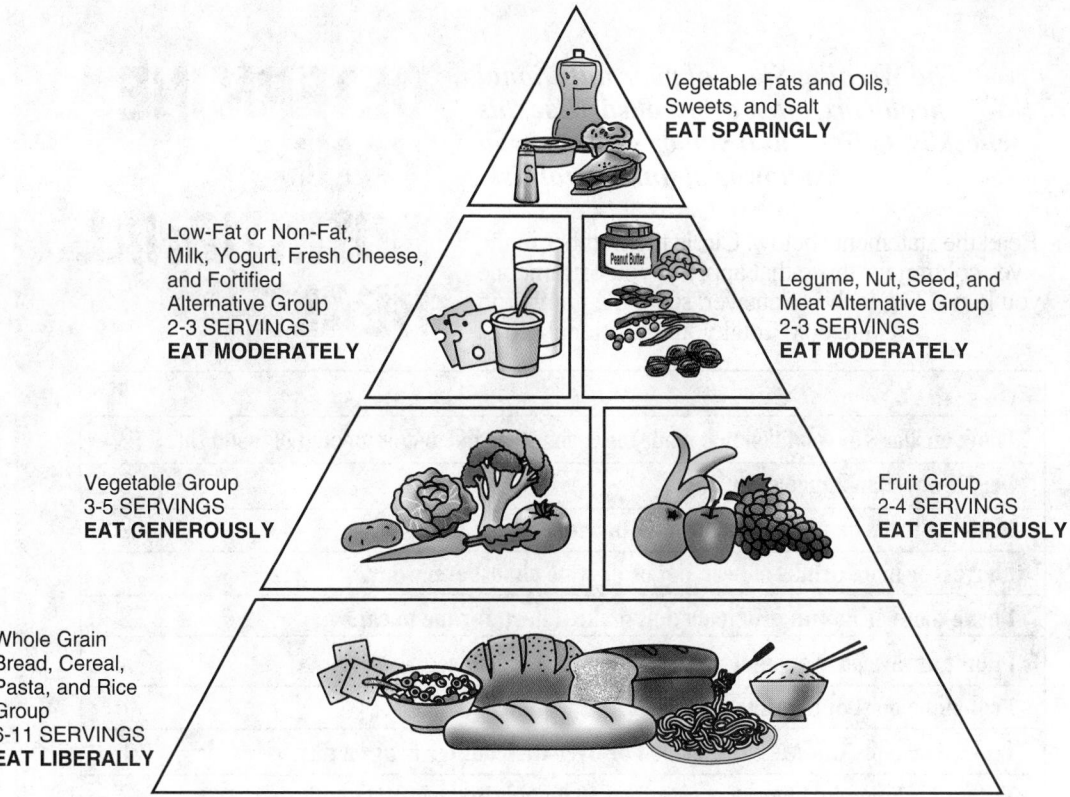

Figure 64–3. Food pyramid for a vegetarian diet. (Courtesy of the Health Connection.)

Chart 64–1

Nursing Care Highlight: Initial Nutrition Screening Assessment

The presence of one or more of the following conditions should alert the nurse that the client is at risk for malnutrition or has had a condition in the past requiring special nutritional care.

General

- Does the client have any conditions that cause nutrient loss, such as malabsorption syndromes, draining abscesses, wounds, fistulas, or protracted diarrhea?
- Does the client have any conditions that increase the need for nutrients, such as fever, burn, injury, sepsis, or antineoplastic therapies?
- Has the client been NPO for 3 days or more?
- Is the client receiving a modified diet or a diet restricted in one or more nutrients?
- Is the client being enterally or parenterally fed?
- Does the client describe food allergies, lactose intolerance, or limited food preferences?
- Has the client experienced recent unexplained weight loss?

Gastrointestinal

- Does the client complain of nausea, indigestion, vomiting, diarrhea, or constipation?
- Does the client exhibit glossitis, stomatitis, or esophagitis?
- Does the client have difficulty chewing or swallowing?
- Does the client have a partial or total GI obstruction?
- What is the client's state of dentition?

Cardiovascular

- Does the client have ascites or edema?
- Is the client able to perform activities of daily living?
- Does the client have congestive heart failure?

Genitourinary

- Does fluid input approximately equal fluid output?
- Does the client have an ostomy?
- Is the client hemodialyzed or peritoneally dialyzed?

Respiratory

- Is the client receiving mechanical ventilatory support?
- Is the client receiving oxygen via nasal prongs?
- Does the client have chronic airway limitation?

Integumentary

- Does the client have nail or hair changes?
- Does the client have rashes or dermatitis?
- Does the client have dry or pale mucous membranes or decreased skin turgor?
- Does the client have pressure areas on the sacrum, hips, or ankles?

Extremities

- Does the client have pedal edema?
- Does the client exhibit cachexia?

Adapted with permission of Ross Products Division, Abbott Laboratories, Columbus, OH.

The Warning Signs of poor nutritional health are often overlooked. Use this checklist to find out if you or someone you know is at nutritional risk.

Read the statements below. Circle the number in the yes column for those that apply to you or someone you know. For each yes answer, score the number in the box. Total your nutritional score.

DETERMINE YOUR NUTRITIONAL HEALTH

	YES
I have an illness or condition that made me change the kind and/or amount of food I eat.	2
I eat fewer than 2 meals per day.	3
I eat few fruits or vegetables, or milk products.	2
I have 3 or more drinks of beer, liquor or wine almost every day.	2
I have tooth or mouth problems that make it hard for me to eat.	2
I don't always have enough money to buy the food I need.	4
I eat alone most of the time.	1
I take 3 or more different prescribed or over-the-counter drugs a day.	1
Without wanting to, I have lost or gained 10 pounds in the last 6 months.	2
I am not always physically able to shop, cook and/or feed myself.	2
	TOTAL

Total Your Nutritional Score. If it's —

0-2   **Good!** Recheck your nutritional score in 6 months.

3-5   **You are at moderate nutritional risk.** See what can be done to improve your eating habits and lifestyle. Your office on aging, senior nutrition program, senior citizens center or health department can help. Recheck your nutritional score in 3 months.

6 or more **You are at high nutritional risk.** Bring this checklist the next time you see your doctor, dietitian or other qualified health or social service professional. Talk with them about any problems you may have. Ask for help to improve your nutritional health.

Remember that warning signs suggest risk, but do not represent diagnosis of any condition. Turn the page to learn more about the Warnings Signs of poor nutritional health.

These materials developed and distributed by the Nutrition Screening Initiative, a project of:

 AMERICAN ACADEMY OF FAMILY PHYSICIANS

 THE AMERICAN DIETETIC ASSOCIATION

 NATIONAL COUNCIL ON THE AGING, INC.

Figure 64–4. The "Determine Your Nutritional Health" checklist used to alert older adults to the warning signs of poor nutritional health. (Courtesy of the Nutrition Screening Initiative, Washington, D.C.)

- The *DETERMINE* Your Nutritional Health Checklist to alert older adults about the warning signs for poor nutritional health (Fig. 64–4).
- The Level I screen developed for use by professionals in health or social service settings such as adult day-care

centers, congregate meal programs, and assisted-living facilities.
- The Level II screen developed for use in medical settings such as acute care hospitals, physicians' offices, and long-term care facilities.

The Nutrition Checklist is based on the Warning Signs described below.
Use the word <u>DETERMINE</u> to remind you of the Warning Signs.

DISEASE

Any disease, illness or chronic condition which causes you to change the way you eat, or makes it hard for you to eat, puts your nutritional health at risk. Four out of five adults have chronic diseases that are affected by diet. Confusion or memory loss that keeps getting worse is estimated to affect one out of five or more of older adults. This can make it hard to remember what, when or if you've eaten. Feeling sad or depressed, which happens to about one in eight older adults, can cause big changes in appetite, digestion, energy level, weight and well-being.

EATING POORLY

Eating too little and eating too much both lead to poor health. Eating the same foods day after day or not eating fruit, vegetables, and milk products daily will also cause poor nutritional health. One in five adults skip meals daily. Only 13% of adults eat the minimum amount of fruit and vegetables needed. One in four older adults drink too much alcohol. Many health problems become worse if you drink more than one or two alcoholic beverages per day.

TOOTH LOSS/ MOUTH PAIN

A healthy mouth, teeth and gums are needed to eat. Missing, loose or rotten teeth or dentures which don't fit well or cause mouth sores make it hard to eat.

ECONOMIC HARDSHIP

As many as 40% of older Americans have incomes of less than $6,000 per year. Having less--or choosing to spend less--than $25-30 per week for food makes it very hard to get the foods you need to stay healthy.

REDUCED SOCIAL CONTACT

One-third of all older people live alone. Being with people daily has a positive effect on morale, well-being and eating.

MULTIPLE MEDICINES

Many older Americans must take medicines for health problems. Almost half of older Americans take multiple medicines daily. Growing old may change the way we respond to drugs. The more medicines you take, the greater the chance for side effects such as increased or decreased appetite, change in taste, constipation, weakness, drowsiness, diarrhea, nausea, and others. Vitamins or minerals when taken in large doses act like drugs and can cause harm. Alert your doctor to everything you take.

INVOLUNTARY WEIGHT LOSS/GAIN

Losing or gaining a lot of weight when you are not trying to do so is an important warning sign that must not be ignored. Being overweight or underweight also increases your chance of poor health.

NEEDS ASSISTANCE IN SELF CARE

Although most older people are able to eat, one of every five have trouble walking, shopping, buying and cooking food, especially as they get older.

ELDER YEARS ABOVE AGE 80

Most older people lead full and productive lives. But as age increases, risk of frailty and health problems increase. Checking your nutritional health regularly makes good sense.

The Nutrition Screening Initiative • 1010 Wisconsin Avenue, NW • Suite 800 • Washington, DC 20007
The Nutrition Screening Initiative is funded in part by a grant from Ross Laboratories, a division of Abbott Laboratories.

Figure 64–4. *Continued*

Anthropometric Measurements

Anthropometric measurements provide noninvasive methods to evaluate the client's nutritional status. These include height and weight and assessment of body fat.

Measurement of Height and Weight

Height and weight provide a baseline determination of nutritional status. The nurse or assistive nursing personnel obtains accurate measurements because clients who report their own height and weight tend to overestimate height and underestimate weight. Subsequent measurements may indicate an early change in nutritional status.

Height

Clients should be measured and weighed while wearing minimal clothing and no shoes. The nurse or assistive nursing personnel determines the client's height in inches or centimeters with the measuring stick of a weight scale. The client should stand erect, with heels together and arms at the sides, looking straight ahead.

Implications for the Elderly. Elderly clients may have difficulty standing erect, and their actual height may be less than their height on recall. If height cannot be measured directly, it should be estimated by arm span or with use of a knee-height caliper, which provides a more precise height estimate.

Weight

The nurse or assistive nursing personnel weighs ambulatory clients with an upright balance beam scale. Nonambulatory clients can be weighed with a movable wheelchair balance beam scale or a bed scale. The manufacturer should calibrate weight scales twice yearly to ensure accurate readings. For daily or sequential weights, the nurse or assistive personnel notes the time and obtains the weight at the same time each day. Such conditions as heart failure and renal disease affect fluid balance and therefore weight.

Normal weights for adult men and women are shown in the Metropolitan Life tables (Table 64–3). The latest of the U.S. Department of Agriculture (USDA) and the Department of Health and Human Services (DHHS) Dietary Guidelines contain weight guidelines that emphasize both weight maintenance and weight loss. The same healthy weight guideline applies to all adults. Older adults are no

TABLE 64–3

Metropolitan Life Height and Weight Tables				
Height*		**Weight†**		
Feet	Inches	Small Frame	Medium Frame	Large Frame
Men				
5	2	128–134	131–134	138–150
5	3	130–136	133–143	140–153
5	4	132–138	135–145	142–156
5	5	134–140	137–148	144–160
5	6	136–142	139–151	146–164
5	7	138–145	142–154	149–168
5	8	140–148	145–157	152–172
5	9	142–151	148–160	155–176
5	10	144–154	151–163	158–180
5	11	146–157	154–166	161–184
6	0	149–160	157–170	164–188
6	1	152–164	160–174	168–192
6	2	155–168	164–178	172–197
6	3	158–172	167–182	176–202
6	4	162–176	171–187	181–207
Women				
4	10	102–111	109–121	118–131
4	11	103–113	111–123	120–134
5	0	104–115	113–126	122–137
5	1	106–118	115–129	125–140
5	2	108–121	118–132	128–143
5	3	111–124	121–135	131–147
5	4	114–127	124–138	134–151
5	5	117–130	127–141	137–155
5	6	120–133	130–144	140–159
5	7	123–136	133–147	143–163
5	8	126–139	136–150	146–167
5	9	129–142	139–153	149–170
5	10	132–145	142–156	152–173
5	11	135–148	145–159	155–176
6	0	138–151	148–162	158–179

Reprinted courtesy of Metropolitan Life Insurance Company, 1983.
*Shoes with 1-inch heels.
†Weight in pounds. Men: allow 5 pounds of clothing. Women: allow 3 pounds of clothing

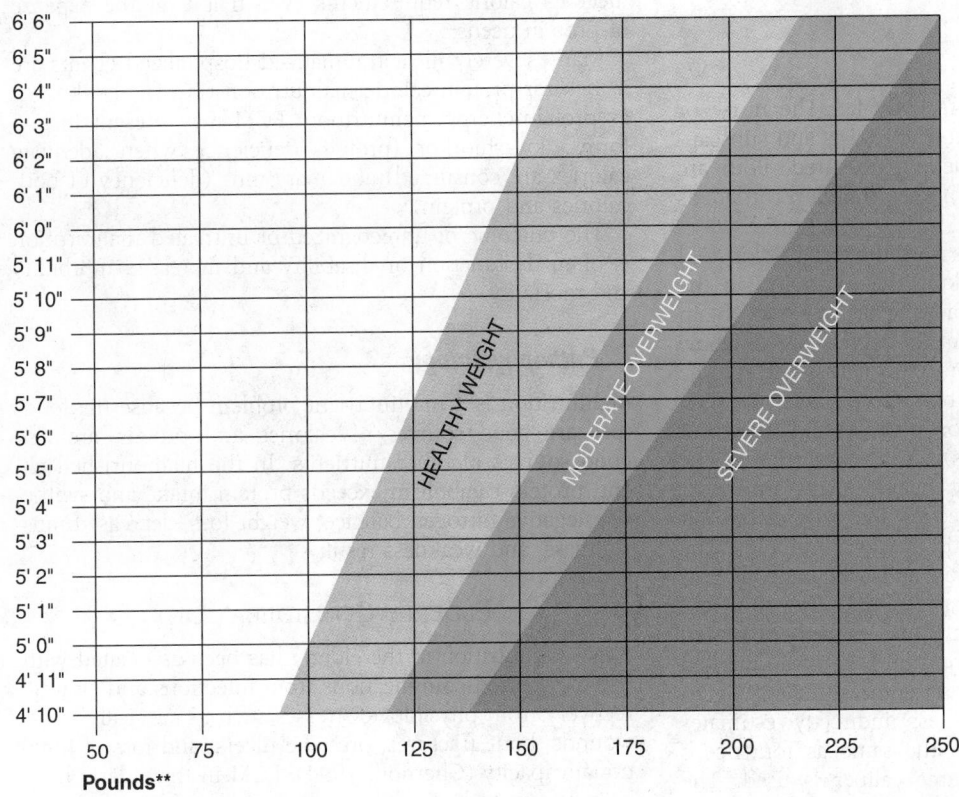

Figure 64–5. USDA/DHHS guidelines for determining proper weight or degree of obesity. (Redrawn from http://www.nalusda.gov/fnic/Dietary/9dietgui.htm.).

* Without shoes.

** Without clothes. The higher weights apply to people with more muscle and bone, such as many men.

longer permitted a higher weight standard. The weight range appears in the guidelines as a chart with three categories: healthy weight, moderate overweight, and severe overweight (Fig. 64–5). Either the Metropolitan Life tables or the New Weight Guidelines from the USDA and the DHHS may be used for comparison with a client's height and weight. Some health care professionals prefer the Metropolitan Life tables because they take body build differences into account by gender.

Changes in body weight can be expressed by three different formulas:

1. Weight as a percentage of ideal body weight (IBW):

   % IBW = current weight × 100/ideal weight

2. Current weight as a percentage of usual body weight (UBW):

   % UBW = current weight × 100/usual weight

3. Change in weight:

$$\text{weight change} = \frac{\text{usual weight} - \text{current weight}}{\text{usual weight}} \times 100$$

An involuntary weight loss of 10% at any time significantly affects nutritional status. Weights may need to be taken daily, several times a week, or weekly for monitoring status and the effectiveness of nutritional support.

Assessment of Body Fat
Body Mass Index

The body mass index (BMI), or Quetelet index, is a measure of nutritional status that does not depend on frame size. The BMI indirectly estimates total fat stores within the body by the relationship of weight to height, or

$$\text{BMI} = \text{weight (kg)/height}^2 \text{ (m}^2)$$

A simpler calculation for estimating BMI, which can be programmed into hand-held computers, is

$$\text{BMI} = \text{(pounds divided by inches squared)} \times 705$$

BMI can also be determined using a nomogram. The least risk of death from malnutrition is associated with scores between 20 and 25 (Mahan & Escot-Stump, 1996). BMIs above and below these values are associated with increased health risks. However, older, healthy adults should have a BMI between 24 and 27 (Nutrition Screening Manual, 1991).

Skin Fold Measurements

Skin fold measurements estimate body fat. The nurse or dietitian may measure the client. The triceps and subscapular skin folds are most frequently measured. Both are compared with standard measurements and recorded as percentiles.

The nurse or dietitian can measure the triceps skin fold thickness by locating and marking the midpoint on the client's upper arm with use of a tape measure. To obtain the midpoint, the left arm is bent 90 degrees at the elbow and the forearm is placed palm down across the middle of the body. The midpoint is half the distance between the tip of the shoulder (acromion process) and the tip of the elbow (olecranon process). The skin should be marked at this point before any measurements are made. The triceps skin fold is measured on the back of the left arm over the triceps muscle at the marked midpoint. The nurse holds a double fold of skin and subcutaneous adipose tissue between the fingers and thumb. The skin fold is held until the jaws of the skin fold caliper are placed perpendicular to the length of the skin fold at the marked midpoint. The nurse then records the measurement.

Subscapular skin fold thickness indirectly estimates body fat. The body position is the same as for triceps skin fold thickness, and the same caliper is used. The nurse holds a double fold of skin and subcutaneous adipose tissue in a line from the inferior angle of the left scapula to the left elbow, applies the calipers, and records the measurement.

Arm Circumference

The mid-arm circumference (MAC) can be obtained to measure muscle mass and subcutaneous fat. To measure MAC, the nurse or dietitian places a flexible tape around the arm at the same marked midpoint used to measure skin fold thickness, taking care to hold the tape firmly but gently to avoid compressing the tissue. The measurement is recorded in centimeters. The mid-arm muscle mass (MAMM) measures the amount of muscle in the body and is a more sensitive indicator of protein reserves. It can be computed from the MAC and the triceps skin fold measure.

Malnutrition

Overview

Carbohydrates, protein, and fat supply the body with energy. Under healthy conditions, the majority of this energy undergoes digestion and is absorbed from the gastrointestinal tract. Food energy is used to maintain body temperature, respiration, cardiac output, muscle function, protein synthesis, and storage and metabolism of food sources.

Energy balance refers to the relationship between energy expended and energy stored. When energy expended exceeds energy stored, energy balance is disrupted, and weight loss occurs. Body proteins are used for energy when calorie intake is insufficient. The body attempts to meet its calorie requirements even if it is at the expense of protein needs.

Many severely ill or traumatized hospitalized clients are at risk for protein-calorie malnutrition (PCM), also known as protein-energy malnutrition. PCM may present in two forms: kwashiorkor (protein deficiency when adequate calories are consumed) and marasmus (deficiency of both calories and protein).

The outcome of unrecognized or untreated malnutrition is often dysfunction or disability and increased morbidity and mortality.

Pathophysiology

Malnutrition is a multinutrient problem because the foods that are good sources of calories and protein are also good sources of other nutrients. In the malnourished client, protein catabolism exceeds protein intake and synthesis; negative nitrogen balance, weight loss, decreased muscle mass, and weakness result.

ELDERLY CONSIDERATIONS

Malnutrition in the elderly has been associated with increased complications from infections and slower recovery from physiologic stresses such as surgical wounds, bone fractures, pressure ulcers, and loss of functional capacity (Chernoff, 1994). PCM in the elderly has been shown to be a strong independent risk factor for 1-year post-hospital discharge mortality.

The functional ability of the liver, heart, lungs, gastrointestinal tract, and immune system diminishes in the client with malnutrition. A decrease in serum proteins (hypoproteinemia) occurs as protein synthesis in the liver decreases. Vital capacity is also reduced as a result of respiratory muscle atrophy; cardiac output diminishes. Malabsorption occurs because of atrophy of gastrointestinal mucosa and loss of intestinal villi.

Other complications of severe malnutrition in adults include

- Leanness and cachexia
- Decreased effort tolerance
- Lethargy
- Intolerance to cold
- Ankle edema
- Dry, flaking skin and various types of dermatitis
- Poor wound healing and a higher than usual number of infections, particularly postoperative infection

Etiology

Malnutrition results from inadequate nutrient intake, increased nutrient losses, and increased nutrient requirements. Inadequate nutrient intake can be linked to poverty, lack of education, substance abuse, and poor availability of food. Infectious diseases, such as tuberculosis and human immunodeficiency virus (HIV) infection, are precipitating factors in PCM. Diseases that produce diarrhea and respiratory and other infections result in negative calorie and protein balance because anorexia leads to poor food intake. Vomiting leads to decreased absorption with increased nutrient losses. In addition, catabolic processes increase nutrient requirements and metabolic losses.

Incidence/Prevalence

Malnutrition is present in many hospitalized clients (Bowers, 1996; Grindel & Costello, 1996). In a review of eight studies with more than 1347 hospitalized adults, 40% to 55% were determined to be malnourished or at risk for malnutrition and up to 12% were severely malnourished. Malnourished clients have slower healing, suffer more complications, and have a higher mortality rate. Surgical clients with the likelihood of malnutrition were two to three times more likely to experience minor and major complications and excess mortality. Length of hospitalization stay in malnourished medical-surgical clients can be extended by as much as 90%, which clearly increases health care costs (Gallagher-Allred et al., 1996).

The prevalence of PCM in long-term care facilities has been reported to range from 17% to 65% (Morley & Silver, 1995). In one study, the prevalence of malnutrition in 100 clients admitted consecutively to a skilled nursing facility was 39%. The highest prevalence of malnutrition was found in those clients who were admitted from acute care hospitals (Nelson et al., 1993).

Acute PCM may develop in clients who were adequately nourished before hospitalization if they experience starvation while in a catabolic state from infection, stress, or injury. *Chronic* PCM can occur in clients who have cancer, end-stage renal or hepatic disease, or chronic neurologic disease.

WOMEN'S HEALTH CONSIDERATIONS

 In the general elderly population, as many as 25% may be malnourished, most of them women (Wellman, 1997). Elderly women are particularly at risk for PCM (Chart 64–2) because of

- Acute and chronic disease
- Processes that lead to reduction of food intake
- Malabsorption and maldigestion
- Decreased efficiency of nutrient use
- Multiple medication therapy
- Poverty
- Social isolation
- Dependency/disability

TRANSCULTURAL CONSIDERATIONS

In Western countries, cultural factors do not seem to have a major influence on the development of malnutrition. However, newly arriving immigrants from developing countries may be at risk for malnutrition because of limited food supplies, poverty, and eating habits.

In the Native-American population of the United States, poor nutrition has also been directly related to several leading causes of death, including heart disease and cirrhosis of the liver. The diets of many Native-American tribes continue to be inadequate in protein, calcium, and vitamins A and C. These deficiencies may result from

---

| Chart 64–2 |

Nursing Focus on the Elderly: Risk Assessment for Malnutrition

- Recognize that clinical manifestations of malnutrition may not be apparent because they are similar to physiologic changes associated with aging (e.g., dry skin, decreased muscle tone, dry hair).
- Assess body weight and compare it with the usual body weight or the ideal body weight.
- Be aware that multiple chronic diseases predispose the client to malnutrition, especially gastrointestinal disorders such as malabsorption syndromes.
- Assess the client's financial ability to buy healthy food.
- Assess the client's physical and mental ability to prepare food.
- Inspect the client's oral cavity for the presence of teeth or dentures, gum disease, or oral lesions that could affect food intake.
- Review the client's medications, including prescription and over-the-counter (OTC) drugs. Many drugs interact with food or cause anorexia or nausea.
- Use the DETERMINE checklist and Level I or II screen if appropriate.

---

unavailability or lack of money to purchase foods that are high in these nutrients (Giger & Davidhizar, 1995).

Collaborative Management

Assessment

➤ History

The nurse reviews the medical history to determine diagnosis, possibility of increased metabolic needs or nutritional losses, chronic disease, recent surgery of the gastrointestinal tract, drug and alcohol abuse, and recent, significant weight loss. Each of these conditions can contribute to malnutrition. For elderly clients the nurse also explores mental status deterioration, poor eyesight or hearing, diseases affecting major organs, constipation or incontinence, slowed reactions, review of prescription and over-the-counter medications taken, and physical disabilities.

For clients who live independently, the nurse assesses the performance of instrumental activities of daily living (IADL). Functional status can best be evaluated for institutionalized clients by assessing performance of activities of daily living (ADL). Inability to perform any of the eight IADLs or any of the six ADLs indicates a high level of dependence and the potential of disease and poor nutritional status (Nutrition Screening Manual, 1991). When functional status is evaluated with nutritional status, there appears to be a strong predictability of infections and complications among institutionalized adults. Chapter 13 describes functional assessment in detail.

The nurse interviews the client to obtain information about the client's usual daily food intake, eating behaviors, change in appetite, and recent weight changes. The client is asked to describe the usual foods eaten daily and the times of meals and snacks. The nurse compares this information with the Food Guide Pyramid and assesses gross deficiencies. The dietitian can more thoroughly analyze the diet, if necessary.

The nurse explores with the client any changes in eating habits as a result of illness. Any change in appetite and involuntary weight loss is recorded. The nurse notes any changes in taste. Difficulty or pain in chewing or swallowing is also assessed. The nurse asks the client

whether any foods are avoided and why. The occurrence of nausea, vomiting, heartburn, and any other symptoms of discomfort with eating are also recorded. Finally, the nurse asks the client about dental health problems, including the presence of dentures. Dentures or partial plates that do not fit well interfere with food intake.

➤ *Physical Assessment/Clinical Manifestations*

The nurse assesses for signs and symptoms of various nutrient deficiencies (Table 64–4). The nurse inspects the

TABLE 64–4

Signs and Symptoms of Nutrient Deficiencies

Area of Examination	Sign/Symptom	Potential Nutrient Deficiency
Hair	• Alopecia • Easy pluckability • Lackluster • "Corkscrew" hair • Decreased pigmentation	• Zinc, essential fatty acids • Protein, essential fatty acids • Protein, zinc • Vitamin C, vitamin A • Protein, copper
Eyes	• Xerosis of conjunctiva • Corneal vascularization • Keratomalacia • Bitot's spots	• Vitamin A • Riboflavin • Vitamin A • Vitamin A
Gastrointestinal tract	• Nausea, vomiting • Diarrhea • Stomatitis • Cheilosis • Glossitis • Magenta tongue • Swollen, bleeding gums • Fissured tongue • Hepatomegaly	• Pyridoxine • Zinc, niacin • Pyridoxine, riboflavin, iron • Pyridoxine, iron • Pyridoxine, zinc, niacin, folic acid, vitamin B_{12} • Riboflavin • Vitamin C • Niacin • Protein
Skin	• Dry and scaling • Petechiae/ecchymoses • Follicular hyperkeratosis • Nasolabial seborrhea • Bilateral dermatitis	• Vitamin A, essential fatty acids, zinc • Vitamin C, vitamin K • Vitamin A, essential fatty acids • Niacin, pyridoxine, riboflavin • Niacin, zinc
Extremities	• Subcutaneous fat loss • Muscle wastage • Edema • Osteomalacia, bone pain, rickets • Arthralgia	• Calories • Calories, protein • Protein • Vitamin D • Vitamin C
Hematologic	• Anemia • Leukopenia, neutropenia • Low prothrombin time, prolonged clotting time	• Vitamin B_{12}, iron, folic acid, copper, vitamin E • Copper • Vitamin K, manganese
Neurologic	• Disorientation • Confabulation • Neuropathy • Paresthesia	• Niacin, thiamine • Thiamine • Thiamine, pyridoxine, chromium • Thiamine, pyridoxine, vitamin B_{12}
Cardiovascular	• Congestive heart failure, cardiomegaly, tachycardia • Cardiomyopathy	• Thiamine • Selenium

Used with permission of Ross Products Division, Abbott Laboratories, Columbus, OH.

client's hair, eyes, oral cavity, nails, and musculoskeletal and neurologic systems. The condition of the skin, including any reddened or open areas, is observed. The nurse may obtain the anthropometric measurements previously described. The nurse or assistive personnel monitors all food and fluid intake, observes the client at mealtime, and notes any mouth pain or difficulty in chewing or swallowing.

➤ Psychosocial Assessment

The psychosocial history provides information about the client's economic status, occupation, educational level, living and cooking arrangements, and mental status. The nurse determines whether financial resources are adequate for providing the necessary food. If resources are inadequate, the social worker may refer the client to available community services.

➤ Laboratory Assessment

Routine laboratory tests provide additional information about nutritional status. These tests supply objective data that can support subjective data and identify preclinical deficiencies. Laboratory tests must be carefully interpreted with regard to the total client; an isolated value may yield an inaccurate conclusion.

Hematology. Hemoglobin is measured to detect iron deficiency anemia. A low hemoglobin level may indicate anemia, recent hemorrhage, or hemodilution caused by fluid retention. Hemoglobin may be low secondary to such conditions as low serum albumin, infection, catabolism, or cancer.

High hemoglobin levels may indicate hemoconcentration or dehydration, or they may be secondary to liver disease.

Hematocrit, a measure of cell volume, indicates iron status. A low hematocrit may reflect anemia, hemorrhage, excessive fluid, renal disease, or cirrhosis

High hematocrit levels may indicate dehydration or hemoconcentration.

Protein Studies. Serum albumin, transferrin, and thyroxine-binding prealbumin can be measured in the laboratory. Serum albumin indicates the body's protein status

TABLE 64–5

Method of Assessing Visceral Protein Mass	
When Serum Albumin (mg/dL) Is	**The Level of Visceral Protein Depletion Is**
>3.5	None
2.8–3.5	Mild
2.1–2.7	Moderate
<2.1	Severe

Adapted with permission of Ross Products Division, Abbott Laboratories, Columbus, OH.
Note: Because the half-life of serum albumin is relatively long, about 20 days, albumin indicates initial visceral protein status but is not sensitive enough for detecting early changes in nutritional status.

TABLE 64–6

Method of Assessing Visceral Protein Mass	

Serum transferrin is measured or calculated from total iron-binding capacity (TIBC) by the equation

$$\text{calculated transferrin} = (0.68 \times \text{TIBC}) + 21$$

When Serum Transferrin (mg/dL) Is	**The Level of Visceral Protein Depletion Is**
>200	None
151–200	Mild
100–150	Moderate
<100	Severe

Adapted with permission of Ross Products Division, Abbott Laboratories, Columbus, OH.
Note: Serum transferrin has a half-life of approximately 8 days and therefore reflects acute changes in visceral protein status. The disadvantage of measuring serum transferrin is that the test is not routinely available in many clinical laboratories. Several formulas have been derived that can calculate serum transferrin from TIBC, a measurement that is more readily available. However, measured transferrin is more accurate and is preferable when possible.

but is not sensitive enough for the detection of early changes in nutritional status. The normal serum albumin level for men and women is greater than 3.5 g/dL. Table 64–5 indicates the level of protein depletion based on the serum albumin level.

Serum transferrin, an iron-transport protein, can be measured directly or calculated as an indirect measurement of total iron-binding capacity (TIBC), as follows:

$$\text{calculated transferrin} = (0.68 \times \text{TIBC}) + 21$$

With a shorter half-life of 8 to 10 days, serum transferrin is a more sensitive indicator of protein status than is albumin. Table 64–6 indicates the level of protein depletion based on serum transferrin level.

Thyroxine-binding prealbumin (PAB) provides a more sensitive indicator of protein deficiency because of its short half-life of 2 days. The normal PAB range is 10 to 40 mg/dL. PAB can also assess improvement in nutritional status with refeeding; levels can increase by 1 mg/dL/day with adequate nutritional support. This test is expensive, however, and its cost may be prohibitive except at large facilities.

Serum Cholesterol. Cholesterol levels normally range between 160 and 200 mg/dL in adult men and women. Values are typically low in malabsorption, liver disease, pernicious anemia, terminal stages of cancer, sepsis, or stress. A cholesterol level below 160 mg/dL has been identified as a possible indicator of malnutrition.

Other Laboratory Tests. Total lymphocyte count (TLC) can be used to assess immune function. Malnutrition suppresses the immune system and leaves the client more vulnerable to infection. When a client is malnourished, the TLC is usually decreased.

Analysis

➤ Common Nursing Diagnoses and Collaborative Problems

The most common diagnosis for the client with malnutrition is Altered Nutrition: Less Than Body Requirements related to inadequate food intake or increased nutrient requirements.

➤ Additional Nursing Diagnoses and Collaborative Problems

In addition to the common nursing diagnosis, some clients may have one or more of the following problems associated with malnutrition:

- Risk for Impaired Skin Integrity related to depleted protein stores
- Risk for Infection related to suppressed immune system
- Risk for Body Image Disturbance related to physical changes from weight loss

The following collaborative problems may also result from malnutrition:

- Potential for anemia
- Potential for an immunocompromised state

Planning and Implementation

➤ Altered Nutrition: Less Than Body Requirements

Planning: Expected Outcomes. The client is expected to have an adequate intake of all required nutrients on a daily basis, and experience no further weight loss or will have a weight increase.

Interventions. The preferred route for feeding is through the gastrointestinal tract because it is safer, easier, less expensive, and more physiologically sound and enhances the immune system (Bowers, 1996). In collaboration with the health care provider and dietitian, the nurse provides high-calorie, high-protein foods, such as milkshakes. A feeding schedule of six small meals benefits many clients. If the client has difficulty chewing or is edentulous, a puréed or dental soft diet may facilitate food intake.

Malnourished ill clients often need encouragement to eat. The nurse provides a quiet environment, which is conducive to eating. The client may take a long time to eat, even with small quantities of food, especially the elderly.

Partial Enteral Nutrition. The dietitian calculates the nutrients required daily and translates these requirements into meals for the client. If the client cannot ingest sufficient nutrients as food, partial enteral nutrition with fortified nutritional supplements, such as Ensure or Carnation Instant Breakfast, may be given. Many commercial enteral products are available. For clients with medical diagnoses such as liver and renal disease, special products that meet the needs of these clients are also available. The client must enjoy the taste of the product for acceptability and optimal intake.

Nutritional supplements are supplied as liquid formulas, powders, and puddings in a variety of flavors. They come in different degrees of sweetness and are also available as modular supplements, which provide single nutrients. Examples of modular supplements are Polycose for carbohydrates and ProPac for protein. Carbohydrate modulars are useful only if additional calories are needed. Protein modulars are indicated when metabolic stress causes a need for higher protein intake.

The nurse bases adequate daily fluid intake on 30 mL of fluid per kilogram of body weight. This recommendation is *not* for clients with severe cardiac problems or fluid restrictions. The health care provider may also prescribe vitamin and mineral supplements.

The nurse or assistive nursing personnel maintains a daily calorie count and fluid intake to assess whether the client can meet the goals of nutritional therapy. The dietitian usually asks the nursing staff to keep the food intake record for at least 3 consecutive days. Accurate daily or weekly weights, depending on the amount of depletion, are also essential.

Total Enteral Nutrition. The client often cannot meet the goals of nutritional therapy through usual oral intake because of increased metabolic demands or decreased ability to eat. In such cases, enteral feeding by tube may be necessary to supplement oral intake or provide total nutritional support.

Candidates for Total Enteral Nutrition. Clients likely to receive total enteral nutrition (TEN) can be divided into three groups:

- Clients who can eat but cannot maintain adequate nutrition by oral intake of food alone
- Clients who have permanent neuromuscular impairment and cannot swallow
- Clients who do not have permanent neuromuscular impairment but are critically ill and cannot eat because of their condition

Clients in the first group are often elderly clients or clients receiving cancer treatment who cannot meet calorie and protein needs. Clients in the second group usually have permanent swallowing problems and require some type of feeding tube for delivery of the enteral product on a long-term basis. Examples of conditions that can cause permanent swallowing problems are cerebrovascular accident, severe head trauma, and advanced multiple sclerosis. Clients in the third group receive enteral nutrition for as long as their illness lasts. When the client improves and can eat again, the feeding is discontinued.

Total enteral nutrition is contraindicated for clients with diffuse peritonitis, severe pancreatitis, intestinal obstruction, intractable vomiting or diarrhea, and paralytic ileus (Bowers, 1996).

Types of Enteral Products. Many commercially prepared enteral products are available. An appropriate combination of carbohydrates, fat, vitamins, minerals, and trace elements is available in liquid form. Differences among products allow the dietitian to select the right formula for each client. An order from the health care provider is required for enteral nutrition, but the dietitian usually makes the recommendation and computes the amount and type of product needed for each client.

Methods of Administration of Total Enteral Nutrition. Total enteral nutrition is administered as "tube feedings" through one of the available gastrointestinal tubes, either via a nasoenteric tube (NET) or an enterostomal tube.

Types of Tubes. A nasoenteric tube is any feeding tube inserted nasally and then advanced into the gastrointestinal tract. Commonly used NETs include the nasogastric tube (NGT) and the nasoduodenal tube (NDT). A nasojejunal tube (NJT) is also available but used less often than the other NETs.

NETs are used for delivering short-term enteral feedings because they are easy to use and are safe for the client at risk for aspiration *if* the tip of the tube is placed below the pyloric sphincter of the stomach. Small-bore polyurethane or silicone tubes are preferred over large-bore plastic or latex tubes. The smaller tubes are more comfortable and less likely to cause complications such as nasal irritation, sinusitis, tissue erosion, and pulmonary compromise (AGA, 1995).

Enterostomal feeding tubes are used for clients needing long-term enteral feeding. The most common types are gastrostomies and jejunostomies. The physician directly accesses the gastrointestinal tract using various surgical, endoscopic, and laparoscopic techniques.

A gastrostomy is a stoma created from the abdominal wall into the stomach through which a short feeding tube is inserted by the physician. The gastrostomy may require a small abdominal incision or may be placed endoscopically, called a percutaneous endoscopic gastrostomy (PEG). The PEG does not require general anesthesia and is more secure and more durable than traditional gastrostomies (Bowers, 1996). An alternative to either device is the low-profile gastrostomy device (LPGD). This device is less irritating to the skin, longer lasting, more cosmetically pleasing, and allows greater client independence. However, skin-level devices do not allow easy access for checking residuals (Bowers, 1996).

Jejunostomies are used less often than gastrostomies. A jejunostomy is used for long-term feedings when it is desirable to bypass the stomach, such as gastric disease, upper GI obstruction, and abnormal gastric or duodenal emptying.

Types of Feedings. Tube feedings are administered by bolus feeding, continuous feeding, and cyclic feeding.

Bolus feeding is an intermittent feeding of a specified amount of the enteral product at specified times during a 24-hour period, typically every 4 hours. This method can be accomplished manually or by infusion through a mechanical pump or controller device. A more popular method of tube feeding is continuous enteral feeding. *Continuous* feeding is similar to intravenous therapy in that small amounts are continuously infused (by gravity drip or by a pump or controller device) throughout a specified time. *Cyclic* feeding is the same as continuous feeding, except that the infusion is stopped for a specified time, usually 6 to 10 or more hours ("down time") in each 24-hour period. The down time is typically in the

morning to allow bathing, bed making, and other treatments.

Infusion rates for continuous and cyclic feedings (and to some extent for intermittent bolus feeding) vary with the total amount of solution to be infused, the specific composition of the product, and the response of the client to the procedure.

The health care provider and dietitian usually decide the type, rate, and method of tube feeding as well as the amount of additional water needed. If the client can swallow small amounts of food, he or she may also eat orally while the tube is in place.

The nurse is responsible for the care and maintenance of the feeding tube and the enteral feeding. Chart 64–3 lists the major nursing interventions for the client receiving enteral feeding.

Complications of Total Enteral Nutrition. The nurse is responsible for prevention, assessment, and management

---

Chart 64–3

Nursing Care Highlight: Tube Feeding Care and Maintenance

- If nasogastric or nasoduodenal feeding is ordered, use a soft, flexible, small-bore feeding tube (smaller than 10 French). Initial placement should be confirmed by x-ray.
- Check tube placement by x-ray when the correct position of the tube is in question; an x-ray is the only reliable method. Checking pH of the aspirant may be a useful adjunct. Other traditional methods for determining tube placement have not proved to be reliable.
- If a gastrostomy or jejunostomy tube is used, assess the insertion site for signs of infection, such as excessive redness and drainage. Cover the site with a dry sterile dressing that is changed at least daily.
- Check and record residual volume every 4 hours by aspirating stomach contents into a syringe. If residual feeding is obtained, check the physician's order for the appropriate intervention (usually to slow or stop the feeding for a time).
- Check the feeding pump or controller device (if used) to ensure proper mechanical operation.
- Ensure that the prescribed enteral product is infused at the ordered rate (mL/hr).
- Change the feeding bag and tubing every 24 hours; label the bag with the date and time of the change. Use an irrigation set for no more than 24 hours.
- For continuous or cyclic feeding, add only 4 hours of product to the bag each time to prevent bacterial growth; a closed system may be used for 24 hours.
- During the feeding and for 1 hour after feeding, keep the head of the bed elevated at least 30 degrees to prevent aspiration.
- Monitor laboratory values, especially blood urea nitrogen (BUN), serum electrolytes, hematocrit, and glucose.
- Monitor for complications of tube feeding, especially diarrhea.
- Monitor and carefully record the client's intake and output.

Chart 64-4

Nursing Care Highlight: Maintaining a Patent Feeding Tube

- Flush the tube with 30 to 60 mL of water (amount usually ordered by the health care provider or dietitian):
  - At least every 4 hours during a continuous tube feeding
  - Before and after each intermittent tube feeding
  - Before and after medication administration (use warm water)
  - After checking residual volume
- If the tube becomes clogged, use 30 mL of water for flushing, applying gentle pressure with a 50-mL piston syringe.
- Avoid the use of carbonated beverage except for existing clogs *when water is not effective.*
- Whenever possible, use liquid medications instead of crushed tablets.
- Do not mix medications with the feeding product. Crush tablets as finely as possible and dissolve in warm water.
- Consider use of automatic flush feeding pump such as Flexiflo, Quantum, or Kangaroo Entri-Flush.

of complications associated with tube feeding. Some of the complications of therapy result from the type of tube used to administer the feeding; other complications result from the enteral product. The most common problem associated with feeding tubes is the development of a clogged tube (Bockus, 1993). Chart 64-4 lists nursing interventions for maintaining a patent tube.

A less common but more serious complication is dislodgement of the tube. Several techniques should be used to confirm proper placement. X-ray is the most accurate confirmation method that should always be done on initial tube insertion. After initial placement is confirmed, the nurse checks placement before each intermittent feeding or at least every 8 hours during continuous or cyclic feeding.

The traditional auscultatory method is not reliable, especially for clients with small-bore tubes (see Research Applications for Nursing). In this method, the nurse instills 20 to 30 mL of air into the tube while listening over the stomach with a stethoscope. The whooshing sound that results does not guarantee correct tube placement. Instead, the nurse should aspirate a sample of the gastrointestinal content, observe its color, and test its pH. When aspirating fluid, the nurse waits at least 1 hour following medication administration, then flushes the tube with 20 mL of air to clear it. The aspirate is collected and then tested using pH paper. The pH of gastric fluid ranges from 0 to 4.0. If the tube has migrated down into the intestines, the pH will be between 7.0 and 8.0. If the tube is in the lungs, the pH will be greater than 6.0 (Viall, 1996).

Fluid Imbalances. Clients receiving enteral nutrition therapy are at an increased risk for fluid imbalances. Clients who receive this therapy are often elderly or de-

bilitated and may have cardiac or renal problems as well. Fluid imbalances associated with enteral nutrition are usually related to the body's response to increased serum osmolarity.

Increased Osmolarity. Osmolarity is the amount or concentration of particles dissolved in solution. This concentration exerts a specific osmotic pressure within the solution. Normal osmolarity of the extracellular fluid (ECF) ranges between 270 and 300 mOsm. Enteral feeding products range in osmolarity from isotonic (about 300 mOsm) to extremely hypertonic (<600 mOsm). Electrolytes (including sodium) contribute to this hypertonicity, but more of the osmolarity is determined by the concentration of proteins and sugar molecules in the enteral product. Even when the product is isotonic, the ECF can become hyperosmolar unless some hypotonic fluids are also administered to the client. This situation is most likely to develop in clients who are unconscious, unable to respond to the thirst reflex, on fluid restrictions, or receiving hyperosmotic enteral preparations.

An increase in the osmolarity of the plasma increases the osmotic pressure of the plasma. Because this increased osmolarity is largely a result of extra glucose and proteins (which tend to remain in the plasma rather than move to interstitial spaces), the plasma osmotic pressure (water-pulling pressure) is increased. In this situation, intracellu-

▷ Research Applications for Nursing

What's the Best Way to Determine Whether a Nasogastric Tube Is in the Right Place?

Metheney, N., Smith, L., Wehrle, M. A., et al. (1998). pH, color, and feeding tubes. RN, 61 (1), 25–27.

The researchers aspirated gastrointestinal (GI) fluid from more than 1000 feeding tubes in acutely ill clients with new tubes. Next to x-ray, testing pH of the aspirate is the most dependable method of confirming tube placement. The pH of gastric contents ranged between 0 and 4. When the tube was in the small intestine, the pH increased to 7. The researchers also found that the color of gastric contents was different from aspirates from the pulmonary system or intestines. Gastric fluid was green, tan, off-white, bloody, or brown. Duodenal samples were a medium to golden yellow; aspirates from the tracheobronchial tree in clients whose tubes were malpositioned were off-white and heavily tinged with mucus.

Critique. The primary author has been researching the most reliable methods for confirming proper placement of nasogastric tubes for over 10 years. This study replicated previous findings and added the assessment of color as another tool. A large sample of homogeneous clients was used to help generalize conclusions.

Possible Nursing Implications. The researchers clearly demonstrated that pH and color are more reliable indicators for ensuring proper placement of nasoenteric tubes than the auscultatory method, although the latter is common practice in clinical agencies. Nurses should use all of these methods to prevent enteral feeding into the lungs.

lar and interstitial water move into and expand the plasma volume. This volume expansion results in an increased renal excretion of water (among clients with normal renal function) and leads to osmotic dehydration. If clients do not have normal renal and cardiac function, the expansion of the plasma volume can lead to circulatory overload and the formation of pulmonary edema, especially in the elderly. The nurse assesses for signs and symptoms of circulatory overload and collaborates with the dietitian and physician in planning the correct amount of fluid to be provided to the client.

Dehydration. When hyperosmolar enteral preparations are delivered quickly, excessive diarrhea may develop. This situation can also lead to dehydration through excessive water loss. The nurse consults with the health care provider and dietitian for recommendations to prevent diarrhea.

First, the strength of the feeding may be changed. Some clients need to begin at half-strength feeding (half water and half enteral feeding product). This may be slowly increased to three-quarter strength before full strength is tried. In addition, the rate of the feeding is usually slow at first and then increased over time as the client tolerates the feeding. If these measures are ineffective in preventing diarrhea, a different product with lower osmolarity may be used. In severe cases, the physician may also prescribe loperamide (Imodium, Imodium A-D) until diarrhea is controlled.

Another cause of diarrhea-related fluid imbalance among clients receiving enteral feeding preparations is lactose intolerance. Clients receiving milk-based enteral feeding preparations may become lactose intolerant. Most enteral products, such as Ensure, are lactose free.

A comprehensive review of research on diarrhea related to tube feeding was conducted by Vines et al. (1992). The authors concluded that diarrhea often results from bacterial contamination and therefore implemented interventions for decreasing this risk. Another more recent study suggests that added fiber can help minimize diarrhea (Reese et al., 1996).

Electrolyte Imbalances. Depending on the client's state of health, some electrolyte imbalances can be avoided. This is achieved by use of enteral preparations with lower concentrations of the electrolytes the client cannot handle well.

In addition to the client's specific electrolyte imbalances, the two most common electrolyte imbalances associated with enteral nutrition therapy are hyperkalemia and hypernatremia. Both of these conditions may be related to hyperglycemia-induced hyperosmolarity of the plasma and the resultant osmotic diuresis. (Electrolyte imbalances are discussed in detail in Chapter 16.)

Parenteral Nutrition. When a client cannot effectively use the gastrointestinal tract for nutrition, parenteral nutrition therapy may maintain or improve the client's nutritional status. This form of intravenous (IV) therapy differs from standard IV therapy in that *all* nutrients (carbohydrates, proteins, fats, vitamins, minerals, and trace elements) are delivered to the client. One liter of fluid containing 5% dextrose, often used standard IV therapy,

provides only 170 kcal. A hospitalized client typically receives 3 or 4 L a day for a total number of calories ranging between 500 and 700 a day. This calorie intake is not sufficient when the client requires IV therapy for a prolonged period and cannot eat an adequate diet or has increased calorie needs for tissue repair and building.

Parenteral nutrition (hyperalimentation, or "hyperal") is subdivided into two categories:

- Partial parenteral nutrition (PPN), or peripheral parenteral nutrition
- Total parenteral nutrition (TPN), or central parenteral nutrition

As suggested by the names, these categories differ by the site of administration and the content of the solutions.

Partial Parenteral Nutrition. Partial parenteral nutrition (PPN) is typically prescribed for clients who can take oral feedings but not in adequate amounts to meet the required nutrition level. PPN is usually delivered peripherally through a cannula or catheter in a large distal vein of the arm. Two types of solutions are commonly used in various combinations for PPN: lipid (fat) emulsions and amino acid–dextrose solutions.

Most lipid emulsions (20%) are isotonic, but the tonicity of commercially prepared amino acid–dextrose solutions ranges from 300 mOsm to nearly 1200 mOsm. The amino acid–dextrose solutions are considered more stable than the lipid emulsions, however, so additives (such as vitamins, minerals, electrolytes, and trace elements) tend to be given with the amino acid–dextrose solutions. The amino acid–dextrose solution must be delivered through an in-line filter. Lipids and amino acid–dextrose solutions are administered by a pump or controller device for accuracy and constancy in delivery rate.

A newer product for PPN is a *mixture* of lipids (10% or 20% fat emulsion) and an amino acid–dextrose (usually 10%) solution (Booker & Ignatavicius, 1996) This mixture of three types of nutrients is referred to as a 3:1, total nutrient admixture (TNA), or triple-mix solution; it is available in 3-L bags.

Total Parenteral Nutrition. When the client requires intensive nutritional support (in excess of 2500 kcal/day) for an extended time, the health care provider prescribes centrally administered total parenteral nutrition (TPN). TPN is delivered through access to central veins, usually the subclavian or internal jugular veins. (Central venous catheters and associated nursing care are described in detail in Chapter 17.)

Total parenteral nutrition solutions contain high concentrations of dextrose and proteins, usually in the form of synthetic amino acids or protein hydrolysates (3% to 5%). These solutions are hyperosmotic (three to six times the osmolarity of normal blood). The base solutions are available as commercially prepared solutions. The hospital or community pharmacist adds components (specific electrolytes, minerals, trace elements, and insulin) on the basis of the nutritional needs of the client. This therapy provides needed calories and spares body protein from catabolism for energy requirements.

Total parenteral nutrition solutions are administered with a pump or an infusion controller device. The osmolarity of the fluid and the concentrations of the specific components make controlled delivery essential.

Complications of Parenteral Nutrition. Clients receiving PPN or TPN are at risk for a wide variety of serious and potentially life-threatening complications. Complications may result from the PPN and TPN solutions or from the central venous catheter. This discussion is limited to the complications of PPN and TPN that involve fluid or electrolyte balance. (Complications of intravenous cannulas and central venous catheters are discussed in Chapter 17.)

Fluid Imbalances. Clients receiving PPN or TPN are at increased risk for fluid imbalance. Not only is fluid delivered directly into the venous system, but the extreme hyperosmolarity of the solutions stimulates fluid shifts between body fluid compartments.

The hyperosmolarity of parenteral nutrition solutions is caused by their amino acid and dextrose concentrations. Increased dextrose causes hyperglycemia. As a result, some of the dextrose moves into the interstitial and intracellular spaces, where it is metabolized. However, when the solutions are administered too rapidly, without enough insulin coverage, or in the presence of hyponatremia and hypokalemia, the dextrose remains in the plasma volume. The result is a shift of water from the interstitial and intracellular spaces into the plasma. Expansion of the plasma volume together with hyperglycemia can cause osmotic diuresis and lead to serious dehydration and hypovolemic shock. If the client has an accompanying cardiac or renal dysfunction, the situation can lead to overhydration, congestive heart failure, and pulmonary edema.

The nurse monitors for these complications by recording accurate intake and output while the client is receiving parenteral nutrition and by taking daily weights. Serum glucose and electrolyte values are also monitored (Chart 64–5). Any major changes or abnormalities are reported to the health care provider.

Electrolyte Imbalances. Clients receiving either PPN or TPN are at an increased risk for many different electrolyte imbalances, depending on the electrolyte composition of the solution and whether a fluid imbalance occurs. Therefore, the health care provider usually orders daily determinations of serum electrolyte levels to detect imbalances. The risk of metabolic and electrolyte complications is reduced when the rate of administration is carefully controlled and clients are closely monitored for response to treatment. Potassium and sodium imbalances are common among clients receiving PPN and TPN, especially when insulin is also administered as part of the therapy. Calcium imbalances, especially hypercalcemia, are associated with PPN and TPN, although immobility may play a role in the development of this imbalance more than the actual parenteral therapy.

Drug Therapy. There is no specific drug therapy for malnutrition, although multivitamins and an iron preparation may be prescribed for treatment or prevention of anemia. The nurse carefully reviews the client's medications because of food-medication interactions. Medications can affect nutritional status, and the foods ingested can affect the efficacy of medications.

Chart 64–5

Nursing Care Highlight: Care and Maintenance of Total Parenteral Nutrition

- Check each bag of total parenteral nutrition (TPN) solution for accuracy by comparing with the physician's order.
- Monitor the IV pump for accuracy in delivering the prescribed hourly rate.
- If the TPN solution is temporarily unavailable, give 10% dextrose/water (D/W) or 20% D/W until it can be obtained.
- If the TPN administration is not on time ("behind"), do not attempt to "catch up" by increasing the rate.
- Monitor the client's weight daily or according to agency protocol.
- Monitor serum electrolytes and glucose daily or per agency protocol. (Some agencies require fingerstick blood sugars [FSBSs] every 4 hours, especially if the client is receiving insulin. Urine testing for ketones may also be ordered.)
- Monitor and carefully record the client's intake and output.
- Assess the client's IV site for signs of infection or infiltration (see Chap. 17).
- Change the IV tubing every 24 hours or per agency protocol.
- Change the dressing around the IV site every 48 to 72 hours or per agency protocol.

 Continuing Care

Malnourished clients can be cared for in a variety of settings, including the acute care hospital, subacute unit, nursing home, or own home. Malnutrition is often diagnosed when the client is admitted to the acute care hospital or as a consequence of events that occur after hospitalization such as poor wound healing or sepsis. If the client is severely compromised, he or she may require admission to a subacute unit or traditional nursing home for either transitional or long-term care. If adequate home support is available, the client may be discharged to home in the care of a family member significant other, or other caregiver. Home care nurses and aides may direct the care.

➤ Health Teaching

The dietitian instructs the malnourished client and the family about the high-calorie, high-protein diet and nutritional supplements. The pharmacist reviews any parenteral solutions with the client and family or significant others.

The nurse reinforces the importance of adhering to the diet and reviews any medications the client may be taking. If the client takes an iron preparation, the nurse teaches the importance of taking the medication immediately before or during meals. The nurse also cautions the client that iron tends to cause constipation.

ELDERLY CONSIDERATIONS

 For the elderly client already susceptible to constipation, the nurse stresses measures for prevention, including adequate fiber intake, adequate fluids, and exercise.

➤ Home Care Management

The malnourished client needs a variety of resources at home to continue aggressive nutrition support. If the client can consume food by the oral route, the social worker or other discharge planner determines whether financial resources are adequate for providing the necessary food and nutrition supplements. If the hospital provides outpatient nutrition counseling services, the client is scheduled for follow-up after discharge for assessment of weight gain. Additional anthropometric measurements may be compared with previous ones during hospitalization to assess progress with nutrition therapy. The nurse assesses the ability of the client and family to comply with instructions.

The malnourished client discharged home on enteral or parenteral nutrition support needs the specialized services of a home nutrition therapy team. This team generally consists of the physician, nurse, dietitian, pharmacist, and social worker. Several commercial companies supply these services to clients in addition to the feeding supplies and formulas.

➤ Health Care Resources

The malnourished client may need help from community resources. Once nutrition therapy has progressed, the client may be discharged to the home setting or to a long-term care facility. The nurse collaborates with the case manager or discharge planner to find the best placement for each client. If the client is discharged home, a home health nurse may visit until the client is stable.

Whether the client is discharged home or to another facility, the dietitian provides written instructions about the diet and nutritional supplements. Communication with the new care provider is ideal for continuity of care.

Evaluation

On the basis of the identified nursing diagnoses, the nurse evaluates the care of the malnourished client. Outcomes include that the client is expected to

- Have an adequate intake of all required nutrients on a daily basis
- Experience no further weight loss or have a weight increase

Obesity
Overview

The terms *obesity* and *overweight* are often used interchangeably, but they refer to different conditions. Overweight is an increase in body weight for height compared with a reference standard, such as the Metropolitan Life height and weight tables (see Table 64–3) or 10% greater than ideal body weight. However, this weight may not reflect excess body fat. It is possible for well-developed athletes to appear overweight because of increased muscle mass; the proportion of muscle to fat is greater than average.

An obese person weighs at least 20% more than ideal body weight. *Morbid* obesity refers to a weight that negatively affects a person's health, usually more than 100% above ideal body weight.

Pathophysiology

Obesity refers to an excess amount of body fat. It is possible to be obese at a weight within normal range, according to a reference standard. The normal amount of body fat in *men* is between 15% and 20% of body weight. Obese young men have body fat greater than 22%, and older obese men have body fat greater than 25%. For *women,* the normal amount of body fat is 18% to 32% Obese young women have body fat greater than 35% (Bray, 1992). Body fat can be measured in several ways. However, height and weight are the easiest and most practical anthropometric measurements for determining degree of overweight.

Obesity Indices

To establish percentage of ideal body weight (IBW), the height and weight of the client are compared with the midpoint for medium frame/desirable weight of the appropriate sex in the Metropolitan Life height and weight tables. The body mass index (BMI), as described previously under Nutritional Assessment, is a measure of heaviness and is only indirectly an indicator of body fat. It reflects the combined effects of body build, proportions, lean body mass, and body fat. However, BMI has exhibited substantial correlations with fat mass for adult men and women and has been validated as a risk factor for cardiovascular disease (Borecki et al., 1994). As a general rule, a BMI of 27 indicates obesity and an increased risk of health problems. Arm circumference and skin fold measurements more completely define body composition and adiposity.

The distribution of excess body fat rather than the degree of obesity has been used to predict increased health risks. The waist-to-hip ratio (WHR) or abdominal/gluteal ratio (AGR) differentiates a predominantly peripheral (gynoid) lower body obesity from a central (android) upper body obesity. A WHR of 0.95 or greater in men (0.8 or greater in women) indicates android obesity with excess fat at the waist and abdomen; this pattern carries the greatest health risk. Two risk groups have since been identified by location of the abdominal fat: one with subcutaneous fat and one with intra-abdominal fat. The group with subcutaneous fat had fewer complications than did those with excess intra-abdominal fat. Cross-sectional studies have shown that increased abdominal fat has been related to stroke, insulin resistance, hyperinsulinemia, and frank diabetes mellitus. Excessive abdominal fat may also enhance the risk for gallbladder disease (Pi-Sunyer, 1993).

Complications of Obesity

Obesity is a major public health problem associated with many complications. Complications of obesity that improve with weight loss are

- Diabetes mellitus
- Hypertension
- Altered lipid metabolism resulting in hyperlipidemia
- Cardiac disease
- Sleep apnea
- Cholelithiasis
- Chronic back pain
- Early degenerative arthritis
- Certain types of cancer

Obese people are also more susceptible to infectious diseases than are thinner people.

Classification

Bray (1994) has developed a classification of obesity based on BMI with the corresponding risk for disease associated with obesity (Table 64–7). This classification system eliminates describing obesity in unflattering and prejudicial terms such as *morbid* or *gross*.

Etiology

The cause of obesity involves complex interrelationships of many factors, including

- Genetic
- Environmental
- Psychological
- Social
- Cultural
- Pathologic
- Physiologic

Five major causes of both human and animal obesity have been identified (Bray, 1994). The first, neuroendocrine causes, include injury to the hypothalamus, Cushing's disease, polycystic ovary failure, hypogonadism, and growth hormone deficiency and insulinoma.

A second cause is dietary obesity associated with high-fat diets. Data suggest that obesity associated with a high-

fat diet is more pronounced when the diet contains a significant amount of saturated fat.

Genetic factors are being studied as a third cause. They are found in clinically uncommon states, such as Prader-Willi syndrome. Genetic composition may predispose some people to obesity but not others. Researchers have recently identified the *ob* gene in mice that helps to regulate energy balance. Leptin, the hormone encoded by the *ob* gene, appears to send a message to the brain that the body has stored enough fat, which serves as a signal to stop eating. For obese humans, a variant in this gene may mean that the body does not receive the signal to stop eating (Zhang et al., 1994). More recent evidence suggests that energy balance and adiposity are regulated not only by the hormonal action of leptin and its receptors but also by the interaction of leptin and insulin with the hypothalamic neuropeptide Y system (Schwartz, 1997).

The fourth cause is drug treatment. Drugs that promote obesity include

- Corticosteroids
- Estrogens
- Nonsteroidal anti-inflammatory drugs
- Antihypertensives
- Antidepressants
- Antiepileptics
- Phenothiazines

Physical inactivity has been identified as the fifth cause.

Incidence/Prevalence

The third National Health and Nutrition Examination Survey (NHANES III), phase 1, conducted between 1988 and 1991, concluded that 58 million adults in the United States were overweight. This figure represents 33.4% of Americans. "Overweight" in this study was a BMI equal to or greater than 27.8 for men (which represents approximately 124% of ideal body weight) and a BMI equal to or greater than 27.3 for women (which represents approximately 120% of ideal body weight (Kuczmarski et al., 1994).

Familial and genetic factors play an important role in obesity. When both parents are overweight, approximately 80% of their children will be overweight. However, if neither parent is overweight, fewer than 10% of the children will be overweight. In studies of identical twins, nonidentical twins, and parent-sibling relationships, about 50% of the difference in body fatness is transmitted to children and approximately 50% of this amount is genetically controlled (Bouchard et al., 1988). Some types of obesity have a genetic component as high as 67% in studies of twins and adoptees (Stunkard et al., 1990). In genetically predisposed people, the combination of improper diet and lack of physical activity produces obesity.

TRANSCULTURAL CONSIDERATIONS

Race seems to be a factor in the prevalence of obesity. The prevalence of obesity among ethnic minorities, including African-Americans, Hispanic-Americans, Asian-Americans and Pacific Islanders, Native Americans, and Native Alaskans and Native Hawaiians, is substantially higher than in Caucasians, especially among women

TABLE 64–7

Classification of Obesity Based on Body Mass Index (BMI)

BMI	Class	Risk for Disease Associated with Obesity
20–25	0	Low (not obese)
25–30	1	Low
30–35	2	Moderate
35–40	3	High
40+	4	Very high risk

Data from Bray, G. A. (1994). Etiology and prevalence of obesity. In C. Bouchard (Ed.). *The genetics of obesity* (pp. 17–33): Boca Raton: CRC Press.

(Kumanyika, 1993). The percentage of overweight and obese African-American women (49.8%) is almost double that of Caucasians (27.5%) and more African-American women are severely overweight (Conway, 1995). Obesity is viewed more favorably in cultures where it is associated with robustness and freedom from hunger.

Collaborative Management

 Assessment

➤ History

The nurse or dietitian collects information about the client's

- Economic status
- Usual food intake
- Eating behavior
- Cultural background
- Attitude toward food
- Appetite
- Chronic diseases
- Medications
- Physical activity

A diet history usually incorporates a 24-hour recall of food intake and the frequency with which foods are consumed. The nurse or dietitian is objective but understanding of the personal nature of these questions. The adequacy of the diet can be rapidly evaluated by comparison of the amount and types of foods consumed daily with the Dietary Guidelines for Americans (see Fig. 64–1). Gross inadequacies for specific nutrients can be identified with this approach. The dietitian can provide a more detailed analysis of dietary intake.

WOMEN'S HEALTH CONSIDERATIONS

Women are at unique risk for nutrition-related diseases and conditions and weight-related problems due to biological, social, and political factors. The American Dietetic Association (ADA, 1995) and the Canadian Dietetic Association (CDA) recently issued a joint position paper on women's health and nutrition. Five of the leading causes of morbidity and mortality in North American women are cardiovascular disease, cancer, osteoporosis, diabetes, and weight. Women are vulnerable to several weight-related health risks associated with being overweight. Recent estimates of North American women who are overweight range from 25% to 33%, with certain native and ethnic populations reporting even higher percentages.

Being overweight adds many risks for women, especially if the fat stores are located in the abdominal or truncal areas of the body. A waist/hip ratio of 0.85 puts women at higher risk for coronary heart disease, hypertension, dyslipidemia, diabetes, gallstone formation, and cancer of the reproductive organs. In addition to these medical risks, women are vulnerable to the social, economic, and emotional pressures associated with being overweight. Overweight women may find it difficult to feel good about themselves when challenged by society's discrimination against the overweight. The constant struggle for many women to lose weight often ends in failure and leads to patterns of weight cycling or disordered eating patterns. Prevention and early intervention programs for overweight women and their families remain a critical need. The ADA and the CDA will continue their efforts to include nutrition in clinical and preventive services for women because it is such a critical component of both risk reduction and treatment for the weight-associated conditions.

➤ Physical Assessment/Clinical Manifestations

The nurse, in collaboration with the dietitian, accurately obtains the client's height and weight and calculates the percentage of ideal body weight (% IBW) and the body mass index (BMI).

- Calculates the waist/hip ratio
- Makes the necessary skin fold measurements and records them in the chart

The nurse also examines the skin of the obese client for reddened or open areas; these may not be easily visible because of excess fat.

➤ Psychosocial Assessment

The nurse obtains a psychosocial history to determine the client's circumstances and the emotional factors that might prevent success of therapy or be worsened by it. The nurse or social worker interviews the client to determine the client's perception of current weight. The client may or may not view weight as a problem, which will affect treatment and outcome.

The nurse explores the client's past history to assess

- Cause and duration of weight gain
- Family history of obesity
- Past attempts at weight reduction and outcomes

The nurse asks the client about

- Current reasons for wanting to lose weight
- Stressors (such as home, employment, personal, financial, or community) that might prevent success
- Exercise patterns
- Medications currently used
- Perceptions of self-worth

The diet history provides a detailed analysis of the client's eating habits.

The nurse as a member of the medical team can evaluate the data to coordinate an interdisciplinary approach incorporating diet, exercise, behavior modification, and psychological support. The nurse may refer the client to a community support group if one is available.

➤ Laboratory Assessment

There are no significant laboratory tests for obesity. However, the nurse should review all laboratory test results to assess the nutritional status of the client.

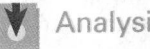 Analysis

➤ Common Nursing Diagnoses and Collaborative Problems

The most common nursing diagnoses pertinent to the client with obesity or overweight are

1. Altered Nutrition: More Than Body Requirements related to dysfunctional eating pattern or neuroendocrine disorder
2. Activity Intolerance related to a sedentary lifestyle

➤ *Additional Nursing Diagnoses and Collaborative Problems*

In addition to the common nursing diagnoses, the client may have one or more secondary problems associated with obesity and overweight. These include
- Self Esteem Disturbance related to guilt associated with eating style
- Body Image Disturbance related to physical appearance
- Altered Thought Processes related to depression

Collaborative problems that the obese client may experience include
- Potential for diabetes mellitus
- Potential for cardiovascular disease
- Potential for hypertension

 ## Planning and Implementation

Altered Nutrition: More Than Body Requirements

Planning: Expected Outcomes. The outcome is that the client is expected to establish a lasting, healthful dietary pattern that will result in permanent, sustained weight loss.

Interventions. Weight is lost only when energy expended is greater than intake. It may be accomplished by dietary restriction with or without the aid of drugs. Clients who are candidates for surgical treatment
- Repeatedly fail at nonsurgical techniques
- Have a BMI equal to or greater than 40 (class IV)
- Weigh more than 100% above ideal body weight
- Have medically significant obesity

Nonsurgical Management. The first clinical practice *Guidelines for Treatment of Adult Obesity* outline treatment decisions based on risk assessment. Recommendations for appropriate weight reduction strategies or weight maintenance to prevent further weight gain are also included (Shape Up America and American Obesity Association, 1996). Various diet programs have attempted to help obese clients achieve permanent weight loss.

Diet Programs. Modalities for helping people lose weight include fasting, very-low-calorie diets, balanced and unbalanced low-energy diets, and novelty diets.

Fasting. Short-term fasting programs have not been successful in treating morbidly obese clients, and prolonged fasting does not produce permanent benefits. Most clients regain the weight that was lost. In addition, the risks associated with fasting, such as severe ketosis, require close medical supervision.

Very-Low-Calorie Diets. Very-low-calorie diets generally provide 200 to 800 calories per day. Two types of very-low-calorie diets are the *protein-sparing modified fast* and the *liquid formula diet*.

The protein-sparing modified fast provides protein of high biological value (1.5 g/kg of desirable body weight/day) within a limited number of calories. The diet produces rapid weight loss while preserving lean body mass.

The liquid formula diet provides between 33 and 70 g of protein daily. For both diets, an initial cardiac evaluation, supervision by an interdisciplinary health team with monitoring by a physician, nutrition counseling by a registered dietitian, and supplementation with vitamins and minerals are required. These diets are only one part of a weight reduction program. Clients on these diets should receive nutrition education, psychological counseling, exercise, and behavior therapy. Comparable weight losses have been achieved by people following both diets, but most clients do not sustain the weight loss and thus regain the weight.

Balanced and Unbalanced Low-Energy Diets. Nutritionally balanced diets generally provide 1200 calories/day with a conventional distribution of carbohydrate, protein, and fat. Vitamin and mineral supplements may be necessary if energy intakes fall below 1200 calories for women and 1800 calories for men. This diet provides conventional foods that are economical and easy to obtain; thus, the goal of weight loss is facilitated, and that loss is maintained.

Unbalanced low-energy diets, such as the low-carbohydrate diet, restrict one or more nutrients. No evidence supports the claim that the restricted nutrient increases or decreases weight loss beyond the calorie deficit it produces.

Novelty Diets. Novelty diets, such as the grapefruit diet, are often nutritionally *inadequate*. This type of diet implies that a certain food increases metabolic rate or accelerates oxidation of body fat. Weight loss is achieved because energy is restricted by food choice, but clients do not sustain weight loss after terminating the diet.

Diet Therapy. Diet recommendations for each client should be developed through close interaction between the client, physician, and dietitian. The diet should meet the client's needs and habits and should be realistic.

The dietitian develops a diet plan and instructs the client. At a minimum, the diet should
- Have a scientific rationale
- Be nutritionally adequate for all nutrients except energy
- Have a low risk/benefit ratio
- Be practical and conducive to long-term success

Calorie estimates are easily calculated by use of a formula. Resting metabolic rate is determined using a sex-specific formula that incorporates the appropriate activity factor. This figure reflects the total calories needed daily for maintaining current weight. To encourage weight loss of 1 pound (2.2 kg) a week, the dietitian subtracts 500 calories/day. To encourage weight loss of 2 pounds (4.4 kg) a week, the dietitian subtracts 1000 calories/day. The amount of weight lost varies with the client's food intake, level of physical activity, and water losses. Carbohydrate, protein, and fat can be calculated as in Table 64–8. A reasonable goal of 5% to 10% loss of body weight has been shown to improve glycemic control and

TABLE 64-8

Nutrient Needs During Weight Reduction				
Calorie Level	**Protein**	**Carbohydrate**	**Fat**	**Multivitamin and Mineral Supplement**
<600	• 1.5 g/kg/day*	• 50 g/day minimum	• 3–6 g/day linoleic acid minimum	• Yes 100% of RDA or RNI
600–1200	• 1–1.5 g/kg/day	• ≥55% of calories	• ≤30% of calories	• Yes 100% of RDA or RNI
>1200	• 0.8–1.5 g/kg/day	• ≥55% of calories	• ≤30% of calories	• Optional
Minimum at all calorie levels: Na, 500 mg/day; K, 2000 mg/day; Ca, 800 mg/day; Fe, 15 mg/day; 2 L/day noncaloric fluids.				

Adapted from Dwyer, J. T. (1991). Nutrient needs in weight management. *Contemporary Management of the Overweight Patient, 3,* 1–8.
*This requirement may necessitate more than 600 calories/day. Protein needs are based on ideal body weight.
RDA = Recommended Dietary Allowances: RNI = Recommended Nutrient Intakes of Canada.

reduce cholesterol and blood pressure (Goldstein, 1992), and these benefits continue if the weight loss is sustained (Wing & Jeffery, 1995).

Drug Therapy. Clients with a BMI > 30, or a BMI > 27 with comorbidities, is one indicator for the use of drug therapy (Shape Up America and American Obesity Association, 1996). Anorectic drugs suppress appetite, which reduces food intake and over time may result in weight loss. These drugs play a valuable role in a comprehensive weight reduction program but should only be used as part of such a program. Currently available drugs used to treat obesity act on either the noradrenergic or serotonergic systems in the central nervous system. The most commonly used anorectic drugs for the treatment of obesity include diethylpropion, phentermine, mazindol, fluoxetine, and sibutramine (Merida). All of these drugs have side effects that must be evaluated in risk/benefit analysis. In an extensive review of pharmacologic agents used in the treatment of weight loss, Goldstein and Potvin (1994) found that drugs were just as good as intensive diet therapy with or without behavior therapy for the first 6 months. About one-third of the clients lost 5% to 10% of their body weight. However, if drug therapy was not continued, these clients quickly returned to their starting weight. Other drugs are being investigated that alter thermogenesis, increase lipolysis, moderate insulin sensitivity, and act as digestion or absorption inhibitors (Bray, 1992).

Behavioral Treatment. Behavioral treatment of obesity consists of various strategies to change daily eating habits to achieve weight loss. This ongoing process should produce a change in behavior. Self-monitoring techniques used include keeping a record of foods eaten (food diary), exercise patterns, and emotional and situational factors. Stimulus control involves controlling the external cues that promote overeating. Reinforcement techniques are used to self-reward the behavior change. Cognitive restructuring involves modifying negative beliefs through learning positive coping self-statements (Brownell & Kramer, 1994).

Fairburn and Cooper (1996) have developed a new cognitive behavioral approach to the acquisition of weight maintenance behavior skills. Clients are encouraged to accept modest weight loss goals and are further discouraged from losing more weight. The treatment focuses on the acquisition of weight maintenance skills and on cognitive factors and any tendency to evaluate self-worth in terms of body size. The client's focus is shifted from physical appearance to a concern for health.

Surgical Management. Clients who do not respond to traditional dietary intervention may be considered for a surgical procedure aimed at producing permanent weight loss. All clients with a BMI ≥ 40, or a BMI ≥ 35 with additional risk factors, should be considered for surgery (Shape Up American and American Obesity Association, 1996). Most surgical procedures fall into three categories:

- Mechanical or physical (adipose tissue removal or intake restriction)
- Malabsorptive (bypass of the gastrointestinal tract)
- Regulatory (directly affecting hunger or thirst)

Preoperative Care. The nurse reinforces health teaching before the client has surgery. Preoperative care is similar to that for any client undergoing abdominal surgery (see Chap. 20).

Operative Procedures. Surgical procedures that physically restrict intake of food include

- Maxillomandibular fixation (jaw wiring)
- Esophageal banding
- Gastroplasty (banding or stapling the stomach)
- Intestinal bypass, in which the stomach and jejunum are connected

One of the most common procedures is gastroplasty, which decreases the size of the stomach. Stapling horizontally across the top of the stomach leaves only a small opening (0.8 to 1 cm) into the distal stomach. However, the fundic pouch created is often stretched too much and inhibits weight loss. The vertical banded gastroplasty evolved from earlier forms of gastroplasty. It is designed with a less distensible vertical pouch that reduces the capacity for a meal by 100-fold. The small pouch outlet delays emptying and provides an internal cue for satiety

(Mason & Doherty, 1993). These gastric restrictive operations sometimes produce maladaptive eating behaviors, such as

- "Soft calorie syndrome" (consumption of excessive amounts of soft or liquid calorically dense foods)
- Vomiting from inadequate chewing
- Inappropriate consumption of liquids after solids

Intestinal bypass reduces the size of the stomach with stainless steel staples but connects a small opening in the upper portion of the stomach to the small intestine by means of an intestinal loop (Fig. 64–6). Complications of the intestinal bypass include bloating of the pouch. Incidence of nausea and vomiting is similar to that with gastroplasty, but intestinal bypass usually leads to greater weight loss, in part because of dumping syndrome as use of the lower part of the stomach is omitted. Intestinal bypass operations have been modified to avoid blind loop bacterial overgrowth syndromes and are now performed as biliointestinal bypass, jejunoileal bypass with ileogastrostomy, or duodenoileal bypass.

Surgical treatment of clinically severe obesity by either vertical banded gastroplasty or Roux-en-Y gastric bypass is a viable option for selected clients (NIH Consensus Development Conference Panel, 1991). Maximum weight loss from these procedures generally occurs 18 to 24 months after surgery. Two years after surgery, Roux-en-Y clients lost 60% to 70% while gastroplasty clients lost 40% to 60%.

Postoperative Care. Immediately after gastroplasty or intestinal bypass, the client has a nasogastric tube (NGT) in place. In gastroplasty, the NGT drains both the proximal pouch and the distal stomach. The nurse closely monitors the tube for patency. The nurse never repositions the tube because tube movement can disrupt the suture line.

The NGT is removed on the third day if the client has bowel sounds and is passing flatus. The nurse gives the client 1 ounce (30 mL) of water in a 1-ounce medicine cup and instructs the client to sip it slowly over 1 hour. Clear liquids are given if the client can tolerate water, and

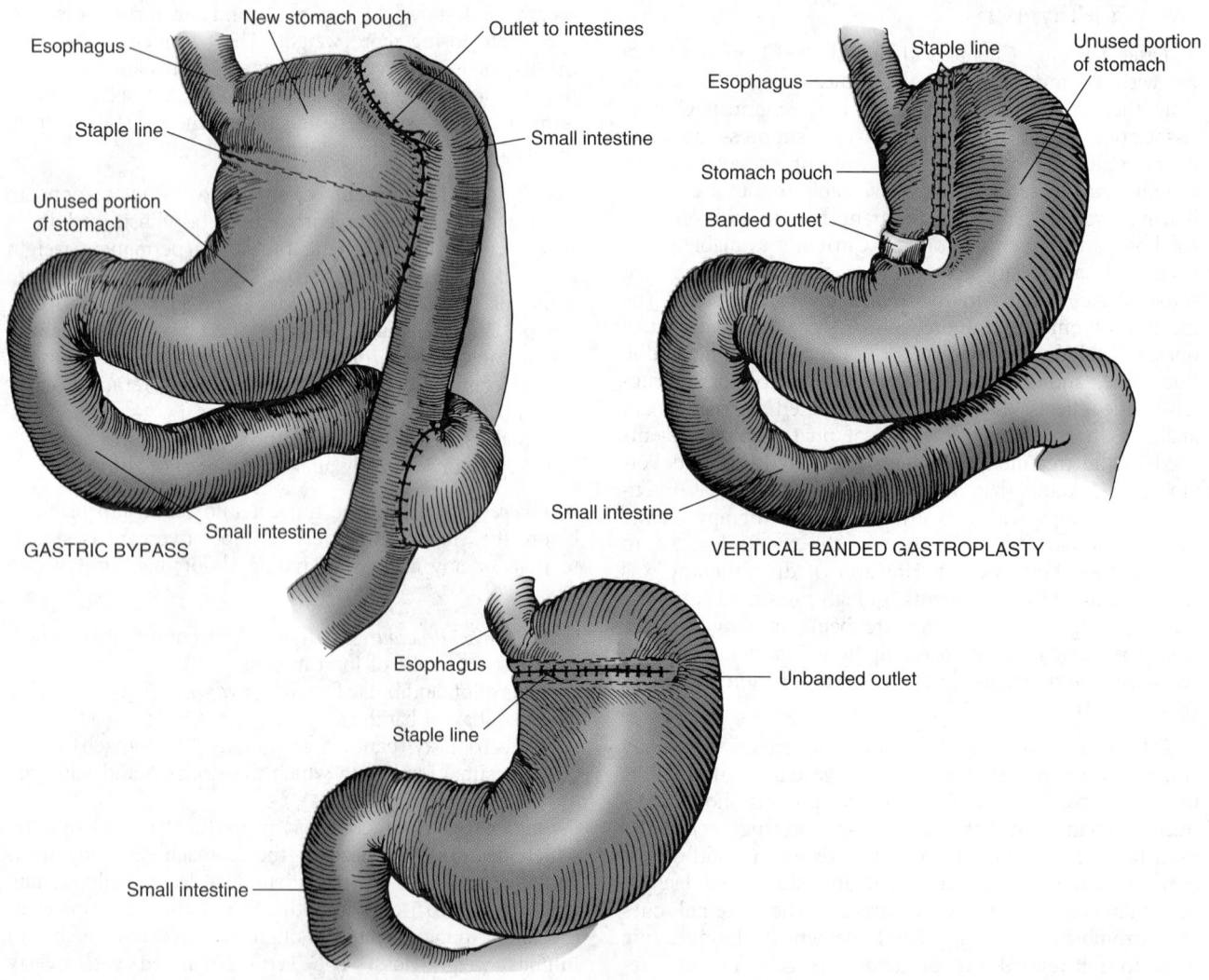

Figure 64–6. Surgical procedures for obesity. (Redrawn from Mahan, L. K., & Escott-Stump, S. [1996], *Krause's Food, Nutrition, & Diet Therapy* [9th ed]. Philadelphia, W. B. Saunders Co.).

1-ounce cups are used for each serving. Puréed foods, juice, and soups thinned with broth, water, or milk are added to the diet 24 to 48 hours after clear liquids are tolerated. The client can increase the volume to 1 ounce over 5 minutes or until satisfied, but the diet is limited to liquids or puréed foods for 6 weeks. The client then progresses to three meals a day, with emphasis on nutrient-dense foods. Nausea, vomiting, or discomfort occurs if too much liquid is ingested.

Before the client is discharged from the hospital, the nurse instructs the client to take liquid or chewable multivitamins daily and to consume adequate protein to promote wound healing. To avoid blockage of the pouch opening, clients are encouraged to eat slowly, chew foods well, and avoid swallowing chunks of food that cannot be liquefied completely.

Activity Intolerance

Planning: Expected Outcomes. The client is expected to slowly increase the amount of physical exercise to aid in promoting weight loss and to incorporate daily exercise into his or her lifestyle.

Interventions. Management of the overweight or obese client is an interdisciplinary effort. The nurse collaborates with the physician, dietitian, and physical therapist or exercise physiologist to meet the goal of improving physical activity tolerance. The major intervention is to increase the kind and amount of daily exercise to create a calorie deficit along with modification of eating habits. Adding exercise to a diet intervention produces more weight loss than just dieting alone. More of the weight lost is fat, preserving lean body mass. An increase in exercise will produce a reduction in the waist/hip ratio (Blair, 1993).

Increasing and maintaining physical activity levels is important in maintaining weight loss. Many overweight or obese clients are so unfit that it may take several months of conditioning before they can exercise sufficiently to achieve weight loss.

First, the nurse or physical therapist or exercise physiologist obtains a clinical exercise history. It is important to determine the client's exercise habits over a lifetime and the client's current exercise pattern. The client should understand the importance of an exercise component in a weight loss program. The nurse also ascertains the client's desire to participate in an exercise program and which types of exercise are preferred.

The physician evaluates the client by an exercise stress test. Not all clients need a stress test, but those with chronic disease may need a stress test and more specific exercise recommendations. The nurse counsels clients about unusual signs and symptoms during exercise (e.g., chest pain) and what to do if they occur. The physical therapist or exercise physiologist emphasizes the importance of exercising consistently first, then stresses duration, intensity, and frequency. A minimal level work-out should be developed for the client so that consistency can be achieved. The goal for the client is to maintain a lifetime of increased physical activity. With a low-intensity, short-duration program, the client is apt to be less

fatigued and discouraged (Zelasko, 1995). Sedentary clients are encouraged to increase their activity by walking 30 to 40 minutes daily (15 to 20 minutes/mile) or the equivalent. The activity may be performed all at once or divided over the course of the day. The nurse teaches the client to exercise only under the supervision of the physician. All members of the interdisciplinary team should provide encouragement and support for any increase in physical activity.

 Continuing Care

Obese clients can be cared for in a variety of settings, including the acute care hospital and subacute unit, particularly following surgical treatment for obesity, or in their own home. Obesity is a chronic, lifelong problem. Diets, drug therapy, exercise, and behavior modification can produce short-term weight losses with reasonable safety. However, most clients who do lose weight often will regain the weight. Treatment of obesity should focus on the long-term reduction of health risks and medical problems associated with obesity, improving the quality of life and promoting a health-oriented lifestyle. The interdisciplinary team members need to provide the obese client with a nonjudgmental, supportive atmosphere that encourages the client to increase physical activity, decrease fat intake and reliance on medication use, establish a normal eating pattern in response to physiologic hunger and address psychological problems. Frequent, long-term outpatient follow-up is essential for successful treatment.

➤ Health Teaching

The most important features of client education focus on health-related behavior patterns. The dietitian counsels the client on a healthful eating pattern. The nurse reinforces the importance of maintaining a healthful eating pattern and provides support. The physical therapist or exercise physiologist recommends an appropriate exercise program. A psychologist recommends cognitive restructuring approaches that help alter dysfunctional eating patterns.

➤ Home Care Management

The overweight or obese client needs proper weighing devices and measuring utensils to follow the diet prescribed by the physician. No other home care preparation is needed.

➤ Health Care Resources

The chances for success in a weight control program are enhanced if additional support is available. The nurse provides the client with a list of available community resources, such as Weight Watchers, Overeaters Anonymous, Take Off Pounds Sensibly (TOPS), comprehensive interdisciplinary treatment programs, and a list of professionals including a registered dietitian, psychologist, and exercise physiologist who may provide frequent follow-up in an ambulatory care setting.

Evaluation

On the basis of the identified nursing diagnoses, the nurse evaluates the care of the obese client. Outcomes include that the client is expected to

- Establish a lasting, healthful dietary pattern that will result in permanent, sustained weight loss
- Slowly increase the amount of physical exercise to aid in promoting weight loss
- Incorporate daily exercise into lifestyle

SELECTED BIBLIOGRAPHY

*American Dietetic Association. (1990). Position of the American Dietetic Association: Very low-calorie weight loss diets. *Journal of the American Dietetic Association, 90,* 722.

American Dietetic Association. (1997). Position of the American Dietetic Association: Vegetarian diets. *Journal of the American Dietetic Association, 97,* 1317.

American Dietetic Association. (1995). Position of the American Dietetic Association and the Canadian Dietetic Association: Women's health and nutrition. *Journal of the American Dietetic Association, 95,* 362–366.

Andris, D. A. (1998). Total parenteral nutrition in surgical patients. *MEDSURG Nursing, 7*(2), 76–83.

*A.S.P.E.N. (1993). Section II: Rationale for adult nutrition support guidelines. *Journal of Parenteral and Enteral Nutrition, 17*(4), 5SA–6SA.

Bass, J. D., Forman, L. P., Abrams, S. E., & Hsueh, A. M. (1996). The effect of dietary fiber on tube-fed elderly patients. *Journal of Gerontology Nursing, 22*(10), 37–44.

*Blair, S. N. (1993). Evidence for success of exercise in weight control and loss. *Annals of Internal Medicine, 119,* 702–706.

*Bockus, S. (1991). Troubleshooting your tube feedings. *American Journal of Nursing, 91*(5), 24–30.

*Bockus, S. (1993). When your patient needs tube feedings: Making the right decisions. *Nursing, 23*(7), 34–43.

Booker, M., & Ignatavicius, D. (1996). *Infusion therapy for nurses.* Philadelphia: W. B. Saunders.

Borecki, I. B., Province, M. A., Bouchard, C., & Rao, D. C. (1994). Genetics of obesity: Etiologic heterogeneity and temporal trends. In C. Bouchard (Ed.), *The genetics of obesity* (pp. 109–123). Boca Raton: CRC Press.

*Bouchard, C., et al. (1988). Inheritance of the amount and distribution of human body fat. *International Journal of Obesity, 12,* 205–215.

Bowers, S. (1996). Tubes: A nurse's guide to enteral feeding devices. *MEDSURG Nursing, 5*(5), 313–324.

*Bray, G. A. (1992). Overview of obesity 1992: Classification of subtypes. In *Obesity: The disease. Current status and future treatment.* Ninth Annual Virginia Nutrition Conference, Hampton, VA, March 5–7.

Bray, G. A. (1994). Etiology and prevalence of obesity. In C. Bouchard (Ed.), *The genetics of obesity* (pp. 17–33). Boca Raton: CRC Press.

Brownell, K. D., & Kramer, F. M. (1994). Behavioral management of obesity. In G. L. Blackburn & B. S. Kanders (Eds.), *Obesity: Pathophysiology, psychology and treatment* (pp. 231–252). New York: Chapman & Hall.

Chernoff, R. (1994). Meeting the nutritional needs of the elderly in the institutionalized setting. *Nutrition Reviews, 52,* 132–136.

Conway, J. M. (1995). Ethnicity and energy stores. *American Journal of Clinical Nutrition, 62*(suppl), 1067S–1071S.

Costello, M. C. (1996). Home health nutrition. *MEDSURG Nursing, 5*(4), 229–239.

Davidhizar, R. N., & Dunn, C. (1996). Malnutrition in the elderly. *Home Healthcare Nurse, 14*(12), 948–956.

Fairburn, C. G., & Cooper, Z. (1996). New perspectives on dieting and behavioural treatments for obesity. *International Journal of Obesity, 20*(suppl 1), S9–S13.

Food and Nutrition Board, Institute of Medicine, National Academy of Sciences (1997). Dietary reference intakes: Calcium, phosphorus, magnesium, vitamin D, and fluoride. Washington, DC: National Academy Press.

*Food and Nutrition Board, National Research Council/National Academy of Sciences. (1989). *Recommended dietary allowances* (10th ed.). Washington, DC: National Academy Press.

Gallagher-Allred, C. R., et al. (1996). Malnutrition and clinical outcomes: The case for medical nutrition therapy. *Journal of the American Dietetic Association, 96,* 366–369.

Giger, J. N., & Davidhizar, R. E. (1995). *Transcultural nursing: Assessment and intervention* (2nd ed.). St. Louis: C. V. Mosby.

Goff, K. L. (1997). The nuts and bolts of enteral infusion pumps. *MEDSURG Nursing, 6*(1), 9–16.

*Goldstein, D. J. (1992). Beneficial health effects of modest weight loss. *International Journal of Obesity and Related Metabolic Disorders, 16,* 397–415.

Goldstein, D. J. & Potvin, J. H. (1994). Long-term weight loss: The effect of pharmacologic agents. *American Journal of Clinical Nutrition, 60,* 647–657.

Grindel, C. G., & Costello, M. C. (1996). Nutrition screening: An essential assessment parameter. *MEDSURG Nursing, 5*(3), 145–156.

Jones, S. A., & Guenter, P. (1997). Automatic flush feeding pumps. *Nursing97, 27*(2), 56–59.

Kennedy, E., Meyers, L., & Layden, W. (1996). The 1995 dietary guidelines for Americans: An overview. *Journal of the American Dietetic Association, 96,* 234–237.

Kuczmarski, R. J., et al. (1994). Increasing prevalence of overweight among U.S. adults: The National Health and Nutrition Examination Surveys, 1960–1991. *Journal of the American Medical Association, 272,* 205–211.

*Kumanyika, S. (1993). Special issues regarding obesity in minority populations. *Annals of Internal Medicine, 119,* 650–654.

Lord, L. M., Lipp, J., & Stull, S. (1996). Adult tube feeding formulas. *MEDSURG Nursing, 5*(6), 407–420.

Lyman, B., & Marquardt, P. (1997). Nutrition screening tool development and utilization for home care patients. *Home Healthcare Nurse, 15*(12), 835–842.

Mahan, L. K., & Escot-Stump, S. (1996). *Krause's food, nutrition and diet therapy* (9th ed.). Philadelphia: W. B. Saunders.

*Metheney, N., et al. (1990). Effectiveness of the auscultatory method in predicting feeding tube location. *Nursing Research, 39,* 262–267.

Metheney, N., Smith, L., Wehrle, M. A., Wierdema, L., & Clark, J. (1998). pH, color, and feeding tubes. *RN, 61*(1), 25–27.

*Mitchell, C. O., & Lipschitz, D. A. (1982). Arm length measurement as an alternative to height in nutritional assessment in the elderly. *Journal of Parenteral and Enteral Nutrition, 6,* 226.

Morley, J. E., & Silver, A. J. (1995). Nutritional issues in nursing home care. *Annals of Internal Medicine, 123,* 850–859.

*Nelson, K. J., Coulston, A. M., Sucher, K. P., & Tseng, R. Y. (1993). Prevalence of malnutrition in the elderly admitted to long-term care facilities. *Journal of the American Dietetic Association, 93,* 459–461.

*NIH Consensus Development Conference Panel. (1991). Gastrointestinal surgery for severe obesity. *Annals of Internal Medicine, 115,* 956–961.

Nutrition and your health: Dietary guidelines for Americans (4th ed). (1995). Washington, DC: U.S. Department of Agriculture and U.S. Department of Health and Human Services (Home and Garden Bulletin No. 232).

Nutrition Screening Manual for Professionals Caring for Older Americans: Nutrition Screening Initiative. (1991). Washington, DC: Greer, Margois, Mitchell, Grunwald & Associates. (Available from The Nutrition Screening Initiative, 2626 Pennsylvania Ave., N.W., Suite 301, Washington, D.C. 20037.)

*Pi-Sunyer, F. X. (1993). Medical hazards of obesity. *Annals of Internal Medicine, 119,*(7, pt. 2), 655–660.

Pontieri-Lewis, V. (1997). The role of nutrition in wound healing. *MEDSURG Nursing, 6*(4), 187–192.

Reese, J. L., Means, M. E., Hanrahan, K., et al. (1996). Diarrhea associated with nasogastric feedings. *Oncology Nursing Forum, 23*(1), 59–66.

*Scientific Review Committee and Communications/Implementation Committee, Minister of National Health and Welfare. (1990). *Nutrition recommendations. A call for action* (Cat. No. H39—162, 1990E). Ottawa: Minister of Supply and Services.

Schwartz, M. W., & Seeley, R. J. (1997). The new biology of body weight regulation. *Journal of the American Dietetic Association, 97,* 54–58.

Shape Up America and American Obesity Association (1996). *Guidelines for Treatment of Adult Obesity*. Bethesda, MD: Shape Up America.

*Stunkard, A. J., et al. (1990). The body-mass index of twins who have been reared apart. *New England Journal of Medicine, 322,* 1483.

Vegetarian food pyramid. (1994). *Vegetarian Journal, 13,* 21.

Viall, C. D. (1996). Location, location, location. *Nursing96, 26*(9), 43–45.

*Vines, S. W., et al. (1992). Research utilization: An evaluation of the research related to causes of diarrhea in tube-fed patients. *Applied Nursing Research, 5,* 164–173.

*Webber-Jones, J., et al. (1992). How to declog a feeding tube. *Nursing, 22*(4), 62–64.

*Weinstein, S. M. (1993). *Plumer's principles and practice of intravenous therapy* (5th ed.). Philadelphia: J. B. Lippincott.

Wellman, N. S. (1997). A case manager's guide to nutrition screening and intervention. *The Journal of Care Management, 3*(2), 12–27.

Wing, R. R. & Jeffery, R. W. (1995). Effect of modest weight loss on changes in cardiovascular risk factors: Are there differences between men and women or between weight loss and maintenance? *International Journal of Obesity, 19,* 67–73.

Zelasko, C. J. (1995). Exercise for weight loss: What are the facts? *Journal of the American Dietetic Association, 95,* 1414–1417.

Zhang, Y., et al. (1994). Positional cloning of the mouse obese gene and its human homologue. *Nature, 372,* 425–432.

SUGGESTED READINGS

Davidhizar, R., & Dunn, C. (1996). Malnutrition in the elderly. *Home Healthcare Nurse, 14*(12), 948–956.

This excellent article first discusses risk factors that contribute to malnutrition in the elderly. Then, the authors list and describe 13 interventions that home care nurses can use to prevent and manage anorexia. A quiz for continuing education credit follows the article.

Lyman, B., & Marquardt, P. (1997). Nutrition screening tool development and utilization for home care patients. *Home Healthcare Nurse, 15*(12), 835–842.

The authors describe the nutrition screening tools that they developed for their home health agency clients and discuss how they use these assessments to identify clients needing interventions. The Level I screen is used for all clients; the Level II screen is used for clients identified at nutritional risk from the Level I tool and for clients receiving parenteral or enteral nutrition.

Wellman, N. S. (1997). A case manager's guide to nutrition screening and intervention. *The Journal of Care Management, 3*(2), 12–27.

This comprehensive article describes how case managers can easily incorporate nutrition screening into their assessments. The DETERMINE nutritional assessment is included and discussed as a valuable screening tool. The article ends with a list of resources available from the Nutrition Screening Initiative.

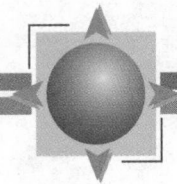

UNIT 13

Problems of Regulation

and Metabolism:

Management of Clients

with Problems of the

Endocrine System

ASSESSMENT OF THE ENDOCRINE SYSTEM

The endocrine system is diverse and has complex interrelationships with the nervous, immune, and other systems. The term "endocrine" simply refers to the internal secretion of biologically active substances known as *hormones*. Key components in endocrine function include neuroregulatory mechanisms in the hypothalamus and the sympathetic nervous system. Also included are other molecules not usually considered hormones that can act as hormones and tissues not considered endocrine glands that may produce and release hormones. The specific glands and structures of the endocrine system (Fig. 65–1) are the

- Pituitary gland
- Adrenal glands
- Thyroid gland
- Islet cells of the pancreas
- Parathyroid glands
- Gonads

Hormones usually travel through the bloodstream and affect distant parts of the body by regulating the function of target tissues. Actions at the target tissues are mediated by binding of the hormone to specific receptor sites. The hormones produced by the endocrine glands regulate a wide variety of physiologic processes (Table 65–1).

Disorders of the endocrine system are related to either an excess or a deficiency of a specific hormone or to a defect at its receptor site. The onset of these disorders can be slow and insidious or abrupt and life-threatening, and the age of onset can range from infancy to old age. Some disorders may not be diagnosed until postmortem examination.

The nurse's observation and interviewing skills are especially important in endocrine system assessment. Except for the thyroid gland and the testicles, the endocrine glands cannot be examined directly. Knowledge of the anatomy and physiology of the endocrine system together with data obtained from the history and laboratory diagnostic tests is essential in assessing the endocrine system.

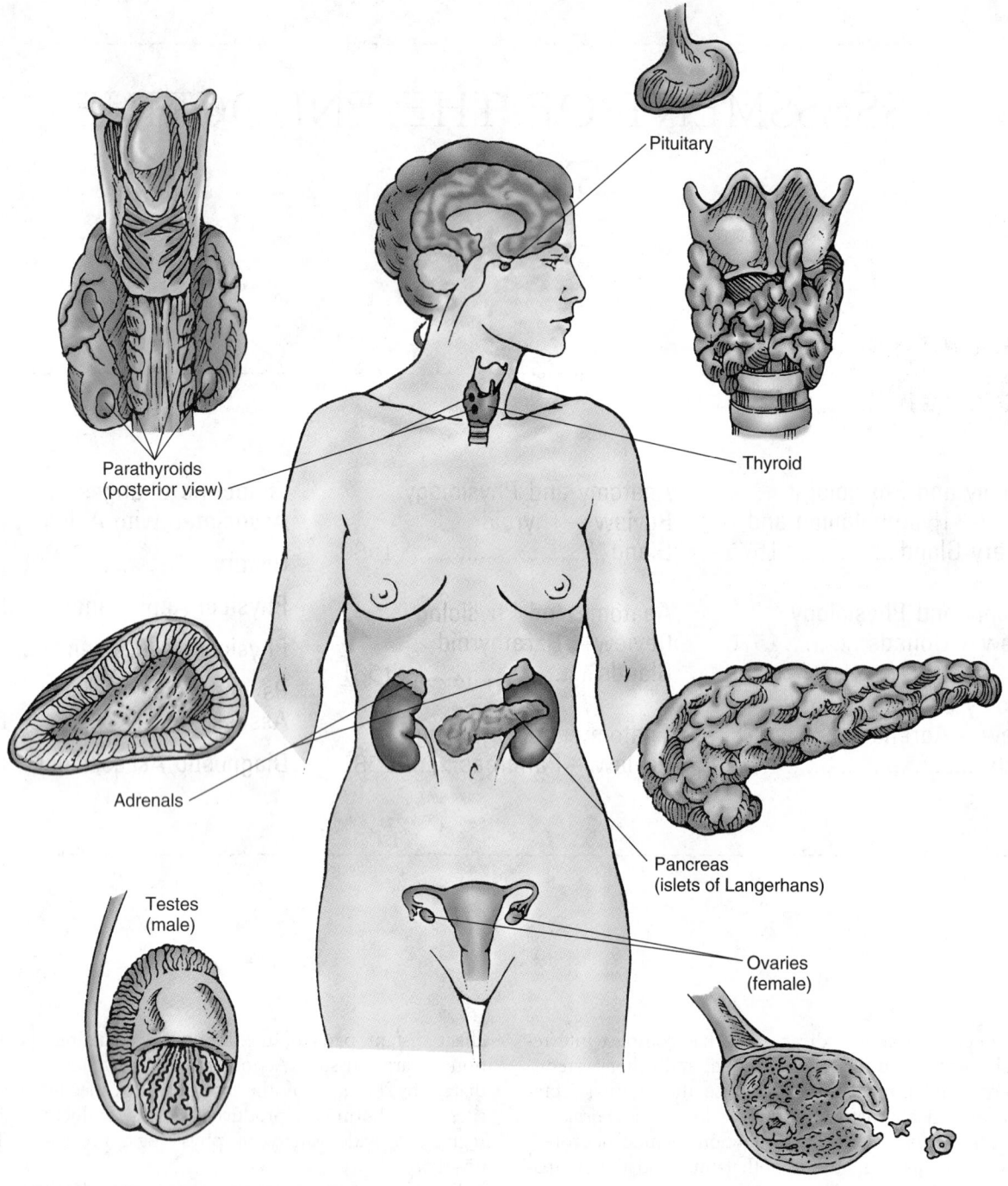

Figure 65–1. The endocrine system.

ANATOMY AND PHYSIOLOGY REVIEW

The control of cellular function by any hormone depends on a series of reactions. Synthesis of the hormone in the endocrine cell begins the sequence of events that ends with feedback control systems acting on that cell. This series of reactions integrates the neuroregulatory mechanisms to bring about homeostasis as follows:

- The central nervous system receives and reacts to various stimuli transmitted to the hypothalamus.
- The hypothalamus responds to the stimuli with the production and release of either releasing or inhibiting factors, which are transported to the pituitary.
- In the pituitary gland, the releasing or inhibiting factors either stimulate or inhibit the release of specific hormones.
- The anterior pituitary responds to these hormones by

TABLE 65–1

Principal Hormones of the Endocrine Glands

Gland	Hormones
Anterior pituitary	• Thyroid-stimulating hormone (TSH) • Adrenocorticotropic hormone (ACTH, corticotropin) • Luteinizing hormone (LH) • Follicle-stimulating hormone (FSH) • Prolactin (PRL) • Growth hormone (GH) • Melanocyte-stimulating hormone (MSH)
Posterior pituitary	• Vasopressin (antidiuretic hormone [ADH]) • Oxytocin
Thyroid	• Triiodothyronine (T_3) • Thyroxine (T_4) • Calcitonin
Parathyroids	• Parathyroid hormone
Adrenal cortex	• Glucocorticoids (cortisol) • Mineralocorticoids (aldosterone)
Ovary	• Estrogen • Progesterone
Testes	• Testosterone
Pancreas	• Insulin • Glucagon • Somatostatin

controlling the secretion of hormones from target organs or tissue.

This type of control is demonstrated by the interaction of the hypothalamus and the anterior pituitary with a target organ (e.g., the thyroid, the adrenal cortex, or the gonads; Fig. 65–2). Each hormone's maintenance level range is well defined, and deviation in either direction leads to pathologic conditions.

Hypothalamus and Pituitary Glands

Structure

The hypothalamus plays a major role in regulating endocrine function. The hypothalamus consists of nervous tissue located beneath the cerebral hemispheres and thalamus on each side of the third ventricle in the brain. Nerve fibers connect the hypothalamus to the rest of the central nervous system. Blood from the internal carotid arteries flows to the superior hypophysial arteries and then to a capillary plexus in the *anterior* pituitary. This venous portal system is called the hypothalamic-hypophysial portal system.

The pituitary gland is located in the sella turcica, an indentation of the sphenoid bone at the base of the brain (see Fig. 65–1). The oval gland, which has a diameter of approximately ⅓ inch (1 cm), is divided into three lobes (Fig. 65–3). The anterior lobe, or *adenohypophysis,* consti-

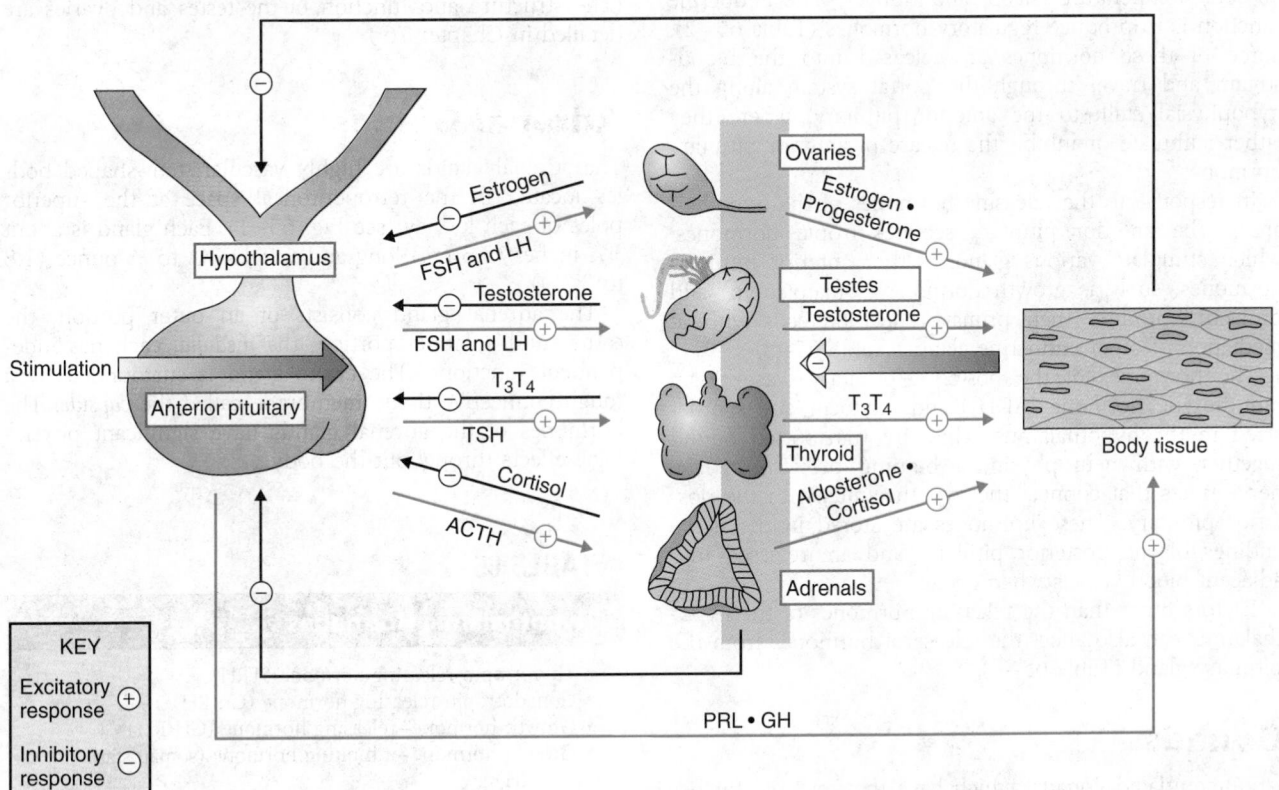

Figure 65–2. The feedback system of the hypothalamic-pituitary-target gland axis. (ACTH, adrenocorticotropic hormone; TSH, thyroid-stimulating hormone; T_3, triiodothyronine; T_4, thyroxine; FSH, follicle-stimulating hormone; LH, luteinizing hormone; PRL, prolactin; GH, growth hormone.)

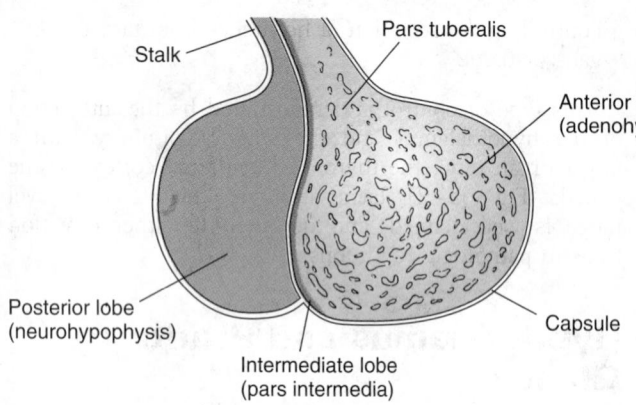

Figure 65–3. The pituitary gland.

tutes about 70% of the gland. The posterior lobe, or *neurohypophysis*, stores hormones produced in the hypothalamus. Nerve fibers in the hypophysial stalk, a structure extending from the hypothalamus, connect the hypothalamus to the posterior pituitary. The area between the anterior and posterior lobes is the intermediate lobe (*pars intermedia*). Under normal circumstances, this lobe does not seem to be significant, but further study is necessary.

Function

The hypothalamus has both endocrine and nonendocrine functions. Nonendocrine functions include the regulation of body temperature, sleep, and hunger. The endocrine function is to produce regulatory hormones (Table 65–2). Some of these hormones are released into the bloodstream and travel through the portal system along the hypophysial stalk to the anterior pituitary, where they either stimulate or inhibit the release of anterior pituitary hormones.

In response to the releasing hormones of the hypothalamus, the anterior pituitary secretes tropic hormones, which stimulate various glands. Other anterior pituitary hormones, such as growth hormone (somatotropin) and prolactin, produce their primary effect on cells without mediation of other endocrine glands (Table 65–3).

The hormones of the posterior pituitary, vasopressin (antidiuretic hormone [ADH]) and oxytocin, are synthesized in the hypothalamus. They are transported bound together with neurophysin, a binding protein, by the nerve tracts that connect the hypothalamus with the posterior pituitary. These hormones are stored in the nerve endings of the posterior pituitary and are released into adjacent blood vessels when needed.

Factors other than the releasing hormones of the hypothalamus can also affect the release of hormones from the pituitary gland (Table 65–4).

Gonads

Undifferentiated gonads, which have the potential for becoming male testes or female ovaries, appear in the embryo during the fifth week of gestation. Differentiation, precipitated by the fetal testosterone level, occurs between the seventh and eighth weeks of gestation. The placenta secretes human chorionic gonadotropin (hCG), which stimulates testosterone to develop the vas deferens, epididymis, and seminal vesicles. Development of the prostate, urethra, and external genitalia is stimulated by dehydrotestosterone, a metabolite of testosterone.

Without the stimulation of testosterone, the maternal hormones influence the developing gonad to differentiate into an ovary. Maternal hormones then cause regression of male genitalia structures and permit initial development of female internal and external genitalia structures.

During puberty, increased secretion of gonadotropins stimulates maturation of the testes and external genitalia. (The structure and function of the testes and ovaries are detailed in Chapter 76.)

Adrenal Glands

The adrenal glands are highly vascular, tent-shaped bodies located in the retroperitoneal space at the superior poles of each kidney (see Fig. 65–1). Each gland is about 1½ inches (3.3 cm) long and weighs 1/16 to 1/8 ounce (1.8 to 3.5 g).

The adrenal gland consists of an outer portion, the *cortex*, and an inner portion, the *medulla;* each has independent functions. The entire gland is surrounded by a tough connective tissue membrane called the *capsule.* The hormones of the adrenal glands have significant physiologic effects throughout the body.

TABLE 65–2

Hypothalamic Hormones

- Thyrotropin-releasing hormone (TRH)
- Gonadotropin-releasing hormone (Gn-RH)
- Growth hormone–releasing hormone (GH-RH)
- Growth hormone–inhibiting hormone (somatostatin) (GH-IH)
- Corticotropin-releasing hormone (CRH)
- Prolactin-inhibiting hormone (PIH)
- Melanocyte-inhibiting hormone (MIH)

TABLE 65-3

Pituitary Hormones: Target Tissues and Subsequent Actions

Hormone	Target Tissue	Actions
Anterior Pituitary		
TSH (thyroid-stimulating hormone)	• Thyroid	• Stimulates synthesis and release of thyroid hormone
ACTH (adrenocorticotropic hormone, corticotropin)	• Adrenal cortex	• Stimulates synthesis and release of corticosteroids and adrenocortical growth
LH (luteinizing hormone)	• Ovary • Testes	• Stimulates ovulation and progesterone secretion • Stimulates testosterone secretion
FSH (follicle-stimulating hormone)	• Ovary • Testes	• Stimulates estrogen secretion and follicle maturation • Stimulates spermatogenesis
PRL (prolactin)	• Mammary glands	• Stimulates breast milk production
GH (growth hormone)	• Bone and soft tissue	• Promotes growth through lipolysis, protein anabolism, and insulin antagonism
MSH (melanocyte-stimulating hormone)	• Melanocytes	• Promotes pigmentation
Posterior Pituitary*		
Vasopressin (antidiuretic hormone [ADH])	• Kidney	• Promotes water reabsorption
Oxytocin	• Uterus and mammary glands	• Stimulates uterine contractions and ejection of breast milk

*These hormones are synthesized in the hypothalamus and are stored in the posterior pituitary gland. They are transported from the hypothalamus to the posterior pituitary while bound to neurophysins.

TABLE 65-4

Factors Affecting Release of Selected Hormones from the Pituitary

Factor	Hormone	Effect on Release
Congestive heart failure	• Vasopressin	• Increase
Hemorrhage		• Increase
Diuretic use		• Increase
Opiate use		• Increase
Alcohol use		• Decrease
Chlorpropamide (Diabinese, Novopropamide✤)		• Increase
Clofibrate (Atromid-S, Claripex✤)		• Increase
Surgical stress		• Increase
Hypoxia		• Increase
Prostaglandins		• Increase
High-protein diet	• Growth hormone	• Increase
Exercise		• Increase
Hypoglycemia		• Increase
Stress		• Increase
Levodopa use		• Increase
Hyperglycemia		• Decrease
Stress	• Prolactin	• Increase
Sucking at breast		• Increase
Estrogen use		• Increase
Use of dopamine antagonists		• Increase
Chlorpromazine (Thorazine, Chlorpromanyl✤)		• Increase
Sucking at breast	• Oxytocin	• Increase
Sexual activity (orgasm)		• Increase
Stress		• Decrease

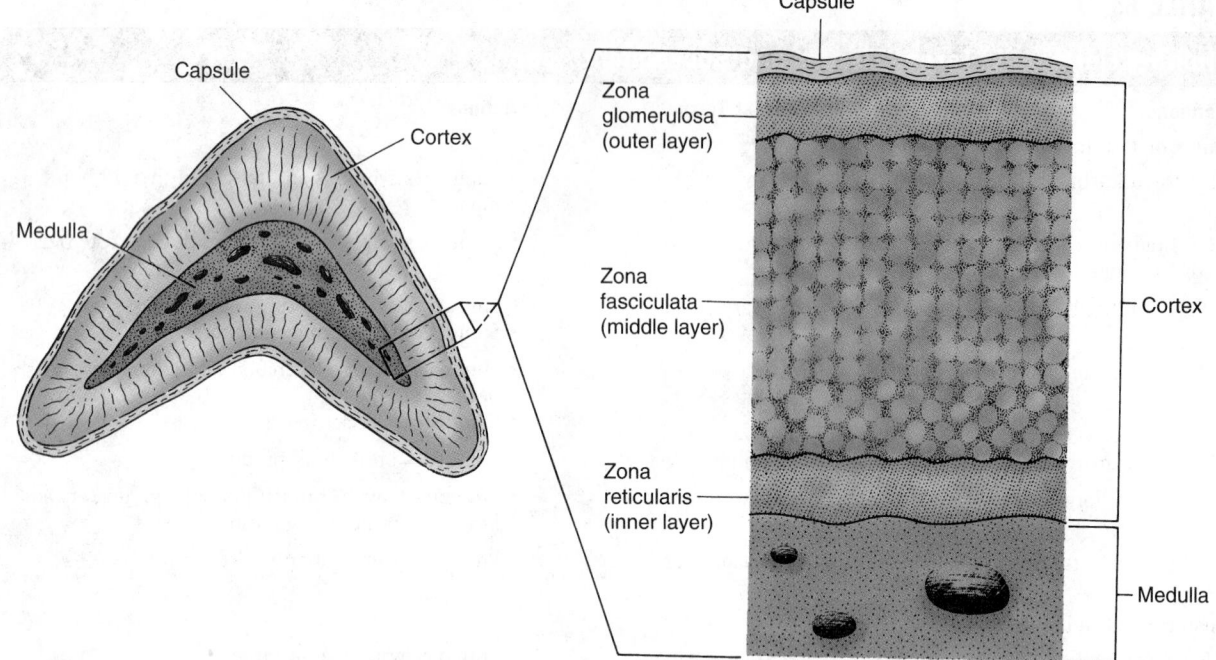

Figure 65–4. The structural detail of the adrenal gland.

Adrenal Cortex

Structure

The adrenal cortex constitutes approximately 90% of the adrenal gland. It consists of cells divided into three zonal layers (Fig. 65–4). Mineralocorticoids are produced in the zona glomerulosa; glucocorticoids, androgens, and estrogens are produced in the zona fasciculata and the zona reticularis. The hormones synthesized and secreted by the cortex are frequently called adrenal steroids or corticosteroids.

Function

Mineralocorticoids

The adrenal cortex maintains life-sustaining physiologic activities. *Aldosterone,* the chief mineralocorticoid produced by the adrenal cortex, plays a vital role in the maintenance of adequate extracellular fluid volume. Aldosterone promotes sodium and water reabsorption and potassium excretion in the distal convoluted tubules of the kidney. Secretion of aldosterone is regulated primarily by the renin-angiotensin system but also by serum potassium ion concentration and adrenocorticotropic hormone (ACTH or corticotropin).

Renin is produced by the juxtaglomerular cells of the renal afferent arterioles. Its release is stimulated by a decrease in extracellular fluid volume as can occur from blood loss, sodium loss, or changes in posture. Renin acts to convert angiotensinogen, a plasma protein from the liver, to angiotensin I. Angiotensin I undergoes a reaction catalyzed by a converting enzyme to form angiotensin II, the active form of angiotensin. In turn, angiotensin II stimulates the secretion of aldosterone. (Chapters 14 [Fig. 14–6], 15 [Fig. 15–2], and 72 further describe the renin-angiotensin system.)

Serum potassium ion concentration also has a regulatory effect on aldosterone secretion. The adrenal cortex secretes aldosterone when the ratio of serum potassium ions to serum sodium ions increases. The increased serum potassium concentration then directly stimulates the adrenals to release mineralocorticoids.

ACTH has a weak stimulatory effect on aldosterone secretion. When ACTH is administered, aldosterone secretion rapidly rises during the first hour, then decreases rapidly to basal levels.

Glucocorticoids

The principal glucocorticoid secreted by the adrenal cortex is *cortisol.* Cortisol

- Affects carbohydrate, protein, and fat metabolism
- Plays a role in the body's response to stress
- Maintains emotional stability
- Affects immune function

Cortisol has a permissive effect on other physiologic processes. This means that cortisol must be present for other physiologic processes to occur, such as catecholamine action and maintenance of normal excitability of the myocardium. Glucocorticoid functions are summarized in Table 65–5.

The release of glucocorticoids is regulated directly by the anterior pituitary hormone ACTH and indirectly by the hypothalamic corticotropin-releasing hormone (CRH). The release of CRH and ACTH is affected by the serum concentration of free cortisol, the diurnal sleep-wake cycle, and stress.

When levels of serum cortisol are low, the hypothalamus secretes CRH, which stimulates the pituitary to release ACTH. ACTH then stimulates the adrenal cortex to secrete cortisol. Conversely, adequate or elevated levels of circulating free cortisol *inhibit* the release of CRH and

TABLE 65–5

Functions of Glucocorticoid Hormones

- Maintain blood glucose level by increasing hepatic gluconeogenesis and inhibiting peripheral glucose use
- Increase lipolysis, releasing glycerol and free fatty acids
- Increase protein catabolism
- Degrade collagen and connective tissue
- Increase the number of polymorphonuclear leukocytes released from bone marrow
- Exert anti-inflammatory effects that decrease migration of inflammatory cells to sites of injury
- Maintain behavior and cognitive functions

ACTH. This inhibitory effect is an example of a negative feedback system.

Glucocorticoid release peaks in the morning and reaches its lowest level 12 hours before and after each peak. Emotional, chemical, or physical stress results in increased release of glucocorticoids.

Sex Hormones

Small amounts of androgens and estrogens are secreted by the adrenal cortex in both sexes. Adrenal secretion of these hormones is usually physiologically insignificant because the gonads (ovaries and testes) secrete large amounts of estrogens and androgens. In women, however, the adrenal gland is the major source of androgens. With adrenal insufficiency or surgical removal of the adrenals, women may need a small amount of testosterone replacement.

Adrenal Medulla

Structure

The adrenal medulla arises embryonically from the neural crest. It is a sympathetic ganglion with glandular secretory cells.

Stimulation of the sympathetic nervous system results in the release of adrenal medullary hormones, the *catecholamines*. Catecholamines travel to all areas of the body through the bloodstream and exert their effects on target cells. The adrenal medullary hormones are not essential for life but play a role in the physiologic stress response.

Function

The adrenal medulla secretes two catecholamines, norepinephrine (NE) and epinephrine, in the proportions of 85% and 15%, respectively. The effects of catecholamines vary, depending on the specific receptor in the cell membranes of the target tissue.

These receptors are of two types: alpha adrenergic and beta adrenergic. Both types of receptors are further classified as alpha$_1$- and alpha$_2$-receptors and beta$_1$-, beta$_2$-, and beta$_3$-receptors. NE acts primarily on alpha-adrenergic receptors; epinephrine most often stimulates beta-adrenergic receptors.

Catecholamines exert actions on many target organs. Table 65–6 summarizes the effects of adrenal medullary hormone stimulation on body tissues and organs.

Activation of the sympathetic nervous system, with the subsequent release of adrenal medullary catecholamines, is an important component of the body's response to stress. Catecholamines are secreted in small amounts at all

TABLE 65–6

Catecholamine Receptors and Effects of Adrenal Medullary Hormone Stimulation on Selected Organs and Tissues

Organ or Tissue	Receptors	Effects
Heart	• Beta$_1$	• Chronotropic action • Inotropic action
Blood vessels	• Alpha • Beta$_2$	• Vasoconstriction • Vasodilation
Gastrointestinal tract	• Alpha • Beta	• Increased sphincter tone • Decreased motility
Kidney	• Beta$_2$	• Increased renin release
Bronchioles	• Beta$_2$	• Relaxation; dilation
Bladder	• Alpha • Beta$_2$	• Sphincter contractions • Relaxation of detrusor muscle
Skin	• Alpha	• Increased sweating
Fat cells	• Beta	• Increased lipolysis
Liver	• Alpha	• Increased gluconeogenesis and glycogenolysis
Pancreas	• Alpha • Beta	• Decreased glucagon and insulin release • Increased glucagon and insulin release
Eyes	• Alpha	• Dilation of pupils

times to maintain homeostasis. Severe physical or psychological stress triggers increased secretion of catecholamines. This sympathetic activation results in the "fight-or-flight" response, a state of heightened physical and emotional awareness. (See Chapter 8 for more information on stress and Chapter 43 for more information on the sympathetic [adrenergic] nervous system.)

Thyroid Gland

Structure

The thyroid gland is located anteriorly in the neck, directly below the cricoid cartilage (Fig. 65–5). In the average adult, the thyroid weighs approximately ³/₅ ounce (18 g). It has two lobes joined by a thin isthmus that lies in front of the trachea.

The thyroid gland is highly vascular and receives its blood supply from the superior thyroid artery (a branch of the external carotid artery) and the inferior thyroid artery (a branch of the subclavian artery). The right lobe has a greater blood supply and is often larger than the left lobe. Nervous innervation of the thyroid gland is by the adrenergic and cholinergic nervous systems. Adrenergic stimulation arises from the cervical ganglia; cholinergic stimulation comes from the vagus nerve.

The thyroid is composed of follicular and parafollicular cells. Follicular cells produce and secrete the thyroid hormones thyroxine (T_4) and triiodothyronine (T_3). Parafollicular cells produce and secrete thyrocalcitonin (calcitonin), which plays a role in calcium regulation.

Function

Regulation of Basal Metabolic Rate

Both T_3 and T_4 increase the basal metabolic rate, which is associated with an increase in oxygen consumption and heat production. This effect does not occur in the brain, spleen, lungs, or gonads.

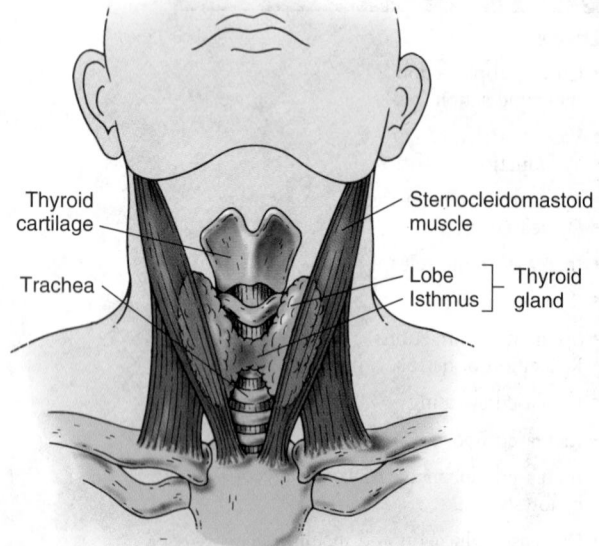

PERTINENT ANATOMY

Figure 65–5. Anatomic location of the thyroid gland.

TABLE 65–7

Functions of Thyroid Hormones

- Fetal development, particularly neural and skeletal systems
- Control metabolic rate of all cells
- Promote sufficient pituitary secretion of GH and gonadotropins
- Regulate protein, carbohydrate, and fat metabolism
- Exert chronotropic and inotropic cardiac effects
- Increase red blood cell production
- Affect respiratory rate and drive
- Increase bone formation and resorption
- Act as insulin antagonists

GH = growth hormone.

The two hormones differ not in function but rather in structure. Approximately 99.5% of circulatory T_4 and T_3 is bound to plasma proteins, including prealbumin, albumin, and thyroid-binding globulin, but the proportion of bound hormone is in equilibrium with the free hormone. The free hormone is transported into the cell, where it binds to a specific receptor in the cell nucleus. Once in the cell, T_4 is converted to T_3. T_3 is the most active form of the hormone, suggesting that T_4 may be a prohormone. The cellular conversion of T_4 to T_3 is impaired by a number of factors including stress, starvation, radiopaque dyes, beta-blockers, and propylthiouracil (PTU), whereas cold temperatures seem to increase conversion. Table 65–7 summarizes thyroid hormone function.

Secretion of T_3 and T_4 is regulated by a hypothalamic-pituitary-thyroid gland axis, or feedback mechanism. The anterior pituitary secretes thyroid-stimulating hormone (TSH), which stimulates the thyroid gland to release thyroid hormone. The circulating level of thyroid hormone is the major factor regulating the release of TSH: if the thyroid hormone levels are high, TSH release is inhibited; if low, TSH release is increased. This is a classic example of a negative feedback system. Secretion of TSH is also affected by the hypothalamic secretion of thyrotropin-releasing hormone (TRH). Cold and stress are two factors that cause the hypothalamus to secrete TRH, which then stimulates the anterior pituitary to secrete TSH.

The synthesis of thyroid hormones involves a series of steps. Sufficient dietary intake of protein and iodine in food and water is essential to produce thyroid hormones. Iodine is absorbed from the gastrointestinal tract as iodide, and the thyroid gland withdraws iodide from circulation where it is concentrated. After its transport within the thyroid, iodide enters into a sequence of reactions resulting in the formation of T_4 or T_3. The hormones, bound to thyroglobulin, are stored in the follicular cells. With stimulation, T_4 and T_3 break off from thyroglobulin and are released into circulation.

Calcium and Phosphate Regulation

Calcitonin is another thyroid hormone produced in the medullary portion of the thyroid. Calcitonin lowers serum calcium and serum phosphate levels by inhibiting bone

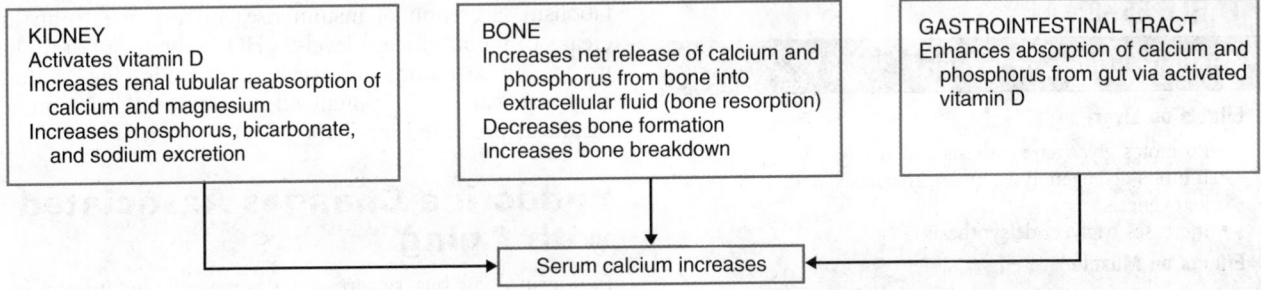

Figure 65–6. Effects of parathyroid hormone on target organs.

resorption (breakdown). It is the physiologic antagonist of parathyroid hormone (PTH).

The primary factor influencing calcitonin secretion is the serum calcium level. Low serum calcium levels suppress the release of calcitonin; elevated serum calcium levels increase its secretion. Additional factors that cause increased release of calcitonin are pregnancy, a high-calcium diet, and increased secretion of gastrin.

Parathyroid Glands

Structure

The parathyroid glands consist of four small glands located close to, embedded in, or attached to the posterior surface of the thyroid gland (see Fig. 65–1). The parathyroid glands are composed of two types of cells: chief and oxyphil. The chief cell, the major cell of the parathyroid gland, synthesizes and secretes parathyroid hormone (PTH). Oxyphil cells, also called Hürthle cells, are large eosinophilic cells sometimes found in the thyroid gland.

Function

PTH regulates calcium and phosphate metabolism as a result of its effect on three target organs (Fig. 65–6): bone, kidney, and the gastrointestinal (GI) tract. Bone is the primary reservoir of calcium in the body. PTH promotes increased bone resorption, thus increasing serum calcium. In the renal tubules, PTH activates vitamin D and increases the absorption of calcium and phosphate from the GI tract.

Calcium is the major controlling factor of PTH secretion. When the serum calcium level is elevated, secretion of PTH decreases; it increases in the presence of low serum calcium levels. Serum phosphate levels also affect PTH secretion, most likely because of its effect on serum calcium levels. PTH and calcitonin work in concert to maintain a normal level of ionic calcium in the extracellular fluid.

Pancreas

Structure

The pancreas lies retroperitoneally behind the stomach and has endocrine and exocrine functions. The *islets of Langerhans* perform the pancreas' endocrine functions (Fig. 65–7). There are approximately 1 million islet cells throughout the pancreas.

The islets of Langerhans are composed of three distinct cell types:

- Alpha cells, which secrete *glucagon*
- Beta cells, which secrete *insulin*
- Delta cells, which secrete *somatostatin*

Glucagon and insulin have a significant effect on carbohydrate, protein, and fat metabolism. Somatostatin, secreted not only in the pancreas but also in the gut and the brain, inhibits the release and action of glucagon and insulin from the pancreas and also inhibits the release and action of gastrin, secretin, and other peptides in the gut.

Function

The exocrine function of the pancreas involves the secretion of digestive enzymes through ducts emptying into the duodenum (see Chap. 55). The primary endocrine function of the pancreas is to regulate blood glucose (sugar).

Glucagon increases blood glucose levels. Glucagon is stimulated by a decrease in blood glucose levels and an increase in blood amino acid levels. In conjunction with

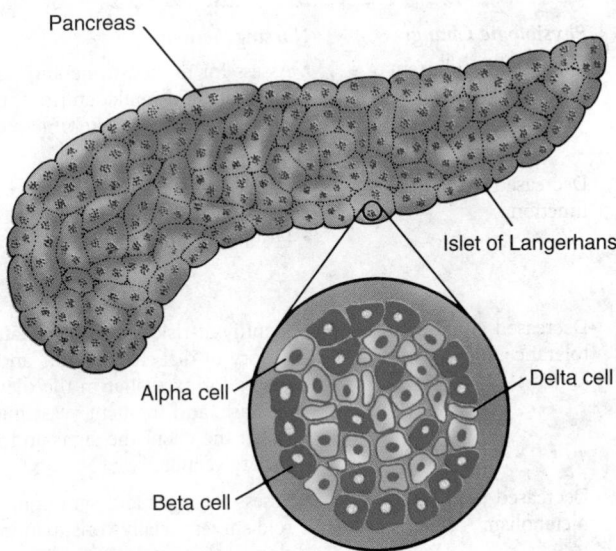

Figure 65–7. The islets of Langerhans of the pancreas.

TABLE 65–8

Anabolic Effects of Insulin

Effects on Liver

- Promotes glycogen synthesis and storage
- Inhibits glycogenolysis, gluconeogenesis, and ketogenesis
- Increases triglyceride synthesis

Effects on Muscle

- Promotes protein synthesis
- Increases amino acid transport
- Promotes glycogenesis

Effects on Fat

- Increases fatty acid synthesis
- Promotes triglyceride storage
- Decreases lipolysis

epinephrine, growth hormone (GH), and the glucocorticoids, glucagon maintains blood glucose levels. In the liver, the primary target organ of glucagon, glucagon promotes glycogenolysis (the conversion of glycogen to glucose). In addition, glucagon enhances amino acid transport from muscle and promotes gluconeogenesis (the conversion of amino acids and fatty acids to glucose). In fat metabolism, glucagon enhances lipolysis and subsequent ketone formation.

Insulin, primarily an anabolic hormone, promotes synthesis and storage in carbohydrate (CHO), protein, and fat metabolism (Table 65–8). Insulin lowers blood glucose levels by promoting glucose diffusion across cell membranes in most tissues. Basal levels of insulin are secreted continuously in the fasting state to control me-

tabolism. Secretion of insulin rises in response to an increase in blood glucose levels. CHO is the major stimulus for insulin secretion; however, amino acids may produce a similar but not as potent effect. (More information on insulin is presented in Chapter 68.)

Endocrine Changes Associated with Aging

Endocrinology has progressed dramatically in its application to the elderly population, but the effects of aging on the endocrine system vary considerably. It is difficult to distinguish normal from abnormal endocrine activity because of such age-related variables as

- Acute and chronic illnesses
- Alterations in diet, activity, and lean body mass/fat ratio
- Disturbances in sleep patterns
- Decreased metabolic clearance rate of hormones

The nurse considers these variables when assessing the client with endocrine dysfunction.

The nurse encourages the elderly client to participate in regular screening examinations, including fasting and postprandial blood glucose checks; calcium level determinations; and thyroid function testing. Chart 65–1 summarizes the endocrine changes that occur in the elderly and lists related nursing interventions.

HISTORY

The nurse develops a systems approach for taking the history of the client with a suspected endocrine problem. This approach can be difficult because of the variety and combination of clinical symptoms. The information gathered from the history provides a basis for physical assess-

Chart 65–1

Nursing Focus on the Elderly: Changes in the Endocrine System Related to Aging

Physiologic Change	Nursing Actions	Rationale
Increased antidiuretic hormone (ADH)	• Assess for diluted urine and polyuria. • Monitor fluid intake and output. • Encourage fluid intake unless contraindicated.	• Ongoing assessment helps to detect early signs of complications. • A sufficient fluid intake may help prevent dehydration.
Decreased ovarian function	• Teach the client the signs and symptoms of estrogen deficiency. • Promote exercise and calcium intake.	• The client's ability to cope with changes may be enhanced with knowledge. • Sufficient exercise and calcium intake delay bone loss and prevent osteoporosis.
Decreased glucose tolerance	• Identify at-risk clients by obtaining a family history of diabetes mellitus and obesity. • Assess for excess fat in the diet, little physical exercise, and frequent yeast infections. • Teach the client the signs and symptoms of hyperglycemia.	• Identification of at-risk clients helps in early detection of complications and such conditions as diabetes. • Knowledge helps improve the client's ability to recognize hyperglycemia.
Decreased peripheral metabolism	• Assess for signs and symptoms of hypothyroidism, especially constipation, lethargy, dry skin, and mental deterioration.	• Ongoing assessment helps differentiate hypothyroidism from the clinical features of aging.

ment and for planning care. The nurse identifies the client's response to actual or perceived changes and discusses the potential diagnostic and treatment plan. The nurse then combines these data with physical, psychosocial, and laboratory findings for a comprehensive assessment of the endocrine system.

Demographic Data

The age and gender of the client provide essential baseline assessment data. Certain disorders are seen more frequently in older than in younger clients, such as hyperosmolar states, loss of ovarian function, and decreased thyroid and parathyroid function.

Manifestations of endocrine disorders can be gender-related, such as the sexual effects of hyperpituitarism and hypopituitarism (see Chap. 66).

Personal and Family History

In the initial interview, the nurse obtains a family history of endocrine dysfunction. The nurse asks about any family history of obesity, growth or development difficulties, diabetes mellitus, infertility, or thyroid disorders. The nurse further assesses the client for a history of

- Endocrine dysfunction
- Signs or symptoms that could indicate an endocrine disorder
- Hospitalizations

The nurse asks about and carefully records past and current medications, such as hydrocortisone, levothyroxine, oral contraceptives, and antihypertensive drugs.

Diet History

Nutritional changes or gastrointestinal tract disturbances may reflect a variety of endocrine problems. The nurse assesses for a history of nausea, vomiting, and abdominal pain. An increase or decrease in food or fluid intake may also indicate specific disorders such as

- Diabetes insipidus, characterized by excessive thirst
- Primary adrenal hypofunction, characterized by salt craving

Hunger and thirst may also be increased in diabetes mellitus. Rapid changes in weight without accompanying changes in diet can signal the onset of a number of endocrine disorders, including diabetes mellitus and thyroid dysfunction.

Socioeconomic Status

Because the client's socioeconomic status can be a sensitive issue, the nurse explores with the client whether his or her resources are adequate to maintain a healthy diet, purchase needed medications, and seek consistent health care follow-up. This initial determination of socioeconomic status allows the nurse to involve social service and home care agencies at an early stage.

Current Health Problems

The nurse focuses on the client's reason for seeking health care, asking such questions as

- Did the client's symptoms occur gradually, or was the onset sudden?
- Has the client been treated for this problem in the past?
- How have the current symptoms interfered with activities of daily living?

Such questioning provides clues to specific endocrine disorders. The nurse also explores changes in energy levels, elimination patterns, sexual and reproductive functions, and physical characteristics.

Energy Levels

Changes in energy levels are associated with a number of endocrine problems, particularly of the thyroid (see Chap. 67) and adrenal glands (see Chap. 66). The nurse asks the client about any change in ability to perform daily activities and assesses the client's current energy level. Has the client been sleeping longer or experiencing fatigue or generalized weakness, for instance? The nurse incorporates this information into planning activities and rest periods.

Elimination

Elimination patterns are also affected by the endocrine system. The nurse identifies the client's past pattern of elimination to determine deviations from the normal routine. The nurse questions the client about urinary frequency and amount. Does the client wake during the night to urinate (nocturia) or experience pain on urination (dysuria)? Information about the frequency of bowel movements, their consistency and color, may provide clues to problems in fluid balance.

Sex and Reproduction

Sexual and reproductive functions are greatly affected by disturbances in the endocrine system. The nurse asks women about any changes in the menstrual cycle such as

- Increased flow, duration, and frequency of menses
- Pain or excessive cramping
- Recent change in the regularity of menses

The nurse asks men whether they have experienced impotence. The nurse questions both men and women about a change in libido or any fertility problems.

Physical Appearance

The nurse discusses any changes in physical characteristics the client perceives. Overt changes are identified during the physical assessment; however, clients may be able to describe subtle changes that the nurse might miss. The nurse questions the client about changes in

- Hair texture or distribution
- Facial contours
- Voice quality

- Body proportions
- Secondary sexual characteristics

For example, the nurse might ask a man if he is shaving less often or a woman if she has noticed an increase in facial hair. These changes may be associated with pituitary, thyroid, parathyroid, or adrenal dysfunction.

PHYSICAL ASSESSMENT

Inspection

Dysfunction of the endocrine system can result in characteristic physical changes because of its effect on growth and development, regulation of sex hormone levels, fluid and electrolyte balance, and the body's use of nutrients. The nurse should be cautious, however, as many different clinical findings can be associated with multiple endocrine disorders or with nonendrocrine pathologic processes.

When performing the physical assessment, the nurse uses a systems approach to avoid losing valuable data. Inspection of the client with a head-to-toe approach is often effective. The nurse initially observes the client's general appearance and assesses (in relation to age)

- Height
- Weight
- Fat distribution
- Muscle mass

The nurse remembers that heredity and age rather than a pathologic condition may be responsible for significant deviations (e.g., short stature).

When examining the head, the nurse focuses on abnormalities of facial structure, features, and expression such as

- Prominent forehead or jaw
- Round or puffy face
- Dull or flat expression
- Exophthalmos (protruding eyeballs and retracted upper lids)

The nurse initially observes the lower half of the client's neck for a visible enlargement of the thyroid gland. In most instances, however, thyroid tissue cannot be observed. The isthmus may be noticeable when the client swallows. Jugular vein distention may be noted on inspection of the neck and can indicate fluid overload (see Chap. 15).

Skin abnormalities may reflect dysfunction of specific endocrine glands. The nurse observes skin color and notes areas of hypo- or hyperpigmentation. Fungal skin infections, slow wound healing, bruising, and petechiae are often seen in clients with adrenocortical hyperfunction. In secondary hypofunction of the adrenal glands, skin over finger joints, elbows, and knees and any scar tissue may show increased pigmentation due to increased levels of ACTH and melanocyte-stimulating hormone.

Vitiligo (patchy areas of depigmentation with increased pigmentation at the edges), seen in primary hypofunction of the adrenal glands, is due to autoimmune destruction of melanocytes in the skin. Areas of decreased pigmentation most often occur on the face, neck, and extremities.

Mucous membranes can exhibit large areas of pigmentation. For all skin discolorations and lesions, the nurse documents

- Location
- Distribution
- Color
- Size

The nurse inspects the client's nails for malformation, thickness, or brittleness, all of which may suggest thyroid gland difficulties. The nurse also examines the extremities and the base of the spine for edema, which suggests a disturbance in fluid and electrolyte balance.

A visual examination of the trunk can show signs of specific endocrine dysfunction. The nurse notes any abnormalities in size and symmetry of the chest. Truncal obesity, supraclavicular fat pads, and a "buffalo hump" may indicate adrenocortical excess. Hormonal imbalance may change secondary sexual characteristics as well. The nurse inspects the breasts (of men and women) for size, symmetry, pigmentation, and discharge. Striae (usually reddish purple) on the breasts or abdomen are frequently seen with adrenocortical excess.

The nurse assesses the client's hair distribution for indications of endocrine gland dysfunction, including

- Hirsutism (abnormal growth of body hair, especially on the face, chest, and the linea alba of the abdomen of women)
- Excessive hair loss
- Changes in hair texture

Examination of the genitalia may reveal a dysfunction in hormone secretion. The nurse notes the size of the scrotum and penis and labia and clitoris in relation to standards for the client's age. Distribution and quantity of pubic hair are often affected in hypogonadism, and the nurse documents any abnormalities.

Palpation

The thyroid gland and the testes can be examined by palpation. (Chapters 72 and 79 discuss examination of the testes, and Chart 79–8 reviews testicular self-examination.) A specially trained nurse palpates the thyroid gland during initial assessment for size, symmetry, general shape, and the presence of nodules or other irregularities.

The nurse palpates the thyroid gland by standing either behind or in front of the client (Fig. 65–8); the posterior approach may be easier. Offering the client sips of water to promote swallowing during the examination helps the nurse palpate the thyroid gland.

The nurse asks the client to be seated and to lower the chin. Using the posterior approach, the nurse places the thumbs of both hands on the back of the client's neck, with the fingers curved around to the front of the client's neck on either side of the trachea. The client is requested to swallow, and the nurse locates the isthmus of the thyroid and feels it rising. The nurse also identifies the anterior surface of the thyroid lobe. To examine the right lobe, the nurse

- Turns the client's head to the right

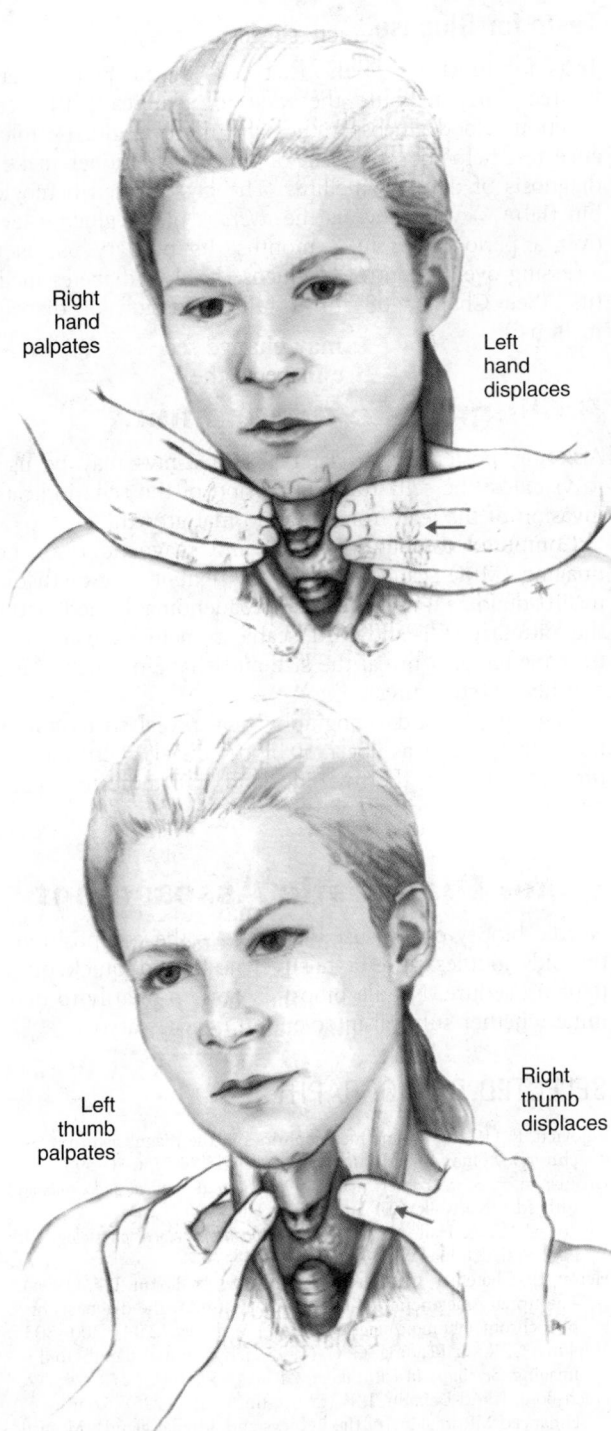

Right
hand
palpates

Left
hand
displaces

Left
thumb
palpates

Right
thumb
displaces

Figure 65–8. Palpation of the thyroid gland.

- Displaces the thyroid cartilage to the right with the fingers of the left hand
- Palpates the right lobe with the right hand

The procedure is reversed for examination of the left lobe.

Auscultation

The nurse auscultates the client's chest to establish baseline vital signs and to determine irregularities in cardiac rate and rhythm. A variety of endocrine disturbances can cause dehydration and volume depletion. Therefore, the nurse documents any difference in the client's blood pressure and pulse in lying, standing, or sitting positions (orthostatic vital signs).

If an enlarged thyroid gland is palpated, the nurse auscultates the area of enlargement for bruits. Hypertrophy of the thyroid gland causes an increase in vascular flow, which may result in bruits.

PSYCHOSOCIAL ASSESSMENT

Information obtained from the history and physical examination aids the nurse in identifying potential or actual psychosocial problems. The nurse assesses the client's coping skills, support systems, and health-related beliefs.

A number of endocrine disorders seriously affect the client's perception of self. For example, body characteristics can change significantly in disorders of the pituitary, adrenal, and thyroid glands. Infertility, impotence, and other changes in sexual functioning may result from endocrine dysfunction. The nurse addresses any difficulty in coping with such changes. Additional support from social or counseling services may be appropriate when care is being planned.

Clients with endocrine problems may require lifelong medication and follow-up care. The nurse assesses the client's readiness to learn and ability to carry out specific self-management skills. Clients may also face financial difficulties resulting from a prolonged medical regimen or interruption of employment. A referral to social service agencies may be necessary.

DIAGNOSTIC ASSESSMENT
Laboratory Tests

For the client with suspected endocrine dysfunction, laboratory tests are an essential part of the diagnostic process. (The highly specialized testing for specific disorders is described in Chapters 66 to 68.) Some generalizations can be made, however. Nursing responsibilities are listed in Chart 65–2.

Stimulation/Suppression Tests

Measurement of specific hormone levels does not always distinguish between the normal and the abnormal. The wide normal range for some hormones makes it necessary to elicit responses by stimulation or suppression tests.

In the client with suspected underactivity of an endocrine gland, a stimulus may be provided to determine whether the gland is capable of normal hormone production. This method is called *stimulation testing*. Measured amounts of selected hormones are given to stimulate the target gland to maximal production. Hormone levels are then measured and interpreted against a given norm. Failure of the hormone level to rise with stimulation denotes hypofunction.

Suppression tests are used when hormone levels are high or in the upper range of normal. Failure of hormone production to be suppressed during standardized testing

Chart 65-2

Nursing Care Highlight: Endocrine Testing

- Explain the procedure to the client.
- Emphasize the importance of taking a medication prescribed for the test on *time*. Tell the client to set an alarm if the medication is to be taken during the night.
- Instruct the client to begin the urine collection (whether for 2, 4, 8, 12, or 24 hours) by emptying his or her bladder. Tell the client *not* to save the urine specimen that begins the collection. It is after this specimen that the timing for the urine collection begins. To end the collection, the client empties his or her bladder at the end of the timed period and adds that urine to the collection.
- Make sure that the preservative has been added to the collection container at the beginning of the collection, if necessary. Tell the client of its presence in the container.
- Check your laboratory's method of handling hormone test samples. Blood samples drawn for certain hormones (e.g., catecholamines) must be placed on ice and taken to the laboratory immediately.
- If you are drawing blood samples from a line, clear the intravenous line thoroughly. Do not use a double- or triple-lumen line to obtain samples; contamination or dilution from another port is possible.

indicates hyperfunction. (See specific tests in Chapters 66 and 67.)

Radioimmunoassay

Radioimmunoassay is a competitive binding assay in which radioactively labeled amounts of hormone (antigen) compete with unlabeled hormones from the plasma or serum for antibody binding sites. Various techniques measure the amount of unbound and bound hormone, which are identified as such. The unbound hormone is the active hormone.

Urine Tests

In addition to the measurement of hormones in the blood, hormone levels and the metabolites of specific hormones in the urine are frequently measured. Because many of the endocrine hormones are secreted in a pulsatile fashion, measurement of a specific hormone in a 24-hour urine collection better reflects the overall function of certain glands, such as the adrenal. The nurse teaches the client how to collect a 24-hour urine sample (see also Chart 65-2).

Certain hormones require additives in the container at the beginning of the collection. The nurse instructs the client not to discard the preservative from the container and to use caution when handling it because some solutions are caustic. The client is also reminded that this collection is timed for *exactly* 24 hours. The nurse instructs the client to avoid taking any unnecessary medications during endocrine testing; drugs may interfere with the laboratory assays.

Tests for Glucose

Tests for functions of the islet cells of the pancreas are indirect; they measure the *result* of pancreatic islet cell function. Blood glucose values and the oral glucose tolerance test help the physician or nurse practitioner make a diagnosis of diabetes mellitus. The glycosylated hemoglobin (HbA_{1C}) value reveals the *average* blood glucose level over a period of 2 to 3 months. Its primary use is in assessing overall control of glucose level in diabetes mellitus. (See Chapter 68 for a full discussion of diabetes mellitus.)

Radiographic Assessment

Anterior, posterior, and lateral skull x-rays may be used to visualize the sella turcica. Erosion of the sella indicates invasion of the wall from an abnormal growth.

Computed tomography (CT) and magnetic resonance imaging (MRI) scans can show the extent of growth of a macroadenoma or locate a microadenoma buried within the pituitary. CT and MRI scans, sometimes using contrast media, also reveal the size and shape of other glands and nearby structures.

Angiography and venography may reveal structural abnormalities, such as aberrant blood vessels. Ultrasonography, especially of the thyroid gland, can indicate whether nodules or masses are solid or cystic.

Other Diagnostic Assessment

Needle biopsy can be used to indicate the composition of thyroid nodules. It is a relatively safe and quick outpatient procedure. Needle biopsy is done primarily to determine whether surgical intervention is necessary.

SELECTED BIBLIOGRAPHY

Elijovich, F. (1996). Plasma metanephrines in the diagnosis of pheochromocytoma. *Annals of Internal Medicine, 124*(7), 694–695.

Greenspan, F. S., & Baxter, J. D. (1994). *Basic & clinical endocrinology* (4th ed.). Norwalk, CT: Appleton & Lange.

Guyton, A. C., & Hall, J. E. (1996). *Textbook of medical physiology* (9th ed.). Philadelphia: W. B. Saunders.

Heron, E., Chatellier, G., Billaud, E., Foos, E., & Plouin, P.F. (1996). The urinary metanephrine-to-creatinine ratio for the diagnosis of pheochromocytoma. *Annals of Internal Medicine, 125*(4), 300–303.

Hopkins, C. R., & Reading, C. C. (1995). Thyroid and parathyroid imaging. *Seminars in Ultrasound, CT and MRI, 16*(4), 279–295.

Huch-Boni, R. A., Debatin, J. F., & Krestin, G. P. (1996). Contrast-enhanced MR imaging of the kidneys and adrenal glands. *Magnetic Resonance Imaging Clinics of North America, 4*(1), 101–131.

Kelley, W. (Ed.). (1997). *Textbook of internal medicine,* (3rd ed.) Philadelphia: Lippincott-Raven.

Ladenson, P. W. (1996). Optimal laboratory testing for diagnosis and monitoring of thyroid nodules, goiter, and thyroid cancer. *Clinical Chemistry, 42*(1), 183–187.

Locker, F. (1996). Hormonal regulation of calcium homeostasis. *Nursing Clinics of North America, 31*(4), 797–803.

Loriaux, T. (1996). Endocrine assessment: Red flags for those on the front lines. *Nursing Clinics of North America, 31*(4), 695–713.

McFarland, K. (1996). The thyroid: Keeping the body in balance. *Women's Health Digest, 2*(1), 12–14.

Mettler, F. A. (1996). *Essentials of radiology.* Philadelphia: W. B. Saunders.

Miller, M. (1996). Endocrine disorders: New technology allows quick, accurate diagnosis. *Geriatrics, 51*(1), 52–54, 57–58.

Mooradian, A. (1995). Normal age-related changes in thyroid hormone economy. *Clinics in Geriatric Medicine, 11*(2), 159–169.

Peaston, R. T., Lennard, T. W., & Lai, L. C. (1996). Overnight excretion of urinary catecholamines and metabolites in the detection of pheochromocytoma. *Journal of Clinical Endocrinology and Metabolism, 81*(4), 1378–1384.

Roberts, A. (1996). Systems of life: Endocrine function of the pancreas. *Nursing Times, 92*(37), 38–40.

Shilo, S., & Rosler, A. (1995). Single intravenous bolus of dexamethasone for the differential diagnosis of Cushing's syndrome. *Journal of Pediatric Endocrinology and Metabolism, 8*(1), 27–33.

Toto, K. (1994). Endocrine physiology: A comprehensive review. *Critical Care Nursing Clinics of North America, 6*(4), 637–659.

Walker, I. A. (1996). Selective venous catheterization and plasma catecholamine analysis in the diagnosis of phaeochromocytoma. *Journal of the Royal Society of Medicine, 89*(4), 216–218.

Winger, J., & Hornick, T. (1996). Age-associated changes in the endocrine system. *Nursing Clinics of North America, 31*(4), 827–844.

SUGGESTED READINGS

Loriaux, T. (1996). Endocrine assessment: Red flags for those on the front lines. *Nursing Clinics of North America, 31*(4), 695–713.

This article provides a comprehensive guide to the identification of clinical manifestations associated with endocrine dysfunction. An endocrine assessment tool is included. Photographs of changes associated with specific endocrine dysfunctions are provided.

McFarland, K. (1996). The thyroid: Keeping the body in balance. *Women's Health Digest, 2*(1), 12–14.

This basic article describes thyroid function in clear, simplistic language. It is an appropriate article for nurses to give to clients and families wanting more information on thyroid function.

Toto, K. (1994). Endocrine physiology: A comprehensive review. *Critical Care Nursing Clinics of North America, 6*(4), 637–659.

This article describes in detail the physiologic functioning and interactions between the endocrine glands. The concept of negative feedback control is reviewed. The influence of systemic and local hormones on nonendocrine organs is discussed.

Winger, J., & Hornick, T. (1996). Age-associated changes in the endocrine system. *Nursing Clinics of North America, 31*(4), 827–844.

The excellent article presents information about how hormone secretion changes as a result of the aging process. Secretion of some hormones does not change with age, whereas secretion of others increases or decreases as a direct result of the aging process. The authors describe clinical manifestations of endocrine disorders unique to the older client.

Chapter 66

INTERVENTIONS FOR CLIENTS WITH PITUITARY AND ADRENAL GLAND PROBLEMS

Too much or too little of a specific hormone leads to pituitary or adrenal gland dysfunction. Problems can also arise as a result of specific receptor sites' inability to respond to the hormone. Hormones secreted from the anterior pituitary gland regulate growth, metabolic activity, and sexual development. Posterior pituitary dysfunction involves a deficiency or an excess of vasopressin, commonly known as antidiuretic hormone (ADH). Disorders of the adrenal gland can be caused by too much or not enough adrenocorticotropic hormone (ACTH) from the anterior pituitary or from a disorder of the adrenal gland itself. Regardless of the cause, the result is hyposecretion or hypersecretion of the adrenal hormones.

The clinical course and quality of life of clients can be influenced by nursing interventions. The nursing care for clients with pituitary and adrenal gland disorders includes

- Performing a careful assessment
- Educating clients
- Evaluating responses to therapy
- Providing psychosocial support

A complete history and physical are performed during the assessment to detect characteristic clinical findings. Clients also often undergo a variety of diagnostic tests that necessitate specific instructions and explanations from the nurse. Surgical intervention may be indicated. Further, adrenal and pituitary disorders may result in characteristic physical changes, and clients often need hormone replacement therapy for the rest of their lives. The nurse identifies difficulties in the client's coping skills and works with all members of the health care team to support the client. Psychosocial support is critical.

DISORDERS OF THE PITUITARY GLAND

Primary pituitary dysfunction is a disturbance in the pituitary gland itself and can result in hypo- or hypersecretion of one or more of the pituitary hormones. Secondary pituitary dysfunction results from a problem in the hypothalamus, which then causes either excess or deficient amounts of pituitary hormones.

Disorders of the Anterior Pituitary Gland

The anterior pituitary gland (adenohypophysis) regulates growth, metabolic activity, and sexual development. The effects of oversecretion or undersecretion of hormones from the anterior pituitary gland occur throughout the body. These hormones are

- Growth hormone (GH; somatotropin)
- Prolactin (PRL)
- Thyrotropin (thyroid-stimulating hormone [TSH])
- Corticotropin (adrenocorticotropic hormone [ACTH])
- Follicle-stimulating hormone (FSH)
- Luteinizing hormone (LH)
- Melanocyte-stimulating hormone (MSH)

Hypopituitarism

Overview

A person with hypopituitarism has a deficiency of one or more anterior pituitary hormones. Adults experience metabolic abnormalities and sexual dysfunction. Partial or total failure of production of *all* of the anterior pituitary hormones is an extremely rare condition known as *panhypopituitarism.*

More commonly, a marked decrease in the secretion of one hormone and a lesser decrease in others occur. Deficiencies of ACTH and TSH are the *most* life-threatening because they result in insufficient stimulation of the target glands, the adrenal glands and the thyroid, to produce adrenal hormones and thyroid hormones. Adrenal hypofunction is discussed later in this chapter; hypothyroidism is discussed in Chapter 67.

Deficiency of LH and FSH in males results in testicular failure, with decreased testosterone production from the Leydig cells and decreased or absent spermatogenesis from the seminiferous tubules. Decreased testosterone levels cause delayed onset of puberty and sterility in men.

In females, a deficiency or absence of gonadotropins results in ovarian failure. The loss of follicular stimulation, ovulation, and corpus luteum formation and maintenance result in amenorrhea and sterility.

A GH deficiency is a problem in synthesis, release, or use of GH, or a lack of tissue response to somatomedin. Somatomedin C (insulin-like growth factor 1 [IGF-1]), a hormone produced in the liver under direct stimulation of GH, is sometimes absent. This substance directly promotes bone and cartilage growth, and GH or somatomedin deficiency in children results in either growth retardation or short stature. GH deficiency in adults produces no observable clinical manifestations.

The etiology of hypopituitarism is extremely varied. Nonsecreting pituitary tumors cause compression and destruction of pituitary tissue. Craniopharyngioma is the most common brain tumor causing hypopituitarism. Pituitary gland function can be impaired by severe malnutrition or rapid loss of body fat, such as in people with anorexia nervosa. Other causes of primary and secondary hypopituitarism are listed in Table 66–1. Idiopathic hypopituitarism is usually the result of an isolated hormone deficiency, and often the cause is unknown.

TABLE 66–1

Causes of Hypopituitarism
Causes of Primary Hypopituitarism
• Pituitary tumor (craniopharyngioma)
• Partial or total surgical hypophysectomy
• Radiation
• Infarction
• Metastatic disease
• Granulomatous process
• Trauma
Causes of Secondary Hypopituitarism
• Infection
• Trauma
• Brain tumor
• Congenital defects

Postpartum hemorrhage is the most common cause of pituitary infarction. This clinical entity is referred to as *Sheehan's syndrome.* The pituitary normally hypertrophies during pregnancy, and when hypotension results from hemorrhage, ischemia and necrosis of the gland occur. This condition may develop immediately postpartum or several years after delivery.

Collaborative Management

 Assessment

Gonadotropin (LH and FSH) deficiency results in the loss of secondary sex characteristics in adult males and females. While assessing the male client, the nurse notes the key signs and symptoms of facial and body hair loss. The nurse asks about episodes of impotence and decreased libido. Female clients may report primary amenorrhea, painful intercourse, difficulty in achieving pregnancy, and decreased libido. While examining the female client, the nurse checks for dry skin, breast atrophy, and decreased amount or absence of axillary and pubic hair. Gonadotropin deficiency does *not* cause other appreciable clinical manifestations in the adult.

Neurologic manifestations of hypopituitarism due to tumor growth are often observed initially as visual disturbances. During the physical assessment, the nurse evaluates the client's visual acuity, particularly peripheral vision. Bilateral temporal headaches are a common finding. Cranial nerves III, IV, and VI are sometimes affected by pituitary tumor growth, which results in diplopia and ocular muscle paralysis. (Chapter 43 covers neurologic assessment.)

Laboratory findings may vary widely in people with hypopituitarism. Basal levels of some target organ hormones can be measured easily, such as triiodothyronine (T_3) and thyroxine (T_4) from the thyroid, as well as testosterone and estradiol from the gonads. If levels of one or all of these hormones are low or in the low-normal range, and the health care team strongly suspects hypopituitarism (e.g., the client has a hypothalamic tumor), further evaluation is necessary. Levels of pituitary gonadotropins (LH and FSH) and TSH are sufficient if function of the target organ is apparent. ACTH levels may be normal or low, and prolactin (PRL) levels are low to high.

In some cases, pituitary reserve cannot be assessed without stimulation tests. The insulin tolerance test is performed to assess ACTH and GH reserves. Regular insulin (0.05–1 unit/kg of body weight) is injected to induce hypoglycemia, which acts as a stimulus to release GH and ACTH. ACTH levels can be determined directly, or indirectly by measuring the effect on the adrenal gland. Thyrotropin-releasing hormone (TRH) is given to stimulate the production of TSH from the pituitary. The normal value for PRL is less than 25 mg/mL, but PRL levels rise in response to TRH stimulation. Gonadotropin-releasing hormone (GnRH) is given to stimulate the production of LH and FSH. Normal results are based on a peak response occurring between 15 and 45 minutes after administration of GnRH.

Conventional skull x-rays can reveal certain abnormalities of the sella turcica, including enlargement, erosion, and calcifications in the area of the sella from pituitary tumors. Computed tomography (CT) and magnetic resonance imaging (MRI) can define intrasellar and suprasellar lesions. Some diagnosticians also use angiography to rule out an aneurysm or congenital vascular malformations before any surgical intervention.

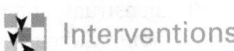 Interventions

Management of the adult with hypopituitarism focuses on replacement of deficient hormones. Elderly clients or those with a chronic disease often require a lower amount of hormone replacement. Postpubertal males who have gonadotropin deficiency are treated with androgens (testosterone). The most widely used and most effective route of administration is intramuscular (IM), although the recent development of transdermal testosterone shows promise. The nurse instructs the client in self-administration. Therapy is usually initiated with high-dose testosterone derivatives and continued until virilization is achieved. The dose may then be decreased, but therapy continues throughout life.

Androgen therapy is contraindicated in men with prostate cancer. Side effects of testosterone therapy include gynecomastia (the development of breast tissue in men), baldness, and prostatic hypertrophy. Maximal effects of treatment include increases in penis size, libido, muscle mass, bone size, and bone strength. Chest, facial, pubic, and axillary hair growth also increase, and the client's voice deepens. Clients usually report improved self-esteem and body image after therapy is initiated.

Achieving fertility in these clients is difficult and requires additional parenteral gonadotropin therapy. The nurse educates the client about the course of additional therapy and supports the client and family members emotionally because the outcome of fertility treatment is uncertain.

Female clients beyond puberty receive hormone replacement with a combination of estrogen and progesterone administered at their menstrual cycle, which causes withdrawal bleeding. Caution must be exercised if the client has not achieved full growth potential because these hormones also may cause premature closure of the epiphyses. Clients must be aware of the risk for hypertension or thrombophlebitis associated with estrogen therapy, and the nurse emphasizes measures to reduce risk and the need for regular health visits. For female clients who wish to become pregnant, clomiphene citrate (Clomid) may be given to induce ovulation. Menotropins in conjunction with human chorionic gonadotropin (hCG) are used to stimulate ovulation when therapy with clomiphene citrate has failed.

Adult clients who have isolated GH deficiency may be treated with exogenous GH, although this treatment is rare. Adrenal hypofunction is discussed later in this chapter, and thyroid replacement therapy is discussed in Chapter 67.

Hyperpituitarism
Overview

Hyperpituitarism is a pathologic state that occurs when a client has pituitary tumors or hyperplasia not associated with the absence of the normal regulatory feedback mechanisms. Tumors usually arise from the somatotropic cells (GH), the lactotropic cells (PRL), and the corticotropic cells (ACTH) located in the anterior pituitary (adenohypophysis). The major exception is the overproduction of PRL, which may be associated with tumors that produce other hormones, such as GH and ACTH. Hypersecretion of ACTH is sometimes associated with increased secretion of MSH. Tumors producing TSH or LH and FSH are so rare that only a few cases have been documented.

Pathophysiology

A common reason for hyperpituitarism is the presence of a pituitary adenoma, a benign epithelial tumor. Adenomas are classified by size, degree of invasiveness, and the hormone secreted. An invasive pituitary adenoma involves a portion or all of the sella turcica. When the sella turcica is not involved, the adenoma is "enclosed."

Changes in neurologic function may occur as adenomas grow and compress surrounding structures. Neurologic manifestations vary and may include visual defects, headache, and increased intracranial pressure. PRL-secreting tumors are the most common of the pituitary adenomas. Excessive PRL secretion inhibits the secretion of gonadal steroids and gonadotropins in males and females, resulting in galactorrhea, amenorrhea, and infertility.

Overproduction of GH results in *gigantism* (Fig. 66–1) or *acromegaly* (Fig. 66–2). The onset of the disease may be insidious, and frequently the disorder is present for years before the diagnosis. Early detection and treatment are essential to prevent irreversible changes in the soft tissues, such as those of the face, hands, feet, and skin. These changes are, to a certain extent, reversible after treatment, but skeletal changes are permanent.

In those with gigantism, onset of GH hypersecretion occurs *before* closure of the epiphyses and puberty, which causes rapid proportional growth in the length of all bones. In those with acromegaly, excessive GH secretion in adults produces increased skeletal thickness, hypertrophy of the skin, and enlargement of visceral organs.

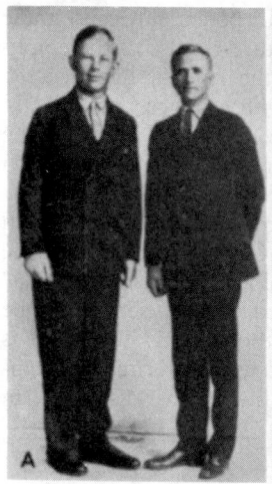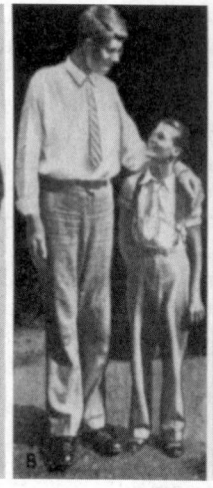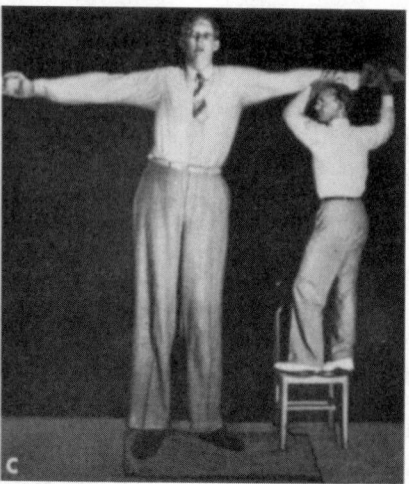

Figure 66–1. The clinical features of GH excess. Robert Wadlow, the "Alton giant," weighed 9 pounds at birth but grew to 30 pounds by the time he was 6 months old. By his first birthday, he had reached 62 pounds. At the time of his death at age 22 from cellulitis of the feet, he was 8 feet 11 inches tall and weighed 475 pounds.

In adults, bony changes related to excessive GH occur slowly and include cortical thickening, tufting of terminal phalanges (arrowhead fingertips), and bone-cell proliferation. Degeneration of joint cartilage and hypertrophy of ligaments, vocal cords, and eustachian tube mucosa are common. Nerve entrapment occurs because of tissue overgrowth, with demyelinization of peripheral nerves. Because GH is an insulin antagonist, glucose intolerance is also common.

Hypersecretion of ACTH results in overstimulation of the adrenal cortex. This produces excessive amounts of glucocorticoids, mineralocorticoids, and androgens, which leads to the development of Cushing's disease (see the section on Hypercortisolism).

Etiology

Most cases of hyperpituitarism result from hormone-secreting adenomas arising from their respective cell types. Hyperpituitarism can also be due to hypothalamic dysfunction.

Adenomas usually develop in clients without a family history or as part of a syndrome known as *multiple endocrine neoplasia*. This familial disorder is transmitted as an autosomal dominant trait and may include parathyroid and pancreatic tumors.

Incidence/Prevalence

The most common secretory tumors are prolactinomas, followed by GH-producing adenomas. Tumors secreting gonadotropin or TSH are the least common. Of all tumors for which surgery is performed, approximately 70% secrete one or more hormones. Hyperpituitarism in the general population is rare.

Collaborative Management

 Assessment

➤ History

The symptoms of hyperpituitarism vary, depending on the hormone produced in excess. The nurse obtains data about the client's age, gender, and family history. Also, the nurse asks the client about any change in hat, glove, ring, or shoe size. The client may report fatigue and lethargy. Clients with excessively high GH levels describe discomfort, such as backache and arthralgias. The nurse notes reports of visual difficulties and headaches.

Clients with hypersecretion of PRL (hyperprolactinemia) often report difficulties in sexual functioning. The nurse asks the female client about menstrual changes (e.g., amenorrhea, irregular menses, and difficulty in achieving pregnancy) and about decreased libido or dyspareunia (painful intercourse). Male clients may report decreased libido and impotence.

➤ Physical Assessment/Clinical Manifestations

Initial manifestations of GH hypersecretion are changes in the facial features, including increases in lip and nose size; in head, hand, and foot sizes; and a prominent supraorbital ridge. Prognathism, a projection of the jaw beyond the facial features, becomes marked. The nurse assesses the client for difficulty in chewing and for dentures that no longer fit. Arthritic changes causing joint pain and decreased mobility may also be noted. The nurse observes fingers and toes for an "arrowhead" or tufted shape on x-rays and a thickened appearance. At onset, acromegaly is characterized by increased metabolism and strength. As the disease progresses, these manifestations are replaced with lethargy and weakness.

The nurse assesses the client's vision for any changes related to compression on the optic nerves. The nurse also notes any increased perspiration and oil secretion on the client's skin. Other prominent features include

- Organomegaly (cardiac or hepatic)
- Hypertension
- Dysphagia from an enlarged tongue
- Deepening of the voice caused by hypertrophy of the larynx

Hypersecretion of PRL is often observed together with hypogonadism and galactorrhea. Galactorrhea (spontaneous milk flow from the nipples) may be present in either gender but is predominant in females.

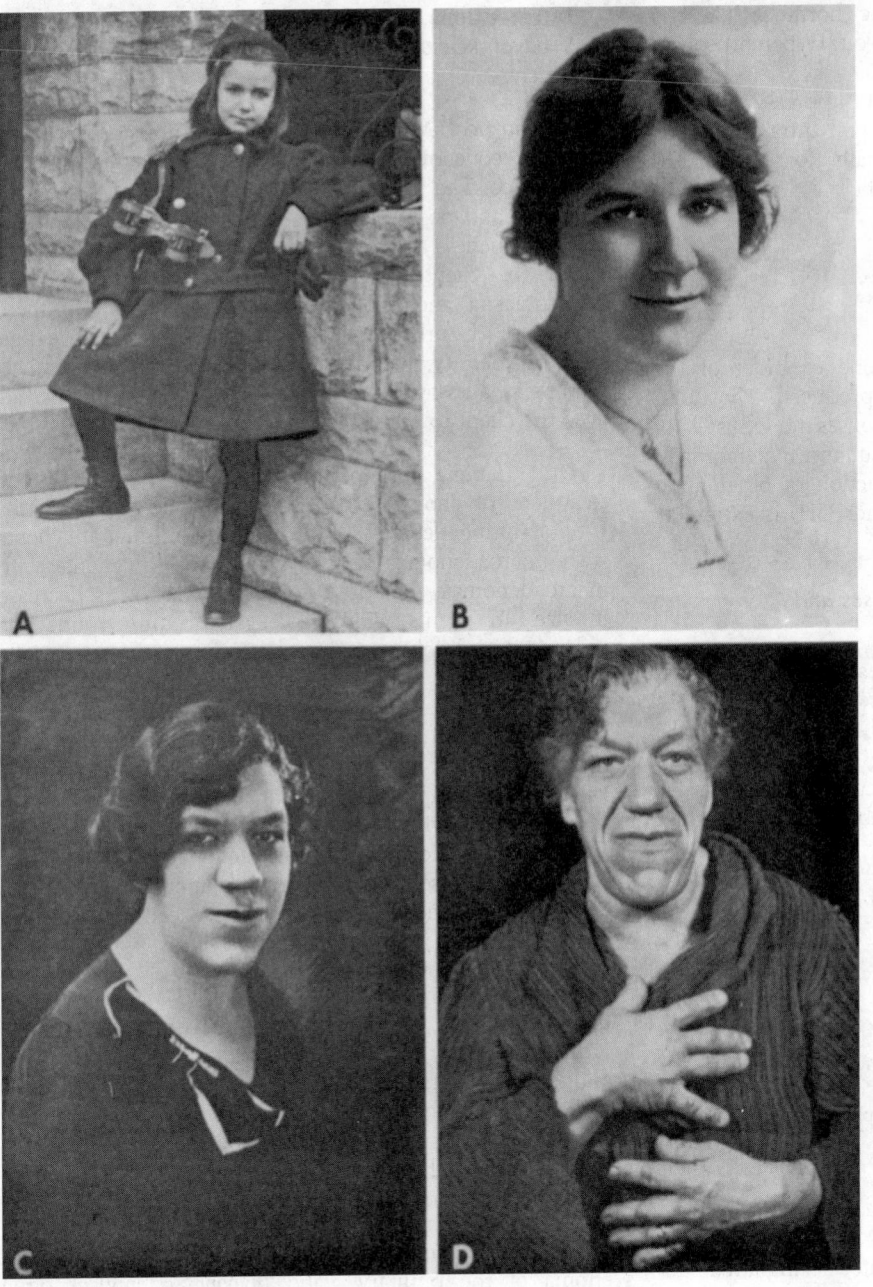

Figure 66–2. The progression of acromegaly.

➤ Psychosocial Assessment

Clients with hyperpituitarism often seek health care because of dramatic changes in their physical appearance. The nurse assesses the impact of these physical changes on the client's interpersonal relationships.

In clients who are disturbed by an inability to conceive, the nurse identifies symptoms of emotional distress, such as crying, reports of depression, irritability, and hostility. Because intracranial lesions are often an etiologic factor in hyperpituitarism, clients may express fear of this diagnosis, subsequent surgery, and prognosis.

➤ Laboratory Assessment

In a person with hyperpituitarism, usually only one hormone is produced in excess, the most common being PRL, ACTH, or GH. Tumors producing TSH, LH, or FSH are extremely rare. Elevated levels of any of these hormones demand further investigation, but LH and FSH are normally elevated in the postmenopausal and climacteric adult.

➤ Radiographic Assessment

Radiographic evaluation of the client with hyperpituitarism is identical to that for a client with hypopituitarism. Conventional skull x-rays are made to identify abnormalities of the sella turcica. Computed tomography and magnetic resonance imaging can define intrasellar and suprasellar lesions, and angiography can rule out an aneurysm or congenital vascular malformations.

➤ Other Diagnostic Assessment

Suppression tests are helpful in the diagnosis of hyperpituitarism. Dexamethasone suppression tests determine the suppressibility of adrenocorticotropic hormone (ACTH) from the pituitary (see the section on Hypercortisolism [Cushing's syndrome]).

In a glucose tolerance test for GH suppression, 100 g oral glucose or 0.5 g/kg of body weight intravenously is given. GH levels are measured serially for up to 120 minutes. GH levels that do not fall below 5 ng/mL indicate a positive (abnormal) result.

 Analysis

When hyperpituitarism is present, one or more of the anterior pituitary hormones are overproduced. The nursing diagnoses focus on clients' responses to excesses of PRL and GH. An excess of ACTH results in hypercortisolism (described later). The overproduction of other anterior pituitary hormones (TSH, LH, and FSH) is extremely rare.

➤ *Common Nursing Diagnoses and Collaborative Problems*

The most common nursing diagnoses seen in the client with hyperpituitarism are
1. Body Image Disturbance related to altered physical appearance
2. Sexual Dysfunction related to actual limitation imposed by disease (e.g., loss of libido, infertility, impotence)

➤ *Additional Nursing Diagnoses and Collaborative Problems*

The client with hyperpituitarism may also have the following nursing diagnoses:
- Pain (e.g., discomfort, headache) related to compression of tissues by tumor, backache, or arthralgia related to the effects of excessive GH levels, and dyspareunia related to excessive PRL levels
- Fear related to a perceived threat of death from intracranial mass
- Anxiety related to a threat of or a change in health status
- Ineffective Individual Coping related to impaired self-concept and loss of control over the body
- Activity Intolerance related to the effects of excessive GH levels (e.g., pain or discomfort, lethargy, and weakness)
- Sensory/Perceptual Alterations (Visual) related to altered nerve transmission as a consequence of nerve compression from tumor or surrounding structures
- Knowledge Deficit (diagnosis and treatment regimen) related to unfamiliarity with information

 Planning and Implementation

➤ *Body Image Disturbance*

Planning: Expected Outcomes. The primary outcome is that the client is expected to experience an improvement in body image.

Interventions. The client who has excessive GH levels may have skeletal changes that cannot be reversed with treatment.

Nonsurgical Management. Clients are encouraged to verbalize concerns and fears about their altered physical appearance. The nurse helps the client identify his or her strengths and positive characteristics, reinforcing each client's uniqueness and importance.

For the client with hyperprolactinemia, galactorrhea, gynecomastia, and difficulties in sexual functioning, these can cause disturbances in the client's body image and personal identity. The nurse reassures the client that treatment may alleviate some of these symptoms and encourages the client to discuss his or her feelings.

Drug Therapy. Bromocriptine mesylate (Parlodel) is the treatment of choice for clients with hyperprolactinemia. Bromocriptine decreases PRL levels to normal in clients with microadenomas and to about 90% in clients with macroadenomas; in most cases, macroadenomas decrease in size. In clients with acromegaly, bromocriptine has reduced GH levels and decreased tumor size, especially when GH levels remain high after surgery or before the full effect of radiation therapy has occurred.

Side effects of bromocriptine include orthostatic (postural) hypotension, gastric irritation, nausea, headaches, abdominal cramps, and constipation. The nurse gives bromocriptine with a meal or a snack to help alleviate some of these side effects. Treatment is usually initiated with a low dose and is gradually increased until the desired level (usually 7.5 mg/day) is reached. If pregnancy occurs, the drug is stopped immediately.

Radiation Therapy. Radiation therapy is not useful in the management of acute hyperpituitarism. Conventional radiation therapy regimens take a long time to complete, and several years pass before any therapeutic effect is evident. Proton beam or alpha particle radiation is effective, but the response is slow. Side effects of radiation therapy include hypopituitarism, optic nerve damage, oculomotor dysfunction, and visual field defects.

Surgical Management. Surgical removal of a microadenoma of the pituitary gland (*hypophysectomy*) is often indicated for clients with hyperpituitarism.

Preoperative Care. The nurse explains that hypophysectomy decreases hormone levels, relieves headaches, and may reverse changes in sexual functioning. Body changes, visceral enlargement, and visual changes are not usually reversible. The nurse explains that because nasal packing is present for 2–3 days postoperatively, it will be necessary to breathe through the mouth, and a "mustache" dressing ("drip" pad) will be placed under the client's nose. The nurse tells the client not to brush his or her teeth, cough, sneeze, blow the nose, and bend forward after surgery. These activities can hinder healing of the incision, disrupt the muscle graft, and cause momentary increases in intracranial pressure.

The nurse explains preoperative diagnostic tests, neuroradiologic examinations (see Chap. 43), endocrine testing, and visual field examinations. Nasal and oral mucous

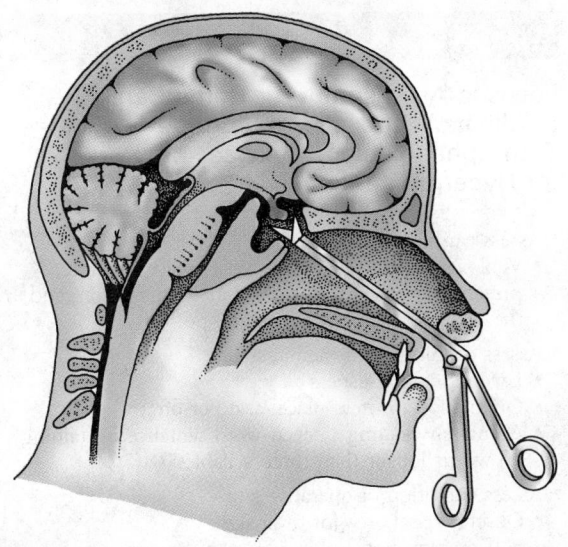

Figure 66–3. The transsphenoidal surgical approach to the pituitary gland. Selective adenomectomy leaves normal pituitary tissue undisturbed.

membrane swab specimens for bacterial culture and sensitivity are obtained preoperatively.

Operative Procedure. A transsphenoidal approach to the pituitary gland is most commonly used. Transsphenoidal hypophysectomy is microscopic surgery performed with the client under general anesthesia and in a semi-sitting position. The surgeon makes the initial incision at the inner aspect of the upper lip and enters the sella turcica via the sphenoid sinus (Fig. 66–3). After the gland is removed, a muscle graft is taken, often from the anterior thigh, to pack the dura and to prevent leakage of cerebrospinal fluid (CSF). The surgeon inserts nasal packing after the incision is closed and applies a mustache dressing to prevent the packing from dislodging. If the tumor is inaccessible by this route, a transfrontal craniotomy may be indicated (see Chap. 47).

Postoperative Care. The nurse monitors the client's neurologic response and notes any changes in vision, disorientation, altered level of consciousness, or decreased strength of the extremities. The nurse also observes the client for postoperative complications (e.g., transient diabetes insipidus [DI]).

The nurse monitors the intake of intravenous (IV) fluid, encourages fluid intake in response to thirst, and administers vasopressin as indicated. In a client with diabetes insipidus, urine specific gravity measurements are low, and he or she is polyuric. A urinary catheter may be inserted for accurate measuring of urine output, and daily weights are taken.

The nurse instructs the client to report any postnasal drip, which might indicate leakage of CSF. The head of the bed is elevated postoperatively. The nurse assesses nasal drainage for quantity, quality, and the presence of glucose (which indicates that the fluid is CSF). A light-yellow color at the edge of the clear drainage on the dressing is called the "halo sign" and indicates CSF. If the

client complains of persistent, severe headaches, CSF fluid may have leaked into the sinus area. Most CSF leaks resolve with bed rest. If the CSF leak persists, the physician may perform a spinal tap to reduce CSF pressure. Surgical intervention is rarely necessary.

Coughing is *not* encouraged postoperatively because it increases pressure in the incisional area and may lead to a CSF leak. The nurse reminds the client to practice frequent deep breathing exercises to prevent pulmonary complications. Clients may also experience mouth dryness as a result of mouth breathing. The nurse or assistive nursing personnel performs frequent oral rinses and applies petroleum jelly to dry lips.

Infection can occur postoperatively as well. The nurse is particularly alert for symptoms of meningitis, such as headache, elevated temperature, and nuchal (neck) rigidity. The physician may prescribe antibiotics, analgesics, and antipyretics.

If the entire pituitary gland has been removed, thyroid hormones and glucocorticoids must be replaced. (Gonadotropin deficiency is also noted in male and female clients.) Postoperative care is reviewed in Chart 66–1.

➤ *Sexual Dysfunction*

Planning: Expected Outcomes. The primary outcome is that the client is expected to achieve a personal desired level of sexual functioning.

Interventions. The nurse identifies the specific problems that the client is experiencing and encourages the client to discuss any effect that sexual dysfunction has had on his or her sexual partner. Drug therapy with bromocriptine can decrease prolactin (PRL) levels in clients with PRL-secreting tumors. After PRL levels are decreased, gonadotropin function often returns to normal.

Chart 66–1

Nursing Care Highlight: The Client Who Has Undergone Hypophysectomy

- Monitor the client's neurologic status.
- Monitor fluid balance, especially for output greater than intake, because transient diabetes insipidus can occur.
- Encourage the client to maintain pulmonary hygiene through deep breathing exercises.
- Instruct the client *not* to cough, blow the nose, or sneeze.
- Instruct the client to use dental floss and oral mouth rinses because brushing the teeth is not permitted until the incision heals sufficiently.
- Instruct the client to avoid bending at the waist for any reason.
- Monitor the nasal drip pad for type and amount of drainage. The presence of the halo sign may indicate a CSF leak.
- Monitor bowel movements to prevent constipation and subsequent "straining."
- Teach the client self-administration of the prescribed hormones.

Clients requiring hypophysectomy for hyperpituitarism may experience sexual dysfunction as a result of postsurgical gonadotropin deficiency (see hormone replacement in the preceding section on Hypopituitarism).

 Continuing Care

Clients who have advanced acromegaly may experience arthritic changes. The nurse assesses the degree of mobility impairment and identifies appropriate adaptations, such as the use of ambulatory aids (cane or walker) and the accessibility of bathroom facilities.

➤ *Health Teaching*

After a transsphenoidal hypophysectomy, the nurse advises the client to avoid activities that might interfere with healing. Clients must avoid bending over from the waist to pick up objects or tie shoes because doing so increases intracranial pressure. The nurse instructs the client to bend the knees and then lower the body to retrieve fallen objects. Intracranial pressure also increases when clients strain to have a bowel movement, and clients are encouraged to prevent constipation by eating high-fiber foods, drinking additional fluids, and using stool softeners or laxatives. Both bending and straining with defecation should be avoided for up to 2 months after surgery.

The nurse encourages clients to use mouthwash or dental floss for 1–2 weeks until the incision has healed and they can resume brushing their teeth. Transient numbness in the area of the incision and a decreased sense of smell are usual and last 3–4 months. Because of reduced sensation, the nurse advises the client to use a mirror to check the gums for bleeding.

After hypophysectomy, hormone replacement may be necessary to maintain fluid balance. (See the discussion of vasopressin replacement in clients with diabetes insipidus in the next section.) If the anterior portion of the pituitary gland is removed, clients may require instruction in cortisol, thyroid, and gonadal hormone replacement. The nurse instructs the client to report the return of any symptoms of hyperpituitarism immediately to the primary health care provider.

➤ *Home Care Management*

After treatment, clients who have hyperpituitarism may need daily self-management regimens and frequent checkups. The client may also need to develop strategies to minimize stress to prevent alterations of hormone production. The nurse performs a focused assessment during the first several home visits to a client who has had a hypophysectomy (Chart 66–2). Medication regimens, signs and symptoms of infection, and cerebral edema are reviewed with the family.

➤ *Health Care Resources*

Clients with decreased mobility related to acromegaly or clients who have had recent surgery may require a home

> **Chart 66–2**
>
> **Focused Assessment for Home Care of Clients Who Have Undergone Transsphenoidal Hypophysectomy for Hyperpituitarism**
>
> - Assess cardiovascular status
>   - Vital signs including apical pulse, pulse pressure, presence or absence of orthostatic hypotension, and the quality/rhythm of peripheral pulses
> - Assess cognition and mental status
>   - Level of consciousness
>   - Orientation to time, place, and person
>   - Accurately reading a seven-word sentence containing no words longer than three syllables
> - Assess condition of operative site
>   - Observe nasal area for drainage
>   - If present, note color, clarity, and odor
>   - Test clear drainage for the presence of glucose
> - Assess neuromuscular status
>   - Reactivity of patellar and biceps reflexes
>   - Oral temperature
>   - Handgrip strength
>   - Steadiness of gait
>   - Visual fields
>   - Distant and near visual acuity
>   - Pupillary responses to light
> - Assess renal system
>   - Observe urine specimen for color, odor, cloudiness, and amount
> - Ask about:
>   - Headaches or visual disturbances
>   - Ease of bowel movements
>   - 24-hour fluid intake and output
>   - 24-hour diet recall
>   - 24-hour activity recall
>   - Over-the-counter and prescribed medications taken
> - Assess client's understanding of illness and compliance with treatment
>   - Signs and symptoms to report to health care provider
>   - Medication plan (correct timing and dose)

health aide or nurse to help maintain activities of daily living (ADL). In addition, clients with hyperpituitarism must continue to have hormone levels monitored at regular intervals to detect any recurrence of tumor. Access to the physician and other health care team members is essential.

 Evaluation

The expected outcomes based on the common nursing diagnoses for hyperpituitarism and its treatment include that the client will
- Experience an improvement in body image
- Achieve a personal desired level of sexual functioning

DISORDERS OF THE POSTERIOR PITUITARY GLAND

Disorders of the posterior pituitary (neurohypophysis) are directly related to a deficiency or excess of the hormone vasopressin (antidiuretic hormone [ADH]). Two disorders associated with ADH deficiency or excess are diabetes insipidus and the syndrome of inappropriate antidiuretic hormone (SIADH).

Diabetes Insipidus

Overview

Diabetes insipidus is a disorder of water metabolism caused by a deficiency of ADH—either a decrease in ADH synthesis or an inability of the kidney to respond appropriately to ADH. ADH deficiency results in the excretion of large volumes of dilute urine. The permeability of water in the distal tubules and collecting ducts of the kidneys is severely impaired by a deficiency of ADH, causing an excessive loss of free water and polyuria.

Dehydration accompanying this massive diuresis results in an increase in plasma osmolality, which stimulates the osmoreceptors to relay a sensation of thirst to the cerebral cortex. Normally, thirst promotes increased fluid intake and aids in maintaining water homeostasis. If the thirst compensatory mechanism is inadequate or absent, or if the person is unable to obtain water, dehydration becomes progressively more severe.

ADH deficiency can be classified as

- Nephrogenic
- Drug-related
- Primary
- Secondary

Nephrogenic diabetes insipidus is an inherited defect. The renal tubules do not respond to the actions of ADH, which results in inadequate water reabsorption by the kidney. The amount of hormone is not deficient.

Primary diabetes insipidus is caused by a familial or idiopathic defect in the pituitary gland. Secondary diabetes insipidus results from tumors in the hypothalamic-pituitary region, head trauma, infectious processes, surgical procedures (hypophysectomy), or metastatic tumors, usually from the lung or the breast. Less frequently, it is caused by cerebrovascular hemorrhage, granulomatous disease, or cerebral aneurysm.

Drug-related ADH deficiency is caused by the administration of lithium carbonate (Eskalith, Lithobid, Carbolith✦) and demeclocycline (Declomycin). These agents can interfere with the renal response to ADH.

Collaborative Management

 Assessment

The nurse notes the key symptoms of an increase in the frequency of urination and excessive thirst. The nurse also notes a history of any known etiologic factors, such as recent surgery, head trauma, and medication use (e.g., lithium). Although increased fluid intake usually prevents serious dehydration and volume depletion, clients deprived of fluids or clients who cannot increase their oral fluid intake may experience circulatory collapse caused by fluid loss and neurologic changes related to plasma hyperosmolality. Signs of dehydration, such as poor skin turgor and dry or cracked mucous membranes or skin, may be present in varying degrees. (See Chapter 15 for further discussion of clients with dehydration.)

Loss of free water produces characteristic changes in blood and urine tests. The initial step in diagnosis is to measure 24-hour fluid intake and output. The amount of the client's food and fluid is not restricted during this measurement. Urine output must be more than 4 L during this period for diabetes insipidus to be diagnosed. The amount of urine excreted in 24 hours may vary from 4 to 30 L/day. Urine is dilute and therefore has a low specific gravity (less than 1.005) and low osmolality (50–200 mOsm/kg). Fluid deprivation and hypertonic saline tests are also used for differential diagnosis (Table 66–2).

 Interventions

Medical management is aimed at controlling the symptoms of disease by drug therapy (Chart 66–3). If only a partial deficit of ADH is present, effective control can be achieved by oral chlorpropamide (Diabinese, Novo-Propamide✦) or clofibrate (Atromid-S, Claripex✦). These drugs augment the action of existing ADH and possibly have a direct stimulating effect on the synthesis of ADH in the hypothalamus. However, because of the side effects of these drugs, they are not used as often as synthetic vasopressin.

When ADH deficiency is severe, ADH is replaced in amounts sufficient to maintain water balance. Desmopressin acetate (DDAVP) is a synthetic analog of vasopressin administered intranasally in a metered spray and is the drug of choice. The frequency of administration varies in different clients. Each metered spray delivers 10 μg, and clients with mild DI may require only 1–2 doses in 24 hours. For clients with more severe DI, 1–2 metered doses 2–3 times per day may be needed. Lypressin [Diapid] is an older form of the drug, given by nasal spray or subcutaneously when short-acting therapy is indicated. Subcutaneous injections last only 3–6 hours. During hospitalization, ADH may be given intravenously or intramuscularly. Ulceration of the mucous membranes, allergy, a sensation of chest tightness, and inhalation of the spray, which precipitates pulmonary problems, may occur with use of the intranasal preparations. If side effects occur or if the client has an upper respiratory tract infection, subcutaneous vasopressin is used.

Nursing management is aimed at the early detection of dehydration and the maintenance of adequate hydration. Interventions include

- Accurately measuring fluid intake and output
- Checking urine specific gravity
- Recording the client's weight daily

TABLE 66-2

Care of the Client Undergoing Special Tests for Diabetes Insipidus

Test	Nursing Interventions	Rationale
Fluid deprivation test (to identify the cause of polyuria)	• Obtain baseline vital signs; then check them hourly. • Deprive the client of fluid. • Observe the client for compliance with fluid restriction. • Measure urinary output, specific gravity, and osmolality hourly. • Weigh the client hourly. • Give 5 units of aqueous vasopressin (subcutaneously), as ordered. • Continue hourly urinary measurements.	• Assessment permits the nurse to detect changes, especially postural hypotension and tachycardia. • Fluid restriction must be maintained for test results to be of diagnostic importance. • Urine testing results determine whether testing can proceed. Testing can proceed if urinary osmolality stabilizes for three samples and 3% weight loss is noted. • Vasopressin triggers—and ongoing assessment detects—changes in urinary specific gravity and osmolality. Specific gravity and osmolality decrease with primary and secondary diabetes insipidus. No response is seen with nephrogenic diabetes insipidus.
Hypertonic saline test (to stimulate release of ADH)	• Administer a normal water load to the client, followed by infusion of hypertonic saline. • Measure urinary output hourly.	• The procedure detects ADH release. A sudden decrease in urinary output is a sign of ADH release.

Chart 66-3

Drug Therapy for Diabetes Insipidus

Drug	Usual Dosage	Nursing Interventions	Rationale
Lypressin (Diapid)	• 4–8 sprays (5–10 pressor units) (nasal spray) in divided doses	• Monitor for upper respiratory tract infections or allergy.	• The effectiveness of nasal sprays is affected by upper respiratory tract infections.
Desmopressin (DDAVP)	• 0.1–0.4 mL in single or divided dose (nasal spray)	• Teach the client the proper method of administration.	• Some clients may have difficulty with measuring and inhaling.
Aqueous vasopressin (Pitressin)	• 5–20 units in divided doses (SC, IM, or nasal spray)	• Instruct the client to sit upright when spraying. • Instruct the client to hold his or her breath when using nasal spray. • Monitor the client's intake and output. • Have the client space fluid intake during waking hours. • Monitor the client frequently (q3–4h) for a recurrence of symptoms. • Monitor the client's weight.	• An upright position promotes effective absorption in the nasal mucosa. • Holding one's breath prevents nasal spray from entering lungs and potentially causing pneumonia. • Intake and output measurement helps to guide dosage regulation. • Extra fluid intake at night can cause nocturia. • Monitoring detects the need for additional doses of these short-acting medications. • Water retention can be detected by weight gain.
Clofibrate (Atromid-S, Claripex✦)	• 1.5–2 g in 4 doses PO OD	• Watch for signs of SIADH.	• The drug can potentiate the action of vasopressin.
Chlorpropamide (Diabinese, Novopropamide✦)	• 125–250 mg PO OD • **Elderly:** 100–125 mg PO OD	• Monitor the client for signs and symptoms of hypoglycemia.	• Hypoglycemia is a potentially severe side effect.

The nurse encourages the client to consume amounts of oral fluids approximately equal to urine output. If fluids are administered intravenously, the nurse ensures the patency of the access catheter and pays meticulous attention to the amount infused each hour.

Clients with permanent diabetes insipidus require life-long vasopressin therapy; the nurse must assess the client's ability to follow instructions and willingness to participate in health care. Clients using vasopressin preparations are also instructed to recognize polyuria and polydipsia as signals for another dose of medication. All clients taking vasopressin need to record daily weight measurements to identify weight gain. The nurse emphasizes the importance of using the same scale and weighing at the same time of day while wearing a similar amount of clothing. If weight gain occurs, clients are encouraged to notify their health care providers. Clients with diabetes insipidus should also wear a medical alert (Medic-Alert) bracelet identifying the disorder and current medication.

Syndrome of Inappropriate Antidiuretic Hormone Secretion

Overview

Syndrome of inappropriate antidiuretic hormone (SIADH) occurs when vasopressin (ADH) is secreted in the presence of low plasma osmolality. A decrease in plasma osmolality normally inhibits ADH production and secretion. SIADH is also known as the Schwartz-Bartter syndrome. (SIADH is also discussed in Chapter 27 as a complication of cancer and cancer therapy.)

Pathophysiology

In clients with SIADH, the feedback mechanisms that regulate ADH do not function properly. ADH continues to be released even when plasma is hyposmolar. Water is *retained,* which results in dilutional hyponatremia (a decreased serum sodium level due to dilution) and expansion of the extracellular fluid volume. The increase in plasma volume causes an increase in the glomerular filtration rate and inhibits the release of renin and aldosterone. The combined effect is an increased sodium loss in urine, further contributing to hyponatremia.

Etiology

SIADH is associated with a variety of pathologic conditions and specific drugs. Table 66–3 lists common causes of SIADH.

Collaborative Management

 Assessment

➤ *History*

The nurse asks about the client's medical history, which may reveal conditions associated with the development

of SIADH. The nurse pays particular attention to a history of

- Recent trauma
- Cerebrovascular disease
- Tuberculosis or other pulmonary disease
- Cancer
- All past and current medication use

➤ *Physical Assessment/Clinical Manifestations*

Initially, the symptoms of SIADH are related to water retention: gastrointestinal disturbances, such as loss of appetite, nausea, and vomiting. The nurse weighs the client and documents any recent weight gain. The nurse also checks the client's extremities for edema. In clients with SIADH, free water, not salt, is retained, and edema is not usually present.

Water retention, hyponatremia, and resulting fluid shifts affect central nervous system function, especially when the serum sodium level drops below 115 mEq/L. The client may experience episodes of lethargy, headaches, hostility, uncooperativeness, and disorientation. A change in the client's level of consciousness is an early sign of SIADH. Neurologic symptoms can progress from lethargy and headaches to decreased responsiveness, seizures, and coma. The nurse assesses deep tendon reflexes, which are often decreased or sluggish.

Vital sign changes include tachycardia associated with increased fluid volume and hypothermia associated with

TABLE 66–3

Conditions Causing SIADH	
Malignancies	• Small cell carcinoma of the lung • Pancreatic, duodenal, and GU carcinomas • Thymoma • Ewing's sarcoma • Hodgkin's lymphoma • Non-Hodgkin's lymphoma
Pulmonary Disorders	• Viral and bacterial pneumonia • Lung abscesses • Active tuberculosis • Pneumothorax • Chronic lung diseases • Mycoses • Positive pressure ventilation
CNS Disorders	• Trauma • Infection • Tumors (primary or metastatic) • Cerebrovascular accidents • Porphyria • Systemic lupus erythematosus
Drugs	• Exogenous ADH • Chlorpropamide • Vincristine • Cyclophosphamide • Carbamazepine • Opioids • Tricyclic antidepressants • General anesthetics

Client Care Plan

The Client with Syndrome of Inappropriate Antidiuretic Hormone

Nursing Diagnosis No. 1: Fluid Volume Excess related to compromised regulatory mechanism and excess antidiuretic hormone

Expected Outcomes	Nursing Interventions	Rationale

The client's fluid balance is expected to be restored.
The client's serum sodium levels are expected to be within normal ranges.
	▪ Maintain fluid restriction as ordered.
	▪ Prohibit all water intake:
	  ▪ Prohibit ice chips or drinking water.
	  ▪ Irrigate tubes and mix medications with normal saline solution rather than water.
	▪ Maintain accurate intake and output measurements.
	
	▪ Weigh the client daily.
	
	▪ Monitor the client's serum sodium level.
	
	▪ Administer IV hypertonic saline (3%), diuretics, and demeclocycline as ordered.
		▪ Fluid is restricted to prevent worsening of the condition.
		▪ Water excess is the hallmark of the condition.
		
		▪ Mixing medications with saline helps to replace some sodium.
		
		▪ Output should be greater than intake while excessive fluid is removed.
		▪ Weight loss of 1 kg means 1 L of body fluid has been removed.
		▪ As the client responds to treatment, the serum sodium level should return to the normal range.
		▪ Hypertonic saline and demeclocycline help to correct the serum sodium level.
		▪ Diuretics help rid the body of excessive fluid.

Nursing Diagnosis No. 2: High Risk for Injury related to altered level of consciousness, confusion, and the possibility of seizures

Expected Outcomes	Nursing Interventions	Rationale
The client is expected to remain free from injury.	▪ Assess the client's level of consciousness and mental status ▪ Assess for muscle twitching or other signs and symptoms of seizures. ▪ Maintain the neurologic observation check sheets as ordered. ▪ Implement basic safety measures in the client's environment.	▪ Decreased level of consciousness and seizures are complications of the low serum sodium level related to SIADH. ▪ Frequent assessment helps to detect early signs of complications. ▪ Basic safety measures help to prevent injury.

central nervous system disturbance. (Chapter 16 presents other findings associated with hyponatremia.)

➤ Diagnostic Assessment

Water retention changes both plasma and urine osmolality. Plasma osmolality is decreased, and the urine is hy-

perosmolar in relation to the plasma. Elevated urine sodium levels and specific gravity reflect increased urine concentration. Serum sodium levels are decreased, often as low as 110 mEq/L, because of volume expansion and increased sodium excretion.

Radioimmunoassay of ADH can diagnose SIADH when

levels are inappropriately elevated in relation to plasma osmolality. When plasma osmolality is normal or decreased, ADH hormone levels should be low.

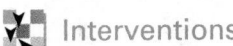 Interventions

Interventions to treat SIADH are presented in the Client Care Plan. The interventions focus on restricting fluid intake, promoting the excretion of water, replacing lost sodium, interfering with the action of ADH, and preventing injury if the client experiences increased cranial pressure or seizures.

➤ Fluid Restriction

Fluid restriction is essential in the management of the client with SIADH. In some cases, fluid intake may be kept as low as 500–600 mL/24 hours. The nurse prohibits any free water intake because this further dilutes the serum sodium concentration. The physician orders that tube feedings be diluted with a solution other than water and orders saline to irrigate gastrointestinal (GI) tubes. The nurse also mixes any medications for GI tube administration with saline.

Measurement of intake, output, and daily weights determines the degree of fluid restriction necessary. A weight gain of 2 pounds (1 kg) or more per day or a gradual increase over several days is cause for concern. A 1-kg weight increase is equivalent to a 1000-mL fluid retention (1 kg = 1 L). Clients are often uncomfortable during fluid restriction, and the nurse keeps mucous membranes moist by frequent oral rinsing, reminding the client not to swallow these rinses.

➤ Drug Therapy

Diuretics are sometimes used to treat clients with SIADH, particularly if congestive heart failure results from fluid overload. The nurse must be aware of the potential effect of electrolyte losses; sodium loss can be potentiated, further contributing to the clinical picture of SIADH.

Hypertonic saline (i.e., 3% sodium chloride [3% NaCl]) treats SIADH. IV saline is given cautiously because it may contribute to existing fluid overload and precipitate an episode of congestive heart failure. If the client needs routine IV fluids, the physician orders a saline solution rather than a water solution.

The administration of certain drugs, such as lithium carbonate (Eskalith, Lithobid, Carbolith✦) and demeclocycline (Declomycin), is associated with the development of diabetes insipidus. Their use, therefore, has been explored in the treatment of SIADH. Lithium has not been used successfully because of its toxicity, but demeclocycline is promising.

➤ Providing a Safe Environment

The nurse carefully notes changes in the client's neurologic status. The nurse attempts to detect subtle changes, such as muscle twitching, before they progress to seizures or coma. The nurse also checks the client's orientation to time, place, and person because disorientation may be

present. Confusion is another neurologic sign, and the nurse reduces environmental stimuli and explains interventions in simple terms.

Flow sheets containing ongoing information about the level of consciousness, motor and sensory neurologic assessments, and pertinent laboratory data are helpful in detecting neurologic trends. The frequency of neurologic checks depends on the status of the client: for the client with SIADH who is hyponatremic but alert, awake, and oriented, neurologic checks every 4 hours are sufficient. For the client who has had a change in level of consciousness, neurologic checks take place at least every hour. The nurse also inspects the environment at regular intervals, making sure that basic safety measures, such as side rails securely in place, are observed.

DISORDERS OF THE ADRENAL GLAND

Hypofunction of the Adrenal Gland

Overview

Production of adrenocortical steroids may decrease as a result of inadequate secretion of ACTH, dysfunction of the hypothalamic-pituitary control mechanism, and complete or partial destruction of the adrenal glands. Manifestations may develop gradually or accelerate quickly with stress. In acute adrenocortical insufficiency (adrenal crisis), life-threatening manifestations may appear without warning. Figure 66–4 outlines the normal pathway for adrenocortical hormone synthesis.

Loss of the adrenal medulla, unlike that of the cortex, does not upset the maintenance of homeostasis. This is because catecholamines also are synthesized and released from other areas in the sympathetic nervous system.

Pathophysiology

Insufficiency of adrenocortical steroids causes defects associated with the loss of mineralocorticoid (aldosterone) and glucocorticoid (cortisol) action. Impaired secretion of cortisol results in decreased gluconeogenesis, with depletion of liver and muscle glycogen and thus hypoglycemia. Glomerular filtration rate and gastric acid production decrease, leading to a reduction in urea nitrogen excretion, anorexia, and weight loss.

Reduced aldosterone secretion disturbs potassium, sodium, and water excretion in the kidney. Potassium excretion is decreased, causing hyperkalemia; sodium and water excretion is increased, causing hyponatremia and hypovolemia. Potassium retention also promotes reabsorption of hydrogen ions, which can ultimately lead to metabolic acidosis.

Lower adrenal androgen levels result in the decrease or loss of body, axillary, and pubic hair, especially in females, because the adrenals produce most of the androgens. The severity of symptoms is related to the degree of deficiency in hormone secretion.

Acute adrenal insufficiency, or Addisonian crisis, is a life-threatening event in which a client's physiologic re-

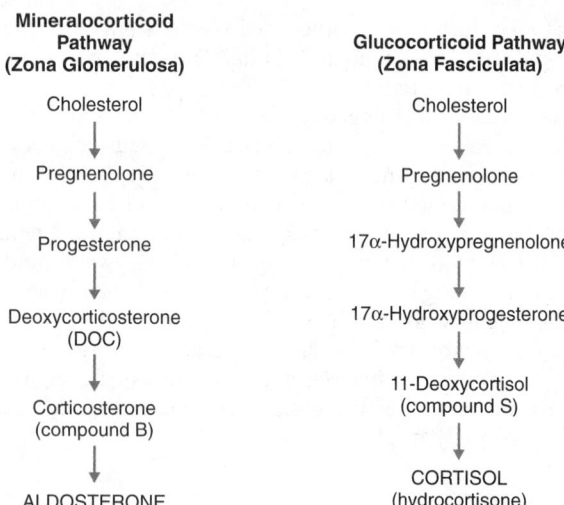

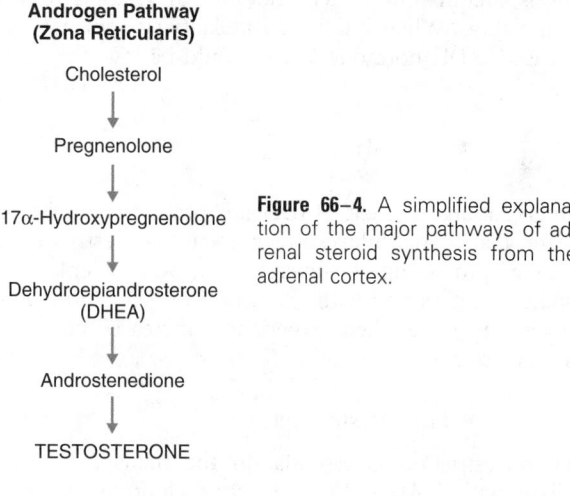

Figure 66–4. A simplified explanation of the major pathways of adrenal steroid synthesis from the adrenal cortex.

quirement for glucocorticoid and mineralocorticoid hormones exceeds the available supply. In most cases, acute adrenal insufficiency is precipitated by a stressful event (e.g., surgery, trauma, or severe infection) and when adrenal hormone output is already compromised. The pathophysiology of acute adrenal crisis is almost the same as that of chronic insufficiency: the one difference occurs in clients with acute adrenal crisis related to bilateral adrenal hemorrhage. These clients may have normal sodium and potassium levels because the time between the initial incident and the presentation may be too short for a change to occur. Unless intervention is initiated promptly, however, sodium levels fall, and potassium levels rise rapidly. More severe hypotension results from intravascular volume depletion associated with the loss of mineralocorticoid. Emergency care for clients with acute adrenal insufficiency (Addisonian crisis) is outlined in Chart 66–4.

Etiology

Adrenal insufficiency may be classified as primary or secondary. Causes of primary and secondary adrenal insufficiency are listed in Table 66–4. *One of the most frequent causes of secondary adrenal insufficiency is the sudden cessation of long-term, high-dose glucocorticoid therapy.* This therapy suppresses the hypothalamic-pituitary-adrenal (HPA) axis and must be withdrawn gradually to allow for pituitary production of ACTH and adrenal production of cortisol.

Collaborative Management

 Assessment

➤ History

While taking a history from the client with suspected adrenal hypofunction, the nurse asks questions about symptoms and factors contributing to adrenal hypofunction. The nurse also asks about any change in activity level because lethargy, fatigue, and muscle weakness are often present. Questions about salt intake are included

because salt craving is often a symptom of adrenal hypofunction.

Gastrointestinal problems, such as anorexia, nausea, vomiting, diarrhea, and abdominal pain, often occur. The nurse asks about weight loss during the past weeks or months. Female clients report menstrual changes related to weight loss, and males may report impotence.

The medical history identifies potential causes of adrenal hypofunction. The nurse asks whether the client has had radiation to the abdomen or head. The nurse also documents significant medical problems, such as tuberculosis and previous intracranial surgery, and all past and current medications, particularly steroids, anticoagulants, or cytotoxic drugs.

➤ Physical Assessment/Clinical Manifestations

The clinical manifestations of adrenal hypofunction vary. The severity of symptoms is related to the degree of

---

Chart 66–4

Nursing Care Highlight: Acute Adrenal Insufficiency (Addisonian Crisis)

- Before initiating treatment, obtain a complete blood count and electrolyte, blood urea nitrogen, and plasma cortisol levels as ordered by the physician.
- Give an initial dose of hydrocortisone sodium succinate (Solu-Cortef), 100–300 mg IV; then infuse 100 mg during 8 hr, as ordered by the physician.
- Give concomitant doses of hydrocortisone, 50 mg IM every 12 hr, as ordered by the physician.
- After resolution of the crisis, adjust the dosage of medications as ordered by the physician:
  - Give oral glucocorticoids (e.g., hydrocortisone)
  - Decrease the dosage of oral glucocorticoids during several days as maintenance levels are reached.
- Give supplemental mineralocorticoids, such as fludrocortisone (Florinef), as the glucocorticoid dosage is tapered.

TABLE 66–4

Causes of Primary and Secondary Adrenal Insufficiency

Primary	• Idiopathic (autoimmune) disease* • Tuberculosis • Metastatic cancer • Fungal lesions • AIDS • Hemorrhage • Gram-negative sepsis (Waterhouse-Friderichsen syndrome) • Adrenalectomy • Abdominal radiation therapy • Drugs and toxins (mitotane)
Secondary	• Pituitary tumors • Postpartum pituitary necrosis (Sheehan's syndrome) • Hypophysectomy • High-dose pituitary radiation • High-dose whole brain radiation

* Most common cause.

hormone deficiency. In clients with primary adrenal hypofunction, plasma ACTH and melanocyte-stimulating hormone (MSH) levels are elevated because of the loss of the adrenal-hypothalamic-pituitary feedback system. Elevated MSH levels result in areas of increased pigmentation (Fig. 66–5). In clients who have a primary autoimmune disease, areas of decreased pigmentation may occur because of destruction of pigment-producing cells in the skin (melanocytes). Body hair may also be decreased. In secondary disease, there is no increase in skin pigmentation.

The nurse assesses the client for symptoms of hypoglycemia (e.g., sweating, headaches, tachycardia, and tremors) and volume depletion (postural hypotension and de-

hydration). Hyperkalemia can cause dysrhythmias with an irregular heart rate and result in cardiac arrest.

➤ Psychosocial Assessment

Depending on the degree of metabolic imbalance, clients may appear lethargic, apathetic, depressed, confused, and even psychotic. The nurse observes the client and checks his or her orientation to person, place, and time. Families may report that the client has a decreased energy level, is emotionally labile, and is forgetful.

➤ Diagnostic Assessment

Laboratory findings may include low serum cortisol, decreased fasting blood glucose, low sodium, elevated potassium, and increased serum blood urea nitrogen (BUN) levels (Chart 66–5). In primary disease, the eosinophil count and ACTH level are elevated. Plasma cortisol levels fail to rise during stimulation tests.

Urinary 17-hydroxycorticosteroids are the glucocorticoid metabolites, and 17-ketosteroid levels reflect the adrenal androgen metabolites. Both levels are in the low or low-normal range in adrenal hypofunction. Table 66–5 lists drugs that can interfere with test results.

Skull x-rays, computed tomography (CT), magnetic resonance imaging, and arteriography may aid in the search for an intracranial lesion impinging on the pituitary gland, adenomas of the gland itself, aneurysms, or an empty sella turcica.

Noninvasive procedures of the adrenal gland, such as CT scans without dye, may occasionally show atrophy of the gland. Although never considered diagnostic by itself, CT scans may help determine adrenal hypofunction.

An ACTH (cosyntropin [Cortrosyn], synthetic ACTH) stimulation test is necessary for a definitive workup of adrenal insufficiency. A rapid ACTH stimulation test may be administered on an outpatient basis. Cosyntropin, 0.25 to 1 mg, is given intramuscularly or intravenously, and plasma cortisol levels are obtained at 30-minute and 1-hour intervals after the baseline value is established. In

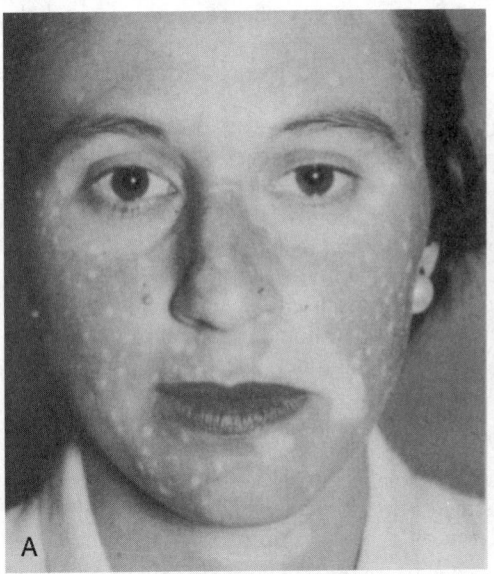 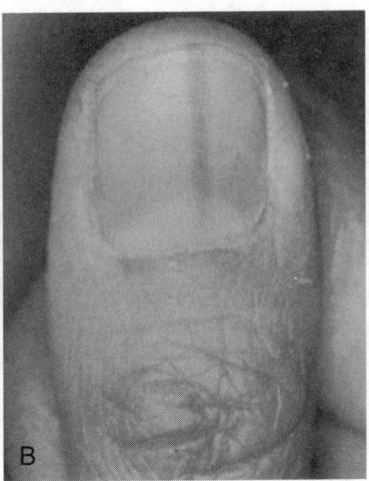

A   B

Figure 66–5. The increased pigmentation seen in primary adrenocortical insufficiency.

Chart 66–5

Laboratory Profile: Adrenal Gland Assessment

		Significance of Abnormal Findings	
Test	Normal Range for Adults	Hypofunction of the Adrenal Gland	Hyperfunction of the Adrenal Gland
Sodium	• 136–145 mEq/L	• Decreased	• Increased
Potassium	• 3.4–4.5 mEq/L	• Increased	• Decreased
Glucose	• 74–106 mg/dL • **Elderly:** slightly increased	• Normal to decreased	• Normal to increased
Calcium	• 8.6–10.0 mg/dL (total) • 4.6–5.08 mg/dL (ionized) • **Elderly:** slightly decreased	• Increased	• Decreased
Leukocytes	• 20%–40%	• Normal	• Increased
Eosinophils	• 1%–4%	• Increased	• Decreased
Bicarbonate	• 22–29 mEq/L	• Increased	• Decreased
BUN	• 6–20 mg/dL • **Elderly:** may be slightly higher	• Increased	• Normal
Cortisol	• 6 AM–8 AM 5–23 µg/dL or 138–635 SI units (nmol/L) • 4 PM–6 PM 3–16 µg/dL or 83–441 SI units (nmol/L)	• Decreased	• Increased

---

primary insufficiency, the cortisol response is absent or markedly decreased; in secondary insufficiency, it is decreased.

A longer ACTH stimulation test involves a continuous

TABLE 66–5

Some Drugs that Interfere with Tests for Urinary 17-Hydroxycorticosteroids and Urinary 17-Ketosteroids

- Acetaminophen
- Acetazolamide
- Acetylsalicylic acid
- Amphetamines
- Ascorbic acid
- Barbiturates
- Calcium gluconate
- Carbon disulfide
- Chloral hydrate
- Chlordiazepoxide
- Chlormerodrin
- Chlorothiazide
- Chlorpromazine
- Chlorthalidone
- Colchicine
- Corticotropin
- Cortisone
- Dexamethasone
- Diazepam
- Digitoxin
- Digoxin
- Diphenhydramine
- Diphenylhydantoin
- Erythromycin
- Estrogens
- Fructose
- Glutethimide

- Hydralazine
- Iodides
- Medroxyprogesterone
- Meperidine
- Meprobamate
- Metyrapone
- Mitotane
- Morphine
- Nalidixic acid
- Oral contraceptives
- Paraldehyde
- Penicillin
- Pentazocine
- Perphenazine
- Phenobarbital
- Phenothiazines
- Phenylbutazone
- Promazine
- Propoxyphene
- Quinidine
- Quinine
- Reserpine
- Secobarbital
- Spironolactone
- Testosterone
- Vitamin K

infusion of 50 units of ACTH in saline for 24 hours, or an 8-hour infusion daily for 4–5 days, with simultaneously collected 24-hour urine samples. Levels of urinary 17-hydroxycorticosteroids and urinary free cortisol are also measured. In clients with primary adrenal insufficiency, the response is low or absent; in those with secondary insufficiency, the value for 17-hydroxycorticosteroids fails to rise above 20 mg per total volume.

 Interventions

The nurse promotes fluid balance and carefully monitors for a fluid deficit. The nurse or assistive personnel do so by weighing the client daily and recording intake and output. The nurse also checks the client's vital signs every 1–4 hours, depending on the client's condition and the occurrence of dysrhythmias or postural hypotension. Laboratory values are monitored to identify hemoconcentrations (e.g., increased hematocrit or BUN). (Chapter 15 discusses fluid volume deficit in detail.)

Glucocorticoid and mineralocorticoid deficiencies are completely corrected by replacement therapy. Hydrocortisone corrects glucocorticoid deficiency (Chart 66–6). Glucocorticoid replacement regimens vary. Generally, divided doses are given, with two thirds in the morning and one third in the late afternoon to mimic the normal diurnal adrenal rhythm. Although the majority of clients do well on this regimen, other clients may not tolerate the dosage or may need more.

An additional mineralocorticoid hormone may be needed, such as fludrocortisone (Florinef), to maintain correct electrolyte balance (especially sodium and potassium). Adjustments in dosage may be necessary in hot weather when additional sodium is lost due to excessive perspiration. Salt restriction or diuretic therapy should

---

Chart 66–6

Maintenance Drug Therapy for Hypofunction of the Adrenal Gland

Drug	Usual Dosage	Nursing Interventions	Rationale
Cortisone	• 25–50 mg PO daily either once daily in AM or daily in divided doses	• Instruct the client to take the drug with meals or a snack. • Instruct the client to report the following signs or symptoms of excessive drug therapy: • Rapid weight gain • Round face • Fluid retention	• Gastrointestinal irritation can occur • Cushing's syndrome, which indicates a need for dosage adjustment, can occur.
Hydrocortisone (Cortef, Hycort❖)	• 20–50 mg PO daily either once daily in AM or daily in divided doses	• Instruct the client to report illness, such as: • Severe diarrhea • Vomiting • Fever	• Other conditions may indicate a need for dosage change. The usual daily dosage may not be adequate during periods of illness or severe stress
Prednisone (Winpred❖)	• 5–10 mg PO daily either once daily in AM or daily in divided doses		
Fludrocortisone (Florinef)	• 0.05–0.2 mg PO daily	• Monitor the client's blood pressure. • Instruct the client to report weight gain or edema.	• Hypertension is a potential side effect. • Sodium-related fluid retention is possible.

---

not be started without consideration of precipitating an adrenal crisis.

Hyperfunction of the Adrenal Gland

Hypersecretion by the adrenal cortex may result in excessive amounts of glucocorticoids, leading to

- Hypercortisolism (e.g., Cushing's syndrome)
- Excessive mineralocorticoid production, which leads to hyperaldosteronism
- Excessive androgen production, in generalized cortical hyperplasia or in the congenital and acquired enzyme deficiency states

Hypersecretion by the adrenal medulla (*pheochromocytoma*) results in excessive secretion of catecholamines, of which 80% is epinephrine and the remainder is norepinephrine.

Hypercortisolism (Cushing's Syndrome)

Overview

Pathophysiology

Cushing's syndrome exaggerates the normal physiologic action of glucocorticoids, causing widespread abnormalities. Adrenocortical hyperplasia caused by excessive stimulation by ACTH of either pituitary or ectopic origin results in

- Loss of normal diurnal rhythms
- Decreased responsiveness of prolactin, thyrotropin, and gonadotropin to their respective releasing hormones
- Abnormal sleep patterns

Some of these changes are due to excessive amounts of glucocorticoids, but others are linked to undefined hypothalamic abnormalities.

Clients who have Cushing's syndrome exhibit alterations of nitrogen, carbohydrate, and mineral metabolism. An increase in total body fat results from a depressed turnover of plasma fatty acids, and a redistribution of bulk produces the typical centripetal (truncal) pattern (Fig. 66–6). Moderate-to-marked increases in the breakdown of tissue protein and a marked increase in urine nitrogen level also occur, resulting in

- Decreased muscle mass with a proximal myopathy
- Atrophic (thin) skin
- Decreased bone matrix with a loss of total skeletal calcium levels

High levels of corticosteroids kill lymphocytes and shrink organs containing lymphocytes, such as the liver, the spleen, and the lymph nodes. Thus, the protection of the inflammatory and immune responses is reduced.

In most cases, corresponding increased androgen production causes acne, hirsutism (increased hair growth), and, rarely, clitoral hypertrophy. Increased androgen production can also interrupt the normal pituitary-ovarian axis, decreasing the ovary's production of estrogens and progesterone and causing oligomenorrhea (scant or infrequent menses).

Etiology

Cushing's syndrome is a group of clinical problems caused by an excess of cortisol, secreted by the adrenal cortex (endogenous) or administered for another clinical disorder (exogenous or iatrogenic). Table 66–6 lists causes of endogenous and exogenous secretion of cortisol. Women are affected eight times more frequently than are men.

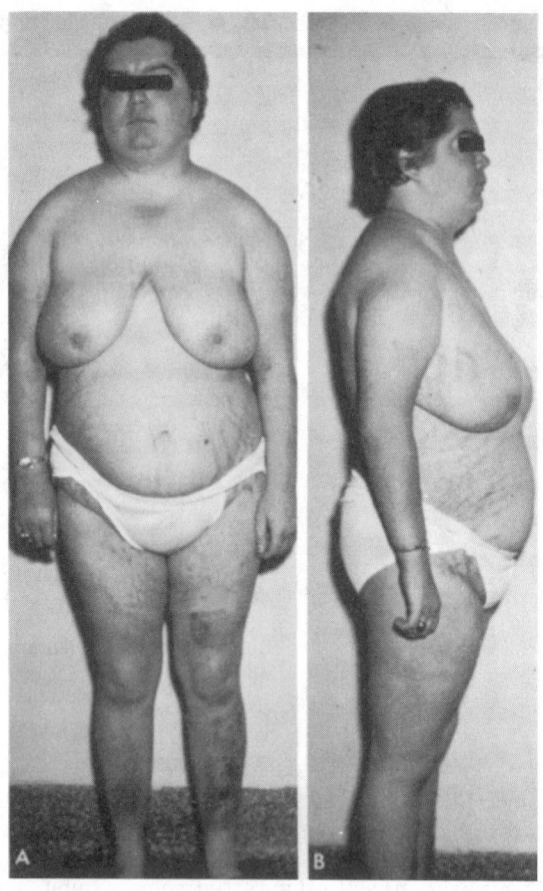

Figure 66–6. The characteristic changes in a client with adrenal hyperfunction.

➤ *Physical Assessment/Clinical Manifestations*

The client with hypercortisolism has characteristic physical changes (see Fig. 66–6). The nurse observes the general appearance of the client. Changes in fat distribution may result in a buffalo hump, truncal obesity, supraclavicular fat pads, and a round face (moon face). The nurse notes a large trunk with thin legs and arms, generalized muscle wasting, and weakness.

The nurse also inspects the client for skin changes resulting from increased blood vessel fragility, such as bruises, thin or translucent skin, and wounds that have not healed properly. Reddish-purple striae are often present on the abdomen and upper thighs because of cortisol's degradative effect on collagen.

Excessive cortisol secretion may result in a fine coating of hair over the face and body and in acne. In the female client, the nurse looks for the presence of hirsutism, clitoral hypertrophy, and male-pattern balding related to androgen excess.

Elevations in blood glucose levels are also a frequent finding. While assessing vital signs, the nurse notes elevated blood pressure, another common finding.

➤ *Psychosocial Assessment*

Because hypercortisolism can result in emotional lability, the nurse questions the client about mood swings, irritability, confusion, or depression. The client can become neurotic or psychotic as a result of changes in blood cortisol levels.

Collaborative Management

 Assessment

A thorough history and physical assessment aid in detecting clinical features of hypercortisolism, which result from glucocorticoid excess.

➤ *History*

Clients who have hypercortisolism have varied complaints because of the widespread effect of excessive cortisol levels in the body. The nurse asks the client about changes in activity or sleep patterns, fatigue, and muscle weakness. Osteoporosis is common in hypercortisolism; the nurse asks clients about bone pain or a history of fractures. The nurse also questions the client about a history of frequent infections and easy bruising, which suggest hypercortisolism. Female clients may report a cessation of menses. Gastrointestinal complaints may indicate ulcer formation from increased hydrochloric acid secretion.

The nurse also refers to the client's medical history. Steroid or alcohol abuse can produce the clinical and biochemical features of Cushing's syndrome.

TABLE 66–6

Conditions Causing Increased Cortisol Secretion	
Endogenous secretion	• Bilateral adrenal hyperplasia*
	• Pituitary adenoma increasing the production of ACTH (pituitary Cushing's syndrome)
	• Malignancies: carcinomas of the lung, gastrointestinal tract, pancreas
	• Adrenal adenomas or carcinomas
Exogenous secretion	• Therapeutic use of ACTH or glucocorticoids—most commonly for treatment of
	• Asthma
	• Autoimmune disorders
	• Organ transplantation
	• Cancer chemotherapy
	• Allergic responses
	• Chronic fibrosis

* Most common cause.

➤ *Diagnostic Assessment*

Plasma cortisol levels are elevated in clients with hypercortisolism. Blood for cortisol assays is obtained at the same time of day because levels vary throughout the day. Further diagnostic testing is performed to confirm the diagnosis of hypercortisolism because an increase in cortisol level is also seen in acute illness and trauma. Plasma ACTH levels vary, depending on the cause of hypercortisolism. In ectopic (ACTH-producing) syndromes, the ACTH level is elevated. In Cushing's syndrome (primary disease of the adrenal gland), ACTH levels are low to immeasurable. Additional laboratory findings may include

- Increased blood glucose level
- Elevated white blood cell count
- Elevated lymphocyte count
- Increased sodium level
- Decreased serum calcium level
- Decreased serum potassium level

Urine is tested to measure levels of free cortisol and the adrenal metabolites of cortisol and androgens (17-hydroxycorticosteroids and 17-ketosteroids). Clients must be reminded to save *all* their urine for 24 hours. Basal levels of urinary free cortisol, 17-ketosteroids, and 17-hydroxycorticosteroids are all elevated as are levels of urinary calcium, potassium, and glucose.

Radiographic studies, CT scans, MRI, and arteriography may identify lesions of the adrenal or pituitary glands, lung, GI tract, or pancreas in a client with clinical manifestations of cortisol hypersecretion.

The *overnight dexamethasone suppression test* is an initial screening method for Cushing's syndrome. The client is instructed not to take any medications (phenytoin [Dilantin] and phenobarbital, in particular) for at least 2 days before the test. Normally, plasma cortisol levels are lower than 5 μg/dL. If higher, further definitive testing is necessary.

For the *3-day, low-dose* dexamethasone suppression test, if possible, the client must take no medications for at least 2 days before this test, and no stressful procedures (e.g., barium enema, myelogram, or an intense physical therapy session) should be performed during the test. Table 66–5 lists drugs that interfere with testing. A baseline 24-hour urine sample is collected on day 1. Dexamethasone, 0.5 mg, is administered every 6 hours on days 2 and 3, with concomitant 24-hour urine collections. The 24-hour urine collections are tested for 17-ketosteroids, 17-hydroxycorticosteroids, creatinine, and urinary free cortisol. Normally, urinary 17-hydroxycorticosteroid excretion and free cortisol levels are suppressed by dexamethasone, and Cushing's syndrome is ruled out. If these levels are not suppressed, an additional higher-dose dexamethasone test is performed.

The *high-dose* (8-mg) dexamethasone suppression test distinguishes between bilateral adrenocortical hyperplasia (e.g., Cushing's syndrome) and adrenocortical neoplasm as a cause of hypercortisolism. This test can be performed as an overnight test or a 2-day test and is similar to the tests previously discussed but uses higher doses of dexamethasone. In the overnight high-dose test, the client with Cushing's disease will have a reduced plasma cortisol level, less than 50% of baseline. This test is more reliable than the 2-day, high-dose test.

 Interventions

Specific nursing interventions and drug therapy address the problems of clients who have hypercortisolism. Preoperative and postoperative nursing care is an integral part of the management of the client with endogenous hypercortisolism because surgical intervention is usually necessary for the relief of symptoms.

➤ *Nonsurgical Management*

The nurse weighs the client daily and monitors the client's intake and output to assess the accumulation of excessive fluid. Restriction of fluid intake is sometimes necessary to maintain fluid balance.

Drug Therapy. Most clients with endogenous hypercortisolism undergo surgery. However, drugs that interfere with ACTH production or adrenal hormone synthesis may be used for palliation. Mitotane (Lysodren) is an adrenal cytotoxic agent used for inoperable adrenal tumors. Aminoglutethimide (Elipten, Cytadren) is an adrenal enzyme inhibitor that decreases cortisol production. Trilostane (Modrastane), also an enzyme inhibitor, has not always been effective. Cyproheptadine (Periactin) is less commonly used to treat clients with adrenal hyperfunction resulting from pituitary-related Cushing's disease because it interferes with ACTH production. During all drug therapy, the nurse assesses the client for symptoms of side effects or toxicity.

Radiation Therapy. Radiation may be used to treat hypercortisolism resulting from pituitary adenomas. Radiation, applied internally (transsphenoidal implantation) or externally, is not always effective and may destroy normal tissue. The nurse notes any changes in the client's neurologic status, such as headache, elevated blood pressure or pulse, disorientation, and changes in pupil size or reaction. Clients may experience skin dryness, redness, flushing, or alopecia at the radiation site. The nurse reviews these possible side effects with the client. Chapter 47 specifically discusses radiation therapy to the head.

➤ *Surgical Management*

The surgical treatment of adrenocortical hypersecretion depends on the cause of the disease. When adrenal hyperfunction is due to increased pituitary secretion of ACTH, a transsphenoidal removal of an adenoma may be attempted. In many instances, small adenomas cannot be localized and *hypophysectomy* (surgical resection of the pituitary gland) is indicated. Hypophysectomy is performed via the transsphenoidal or transfrontal craniotomy route. See earlier in this chapter for a discussion of hypophysectomy and Chapter 47 for nursing care of clients undergoing craniotomy.

If hypercortisolism is caused by adrenal adenomas or carcinomas, an *adrenalectomy* (removal of the adrenal gland) is indicated.

Preoperative Care. Electrolyte imbalances are corrected before surgery, and the nurse monitors potassium, sodium, and chloride values. Dysrhythmias from potassium imbalance may occur; cardiac monitoring may be indicated. Hyperglycemia, if present, is controlled before surgery, and the nurse monitors blood glucose levels. Clients with hypercortisolism are susceptible to complications, such as infections and fractures, and the nurse and other assistive nursing personnel attempt to prevent infection with hand-washing and aseptic technique. The risk for falls is decreased by raising the side rails of the bed and encouraging the client to ask for assistance when getting out of bed. The physician orders a high-calorie, high-protein diet before surgery.

The nurse administers a glucocorticoid preparation as ordered. The client continues to receive glucocorticoids throughout the operative procedure to prevent adrenal crisis. The removal of the tumor results in a sudden drop in cortisol levels. The nurse discusses postoperative care and long-term medication therapy during preoperative teaching.

Operative Procedure. A unilateral adrenalectomy is performed when one gland is involved. A bilateral adrenalectomy is necessary when ectopic ACTH-producing tumors cannot be treated by other means or when both adrenal glands are diseased.

Surgery can be transabdominal or through the lateral flank. Transabdominal surgery causes a higher degree of illness, accompanied by all the risks inherent in abdominal surgery. In the flank approach—the preferred approach—the abdominal cavity is not entered, and the morbidity and mortality rates are reduced. A new approach, laparoscopic adrenalectomy, may reduce the incidence of some postoperative complications (see the accompanying Research Applications for Nursing feature).

Postoperative Care. After an adrenalectomy, the client is usually sent to a critical care unit. In the immediate postoperative period, the nurse assesses the client frequently to identify symptoms of cardiovascular collapse or shock due to possible insufficient glucocorticoid replacement, such as hypotension, a rapid, weak pulse, and a decreasing urinary output. The nurse monitors ongoing vital signs and other hemodynamic variables (central venous pressure, pulmonary wedge pressure), intake and output, daily weights, and serum electrolyte levels.

After a bilateral adrenalectomy, clients require lifelong glucocorticoid and mineralocorticoid replacement. The nurse administers glucocorticoid preparations as ordered. In unilateral adrenalectomy, glucocorticoid replacement continues for up to 2 years after surgery until the remaining gland regains function.

➤ Preventing Complications

Clients who have hypercortisolism are prone to injury from skin breakdown, pathologic bone fractures, and gastrointestinal bleeding. Prevention of such injuries is a major nursing care focus.

Skin Breakdown. The nurse assesses the client's skin to detect reddened areas, excoriation, breakdown, and

➤ Research Applications for Nursing

Laparoscopic Adrenalectomy May Reduce Postoperative Complications

Brunt, L. M., Doherty, G. M., Norton, J. A., Soper, N. J., Quasebarth, M. A., & Moley, J. F. (1996). Laparoscopic adrenalectomy compared to open adrenalectomy for benign adrenal neoplasms. Journal of the American College of Surgeons, 183(1), 71–77.

This retrospective descriptive study compared the outcomes of clients who had either laparoscopic or open adrenalectomy. The researchers reviewed the charts of 66 consecutive clients with benign adrenal neoplasms who underwent adrenalectomy from 1988 to 1995. The sample consisted of 3 groups of subjects: Group I (n = 25) had an open anterior transabdominal surgical approach, group II (n = 17) had an open posterior retroperitoneal surgical approach, and Group III (n = 24) had a laparoscopic transabdominal flank approach. The subjects who underwent laparoscopic adrenalectomy had significantly less blood loss, needed less postoperative pain medication, and resumed eating sooner. The length of stay was also significantly shorter in this group, with less total hospital charges. The subjects who underwent laparoscopic surgery were able to return to work an average of 6 days before those in the other two groups.

Critique. Although the group who underwent the laparoscopic surgery had a shorter length of stay and needed less pain medication postoperatively, there was no mention of other variables that might account for this difference. Some of these variables might include the clients' general health preoperatively and level of physical fitness. Another possible explanation for group III's ability to return to work an average of 6 days earlier might be these clients' occupations.

Possible Nursing Implications. Laparoscopic surgical procedures are increasingly common, and the length of stay of these clients will be less than those in whom the traditional surgical approach is used. As medicine uses this technique for more serious conditions, the nurse will be challenged to include all the education about medications and activities that the client requires in a much shorter period of time. More emphasis will be placed on education in the home and home care follow-up.

edema. If mobility is decreased, the nurse turns the client frequently and pads bony prominences to prevent skin breakdown.

The nurse instructs the client to avoid activities that can result in skin trauma. To minimize tissue injury, the client may use a soft toothbrush and electric razor. Proper hygiene is important, and clients are instructed to keep the skin clean and to dry it thoroughly after washing. The client can prevent excessive dryness by using a moisturizing lotion.

Adhesive tape frequently causes breakdown of the client's skin. The client should use tape sparingly and should exercise extreme caution when removing it. After venipuncture or arterial puncture, clients may experience an increase in bleeding because of blood vessel fragility. The nurse may need to exert pressure over the site for longer than normal to prevent excessive bleeding and ecchymosis (bruising).

Pathologic Fractures. Hypercortisolism results in demineralization of bone, which, if it persists, may lead to osteoporosis. The nurse instructs the client about safety issues and dietary needs. Clients with osteoporosis are susceptible to fractures as a result of accidental falls or bumps. The nurse instructs the client to call for assistance when ambulating. The nurse also reviews the use of ambulatory aids (walkers or canes), if needed, with the client. Rooms should be kept free from extraneous objects that might cause a fall. When assisting with daily activities, the nurse prevents the client from bumping into hard objects.

The nurse enlists a dietitian to counsel the client about diet therapy. A high-calorie diet is ordered, including items from all the major food groups and increased amounts of calcium and vitamin D. Generous amounts of milk, cheese, yogurt, and green leafy and root vegetables add considerable amounts of calcium to the diet. The nurse advises the client to avoid substances containing caffeine and alcohol.

Gastrointestinal Bleeding. Interventions are aimed at minimizing gastric irritation, usually through drug therapy. Drug therapy involves two different types of agents, those that protect the GI mucosa and those that decrease the secretion of hydrochloric acid.

Agents Protecting the GI Mucosa. Antacids are prescribed to buffer stomach acids and to protect the GI mucosa. The nurse teaches the client that these drugs should be taken on a regular schedule, not PRN.

Agents Inhibiting the Secretion of Hydrochloric Acid. The most effective agents are those that block the H_2 receptor site in the gastric mucosa. When histamine binds to this receptor site, a series of membrane actions occur that result in the release of hydrochloric acid. Drugs that block the H_2 receptor site include cimetidine (Tagamet, Peptol, Novocimetine✚), ranitidine (Zantac, Apo-Ranitidine✚), famotidine (Pepcid), and nizatidine (Axid). Omeprazole (Losec✚, Prilosec) inhibits the gastric proton pump and prevents the formation of hydrochloric acid.

Prevention of Irritation. Clients are encouraged to reduce or eliminate habits that contribute to gastric irritation, such as consuming alcohol or caffeine, smoking, and fasting. The nurse discusses with the client other prescribed and over-the-counter medications the client may be taking. Nonsteroidal anti-inflammatory drugs and drugs that contain aspirin or other salicylates can cause gastritis and intensify any bleeding episode.

➤ Health Teaching

After bilateral adrenalectomy, the client depends on lifelong exogenous adrenal hormone replacement. The nurse educates the client and family members about compliance with the medication regimen and its side effects. Wearing a medical alert bracelet is essential. Education of clients

---

> **Chart 66–7**
>
> ## Education Guide: Cortisol Replacement Therapy
>
> - Take your medication in divided doses, the first dose in the morning and the second dose between 4 and 6 PM.
> - Take your medication with meals or snacks.
> - Weigh yourself daily.
> - Increase your dosage as directed for increased physical stress or severe emotional stress, including surgery, dental work, influenza, fever, pregnancy, and family problems.
> - Never skip a dose of medication. If you have persistent vomiting or severe diarrhea and cannot take your medication by mouth for 24–36 hr, call your physician. If you cannot reach your physician, go to the nearest emergency room. You may need an injection to take the place of your usual oral medication.
> - Always wear your medical alert (Medic-Alert) bracelet or necklace.
> - Make regular visits for health care follow-up.
> - Learn how to give yourself an intramuscular injection of hydrocortisone.

---

after bilateral adrenalectomy and hypophysectomy is the same as that for clients undergoing cortisol replacement (see Chart 66–7).

Hyperaldosteronism
Overview

In clients with hyperaldosteronism, increased secretion of aldosterone results in mineralocorticoid excess. *Primary* hyperaldosteronism (Conn's syndrome) is due to excessive secretion of aldosterone from one or both adrenal glands, most commonly caused by an adenoma. In a person with *secondary* hyperaldosteronism, the continuous excessive secretion of aldosterone results from higher levels of angiotensin II because of high plasma renin activity. The principal causes of this renin activation are renal hypoxemia and thiazide diuretics.

Increased aldosterone levels primarily affect the renal tubular epithelial cells and cause sodium retention with potassium and hydrogen ion excretion from the extracellular fluid. Hypernatremia, hypokalemia, and metabolic alkalosis result. Sodium retention increases extracellular fluid volume, which elevates blood pressure and suppresses renin production. The elevated blood pressure may cause cerebrovascular accidents and renal damage. Peripheral edema occurs rarely because of the "renal escape mechanism," in which the proximal tubule decreases sodium reabsorption. However, no compensatory mechanism exists to stop or reverse the loss of potassium. (See Chapter 16 for further discussion of electrolyte imbalances.)

Hyperaldosteronism occurs three times more frequently

in women than in men and is most prevalent in clients between 30 and 60 years of age.

Assessment

Symptoms related to hypokalemia and elevated blood pressure are the most common presenting complaints of clients who have hyperaldosteronism. The history may reveal a variety of nonspecific findings, such as headache, fatigue, muscle weakness, nocturia, and loss of stamina. Polydipsia and polyuria occur less frequently. Paresthesias may occur if potassium depletion is severe. Clients may note visual changes related to hypertension.

The diagnosis of primary hyperaldosteronism is made on the basis of laboratory studies and radiographic findings. Serum potassium levels are decreased, and sodium levels are elevated. Plasma renin levels are low; aldosterone levels are elevated. Increased hydrogen ion secretion results in metabolic alkalemia (elevated blood pH). Urine studies demonstrate low specific gravity and elevated aldosterone levels. Computed tomography scans reveal the presence and location of adrenal adenomas.

Interventions

Surgery is the treatment of choice for hyperaldosteronism if identified in its early stages. Adrenalectomy may be unilateral or bilateral. Surgery is not performed, however, until the client's potassium levels are normal. The physician orders spironolactone (Aldactone A, Sincomen✦), a potassium-sparing diuretic and aldosterone antagonist, to promote fluid balance. Potassium supplements may be ordered to increase potassium levels before surgery. Clients may also benefit from a low-sodium preoperative diet, but no dietary restrictions are needed after surgery because aldosterone levels should return to normal.

Clients undergoing unilateral adrenalectomy may require temporary glucocorticoid replacement, and clients undergoing bilateral adrenalectomy need lifelong replacement. Glucocorticoids are administered before surgery to prevent adrenal hypofunction. Clients receiving long-term replacement therapy should wear a medical alert band. (See the discussion of adrenalectomy in the section on Hypercortisolism [Cushing's syndrome] for further postoperative care and client education.)

When surgery is inadvisable, spironolactone therapy is continued to control the symptoms of hypokalemia and hypertension. Because spironolactone is a potassium-sparing diuretic, hyperkalemia can occur in clients who have impaired renal function or excessive potassium intake. The nurse advises the client to avoid potassium supplements and foods rich in potassium. Because hyponatremia can occur with spironolactone therapy, clients may require increased dietary sodium. The nurse instructs clients to note symptoms of hyponatremia, such as dryness of the mouth, thirst, lethargy, or drowsiness, and advises clients to avoid other potassium-sparing diuretics. The nurse alerts clients to report any additional side effects of spironolactone therapy, which include gynecomastia, diarrhea, drowsiness, headache, rash, urticaria (hives), confusion, inability to maintain an erection, hirsutism, and amenorrhea.

Pheochromocytoma

Overview

Pheochromocytoma is a catecholamine-producing tumor that arises in chromaffin cells. Pheochromocytomas usually occur as single, unilateral lesions on the right side; approximately 10% are bilateral lesions, and another 10% are found in the abdomen. Pheochromocytomas are most often benign, but approximately 10% are malignant. The tumors produce and store catecholamines much like normal medullary tissue, but little is known about how these stored hormones are released excessively.

Pheochromocytomas synthesize the catecholamines epinephrine and norepinephrine (NE). Excessive epinephrine and NE stimulate alpha-receptors and beta-receptors and can have wide-ranging adverse effects mimicking stimulation of the sympathetic division of the autonomic nervous system.

Causes are unknown, but some are associated with inherited disorders, such as neurofibromatosis and multiple endocrine neoplasia type II syndrome. Pheochromocytomas are seen in 0.1% of the hypertensive population and are slightly more common in women. Pheochromocytomas can occur at any age but appear most commonly in clients between 40 and 60 years old.

Collaborative Management

Assessment

The history may reveal paroxysmal hypertensive episodes or attacks that vary in length from a few minutes to several hours. During these episodes, clients experience severe headaches, palpitations, profuse diaphoresis, flushing, apprehension, or a feeling of impending doom. Pain in the chest or abdomen, with nausea and vomiting, can also occur. Certain stimuli, such as increased abdominal pressure, micturition, and vigorous abdominal palpation, can provoke a hypertensive crisis. Clients may also report heat intolerance, weight loss, and tremors.

Diagnostic tests include 24-hour urine collections for vanillylmandelic acid (VMA) (a product of catecholamine metabolism), metanephrine, and free catecholamines, all of which are elevated in pheochromocytoma. The nursing care associated with the VMA test is covered in Chart 66–8. Basal plasma catecholamine levels are elevated after the client has been at rest for at least 30 minutes. The clonidine suppression test involves oral administration of clonidine hydrochloride (Catapres, Dixarit✦), which blocks sympathetic nervous system activity. The drug does not suppress plasma catecholamine levels in clients

---

Chart 66–8

Nursing Care Highlight: The Client Having a Vanillylmandelic Acid (VMA) Test

- Describe the test to the client and explain that his or her participation is needed for accurate test results.
- Instruct the client on the special VMA-restricted diet that starts 2 or 3 days before the 24-hr urine collection.
- Restricted foods include those containing caffeine (coffee, tea, cola, and chocolate or cocoa), certain fruits (citrus fruits and bananas), vanilla-containing foods, and licorice. Check your laboratory for a more inclusive food list.
- Confer with the physician about which medications should not be given during the 3- or 4-day test. Medications usually withheld include aspirin and antihypertensive agents.
- Be aware that strenuous physical activity, stress, and starvation can increase VMA levels; monitor, intervene, and teach the client as appropriate.
- Instruct the client about how to collect an accurate 24-hr urine sample: the collection is started with an empty bladder, and then all urine formed over the next 24 hr is collected in one container. At the end of the 24-hr period, the client voids and adds that urine to the collection.
- Obtain a urine collection container with preservative from the laboratory. Check with the laboratory about keeping the collection on ice.
- When the collection is complete, send the urine to the laboratory promptly.
- Help the client understand the test results; normal VMA excretion in 24 hr is 2–7 mg, or 10–35 μmol.

---

who have pheochromocytoma. Catecholamine stimulation of glycogenolysis and suppression of insulin may cause hyperglycemia and glycosuria, revealed by blood and urine studies.

After the diagnosis is established, CT scans of the adrenal glands locates intra-adrenal tumors. Chest x-rays and tomograms can locate lesions of the thoracic area; arteriograms can locate intra-abdominal tumors.

 Interventions

Surgery is the treatment of choice for pheochromocytoma. One or both adrenal glands are removed (if tumor is bilateral). Preoperatively, the nurse focuses on adequate tissue perfusion, nutritional needs, and comfort measures.

Hypertension is the hallmark of the disease. The nurse monitors the client's blood pressure regularly and places the cuff consistently on the same arm, with the client in lying and standing positions. The nurse also identifies stressors that may precede a hypertensive crisis and attempts to minimize them. The nurse instructs the client

not to smoke, drink caffeine-containing beverages, or change position suddenly. The client's abdomen *should not be palpated*. A diet rich in calories, vitamins, and minerals is provided.

Clients often benefit from preoperative hydration therapy because inadequate extracellular fluid volume increases the risk of intraoperative and postoperative hypotension. The nurse assesses the client's hydration status and notes symptoms of dehydration or fluid overload.

Because clients with pheochromocytoma can experience incapacitating headaches, the nurse provides a calm, restful environment. The nurse instructs the client to limit activity. A private, darkened room helps to promote rest. If the client is sleeping, interruptions are avoided if possible.

The physician stabilizes the client with alpha-adrenergic blocking agents before surgery because the client is at increased risk for hypertension during surgery. Anesthetic agents and manipulation of the tumor during surgery can produce a release of catecholamines. The physician orders the short-acting alpha-adrenergic blocker phentolamine (Regitine, Rogitine✦) via IV bolus or drip for a hypertensive crisis. Oral phenoxybenzamine hydrochloride (Dibenzyline) produces long-acting alpha-adrenergic blockade and is most suitable for preoperative management of hypertension and prevention of hypertensive crisis. It is also a drug of choice for long-term management of the client who is not a candidate for surgery.

The physician adjusts drug dosages for 2–3 weeks until blood pressure is controlled and no further hypertensive attacks occur. The contracted plasma expands, and blood pressure with the client in the supine position returns to normal. The alpha-blocker prazosin hydrochloride (Minipress) is used less frequently for the preoperative client because of its shorter duration of action.

The physician never uses beta-receptor blocking agents in clients with suspected or confirmed pheochromocytoma until after alpha-adrenergic blockade has been initiated because these drugs may cause blood pressure to rise. After alpha-adrenergic blockade, low doses of propranolol hydrochloride (Inderal, Detensol✦) may be used to treat tachycardia and dysrhythmias.

Postoperative nursing care is similar to that for the client undergoing adrenalectomy (see Hypercortisolism [Cushing's Syndrome]). The nurse closely monitors the client for hypotension related to the sudden decrease in catecholamine level and hypovolemia, especially the client who is inadequately prepared for surgery. Hemorrhage and shock are possible, and the nurse administers plasma expanders and fluids as prescribed. The nurse monitors the client's vital signs frequently and carefully records fluid intake and output. If opioids are administered, the nurse observes their effect on blood pressure.

Infrequently, tumors may be inoperable because of disseminated malignancy or concurrent illness. Treatment in these cases is medical, with alpha-adrenergic and beta-adrenergic blocking agents, because these tumors do not respond well to chemotherapy or radiation therapy. For clients who are medically managed, self-measurement of blood pressure with home monitoring equipment is essential.

Case Study for the Client with Acromegaly and Hypophysectomy

■ A 56-year-old man with acromegaly is scheduled to have a transsphenoidal hypophysectomy. He has reported an increase in his hat, glove, and shoe size. He also discloses that he has had a problem with impotence. He is hypertensive and has hepatomegaly.

QUESTIONS:

1. What information should you give this client before surgery?
2. During the postoperative period, what should you assess?
3. What are the possible complications of this surgery that you should be alert to?
4. What teaching should you give to this client before he goes home?
5. What expected outcomes are specific to this situation?

SELECTED BIBLIOGRAPHY

Batcheller, J. (1994). Syndrome of inappropriate antidiuretic hormone secretion. *Critical Care Nursing Clinics of North America,* 6(4), 687–691.

Baxter, M. A. (1994). Acromegaly and transsphenoidal hypophysectomy: A case report. *AANA Journal,* 62(2), 182–185.

Bell, T. N. (1994). Diabetes insipidus. *Critical Care Nursing Clinics of North America,* 6(4), 675–685.

Braunstein, G. (1994). Testes. In F. S. Greenspan & J. D. Baxter, *Basic & clinical endocrinology* (4th ed.) Norwalk, CN: Appleton & Lange.

Brunt, L. M., Doherty, G. M., Norton, J. A., Soper, N. J., Quasebarth, M. A., & Moley, J. F. (1996). Laparoscopic adrenalectomy compared to open adrenalectomy for benign adrenal neoplasms. *Journal of the American College of Surgeons,* 183(1), 1–10.

Bryce, J. (1994). Action stat! S.I.A.D.H. *Nursing 94,* 24(4), 33.

Celen, O., O'Brien, M. J., Melby, J. C., & Beazley, R. M. (1996). Factors influencing outcome of surgery for primary aldosteronism. *Archives of Surgery,* 131(6), 646–650.

Davis-Martin, S. (1996). Pearls for practice: Disorders of the adrenal glands. *Journal of the American Academy of Nurse Practitioners,* 8(7), 323–326.

Foo, M., Burton, B. J., & Ahmed, R. (1995). Phaeochromocytoma. *British Journal of Hospital Medicine,* 54(7), 318–321.

Frohman, L. A. (1996). Acromegaly: what constitutes optimal therapy? *Journal of Clinical Endocrinology and Metabolism,* 81(2), 443–445.

Greenspan, F. S., & Baxter, J. D. (1994). *Basic & clinical endocrinology* (4th ed.). Norwalk, CT: Appleton & Lange.

Gumowski, J., & Loughran, M. (1996). Diseases of the adrenal gland. *Nursing Clinics of North America,* 31(4), 747–767.

Heron, E., Chantellier, G., Gillaud, E., Foos, E., & Plouin, P. (1996). The urinary metanephrine-to-creatinine ratio for the diagnosis of pheochromocytoma. *Annals of Internal Medicine,* 125(4), 300–303.

Kelley, W. (Ed.) (1997). *Textbook of internal medicine* (3rd ed). Philadelphia: Lippincott-Raven.

Litchfield, W. R., & Dluhy, R. G. (1995). Primary aldosteronism. *Endocrinology and Metabolism Clinics of North America,* 24(3), 593–612.

Lopez, E., Piedrola, G., & Villalon, L. (1995). Bilateral adrenal masses. *Postgraduate Medical Journal,* 71(839), 567–568.

McEwen, D. (1995). Transsphenoidal adenomectomy. *AORN Journal,* 61(2), 321–326.

Melmed, L., Ho, K., Klibanski, A., Reichlin, S., & Thorner, M. (1995). Clinical review 75: Recent advances in pathogenesis, diagnosis, and management of acromegaly. *Journal of Clinical Endocrinology and Metabolism,* 80(12), 3395–3402.

O'Donnell, M. (1997). Addisonian crisis. *American Journal of Nursing,* 97(3), 41.

Roberts, A. (1995). Growth hormone and prolactin. *Nursing Times,* 91(28), 33–35.

Romeo, J. (1996). Hyperfunction and hypofunction in the anterior pituitary. *Nursing Clinics of North America,* 31(4), 769–777.

Rusterholtz, A. (1996). Interpretation of diagnostic laboratory tests in selected endocrine disorders. *Nursing Clinics of North America,* 31(4), 715–724.

Sassolas, G. (1995). Medical therapy with somatostatin analogues for acromegaly. *European Journal of Endocrinology,* 133(6), 686–690.

Stewart, P. M., Kane, K. F., Stewart, S. E., Lancranjan, I., & Sheppard, M. C. (1995). Depot long-acting somatostatin analog (Sandostatin-LAR) is an effective treatment for acromegaly. *Journal of Clinical Endocrinology and Metabolism,* 80(11), 3267–3272.

Tormey, W. P. (1995). Phaeochromocytoma diagnosis [letter]. *Annals of Clinical Biochemistry,* 32(6), 595–597.

SUGGESTED READINGS

Batcheller, J. (1994). Syndrome of inappropriate antidiuretic hormone secretion. *Critical Care Nursing Clinics of North America,* 6(4), 687–691.

This article describes the pathophysiology of SIADH. A large portion explores the many causes of SIADH and its clinical manifestations, including the fact that many of the drugs causing SIADH are commonly taken agents, such as nicotine and diuretics. Diagnosis is made by the simultaneous occurrence of plasma hyponatremia and hypo-osmolality with very dilute urine.

Bell, T. N. (1994). Diabetes insipidus. *Critical Care Nursing Clinics of North America,* 6(4), 675–685.

This article discusses in depth the physiologic regulation of water balance, particularly as influenced by ADH. The pathophysiology of central diabetes insipidus as well as nephrogenic causes are detailed. After presenting the clinical manifestations and the treatment of diabetes insipidus, a case study is presented that illustrates the material in the article.

Davis-Martin, S. (1996). Pearls for practice: Disorders of the adrenal glands. *Journal of the American Academy of Nurse Practitioners,* 8(7), 323–326.

This article begins with a case study and then presents the basic anatomy and physiology of the adrenal glands. Pathologies for adrenocortical hypofunction and hyperfunction are discussed. Disorders of the adrenal medulla and disorders of aldosterone secretion are also covered, with implications for practice.

Chapter 67

INTERVENTIONS FOR CLIENTS WITH PROBLEMS OF THE THYROID AND PARATHYROID GLANDS

Clients with thyroid and parathyroid gland disturbances have symptoms that reflect the widespread effects that hormones from these glands have on many body systems. The symptoms may be very subtle or can progress to life-threatening emergencies. The nurse can be instrumental in preventing such complications.

THYROID DISORDERS
Hyperthyroidism

Overview

Excessive thyroid hormone secretion results in hyperthyroidism. *Thyrotoxicosis* refers to the signs and symptoms that appear when body tissues are stimulated by increased thyroid hormones. Thyroid hormones affect virtually all metabolic processes in all body organs and will, therefore, produce numerous and varied clinical manifestations. Hyperthyroidism can be transient or permanent depending on the cause.

Pathophysiology

In a person with hyperthyroidism, the normal regulatory controls of thyroid hormone secretion fail. Because thyroid hormones stimulate most body systems, excessive thyroid hormones produce a state of hypermetabolism, with increased sympathetic nervous system activity. Many of the clinical manifestations of hyperthyroidism (Chart 67–1) are caused by the body's attempt to respond to the demands of hypermetabolism.

Excessive amounts of thyroid hormones directly stimulate the heart. The increased heart rate and stroke volume cause an increase in cardiac output and peripheral blood flow, a hyperdynamic circulatory state that results from an increase in adrenergic responsiveness. Beta-adrenergic receptor sites in the heart increase in response to thyroid hormones.

Elevated levels of thyroid hormones profoundly affect protein, carbohydrate, and lipid metabolism. Protein synthesis (build-up) and degradation (breakdown) are increased, but degradation exceeds synthesis, resulting in a negative nitrogen balance. Glucose tolerance may be slightly to markedly decreased. Mobilization, synthesis, and breakdown of triglycerides are increased, with a net effect of lipid depletion. A state of chronic nutritional and caloric deficiency also results.

The secretion and metabolism of hypothalamic, pituitary, and gonadal steroids are altered. If hyperthyroidism

---

Chart 67–1

Key Features of Hyperthyroidism

Integumentary Manifestations
- Diaphoresis
- Fine, soft, silky hair
- Smooth, moist skin

Pulmonary Manifestations
- Dyspnea with or without exertion

Cardiovascular Manifestations
- Palpitations
- Chest pain
- Increased systolic blood pressure
- Widened pulse pressure
- Tachycardia
- Dysrhythmias

Gastrointestinal Manifestations
- Weight loss
- Increased appetite
- Diarrhea

Musculoskeletal Manifestations
- Proximal muscle weakness

Neurologic Manifestations
- Blurred or double vision
- Eye fatigue
- Insomnia
- Corneal ulcers or infections
- Increased tears
- Injected (red) conjunctiva
- Photophobia
- Eyelid retraction, eyelid lag
- Globe lag
- Hyperactive deep tendon reflexes
- Tremors

Metabolic Manifestations
- Increased basal metabolic rate
- Heat intolerance
- Low-grade fever

Psychological/Emotional Manifestations
- Decreased attention span
- Restlessness
- Irritability
- Emotional lability
- Manic behavior

Reproductive Manifestations
- Amenorrhea
- Decreased menstrual flow
- Increased libido

Other Manifestations
- Goiter
- Wide-eyed (startled) appearance
- Weakness, fatigue

---

is present before the onset of puberty, sexual development is delayed in both males and females. If hyperthyroidism develops after puberty, females experience menstrual irregularities and decreased fertility. Both males and females experience increased libido.

Etiology

The causes of hyperthyroidism are numerous (Table 67–1). The most common cause is *Graves' disease* (toxic diffuse goiter). However, not all clients with a goiter have hyperthyroidism. Some goiters result in hypothyroidism. Graves' disease is characterized by hyperthyroidism, goiter (enlargement of the thyroid gland), exophthalmos (abnormal protrusion of the eyes), and pretibial myxedema.

Graves' disease is thought to be an autoimmune disorder. Immunoglobulins, or antibodies, known as thyroid-stimulating immunoglobulins (TSIs) bind to the thyroid gland, causing it to enlarge and oversecrete thyroid hormone. In addition to the expected cellular hyper-

---

TABLE 67–1

Causes of Hyperthyroidism

Cause	Mechanism
Graves' disease (toxic diffuse goiter)	• Probably autoimmune in nature. Immunoglobulins cause stimulation of the thyroid gland.
Toxic multinodular goiter	• Multiple thyroid nodules, resulting in thyroid hyperfunction.
Thyroid adenoma	• Autonomous functioning of adenoma of follicular cells.
Pituitary hyperthyroidism	• Pituitary adenoma resulting in excessive TSH secretion.
Thyroiditis (radiation-induced)	• T_3 and T_4 secretion increased before destruction of gland. Hyperthyroid state usually transient.
T_3 thyrotoxicosis	• Increase in thyroid secretion of T_3. Cause unknown.
Factitious hyperthyroidism	• Ingestion of excessive amounts of thyroid hormone.
Jodbasedow (iodine induced)	• Administration of iodine to an individual with endemic goiter (see p. 1622), resulting in excessive production of thyroid hormone.
Struma ovarii	• Dermoid tumor of the ovary that secretes thyroid hormone.
Thyroid carcinoma	• Uncommon, usually occurs with large follicular carcinomas.
Trophoblastic tumors	• Choriocarcinoma, hydatidiform mole, and embryonal carcinoma with high concentrations of chorionic gonadotropins that stimulate T_3 and T_4 secretion.

T_3 = triiodothyronine; T_4 = thyroxine; TSH = thyroid-stimulating hormone.

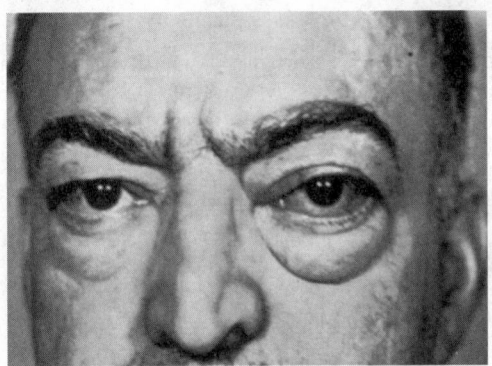

Figure 67–1. Ophthalmopathy. The client has proptosis.

metabolism, exophthalmos and pretibial myxedema are associated with Graves' disease. Pretibial myxedema is characterized by a dry, waxy swelling on the anterior surface of the lower legs. TSI activity is present in 80% of clients with Graves' disease.

Hyperthyroidism caused by multiple thyroid nodules is termed *toxic multinodular goiter*. Affected people usually have had nontoxic multinodular goiter for years. The overproduction of thyroid hormone is usually milder than that seen in Graves' disease and is not associated with exophthalmos or pretibial edema.

Additionally, hyperthyroidism can be caused by over-medication with thyroid hormone (exogenous). Thyroid hormone has been abused by people seeking to control weight or to increase their energy levels.

When hyperthyroidism is untreated or inadequately treated or when the client is severely stressed, a condition called *thyroid storm* or *thyroid crisis* can occur. This condition is an extreme state of hyperthyroidism in which all clinical manifestations are more severe and life threatening. Even when treated, thyroid storm has a 20% to 25% mortality rate.

Incidence/Prevalence

Graves' disease can occur at any age, but the peak incidence is between 20 and 40 years of age, primarily in women. The true incidence is unknown. Toxic multinodular goiter usually occurs after the age of 50 and affects women four times more frequently than men. Overall, hyperthyroidism is a common endocrine disorder.

Collaborative Management

 Assessment

➤ History

The client's history provides essential information to detect hyperthyroidism. Because hyperthyroidism can affect numerous body systems, the client usually has a wide array of subjective complaints.

The nurse documents the client's age, gender, and usual weight. The client may report recent weight loss and increased appetite. The client may report diarrhea

when the nurse asks about any noticeable change in the frequency or consistency of bowel movements.

A hallmark of hyperthyroidism is heat intolerance. The nurse determines whether the client has experienced diaphoresis or has been wearing lighter clothing in cold weather. As a result of the cardiovascular effects of hyperthyroidism, the client may also report palpitations or chest pain. The nurse asks about changes in breathing patterns, because dyspnea, with or without exertion, is common.

Visual difficulties in the hyperthyroid client result from ophthalmopathy (Fig. 67–1). The nurse asks about changes in vision, such as blurring or double vision and tiring of the eyes.

The nurse inquires whether the client has noticed a change in his or her ability to perform activities of daily living (ADLs). Complaints of fatigue, weakness, and insomnia are recorded. Family and friends may report that the client has become more irritable or depressed.

The nurse asks women about changes in menses, because amenorrhea or a decreased menstrual flow is common. Initially, both men and women may experience an increase in libido.

The nurse explores the client's medical history. A history of thyroid surgery or radiation therapy to the neck can be significant, because some people remain hyperthyroid after surgery or are resistant to radiation therapy. The nurse asks about past or current medications, noting the use of thyroid hormone replacement or antithyroid drugs.

➤ *Physical Assessment/Clinical Manifestations*

The nurse notes the client's general appearance. Two types of ophthalmopathy are common in people with hyperthyroidism: eyelid retraction (eyelid lag) and globe (eyeball) lag. Eyelid lag occurs in all forms of thyrotoxicosis. The upper eyelid fails to descend promptly and steadily when the client gazes slowly downward. In globe lag, the upper eyelid pulls back faster than the eyeball when the client gazes upward. The nurse asks the client to look down and then up and observes the response.

Infiltrative ophthalmopathy, leading to exophthalmos (Fig. 67–2), is common in the client with Graves' disease. The wide-eyed, or "startled" look is due to edema in the extraocular muscles and increased retro-orbital fat,

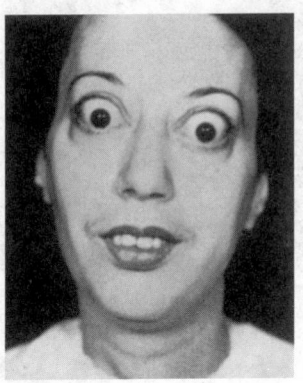

Figure 67–2. Exophthalmos.

which pushes the globe forward. Pressure on the optic nerve may impair vision. Swelling and shortening of the muscles may cause problems with focusing. If the eyelid fails to close completely and the eye is unprotected, corneal ulcerations and infections can result. The nurse observes the client's eyes for excessive tearing and a bloodshot appearance and asks about sensitivity to light (photophobia).

The nurse palpates the thyroid gland to determine the presence of a mass or general enlargement, observing the size and symmetry of the gland. In goiter (Fig. 67–3), a generalized thyroid enlargement in people with Graves' disease, the thyroid gland may increase to four times its normal size. *Bruits* (turbulence from increased blood flow) may be heard with a stethoscope. (See Chapter 65 for full discussion of thyroid palpation and auscultation.)

The nurse inspects the client's hair and skin. Fine, soft, silky hair and smooth, moist skin are common in people with hyperthyroidism. Clients may experience extremity muscle weakness, hyperactive deep tendon reflexes, or tremors. The nurse observes the client's gross motor movements, checks reflexes, and notes any fine hand tremors. The client may appear extremely restless, irritable, and fatigued.

➤ *Psychosocial Assessment*

Clients with hyperthyroidism frequently experience emotional lability (instability), irritability, decreased attention span, and manic behavior. Moods fluctuate, resulting in a chaotic emotional condition. Mild to severe hyperactivity often leads to a state of fatigue because of the inability to sleep well. The nurse asks the client whether he or she has been crying or laughing inappropriately or has had difficulty concentrating. The nurse must include family or significant others when identifying these problems. Often, the client's family members report these changes in mental or emotional status.

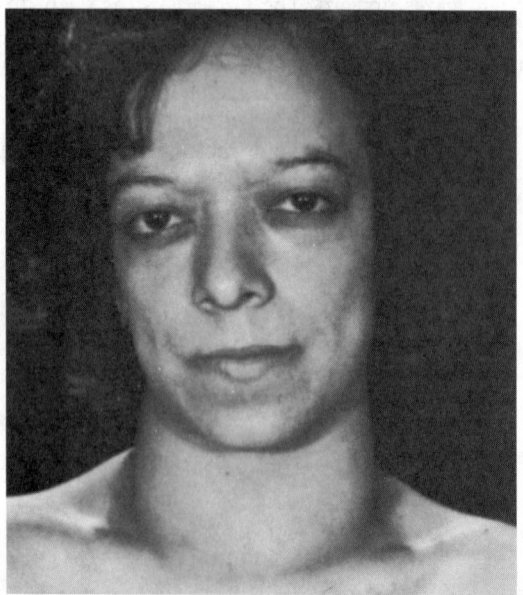

Figure 67–3. Goiter.

➤ *Laboratory Assessment*

The diagnostic work-up for hyperthyroidism includes measurement of the following serum values: triiodothyronine (T_3), thyroxine (T_4), T_3 resin uptake (T_3RU), and thyroid-stimulating hormone (TSH). Further evaluation may include the thyrotropin-releasing hormone (TRH) stimulation test and the thyroid suppression test. Laboratory findings in clients with hyperthyroidism are summarized in Chart 67–2.

➤ *Other Diagnostic Assessment*

Thyroid Scan. The thyroid scan evaluates the position, size, and functioning of the thyroid gland. Radioactive iodine (RAI, ^{123}I) is given by mouth, and the uptake of iodine by the thyroid gland (RAIU) is measured. Normally, the thyroid has an uptake of 5% to 35% of the administered dose when measured at 24 hours. In the hyperthyroid client, the RAIU is increased. RAI not used by the thyroid is excreted by the kidney. The half-life of ^{123}I is short, and no radiation precautions are necessary. However, pregnancy should be ruled out before the scan is done.

The nurse assesses whether the client has had procedures or medication that might affect the results of the scan. Any procedure, such as an intravenous pyelogram (IVP), that uses contrast material containing iodine should not be done for at least 4 weeks before a thyroid scan. The administration of any medication containing iodine should be discontinued for 1 week before the scan.

Ultrasonography. Ultrasonography of the thyroid gland can determine size of the thyroid gland and evaluate masses or nodules. The nurse reassures the client that this procedure is painless; it takes approximately 30 minutes to perform.

Electrocardiography. An electrocardiogram (ECG) may show tachycardia, atrial fibrillation, and alterations in P and T waveforms.

 Interventions

Because Graves' disease is the most common form of hyperthyroidism, the following interventions include those for infiltrative ophthalmopathy as well as for all types of hyperthyroidism.

➤ *Hyperthyroidism*

Because clients with hyperthyroidism can have increased systolic blood pressure, a widened pulse pressure, tachycardia, and other dysrhythmias, the goals of nonsurgical management are to decrease the effect of thyroid hormone on peripheral tissues and to reduce thyroid hormone secretion. Surgery may be necessary when nonsurgical interventions are unsuccessful.

Nonsurgical Management

The nurse monitors the client's apical pulse, blood pressure, and temperature at least every 4 hours. The nurse

Chart 67–2

Laboratory Profile: Thyroid Function

Test	Normal Range for Adults	Significance of Abnormal Findings	
		Hyperthyroidism	*Hypothyroidism*
Serum T_3	• 110–230 ng/dL, or 1.2–1.5 SI units	• Increased	• Decreased
Serum T_4	• 4.6–11 μg/dL, or 59–142 SI units	• Increased	• Decreased
Free T_4 index	• 0.8–2.8 ng/dL, or 10–30 SI units	• Increased	• Decreased
T_3 resin uptake	• 25%–35% (varies with different laboratories)	• Increased	• Decreased
TRH stimulation test	• Doubling of baseline TSH 30 minutes after IV injection of 500 μg TRH (women have greater response)	• Little or no TSH response	• Delayed or poor TSH response in secondary hypothyroidism (pituitary failure) • Elevated two or more times the normal in primary hypothyroidism (thyroid gland failure)
Thyroid suppression test	• N/A	• Fails to suppress RAIU or T_4 levels	• No change in RAIU or T_4 levels
TSH stimulation test (thyroid stimulation test)	• >10% in RAIU or >1.5 μg/dL	• N/A (test differentiates primary from secondary hypothyroidism)	• No response in primary hypothyroidism • Normal response in secondary hypothyroidism
Thyroid antibodies (anti-thyroglobulin antibody)	• Titer <1:100	• High titer of antithyroglobulin antibodies	• Increased titers

TSH = thyroid-stimulating hormone; RAIU = radioactive iodine uptake; N/A = not applicable; T_3 = triiodothyronine; T_4 = thyroxine; TRH = thyrotropin-releasing hormone.

instructs the client to report any palpitations, dyspnea, vertigo, or chest pain immediately.

The nurse and other assistive nursing personnel minimize the client's discomfort from the clinical effects of hyperthyroidism. Because activity intolerance and fatigue are common, the nurse encourages the client to rest and provides as quiet an environment as possible. Frequent bed linen changes, sponge baths, and a cool environment decrease discomfort caused by diaphoresis and heat intolerance.

Drug Therapy. The most frequently ordered antithyroid drugs are the thionamides, including propylthiouracil (PTU) and methimazole (Tapazole), which block thyroid hormone synthesis (Chart 67–3).

Iodine preparations inhibit synthesis and release of thyroid hormone. Iodine achieves its effect by decreasing vascularity and increasing firmness in the gland.

Lithium carbonate also inhibits thyroid hormone release. However, its use is limited because of certain side effects, such as depression, nephrogenic diabetes insipidus, tremors, nausea, and vomiting. Lithium may be prescribed when a client cannot tolerate other antithyroid drugs.

Beta-adrenergic blocking drugs, such as propranolol (Inderal, Detensol✱), relieve diaphoresis, anxiety, tachycardia, and palpitations.

Radioactive Iodine Therapy. The client with hyperthyroidism may receive oral [131]I. The dosage depends on the thyroid gland's size and degree of radiosensitivity. The thyroid gland picks up the RAI, and some of the cells that synthesize thyroid hormone are destroyed by the local radiation. Because the thyroid gland stores thyroid hormone to some degree, the client may not experience symptom relief until 6 to 8 weeks after RAI therapy. During the first few weeks after treatment, the client may still require supportive drug therapy.

Radioactive iodine therapy usually entails one dose and can be performed on an outpatient basis. Occasionally, a client requires a second or third dose. Unless the dosage is extremely high, no radiation precautions are required. The nurse reassures the client that the radioactivity quickly dissipates. Hypothyroidism is one of the most frequent complications of this therapy and can occur several years after treatment. The client then needs lifelong thyroid hormone replacement.

Radioactive iodine therapy is contraindicated in pregnant

Chart 67–3

Drug Therapy for Hyperthyroidism

Drug	Usual Dosage	Nursing Interventions	Rationale
Propylthiouracil (PTU, Propyl-Thyracil♣)	• 100–150 mg tid PO	• Give at 8-hr intervals around the clock	• Spreading out dosage helps maintain suppression of hormone.
Methimazole (Tapa-zole)	• 5–15 mg tid PO	• Monitor vital signs. • Weigh the client weekly. • Observe for sore throat, fever, headache, and skin eruptions.	• Changes in vital signs or weight and appearance or other signs and symptoms may indicate adverse reactions, which may necessitate discontinuation of drug use.

Iodine products
  Strong iodine (Lugol's) solution
  Saturated solution of potassium iodide (SSKI)
  Potassium iodide tablets, solution, and syrup
	• Dosage varies, depending on the type of iodine prescribed, the manufacturer, and the form supplied (tablet, solution, or syrup)	• Give in fruit juice or water.
		• Observe for fever, rash, metallic taste, sore mouth, severe GI distress, and burning mouth and throat.
		• Instruct the client to take tablets after meals.
			• Giving in fruit juice or water improves taste.
			• Signs of iodism may necessitate discontinuation of drug use.
			• Taking after meals enhances absorption.

Lithium carbonate (Lithobid, Carbolith♣, Lithizine♣)	• Individualized, 900–1200 mg/day PO in divided doses	• Observe for signs of hypothyroidism. • Instruct the client to drink 10–12 glassfuls of fluid a day • Instruct the client to maintain normal sodium intake.	• Signs of hypothyroidism may indicate drug-induced thyroid enlargement. • Extra fluid intake helps to prevent dehydration. • Reduced sodium intake can cause retention of the drug.
Propranolol (Inderal, Detensol♣)	• 20 mg/day qid in divided doses	• Weigh the client daily. • Measure intake and output. • Instruct the client to take propranolol with food. • Instruct the client to avoid smoking. • Monitor the client's pulse.	• Increased weight and decreased output may indicate congestive heart failure. • Taking the drug with food enhances absorption. • The drug's effect is reduced by smoking. • Tachycardia is a sign of hyperthyroidism.

GI = gastrointestinal; PO = orally; tid = three times a day; qid = four times a day.

women because ¹³¹I crosses the placenta and can adversely affect the fetal thyroid gland.

Surgical Management

Antithyroid drugs and RAI therapy have become the treatments of choice for clients with hyperthyroidism. Clients who have large goiters causing tracheal or esophageal compression or who are unresponsive to antithyroid drugs may be candidates for surgery to remove all or part of the thyroid gland. Removal of all (total thyroidectomy) or part (subtotal thyroidectomy) of the thyroid tissue results in a decreased level of thyroid hormones. Clients undergoing a total thyroidectomy must take lifelong thyroid hormone replacement. This surgery is indicated in certain types of thyroid cancer.

Preoperative Care. If possible, clients should undergo drug therapy and have near-normal thyroid function (euthyroid) before thyroid surgery. The euthyroid state is achieved with antithyroid drugs that decrease the secretion of thyroid hormone. Iodine preparations are also used to decrease the size and vascularity of the gland, reducing the risk of hemorrhage and the potential for thyroid storm during surgery.

Cardiac problems should be controlled. Clients with

hyperthyroidism are often not at optimal weight, and special attention to adequate nutrition with a high-protein, high-carbohydrate diet is essential.

The nurse instructs clients to perform coughing and deep-breathing exercises and demonstrates how to support the neck when coughing or moving. Placing both hands behind the neck when moving reduces the strain on the suture line. The nurse explains to clients that they may experience hoarseness for a few days as a result of endotracheal tube placement during surgery.

Clients often fear thyroid surgery, perhaps because the incision is in the neck area. The nurse identifies areas of client concern and reassures clients by calmly explaining the surgery and postoperative care in a manner appropriate for their age and educational level.

Operative Procedures. A thyroidectomy is usually performed with the client under general anesthesia. During surgery, the client's neck is extended and the surgeon makes a "collar" incision 1 to 2 cm above the clavicle. The surgeon identifies and avoids the parathyroid glands and recurrent laryngeal nerves to minimize complications and injury.

If a *subtotal thyroidectomy* is performed, the remaining thyroid tissues are sutured to the trachea. If a *total thyroidectomy* is performed, the surgeon leaves the parathyroid glands with an intact blood supply and removes the entire thyroid gland.

Postoperative Care. Care of the client recovering from thyroidectomy is summarized in the Client Care Plan. Initially, the nurse monitors vital signs every 15 minutes until stable and then every 30 minutes. The nurse increases or decreases the frequency of vital sign evaluation depending on changes in the client's condition and the physician's orders.

The nurse assesses the client's level of discomfort. Sandbags or pillows are used to support the client's head and neck. When awake, he or she is placed in a semi-Fowler's position. When positioning the client, the nurse attempts to decrease tension on the suture line. The nurse administers pain medications as needed and as ordered.

Humidification of the air promotes easier respiration and liquefies thick respiratory secretions. The nurse assists the client in coughing and deep breathing every 30 minutes to 1 hour, and suctions oral and tracheal secretions when necessary.

Several complications may arise from thyroid surgery, including hemorrhage, respiratory distress, parathyroid gland injury resulting in hypocalcemia and *tetany* (hyperexcitability of nerves and muscles), damage to laryngeal nerves, and thyroid storm. The nurse is alert to the potential for complications and identifies manifestations early.

Hemorrhage. After surgery, the nurse inspects the neck dressing. A drain may be present with a moderate amount of serosanguineous drainage. Hemorrhage is most likely to occur during the first 24 hours after surgery, and the nurse checks behind the client's neck for blood. Hemorrhage may also be manifested by bleeding at the incision site or by respiratory distress caused by tracheal compression.

Respiratory Distress. Respiratory distress can also result from swelling or tetany. Laryngeal *stridor*—harsh, high-pitched respiratory sounds—is often heard in acute laryngeal obstruction. Equipment for emergency tracheostomy should be easily available, preferably at the client's bedside. The nurse checks that oxygen and suctioning equipment are nearby and in working order. In some instances, nurses are instructed to remove clips or sutures when medical assistance is not immediately available.

Hypocalcemia and Tetany. During thyroid surgery, the parathyroid glands can be damaged or their blood supply impaired. Hypocalcemia and tetany result when parathyroid hormone (PTH) levels decrease. The nurse notes the client's complaints of tingling around the mouth or of the toes and fingers and muscular twitching as signs of calcium deficiency. Calcium gluconate or calcium chloride for intravenous (IV) administration should be available in an emergency situation. (For information on the later signs of hypocalcemia, refer to the later discussion on postoperative care following parathyroidectomy. The care of clients with hypocalcemia is discussed in Chapter 16, and hypoparathyroidism is covered later in this chapter.)

Laryngeal Nerve Damage. If the laryngeal nerve is injured during surgery, hoarseness and a weak voice can result. The nurse assesses the client's voice at 2-hour intervals and notes any changes. The nurse reassures the client that hoarseness is usually temporary.

Thyroid Storm. Thyroid storm (thyroid crisis) is a life-threatening event that occurs in a client with uncontrolled hyperthyroidism attributable to Graves' disease. Signs and symptoms of crisis develop quickly. Usually, the thyroid storm is triggered by a major stressor, such as trauma or infection. Other conditions that can precipitate thyroid storm include vigorous palpation of the goiter, exposure to organic or inorganic iodine, and RAI therapy. In the past, thyroid storm occurred in inadequately prepared clients undergoing thyroid surgery. Today, clients receive antithyroid drugs, beta-blockers, steroids, and iodides before thyroid surgery to avert thyroid crisis.

The characteristic signs and symptoms of thyroid storm result from a rapid increase in the metabolic rate caused by excessive thyroid hormone secretion and include
- Fever
- Tachycardia
- Systolic hypertension

Clients may experience gastrointestinal symptoms, such as abdominal pain, nausea, vomiting, and diarrhea. Typically, clients with thyroid storm experience agitation, tremors, and anxiety. As the crisis progresses, clients may exhibit restlessness, confusion, psychosis, and seizures, leading to coma.

Emergency measures to prevent the client's death vary with the clinical presentation. After the determining cause or event has been identified, the primary concerns (Chart 67-4) are
- Maintaining airway patency
- Providing adequate ventilation
- Stabilizing the hemodynamic status

Client Care Plan

The Client Recovering from Thyroidectomy

Nursing Diagnosis No. 1: Ineffective Airway Clearance related to obstruction from hemorrhage or edema at surgical site, damage to recurrent laryngeal nerves, or injury to parathyroid glands.

Expected Outcomes	Nursing Interventions	Rationale
The client's lungs are expected to be clear. The client's breathing patterns are expected to be within his or her normal limits. The client is expected to be able to speak in his or her usual voice.	■ Monitor the client for signs of respiratory distress, cyanosis, tachypnea, and noisy respirations. ■ Inspect neck dressings every hour during the initial postoperative period, then q4h. ■ Monitor the amount of drainage and frequency of dressing reinforcement. ■ Check with the client regarding sensation of tightness around the incision site. ■ Maintain the client in semi-Fowler's position with an ice-bag to reduce swelling. ■ Ask the client to speak q2h, noting changes in tone or hoarseness. ■ Assess for the presence of Chvostek's and Trousseau's signs. ■ Identify the presence of numbness or tingling of extremities. ■ Monitor serum calcium levels. ■ Keep emergency tracheostomy and suction equipment, oxygen, suture removal kit, and IV calcium readily available.	■ Ongoing monitoring and assessment help to detect and prevent respiratory problems. ■ Surgery in the neck area can result in airway obstruction, primarily owing to postoperative edema. ■ Positioning and ice reduce swelling. ■ Damage to laryngeal nerves during thyroid surgery can cause closure of the glottis. ■ Hypocalcemia, resulting from parathyroid gland damage or removal, can cause tetany and laryngospasm. ■ Being prepared for emergencies helps to ensure prompt treatment and positive outcomes.

Nursing Diagnosis No. 2: High Risk for Decreased Cardiac Output related to hemorrhage

Expected Outcomes	Nursing Interventions	Rationale
The client is expected to remain alert and oriented. Vital signs are expected to be normal for each client.	■ Identify changes in cardiovascular status: ■ Monitor vital signs every 15 minutes in the initial postoperative period, then q1–4h.	■ Ongoing monitoring and assessment help to detect hypovolemia, hypertension, and eventual shock related to excessive blood loss.

Client Care Plan

Expected Outcomes	Nursing Interventions	Rationale
	■ Monitor cardiac rhythm, noting tachycardia or irregularity. ■ Check dressing for excessive bleeding. Check on front, back, and sides of neck, feeling behind neck. ■ Identify changes in level of consciousness or orientation. ■ Administer fluids as ordered.	

Nursing Diagnosis No. 3: Pain related to surgical incision

Expected Outcomes	Nursing Interventions	Rationale
The client is expected to experience minimal pain and discomfort.	■ Assess level of discomfort, using standard pain assessment scales. ■ Assist the client in maintaining correct head and neck position. Place the client in semi-Fowler's position with sandbags or pillows to support the neck. ■ Teach the client to support the head and neck when making position changes. ■ Administer pain medication as ordered. ■ Monitor the client's response to pain medication. ■ Place fluids and call light within easy reach of the client. ■ Maintain a quiet environment, decreasing stress.	■ Assessment helps to determine the need for interventions. Severe pain is uncommon after thyroidectomy, but discomfort occurs owing to difficulty in positioning the head and neck. ■ Proper positioning helps to decrease tension on the suture line. ■ Medication will help to reduce pain and promote comfort. ■ By evaluating the client's response to interventions, the nurse can intervene to make changes in the plan of care as is necessary. ■ Easy accessibility to necessary items promotes compliance and decreases anxiety. ■ A therapeutic environment can promote comfort and reduce the need for pain medication.

➤ *Infiltrative Ophthalmopathy*

Medical therapy for hyperthyroidism does not affect the infiltrative ophthalmopathy of Graves' disease. Treatment of the client with infiltrative ophthalmopathy is symptomatic. When the symptoms are mild, the nurse instructs the client to elevate the head of the bed at night and use an eye lubricant (artificial tears). If photophobia is present, dark glasses or eye patches are often helpful. For the client who cannot close the eyelids completely, the

---

Chart 67–4

Nursing Care Highlight: Emergency Care of the Client During Thyroid Storm

- Maintain a patent airway and adequate ventilation.
- Give antithyroid drugs as ordered: propylthiouracil (PTU, Propyl-Thyracil✦), 300–900 mg/day; methimazole (Tapazole), up to 60 mg/day.
- Administer sodium iodide solution, 2 g/day, IV, as ordered.
- Give propranolol (Inderal, Detensol✦), 1–3 mg IV as ordered. Give slowly over 3 minutes; the client should be connected to a cardiac monitor, and a central venous pressure catheter should be in place.
- Give glucocorticoids as ordered: hydrocortisone, 100–500 mg/day IV; prednisone, 4–60 mg/day IV or IM.
- Monitor continually for cardiac dysrhythmias.
- Monitor vital signs frequently.
- Provide comfort measures, including a cooling blanket.
- Give nonsalicylate antipyretics as ordered.

---

nurse recommends gently taping the lids closed with nonallergenic tape. The physician may suture the eyelids closed in severe cases. These actions prevent further irritation to the eye and are usually sufficient to prevent vision loss and injury. (For more discussion regarding eye protection, see Chapter 49).

In severe cases, the physician prescribes short-term steroid therapy to reduce swelling and halt the infiltrative process. Prednisone (Deltasone, Winpred✦) is often administered in high doses (often 120 mg/day) initially, and then tapered down in accordance with the client's response. The nurse explains the necessity of gradually reducing the prednisone and reviews its side effects with the client.

The physician may prescribe diuretics to decrease periorbital edema. If loss of sight or damage to the eyeball is possible, surgical intervention (orbital decompression) may be necessary.

➤ Health Teaching

The nurse reviews the signs and symptoms of hyperthyroidism and instructs the client to report an increase or recurrence of symptoms. In addition, certain treatments, such as RAI therapy or surgery, can result in hypothyroidism. The nurse reviews the symptoms of hypothyroidism (discussed later) and mentions the corresponding need for thyroid hormone replacement. The nurse reinforces the need for regular health follow-up because hypothyroidism can occur several years after RAI therapy.

If the client has had surgery, the surgeon usually removes the sutures on the third or fourth postoperative day. The nurse instructs the client to inspect the incision area and to report redness, tenderness, drainage, or swelling to a member of the health care team.

The discharged client may continue to be emotionally labile as a result of hyperthyroidism. The nurse explains the reason for emotional lability to the client and family, and reassures them that it will decrease with continued

treatment. The nurse aids the client in identifying coping skills, support systems, and potential stressors.

Hypothyroidism

Overview

Clinical manifestations of hypothyroidism (Chart 67–5) are the result of inadequate peripheral tissue thyroid hormone levels. Hypothyroidism can occur at any time throughout a person's life span. Because clients usually require lifelong thyroid hormone replacements, client education is extremely important.

Pathophysiology

When the production of thyroid hormones is inadequate, the thyroid gland, in response to increasing thyroid-stimulating hormone (TSH) levels, enlarges in an attempt to compensate. Goiter is this enlargement. Simple (nontoxic) goiter is the most common type. Endemic goiter occurs in areas where the soil and water are deficient in iodine. Iodine is necessary to synthesize and secrete thyroid hormones.

Low levels of thyroid hormones result in an overall decrease in the basal metabolic rate, affecting virtually every body system. An insufficient amount of thyroid hormone causes abnormalities in lipid metabolism, with an increase in cholesterol and triglyceride levels. This increase is associated with the development of atherosclerosis and subsequent cardiac disease in the hypothyroid client.

Accumulation of hydrophilic proteoglycans in the interstitial space, which causes an increase in the interstitial fluid, is a characteristic pathologic change. Pleural, cardiac, and abdominal effusions are also results of this process, as is the characteristic mucinous edema (myxedema) (Fig. 67–4).

Myxedema coma is a rare, but serious, presentation of untreated or inadequately treated hypothyroidism. The pathologic basis for myxedema coma is thought to be cardiac in origin. The generalized decrease in metabolism in cardiac tissue causes the heart muscle to become flabby and the chamber size to increase. The result is decreased cardiac output and decreased perfusion to the brain and other vital organs. The decreased perfusion makes the already slowed cellular metabolism worse, resulting in tissue and organ failure. The mortality rate for myxedema coma is extremely high, and it is considered a life-threatening emergency. Myxedema coma can be precipitated by a variety of events or conditions (Table 67–2).

Etiology

Most cases of hypothyroidism occur as a result of thyroid surgery and radioactive iodine (RAI) treatment of hyperthyroidism. Hypothyroidism is also caused by a variety of other conditions and factors listed in Table 67–3.

Incidence/Prevalence

Most cases of hypothyroidism occur in people between 30 and 60 years of age, and occur four times more fre-

Chart 67-5

Key Features of Hypothyroidism

Integumentary Manifestations

- Cool, pale or yellowish, dry, coarse, scaly skin
- Thick, brittle nails
- Dry, coarse, brittle hair
- Decreased hair growth, with loss of eyebrow hair

Pulmonary Manifestations

- Hypoventilation
- Pleural effusion
- Dyspnea

Cardiovascular Manifestations

- Bradycardia
- Dysrhythmias
- Enlarged heart
- Decreased activity tolerance
- Hypotension

Metabolic Manifestations

- Decreased basal metabolic rate
- Decreased body temperature
- Cold intolerance

Musculoskeletal Manifestations

- Muscle aches and pains
- Delayed contraction and relaxation of muscles

Neurologic Manifestations

- Slowing of intellectual functions
  - Slowness or slurring of speech
  - Impaired memory
  - Inattentiveness
- Lethargy or somnolence
- Confusion
- Hearing loss
- Paresthesia (numbness and tingling) of the extremities
- Decreased tendon reflexes

Psychological/Emotional Manifestations

- Apathy
- Agitation
- Depression
- Paranoia
- Withdrawal
- Manic behavior

Gastrointestinal Manifestations

- Anorexia
- Slight weight gain
- Constipation
- Abdominal distention

Reproductive Manifestations

Women

- Changes in menses (amenorrhea or prolonged menstrual periods)
- Infertility
- Anovulation
- Decreased libido

Men

- Decreased libido
- Impotence

Other Manifestations

- Periorbital edema
- Facial puffiness
- Facial coarseness
- Nonpitting edema of the hands and feet
- Hoarseness
- Goiter (enlarged thyroid gland)
- Thick tongue
- Increased sensitivity to opioids and tranquilizers
- Blank expression
- Weakness, fatigue
- Decreased urinary output
- Anemia
- Easy bruising
- Iron deficiency
- Folate deficiency
- Vitamin B_{12} deficiency

quently in women than in men. Endemic goiters frequently occur in people living in iodine-deficient geographic areas. Iodinization of salt or other food products has virtually eliminated this problem in the United States, but endemic goiter is a preventable health problem in other areas.

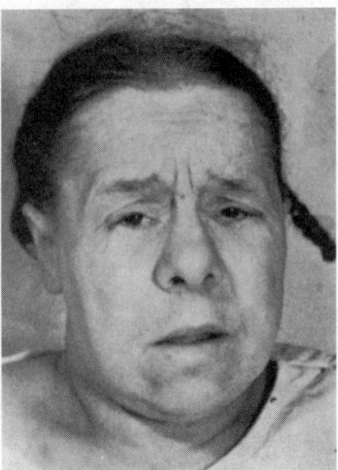

Figure 67-4. Myxedema.

Collaborative Management

 Assessment

➤ *History*

A decrease in thyroid hormone produces a variety of signs and symptoms related to decreased metabolic activity. The nurse asks clients about any change in sleep habits; they usually report an increase in time spent

TABLE 67-2

Conditions or Events Precipitating Myxedema Coma

Acute illness
Anesthesia
Surgery
Hypothermia
Chemotherapy
Sedatives/opioids
Rapid withdrawal of thyroid medications
Untreated hypothyroidism
Inadequately treated hypothyroidism

TABLE 67–3

Causes of Hypothyroidism	
Primary	
Decreased thyroid tissue	Surgical removal of the thyroid
	Radiation-induced thyroid destruction
	Autoimmune thyroid destruction
	Congenital thyroid agenesis
	Congenital thyroid hypoplasia
	Congenital thyroid dysgenesis
	Cancer (thyroidal or metastatic)
Decreased synthesis of thyroid hormone	Endemic iodine deficiency
	Excessive exposure to iodine
	Medications
	Lithium
	Phenylbutazone
	Propylthiouracil
	Sodium or potassium perchlorate
	Aminoglutethimide
Secondary	
Inadequate production of thyroid-stimulating hormone	Pituitary tumors, trauma, infections, or infarcts
	Congenital pituitary defects
	Hypothalamic tumors, trauma, infections, or infarcts

sleeping, sometimes up to 14 to 16 hours/day. Clients may also complain of generalized weakness, anorexia, muscle aches, and paresthesias.

Constipation is common. The nurse asks about the frequency and consistency of bowel movements. Clients often experience cold intolerance; the nurse asks clients whether they have needed more blankets at night or sweaters and extra clothing in warm weather.

Both male and female clients may identify a decrease in libido. In addition, the nurse asks the female client with hypothyroidism if she has had difficulty conceiving or any changes in menses (heavy, prolonged bleeding or amenorrhea). Male clients can experience impotence and fertility problems.

The nurse asks clients about their medical history. Current or previous use of medications, such as lithium, aminoglutethimide, sodium or potassium perchlorate, thiocyanates, or cobalt, can impair the synthesis of thyroid hormone. Clients with a history of hyperthyroidism may have had surgical, radioactive, or medical (drug) treatment, which may have damaged the thyroid gland and provoked hypothyroidism. The nurse determines whether clients are taking any tranquilizers or opioids. Hypothyroid clients have an increased sensitivity to these drugs as a result of metabolic dysfunction.

➤ Physical Assessment/Clinical Manifestations

Initially, the nurse observes the client's overall appearance. Figure 67–5 shows the typical appearance of an adult with untreated congenital hypothyroidism (cretin-

ism). When inspecting the face of a person with adult onset hypothyroidism (see Fig. 67–4), the nurse might note coarse features, edema around the eyes and face, a blank expression, and a thick tongue. The client's overall muscle movement is slow.

A decrease in thyroid hormone levels produces characteristic clinical manifestations in almost every body system. However, some of these clinical manifestations could occur in euthyroid clients. Therefore, additional data obtained from the psychosocial assessment and laboratory testing are essential.

➤ Psychosocial Assessment

The symptoms of hypothyroidism cause major difficulties in psychosocial functioning. Complaints of depression or, less frequently, mania are often given as the reason for seeking medical attention. Family members often bring clients for the initial encounter with the health care team. Clients may be too lethargic, apathetic, or somnolent to recognize changes in their condition. Families may report that clients are withdrawn, but this can also result from simple hearing loss.

The nurse assesses the client's attention span and memory, both of which can be impaired by hypothyroidism. Paranoia and agitation may be additional findings.

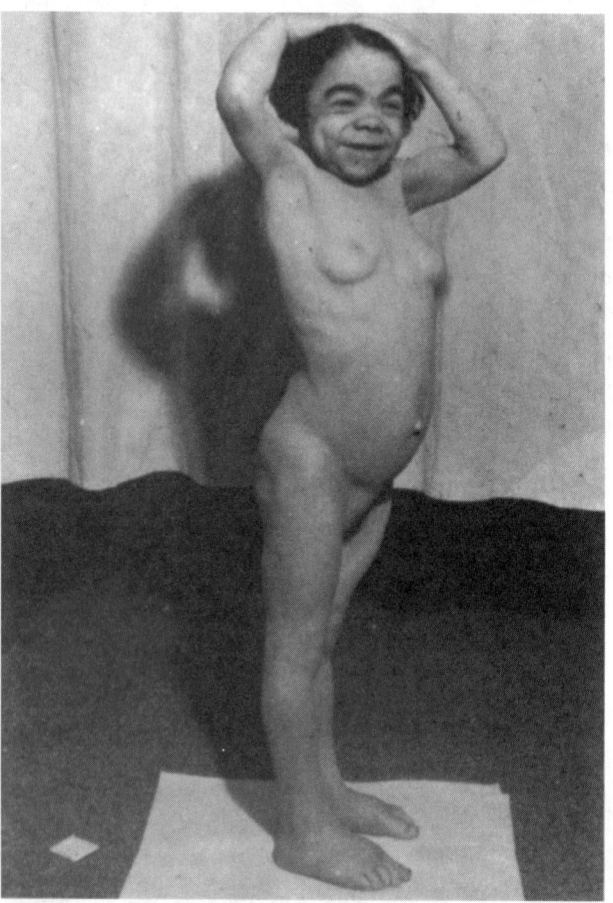

Figure 67–5. This 33-year-old untreated adult cretin exhibits characteristic features: dwarfism (height 44 inches, in this case), underdeveloped breasts, protuberant abdomen, umbilical hernia, widened facial features, and scant axillary and pubic hair.

➤ Laboratory Assessment

The laboratory findings in clients with hypothyroidism are generally the opposite of those with hyperthyroidism. Triiodothyronine (T_3) and thyroxine (T_4) serum levels are decreased, and in primary hypothyroidism, the TSH level is elevated. In clients with secondary and tertiary hypothyroidism, TSH levels can be decreased or near normal. More information is presented in Chart 67–2.

 ## Analysis

➤ Common Nursing Diagnoses and Collaborative Problems

The following nursing diagnoses are common in clients who have hypothyroidism:

1. Decreased Cardiac Output related to decreased stroke volume as a result of electrical or mechanical malfunction from bradycardia and arteriosclerotic coronary artery disease
2. Ineffective Breathing Pattern related to decreased energy, decreased lung expansion, obesity, fatigue, and inactivity
3. Altered Thought Processes related to increased interstitial edema and water retention

The major collaborative problem is the Potential for Myxedema Coma.

➤ Additional Nursing Diagnoses and Collaborative Problems

Clients with hypothyroidism may have the following additional nursing diagnoses:

- Altered Nutrition: More than Body Requirements related to decreased metabolic need
- Hypothermia related to decreased metabolic rate
- Constipation related to decreased motility of the gastrointestinal (GI) tract
- Altered Sexuality Patterns related to the effects of illness, extreme fatigue, and obesity
- Impaired Physical Mobility related to fatigue, decreased strength and endurance, depression, obesity, and muscle aches
- Body Image Disturbance related to changes in physical appearance
- Knowledge Deficit of condition, diagnosis, and treatment related to low energy level and fatigue

Additional collaborative problems for clients with hypothyroidism are the Potential for Paralytic Ileus and Potential for Irreversible Cardiomyopathy.

 ## Planning and Implementation

➤ Decreased Cardiac Output

Planning: Expected Outcomes. The client is expected to maintain normal cardiovascular function.

Interventions. The client with hypothyroidism can have decreased blood pressure, bradycardia, and dysrhythmias. The nurse monitors blood pressure, heart rate, and rhythm, and observes closely for signs of hemodynamic compromise, such as hypotension, decreasing urine output, and mental status changes.

If the hypothyroidism has been chronic, the client may have cardiovascular disease. The nurse instructs the client to report episodes of chest pain or discomfort immediately.

The hypothyroid client requires lifelong replacement of thyroid hormone to relieve associated clinical manifestations. Synthetic hormone preparations are usually prescribed; the most common is levothyroxine sodium (Synthroid, T_4, Eltroxin✦). The physician initiates therapy cautiously, particularly when the client has known cardiovascular problems, and the nurse assesses closely for chest pain and dyspnea. The starting dosage of thyroid hormone is usually low and is then increased every 2 to 3 weeks until the desired response is obtained. The dosage and time required for relief of symptoms vary with each client.

The nurse monitors for and teaches the client signs and symptoms of hyperthyroidism, which can occur with replacement therapy.

➤ Ineffective Breathing Pattern

Planning: Expected Outcomes. The client is expected to maintain normal respiratory function.

Interventions. The nurse observes and records the rate and depth of respirations. The nurse auscultates the lungs and notes any abnormalities, such as a decrease in breath sounds. If hypothyroidism is severe, the client may experience significant respiratory distress, necessitating ventilatory support. Severe respiratory distress is usually associated with myxedema coma.

Sedating a hypothyroid client can contribute to respiratory difficulties and should be avoided, if possible. When a tranquilizer or sedative is needed, the dosage should be reduced because hypothyroidism increases sensitivity to these drugs. The nurse carefully assesses the client for signs of respiratory compromise.

➤ Altered Thought Processes

Planning: Expected Outcomes. Because the client with hypothyroidism experiences a general slowing of all intellectual functions, the outcome is that the client's thought processes are expected to improve.

Interventions. The nurse notes the presence and severity of symptoms, including lethargy, drowsiness, memory deficit, inattentiveness, and difficulty in communicating. With thyroid hormone treatment, symptoms should decrease, and mentation usually returns to normal levels in adults within 2 weeks. In the interim, the nurse

- Orients the client to person, place, and time
- Explains all procedures slowly and carefully
- Provides a safe environment

Family members or significant others may have difficulty coping with the client's symptoms. The nurse encourages them to accept the client's mood changes and mental slowness as manifestations of the disease, which should improve with therapy.

➤ *Myxedema Coma*

Any client with hypothyroidism who has any other health problem or who is newly diagnosed is at risk for myxedema coma. Precipitating factors are listed in Table 67–2. Myxedema coma is characterized by

- Coma
- Respiratory failure
- Hypotension
- Hyponatremia
- Hypothermia
- Hypoglycemia

Untreated myxedema coma leads to ischemic organ damage and death. The nurse is alert to this complication and assesses the client every shift for changes that indicate increasing severity of hypothyroid symptoms, especially changes in cognition and mental status.

The physician institutes treatment quickly, according to the client's clinical presentation and history, without waiting for laboratory confirmation. The nurse provides emergency care as outlined in Chart 67–6.

ELDERLY CONSIDERATIONS

 Metabolic rate and production of thyroid hormone both decrease with advancing age (see Chart 67–7), particularly among people older than 80 years. Until recently, however, data regarding normal levels of T_3 and T_4 were established only for adults between the ages of 20 and 30 years. By such criteria, older people with T_3 and T_4 levels 15% to 20% below "normal levels" (established for a younger population) were considered to have hypothyroidism and therapy with thyroid hormone was initiated. In fact, many of these clients were not truly hypothyroid, and therapy caused pseudohyperthyroidism, stressing many tissues and organs. In addition, daily thyroid hormone therapy decreased the activity of the anterior pituitary gland and the thyroid gland, creating actual hypothyroidism. Health care providers need to assess more than just laboratory data to determine hypothyroidism in the elderly.

➤ Continuing Care

Hypothyroidism is usually a chronic condition that occurs more frequently among the elderly. Clients with hypothy-

---

Chart 67–6

Nursing Care Highlight: Emergency Care of the Client During Myxedema Coma

- Maintain a patent airway.
- Replace fluids as ordered.
- Give levothyroxine sodium IV as ordered.
- Administer glucose IV as ordered.
- Administer corticosteroids as ordered.
- Check the client's temperature frequently.
- Monitor blood pressure.
- Cover the client with warm blankets.
- Monitor for changes in mental status.

Chart 67–7

Nursing Focus on the Elderly: Thyroid Problems

Teach the client the following facts about changes in the thyroid gland related to aging:

- The thyroid gland decreases in size with increasing age.
- Thyroid hormone secretion decreases with age, but the hormone level remains stable because cellular clearance of the hormone also decreases with age.
- The basal metabolic rate decreases with age, usually as a result of decreased activity. This decrease changes the body composition from predominantly muscular to predominantly fatty.
- Elderly clients require lower doses of replacement thyroid hormone. Too large a dose may adversely affect the heart muscle.

---

roidism, once stabilized, are managed on an outpatient basis and may reside in the home, in an assisted-living environment, or in a long-term care facility. Additionally, clients in acute care settings, subacute care settings, and rehabilitation centers may have long-standing hypothyroidism in addition to other acute or chronic health problems. The nurse needs to ensure that clients or whoever is responsible for overseeing daily care is aware of the condition and understands its treatment.

➤ *Health Teaching*

Most of the education needed by the client with hypothyroidism concerns hormone replacement therapy. The nurse emphasizes that the client will need lifelong medication and reviews the signs and symptoms of both hyperthyroidism and hypothyroidism. This information helps the client and family know when to seek medical interventions for dosage adjustment. The nurse reviews all aspects of medication information, including side effects. The nurse also instructs the client not to take any over-the-counter (OTC) medication because thyroid hormone preparations potentiate and interact with many other drugs. Elderly clients may need additional information about the effects of aging on the thyroid gland (see Chart 67–7).

The nurse advises the client to maintain a well-balanced diet with adequate fiber and fluid intake to prevent constipation. Excessive dietary fiber or fiber supplements may interfere with absorption of exogenous thyroid hormone (see Research Applications for Nursing). The client is reminded of the importance of adequate rest periods before resuming a full schedule of daily activities. The nurse encourages family members to voice their concerns to the health care providers.

The nurse discusses the necessity for follow-up care. All clients should wear a Medic-Alert identification bracelet.

The time required for resolution of the symptoms of hypothyroidism varies; the nurse focuses on educating the family to be tolerant of any mental dullness or slowness in their loved one. The nurse encourages the family to

Research Applications for Nursing

Fiber-Enriched Diet May Reduce the Bioavailability of Levothyroxine

Liel, Y., Harman-Boehm, I., & Shany, S. (1996). Evidence for a clinically important adverse effect of fiber-enriched diet on the bioavailability of levothyroxine in adult hypothyroid patients. Journal of Clinical Endocrinology and Metabolism, 81(2), 857–859.

The purpose of this study was to evaluate the effect of dietary fiber supplements on levothyroxine bioavailability in clients who were hypothyroid. The sample consisted of clients requiring high doses of T_4 who had a history of taking dietary fiber supplements. The dosage of levothyroxine remained the same, but the dietary supplementation of fiber was discontinued. Both pre- and post-TSH measurements were taken. The researchers found a reduction in the bioavailability of T_4 when the clients had an intake of dietary fiber supplements. These participants also required a larger than expected dose of T_4 to eliminate the symptoms of hypothyroidism.

Critique. This study should be replicated with a larger sample and with three groups of participants: those who take high-fiber supplements, those who have a high fiber diet, and a control group. There was no control group in this current study. The generalizability of these results would be strengthened by a more carefully controlled study.

Possible Nursing Implications. The possibility that fiber-enriched supplements can adversely affect the bioavailability of thyroid supplementation should direct nurses to specifically address this matter in clients who are hypothyroid and taking medication and in clients who have just been diagnosed as hypothyroid. A complete diet history is imperative.

orient the client frequently and explain everything clearly and simply. Eventually, the client should exhibit interest in the environment, work, family, and friends.

➤ Home Care Management

The client with hypothyroidism does not usually require alterations in the home unless the client has such decreased cognition that he or she poses a danger to self. Activity intolerance and fatigue may necessitate one-floor living for a short time. If symptoms have not cleared before discharge from the hospital, the nurse discusses the need for extra heat or clothing because of cold intolerance. The client who continues to have a decreased attention span may need assistance with medication preparation and administration. The nurse discusses this issue with the family and client and develops a plan for medication administration. One person should be clearly designated as responsible for medication preparation and administration so that doses are neither missed nor duplicated.

➤ Health Care Resources

Immediately after returning home, the client may require a support person to stay and provide more attention than

a visiting nurse or home care aide could. Contact with the health care team is necessary for follow-up and identification of potential problems. When making a home visit to the client being treated for hypothyroidism, the nurse remembers that therapy results are highly individual. The client taking exogenous thyroid medication may show manifestations of hypothyroidism if the dosage is inadequate or hyperthyroidism if is too high. The nurse performs a focused assessment at every home visit on the client under treatment for thyroid disfunction (Chart 67–8).

 Evaluation

On the basis of the identified nursing diagnoses, the nurse evaluates the care of the client with hypothyroidism. The client is expected to

- Maintain normal cardiovascular function
- Maintain normal respiratory function
- Experience improvement in thought processes

Chart 67–8

Focused Assessment for Home Care Clients with Thyroid Dysfunction

- Assess cardiovascular status.
  - Vital signs, including apical pulse, pulse pressure, presence or absence of orthostatic hypotension, and the quality and rhythm of peripheral pulses
  - Presence or absence of peripheral edema
  - Weight gain or loss
- Assess cognition and mental status.
  - Level of consciousness
  - Orientation to time, place, and person
  - Accurately reading a seven-word sentence containing no words greater than three syllables
  - Can the client count backward from 100 by 3s?
- Assess condition of skin and mucous membranes.
  - Moistness of skin, most reliable on chest and back
  - Skin temperature and color
- Assess neuromuscular status.
  - Reactivity of patellar and biceps reflexes
  - Oral temperature
  - Handgrip strength
  - Steadiness of gait
  - Presence or absence of fine tremors in the hand
- Ask about
  - Sleep in the past 24 hours
  - Client warm enough or too warm indoors
  - 24-hour diet recall
  - 24-hour activity recall
  - Over-the-counter and prescribed medications taken
  - Last bowel movement
- Assess client's understanding of illness and compliance with treatment.
  - Signs and symptoms to report to health care provider
  - Medication plan (correct timing and dose)

Thyroiditis

Overview

Thyroiditis is an inflammation of the thyroid gland. There are three types: acute, subacute, and chronic. Chronic thyroiditis (Hashimoto's disease) is the most common type.

Acute Thyroiditis

Acute suppurative thyroiditis, which is caused by bacterial invasion of the thyroid gland, is uncommon. Signs and symptoms include

- Pain
- Neck tenderness
- Malaise
- Elevated temperature
- Dysphagia

Acute thyroiditis is treated symptomatically and usually responds to antibiotic therapy.

Subacute Thyroiditis

Subacute granulomatous thyroiditis results from a viral infection of the thyroid gland, occasionally after an upper respiratory tract infection. It is characterized by

- Fever
- Chills
- Dysphagia
- Muscle and joint pain

The pain can radiate to the ears and the jaw. On palpation, the gland feels hard and moderately enlarged. Thyroid function can remain normal, although hyperthyroidism or hypothyroidism may develop. The client who has mild subacute thyroiditis is managed with rest, fluids, and acetylsalicylic acid (aspirin). In more severe cases, corticosteroids are given to reduce inflammation.

Chronic Thyroiditis

Chronic thyroiditis (Hashimoto's disease) affects females more frequently than males, most commonly clients in their 30s to 50s. Hashimoto's disease is believed to be an autoimmune disorder. The thyroid becomes infiltrated with antithyroid antibodies and lymphocytes, resulting in glandular destruction. Serum thyroid hormone levels are low, and secretion of TSH is increased. Elevated TSH levels result in increased thyroid function and may maintain a euthyroid state for some time, but hypothyroidism eventually develops.

Collaborative Management

Clinical manifestations of Hashimoto's disease include dysphagia and painless enlargement of the gland. Diagnosis is based on the presence of circulating antithyroid antibodies and needle biopsy findings of the thyroid gland. Serum thyroid hormone levels, TSH levels, and radioactive iodine uptake (RAIU) vary, depending on the progress of the disease.

Clients receive thyroid hormone to prevent hypothy-roidism and to suppress TSH secretion, thereby decreasing gland size. If the goiter does not respond to thyroid hormone, is disfiguring, or compresses other structures, surgery (subtotal thyroidectomy) is necessary.

Nursing interventions focus on promoting client comfort and educating the client about hypothyroidism, medications, and surgery. (See discussion of surgical management for hyperthyroidism.)

Thyroid Cancer

Overview

Clients with thyroid cancer experience considerable anxiety and stress. The nurse obtains baseline data from the client relating to knowledge of the disease, coping skills, and family relationships. The nurse encourages the client to verbalize fears and discuss the illness. There are four distinct histologic types of thyroid cancer: papillary, follicular, medullary, and anaplastic.

The initial clinical manifestation of thyroid cancer is a solitary, painless nodule in the thyroid gland. Additional signs and symptoms depend on the presence and location of metastasis (spread of cancer cells).

Papillary Carcinoma

Papillary carcinoma, the most common type of thyroid cancer, is found more frequently in women and in clients younger than 40 years. It is a slow-growing tumor and can be present for years before metastasis to the regional lymph nodes occurs. When the tumor is localized to the thyroid gland, the prognosis is good with a partial or total thyroidectomy.

Follicular Carcinoma

Follicular carcinoma constitutes approximately 25% of all thyroid cancers and primarily affects clients older than 50 years. Follicular carcinoma invades blood vessels and metastasizes to bone and lung tissue. It rarely spreads to regional lymph nodes but can adhere to the trachea, neck muscles, great vessels, and skin, resulting in dyspnea and dysphagia. When the tumor involves the recurrent laryngeal nerves, the client may experience hoarseness. The prognosis is fair when metastasis is minimal at the time of diagnosis.

Medullary Carcinoma

Medullary carcinoma arises from the parafollicular thyroid tissue. It accounts for 5% to 10% of all thyroid cancers and is more common in those older than 50 years. Metastasis occurs via regional lymph nodes and invasion of surrounding structures. This tumor often occurs as part of multiple endocrine neoplasia (MEN) type II, a familial endocrine disorder. There is excessive secretion of calcitonin, adrenocorticotropic hormone (ACTH), prostaglandins, and serotonin.

Anaplastic Carcinoma

Anaplastic carcinoma is a rapid-growing, extremely aggressive tumor that directly invades adjacent structures, causing symptoms of stridor (harsh, high-pitched respiratory sounds), hoarseness, and dysphagia. The prognosis is poor, and most clients die within a year after diagnosis. Clients with anaplastic carcinoma may be treated with palliative surgery, radiation, or chemotherapy.

Collaborative Management

Surgery is the treatment of choice for papillary, follicular, and medullary carcinomas. Usually a total thyroidectomy is performed with a nodal neck dissection if regional lymph nodes are involved. The physician prescribes postoperative suppressive doses of thyroid hormone for 3 months. An RAIU study is performed after medication is withdrawn. If there is RAI uptake, the client is treated with ablative (enough to destroy the tissue) amounts of RAI. If recurrent thyroid cancer does not respond to RAI, a course of chemotherapy is initiated.

PARATHYROID DISORDERS
Hyperparathyroidism

Overview

The parathyroid glands maintain calcium and phosphate homeostasis (Fig. 67–6). Normally, serum calcium concentration is maintained within a narrow range; phosphate levels vary more widely. Increased levels of parathyroid hormone (PTH) act directly on the kidney, causing increased tubular resorption of calcium and phosphate excretion. These processes contribute to hypercalcemia (excessive calcium) and hypophosphatemia (inadequate phosphate) in the client with hyperparathyroidism.

In the bone, excessive PTH levels increase bone resorption by decreasing osteoblastic (bone production) activity and increasing osteoclastic (bone destruction) activity.

TABLE 67–4

Causes of Parathyroid Dysfunction	
Causes of hyperparathyroidism	Parathyroid adenoma Parathyroid carcinoma Congenital hyperplasia Neck trauma or radiation Vitamin D deficiency Chronic renal failure with hypocalcemia Parathyroid hormone-secreting carcinomas of the lung, kidney, or gastrointestinal tract
Causes of hypoparathyroidism	Surgical or radiation-induced thyroid ablation Parathyroidectomy Congenital dysgenesis Idiopathic (autoimmune) hypoparathyroidism Hypomagnesemia

This process results in the release of calcium and phosphate into the circulation and decalcification of bone. When the normal solubility of calcium in the serum is exceeded, as in long-standing hypercalcemia, calcium is deposited in soft tissues.

Although the exact triggering mechanisms are unknown, *primary* hyperparathyroidism results when one or more hyperfunctioning glands is unresponsive to the normal feedback of serum calcium. In 80% to 85% of the cases, the cause is a benign, autonomous adenoma in one parathyroid gland. Table 67–4 lists other causes of hyperparathyroidism.

Collaborative Management

Assessment

The nurse inquires about the client's symptoms and any bone fractures, recent weight loss, arthritis, or psychological distress. Any history of radiation treatment to the head or neck is also obtained. In clients with long-standing disease, the nurse may observe a waxy pallor of the skin and bone deformities in the extremities and back.

There are two types of clinical features:
- Those relating to the effects of excessive PTH
- Those directly relating to the hypercalcemia

Excessive PTH results in renal calculi (kidney stones) and nephrocalcinosis (deposition of calcium in the soft tissue of the kidney). Bone lesions are due to enhanced bone resorption and result in pathologic fractures, bone cysts, and osteoporosis in advanced cases (Fig. 67–7).

Gastrointestinal manifestations, such as anorexia, nausea, vomiting, epigastric pain, constipation, and weight loss, are frequent, particularly when serum calcium levels are high. Hypergastrinemia (elevated serum gastrin levels) results from hypercalcemia and probably accounts for the increased incidence of associated peptic ulcer in hyperparathyroidism. Varying degrees of fatigue and lethargy

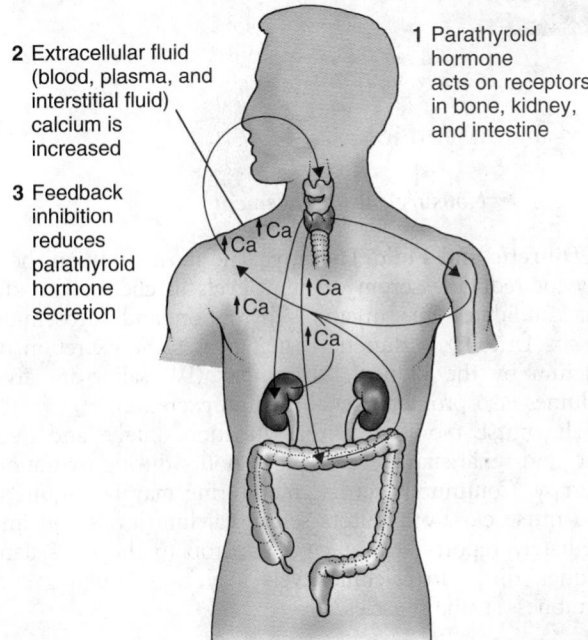

2 Extracellular fluid (blood, plasma, and interstitial fluid) calcium is increased

3 Feedback inhibition reduces parathyroid hormone secretion

1 Parathyroid hormone acts on receptors in bone, kidney, and intestine

Figure 67–6. The physiologic actions of parathyroid hormone.

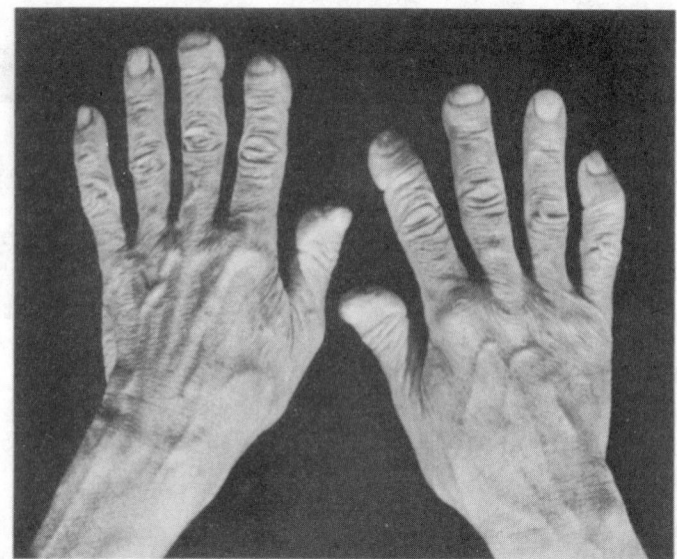

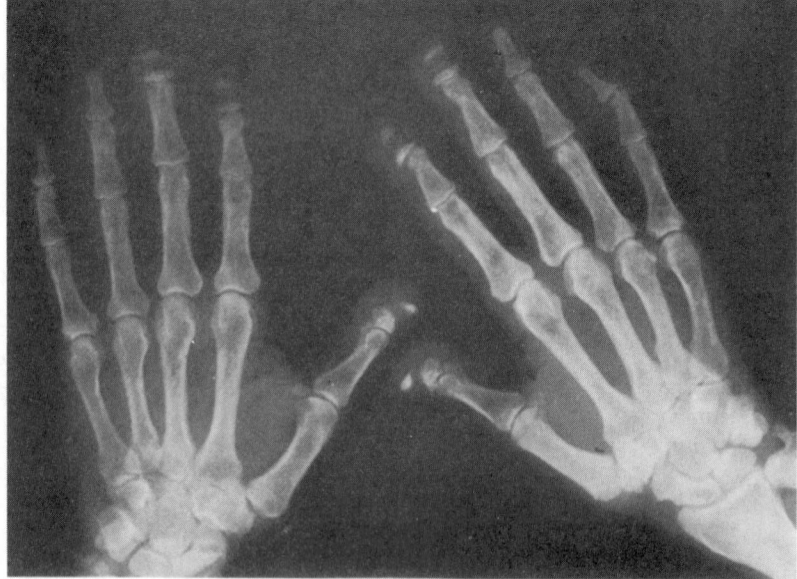

Figure 67–7. Extensive bone erosion resulting from untreated, long-standing hyperparathyroidism. Note the absence of bone at the tips of some fingers, resulting in digital clubbing.

may also be seen and become more severe as the serum calcium levels increase. The clinical course in the client with calcium levels greater than 12 mg/dL includes organic psychosis with mental confusion, leading to coma and death if untreated. (Chapter 16 has more information on the effects of hypercalcemia.)

Serum PTH, calcium, and phosphate measurements and urine cyclic adenosine monophosphate (cAMP) are the most frequently used laboratory tests to detect hyperparathyroidism (Chart 67–9). Radiographic tests demonstrate the presence of renal calculi, nephrocalcinosis, and bone lesions, such as cysts or fractures. Generalized bone demineralization and subperiosteal resorption in long bones occur in the client with chronic hyperparathyroidism. Other diagnostic tests include arteriography, computed tomography (CT), selective venous catheterization of the thyroid veins with sampling of the blood for PTH levels, and ultrasonography. The nurse explains the procedures and cares for the client undergoing diagnostic tests.

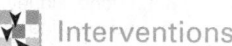 Interventions

➤ *Nonsurgical Management*

Diuretic and Fluid Therapy. The most common therapy for reducing serum calcium levels in clients who are not candidates for surgery is hydration and furosemide (Lasix, Uritol✦), a diuretic that increases the excretion of calcium by the kidney. Intravenous (IV) saline in large volumes also promotes renal calcium excretion.

The nurse monitors cardiac function, intake and output, and renal status every 2 to 4 hours during hydration therapy. Continuous cardiac monitoring may be required. The nurse closely monitors serum calcium levels and immediately reports any precipitous drop to the physician. Sudden drops in calcium levels may cause tingling and numbness in the muscles.

Drug Therapy. When hydration and furosemide cannot reduce hypercalcemia, or if it becomes necessary to

Chart 67–9

Laboratory Profile: Parathyroid Function

Test	Normal Range for Adults	Significance of Abnormal Findings	
		Hyperthyroidism	*Hypothyroidism*
Serum calcium	• Total: 8.6–10.0 mg/dL, or 2.20–2.55 SI units • Ionized (active): 4.64–5.28 mg/dL, or 1.16–1.32 SI units	• Increased in primary hyperparathyroidism	• Decreased
Serum phosphate	• 2.7–4.5 mg/dL, or 0.87–1.45 SI units • **Elderly:** May be slightly lower	• Decreased	• Increased
Serum parathyroid hormone	• <2000 pg/mL	• Increased	• Decreased
Urinary cAMP	• 1–11.5 μmol/dL	• Increased	• Decreased

cAMP = cyclic adenosine monophosphate.

discontinue IV fluids, additional medications can help to reduce the clinical manifestations of hyperparathyroidism, especially those related to hypercalcemia.

Phosphates. Oral phosphates inhibit bone resorption and interfere with calcium absorption. IV phosphates are used only when the serum calcium levels must be lowered rapidly.

Calcitonin. Calcitonin decreases skeletal calcium release and increases the renal clearance of calcium. Because of its short duration of action, calcitonin is not effective when used alone. Its therapeutic effects are greatly enhanced if given in conjunction with glucocorticoids.

Calcium Chelators. Some drugs lower calcium levels by binding (chelating) calcium, reducing the levels of free calcium. Mithramycin, a cytotoxic antibiotic, is the most effective and potent calcium chelator used to lower serum calcium levels. A single IV dose of 10 to 15 μg/kg of body weight via slow infusion can lower serum calcium levels within 48 hours in most clients. The toxic effects, however, limit its use to two or three doses: thrombocytopenia and renal and hepatic toxicity can result after only one dose. The nurse and physician closely monitor liver function studies, blood urea nitrogen and creatinine, and the complete blood count (CBC), along with the serum calcium level. Another calcium chelator is penicillamine (Cuprimine, Pendramine✤).

➤ Surgical Management

Surgical management of hyperparathyroidism is accomplished by parathyroidectomy.

Preoperative Care. Before parathyroidectomy, the client is stabilized and calcium levels are decreased to near normal. If mithramycin has been used to lower serum calcium levels, the physician orders serologic studies to determine bleeding and coagulation times and a CBC to ascertain bone marrow function.

The nurse explains the surgical procedure and advises the client that coughing and deep-breathing exercises should be performed postoperatively and that talking may be painful for the first day or two postoperatively. The nurse demonstrates neck support by having the client place both hands behind the neck to assist in elevating the head.

Operative Procedure. Using general anesthesia with the client's neck hyperextended, the surgeon makes a transverse incision in the lower neck. After the muscles are retracted, both sides of the neck are examined to evaluate all four parathyroid glands. The surgeon visualizes the glands, starting on one side. If only one gland on that side is enlarged, a frozen section is done on both glands. If an adenoma is present in one and the other is normal, the surgeon removes the adenoma and leaves the other side intact.

Postoperative Care. The nurse observes the client for signs of respiratory distress, which may be due to compression of the trachea by hemorrhage or swelling of adjacent tissues. The nurse ensures that emergency equipment, including suction, oxygen, and tracheostomy equipment, is at the bedside. To preserve the airway, the surgeon may need to remove clips from the incision if severe swelling occurs. The nurse monitors vital signs, identifies any change in status, and checks the neck dressing for abnormal amounts of drainage or bleeding. Some serosanguineous drainage (1–5 mL) is normal.

The remaining glands, which may be nonfunctional as a result of PTH overproduction, require several days to several weeks to return to normal function. During this critical period, hypocalcemic crisis can occur. Immediately postoperatively, the serum calcium level is determined and levels are monitored every 4 hours until the initial calcium levels stabilize. The nurse monitors for signs and symptoms of hypocalcemia, such as tingling and twitching in the extremities and face. The nurse checks for Trousseau's and Chvostek's signs, either of which signal potential tetany (see Chap. 16).

Damage to the recurrent laryngeal nerve is rare; however, the nurse assesses the client for persistent changes in voice patterns and hoarseness.

When hyperparathyroidism is due to hyperplasia, usually three glands plus half of the fourth gland are removed; the remaining portion of the fourth gland is tagged to make it easy to find if future surgery is necessary. If all four glands are removed, a small portion of a gland may be implanted in the forearm, where it produces PTH and maintains calcium homeostasis. If all of these maneuvers fail, the client will need lifelong treatment with calcium and vitamin D because the resulting hypoparathyroidism is permanent.

Hypoparathyroidism

Overview

Hypoparathyroidism is an uncommon endocrine disorder. Pathologic findings are directly related to lack of PTH secretion or to decreased effectiveness of PTH on target tissue. Whether the problem is lack of PTH secretion or ineffectiveness of PTH on tissues, the result is the same: hypocalcemia.

Iatrogenic hypoparathyroidism, the most common form, is inadvertently caused by removal of all viable parathyroid tissue during total thyroidectomy or by surgical removal of hyperplastic parathyroid glands.

Idiopathic hypoparathyroidism is a rare condition that can occur spontaneously in children and adults. An autoimmune basis is suspected because antiparathyroid antibodies are present in a significant number of affected clients. In addition, hypoparathyroidism is often associated with the following autoimmune disorders: adrenal insufficiency, hypothyroidism, diabetes mellitus, pernicious anemia, gonadal failure, and vitiligo.

Hypomagnesemia may also cause hypoparathyroidism. Hypomagnesemia is seen in alcoholics and in those with malabsorption syndromes, certain renal diseases, and malnutrition. It causes impairment of PTH secretion and may interfere with PTH effects on target organs (bones and kidneys).

Resistance to PTH (pseudohypoparathyroidism) is a rare hereditary disorder characterized by unresponsiveness of bone, renal tubules, and intestines to PTH, resulting in hypocalcemia and elevated serum phosphate levels. The nurse may observe short stature; facial roundness; a short, thick neck; obesity; and shortened metacarpals and metatarsals, usually the fourth (Fig. 67–8). There may also be evidence of mild to moderate mental retardation.

Collaborative Management

 Assessment

The nurse begins assessment of the client with suspected hypoparathyroidism with a thorough history. The nurse asks about any head or neck surgery or radiation therapy, because these treatments contribute to the development of hypoparathyroidism. The nurse asks the client about the signs and symptoms of hypoparathyroidism, which may range in severity from mild paresthesias to tetany. Perioral tingling and numbness and tingling sensations in the hands and feet reflect mild to moderate hypocalcemia.

Severe muscle cramps, carpopedal spasms, and seizures (with no loss of consciousness or incontinence) reflect a more severe form of the disorder. The client or caregiver may notice mental changes ranging from irritability to frank psychosis.

Physical assessment may reveal characteristic metacarpal, phalangeal, carpal, and elbow flexion, which can signal an impending attack of tetany. The nurse checks for Chvostek's sign and Trousseau's sign; positive responses indicate potential tetany. A parkinsonian-like syndrome may be evident, and the nurse may discover cataracts, denoting chronic hypocalcemia. Bands or pits may encircle the crowns of the teeth, indicating enamel hypoplasia. The roots of the client's teeth may be defective.

Laboratory and other diagnostic tests include electroencephalography (EEG), blood tests, and computed tomography (CT). EEG changes are nonspecific and revert to normal with correction of hypocalcemia. Serum calcium, phosphate, magnesium, vitamin D, and urine cAMP levels may be used in the diagnostic work-up for hypoparathyroidism (see Chart 67–9). CT can show intracranial and basal ganglia calcification, which indicates chronic hypocalcemia.

 Interventions

Medical management of hypoparathyroidism focuses on immediate and long-term correction of hypocalcemia, vitamin D deficiency, and hypomagnesemia. For clients with acute and severe hypocalcemia, IV calcium is administered as a 10% solution of calcium chloride or calcium gluconate 10 to 15 minutes. Acute vitamin D deficiency is treated with calcitriol (Rocaltrol), 0.5 to 2.0 µg/day. Acute hypomagnesemia is corrected with 50% magnesium sulfate in 2-mL doses (up to 4 g/day) intramuscularly or IV. Long-term oral therapy for hypocalcemia involves administration of elemental calcium (0.5–2.0 g/day in divided doses) as lactate, gluconate, or carbonate.

Long-term oral therapy for vitamin D deficiency is 50,000 to 400,000 units of ergocalciferol daily. Dosage is adjusted to keep the client's calcium level in the low-normal range (slightly hypocalcemic), sufficient to prevent symptoms of hypocalcemia. It must also be low enough to prevent hypercalciuria, which can lead to stone formation.

Nursing management includes measures to ensure compliance with the prescribed medication regimen and to alleviate anxiety. The nurse encourages the client to eat foods high in calcium but low in phosphorus; the client is advised to avoid milk, yogurt, and processed cheeses because of their high phosphorus content. The nurse stresses that therapy for hypocalcemia is lifelong. The nurse advises the client of the necessity of some form of identification, such as a Medic-Alert bracelet or a wallet card. The client with severe hypocalcemia may be extremely anxious when leaving the protective atmosphere of the hospital or other facility. The nurse reassures the client that as long as he or she adheres to the prescribed regimen, the calcium level will remain sufficiently high to prevent any crisis.

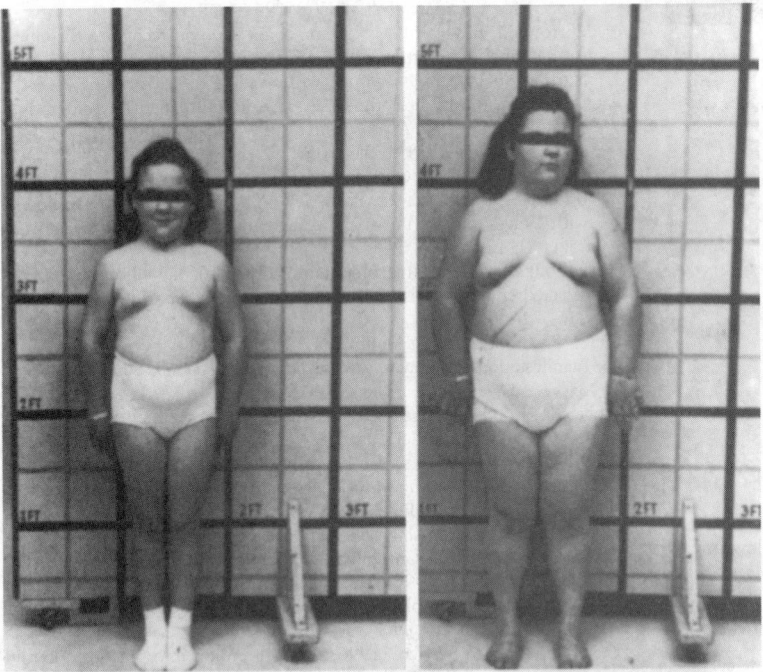

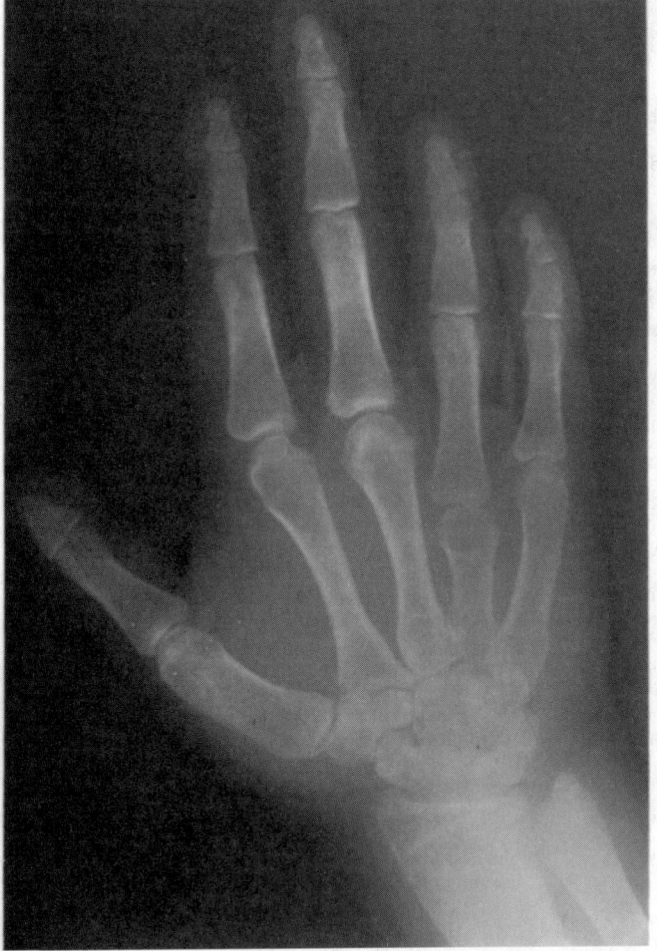

Figure 67–8. The clinical and radiographic features of pseudohypoparathyroidism. Note the short fourth finger in the x-ray.

CASE STUDY for the Client with Graves' Disease

■ A 36-year-old woman returns to your nursing unit after having a subtotal thyroidectomy for Graves' disease. Her vital signs are stable, but she is complaining of circumoral tingling.

QUESTIONS:

1. What laboratory data would you collect?
2. What additional physical assessment techniques would you perform?
3. What safety precautions would you institute?
4. What expected outcomes are specific to this situation?

SELECTED BIBLIOGRAPHY

American Cancer Society (1998). Cancer facts and figures—1998. Atlanta GA: Author, 98-300M-No. 5008.98.

Bartley, G. B., Fatourechi, V., Kadrmas, E. F., Jacobsen, S. J., Ilstrup, D. M., Garrity, J. A., & Gorman, C. A. (1996). Long-term follow-up of Graves ophthalmopathy in an incidence cohort. Ophthalmology, 103(6), 958–962.

Behnia, M., & Gharib, G. (1996). Primary care diagnosis of thyroid disease. Hospital Practice, June 15, 121–134.

Benson, J. W. (1995). Thyroid disorders. In D. Lemcke, J. Pattison, L. Marshall, & D. Cowley (Eds.), Primary care of women (pp. 149–160). Norwalk, CT: Appleton & Lange.

Bianchi, G. P., Marchesini, G., Gueli, C., & Zoli, M. (1995). Thyroid involvement in patients with active inflammatory bowel diseases. Italian Journal of Gastroenterology, 27(6), 291–295.

Coffland, F. I. (1994). Endocrine disorders affecting the cardiovascular system. Critical Care Nursing Clinics of North America, 6(4), 735–745.

Dunn, J. (1996) Seven deadly sins in confronting endemic iodine deficiency, and how to avoid them. Journal of Clinical Endocrinology and Metabolism, 81(4), 1332–1335.

Frizzell, J. (1998). Avoiding lab test pitfalls. American Journal of Nursing, 98(2), 34–37.

Gambert, S. R. (1995). Hyperthyroidism in the elderly. Clinics in Geriatric Medicine, 11(2), 181–188.

Gittoes, N. J., & Franklyn, J. A. (1995). Drug-induced thyroid disorders. Drug Safety, 13(1), 46–45.

Greenspan, F. S., & Baxter, J. D. (Eds.). (1994). Basic & clinical endocrinology (4th ed.). Norwalk, CT: Appleton & Lange.

Healy, P. F. (1995). Self-test. Caring for patients with endocrine disorders. Nursing, 25(9), 22.

Heitman, B., & Irizarry, A. (1995). Hypothyroidism: Common complaints, perplexing diagnosis. Nurse Practitioner, 20(3), 54–56, 58–60.

Jankowski, C. B. (1996). Irradiating the thyroid: How to protect yourself and others. American Journal of Nursing, 96(10), 50–54.

Kahaly, G., Hellermann, J., Mohr-Kahaly, S., & Treese, N. (1996). Impaired cardiopulmonary exercise capacity in patients with hyperthyroidism. Chest, 109(1), 57–61.

Kallner, G., Vitols, S., & Ljunggren, J. G. (1996). Comparison of standardized initial doses of two antithyroid drugs in the treatment of Graves' disease. Journal of Internal Medicine, 239(6), 525–529.

Kelley, W. (Ed.). (1997). Textbook of internal medicine (3rd ed.). Philadelphia: Lippincott-Raven.

Kennedy, L. W., & Caro, J. F. (1996). The ABCs of managing hyperthyroidism in the older patient. Geriatrics, 51(5), 22–24, 27, 31, 32.

Kung, A. W., Pang, R. W., & Janus, E. D. (1995). Elevated serum lipoprotein(a) in subclinical hypothyroidism. Clinical Endocrinology-Oxford, 43(4), 445–449.

Liel, Y., Harman-Boehm, I., & Shany, S. (1996). Evidence for a clinically important adverse effect of fiber-enriched diet on the bioavailability of levothyroxine in adult hypothyroid patients. Journal of Clinical Endocrinology and Metabolism, 81(2), 857–859.

McMorrow, M. E. (1996). Myxedema coma: Do you recognize the clues to this rare complication of hypothyroidism? American Journal of Nursing, 96(10), 55.

Mowschenson, P. M., & Hodin, R. A. (1995). Outpatient thyroid and parathyroid surgery: A prospective study of feasibility, safety, and costs. Surgery, 118(6), 1051–1053.

Ofosu, M. H., Dunston, G., Henry, L., Ware, D., Cheatham, W., Brembridge, A., Brown, C., & Alarif, L. (1996). HLA-DQ3 is associated with Graves' disease in African-Americans. Immunologic Investigation, 25(1–2), 103–110.

Rusterholtz, A. (1996). Interpretation of diagnostic laboratory tests in selected endocrine disorders. Nursing Clinics of North America, 31(4), 715–724.

Sauer, P., Brandes, B., & Mahmarian, R. R. (1995). Lower extremity manifestations of Graves' disease. Journal of Foot and Ankle Surgery, 34(5), 489–497.

Singer, P., Cooper, D., Levy, E., Ladenson, P., Braverman, L., Daniels, G., Greenspan, F., McDougall, R., & Nikolai, T. (1995). Treatment guidelines for patients with hyperthyroidism and hypothyroidism. Journal of the American Medical Association, 273(10), 808–813.

Streff, M., & Pachucki-Hyde, L. (1996). Management of the patient with thyroid disease. Nursing Clinics of North America, 31(4), 779–796.

Trivalle, C., Doucet, J., Chassangne, P., Landrin, I., Kadri, N., Menard, J. F., & Bercoff, E. (1996). Differences in the signs and symptoms of hyperthyroidism in older and younger patients. Journal of the American Geriatric Society, 44(1), 50–53.

U.S. Public Health Service. (1996). Put prevention into practice: Thyroid function. Journal of the American Academy of Nurse Practitioners, 8(10), 495–496.

Wartofsky, L. (1996). The scope and impact of thyroid disease. Clinical Chemistry, 42(1), 121–124.

SELECTED READINGS

Jankowski, C. B. (1996). Irradiating the thyroid: How to protect yourself and others. American Journal of Nursing, 96(10), 51–54.
   This article discusses the indications for iodine-131 treatment and important client and family education. Iodine 131 is used to treat hyperthyroidism resulting from many diseases but most frequently Graves' disease. Some precautions for clients and their families is to limit prolonged exposure to the person being treated with iodine 131, especially children and pregnant women. Also discussed are precautions that nurses and other staff caring for a client must exercise to not exceed the recommended exposure to radiation.

McMorrow, M. E. (1996). Myxedema coma: Do you recognize the clues to this rare complication of hypothyroidism? American Journal of Nursing, 96(10), 55.
   This brief article discusses the emergent nature of myxedemic coma and how to recognize the clues. It is presented in a case study format with supporting pathophysiology.

Streff, M., & Pachucki-Hyde, L. (1996). Management of the patient with thyroid disease. Nursing Clinics of North America, 31(4), 779–796.
   This excellent article provides a comprehensive overview of the physiology, pathology, and treatment of hypo-and hyperthyroidism. Client history, assessment findings, and laboratory findings for each problem are discussed in depth.

U.S. Public Health Service. (1996). Put prevention into practice: Thyroid function. Journal of the American Academy of Nurse Practitioners, 8(10), 495–496.
   This article presents the recommendations of major authorities, such as the American Academy of Family Physicians and the American College of Physicians, regarding screening for thyroid disease in high-risk populations. It discusses the basics of thyroid function screening and describes the implications of the results.

INTERVENTIONS FOR CLIENTS WITH DIABETES

Diabetes mellitus is a common chronic disease affecting many body organs and systems. The nurse encounters clients of all ages with diabetes in all clinical settings, including outpatient and home settings. Often, the client's reason for hospital admission is a complication, or sequela, of diabetes. The interdisciplinary team approach, with central client involvement, is utilized to manage the client's health care. The nurse plans, organizes, and coordinates care among the various health disciplines involved; provides care and education; and promotes the client's health and well-being.

OVERVIEW

Diabetes mellitus has various forms, but all are characterized by insulin deficiency leading to disturbances in carbohydrate, protein, and lipid metabolism. Diabetes mellitus refers to disorders characterized by fasting hyperglycemia or blood glucose levels above defined limits. Diabetes can be life threatening, and in the adult population of the United States it is the seventh leading cause of death (Centers for Disease Control and Prevention [CDC],

1997). Diabetes mellitus is a major risk factor for morbidity and mortality due to coronary disease, cerebrovascular disease, and peripheral vascular disease. The prevalence of these three macrovascular complications is increased two to four times in the diabetic population. These complications are responsible for most of the hospitalizations due to diabetes and account substantially for the $20.4 billion spent annually for diabetes care in the United States.

Although no cure has yet been found, great progress has been made in controlling and managing diabetes. Advances in methods for self-monitoring of blood glucose levels, improved medications, and the formulation of improved nutrition, diet, and exercise guidelines all contribute to extending longevity and improving the quality of life of the diabetic client.

PATHOPHYSIOLOGY
Classification of Diabetes

Diabetes mellitus is classified according to the etiology, presentation, and pathophysiology of the disease. Diabetes mellitus is a disease with insulin-secretion and insulin-

TABLE 68–1

Classification of Diabetes Mellitus

Type 1 Diabetes

- Primary beta-cell destruction leading to absolute insulin deficiency
  - Autoimmune process
  - Idiopathic

Type 2 Diabetes

- Results from insulin resistance with an insulin secretory deficit

Other Specific Types

- Genetic defects of beta-cell function
- Genetic defects in insulin action
- Diseases of the exocrine pancreas such as pancreatitis, trauma, neoplasia, cystic fibrosis, hemochromatosis
- Endocrinopathies such as acromegaly, Cushing's disease, glucagonoma, pheochromotoma, hyperthyroidism, aldosteronoma
- Drug or chemical induced (pentamidine, nicotinic acid, glucocorticoids, thyroid hormone, diazoxide, beta-adrenergic agonists, thiazides, Dilantin, interferon-alpha, others)
- Infections: congenital rubella, cytomegalovirus
- Uncommon forms of immune-related diabetes
- Other genetic syndromes associated with diabetes: Down syndrome, Klinefelter syndrome, Turner syndrome, Huntington's chorea, and others

Gestational Diabetes Mellitus (GDM)

- Carbohydrate intolerance is first recognized during pregnancy
- Children of mothers with GDM are at great risk for neonatal mortality, congenital malformation, and macrosomia (large body size)
- Studies indicate that children of mothers with GDM have an increased risk of obesity and impaired glucose tolerance later in life
- Clients with GDM are at high risk for developing diabetes after pregnancy
- Diagnosis is based on the results of a 100-g oral glucose tolerance test during pregnancy

From American Diabetes Association. (1998a). Position statement: Screening for diabetes. *Diabetes Care, 21*(suppl 1), S20–22; and American Diabetes Association. (1998h). Position statement: Gestational diabetes. *Diabetes Care, 21*(suppl 1), S60–61.

receptor pathology. Table 68–1 outlines the different types of diabetes.

Insulin Physiology

Insulin is an anabolic endocrine hormone made in the beta cells of the islets of Langerhans in the pancreas. Insulin plays a key role in allowing cells of the body to store and utilize carbohydrate, fat, and protein. Several crucial cellular activities that alter the permeability of cell membranes are affected by insulin. Insulin also acts as a catalyst to stimulate the enzymes and chemicals necessary for energy production.

Insulin is formed from *proinsulin,* a precursor that in-

cludes alpha and beta chains, and a peptide fragment designated the C-peptide chain. During the intracellular transport of proinsulin to secretion granules, proinsulin is slowly cleaved to yield insulin and C-peptide (Fig. 68–1). Both insulin and C-peptide are stored in secretion granules. The measurement of C-peptide levels gives an indication of pancreatic beta cell secretory activity.

Several stimuli, including the presence of glucose, are responsible for the regulation of insulin secretion. Insulin is secreted into portal circulation in a biphasic manner. There is an early burst of insulin within 10 minutes of eating, followed by a progressively increasing phase of insulin release that persists as long as the hyperglycemic stimulus is present.

Glucose Homeostasis

The central nervous system depends on glucose as its primary fuel. Because the brain cannot synthesize or store significant amounts of glucose, a continuous supply from the body's circulation is needed. Glucose is the principal carbohydrate used for energy. The principal circulating

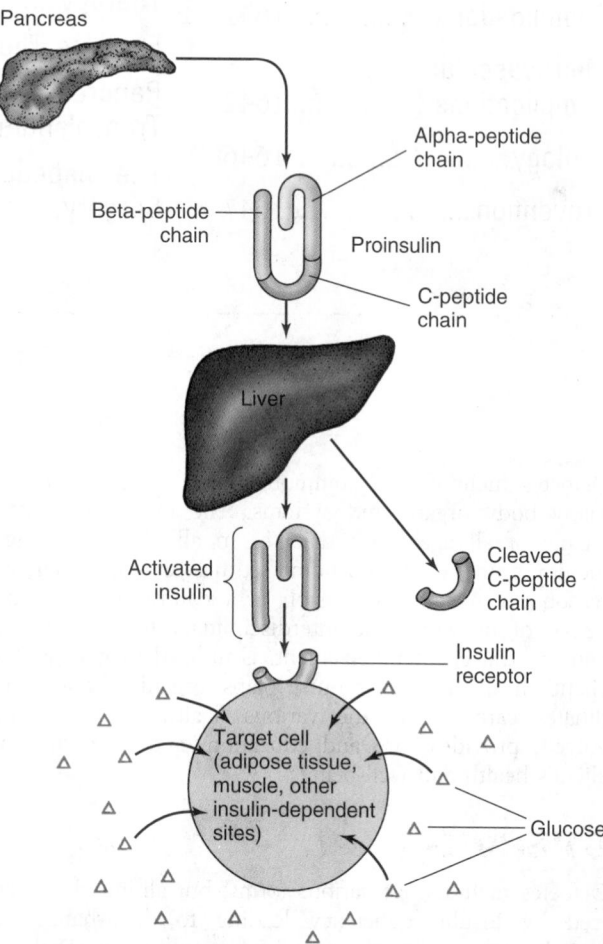

Figure 68–1. Proinsulin, secreted by and stored in the beta cells of the islets of Langerhans in the pancreas, is transformed by the liver into activated insulin. Insulin attaches to receptors on target cells, where it promotes glucose transport into the cells through the cell membranes.

fuels, glucose and free fatty acids, are stored intracellularly as glycogen in the liver and muscles and as triglycerides in adipose tissue. Although protein can be degraded to provide amino acid substrate during periods of starvation, protein is not considered a fuel reservoir.

For adults under the age of 60, the combined actions of insulin and counterregulatory hormones (discussed below) maintain blood glucose within the range of 74 mg/dL (4.1 mmol/L) to 106 mg/dL (5.9 mmol/L) to supply glucose for central nervous system functions. Counterregulatory hormones liberate energy from fuel sources by actions opposite to insulin. Glucagon is the primary counterregulatory hormone and acts by stimulating hepatic glucose production. In type 1 diabetes, glucagon secretion in response to hypoglycemia is lost. This process places the diabetic client in danger of severe hypoglycemic reactions. Additional counterregulatory hormones are catecholamines (epinephrine and norepinephrine), growth hormone, and cortisol.

Absence of Insulin

The lack of insulin in diabetes, either from lack of insulin secretion or from insulin-receptor pathology, prevents insulin-sensitive cells from using glucose as an energy source. Insulin is needed to supply glucose to most of the body's tissues. Without insulin, the body enters a serious state of catabolism. Levels of counterregulatory hormones increase in an attempt to increase the availability of glucose from alternative sources. Table 68–2 outlines the body's response to insufficient insulin.

Without insulin, glucose builds up in the blood, and hyperglycemia results. Hyperglycemia causes a series of fluid and electrolyte imbalances, ultimately resulting in the classic symptoms of diabetes

- Polyuria
- Polydipsia
- Polyphagia

Polyuria (frequent and excessive urination) results from an osmotic diuresis caused by excess excretion of glucose in the urine. As a result of diuresis, sodium chloride and potassium are excreted in the urine in large amounts, accompanied by severe water loss. The resulting dehydration stimulates the thirst mechanism, and polydipsia (excessive thirst) occurs. Because the cells are not receiving any food (glucose), the starvation mechanism results in polyphagia (excessive eating). In spite of ingesting vast amounts of food, the person remains in a state of starvation until adequate amounts of insulin are available to facilitate the movement of glucose into the cells.

When the cells cannot take up glucose as fuel to use for energy generation, alternative fuel sources are used. Conversion of free fatty acids to *ketone bodies* provides a backup energy source. Because ketone bodies (ketones) represent incomplete (and abnormal) degradation products of free fatty acids, they are not further metabolized and may accumulate in the blood and other extracellular fluids when insulin is not available.

Ketones are acid products, and, when ketones accumulate in the blood, acidosis occurs. Urinary excretion of ketones necessitates neutralization by bicarbonate, which generally is available in the body in the form of sodium bicarbonate. Increased urinary excretion of sodium, however, prevents the formation of further bicarbonate, the principal blood buffer for carbonic acid.

Because of the dehydration associated with diabetes mellitus, hemoconcentration and hypovolemia develop, which lead to hyperviscosity and hypoperfusion of tissues, resulting in lactic acidosis and even further contributing to the acidosis. Hypoxic cells are unable to metabolize glucose efficiently; the tricarboxylic acid (Krebs) cycle is blocked; and lactate accumulates. Restoration of tissue perfusion and oxygenation by treating the underlying disorder is essential in halting the production of lactate.

The body attempts to buffer the effects of increasing acidosis. Normal renal mechanisms for acid excretion and bicarbonate conservation become overwhelmed. The increased concentrations of both hydrogen ions and carbon dioxide stimulate the respiratory control areas of the brain to increase the rate and depth of respiration in an attempt to excrete more acid. This type of breathing is known as *Kussmaul's respiration*. Acetone is exhaled, giving the breath a "fruity" odor. When the lungs can no longer offset acidosis, the pH drops. Arterial blood gas studies show the resultant primary metabolic acidosis (decreased arterial bicarbonate [HCO_3] levels) and compensatory respiratory alkalosis (decreased arterial carbon dioxide pressure [$PaCO_2$]). Restoration of pH to a normal level is an essential aspect of therapy.

The absence of insulin causes total body potassium depletion. Because of the increased loss of fluids from hyperglycemia, excessive potassium is excreted in the urine, leading to *low* serum potassium levels. However, *high* serum potassium levels may occur in acidosis because of the shift of potassium from the intracellular to the extracellular fluid compartment. Serum potassium levels in diabetes, then, may be low (hypokalemia), elevated (hyperkalemia), or even normal, depending on the state of hydration, the severity of the acidosis, and the client's response to treatment.

Other minerals, such as calcium, magnesium, and phosphates, are lost in the urine as well. However, the consequences to the body's functioning from these losses are less immediate and less life threatening than those mentioned above.

TABLE 68–2

Physiologic Response to Insufficient Insulin

Decreased glycogenesis (conversion of glucose to glycogen)
Increased glycogenolysis (production of glucose from glycogen)
Increased gluconeogenesis (formation of glucose from noncarbohydrate sources, stimulated by glucocorticoids)
Decreased glycolysis (breakdown of glucose to carbon dioxide and water)
Increased lipolysis (breakdown of fats to ketones, an alternative energy source)

Acute Complications of Diabetes

Three emergencies related to major deviations from normal blood glucose level occur in clients who have diabetes:

- Diabetic ketoacidosis (DKA) is associated with insulin deficiency and ketosis.
- Hyperglycemic hyperosmolar nonketotic syndrome (HHNS) is associated with insulin deficiency, profound dehydration, and the absence of ketosis.
- Hypoglycemia occurs in conditions of insulin excess.

All three conditions need emergency treatment and can result in death if inappropriately treated or not treated at all.

Diabetic Ketoacidosis

DKA occurs in 2% to 5% of all clients with type 1 diabetes mellitus per year. DKA is most often precipitated by concurrent illness, particularly infection. Death can be due to failure or delay in diagnosis, complications such as hypokalemia, or precipitating conditions. Death still occurs in 1% to 10% of these clients. Mortality is highest for clients older than 60 years of age. Most of the deaths in elderly clients occur when the client has a concurrent disease, such as infection, cerebrovascular accident, myocardial infarction, vascular thrombosis, intestinal obstruction, or pneumonia along with DKA.

Metabolic derangements of DKA (Fig. 68–2) result from absolute or relative insulin deficiency combined with the action of counterregulatory hormones. Laboratory diagnosis of DKA is shown in Table 68–3.

DKA is preceded by polyuria, polydipsia, and polyphagia. Central nervous system depression results in changes in consciousness varying from lethargy to coma. Physical examination reveals evidence of dehydration; evaluation of vital signs and hemodynamic monitoring parameters reveals evidence of profound fluid loss. Kussmaul's respiration, abdominal pain, nausea, and vomiting are associated with metabolic acidosis. Initial serum sodium levels may be reduced or within normal limits. The initial potassium levels depend on how long DKA has existed before treatment. After therapy is initiated, serum potassium levels begin to drop quickly. Serum leukocyte counts of 20,000 cells/mm indicate dehydration; counts greater than 30,000 cells/mm may indicate infection. Treatment of DKA is covered later under Potential for Ketoacidosis.

Once DKA has been treated, efforts are directed toward educating the diabetic client about maintenance of target blood glucose levels. Statistics indicate that 80% of the cases of DKA occur in diabetics who are not newly diagnosed (Fish, 1994). This incidence highlights the need to educate the diabetic client about DKA prevention and treatment.

Hyperglycemic Hyperosmolar Nonketotic Syndrome

HHNS is a hyperosmolar state resulting from hyperglycemia of various causes. The resultant pathophysiologic pro-

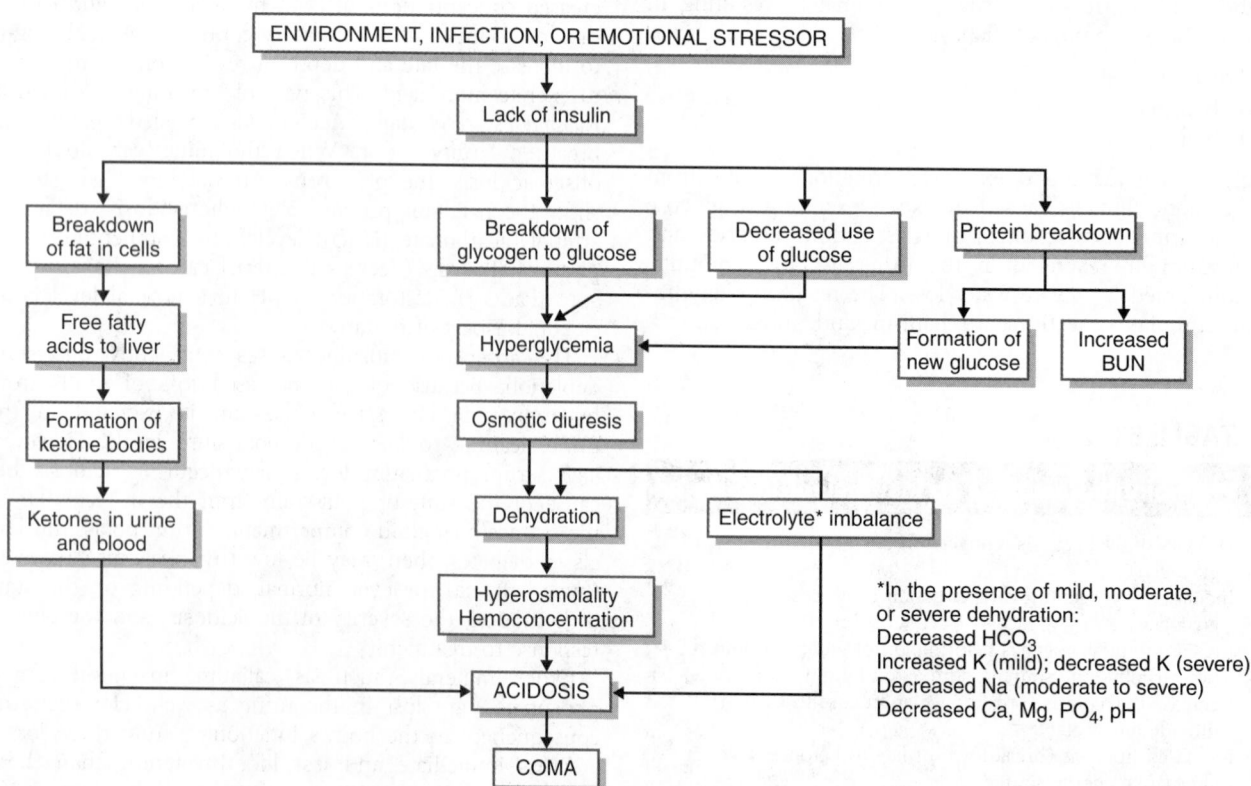

Figure 68–2. The pathophysiologic mechanism of diabetic ketoacidosis.

TABLE 68–3

Differences Between Diabetic Ketoacidosis (DKA) and Hyperglycemic Hyperosmolar Nonketotic Syndrome (HHNS)		
	DKA	**HHNS**
Onset	• Sudden	• Gradual
Precipitating factors	• Infection • Other stressors • Inadequate insulin dose	• Infection • Other stressors • Poor fluid intake
Manifestations	• Ketosis: Kussmaul's respirations (with a "fruity" or sweet smell), nausea, abdominal pain • Dehydration or electrolyte loss; polyuria; polydipsia; weight loss; dry skin; sunken, soft eyeballs; lethargy; coma	• Altered central nervous system function with neurologic symptoms • Dehydration/electrolyte loss: Same as for DKA.
Monitoring variables	• ECG: Hyperkalemia: Peaked T waves, widened QRS complex, prolonged PR interval, flattened or absent P wave • Hypokalemia: Depressed ST segment, flat or inverted T waves, presence of U wave, increased ventricular dysrhythmia	• ECG evidence of hypokalemia as listed with DKA
Laboratory Findings		
Serum glucose	>300 mg/dL (16.7 mmol/L)	>800 mg/dL (44.5 mmol/L)
Osmolality	Variable	>350 mOsm/L
Serum ketones	Positive at 1–2 dilutions	Negative
Serum pH	<7.38	>7.4
Serum HCO_3^-	<15 mEq/L	>20 mEq/L
Serum Na^+	<137 mEq/L	Elevated, normal or low
Serum K^+	Normal Elevated with acidosis Low following hydration	Normal or low
BUN	>20 mg/dL	Elevated
Creatinine	>1.5 mg/dL	Elevated
Urine ketones	Positive	Negative

cesses are outlined in Figure 68–3. HHNS is differentiated from DKA by the absence of significant ketosis and by the presence of higher than average plasma glucose levels and osmolality. By definition, plasma glucose levels should be greater than 800 mg/dL (44.5 mmol/L) and osmolality should be greater than 350 mOsm/L for a diagnosis of HHNS. The biochemical disturbances with HHNS tend to be more severe than those with DKA. Table 68–3 outlines the differences between DKA and HHNS.

HHNS occurs predominately in elderly individuals and almost exclusively in people with type 2 diabetes mellitus, 35% of whom were previously undiagnosed. Mortality rates in elderly clients have been as high as 40% to 70%.

HHNS does not occur in adequately hydrated individuals. Elderly clients with diabetes are at greater risks for dehydration and subsequent HHNS. Because of age-related changes in thirst perception and loss of taste buds and because of poorer urine-concentrating abilities related to aging, elderly clients are more liable to become dehydrated with the onset of concurrent illness. The onset of HHNS is insidious. The elderly client typically seeks medical attention later and is sicker than the younger client.

Conditions such as silent myocardial infarction, sepsis, pancreatitis, and stroke and drugs such as glucocorticoids, diuretics, phenytoin sodium (Dilantin), propranolol (Inderal), and calcium channel blockers may precipitate HHNS. Central nervous system (CNS) findings range from confusion to complete coma. In contrast to clients with DKA, clients with HHNS may present with generalized focal seizures, myoclonic jerking, and reversible hemiparesis.

The development of HHNS rather than DKA in a particular client is thought to be related to residual insulin secretion. The client secretes enough insulin in HHNS to prevent ketosis but not enough to prevent hyperglycemia. The hyperglycemia of HHNS is more severe than that of DKA and results in significant serum hyperosmolality and profound osmotic diuresis. Severe dehydration and electrolyte loss occur; the client may lose 15% to 25% of body fluid. Renal impairment results because of reduced renal blood flow. Glucose, then, is not filtered into the urine and causes even greater hyperglycemia and hyperosmolality. Impairment of the thirst center in the hypothalmus occurs, making it impossible for the client to drink enough fluid to prevent dehydration.

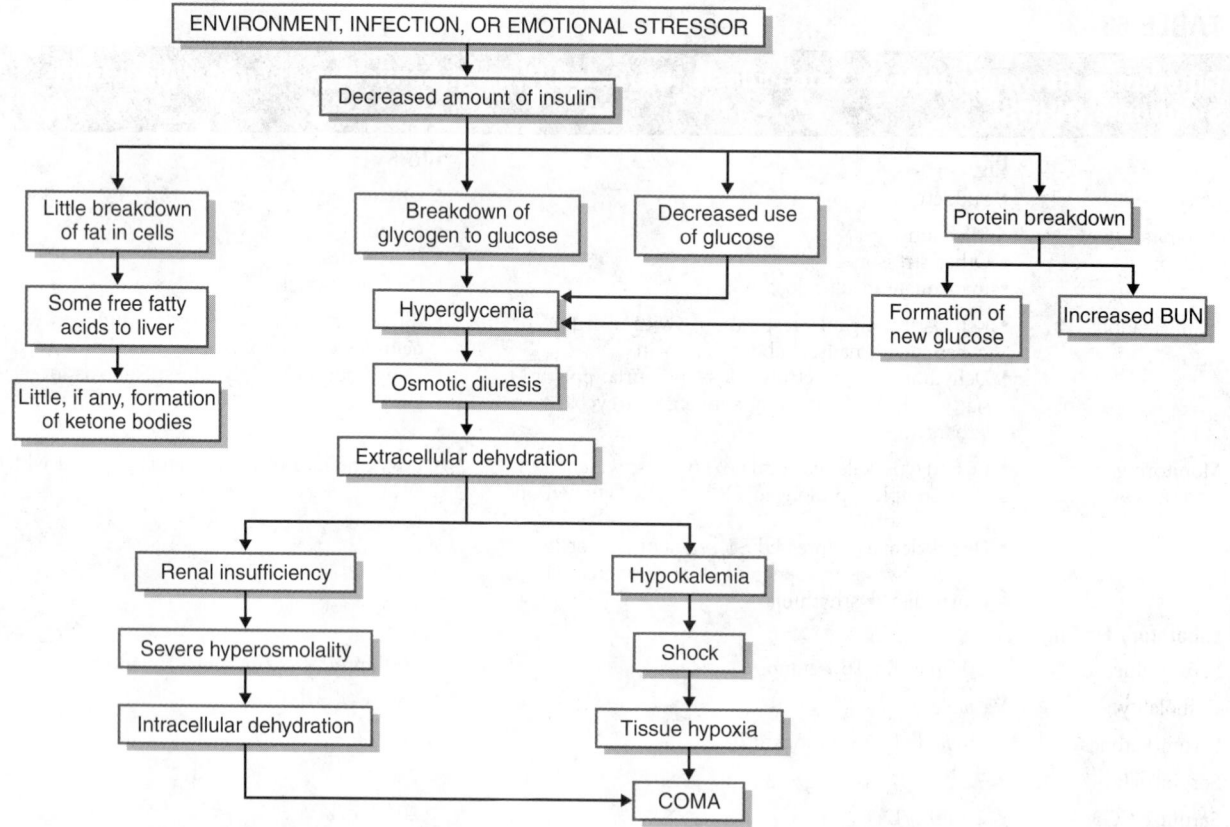

Figure 68–3. The pathophysiologic mechanism of hyperglycemic hyperosmolar nonketotic syndrome.

Hypoglycemia

Preservation of central nervous system function depends on a continuous supply of glucose from circulation. The brain cannot synthesize glucose and stores only a few minutes' supply as glycogen. This continuous supply of glucose cannot be maintained when plasma glucose concentration falls below critical levels.

The first defense against falling plasma glucose in the nondiabetic client is decreased insulin secretion, which normally occurs at a glycemic threshold around 83 mg/dL (4.5 mmol/L). Critical glucose counterregulatory hormones are activated around 68 mg/dL (3.8 mmol/L), a glycemic threshold well above the level for symptoms of hypoglycemia. The primary counterregulatory hormone is glucagon; epinephrine also becomes important when glucagon levels are deficient. Both glucagon and epinephrine raise plasma glucose concentrations by stimulating hepatic glycogenolysis and gluconeogenesis. In addition, epinephrine limits secretion of insulin. Growth hormone and cortisol act largely to limit glucose utilization.

Type 1 diabetes mellitus is characterized by marked abnormalities in the counterregulatory response to hypoglycemia. These changes are evident within 1 to 5 years of diagnosis. Regulation of circulating insulin levels is lost because the source of insulin is the subcutaneous injection site rather than the pancreas. As plasma glucose concentrations fall, insulin levels do not decrease. The ability of alpha cells of the pancreas to secrete glucagon in response to hypoglycemia is lost in individuals with long-standing diabetes. After a few more years of type 1 diabetes, epinephrine response to falling glucose concentrations is also reduced. Epinephrine responses will occur, but at a lower plasma glucose concentration. Diabetic individuals with combined deficiencies of glucagon and epinephrine responses to falling glucose have been found to have a 25-fold increased risk for severe hypoglycemia.

A second syndrome of compromised glucose counterregulation of type 1 diabetes is *hypoglycemic unawareness*. Clients with this syndrome no longer have warning symptoms of impending hypoglycemia that prompt them to take appropriate preventive action. Hypoglycemic unawareness is reported to occur in 50% of all clients with very long-standing (>30 years) type 1 diabetes and in an estimated 25% of clients overall. Hypoglycemic unawareness is thought to be due to the loss of the neurogenic symptoms of impending hypoglycemia.

Symptoms of hypoglycemia are divided into two categories. *Neuroglycopenic* symptoms result directly from brain glucose deprivation and are associated with a more gradual decline in blood glucose. *Neurogenic* symptoms result from autonomic nervous system discharge triggered by hypoglycemia and are associated with an abrupt decline in blood glucose (Table 68–4). Awareness of hypoglycemia is largely the result of perception of neurogenic symptoms.

Clinical severity of hypoglycemia correlates poorly with biochemical measures. Blood glucose levels that elicit symptoms of hypoglycemia vary among diabetic clients.

TABLE 68-4

Symptoms of Hypoglycemia

Neuroglycopenic	Neurogenic
Headache	Adrenergic
Confusion	Shaky/tremulous
Slurred speech	Heart pounding
Behavior changes	Nervous/anxious
Coma	Cholinergic
	Sweaty
	Hungry
	Tingling

Many clients with diabetes identify hypoglycemic symptoms when blood glucose levels are well above 50 mg/dL (2.8 mmol/L), especially if the level has dropped rapidly or if they are accustomed to sustained hyperglycemia. A categorization has been developed to classify hypoglycemia based on clinical rather than biochemical criteria. In cases of mild hypoglycemia, the client with diabetes remains totally alert and is able to treat symptoms. In cases of severe hypoglycemia, neurologic function is so impaired that the assistance of another person is needed for treatment (Peragallo-Dittko et al., 1993).

Chronic Complications of Diabetes

Diabetes mellitus is a major risk factor for morbidity and mortality because of macro- and microvascular complications. *Macrovascular* complications, including coronary heart disease, peripheral vascular disease, and cerebrovascular disease, are responsible for higher mortality rates for diabetic individuals than for the general population. *Microvascular* complications include nephropathy, neuropathy, and retinopathy and involve abnormalities of vessel wall structure and function. Tissues of the retina, kidney, and nerves are all freely permeable to glucose. Three theories have been developed to explain pathogenesis of diabetic vascular complications:

- Chronic hyperglycemia produces irreversible changes in structural and functional proteins resulting in basement membrane thickening, altered extracellular matrix, and loss of functional protein properties leading to organ damage.
- Glucose toxicity directly or indirectly affects functional cell integrity.
- Chronic ischemia in microcirculatory branches results in connective tissue hypoxia and microischemia.

Strong evidence supports the association between chronic hyperglycemia and development of microvascular complications. The association between blood glucose control and macrovascular complications is less clear. The development of macrovascular complications seems more related to factors of hypertension, sedentary lifestyle, lipid abnormalities, and smoking than it does to hyperglycemia. The additional risk factor of obesity is important for people with type 2 diabetes: 80% of clients with type 2 diabetes are obese, and cardiovascular events account for most of their fatalities. Hypertension occurs with increasing frequency with advancing age and is estimated to be responsible for 30% to 70% of diabetic complications (American Diabetes Association [ADA], 1996g).

The National Diabetes Data Group of the National Institutes of Health estimates that the onset of type 2 diabetes may occur 9 to 12 years before clinical diagnosis. During the time that diabetes is not being treated, complications are developing. In one study of type 2 diabetics, up to 21% were found to have retinopathy at the time of first diagnosis (ADA, 1998e). Many elderly diabetic clients do not develop classic signs of hyperglycemia. In these persons, diagnosis of diabetes is made when the person presents for treatment of diabetic complications.

The Diabetes Control and Complications Trial, a prospective study involving 29 medical centers and more than 1400 people with type 1 diabetes, provides convincing evidence that hyperglycemia is a critical factor in the pathogenesis of long-term diabetic complications (Nathan, 1996). Results indicate a 60% reduction in risk between the intensive and standard treatment groups in diabetic retinopathy, nephropathy, and neuropathy. Intensive therapy resulted in delay in onset and a major slowing of progression of these three complications. Clients in the group receiving intensive treatment had a mean blood glucose level of less than 155 mg/dL (8.6 mmol/L) and hemoglobin A1c (HbA1c) concentration of 7.2% (ADA, 1998j).

Similar results were obtained in studies of individuals with type 2 diabetes. The Wisconsin Epidemiologic Study of Diabetic Retinopathy correlated levels of glycated hemoglobin with microvascular complications: The incidence of diabetic neuropathy was higher in subjects with higher baseline levels of HbA1c. A study conducted in Japan among individuals with type 2 diabetes indicated there was no progression of retinopathy or neuropathy with HbA1c levels less than 6.5% (Shamoon, 1996).

Macrovascular Complications
Cardiovascular Disease

Cardiovascular disease is two to four times more common in diabetic than nondiabetic clients. Sixty percent of all diabetic hospitalizations are for treatment of cardiac complications, and up to 75% of deaths are attributed to ischemic heart disease or other heart and vascular diseases. Diabetic clients have increases in both incidence of and fatality rates from acute myocardial infarction and have more extensive disease. Autopsy studies indicated that diabetic individuals have a higher incidence of two- and three-vessel disease and a lower incidence of one-vessel disease than do nondiabetic individuals (Raman & Nesto, 1996). Diabetic clients tend to have a greater risk for congestive heart failure, recurrent infarction, dysrhythmias, and cardiogenic shock and have decreased survival rates once discharged from the hospital. The Multiple Risk Factor Intervention Trial (MRFIT) showed that the presence of hypertension, smoking, or lipid abnormalities with diabetes exaggerated the incidence of cardiovascular disease and mortality (Tschoepe, 1995).

Cardiovascular disease risk factors are commonly found in association with type 2 diabetes, in part related to obesity. Diabetes is often associated with elevated blood pressure. Dyslipidemia, especially hypertriglyceridemia and low levels of high-density lipoprotein cholesterol, is common. Several hemostatic abnormalities involving levels of coagulation factors, platelet dysfunction, and increased blood viscosity are found. The clustering of blood pressure, lipid, and hemostatic abnormalities occurs more often in the diabetic population (Savage, 1996). In addition to being an early indication of nephropathy, albuminuria is a marker of increased cardiovascular morbidity in both type 1 and type 2 diabetes. The finding of microalbuminuria is an indication for screening for vascular disease and aggressive intervention to reduce cardiovascular risk factors (ADA, 1998d).

Diabetes is considered a risk factor for cardiovascular disease. Results from the Honolulu Heart Study indicate that even mild, asymptomatic abnormalities in glucose tolerance increased risk for cardiovascular disease (Savage, 1996). A study conducted in Finland found a significant increase in the risk of coronary heart disease death and all coronary heart disease events in type 2 diabetes subjects with higher levels of hemoglobin A1c than diabetic subjects with lower hemoglobin A1c levels (Kuusisto et al., 1994).

Peripheral Vascular Disease

Peripheral vascular disease is a common complication in diabetes. In diabetes, peripheral arterial disease (PAD) is more common, occurs in younger persons, and progresses more rapidly than in the nondiabetic person. The composition of the atherosclerotic plaque is not different for diabetic versus nondiabetic individuals; however, there are differences in distribution of PAD that have significance for circulation in the lower extremities. Occlusions tend to involve anterior tibial, posterior tibial, and peroneal arteries (LoGerfo & Gibbons, 1996). Arteries supplying the foot (i.e., the dorsalis pedis) tend not to be involved as often.

The status of circulation to the lower extremities is important as it relates to healing of foot ulcers. Diabetic clients with peripheral vascular disease are at risk for amputation. Gangrene, followed by amputation, is 10 to 20 times more likely to occur in diabetic clients.

Cerebrovascular Disease

Diabetes is an established risk factor for atherothrombotic brain infarction. It is second only to hypertension as a major risk factor for stroke, and as many as 25% of clients dying with diabetes have autopsy findings of cerebrovascular disease (Harati, 1996). The presence of other risk factors, such as hyperlipidemia, hypertension, coronary artery disease, nephropathy, peripheral vascular disease, and alcohol and tobacco abuse, substantially increases the risk for stroke. The risk is highest in the female population and greatest for both males and females in their 50s and 60s.

Elevated blood glucose levels at the time of stroke are associated with increased neurologic injury. Studies show that clients with admission serum glucose levels greater

than 120 mg/dL (6.7 mmol/L) have higher morbidity and mortality rates from stroke. Blood glucose fluctuations occurring during acute illness do not seem to affect morbidity as much as does overall blood glucose control.

The physician and nurse carefully evaluate every diabetic client with altered consciousness and a stroke-like syndrome. Hypoglycemia can cause acute neurologic changes and seizure with resultant transient hemiplegia. Focal neurologic findings that disappear with correction of dehydration and hyperglycemia (i.e., seizures and hemiparesis) are features of hyperosmolar nonketotic diabetic syndrome (Bell, 1994).

Microvascular Complications
Ocular Complications

Legal blindness, defined as a corrected visual acuity of 20/200 or less, is 25 times more common in clients with diabetes. In the United States, diabetic retinopathy is the most frequent cause of new cases of blindness among 20- to 74-year-old adults. After 20 years of diabetes, nearly all clients with type 1 diabetes and 60% of those with type 2 diabetes have some degree of retinopathy (ADA, 1998e).

Two major retinal problems cause most of the diabetes-related vision loss: diabetic macular edema and complications from retinal neovascularization. Diabetic macular edema is characterized by edematous thickening of the macula (area of the retina responsible for central vision), which leads to blurred vision. Thickening involving the center of the macula is associated with a high degree of vision loss. With neovascularization, abnormal blood vessels and fibrous tissue "proliferate" from the retina. These vessels may bleed into vitreous fluid, reducing vision.

The pathogenesis of diabetic retinopathy is thought to be related to abnormal vascular permeability, microvascular occlusion, and retinal hypoxia. Nonproliferative retinopathy (NPDR) is caused by years of diabetic vascular damage and has several characteristic features (Fig. 68–4). Hard exudates are lipid or lipoprotein deposits in

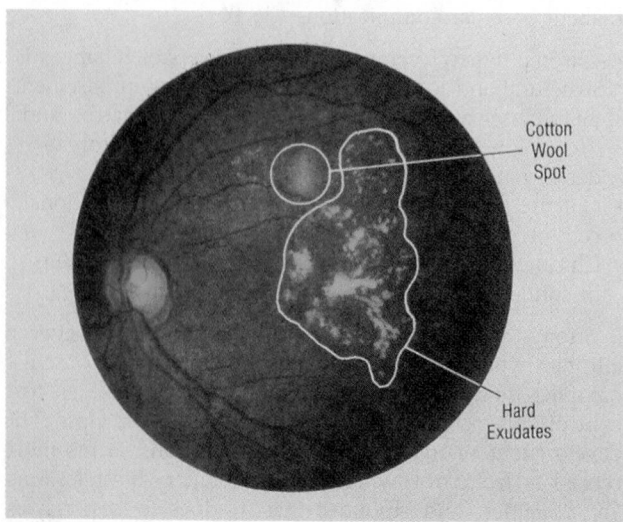

Figure 68–4. Select ophthalmic changes seen in nonproliferative diabetic retinopathy (NPDR).

the outer layers of the retina and are caused by leakage from abnormally permeable capillaries or microaneurysms in the retina. Microaneurysms are small capillary dilations seen as red dots with an ophthalmoscope. Soft exudates, or "cotton wool spots," are areas of nerve fiber ischemia and indicate poor retinal perfusion. They appear as gray or white areas with "soft" or feathery edges and may last for months before disappearing. NPDR develops slowly over time and rarely causes blindness. Diabetic clients with severe NPDR have a 75% chance of progressing to proliferative diabetic retinopathy within 1 year.

Abnormalities of proliferative diabetic retinopathy (PDR) are not contained within the retina. Abnormal new blood vessels and connective tissue erupt through the surface of the retina or optic nerve to grow into the vitreous gel. Hemorrhages result in decreased vision (Fig. 68–5). The appearance of reddish-black particles floating across the field of vision indicates bleeding into vitreous fluid. Fibrous tissue bands, developing in association with neovascularization, cause *retinal detachment* on retraction, with irreversible vision loss.

The benefit of laser photocoagulation for retinopathy was established by the Early Treatment Diabetic Retinopathy Study. Laser photocoagulation prevents further vision loss but does not reverse already diminished visual acuity. The Diabetic Retinopathy Vitrectomy Study (EVS) established the benefit of early vitrectomy in improving visual acuity in clients with recent severe vitreous hemorrhage. *Vitrectomy* involves removing the vitreous fluid and severing the traction bands that lead to retinal detachment.

Several studies have been conducted to determine potential risk for retinopathy. The Diabetes Control and Complications Trial (DCCT) demonstrated that intensive treatment of clients with type 1 diabetes reduced the development of retinopathy by 76% in clients with no retinopathy and slowed progression of retinopathy by 54% in clients with early retinopathy. The risk of retinopathy increases minimally between HbA1c levels of 6% to 8%, whereas risk increases steeply above 8.5%. Studies show that control of blood pressure may reduce the severity and progression of retinopathy. Proteinuria, which

is clearly associated with retinopathy, indicates a more advanced stage of diabetes in which visual loss is more likely. Data from the Early Treatment Diabetic Retinopathy Study demonstrated that elevated levels of serum lipids are associated with both the development and severity of retinal hard exudates and subsequent decreased visual acuity in clients with diabetic retinopathy. Preservation of visual acuity is an important motivator for lowering elevated serum lipids in persons with diabetes.

Vision loss in diabetic clients can occur from several other mechanisms. *Macular degeneration* results in a permanent spot or blur in straight-ahead vision (central vision). The client may report double vision, but peripheral vision is not affected. There is no cure for degeneration of the macula, but laser treatment helps to maintain peripheral vision if the condition is detected in its early stages. There is no known treatment for permanent scarring.

High blood glucose levels change the shape and clarity of the lens, causing *myopia,* and may alter the quality of vision obtained through prescription eyeglasses. The diabetic client may report double vision during periods of hypoglycemia. *Cataracts* occur in diabetic clients at a younger age, progress at a faster rate, and occur with greater frequency than in nondiabetic individuals. Also, open-angle *glaucoma* is more common in diabetic clients. The management and treatment of cataracts and glaucoma are the same as for nondiabetic clients.

ELDERLY CONSIDERATIONS

The elderly diabetic client with retinopathy has the additional effect of visual changes that occur with aging. As a result, the elderly diabetic client's ability to perform self-care activities may be more seriously affected than a younger diabetic. Age-related changes include presbyopia (the inability to focus on close objects); decreased contrast sensitivity (the ability to separate the object from its background); decrease in dark/light adaptation (the inability of the eye to respond to changes in light sensitivity); and delayed glare recovery. In addition, older individuals are more prone to developing cataracts and glaucoma. The ability to discriminate among blues, greens, and violets decreases with normal aging. This deterioration of color perception has implications for clients performing visual blood glucose monitoring.

Diabetic Neuropathy

Diabetic neuropathy is a common and debilitating complication of diabetes, potentially involving all parts of the body. Damage to sensory nerve fibers results in either pain or loss of sensation; damage to motor fibers results in muscular weakness; and damage to nerve fibers in the autonomic nervous system results in loss of function.

Diabetic neuropathy encompasses two distinct groups of disorders (focal and diffuse neuropathies) with different etiologies, progressions, and treatments. The most common neuropathies attributed to complications of diabetes involve diffuse neuropathies. They have slow onset, symmetric distribution, motor and sensory involvement, and a slow progressive course with few spontaneous remissions. Examples include distal symmetric polyneuropathy

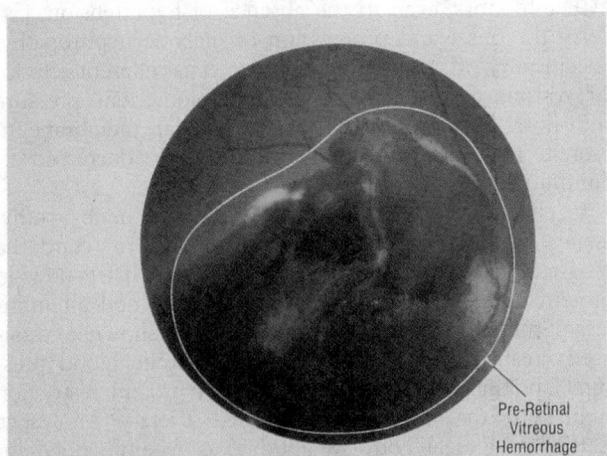

Figure 68–5. Ophthalmic hemorrhage that is possible with proliferative diabetic retinopathy.

Pre-Retinal
Vitreous
Hemorrhage

and autonomic neuropathies (Pfeifer & Schumer, 1995). Late complications of distal symmetric polyneuropathy include foot ulcerations and deformities.

Focal neuropathies are divided into two groups, ischemic and entrapment neuropathies. Ischemic neuropathies result from an acute ischemic event involving a single blood vessel or group of blood vessels to a single nerve or group of nerves. The symptoms tend to be sudden in onset, asymmetric distribution, and self-limiting in duration. Recovery time varies from nerve to nerve. Examples of focal ischemic neuropathies are amyotrophies and cranial neuropathies. Entrapment neuropathies occur because of compression of a nerve within a body compartment. Symptoms tend to be gradual in onset and asymmetric in distribution; they may be bilateral, having a waxing and waning course without spontaneous recovery. Examples of focal entrapment neuropathies are carpal tunnel and tarsal tunnel syndromes.

Insulin deficiency and hyperglycemia are thought to initiate neuropathy. Metabolic and vascular abnormalities result in damage to peripheral and autonomic nerves. Both the axon and its myelin sheath are damaged, resulting in blocked nerve impulse transmission. Vascular abnormalities of diabetes result in reduced blood flow and ischemic damage to neurons. Neuropathy is thought to result from sorbitol accumulation in the nerve. Glucose is converted to sorbitol by the enzyme aldose reductase. The increase in sorbitol is associated with slowed motor nerve conduction velocity.

Cardiovascular autonomic neuropathy, with orthostatic (postural) hypotension and syncope, places the client with diabetes at risk for falling. Orthostatic hypotension can be treated with increasing sodium intake, wearing elastic stockings, and sleeping with the head of the bed elevated. Improvement in blood glucose control with insulin has been shown to eliminate orthostatic hypotension (Doleman et al., 1996).

Hypotonic or neurogenic bladder results in incomplete emptying and can lead to urinary infection and kidney dysfunction. Gastrointestinal symptoms in diabetes are attributed to vagal nerve dysfunction and to sympathetic nerve damage. Dysphagia, heartburn, nausea, and vomiting are common symptoms. Diarrhea caused by diabetes is chronic, can be severe, often occurs at night, and may be associated with anal incontinence. Constipation, the most common gastrointestinal symptom, is intermittent and may alternate with bouts of diarrhea. Gastroparesis (delay in gastric emptying) is a frequent cause of hypoglycemia. Gastroparesis can be treated with drugs that improve gastric motility: metoclopramide (Reglan, Clopra, Octamide, Apo-Metoclop♣, Maxeran♣), erythromycin, and cisapride (Propulsid, Prepulsid♣). Diarrhea resulting from autonomic neuropathy can be treated with tetracycline or, when that is ineffective, with drugs such as diphenoxylate with atropine (Lomotil).

Nursing measures are directed toward assisting the diabetic individual to attain maximum blood glucose control. A major finding of the DCCT was that clinical neuropathy was reduced by 60% with intensive treatment. The nurse can educate the diabetic client with gastroparesis about methods to prevent hypoglycemia and the client with orthostatic hypotension on methods to prevent injury due

to falling. Frequently seen diabetic neuropathies are reviewed in Table 68–5.

Diabetic Nephropathy

Diabetes mellitus is the leading cause of end-stage renal disease (ESRD) in the United States. ESRD is three times more prevalent in African-American clients with diabetes, six times more prevalent in Mexican-Americans, and eight times more prevalent in Native Americans than non-Hispanic whites (ADA, 1996c). Diabetic nephropathy develops in 35% to 45% of clients with type 1 and 5% to 10% of clients with type 2 diabetes. Renal failure represents the most common cause of death in type 1 diabetic clients. Diabetic nephropathy occurs within 15 to 20 years of the onset of diabetes or does not occur at all. Some clients with diabetes seem to be protected against ESRD. Preventing diabetic nephropathy is important because clients with diabetes have a 50% greater rate of mortality once receiving dialysis for ESRD than do clients without diabetes.

Hyperglycemia causes intraglomerular hypertension and renal hyperperfusion. Increased glomerular pressure results in deposition of protein in the mesangium, ultimately leading to glomerulosclerosis and renal failure. The earliest pathological change in the kidney is an increase in the thickness of the glomerular basement membrane. Nodular and diffuse lesions develop as the duration of diabetes increases. The glomerulus becomes unable to function because of the degree of fibrous scarring. *Microalbuminuria* signifies the presence of diabetic nephropathy. Pathologic changes in the composition and structure of the basement membrane are associated with losses of protein. After clinically detectable proteinuria is found, progression to ESRD during the next 7 to 15 years is inevitable.

Renal damage also is related to the mean arterial blood pressure alteration seen as part of cardiovascular disease in diabetic clients. Both systolic and diastolic hypertension markedly accelerate the progression of diabetic nephropathy. Primary care providers frequently assess renal function and focus on blood pressure and glucose control. Angiotensin-converting enzyme (ACE) inhibitors or calcium channel–blocking agents are the drugs of choice for antihypertensive therapy. Recent studies found that ACE inhibitors, even in the absence of hypertension, can delay the onset and progression of diabetic nephropathy. Specifically, ACE inhibitors decrease renal efferent arteriolar resistance and therefore reduce glomerular pressure and flow. Permeability of the glomerular membrane to protein gradually decreases, which leads to decreased albuminuria.

In clients with type 1 diabetes and overt nephropathy, dietary protein restriction has been shown to retard the progression to renal failure (ADA, 1996c). Diets low in protein decrease glomerular perfusion rates and albuminuria. Studies on protein restriction have shown a stabilized creatinine clearance, decreased systolic blood pressure, and increased serum albumin. A protein restriction similar to the adult Recommended Dietary Allowance (0.8 g/kg of ideal body weight/day) is recommended for individuals with evidence of nephropathy (ADA, 1998l).

Nursing measures are directed toward assisting the dia-

TABLE 68-5

Features of Diabetic Neuropathy		
	Complication	**Manifestation**
Diffuse Neuropathies		
Distal symmetric polyneuropathy	• Sensory alterations	• Paresthesia: burning/tingling sensations, polyneuropathy starting in toes, moving up legs • Dysthesiaes: burning, stinging, or stabbing pain • Anesthesia: loss of sensation
	• Motor alterations in intrinsic muscles of foot	• Foot deformities: high arch, claw toes, shift of weight-bearing to metatarsal heads and tips of toes
Autonomic neuropathy	• Anhidrosis	• Lack of perspiration • Drying, cracking of skin
	• Gastroparesis	• Delayed gastric emptying, constipation, nausea, anorexia
	• Diabetic diarrhea • Neurogenic bladder • Impotence • Loss of cardiac reflexes	• Diarrhea and bowel incontinence • Atonic bladder, urinary retention • Erectile dysfunction • Orthostatic hypotension • Resting tachycardia • Defective counterregulation • Loss of warning signs of hypoglycemia
Focal Neuropathies		
Focal ischemic	• Intercostal radiculopathy: pain in root distribution	• Pain radiating across back, side, and front of chest or abdomen with sensory and reflex loss
	• Cranial nerve palsies; cranial nerves III and IV	• Sudden diplopia or strabismus, ptosis
	• Amyotrophy	• Pain, asymmetric weakness, wasting of iliopsoas, quadriceps and adductor muscles
Entrapment	• Median nerve	• Carpal tunnel syndrome neuropathies: weak grasp, numbness, pain
	• Popliteal nerve (knee) • Posterior tibial at tarsal tunnel	• Foot drop • Tarsal tunnel syndrome: sensory impairment in sole of foot; weakness of intrinsic muscles of foot; burning pain and paresthesias at ankle and plantar surface

betic client to attain maximum blood glucose and blood pressure control. The DCCT clearly demonstrated beneficial effects of blood glucose control on the kidney. Subjects receiving intensive therapy in the DCCT had a reduced mean adjusted risk of microalbuminuria of 39%. Recognition of renal disease and treatment at an early stage are important in slowing the progression of disease. Although dialysis and transplantation prevent death from uremia, the 5-year survival rate for the uremic diabetic is only 20%. Pancreatic transplantation is improving the survival rates for diabetic clients.

Male Erectile Dysfunction

Erectile dysfunction, defined as inability to achieve or maintain an erection sufficient for satisfactory sexual performance, occurs at a higher rate and at an earlier age among men with diabetes than the general population. Twenty percent of diabetic persons in a population-based cohort study reported erectile dysfunction (Klein et al., 1996). The prevalence of erectile dysfunction increased with duration of diabetes: Men with 35 years or more of diabetes were 7.2 times as likely to report erectile dysfunction than men with 10 to 14 years of diabetes. Erec-

tile dysfunction was also related to higher glycosylated hemoglobin levels, higher systolic blood pressure, greater body mass index, medically treated hypertension, number of pack-years of cigarettes smoked, and presence of other chronic micro- and macrovascular complications.

The inability to achieve or maintain an erection suitable for sexual intercourse may be caused by neuropathy, vascular disease, or psychogenic factors. Cavernosal artery insufficiency, corporal veno-occlusive dysfunction, and/or autonomic neuropathy are responsible for persistent erectile dysfunction in diabetes (Kahn & Weir, 1994). Depression, anxiety, and relationship problems can impair erectile functioning. Erectile dysfunction from organic causes can be differentiated from psychogenic dysfunction by monitoring nocturnal erections associated with rapid eye movements (REM): Diabetic men have been found to have a decrease in REM-associated erections.

Adjustments in the medication regimen used to treat hypertension may improve sexual function. Thiazide diuretics affect neuroregulation of erectile tissue and are not a good choice in treatment of hypertension for persons with longer duration diabetes. Antihistamines, antipsychotics, opiates, and sedative-hypnotics are also associated with erectile dysfunction.

The presence of diabetic retinopathy or peripheral neuropathy, a history of cardiovascular disease, and lower extremity amputations alert the nurse to the need to discuss erectile dysfunction. Since erectile dysfunction is more prevalent in clients with poorer blood glucose control, measures to achieve tighter blood glucose control and better blood pressure control need to be implemented. The diabetic client may regain sexual function by injection of papaverine into the corpora of the penis, vacuum devices, or penile prosthesis. (Chapter 79 covers erectile dysfunction in more detail.)

ETIOLOGY
Type 1 Diabetes

Type 1 diabetes is an autoimmune disorder in which beta-cell destruction of the islets of Langerhans in the pancreas occurs in a genetically susceptible individual (Table 68–6). This disorder results in destruction of insulin-secreting cells within the islets of Langerhans of the pancreas. Genetically, type 1 diabetic clients have histocompatibility loci patterns HLA-DR3 and/or HLA-DR4 located on the short arm of chromosome 6. There is evidence that viruses (mumps virus, congenital rubella virus, coxsackievirus) represent the environmental factors that initiate autoimmune destruction of pancreatic beta cells.

Markers of immune destruction of the beta cell include islet cell autoantibodies (ICAs), autoantibodies to insulin (IAAs), autoantibodies to glutamic acid decarboxylase (GAD), and autoantibodies to tyrosine phosphates. One, and usually more, of these autoantibodies are present in 85% to 90% of clients when fasting hyperglycemia is initially detected (ADA, 1998a). The presence of ICA and IAA may be of predictive value in determining the onset of type 1 diabetes before clinical diabetes develops.

Risk of developing type 1 diabetes is determined by a genetically recessive HLA gene. Most individuals with this gene do not develop type 1 diabetes; however, 1 in 20 first-degree relatives of individuals with type 1 diabetes *will* develop the disease. It is unclear why genetically susceptible individuals do or do not develop diabetes.

Type 2 Diabetes

The etiology of type 2 diabetes remains unclear. Type 2 diabetes is not a single disease but the result of many conditions that produce hyperglycemia. Three basic abnormalities characterize type 2 diabetes and contribute to hyperglycemia. These abnormalities include excessive glucose production by the liver, impaired insulin secretion, and peripheral insulin resistance primarily occurring in liver, adipose, and muscle tissue (Henry, 1996). Alterations in beta-cell function are found in individuals with type 2 diabetes. Basal insulin secretion is increased; insulin secretion in response to hyperglycemia becomes blunted; and first-phase insulin secretion is lost. Hyperglycemia occurs when the pancreas can no longer produce enough insulin to compensate for insulin resistance.

Studies have shown that insulin resistance, not impaired insulin secretion, initiates the process of type 2 diabetes. Type 2 diabetes is characterized by both fasting and postprandial hyperglycemia. The inability of insulin to lower plasma glucose levels effectively is termed *insulin resistance*. Peripheral tissue is the primary site of insulin resistance. In the early stages insulin is unable to promote glucose uptake and storage as glycogen. Insulin resistance results from decreased insulin receptors (see Fig. 68–1)

TABLE 68–6

Differentiation of Type 1 and Type 2 Diabetes		
Features	**Type 1**	**Type 2**
Former names	Juvenile onset Ketosis prone	Maturity onset Ketosis resistant
Age at onset	Usually under 30 years; occurs at any age	Peaks in 50s, may occur earlier
Symptoms	Abrupt onset, thirst, weight loss	Frequently none; thirst, fatigue, visual blurring, vascular or neural complications
Etiology	Viral	Not known
Pathology	Beta-cell destruction	Insulin resistance Dysfunctional beta cell
Antigen patterns	HLA-DR4, HLA-DR3	None
Antibodies	ICA present at diagnosis	None
Endogenous insulin and C-peptide	None	Low, normal, or high
Inheritance	Recessive	Unknown
Nutritional status	Usually nonobese	60%–80% obese
Insulin	All dependent on insulin	Required for 20%–30%
Sulfonylurea therapy	None	Effective for most clients
Medical nutrition therapy	Mandatory	Mandatory

on cell surfaces (receptor defect) or reduced intracellular response to insulin (postreceptor defect).

The specific genetic basis for type 2 diabetes is not clear. Twin studies have shown that genetic or familial environmental factors play a dominant role in the disease. No single gene locus has been identified for type 2 diabetes.

Other Specific Types of Diabetes: Genetic Defects of the Beta Cell

Formerly referred to as *maturity-onset diabetes of the young,* this type of diabetes is characterized by impaired insulin secretion with little or no defects in insulin action, and it is inherited in an autosomal dominant pattern. This form of diabetes is characterized by onset of mild hyperglycemia, usually occurring before the age of 25 years. Abnormalities on three genetic loci have been identified. The most common form involves mutations on chromosome 12 (Menzel et al., 1995). Genetic abnormalities that result in inability to convert proinsulin to insulin have been identified in a few families (ADA, 1998a).

PREVENTION

Immune-related markers can accurately detect individuals who will develop immune-related type 1 diabetes. Measurement of islet cell antibody (ICA) levels of first-degree relatives of type 1 diabetics identify those at risk for developing the disease. There is no risk for developing type 1 diabetes when levels of ICA and insulin autoantibody (IAA) are negative. There is a 50% risk of developing type 1 diabetes when ICA levels are positive and there is loss of first-phase insulin secretion, as determined by the glucose tolerance test.

Insulin can be administered to susceptible individuals in an attempt to slow destruction of pancreatic beta cells. Sulfonylurea drugs decrease hyperglycemia and stimulate both insulin secretion and insulin action. Metformin (Glucophage) inhibits intestinal absorption of glucose and improves insulin action; this drug has been well tolerated in clinical trials in prevention of type 2 diabetes. Immunosuppressive therapy with azathioprine (Imuran), cyclosporine (Sandimmune), and prednisone (Orasone, Deltasone, Winpred✦) is administered to prolong the person's ability to secrete insulin. Nicotinamide (niacin) decreases the likelihood of diabetes caused by DNA damage.

The risk factors of obesity, physical inactivity, and a high-fat diet for type 2 diabetes can be modified by behavioral changes. Studies have shown that a program of dietary and exercise interventions can substantially reduce the incidence of diabetes in individuals identified as having impaired glucose tolerance (Pan et al., 1997). Increasing physical activity improves insulin sensitivity and may also contribute to weight loss.

INCIDENCE/PREVALENCE

The prevalence of diagnosed and undiagnosed diabetes in the general population over 45 years of age is estimated to be about 6%. Specific subgroups have a much higher prevalence of the disease than the population as a whole. These subgroups have attributes or risk factors that directly cause diabetes or are statistically associated with it (ADA, 1998q). High-risk groups for type 2 diabetes are presented in Table 68–7.

Type 1 diabetes rarely occurs during the first 6 months of life. The incidence begins to increase sharply at about 9 months of age, continues to rise until age 12 to 14 years, and then declines. During the first 30 years of the twentieth century, the incidence rate of type 1 diabetes in the Caucasian population in the United States under age 15 years remained constant. However, over the past three decades, the rate has almost tripled. The data are comparable with those of several other countries.

Incidence data on type 2 diabetes are scarce and unreliable. The incidence of diabetes increases dramatically with age. More than 80% of all diabetic clients are older than 45 years; the disease is present in one in six people at age 65 and in one in four people at age 85. Approximately 10% of clients in whom diabetes mellitus develops are over the age of 70 years. After age 40 years, new-onset diabetes is almost always non–insulin-dependent and ketosis resistant and can be controlled by nutritional therapy, exercise, and possibly oral hypoglycemic agents.

TRANSCULTURAL CONSIDERATIONS

Diabetes is moderately prevalent (3% to 10%) in U.S. non-Hispanic Caucasians and U.S. African-American males. High prevalence rates (11% to 20%) are found in U.S. African-American women and most U.S. Hispanic groups. Mexican-Americans have a prevalence of type 2 diabetes approximately three times higher than non-Hispanic Caucasians. Among non-Hispanic Caucasians, type 2 diabetes is more heavily concentrated in the productive years. In this population, 30% of those with diabetes are elderly, and 23% are younger than 45 years.

Diabetes is found in epidemic proportions in Native American populations. Results of the Strong Heart Study found diabetes rates in the Pima/Maricopa/Papago Indian

TABLE 68–7

Major Risk Factors for Type 2 Diabetes

- Family history of diabetes (parents or siblings)
- Obesity (more than 20% above a person's ideal body weight)
- Origin (African-American, Hispanic-American, Native American, or Asian-American)
- Age older than 45 years plus any of the preceding factors
- Previously identified impaired glucose tolerance or use of certain prescription drugs
- Hypertension (>140/90 mmHg)
- High-density lipoprotein cholesterol level <35 mg/dL (0.90 mmol/L) and triglyceride levels >250 mg/dL (2.82 mmol/L)
- History of gestational diabetes or delivery of babies weighing more than 9 pounds

From American Diabetes Association. (1998q). Position statement: Screening for diabetes. *Diabetes Care, 21*(suppl 1), S20–22.

communities in Arizona of 65% for men and 72% for women. Increasing diabetes in the Native American population may provide support for a genetic link to Native American ancestry (Lee et al., 1995).

In all populations, prevalence of diabetes rises with age. Peak prevalence occurs in the sixth decade of life, followed by a decline in the seventh decade, presumably because of greater mortality of diabetic individuals. Age distributions do not appear to differ across ethnic groups.

There is a strong correlation between relative weight and the prevalence of type 2 diabetes. Diabetes is 2.9 times higher in obese than nonobese people. Prospective studies have shown that higher weight increases the risk of diabetes. The prevalence of obesity is about double for African-American women than Caucasian women. Women whose income is below the poverty line have a much higher incidence of obesity than do women in the non-poverty groups.

Mexican-Americans, African-Americans, and Native Americans are at a higher risk of developing diabetic end-stage renal disease than are non-Hispanic Caucasians. A possible explanation is that social or economic circumstances lead to poorer compliance or poorer access to adequate treatment for diabetes and hypertension.

Collaborative Management

 Assessment

> ### Laboratory Assessment

Blood Tests

The physician uses blood glucose values to diagnose diabetes. The nurse, client, or family member monitors the ongoing status of diabetes by performing capillary blood glucose testing using a blood glucose meter. The physician and nurse assess the overall result of treatment through review of glycosylated hemoglobin and fructosamine levels.

Blood Glucose Tests. Instructions for blood glucose testing are presented in Chart 68–1. The American Dia-

---

---

betes Association (ADA) defines normal blood glucose values as in Chart 68–2 (American Diabetes Association, 1998a). ADA criteria for the diagnosis of adult diabetes mellitus are outlined in Table 68–8.

Oral Glucose Tolerance Test. The oral glucose tolerance test is the most sensitive test for the diagnosis of diabetes. Before the test, the nurse reviews instructions from Chart 68–1 with the client. Carbohydrate intake restriction or bed rest before the test alters glucose tolerance. The client drinks a beverage containing a glucose load of 75 g, and blood samples are collected at 30-minute intervals for 2 hours.

Chart 68–2

Laboratory Profile: Blood Glucose Values

Test	Normal Range for Adults	Significance of Abnormal Findings
Fasting blood glucose	• <110 mg/dL (6.1 mmol/L) • Elderly: Levels rise 10 mg/dL per decade of age	• Elevations >126 mg/dL (7.0 mmol/L) (obtained on 2 occasions) are diagnostic of diabetes, even in older adults
Glucose Tolerance Test (2 hour post-glucose load)	• <140 mg/dL (7.8 mmol/L)	• Levels >140 mg/dL (7.8 mmol/L) and <200 mg/dL (11.1 mmol/L) = IGT (impaired glucose tolerance) • Levels >200 mg/dL diagnostic of diabetes in nonpregnant adults
Glycosylated (glycated) Hemoglobin A1c (HbA1c)	• 4%–6%	• Levels over 8% indicate poor diabetic control with need for adherence to regimen or changes in therapy

TABLE 68–8

Criteria for the Diagnosis of Adult Diabetes

- Symptoms of diabetes plus casual plasma glucose concentration greater than 200 mg/dL (11.1 mmol/L). Casual is defined as any time of day without regard to time since last meal. The classic symptoms of diabetes include polyuria, polydipsia, and unexplained weight loss.

OR

- Fasting plasma glucose greater than 126 mg/dL (7.0 mmol/L). Fasting is defined as no caloric intake for at least 8 hours.

OR

- 2-hour plasma glucose greater than 200 mg/dL during an oral glucose tolerance test. The test should be performed using a glucose load containing the equivalent of 75 g glucose dissolved in water.

Note: Each test must be confirmed, on a subsequent day, under similar circumstances.

From the American Diabetes Association. (1998a). Committee report: Report of the expert committee on the diagnosis and classification of diabetes mellitus. *Diabetes Care, 21*(suppl 1), S5–19.

Capillary Blood Glucose Monitoring. Diabetic clients can monitor their own blood glucose levels by using glucose oxidase-impregnated strips, read either visually or with a reflectance meter. Self-monitoring of blood glucose levels (SMBG) provides information that allows the client to monitor therapy. The nurse teaches the client to use the physician's prescribed formulas to (1) self-adjust diet, exercise, or pharmacologic therapy; (2) identify and properly treat hyper- and hypoglycemia; and (3) improve decision-making and problem-solving (ADA, 1996e).

The ADA recommends SMBG for insulin-treated clients. Knowledge of blood glucose levels is especially important for

- Any diabetic client attempting to maintain glucose levels in the near-normal range
- Pregnant clients
- Clients with a tendency to develop severe ketosis or hypoglycemia
- Clients with hypoglycemic unawareness
- Clients undergoing intensive treatment programs, especially those with portable infusion devices and multiple daily insulin injections

The operating principles of most self-monitoring systems are the same. The finger is pricked, and a drop of blood made to flow over a reagent pad on a testing strip. After a specific interval, the blood is wiped or blotted away, and a color change develops, the intensity of which is proportional to the amount of glucose present. The result can be read visually or by a reflectance meter. In other systems, the electrical current generated by glucose oxidation is measured.

There is some variation between glucose concentration in whole blood measured by SMBG systems and that measured by clinical laboratory procedures. The accuracy of the correlation decreases at both hypo- and hyperglycemic levels. The overall performance of SMBG systems is a combination of accuracy of the specific blood glucose meter, proficiency of the operator, and quality of the test strips. The ADA has set the performance goal to be a total error of no more than 10% at glucose concentrations between 30 mg/dl (1.6 mmol/L) and 400 mg/dL (22.2 mmol/L) (ADA, 1996c). See Research Application for Nursing (Johnson et al., 1995) for evaluation of accuracy and precision of specific blood glucose meters. Results may be influenced by

- The amount of blood on the strip
- The meter's calibration to the strip currently in use
- Environmental conditions of altitude, temperature, and moisture
- Patient-specific conditions of hematocrit level, triglyceride concentration, and presence of hypotension

---

▶ Research Application for Nursing

Accuracy and Precision of Bedside Capillary Blood Glucose Monitoring Devices

Johnson, P. L., Luther, R. J., Hipp, S., et al. (1995). A comparison evaluation of bedside capillary blood glucose monitoring devices designed for hospital use. Diabetes Educator, 21(5), 420–425.

The purpose of this study was to determine the accuracy of four different blood glucose monitors (One Touch II Hospital Meter, Lifescan; Satellite G, Medisense; and Accu-Chek III and Accu-Chek Easy, Boehringer Mannheim Co.) in relation to a standard laboratory reference method. For each blood sample, tests were performed on the capillary blood glucose monitoring devices and the laboratory reference within a 30-minute time period. Testing on the blood glucose monitors was conducted by Certified Diabetes Educators. Pearson (parametric) and Spearman (nonparametric) correlation coefficients were calculated for each device versus the laboratory reference method. In tests of accuracy (closeness to the reference standard), Accu-Chek III and One Touch II showed a high level of correlation with the reference technique in all blood glucose ranges. The Satellite G and the Accu-Chek Easy showed lower correlation coefficients than the other devices. The accuracy of all devices deteriorated in the high and very high blood glucose ranges. In tests of precision (reproducibility of repeated measurements), the One Touch meter had the highest level of performance. Both the Accu-Chek III and the Accu-Chek Easy had variations outside a 5% standard in one of the tested ranges.

Critique. In this study, both accuracy and precision of bedside blood glucose meters were tested in a controlled setting. Previous studies conducted on bedside blood glucose meters support their inaccuracy in very high and very low blood glucose ranges. Because of therapeutic implications made by bedside testing technology, it is essential that meters in use be both precise and accurate. The meter meeting those criteria in this study (One Touch) represents wipeless "technology." Future studies will determine if this technology can provide superior results obtained by previous meters.

Possible Nursing Implications. Nursing staff performing bedside blood glucose testing can obtain accurate and precise results when specific procedures are followed. The nurse needs to teach the diabetic client always to follow the same procedures to obtain precise and accurate measures at home.

Most meters indicate glucose results as a number, but others have voice readouts, display memories, or capabilities for graphic displays on a computer. A client's visual impairments, including color blindness, determine the method of SMBG selected. Several meters used by the general population may be usable by persons with reliable low vision because of large, bold display screens and simple, user-friendly procedures. Voice modules that annunciate the display messages can be added to certain monitors for the individual with visual impairment.

The client and nurse follow Centers for Disease Control and Prevention (CDC) guidelines for infection control during SMBG. The chance of sustaining an infection from blood glucose monitoring processes can be reduced by handwashing prior to monitoring and avoiding reuse of lancets. The nurse instructs clients not to share their monitoring equipment. The meter's surface can be a source of infection. Hepatitis B virus can survive in a dried state for at least 1 week. Infection can be spread in the lancet holder even when the lancet itself has been changed. Small particles of blood can adhere to the device and infection transported between users. Regular meter cleaning is important in infection control. Health care personnel who perform blood glucose testing and family members who assist with testing should wear gloves to provide protection from infection.

Interpretation of Results. The nurse is wary of the accuracy of the client's report of blood glucose measurements. Accuracy may be compromised by errors in technique (Bustamante et al., 1994), equipment failure, or overt misrepresentation. The data obtained from SMBG are evaluated in conjunction with other measures of blood glucose levels (e.g., HbA1c values) or periodic laboratory blood glucose tests. Even when SMBG is performed correctly, the results are affected by hematocrit (anemia falsely elevates, polycythemia falsely depresses results) and may be unreliable in the hypoglycemic or severe hyperglycemic ranges. Laboratory glucose determinations are more accurate than SMBG.

Frequency of Testing. The frequency of monitoring varies with medication schedule complexity and goals of therapy. Diabetic clients with unstable blood glucose levels, as well as those undergoing intensive treatment regimens (continuous subcutaneous insulin infusions with pumps or more than three insulin injections daily), require more frequent monitoring. Clients undergoing minimal treatment regimens designed to prevent symptomatic hyperglycemia and clients with type 2 diabetes receiving oral agents who are at risk for hypoglycemia require less frequent monitoring.

Blood Glucose Therapy Goals. The nurse works with the client to achieve defined goals for blood glucose therapy. Target blood glucose levels are set individually for each client. On the basis of the DCCT results, a diabetes policy group recommends that clients with type 1 diabetes use premeal and bedtime glucose levels of 80 mg/dL (4.4 mmol/L) to 120 mg/dL (6.7 mmol/L) as a goal (Goldstein et al., 1995).

Accuracy of SMBG Results. All meters currently available are reasonably accurate when the manufacturer's di-

rections are followed. Results are technique dependent regardless of whether test strips are read visually or with a meter. The nurse supplies information to assist the diabetic client in selecting a meter on the basis of the cost of meter and strips, ease of use, availability of repair and maintenance service, and ability to discriminate color. The nurse

- Provides training, including an explanation and demonstration of procedure
- Assesses visual acuity; tests for color blindness as indicated
- Checks the learner's ability to accurately perform the procedure through return demonstration

The most common error in SMBG is failure to follow instructions about proper application of blood on the test strip, timing, and removal of the blood samples. Because accuracy of performance tends to deteriorate over time, continued retraining of those performing SMBG is necessary to ensure accurate results.

Assessment of the diabetic client's ability to discriminate between colors is vital for those who do not use a blood glucose meter. In a study of nondiabetic adults, aged 20 to 78 years, all subjects, independent of age, had difficulty reading blood glucose strips accurately. Individuals with poor visual acuity and those who read their strips in less-than-adequate lighting made more errors. Incorrect readings were more frequent with higher blood glucose levels (Laux, 1994).

ELDERLY CONSIDERATIONS

Visual interpretation of blood glucose values is compromised by the normal changes of aging. Color clarity decreases by 25% in the sixth decade and by 50% in the eighth decade. Older persons require three times as much light to see things as they did at age 20. It is more effective to place high-intensity light on the object or surface than to increase light for the entire room (Ebersole & Hess, 1995).

New Technology. Procedures are being developed that can measure blood glucose without piercing the skin. In one procedure, an external light source with wavelengths in the infrared spectrum is directed to or reflected by a body part. Blood glucose results are determined by measuring the amount of light absorption. Another technology under study involves fluid extraction from the skin. In this process, an electric current is applied to the skin. The current pulls out salt, which carries water, which in turn carries glucose. The glucose is extracted from the skin, where it can be absorbed and its concentration measured. Technical problems of accuracy and instrument size must be solved before any of these products become available for commercial use (Klonoff, 1997).

Glycosylated Hemoglobin Assays. Glycosylated hemoglobin (HbA1c) is the best indicator of the diabetic client's average blood glucose level. Because glucose attaches to the hemoglobin molecule, measurement of HbA1c indicates the glucose level during the previous 120 days, the life span of the average red blood cell.

HbA1c testing can be used to assess long-term glycemic control as well as to predict risk for development of chronic complications. Unlike fasting blood glucose, test results cannot be influenced by changing one's eating habits the day before the test. It is recommended that HbA1c testing be performed at time of initial diagnosis, at least quarterly, and as frequently as needed to achieve target blood glucose ranges (Goldstein et al., 1995). Hemolysis, blood loss, and pregnancy all increase red blood cell turnover and cause a reduction in HbA1c levels. Triglycerides and bilirubin interfere with the assay, leading to overestimation of HbA1c levels in individuals with hypertriglyceridemia.

Glycosylated Serum Proteins and Albumin. Because the turnover of human serum albumin is much shorter (14 days), glycosylated serum albumin and glycosylated serum proteins can be used to indicate blood glucose control over a shorter period. These measures are useful when tight control of blood glucose levels is necessary (e.g., during pregnancy) or in short-term follow-up of treatment changes.

Urine Tests

Urine Testing for Ketone Bodies. The presence of urinary ketones may indicate impending ketoacidosis. The ADA recommends urine be tested for ketones during acute illness or stress, when glucose levels are consistently greater than 300 mg/dL (16.7 mmol/L), during pregnancy, or when any symptoms of ketoacidosis (nausea, vomiting, abdominal pain) are present (Goldstein et al., 1995). Ketone testing is recommended for diabetic clients participating in a weight loss program. Ketones are a waste product of fat metabolism. When ketones are present (and blood glucose levels are normal), the diabetic client is assured that weight loss is occurring. The nurse teaches the client, especially those with type 1 diabetes, to test urine for ketones and discusses interventions when results are positive.

Tests for Renal Function. The presence of urine protein in the absence of symptoms may be an indication of microvascular changes in the kidney. Dipstick methods of testing for microalbuminuria can be used in the primary care provider's office. Urinary albumin excretion rates of 20 to 200 μg/minute (30 to 300 mg/hour) are used to define microalbuminuria; rates within this range have been shown to predict progression of diabetic nephropathy. Recent data indicate that even minor elevations of albumin excretion are associated with increased mortality. Treatment is recommended for any diabetic client with albumin excretion levels greater than 10 μg/minute (Alzaid, 1996).

Routine urinalysis should be performed yearly in adults. Clients beyond puberty and with a history of diabetes for at least 5 years should have a timed urine collection (e.g., 24 hours or overnight) once per year. The urine collection is then sent to the laboratory and tested for the presence of microalbumin or for measurement of the albumin/creatinine ratio (ADA, 1998r). Hypertension or an increased serum creatinine level indicates the need for urine evaluation more frequently than yearly (ADA, 1996c).

Once clinical proteinuria has been detected, renal function (e.g., glomerular filtration rate) is assessed by creatinine clearance tests (see Chap. 72). In individuals with established nephropathy, a rise in serum creatinine level is related to both poor glycemic control and hypertension (Bouloux & Rees, 1995).

Urine Testing for Glucose. Indirect measures of blood glucose may be obtained through urinary testing for glucose. The variability of the renal threshold (the point at which the kidneys excrete glucose in the urine) results in less precise monitoring data than does blood glucose testing. Some adults have blood glucose levels of 250 mg/dL (13.8 mmol/L) to 300 mg/dL (16.7 mmol/L) before glucose is found in the urine. As a result of the aging process or kidney damage, the renal threshold rises so that test results correlate even more poorly with blood glucose values. Fluid intake, urine concentration, time interval since last voiding, and certain pharmacologic products alter the results. For clients who cannot or will not perform SMBG, urine glucose testing can be considered an alternative that can provide useful, but limited information. The nurse helps the client understand the limitations of urine glucose testing (ADA, 1998s).

➤ Other Diagnostic Assessment

Immune-related markers can accurately detect people who will develop type 1 diabetes. Measurement of islet cell cytoplasmic antibody (ICA) levels of first-degree relatives of clients with type 1 diabetes identifies those at high risk for diabetes (ADA, 1998o). Insulin autoantibody (IAA) levels correlate with the rate of progression to diabetes and the age at which type 1 diabetes develops (the younger the age at which diabetes develops and/or the faster the progression to diabetes, the higher the level of IAA). Measurement of C-peptide levels indicates beta secretory function of the pancreas. C-peptide levels correlate well with insulin levels.

 Analysis

➤ Common Nursing Diagnoses and Collaborative Problems

Common nursing diagnoses for the diabetic client include
1. Risk for Injury related to hyperglycemia
2. Risk for Injury related to stress of surgery
3. Risk for Injury related to sensory alterations (diabetic neuropathy)
4. Pain related to peripheral nerve dysfunction (diabetic neuropathy)
5. Risk for Injury related to visual sensory-perceptual alterations (diabetic retinopathy)
6. Altered Renal Tissue Perfusion related to the renal effects of vascular abnormalities (diabetic nephropathy)

Primary collaborative problems for the diabetic client include
1. Potential Complication: Hypoglycemia
2. Potential Complication: Diabetic Ketoacidosis

3. Potential Complication: Hyperglycemic Hyperosmolar Nonketotic Syndrome

➤ Additional Nursing Diagnoses and Collaborative Problems

In addition to the common nursing diagnoses and collaborative problems, some clients with diabetes have one or more of the following:

- Altered Nutrition: More than Body Requirements related to an imbalance of food intake and physical activity, lack of knowledge, and ineffective coping skills
- Risk for Fluid Volume Deficit related to fluid shifts, failure of regulatory mechanisms, hyperglycemic osmotic diuresis, polyuria, vomiting, diarrhea, decreased oral intake, and dehydration
- Pain related to insulin injections or capillary blood glucose testing
- Altered Oral Mucous Membranes related to microvascular circulatory changes and uncontrolled blood glucose levels
- Knowledge Deficit related to a lack of familiarity with information resources about disease process, nutrition management, exercise, medications, weight control, and mouth care
- Altered Urinary Elimination with overflow incontinence related to diabetic neuropathy
- Chronic constipation related to diabetic neuropathy
- Diarrhea related to diabetic neuropathy
- Risk for Impaired Skin Integrity related to decreased circulation, increased blood glucose levels, decreased mobility, and decreased sensation
- Risk for Infection related to increased blood glucose levels, decreased tissue perfusion, inadequate primary defenses (e.g., breaks in skin integrity), and the effects of chronic disease
- Risk for Infection related to wounds, urinary tract infection, intravenous access site, or the gums
- Risk for Altered Sexuality Patterns (male) related to autonomic neuropathy, decreased circulation, or psychological considerations
- Risk for Altered Sexuality Patterns (female) related to the physical and psychological stressors of diabetes
- Sexual Dysfunction related to impotence, impaired lubrication, painful intercourse with the changes in neurologic control of genitalia, the effects of actual or perceived limitations imposed by the disease or therapy, and altered self-concept
- Anticipatory Grieving related to perceived loss of body functions as a consequence of diabetes
- Dysfunctional Grieving related to perceived loss of body functions as a consequence of diabetes
- Self Esteem Disturbance related to inability to deal with the self-care demands of the diabetic regimen
- Anxiety related to the diagnosis of diabetes, potential complications of diabetes, and self-care regimens
- Fear related to the diagnosis of diabetes, potential complications of diabetes, and self-care regimens
- Risk for Ineffective Individual Coping related to a chronic disease, a complex self-care regimen, and decreased social support
- Risk for Ineffective Family Coping, Compromised, related to a chronic disease, a complex self-care regimen, and decreased social support
- Powerlessness related to the complications of diabetes (blindness, amputations, renal failure, and neuropathy)
- Social Isolation related to visual impairment or blindness, adoption of a sick role, and a complex self-care regimen
- Risk for Noncompliance with self-care related to the complexity and chronicity of the prescribed regimen
- Risk for Altered Health Maintenance related to insufficient knowledge of nutrition therapy, weight control, weight maintenance, benefits and risks of exercise, self-monitoring of blood glucose, medications, sick-day care, foot care, hypoglycemia, and available resources

 Planning and Implementation

➤ Risk for Injury Related to Hyperglycemia

Planning: Expected Outcomes. The diabetic client is expected to maintain blood glucose levels within the normal range and avoid acute and chronic complications of diabetes.

Interventions. Treatment of diabetes involves dietary interventions, a planned exercise program, and, in some instances, medications to lower blood glucose levels. The nurse, in collaboration with the physician, dietitian, pharmacist, and, in some cases, the physical therapist, plans, organizes, and delivers care to the client. Pancreas transplantation may be considered for select clients with type 1 diabetes.

The American Diabetes Association has proposed HbA1c levels and blood glucose goals for the treatment of individuals with diabetes, including

- HbA1c levels should be maintained at 7% or below.
- The majority of premeal blood glucose levels should be at 80 to 120 mg/dL (4.4 to 6.7 mmol/L).
- Blood glucose values at bedtime should be 100 to 140 mg/dL (5.6 to 7.8 mmol/L) (American Diabetes Association, 1998r)

Implications for the Elderly. The primary aim of therapy in the elderly diabetic client is to attain quality of life by maintaining blood glucose levels in a range that avoids both hypoglycemia and hyperglycemia. In some clients, this precaution may require an aggressive therapy program with insulin in which the effects of uncontrolled hyperglycemia are greater than the risks of hypoglycemia.

Drug Therapy. Medication is indicated when a client with type 2 diabetes cannot achieve blood glucose control with dietary modification, regular exercise, and stress management.

Oral Therapy. The physician prescribes oral agents only when there has been an adequate trial of dietary control.

Sulfonylurea Agents. Sulfonylurea agents are structurally related to thiazide diuretics and sulfonamide antibiotics, but possess no antibacterial activity and are appropriate only for clients with pancreatic beta-cell function. They act by enhancing basal and stimulated insulin secretion, which reduces hepatic glucose output and facilitates peripheral glucose disposal, and by enhancing the number or sensitivity of receptor sites on the cell for interaction with insulin. They do not increase insulin synthesis. The likelihood of achieving desired therapeutic blood glucose levels with only oral therapy declines when the fasting plasma glucose level exceeds 200 mg/dL (11.1 mmol/L). Oral therapy is unlikely to have any benefit when fasting glucose levels are greater than 250 mg/dL (13.8 mmol/L) (Raskin, 1994). Available sulfonylurea agents (Chart 68–3) differ in potency, pharmacokinetics, and metabolism.

Chart 68–3

Drug Therapy for Diabetes Mellitus: Oral Agents

Drug	Usual Dosage and Duration	Nursing Interventions	Rationale
First-Generation Sulfonylurea Agents			
Acetohexamide (Dymelor, Dimelor♣)	250–750 mg q12–24 h Maximum: 1500 mg/day Duration: 12–24 h	Emphasize eating habits and patterns Monitor renal function	There is a high incidence of hypoglycemia in diabetics with renal impairment
Chlorpropamide (Diabinese, Novopropamide♣)	100–500 mg q24 h Maximum: 500 mg/day Duration: 24–60 h	Emphasize eating habits and patterns	The long half-life of the drug is associated with a high incidence of hypoglycemia
Tolazimide (Tolinase)	100–500 mg q12–24 h Maximum: 2000 mg/day Duration: 12–24 h	Administer with meals	Taking with meals helps to avoid gastrointestinal upset
Tolbutamide (Orinase, Mobenol♣)	750–1500 mg q12–24 h Maximum: 3000 mg/day Duration: 6–12 h	Administer 30 minutes before meals	Taking 30 minutes before meals gives the best reduction in postprandial hyperglycemia
Second-Generation Sulfonylurea Agents			
Glipizide (Glucotrol)	2.4–5 mg q12–24 h Maximum: 40 mg/day Duration: 12–24 h	Administer 30 minutes before meals	Taking 30 minutes before meals gives the best reduction in postprandial hyperglycemia
		Emphasize eating habits and patterns	The long half-life of the drug is associated with a high incidence of hypoglycemia
Glyburide (Micronase, DiaBeta, Euglocon♣)	2.5–20 mg q24 h Maximum: 20 mg/day Duration: 16–24 h	Administer with meals	Taking with meals helps to avoid gastrointestinal upset
		Emphasize eating habits and patterns	The long half-life of the drug is associated with a high incidence of hypoglycemia
Glimepiride (Amaryl)	1–4 mg single dose Maximum: 8 mg Duration: 24 h	Take with first main meal Emphasize eating habits and patterns, and blood glucose monitoring results	Clients with impaired renal function are more sensitive to glucose lowering effects of glimepiride
Biguanides			
Metformin (Glucophage)	500 mg q12 h Maximum: 2500 mg/day Duration: 12 h	Administer with morning and evening meals	Taking with meals helps to avoid gastrointestinal upset
Alpha-Glucosidase Inhibitors			
Acarbose (Precose)	25 mg three times/day Maximum: 100 mg three times/day Duration: 4–8 h	Administer with first bite of food	Delays carbohydrate absorption
Thiazolidinedione Antidiabetic Agents			
Troglitazone (Rezulin)	200–600 mg q24 h Maximum: 600 mg/day Duration: 24 h	Administer with meals	Taking with meals increases absorption

Biguanides. Biguanides have no direct effect on insulin secretion; they act by inhibiting hepatic glucose production, increasing peripheral insulin utilization, and reducing intestinal glucose absorption. Metformin (Glucophage) is the only biguanide available in the United States. It is approved for use in diet-failed, non–insulin-dependent diabetes mellitus. Metformin does not cause weight gain as a side effect of reducing hyperglycemia. Because metformin does not affect insulin secretion, hypoglycemia does not occur. Like sulfonylurea agents, the effectiveness of biguanides tends to slowly decline over time (DeFronzo et al., 1995).

Alpha-Glucosidase Inhibitors. Alpha-glucosidase inhibitors reduce postprandial hyperglycemia by slowing digestion and absorption of carbohydrate within the intestine. Acarbose (Precose) inhibits specific enzymes (alpha-glucosidases) in the gut that delay the digestion of carbohydrate, normally accomplished in the jejunum, to the distal jejunum and ileum. The carbohydrate content of the diet is an important factor in the response to alpha-glucosidase inhibitors. The best glycemic response is obtained when the diet is at least 50% carbohydrates. Therapy with acarbose does not cause hypoglycemia. If hypoglycemia occurs for reasons such as insufficient food intake, treatment cannot be given in the form of oral carbohydrates (i.e., sucrose); rather, treatment must be provided in the form of oral glucose (i.e., dextrose).

Thiazolidinedione Antidiabetic Agents. Troglitazone (Rezulin) is an oral antihyperglycemic agent that achieves blood glucose–lowering effects by decreasing insulin resistance. It lowers blood glucose by improving target cell response to insulin. Troglitazone improves sensitivity to insulin in muscle and adipose tissue and inhibits gluconeogenesis. It can be used in combination with a sulfonylurea agent or insulin to improve glycemic control. It may also be used as initial therapy as an adjunct to nutrition therapy and exercise to lower blood glucose in type 2 diabetic individuals. Troglitazone does not stimulate insulin secretion and therefore does not cause hypoglycemia when administered as a single agent. Hypoglycemic potential exists when administered with insulin or other antidiabetic agents.

Drug Administration. To initiate therapy, the physician orders low-dose medication and increases the dose every 1 to 2 weeks until satisfactory glycemic control or maximal dosage is reached. When maximal dosage does not provide control of blood glucose levels, a different oral agent can be used. Insulin therapy is indicated when blood glucose control cannot be achieved after the use of two different oral agents.

Primary drug failure occurs when a client does not respond to initial therapy and generally implies inappropriate treatment with oral agents instead of insulin. *Secondary* drug failure, which develops in 5% to 10% of clients, occurs when glycemic control is achieved and later lost. Secondary failure can occur because of beta-cell exhaustion, which increases insulin resistance. Conditions such as illness, surgery, and severe stress interfere with control of glucose levels and necessitate treatment with insulin. After recovery, oral agents may be successfully reinstituted.

The nurse educates the client about maintaining dietary restrictions and exercise protocols while taking antidiabetic medication. Pharmacologic agents are an adjunct to, rather than a substitute for, dietary modification and exercise. Careful follow-up with the primary care provider during drug therapy initiation is necessary to establish the appropriate dosage. To prevent adverse drug interactions, the nurse teaches the client to consult with the primary care provider before using any over-the-counter drugs.

Complications. Hypoglycemia is the most serious complication of sulfonylurea therapy. In addition to altering cerebral function, hypoglycemia may precipitate stroke, myocardial infarction, or traumatic injury. Hypoglycemic episodes are a particular problem with use of chlorpropamide because of its long duration of action. Cachectic elderly clients with cardiovascular, hepatic, or renal impairment are more susceptible to hypoglycemia.

Sulfonylurea agents are generally well tolerated and produce few side effects; reported effects include

- Hematologic reactions (leukopenia, thrombocytopenia, hemolytic anemia)
- Allergic skin reactions
- Gastrointestinal effects (nausea, epigastric fullness, heartburn)

In addition, many drugs can potentiate or interfere with the actions of sulfonylurea agents (Table 68–9). The nurse, physician, and pharmacist carefully evaluate the client's overall drug regimen.

Metformin (Glucophage) can cause lactic acidosis in diabetic clients with renal insufficiency. The symptoms of lactic acidosis are often subtle and nonspecific. The nurse educates the client to report fatigue, unusual muscle pain, difficulty breathing, unusual or unexpected stomach discomfort, dizziness, light-headedness, or irregular heartbeats to their primary care provider (Hussar, 1995). The nurse cautions against alcohol intake because alcohol potentiates the effects of metformin on lactate metabolism. Gastrointestinal side effects, most commonly diarrhea, occur in about 30% of individuals starting metformin therapy, but generally resolves with time.

Side effects of acarbose (Precose) are related to presence of undigested carbohydrate in the intestinal tract. Flatulence and abdominal discomfort are frequent symptoms. A registered dietitian can provide information on dietary alterations to reduce the gastrointestinal side effects caused by acarbose.

Frequent side effects of troglitazone (Rezulin) include infection, headache, pain, and reversible elevations of liver function tests; it is used cautiously in hepatic dysfunction. Administration of troglitazone and oral contraceptives can result in loss of contraception. Concurrent administration of troglitazone and cholestyramine reduces absorption of troglitazone by 70%. The nurse teaches the client to have serum transaminase levels drawn as recommended and to report liver dysfunction symptoms (e.g., nausea, vomiting, abdominal pain, anorexia, and dark urine) to the physician or nurse.

Drug Selection. The choice of oral agent is determined by the likely compliance of the diabetic client. Sulfonylureas are inexpensive, can be taken once daily, and are associated with few side effects. Metformin (Glucophage)

TABLE 68–9

Drug Interactions with Sulfonylurea Agents

Potentiate Hypoglycemia	Worsen Hyperglycemia
Alcohol	Asparaginase (Elspar)
Androgens (Testoderm)	Beta-adrenergic blocking agents (atenolol,
Angiotensin-converting agents	propranolol)
Captopril (Capoten)	Calcium channel blockers (diltiazem,
Enalapril (Vasotec)	nifedipine, verapamil)
Anticoagulants, coumarin (Coumadin)	Clonidine (Catapres)
Antihyperuricemic agents (allopurinol,	Corticosteroids (prednisone)
probenecid, Anturane)	Diazoxide, parenteral (Hyperstat)
Barbiturates (phenobarbital)	Diuretics, thiazides (hydrochlorothiazide)
Beta-adrenergic blocking agents (atenolol,	Estrogen (Estrace, Premarin)
propranolol)	Estrogen-progesterone–containing oral
Chloramphenicol (Chloromycetin)	contraceptives (Brevicon, Depo-Provera,
Cimetidine (Tagamet)	Estrostep)
Ciprofloxacin (Cipro)	Furosemide (Lasix)
Clofibrate (Atromid-S)	Glucagon
Disopyramide (Norpace)	Isoniazid
Guanethidine (Ismelin)	Lithium (Eskalith, Lithane, Lithobid)
MAO inhibitors (Nardil)	Morphine
NSAIDs (Indocin, Advil)	Nicotinic acid (Nicolar)
Octreotide (Sandostatin)	Phenothiazines (Compazine, Stelazine)
Pentamidine (NebuPent, Pentam)	Phenytoin (Dilantin)
Phenylbutazone (Butazolidin❈)	Rifampin (Rifadin)
Quinidine (Quinidex)	Thyroid hormones (Cytomel, Levothroid,
Salicylates, in large doses (aspirin)	Synthroid)
Ranitidine (Zantac)	
Sulfonamides (Bactrim, Gantrisin)	
Tetracycline (Sumycin)	
Theophylline (Slo-Bid, Theo-Dur)	
Vitamin B_6 (pyridoxine)	

USPDI, 1997.

is more expensive than sulfonylurea agents, does not cause hypoglycemia, and is associated with gastrointestinal side effects. Acarbose must be taken prior to each meal, potentially reducing compliance (ADA, 1996d).

Selection is also determined by the client's nutritional and physical condition. Clients who skip meals are more vulnerable to hypoglycemia. Oral agents have adverse interactions with many medications commonly prescribed for elderly clients. Both first- and second-generation sulfonylurea agents induce severe and prolonged hypoglycemia. Clients with impaired renal function are susceptible to hypoglycemia caused by chlorpropamide and acetohexamide and to lactic acidosis caused by metformin. Clients with hypertension or congestive heart failure may experience excessive fluid retention because of chlorpropamide's antidiuretic hormone activity.

Beta-cell function tends to deteriorate with time, reducing effectiveness of the oral hypoglycemic medications. Treatment may eventually require insulin therapy either alone or combined with oral agents to achieve the goal of euglycemia (normal blood glucose values).

Insulin Therapy. Insulin therapy is necessary for type 1 diabetes and for moderate-to-severe type 2 diabetes. The success of insulin therapy in elderly clients may be affected by decreasing visual acuity, mobility, memory, or coordination. There are numerous types of insulin avail-

able and numerous regimens possible, all aimed at achieving euglycemia.

Types of Insulin. Insulin is obtained from beef or pork pancreas. Semisynthetic human insulin is prepared by a process that substitutes an alanine residue at position B29 of pork insulin with threonine, resulting in an insulin molecule with an amino acid sequence identical to that of human insulin (Shannon, 1995). Biosynthetic human insulin is obtained from cultures of *Escherichia coli* genetically modified by recombinant deoxyribonucleic acid (DNA) technology. Humalog is synthesized by adding the gene for insulin lispro in a nonpathogenic strain of *E. coli* bacteria.

In many parts of the world human insulin is replacing animal-source insulin. Clients changing from animal-source insulin to human insulin must be alerted to the differences in time action profiles of human insulins. Human insulin tends to have a more rapid onset of action, a shorter peak action, and a shorter duration of action than animal-source insulin. Human insulin is preferred for pregnant women or women considering pregnancy, clients with allergies or immune resistance to animal-derived insulins, clients initiating insulin therapy, and clients expected to use insulin only intermittently (ADA, 1998k).

Insulin is available in rapid-, short-, intermediate-, and long-acting forms that may be injected separately or

TABLE 68–10

Insulin Preparations

Type	Source	Onset* (hr)	Peak* (hr)	Duration*
Rapid-Acting Insulin				
Insulin analog (insulin lispro)				
Humalog (Lilly)	DNA technology	0.3–0.5	0.5–2.5	3.0–4.3
Short-Acting Insulins				
Insulin injection (regular crystalline insulin)				
Iletin II R (Lilly)	Pork (purified)	0.5–1	2–4	6–8
Regular (Novo Nordisk)	Pork	0.5	2.5–5	8
Humulin R (Lilly)	DNA technology	0.5–1	2–4	6–8
Novolin R (Novo Nordisk)	DNA technology	0.5	2.5–5	5–8
Velosulin BR (Novo Nordisk)	Semisynthetic	0.5	1–3	8
Iletin II U-500 (Lilly)	Pork (purified)	0.5	—	24
Intermediate-Acting Insulins				
Isophane Insulin Suspension (NPH Insulin)				
Iletin II (Lilly)	Pork (purified)	2	6–12	18–26
NPH (Novo Nordisk)	Beef	1.5	4–12	24
NPH Pork (Novo Nordisk)	Pork (purified)	1.5	4–12	24
Humulin N (Lilly)	DNA technology	1–2	6–12	18–24
Novolin N (Novo Nordisk)	DNA technology	1.5	4–12	18–24
Insulin Zinc Suspension (Lente Insulin)				
Iletin II (Lilly)	Pork (purified)	2–4	6–12	18–24
Lente (Novo Nordisk)	Beef	2.5	7–15	24
Lente Pork (Novo Nordisk)	Pork (purified)	2.5	7–15	22
Humulin L (Lilly)	DNA technology	1–3	6–12	18–24
Novolin L (Novo Nordisk)	DNA technology	2.5	7–15	18–24
Fixed Combination Insulins				
Humulin 70/30 (Lilly)	DNA technology	0.5	2–12	24
Humulin 50/50 (Lilly)	DNA technology	0.5	3–5	24
Novolin 70/30 (Novo Nordisk)	DNA technology	0.5	2–12	24
Long-Acting Insulins (Ultralente)				
Humulin U (Lilly)	DNA technology	4–6	8–20	24–28
Buffered Insulins for Use in External Pumps				
Humulin BR (Lilly)	DNA technology	0.5–1		
Velosulin R (Novo Nordisk)	Pork (purified)	0.5		

*For subcutaneous administration.

mixed in the same syringe. Insulin preparations with a predetermined amount of neutral protamine Hagedorn (NPH) mixed with regular, such as 70% NPH to 30% regular and a 50:50 mixture of NPH and regular insulins, are considered intermediate acting. Insulin is available in concentrations of 100 U/mL (U-100) and 500 U/mL (U-500). U-500 is used only in rare cases of insulin resistance. U-500 and insulin lispro are the only insulins that require a prescription. Velosulin BR and Velosulin Human✱, both U-100 insulins, contain phosphate buffers

for use with external insulin pumps. U-400 is being used in some implantable pumps on an experimental basis.

The nurse teaches the client that insulin type and species, site of injection, and individual response can all affect absorption, onset, degree, and duration of insulin activity. The nurse reinforces that changing insulins may affect blood glucose control and should be done only under careful supervision. Table 68–10 reviews available insulin preparations, and Table 68–11 outlines the time activity of subcutaneous insulin.

TABLE 68–11

Time Activity (Hours) of Subcutaneous Humulin Insulin

	Rapid-Acting Lispro	Short-Acting Regular	Intermediate-Acting			Long-Acting Ultralente
			70/30	NPH	Lente	
Onset	0.3–0.5	0.5–1	0.5	1–4	1–3	4–6
Peak	0.5–2.5	1–5	2–12	6–12	6–15	16–20
Duration	3.0–4.3	5–8	24	18–26	18–24	24–36

Insulin Regimens. Insulin regimens attempt to duplicate the normal secretory pattern of endogenous insulin. The pancreas produces a constant *(basal)* amount of insulin that balances hepatic glucose production with glucose utilization and maintains normal blood glucose levels between meals. The pancreas also produces additional *(prandial)* insulin in anticipation of a meal that prevents postmeal blood glucose elevations. The insulin dose required for satisfactory blood glucose control varies considerably among clients. A usual starting dose is between 0.5 and 1 U/kg of body weight per day. For multiple-dose regimens or continuous subcutaneous insulin infusion (CSII), basal insulin requirements comprise 40% to 50% of the total daily dosage, with the remainder divided into premeal doses of regular insulin. Adjustments are based on blood glucose monitoring. Because the rate of absorption is slowed by increasing the dosage, adjustments in dosage should be made no more often than every 3 to 4 days.

Most insulin regimens are based on NPH insulin as a basis for basal insulin coverage. Humulin U ultralente insulin provides a lower basal rate and may be used when frequent hypoglycemic episodes occur, but may not provide enough basal coverage during the night to suppress hepatic production of glucose. The diabetic client determines the effect of long-acting insulin by monitoring fasting blood glucose values. Different insulin regimens are shown in Figure 68–6.

Single Daily Injection. Many clients take only one insulin injection daily. This regimen may include only intermediate-acting insulin or a combined dose of short-

and intermediate-acting insulin. A single dose of intermediate-acting insulin may not match the plasma insulin level and food intake. When fasting glucose levels become elevated, a multiple-injection protocol should be considered.

Two-Dose Protocol. A protocol of twice-daily injections of mixtures of short- and intermediate-acting insulin is considered conventional therapy. Two-thirds of the daily dose is given before breakfast and one-third before the evening meal. As a starting point, intermediate-acting and regular insulin are usually given in a 2:1 ratio, whereas the evening (or bedtime) dose is given in a 1:1 ratio. Changes in these ratios are then based on results of blood glucose monitoring. Disadvantages of this protocol are that night-time hypoglycemia is common, and the blood glucose value prior to noon is higher than desired.

Three-Dose Protocol. A combination of short- and intermediate-acting insulin is given before breakfast, short-acting insulin is given before the evening meal, and intermediate-acting insulin is given at bedtime. Administration of intermediate-acting insulin at bedtime results in lower fasting and post-breakfast blood glucose levels. This protocol avoids night-time hypoglycemia but might not provide coverage for the noon meal.

Four-Dose Protocol. Prandial insulin availability is best provided by administering short-acting insulin 30 minutes before meals. Basal insulin is provided by twice-daily administration of intermediate-acting insulin or the administration of long-acting insulin at bedtime. The administration of premeal short-acting insulin based on anticipated

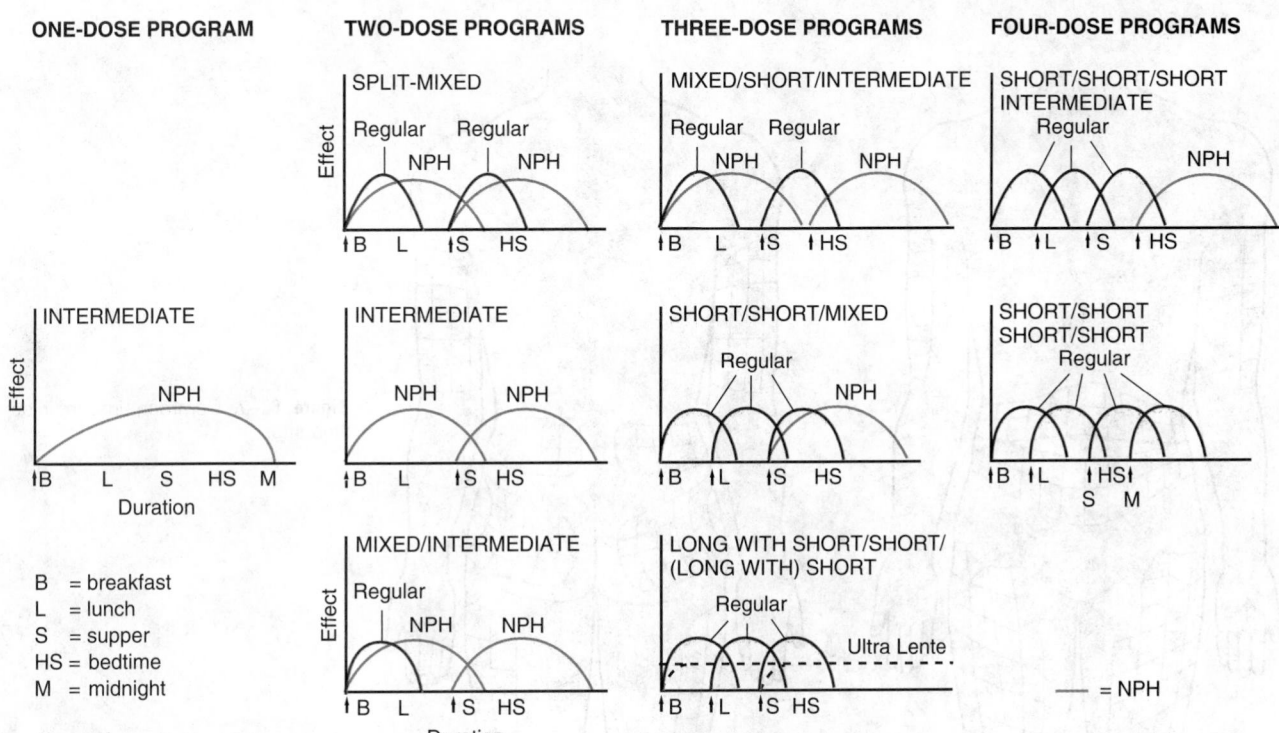

Figure 68–6. Insulin regimens. One injection a day of short-acting or intermediate-acting insulin may be enough to control blood glucose levels. However, split doses (two, three, or four injections of the daily dose) or split mixed doses (a mixture of short-acting and longer acting insulins) may give better control.

carbohydrate intake allows some highly motivated clients with type 1 diabetes flexibility in meal timing and size. Insulin lispro should be given within 15 minutes of eating a meal; peak action is usually obtained within 30 to 90 minutes. Because of its short duration of action, individuals taking insulin lispro also require a longer acting insulin to provide for basal insulin requirements.

Combination Therapy. A combination of sulfonylurea agents and intermediate-acting insulin is given to clients with type 2 diabetes in whom reasonable control of blood glucose levels cannot be achieved. Studies indicate that obese diabetic individuals with higher fasting C-peptide levels may be more likely to respond to combination therapy.

Intensified Insulin Regimens. Intensified regimens are composed of a basal insulin dose of intermediate-acting insulin and bolus doses of short-acting insulin designed to bring the next blood glucose value into the target range. Dosages of insulin are based on the individual's blood glucose patterns. Frequency of blood glucose monitoring is based on the timed action of short- and intermediate-acting insulins and may be required as many as eight times daily. Blood testing 1 hour postprandially and just before the next meal helps determine the adequacy of bolus insulin doses. The diabetic client determines the effects of basal insulin doses by monitoring pre-dinner (evening) and fasting blood glucose values. Blood glucose values at 3 AM detect night-time hypoglycemia and indicate adequacy of both short- and intermediate-acting insulin doses. Goals for glycemic control in an intensified regimen (Hollander, 1994) are

- Fasting blood glucose: 60 to 110 mg/dL (3.4 to 6.2 mmol/L)
- Preprandial blood glucose: 60 to 120 mg/dL (3.4 to 6.7 mmol/L)
- Postprandial blood glucose: < 200 mg/dL (11.1 mmol/L)
- Hemoglobin Alc: 4% to 6%

Clients on intensified insulin regimens need extensive education to achieve target blood glucose values. The client needs to understand clearly how to self-adjust insulin doses and must understand medical nutritional therapy so that dietary flexibility can be maintained within target blood glucose values. Clients must also commit to performing blood glucose monitoring with precision so that therapeutic decisions can be based on accurate data. Frequent contact between the diabetic client and the health care provider is essential.

Pharmacokinetics of Insulin. When insulin is injected, glucose availability to the cells depends on various factors.

Injection Site. Figure 68–7 shows common insulin injection sites. The speed of insulin absorption varies with anatomic site. Absorption is fastest in the abdomen, followed by the upper arm, thigh, and buttocks. Rotation of the injection site is important in preventing lipohypertrophy or lipoatrophy. Rotation *within* one anatomic site is preferable to rotation from one anatomic site to another to prevent day-to-day variation in absorption. The abdomen (except for a 2-inch radius around the navel) is the preferred site of injection because it provides the most rapid insulin absorption.

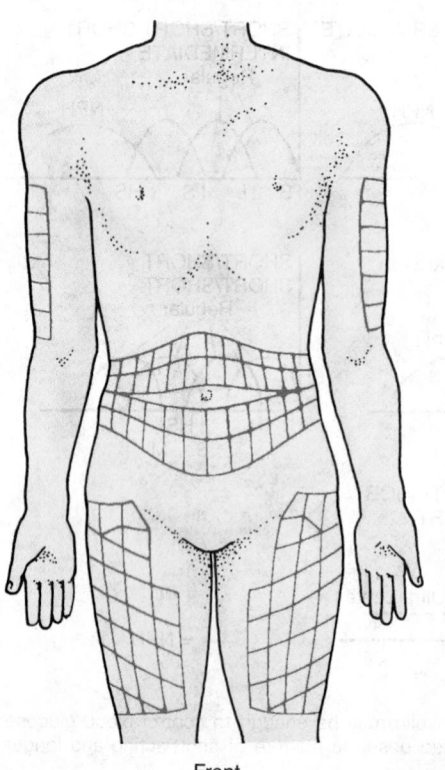
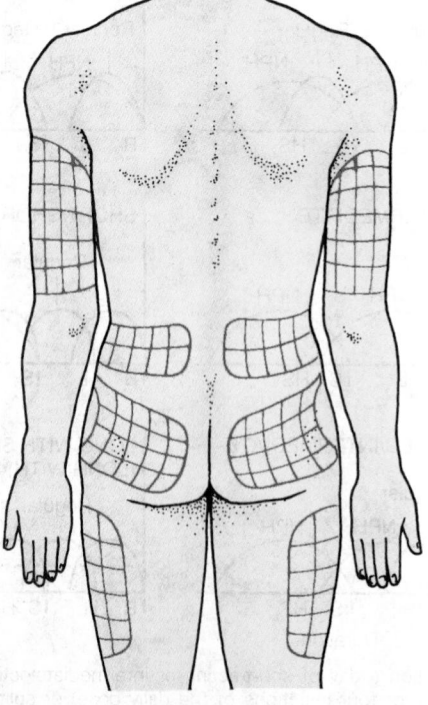

Figure 68–7. Common insulin injection sites.

Front

Back

Absorption Rate. Factors that increase blood flow from the injection site, such as local application of heat, massage of the area, and exercise of the injected area, increase insulin absorption. Scarred sites often become favorite injection sites because they are relatively anesthetic, but injection into scar tissue may delay absorption. Lipodystrophy apparently does not delay the rate of insulin absorption.

Injection Depth. Usually injections are made into the subcutaneous tissue. Most individuals are able to lightly grasp a fold of skin and inject at a 90-degree angle. Routine aspiration for blood is not necessary. Thin people or children may need to pinch the skin and inject at a 45-degree angle to avoid intramuscular (IM) injection. IM injection produces a slightly faster absorption than does subcutaneous injection, but is not recommended for routine insulin administration. The nurse assesses the elderly client's ability to administer insulin and arranges for assistance when self-care is no longer possible.

Time of Injection. The administration of insulin 30 minutes before eating provides a greater amount of plasma-free insulin at mealtime. Eating within a few minutes after (or before) injecting short-acting insulin reduces the ability of insulin to prevent rapid rises in postmeal blood glucose and may increase the risk of delayed hypoglycemia. Insulin lispro should be given within 15 minutes before a meal.

Mixing Insulins. Mixtures of short- and intermediate-acting insulins produce more normal blood glucose levels in some clients than use of a single dose of insulin, but the client's response to mixed insulin may differ from when the insulins are given separately. Chemical changes in the mixture may also occur either immediately on mixing or with time.

When rapid (insulin lispro) or short-acting (regular) insulin is mixed with a longer acting insulin, the shorter acting insulin dose is drawn into the syringe first. This procedure prevents contamination of the shorter acting insulin vial with the longer acting insulin. The injection should be given immediately after mixing; when insulin lispro is mixed, the injection is given within 15 minutes of eating a meal. The nurse follows ADA guidelines for mixing insulins (Table 68–12).

Complications of Insulin Therapy. Hypoglycemia, the result of excessive insulin levels, has a variety of causes. Manifestations and treatment of hypoglycemia are discussed earlier and under Potential Complication: Hypoglycemia.

Hypertrophic lipodystrophy is a spongy swelling at or around the injection site. The condition occurs because of repeated injections in the same area. The overlying skin becomes anesthetic, and the area can become large and unsightly. Treatment consists of rotating the injection site. *Lipoatrophic lipodystrophy* is a loss of fat at or distant to the injection site and occurs as an immunologic reaction to beef or pork insulin. Treatment consists of injection of purified pork or human insulin at the edge of the lipoatrophic area.

Two conditions of fasting hyperglycemia can occur (Fig. 68–8). *Dawn phenomenon* is thought to result from a nocturnal release of growth hormone secretion that may cause blood glucose elevations at about 5 to 6 AM. Dawn phenomenon is treated by providing more insulin for the overnight period (e.g., administering the evening dose of intermediate-acting insulin at 10 PM). *Somogyi's phenomenon* is morning hyperglycemia due to effective counter-regulatory response to night-time hypoglycemia. Somogyi's phenomenon is treated by ensuring adequate dietary intake at bedtime and evaluation of insulin dose and exercise programs to prevent conditions that precipitate hypoglycemia. Both phenomena are diagnosed by blood glucose monitoring conducted during the night. The nurse helps to identify these phenomena and provides pertinent client and family teaching.

Alternative Methods of Insulin Administration

Continuous Subcutaneous Infusion of Insulin. Continuous subcutaneous infusion of a basal dose of insulin (CSII) with meal-associated increases in insulin seems to

---

TABLE 68–12

American Diabetes Association Guidelines for the Mixing of Insulins

- Clients who are well controlled on a particular mixed-insulin regimen should maintain their standard procedure for preparing insulin doses
- No other medication or diluent should be mixed with any insulin product unless approved by the prescribing physician
- Commercially available premixed insulins may be used if the insulin ratio is appropriate to the client's insulin requirements
- Currently available NPH and short-acting insulin formulations may be used immediately or stored for future use
- When rapid-acting and Ultralente insulins are mixed, there is no blunting of the onset of action of the rapid-acting insulin. A slight decrease in the absorption rate is seen when rapid-acting insulin and protamine-stabilized insulin (NPH) are mixed. When rapid-acting insulin is mixed with either an intermediate- or long-acting insulin, the mixture should be injected 15 min before a meal
- Mixing of short-acting and Lente insulin is not recommended, except for a few clients already controlled on this mixture
- On mixing, zinc present in Lente preparations binds with the regular insulin and delays its onset of action
- Clients using Lente mixed with regular insulin should standardize the interval between mixing and injecting
- Phosphate-buffered insulins (NPH) should not be mixed with Lente insulins. Zinc phosphate, present in NPH insulin, may precipitate and convert the longer-acting insulin to a short-acting insulin, with unpredictable results
- There is no rationale for mixing animal with human insulins

From American Diabetes Association. (1998k). Position statement: Insulin administration. *Diabetes Care, 21*(suppl 1), S72–75.

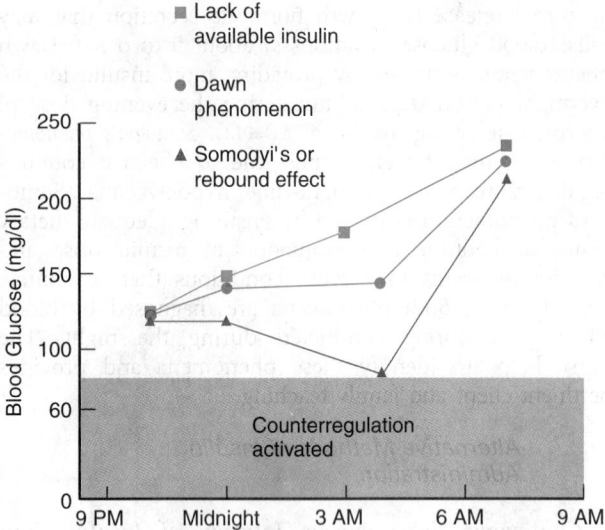

Figure 68-8. Three blood glucose phenomena in diabetic clients.

be more effective than a multiple-injection protocol in providing metabolic control. CSII allows for total flexibility in meal timing because when a meal is skipped the prandial dose of insulin is not administered. CSII is administered by an externally worn pump containing a syringe and reservoir with regular insulin connected to the client by an infusion set. The nurse teaches the client to adjust the amount of insulin received based on data from blood glucose monitoring.

Skin infections may occur when the infusion site is not cleaned every 48 hours or the needle placement is not changed every 3 days. Because the client is euglycemic (blood glucose values in the normal range) and is receiving regular insulin, cessation of insulin administration quickly results in hyperglycemia. CSII is associated with a higher rate and more severe ketoacidosis than with other methods of insulin administration. Ketoacidosis is related to the client's or provider's inexperience in using the pump, concurrent infection, or accidental cessation of insulin infusion, infusion set obstruction, or mechanical problems related to the pump. Buffered insulin is used to prevent the precipitation of insulin crystals within the catheter. The nurse stresses the importance of regular urine testing for presence of ketones.

Intensive education is necessary for clients using CSII. Because of potential hypo- and hyperglycemia, the client must be motivated to perform all necessary functions to ensure accurate insulin administration. The nurse teaches the client to operate the pump, make adjustments in settings, and investigate alarms. Removal of the pump for any length of time can result in hyperglycemia. The nurse provides the client with supplemental insulin schedules for times when the pump is not operational. CSII is expensive; not all costs are covered by insurance.

Closed-Loop Insulin Delivery. Maintenance of euglycemia is useful during surgery, labor and delivery, and dialysis procedures in certain clinical conditions. This can be accomplished by use of an "artificial pancreas," which provides continuous glucose monitoring and delivers insulin based on blood glucose concentrations. In closed-loop systems, a glucose sensor measures blood glucose levels each minute and adjusts the insulin and glucose infusions to maintain a predetermined glucose value. The system utilizes large intravenous catheters for blood withdrawal and for dextrose, insulin, and heparinized saline infusions as needed.

Implanted Insulin Pumps. Insulin pumps are implanted in the peritoneal cavity, where insulin can be absorbed in a more physiologic manner. The peritoneum provides constant and reproducible insulin absorption. Absorption of insulin into the portal circulation is believed to have beneficial effects in reducing peripheral hyperinsulinemia. Because mechanical problems associated with the pump, catheter, and insulin delivery have not been solved, the implantable pump is not widely available.

Injection Devices. With an injection device, the needle is replaced by an ultrathin liquid stream of insulin forced through the skin under high pressure. Insulin administered by jet injection is absorbed at a faster rate, with a resulting shorter duration of insulin action. How these changes affect overall metabolic control is yet to be determined. Cost is a primary drawback to this system.

Pen-type injectors hold small-sized, light-weight, prefilled insulin cartridges. They are easy to carry and make intensive insulin therapy with multiple injections easier to accomplish. These devices may improve accuracy for visual or neurologically impaired diabetic clients. The nurse discusses methods of maintaining the insulin cartridges at an appropriate temperature when vacationing or traveling.

New Technology. A nasal spray, administered via nebulizer, is one new technology for insulin administration. Absorption across the nasal mucosa is rapid; however, only a small amount of insulin is actually absorbed, making glycemic control inconsistent. Studies are also underway to evaluate the effects of aerosolized insulin given by nebulizer. Regular insulin (U-500) is delivered in an inhaler during inspiration. The lungs provide a large surface for absorption of insulin.

Client Education. The nurse provides specific instructions to the client undergoing insulin therapy.

Storage. Insulin not in use should be refrigerated; refrigeration minimizes loss of potency, prevents exposure to sunlight, and inhibits bacterial growth. Insulin in use may be kept at room temperature to limit local irritation at the injection site, which may occur when cold insulin is used.

To prevent loss of potency, the nurse teaches the client to avoid subjecting human and pork insulin to temperature extremes (less than 2.2° C [36° F] or greater than 30° C [86° F]) or to excessive agitation. Insulin lispro should be stored in a refrigerator (2° to 8° C [36° to 46° F]), but not in the freezer. If refrigeration is not possible, the vial or cartridge of insulin lispro can be unrefrigerated for up to 28 days, as long as it is kept as cool as possible (not greater than 30° C [86° F]) and away from direct heat and light.

The nurse instructs the client always to have available a spare bottle for each type of insulin used. Although the expiration date is stamped on each vial of insulin, a slight loss in potency may occur after the bottle has been in use for more than 30 days. When refrigerated, prefilled syringes are stable up to 30 days. If possible, the syringes should be stored in the vertical position, with the needle pointing upward so that suspended insulin particles do not clog the needle. The predrawn syringe should be rolled between the hands before administration. A quantity of syringes may be premixed and stored. The effect of premixing insulins on glycemic control should be assessed by the primary care provider on the basis of blood glucose monitoring.

Dose Preparation. The person administering the insulin inspects the bottle before each use for changes (e.g., clumping, frosting, precipitation, or change in clarity or color) that may signify loss in potency. Visual examination should reveal rapid- and short-acting insulins to be clear and all other types of insulin to be uniformly cloudy after rolling gently between the hands. If uncertain about the potency of a vial of insulin, the person should replace the vial in question with another of the same type of insulin.

Syringes. Conventional insulin administration involves subcutaneous injection with syringes marked in insulin units. Differences in the way units are indicated depend on the size of the syringe and manufacturer. Some syringes are marked in 1-U increments, and other syringes are marked in 2-U increments. Syringes are manufactured in 0.25-, 0.3-, 0.5-, and 1-mL capacities. Two lengths of needles are available: short, 8-mm, and long, 12.7-mm. Short needles are not indicated for obese individuals because of variability of insulin absorption. To ensure accurate insulin measurement, the nurse instructs the client to be cautious when purchasing syringes. Most insulin preparations have bacteriostatic additives that inhibit growth of bacteria commonly found on the skin. Studies of insulin syringe reuse have not found an increased rate of skin infections at the injection site. Charts 68–4 and 68–5 review instructions for drawing a single insulin injection and for mixing regular and NPH insulin in the same syringe (ADA, 1998k).

Other Drug Therapy. The onset of type 1 diabetes can be predicted using autoantibody assays and metabolic testing. Several treatment methods are being tested to determine if the onset of diabetes can be allayed or even prevented. In an attempt to slow the destruction of pancreatic beta cells, low-dose insulin is administered to clients at high risk for type 1 diabetes. The physician also may order azathioprine (Imuran), cyclosporine (Neoral, Sandimmune), and prednisone (Winpred✱) for these clients. Animal studies are underway to determine if type 2 diabetes can be prevented by monoclonal antibody therapy directed against T lymphocytes.

Medical Nutritional Therapy. Effective self-management of diabetes requires a client-specific meal plan, education, and counseling program. Because of the complexity of nutritional issues, a registered dietitian, knowledgeable and skilled in implementing current principles and recommendations for diabetes, should be a member of the treatment team. The nurse and dietitian work to-

---

Chart 68–4

Education Guide: Subcutaneous Insulin Administration

- Wash your hands.
- Inspect the bottle for the type of insulin and the expiration date.
- Gently roll the bottle of intermediate-acting insulin in the palms of your hands to mix it.
- Clean the rubber stopper with an alcohol swab.
- Remove the needle cover and pull back the plunger to draw air into the syringe. The amount of air should be equal to the insulin dose. Push the needle through the rubber stopper and inject the air into the insulin bottle.
- Turn the bottle upside down and draw the insulin dose into the syringe.
- Remove air bubbles in the syringe by tapping on the syringe or injecting air back into the bottle: Redraw the correct amount.
- Make certain the tip of the plunger is on the line for your dose of insulin. Magnifiers are available to assist in measuring accurate doses of insulin.
- Remove the needle from the bottle. Recap the needle if the insulin is not to be given immediately.
- Select a site within your injection area that has not been used in the past month.
- Clean your skin with an alcohol swab. Lightly grasp an area of skin and insert the needle at a 90-degree angle.
- Push the plunger all the way down. This will push the insulin into your body. Release the pinched skin.
- Pull the needle straight out quickly. Do not rub the place where you gave the shot.
- Dispose of the syringe and needle without recapping in a puncture-proof container.

From American Diabetes Association (1998k). Position statement: Insulin administration. *Diabetes Care, 21*(suppl 1), S72–75.

---

gether with the client and family members on all aspects of the meal plan. To encourage compliance with nutrition therapy, the client's meal plan must be realistic and should provide as much flexibility as possible.

Goals of Medical Nutritional Therapy. Nutritional therapy for diabetes focuses on the following goals:

- Maintenance of as near-normal blood glucose levels as possible
- Achievement of optimal serum lipid levels: low-density lipoprotein cholesterol less than 130 mg/dL (< 3.35 mmol/L); the goal for diabetic clients with known cardiovascular disease is to lower low-density lipoprotein cholesterol to less than 100 mg/dL (2.60 mmol/L) and triglycerides to less than 200 mg/dL (< 2.30 mmol/L) (ADA, 1998r)
- Achievement of optimal blood pressure goals, usually less than 140/90
- Provision of adequate calories for achieving reasonable weight for adults, normal growth and development in children and adolescents, increased metabolism during pregnancy and lactation, or recovery from catabolic illness, as needed
- Prevention and treatment of acute complications of

Chart 68–5

Education Guide: How To Mix a Prescribed Dose of 10 U of Regular Insulin and 20 U of NPH Insulin

- Wash your hands.
- Inspect the bottles for the type of insulin and the expiration date.
- Gently roll the bottle of intermediate-acting insulin in the palms of your hands to mix it.
- Clean the rubber stopper with an alcohol swab.
- Inject 20 U of air into the NPH insulin bottle. The amount of air should be equal to the dose of insulin needed. Always inject air into the intermediate-acting insulin first. Withdraw the syringe.
- Inject 10 U of air into the regular insulin bottle. The amount of air is equal to the dose of insulin desired.
- Withdraw 10 U of regular insulin. Be sure that the syringe is free of air bubbles. Always withdraw the shorter acting insulin first.
- Withdraw 20 U of NPH insulin with the same syringe, being careful not to inject any short-acting insulin into the bottle. (A total of 30 U should be in the syringe.)

From American Diabetes Association (1998k). Position statement: Insulin administration. *Diabetes Care, 21*(suppl 1), S72–75.

---

hypoglycemic medications, short-term illness, and exercise-related problems
- Prevention and treatment of chronic complications of diabetes such as renal disease, autonomic neuropathy, and cardiovascular disease
- Improvement of overall health through optimal nutrition and healthy food choices (Franz et al., 1994)

Principles of Good Nutrition in Diabetes. The dietitian formulates a meal plan based on the individual's usual food intake. Day-to-day consistency in timing and amount of food is important in maintaining blood glucose control. Individuals on insulin therapy need to eat at consistent times synchronized with the time of insulin action. Individuals on intensive insulin therapy can be taught to adjust premeal insulin to compensate from departures in their meal plan.

Protein. At present, data are insufficient to recommend protein intake either higher or lower than what is recommended for the general population (i.e., that 10% to 20% of total caloric intake come from protein). A dietary protein intake of 10% of calories (0.8 g/kg) is recommended for individuals with evidence of nephropathy.

Fat/Carbohydrate. The amount of calories from fat and carbohydrates (CHO) is based on individualized nutritional goals. Of the remaining 80% to 90% of caloric intake, less than 10% should be from saturated fat and up to 10% from polyunsaturated fat. The remaining 60% to 70% of calories are obtained from monounsaturated fats and CHO.

Reduction of dietary fat intake, combined with an exercise program, is an effective way to achieve weight loss. Further dietary fat restrictions for individuals with diabe-

tes are determined by a dietitian based on specific lipid abnormalities. Adults with diabetes should be tested for lipid abnormalities annually with a fasting serum cholesterol, triglycerides, high-density lipoprotein cholesterol, and calculated low-density lipoprotein cholesterol (ADA, 1998r).

Fiber. High-fiber diets seem to improve CHO metabolism and lower total cholesterol and low-density lipoprotein cholesterol levels. The nurse teaches the client to select foods with moderate-to-high amounts of dietary fiber (e.g., legumes, lentils, roots, green leafy vegetables or other raw vegetables, all types of whole-grain cereals, and raw fruits). About 20 to 35 g of dietary fiber per day is ideal.

The nurse teaches the client that abdominal cramping, discomfort, loose stools, and flatulence can be minimized by incorporating high-fiber foods into the diet gradually. An increase in fluid intake should accompany increased fiber intake. The nurse and the client pay careful attention to plasma glucose levels because hypoglycemia can result when there is a significant change in dietary fiber intake.

Non-Nutritive Sweeteners. The use of products to enhance the taste of food, while not compromising blood glucose control, is desirable. Three non-nutritive sweeteners have been approved for use by the Food and Drug Administration (FDA): saccharin, aspartame, and acesulfame K.

Saccharin is 300 times sweeter than sucrose. Despite an association with bladder cancer with consumption of high doses of saccharin by laboratory animals, the use of saccharin is considered safe for humans. Recommended limits are 500 mg/day for children and 1000 mg/day for adults. One teaspoon contains 14 to 20 mg of saccharin (ADA, 1993). Saccharin is not affected by cooking. Aspartame is 180 times sweeter than sucrose. The FDA has established a level of 50 mg/kg per day as the lifetime limit for aspartame. The usual level of intake is well below this level. Aspartame is not stable to heat but can be added to foods that have completed the cooking process. Acesulfame K is 200 times sweeter than sucrose. It is water soluble and stable at temperatures up to 225° C (400° F). Acceptable daily limits set by the FDA are 0 to 15 mg/kg of body weight.

Fat Replacers. Fat replacers are introduced into food processing to create good-tasting, lower fat foods, but may have increased carbohydrate (CHO) content. The dietitian and nurse provide self-management training to persons with diabetes on how to incorporate fat replacer foods into their meal plan. General guidelines for the use of fat replacers include
- Less than 20 calories or less than 5 g of CHO per serving if it is a "free food." Limit to three servings per day
- From 6 to 10 g of CHO per serving is one-half of a carbohydrate choice
- From 11 to 20 g of CHO per serving is one carbohydrate choice (ADA, 1998p)

Alcohol. Under normal circumstances, blood glucose levels will not be affected by *moderate* use of alcohol when diabetes is well controlled. The nurse teaches the clients using insulin that two alcoholic beverages (one alcohol beverage = 12 oz of beer, 5 oz wine, or 1.5 oz of distilled spirits) for men and one for women can be ingested with and in addition to the usual meal plan. Because of the potential for alcohol-induced hypoglycemia, the nurse instructs the diabetic person to ingest alcohol only with or shortly after meals. Because alcohol elevates plasma triglycerides, reduction of or abstention from alcohol intake may be recommended for diabetic people with dyslipidemia or alcohol abuse or during pregnancy (Bell, 1996). One alcoholic beverage is substituted for two fat exchanges when caloric intake is calculated (ADA, 1998l).

Food Labeling. Food labels provide nutrient and ingredient information to help clients make appropriate food choices and to select suitable portion sizes. For persons with diabetes, foods containing sucrose and other sugars are not restricted. These foods should be used sparingly and substituted for other CHO in the individual meal plan. The dietitian and nurse educates the client to utilize food labels to determine CHO content to aid in glycemic control (ADA, 1998f).

Nutritional Counseling. The 1994 Nutrition Recommendations for Diabetes recognized that no one single meal plan is appropriate for all diabetics. The current nutrition recommendations are assessment based. Data for the assessment comes from blood glucose monitoring results, blood lipid levels (total cholesterol, low-density lipoprotein cholesterol, high-density lipoprotein cholesterol, and triglycerides), and glycated hemoglobin. Results from self-monitoring of blood glucose provide direction in determining whether current patterns of meals and exercise need any adjustment or whether present habits need reinforcement. An individual dietary prescription is then developed for each diabetic client (Tinker, 1994).

The nurse supports and reinforces nutrition information provided by the dietitian. The client needs to understand how to make adjustments in nutritional intake during illness, planned exercise, and social occasions such as restaurant meals where the usual time of eating is delayed. The client may be unable to follow the prescribed diet because of an inability to see, read, or understand printed materials. The reading level of the material should be geared to the client's educational level. The nurse and the dietitian also share dietary information with the person who prepares the meals. The dietitian sees the client at least yearly to note subtle changes in lifestyle and make appropriate nutritional therapy changes. Some clients, especially those with weight control problems, may require more frequent evaluation and counseling.

Meal Planning Strategies. A variety of meal planning approaches is available. Each approach emphasizes different aspects of nutrition.

Exchange System. The exchange system is based on three food groups: carbohydrate, meat and meat substitutes, and fat. The client is given a prescription of how many items from each food group are to be eaten at a meal or snack. Table 68–13 provides an example of the exchange system of diet therapy. The exchange list for

meal planning assumes that foods with similar nutrient content have similar effects on postprandial plasma glucose concentrations. Studies conclude that diets based on the exchange system produce predictable blood glucose responses.

Carbohydrates. Carbohydrate (CHO) counting provides a simple approach to meal planning. Because fat and protein have little effect on postprandial blood glucose, CHO counting places emphasis on the nutrient that has the greatest impact on postprandial blood glucose. As a result of passage of the Nutrition Labeling and Education Act of 1990 (ADA, 1997e), the nutritional contents of many items are listed on labels. CHO counting uses total grams of CHO, regardless of food source. The dietitian determines the number of CHO grams to be eaten at each meal and snack and assists the client in making appropriate food choices. CHO counting is effective in achieving overall blood glucose control. Acceptable glycemic control is facilitated by consistent CHO intake from day to day. Clients who are on intensive insulin or pump therapies can use CHO counting to determine insulin coverage. After the amount of insulin needed to cover the usual meal is determined, insulin may be added or subtracted for changes in CHO intake. The usual formula is 1 U of regular insulin for each 15 g of CHO (Gregory & Davis, 1994).

Special Consideration for Type 1 Diabetes. A meal plan based on the client's usual food intake should be determined and insulin therapy integrated into the usual eating and exercise patterns. To prevent wide swings in blood glucose levels, day-to-day consistency in the timing and amount of food is important for clients receiving conventional insulin therapy (one to two daily insulin injections). To match the effects of insulin administration, the daily energy intake is distributed among three main meals, a bedtime snack, and one or more between-meal snacks. Clients on intensified insulin therapy with multiple daily injections of insulin or an insulin pump have considerable flexibility in the choice and timing of meals and snacks.

A secondary goal for the treatment of clients with type 1 diabetes is to avoid undesirable weight gain. Hyperinsulinemia, which can occur with intensive treatment protocols, may result in weight gain. It may be more appropriate to treat hyperglycemia by caloric restriction than by increases in insulin dosage. Potential for weight gain can be minimized by focusing on food choices, portion control, and appropriate treatment of hypoglycemia (Franz et al., 1994).

Special Considerations for Type 2 Diabetes. With type 2 diabetes, nutritional therapy directed toward weight reduction and improvement in blood glucose and lipid levels has the greatest effect on morbidity and mortality. For diabetic clients for whom caloric reduction and exercise have not been successful in achieving long-term weight loss, emphasis should be on achieving blood glucose and lipid reduction goals. A moderate caloric restriction (250 to 500 kcal less than average daily intake) and an increase in physical activity may lead to improved diabetic control and weight control. Mild-to-moderate

TABLE 68–13

Exchange System for Medical Nutrition Therapy

Food Content Examples	Carbohydrate (g)	Protein (g)	Fat (g)	Calories
Carbohydrates 1 slice bread, ½ bagel, ½ hamburger bun, ½ cup corn, ½ cup mashed potato	15	3	1 or less	80
Fruit 1 Apple, ½ banana, ½ grapefruit	15	—	—	60
Milk				
Skim 1 cup skim milk	12	8	0–3	90
Low-fat 1 cup 2% milk	12	8	5	120
Whole 1 cup whole milk	12	8	8	150
Other 1 glazed donut, 1 bar granola, 1 sweet roll	Varies	Varies	Varies	Varies
Vegetables Carrots, green beans, and spinach; ½ cup cooked, 1 cup raw, 1 large tomato	5	2	—	25
Meat/Meat Substitutes				
Very lean 1 oz white meat chicken, no skin; 1 oz. fat free cheese	—	7	0–1	35
Lean 1 oz lean beef, chicken (skinless), or fish; ¼ cup cottage cheese	—	7	3	55
Medium-fat 1 oz most beef, pork, lamb, and chicken (with skin) products; ¼ cup tuna fish	—	7	5	75
High-fat 1 oz pork sausage, 1 tbsp peanut butter, 1 oz regular cheese	—	7	8	100
Fat 1 tsp butter or margarine, 1 strip bacon			5	45

Courtesy of Carole Colebank, R.D., C.D.E., Veterans Administration Medical Center.

weight loss of 10 to 20 pounds has been shown to improve diabetes control, even when weight loss goals have not been met.

The most frequent lipid abnormalities in individuals with type 2 diabetes are hypertriglyceridemia, increased very-low-density lipoprotein cholesterol, and reduced high-density lipoprotein cholesterol. A reduction in high dietary intakes of cholesterol-raising fatty acids is important in reducing the risk of cardiovascular disease.

ELDERLY CONSIDERATIONS

The overall goals of nutrition therapy for the elderly are the same as for persons with diabetes. The elderly are at increased risk for malnutrition and hypoglycemia and are particularly prone to developing dehydration, a factor in the development of the hyperglycemic hyperosmolar nonketotic syndrome. Malnutrition is often a multifactorial process. Elderly clients who prepare their own food or who have tooth loss or poorly fitting dentures might not eat enough food. Autonomic neuropathy with gastric retention or diarrhea compounds poor food intake. Impaired cognition and depression may alter compliance with self-management. Socioeconomic factors play an important role in nutrition therapy. Clients may have a marginal food supply because of inadequate income, may have poor understanding of meal planning goals, or may live alone and have reduced incentive to prepare or eat proper meals. They may eat in restaurants or live in situations where they have little control over meal preparation. Regular visits by home health care nurses can assist the elderly client in following a diabetic meal plan.

A realistic approach to diet therapy is essential for the elderly diabetic client. Changing eating habits of 60 to 70 years is difficult. The nurse and dietitian assess the client's usual eating patterns. The nurse helps the elderly client taking hypoglycemic medications to understand the importance of

- Eating meals and snacks at the same time every day
- Eating the same amount of food from day to day
- Eating all food allowed on the diet

The nurse reinforces measures that maintain overall blood glucose control for the diabetic client.

Exercise Therapy. Regular physical exercise is a recommended component of a comprehensive diabetic treatment plan. Although exercise programs alone do not improve glycemic control, exercise is encouraged because of its potential to improve cardiovascular fitness and psychological well-being (ADA, 1998c). The beneficial effect of exercise on blood glucose control seems to reverse insulin resistance.

The response to exercise depends on insulin availability at the onset of exercise. Physical activity by the client with type 1 diabetes may lead to improvement or deterioration of metabolic control. With sufficient insulin, energy is obtained from the breakdown of muscle glycogen, hepatic glucose production, gluconeogenesis, and the use of free fatty acids (FFA). During the first 40 minutes of exercise, energy is provided by hepatic glucose production. Fat provides energy for exercise sessions lasting longer than 120 minutes. Exercise potentiates the action of insulin, resulting in an increased risk of hypoglycemic reactions during and after exercise.

In the uncontrolled diabetic client without adequate insulin, cells are unable to receive glucose, the preferred fuel, despite high blood glucose levels. Low insulin levels allow glucagon to increase hepatic glucose production, further raising blood glucose levels, with no means of using glucose at the muscle site. FFAs become the source of energy. Exercise in this client results in further hyperglycemia and ketone formation.

Clients with good metabolic control may have sustained hyperglycemia after vigorous exercise periods. Hepatic glucose production increases to provide the energy needs for exercise. In nondiabetic clients, this increased glucose production is balanced by an increase in plasma insulin secretion so that major fluctuations in blood glucose levels are avoided. The client with type 1 diabetes is unable to increase plasma insulin levels, and post-exercise hyperglycemia develops. This occurrence is thought to result from hepatic glucose production at a greater rate than peripheral glucose uptake.

Benefits of Exercise. Moderate sustained exercise helps regulate blood glucose levels on a day-to-day basis and results in lowered insulin requirements for clients with type 1 diabetes. Regular exercise improves diabetic control by increasing insulin sensitivity, improving glucose clearance, and promoting weight loss.

Regular exercise decreases risk factors for cardiovascular disease, such as hyperlipidemia, coagulation abnormalities, hypertension, glucose intolerance, and obesity. In response to exercise training, clients with type 1 diabetes have decreases in total cholesterol, low-density lipoproteins, and triglyceride levels and an increase in high-density lipoproteins (Wasserman & Zinman, 1994). Exercise decreases systolic and diastolic blood pressures and improves cardiovascular function. Regular vigorous physi-cal activity appears to have an important role in the prevention of type 2 diabetes through its association with reduced body weight and through independent effects on insulin resistance and glucose intolerance.

Risks Related to Exercise. Prolonged alterations in blood glucose levels can occur, particularly after sustained high-intensity activity. Hypoglycemia can occur 6 to 15 hours after exercise and may persist for 24 hours. Hyperglycemia, occurring even in clients with well-controlled diabetes, can persist for several hours after exercise is completed.

Several complications of diabetes can be aggravated by exercise. The nurse and the physician advise clients with proliferative retinopathy to avoid activities that increase blood pressure or are associated with the Valsalva maneuver. Heavy lifting, rapid head motion, or jarring activities can precipitate vitreous hemorrhage or retinal detachment. Exercise is associated with increased proteinuria in clients with diabetic nephropathy. The risk of foot and joint injury is increased for clients with peripheral neuropathy. Autonomic neuropathy can cause post-exercise (orthostatic) hypotension.

Screening Before Initiating an Exercise Program. The nurse advises the client to have a complete history and physical examination before initiating a physical activity program. Regular activity increases the risk of both musculoskeletal injury and life-threatening cardiovascular events. Several risk factor assessment scales are in use, but all base recommendations for exercise on the results of exercise stress tests. The ability of the heart to respond to increasing levels of exercise on a treadmill and the presence of other risk factors form the bases of the exercise prescription. For diabetic clients unable to perform vigorous exercise, the heart's ability to exercise is tested with cardiac stressor drugs (e.g., coronary vasodilators, dipyridamole thallium scans) (Fleg, 1995). The client also is carefully evaluated for diabetic complications (e.g., proliferative retinopathy and autonomic or peripheral neuropathy) to determine specifics of the exercise prescription.

Guidelines for Exercise. The client determines blood glucose levels before exercise. When levels are greater than 250 mg/dL (13.8 mmol/L), the client tests urine for ketones. The absence of urinary ketones suggests that adequate insulin is available to promote intracellular glucose transport and utilization and that exercise should be effective in lowering blood glucose levels. Ketones, a contraindication to exercise, indicates that current insulin levels are inadequate and exercise would lead to further elevation in blood glucose levels.

Aerobic exercise is performed with energy (ATP) produced from oxidation of amino acids, fatty acids, and glucose via the Krebs cycle. When recommending exercises appropriate for diabetic clients, the nurse understands that less intense aerobic exercise for longer durations is effective in achieving desired health effects. Aerobic exercise is characterized by slow, submaximal effort, continues for greater than 12 to 15 minutes, is rhythmic in nature, and results in a moderately elevated heart rate (above 50 maximal heart rate). Aerobic exercise has been shown to improve cardiac output (blood volume and stroke volume). Examples of aerobic activities include walking briskly, running, jogging, stationary or regular bicycling, swimming, calisthenics, aerobic dancing, rowing, and cross-country skiing.

For individuals with type 1 diabetes, duration of aerobic exercise should be 20 to 40 minutes, with a recommended frequency of 4 to 7 days per week. A 5- to 10-minute warm-up period consisting of static stretching and low-intensity exercise, with a 5- to 10-minute cool-down period reduces the risk of post-exercise dysrhythmias. The intensity and duration of exercise for individuals with type 2 diabetes is based on results of stress testing. Exercise should be undertaken at least four times a week. Daily exercise will increase total energy expenditure and facilitate weight loss. Daily exercise is also preferred for individuals taking insulin because of improved blood glucose control with the combination of exercise and insulin injections.

Special Precautions Related to Exercise. The nurse instructs the client to always use proper footwear with good traction and cushioning to help prevent falls. The client examines the feet daily and after exercise. The nurse advises the client to avoid exercise in extreme heat or cold or during periods of poor control of diabetes and to maintain hydration, especially during and after exercise in a warm environment.

The nurse teaches the client not to exercise within 1 hour of insulin injection or at the peak time of insulin action. Physical activity can increase absorption of insulin from the injection site, with a resultant increase in plasma insulin concentration. The potential for hypoglycemia increases when insulin is injected into an area that is exercised.

The nurse makes certain that all diabetic clients engaging in exercise, whether on a planned or sporadic basis, are aware of the potential for hypoglycemia and teaches preventive measures. Clients taking oral medications or insulin should perform blood glucose monitoring to determine effects of their exercise program. The nurse teaches the client that supplemental snacks of rapidly absorbable carbohydrates (CHO) may be taken before and during exercise to maintain blood glucose levels within normal ranges. Additional CHO may be taken for up to 24 hours after exercise to replenish muscle and liver glycogen stores and to prevent post-exercise hypoglycemia. The amount of additional CHO intake is directed by the results of blood glucose monitoring. The nurse instructs the client to decrease insulin dosage before planned exercise according to primary care provider direction.

Clients with type 1 diabetes should undertake vigorous exercise only if blood glucose levels are in the range of 80 mg/dL (4.4 mmol/L) to 250 mg/dL (13.8 mmol/L) and if there are no ketones (Wasserman & Zinman, 1995). In the nonobese client who is taking insulin, the nurse recommends a CHO-containing snack if at least 1 hour has elapsed since the last food was eaten or if high-intensity exercise is planned. The nurse explains that there is no need for additional CHO intake when the blood glucose level is greater than 100 mg/dL (5.6 mmol/L) before exercise and the planned activity is of low intensity and short

duration. When vigorous activity of long duration is planned, the client should eat an additional 15 to 30 g of CHO for every 30 to 60 minutes of exercise. Snacks such as fruit, fruit juice, bread products, and whole milk are effective in preventing hypoglycemia. The nurse teaches the client to carry a simple sugar (hard candy) to take for symptomatic hypoglycemia. Intake of a rapidly absorbed CHO causes a greater increase in plasma glucose concentration. The nurse also instructs the client to carry identifying information about being a diabetic.

ELDERLY CONSIDERATIONS

With age, ability of the heart and lungs to deliver oxygen to the periphery, as measured by oxygen use during exercise testing (VO_2 max), declines. Studies show these changes may be due more to decline in muscle mass than to alterations in cardiac output. Healthy elderly clients are able to maintain cardiac output by compensatory changes in stroke volume during exercise. Aerobic activities are thought to be important in maintaining muscle mass.

Specific exercise programs are beneficial for the *frail elderly*, who, because of weak muscles and poor balance, are at greater risk for falls and fractures. Clients who are limited to low-intensity programs can achieve benefits when exercise is performed frequently. Leg-lifting exercises, performed three times a week, has resulted in improved muscle size and better functional abilities in nursing home residents.

Whole Pancreas Transplantation. Pancreas transplantation can be an alternative to continued insulin therapy in type 1 diabetic clients with end-stage renal disease who plan to have a kidney transplant. Quality of life is improved when clients no longer have to take insulin injections and are free from diabetic dietary restrictions. However, no evidence currently indicates that pancreas transplantation can prevent or retard development and/or progression of long-term complications of diabetes, nor does evidence suggest that transplantation can prolong the life of the diabetic individual (ADA, 1998n).

More than 6000 pancreas transplants had been reported to the International Pancreas Transplant Registry by mid-1995 (Sutherland & Gruessner, 1995). In the United States, the overall 1-year survival rate for all types of pancreas transplant is 91% and the pancreas-graft survival rate (independent of need for exogenous insulin) is 72% (Larsen et al., 1994). Most transplanted pancreas glands are from cadaver donors. HLA-DR matching or mismatching affects the results. Pancreas transplantation can be performed in one of three situations: pancreas transplantation alone in the pre-uremic client, pancreas transplantation after successful kidney transplantation, and simultaneous pancreas-kidney transplantation (SPK). The procedure of choice for the diabetic uremic client is SPK.

Surgical Procedure. The SPK procedure with drainage of exocrine secretions into the urinary bladder has the highest graft survival rate. Data from the International Pancreas Transplant Registry indicated 1-year survival rates of 76% with simultaneous procedures and 50%

when the procedure was performed after the kidney transplant or in the pre-uremic diabetic individual (Sollinger & Geffner, 1994). Recently there has been renewed interest in the surgical technique of anastomosing the transplanted pancreas to the duodenum. Exocrine secretions are then absorbed as normal through the gastrointestinal tract, thereby preventing the dehydration that is common with bladder-drained transplantation.

Rejection Management. Immunosuppressive therapy with monoclonal antibodies (OKT3) or polyclonal antibody preparations (antithymocyte serum [Atgam]), azathioprine (Imuran), cyclosporine (Neoral, Sandimmune), tacrolimus (Prograf), and prednisone (Winpred♣), is given to prevent rejection of the transplanted pancreas. Cyclosporine is started when adequate kidney function has been established and serum creatinine is less than 3 mg/dL. High-dose steroids are used as initial treatment for graft rejection, with severe rejection requiring additional OKT3. Azathioprine therapy is based on degree of bone marrow suppression: white blood cell levels less than $5000/\mu L$ indicate a need for dosage reduction (Villagomez, 1995).

Successful pancreatic transplantation is indicated by improvement in blood glucose control as measured by glucose tolerance tests and glycosylated hemoglobin determinations, as well as by measurements of C-peptide levels. In nearly 90% of rejection episodes, kidney dysfunction manifests itself earlier than pancreatic dysfunction. In diabetic clients with urinary drained solitary pancreatic transplants, a decrease in urine amylase level by 25% is used as an indication to treat rejection. Hyperglycemia is a later marker of rejection and usually indicates irreversible graft failure.

Long-Term Effects. Long-term concerns include the effects of immunosuppression and hyperinsulinemia. Long-term immunosuppressive therapy is associated with increased risk of infections, secondary malignant lesions, and atherosclerosis. The transplanted pancreas approximates but does not duplicate the functions of a normal pancreas. Because the pancreas is transplanted into the peritoneal cavity, insulin drains into systemic rather than portal circulation, with elevations in circulating insulin levels. Hyperinsulinemia is a risk factor for both hypertension and macrovascular disease.

Complications of Pancreas Transplantation. Complications are to be anticipated in clients receiving organ transplants and requiring long-term immunosuppressive therapy. Major complications of pancreas transplant include venous thrombosis, rejection, and infection. Sollinger & Geffner (1994) indicate that 80% of individuals receiving SPK transplant had at least one episode of acute rejection, and 81.4% suffered at least one episode of infection. Careful monitoring of laboratory values, fluid and electrolyte status, physical signs and symptoms, and vital sign changes can alert the nurse to possible complications and the need to notify the physician for therapy. Early removal of invasive intravascular lines, sterile technique with dressing changes and catheter irrigations, strict hand washing by health care personnel, and vigorous pulmonary toilet all help prevent infection.

Thrombosis of vessels supplying the pancreas has occurred in as many as 30% of the transplant population. Changes in surgical technique have reduced the incidence of this complication. The nurse observes for and reports to the physician any sharp and sudden drop in urine amylase levels, rapid increases in serum glucose, gross hematuria, severe pain in the iliac fossa, and tenderness in the graft area (Villagomez, 1995).

The nurse assesses the diabetic client for signs and symptoms of acute and chronic graft rejection. Deterioration in renal function is reflected by increased serum creatinine and blood urea nitrogen, decreased urine output, hypertension, increased weight, graft tenderness, and fever. Proteinuria is often the first indicator of chronic graft rejection. The nurse observes for signs and symptoms of pancreatic rejection: decreased urinary amylase, graft tenderness, hyperglycemia, and fever. It is especially important to assess for signs and symptoms of infection and initiate appropriate treatment. Fever can be a sign of both infection and rejection.

The nurse monitors for side effects of immunosuppressive drugs. Cyclosporine (Neoral) is nephrotoxic: symptoms of toxicity include a rise in creatinine and possibly a decrease in urine output. White blood counts are monitored daily because azathioprine (Imuran) is associated with myelosuppression. Prednisone has multiple side effects, including steroid-induced diabetes. Hypertension is a common adverse effect of tacrolimus (Prograf).

The client's quality of life is improved as a result of freedom from the need for insulin, a less restricted lifestyle, and a return to normal diet. The nurse must stress, however, the potential for future insulin injections to treat hyperglycemia caused by immunosuppressive drugs.

Islet Cell Transplantation. Islet cell transplantation in rodents and canines successfully eliminates the requirement for exogenous insulin administration and protects the recipients from the complications of diabetes. Transplantation of islet cells into humans has been limited by the technical inability to obtain a sufficient number of islet cells. HLA-matched cadaver pancreas glands are used, and isolated islet cells are injected into the portal vein or implanted beneath the renal capsule or into the splenic parenchyma. Successful transplantation has occurred in a small number of clients. Islet cell transplantation is currently considered to be an experimental procedure.

➤ Risk for Injury Related to Stress of Surgery

Planning: Expected Outcomes. The diabetic client undergoing a surgical procedure is expected to have a satisfactory and complete postoperative recovery without complications.

Interventions. Surgery is a physical and emotional stressor, and the diabetic client is at more-than-average risk for intraoperative and postoperative complications. Acute stress increases the supply of glucose through the action of the various counterregulatory hormones. These hormones suppress the action of insulin, predisposing the client to ketoacidosis and metabolic acidosis. Postoperative fasting contributes to the development of ketoacidosis. Osmotic diuresis, resulting from hyperglycemia, can cause severe dehydration with loss of electrolytes.

Atherosclerotic disease, diabetic nephropathy, and autonomic neuropathy further increase the risk of surgical complications. Postoperative mortality has been reported to be 50% higher in clients with cerebrovascular disease and diabetes. Diabetic nephropathy makes fluid management more difficult. Cardiac dysrhythmias may result from the combined effect of anesthesia and autonomic neuropathy on the cardiovascular system. Autonomic neuropathy may cause postoperative complications of ileus formation and urinary retention.

Glycemia must be controlled to prevent acute complications of hypoglycemia, diabetic ketoacidosis, and hyperglycemic hyperosmolar nonketotic syndrome. Glycemic control is also necessary to reduce infection and ensure postoperative wound healing. Perioperative blood glucose levels between 120 mg/dL (6.7 mmol/L) and 200 mg/dL (11.1 mmol/L) have been found to prevent hypoglycemia, reduce infection, and ensure postoperative wound healing (Hirsh & Paauw, 1997). Surgical procedures that can be performed on a nonemergent basis have better outcomes. A period of 12 to 16 hours may be needed to achieve good metabolic control in clients requiring emergency surgery. In cases of sepsis, delay in operation only increases surgical risk. Insulin resistance and metabolic decompensation associated with infection respond only after the source of infection has been properly treated.

Preoperative Care. The physician should discontinue chlorpropamide (Diabinese) for at least 36 hours before surgery. Metformin (Glucophage) should be discontinued 48 hours prior to the surgical procedure and reinstituted only after renal function has been re-evaluated and found to be normal (Hirsh & Paauw, 1997). All other oral agents should be discontinued the day of surgery. Adjustments in insulin therapy are based on preoperative blood glucose levels. Upon admission, the nurse starts intravenous fluids as ordered to maintain hydration, monitors blood glucose results, and administers insulin as ordered. Preoperative blood glucose management may promote optimal nutritional status of the diabetic, promoting the inflammatory response and collagen synthesis.

Operative procedures for individuals with type 1 diabetes performed early in the day will cause the least disruption in metabolic control. Stable blood glucose levels can be achieved by administration of intravenous insulin when operative procedures are scheduled later in the day. Withholding normal insulin doses can cause significant hyperglycemia and ketonemia, resulting in electrolyte abnormalities. Administering a portion of the normal subcutaneous insulin dose involves guesswork and may cause a large, unexpected release of depot insulin after surgery is underway (Hirsh & Paauw, 1997). The nurse performs frequent blood glucose monitoring to determine the need for supplemental insulin.

Plans for postoperative pain control need to be made in the preoperative period. Pain stimulates the release of counterregulatory hormones with resultant hyperglycemia and corresponding increased insulin requirements. The older patient who receives opioid analgesic medication may be more susceptible to complications such as confu-

sion, ileus, hypoventilation, and hypotension. The effects of opioid analgesics on retarding gastrointestinal motility and the subsequent effects on blood glucose levels needs to be considered. Many individuals with long-standing diabetes have gastroparesis. Compared with intramuscular injections of opioids, patient-controlled analgesia systems are associated with fewer respiratory complications and a lower incidence of confusion. (See Chapter 9 for interventions related to pain and Chapter 20 for general preoperative care.)

Intraoperative Care. The frequency of intraoperative assessments of blood glucose depends in part on the type of anesthetic agent used. Epidural anesthesia has minimal effects on glucose metabolism. During general anesthesia, glucose levels increase early and remain elevated throughout the operative period. Operative procedures lasting 3 to 5 hours or longer produce considerable hyperglycemia, with these clients requiring supplemental short-acting insulin.

Intraoperative intravenous administration of short-acting insulin in 5% to 10% glucose is recommended for all insulin-treated clients, as well as for poorly controlled drug- or diet-treated clients who are undergoing general anesthesia. Blood glucose levels less than 200 mg/dL at the time of tissue injury may also promote leukocyte function and reduce the incidence of wound infection. Because of insulin resistance created by counterregulatory hormones, larger-than-normal doses of insulin may be necessary. The physician orders insulin/glucose infusion rates based on results of hourly intraoperative capillary blood glucose tests.

In addition to monitoring blood glucose values, the nurse monitors the client's temperature. Body temperature is deliberately lowered in some operative procedures and inadvertently in others. The physical temperature of the operating room and the size of the surgical incision create conditions that help lower body temperature. Hypothermia decreases metabolic needs, depresses heart rate and myocardial contractility causes peripheral vasoconstriction, and impairs insulin release with resultant hyperglycemia. In addition, the nurse and the anesthesiologist monitor arterial blood gas values for acidosis.

Postoperative Care. The nurse continues glucose and insulin infusions as ordered until the client is stable and able to tolerate oral feedings. Supplemental short-acting insulin, with the dosage based on blood glucose monitoring, may be needed to control hyperglycemia until the client's usual medication regimen can be restarted. Short-term insulin therapy may be necessary for the client receiving oral agents alone, or changes in the usual insulin dosage may be needed until the stress of surgery subsides. Only human insulin should be used for short-term therapy to prevent the potential for subsequent insulin allergy.

Postoperative Monitoring. Clients with autonomic neuropathy or vascular disease require careful monitoring to avoid hypotension or respiratory arrest. Clients whose hypertension is well controlled with the administration of beta-blockers must be monitored carefully for asymptomatic hypoglycemia. Clients with azotemia (increased nitrogen waste products in the blood) may have problems with fluid management. The nurse monitors central venous pressure or pulmonary artery pressure as necessary.

Hyperkalemia is often seen in clients with mild to moderate kidney failure and can precipitate an acute cardiac dysrhythmia. In other clients, hypokalemia may be present and is aggravated by insulin and glucose therapy given during surgical treatment. The nurse monitors the client's cardiac rhythm and serum potassium values as ordered.

Cardiovascular Assessment. Serial postoperative electrocardiograms (ECG) are recommended for older diabetic clients, those with long-standing type 1 diabetes, and clients with known heart disease. Diabetic clients have a high incidence of postoperative myocardial infarctions that are associated with a high mortality rate. Alterations in ECG or in potassium levels may indicate a silent myocardial infarction.

Renal Assessment. Careful monitoring of fluid balance helps detect acute kidney failure. Diagnosis of renal impairment may require the use of x-rays with iodinated contrast material. Treatment of infections may necessitate the use of nephrotoxic antibiotics. The physician and nurse ensure adequate hydration of the client when these drugs are used. The nurse monitors for impending renal failure by careful evaluation of the client's fluid and electrolyte status.

Nutritional Care. The use of total parenteral nutrition (TPN) in diabetic clients can result in severe metabolic challenges. Frequent capillary blood glucose monitoring determines the need for supplemental short-acting insulin. After a stable dose of insulin is reached, insulin can be added to the TPN solution and the frequency of capillary blood glucose determinations decreased.

Returning to a normal meal plan as soon as possible postoperatively promotes healing and re-establishes homeostasis. After the client is tolerating oral foods, the nurse ensures that the client takes at least 150 to 200 g of carbohydrate daily to prevent hypoglycemia and ketosis due to starvation.

> ➤ *Risk for Injury Related to Sensory Alterations*

Planning: Expected Outcomes. The client will
- Identify factors that increase potential for injury
- Practice proper foot care to prevent injury
- Maintain intact skin on feet

Interventions. Foot disease is the most common complication of diabetes leading to hospitalization. Diabetes is associated with more than 51% of nontraumatic lower-limb amputations. The overall risk of amputation is 15-fold greater in diabetic clients than in nondiabetic people. In a study of amputations on type 2 diabetes clients, 77% of the amputations were indicated for the treatment of gangrene. After gangrene, the secondary reason for amputation was nonhealing ulcerations. For those clients who have had a previous amputation, the risk of amputation in the second leg is 10 to 20 times greater than the risk of amputation in the general population.

Studies support the need for intensive education about foot care in diabetic populations. Seventy-three percent of

lower-extremity amputations in one study were caused by trauma that resulted in tissue injury. Thirty percent of these were due to ill-fitting shoes, and another 18% were due to accidental cuts and thermal burns. The importance of glycemic control was emphasized in a study by Lehto et al. (1996). Decreasing levels of high-density lipoprotein cholesterol, increasing levels of plasma glucose and HbAlc, and increasing duration of diabetes were associated with elevated risk of amputation.

Sensory neuropathy, ischemia, and infection are the leading pathogenic factors in foot disease associated with diabetes. Peripheral neuropathy is present in more than 80% of diabetic individuals with foot lesions. Loss of sensation in the foot increases the chance of injury and development of ulcerations. Impaired blood flow to the foot limits healing of the wound.

Foot deformities due to peripheral neuropathy frequently lead to ulceration. Foot deformities occur because of motor nerve loss to the interosseous muscles. The imbalance of these muscles results in claw toes or hammer toes. The toes become ulcerated because of increased pressure from the top of the shoe and/or from the insole. There is also a thinning or shifting of the fat pad under the first metatarsal head, which predisposes this area to calus formation, ulceration, and infection. Figure 68–9 illustrates hallux valgus (turning of the great toe), and Figure 68–10 illustrates hammer toes. Ulcerations on the dorsum of the foot are most likely caused by trauma; those on the side of the foot are most likely due to an ill-fitting shoe (Levin, 1996).

The Charcot foot is another example of a diabetic foot deformity. The Charcot foot is warm, swollen, and somewhat painful. Continued ambulation results in collapse of the arch, shortening of the foot, and rocker bottom shape to the foot. The client feels these changes because of autonomic nervous system involvement.

Although sensory neuropathy may be manifested as tingling or burning, it is more often evident as numbness and reduced sensation. Many clients have autonomic neuropathy that causes dry and atrophic skin. Cracks and fissures in the skin predispose the client to infection.

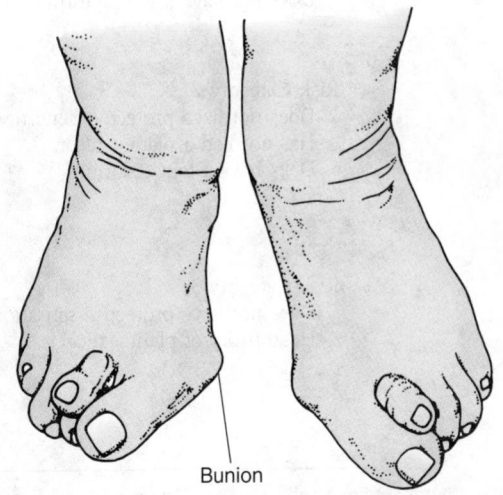

Bunion

Figure 68–9. The appearance of hallux valgus with a bunion.

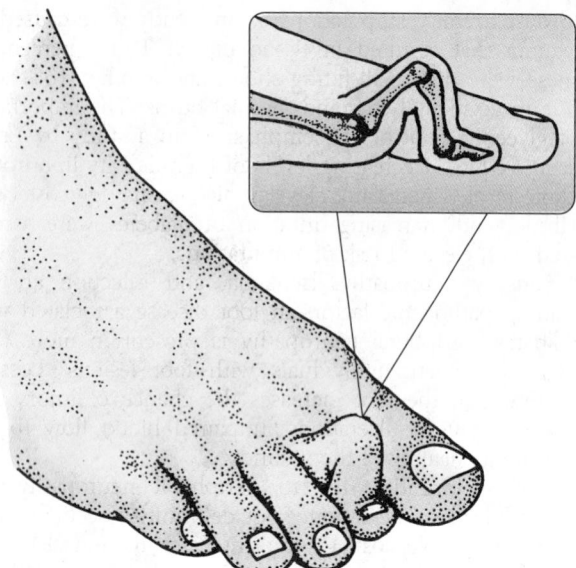

Figure 68–10. Hammer toe of the second metatarsophalangeal (MTP) joint.

The progressive loss of sensation allows prolonged painless trauma to cause major foot problems. Because sensation is absent, the client does not notice mechanical, thermal, or chemical injuries to the foot. Thus, the client does not take measures to treat the injuries. Foot injuries can be caused by walking barefoot, wearing ill-fitting shoes, sustaining thermal injuries from hot water (e.g., hot water bottles, heating pads, and baths), and receiving caustic burns caused by over-the-counter medications to treat corns. Because vascular supply to the diabetic foot is compromised, these injuries sometimes lead to amputation.

Importance of Blood Glucose Control. Selby and Zhang (1995) found a strong association between overall blood glucose control and the incidence of lower-extremity amputations. Both fasting and random blood glucose values were higher in those clients undergoing amputation. This study highlights the need to educate the client about measures to achieve and maintain blood glucose control.

Foot Screening. A comprehensive vascular, neurologic, musculoskeletal, and skin and soft-tissue evaluation should be done at least annually to determine risk for foot-related problems (ADA, 1998g) (Table 68–14). Sensory examination with Semmes-Weinstein monofilaments remains the single most practical measure of the risk for foot ulcers (McNeely et al., 1995). The nylon filament is pressed against the skin until it buckles. Inability to feel the 5.07 Semmes-Weinstein monofilament indicates high risk for injury. See Research Application for Nursing regarding assessment of the diabetic foot "at risk" for injury.

TABLE 68–14

Foot Risk Categories

Risk Categories	Management Categories
Risk Category 0 Has disease that leads to insensitivity Has protective sensation Has not had a plantar ulcer	Management Category 0 Examine feet at each visit, at least 4 times per year Foot clinic once a year Client education
Risk Category 1 Does not have protective sensation Has not had a plantar ulcer Does not have a foot deformity	Management Category 1 Examine feet at each visit, at least 4 times per year Foot clinic visit every 6 months Soft insoles Client education
Risk Category 2 Does not have protective sensation Has not had a plantar ulcer Does have a foot deformity	Management Category 2 Examine feet at each visit, at least 4 times per year Foot clinic visit every 3–4 months Custom-molded insoles Prescription footwear Client education
Risk Category 3 Does not have protective sensation Has history of plantar ulcer	Management Category 3 Examine feet at each visit, at least 4 times per year Foot clinic visit every 1–2 months Custom-molded insoles Prescription footwear Client education

From Gillis W. Long Hansen's Disease Center Rehabilitation Branch (1992). *Foot screening: Care of the foot in diabetes, the Carville approach.* Carville, LA: Department of Health and Human Services.

Research Application for Nursing

Identifying the Diabetic Foot "At Risk" for Injury

Collier, J. H., & Brodbeck, C. A. (1993). Assessing the diabetic foot: Plantar callus and pressure sensation. Diabetes Educator, 19(6), 503–508.

Pressure sensation measurement is considered an appropriate way to identify individuals at risk for diabetic foot ulceration. Plantar calluses forming on the prominent weight-bearing point of the foot are considered one of the most common precursors of plantar ulceration. The purpose of the study was to determine the relationship between loss of protective pressure sensation in the foot and formation of plantar calluses.

Data were collected on 102 diabetics referred for diabetes education. Pressure sensation was measured at nine points on each foot using Semmes-Weinstein monofilaments. The monofilament was applied perpendicular to the skin, pinning the free end on the skin and keeping the handle end directly above the free end until lateral bending occurred. Filaments were applied at the rate of 1-second touch, 1-second hold, and 1-second lift, with care taken not to slide the filament across the skin. Subjects were tested in a quiet area, wearing covered glasses to prevent them from seeing application of the filaments. Filaments were applied in ascending order of 1 g (4.17), 10 g (5.07), and 75 g (6.10). The location of calluses was recorded on a data sheet. Plantar calluses were measured to the nearest millimeter with a flexible centimeter ruler by identifying the lateral edges of the callus and recording the length and width of the callus at its longest and widest points. Subjects were defined as insensitive if they were unable to perceive application of the Semmes-Weinstein 10-g (5.07) monofilament on any one or more of six plantar sites tested on each foot.

The 67 persons found to have protective sensation had a mean duration of diabetes of 4.4 years, while the 35 insensitive subjects had a mean duration of diabetes of 11.6 years. Those with protective sensation were younger with an average age of 53.9, while those in the insensitive group had an average age of 60.3 years.

Problems were encountered while attempting to measure thickness of the callus.

Critique. Plantar calluses occur in both diabetic and non-diabetic populations. Because they are difficult to measure in a consistent and predictable way, their use as a predictive tool for diabetic foot care may be limited. Assessment of pressure sensation with Semmes-Weinstein monofilaments identified diabetic individuals at risk for foot injury as long as specific procedures were followed.

Possible Nursing Implications. Use of the Semmes-Weinstein monofilaments is an efficient way of identifying individuals at risk for diabetic foot injuries, particularly in populations with long-standing diabetes. This is a procedure that can be easily performed and can assist the nurse to determine the type of education needed by the diabetic client and the frequency of follow-up foot care that is required to prevent foot injury.

The nurse completes a full assessment of the diabetic foot as outlined in Chart 68–6.

Preventive Foot Care. All diabetic clients require education in preventive foot care and an examination of feet and legs at each visit to a health care provider. Clients with diabetes must understand the importance of proper foot care (ADA, 1998g). The nurse instructs *low-risk* clients about

- Foot hygiene
- Proper footwear
- Avoidance of foot trauma
- The need to stop smoking
- Actions to take if problems develop

In addition, clients determined to be at "high risk" for foot injury are taught to inspect their feet daily. Chart 68–7 outlines foot care instructions.

Footwear. All diabetic clients need to wear shoes that protect the foot from injury. Shoes need to be fit to the client by an experienced shoe fitter, such as a certified podiatrist. The shoe should be ½ to ⅝ inches longer than the longest toe. Heels greater than 2 inches in height shift the body weight toward the forefoot, onto the first and second metatarsal heads. The shift of weight increases pressure under the metatarsal heads, increasing the risk of foot ulcerations. Pressure from shoes that are too tight will cause tissue damage when maintained for 4 hours or more with no relief. The nurse teaches diabetic clients to

---

Chart 68–6

Focused Physical Assessment: The Diabetic Foot

- Assess the client for risk of diabetic foot problems
  - History of previous ulcer
  - History of previous amputation
- Assess the foot for evidence of deformity
  - Absence of pedal, popliteal, or femoral pulses
  - Prolonged capillary filling time (>3–4 seconds)
  - Decreased skin temperature
  - Toe deformity: Clawed toes, hammer toes, or unusual angulation of the toes
  - Prominent metatarsal heads: Metatarsal head is easily felt under the skin
  - Hallux valgus or bunions
  - Calluses, corns
  - Dry, cracked, fissured skin
  - Ulcers
  - Toenails: Thickened, long nails, ingrown nails, crumbling toenails
  - Charcot ("rocker bottom") foot
- Assess the foot for loss of strength
  - Limited ankle joint range of motion
  - Limited motion of great toe
- Assess the foot for loss of protective sensation
  - Numbness, burning, tingling
  - Semmes-Weinstein monofilament testing at 10 points on each foot
- Assess the foot for status of circulation
  - Presence/absence of dorsalis pedis or posterior tibial pulse

Education Guide: Foot Care Instructions

- Inspect your feet daily, especially the area between the toes.
- Wash your feet daily with lukewarm water and soap. Dry thoroughly.
- Apply moisturizing cream to your feet after bathing. Do not apply to the area between your toes.
- Change into clean, cotton socks every day.
- Do not wear the same pair of shoes 2 days in a row, and wear only leather shoes.
- Check your shoes for foreign objects (nails, pebbles) before putting them on: Check inside the shoes for cracks or tears in the lining.
- Purchase shoes that have plenty of room for your toes. Buy shoes later in the day when feet are normally larger. Break in new shoes gradually.
- Wear socks to keep your feet warm.
- Trim your nails straight across with a nail clipper. Smooth the nails with an emery board.
- See your physician or nurse immediately if you have blisters, sores, or infections. Protect area with a dry, sterile dressing. Do not use adhesive tape to secure dressing.
- Do not treat blisters, sores, or infections with home remedies.
- Do not smoke.
- Do not step into the bathtub without checking the temperature of the water with your wrist. Optimal temperature is 29.4°–35° C (95° F).
- Do not use very hot or cold water. Never use hot water bottles, heating pads, or portable heaters to warm your feet.
- Do not treat corns, blisters, bunions, calluses, or ingrown toenails yourself.
- Do not go barefooted.
- Do not wear sandals with open toes or straps between the toes.
- Do not cross your legs or wear garters or tight stockings that constrict blood flow.
- Do not soak your feet.

change their shoes by midday and again in the evening. Socks or stockings need to fit properly and be appropriate for planned activity. Stockings should feel soft and not have thick seams, creases, or holes that can irritate the skin. Stockings should provide padding for the foot and be able to absorb excess moisture. Stockings that are tight or have constricting bands are to be avoided. Diabetic clients with toe deformities need to purchase custom shoes with high, wide toe boxes and extra depth features. Clients with markedly deformed feet, such as Charcot feet, need specially molded shoes. All newly purchased shoes should have a slow break-in period, with periodic self-inspection of both feet for signs of irritation or blistering.

Wound Care. Wound care involves treatment of any localized infection, debridement of devitalized tissue, provision of a suitable environment for wound healing, and modification of weight bearing of the plantar surface of the foot. No controlled studies have yet determined the most appropriate topical solution to apply to a diabetic ulcer, but some controversy surrounds the effects of povidone-iodine, peroxide, or other antiseptics on wound healing. Treatment with these products is reported to kill fibroblasts within the wound and can dry and crack the surrounding skin. In cases of granulating wounds, which are more resistant to infection, the application of wet-to-dry saline dressings twice daily keeps the wound moist and provides gentle debridement. Promising results are being obtained with the application of platelet-derived growth factor directly to the wound.

The elimination of pressure on an infected area is essential to wound treatment. Pressure is reduced through specialized orthotic devices, custom-molded shoe inserts, or shoe sole modifications that redistribute weight as ordered by a podiatrist. Weight-bearing hinders the healing process, and simply telling the client to not walk does not produce compliance. The use of contact casting reduces pressure and still permits ambulation. The cast is minimally padded and carefully molded to the shape of the foot and leg, with a heel for walking. It is designed to distribute weight over the entire surface of the foot and leg, thereby protecting the ulcer site. The cast is removed 24 to 48 hours after application and weekly thereafter until the ulcer is healed. Discussing care after wound healing is essential. The client must understand that unless measures are taken to redistribute weight on a permanent basis, foot ulcers will recur. Clients, therefore, cannot wear their old, comfortable shoes.

Administration of Growth Factors. Topical application of growth factors accelerates tissue healing and results in a thick, durable scar. Six ounces of peripheral blood provide enough growth factor for topical application to a wound twice a day for 8 weeks. Because the treatment is expensive and based on having other aspects of diabetes controlled, this treatment is generally administered in comprehensive treatment centers. Long-standing diabetic foot ulcers are being healed with this treatment.

➤ *Pain Related to Peripheral Nerve Dysfunction*

Planning: Expected Outcomes. The client is expected to experience relief of pain and identify measures that increase comfort.

Interventions. Hyperglycemia is important not only in the pathogenesis of neuropathy but also in its treatment. Normalizing blood glucose levels may relieve symptoms of acute nerve dysfunction. However, many of the neuropathies result from irreversible structural change. Antidepressants, particularly amitriptyline hydrochloride (Elavil, Levate✦), are beneficial in treating pain caused by neuropathy. These drugs have an analgesia effect as a result of increases in norepinephrine and serotonin at the nerve synapse. Smaller doses are required for analgesia than for antidepressant effects. Capsaicin cream 0.075% (Axsain✦, Zostrix-HP), a derivative of the pepper plant, is used to relieve painful neuropathy. Capsaicin promotes depletion of pain-modulating substance P from terminals of small sensory neurons (Clark & Lee, 1995). Topical applications four times daily are needed for several weeks before relief is achieved. Clients may not tolerate the side effects of burning that occur during application to the skin. Trauma prevention is a major nursing intervention for diabetic clients with sensory peripheral neuropathy.

➤ Risk for Injury Related to Visual Sensory-Perceptual Alterations

Planning: Expected Outcomes. The client is expected to maintain optimal vision and be free from injury related to decreased visual acuity.

Interventions. Hyperglycemia, proteinuria, diastolic hypertension, and longer duration of diabetes are associated with the development of diabetic retinopathy. The DCCT demonstrated that retinopathy can be markedly reduced with good control of serum glucose. Three prospective randomized clinical trials have shown that vision loss from diabetes can be avoided with appropriate laser surgery or vitrectomy surgery.

Two major retinal problems cause most of the diabetes-related vision loss: diabetic macular edema and complications from retinal neovascularization (Murphy, 1995). Because these complications frequently do not cause visual symptoms, periodic dilated eye examinations are required. Studies show that as many as 21% of diabetics have retinopathy at the time of diagnosis.

The Diabetic Retinopathy Vitrectomy Study established the benefit of early vitrectomy in improving visual acuity in clients with recent severe vitreous hemorrhage. *Vitrectomy* involves removing the vitreous fluid and severing the traction bands that lead to retinal detachment.

The Early Treatment Diabetic Retinopathy Study established the benefit of focal laser photocoagulation in eyes with macular edema and scatter photocoagulation for severe retinopathy. Laser photocoagulation is beneficial in preventing further vision loss but not in reversing already diminished visual acuity. Macular edema is treated by placing laser spots in a grid pattern to stabilize visual acuity. Fragile blood vessels develop on the retina in response to a neovascular growth factor caused by hypoxia. Laser photocoagulation destroys the ischemic retina that produces the hypoxic stimulus for new vessel development. Expected side effects of laser therapy include decreased peripheral field vision, problems with night vision (nyctalopia), and subtle changes in color perception. Laser therapy applied to large vessels can be associated with vitreous hemorrhage (Aiello et al., 1996). A local anesthetic agent is usually injected before panretinal photocoagulation therapy.

The nurse helps relieve discomfort from the procedure by offering an ice pack and administering an ordered analgesic. One complication of laser therapy is macular edema, with resultant decrease in vision. The nurse explains that the blurred vision may persist for a few weeks and that it may take several months for visual improvement to occur. The diabetic client is instructed to avoid heavy lifting and straining for a few days.

The nurse stresses the need for evaluation of visual status according to ADA Standards of Care. A comprehensive dilated eye and visual examination should be performed annually by an ophthalmologist or optometrist for all diabetic clients over the age of 10 years who have had

diabetes for 3 to 5 years, all diabetic individuals over the age of 30 years, and any diabetic with visual symptoms and/or abnormalities (ADA, 1998r). Diabetic clients with persistently elevated serum glucose levels or proteinuria should be evaluated yearly for retinopathy (ADA, 1998e). Clients who have identified retinopathy, and particularly those who have received laser treatment, should be under the care of a retinal specialist and are encouraged to keep follow-up appointments. Information for receiving eye examinations at reduced cost for clients over the age of 65 years can be obtained by calling 1-800-222-EYES. An informational kit to help nurses advise clients about the dangers of blindness arising from diabetes can be obtained from the National Eye Health Education Program, 1-800-869-2020.

Only about 10% of all individuals with visual impairment are totally blind. The remainder have decreased visual abilities. In addition to regular eye examinations to evaluate retinopathy, the nurse encourages the client with diabetes and visual impairment to be examined by an optometrist or ophthalmologist for assessment of functional vision and prescription of appropriate eyewear. A functional vision assessment, performed by a low-vision technician, rehabilitation teacher, or diabetes educator, is a task-specific evaluation that determines the client's use of lighting, contrast, nonoptical and low-vision devices, and large-print options. Included in the functional vision assessment is whether the client uses central or peripheral vision. Diabetic clients with macular edema have loss of central vision. This process causes difficulties with detail discrimination, reading printed materials, preparing insulin syringes for injection, or performing self-monitoring of blood glucose.

Not all diabetics with visual impairment require use of special optical devices. Manipulation of lighting, contrast, color, distance, size, and eye movement will often improve visual abilities. The nurse recommends that the client improve vision by supplementing overhead fluorescent lighting with an incandescent lamp directed toward the work space. Placing dark equipment against a white or yellow background (or vice versa) provides contrast that will enhance vision. Coding objects such as vials of insulin with bright colors or with felt-tipped markers will aid in identification of the correct bottle to use. Bringing the blood glucose lancet or insulin syringe close to the eye makes it easier to see. The nurse directs the client to sources of materials printed with an enlarged typeface to enhance ability to read. The nurse helps the client learn to use peripheral fields of vision by learning to move the eye to maximize vision.

Visually adapted devices make it possible for the diabetic client to self-administer reliable insulin doses independently. Pre-set dose gauges (used to measure the space between the ends of the syringe barrel and plunger) allow an individual to draw the correct amount of insulin by touch. Variable dose gauges draw insulin in variable and mixed doses of 1-, 2-, and 10-U increments. The client obtains the desired dose by pressing a lever or turning a screw on the device. Pen-like devices dispense insulin from a cartridge after the client presses the plunger. Critical points to stress when teaching the client to use an adaptive device include the following:

- Different types of insulin need to be identified by an added tactile label. The label needs to be attached so that the type of insulin and expiration date are easily identified.
- Proper placement of the device on the syringe is essential for correct measurements.
- The insulin bottle needs to be held upright when measuring insulin.
- Air can be expelled from the syringe by pulling a small amount of insulin into the syringe, moving the plunger in and out three times, and measuring insulin on the fourth draw.
- A system to determine how many doses can be drawn from a bottle of insulin needs to be established so that the client does not inject air from an empty bottle rather than insulin (Cleary, 1994).

The nurse needs to assist the diabetic with visual impairment to maintain blood glucose control to limit the amount of functional vision change that normally occurs with hypo- and hyperglycemia.

➤ Altered Renal Tissue Perfusion

Planning: Expected Outcomes. The client is expected to maintain optimal urinary output.

Interventions. Strict control of blood glucose levels may reverse microalbuminuria in clients with type 1 diabetes. Results of the DCCT showed that intensive metabolic control reduced the incidence of microalbuminuria and reduced the progression of renal disease. Persistent microalbuminuria is shown to increase by about 20% per year in some clients and greater than 60% in others when blood pressure remains elevated. Treating hypertension does not arrest the progression to proteinuria but seems to slow the rate of decline in the glomerular filtration rate (Carella et al., 1994).

Control of blood pressure and blood glucose levels depends on the participation and cooperation of the patient. Prescribed medications must be taken according to schedules and dietary restriction maintained. All diabetic clients must be aware of the roles of blood pressure and blood glucose level in the development of renal disease. Nursing measures are directed toward assisting the diabetic client to maintain normal blood glucose and blood pressure levels below 130/85 mmHg (ADA, 1996e). Additionally, the nurse stresses the need for yearly screening for microalbuminuria.

The nurse stresses the need for yearly evaluation of renal status according to ADA Standards of Care. Routine urinalysis should be performed yearly in adults. In diabetic clients beyond the age of puberty with a history of diabetes for at least 5 years, a timed urine collection (e.g., 24 hours or overnight) should be tested for the presence of microalbumin, or the albumin/creatinine ratio should be measured yearly (ADA, 1998r). The development of hypertension or a rise in serum creatinine level indicates the need for more frequent evaluation. The nurse explains the implications of the test and assists the client in collecting the specimen if necessary.

Restriction of dietary protein to 0.8 g/kg body weight/day is recommended for individuals with evidence of microalbuminuria. In diabetic clients with overt diabetic nephropathy, restriction of dietary protein has been shown to retard progression to renal failure (ADA, 1998l). Because of the difficulty in maintaining lifelong dietary restrictions, the nurse provides ongoing education to assist with dietary compliance.

The nurse educates the client about the signs and symptoms of urinary tract infection. Because studies have shown that many clients do not complete their prescribed course of antibiotics for treatment of urinary tract infections, the nurse instructs the diabetic client to take medications exactly as prescribed, making certain that the course of treatment is completed. The client needs to see the physician or nurse for follow-up urine cultures as directed to reduce the risk of renal damage. In particular, aminoglycosides should be administered cautiously to clients with impaired renal function, in particular, and to diabetic clients, in general, to avoid nephrotoxicity. The administration of nonsteroidal anti-inflammatory drugs should be avoided. Diabetic clients are cautioned not to take unapproved over-the-counter medications.

Dialysis treatment for diabetics with renal failure is the same as for clients without diabetes. The dosage of insulin needs to be adjusted when dialysis is started.

➤ Potential Complication: Hypoglycemia

Planning: Expected Outcomes. The client is expected to have an optimal level of mental status functioning (e.g., be alert and oriented to person, place, and time, with a Glasgow Coma Scale score greater than 7) and have decreased episodes of hypoglycemia.

Interventions. Many diabetic clients will experience symptoms of hypoglycemia at levels above the biochemical definition of 50 mg/dL. A blood glucose level below 70 mg/dL should alert the nurse to assess for signs and symptoms of hypoglycemia (Table 68–15; see also Table 68–4).

Monitoring. The nurse monitors blood glucose levels before administering hypoglycemic agents, before meals, and before the hour of sleep, or when the client is symptomatic. All clients with diabetes who take insulin or sulfonylurea agents to lower blood glucose levels are at risk for hypoglycemia. Clients who take sulfonylurea agents are at risk for hypoglycemia

- If they are elderly
- If they have renal or hepatic impairment
- If they are receiving medication that potentiates the effects of oral agents

Treating Hypoglycemia. When the client is determined to be hypoglycemic, the nurse initiates treatment with carbohydrate replacement per physician orders or standing protocols. When the client can swallow, a liquid form of carbohydrate is administered, although virtually any low-fat source of carbohydrate can be used to treat hypoglycemia. Specific treatment recommendations are listed in Chart 68–8. The level of blood glucose being treated may determine the form of glucose to be used. Fluid is absorbed much more quickly from the gastrointestinal tract than solids. Sweetened fluids that are too concentrated may retard absorption. Commercially available products provide predictable amounts of glucose.

TABLE 68–15

Differentiation of Hypoglycemia and Hyperglycemia

Feature	Hypoglycemia	Hyperglycemia
Skin	Cool, clammy	Hot, dry*
Dehydration		Present
Perspiration	Profuse*	
Respirations		Rapid, deep* Kussmaul breathing Acetone odor to breath
Mental status	Anxious Nervous* Behavior change Irritable Mental confusion* Seizures Coma	Altered level of consciousness Lethargic* Stupor Coma
Symptoms	Weakness* Double vision Blurred vision Hunger Tachycardia Palpitations	Nausea and vomiting Abdominal cramps
Glucose	50 mg/dL (2.8 mmol/L)	>250 mg/dL (13.8 mmol/L)
Ketones	Negative	May be positive

*Classic symptoms.

Glucagon administered subcutaneously or intramuscularly and 50% dextrose administered intravenously are given to diabetic clients who are unable to swallow. Glucagon acts by converting liver glycogen to glucose and is not effective in severely starved patients. The nurse or assistive personnel take care to prevent aspiration in clients receiving glucagon, as it often causes vomiting. The nurse gives 50% dextrose carefully to avoid extravacation. The effects of glucagon and dextrose are temporary, and, after the client responds, the nurse administers a simple sugar followed by a small snack or meal.

The nurse evaluates the results of treatment by monitoring blood glucose levels for several hours. Blood glucose values provide more accurate assessment data for responses to treatment than do physical symptoms of the client. Posthypoglycemic adrenergic and neuroglycopenic symptoms may persist for 1 hour or more after treatment of hypoglycemia. A target blood glucose level is 70 mg/dL (3.9 mmol/L) to 110 mg/dL (6.2 mmol/L).

Preventing Hypoglycemia. The nurse teaches the diabetic client how to prevent future episodes of hypoglycemia. Four common causes of hypoglycemia are (1) excess insulin, (2) deficient intake or absorption of food, (3) exercise, and (4) alcohol. There are substantial variations in insulin absorption in any one individual diabetic. Even when insulin is injected in a consistent manner in a nonexercised body area, variations in insulin absorption can cause hypoglycemia. Excess insulin can be a consequence of lowered insulin resistance, which occurs with termination of pregnancy, resolution of an infection, or increased insulin sensitivity, which occurs with weight loss or exercise programs. The nurse instructs the diabetic individuals taking insulin not to change brands or to change from animal source to human insulin without medical supervision. Differences in formulation of insulin can result in hypoglycemia.

Inadequate or incorrectly timed dietary intake can result in hypoglycemia. Irregularities in gastric absorption sometimes cause hypoglycemia in patients with autonomic neuropathy. Gastroparesis is more common in patients with longer duration diabetes, is more pronounced with solid than with liquid meals, and may be temporarily aggravated by illness or poor metabolic control. The nurse instructs the diabetic client about the importance of regularity and consistency in timing and quantity of food eaten.

Blood glucose levels commonly decline during exercise in an individual with type 1 diabetes. With severe and prolonged exercise, increased rates of glucose utilization persist for several hours after the exercise has been completed. The nurse instructs the diabetic client in blood glucose monitoring and carbohydrate supplementation during exercise. Client-specific protocols, developed in consultation with the physician, assist the diabetic client to make appropriate adjustments in insulin dosage. The nurse ensures that the client understands specifics of the protocols and can make insulin adjustments safely.

Alcohol interferes with gluconeogenesis, the process by which blood glucose is maintained when food is not being absorbed. Alcohol cannot be converted to glucose and interferes with counterregulatory responses to insulin-in-

Chart 68-8

Education Guide: Treatment of Hypoglycemia at Home

For *mild* hypoglycemia (hungry, irritable, shaky, weak, headache, fully conscious, blood glucose usually less than 60 mg/dL [3.4 mmol/L]):

- Treat the symptoms of hypoglycemia with 10 to 15 g of carbohydrate. You can use one of the following:
  - 2–3 glucose tablets
  - ½ cup of orange or grape juice
  - ½ cup of regular soft drink
  - 8 oz of skim milk
  - 6–10 hard candies
  - 4 cubes of sugar
  - 2 packets of sugar
  - 6 saltines
  - 3 graham crackers
- Retest blood glucose in 15 minutes.
- Repeat this treatment if symptoms do not resolve.
- Take some food or the next scheduled meal within 15 to 30 minutes.

For *moderate* hypoglycemia (pale, cold and clammy skin, rapid pulse, rapid and shallow respirations, marked change in mood, drowsiness, blood glucose usually less than 40 mg/dL [2.2 mmol/L]):

- Treat the symptoms of hypoglycemia with 15 to 30 g of rapidly absorbed carbohydrate.
- Take additional food, such as low-fat milk or cheese, after 10 to 15 minutes.

For *severe* hypoglycemia (unable to swallow, unconsciousness or convulsions, blood glucose usually less than 20 mg/dL [1.0 mmol/L]), treatment administered by family members:

- Administer 1 mg of glucagon as intramuscular or subcutaneous injection.
- Administer a second dose in 10 minutes if the person remains unconscious.
- Notify a primary care provider immediately and follow instructions.
- If still unconscious, transport the person to the emergency department.
- Give a small meal when the person wakes up and is no longer nauseated.

normal rates of gluconeogenesis needed to prevent nighttime hypoglycemia) (Bell, 1994).

The cause of hypoglycemia may be subtle. At the onset of menses, a fall in progesterone level may decrease insulin requirements and contribute to hypoglycemia. When clients switch to a new bottle of insulin, hypoglycemia may be noted because the old bottle of insulin had lost its potency. Some clients report hypoglycemia when they change injection sites. Drugs, such as propranolol hydrochloride (Inderal, Detensol◆) or other beta-adrenergic blockers, may mask the early adrenergic warning signs and thus predispose clients to severe hypoglycemia. Some episodes of hypoglycemia occur without an obvious cause, and many are due to the erratic absorption of insulin, a problem that is not eliminated even in the most careful client.

The nurse can help each diabetic client develop a personally calibrated treatment plan for hypoglycemia. Routine administration 10 to 15 g of carbohydrate results in overtreatment of hypoglycemic episodes in some individuals and undertreatment in others. The exact glucose rise produced by a given amount of carbohydrate varies among individuals. Using the estimate that each 5 g of carbohydrate raises blood glucose about 20 mg/dL, a personal treatment plan can be developed that will provide direction for treatment of specific blood glucose levels. As an example, the diabetic can be directed to take

- 30 g of carbohydrate for a blood glucose level less than 40 mg/dL (2.2 mmol/L)
- 25 g for a blood glucose level from 40 to 50 mg/dL (2.2 to 2.8 mmol/L)
- 20 g for a blood glucose level of 51 to 60 mg/dL (2.8 to 3.4 mmol/L)
- 15 g for a blood glucose level of 61 to 80 mg/dL (3.4 to 4.4 mmol/L) (Farkas-Hirsh, 1995)

The parameters of the treatment plan are revised or reinforced by blood glucose monitoring results.

The nurse or assistive personnel instructs clients to wear an identification bracelet to advise others of their diabetic status. The bracelet is helpful if clients become hypoglycemic and are unable to provide self-care. The nurse also assists the client in obtaining the medical alert bracelet.

The nurse teaches the client and family about the signs and symptoms of hypoglycemia. Clients and family members must know that delaying a meal for more than 30 minutes carries the risk of hypoglycemia. The client should have a carbohydrate source available at all times.

The cause of all episodes of hypoglycemia should be determined and measures taken to prevent recurrence. Hypoglycemia is a major risk factor associated with exercise programs for clients receiving intensive insulin protocols. Nightmares or headaches on days after prolonged or severe exercise are associated with hypoglycemia, and this possibility should be understood by the client and family.

duced hypoglycemia (Farkas-Hirsh, 1995). The major problem with alcohol is the induction and masking of hypoglycemia from other causes. Hypoglycemia most commonly occurs when fasting takes place in conjunction with depletion of hepatic glycogen stores. Alcohol may also impair glycogenolysis and have a potentiating effect on exercise-induced hypoglycemia or the hypoglycemia induced by drugs such as beta-blockers (Bell, 1994). The nurse instructs the diabetic person to ingest alcohol according to ADA guidelines (ADA, 1998l) only with, or shortly after, eating a meal with sufficient carbohydrate to negate the hypoglycemic effects of alcohol. Additionally, the nurse cautions the diabetic about the dangers of excesses of alcohol at bedtime (i.e., alcohol interferes with

Establishing Treatment Plans. Blood glucose monitoring provides information on successful treatment of specific hypoglycemic episodes. The nurse will continue treatment per protocol until desired blood glucose results have been achieved and maintained. Once treatment has been provided and blood glucose control is regained, the specific cause of each hypoglycemic episode must be determined and measures taken by the diabetic client to prevent further recurrences.

➤ Potential Complication: Ketoacidosis

Planning: Expected Outcomes. The client is expected to maintain a normal blood glucose level and have minimized episodes of hyperglycemia.

Interventions. The nurse monitors for signs and symptoms of diabetic ketoacidosis (DKA) (see Table 68–3 and Fig. 68–2). In the initial phases of treatment, the nurse checks the client's blood pressure, pulse, and respiration every 15 minutes until stable. The nurse records urine output, temperature, and mental status every hour. When the physician has placed a central venous catheter, the nurse assesses central venous pressure as ordered, usually every 30 minutes. Assessing the client's level of consciousness, hydration status, status of fluid and electrolyte replacement, and levels of blood glucose are primary nursing measures, as are maintaining a patent airway and intact skin. After treatment is underway and these variables are stable, recording values every 4 hours is acceptable. Hourly determination of blood glucose values can be achieved by either laboratory or bedside glucose monitoring. Results indicate the adequacy of insulin replacement and establish the time to switch from saline to dextrose-containing solutions.

Fluid Therapy. Diligent assessment of the *fluid status* of the diabetic client is essential. The kidneys are less able to respond to changes in pH or fluid and electrolyte balance, to concentrate urine, or to selectively regulate osmolarity. The risk of kidney failure also rises with age. Impaired bicarbonate reabsorption and net acid excretion resulting from poorly functioning renal tubules can progress to acidosis. Cardiovascular disease can cause fluid retention. The dehydrated client's lips and mouth may appear dry and the tongue furrowed. Body temperature is often elevated. Because of age-related skin changes, such as loss of elasticity and dryness, skin turgor is a poor sign of dehydration in the elderly. In clients with poor renal function and excess fluid volume, the nurse observes for periorbital and extremity edema, increasing abdominal girth, blood pressure and pulse volume increases, jugular venous distention, and orthostatic hypotension. Daily weights and measurement of the abdomen provide a good indication of fluid retention (O'Donnell, 1995).

Upon physician orders, the nurse initiates treatment to correct fluid volume deficit. The initial goal of fluid therapy is to restore circulating volume and protect against cerebral, coronary, or renal hypoperfusion. The nurse administers 1 L of isotonic saline in 30 to 60 minutes, followed by a second liter in the next hour, or as ordered. The second objective of fluid therapy is to replace total body and intracellular losses and is achieved more slowly. The physician usually orders 0.45% saline at this time. When blood glucose levels reach 250 mg/dL (13.8 mmol/L), 5% dextrose in 0.45% saline is administered. This measure prevents hypoglycemia and the development of cerebral edema, which can occur when serum osmolality is reduced too rapidly.

During the first 24 hours of treatment, the client needs sufficient fluids, perhaps as much as 6 to 10 L, to replace both the volume deficit and ongoing losses. The nurse monitors for signs of congestive heart failure and pulmonary edema with infusion rates of this magnitude. To assess the affects of rapid intravenous therapy on the client's cardiac status, the physician may order central venous pressure monitoring in elderly clients and those with myocardial disease.

Drug Therapy. The goal of insulin therapy is to lower the serum glucose level by approximately 75 to 150 mg/dL/hr. Considerable controversy exists about the best insulin protocol to accomplish this goal. Current "low-dose" insulin therapy is associated with less incidence of hypokalemia and hypoglycemia than is seen with "high-dose" regimens. Although both intramuscular and intravenous (IV) administration have been used, most protocols for treating DKA recommend continuous IV administration of regular insulin because absorption from intramuscular or subcutaneous sites may be erratic. A steady-state level of insulin can be reached in 25 to 30 minutes. Effective concentrations can be achieved almost immediately when an IV bolus dose is given at the start of the infusion. As ordered, the nurse gives an initial IV bolus dose of 0.1 U/kg of regular insulin, followed by an IV drip of 0.1 U/kg/hour. Continuous infusion of insulin is required because of the 4-minute half-life of IV insulin. There is disagreement as to the availability of insulin after binding with the plastic of IV tubing. Subcutaneous insulin is started when the client can take oral nourishment and ketosis has stopped (Urban, et al, 1995).

Regardless of the initial potassium value, there is a large total body potassium deficit. With insulin therapy, the serum potassium level falls rapidly as potassium shifts to the intracellular space. The nurse monitors the client for signs of hypokalemia: muscle weakness, abdominal distention or paralytic ileus, hypotension, and weak pulse. An electrocardiogram shows cardiac conduction changes related to potassium. Hypokalemia remains a significant cause of mortality in the treatment of DKA. Prior to administration of IV potassium, the nurse ensures that the client's urinary output is at least 30 mL/hour.

Bicarbonate therapy is indicated only for *severe* acidosis. Inappropriate use of bicarbonate may reverse acidosis too rapidly and result in severe hypokalemia, which can produce fatal cardiac dysrhythmias. Rapid correction of acidosis can result in worsening of the client's mental status. Bicarbonate diffusion through the blood-brain barrier lowers cerebrospinal pH, causing central nervous system acidosis, with resultant respiratory depression and worsening of coma.

DKA carries a significant risk of thrombosis, especially in elderly, unconscious, or severely hyperosmolar clients. Subcutaneous heparin doses of 5000 U every 8 hours is a valuable preventive measure (Fish, 1994).

After metabolic disturbances have been corrected, the health team's efforts are directed toward determining the cause of DKA. Infection is the most common precipitating cause.

Client Education. Investigation of the factors precipitating DKA directs the nurse's educational efforts with the client. After the client is discharged from the hospital, blood glucose monitoring and attention to physical symptoms help the client detect impending hyperglycemia and institute appropriate action. The nurse teaches the client to perform self-monitoring of blood glucose levels (SMBG) every 4 to 6 hours as long as symptoms such as anorexia, nausea, and vomiting are present and as long as SMBG results are greater than 250 mg/dL (13.8 mmol/L). The client checks urinary ketone levels when blood glucose levels are higher than 240 mg/dL (13.3 mmol/L).

Minimizing Dehydration. The nurse teaches the client to minimize the risk of dehydration by maintaining food and fluid intake. With nausea, the nurse instructs the client to take liquids containing both glucose and electrolytes (e.g., soda pop, diluted fruit juice, and sports drinks [Gatorade]). Small amounts of fluid may be tolerated even when vomiting is present. The client should take 8 to 12 oz (240 to 360 mL) of fluid every hour while awake.

Liquids containing carbohydrates can be taken when the diabetic client is unable to eat solid food. The risk of starvation ketosis is reduced by a minimum daily carbohydrate intake of 100 to 150 g. After consulting with the primary care provider, the nurse may instruct the client to take additional regular insulin based on SMBG results.

Preventing Future Episodes of Diabetic Ketoacidosis. The nurse instructs the client to consult the primary care provider

- When SMBG results are greater than 250 mg/dL (13.8 mmol/L)
- When ketonuria is present for more than 24 hours
- When unable to take food or fluids
- When illness persists for more than 1 to 2 days

The nurse also instructs the client or the primary caregiver to detect hyperglycemia by performing SMBG when the client is ill. Significant illness can result in dehydration with DKA, hyperglycemic hyperosmolar nonketotic syndrome, or both. The nurse helps the client understand that adjustments in the management of diabetes beyond the scope of self-management are necessary. The sooner the client seeks treatment, the less severe is the degree of metabolic alteration. Chart 68–9 reviews guidelines for the client to follow.

➤ Potential Complication: Hyperglycemic Hyperosmolar Nonketotic Syndrome

Planning: Expected Outcomes. The client is expected to maintain a normal blood glucose level and have minimized episodes of hyperglycemia.

Interventions. The nurse monitors for signs and symptoms of hyperglycemic hyperosmolar nonketotic syndrome (HHNS) (see Tables 68–3 and 68–15 for symptoms of hyperglycemia). The nurse performs ongoing assessment of fluid status.

Fluid Therapy. The most critical element in the management of HHNS is the choice of fluid replacement and the rate of administration. The goal of therapy is to complete rehydration and normalize serum glucose levels within 36 to 72 hours. The degree of central nervous

***

> **Chart 68–9**
>
> ### Health Promotion Guide: Sick Day Rules
>
> - Notify your health care provider that you are ill.
> - Monitor your blood glucose at least every 4 hours.
> - Test your urine for ketones when your blood glucose level is greater than 240 mg/dL (13.8 mmol/L).
> - Continue to take insulin or oral hypoglycemic agents.
> - To prevent dehydration, drink 8 to 12 oz of sugar-free liquids every hour that you are awake.
> - Continue to eat meals at regular times.
> - If unable to tolerate solid food because of nausea, consume more easily tolerated foods or liquids equal to the carbohydrate content of your usual meal.
> - Treat your symptoms (e.g., diarrhea, nausea, vomiting, and fever) as directed by your physician or advanced nurse clinician.
> - Get plenty of rest.

***

system abnormality in HHNS correlates with the level of hyperosmolarity, which reflects intracellular dehydration. The difficulty in achieving intracellular brain hydration explains why many clients do not recover baseline central nervous system function until several hours after plasma glucose levels have returned to normal values.

As with DKA, the *initial* objective for fluid replacement in HHNS is to raise circulating blood volume. The volume deficit is corrected with intravenous saline at a rate of 1 L/hour until central venous pressure or pulmonary capillary wedge pressure begins to rise or until the blood pressure and urine output are acceptable. The rate is then reduced to 100 to 200 mL/hour. The physician calculates for half of the estimated water deficit to be replaced in the first 12 hours and the remainder to be given during the next 36 hours. When the blood glucose level reaches 250 mg/dL (13.8 mmol/L), 5% dextrose is added to the infusion. The rate of fluid administration is determined by body weight, urine output, kidney function, and the presence or absence of pulmonary congestion and jugular venous distention. In clients with prior congestive heart failure or renal insufficiency or in those with acute kidney failure associated with HHNS, central venous pressure monitoring is indicated. The nurse assesses the client's level of consciousness hourly. The nurse reports changes in pupillary size or reaction to light to the physician immediately. Failure of the client to show any improvement in level of consciousness may indicate inadequate rates of fluid replacement or inadequate reduction in plasma osmolarity. Regression after initial improvement may indicate too rapid a reduction in plasma osmolarity. A slow but steady improvement in central nervous system function is the best evidence that fluid management is satisfactory.

Other Therapy. Intravenous insulin should be given at a rate of 10 U/hour. Although fluid replacement has a major impact on hyperglycemia, it should not be solely relied on to reduce glucose levels. Potassium depletion occurs in HHNS, although not to the degree that it does in DKA. Because initial oliguria occurs, potassium replacement may not be needed at the onset of therapy. Client education and interventions to minimize dehydration are similar to those of ketoacidosis.

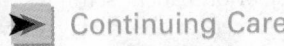

Continuing Care

➤ Health Teaching

Assessing Learning Needs

To attain blood glucose control, education must begin at the time of diagnosis of diabetes. Education is conducted in a hospital or outpatient setting, clinic, or primary care provider's office and involves the coordinated efforts of physicians, dietitians, nurses, pharmacists, social workers, and psychologists. Although some education can be conducted in group settings, most will need to be done on a one-to-one basis. Continuing education will need to take place over time to master the knowledge, skills, and flexibility required to maintain long-term blood glucose control.

The client's awareness of diabetes and the needs of the person and his or her family must be assessed before the educator initiates teaching (Brink et al., 1995). This assessment includes

- Age, occupation
- Likes, dislikes, fears
- Current lifestyle
- Evaluation of general health, attitudes about health, self-care behaviors
- Learning ability and style, willingness to learn
- Acceptance of diabetes, current knowledge of diabetes
- Skills needed, attitudes, goals
- Ethnic background, language
- Home situation

Before beginning actual diabetic education, the nurse assesses the client's baseline knowledge of diabetes and its treatment. Adult learners are interested in information that applies directly to their situation. It is appropriate to ask what the client wants to learn. Starting with what the client already knows and building on that base are good ways to increase knowledge and correct any errors in information that the diabetic client may have. To capture interest and motivate for further learning, the nurse presents material important to the client's first questions. Because they will be required to manage their own care after discharge, clients tend to focus on narrow issues most important to them. Teaching about treatment measures that need to be implemented soon after diagnosis may be of more interest to the diabetic client than long-term control.

The client's physical condition dictates when teaching is appropriate. When blood glucose levels are fluctuating, the client does not have the energy to learn complex information. To emphasize the importance of compliance with recommendations, the nurse can cite the improved sense of well-being that comes with control of blood glucose levels. The nurse initiates an informal teaching program until the client feels able to attend a formal class. The nurse observes technique for injections and blood glucose monitoring.

Individual clients learn in individual ways. A successful diabetic education program combines several different teaching methods. Some clients learn better when they read pamphlets, others when they watch videotapes. Learning is enhanced when

- The equipment is handled
- Techniques are practiced
- Success is rewarded
- Errors are corrected immediately

Assessing Physical, Cognitive, and Emotional Limitations

The nurse assesses the educational and reading levels of the client to determine what level of information to present. The nurse also determines the client's visual abilities in reading printed information. In addition, the client taking insulin needs to be able to read the labels and markings on syringes and equipment. Many clients with type 2 diabetes have presbyopia (farsightedness) and baseline visual difficulty that is made worse by blurred vision caused by fluctuating blood glucose levels. The client must be able to understand the printed material that is presented. Even highly educated clients do not want to read complicated information when they are sick. Much of the printed material from drug companies is printed at the sixth- or seventh-grade level. The International Diabetes Center prepares printed diabetic education material at the second- and third-grade levels. The nurse develops creative teaching strategies for the client who cannot read.

The nurse also assesses the client's ability to conceptualize. The adjustment of insulin dosage on the basis of blood glucose monitoring is a difficult concept to understand and may not be appropriate for clients who are unable to understand the concepts involved. Self-management of medication, exercise, and diet is considered complex.

The nurse assesses manual dexterity and any physical limitations that may alter the teaching plan. A history of hand injury, the presence of hand tremors, or severe arthritis necessitates modifications in insulin preparation instruction.

Information is best learned when the client is ready. Clients with newly diagnosed diabetes are facing a life crisis. Some may be more motivated to learn information that will help them change lifelong behaviors. Others may grieve the loss of their previous lifestyle and use denial as a means of coping with the diagnosis. In this instance, the client may not be able to learn needed information.

Explaining Survival Skills

The initial phase of diabetic education involves basic survival skills. The basic pathologic changes of diabetes and the relationship of nutrition, medication, and exercise to overall metabolic control are important.

A dietitian provides the initial diet instruction. The diabetic client needs to understand what food is to be eaten, how much food is to be eaten, and when the food is to be eaten. The nurse stresses the importance of eating meals on time, as well as the dangers of skipping meals. The client must be able to explain how to maintain food intake during illness. The nurse reinforces dietary instruction, answers questions, and refers questions to the dietitian or physician as indicated.

After the nurse provides medication instruction, the client should be able to identify the specific medication required for control of blood glucose levels. When insulin administration is needed, the client must be able to prepare and administer the ordered dose with accuracy and with sterile technique. The client must also be able to verbalize when insulin injections are to be taken, where insulin is to be injected, and how insulin is to be stored. The nurse stresses the dangers of omitting insulin doses. All pertinent drug interactions must be carefully reviewed with the diabetic client, particularly elderly individuals on oral hypoglycemic agents.

The diabetic client should be able to state a plan for regular physical activity. The client must be able to verbalize the relationship between exercise and blood glucose control and identify situations when activity is not appropriate. The nurse provides guidelines for additional carbohydrate intake to prevent hypoglycemia as a result of excessive exercise.

The diabetic client also should be able to verbalize, to the nurse, the plan for monitoring blood glucose. The person performing SMBG must be able to do the procedure with accuracy and understanding of the results. The nurse provides guidelines for when SMBG is to be performed, acceptable ranges, and actions to be taken when results are out of these ranges. When the client is unable to perform SMBG, it is important that a resource (e.g., home health agency, health clinic, or primary care provider's office) be available to do monitoring during times of illness.

The client must understand the significance, symptoms, causes, and treatment of hypoglycemia. It is essential for the diabetic client to verbalize the causes of hypoglycemia and the activities needed to prevent recurrence. The diabetic must be able to verbalize appropriate carbohydrate resources to have available and the intent to notify the physician regarding hypoglycemic episodes.

The diabetic client also must understand the significance of hyperglycemia and its relationship to illness. The client must verbalize actions to take during illness and the intent of communicating with the primary care provider.

Most of this survival information is retained when the client is ready to learn. Presentation, however, is a challenge to nurses attempting to provide diabetic education, because clients tend to be hospitalized for shorter periods. All of the diabetic education may be provided in an outpatient setting, where contact with the individual is limited. It becomes necessary to maximize important information into the time frames available. Because of psychological barriers, many clients, regardless of duration of disease, do not progress beyond the survival level.

In-Depth Counseling

The ultimate goal of in-depth counseling is to assist the client to become self-sufficient in diabetes management. Educational sessions with the client and family members to individualize the diabetes regimen to their particular needs, skills, and abilities will be necessary. Education is often provided through the team efforts of a physician, a nurse educator, dietitian, a social worker, a pharmacist, a psychologist, and other health care professionals as needed and occurs in a variety of outpatient settings.

In addition to knowledge gained at the survival level, the diabetic client should be able to discuss the action of insulin in the body and the effects of insulin deficiency on various body systems. The client also should be able to explain the effects of food intake, medication, and activity on control of blood glucose levels. The client should be able to relate the metabolic goals of euglycemia to the prevention of complications and relate variation in SMBG results to the possible need for alteration in insulin dosage.

The diabetic client must be able to describe the meal plan, and to explain that adjustments in dietary intake are made to meet diabetic diet requirements. The diabetic client should state how food intake is altered when increased physical activity is planned and when the client eats in restaurants or at family gatherings. It is essential that the diabetic client list appropriate food to be eaten to prevent and treat hypoglycemia as well as to make adjustments when feeling ill.

Within the physical limitations imposed by baseline health status, the client should be able to perform any desired physical activities. The diabetic client must state SMBG levels that are safe for exercise, the frequency with which to perform SMBG during exercise, the food intake required before exercise, and what food to have available during exercise if symptoms of hypoglycemia occur. The client should be aware of the potential for injury during exercise and explain the importance of protective footwear.

The diabetic client must be able to demonstrate accuracy in insulin preparation and administration. The client should be able to discuss the onset, peak, and duration of the specific insulin preparation. In reviewing insulin administration practices, the nurse stresses the importance of anatomic site selection and injection site rotation. The nurse carefully reviews guidelines for adjustment in insulin dosage based on SMBG results (when permitted by the physician) and that follow-up SMBG documentation is necessary to evaluate the effects of additional insulin. The client should explain the method of protecting insulin when traveling. For diabetic clients with the potential for severe hypoglycemia, the nurse observes a family member's ability to inject glucagon. When the client is taking oral diabetic medications, the nurse asks the client to identify the medication and relate its schedule of administration. Because of the potential for drug interactions, the client must identify over-the-counter drugs that have the potential to cause adverse drug interactions and understand the necessity of informing the primary care provider of the drug regimen.

The goals of in-depth education are for the nurse to assist the diabetic client in solving problems of blood glucose fluctuation through the use of SMBG. The client should be able to identify self-care practices, such as during travel (Chart 68–10), that result in blood glucose fluctuations and to treat these alterations with supplemen-

Chart 68-10

Education Guide: Travel Tips for Diabetic Clients

- Before traveling, visit your primary care provider and diabetes educator:
  - See your physician to make certain you do not have any other health problems.
  - Obtain a letter from your physician that says you have diabetes and lists the medications you are taking.
  - Obtain extra prescriptions from your physician for your medications.
  - Ask about medications for motion sickness, nausea and vomiting, and traveler's diarrhea.
  - Obtain a list of foods from your diabetes educator that you can substitute for food served in restaurants or airplanes.
  - Ask your diabetes educator how to adjust meal patterns to account for changes in time zones or unexpected interruptions in your meal patterns.
- Plan for delays in eating:
  - Eat something every 4 hours.
  - If you are traveling by air, train, or boat, call ahead and request special meals for people with diabetes.
  - Have a supply of fast-acting sugar (such as glucose tablets or gel, hard candy, and sugar cubes), as well as longer acting foods (such as cheese and crackers and peanut butter and crackers) in a travel kit.
  - Drink a glass of water every 2 hours to prevent dehydration.
  - Do not assume that special meals will be available; substitute items you cannot eat with foods you have in your travel kit.
- While traveling:
  - Check your blood glucose level frequently.
  - Stretch and walk around every 2 hours to help your circulation.
  - Check your feet frequently for blisters and sores. You may be doing more walking than usual. Take extra shoes with you, and plan to change shoes often when walking more than normal.
  - Notify airline and hotel personnel that you have diabetes.
  - Always wear medical alert (Medic-Alert) identification and keep your Medic-Alert card in your wallet.
  - Always have your travel kit with you; do not check your kit along with the rest of your luggage.
- Include these items in your travel kit:
  - Medications, extra bottles of insulin, and extra bottles of drugs that you take by mouth
  - Supplies for insulin administration and blood glucose monitoring
  - A letter and extra prescriptions from your physician
  - Food and fast-acting sugar sources
  - A self-monitoring diary to record the impact of the trip on your condition

The diabetic must be able to verbalize a plan for periodic evaluation by the primary care provider of the control of blood glucose levels as well as periodic dental examinations and ophthalmologic evaluations. The client must be able to demonstrate appropriate foot care, wear appropriately fitting shoes, and describe hazards related to foot care. The client must be able to relate plans to reduce specific risk factors, such as cigarette smoking and hypertension.

The diabetic must verbalize that diabetes is a lifelong disease that necessitates lifestyle changes and describe the changes in progress and those that still need to be made. The client should be able to identify stress-producing situations and discuss methods for stress reduction.

Psychosocial Preparation

The diagnosis of diabetes may represent a loss of control. All but a few clients lose flexibility in routines. Life becomes ordered; time schedules and routines must be followed. Certain events surrounding diabetes are predictable. Taking an insulin injection and not eating for several hours causes hypoglycemia. Poorly controlled diabetes leads to debilitating complications and premature death. Results of the Diabetes Control and Complications Trial (DCCT) suggest that good control of blood glucose levels prevents these complications.

The stresses of diabetes are superimposed on the demands of normal daily life. The client must be able to integrate the demands of diabetes into daily and recreational schedules so as not to cause blood glucose alterations.

The nurse assists in healthy psychological adaptation to diabetes by providing successful educational experiences. The mastery of blood glucose monitoring assists the client in assuming control over the disease. Knowledge of the effects of extra activities, or extra food, as well as the result of administration of additional insulin is helpful in making future adjustments in regimens.

The diabetic client's feeling a sense of control over the condition does much to assist in a positive psychological attitude about diabetes. Success in self-injection of insulin provides concrete evidence that the client is able to master the disease. The nurse breaks a task into small, achievable units to ensure mastery of techniques; for example, a client may begin learning how to administer an injection by first obtaining an accurate dose of insulin.

It is appropriate to devote as much time as possible to insulin injection and blood glucose monitoring techniques. Clients with newly diagnosed diabetes are often fearful of giving themselves injections of insulin. After insulin injection technique has been mastered, clients become less anxious and are able to attend to other tasks.

➤ Home Care Management

The maintenance of blood glucose control depends on the client's self-care skills. The nurse teaches all clients with newly diagnosed diabetes basic self-care skills for safe functioning. To determine what additional education is

tal insulin administration, alterations in physical activity levels, or compliance with dietary recommendations. The nurse asks the client to demonstrate appropriate urinary ketone testing techniques and identify the conditions during which urinary ketones should be measured.

needed, the nurse assesses the knowledge level of clients with previously diagnosed diabetes.

The nurse provides information about resources. The client must know who to contact in case of emergency. Elderly clients who live alone must have daily telephone contact with a friend or neighbor. The client may also need assistance with grocery shopping and meal preparation. The client may have limited access to transportation out of the home and may not have sufficient supplies of food, particularly in bad weather. Because of the high frequency of visual problems in older clients, the client may need assistance to prepare insulin syringes for injection or to perform blood glucose monitoring. A referral to a home care or public health agency may be indicated. Chart 68–11 identifies areas for assessment during a home or clinic visit.

➤ Health Care Resources

A wide array of diabetic educational material is available from pharmaceutical companies. The American Diabetes Association will refer a diabetic client to the appropriate agencies or resources (phone 1-800-232-3472 in the United States; 1-703-549-1500 in Canada). The American Association of Diabetes Educators can refer a diabetic individual to a Certified Diabetes Educator in their area for information about diabetes at 1-800-TEAM-UP-4. *Diabetes Forecast* is a patient education booklet published by the ADA that has helpful information. Many aids for diabetic clients with visual impairment are reviewed by Petzinger (1992).

 Evaluation

The ultimate evaluation of success of survival level and in-depth diabetic education is the ability of the client to maintain blood glucose levels within the normal range. Specific outcome criteria for client education are listed below and in Table 68–16.

- Maintain blood glucose levels within the normal range
- Avoid acute and chronic complications of diabetes
- Have a satisfactory and complete postoperative recovery without complications
- Identify factors that increase potential for injury
- Practice proper foot care to prevent injury
- Maintain intact skin on feet
- Experience relief of pain
- Identify measures that increase comfort
- Maintain optimal vision
- Be free from injury related to decreased visual acuity
- Maintain optimal urinary output
- Have an optimal level of mental status functioning
- Have decreased episodes of hypoglycemia
- Have minimized episodes of hyperglycemia

Chart 68–11

Focused Assessment of the Insulin-Dependent Diabetic Client During a Home or Clinic Visit

- Assess overall mental status, wakefulness, ability to converse
- Take vital signs and weight
  - Fever could indicate infection
  - Is blood pressure and weight within target range? Why or why not?
- Question client regarding any change in visual acuity; check current visual acuity
- Inspect oral mucous membranes, gums, and teeth
- Question client about injection areas used; inspect areas being used; assess whether client is utilizing areas and sites appropriately
- Inspect skin for intactness; wounds that have not healed; new sores, ulcers, bruises, or burns. Assess any previously known wounds for infection, progression of healing
- Question client regarding foot care
- Assess lower extremities and feet for peripheral pulses, lack of or decreased sensation, abnormal sensations, breaks in skin integrity, condition of toes and nails
- Question client regarding color and consistency of stools and frequency of bowel movements; assess abdomen for bowel sounds
- Review client's home health diary:
  - Is blood glucose within targeted range? Why or why not?
  - Is glucose monitoring being recorded often enough?
  - Is the client's food intake adequate and appropriate? Why or why not?
  - Is exercise occurring regularly? Why or why not?
- Assess client's ability to perform self-monitoring of blood glucose
- Assess client's procedures for obtaining and storing insulin and syringes, cleaning of equipment, disposing of syringes and needles
- Assess client's insulin preparation and injection technique

---

 CASE STUDY for the Client with Diabetes and Visual Impairment

■ Mr. J.G. has had diabetes mellitus for several years. He takes 30 U of NPH with 10 U of regular insulin in the morning before breakfast and 20 U of NPH insulin before the evening meal. He has recently undergone laser therapy for treatment of diabetic retinopathy. He wants to be independent in insulin administration, and your assessment indicates that he has the intellectual ability to learn the needed skills.

QUESTIONS:

1. List three methods for preventing both hypo- and hyperglycemia that you would stress during your teaching sessions.
2. Discuss four ways of altering the environment to aid in measurement of accurate insulin doses.
3. List five critical points that would be included in a teaching session on adaptive devices for use with insulin syringes.

TABLE 68–16

Outcome Criteria for Diabetic Teaching

Before being discharged home, the diabetic client or the significant other should be able to

- Tell why insulin or an oral hypoglycemic agent is being prescribed
- Name which insulin or oral hypoglycemic agent is being prescribed. Name the dosage and frequency of administration
- Discuss the relationship between meal time and the action of insulin or the oral hypoglycemic agent
- Discuss plans to follow diabetic diet instructions
- Prepare and administer insulin accurately
- Test blood for glucose or state plans for having blood glucose levels monitored
- Test urine for ketones and state when this test should be done
- Verbalize how to store insulin
- List symptoms that indicate a hypoglycemic reaction
- Tell what carbohydrate sources are used to treat a hypoglycemic reaction
- Tell what symptoms indicate hyperglycemia
- Tell what dietary changes are needed during illness
- Verbalize when to call the physician or the nurse: frequent episodes of hypoglycemia, symptoms of hyperglycemia
- Verbalize the procedures for proper foot care

Disease-Specific Outcomes

- Glycosylated hemoglobin within established target range: treatment goal to prevent long-term complication = <7%
- Fasting plasma glucose <120 mg/dL
- SMBG levels within established target ranges
- Achievement of reasonable weight for adults; meeting of weight loss goals where appropriate
- Avoidance of glycemic excursions: take action levels = <80 mg/dL and >140 mg/dL
- Achievement of near-optimal serum lipids: low-density lipoprotein <130 mg/dL, cholesterol and triglyceride levels <200 mg/dL
- Hypoglycemia episodes reduced/eliminated
- Blood pressure for adults 18 or older <130 systolic and <85 diastolic

General Health Outcomes

- Improved sense of well-being

Annual Screening for Diabetic Complications

- Comprehensive dilated eye and visual examination
- Screening for microalbuminuria
- Screening for lipid disorders
- Comprehensive foot examination

Individual Performance Outcomes

- Knowledge
  - Discusses action of medication on blood glucose
  - Discusses relationships among nutrition, exercise, medication, and blood glucose levels
  - Discusses prevention, detection, and treatment of acute complications
  - Discusses prevention, detection, and treatment of chronic complications

- Psychomotor skills
  - Demonstrates appropriate foot care
  - Demonstrates how to perform self-monitoring of blood glucose with appropriate testing material
  - Demonstrates how to perform ketone testing of urine; discusses when this procedure should be done
  - Demonstrates how to prepare and administer insulin correctly

- Compliance
  - Discusses plans to follow nutritional therapy instructions
  - Provides records of self-monitoring of blood glucose to primary care provider

SELECTED BIBLIOGRAPHY

Aiello, L. P., Cavallerano, J., & Bursell, S. E. (1996). Diabetic eye disease. *Endocrinology and Metabolism Clinics of North America, 25*(2), 271–291.

Alzaid, A. A. (1996). Microalbuminuria in patients with NIDDM: An overview. *Diabetes Care, 19*(1), 79–89.

*American Diabetes Association. (1993). Position statement: Use of non-caloric sweeteners. *Diabetes Care, 16*(suppl 2), 30.

American Diabetes Association. (1996a). Consensus statement: Diabetic neuropathy. *Diabetes Care, 19*(suppl 1), 67–71.

American Diabetes Association. (1996b). Consensus statement: The pharmacological treatment of hyperglycemia in NIDDM. *Diabetes Care, 19*(suppl 1), 54–61.

American Diabetes Association. (1996c). Consensus statement: Self-monitoring of blood glucose. Clinical practice recommendations. *Diabetes Care, 19*(suppl 1), 62–66.

American Diabetes Association. (1996d). Consensus statement: Standardized measures in diabetic neuropathy. *Diabetes Care, 19*(suppl 1), 72–92.

American Diabetes Association. (1996e). Consensus statement: Treatment of hypertension in diabetes. *Diabetes Care, 19*(suppl 1), 107–113.

American Diabetes Association. (1997). Position statement: Guide to diagnosis and classification of diabetes mellitus and other categories of glucose intolerance. *Diabetes Care, 20*(suppl 1), S21.

American Diabetes Association. (1998a). Committee report: Report of the expert committee on the diagnosis and classification of diabetes mellitus. *Diabetes Care, 21*(suppl 1), S5–19.

American Diabetes Association. (1998b). Position statement: Continuous subcutaneous insulin infusion. Clinical practice recommendations. *Diabetes Care, 21*(suppl 1), S76.

American Diabetes Association. (1998c). Position statement: Diabetes mellitus and exercise. Clinical practice recommendations. *Diabetes Care, 21*(suppl 1), S40–44.

American Diabetes Association. (1998d). Position statement: Diabetic nephropathy. *Diabetes Care, 21*(suppl 1), S47–49.

American Diabetes Association. (1998e). Position statement: Diabetic retinopathy. *Diabetes Care, 21*(suppl 1), S50–53.

American Diabetes Association. (1998f). Position statement: Food labeling. *Diabetes Care, 21*(suppl 1), S62–63.

American Diabetes Association. (1998g). Position statement: Foot care in patients with diabetes mellitus. Clinical practice recommendations. *Diabetes Care, 21*(suppl 1), S54–55.

American Diabetes Association. (1998h). Position statement: Gestational diabetes. *Diabetes Care, 21*(suppl 1), S60–61.

American Diabetes Association. (1998i). Position statement: Hospital admission guidelines for diabetes mellitus. *Diabetes Care, 21*(suppl 1), S77.

American Diabetes Association. (1988j). Position statement: Implications of the diabetes control and complications trial. *Diabetes Care, 21*(suppl 1), S88–90.

American Diabetes Association. (1998k). Position statement: Insulin administration. *Diabetes Care, 21*(suppl 1), S72–75.

American Diabetes Association. (1998l). Position statement: Nutritional recommendations and principles for individuals with diabetes. *Diabetes Care, 21*(suppl 1), S32–35.

American Diabetes Association. (1998m). Position statement: Management of dyslipidemia in adults with diabetes. *Diabetes Care, 21*(suppl 1), S36.

American Diabetes Association. (1998n). Position statement: Pancreas transplantation for patients with diabetes mellitus. *Diabetes Care, 21*(suppl 1), S79.

American Diabetes Association. (1998o). Position statement: Prevention of type I diabetes. *Diabetes Care, 21*(suppl 1), S83.

American Diabetes Association. (1998p). Position statement: Role of fat replacers in diabetes medical nutrition therapy. *Diabetes Care, 21*(suppl 1), S64–65.

American Diabetes Association. (1998q). Position statement: Screening for diabetes. *Diabetes Care, 21*(suppl 1), S20–22.

American Diabetes Association. (1998r). Position statement: Standards of medical care for patients with diabetes mellitus. *Diabetes Care, 21*(suppl 1), S23–31.

American Diabetes Association. (1998s). Position statement: Tests of glycemia in diabetes. *Diabetes Care, 21*(suppl 1), S69–71.

Atkinson, M. A., & Maclaren, N. K. (1994). The pathogenesis of insulin-dependent diabetes mellitus. *New England Journal of Medicine, 331*(21), 1428–1436.

Bak, L. B., Heard, K. A., & Kearney, G. P. (1996). Tube feeding your diabetic patient safely. *American Journal of Nursing, 96*(12), 47–49.

Ball, K. A. (1995). *Lasers: The perioperative challenge.* St. Louis: C. V. Mosby.

Bell, D. S. (1994). Stroke in the diabetic patient. *Diabetes Care, 17*(3), 213–219.

Bell, D. S. H. (1996). Alcohol and the NIDDM patient. *Diabetes Care, 19*(5), 509–513.

Bernbaum, M., Albert, S., McGinnis, J., et al. (1994). The reliability of self blood glucose monitoring in elderly diabetic patients. *Journal of the American Geriatric Society, 42*(7), 779–781.

Boulox, P. M. G., & Rees, L. H. (1995). *Diagnostic Tests in Endocrinology and Diabetes.* London: Chapman & Hall Medical.

Bove, L. A. (1994). How fluids and electrolytes shift after surgery. *Nursing94, 24*(8), 34–39.

Bridges, R. M., & Deitch, E. (1994). Diabetic foot infections: Pathophysiology and treatment. *Surgical Clinics of North America, 74*(3), 537–555.

Brink, S., Siminerio, L., Hinnen-Hentzen, D., et al. (1995). *Diabetes education goals.* Alexandria, VA: American Diabetes Association.

Brown, D. F., & Jackson, T. W. (1994). Diabetes: "Tight control" in a comprehensive treatment plan. *Geriatrics, 49*(6), 24–34.

Bulat, T., & Kosinski, M. (1995). Diabetic foot: Strategies to prevent and treat complications. *Geriatrics, 50*(2), 46–56.

Burge, M. R., & Schade, D. S. (1997). Insulins. *Endocrinology and Metabolism Clinics of North America, 26*(2), 575–598.

Bustamante, M. A., Hennessey, J. V., Teter, M. L., et al. (1994). Clinical accuracy of capillary blood glucose monitoring in hospitalized patients with diabetes. *Diabetes Educator, 20*(3), 212–215.

Camilleri, M. (1996). Gastrointestinal problems in diabetes. *Endocrinology and Metabolism Clinics of North America, 25*(2), 361–378.

Capriotti, T. (1997). Beyond sulfonylureas: New oral medications in the treatment of NIDDM (type II diabetes). *MEDSURG Nursing, 6*(3), 166–169.

Caputo, G. M., Cavanagh, P. R., Ulbrecht, J. S., et al. (1994). Assessment and management of foot disease in patients with diabetes. *New England Journal of Medicine, 331*(13), 854–860.

Carella, M. J., Gossain, V. V., & Rovner, D. R. (1994). Early diabetic nephropathy: Emerging treatment options. *Archives of Internal Medicine, 154*(6), 625–630.

Carter, T. L. (1994). Age-related vision changes: A primary care guide. *Geriatrics, 49*(9), 37–47.

Centers for Disease Control and Prevention. (1997). Mortality patterns—Preliminary data, United States, 1996. *Morbidity and Mortality Weekly Report, 46*(40), 941–944.

Chaisson, J. L., Josse, R. G., Hunt, J. A., et al. (1994). The efficacy of acarbose in the treatment of patients with non-insulin dependent diabetes mellitus. *Annals of Internal Medicine, 121*(12), 928–935.

Cirone, N. (1996). Diabetes in the elderly, part I: Unmasking a hidden disorder. *Nursing96, 26*(3), 34–39.

Cirone, N., & Schwartz, N. (1996). Diabetes in the elderly, part II: Finding the balance for drug therapy. *Nursing96, 26*(3), 40–45.

Clark, A. P. (1994). Complications and management of diabetes: A review of current research. *Critical Care Nursing Clinics of North America, 6*(4), 723–734.

Clark, C. M., & Lee, D. A. (1995). Prevention and treatment of the complications of diabetes mellitus. *New England Journal of Medicine, 332*(18), 1210–1217.

Cleary, M. E. (Ed.) (1994). *Diabetes and visual impairment: An educator's resource guide.* Chicago: American Association of Diabetes Educators.

*Coleman, W. C. (1993). Footwear in a management program for injury prevention. In M. E. Levin, L. W. O'Neal, & J. H. Bowker (Eds.), *The diabetic foot* (5th ed.). St. Louis: C. V. Mosby, 531–547.

*Collier, J. H., & Brodbeck, C. A. (1993). Assessing the diabetic foot: Plantar callus and pressure sensation. *Diabetes Educator, 19*(6), 503–508.

Coniff, R. F., Shapiro, J., Seaton, T. B., et al. (1995). A double blind placebo controlled trial evaluating the safety and efficacy of acarbose for the treatment of patients with insulin requiring type II diabetes. *Diabetes Care, 18*(7), 928–932.

Cryer, P. E. (1994). Hypoglycemia: The limiting factor in the management of NIDDM. *Diabetes, 43*(11), 1378–1389.

Cryer, P. E., Fisher, J. N., & Shamoon, H. (1994). Hypoglycemia. *Diabetes Care, 17*(7), 734–755.

Deakins, D. A. (1994). Teaching elderly patients about diabetes. *American Journal of Nursing, 94*(4), 38–43.

*DeFronzo, R. A., Bonadonna, R. C., & Ferrannini, E. (1992). Pathogenesis of NIDDM. *Diabetes Care, 15*(3), 318–353.

DeFronzo, R. A., Goodman, A. M., and the Multicenter Metformin Study Group. (1995). Efficacy of metformin in patients with non-insulin dependent diabetes mellitus. *New England Journal of Medicine, 333*(9), 541–549.

Doleman, C. J. A., Oude Elberink, J. G. G., Miedema, K., et al. (1996). Orthostatic hypotension in poorly regulated NIDDM. *Diabetes Care, 19*(5), 542.

Dorgan, M. B., Birke, J. A., Moretto, J. A., et al. (1995). Performing foot screening for diabetic patients. *American Journal of Nursing, 95*(11), 32–37.

Drass, J. A. & Peterson, A. (1996). Type II diabetes: Exploring treatment options. *American Journal of Nursing, 96*(11), 45–49.

Ebersole, P., & Hess, P. (1995). *Toward healthy aging.* St. Louis: C. V. Mosby.

Elbein, S. C., Hoffman, M. D., Bragg, K., et al. (1994). The genetics of IDDM. *Diabetes Care, 17*(12), 1523–1533.

Farkas-Hirsh, R. (Ed.). (1995). *Intensive diabetes management.* Alexandria, VA: The American Diabetes Association.

Ferris, F. L., Chew, E. Y., & Hoogwerf, B. J. (1996). Serum lipids and diabetic retinopathy. *Diabetes Care, 19*(11), 1291–1293.

Fish, L. H. (1994). Diabetic ketoacidosis. *Postgraduate Medicine, 96*(3), 75–96.

Fishman, T. D., Freedline, A. D., & Kahn, D. (1996). Putting the best foot forward. *Nursing96, 26*(1), 58–60.

Fleg, J. L. (1995). Diagnostic and prognostic value of stress testing in older persons. *Journal of American Geriatrics Society, 43*(2), 190–194.

Frank, R. N. (1994). The aldose reductase controversy. *Diabetes, 43*(2), 169–172.

Franz, M. J., Horton, E. S., Bantle, J. P., et al. (1994). Nutrition principles for the management of diabetes and related complications. *Diabetes Care, 17*(5), 490–518.

Friedman, E. A. (1996). Renal syndromes in diabetes. *Endocrinology and Metabolism Clinics of North America, 25*(2), 293–324.

*Galloway, J. A. (1993). New directions in drug development. Mixtures, analogues and modeling. *Diabetes Care, 16*(suppl 3), 16–23.

*Gillis, W. Long Hansen's Disease Center Rehabilitation Branch. (1992). *Care of the foot in diabetes, the Carville approach.* Carville, LA: Department of Health and Human Services.

Gold, A. E., MacLeod, K. M., & Frier, B. M. (1994). Frequency of severe hypoglycemia in patients with type I diabetes with impaired awareness of hypoglycemia. *Diabetes Care, 17*(7), 697–703.

Goldhahn, R. E. (1996). I'm a born-again diabetic. *RN, 59*(12), 33–35.

Goldstein, D. E., Little, R. R., Lorenz, R. A., et al. (1995). Tests of glycemia in diabetes. *Diabetes Care, 18*(6), 896–909.

Green, S. E., & Fischer, R. G. (1996). Diabetic peripheral neuropathy. *ADVANCE for Nurse Practitioners, 4*(10), 30–33.

Gregory, R. P., & Davis, D. (1994). Use of carbohydrate counting for meal planning in type I diabetes. *Diabetes Educator, 20*(5), 406–409.

Harati, Y. (1996). Diabetes and the nervous system. *Endocrinology and Metabolism Clinics of North America, 25*(2), 325–359.

Harris, M., & Robbins, D. C. (1994). Prevalence of adult-onset IDDM in the U.S. population. *Diabetes Care, 17*(11), 1337–1340.

Hefland, A. E. (1996). What you need to know about therapeutic footwear. *Practical Diabetology, 15*(4), 4–9.

Henry, R. R. (1996). Glucose control and insulin resistance in non-insulin-dependent diabetes mellitus. *Annals of Internal Medicine, 124*(1, pt 2), 97–103.

Henry, R. R. (1997). Thiazolidinediones. *Endocrinology and Metabolism Clinics of North America, 26*(2), 553–573.

Hermann, L. S., Schersten, Bitzen, P. O., et al. (1994). Therapeutic comparisons of metformin and sulfonylurea, alone and in various combinations. *Diabetes Care, 17*(10), 1100–1109.

Hirsh, C. H. (1995a). When your patient needs surgery: Weighing risks versus benefits. *Geriatrics, 50*(1), 26–31.

Hirsh, C. H. (1995b). When your patient needs surgery: How planning can avoid complications. *Geriatrics, 50*(2), 39–44.

*Hirsh, I. B., & Farkas-Hirsh, R. (1993). Type I diabetes and insulin therapy. *Nursing Clinics of North America, 28*(1), 9–23.

Hirsh, I. B., Paauw, D. S., & Brunzell, J. (1997). Diabetes management in special situations. *Endocrinology and Metabolism Clinics of North America, 26*(2), 631–645.

Hirsh, I. B., Paauw, D. S., & Brunzell, J. (1995). Inpatient management of adults with diabetes. *Diabetes Care, 18*(6), 870–878.

Hollander, P. (1994). Intensified insulin regimens: Should they be used in all patients with type I diabetes? *Postgraduate Medicine, 96*(3), 63–72.

Hollander, P. A. (1995). New oral agents for type II diabetes. *Postgraduate Medicine, 98*(6), 110–126.

Howey, D. C., Bowsher, R. R., Brunelle, R. L., et al. (1994). [Lys (B28), Pro (B29)]–human insulin. A rapidly absorbed analogue of human insulin. *Diabetes, 43*(3), 396–402.

Humphrey, L. L., Palumbo, P. J., Butters, M. A., et al. (1994). The contribution of non-insulin diabetes to lower-extremity amputation in the community. *Archives of Internal Medicine, 154*(8), 885–892.

Hussar, D. A. (1995). New drugs: Learn more about the 15 new drugs marketed in the first half of 1995. *Nursing95, 25*(12), 50–51.

Johnson, M. D., White, J. R. Campbell, R. K. (1996). Insulin therapy in the era of insulin analogs. *U.S. Pharmacist, 21*(11), HS35–HS42.

Johnson, P. L., Luther, R. J., Hipp, S., et al. (1995). A comparative evaluation of bedside capillary blood glucose monitoring devices designed for hospital use. *Diabetes Educator, 21*(5), 420–425.

Jones, T. L. (1994). From diabetic ketoacidosis to hyperglycemic hyperosmolar nonketotic syndrome: The spectrum of uncontrolled hyper-

glycemia in diabetes mellitus. *Critical Care Clinics of North America, 6*(4), 703–720.

Kahn, C. R., & Weir, G. C. (Eds.) (1994). *Joslin's diabetes mellitus* (13th ed.). Philadelphia: Lea & Febiger.

Karas, B. S., & Alpuche, A. (1995). Refilling an implantable pump. *American Journal of Nursing, 95*(11) 57–61.

Karlsson, E. O., & Garber, A. J. (1995). Metformin comes to America: What to do now. *Clinical Diabetes, 13*(6), 78–83.

Kasden, F. (1997). Teaching diabetes survival skills. *ADVANCE for Nurse Practitioners, 5*(5), 51–54.

Keen, H. (1994). Insulin resistance and the prevention of diabetes mellitus. *New England Journal of Medicine, 331*(18), 1226–1227.

Kestel, F. (1994). Are you up to date on diabetes medications? *American Journal of Nursing, 94*(7), 48–52.

Kitabchi, A. E., & Bryer-Ash, M. (1997). NIDDM: New aspects of management. *Hospital Practice, March 15*, 135–138, 143–144, 149–151, 155–156, 162–164.

Kitabchi, A. E., & Wall, B. M. (1995). Diabetic ketoacidosis. *Medical Clinics of North America, 79*(1), 9–37.

Klein, R. (1995). Hyperglycemia and microvascular and macrovascular diseases in diabetes. *Diabetes Care, 18*(2), 258–268.

Klein, R. K., Klein, B. E. K., Lee, K. E., et al. (1996). Prevalence of self-reported erectile dysfunction in people with long-term IDDM. *Diabetes Care, 19*(2), 135–141.

Klein, R., Klein, E. K., Moss, S. K., et al. (1994). Relationship of hyperglycemia to the long-term incidence and progression of diabetic retinopathy. *Archives of Internal Medicine, 154*(19), 2169–2178.

Klonoff, D. C. (1997). Noninvasive blood glucose monitoring. *Diabetes Care, 20*(3), 433–437.

Knowler, W. C., Narayan, K. M. V., Hanson, R. L., et al. (1995). Preventing non-insulin-dependent diabetes. *Diabetes, 44*(5), 483–488.

Krolewski, A. S., Warram, J. H., & Freire, M. B. (1996). Epidemiology of late diabetic complications: A basis for the development and evaluation of prevention programs. *Endocrinology and Metabolism Clinics of North America, 25*(2), 217–242.

Kuusisto, J., Mykkanen, L., Pyorala, K., et al. (1994). NIDDM and its metabolic control predict coronary heart disease in elderly subjects. *Diabetes, 43*(8), 960–967.

Larsen, J., Duckworth, W. C., & Stratta, R. J. (1994). Pancreas transplantation for type I diabetes mellitus. *Postgraduate Medicine, 96*(3), 105–111.

Laux, L. (1994). Visual interpretation of blood glucose test strips. *Diabetes Educator, 20*(1), 41–44.

Lebovitz, H. E. (1997). Alpha-glucosidase inhibitors. *Endocrinology and Metabolism Clinics of North America, 26*(2), 539–551.

Lee, E. T., Howard, B. V., Savage, P. J., et al. (1995). Diabetes and impaired glucose tolerance in three American Indian populations aged 45–74 years. *Diabetes Care, 18*(5), 599–610.

Lehto, S., Ronnemaa, T., Pyorala, K., et al. (1996) Risk factors predicting lower extremity amputation in patients with NIDDM. *Diabetes Care, 19*(6), 601–612.

LeMone, P. (1996). Differentiating and treating altered glycemic responses. *MEDSURG Nursing, 5*(4), 257–268.

Lerman, I., Perez, F. J. G., Aguilar-Salinas, C. A., et. al. (1996). Acarbose: In search for its real indications in current medical practice. *Diabetes Care, 19*(1), 94–95.

Levin, M. E. (1995). Preventing amputation in the patient with diabetes. *Diabetes Care, 18*(10), 1383–1394.

Levin, M. E. (1996). Foot lesions in patients with diabetes mellitus. *Endocrinology and Metabolism Clinics of North America, 25*(2), 447–462.

*Levin, M. E., O'Neal, L. W., & Bowker, J. H. (Eds.) (1993). *The diabetic foot* (5th ed.). St. Louis: C. V. Mosby.

LoGerfo, F. W., & Gibbons, G. W. (1996). Vascular disease of the lower extremities in diabetes mellitus. *Endocrinology and Metabolism Clinics of North America, 25*(2), 439–445.

Lorber, D. (1995). Nonketotic hypertonicity in diabetes mellitus. *Medical Clinics of North America, 79*(1), 39–52.

Maffeo, R. (1997). Helping families cope with type I diabetes. *American Journal of Nursing, 97*(6), 36–39.

McNeely, M. J., Boyko, E. J., Ahroni, J. H., et al. (1995). The independent contribution of diabetic-neuropathy and vasculopathy in foot ulceration: how great are the risks? *Diabetes Care, 18*(2), 216–219.

Menzel, S., Yamagata, K., Trabb, J. B., et al. (1995). Localization of

MODY3 to a 5-cM region of human chromosome 12. *Diabetes, 44*(12), 1408–1413.

Mogensen, C. E. (1997). How to protect the kidney in diabetic patients. *Diabetes, 46*(suppl 2), S104–111.

Mueller, M. J. (1996). Identifying patients with diabetes mellitus who are at risk for lower-extremity complications: Use of Semmes-Weinstein monofilaments. *Physical Therapy, 76*(1), 68–71.

Murphy, R. P. (1995). Management of diabetic retinopathy. *American Family Physician, 51*(4), 785–795.

*Nathan, D M. (1993a). Diabetes Control and Complications Trial Research Group: The effect of long-term intensified insulin treatment on development of microvascular complications of diabetes. *New England Journal of Medicine, 329*(14), 977–986.

*Nathan, D. M. (1993b). Long-term complications from diabetes mellitus. *New England Journal of Medicine, 328*(23), 1676–1685.

Nathan, D. M. (1996). The pathophysiology of diabetic complications: How much does the glucose hypothesis explain? *Annals of Internal Medicine, 124*(1, part 2), 86–89.

O'Donnell, M. E. (1995). Assessing fluid and electrolyte balance in elders. *American Journal of Nursing, 95*(11), 41–46.

Pan, X., Li, G., et al. (1997). Effects of diet and exercise in preventing NIDDM in people with impaired glucose tolerance. *Diabetes Care, 20*(4), 537–544.

Partanen, J., Niskanen, L., Lehtinen, J., et al. (1995). Natural history of peripheral neuropathy in patients with non-insulin dependent diabetes mellitus. *New England Journal of Medicine, 333*(2), 89–94.

*Peragallo-Dittko, V., Godley, K., & Meyer, J. (1993). *A core curriculum for diabetes education* (2nd ed.). Chicago: American Association of Diabetes Educators.

Perkins, A. T., & Morgenlander, J. C. (1997). Endocrinologic causes of peripheral neuropathy. *Postgraduate Medicine, 102*(3), 81–82, 90–92, 102–106.

*Petzinger, R. A. (1992). Diabetes aids and products for people with visual or physical impairment. *Diabetes Educator, 18*(2), 121–138.

Pfeifer, M. A., & Schumer, M. P. (1995). Clinical trials of diabetic neuropathy: past, present and future. *Diabetes, 44*(12), 1355–1361.

Purnell, J. Q. & Hirsch, I. B. (1997). New oral therapies for type 2 diabetes. *American Family Physician, 56*(7), 1835–1842.

Raman, M., & Nesto, R. W. (1996). Heart disease in diabetes mellitus. *Endocrinology and Metabolism Clinics of North America, 25*(2), 425–438.

Raskin, P. (Ed.) (1994). *Medical-management of non-insulin dependent (type II) diabetes.* Alexandria, VA: American Diabetes Association, Inc.

Reiber, G. E. (1994). Who is at risk of limb loss and what to do about it? *Journal of Rehabilitation Research and Development, 31*(4), 357–362.

Reising, D. L. (1995a). Acute hyperglycemia. *Nursing95, 25*(2), 33–40.

Reising, D. L. (1995b). Acute hypoglycemia: Keeping the bottom from falling out. *Nursing95, 25*(2), 41–48.

Rolih, C. A., Ober, K. P. (1995). The endocrine response to critical illness. *Medical Clinics of North America, 79*(1), 211–224.

*Rooney, E. M. (1993). Exercise for older patients: Why it's worth your effort. *Geriatrics, 48*(11), 68–77.

Saulie, B., White, J., & Campbell, K. (1995). Metformin in the treatment of non-insulin dependent diabetes. *Diabetes Educator, 21*(5), 441–445.

Savage, P. J. (1996). Cardiovascular complications of diabetes mellitus: What we know and what we need to know about their prevention. *Annals of Internal Medicine, 124* (1, pt 2), 123–126.

Savinetti-Rose, B., & Bolmer, L. (1997). Understanding continuous subcutaneous insulin infusion therapy. *American Journal of Nursing, 97*(3), 42–49.

Selby, J. V., & Zhang, D. (1995). Risk factors for lower extremity amputation in persons with diabetes. *Diabetes Care, 18*(4), 509–515.

Service, J. F. (1995). Hypoglycemia. *Medical Clinics of North America, 79*(1), 1–8.

Shamoon, H. (1996). The relationship between hemoglobin A1c levels and the long-term complications of diabetes. *Drug Benefit Trends, 8*(suppl E), 10–17.

Shannon, M. T., Wilson, B. A., & Stang, C. L. (1995) *Drugs and nursing implications* (8th ed.) Norwalk, CT: Appleton & Lange.

Shaw, J. E., Boulton, A. J. M. (1997). The pathogenesis of diabetic foot problems. *Diabetes, 46*(suppl 2), S58–61.

*Siegel, J. (1993). Teaching infection control in blood glucose monitoring. *Diabetes Educator, 19*(6), 489–495.

Singh, I., & Marshall, M. C. (1995). Diabetes mellitus in the elderly. *Endocrinology and Metabolism Clinics of North America, 24*(2), 255–272.

Sollinger, H. W., & Geffner, S. R. (1994). Pancreas transplantation. *Surgical Clinics of North America, 74*(5), 1183–1195.

Stanford, G. G. (1994). The stress response to trauma and critical illness. *Critical Care Clinics of North America, 6*(4), 702.

Stockley, I. H. (1995). *Drug interactions.* Oxford: Blackwell Scientific.

Sutherland, D. E. R., & Gruessner, A. (1995). Long-term function (>5 years) of pancreas grafts from the Internal Pancreas Transplant Registry database. *Transplantation Proceedings, 27*(6), 2977–2980.

Tanja, J. J., Langlass, T. M. (1995). Metformin: A biguanide. *Diabetes Educator, 21*(6), 509–513.

Tinker, L., Heins, J. M., & Holler, H. J. (1994). Commentary and translation: 1994 nutritional recommendations for diabetes. *Journal of the American Dietetic Association, 94*(5), 507–511.

Tomky, D. (1997). Diabetes. *Nursing97, 27*(11), 41–46.

Tschoepe, D. (1995). The activated megakaryocyte-platelet-system in vascular disease: Focus on diabetes. *Seminars in Thrombosis and Hemostasis, 21*(2), 152–159.

Turner, R., Cull, C., Holman, R., et al. (1996). United Kingdom prospective diabetes study 17: A 9 year update of a randomized, controlled trial on the effect of improved metabolic control on complications of non-insulin-dependent diabetes mellitus. *Annuals of Internal Medicine, 124*(1, pt 2), 136–145.

Villagomez, E. (1995). Pancreas transplantation. *Critical Care Nursing Quarterly, 17*(4), 15–26.

Ulak, L. J. (1995). Sulfonylurea overdose. *MEDSURG Nursing, 4*(5), 403–404.

United States Pharmacopeial Convention, Inc. (1997). *USP DI, Vol. I: Drug information for the health care professional* (17th ed.). Taunton, MA: Rand McNally.

Urban, N., Greenlee, K. K., Krumberger, J., et al. (1995). *Guidelines for Critical Care Nursing.* St. Louis: C. V. Mosby.

Wasserman, D. H., & Zinman, B. (1994). Exercise in individuals with IDDM. *Diabetes Care, 17*(8), 924–937.

Williams, A. S. (1994). Recommendations for desirable features of adaptive diabetes self-care equipment for visually impaired persons. *Diabetes Care, 17*(5), 451–452.

Wilson, J., Beller, B., Cohen, L., et al. (1995). *Guide to teaching diabetes survival skills.* Chicago: American Association of Diabetes Educators and the Metropolitan New York Association of Diabetes Educators.

Yarborough, P. (1995). Diabetic eye disease. *U.S. Pharmacist, 20*(11), 46–66.

Zimmet, P. Z. (1995). The pathogenesis and prevention of diabetes in adults: Genes, autoimmunity and demography. *Diabetes Care, 18*(7), 1050–1604.

SUGGESTED READINGS

Bak, L. B., Heard, K. A., & Kearney, G. P. (1996). Tube feeding your diabetic patient safely. *American Journal of Nursing, 96*(12), 47–49.

The article begins by reviewing concerns related to tube feedings in general and then focuses those concerns on the client receiving tube feedings who also has diabetes. Reasons why the diabetic client may be placed on Osmolite HN, Jevity, or Glucerna and how to administer anti-diabetic medication related to the tube feedings is discussed. Case examples are included for the type 1 and the type 2 diabetic.

Capriotti, T. (1997). Beyond sulfonylureas: New oral medications in the treatment of NIDDM (type II diabetes). *MEDSURG Nursing, 6*(3), 166–169.

The article begins with a review of type II diabetes (now called type 2), including incidence, pathophysiology, insulin resistance, symptoms, complications, and treatment. The remainder of the article discusses oral medications used in the management of type 2 diabetes. Reasons why the sulfonylureas become ineffective after 5 to 10 years of therapy are discussed. The newest sulfonylurea, glimepiride (Amaryl), the biguanides, and the alpha-glucosidase inhibitors are discussed, as are drugs being researched at the time of publication. The article concludes with a section on nursing implications.

Tomky, D. (1997). Diabetes. *Nursing97, 27*(11), 41–46.

This article begins by reviewing the new terminology and classification of diabetes. Drawings to help understand the pathophysiologies of types 1 and 2 are included. Both screening and diagnostic criteria are covered. A continuing education test completes the article.

UNIT 14

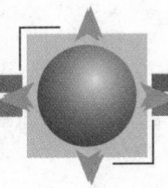

Problems of Protection:

Management of Clients

with Problems of the

Integumentary System

ASSESSMENT OF THE SKIN, HAIR, AND NAILS

The skin, hair, and nails comprise the integumentary system, which continually shields the inner organs from the external environment. The skin is the largest organ of the body and regulates many physiologic functions, such as body temperature and fluid and electrolyte balance. It also is a physical barrier to invasion by microorganisms. The appearance and functioning of the skin may be altered by a number of factors throughout a person's lifetime. Such factors include the aging process, emotional stress, skin injury, and skin or systemic disease.

For the nurse, an important characteristic of the skin is its ability to communicate information. The appearance and texture of the skin, as well as subjective reports of pain, itching, heat, cold, and pressure, can provide clues about a client's well-being. The sensory function of the skin allows the nurse to use touch as a therapeutic intervention to comfort, relieve pain, and communicate caring.

ANATOMY AND PHYSIOLOGY REVIEW
Structure of the Skin

As shown in Figure 69-1, skin has three distinct anatomic layers: fat, dermis, and epidermis. Each layer has unique characteristics that contribute to the skin's ability to maintain its complex functions.

Subcutaneous Fat (Adipose Tissue)

The innermost layer of skin overlying muscle and bone is the major site for fat formation and storage. Fat cells act as a thermal insulator for the body. They absorb shock and protect against mechanical injury by padding internal structures. The distribution of fat varies with anatomic area, age, and gender. Numerous blood vessels perforate the fatty layer and extend into the dermal layer, forming capillary networks that supply nutrients and remove waste products.

Dermis (Corium)

Above the subcutaneous fat lies the dermis, a layer of noncellular connective tissue. The dermis is composed of interwoven collagen and elastic fibers that give the skin both flexibility and mechanical strength.

Collagen, the main fibrous component of dermal tissue, is a protein formed by dermal cells called fibroblasts. The production of collagen increases in areas of tissue injury and helps form scar tissue. Fibroblasts also produce

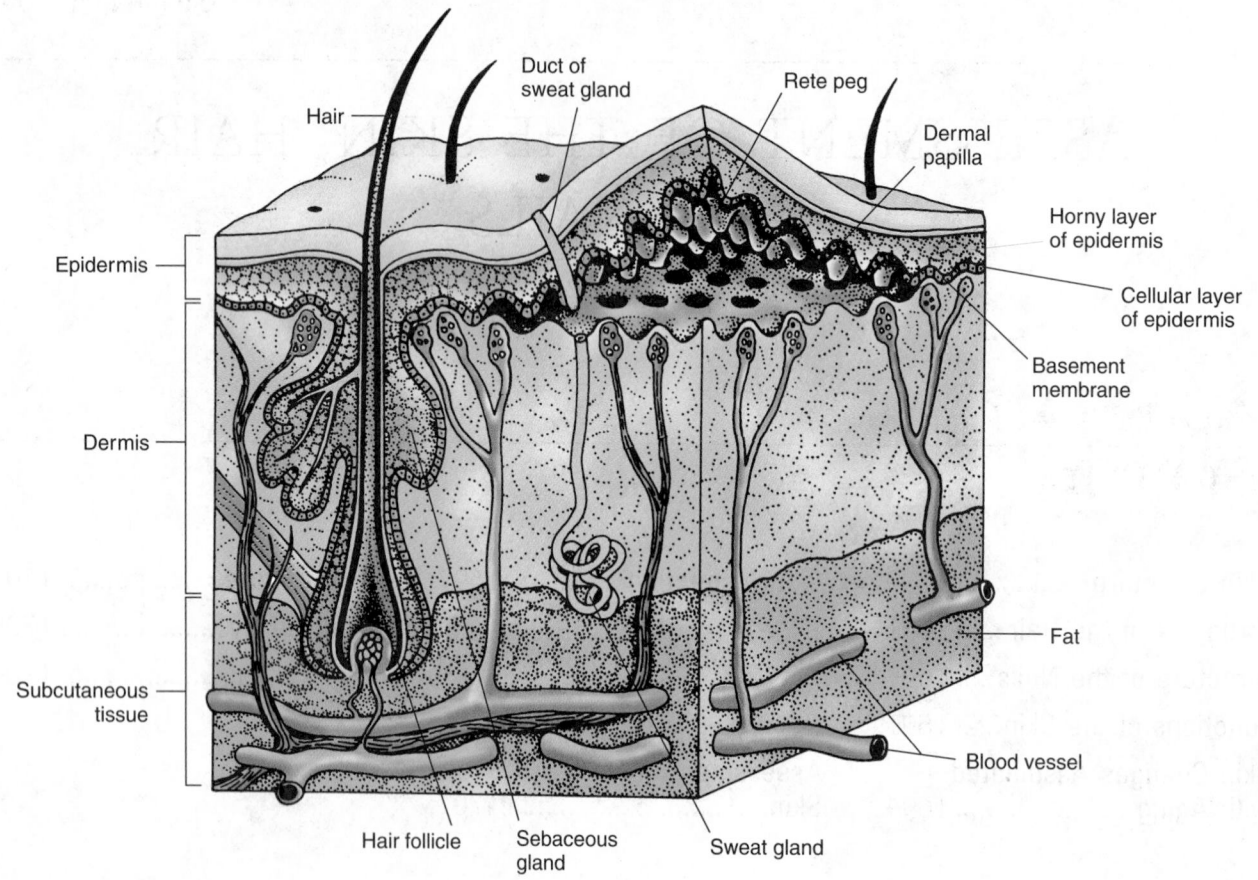

Figure 69–1. Anatomy of the skin.

ground substance, a lubricating mucopolysaccharide material (composed of protein and sugar groups) that surrounds the dermal cells and fibers and contributes to the skin's normal suppleness and turgor.

The elasticity of the skin depends on both the quantity and quality of the elastic fibers, which are interspersed among the collagen fibers. The major component of the elastic fiber is *elastin.*

The dermis houses a network of capillaries and lymph vessels in which the exchange of oxygen and heat takes place. The dermis is also rich in sensory nerves that transmit the sensations of touch, pressure, temperature, pain, and itch.

Epidermis

Anchored to the dermis by finger-like projections of dermal tissue (dermal papillae) is the outermost layer of skin: the epidermis. The corresponding interlocking fingers of epidermal tissue are called rete pegs. The epidermis is less than 1 mm thick; however, it provides the protective barrier between the body and noxious stimuli in the environment.

The epidermis lacks a blood supply. It receives its nutrients by diffusion from the highly vascular dermal layer through a porous basement membrane at the dermal-epidermal junction. Attached to the basement membrane are the functional cells (keratinocytes). Through the

process of mitosis, the basal cells (those keratinocytes capable of cell division and located closest to the basement membrane) continuously divide to form new cells. Older keratinocytes are pushed upward to form the characteristic stratified layers of the epithelium (malpighian layers). As keratinocytes move toward the surface, they flatten and eventually die. The outermost skin layer, the stratum corneum (horny layer), is composed of these dead cells. *Keratin,* the chemical protein produced by keratinocytes, makes the horny layer relatively waterproof. A keratinocyte takes about 28–45 days to move from the basement membrane to the skin surface, where it is shed, or exfoliated.

The final synthesis of vitamin D occurs primarily within the stratified epidermal layer. Vitamin D is activated by ultraviolet (UV) light.

Melanocytes are found at the level of the basement membrane in a ratio of about 1 melanocyte for every 10 keratinocytes. These pigment-producing cells give color to the skin and account for the racial differences in skin tone. The darker skin tones are not caused by increased numbers of melanocytes; rather, the size of the pigment granules (melanin) contained in each cell determines color. UV light stimulates the production of melanin, which protects against the harmful effects of sun exposure. Melanin production increases locally in response to endocrine changes or inflammation.

Structure of the Skin Appendages

Hair

Hair, a remnant of the thick protective pelt worn by most mammals, serves primarily as an adornment to modern humans. Hair growth varies with race, gender, age, and genetic predisposition. Individual hairs can differ in both structure and rate of growth, depending on body location.

Hair follicles are located in the dermal layer of the skin (see Fig. 69-1) but are actually extensions of the epidermal layer. Within each hair follicle, a cylindrical column of keratin forms the mature hair shaft. The increased sulfur content of hair keratin (in contrast to that of keratin found in the cells of the stratum corneum) contributes to the toughness of the hair shaft as it is formed. Hair color is genetically determined by the person's rate of melanin production.

Hair growth occurs in cycles; a growth phase (anagen) is followed by a resting phase (telogen). Local and systemic stressors can alter the growth cycle and result in temporary hair loss. Permanent baldness, such as common male pattern baldness, is genetic in origin and is seldom influenced by personal or environmental factors.

Nails

Well-groomed fingernails and toenails have cosmetic value and serve as useful tools with which to scrape and grasp. Like hair follicles, the nail appendages are extensions of the keratin-producing epidermal layers of the skin.

The white crescent-shaped portion of the nail at the proximal end of the nail plate (the lunula) reflects the underlying nail matrix, where nail keratin is formed and nail growth begins (Fig. 69-2). Unlike hair growth, which is cyclic, nail growth is a continuous but slow process. Total replacement of a fingernail from the matrix to the end of the finger requires 3-4 months. Total replacement of a toenail may take up to 12 months.

The *cuticle,* a layer of keratin produced by the epithelial cells of the proximal nail fold, attaches the nail plate to the soft tissue of the nail fold. The nail body is largely translucent; the pinkish hue reflects a rich capillary blood supply beneath the nail surface. Nail growth and appearance are frequently altered during systemic disease or serious illness.

Glands

Sebaceous Glands

Sebaceous glands are distributed over the entire skin surface, except for the palms and soles. Most sebaceous glands are structurally connected to the hair follicles (Fig. 69-3). Sebaceous glands of the eyelids, nipple areolae, and genitalia are freestanding.

Sebaceous glands continuously produce *sebum,* a mildly bacteriostatic lipid-containing substance. Sebum lubri-

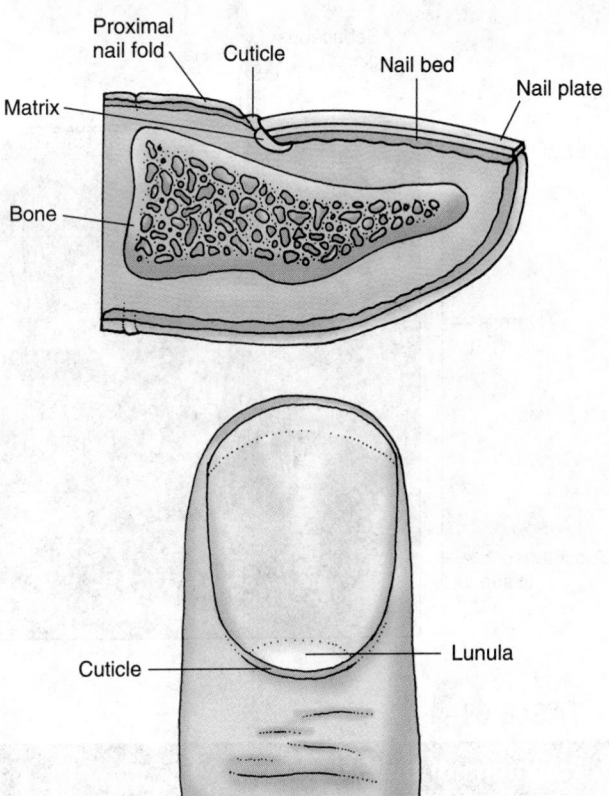

Figure 69-2. Anatomy of the nail.

cates the skin and reduces water loss from the skin surface.

Sweat Glands

The sweat glands of the skin are of two types: eccrine and apocrine. Eccrine sweat glands originate from epithelial cells. They are found over the entire skin surface and are not associated with the hair follicle. The odorless, colorless, isotonic secretions of the eccrine glands are the single most important factor in the regulation of body temperature. Stimulation of the eccrine sweat glands and the resultant evaporative water loss enable the body to lose as much as 10-12 L of fluid in a single day.

Apocrine sweat glands communicate directly with the hair follicle. They occur primarily in the areas of the axillae, the perineum, the nipple areolae, and the periumbilicus. Interaction of skin bacteria with the secretions of the apocrine glands causes the characteristic body odor.

Functions of the Skin

The skin is a complex organ responsible for the regulation of many body functions throughout the life span (Table 69-1). Although the skin has mainly protective and regulatory functions, the dynamic interrelationship between the skin and the outside world makes it an important vehicle for communication of a client's state of health and body image.

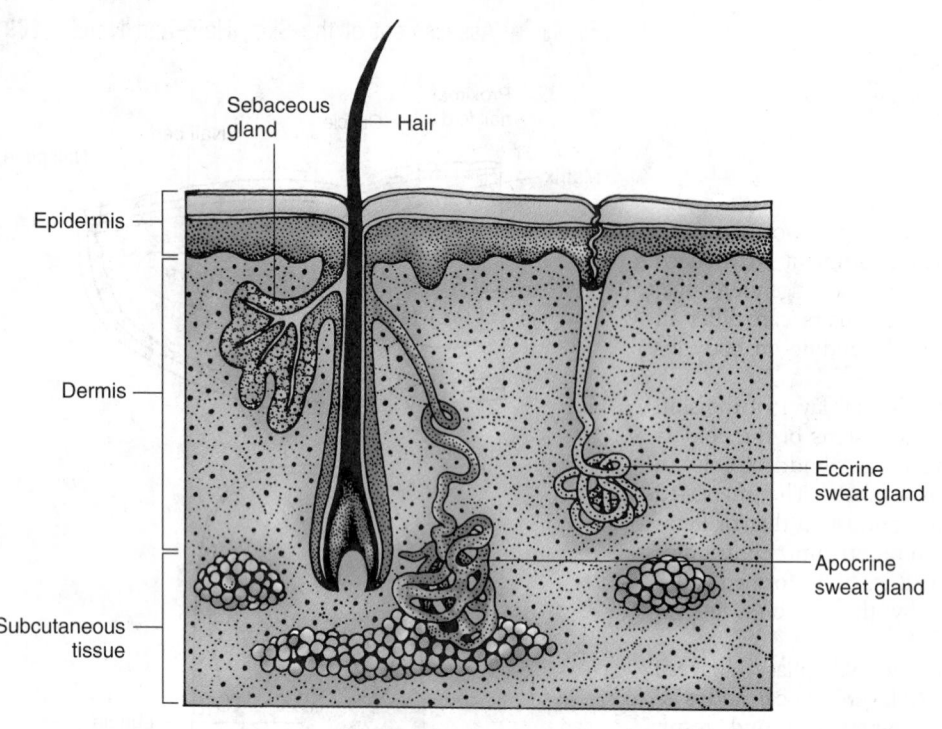

Sebaceous gland

Hair

Epidermis

Dermis

Eccrine sweat gland

Apocrine sweat gland

Subcutaneous tissue

Figure 69–3. Anatomy of the hair follicle and sebaceous and sweat glands.

TABLE 69–1

Functions of the Skin

Epidermis	Dermis	Subcutaneous Tissue
Protection		
Keratin provides protection from injury by corrosive materials	• Provides fibroblasts for wound healing	• Mechanical shock absorber

Inhibits proliferation of microorganisms because of dry external surface	• Provides mechanical strength
	  • Collagen fibers
	  • Elastic fibers
	  • Ground substance	

Mechanical strength through intracellular bonds	• Lymphatic and vascular tissues respond to inflammation, injury, and infection	
Homeostasis (Water Balance)		
Low permeability to water and electrolytes prevents systemic dehydration and electrolyte loss		
Temperature Regulation		
The eccrine sweat glands allow dissipation of heat through evaporation of sweat secreted onto the skin surface	• Cutaneous vasculature, through dilation or constriction, promotes or inhibits heat conduction from the skin surface	• Fat cells act as insulators and assist in retention of body heat
Sensory Organ		
Transmits a variety of sensations through the neuroreceptor system	• Encloses an extensive network of free and encapsulated nerve endings for relaying sensations to the brain	• Contains large pressure receptors
Vitamin Synthesis		
7-Dehydrocholesterol is present in large concentrations in malpighian cells; photoconversion to vitamin D takes place		
Psychosocial		
Body image alterations with many epidermal diseases, such as generalized psoriasis	• Body image alterations with many dermal diseases, such as scleroderma	• Body image alterations may result from increases, decreases, and redistribution of body fat stores

Chart 69–1

Nursing Focus on the Elderly: Changes in the Integumentary System Related to Aging

Physical Changes	Clinical Findings	Changes in Functional Ability
Epidermis		
Decreased thickness in epidermal layer	• Increased skin transparency and fragility	
Decreased epidermal mitotic activity	• Delayed wound healing	• Decreased cell replacement
Decreased epidermal mitotic homeostasis	• Skin hyperplasia, such as hyperkeratoses and skin cancers (especially in sun-exposed areas)	
Increased epidermal permeability	• Increased susceptibility to irritant reactions	• Decreased barrier function
Decreased number of Langerhans cells	• Decreased cutaneous inflammatory response	• Decreased injury response
Decreased number of active melanocytes	• Increased sensitivity to sun exposure	
Hyperplasia of melanocytes at the dermal-epidermal junction (especially in sun-exposed areas)	• Mottled hyperpigmentation and hypopigmentation (e.g., liver spots and age spots)	
Decreased vitamin D production	• Increased susceptibility to osteomalacia	• Decreased vitamin D production
Flattening of the dermal-epidermal junction	• Increased susceptibility to shearing forces, with resultant blisters, purpura, skin tears, and pressure-related skin problems	
Dermis		
Decreased dermal blood flow	• Increased susceptibility to dry skin (xerosis)	• Decreased chemical clearance
Decreased vasomotor responsiveness	• Increased thermoregulatory alterations (predisposition to heat stroke and hypothermia)	• Decreased vascular responsiveness
Decreased dermal thickness	• Paper-thin, transparent skin with an increased susceptibility to trauma	• Decreased injury response
Degeneration of elastic fibers	• Decreased tone and elasticity (wrinkles)	• Body image alterations
Benign proliferation of capillaries	• Cherry hemangiomas	
Abnormal nerve endings	• Alterations in sensory perception	• Decreased sensory perception
Subcutaneous Layer		
Redistribution of adipose tissue	• "Bags," cellulite, double chin, abdominal apron	• Body image alterations
Thinning of subcutaneous fat layer	• Increased susceptibility to hypothermia	• Decreased thermoregulation
	• Decreased resistance to mechanical injury (especially pressure necrosis)	• Decreased injury response
Hair		
Decreased number of hair follicles and rate of growth	• Increased hair thinning	• Decreased cell replacement
Decreased number of active melanocytes in follicle	• Gradual loss of hair color (graying)	• Body image alterations
Nails		
Decreased rate of growth	• Increased susceptibility to fungal infections	• Decreased cell replacement
Decreased blood flow beneath the nail bed	• Longitudinal nail ridges	
Glands		
Decreased sebum production, despite sebaceous gland hyperplasia	• Increased size of pores (especially on nose); large comedones in malar region	• Decreased sebum production
Decreased eccrine and apocrine gland activity	• Increased susceptibility to dry skin	• Decreased sweat production
	• Decreased perspiration, leading to decreased cooling effect	• Decreased thermoregulation
	• Decreased need for antiperspirants	

Skin Changes Associated with Aging

The process of aging begins at birth. As changes in physiologic processes progress with aging, the skin also undergoes age-related alterations in both structure and function (Chart 69–1). Figures 69–4 through 69–15 show some common age-related skin changes.

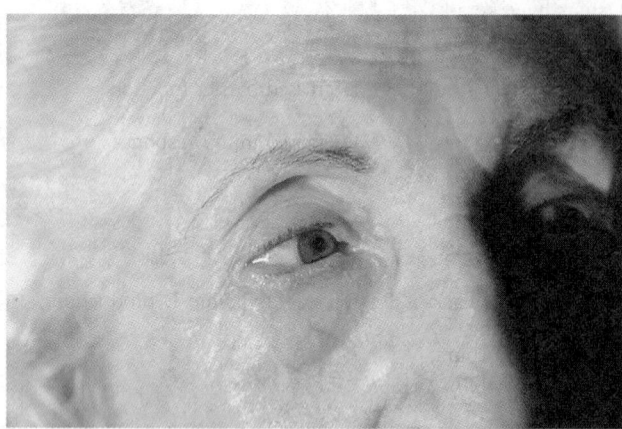

Figure 69–4. Eyelid eversion.

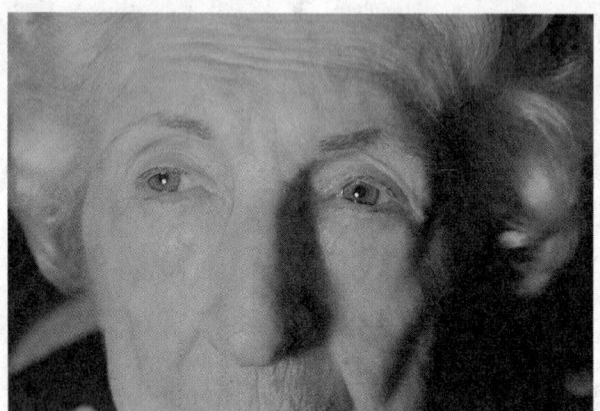

Figure 69–5. Deepening of the orbit.

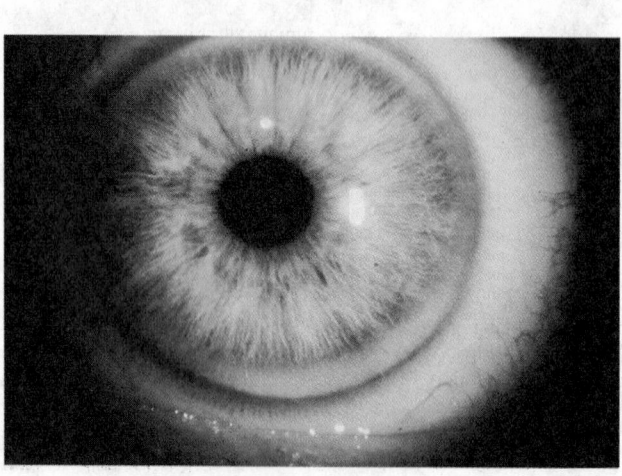

Figure 69–6. Arcus senilis of the iris.

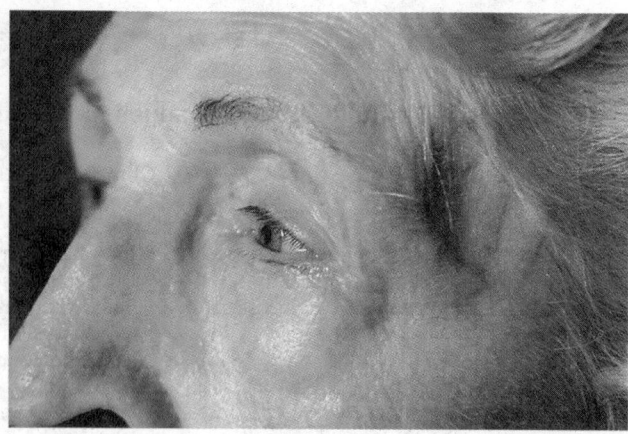

Figure 69–7. Changes in the body contour: "bags" under the eyes.

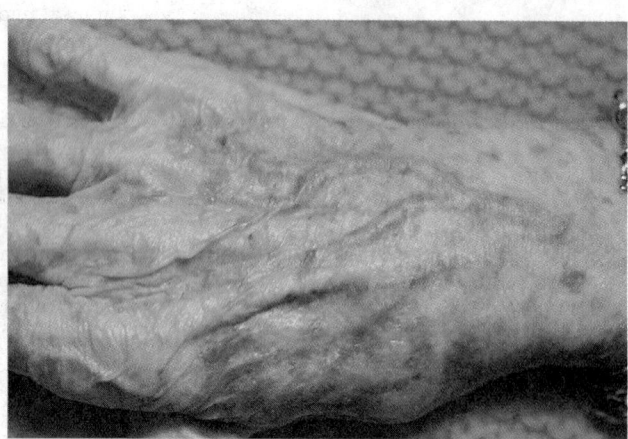

Figure 69–8. Paper-thin, transparent skin.

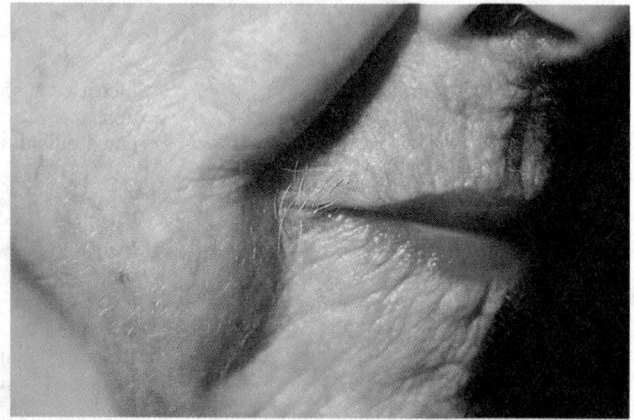

Figure 69–9. Wrinkles.

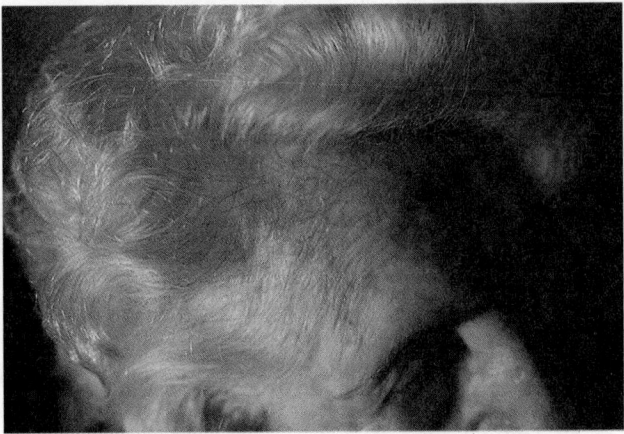

Figure 69–10. Graying and thinning of the hair.

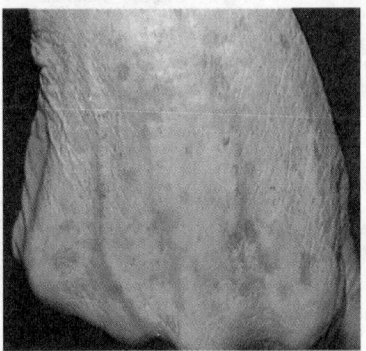

Figure 69–13. Actinic lentigo (liver spots).

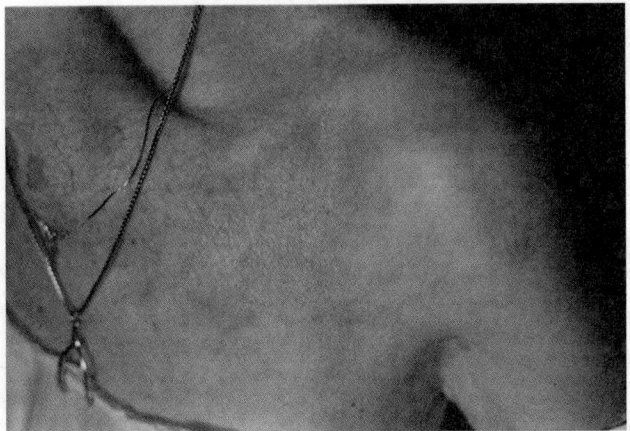

Figure 69–11. Xerosis (dry skin).

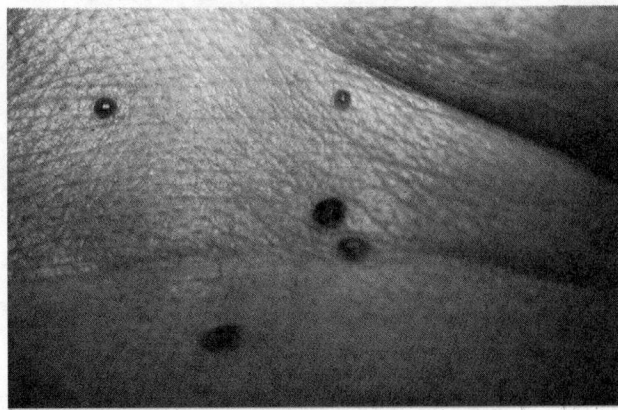

Figure 69–14. Senile (cherry) angiomas.

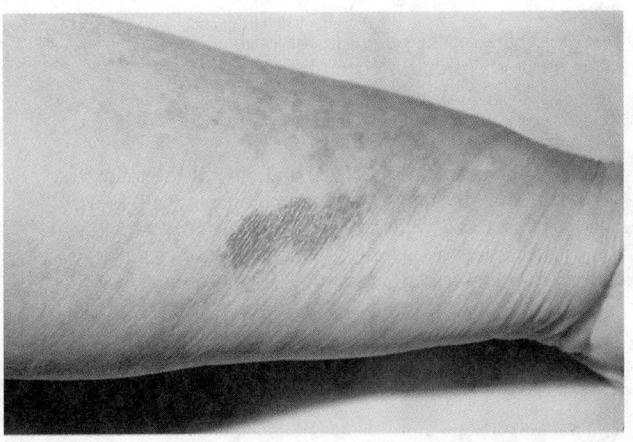

Figure 69–12. Actinic purpura.

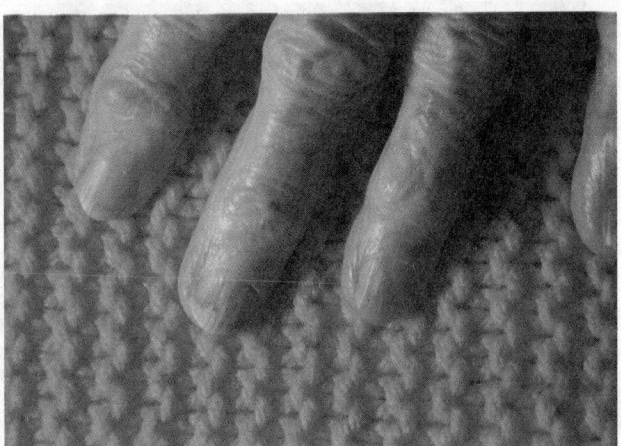

Figure 69–15. Nail changes, longitudinal ridges and thickening.

There are individual differences in how quickly and to what degree the skin ages. Although genetic background, hormonal changes, and systemic disease may greatly contribute to changes in the appearance of the skin over time, chronic sun exposure is the single most important factor leading to degeneration of the skin components (Fig. 69–16).

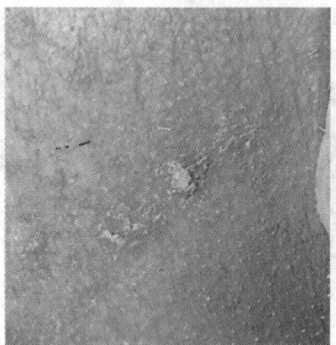

Figure 69–16. Actinic (solar) keratosis.

ASSESSMENT OF THE SKIN, HAIR, AND NAILS
History

Before examining the skin, the nurse obtains an accurate history from the client so that actual and potential skin problems can be readily identified (Chart 69–2). The nurse begins by gathering information about integumentary changes and current skin care practices.

Demographic Data

The nurse obtains demographic data from clients with actual or potential skin disorders. Age is important because many changes in the integumentary system are normal manifestations of the aging process.

Race and nationality can also be important. Some variations in skin appearance are normal cutaneous manifestations among clients of specific races and nationalities and are abnormal for clients of other races or nationalities.

Information regarding the client's occupation and hobbies can provide clues to chronic skin exposure to chemicals, irritants, abrasive substances, and other environmental factors that may contribute to skin problems.

Personal and Family History

The nurse obtains the client's medical history, including previous or current illnesses and surgical procedures. This information helps the nurse determine whether skin changes are a manifestation of an underlying systemic disorder.

Because predisposition to many skin diseases is genetically determined, the nurse explores any family tendency toward chronic skin problems. In addition, an examination of the immediate family's current health status may identify a communicable disease that has been transferred between family members.

Medication History

Because skin reactions to systemic medications are common, the nurse asks the client about recent use of prescription and over-the-counter (OTC) preparations, such as laxatives, antacids, and cold remedies. The nurse determines when each medication was started, the dose and frequency of the medication, and the time the last dose was taken. A medication history also helps identify skin changes that result from the treatment of other medical

---

Chart 69–2

Nursing Care Highlight: Important Points in the Nursing History of Clients with Skin Problems

Medical-Surgical History
- Does the client have any current or previous medical problems?
- Has the client undergone any recent or previous surgical procedures?

Family History
- Is there any family tendency toward chronic skin problems?
- Do any members of the immediate family have recent skin complaints?

Medication History
- Is the client allergic to any systemic or topical medication? If so, have the client describe the reaction.
- What prescription drugs has the client taken recently? When was the drug started? What is the dose or frequency of administration? When was the last dose taken?
- What over-the-counter drugs has the client taken recently? When was the drug started? What is the dose or frequency of administration? When was the last dose taken?

Social History
- What is the client's occupation?
- What recreational activities does the client enjoy?
- Has the client traveled recently?
- What is the client's nutritional status?

Current Health Problem
- When did the client first notice the skin problem?
- Where on the body did the problem begin?
- Has the problem gotten better or worse?
- Has a similar skin condition ever occurred before? If so, have the client describe the typical course and how it was treated.
- Is the problem associated with any of the following: itching, burning, stinging, numbness, pain, fever, nausea and vomiting, diarrhea, sore throat, cold, stiff neck, new foods, new soaps or cosmetics, new clothing or bed linens, or stressful situations?
- Does anything seem to make the problem worse (e.g., sun exposure, medications, heat or cold, and menses)?
- Does anything seem to make the problem better?

problems, such as the changes that occur with long-term steroid or anticoagulant therapy.

Diet History

The nurse notes the client's weight, height, body build, and food preferences. Poor nutrition, especially protein deficiencies, vitamin deficiencies, and obesity, can predispose a client to skin lesions and delay wound healing. Fat-free diets and chronic alcoholism can lead to fatty acid deficiencies and related skin changes. Some skin diseases, such as chronic urticaria and acne, may become worse by certain foods or food additives.

Socioeconomic Status

The nurse seeks information about a client's social and economic background as a means of identifying environmental factors that might contribute to skin disease. Recent travel may be a source of skin infections or unusual lesions.

If the client is well tanned, the nurse inquires about the amount of time spent in the sun and tanning booths and whether the client has had any skin problems associated with sun exposure.

Skin problems related to poor hygiene are common. The nurse questions the client about living conditions, bathing practices, and the availability of running water.

Current Health Problem

If a skin problem is identified, the nurse elicits additional information about the specific complaint:

■ When did the client first notice the rash?
■ Where on the body did the rash begin?
■ Has the problem improved or become worse?

If a similar problem has occurred before, the nurse asks the client to describe the course of the skin lesion and how it was treated. The nurse tries to link the problem with specific symptoms, such as itching, burning, numbness, pain, fever, sore throat, stiff neck, or nausea and vomiting. The nurse asks the client to identify anything that seems to make the problem better or worse.

Physical Assessment
Skin Inspection

Skin changes may be related to specific skin diseases and may also reflect an underlying systemic disorder. By using skin assessment skills, the nurse is in a unique position to identify obvious and subtle clues about a client's state of wellness.

A thorough assessment of the skin is best accomplished with the client partially or completely disrobed. The nurse integrates monitoring for actual or potential impairments in skin integrity as a routine part of daily care during bathing of the client or while assisting the client with other hygiene measures.

The nurse inspects the client's skin surfaces in a well-lighted room; natural or bright fluorescent lighting enhances visibility of subtle skin changes. Although no special equipment is needed, a penlight is often helpful for close inspection of lesions and can illuminate the oral cavity.

During the physical examination, the nurse systematically inspects each skin surface, including the scalp, hair, nails, and mucous membranes. Particular attention is given to the skin fold areas. The moist, warm environment of skin folds can harbor opportunistic microorganisms, such as yeast or bacteria. The nurse notes

■ Obvious changes in color and vascularity
■ The presence or absence of moisture
■ Edema
■ Skin lesions

In addition, the cleanliness of the various body areas may indicate a need for further evaluation of self-care activities.

Color

Skin color is affected by a number of factors, including blood flow, oxygenation, body temperature, and pigment production. In addition to these factors, the wide variability in natural skin tones often makes color assessment difficult, especially in the client with darker skin. (For suggestions for assessment of darker skin see Transcultural Considerations.)

Changes in skin color are described by their appearance (Table 69–2). The nurse documents the observable alterations in color and notes whether the distribution is generalized or localized. Inspection of the areas of least pigmentation, such as the buccal mucosa, the sclera, the nail beds, and the palms and soles, where color changes are accentuated, may help confirm more subtle color alterations of general body areas.

Lesions

Skin disease is clinically described in terms of primary and secondary lesions (Fig. 69–17).

■ Primary lesions represent the initial reaction to an underlying problem that alters one of the structural components of the skin.
■ Secondary lesions are changes in the appearance of the primary lesion. They occur with normal progression of the underlying disease or in response to therapeutic intervention in the form of topical or systemic treatment.

For example, acute dermatitis frequently occurs as primary vesicles with associated pruritus. Secondary lesions in the form of crusts become evident as the vesicles are disrupted and the serous exudate dries. In a person with chronic dermatitis, the skin often becomes lichenified (thickened) owing to the client's continual rubbing of the epidermis to relieve the pruritus.

In addition to the primary and secondary classification, the nurse describes the lesions in terms of their color, size, location, and configuration. The nurse notes whether the lesions occur as isolated changes or are grouped to form a distinct pattern. Table 69–3 defines terms commonly used to describe lesion configurations.

PRIMARY LESIONS

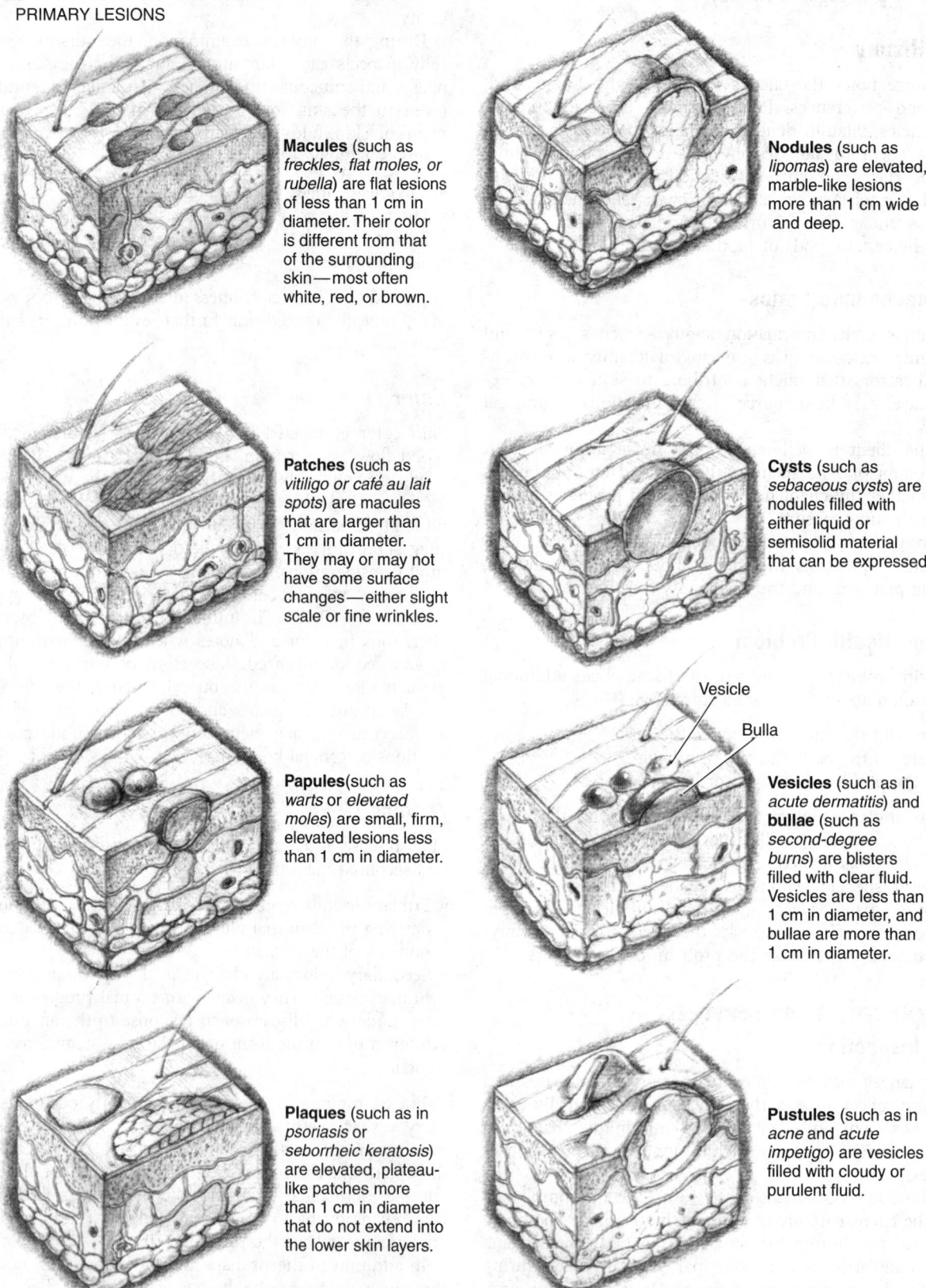

Macules (such as *freckles, flat moles, or rubella*) are flat lesions of less than 1 cm in diameter. Their color is different from that of the surrounding skin—most often white, red, or brown.

Nodules (such as *lipomas*) are elevated, marble-like lesions more than 1 cm wide and deep.

Patches (such as *vitiligo or café au lait spots*) are macules that are larger than 1 cm in diameter. They may or may not have some surface changes—either slight scale or fine wrinkles.

Cysts (such as *sebaceous cysts*) are nodules filled with either liquid or semisolid material that can be expressed.

Papules (such as *warts* or *elevated moles*) are small, firm, elevated lesions less than 1 cm in diameter.

Vesicle

Bulla

Vesicles (such as in *acute dermatitis*) and **bullae** (such as *second-degree burns*) are blisters filled with clear fluid. Vesicles are less than 1 cm in diameter, and bullae are more than 1 cm in diameter.

Plaques (such as in *psoriasis* or *seborrheic keratosis*) are elevated, plateau-like patches more than 1 cm in diameter that do not extend into the lower skin layers.

Pustules (such as in *acne* and *acute impetigo*) are vesicles filled with cloudy or purulent fluid.

Figure 69–17. Classification of skin lesions.

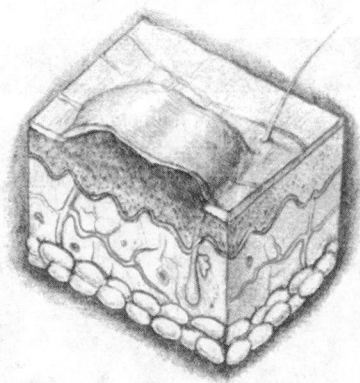

Wheals (such as *urticaria* and *insect bites*) are elevated, irregularly shaped, transient areas of dermal edema.

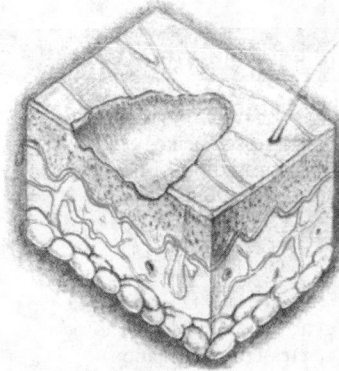

Erosions (such as in *varicella*) are wider than fissures but involve only the epidermis. They are often associated with vesicles, bullae, or pustules.

SECONDARY
LESIONS

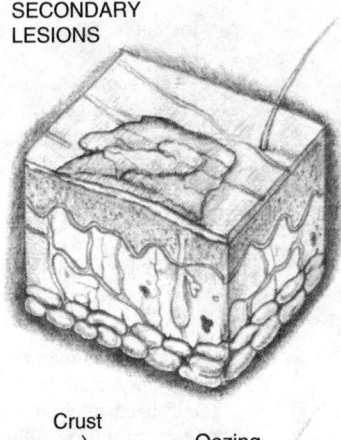

Scales (such as in *exfoliative dermatitis* and *psoriasis*) are visibly thickened stratum corneum. They appear dry and are usually whitish. They are seen most often with papules and plaques.

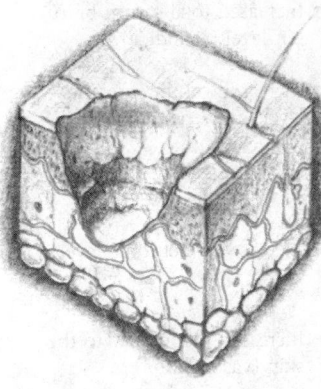

Ulcers (such as *stage 3 pressure sores*) are deep erosions that extend beneath the epidermis and involve the dermis and sometimes the subcutaneous fat.

Crust

Oozing

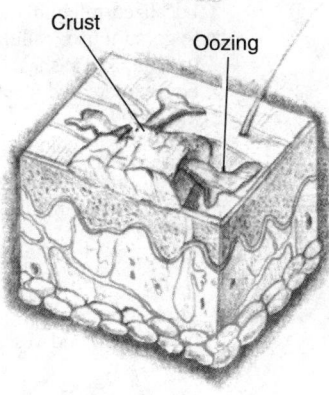

Crusts and oozing (such as in *eczema* and *late-stage impetigo*) are composed of dried serum or pus on the surface of the skin, beneath which liquid debris may accumulate. Crusts frequently result from broken vesicles, bullae, or pustules.

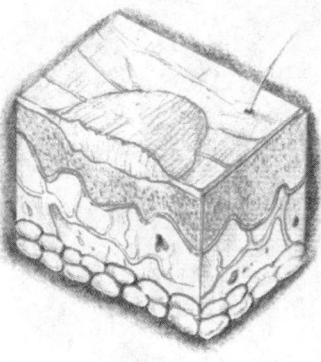

Lichenifications (such as in *chronic dermatitis*) are palpably thickened areas of epidermis with accentuated skin markings. They are caused by chronic rubbing and scratching.

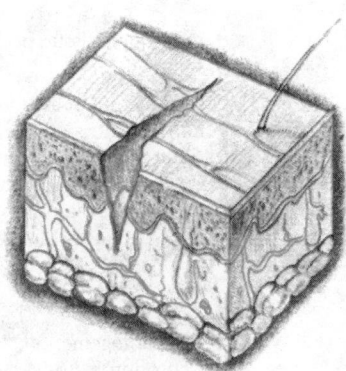

Fissures (such as in *athlete's foot*) are linear cracks in the epidermis, which often extend into the dermis.

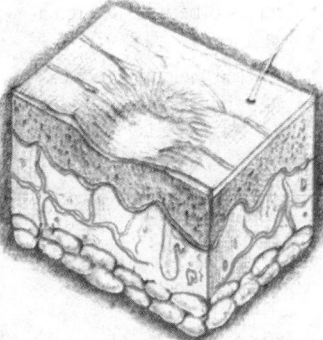

Atrophy (such as *striae* [stretch marks] and *aged skin*) is characterized by thinning of the skin surface with loss of skin markings. The skin is translucent and paper-like. Atrophy involving the dermal layer results in skin depression.

Figure 69–17. *Continued*

TABLE 69–2

Common Alterations in Skin Color

Alteration	Underlying Cause	Location	Significance
White (pallor)	• Decreased hemoglobin level • Decreased blood flow to the skin (vasoconstriction)	• Conjunctivae • Mucous membranes • Nail beds • Palms and soles • Lips	• Anemia • Shock or blood loss • Chronic vascular compromise • Sudden emotional upset • Edema • Albinism
	• Genetically determined defect of the melanocyte (decreased pigmentation) • Acquired patchy loss of pigmentation	• Generalized • Localized	 • Vitiligo; tinea versicolor
Yellow-orange	• Increased total serum bilirubin level (jaundice) • Increased serum carotene level (carotenemia) • Increased urochrome level	• Generalized • Mucous membranes • Sclera • Perioral • Palms and soles • Absent in sclera and mucous membranes • Generalized • Absent in sclera and mucous membranes	• Increased hemolysis of red blood cells • Liver disorders • Increased ingestion of carotene-containing foods (carrots) • Pregnancy • Thyroid deficiency • Diabetes • Chronic renal failure (uremia)
Red (erythema)	• Increased blood flow to the skin (vasodilation)	• Generalized • Localized (to area of involvement) • Face, cheeks, nose, and upper chest • Area of exposure	• Generalized inflammation (e.g., erythroderma) • Localized inflammation (e.g., sunburn, cellulitis, trauma, and rashes) • Fever; increased alcohol intake • Exposure to cold

Blue	• Increase in deoxygenated blood (cyanosis)
	
	• Bleeding from vessels into tissue:
	  • Petechiae (1–3 mm)
	  • Ecchymosis (>3 mm)
		• Nail beds
		• Mucous membranes
		• Generalized
		
		• Localized
			• Cardiopulmonary disease
			• Methemoglobinemia
			
			• Thrombocytopenia
			• Increased blood vessel fragility

Reddish blue	• Increased overall amount of hemoglobin • Decreased peripheral circulation	• Generalized • Distal extremities, nose	• Polycythemia vera • Inadequate tissue perfusion
Brown	• Increased melanin production • Café au lait spots (tan-brown patches) <6 spots >6 spots • Melanin and hemosiderin deposits (bronze or grayish-tan color)	• Localized (to area of involvement) • Pressure points, areolae, palmar creases, and genitalia • Face, areolae, vulva, and linea nigra • Localized • Generalized • Distal lower extremities • Exposed areas or generalized	• Chronic inflammation • Exposure to sunlight • Addison's disease • Pregnancy; oral contraceptives (melasma) • Nonpathogenic • Neurofibromatosis • Chronic venous stasis • Hemochromatosis

TABLE 69–3

Terms Commonly Used to Describe Skin Lesion Configurations

- Annular: ring-like with raised borders around flat, clear centers of normal skin
- Circinate: circular
- Circumscribed: well defined with sharp borders
- Clustered: several lesions grouped together
- Coalesced: lesions that merge with one another and appear confluent
- Diffuse: widespread, involving most of the body with intervening areas of normal skin; generalized
- Linear: occurring in a straight line
- Serpiginous: with wavy borders, resembling a snake
- Universal: all areas of the body involved, with no areas of normal-appearing skin

The nurse assesses each lesion for the "ABCD" characteristics associated with skin cancer:

- A: Asymmetry of shape
- B: Border irregularity
- C: Color variation within one lesion
- D: Diameter greater than 5 mm

A dermatologist or surgeon evaluates any lesion demonstrating one or more of the ABCD characteristics.

In describing the location of lesions, the nurse notes whether the lesions are generalized or localized. If the lesions are localized, the nurse identifies the specific body regions involved. This information is important because some diseases are associated with a specific pattern of skin lesions. Involvement of only the sun-exposed areas of the body is important information when a possible cause is being considered. Rashes limited to the skin fold areas (e.g., on the axillae, beneath the breasts, in the groin) alert the nurse to problems associated with friction, heat, and excessive moisture.

Edema

The presence of edema causes the skin to appear shiny, taut, and paler than uninvolved skin. During skin inspection, the nurse notes the location, distribution, and color of any areas of edema.

Skin elasticity is also affected by edema. The nurse places the tip of the index finger against edematous tissue with moderate pressure to determine the degree of indentation, or pitting (see Chaps. 14 and 15).

Moisture

The nurse carefully examines the skin for moisture content. Normally, increased moisture in the form of perspiration can be expected with increased activity or elevated environmental temperatures. Dampness of the skin fold areas is common because of decreased air circulation where the skin surfaces touch. However, in bedridden and debilitated clients, excess moisture can contribute to maceration and eventual skin breakdown.

Overly dry skin can be caused by such factors as a dry environment, improper skin lubrication, inadequate fluid intake, and the normal processes of aging. Dry skin is characterized by scaling of the stratum corneum. In areas of limited circulation, such as the distal lower extremities, dry skin may be especially marked. Dry skin becomes a problem for most adults during the winter months, when the air contains less moisture, and in the hospital environment, where humidity is often poorly controlled. (See Research Applications for Nursing.)

Vascular Markings

Vascular changes are classified as normal or abnormal depending on the cause. Normal vascular markings include birthmarks, cherry angiomas (Fig. 69–14), spider angiomas, and venous stars (Table 69–4). Bleeding from the vasculature into the tissue results in purpuric lesions: petechiae and ecchymosis.

▷ Research Applications for Nursing

Increased Bathing May Reduce Skin Dryness

Hardy, M. (1996). What can you do about your patient's dry skin? Journal of Gerontological Nursing, 22(5), 10–18.

This study of 160 older adults living independently, in assisted-living quarters, and in long-term care institutions sought to determine the effects of a dry skin intervention (bathing and skin care protocol) on prevention/correction of xerosis. The interactive effects of age, gender, disease history, fluid intake, and humidity on the effectiveness of the intervention also were examined. The intervention consisted of the use of Dove soap for bathing, maintaining bath/shower water temperature between 90° and 105° F, 10 minutes of direct water contact per bathing episode, patting skin dry with a cotton towel, application of mineral oil to all body parts, and use of cotton clothing and well-rinsed linens not exposed to fabric softeners. Baseline data on all participants were obtained for 6 weeks; the intervention was implemented for 6 weeks; and the participants were re-examined 6 weeks after the intervention ceased.

All groups of participants had less xerosis during the intervention period. Women overall were found to have drier skin with more scaling and redness than men, and women responded less well to the intervention. Participants in higher-humidity environments (>60%) responded more favorably to the intervention as did those with daily fluid intake greater than 2000 mL. Contrary to popular opinion, participants who bathed/showered more frequently had less dry skin.

Critique. This clinical study was well designed and implemented. The study could be strengthened using a control group and random assignment.

Possible Nursing Implications. Many people, nurses included, believe that frequent bathing increases skin dryness. The results of this study refute that belief. It is known that contact with water is the factor that softens skin and that moisture retention in skin cells decreases dryness. Perhaps greater exposure to water, with or without soaps, may prove beneficial to all clients with dry skin, particularly the elderly.

TABLE 69–4

Common Vascular Skin Lesions

Lesion	Clinical Findings	Location	Significance
Cherry angioma (senile angioma)	• Bright to dusky red, dome-shaped papule 2–5 mm in diameter • Adjacent lesions may vary in size and color • Partial blanching on palpation	• Chest and back	• Normal skin change with aging
Spider angioma	• Bright red, star-like lesion varying in size from small to 2 cm • Center of "star" is sometimes raised and may pulsate when palpated	• Face, neck, and upper trunk	• Associated with liver disease, pregnancy (change in estrogen level), and vitamin B deficiency • May be normal finding
Telangiectasia	• Reddish blue linear or star-like lesion caused by enlargement of the superficial blood vessels	• Face and trunk	• Associated with sun exposure and prolonged alcohol intake • May be seen in systemic scleroderma and after continued use of potent topical steroids
Venous star	• Spider-like, blue marking varying in size from small to several inches • May have a "cascading" appearance • Does not blanch with pressure	• Legs (near veins) and anterior chest	• Associated with increased pressure in superficial veins (varicose veins)
Port-wine stain	• Large dark red to purple area of discoloration • Does not blanch with pressure	• Face, scalp, and groin	• Congenital abnormality • If on the face, may be associated with neurologic disorders and ocular abnormalities

Petechiae are small, nonblanchable vascular lesions smaller than 0.5 mm in diameter (Fig. 69–18). They frequently indicate increased capillary fragility. Petechiae of the lower extremities are commonly associated with stasis dermatitis, a condition frequently seen in clients who have a history of chronic venous insufficiency.

Ecchymoses (bruises) are larger areas of hemorrhage that range in size from several millimeters to many centimeters. In elderly people, bruising is common after minor trauma to the skin, especially on sun-exposed areas of the body.

Integrity

The nurse thoroughly examines those areas with actual breaks in skin integrity. For example, as a result of a flattening of the dermal-epidermal junction with aging, skin tears are a common finding in elderly people. The thin, fragile skin is easily disrupted by the application of friction or shearing forces, especially if areas of ecchymosis are already present. The nurse looks for skin tears

■ In areas where constricting clothing rubs against the skin surface
■ On the upper extremities where one often grasps the skin in assisting a client to ambulate

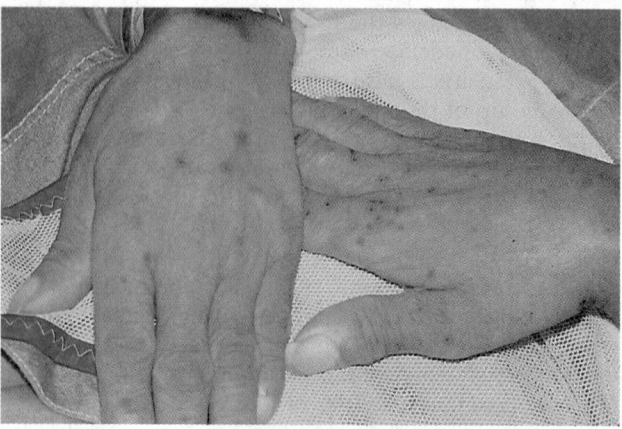

Figure 69–18. Petechiae.

- In areas where adhesive tapes or dressings have been applied and removed

The nurse remains alert to the presence of multiple abrasions or early pressure-related skin changes. These may signal previously unrecognized impairments in physical mobility or alterations in sensory perception.

Breaks in the integrity of the skin are described by their location, size, color, distribution, and the presence of drainage or any signs of infection. (Evaluation of partial-thickness and full-thickness wounds, including objective criteria that describe progress toward healing, is discussed in Chapter 70.)

Cleanliness

The nurse evaluates the cleanliness of the skin to gain information about health maintenance needs. The hair,

nails, and skin are inspected closely for excessive soiling and offensive odor. Depending on a client's degree of self-care deficit, hard-to-reach areas (e.g., the perirectal and inguinal skin folds, the axillae, and the feet) may be less clean than other skin surface areas.

Skin Palpation

Because skin inspection alone can be misleading, the nurse performs palpation (Table 69-5) concurrently with the inspection to gather additional information about skin lesions, moisture, temperature, texture, and turgor.

Palpation confirms the size of the lesions and determines whether they are flat or slightly raised. The consistency of larger lesions can vary from soft and pliable to firm and solid. With eyes closed, the nurse can detect more subtle changes, such as the difference between a

TABLE 69-5

Common Clinical Findings in Skin Palpation

Clinical Findings	Cause	Location	Examples of Predisposing Conditions
Edema			
Localized	• Inflammatory response	• Area of injury or involvement	• Trauma
Dependent or pitting	• Fluid and electrolyte imbalance	• Ambulatory: dorsum of foot and medial ankle	• Congestive heart failure
	• Venous and cardiac insufficiency	• Bedridden: buttocks, sacrum, and lower back	• Renal disease
			• Hepatic cirrhosis
			• Venous thrombosis or stasis
Nonpitting	• Endocrine imbalance	• Generalized, but more easily seen over the tibia	• Hypothyroidism (myxedema)
Moisture			
Increased	• Autonomic nervous system stimulation	• Face, axillae, skin folds, palms, and soles	• Fever, anxiety, activity
Decreased	• Dehydration	• Buccal mucous membranes with progressive involvement of other skin surfaces	• Hyperthyroidism
	• Endocrine imbalance		• Fluid loss
			• Postmenopausal status
			• Hypothyroidism
			• Normal aging
Temperature			
Increased	• Increased blood flow to the skin	• Generalized	• Fever, hypermetabolic states
		• Localized	• Inflammation
Decreased	• Decreased blood flow to the skin	• Generalized	• Impending shock, sepsis, anxiety
			• Hypothyroidism
		• Localized	• Interference with vascular flow
Turgor			
Decreased	• Decreased elasticity of the dermis (tenting when pinched)	• Abdomen, forehead, or radial aspect of the wrist	• Severe dehydration
			• Sudden severe weight loss
			• Normal aging
Texture			
Roughness or thickness	• Irritation, friction	• Pressure points (e.g., soles, palms, and elbows)	• Calluses
			• Chronic eczema
			• Atopic skin diseases
	• Sun damage	• Areas of sun exposure	• Normal aging
	• Excessive collagen production	• Localized or generalized	• Scleroderma
			• Keloids
Softness or smoothness	• Endocrine disturbances	• Generalized	• Hyperthyroidism

fine macular (flat) and a papular (raised) rash. The nurse notes whether the client experiences pain or tenderness during palpation of the skin.

The nurse touches areas of excess moisture to determine the thickness and consistency of secretions. In areas of excess dryness, the nurse rubs a finger against the skin surface to determine the degree of flaking or scaling.

The nurse detects both generalized and localized changes in skin temperature by placing the back of a hand on the skin surface. Before assessing for changes in skin temperature, the nurse makes certain to have warm hands. Cold hands interfere with accurate assessment and are uncomfortable for the client.

The nurse palpates the skin surfaces to assess texture, which differs according to body region and exposure to environmental irritants. For example, areas of long-term sun exposure have a rougher texture than that of protected skin surfaces. The client whose occupation requires repeated exposure to harsh soaps or chemicals may show skin changes related to the exposure. An increase in thickness of the skin from scarring, lichenification, or edema usually decreases elasticity.

Turgor indicates the amount of skin elasticity. The turgor of the skin can be altered by a number of factors, including water content and age. The nurse pinches the skin gently between a thumb and forefinger and then releases it. If skin turgor is normal, the skin immediately returns to its original state when released. Poor skin turgor is evidenced by "tenting" of the skin, with gradual return to the original state (see Chap. 14). Normal loss of elasticity with aging makes assessment of skin turgor difficult in the elderly client. If the client is in a supine position, the forehead or chest tissue gives the best indication of skin hydration.

Hair Assessment

During the skin assessment, hair is inspected and palpated for cleanliness, distribution, quantity, and quality. Hair is normally found in an even distribution over most of the body surfaces; hair on the scalp, in the pubic region, and in the axillary folds is thicker and coarser than hair on the trunk and extremities. Although color and growth patterns vary widely, sudden or marked changes in hair characteristics may reflect an underlying disease process. As with skin changes, the nurse investigates any abnormal findings by obtaining an in-depth history of the circumstances surrounding any change.

How well the hair is groomed, including the cleanliness of areas of thicker hair growth, can confirm information already gathered about a client's social history and health care needs. If the client has intense itching or scratches continually, the nurse carefully examines the scalp and pubis for lice and nits (lice eggs). The nurse also inspects the scalp for excessive scaling, redness, lesions, excoriation, crusting, and tenderness.

Dandruff is common; an accumulation of patchy or diffuse white or gray scales appears on the surface of the scalp. Although dandruff is mainly a cosmetic problem, inflammatory changes can occur if the scalp is excessively oily, with resultant erythema and pruritus. Severe inflam-

matory dandruff can extend to involve the eyebrows as well as the skin of the face and neck. *If severe dandruff is not treated, hair loss can occur.*

Although gradual hair loss is associated with aging, sudden asymmetric or patchy hair loss at any age is of concern. The nurse assesses the scalp for distribution and thickness of the hair and notes variations.

Increased hair growth across the face and anterior chest in women is a sign of hirsutism. Hirsutism is one manifestation of hormonal imbalance. If hirsutism is apparent, the nurse looks for

▪ Associated changes in fat distribution and capillary fragility, which can occur in Cushing's disease
▪ Clitoral enlargement and deepening of the voice, which may indicate ovarian dysfunction

Assessment of the Nails

Dystrophic (abnormal) nails often reflect serious systemic illness or local skin disease involving the epidermal keratinocytes. The nurse evaluates the fingernails and toenails for color, shape, thickness, texture, and the presence of lesions.

Many variations in color, texture, and grooming of the nails are influenced by factors unrelated to disease, such as occupation. When assessing the elderly client, the nurse notes minor variations associated with the aging process (see Fig. 69–15), such as gradual thickening of the nail plate, the appearance of longitudinal ridges, or a yellowish-gray discoloration.

Color

The color of the nail plate depends on many factors (Table 69–6), including thickness and transparency of the nail, blood composition, adequacy of arterial blood flow, and pigment deposits. Figure 69–19 shows normal variations in nail color. Changes in color can be attributed to external factors, such as the chemical damage encountered in some occupations and the long-term use of nail polish.

During examination, the client's fingers and toes should be free of any surface pressure that might interfere with local blood flow or alter the appearance of the digits. To differentiate between color changes attributable to the underlying vascular supply and those resulting from pigment deposition, the nurse blanches the nail bed to see whether a significant color change occurs with pressure. The nurse gently squeezes the end of the finger or toe, exerts downward pressure on the nail bed, and then releases the pressure. Color caused by vascular alterations changes as pressure is applied and returns to the original state when pressure is released. Color caused by pigment deposition remains unchanged.

Shape

Nail shape may indicate early or late changes consistent with systemic disease. For example, fingernail clubbing is diagnostic for impaired gas exchange.

The nurse evaluates nail shape by examining the curva-

TABLE 69–6

Common Alterations in Nail Color

Alteration	Clinical Findings	Significance
White	• Horizontal white banding or areas of opacity	• Chronic hepatic or renal disease (Hypoalbuminemia)
	• Generalized pallor of nail beds	• Shock
		• Anemia
		• Early arteriosclerotic changes (toenails)
		• Myocardial infarction
Yellow-brown	• Diffuse yellow to brown discoloration	• Jaundice
		• Peripheral lymphedema
		• Bacterial or fungal infections of the nail
		• Psoriasis
		• Diabetes
		• Cardiac failure
		• Staining from tobacco, nail polish, or dyes
		• Long-term tetracycline therapy
		• Normal aging (yellow-gray color)
	• Vertical brown banding extending from the proximal nail fold distally	• Normal finding in African-American clients
		• Nevus or melanoma of nail matrix in Caucasian clients
Red	• Thin, dark red vertical lines 1–3 mm in length (splinter hemorrhages)	• Bacterial endocarditis
		• Trichinosis
		• Trauma to the nail bed
		• Normal finding in some clients
	• Red discoloration of the lunula	• Cardiac insufficiency
	• Dark red nail beds	• Polycythemia vera
Blue	• Diffuse blue discoloration that blanches with pressure	• Respiratory failure
		• Methemoglobinuria
		• Venous stasis disease (toenails)

ture of the nail plate and surrounding soft tissue from all angles. The nurse palpates the fingertips to define areas of sponginess, tenderness, or marked edema. Table 69–7 describes common variations in nail shape.

Thickness

The nail plate can thicken as a result of trauma, chronic dermatologic disease, or decreased arterial blood flow. If the client is elderly, the nurse looks for a "heaped-up" appearance of the toenails, which is commonly associated with fungal infection (*onychomycosis*).

Consistency

Nail consistency is described as hard, soft, or brittle. Nail plates may become hard, with increased thickening. A warm-water soak or lubrication with petroleum jelly is

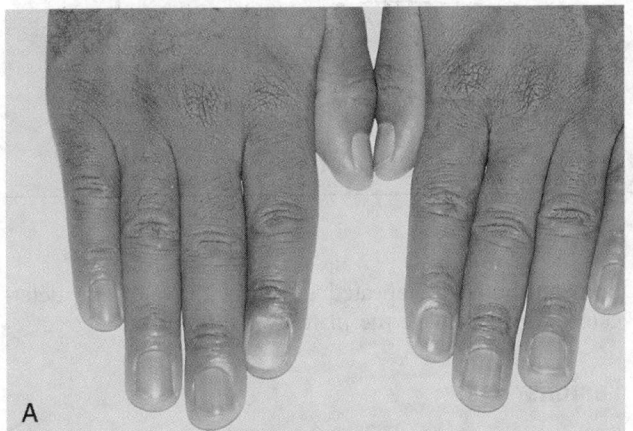
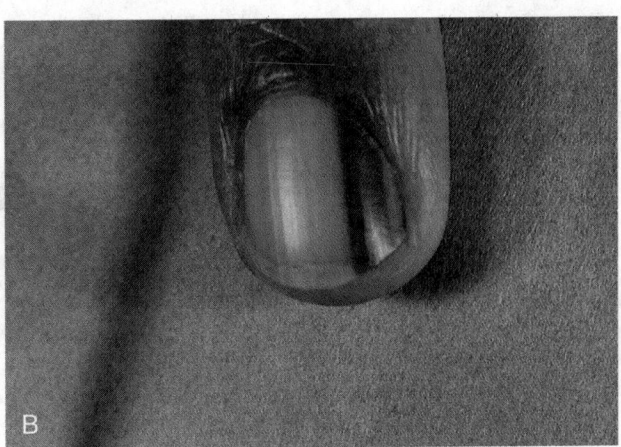

Figure 69–19. *A,* Diffuse nail pigmentation. *B,* Linear nail pigmentation.

TABLE 69-7

Common Variations in Nail Shape

Nail Shape	Clinical Findings		Significance
Normal	• Angle of 160 degrees between the nail plate and the proximal nail fold • Nail surface slightly convex • Nail base firm when palpated		• Normal finding
Clubbing Early clubbing	• Straightening of angle between the nail plate and the proximal nail fold to 180 degrees • Nail base spongy when palpated		• Hypoxia • Lung cancer
Late clubbing	• Angle between the nail plate and the proximal nail fold exceeds 180 degrees • Nail base visibly edematous and spongy when palpated • Enlargement of the soft tissue of the fingertips gives a "drumstick" appearance when viewed from above		• Prolonged hypoxia • Advanced lung cancer
Spoon nails (koilonychia) Early koilonychia	• Flattening of the nail plate with an increased smoothness of the nail surface		• Iron deficiency (with or without anemia) • Poorly controlled diabetes >15 yr in duration
Late koilonychia	• Concave curvature of the nail plate		• Local injury • Psoriasis • Chemical irritants • Developmental abnormality
Beau's grooves	• 1-mm wide horizontal depressions in the nail plates caused by growth arrest (involves all nails)		• Acute, severe illness • Prolonged febrile state • Isolated periods of severe malnutrition
Pitting	• Small, multiple pits in the nail plate • May be associated with plate thickening and onycholysis • Most often involves the fingernails, several or all		• Psoriasis • Alopecia areata

required to soften the nail plates before they can be trimmed.

Soft nail plates, which are thin and bend easily with pressure, have been associated with malnutrition, chronic arthritis, myxedema, and peripheral neuritis. Brittle or friable nails can split, as in the client with onychomycosis or advanced psoriasis. Splitting of the nail plate has also been attributed to repeated exposure to water and detergents, which damage the plate over time.

Lesions

Separation of the nail plate from the nail bed (*onycholysis*) creates an air pocket beneath the nail plate. The pocket appears initially as a grayish-white opacity. The color may change as dirt and keratin collect in the pocket and the area becomes malodorous. Onycholysis is common with fungal infections and after trauma. Separation of the nail plate may also occur with psoriasis or as a result of prolonged contact with chemical irritants.

The nurse inspects the soft-tissue folds around the nail plate for localized redness, heat, swelling, and tenderness. Inflammation of the skin around the nail (*acute paronychia*) is usually associated with a torn cuticle or an ingrown toenail. If acute paronychia occurs in an immunocompromised client, an opportunistic infection caused by *Staphylococcus* is probable.

Chronic paronychia is more common and is characterized by inflammation that persists for months. People thought to be at high risk for chronic paronychia are men and women with frequent intermittent exposure to water, such as homemakers, bartenders, and laundry workers.

TRANSCULTURAL CONSIDERATIONS

Pallor, erythema, cyanosis, and other color changes reflective of a client's physical state are more difficult to recognize in people with naturally dark skin tones. Although physiologic processes are the same for both light-skinned and dark-skinned clients, the amount of skin pigmentation greatly alters how the skin appears in response to physiologic alterations. Consequently, the nurse develops assessment skills to detect the more subtle color changes. The nurse becomes familiar with the normal appearance of a dark-skinned client's mucous membranes, nail beds, and skin tone so that variations from normal can be identified.

Assessment of Pallor in Dark-Skinned Clients. To detect generalized pallor, the nurse inspects the mucous membranes for an ash-gray color. If the lips and the nail beds are not heavily pigmented, they appear paler than normal for that client. The nurse examines the skin under appropriate lighting for the absence of the underlying red tones that normally give heavily pigmented skin a healthy glow. With generalized decreased blood flow to the skin, brown skin appears yellow-brown, and very dark brown skin is ash gray.

Assessment of Cyanosis in Dark-Skinned Clients. Cyanosis is even more difficult to detect than pallor. If impaired gas exchange is anticipated, the nurse examines the lips, tongue, nail beds, conjunctivae, and palms and soles at regular intervals for subtle color changes. In a client with cyanosis, the lips and tongue are gray; the palms, soles, conjunctivae, and nail beds have a bluish tinge. To support these observations, the nurse assesses for the more obvious manifestations of hypoxia, including tachycardia, hypotension, changes in respiratory rate or rhythm, decreased breath sounds, changes in level of consciousness, and any increase in amount or viscosity of secretions.

Assessment of Inflammation in Dark-Skinned Clients. If areas of acute inflammation are suspected, the nurse uses the back of the hand to palpate for the increased warmth that occurs when blood flow to the skin increases. With the fingertips, the nurse palpates for hardened areas deep in the tissue, which may give the skin a "woody" feeling. Inflamed skin is tender and edematous. If edema is extensive, the skin is taut and shiny.

Areas of the body where inflammation, such as an inflammatory rash or cellulitis, has recently resolved appear darker than the normal skin tone. This is due to stimulation of the melanocytes during the inflammatory process and to increased pigment production, which continues after inflammation subsides. More extensive injury to the skin, with destruction of melanocytes (such as a deep ulcer or a full-thickness burn), may heal with color changes that are lighter than the normal skin tone. Unlike acute changes, chronic inflammatory changes seldom produce tenderness on palpation. If scar tissue is present, the skin may feel less supple, especially over joints. If chronic inflammatory changes are suspected, the nurse asks the client about a history of skin problems in that area of the body.

Assessment of Jaundice in Dark-Skinned Clients. The nurse can best observe jaundice by inspecting the oral mucosa, especially the hard palate, for yellow discoloration. Inspection of the conjunctivae and adjacent sclera may be misleading because normal deposits of subconjunctival fat produce a yellowish hue visible in contrast to the dark periorbital skin. Therefore, the nurse examines the sclera closest to the cornea for a more accurate determination of jaundice. The palms and soles of dark-skinned clients may appear yellow if they are callused; callus should not be mistaken for jaundice.

Assessment of Purpura and Purpuric Lesions in Dark-Skinned Clients. Purpuric lesions may be difficult to detect, depending on the degree of skin pigmentation. Areas of ecchymosis appear darker than normal skin; they may be tender and easily palpable, depending on whether hematoma is present. In most cases, the client relates a history of trauma to the area that confirms the assessment. Petechiae are rarely visible in dark skin and may be evidenced only in the oral mucosa and conjunctiva.

Psychosocial Assessment

Actual impairments in skin integrity are commonly associated with altered perceptions in body image, especially with involvement of the more visible skin surfaces, such as the face, the hair, or the hands. The nurse assesses the client's body language for clues indicating a disturbance in self-concept. For example, avoidance of eye contact or the use of garments to cover the affected areas communicates concern about physical appearance. Clients with chronic skin diseases often relate a history of social isolation, attributable to fear of rejection by others or a belief that the skin problem is contagious.

Skin changes linked to poor hygiene are common in clients from low socioeconomic backgrounds. The nurse assesses overall appearance for excessive soiling, matted hair, body odor, or other self-care deficits. The nurse confirms unsanitary living conditions by obtaining a social history. Clients may relate similar skin problems among family members, friends, and sexual contacts.

If skin problems related to poor hygiene are identified in elderly clients, the nurse also evaluates any physical limitations that may be contributing to poor health maintenance. For example, visual problems or limited mobility can make it difficult for clients to see or reach skin surfaces to clean them.

Diagnostic Assessment

Laboratory Tests

When a fungal, bacterial, or viral pathogen is suspected as the cause of certain skin changes, confirmation by microscopic examination is necessary.

Cultures for Fungal Infections

When superficial fungal (dermatophyte) infections are suspected, scales are gently scraped from the skin lesions into a Petri dish or a similar clean container and transported to the diagnostic laboratory for implantation into a suitable culture medium. Fingernail clippings and hair are collected in a similar manner. Unfortunately, waiting for culture results can delay treatment of superficial fungal infection. For this reason, the specimen is also stained with a potassium hydroxide (KOH) preparation and examined microscopically.

For deeper fungal infections, a piece of tissue is obtained for culture. The physician obtains the specimen by punch biopsy (see Skin Biopsy). The biopsy specimen may be sent for histopathologic analysis and special fungal stains; the tissue specimen is bisected, or two separate biopsy specimens are obtained.

Cultures for Bacterial Infections

Specimens for bacterial culture are obtained from intact primary lesions (bullae, vesicles, or pustules), if possible. Material is expressed from the lesion, collected with a cotton-tipped applicator, and placed in a bacterial culture medium. For intact lesions, unroofing (lifting or puncturing of the outer surface) may be required with a sterile small-gauge needle before material can be easily expressed. If secondary lesions in the form of crusts are present, the nurse removes the crusts and swabs the underlying exudate.

Biopsy of deep bacterial infections may be required to obtain a specimen for culture. If bacterial cellulitis is suspected, nonbacteriostatic saline can be injected deep into the tissue and aspirated; the aspirant is sent for culture.

Cultures for Viral Infections

Viral cultures are indicated if herpesvirus infection is suspected. With a cotton-tipped applicator, the physician obtains vesicle fluid from intact lesions. Unlike bacterial and fungal specimens, which can remain at room temperature until transport to the laboratory, viral culture tubes are placed in ice immediately after the specimen is obtained and transported to the laboratory as soon as possible.

Other Diagnostic Tests

Skin Biopsy

To establish an accurate diagnosis or assess the effectiveness of a therapeutic intervention, the physician must often obtain a small piece of skin tissue for histopathologic study. Depending on the size, depth, and location of the skin changes, the physician may perform punch biopsy, shave biopsy, or scalpel excision (excisional biopsy). Before preparing the client, the nurse checks with the physician to determine the number, location, and type of skin biopsies to be performed.

PUNCH BIOPSY. The punch biopsy is the most basic technique. A small circular cutting instrument, or punch, ranges in diameter from 2 to 6 mm. After the site is injected with a local anesthetic, a cylindric plug of tissue is cut to the depth of the subcutaneous fat and removed with forceps and scissors. The biopsy site may be closed with one or two sutures if it is on the face or lower extremity. Some physicians allow the biopsy site to heal without suturing.

SHAVE BIOPSY. A shave biopsy removes only that portion of the skin elevated above the plane of the surrounding tissue by injection of the local anesthetic. A scalpel or razor blade is moved parallel to the skin surface to remove the tissue specimen. Shave biopsies are usually indicated for superficial or raised lesions. Suturing is not necessary.

EXCISIONAL BIOPSY. In rare instances, larger or deeper specimens are obtained by excision with a scalpel. Deep incisions are made and then sutured after the specimen is removed. In contrast to punch and shave biopsies, excisional biopsies usually involve more discomfort for the client while the site is healing.

CLIENT PREPARATION. As with any invasive procedure, the nurse prepares the client for a biopsy by briefly explaining what to expect. The nurse emphasizes that a biopsy is a minor procedure with few, if any, complications. If a punch or shave biopsy is planned, the nurse reassures the client that scarring is minimal because of the small size of the tissue removed. If an excisional biopsy is planned, the nurse tells the client to expect a cosmetic result similar to that of a healed surgical incision.

PROCEDURE. The nurse establishes a sterile field and assembles all necessary supplies and instruments. A syringe with the physician's choice of local anesthetic is available. A small-gauge needle (no. 25) is attached to the syringe to minimize discomfort during injection. Although preparation of the biopsy site differs according to the physician's preference, in most cases the skin is simply wiped with alcohol.

The most uncomfortable time for the client is during the injection of a local anesthetic agent, which produces a burning or stinging sensation. The nurse reassures the client that the discomfort will subside as anesthesia takes effect. Talking the client through the procedure with a quiet voice, combined with gentle touch, has a calming effect.

After removal, tissue specimens for routine pathologic study are placed directly in 10% formalin for fixation. Specimens for culture are placed in sterile saline solution. Bleeding of the biopsy site is sometimes controlled with Monsel's solution, a topical hemostatic agent. If topical treatment does not stop the bleeding, suturing is considered.

FOLLOW-UP CARE. After bleeding is under control and any sutures have been placed, the site is covered with an adhesive bandage or a dry gauze dressing. The nurse instructs the client to keep the dressing dry and in place for a minimum of 8 hours. After the dressing is removed, the site is cleaned once a day with tap water or saline to remove any dried blood or crusts. The physician may also prescribe an antibiotic ointment to minimize local bacterial colonization. The biopsy site may be left open unless a covering is preferred for cosmetic reasons or because the site is an area frequently soiled. The nurse instructs the client to report any erythema or excessive drainage at the site. Sutures are usually removed 7–10 days after biopsy.

Wood's Light Examination

A hand-held, long-wavelength ultraviolet (black) light or Wood's light is sometimes used during physical examination. Areas of blue-green or red fluorescence are associated with certain skin infections. Hypopigmented skin becomes more prominent when it is viewed under black light, which greatly facilitates evaluation of pigment changes in fair-skinned clients.

Examination of the skin under a Wood's light is always carried out in a darkened room. The nurse reassures the client that no discomfort is associated with Wood's light examination.

Diascopy

Diascopy is a noninvasive and painless technique that eliminates erythema caused by increased blood flow to the skin, thereby facilitating the inspection of skin lesions. A glass slide or lens is pressed down over the area to be examined, blanching the skin and revealing the shape of the underlying lesions.

Skin Testing

PATCH TESTING. If a client's rash is thought to be an allergic contact dermatitis, patch testing may identify the responsible allergen. Contact with a substance to which the client is allergic results in a delayed hypersensitivity reaction, which develops in 48–96 hours.

Test chemicals are applied to uninvolved skin under occlusive tape patches. After the patches are removed, the skin areas in contact with the chemical are examined closely for indications of a cutaneous allergic response (localized erythema, swelling, and vesicular eruption). For a positive patch test result to have clinical relevance, a history of exposure to substances containing the chemical is also required.

Client Preparation. To prevent suppression of the inflammatory response to an allergen, the physician discontinues administration of systemic corticosteroids or antihistamine for at least 48 hours before the test. Topical steroid therapy may be continued as long as the agent is not applied on the area to be tested. To allay anxiety, the nurse explains that patch testing does not involve pricking the skin with needles. The nurse informs the client that testing will involve three separate visits to the dermatologist:

- One to apply the test patches
- The second for an initial reading
- The third for detection of any delayed hypersensitivity reactions

Procedure. The preferred site for application of test patches is the upper back. After the client has disrobed, the back is inspected for evidence of rash and the presence of hair. If rash is present, alternative test sites are the flanks, the lower back, and the upper arms. Any hair is shaved to prevent poor contact and subsequent false-negative results. Removal of skin oils with alcohol promotes adhesiveness of the patches.

Small quantities of chemicals and solutions in standardized concentrations are placed in separate metal chambers backed with hypoallergenic adhesive tape. The tape is then carefully applied to the skin so that each chemical is held in contact with the skin surface. Each chamber is marked for later identification. As many as 60 or more chemicals may be tested simultaneously.

The nurse instructs the client to keep the test sites dry at all times. If the client is accustomed to taking showers, baths are substituted until testing is complete. The nurse emphasizes that the client must use caution when washing the hair to avoid getting the patches wet. The nurse also discourages excessive physical activity that will result in sweating. If the client reapplies patches that come loose, this can interfere with an accurate interpretation of true allergic reactions. The nurse reinforces the necessity of removing loose or nonadherent test patches for reapplication by the physician or nurse at a later date.

The initial reading is performed 2 days after application. The tape containing the chemical-filled chambers is peeled away from the skin, and each area of contact is marked with indelible ink for future reading. The nurse notes any initial allergic or irritant reactions in the client's medical record. The final reading of the test results is done 2–5 days later.

Follow-Up Care. If a potential allergen is identified, the client is given a list of items containing that chemical; these are to be avoided. Follow-up visits to the dermatologist are necessary to monitor the progress of the rash.

SCRATCH TESTING. A scratch or prick test differs from a patch test in that it evokes an immediate hypersensitivity reaction to an allergen. Scratch tests are used in routine allergy testing to determine the possible cause of urticaria (hives). Allergens introduced to the skin through a superficial scratch or prick cause a localized reaction (wheal) when the test result is positive.

Client preparation and follow-up for scratch testing are similar to those for patch testing. However, an inadvertent intradermal injection of solutions used for scratch testing may induce an anaphylactic reaction. The nurse ensures that emergency equipment is readily available during a scratch test.

SELECTED BIBLIOGRAPHY

*Arnold, H., Odum, R., & James, W. (1990). *Diseases of the skin: Clinical dermatology* (2nd ed.). Philadelphia: W. B. Saunders.

*Bryant, R. (1988). Saving the skin from tape injuries. *American Journal of Nursing, 88,* 189–191.

*Cuzzell, J. (1990a). Derm detective clues: Itching and burning, in skin folds. *American Journal of Nursing, 90*(1), 23–24.

*Cuzzell, J. (1990b). Derm detective clues: Pain, burning, and itching. *American Journal of Nursing, 90*(7), 15–16.

*Fenske, N., Grayson, L., & Newcomer, V. (1992). Tips for treating aging skin. *Patient Care, 26*(6), 61–64, 67, 70, 71.

*Gaskin, F. C. (1986). Detection of cyanosis in the person with dark skin. *Journal of the National Black Nurses Association, 1*(1), 52–60.

Guyton, A., & Hall, J. (1996). *Textbook of medical physiology* (9th ed.). Philadelphia: W. B. Saunders.

Hardy, M. (1996). What can you do about your patient's dry skin? *Journal of Gerontological Nursing, 22*(5), 10–18.

Jarvis, C. (1996). *Physical examination and health assessment* (2nd ed.). Philadelphia: W. B. Saunders.

Jubeck, M. (1994). Teaching the elderly: A commonsense approach. *Nursing94, 24*(5), 70–71.

*Lookingbill, D. P., & Marks, J. G., Jr. (1993). *Principles of dermatology* (2nd ed.). Philadelphia: W. B. Saunders.

Matteson, M. (1997). Age-related changes in the integument. In M. Matteson, E. McConnell, & A. Linton (Eds.), *Gerontological nursing: Concepts and practice* (2nd ed., pp. 174–195). Philadelphia: W. B. Saunders.

*Roach, L. B. (1977). Color changes in dark skins. *Nursing77, 7,* 48–51.

Skewes, S. (1996). Skin care rituals that do more harm than good. *American Journal of Nursing, 96*(10), 33–35.

White, M., Karam, S., & Cowell, B. (1994). Skin tears in frail elders: A practical approach to prevention. *Geriatric Nursing, 15*(2), 95–99.

SUGGESTED READINGS

*Gaskin, F. C. (1986). Detection of cyanosis in the person with dark skin. *Journal of the National Black Nurses Association, 1*(1), 52–60.
This classic article presents tips and clues for assessing cyanosis in clients with darker skin that are still applicable for today's practitioners. Assessment of subtle changes in skin color that reflect life-threatening physiologic alterations is much more difficult in dark-skinned clients. Helpful techniques for accurately detecting cyanosis in the client with dark skin are described.

Skewes, S. (1996). Skin care rituals that do more harm than good. *American Journal of Nursing, 96*(10), 33–35.
The author lists many "skin care rituals" carried out by nurses and assistive nursing personnel. Research-based arguments against the indiscriminate implementation of these rituals are presented. This article encourages the reader to use judgment in the use of any skin care or wound care technique.

INTERVENTIONS FOR CLIENTS WITH SKIN PROBLEMS

Skin problems may arise as a result of skin disease or injury or may be a manifestation of another type of health problem. Many drugs and other medical or surgical treatments can trigger a skin reaction or skin infection and can delay wound healing. The elderly client is at particular risk for skin problems associated with age-related skin changes as well as problems arising from immobility, debility, and chronic disease.

MINOR IRRITATIONS

Dryness

Overview

Dry skin is a common problem, especially in elderly clients. Dry skin is seen as a fine flaking of the stratum corneum (outermost skin layer), which is more pronounced over the distal lower extremities. Severe dehydration of the stratum corneum (*xerosis*) is often accompanied by a generalized pruritus (itching). In clients with chronic skin conditions, unrelieved pruritus may result in secondary skin lesions, excoriations, lichenification (thickening), and infection as they scratch and rub the skin in an attempt to relieve the intense itching.

Xerosis is exacerbated in dry climates. Central heating and air conditioning reduce the available humidity in the air and increase skin dryness. Wind, cold, and sunlight also contribute to the problem. Frequent bathing with harsh soap and hot water further dries the skin; however, frequent bathing with moisturizing soaps, oils, and lotions may reduce dryness (see Research Applications for Nursing in Chapter 69).

Collaborative Management

Immediate nursing intervention is aimed at rehydration of the skin and relief of any associated pruritus. A 20-minute soak in a tepid bath, followed by application of an emollient cream or lotion, is often sufficient to rehydrate the stratum corneum and promote comfort. If the client is bedridden or if tub baths are contraindicated, the trunk and extremities can be wrapped in warm, moist towels covered by plastic sheeting and additional blankets to prevent chilling. The nurse always applies skin creams or lotions to slightly damp skin after these procedures or within 2 to 3 minutes after routine bathing.

Contrary to popular belief, the cream or lotion is not what makes the skin soft and supple. Water is the agent that softens the outer skin layers. Lubricating creams and lotions seal in the moisture provided by water, promoting suppleness and preventing flaking. Some skin lotions are hydrophilic and actually draw moisture from the skin and contribute to the dryness if they are not applied directly to damp skin.

Health Promotion Guide: Prevention of Dry Skin

- Use a room humidifier during the winter months or whenever the furnace is in use.
- Take a complete bath or shower only every other day (wash face, axillae, perineum, and any soiled areas daily).
- Use tepid water.
- Use a superfatted, nonalkaline soap instead of deodorant soap.
- Rinse the soap thoroughly from your skin.
- If you like bath oil, add the oil to the water at the end of the bath.
- Pat rather than rub skin surfaces dry.
- Avoid clothing that continuously rubs the skin, such as tight belts, nylon stockings, or panty hose.
- Maintain a daily fluid intake of 3000 mL unless contraindicated for another medical condition.
- Do not apply rubbing alcohol, astringents, or other drying agents to the skin.
- Avoid caffeine and alcohol ingestion.

The nurse also educates clients or significant other in measures to maintain healthy skin. Chart 70–1 lists ways to avoid drying the skin.

Pruritus

Overview

Pruritus, or itching, is a distressing cutaneous symptom that may or may not be associated with skin disease. Pruritus is caused by stimulation of itch-specific nerve fibers at the dermal-epidermal junction. Physical or chemical agents act directly on either these nerve fibers or activate chemical mediators, such as histamine, which act on the itch receptors.

As a subjective sensation similar to pain, pruritus varies among clients in distribution and severity. Regardless of the underlying cause, clients usually report that pruritus is worse at night. Pruritus can be exacerbated by poor skin hydration, increased skin temperature, perspiration, and emotional stress.

Collaborative Management

Clients usually seek relief from pruritus by scratching or rubbing the skin, a reflex response that further stimulates the itch receptors and initiates a pattern referred to as the itch-scratch-itch cycle. When the pruritus is associated with skin lesions, effective relief can usually be obtained by treatment of the underlying dermatologic disorder with appropriate topical and systemic medications. Systemic diseases, such as liver and venous disorders, can also result in pruritus without the presence of skin lesions.

The nurse plans care to promote comfort and prevent alterations in skin integrity that can result from vigorous scratching. Because dry skin is often a contributing factor, the nurse emphasizes proper bathing and skin lubrication

techniques (see Chart 70–1). The nurse encourages clients to keep the fingernails trimmed short, with rough edges filed, to minimize excoriation. Clients might wear mittens or splints at night to prevent inadvertent scratching during sleep.

A cool sleeping environment combined with the administration of a larger dose of sedating antihistamines at bedtime (when the associated drowsiness is welcome) may be sufficient to provide an uninterrupted night's sleep. Therapeutic baths (*balneotherapy*) containing colloidal oatmeal preparations or tar extracts may provide temporary relief (Table 70–1).

If the physician orders antihistamines, the nurse closely monitors clients' response to therapy so that the dosage can be adjusted as needed. The antiinflammatory properties of many topical steroid preparations can be maximized if the nurse applies the ointment or cream to slightly damp skin.

Sunburn

Overview

Sunburn is a first-degree burn and one of the most common skin injuries. Excessive exposure to ultraviolet (UV) light results in injury to the superficial dermis, with subsequent dilation of the capillaries, erythema, tenderness, edema, and occasional blister formation. Involvement of large areas of the body may also produce systemic symptoms, such as headache, nausea, and fever.

Collaborative Management

Erythema and discomfort begin within a few hours after sunburn has occurred and gradually increase in intensity for 1 to 2 days before subsiding. Treatment is directed toward symptomatic relief of discomfort and includes cool baths and soothing lotions, such as bland lubricants or refrigerated moisturizing lotions. Antibiotic ointments are indicated only if blistering of the skin results in secondary infection. If discomfort is severe, the use of topical corticosteroids may decrease the inflammation temporarily.

Urticaria

Overview

Urticaria (hives) is characterized by white or red edematous papules or plaques of varying sizes. Urticaria generally results from exposure to a specific noxious stimulus, which causes the release of histamine in the dermal tissue, vasodilation, and subsequent leakage of plasma protein to form the characteristic lesions, or wheals. Unfortunately, a definitive cause of urticaria is identified in only a small number of cases. The following factors have been implicated: drugs, food products, infections, autoimmune diseases, malignancies, physical stimuli, and psychogenic responses.

Collaborative Management

Treatment is aimed at removal of the potentially harmful stimulus and relief of any associated symptoms. Because the skin reaction is associated with histamine release, antihistamines are the drugs of choice. The nurse instructs

TABLE 70-1

Uses of Therapeutic Baths

Agents	Disease	Purpose
Antibacterial Baths		
Potassium permangenate (1:32,000; 1:64,000)	• Infected eczema • Pemphigus • Multiple infected ulcerations	• To lower skin bacterial load
Colloidal Baths		
Starch and baking soda (1 cup each/tub) Aveeno colloidal oatmeal (1 cup/tub) Aveeno oilated colloidal oatmeal	• Atopic eczema • Psoriasis • Chickenpox	• To relieve itching • To soothe • To lubricate
Emollient Baths*		
Bath oils; Alpha Keri Lubath Mineral oil	• Any dry skin condition	• To clean and hydrate the skin
Tar Baths*		
Bath oils with tar: Balnetar, Zetar, Polytar Coal tar concentrate (liquor carbonis, detergents)	• Scaly dermatosis • Psoriasis • Eczema	• To loosen scale • To relieve itching • To potentiate ultraviolet A or ultraviolet B light therapy

Modified from Rosen, T., Lanning, M. B., & Hill, M. J. (1983). *The nurse's atlas of dermatology* (p. 176). Copyright © 1983 by Theodore Rosen and Marilyn B. Lanning. Reprinted by permission of Little, Brown & Co., Boston.
* For emollient and tar baths, add 3 to 6 capfuls of therapeutic agent per standard bathtub.

the client to avoid overexertion, alcohol consumption, and warm environments, which may contribute to vasodilation and exacerbate the symptoms.

Trauma

Overview

Skin trauma can vary from a neat, aseptic surgical incision performed in a controlled environment to a grossly infected, draining pressure ulcer with significant tissue destruction. Injury to the skin results in a predictable series of events aimed at repairing the defect and thus reestablishing the continuity of the body's protective barrier.

Phases of Wound Healing

Wound healing occurs in three phases: the inflammatory, or "lag," phase; the fibroblastic, or connective tissue repair phase; and the maturation, or remodeling, phase. Table 70-2 summarizes the key events involved in the normal phases of wound healing. The length of each phase depends on the circumstances surrounding the injury and

TABLE 70-2

Normal Wound Healing

Phase	Events/Characteristics
Inflammatory phase	• Begins at the time of injury or cell death and lasts 3-5 days. • Immediate responses are vasoconstriction and clot formation. • After 10 minutes, vasodilation with increased capillary permeability and leakage of plasma (and plasma proteins) into the surrounding tissue. • Migration of white blood cells (especially macrophages) into the wound. • Clinical manifestations of local edema, pain erythema, and warmth.
Fibroblastic phase	• Begins about the 4th day after injury and lasts 2-4 weeks. • Fibrin strands form a scaffold or framework. • Mitotic fibroblast cells migrate into the wound, attach to the framework, divide, and stimulate the secretion of collagen. • Collagen, together with ground substance, builds tough and inflexible scar tissue. • Capillaries in areas surrounding the wound form "buds" that grow into new blood vessels. • Capillary buds and collagen deposits form the "granulation" tissue in the wound, and the wound contracts. • Epithelial cells grow over the granulation tissue bed.
Maturation phase	• Begins as early as 3 weeks after injury and may continue for a year. • Collagen is reorganized to provide greater tensile strength. • Scar tissue gradually becomes thinner and paler in color. • The mature scar is firm and inelastic when palpated.

The Process of Wound Healing

 Healing by First Intention

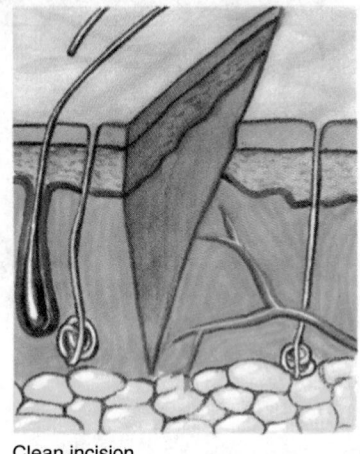

Clean incision

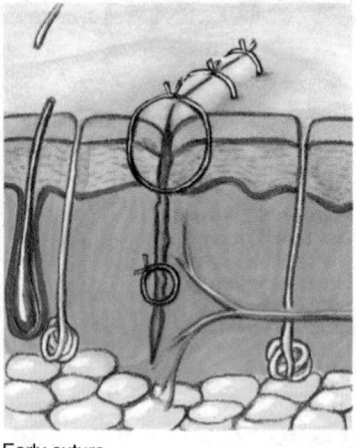

Early suture

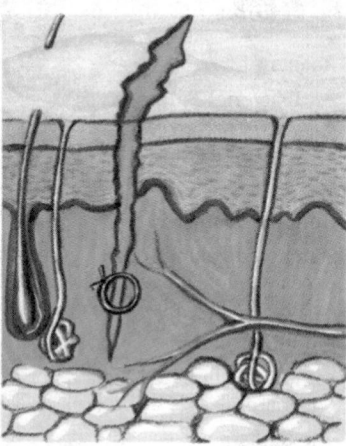

"Hairline" scar

An aseptically made wound with minimal tissue destruction and minimal tissue reaction begins to heal as the edges are approximated by close sutures or staples. No open areas or dead spaces are left to serve as potential sites of infection.

Healing by Second Intention (Granulation) and Contraction

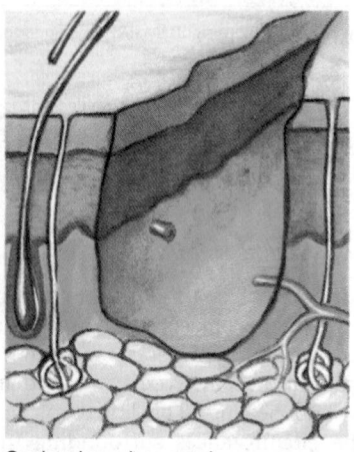

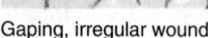
Gaping, irregular wound

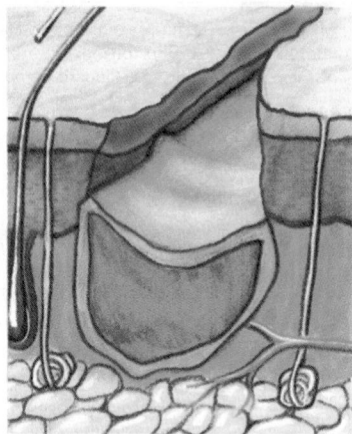

Granulation and contraction

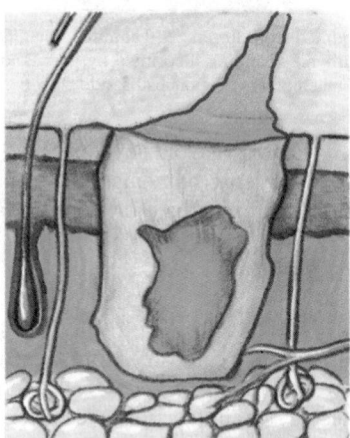

Growth of epithelium over scar

An infected or chronic wound or one with tissue damage so extensive that the edges cannot be smoothly approximated is usually left open and allowed to heal from the inside out. The nurse periodically cleans and assesses the wound for healthy tissue production. Scar tissue is extensive, and healing is prolonged.

Healing by Third Intention (Delayed Closure)

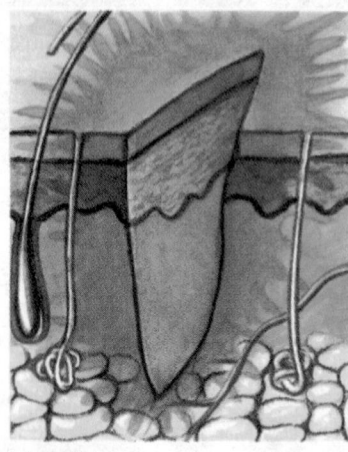

Infected wound

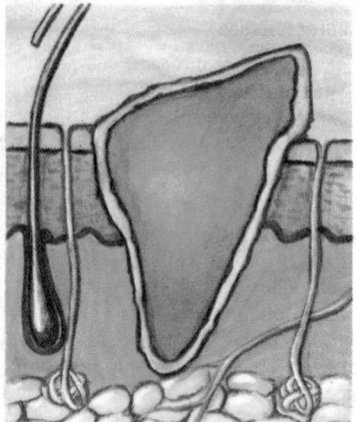

Granulation

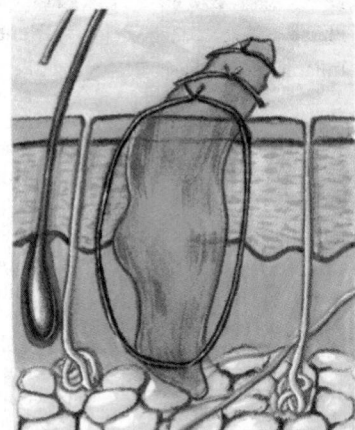

Closure with wide scar

A potentially infected surgical wound may be left open for several days. If no clinical signs of infection occur, the wound is then closed surgically.

Figure 70–1. The process of wound healing.

whether the wound is allowed to heal by first, second, or third intention (Fig. 70–1).

A wound without tissue loss, such as a clean laceration or a surgical incision, can be closed with sutures or staples. The wound edges are brought together, with the skin layers approximated and held in place until healing is complete. Because the defect can be easily corrected and dead space eliminated, healing by *first intention* shortens the phases of tissue repair considerably. Inflammation resolves quickly, and connective tissue repair is minimal, resulting in a thin scar.

Deeper tissue injuries or those wounds with tissue loss, such as a chronic pressure ulcer or venous stasis ulcer, result in a cavity-like defect that requires gradual filling in of the dead space with connective tissue. Consequently, healing by *second intention* prolongs the repair process.

Wounds with a high potential for infection, such as surgical incisions that enter a nonsterile body cavity or traumatic wounds that occur under unclean conditions, may be intentionally left open for several days. After debris and exudate have been removed and inflammation has subsided, the wound is closed by first intention. Healing by delayed primary closure, or *third intention*, results in a scar similar to that found in wounds that heal by first intention. As shown in Table 70–3, healing can be impaired by a number of stressors.

Mechanisms of Wound Healing

The body restores skin integrity through the processes of *epithelialization* and *contraction*. The degree to which these processes achieve wound closure depends on the depth of injury and the extent of tissue loss. The mechanisms of epithelialization and contraction can be easily understood if two categories of injury are considered: partial-thickness and full-thickness wounds.

Partial-Thickness Wounds

Partial-thickness, or superficial, wounds heal by *epithelialization*, the reproduction of new skin cells by epithelial cell remnants in the dermal layer of the skin and at the base of the epidermal appendages (Fig. 70–2). On injury, a fibrin clot forms. Undamaged epithelial cells at the level of the basement membrane and at the base of the hair follicles and glands undergo a burst of cell division. Movement of the new skin cells is directed into "cell-free" spaces on the wound surface, where the fibrin clot acts as a scaffold. Resurfacing, initially only one cell layer thick, proceeds with thickening or restratification of the new epidermis and, eventually, rete peg formation and keratin production.

In a healthy client, healing of a partial-thickness wound by epithelialization takes 5 to 7 days. Epithelialization occurs best in tissue that is well hydrated, is well oxygenated, and has few microorganisms.

Full-Thickness Wounds

In a client with a deeper or full-thickness wound, most—if not all—of the epithelial remnants have been destroyed, except those remaining at the wound margins. For a full-thickness wound to heal, the nonviable tissue

TABLE 70–3

Causes of Impaired Wound Healing

Cause	Mechanism
Altered Inflammatory Response	
Local	
Arteriosclerosis	• Altered local tissue circulation, resulting in ischemia, impaired leukocytic response to wounding, and increased probability of wound infection
Diabetes	
Vasculitis	
Thrombosis	
Venous insufficiency	
Lymphedema	
Pharmacologic vasoconstriction	
Irradiated tissue	
Crush injuries	
Primary closure under tension	
Systemic	
Leukemia	• Systemic inhibition of leukocytic response, resulting in impaired host resistance to infection
Prolonged administration of high-dose anti-inflammatory drugs	
Corticosteroids	
Aspirin	
Impaired Cellular Proliferation	
Local	
Wound infection	• Prolonged inflammatory response, which can result in low tissue oxygen tension and further tissue destruction
Foreign body	
Necrotic tissue	
Repeated injury or irritation	
Movement of wound (e.g., across a joint)	
Wound desiccation or maceration	
Systemic	
Aging	• Impaired cellular proliferation and collagen synthesis
Chronic stress	
Nutritional deficiencies	• Decreased wound contraction
Calories	
Protein	
Vitamins	
Minerals	
Water	
Impaired oxygenation	
Pulmonary insufficiency	
Heat failure	
Hypovolemia	
Cirrhosis	
Uremia	
Prolonged hypothermia	
Coagulation disorders	
Cytotoxic drugs	

must be removed so that gradual filling in of the defect with granulation tissue can progress.

Occurring at the same time as collagen synthesis and wound revascularization is the drawing together of the wound edges, a mechanism of healing known as *contraction* (see Fig. 70–1). Unlike epithelialization, in which new tissue is formed, the phenomenon of wound contraction decreases the surface area of a full-thickness wound by stretching and thinning the existing tissue surrounding

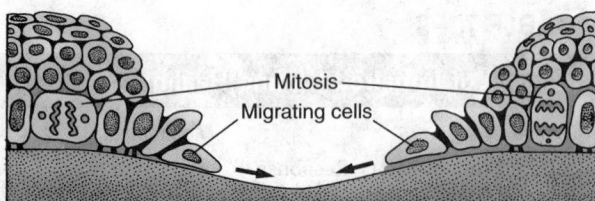

Skin cells at the edge of the wound begin multiplying and migrate toward the center of the wound.

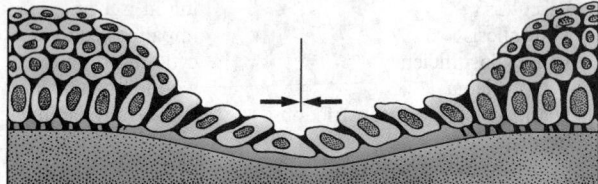

Once advancing epidermal cells from the opposite sides of the wound meet, migration halts.

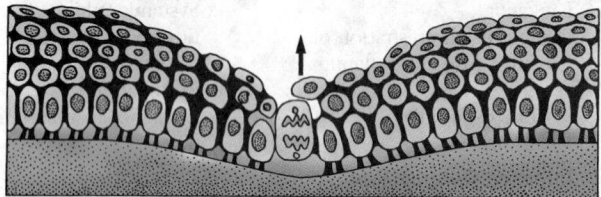

Epithelial cells continue to divide until the thickness of the new skin layer approaches normal.

Figure 70–2. Epithelialization (Modified from Swaim, S. F. [1980]. *Surgery of traumatized skin.* Philadelphia, W.B. Saunders Co.)

the wound. Contractile fibroblasts in the wound bed exert a mechanical force on the wound edges, causing the wound to decrease in size at a uniform rate of about 0.6 to 0.75 mm/day. Complete closure of a wound by contraction depends on the dermal mobility of the surrounding skin as tension is applied to it. Necrotic tissue provides a physical obstacle to wound contraction and must be removed for healing to occur.

If tension in the surrounding skin meets or exceeds the force of contraction, wound closure ceases, and the wound remains open until epithelial cells at the wound edges eventually bridge the remaining defect. Unlike epithelialization in partial-thickness wounds, in which the skin integrity soon returns to normal, the migration of epithelial cells from wound margins over fibrous connective tissue results in an unstable epithelial surface that is poorly attached to the underlying tissue and thus is susceptible to reinjury. A venous stasis leg ulcer is one example of a skin defect in an area where effective movement of the surrounding skin is usually not sufficient to allow wound healing by contraction. As a result, the thin epithelial covering cannot withstand environmental hazards and abrades easily.

The mechanisms of epithelialization and contraction do not continue indefinitely. Natural healing processes can slow down or even be halted by the presence of infection, pressure, or mechanical obstacles, such as a poorly applied dressing. In the case of chronic wounds, healing can cease spontaneously and without a clearly defined cause.

Collaborative Management

Specific treatment of skin trauma varies with the depth and circumstances of the injury. The focus of all treatment for any type of skin trauma is to enhance wound healing, prevent infection, and restore function to the area. Management for pressure ulcers presents common interventions as does treatment for burns (see Chap. 71).

Pressure Ulcers

Overview

Pressure ulcers are a specific type of skin trauma that occurs almost exclusively in people with limited mobility. Once formed, pressure ulcers are slow to heal, requiring weeks to years, and result in increased morbidity and health care costs. The term *pressure ulcer* matches the guidelines provided by the Agency for Health Care Policy and Research, U.S. Department of Health and Human Services.

Pathophysiology

Mechanical forces exerted to or on the skin are the mechanisms that lead to the formation of pressure ulcers. These forces—pressure, friction, and shear—lead to direct and ischemic tissue damage. Although injury occurs more often to skin over bony prominences, pressure ulcers may occur anywhere. Excessive skin moisture increases the susceptibility of the skin to damage when mechanical forces are exerted.

Pressure

Pressure occurs as a result of gravity. Dependent tissues in contact with a fixed surface experience varying degrees of pressure. Pressure is determined by the amount of weight exerted at the point of contact, the distribution of weight at the point of contact, and the density of the contacting surface. Excessive or prolonged pressure can compress blood vessels at the point of contact, leading to ischemia, inflammation, and tissue necrosis. Pressure occurs when the client is positioned on hard, unyielding surfaces that do not diffuse the weight or when the client remains in the same position too long.

Friction

Friction occurs when external surfaces rub the skin surface and irritate or directly pull off epithelial tissue. Such forces are generated when the client is dragged or pulled across bed linen.

Shear

Shear or shearing forces are generated when the skin itself remains stationary and the tissues below the skin (such as fat and muscle) shift or move (Fig. 70–3). The movement of the deeper tissue layers diminishes the blood supply to the skin, leading to skin hypoxia, anoxia, ischemia, inflammation, and necrosis.

Gravity plays a role in the development of shear forces. A shear injury commonly occurs when a client is in bed

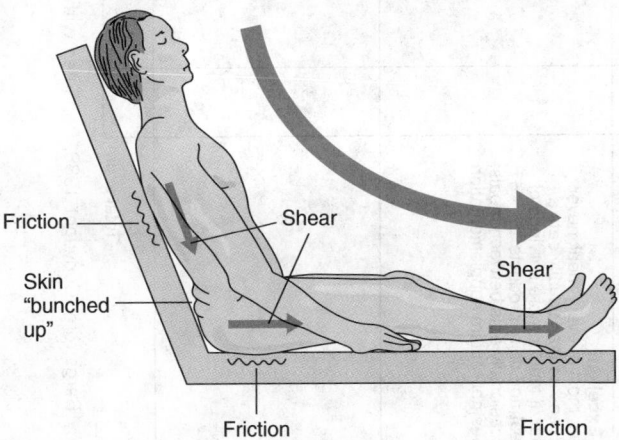

Figure 70–3. Shearing forces pulling skin layers away from deeper tissue. The skin is "bunched up" against the back of the mattress while the rest of the bone and muscle in the area press downward on the lower part of the mattress. Blood vessels become kinked, obstructing circulation and leading to tissue death.

in a semisitting position and gradually slides downward. Often, the skin over the sacrum does not slide down at the same pace as the deeper tissues; thus, the skin is mechanically "sheared," causing blood vessels to stretch and leading to soft-tissue ischemia, although no break in external skin integrity is observed.

Etiology

Pressure ulcers occur as a result of mechanical trauma and tissue anoxia.

ELDERLY CONSIDERATIONS

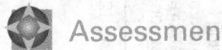 Elderly clients are at particular risk for pressure ulcers because of the presence of age-related skin changes. Progressive flattening of the dermal-epidermal junction predisposes older people to skin tears from mechanical shearing forces, such as the removal of adhesive tape and friction from tightly applied restraints. In addition, skin moisture and irritation from incontinence and friction over bony prominences can lead to partial-thickness skin destruction and early pressure ulcer formation. *If pressure is unrelieved, tissue destruction progresses to full-thickness injury.*

Collaborative Management

Assessment

➤ History

When taking a history from clients with pressure ulcers, the nurse attempts to identify the underlying cause of skin loss as well as factors that may impair healing. The nurse investigates the specific circumstances of the skin loss. In general, clients with chronic pressure ulcerations usually relate a history of delayed healing or recurrence of the ulcer after healing has occurred. Because pressure-related skin loss is common among the severely debili-

tated, the nurse remains alert to contributing factors, such as

- Prolonged bed rest
- Immobility
- Incontinence
- Inadequate nutrition or hydration
- Altered mental status (decreased sensory perception)

➤ *Physical Assessment/Clinical Manifestations*

The nurse assesses clients' risk for pressure ulcers. Several assessment tools have been developed to assess the risk. The Braden Scale for predicting pressure sore risk has been well tested and is widely used (see Fig. 70–4 and the Research Applications for Nursing about the Braden Scale). The nurse inspects the entire body, including the back of the head, for areas of skin injury or pressure. Special attention is given to bony prominences such as heels, the sacrum, elbows, trochanter, posterior and anterior iliac spines, and areas that are vulnerable to excessive moisture.

The physical appearance of pressure ulcers changes

▷ Research Applications for Nursing

Braden Scale Rating Compared with Clinical Judgment in Risk for Pressure Ulcer Formation

VandenBosch, T., Montoye, C., Satwicz, M., Durkee-Leonard, K., & Boylan-Lewis, B. (1996). Predictive validity of the Braden Scale and nurse perception in identifying pressure ulcer risk. Applied Nursing Research, 9(2), 80–86.

This prospective study of 103 hospitalized clients had two purposes: (1) to establish validity and reliability data for the Braden Scale and (2) to compare the accuracy of clinical judgment and the Braden Scale in predicting pressure ulcer risk. The Braden Scale was administered for these randomly assigned participants six times over a 2-week hospitalization period. During the same period, each participant was reviewed by bedside nurses and evaluated by clinical judgment for risk of pressure ulcer formation.

During the study period, one or more pressure ulcers developed in 29 of the 103 participants. Nurses' clinical judgments were not accurate in predicting high risk or low risk for pressure ulcer formation. The Braden Scale demonstrated significant accuracy ($P = .0038$) in predicting high and low risk for pressure ulcer formation.

Critique. This study was well designed. The methods of the study were appropriate for the research questions asked. Interrater reliability for the multiple data collectors was set at 90% to 100%. The two limitations of the study were (1) that some clients were on pressure ulcer prevention precautions, and (2) knowledge of the ongoing study at the institution may have contaminated the clinical judgments of the bedside nurses by heightening their awareness of pressure ulcer risk.

Possible Nursing Implications. The Braden Scale has demonstrated reliability, validity, sensitivity, and specificity in predicting pressure ulcer risk. This scale should be used by all nurses caring for clients who are expected to be in an institutional environment for 5 days or longer.

Client's name _____ Evaluator's name _____ Date of assessment

Sensory perception Ability to respond meaningfully to pressure-related discomfort	**1. Completely limited** Unresponsive to painful stimuli (does not moan, flinch, or grasp) because of diminished level of consciousness or sedation OR limited ability to feel pain over most of body surface	**2. Very limited** Responds only to painful stimuli; cannot communicate discomfort except by moaning or restlessness OR has a sensory impairment that limits the ability to feel pain or discomfort over half of the body	**3. Slightly limited** Responds to verbal commands but cannot always communicate discomfort or need to be turned OR has some sensory impairment that limits ability to feel pain or discomfort in one or two extremities	**4. No impairment** Responds to verbal commands; has no sensory deficit that would limit ability to feel or voice pain or discomfort
Moisture Degree to which skin is exposed to moisture	**1. Constantly moist** Skin is kept moist almost constantly by perspiration, urine; dampness is detected every time the client is moved or turned	**2. Very Moist** Skin is often but not always moist; linen must be changed at least once a shift	**3. Occasionally moist** Skin is occasionally moist, requiring an extra linen change approximately once a day	**4. Rarely moist** Skin is usually dry; linen requires changing only at routine intervals
Activity Degree of physical activity	**1. Bedfast** Confined to bed	**2. Chairfast** Ability to walk severely limited or nonexistent; cannot bear own weight and must be assisted into chair or wheelchair	**3. Walks occasionally** Walks occasionally during the day but for very short distances, with or without assistance; spends the majority of each shift in bed or chair	**4. Walks frequently** Walks outside the room at least twice a day and inside the room at least once every 2 hours during waking hours
Mobility Ability to change or control body position	**1. Completely immobile** Does not make even slight changes in body or extremity position without assistance	**2. Very limited** Makes occasional slight changes in body or extremity position but unable to make frequent or significant changes independently	**3. Slightly limited** Makes frequent though slight changes in body or extremity position independently	**4. No limitations** Makes major and frequent changes in position without assistance
Nutrition Usual food intake pattern	**1. Very poor** Never eats a complete meal; rarely eats more than a third of any food offered; eats two servings or less of protein (meat or dairy products) per day; takes fluids poorly; does not take a liquid dietary supplement OR is NPO or maintained on clear liquids or IV for more than 5 days	**2. Probably inadequate** Rarely eats a complete meal and generally eats only about half of any food offered; protein intake includes only three servings of meat or dairy products per day; occasionally will take a dietary supplement OR receives less than optimal amount of liquid diet or tube feeding	**3. Adequate** Eats over half of most meals; eats a total of four servings of protein (meat, dairy products) each day; occasionally will refuse a meal, but will usually take a supplement if offered OR is receiving tube feeding or total parenteral nutrition, which probably meets most nutritional needs	**4. Excellent** Eats most of every meal; never refuses a meal; usually eats a total of four or more servings of meat and dairy products; occasionally eats between meals; does not require supplementation
Friction and shear	**1. Problem** Requires moderate to maximum assistance in moving; complete lifting without sliding against sheets is impossible; frequently slides down in bed or chair, requiring frequent repositioning with maximum assistance; spasticity, contractures, or agitation leads to almost constant friction	**2. Potential problem** Moves feebly or requires minimum assistance during a move; skin probably slides to some extent against sheets, chair, restraints, or other devices; maintains relatively good position in chair or bed most of the time but occasionally slides down	**3. No apparent problem** Moves in bed and in chair independently and has sufficient muscle strength to lift up completely during move; maintains good position in bed or chair at all times	

Total score

Scoring system: 15–16 = mild risk, 12–14 = moderate risk, <11 = severe risk

Figure 70–4. The Braden Scale for predicting pressure ulcer risk. IV = intravenous; NPO = nothing by mouth. (From Barbara Braden and Nancy Bergstrom. Copyright 1988. Reprinted with permission.)

Chart 70–2

Key Features of Pressure Ulcers*

Stage I

- Skin is intact.
- Area is red and does not blanch with external pressure.
- For clients with darker skin that does not blanch†:

Observable pressure-related alteration of intact skin—changes are compared with an adjacent or opposite area and include one or more of the following:
  - Skin temperature (warmth or coolness)
  - Tissue consistency (firm or boggy)
  - Sensation (pain, itching)

The ulcer appears as a defined area of persistent redness in lightly pigmented skin, whereas in darker skin tones, the ulcer may appear with persistent red, blue, or purple hues.

Stage II

- Skin is not intact.
- There is partial-thickness skin loss of the epidermis or dermis.
- Ulcer is superficial and may be characterized as an abrasion, a blister, or a shallow crater.

Stage III

- Skin loss is full thickness.
- Subcutaneous tissues may be damaged or necrotic.
- Damage extends down to but not through the underlying fascia.
- There is a deep crater-like appearance or eschar present.
- Undermining may or may not be present.

Stage IV

- Skin loss is full thickness with extensive destruction, tissue necrosis, or damage to muscle, bone, or supporting structures.
- Undermining is present.
- Sinus tracts may develop.

Data from U.S. Department of Health and Human Services. (1992). *Pressure ulcers in adults: Prediction and prevention* (Clinical Practice Guideline, No. 3). Rockville, MD: Agency for Health Care Policy and Research.

† From Henderson, C., Ayello, E., Sussman, C., Leiby, D., Bennett, M., Dungog, E., Sprigle, S., & Woodruff, L. (1997). Draft definition of stage I pressure ulcers: Inclusion of persons with darkly pigmented skin. *Advances in Wound Care, 10*(5), 16–19.

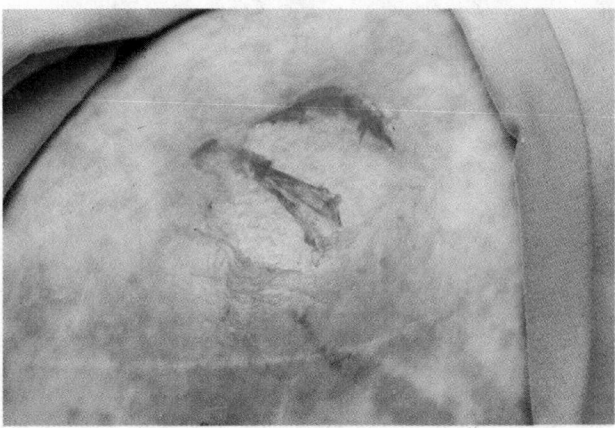

Figure 70–6. A stage II pressure ulcer.

with the depth of the injury. Chart 70–2 lists the characteristics of the four stages of pressure ulceration, and Figures 70–5 to 70–8 show examples. These guidelines include a proposed change in the definition of a stage I pressure ulcer to accommodate changes observed in darker skin. This new definition has been proposed by the National Pressure Ulcer Advisory Panel (NPUAP).

The nurse inspects the wound margins for *cellulitis* (inflammation of the skin cells) extending well beyond the area of injury. Progressive tissue destruction, as reflected by an increase in the size or depth of the ulcer, usually indicates an impairment in the client's ability to resist infection if proper measures have been taken to relieve pressure.

The nurse inspects the wound for the presence or absence of necrotic tissue. Because of the depth of tissue destruction, a full-thickness pressure ulcer is initially covered by a layer of black or brown, nonviable, denatured collagen, called wound *eschar*.

In the early stages of wound healing, the eschar is dry, leathery, and firmly attached to the wound surface. As the inflammatory phase of wound healing begins and removal of wound debris progresses, the eschar starts to lift up and separate from the tissue beneath. When disrupted, this nonviable eschar serves as an excellent culture medium for bacteria normally found on the skin surface as

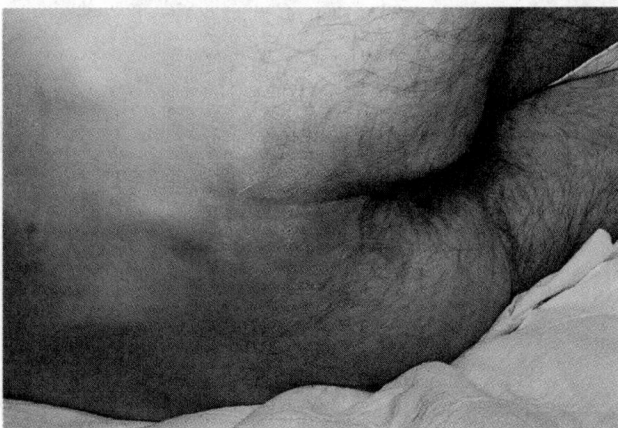

Figure 70–5. A stage I pressure ulcer.

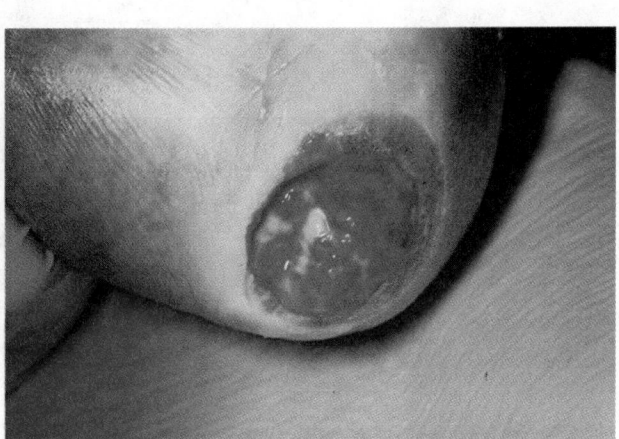

Figure 70–7. A stage III pressure ulcer.

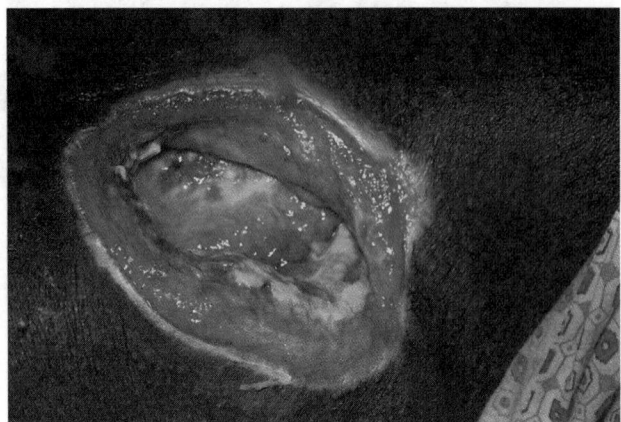

Figure 70–8. A stage IV pressure ulcer.

well as those inadvertently introduced by other means. As bacteria increase in number, they release enzymes, which further hasten the liquefaction of necrotic tissue. This tissue becomes softer in consistency and more yellow in color. In the presence of bacterial colonization, wound exudate increases substantially; the color and odor of wound exudate indicate the predominant microorganism present. The characteristics of wound exudate are presented in Table 70–4.

Beneath the separating necrotic material, granulation tissue appears. Early granulation is pale pink, progressing to a beefy-red color as it grows and fills the wound defect. A wound with inadequate local arterial blood supply appears dry, with pale immature granulation tissue present. Conversely, venous obstruction results in an excessively moist ulcer surface with a deep-red color reflective of the deoxygenated blood beneath the ulcer surface.

The nurse palpates the ulcerated area or wound to determine the texture of the mature granulations. Healthy granulations have a slightly spongy texture. Pressure ulcers may involve more extensive tissue destruction than is first evident on inspection. The nurse palpates the bony prominences for deep hardening of the surrounding soft tissue, which often suggests tissue ischemia well beneath the surface of the skin.

After ischemia has occurred, continued pressure over the area of injury results in progress of tissue destruction from the deep tissue layers toward the surface. This "hidden" wound may first appear as a small opening in the skin through which purulent drainage exudes. If such an opening is observed, the nurse uses a cotton-tipped applicator to probe gently for a much larger pocket of necrotic tissue beneath.

► *Psychosocial Assessment*

The client with pressure ulcers may have an altered body image. Ineffective coping patterns emerge as the client or significant other strives to comply with changes in lifestyle necessary to facilitate healing. In addition, chronic, slow-healing ulcers are often painful and costly to treat.

The nurse assesses the client's or significant other's knowledge of the treatment goals at each stage of the healing process as well as the client's compliance with the prescribed treatment regimen. The nurse further assesses the client's skills in cleaning the wound and applying a dressing. Noncompliance with pressure ulcer care procedures may reflect a client's inability to accept the diagnosis or to cope with the pain, cost, or potential scarring associated with prolonged healing. Depending on the client's activity level and location of the ulcer, the client may need the assistance of a family member or visiting nurse to care adequately for the pressure ulcer at home.

The nurse explores with the client specific changes in activities of daily living (ADLs) that are needed to relieve pressure and promote healing. Increased activity is promoted whenever possible to enhance circulation to the affected tissue. Frequent bed rest with elevation of the legs may be necessary for healing when ulcers occur on the lower legs, particularly in the client with venous insufficiency and lower-leg edema. When the client is bedridden, frequent repositioning to relieve pressure (every 2 hours in bed; every 1 hour in chair) can be labor intensive. In the home environment, repositioning, incontinence management, and dressing changes are often required around the clock, disrupting family routines and contributing to stress.

► *Laboratory Assessment*

Bacterial specimens are obtained for culture and sensitivity studies to identify the causative microorganism in suspected ulcer infection. When interpreting culture results,

TABLE 70–4

Types of Wound Exudate

Type	Characteristics	Significance
Serosanguineous	• Blood-tinged amber fluid consisting of serum and red blood cells	• Normal for first 48 hr after injury • Sudden increase in amount precedes wound dehiscence in wounds closed by first intention
Purulent	• Creamy yellow pus • Greenish-blue pus, causing staining of dressings and accompanied by a "fruity" odor • Beige pus with a "fishy" odor • Brownish pus with a "fecal" odor	• Colonization with *Staphylococcus* • Colonization with *Pseudomonas* • Colonization with *Proteus* • Colonization with aerobic coliform and *Bacteroides* (usually occurs after intestinal surgery)

the nurse must understand the difference between bacterial colonization of a wound and true wound infection. All wounds allowed to heal by second intention become colonized by bacterial flora on the skin and in the environment. In most cases, local tissue defenses are adequate to keep the numbers of bacteria at a minimum.

If wounds are extensive, if the client is severely immunocompromised, or if local blood supply to the wound is impaired, bacterial growth may exceed the body's ability to defend against invasion into deeper tissue layers. The result is deep wound infection and, eventually, bacteremia and sepsis (systemic infection).

Swab cultures are helpful only in identifying the types of bacteria present on the ulcer surface but do not reflect the relative concentration of bacteria in the underlying tissues. Tests such as quantitative wound biopsies allow the numbers of bacteria to be analyzed. Unfortunately, these tests are time consuming, costly, and rarely indicated except for large, extensive wounds. Therefore, the clinical indicators of infection—cellulitis, progressive increase in ulcer size or depth, changes in the quantity and quality of exudate, and systemic signs of bacteremia—are important criteria in the diagnosis and subsequent treatment of an infection.

➤ Other Diagnostic Assessment

Any additional laboratory studies are performed on the basis of the suspected cause of the wound. For pressure ulcers to show progress toward healing, the underlying factors contributing to delayed healing must be diagnosed and treated. For example, noninvasive and invasive arterial blood flow studies are indicated if arterial occlusion is suspected in delayed healing of a pressure ulcer on the heel or ankle. Similarly, blood tests to establish specific nutritional deficiencies are helpful in treating the debilitated, malnourished client with a pressure ulcer.

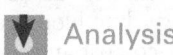 Analysis

➤ Common Nursing Diagnoses and Collaborative Problems

The nursing diagnosis most commonly found in the client with pressure ulcers is impaired skin integrity related to vascular insufficiency and traumatic circumstances.

The most common collaborative problem for the client with pressure ulcers is risk for infection and wound extension related to disruption of the skin's protective barrier and impaired local blood supply.

➤ Additional Nursing Diagnoses and Collaborative Problems

The client may have one or more of the following additional diagnoses or collaborative problems, depending on the cause of the skin loss:

- Pain related to skin trauma, wound infection, and wound treatment
- Body Image Disturbance related to loss of skin and altered appearance
- Ineffective Individual Coping related to the chronic-

ity of the ulcer, alteration in body image, and changes in lifestyle required to promote healing
- Altered Nutrition: Less than Body Requirements related to inadequate intake of calories, protein, vitamins, and minerals
- Altered (Peripheral) Tissue Perfusion related to vascular disease and prolonged alterations in fluid volume
- Knowledge Deficit related to lack of information about or unclear explanation of the treatment regimen

 Planning and Implementation

➤ Impaired Skin Integrity

Planning: Expected Outcomes. The desired outcomes are that the client is expected to
- Protect the viable cells on the wound surface until healing is completed
- Experience complete ulcer healing
- Not experience the formation of other pressure ulcers

Interventions. Wound care techniques for pressure ulcers vary according to each client's needs and the physician's preference. Although aggressive removal of necrotic tissue by surgical excision may be indicated in a severely immunosuppressed client who is susceptible to a life-threatening wound infection, a nonsurgical approach to ulcer debridement is preferred for an elderly client who has adequate host defenses but is too ill or debilitated to undergo surgery.

Nonsurgical Management. Nonsurgical intervention of pressure ulcers is often left to the discretion of the nurse, who selects a method of wound dressing on the basis of the identified goal of wound management.

Dressings. A properly designed dressing can expedite healing by removing unwanted debris from the ulcer surface, protecting exposed viable tissues, and re-establishing a temporary barrier between the body and the environment until ulcer closure is complete. For a client with a draining, necrotic ulcer, the dressing must be designed to remove excessive exudate and loose debris without damaging migrating epithelial cells or newly formed granulation tissue. If necrosis is extensive and the eschar is thick, nonviable tissue must be surgically removed before further debridement with dressings proves effective. Depending on the dressing material used, dressings help to remove debris either through mechanical entrapment and detachment of dead tissue or by creating an environment that promotes self-digestion of necrotic material by the bacterial enzymes (Table 70–5).

After all of the nonviable tissue has been removed, protection of any exposed vital structures, such as tendon, bone, and newly formed collagen, becomes a primary objective of pressure ulcer care. The ideal environment for healing by epithelialization and contraction is a clean, *slightly* moist ulcer surface with minimal bacterial colonization. Heavy moisture from an excessively secret-

TABLE 70–5

Common Dressing Techniques for Wound Debridement

Technique	Mechanism of Action
Wet-to-dry saline-moistened gauze	• Dry, necrotic debris is softened by the saline, allowing it to become more effectively entrapped in the interstices as the gauze dries and shrinks. Dressing may also entrap healing tissue.
Wet-to-damp saline-moistened gauze	• As with the wet-to-dry technique, necrotic debris is mechanically removed, but with less trauma to healing tissue.
Continuous wet gauze	• The wound surface is continually bathed with a wetting agent of choice, promoting dilution of viscous exudate and softening of dry eschar.
Topical enzyme preparations	• Proteolytic action on thick, adherent eschar causes breakdown of denatured protein and more rapid separation of necrotic tissue.
Moisture-retentive dressing	• Spontaneous separation of necrotic tissue is promoted by autolysis.

ing ulcer or a too-wet dressing can interfere with healing by promoting the growth of microorganisms and causing maceration of healthy tissue. Likewise, if a clean ulcer surface is exposed to air or if highly absorbent dressing materials are used for prolonged periods, the subsequent drying effect can lead to dehydration of viable surface cells, scab formation, or conversion to a deeper injury.

The nurse assesses the ulcer for the presence or absence of nonviable tissue and the quantity of exudate. A dressing material with properties that promote an optimal environment for healing is selected (Table 70–6). For example, a material that is nonadherent to the wound surface and does not remove fragile epithelial cells when it is changed is the dressing of choice for protecting new tissue. Depending on the amount of drainage, the nurse selects either a hydrophobic or a hydrophilic material:

- A *hydrophobic* (nonabsorbent, waterproof) material is beneficial when the wound is relatively free of drainage and the objective is to protect the ulcer from external contamination, such as urine or feces.
- A *hydrophilic* (absorbent) material draws excessive drainage away from the ulcer surface, preventing maceration.

A variety of synthetic materials with hydrophilic and hydrophobic properties are available. Unlike cotton gauze dressings, these may be left intact for extended periods. Some biological skin substitutes can also prevent tissue dehydration and provide an environment conducive to healing (see Chap. 71). These substances include homograft (human cadaver skin), heterograft (pigskin), collagen materials, amniotic membrane, and cultured epithelium.

The frequency of dressing changes depends on the amount of necrotic material or exudate. Dry gauze dressings are changed when "strike through" occurs or when the outer layer of the dressing first becomes saturated with exudate. Gauze dressings used for debridement, such as those placed on a wound wet, allowed to dry, and then removed, are changed frequently enough to take off actively any loose debris or exudate, usually every 4 to 6 hours. Synthetic dressings are changed when accumulation of exudate causes the adhesive seal to break and leakage to occur.

Before reapplying any dressing, the nurse gently cleans

the ulcer surface with saline or a nontoxic wound cleanser as prescribed. If an antibacterial cleanser is ordered, the nurse dilutes the agent to minimize tissue toxicity and then rinses and dries the surface thoroughly before applying the dressing.

Physical Therapy. As an adjunct to the use of dressings for ulcer debridement, the use of daily whirlpool treatments can facilitate mechanical removal of dead tissue. The ulcerated area is immersed in warm tap water to which an antibacterial cleansing agent has been added. Continuous agitation of the water mechanically loosens the debris and washes away exudate and particulate matter. During treatment, the ulcer surface is cleaned with a gauze pad. After treatment, the therapist or certified nurse often uses instruments to trim away any obvious bits of dead tissue that are still loosely attached to the ulcer surface.

Drug Therapy. Clean, healthy granulation tissue is highly vascular and capable of providing white blood cells and antibodies to the ulcer surface to combat infection. However, if extensive necrosis is present or local tissue defenses are impaired, topical antibacterial agents are often indicated to control bacterial growth. (Chapter 71 details the advantages and uses of topical antimicrobial agents.) In the absence of established ulcer infection, prophylactic antibiotics are usually avoided because of the danger of the development of resistant strains of bacteria.

Diet Therapy. Successful healing of pressure ulcers depends on adequate nutritional stores of calories, protein, vitamins, minerals, and water. Nutritional deficiencies are common among the elderly and chronically ill clients. Such deficiencies contribute to an increased risk of skin breakdown and delayed healing of wounds already present. Severe protein deficiency inhibits all stages of the healing process and impairs local host defenses against bacterial invasion.

To promote healing, the nurse encourages the client to eat a well-balanced diet, emphasizing foods containing nutrients vital to epidermal proliferation and collagen synthesis (Table 70–7). If the client cannot orally ingest sufficient amounts of food, nasogastric feedings and hyperalimentation via central venous catheter may be needed to increase protein and calorie intake. Vitamin and mineral supplements also are indicated.

Surgical Management. Surgical management of a pressure ulcer includes sharp debridement of nonviable tissue and skin grafting to re-establish skin integrity in wounds that cannot heal by epithelialization and contraction.

Preoperative Care. Preoperative care is focused on preparing the ulcer to accept a skin graft. The nurse carefully monitors potential donor sites, taking care to maintain the integrity of the donor skin and to avoid minor injuries that may result in infection and graft loss.

Operative Procedure. The operative procedures commonly used for surgical management of pressure ulcers include debridement, grafting, or both.

Debridement, or sharp excision of thick, adherent wound eschar using a scalpel or scissors, is sometimes undertaken to hasten the removal of the devitalized tissue, a potential source of infection. Surgical debridement is indicated for severely immunosuppressed clients or those with large full-thickness ulcers, because the extensive time required for spontaneous separation of eschar places the client at risk for systemic sepsis or prolonged hospitalization. Depending on the size and depth of the ulcer and the projected blood loss, the surgeon can perform the excision at the bedside, in the treatment room, or in an operating room.

Grafting or autografting is indicated for satisfactory wound closure when full-thickness ulcers cannot close by second intention because of the extent of the injury or forces inhibiting contraction and when natural healing results in loss of joint function, unacceptable cosmetic appearance, or high potential for wound recurrence. Successful grafting of skin requires a clean granulating or freshly excised ulcer bed. Partial-thickness (split-thickness) or full-thickness strips of skin are removed from a donor area (Fig. 70–9), transferred to the ulcer, and sutured or stapled in place. Full-thickness free grafts and myocutaneous flaps are used to cover deep, massive ulcers or ulcers in which vital structures, such as bone or tendon, are exposed.

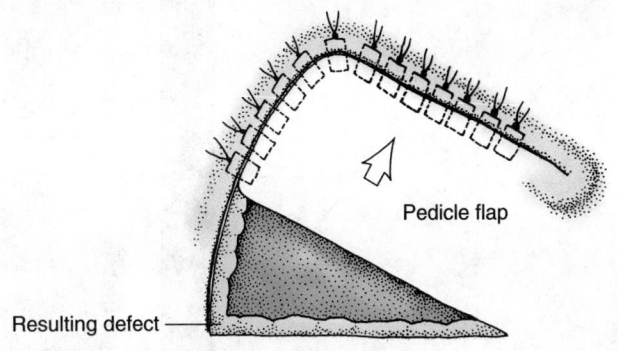

Figure 70–10. A full-thickness pedicle flap of skin is separated and rotated to cover the wound. Blood vessels are left intact. The resultant defect is either primarily closed or covered with skin grafts. The flap is held in place with staples or sutures.

Unlike free grafts, a pedicle flap is a full-thickness flap of skin that is raised and rotated to cover the defect, with one edge of the flap still attached to the site of origin to provide a blood supply (Fig. 70–10). Because all skin layers are removed, full-thickness donor sites are closed primarily or covered with additional split-thickness skin grafts. Partial-thickness donor sites heal by epithelialization if secondary infection is avoided.

Postoperative Care. Postoperative graft sites are immobilized with bulky cotton pressure dressings for 3 to 5 days to allow vascularization, or "take," of the newly grafted skin. The nurse does not disturb the dressing and encourages elevation and complete rest of the grafted area. Any activity that might cause movement of the dressing against the body and separation of the graft from the wound is prohibited.

After dressings are removed, the nurse monitors the graft for a sign of failure to vascularize: nonadherence to the wound or graft necrosis. If a pedicle flap has been used to cover the wound, the nurse inspects the edges of the flap frequently for changes in color. A pale flap with delayed capillary filling when blanched may have inadequate arterial perfusion. A dusky color or sharp line of color demarcation suggests inadequate venous or lymphatic drainage. Other techniques to monitor trends of blood flow in the graft, depending on location, include pulse oximetry, Doppler ultrasonography, and transcutaneous oxygen determination.

Postoperative care of donor sites aims to protect the area from injury and infection until healing can occur and promote client comfort. The client usually returns from surgery with a pressure dressing in place over the donor area to promote hemostasis. After 24 to 48 hours, this outer dressing is removed, revealing a single wound contact layer of fine-mesh gauze.

If the donor site is treated with dry exposure, the nurse promotes air circulation to the wound by positioning the client to avoid pressure on the site and using an overbed cradle to tent the sheets. When heat lamps are ordered, the nurse places the bulb (60–100 W) at least 2 feet from the wound to prevent thermal injury to the skin. After the dressing has dried and formed a "scab," the

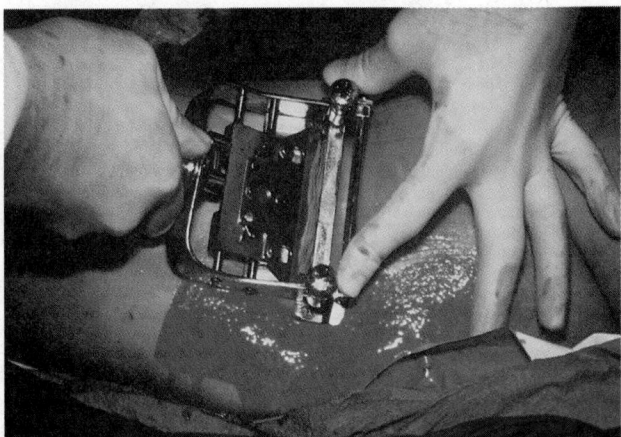

Figure 70–9. Removal of a partial-thickness (split-thickness) skin graft.

TABLE 70–6

Commonly Used Dressing Materials

Dressing Type	Alginates	Biological Dressings	Cotton Gauze Dressing	Foams	Hydrocolloidal Wafers	Hydrogel Dressing	Transparent Films
Examples	• Curasorb • Sorbsan • Kaltostat	• Collagen • Porcine heterograft • Cadaver homograft • Amnion • Cultured Epithelium	• Continuous dry • Continuous wet • Wet to damp • Wet to dry	• Epilock • Flexzan • LYOFOAM	• Comfeel Plus • Cutinova hydro • DuoDerm CGF	**Sheets** • Vigilon • Nu-Gel **Amorphous** • Carrasyn • Intra Site Gel	• Bioclusive • Op-Site • Tegaderm
Indications	• Absorption • Protection	• Debridement after eschar removal* • Protection • Test before skin grafts (pigskin and cadaver skin)	**Continuous Dry** • Absorption • Protection (non-adherent contact layer) **Continuous Wet** • Delivery of topical agent • Debridement (autolysis) • Protection **Wet to Damp** • Atraumatic mechanical debridement **Wet to Dry** • Agressive mechanical debridement	• Absorption • Protection	• Debridement* • Absorption • Protection	• Debridement* • Absorption • Protection	• Debridement* • Protection (partial-thickness lesions) • Secondary (cover) dressing

Advantages	• Highly absorbent • Biodegradable • Easy application • Nonadhesive • Can be used as packing for deep wounds • Can be used for infected wounds	• Most "natural" wound covering • Reduces pain • Conforms to uneven wound surfaces • Available in a variety of sizes and types	• Readily available • Good mechanical debridement if *used properly* • Effective delivery of topical agents	• Absorbent • Insulates wound • Easy application • Nonadhesive (most products) • Conforms to uneven wound surfaces	• Absorbent • Excludes bacteria • Waterproof • Reduces pain • Easy application • Easy to store	• Absorbent • Nonadhesive • Reduces pain • Conductive to use with topical agents • Conforms to uneven wound surfaces • Amorphous form can be used as a filler • Easy to store	• Wound visualization • Good adhesion • Waterproof • Reduces pain • Cost effective • Easy to store
Disadvantages	• Requires secondary dressing to secure • Can cause desiccation of tissue if drainage is minimal	• Requires secondary dressing to secure • Time consuming to apply • Potential allergen • Very expensive	• Delayed healing if used improperly • Pain or removal • Requires frequent dressing changes	• Poor barrier function • Requires secondary dressing to secure	• Nontransparent • Softening and loss of shape with pressure, heat, and friction • Odor with dressing removal • Expensive • Requires use of "fillers" for deep, draining lesions	• Poor barrier function • Only partial wound visualization • Requires secondary dressing to secure • Can promote growth of *Pseudomonas* and other microorganisms	• Difficult to apply properly • Nonabsorbent • Adhesive to normal and healing tissue • Limited to superficial lesions
Dressing changes	• When dressing is saturated (q3–5 days) or more frequently	• Every 24 hours until adherent, then every 5–7 days as needed	• Necrotic base: q4–6h • Clean base: q12–24h	• When dressing is saturated or more frequently	• Necrotic base: q24h • Clean base: on leakage of exudate	• Necrotic base: q6–8h • Clean base: q24h	• Necrotic base: q24h • Clean base: on leakage exudate

* Use with caution in patients with leukopenia or vascular disease.

TABLE 70–7

Foods That Promote Wound Healing

Food	Function	Food	Function
Protein Sources		**Iron Sources*** *Continued*	
Meat Fish Poultry Milk Cheese Eggs Soybeans Legumes Nuts Nutritional supplements	• Maintenance and healing of body tissues • Antibody production • Energy	Eggs Dark green leafy vegetables Blackstrap molasses Whole grain breads and cereals	
		Sources of Vitamin B₁₂	
Carbohydrate Sources		Liver Organ meats Muscle meats Fish Eggs Shellfish Milk Yogurt Cheese	• Protein synthesis
Whole grains (preferable to enriched because of higher nutritional and fiber content) Enriched grain and cereal products Fruit Juices Vegetables (especially starchy ones: corn, peas, potatoes) Milk Desserts and sweets	• Energy • Sparing of protein (if diet does not contain sufficient nonprotein calories, protein from body tissues will be broken down to supply energy) • Wound healing		
		Sources of Vitamin B₆	
Sources of Vitamin C		Meats Liver Some vegetables (including potatoes) Wheat germ Wheat bran Whole grain cereals and breads Fish Brewer's yeast Dried beans	• Amino acid metabolism
Berries Broccoli Brussels sprouts Cabbage Citrus fruits and juices Green peppers Kale Melons Spinach and dark green vegetables Tomatoes Vitamin C–enriched juices	• Collagen synthesis • Immunity		
		Folate Sources	
		Liver Yeast Leafy vegetables Dried beans Green vegetables Nuts Fresh oranges Whole wheat cereals and breads	• Protein synthesis
Zinc Sources		**Water Sources**	
Same as protein sources Beef Organ meat Shellfish Salmon Poultry Cheese Whole grains Dried beans	• Tissue repair (zinc-deficient diet causes poor wound healing, decreased ability to taste, and poor appetite) • Protein synthesis	Water Milk Juices Gelatin Tomatoes Citrus fruit Melons Vegetables Berries Broths Soups Tea Coffee Carbonated beverages	• Maintain condition of the skin (dehydration can lead to tissue breakdown, poor appetite, and constipation)
Iron Sources*			
Liver Meat Baked beans Dried fruits Legumes	• Cellular respiration • Hemoglobin synthesis		

From Ross, R., & Noe, J. (1983). *Chronic problem wounds* (p. 60). Boston: Little, Brown & Co. Used with permission.
* Iron cooking utensils add iron to the diet.

wound is kept dry and left undisturbed until healing is evident (10–14 days). As the donor site heals, the gauze and dried blood lift away from the new epithelium beneath. Trimming the separating gauze close to the skin surface minimizes the chance of the client's catching the loose end of the dressing on an object and removing the still-adherent gauze before healing is complete. Some surgeons may prefer to dress donor sites with moisture-retentive dressing instead of the traditional dry exposure method of treatment (see Table 70–6).

Because exposed donor sites are initially more painful than graft sites, the nurse administers pain medication as ordered and provides other comfort measures as needed. The nurse repositions the client during the immediate postoperative period to promote comfort only if movement of the graft site can be avoided. The nurse may offer back rubs to help relieve muscle spasms that occur with bed rest and immobility. Attention must also be paid to relieving pressure over unaffected bony prominences that may lead to additional ulcers.

Graft and donor sites involving the posterior body surfaces present a particular problem. For the graft or flap to become fully vascularized or for the donor sites to dry, the client must be immobilized in a side-lying or prone position for 7 to 10 days.

An alternative to difficult positioning is the use of special low-pressure or air-fluidized beds, which not only minimize ischemia of the graft or flap while the client is supine but also help prevent breakdown of intact skin. A major limitation to use of these beds is cost, which is usually outweighed by the potential for decreased morbidity and length of hospital stay.

➤ Risk for Infection and Wound Extension

Planning: Expected Outcomes. The client is expected to remain free of wound infection or systemic sepsis and to experience healing of the pressure ulcer.

Interventions. Because of the many intrinsic factors that can affect a client's resistance to infection, the nurse closely monitors the ulcer's progress so that timely treatment with topical and systemic antibiotics can be initiated if ulcer deterioration occurs. Steps are taken to minimize introduction of pathogenic organisms to the ulcer through direct contact.

Monitoring Ulcer Progress. Frequent monitoring of ulcer appearance using objective criteria allows the nurse to evaluate response to treatment and recognize early signs of impending infection. If an ulcer shows no progress toward healing within 3 weeks, the treatment plan should be reevaluated. Table 70–8 outlines objective indicators of local infection for wounds with and without tissue loss. Clients who are at highest risk for infection may exhibit a reduced inflammatory response to infection. These clients include those who are elderly, have white blood cell disorders, are receiving steroid therapy, or have wounds with a compromised blood supply.

Prevention of Infection and Extension. Complications of infection and wound extension are avoided by diligent monitoring of ulcer progress and prevention of new ulcer

---

Chart 70–3

Nursing Care Highlight: Interventions to Prevent Pressure Ulcers

Positioning

- Pad contact surfaces with foam, silicon gel, or air pads.
- Do not keep the head of the bed elevated above 30 degrees.
- Use a lift sheet to move client in the bed. Avoid dragging or sliding the client.
- When positioning a client on his or her side, do not position directly on the trochanter.
- Reposition an immobile client every 2 hours while in bed and every 1 hour while sitting in a chair.
- Do not place a rubber ring or doughnut under the client's sacral area.
- When moving an immobile client from a bed to another surface, use a designated slide board well lubricated with talc.
- Place pillows or foam wedges between two bony surfaces.
- Keep the client's skin directly off plastic surfaces.
- Keep the client's heels off the bed surface.

Nutrition

- Ensure a fluid intake between 2000 and 3000 mL/day.
- Help the client maintain an adequate intake of protein and calories.

Skin Care

- Use moisturizers daily on dry skin; and apply when skin is damp.
- Keep moisture from prolonged contact with skin.
  - Dry areas where two skin surfaces touch, such as the axilla and under the breasts.
  - Place absorbent pads under areas where perspiration collects.
  - Use moisture barriers on skin areas where wound drainage or incontinence occurs.
- Do not massage bony prominences.
- Humidify the room.

Skin Cleaning

- Clean the skin as soon as possible after soiling occurs and at routine intervals.
- Use a mild, heavily fatted soap.
- Use tepid rather than hot water.
- While cleaning, use the minimal scrubbing force necessary to remove soil.
- Gently pat rather than rub the skin dry.

---

formation. The nurse reports the following signs to the physician:

- Sudden deterioration of the ulcer, as evidenced by an increase in the size or depth of the lesion
- Changes in the color or texture of the granulation tissue
- Changes in the quantity, color, or odor of exudate

The nurse also remains alert for the classic signs of wound infection: increased erythema, edema, purulent and malodorous drainage, and tenderness of the wound margins, which may or may not be accompanied by clini-

TABLE 70–8

Monitoring Wound Infection

Variable	Frequency of Assessment	Rationale
Wounds Without Tissue Loss		
Examples		
Surgical incisions and clean lacerations closed primarily by sutures or staples		
Observations (Using First Postoperative Dressing Change as Baseline)		
Check for the presence or absence of increased: Localized tenderness Swelling of the incision line Erythema of the incision line >1 cm on each side of wound Localized heat	• At least every 24 hr until sutures or staples are removed	• To detect cellulitis (bacterial infections)*
Check for the presence or absence of: Purulent drainage from any portion of the incision site Localized fluctuance (from fluid accumulation) and tenderness beneath a *portion* of the wound when palpated	• At least every 24 hr until sutures or staples are removed	• To detect abscess formation related to presence of foreign body (suture material) or deeper wound infection*
Check for the presence or absence of approximation (sealing) of wound edges with or without serosanguineous drainage.	• At least every 24 hr until sutures or staples are removed	• To detect potential for wound dehiscence
Wounds with Tissue Loss		
Examples		
Partial- or full-thickness skin loss caused by pressure necrosis, vascular disease, trauma, etc. and allowed to heal by secondary intention		
Observations		
Wound Size		
Measure wound size at greatest length and width using a metric ruler or, for asymmetric ulcers, by tracing the wound onto a piece of plastic film or sheeting (plastic template). Compare all subsequent measurements against the initial measurement.	• At least every week	• To detect increase in wound size and depth secondary to infectious process
Ulcer Base		
Check for the presence or absence of Necrotic tissue (loose or adherent) Presence or absence of foul odor from wound when dressing is changed Note the frequency of dressing changes or dressing reinforcements owing to drainage.	• At least every 24 hr	• To detect the need for debridement or the response to treatment (necrotic tissue) and the detect local wound infection (frequent dressing changes and foul odor)
Wound Margins		
Check for the presence or absence of Erythema and swelling extending outward >1 cm from wound margins Increased tenderness at wound margins	• At least every 24 hr or at each dressing change	• To detect wound infection*
Systemic Response		
Check for the presence or absence of elevated body temperature, WBCs, or positive blood culture	• PRN	• To detect bacteremia

WBCs = white blood cells; PRN = as needed.
* The wounds of clients who are severely immunosuppressed or those wounds with compromised blood supply may not exhibit a typical inflammatory response to local wound infection.

cal signs of bacteremia, such as fever, elevated white blood cell count, and positive blood cultures. The nurse uses appropriate interventions to prevent the formation of new pressure ulcers and to prevent early-stage ulcers from progressing to deeper wounds (Chart 70–3).

Maintaining a Safe Environment. Because of the variety of microorganisms in the hospital environment, keeping an ulcer totally free of bacteria is impossible. Therefore, optimal ulcer management is based on maintaining acceptably low levels of microorganisms through meticulous local wound care and minimizing contamination with pathogenic organisms. The nurse and assistive nursing personnel use standard precautions to prevent direct contact with ulcer secretions and cross-contamination among clients. All health care providers and assistive personnel practice thorough hand washing before and after dressing changes and properly dispose of soiled dressings and linens.

 Continuing Care

Clients with pressure ulcers may be in acute care, subacute care, long-term care, or home care settings. If pressure ulcer therapy requires hospitalization, most clients with pressure ulcers are discharged before complete wound closure is obtained. Discharge may be to the home setting or to a long-term care facility, depending on the degree of debilitation and other client factors.

▶ Health Teaching

Before the client is discharged, the client or family member who will be performing the wound care should demonstrate facility in removing the dressing, cleaning the wound, and applying the dressing. When choosing a dressing to be used at home, the nurse considers the client's or family member's ability to apply the dressing properly. If the client's finances are limited, the nurse also addresses the cost of the dressing material. Some dressings may be easier to apply and less expensive than other materials. At times, the more expensive dressing materials that require less frequent changing may be preferred. The nurse explains the signs and symptoms of wound infection.

The nurse encourages the client to eat a balanced diet, with frequent high-protein snacks. The nurse discusses diet preferences with the client and suggests foods that promote wound healing (see Table 70–7). The physician may order vitamin and mineral supplements if there are dietary deficiencies.

If the client is incontinent, the nurse emphasizes the need to keep the skin clean and dry. If bowel and bladder training are not possible, the use of absorbent underpads, briefs, and topical moisture barrier creams and ointments are discussed as methods to reduce skin exposure to urine and feces.

▶ Home Care Management

Care of the ulcer in the client's home is similar to care in the hospital. Most dressing supplies and pressure relief devices can be easily obtained at the local pharmacy or medical supply store. If mechanical debridement of the ulcer is still needed, a hand-held shower device or forceful irrigation of the wound with a 35-mL syringe and 19-gauge angiocatheter can be substituted for whirlpool therapy.

Clients with chronic pressure ulcers are often depressed about their debilitated state, which may affect their compliance with wound care measures. Many clients cannot change their own dressings because of distress over altered body image or the pain experienced with dressing removal. Others are totally dependent on family members or support personnel because of limited physical mobility or inability to reach the wound.

For some clients, drastic changes in daily activities are necessary to promote healing. Clients with pressure ulcers on the lower extremities may need frequent rest periods with leg elevation to minimize edema. Immobile clients with pressure ulcers require around-the-clock repositioning as often as every 2 to 4 hours to prevent further breakdown, which takes its toll on family members or caregivers. The nurse explains the rationale for activity changes to the client and family and explores alternative ways of coping with these changes.

▶ Health Care Resources

A home care nurse may be needed to follow wound progress after the client is discharged. The hospital nurse provides details of ulcer size and appearance and any special wound care needs to the nurse in the home, who can then accurately judge changes in ulcer appearance. Chart 70–4 provides a guideline for focused assessment of the client with pressure ulcers.

To minimize waste and to help decrease the overall cost of treatment, the nurse emphasizes proper use of dressing materials. Clean tap water and nonsterile supplies are acceptable for treatment of chronic wounds in the home and are less costly than sterile products. Nonsterile dressing materials can often be purchased in bulk from a local medical supply store at reduced cost.

The client with activity restrictions may require daily assistance from a home care aide. A physical therapy consult may be appropriate to help the client and family continue rehabilitation efforts in the home.

 Evaluation

On the basis of the identified nursing diagnoses, the expected outcomes for the client with a pressure ulcer may include that the client should be able to

- Demonstrate skills necessary to care for the wound in the home environment
- Incorporate modifications of lifestyle related to promotion of healing in activities of daily living (ADLs)
- List the signs and symptoms of wound infection
- Make the necessary changes in dietary intake to correct any nutritional deficiencies
- Demonstrates an understanding of measures needed to prevent future episodes of skin breakdown and pressure ulcer formation.

Focused Assessment for Home Care Clients at Risk for Pressure Ulcer

- Assess cardiovascular status.
  - Presence or absence of peripheral edema
  - Hand vein filling in the dependent position
  - Neck vein filling in the recumbent and sitting positions
  - Weight gain or loss
- Assess cognition and mental status.
  - Level of consciousness
  - Orientation to time, place, and person
  - Can the client accurately read a 7-word sentence containing no words greater than three syllables?
- Assess condition of skin.
  - Assess general skin cleanliness.
  - Observe all skin areas, paying particular attention to bony prominences and those areas in greatest contact with bed and other firm surfaces.
  - Measure and record any areas of redness or loss of integrity.
  - If possible, photograph areas of concern.
  - Note presence or absence of skin tenting over the sternum or the forehead.
  - Note moistness of skin and mucous membranes.
  - If wounds are present, remove dressings (noting condition of dressings), cleanse the wound, compare with previous notations of wound condition.
    - Presence, amount, and nature of exudate
    - Use a ruler to measure wound diameter and depth
    - Amount (%) and type of necrotic tissue
    - Presence of granulation/epithelium
    - Presence/absence of cellulitis
    - Presence/absence of odor
- Take the client's temperature.
- Assess client's understanding of illness and compliance with treatment.
  - Signs and symptoms to report to health care provider
  - Medication plan (correct timing and dose)
  - Ambulation or positioning schedule
  - Dressing changes/skin care
  - Diet modifications (24-hour diet recall)
- Assess client's nutritional status.
  - Change in muscle mass
  - Lackluster nails, sparse hair
  - Recent weight loss >10% of usual weight
  - Impaired oral intake
  - Difficulty swallowing
  - Generalized edema

COMMON INFECTIONS

Bacterial Infections

Overview

Typical primary bacterial lesions involve the hair follicle, where bacteria easily accumulate and flourish in the warm, moist environment. Folliculitis is a superficial infection involving only the upper portion of the follicle and is usually caused by *Staphylococcus* (Fig. 70–11). Furuncles (boils) are also caused by *Staphylococcus*, but the infection is much deeper in the follicle (Fig. 70–12). Cellulitis is a generalized nonfollicular infection with either *Staphylococcus* or *Streptococcus* and involves the deeper connective tissue.

Minor skin trauma usually precedes the appearance of folliculitis and furuncles and may or may not be associated with the development of cellulitis. Clients may spread the infection to other parts of their bodies by scratching or rubbing the skin with fingernails that have microorganisms under them. Furuncles are more likely to occur in the presence of heat and moisture, such as in the hair-bearing skin fold areas. Cellulitis can occur as a result of secondary bacterial infection of an open wound, or it may be unrelated to skin trauma.

Viral Infections

Herpes Simplex Virus

Herpes simplex virus (HSV) infection is the most common viral infection of adult skin. HSV infections are of two types. Type 1 (HSV 1) infections cause the classic recurring cold sore. The severity of the disease increases with age and immunosuppression. Genital herpes, caused by type 2 (HSV 2), is also recurrent (see Chap. 80).

After a primary infection, the virus resides in a dormant state in the nerve ganglia, and the client is asymptomatic. Reactivation of the infection stimulates the virus to travel the pathway of sensory nerves to the skin, where lesions reappear. In healthy people, recurrence of herpes simplex virus infection is triggered by physical or psychological stressors, such as sunburn, trauma, fever, menses, and fatigue. The virus can also be spread by direct contact between an actively infected person and a susceptible host. *Autoinoculation*, or transfer of either viral type from one part of the body to another, is also possible.

The time span between episodes and the severity of individual attacks varies. Outbreaks of oral herpes simplex usually last 3 to 10 days, and active shedding of the virus and contagion are possible for the first 3 to 5 days. The client may experience tingling or burning of the lip before any lesion is evident.

The most typical clinical presentation of HSV 1 infection is isolated or grouped vesicles on an erythematous

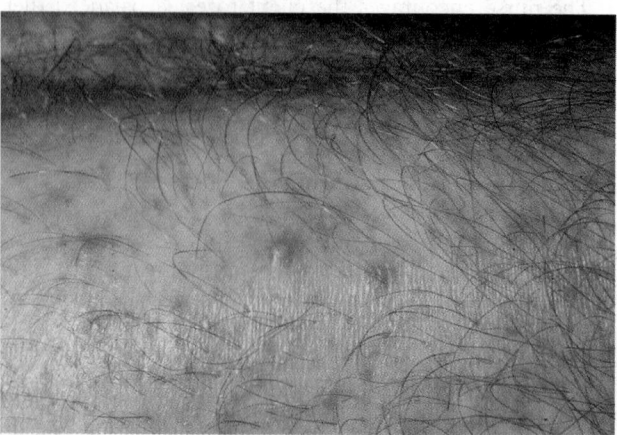

Figure 70–11. Folliculitis.

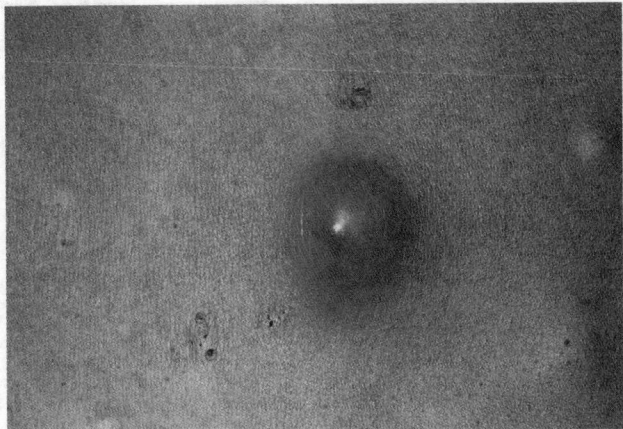

Figure 70–12. A furuncle.

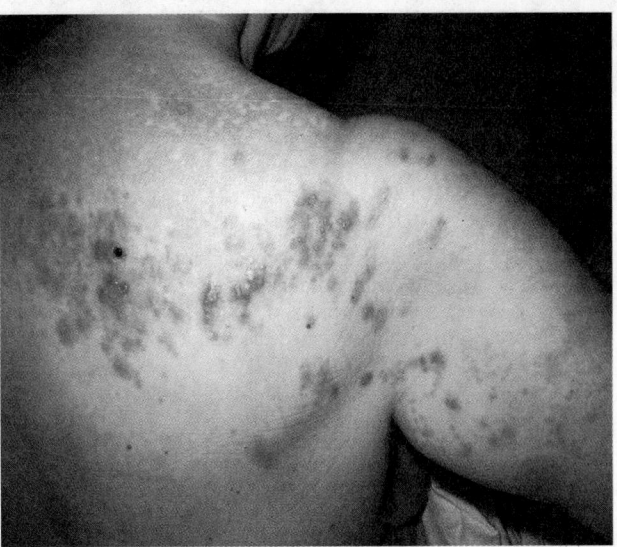

Figure 70–14. Herpes zoster.

base (Fig. 70–13). The infection can occur anywhere on the skin and may be spread by respiratory droplets or by direct contact with an active lesion or virus-containing fluid (such as saliva).

Herpetic whitlow is a form of herpes simplex infection occurring on the fingertips of medical personnel who have come in contact with viral secretions. This form of herpes is a potential source of client inoculation. Immunosuppressed clients are at a particular risk for severe and persistent eruptions that can lead to life-threatening complications.

Herpes Zoster

Herpes zoster (shingles) is caused by reactivation of the latent varicella-zoster virus in clients who have previously had chickenpox. The dormant virus resides in the dorsal root ganglia of the sensory cranial and spinal nerves. The individual lesions of herpes zoster infections are similar to those of herpes simplex, but they have a different distribution pattern (Fig. 70–14). Multiple lesions occur in a segmental distribution on the skin area innervated by the infected nerve. Herpes zoster eruptions are preceded by several days of discomfort, which may vary from minor irritation and itching to severe, deep pain. The course of

eruption usually lasts several weeks. Postherpetic neuralgia, pain persisting after the lesions have resolved, is a common complication in elderly clients.

Herpes zoster is essentially a disease of immunosuppression, occurring with increased frequency and severity in elderly people as a result of age-related alterations in host resistance. Dissemination of the virus can be accompanied by fever and malaise, often progressing to visceral involvement. Herpes zoster is contagious to people who have not been previously exposed to chickenpox.

Complications can include full-thickness skin necrosis, Bell's palsy, or ophthalmic infection and scarring if the virus is introduced into the eye.

Fungal Infections

Superficial fungal (dermatophyte) infections can differ in lesion appearance, anatomic location, and species of the infecting organism. The term *tinea* is used to describe dermatophytoses. Table 70–9 lists the corresponding anatomic locations of the various categories of infection.

Depending on the species, dermatophytes reside predominantly in the soil, on animals, and on humans. Superficial infection can be initiated only if suitable conditions exist for inoculation and maintenance of the organism in the outer layers of the skin. Predisposing factors for dermatophytosis include impairment of the

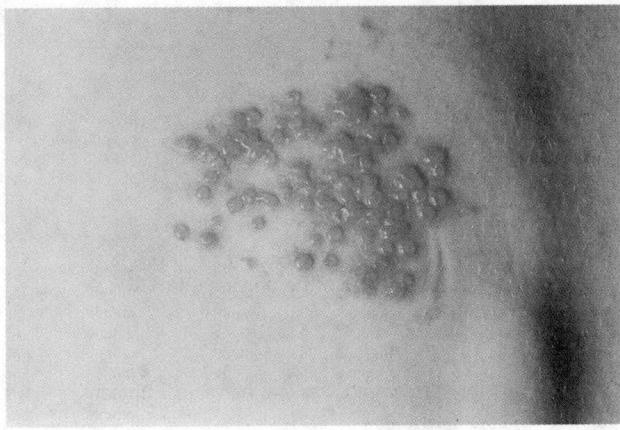

Figure 70–13. Herpes simplex.

TABLE 70–9

Tinea Infections	
Infection	**Location**
Tinea pedis	• Feet (athlete's foot)
Tinea manus	• Hands
Tinea cruris	• Groin (jock itch)
Tinea corporis	• Smooth skin surfaces (ringworm)
Tinea capitis	• Scalp
Tinea barbae	• Beard

Chart 70–5

Key Features of Common Skin Infections

Clinical Manifestations	Distribution
Bacterial Infections	
Folliculitis	
• Isolated erythematous pustules occur singly or in groups; hairs grow from centers of many of the lesions. • Occasional papules are present. • There is little or no associated discomfort. • There is no residual scarring.	• Areas of hair-bearing skin, especially buttocks, thighs, beard area, and scalp
Furuncle	
• Small, tender erythematous nodules become pus filled and more tender over time. • Lesions may be single or multiple and also recurrent. • Regional lymphadenopathy is sometimes present; fever is rare. • Occasional scarring results.	• Areas of hair-bearing skin, especially buttocks, thighs, abdomen, posterior neck regions, and axillae
Cellulitis	
• Localized area of inflammation may enlarge rapidly if not treated. • Redness, warmth, edema, tenderness, and pain are present. • On rare occasions, blisters are present. • Cellulitis is often accompanied by lymphadenopathy and fever.	• Lower legs, areas of persistent lymphedema, and areas of skin trauma (leg ulcer, puncture wound, and so forth)
Viral Infections	
Herpes Simplex	
• Grouped vesicles are present on an erythematous base. • Vesicles evolve to pustules, which rupture, weep, and crust. • Older lesions may appear as punched-out, shallow erosions with well-defined borders. • Lesions are associated with itching, stinging, or pain. • Secondary bacterial infection with necrosis is possible in immunocompromised clients.	• Type 1 classically on the face and type 2 on the genitalia, but either may develop in any area where inoculation has occurred. Recurrent infections occur repeatedly in the same skin area.
Herpes Zoster	
• Lesions are similar in appearance to herpes simplex and also progress with weeping and crusting. • Grouped lesions present unilaterally along a segment of skin following the pathway of a spinal or cranial nerve (dermatomal distribution). • Eruption is preceded by deep pain and itching. • Postherpetic neuralgia is common in the elderly. • Secondary infection with necrosis is possible in immunocompromised clients.	• Anterior or posterior trunk following involved dermatome; face, sometimes involving trigeminal nerve and eye
Fungal Infections	
Dermatophytosis	
• Annular or serpiginous patches are present with elevated borders, scaling, and central clearing. • Pruritus is common. • Lesions may be single or multiple.	• Anywhere on the body
Candidiasis	
• Erythematous macular eruption occurs with isolated pustules or papules at the border (satellite lesions). • Candidiasis is associated with burning and itching. • Oral lesions (thrush) appear as creamy-white plaques on an inflamed mucous membrane. • Cracks or fissures at the corners of the mouth may be present.	• Skin fold areas: perineal and perianal region, axillae, beneath breasts, and between the fingers; under wet or occlusive dressings • Lesions possibly present on the oral or vaginal mucous membranes

barrier function of the stratum corneum in warm, humid environments, followed by minor skin trauma.

Dermatophyte infections occur when the infecting organism comes in contact with an impaired skin surface in a susceptible host. Most infections are spread by direct contact with infected humans or animals. Certain types of dermatophytoses, such as tinea capitis and tinea corporis, can be transmitted by means of inanimate objects. For example, tinea capitis is associated with poor personal hygiene and the subsequent sharing of contaminated combs, brushes, hats, pillowcases, and similar objects.

Collaborative Management

 Assessment

➤ History

The clinical manifestations of the skin infection provide direction for collection of data to confirm a suspected diagnosis. To differentiate among the possible causes of the lesions, the nurse concentrates on risk factors associated with each type of infection. If the location and appearance of lesions suggest a bacterial infection, the nurse explores any recent history of skin trauma as well as past or current staphylococcal or streptococcal infections. The nurse also notes associated symptoms of fever and malaise.

Lesions appearing on the lips, in the oral cavity, or in the genital region alert the nurse to a possible viral infection. The nurse seeks information about the following:

- A history of similar lesions in the same location
- Signs of burning, tingling, or pain
- Recent stress factors that may have precipitated the outbreak
- Recent contact with an infected person

Acknowledgment by the client of the recurrent nature of lesions is often important in helping to differentiate viral from bacterial lesions. If herpes zoster is suspected, the nurse confirms *previous exposure to chickenpox* and inquires whether the client has a history of shingles.

The type of information asked of a client with probable dermatophyte infection depends on the anatomic location of the lesions. The presence of tinea corporis and tinea capitis requires further assessment of social and environmental factors that may have contributed to inoculation, such as direct contact with an infected person, poor personal hygiene practices, or frequent contact with animals. If tinea cruris and tinea pedis are suspected, the nurse asks the client about the type and frequency of athletic activities.

➤ Physical Assessment/Clinical Manifestations

Because most skin infections are contagious, the nurse takes necessary precautions to prevent the spread of infection when performing a physical assessment. Chart 70–5 lists the clinical manifestations of common skin infections.

➤ Laboratory Assessment

When pustules are present in bacterial infections, the infecting organism is confirmed by swab culture of the purulent material. Blood cultures may prove helpful, especially if the client is showing clinical signs of bacteremia.

Viral infections are confirmed by *Tzanck's smear* and viral culture. Tzanck's smear is a cytologic examination in which cells from the base of a lesion are examined under a microscope. The presence of multinucleated giant cells confirms a viral infection.

Fungal infections are confirmed by a potassium hydroxide (KOH) test. Scrapings of scales from the lesions are obtained and, after preparation with KOH, examined under a microscope. The presence of fungal hyphae confirms the diagnosis. In addition to a KOH test, a fungal culture is sometimes indicated. Occasionally, a skin biopsy is performed to obtain microorganisms for identification.

 Interventions

Most skin infections heal well with nonsurgical management. Surgical intervention may be required when an infectious agent is present in deep tissue layers.

➤ Nonsurgical Management

The nurse is concerned with meticulous skin care to the involved areas to facilitate resolution of lesions and adherence to general isolation precautions. In some instances, drug therapy is also warranted.

Skin Care. Clients with bacterial infections should bathe daily with an antibacterial soap. The nurse instructs the client to remove any pustules or crusts gently so that topical medications are more easily absorbed. Application of warm compresses twice a day to furuncles or areas of cellulitis often increases the client's comfort.

Application of astringent compresses, such as Burow's solution, to viral lesions for 20 minutes three times a day promotes crust formation and healing. Compresses also relieve the irritation and pain associated with herpetic infection. The nurse instructs the client to avoid constricting garments that might rub the lesions and increase irritation.

Most superficial skin infections resolve more quickly if the involved skin is allowed to dry between treatments. Excessive moisture, especially under occlusion, promotes growth of microorganisms. If the client is bedridden, the nurse or other assistive personnel positions the client for optimal air circulation to the area and avoids occlusive dressings or garments.

Isolation Precautions. The nurse takes precautions to minimize the spread of pathogenic organisms to other people. For most superficial bacterial infections, attention to proper hand washing is sufficient to prevent cross-contamination. However, when hospitalized clients are colonized with *Staphylococcus* that is resistant to antibiotic therapy, strict adherence to isolation procedures is necessary.

Of the dermatophyte infections, tinea capitis, tinea corporis, and tinea pedis show the highest rates of cross-transmission. The nurse instructs clients to avoid sharing potentially contaminated personal items, such as hairbrushes, articles of clothing, or footwear. Repeated infections transmitted by dogs or cats may mean that clients might have to get rid of a family pet to control infections.

Drug Therapy. Commonly used topical medications for the treatment of bacterial, viral, and fungal skin infections are listed in Chart 70–6.

Mild bacterial infections of the skin usually resolve with topical antibacterial treatment. Clients with extensive infections, including those with associated fever or lymphadenopathy, require systemic antibiotic therapy.

Acyclovir (Zovirax) is the drug of choice for the treatment of viral infections. Topical acyclovir ointment decreases the numbers of active virus on the skin surface and reduces pain in primary herpetic infections and localized lesions in immunocompromised clients. Topical treatment is of little benefit in recurrent infection. Intravenous (IV) administration is limited to severe primary infections and immunosuppressed clients with symptoms of systemic involvement.

Topical antifungal agents are indicated for clients with dermatophyte and yeast infections. An imidazole cream is applied to the infected skin at least twice a day until the lesions have cleared. To discourage recurrence, the therapy is usually continued for 1 to 2 weeks after clearing. In some instances, antifungal powders may also help to suppress fungal growth. For widespread or resistant fungal infections, systemic antifungal agents, such as ketoconazole (Nizoral), are administered.

➤ Surgical Management

Surgery is not usually performed for a superficial skin infection, except for incision and drainage of furuncles. In severely immunocompromised clients, superficial lesions can progress to full-thickness wounds requiring surgical excision.

Chart 70–6

Drug Therapy for Skin Disorders

Drug	Usual Dosage	Nursing Interventions	Rationale
Antibacterial Drugs			
Ointments			
Neomycin sulfate Combination antibiotics (Neosporin, Bacitracin, Polysporin, Mycitracin) Gentamicin (Garamycin) Chloramphenicol (Chloromycetin) Povidone-iodine (Betadine) Bactroban	• Apply a thin layer to the affected area tid. Dressing is optional.	• Gently clean affected areas with saline, half-strength peroxide, or tap water before applying ointments. • Avoid rubbing ointment into skin. Apply with downward strokes in direction of hair growth. • Assess for worsening of problem in spite of topical therapy. Discontinue use if rash appears.	• Atraumatic cleaning promotes healing by preventing further injury to skin cells. Cleaning helps to remove exudate, crusts, and residual medication and increases the effectiveness of therapy. • Ointments can irritate hair follicles and lead to folliculitis. • Client may become allergic to active ingredients, the ointment base, or added preservatives.
Creams			
Silver sulfadiazine (Silvadene, SSD, Flamazine✤)	• Apply in layer approximately ¹⁄₁₆-inch thick to affected areas tid and PRN. Dressing is optional.	• Assess for allergy to sulfa drugs. • Gently clean affected areas with saline, half-strength hydrogen peroxide, or tap water before reapplying. • If affected areas are left open without dressings, reapply cream PRN between cleanings to maintain a layer of cream at all times. • Monitor white blood cell count for drop to <5000/mm³.	• Use should be avoided in clients with a suspected or known sulfa allergy. • Cleaning removes crusts, exudate, and caked-on medication while promoting percutaneous absorption of drug. • Cream base melts with increase in body or room temperature and is easily rubbed off with movement if left uncovered. • Use of silver sulfadiazine over large skin surface areas has been associated with a transient leukopenia (cause unknown).

Chart 70–6. Drug Therapy for Skin Disorders   Continued

Drug	Usual Dosage	Nursing Interventions	Rationale
Antifungal Drugs			
Ointments and Creams			
Clotrimazole (Lotrimin, My-celex canesten✦) Nystatin (Mycolog, Myco-statin, Nilstat) Ciclopirox olamine (Loprox) Miconazole nitrate (Monistat-Derm 2%) Econazole (Spectazole, Ecostatin✦) Tolnaftate (Tinactin, Pitrex✦) Haloprogin (Halotex✦) Undecylenic acid (Desenex) Ketoconazole (Nizoral)	• Apply a thin layer to the affected area tid.	• Teach the importance of thoroughly drying the skin before applying medication. • Position bedridden clients for maximal air circulation to involved areas. • Emphasize wearing of non-constricting cotton garments to absorb perspiration.	• Moist environment promotes the growth of fungal organisms. • Increasing air circulation to the affected areas promotes drying. • Cream base is easily removed with perspiration, decreasing the effectiveness of therapy.
Powders			
Nystatin (Mycostatin) Tolnaftate (Zeosorb-AF 1%)	• Apply a thin dusting of powder to the affected area tid.	• Teach the client to thoroughly dry skin before applying powder.	• In addition to discouraging the growth of fungal organisms, a dry skin surface minimizes caking of powder in skin fold areas.
Oral Preparations			
Nystatin (Mycostatin oral suspension, Nilstat oral suspension)	• Rinse the mouth qid with 4–6 mL (400,000–600,000 units) and swallow.	• Teach the client to coat the entire oral cavity with medication and hold the suspension in mouth for several minutes before swallowing.	• Effectiveness of medication is dependent on good contact of medication with mucous membrane surfaces.
Clotrimazole (Mycelex troche)	• Take 1 troche five times daily.	• Teach the client to let troche dissolve slowly in the mouth.	
Anti-inflammatory Drugs			
Steroid Preparations			
Potent Fluorinated Clobetasol propionate (Temovate 0.05%) Triamcinolone acetonide (Aristocort 0.5%, Kenalog 0.5%, Triaderm✦ 0.5%) Amcinonide (Cyclocort 0.1%) Betamethasone dipropionate (Diprosone 0.05%, Betaderm✦ 0.5%) Diflorasone diacetate (Maxiflor 0.05%, Florone 0.05%) Halcinonide (Halog 0.025%) Fluocinonide (Lidex 0.05%, Topsyn gel 0.05%, Lidemol✦ 0.05%, Topsyn✦ 0.05%) Fluocinolone acetonide (Syn-alar-HP 0.2%, Fluoderm✦ 0.2%) Desoximetasone (Topicort 0.25%) Betamethasone benzoate (Uticort 0.025%, Novobetamet✦ 0.025%)	• Apply a small amount to affect areas no more than four times in 24 hr.	• Teach the client to use the least amount of medication possible to cover the treatment site and to use the medication *only* under the direction of a physician. • Never apply highly potent steroid preparations to the face, genital area, or skin fold areas.	• Overuse of topical steroid preparations can cause serious side effects, including skin thinning (atrophy), superficial dilated blood vessels (telangiectasia), acne-like eruptions, and adrenal suppression. The incidence of side effects increases proportionately with the potency of the steroid and is most common with prolonged widespread use of the high-potency preparations. • Absorption of topical steroids is much higher in these areas, and the associated side effects are more severe.

Continued

Chart 70–6. Drug Therapy for Skin Disorders   Continued

Drug	Usual Dosage	Nursing Interventions	Rationale
Medium-Potency Fluorinated			
Triamcinolone acetonide (Kenalog 0.025%, 0.1%; Aristocort 0.025%, 0.1%)			
Flurandrenolide (Cordran 0.5%, 0.025%)			
Fluocinolone acetonide (Fluonid 0.025%, Synalar 0.025%)			
Desoximetasone (Topicort LP 0.05%)			
Betamethasone valerate (Valisone 0.1%)			
Low-Potency Nonfluorinated		• Teach the client to hydrate the skin before applying a topical steroid.	• Skin hydration increases percutaneous absorption and maximizes the effectiveness of topical treatment.
Hydrocortisone 0.5%, 1.0%, 2.5%			
Desonide (Tridesilon)			
Hydrocortisone valerate (Westcort)			
Antiviral Drugs			
Ointments			
Acyclovir (Zovirax)	• Apply to affected areas six times a day.	• Teach the client to use topical acyclovir only under the direction of a physician for primary infections. • Emphasize precautionary measures to prevent transmission of infection while the lesion is present.	• Topical acyclovir has no proven clinical benefit in the prevention or treatment of recurrent infections. • There is no evidence that topical treatment prevents transmission of infection.

tid = three times a day; PRN = as needed.

PARASITIC DISORDERS

Parasitic skin disorders are most often associated with poor hygiene and substandard living conditions. The nurse examines clients who show obvious signs of a self-care deficit for these contagious parasitic infections.

Pediculosis

Overview

Pediculosis refers to infestation by human lice: pediculosis capitis (head lice), pediculosis corporis (body lice), and pediculosis pubis (pubic or crab lice). Human lice are oval and measure approximately 2 to 4 mm. The female louse lays hundreds of eggs called *nits*, which are deposited at the base of the hair shaft in hair-bearing areas.

Collaborative Management

The most prominent symptom of pediculosis is pruritus, which may or may not be accompanied by excoriation. In addition to causing discomfort, these parasites can also be vectors of systemic disease, such as typhus and recurrent fever.

 Assessment

Pediculosis capitis occurs more commonly in women than men, especially on the sides and back of the scalp. Pruritus, the result of biting of the scalp by the parasites, is intense. With severe infestation, it is possible for a secondary infection to develop from scratching.

Because the louse is difficult to see on inspection, the nurse examines the scalp for visible white flecks, the nits of the female louse. Matting and crusting of the scalp accompanied by a foul odor alert the nurse to the probability of secondary infection.

Pediculosis corporis is caused by lice that live and lay eggs in the seams of clothing. The parasites also cause itching. The only visible sign of infestation may be excoriations on the trunk, abdomen, or extremities.

Pediculosis pubis causes intense pruritus of the vulvar or perirectal region. Pubic lice, which are more compact and crab-like in appearance than body lice, can be contracted from infested bed linen or during sexual intercourse. Although the louse is usually confined to the genital region, it can also infest the axilla, the eyelashes, and the chest.

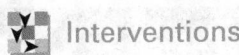 Interventions

The treatment of pediculosis is chemical killing of the parasites with agents such as lindane (Bio-Well, Kwell, Kwellada✦) or topical malathion (Ovide, Prioderm). In the case of pediculosis capitis, areas where the client's head has rested (such as on pillows or chair backs) should also be treated. Clothing and bed linens should be washed in hot water or dry cleaned. The use of a fine-toothed comb can help remove nits from an infested scalp. In all cases of louse infestation, social contacts are treated when possible.

Scabies

Overview

Scabies is a contagious skin disease caused by mite infestations. Scabies infections are transmitted by close and prolonged contact with an infested companion or infested bedding. Infestation is common among clients of lower socioeconomic status. The scabies mite is also carried by pets and is found among schoolchildren and institutionalized elderly clients.

Collaborative Management

Scabies is characterized by epidermal curved or linear ridges and follicular papules. The pruritus experienced by clients with scabies infestation is more intense than in those with pediculosis, and clients frequently report that the itching becomes unbearable at night.

The visible white epidermal ridges are formed by burrowing of the mite into the outer skin layers. The nurse closely examines the skin between the fingers and on the palms and volar aspects of the wrists, where these ridges are most common. A hypersensitivity reaction to the mite results in excoriated erythematous papules, pustules, and crusted lesions found primarily on the elbows, nipples, lower abdomen, buttocks, and thighs and in the axillary folds. Male clients can also have excoriated papules on the penis.

Suspected infestation is confirmed by taking a scraping of a lesion and examining it under the microscope for mites and eggs. Close contacts are also monitored for the possibility of infestation.

Treatment consists of chemical disinfection with scabicides, such as lindane (Kwell, Kwellada✦) or topical sulfur preparations, with one or two daily applications. Clothes and personal items are laundered but do not need to be disinfected.

COMMON INFLAMMATIONS

Overview

The inflammatory skin conditions are characterized by a variety of nonspecific epidermal manifestations, including marked pruritus, lesions with indistinct borders, and different distribution patterns. The cause of the eruption may or may not be identifiable. Inflammatory rashes can evolve from acute to chronic conditions.

Most inflammatory rashes are related to allergic immune responses. The responses may be triggered by external skin exposure to allergens or by exposure of the internal environment to allergens and irritants. The result is tissue destruction or epidermal alteration induced by antibodies or cellular mediators of the immune system. (A more detailed description of these immune mechanisms is presented in Chapter 23.)

The specific cause of inflammatory rashes is not always known. When this is the case, the catchall diagnosis of nonspecific eczematous dermatitis, or *eczema*, is often used.

Contact dermatitis is an acute or chronic eczematous rash caused by either direct contact with an irritant substance, resulting in toxic injury to the skin or contact with an allergen, resulting in a cell-mediated immune reaction.

Atopic dermatitis is a chronic rash associated with genetic predisposition to respiratory allergies and atopic skin disease. Although the exact mechanism is unknown, atopic dermatitis is exacerbated by a number of factors, including dry or irritated skin, food allergies, chemicals, or stress. Chapter 25 describes atopic inflammatory reactions.

Collaborative Management

 Assessment

Because all of the inflammatory skin eruptions have similar clinical presentations, data collected from the client are often the determining factor in identifying the cause. Although the clinical appearance of eczematous dermatitis lesions is similar, the chronicity of the disease, the distribution of lesions, and associated symptoms may vary. Chart 70–7 lists the clinical manifestations of the various types of inflammatory skin conditions. Diagnosis is based on historical and clinical data.

 Interventions

If the cause of the rash is identified, avoidance therapy is used in an attempt to reverse the reaction and clear the rash. Even when the cause is unclear, certain irritants in the environment may cause the rash to worsen and increase the client's discomfort. Additional interventions are aimed at promoting comfort through suppression of the inflammatory response.

➤ *Steroids*

Topical, intralesional, or systemic steroids are prescribed to suppress inflammation. The vehicle used to deliver a topical steroid generally depends on the body area involved. Because a side effect of oral corticosteroid administration is adrenal suppression, clients receiving long-term therapy must taper their drug dosages rather than come to an abrupt halt.

Corticosteroids never cure. During active disease, these agents keep the disease from manifesting itself and relieve associated discomfort. The nurse can moisten dressings

---

Chart 70–7

Key Features of Common Inflammatory Skin Conditions

Clinical Manifestations	Distribution
Nonspecific Eczematous Dermatitis	
• Evolution of lesions from vesicles to weeping papules and plaques. Lichenification occurs in chronic disease.	• Anywhere on the body; localized eczema commonly involves the hands or feet
• Oozing, crusting, fissuring, excoriation, or scaling may be present.	
• Pruritus is common.	
Contact Dermatitis	
• Localized eczematous eruption with well-defined, geometric margins that is consistent with contact by an irritant or allergen.	• Cosmetic/perfume allergy: head and neck
	• Hair product allergy: scalp
• Usually seen in the acute form, but may become chronic if exposure is repeated.	• Shoe/rubber allergy: dorsum of feet
	• Nickel allergy: ear lobes
• Allergy to plants (e.g., poison ivy or oak) classically occurs as linear streaks of vesicles or papules.	• Mouthwash/toothpaste allergy: perioral region
	• Airborne contact allergy (e.g., paint and ragweed): generalized
Atopic Dermatitis	
• Hallmark in adults is lichenification with scaling and excoriation.	• Face, neck, upper chest, and antecubital and popliteal fossae
• Extremely pruritic.	
• Face involvement is seen as dry skin with mild to moderate erythema, perioral pallor, and skin folds beneath the eyes (Dennie-Morgan lines).	
• Associated with linear markings on the palms.	
Drug Eruption	
• Bright red erythematous macules and papules are found. Skin blisters in extreme cases.	• Generalized
• Lesions tend to be confluent in large areas.	
• Moderately pruritic.	• Involvement begins on trunk, proceeds distally (legs are the last to be involved)
• Fever is rare.	
• Dehydration and hypothermia can occur with extensive involvement.	
• Condition clears only after offending medication has been discontinued.	

---

with warm tap water to place over topical steroid preparations for short periods to facilitate absorption.

➤ Oil-Based Products

Oil-based ointments and pastes are not applied in the sweaty skin fold areas because increased maceration and blocking of pores may result in folliculitis. Instead, water-soluble creams are the vehicle of choice for these areas. Lotions and gels prevent matting of the hair and are more appropriate for hairy areas, such as the scalp. Finally, stiff pastes are used to apply therapy to localized areas because this vehicle clings to the skin where it is applied and resists spreading to uninvolved skin.

Cream preparations are indicated in clients with acute dermatitis with oozing and weeping. Chronic dermatitis responds more favorably to oil-based ointments that seal in moisture and help combat dryness and scaling.

➤ Antihistamines

Antihistamines provide some relief of pruritus but may fail to keep the client totally symptom free. The sedative effects of antihistamines can be minimized if the client takes most of the daily dose near bedtime.

➤ Compresses and Baths

Cool, moist compresses and tepid baths with bath additives have a soothing effect, decrease inflammation, and help debride crusts and scales. Colloidal oatmeal preparations, tar extracts, cornstarch, or oils are often added to baths to relieve pruritus (see Table 70–1).

PSORIASIS

Overview

Psoriasis is a lifelong disorder characterized by exacerbations and remissions. Even though psoriasis cannot be cured, clients can usually achieve control of symptoms with proper treatment.

Pathophysiology

Psoriasis is a scaling disorder with underlying dermal inflammation. Pathogenesis involves an abnormality in the proliferation of epidermal cells in the outer skin layers. Normally, cells at the basement membrane of the epidermis take about 27 days to reach the outermost stratum corneum, where they are shed. In a person with psoriasis, the rate of cell division is speeded up so that cells are shed every 4 to 5 days.

Etiology

The cause of psoriasis is not known. A genetic predisposition has been recognized in some cases; however, often there is no family history of the disease. Many environmental factors precipitate outbreaks and influence the severity of clinical symptoms, but these vary significantly from person to person. Triggering factors may be local or systemic. A psoriatic lesion may appear after skin trauma (Koebner's phenomenon), such as surgery, sunburn, or excoriation.

Clients with psoriasis seem to improve in warmer climates, where there is more exposure to sunlight. Systemic factors that can aggravate the disease include infections (severe streptococcal throat infection, *Candida* infection, upper respiratory tract infection), hormonal changes (during puberty and menopause), psychological stress, drugs (lithium, beta-blocking agents, indomethacin, antimalarials), obesity, and the presence of other diseases.

Incidence/Prevalence

The initial outbreak of psoriasis may occur at any age; the average age at onset is about 27 years. Psoriasis occurs equally among women and men, although the incidence is lower in darker-skinned races.

Collaborative Management

 Assessment

➤ History

In addition to collecting routine epidemiologic data, the nurse asks the client about any family history of psoriasis, including age at onset, a description of disease progression, and the pattern of recurrences. The nurse asks the client to describe the current flare of psoriasis, including whether the onset was gradual or sudden, where the lesions first appeared, whether the client observed any changes in severity over time, and whether associated symptoms (e.g., fever and pruritus) are present. Possible precipitating factors are explored, including recent skin trauma, upper respiratory tract infection, recent surgeries, menopause status, past and current use of medication, and recent stress-provoking occurrences. Finally, the nurse investigates previous treatment modalities and the effectiveness of each in initiating and maintaining remission of the disease.

➤ *Physical Assessment/Clinical Manifestations*

The appearance of psoriasis and its course vary among clients. Typically, during flares of the disease, lesions thicken and extend to involve new areas of the body. As psoriasis responds to treatment, individual lesions become thinner with less scaling.

Psoriasis Vulgaris. Psoriasis vulgaris, the most common presentation of psoriasis, is characterized by thick erythematous papules or plaques surmounted by silvery-white scales (Fig. 70–15*A*, *B*). Borders between the lesions and normal skin are sharply defined. As a result of maceration from perspiration, patches appear less red and more moist in skin fold areas. Lesions are usually distributed symmetrically; the more common sites are the scalp, elbows, trunk, knees, sacrum, and extensor surfaces of the limbs. The facial skin is rarely affected. The client may have only a few isolated lesions, or the entire skin surface may be affected.

Exfoliative Psoriasis. Exfoliative psoriasis (erythrodermic psoriasis) is an explosively eruptive form of the disease characterized by generalized erythema and scaling without obvious lesions. The nurse examines for signs of dehydration and hypothermia or hyperthermia related to this severe inflammatory reaction. The vasodilation and increased blood flow to the skin that occur with inflammation can alter fluid volume as a result of increased evaporative water loss from the skin surface.

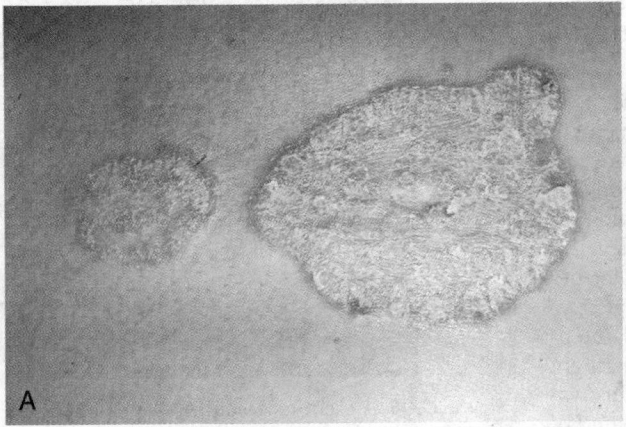
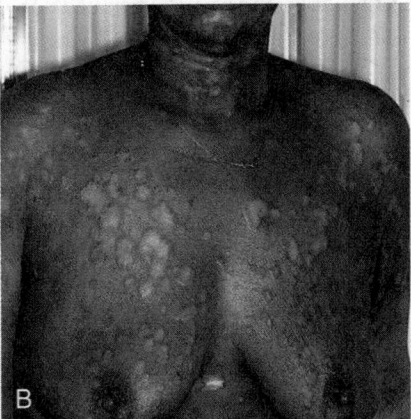

Figure 70–15. A. Psoriasis vulgaris in a Caucasian client. B. Psoriasis vulgaris in an African-American client.

✦ Interventions

The several approaches to therapy are based on the physician's preference and resistance of psoriasis to treatment. Therapy is aimed at decreasing epidermal proliferation and underlying inflammation.

➤ *Topical Therapy*

The pharmacologic and physical topical agents used to treat psoriasis are topical steroids, topical tar and anthralin preparations, and ultraviolet (UV) light.

Topical Steroids. Corticosteroids have antiinflammatory properties. When they are applied to psoriatic lesions, they suppress mitotic activity. The effectiveness of a topical steroid depends on its potency and ability to be absorbed into the skin. The more potent preparations are generally used to treat clients with psoriasis.

A simple procedure for enhancing the percutaneous penetration of these agents is for the steroid to be applied directly to the skin. This step is followed by warm, moist dressings and an occlusive outer wrap of plastic film, plastic gloves, booties, or similar garments. When large surface areas are involved, occlusive therapy is limited to 12 hours per day because of the increased risk of local and systemic side effects.

Tar Preparations. When a tar preparation is applied to the skin, it suppresses mitotic activity and produces an antiinflammatory effect. Preparations containing crude coal tar and derivations of crude coal tar are available as solutions, ointments, lotions, gels, and shampoos. The use of crude coal tar ointments is usually limited to inpatient care and specialized outpatient treatment clinics because they are messy, cause staining, and have an unpleasant odor.

Topical therapy with anthralin (Anthraforte✦, Drithocreme, Lasan), a hydrocarbon with action similar to that of tar, also relieves chronic psoriasis. Topical therapy is used in a variety of potencies alone and in combination with coal tar baths and UV light.

The nurse applies high-potency anthralin, suspended in a stiff paste, to individual lesions for short periods, not exceeding 2 hours. Because anthralin is a strong irritant and can cause chemical burns, the nurse observes for local tissue reaction and prevents inadvertent contact with uninvolved skin. Anthralin is not indicated for the treatment of acute, spreading psoriasis because it tends to induce Koebner's phenomenon (see Skin Cancer).

Ultraviolet (UV) Light Therapy. UV radiation is a physical agent commonly used as a topical treatment in many skin conditions, including psoriasis. Ultraviolet B (UVB) light, which produces more energy, is responsible for the obvious biological effects of the sun, such as burning. Ultraviolet A (UVA) light emits a lower level of energy, requiring longer exposure time before cellular destruction occurs. Although the sun is the least expensive source of UV radiation, control of availability and intensity in skin treatment are best obtained with artificial light sources. These sources include high-intensity mercury vapor lamps or specially constructed cabinets containing UV tubes.

In general, UV therapy is governed by the potency and distance of the source from the skin as well as the exposure time. Potency and distance remain constant, and the time of exposure is gradually increased to achieve a mild sunburn effect without burning or tenderness. Skin type, ranging from fair to darkly pigmented, reflects the client's susceptibility to burning and determines the initial and subsequent exposure times. Because of the extremely high intensity of most artificial UVB light sources, daily treatments are measured in seconds of exposure; clients must wear eye protection during treatment.

The nurse teaches clients to inspect the skin carefully each day for signs of overexposure. If clients complain of tenderness on palpation and have clinical signs of severe erythema or vesicle and bullae formation, the physician must be notified promptly before therapy is resumed.

Psoralen and UVA (PUVA) treatments are more common on an outpatient basis (Fig. 70–16). Clients ingest psoralen, a photosensitizing agent, 2 hours before exposure to UVA light. Because UVA light produces less energy than UVB light, the onset of erythema and pigmentation may be delayed as long as 96 hours after exposure. Treatments are limited to two to three times a week and are not given on consecutive days. Exposure is gradually increased until tanning occurs. As with UVB exposure, dosage corrections are adjusted according to the erythema reaction of normal skin as well as the response of psoriatic lesions.

The nurse observes for generalized erythema with edema and tenderness. Treatment must be interrupted until symptoms subside. Because of the strong photosen-

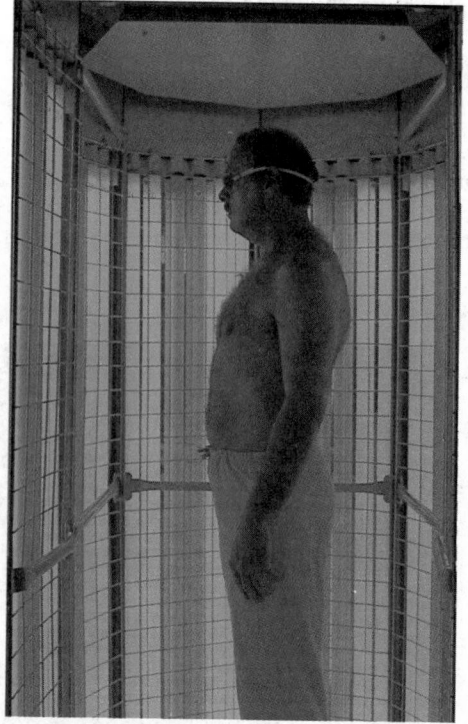

Figure 70–16. A client receiving PUVA treatment. (Courtesy of the Department of Dermatology, Baylor College of Medicine, Houston, TX.)

sitizing properties of psoralen, clients must wear dark glasses during treatment and for the remainder of the day.

Long-term side effects of both UVB and PUVA therapies include premature aging of the skin, actinic keratosis, and increased incidence of skin cancer.

➤ Systemic Therapy

Some clients have severe psoriasis that is resistant to topical therapy. In these instances, systemic treatment with a cytotoxic agent, such as methotrexate (Folex, Mexate), is warranted. Because of the hepatotoxic side effects of methotrexate, a liver biopsy is indicated before therapy is initiated and yearly thereafter. Relatively small doses are required to obtain clearing of lesions. This treatment of last resort is contraindicated if clients have liver damage, bone marrow suppression, or impaired renal function.

Because psoriasis has an autoimmune basis, some systemic agents that induce immunosuppression are used occasionally when lesions do not respond to other therapies. Such agents include cyclosporin (Sandimmune) and azathioprine (Imuran). The many health risks associated with these therapies must be considered along with the potential benefits.

➤ Emotional Support

Often clients' self-esteem suffers not only because of the presence of skin lesions but also because of the unpleasantness associated with some of the treatment modalities. Tar not only looks dirty but also has a very unpleasant odor. Bed linen and pajamas become stained, further discouraging social interaction.

The nurse encourages contact with other clients who have similar problems. Group discussions involving family members can increase the socialization process.

In addition, the use of touch takes on an added significance for clients with psoriasis. For example, the nurse shakes the client's hand during an introduction or places a hand on the client's shoulder when explaining a procedure. The nurse does not wear gloves during these social interactions. Touch, more than any other gesture, communicates acceptance of the person and the skin problem.

BENIGN TUMORS

Cysts

Overview

Cysts are firm, flesh-colored nodules that contain liquid or semisolid material. Unlike malignant growths, which are hard and firmly attached to underlying structures, a cyst is characterized by fluctuance and mobility on palpation. Often there is a central pore through which the material can be expressed if the lesion is squeezed.

The most common cyst is an epidermal inclusion cyst. These benign growths often occur spontaneously and are asymptomatic. They can be located anywhere on the body but occur most frequently on the head and trunk (Fig. 70–17). The most common cyst on the scalp is the sebaceous, or pilar, cyst.

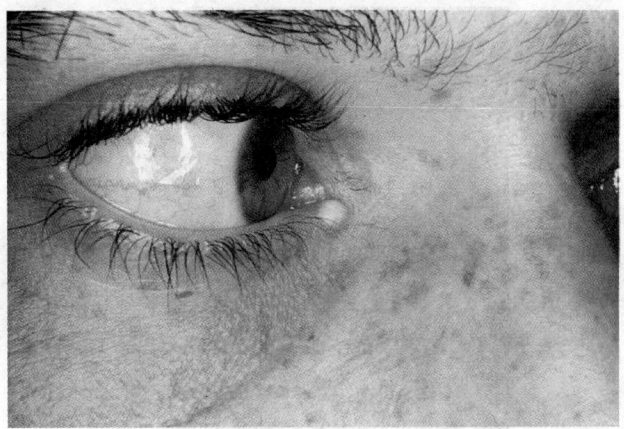

Figure 70–17. An epidermal inclusion cyst.

Collaborative Management

Therapy to remove cysts is rarely indicated. If the client prefers that the cyst be removed, surgical excision with primary closure is performed with a local anesthetic agent. The surgeon removes the entire cyst wall during excision to prevent recurrence.

A pilonidal cyst is a lesion of the sacral area that is often associated with a sinus track extending into deeper tissue structures. Because the lesion's proximity to the perineum may result in secondary infection, surgical incision and drainage are necessary.

Seborrheic Keratoses

Overview

Seborrheic keratoses are a common malady of older people. These benign epidermal neoplasms are gradually acquired after middle age and are often mistaken for actinic keratoses or pigmented skin cancers. These growths may occur anywhere on the body but are more commonly found on the face, neck, upper trunk, and arms.

Collaborative Management

On inspection, seborrheic keratoses appear as multiple "pasted-on" papules or plaques ranging in color from flesh tones to brown or black. The surface of the lesion has a rough, greasy, wart-like texture on palpation.

Seborrheic keratoses should be removed only for cosmetic reasons or if a lesion becomes irritated from friction or excoriation. Cryosurgery or curettage with or without local anesthetic is performed.

Keloids

Overview

A keloid is overgrowth of a scar resulting from an excessive accumulation of collagen and ground substance after skin trauma. Keloids are more common in darker-skinned people and often arise at sites of surgical incisions, burns, and ear piercing (Fig. 70–18).

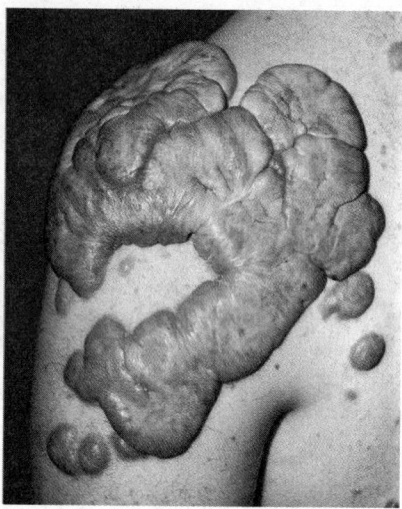

Figure 70–18. A keloid.

Collaborative Management

On physical examination, a keloid appears as an elevated, protruding lesion that extends well beyond the boundaries of the original injury. Treatment of these cosmetically disfiguring lesions is difficult and not always successful. Because surgical excision alone can result in a larger, more protuberant scar, surgery is usually combined with another form of therapy, such as intralesional steroid injections or low-dose radiotherapy. Pressure dressings or elastic garments worn over the skin for 1 year after excision or steroid injection may also help to keep the lesion flat.

Nevi

Overview

A nevus, or mole, is a benign neoplasm of the pigment-forming cells. These lesions are classified according to their location within the layers of the skin.

Collaborative Management

Normal nevi have regular, well-defined borders and are uniform in color, ranging from light colors to dark brown. The lesion's surface may be rough or smooth. Because about 50% of malignant melanomas arise from moles, nevi with irregular or spreading borders and those with variegated colors should be considered highly suspicious. Other abnormal findings include sudden changes in size of the lesion and complaints of itching or bleeding.

Unsightly nevi or those subject to repeated irritation or trauma can be removed. Biopsy of any suspicious lesions is performed to rule out malignancy.

Warts

Overview

Warts, or verrucae, are small tumors caused by papillomavirus infection of the skin cells. They may occur singly or in groups and are classified according to their anatomic location.

Common warts are raised, flesh-colored papules with a rough surface (Fig. 70–19). Although they may grow anywhere on the skin surface, they often occur on the hands and fingers.

Flat warts range in size from 2 to 4 mm. They appear as slightly elevated reddish-brown or flesh-colored papules with flat tops and minimal scale. These warts often multiply and affect the hands and the face.

An often painful wart occurring on the bottom of the foot is the plantar wart. Plantar warts are covered with a thick callus that, when removed, reveals tiny black dots (thrombosed capillaries).

Collaborative Management

The treatment of warts is aimed at destroying the skin cells containing the virus, a process that can be destructive and painful. Treatment modalities include surgical excision, electrodesiccation and curettage, and cryosurgery. Cryosurgery is usually preferred because local anesthetic is not required and scarring is less likely. Topical caustic agents, including salicylic acid and lactic acid, are also used. These agents are painted onto the surface of the lesion and result in destruction of the cells and peeling of the infected skin area.

Hemangiomas

Hemangiomas (angiomas) are vascular neoplasms and represent one of the most common of the benign tumors. The clinical presentation varies, from lesions that appear shortly after birth and gradually regress to those that are present at birth and gradually expand in size with growth.

Nevus flammeus is a congenital vascular hemangioma involving the mature capillaries. These lesions favor the face and the upper body and occur as well-demarcated macular patches ranging in color from pink to bluish-purple. Although nevus flammeus may gradually fade during the first years of life, a form of this neoplasm—the port-wine stain—grows proportionately with the child and remains unchanged in adult life. Port-wine

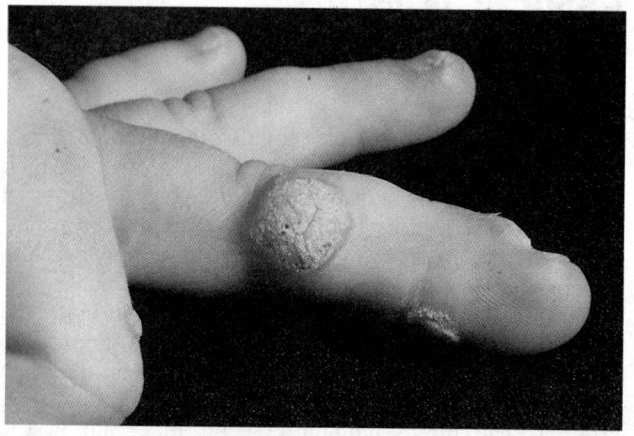

Figure 70–19. A common wart.

stains usually occur as solitary lesions but may vary in size.

The significance of nevus flammeus is cosmetic. Depending on the size of the lesion, surgical excision with or without skin grafting may be indicated. Treatment with laser therapy also is an alternative to surgery. Noninvasive treatment consists of masking the lesion by covering it with an opaque make-up.

The cherry hemangioma is often seen in elderly clients. These lesions are small, dome-shaped papules ranging in color from red to purple (see Fig. 69–14). Treatment is not indicated except for cosmetic reasons.

SKIN CANCER

Overview

Overexposure to sunlight is the major cause of skin cancer, although other factors also are associated. Because sun damage is an age-related skin finding, screening for suspicious lesions is an integral part of routine physical assessment of the elderly. The most common skin cancers are actinic or solar keratosis, squamous cell carcinoma, basal cell carcinoma, and melanoma.

Pathophysiology

Actinic keratoses are premalignant lesions involving the cells of the epidermis. These lesions are common in people with chronically sun-damaged skin (see Figure 69–16). Progression to squamous cell carcinoma may occur if lesions are untreated.

Squamous cell carcinomas are malignant neoplasms of the epidermis. They can invade locally and are potentially metastatic. Lesions on the ear, lip, and external genitalia are more likely to invade and metastasize than those found elsewhere on the body (Fig. 70–20). Chronic skin damage from repeated injury or irritation also predisposes to this malignancy.

Basal cell carcinomas arise in the basal cell layer of the epidermis (Fig. 70–21). Early malignant lesions often go unnoticed, and although metastasis is rare, underlying tissue destruction can progress to include vital structures. Genetic predisposition and chronic irritation are risk factors; however, ultraviolet (UV) radiation remains the primary carcinogen.

Melanomas are pigmented malignant lesions originating

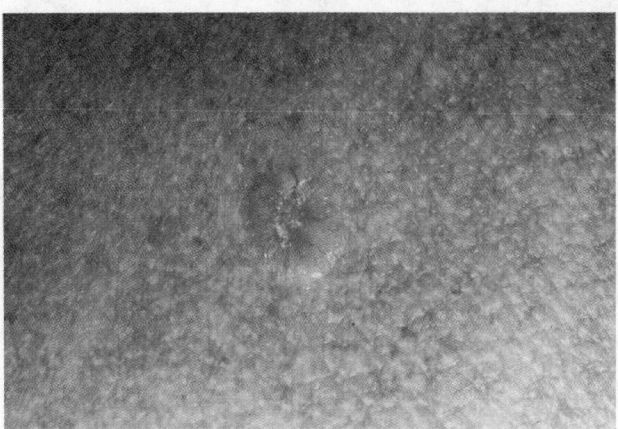

Figure 70–21. Basal cell carcinoma.

in the melanin-producing cells of the epidermis (Fig. 70–22). Risk factors include genetic predisposition, excessive exposure to UV light, and the presence of one or more precursor lesions that resemble unusual moles. *This skin cancer is highly metastatic, and a person's survival depends on early diagnosis and treatment.*

Incidence/Prevalence

The incidence of skin cancer is highest among light-skinned races and people older than 60 years (American Cancer Society, 1998). The incidence is higher among people who work outdoors and live at higher altitudes or lower latitudes. Occupational exposure to arsenic or other chemical carcinogens also increases risk. The incidence of malignant melanoma has rapidly increased during the past 30 years, accounting for 2% of all cancers and 1% of all cancer deaths (American Cancer Society, 1998).

The single most effective prevention strategy for skin cancer is avoiding or reducing skin exposure to sunlight. However, even when people understand the cause of skin cancer and the seriousness of the disease, preventive behaviors are not always practiced (see Research Applications for Nursing about risk beliefs).

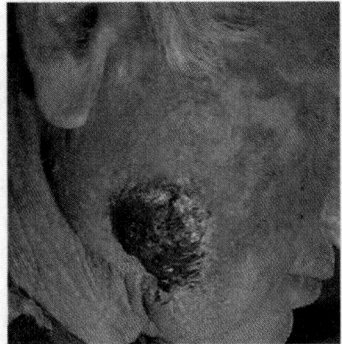

Figure 70–20. Squamous cell carcinoma.

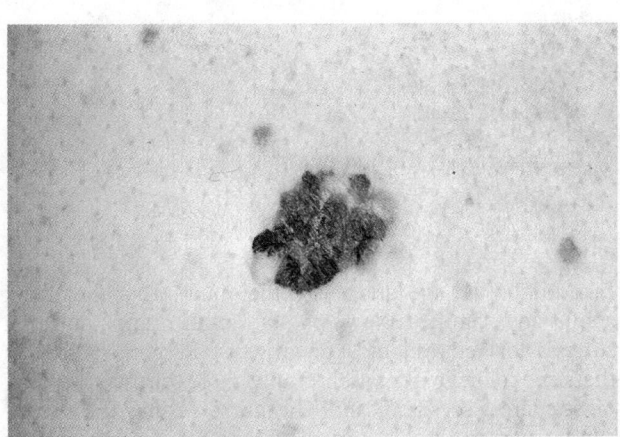

Figure 70–22. Melanoma.

▷ Research Applications for Nursing

Risk Beliefs and Preventive Practices in Conflict

Marlenga, B. (1995). Health beliefs and skin cancer prevention practices of Wisconsin dairy farmers. Oncology Nursing Forum, 22(4), 681–686.

This descriptive study of 202 male dairy farmers at high risk for skin cancer through occupational sun exposure revealed a conflict between preventive practices and health beliefs. Most farmers responding to the survey indicated that they knew that sun exposure is a major cause of skin cancer, that skin cancer was serious, that they had an increased risk for skin cancer because of their outdoor occupation, and that sun protection measures could be effective in reducing skin cancer. However, most of the participants indicated that they did not use precautions on a regular basis. Reasons cited for not taking precautions included that it was too hot or inconvenient, they forgot, and tanned skin was attractive. The investigator concluded that the perceived barrier was the only predictor of why dairy farmers did not practice sun protection and that perhaps an additional framework might provide a better explanation.

Critique. The study was appropriately designed for acquiring descriptive data, an important step before hypothesizing interventions. It is possible that the investigator may be misinterpreting the issue regarding participants' knowledge levels, an important component of the health belief model. Although the overall responses indicated that most participants knew that sun exposure increased the risk for skin cancer and considered skin cancer a serious problem, most did not know that melanoma is a type of skin cancer and could be fatal. In addition, most participants, while acknowledging an increased risk for skin cancer, were unaware that their lifetime skin cancer risk was as high as 1 in 4. Therefore, it is possible that such knowledge deficits contributed to a less strong belief in the seriousness of the problem.

Possible Nursing Implications. With a preventable cancer, the greatest impact nurses can have is encouragement of preventive practices. More information regarding personal risk and the degree of seriousness should be stressed. The investigator recommended strategies to increase awareness among farmers by including skin cancer education at rural high schools and making informational materials available at feed stores and other places frequented by dairy farmers.

Collaborative Management

 Assessment

In addition to age and race, the nurse asks the client about any family history of skin cancer and any past surgery for removal of skin growths. Recent changes in the size, color, or sensation of any mole, birthmark, wart, or scar are also significant. The nurse verifies the role of sun exposure by inquiring about geographic regions where the client has lived and currently resides and about

occupational and recreational activities in relation to sun exposure. Finally, the nurse explores an occupational history of exposure to chemical carcinogens (e.g., arsenic, coal tar, pitch, radioactive waste, and radium). The nurse also asks the client about any skin growths that are repeatedly irritated by the rubbing of clothes against them.

The skin cancers vary in their appearance and distribution. Although most of the cancerous lesions appear in sun-exposed areas of the body, the nurse inspects the entire skin surface. The nurse systematically examines the skin for any unusual lesions, particularly moles, warts, birthmarks, and scars. Hair-bearing areas of the body, such as the scalp and genitalia, are also examined. The nurse palpates lesions to determine their surface texture. The location, size, color, and surface characteristics of all lesions are documented as are any subjective reports of associated tenderness or itching.

Table 70–10 summarizes important facts about common skin cancers. Chart 70–8 lists activities that clients can use to reduce their risk for skin cancer.

Punch, shave, or excisional biopsy of suspicious lesions is necessary to confirm the diagnosis of a malignancy.

 Interventions

Nonsurgical and surgical interventions are combined for the most effective management of skin cancer. Specific treatment is determined by the size and severity of the malignancy, location of the lesion, and the age and general health of the client.

➤ Nonsurgical Management

Drug Therapy. Topical chemotherapy with 5-fluorouracil cream is reserved for treatment of clients with multiple actinic keratoses or, in rare instances, widespread superficial basal cell carcinoma that would require several surgical procedures to eradicate. Therapy is continued for several weeks; during this time, the treated areas become increasingly tender and inflamed as the lesions crust, ooze, and erode. The nurse prepares the client for an unsightly appearance during therapy and reassures the client that the cosmetic result is positive.

After treatment is discontinued, cool compresses and topical corticosteroid preparations help to decrease inflammation and promote comfort.

Systemic chemotherapeutic agents are rarely indicated in the treatment of cutaneous malignancy. These agents may be used, however, when the prognosis is poor, as in advanced metastatic melanoma.

Radiation Therapy. Radiation therapy for malignant skin lesions is limited to elderly clients with large, deeply invasive basal cell tumors and those clients who are poor risks for surgery. Primary malignant melanoma is resistant to radiation therapy; however, radiation therapy has proved of some value for clients with metastatic disease when used in combination with systemic corticosteroids.

Immunotherapy. An experimental treatment available at some centers for clients with melanoma that has metastasized to distant sites is a melanoma vaccine. This treat-

TABLE 70–10

Common Skin Cancers

Skin Cancer	Clinical Manifestations	Distribution	Course
Actinic keratosis (premalignant)	• Small (1–10 mm) macule or papule with dry, rough, adherent yellow or brown scale • Base may be erythematous • Associated with yellow, wrinkled weatherbeaten skin • Thick, indurated keratoses more likely to be malignant	• Cheeks, temples, forehead, ears, neck, backs of hands, and forearms	• May disappear spontaneously or reappear after treatment. • Slow progression to squamous cell carcinoma is possible.
Squamous cell carcinoma	• Firm, nodular lesion topped with a crust or with a central area of ulceration • Indurated margins • Fixation to underlying tissue with deep invasion	• Sun-exposed areas, especially head, neck, and lower lip • Sites of chronic irritation or injury (e.g., scars, irradiated skin, burns, and leg ulcers)	• Rapid invasion with metastasis via the lymphatics occurs in 10% of cases. • Larger tumors are more prone to metastasis.
Basal cell carcinoma	• Pearly papule with a central crater and rolled, waxy borders • Telangiectasias and pigment flecks visible on close inspection	• Sun-exposed areas, especially head, neck, and central portion of face	• Metastasis is rare. • May cause local tissue destruction. • 50% recurrence rate related to inadequate treatment.
Melanoma	• Irregularly shaped, pigmented papule or plaque • Variegated colors, with red, white, and blue tones	• Can occur anywhere on the body, especially where nevi (moles) or birthmarks are evident • Commonly found on upper back and lower legs • Soles of feet and palms in Asians and African-Americans	• Horizontal growth phase followed by vertical growth phase. • Rapid invasion and metastasis with high morbidity and mortality.

Chart 70–8

Health Promotion Guide: Prevention of Skin Cancer

• Avoid sun exposure between 11:00 AM and 3:00 PM.
• Use sunscreens with the appropriate skin protection factor for your skin type.
• Wear a hat, opaque clothing, and sunglasses when you are out in the sun.
• Examine your body monthly for possibly cancerous or precancerous lesions.
• Seek medical advice if you note any of the following:
  • A change in the color of a lesion, especially if it darkens or shows evidence of spreading
  • A change in the size of a lesion, especially rapid growth
  • A change in the shape of a lesion, such as a sharp border becoming irregular or a flat lesion becoming raised
  • Redness or swelling of the skin around a lesion
  • A change in sensation, especially itching or increased tenderness of a lesion
  • A change in the character of a lesion, such as oozing, crusting, bleeding, or scaling

ment takes advantage of distinctive cell surface proteins found on some melanomas that can act like antigens. Although this form of cancer therapy is new and, as yet, unapproved, it shows promise for this type of cancer (see Research Applications for Nursing about melanoma vaccine).

➤ Surgical Management

Surgical intervention ranges from local treatment of individual lesions, with minimal discomfort and positive cosmetic results, to massive excision of large areas of the skin.

Cryosurgery. Cryosurgery involves the local application of liquid nitrogen (−200° C) to isolated lesions, causing cell death and tissue destruction. Local anesthesia is seldom needed because clients experience only minor discomfort during the procedure. The nurse prepares clients for swelling and increased tenderness of the treated area when the skin thaws. Tissue freezing is followed in 1 or 2 days by hemorrhagic blister formation. The nurse instructs clients to clean the treatment sites with hydrogen peroxide to prevent infection. A topical antibiotic may also be ordered.

► Research Applications for Nursing

Can a Vaccine Control Melanoma?

Morton, D., & Barth, A. (1996). Vaccine therapy for malignant melanoma. CA: A Cancer Journal for Clinicians, 46(4), 225–244.

This 8-year clinical study of 75 clients with metastatic melanoma involved treatment with a living, whole-cell melanoma vaccine called CancerVax. The survival time and response rates for these clients were compared with those of 1,275 historical controls. Overall, clients who received the vaccine had a mean survival time of 23 months compared with 7.5 months mean survival time for the historical controls. More than 25% of clients receiving the vaccine survived 5 years or longer. Only 6% of historical controls survived up to 5 years after diagnosis. The creation of the vaccine was based on the fact that different proteins on the surface of melanoma cells were found to be capable of stimulating an immunologic response.

Critique. This study represents early clinical work. Much more testing using larger samples, double-blind methodologies, and randomization are needed.

Possible Nursing Implications. The results of this study are encouraging and may represent a new treatment modality for metastatic melanoma. Nurses may be able to instill hope to those clients with metastatic melanoma that research for their problem continues and progress is being made.

Curettage and Electrodesiccation. For clients who have small lesions with well-defined borders, curettage and electrodesiccation are used to destroy the cancerous cells while minimizing damage to the surrounding uninvolved tissue. After a local anesthetic is administered, the surgeon uses a semisharp dermal curette to scrape away the cancerous tissue. After curettage is complete, the surgeon places an electric probe on the wound surface, and malignant remnants of the tumor are destroyed by thermal and mechanical energy.

Wounds treated by curettage and electrodesiccation are allowed to heal by second intention. Scarring is usually minimal. The nurse instructs clients in caring for the wound, including cleaning the wound, using prescribed antibacterial medications, and applying prescribed dressings.

Excision. For clients with large or poorly defined skin cancers, recurrent tumors, and deeply invasive cancers, wide excision is required to remove the malignancy. If the size and location of the lesion permit, surgical excision with primary closure is the procedure of choice. If the tumor has already been removed several times or if radiation therapy has damaged the surrounding skin, healing by second intention is indicated. This procedure allows the wound to be carefully monitored for cancer recurrence. Skin grafts and flaps are used to repair large defects with deep-tissue destruction.

A specialized form of excision, Mohs' surgery, is used to treat basal and squamous cell carcinomas. The cancerous tissue is sectioned horizontally in layers, and each layer is examined histologically to determine the exact location of residual tumor cells. Although the procedure is long and tedious, cure rates are higher, and there is less sacrifice of healthy tissue compared with other surgical methods.

PLASTIC OR RECONSTRUCTIVE SURGERY

Overview

The aim of plastic or reconstructive surgery is to correct functional defects and alter physical appearance, processes that directly influence a person's concept of self. Unlike a medical illness that is unexpected, plastic surgery is usually an elective procedure. Surgical intervention is sought by clients who cannot perform activities of daily living (ADLs) as a result of an anatomic malformation or by those who are unsatisfied with their body image. In the United States, the decision to undergo plastic surgery is frequently a response to established social and cultural norms. Clients become self-conscious about unsightly scars, obvious facial lesions, disproportionate anatomic features, or changes in physical features associated with aging. In some instances, severe trauma or extensive surgical excision of soft tissue leads to acquired functional defects that warrant surgical correction. For example, breast reconstruction is commonly performed after radical mastectomy. This type of surgery not only serves an aesthetic purpose for some clients but also replaces lost anatomy and negates the need for a prosthesis.

Clients may request plastic surgery as a remedy for the normal changes in skin appearance that occur with aging. Loss of skin elasticity and redistribution of adipose tissue is progressive and especially noticeable around the eyes, near the cheeks, and on the neck. Fine facial wrinkles around the eyes and mouth are one of the first signs of aging, followed by gradual stretching and downward displacement of the soft tissue of the lower two thirds of the face. Similar changes in skin texture contribute to wrinkling and flaccidity of skin on the upper extremities, the chest, the abdomen, buttocks, and thighs, a problem also seen after dramatic weight loss. Gradual appearance of skin lesions associated with chronic sun exposure may trouble the aging client.

Collaborative Management

 Assessment

► History

When taking a history from a client who elects to have plastic surgery, the nurse uses a nonjudgmental approach and is careful not to assume the reason for surgery on the basis of physical appearance. Often what might appear to be unsightly to the nurse is of little concern to the client, who wishes to change something else. The nurse also observes for any nonverbal communication that might establish the emotional state of the person or reveal feelings of embarrassment or guilt. The nurse encourages the client to describe the problem, including why it is bothersome and what the client expects as a result of the change. The client is asked about both health history and recent medical problems, including obesity and trauma, to predict the amount of surgery needed to correct the defect and potential complications.

➤ *Physical Assessment/Clinical Manifestations*

The client seeking plastic surgery may have alterations in appearance ranging from minor to significant deformity. Depending on the location of the deformity, the client may need to disrobe before the examination. The client may be embarrassed by the problem, and the nurse ensures privacy.

The nurse begins the physical assessment by closely examining the area of involvement to determine the extent of the deformity or problem. Having the client assume different normal sitting and standing postures may provide better visibility of nonfacial defects. The nurse notes any asymmetry of anatomic features, wrinkling or skin redundancy, scars or disfiguring skin marks, and any obvious skin lesions.

➤ *Psychosocial Assessment*

The nurse addresses the client's expectations of plastic surgery. Often people who seek plastic surgery have unrealistic expectations or are uncertain about what they actually want. For example, the client with minor deformities who is seeking perfection is sure to be disappointed. The client who wants an operation mainly to please the spouse or partner is also a poor candidate. The client's psychological outlook before surgery should be positive if results are to be therapeutic.

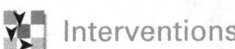 Interventions

➤ *Surgical Management*

Depending on the planned intervention, surgery is performed either in the outpatient setting under local anesthesia or in the hospital. Most clients scheduled for plastic surgery will have had several office consultations with their physician to discuss the planned intervention, possible complications, and postoperative expectations. The indications and complications of common cosmetic procedures are summarized in Table 70–11.

Many plastic surgeons use photography both as a visual aid when discussing clients' problems and as a means of documentation before and after surgical intervention. Pictures taken of clients are confidential. Showing clients pictures of other clients is done only after proper consent is obtained.

Preoperative Care. Because of the large amount of blood loss associated with skin (particularly facial) surgery, the nurse instructs the client to avoid ingestion of salicylates for several weeks before and after the procedure. Immediate preoperative care is focused on collection of any routine laboratory test data required before general anesthesia and preparation of the operative site. In most cases, the procedure for shaving and washing the skin is dictated by physician's preference.

Clients undergoing facial surgery, specifically rhytidectomy (face-lift), are frequently asked to wash their hair several times with antibacterial soap to decrease bacterial flora near the incision site. The nurse instructs clients to remove any make-up and avoid using face creams before surgery. If a rhinoplasty (reconstruction of the nose) is scheduled, the nurse prepares clients for the early postoperative period by explaining the need for nasal packing to control bleeding and by reviewing mouth-breathing techniques.

Operative Procedure. Reconstructive procedures vary extensively depending on the location, purpose, and extent of reconstruction. Ironically, in performing plastic surgery, the surgeon must inflict a potentially disfiguring wound to correct existing skin deformities.

Postoperative Care. Postoperative care focuses on monitoring for complications associated with surgical intervention (see Chap. 21). Pressure dressings may be applied at the time of surgery and left in place for several days to control hemorrhage and edema formation. The nurse checks dressings and any nasal packing for bright-red bleeding and monitors changes in vital signs and level of consciousness indicating active hemorrhage.

Repeated swallowing followed by belching after rhinoplasty is a sign of postnasal bleeding, and the nurse reports such a sign immediately to the surgeon. The client who has had breast surgery may have drains in place postoperatively, and the nurse monitors the amount and color of drainage. If a rhytidectomy, blepharoplasty (removal of "bags" around the eyes), or rhinoplasty has been performed, the nurse places the client in a semi-Fowler's position to minimize edema and promote comfort.

Additional comfort measures, such as the application of ice packs or cold compresses, are instituted as ordered. Special support garments are often indicated after breast augmentation surgery to minimize edema and tension on the suture line from the weight of the breast tissue.

The nurse monitors for signs and symptoms of wound infection and progress toward healing. Of particular concern are any areas of skin necrosis or eschar formation near the operative site, a complication related to excessive tension on the suture line from edema and subsequent obstruction of microcirculation. (For a description of criteria used to monitor wound infection, see Table 70–8.)

Regardless of the planned procedure, the nurse prepares the client preoperatively for edema and discoloration of the operative site. Swelling and ecchymosis alter the facial features and may not resolve for several weeks after surgery. The nurse reminds the client that the true results of surgery will not be visible until healing is complete, usually 6 months to a year or longer postoperatively.

TABLE 70–11

Common Plastic Surgical Procedures

Procedure	Description	Indications	Complications
Blepharoplasty	• Excision of bulging fat and redundant skin of the periorbital area with primary closure	• Bags under the eyes	• Hematoma • Ectropion • Corneal injury • Visual loss (rare) • Wound infection (rare)
Breast augmentation (augmentation mammaplasty)	• Insertion of synthetic breast-shaped implants through a skin incision	• Inadequate breast volume or contour	• Hematoma or hemorrhage • Wound infection (with gram-positive organisms) • Phlebitis
Breast reduction (reduction mammaplasty)	• Excision of excessive breast tissue and skin with primary closure	• Hypertrophy of breast tissue caused by elevated hormone levels, endocrine abnormalities, or obesity	• Hematoma or hemorrhage • Nipple, areola, and skin flap necrosis • Wound infection • Fat necrosis • Wound dehiscence
Dermabrasion	• Abrasive removal of the facial epidermis and a portion of the dermis followed by healing by second intention	• Moderate to severe acne scars • Deep wrinkling • Multiple actinic keratoses • Hyperpigmentation (postinflammatory or after the use of estrogens)	• Hypertrophic scarring • Altered skin pigmentation • Acne flare • Wound infection (rare)
Rhinoplasty	• Removal of excessive cartilage and tissue from the nose with correction of septal defects if indicated	• Disproportionate nasal anatomy • Post-traumatic nasal deformity	• Hematoma or hemorrhage • Ecchymosis and edema (temporary) • Wound infection (with gram-positive organisms) • Septal perforation • Minor skin irritation
Rhytidectomy (face-lift)	• Removal of excess skin and tissue from the face at the level of the hairline followed by primary closure	• Excessive wrinkling or sagging of facial skin	• Hematoma or hemorrhage • Facial nerve damage (temporary or permanent) • Wound infection • Ecchymosis and edema (temporary) • Skin necrosis • Hair loss
Liposuction (suction lipectomy)	• Removal of subcutaneous fat from localized areas of accumulation such as the hips, abdomen, neck and arms	• Disproportionate distribution of adipose tissue	• Hematoma • Severe pain • Infection • Emboli • Sagging of skin (if skin is not elastic enough to contract after fat removal)

OTHER SKIN DISORDERS

Acne

Overview

Acne is a red pustular eruption affecting the sebaceous glands of the epidermis. It is a common condition that, despite popular belief, is not confined to adolescents. Lesions result from increased sebum production, stimulated by elevated androgenic hormones and obstruction of the sebaceous canal outlet. Accumulation of debris leads to proliferation of bacteria and eventual rupture of the sebaceous gland into the surrounding dermis with inflammation.

Collaborative Management

Acne is a progressive disorder that results in the clinical appearance of several types of lesions, including noninflammatory comedones (blackheads and whiteheads), inflammatory papules, pustules, and cysts. Distribution of lesions is usually limited to the face and upper trunk (Fig. 70–23).

Control of the disorder is possible, with spontaneous remission occurring over time. However, severe eruptions or chronic inflammation can lead to extensive scarring.

For clients with superficial lesions and comedones, topical agents (retinoic acid, benzoyl peroxide, antibiotic solutions) are used. Systemic antibiotics, with tetracycline the drug of choice, are indicated for those with inflammatory disease. Clients with severe acne have undergone dramatic improvement after receiving isotretinoin (Accutane, Accutane Roche✦). Side effects include elevated liver function test results and dry, chapped skin. The most important concern, however, is the teratogenic effect of systemic retinoic acid. A pregnancy test is required before therapy, and strict birth control measures are used during therapy.

Lichen Planus

Overview

Lichen planus is a fairly common skin disorder characterized by purple, flat-topped papules that are pruritic. Al-

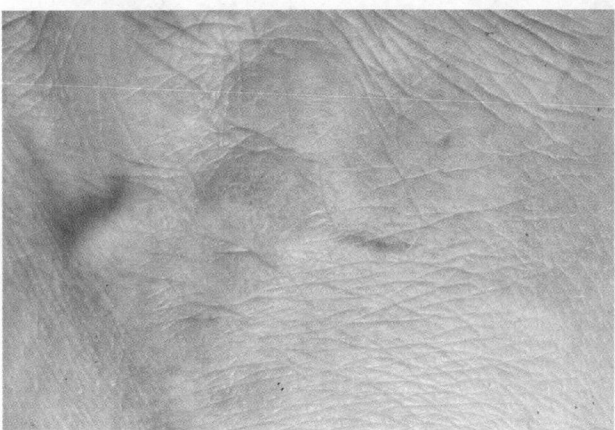

Figure 70–24. Lichen planus.

though viral infections and emotional stress may be possible causes, lichen planus remains an idiopathic disorder. The course of the disease can be chronic, or it can resolve spontaneously.

Collaborative Management

Lesions of lichen planus are usually distributed over the wrists and the inner surfaces of the forearms, but they may also be present on the lower legs, genitalia, and other body areas. Oral lesions may occur alone or in combination with skin changes. Unlike the skin lesions, mucosal lesions have a characteristic white lace-like appearance, usually on the buccal mucosa and are often confused with thrush (Fig. 70–24).

Treatment is symptomatic. Topical steroids help to reduce inflammation, and antihistamines help to relieve pruritus. Occasionally, systemic steroids are warranted when involvement is widespread, but long-term use is avoided because of the associated toxicity.

Pemphigus Vulgaris

Overview

Pemphigus vulgaris is a rare, chronic blistering disease with high morbidity and mortality. It is caused by an autoimmune disorder that occurs predominantly during middle and old age.

Collaborative Management

The acute lesions of pemphigus vulgaris occur on non-erythematous, normal-appearing skin or mucous membrane surfaces as fragile, flaccid bullae (Fig. 70–25). Disruption of the bullae leaves partial-thickness wounds that bleed, weep, and eventually form crusts.

Distribution is generalized; the initial lesions usually occur on the oral mucosa; later lesions form on the trunk. Spread of the disease is characterized by the appearance of new lesions, particularly on the face and in skin fold areas, whereas older lesions are in the process of

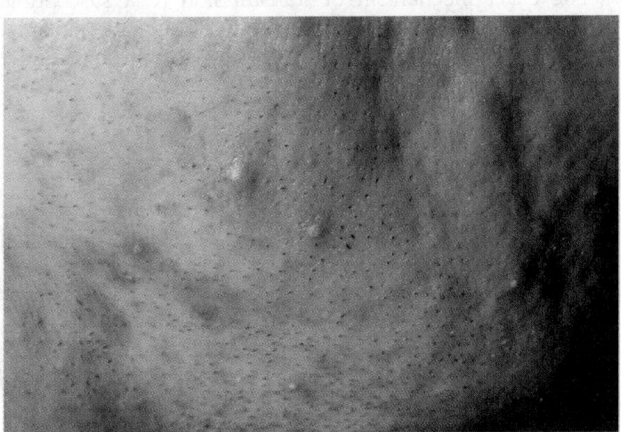

Figure 70–23. Acne.

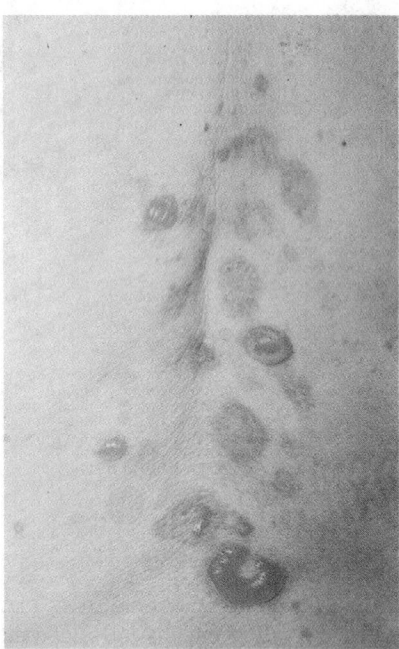

Figure 70–25. Pemphigus vulgaris.

healing. Oral lesions are common and can interfere with chewing and swallowing.

Treatment of pemphigus vulgaris is aimed at suppressing the immune response that causes the blister formation. Systemic steroids and cytotoxic agents are used to bring about remission. Topical antibiotic creams or ointments are used to minimize bacterial infection of the unhealed lesions.

Toxic Epidermal Necrolysis

Overview

Toxic epidermal necrolysis (TEN) is a rare, acute drug reaction of the skin characterized by diffuse erythema and bullae formation. Mucous membranes are often involved, and marked systemic toxicity is evident. The drugs most frequently implicated in triggering this disease are sulfonamides, pyrazolones, barbiturates, and antibiotics. Removal of the offending agent is usually followed by gradual healing in 2 to 3 weeks, with widespread peeling of the epidermis.

Collaborative Management

The drug thought to be causing a toxic reaction is discontinued, and therapy is aimed at systemic support and prevention of secondary infection. Clients with TEN are often admitted to burn units where fluid and electrolyte balance, caloric intake, and potential problems with hypothermia can be closely monitored. Topical antibacterial agents are used to suppress bacterial growth until healing occurs. Systemic steroids are not beneficial in the treatment of clients with TEN and, because of the increased risk for infection, are avoided.

Frostbite

Overview

Cold injury of the skin depends on the intensity of the external temperature, the duration of exposure to cold temperatures, and the relative hypoxia of the tissues at the time of exposure. Cell death occurs as a result of inadequate tissue oxygenation owing to cold-induced blood vessel constriction. With continued exposure to the cold, vascular necrosis and gangrene are imminent. Factors that increase the risk for cold injury are age, immobility, alcohol use, vascular disease, and psychiatric disorders.

Collaborative Management

Acute frostbite is ideally treated in the hospital setting, with rapid and continuous rewarming of the tissue in a water bath (90°–107° F; 32°–42° C) for 15 to 20 minutes or until flushing of the skin occurs. Slow thawing or interrupted periods of warmth are avoided because they can contribute to increased cellular damage. Thawing can cause considerable pain, and the nurse administers analgesics as ordered.

After thawing, the extremity is left exposed so that local tissue changes can be monitored. Blisters are left intact. With time, the degree of actual tissue destruction becomes evident as an eschar forms. After an eschar is evident, local care of the wound is similar to that for skin trauma. Complications of cold injury include amputation, scarring, depigmentation, and thickened nail plates.

Leprosy

Overview

Leprosy (Hansen's disease) is a chronic, contagious, systemic mycobacterial infection of the peripheral nervous system with secondary skin involvement. The clinical course of the disease is either progressive or self-limiting, depending on the immunologic status of the host. Although often thought to be extinct, Hansen's disease is found in the United States; most cases are reported in Florida, Louisiana, Texas, New York, California, and Hawaii.

The exact mechanism of transmission to a susceptible host remains unknown. Clinical studies suggest transmission via the airborne route, by insects, or through direct contact with skin lesions.

Collaborative Management

Clinical manifestations of leprosy, including any skin changes, are directly related to the degree of individual resistance to the mycobacteria:

- Localized (high-immunity) leprosy is characterized by one or two isolated, erythematous, anesthetic plaques that are hairless and sometimes scaly in texture.
- Generalized (low-immunity) leprosy involves widespread faintly erythematous macules, papules, nodules, and plaques.

Varying degrees of diminished skin sensation of the lesions are caused by the concomitant peripheral nerve damage.

Modern treatment is available on an outpatient basis. The aim is to control bacterial proliferation and minimize associated physical deformities. The drug of choice is dapsone (DDS, Avlosulfon✱), a sulfone with relatively few side effects that clients must take for life. In clients with sulfone-resistant disease, other antibacterial drugs are indicated.

NAIL DISORDERS

Ingrown Toenail

Overview

Although seemingly a minor problem, an ingrown toenail (unguis incarnatus) can be troublesome. Pain and local infection result when the edge of the nail plate grows into the soft pulp of the toe.

Collaborative Management

Conservative management is aimed at controlling local infection while encouraging the nail edges to grow beyond the level of the pulp, where the nail plate can be trimmed transversely. The client soaks the foot in warm water (to which an antiseptic has been added) for 20 to 30 minutes. The softened nail plate is gently lifted, and a small piece of gauze is inserted between the nail and the flesh on each side. This procedure is repeated twice daily until the nail has grown beyond the flesh so that it can be cut.

An ingrown toenail can be treated more aggressively with a surgical wedge excision of the nail plate. However, the pain of surgical removal can be severe, and recurrence is possible if the nail bed is not completely destroyed.

Hypertrophy

Thickening of the nail plate (onychauxis) is associated with a number of disorders, including fungal infections, psoriasis, lichen planus, and chronic dermatitis. Because topical preparations, such as antifungal agents, cannot penetrate the thickened nail plate, oral antifungal agents are the treatment of choice if fungus is a problem. Local psoralen and ultraviolet A (PUVA) treatments and oral vitamin A can relieve hypertrophy caused by psoriasis; however, response to any treatment (regardless of the underlying cause) is slow.

⊕ CASE STUDY for the Client with a *Candida* Skin Infection

■ You are assigned to make a home visit and perform an initial nursing assessment on a 92-year-old white female with a diagnosis of right lower lobe pneumonia. The client is bedridden and confused, requiring the constant care of her 68-year-old daughter, who lives with the client. While you are completing a head-to-toe skin assessment, the daughter explains that the mother "can't control her urine." On removing the adult briefs, you note that the client grimaces. The perineal area is inflamed with denuded areas of skin that are open and weeping. A red papular rash is also observed in the gluteal fold and groin areas.

QUESTIONS:

1. What assessment information do you need to document?
2. What additional skin assessment data do you need to collect and document?
3. What priority nursing actions do you need to implement?
4. What expected outcomes would be specific to this situation?

SELECTED BIBLIOGRAPHY

American Cancer Society. (1998). *Cancer facts and figures*. Atlanta: Author.

Anderson, R., & Muksad, D. (1994). Psychologic adjustments to reconstructive surgery. *Nursing Clinics of North America, 29*(4), 711–724.

*Arnold, H., Odum, R., & James, W. (1990). *Diseases of the skin: Clinical dermatology* (2nd ed.). Philadelphia: W. B. Saunders.

Barr, J. (1995). Physiology of healing: The basis for the principles of wound management. *MedSurg Nursing, 4*(5), 387–392.

Barr, J., & Cuzzell, J. (1996). Wound care clinical pathway: A conceptual model. *Ostomy/Wound Management, 42*(7), 18–26.

Benbow, M. (1995a). Intrinsic factors affecting the management of chronic wounds. *British Journal of Nursing, 4*(7), 407–410.

Benbow, M. (1995b). Parameters of wound assessment. *British Journal of Nursing, 4*(11), 647–651.

Bjorgen, S. (1998). Clinical snapshot: Herpes zoster. *American Journal of Nursing, 98*(2), 46–47.

Black, J. (1994). Surgical management of pressure ulcers. *Nursing Clinics of North America, 29*(4), 801–808.

Black, J. (1996). Surgical options in wound healing. *Critical Care Nursing Clinics of North America, 8*(2), 169–182.

Camisa, C. (1995). Treatment of severe psoriasis with systemic drugs. *Dermatology Nursing, 7*(2), 107–120.

Cassidy, S. (1996). Pressure ulcers: Prevention and treatment. *The Journal of Care Management, 2*(Suppl.), 3–10.

Cuzzell, J. (1995). Wound healing: Translating theory into clinical practice. *Dermatology Nursing, 1*(2), 127–131.

Cuzzell, J., & Krasner, D. (1995). Wound dressings. In P. Gogia (Ed.), *Clinical wound management* (pp. 131–145). Thorofare, NJ: SLACK, Inc.

Dealey, C. (1995). Common problems in wound care: Caring for the skin around wounds. *British Journal of Nursing, 4*(1), 43–44.

Erwin-Toth, P., & Hocevar, B. (1995). Wound Care: Selecting the right dressing. *American Journal of Nursing, 95*(2), 46–51.

Fenske, N., Grayson, L., & Newcomer, V. (1992). Tips for treating aging skin. *Patient Care, 26*(6), 61–64, 67, 70, 71.

*Fewkes, J., & Mohs, F. E. (1987). Dermatologic surgery: Microscopically controlled surgical excision (the Mohs technique). In T. B. Fitzpatrick, A. Z. Eisen, K. Wolff, I. M. Freedberg, & K. F. Austen (Eds.), *Dermatology in general medicine* (3rd ed., pp. 2557–2563). New York: McGraw-Hill.

Fowler, M. (1994). Body contouring surgery. *Nursing Clinics of North America, 29*(4), 753–761.

Frankel, E. (1995). Psoriasis. *Journal of the American Academy of Nurse Practitioners, 7*(5), 237–240.

Guyton, A., & Hall, J. (1996). *Textbook of medical physiology* (9th ed.). Philadelphia: W. B. Saunders.

Hanson, D., Langemo, D., Olson, B., Hunter, S., & Burd, C. (1996). Decreasing the prevalence of pressure ulcers. *Home Healthcare Nurse, 14*(7), 525–531.

Hardy, M. (1996). What can you do about your patient's dry skin? *Journal of Gerontological Nursing, 22*(5), 10–18.

Henderson, C., Ayello, E., Sussman, C., et al. (1997). Draft definition of stage I pressure ulcers: Inclusion of persons with darkly pigmented skin. *Advances in Wound Care, 10*(5), 16–19.

Jubeck, M. (1994). Teaching the elderly: A commonsense approach. *Nursing94, 24*(5), 70–71.

Krasner, D., & Cuzzell, J. (1995). Pressure ulcers. In P. Gogia (Ed.), *Clinical wound management*. Thorofare, NJ: Slack, Inc.

Kravitz, M. (1996). Outpatient wound care. *Critical Care Nursing Clinics of North America, 8*(2), 217–223.

*Lookingbill, D. B., & Marks, J. G., Jr. (1993). *Principles of dermatology* (2nd ed.). Philadelphia: W. B. Saunders.

Maklebust, J. (1995). Pressure ulcers: What works. *RN, 58*(9), 46–51.

*Marks, R. (1987). *Skin disease in old age*. Philadelphia: J. B. Lippincott.

Marlenga, B. (1995). Health beliefs and skin cancer prevention practices of Wisconsin dairy farmers. *Oncology Nursing Forum, 22*(4), 681–686.

Matteson, M. (1997). Age-related changes in the integument. In M. Matteson, E. McConnell, & A. Linton (Eds.), *Gerontological nursing: Concepts and practice* (2nd ed., pp. 174–195). Philadelphia: W. B. Saunders.

*McGovern, M., & Kuhn, J. (1992). Skin assessment of the elderly client. *Journal of Gerontologic Nursing, 18*(4), 39–43.

Milward, P. (1995). Common problems associated with necrotic and sloughy wounds. *British Journal of Nursing, 4*, 896–900.

Morton, D., & Barth, A. (1996). Vaccine therapy for malignant melanoma. *CA: A Cancer Journal for Clinicians, 46*(4), 225–244.

Motta, G. (1995). Moistening up for good healing. *Nursing95, 25*(4), 32H–32J.

Murray, M., & Blaylock, B. (1994). Maintaining effective pressure ulcer prevention programs. *MedSurg Nursing, 3*(2), 85–92.

Netscher, D., & Clamon, J. (1994). Methods of reconstruction. *Nursing Clinics of North America, 29*(4), 725–739.

Nichols, P. (1994). When your resident has scabies. *Geriatric Nursing, 15*(5), 271–273.

Pontieri-Lewis, V. (1995a). Pressure ulcers: Assessment to evaluation. *MedSurg Nursing, 4*(3), 220–221.

Pontieri-Lewis, V. (1995b). Therapeutic beds: An overview. *MedSurg Nursing, 4*(4), 323–324, 330.

Skewes, S. (1996). Skin care rituals that do more harm than good. *American Journal of Nursing, 96*(10), 33–35.

Smith, L., Booth, N., Douglas, D., Robertson, W., Walker, A., Durie, M., Fraser, A., Hillan, E., & Swaffield, J. (1995). A critique of "at risk" pressure sore assessment tools. *Journal of Clinical Nursing, 4*(3), 153–159.

Spencer, K. (1994). Selection and preoperative preparation of plastic surgery patients. *Nursing Clinics of North America, 29*(4), 697–710.

Urist, M. (1996). Surgical management of primary cutaneous melanoma. *CA: A Cancer Journal for Clinicians, 46*(4), 217–224.

*U.S. Department of Health and Human Services. (1992a). *Pressure ulcers in adults: Prediction and prevention* (Clinical Practice Guideline No. 3). Rockville, MD: Agency for Health Care Policy and Research.

*U.S. Department of Health and Human Services. (1992b). *Preventing pressure ulcers: A patient's guide* (Clinical Practice Guideline No. 3). Rockville, MD: Agency for Health Care Policy and Research.

VandenBosch, T., Montoye, C., Satwicz, M., Durkee-Leonard, K., & Boylan-Lewis, B. (1996). Predictive validity of the Braden Scale and nurse perception in identifying pressure ulcer risk. *Applied Nursing Research, 9*(2), 80–86.

Viehbeck, M., McGlynn, J., & Harris, S. (1995). Pressure ulcers and wound healing: Educating the spinal cord injured individual on the effects of cigarette smoking. *SCINursing, 12*(3), 73–76.

White, M. (1996). Surgical management of melanoma. *Allegheny General Hospital Oncology Journal,* Summer, 5–12.

Williams, L. (1994). Facial rejuvenation. *Nursing Clinics of North America, 29*(4), 741–751.

Young, T. (1995a). Common problems in wound care: Cleansing. *British Journal of Nursing, 4*(5), 286, 288, 289.

Young, T. (1995b). Common problems in wound care: Overgranulation. *British Journal of Nursing, 4*(3), 169–170.

SUGGESTED READINGS

Barr, J. (1995). Physiology of healing: The basis for the principles of wound management. *MedSurg Nursing, 4*(5), 387–392.

This excellent article provides a comprehensive view of the physiology of wound healing. Suggestions for wound cleansing and wound dressing are based on the specific characteristics of the wound.

Cuzzell, J. (1995). Wound healing: Translating theory into clinical practice. *Dermatology Nursing, 1*(2), 127–131.

This article uses outstanding photographs to present specific skin problems graphically. Nursing actions, both protective and therapeutic, are described clearly and appropriate to the problems presented.

Frankel, E. (1995). Psoriasis. *Journal of the American Academy of Nurse Practitioners, 7*(5), 237–240.

The article is an excellent review of the types of presentation and clinical manifestations associated with psoriasis and those that are frequently misdiagnosed as psoriasis. Color photos enhance the article. Self-assessment questions are attached.

Motta, G. (1995). Moistening up for good healing. *Nursing95, 25*(4), 32H–32J.

A comprehensive discussion of the effects of moisture-retentive dressings is provided in concise language. The article contains a table to guide the reader in selecting an appropriate dressing for a specific wound.

Williams, L. (1994). Facial rejuvenation. *Nursing Clinics of North America, 29*(4), 741–751.

This article reviews common types of plastic surgery for facial aging or scarring. Explanations of the operative procedures are provided as are descriptions of the expected postoperative courses.

INTERVENTIONS FOR CLIENTS WITH BURNS

Clients with burns of the skin and other tissues experience many physiologic, metabolic, and psychological changes. These injuries, regardless of cause, can range from loss of small segments of the outermost layers of the skin to an injury involving loss to all layers of the skin with complex involvement of all body systems. To assist burn clients, nurses need a thorough understanding of the pathophysiologic changes and treatment modalities throughout the phases of injury and healing. In addition, collaboration with a multidisciplinary team of health care providers is essential to ensure optimal care and improve client outcomes.

PATHOPHYSIOLOGY OF BURN INJURY

The tissue destruction caused by a burn injury may result in many local and systemic disturbances, including fluid and protein losses, sepsis, and abnormalities of the metabolic, endocrine, respiratory, cardiac, hematologic, and immune systems. The extent of local and systemic disruption is related to many factors, including age, general health status, and the extent and depth of injury. Even

after healing, the burn injury can cause late complications such as contracture and hypertrophic scarring. Burn wound healing and prevention of infection are vitally important. Lack of or delay in healing is the key mediator of all systemic disturbances and the major factor in morbidity and mortality among burn victims.

Integumentary Changes Resulting from Burn Injury

Anatomic Changes

The skin is the largest organ of the body (see Chap. 69). Each of its two major layers, the epidermis and dermis, has several sublayers. The epidermis, the outer layer of skin, is a superficial layer of stratified epithelial tissues, approximately 0.15 mm thick (somewhat thinner in the older adult). This layer can regenerate continually after a significant injury because epidermal cells surrounding hair follicles and sweat and oil glands extend into dermal tissue and are responsible for healing of partial-thickness wounds. The epidermis has no blood vessels and receives nutrients by diffusion of fluid from the second layer of skin, the dermis.

TABLE 71–1

Comparison of Burn Depth Classification Systems

Characteristic	Classification by Burn Degree				Classification by Burn Thickness				
	First-Degree	Second-Degree	Third-Degree	Fourth-Degree	Superficial	Partial-Thickness Superficial	Partial-Thickness Deep	Full-Thickness	Deep Full-Thickness
Color	Pink to red	Red	Red, white, brown, yellow, black	Black	Pink to red	Pink to red	Red to white	Black, brown, yellow, white, red	Black
Edema	Mild	Moderate	Severe	Absent	Mild	Mild to moderate	Moderate	Severe	Absent
Pain	Yes	Yes	Usually absent	Absent	Yes	Yes	Yes	Yes and no	Absent
Blisters	No	Yes	No	No	No	Yes	Rare	No	No
Eschar	No	No	Yes, hard and inelastic	Yes, hard and inelastic	No	No	Yes, soft and dry	Yes, hard and inelastic	Yes, hard and inelastic
Healing time	3–5 days	2–6 wk	Weeks to months	Weeks to months	3–5 days	~2 wk	2–6 wk	Weeks to months	Weeks to months
Grafts required	No	Can be used if healing is prolonged	Yes	Yes	No	No	Can be used if healing is prolonged	Yes	Yes
Example	Sunburn, flash burns	Scalds, flames, brief contact with hot objects	Scalds; flames; prolonged contact with hot objects, tar, grease, chemicals	Scalds; flames; prolonged contact with hot objects, tar, grease, chemicals, electricity	Sunburn, flash burns	Scalds, flames, brief contact with hot objects	Scalds; flames; prolonged contact with hot objects, tar, grease, chemicals	Scalds; flames; prolonged contact with hot objects, tar, grease, chemicals, electricity	Flames, electricity, grease, tar, chemicals

The basement membrane, a thin noncellular protein surface, separates the dermis from the epidermis. The dermis is sometimes called the "true skin" because it is not constantly shed and replaced; it is thicker than the epidermis and ranges from 0.60 to 1.2 mm. The dermis makes up the bulk of the skin and is composed of collagen meshes, fibrous connective tissue, and elastic fibers. Within the dermis are the functional elements of the skin:

- Blood vessels
- Sensory nerves
- Hair follicles
- Lymph system
- Sebaceous glands and sweat glands

When burn injury occurs, the skin can regenerate as long as parts of the dermis are present. When the entire layer of dermis is burned, all epithelial cells or elements are destroyed, and the skin can no longer regenerate spontaneously. The subcutaneous tissue, or superficial fascia, varies in thickness and lies below the dermis. With deep burns, the subcutaneous tissue may be damaged, leaving bones, tendons, and muscles exposed.

Functional Changes

The skin serves various functions (see Table 69–1). The skin is primarily a protective barrier against injury and microbial invasion from the environment. This barrier is broken when a burn injury occurs, greatly increasing the client's risk for infection.

The skin also maintains the delicate fluid and electrolyte balance essential for life. After a burn injury, massive fluid loss through evaporation occurs. Water vapor can evaporate through burn-injured skin four times as rapidly as from intact skin. This rate is proportional to the extent and depth of the injury.

Skin is important in thermoregulation. Normally, the body can adjust to normal fluctuations in environmental temperatures because subcutaneous fat provides insulation, and blood flow to the skin changes with fluctuations in environmental temperature. When the skin is damaged, the body cannot adjust to the loss of heat as readily, and body temperature tends to decrease.

The skin is an excretory organ allowing perspiration. When deep burns occur, the sweat glands are destroyed and this excretory ability is lost.

The skin also functions as the largest sensory organ of the body. Pain, pressure, temperature, and touch are sensed on the skin in normal daily activities, allowing a person to react to the environment and to respond to danger. With partial-thickness burns, nerve endings are exposed to the surface; sensitivity and sensory stimulation on these areas increase. With full-thickness burns, nerve endings are destroyed, and sensation is thought to be lost. However, this is an area of controversy because many clients with full-thickness wounds do experience pain.

Skin exposed to sunlight produces vitamin D. The conversion of cholesterol derivatives into the active form of vitamin D is completed in the skin. In a person with partial-thickness burns, this function is diminished; in a person with full-thickness burns, it is completely lost.

The skin is an important determinant of physical identity. The skin's cosmetic quality contributes to each person's unique appearance. With a change in appearance through a major burn, severe psychological problems may develop.

Temperature

The temperature of the body's internal environment falls within a narrow range (approximately 29° to 43° C [84.2° to 109.4° F]) compared with the wide fluctuations the external environment inflicts on body surfaces. The body has several mechanisms to compensate for the wide variations in external temperature. Circulating blood both provides and dissipates heat. Dissipation of heat is efficient under normal conditions. When heat is applied to the skin, the temperature of the immediate subdermal layer rises rapidly. As soon as the heat source is removed, the body's compensatory mechanisms can return the area to a normal temperature quickly. If the heat source is not removed, or if it is applied at a rate or level that exceeds the skin's capacity to dissipate it, cells are destroyed.

The skin can tolerate temperatures up to 40° C (104° F) without sustaining injury. At temperatures of 70° C (158° F) and above, cell destruction is so rapid that brief periods of exposure damage the skin down to and including the subcutaneous level. Figure 71–1 shows the relationship between temperature and exposure time for burn injury.

Depth of Burn Injury

The magnitude of the injury is based on the depth and extent of the total body surface burn. The depth of tissue destruction is determined by the nature of the burning agent as well as by the temperature and the duration of exposure to the heat source.

Variations in skin thickness over different parts of the body also influence burn depth. In areas where the epidermis and dermis are thin (such as the eyelids, ears, nose, genitalia, medial portions of the upper extremities, fingers, and toes), a short exposure to extreme temperatures can result in a deep burn injury. The skin is thinner in the elderly, and thinner skin predisposes them to more severe burns with exposure at lower temperatures and of shorter durations.

In the past, burns were classified into first-, second-, third-, and fourth-degree injuries. This classification is rarely used in clinical settings. Instead, the American Burn Association (ABA) advocates a more functional and precise descriptive classification, categorizing the burn injury according to the depth of tissue destruction. Burn wounds are now classified as superficial-thickness wounds, partial-thickness wounds, full-thickness wounds, and deep full-thickness wounds. The partial-thickness wounds are further separated into superficial and deep subgroups. Table 71–1 compares the two classification systems.

The ABA further describes burns as minor, moderate, or major, depending on the depth, extent, and location of injury (Table 71–2). Figure 71–2 illustrates involvement of specific tissues with different depths of injury.

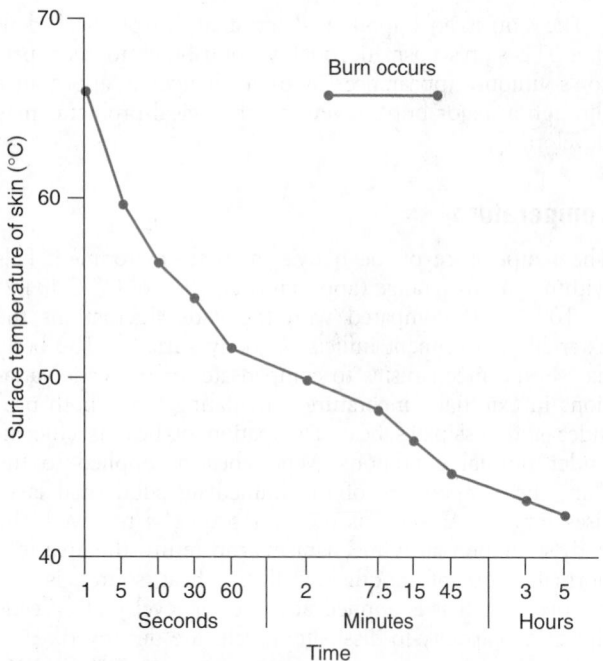

Figure 71–1. Relationship between intensity of heat and the duration of exposure. Exposure for prolonged periods causes burns, even with milder temperatures. At more extreme temperatures, tissue damage results after only seconds. (Modified from Moritz, A. R. [1947]. Studies of thermal injuries. II: The relative importance of time and surface temperature in causation of cutaneous burns. *American Journal of Pathology, 23,* 695.)

Superficial-Thickness Wounds

Of all burn types, superficial-thickness wounds reflect the least destruction because the epidermis is the only portion of the skin that is injured. The basal epithelial cells and basement membrane, structures necessary for total regrowth of epithelial cells, are present.

Superficial-thickness wounds frequently result from prolonged exposure to low-intensity heat (e.g., sunburn) or short (flash) exposure to high-intensity heat. Erythema with mild edema, pain, and increased sensitivity to heat is the result. Peeling of dead skin (desquamation) occurs for 2–3 days after the burn, and the area rapidly heals in 3–5 days without a scar. No significant clinical consequences occur at this level of injury.

Partial-Thickness Wounds

A partial-thickness wound involves the entire epidermis and varying depths of the dermis. Depending on the amount of dermal tissue damaged, partial-thickness wounds are further subdivided into superficial partial-thickness and deep partial-thickness injuries.

Superficial Partial-Thickness Wounds

Superficial partial-thickness wounds result from either increased duration or increased intensity of exposure. These wounds are typically erythemic and moist (Fig. 71–3). The classic *vesicle* (blister) forms as the stratum corneum

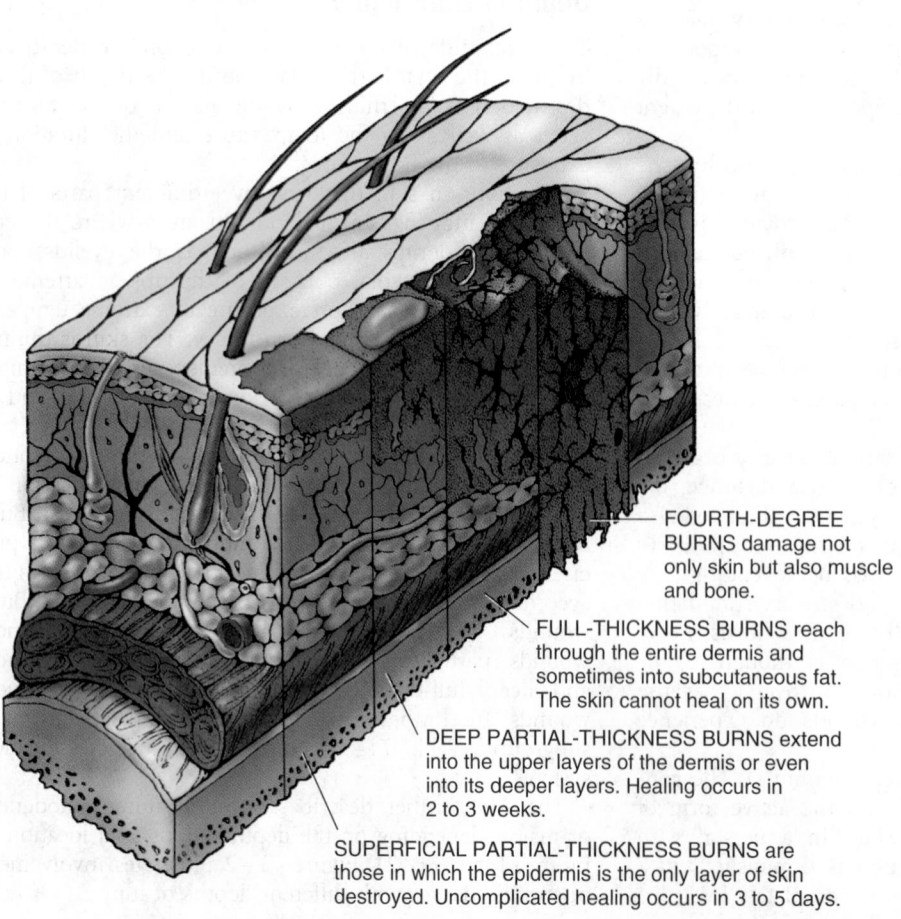

Figure 71–2. The tissues involved in burns of various depths.

FOURTH-DEGREE BURNS damage not only skin but also muscle and bone.

FULL-THICKNESS BURNS reach through the entire dermis and sometimes into subcutaneous fat. The skin cannot heal on its own.

DEEP PARTIAL-THICKNESS BURNS extend into the upper layers of the dermis or even into its deeper layers. Healing occurs in 2 to 3 weeks.

SUPERFICIAL PARTIAL-THICKNESS BURNS are those in which the epidermis is the only layer of skin destroyed. Uncomplicated healing occurs in 3 to 5 days.

TABLE 71–2

Classification of Burn Injury and Burn Center Referral Criteria

Burn Class	Characteristics	Comments
Minor burns	Deep partial-thickness burns <15% TBSA Full-thickness burns <2% TBSA No burns of eyes, ears, face, hands, feet, or perineum No electrical burns No inhalation injury No complicated concomitant injury Patient is under 60 yr and has no chronic cardiac, pulmonary, or endocrine disorder	Clients in this category should receive emergency care at the scene and be taken to a hospital emergency department. Special expertise hospital or designated burn center is not necessary
Moderate burns	Deep partial-thickness burns 15%–25% TBSA Full-thickness burns 2%–10% TBSA No burns of eyes, ears, face, hands, feet, or perineum No electrical burns No inhalation injury No complicated concomitant injury Patient is under 60 yr and has no chronic cardiac, pulmonary, or endocrine disorder	Clients in this category should receive emergency care at the scene and be transferred either to a special expertise hospital or to a designated burn center
Major burns	Partial-thickness burns >25% TBSA Full-thickness burns >10% Any burn involving the eyes, ears, face, hands, feet, perineum Electrical injury Inhalation injury Client over 60 yr of age Burn is complicated with other injuries (e.g., fractures) Client has cardiac, pulmonary, or other chronic metabolic disorders	Clients who meet *any one* of the criteria for a major burn should receive emergency care at the nearest emergency department and then be transferred as soon as possible to a designated burn center

and stratum granulosum are destroyed. When intact, the blister forms a sterile environment, protecting the wound from potential infection and excess water loss. However, when blisters are large or numerous, they are opened to promote healing and prevent changes in leukocyte function.

People who have a superficial partial-thickness wound experience increased pain sensation. Nerve endings are exposed to the surface, and any stimulation (touch or temperature changes) causes intense pain. These burns heal in 10–14 days with no scar, although some minor pigment changes may occur.

Deep Partial-Thickness Wounds

Deep partial-thickness wounds extend deeper into the dermal layer of the skin, and fewer epidermal cells are viable. The area usually appears red and waxy-white without blisters (Fig. 71–4). Edema is moderate, and pain is present, but to a lesser degree than with superficial burns because more of the nerve endings have been destroyed. Blisters are absent because the dead tissues adhere to the underlying dermal collagen fibers.

Because the remaining blood supply to these areas is marginal, the potential for progression to a deeper injury can occur through hypoxia and ischemia. Adequate hydration, nutrients, and oxygen are necessary for spontaneous re-epithelialization of the wound and prevent deeper burns. Because partial-thickness wounds can convert to full-thickness wounds as a result of tissue damage from infection, the client must remain free of infection. Deep partial-thickness wounds generally heal in 3–6 weeks, but a large amount of scar formation results. If healing will be prolonged, surgical intervention with skin grafting is required.

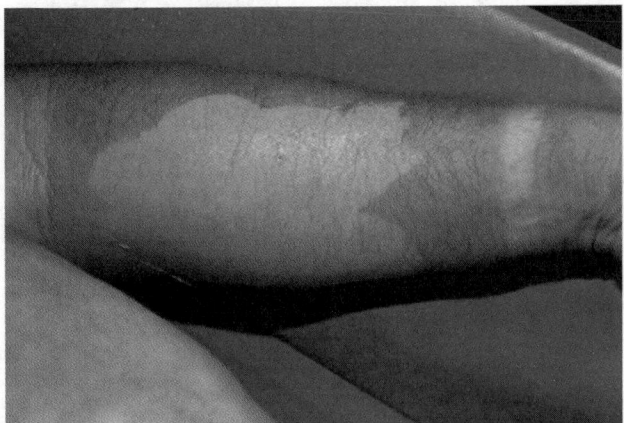

Figure 71–3. The typical appearance of a superficial partial-thickness burn injury.

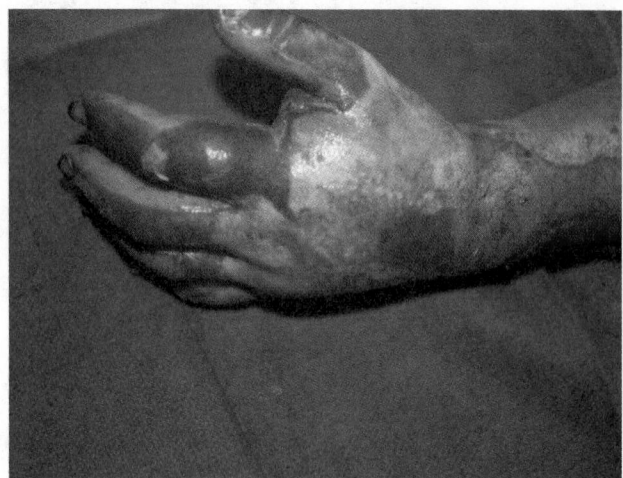

Figure 71–4. The typical appearance of a deep partial-thickness burn injury.

Full-Thickness Wounds

A full-thickness wound involves the entire epidermal and dermal layers of the skin (Fig. 71–5). No epidermal cells are present for re-epithelialization, and skin grafts are required in areas larger than approximately 12–16 cm². In smaller areas, secondary wound closure occurs by the growth of collagen-based scar tissue from the unburned edges inward (see Chap. 70).

The area of full-thickness injury is characterized by a hard, dry, leathery eschar that forms from coagulated particles of destroyed dermis. The eschar is dead tissue; it must slough off or be removed from the burn wound before healing can occur. The thick, coagulated particles often adhere to the subcutaneous layer by collagen fibers, which makes removal of eschar difficult. Edema in a full-thickness wound is pronounced; when the injury totally surrounds an extremity or the thorax (circumferential), circulation and respiration may be compromised by tight eschar. Escharotomies (incisions through the eschar) or fasciotomies (incisions through eschar and fascia) may be required to relieve pressure and allow normal circulation and breathing (see Altered Tissue Perfusion, Surgical Management).

The color of the burn wound varies from waxy-white, deep red, yellow, or brown to black. Thrombosed vessels may be present beneath the surface of the burn because the dermal blood vessels are heat coagulated, resulting in avascular tissue. Sensation is minimal or absent in these areas of injury because the nerve endings have been destroyed. Healing time depends on the re-establishment of an adequate vascular bed within the injured areas and can range from weeks to months.

Deep Full-Thickness Wounds

Deep full-thickness wounds extend beyond the skin into underlying fascia and have also been termed "fourth-degree burns." These deep injuries damage muscle, bone, and tendons and leave them exposed to the surface

(Nuchtern et al., 1995). These burns occur with deep flame, electrical, or chemical injuries. The wound is blackened and depressed, and sensation is completely absent (Fig. 71–6). When an extremity is involved, amputation may be required.

Vascular Changes Resulting from Burn Injuries

Immediately after a burn injury, major circulatory destruction occurs at the burn site. The vessels supplying the burned skin are occluded, and blood flow through the arterial and venous channels decreases or completely ceases. Damaged macrophages within the tissues release chemical substances that initially produce vasoconstriction. Peripheral vessel thrombosis may occur; this decrease in tissue perfusion can produce necrosis, which can lead to deeper injuries in the involved areas.

Fluid Shift

After the initial vasoconstriction, adjacent vessels to the burn injury dilate, which leads to increased capillary hydrostatic pressure, accompanied by an increased capillary permeability (Fig. 71–7). This fluid shift, also known as *third spacing* or *capillary leak syndrome,* is a continuous leak of plasma from the intravascular space into the interstitial space. The loss of plasma fluids and proteins results in a decreased colloid osmotic pressure in the vascular compartments. Leakage of fluid and electrolytes from the vascular compartment continues, resulting in additional edema formation. Fluid shift is most prevalent in the first 12 hours after the burn but can continue for 24 to 36 hours.

The amount of plasma to interstitial fluid shifted depends on the extent and severity of injury. When tissue damage is extensive (20% to 30% total body surface area [TBSA] or greater), vascular changes can occur in unburned as well as burned tissues. As the protein-rich fluids, plasma, and electrolytes escape into the interstitial space, peripheral edema develops. Tissue colloidal osmotic pressure increases as a result of this movement of proteins, further increasing the third-spacing fluid shift.

As a result of the fluid shift and other physiologic

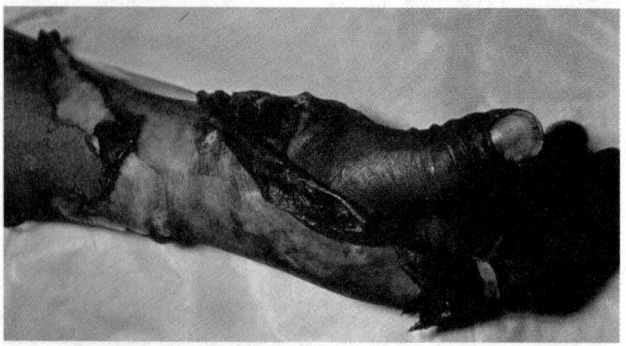

Figure 71–5. The typical appearance of a full-thickness burn injury.

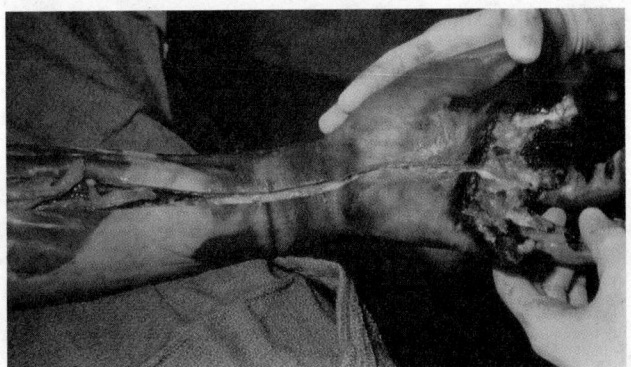

Figure 71–6. The typical appearance of a deep full-thickness burn injury.

disruptions caused by injury, profound imbalances of fluid, electrolytes, and acid-base occur. These imbalances usually include hypovolemic shock, metabolic acidosis, hyperkalemia, and hyponatremia. Hemoconcentration develops from the circulatory dehydration, increasing the viscosity of the blood, which reduces flow through small vessels. Adequate fluid resuscitation minimizes damage from hemoconcentration and restores electrolyte and acid-base balance.

Fluid Remobilization

The inflammatory responses halt 24 to 36 hours after the injury, and the plasma to interstitial fluid leak ceases. Fluid shifts back into the intravascular compartment. This "fluid remobilization" phase restores fluid and electrolyte levels and renal blood flow, resulting in increased urine formation and diuresis. Body weight returns to normal as peripheral edema subsides.

During this phase, hyponatremia is likely to develop because of increased renal sodium excretion and evaporative losses of sodium from wounds. Hypokalemia can occur as potassium returns to the intracellular compartment. As a result of hemodilution, anemia frequently develops, but it is generally not severe enough to require blood transfusions. Transfusions are indicated if the client's hematocrit is less than 25% and hypoxic changes are present.

Cardiac Function Changes Resulting from Burn Injury

Because of the initial fluid shifts and hypovolemic shock that occur after a burn injury, cardiac output decreases in spite of an increased heart rate. Cardiac output may remain depressed until 18–36 hours after the burn. The cardiac output increases with adequate fluid resuscitation and reaches normal levels before plasma volume has been restored completely. Appropriate fluid resuscitation and support with adequate oxygenation prevent further complications.

Pulmonary Changes Resulting from Burn Injury

Respiratory insufficiency (inhalation injury) rarely occurs from direct contact with flames. Rather, respiratory insufficiency is caused by superheated air, steam, toxic fumes, or smoke and is a major cause of morbidity and mortality in thermally injured clients. Respiratory failure associated with burn injuries can also result from airway edema through overhydration during fluid resuscitation, increased alveolar capillary permeability, circumferential chest burns that compromise breathing, and carbon monoxide poisoning. Damage to the respiratory system from inhalation injury can occur in the upper and major airways and the parenchyma. The upper airway is affected when inhaled smoke or irritants cause edema and obstructive closure of the trachea. When these irritants come in contact with the upper airway, a reflex closure of the vocal cords occurs, causing a decrease in the amount of smoke and toxic gases entering the major airways. Although air is a poor conductor of heat, some heat does reach the upper airway, causing an inflammatory response that leads to oropharyngeal edema and potentially dangerous airway obstruction.

Major airway injury results from chemicals and toxic gases, rather than heat, that are produced from incomplete combustion. Normally, the ciliated, mucus-secreting epithelial cells lining the trachea trap bacteria and foreign materials. Smoke and products of combustion slow this activity, which allows foreign particles to enter the bronchi. The lining of the trachea and bronchi may slough

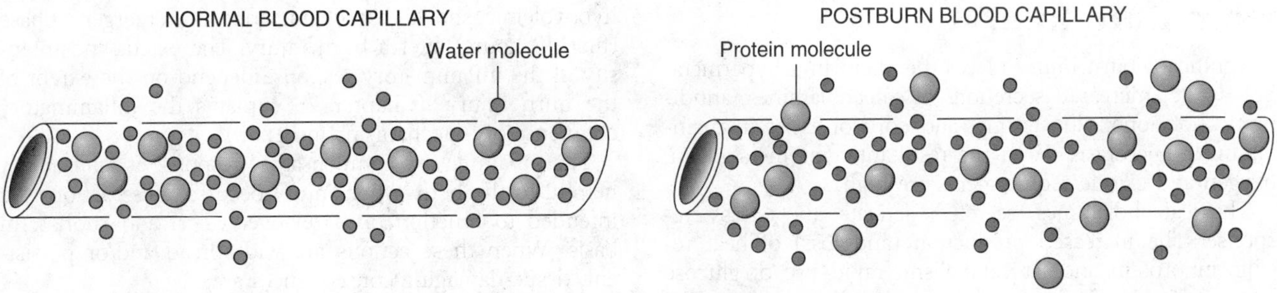

NORMAL BLOOD CAPILLARY

Water molecule

POSTBURN BLOOD CAPILLARY

Protein molecule

Water is the smallest molecule that can pass through the capillary pores.

Permeability is drastically increased, which allows large molecules such as proteins to pass through the capillary pores easily.

Figure 71–7. The vascular capillary response to burn injury (early phase).

48–72 hours after injury, enter the airway, and narrow the tracheal lumen, resulting in obstructive edema and pulmonary parenchymal damage.

Parenchymal injuries result from damage to the alveolar epithelium and capillary endothelium by toxic irritants (Sadowski, 1989). Increased alveolar-capillary membrane permeability results in intra-alveolar edema. This edema can occur immediately or as late as 1 week after injury. The fluid that diffuses across the membrane settles in the interstitial spaces; eventually, fibrinous membranes form, which leads to respiratory distress. Progressive pulmonary failure develops with acute pulmonary insufficiency and infection.

Gastrointestinal Changes Resulting from Burn Injury

Because of the fluid shifts that occur after injury and the decreased cardiac output, blood flow is shifted to the brain, heart, and liver. Consequently other organs, including the gastrointestinal tract, have decreased perfusion. Gastric motility is impaired. The sympathetic nervous system stress response causes increased secretion of catecholamines (especially epinephrine and norepinephrine), which inhibit gastrointestinal motility and reduce the flow of blood to the area. Peristalsis ceases, and a paralytic ileus is present. Mucosal secretions and gases accumulate in the intestines and stomach, causing abdominal distention.

Curling's ulcer, or acute ulcerative gastroduodenal disease, may develop within 24 hours after a severe burn injury because of compromised gastrointestinal perfusion and mucosal damage. The mucosal membrane normally acts as a barrier to the absorption of hydrogen ions that are secreted into the gastric lumen. With an alteration in gastric mucosal function, this barrier is compromised, and hydrogen ion production is increased. As a result, ulcerations may develop. This problem is now rarely seen in burn centers because of the early intervention of preventive measures. These measures include drug therapy with proton pump inhibitors such as omeprazole (Prilosec, Losec✦), H_2-histamine blockers such as cimetidine (Tagamet) and ranitidine (Zantac), and mucoprotectants such as sucralfate (Carafate). The institution of early enteral feeding also helps prevent Curling's ulcer.

Metabolic Changes Resulting from Burn Injury

A significant burn injury places the client in a hypermetabolic state. Increased secretions of catecholamines, antidiuretic hormone, aldosterone, and cortisol assist in maintaining homeostasis. With the resultant hypermetabolism, oxygen and calorie requirements are high.

The catecholamines secreted activate the stress response. The increased production (and loss) of heat results in protein and fat catabolism, rapid use of glucose and calories, and increased urinary nitrogen losses. The evaporated heat and water from the burn also increase metabolic and catabolic rates, which increase calorie expenditure. Depending on the extent of injury, the client's calorie requirements may be double or triple normal en-

ergy needs. These increased rates peak 4–12 days after the burn and can remain for months after injury until all wounds are closed and all body system functions are restored to normal.

The hypermetabolic condition also results in an increase in core body temperature. The client loses heat through the burned skin surfaces because the protective barrier is lost. Core body temperature increases as a response to the adjustment in the hypothalamus. The central thermoregulation is altered to compensate for the hypermetabolic state. There is an impaired shift in temperature; a low-grade fever can develop, which is normal for clients with burn injuries.

Immunologic Changes Resulting from Burn Injury

A thermal injury results in loss of the protective barrier of the skin, which increases the chance of infection. The burn injury activates the inflammatory response but can also compromise immune function (see Chap. 23). Antibody-mediated immunity and cell-mediated immunity are both suppressed. All immune responses are therefore reduced (Trofino, 1996).

Topical antimicrobial agents, systemic antibiotics, general anesthesia, and the stress of surgical procedures further compromise immune function.

Compensatory Responses to Burn Injury

Any tissue injury is a threat to homeostasis and a physiologic stressor. Two compensatory responses have immediate benefit, the inflammatory response and the sympathetic nervous system stress response. Together, these compensatory responses cause the physiologic changes that result in many of the clinical manifestations in the first 2 to 3 days after the burn injury.

Inflammatory Compensation

The inflammatory compensatory response initiates healing in the injured tissues. Inflammatory compensation causes blood vessels to leak fluid into the interstitial space and white blood cells to release chemicals that generate local tissue reactions. The inflammatory compensatory mechanisms cause the massive fluid shift, edema formation, and hypovolemic shock that characterize the emergent phase (first 48 hours) after a burn injury. The extent and intensity of the inflammatory response depend on the extent of the burn injury. (Chapter 23 explains the inflammatory compensatory mechanisms in detail.)

The inflammatory compensatory response is *immediately* helpful to the body when injury occurs. These actions are intended to function on a relatively local and short-term basis. When these actions are widespread and/or persistent, tissue-damaging consequences are severe.

Sympathetic Nervous System Compensation

The sympathetic nervous system stress response is generated by the sympathetic division of the autonomic ner-

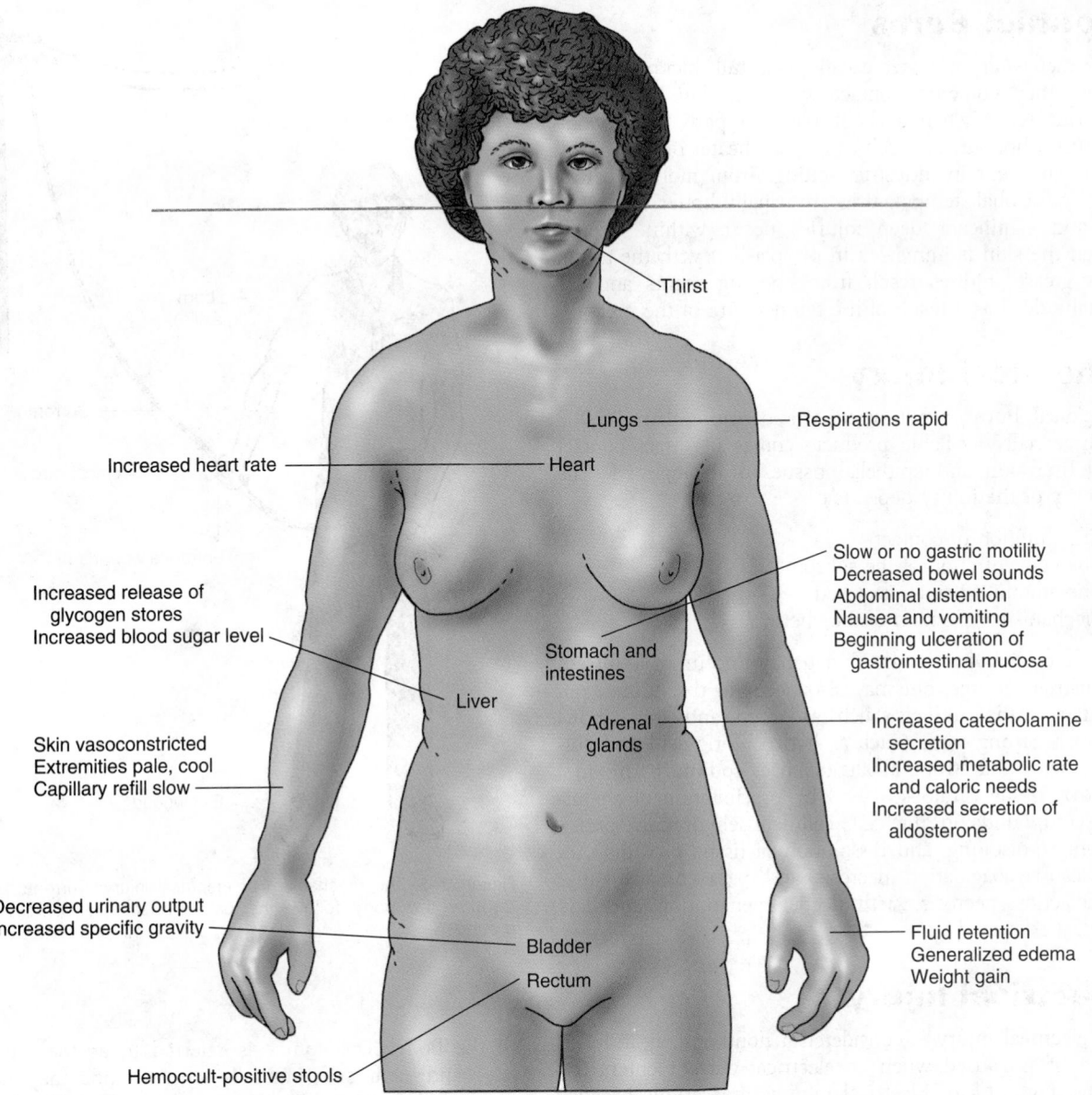

Thirst

Lungs — Respirations rapid

Increased heart rate — Heart

Slow or no gastric motility
Decreased bowel sounds
Abdominal distention
Nausea and vomiting
Beginning ulceration of
gastrointestinal mucosa

Increased release of
glycogen stores
Increased blood sugar level

Stomach and
intestines

Liver

Adrenal
glands

Increased catecholamine
secretion
Increased metabolic rate
and caloric needs
Increased secretion of
aldosterone

Skin vasoconstricted
Extremities pale, cool
Capillary refill slow

Decreased urinary output
Increased specific gravity

Bladder

Rectum

Fluid retention
Generalized edema
Weight gain

Hemoccult-positive stools

Figure 71–8. The physiologic actions of the sympathetic nervous system compensatory responses to burn injury (early phase).

vous system and some components of the endocrine system when any physical or psychological stressors are present. Changes resulting from sympathetic compensation are most evident in the cardiovascular, respiratory, and gastrointestinal systems. Figure 71–8 summarizes the physical consequence of sympathetic nervous system compensation.

ETIOLOGY OF BURN INJURY

Burn injuries are caused by a variety of sources, including dry heat (flame), moist heat (scald), contact with hot surfaces, chemicals, electricity, and ionizing radiation. The causative agent of the injury affects both prognosis and treatment.

Dry Heat

Dry heat injuries are caused by open flame. The most common causes of flame injuries are house fires and explosions. Ignition of clothing from an open flame accounts for most of the injuries. Explosions usually result in flash burns because they produce brief exposure to very high temperatures.

Moist Heat

Moist heat (scald) injuries are caused by contact with hot liquids. Scald injuries are most common among adults older than 65 years. Hot liquid spills usually burn the upper, frontal surfaces of the body. Immersion scald injuries usually involve the lower portions of the body.

Contact Burns

Hot metal, tar, and grease can cause full-thickness burns when they come in contact with the skin. Hot metal injuries occur when a client places a part of the body against a hot surface, such as a space heater or iron. They also can occur in industrial settings from molten metals. Tar and asphalt temperatures are usually hotter than 400° F, and significant deep injuries occur within seconds when the skin is immersed in or splashed with the agent. Hot grease injuries result from cooking agents and are usually deep as a result of the temperature of the grease.

Chemical Injury

Chemical burns result when one of more than 25,000 commercially available products comes in direct contact with the skin and epithelial tissues or is ingested. The severity of the injury depends on

- The duration of contact
- The concentration of the substance
- The amount of tissue exposed
- Mechanisms of action of the chemical

Chemical burns to the skin usually occur in adults in industrial settings, but may also occur in the home from contact with products such as drain and toilet bowl cleaner. Strong acids (such as hydrochloric acid and sulfuric acid) and strong alkalis (such as sodium hydroxide) destroy tissue (Bullock, 1996) by precipitation of chemical compounds in the cell, cellular dehydration, protoplasmic poisoning, and dissolution of tissue proteins. Acids cause coagulation necrosis and pain. Alkalis cause liquefaction necrosis, with deeper penetration and less pain.

Electrical Injury

An electrical injury is considered a nonthermally induced burn; it is caused when an electrical current enters the body (Fig. 71–9). Electrical injuries are serious because they damage deep structures and organs and can even result in the loss of one or more limbs. The amount of damage depends on amperage, voltage, resistance to flow, type of current, duration of contact, and the current's course through the body.

Resistance, the impedance to flow, varies in different parts of the body. Nerve, muscle, and blood vessels have very low resistance and are susceptible to deep injuries. Tendons, fat, and bone have the most resistance. Skin has intermediate resistance. Wet skin has less resistance than do dry, calloused areas. The higher the resistance, the greater the heat generated by the current flow and the greater the potential for soft-tissue injury.

The longer the electricity is in contact with the body, the more damage occurs due to the greater current flow and heat generated. The duration of contact may be increased by tetanic contractions of the strong flexor group in the forearm; the person cannot release the live wire or pole. Damage is usually severe to the extremity and may result in the loss of a limb.

It is difficult to know the exact course a current takes

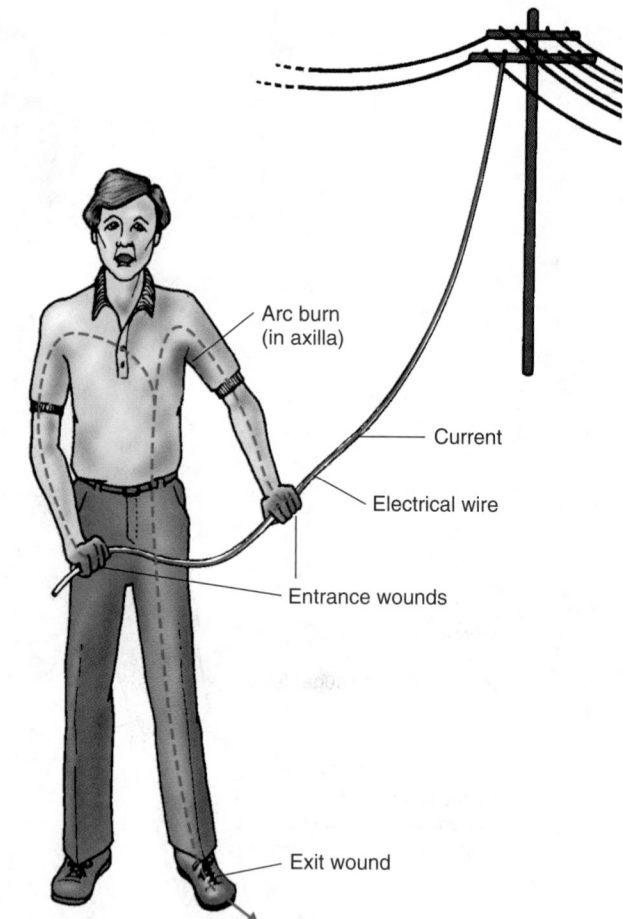

Figure 71–9. The mechanism of electrical injury: Currents passing through the body follow the path of least resistance to the ground.

Arc burn (in axilla)

Current

Electrical wire

Entrance wounds

Exit wound

in the body. The course is referred to as the "entrance site" and "exit site." Initially, the wounds may not be obvious. When visible, the entrance site is usually well defined and rounded. The exit site is usually explosive and surrounded by charred tissue.

Burn injuries from electricity can occur in one of three ways: *thermal burns, external burns,* or *true electrical injury.* Thermal burns may occur when clothes ignite from heat or flames produced by electrical sparks. External burn injuries can occur when the electrical current jumps, or "arcs," between two charged surfaces. These injuries are usually severe and deep and are associated with high-tension current. True electrical injury can occur when direct contact of the body is made with an electrical source. Internal damage results, and the injuries are devastating. Damage starts on the inside and goes out; deep-tissue destruction may not be apparent initially after injury. Organs in the path of the current may become ischemic and necrotic.

Radiation Injury

Clients incur radiation injuries when they are exposed to large doses of radioactive material. The most common type of radiation exposure leading to tissue injury occurs in conjunction with therapeutic radiation. This injury is usually minor and rarely causes extensive skin damage.

Radiation exposure is more serious in industrial settings where radioactive energy is produced or radioactive isotopes are used. The injury depends on the amount and type of energy deposited over time. (Chapter 27 discusses the penetrating ability and potential for tissue damage of alpha, beta, and gamma radiation.)

The severity of injury is determined by factors that include

- Type of radiation
- Distance from the source
- Duration of exposure
- Absorbed dose
- Depth of penetration into the body

INCIDENCE/PREVALENCE OF BURN INJURY

Each year in the United States, approximately 2 million burn injuries occur, and half of these require medical attention. Approximately 70,000 of those clients seeking medical attention suffer potentially life-threatening injuries, either from the high percentage of skin area involved or from complications of smoke inhalation and other concomitant injuries. Of the other 1 million people with burns who do not seek medical attention, about 5670 die at the scene of the accident (Rice & McKenzie, 1989). The rest of the injuries are minor, and treatment with basic first aid at home is adequate.

Burns are the sixth leading cause of accidental deaths in the United States. Causes vary among different age groups (Table 71–3). The highest risk is among those 75 years and older. Males are at slightly higher risk for both fatal and nonfatal injuries resulting from fires and burns (Rice & McKenzie, 1989).

WOMEN'S HEALTH CONSIDERATIONS

Burn injury during pregnancy has adverse effects on both maternal and fetal survival. The problems affecting the fetus include spontaneous uterine activity and an increase in intrauterine fetal death due to compro-

mised circulation. Signs of shock may not be evident until 30%–35% of circulating blood volume is lost. Placental fetal perfusion depends on maternal blood pressure. Therefore, if the mother has sustained a significant burn injury and is in hypovolemic shock, fetal circulation is decreased. Fetal monitoring is then necessary to determine fetal response.

In addition, respiratory injuries to the mother add additional trauma to the fetus due to the respiratory-exchange disturbances across the placental barrier leading to hypoxia. Cesarean delivery may be indicated, depending on the condition of the mother and the fetus. Each case is different, and the decision must be based on the gestational age of the fetus and available data obtained through complete assessments of both the mother and fetus.

Emergent Phase of Burn Injury

Overview

Burns are one of the most severe forms of trauma that can be sustained by the body. These injuries are often referred to as the most devastating and dehumanizing experiences a person can endure. Events within the first hour after injury can make the difference between life and death in a thermally injured client. Immediate care focuses on limiting the extent of injury and maintaining the function of vital organs. Chart 71–1 outlines emergency management of burn injury.

The emergent phase is the first phase of burn injury and occurs from the onset of injury to approximately 48 hours later. During this phase the injury is evaluated, and immediate problems resulting from the burn, including fluid loss, edema formation, and potential for peripheral circulatory impairment, are assessed and interventions are taken to resolve and/or prevent potential complications.

Collaborative Management

 Assessment

➤ *History*

During the emergent phase, the nurse obtains a history and other pertinent information from a client or the signif-

TABLE 71–3

Percentage of Burn Injuries by Age in the United States						
Age	Dry Heat (Flame)	Moist Heat (Scalds)	Contact	Chemical	Electrical	Ionizing Radiation
Birth–23 mo	10	72	15	1	2	<1
2–4 yr	34	54	8	1	3	<1
5–12 yr	70	23	4	1	2	<1
13–18 yr	69	20	5	2	4	<1
19–35 yr	56	26	10	4	4	<1
36–54 yr	44	33	13	4	6	<1
55 yr and older	73	21	4	1	1	<1

Chart 71–1

Nursing Care Highlight: Emergency Management of Burns

General Management for All Types of Burns

- Assess for airway patency.
- Administer oxygen as needed.
- Cover the client with a blanket.
- Keep the client on NPO status.
- Elevate the extremities if no fractures are obvious.
- Obtain vital signs.
- Initiate an intravenous line and begin fluid replacement.
- Administer tetanus toxoid for prophylaxis.
- Perform a head-to-toe assessment.

Specific Management

Flame Burns

- Smother the flames.
- Remove smoldering clothing and all metal objects.

Chemical Burns

- Brush off any dry chemicals present on the skin or clothing.
- Remove the client's clothing.
- Ascertain the type of chemical causing the burn.
- Do not attempt to neutralize the chemical unless the chemical has been positively identified and the appropriate neutralizing agent is available.

Electrical Burns

- At the scene, separate the client from the electrical current.
- Smother any flames that are present.
- Initiate cardiopulmonary resuscitation.
- Obtain an ECG.

Radiation Burns

- Remove the client from the radiation source.
- If the client has been exposed to radiation from an unsealed source, remove the client's clothing (using tongs or lead protective gloves).
- If the client has radioactive particles on his or her skin, send the client to the nearest designated radiation decontamination center.
- Help the client to bathe or shower.

---

icant other of a client who has experienced a burn as early as possible after the injury. If information cannot be obtained from the client, the nurse questions significant others and those present at the scene of the injury. The nurse obtains information about the circumstances of the injury, demographic data, health history (including pre-existing illness), and the presence of concomitant injuries and pain. The nurse keeps in mind the potential complications associated with burn injuries. Pertinent information about the circumstances of the injury includes time of injury, source and cause of injury, detailed description of how the burn occurred, and the events occurring from the time of injury until help arrived. The nurse notes the specific physical environment where the injury occurred.

Demographic data include age, weight, and height. The

rate of serious complications and death from burn injuries is greatly increased among adults over 50 years old. Chart 71–2 summarizes the age-related differences in the elderly in response to a burn injury (Cadier & Shakespear, 1995; Covington et al., 1996). The client's pre-burn weight is used to calculate fluid rates, energy requirements, and drug doses. Calculations based on a weight obtained after initiation of fluid replacement are not accurate because of water-induced weight gain. Height is important in determining body surface area (BSA), which is used to calculate nutritional needs.

A health history, including any pre-existing illness, must be known for appropriate treatment to be given. The nurse specifically inquires about heart or kidney impairment and diabetes mellitus; any of these problems will influence fluid resuscitation. The nurse asks the client about known allergies and the current use of any medications. The dose and the last time the medication was taken are determined. The nurse ascertains whether the client is a smoker or ingests alcohol daily; these factors can influence treatment and physical responses.

Other injuries may have occurred at the time of the burn. Such injuries often affect the morbidity and mortality of the client. The nurse determines whether additional injuries such as fractures, chest injuries, and abdominal trauma are causing pain or discomfort.

➤ Physical Assessment/Clinical Manifestations

Physical assessment findings in the emergent phase may vary greatly from findings later in the course of the injury. Expected assessment findings are discussed with a systems approach. The systems assessed first are those

---

Chart 71–2

Nursing Focus on the Elderly: Age-Related Changes That Increase Mortality and Morbidity from Burns

- The skin of an elderly person is thinner and more easily damaged than that of a younger person. Therefore, burn injuries tend to be more extensive in elderly clients even when exposure to causative agents is short.
- Healing time is slower in the elderly, which increases the risk for infection and other complications.
- Cardiac impairment in the elderly client with burns limits the amount and type of fluids used in resuscitation. As a result, elderly clients are more likely to develop complications from hypovolemic shock and inadequate renal perfusion.
- The immune responses of the older client may be reduced, which increases the risk for infection and sepsis. In addition, the elderly client may not have a fever when an infection is present.
- The elderly are more likely to have a pre-existing medical condition (such as diabetes mellitus, cardiovascular disorders, pulmonary or renal impairment, or immunosuppression) that may further compromise vital organ function or interfere with resuscitation and treatment.

Chart 71-3

Key Features of Upper Airway Obstruction and Inhalation Injury

Upper Airway Obstruction

- Edema, erythema, and ulceration of airway mucosa, especially posterior pharynx
- Increased hoarseness
- Stridor
- Any face or neck burn with edema formation
- Heat-induced intraoral injury

Inhalation Injury

- Airway injury
- Carbonaceous sputum
- Singed nasal hairs
- Bronchorrhea
- Wheezing
- Pulmonary vasoconstriction
- Reduced cardiac output
- Bronchospasm

that can have immediate, life-threatening alterations in function.

Respiratory Assessment. Clients with major burn injuries and those with inhalation injury are at risk for respiratory complications. Respiratory manifestations commonly associated with a burn injury are presented in Chart 71-3.

Direct Airway Injury. The degree of inhalation damage depends on fire source, temperature, environment, and types of toxic gases generated. Therefore, the nurse obtains information about the source of the fire and the duration of exposure. The nurse initially assesses the client's respiratory system by visually inspecting the mouth, nose, and pharynx. Burns of the lips, face, ears, neck, eyelids, eyebrows, and eyelashes are strong indicators of exposure to flames; these burns increase the possibility of an inhalation injury. Intraoral burns and singed nasal hairs indicate potentially serious injuries. Black carbon particles in the nose and mouth, along with congestion and edema of the nasal septum, indicate smoke inhalation.

Other indicators of possible impending pulmonary complications are alterations in breathing patterns. The client may

- Become progressively hoarse
- Exhibit a brassy cough
- Drool or have difficulty swallowing
- Have expiratory sounds that include grossly audible wheezes, crowing, and stridor

Upper airway edema and inhalation burn damage are most notable in the trachea and mainstem bronchi. The nurse auscultates these areas, listening for wheezes as a sign of obstruction. Clients with severe inhalation injuries may sustain such progressive obstruction that in a short time they cannot force air through the narrowed airways. As a result, the wheezing sounds disappear. This finding

indicates almost complete airway obstruction and demands immediate intubation.

Carbon Monoxide Poisoning. Carbon monoxide is a colorless, odorless, tasteless gas produced in almost every fire. Clients with any degree of inhalation injury are at risk for concomitant carbon monoxide poisoning.

When carbon monoxide is inhaled, it binds to the hemoglobin molecule at a rate 200 to 250 times more tightly than oxygen, forming carboxyhemoglobin (CoHb). This situation shifts the oxyhemoglobin curve to the left and impairs tissue oxygen availability. CoHb reduces the oxygen-carrying capacity of hemoglobin, which results in

- Impaired oxygen transport
- Decreased oxygen delivery
- Inability of the cells to use oxygen

Even though the oxygen-carrying capacity of the hemoglobin is reduced, the partial pressure of oxygen dissolved in the arterial blood (PaO_2) is normal. The vasodilating action of carbon monoxide causes the "cherry-red" color in these clients. Clinical manifestations vary with the concentration of CoHb. Table 71-4 summarizes the physiologic effects of carbon monoxide poisoning.

Thermal (Heat) Injury. Thermal injury to the respiratory tract results from the inhalation of superheated air or

TABLE 71-4

Physiologic Effects of Carbon Monoxide Poisoning

Carbon Monoxide Level	Physiologic Effects
1%–10% (normal)	Increased threshold to visual stimuli Increased blood flow to vital organs
11%–20% (mild poisoning)	Headache Decreased cerebral function Decreased visual acuity Slight breathlessness
21%–40% (moderate poisoning)	Headache Tinnitus Nausea Drowsiness Vertigo Altered mental state Confusion Stupor Irritability Decreased blood pressure and increased heart rate Depressed ST segment on electrocardiogram and dysrhythmias on palpation Pale to reddish purple skin
41%–60% (severe poisoning)	Coma Convulsions Cardiopulmonary instability
61%–80% (fatal poisoning)	Death

steam. The client inhales the hot air, which is rapidly cooled by the upper airway. Therefore, the most severe damage from superheated air is confined to the upper airway.

Inhaled steam can injure the lower respiratory tract because water holds heat better than dry air does. The entire respiratory tract, up to the major bronchioles, can be damaged by steam. Ulcerations, erythema, and edema of the mouth and epiglottis are usually the first manifestations, with rapid edema formation progressing to upper airway obstruction. Stridor, hoarseness, and shortness of breath result.

Smoke Poisoning. Smoke poisoning, or chemical injury from the inhalation of products of combustion, is the most common mechanism of inhalation injury. Toxic by-products are produced when various structural materials (especially plastics) or home furnishings are burned. The most significant effects of smoke poisoning are atelectasis, pulmonary edema, and tissue anoxia.

Pulmonary Fluid Overload. Pulmonary edema can result even when the lung tissues have not sustained any direct damage. Instead, other damaged tissues release such large quantities of vasoactive amines, leading to increased capillary permeability, that even pulmonary capillaries leak fluid into the pulmonary interstitial spaces.

Circulatory overload from fluid resuscitation may cause left-sided congestive heart failure. The circulatory overload creates such high hydrostatic pressure within pulmonary vessels that even more fluid is lost from the pulmonary vascular space into the interstitial spaces. Excess interstitial fluid makes gas exchange difficult. The client is extremely short of breath and experiences increased dyspnea in the supine position. Crackles are heard on auscultation.

External Factors. Clients with burn injuries may have respiratory difficulties as a result of external factors in addition to pulmonary problems. The most common external factor affecting respiration is tight eschar from deep circumferential chest burns. The eschar either restricts chest movement or compresses anatomic structures in the neck and throat to such an extent that ventilation is impaired. The nurse visually assesses the ease of respiration and the amount of chest movement as well as the rate and effort required to breathe.

Cardiovascular Assessment. Changes in the cardiovascular system begin immediately after the burn injury and include shock from various causes. Shock is a common cause of death in the immediate post-burn period in clients with significant injuries. (Chapter 39 discusses the pathophysiologic and compensatory mechanisms for all types of shock.)

The initial cardiovascular clinical manifestations reflect hypovolemia and decreased cardiac output. The nurse notes the presence of edema and assesses cardiovascular status by measuring central and peripheral pulses, blood pressure, capillary refill, and pulse oximetry. Initially, tachycardia, decreased blood pressure, and diminished peripheral pulses are present. As tissue perfusion decreases, peripheral capillary refill is slow or absent. With fluid resuscitation in the initial post-burn period, peripheral edema increases, as does the client's body weight.

Electrocardiographic (ECG) changes indicate electrical damage to the heart. These changes are frequently associated with electrical burn injuries or with situational stress that induces a myocardial infarction. The nurse obtains baseline ECG tracings at the time of the client's admission to the hospital or burn center.

Renal/Urinary Assessment. Changes in renal function with burn injury are related to the secondary alterations of renal perfusion and to the presence of cellular debris. During the fluid shift of the emergent period, perfusion may not be adequate for glomerular filtration. As a result, urinary output is greatly diminished compared with intravenous fluid intake. The urine is highly concentrated and has a high specific gravity.

As a result of specific tissue damage, other substances may be present in the blood that perfuses the kidney. Destroyed red blood cells release hemoglobin and potassium. When muscle damage occurs from a major burn or electrical injury, a large oxygen-carrying protein called *myoglobin* is released from damaged muscle and circulates to the kidney. Most damaged cells release protein products that form uric acid. All of these large molecules in the blood may precipitate in the kidney tubular system. This precipitation blocks filtrate flow and may contribute to severe renal dysfunction.

The nurse assesses renal function by accurately measuring urine output and comparing this value with fluid intake. During the first 24 hours of the emergent phase, urine output is decreased. The rate of resuscitation fluid administration should maintain adult urine output at 30–50 mL/hour. Adequate response to fluid resuscitation is further assessed by measurement of urine specific gravity and blood urea nitrogen (BUN), serum creatinine, and serum sodium levels. The nurse examines the urine for color, odor, and the presence of particulate matter or foam.

Integumentary Assessment. The nurse assesses skin to determine the size and depth of the injury. The size of the injury is first estimated in comparison to the total body surface area (TBSA). For example, a burn that involves 40% of the TBSA is a "40% burn." The size of the injury is important not only for diagnosis and prognosis but also for calculating specific therapeutic parameters, such as drug dose, fluid replacement volumes, and calorie needs.

The nurse inspects the skin visually for changes in color and appearance and to delineate injured areas. Except for electrical burns, this initial size assessment can usually be made accurately with specific assessment tools and charts.

The most rapid method for calculating the size of a burn injury in adult clients whose weights are in normal proportion to their heights is the *rule of nines* (Fig. 71–10). The body is divided into areas that are multiples of 9%. Although the rule of nines is useful at the site of injury and in emergency departments, it is not accurate for estimating the percentage of TBSA for adults who are short, extremely thin, or obese. In addition, even among

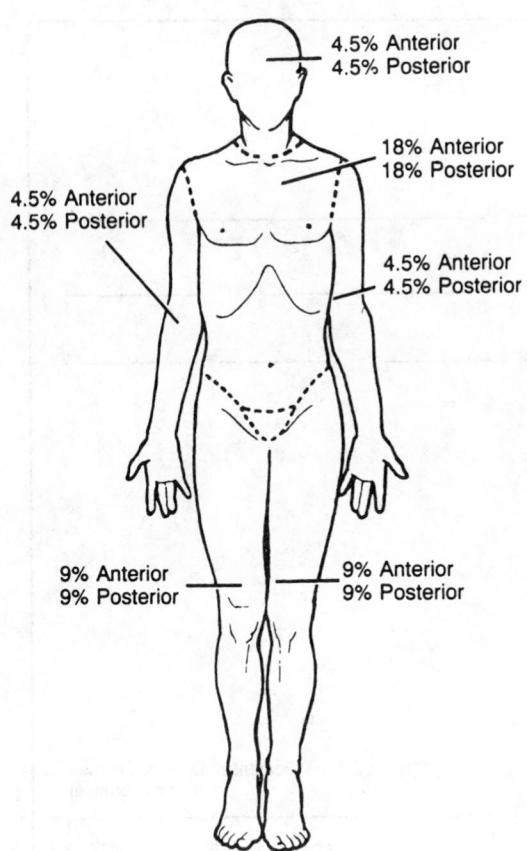

Figure 71–10. The rule of nines for estimating burn percentage.

4.5% Anterior
4.5% Posterior

18% Anterior
18% Posterior

4.5% Anterior
4.5% Posterior

4.5% Anterior
4.5% Posterior

9% Anterior
9% Posterior

9% Anterior
9% Posterior

average-sized adults there is a tendency to overestimate TBSA with this method.

The Lund-Browder method (also known as the Berkow method; Fig. 71–11) is more accurate for evaluation of the size of injury. This method takes into account changes in body surface area throughout the life span (Lund & Browder, 1944).

Because specific treatments are related to the depth of the burn injury, initial assessment of the integumentary system includes estimations of burn depth. Criteria for establishing depth of injury are based on appearance and associated characteristics (see Depth of Burn Injury).

Gastrointestinal Assessment. Although the gastrointestinal (GI) tract usually is not directly injured in most burn clients (except in chemical burns), alterations in GI function are expected. The decreased blood flow during the emergent phase results in loss of GI motility and paralytic ileus. The nurse auscultates the abdomen for bowel sounds to assess GI motility. Bowel sounds are diminished or absent in the client with severe burns. Associated clinical manifestations include nausea, vomiting, and abdominal distention. To prevent complications, a nasogastric tube (NG) is placed. The nurse assesses the nasogastric tube for proper placement and patency.

Because of the potential for ulcer formation in the GI tract, the nurse examines the stool and the vomitus for the presence of gross blood or material indicative of par-

tially digested blood. In addition, tests for the presence of occult blood are performed.

➤ *Laboratory Assessment*

Alterations in laboratory test values are found in different phases of post-burn recovery and usually indicate direct tissue damage and expected compensatory mechanisms. However, other alterations in specific laboratory findings suggest complications.

During the emergent phase, before the initiation of fluid resuscitation, venous blood analysis reflects the fluid shift and direct tissue damage. Baseline laboratory test values and early post-burn variations are presented in Chart 71–4.

Changes in the total white blood cell (WBC) count and differential count reflect immune function responses to the trauma of burn injury. The burn client's total WBC count, especially the neutrophil percentage, initially rises and then drops precipitously with a "left shift" (see Chap. 23) as the immune system becomes unable to sustain its defenses. If sepsis occurs, the total WBC count may be as low as 2000 cells/mm^3.

Additional laboratory tests that provide useful information about the burn client's status may include urine electrolyte assays, urine cultures, liver enzyme studies, and clotting studies. Drug and alcohol screens are obtained if drug or alcohol intoxication is suspected.

TRANSCULTURAL CONSIDERATIONS

For African-American clients, a sickle cell preparation may be appropriate if the client's sickle status is unknown because trauma often triggers a sickle cell crisis in clients who have the disease and in those who carry the sickle cell trait.

➤ *Radiographic Assessment*

Standard x-rays and scans do not provide direct assessment data about the burn wound. Such assessment is not performed unless additional trauma is suspected.

➤ *Other Diagnostic Assessment*

In addition to routine laboratory tests and examinations, specific studies of involved organs are performed. For example, when burn injuries involve the eye, ophthalmic evaluation detects corneal damage. (Chapters 48 and 49 describe specific ophthalmic evaluation procedures.)

When visceral organ trauma is suspected, specific diagnostic examinations can be performed. They include intravenous pyelography (IVP), computed tomography (CT), ultrasonography, bronchoscopy, and magnetic resonance imaging (MRI) studies.

 Analysis

The burned client experiences dramatic changes not only in the directly damaged tissues but also in many other body systems. Most burn clients experience all of the common and many of the additional nursing diagnoses during the course of the illness.

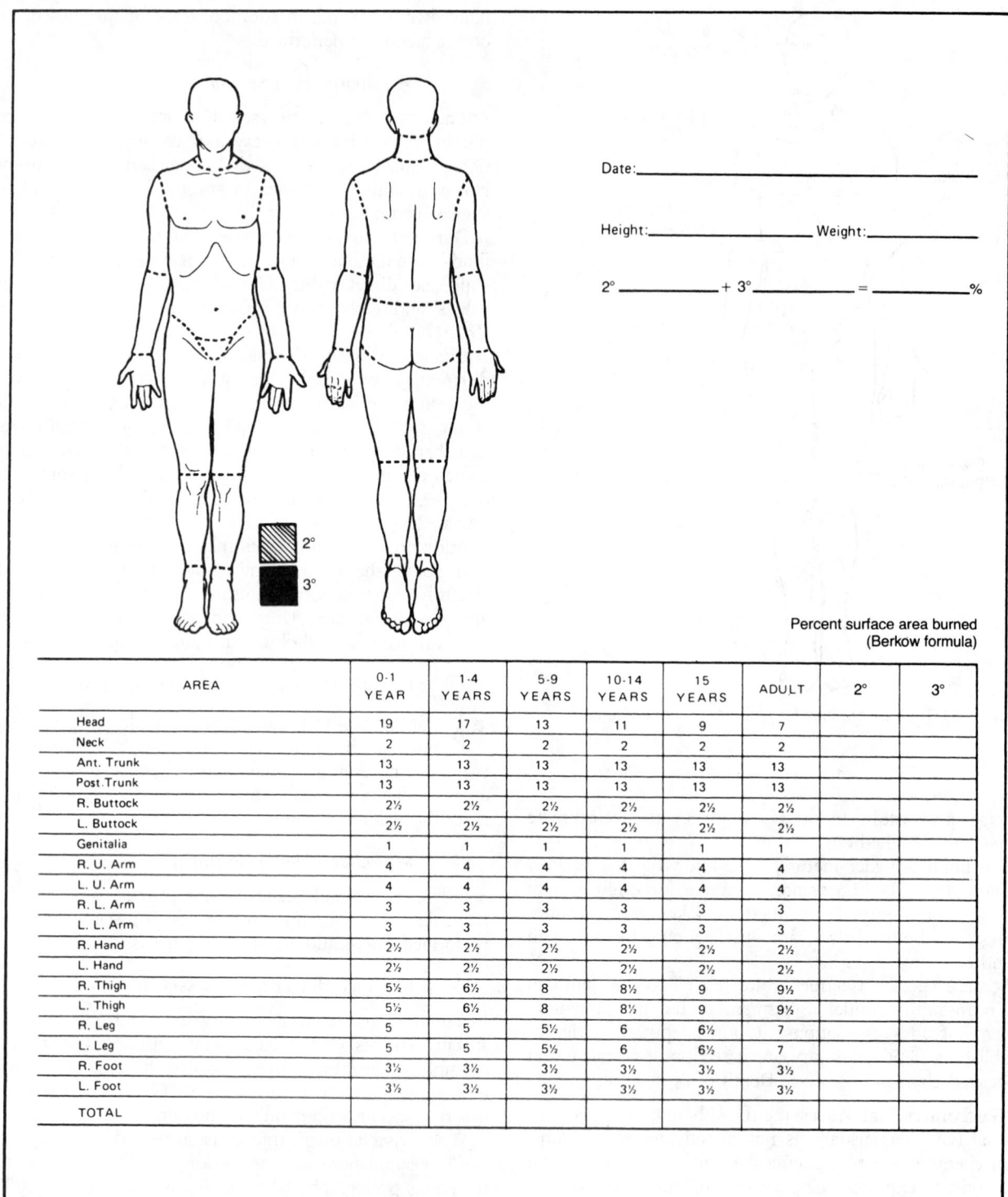

Date:_____

Height:_____ Weight:_____

2° _____ + 3° _____ = _____%

Percent surface area burned
(Berkow formula)

AREA	0-1 YEAR	1-4 YEARS	5-9 YEARS	10-14 YEARS	15 YEARS	ADULT	2°	3°
Head	19	17	13	11	9	7		
Neck	2	2	2	2	2	2		
Ant. Trunk	13	13	13	13	13	13		
Post.Trunk	13	13	13	13	13	13		
R. Buttock	2½	2½	2½	2½	2½	2½		
L. Buttock	2½	2½	2½	2½	2½	2½		
Genitalia	1	1	1	1	1	1		
R. U. Arm	4	4	4	4	4	4		
L. U. Arm	4	4	4	4	4	4		
R. L. Arm	3	3	3	3	3	3		
L. L. Arm	3	3	3	3	3	3		
R. Hand	2½	2½	2½	2½	2½	2½		
L. Hand	2½	2½	2½	2½	2½	2½		
R. Thigh	5½	6½	8	8½	9	9½		
L. Thigh	5½	6½	8	8½	9	9½		
R. Leg	5	5	5½	6	6½	7		
L. Leg	5	5	5½	6	6½	7		
R. Foot	3½	3½	3½	3½	3½	3½		
L. Foot	3½	3½	3½	3½	3½	3½		
TOTAL								

Figure 71–11. Estimation of the extent of burn injury by the Berkow method. Ant., anterior; Post., posterior; R., right; L., left; R.U., right upper; L.U., left upper; R.L., right lower; L.L., left lower.

➤ *Common Nursing Diagnoses and Collaborative Problems*

The following nursing diagnoses are common to clients in the emergent phase who have sustained a burn injury greater than 25% of the total body surface area (TBSA):

1. Decreased Cardiac Output related to increase in capillary permeability
2. Fluid Volume Deficit related to electrolyte imbalance, loss of plasma volume, and inadequate fluid resuscitation

Chart 71–4

Laboratory Profile: Burn Assessment During the Emergent Period

Test	Normal Range for Adults	Significance of Abnormal Findings
Serum Studies		
Hemoglobin	• 11.7–15.3 g/dL (women) • 13.2–17.3 g/dL (men)	Elevated as a result of fluid volume loss
Hematocrit	• 35%–47% (women) • 39%–50% (men)	Elevated as a result of fluid volume loss
Urea nitrogen	• 6–20 mg/dL	Elevated as a result of fluid volume loss
Glucose	• 74–106 mg/dL	Elevated as a result of the stress response and increased uptake across injured tissues
Electrolytes		
Sodium	• 136–145 mEq/L (mmol/L)	Decreased; sodium is trapped in edema fluid and lost through plasma leakage
Potassium	• 3.5–5.1 mEq/L (mmol/L)	Elevated as a result of disruption of the sodium-potassium pump, tissue destruction, and red blood cell hemolysis
Chloride	• 98–107 mEq/L (mmol/L)	Elevated as a result of fluid volume loss and reabsorption of chloride in urine
Arterial Blood Gas Studies		
PaO_2	• 83–108 mmHg	Slightly decreased
$PaCO_2$	• 32–48 mmHg	Slightly increased from respiratory injury
pH	• 7.35–7.45	Low as a result of metabolic acidosis
Carboxyhemoglobin	• 0%–10%	Elevated as a result of inhalation of smoke and carbon monoxide
Other		
Total protein	• 6–8.3 g/dL	Low; protein exudate is lost through the wound
Albumin	• 3.4–4.8 g/dL	Low; protein is lost through the wound and through vascular membranes because of increased permeability

Normal values are from Tietz (1995).

3. Altered Tissue Perfusion (Cerebral, Cardiopulmonary, Renal, Gastrointestinal, and Peripheral) related to decreases in cardiac output, extravascular fluid shifts, hypovolemia, constriction of eschar, and edema
4. Ineffective Breathing Pattern related to respiratory distress from upper airway edema, pulmonary edema, airway obstruction, or pneumonia
5. Pain related to damaged or exposed nerve endings, debridement, dressing changes, invasive procedures, and donor sites

The primary collaborative problems are
1. Potential for Pulmonary Edema
2. Potential for Adult Respiratory Distress Syndrome (ARDS)

➤ *Additional Nursing Diagnoses and Collaborative Problems*

The client with burn injuries in the emergent phase may present with one or more of the following nursing diagnoses and collaborative problems:
  ▪ Fluid Volume Excess related to massive intravenous fluid administration

  ▪ Risk for Altered Body Temperature related to loss of protective barrier and hypermetabolism
  ▪ Sensory/Perceptual Alterations related to periorbital edema or ulcerations, hospital environment, noise, infections, and dressings
  ▪ Anxiety related to initial burn trauma, threat of death, situational crisis, painful procedures, unfamiliar environment, separation from significant others, and loss of control
  ▪ Fear related to pain, knowledge deficit, therapeutic procedures, hospitalization, separation, and social reentry

 Planning and Implementation

➤ *Decreased Cardiac Output: Fluid Volume Deficit; Altered Tissue Perfusion*

Planning: Expected Outcomes. Following appropriate intervention, the client is expected to
  ▪ Have cardiac output restored to normal
  ▪ Maintain adequate oxygenation and circulation to all vital organs

Interventions. Interventions are aimed at increasing vascular fluid volume, supporting compensatory mechanisms, and preventing complications. Nonsurgical management is often sufficient for achieving these aims. Surgical management is required most frequently for full-thickness burns.

Nonsurgical Management. Restoration of fluid volume and tissue perfusion can be accomplished through intravenous fluid therapy, plasma exchange therapy, and drug therapy.

Intravenous Fluid Therapy. Appropriate infusion of intravenous fluids maintains a circulating volume sufficient for normal cardiac output, mean arterial pressure, and tissue oxygenation. Many formulas for calculating fluid requirements exist. Table 71–5 summarizes the formulas most commonly used for therapy of adult clients. Although the types and amounts of electrolytes, crystalloids, and colloids vary, the ultimate purpose of all of these formulas is to prevent shock by maintaining an adequate circulating fluid volume. The optimal formula and administration schedule are controversial issues.

The client being resuscitated from a severe burn receives large fluid loads in a short time. The Parkland formula suggests that the nurse administer half of the calculated fluid in the first 8 hours after the burn. The nurse administers the other half over the next 16 hours, for a total of 24 hours. In the second 24-hour period after a burn injury, the volume and content of the intravenous fluids are based on the client's specific volume and electrolyte imbalances and the client's response to treatment.

Most fluid replacement formulas are calculated from the time of injury and not from the time of arrival at the hospital. For example, if a client was burned at 8 AM but admitted to the hospital at 10 AM, the client's first 8-hour period would be completed at 4 PM, or 8 hours after the injury. Thus, if resuscitation were delayed until admission to the hospital, calculated fluids would need to be administered over a 6-hour period rather than an 8-hour period.

For clients with extensive burns, a large-bore central venous catheter is inserted so that massive fluid loads can be administered. At times, peripheral lines may easily become dislodged or the fluid flow cut off because of massive peripheral edema.

Plasma Exchange Therapy. Shock may persist in the post-burn period despite adequate fluid resuscitation. Although the cause of this persistent shock is unknown, numerous toxic serum factors have been suggested. Plasma exchange can reverse this condition.

The plasma exchange process either removes the client's plasma and replaces it with fresh frozen plasma (*plasmapheresis*) or removes the client's blood and replaces it with whole banked blood (*exchange transfusion*). Plasma exchange can assist with decreasing the amount of required fluid and increasing urinary output; thus, those clients who do not respond to conventional fluid therapy are helped (Kravitz et al., 1989).

Monitoring. The nurse monitors criteria to determine the adequacy of fluid resuscitation. These parameters are indications of hydration and adequate tissue perfusion to the brain, heart, and kidneys. During resuscitation, deviation from any of the desirable parameters suggests an inadequate or excessive amount of fluid.

Urine output is the most common and most sensitive noninvasive assessment parameter for cardiac output and tissue perfusion (see Chaps. 14 and 39). Regardless of the total amount of fluid calculated as appropriate to meet the fluid needs of the client, the amount of fluid administered depends on how much intravenous fluid per hour is required to maintain urine output at 1 mL/kg/% burn (up to 30 mL/hour). Adjustment of the rate of administration of intravenous fluid on the basis of urinary output plus serum electrolyte values is known as *titration* of fluid to meet the perfusion needs of the client. In clients with burns larger than 35% TBSA, the use of urine output and vital signs to guide resuscitation may be insufficient. Additional invasive monitoring of cardiopulmonary function is necessary to ensure optimal fluid resuscitation.

TABLE 71–5

Common Fluid Resuscitation Formulas for the First 24 Hours After a Burn Injury			
	Formula	**Solution**	**Rate of Administration**
Modified Brooke	• 0.5 mL/kg/% BSA burn • 1.5 mL/kg/% BSA burn	• Protenate or 5% albumin in isotonic saline • Lactated Ringer's without dextrose	• ½ given in first 8 hr ½ given in next 16 hr
Parkland (Baxter)	• 4 mL/kg/% BSA burn for 24-hr period	• Crystalloid only (lactated Ringer's)	• ½ given in first 8 hr ½ given in next 16 hr
Monafo		• Crystalloid (hypertonic saline: sodium = 250 mEq/L)	• Adjust to maintain urinary output of 30 mL/hr
Modified Parkland	• 4 mL/kg/% BSA burn + 15 ml/m² of BSA	• Crystalloid only (lactated Ringer's)	• ½ given in first 8 hr ½ given in next 16 hr
Winski	• 2 mL/kg/% burn + maintenance fluid	• Crystalloid only (lactated Ringer's)	• ½ given in first 8 hr ½ given in next 16 hr

Burn clients are often in severe shock and require invasive cardiac monitoring. With use of modern electronic equipment (see Chap. 39), nurses monitor vital parameters, such as central venous pressure, pulmonary artery pressures, and cardiac output. Because an adequately functioning cardiovascular system is imperative, the nurse monitors the electrocardiographic activity of clients who have sustained large burns. Rhythms that affect the mechanics of the heart, such as atrial fibrillation, are often present in the elderly client.

Drug Therapy. A frequent mistake in treatment is to administer diuretics to increase urinary output rather than to change the amount and rate of fluids administered to the client. Diuretics do not increase cardiac output; they actually decrease circulating volume and cardiac output by pulling fluid from the circulating blood volume to enhance diuresis. This effect can cause a dangerous reduction in perfusion to other vital organs (especially the heart, lungs, and brain) and greatly increases the risk of shock. Therefore, diuretics are not generally used to improve urinary output for burn clients. An exception is the client with a burn injury caused by electrical energy. Muscle and deep tissue damage can cause the release of large protein molecules (myoglobin), which precipitate in and obstruct the renal tubules. Although the diuretic mannitol (Osmitrol✦) is often used in this situation, it should always be given after adequate urinary output has been established and is accompanied with alkalinization of urine with sodium bicarbonate supplementation.

In some clients, particularly the elderly or those with a history of cardiac disease, a complicating factor in reduced cardiac output may be congestive heart failure or myocardial infarction. Drugs that increase cardiac output, such as dopamine (Intropin, Revimine✦), or that strengthen the force of myocardial concentration, such as digoxin (Lanoxin, Novodigoxin✦), may be used in conjunction with fluid therapy.

Surgical Management. The primary surgical procedure for treatment of inadequate tissue perfusion is *escharotomy*. An incision into the burn eschar with an electrocautery or scalpel relieves pressure caused by the restricting force of circumferential burns on the extremity or chest and improves circulation. If the pressure is not relieved, arterial compression can occur with resultant compromise of extremity perfusion, ischemia, and possibly necrosis. The incisions are made along the medial and lateral sides of the extremity and extend into subcutaneous tissue (Figs. 71–6, 71–12). This procedure breaks the tourniquet effect of the eschar. If tissue measurements remain elevated after the escharotomies, a *fasciotomy* (an incision extending through the subcutaneous tissue and fascia) is performed.

Escharotomies and fasciotomies are frequently performed at the bedside. No anesthesia is required because nerve endings have been destroyed by the burn injury, but sedation and analgesia are commonly given to reduce anxiety. The nurse prepares clients by assuring them that they will be made as comfortable as possible. The nurse removes the dressings and thoroughly cleans the areas to be incised. After the procedure, the nurse applies topical

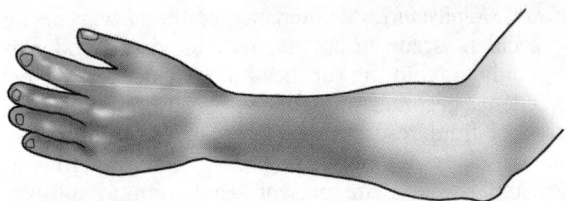

Tight, circumferential eschar restricting outward swelling as edema forms in the tissues beneath the eschar. Edema compresses blood vessels, which inhibits blood flow to the distal extremity.

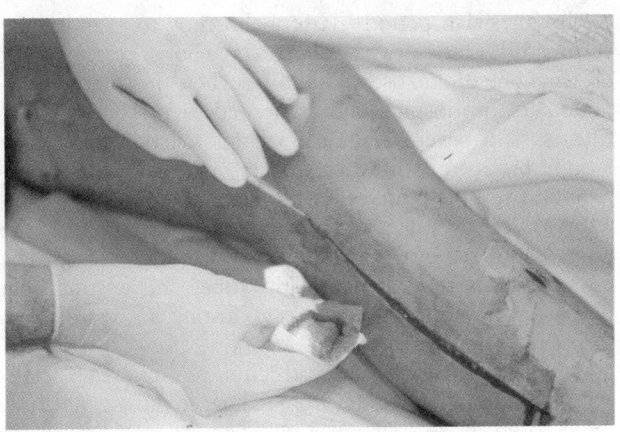

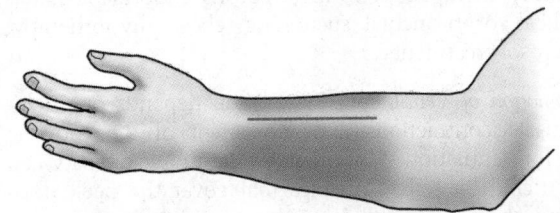

An escharotomy incision allows outward swelling of edematous tissues. Restricted blood flow through the vessels to the distal extremity is relieved.

Figure 71–12. Escharotomy to release circumferential burn eschar and improve circulation to a distal extremity.

antimicrobial agents and dressings to the area and monitors the escharotomy sites for bleeding.

> *Ineffective Breathing Pattern*

Planning: Expected Outcomes. With appropriate intervention, the client is expected to
- Maintain a patent airway
- Have an effective breathing pattern

Interventions. Interventions are aimed at supporting normal pulmonary mechanisms and preventing pulmonary problems. Specific plans for pulmonary management depend on the cause of the insult and the status of the respiratory tract.

Nonsurgical Management. Appropriate interventions include airway maintenance, promotion of ventilation, monitoring gas exchange, oxygen therapy, drug therapy, and positioning and deep breathing.

Airway Maintenance. Maintenance of the airway begins at the accident scene in an unconscious victim and may involve only a chin lift or head tilt maneuver. Upper airway edema becomes pronounced 8–12 hours after the initiation of fluid resuscitation. These clients require immediate nasal or oral intubation once signs of crowing, stridor, and dyspnea are present. Hesitation to intubate clients often leads to an emergency, as the airway becomes completely obstructed and surgical intervention is required. Therefore, intubation is often done prophylactically.

The physician performs a bronchoscopy to examine the vocal cords and airways of clients who are at risk for obstruction. Bronchoscopy is done when the client is admitted to the hospital and as needed to prevent a crisis. Clients with severe smoke inhalation or poisoning may require bronchoscopy when they are admitted to the hospital and routinely thereafter for examination of the respiratory tract, accurate diagnoses, deep suctioning of the lungs, and removal of sloughing necrotic tissue. The nurse assesses the patency of the tubes and ensures that proper positioning is maintained during respiratory assessment of intubated clients.

Other causes of airway obstruction are excessive secretions and sloughed tissue from damaged lungs. As indicated based on assessment or clinician order, the nurse or respiratory therapist performs vigorous endotracheal, nasotracheal, or bronchial suctioning, chest physiotherapy, and aerosol treatments.

Promotion of Ventilation. Respiration depends on skeletal muscle contractions and movement of the thoracic cavity for ventilation. Movement of the thoracic cavity can be restricted by tight dressings that cover the neck, thorax, and abdomen. The nurse observes the client for ease and effectiveness of respiratory movements and loosens tight dressings as needed to assist with ventilation.

Monitoring Gas Exchange. The nurse monitors the effectiveness of gas exchange by using laboratory tests, such as arterial blood gas and carboxyhemoglobin levels, as well as by noting physical signs, such as cyanosis, disorientation, and increased pulse rate. Other data to monitor for effectiveness of gas exchange in critically ill clients include chest x-rays, Swan-Ganz catheters, and central venous pressure measurement.

Oxygen Therapy. Management of impaired breathing patterns includes the administration of humidified oxygen to the client by face mask, cannula, or hood. Arterial oxygenation less than 60 ($PaO_2 < 60$ mmHg) is an indication for intubation, and mechanical ventilation is instituted. So that time is not wasted in securing the equipment needed in an emergency, the nurse ensures that respiratory equipment is located at or near the client's bedside, including

- Oxygen
- Masks
- Cannulas
- Ambu bags
- Laryngoscope
- Endotracheal tubes
- Materials for tracheostomy

(Chapter 34 addresses specific nursing actions for clients during mechanical ventilation.)

Drug Therapy. When pneumonia or other pulmonary infections further impair breathing, the physician prescribes antibiotics. Impaired breathing patterns that result from cardiac failure and increased pulmonary pressures may be treated with drugs that improve cardiac output and enhance renal excretion.

When a client's activity severely compromises respiratory mechanics, it may be necessary to use a paralytic drug, such as pancuronium bromide (Pavulon). Paralytic agents remove all ventilatory control from the client and allow uninterrupted administration of artificial ventilation. However, these drugs do not prevent the client from seeing and hearing or experiencing fear, pain, and loss of control. Any client receiving neuromuscular blockade drugs should also receive agents for sedation, analgesia, and antianxiety. The nurse ensures that all alarms are operative because the client cannot call for help.

Positioning and Deep Breathing. To improve breathing patterns, the nurse turns the client frequently, helps the client out of bed, encourages as much movement as possible, and teaches the use of incentive spirometry, coughing, and deep breathing. Chest physiotherapy is performed by the nurse or respiratory therapist according to the client's need and the clinician's prescription.

Surgical Management. A tracheostomy may be necessary in clients for whom long-term intubation is expected. Tracheostomy carries a greater risk of infection in burn clients than in nonburned clients. Emergency tracheostomies are performed when an airway becomes occluded and oral or nasal intubation cannot be achieved.

Other common surgical procedures for improving the burn client's breathing pattern include insertion of chest tubes and the performance of escharotomy. Chest tubes are used to re-expand the lung when pneumothorax or hemothorax has occurred (see Chap. 32).

Tight eschar on the neck, chest, or abdomen can restrict respiratory movement. Escharotomies (described earlier) can relieve this restriction and permit greater respiratory movement.

➤ Pain

Pain associated with burn injuries is both chronic and acute. Many factors contribute to burn pain, and these factors are manipulated to alter the response to pain. Pain from the actual injury is compounded when painful procedures are performed. Accurate assessment of the client's pain before and during procedures is an essential part of pain management (see Research Applications for Nursing).

Planning: Expected Outcomes. The client's pain is expected to be alleviated or reduced.

Interventions. The plan for pain management is tailored to the client's tolerance for pain, coping mechanisms, and physical status.

Nonsurgical Management. Interventions for the client experiencing pain (Latarjet & Choinere, 1995; Kealey, 1995a, b; Patterson, 1995) include drug therapy, comple-

Research Applications for Nursing

Client and Nurse Assessments of Pain Do Not Agree

Geisser, M., Bingham, H., & Robinson, M. (1995). Pain and anxiety during burn dressing changes: Concordance between patients' and nurses' ratings and relation to medication administration and patient variables. Journal of Burn Care and Rehabilitation, 16, 165–171.

This study examined the relationship between clients' and nurses' ratings of client pain and anxiety during burn dressing changes. Eleven clients undergoing 107 dressing changes were asked to rate their average and maximum levels of pain during the dressing changes using a 10-cm visual analog scale. At least one nurse per dressing change was to do the same. The percentage agreement between the clients and nurses for overall and worse pain was 25% and 27%, respectively. The percentage agreement for tension before dressing changes was 35.4% and during dressing changes was 37.4%. As a result, the agreement between clients' and nurses' ratings of pain and tension were generally low. In addition, the nurses' ratings of clients' pain were positively related to the clients' report of pain and to the amount of analgesic administered.

Critique. No indications were given to control for within-subject variances. This lack of control may account for the lower correlations between the nurses' and the clients' ratings. In addition, the reliability of the scale utilized was poor and may account for lower correlations between the clients and the nurses.

Possible Nursing Implications. Because pain is such a subjective phenomenon, nurses' ratings of the clients' pain during the administration of anagelsic medication may not be the best method to utilize. Nurses should not depend solely on their assessments but rather on feedback from the client whenever possible. In addition, because tension and anxiety tend to relate to increased pain during dressing changes, interventions aimed at reducing anxiety before and during dressing changes may be a more effective method of managing procedural pain in burn clients.

mentary therapy measures, and environmental manipulation.

Drug Therapy. Opioid and nonopioid analgesics, such as morphine sulfate, meperidine (Demerol), and nalbuphine (Nubain), are given with relative frequency throughout hospitalization. These drugs rarely offer more than moderate relief during acutely painful procedures, however, and they produce side effects of respiratory depression and diminished gastrointestinal motility. During the emergent post-burn phase, these agents are administered intravenously because the fluid shift significantly limits absorption from the subcutaneous and intramuscular spaces; thus, agents administered by these routes remain in the spaces and do not relieve pain. In addition, when edema is present, cumulative subcutaneous or intramuscular doses are rapidly reabsorbed when the fluid shift is resolving. This delayed reabsorption can result in lethal blood levels of analgesics.

Anesthetic agents, such as ketamine (Ketalar), pentobar-

bital sodium (Nembutal, Novopentobarb✤), and nitrous oxide, also reduce pain. Extreme care must be taken during their administration, and the presence of an anesthesiologist, nurse anesthetist, or specially trained medical personnel is required.

Complementary Therapy. Complementary therapy measures include relaxation techniques, meditative breathing, guided imagery, music therapy, massage, and therapeutic or healing touch. Hypnosis and autohypnosis of lucid, cooperative clients can be attempted by trained therapists. Therapeutic touch, acupuncture, and acupressure are used to a limited extent for burn clients with variable results. (Nontraditional and complementary therapy types of pain intervention are detailed in Chapter 9.)

Environmental Manipulation. The nurse can increase the client's comfort by providing a quiet environment, using nonpainful tactile stimulation, and increasing the client's control. Increasing the client's sleep or rest time in a quiet environment helps reduce the adverse effects of sleep deprivation, replenishes catecholamine stores, helps prevent critical care unit psychosis, and restores diurnal effects of endorphins. The nurse and assistive personnel attempt to perform as many procedures as possible during the client's waking hours.

Tactile stimulation can reduce pain. The nurse changes the client's position routinely to reduce pressure on any specific area; repositioning improves circulation to painful areas and reduces pain. Massaging nonburn areas may reduce pain transmission on thick pain-sensory nerve fibers by stimulating an increased release of endorphins. Applying heat and maintaining warm room temperatures prevent the client from shivering and stimulate the production of serotonin, which has been associated with triggering of the relaxation response.

To reduce anxiety and increase feelings of confidence and independence, the nurse encourages the client's participation in pain control measures. For example, the nurse and client make a contract that specifies how long a painful procedure will last. This helps clients deal with the pain for that particular period. Patient-controlled analgesia (PCA) also reduces pain in burned clients.

Surgical Management. A technique of early surgical excision of the burn wound is used in many burn centers (see Impaired Skin Integrity, Surgical Excision). Early excision under anesthesia can reduce the pain associated with daily debridement at the bedside or during hydrotherapy.

➤ Potential for Pulmonary Edema

Planning: Expected Outcomes. With intervention, the client is expected to be free of pulmonary edema.

Interventions. Pulmonary edema can arise from pulmonary injury; however, pulmonary edema in the emergent phase is associated with fluid resuscitation and myocardial overload. Even a young healthy person may have some degree of ventricular insufficiency. Usually, these clients receive digoxin or another inotropic agent to improve left ventricular function and prevent or treat pulmonary edema. Diuretics, a mainstay of therapy for pulmonary edema from other causes, may or may not be used in the emergent phase depending on the client's vascular hydration status and renal function.

➤ *Potential for Adult Respiratory Distress Syndrome*

Planning: Expected Outcomes. The client is expected to

- Have arterial blood gases (ABGs) within normal limits
- Maintain normal lung compliance
- Be free of respiratory distress

Interventions. Clients who have developed ARDS as a result of burn injury require thorough assessments and interventions. The interventions aim at increasing lung compliance and improving PaO_2 levels.

In collaboration with the physician and respiratory therapist, the client will receive positive end-expiratory pressure (PEEP) to augment the decreased lung volume by providing a continuous positive pressure in the airways and alveoli (Roberts, 1996). This procedure optimizes diffusion of oxygen across the alveolar-capillary membrane. PEEP can be combined with intermittent mandatory volume (IMV) to enhance the therapeutic potential of PEEP.

The client's response is assessed and documented so that appropriate ventilator changes can be made. Any signs of respiratory distress and changes in respiratory patterns are documented and reported to the physician. Pulse oximetry and ABG levels are also monitored for changes in respiratory status.

Neuromuscular blocking agents (pancuronium bromide) can be used in clients requiring mechanical ventilation to reduce or eliminate spontaneous breathing efforts and to reduce oxygen consumption (see specific nursing care under Ineffective Breathing Pattern, Drug Therapy).

Acute Phase of Burn Injury

Overview

The acute phase of burn injury begins approximately 48 hours after injury and lasts until wound closure is complete. During this phase, an intense collaborative approach to care is directed toward continued assessment and maintenance of the cardiovascular and respiratory systems, as well as gastrointestinal and nutritional status, burn wound care, pain control, and psychosocial interventions.

Collaborative Management

 Assessment

➤ *Physical Assessment/Clinical Manifestations*

Cardiopulmonary Assessment. The physical assessment findings in the acute phase of burn injury related to the cardiovascular and respiratory systems are directed at maintenance of these systems as well as treating potential complications as they occur. Although airway injuries should be resolved, the client may experience pneumonia

that can compromise the airway and result in respiratory failure requiring mechanical ventilation (Miller et al., 1994). The cardiovascular system problems should also be resolved. However, the client is at risk for infection, which can lead to septic shock and affect cardiovascular function. The assessment and clinical interventions undertaken in the emergent phase should also be used in these isolated clinical situations.

Neuroendocrine Assessment. The increased metabolic demands placed on the body after a severe burn injury can severely compromise the client's nutritional status (Rodriguez, 1996). The nurse weighs the client daily and compares the findings with the client's pre-burn weight. The client is weighed without dressings or splints, if possible. A loss of 2% in body weight indicates a mild deficit; a weight loss of 10% or more is a significant deficit and requires evaluation of calorie and fluid intake and appropriate modifications.

Some burn units use indirect calorimetry to obtain accurate calorie requirements for burn clients. This technique determines kilocalories of energy expenditure by measurement of oxygen consumption (VO_2) and carbon dioxide production (VCO_2). Measurements are performed while the client is at rest and, preferably, when dressing changes or other stressful procedures have not been done for at least 30 minutes. If available, indirect calorimetry is performed on admission and at least once each week until the wounds are closed (Mayes et al., 1997).

Immunologic Assessment. As a result of the inflammatory response and the compromise in immune function, the client is susceptible to infection. Burn wound sepsis is a serious complication of burn injury, and infection remains the leading cause of morbidity and mortality during the acute phase of recovery (Green et al., 1994; Law et al., 1994). The nurse continually assesses the client for signs of local and systemic infections (Table 71–6), including changes in wound appearance, changes in neurologic and gastrointestinal function, and subtle changes in vital signs. Gram-positive, gram-negative, and fungal infections produce a variety of clinical signs and symptoms, and the nurse monitors the client for these differences (Table 71–7). The nurse and other assistive personnel use meticulous hand washing and aseptic technique in caring for wounds and during invasive monitoring or therapy.

Musculoskeletal Assessment. Burned clients are at risk for musculoskeletal problems as a result of other injuries, immobility, healing processes, and treatment. The nurse initially evaluates the client's musculoskeletal status within the first few hours after admission to the hospital or burn center and throughout the acute phase of injury. The nurse assesses the client's active and passive range of motion for all joints, including the neck. Special attention is given to joints within the burn area. Ranges and limitations are noted for future reference.

 Analysis

During the acute phase of the burn injury, the burned client has resolution of some earlier problems, may have

TABLE 71-6

Local and Systemic Signs of Infection

Local

- Conversion of a partial-thickness injury to a full-thickness injury
- Ulceration of healthy skin at the burn site
- Erythematous, nodular lesions in uninvolved skin and vesicular lesions in healed skin
- Edema of healthy skin surrounding the burn wound
- Excessive burn wound drainage
- Pale, boggy, dry, or crusted granulation tissue
- Sloughing of grafts
- Wound breakdown after closure
- Odor

Systemic

- Altered level of consciousness
- Changes in vital signs (tachycardia, tachypnea, temperature instability, hypotension)
- Increased fluid requirements for maintenance of a normal urinary output
- Hemodynamic instability
- Oliguria
- Gastrointestinal dysfunction (diarrhea, vomiting, abdominal distention, paralytic ileus)
- Hyperglycemia
- Thrombocytopenia
- Change in total white blood cell count (above normal or below normal)
- Metabolic acidosis
- Hypoxemia

initial problems extend into the acute phase, and experiences new problems in many body systems.

➤ Common Nursing Diagnoses and Collaborative Problems

The following nursing diagnoses are common to clients in the acute phase who have sustained a burn injury greater than 25% of the total body surface area (TBSA):

1. Impaired Skin Integrity related to burn wound, graft site, or donor site
2. Risk for Infection related to impaired skin integrity,

presence of multiple invasive catheters, compromise in immune function, and nutritional compromise
3. Altered Nutrition: Less than Body Requirements related to increased metabolic rate; reduced calorie intake; altered glucose, fat, and protein metabolism; and increased urinary nitrogen losses
4. Impaired Physical Mobility related to open burn wounds, pain, and scar and contracture
5. Body Image Disturbance related to change in physical appearance, change in lifestyle, and alterations in sensory and motor function

The primary collaborative problem is Wound Care Management

➤ Additional Nursing Diagnoses and Collaborative Problems

The client with burn injuries in the acute phase may present with one or more of the following nursing diagnoses and collaborative problems:

- Anticipatory Grieving related to loss of significant others, loss of possessions, physical disfigurement, and changes in body image
- Ineffective Family Coping related to loss of home, family, or significant others; crisis resulting from burn injury; disturbances in normal functions; role changes; and prolonged hospitalization and rehabilitation
- Ineffective Individual Coping related to situational crises, disfigurement, separation, and sensory overload
- Self Care Deficit related to pain; contractures; and loss of function in hands, extremities, and other body parts
- Sexual Dysfunction related to perineal, genital, and breast burns; immobility, fatigue, and depression; and disturbance in body image
- Sleep Pattern Disturbance related to pain, treatment regimen, and environmental noise
- Social Isolation related to protective isolation treatment regimen and alterations in physical appearance
- Knowledge Deficit related to treatment regimen and healing process
- Potential for Pneumonia
- Potential for Septicemia

TABLE 71-7

Signs and Symptoms of Sepsis Caused by Different Organisms

Sign/Symptom	Gram-Positive	Gram-Negative	Fungal
Onset	• Insidious, 2–6 days	• Rapid, 12–36 hr	• Delayed
Sensorium	• Severe disorientation and lethargy	• Mild disorientation	• Mild disorientation
Ileus	• Severe	• Severe	• Mild
Diarrhea	• Rare	• Severe	• Occasional
Temperature	• Hyperpyrexia	• Hypothermia	• Hyperpyrexia
Hypotension	• Late	• Early	• Late
White blood cell count	• Neutrophilia	• Neutropenia	• Neutrophilia
Platelets	• Normal	• Low	• Low

Planning and Implementation

➤ Impaired Skin Integrity; Wound Care Management

Planning: Expected Outcomes. With appropriate intervention, the client is expected to

- Experience no further loss of skin integrity
- Have skin integrity restored without complications

Interventions. Interventions aim at preserving the integrity of nonburned skin, enhancing wound healing of burned skin, and preventing complications.

Nonsurgical Management. Nonsurgical burn wound management, or conservative treatment, involves removing exudates and necrotic tissue, cleaning the area, stimulating granulation and revascularization, and applying dressings. Restoration of skin, whether by natural healing or by grafting, starts with removal of eschar and other cellular debris from the burn wound. This removal is called *debridement*. Conservative treatment allows noninvasive debriding of the wound through mechanical and enzymatic actions that stimulate the separation of eschar over time. The goal is to have the wound slowly prepare itself for grafting and wound closure by a natural process.

Mechanical Debridement. Burn wounds are debrided and cleaned a minimum of once, and usually two to three times, each day during hydrotherapy (the application of water for treatment). Nurses, assistive nursing personnel, and physiotherapists perform hydrotherapy daily to debride necrotic tissue and to examine the wounds. Hydrotherapy can be accomplished by immersing the client in a tub, showering the client on a specially designed table, or successively washing only small areas of the wound at the bedside if the client is too unstable to be moved. Showering enhances visualization of the wounds and allows water temperature to be kept constant.

Nurses and skilled technicians use forceps and scissors to remove loose, nonviable tissue during hydrotherapy. The management of intact blisters is controversial. At most institutions, small blisters are left alone because they serve as a protective barrier that assists with wound healing and re-epithelialization. Because the protein-filled fluid within blisters can cause some degree of immunosuppression, many institutions open larger blisters. Washcloths or gauze sponges can also facilitate debridement of "cheesy" eschar or pseudoeschar. During hydrotherapy, the burn areas are washed thoroughly and gently with mild soap or detergent and water. The areas are then rinsed with normal saline or water at room temperature.

Enzymatic Debridement. Enzymatic debridement can occur naturally by *autolysis* or artificially by application of exogenous agents. Autolysis is the spontaneous disintegration of tissue by the action of the client's own cellular enzymes. This process is seldom used in North America for larger burns because it is slow and results in prolonged hospital stay.

Exogenous agents, such as collagenase (Santyl), is a topical enzyme used for rapid wound debridement. When this agent is applied directly to the burn wound in a once a day dressing change, the enzyme digests native and denatured collagen in necrotic tissues (Hansbrough et al., 1995). Because collagen accounts for 75% of the dry weight of skin tissue, the ability of collagenase (Santyl) to digest collagen in the physiologic pH range makes it an important debriding agent for burn wounds. Polysporin powder is frequently used with this topical agent to prevent infection.

Dressing the Burn Wound. After burn wounds are cleaned and debrided, the nurse applies topical antibiotics to prevent infection (see Risk for Infection). Some type of dressing is then applied to the burn wound. Burn dressings include standard wound dressings, biologic dressings, and synthetic dressings and artificial skin. (Table 70–6 describes the characteristics of many types of dressings.)

Standard Wound Dressings. Standard wound dressings are multiple layers of gauze that are applied over the topical agent or antibiotic on the burn wound. The number of gauze layers depends on

- The depth of the injury
- The amount of drainage expected
- The area injured
- The client's mobility
- The frequency of dressing changes

The gauze layers are held in place with roller-type gauze bandages applied in a distal to proximal direction or with circular net fabrics. On the client's extremities, the nurse covers gauze dressings with elastic wraps, especially if the client is ambulatory. Based on assessed needs or clinician orders, the nurse or assistive nursing personnel changes and reapplies the dressings every 8–12 hours after thoroughly cleaning the areas.

Biologic Dressings. Biologic dressings are materials obtained from living or deceased humans (homograft or allograft) or animals (heterograft or xenograft). When applied over open wounds, a biologic dressing rapidly adheres and promotes healing or prepares the wound for permanent autograft coverage.

Biologic materials are used on healing partial-thickness and granulating full-thickness wounds that are clean and free of eschar. Table 71–8 outlines the advantages and disadvantages of biologic dressings. The type of biologic dressing selected depends on the type of wound to be covered and the availability of the material.

Homograft. Skin for a homograft (allograft) is usually obtained from a cadaver and provided through a skin bank. It is fresh or frozen; frozen skin is thawed in a warm bath of sterile normal saline before application. Disadvantages to the use of homograft are the excessive costs ($750 to $1000 per square foot) and the risk of transmitting a bloodborne infection.

Heterograft. Skin for a heterograft (xenograft) is obtained from another species. Pigskin is the most common heterograft because of its relative compatibility with human skin. The pigskin is replaced on a continual basis until the wound heals naturally or is closed with autograft. Because pigskin does not control bacterial proliferation, it is changed frequently.

Amniotic Membrane. Amniotic membrane is another form of biologic dressing used on burn wounds. Its large

TABLE 71-8

Biologic Dressings

Uses

- Debridement of untidy wounds after separation of eschar
- Promotion of re-epithelialization of deep partial-thickness wounds
- Temporary coverage after excision of the burn wound
- Protection of granulation tissue between autografts
- Test graft before autografting

Advantages

- Early adherence to the wound
- Reduction of evaporative heat loss
- Reduction of evaporative water loss
- Prevention of desiccation of granulation tissue
- Reduction of exudate protein losses
- Reduction of pain
- Assistance in wound debridement
- Enhancement of healing with partial-thickness injuries
- Protection of exposed neovascular tissue
- Inhibition of bacterial proliferation

Disadvantages

- Early lysis resulting in bacterial proliferation
- Expensive
- Rejection responses
- Possible burn wound sepsis if applied over eschar
- Not readily available
- Storage (some may require refrigeration)
- Possible transmission of diseases, such as hepatitis

size, low cost, and availability have helped with its success. In full-thickness injuries, the amniotic membrane immediately adheres to the wound. With partial-thickness areas, the amniotic membrane is effective as a dressing until re-epithelialization takes place. The membrane may require frequent changes because it does not vascularize and has the tendency to disintegrate in 48 hours.

Cultured Skin. Cultured skin can be grown from a small biopsy specimen of epidermal cells from an unburned portion of the client's body. The cells are grown in a laboratory to produce larger epithelial sheets that can be grafted on the client to generate a permanent epidermal surface. The length of time for culturing and growing the skin is prolonged, and the epithelial sheets are not durable (Still et al., 1994). Care is taken when these sheets are applied to ensure adherence and prevent sloughing.

Artificial Skin. Artificial skin, first developed in 1980, is an alternative approach to closure of the burn wound. This substance has two layers composed of a Silastic epidermis and a porous dermis made from bovine hide collagen and shark cartilage (Cooper & Spielvogel, 1994).

After the artificial skin is applied to a clean, excised wound surface, fibroblasts move into the collagen part of the artificial skin and create a fibrinous structure similar to normal dermis. The artificial dermis slowly dissolves and is replaced with normal blood vessels and connective

tissue (*neodermis*). The neodermis will support a standard split-thickness autograft that is placed over it when the Silastic layer is removed.

Synthetic Dressings. Synthetic dressings consisting of solid silicone and plastic membranes, such as polyvinyl chloride and polyurethane, may be substituted for antimicrobial, standard, or biologic dressings. Synthetic dressings are applied directly to the surface of a clean or surgically prepared wound and remain in place until they fall off or are removed due to nonadhesion. Because many of these dressings are transparent or translucent, the nurse can inspect the wound without removing the dressing. The client experiences pain reduction at the site because these agents also prevent contact of the wound with air.

Surgical Management. Surgical management of burn wounds focuses on surgical excision and wound covering. Surgical excision usually occurs early in the post-burn period. Grafting procedures for skin covering may be performed throughout the acute phase as burn wounds are made ready and donor sites are available. In the rehabilitative phase, grafting may improve function or appearance.

Wound covering is achieved through *autografting,* the transplantation of viable skin from an area of the client's intact, healthy skin to the full-thickness burn wound.

Surgical Excision. Surgical excision is a widely used method for managing full-thickness injuries; it is the treatment of choice for most deep partial-thickness wounds. The client is taken to the operating room as early as possible within the first 5 days after injury and as needed until complete permanent coverage has been achieved.

The burn wound is excised by either a tangential or a fascial excision technique. For the tangential techniques the surgeon excises very thin layers of the necrotic burn surface until bleeding tissue is encountered. Bleeding indicates that a viable bed of dermis or subcutaneous fat has been reached for application of the graft.

With the fascial technique, the surgeon excises the burn wound to the level of superficial fascia. Fascial excision is usually reserved for very deep and extensive burns. Blood loss is minimal, and grafting is usually successful.

Wound Covering. Permanent skin coverage for extensive full-thickness injuries is achieved through the application of an autograft. Skin for an autograft is taken from the client's own body. The surgeon usually removes a piece of skin from a remote area of the body that is unburned and transplants it to cover the burn wound. Skin grafts are generally of split thickness (0.015 inch); a partial-thickness injury is formed at the site of surgical removal, the donor site. Grafts are placed either on a clean granulated bed or over a surgically excised area of burn (see also Chap. 70).

The availability of donor sites for larger burns is small. Clients with burns of a large surface area may have a mere 5% to 20% of the skin surface available to cover the 80% to 95% burned area. Coverage is accomplished by

- Successive reharvesting of the available donor site, with time allowed between harvests for re-epithelialization and healing
- Meshing the split-thickness skin grafts (Fig. 71–13)

Meshing allows a small graft to cover a larger area, although small open spaces (interstices) are present uniformly throughout the graft. Healing time is slower for a meshed graft because the skin must fill in the interstices as well as attach to the granulation bed.

> ### Risk for Infection

Burn wound infection occurs through *autocontamination,* in which the client's own normal flora overgrows and penetrates the internal environment, and *cross-contamination,* in which microorganisms from another person or the environment are transferred to the client.

Planning: Expected Outcomes. The client is expected to

- Remain free from infection by cross-contamination
- Not experience septicemia

Interventions. Interventions aim at prevention of infection and removal of infected tissue.

Nonsurgical Management. Nonsurgical management of clients at high risk for infection consists of minimizing exposure of the burn client to exogenous microorganisms, reducing the risk of autocontamination, and recognizing signs and symptoms of infection early. Drug therapy, isolation therapy, and environmental manipulation are appropriate strategies for preventing and managing infection.

Drug Therapy for Infection Prevention. Burn wound conditions favor the growth of *Clostridium tetani.* All burn clients are considered at risk for this often fatal infectious complication. Tetanus toxoid, 0.5 mL administered intramuscularly, enhances previously acquired immunity to *C. tetani;* this is a routine prophylactic procedure when the client is admitted to the hospital. The additional administration of tetanus immune globulin (human) (Hyper-Tet) is recommended when the history of tetanus immunization is questionable.

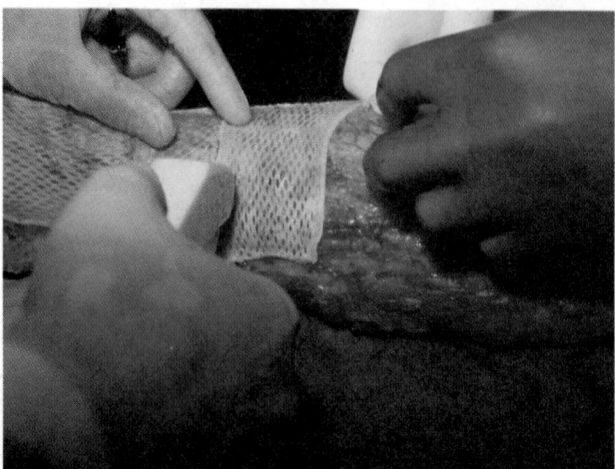

Figure 71–13. The typical appearance of meshed autografts.

The use of topical antimicrobial agents is one of the most important interventions for infection prevention in burn wounds (Greenfield & McManus, 1997). The primary goal of topical antimicrobial therapy is to minimize bacterial proliferation in the wound.

The nurse applies topical antibiotics by either the *open* or the *closed* technique. With the open technique, the nurse directly applies the agent to the burn wound, using either aseptic or clean methods, without further dressing the wound. The nurse cleans the wound every 8–12 hours and applies fresh antimicrobial agents. With the closed technique, which is more commonly used, the nurse dresses the burn wound after applying the topical agents.

Topical antimicrobial drugs are not applied to freshly grafted areas because many of these agents inhibit cell growth. Chart 71–5 summarizes characteristics of various topical antimicrobial agents; two of the more commonly used are silver sulfadiazine (Silvadene, Flamazine✲) and mafenide acetate (Sulfamylon).

Drug Therapy for Treatment of Infection. When burn clients experience symptoms of an actual infection, including septicemia, systemic antibiotics are ordered. Broad-spectrum antibiotics are administered until the results of blood cultures and sensitivity status are available. At that time, more specific antibiotics, including the aminoglycosides and cephalosporins, are used. Because of increased metabolism, burn clients generally require a larger than normal dose of these drugs for therapeutic serum levels to be maintained. If aminoglycosides are used, serial peak and trough serum levels are obtained to monitor the efficacy of treatment.

Isolation Therapy. Some clinicians believe that isolation therapy significantly reduces the incidence of cross-contamination; however, methods of isolation are varied and controversial. In some burn care units, virtually no isolation is practiced; in others, total sterile conditions preside. All isolation methods for the client with burns emphasize proper and consistent hand washing as the single most effective technique for preventing the transmission of infection.

Environmental Manipulation. The nurse wears gloves during all contact with open wounds. The use of sterile versus clean gloves for noninvasive, routine wound care procedures varies by agency and is a matter of debate (Sadowski, 1988). Regardless of sterility, the nurse changes gloves when handling wounds on different areas of the body and between handling old and new dressings.

Equipment on burn units is not shared among clients. Disposable items (e.g., pillows, syringes, and dishes) are used as much as possible. The nurse assigns equipment used in daily routine care to each client (e.g., thermometers, blood pressure cuffs, and stethoscopes). Daily cleaning of the equipment and general housekeeping are essential for environmental infection control. All equipment must be cleaned after use on one client and before use on another. Because *Pseudomonas* has been shown to sequester in plants, the presence of plants and flowers is prohibited. Some burn units do not permit clients to eat raw foods (such as salads, fruit, and pepper) so that exposure

Chart 71–5

Topical Drug Therapy for Burns

Agent	Description	Action	Advantages	Disadvantages	Interventions
Silver sulfadiazine (Silvadene, Flamazine✤)	• Nontoxic salt of silver sulfadiazine in water-based cream	• Binds to bacterial cell membranes and interferes with DNA synthesis	• Does not cause hypochloremia, hyponatremia, electrolyte imbalance, or kidney disease • Painless • Wide-spectrum antimicrobial action against gram-positive and gram-negative organisms • Long shelf life • Delays eschar separation less than many other topical agents do	• Absorbed into eschar less than other agents • May cause rash, pruritus, burning, and leukopenia • Not consistently effective for burns covering more than 60% of the body • Not effective against *Pseudomonas*	• Watch for signs of infection, such as soupiness of wound area. • Watch for allergic reaction causing drop in white blood cell count. • Do not use if reaction to sulfonamide has occurred.
Collagenase (Santyl) with polysporin powder	• Topical enzymatic debriding agent with 250 collagenase u/g of white petroleum	• Digests collagen in necrotic tissue	• Painless • Qd dressing changes • No side effects • Quick debridement action • Easy to apply	• Expensive • Use only on partial-thickness injuries	• Apply only qd
Mafenide acetate (Sulfamylon)	• Soft, white, nonstaining water-based cream	• Bacteriostatic action against many gram-positive and gram-negative organisms	• Effective against *Pseudomonas* • Long shelf life • Excellent for treating electrical burns • Penetrates thick eschar	• May lead to infection • May cause metabolic acidosis, hyperpnea, and rash • When applied, may cause pain that lasts 30–40 min	• Premedicate for pain before application. • Monitor blood gas and serum electrolyte levels. • Do not use if sulfa drug allergy or respiratory or kidney disease is present.
Nitrofurazone (Furacin)	• Cream, solution, or water-soluble powder	• Wide-spectrum anti-bacterial	• Effective against *Staphylococcus aureus* and some antibiotic-resistant organisms • Causes neither pain nor maceration	• May cause contact dermatitis (rare) • Messy to apply in cream form • May cause renal problems if used on clients with extensive burns	• Observe carefully for signs of allergic reaction and evidence of super-infections.

Continued

to exogenous microorganisms is minimized. Rugs and upholstered articles are difficult to clean and may harbor organisms; their use is also restricted.

Visitors are restricted when the client is immunosup-pressed. Ill people, small children, and other clients should not come into direct contact with the burn client. Some burn units recommend that all visitors wear protective clothing (gowns, gloves, masks, and shoe and hair

CHART 71–5. Topical Drug Therapy for Burns Continued

Agent	Description	Action	Advantages	Disadvantages	Interventions
Povidone-iodine (Betadine)	• Iodine complex available as solution, ointment, or foam	• Microbicidal against gram-positive and gram-negative organisms	• Effective against many infections not well controlled by silver sulfadiazine	• May cause metabolic acidosis and elevated serum iodine levels • May form crusts if burns are not cleaned properly • Causes rash and burning in some clients • Stains clothes and linen • Deactivated by wound proteins	• Check serum electrolyte and serum iodine levels frequently.
Gentamicin sulfate (Garamycin, Gentamar)	• Available as cream or solution for topical use	• Antibiotic action against organisms resistant to other agents	• Effective against *Pseudomonas* • Does not cause pain	• May have ototoxic and nephrotoxic effects • May result in resistance to certain organisms	• Use with caution in clients with decreased renal function. • Monitor serum and urine creatinine clearance before and during treatment.
Polymyxin B–bacitracin	• Topical cream	• Wide-spectrum antibacterial	• Painless • Effective against many gram-positive and gram-negative organisms • Can be used on the face • Can be placed on healed grafts to lubricate	• May cause urticaria, burning, and inflammation • Does not penetrate eschar	• Apply q2–8h to keep areas moist.

covers) in the room of the immunosuppressed client; however, no conclusive data support this approach.

Secondary Prevention/Early Detection. The nurse monitors the burn wounds on admission and at each dressing change. The nurse examines the wounds for the following signs of infection:

- Pervasive odor
- Color changes
- Change in texture
- Purulent drainage
- Exudate
- Sloughing grafts
- Redness at the wound edges extending to nonburned skin

Laboratory cultures and biopsies are recommended. Quantitative biopsies of the eschar and granulation tissue are performed routinely and as needed to monitor prolif-

eration of organisms and are considered the "gold standard" for wound monitoring.

Surgical Management. Infected burn wounds with colony counts of or approaching 10^5 colonies per gram of tissue are life threatening, even with antibiotic therapy. Aggressive surgical excision of the burn wound may be necessary.

➤ *Altered Nutrition: Less Than Body Requirements*

Planning: Expected Outcomes. The client is expected to maintain adequate nutritional intake for meeting the body's calorie requirements.

Interventions. Interventions aim at calculating the client's calorie needs and providing an adequate daily source of calories and nutrients that the client can ingest and metabolize.

Diet therapy begins with calculation of the client's current daily metabolic needs and calorie requirements. Several formulas and charts are used for this calculation. Nutritional requirements for clients with a relatively large burn area can exceed 5000 kcal/day. In addition to a high-calorie intake, the burn client requires a diet high in protein for wound healing. The nurse collaborates with the dietitian and the client to plan alternatives to conventional nutritional patterns.

Oral diet therapy may be delayed for several days after the injury until the client has sufficient gastrointestinal motility. As a result, nasoduodenal tube feedings are initiated. This type of nutritional supplement prevents nutritional deficits in critically burned clients.

The nurse encourages clients who can eat solid foods to ingest as many calories as possible. The client's preferences are taken into consideration for diet planning and food selection. Clients are encouraged to request food whenever they feel they can eat, not just according to the hospital's standard meal schedule. The nurse also offers frequent high-calorie, high-protein supplemental feedings. Care is taken to keep an accurate calorie count for foods and beverages that are actually ingested by the client.

Clients who cannot swallow but who have adequate gastric motility may meet calorie and nutrition needs through enteral tube feedings (see Chap. 64). When the gastrointestinal tract is not functional or when the client's nutritional requirements cannot be met by oral and enteral feeding, parenteral nutrition may be administered by the intravenous route. This method is used as a last resort because it is invasive and can lead to infectious and metabolic complications.

➤ *Impaired Physical Mobility*

Planning: Expected Outcomes. The client is expected to regain and maintain optimal physical mobility.

Interventions. Interventions aim to maintain the client's pre-burn range of joint motion and prevent contracture formation.

Nonsurgical Management. Nonsurgical management includes positioning, range-of-motion exercises, ambulation, and pressure dressings.

Positioning. Positioning is critical for clients with burn injuries because the position of comfort for the client is often one of joint flexion, which predisposes to the development of contractures. The nurse takes care to maintain the client in a neutral body position with minimal flexion. Recommended positions for the prevention of contracture are presented in Chart 71-6. Splints and other conforming devices may assist in maintaining position. These devices are used most frequently on joints of the hands, elbows, knees, neck, and axillae.

Range-of-Motion Exercises. Range-of-motion exercises are performed actively at least three times a day. If the client cannot move a joint actively, the nurse performs passive range-of-motion exercises. Burned hands are given special attention. The nurse encourages the client to perform active range-of-motion exercises for the hand, thumb, and fingers every hour while awake.

Ambulation. For clients who have not sustained fractures or other serious injuries to the legs and feet, ambulation is started as soon as possible after the fluid shift

---

Chart 71-6

Nursing Care Highlight: Positioning to Prevent Contractures

Affected Body Part	Position of Function	Interventions
Head and neck	• Hyperextension	• Place a towel roll under the client's neck or shoulder, or use a double mattress.
Posterior neck	• Flexion	• Have the client turn the head from side to side.
Upper chest and chest	• Shoulder retraction	• Place the client supine. Do not allow pillows. Place a folded towel under the spine between the scapulae.
Lateral trunk	• Flexion to uninvolved side	• Place the client supine with the arm on the affected side up over the head.
Anterior shoulder	• Abduction and external rotation	• Maintain the upper arm at 90 degrees of abduction from the lateral aspect of the trunk.
Posterior shoulder	• Slight flexion and interior rotation	• Keep the arm slightly behind the midline.
Elbow	• Extension and supination	• Keep the joint in the extended position.
Wrist	• 30–45 degrees of extension	• Use a splint.
Fingers		
MP joints	• 70–90 degrees of flexion	• Use a splint.
PIP and DIP joints	• Extended	• Use a splint.
Ankle	• 90 degrees of dorsiflexion	• Use a footboard or splint.
Legs	• 15–20 degrees of abduction	• Place a small pillow between the legs.

MP = metacarpal-phalangeal; PIP = proximal interphalangeal; DIP = distal interphalangeal.

has resolved. Clients with a variety of attached equipment (intravenous catheters, nasogastric tubes, electrocardiographic leads, extensive dressings) can ambulate with preparation and assistance. Ambulation is performed two or three times a day and progresses in length each time. Ambulation inhibits loss of bone density, strengthens muscles, stimulates immune function, promotes ventilation, and prevents a wide variety of complications.

Pressure Dressings. After the graft heals, pressure dressings prevent the formation of contractures and tight hypertrophic scars, which can inhibit mobility. These dressings also inhibit venous engorgement and edema formation in areas with decreased lymphatic outflow. Pressure dressings may be elastic wraps or specially designed, custom-fitted, elasticized clothing that provide continuous and uniform pressure over burned surfaces. Figure 71–14 illustrates such garments. For maximal effectiveness, pressure garments must be worn at least 23 hours a day, every day, until the scar tissue is mature (12–24 months). The nurse reinforces that wearing pressure garments is extremely beneficial in maintaining mobility and reducing hypertrophic scarring, although increased warmth and itchiness may cause the client some discomfort.

Surgical Management. Surgical management is restorative rather than preventive. Surgical techniques for contracture release are most commonly performed in the neck, axilla, elbow flexion areas, and hand. Specific surgical procedures to improve movement vary for each client.

Postoperative nursing responsibilities include the non-

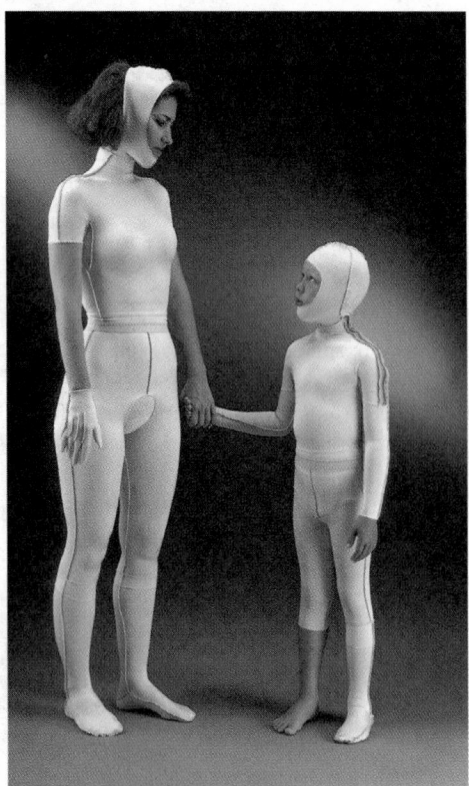

Figure 71–14. Models wearing pressure garments. (Courtesy of Beiersdorf-Jobst, Inc, Charlotte, NC.)

surgical interventions to prevent contractures from reforming as well as care of new grafts and suture lines. The nurse constantly reinforces the need for the client to comply with exercise and splinting regimens to prevent recurrence of joint immobility.

➤ Body Image Disturbance

Planning: Expected Outcomes. Following intervention, the client is expected to
- Accept his or her altered appearance
- Successfully progress through the grieving process
- Use support systems

Interventions. Nonsurgical and surgical interventions can assist clients who experience body image disturbances as a result of burn injury.

Nonsurgical Management. Understanding the stages of grief is helpful for the client, family, and nurse. The nurse assesses which stage of grief the client is currently experiencing and helps interpret the client's behaviors. Clients are frequently unaware of or confused by their feelings. The nurse reassures the client that feelings of grief, loss, anxiety, anger, fear, and guilt are normal. The client may be grieving for losses of body parts, appearance, role identity, and social identity. The nurse seeks the help of other health care team members (e.g., psychologist, psychiatrist, social worker, or clergy or religious leader) in addressing these problems.

The nurse accepts the physical and psychological characteristics of the client. Clients and families are presented with realistic expected outcomes for the client's functional capacity and physical appearance (Blalock et al., 1994). Information sessions and counseling for the family or significant others can identify previous and current patterns of support that are effective for the client and family. The nurse facilitates the client's and family's use of these systems and the development of new support systems, making referrals to specific support groups. To identify the effectiveness of such assistance and possible gaps in support, the nurse continually evaluates support resources for the client and family throughout the course of illness.

Engaging in decision-making and independent activities fosters feelings of self-worth, which are closely linked to body image. To this end, the nurse plans and encourages the client's participation in self-care activities. The nurse assists family members to understand that it is more beneficial for the client to perform these activities than to have them done by someone else. Families are encouraged to include the client in family decision-making to the same degree that the client had participated in this process before the injury.

Surgical Management. Reconstructive and cosmetic surgery can be performed for many years after the burn injury. Restoration of function and improvement of physical appearance through surgical techniques often increase the client's feelings of self-worth and promote a positive body image. Many clients may have unrealistic expectations of reconstructive surgery and envision an appearance identical with or equal in quality to the pre-burn state. The nurse educates the client and family about expected cosmetic outcomes.

Rehabilitative Phase of Burn Injury

Overview

Although rehabilitation efforts are started from the time of admission, the technical rehabilitative phase begins with wound closure and ends when the client returns to the highest level of functioning possible. The emphasis during this phase is the psychosocial adjustment of the client, the prevention of scars and contractures, and the resumption of pre-burn activity, including work, family, and social roles. This phase may take years or even last a lifetime as clients adjust to permanent limitations that may not be apparent until long after the initial injury.

Collaborative Management

Although attention is initially placed on physical interventions for and clinical manifestations of the burn injury, psychological care is equally important. The nurse provides psychosocial support to the client and family throughout hospitalization, but more extensively throughout the rehabilitative phase.

Information from the client and family aids in the assessment and diagnosis of psychological problems and allows treatment to be instituted. The nurse explores the client's feelings about the burn injury (Baker et al., 1996). It is extremely difficult for clients to concentrate on the many tasks before them when such obstacles as guilt and grief are in the forefront.

The nurse asks the client or family whether there is a history of psychological or organic impairment. The nurse asks what type of coping mechanisms the client has used successfully during times of stress and documents these findings to assist with a future plan of care. The nurse also assesses the client's family unit and the family members' history of interaction. The nurse determines cultural and ethnic factors and takes these into consideration when planning psychosocial interventions.

Throughout the hospitalization the client progresses through a variety of stages and exhibits myriad feelings, including denial, regression, and anger. The nurse accurately assesses the client's feelings during each stage so that appropriate plans of care can be made.

► Continuing Care

Discharge planning for the client who has a burn injury begins at the time of admission to the hospital or burn center. In most burn centers, the multidisciplinary team meets regularly to plan for the client's discharge. In assisting the client to reach mutually established discharge goals, the team evaluates the progress of each discipline. Table 71–9 summarizes the usual discharge needs of the client with burns.

► Psychosocial Preparation

Clients with severe burn injuries are likely to experience psychological problems during the recovery period and for some time after discharge from the hospital that may require psychosocial assistance. Problems include post-

TABLE 71–9

Needs To Be Addressed Before Discharge of the Client with Burns

- Early client assessment
- Financial assessment
- Evaluation of family resources
- Weekly discharge planning meeting
- Psychological referral
- Client and family teaching (home care)
- Designation of principal learners (specific family members or significant others who will help with care)
- Development of teaching plan
- Training for wound care
- Rehabilitation referral
- Home assessment (on-site visit)
- Medical equipment
- Public health nursing referral
- Evaluation of community resources
- Visit to referral agency
- Re-entry programs for school or work environment
- Nursing home placement
- Environmental interventions
- Auditory testing
- Speech therapy
- Prosthetic rehabilitation

traumatic stress disorder, sexual dysfunction, and severe depression. Assistance is coordinated with the client, family, and health care team. Psychosocial assistance is best provided by a professional counselor with previous experience in helping burn clients.

One specific area to be addressed with the client who has been burned is the reaction of others to the sight of healing wounds and disfiguring scars. Clients with facial burns are especially subjected to stares and other forms of disquieting behavior from the general public. Visits from friends and short public appearances before discharge may help the client begin adjusting to this problem. Community reintegration programs can assist the psychosocial and physical recovery of the client with serious burns.

► Home Care Management

The client with severe burns is frequently discharged from the acute care setting when life-threatening complications are resolved and minimal wound areas remain open. During the initial weeks at home after discharge, the client usually continues to require extensive daily wound care, rehabilitative therapy, nutritional support, symptom management, and drug therapy.

Although the client usually views the prospect of going home positively, the difficulties associated with physical care and the psychological stresses associated with changes in appearance, role, function, and lifestyle are numerous and may overwhelm the client and family. Successful discharge depends on extensive planning and preparation of the client, family, and home environment through education and appropriate support agencies and services (Dattolo et al., 1996).

Preparation for discharge includes assessment of the family and home care situation from physical and social perspectives. The nurse considers the needs of the client when evaluating the environment for cleanliness; access to bathing facilities, electricity, and running water; stairways; number of occupants; temperature control; and safety. If the burn injuries are a result of a fire at home, a new residence may need to be established.

➤ Health Teaching

Education about burn care and living with the consequences of burn injuries begins when the client is admitted to the hospital or burn center. A weekly plan for client education is outlined; the primary goal is progression toward independence for the client and family. Critical for this goal is teaching clients, family members, or significant others to perform specific care tasks, such as dressing changes. Clients and family members first observe the nurse changing the dressings, then assist the nurse or assistive nursing personnel in performing the changes, and finally change the dressings independently under the supervision of the burn care nurse.

Before discharge, all people who will be involved in the client's home care participate in discharge planning and teaching sessions. In addition to details about dressing changes, the nurse explains

- Signs and symptoms of infection
- Medication regimens
- Proper use of prosthetic and positioning devices
- Correct application and care of pressure garments
- Comfort measures to reduce pruritus

➤ Health Care Resources

The nurse and health care team evaluate the family in terms of capacity and willingness to assist in providing care to the client after discharge. A visiting nurse or case manager referral benefits the family with care problems arising at home. In addition, the visiting nurse can help the family determine what special equipment, supplies, or services will be needed. The frequency of home visits depends on the client's condition and the ability of family members to function as care providers.

Home care of a client after an extensive burn frequently involves daily physical therapy and rehabilitation sessions at special centers. Transportation problems are addressed and resolved before the client is discharged. In some instances, the burn center has arrangements for transportation. Some community volunteer agencies provide transportation by private car.

When rehabilitation is expected to be prolonged, the client may be discharged to a special rehabilitation facility. Before this point, the burn care nurse consults with the rehabilitation nurse or team and provides them with copies of the care and teaching plans that have been used with the client.

 Evaluation

On the basis of the identified nursing diagnoses, the expected outcomes for the client with burn injuries may include that the client will

- Have cardiac output restored to normal
- Maintain adequate oxygenation and circulation to all vital organs
- Maintain a patent airway
- Have an effective breathing pattern
- Have pain alleviated or reduced
- Experience no further loss of skin integrity
- Have skin integrity restored without complications
- Remain free from infection by cross-contamination
- Not experience septicemia
- Maintain an oral intake sufficient for meeting the body's calorie requirements
- Regain and maintain optimal physical mobility
- Accept altered appearance as a result of the burn injury
- Successfully progress through the grieving process
- Use support systems
- Have ABGs within normal limits
- Have normal lung compliance
- Be free of respiratory distress
- Be free of pulmonary edema
- Be free of visceral organ damage
- Maintain stable cardiac rhythms

⏻ CASE STUDY for the Client with a Burn Injury

■ A 45-year-old male is admitted to the burn unit after rescue from a house fire. He is incoherent with burns of the face, head, neck, circumferential bilateral arms and legs, and one-half of the anterior chest. Carbon particles are present around the nose and mouth. He is short of breath and complains of pain in the face and arms.

QUESTIONS:

1. What initial physical assessment techniques and interventions should be done during the primary survey?
2. Once the patient is stabilized, what ongoing assessment parameters should be undertaken during the emergent phase of injury?
3. Discuss actual and potential problems with interventions that may be done during the acute phase of burn injury.
4. During the rehabilitation phase of burn injury, what teaching parameters should be implemented for the patient and family?

SELECTED BIBLIOGRAPHY

Akhtar, M. A., Mulawkar, P., & Kulkarni, H. (1994). Burns in pregnancy: Effect on maternal and fetal outcomes. *Burns, 20*(4), 351–355.

Ashburn, M. A. (1995). Burn pain: The management of procedure-related pain. *Journal of Burn Care and Rehabilitation, 16*(3), 365–371.

Baker, R. A. U., Jones, S., Sanders, C., Sadinski, C., Martin-Duffy, K., Berchin, H., & Valentine, S. (1996). Degree of burn, location of burn, and length of hospital stay as predictors of psychosocial status and physical functioning. *Journal of Burn Care and Rehabilitation, 17,* 327–333.

*Baxter, C., & Shires, G. (1968). Physiological response to crystalloid resuscitation of severe burns. *Annals of the New York Academy of Sciences, 150,* 874–880.

Blalock, S., Bunker, B., & DeVellis, R. (1994). Psychological distress among survivors of burn injury: The role of outcome expectations and perceptions of importance. *Journal of Burn Care and Rehabilitation, 15*(5), 421–427.

Bullock, B. (1996). Alterations in skin integrity. In B. L. Bullock (Ed.), *Pathophysiology: Adaptations and alterations in function* (4th ed.). Philadelphia: Lippincott.

Byers, J., & Flynn, M. (1996). Acute burn injury: A trauma case report. *Critical Care Nurse, 16*(4), 55–66.

Cadier, M., & Shakespear, P. (1995). Burns in octogenarians. *Burns, 21*(3), 200–204.

Cianci, P., & Sato, R. (1994). Adjunctive hyperbaric oxygen therapy in the treatment of thermal burns: A review. *Burns, 20*(1), 5–14.

Cooper, M., & Spielvogel, R. (1994). Artificial skin for wound healing. *Clinics in Dermatology, 12*(1), 183–191.

Covington, D., Wainwright, D., & Parks, D. (1996). Prognostic indicators in the elderly patient with burns. *Journal of Burn Care and Rehabilitation, 17*(3), 222–230.

Cram, E. (1994). Burn unit survival strategies in changing economic times: Changes in burn nursing. *Journal of Burn Care and Rehabilitation, 15*(4), 372–373.

Dattolo, J., Trout, S., & Connolly, M. (1996). Home health care and burn care: An educational and economical program. *Journal of Burn Care and Rehabilitation, 17*(2), 182–187.

Davis, S., & Sheely-Adolphson, P. (1997). Psychosocial interventions: Pharmacologic and psychologic modalities. *Nursing Clinics of North America, 32*(2), 331–342.

Farrell, K., & Bradley, S. (1994). Estimation of nitrogen requirement in patients with burns. *Journal of Burn Care and Rehabilitation, 15*(2), 174.

Foertsch, C., O'Hara, M., Kealey, G., Foster, L., & Schumacher, E. (1995). A quasi-experimental, dual-center study of morphine efficacy in patients with burns. *Journal of Burn Care and Rehabilitation, 16*(2), 118–126.

Geisser, M., Bingham, H., & Robinson, M. (1995). Pain and anxiety during burn dressing changes: Concordance between patients' and nurses' ratings and relation to medication administration and patient variables. *Journal of Burn Care and Rehabilitation, 16*(2), 165–171.

Gordon, M., & Goodwin, C. (1997). Initial assessment, management, and stabilization. *Nursing Clinics of North America, 32*(2), 237–249.

Green, D., Still, J. M., & Law, E. J. (1994). *Candida parapsilosis* sepsis in patients with burns: Report of six cases. *Journal of Burn Care and Rehabilitation, 15*(3), 240–243.

Greenfield, E., & Jordan, B. (1996). Advances in burn wound care. *Critical Care Nursing Clinics of North America, 8*(2), 203–215.

Greenfield, E., & McManus, A. (1997). Infectious complications: Prevention and strategies for their control. *Nursing Clinics of North America, 32*(2), 297–309.

Hansbrough, J., Achauer, B., Dawson, J., Himel, H., Luterman, A., Slater, H., Levenson, S., Salzberg, A., Hansbrough, W., & Dore, C. (1995). Wound healing in partial-thickness burn wounds treated with collagenase ointment versus silver sulfadiazine cream. *Journal of Burn Care and Rehabilitation, 16*(3), 241–247.

Herdon, D. (1994). Accepting the challenge. *Journal of Burn Care and Rehabilitation, 15*(6), 463–469.

Hopkins, A. (1994). The trauma nurse's role with families in crisis. *Critical Care Nursing, 14*, 35–43.

Jordan, B., & Harrington, D. (1997). Management of the burn wound. *Nursing Clinics of North America, 32*(2), 251–273.

Kealey, G. (1995a). Pharmacologic management of background pain in burn victims. *Journal of Burn Care and Rehabilitation, 16*(3), 358–362.

Kealey, G. (1995b). Opioids and analgesia. *Journal of Burn Care and Rehabilitation, 16*(3), 363–364.

*Kravitz, M., Warden, G., Sullivan, J., & Saffle, J. (1989). A randomized trial of plasma exchange in the treatment of burn shock. *Journal of Burn Care and Rehabilitation, 10*(1), 17–26.

Latarjet, J., & Choinere, M. (1995). Pain in burn patients. *Burns, 21*(5), 344–348.

Law, E. J., Blecher, K., & Still, J. (1994). Enterococcal infections as a cause of mortality and morbidity in patients with burns. *Journal of Burn Care and Rehabilitation, 15*(3), 236–239.

*Lund, C., & Browder, N. C. (1944). The estimation of areas of burns. *Surgery, Gynecology and Obstetrics*, 352–358.

Mayes, T., Gottschlich, M., & Warden, G. (1997). Clinical nutrition protocols for continuous quality improvements in the outcomes of patients with burns. *Journal of Burn Care and Rehabilitation, 18*(4), 365–368.

McCain, D., & Sutherland, S. (1998). Skin grafts for patients with burns. *American Journal of Nursing, 98*(7), 34–38.

McKenna, S., Latenser, B., Jones, L., Barrette, R., Sherman, H., & Varcelotti, J. (1995). Serious silver sulphadiazine and mafenide acetate dermatitis. *Burns, 21,* 310–312.

Mertens, D., Jenkins, M., & Warden, G. (1997). Outpatient burn management. *Nursing Clinics of North America, 32*(2), 343–364.

Miller, J., Bunting, P., Burd, D., & Edwards, J. (1994). Early cardiorespiratory patterns in patients with major burns and pulmonary insufficiency. *Burns, 20,* 542–546.

Monafo, W. (1995). Physiology of pain. *Journal of Burn Care and Rehabilitation, 16*(3), 345–347.

*Monafo, W., Chuntrasakul, C., & Ayvazian, V. (1973). Hypertonic sodium solutions in the treatment of burn shock. *American Journal of Surgery, 126,* 778–783.

*Moritz, A. R. (1947). Studies of thermal injuries. II: The relative importance of time and surface temperature in the causation of cutaneous burns. *American Journal of Pathology, 23,* 695.

Murphy, P. A. (1994). The nurse's role in end-of-life decisions. *Journal of Burn Care and Rehabilitation, 15*(1), 84–85.

Nath, S., Erzingatsian, K., & Simonde, S. (1994). Management of postburn contracture of the neck. *Burns, 20,* 438–441.

*Nebraska Burn Institute. (1993). Advanced Burn Life Support Curriculum. (1993). Lincoln: Nebraska Burn Institute.

Nuchtern, J., Engrav, L., Nakamura, D., Dutcher, K., Heibach, D., & Vedder, N. (1995). Treatment of fourth-degree hand burns. *Journal of Burn Care and Rehabilitation, 16*(1), 36–42.

Patterson, D. (1995). Non-opioid based approaches to burn pain. *Journal of Burn Care and Rehabilitation, 16*(3), 372–376.

Pessina, M., & Ellis, S. (1997). Rehabilitation. *Nursing Clinics of North America, 32*(2), 365–373.

*Rice, D., & McKenzie, E., and Associates (1989). *Cost of injury in the United States: A report to Congress.* San Francisco: Institute for Health & Aging, University of California and Injury Prevention Center, The Johns Hopkins University.

Roberts, S. L. (1996). *Critical care nursing: Assessment and intervention.* Stamford, CT: Appleton & Lange.

Rodriguez, D. (1996). Nutrition in patients with severe burns: State of the art. *Journal of Burn Care and Rehabilitation, 17*(1), 62–70.

*Sadowski, D. (1988). Use of nonsterile gloves for routine noninvasive procedures in the thermally injured patient. *Proceedings of the American Burn Association, 20,* 111.

*Sadowski, D. (1989). Smoke inhalation/carbon monoxide poisoning. In M. S. Sommers (Ed.), *Difficult diagnoses in critical care nursing* (pp. 142–162). Rockville, MD: Aspen Publishers.

Still, M., Orlet, H., & Law, E. (1994). Use of cultured epidermal autografts in the treatment of large burns. *Burns, 20,* 539–541.

Tietz, N. (1995) *Clinical guide to laboratory tests* (3rd ed.). Philadelphia: W. B. Saunders.

Trofino, R. (1996). Nursing management of the patient with burns. In S. Ruppert, J. Kernicki, & J. Dolan (Eds.), *Dolan's critical care nursing: Clinical management through the nursing process* (pp. 941–959). Philadelphia: F. A. Davis.

Valentino, L. (1996). Burns. In L. Urden, M. Lough, & K. Stacy (Eds.), *Priorities in critical care nursing* (pp. 415–425). St. Louis, MO: Mosby-Year Book.

Wurtz, R., Karajovic, M., Dacumos, E., Jovanovic, B., & Hanumadass, M. (1995). Nosocomial infections in a burn intensive care unit. *Burns, 21,* 181–184.

SUGGESTED READINGS

Cram, E. (1994). Burn unit survival strategies in changing economic times: Changes in burn nursing. *Journal of Burn Care and Rehabilitation, 15*(4), 372–373.

This article looks at changes in burn care resulting from new policies and the challenges and opportunities presented to nurses by the necessity of reducing hospital costs. It identifies strategies burn unit nurses may use to position themselves for success in the changing health care environment. Options for Advanced Practice Nurses and case managers are also discussed in relationship to cost reduction and improved client satisfaction.

Greenfield, E., & Jordan, B. (1996). Advances in burn wound care. *Critical Care Nursing Clinics of North America, 8*(2), 203–215.
This excellent article provides in-depth information about burn wound care. The advantages and disadvantages of different management approaches are presented.

Mertens, D., Jenkins, M., & Warden, G. (1997). Outpatient burn management. *Nursing Clinics of North America, 32*(2), 343–364.
This article describes a team approach to burn management in the outpatient setting. Care needs are divided by stages into acute burn management, rehabilitation burn management, and reconstructive burn management. Client selection criteria for outpatient management are discussed.

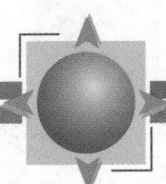

Problems of Excretion:

Management of Clients

with Problems of the

Renal/Urinary System

ASSESSMENT OF THE RENAL/URINARY SYSTEM

The kidneys filter metabolic waste products and excess fluid out of the blood; the ureters, bladder, and urethra provide a drainage route for the excretion of urine. The integrity and function of the renal/urinary system is critical to maintaining overall homeostasis and health. Structural or functional alterations in any part of the renal or urinary tract may be life threatening.

The nurse assesses the client at risk for or with actual problems of the renal or urinary system and pays special attention to the history and physical examination findings. A variety of diagnostic tests provide information about the structure and function of the renal/urinary tract, although some tests may pose increased risks for the client with confirmed renal deterioration. The nurse helps the client understand the purpose of the diagnostic tests, teaches about the procedures, and physically and emotionally prepares the client for them.

ANATOMY AND PHYSIOLOGY REVIEW

Kidneys

Structure

Gross Anatomy

Normally, two kidneys are located in the retroperitoneal space, one on either side of the vertebral column (Fig. 72–1). When the client is in a supine position, the kidneys are located between the twelfth thoracic and third lumbar vertebrae. The upper poles of each kidney are partially protected by the lower portion of the rib cage. When the client is standing, the kidneys may descend to the top of the sacroiliac crest. The adult kidney is 4–5 inches (11–13 cm) long, 2–3 inches (5–7 cm) wide, and

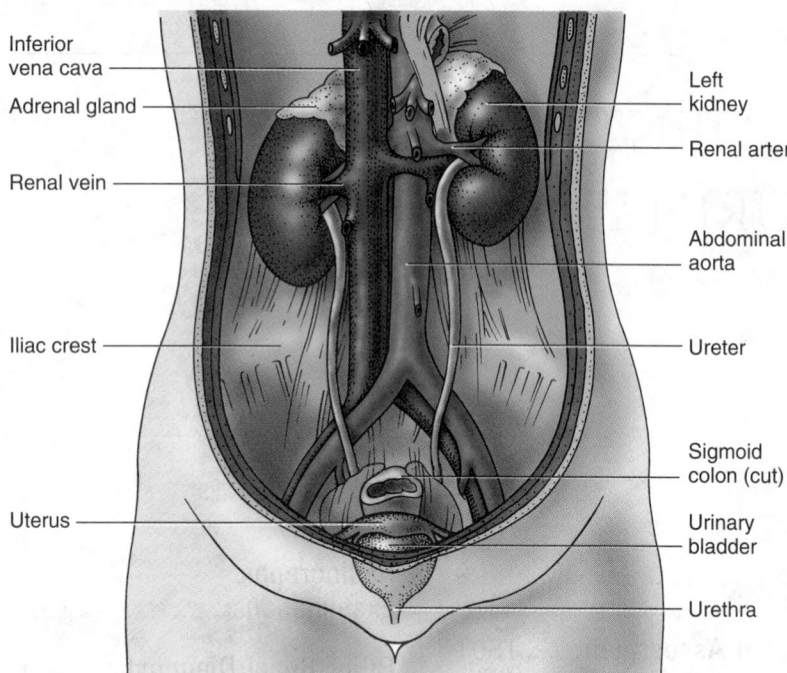

Inferior
vena cava

Adrenal gland

Renal vein

Iliac crest

Uterus

Left
kidney

Renal artery

Abdominal
aorta

Ureter

Sigmoid
colon (cut)

Urinary
bladder

Urethra

Figure 72–1. Anatomic location of organs of the renal/urinary system.

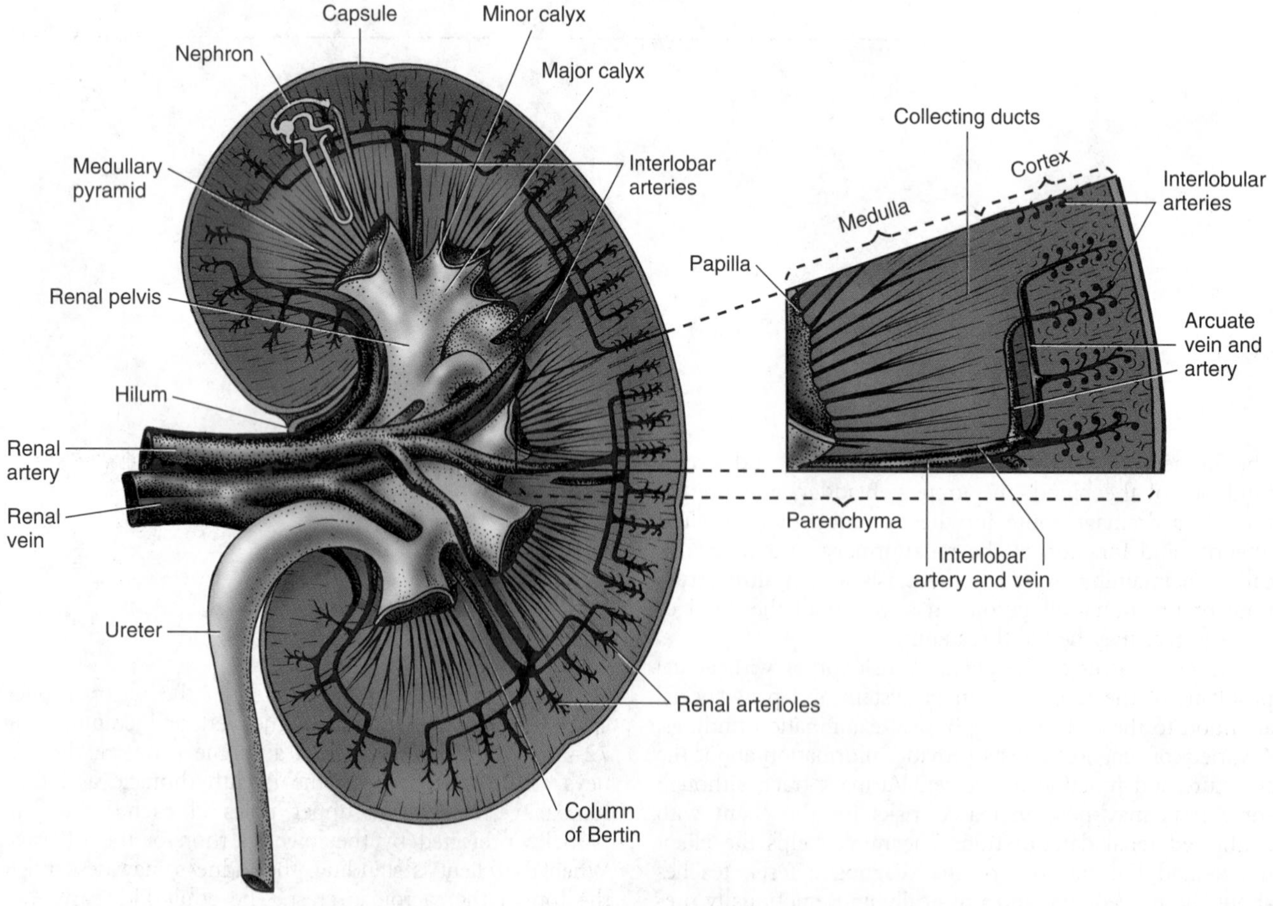

Capsule

Minor calyx

Nephron

Major calyx

Medullary
pyramid

Interlobar
arteries

Renal pelvis

Hilum

Renal
artery

Renal
vein

Ureter

Renal arterioles

Column
of Bertin

Collecting ducts

Cortex

Medulla

Interlobular
arteries

Papilla

Arcuate
vein and
artery

Parenchyma

Interlobar
artery and vein

Figure 72–2. Bisection of the kidney showing the major structures of the kidney.

about 1 inch (2.5–3 cm) thick. It weighs about 8 ounces (250 g). The left kidney is slightly longer and narrower than the right kidney.

The kidneys are surrounded by several layers of protective, supportive tissue. On the outer surface of the kidney is a layer of fibrous tissue called the *renal capsule* (Fig. 72–2). The capsule covers all aspects of the kidney, except the *hilum,* the area where the renal artery enters and the renal vein and ureter exit. The renal capsule is surrounded by layers of perirenal fat and Gerota's fascia. External to these layers are the muscles of the back, flank, and abdomen, as well as layers of fat, subcutaneous tissue, and skin.

Lying beneath the capsule is functional renal tissue, the parenchyma. The renal parenchyma is composed of two distinct structural sections, the cortex and the medulla. The renal cortex is in direct contact with the capsule. The medulla, or medullary tissue, is below the cortex. The medullary tissue lies within the kidney and is in the shape of many fans. Each "fan" is called a *pyramid.* There are 12 to 18 pyramids per kidney. The renal *columns* (columns of Bertin) are cortical tissue that descends into the interior of the kidney, separating the pyramids. The tip, or end, of each pyramid is called the *papilla.*

The papillae funnel formed urine into the collecting system. Structurally, a *minor* calyx cups the papilla of each pyramid. Several minor calices merge to form a *major* calyx. The major calices merge to form the *renal pelvis,* which narrows to become the ureter.

The blood supply to the kidneys (Table 72–1) is usually delivered by a single *renal artery,* which is a major branch of the abdominal aorta. The longer *right* renal artery extends below the inferior vena cava to the right kidney. The *left* renal artery is shorter because the aorta is closer to the left kidney. Each renal artery separates into progressively smaller arteries, supplying all areas of the renal parenchyma. The kidneys receive 20% to 25% of the total resting cardiac output. Renal blood flow varies widely from approximately 600 to 1300 mL/min.

Renal venous blood flow generally parallels that of the arterial system. Venules in the cortex become progres-

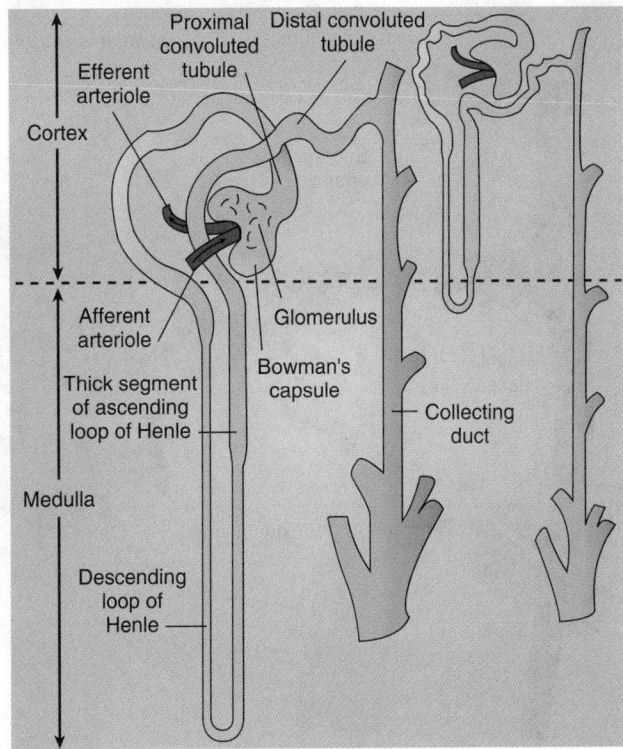

Figure 72–3. Anatomy of the nephron, the functional unit of the kidney. Note that the particular nephron labeled here is a juxtamedullary nephron.

sively larger and return blood via the right and left renal veins to the inferior vena cava. The left renal vein is longer than the right because it traverses anteriorly over the aorta.

The kidneys have some lymphatic vessels and nerve supply. Lymphatics for renal parenchyma drain into aortic lymph nodes. The nerve supply to the kidneys is derived from the lesser splanchnic (i.e., visceral) nerves and primarily influences renal circulation.

Microscopic Anatomy

The *nephron* (Fig. 72–3) is the functional unit of the kidney. There are 1–1.25 million nephrons per kidney. Each nephron can function as an independent unit. Structurally, the nephrons are contained within the renal cortex and the renal medulla.

The two types of nephrons are cortical nephrons and juxtamedullary nephrons. Each nephron has two major components, a vascular system and a tubular system. The cortical nephrons are shorter than the juxtamedullary nephrons, with all vascular and part of the tubular components located in the renal cortex. The vascular components of the juxtamedullary nephrons are deeper in the cortex, and tubular components extend deeply into the medulla.

Blood supply to the nephron is delivered via the *afferent arteriole,* the smallest, most distal portion of the renal artery. From the afferent arteriole, blood flows into the *glomerulus,* a series of specialized capillary loops. Blood exits the glomerulus via the *efferent arteriole.* From the

TABLE 72–1

The Sequence of Renal Blood Flow from the Renal Artery to the Renal Vein
1. Renal artery
2. Interlobar artery
3. Arcuate artery
4. Interlobular artery
5. Afferent arteriole
6. Glomerulus
7. Efferent arteriole
8. Peritubular capillaries or vasa recta
9. Stellate vein
10. Interlobular vein
11. Arcuate vein
12. Interlobar vein
13. Renal vein

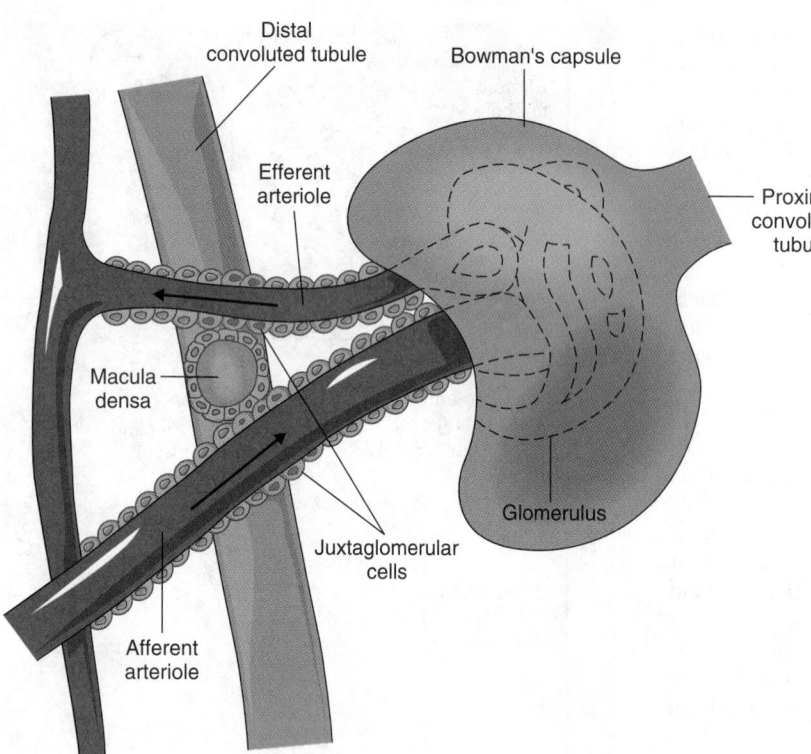

Figure 72-4. The juxtaglomerular complex showing juxtaglomerular cells and the macula densa.

efferent arteriole, blood exits into one of two additional capillary systems:

- The *peritubular capillaries* around the tubular component of cortical nephrons
- The *vasa recta* around the tubular component of juxtamedullary nephrons

The tubular component of the nephron begins with *Bowman's capsule,* a sac-like concave structure that surrounds the glomerulus. The tubular tissue of Bowman's capsule narrows into the *proximal convoluted tubule* (PCT). The PCT twists and turns, finally straightening into the descending limb of the *loop of Henle.* The descending loop of Henle dips in the direction of the medulla but forms a hairpin loop and is redirected toward the cortex.

As the loop of Henle changes direction, two segments are identified in the ascending limb of the loop of Henle, the thin and thick segments. From the thick segment of the ascending limb of the loop of Henle, the *distal convoluted tubule* (DCT) is identified. The DCTs of several nephrons terminate in one of many *collecting ducts,* located in the renal parenchyma. The collecting ducts pass through the papillae and empty into the caliceal system of the renal pelvis.

A series of specialized cells, located in the afferent arteriole, the efferent arteriole, and the DCT, are collectively known as the *juxtaglomerular complex* (Fig. 72-4). The modified smooth muscle cells of the afferent and efferent arterioles are called the *juxtaglomerular cells* (JGCs). These cells synthesize and store renin in its inactive form, prorenin. Renin is a hormone that helps to regulate blood flow, glomerular filtration rate (GFR), and systemic blood pressure. The area in the DCT where epithelial cells are more dense is the *macula densa.* The

macula densa contains receptors sensitive to volume and pressure changes. It lies adjacent to the JGCs of both afferent and efferent arterioles.

Microscopically, the glomerular capillary wall has three distinct layers (Fig. 72-5): the endothelium, the basement membrane, and the epithelium. The endothelial and epithelial cells lining the glomerular capillary are separated by pores through which certain molecular substances may pass from the blood into Bowman's capsule, thus becoming *filtrate.* The tubular lumen is lined with cells of varying sizes and characteristics. These variations promote or delay molecular movement. The capillary loops of the glomerulus also contain *mesangial cells,* which provide some structural support. The glomeruli and tubules are surrounded by interstitial tissue.

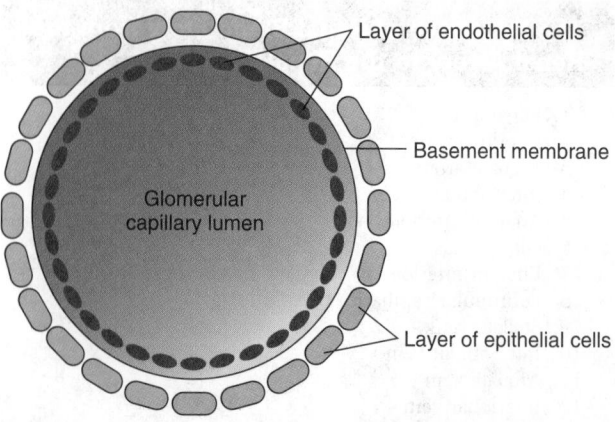

Figure 72-5. Glomerular capillary wall.

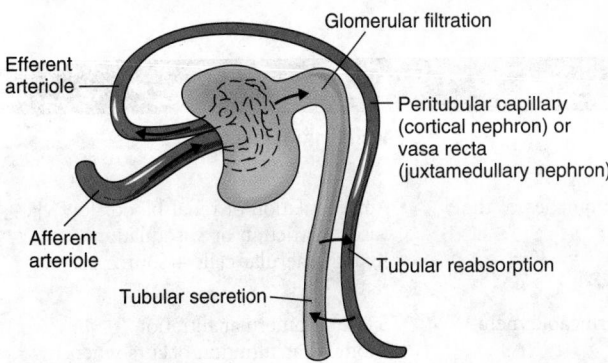

Figure 72–6. Glomerular filtration, tubular reabsorption, and tubular secretion.

Function

The kidneys perform various essential functions, including removing nitrogenous and toxic waste products and regulating fluid, electrolyte, and acid-base balance. The kidneys produce several hormones that significantly affect the client's physiologic well-being and help to regulate blood pressure.

Regulatory Functions

The physiologic processes responsible for the preservation of the body's internal environment include glomerular filtration, tubular reabsorption, and tubular secretion (Fig. 72–6). These processes are accomplished through filtration, diffusion, active transport, and osmosis. Table 72–2 summarizes the functional activities of vascular and tubular components of the nephron.

Glomerular Filtration

Glomerular filtration is the initial process in urine formation. As blood passes from the afferent arteriole into the glomerulus, water, electrolytes, and solutes (e.g., creatinine, urea nitrogen, and glucose) are filtered across the glomerular membrane into Bowman's capsule to form *glomerular* filtrate. Electrolytes and nonelectrolytes are transported into the glomerular filtrate by a mechanism referred to as *solute drag*. As the filtrate enters the proximal convoluted tubule (PCT), it is called *tubular* filtrate.

Substances with molecular weights greater than 69,000 are too large to pass through the glomerulus and are subject to electrostatic repulsion by the basement membrane of the glomerular capillary. Examples of high-molecular-weight substances are the protein molecules albumin and globulin and red blood cells (RBCs). These substances, therefore, are not normally present in the filtrate.

The creation of a net positive pressure is responsible for glomerular filtration. Hydrostatic pressure (blood pressure) is the primary force promoting ultrafiltration of the blood. Forces opposing glomerular filtration include the plasma oncotic pressure of the blood in the glomerulus and the tubular filtrate pressure of the filtrate in Bowman's capsule. When the hydrostatic pressure exceeds the sum of the two opposing pressures (plasma oncotic and tubular filtrate pressures), a net pressure in favor of filtration exists.

Approximately 180 L of glomerular filtrate is formed each day. The rate of filtration is often expressed in milliliters per minute. A normal glomerular filtration rate (GFR) averages 125 mL/minute. If all filtrate were excreted as urine, death would promptly ensue from massive fluid and electrolyte depletion. Actually, only about 1–2 L are excreted each day as urine.

The ability of the kidneys to autoregulate renal blood pressure and renal blood flow promotes a relatively constant GFR. Smooth muscle fibers of the afferent and efferent arterioles are responsible for this autoregulation. Although increased systemic blood pressure can greatly increase GFR, vasodilation of the afferent arteriole decreases the blood pressure in the kidney and thus maintains a fairly constant GFR. Similarly, with a relatively low systemic blood pressure, vasoconstriction of the smooth muscles of the efferent arterioles raises the renal blood pressure, allowing glomerular filtration to continue without major alteration. Autoregulation occurs as long as systolic blood pressure is maintained between 75 and 160 mmHg.

Tubular Reabsorption

Tubular reabsorption is the second process involved in urine formation. As the filtrate passes through the tubular component of the nephron, variable quantities of water, electrolytes, and other solutes are reabsorbed by the body. Reabsorption occurs *from the filtrate* across the tubular lumen of the nephron into the plasma of the peritubular capillaries or vasa recta. The PCT reabsorbs approximately 65% of the total glomerular filtrate.

Water Reabsorption

The tubules reabsorb more than 99% of all filtered water back into the body (Fig. 72–7). Most water reabsorption from the filtrate into the plasma occurs as the filtrate passes through the PCT. As the filtrate flows down the descending loop of Henle, water reabsorption continues. The thin segment of the ascending loop of Henle is *not* permeable to water.

As the filtrate continues to flow through the tubule and enters the distal convoluted tubule (DCT), water reabsorption occurs because the membrane is potentially permeable to water. The membrane of the DCT may be made more permeable to water through the influence of vasopressin (antidiuretic hormone [ADH]) and aldosterone. ADH increases the permeability of the membrane to water and enhances water reabsorption. Aldosterone promotes the reabsorption of sodium in the DCT; water reabsorption occurs as a result of the movement of sodium.

The ability of the kidneys to produce variations in the volume or concentration of urine helps regulate water balance. The medullary interstitium becomes hypertonic as sodium and chloride are actively reabsorbed from the ascending thin segment of the loop of Henle. The location of the tubular components of the juxtamedullary neph-

TABLE 72–2

Vascular and Tubular Components of the Nephron

Structure	Anatomic Features	Physiologic Aspects
Vascular Components		
Afferent arteriole	• Delivers arterial blood from the branches of the renal artery into the glomerulus	• Autoregulation of renal blood flow via vasoconstriction or vasodilation • Juxtaglomerular cells—source of renin
Glomerulus	• Capillary loops with thin semipermeable membrane	• Site of glomerular filtration • Glomerular filtration occurs when hydrostatic pressure (blood pressure) is greater than opposing forces (tubular filtrate and oncotic pressure)
Efferent arteriole	• Delivers arterial blood from the glomerulus into the peritubular capillaries or the vasa recta	• Autoregulation of renal blood flow via vasoconstriction or vasodilation
Peritubular capillaries (PTCs) and vasa recta (VR)	• PTCs: surround tubular components of cortical nephrons • VR: surround tubular components of juxtamedullary nephrons	• Tubular reabsorption and tubular secretion allow movement of water and solutes to or from the tubules, interstitium, and blood.
Tubular Components		
Bowman's capsule (BC)	• Thin membranous sac surrounding ⅞ of the glomerulus	• Collects glomerular filtrate (GF) and funnels GF into the tubule
Proximal convoluted tubule (PCT)	• Evolves from, and is continuous with, Bowman's capsule • Specialized cellular lining facilitates tubular reabsorption	• Site for reabsorption of sodium, chloride, water, glucose, amino acids, potassium, calcium, bicarbonate, phosphate, and urea
Loop of Henle Descending limb (DL)	• Continues from PCT • Juxtamedullary nephrons dip deep into the medulla • Permeable to water, urea, and sodium chloride	• Regulation of water balance via the countercurrent multiplying and exchange system
Ascending limb (AL)	• Emerges from DL as it turns and is redirected up toward the renal cortex	• Potassium and magnesium reabsorption in the thick segment • Thin segment is impermeable to water
Distal convoluted tubule (DCT)	• Evolves from AL and twists so that the macula densa cells lie adjacent to the juxtaglomerular cells of afferent arteriole	• Site of additional water and electrolyte reabsorption, including bicarbonate • Potassium and hydrogen secretion
Collecting ducts	• Collects formed urine from several tubules and delivers it into the renal pelvis	• Antidiuretic hormone regulation of water balance

rons deep within the hypertonic medullary interstitium enables wide variations in the osmolality of the urine produced. The high concentrations of sodium, chloride, and urea in the medullary interstitium and the countercurrent directional flow of filtrate and plasma allow the formation of a large, dilute volume of urine or a smaller, concentrated volume of urine (see Chapter 14 for additional information on fluid balance).

Solute Reabsorption

Most sodium, chloride, and water reabsorption occurs in the PCT. The collecting ducts are the other major site of sodium, chloride, and water reabsorption, which usually occurs under the stimulation of aldosterone. Potassium is also primarily reabsorbed in the PCT, with 20%–40%

of potassium reabsorption occurring in the thick segment of the ascending loop of Henle.

Bicarbonate, calcium, and phosphate are primarily reabsorbed in the PCT with additional reabsorption occurring in the ascending loop of Henle and the DCT. The reabsorption of bicarbonate provides base for the neutralization of acids in the plasma and helps to maintain a normal serum pH. Calcium reabsorption and excretion is influenced by circulating calcitonin and parathyroid hormone (PTH) levels. Magnesium is primarily reabsorbed in the thick segment of the ascending loop of Henle. A smaller percentage is reabsorbed in the PCT.

The usual renal threshold for glucose is at serum glucose levels of approximately 220 mg/dL. Normally, almost all glucose and any filtered amino acids or proteins are reabsorbed. About 50% of all urea present in the glome-

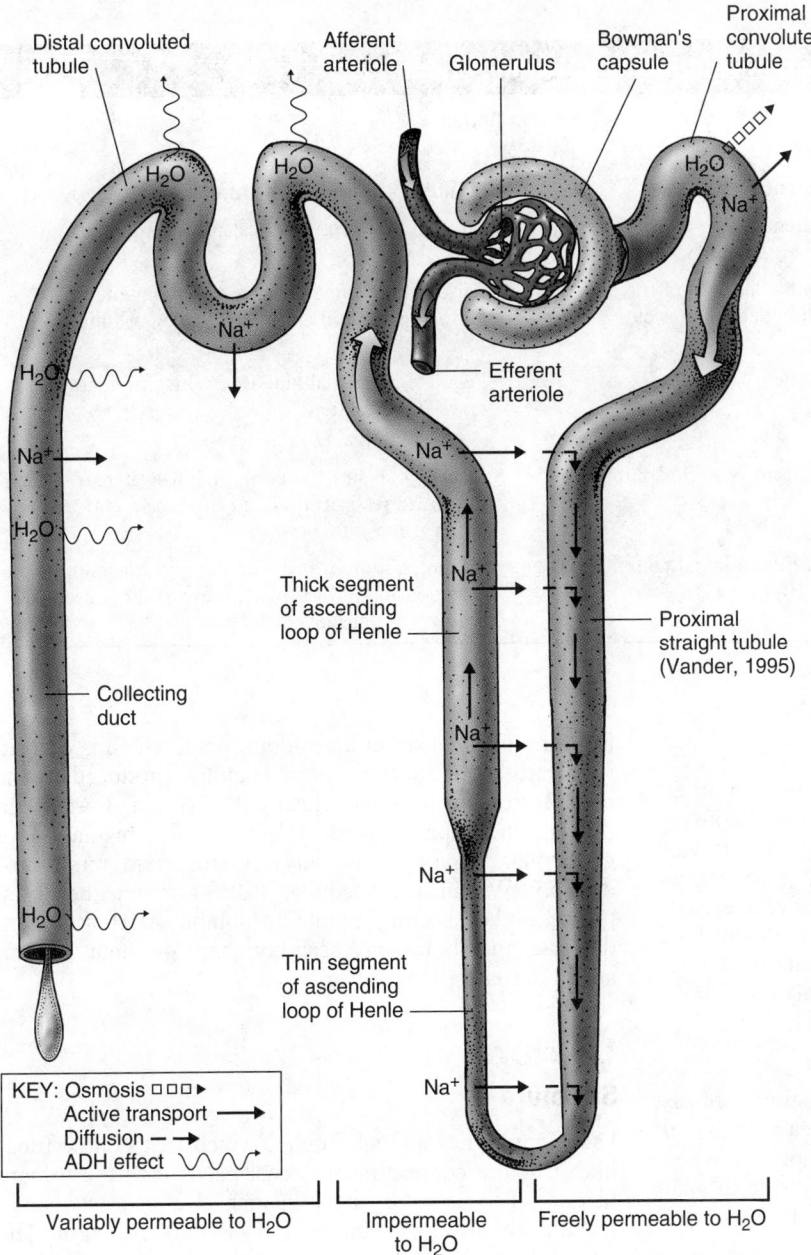

Figure 72–7. Sodium and water reabsorption by the tubules of a cortical nephron.

rular filtrate is reabsorbed, but virtually no creatinine is reabsorbed.

Tubular Secretion

Tubular secretion is a third process involved in urine formation. Like glomerular filtration, it is a process by which substances may move *from the plasma* into the tubular filtrate. During tubular secretion, molecules pass from the peritubular capillaries across capillary membranes into the cells that line the tubules. A constant exchange of molecules and the corresponding chemical reactions permit the removal of hydrogen (via ammonium chloride) and potassium excesses from the body and contribute to the regeneration of bicarbonate.

Hormonal Functions

The kidneys produce erythropoietin, activated vitamin D, renin, and prostaglandins (Table 72–3). Other secretions, such as the kinins, influence renal blood flow and capillary permeability. The kidneys also have a role in the breakdown and excretion of insulin.

Erythropoietin Production

Erythropoietin is produced and released in response to decreased oxygen tension in the renal blood supply. Erythropoietin stimulates red blood cell (RBC) production in the bone marrow. As the renal parenchymal mass decreases, erythropoietin production decreases.

TABLE 72–3

Renal Hormone Production and Hormones Influencing Renal Function		
	Site	Action
Renal Hormone Production		
Erythropoietin	• Renal parenchyma	• Stimulates bone marrow to make red blood cells
Activated vitamin D	• Renal parenchyma	• Promotes absorption of calcium in the gastrointestinal tract
Renin	• Juxtaglomerular cells of the afferent and efferent arterioles	• Raises blood pressure as result of angiotensin (vasoconstriction) and aldosterone (volume expansion) secretion
Prostaglandins	• Renal tissues	• Regulate intrarenal blood flow by vasodilation or vasoconstriction
Hormones Influencing Renal Function		
Antidiuretic hormone (ADH)	• Released from posterior pituitary	• Makes DCT and CD permeable to water to maximize reabsorption and produce a concentrated urine
Aldosterone	• Released from adrenal cortex	• Promotes sodium reabsorption and potassium secretion in DCT and CD; water and chloride follow sodium movement

DCT = distal convoluted tubule; CD = collecting ducts.

Vitamin D Activation

A series of metabolic changes are necessary for vitamin D, a hormone, to achieve an active form. Metabolic conversions take place in the skin through exposure to ultraviolet light and then in the liver. From there, vitamin D is converted to its active form (1,25-dihydroxycholecalciferol) in the kidney (see Chap. 53). Activated vitamin D is necessary to absorb calcium in the gastrointestinal tract and is critical in the regulation of calcium balance.

Renin Production

Renin assists in the regulation of blood pressure. Renin is formed and released when there is a decrease in blood flow, volume, or pressure through the arterioles or when a decrease in the sodium ion concentration of the tubular filtrate is detected through the receptors of the juxtaglomerular complex.

The release of renin stimulates the production of *angiotensin II* through a series of metabolic steps. Angiotensin II increases systemic blood pressure through powerful vasoconstrictive effects and stimulates the release of aldosterone from the adrenal cortex. *Aldosterone,* a mineralocorticoid, promotes increased reabsorption of sodium in the distal tubule of the nephron. Therefore, more water is reabsorbed and blood pressure is increased because of increases in intravascular volume expansion. This system of blood pressure regulation—the renin-angiotensin-aldosterone system—influences the autoregulatory blood pressure processes within the nephron as well as systemic blood pressure when renal blood flow is diminished (see also Chap. 14 and Fig. 14–8).

Prostaglandin Production

Prostaglandins are produced in a variety of tissues, including the renal parenchyma. Prostaglandins are formed from the metabolism of arachidonic acid, which is derived from fatty acids. Specific prostaglandins produced in the renal cortex are prostaglandin E_2 (PGE_2) and prostacyclin (PGI_2). These prostaglandins facilitate the regulation of glomerular filtration, vascular resistance, and renin production. Within the medulla, PGE_2 acts on the distal tubule and collecting tubule to inhibit ADH secretion, decrease membrane permeability, and promote sodium and water excretion.

Ureters
Structure

Each kidney has a single ureter, which is a hollow tube-like structure connecting the renal pelvis with the urinary bladder. The ureter is about ½ inch (1.25 cm) in diameter and about 12–18 inches (30–45 cm) in length. The ureters lie within the retroperitoneal space.

The diameter of the ureter narrows in three distinct areas:

- In the upper third of the ureter, at the point where the renal pelvis becomes the ureter, is a narrowing known as the *ureteropelvic junction* (UPJ).
- The ureter also narrows as it arches toward the anterior abdominal wall traversing beneath the iliac vessels (aortoiliac bend).
- Each ureter then narrows on entering the posterior wall of the urinary bladder at an oblique angle, at a point referred to as the *ureterovesical junction* (UVJ).

The ureter tunnels through bladder tissue for a few centimeters before opening into the bladder in an area referred to as the *trigone* (Fig. 72–8).

The ureter is composed of three layers: an inner lining of mucous membrane (urothelium), a middle layer of smooth muscle fibers, and an outer layer of fibrous tissue.

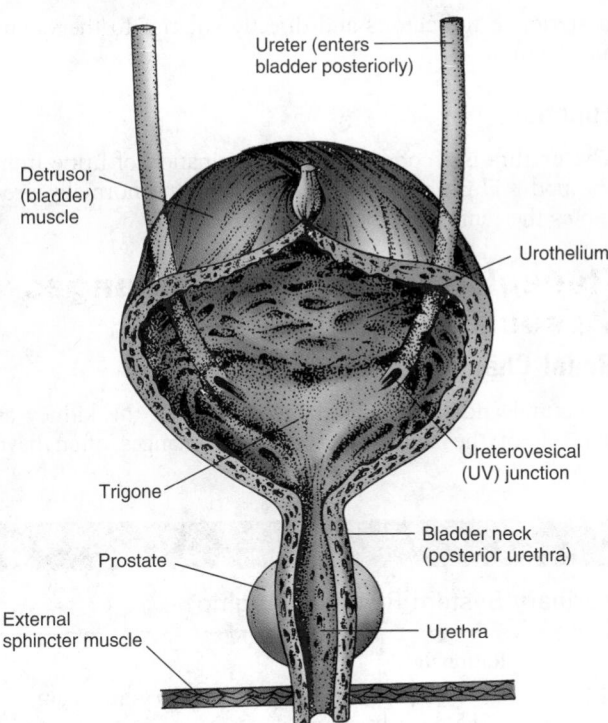

Figure 72–8. Gross anatomy of the urinary bladder.

The outer layer of the ureter contains the blood supply, which is derived primarily from the ureteral artery, a branch of the renal artery. Branches from other vessels, such as the aorta and the internal spermatic, iliac, uterine, vaginal, hemorrhoidal, and superior vesical arteries, may also supply the ureter. The middle layer of ureteral tissue contains longitudinal and circular muscle fibers. These muscle fibers are under the control of a variety of nerve pathways from the sacroiliac branches.

Function

Rapid peristaltic contractions of the smooth muscle fibers of the ureter transport urine from the renal pelvis of the kidney to the urinary bladder. The normal regulator for ureteral peristalsis is the stretch receptors from urine in the renal pelvis. These stretch receptors may be mediated by pacemaker cells located in or near the calyx.

Urinary Bladder
Structure

The urinary bladder is a muscular sac. The superior surface is adjacent and exterior to the peritoneal cavity. In men, the bladder is anterior to the rectum. In women, the bladder is anterior to the vagina. The bladder lies directly behind the pubic symphysis, the connecting point for pelvic bone structures.

The bladder is composed of the *body,* the rounded sac portion, and the *bladder neck,* or posterior urethra, which connects to the bladder body. The bladder has three linings, including an inner lining of epithelial cells known as the *urothelium,* middle layers of smooth muscle (the *detru-*

sor muscle), and an outer lining. The trigone is an anatomic landmark on the inner aspect of the posterior bladder wall formed by the points of ureteral entry (ureterovesical junctions [UVJs]) and the urethra.

The *internal urethral sphincter* is composed of the smooth detrusor muscle of the bladder neck and elastic tissue. The *external urethral sphincter* is composed of skeletal muscle that surrounds the urethra. In men, the external sphincter surrounds the urethra at the base of the prostate gland. In women, the external sphincter is at the base of the bladder. The urinary bladder receives blood supply from the internal iliac arteries. The pudendal nerve from spinal cord segments S-2 and S-3 transmits motor impulses to the external sphincter.

Function

The urinary bladder provides a site for the temporary storage of urine. The urinary bladder also provides continence and enables micturition (voiding). Secretions of the bladder lining resist bacteria.

Bladder continence is achieved during filling through the combination of detrusor muscle relaxation, internal sphincter muscle tone, and external sphincter contraction. As the bladder fills with urine, neuroreceptors transmit the stretch sensations to segments of spinal sacral nerves S-2 and S-3.

Maintaining Continence

Continence is maintained by the interaction of nerves that control muscles of the bladder, bladder neck, urethra, and pelvic floor and factors that close the urethra. During bladder filling, the sympathetic nervous system fibers dominate and override detrusor muscle contraction. These control centers are located in the cerebral cortex as well as in nuclei in the pons and the sacral part of the spinal cord. For urethral closure to be adequate for continence, the mucosal surfaces must be in contact and must be adhesive. Contact depends on the structural and functional integrity of the involved nerves and muscles. Adhesion depends on adequate secretion of mucus-like substances.

Micturition

Micturition is a reflex of parasympathetic control that stimulates detrusor muscle contraction with the simultaneous relaxation of the external sphincter and the muscles of the pelvic floor. With detrusor muscle contraction, the UVJ of the ureter closes, and the normally round bladder assumes the shape of a funnel. Voiding becomes a voluntary act as a result of a learned response controlled by the cerebral cortex and the brain stem. Tonic contractions of the external sphincter inhibit the micturition reflex and prevent voiding.

Urethra
Structure

The urethra is a narrow tube-like structure lined with mucous membrane and epithelial cells. The *urethral mea-*

tus, or opening, is the terminal point of the urethra. In men, the urethra is about 6–8 inches (15–20 cm) long, and the urethral meatus is located at the tip of the penis. Three sections make up the male urethra:

- The prostatic urethra traverses the prostate gland from the urinary bladder.
- The membranous urethra traverses the wall of the pelvic floor.
- The cavernous urethra is external and extends through the length of the penis.

In women, the urethra is about 1–1½ inches (2.5–3.75 cm) long and exits the urinary bladder through the pelvic floor. The urethral meatus is located slightly posterior to the clitoris and directly anterior to the vagina and rectum.

Function

The urethra is a conduit for the elimination of urine from the body. Flushing by the passing of urine normally promotes the removal of bacteria.

Renal/Urinary System Changes Associated with Aging
Renal Changes

Structural and functional changes occur in the kidney as a result of the aging process. These changes often have

---

Chart 72–1

Nursing Focus on the Elderly: Changes in the Renal/Urinary System Related to Aging

Physiologic Change	Nursing Implications	Rationale
Decreased glomerular filtration rate (GFR)	• Monitor hydration status. • Ensure adequate fluid intake. • Administer potentially nephrotoxic agents or medications carefully.	• With aging, the ability of the kidneys to regulate water balance is decreased. • The kidneys are less able to conserve water when necessary. • Dehydration results in decreased renal blood flow and increases the nephrotoxic potential of many agents. Acute or chronic renal failure may result.
Nocturia	• Ensure adequate nighttime lighting and a hazard-free environment. • Ensure the availability of a toilet, bed pan, or urinal. • Discourage excessive fluid intake for 2–4 hr before the client retires for the evening.	• Nocturia may occur from decreased renal concentrating ability associated with aging. • The desire to maintain continence prompts individuals to seek the bathroom. Falls and injuries are common among older clients seeking bathroom facilities. • Excessive fluid intake at nighttime may increase nocturia.
Decreased bladder capacity	• Encourage the client to use the toilet, bed pan, or urinal at least q2h. • Respond as soon as possible to the client's indication of the need to void.	• By emptying the bladder on a regular basis, urinary incontinence from overflow may be avoided.
Weakened urinary sphincter muscles and shortened urethra in women	• Respond as soon as possible to the client's indication of the need to void. • Provide thorough perineal care after each voiding.	• A quick response may alleviate episodes of urinary stress incontinence. • The shortened urethra increases the potential for bladder infections. • Good perineal hygiene may prevent skin irritations and urinary tract infection. (UTI).
Tendency to retain urine	• Observe the client for urinary retention (e.g., bladder distention) or urinary tract infection (e.g., dysuria, foul odor, confusion). • Provide privacy, assistance, and voiding stimulants such as warm water over the perineum as needed.	• Urinary stasis may result in a UTI. UTIs may become bloodstream infections, resulting in septicemia or septic shock. • Nursing interventions can help to initiate voiding.

clinical significance. Loss of renal cortex mass accounts for a decrease in renal mass to 180–200 g by age 80 years. Cortex changes are most likely related to changes in renal blood flow. The renal medulla appears not to be affected by aging, and the juxtamedullary nephrons are generally preserved. In the nephron, a thickening of the glomerular and tubular basement membranes is observed on microscopic examination. Both the number of glomeruli and their surface area decrease with aging. The length of the tubules decreases proportionately.

Kidney function also changes with aging (Chart 72–1). Blood flow to the kidney decreases approximately 10% per decade as blood vessels become thickened and more rigid. Hypertrophy does not occur as it does in a younger person who has had one kidney removed. GFR decreases with advancing age, more rapidly after age 45 years. By age 65 years, the GFR decreases to approximately 65 mL/min (roughly half the rate in a young adult). The decline is more rapid in clients with diabetes or hypertension.

Tubular changes with aging are shown by the inability to concentrate urine, resulting in nocturia. The excretion and regulation of solutes (e.g., sodium, acids, bicarbonate) remain effective but less efficient because homeostasis is slower. These changes, along with an age-related impairment in the thirst mechanism, may be associated with the increased incidence of volume depletion and hypernatremia in the elderly (Brenner, 1996). Renal endocrine changes include a decrease in renin secretion, aldosterone levels, and the activation of vitamin D.

TRANSCULTURAL CONSIDERATIONS

African-Americans have more rapid age-related decreases in GFR than Caucasians (Brenner, 1996). Renal excretion of sodium is less effective in hypertensive African-Americans who have high sodium intake, and the kidneys have approximately 20% less blood flow from anatomic changes in small renal vessels (Shulman & Hall, 1991).

Urinary Changes

Changes in the elasticity of the detrusor muscle may cause decreased bladder capacity and a decreased ability to retain urine. The sensation of the urge to void may necessitate immediate bladder emptying because the urinary sphincters lose muscle tone and often become weaker with age. In women, weakening muscles shorten the urethra, which further contributes to stress incontinence. In men, prostatic hypertrophy results in difficulty starting the urine stream and may cause urinary retention.

HISTORY
Demographic Data

Age, gender, race, and ethnicity are important in the overall history of the client with suspected renal or urinary dysfunction. A sudden onset of hypertension in clients older than 50 years suggests a secondary origin (e.g., renovascular disease). Clinical evidence of adult polycystic kidney disease typically occurs in clients in their 40s or 50s. In men older than 50 years, altered urinary patterns suggest prostatic disease.

Anatomic gender differences may potentiate specific disorders. For example, men rarely have urinary tract infections unless there are structural abnormalities, such as ureteral reflux or prostatic involvement. Women, who have a shorter urethra, frequently experience cystitis, because bacteria pass more readily into the bladder.

TRANSCULTURAL CONSIDERATIONS

End-stage renal disease (ESRD) is three to four times more common in African-Americans, Native Americans, and Mexican-Americans than in Caucasian Americans. A history of hypertension or diabetes mellitus is also common in these groups.

Personal and Family History

The family history of the client with a suspected renal or urologic problem is significant because some disorders are genetically transmitted or have a familial inheritance pattern. The nurse asks whether the client's siblings, parents, parents' siblings, or grandparents have had renal problems. Terms used in the past for renal disease include Bright's disease, nephritis, and nephrosis. Clients may use these terms to describe the diseases of the kidney as they were known by parents or grandparents in the earlier part of the 20th century. Adult polycystic kidney disease can be transmitted to children as a result of an autosomal dominant genetic defect from a parent of either sex.

The nurse asks the client about any previous renal or urologic disorders, including tumors, infections, stones, or urologic surgical interventions. A history of any chronic health problems, such as diabetes mellitus, hypertension, and arthritis, also is important in renal or urologic assessment.

The nurse identifies all prescription medications taken by the client, including drugs taken routinely and those taken as needed. The nurse inquires about the duration of use and whether any recent changes in medications have been prescribed. Medications prescribed for diabetes mellitus, hypertension, cardiac disorders, hormonal disorders, cancer, and arthritis are potential causes of renal dysfunction. Antibiotics, such as gentamicin (Garamycin, Cidomycin✦), taken for infections may also produce sudden renal dysfunction.

In addition, the nurse asks about over-the-counter (OTC) medications or agents, including vitamin and mineral supplements and replacements, laxatives, analgesics, and nonsteroidal anti-inflammatory drugs (NSAIDs). Many of these medications can influence renal function. Long-term analgesic intake, especially combination agents, can also affect renal function. The nurse asks the client to describe medication intake in as much detail as possible.

The nurse inquires about the results of previous physical examinations, such as for school, employment, insurance eligibility, or military induction. Occasionally, the nurse's questions regarding "protein or albumin in the urine" prompt the client's recall of problems not previously remembered or identified as renal related. The question "Have you ever been told that your blood pressure was high?" may prompt a vastly different response than "Do you have high blood pressure?" Recall of earlier physical or health examinations may also help the client remember previous reports of elevated blood pressures, which may suggest a correlation with current problems. The nurse also asks female clients about health problems associated with pregnancy (e.g., proteinuria, high blood pressure, and urinary tract infections).

The nurse inquires about

- Chemical or environmental toxin exposure in occupational or other settings
- Recent travel to geographic regions posing infectious disease risks
- Recent physical injuries
- Trauma
- Sexual contacts
- A history of altered patterns of urinary elimination

Answers to any of these questions may provide information significant to the urologic assessment.

Diet History

The nurse asks the client with known or suspected renal or urologic disorders about his or her usual dietary intake. The nurse seeks information describing any recent changes in the dietary pattern. The nurse notes the excessive intake or omission of certain categories of foods. The diet history includes fluid intake as well as food items. Changes in appetite, alterations in taste acuity, and the inability to discriminate tastes are important. These symptoms are associated with the accumulation of nitrogenous waste products from renal failure. In addition, if the client has followed a diet for weight reduction, the details of the diet plan are pertinent. A high-protein intake can result in transient renal problems. Clients susceptible to calculi formation who ingest increased amounts of calcium-containing products or have an insufficient fluid intake may form new stones. Changes in thirst or fluid intake may also produce changes in urine output or other evidence of urologic disorders. Endocrine disorders may also produce changes in thirst, fluid intake, and urine output (see Chap. 66).

Socioeconomic Status

The socioeconomic status of the client may influence health care practices. People with limited income or no health insurance often ignore physical ailments or delay seeking health care because they lack funds to pay for diagnostic tests or treatment. They may also have difficulty following medical advice, having prescriptions filled, and keeping follow-up appointments.

The information that a client has about the disease and its symptoms may relate to educational level. A client's educational level also may affect health-seeking practices. Recurring urinary tract infections often result from inadequate or incomplete treatment, including lack of follow-up to ensure eradication. The lack of money to pay for antibiotics or nutritious foods or the lack of knowledge or motivation to select healthful foods may inhibit full recovery.

The client's health belief model affects the approach to health and illness (see Chap. 1). Cultural background or religious affiliation may influence the belief system. The nurse assesses the client's belief model and identifies the importance of culture or religion to the client.

The language used by clients may be different from that of the health care professional. Anatomic or medical terminology may have no meaning for the client. When obtaining a history, the nurse listens to and explores terminology used by the client. By using the client's own terms or language, the nurse may enable the client to provide a more complete and thorough description of the problems being experienced. This technique may increase the amount of information communicated and decrease the client's discomfort when discussing bodily functions.

Current Health Problem

Because the effects of renal failure result in changes in all body systems, the nurse thoroughly documents all the client's current health problems. The nurse asks the client for a complete list of perceived current health problems. The nurse encourages the client to describe all concerns because some renal and urologic disorders are associated with symptoms that are related to other body systems or occur as generalized problems. The client is often prompted to seek health care when experiencing severe discomfort associated with urination or noticing the appearance or quantity of urinary output change.

Specifically, the nurse inquires about any changes in the appearance (color, odor, clarity) of the urine, pattern of urination, ability to initiate or control voiding, and other unusual symptoms. Urine that is reddish, dark brown or black, greenish, or any deviation from the usual yellowish, straw color urine usually prompts the client to seek health care assistance. Typically, urine has a mild but distinctive odor suggestive of ammonia. An increase in the intensity or a change in the quality of the odor or a decrease in clarity may suggest infection.

The nurse asks about changes in the pattern of urination such as waking during the night to void (nocturia), a change in frequency (an increase or decrease in the number of times per day that urine is passed), and an increase or decrease in the quantity of urine. The normal urinary output for adults is 1 mL/kg per hour, or approximately 1500–2000 mL/day. The client generally does not have information about the specific quantity of urine produced. The nurse interprets the client's answers by understanding equivalent health care terminology (Table 72–4).

The nurse also inquires

- Whether any difficulties are encountered in initiating the flow of urine
- Whether a burning sensation or other discomfort is associated with the urinary flow
- Whether there is a decrease in the force of the urinary stream in men

The nurse asks about any loss of urinary continence. Situations that increase intra-abdominal pressure (e.g., coughing and sneezing) may result in the involuntary passage of urine. Clients may also report persistent dribbling of urine.

TABLE 72–4

Commonly Used Renal and Urinary Terms

Dysuria—Discomfort or pain associated with micturition

Frequency—Feeling the need to void often, usually voiding small amounts of urine each time; may void every hour or even more frequently than hourly

Hesitancy—Difficulty in initiating the flow of urine, even when the bladder has sufficient urine to initiate a void and the sensation of the need to void is present

Micturition—The act of voiding

Nocturia—Awakening prematurely from sleep because of the need to empty the bladder

Urgency—A sudden onset of the feeling of the need to void immediately; may result in incontinence if the client is unable to locate or get to toileting facilities quickly

Anuria—Total urinary output of less than 100 mL in 24 hr

Oliguria—Decreased urinary output; total urinary output between 100 and 400 mL in 24 hr

Polyuria—Increased urinary output; total urinary output usually greater than 2000 mL in 24 hr

Azotemia—Increased blood urea nitrogen and serum creatinine levels suggestive of renal impairment, but without outward symptoms of renal failure

Uremia—Full-blown signs and symptoms of renal failure; sometimes referred to as the uremic syndrome, especially if the cause of the renal failure is unknown

The onset of pain in the flank, the lower abdomen or pelvic region, or the perineal area is often of great concern and usually prompts the client to seek assistance. The nurse inquires about the onset, intensity, and duration of pain, its location, and its association with any activity or event.

The pain may be sharp or dull, localized or diffuse. Pain associated with renal or ureteral irritation is often severe and spasmodic. When the pain radiates into the perineal area, groin, scrotum, or labia, it is described as *renal colic*. Renal colic pain is usually associated with distention or spasm of the ureter, as in obstruction or the passing of a stone, and may be intermittent.

Pain associated with the descent of a stone through the ureter is excruciating and can have a dramatic presentation. As a result of sympathetic nervous system stimulation, the client may exhibit a shock-like condition with pallor, diaphoresis (profuse perspiration), and hypotension. In addition, the client may have gastrointestinal (GI) symptoms, such as nausea, vomiting, and diarrhea. These symptoms occur because of the proximity of nerve tracts associated with the kidneys, the ureters, and internal abdominal organs.

Recent upper respiratory tract problems, generalized musculoskeletal discomfort, or GI problems may be related to systemic conditions that can influence renal function. GI symptoms, such as anorexia, nausea, and vomiting, are classic manifestations of uremia but may be present with other pathologic conditions as well. Because the kidneys are close to the GI organs and the nerve pathways are similar, GI symptoms may be part of the client's presenting history. These *renointestinal reflexes* commonly complicate the detailed description of the renal problem.

Uremia refers to the clinical symptoms associated with the accumulation of nitrogenous waste products in the blood, an effect of renal failure. These symptoms include anorexia, nausea and vomiting, muscle cramps, pruritus (itching), fatigue, and lethargy.

PHYSICAL ASSESSMENT

Physical assessment of the client with a known or suspected renal or urologic disorder includes

- An assessment of general appearance
- A general review of body systems
- Specific consideration of the organs and functions of the renal and urinary systems

The nurse assesses the general appearance of the client and checks for a yellowish skin color and the presence of any rashes, ecchymoses, or other discoloration. The skin and tissues may show evidence of edema, which, with renal disorders, may be detected in the pedal, pretibial, presacral, and periorbital tissues. The nurse auscultates the lungs to determine whether fluid is present. Weight and blood pressure measurements are obtained for comparison purposes.

The nurse also assesses the client's general level of consciousness, noting deficits in concentration, thought processes, or memory, and level of alertness. Family members may report subtle changes.

Assessment of the Kidneys, Ureters, and Bladder

Assessment of the kidneys, ureters, and bladder is performed in conjunction with abdominal assessment. Auscultation precedes percussion and palpation because the nurse needs to auscultate for abdominal bruits before enhancing bowel sounds by abdominal palpation or percussion.

Inspection

The nurse inspects the abdomen and the flank regions with the client in both supine and sitting positions. The nurse observes for asymmetry (e.g., swelling) or discoloration (e.g., ecchymoses or redness) in the flank region, known as the *costovertebral angle* (CVA). The CVA is defined by the lower portion of the 12th rib and the vertebral column (Fig. 72–9).

Auscultation

After inspection, the nurse listens for a bruit over each renal artery on the mid-clavicular line. A *bruit* is an audible swishing sound produced when the volume of blood or the diameter of the blood vessel is changed. A bruit over an artery is usually associated with blood flow through a narrowed vessel, as in renal artery stenosis.

Palpation

After auscultation, the nurse lightly palpates all quadrants of the abdomen. The nurse inquires about areas of tenderness or discomfort and examines nontender areas first. In clients with severe bladder distention, the outline of the bladder may be identified as high as the umbilicus. When the client's bladder is distended, abdominal palpation to locate and examine the kidneys produces discomfort and may be impossible. Although the ureters are not palpable, a spasm of the ureteral musculature results in flank or low abdominal pain that is severe, excruciating, and similar to colic. The sensations spread to the scrotum in men and the labia in women.

Renal palpation identifies masses and areas of tenderness in or around the kidney. Special training and practice under the guidance of a qualified practitioner are necessary; therefore appropriate education is essential before attempting the procedure. If tumor or aneurysm is suspected, palpation may harm the client.

Because the kidneys are deep, posterior structures, palpation is more readily accomplished in thinner clients. When the kidneys are of normal size and position, only the lower poles are palpable. In clients with strong abdominal muscles or significant adipose tissue or abdominal fluid, it may be difficult or impossible to palpate the kidneys. The nurse helps the client assume a supine position.

To palpate the right kidney, the nurse places one hand under the right flank and the other hand over the abdomen below the lower right part of the rib cage. The lower hand raises the flank, and the upper hand depresses the anterior abdomen (Fig. 72–10) as the client takes a deep breath. The left kidney is deeper and rarely palpable. A transplanted kidney is readily palpable in either the lower right or left abdominal quadrant.

The kidney should feel smooth, firm, and nontender. If the kidneys are enlarged because of polycystic kidney disease or the presence of other renal conditions, the nurse palpates gently to avoid increasing the client's discomfort.

Percussion

A distended urinary bladder sounds dull when percussed. After gently palpating to determine the general outline of

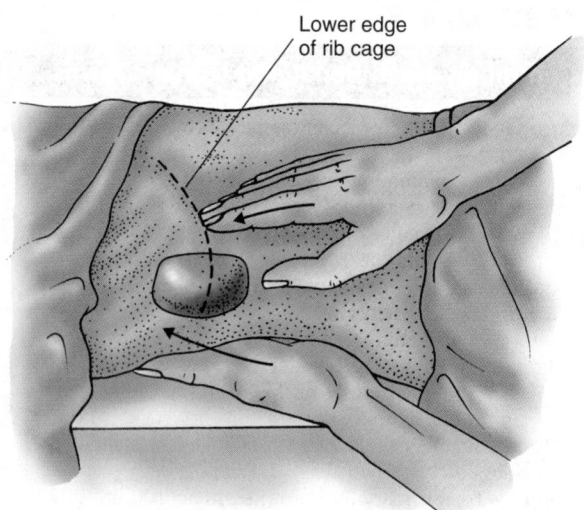

Figure 72–10. Advanced technique for palpation of the kidney.

the distended bladder, the nurse begins percussion on the skin of the lower abdomen and continues in the direction of the umbilicus until dull sounds are no longer produced.

Clients with inflammation or infection in the kidney or adjacent structures may describe their pain as severe or as a constant, dull ache. If the client identifies flank pain or tenderness, the specially trained nurse first percusses the nontender CVA. The client assumes a sitting, side-lying, or supine position, and the nurse forms one hand into a clenched fist. The heel of the hand and the little finger form a flat area, with which a firm thump to the CVA area can be quickly administered. Costovertebral tenderness during this technique is highly suggestive of kidney infection or inflammation.

Assessment of the Urethra

Using a good light source and wearing gloves, the nurse inspects the urethra by examining the meatus and surrounding tissues. The nurse notes any unusual discharge, such as blood, mucus, and purulent drainage. The nurse inspects the skin and mucous membranes of surrounding tissues and notes the presence of lesions, rashes, or other abnormalities of the penis or scrotum or of the labia or vaginal orifice. Urethral irritation is suspected when the client reports discomfort with urination.

PSYCHOSOCIAL ASSESSMENT

Concerns about the urologic system may evoke fear, anger, embarrassment, anxiety, guilt, or sadness in the client. Childhood learning often includes privacy with regard to habits associated with urination. Urologic disorders may stimulate previously forgotten memories of difficult toilet training or bed-wetting. The client may deny symptoms or delay seeking health care.

Emotional responses to problems of the urologic system may occur because of general anxieties about body image, fear of sexual dysfunction, or fear of death. The

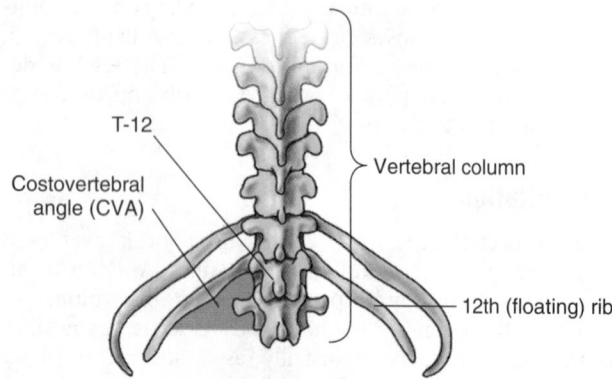

Figure 72–9. Posterior view of the costovertebral angle *(shaded)*.

client may irrationally link symptoms of the urogenital system to natural body-exploring childhood activities. Similarly, adult sexual practices may also evoke anxieties and other emotional responses.

Other memories, such as those of the deaths of relatives or friends with diseases known to cause kidney disease, often provoke a fear of death. Past experiences, as well as daily media discussions of causes of death and disease, can stimulate anxiety.

DIAGNOSTIC ASSESSMENT
Laboratory Tests
Blood Tests
Serum Creatinine

Serum creatinine determination is a measurement of the end-product of muscle and protein metabolism. Creatinine is filtered by the kidneys and excreted in urine. Because muscle mass and metabolism are relatively constant, the serum creatinine level is an excellent indicator of renal function. The normal serum creatinine level is expressed as a range of normal values, reflective of differing muscle mass composition. For adult men, the normal serum creatinine value is slightly higher than for adult women (Chart 72–2). Men generally have a larger muscle mass than do women, but there are exceptions. As a person ages, muscle mass and the amount of creatinine produced diminish. Yet, because of decreased rates of creatinine clearance, the serum creatinine level remains relatively constant in older people, unless renal disease is present.

No common pathologic condition other than renal disease results in an increase in serum creatinine level. Because the serum creatinine level is not increased until at least 50% of the renal function is lost, *any* elevation of serum creatinine values is important.

Blood Urea Nitrogen

Blood urea nitrogen (BUN) measures the renal excretion of urea nitrogen. Urea nitrogen is a byproduct of the hepatic metabolism of protein. Urea nitrogen is produced primarily from food sources of protein, which undergo biotransformation by the liver. The kidneys filter urea nitrogen from the blood and excrete the nitrogenous waste in urine; BUN levels indicate the extent of renal clearance of this nitrogenous waste product.

Because other factors may influence the BUN level, an elevation of BUN level does not always represent renal disease (see Chart 72–2). For example, rapid cell destruction from infection or steroid therapy may also produce an elevated BUN level. In addition, blood is a protein. Therefore, if there is blood in body tissues, the reabsorption of the blood protein is processed by the liver, resulting in an increased BUN level.

The liver must function properly to produce urea nitrogen. When hepatic and renal dysfunction are both present, urea nitrogen levels are actually decreased, reflecting hepatic failure but not renal failure. Therefore, the BUN level is not always elevated with renal disease and is not the most reliable indicator of renal function. However, an elevated BUN level is highly *suggestive* of renal dysfunction.

Chart 72–2

Laboratory Profile: Renal Function Blood Studies

Test	Normal Range for Adults	Significance of Abnormal Findings
Serum creatinine	• Males: 0.9–1.3 mg/dL (80—115 mmol/L) • Females: 0.6–1.1 mg/dL (53–97 mmol/L) • **Elderly:** may be decreased	• An *increased level* indicates renal impairment or a diet high in meat. • A *decreased level* may be caused by a decreased muscle mass.
Blood urea nitrogen (BUN)	• 6–20 mg/dL (2.1–7.1 mmol/L) • **Elderly:** 60–90 yr: 8–23 mg/dL (2.9–8.2 mmol/L); over 90 yr: 10–31 mg/dL (3.6–11.1 mmol/L)	• An *increased level* may indicate hepatic or renal disease, dehydration or decreased renal perfusion, a high-protein diet, infection, stress, steroid use, GI bleeding, or other situations in which there is blood in body tissues. • A *decreased level* may indicate malnutrition, fluid volume excess, or severe hepatic damage.
BUN/creatinine ratio	• Mass ratio: 12:1 to 20:1; mole ratio: (48.5:1 to 80.8:1)	• An *increased ratio* may indicate fluid volume deficit, obstructive uropathy, catabolic state, or high protein diet. • A *decreased ratio* may indicate fluid volume excess or acute renal tubular acidosis. • *No change* in the ratio with increases in both the BUN and creatinine levels indicates renal impairment.

Ratio of Blood Urea Nitrogen to Serum Creatinine

The BUN/creatinine ratio determines whether factors such as dehydration or lack of renal perfusion are causing the elevated BUN level. When an intravascular fluid volume deficit or hypoperfusion exists, the BUN level rises more rapidly than the serum creatinine level. As a result, the ratio of BUN to creatinine is *increased*. This situation is considered potentially correctable; thus, the BUN/serum creatinine ratio is restored when renal perfusion is stabilized.

When both the BUN and serum creatinine levels increase at the same rate, the BUN/creatinine ratio remains normal. However, the elevated serum creatinine and BUN levels suggest renal dysfunction, which is not related to acute volume depletion or hypoperfusion.

Urine Tests
Urinalysis

Urinalysis (Chart 72–3) is a usual component of any complete physical examination but is particularly informative for clients with suspected renal or urologic disorders. Ideally, the urinalysis specimen is collected at the first morning's voiding; specimens obtained at other times may not provide sufficient concentration or acidity. The specimen may be collected by several techniques (Table 72–5).

Color, Odor, and Turbidity

The color of urine is derived from urochrome pigment. Variations in color may result from increased levels of urochrome or other pigments, changes in the concentration or dilution of the urine, and presence of medication metabolites in the urine. Urine smells faintly like ammonia because of the breakdown of urea. Turbidity describes cloudiness, but urine is normally clear on inspection without cloudiness or haziness.

Specific Gravity

The specific gravity of urine measures the relative concentration, or density, of urine relative to water. The specific gravity of water is 1.000. If renal function is normal, a change in the specific gravity of urine occurs when there is a need to excrete more or less water to normalize the serum. Changes from what would be expected reflect a disturbance in the concentrating and diluting function of the tubules.

An *increase* in specific gravity occurs with insufficient fluid intake, decreased renal perfusion, or the presence of antidiuretic hormone (ADH). ADH production is normally increased with stress, surgery, anesthetic agents, and certain drugs, such as morphine and oral hypoglycemic agents. In each of these situations, the expected renal response is to reabsorb water and decrease urinary output. Consequently, the urine produced is more concentrated.

A *decrease* in specific gravity occurs with increased fluid intake, diuretic administration, and diabetes insip-

idus. In each of these situations, the normal renal response is to excrete more water; thus, urinary output is increased. In renal disease, the specific gravity decreases because of less solute and does not vary with changes in plasma osmolality (e.g., becomes fixed).

pH

A pH value less than 7 is considered acidic; a value greater than 7, alkaline. Various factors influence the acidity or alkalinity of urine. A diet high in certain fruits and vegetables, for example, results in a more alkaline urine, whereas a high-protein diet produces a more acidic urine. The presence of *Escherichia coli* in the urine also results in an acidic urine.

Urine specimens become more alkaline under the following circumstances:

- If allowed to stand unrefrigerated, especially for more than 1 hour
- If urea-splitting bacteria are present
- If a specimen is left uncovered

An alkaline urine promotes cellular breakdown; thus, abnormal urinary sediment (e.g., red blood cells) may be missed on analysis. The nurse ensures that urine specimens are covered and delivered to the laboratory promptly or refrigerated. During systemic processes involving acidosis or alkalosis (metabolic or respiratory), the kidneys, along with blood buffers and the lungs, should respond appropriately to maintain a normal serum pH.

Respiratory Acidosis

During respiratory acidosis (retention of volatile acids), the kidneys increase the excretion of hydrogen ions, contributing to a more acidic urinary pH.

Respiratory Alkalosis

During respiratory alkalosis (loss of volatile acids), the kidneys conserve hydrogen, and the urine becomes alkaline.

Metabolic Alkalosis

During metabolic alkalosis, systemic processes produce an excess of bicarbonate; therefore, the renal response expected is an alkaline urine attributable to the excretion of bicarbonate. Yet the kidneys have an obligatory load of hydrogen to excrete, and this requirement results in a more acidic urine than expected.

Metabolic Acidosis

During metabolic acidosis, systemic processes produce excess hydrogen, and available bicarbonate is used as a blood buffer. The urine is expected to be acidic if the kidneys are properly excreting the increased acid load. In clients with renal failure, a frequent cause of metabolic acidosis, the kidneys cannot excrete hydrogen or regenerate adequate bicarbonate for buffering. Thus, the urine of a client who has metabolic acidosis from renal failure is less acidic than expected. (Chapters 18 and 19 discuss acid-base balance and imbalance.)

Chart 72-3

Laboratory Profile: Urinalysis

Test	Normal Range for Adults	Significance of Abnormal Findings
Color	• Pale yellow	• *Dark amber* indicates concentrated urine. • *Very pale yellow* indicates dilute urine. • *Dark red or brown* indicates blood in the urine; brown also may indicate increased urinary bilirubin level; red may also indicate the presence of myoglobin. • *Other color changes* may result from diet or medications.
Odor	• Specific aromatic odor, similar to ammonia	• *Foul smell* indicates possible infection, dehydration, or ingestion of certain foods or drugs.
Turbidity	• Clear	• *Cloudy urine* indicates infection or sediment or high levels of urinary protein.
Specific gravity	• Usually 1.015–1.025; possible range 1.002–1.030; after 12-hr fluid restriction >1.025 • **Elderly:** Decreased because of decreased concentrating ability	• *Increased* in decreased renal perfusion, inappropriate antidiuretic hormone secretion, or congestive heart failure. • *Decreased* in chronic renal insufficiency, diabetes insipidus, malignant hypertension, diuretic administration, and lithium toxicity.
pH	• Average 5–6; possible range 4.5–8	• *Changes* are caused by diet, the administration of medications, infection, freshness of the specimen, acid-base imbalance, and altered renal function.
Glucose	• <15 mg/dL (0.1–0.8 mmol/L)	• *Presence* reflects hyperglycemia or a decrease in the renal threshold for glucose.
Ketones	• None	• *Presence* reflects incomplete metabolism of fatty acids, as in diabetic ketoacidosis, prolonged fasting, anorexia nervosa.
Protein	• 1–14 mg/dL (10–140 mg/L)	• *Increased amounts* may indicate stress, infection, recent strenuous exercise, or glomerular disorders.
Bilirubin (urobilinogen)	• None	• *Presence* suggests hepatic or biliary disease or obstruction.
Red blood cells (RBCs)	• 0–2 per high-power field	• *Increased* amounts are normal with indwelling or intermittent catheterization or menses but may reflect tumor, stones, trauma, glomerular disorders, cystitis, or bleeding disorders.
White blood cells (WBCs)	• Males: 0–3 per high-power field • Females: 0–5 per high-power field	• *Increased* amounts may indicate an infectious or inflammatory process anywhere in the renal/urinary tract, renal transplant rejection, fever, or exercise.
Casts	• A few or none, composed of RBC or WBC, protein, or tubular cell casts	• *Increased amounts* indicate the presence of bacteria or protein, which is seen in severe renal disease and could also indicate urinary calculi.
Crystals	• None	• *Presence* of normal or abnormal crystals may indicate that the specimen has been allowed to stand.
Bacteria	• <1000 colonies/mL	• *Increased amounts* indicate the need for urine culture to determine the presence of urinary tract infection.
Parasites	• None	• *Presence* of *Trichomonas vaginalis* indicates infection, usually of the urethra, the prostate, or the vagina.
Nitrates	• None	• *Presence* suggests bacteria, usually *Escherichia coli.*

TABLE 72–5

Collection of Urine Specimens

Type of Specimen	Nursing Interventions	Rationale
Voided urine	• Collect the first specimen voided in the morning. • Send the specimen to the laboratory as soon as possible. • Refrigerate the specimen if a delay is unavoidable.	• Urine is more concentrated in the early morning. • After urine is collected, cellular breakdown results in more alkaline urine. • Refrigeration delays the alkalinization of urine. Bacteria are more likely to multiply in an alkaline environment.
Clean catch specimen	• Explain the purpose of the procedure to the client. • Instruct the client to self-clean before voiding. • Instruct the female client to separate the labia and use the sponges and solution provided to wipe with three strokes over the urethra. The first two wiping strokes are over each side of the urethra; the third wiping stroke is centered over the urethra (from front to back). • Instruct the male client to retract the foreskin of the penis and to similarly clean the urethra, using three wiping strokes with the sponge and solution provided (from the head of the penis downward). • Instruct the client to initiate voiding after cleaning. The client then stops and resumes voiding into the container. Only 1 ounce (30 mL) is needed; the remainder of the urine may be discarded into the commode. • Ensure that the client understands the procedure. • Assist the client as needed.	• Correct technique is needed to obtain a valid specimen. • Surface cleaning is necessary to remove secretions or bacteria from the urethral meatus. • A mid-stream collection further removes secretions and bacteria because urine flushes the distal portion of the internal urethra. • An improperly collected specimen may result in inappropriate or incomplete treatment. • The client's understanding and the nurse's assistance ensure proper collection.
Catheterized specimen	• For nonindwelling (straight) catheters: • Avoid routine use. • Follow the facility's procedures for catheterization technique.	• The one-time passage of a urinary catheter may be necessary to obtain an uncontaminated specimen for analysis or to measure the volume of residual urine. • These procedures minimize bacterial entry.

Glucose

Glucose is filtered at the glomerular level and reabsorbed in the proximal tubule in the nephron. Usually, when the blood glucose level rises above a certain level (greater than 220 mg/dL), the renal threshold for reabsorption is exceeded, and glucose is excreted in the urine. Variations in the renal threshold for glucose occur in clients who have had diabetes mellitus for a number of years. It is possible that their serum glucose level may be high (e.g., greater than 400 mg/dL), and glucose may still not be present in the urine.

Ketone Bodies

Three types of ketone bodies are acetone, acetoacetic acid, and beta-oxybutyric acid. Ketone bodies are byproducts of incomplete metabolism of fatty acids. Normally, there are no ketones in urine. Ketone bodies are produced when there is a deficiency of insulin and when alternative metabolic pathways (gluconeogenesis) are utilized to convert fat sources to glucose and provide cellular energy. When ketones are present in the serum, glomerular filtration results in a partial urinary excretion of these ketones.

Protein

Protein, such as albumin, is not normally present in the urine. Levels greater than 300 mg/24 hours, or 200 μg/minute, are abnormal. The glomerular membrane is semipermeable to small molecules; protein molecules are too large to pass through this semipermeable membrane. When permeability of the glomerular membrane is increased, the protein molecules pass through and are excreted in the urine. An increased glomerular membrane permeability may be caused by infection or inflammation

TABLE 72–5

Collection of Urine Specimens *Continued*

Type of Specimen	Nursing Interventions	Rationale
	• For indwelling catheters:	• Collection of urine from an indwelling catheter or tubing is performed when clients have catheters for continence or long-term urinary drainage.
	• Apply a clamp to the drainage tubing, distal to the injection port.	• Clamping allows urine to collect in the tubing at the location where the specimen is obtained.
	• Clean the injection port cap of the catheter drainage tubing with an appropriate antiseptic. Povidone-iodine solution or alcohol is acceptable.	• Surface contamination is prevented by following the cleaning procedures.
	• Insert a sterile 5-mL syringe into the port and aspirate the quantity of urine required.	• A minimum of 5 mL is needed for culture and sensitivity (C&S) testing.
	• Inject the urine sample into a sterile specimen container.	• A sterile container is used for C&S specimens.
	• Remove the clamp to resume drainage.	
	• Properly dispose of the syringe.	
24-hr urine collection	• Instruct the client thoroughly.	• A 24-hr collection of urine is necessary to quantify or calculate the rate of clearance of a particular substance.
	• Provide written materials to assist in instruction.	• Instructional materials for clients, signs, and so on, remind clients and staff to ensure that the total collection is completed.
	• Place signs appropriately.	
	• Inform all personnel or family caregivers of test in progress.	
	• Check laboratory or procedure manual on proper technique for maintaining the collection (e.g., on ice, in a refrigerator, or with a preservative).	• Proper technique prevents breakdown of elements to be measured.
	• On initiation of the collection, ask the client to void, discard the urine, and note the time.	• Proper techniques ensure that *all* urine formed within the 24-hr period is collected.
	• Collect all urine for the next 24 hr.	
	• 24 hr after initiation, ask the client to empty the bladder and add that urine to the container.	
	• Do not remove urine from the collection container for other specimens.	• Urine in the container is not considered a "fresh" specimen and may be mixed with preservative.

and associated immunologic mechanisms. Certain systemic processes result in the production of abnormal proteins, such as globulin. These proteins are not detected with routine urinalysis procedures; urine protein electrophoresis or other tests are necessary to detect these unusual proteins.

A random finding of proteinuria followed by a series of negative (normal) findings does not imply renal disease. If infection is suspected to be the cause of the proteinuria, urinalyses after eradication of the infection should be negative for protein. Persistent proteinuria needs further investigation. Usually, a 24-hour urine collection for total protein determination is indicated. Protein in the urine is associated with glomerular disease, usually as a result of immunologic mechanisms.

Microalbuminuria is the presence of albumin in the urine that is not measurable by urinary dipstick or conventional urinalysis procedures. Specialized immunoassay tests can analyze quickly a freshly voided urine specimen for microscopic levels of albumin. Levels of 30–300 mg/24 hours, or 20–200 μg/min, indicate microalbuminuria.

Sediment

Urinary sediment refers to particles present in the urine. These include cells, casts, crystals, and bacteria.

Cells

Types of cells abnormally present in the urine may include tubular cells (from the tubule of the nephron), epithelial cells (from the urothelial lining of the urinary tract), red blood cells (RBCs), and white blood cells (WBCs).

Casts

Casts are structures formed around other particles. There may be casts of cells, bacteria, or protein. When casts are formed, there is a clumping or agglutination of the element, and gelatinous substances form the surrounding structure, a cast. Casts are described by the type of element in the structure (e.g., RBC cast, WBC cast, tubular epithelial cast) or the stage of degeneration. The degeneration of casts refers to the stage of breakdown of the internal element. Casts are described as "granular" (coarse or fine) and "waxy."

Crystals

Crystals in the urine come from various salts. These particles may be from components of the diet, drugs, or disease. The salts may be composed of calcium, oxalate, urea, phosphate, magnesium, or other substances. Certain drugs, such as the sulfates, also can produce crystals.

Bacteria

Bacteria in a urine sample multiply quickly, so the specimen must be analyzed promptly.

Urine for Culture and Sensitivity

The nurse may collect a sample of urine for laboratory determination of the number and types of pathogens present. The presence of clinical symptoms and unexplained bacteria in a urinalysis specimen are indications for urine culture and sensitivity testing. After the culture specimen is incubated for 24 to 48 hours, the colonies are inoculated onto plates with various antimicrobial agents. Those antibiotics to which the microorganisms are sensitive or resistant are reported to guide decisions about needed therapy. A clean-catch or catheter-derived specimen is always preferred for culture and sensitivity testing.

Composite Urine Collections

When ordered, urine collections are made for a number of hours (e.g., 2–24 hours) for laboratory quantitative and qualitative analysis of one or more substances. Collections are often ordered for the measurement of levels of urinary creatinine or urea nitrogen, sodium, chloride, calcium, catecholamines, or other components (Chart 72–4). For a composite urine specimen, *all* urine within the designated time frame must be collected (see Table 72–5). If other voided or catheterized specimens must be obtained while the collection is in progress, the nurse measures and appropriately documents the amount collected, but not added to the timed collection.

If the client has a Foley catheter in place, the nurse empties the catheter, the tubing, and the drainage bag at the designated start time. From the start time until the defined period has elapsed, all urine produced is col-

lected, measured, and stored in a specific container, depending on the reason for the urine collection. The urine collection may need to be refrigerated or stored on ice to prevent changes in the urine during the collection time. The nurse follows the procedure from the laboratory for urine storage.

The nurse explains that the urine collection must be free from fecal contamination. Menstrual blood and toilet tissue also contaminate the specimen and can invalidate the results. If the client has a Foley catheter, the nurse remembers to empty the catheter, tubing, and drainage bag at the ending time.

The collection of urine for a 24-hour period is often more difficult than it seems. In hospitalized clients, the cooperation of staff personnel, the client, family members, and visitors is essential. Any person who might forget and discard collected urine contributes to sources of error during the collection. Placing signs in the bathroom, instructing the client and family, and emphasizing the need to save the urine are helpful.

Creatinine Clearance Test

Creatinine clearance is a calculation of glomerular filtration rate. It is the best indication of overall renal function. The amount of creatinine cleared from the blood (e.g., filtered into the urine) is measured in the total volume of urine excreted in a defined period. A urine specimen for a creatinine clearance test is usually collected for 24 hours, but it can be collected for shorter periods (e.g., 8 or 12 hours). The calculation entails comparison with the serum creatinine level, so a blood specimen for creatinine must also be collected.

The laboratory or the physician calculates the creatinine clearance. Because the client's age, sex, height, weight, diet, and activity level influence the expected amount of creatinine to be excreted, these variables are considered in the interpretation of creatinine clearance test results. Knowledge of the total grams of creatinine excreted into the urine collection assists in determining the adequacy of the collection. The nurse interprets the test results to provide a basis for care planning and client education.

The formula for the calculation of creatinine clearance is

$$\text{creatinine clearance} = U \times V/P \times T$$

where U is creatinine in urine (mg/dL), V is volume of urine (mL/24 hours), P is creatinine in plasma (mg/dL), and T is time in minutes.

The rate of creatinine clearance is expressed as milliliters per minute per 1.73 m^2 of body surface area. This formula also is corrected for estimated variations in surface area. The normal creatinine clearance range for adult males is 95–135 mL/min; for adult females, the normal range is 85–125 mL/min.

To determine the client's existing renal function, creatinine clearance measurements are necessary. Decreases in the creatinine clearance rate may necessitate modification of drug dosing or signify the need for further investigation of the cause of renal deterioration.

Chart 72–4

Laboratory Profile: 24-Hour Urine Collections

Component	Normal Range for Adults	Significance of Abnormal Findings
Creatinine	• 0.8–2 g/24 hr • Males: 1–2 g/24 hr or 14–26 mg/kg/24 hr (124–230 μmol/kg/24 hr or 7.1–17.7 mmol/24 hr) • Females: 0.6–1.8 g/24 hr or 11–20 mg/kg/24 hr (97–177 μmol/kg/24 hr or 5.3–15.9 mmol/24 hr) • **Elderly:** 10 mg/kg/24 hr (88.4 μmol/kg/24 hr) at 90 yr	• *Decreased amounts* indicate a deterioration in renal function caused by renal disease, shock, hypovolemia, or any condition affecting muscle. • *Increased amounts* occur with infections, exercise, diabetes mellitus, and meat meals.
Urea nitrogen	• 12–20 g/24 hr (0.43–0.71 mmol/24 hr)	• *Decreased amounts* occur when renal damage or liver disease is present. • *Increased amounts* commonly result from a high-protein diet, dehydration, trauma, or sepsis.
Sodium	• 40–220 mEq/24 hr (40–220 mmol/24 hr)	• *Decreased amounts* are seen in hemorrhage, shock, hyperaldosteronism, and prerenal acute renal failure. • *Increased amounts* are common with diuretic therapy, excessive salt intake, hypokalemia, and acute tubular necrosis.
Chloride	• 110–250 mEq/24 hr (110–250 mmol/24 hr) • **Elderly:** 95–195 mEq/24 hr (95–195 mmol/24 hr)	• *Decreased amounts* are seen in certain renal diseases, malabsorption syndrome, pyloric obstruction, prolonged nasogastric tube drainage, diarrhea, diaphoresis, congestive heart failure, and emphysema. • *Increased amounts* are seen with hypokalemia, adrenal insufficiency, and massive diuresis.
Calcium	• 50–300 mg/24 hr (1.25–7.50 mmol/kg/24 hr)	• *Decreased amounts* are often associated with hypocalcemia, hypoparathyroidism, nephrosis, and nephritis. • *Increased amounts* are commonly seen with calcium renal stones, hyperparathyroidism, sarcoidosis, certain cancers, immobilization, and hypercalcemia.
Total catecholamines*	• <100 μg/24 hr (<591 mmol/24 hr)	• *Increased amounts* occur with pheochromocytoma, neuroblastomas, stress, or strenuous exercise.
Protein	• 1–14 mg/dL (10–140 mg/L) or 50–80 mg/24 hr at rest	• *Increased amounts* indicate glomerular disease, nephrotic syndrome, diabetic nephropathy, urinary tract malignancies, and irritations.

* Epinephrine and norepinephrine only; dopamine is not measured.

Urinary Electrolytes

The nurse may collect a sample of urine as ordered for analysis of urinary electrolyte levels (e.g., sodium and chloride). Normally, the amount of sodium excreted in the urine is nearly equal to that consumed. Urinary sodium levels are measured to assist with the medical differential diagnosis of prerenal azotemia from lack of renal perfusion versus acute tubular necrosis (ATN). Urinary sodium levels of less than 10 mEq/L indicate that the tubules are functioning to conserve (reabsorb) sodium.

Osmolality

Osmolality is a measure of the concentration of particles in solution, in this case the concentration of solutes in urine. These solutes include electrolytes and solutes such as glucose, urea, and creatinine.

Plasma Osmolality

The kidneys excrete or reabsorb water to maintain a plasma osmolality in the range of 275–295 mOsm/kg of

TABLE 72–6

Common Radiologic and Special Diagnostic Tests for Clients with Disorders of the Renal/Urinary System

Test	Purpose	Comments
Radiography of kidneys, ureters, and bladder (KUB) (plain film of abdomen)	• To screen for the presence of two kidneys • To measure the kidneys' size • To detect gross obstruction	
Excretory urography	• To measure the kidneys' size • To detect obstruction • To assess parenchymal mass	• Radiopaque contrast media may cause an allergic (hypersensitivity) reaction in iodine-sensitive clients. • Contrast agent is also hypertonic and increases the risk of acute renal failure in adults with serum creatinine levels greater than 1.5 mg/dL, diabetes mellitus, multiple myeloma, or dehydration. • Nephrotoxic complications can be prevented by parenteral fluid administration, the use of mannitol, and daily monitoring of serum creatinine levels.
Nephrotomography	• To assess various planes of kidney tissue for cysts, tumors, or calculi	• Same as for excretory urogram.
Computed tomography (CT)	• To measure the size of the kidneys • To evaluate contour to assess for masses or obstruction	• Contrast medium may provoke acute renal failure. • See comments with excretory urography for high-risk clients and preventive measures related to contrast. • May be performed without contrast medium and still obtain adequate visualization.
Cystography and cystoscopy	• To identify abnormalities of the bladder wall and urethral and ureteral occlusions • To treat small obstructions or lesions via fulguration, lithotripsy, or removal with a stone basket	• Instrumentation of the urinary tract increases the risk of infection. • Monitor for infection for 48–72 hr after the procedure.
Voiding cystourethrography (VCUG)	• To outline the bladder's contour and to detect urinary reflux from vesicourethral junctions	• The risk of infection is similar to that in cystography because urinary catheterization is necessary. • Monitor for post-procedure infection.
Renal arteriography	• To identify vascular abnormalities within each kidney and adjacent aorta	• Contrast medium may provoke acute renal failure. • See comments with excretory urography for high-risk clients and preventive measures related to contrast. • Essential for diagnosis and treatment of some vascular abnormalities, such as renal artery stenosis. • Monitor for bleeding after the procedure.
Ultrasonography (US)	• To identify the size of the kidneys or obstruction in the kidneys or the lower urinary tract • May detect tumors or cysts	• Ultrasonography entails minimal risk to the client. • Ultrasonography is a good alternative to excretory urography.

extracellular water. The value in the elderly is slightly higher, 280 to 301 mOsm/kg of extracellular water. When plasma osmolality is decreased, ADH release is inhibited. Without ADH, the distal tubule and collecting ducts are *not* permeable to water. Therefore, water is *excreted,* not reabsorbed. When the plasma osmolality is increased, ADH is produced. With ADH production, the distal tubule is made permeable to water. Consequently, water is reabsorbed, and less urine is excreted. Thus, increased urine osmolality reflects a concentrated urine with less water than solutes. A decreased urine osmolality value reflects a dilute urine with more water than solutes.

Urinary Osmolality

Urinary osmolality can vary from 50 to 1200 mOsm/kg water, depending on the clinical and hydration status of the client and the functional status of the kidneys. With average fluid intake, the urine osmolality range is 300–900 mOsm/kg water. The fixed acids and other wastes that are continually produced constitute a solute load that must be excreted in the urine on a regular basis. This is referred to as *obligatory solute excretion.* If the client has lost excessive fluids, the renal response is to conserve water, preserve plasma osmolality, and excrete a small-volume, highly concentrated urine. Many factors, such as diet, medications, and activity, can influence the urine osmolality.

Radiographic Examinations

Radiographic and other special procedures are used to diagnose structural and functional abnormalities within the genitourinary system (Table 72–6). As with other diagnostic tests, the nurse explains the procedures thoroughly to the client, prepares the client, and provides post-procedural care.

Kidney, Ureter, and Bladder (KUB) X-Ray

Radiographic examination of the kidneys, ureters, and bladder (KUB) is a plain film of the abdomen taken without any specific client preparation. The KUB study shows gross anatomic features. It may show obvious stones, strictures, calcifications, or obstructions in the urinary tract. The test identifies the organs' shape, size, and relationship to other parts of the urinary tract. Other tests are necessary for definitive diagnosis of functional or structural abnormalities.

The nurse advises the client that there is no discomfort or risk from the procedure. The nurse tells the client that the films will be taken while the client is in a supine position. Excessive flatus in the colon may distort the results. No specific post-procedure care is necessary.

Intravenous Urography

Other names for intravenous urography include excretory urography and (the older term) intravenous pyelography (IVP).

Client Preparation

Before urography, the nurse assesses the client (Chart 72–5), institutes bowel preparation to promote adequate visualization of the renal system, and teaches the client. The nurse reports allergy information to the physician. Contrast reactions can be minor (nausea and vomiting, urticaria, itching, sneezing), moderate (nephrotoxic effects, congestive heart failure, pulmonary edema), or severe (bronchospasm, anaphylactoid). If the diagnostic test is still to be performed, the physician orders pre-procedural medications such as a steroid (methylprednisone or prednisone), an antihistamine (diphenhydramine hydrochloride [Benadryl, Allerdryl♣]), and possibly an H_2 blocker (cimetidine [Tagamet] or ranitidine [Zantac]) to suppress the allergic response (Cohan & Ellis, 1997). The nurse explains the rationale to the client.

Procedures to ensure that films provide adequate visualization vary, depending on the radiologist's preferences. Some radiologists recommend a light evening meal or clear liquids, then fasting (NPO status) from midnight on the night before the procedure. Others recommend liberal fluid intake to prevent dehydration up until the time of the procedure. Because of the possibility of a vomiting reaction to the intravenous (IV) contrast, however, the physician may prefer that the client remain NPO at least a few hours before the procedure. The physician orders hydration with IV fluids as indicated.

The physician orders a bowel preparation to remove fecal contents, fluid, and air from the gut, which permits an adequate outline of the lower poles of the kidneys, ureters, and bladder. Bowel preparation procedures vary but usually include the administration of laxatives the day before the procedure. Enemas also may be prescribed but are controversial because air and fluid can be introduced with inadequate expulsion of fecal contents. Bowel preparation procedures contribute to potential dehydration, especially in elderly clients. To help prevent dehydration, the nurse contacts the testing department and requests that urograms be scheduled early in the day for elderly clients.

The contrast medium is potentially nephrotoxic. The risk for *contrast-induced renal failure* is greatest in clients who are elderly or dehydrated, who have some renal insufficiency (e.g., serum creatinine level greater than 1.5 mg/dL), or who are receiving other potentially nephrotoxic medications. The physician may order IV fluid administration before the procedure to maintain hydration and to decrease the nephrotoxic potential. To maximize excretion of the potentially toxic agent, the physician may prescribe IV administration of mannitol (Osmitrol♣) immediately after injection of the contrast agent.

The nurse instructs the client in the preparation procedures for the urogram and explains the procedure so the client knows what to expect in the examination room (Chart 72–6). The nurse allows time for questions and refers questions beyond his or her expertise to the appropriate staff. The nurse intervenes on behalf of the client to ensure that questions are answered *before* the procedure.

Chart 72–5

Focused Assessment for the Client About to Undergo a Diagnostic Test or Interventional Procedure Using Contrast Media

Prior to the procedure:

- Ask the client if he or she has ever had a reaction to contrast media. (Such a client has the highest risk for having another reaction.)
- Ask the client about a history of asthma. (Asthmatics have been shown to be at greater risk for contrast reactions than the general public; and, when reactions do occur, they are more likely to be severe.)
- Ask the client about known hay fever or food or medication allergies, especially to seafood, eggs, milk, or chocolate. (Contrast reactions have been reported to be as high as 15% in these clients.)
- Ask the client to describe any specific allergic reactions (e.g., hives, facial edema, difficulty breathing, bronchospasm).
- Assess for history of renal insufficiency and for conditions that have been implicated in increasing the chance of developing renal failure after contrast media (e.g., diabetic nephropathy, class IV heart failure, dehydration, concomitant use of potentially nephrotoxic medications such as the aminoglycosides or NSAIDs, and cirrhosis).
- Ask the client if he or she is taking metformin (Glucophage). (Metformin must be discontinued at least 48 hours before any study using contrast media because the life-threatening complication of lactic acidosis, although rare, could occur.)
- Assess hydration status by checking blood pressure, heart and respiratory rates, mucous membranes, skin turgor, urine concentration.
- Ask the client when he or she last ate or drank anything.

From Cohan, R. H., & Ellis, J. H. (1997). Iodinated contrast material in uroradiology: Choice of agent and management of complications. *Urologic Clinics of North America, 24*(3), 471–491.

Procedure

A radiopaque contrast medium is intravenously injected as a bolus or an infusion with the client in a supine position. As blood (with the contrast medium) rapidly circulates into the renal vasculature and is filtered by the glomeruli, the contrast medium is excreted in the urine. A series of x-rays are taken at various times after injection. When ordered, nephrotomograms are taken at the same time as the urogram. Tomograms provide images of different planes of tissue, showing any abnormalities present at varying depths. The technologist then asks the client to empty the bladder and return for a few more films. An outline of the kidneys, ureters, and bladder results as urine containing the contrast medium is excreted. The urogram provides information about

- The number, size, shape, and location of the kidneys
- The adequacy of uptake (filling) and the rate of excretion of contrast medium

- The number, size, location, appearance, and patency of the calices, pelves, and ureters
- The size, location, and nature of the urinary bladder

Follow-Up Care

After the urogram, the nurse monitors the client for altered renal function and other effects from the contrast medium. The nurse ensures adequate hydration by encouraging the client to take fluid orally or administering parenteral fluids at the prescribed rate. Hydration minimizes the potential for renal deterioration. The nurse and the physician monitor serum creatinine levels. Elevations may be due to acute renal failure induced by contrast media. The nurse monitors urinary output but realizes that an elevation of the serum creatinine level may occur

---

Chart 72–6

Education Guide: Excretory Urogram

- The urogram outlines your urinary tract and helps determine any problems there.
- Notify your nurse or physician if you have had any reactions (allergic or otherwise) to any food or drugs, especially shellfish (shrimp, scallops, crab, lobster, and so on) or iodine, or to x-ray "dyes" such as contrast media; if you have a history of asthma; or if you are taking metformin (Glucophage).
- The day before the test, follow the instructions about changes in your diet and fluid intake to be sure that as much information as possible is gained from the test.
- After you start the bowel preparation, you may need to be close to toileting facilities. The preparation medications usually work quickly.
- You will be lying on an x-ray table with the x-ray machine above you for most of the procedure.
- A pressure band, similar to a large blood pressure cuff, may be placed around your stomach or abdomen to help obtain better x-ray pictures.
- If you do not already have an intravenous access site, one will be started to give you the contrast agent.
- After the contrast is injected, you may feel a sense of warmth or heat as it travels throughout your body. You also may have a taste in your mouth that is sometimes described as metallic. These sensations last only a few seconds or minutes.
- When the pressure band is inflated, you may feel some tightness around your abdomen. The sensation is similar to the feeling on your arm when you have your blood pressure taken.
- A series of x-ray pictures will be taken. You may be asked to empty your bladder and return to the table for more films. You may be asked to have a standing film taken as well.
- After the test is completed, you are usually able to resume your normal activities and diet.
- The contrast will be excreted normally in your urine. You will not notice any change in the color or characteristics of your urine.
- Please do not hesitate to ask your nurse, physician, or x-ray technologist any question you have, no matter how slight the question may seem to you. It is important for you to have as much understanding as possible.

despite normal urinary output (nonoliguric acute renal failure).

Computed Tomography
Client Preparation

The nurse informs the client that computed tomography (CT) is performed to provide three-dimensional information about the structures of the abdomen, including the kidneys, the ureters, the bladder, and surrounding tissues. CT usually performed after other diagnostic procedures and yields definitive information about tumors, cysts, abscesses, or other masses, as well as obstruction or some vascular abnormalities.

Client preparation includes a bowel preparation with laxatives or an enema and a light meal the evening before the procedure. The client is maintained on nothing by mouth (NPO) status after midnight on the night preceding the examination. For clients having the CT scan with contrast medium, the physician orders pre-procedural IV hydration as for clients undergoing a urogram. The nurse assesses for sensitivity or allergy to contrast and intervenes as with a urogram.

Procedure

The CT scan is performed in a special room, usually located in the radiology department. An IV injection of radiopaque contrast media may be administered before the initiation of imaging procedures. The use of contrast media may be eliminated in clients at risk for contrast media–induced acute renal failure, but the images produced are less distinct. Tomograms (images obtained from cross-sectional angles) are obtained at various levels.

Follow-Up Care

No special follow-up care is necessary unless a contrast medium was used. In that case, the follow-up care is the same as for clients after a urogram.

Cystography and Cystourethrography
Client Preparation

The nurse explains the procedure to the client who requires cystography or cystourethrography. The nurse explains that a urinary catheter is temporarily needed to instill a contrast medium. The contrast medium is necessary for visualization of the lower urinary tract.

Procedure

In both cystography and cystourethrography, contrast medium is instilled into the bladder via a urethral catheter. After bladder filling, a variety of films are obtained from anterior, posterior, and oblique positions. For the voiding cystourethrogram (VCUG), the client is requested to void and films are taken during the voiding. A VCUG is obtained to determine whether vesicoureteral reflux is present. The cystogram is often indicated in cases of trauma when urethral or bladder injury is suspected.

Follow-up Care

The nurse monitors for the development of infection as a result of urinary catheterization. The contrast medium is not nephrotoxic (it is not injected into the bloodstream). The nurse encourages fluid intake to dilute the urine and reduce the burning sensation from catheter irritation after removal. Because pelvic or urethral trauma may be present, the nurse also monitors the client for changes in urinary output that can result from the disruption of urinary tract patency.

Other Diagnostic Tests
Other Renal Diagnostic Tests
Renal Arteriography (Angiography)
Client Preparation

The nurse informs the client that arteriography is performed to assess the arterial blood supply of the kidneys. The nurse explains that, before the examination, a bowel preparation is given to remove fecal contents, gas, and fluid. A light evening meal is given, and the client is maintained on NPO until after the procedure. An IV access site may be placed before the procedure. Often, orders for IV fluid administration are provided to ensure adequate hydration because a contrast medium is used as part of the procedure.

The nurse reviews the procedure for the test with the client, answers questions, and reviews the client's medication regimen and blood study results as indicated. For example, the nurse reviews the prothrombin time if the client has been taking warfarin sodium (Coumadin, Warfilone✦). The client also signs a form indicating informed consent. Renal arteriography is performed to explore suspected causes of decreased renal function such as renovascular hypertension, other vessel abnormalities, and bleeding from trauma.

Procedure

The injection of a radiopaque contrast medium into the renal arteries necessitates entry into the arterial vasculature, usually the femoral artery in the groin. After the client is sedated and the skin is prepared and draped, the radiologist injects a local anesthetic. The physician then performs an arterial puncture through which the angiographic catheter is inserted.

The movement of the catheter is guided (by the radiologist) fluoroscopically into the abdominal aorta and orifices of the renal arteries. When the tip of the catheter is positioned at the renal arteries, the radiologist injects contrast medium into each artery, and films are taken at specified time intervals. The speed of distribution of the contrast medium is noted, along with any areas of vascular narrowing. Arterial blockage is noted when there is failure of contrast medium uptake. Extravasation (infiltration) of contrast medium into surrounding tissue indicates vessel rupture, which could be present after trauma.

By using a digital subtraction technique, visualization of renal vessels can be improved. In the digital subtraction arteriogram (DSA), a computer is used to "subtract out" loops of bowel, ribs, and so on that are normally seen on the x-ray. As a result, even the small-vessel images are improved. In addition, a lesser amount of contrast medium means less risk of nephrotoxicity. When used without full arteriography, DSA procedures may not provide sufficient detail for surgical intervention.

Follow-Up Care

Bleeding from the catheter insertion site and contrast medium–induced reactions are the two most common complications of renal arteriography. The nurse monitors the catheter insertion site for signs of bleeding or swelling. A pressure dressing may have been placed as a preventive measure before the client returned to the nursing area. The nurse ensures that a 5-pound sandbag and ice are available in case of emergency.

The nurse measures and records the client's vital signs as per order or according to the agency's policy. A typical protocol specifies that vital signs be determined every 15 minutes for 1 hour, every 30 minutes for 2 hours, every hour for 4 hours, then every 4 hours. The nurse checks the temperature and color of the extremities and distal pulses. Sudden absence of pulses may reflect hematoma formation or embolization. Hemoglobin and hematocrit levels are measured closely for 24 hours after the procedure, usually every 6 hours.

The period of absolute bed rest (to prevent bleeding) after arteriography varies. In general, bed rest is maintained for at least 6 hours. The nurse instructs the client on the importance of maintaining the procedural leg in a straight position for those 6 hours. With the client's consent, a restraint may be used on the leg. The nurse encourages ankle flexing and weight shifting to prevent deep venous thrombosis. After 6 hours, if there is no evidence of bleeding, the client may be permitted to stand to void or use a bedside commode.

The physician orders serum creatinine tests for several days after the arteriogram to determine whether the procedure has caused further deterioration in renal function. For some clients with renal insufficiency, the administration of contrast media may provoke an episode of acute renal failure sufficient to necessitate short-term dialysis. Because the test is used to provide definitive information that may permit interventions to restore blood flow and thus preserve renal function, many clients are willing to accept the risk of short-term dialysis to prevent the need for permanent dialysis. With the physician's order, the nurse encourages the client to drink fluids after the procedure to ensure adequate excretion of the contrast medium.

Renal Biopsy

Client Preparation

The nurse explains that a biopsy of the kidney is performed to determine a pathologic reason for unexplained renal dysfunction and to direct or change a course of therapy. The client signs an informed consent or operative permit (see Chap. 20).

The physician obtains renal tissue samples percutane-ously (closed biopsy) or surgically (open biopsy). Factors to consider include the number of kidneys, the ability of the client to participate cooperatively, and the necessity for abdominal surgical exploration. If a percutaneous biopsy is selected, the client must have two kidneys, be able to breathe comfortably in a prone position for 30–45 minutes, and be able to suspend breathing on request for several seconds. Percutaneous biopsy of a transplanted kidney entails less client cooperation because the client is in a supine position for the anterior abdominal percutaneous approach. The client is maintained on NPO status for 4 to 6 hours before the procedure in case a major complication necessitates immediately going to the operating room.

An open renal biopsy is performed when the client has only one kidney, cannot participate by suspending breathing, is unable to tolerate a prone position, or when a malignancy is suspected. If abdominal surgery is necessary for other reasons and a renal biopsy is also needed, the nephrologist may request the surgeon to perform the biopsy, thus eliminating a second procedure via the percutaneous route. If an open biopsy is performed, client preparation is as for general surgery and anesthesia (see Chap. 20).

Because of the risk for post-procedure bleeding, the physician orders coagulation studies such as platelet count, activated partial thromboplastin time (aPTT), prothrombin time (PT), and bleeding time. The physician may order a blood transfusion to correct a low hemoglobin level before biopsy. Hypertension and uremia increase the risk for bleeding so the physician may order antihypertensive medications or dialysis before a biopsy.

Procedure

Immediately prior to percutaneous biopsy, the nurse asks the client to void to decrease the possibly of puncturing the bladder. The left kidney is biopsied because it is closer to the skin and is not adjacent to the liver. The exact position of the kidney is determined via fluoroscopic or ultrasonographic examination or by radionuclide scan. For some clients, the nephrologist may locate the kidney by landmarks from previous images. For other clients, the closed biopsy is performed directly during fluoroscopy or ultrasonographic examination. The biopsy technique varies with the nephrologist's training and preference.

During the closed biopsy, the client is placed in a prone position. A roll of padding is placed under the client's abdomen to angle the kidney closer to the skin. The client's skin is prepared and draped, and a local anesthetic is injected. The depth of the kidney is identified by the insertion of a thin-gauge spinal needle. Movement of the spinal needle with breathing helps to determine that the capsule of the kidney has been located. A specially designed trocar is inserted in the path established by the spinal needle. While the client suspends breathing, a specimen of tissue is obtained by insertion of the biopsy needle through the trocar and capsule into the renal cortex. Newer automated spring-loaded and smaller biopsy needles have improved the tissue samples obtained. Ideally, three tissue specimens are obtained.

Follow-Up Care

After a closed percutaneous biopsy, the major risk is bleeding from the biopsy site. For 24 hours after the biopsy, the nurse monitors the dressing site, vital signs, urinary output, hemoglobin level, and hematocrit (as for postarteriography protocols). Even if the dressing is dry and there is no hematoma, the client could be bleeding from the site. A retroperitoneal bleed is not readily visible but is suspected with flank pain, a decreasing blood pressure, decreasing urinary output, or other signs of hypovolemia or shock.

The client follows a plan of strict bed rest, lying in a supine position with a back roll for additional support for at least 6 hours after the biopsy. The head of the bed may be elevated, and the client may resume oral intake of food and fluids. After 6 hours, if there is no evidence of bleeding, the client may be permitted to have limited bathroom privileges.

The nurse monitors for hematuria, the most common complication. Hematuria occurs microscopically in almost all clients, while 5%–9% have gross hematuria. Usually this problem resolves spontaneously in 48–72 hours after biopsy but could persist for 2–3 weeks. In rare cases, transfusions and surgery are required (Brenner, 1996). There should be no obvious blood clots in the urine.

After the percutaneous renal biopsy, the client may experience some local discomfort. If aching originates at the biopsy site and begins to radiate to the flank and around the front of the abdomen, the nurse suspects an onset of bleeding or perinephric hematoma. This typical pattern of discomfort with bleeding occurs because blood in the perirenal tissues and musculature increases the pressure on local nerve tracts. If bleeding occurs, the administration of IV fluid, packed RBCs, or both may be necessary to restore blood pressure. Generally, a small amount of bleeding creates sufficient pressure to compress bleeding sites; this is termed *tamponade effect.* If tamponade does not occur and bleeding becomes extensive, surgical intervention for hemostasis or even nephrectomy may be necessary. A perinephric hematoma may become infected, requiring treatment with antibiotics and surgical drainage.

If no bleeding occurs, the client can resume general activities after 24 hours. The nurse instructs the client to avoid lifting heavy objects, exercising, or performing other strenuous activities for 1–2 weeks after the biopsy procedure. The physician may also restrict the client's driving.

For the follow-up care of a client undergoing an open renal biopsy, refer to Chapter 22 for general postoperative care.

Renography (Kidney Scan)

Client Preparation

The nurse explains to the client that a kidney scan is performed to provide general information about renal blood flow. The nurse explains the injection of the radionuclide and reassures the client that there is generally no danger from the small amount of radioactive material present in the agent.

Procedure

For a kidney scan, the radionuclide is injected intravenously. After injection of the agent, its uptake in the renal parenchyma is measured by a scintillator. A specially designed camera records the emissions, or scintillations, provided by the radionuclide to produce an image. Simultaneously, the rate and location of the emissions are recorded by computer, and information about renal blood flow, or glomerular filtration, is provided.

A kidney scan demonstrates only the relative amount of radionuclide uptake (renal blood flow) into each kidney, thus providing primarily structural information. On the other hand, the renogram provides some functional information by noting the amount of radionuclide excreted. The renogram thus measures glomerular filtration and tubular secretion, in addition to perfusion.

Follow-Up Care

If the client is able, urination into a commode is acceptable without risk from the small amount of radioactive material to be excreted. If the client is incontinent, the nurse changes the bed linens promptly and wears gloves to maintain body secretion precautions and prevent unnecessary skin contact.

Ultrasonography

Client Preparation

The nurse informs the client that ultrasonography does not cause discomfort and is without risk. The nurse explains that, by applying sound waves to structures of different densities, images of the kidneys, ureters, and bladder and surrounding tissues may be produced. The physician uses sonograms (echograms) to assess kidney size, cortical thickness, and status of the calices. Ultrasonography can identify obstruction in the urinary tract, tumors, cysts, and other masses. It does not necessitate the administration of potentially harmful nephrotoxic agents.

Procedure

The client undergoing renal ultrasound is usually placed on a table in a prone position. A gel such as mineral oil is applied to the skin over the back and flank areas to promote the conduction of sound waves. A transducer, in contact with and moving across the skin, delivers sound waves and measures the echoes. Images of the internal structures are produced.

Follow-Up Care

Skin care to remove the gel is all that is necessary after ultrasonography.

Other Urinary Tract Diagnostic Tests

Cystoscopy and Cystourethroscopy

Client Preparation

The nurse provides a complete description of and reasons for the procedure. The nurse completes a preoperative checklist and ensures that consent has properly been obtained (see Chap. 20). Cystoscopy may be performed for diagnosis or treatment. Diagnostic indications include examination for bladder trauma (cystoscopy) or urethral trauma (cystourethroscopy) and identification of the causes of urinary tract obstruction from stones or tumors. Cystoscopy may be indicated to remove bladder tumors or an enlarged prostate gland.

Cystoscopy may be performed under general or local anesthesia with sedation. The client's age and general health and the expected duration of the procedure are some of the considerations in the decision about anesthesia (also see Chaps. 20 and 21). The physician orders a light evening meal for the client and then places the client on NPO status after midnight on the night preceding the cystoscopy. The nurse institutes bowel preparation as ordered with laxatives or enemas the evening before the procedure.

Procedure

The cystoscopic examination is performed in a specially designed cystoscopic examination room. If it is performed in a surgical suite under general anesthesia, traditional surgical support personnel are present, including an anesthesiologist or nurse anesthetist, circulating and scrub nurses, and a surgical assistant. Increasingly, the procedure is performed in outpatient settings, such as a clinic, an ambulatory surgery or short-procedure unit, or a urologist's office.

The nurse assists the client onto a table and, after the client is sedated, into the lithotomy position. After the administration of anesthesia, skin cleaning, and draping, a cystoscope is inserted via the urethra into the urinary bladder. If visualization of the urethra is also indicated, a urethroscope is used. Commonly, examinations include the use of both the cystoscope and the urethroscope.

Follow-Up Care

After cystoscopic examination with general anesthesia, the client is returned to a postanesthesia care unit (PACU) or area. If local anesthesia and sedation were administered, the client may be returned directly to the hospital room. Clients having cystoscopic examinations as outpatients are transferred to an area for monitoring before discharge home. The nurse monitors the client for airway patency and breathing, alterations in vital signs (including temperature), and changes in urinary output. The nurse also observes for the major complications of bleeding and infection.

After cystoscopy, a catheter may or may not be present. The client without a catheter has urinary frequency due to irritation from the catheter. The urine may be pink tinged, but gross bleeding is not expected. Bleeding, or the presence of clots, may result in catheter obstruction and decreased urinary output. The nurse monitors the client's urinary output and notifies the physician of obvious blood clots or a decreased or ceased urinary output. The nurse irrigates the Foley catheter with sterile saline, as ordered, when permitted by the agency's policy. The

nurse also notifies the physician if the client has fever, with or without chills, and an elevated WBC count, which suggests infection. The nurse encourages the client to take oral fluids and increases IV fluid administration as ordered to promote adequate urinary output (which helps prevent clotting) and to reduce a burning sensation on urination.

Retrograde Procedures
Client Preparation

The client is prepared for retrograde procedures (retrograde pyelography, retrograde cystography, and retrograde urethrography) in a manner similar to that for the cystoscopic examination. Retrograde means going against the normal flow of urine. The nurse explains that the retrograde examination of the ureters and pelves (pyelogram), the bladder (cystogram), and the urethra (urethrogram) involves the direct injection of radiopaque contrast medium into the lower urinary tract. Because the contrast medium is instilled directly to obtain an outline of the structures desired, the contrast medium does not enter the bloodstream. Consequently, the client is not at risk for contrast medium–induced acute renal failure or an allergic response.

Procedure

Retrograde films are obtained during the cystoscopic examination. After the placement of the cystoscope by the urologist, catheters are placed into each ureter, and contrast medium is instilled into each ureter and renal pelvis. The catheters are removed by the urologist, and films by the radiology technician are taken to outline these structures as the contrast medium is excreted. The procedure identifies any obstruction or structural abnormality.

For clients undergoing retrograde cystoscopy or urethrography, contrast medium is instilled similarly into the bladder or the urethra. Cystography and urethrography also identify structural abnormalities, such as fistulas, diverticula, and tumors.

Follow-Up Care

After retrograde procedures, the nurse monitors the client for the development of infection as a result of instrumentation of the urinary tract. Because these procedures are performed during cystoscopic examination, the follow-up care is the same as that for cystoscopy.

Urodynamic Studies

Urodynamic studies are procedures to describe the processes of voiding and include

- Tests of bladder capacity, pressure, and tone
- Studies of urethral pressure and urinary flow
- Examination of the function of voluntary muscles of the perineum

These tests are often used along with excretory urographic or cystoscopic procedures to evaluate problems with urinary flow.

Cystometrography

Client Preparation

The nurse explains that the purpose of a cystometrogram (CMG) is to determine the effectiveness and sensitivity of the bladder wall (detrusor) muscle. With these measurements of detrusor muscle quality, determinations about bladder capacity, bladder pressure, and voiding reflexes may be made. The nurse informs the client that a urinary catheter may be necessary temporarily during the procedure.

Procedure

Initially, the nurse requests the client to void normally; the nurse records measurements of the amount, rate of flow, and time of voiding. The nurse then inserts a urinary catheter to measure the residual bladder urine volume. The cystometer is attached to the catheter, and fluid is instilled via the catheter into the bladder. The point at which the client notes a feeling of the urge to void is recorded, as well as the point at which the client notes a strong urge to void. Readings of bladder capacity and bladder pressure are recorded graphically. The client is requested to void when the bladder instillation is complete (about 500 mL). The urinary residual after voiding is noted, and the catheter is removed. Electromyography of the perineal muscles may also be performed during the cystometric examination.

Follow-Up Care

As with any any instrumentation of the urinary tract, the nurse monitors for infection. The nurse measures and records the client's temperature, notes the characteristics and amount of urinary output, and observes for an increased WBC count, which suggests infection.

Urethral Pressure Profile

Client Preparation

The nurse explains that a urethral pressure profile (also called urethral pressure profilometry [UPP]) is potentially informative about the nature of urinary incontinence or urinary retention. A urinary catheter may be temporarily placed during the procedure.

Procedure

A special catheter with pressure-sensing capabilities is inserted into the bladder. As the catheter is slowly withdrawn, variations in the pressure of the smooth muscle of the urethra are recorded.

Follow-Up Care

As with other studies involving instrumentation of the urinary tract, the client is monitored for the development of infection.

Electromyography

Client Preparation

The nurse explains that electromyography (EMG) of the perineal muscles may be useful in evaluating the quality of the function of voluntary muscles involved in voiding. The information may assist in identifying methods of improving continence. The nurse informs the client that some temporary discomfort may accompany the placement of the electrodes.

Procedure

In EMG of the perineal muscles, electrodes are placed in either the rectum or the urethra to measure muscle contraction and relaxation (see Chap. 52).

Follow-Up Care

After completion of EMG, the nurse administers analgesics to promote the client's comfort. Any discomfort is usually mild and of short duration.

Urine Stream Test

Client Preparation

The nurse explains that a urine stream test evaluates pelvic muscle strength and the effectiveness of pelvic musculature in interrupting the flow of urine. It is useful in evaluating urinary incontinence.

Procedure

Three to five seconds after micturition is initiated, the examiner gives the client a signal to stop urine flow. The length of time required to interrupt the flow of urine is recorded.

Follow-Up Care

Cleansing of the perineal area, as after any voiding, is all that is necessary after the urine stream test.

SELECTED BIBLIOGRAPHY

Brenner, B. M. (Ed.). (1996). *Brenner & Rector's the kidney* (5th ed.). Philadelphia: W. B. Saunders.
*Carnevali, D. L., & Patrick, M. (Eds.). (1993). *Nursing management for the elderly* (3rd ed.). Philadelphia: J. B. Lippincott.
*Chmielewski, C. (1992). Renal anatomy and overview of nephron function. *American Nephrology Nurses' Association Journal, 19*(1), 34–38.
Cohan, R. H., & Ellis, J. H. (1997). Iodinated contrast material in uroradiology: Choice of agent and management of complications. *Urologic Clinics of North America, 24*(3), 471–491.
*Cooper, C. (1993). What color is that urine specimen? *American Journal of Nursing, 93*(8), 37.
Driver, D. S. (1996). Renal assessment: Back to basics. *American Nephrology Nurses' Association Journal, 23*(4), 361–368.
Guyton, A. C., & Hall, J. E. (1996). *Textbook of medical physiology* (9th ed.). Philadelphia: W. B. Saunders.
*Holechek, M. J. (1992). Glomerular filtration and renal hemodynamics. *American Nephrology Nurses' Association Journal, 19*(3), 237–245.
Jarvis, C. (1996). *Physical examination and health assessment* (2nd ed.) Philadelphia: W. B. Saunders.
*Kee, C. C. (1992). Age-related changes in the renal system: Causes, consequences, and nursing implications. *Geriatric Nursing, 13*(2), 80–83.

UNIT 15 ■ Problems of Excretion: Management of Clients with Problems of the Renal/Urinary System

Lancaster, L. E. (Ed.). (1995). *Core curriculum for nephrology nursing* (3rd ed.). Pitman, NJ: A. J. Janetti.

*Ludlow, M. (1993). Renal handling of potassium. *American Nephrology Nurses' Association Journal, 20*(1), 52–56.

*Porcush, J. G., & Faubert, P. F. (1991). *Renal disease in the aged.* Boston: Little, Brown.

*Preisig, P. (1992). Urinary concentration and dilution. *American Nephrology Nurses' Association Journal, 19*(4), 351–354.

*Preisig, P. (1994). Renal acidification. *American Nephrology Nurses' Association Journal, 21*(4), 251–257.

*Radke, K. J. (1994). The aging kidney: Structure, function, and nursing practice implications. *American Nephrology Nurses' Association Journal, 21*(4), 181–193.

*Rostand, S. G. (1992). U.S. minority groups and end-stage renal disease: A disproportionate share. *American Journal of Kidney Diseases, 19*(5), 411–413.

*Shulman, N. B., & Hall, W. D. (1991). Renal vascular disease in African-Americans and other racial minorities. *Circulation, 83*(4), 1477–1479.

Tietz, N. W. (Ed.). (1995). *Clinical guide to laboratory tests.* Philadelphia: W. B. Saunders.

U. S. Renal Data Systems. (1995). *USRDS 1995 Annual Data Report.* Bethesda, MD: National Institutes of Health, National Institute of Diabetes and Digestive and Kidney Diseases.

Valtin, H., & Schafer, J. A. (1995). *Renal function* (3rd ed.). Boston: Little, Brown.

Vander, A. J. (1995). *Renal physiology* (5th ed.). New York: McGraw-Hill.

*Yucha, C. (1993). Renal control of calcium, phosphorus and magnesium. *American Nephrology Nurses' Association Journal, 20*(4), 440–450.

Yucha, C., & Keen, M. (1996). Renal regulation of extracellular fluid volume and osmolality. *American Nephrology Nurses' Association Journal, 23*(5), 487–497.

SUGGESTED READINGS

Cohan, R. H., & Ellis, J. H. (1997). Iodinated contrast material in uroradiology: Choice of agent and management of complications. *Urologic Clinics of North America, 24*(3), 471–491.

This article begins with a discussion of ionic (such as Renografin) and nonionic (such as Omnipaque) contrast agents. Contrast reactions are described in detail, differentiating between idiosyncratic (anaphylactoid) and nonidiosyncratic (dose-dependent) reactions. Specific protocols for the administration of corticosteroids, antihistamines, and H_2 blockers as pretreatment to reduce adverse reactions to ionic agents are included.

Yucha, C., & Keen, M. (1996). Renal regulation of extracellular fluid volume and osmolality. *American Nephrology Nurses' Association Journal, 23*(5), 487–497.

This comprehensive article discusses the renal mechanisms of sodium filtration, sodium reabsorption, and water excretion in detail. The role of baroreceptors, renin, arterial oncotic pressure, aldosterone, atrial natriuretic hormone, and antidiuretic hormone are reviewed. The cellular handling of sodium, chloride, water, potassium, and bicarbonate for each segment of the nephron is included.

Chapter 73

INTERVENTIONS FOR CLIENTS WITH URINARY PROBLEMS

Once urine leaves the kidney, structural or functional disorders of the urinary tract can affect the storage or elimination of urine. Infections, the most common problem, are easily treated in the ambulatory care setting and rarely cause serious complications. Cancer and trauma are less common problems but can be life threatening. Incontinence of urine often creates feelings of shame and embarrassment for clients and their families, resulting in serious social and psychological consequences. Nursing interventions are directed toward prevention, detection, and management of urologic disorders.

INFECTIOUS DISORDERS

Infections in the urinary tract are described by the primary structure or site of the infectious process. Acute infections in the lower urinary tract include urethritis (urethra), cystitis (bladder), and prostatitis (prostate gland). Acute pyelonephritis is an upper urinary tract (kidney) infection.

Symptoms of urinary tract infection (UTI) account for more than 5 million health care visits annually in the United States and more than 100,000 hospitalizations. UTIs are the leading cause of nosocomial infection in hospitals. Infections of the pelvis, vulva, vagina, and prostate may produce symptoms similar to a UTI. The clinician identifies both the site (locus) of infection and the specific bacterial species. The site of infection is the most critical determinant of treatment. Acute pyelonephritis (covered in Chapter 74) is more often treated in the hospital; other infections are treated in the ambulatory setting unless complications occur.

Cystitis

Overview

Infectious cystitis is an inflammation of the urinary bladder caused by bacteria, viruses, fungi, or parasites. Noninfectious cystitis is caused by chemicals or radiation. Interstitial cystitis is an inflammatory process of unknown etiology. A number of factors, such as structural or functional abnormalities of the urinary tract and characteristics of the urine, are thought to predispose clients to UTIs (Table 73–1).

Pathophysiology

Infectious agents, most commonly bacteria, typically ascend the urinary tract from the external urethra to the bladder, although hematogenous and lymphogenous spread can occur. Once bacteria enter the system, several factors (Table 73–2) influence the outcome.

There is considerable debate about the potential for renal parenchymal damage and subsequent kidney failure as a result of bacteria ascending from the bladder to the kidney. Most experts believe that severe deterioration of

TABLE 73–1

Factors Contributing to Urinary Tract Infections

Factor	Mechanism	Interventions
Obstruction	• Incomplete bladder emptying creates a continuous pool of urine where bacteria can grow, prevents flushing out of bacteria, and allows bacteria to ascend more easily to higher structures.	• Relieve or bypass the obstruction to promote complete bladder emptying.
	• Bacteria have a greater chance of multiplying the longer they remain in residual urine.	• Increase liquids to dilute urine and encourage more frequent voiding.
	• Overdistention of the bladder damages the mucosa and allows bacteria to invade the bladder wall.	• Use intermittent catheterization to keep the bladder from becoming distended.
Calculi	• Large calculi can cause obstruction to urine flow.	• Remove calculi and/or treat the underlying condition that causes the calculi to form.
	• The rough surface of a calculus irritates mucosal surfaces and creates a spot where bacteria can establish and grow.	
	• Bacteria can live within calculi and cause reinfection.	
Vesicoureteral reflux	• Bacteria-laden urine is forced backward from the bladder up into the ureters and kidneys, where pyelonephritis can develop.	• The affected ureters may be able to be surgically reimplanted in the bladder to eliminate the reflux.
	• Reflux of sterile urine can cause renal scarring, which may promote renal dysfunction.	
Diabetes mellitus	• Excess glucose in urine provides a rich medium for bacterial growth.	• Maintain good glucose control in clients with diabetes.
	• Peripheral neuropathy affects bladder innervation and leads to a flaccid bladder and incomplete bladder emptying.	
Characteristics of urine	• Acidic urine and high osmolality in acidic urine inhibit bacterial growth.	• Acidify urine by taking vitamin C tablets, not citrus fruits. Such fruits make the urine alkaline.
	• Dilute urine inhibits bacterial growth.	• Increase urine volume by increasing fluid intake.
Gender	• Female clients are susceptible to periurethral and vaginal colonization with coliform bacteria.	• Explain the importance of perineal hygiene (wiping front to back) to prevent large amounts of coliform bacteria from remaining in the perineal area.
	• Pregnancy predisposes women to cystitis and the development of pyelonephritis.	• Frequent and routine monitoring of pregnant women for UTIs prevents complications.
	• A diaphragm or pessary that is too large can cause an obstruction to urine flow or trauma to the urethra.	• Be sure diaphragms and pessaries are properly fitted.
	• Prostatic secretions inhibit bacterial growth in young men.	
Age	• Obstruction may be caused by incomplete bladder emptying as a result of an enlarged prostate in men and cystocele and prolapse in women.	• Do not rush elderly clients during toileting; provide regular and private toileting times to promote complete bladder emptying.
	• Neuromuscular conditions that cause incomplete bladder emptying, such as Parkinson's disease and strokes, affect the elderly more frequently.	• Straight cath for residual and Credé to promote more complete emptying upon order.
	• The frequent use of anticholinergic medications in the elderly contributes to delayed bladder emptying.	• Monitor and report this medication side effect.
	• Fecal incontinence contributes to poor perineal hygiene when clients remain in wet and soiled clothes for long periods.	• Promptly clean clients after episodes of incontinence.
	• Hypoestrogenism in elderly women adversely affects the cells of the vagina and urethra, making them more susceptible to infections.	• Give vaginal estrogen cream as directed to improve the health of the client's vaginal and urethral cells.

TABLE 73-2

Important Factors Influencing the Outcome of UTIs

Factor	Facilitating Aspects	Protective Aspects
Anatomy	Females: Short length of the urethra and its proximity to the vagina and rectum facilitate colonization of coliform bacteria. Males: With age, the prostate enlarges and may obstruct the normal flow of urine, producing stasis.	Males: Long length of the urethra and its distance from rectum provide protection from colonization with coliform bacteria.
Physiology	Females: Pregnancy predisposes a woman to ureteral reflux and subsequent pyelonephritis; with age the decline in estrogen facilitates colonization of E. coli. Males: With age, prostatic secretions lose their antibacterial characteristics and predispose to bacterial proliferation in the urine.	Females: Well-estrogenized mucosa in the urethra and trigone may inhibit bacterial colonization. Males: Normal prostatic secretions inhibit bacterial growth. Both males and females: Mucin is produced by urothelial cells lining the bladder—this helps to maintain mucosal integrity and prevent cellular damage; mucin may also prevent bacteria from adhering to urothelial cells.
Trauma	Females: Vaginal penetration with sexual intercourse may traumatize the urethra and bladder base, leading to postcoital (or honeymoon) cystitis; a vaginal diaphragm that is too large can place pressure on the urethra, causing trauma; vaginal childbirth can cause permanent damage to the urethra. Males: Sexually transmitted diseases may cause urethral strictures that obstruct the flow of urine and predispose to urinary stasis. Both males and females: Urethral instrumentation (such as catheterization) may disturb the urothelial surface and predispose to adherence of bacteria that would ordinarily not be pathogenic.	Females: Adequate lubrication, either natural or artificial, with intercourse may prevent any trauma.
Infectious agent	Virulent organisms are better able to adhere to host cells and secrete substances that induce inflammation.	A small inoculum (number of microorganisms introduced into the body) is more easily flushed away by the forces of urine flowing through the system.

renal function is a rare complication without one or more predisposing factors, such as anatomic abnormalities, pregnancy, obstruction, reflux, calculi, or diabetes mellitus. Other complications from spread of the infectious agent include bacteremia, sepsis (often termed urosepsis), and septic shock.

Asymptomatic bacteriuria is more common in the elderly and is generally considered a benign condition. No studies have demonstrated a relationship between asymptomatic bacteriuria and progression to acute infection or renal insufficiency in clients without obstructive conditions, reflux, calculi, or diabetes mellitus (Gray & Malone-Lee, 1995).

Etiology

Infectious causes of cystitis include bacteria, viruses, fungi, and parasites. Coliform bacteria, normally found in the gastrointestinal tract, account for most cases (90%) of bacterial cystitis (Mahon & Manuselis, 1995). Infection ascends from the urethral entry point. *Escherichia coli*, the

most common of these gram-negative organisms, accounts for 70% to 80% of cases. Although it is the most common infecting organism, *E. coli* has many serotypes. Symptoms therefore vary from mild to life threatening, and the virulence of any one type depends on many factors. Other infecting organisms include *Enterococcus, Klebsiella, Proteus, Serratia, Pseudomonas,* and *Staphylococcus.*

Bacteria may be introduced during genitourinary surgery or instrumentation of the urinary tract. Long-term urethral catheterization is an important source of gram-negative bacteremia in hospitals (Gray & Malone-Lee, 1995). Catheters are the most common predisposing factor for gram-negative sepsis in the elderly (Duffield, 1997). Catheterization should be limited as much as possible to reduce this risk. Indications for catheter use are listed in Table 73-3.

Fungal infections, such as those caused by *Candida,* develop during long-term antibiotic therapy; antibiotics alter normal flora. Clients who are severely immunocompromised and have decreased resistance to infection, are

TABLE 73–3

Reasons for the Use of Indwelling Urinary Catheters

Short-Term Use (2–3 days)
- Indwelling urinary catheters allow accurate measurement of urinary output during acute illness or postoperatively.
- Catheters are placed during or before surgery to keep the bladder empty or to prevent postoperative retention.

Long-Term Use (>3 days)
- Indwelling urinary catheters are used in cases of chronic urinary retention and urinary incontinence in selected situations.

receiving glucocorticosteroids or other immunosuppressive agents, or have diabetes mellitus or AIDS are also at risk for fungal UTIs or fungemia.

Viral and parasitic infections are rare and are generally presumed to accompany an infection in another site. For example, *Trichomonas,* a parasite found in the vagina, can also be found in the urine. Treatment of the vaginal infection (see Chap. 78) is sufficient to treat the organisms in the urine.

Noninfectious cystitis may result from chemical exposure, such as to drugs (e.g., cyclophosphamide [Cytoxan, Procytox✦]), radiation therapy, and immunologic responses, as with systemic lupus erythematosus (SLE). Interstitial cystitis (IC) is a relatively rare, chronic inflammation of the bladder. The condition affects women predominantly (in a 12:1 ratio), and the diagnosis is difficult to make. The symptoms are identical to those of simple cystitis, but the urgency and bladder pain are more intense (Thompson & Christmas, 1996).

Incidence/Prevalence

The incidence of UTI is second only to that of upper respiratory infections in primary care. Clients who have the triad of frequency, dysuria, and urgency account for more than 5 million health care visits annually. Approximately 50% of those clients will have a confirmed UTI. Recurrent infections account for an unknown number of those visits, particularly by women.

The prevalence of UTIs varies with age and gender, correlating with the pathophysiologic processes of obstruction, reflux, and changes in host defense mechanisms. Generally, women are more commonly affected with UTIs than men. In men 65 to 70 years old, the incidence of UTI is 3%; after age 70, however, the incidence is 20%. In elderly women over the age of 80, the prevalence rises from 20% to 50% (Gray & Malone-Lee, 1995; Duffield, 1997).

Collaborative Management

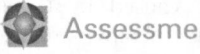 Assessment

Frequency, urgency, and dysuria are the primary clinical manifestations of a UTI, but other signs and symptoms

may be present (Chart 73–1). Elderly clients are at greater risk for an overwhelming and generalized infection called *urosepsis,* caused by a gram-negative bacteremia. Urosepsis is a serious condition that can develop rapidly; it has a mortality rate of 15%.

Before performing the physical assessment, the nurse asks the client to void so that the urine can be examined and the bladder emptied before palpation. The nurse assesses the client's vital signs to help rule out sepsis, inspects the lower abdomen, and palpates the urinary bladder. Distention after voiding indicates incomplete bladder emptying. Costovertebral angle (see Fig. 72–9) tenderness may indicate pyelonephritis.

Using Standard Precautions (see Chap. 28), the nurse notes inflammation and any skin lesions around the urethral meatus and vaginal introitus (opening). Female clients frequently report "burning with urination" when normal, acidic urine touches labial tissues inflamed and ulcerated by vaginal infections or sexually transmitted diseases. The nurse maintains the client's privacy with drapes during the examination.

The prostate is palpated by rectal examination for size, alteration in contour, and any evidence of tenderness. The physician or advanced nurse clinician performs the rectal prostate assessment.

Chart 73–1

Key Features of Urinary Tract Infection

Common Clinical Manifestations
- Frequency
- Urgency
- Dysuria
- Hesitancy or difficulty in initiating urine stream
- Low back pain
- Nocturia
- Incontinence
- Retention
- Suprapubic tenderness or fullness
- Feeling of incomplete bladder emptying

Rare Clinical Manifestations
- Fever
- Chills
- Nausea
- Vomiting
- Malaise
- Flank pain

Unusual Clinical Manifestations That May Occur in the Elderly
- The only symptom may be something as vague as increasing mental confusion or frequent, unexplained falls
- A sudden onset of incontinence or a worsening of incontinence may be the only symptom of an early UTI
- Fever, tachycardia, tachypnea, and hypotension, even without any urinary symptoms, may be signs of urosepsis
- Loss of appetite, nocturia, and dysuria are common symptoms

⊳ Research Applications for Nursing

Specific Techniques for Obtaining Urine Specimens for Culture Will Reduce Costs and Expediate Treatment

Brazier, A., & Palmer, M. (1995). Collecting clean-catch urine in the nursing home: Obtaining the uncontaminated specimen. Geriatric Nursing, 16(5), 217–224.

The purpose of this study was to describe the best technique for obtaining clean-catch urine specimens from impaired clients. The sample consisted of 28 specimens from 17 incontinent and 11 continent nursing home residents (21 female specimens), all of whom were at least 60 years old and had been admitted to the facility in the past 12 months. The specimens were collected early in the morning, if possible, and each client was assisted into an upright position, preferably in the bathroom. The clients received perineal cleansing with liquid soap followed by cleansing of the area around the urinary meatus with antiseptic solution. For women clients, one of the most important techniques was in holding the labia apart until the specimen was obtained. The average time it took to obtain the specimen was 10.2 minutes (range, 2–50 minutes).

Critique. The study provides initial data that can be used to help nurses collect urine specimens. The small sample size and lack of controls limit broad research-based application of these techniques without further study. Much of the article was written as a general nursing informational article rather than as a research article.

Possible Nursing Implications. The authors have described some innovative techniques for collecting clean-catch urine specimens. For example, they describe how sitting on the toilet *facing* the tank or straddling the *wide* part of the bedpan will better separate labia. For the most difficult-to-obtain specimens, they describe the application of an external female urinary pouch manufactured by Hollister, Inc., which adheres to the perineum *with the labia separated* until urine is obtained. They also suggested using a wide-mouthed sterile utility bowl initially for easier collectability and then transferring the specimen into the usual laboratory container.

⊳ Laboratory Assessment

A urinalysis is performed on a clean-catch midstream specimen (see Research Applications for Nursing). When infection occurs, several abnormalities, including bacteria, white blood cells (WBC), and red blood cells (RBC), may be present. If the infection is bacterial, urine culture confirms the type of microorganism and the number of colonies. Sensitivity testing is not done routinely because most infecting organisms are sensitive to many antiseptics and antibiotics. However, when a complicating factor (such as calculi or recurrent infection) is present or when the client is elderly, sensitivity testing is mandatory. If the client cannot produce a clean-catch specimen, the nurse may need to obtain the specimen with a small-caliber (6 French) urethral catheter; in rare cases, the physician or

an advanced nurse clinician may perform a suprapubic aspiration. For a routine urinalysis, 10 mL of urine is required; smaller quantities are sufficient for culture.

A urine specimen properly obtained (without contamination) should not contain colony-forming units (CFU) of bacteria. Significant bacteriuria is usually defined as more than 100,000 CFU/mL. Urine cultures that show more than 10,000 CFU/mL but less than 100,000 CFU/mL, however, may be considered significant because bacteria are in the process of multiplying. When another urine specimen for culture is obtained in 6 hours, bacterial multiplication is confirmed. Factors that contribute to the variable multiplication rate of the bacteria include growth rates of the bacterial species, pH and concentration of the urine, time lapsed since last voiding, and incomplete emptying of the bladder. Multiple organisms in low colony counts generally indicate a contaminated specimen.

It takes 24 to 48 hours for a culture to grow, whereas microscopic analysis of a centrifuged sample of urine provides a quick determination of the likelihood of infection. The presence of bacilli in the centrifuged urine correlates well with culture results. Clients who have symptoms of acute cystitis are frequently treated with antibiotics before final confirmation of urine culture results. This practice has led some to question the value of pretreatment urine cultures or to recommend them only for the first infection or under other unusual circumstances.

Occasionally, the serum WBC count may be elevated, with the differential WBC count showing "a shift to the left." This shift indicates that the number of immature WBCs is increasing in response to the infectious organisms. Consequently, the number of bands, or immature WBCs, is elevated. Left shift most commonly occurs with urosepsis and rarely occurs with uncomplicated cystitis.

⊳ Other Diagnostic Assessment

The clinician usually bases the diagnosis of cystitis on the history, physical examination, and laboratory data. If urinary retention and obstruction to urinary outflow are suspected, excretory urography, abdominal sonography, or computed tomography (CT) helps determine the site of obstruction or the presence of calculi. Voiding cystourethrography (see Chap. 72) is used for the diagnosis of suspected cases of vesicoureteral reflux.

Cystoscopy (see Chap. 72) is often performed when there is a history of recurrent (more than three or four a year) UTIs. The urine is sterilized with antibiotic therapy before the procedure so that the risk of sepsis is not increased. Cystoscopy can identify abnormalities that may have contributed to the development of cystitis. These abnormalities include bladder calculi, bladder diverticula, urethral strictures, foreign bodies (such as sutures from previous surgery), and trabeculation (an abnormal thickening of the bladder wall caused by urinary retention and obstruction).

Retrograde pyelography accompanies the cystoscopic examination, producing outlines and images of the drainage tract. Areas of obstruction or malformation and the presence of reflux are thus identifiable.

Cystoscopy is the only means of accurately diagnosing interstitial cystitis. Classic findings in interstitial cystitis include a small-capacity bladder, the presence of Hunner's ulcers (a type of bladder lesion), and petechial hemorrhages after bladder distention.

Interventions

The client with cystitis usually has the common nursing diagnosis of Pain related to the inability to void, dysuria, or bladder spasm secondary to physical (distention) and biologic (inflammation, infection, spasm) agents. Interventions for the management of the discomfort accompanying cystitis include medication and fluid administration. Increased fluid intake has two purposes:

- The increased dilution of the growth medium (urine) inhibits bacterial growth.
- The increased volume causes more frequent flushing of the bacteria out of the bladder and urethra.

Drug Therapy

Medications prescribed to promote comfort in the client with cystitis include analgesics, urinary antiseptics or antibiotics, and antispasmodics. The antispasmodic agents (anticholinergics) decrease bladder spasm and promote complete bladder emptying. The clinician prescribes antibiotics (Chart 73–2) to treat any infection. Antifungal agents are administered when the infecting organism is a fungus; amphotericin B is most often given in daily bladder instillations, and ketoconazole (Nizoral) is given in oral or parenteral form.

Research has demonstrated satisfactory antibiotic treatment of simple, acute bacterial cystitis in healthy, ambulatory clients with a 3-day course of therapy. Although these shorter courses increase compliance and reduce cost, controversy continues about their effectiveness in reducing recurrent infections. Treatment failures and recurrences may indicate a more complicated infection and the need for further diagnostic evaluation. Longer treatment regimens (at least 7–10 days) of oral or parenteral antibiotics are required for hospitalized clients; those with complicating factors, such as indwelling catheters or calculi; and those with a history of diabetes or immunosuppression.

Pregnant women require vigorous intervention when bacteriuria is identified because of the tendency of simple cystitis to evolve into acute pyelonephritis. Pyelonephritis in pregnancy is associated with preterm labor and deleterious effects on the fetus. Studies have recommended long-term or postcoital prophylaxis during pregnancy for prevention of recurrent pyelonephritis (Kunin, 1996).

Long-term antibiotic therapy is frequently recommended for the treatment of chronic, recurring infections caused by structural abnormalities or calculi. Trimethoprim 100 mg daily may be prescribed for long-term management of the elderly client with frequent UTIs (Duffield, 1997). For women who experience recurrent UTI associated with sexual intercourse, one low-dose tablet of nitrofurantoin (Macrodantin, Nephronex✦, Novofuran✦) after coitus is often recommended.

Diet Therapy

The diet should represent intake from all food groups and include an adequate number of calories for the increased metabolic processes associated with infection. Unless medically contraindicated, fluid intake needs to be at least 2 to 3 L/day for adequate flushing of urine through the system. Evidence suggests that cranberry juice reduces bacteriuria in some clients (Fleet, 1994).

Other Pain Relief Measures

A warm sitz bath taken two or three times a day for 20 minutes may provide comfort and some relief of local symptoms. If burning with urination is severe or urinary retention occurs, the nurse instructs the client to sit in the sitz bath and urinate into the warm water.

Surgical Management

Surgical interventions for clients with cystitis are limited to treatment of conditions that predispose to recurrent UTIs (e.g., removal of obstructions, treatment of calculi, and repair of vesicoureteral reflux). Procedures may include cystoscopy (see Chap. 72) to identify and remove calculi or obstructions. During cystoscopy examination, manipulation or pulverization of the stone removes the obstruction.

 Continuing Care

The nurse assesses the client's level of understanding from the client's description of the problem. The client's knowledge about factors contributing to the development of cystitis is the basis on which further teaching interventions are planned.

The nurse instructs the client in self-administration of medications, stresses appropriate spacing of doses throughout the day, and emphasizes the need to complete all of the prescribed medication. If the medication will change the color of the urine, as it does with phenazopyridine (Pyridium, Pyronium✦), the nurse informs the client to expect this occurrence. The nurse offers techniques for remembering the medication schedule, such as the use of a daily calendar or the association of medications with usual activities (e.g., mealtimes).

Clients may associate symptoms of discomfort with sexual activities and experience feelings of guilt and embarrassment. Frank and sensitive discussions with a woman who experiences frequent recurrences of UTI after sexual intercourse can help her find appropriate techniques to handle the problem. The nurse explores with her the factors that contribute to her postcoital infections, such as diaphragm use and her general resistance to infection. The nurse also discusses her feelings about the problem. The client should understand that vigorous cleaning of the perineum with harsh soaps and vaginal douching does not eliminate the tendency to infection. More helpful techniques include adequate lubrication during intercourse, voiding after intercourse, and prompt attention to vaginal or urinary symptoms. At the client's request, the

Chart 73–2

Drug Therapy for Urinary Tract Infection

Drug	Usual Dosage	Nursing Interventions	Rationale
Quinolones Norfloxacin (Noroxin)	• 400 mg bid PO × 3, 7 or 10 days	• Avoid caffeinated beverages and use with caution in clients receiving theophylline.	• Quinolones prolong the half-life of caffeine and theophylline.
Ciprofloxacin (Cipro)	• 250 mg bid PO × 3, 7 or 10 days	• Avoid aluminum- or magnesium-containing antacids.	• Aluminum and magnesium interfere with absorption of the drug.
Nitrofurantoin (Macrodantin, Nephronex✦, Novofuran✦)	• 50–100 mg qid PO × 7–10 days • 50 mg hs PO × 6 mo • 50 mg PO after coitus	• Give with food or milk. • Monitor for flu-like symptoms in the elderly and in clients with pulmonary problems.	• Nitrofurantoin can cause GI irritation. Food or milk helps decrease this problem. • Rare cases of interstitial pneumonitis have been seen in susceptible clients receiving nitrofurantoin.
Trimethoprim/sulfamethoxazole (Bactrim, Septra, Apo-Sulfatrim✦, Roubac✦)	• 160/800 mg hs PO × one dose • 160/800 mg bid PO × 3, 7, or 10 days • 80/400 mg PO after coitus • **Note:** DS or DF means double-strength, which is 160/800 mg	• Provide an adequate fluid intake and avoid ascorbic acid and ammonium chloride, which will acidify the urine. • Use with caution in clients with asthma, G6PD deficiency, and multiple allergies.	• Sulfa has a tendency to crystallize, especially in acidic or concentrated urine. • Sulfa allergies are common in these clients.
Amoxicillin/clavulanic acid (Augmentin, Clavulin✦)	• 250 mg q8h PO × 7–10 days	• Give with food. • Do not substitute half of a 500-mg tablet for a 250-mg tablet.	• Augmentin can cause GI irritation. Food helps decrease this problem. • Both 250-mg and 500-mg tablets contain 125 mg clavulanic acid
Cephalosporins: Cefuroxime (Ceftin)	• 250 mg has PO × one dose • 250 mg q12h PO × 3, 7, or 10 days	• Inquire about history of penicillin allergy. • Give with food.	• Cross-sensitivity with penicillin is possible. • Absorption is enhanced in the presence of food.
Phenazopyridine (Pyridium, Phenzo✦, Pyronium✦)	• 100–200 mg PO tid × 2 or 3 days until pain is relieved	• Give with food. • Notify the client that the urine will become red or orange in color. • Inform the client that the drug is a urinary mucosal anesthetic.	• Food helps reduce GI distress. • Urine discoloration is normal. • The client may think the drug is an antibiotic.
Amoxicillin (Amoxil)	• 3 g PO × one dose • 500 mg PO tid × 3, 7, or 10 days	• Inquire about history of penicillin allergy. • Give with food.	• Amoxicillin is a penicillin. • Food helps reduce GI distress.

nurse is prepared to discuss the problem with the client and her partner to help them find ways of maintaining their intimate relationship. Chart 73–3 gives other specific instructions for preventing UTIs.

Educational materials about cystitis may be obtained from medical, health education, or community libraries that have special collections for clients with health-related concerns. In addition, the National Kidney Foundation chapters and affiliates have some basic pamphlets and brochures. The Interstitial Cystitis Foundation provides a newsletter and ongoing mailings of items of interest for affected clients. Nurses in urologic practice can be contacted through the Society of Urologic Nurses and Associates.

Chart 73–3

Health Promotion Guide: Preventing a Urinary Tract Infection

- Drink 2–3 L of fluid every day.
- Drink cranberry juice to acidify your urine.
- Be sure to get enough sleep, rest, and nutrition daily.
- [For women] Clean your perineum (the area between your legs) from front to back.
- [For women] Avoid irritating substances, such as bubble bath, nylon underwear, and scented toilet tissue. Wear loose-fitting cotton underwear.
- If you experience burning when you urinate, if you have to urinate frequently, or if you find it difficult to begin urinating, notify your physician or other health care provider right away, especially if you have a chronic medical condition (such as diabetes).
- Empty your bladder as soon as you feel the urge to urinate.
- Empty your bladder regularly (e.g., every 4 hours), even if you do not feel the urge to urinate.
- You may try home therapies such as
  - Apple cider vinegar, 2 tablespoons three times per day in juice.
  - Echinacea (herb), one dropperful three times per day in juice or herbal tea (Duffield, 1997).
- To prevent recurrent infection:
  - Take your medication as directed even after the symptoms go away.
  - Schedule a follow-up appointment for 10–14 days after you finish taking your medication. At your follow-up visit, another urine sample may be taken for culture.

Urethritis

Overview

Urethritis is an inflammation of the urethra that causes symptoms similar to urinary tract infection (UTI). In male clients, signs and symptoms of urethritis are burning or difficulty with urination and usually a discharge from the urethral meatus. The most common cause of urethritis in men is sexually transmitted diseases (STD): gonorrhea or nonspecific urethritis caused by *Ureaplasma* (a gram-negative bacterium), *Chlamydia* (a prevalent sexually transmitted gram-negative bacterium), or *Trichomonas vaginalis* (a protozoan found in both the male and female genital tract).

In female clients, urethritis mimics cystitis of bacterial origin. Urethritis is known by several synonyms:

- The pyuria-dysuria syndrome
- The frequency-dysuria syndrome
- Trigonitis syndrome
- Urethral syndrome

Urethritis is most common in postmenopausal women and is probably caused by tissue changes related to low estrogen levels.

Collaborative Management

 Assessment

The nurse asks the client about a history of sexually transmitted disease, painful or difficult urination, discharge from the penis or vagina, and internal discomfort in the lower abdomen. Urinalysis may show white blood cells (pyuria) without a significant number of bacteria; however, results of urethral culture may indicate a sexually transmitted disease. In female clients, the diagnosis may be made by exclusion when urinalysis and urethral culture are negative for bacteria and symptoms persist. In such cases, pelvic examination may provide evidence of hypoestrogenism in the vagina; cystourethroscopy may show hypoestrogenism with inflammation of urethral tissues.

 Interventions

Sexually transmitted diseases (STDs) are treated with appropriate antibiotic therapy:

- Penicillin or ceftriaxone (Rocephin) for gonorrhea
- Doxycycline (Vibramycin) for *Ureaplasma* and *Chlamydia* infection
- Metronidazole (Flagyl, Neo-Metric✦) for *Trichomonas* infection

(Chapter 80 has more information on STDs.)

Postmenopausal women with urethral syndrome frequently experience improvement in their urethral symptoms with the use of estrogen vaginal cream. Estrogen cream applied locally to the vagina increases the amount of estrogen in the urethra as well; thus, irritative symptoms are reduced.

Urethral Strictures

Overview

Urethral strictures may result from complications of an STD (usually gonorrhea) and from trauma during catheterization, urologic instrumentation, or childbirth. Strictures occur more often in men than in women and may be an important predisposing factor in other urologic conditions, such as recurrent UTI, urinary incontinence, and urinary retention.

Collaborative Management

 Assessment

The most common symptom of urethral stricture is obstruction to the flow of urine; strictures rarely cause pain. Because stasis of urine can result when flow is obstructed, the client with a stricture is more likely to contract a UTI and, potentially, experience overflow incontinence. Overflow incontinence refers to the involuntary loss of urine associated with overdistention of the bladder. The nurse assesses the client for these two problems.

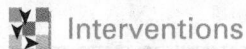 Interventions

A urethral stricture is usually treated surgically. Dilation of the urethra (with use of a local anesthetic) is a temporary measure, not a curative one. The best chance of long-term cure is with *urethroplasty,* a surgical procedure in which the affected area is excised or grafted to create a larger opening for the passage of urine. The recurrence rate is still high with surgical interventions, and most clients need repeated procedures.

Urinary Incontinence

Overview

Continence of urine is a unique accomplishment of humans and certain domestic animals. Continence is a learned behavior whereby a person can suppress the physiologic urge to urinate until a socially appropriate (culturally prescribed) location is available (e.g., a toilet). Efficient bladder emptying, that is, coordination between bladder contraction and urethral relaxation, is also a prerequisite for continence. Continence is learned in early childhood through toilet training and is generally accomplished by age 5 years.

Incontinence is the involuntary loss of urine severe enough to cause social or hygienic problems. Incontinence is not, as some assume, a normal consequence of aging or childbirth. Because of the stigma associated with incontinence and the belief that it is normal in the elderly, incontinence is one of the most underreported health problems. Many people suffer in silence, socially isolated and unaware that treatment is available.

The National Institutes of Health convened a consensus panel in 1988 to address the problem of incontinence. The panel determined that

- The psychosocial burden of incontinence is great.
- The monetary costs associated with the condition are high. (Treatment in the United States has risen to $16 billion annually, and the public spends approximately $1.5 billion per year on incontinence products [Peters, 1997]).
- Incontinence can be cured or significantly improved in most cases.

Subsequently, the Agency for Health Care Policy and Research (AHCPR) chose urinary incontinence as one of its first topics for Clinical Practice Guidelines. The agency's goal is to educate the public and health professionals about assessment and management of this condition (U. S. Department of Health and Human Services [USDHHS], 1992; revised, 1996). These guidelines are available for the consumer from the AHCPR.

Pathophysiology

Continence is maintained when pressure in the urethra is greater than pressure in the bladder. For normal voiding to occur, the urethra must relax, and the bladder must sustain a contraction of sufficient pressure and duration to empty completely. Voiding should occur in a smooth and coordinated way under a person's conscious, volitional (willing) control. The pathophysiologic process of urinary incontinence (Table 73–4) is complex and involves

- Abnormalities of bladder contraction
- Abnormalities of urethral relaxation
- Abnormalities outside the bladder and urethra

Abnormalities of Bladder Contraction

Bladder contractions are perceived as an urge to urinate. When the bladder is full, contraction of the smooth muscle fibers of the *detrusor* muscle (bladder) normally signals the brain that it is time to urinate. Continent persons override that signal and relax the detrusor muscle for the time it takes to locate a toilet. Those who suffer from *urge incontinence* cannot suppress the signal. Abnormal detrusor contractions may result from neurologic abnormalities, or there may be no associated neurologic abnormality.

When the detrusor muscle is unresponsive, the bladder becomes overdistended. *Reflex (overflow) incontinence* occurs when the bladder has reached its absolute maximal capacity and some urine must leak out to prevent bladder rupture. Causes for the underactive or acontractile bladder may or may not be determined.

Abnormalities of Urethral Relaxation

The urethra can be relaxed and tightened under conscious control because it is surrounded by skeletal muscles of the pelvic floor. When a person feels the urge to urinate, the conscious contraction of the urethra can override a bladder contraction if the urethral contraction is strong enough.

Clients who suffer from *stress incontinence* cannot tighten the urethra sufficiently to overcome the increased detrusor pressure. Stress incontinence is common after childbirth, when the pelvic muscles are stretched and weakened from pregnancy and delivery. The weakened pelvic floor contributes to a significant hypermobility and displacement of the urethra during exertion. If the pelvic muscles are not properly strengthened, this condition continues. Decreasing amounts of estrogen postmenopause also contributes to stress incontinence. Vaginal, urethral, and pelvic floor muscles become thin and weaken without estrogen. Stress incontinence is the most common form of incontinence in women.

The urethra can also be obstructed so that it fails to relax sufficiently to allow urine to flow. The most common causes of outflow obstruction are external to the mechanism of the urethra. Incomplete bladder emptying or complete urinary retention due to urethral obstruction results in *overflow incontinence.*

Abnormalities Outside the Bladder and Urethra

Factors other than the abnormal function of the bladder and urethra also result in a significant number of cases of *functional incontinence.* The most common factor is a loss of cognitive function in clients affected by dementia. To

TABLE 73-4

Types of Urinary Incontinence

Type	Definition/Description	Causes	Clinical Manifestations
Abnormalities of Bladder Contraction			
• Urge incontinence	• The involuntary loss of urine associated with a strong desire to urinate • Clients cannot suppress the signal from the bladder muscle to the brain that it is time to urinate		• An abrupt and strong urge to void • May have loss of large amounts of urine with each occurrence
• Detrusor hyperreflexia (reflex incontinence)	• The abnormal detrusor contractions result from neurologic abnormalities	• Stroke, multiple sclerosis, and parasacral spinal cord lesions	• Post-void residual usually >50 mL
• Detrusor instability	• No associated neurologic abnormality		• Post-void residual usually ≤50 mL
• Overflow incontinence	• The involuntary loss of urine associated with overdistention of the bladder when the bladder's capacity has reached its maximum • The detrusor muscle is underactive and does not send signals to the brain that the bladder is full; overdistention results, and some urine must leak out to prevent bladder rupture	• Diabetic neuropathy, side effect of medication, after radical pelvic surgery or spinal cord damage, outlet obstruction	• Bladder distention, often up to the level of the umbilicus • Constant dribbling of urine
Abnormalities of Urethral Relaxation			
• Stress incontinence	• The involuntary loss of urine during activities that increase abdominal and detrusor pressure • Clients cannot tighten the urethra sufficiently to overcome the increased detrusor pressure; leakage of urine results	• After childbirth • Intrinsic sphincter deficiency caused by such congenital conditions as epispadias (abnormal location of the urethra on the dorsum of the penis) or myelomeningocele (protrusion of the membranes and spinal cord through a defect in the vertebral column) • Acquired conditions, such as repeated incontinence surgery, prostatectomy, radiation therapy, and trauma	• Urine loss with physical exertion, cough, sneeze, or exercise • Usually only small amounts of urine are lost with each exertion • Normal voiding habits (≤8 times per day, 2 or fewer times per night) • Post-void residual usually ≤50 mL • Pelvic examination generally shows hypermobility of the urethra or bladder neck with Valsalva maneuvers • Pelvic or rectal examination shows weak pelvic muscles
• Overflow incontinence	• The urethra is obstructed, so it fails to relax sufficiently to allow urine to flow • Urethral obstruction usually results in incomplete bladder emptying or complete urinary retention, causing overflow incontinence	• Causes external to the mechanism of the urethra include an enlarged prostate (male clients) and large genital prolapse (female clients) • When the cause is intrinsic to the urethra, abnormal contraction of the skeletal muscle occurs, causing obstruction; this condition, called *detrusor sphincter dyssynergia,* is commonly caused by neurologic abnormalities, such as spinal cord injuries and multiple sclerosis	• Same as overflow incontinence (above)

TABLE 73–4

Types of Urinary Incontinence *Continued*

Type	Definition/Description	Causes	Clinical Manifestations
Abnormalities Outside the Bladder and Urethra			
• Functional incontinence	• Leakage of urine caused by factors other than disease of the lower urinary tract		• Quantity and timing of urine leakage vary; patterns are difficult to discern
• Transient causes	• Transient causes will improve with treatment of the underlying condition	• Loss of cognitive functioning • Loss of awareness that urination is to occur in a socially acceptable place	• Altered mental state, as in delirium, confusion, depression, dementia, sepsis, mental illness, or severe psychologic stress
		• Abnormal openings in the urinary tract, such as a fistula or diverticulum	• Urinary drainage noted from areas other than the urinary meatus
		• Medications, such as sedatives, hypnotics, diuretics, anticholinergics, decongestants, antihypertensives, and calcium channel blockers	• Some medications cause altered mental state; others cause increased urine production
		• Diabetes insipidus or psychogenic polydipsia • Inability to get to toileting facilities	• Increased urinary output
		• Direct bladder pressure or urethral obstruction	• Restraints, restricted mobility
• Permanent causes	• Permanent causes are organic but may be improved with treatment	• Cognitive impairment • Traumatic or surgical effects	• Constipation or fecal impaction
		• Those factors contributing to stress incontinence, urge incontinence, and overflow incontinence	• Clinical manifestations depend on the cause
		• Structural or functional defects of the bladder or the sphincters	
		• Injuries or diseases of the spinal cord, brain stem, or cerebral cortex (neurogenic bladder)	
		• Congenital defects, including exstrophy of the bladder (bladder turned "inside out") and spina bifida	

maintain continence, a person must be aware that urination needs to occur in a socially acceptable place; clients with dementia may not have that awareness.

Transient causes of incontinence are usually external to the urinary tract and involve no significant disorder of the urinary tract itself. Incontinence can also be caused by a combination of factors.

Etiology

Incontinence may have transient or permanent causes. Evaluation of the incontinent client means considering all possible causes, beginning with those that are transient (correctable). Surgical and traumatic causes of urinary incontinence typically relate to procedures or events that necessitate surgical interventions in the lower pelvic structures, areas that are richly supplied by complex nerve pathways. Radical urologic, prostatic, and gynecologic

procedures associated with malignant pelvic neoplasms may result in postsurgical urinary incontinence. Trauma that injures sacral segments S2–4 of the spinal cord may cause incontinence from interruption of normal nerve pathways.

Inappropriate bladder contraction may result from

■ Disorders of the brain and nervous system
■ Bladder irritation from chronic infection, stones, chemotherapy, or radiation therapy

Failure of bladder contraction accompanies the autonomic neuropathy associated with diabetes mellitus and syphilis.

ELDERLY CONSIDERATIONS

Numerous factors contribute to urinary incontinence in the elderly (Chart 73–4). An elderly person may have decreased mobility from disease, neurologic dysfunc-

---

Chart 73–4

Nursing Focus on the Elderly: Factors Contributing to Urinary Incontinence

Medications

- Central nervous system depressants, such as opioid analgesics, decrease the client's level of consciousness and the urge to void, and they contribute to constipation.
- Diuretics cause frequent voiding, often of large amounts of urine.
- Multiple medications can contribute to changes in mental status or mobility.

Disease

- Cerebrovascular accidents and other neurologic disorders decrease mobility, sensation, or cognition.
- Arthritis decreases mobility and causes pain.
- Parkinson's disease causes muscle rigidity and an inability to initiate movement.

Depression

- Depression decreases the energy necessary to maintain continence.
- Decreased self-esteem and feelings of self-worth decrease the importance to the client of maintaining continence.

Inadequate Resources

- Clients who have glasses or use a cane, walker, or slippers may be afraid to ambulate.
- Products that help clients manage incontinence are often costly.
- No one may be available to assist the client to the bathroom or help with incontinence products.

These factors are in addition to the physiologic changes of aging given in Chapter 5.

---

tion, or musculoskeletal degeneration. In the hospital or extended care setting, mobility is further limited when the older client is restrained or placed on bed rest. Vision and hearing impairments may also prevent the client from locating a call bell to notify the nurse or assistive personnel of the need to void. The nurse assesses for these factors and, if possible, minimizes them to prevent urinary incontinence.

Incidence/Prevalence

Urinary incontinence is a significant health problem that affects more than 13 million people of all ages in the United States (AHCPR, 1996); about 85% are women. The elderly are predisposed to incontinence, and estimates suggest that up to 35% of community-dwelling elderly are incontinent. More than 50% of all nursing home residents are incontinent; these clients usually have multiple episodes every day. Up to 30% of hospitalized clients are affected by incontinence (Thayer, 1994).

In adult clients under 65 years old, urinary incontinence occurs twice as frequently in women as in men. Incontinence in women of this age may occur after one or more pregnancies. Men in this age group rarely experi-

ence urinary incontinence unless they have prostate disease or a spinal cord injury.

Collaborative Management

 Assessment

➤ History

The nurse asks, "Do you ever leak urine?" If the answer is yes, the nurse proceeds with a focused assessment (Chart 73–5). Incontinence may be underreported because health professionals do not question their clients about urine loss. It is not safe to assume that clients will volunteer the information without specifically being asked.

➤ Physical Assessment/Clinical Manifestations

The nurse palpates the abdominal area for evidence of urinary distention or discomfort, then gently palpates a distended bladder to determine whether tenderness is present or loss of urine occurs. When the nurse percusses a distended bladder, the sound is dull compared with the resonance of the air-filled bowel. If the client has a full bladder and can stand, the nurse observes for leakage of urine while the client strains by coughing or bearing down in the standing position. With a physician's order, the nurse determines the amount of post-void residual urine by catheterizing the client immediately after voiding. In some facilities, the nurse may also estimate the post-void residual amount with a pelvic ultrasonographic scanner (AHCPR, 1996).

For women, the nurse inspects the external genitalia to determine whether there is apparent urethral or uterine prolapse, cystocele (when the bladder herniates into the vagina), or rectocele; these conditions occur because of pelvic floor muscle weakness. An advanced practice nurse puts on an examination glove and inserts two fingers into the vagina to assess the strength of those muscles. Strength is described as weak, adequate, or strong on the basis of the amount of pressure felt by the nurse as the client tightens her vaginal muscles. The nurse describes the color, consistency, and odor of any secretions from the genitourinary orifices. The urine stream interruption test (see Chap. 72) is another method of determining pelvic muscle strength. For men, the nurse inspects the urethral meatus for any discharge; color and other characteristics are noted.

The physician or advanced practice nurse performs a digital rectal examination of both male and female clients. The digital rectal examination may provide information about the integrity of the nerve supply to the bladder. The examiner determines whether there is tactile sensation in the anorectal area by noting whether the rectal sphincter is relaxed or contracted on digital insertion. Because nerve supply to the bladder and rectum is similar, the presence of tactile sensation and a rectal sphincter that contracts suggest that the nerve supply to the bladder is intact. During rectal examination, the nurse also notes any fecal impaction; enlargement of the prostate is assessed in men.

Chart 73–5

Focused Assessment of the Client with Urinary Incontinence

- Note the client's gender, age, and, if female, menopausal status.
- Review the client's past or current medical history for diabetes mellitus or any neurologic disease process, such as Parkinson's disease, Alzheimer's disease, or multiple sclerosis.
- Ascertain whether the client has had any gynecologic or urologic surgical procedures or urologic or spinal cord trauma.
- If female, has the client had any pregnancies?
- Assess the client's current medication history (prescription and over the counter).
- Assess for symptoms by asking the following questions:
  - Tell me about the problems you are having with your bladder.
  - How often do you lose urine when you don't want to?
  - When was the first time you remember leaking urine? (Is the onset recent or long ago?)
  - When do you lose urine—during physical activities such as exercise, coughing, sneezing, laughing, or when trying to make it to the bathroom?
  - Do you lose urine when standing in lines at the bathrooms, when you hear the sound of water, or when washing your hands?
  - Do you sometimes wet the bed (occurring during sleep)?
  - Have you ever had an accident during intercourse?
  - Do you have warning signals such as bladder pressure, fullness, or spasm before the leakage occurs?
  - Have you noticed a decrease in the amount of urine (quantity) each time you urinate?
  - Have you noticed an increase in the number of times (frequency) you urinate?
  - How often do you wear a pad or protective device?
  - What type of activities have you given up because of incontinence? (Social excursions may be curtailed out of fear of embarrassing incidents of incontinence or limited to places with accessible toilets. The client may hesitate to hug, pick up a child, or kiss because of fear of odor or incontinence.)
  - Do you dream about going to the bathroom?
  - Are you having any problem with your bowels?
  - Do you have any stresses or concerns associated with work, family, or financial affairs?
  - Do you feel anxious, depressed, or feel as though lately your mind hasn't been the way it usually is?
  - How has the leaking of urine affected your relationship with family or friends?
  - Has your sexual functioning or the relationship with your sexual partner been affected?

Adapted, in part, from Peters, S. (1997). Don't ask, don't tell: Breaking the silence surrounding female urinary incontinence. *ADVANCE for Nurse Practitioners*, 5(5), 41–44.

► Laboratory Assessment

A urinalysis is inexpensive and useful to rule out infection; it should be the first step in the assessment of incontinent clients of any age. The presence of red blood cells (RBC), white blood cells (WBC), leukocyte esterase, or nitrites is an indication for culturing the urine. Any infection is treated before further assessment of incontinence.

► Radiographic Assessment

Radiographic assessment is rarely indicated unless surgery is contemplated. Excretory urography is the most useful for precise localization of the kidneys and ureters. A voiding cystourethrogram (VCUG) may be performed to

- Assess the size, shape, support, and function of the bladder
- Look for obstruction (especially prostate obstruction in men)
- Assess for post-voiding residual (PVR) with a post-voiding film

An assessment of PVR also can be made with a portable ultrasonographic bladder scanner.

► Other Diagnostic Assessment

Clients who have unusual symptoms, medical complications, or a history of failed incontinence surgery often undergo a more complete diagnostic procedure (urodynamic studies) to determine the cause of their incontinence. A urodynamic evaluation is not a standardized procedure and may consist of any combination of the following tests:

- Cystourethroscopy to examine the inside of the bladder and urethra directly
- Cystometrogram (CMG) to measure the pressure inside the bladder as it fills
- Urethral pressure profilometry (UPP) to measure the pressure in the urethra in relation to the bladder pressure during various activities
- Uroflowmetry to measure speed and completeness of bladder emptying

Testing may take several hours and more than one visit (see Chap. 72).

Electromyography (EMG) of the pelvic muscles may be a part of the urodynamic studies. A perineometer is a tampon-shaped instrument inserted into the vagina to measure the strength of pelvic muscle contractions. The graph can be used to demonstrate the amplitude of muscle contraction to the client as a method of biofeedback.

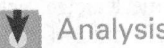 Analysis

► Common Nursing Diagnoses

The nurse and physician carefully analyze the assessment data to make the appropriate diagnosis or diagnoses. Diagnoses may include the following (AHCPR, 1996):

- Stress Incontinence related to weak pelvic muscles and structural supports
- Urge Incontinence related to decreased bladder capacity, bladder spasms, and neurologic impairment (also termed reflex incontinence)
- Overflow Incontinence related to incomplete bladder emptying

- Functional (or Chronic Intractable) Incontinence related to cognitive, motor, or sensory deficits

Nursing diagnoses related to incontinence are confusing because they are not consistent with the terminology of the Clinical Practice Guidelines of the Agency for Health Care Policy and Research (AHCPR). For example, the AHCPR includes reflex incontinence as a type of urge incontinence and addresses overflow incontinence separately. Also, more than one diagnosis may be made, particularly in women and the elderly. For example, a woman might have stress incontinence related to weak pelvic muscles after childbirth and urge incontinence related to decreased bladder capacity. Incontinence with more than one cause is frequently called a *mixed incontinence* (which generally refers to a combination of stress and urge incontinence). It may not be possible to prioritize the common nursing diagnoses for incontinence because a client may have one or several concurrently. The priority will sometimes be to investigate transient factors related to functional incontinence.

➤ Additional Nursing Diagnoses

In addition to the common diagnoses, the incontinent client may also have the following additional nursing diagnoses:

- Social Isolation related to altered state of wellness, fear of embarrassment
- Risk for Impaired Skin Integrity related to external risk factors, such as urinary excretions
- Body Image Disturbance related to odor, need to alter clothing selections, or need to wear protective briefs or supplies
- Risk for Infection related to retained or refluxing urine

 Planning and Implementation

Stress Incontinence

Planning: Expected Outcomes. The client should have fewer episodes of stress incontinence or a decreased amount of urine lost with each episode.

Interventions. Initial interventions for clients with stress incontinence include diary keeping, behavioral interventions, and medications. Surgery is reserved as a last resort. The nurse explains the purpose of a detailed diary in which the client records times of urine leakage, activities, and foods eaten. The diary is then utilized by the health care practitioner to plan interventions. Collection devices, absorbent pads, and undergarments may be used temporarily throughout the sometimes lengthy process of assessment and treatment and by those clients who elect not to pursue further interventions.

Nonsurgical Management. Drug therapy and behavioral interventions (primarily diet and exercise) for stress incontinence involve a significant amount of participation on the part of the client. The ongoing availability of a nurse to provide encouragement, clarification, and support is extremely valuable for maximizing the effects of all interventions.

Exercise Therapy. Kegel exercises for female clients with stress incontinence are designed to strengthen the muscles of the pelvic floor (circumvaginal muscles). These muscles become strengthened (just as any other skeletal muscle in the body does) by frequent, systematic, and repeated contractions.

The most important step in teaching pelvic muscle exercises is to help the client establish an awareness of the proper muscle to exercise. During the pelvic examination in women and the rectal examination in men or women, the nurse instructs the client to tighten the pelvic muscles around the examiner's fingers. The nurse then provides feedback about the adequacy of the contraction. Biofeedback devices, such as electromyography (EMG) or perineometers (see Other Diagnostic Assessment related to incontinence), measure the strength of contraction. Retention of a vaginal weight is also evidence that the client has identified the proper muscle. The ability to start and stop the urine stream or stop the passage of flatus is further evidence that the client has correctly identified the pelvic muscles.

Instructions for the pelvic muscle exercises are given in Chart 73–6. Although improvement may take several weeks, most clients notice significant benefit after 6 weeks; maximal improvement is achieved by 3 months.

Chart 73–6

Education Guide: Pelvic Muscle Exercises

- The pelvic muscles are composed of a sling of muscles that support your bladder, urethra, and vagina. Like any other muscles in your body, you can make your pelvic muscles stronger by alternately contracting (tightening) and relaxing them in regular exercise periods. By strengthening these muscles, you will be able to stop your urine flow more effectively.
- *To identify your pelvic muscles,* sit on the toilet with your feet flat on the floor about 12 inches apart. Begin to urinate, then try to stop the urine flow. Do not strain down, lift your bottom off the seat, or squeeze your legs together. When you start and stop your urine stream, you are using your pelvic muscles.
- *To perform pelvic muscle exercises,* tighten your pelvic muscles for a slow count of 10, then relax for a slow count of 10. Do this exercise 15 times while you are lying down, sitting up, and standing (a total of 45 exercises). This should take no more than 10 to 12 minutes for all three positions, or 3.5 to 4 minutes for each set of 15 exercises.
- Begin with 45 exercises a day in three sets of 15 exercises each. You will notice faster improvement if you can do this twice a day, or a total of 20 minutes each day. Remember to exercise in all three positions so your muscles learn to squeeze effectively despite your position. At first, it is helpful to have a designated time and place to do these exercises because you will have to concentrate to do them correctly. After you have been doing them for several weeks, you will notice improvement in your control of urine; however, many people report that improvement may take as long as 3 months.

Clients may need to continue the exercises to maintain the improvement (AHCPR, 1996).

Diet Therapy. A diet plan to encourage weight reduction is indicated for obese clients because stress incontinence is aggravated by increased abdominal pressure from obesity. The nurse instructs the client to avoid alcohol and caffeine (bladder stimulants) and refers the client to the dietitian as needed.

Drug Therapy. Because bladder pressure exceeds urethral resistance in clients with stress incontinence, medications may be prescribed to increase the resistance of the urethra (Chart 73–7). Beta-adrenergic–blocking agents, such as propranolol (Inderal, Detensol✣), have not been adequately tested in controlled trials and thus are not recommended for the treatment of incontinence (AHCPR, 1996).

Estrogen is used to treat postmenopausal women with stress incontinence, although its exact mechanism of action is unknown. Estrogen may increase the vascularity and tone of the circumvaginal and periurethral muscles and thus improve the client's ability to contract those muscles during times of increased intra-abdominal stress.

Vaginal Cone Therapy. Vaginal cones are a set of five small, cone-shaped weights. They are of equal size but varying weights and are used as an adjunct to pelvic muscle exercise. The woman inserts the lightest cone, labeled 1, into her vagina (Fig. 73–1), with the string to the outside, for a 1-minute test period. If she can hold the first cone in place without it slipping out while she walks around, she proceeds to the second cone, labeled 2, and repeats the procedure. She begins her treatment with the heaviest cone she can comfortably hold in her vagina for the 1-minute test period; treatment periods are 15 minutes twice a day. When she can comfortably hold the cone in her vagina for the 15-minute period, she progresses to the next heaviest weight. Treatment is completed with the cone labeled 5.

Several studies have shown weighted vaginal cones to be of benefit in strengthening the pelvic muscles and decreasing stress incontinence (AHCPR, 1996). Further research is needed, however, before recommending the weights to certain populations, such as postmenopausal women or those with pelvic prolapse. Vaginal cones are available without prescription; the cost may be reimburseable by some health insurance companies.

Chart 73–7

Drug Therapy for Urinary Incontinence

Drug	Usual Dosage	Nursing Interventions	Rationale
Alpha-adrenergic agonists Phenylpropanolamine (Nolamine)	• 25–75 mg bid PO	• Monitor BP and HR for elevations. • Report headache, anxiety, insomnia, or agitation.	• Alpha-agonists stimulate the sympathetic nervous system and may cause elevations in HR and BP, headache, anxiety, insomnia, and agitation.
Estrogen (Premarin, C.E.S.✣)	• 0.3–1.25 mg PO daily • 1–2 g qod per vagina	• Report any unusual vaginal bleeding or calf pain.	• Estrogen use can increase the risk of endometrial cancer and thrombophlebitis.
Anticholinergics/antispasmodics Propantheline (Pro-Banthine, Propanthel✣)	• 7.5–30 mg PO tid/qid	• Check the client's intraocular pressure before starting the regimen.	• Anticholinergics can increase intraocular pressure and are contraindicated in the presence of narrow-angle glaucoma.
Oxybutynin (Ditropan)	• 2.5–5 mg PO tid/qid	• Offer fluids and hard candy to moisten the mouth.	• Anticholinergics cause extreme dryness of the mouth.
Dicyclomine hydrochloride (Bentyl, Di-Spaz, Bentylol✣, Formulex✣, Lomine✣)	• 10–20 mg PO tid	• Give the drug between meals. • Increase fluids and fiber in the client's diet.	• Food interferes with absorption of the drug. • Anticholinergics decrease GI motility and can cause constipation.
Tricyclic antidepressants Imipramine (Tofranil, Novo-Pramine✣)	• 25–100 mg PO daily	• Administer the full dose hs if possible and warn clients that dizziness may occur on arising in the morning.	• Tricyclics have a high potential to cause postural hypotension.
Desipramine (Norpramin)	• 10–25 mg PO tid	• Warn clients about other anticholinergic and alpha-adrenergic side effects.	• Tricyclics have a combination of anticholinergic and alpha-adrenergic effects.
Nortriptyline (Pamelor)	• 10–25 mg PO tid		

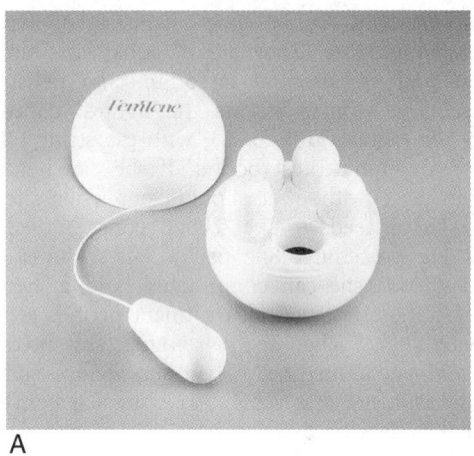

A

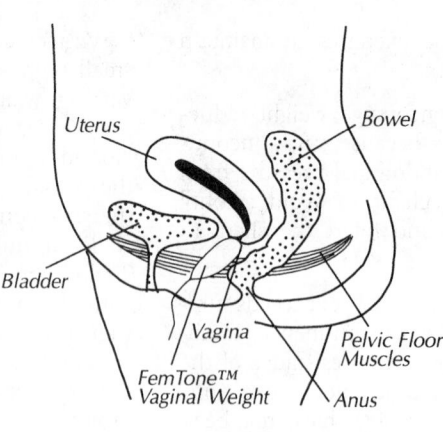

B

Figure 73–1. *A,* FemTone vaginal weights, or cones. The number on the top of each cone represents increasing weight up to the heaviest cone, a 5. *B,* Diagram showing the correct positioning of a vaginal weight, or cone, in place. (*A,* courtesy of Convatec, A Bristol-Myers Squibb Company, a Division of E. R. Squibb & Sons, Inc., Princeton, NJ; *B,* from Convatec. [1996]. *FemTone vaginal weights: A training aid for pelvic floor exercises* [brochure]. Princeton, NJ: Author.)

Other Therapy. Other types of behavioral interventions for stress incontinence include behavior modification, psychotherapy, and electrical stimulation devices to strengthen urethral contractions. A variety of intravaginal and intrarectal electrical stimulation devices have been used to treat neurologically and non-neurologically impaired clients with varying degrees of success. More research is needed to determine the ideal parameters for stimulation and methods of reducing the associated discomfort before electrical stimulation becomes a standard treatment for incontinence.

A new product, the Reliance insert, is like a tiny tampon the client inserts into the urethra. After insertion, the client inflates a tiny balloon, which rests at the bladder neck and prevents the flow of urine. To void, the client pulls a string to deflate the balloon and removes the device. The applicator is reusable; the tampon part is disposed of after each void (Peters, 1997).

Surgical Management. Stress incontinence may be surgically corrected by vaginal, abdominal, or retropubic procedures. Success rates are difficult to evaluate because of the varying definitions of "cure" in the studies; in addition, complication rates are not always presented.

Preoperative Care. The nurse instructs the client about the surgical procedure and clarifies events surrounding the surgery. Extensive urodynamic testing (see Chap. 72) is frequently performed before surgery, and the need for such thorough assessment should be explained to the client.

Operative Procedures. The surgical procedures used for women (Table 73–5) are designed to
- Elevate the bladder and urethra into a normal intra-abdominal position
- Increase the length of the urethra
- Decrease hypermobility of the bladder neck

Treatment of intrinsic urethral sphincter defects requires
- Implantation of an artificial urinary sphincter
- Injection of a collagen material around the urethra to increase urethral compression (this procedure is often done in an ambulatory care setting)
- Placement of a sling of fascia or artificial material under the urethrovesical junction and anchoring it to abdominal structures

Postoperative Care. After surgery, the nurse assesses for and intervenes to prevent or detect complications. For prevention of unnecessary movement or traction on the bladder neck, the urethral catheter is secured with tape or a tube holder. If a suprapubic catheter is present instead of a urethral catheter, the nurse monitors the dressing for leakage of urine as well as serosanguineous drainage. Catheters are usually in place until the client can urinate easily and has post-voiding residual urine of less than 50 mL.

(See Chapters 20 and 22 for a thorough discussion of general preoperative and postoperative care.)

Urge Incontinence

Planning: Expected Outcomes. The client is expected to use techniques to prevent or manage urge incontinence.

Interventions. Interventions for clients with urge incontinence include behavioral interventions and medications; surgery is not recommended for treatment of this condition (AHCPR, 1996). As with stress incontinence, collection devices and absorbent pads and undergarments may be used.

Drug Therapy. Because the hypertonic bladder contracts involuntarily in clients with urge incontinence, medications that relax the smooth muscle and increase the bladder's capacity are prescribed (see Chart 73–7).

The most effective medications are anticholinergics, such as propantheline (Pro-Banthine, Propanthel✦), and anticholinergics with smooth muscle relaxant properties, such as oxybutynin (Ditropan) and dicyclomine hydrochloride (Bentyl, Formulex✦, Spasmoban✦, Viscerol✦). Anticholinergics have serious side effects in the dosages required to relax the bladder and are therefore used in conjunction with behavioral interventions. These agents inhibit the cholinergic fibers that stimulate bladder contraction. Tricyclic antidepressants with anticholinergic and alpha-adrenergic agonist activity, such as imipramine (Tofranil, Novo-Pramine✦), have been used successfully. Other drugs, such as flavoxate (Urispas), and the antihistamines, nonsteroidal anti-inflammatory agents, beta-adrenergic agonists, and calcium channel blockers, have not

TABLE 73–5

Surgical Procedures for Stress Incontinence

Procedure	Purpose	Cure Rate	Complication Rate	Nursing Considerations
Anterior vaginal repair (colporrhaphy)	• Elevates the urethral position and repairs any cystocele	• 36%–69% (poor long-term cure rates)	• 14%	• Because the operation is performed by vaginal incision, it is often done in conjunction with a vaginal hysterectomy. Recovery is usually rapid, and a urethral catheter is in place for 24–48 hr.
Retropubic suspension (Marshall-Marchetti-Krantz or Burch colposuspension)	• Elevates the urethral position and provides longer lasting results	• 71%–98%	• 18%	• The operation requires a low abdominal incision and a urethral or suprapubic catheter for several days postoperatively. Recovery takes longer, and urinary retention and detrusor instability are the most frequent complications.
Needle bladder neck suspension (Pereyra or Stamey procedure)	• Elevates the urethral position and provides longer lasting results without a long operative time	• 40%–94% (long-term rates probably decline)	• 2%–60%	• The combined vaginal approach with a needle and a small suprapubic skin incision does not allow direct vision of the operative site; however, the high complication rates may be due to the selection of clients who, because of their medical condition, are not good candidates for longer retropubic procedures.
Pubovaginal sling procedures	• A sling made of synthetic or fascial material is placed under the urethrovesical junction to elevate the bladder neck	• 62%–81%	• 17%–22%	• The operation uses an abdominal, vaginal, or combined approach to treat intrinsic sphincter deficiencies. Temporary or permanent urinary retention is common postoperatively.
Artificial sphincters	• A mechanical device to open and close the urethra is placed around the anatomic urethra	• 82%–92%	• 32%	• The operation is done more frequently in men. The most common complications include mechanical failure of the device, erosion of tissue, and infection.
Periurethral injection of collagen or siloxane	• Implantation of small amounts of an inert substance through several small injections provides support around the bladder neck	• 64%–93% (short term only)	• Unknown, but probably quite low	• The procedure can be done in an ambulatory care setting and can be repeated as often as necessary. Certain compounds may migrate after injection; an allergy test to bovine collagen must be performed before implantation.

Data from Smith, D. J., Chapple, C. R, Kreder, K. J. (1995). The contemporary clinical treatment of female stress incontinence. *International Urogynecology Journal, 5,* 112–118.

been studied well enough for their use to be recommended (AHCPR, 1996).

Diet Therapy. The nurse instructs the client to avoid foods that have a direct bladder-stimulating or diuretic effect, such as caffeine and alcohol. Spacing fluids at regular intervals throughout the day (e.g., 120 mL every hour or 240 mL every 2 hours) and limiting fluids after the dinner hour (e.g., only 120 mL at bedtime) help avoid placing a fluid overload on the bladder and allow urine to accumulate at a steady pace.

Behavioral Interventions. Behavioral interventions for urge incontinence include bladder training, habit training, exercise therapy, and electrical stimulation.

It can be difficult for clients to understand these interventions, as they involve a significant amount of participation on the part of the client. The ongoing availability of a nurse to provide encouragement, clarification, and support is extremely valuable for maximizing the effects of all interventions. Behavioral interventions are often combined with drug therapy for maximal effect.

Bladder Training. Bladder training is primarily an education program for the client that begins with a thorough explanation of the problem of urge incontinence. Instead of the bladder being in control of the client, the client learns to control the bladder. For the program to succeed, the client must be alert, aware, and able to resist the urge to urinate.

A regular schedule for voiding is established, beginning with the longest interval that is comfortable for the client, even if the interval is only 30 minutes. The nurse instructs the client to void every 30 minutes and ignore any urge to urinate between the mandated intervals. Once the client is comfortable with the initial schedule, the interval is increased by 15–30 minutes; the new schedule is followed until the client again achieves success. As the client progressively increases the voiding interval, the bladder gradually tolerates more volume. The nurse teaches the client relaxation and distraction techniques to maximize success in the retraining. The nurse provides positive reinforcement for maintaining the prescribed schedule.

Habit Training. Habit training (scheduled toileting) is a variation on bladder training that has been successful in reducing incontinence in cognitively impaired clients. To use habit training, caregivers assist the client to void at specific times (e.g., every 2 hours on the even hours) in an effort to get the client to the toilet before incontinence can occur. There is no effort to increase bladder capacity by gradually lengthening the voiding intervals.

Prompted voiding, a supplement to habit training, attempts to increase the client's awareness of the need to void and to prompt the client to ask for toileting assistance. Habit training, otherwise, relies completely on a time schedule.

Exercise Therapy. Pelvic muscle exercises for urge incontinence have been helpful and are taught in the same way as for stress incontinence (see Chart 73–6). Improved urethral resistance enhances the client's ability to overcome abnormal detrusor contractions long enough to get to the toilet.

Electrical Stimulation. A variety of intravaginal and intrarectal electrical stimulation devices have been used to treat both urge and stress incontinence.

Overflow Incontinence

Planning: Expected Outcomes. The client should achieve continence by keeping urine volume in the bladder within normal limits; thus, the bladder is not overdistended.

Interventions. Interventions for the client with overflow incontinence caused by obstruction of the bladder outlet may include surgery to relieve the obstruction. The most common surgical procedures are removal of the prostate (see Chap. 79) and repair of genital prolapse (see Chap. 78). For overflow incontinence related to detrusor muscle inadequacy, the most effective method of treatment is intermittent catheterization. Medications have generally not proved effective (AHCPR, 1996). Behavioral interventions, such as bladder compression and intermittent self-catheterization, are the primary management techniques for urinary retention leading to overflow incontinence.

Drug Therapy. Medications are prescribed for short-term management of urinary retention, often postoperatively. They are not indicated in long-term management of the hypotonic bladder resulting in overflow incontinence. The most commonly used medication is bethanechol chloride (Urecholine), a cholinergic agent that increases bladder pressure.

Behavioral Interventions

Bladder Compression. Techniques that promote bladder emptying include the Credé method, the Valsalva maneuver, double-voiding, and splinting.

In the Credé method (see also Chap. 13), the nurse instructs the client in external compression of the urinary bladder; this technique manually assists the bladder to empty. In the Valsalva maneuver, breathing techniques increase intrathoracic and intra-abdominal pressure; this increased pressure is then directed toward the bladder during exhalation. With the technique of double-voiding, the client empties the bladder and then, within a few minutes, consciously attempts a second bladder emptying.

For women who have a severe cystocele (prolapse of the bladder through the vaginal introitus), a technique called *splinting* both compresses the bladder and moves the obstruction out of the way. The woman inserts her own fingers into her vagina, gently pushes the cystocele back into the vagina, and begins to urinate.

Intermittent Self-Catheterization. The nurse teaches intermittent self-catheterization to clients with long-term problems of incomplete bladder emptying. Techniques of self-catheterization are well established and can be learned fairly easily. The nurse remembers the following important points in teaching this technique:
- Proper hand washing and cleaning of the catheter reduce the frequency of infection
- A small lumen and adequate lubrication of the catheter prevent urethral trauma

■ A regular schedule for bladder emptying prevents overdistention of the bladder with subsequent mucosal trauma

Suitable candidates for training are able to comprehend instructions and have the manual dexterity to manipulate the catheter. Caregivers or family members in the home can also be taught to perform straight catheterization.

Functional Incontinence

Planning: Expected Outcomes. The client should use methods of urine containment or collection that ensure dryness until the underlying cause of the incontinence is treated.

Interventions. Causes of functional incontinence vary greatly; some are reversible, and others are not. The primary focus of intervention is treatment of reversible causes. When incontinence is not reversible, containment of the urine and protection of the client's skin are the priorities to be addressed. Nonsurgical interventions include applied devices, containment, and urinary catheterization.

Applied Devices. Applied devices include intravaginal pessaries for women and penile clamps for men. The intravaginal pessary supports the uterus and vagina and helps maintain the correct position of the bladder. (See Chapter 78 for further discussion of pessaries.) The penile clamp is applied externally to compress the urethra and to prevent leakage of urine.

The dangers of pessaries and penile clamps include damage to the tissues and subsequent infection from constant pressure in sensitive areas. Both require a client who has manual dexterity or a caregiver who applies and removes the device. The clinician prescribes the device, and the nurse instructs the client or the client's caregivers in its use. Male clients may use an external collecting device, such as a condom catheter; design of a suitable external collecting device for women has not been as successful.

Containment. Absorbent pads and briefs are designed to collect urine and keep the client's skin and clothing dry. A variety of types and sizes of pads are available:

■ Shields or liners inserted inside a panty
■ Undergarments consisting of full-sized pads with waist straps
■ Plastic-lined protective underpants with or without elastic legs
■ Combination pad and pant systems
■ Absorbent bed pads

A major concern with the use of protective pads is the risk that skin breakdown will occur. Materials and costs vary; some are reusable, and others are disposable. The disposal of these products raises ecologic concerns. Newer, more absorbent products are coming on the market as manufacturers take advantage of the growth of the "adult diaper" market. The nurse avoids use of the word "diaper," however, because of the usual association of diapers with a baby.

Urinary Catheterization. Catheterization for the control of incontinence may be intermittent or involve placement of an indwelling catheter. Intermittent self-catheterization is preferred to placement of an indwelling catheter because of the decreased likelihood of infection. Indwelling urinary catheters should be used minimally, temporarily, and only when all other alternatives have been tried and have been unsuccessful. An indwelling urinary catheter is appropriate for

■ Clients with skin breakdown who need a dry environment for healing
■ Clients who are terminally ill and deserve comfort
■ Clients who are acutely or critically ill and need careful measurement of urinary output

 ## Continuing Care

Continuing care for the client with urinary incontinence considers the personal, physical, emotional, and social resources of the client. Important personal resources for self-care include mobility, vision, and manual dexterity. The nurse considers who will be the primary caregiver and what environmental circumstances or factors will influence the effectiveness of the plan.

➤ Health Teaching

The nurse teaches the client and family about the cause of the identified type of urinary incontinence and discusses treatment options available for its management. The teaching plan addresses the prescribed medications (purpose, dosage, method and route of administration, and expected and potential side effects). The nurse also teaches the client and family about the importance of weight reduction and dietary modification to assist with control of urinary incontinence.

When external devices or protective pads are needed, the nurse

■ Describes the possible options
■ Discusses the advantages and disadvantages of each
■ Helps the client make a selection that considers lifestyle and resources

For clients who will use intermittent catheterization or those with artificial urinary sphincters, the nurse demonstrates the appropriate technique to the client or caregiver. The nurse evaluates return demonstrations for correct technique. Chart 73–8 also addresses teaching.

The embarrassment experienced by incontinent clients is potentially devastating to their self-esteem, body image, and interpersonal relationships. The unpredictability of incontinence creates anxiety. Clients are often embarrassed to seek help, and even when resources are identified clients may need assistance to feel comfortable in using the resources. Even purchasing supplies in the local drugstore or grocery store can be perceived as a threat to their privacy.

The nurse assists in psychosocial preparation by accepting and acknowledging the personal concerns of the client and caregiver. These concerns must never be minimized or made to seem trivial. The nurse helps the client learn methods of controlling or managing the fear or anxiety. As the client learns the specifics of the plan that will allow control of urinary incontinence, the confidence to resume psychosocial interactions should return.

Chart 73-8

Education Guide: Urinary Incontinence

- Maintain a normal body weight to reduce the pressure on your bladder.
- Do not try to control your incontinence by limiting your fluid intake. Adequate fluid intake is necessary for kidney function and health maintenance.
- If you have a catheter in your bladder, follow the instructions given to you about maintaining the sterile drainage system.
- If you are discharged with a suprapubic catheter in your bladder, inspect the entry site for the tube daily, clean the skin around the opening gently with warm soap and water, and place a sterile gauze dressing on the skin around the tube. Report any redness, swelling, drainage, or fever to your physician.
- Do not put anything into your vagina, such as tampons, medications, hygiene products, or exercise weights, until you check with your physician at your 6-week checkup after surgery.
- Do not have sexual intercourse until after your 6-week postoperative checkup.
- Do not lift or carry anything heavier than 5 pounds or participate in any strenuous exercise until your physician gives you postoperative clearance. In some cases, this could be as long as 3 months.
- Avoid exercises, such as running, jogging, step or dance aerobic classes, rowing, cross-country ski or stairclimber machines, and mountain-biking. Brisk walking without any additional hand, leg, or body weights is allowed. Swimming is allowed after all drains and catheters have been removed and your incision is completely healed.
- If Kegel exercises are recommended, ask your nurse for specific instructions.

➤ Home Care Management

The home environment is assessed for barriers that impede access to the toileting facilities. Environmental hazards that might slow walking or contribute to injury should be eliminated. These hazards might include

- Small area rugs (throw rugs)
- Tables or chairs with legs that extend into the walking area
- Slippery waxed or polished floors
- Inadequate lighting

If the client must climb stairs to reach a bathroom, hand railings should be installed and stairs should be kept free of obstacles. Toilet seat extenders may help provide the appropriate level of seating so that maximal abdominal pressure may be applied to encourage voiding. Portable commodes may be obtained for homes in which ambulatory access to toilets is impractical or impossible. Physical and occupational therapists are valuable adjunctive resources for assisting with home care management.

➤ Health Care Resources

Referral to home care agencies for assistance with personal care and to continence clinics that specialize in evaluation and treatment may be helpful. In many conti-

nence clinics, nurses collaborate with physicians and other health care professionals to evaluate and manage clients. The treatment plan is specific for each client; supplies and products are custom selected.

Clients benefit emotionally from education and from the support of others who experience similar concerns. The National Association for Continence (NAFC) and the Simon Foundation for Continence publish newsletters with informative articles and educational materials written with simple, easy-to-understand explanations. Several books that explain incontinence in detail and include management options are now available for the lay person. The AHCPR has also published a caregiver guide (Publication No. 96-0683) for the public that is available on the Internet or by calling 1-800-358-9295. Local hospitals, in collaboration with NAFC, may conduct local support groups.

 Evaluation

The nurse evaluates the effectiveness of the interventions on the basis of the expected outcomes. Desired outcomes include that the client can

- Describe the type of urinary incontinence experienced
- Demonstrate knowledge of proper use of medications and correct procedures for self-catheterization, use of the artificial sphincter, or care of an indwelling urinary catheter
- Demonstrate effective use of the selected exercise or bladder training programs
- Select and appropriately use incontinence devices and products
- Demonstrate a reduction in the number of incontinence episodes

Urolithiasis

Overview

Urolithiasis refers to the presence of calculi (stones) in the urinary tract. Calculi are generally asymptomatic until they pass into the lower urinary tract; this movement can cause excruciating pain. The term *nephrolithiasis* describes a condition in which calculi form in the renal parenchyma. Formation of calculi in the ureter is referred to as *ureterolithiasis*. Often, the location of the stone is identified by the section of the urinary tract it occupies (i.e., in the proximal or upper third, middle third, or distal or lower third).

Pathophysiology

Urologic calculi result from a variety of metabolic disorders. However, the exact mechanism of calculus formation, commonly referred to as stone disease, is not entirely understood. Everyone excretes crystals in the urine at some time, but fewer than 10% of people form calculi. About 75% of calculi contain calcium as one component of the stone complex, which may be calcium oxalate or calcium phosphate (Hruska, 1996). Struvite (15%), uric acid (8%), and cystine (3%) make up the less common stones (Balaji and Menon, 1997).

Formation of stones seems to involve three conditions:

- Alteration in urine flow, resulting in supersaturation of the urine with the particular element (such as calcium) that first becomes crystallized and later becomes the stone
- Epithelial damage to the lining of the urinary tract (i.e., from crystals)
- Decreased inhibitor substances in the urine which would otherwise prevent supersaturation and crystal aggregation (Balaji and Menon, 1997).

High urine acidity (as with uric acic and cystine stones) or alkalinity (as with calcium phosphate and struvite stones) also contributes to stone formation.

One example of a metabolic deficit causing stone formation begins when excessive amounts of calcium are absorbed through the intestinal tract (the most common cause of hypercalciuria). As blood circulates through the kidneys, the excess calcium is filtered into the urine, causing supersaturation of calcium in the urine. If fluid intake is inadequate, such as when a client is dehydrated, supersaturation is more likely to occur, and there is an increased probability of calcium complexing (combination of calcium with another compound to form a larger molecule). The calcium complex often serves as a nidus (breeding site) for additional deposition, and eventually a calculus forms. In addition, urinary inhibitors to the formation of both calcium oxalate and calcium phosphate have been identified; therefore, for one of these types of stones to form, the client has insufficient amounts of these inhibitors.

Calculi that form in the kidney and subsequently pass into the ureter often lodge in the ureteropelvic angle, the aortoiliac bend, or the ureterovesical angle (see also Chap. 72). When the calculus occludes the ureter and blocks the flow of urine, the ureter dilates. An enlargement of the ureter is called *hydroureter.*

The pain associated with ureteral spasm is excruciating and may cause the client to go into shock from sympathetic stimulation. In addition, hematuria may result from damage to the urothelial lining. If the obstruction is not removed, urinary stasis may result in infection and subsequently impair renal function on the side of the blockage. As the blockage persists, hydronephrosis (enlargement of the kidney) and irreversible kidney damage, although rare, may develop.

Etiology

The cause of urolithiasis is unknown, although several hypotheses have been suggested. At least 90% of clients with calculi have an identifiable metabolic risk factor. Table 73–6 summarizes the known metabolic defects that commonly cause stone formation.

A diet high in calcium is not believed to result in renal calculi unless a metabolic defect or renal tubular defect already exists. Even in clients with a history of nephrolithiasis, supplementation with calcium citrate does not cause new stone formation (Levine et al., 1994). Urinary stasis, urinary retention, immobilization, and dehydration all contribute to a calculus-forming environment. Except for the use of the thiazides for calcium oxalate stones,

TABLE 73–6

Metabolic Defects That Commonly Cause Calculi	
Metabolic Deficit	**Etiology**
Hypercalcemia	
Primary	Absorptive: increased intestinal calcium absorption
	Renal: impaired renal tubular resorption of calcium
Secondary	Resorptive: hyperparathyroidism, vitamin D intoxication, renal tubular acidosis, prolonged immobilization
Hyperoxaluria	
Primary	Genetic: autosomal recessive trait resulting in high oxalate production
Secondary	Dietary: excess oxalate from foods such as spinach, rhubarb, Swiss chard, cocoa, beets, wheat germ, pecans, peanuts, okra, chocolate, and lime peel
Hyperuricemia	
Primary	Gout is an inherited disorder of purine metabolism (20% of clients with gout have uric acid calculi)
Secondary	Increased production or decreased clearance of purine from myeloproliferative disorders, thiazide diuretics, carcinoma
Struvite	Made of magnesium ammonium phosphate and carbonate apatite. Formed by urea splitting by bacteria, most commonly, *Proteus mirabilis.* Needs an alkaline urine to form
Cystinuria	Autosomal recessive defect of amino acid metabolism that precipitates insoluble cystine crystals in the urine

diuretics can cause volume depletion and thus may promote the formation of calculi.

Incidence/Prevalence

The incidence of stone disease in the adult population is relatively high and varies with geographic location, race, and family history. Approximately 12% of the U.S. adult population will have at least one episode of renal stone disease. Overall, the incidence is higher in men; however, struvite calculi are twice as common in women. Recurrence rates vary depending on type of treatment. The recurrence rate of untreated calcium oxylate stones is 35% to 50% in 5 to 10 years. A higher recurrence of stones is found in those with a family history of stone disease and those who had their first occurrence by age 25 years.

TRANSCULTURAL CONSIDERATIONS

There is a definite increased incidence of stone disease in the southeastern United States and a rising incidence in Japan and Western Europe. Calcium stone disease is more common in men than women and tends to occur in young adults or during early middle adulthood. Stone disease in African-Americans is uncommon (Hruska, 1996). Cystinuria is more common among Jews of Libyan extraction (Rutchik & Resnick, 1997).

Collaborative Management

 Assessment

➤ History

The nurse inquires about a personal or family history of urologic calculi and obtains a diet history. If the client has a history of calculus formation, the nurse asks whether chemical analysis of the stone was performed and what preventive measures the client follows. In addition, the nurse asks about past treatments for stone disease.

➤ Physical Assessment/Clinical Manifestations

The major clinical manifestation of calculi is severe pain, commonly called *renal colic.* Flank pain suggests localization of the calculi in the kidney or upper ureter; flank pain that radiates abdominally or into the scrotum and testes or the vulva suggests that calculi are in the ureters or bladder. Pain is most intense when the stone is moving or when obstruction of the ureter is present (Presti et al., 1994).

Renal colic begins suddenly and is usually described as "unbearable." Nausea, vomiting, pallor, and diaphoresis frequently accompany the pain. A large stationary stone in the kidney (staghorn calculus), however, rarely causes much pain. Frequency and dysuria occur when a stone reaches the bladder.

Hematuria is a common finding; blood may make the urine appear smoky or rusty. Increased turbidity and odor are associated with infectious processes that may accompany urolithiasis. Oliguria (scant urinary output) or anuria (absence of urinary output) suggests obstruction, possibly at the bladder neck or urethra. Obstruction of the urinary tract is an emergency and must be treated immediately to preserve kidney function.

The nurse examines the client to detect bladder distention. The physical examination may reveal pale, ashen, diaphoretic skin; the client may suffer from excruciating pain. The nurse measures vital signs, which are moderately elevated with pain; temperature and pulse are elevated with infection. Blood pressure may decrease markedly if the severe pain causes shock.

➤ Laboratory Assessment

Urinalysis may show red blood cells (RBC), white blood cells (WBC), and bacteria. Red blood cells are most likely the result of direct trauma caused by the calculus in the endothelial lining of the ureter, bladder, or urethra. White blood cells and bacteria may be present as a result of urinary stasis. Urine culture reveals infection (associated with struvite stones); sensitivity studies of the culture identify antibiotic effectiveness. Microscopic examination of the urine may identify crystals from which calculi could form. Urinary pH is measured to determine acidity or alkalinity.

The serum WBC count is elevated with infection; the differential count indicates an increased number of immature WBCs, such as bands, if the infection is recent and acute. Increases in the serum calcium, serum phosphate, or serum uric acid levels suggest that excess minerals are present and may contribute to calculus formation.

➤ Radiographic Assessment

Calculi are easily seen on x-rays of the kidneys, ureters, and bladder (KUB), intravenous urograms, or computed tomographic (CT) scans. The primary purpose of these radiographic procedures is to confirm the presence and location of the calculi.

The urogram is useful for identifying whether urinary tract obstruction is present; however, because of the risk of acute renal failure induced by contrast media, other diagnostic tests may be chosen for high-risk clients (the elderly and clients who have diabetes mellitus, multiple myeloma, or elevated serum creatinine levels). CT is generally required to visualize cystine or uric acid stones, neither of which are visible on x-ray.

➤ Other Diagnostic Assessment

Renal ultrasonography produces images from sound waves. Structures of varying density are reproduced. Solid structures, such as calculi, are extremely dense; therefore, the images of calculi are obvious. With renal ultrasonography, the visualization of small calculi and their exact location may not be as precise as desired.

 Analysis

➤ Common Nursing Diagnoses

The priority nursing diagnoses are
1. Pain related to physical injury agents (i.e., the presence or movement of the calculus)
2. Risk for Infection related to urinary stasis and the presence of a foreign object (calculus)
3. Risk for Injury related to internal risk factors (risk of urinary obstruction)

➤ Additional Nursing Diagnoses and Collaborative Problems

Additional nursing diagnoses for the client with urolithiasis include
- Anxiety related to threat to self-concept, threat to or change in health status, or fear of severe discomfort
- Knowledge Deficit regarding prevention of recurrences related to lack of information

A collaborative problem is Potential for Hydronephrosis and Subsequent Renal Failure.

 Planning and Implementation

Pain

Planning: Expected Outcomes. The client should achieve acceptable comfort levels.

Interventions. The majority of clients will be able to expel the calculus without invasive procedures. The most important factors regarding whether a stone will pass on its own are its composition, size, and location. The larger the stone and the higher up in the urinary tract it is, the less likely it is to be passed. Other interventions may be necessary when the client does not pass the stone spontaneously (Fig. 73–2).

Nonsurgical Management. Nonsurgical interventions for altered comfort include drug therapy and pain relief measures. Pain is most severe in the first 24–36 hours. Avoiding overhydration in the acute phase helps to make the spontaneous passage of a stone less painful (Singal & Denstedt, 1997). The nurse strains the urine to monitor for excretion of the calculus. Any calculi obtained are sent to the laboratory for analysis; preventive therapy is based on stone composition.

Drug Therapy. Opioid analgesics are frequently required to control the moderately severe to severe pain caused by calculi in the urinary tract. Opioid agents, such as morphine sulfate (Statex✤), are often administered intravenously so that prompt and adequate absorption is ensured. Nonsteroidal anti-inflammatory drugs such as ketorolac (Toradol) in the acute phase may be quite effective.

Control of pain is more effective when medications are given at regularly scheduled intervals or via a constant delivery system (e.g., skin patch) instead of as needed. Spasmolytic agents, such as oxybutynin chloride (Ditropan) and propantheline bromide (Pro-Banthine, Propanthel✤), are extremely important for the relief and control of pain (see Chart 73–7). The nurse administers the medication and assesses the client's response by asking the client to rate the discomfort on a rating scale.

Other Pain Relief Measures. Relaxation techniques, such as hypnosis and imagery, therapeutic or healing touch, and acupuncture, can relieve pain. Clients often have great difficulty finding a comfortable position in which to relax; assisting the client with positioning can often aid in relaxation. Breathing techniques, such as those used in childbirth education, labor, and delivery, can also assist clients to relax.

Extracorporeal Shock Wave Lithotripsy (ESWL). Lithotripsy is the application of sound (ultrasound) or dry shock wave energies (electrohydraulic, electromagnetic, or piezoelectric) to fragment the calculus. The client receives conscious sedation and lies on a flat x-ray type table with the lithotriptor aimed at the calculus, which is visualized by fluoroscopy. A local anesthetic cream is applied to the skin focal site, but should be applied 45 minutes before the procedure. Older lithotriptors require the client to be submerged in a water bath under epidural or general anesthesia.

During the procedure, cardiac rhythm is monitored by electrocardiography, and the shock waves are administered in synchrony with the R wave; 500 to 1500 shock waves are administered in 30 to 45 minutes. Continuous electrocardiographic monitoring for ectopy and fluoroscopic observation for disintegration of the calculus are maintained.

After lithotripsy, the nurse may strain the urine to monitor the elimination of calculus fragments. Some ecchymosis may be noted on the flank of the affected side after extracorporeal shock wave lithotripsy.

Occasionally, ESWL is preceded by the placement of a stent in the ureter to facilitate passage of the stone fragments. Cystine stones are generally resistant to ESWL.

Surgical Management. Various minimally invasive surgical and open surgical procedures are indicated if urinary

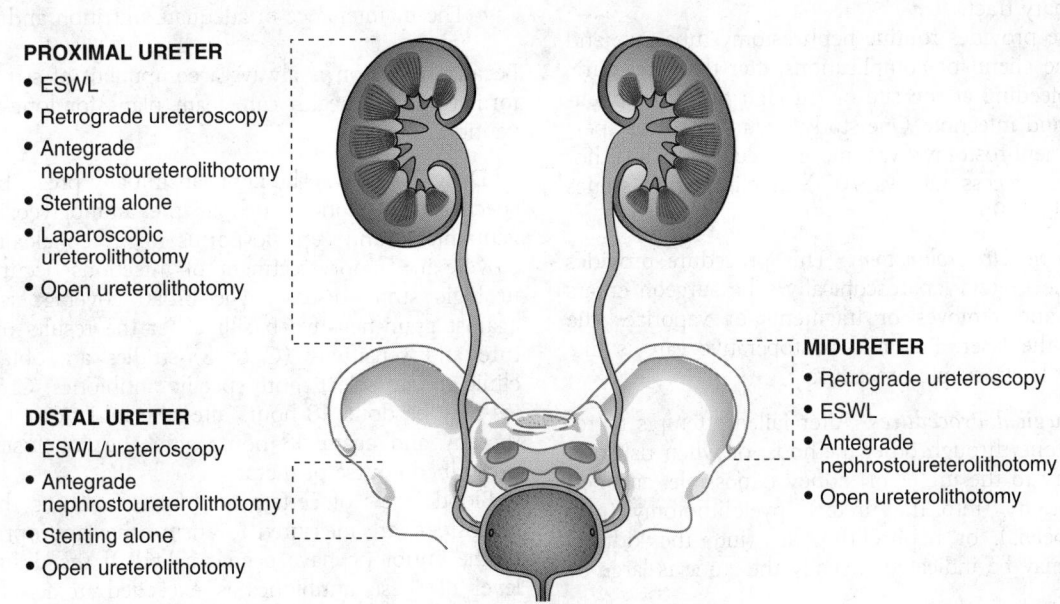

PROXIMAL URETER
- ESWL
- Retrograde ureteroscopy
- Antegrade nephrostoureterolithotomy
- Stenting alone
- Laparoscopic ureterolithotomy
- Open ureterolithotomy

DISTAL URETER
- ESWL/ureteroscopy
- Antegrade nephrostoureterolithotomy
- Stenting alone
- Open ureterolithotomy

MIDURETER
- Retrograde ureteroscopy
- ESWL
- Antegrade nephrostoureterolithotomy
- Open ureterolithotomy

ESWL=Extracorporeal Shock Wave Lithotripsy

Figure 73–2. Treatment options for ureteral stones. (From Singal, R. K. & Denstedt, J. D. [1997]. Contemporary management of ureteral stones. *The Urologic Clinics of North America, 24*[1], 59–70.)

obstruction occurs or if the calculus is too large to be passed spontaneously.

Minimally Invasive Surgical Procedures. Minimally invasive surgical (MIS) procedures include stenting, retrograde ureteroscopy, percutaneous antegrade nephrostoureterolithotomy, and laparoscopic ureterolithotomy.

Stenting. A stent is a small tube placed in the ureter through the endoscopic procedure of ureteroscopy. The stent dilates the ureter and creates a passageway for the stone or stone fragments. This procedure prevents the passing stone from coming in contact with the ureteral mucous, thereby reducing pain. A Foley catheter also may be placed to facilitate passage of the stone through the urethra.

Retrograde Ureteroscopy. Retrograde ureteroscopy is an endoscopic procedure. The ureteroscope is passed through the urethra and bladder into the ureter. Once the stone is visualized, it can be extracted using grasping baskets, forceps, or loops. Through the ureteroscope, intraluminal lithotripsy also can be performed using the energies of ESWL or laser. A Foley catheter also may be placed to facilitate passage of the stone fragments through the urethra.

Percutaneous Antegrade Nephrostoureterolithotomy. In this procedure the client lies prone, or laterally, and receives general anesthesia. The physician identifies the ideal renal entry point with fluoroscopy, then passes a needle into the collecting system of the kidney. Once a tract has been made in the kidney, other equipment, such as an intracorporeal (inside the body) ultrasonic or laser lithotriptor, can be utilized to facilitate stone fragmentation and removal. An endoscope with a special attachment to grasp and extract the stone also could be used. Frequently a nephrostomy tube is left in place initially to prevent the stone fragments from passing through the normal urinary tract.

The nurse provides routine nephrostomy tube care and monitors the client for complications after the procedure, including bleeding at the site or through the tube, pneumothorax, and infection. One study documented that percutaneous nephrostomy was more effective than lithotripsy (96% success rate vs 70%) in eliminating stones (Jewett et al., 1995).

Laparoscopic Ureterolithotomy. This procedure provides access to the ureters laparoscopically. The surgeon enters the ureter and removes or fragments or vaporizes the stone with the laser. Pre- and postoperative care is like that for any laparoscopic procedure.

Open Surgical Procedures. After failed attempts to remove the stone through other methods, or when risk of a lasting injury to the ureter or kidney is possible, an open ureterolithotomy (into the ureter), pyelolithotomy (into the renal pelvis), or nephrolithotomy (into the kidney) procedure may be indicated. Usually the stone is large or impacted.

Preoperative Care. The nurse prepares the client for the selected procedure by explaining how, when, and where the procedure will be performed. The nurse describes what the client can expect before and after the procedure. Written materials are provided as available. The client receives nothing by mouth and also receives preoperative bowel preparation. (Chapter 20 discusses routine preoperative care.)

Operative Procedures. The retroperitoneal area is entered through a large flank incision as for nephrectomy (see Chap. 74), for pyelolithotomy, or for nephrolithotomy and through a lower abdominal incision for ureterolithotomy. The urinary tract is entered surgically and the stone removed. Before closure, various tubes and drains may be placed (e.g., nephrostomy tube, ureteral stent, Penrose or other wound drainage device, and Foley catheter).

Postoperative Care. The nurse follows routine procedures for assessment of the client who has received anesthesia. (Chapter 22 discusses routine postoperative care.)

The nurse's primary concerns after urologic surgery are
- Monitoring the amount of bleeding from incisions and wounds and through the urine (hematuria)
- Maintaining adequate urinary output
- Straining the urine to monitor the elimination of calculus fragments
- Preventing future stones through dietary modification

Risk for Infection

Planning: Expected Outcomes. The client should have no new infections and be free of previously acquired infections.

Interventions. Control of infections before invasive and noninvasive procedures is critical for the prevention of urosepsis. Interventions include
- The administration of appropriate antibiotics, either to eliminate an existing infection or to prevent new infections
- The maintenance of adequate nutrition and fluid intake

Because infection is always a component of struvite stone formation, the health care team plans for long-term prevention.

Drug Therapy. The clinician initially prescribes broad-spectrum antibiotics, such as the aminoglycosides (e.g., gentamicin) and cephalosporins (e.g., cephalexin [Keflex, Novolexin✦]), for treatment of infections occurring with urologic stone disease. The broad coverage is effective against gram-negative bacilli. After the results of the culture and sensitivity (C & S) studies are obtained, the clinician can select more specific antibiotics. C & S studies may be done 48 hours after the initiation of antibiotic therapy and again 48 hours after the conclusion of the prescribed course of therapy.

Blood levels of certain antibiotics, such as the aminoglycosides, are measured to ensure that appropriate levels of the antibiotic have been reached. If the desired blood level of these antibiotics is exceeded, toxic effects and kidney damage may result. If the blood level of the antibiotic is inadequate, bactericidal or fungicidal effects will not be achieved. New clinical evidence of an infection (such as chills, fever, or altered mental status) warrants the collection of a urine sample for repeated culture and sensitivity tests.

For the client with struvite stones, the primary care provider will prescribe periodic and long-term monitoring of the urine for infection. Commonly, urine cultures are ordered monthly for 3 months, then quarterly for 1 year. Drugs that prevent bacteria from splitting urea, such as acetohydroxamic acid (Lithostat) and hydroxurea (Hydrea), often are prescribed on a long-term basis for clients with struvite calculi. The primary care provider monitors the serum creatinine with acetohydroxamic acid; its administration is contraindicated for levels above 2 mg/dL.

As was covered with cystitis, the nurse reviews interventions aimed at preventing urinary tract infection.

Diet Therapy. The client's diet ideally includes adequate calorie intake representing a balance of all food groups. Unless medically contraindicated, the nurse encourages fluid intake of 2 to 3 L/day.

Risk for Injury

Planning: Expected Outcomes. The client should remain free of urinary obstruction.

Interventions. Measures to prevent urinary obstruction by calculi include a high intake of fluids (3 L/day or more) and careful measures of intake and output. A liberal fluid intake assists in preventing dehydration, promotes the flow of urine, and decreases the chance of crystals precipitating into calculi. Interventions also depend on the type of calculus. Medications, diet modification, and fluid intake are the major strategies available.

Drug Therapy. The selection of drugs for the prevention of obstruction depends on the problem promoting formation of calculi and the type of calculus formed. The nurse teaches the client the reason for the medication and assesses for side effects or adverse drug reactions.

Calcium-containing Calculi. Medications to treat hypercalciuria may include thiazide diuretics (e.g., chlorothiazide [Diuril] or hydrochlorothiazide [HydroDIURIL,

Natrimax♣, Urozide♣]), orthophosphate, and sodium cellulose phosphate. The thiazide diuretics promote calcium resorption from the renal tubules back into the body, thereby preventing excess calcium loads in the urine. Orthophosphate affects normal calcium-phosphorus metabolism, resulting in decreased urinary saturation of calcium oxalate. Sodium cellulose phosphate reduces intestinal absorption of calcium.

Oxalate-containing Calculi. For clients with hyperoxaluria, allopurinol (Zyloprim) and vitamin B_6 (pyridoxine) are used.

Uric acid-containing calculi. For clients with chronic gout, allopurinol helps prevent the formation of urate (uric acid) stones. To alkalinize the urine, medications such as potassium citrate, 50% sodium citrate, and sodium bicarbonate may be used. The desired urinary pH is 6 to 6.5. Because the normal urinary pH averages 5 to 6, these desired values are termed "alkaline."

Cystine-containing Calculi. For clients with cystinuria, alpha-mercaptopropionylglycine (AMPG) and captopril (Capoten) have both been found to lower urinary cystine levels. Their use is reserved for when hydration and alkalinazation of the urine has not been successful.

Diet Therapy. As with medications, diet modification depends on the type of calculus formed (Table 73–7). The nurse consults the dietitian to plan the appropriate diet for the client.

If the client forms calculi containing calcium (calcium phosphate or calcium oxalate), the diet may be modified to limit calcium-containing foods. With limitation of dairy foods and others high in calcium, the dietary calcium intake is approximately 400–600 mg/day. In some clients who decrease their dietary calcium intake, oxalate production increases. Consequently, sources of oxalate may also need to be limited; oxalate is found in dark-green foods, such as spinach. Absorption of oxalate increases when calcium intake decreases.

For clients who form uric acid calculi, a reduced intake of foods containing purines, such as boned fish and organ

TABLE 73–7

Dietary Treatment for Renal Stones		
Stone Type	**Dietary Interventions**	**Rationale**
Calcium oxalate	• Avoid oxalate sources, such as spinach (also see Table 73–6).	• Reduction of urinary oxalate content may help prevent these stones from forming. Urinary pH is not a factor.
Calcium phosphate	• Decrease intake of foods high in calcium, such as milk and other dairy products.	• Reduction of urinary calcium content may help prevent these stones from forming.
Struvite (magnesium ammonium phosphate)	• Limit high-phosphate foods, such as dairy products, red and organ meats, and whole grains.	• Reduction of urinary phosphate content may help prevent these stones from forming.
Uric acid (urate)	• Decrease intake of purine sources, such as organ meats, poultry, fish, gravies, red wines, and sardines.	• Reduction of urinary purine content may help prevent these stones from forming.
Cystine	• Encourage PO fluids, up to 3 L/day.	• Increased fluid helps dilute the urine and prevent the cystine crystals from forming.

meats, is encouraged. The client should avoid rich foods, such as organ meats, red wines, and gravies.

Acidity of the urine can be increased by providing an acid ash diet. A more acidic urine helps prevent calcium and struvite stones from forming. Other stones, such as uric acid or cystine stones, form more readily in acidic urine. The alkaline ash diet will promote a more alkaline urine.

Other Measures. The nurse encourages the client to ambulate frequently. Ambulation promotes passage of the calculi and reduces the possibility of calcium resorption from the bones. The nurse checks the pH of the urine daily and strains the urine with filter paper to collect passed fragments of calculi.

 Continuing Care

> ### ➤ *Health Teaching*

Key points of health teaching are described in Chart 73–9. The client often experiences tremendous anxiety and fear that a calculus and its related pain may recur. In addition to anxiety about the pain, the possibility of repeated surgical interventions or permanent and serious kidney damage is of tremendous concern. Although the memories of the pain are blunted over time, the intensity of the experience is not forgotten.

Psychosocial preparation is generally enhanced when clients know what to expect and what actions to take should the unexpected develop. The nurse reassures the

---

Chart 73–9

Education Guide: Urinary Calculi

- Finish your entire prescription of antibiotics to ensure that you will not get a urinary tract infection.
- You may resume your usual daily activities.
- Remember to balance regular exercise with sleep and rest.
- You may return to work 2 days to 6 weeks after surgery, depending on the type of intervention, your personal tolerance, and your physician's directives.
- Depending on the type of stone you had, your diet may be restricted to prevent further stone formation.
- Remember to drink at least 3 L of fluid a day to dilute potential stone-forming crystals, prevent dehydration, and promote urine flow.
- Monitor urine pH as directed, may be up to three times per day.
- You can expect bruising after lithotripsy. The bruising may be quite extensive and may take several weeks to resolve.
- Your urine may be bloody for several days after surgery.
- Pain in the region of the kidneys or bladder may signal the beginning of an infection or the formation of another stone. Report any pain, fever, chills, or difficulty with urination immediately to your physician or nurse.
- Keep follow-up appointments to check on infection, have repeat cultures done, and so forth.

---

client that preventive and health promotion activities are designed to prevent recurrence.

> ### ➤ *Home Care Management*

If the client has the support of family or a significant other, the nurse includes these people in the assessment and planning for home care. In many instances, no additional home care is necessary. The nurse may suggest that home care assistance be considered by clients who live alone or whose families or significant others are not available or cannot provide the supportive care.

> ### ➤ *Health Care Resources*

Health care resources that may be of interest to the client include the National Kidney Foundation, which has local chapters and affiliates. This organization has literature written specifically for client education. Other resources include hospital and community libraries. Clinical nurse specialists provide education and counseling. Kidney stone treatment centers in hospitals are becoming more prevalent and may offer extensive resources for clients.

 Evaluation

Evaluating the care of the client with urolithiasis, the nurse expects the client will

- Explain preventive health actions related to diet modification, fluid intake, and medication administration
- Follow self-care routines necessary for return to usual activities of daily living
- State the symptoms of infection and obstruction to urine flow
- Describe measures for minimizing discomfort and seeking medical attention, as appropriate

Urothelial Cancer
Overview

Urothelial cancer refers to malignant neoplasms of the urothelium, which is the lining of transitional cells in the renal pelvis, ureters, urinary bladder, and urethra. Most urothelial tumors occur in the urinary bladder. Consequently, bladder cancer is a general term that is sometimes used to describe this pathologic condition.

Pathophysiology

A national study (Lynch & Cohen, 1994) on urinary tract cancers revealed that 72% were transitional cell carcinomas and primarily occurred in the bladder. The second most common site of cancer in the urinary tract was the kidney and renal pelvis (27%), most of which were adenocarcinomas. Squamous cell carcinoma accounted for approximately 5% of all bladder cancers.

Urothelial tumors are generally low grade, polypoid in appearance, multifocal, and recurrent. Once lesions spread beyond the transitional cell layer they tend to be highly invasive and metastatic. Because of the multifocal, recurrent nature of the disease, clients with superficial tumors may experience recurrence after 10 years of being tumor free (Morris et al., 1995). Long-term surveillance of these clients is therefore an important consideration.

Table 73–8 displays the staging of bladder cancer. Tumors confined to the mucosa are treated by simple excision, whereas carcinoma in situ (CIS), or stage TIS, is generally treated with excision plus intravesical (inside the bladder) chemotherapy. Disease that has progressed beyond CIS is treated with more extensive resection, often a radical cystectomy with urinary diversion. Chemotherapy and radiotherapy are used as adjunctive treatment.

When the tumor remains unchecked, it can invade surrounding structures (i.e., uterus, cervix, prostate). When lymphatic metastasis occurs, it is generally to the liver, lung, and bone.

Etiology

Exposure to environmental toxins, particularly the aromatic amines used in the rubber, paint, electric, cable, and textile industries, is highly associated with bladder cancer. In developed countries such occupational exposures have been largely eliminated through improved

TABLE 73–8

Staging of Bladder Cancer	
Primary tumor (T)	
TX	Primary tumor cannot be assessed
T0	No evidence of primary tumor
TIS	Carcinoma in situ: "flat tumor"
T1	Tumor invades submucosa (subepithelial connective tissue)
T2	Tumor invades superficial muscle (inner half)
T3	Tumor invades deep muscle or perivesical fat
T3a	Tumor invades deep muscle (outer half)
T3b	Tumor invades perivesical fat
T4	Tumor invades any of the following: prostate, uterus, vagina, pelvic wall, abdominal wall
T4a	Tumor invades prostate, uterus, vagina
T4b	Tumor invades pelvic or abdominal wall
Lymph node (N)	
NX	Regional lymph nodes cannot be assessed
N0	No regional lymph node metastasis
N1	Metastasis in a single lymph node, 2 cm or less in greatest dimension
N2	Metastasis in a single lymph node, more than 2 cm, but not more than 5 cm in greatest dimension, or multiple lymph nodes, none more than 5 cm in greatest dimension; pelvic only
Distant metastasis (M)	
MX	Presence of distant metastasis cannot be assessed
M0	No distant metastasis
M1	Distant metastasis or nodes positive above aortic bifurcation

Adapted from American Joint Committee on Cancer. (1992). In O. H. Beahrs (Ed.), *Manual for staging of cancer* (4th ed.). Philadelphia: Lippincott-Raven; and Bennett, J. C., & Plum, F. (Eds.). (1996). *Cecil textbook of medicine* (20th ed.). Philadelphia: W. B. Saunders.

safety practices. The greatest unregulated risk factor in the United States remains tobacco use. Other risks include (Shapiro, 1996)

- Schistosoma haematobium (a parasite)
- Excessive use of phenacetin compounds
- Long-term administration of cyclophosphamide (Cytoxan, Procytox✶)

Incidence/Prevalence

There are approximately 54,500 new cases of bladder cancer diagnosed each year in the United States and approximately 11,700 deaths per year from the disease (Parker et al., 1997). The condition is rare in adults younger than age 40 and there is a substantial increase in incidence after age 60.

TRANSCULTURAL CONSIDERATIONS

 Bladder cancer is primarily a disease of Caucasian men. In all racial groups, however, it affects men two to four times more often than women. It is the second most common genitourinary cancer in men and women. Survival rates for Caucasians are significantly better than for African-Americans. African-American females have the lowest survival rates.

Collaborative Management

Assessment

➤ History

The nurse inquires about the client's perception of general health. The sex and age of the client are documented. The nurse inquires about active and passive exposure to cigarette smoke. To detect potentially harmful environmental agents, the nurse describes the client's occupation in detail. The nurse also asks the client specifically to describe any change in the color, frequency, or amount of urine and any abdominal discomfort.

➤ Physical Assessment/Clinical Manifestations

The nurse observes the overall appearance of the client, noting skin color and general nutritional status. The nurse inspects, percusses, and palpates the abdomen for asymmetry, tenderness, and bladder distention.

The nurse also observes the urine for color and clarity. Hematuria is the predominant sign associated with bladder cancer; it may be gross or microscopic and is usually painless and intermittent. Dysuria, frequency, and urgency are usual symptoms when infection or obstruction is also present.

The nurse assesses the client's emotional response to known or suspected bladder cancer and notes anxiety, fear, sadness, anger, or guilt. Early symptoms are painless, and many clients deny hematuria because it is often intermittent. Clients may also be reluctant to seek treatment because they suspect a sexually transmitted disease. Consequently, clients may experience guilt or anger about their own delays in seeking medical attention.

The nurse assesses the client's personal methods of

coping and the degree of support evident from family or significant others. Social interaction and active role relationships with others may provide support and motivation for coping with convalescence.

➤ *Laboratory Assessment*

The only significant finding on a routine urinalysis is generally gross or microscopic hematuria. Cytologic testing on voided urine specimens is not uniformly reliable; bladder-wash specimens and bladder biopsies via cystoscope are the most sensitive and specific tests for diagnosis (Sack et al., 1995).

➤ *Radiographic Assessment*

Cystoscopy with retrograde pyelography is the primary method for evaluation of painless hematuria. A transurethral biopsy of a visible bladder tumor can be performed during cystoscopy. This is essential for staging and is usually accomplished in a day-surgery unit prior to admission to the hospital for treatment. Excretory urography is particularly informative in delineating obstructions, especially at the ureterovesical junction. The computed tomographic (CT) scan shows tumor invasion of surrounding tissues.

➤ *Other Diagnostic Assessment*

Ultrasonography shows masses but is less valuable for tumor staging. Magnetic resonance imaging (MRI) may help in the assessment of deep, invasive tumors.

 Analysis

➤ *Common Nursing Diagnosis*

The common nursing diagnosis is Risk for Injury related to urinary obstruction and metastasis or recurrence of the cancer.

➤ *Additional Nursing Diagnoses and Collaborative Problems*

Other possible nursing diagnoses include
- Knowledge Deficit regarding diagnostic and treatment procedures related to lack of information resources
- Fear related to possible death
- Altered Nutrition: Less than Body Requirements related to increased metabolic needs
- Anxiety related to concern for changes in body image, changes in body functioning, and fear of death

A common collaborative problem is Potential for Sepsis related to tumor invasion of surrounding tissues.

 Planning and Implementation

Risk for Injury

Planning: Expected Outcomes. The client should not experience urinary obstruction, cancer recurrence, or tumor metastasis.

Interventions. Therapy for the client with bladder cancer usually begins with a surgical resection of the lesions for definitive diagnosis and staging of disease. For lesions extending beyond the mucosa, the initial resection will be followed by intravesical chemotherapy or immunotherapy. High-grade or recurrent lesions will be treated with more radical surgery plus intravesical chemotherapy and/or radiotherapy. Systemic chemotherapy is reserved for clients with distant metastases. (See Chapter 27 for general care of the client receiving chemotherapy or radiation therapy.)

Nonsurgical Management. Prophylactic immunotherapy with intravesical instillation of bacille Calmette-Guérin (BCG), a compound used to vaccinate against tuberculosis in some countries, is used to prevent tumor recurrence of superficial cancers (stage T1 or lower). This procedure has been more effective than single agent chemotherapy; side effects, however, are comparable (Shapiro et al., 1996).

Multiagent systemic chemotherapy is successful in prolonging life after distant metastasis has occurred but is rarely curative. Radiation therapy has also been successful in prolonging life.

Surgical Management. The type of surgical management for bladder cancer depends on the type and stage of the cancer and the client's general health status. Complete cystectomy with extensive surgical dissection of surrounding muscle and tissue offers the best chance of a cure for large, invasive bladder cancers.

Preoperative Care. Specific client education depends on the type and extent of the planned surgical procedure. The nurse coordinates preoperative education with the physician and enterostomal (ET) therapist. The nurse discusses the type of urinary diversion and the selection of a site for the stoma. The goal is for the client to have a positive attitude about body image and a positive self-image. The nurse intervenes with educational counseling to ensure accurate understanding about self-care practices, methods of pouching, control of urinary drainage, and minimization of odor.

The site selected for the stoma should be visible and should avoid folds of skin, bones, and scar tissue. The client's waistline or belt area is ideally avoided. The nurse prepares the client for the number and type of drains that will be present postoperatively. (General preoperative care is discussed in Chapter 20.)

Operative Procedures. Transurethral resection of the bladder tumor (TURBT) or partial cystectomy is performed for small, early, superficial tumors. In a partial (segmental) cystectomy, a portion of the urinary bladder is removed. This procedure is generally reserved for treatment of a solitary isolated bladder tumor.

When the entire cancerous bladder must be removed (complete cystectomy), the ureters must be diverted into a collecting reservoir. Techniques for urinary diversion are illustrated in Figure 73–3. With an ileal conduit the ureters are surgically implanted in a portion of the ileum, and urine is collected in a pouch on the skin around the

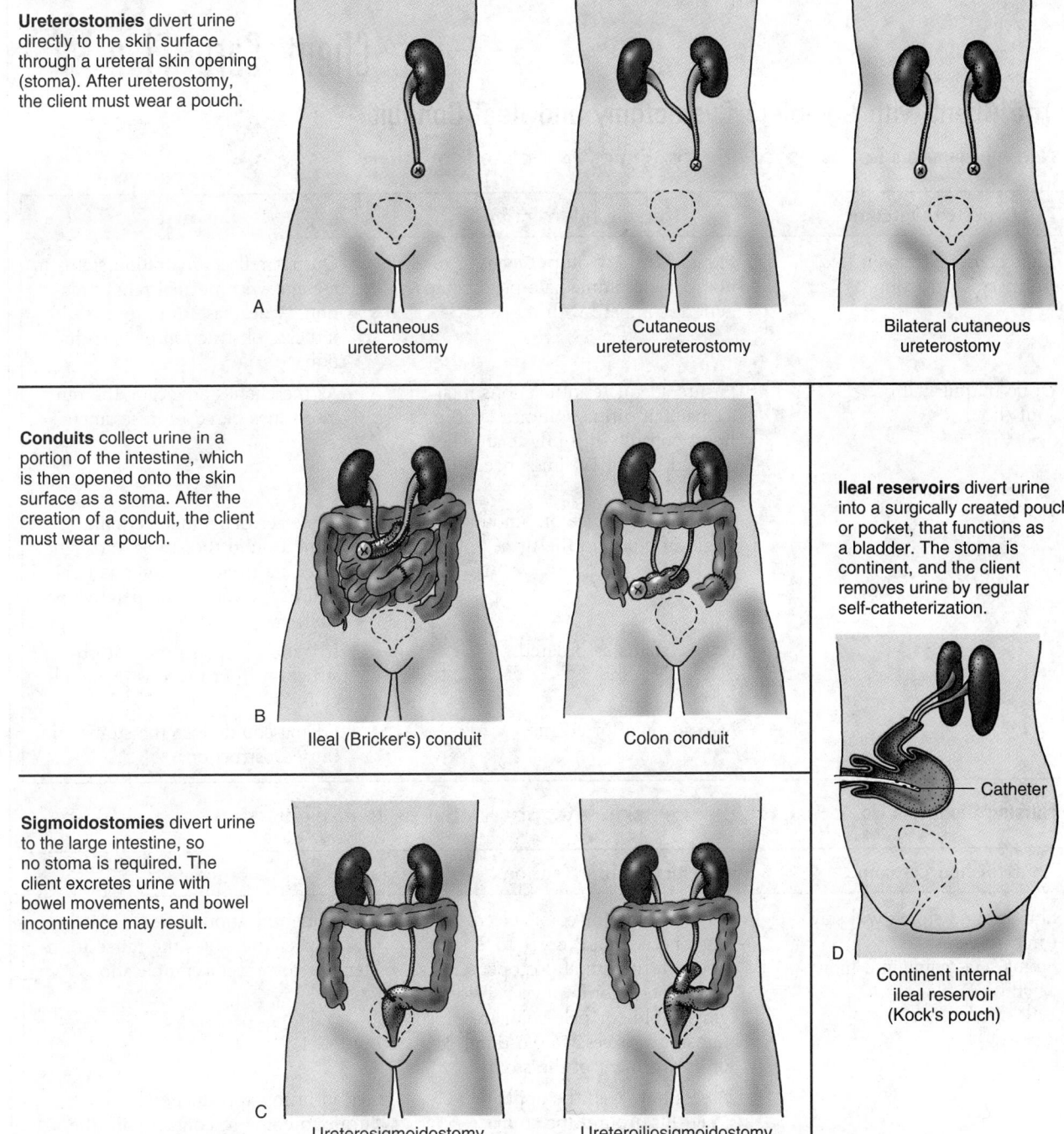

Ureterostomies divert urine directly to the skin surface through a ureteral skin opening (stoma). After ureterostomy, the client must wear a pouch.

A

Cutaneous ureterostomy

Cutaneous ureteroureterostomy

Bilateral cutaneous ureterostomy

Conduits collect urine in a portion of the intestine, which is then opened onto the skin surface as a stoma. After the creation of a conduit, the client must wear a pouch.

B

Ileal (Bricker's) conduit

Colon conduit

Ileal reservoirs divert urine into a surgically created pouch, or pocket, that functions as a bladder. The stoma is continent, and the client removes urine by regular self-catheterization.

Catheter

Sigmoidostomies divert urine to the large intestine, so no stoma is required. The client excretes urine with bowel movements, and bowel incontinence may result.

C

Ureterosigmoidostomy

Ureteroiliosigmoidostomy

D

Continent internal ileal reservoir (Kock's pouch)

Figure 73–3. *A–D,* Urinary diversion procedures used in the treatment of bladder cancer.

stoma. Increasingly, continent reservoirs are being used. With cutaneous ureterostomy or ureteroureterostomy, the ureter opening is brought out onto the skin. The cutaneous ureterostomies may be located on either side of the abdomen or side by side.

Postoperative Care. The Client Care Plan outlines postoperative care of the client who has an ileal conduit. After cutaneous ureterostomy, as with the ileal conduit, an external pouch covers the ostomy to collect urine. The

nurse collaborates with the enterostomal therapist and focuses care on the wound, the skin, and urinary drainage. (See Chapters 59 and 60 for ostomy care.)

The client with a Kock's pouch, a continent reservoir, may have a Penrose drain and a plastic Medena catheter in the stoma. The drain removes lymphatic fluid or other secretions; the catheter ensures urinary drainage so that suture lines may heal. The physician orders irrigation of the catheter to ensure patency. (General postoperative care is discussed in Chapter 22.)

Client Care Plan

The Client with Complete Cystectomy and Ileal Conduit

Nursing Diagnosis No. 1: Altered urinary elimination related to urinary diversion.

Expected Outcomes	Nursing Interventions	Rationale
The client will remain free of urinary obstruction.	■ Monitor urinary output every 1 to 2 hours in the immediate postoperative period; compare with intake.	■ Output reflects hydration status in a client with normal renal function. A decrease in output could indicate obstruction or dehydration.
Urine output will be > 30 mL/hour.	■ Ensure adequate intravenous intake to maintain urine volumes > 30 mL/hour; consult with physician when ordered rate of IV fluids needs to be changed.	■ As the client's advocate, the nurse intervenes based on assessment.
	■ Assess for presence of, amount, and origin of blood in the urine.	■ Some serosanguineous drainage from around the stoma and light bleeding from the stoma is normal in the early postoperative period.
	■ Irrigate stents as ordered.	■ Irrigation helps to prevent obstruction from mucous or blood clots.
	■ Assess stoma for edema.	■ Edema could close the stoma and cause obstruction.

Nursing Diagnosis No. 2: Risk for impaired skin integrity related to urinary diversion.

Expected Outcomes	Nursing Interventions	Rationale
Skin around stoma will stay intact. Stoma will maintain a moist, light red color.	■ Assess stoma for color, bleeding, and edema every 1 to 2 hours in the initial postoperative period; notify physician for grayish-blue or pale color to the stoma, excessive bleeding, or enlargement of the stoma.	■ Early identification of deviations from the expected enables the nurse to intervene to prevent complications.
	■ Assess how well the appliance (bag) fits around the stoma.	■ An ill-fitting appliance will allow urine to come in contact with the skin, causing skin breakdown.
Incision will heal without complications.	■ Assess skin around the stoma for any breakdown.	■ Ongoing assessment helps to detect early signs of complications.
	■ Clean skin around the stoma with each appliance change and around the appliance at other times.	■ Cleaning removes the medium in which bacteria can grow and helps to prevent breakdown from moisture.
	■ Assess incision for redness, pain, swelling, drainage.	■ Ongoing assessment helps to detect early signs of complications.

Client Care Plan

Nursing Diagnosis No. 3: Risk for infection related to loss of normal drainage and storage for urine.

Expected Outcomes	Nursing Interventions	Rationale
Urinary tract, including kidneys, will remain infection free.	■ Assess urine for color and odor.	■ Because of mucous secretion by the ileal segment, the urine will appear slightly cloudy; turbidity and a foul smell could indicate infection.
	■ Collect urine specimens from the stoma rather than the appliance.	■ Urine that is allowed to stand will grow bacteria. A fresh urine specimen will yield the most accurate results.
	■ Monitor client's temperature.	■ Fever could indicate infection.
	■ Ensure adequate hydration through intake and output assessment and hydration assessment.	■ Adequate fluid intake promotes the flow of urine.
	■ Maintain sterile asepsis for all care around the urinary diversion.	■ The stoma provides the ureters a direct access to the environment. The shorter proximity of the ureters to the kidney makes the kidney more at risk for infection.

 Continuing Care

➤ Health Teaching

The nurse educates the client and family about medications, diet and fluid therapy, the use of external pouching systems, and the technique for catheterization of a continent reservoir.

With some procedures, the client may require electrolyte replacements to prevent long-term deficits. The nurse instructs the client to avoid foods that are known to produce gas if the urinary diversion is into the gastrointestinal tract. When the intestinal production of gas is minimized, flatus will not result in incontinence.

The nurse also instructs the client and the family or significant other about any alterations in self-care activities related to the urinary diversion. In conjunction and collaboration with the enterostomal therapist, the nurse demonstrates external pouch application, local skin care, pouch care, methods of adhesion, and drainage mechanisms. If Kock's pouch has been created, the nurse instructs the client about the technique of catheterization.

Preoperative education can shorten the time for postoperative learning. For all modules of instruction, the nurse observes at least one return demonstration by the client or the family caregiver. The client ideally assumes responsibility for self-care before discharge.

The nurse assists the client to prepare psychologically for the impact of urinary diversion on self-image, body image, sexual functioning, and self-esteem. Counseling provides information and support so that the feelings of powerlessness may be minimized.

By discussions with the client about typical social situations, the nurse helps the client gain control over new toileting practices. Men with a urinary diversion into the sigmoid colon need to learn a new habit of sitting to urinate. For clients of either sex, the nurse promotes confidence in social situations by encouraging frequent emptying of urinary collection devices before traveling or attending social functions or events. Resumption of sexual activity is a major concern for many adult clients, regardless of age; this topic needs to be addressed openly and with sensitivity. Cystectomy causes physiologic impotence in men, but treatment is available (see Chap. 79).

➤ Home Care Management

Preparation for home care considers the client's self-care abilities and limitations and the family's ability and willingness to assist in care. The long-term need for stoma care and skin protection is a primary consideration for those clients who have had surgical intervention.

➤ Health Care Resources

The United Ostomy Association and the American Cancer Society affiliates and chapters have educational materials that may be useful to clients. In some areas, local support groups have meetings to assist others and to send visitors to provide peer counseling and support to clients. Home care personnel may assist with follow-up, easing the transition from hospital to home. The Wound, Ostomy, and Continence Nurses Society provides educational programs and a journal devoted to the care of clients with ostomies.

 Evaluation

The nurse evaluates the effectiveness of the interventions and the plan of care by identifying the outcomes. Expected outcomes indicate that the client will
- Demonstrate the ability to apply an external pouch, to provide skin care, and to empty the device or to catheterize the Kock's pouch correctly and at appropriate intervals
- Explain the role of fluid and food intake in preventing infections and promoting urinary health
- Demonstrate self-confidence by proceeding with social interactions and avoiding self-isolation
- Verbalize positive comments about self-esteem and body image during the adjustment phase

Bladder Trauma
Overview

Bladder trauma results from penetrating or blunt injury to the lower abdomen. Penetrating lower abdominal injury may occur by stabbing, gunshot wound, or other trauma in which objects pierce the abdominal wall. A fractured pelvis with puncture of the bladder by bone fragments is the most common cause of bladder trauma. Bladder trauma may also be a result of sexual assault.

Blunt trauma compresses the abdominal wall and the bladder. A seat belt may sufficiently compress the bladder to cause injury, especially if the bladder is full or distended.

Collaborative Management

 Assessment

Clients with a penetrating bladder wound often have anuria or hematuria. In the emergency department, initial assessment includes inspection of the urinary meatus for blood.

Diagnostic tests include cystography and voiding cystourethrography (VCUG). If renal or ureteral trauma is suspected, intravenous urography is scheduled before cystography so that any leakage of bladder contrast medium does not mask the outlines of the kidneys or ureters. The cystogram shows whether there is a defect in bladder filling; the voiding cystourethrogram defines bladder emptying.

 Interventions

Bladder trauma, other than a simple contusion, requires surgical intervention. Stabilization of any fractures usually

precedes bladder repair. Surgical interventions include procedures to repair the anterior or posterior bladder wall and peritoneal membrane. In general, repairs of the bladder are accomplished by closure procedures.

The client with an anterior bladder wall injury commonly has a Penrose drain and a Foley catheter in place postoperatively; the client with a posterior bladder wall injury has a Penrose drain and Foley or suprapubic catheter. In some instances, vaginal or rectal fistulas may also require repair.

Psychosocial support is critical for clients who have sustained traumatic injuries. The nurse refers the client to appropriate resources to assist in dealing with potential psychosocial issues.

 CASE STUDY for the Client with Incontinence

■ Mrs. Piley, a frail 88-year-old woman, is in the hospital for pneumonia. She is responding well to antibiotic therapy, but you notice she only makes small amounts of concentrated urine; often she is incontinent. When you try to encourage her to drink (as prescribed), she says, "Oh honey, I can't drink that. If I do I won't be able to get to the bathroom in time."

QUESTIONS:
1. What is Mrs. Piley thinking that led her to the response she gave you?
2. How important is it for Mrs. Piley to force fluids? Why?
3. Other than explaining why she needs an increased fluid intake, what other interventions could you discuss with Mrs. Piley?

SELECTED BIBLIOGRAPHY

Adams, D. H., & Abernathy, B. B. (1996). Laser ureterolithotripsy for cystine calculi. *AORN Journal, 64*(6), 924, 926–927, 929–930.
Balaji, K. C., & Menon, M. (1997). Mechanism of stone formation. *The Urologic Clinics of North America, 24*(1), 1–11.
Brazier, A., & Palmer, M. (1995). Collecting clean-catch urine in the nursing home: Obtaining the uncontaminated specimen. *Geriatric Nursing, 16*(5), 217–224.
Connor, P. A., & Kooker, B. M. (1996). Nurses' knowledge, attitudes, and practices in managing urinary incontinence in the acute care setting. *MEDSURG Nursing, 5*(2), 87–92, 117.
*Cubler-Goodman, A., Devlin, M. A., & Dinatale, R. (1993). Endoscopic lithotripsy for urinary calculi: Treatment alternatives. *AORN Journal, 58*(5), 954–956, 958–960.
Czarapata, B. J. R. (1996). Interstitial cystitis and vulvodynia. *ADVANCE for Nurse Practitioners, 4*(10), 21–24.
Duffield, P. (1997). Urinary tract infections in the elderly. *ADVANCE for Nurse Practitioners, 5*(4), 30–32.
Faller, N. A., & Lawrence, K. G. (1994). Obtaining a urine specimen from a conduit urostomy. *American Journal of Nursing, 94*(1), 37.
Fleet, J. C. (1994). New support for a folk remedy: Cranberry juice reduces bacteriuria and pyuria in elderly women. *Nutrition Review, 52*(5), 168–170.
Goshorn, J. (1996). Kidney stones. *American Journal of Nursing, 96*(9), 40.
Gray, R., & Malone-Lee, J. (1995). Review: Urinary tract infection in elderly people—time to review management? *Age and Ageing, 24,* 341–345.
Hanno, P. M. (Ed.). (1994). Interstitial cystitis. *The Urologic Clinics of North America, 21* (1).

Hruska, K. (1996). Renal calculi. In J. C. Bennett & F. Plum (Eds.), *Cecil textbook of Medicine.* Philadelphia: W. B. Saunders.

Jackson, B. J., & Hicks, L. E. (1997). Effect of cranberry juice on urinary pH in older adults. *Home Healthcare Nurse, 15*(3), 199–202.

*Jeter, K., Faller, N., & Norton, C. (1990). *Nursing for continence.* Philadelphia: W. B. Saunders.

Jewett, M., Bombardier, C., & Menchions, C. W. (1995). Comparative costs of the various strategies of urinary stone disease management. *Urology, 46*(suppl 3A), 15–22.

Karlowicz, K. A. (Ed.) (1995). *Urologic nursing: Principles and practice.* Philadelphia: W. B. Saunders.

Kirton, C. A. (1997). Assessing for bladder distension. *Nursing97, 27*(4), 64.

*Koch, M. O. (1989). Bladder substitution with intestine: Past and present. *Journal of Urological Nursing, 8,* 610–617.

Kreder, K. J., & Nygaard, I. E. (1994). Treatment of stress urinary incontinence with artificial urinary sphincter. *International Urogynecology Journal, 5,* 168–174.

Kunin, C. M. (1996). Urinary tract infections and pyelonephritis. In J. C. Bennett & F. Plum (Eds.), *Cecil textbook of medicine* (20th ed.). Philadelphia: W. B. Saunders.

Levine, B. S., Rodman, J. S., Wienerman, S., Bockman, R. S., Lane, J. M., & Chapman, D. S. (1994). Effect of calcium citrate supplementation on urinary calcium oxalate saturation in female stone formers: Implications for prevention of osteoporosis. *American Journal of Clinical Nutrition, 60,* 592–596.

*Lowe, A., & Gabriel, L. S. (1993). Laser lithotripsy: Patient care, staff education. *AORN Journal, 58*(5), 961–964, 966, 968–969.

Lynch, C. F., & Cohen, M. B. (1995). Urinary system. *Cancer, 75*(1) (suppl), 316–329.

Mahon, C. R., & Manuselis, G. (1995). *Textbook of diagnostic microbiology.* Philadelphia: W. B. Saunders.

Malarkey, L. M., & McMorrow, M. E. (1996). *Nurse's Manual of Laboratory Tests and Diagnostic Procedures.* Philadelphia: W. B. Saunders.

*Moore, S., Newton, M., & Yancey, R. (1993). How to irrigate a nephrostomy tube. *American Journal of Nursing, 93*(7), 63–67.

Morris, S. B., Gordon, E. M., Shearer, R. J., & Woodhouse, C. R. (1995). Superficial bladder cancer: For how long should a tumor-free patient have check cystoscopies? *British Journal of Urology, 75,* 193–196.

Palmer, M. (1996). *Urinary continence: Assessment and promotion.* Baltimore, Maryland: Aspen Publications.

Parker, S. L., Tong, T., Bolden, S., & Wingo, P. A. (1997). Cancer statistics, 1997. *CA: A Cancer Journal for Clinicians, 47*(1), 5–27.

*Peattie, A. B., Plevnik, S., & Stanton, S. L. (1988). Vaginal cones: A conservative method of treating genuine stress incontinence. *British Journal of Obstetrics and Gynaecology, 95*(10), 1049–1053.

Peters, S. (1997). Don't ask, don't tell: Breaking the silence surrounding female urinary incontinence. *ADVANCE for Nurse Practitioners, 5*(5), 41–44.

Presti, J. C., Stoller, M. L., & Carroll, P. R. (1994). Genitourinary tract. In L. M. Tierney, S. J. McPhee, & M. A. Papadakis (Eds.), *Current medical diagnosis and treatment* (pp. 736–778). Norwalk, CT: Appleton & Lange.

*Resnick, B. (1993). Retraining the bladder after catheterization. *American Journal of Nursing, 93*(11), 46–49.

Resnick, M. I. (Ed.). (1997). Urolithiasis. *Urologic Clinics of North America, 24*(1).

Ruml, L. A., Pearle, M. S., & Pak, C. Y. C. (1997). Medical therapy: Calcium oxalate urolithiasis. *Urologic Clinics of North America, 24*(1), 117–133.

Rutchik, S. D., & Resnick, M. I. (1997). Cystine calculi. *Urologic Clinics of North America, 24*(1), 163–171.

Sack, M. J., Artymyshym, R. L., Tomaszewski, J. E., & Gupta, P. K. (1995). Diagnostic value of bladder wash cytology, with special reference to low grade urothelial neoplasms. *Acta Cytologia, 39*(2), 187–194.

*Sampselle, C. M., & DeLancey, J. O. (1992). The urine stream interruption test and pelvic muscle function. *Nursing Research, 41*(2), 73–77.

Shapiro, C. L., Garnick, M. B., & Kantoff, P. W. (1996). Tumors of the kidney, ureter, and bladder. In J. C. Bennett & F. Plum (Eds.), *Cecil textbook of medicine* (20th ed.). Philadelphia: W.B. Saunders.

Singal, R. K., & Denstedt, J. D. (1997). Contemporary management of ureteral stones. *Urologic Clinics of North America, 24*(1), 59–70.

Smith, D. J., Chapple, C. R., & Kreder, K. J. (1994). The contemporary clinical treatment of female stress incontinence. *International Urogynecology Journal, 5,* 112–118.

Strangio, L. (1997). Interventional uroradiologic procedures. *AORN Journal, 66*(2), 286–290, 292–294.

Strasinger, S. K. (1994). *Urinalysis and body fluids.* Philadelphia: F. A. Davis.

Thayer, D. (1994). How to assess and control urinary incontinence. *American Journal of Nursing, 94*(10), 42–48.

Thompson, A. C., & Christmas, T. J. (1996). Interstitial cystitis—an update. *British Journal of Urology, 78,* 813–820.

*U. S. Department of Health and Human Services, Agency for Health Care Policy and Research. (1992). *Urinary incontinence in adults: Clinical practice guidelines* (AHCPR Publication No. 92-0038), revised, 1996. *Urinary incontinence in adults: Acute and chronic management.* (AHCPR Publication No. 96-0682). Rockville, MD: U. S. Department of Health and Human Services.

*Wyman, J. F., Harkins, S. W., & Fantl, J. A. (1990). Psychosocial impact of urinary incontinence in the community-dwelling population. *Journal of the American Geriatrics Society, 38*(3), 282–288.

Zagoria, R. J. (Ed.). (1997). Uroradiology. *Urologic Clinics of North America, 24*(3).

SUGGESTED READINGS

Czarapata, B. J. R. (1996). Interstitial cystitis and vulvodynia. *ADVANCE for Nurse Practitioners, 4*(10), 21–24.

The author first focuses on the treatment of any infection associated with interstitial cystis. She then discusses interventions for relief of the "bladder" pain, which may actually be referred pain. She describes therapy with ice, then hot wet towels on trigger points for the piriformis and rectus abdominus muscles, and biofeedback for the pelvic floor muscles. Specific bladder irritating foods to avoid are listed. Bowel and bladder training, fluid intake, and intervention during an acute episode are included.

Palmer, M. (1996). *Urinary continence. Assessment and promotion.* Baltimore: Maryland: Aspen Publications.

This comprehensive book addresses the nurse's role in promoting continence in a variety of settings. Several tools for assessing continence are presented, along with tips on incorporating their use into nursing practice. The terminology conforms to the standards set by the AHCPR.

*U. S. Department of Health and Human Services, Agency for Health Care Policy and Research. (1992). *Urinary incontinence in adults: Clinical practice guidelines* (AHCPR Publication No. 92-0038), revised, 1996. *Urinary incontinence in adults: Acute and chronic management.* (AHCPR Publication No. 96-0682). Rockville, MD: U. S. Department of Health and Human Services.

A panel of experts who reviewed the current literature on incontinence developed these comprehensive guidelines. Recommendations for management are based on scientific evidence. The guidelines also promote uniform terminology in dealing with incontinence. (All terms used in this chapter conform to the recommended definitions.) Both panels of experts were co-chaired by a nurse/physician team and contained experts from a variety of professions with interest and expertise in treating urinary incontinence. The guidelines, along with a small client education brochure, are free and available by calling 1-800-358-9295.

Chapter 74

INTERVENTIONS FOR CLIENTS WITH RENAL DISORDERS

Renal disorders may be a primary condition or develop secondarily to another disease or disorder. For example, renal cell cancer and polycystic kidney disease are primary diseases, whereas diabetic nephropathy develops due to diabetes mellitus and nephrosclerosis due to hypertension. If appropriate diagnosis and treatment are not implemented, consequences can be serious and even life threatening.

Advances in electron microscopy, immunology, and biology have increased our knowledge of many renal disorders. Although information on the sites, mechanisms, and potential causes of various renal disorders has expanded, the nomenclature and classification of many of these syndromes is increasingly confusing, and, because of ongoing scientific findings overlapping or combined terminology, statistical data on renal disorders are not readily available. For example, in 1993, the eighth cause of death for people over age 64 years in the United States is listed only as "nephritis, nephrotic syndrome, and nephrosis" (National Center for Health Statistics, 1996). Nursing interventions aim to prevent, detect, and manage renal disorders.

CONGENITAL DISORDERS

Polycystic Kidney Disease

Overview

Polycystic kidney disease (PKD) is typically an inherited kidney disorder. A phenomenon described as *spontaneous mutation* accounts for the 5% to 10% incidence of PKD in clients with no family history.

PKD is one of the most common inherited disorders, affecting 400,000 to 600,000 people in the United States. PKD and other cystic kidney diseases are the fourth leading cause of end-stage renal disease (ESRD) in the United States (U.S. Renal Data Systems, 1995). The general public is more aware, however, of other less common inherited disorders, such as cystic fibrosis. PKD is more common in Caucasians than in African-Americans.

Pathophysiology

Polycystic kidney disease affects the renal parenchyma and occurs bilaterally. Although PKD is viewed as a kidney disease, the cysts also occur frequently in other tissues, such as the liver, cerebral blood vessels, and cardiac blood vessels.

In the kidney, the nephron is the primary site of pathophysiologic damage. Cysts can develop anywhere throughout the glomeruli and/or the tubules, while many nephrons remain free of the disorder. Over time, small cysts become progressively larger (up to a few centimeters in diameter) and more diffusely distributed; the glomerular and tubular membranes are damaged; then, as the cysts become filled with tubular filtrate, glomerular filtration, tubular reabsorption, and tubular secretion become less effective.

Eventually, the renal parenchymal tissue is replaced by nonfunctioning cysts, which look like a cluster of grapes (Fig. 74–1). The kidneys are grossly enlarged; each cystic kidney may enlarge to two or three times its normal size, becoming as large as a football. Other abdominal organs are displaced, and the client experiences considerable discomfort. The fluid-filled cysts are also prone to infection, rupture, and bleeding.

More than 60% of clients with PKD have high blood pressure, which may be present before PKD is diagnosed. The hypertension's cause is thought to be related to renal ischemia from the enlarging cysts. As the vessels are compressed, the renin-angiotensin system is activated, and blood pressure increases. Control of hypertension is a top priority because it also can affect renal function.

Cysts also may alter liver function or result in spontaneous rupture of vascular cysts (*berry aneurysms*) in the brain, causing sudden death. For reasons as yet unknown, kidney stones occur in 8% to 36% of the clients with PKD. Heart valve abnormalities (e.g., mitral valve prolapse), left ventricular hypertrophy (Research Applications for Nursing), and colonic diverticuli are more prevalent in clients with PKD.

Etiology

PKD has at least three autosomal dominant forms. Because the gene responsible for PKD is not located on the

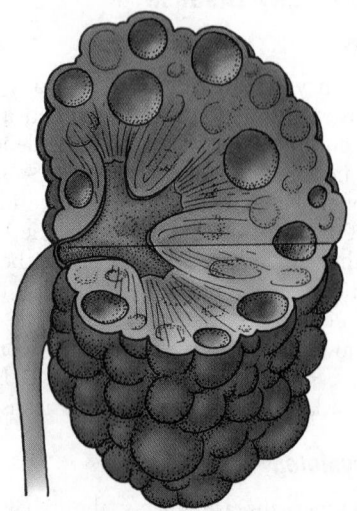

Figure 74–1. Polycystic kidney.

▷ Research Applications for Nursing

Left Ventricular Hypertrophy Is More Common in Polycystic Kidney Disease

Chapman, A. B., Johnson, A. M., Rainguet, S., et al. (1997). Left ventricular hypertrophy in autosomal dominant polycystic kidney disease. Journal of the American Society of Nephrology, 8, 1292–1297.

With cardiovascular complications being the major cause of death in polycystic kidney disease (PKD), these researchers studied 116 people with PKD and 77 control subjects to determine the relative presence of left ventricular hypertrophy (LVH). They examined the variables of severity and duration of hypertension, age, sex, renal function, renal volume, and hematocrit in those with PKD. LVH was determined by echocardiography. Hypertension was defined as greater than or equal to 140/90.

When compared with controls, those with PKD had significantly higher blood pressures as well as an increased frequency of LVH. LVH was found in 47% of males and 37% of females with PKD. The PKD subjects with LVH were significantly older, heavier, and had a greater prevalence of hypertension than the PKD subjects without LVH. Forty-eight percent of those with hypertension and PKD demonstrated LVH, whereas LVH is usually found in 12% to 30% of those with essential hypertension. Men with PKD and LVH also had higher serum creatinine levels and lower hematocrits than men with PKD, but without LVH. Women with PKD and LVH had a longer duration of hypertension than women with PKD, but without LVH.

The researchers conclude that blood pressure is a contributing factor in the development of LVH because of earlier onset of hypertension in PKD and because treatment for hypertension in PKD may be inadequate.

Critique. The PKD subjects were older and had larger body surface areas than the control subjects; this variation could affect interpretation of the results. Even though the researchers studied a number of correlating factors, there may be other factors, such as anemia, obesity, sodium intake, and genetic factors, that they did not study.

Possible Nursing Implications. The study emphasizes the importance of adequate blood pressure management in PDK. The nurse plays a large role in education about the importance of blood pressure control and also working closely with clients to help with compliance issues, which may require lifestyle changes.

sex chromosomes, men and women have an equal chance of inheriting the disease: The offspring of parents who have PKD have a 50% probability of inheriting the gene that causes the disease. The gene causing PKD-1 occurs on the short arm of chromosome 16 and accounts for 85% to 95% of the cases. PKD-2 maps to the short arm of chromosome 4 and accounts for almost all remaining genetically transmitted cases (Germino, 1997). Little is known about PKD-3.

Although there is evidence of cyst formation even in utero, clinical evidence of the disease usually does not appear until well into adulthood. Half will develop renal failure by age 50 years. PKD-1 is the most severe form both in disease progression and in mortality. In PKD-2 there is a slower rate of progression, and people experience renal failure and other complications a decade later.

At present, there is no way to prevent PKD, although early detection and management of hypertension may retard the progression of renal impairment. For adults who have one or both parents with PKD, genetic counseling and evaluation have limited use. Because clinical evidence may not be present until a client's 30s, 40s, or even 50s, the childbearing years have passed for many people. Prenatal genetic testing can identify whether the fetus has the genetic composition that will cause PKD, but this knowledge presents ethical problems.

Collaborative Management

 Assessment

➤ History

The nurse explores the family history of a client with suspected or actual PKD. The nurse asks whether either parent was known to have PKD and whether there is any family history of kidney disease. The age at which signs and symptoms developed in the parent and any related complications may have prognostic significance. The nurse also asks the client about constipation, abdominal discomfort, a change in urine color or frequency, high blood pressure, headaches, and a family history of sudden death from a stroke-like phenomenon. The nurse obtains this information with sensitivity and concern for the client's fears and anxieties.

➤ Physical Assessment/Clinical Manifestations

Chart 74–1 lists key features of PKD. Pain is the presenting symptom in 20% to 30% of clients and is noted in at least 60%. The nurse inspects the abdomen. A protruding and distended abdomen is common as the cystic kidneys swell and push abdominal contents forward. Polycystic kidneys are readily palpated because of their increased size. The nurse proceeds with *gentle* abdominal palpation because the cystic kidneys and nearby tissues may be tender and uncomfortable.

The client also may experience flank pain, reported as a dull ache or as sharp and intermittent. Sharp, intermittent pain may be the result of a ruptured cyst or the presence of a stone. The dull and aching pain may result

from increased kidney size with distention or from infection within the cyst. When a cyst ruptures, the client may notice bright red or cola-colored urine. If the urine is cloudy or foul smelling or if there is dysuria, the nurse suspects infection.

Nocturia may be an early disease sign and occurs because of decreased renal concentrating ability. As renal function further deteriorates, the client may experience increasing hypertension, edema, and obvious uremic symptoms, such as anorexia, nausea, vomiting, pruritus, and fatigue (see Chap. 75). Because berry aneurysms occur frequently in clients with PKD, a severe headache with or without neurologic or vision alterations deserves particular attention.

➤ Psychosocial Assessment

As a familial transmitted disease, polycystic kidney disease may cause complex psychosocial responses. The client frequently has had direct experience with the effects and consequences of the disease in other close family members. The person may have had a parent who died or other siblings or parent who required dialysis or transplantation. As the family history is obtained, the nurse listens carefully for spoken and unspoken feelings of anger, resentment, hostility, futility, sadness, or anxiety, which the nurse may explore further. The focus may be one or both parents or the process of diagnosis and treatment. Feelings of guilt and concern for the client's own children may further complicate adjustment.

➤ Diagnostic Assessment

Urinalysis usually reveals proteinuria once the glomeruli are involved. Hematuria may be gross or microscopic. Bacteria in the urine suggests an infection, usually in the cysts. A urine sample for culture and sensitivity testing is obtained when there is clinical or laboratory evidence of potential infection. As renal function deteriorates, serum creatinine and blood urea nitrogen (BUN) levels rise. With worsening renal function, the 24-hour creatinine clearance decreases. Renal handling of sodium may include increased sodium losses or sodium retention.

Diagnostic studies include renal sonography, computed tomography (CT), and magnetic resonance imaging (MRI). Small cysts are detectable by sonography, CT, or MRI. Renal sonography provides diagnostic evidence of PKD with minimal risk in most cases. Improvements in sonography make this a useful test for identifying even small cysts.

Interventions

Common nursing diagnoses for the client with PKD include Pain; Knowledge Deficit regarding medications, diet, and other therapies; Risk for Constipation; and Anxiety. Common collaborative problems include Potential for Infection, Hypertension, Stone Formation, or Renal Failure.

➤ Pain

Comfort strategies include chemical, physical, and psychosocial approaches. A combination may be most

---

Chart 74–1

Key Features of Polycystic Kidney Disease

- Abdominal or flank pain
- Hypertension
- Nocturia
- Increased abdominal girth
- Constipation
- Bloody or cloudy urine
- Kidney stones

Chart 74–2

Drug Therapy: Diuretics Used to Increase Urine Output

Drug	Usual Dosage	Indication	Nursing Interventions	Rationale
Osmotic diuretics (act on proximal convoluted tubule)				
Mannitol (Osmitrol♣), urea	• 50–100 g IV as a 5%–25% solution	• Causes rapid diuresis (e.g., after contrast media infusion)	• Measure fluid intake and output. • Check vial for crystals • If crystals are present, warm vial between the hands. • Administer through a filter.	• Severe dehydration is possible. • Mannitol may crystallize while on the shelf. • Crystals will dissolve with body warmth. • This will prevent remaining crystals from entering the body.
Thiazide and Thiazide-like Diuretics (act on cortical diluting site of ascending limb of loop of Henle)				
Chlorothiazide (Diuril)	• 250 mg PO, IV once to four times/day	• Hypertension	• Observe for signs and symptoms of electrolyte imbalance.	• Common complications include hypokalemia and hypercalcemia.
Hydrochlorothiazide (HydroDIURIL, Apo-Hydro♣, Urozide♣)	• 25–100 mg PO once or twice daily	• Congestive heart failure (CHF) with edema	• Monitor heart sounds for S_3, lung sounds for crackles and other signs of CHF.	• Ongoing monitoring detects complications and helps ensure prompt treatment.
Chlorthalidone (Hygroton, Uridon♣)	• 25–100 mg PO daily	• Edema, hypertension	• Do not give with NSAIDs*.	• An increased diuretic effect is seen with concomitant use of NSAIDs.
Metolazone (Zaroxolyn)	• 5–20 mg PO daily	• Edema, hypertension	• Do not give with NSAIDs.	
Loop Diuretics (act on ascending limb of loop of Henle)				
Furosemide (Lasix, Furoside♣)	• 20–80 mg PO, IV once or twice daily, maximum dose 600 mg/day	• Hypertension	• Observe for orthostatic hypotension.	• An early sign of rapid fluid volume depletion may be orthostatic hypotension.
Bumetanide (Bumex)	• 0.5–2 mg PO daily	• CHF	• Monitor for possible hyponatremia and hypokalemia.	• These agents increase excretion of both sodium and potassium.
Ethacrynic acid (Edecrin)	• 50–200 mg PO daily	• Edema (when creatinine clearance is <25–50 mL/min)	• Monitor elderly clients closely for excessive diuresis.	• Elderly are susceptible to the effects of rapid fluid changes.
Potassium-Sparing Diuretics (act on distal convoluted tubule)				
Spironolactone (Aldactone, Novo-spiroton♣)	• 25–200 mg PO once or twice daily	• Primary aldosteronism	• Observe for signs and symptoms of electrolyte imbalance.	• Hyperkalemia with cardiac manifestations is a common complication.
Triamterene (Dyrenium)	• 25–100 mg once or twice daily, maximum dose 300 mg/day	• Hypertension (with other drugs to decrease potassium loss)	• Teach client to avoid unprotected sun exposure.	• Photosensitivity reactions are possible.
Amiloride (Midamor♣)	• 5–10 mg daily	• Edema, hypertension	• Give with food or milk.	• Stomach upset is possible.

* NSAID = nonsteroidal anti-inflammatory drug.

effective. Analgesics, such as acetaminophen (Tylenol, Campain✦, Exdol✦, Robigesic✦), may be prescribed to promote comfort, but aspirin-containing compounds are avoided to prevent increased potential for bleeding. Nonsteroidal anti-inflammatory drugs (NSAIDs) should be avoided because of their tendency to adversely affect renal function.

If renal cyst infection is the cause of discomfort, the physician orders a lipid-soluble antibiotic such as trimethoprim/sulfamethoxazole (Bactrim, Septra, Trimpex) or ciprofloxacin (Cipro), which penetrates the cyst wall (Beebe, 1996). Monitoring of renal function through assay of serum creatinine prevents nephrotoxicity resulting from antibiotic therapy. Application of dry heat to the abdomen or flank may promote comfort when renal cysts are infected. When pain is severe or debilitating, cysts can be decompressed with percutaneous needle aspiration and drainage (Beebe, 1996).

The nurse teaches the client methods of enhancing relaxation and promoting comfort via deep breathing, guided imagery, or other relaxation strategies. The overall goal is client self-management. (See Chapter 9 for pain management.)

➤ Constipation

The nurse also teaches the client how to prevent constipation. The teaching plan covers adequate fluid intake, the role of increased dietary fiber when fluid intake is more than 2500 mL/24 hr, and the need for regular exercise to achieve regular bowel elimination. The nurse explains that as the polycystic kidneys increase in size, pressure on the large intestine may further impede normal peristalsis. Consequently, the client should know that these recommendations for bowel management may change. Furthermore, when renal failure develops, the nurse assists the client in modifying the bowel management program. These modifications depend on the dialysis selected and the need to avoid excessive fluid volume and hyperkalemia. The nurse may also advise about appropriate use of stool softeners and bulk agents, including the monitored use of laxatives, necessary to prevent complications related to chronic constipation.

➤ Anxiety

Concerns related to future or current needs for dialysis and transplantation may be overwhelming, even though the client may have anticipated this outcome for years. The statement that one actually needs dialysis or transplantation creates a difficult new reality, and adjustment must begin anew. Referral to dialysis support groups may help the client cope effectively with this new challenge.

➤ Hypertension and Renal Failure

Blood pressure control is necessary to minimize cardiovascular consequences and retard the progression of renal dysfunction. Nursing interventions include education to promote self-management and understanding (see Chap. 38 for more on hypertension). When renal impairment is evident through a decreased concentrating ability (e.g., nocturia, low urine specific gravity), the nurse encourages the client to drink at least 2 L of fluid per day to prevent fluid volume deficit, which could further affect renal function. Blood pressure may be controlled by restricting excess dietary sodium intake. Fluid volume intake is not restricted so intravascular volume depletion and decreased renal perfusion do not occur.

Medications prescribed for blood pressure control include antihypertensive agents and diuretics. Antihypertensive agents include angiotensin-converting enzyme (ACE) inhibitors, calcium channel blockers, beta-blockers, and vasodilators (see Chart 38–2). Mild diuretics (Chart 74–2) may be effective for clients with some decrease in kidney function. As renal function decreases, ACE inhibitors will not be able to be continued, and more potent diuretics may be needed. When the disease progresses to the point that urine output is unresponsive to diuretics, fluid and sodium must be restricted.

The nurse teaches the client, family, or significant other how to measure and record blood pressure. The nurse also helps the client establish a schedule for self-administering medications, monitoring daily weights, and blood pressure record-keeping (Chart 74–3). The nurse also explains potential side effects of the medications. The nurse makes written materials, such as medication teaching cards and booklets, available.

A low-sodium diet is frequently prescribed to control the hypertension that usually accompanies PKD. Some clients may experience a salt-wasting phenomenon, however, and not require a sodium-restricted diet. As the disease progresses, the physician may limit the client's protein intake to retard the development of renal failure. The nurse assists the client, family, or significant other in understanding the recommended diet plan and clarifies its rationale. The nurse works closely with the dietitian to foster the client's understanding. The nurse may also initiate a referral for nutritional counseling.

➤ Potential for Infection or Stones

See Chapter 73 for information and treatment of urinary tract infections and urinary calculi (stones).

Chart 74–3

Education Guide: Polycystic Kidney Disease

- Measure and record your blood pressure daily.
- Take your temperature if you suspect you have a fever.
- Weigh yourself every day at the same time of day with the same amount of clothing; notify your physician or nurse if you have a sudden weight gain.
- Limit your intake of salt to help control your blood pressure.
- If your urine is foul smelling or if there is blood in your urine, notify your physician or nurse.
- Notify your physician or nurse if you have a headache that does not go away or if you have visual disturbances.
- Monitor bowel movements to prevent constipation.

➤ *Health Care Resources*

The Polycystic Kidney Research Foundation was formed to promote research and education about PKD. Many publications are available on request; for some materials, there is a fee. Chapters of the National Kidney Foundation (NKF) and the American Association of Kidney Patients (AAKP) may also provide resources for client information and support.

OBSTRUCTIVE DISORDERS

Hydronephrosis, Hydroureter, and Urethral Stricture

Overview

Hydronephrosis and hydroureter are disorders usually associated with obstruction of urine outflow. Urethral strictures also obstruct outflow. Prompt recognition and treatment are crucial to prevent permanent renal damage.

In *hydronephrosis*, the kidney becomes enlarged as urine accumulates in the pelvis and calyceal system. Because the capacity of the renal pelvis is normally 5 to 8 mL, obstructions within it or at the ureteropelvic junction (UPJ) quickly result in renal pelvic distention. As the volume of urine increases, the calix dilates and the medulla endures increasing pressure. Over time, which might be a matter of hours, the vasculature and renal tubules can be damaged extensively (Fig. 74–2).

In clients with *hydroureter,* the pathophysiologic effects are similar, but the obstruction is lower in the urinary tract. The ureter is most likely to become obstructed where the iliac vessels cross or at the ureterovesical entry. Dilation of the ureter proximal to the point of obstruction

results in enlargement as urine continues to accumulate (see Fig. 74–2).

In a client with a *urethral stricture,* the obstruction is most distal in the urinary tract. Bladder distention, then, occurs before hydroureter and hydronephrosis. The pathologic consequences may be similar, however, without prompt treatment (also see Chap. 73).

A urinary obstruction can cause structural damage when pressure builds up directly on tissue. Within the nephron, the tubular filtrate pressure also increases as drainage through the collecting system is impaired. With this added pressure, the force opposing glomerular filtration is enhanced, glomerular filtration decreases or ceases, and renal failure results. Nitrogenous waste products (urea, creatinine, and uric acid) and electrolytes (sodium, potassium, chloride, and phosphorus) are retained in the serum, and renal regulation of acid-base balance is impaired.

Disorders that can cause hydronephrosis or hydroureter include tumors, stones, trauma, congenital structural defects, and retroperitoneal fibrosis. Treatment can prevent hydronephrosis and hydroureter and thus prevents permanent renal damage. The specific time needed to prevent permanent damage is uncertain and depends on the client's underlying renal status. For some clients, permanent damage may occur in less than 48 hours; for others, it may occur after several weeks.

Collaborative Management

 Assessment

The nurse obtains a history from the client, focusing on known renal or urologic disorders. A history of childhood urinary tract problems may signal that structural defects are present that have not been identified previously. The nurse inquires about the client's pattern of urination, especially its amount, frequency, color, clarity, and odor. The nurse also asks about recent flank or abdominal pain. Chills, fever, and malaise may be present with a urinary tract infection (UTI).

The nurse inspects each flank to identify asymmetry, which may occur with a renal mass, and *gently* palpates the client's abdomen to identify any areas of tenderness. The nurse also palpates and percusses the urinary bladder to detect distention. Gentle pressure on the abdomen may cause urine leakage, which reflects a full urinary bladder and possible obstruction of the bladder/urethral junction.

Urinalysis may show bacteria or white blood cells if infection is present. When urinary tract obstruction is prolonged, microscopic examination may reveal tubular epithelial cells. The chemical analysis of serum is normal unless decreased glomerular filtration has occurred; with a decreased glomerular filtration rate (GFR), serum creatinine and BUN levels increase. Serum electrolyte levels may also be altered and indicate hyperkalemia, hyperphosphatemia, hypocalcemia, and metabolic acidosis (bicarbonate deficit).

Intravenous urography reveals ureteral or renal pelvis dilation. Urinary outflow obstruction may be revealed by sonography (renal echography) or computed tomography (CT).

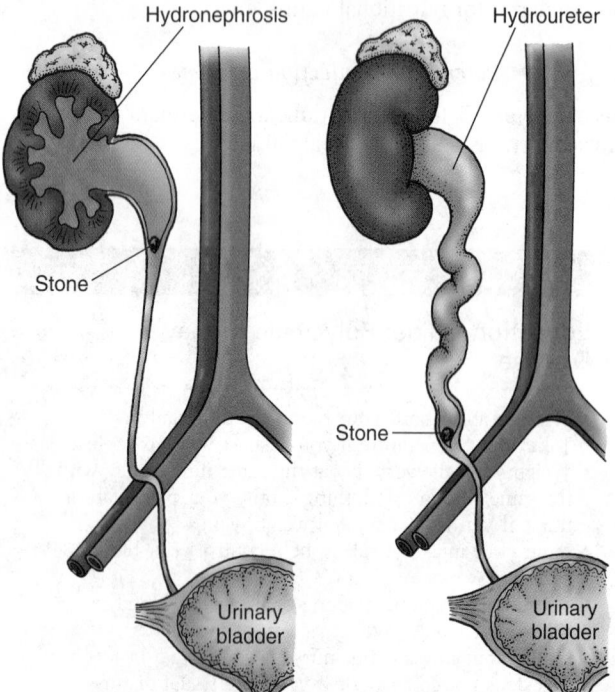

Figure 74–2. Hydronephrosis is caused by obstruction in the upper part of the ureter; hydroureter is caused by obstruction in the lower part of the ureter.

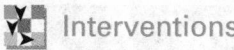 Interventions

Urinary retention and potential for infection are the primary problems. Failure to treat the cause of urinary obstruction may lead to infection and renal failure. (See Infectious Disorders below and Chapter 75 for renal failure.)

INFECTIOUS DISORDERS

Normally, the urinary system is one in which a sterile body fluid (urine) is excreted. The unobstructed and complete passage of urine from the renal and urinary systems is critical to the sterility of the urinary tract. When a structural abnormality, either congenital or acquired, is present, the potential for degenerative changes from infection is dramatically increased. *Urinary tract infection* (UTI) usually refers to infections in this sterile system. Pyelonephritis traditionally refers to bacterial infection within the kidney and renal pelvis, the *upper* urinary tract. (Infections within the *lower* urinary tract are described in Chapter 73.)

Pyelonephritis
Overview

With improved diagnostic techniques and a more precise understanding of the inflammatory response, pyelonephritis has come to refer to active microorganisms or the remaining effects of previous kidney infections. *Acute* pyelonephritis describes the condition resulting from an active bacterial infection, *chronic* pyelonephritis from repeated or continued upper urinary tract infections. Chronic pyelonephritis is usually superimposed on an anatomic urinary tract anomaly, urinary obstruction, or, most commonly, vesicoureteral reflux (Rubin et al., 1996). The vesicoureteral junction is the point where the ureter joins the bladder. Reflux refers to reverse (e.g., backward, upward, ascending) flow of urine toward the renal pelvis and kidney.

Pathophysiology

In pyelonephritis, microorganisms usually ascend from the lower urinary tract into the renal pelvis. Infection from organisms carried in the blood (hematogenous or blood-borne infection) may occur, but with much less frequency. Bacteria activate the inflammatory response, which mobilizes the white blood cells, specifically polymorphonuclear leukocytes and monocytes. As with any inflammatory response, local edema results.

In acute pyelonephritis, there is acute interstitial inflammation, tubular cell necrosis, and a tendency for abscess formation. Abscesses, pockets of localized infection, can appear in the capsule, cortex, or medulla. The pattern of infection within the kidney is not a uniform one; therefore, normal tissue and tubules lie adjacent to infected areas. As the inflammatory process subsides, fibrosis or scar tissue develops. The calices become blunted, and scars develop in the interstitial tissue.

Vesicoureteral and intrarenal reflux of infected urine are the major mechanisms responsible for chronic pyelonephritis. Some papillae in the kidney do not close with increased intracaliceal pressure, causing intrarenal reflux. These refluxing papillae are most often located in the upper and lower poles of the kidney and therefore are more susceptible to chronic pyelonephritis. Inflammation, fibrosis, and deformity of the renal pelvis and calices, especially in the upper and lower poles, is evident. Repeated infectious episodes or ongoing infection produce additional scar tissue. Vascular, glomerular, and tubular changes within the scars can occur. Eventually, glomerular function, tubular reabsorption, and secretion become impaired, and renal function diminished (Fig. 74–3).

Etiology

Single episodes of *acute* pyelonephritis may result from the entry of bacteria associated with pregnancy, obstruction, or reflux. *Chronic* pyelonephritis is usually associated with structural abnormalities and/or obstruction with reflux. Vesicoureteral reflux or obstruction leading to chronic pyelonephritis is often due to stones, obstruction, or neurogenic impairment involving the voiding mechanism. Reflux is more common in children, who as adults display scarring indicative of chronic pyelonephritis. Clients who develop chronic pyelonephritis without having reflux as a child are adults with a history of spinal cord injury, bladder tumor, prostatic hypertrophy, or urinary tract stones.

Acute or chronic pyelonephritis is more likely to occur in clients who have had instrumentation of the urinary tract (such as placement of a urinary catheter), those who have diabetes mellitus or chronic renal calculi, or those who overuse analgesics. For clients who have diabetes mellitus, the development and progression of autonomic neuropathy and subsequent bladder atony increase the tendency to acute and/or chronic pyelonephritis. Similarly, in clients with chronic stone disease, the calculi provide a site for ongoing infection and resultant renal scarring, and analgesic use has been associated with papillary necrosis, which then permits reflux.

Although many organisms can cause lower urinary tract infections, the most common pyelonephritis-causing orga-

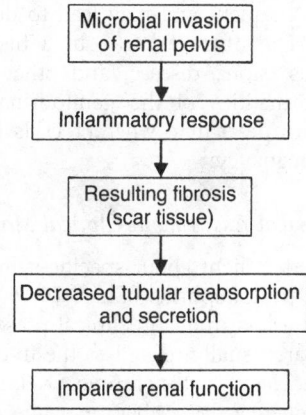

Figure 74–3. Pathophysiology of pyelonephritis.

nism is *Escherichia coli. Enterococcus faecalis* is common in hospitalized clients. Both are common organisms of the gastrointestinal tract. Non–*E. coli* organisms such as *Proteus mirabilis, Klebsiella,* and *Pseudomonas aeruginosa* and the more antibiotic-resistant organisms are also common in hospitalized clients. When the infection is blood borne, common infecting organisms include *Staphylococcus aureus,* the *Candida* and *Salmonella* species, and *P. aeruginosa.*

Theories of noninfectious or idiopathic causes of intrarenal scarring and eventual outcome of the pyelonephritis include an antibody reaction, cell-mediated immunity against the bacterial antigens, or an autoimmune reaction.

Incidence/Prevalence

The exact incidence and prevalence of pyelonephritis, acute or chronic, are not known. Lower urinary tract infections are more common in women; hence women overall have more cases of pyelonephritis. After age 65 years, however, rates for men increase greatly because of the increased incidence of prostatitis. The peak incidence of obstructive uropathy as a cause of end-stage renal disease (ESRD) occurs at age 75 to 79 years, with more men being affected than women (U.S. Renal Data Systems, 1995).

The rate of "kidney infections" is reported as 8.1 per 100,000 for those aged 18 to 44 years, 7.4 for those aged 45 to 74 years, and 12.1 for those older than 75 years (Collins, 1993). Overlapping definitions and lack of clarity in specific etiology (e.g., is the disorder from obstruction or infection?) are evident in the statistics reported for the causes of ESRD. Approximately 2% of ESRD cases result from disorders related to "obstructive nephropathy" (U.S. Renal Data Systems, 1995). Acute and chronic pyelonephritis and reflux nephropathy diagnoses are included in these categories, as are other causes.

Collaborative Management

 Assessment

➤ History

The nurse asks the client about any previous experiences with pyelonephritis and of similar symptoms in the past. Recurrences are frequent and may lead to deterioration of renal function. The nurse asks about a history of UTIs, diabetes mellitus, stone disease, and other structural or functional abnormalities of the genitourinary tract. The nurse attempts to determine whether UTIs have been associated with pregnancy.

➤ Physical Assessment/Clinical Manifestations

The nurse asks the client about specific symptoms associated with acute pyelonephritis (Chart 74–4). Chronic pyelonephritis has a less dramatic clinical presentation; signs and symptoms are usually related to the infection or renal impairment associated with chronic pyelonephritis. The nurse asks the client to describe any vague or nonspecific urinary symptoms or abdominal discomfort and inquires

---

> ### Chart 74–4
>
> ## Key Features of Acute Pyelonephritis
>
> - Fever
> - Chills
> - Tachycardia and tachypnea
> - Flank, back, or loin pain
> - Tender costal vertebral angle (CVA)
> - Abdominal, often colicky, discomfort
> - Nausea and vomiting
> - General malaise or fatigue
> - Burning, urgency, or frequency of urination
> - Nocturia

---

about any history of repeated, low-grade fevers. Often the client with chronic pyelonephritis will have asymptomatic bacteremia. Chart 74–5 outlines the renal effects of chronic pyelonephritis.

The nurse inspects the flanks and gently palpates in the costovertebral angle (CVA) (see Fig. 72–9). The nurse inspects each CVA to determine any enlargement or asymmetry, edema, or erythema, possible manifestations of inflammation. If there is no local tenderness to light palpation in either CVA, a specially trained nurse firmly percusses each area. Tenderness or discomfort reflects evidence of infection or inflammation.

➤ Psychosocial Assessment

As with any disorder associated with the genitourinary tract, the client may have feelings of anxiety, embarrassment, or guilt. The nurse listens carefully to the client's description for evidence of generalized anxiety or specific fears and prevents embarrassment during assessment. Feelings of guilt, often associated with sexual habits or practices, may be masked through denial, such as delay in seeking treatment, or vague, nonspecific responses to specific or direct questions. The nurse encourages clients to tell their own story in familiar, comfortable language. This approach is extremely valuable in promoting the rapport and trust necessary for more in-depth interviewing.

➤ Laboratory Assessment

A urinalysis shows white blood cells and bacteria. The urine should be analyzed by Gram's stain procedures to determine whether gram-positive or -negative organisms are responsible. The urine sample for culture and sensitivity testing, obtained by the clean-catch method, reveals the bacterial species and susceptibility or resistance of the specific organism to various antibiotics. In clients with recurrent episodes of pyelonephritis or upper UTIs, more specific testing of bacterial antigens and antibodies may help determine whether the same organism is responsible for the recurrent infections.

Blood cultures are examined for specific pathogenic microorganisms. Nonspecific serologic tests include the C-reactive protein and erythrocyte sedimentation rate often elevated in infection.

Chart 74–5

Key Renal Features of Chronic Pyelonephritis

- Hypertension
- Inability to conserve sodium
- Decreased concentrating ability (nocturia)
- Tendency to develop hyperkalemia and acidosis

➤ Radiographic Assessment

X-ray examination of the kidneys, ureters, and bladder (KUB) and intravenous urography are performed initially to determine the presence of stones or obstructions. For many clients, a cystourethrogram is also indicated, at least for the first episode. These radiographic procedures define urinary tract structures and identify any structural defects. Specific defects to be identified include foreign bodies, such as stones; obstruction to the outflow of urine, such as tumors, structural defects, or prostate enlargement; and urine reflux, associated with incompetent ureterovesical valve closure.

See Chapter 72 for more information on radiographic diagnostic assessment.

➤ Other Diagnostic Assessment

Several other diagnostic tests are currently being researched, including examining antibody-coated bacteria in urine; certain enzymes, such as lactate dehydrogenase isoenzyme 5; and radionuclide scintillation (e.g., the gallium scan). Examining urine for antibody-coated bacteria is not useful for therapy. Its primary value is apparently in identifying clients who may need long-term antibiotic therapy. High-molecular-weight enzymes in urine, such as lactate dehydrogenase isoenzyme 5, is also not specific. These enzymes are present with any process associated with renal tissue deterioration. The gallium scan, however, can identify active pyelonephritis or abscesses in the perinephric region.

 Analysis

➤ Common Nursing Diagnoses and Collaborative Problems

The primary common nursing diagnosis for the client with pyelonephritis is Pain (flank and abdominal) related to inflammation and infection. A common collaborative problem is Potential for Renal Failure.

➤ Additional Nursing Diagnoses and Collaborative Problems

The client with pyelonephritis may have the following additional nursing diagnoses:
- Infection or Risk for Infection related to inadequate primary defenses (urinary stasis) or instrumentation
- Knowledge Deficit regarding medical diagnosis and therapy related to lack of information resources

- Activity Intolerance related to fatigue, debilitation, and generalized weakness associated with the infection
- Fear of development of chronic renal failure related to inability to control recurrent infections
- Hyperthermia related to increased metabolic rate from infection

An additional collaborative problem is Potential for Sepsis and Septic Shock.

 Planning and Implementation

Pain

Planning: Expected Outcomes. The client should indicate that he or she has achieved a state of comfort allowing for adequate rest, nutrition, and activity.

Interventions. Interventions may be nonsurgical or surgical methods. However, the availability and success of several noninvasive techniques that result in stone crushing, such as extracorporeal shock wave lithotripsy and percutaneous ultrasonic pyelolithotomy (see Chap. 73), have decreased the need for surgery. Surgical interventions may be necessary to correct structural defects or control infection.

Nonsurgical Management. Nonsurgical interventions include the use of medications, diet and fluid therapy, and educational counseling to ensure the client's understanding about the treatment.

Drug Therapy. The physician orders analgesic and urinary antiseptic medications (such as nitrofurantoin [Macrodantin]) to provide comfort and antibiotics to definitively treat the infection, the source of discomfort. Initially, the antibiotics are broad spectrum. After urine and blood culture and sensitivity reports are obtained, the physician may order a more specific antibiotic.

Diet Therapy. For healing to occur, the client's nutritional intake must include adequate numbers of calories and all food groups. Fluid intake is recommended at 2 to 3 L/day unless medically contraindicated.

Surgical Management. Surgical interventions may be needed to correct structural abnormalities causing urinary reflux or obstruction of urinary outflow or to eradicate the source of intractable infection.

Preoperative Care. Antibiotics are given, usually intravenously, to achieve adequate blood levels or sterile blood culture results. The nurse also teaches the client the nature and purpose of the proposed surgery, the expected outcome, and expectations of how the client can participate.

Operative Procedures. The surgical procedures may be one of the following:
- Pyelolithotomy (stone removal from the renal pelvis)
- Nephrectomy (removal of the kidney)
- Ureteral diversion
- Reimplantation of ureter to restore the bladder drainage mechanism

A pyelolithotomy is indicated for removal of a large calculus in the renal pelvis that blocks urinary flow and causes infection. Nephrectomy is considered a last resort when all other measures to eradicate infection have failed. For clients with incompetent ureterovesical valve closure or dilated ureters, ureteroplasty (repair or revision) or ureteral reimplantation (through another site in the posterior bladder wall) preserves renal function and eliminates infections.

Postoperative Care. See Chapter 73 for specific postoperative nursing care for the client undergoing urologic surgery.

Potential For Renal Failure

Planning: Expected Outcomes. It is expected that the client under treatment will conserve existing renal function for as long as possible and then, once the process of renal failure begins, to retard the progression of renal failure.

Interventions. The physician or nurse practitioner orders specific antibiotics to treat the infection. The nurse explains the importance of taking all the medication as directed. The nurse also discusses with the client and family the importance of regular follow-up examinations and completing diagnostic tests as recommended.

As with polycystic kidney disease, control of blood pressure is necessary to prevent and retard the progression of renal dysfunction. When renal impairment is evident through a decreased concentrating ability (e.g., nocturia, low urine specific gravity), the nurse encourages the client to drink at least 2 L of fluid per day to prevent fluid volume deficit, which could further affect renal function. When dietary protein is restricted to delay the onset of renal failure, the nurse refers the client to the dietitian as needed. Other interventions related to the progression of chronic renal failure are covered in Chapter 75.

 Continuing Care

Pyelonephritis, acute or chronic, provokes fear and anxiety in the client and family. The severity of the acute process and its potential to develop into a chronic process are quite frightening. Both the client and the family require emotional reassurance that treatment and attention to preventive measures can be accomplished.

➤ Health Teaching

After assessing the client's and family's understanding of pyelonephritis and the suggested treatment, the nurse explains
- Medication administration (purpose, timing, frequency, duration, and possible side effects)
- The role of nutrition and adequate fluid intake
- The need for a balance between rest and activity, including any limitations after surgery
- The signs and symptoms of disease recurrence
- Using previously successful coping mechanisms

The nurse advises the client to complete all prescribed

antibiotic regimens. The nurse also encourages the client to report any side effects or unusual symptoms to the prescribing health team member rather than suspend the regimen. The nurse refers the client and family for nutritional counseling as needed, because many clients have special nutritional requirements, such as those caused by diabetes mellitus or pregnancy.

➤ Home Care Management

The client with pyelonephritis often needs hospitalization, which may include medical or surgical intervention or both. If no surgery is performed, the client may need assistance with self-care, nutrition, and medication administration at home. If surgical intervention is necessary, the client may require help with incision care, self-care, and transportation for follow-up medical appointments.

➤ Health Care Resources

The client may also briefly need a community health nurse to help administer medications or nutrition at home. Housekeeping services may also be helpful while the client is regaining strength.

 Evaluation

The nurse evaluates the effectiveness of the interventions based on the identified nursing diagnoses. Expected outcomes may include that the client will
- Demonstrate methods of enhancing comfort
- Describe the role of antibiotics and self-administration of medications
- Explain and offer techniques to ensure adequate nutrition and hydration
- Describe the plan for post-treatment follow-up, including knowledge of recurrent symptoms

Renal Abscess

An *abscess* is a collection of fluid and cells caused by the inflammatory response to bacteria. An abscess may occur within the renal parenchyma (renal abscess), in the renal and Gerota's fascia (perinephric abscess), or in the flank. Abscess is suspected when fever and symptoms are not relieved promptly by antibiotic therapy.

Diagnosis of a renal or perirenal abscess is readily accomplished via sonography or computed tomography (CT). Arteriography and radionuclide scintillation methods (e.g., gallium scan) also may be diagnostic. Symptoms of a renal abscess include fever, flank pain, and general malaise. Local flank edema and erythema may be observed.

Drainage by surgical incision or needle aspiration is often necessary. Appropriate broad-spectrum antibiotics are also prescribed.

Renal Tuberculosis

The genitourinary tract is the most common extrapulmonary site of tuberculosis. Approximately 10% of new tuberculosis cases are extrapulmonary (Rubin et al., 1996). Tuberculosis of the kidney is sometimes called *granulomatous nephritis.* After *Mucobacterium tuberculosis* invades the kidneys, usually by a blood-borne route, an inflammatory response is activated that forms scar tissue (granuloma) that replaces renal parenchyma. Clinically, clients may experience urinary frequency, dysuria, hematuria and/or proteinuria, flank pain or renal colic secondary to the passage of clots or stones, pyuria, and hypertension. Skin test (e.g., purified protein derivative, or PPD) or chest x-ray film evidence of tuberculosis may or may not be present.

Clients with current or previous pulmonary tuberculosis who show signs of unexplained fever, hematuria, and sterile pyuria are at high risk for renal tuberculosis. The diagnosis is made through urine culture of three clean-catch, first-morning specimens. Other genitourinary sites for tuberculosis include the prostate, epididymis, ureters, testes, bladder, and seminal vesicles.

Chemotherapy is the primary treatment. Current recommendations include a 2-month course of rifampin, isoniazid, and pyrazinamide, followed by 4 months of rifampin and isoniazid. Three to six more months of rifampin and isoniazid may be recommended for men who may be harboring the organism in the prostate (Rubin et al., 1996).

Complications include loss of renal function, nephrolithiasis, obstructive uropathy, and bacterial superinfection of the urinary tract. Surgical excision of diseased tissue may be indicated to preserve renal function.

GLOMERULAR DISORDERS

Both primary and secondary diseases or syndromes result in glomerular injury (Glassock et al., 1996; Adler et al., 1996). In primary disease (Table 74–1), the glomeruli are the predominant tissue involved; extrarenal effects of primary disease stem from the glomerular injury. Most primary diseases and syndromes have an immunologic component and are discussed in the next section. Many primary diseases also have an underlying genetic basis. Secondary glomerular disease refers to the situation where glomerular involvement is part of another disease. For example, certain systemic diseases and infections can have renal effects and cause glomerular injury (Table 74–2).

Each primary or secondary disease or syndrome has a specific pathophysiology and associated clinical manifestations. Their *glomerular* effects, however, are caused by injury to the glomeruli and result in proteinuria, hematuria, decreased glomerular filtration rate (GFR), edema, and hypertension due to sodium retention. The extent and

TABLE 74–1

Primary Glomerular Diseases and Syndromes
• Acute glomerulonephritis
• Rapidly progressive glomerulonephritis (RPGN)
• Chronic glomerulonephritis
• Nephrotic syndrome
• Persisting urinary abnormalities with few or no symptoms

TABLE 74–2

Secondary Glomerular Diseases and Syndromes
• Systemic lupus erythematosus (SLE)
• Schönlein-Henoch purpura
• Goodpasture syndrome
• Systemic necrotizing vasculitis
• Wegener granulomatosis
• Periarteritis nodosa (also called polyarteritis nodosa)
• Amyloidosis
• Diabetic glomerulopathy
• HIV-associated nephropathy
• Alport syndrome
• Multiple myeloma
• Viral hepatitis B
• Viral hepatitis C
• Cirrhosis
• Sickle-cell disease
• Nonstreptococcal postinfectious acute GN
• Infective endocarditis
• Hemolytic-uremic syndrome
• Thrombotic thrombocytopenic purpura (TTP)

duration of renal injury, prognosis, and specific known cause vary considerably among these syndromes.

Most conditions causing secondary glomerular disease are beyond the scope of this chapter. Some of the conditions are discussed elsewhere (e.g., systemic lupus erythematosus in Chapter 24). Diabetic nephropathy is discussed later in this chapter and in Chapter 68.

IMMUNOLOGIC DISORDERS

Immunologic changes may result in injury to the glomeruli, interstitium, and/or tubules; effects may be acute or chronic. Both humoral and cellular immune responses are involved. The resultant renal disorder may be localized in the kidneys or be a systemic disease.

Immunologic Glomerular Disorders

"Glomerulonephritis," an inconsistently described term, is the third leading cause of ESRD. Approximately 16% of all ESRD cases are attributed to one of the primary or secondary causes of glomerulonephritis (U.S. Renal Data Systems, 1995).

Most forms of glomerulonephritis are associated with accumulation of immune complexes in the glomeruli. An immune complex is made up of antigen and antibody. The antigen can be normal kidney tissue such as the glomerular basement membrane, tubular basement membrane, or mesangium or could be dissolved in a body fluid (e.g., blood). Bacteria and viruses are also examples of antigens. Increasingly, exposure to bacteria, viruses, drugs, or other toxins is believed to be the trigger for glomerular injury.

Antibody reaction with antigen can lead to immune complex formation either directly in, or deposited in, glomerular tissue. The immune complexes activate many mediators, including complement, leukocytes, and coagulation proteins, responsible for the resultant renal tissue injury. Some of the major responses promoting tissue injury include disruption of cell membranes, local edema, movement of macrophages and neutrophils to the site of inflammation, and activation of platelets.

Acute Glomerulonephritis

Overview

An infection frequently precedes the renal manifestations of acute glomerulonephritis (GN). The onset of symptoms is usually sudden (averaging 10 days from time of infection); recovery is usually complete and quick, although a broad range of severity of illness exists. The term *acute nephritic syndrome* also describes this disorder.

Most causes are postinfectious (Table 74–3) or related to other multisystem diseases (see Table 74–2). The incidence of acute GN is unknown, but post-streptococcal GN is more common in males.

Collaborative Management

 Assessment

➤ *History*

The nurse inquires about recent infections, particularly of the skin or upper respiratory tract, and about recent travel or other activities with possible exposure to viruses, bacteria, fungi, or parasites. Recent illnesses, surgery, or other invasive procedures may suggest infections. The nurse also inquires about any known systemic diseases, such as systemic lupus erythematosus (SLE), which could cause acute GN.

TABLE 74–3

Infectious Causes of Acute Glomerulonephritis

- Group A beta-hemolytic *Streptococcus*
- Staphylococcal or gram-negative bacteremia or sepsis
- Pneumococcal, *Mycoplasma,* or *Klebsiella* pneumonia
- Syphilis
- Visceral abscesses
- Infective endocarditis
- Hepatitis B
- Infectious mononucleosis
- Measles
- Mumps
- Rocky Mountain Spotted Fever
- Cytomegaloviral (CMV) infection
- Histoplasmosis
- Toxoplasmosis
- Varicella
- *Chlamydia psittaci* infection
- Coxsackievirus infection
- Any bacterial, parasitic, fungal, or viral infection (potentially)

➤ *Physical Assessment/Clinical Manifestations*

The nurse inspects the client's skin for lesions or recent incisions and the face, eyelids, hands, and other peripheral tissues for edema (present in approximately 75% of the clients with acute GN). In assessing for circulatory congestion and fluid overload, which frequently accompanies the sodium and fluid retention associated with acute GN, the nurse inquires about any difficulty in breathing, nocturnal or exertional dyspnea, or orthopnea. The nurse also assesses for neck vein distention, an S_3 heart sound (gallop rhythm), and crackles in the lung fields.

The nurse also asks about changes in urination pattern and notes any change in urine color. Gross hematuria may occur, but microscopic hematuria occurs up to 66% of the time, and clients frequently describe it as smoky, reddish-brown, rusty, or cola colored. The nurse asks the client about dysuria (common), or oliguria, a decrease in urine produced, which occurs occasionally. The nurse weighs the client because changes in urinary output may result in fluid retention.

The nurse measures blood pressure and compares results with the client's baseline blood pressure. Mild to moderate hypertension frequently accompanies acute GN due to sodium and fluid retention. The client may have symptoms of fatigue, lack of energy, anorexia, nausea, and/or vomiting if uremia from renal failure is present.

ELDERLY CONSIDERATIONS

The less common signs are especially frequent in the elderly. Circulatory congestion often dominates the elderly client's clinical picture. Acute GN is easily confused with congestive heart failure.

➤ *Laboratory Assessment*

Urinalysis reveals red blood cells (hematuria) and protein (proteinuria). Microscopic examination of an early morning specimen of urine is preferred because the urine is most acidic and formed elements are more intact at that time. Further microscopic examination, usually performed personally by the physician or consulting nephrologist, often reveals red blood cell casts. Renal tubular epithelial cells, leukocytes, white blood cell casts, granular casts, or hyaline casts also may be present in the urine. There is usually a positive urinary sediment assay.

The glomerular filtration rate (GFR), measured by the 24-hour urine test for creatinine clearance, may be decreased to 50 mL/minute. Yet serum creatinine levels may be normal or at the upper limits of normal. Serum urea nitrogen levels, however, are usually increased. The elderly client may have a more pronounced decline in GFR.

A 24-hour urine collection for total protein assay is also obtained. The protein excretion value for clients with acute GN may be increased to 500 mg to 3 g/24 hr in more than 75% of clients. Serum albumin levels may be decreased because of the large amount of protein lost in the urine and because of fluid retention (dilutional value).

Specimens from blood, skin, or throat are obtained for culture, if indicated. Other serologic tests include
- Antistreptolysin O titers
- C3 complement levels

- Cryoglobulins (IgG)
- Antinuclear antibodies (ANA)
- Circulating immune complexes

Antistreptolysin O titers are increased after group A beta-hemolytic *Streptococcus* infections. Complement levels are decreased when the complement system is activated; a variety of causes may be implicated, such as SLE and postinfectious factors. Type III cryoglobulins may be found during acute illness. Antinuclear antibodies suggest an autoimmune response, and SLE is only one possibility. Circulating immune complexes containing IgG and C3 are frequently detected.

➤ *Other Diagnostic Assessment*

A percutaneous renal biopsy (see Chap. 72) may provide a precise diagnosis of the pathologic condition, assist in determining the prognosis, and help outline treatment. The specific tissue morphology is determined by light microscopy, immunofluorescent stains, and electron microscopy to identify

- The type of cellular proliferation (light microscopy)
- The presence of immunoglobulins (immunofluorescence)
- The specific type of tissue deposits (electron microscopy)

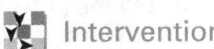 Interventions

Common nursing diagnoses include Altered Nutrition: Less than Body Requirements related to increased metabolic demands and anorexia and Risk for Activity Intolerance related to fatigue, fluid volume excess, and loss of energy. Potential for Renal Failure is a common collaborative problem.

Treatment for cases of acute GN with an infectious cause would be the appropriate anti-infective. In poststreptococcal GN, penicillin, erythromycin, or azithromycin are usually prescribed. The nurse checks the client's known allergies before administering any medication. To prevent infection spread, the physician also may order anti-infective drugs for persons in immediate close contact with the client. The nurse stresses personal hygiene and basic infection control principles such as handwashing to prevent spread of the organism.

For clients with circulatory congestion, hypertension, and edema, the physician orders sodium and water restriction along with diuretics. Antihypertensive medications (see Chart 38–2) may be needed to control hypertension. The usual fluid allowance is equal to the 24-hour urinary output plus 500 to 600 mL for insensible fluid losses. Clients with oliguria also usually have urinary retention of potassium and blood urea nitrogen (BUN) level elevation. Potassium and protein intake may be restricted to prevent hyperkalemia and additional uremic manifestations of the elevated BUN. Nausea, vomiting, or anorexia indicates that uremia is interfering with nutrition. If uremic symptoms or fluid volume excess cannot be controlled, dialysis (see Chap. 75) will be necessary. Plasmapheresis also may be attempted (see Chap. 46); steroids are not usually helpful.

To conserve and maintain the client's energy, the nurse

encourages and promotes a restful environment by eliminating unnecessary intrusions, spacing activities, and coordinating necessary assessments and treatments. The nurse demonstrates energy conservation techniques by alternating active periods with rest periods. The client also needs to minimize emotional stress, and the nurse encourages the client to practice relaxation techniques and participate in diversional activities (see Chap. 8).

The nurse also instructs the client, family, or significant other about the purpose and desired effects of prescribed medications, the dosage and route of administration, and potentially adverse side effects. The nurse ensures that the client and family understand dietary or fluid modifications, including methods of detecting fluid retention. The nurse advises the client to

- Measure weight and blood pressure daily at the same time each day
- Notify primary care provider of sudden increases in weight or any increase in blood pressure
- Perform regular exercise, as tolerated
- Schedule extra rest and sleep periods

If short-term dialysis is required for control of fluid volume excess or uremic symptoms, the nurse explains peritoneal or vascular access care and dialysis schedules and routines (also see Chap. 75).

Rapidly Progressive Glomerulonephritis

Rapidly progressive glomerulonephritis (RPGN), a variant of acute nephritis, is also called *crescentic glomerulonephritis* because of the usual accumulation of crescent-shaped cells in Bowman's space. RPGN develops over several weeks or months and is associated with significant loss of renal function. Clients can become quite ill quickly, with signs and symptoms of renal failure:

- Fluid volume excess with hypertension and oliguria
- Electrolyte imbalances
- Uremic symptoms

A prior infection or association with multisystem disease such as systemic lupus erythematosus (SLE) is sometimes identified in the client's recent history. The renal deterioration often progresses to nonreversible end-stage renal disease (ESRD).

Chronic Glomerulonephritis

Overview

Chronic glomerulonephritis, or *chronic nephritic syndrome,* refers to renal deterioration or failure that develops over 20 to 30 years or even longer. The exact onset of the disorder is rarely identified. In many instances, the cause of the disease is not known because the kidneys are atrophied and tissue is not available for biopsy or diagnosis. Mild proteinuria and hematuria, hypertension, and occasional edema are often the only manifestations, resulting in ESRD.

Although the exact pathogenesis is not known, changes in the renal parenchyma may result from

- Hypertension
- Intermittent or recurrent parenchymal infections and inflammation
- Altered metabolism and hemodynamics

Kidney tissue atrophies, and the functional mass of nephrons decreases significantly. The cortex of the parenchyma is thinned, but the calices and pelves are normal. Tissue, if obtained by renal biopsy in the late stages of atrophy, may reveal hyalinization of the glomeruli, loss of tubules, and fibrosis of the interstitium. Immunofluorescent examination and electron microscopy may reveal residual effects of immune complex deposition.

The loss of nephrons (the functional units of the renal parenchyma) results in decreased glomerular filtration. Commonly, hypertension with sclerosis of renal arterioles is present. The glomerular injury also results in proteinuria because of increased permeability of the glomerular basement membrane. Eventually, chronic glomerulonephritis results in chronic renal failure (see Chap. 75).

The cause usually remains unknown. Renal manifestations of systemic diseases, such as SLE, amyloid disease, or diabetes mellitus, resemble those of chronic glomerulonephritis. In ESRD, scar tissue replaces normal renal tissue so further diagnosis is not possible. Chronic glomerulonephritis is a primary cause of ESRD, resulting in dialysis or transplantation.

Collaborative Management

 Assessment

The nurse asks the client about previously identified health problems, including systemic diseases and prior renal or urologic disorders. The nurse notes childhood infectious diseases (such as streptococcal infections) and recent exposures to infections. The nurse inquires about the client's perception of overall health status and documents increasing fatigue and lethargy.

The client's pattern of voiding is noted; the nurse asks whether the frequency of voiding has increased or the quantity of urine has decreased. The nurse asks the client about changes in urine color, odor, or clarity.

Because edema can result from oliguria and fluid volume excess, the nurse also inquires about the client's general comfort and any dyspnea at rest or with exertion.

The nurse asks about and observes changes in mental functioning, such as irritability, frequent interruptions of others' conversations, the ability to read, perform job-related functions, or other processes requiring mental concentration. Changes in memory or the ability to concentrate occur with the waste product accumulation that accompanies renal failure.

The nurse inspects the client's skin for a yellowish color, texture, ecchymoses, rashes, or eruptions. The nurse notes areas of dryness and breaks that may have resulted from scratching. The nurse also assesses the cardiovascular and peripheral tissues for fluid retention by measuring blood pressure and weight and by auscultating the heart to describe rate, rhythm, and the presence of an S_3 heart sound.

The nurse auscultates the lung fields to detect rales or crackles and observes the rate and depth of breathing. The nurse inspects the neck veins to identify venous engorgement and checks for edema in the pedal, pretibial, and presacral tissues. The nurse notes whether the client has slurred speech, ataxia, tremors, or asterixis (flapping tremor of the fingers, or the inability to maintain a fixed posture with the arms extended and wrists hyperextended).

Urinary output may decrease, but gross visual changes in urine are not usual unless there is an associated urinary tract infection (UTI). Urinalysis commonly reveals proteinuria, usually less than 2 g in a 24-hour collection; the specific gravity is usually fixed at a constant level of dilution, around 1.010. There may be red blood cells and casts (hyaline, waxy, or granular) in the urine, suggesting chronic renal disease processes.

The glomerular filtration rate (GFR), measured by creatinine clearance, is reduced from the normal range of 105 to 120 mL/minute. In clients with ESRD, the creatinine clearance value is less than 5 to 10 mL/min. The serum creatinine level is elevated and varies, depending on the client's muscle mass. Serum creatinine levels are usually greater than 6 mg/dL but may be as high as 30 mg/dL or more. Blood urea nitrogen (BUN) is increased and varies in relation to the dietary protein intake; BUN levels are often between 100 and 200 mg/dL.

Serum electrolyte levels also reveal deterioration of renal function. Sodium retention is common, but dilution of the plasma from excess fluid results in an apparently normal serum sodium level (135 to 145 mEq/L) or a dilutional hyponatremia (<135 mEq/L). When oliguria develops, potassium retention occurs; hyperkalemia is present when levels exceed 5.4 mEq/L. Hyperphosphatemia develops, and levels are higher than 4.7 mg/dL. Serum calcium levels are usually at the lower end of the normal range or slightly below normal.

A base deficit is noted by the decrease in serum carbon dioxide (CO_2) or CO_2 combining power to less than the normal range of 24 to 32 mEq/L. Respiratory compensation for this metabolic acidosis is accomplished by hyperventilation to lower the partial pressure of CO_2 ($PaCO_2$) of arterial blood.

If respiratory compensation is present, the pH of arterial blood is between 7.35 and 7.45. Metabolic acidemia, a pH of less than 7.35, signifies inadequate respiratory compensation for metabolic acidosis.

In clients with chronic glomerulonephritis, the kidneys appear to be small when observed by radiography (KUB) or intravenous urography and when measured by sonography or computed tomography (CT).

A renal biopsy (percutaneous or open) is rarely performed for clients with ESRD because the kidneys are too small to obtain tissue. In the early stages of GN, when proteinuria or hematuria is initially identified, a diagnostic renal biopsy is important. Changes include an increase in the number and types of cells infiltrating the glomerular tissue, deposition of immune complexes, and vessel sclerosis.

[image] Interventions

Nursing diagnoses depend on the stage of renal deterioration. After glomerular injury has occurred, disease progression is predictable and difficult to prevent. In some situations, early recognition and treatment may bring about remission or delay progression. Consistent follow-up by clients to control hypertension, reduce dietary protein and phosphate intake, and avoid nephrotoxic agents and salt depletion may delay the onset of ESRD.

Treatment may be conservative, consisting of dietary modification, fluid intake sufficient to prevent reduced blood flow volume to the kidneys, and medication therapy to temporarily control the symptoms of uremia. Eventually, the client requires dialysis or transplantation to prevent death from the numerous potential systemic effects of uremia. (Nursing care for the client with ESRD requiring dialysis or transplantation is discussed in Chapter 75.)

Nephrotic Syndrome

Overview

Nephrotic syndrome (NS) results in massive proteinuria, edema, and hypoalbuminemia. As one of the primary glomerular syndromes, multiple and diverse causative agents, diseases, and physiologic processes are implicated or associated with NS.

Immunologically mediated glomerular membrane changes permit protein loss into urine. With this loss, plasma albumin levels decrease and edema develops. Increased liver activity results in elevated lipid production.

Collaborative Management

The primary feature of nephrotic syndrome is severe proteinuria (>3.5 g of protein in 24 hours). Clients diagnosed with NS also often have hypoalbuminemia (serum albumin <3 g/dL), hyperlipidemia, lipiduria, edema, and hypertension (Chart 74–6). Renal vein thrombosis often occurs concomitantly as either a cause or effect. Thromboembolic phenomena development is not clearly understood, but abnormalities in clotting studies may be detected. NS may progress to ESRD, but progression is not inevitable.

Treatment varies, depending on the specifics of the glomerulopathy identified by renal biopsy. Some immunologic processes may respond to steroids or cytotoxic agents. Dietary modification is also frequently prescribed. If the glomerular filtration rate (GFR) is normal, proteins should contain all essential amino acids; if decreased, dietary protein intake is decreased. Mild diuretics (see Chart 74–2) and dietary sodium restriction may be pre-

scribed to control edema and hypertension. The nurse assesses the client to ensure that intravascular volume depletion does not occur; hemodynamic changes and acute renal failure may be avoided if renal perfusion can be maintained. In clients with NS, the effects of hyperlipidemia on the development of atherosclerosis are unclear, as are the effects of dietary modifications.

Urinary Abnormalities

Immunologic glomerular disorders described as urinary abnormalities with hematuria and proteinuria are also referred to as:

- Asymptomatic proteinuria and/or hematuria
- Persisting urinary abnormalities with few or no symptoms

In these clients, blood pressure is typically normal, renal function has not decreased, and edema is not present.

Immunologic Interstitial and Tubulointerstitial Disorders

Interstitial and tubulointerstitial disorders in the kidney may be immunologically mediated; renal changes may be acute or chronic. These effects are often associated acutely with medications such as penicillin-like antibiotics, sulfonamides, or nonsteroidal anti-inflammatory drugs. Chronic interstitial nephritis has many causes, including analgesic nephropathy, the medication cyclosporin, polycystic kidney disease, systemic lupus erythematosus, sarcoidosis, multiple myeloma, sickle cell disease, obstructive disorders, and radiation nephritis. Drug-induced lesions are often associated with rash or eosinophilia; fever is common in idiopathic forms of interstitial nephritis.

Unless an offending agent can be identified and removed, progression to ESRD is likely. Spontaneous resolution may occur in cases of idiopathic interstitial nephritis, but more than 50% of clients are left with residual renal dysfunction (Kelly & Neilson, 1996). Acute and chronic interstitial nephritis make up one of the leading causes of end-stage renal disease (U.S. Renal Data Systems, 1995).

DEGENERATIVE DISORDERS

Degenerative disorders that cause changes in renal function are usually associated with the pathophysiologic effects of a multisystem disorder. Because the renal parenchyma is extremely vascular, many of these degenerative disorders result from changes in the renal vasculature.

Nephrosclerosis

Overview

Nephrosclerosis refers to changes in the nephron, specifically the afferent and efferent arterioles and the glomerular capillary loops. The vessel walls thicken, and the vessel lumen narrows. As a result, renal blood flow is decreased and interstitial tissue changes occur. Over time, ischemia and fibrosis develop.

Chart 74–6

Key Features of Nephrotic Syndrome

- Massive proteinuria
- Hypoalbuminemia
- Edema
- Hyperlipidemia
- Increased coagulation
- Infection

Nephrosclerosis is associated with benign essential hypertension or malignant hypertension, atherosclerosis, and a history of diabetes mellitus. Malignant hypertension is characterized by severe accelerating hypertension with neuroretinopathy or papilledema of the optic nerves and by evidence of renal damage (Laragh & Blumenfeld, 1996). Because of individual variations in vessel response to elevated blood pressures, no specific blood pressure readings can define malignant hypertension. The condition is rarely seen, however, below 160/110 mmHg. When malignant hypertension occurs, ischemia and necrosis may develop quickly. The changes associated with malignant hypertension may be reversible or progress to ESRD within months or years.

"Hypertension" is the second leading cause of ESRD. Approximately 30% of clients requiring a renal replacement therapy (e.g., dialysis or transplantation) for the maintenance of life have hypertension as the cause of their renal failure (U.S. Renal Data Systems, 1995).

TRANSCULTURAL CONSIDERATIONS

 Hypertension is more common in African-Americans, and the risks of end-stage renal disease (ESRD) from hypertension are also greater for African-Americans (Saunders, 1990). For people between the ages of 25 and 45 years, the ratio of African-Americans to Caucasians at risk for ESRD from hypertension is nearly 20:1 (Luke, 1992). These findings do not suggest that ESRD from nephrosclerosis does not occur in Caucasians, but that affected Caucasians are likely to be older.

Collaborative Management

Treatment aims to control high blood pressure and preserve renal function. Although many antihypertensive agents may lower blood pressure, the client's response is significant in ensuring long-term adherence to the prescribed therapy.

The nurse inquires about medication tolerance and any unusual or bothersome side effects. Agents that produce unusual fatigue, drowsiness, or impotence are likely not being taken as prescribed. The cost of some medications may also be prohibitive. Doses taken several times a day are often missed, and blood pressure control may thus be erratic and inadequate.

Lack of basic knowledge about hypertension or sheer misinformation poses additional challenges to nurses and all health care providers working with hypertensive clients. When evidence of renal disease occurs, adherence to therapy is even more important to preserve the client's health. Factors promoting adherence include regimen simplicity (e.g., once-a-day dosing), low cost, and minimal side effects.

Many medications can control high blood pressure (see Chart 38–2); more than one agent may be necessary. Calcium channel blockers and angiotensin-converting enzyme (ACE) inhibitors seem to produce fewer side effects and can be used while the client still has good renal function. Potent diuretics (e.g., furosemide or Zaroxolyn) in increasingly higher doses or in combination may be required as renal function deteriorates. Extreme caution is required to prevent hyperkalemia when potassium-sparing diuretics (e.g., triamterene or spironolactone) or combination agents containing a potassium-sparing diuretic are used for clients with known renal disease.

Renovascular Disease
Overview

Pathologic processes affecting the renal arteries may result in severe lumen narrowing and drastically reduced blood flow to the renal parenchyma. Uncorrected renovascular disease, such as renal artery stenosis or thrombosis, results in ischemia and atrophy of renal tissue.

Renovascular disease is suspected with a sudden onset of hypertension, particularly in clients older than 50 years. Clients with high blood pressure but with a negative family history for hypertension may also be considered potential candidates for renal artery stenosis (RAS).

RAS from atherosclerosis or fibromuscular hyperplasia (increased amount of tissue) is the primary cause of renovascular disease. Other causes include thrombosis and renal aneurysms.

Atherosclerotic changes in the renal artery are frequently associated with corresponding aortic and other major vessel disease. Changes in the renal artery are usually within a centimeter of where the renal artery and aorta meet. Fibromuscular changes of the vessel wall occur throughout the length of the renal artery between the aortic junction and the points of branching into the renal segmental arteries.

Collaborative Management

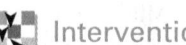 Assessment

Key features of renovascular disease are listed in Chart 74–7. Usually, the onset of hypertension is after age 40 to 50 years, and the family history is frequently negative for hypertension. Diagnosis is made by renal arteriography; measurement of renal vein renin levels provides additional evidence, but may not be confirmatory. A renal arteriogram visualizes the renal vasculature and offers critical information for invasive treatment. The comparison of renal vein renin levels *may* reveal which kidney is producing more renin.

Interventions

Excellent visualization of the type of defect, extent of narrowing, and surrounding vasculature is critical to de-

---

Chart 74–7

Key Features of Renovascular Disease

- Significant, difficult to control blood pressure
- Elevated serum creatinine
- Decreased creatinine clearance

cide treatment intervention. The client's overall condition and the size of the atrophied kidney further influence decisions about therapeutic intervention.

RAS may be treated by medications to control high blood pressure and by percutaneous transluminal balloon angioplasty or by surgical bypass procedures to restore renal blood supply. Medications may control high blood pressure but may not preserve kidney function long term. In young and middle-aged adults, a lifetime of treatment with multiple agents for high blood pressure may make treatment difficult; preservation of renal function is also a concern.

Balloon angioplasty technique (see Chap. 40) is considered less risky and requires much less time for recovery than renal artery bypass surgery. Renal artery bypass surgery is a major procedure, involving 2 months or more for convalescence. Bypass may be performed for either one or both renal arteries. The surgeon inserts a synthetic graft that redirects blood flow from the abdominal aorta into the renal artery, beyond the area of stenosis. Increasingly, splenorenal bypass procedures can also restore renal blood flow. Technically, the process is similar to other arterial bypass procedures (see Chap. 38).

For clients with RAS, the diagnostic and treatment alternatives present tremendous decisional conflict. Often, clients experience deterioration of renal function, as noted by elevated serum creatinine levels and decreased creatinine clearance. These clients are at increased risk for acute renal failure from the administration of nephrotoxic agents such as radiopaque contrast media and from possible intraoperative hypotensive episodes. No treatment, however, probably means that dialysis is inevitable.

Diabetic Nephropathy

Overview

Diabetes mellitus is the leading cause of end-stage renal disease (ESRD) in the United States among Caucasians. Approximately 36% of clients requiring dialysis or renal transplantation have diabetes mellitus as their primary etiologic feature. Diabetic nephropathy may result from type 1 diabetes mellitus (formerly, insulin-dependent or IDDM) or type 2 diabetes mellitus (formerly, non–insulin-dependent or NIDDM).

About 50% of clients with type 1 diabetes will progress to ESRD within 5 years after the onset of proteinuria. Proteinuria is usually present within 16 to 21 years after the onset of diabetes mellitus.

As many as 60% of clients with type 2 diabetes mellitus will progress to ESRD. Diabetic renal manifestations in these clients is associated with aging. Diabetic renal disease is influenced by the extent, duration, and effects of atherosclerosis and hypertension and those of autonomic neuropathy, which promotes bladder atony, urinary stasis, and urinary tract infections.

Immunologic response mechanisms have also been implicated in glomerular basement membrane thickening and other changes in clients with diabetic renal disease. Investigations continue to explore if defects are the result of genetic or metabolic disturbances.

Collaborative Management

Diabetic nephropathy is a *microvascular* complication of diabetes defined by persistent albuminuria, as shown by dipstick or a urinary albumin excretion rate above 0.3 g/dL, without evidence of other renal disease. A diagnosis of renal disease in clients with diabetes mellitus is often presumptive, given the history and clinical examination. Diabetic renal disease is progressive (Table 74–4).

Structural and functional changes occur in the kidneys of diabetic clients. Initially, kidney size is slightly increased and glomerular filtration rates (GFR) are higher than normal. Radioimmunoassay of urine detects the microlevels of albumin associated with albuminuria. Progressive renal damage occurs before dipstick procedures can detect protein in the urine. For most clients, the proteinuria (albuminuria) necessitates a renal biopsy for further diagnosis. For the client with diabetes, however, a funduscopic examination of the retina showing capillary leakage, fibrosis, and the characteristic changes of diabetic retinopathy eliminates the need for a risky renal biopsy.

Proteinuria may be mild, moderate, or severe, as in nephrotic syndrome. Clients with diabetes mellitus are always considered to be at risk for renal failure. If possible, nephrotoxic agents (such as radiopaque contrast media or aminoglycosides) and fluid volume deficit must be avoided. Clients with worsening renal function may begin to have frequent hypoglycemic episodes and a decreased need for insulin or oral antihyperglycemic agents. The nurse explains to the client that the kidneys metabolize and excrete insulin. Consequently, when renal function deteriorates, the insulin is available longer and less insulin is needed. Unfortunately, many clients believe that their diabetes mellitus is improving. The result is often ESRD, with the client requiring chronic dialysis or transplantation. (See Chapter 68 for more information on diabetic nephropathy.)

TABLE 74–4

The Stages of Progression of Type 1 Diabetic Renal Disease

- *Stage I, at the time diabetes is diagnosed:* Kidney size and glomerular filtration rate are increased. Blood sugar control can reverse the changes.
- *Stage II, 2–3 yr after diagnosis:* Glomerular and tubular capillary basement membrane changes result in microscopic changes, with loss of filtration surface area and scar formation. Glomerular changes are referred to as glomerulosclerosis.
- *Stage III, 7–15 yr after diagnosis:* Microalbuminuria is present. The glomerular filtration rate (GFR) may still be normal or may be increased.
- *Stage IV:* Albuminuria is detectable by dipstick. GFR is decreased. Blood pressure is increased, and retinopathy is present.
- *Stage V:* GFR decreases at an average rate of 10 mL/min/yr.

TUMORS

Cysts and Benign Tumors

Benign urinary tract growths include cysts and benign tumors of the renal parenchyma or urinary bladder. Because malignant growths may occur within cystic structures, thorough evaluation is essential.

A simple renal cyst grows out of renal parenchymal tissue, usually the *cortical* tissue. The cyst is filled with fluid; as it enlarges, it can cause local tissue destruction. Many cysts cause no symptoms and are discovered accidentally during fluoroscopic examination or autopsy.

Although the exact cause is unknown, cysts are usually considered an embryonic developmental defect. The etiology and incidence of benign tumors is also unknown. Thus far, there are no recognized methods of prevention.

Diagnosis of a simple renal cyst involves intravenous urography, sonography, and computed tomography (CT). If the cyst appears to be filled with fluid at urographic examination, sonography is generally recommended; if the cyst appears more dense, a CT scan is needed.

Treatment may consist of percutaneous aspiration of a fluid-filled cyst or surgical exploration with the potential for total or subtotal nephrectomy.

Renal Cell Carcinoma

Overview

Renal cell carcinoma is also referred to as *adenocarcinoma* or *hypernephroma,* an outdated but frequently used term. As with other malignant neoplasms, the healthy functional tissue of the kidney is replaced and displaced by abnormal, nonfunctional cells. Although the exact mechanism is not known, the tumor cells probably originate in the proximal convoluted tubules of the nephron.

Systemic, concomitant pathophysiologic effects are called *paraneoplastic syndromes* and include

- Anemia
- Erythrocytosis
- Hypercalcemia
- Liver dysfunction, with elevated liver enzymes
- Hormonal effects
- Increased sedimentation rate
- Hypertension

Anemia and erythrocytosis may appear contradictory: There is some blood loss from hematuria, but the amount is not considered consistent with the degree of anemia. Erythrocytosis may originate from erythropoietin production from the tumor cells. Hypertension may result from increased renin.

Parathyroid hormone produced by tumor cells may be the cause of hypercalcemia; other hormone alterations include increased renin levels, potentially accounting for hypertension, and increased human chorionic gonadotropin (hCG) levels, which are accompanied by decreased libido and changes in secondary sex characteristics. The cause of the increased sedimentation rate and changes in liver function studies is not known.

Renal tumors are categorized into four stages (Table

TABLE 74–5

Staging Renal Tumors
• *Stage I:* Tumors of up to 2.5 cm within the capsule of the kidney; the renal vein, perinephric fat, and adjacent lymph nodes have no tumor.
• *Stage II:* Tumors are larger than 2.5 cm and extend beyond the capsule but are within Gerota's fascia; the renal vein and lymph nodes are not involved.
• *Stage III:* Tumors extend into the renal vein and/or lymph nodes.
• *Stage IV:* Tumors include invasion of adjacent organs beyond Gerota's fascia or metastasis to distant tissues.

74–5). Complications include metastasis and urinary tract obstruction. Metastasis usually occurs via the blood or lymph to the ipsilateral adrenal gland, liver, lungs, long bones, or contralateral kidney. Direct tumor invasion surrounding the ureter may result in hydroureter and urinary tract obstruction.

The exact cause of renal cell carcinoma is unknown, but links to tobacco use and exposure to such chemicals as lead, phosphate, and cadmium have been observed. Other studies explore the possibility of genetic transmission and the meaning of observed chromosome translocations.

Renal malignancies account for approximately 2% of reported cancers, with about 28,800 new cases and 11,300 deaths annually in the United States. The 5-year survival rates for 1986–1992 for Caucasians and African-Americans were 60% and 55%, respectively (Parker et al., 1997). The usual age of presentation is between 55 and 60 years.

Collaborative Management

 Assessment

➤ History

The nurse asks the client for specific information, including age, known risk factors such as smoking or environmental exposures, history of weight loss, changes in urine color, abdominal or flank discomfort, and fever. The fever's cause is unknown, but pyrogens produced by the tumor cells have been implicated.

➤ Physical Assessment/Clinical Manifestations

Classic presentations (seen only in 5% to 10% of clients) include flank pain, gross hematuria, and a palpable renal mass. The nurse inquires into the nature of the flank or abdominal discomfort; clients typically describe the pain as dull and aching. If bleeding into the tumor occurs, the pain may be more intense. The nurse inspects the flank, noting asymmetry or obvious protrusions. An abdominal mass may be detected through *gentle* palpation. A renal bruit may be heard on auscultation.

Hematuria is a *late,* frequently observed sign. Blood in the urine may be grossly observable as bright red flecks or clots, or the urine may appear smoky or cola colored. In the absence of gross hematuria, microscopic examination may or may not reveal red cells.

The nurse inspects the skin for pallor, increased areolar pigmentation, and gynecomastia. Other findings may include muscle wasting, weakness, generally poor nutritional status, and weight loss. All tend to occur late in the disease.

Anxiety and fear should be expected in clients with known or suspected neoplasms. The client may also have denied or minimized symptoms, and guilt related to a delay in seeking medical attention is common. The client may fear death and have anxieties about the potential effects of treatment, such as chemotherapy or radiation, or the possibility of renal failure.

➤ Diagnostic Assessment

Urinalysis may reveal red blood cells. The nurse reviews laboratory results, which may reveal many paraneoplastic syndromes. Hematologic studies reveal decreased hemoglobin and hematocrit values, hypercalcemia, and increased erythrocyte sedimentation rate and adrenocorticotropic hormone, hCG, cortisol, renin, and parathyroid hormone levels.

Renal masses may be detected incidentally by surgical exploration, intravenous urogram with nephrograms, or sonography. The mass and surrounding structures may be further delineated by CT with contrast or magnetic resonance imaging (MRI). Staging or determining the extent of tumor spread is best accomplished with renal arteriography and renal venography.

Interventions

Common nursing diagnoses for the client with renal cell carcinoma are

1. Risk for Injury related to possible metastases or recurrence of cancer
2. Anxiety and Fear related to diagnostic and therapeutic options

Nonsurgical Management. Chemotherapy with a variety of agents, singly and in combination, have had limited effectiveness. The U.S. Food and Drug Administration (FDA) has approved expanded clinical trials for the study of interleukin-2 (IL-2). One protocol gives 600,000 IU/kg by intravenous bolus every 8 hours for 5 days, followed by a second cycle 1 week later (Haas et al., 1993). Another protocol outlines 28 doses, at 0.037 mg/kg, over two 1-week administration periods (Letizia & Conway, 1996). Interferon and tumor necrosis factor are also being used investigationally.

Hormonal agents (e.g., progesterone and estrogen) have also not been effective in controlling tumor cell growth. Interferons produced using recombinant DNA technique are beginning to show promising results, however, especially interferon-alpha. Studies with lymphokine-activated killer (LAK) cells and tumor-infiltrating lymphocytes (TIL) are in the clinical trial stage.

Surgical Management. Renal cell carcinoma is usually treated surgically by *nephrectomy* (kidney removal), the surgical procedure of choice when pain, bleeding, or tumor spread cannot be controlled otherwise. The decision to remove a single kidney is difficult. Even in clients with diseased kidneys, usually some production of erythropoietin and urine provides physiologic benefits. Therefore, a decision to proceed is often delayed until other treatment options have been exhausted.

Preoperative Care. The nurse advises the client about surgical routines (see Chaps. 20–22). The nurse explains the probable site of incision and the postoperative dressings, drains, or other equipment needed, reassuring the client of pain relief. Preoperative care includes administration of blood and fluids to achieve hemodynamic stabilization. Because blood provides an excellent medium for bacteria proliferation, the nurse expects antibiotics to be administered preoperatively.

Surgical Procedure. The nurse places the client in the lateral position with the operative kidney uppermost; after positioning of the arms and legs, the kidney rest is raised to flex the client's trunk area. The surgeon makes the incision through skin, fat, fascia, and muscle. Often, the 11th or 12th rib is removed to provide better access to the kidney. The surgeon removes the entire kidney and adjacent adrenal gland, renal artery and vein, and surrounding Gerota's fascia after ligation of the ureter. The adrenal gland is left intact. A drain may be placed in the wound before closure.

When a *radical* nephrectomy is performed, the periaortic lymph nodes are also removed. Surgical approach may be transthoracic (as discussed above), lumbar, or transabdominal, depending on the size and location of the lesion. Radiation therapy may follow radical nephrectomy. Studies are ongoing to identify adjuvant therapy (e.g., chemotherapy) effectiveness.

Postoperative Care. The Client Care Plan summarizes priority nursing diagnoses and potential complications for the client who has had a nephrectomy. The nurse observes the client's abdomen for distention from bleeding and symptoms of adrenal insufficiency. The nurse observes bed linens under the supine client, because bleeding may be present. Hemorrhage or adrenal insufficiency may be accompanied by hypotension, decrease in urinary output, and altered level of consciousness.

A decrease in blood pressure is one of the earliest signs of both hemorrhage and adrenal insufficiency; however, in clients with hypotension, urinary output also decreases immediately. In clients with adrenal insufficiency, large water and sodium losses in the urine occur; consequently, a large urinary output is followed by hypotension and subsequent oliguria (< 400 mL/24 hr or less than 25 mL/hr). The physician may prescribe intravenous replacement of fluids and administration of packed red blood cells.

The second kidney is expected to provide adequate renal function. The nurse assesses urinary output hourly for the first 24 hours postoperatively; a urine flow of

Client Care Plan

The Client Who Has Had a Nephrectomy

Nursing Diagnosis No. 1: Ineffective Airway Clearance related to pain, ineffective cough, fatigue

Expected Outcomes	Nursing Interventions	Rationale
The client's lung sounds will be clear to auscultation in all lung fields or at client's baseline.	■ Assess and document lung sounds every 4 to 6 hours. ■ Assure vigorous pulmonary toilet with incentive spirometer, coughing, turning, and deep breathing exercises every 1 to 2 hours. ■ Assist the client to be out of bed by the first postoperative day unless medically contraindicated. ■ Assist the client with early ambulation, starting with a few steps at a time. ■ Monitor client's temperature every 4 hours initially, then every 8 hours.	■ Ongoing assessment promotes early detection and treatment of complications. ■ Pulmonary hygiene promotes lung expansion and clearance of secretions and helps to prevent atelectasis and pneumonia. ■ Getting out of bed promotes lung expansion and clearance of secretions and helps to prevent atelectasis and pneumonia. ■ Ambulation promotes lung expansion and clearance of secretions and helps to prevent atelectasis and pneumonia. ■ An increased temperature could indicate atelectasis or pneumonia.

Nursing Diagnosis No. 2: Pain related to intraoperative positioning, surgical procedure, and location of incision

Expected Outcomes	Nursing Interventions	Rationale
The client will be as pain free and as alert as possible.	■ Perform a complete pain assessment using designed pain level scale every 2 to 4 hours. ■ Administer analgesics as ordered, preferably with patient-controlled analgesia (PCA) or epidural analgesics. ■ Plan activities such as getting out of bed or ambulation to coincide with peak of analgesic effectiveness. ■ Teach patient how to splint the incision during pulmonary exercises or activities. ■ Provide and encourage the use of complementary therapies such as diversion, aroma therapy, relaxation techniques, and uninterrupted rest time. ■ Monitor the client's respiratory rate and depth and pulse oximetry reading every 2 to 4 hours while receiving analgesic medication.	■ Ongoing assessment helps to determine the effectiveness of pain management interventions. ■ PCA or epidural administration provides more constant drug levels, therefore increasing the effectiveness of the medication. ■ The client's ability to perform beneficial activities will be increased with effective pain management. ■ Splinting reduces stretch on the surgical area, which otherwise can cause pain and discomfort. ■ Supplemental interventions enhance effectiveness of analgesic medication, help to conserve and maintain energy, and help to reduce mental and physical stress. ■ Respiratory depression can occur with opioid analgesics.

Client Care Plan

Nursing Diagnosis No. 3: Impaired Skin and Tissue Integrity related to surgical procedure

Expected Outcomes	Nursing Interventions	Rationale
The client's operative site will heal without complications within the expected time frame.	■ Assess the surgical dressing for evidence of drainage at least once every shift. ■ Mark the edges of any drainage on the dressing with a pen, noting the date and time. ■ Use sterile asepsis during dressing changes. ■ Assess incision site at each dressing change for redness, swelling, pain, drainage, and closure; document your findings.	■ Ongoing assessment promotes early detection and treatment of complications. ■ Markings show how much drainage has occurred between assessments. ■ Sterile asepsis prevents the introduction of organisms that could cause infection. ■ Ongoing assessment promotes early detection and treatment of complications; documentation provides a basis for comparison of data.

Potential Complication No. 1: Potential Complication: Renal Failure related to fluid volume deficit, inadequate drainage of urine

Expected Outcomes	Nursing Interventions	Rationale
The client will attain or maintain a urinary output of >30 mL/hour.	■ Monitor urinary output every 1 to 2 hours initially. ■ Assess overall hydration status (i.e., check blood pressure, review intake and output, monitor heart rate and quality, and assess neck veins and central venous pressure readings) every 2 to 4 hours initially. ■ Assure adequate hydration, usually 2000–2500 mL/24 hours. ■ Assess wound site and drains, and check underneath the client for excessive bleeding or drainage. ■ Check to be sure the Foley catheter is not kinked or disconnected and is draining properly.	■ Ongoing assessment promotes early detection and treatment of complications. ■ Ongoing assessment promotes early detection and treatment of complications. ■ Adequate hydration helps to prevent fluid volume deficit. ■ Bleeding or excessive drainage can cause fluid volume deficit. ■ Foley patency is important to help prevent back-up of urine, which could cause renal failure.

30 to 50 mL/hour is acceptable. Flow rates of less than 25 to 30 mL/hour suggest a decrease in renal perfusion. Initially postoperatively, hemoglobin level, hematocrit values, and white blood cell count may be measured every 6 to 12 hours.

The nurse monitors the client's temperature, pulse rate, and respiratory rate at least every 4 hours; careful measurement and recording of fluid intake and output are critical. The client is weighed daily.

The client may be in a special care unit for 24 to 48 hours postoperatively for monitoring of bleeding and/or adrenal insufficiency. The drain placed near the site of incision ensures residual fluid removal. Because of the discomfort associated with lung expansion, the client is susceptible to atelectasis. Fever, chills, thick sputum, or decreased breath sounds suggest pneumonia.

Postoperative Drug Therapy. After surgery, opioid analgesics (such as meperidine [Demerol], hydromorphone [Dilaudid], and morphine sulfate [Statex♣]) are given parenterally. Acute pain control is more effective when sedatives such as promethazine hydrochloride (Phenergan) or hydroxyzine pamoate (Vistaril) are combined with the opioid analgesic. Concerns about respiratory depression and addiction are usually not warranted. The incision site, in which the major muscle groups associated with breathing and movement are involved, necessitates the liberal use of analgesic agents. The nurse expects these medications may be required for 3–5 days. When the client is permitted to consume food and fluids orally, oral analgesic agents may be considered.

One or more antibiotics may be prescribed for intraoperative and postoperative prophylaxis. Usually, these agents are given as single-dose prescriptions. The need for additional antibiotics is based on clinical and laboratory evidence of infection. Steroid replacements may be necessary in adrenal insufficiency.

RENAL TRAUMA

Overview

Trauma to one or both kidneys is always a concern in penetrating wounds or blunt injuries to the back, flank, or abdomen. Injury to the kidney can be minor, major, or pedicle (Fig. 74–4).

MINOR. Minor injuries include contusions, small lacerations, and disruption of the integrity of the parenchyma and the calyx (forniceal disruption). In a person with a contusion, one or both kidneys sustained a bruise because

MINOR TRAUMA

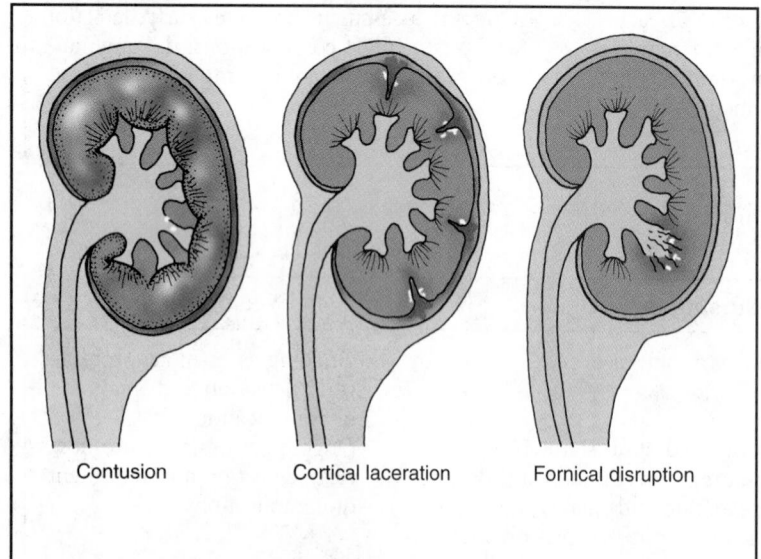

Contusion

Cortical laceration

Fornical disruption

PEDICLE INJURY

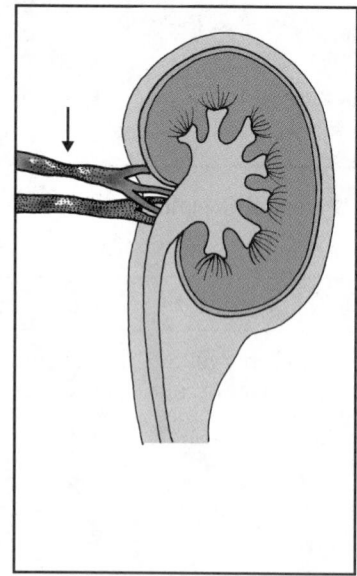

MAJOR TRAUMA

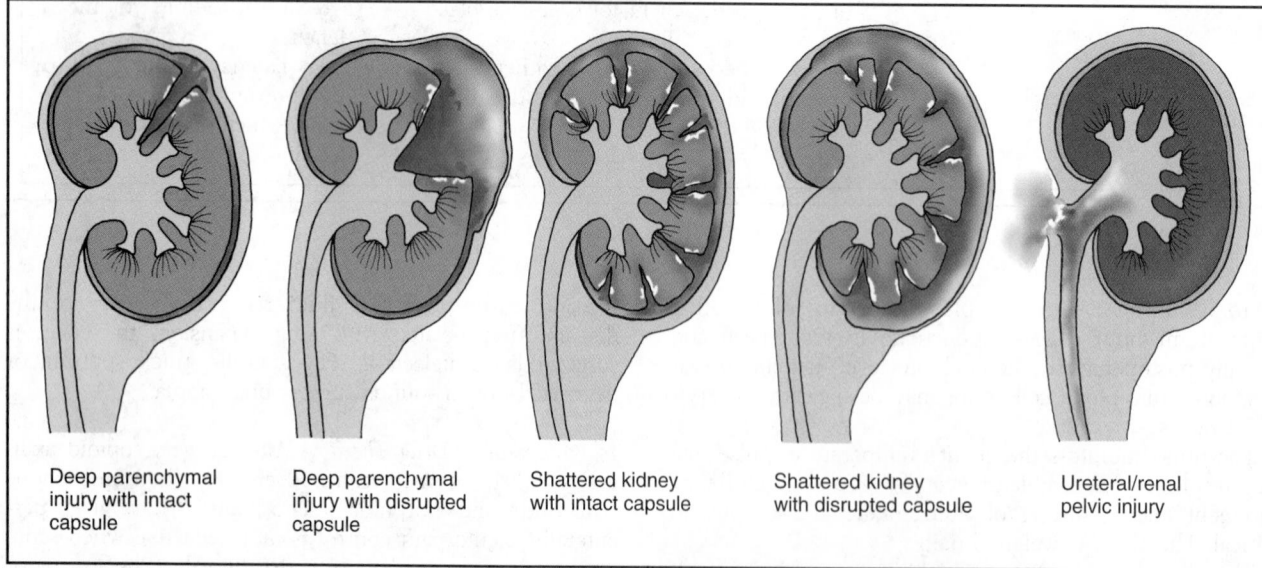

Deep parenchymal injury with intact capsule

Deep parenchymal injury with disrupted capsule

Shattered kidney with intact capsule

Shattered kidney with disrupted capsule

Ureteral/renal pelvic injury

Figure 74–4. Common types and locations of renal trauma.

of the major impact. Small blood vessels may be damaged, causing some hematuria. One or more small lacerations may result in small, localized hematomas. There may also be a small hematoma at the site of forniceal disruption.

MAJOR. Major injuries involve lacerations to the cortex, medulla, or one of the segmental branches of the renal artery or vein. Deep parenchymal injuries may extend throughout the kidney and result in hematomas contained within or disrupting the capsule. Other parenchymal injuries involve the cortex and cause shattering of tissue, resulting in either an intact or a disrupted capsule.

A major injury is most likely to follow a penetrating abdominal, flank, or back wound. Bleeding is extensive, and surgical exploration is often required. Because of the hemorrhage, hypoperfusion of renal parenchyma can produce short- or long-term renin-induced hypertension.

PEDICLE. Pedicle injuries involve a laceration or disruption of the renal artery and/or renal vein. Hemorrhage is extensive and rapid, and death may ensue quickly unless diagnosis and intervention are prompt. Even with rapid surgical repair, renin-induced hypertension easily results; consequently, management of hypertension becomes a lifetime health problem.

Etiology

The causes of renal trauma are diverse. *Penetrating* wounds of the abdomen, flank, or back are typically gunshot wounds or knife injuries. Clients thrown from vehicles may sustain penetrating abdominal wounds that injure the kidneys.

Blunt causes of renal trauma include automobile, motorcycle, snowmobile, sled, and pedestrian accidents in which the person is thrown from the vehicle or to the ground. Accidents that propel the person into the air usually involve significant force; these forces are referred to as *acceleration/deceleration* forces and are most likely to create pedicle injuries. Blunt trauma suffered during contact sports (football, soccer, rugby, hockey, basketball, baseball, snow or water-skiing) also causes renal injury. Falls of all types can result in contusion or laceration of the renal parenchyma.

Prevention of trauma is reviewed in Chart 74–8.

Collaborative Management

 Assessment

The nurse obtains a history of the client's personal health status and the events surrounding the trauma from the client, a witness, or emergency personnel. Critical assessment information includes a history of renal or urologic disease, surgical intervention, or systemic health problems (such as diabetes mellitus or hypertension).

Ureteral and/or renal pelvic injury may cause diffuse abdominal pain, local collections of urine, and infection.

The nurse questions the client about pain, specifically flank or abdominal pain. The nurse solicits a description: Is the pain dull? Sharp? Constant? Intermittent? Aggravated by coughing?

The nurse measures the client's blood pressure and apical and peripheral pulse rates, respiratory rate, and temperature. The nurse also inspects the right and left flanks to determine asymmetry, or penetrating injuries of the lower thorax or back. Similarly, the nurse inspects and percusses the abdomen for ecchymoses and abdominal distention, respectively, and for penetrating wounds. The nurse also inspects the urethra for gross bleeding.

Urinalysis commonly reveals hemoglobin or red blood cells from the rupture of small or large renal blood vessels. Microscopic examination of the urine may also show red blood cell casts, which suggest tubular damage. Hemoglobin and hematocrit values decrease with blood loss; the white blood cell count is elevated with inflammation if the trauma occurred several days previously.

Fluoroscopic procedures include intravenous urography, renal arteriography, and computed tomography (CT). Urogram reveals the number of kidneys and the integrity and patency of the collecting system. Renal sonography is an alternative diagnostic procedure to a urogram that allows radiopaque contrast media to be avoided in clients with elevated serum creatinine levels.

Renal arteriography also reveals the number of kidneys but, more specifically, the blood supply to each. In clients with pedicle injuries, the contrast media used in arteriography extravasates from the ruptured vessels, and the renal parenchyma is not visualized. The CT scan shows the location of the injury and vascular and tissue integrity. Intracapsular and extracapsular hematomas are readily observable on the CT scan.

 Interventions

Nursing diagnoses for the client with renal trauma include Altered (Renal) Tissue Perfusion, Anxiety, Pain, Altered Urinary Elimination, Post-Trauma Response, and Risk for Infection. Interventions include medications for vascular support, fluids to restore fluid volume, and surgery when indicated.

Drug Therapy

The physician prescribes medications, such as dopamine (Revimine♦), to support renal perfusion, promote peripheral vasoconstriction, and possibly elevate blood pressure. Low doses of dopamine also enhance renal blood flow.

Fluids

Fluid administration to restore circulating blood volume is critical for renal tissue perfusion. *Crystalloid* solutions replace water and some electrolytes and include 0.9% sodium chloride (NSS), 5% dextrose in 0.45% sodium chloride, and Ringer's solution. When significant bleeding has occurred, whole blood or packed red cell replacement restores the oxygen-carrying capacity of hemoglobin. *Plasma volume expanders,* such as dextran or albumin, help re-establish plasma oncotic pressure and minimize fluid shift from the intravascular to the interstitial fluid space.

During fluid resuscitation or restoration, the nurse administers fluid at the prescribed rate and monitors the client for hemodynamic instability. The nurse also monitors vital signs as often as every 5 to 15 minutes and measures and records urinary output hourly. Urinary output should be no less than 25 to 30 mL/hour. The physician may detail guidelines for specific urinary flow.

Surgery

Surgical interventions may include nephrectomy and partial nephrectomy. For clients with major vascular tearing, the kidney may be surgically removed, repaired through revascularization techniques, and then reimplanted. The repair of kidney tissue outside the client is called *bench surgery.* Autotransplantation is transplantation of one's own kidney.

 Continuing Care

The nurse instructs the client, family, or significant other about the injury's effects and how to assess for infection or other complications, such as the onset of bleeding or urinary retention. The nurse instructs the client to observe the pattern and frequency of urination and to note whether the color, clarity, and amount appear normal. The nurse also instructs the client to seek medical attention if these characteristics change significantly and if a feeling of bladder distention or inadequate bladder emptying occurs, suggesting an obstruction. Chills, fever, lethargy, and/or cloudy, foul-smelling urine may suggest a urinary tract infection. The nurse warns the client not to ignore these symptoms and to seek medical care promptly if they occur.

CASE STUDY For the Client with Diabetic Nephropathy

■ Mrs. Adams has had diabetes for 15 years and has recently been diagnosed with diabetic nephropathy. She tells you, "Well, now I got the disease in my kidneys. There isn't anything I can do now . . . I may as well give up. Dialysis, here I come, ready or not!"

QUESTIONS:

1. How would you initially respond to her?
2. What would you say to her about dialysis?
3. What resources could you refer her to?

SELECTED BIBLIOGRAPHY

Adler, S. G., Cohen, A.H., & Glassock, R. J. (1996). Secondary glomerular diseases. In B. M. Brenner (Ed.), *Brenner & Rector's the kidney* (5th ed., pp. 1498–1596). Philadelphia: W. B. Saunders.

Beebe, D. K. (1996). Autosomal dominant polycystic kidney disease. *American Family Physician, 53*(3), 925–931, 935–936.

Boam, W. D., & Miser, W. F. (1995). Acute focal bacterial pyelonephritis. *American Family Physician, 52*(3), 919–924.

Brenner, B. M. (Ed.). (1996). *Brenner & Rector's the kidney* (5th ed.). Philadelphia: W. B. Saunders.

Chapman, A. B., Johnson, A. M., Rainguet, S., et al. (1997). Left ventricular hypertrophy in autosomal dominant polycystic kidney disease. *Journal of the American Society of Nephrology, 8,* 1292–1297.

*Clayman, R. V., Kavoussi, L. R., Soper, N. J., et al. (1991). Laparoscopic nephrectomy: Initial case report. *The Journal of Urology, 146,* 278–282.

*Collins, J. G. (1993). *Prevalence of selected chronic conditions: United States, 1986–88.* National Center for Health Statistics. Vital Health Stat 10(182). DHHS Pub. No. (PHS) 93–1510. p. 52. Hyattsville, MD: U.S. Department of Health and Human Services.

*Davidson, J. A. (1991). Diabetes care in minority groups. *Postgraduate Medicine, 90*(2), 153–168.

*deGuzman, L., & Joyce, K. (1991). Case study of a patient with severe nephrotic syndrome. *American Nephrology Nurses' Association Journal, 18*(5), 502–503.

*Duley, I., & Gabow, P. (1990). *PKD patient's manual: Understanding and living with autosomal dominant polycystic kidney disease.* Kansas City, MO: PKD Foundation.

Dunfee, T. P. (1995). The changing management of diabetic nephropathy. *Hospital Practice, 30*(5), 45–49, 53–55.

*Feldman, H. I., Klag, M. J., Chiapella, A. P., & Whelton, P. K. (1992). End-stage renal disease in U.S. minority groups. *American Journal of Kidney Diseases, 19*(5), 397–410, 411–413.

*Gabow, P. A., & Grantham, J. J. (1993). Polycystic kidney disease. In R. W. Schrier & C. W. Gottschalk (Eds.), *Diseases of the kidney* (5th ed., pp. 535–569). Boston: Little, Brown & Company.

Garnick, M. B., & Richie, J. P. (1996). Renal neoplasia. In B. M. Brenner (Ed.), *Brenner & Rector's the kidney* (5th ed., pp. 1959–1977). Philadelphia: W. B. Saunders.

Germino, G. G. (1997). Autosomal dominant polycystic kidney disease: A two-hit model. *Hospital Practice, 32*(3), 81–82, 85–88, 91–92, 95–97, 102.

Glassock, R. J., Cohen, A. H., & Adler, S. G. (1996). Primary glomerular diseases. In B. M. Brenner (Ed.), *Brenner & Rector's the kidney* (5th ed., pp. 1392–1497). Philadelphia: W. B. Saunders.

Grantham, J. J. (1995). Polycystic kidney disease: Etiology, pathogenesis, and treatment. *Disease-A-Month, 41,* 693–765.

*Haas, G. P., Hillman, G. G., Redman, B. G., & Pontes, J. E. (1993). Immunotherapy of renal cell carcinoma. *CA: A Cancer Journal for Clinicians, 43*(3), 177–185.

*Hahn, B. H. (1990). Lupus nephritis: Therapeutic decisions. *Hospital Practice, 25*(3A), 89–93, 96–97, 103–104.

Holcomb, S. S. (1997). Understanding the ins and outs of diuretic therapy. *Nursing97, 27*(2), 34–40, 47.

*Humphrey, L. L., & Ballard, D. J. (1990). Renal complications in non–insulin-dependent diabetes mellitus. *Clinics in Geriatric Medicine, 6*(4), 807–825.

Kelly, C. J., & Neilson, E. G. (1996). Tubulointerstitial diseases. In B. M. Brenner (Ed.), *Brenner & Rector's the kidney* (5th ed., pp. 1655–1697). Philadelphia: W. B. Saunders.

Lancaster, L. E. (Ed.). (1995). *Core curriculum for nephrology nursing* (3rd ed.). Pitman, NJ: A. J. Jannetti.

Laragh, J. H., & Blumenfeld, J. D. (1996). Essential hypertension. In B. M. Brenner (Ed.), *Brenner & Rector's the kidney* (5th ed., pp. 2071–2105). Philadelphia: W. B. Saunders.

Letizia, M., & Conway, A. M. (1996). Interleukin-2 therapy for renal cell cancer. *Critical Care Nurse, 16*(5), 20–26, 30–32, 34–35.

*Luke, R. G. (1992). Can we prevent end-stage renal disease due to hypertension or diabetes? *Journal of the American Medical Association, 268*(21), 3119–3120.

McKinney, B. (1996). When this rare cancer strikes . . . renal cell carcinoma. *RN, 59*(12), 36–41, 51.

McCarthy, S., & McMullen, M. (1997). Autosomal dominant polycystic kidney disease: Pathophysiology and treatment. *American Nephrology Nurses' Association Journal, 24*(1), 45–53.

Meeker, M. H., & Rothrock, J. (Eds.). (1995). *Alexander's care of the patient in surgery* (10th ed.). St. Louis: Mosby Year Book.

*Morgensen, C. E., & Schmitz, O. (1988). The diabetic kidney: From hyperfiltration and microalbuminuria to end-stage renal failure. *Medical Clinics of North America, 72*(6), 1465–1492.

National Center for Health Statistics. (1996). *Health, United States, 1995*. DHHS Pub. No. (PHS) 96-1232. Hyattsville, MD: Public Health Service.

Parker, S. L., Tong, T., Bolden, S., et al. (1997). Cancer statistics, 1997. *CA: A Cancer Journal for Clinicians, 47*(1), 5–27.

*Pasternack, M. S., & Rubin, R. H. (1993). Urinary tract tuberculosis. In R. W. Schrier & C. W. Gottschalk (Eds.), *Diseases of the kidney* (5th ed., pp. 909–928). Boston: Little, Brown & Company.

*Ravine, D., Gibson, R. N., Walker, R. G., et al. (1994). Evaluation of ultrasonographic diagnostic criteria for autosomal dominant polycystic kidney disease. *Lancet, 343*, 824–827.

*Rosmarin, P. C. (1989). Secondary hypertension. *Clinics in Geriatric Medicine, 5*(4), 753–768.

*Rostand, S. G. (1992). U.S. minority groups and end-stage renal disease: A disproportionate share. *American Journal of Kidney Diseases, 19*(5), 411–413.

Rubin, R. H., Cotran, R. S., & Tolkoff-Rubin, N. E. (1996). Urinary tract infection, pyelonephritis, and reflux nephropathy. In B. M. Brenner (Ed.), *Brenner & Rector's the kidney* (5th ed., pp. 1597–1654). Philadelphia: W. B. Saunders.

Saklayen, M. G. (Ed.). (1997). Renal disease. *Medical Clinics of North America, 81*(3).

*Saunders, E. (1990). Tailoring treatment to minority patients. *American Journal of Medicine, 88*(Suppl. 3B), 215–235.

*See, W. A., & Williams, R. D. (1992). Tumors of the kidney, ureter, and bladder. *Western Journal of Medicine, 156*(5), 523–534.

*Smith, M. F. (1990). Renal trauma: Adult and pediatric considerations. *Critical Care Nursing Clinics of North America, 2*(10), 67–77.

*Sommers, M. S. (1990). Blunt renal trauma. *Critical Care Nurse, 10*(3), 38–49.

Teichman, J. M. H., & Hulbert, J. C. (1995). Laparoscopic marsupialization of polycystic kidney. *Journal of Urology, 153*, 1105–1107.

Torres, V. E. (1996). Polycystic kidney disease: Guidelines for family physicians. *American Family Physician, 53*(3), 847, 848, 850.

U.S. Renal Data Systems. (1995). *USRDS 1995 annual data report*. Bethesda, MD: The National Institutes of Health, National Institute of Diabetes and Digestive and Kidney Diseases.

*Walker, W. G., Neaton, J. D., Cutler, J. A., Neuwirth, R., & Cohen, J. D. (1992). Renal function change in hypertensive members of the multiple risk factor intervention trial. *Journal of the American Medical Association, 268*(21), 3085–3091.

Watson, M., & Torres, V. (Eds.). (1996). *Polycystic kidney disease*. New York: Oxford University Press.

*Wiseman, K. C. (1991). Nephrotic syndrome: Pathophysiology and treatment. *American Nephrology Nurses' Association Journal, 18*(5), 469–478, 504.

*Working Group on Renovascular Hypertension. (1987). Detection, evaluation, and treatment of renovascular hypertension: Final report. *Archives of Internal Medicine, 147*, 820–829.

SUGGESTED READINGS

Holcomb, S. S. (1997). Understanding the ins and outs of diuretic therapy. *Nursing97, 27*(2), 34–40, 47.
This article begins with a review of fluid balance in the kidney, including the effects of aldosterone, antidiuretic hormone, and atrial natriuretic factor on the kidney. A detailed description of the five classes of diuretics follows. These classes include loop diuretics, thiazides, potassium-sparing diuretics, carbonic anhydrase inhibitors, and osmotic diuretics. Actions, indications, contraindications, adverse effects, and nursing implications are covered. A continuing education test is included.

Letizia, M., & Conway, A. M. (1996). Interleukin-2 therapy for renal cell cancer. *Critical Care Nurse, 16*(5), 20–26, 30–32, 34–35.
This article reviews renal cell carcinoma and then discusses the immune system effects of interleukin-2 (IL-2), the use of IL-2 (Proleukin) as treatment for advanced renal cell carcinoma, its dosages, and its side effects. Nursing diagnoses related to common side effects are identified. Comprehensive discharge information for clients receiving IL-2 is presented in table format.

McCarthy, S., & McMullen, M. (1997). Autosomal dominant polycystic kidney disease: Pathophysiology and treatment. *American Nephrology Nurses' Association Journal, 24*(1), 45–53.
This comprehensive article on polycystic kidney disease (PKD) covers all aspects of the disease. The three different genotypes causing the three different types of PKD are explained, as are the pathophysiologic mechanisms of cyst formation. Pathophysiology, treatment, and nursing implications for the renal and extrarenal manifestations of PKD are discussed. Diagnostic studies, including DNA linkage studies and genetic screening, are included. There is a comprehensive reference list and a continuing education test.

Chapter 75

INTERVENTIONS FOR CLIENTS WITH CHRONIC AND ACUTE RENAL FAILURE

CHAPTER

HIGHLIGHTS

In the United States, kidney disease remains a major cause of morbidity, afflicting millions of people annually and placing a financial burden on the health care system. Infections and obstructive conditions have been implicated in the development of renal failure. With advances such as dialysis and renal transplantation, however, many people with renal failure have increased life spans. This aspect of improved care does contribute to the increased morbidity statistics and incurs costs of approximately 10 billion dollars annually.

The functions of the kidney are excretion of waste, water and salt regulation, maintenance of acid balance, and hormone secretion. When renal function deteriorates gradually, as occurs with most causes of chronic renal failure, 90% to 95% of the nephrons must be destroyed before significant renal failure is evident. The client may have many years of decreased renal reserve and chronic renal insufficiency before the uremia of end-stage renal failure develops. During this time of decreased renal reserve or chronic renal insufficiency, the client is at increased risk for acute renal failure due to the diminished availability of functioning nephrons.

When renal deterioration is sudden, the capacity of the functioning nephrons is exceeded more quickly, and thus renal failure may develop with the loss of only 50% of functioning nephrons. Acute and chronic renal failure are compared in Table 75–1. Acute renal failure affects *many* body systems; chronic renal failure affects *every* body system. The abnormalities are primarily related to the effects of

- Fluid volume excess
- Electrolyte and acid-base abnormalities
- Accumulated nitrogenous wastes
- Hormonal inadequacies

When renal function decreases to the point that the kidneys can no longer meet the body's homeostatic demands, renal replacement therapy is required to prevent death from potentially life-threatening consequences.

Chronic Renal Failure

Overview

Chronic renal failure (CRF) is a clinical syndrome of progressive, irreversible kidney injury. When kidney function is inadequate for sustaining life, chronic renal failure is

TABLE 75–1

Characteristics of Acute and Chronic Renal Failure		
Characteristic	**Acute Renal Failure**	**Chronic Renal Failure**
Onset	• Sudden (hours to days)	• Gradual (months to years)
Percentage of nephron involvement	• ~50%	• 90%–95%
Duration	• 2–4 weeks; less than 3 months	• Permanent
Prognosis	• Good for return of renal function with supportive care; high mortality in some situations	• Fatal without a renal replacement therapy such as dialysis or transplantation

referred to as end-stage renal disease (ESRD). Terms associated with renal failure include *azotemia* (the accumulation of nitrogenous waste products in the bloodstream), *uremia* (azotemia with clinical symptoms [Chart 75–1]), *uremic syndrome* (the diverse systemic clinical and laboratory manifestations associated with ESRD), and *renal replacement therapy* (hemodialysis, peritoneal dialysis, renal transplantation; necessary to sustain life in clients with renal failure).

Pathophysiology

Stages of Renal Failure

The kidneys tend to fail in an organized fashion. The client's progression toward ESRD (Table 75–2) usually begins with a gradual decrease in renal function. Initially, there is a *diminished renal reserve.* A 24-hour urine specimen for monitoring creatinine clearance is necessary to detect that renal reserve is less than normal. In this stage, reduced renal function occurs without any measurable accumulation of metabolic wastes in the serum because of the ability of the unaffected nephrons to compensate for the decreased functioning of the diseased nephrons. Renal damage is accompanied by an elevation in the systemic blood pressure, resulting in an increase in the pressure within the glomerular apparatus and the remaining unaffected nephrons. Eventually, the unaffected nephrons may be damaged by long-term exposure to this increased pressure, leading to the progressive renal damage characteristic of chronic renal failure (CRF).

In the next stage, *renal insufficiency,* metabolic wastes begin to accumulate in the blood because the healthier

kidney tissue can no longer compensate for the loss of nonfunctioning nephrons. Levels of blood urea nitrogen (BUN), serum creatinine, uric acid, and phosphorus are increasingly elevated in relation to the degree of renal function loss. Careful nursing and medical management of fluid volume, blood pressure, electrolytes, dietary intake, and medication administration may slow the progression of renal failure.

Many clients ultimately progress to *end-stage-renal disease.* Excessive amounts of nitrogenous wastes, such as urea and creatinine, accumulate in the blood, and the kidneys cannot maintain homeostasis. Initially, severe fluid overload and electrolyte and acid-base imbalances occur. Without renal replacement therapy, fatal complications are likely.

TABLE 75–2

Progression Toward Chronic Renal Failure
Stage I: Diminished Renal Reserve
• Renal function is reduced, but no accumulation of metabolic wastes occurs.
• The healthier kidney compensates for the diseased kidney.
• Ability to concentrate urine is decreased, resulting in nocturia and polyuria.
• A 24-hour urine for creatinine clearance is necessary to detect that renal reserve is less than normal.
Stage II: Renal Insufficiency
• Metabolic wastes begin to accumulate in the blood because the unaffected nephrons can no longer compensate.
• Responsiveness to diuretics is decreased, resulting in oliguria and edema.
• The degree of insufficiency is determined by decreasing GFR and is classified as mild, moderate, or severe.
• Treatment is medical.
Stage III: End-Stage Renal Disease
• Excessive amounts of metabolic wastes such as urea and creatinine accumulate in the blood.
• The kidneys are unable to maintain homeostasis.
• Treatment is by dialysis or other renal replacement therapy.

GFR = glomerular filtration rate.

Chart 75–1

Key Features of Uremia

• Metallic taste in the mouth	• Fatigue and lethargy
• Anorexia	• Hiccups
• Nausea	• Edema
• Vomiting	• Dyspnea
• Muscle cramps	• Muscle cramps
• Itching	• Paresthesias

Pathologic Alterations

Renal dysfunction causes multiple pathologic situations, including disruptions in the glomerular filtration rate (GFR), abnormalities of urine production and water excretion, electrolyte imbalances, and metabolic abnormalities. The kidneys can maintain an effective GFR until 70% to 80% of renal function is lost. Homeostasis is maintained until late in the course of renal failure. When less than 20% of the nephrons are functional, the GFR is altered despite hypertrophy of the remaining nephrons. This alteration occurs because the hypertrophied nephrons can maintain the excretion of solutes or waste products only by decreasing water reabsorption. As a result, *hyposthenuria* (the loss of urine concentrating ability) and *polyuria* (increased urinary output) occur. Both hyposthenuria and polyuria are early signs of CRF and, if untreated, can cause severe dehydration.

As the disease progresses, the ability to dilute the urine is increasingly diminished, resulting in urine with a fixed osmolality (*isosthenuria*). As renal function continues to diminish, the concentration of urea is increased in the blood, and urinary output decreases. When renal function deteriorates to this level, the client is at risk for fluid overload due to loss of adequate urinary output.

Metabolic Alterations

UREA AND CREATININE.
Renal failure also causes disturbances in urea and creatinine excretion. Creatinine is derived from creatine and phosphocreatine, which are present in skeletal muscle. The normal rate of creatinine excretion depends on muscle mass, physical activity, and diet. Without *major* alterations in diet or physical activity, the serum creatinine level remains relatively constant. Creatinine is partially excreted by the renal tubules, and a decrease in renal function leads to a build-up of serum creatinine. Urea is the primary product of protein metabolism and is excreted by the kidneys. The BUN level normally varies directly with protein intake.

An important method for accurately estimating the GFR is monitoring the creatinine clearance of the kidneys. As renal function and glomerular filtration diminish, creatinine clearance decreases, and the serum creatinine level rises (see Chap. 72).

SODIUM.
In addition to decreased BUN and creatinine excretion, alterations in sodium excretion are common. Early in CRF, the client is particularly susceptible to hyponatremia (sodium depletion) because, although a diminishing number of nephrons are reabsorbing sodium at their maximal ability, there is an obligatory loss of sodium in urine production. Thus, the polyuria often seen in early renal failure also causes sodium depletion.

In the later stages of renal failure, the capacity of the kidneys to excrete sodium diminishes as urine production decreases. As a result, sodium retention can occur with only modest increases in dietary sodium intake and can lead to severe fluid and electrolyte imbalances (see Chaps. 15 and 16). Sodium retention manifests as hypertension and edema.

Despite the sodium retention, the concurrent retention of water results in an *apparently* normal serum sodium level; dilutional hyponatremia is likely, as fluid volume excess develops (Table 75–3).

POTASSIUM.
The kidney is the primary organ responsible for potassium excretion. Any increase in potassium load during the later stages of renal disease can lead to hyperkalemia (excessive potassium retention). Normal serum potassium levels of 3.5 to 5 mEq/L are maintained until the 24-hour urinary output falls below 500 mL, with a decreased GFR. When hyperkalemia develops, serum levels are quickly elevated and may be 7 to 8 mEq/L or higher. Severe electrocardiographic (ECG) changes result from this elevation, increasing the risk of fatal dysrhythmias. Other factors contributing to hyperkalemia in renal failure include ingestion of potassium in medications, failure to restrict potassium in the diet, blood transfusions, and excessive bleeding or hemorrhage. (See Chapter 16 for discussion of hyperkalemia.)

ACID-BASE BALANCE.
In the early stages of renal disease, loss of functioning nephrons causes little change in blood pH because the remaining nephrons increase their rate of acid excretion. As the loss of nephrons continues, the kidneys cannot compensate, and acid excretion is restricted; a *bicarbonate deficit* or *metabolic acidosis* results (see Chap. 19).

Numerous factors contribute to metabolic acidosis in renal failure. First, the kidney becomes unable to excrete excessive hydrogen ions. Normally, renal tubular cells secrete hydrogen ions into the tubular lumen for excretion, but ammonia and bicarbonate are required for excretion to take place. In clients with renal failure, the kidney's ability to produce ammonia is decreased, and the normal reabsorption of filtered bicarbonate does not occur. This process leads to a build-up of hydrogen ions for which the supply of bicarbonate and other buffering bases is inadequate. As a result, there is a base (bicarbonate) deficit in an environment with excess acid. In the presence of hyperkalemia, renal ammonium production and excretion are inhibited further.

As renal failure advances and acid retention increases, respiratory compensation is essential for maintenance of a blood pH compatible with life. The respiratory system compensates for the decreased pH by increasing the rate and depth of breathing to excrete carbon dioxide through the lungs. This pattern of breathing, called *Kussmaul respirations,* is increasingly apparent with worsening renal failure results in respiratory alkalosis. Serum bicarbonate measures the extent of metabolic acidosis (bicarbonate deficit). Individuals with CRF usually require treatment with alkali replacement to counteract acidosis.

CALCIUM AND PHOSPHATE.
A complex, balanced reciprocal relationship between calcium and phosphate is influenced by vitamin D (see Chap. 16). Vitamin D facilitates calcium absorption in the intestines, and the kidney produces 1,25-dihydroxycholecalciferol, a hormone needed to create active vitamin D.

In renal failure, phosphate retention and a deficiency of active vitamin D contribute to the disruption in calcium and phosphate balance and metabolism. Normally, excessive dietary phosphate is excreted by the kidneys in the

TABLE 75–3

Effects of Renal Failure on Electrolyte Balance

Electrolyte	Effects of Renal Failure	Problems	Treatments
Potassium	• Retained with oliguria	• Hyperkalemia 　• Cardiac dysrhythmias 　• Asystole	• Kayexalate, PO or rectal • Regular IV insulin with 5% to 50% dextrose • IV calcium gluconate • Dialysis
Sodium	• Retained	• Dilutional hyponatremia • Fluid volume excess • Hypertension • Congestive heart failure • Pulmonary edema	• Diuretics, until no longer responsive • Dialysis • Fluid restriction • Sodium restriction
Phosphate	• Retained	• Hyperphosphatemia • Metastatic calcium phosphate deposits • Renal bone disease	• Phosphate-binding agents • Limit phosphorus intake • Vitamin D analogs
Calcium	• Decreased gastrointestinal absorption • Binds to phosphate	• Bone demineralization • Pathologic fractures	• Replace vitamin D • Calcium supplements
Hydrogen	• Retained	• Binds with bicarbonate for excretion through respiratory compensation	• Dialysis • Bicarbonate supplements
Bicarbonate	• Depleted	• Used for blood buffering to prevent metabolic acidemia	• Dialysis • Bicarbonate supplements
Magnesium	• Retained	• Potential for hypermagnesemia	• Avoid magnesium-containing antacids and laxatives

urine. Parathyroid hormone (PTH) regulates the amount of phosphate in the blood by causing tubular excretion of phosphate when there is a serum phosphate excess. One of the initial effects of decreased renal function is decreased phosphate excretion due to a diminished GFR (Fig. 75–1). As plasma phosphate levels increase (causing hyperphosphatemia), calcium levels decrease (causing hypocalcemia). Chronic hypocalcemia results in chronic stimulation, hyperplasia, and hypertrophy of the parathyroid glands. Under the influence of additional PTH, calcium is released from storage areas in bones (bone resorption), which results in demineralization. The additional calcium is needed to compensate, or balance, excess plasma phosphate concentration. The problem of hypocalcemia is compounded because decreased renal function also causes decreased production of active vitamin D. Thus, less calcium is absorbed through the intestinal mucosa in the absence of sufficient vitamin D.

The pathologic process in bone metabolism and structure caused by hypocalcemia and hyperphosphatemia is called *renal osteodystrophy*. Skeletal demineralization resulting from hyperparathyroidism may be manifested as bone pain, sclerosis of the spine, pseudofractures, demineralization of parts of the skull, osteomalacia, resorption of bone, or loss of the lamina dura in the teeth.

Metastatic calcifications, crystals formed from excessive calcium phosphate, may precipitate in various parts of the body. When the plasma concentration of the calcium-phosphate product (serum calcium concentration × serum phosphate concentration) exceeds 70 mg/100 mL,

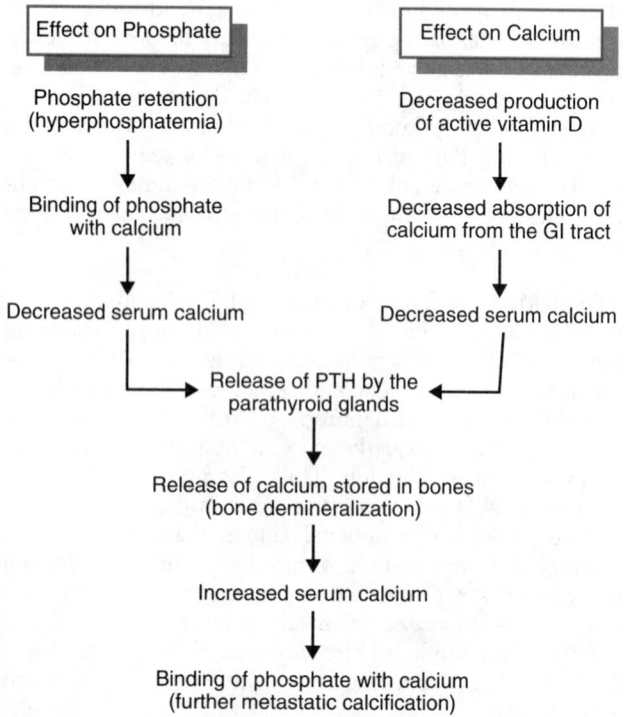

Figure 75–1. The effects of renal failure on phosphate and calcium balance.

the crystals may lodge in the kidneys, heart, lungs, major blood vessels, joints, eyes (causing conjunctivitis), and brain. Uremic pruritus is also believed to be the result of calcium-phosphate imbalances and excess PTH production.

Cardiac Alterations

Chronic renal failure (CRF) also disrupts the cardiovascular system. The more common manifestations are hypertension, congestive heart failure (CHF), and uremic pericarditis.

HYPERTENSION. Approximately 80% to 90% of clients with CRF have hypertension. Hypertension may be either the cause or the result of CRF. The elevation in blood pressure results from fluid and sodium overload and the malfunction of the renin-angiotensin-aldosterone system. The retention of sodium and water in renal disease causes circulatory overload, which leads to elevated blood pressure (BP). The kidneys respond to a decrease in renal blood flow or low serum sodium levels by trying to improve renal blood flow. The release of renin further stimulates the production of angiotensin and aldosterone. Angiotensin causes vasoconstriction and an elevation of blood pressure. Aldosterone, a mineralocorticoid released by the adrenal glands, stimulates the distal convoluted tubule to reabsorb sodium and water. Consequently, plasma volume is expanded, and BP is elevated. As a result of this malfunction of the renin-angiotensin-aldosterone system, BP is elevated either by vasoconstriction or by volume expansion. The kidneys do not recognize the increase in BP and continue to produce renin. The result is severe hypertension that is difficult to treat and that ultimately worsens renal function.

CONGESTIVE HEART FAILURE. Many clients with renal failure have some form of myocardial dysfunction. CRF causes an increased workload on the heart because of anemia, hypertension, and fluid overload. Left ventricular hypertrophy and CHF are common manifestations of late end-stage renal disease (ESRD). Uremia itself may cause uremic cardiomyopathy, the uremic toxin effect on the myocardium. CHF is also common in these clients because of the presence of hypertension and coronary artery disease. Cardiac disease is the leading cause of death in clients with ESRD (U.S. Renal Data System [USRDS], 1996).

UREMIC PERICARDITIS. Pericarditis also occurs in clients with CRF. If it is not carefully treated, this inflammation of the pericardium can lead to pericardial effusion, cardiac tamponade, and death. The pericardial sac becomes inflamed and irritated by uremic toxins or infection. Signs and symptoms include localized, severe chest pain, increased pulse rate, low-grade fever, and an intermittent and transient pericardial friction rub that can be heard on auscultation.

As the pericarditis continues and the pericardial effusion worsens, dysrhythmias may develop: Heart tones become softer and less audible; BP decreases; and the client may experience shortness of breath. Progressive pericardial effusion results in cardiac tamponade, a medical and surgical emergency in which pulse pressure diminishes and bradycardia or asystole results. Treatment of pericardial tamponade involves removal of pericardial fluid by placement of a needle, catheter, or drainage tube into the pericardium or pericardiectomy with pericardial drainage.

Hematologic Alterations

Anemia is the primary hematologic abnormality in clients with chronic renal failure. The causes include decreased erythropoietin level with resulting decreased red blood cell (RBC) production, decreased RBC survival time resulting from uremia, iron and folic acid deficiencies, and impaired platelet function as a result of uremic toxins.

Gastrointestinal Alterations

Uremia can affect all levels of the GI system. The normal flora of the oral cavity is altered in uremia. The mouth normally contains the enzyme urease that hydrolyzes urea. The ammonia generated from this reaction contributes to uremic halitosis and may also cause uremic stomatitis (mouth inflammation).

Anorexia, nausea, vomiting, and hiccups are relatively common in clients with uremia. The specific cause of these symptoms is uncertain but may be related to increased nitrogenous waste levels (i.e., BUN and creatinine) and metabolic acidosis.

Uremic colitis with profound watery diarrhea or constipation may also be present in clients with uremia. Ulcerations may occur in the stomach or small or large intestines, causing erosion of blood vessels. The blood loss caused by these erosions may result in melena or, in more serious cases, may progress to hemorrhagic shock from severe GI bleeding.

Etiology

The etiology of CRF is complex (Table 75–4). More than 100 different disease processes can cause progressive loss of renal function (see also Chap. 74). The overlapping nature of the causes of CRF are related to a variety of classification schemes used to organize the disorders. Improved diagnostic techniques have created new perspectives about the nature of CRF.

Incidence/Prevalence

The number of clients with CRF is continually increasing. As people age and live longer, irreversible (chronic) renal failure from diabetes mellitus and hypertension is more apparent. Because information on the incidence of CRF was not available, the U.S. Renal Data System was created in 1988 to centralize data and provide information about the incidence, prevalence, causes, mortality, and morbidity associated with ESRD. The 1996 United States Renal Data Systems Annual report suggests that over 242,757 people in the United States are receiving treatment for end-stage renal disease. In 1996, the reported incidence of renal disease (i.e., new clients requiring renal replacement therapy) was 54,586. There were 37,106 deaths in 1994 related to ESRD. Three primary causes of ESRD

TABLE 75–4

Selected Causes of Chronic Renal Failure

Morphologic

Glomerular Disease

- Glomerulonephritis
- Basement membrane disease
- Goodpasture syndrome
- Intercapillary glomerulosclerosis

Tubular Disease

- Chronic hypercalcemia
- Chronic potassium depletion
- Fanconi syndrome
- Heavy metal (lead) poisoning

Vascular Disease of the Kidney

- Ischemic disease of the kidney
- Bilateral renal artery stenosis
- Nephrosclerosis
- Hyperparathyroidism

Urinary Tract Disease

- Obstructive uropathy

Congenital Anomalies

- Hypoplastic kidneys
- Medullary cystic disease
- Polycystic kidney disease

Etiologic

Infection

- Pyelonephritis
- Tuberculosis

Systemic Vascular Disease

- Intrarenal renovascular hypertension
- Extrarenal renovascular hypertension

Metabolic Renal Disease

- Amyloidosis
- Gout (hyperuricemic nephropathy)
- Diabetic nephropathy
- Milk-alkali syndrome
- Sarcoidosis

Connective Tissue Disease

- Progressive systemic sclerosis
- Systemic lupus erythematosus
- Polyarteritis

Note: List is not all-inclusive.

include diabetes mellitus (26%), hypertension (24%), and glomerulonephritis (19%) (U.S. Renal Data System, 1996). The annual growth rate is about 10% per year. The greatest increase in ESRD is among those 65 years old and older. More than 186,822 people were estimated to be receiving renal replacement therapy in the United States in 1994 (U.S. Renal Data System, 1996). Chart 75–2 addresses *prevention* of renal failure.

The ability to extend and maintain life with dialysis or transplantation has evolved in the past 20 to 25 years. Before 1973, many people with ESRD did not have access to the technology that was developing in university-based or affiliated research centers; the treatments were also expensive, and long-term therapy was not realistic for most. Consequently, most clients died from the disorder. The passage in 1973 of Public Law 92–603, an amendment to the Social Security legislation, created a special provision of Medicare for people of any age with ESRD. As a result of this and subsequent legislation, federal reimbursement for many, but not all, expenses for renal replacement therapy has extended the lives of thousands of people.

Collaborative Management

 Assessment

➤ History

When taking a history from a client with suspected chronic renal failure (CRF), the nurse remembers the signs and symptoms of CRF. The nurse notes the client's age and gender. The nurse obtains accurate weight and height measurements and inquires about usual weight and recent weight gain or loss. Weight gain may indicate cardiovascular overload and fluid retention caused by poorly functioning kidneys. Weight loss may be the result of anorexia associated with the uremic syndrome. The nurse ascertains the client's blood pressure if known.

Chart 75–2

Health Promotion Guide: Prevention of Renal and Urinary Problems

- Be alert to the general appearance of your urine. Note any changes in its color, clarity, or odor.
- Changes in the frequency or volume of urine passage occur with changes in fluid intake. More frequent, or infrequent, voiding not associated with changes in fluid intake may signal potential problems.
- Any discomfort or distress with the passage of urine is not normal. Pain, burning, urgency, aching, or difficulty with initiating urine flow or complete bladder emptying is of some concern.
- The kidneys need 1½ to 2 quarts of fluid a day to flush out your body wastes. Water is the ideal flushing agent.
- Changes in kidney function are often silent for many years. Periodically ask your health care provider to measure your kidney function with a blood test (serum creatinine) and a urinalysis.
- If you have a history of renal disease, diabetes mellitus, or hypertension (high blood pressure) or a family history of kidney disease, you should know your serum creatinine level and your 24-hour creatinine clearance. At least one checkup per year that includes laboratory blood and urine testing of kidney function is recommended.
- If you are identified as having decreased kidney function, ask about whether any prescribed medication, diet, diagnostic test, or therapeutic procedure will present a risk to your current kidney function. Check out all nonprescription medications with your physician or pharmacist before using them.

The nurse also obtains a complete history of known renal or urologic disorders, long-term health problems, medication use, and current health conditions. The client is asked about any knowledge of existing renal disease or family history of renal disease, which might indicate a hereditary disorder. A history of kidney infection or renal calculi could imply past kidney damage. It is important to explore long-term health problems because illnesses such as hypertension, diabetes, systemic lupus erythematosus, arthritis, cancer, and tuberculosis can contribute to decreased renal function.

The nurse documents medication use, both prescription and over the counter, because many medications are potentially nephrotoxic and can cause renal damage.

The nurse examines the client's dietary or nutritional habits and discusses any present GI problems. A change in the taste of foods often accompanies renal failure. Clients may note that sweet foods are not as appealing or that certain foods, especially meats, leave a metallic taste in the mouth. The nurse specifically assesses the client for a history of GI problems, such as nausea, vomiting, anorexia, hiccups, diarrhea, or constipation. Any of these manifestations can be the result of the build-up of nitrogenous or other metabolic wastes that the body cannot excrete because of renal malfunction.

The nurse questions the client about his or her current energy level and any recent injuries or bleeding. The nurse explores and notes changes in the client's daily routine as a *result* of physical fatigue. Weakness, drowsiness, and shortness of breath are typical and suggest impending pulmonary edema or neurologic degeneration. The nurse asks specifically about abnormal bruising or bleeding, which may be the result of hematologic changes associated with uremia.

The nurse discusses the client's urinary elimination in detail, including frequency of urination, appearance of the urine, and any difficulty starting or controlling urination. This information can help identify existing urologic disorders that may influence the preservation of existing renal function.

➤ *Physical Assessment/Clinical Manifestations*

Chronic renal failure (CRF) results in many multisystem manifestations (Chart 75-3). Clinical manifestations of CRF or uremia are associated with changes in fluid volume and chemical composition. The specific causes of many of these manifestations are not known.

Neurologic Manifestations. Neurologic manifestations of the uremic syndrome of CRF are numerous (see Chart 75-3) and vary widely, depending on nitrogenous waste products, acid-base imbalances, and electrolyte imbalances. The nurse observes for neurologic signs, ranging from lethargy to seizures or coma, indicating uremic encephalopathy. In addition, the nurse assesses for sensory changes that generally appear in a glove and stocking distribution over the lower extremities and examines for weakness in the upper or lower extremities (i.e., uremic neuropathy).

If untreated, uremic encephalopathy progresses to seizures and coma. Dialysis is the treatment of choice for neurologic disturbances associated with CRF. The mani-

festations of uremic encephalopathy resolve with the initiation of dialysis. However, improvement in uremic neuropathy is limited if the neuropathy is severe and motor function is already impaired.

Cardiovascular Manifestations. The clinical manifestations of CRF and uremia lead to specific cardiovascular abnormalities of fluid volume excess, hypertension, congestive heart failure (CHF), uremic pericarditis, and cardiac dysrhythmias associated with hyperkalemia. The nurse assesses for signs of a diminished ability to excrete salt and water. The resulting circulatory fluid overload, if untreated, can lead to CHF, pulmonary edema, peripheral edema, and hypertension.

The nurse assesses heart rate and rhythm, listening for extra beats (particularly an S_3), irregular patterns, or a pericardial friction rub. Unless a hemodialysis vascular access has been previously created, blood pressure is measured in each arm. The nurse inspects the jugular veins for distention and assesses for pedal, pretibial, presacral, and periorbital edema. Shortness of breath with exertion and paroxysmal nocturnal dyspnea (PND) suggest fluid volume excess.

Respiratory Manifestations. Respiratory manifestations of CRF vary widely among clients (for example, breath that smells like urine [*uremic fetor* or uremic halitosis], deep sighing, yawning, shortness of breath). The nurse notes the rhythm, rate, and depth of breathing. Tachypnea (increased rate of breathing) and hyperpnea (increased depth of breathing) are respiratory compensation mechanisms for worsening metabolic acidosis.

With severe metabolic acidosis, the nurse may observe extreme hyperventilation or Kussmaul respirations. A few clients have hilar pneumonitis, or *uremic lung*. In these clients, the nurse assesses for thick sputum, minimal coughing, increased respiratory rate, and an elevated temperature. A pleural friction rub may be heard with a stethoscope. Clients often have pleuritic pain with breathing. The nurse auscultates the lungs for crackles, which indicate fluid volume overload.

Hematologic Manifestations. Hematologic abnormalities include anemia and abnormal bleeding. The nurse notes indicators of anemia, including fatigue, pallor, lethargy, weakness, shortness of breath, and dizziness. The nurse assesses for abnormal bleeding by noting bruising, petechiae, purpura, ecchymoses (confluent bruises), mucous membrane bleeding in the nose or gums, abnormal vaginal bleeding, or gastrointestinal (GI) bleeding (often demonstrated by black tarry stools [melena]).

Gastrointestinal Manifestations. The nurse assesses for a foul odor to the breath, mouth ulceration, or mouth inflammation and notes any vomiting. Abdominal pain or cramping may be associated with uremic colitis. Stools may test positive for blood.

Urinary Manifestations. The urinary findings in renal failure reflect the kidneys' decreasing functioning. At first, changes occur in the amount, frequency, and appearance of the urine. Many etiologic features of chronic renal disease result in proteinuria; some cause hematuria.

The quantity and composition of the urine change as

Chart 75–3

Key Features of Chronic Renal Failure

Neurologic Manifestations
- Lethargy and daytime drowsiness
- Inability to concentrate or decreased attention span
- Seizures
- Coma
- Slurred speech
- Asterixis
- Tremors, twitching, or jerky movements
- Myoclonus
- Ataxia (alteration in gait)
- Paresthesias

Cardiovascular Manifestations
- Cardiomyopathy
- Hypertension
- Peripheral edema
- Congestive heart failure
- Uremic pericarditis
- Pericardial effusion
- Pericardial fraction rub
- Cardiac tamponade

Respiratory Manifestations
- Uremic halitosis
- Tachypnea
- Deep sighing, yawning
- Kussmaul respirations
- Uremic pneumonitis
- Shortness of breath
- Pulmonary edema
- Pleural effusion
- Depressed cough reflex
- Crackles

Hematologic Manifestations
- Anemia
- Abnormal bleeding and bruising

Gastrointestinal Manifestations
- Anorexia
- Nausea
- Vomiting
- Metallic taste in the mouth
- Changes in taste acuity and sensation
- Uremic colitis (diarrhea)
- Constipation
- Uremic gastritis (possible GI bleeding)
- Uremic fetor
- Stomatitis
- Diarrhea

Urinary Manifestations
- Polyuria, nocturia (early)
- Oliguria, anuria (later)
- Proteinuria
- Hematuria
- Diluted, straw-like appearance

Integumentary Manifestations
- Decreased skin turgor
- Yellow-gray pallor
- Dry skin
- Pruritus
- Ecchymosis
- Purpura
- Soft-tissue calcifications
- Uremic frost (late, premorbid)

Musculoskeletal Manifestations
- Muscle weakness and cramping
- Bone pain
- Pathologic fractures
- Renal osteodystrophy

Reproductive Manifestations
- Decreased fertility
- Infrequent or absent menses
- Decreased libido
- Impotence

---

renal function deteriorates. With the onset of end-stage renal disease (ESRD), the urine may become more dilute and clearer, reflecting a diminished glomerular filtration rate (GFR). The nurse must be aware that the actual urinary output in a client with CRF varies with the amount of remaining renal function. The client with ESRD usually has oliguria (urinary output of 400–500 mL/24 hours), but some clients will remain relatively nonoliguric, producing 1 L or more per 24 hours. Urine volume produced per day will probably change again after dialysis is initiated.

Integumentary Manifestations. There are several dermatologic manifestations of CRF. In clients with uremia, deposition of urochrome pigment in the skin results in a yellowish coloration. Some African-American clients report a darkening of the skin. The anemia of CRF causes a sallowness to the quality of the color, which some people describe as a faded suntan. This is most noticeable in lighter skinned clients.

Skin oils and turgor are decreased in clients with uremia. One of the most uncomfortable problems of uremia is severe pruritus (itching). The nurse also assesses for bruises (ecchymoses), purple patches (purpura), and, occasionally, drug-induced rashes.

Uremic frost, a layer of urea crystals from evaporated perspiration, may appear on the face, eyebrows, axilla, and groin in clients with advanced uremic syndrome.

➤ Psychosocial Assessment

Chronic renal failure (CRF) and its treatment disrupt more aspects of a client's life than almost any other illness. Nurses are in a unique position to evaluate the client with newly diagnosed renal failure and to assist with these adjustments.

Psychosocial assessment and support are part of the nurse's role from the time that CRF is first diagnosed. Initially, the nurse asks about the client's understanding of the diagnosis and its implications for treatment regimens (e.g., diet, medication, and dialysis). The nurse assesses for any signs of anxiety and for the coping mechanisms used by the client or family members. Some of the psychosocial aspects altered by CRF include family relations, social activity, work patterns, body image, and sexual activity. The chronicity of ESRD, the variety of treatment options, and the uncertainties surrounding the course of the disease and its treatment necessitate an ongoing psychosocial assessment.

➤ Laboratory Assessment

Chronic renal failure results in serious abnormalities in many laboratory values (Chart 75–4). The following blood values are routinely monitored in CRF clients: creatinine, blood urea nitrogen, sodium, potassium, calcium, phosphate, bicarbonate, hemoglobin, and hematocrit.

Initially, a urinalysis is performed, and a 24-hour urine specimen for creatinine and urea clearance is obtained. In the early stages of renal insufficiency, urinalysis can reveal key indicators of kidney function. Urinalysis may show excessive protein, glucose, red blood cells (RBCs), white blood cells (WBCs), and decreased or fixed specific gravity. Urine osmolality is usually decreased. A 24-hour creatinine clearance is calculated after serum and urinary creatinine levels are collected and quantified. These data, along with information on body weight and height, are used to calculate renal creatinine clearance. As renal failure progresses, the urinary output may decrease dramatically.

Trends in renal function and progressive deterioration are typically monitored by measurements of the serum creatinine and BUN levels. Serum creatinine levels may increase gradually over a period of years, reaching levels of 15 to 30 mg/dL or more, depending on the client's muscle mass. Urea nitrogen levels are directly related to dietary protein intake. Without dietary protein restriction, BUN levels are typically 10 to 20 times that of the serum creatinine level. As dietary protein is increasingly restricted in an attempt to slow the rate of progression of renal failure, BUN levels remain elevated but less than the 10:1 to 20:1 ratio of nonprotein-restricted clients. Other factors affect the level of BUN, and the nurse must consider these for a complete client assessment. (Chapter 72 describes the factors influencing BUN levels as well as the interpretation of serum creatinine and creatinine clearance.)

➤ Radiographic Assessment

X-ray findings in clients with CRF are few. Bone radiographs of the metacarpals and phalanges of the hand can reveal the presence of renal osteodystrophy. With established ESRD, the kidneys are atrophic and may be 8 to 9 cm or less. This diminished size is usually the result of renal tubular atrophy and fibrosis. If obstructive uropathy is a possible factor contributing to more rapid than expected deterioration of renal function, a renal ultrasound or computed tomographic (CT) scan without contrast media may be obtained. (See Chapter 72 for a complete description of renal diagnostic tests.)

 Analysis

The client with CRF has usually experienced a progressive degeneration of renal function and is frequently hospitalized for evaluation and modification of the treatment plan. The focus of care is to control or manage symptoms and prevent complications.

➤ Common Nursing Diagnoses and Collaborative Problems

The following nursing diagnoses are applicable to all clients with chronic renal failure:
1. Altered Nutrition: Less than Body Requirements related to nausea and vomiting, decreased appetite, effects of a catabolic state, decreased level of consciousness, altered taste sensations, or dietary restrictions
2. Fluid Volume Excess related to compromised regulatory mechanisms (the inability of the kidney to maintain body fluid balance)
3. Decreased Cardiac Output related to reduction in stroke volume as a result of electrical malfunction (dysrhythmias) and mechanical malfunction (increased preload [volume excess] and increased afterload [increased peripheral vascular resistance])
4. Risk for Infection related to inadequate primary defenses (broken skin), chronic disease, or malnutrition
5. Risk for Injury related to internal biochemical risk factors associated with renal failure (increased susceptibility to bleeding, falls, and pathologic fractures) and external risk factors, such as drugs
6. Fatigue related to altered metabolic energy production, imbalance between oxygen supply and demand, and anemia
7. Anxiety related to threat to or change in health status, socioeconomic status, relationships, role functioning, support systems, or self-concept; situational crisis; threat of death; lack of knowledge (procedures, diagnostic tests, disease process, renal replacement therapy); loss of control; feelings of failure; or disrupted family life

The primary collaborative problem is Potential for Pulmonary Edema.

➤ Additional Nursing Diagnoses and Collaborative Problems

The client may also exhibit one or more of the following diagnoses and collaborative problems:
- Diarrhea related to chemical or electrolyte imbalances, fear, anxiety, or side effects of medications
- Altered Oral Mucous Membrane related to parotid gland changes, limited fluid intake, malnutrition, and elevated levels of uremic toxins
- Impaired Skin Integrity related to altered chemical balance and uremic toxins

Chart 75–4

Laboratory Profile: Renal Failure

Test	Normal Range for Adults	Values in Renal Failure	Comments
Tests to Evaluate Removal of Nitrogenous Wastes			
Serum creatinine	• 0.6–1.1 mg/dL (women) • 0.9–1.3 mg/dL (men) • **Elderly:** Decreased	*In Chronic Renal Failure* • May increase by 0.5–1.0 mg/dL every 1–2 yr • May be as high as 15–30 mg/dL *before* symptoms of CRF are present *In Acute Renal Failure* • Gradual increase of 1–2 mg/dL every 24–48 hr • May increase 1–6 mg/dL in 1 wk or less	• Consistently elevated levels indicate decreased renal function. • Serum creatinine levels are used to evaluate the effectiveness of dialysis treatments.
Blood urea nitrogen	• 6–20 mg/dL • **Elderly:** May be slightly increased	*In Chronic Renal Failure* • May reach 180–200 mg/dL *before* symptoms develop *In Acute Renal Failure* • Often increases by 10–20 mg/dL at same pace as serum creatinine level • May reach 80–100 mg/dL within 1 wk	• Increases depend on protein intake and other factors (see text). • Rate of increase is controlled by limiting protein intake. This intervention is believed to decrease the rate of onset of systemic symptoms, such as anorexia, nausea, and vomiting. • Elevations have multiple causes, including diminished renal function, excessive protein intake, sepsis, GI bleeding, dehydration, and tissue catabolism.
Electrolyte Studies			
Serum sodium	• 132–146 mEq/L; 136–145 mmol/L (SI units)	• Normal or decreased	• Clients with renal failure retain sodium. • With associated water retention, serum sodium levels seem normal. • With excessive water retention, serum sodium levels seem decreased owing to hemodilution. • Assess the client for evidence of fluid volume excess: edema, weight increase, or elevation of diastolic blood pressure. • Limit fluid intake as directed. • Avoid excessive sodium intake. • Monitor for signs of hypernatremia: dry skin, excessive thirst, dry mucous membranes, elevated body temperature, and flushed skin. • Client may need diuretics or dialysis.

■ Social Isolation related to illness or alterations in physical appearance
■ Altered Family Processes related to situational crisis, reduced income, unemployment, or effects of chronic illness
■ Sexual Dysfunction related to altered body function

(decreased libido and/or impotence) from disease and/or effects of medications, depression, or disturbance in self-esteem or body image
■ Altered Thought Processes related to irritation, CNS depression, side effects of medications, sleep deprivation, or clinical depression

Chart 75-4. Laboratory Profile: Renal Failure   Continued

Test	Normal Range for Adults	Values in Renal Failure	Comments
Serum potassium	• Male 3.5–4.5 mmol/L (SI units); female 3.4–4.4 mmol/L (SI units)	• Increased	• Advise the client to avoid salt substitutes and to limit potassium-containing foods. • Monitor for rapidly increasing serum potassium levels in ARF. • ECG changes occur with serum potassium levels of ≥6.5. • Monitor for signs of hyperkalemia; dizziness, weakness, cardiac irregularities, muscle cramps, diarrhea, and nausea. • May require administration of sodium polystyrene sulfonate (Kayexalate) or other treatment.
Serum phosphorus (phosphate)	• 2.7–4.5 mg/dL; 0.87–1.45 mmol/L (SI units) • **Elderly:** May be slightly decreased	• Increased	• Short-term increases have potential to cause rapid decrease in serum calcium level and cardiac rhythm disturbances. • Long-term increases demineralize bones of calcium and enhance fracture potential. • Phosphate-binding medications help control hyperphosphatemia and prevent calcium depletion from the bones.
Serum calcium	• Total calcium: 9.0–10.5 mg/dL; 2.25–2.75 mmol/L (SI units) • Ionized calcium: 4.60–5.08 mg/dL; 1.15–1.27 mmol/L (SI units) • **Elderly:** Slightly decreased	• Decreased	• Decreases in ARF may necessitate replacement. • Decreases in CRF may only be slight and may or may not necessitate replacement. As the serum phosphate level increases, the serum calcium level decreases. • Chronic calcium deficiency leads to renal osteodystrophy. • Control of phosphate excess is usually essential before calcium replacement is initiated. • Monitor for signs and symptoms of hypocalcemia: abdominal cramps, hyperactive reflexes, tingling in fingertips, and spasms in feet and wrists (see also Chap. 16).
Serum magnesium	• 1.6–2.6 mEq/L; 0.66–1.07 mmol/L (SI units)	• Increased	• Advise the client to avoid compounds containing magnesium (e.g., laxatives).
Serum carbon dioxide combining power (bicarbonate)	• 23–29 mEq/L (venous); 23–29 mmol/L (SI units)	• Decreased	• Replace bicarbonate. • Monitor respiratory rate and depth. • Monitor for decreased orientation.

Continued

- Knowledge Deficit (disease process, care regimen, and follow-up care) related to lack of informational resources and magnitude of the care issues
- Potential for Sepsis
- Potential for Malnutrition
- Potential for Electrolyte Imbalances
- Potential for Metabolic Acidosis
- Potential for GI Bleeding

 Planning and Implementation

Altered Nutrition: Less than Body Requirements

Planning: Expected Outcomes. With intervention, the client is expected to attain and maintain

Chart 75–4. Laboratory Profile: Renal Failure   Continued

Test	Normal Range for Adults	Values in Renal Failure	Comments
Tests of Acid-Base Balance			
Arterial blood pH	• 7.31–7.42	• Decreased (in metabolic acidosis) or normal	• The respiratory system attempts to compensate by hyperventilation (increased rate and depth of respiration). • Values are within the normal range if blood buffers and lungs can compensate. • Monitor breathing rate and depth. Monitor level of consciousness.
Arterial blood bicarbonate (HCO_3^-)	• 21–28 mEq/L	• Decreased	• Provide replacement PO, IV, or by hemodialysis or peritoneal dialysis.
Arterial blood $PaCO_2$	• Male 35–48 mmHg • Female 32–45 mmHg	• Decreased	• Monitor for respiratory fatigue (the client breathes more rapidly and deeply to "blow off" carbon dioxide).
Other Blood Studies			
Hemoglobin	• 11.7–15.5 g/dL (women); 7.4–9.9 mmol/L (SI units) • 13.2–17.3 g/dL (men); 8.7–11.2 mmol/L (SI units) • **Elderly:** Slightly decreased	• Decreased	• Decreased levels indicate anemia. • Monitor for pallor, weakness, lethargy, dizziness, possible shortness of breath, and activity intolerance.
Hematocrit	• 35%–45% (women) • 39%–49% (men) • **Elderly:** May be slightly decreased	• Decreased to 20%	• Same as for hemoglobin. • With EPO therapy, may be able to obtain levels as high as 36%.
Urinalysis*			
Specific gravity	• Usually 1.016–1.022; possible range: 1.001–1.035	• Usually decreased and fixed	• Reflects inability of the tubules to produce a concentrated or diluted urine in response to changes in plasma osmolality. • Monitor for fluid volume deficit or excess.
pH	• Average 5.5–6; possible range: 4.5–8	• May be fixed; pH does not change with dietary changes	• Collect a freshly voided specimen for testing.
Glucose	• None or <15 mg/100 mL • Usually detectable in urine of nondiabetics when blood level is 160–180 mg/dL	• Increased	• The renal threshold is often increased; therefore the blood glucose level may be >160–180 mg/dL before glucose is detectable in the urine. • Monitor *blood* glucose levels.

■ An adequate nutritional status
■ Ideal body weight for age, height, and body build
■ Laboratory values within safe levels

Interventions. The nutritional requirements of the client with renal failure vary according to the degree of decrease in renal function and the type of dialysis performed, if any (Table 75–5). Dietary restrictions include regulation of protein intake, limitation of fluid intake, restriction of potassium, sodium, and phosphorus intake, administration of appropriate vitamin and mineral supplements, and provision of adequate calories to meet metabolic demand.

If adequate calories are not supplied, the body will use tissue protein for energy, which leads to negative nitrogen balance and malnutrition. The diet prescribed for each

Chart 75–4. Laboratory Profile: Renal Failure   Continued

Test	Normal Range for Adults	Values in Renal Failure	Comments
Protein	• 2–8 mg/100 mL	• Increased when there is glomerular damage or disease	• Increases may be an incidental and benign finding. Transient increases occur with extreme exercise, fever, stress, or infection. • Persistent proteinuria requires 24-hr collection for determination of total quantity excreted. • Persistent proteinuria may indicate a serious renal problem. • Instruct the client about the need for follow-up. • Instruct the client in the correct procedure for collection of 24-hr specimen (see Chap. 72).
Occult blood	• No RBCs or occasionally 2 or 3 RBCs per high-power field • No hemoglobin	• More than 2 or 3 RBCs per high-power field • Detectable hemoglobin	• Hemoglobin is detectable when hemolysis of RBCs has occurred. • Intact RBCs are only detectable with microscopic examination. • Collect a freshly voided specimen for testing.
WBCs	• 0–5 per high-power field	• Increased in urinary tract infection	• Often indicates need for urine culture.
Bacteria	• Less than 1000 colonies/mL	• Increased in the presence of infection, with or without an increase in WBCs	• Obtain urine culture.
Casts	• None or a few; composed of RBCs, WBCs, protein, or tubular cell casts such as hyaline	• Casts present	• Casts may be a benign occurrence or may signify that some renal injury or disease is present. • Collect a freshly voided specimen for direct microscopic examination.
Creatinine clearance	• 97–137 mL/min (men) • 88–128 mL/min (women) • **Elderly:** Progressively decreased with advancing age	• Decreased	• Change reflects decreases in GFR. • Creatinine clearance is determined from a 24-hr urine collection, and a serum creatinine value.

*Urine may become cloudy with heavy sediment. Urinary output and appearance vary, depending on remaining renal function.

ARF = acute renal failure; ECG = electrocardiogram; CRF = chronic renal failure; RBCs = red blood cells; WBCs = white blood cells; GFR = glomerular filtration rate.

client should also consider the nutritional needs dictated by age, height, body build, and level of activity. Collaboration with a registered dietitian, nutrition support service, and physician is necessary to assist the client in maintaining adequate nutrition.

Protein Restriction. Preliminary research indicates that early implementation of a protein-restricted diet prevents some of the symptoms associated with CRF and may preserve kidney function. Because accumulation of waste products from protein metabolism is the primary cause of uremia, protein in the diet is restricted on the basis of the degree of renal insufficiency and the severity of the symptoms associated with nitrogen retention.

The glomerular filtration rate (GFR) is often used as an indicator of renal function and can be a guide to safe levels of protein consumption. A client with a severely reduced GFR who is not undergoing dialysis is usually permitted 0.55 to 0.60 g of protein per kilogram of body weight (e.g., 40 g of protein daily for a 150-pound [70-kg] adult). If proteinuria is present, protein is added to the diet in amounts equal to that lost in the urine, as determined by a 24-hour urine collection. The calculation for protein requirement is based on actual body weight (corrected for edema), not ideal body weight. The client receiving dialysis requires more protein because of losses incurred as a result of the therapy. Hemodialysis (HD) clients have their protein requirements individually tailored and based on the client's postdialysis or "dry weight." Typically, HD client's are allowed 1 to 1.2 g of protein per kilogram daily; peritoneal dialysis (PD) clients are allowed 1.2 to 1.4 g of protein per kilogram daily because protein is lost with each exchange (Nelson et al., 1994; Levine, 1997).

TABLE 75–5

Dietary Restrictions for the Client with Renal Failure			
Dietary Component	**With Chronic Uremia**	**With Hemodialysis**	**With Peritoneal Dialysis**
Protein	• 0.55–0.60 g/kg of body weight per day	• 1.0–1.2 g/kg of body weight per day	• 1.2–1.4 g/kg of body weight per day
Fluid	• Depends on urinary output, but may be as high as 1500–3000 mL/day	• 500–700 mL/day plus amount of urinary output	• Restriction based on fluid weight gain and blood
Potassium	• 60–70 mEq/day	• 70 mEq/day	• Usually no restriction
Sodium	• 1–3 g/day	• 2–4 g/day	• Restriction based on fluid weight gain and blood pressure
Phosphorus	• 700 mg/day	• 700 mg/day	• 800 mg/day

Three-fourths of the protein should be of high biologic value, such as milk, meat, or eggs. If protein intake is inadequate, a negative nitrogen balance develops and causes muscle wasting. Serum albumin and BUN levels are used to monitor the adequacy of protein consumption. Decreases in serum albumin levels indicate inadequate protein intake and malnutrition. Excessive protein intake can dramatically increase BUN levels in clients with renal failure.

Sodium Restriction. The nurse closely monitors fluid and sodium intake. In clients with little or no urinary output, fluid and sodium retention can cause edema, hypertension, and congestive heart failure (CHF). Most clients with renal failure retain sodium; a few cannot conserve sodium.

The client's status of fluid and sodium retention can be estimated by monitoring body weight and blood pressure. In nondialyzed uremic clients, sodium is limited to 1 to 3 g daily, and fluid intake depends on urinary output. In oliguric clients receiving dialysis, the sodium restriction is 2 to 4 g daily; fluid intake is limited to 500 to 700 mL plus the amount of any urinary output. The client should know not to add salt at the table or during food preparation. Clients should consume foods with a high sodium content (processed foods, fast foods, potato chips, pretzels, pickles, ham, bacon, and sausage) in moderation.

Potassium Restriction. The nurse carefully monitors potassium intake because hyperkalemia can cause dangerous cardiac dysrhythmias. The nurse monitors the client's cardiac rhythm for the tall, peaked T waves characteristic of hyperkalemia; the serum potassium level is also documented. In conjunction with the physician's orders and dietary instruction, the nurse instructs clients with advanced chronic renal failure (CRF) to limit their potassium intake to 60 to 70 mEq/day. The labels of seasoning agents are carefully inspected for sodium and potassium content. Clients are instructed to avoid salt substitute agents, many of which are composed of potassium chloride, if oliguria is present. Clients receiving PD or who are producing urine may not need dietary potassium restrictions.

Phosphorus Restriction. To avoid osteodystrophy, the control of phosphate levels is begun early in renal failure. The nurse monitors serum phosphate levels, and the physician may order dietary phosphorus restrictions and medications to assist with phosphate control. Phosphate binders must be taken at mealtime. Most clients with kidney disease already restrict their protein intake, and, because high-protein foods are high in phosphorus, their phosphorus consumption is also reduced. (Chapter 16 lists foods high in potassium, sodium, and phosphorus.)

Vitamin Supplementation. Most clients with renal failure require daily vitamin and mineral supplementation. Low-protein diets are usually deficient in vitamins, and water-soluble vitamins are removed from the blood during dialysis. In addition, anemia is a chronic problem in clients with renal failure because of the limited iron content of low-protein diets and decreased erythropoietin production by the kidneys, necessitating supplemental iron administration. Calcium and vitamin D supplements may also be required if the client's serum levels and bone status warrant.

Individualization of the Diet. Clients undergoing peritoneal dialysis (PD) require a slightly different diet from those undergoing hemodialysis (HD). Because protein is lost with the dialysate in PD, a major nutritional problem for these clients is compensating for this protein loss. In many cases, 100 to 120 g of protein daily is recommended. Because of the anorexia that often accompanies advanced renal disease, many clients require high-protein, high-calorie enteral supplements. The amount of sodium restriction varies with fluid weight gain and blood pressure. There is usually no need to restrict dietary potassium because the dialysate is potassium free. The potassium restriction, if any, is determined by the client's serum potassium level.

The nurse plays a vital role in managing the client's diet. In collaboration with the dietitian, the nurse provides teaching and performs ongoing assessments of the client's comprehension of and compliance with dietary regimens. The nurse can help clients adapt the diet to their budget, ethnic background, and food preferences to maximize calorie intake within the diet's restrictions.

Fluid Volume Excess

Planning: Expected Outcomes. With intervention, the client is expected to
- Achieve and maintain an acceptable fluid balance
- Minimize the risk of complications from fluid imbalances

Interventions. Management of the client with CRF includes drug therapy, diet therapy, fluid restriction, and dialysis. (Diet therapy is discussed under Altered Nutrition, and dialysis is discussed under Renal Replacement Therapies.)

Drug Therapy. Diuretics (see Chart 74–2) are prescribed for clients with renal insufficiency when needed for treatment of fluid retention or as an adjunct to the control of high blood pressure. The diuresis produced from these drugs is useful in treating fluid overload in clients who still have some urinary output. Diuretics are seldom used in clients with end-stage renal disease (ESRD) after dialysis has been initiated because, as kidney function diminishes, these drugs can have harmful side effects, including nephrotoxic and ototoxic effects.

The nurse uses daily weight measurements and intake and output records as important sources of assessment data. Increasing body weight on a daily basis generally indicates fluid retention rather than body weight gain. The nurse estimates the amount of fluid retained: 1 kg of weight equals approximately 1 L of fluid retained. The nurse ensures that daily weights are taken at the same time each day, on the same scale, with the client wearing the same amount of clothing, and after the bladder has been emptied if the client is not anuric.

Fluid Restriction. The amount of fluid restriction ordered is discussed above under Sodium Restriction. The nurse considers all forms of intake, including by mouth (PO), intravenous (IV) admixture (for medications), and fluid administration through gastrointestinal tubes as with medication administration, when calculating fluid intake.

Decreased Cardiac Output

Planning: Expected Outcomes. The client is expected to attain and maintain normal sinus rhythm, adequate cardiac output, and blood pressure (BP) within normal limits.

Interventions. Many clients with long-standing hypertension have renal insufficiency, and some progress to CRF and ESRD. Therefore, the control of hypertension is an essential factor in preservation of renal function. To control hypertension, the physician may order calcium channel blockers, angiotensin-converting enzyme (ACE) inhibitors, alpha- and beta-adrenergic blockers, and vasodilators. Recent studies have documented the effectiveness of ACE inhibitors in slowing the progress of renal failure compared with other antihypertensives (Levine, 1997). (More information on the specific medications can be found in Chart 38–2.) Indications vary, depending on the client, and these drugs are used carefully to avoid hyperkalemia and hypotension. Various combinations and doses may be tried until control of BP is adequate and

side effects are minimized. Calcium channel blockers seem to improve GFR and renal blood flow.

The nurse instructs the client and significant other to measure BP. The nurse evaluates the client's ability to measure and record BP accurately with use of the client's own equipment. The nurse periodically rechecks measurement accuracy. In addition to accurate measurement of BP, the client and significant other must understand the relationship of BP control and regulation to diet and medication therapy. The nurse further instructs the client to measure weight daily and to bring records of blood pressure measurements and weights for discussion with the physician, nurse, or dietitian.

The nurse assesses and monitors, on an ongoing basis, for signs and symptoms of decreased cardiac output, heart failure, congestive heart failure, and dysrhythmias. (Chapters 35 to 37 cover these topics.)

Risk for Infection

Planning: Expected Outcomes. The client is expected to remain free from infection.

Interventions. The nurse and assistive personnel provide meticulous care to any areas where the integrity of the skin has been broken (incisions, site of drains, puncture sites, cracked or excoriated skin, pressure sores) and provide good basic preventive skin care. For clients receiving dialysis, the nurse also inspects the vascular access site or PD catheter insertion site. The nurse assesses these areas on an ongoing basis for redness, swelling, pain, and drainage and monitors vital signs, notifying the physician promptly if any signs or symptoms of infection occur.

Risk for Injury

Planning: Expected Outcomes. The client is expected to remain free from injury (will not fall or experience injury from a fall and will not experience pathologic fractures, bleeding, or toxic effects of medications administered in the presence of chronic renal failure).

Interventions. Managing drug therapy in clients with CRF is a complex and ongoing clinical problem. Many over-the-counter agents contain ingredients that may affect renal function. Therefore, it is important to obtain a detailed drug history from the client. The nurse must be aware of the use of each drug, its side effects, and the site of metabolism. The nurse, in conjunction with the physician and pharmacist, monitors the client closely for drug-related complications and adjusts dosages accordingly.

Certain medications must be avoided, and the dosages of others must be adjusted according to the degree of remaining renal function. As the client's renal function decreases, repeated dosage adjustments are necessary. The nurse assesses the client for side effects and signs of drug toxicity and notifies the physician as appropriate.

A number of medications are routinely administered to clients with renal failure (Chart 75–5). The nurse giving these medications understands the rationale for administration and the nursing interventions for each drug. Many clients have some degree of cardiac disease and may require cardiotonic drugs, such as digoxin. The nurse is aware that clients with decreased renal function are par-

Drug Therapy for Renal Failure

Drug	Usual Dosage	Indications	Nursing Interventions	Rationale
Cardiotonics				
Digoxin (Lanoxin, Novodigoxin♣)	• 0.125–0.25 mg PO or IV daily or every other day • **Elderly:** 0.0625–0.125 PO or IV daily or every other day	• Decreased stroke volume • Decreased strength of cardiac contractions	• Monitor for signs of digoxin toxicity and hypokalemia. • Monitor for bradycardia (pulse <50–60 beats per minute). • Monitor serum drug levels.	• Digoxin remains in the body longer when renal function is impaired. • Bradycardia is a sign of digoxin toxicity. • A toxic digoxin level is >2.5 ng/mL.
Vitamins and Minerals				
Folic acid (vitamin B_9, Folvite, Novofolacid♣) Ferrous sulfate (Feosol, Fero-Grad♣, Novo-ferrosulfa♣)	• 0.1 mg PO, SC, or IM daily • 325 mg PO tid or qid	• Dietary supplement • Anemia	• Usually given after dialysis. • Monitor for constipation. • Note any change in the stools, which normally become blackish-green.	• Water-soluble vitamins are removed during dialysis. • Constipation is a frequent and uncomfortable side effect associated with oral iron supplements. • The color is caused by the presence of unabsorbed iron and is harmless.

ticularly susceptible to digoxin toxicity because the drug is excreted by the kidneys. The nurse caring for clients with CRF who are receiving any digitalis derivative, including digoxin, monitors for signs of toxicity, such as nausea, vomiting, anorexia, visual disturbances, restlessness, headache, fatigue, confusion, cardiac irregularities (particularly bradycardia [pulse rate <50–60 beats per minute] and tachycardia [pulse rate >100 beats per minute]), and serum drug levels above therapeutic range. In addition, the nurse and physician closely monitor serum levels of electrolytes, such as potassium, in any client receiving cardiotonic medications.

Agents to control an excessively high phosphate level include phosphate-binding compounds. Calcium acetate, calcium carbonate, and aluminum hydroxide are used as phosphate-binding agents in clients with renal failure. These drugs treat the metabolic complications that, if untreated, may lead to renal osteodystrophy and related injuries. To prevent further complications, the nurse stresses the importance of these—and all—medications.

Hypercalcemia (excessively high calcium levels) is a possible complication for clients taking calcium-containing compounds to control phosphate excess. Hypophos-

phatemia is also a possible outcome of phosphate binding but is typically also associated with phosphate depletion in clients who are not eating adequately but are continuing to take phosphate-binding medications. In clients taking aluminum-based phosphate binders for prolonged periods, retention and deposition of aluminum may cause bone disease or neurologic manifestations that may not be reversible. The nurse monitors for evidence of muscle weakness, anorexia, malaise, tremors, and bone pain.

Clients with renal disease should avoid antacid compounds containing magnesium. Clients in renal failure cannot excrete magnesium and thus should avoid additional intake.

In addition to the drugs used to treat renal failure, clients taking other medications require special consideration. These medications include antibiotics, opioids, antihypertensives, diuretics, insulin, and heparin.

Many antibiotics are safe for clients with renal failure, but those excreted primarily by the kidney require dose modification. To prevent complications of bloodstream infections from oral cavity bacteria, prophylactic antibiotic treatment is routinely given to clients with CRF before any dental procedures. The antibiotic and protocol used

Chart 75–5. Drug Therapy for Renal Failure Continued

Drug	Usual Dosage	Indications	Nursing Interventions	Rationale
Phosphate Binders				
Aluminum hydroxide gel (Amphojel, AlternaGEL, Alu-Cap, Nephrox) Aluminum carbonate gel (Basaljel)	• 500 mg–2 g PO bid–qid as tablets, capsules, or oral suspension	• Phosphate binder • Prevention of renal osteodystrophy	• Monitor for constipation, which occurs frequently. • Monitor for signs of hypophosphatemia. • Monitor serum aluminum levels.	• Constipation is a frequent side effect of many drugs that bind phosphorus. • These drugs can prevent intestinal absorption of phosphorus to the extent that the client develops hypophosphatemia. • Aluminum toxicity may cause bone disease and dementia.
Calcium carbonate (Tums, Os-Cal, Calci-Chew)	• 1–3 PO daily in divided doses tid or qid	• Dietary supplement • Phosphate binder	• Give only when serum phosphate levels are normal. • Monitor for hypercalcemia, constipation, and soft-tissue calcifications. • Give after meals.	• Calcium supplements may cause a *decrease* in the serum phosphate levels because these two minerals exist in the blood in a balanced, *reciprocal* relationship. • Giving binders after meals enhances binding capacity.
Stool Softeners and Laxatives				
Docusate sodium (Colace) Bisacodyl (Dulcolax, Bisco-Lax, Laxit✱)	• 100–300 mg daily • 5–10 mg PO or PR daily or every other day	• Prevention of constipation caused by limited fluid intake, iron supplements, and phosphate binders	• Observe for abdominal cramps and diarrhea. • Monitor bowel movements.	• These GI effects indicate drug overdose. • Monitoring bowel movements is a way of determining medication effectiveness.

vary with the client's needs and the physician's preference.

The nurse administers opioid analgesics cautiously in clients with renal failure because the effects often last much longer than in people with healthy kidneys. Uremic clients are particularly sensitive to the respiratory depressant effects of these drugs. Because opioids are metabolized by the liver and not the kidneys, the dose recommendations are often the same regardless of the level of renal function. The nurse monitors these clients closely after opioid administration and evaluates the need for additional administration on the basis of the client's reaction to the drug.

As renal disease progresses, the client with diabetes mellitus often requires modification of an insulin or oral agent dose because of decreased insulin metabolism by failing kidneys. Frequent blood glucose determinations are obtained to evaluate the client's insulin or oral agent needs. Urinary glucose measurements are less accurate when renal disease is present.

Because of defective platelet function and capillary fragility in renal failure, heparin and other anticoagulants are used cautiously.

Fatigue

Planning: Expected Outcomes. The client is expected to be able to perform self-care and activities of daily living.

Interventions. All clients with renal dysfunction are given some type of vitamin and mineral supplement. As a result of diet restrictions and vitamin losses associated with both peritoneal dialysis (PD) and hemodialysis (HD), water-soluble vitamins must be replaced. The nurse avoids giving the client these vitamin supplements before HD treatment because they will be dialyzed out of the body and the client will receive no benefit.

The anemic client with chronic renal failure is treated with recombinant erythropoietin (epoetin alfa [Epogen, Procrit]). For erythropoietin to stimulate bone marrow to produce red blood cells, clients must have adequate iron stores. In addition, chronic administration of erythropoietin can deplete iron stores, necessitating iron supplementation. Many clients who receive epoetin alfa report improved appetite and sexual function along with decreased fatigue; in some clients hypertension associated with a rise in hematocrit has been reported. The improved appetite may challenge clients to maintain dietary protein, potassium, and fluid restrictions and necessitates additional client education.

Anxiety

Planning: Expected Outcomes. The client is expected to display
- Reduced anxiety by an absence of physical cues indicating increased anxiety
- An ability to describe the renal failure process
- An awareness of the purpose and procedures for all treatments and tests

Interventions. The nurse has the most frequent contact with the client with chronic renal failure (CRF) when the client is hospitalized or undergoing in-center dialysis treatments. Thus, nurses perform an ongoing assessment of the client's anxiety level to determine the level of nursing intervention required for each client. The nurse observes the client's behavior for physical cues indicating anxiety, for example, an anxious facial expression or gestures and an increased pulse rate. In addition, the nurse evaluates the client's support systems, as evidenced by the involvement of family and friends with the client's care.

Unfamiliar settings and situations and lack of knowledge about treatments and tests can increase the client's anxiety level. The nurse explains all procedures, tests, and treatments. The nurse identifies the client's knowledge deficits concerning normal renal function and renal failure. Evaluating the client's current knowledge avoids needless repetition during teaching sessions. The nurse provides instruction appropriate to the client's needs and ability to understand. By explaining the disease process, the nurse enhances the client's acceptance and decreases anxiety.

The nurse provides continuity of care, whenever possible, to establish a consistent nurse-client relationship to decrease anxiety and promote discussions of client and family concerns. As the nurse-client relationship develops, the nurse encourages the client to discuss current problems or concerns. A multidisciplinary team of professionals participates to provide support and counseling for the client and family, often over many years of treatment.

Finally, the nurse encourages the client to ask questions and discuss fears about the diagnosis of renal failure. An open atmosphere that allows for discussion can decrease the client's anxiety level. Nurses also facilitate discussions with family members concerning the client's prognosis and the potential impact on the client's lifestyle. This process allows the nurse to provide support to the family and may also facilitate discharge planning.

Potential for Pulmonary Edema

Planning: Expected Outcomes. The primary outcome for the client is to be free of pulmonary edema. A secondary outcome for the client with chronic renal failure is to maintain optimum fluid volume balance through dialysis and pharmacologic measures, thus preventing the onset of pulmonary edema.

Interventions. In the client with chronic renal failure, pulmonary edema can result from two distinct mechanisms: left-sided heart failure or microvascular injury. In left-sided heart failure, the heart is unable to adequately eject blood from the left ventricle, leading to an increase in hydrostatic pressure. The increased pressure allows fluid to cross the capillaries into the pulmonary interstitium. Pulmonary edema can also occur from injury to the vascular endothelium or alveolar epithelial cells secondary to uremia. Fluids then leak into the interstitial space and ultimately into the alveoli.

The nurse assesses the client for early signs of pulmonary edema, such as restlessness, heightened anxiety, tachycardia, dyspnea, and crackles that begin at the bases of the lungs. As pulmonary congestion worsens, the level of fluid in the lung rises. Auscultation will reveal increased rales, decreased air exchange, and dullness to percussion at the upper limits of fluid collection. The client may expectorate frothy, blood-tinged sputum. With further cardiac and respiratory compromise, the client can become diaphoretic and cyanotic.

The client who develops pulmonary edema is frequently admitted to the intensive care unit for aggressive treatment, which includes continuous cardiac monitoring. The client is placed in a high-Fowler's position and on oxygen to maximize lung expansion and improve gas exchange. Pharmacologic management of the client with renal failure and pulmonary edema is difficult at best due to the potential adverse effects of drugs on the kidney. Treatment of pulmonary edema involves the administration of potent loop diuretics, such as furosemide (Lasix). Furosemide dosing usually begins at 40 mg IV, administered over 1 to 2 minutes. This dose may be repeated in 30 minutes if no response is elicited. For clients already receiving maintenance doses of furosemide, an IV dose equivalent to the PO maintenance dose is given; it is doubled in 30 minutes if no response is seen (McCormack et al., 1996). Renal impairment multiplies the risk of ototoxicity with the use of furosemide: thus delivery of IV doses are done cautiously.

Morphine sulfate 1 to 2 mg IV is usually prescribed to reduce myocardial oxygen demand by reducing ventricular preload and to provide vasodilation and sedation. The dose is adjusted to achieve the desired response, but the potential for respiratory depression exists. Therefore, the nurse monitors the client's respiratory rate and blood pressure closely. To further decrease hydrostatic pressure, a continuous infusion pump may administer a vasodilator, such as nitroglycerine. The nurse monitors vital signs vigilantly, as these drugs in combination may result in severe hypotension.

Nursing interventions include Foley catheter placement and frequent assessment of urinary output to gauge the effectiveness of diuretic therapy. The nurse can expect diuresis to begin within 5 minutes of administration of IV furosemide. Urinary output is measured every 15–30 minutes during the acute episode and every hour thereafter until the client is stabilized. In addition, the nurse assesses breath and heart sounds for improvement in rales and for the presence of an S_3, indicating fluid overload.

The nurse monitors serum chemistry results for electrolyte imbalances and reports abnormalities to the appropriate health care provider so that correction of imbalances can be initiated. The nurse initiates continuous cardiac monitoring to identify potential dysrhythmias. The nurse also monitors oxygen saturation levels by means of pulse oximetry and arterial blood gas values. The oxygen delivery system is adjusted to maintain adequate oxygen saturation levels. The nurse monitors the client for deterioration, manifested as increasing pulmonary congestion and hypoxemia. It may be necessary to intubate and mechanically ventilate the client at this point to prevent mortality.

Clients with chronic renal failure are at increased risk of developing pulmonary edema as they may present with precipitating fluid volume overload and existing cardiac compromise secondary to hypertension and volume overload. Such clients are less likely to respond quickly to treatment and are more likely to develop adverse effects from pharmacologic agents due to renal impairment. Occasionally, ultrafiltration may be employed to further reduce fluid volume.

Renal Replacement Therapies

Renal replacement therapy is required only when the clinical and laboratory manifestations of renal failure present complications that are potentially life threatening or that pose continuing discomfort to the client. When the client can no longer be managed with conservative therapies, such as diet, medication, and fluid restriction, dialysis is indicated. Transplantation may be discussed at any time.

Hemodialysis. Hemodialysis (HD) is one of several renal replacement therapies for the treatment of renal failure (Table 75–6). Dialysis removes excess fluids and waste products and restores chemical and electrolyte balance. HD involves the extracorporeal (outside of the body) passage of the client's blood through a semipermeable membrane that serves as an artificial kidney.

Client Selection. Any client may be considered for hemodialysis therapy. Initiation of renal replacement therapy depends on the symptoms of the client, not on the creatinine clearance (Albee et al., 1996). Dialysis is initiated immediately for clients who exhibit the following: fluid overload refractory to diuretics, presence of pericarditis, uncontrolled hypertension, neurologic manifestations, and the development of bleeding diathesis. More commonly, dialysis is initiated when clients have signs of symptom progression, such as nausea and vomiting, decreased attention span, decreased cognition, worsening anemia, and pruritis (Levine, 1997).

The duration of survival after HD depends on the client's age, the cause of renal failure, and the presence of other diseases, such as coronary artery disease, hypertension, and diabetes. General guidelines for appropriate client selection for HD include

- The presence of fatal, irreversible renal failure when other therapies are unacceptable
- The absence of illnesses that would prevent or seriously complicate hemodialysis
- The expectation of rehabilitation
- The client's acceptance of the regimen

Dialysis Settings. Clients may receive HD treatments in any of several settings, depending on specific needs. They may be dialyzed in an acute care (hospital-based) center if they have recently begun treatment or have complicating conditions that require close nursing or medical supervision. Stable CRF clients may be hemodialyzed in a free-standing HD center in the community when they no longer require intensive supervision. Stable clients may participate in complete or partial self-care in an outpatient center or in-home hemodialysis.

In-home hemodialysis offers the least disruptive form of therapy and allows for the most adaptation of the regimen to the client's lifestyle. Unfortunately, many clients cannot participate in home dialysis because they lack a reliable and consistent partner to administer the therapy and manage the dialysis machine. For some clients and partners, the responsibilities of in-home dialysis are extremely stressful so that this option is less desirable. In addition, a water treatment system must be installed in the home to provide a safe, clean water supply for the dialysis process.

Regardless of the setting for therapy, the client needs ongoing nursing support and intervention to maintain this complex and life-saving treatment.

Procedure. The principles of hemodialysis are based on the passive transfer of toxins, which is accomplished by diffusion. *Diffusion* is the movement of molecules from an area of higher concentration to an area of lower concentration. The rate of diffusion is affected by numerous factors. *Diffusion* during dialysis occurs more rapidly when the membrane pores are large, there is a large surface area of membrane, the temperature of the solutions is higher, and there is a greater difference in the solute concentrations. Molecules that are too large, such as RBCs and plasma proteins, cannot pass through the membrane.

When HD is initiated, blood and dialysate flow in opposite directions from their respective sides of an enclosed semipermeable membrane. The dialysate is a balanced mix of electrolytes and water that closely resembles human plasma. On the other side of the membrane is the client's blood, which contains metabolic waste products, excess water, and excess electrolytes. During HD, the waste products move from the blood into the dialysate because of the difference in their concentrations (diffusion). Excess water is also removed from the blood into the dialysate (osmosis). Electrolytes can move in either direction, as needed, and take some fluid with them. Potassium and sodium typically move out of the plasma into the dialysate, whereas bicarbonate and calcium move

TABLE 75–6

A Comparison of Hemodialysis and Peritoneal Dialysis as Renal Replacement Treatment Options	
Hemodialysis	**Peritoneal Dialysis**
Advantages	
• More efficient clearance	• Easy access
• Short time needed for treatment	• Few hemodynamic complications
Complications	
• Disequilibrium syndrome	• Protein loss
• Muscle cramps	• Peritonitis
• Hemorrhage	• Hyperglycemia
• Air embolus	• Respiratory distress
• Hemodynamic changes (hypotension, cardiac dysrhythmias, and anemia)	• Bowel perforation
Contraindications	
• Hemodynamic instability	• Extensive peritoneal adhesions
	• Peritoneal fibrosis
	• Recent abdominal surgery
Access	
• Vascular access route	• Intra-abdominal catheter
Procedure	
• Complex	• Simple
• Specially trained registered nurses required	• Training less complex than for hemodialysis
Nursing Implications	
• Vascular access care	• Abdominal catheter care
• Restrict diet	• More flexible diet

from the dialysate into the plasma. This process continues as the blood and the dialysate are circulated past the membrane for a pre-set length of time. Water volume may be removed from the plasma by applying positive or negative pressure to the system.

The components of a hemodialysis system include a dialyzer, dialysate, vascular access routes, and a hemodialysis machine. The artificial kidney, or *dialyzer*, is available in several designs (Fig. 75–2). All dialyzers have four components: a blood compartment, a dialysate compartment, a semipermeable membrane, and an enclosed structure to support the membrane.

Dialysate is made from clear water and chemicals and is free from any metabolic waste products or drugs. Because bacteria and other microorganisms are too large to pass through the membrane, dialysate does not need to be sterile. The water used in dialysate must meet specific standards, and water treatment systems are used to ensure a safe water supply. The dialysate's composition may be altered according to the client's needs for treatment of electrolyte imbalances. During HD, the dialysate is warmed to approximately 37.8° C (100° F) to increase the efficiency of diffusion and to prevent a decrease in the client's blood temperature.

An essential function of a hemodialysis machine is the monitoring for potential problems, including

- Changes in dialysate temperature
- The presence of air in the blood tubing
- A blood leak in the dialysate compartment
- Changes in the pressures or composition within the blood and the dialysate compartments

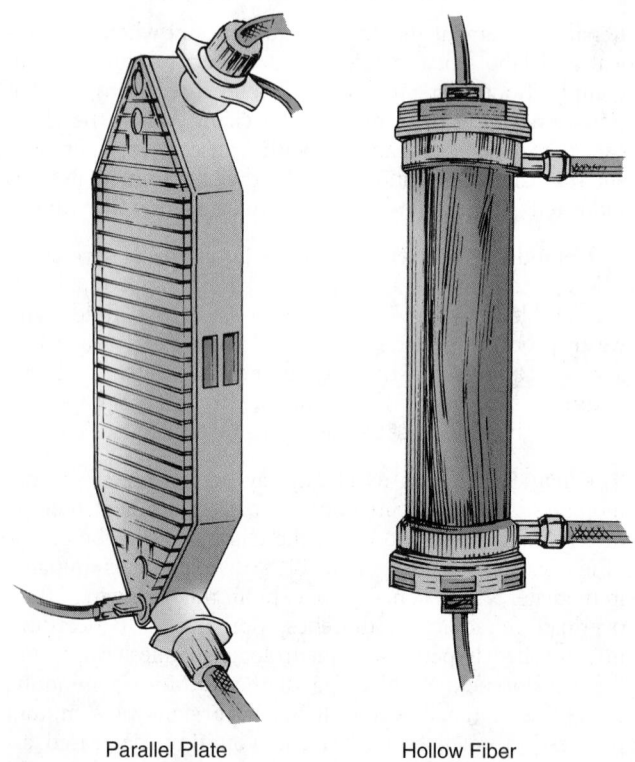

Parallel Plate
Dialyzer

Hollow Fiber
Dialyzer

Figure 75–2. Artificial kidneys (dialyzers) used in hemodialysis.

If any of these problems is detected, an alarm alerts the nurse. The monitoring systems protect the client from life-threatening complications that can result if these technical problems are not corrected.

All models of HD machines function, in principle, as illustrated in Figure 75-3. Figure 75-4 shows one type of machine. The duration and frequency of HD treatments depend on the amount of metabolic waste to be cleared, the clearance capacity of the dialyzer, and the amount of fluid to be removed. Most dialyzers provide sufficient clearance to limit the total number of hours of dialysis to around 12 hours a week. This time is usually divided into three 4-hour treatments a week. For clients with less muscle or more ongoing urine production, two 5- to 6-hour treatments a week may be adequate. If the client gains large amounts of fluid weight, a longer treatment time may be needed to remove the fluid without hypotension or severe side effects.

Anticoagulation. To prevent blood clots from forming within the dialyzer membrane and the blood tubing, anticoagulation with heparin is necessary during HD treatments. Heparin, a short-acting anticoagulant, inhibits the tendency of blood to clot when it comes in contact with foreign surfaces. There is considerable variability among clients in their anticoagulation response and elimination of heparin. The heparin dose must be adjusted on the basis of each client's need. Clients receiving erythropoietin may need more heparin.

Because heparin remains active in the body for 4 to 6 hours after administration, the client is at risk for hemorrhage during and immediately after HD treatments. The client must avoid any invasive procedures during that time. Thus, the nurse monitors clients closely for any signs of bleeding or hemorrhage. Clotting tendencies can be monitored during HD with a bedside machine (such as the Hemochron), by whole-blood clotting times (Lee-White clotting test), or by activated partial thromboplastin (aPTT) times during and after HD. Protamine sulfate is given as an antidote to neutralize heparin's anticoagulant activity when necessary.

Vascular Access. For HD to be performed, a vascular access route is required (Table 75-7). Dialysis treatments necessitate the easy availability of a large amount of blood flow, at least 250 to 300 mL/minute, usually for a period of 3 to 4 hours. Normally, the body cannot provide this type of circulatory access without surgical revision of blood vessels.

Long-Term Vascular Access. An internal access is preferred for most clients undergoing long-term HD (see Table 75-7). There are two common choices, an internal arteriovenous (AV) fistula and an AV graft (Fig. 75-5).

AV fistulas are formed by the anastomosis of an artery to a vein. The most commonly used vessels are the radial or brachial artery and the cephalic vein of the nondominant arm. This process increases the blood flow through the vein to 250 to 400 mL/minute, the amount required for dialysis to be effective.

Some time is necessary for an AV fistula to develop, and the amount of time required for the fistula to "mature" varies. Primary AV fistulas may not be suitable for use for as long as 4 months. Therefore, vascular access

must be planned accordingly. As the fistula matures, the increased pressure of the arterial blood flow into the vein causes the vessel walls to thicken. This thickening increases their strength and suitability for repeated cannulation.

To obtain access to a fistula, the nurse cannulates it or inserts two needles, one toward the venous blood flow and one toward the arterial blood flow. This procedure allows the HD machine to draw the blood out through the arterial needle and return it through the venous needle. The client may require a temporary vascular access (AV shunt or HD catheter) for HD treatments until the fistula is ready for use.

AV grafts are used when the AV fistula does not develop or when complications of the AV fistula limit continued use. The polytetrafluoroethylene (PTFE) graft is a synthetic material (Gore-Tex). This type of graft is used commonly among the elderly undergoing hemodialysis (see Research Applications for Nursing).

Precautions. Several precautions must be observed to ensure the functioning of an internal AV fistula or AV graft. First, the nurse assesses for adequate circulation in the fistula or graft as well as in the distal portion of the extremity. The nurse checks for a bruit or a thrill by auscultation or palpation over the access site. Because repeated compression can result in the loss of the vascular access, the nurse avoids taking the BP in the arm with the vascular access unless absolutely necessary. The AV fistula or graft is *not* used for administration of IV fluids; venipuncture is avoided anywhere in the arm used for hemodialysis access (Chart 75-6).

Complications. Complications can occur regardless of the type of access. The most common problems include thrombosis or stenosis, infection, aneurysm formation, ischemia, and high-output heart failure.

Thrombosis, or clotting, is the most frequent complication. Some clients are more susceptible to clotting than are others and may be given anticoagulants. Surgical declotting or revision of stenotic areas is typically performed in the surgical suite with use of local anesthesia.

Most infections that occur in clients undergoing long-term hemodialysis involve the vascular access. The most common organism causing infection is *Staphylococcus aureus,* which can be introduced by punctures for dialysis access. The nurse limits the incidence of infections by using careful sterile technique before needle cannulation (Table 75-8).

Aneurysms can form in any internal fistula and are caused by repeated needle punctures at the same site. Aneurysms that appear to be increasing in size may cause loss of the fistula's function and require surgical repair.

Ischemia occurs in a few clients with vascular accesses when the formation of the fistula causes a decrease in arterial blood flow to areas distal to the fistula. Ischemic symptoms (*steal syndrome*) vary from cold or numb fingers to gangrene. If the collateral circulation is inadequate, the fistula may have to be ligated and placed in another area for circulation to be preserved in the extremity.

Finally, the shunting of blood directly from the arterial system to the venous system, through the fistula, can

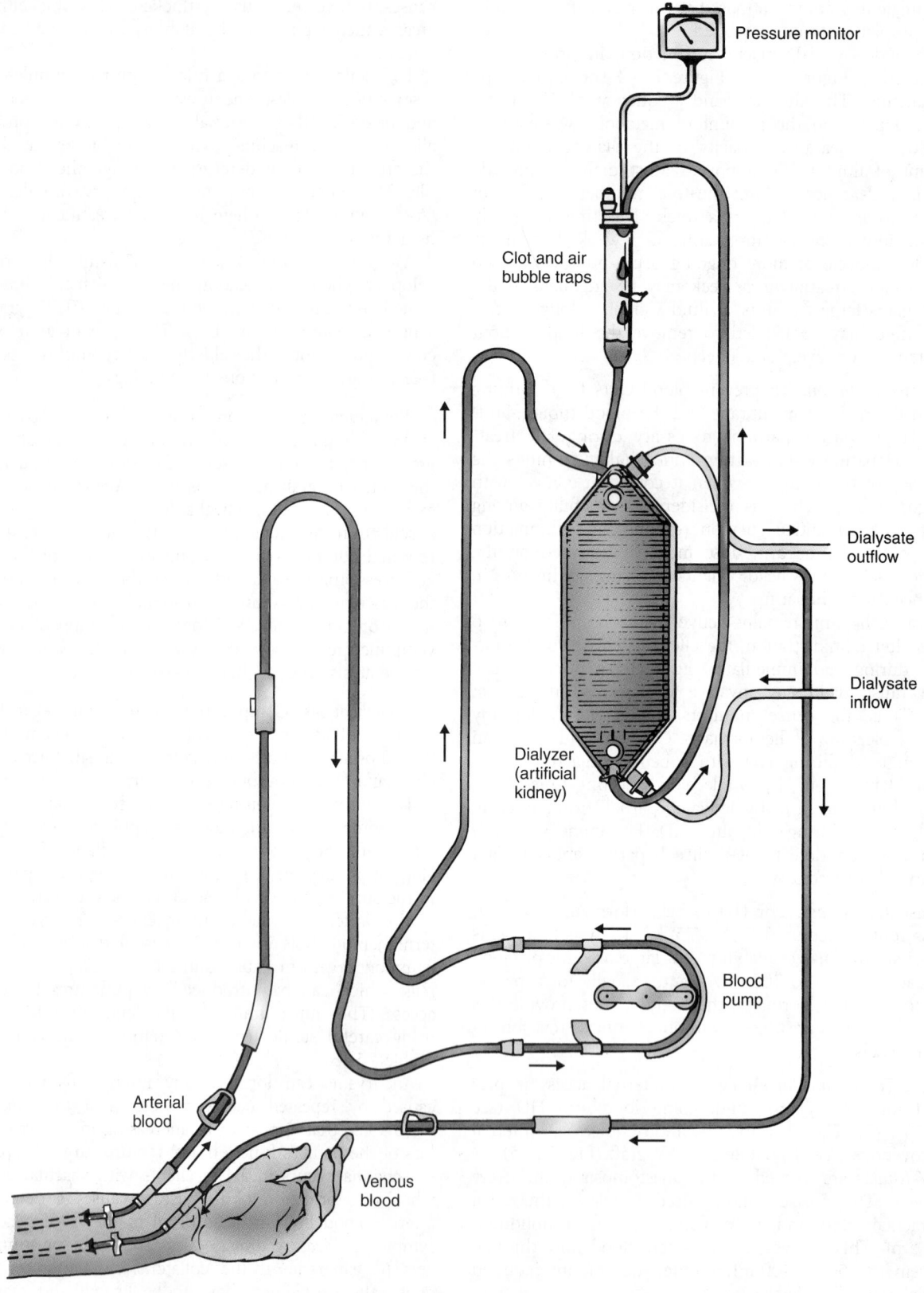

Figure 75–3. A hemodialysis circuit.

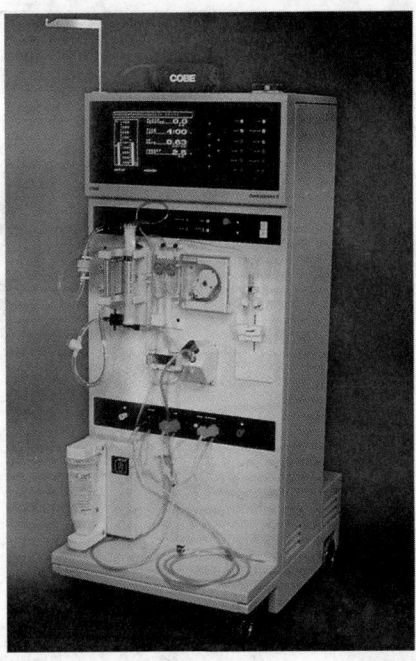

Figure 75–4. A hemodialysis machine. (Courtesy of GAMBRO Healthcare.)

cause high-output heart failure in clients with a limited cardiac reserve (see Chap. 37). This complication occurs rarely, but if it does, the fistula may need to be revised to decrease the blood flow from the arterial supply.

Temporary Vascular Access. The first type of vascular access developed was the external *arteriovenous (AV) shunt* (Fig. 75–6; see also Table 75–7), but it is rarely used today. To create a shunt, the surgeon places a piece of silicon rubber (Silastic) tubing into an artery and a second piece into an adjacent vein. The tubings are connected externally to provide a readily available vascular access. The arterial limb is used to obtain the blood for passage through the artificial kidney (dialyzer membrane), and the venous limb is used to return the blood to the client's body after each pass through the dialyzer.

Temporary vascular access with special catheters has replaced the use of the AV shunt for most clients requiring immediate HD. A catheter designed for HD may be inserted into the subclavian, internal jugular, or femoral vein if no permanent vascular access is available for use (see Acute Renal Failure).

Postdialysis Nursing Care. The nurse closely monitors the client immediately after dialysis and for several hours

TABLE 75–7

Types of Vascular Access for Hemodialysis			
Access Type	**Description**	**Location**	**Initial Use**
Permanent			
AV fistula	• An internal anastomosis of an artery to a vein	• Forearm	• 2–4 months or longer
AV graft	• Synthetic vessel tubing tunneled beneath the skin, connecting an artery and a vein	• Forearm • Upper arm • Inner thigh	• 1–2 weeks
Dual-lumen hemodialysis catheter	• An extended-use catheter, surgically tunneled under the skin with a barrier cuff	• Subclavian vein	• Immediately post-operatively and after x-ray confirmation of placement
Temporary			
Hemodialysis catheter (dual- or triple-lumen)	• A specially designed catheter with two or three lumens • Two lumens are for blood outflow and inflow for hemodialysis; a third lumen allows venous access without accessing dialysis lumens	• Subclavian, internal jugular, or femoral vein	• Immediately after insertion and x-ray confirmation of placement
AV shunt (relatively uncommon)	• An external loop of Silastic tubing connecting an artery and a vein • Each section of tubing is sutured into a vessel and brought through a skin stab wound	• Forearm	• Immediately after insertion

AV = arteriovenous.

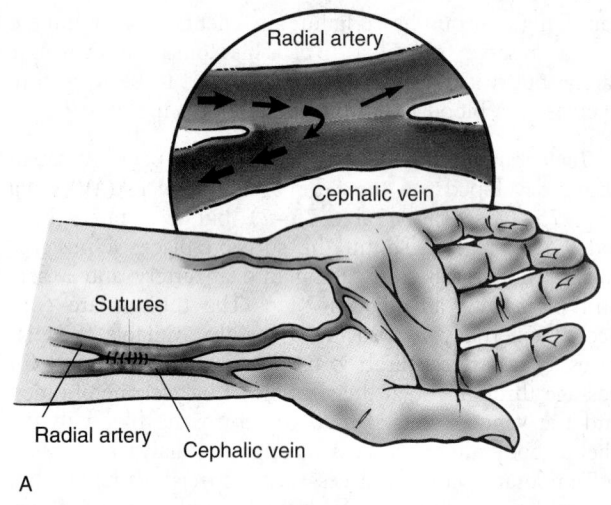

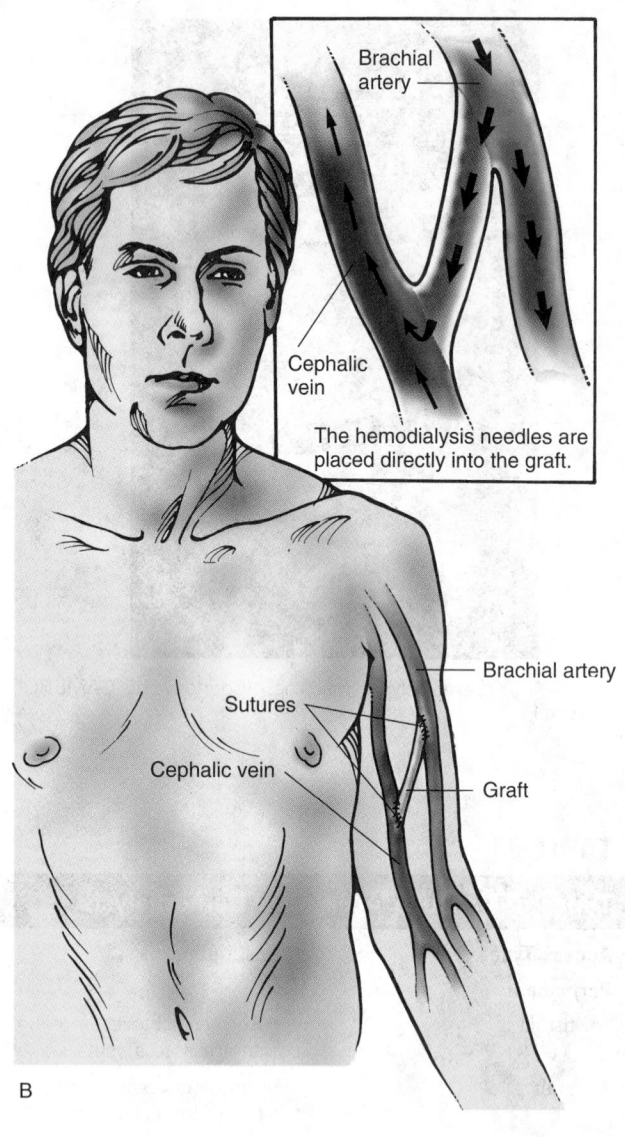

Figure 75–5. Options for long-term vascular access for hemodialysis. *A,* A surgically created venous fistula. The increased pressure from the artery forces blood into the vein. This process causes the vein to dilate enough for fistula needles to be placed for hemodialysis. When the vein dilates in this manner, the fistula is said to be "developed." *B,* A surgically placed straight vascular graft in the upper arm. The graft creates a shunt between arterial and venous blood.

afterward for any side effects from the treatment. The more common clinical manifestations of complications include hypotension, headache, nausea, malaise, vomiting, dizziness, and muscle cramps.

The nurse obtains vital signs and weight for comparison with predialysis measurements. Blood pressure and weight are expected to be reduced because of fluid removal. Excessive hypotension may require rehydration with IV fluids, such as normal saline. The client's temperature may also be elevated because the dialysis machine warms the blood slightly. If the temperature is elevated excessively, sepsis is suspected and a blood sample is obtained, as ordered, for culture and sensitivity determinations.

The heparinization required for hemodialysis increases the clotting time and thus the risk for excessive bleeding. All invasive procedures must therefore be avoided for 4 to 6 hours after dialysis, and the nurse continually monitors

the client for signs of hemorrhage during dialysis and for 1 hour after dialysis (Chart 75–7).

Complications of Hemodialysis. A variety of fluid-related and infectious complications can occur from hemodialysis. The most common complications include disequilibrium syndrome and aquisition of viral infections.

Dialysis disequilibrium syndrome may develop during hemodialysis (HD) or after HD has been completed. The cause is unknown but may be due to the rapid decrease in BUN levels during hemodialysis. These changes in urea levels can cause cerebral edema, which leads to increased intracranial pressure. Neurologic complications result (headache, nausea, vomiting, restlessness, decreased level of consciousness, seizures, coma, and death).

Early recognition by the nurse of the signs of the syndrome and appropriate treatment with anticonvulsant medications and barbiturates may prevent a life-threaten-

▷ Research Applications for Nursing

Are There Differences in Vascular Access and Outcome in Patients Less Than 65 Years and Those 65 Years or Older?

Culp, K., Taylor, L., & Hulme, P. (1996). Geriatric hemodialysis patients: A comparative study of vascular access. American Nephrology Nurses' Association Journal, *23(6), 583–591.*

This study utilized a descriptive, longitudinal design over 1 year to examine vascular access problems, particularly those related to type of access, location, co-morbid conditions, and outcomes. The study sample was stratified from 46 dialysis facilities and enrolled 267 patients. Information gathered included documentation of maturity of grafts at the time of first dialysis and first vascular access thrombosis (VAT). The sample was equivalent with regard to medication and anticoagulant usage. There was significantly more atherosclerosis and peripheral vascular disease among the 65 and older age group, and this group had more polytetrafluoroethylene (PTFE) grafts, while the under 65 age group had more arteriovenous fistulas (AVF) placed.

Critique. This study represents beginning knowledge development concerning the special needs of the geriatric hemodialysis client. Recommendations for future research include defining age groups more specifically and examining gender and differences in the geriatric hemodialysis population.

Possible Nursing Implications. To reduce the risk of VAT, use of AVF should be postponed for a minimum of 30 days after placement. Upper-arm placement of access devices in geriatric patients was associated with less VAT, and this location should be used where appropriate.

Chart 75–6

Nursing Care Highlight: The Client with an AV Fistula, AV Graft, or AV Shunt

- Do not take blood pressure readings using the extremity in which the vascular access is placed.
- Do not perform venipunctures or start IVs in the extremity in which the vascular access is placed.
- Palpate for thrills and auscultate for bruits every 4 hours while the client is awake.
- Assess the client's distal pulses and circulation.
- Elevate the affected extremity postoperatively.
- Encourage routine range-of-motion exercises.
- Check for bleeding at needle insertion sites or shunt tubing insertion sites. (Keep small clamps handy on the dressing of the AV shunt.)
- Assess for signs and symptoms of infection at needle sites and shunt tubing insertion sites.
- Instruct the client not to carry heavy objects or anything that compresses the extremity in which the vascular access is placed.
- Instruct the client against sleeping with his or her body weight on top of the extremity in which the vascular access is placed.

---

ing situation. Dialysis disequilibrium syndrome may be avoided, or minimized, by introducing HD for short periods initially with low blood flows so that rapid changes in plasma composition are avoided.

Infectious diseases transmitted by blood transfusion constitute another serious complication associated with long-term HD. Two of the most serious blood-transmitted infections are hepatitis and human immunodeficiency virus (HIV).

Hepatitis infection among clients with CRF has decreased in recent years paralleling the decrease in blood transfusion requirement for these clients because of the availability of recombinant erythropoietin. Yet because of the blood access and the risk of microscopic exposure, hepatitis continues to be a problem for clients undergoing HD. The hepatitis B virus can be transmitted through use of contaminated needles or instruments, by entry of contaminated blood through open wounds in the skin or

---

TABLE 75–8

Nursing Measures for Prevention of Complications in Hemodialysis Vascular Access

Access Type	Bleeding	Infection	Clotting
AV fistula or AV graft	• Apply pressure to the needle puncture sites.	• Ensure adequate site cleaning before cannulation.	• Avoid constrictive devices. • Rotate needle insertion sites with each hemodialysis treatment. • Assess for thrill and bruit.
AV shunt	• Keep clamps available.	• Perform exit site care three times a week.	• Avoid constrictive devices. • Assess for thrill and bruit.
Hemodialysis catheters (temporary and permanent)	• Monitor the access site.	• Use aseptic technique. • Change the dressing three times a week.	• Place a heparin or heparin/saline dwell solution after hemodialysis treatment. • Not used between treatments.

AV = arteriovenous.

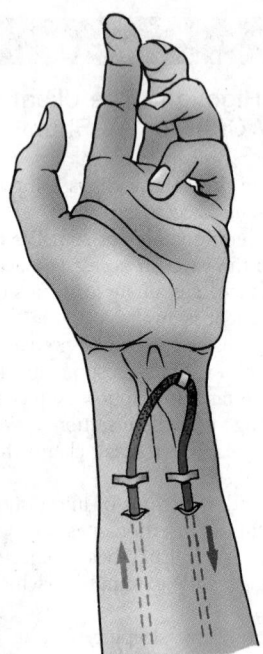

Figure 75–6. An arteriovenous shunt in the forearm. One part of the shunt cannula is placed in an artery; the other part in a vein. The ends of the shunt cannula are joined when dialysis is not in progress.

mucous membranes, and through transfusion of blood contaminated with the virus.

The incubation period for acute hepatitis is 6 weeks to 6 months. Thus, the nurse continually monitors the client undergoing HD who is receiving frequent transfusions for signs of hepatitis virus infection (see Chap. 61).

Human immunodeficiency virus infection (HIV) is a blood- and body fluid-borne virus with some potential threat to clients undergoing HD. Fortunately, the risks of HIV transmission are minimized by the consistent practice of Standard Precautions (blood and body fluids), routine screening of donated blood for HIV, and the decreased blood transfusions for clients with ESRD. Despite this progress, however, an unknown number of clients may have already been infected with the HIV virus. Clients who have been undergoing HD and who received frequent transfusions during the early to mid-1980s are at risk for acquired immunodeficiency syndrome (AIDS) (see also Chap. 25).

ELDERLY CONSIDERATIONS

There is greater occurrence of ESRD among those over 65 years of age. In 1993, the Health Care Financing Administration (HCFA) reported that 40.1% of dialysis patients were age 65 and older, and 14.1% were age 75 and older. In addition, clients over age 65 who are receiving dialysis treatments are more at risk of dialysis-induced hypotension.

Peritoneal Dialysis. Peritoneal dialysis (PD) takes place within the client's peritoneal cavity. PD is slower than HD, however, and more time is needed for the same effect to be obtained.

Client Selection. Most clients with CRF can select either HD or PD. For clients who are hemodynamically unstable and for those who cannot tolerate systemic anticoagulation, PD is less hazardous than HD. The lack of vascular access due to inadequate vessels may eliminate HD as an option. In addition, some clients with a new arteriovenous (AV) fistula receive PD while waiting for the access to mature for HD. PD is also often the treatment of choice in the elderly and pediatric populations because it offers more flexibility if the client's status changes frequently.

In some relatively rare situations, peritoneal dialysis cannot be performed, usually because of peritoneal adhesions or intra-abdominal surgery in the peritoneal cavity. In these cases, the peritoneal membrane's surface area has been reduced too much to allow for adequate dialysis exchange. In other cases, peritoneal membrane fibrosis may occur after repeated infections, which decreases membrane permeability despite adequate surface area.

Procedure. The surgical insertion of a siliconized rubber (Silastic) catheter into the abdominal cavity is required to allow the infusion of dialyzing fluid (dialysate) (Fig. 75–7). According to the physician's order, 1 to 2 L of dialysate is infused by gravity (*fill*) into the peritoneal space over 10 to 20 minutes, according to the client's tolerance. The fluid *dwells* in the cavity for a specified time ordered by the physician. The fluid then flows out of the body (*drain*) by gravity into a drainage bag. The peritoneal outflow contains the dialysate in addition to the excess water, electrolytes, and nitrogenous waste products that have accumulated in the client's body. The dialyzing fluid is called peritoneal *effluent* upon outflow. The three phases of the process (infusion or "fill," dwell, and outflow or drain) are considered one PD exchange. The number and frequency of PD exchanges are prescribed by the physician, depending on the client's clinical manifestations and laboratory data.

Process. Peritoneal dialysis occurs through diffusion and osmosis across the semipermeable peritoneal mem-

---

Chart 75–7

Nursing Care Highlight: The Client Undergoing Hemodialysis

- Weigh the client before and after dialysis.
- Know the client's dry weight.
- Discuss with the physician whether any of the client's medications should be withheld until after dialysis.
- Be aware of events that occurred during the dialysis treatment.
- Measure blood pressure, pulse rate, respirations, and temperature.
- Assess for symptoms of orthostatic hypotension.
- Assess the vascular access site.
- Observe for bleeding.
- Assess the client's level of consciousness and assess for headache, nausea, and vomiting.

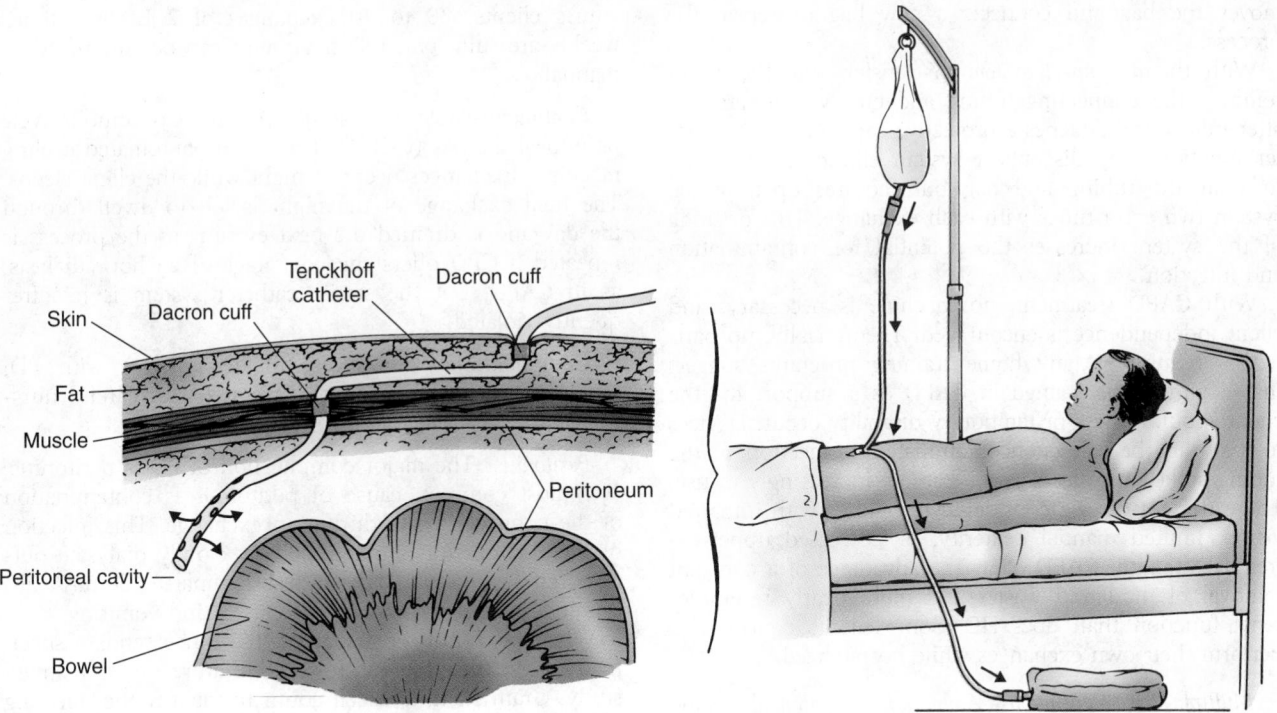

Figure 75–7. Manual peritoneal dialysis via an implanted abdominal catheter (Tenckhoff catheter).

brane and adjacent capillaries. The peritoneal membrane is large and porous. It allows solutes, which carry fluid with them, to move by an osmotic gradient from an area of higher concentration in the body (blood) to an area of lower concentration in the dialyzing fluid.

The peritoneal cavity is rich in capillaries and provides a ready access to the blood supply. The fluid and waste products dialyzed from the client move through the blood vessel walls, the interstitial tissues, and the peritoneal membrane and are removed when the dialyzing fluid is drained from the body.

The efficiency of PD can be affected by numerous situations, such as changes in the peritoneal membrane's permeability caused by infection or irritation and changes in capillary blood flow resulting from vasoconstriction, vascular disease, or decreased perfusion of the peritoneum. Excess water removal (ultrafiltration) in HD is accomplished by use of hydrostatic positive pressure or transmembrane negative pressure on the dialysis machine. In PD, the amount of water removed from the client depends on the concentration of the dialysate. Increasing the glucose concentration of the dialysate makes the solution increasingly more hypertonic. The more hypertonic the solution, the greater the osmotic pressure for ultrafiltration and thus the greater the amount of fluid removed from the client during an exchange. The physician orders the dialysate concentration on the basis of the client's fluid status.

Medication Additives. Heparin may be added to the dialysate to prevent fibrin clot formation in the catheter or tubing; this intraperitoneal (IP) heparin administration is necessary only after new catheter placement or with the occurrence of peritonitis. There is no systemic absorption of heparin with IP administration, so clotting studies are not needed.

Other agents that may be administered by the IP route include potassium chloride (KCl) and antibiotics. Commercially prepared dialysate does not contain potassium chloride. Some clients will need KCl added to dialysate so that the dialysate does not excessively deplete potassium from the plasma. Oral potassium supplements may be prescribed in selected clients. The physician may order IP administration of antibiotics (e.g., gentamicin, vancomycin, cephalosporins) when peritonitis is present or suspected. The combination of KCl and antibiotics in the same bag of dialysate is not recommended because chemical interactions may limit effectiveness.

Types of Peritoneal Dialysis. Many types of peritoneal dialysis are available, including continuous ambulatory peritoneal dialysis, multiple-bag continuous ambulatory peritoneal dialysis, automated peritoneal dialysis, intermittent peritoneal dialysis, and continuous-cycle peritoneal dialysis. Selection of type depends on client ability and lifestyle.

Continuous Ambulatory Peritoneal Dialysis (CAPD). The client performs self-dialysis by infusing four 2-L exchanges of dialysate into the peritoneal cavity, where the dialysate remains for 4 to 8 hours, 7 days a week. During the dwell period, the client can choose a continuous *connect* system or a *disconnect* system.

With the continuous connect system (straight transfer set), the dialysate bag is usually attached to the catheter by 48-inch (122-cm) tubing; the empty bag and tubing are folded and worn beneath the client's clothing until they are used for outflow. After draining, the client removes the bag and connects a new bag to repeat the process.

With the *disconnect system* (Y-transfer set), the client removes the connecting tubing and empty dialysate bag after inflow and attaches a protective cap to the PD catheter junction. The disconnect system eliminates the need to wear the tubing and bag but requires opening the system two extra times with each exchange. This opening of the system increases the potential for contamination and infection.

With CAPD treatment, no machine is necessary, and client independence is encouraged. Theoretically, no partner is required. Many home training programs suggest that a partner be trained in CAPD as a support for the client should illness or temporary disability occur. Devices to assist in the safe, noncontaminated connection of the tubing spike into the dialysate bag are increasingly in use. These devices can be considered for clients with impaired vision, limited manual dexterity, or decreased upper-extremity strength. CAPD offers the advantage of a constant removal of fluid and wastes and more nearly resembles renal function than does HD. Some clients continue to perform their own exchanges while hospitalized.

Multiple-Bag Continuous Ambulatory Peritoneal Dialysis. For those who are unable to perform self-CAPD in the acute care setting, a multiple-bag CAPD (MB-CAPD) system allows continuation of CAPD. With MB-CAPD, a manifold of tubing connected to dialysate and hanging on a portable pole is attached to the PD catheter by connecting tubing (see Fig. 75–7). The nurse inflows the dialysate at the prescribed time, allows the dwell, and initiates the outflow for each exchange. The MB-CAPD system permits mobility for the ambulatory client and provides for continuous peritoneal dialysis.

Automated Peritoneal Dialysis. An automated cycling machine that provides for dialysate inflow, dwell, and outflow according to pre-set times and volumes may be used. A warming chamber for dialysate is part of the machine. Automated peritoneal dialysis (APD) may be used in the acute care setting, the outpatient dialysis center, or the client's home. The functions are performed in response to machine programming that can be individualized for the client's specific needs. A typical prescription calls for 30-minute exchanges (10/10/10 for inflow, dwell, and outflow) for a period of 8 to 10 hours. The machines have numerous safety monitors and alarms and are relatively simple to learn to use.

APD has several distinct advantages. APD permits the performance of home dialysis while the client sleeps, allowing the client to be dialysis free during waking hours. Also, because the number of connections and disconnections are fewer using APD, the rate of peritonitis has been reduced. Lastly, APD provides a means by which increased volumes of dialysis solution can be administered to clients who require higher clearances (Levine, 1997).

Intermittent Peritoneal Dialysis. Intermittent peritoneal dialysis (IPD) combines the principles of an osmotic pressure gradient and true dialysis. The client usually requires exchanges of 2 L of dialysate at 30- to 60-minute intervals, allowing 15 to 20 minutes of drain time. For most anuric clients, 30 to 40 exchanges of 2 L three times weekly are sufficient. IPD treatments can be automated or manual.

Continuous-Cycle Peritoneal Dialysis. Continuous-cycle peritoneal dialysis (CCPD) also uses an automated cycling machine. Exchanges occur at night while the client sleeps. The final exchange of the night is left to dwell through the day and is drained the next evening as the process is repeated. CCPD offers the advantage of 24-hour dialysis, as in CAPD, but the sterile catheter system is less frequently violated.

Complications. Complications are possible with PD, but many can be treated or prevented with careful nursing care.

Peritonitis. The major complication of PD is peritonitis. The most common cause of peritonitis is contamination of the connection site during an exchange. This infection of the peritoneum is manifested by cloudy dialysate outflow (effluent), fever, rebound abdominal tenderness, abdominal pain, general malaise, nausea, and vomiting.

When peritonitis is suspected, the nurse sends a specimen of the dialysate outflow for culture and sensitivity study, Gram stain, and cell count to identify the infecting organism so an appropriate antibiotic can be ordered. Procedures for routine or periodic culturing of PD effluent vary with institutional practice. In today's era of cost containment, routine practices are less likely to be the norm. Cloudy or opaque effluent is the earliest sign of peritonitis. Thus, nursing observations are key to the detection and identification of peritonitis. The best treatment of peritonitis is prevention. The nurse must maintain meticulous sterile technique when caring for the PD catheter and when hooking up or clamping off dialysate bags (Chart 75–8).

Pain. Pain during the inflow of dialysate is common during the first few exchanges because of peritoneal irritation; however, it disappears after a week or two. Cold

---

Chart 75–8

Nursing Care Highlight: The Client with a Peritoneal Dialysis Catheter

1. Mask yourself and your client. Wash your hands.
2. Put on sterile gloves. Remove the old dressing. Remove the contaminated gloves.
3. Assess the area for signs of infection, such as swelling, redness, or discharge around the catheter site.
4. Use *aseptic technique.*
   a. Open the sterile field on a flat surface and place two pre-cut 4- × 4-inch gauze pads on the field.
   b. Place three cotton swabs soaked in povidone-iodine on the field. Put on sterile gloves.
5. Use cotton swabs to clean around the catheter site. Use a circular motion starting from the insertion site and moving away toward the abdomen. Repeat with all three swabs.
6. Apply pre-cut gauze pads over the catheter site. Tape only the edges of the gauze pads.

dialysate aggravates discomfort. Thus, the dialysate bags should be warmed before instillation by use of a heating pad to wrap the bag or the warming chamber of the automated cycling machine. Microwave ovens for the warming of dialysate are not recommended because of their unpredictable warming patterns and temperatures.

Exit Site and Tunnel Infection. The normal exit site from a peritoneal dialysis catheter should be clean, dry, and without pain or evidence of inflammation. Exit-site infections (ESI) are associated with all types of peritoneal dialysis catheters. Such infections can be difficult to treat and can become chronic. ESI and tunnel infections cause increased morbidity, as they can lead to peritonitis, catheter failure, and hospitalization. Dialysate leakage and pulling or twisting of the catheter can predispose the client to ESI. Exit sites with purulent drainage should have a Gram stain and culture performed.

Tunnel infections occur in the path of the catheter from the skin to the cuff. Signs of infection include redness, tenderness, and pain. ESI infections are treated with antimicrobials; however, deep cuff infections usually require catheter removal.

Insufficient Flow of the Dialysate. Constipation is the primary cause of inflow and outflow problems. To prevent constipation, the physician orders a bowel preparation before placing the PD catheter. Colon evacuation before the initiation of PD may also prevent constipation. A high-fiber diet and stool softeners are often needed for ongoing prevention. Other causes of inflow/outflow difficulty include kinking or clamped connection tubing, the client's positioning, fibrin clot formation, and PD catheter migration.

Because outflow drainage is by gravity, the nurse ensures that the drainage bag is lower than the client's abdomen. The nurse inspects the connection tubing and PD system for kinking or twisting and rechecks to make sure that clamps are open. If inflow or outflow drainage is still inadequate, the nurse attempts to stimulate inflow or outflow by repositioning the client. Turning the client to the other side or making sure that the client is in good body alignment may help. Having the client in a supine low-Fowler's position seems to minimize the build-up of intra-abdominal pressure. Increased intra-abdominal pressure that occurs in the sitting or standing position, or with coughing, contributes to leakage at the PD catheter site.

Fibrin clot formation may occur after PD catheter placement or with the onset of peritonitis. Careful milking of the tubing may dislodge the fibrin clot and facilitate inflow and outflow. Radiographic examination is needed to identify PD catheter migration out of the pelvic area. If migration has occurred, the physician repositions the PD catheter.

Dialysate Leakage. When dialysis is initiated, small volumes of dialysate are used. It may take clients 1 to 2 weeks to tolerate a full 2-L exchange without leaking around the catheter site. Leakage tends to occur most often in obese or diabetic clients, the elderly, and those on long-term steroid therapy (Levine, 1997). Dialysate leakage presents as clear fluid emitting from the catheter

exit site. During this time, clients may require hemodialysis support.

Other Complications. The PD effluent (outflow drainage) is expected to be relatively clear and light yellow. The nurse notes any change in the color of the outflow. With the initial exchanges, the outflow may be bloody. The physician may order several in-and-out exchanges of unwarmed dialysis solution in an effort to clear the dialysate of blood. In these cases, the client's hematocrit, pulse, and blood pressure are closely monitored. If the drainage return is brown, a bowel perforation must be suspected. Similarly, if the outflow is the same color as urine and has the same glucose concentration, a possible bladder perforation should be investigated. If the drainage is cloudy or opaque, an infection is suspected.

Nursing Care During Peritoneal Dialysis. In the hospital setting, peritoneal dialysis (PD) is routinely initiated and monitored by the nursing staff. Before the treatment, the nurse evaluates baseline vital signs, including blood pressure, apical and radial pulse rates, temperature, quality of respirations, and breath sounds. The client is weighed, always on the same scale, before beginning the procedure and at least every 24 hours while receiving treatment. Baseline laboratory value determinations, such as electrolyte and glucose levels, are also essential and are repeated at least daily during the PD treatment.

During PD, the nurse continually monitors the client. Vital signs are taken regularly and recorded on a flow sheet. For the first few exchanges, the nurse records the vital signs every 15 minutes. The nurse also performs an ongoing assessment of the client for signs of respiratory distress, pain, or discomfort. The nurse also regularly checks the abdominal dressing around the catheter exit site for wetness. The nurse monitors dwell time and initiates outflow. The physician orders dwell time according to the client's needs for fluid removal and electrolyte balance.

For hourly exchanges, dwell time usually ranges from 20 to 40 minutes. Glucose absorption may occur in some clients, and blood glucose assessment is necessary. The outflow should be a continuous stream after the clamp is completely open. The total amount of outflow is recorded accurately after each exchange. The nurse maintains accurate inflow and outflow records when providing hourly peritoneal dialysis exchanges. When outflow is less than inflow, the difference is equal to the amount absorbed or retained by the client during dialysis and should be counted as intake. For clients performing self-CAPD, or when the MB-CAPD system is used, a daily weight is used to monitor fluid status. A visual inspection of the outflow bag and daily weights may be sufficient to note the adequacy of the return.

Renal Transplantation. Dialysis and transplantation are life-sustaining treatments for end-stage renal disease (ESRD); transplantation is not considered a "cure." It is up to each client, in consultation with nephrology personnel, to determine which type of therapy is best suited to that client's physical condition and lifestyle. In 1994, 11,312 kidney transplants were performed. Currently, more than 31,000 people are awaiting renal transplantation in the United States alone (U.S. Renal Data Report, 1996).

Preoperative Care. Many issues must be decided before transplantation. Some issues are related to client health and others to the actual transplant procedures.

Immunologic Studies. The major barrier to successful renal transplantation after a suitable donor kidney is available is the body's ability to identify and reject tissue that is not its own. This immunologic process attacks the transplanted kidney and renders it nonfunctional. For immunologic contraindications to be overcome, in-depth tissue typing is done on all candidates for transplantation. These studies include simple ABO blood group typing for compatible blood transfusions and human leukocyte antigen (HLA) studies as well as other tests. The HLAs have become the principal histocompatibility system used to match transplant recipients with compatible donors. The more similar the antigens of the donor are to those of the recipient, the more likely it is that the transplant will be successful and immunologic rejection will be avoided. Research is ongoing in immunology, and new information in this area could increase the success rate of organ transplantations in the future (see Chap. 23 on immunity).

Candidates. Candidates for transplantation must be free from medical problems that might increase the risks associated with the procedure. The usual age range for clients undergoing transplantation is 4 to 70 years. In clients older than 70 years, the risk of complications increases, but clients older than 70 years are considered on an individual basis. A thorough body systems assessment of the client is performed before the client is considered for transplantation. The process of transplantation can place a life-threatening stress on the cardiac system in clients with advanced, uncorrectable cardiac disease. Thus, these clients are usually excluded from consideration for transplantation. Other contraindications include active infection, IV drug abuse, malignant neoplasms, severe obesity, active vasculitis, and severe psychosocial problems. In addition, long-standing disease of the pulmonary system increases the risk of morbidity and mortality owing to respiratory tract infections after transplantation. Clients with diseases of the gastrointestinal (GI) system may require treatment before consideration for transplantation. Such problems as peptic ulcer and diverticulosis can be severely aggravated by the large doses of steroids used after transplantation.

The urinary system must be completely evaluated to ensure its ability to manage normal urine flow. Many clients with ESRD have not used their lower urinary tract for extended periods, and ureteral or bladder abnormalities may require surgical correction before renal transplantation.

Metabolic diseases, such as diabetes mellitus, gout, and hyperparathyroidism, cause even greater risks. These clients can still accept a renal transplant, but careful observation and management are necessary to limit complications. Other conditions that may complicate transplantation include malignant neoplasm and inflammatory disease. Clients with a recent history of malignant tumor are usually treated with dialysis because of the shortage of donor organs, the possibility that the cancer could attack the transplanted kidney, and the limited life expectancy of these clients. In addition, the immunosuppressive agents used after transplantation increase the risk of cancer recurrence. If more than 1 year has passed since eradication of the cancer, the client can again be considered for a transplant.

Other complicating conditions are considered on an individual basis, depending on the client's current health status. Renal transplantation can be considered for most of those with ESRD and may prove to be the optimal therapy for many people.

Donors. The sources of donor kidneys are living related donors and cadaver donors. Some centers are using living *unrelated* donors who meet stringent eligibility requirements. The available kidneys are matched on the basis of immunologic similarity between the donor and the recipient. Clients and donors do not need to be matched for age, race, or gender. To minimize injury to the donor kidney, the preoperative work-up must be done quickly if a cadaver donor is used.

The size of the kidney is seldom a problem except in the youngest pediatric clients. Pediatric cadaver kidneys hypertrophy to accommodate adult needs within a few months; an adult kidney shrinks after placement in a child's abdominal cavity and then increases in size as the child grows.

Organs from living *related* donors (LRD) provide the highest rates of renal graft survival (90%). Donors are usually at least 18 years old because of legal requirements and are seldom older than 65 years. General physical criteria for donors include

- The absence of systemic disease and infection
- No history of cancer
- The absence of hypertension and renal disease
- Adequate renal function as evidenced by diagnostic studies

In addition, living related donors must express a clear understanding of the associated surgery and a willingness to give up a kidney. Some transplant centers also require a psychiatric evaluation to determine the motivation of the donor.

The *cadaver* donor is usually a child or young adult who has been the victim of trauma or other cerebral injury. The person must be diagnosed as brain dead by a physician on the basis of specific criteria, which may vary from state to state. Cadaver donors must meet all the physical criteria that living related donors meet, and the deceased's family must give written consent to organ donation in the absence of a signed uniform donor card. These cards express the client's wish to serve as a donor, but transplant centers still request agreement from the next of kin. The brain-dead person's body is kept functioning by technical means until immediately before the kidneys are removed. The kidneys are then specially preserved and transported immediately to recipients waiting in another operating room or in another hospital. Because of advances in immunosuppressant therapy and medical management, the United Network of Organ Sharing reported 1-year renal transplant graft survival to be 83% to 90% for all centers in the United States. Almost one-half of all cadaver donor recipients will retain allograft function 10 years after surgery (Levine, 1997).

Surgical Team. The surgical team is a group of specialists trained in transplantation procedures. The team includes operating room nurses (circulating and scrub nurses), clinical nurse specialists, and preoperative nurses as well as transplant surgeons, anesthesiologists, and nephrologists. The role of the preoperative nurse includes

- Teaching about the procedure and postoperative care
- In-depth client assessment
- Coordination of diagnostic tests
- Development and implementation of treatment plans

The transplant recipient usually requires dialysis within 24 hours of the surgery. In addition, the recipient often receives a blood transfusion before surgery. Current research favors donor-specific transfusions, in which blood from the kidney donor is transfused into the recipient. This procedure has resulted in increased graft survival, especially of organs from living related donors.

Operative Procedure. The donor nephrectomy procedure varies between the cadaver donor and LRDs. The cadaver donor nephrectomy is conducted as a sterile autopsy in the operating room. All arterial and venous vessels and as long a piece of ureter as possible are carefully preserved. After removal, the kidneys are preserved until time for implantation into the recipient. The technique for kidney removal from LRDs requires greater surgical care and is a delicate procedure lasting 3–4 hours. A flank incision is used, and care is taken to avoid scarring. Donors usually experience more pain than do recipients. They also need special nursing care and support for the psychological adjustment to loss of a body part.

The transplantation surgery usually takes 4–5 hours. The transplanted kidney is usually placed in the right anterior iliac fossa (Fig. 75–8) instead of the usual anatomic position. This placement allows easier anastomosis of the ureter and the renal artery and vein, and it also allows for assessment by palpation. The recipient's own nonfunctioning kidneys are not usually removed unless chronic infection in one or both kidneys would compromise overall recovery. The client is then taken to the postanesthesia unit and then, when stable, to a designated surgical unit in the transplant center or in a critical care unit.

Postoperative Care. Postoperative care of the kidney transplant recipient requires that nurses be knowledgeable about the expected clinical findings and potential complications unique to this population (see the Clinical Pathway). Nursing care includes ongoing physical assessment, with an emphasis on evaluation of renal function. The transplant recipient requires particularly close attention because the immunosuppressive drug therapy to prevent tissue rejection causes impaired healing and an increased susceptibility to infection. Careful urologic management is essential to graft success. These clients always have a large indwelling (Foley) catheter for accurate measurements of urinary output and decompression of the bladder and to prevent stretch on suture and anastomosis sites on the bladder. An abrupt decrease in urine output is significant, as it can herald the onset of complications such as rejection, acute tubular necrosis, thrombosis, or obstruction. The urine color is carefully monitored (usually hourly). The urine is initially pink and bloody, but it gradually returns to normal during several days to several weeks, depending on renal function. A continuous bladder irrigation is occasionally prescribed to decrease the formation of blood clots, which could increase pressure in the bladder and jeopardize the graft. Routine catheter care is performed to minimize contamination of the catheter; the nurse adheres to the agency's policy. The catheter is removed as soon as possible to avoid infection, usually 3–7 days postoperatively. The nurse is also responsible for obtaining daily urine tests, including urinalysis, glucose determinations, the presence of acetone, culture, and specific gravity measurement.

During the postoperative period, the function of the transplanted kidney (renal graft) can result in either oliguria or diuresis. Oliguria may occur as a result of ischemia and acute tubular necrosis (ATN), rejection, and other complications. To increase urinary output, the physician may order diurectics and osmotic agents, such as mannitol. The nurse and the physician carefully monitor the client's fluid status because fluid overload can cause hypertension, congestive heart failure (CHF), and pulmonary edema. Daily weight measurement, frequent BP readings, and careful intake and output measurements are required to evaluate fluid status.

Instead of oliguria, the client may have diuresis, especially with a living related transplanted kidney. The nurse carefully monitors fluid intake and output and observes for electrolyte imbalances, such as hypokalemia and hyponatremia. Hypovolemia from excessive diuresis may cause hypotensive episodes. The nurse strives to prevent this situation because decreased blood pressure also decreases the oxygen and blood supply to the new kidney, which can threaten graft survival.

Complications. Unfortunately, numerous potential complications are associated with transplantation surgery.

Rejection. The most common and the most threatening complication of renal transplantation is rejection. Rejec-

Text continued on page 1914

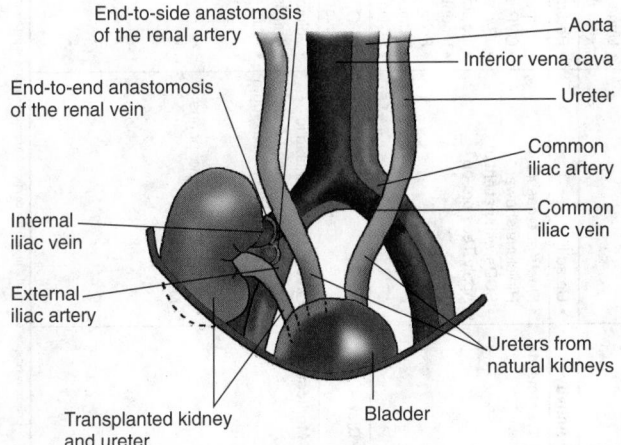

Figure 75–8. Placement of a transplanted kidney in the right iliac fossa.

End-to-side anastomosis of the renal artery

End-to-end anastomosis of the renal vein

Internal iliac vein

External iliac artery

Transplanted kidney and ureter

Aorta

Inferior vena cava

Ureter

Common iliac artery

Common iliac vein

Ureters from natural kidneys

Bladder

University Hospitals
of Cleveland

CARE PATH NAME: KIDNEY TRANSPLANT

DRG: ____ ELOS: 7 Days
Expected Disposition: Home
Surgery Date: __/__/__
Pre-Op Dry Weight: ____ Kg

Collaborative Problem List
1. Impaired Home Maintenance Management
2. Potential for Infection
3. Knowledge Deficit
4. Fluid and Electrolyte Imbalance
5. Plan Management
6.
7.

Focus	Pre-Op Date: __/__/__	Day of Surgery Date: __/__/__	Post-Op to Day 1 Date: __/__/__	Post-Op to Day 2 Date: __/__/__	Post-Op to Day 3 Date: __/__/__	Post-Op to Day 4 Date: __/__/__
Laboratory Tests/ Procedures	• Chem 23 • CBC + Diff • PT/PTT • Urine C&S • T&C 2u PRBC • Check CMV status • Chemstick of diabetic • CMV IgG quantitative	• Immediately post-op: Chem 7, CBC • 8 hours post-op: Chem 7, CBC • CXR on arrival to PACU	• CBC + Diff • Chem 23 • CD3 level if on OKT3 • CXR • Ultrasound as indicated per protocol	• Chem 7 • Urine for bacteria/fungus • CBC (Diff if on OKT3) • CD3 level if on OKT3 • CYA level starting day 2 of therapy		• Chem 23
Consults/ Referrals			• Consider PT Consult • Dietary screen and evaluation			
Physical Assessment	• VS q 4 h • Weight • Baseline skin assessment • Renal assessment regarding need for dialysis	• BP, AP, Rq 1/2 h until stable then q 2 h-q 4 h then q 4 h prn • Temp. immediately and q 2 h x 16 h then q 4 h • CVP q 2-4 x 16 h then q 4 h • Pulse ox baseline and prn • Urine output q 1 h x 24 h then q 4 h x 24 then qs	• VS q 4 h with CVP • Urine output q 4 h weight • Bowel sounds	• VS q 4 h • I&O q shift • Weight • Pulse ox x 2	• VS q shift	
Activity	• Up ad lib	• Bed rest	• Out of bed → chair		• Out of bed ad lib	
Treatments	• Fleets enemas x 2 • Hibiclens shower • SCDs with patient to OR • Apply Teds pre-op	• O2 per order, wean as tolerated • CVP dressing • JP dressing • Incision dressing • Incentive spirometry q 1 h W/A • Foley care • Guaiac stools • SCDs and Teds	• D/C O2 if RA pulse ox > 92% • Incision care	• Up with assistance • CVP dressing • D/C JP if output < 30 cc • Remove incision dressing	• Incentive spirometry q 2 h W/A	• CVP dressing • D/C Foley
Diet	• NPO	• NPO, ice chips • Advance as tolerated	• Diabetic/or any other diet restrictions as indicated			
Medications	• On call to OR: Antibiotic Solumedrol 250 mg IV Imuran 5 mg/kg IV maximum dose — 500 mg • Induction options: OKT3, ATG, Cyclosporine, MMF, Neoral	• Solumedrol 60 mg q 6 h IV • Antibiotic • Fluid replacements	• Imuran or Mycophenolate • OKT3, ATG, Cyclosporine, Neoral • Gancyclovir 2.5 mg/kg qd if CMV (+) or CMV (−) receiving (+) organ • MSO4 PRN	• Solumedrol 60 mg IV q 8 h • OKT3, ATG, Cyclosporine, Neoral • Gancyclovir • Bactrim ss or Trimethoprim qd • Colace • Clotrimazole • Acyclovir • Zantac	• Solumedrol 60 mg IV q 12 h • Tylenol #3 • CytoGam if donor CMV (+) and recipient (−)	• Prednisone 1 mg/kg/day • OKT3, CYA, or ATG • Tylenol or Darvon

Focus	Pre-Op Date: _/_/_	Day of Surgery Date: _/_/_	Post-Op to Day 1 Date: _/_/_	Post-Op to Day 2 Date: _/_/_	Post-Op to Day 3 Date: _/_/_	Post-Op to Day 4 Date: _/_/_
Patient/Family Teaching	• View pre-op transplant video • Orient to Tower 9		• Give teaching materials to patient • Renal transplant booklet • Preprinted cards • I&O sheet • Outcome criteria form	• Review of meds and teaching material with patient/family		• Continued review and if ready, take test
Discharge Planning		• Social Worker review notes from information appointments	• Review chart, interview RN and patient • Collect psychosocial data (insurance, financial issues discharge needs)	• Psychosocial assessment, support and education/ information	• Initial note in chart • Discuss prescription plan	• Arrange financial applications • Begin arranging prescription plans • Meet/talk with family prn • Consult/refer to other disciplines prn • For patients using mail order program, arrange forms with physicians
Intermediate Outcomes	1. Viewed video 2. Negative crossmatch	1. Hemodynamically stable 2. CVP 10-12 3. Euvolemic with fluid replacements 4. Vital signs returned to baseline 5. K + < 6.0 6. Equal and clear breath sounds 7. Pain controlled	1. Hemodynamically stable 2. CVP 10-12 3. Euvolemic with or without fluid replacements 4. Vital signs at baseline 5. Decrease in BUN and Cr from pre-op 6. Equal and clear breath sounds 7. Pain controlled 8. Teaching material given to patient/family 9. Immunosuppression dosages adjusted	1. Hemodynamically stable 2. Euvolemic without fluid replacements 3. Decrease in BUN and Cr 4. Electrolytes WNL 5. Equal and clear breath sounds 6. Pain controlled 7. Ambulating 8. Tolerating oral meds and diet 9. Teaching begun 10. JP removed if drainage is < 30 cc for 24 h 11. Immunosuppression dosages adjusted 12. Wound dry and approximated	1. Hemodynamically stable 2. Euvolemic 3. Decrease in BUN and Cr 4. Electrolytes WNL 5. Equal and clear breath sounds 6. Pain controlled 7. Actively participates in ADLs 8. Ambulates at baseline 9. Has bowel movement 10. Initial Social Worker note in chart 11. Teaching continues 12. JP removed if drainage is < 30 cc for 24 h 13. Immunosuppression dosages adjusted 14. Wound dry and approximated	1. Hemodynamically stable 2. Euvolemic 3. Decrease in BUN and Cr 4. Electrolytes WNL 5. Equal and clear breath sounds 6. Actively participates in ADLs 7. Pain controlled 8. Ambulates at baseline 9. Has bowel movement 10. Teaching continues 11. Foley discontinued 12. JP removed if drainage is < 30 cc for 24 h 13. Immunosuppression dosages adjusted 14. Wound dry and approximated 15. Financial and prescription arrangements made
Intermediate Outcomes RN Signature Days	☐ Met ☐ Not Met (see notes) #s not met ____ Signature ____	☐ Met ☐ Not Met (see notes) #s not met ____ Signature ____	☐ Met ☐ Not Met (see notes) #s not met ____ Signature ____	☐ Met ☐ Not Met (see notes) #s not met ____ Signature ____	☐ Met ☐ Not Met (see notes) #s not met ____ Signature ____	☐ Met ☐ Not Met (see notes) #s not met ____ Signature ____
Intermediate Outcomes RN Signature Evenings	☐ Met ☐ Not Met (see notes) #s not met ____ Signature ____	☐ Met ☐ Not Met (see notes) #s not met ____ Signature ____	☐ Met ☐ Not Met (see notes) #s not met ____ Signature ____	☐ Met ☐ Not Met (see notes) #s not met ____ Signature ____	☐ Met ☐ Not Met (see notes) #s not met ____ Signature ____	☐ Met ☐ Not Met (see notes) #s not met ____ Signature ____
Intermediate Outcomes RN Signature Nights	☐ Met ☐ Not Met (see notes) #s not met ____ Signature ____	☐ Met ☐ Not Met (see notes) #s not met ____ Signature ____	☐ Met ☐ Not Met (see notes) #s not met ____ Signature ____	☐ Met ☐ Not Met (see notes) #s not met ____ Signature ____	☐ Met ☐ Not Met (see notes) #s not met ____ Signature ____	☐ Met ☐ Not Met (see notes) #s not met ____ Signature ____

University Hospital's carepaths have been developed to assist clinicians in patient management and clinical decision-making. The carepaths are intended to meet the needs of patients in most circumstances. They are not intended to replace a clinician's judgment or establish a protocol for all patients with this diagnosis.
SP-9601 (01/05/96)

Focus	Post-Op Day 5 Date: __/__/__	Post-Op Day 6 Date: __/__/__	Post-Op Day 7 Date: __/__/__
Laboratory/ Tests/ Procedures	• CBC (Diff on OKT3) → • Chem 7 → • CD 3 level if on OKT3 → • CYA level →		
Consults/ Referrals	• Consider Home Team referral		
Physical Assessment	• VS qs → • I&O qs → • Weight →		
Activity	• OOB ad lib →		
Treatments	• Guaiac stools • Incentive spirometry q 2 h W/A	• CVP dressing	• D/C central line
Diet	• Diabetic or any other diet restriction as indicated →		
Medications	• Prednisone — taper as indicated → • Imuran or Mycophenolate → • OKT3, ATG, Neoral, or Cyclosporine → • Gancyclovir → • Bactrim → • Colace → • Clotrimazole → • Acyclovir → • T3 or Darvon → • Zantac →		• D/C Ganciclovir • Acyclovir **SrCr** **Dosage** < 1.4 800 mg po q 6 h 1.5-2.5 800 mg po q 8 h 2.6-4.5 800 mg po q 12 h > 4.5 800 mg po q 24 h HD 800 mg po q 48 h

Focus	Post-Op Day 5 Date: ___/___/___	Post-Op Day 6 Date: ___/___/___	Post-Op Day 7 Date: ___/___/___
Patient/ Family Teaching	• Take test • Diet teaching prn	• Review material as needed and retake test if needed	• Review homegoing med dosages, clinic and lab test follow-up appointments
Discharge Planning	• Arrange financial applications • Arrange prescription plans • Meet/talk with family prn • Consult/refer to other disciplines prn • Other D/C plans • Psychosocial assessment, support, and education/information	• Transportation arrangements prn • Other D/C plans carried out prn • Final note in chart with D/C plan Psychosocial assessment, support, and education/information	
Homegoing Medications	• Mail order prescription forms completed and faxed by 2:00 PM. (If weekend/ holiday D/C anticipated must do this by 2:00 PM, Friday)	• Delivery of medications prn	
Intermediate Outcomes	1. Hemodynamically stable 2. Euvolemic 3. Electrolytes WNL 4. Independent in ADLs and ambulation 5. Has bowel movement 6. Test taken and passed with 90% or continue med review 7. Scale and thermometer arranged for home 8. JP removed if drainage is < 30 cc for 24 h 9. Immunosuppression dosage assessed 10. Financial and prescription plans arranged 11. Cyclosporine levels assessed and adjusted	1. Therapeutic cyclosporine level 2. Homegoing meds obtained 3. Test taken and passed with 90%	1. D/C to home with written instructions 2. Medications available to take at home 3. Refer to discharge order form
Intermediate Outcomes RN Signature Days	☐ Met ☐ Not Met (see notes) #s not met _____ Signature _____	☐ Met ☐ Not Met (see notes) #s not met _____ Signature _____	☐ Met ☐ Not Met (see notes) #s not met _____ Signature _____
Intermediate Outcomes RN Signature Evenings	☐ Met ☐ Not Met (see notes) #s not met _____ Signature _____	☐ Met ☐ Not Met (see notes) #s not met _____ Signature _____	☐ Met ☐ Not Met (see notes) #s not met _____ Signature _____
Intermediate Outcomes RN Signature Nights	☐ Met ☐ Not Met (see notes) #s not met _____ Signature _____	☐ Met ☐ Not Met (see notes) #s not met _____ Signature _____	☐ Met ☐ Not Met (see notes) #s not met _____ Signature _____

University Hospital's carepaths have been developed to assist clinicians in patient management and clinical decision-making. The carepaths are intended to assist clinicians in patient management and clinical decision-making. They are not intended to replace a clinician's judgment or establish a protocol for all patients with this diagnosis.

SP-9601 (01/05/96)

tion is the leading cause of graft loss. A reaction occurs between the antigens in the transplanted kidney and the antibodies and cytotoxic T cells in the recipient's blood. These immunologic substances treat the new kidney as a foreign invader and cause tissue destruction, thrombosis, and eventual necrosis of the kidney. The three types of rejection are hyperacute, acute, and chronic. Acute rejection is the most common type in the transplant client. It is treated with increased immunosuppressive therapy and can be reversible. Rejection can be diagnosed by clinical manifestations, renal scan, and renal biopsy. Table 75–9 summarizes the characteristics of the different types; Chapter 23 discusses their pathophysiology and treatment.

Renal Artery Stenosis. Stenosis of the renal artery is detected by identification of hypertension, a bruit over the artery anastomosis site, and decreased renal function. The involved artery must be surgically resected and the kidney anastomosed to another artery. Clients with vascular complications nearly always require surgical intervention. Other vascular problems include vascular leakage or thrombosis, both of which require an emergency transplant nephrectomy.

Other Complications. Other complications may involve the wound or genitourinary tract. Wound complications, such as hematomas, abscesses, and lymphoceles, can become a medium for infection and can place external pressure on the new kidney. Infection is a significant cause of morbidity and mortality in the transplant recipient. Prevention of infection is paramount. Strict aseptic technique and handwashing must be rigorously enforced. Because of immunosuppression, transplant recipients may not present with typical signs of infection. Low-grade fevers, mental status changes, and vague complaints of discomfort may be present prior to sepsis. Nurses play a pivotal role in the early detection of infection.

Genitourinary tract complications include ureteral leak-age, fistula, or obstruction; calculus formation; bladder neck contracture; scrotal swelling; and graft rupture. Surgical intervention may be required.

Immunosuppressive Drug Therapy. The success of renal transplantation depends on changing the client's immunologic response so that the new kidney is not rejected as a foreign organ. The nurse administers and is aware of the immunosuppressive drugs that protect the transplanted organ. These drugs include corticosteroids, antilymphocyte preparations, monoclonal antibodies, and cyclosporine (cyclosporin A). (Chapter 23 discusses the mechanisms of action for these agents and the associated client responses.)

 Continuing Care

➤ Home Care Management

Because of the complex nature of chronic renal failure, its progressive course, and multiple treatment modalities, a case manager may be useful in the planning, coordination, and evaluation of care. As the client's renal disease progresses, the client is seen by a physician or nurse practitioner regularly and may have frequent hospitalizations. The nurse, in conjunction with the dietitian and social worker, evaluates the home environment and determines special equipment needs prior to discharge. Once discharged, home care nurses may direct care and monitor the client's progress (Chart 75–9 provides a focused assessment guideline for the client after renal transplantation).

The nurse provides ongoing health teaching about the diet in renal disease and the pathophysiologic process of renal disease. As CRF approaches end-stage renal disease, one of the following courses of treatment is chosen: hemodialysis, peritoneal dialysis, or transplantation. For each form of treatment, the client must learn the relevant

TABLE 75–9

A Comparison of Hyperacute, Acute, and Chronic Post-transplant Rejection

Hyperacute Rejection	Acute Rejection	Chronic Rejection
Onset		
• Within 48 hr after surgery	• 1 wk to 2 yr postoperatively (most common in first 2 wk)	• Occurs gradually during a period of months to years
Clinical Manifestations		
• Increased temperature	• Oliguria or anuria	• Gradual increase in BUN and serum creatinine levels
• Increased blood pressure	• Temperature over 37.8° C (100° F)	• Fluid retention
• Pain at transplant site	• Increased blood pressure	• Changes in serum electrolyte levels
	• Enlarged, tender kidney	• Fatigue
	• Lethargy	
	• Elevated serum creatinine, BUN, potassium levels	
	• Fluid retention	
Treatment		
• Immediate removal of the transplanted kidney	• Increased doses of immunosuppressive drugs	• Conservative management until dialysis is required

BUN = blood urea nitrogen.

Chart 75–9

Focused Assessment for Home Care Clients with Chronic Renal Failure

Assess cardiovascular and respiratory status, including
  Vital signs, with special attention to blood pressure
  Presence of S_3 and/or pericardial friction rub
  Presence of chest pain
  Presence of edema (periorbital, pretibial, sacral)
  Jugular vein distension
  Presence of dyspnea
  Presence of crackles, beginning at the bases, and
    extending upward
Assess nutritional status, including
  Weight gain or loss
  Presence of anorexia, nausea, or vomiting
Assess renal status, including
  Amount, frequency, and appearance of urine (in
    nonanuric clients)
  Presence of bone pain
  Presence of hyperglycemia secondary to diabetes
Assess hematologic status, including
  Presence of petechiae, purpura, ecchymoses
  Presence of fatigue or shortness of breath
Assess gastrointestinal status, including
  Presence of stomatitis
  Presence of melena
Assess integumentary status, including
  Skin integrity
  Presence of pruritis
  Presence of skin discoloration
Assess neurologic status, including
  Changes in mental status
  Presence of seizure activity
  Presence of sensory changes
  Presence of lower extremity weakness
Assess laboratory data, including
  BUN
  Serum creatinine
  Creatinine clearance
  CBC
  Electrolytes
Assess psychosocial status, including
  Presence of anxiety
  Presence of maladaptive behavior

---

information and procedures and consider personal lifestyle, support systems, and methods of coping. Decision-making about the treatment modality, or even whether to pursue treatment, is very difficult for many clients and their families. Nurses provide information and emotional support to assist clients with these decisions.

Treatment with hemodialysis (HD) necessitates a working knowledge of the dialysis machine and the care of the client's vascular access. If the client chooses in-home HD, the home care nurse makes preparations for installation of the appropriate equipment, including a water treatment system. Regardless of whether the treatment is provided at home or in a center, the nurse provides ongoing physical assessment and health teaching to promote maximal independence at home.

The client receiving peritoneal dialysis (PD) needs ex-

tensive training in the procedures. The client also needs assistance in obtaining equipment and the numerous supplies involved. Home care nurses perform physical assessments, monitor vital signs, assess compliance with drug and diet regimens, and carefully monitor for signs and symptoms of peritonitis.

Finally, the nurse plays a vital role in the long-term care of the client with a renal transplant. This client is usually discharged 3 to 4 weeks after surgery. Meticulous maintenance of prescribed immunosuppressive drug therapy is essential for the survival of the renal graft. Thus, the nurse facilitates the client's acceptance and understanding of this regimen as a part of daily life. The nurse also carefully monitors the client for signs of graft rejection and for complications, such as infection.

➤ Health Teaching

Health teaching is a primary function of nurses caring for clients with any form of renal disease. The home care nurse collaborates with other members of the health care team, especially the dietitian, pharmacist, and physician, to instruct clients and family members in all aspects of diet therapy, necessary drug therapy, and associated renal pathologic changes. Clients and family members are taught to report signs and symptoms of complications, such as fluid overload and infection. When a client requires a more advanced form of therapy, such as dialysis or transplantation, the teaching focuses on the chosen therapeutic intervention.

Hemodialysis is the most complex form of therapy for the client and family to understand. Even if clients receive HD in a dialysis center instead of at home, they are usually expected to have some knowledge of the HD machine. The client or a family member must be taught to care for the vascular access and to report signs of infection and stenosis. The client who plans to have in-home HD will need a partner. Both the client and the partner must be completely educated in the entire process of HD and must be able to perform it independently before the client is discharged from the HD center or hospital HD unit.

Peritoneal dialysis involves extensive client health teaching. This instruction can be given to the client alone or with a family member if the client cannot perform the procedures. The nurse emphasizes sterile technique because peritonitis is the most common complication of PD performed at home. The nurse instructs the client to report the signs and symptoms associated with peritonitis. Clients should report the presence of cloudy effluent and abdominal pain, especially when accompanied by rebound tenderness. Clients are taught that cloudy effluent needs to be analyzed promptly. A specimen is sent by the home care nurse for culture and sensitivity, cell count, and Gram stain to identify the causative organism. The client is taught that peritonitis is treated with antimicrobial therapy, usually given by the intraperitoneal (IP) route. To prevent peritonitis, the client is taught how breaks in aseptic technique can occur, resulting in peritonitis. In addition, to eradicate the infection nurses must educate clients about the importance of completing the antibiotic regimen. Nurses need to teach clients that repeated episodes of peritonitis can result in diminished ultrafiltration capability, which may necessitate transfer to hemodialysis.

The client receiving a renal transplant also needs extensive health teaching. The nurse provides instruction about drug regimens, home monitoring, immunosuppression, signs and symptoms of rejection, infection, and prescribed changes in diet and activity level.

➤ *Psychosocial Preparation*

The nurse provides psychological support for the client and the family. The nurse facilitates the client's adjustment to the diagnosis of renal failure and eventual acceptance of the treatment regimens.

For many clients, the reduction of uremic symptoms in the initial weeks and months of dialysis treatment creates a sense of euphoria and well-being (the "honeymoon" period). Clients feel better physically; their mood may be happy and hopeful; and they tend to overlook the inconvenience and discomfort of frequent dialysis treatments. The nurse realizes that this mood is temporary and uses the time to initiate health care teaching. The nurse stresses that although the client's uremic symptoms have diminished, the client will not return completely to the previous state of well-being. The client and the family may have looked on dialysis as a cure instead of a required lifelong treatment.

Many clients enter a phase of discouragement and disillusionment sometime during the first year of treatment; this may last a few months to a year or longer. The difficulties of incorporating dialysis into daily life are staggering, and clients frequently become disappointed and depressed as the problems become apparent. During this time, the client may struggle against the idea of having to be permanently dependent on a disruptive therapy. The fear of rejection by health staff and family members reinforces feelings of helplessness and dependence. Some people retreat into complete or partial denial of the disease and the need for treatment. They may deny the need for dialysis or may not comply with medication administration and dietary restrictions. Nurses who work with these clients need to monitor any maladaptive behaviors that may contribute to noncompliance and suggest psychiatric referrals. Nurses and family members should focus on the positive aspects of the treatments. The nurse continues health care education with the client as an active participant and decision-maker.

Most clients with chronic renal failure eventually enter a phase of acceptance or, at least, resolution. The prospect of a chronic illness may be devastating for some people, and each person reacts differently. To make this long-term adaptation, the client must adjust to continuous change, but specific concerns depend on the current physical status and particular treatment method.

After clients have accepted or become resigned to the chronicity of their disease, they usually attempt to return to their previous activities. Resuming the previous level of activity, however, may not be possible. The nurse and other health care professionals can help them to establish realistic goals that allow clients to lead active, productive lives.

➤ *Health Care Resources*

Professionals from various disciplines are valuable resources for the client with renal failure. Home care nurses are often required to monitor the client's status and evaluate maintenance of the prescribed treatment regimen (HD or PD). A client with advanced renal failure may need the assistance of a home care aide in performing the activities of daily living. Social services personnel are usually involved because of the complex process of applying for financial aid to pay for the required medical care. To increase the functional capacity of the client, a physical therapist may be beneficial. Consultation with a dietitian will assist the client and family members in understanding the special dietary needs in renal failure. A psychiatric evaluation may be needed to assist with depressive symptoms and maladjustment. Clergy and pastoral care specialists offer spiritual support.

Clients with CRF are routinely observed by a physician, usually a nephrologist. Such organizations as the National Kidney Foundation (NKF), the American Kidney Fund, and the National Association of Patients on Hemodialysis and Transplantation (NAPHT) may be helpful to clients and families.

 Evaluation

Nurses caring for clients with CRF evaluate each person's progress on the basis of the common nursing diagnoses. The client is expected to
- Achieve and maintain appropriate fluid volume
- Maintain serum electrolyte levels within an acceptable range
- Comply with the prescribed dietary regimen
- Maintain an adequate nutritional status
- Experience a reduction in anxiety

Acute Renal Failure
Overview

Acute renal failure (ARF) can be defined as a rapid decrease in renal function, leading to the accumulation of metabolic waste in the body. This situation differs from the much more gradual decline in renal function seen in clients with CRF, although ARF can occur in people with chronic renal insufficiency (CRI). Acute renal failure in clients with CRI may result in end-stage renal disease (ESRD) or may resolve to nearly the pre-ARF level of renal function. Numerous factors contribute to renal insults resulting in ARF, but the acute syndrome, unlike the chronic condition, may be reversible.

Pathophysiology

The pathophysiologic process of ARF is related to the cause of the sudden decrease in kidney function and the site or sites of the kidney involved. Hypoperfusion, exposure to toxins, tubular ischemia, infections, and obstruction have variable pathophysiologic effects. Potential outcomes include a decreased glomerular filtration rate, alterations in renal tubular cell membrane integrity, and tubular lumen obstruction.

With acute hypoperfusion, autoregulatory responses (i.e., renal vasoconstriction, activation of renin-angiotensin-aldosterone, and release of antidiuretic hormone [ADH]) increase blood volume and improve renal perfusion. However, these compensatory mechanisms cause urine volume to fall, resulting in oliguria. Tubular cell injury is more likely to occur from the increasing ischemia related to hypoperfusion. Toxins can provoke vasoconstrictive responses in the kidney, leading to a reduction of renal blood flow and renal ischemia.

Interstitial inflammatory changes from infection, drugs, and infiltrating tumors result in immunologically mediated changes in renal tissue. When tubular damage is extensive, sloughing of tubular cells and other formed elements (e.g., red blood cell casts) may obstruct the tubular lumen and prevent the formation or outflow of urine. Obstruction anywhere within the genitourinary tract eventually results in full or partial obstruction to the formation and outflow of urine.

When intratubular pressure exceeds glomerular hydrostatic pressure, glomerular filtration ceases. This process causes a progressive elevation of the serum BUN and creatinine levels. When the BUN rises faster than the serum creatinine level, the cause is usually related to protein catabolism or volume depletion. When both the BUN and creatinine levels rise and the ratio between the two remains constant, renal failure is present.

Types of Acute Renal Failure

Several syndromes describe the types of ARF. These include prerenal azotemia, intrarenal (intrinsic) acute renal failure, and postrenal azotemia. Table 75–10 summarizes the pathologic changes and causes of acute renal failure.

Prerenal azotemia can be reversed by establishing normal intravascular volume, blood pressure, and cardiac output. Prolonged hypoperfusion can lead to severe ischemic injury and intrarenal failure.

The term *intrarenal acute renal failure* is often shortened to just "acute renal failure" in the clinical setting. Synonyms also include acute tubular necrosis (ATN) and lower nephron nephrosis. Infections (bacteria, viral, and fungal or endotoxins), drugs (especially antibiotics and nonsteroidal anti-inflammatory agents), and infiltrating tumors (e.g., lymphoma and leukemias) can cause acute interstitial nephritis. Inflammation of the glomeruli (glomerulonephritis) or of the small vessels of the kidneys (vasculitis) or a major obstruction to blood flow can also cause intrarenal ARF.

Postrenal azotemia develops from obstruction to the outflow of formed urine anywhere within the genitourinary tract.

Phases of Acute Renal Failure

When a client's renal function has been compromised, the phases of ARF begin (Table 75–11). Increasing numbers of clients have a *nonoliguric* form of acute renal failure.

TABLE 75–10

Causes of the Three Types of Acute Renal Failure

Pathologic Change	Causes
Prerenal	
Decreased blood flow to the kidneys leading to ischemia in the nephrons; prolonged hypoperfusion can lead to tubular necrosis and ARF	• Conditions that cause decreased cardiac output • Shock • CHF • Pulmonary embolism • Anaphylaxis • Pericardial tamponade • Sepsis
Intrarenal (Intrinsic)	
Actual tissue damage to the kidney caused by inflammatory or immunologic processes or from prolonged hypoperfusion	• Acute interstitial nephritis • Exposure to nephrotoxins • Acute glomerulonephritis • Vasculitis • Hepatorenal syndrome • ATN • Renal artery or vein stenosis/thrombosis
Postrenal	
Obstruction of the urinary collecting system anywhere from the calyces to the urethral meatus Obstruction of the bladder must be bilateral to cause postrenal failure unless only one kidney is functional	• Urethral or bladder cancer • Renal calculi • Atony of bladder • Prostatic hyperplasia or cancer • Cervical cancer • Urethral stricture

ARF = acute renal failure; CHF = congestive heart failure; ATN = acute tubular necrosis.

TABLE 75–11

The Phases of Oliguric Acute Renal Failure

Phase	Description	Characteristics	Duration
Onset phase	• Begins with the precipitating event and continues until oliguria develops	• The gradual accumulation of nitrogenous wastes, such as serum creatinine and blood urea nitrogen, may be noted.	• Can last hours to several days
Oliguric phase	• Characterized by a urinary output of 100–400 mL/24 hr that does not respond to fluid challenges or diuretics	• Laboratory data include increasing serum creatinine and BUN levels, hyperkalemia, bicarbonate deficit (metabolic acidosis), hyperphosphatemia, hypocalcemia, and hypermagnesemia. • Sodium retention occurs, but this is masked by the dilutional effects of water retention. • Urinary indices are typically low and fixed; regulation of water balance by the kidneys is impaired, so urine specific gravity and urine osmolality will not vary as plasma osmolality changes.	• Typically lasts 8–15 days but can last for several weeks, especially in older clients or those having pre-existing renal insufficiency
Diuretic phase (high-output phase)	• Often has a prompt onset, with urine flow increasing rapidly over a period of several days • The diuresis can result in an output of up to 10 L/day of dilute urine	• Electrolyte losses typically precede clearance of nitrogenous wastes. • Later in the diuretic phase, the BUN level starts to fall and continues to fall until the level reaches normal limits or reaches a plateau. • Normal renal tubular function is re-established during this phase.	• Usually occurs 2–6 weeks after the onset of oliguric acute renal failure and continues until the BUN level ceases to rise
Recovery phase (convalescent phase)	• In this phase, the client begins to return to normal levels of activity	• The client functions at a lower energy level and has less stamina than before the illness. • Residual renal insufficiency may be noted through regular monitoring of renal function. • Renal function may never return to pre-illness levels, but renal function sufficient for a long and healthy life is likely.	• Renal function may continue to improve for up to 12 months after oliguric acute renal failure began. The client is particularly vulnerable to additional renal injury during this time.

BUN = blood urea nitrogen.

For these clients, there are similarities with the description of the phases, except for references to urinary output. In addition, the treatment of these clients is less complicated because renal replacement therapy is rarely needed. Interventions to restore intravascular volume, improve cardiac output, or re-establish blood pressure may prevent progression of the phases when renal hypoperfusion is present.

Etiology

Many types of renal insults can lead to reduced renal function. Severe hypotension from excessive blood or water loss results in hypoperfusion of blood to the kidneys and can lead to prerenal ARF. Cardiac disease or heart failure also results in decreased renal perfusion. Dehydration causes decreased intravascular volume and thus decreases the blood supply to the kidneys. The client can be oliguric, or even anuric (less than 100 mL/24 hours), if the dehydration or obstruction to renal blood flow is severe. Other conditions that precipitate ARF include

- Nephrotoxic agents (Table 75–12)
- Disseminated intravascular coagulation (DIC)
- Obstruction by thrombosis or stenosis
- Uric acid crystals or other obstructing precipitates
- Acute hemolytic transfusion reactions
- Complications of infection (e.g., endotoxins or sepsis)
- Acute glomerulonephritis
- Vasculitis
- Severe hypertension
- The hepatorenal syndrome of cirrhosis

TABLE 75-12

Some Potentially Nephrotoxic Substances

Drugs

Antibiotics/Anti-Infectives

- Amphotericin B
- Colistimethate
- Methicillin
- Polymyxin B
- Rifampin
- Sulfonamides
- Tetracycline hydrochloride
- Vancomycin

Aminoglycoside Antibiotics

- Gentamicin
- Kanamycin
- Neomycin
- Netilmicin sulfate
- Tobramycin

Antineoplastics

- Cisplatin
- Cyclophosphamide
- Methotrexate

Other Drugs

- Acetaminophen
- Captopril
- Cyclosporine
- Fluorinate anesthetics
- Indomethacin
- D-Penicillamine
- Phenazopyridine hydrochloride
- Quinine

Other Substances

Organic Solvents

- Carbon tetrachloride
- Ethylene glycol

Nondrug Chemical Agents

- Radiographic contrast dye
- Pesticides
- Fungicides
- Myoglobin (from breakdown of skeletal muscle)

Heavy Metals and Ions

- Arsenic
- Bismuth
- Copper sulfate
- Gold salts
- Lead
- Mercuric chloride

Incidence/Prevalence

The incidence of acute renal failure (ARF) depends largely on the underlying disease process and is directly related to the client's age, pre-existing renal function, and the number of situational factors contributing to an increased risk. Volume depletion leading to prerenal azotemia is the most common cause of acute renal deterioration and is reversible in most cases with prompt intervention. It has been reported that critically ill clients with ARF comprise 10% to 20% of the patient population in intensive care units. Acute tubular necrosis and exacerbations of CRI account for 80% of ARF. Of these, 67% have ARF secondary to a combination of sepsis and nephrotoxic drug exposure (Price, 1994).

The mortality associated with ARF remains surprisingly high, at greater that 50%. For clients with ARF requiring dialysis, the mortality rate is between 60% and 90% (Price, 1994). For clients surviving the precipitating event, the opportunity for return of renal function is good. Survival depends on preventing further complications, such as infection. Besides the precipitating event, infection is the major cause of death. The highest mortality occurs with trauma (70%) and surgery; ARF caused by nephrotoxic substances is associated with the lowest rates (10% to 26%). The prognosis for ARF attributable to obstruction or glomerulonephritis is much better.

Complications during the course of ARF can vastly increase mortality. Infection is the most serious and most common complication, often resulting in mortality. Bloodstream infections associated with central and peripheral lines and the pulmonary system are most frequently involved.

Collaborative Management

Prevention

Nurses have an essential role in the prevention of ARF. The nurse notes the signs of impending renal dysfunction through careful physical assessment and close monitoring of laboratory values. Prompt recognition and correction of extrarenal problems usually restore renal function before tissue damage can occur. Careful physical assessment is required to evaluate the client's fluid status. Intake and output records and body weights can assist in identifying trends in fluid balance. If vascular volume is depleted, decreased urinary output, postural hypotension, and tachycardia will be present. Prompt fluid resuscitation for clients in the prerenal stage can prevent intrarenal problems that can lead to renal tissue damage and renal failure.

The nurse also monitors laboratory values for any changes that reflect compromised renal function. Decreased urine specific gravity indicates a loss of urine-concentrating ability and is the earliest sign of renal tubular damage. Other laboratory values that are helpful in monitoring renal function include serum creatinine, urine and serum electrolytes, and blood urea nitrogen (BUN).

The nurse is aware of nephrotoxic substances that the client may ingest or be exposed to (Table 75-12). The nurse questions orders for potentially nephrotoxic drugs, and the ordered dose is validated before the client receives the drug. Antibiotics are the most likely drug group to have nephrotoxic side effects. NSAIDs may cause or potentiate risk for ARF. Combinations of drugs can cause synergistic reactions, further increasing the client's risk for ARF. If a client must receive a potentially nephrotoxic drug, the nurse monitors the client's laboratory values closely and for any clinical manifestations of renal dysfunction.

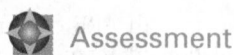 Assessment

➤ History

The accurate diagnosis of ARF, its type, and its cause largely depend on a detailed history. A history must include questions relating to the potential causes of ARF. The nurse questions the client carefully and examines the hospital chart concerning exposure to nephrotoxins, recent surgery or trauma, transfusion, or other factors that might precipitate renal ischemia. In some situations, ARF must be differentiated from chronic renal insufficiency. In these cases, the nurse asks about known renal diseases; systemic diseases, such as diabetes mellitus, systemic lupus erythematosus, and other connective tissue diseases; and chronic malignant hypertension.

To identify possible acute glomerulonephritis, the interviewing nurse includes questions about acute illnesses such as influenza, colds, gastroenteritis, sore throats or pharyngitis, and the presence of cocoa-colored urine (hematuria).

Reversible prerenal azotemia can be suspected after hypotension, hemorrhage or shock, burns, congestive heart failure (CHF), or any situation in which the client experiences intravascular volume depletion. Routine bowel preparations and being allowed nothing by mouth (NPO) preoperatively, when accompanied by fluid losses of most surgical procedures, are sufficient to cause prerenal azotemia in many clients.

Postrenal azotemia can be identified by the nurse's focusing on any history of obstructive disease processes that would be manifested as difficulty in starting the urine stream, changes in amount or appearance of urine, narrowing of the urine stream, nocturia, urgency, and symptoms of renal calculi. The nurse also notes any history of malignant carcinoma that may cause bilateral obstruction.

Because of the widely varied causes and the potentially reversible nature of the illness, the nurse obtains or validates a detailed history when ARF is suspected.

➤ Physical Assessment/Clinical Manifestations

The clinical manifestations of ARF are numerous (Chart 75–10). Specific signs and symptoms noted in a client with suspected ARF depend on the type of renal insult. Signs and symptoms of *prerenal* azotemia are hypotension; tachycardia; decreased urinary output, decreased cardiac output, and decreased central venous pressure (CVP); and lethargy. The general clinical appearance of a client with prerenal azotemia is similar to that of a client with heart failure or dehydration, depending on the cause of the renal compromise.

Intrarenal (intrinsic) acute renal failure usually involves damage to the glomeruli, interstitium, or tubules. Classic manifestations include oliguria (less than 400 mL in 24 hours) or anuria, edema, hypertension, tachycardia, shortness of breath, jugular venous distention, elevated central venous pressure, weight gain, rales or crackles, anorexia, nausea, vomiting, and lethargy or varying level of consciousness. Clinical manifestations of electrolyte abnormalities, such as electrocardiographic changes, may also be present.

Chart 75–10	
Key Features of Acute Renal Failure	
Prerenal azotemia	Hypotension
	Tachycardia
	Decreased cardiac output
	Decreased central venous pressure
	Decreased urine output
	Lethargy
Intrarenal (intrinsic) and postrenal	Renal manifestations
	Oliguria or anuria
	Increased urine specific gravity
	Cardiac manifestations
	Hypertension
	Tachycardia
	Jugular venous distension
	Increased central venous pressure
	ECG changes: tall T waves
	Respiratory manifestations
	Shortness of breath
	Orthopnea
	Rales or crackles
	Pulmonary edema
	Friction rub
	Gastrointestinal manifestations
	Anorexia
	Nausea
	Vomiting
	Flank pain
	Neurologic manifestations
	Lethargy
	Headache
	Tremors
	Confusion
	General manifestations
	Generalized edema
	Weight gain

In clients with *postrenal* azotemia, the nurse monitors for oliguria or intermittent anuria, symptoms of uremia, and lethargy. The nurse reports changes in the character of the urine stream or difficulty starting urination.

➤ Laboratory Assessment

The numerous alterations in laboratory values in the client with acute renal failure (ARF) are similar to those occurring in clients with chronic renal failure (CRF) (see earlier text and Chart 75–4). The oliguric phase of ARF shows many of the same abnormalities in laboratory values as CRF. Serum electrolyte levels (potassium, sodium, calcium, and phosphate) are also consistent with those occurring in CRF. Clients with ARF, however, typically do *not* experience the anemia associated with CRF unless there is hemorrhagic blood loss. However, uremic hemolysis secondary to severe azotemia can develop and may be the cause of anemia in the early phase of ARF.

In the early phases of ARF, urinalysis and microscopic examination of urine may provide diagnostic information.

Urinary sediment (red blood cells, red cell casts, tubular cells), myoglobin or hemoglobin, and electrolyte composition reveal the site and possibly the nature of the ARF. Urinary sodium levels are often less than 10 to 20 mEq/L in clients with prerenal azotemia but are typically 50 to 60 mEq/L or more in clients with established oliguric or nonoliguric acute renal failure.

➤ Radiographic Assessment

X-ray studies help to determine the cause of ARF (see also Chronic Renal Failure). A flat-plate x-ray of the abdomen is obtained to determine the size of the kidneys. In the absence of underlying renal disease, normal-sized kidneys are expected. Enlarged kidneys, possibly due to obstruction, may result from hydronephrosis. This x-ray may also illustrate obstructing calculi in the renal pelvis, ureters, or bladder.

Renal ultrasonography is a noninvasive procedure utilizing high-energy sound waves. It is useful in the diagnosis of urinary tract obstruction. Dilation of the renal calyces and collecting ducts, as well as calculi, can be detected.

Computed tomographic (CT) scans without contrast dye can be obtained to identify obstruction or tumors. Contrast media are usually avoided to prevent further renal damage. A sonogram is generally preferred to the intravenous pyelogram (IVP) to determine kidney size and the patency of the ureters.

Aortorenal angiography may be used to examine renal blood vessels and blood flow. The procedure involves the necessary risk of contrast media but can reveal any occlusion of major renal vessels by thrombus, embolus, or stenosis. Cystoscopy or retrograde pyelography may be indicated to identify possible obstructive lesions in the urinary tract.

➤ Other Diagnostic Assessment

Renal biopsy may be performed if the primary cause is uncertain, an immunologic disease is suspected, or the reversibility of the renal failure needs to be determined after ARF has persisted for an extended period. The nurse assists with many of the diagnostic studies, prepares the client before the test, and provides follow-up care. The nurse must be aware of all test results and understand how they may affect the client's treatment regimen. (For a detailed discussion of renal diagnostic tests, see Chapter 72.)

Interventions

Nursing diagnoses, goals, and interventions for the client with CRF (described earlier) apply to the client with ARF as well, with a few modifications (Client Care Plan). The client with ARF may pass from an oliguric phase (in which fluid and electrolytes are retained) to the diuretic phase. While the client is in the oliguric phase of ARF, the diagnostic procedures and care described for the client with CRF also apply. If the client moves to the diuretic phase, hypovolemia and electrolyte *loss* are the primary problems. As a result, the client in the diuretic

phase of ARF needs a plan of care that focuses on fluid and electrolyte *replacement* and monitoring.

These examples of output variation reflect the continually changing nature of ARF and the need for the plan of care to be constantly updated to reflect the client's movement through the stages of the disease process. Drug therapy, diet therapy, and renal replacement therapy (PD, HD, or hemofiltration) are commonly employed in the management of ARF.

➤ Drug Therapy

As in clients with CRF, clients with ARF receive numerous medications. As kidney function changes, the physician often modifies drug doses. The nurse is knowledgeable about the site of drug metabolism and is especially careful when administering medications. The nurse constantly monitors for possible side effects and interactions of the drugs the client with ARF is receiving (see drug therapy for chronic renal failure and Chart 75–5). Diuretics (see Chart 74–2) may be used to increase urine output.

In clients with prerenal azotemia, fluid challenges and diuretics are frequently used to promote renal perfusion. In prerenal azotemia, the client should respond to the fluid challenge by producing urine soon after the initial bolus. If oliguric renal failure is established, the fluid challenges and diuretics are discontinued. The physician may prescribe dopamine in a small continuous infusion to enhance renal perfusion and/or increase blood pressure (Chart 75–11). These clients frequently require central venous pressure (CVP) monitoring or measurement of pulmonary arterial pressures by means of a Swan-Ganz catheter for a more exact evaluation of their hemodynamic status. They also require constant nursing supervision for assessment of the response to fluid and drug administration. The nurse carefully monitors the client for signs of possible fluid overload.

➤ Diet Therapy

Clients who have acute renal failure often have a high rate of catabolism. The exact mechanism for this state is not well understood. Increases in catabolism may be related to the stress of a critical illness, causing an increase in levels of circulating catecholamines, cortisol, and glucagon, all of which stimulate catabolism. The rate of catabolism is correlated with the severity of uremia and azotemia. This hypercatabolic state causes the breakdown of muscle for protein, which leads to an increase in azotemia and an even more elevated serum BUN level. If the client with ARF has an adequate dietary intake (see Altered Nutrition: Less than Body Requirements in clients with CRF), nutritional support may not be necessary. The nurse continually assesses the client's oral intake to make certain that sufficient calories are consumed.

Many clients with ARF cannot eat sufficient food because of the acuity of their condition or the anorexia of uremia. In these cases, some form of nutritional support (e.g., total parenteral nutrition [TPN] or hyperalimentation) must be initiated to avoid catabolism. The goals of nutritional support in ARF are to provide sufficient nutrients to maintain or improve nutritional status, to preserve

Client Care Plan

The Client with Acute Renal Failure

Nursing Diagnosis No. 1: Altered Renal Tissue Perfusion related to interruption of blood flow, or hypovolemia (fluid volume deficit)

Expected Outcomes	Nursing Interventions	Rationale
The client is expected to have full return of his or her normal renal function.	■ Ensure adequate hydration. ■ Administer fluid challenges and diuretics as ordered. ■ Monitor for fluid volume excess (i.e., check blood pressure, pulse, neck veins, input and output, weight, S_3 heart sound, edema, lung crackles). ■ Administer renal-dose dopamine as ordered. ■ Weigh the client daily. ■ Maintain accurate intake and output. ■ If urinary electrolyte studies are ordered, obtain these before diuretic administration, if possible.	■ Sufficient blood volume must be delivered to the kidney to ensure perfusion. ■ The kidney may begin to function again. ■ If the kidneys do not respond to additional volume, the fluid will be retained. ■ Dopamine in a small dose will dilate renal blood vessels, thereby enhancing renal blood flow. ■ Assessment of weight changes helps determine fluid balance. ■ Review of intake and output helps assess fluid balance. ■ Diuretics alter the electrolyte composition of the urine, making it difficult for the physician to differentiate various causes of acute renal failure.

lean body mass, to restore or maintain fluid balance, and to preserve renal function.

If TPN is administered, the solutions may be formulated to meet the client's specific needs. Because kidney function is unstable in ARF, the nurse constantly monitors the serum electrolyte concentrations and facilitates revisions in the hyperalimentation solution as needed. In addition to TPN, IV fat emulsion (Intralipid) infusions provide a nonprotein source of calories. In uremic clients, fat emulsions can be used in place of glucose to avoid the problems associated with excessive sugars.

➤ *Dialysis*

Hemodialysis (HD) and peritoneal dialysis (PD) can be implemented for clients with ARF, if necessary. The indications for dialysis in ARF include

- Uremia
- Persistent hyperkalemia
- Uncompensated metabolic acidosis
- Fluid volume excess unresponsive to diuretics
- Uremic pericarditis
- Uremic encephalopathy

Immediate vascular access for HD in clients with ARF is readily established by placement of a dual- or triple-lumen catheter specifically designed for HD. For HD that is expected to be necessary for several weeks, the catheter is usually placed into the subclavian or internal jugular vein. If only one or two treatments are believed necessary, as for removal of drugs or toxins by hemoperfusion, a femoral site may be selected. Longer use of the femoral site is generally discouraged because of positioning limitations (i.e., required immobility) and other potential complications, such as hematomas and infection. Repeated cannulation of the femoral site also increases the risk for hematoma formation and makes repeated use of the vein impossible.

The subclavian vein is often preferred to femoral vein cannulation because the catheter can be left in place between dialysis treatments. This placement is also a disadvantage, however, because the longer the catheter is left in place, the greater is the chance of infection. The subclavian dialysis catheter (Fig. 75–9) is inserted at the bedside. A physician performs the sterile procedure, and then the catheter is covered with a sterile dressing. Catheter placement is checked by chest x-ray before its use.

Chart 75–11

Nursing Care Highlight: Administering Renal-Dose Dopamine

- Take an accurate weight because the dose is ordered according to the client's weight.
- Know the hospital's policy regarding who is responsible for calculating the rate of infusion (i.e., physician, pharmacist, or nurse). Renal-dose dopamine is 1 to 5 μ/kg body wt/min but is converted to mL/min for an IV infusion.
- Before hanging the dopamine infusion, double-check the amount of dopamine added to the solution, the total volume of solution (usually 250 mL), and the calculation into mL/minute.
- Do not hang the dopamine infusion until all questions about the calculation are clarified.
- If dopamine is to be infused into a peripheral vein, be sure that the line is intact and secured.
- Once the infusion is started, check the client's blood pressure and pulse per hospital policy or the physician's orders, usually at least every 2 hours.
- Notify the physician of changes in vital signs per policy or the physician's orders.
- Monitor the IV site frequently for clinical manifestations of infiltration.
- If infiltration occurs, stop the infusion but do not discontinue the IV catheter. Prepare for phentolamine (Regitine, Rogitine✤) administration through the IV catheter and subcutaneously into the infiltrated tissue.

HD catheters have two lumens separating the outflow and inflow extensions of the catheter. Consequently, the continuous outflow of blood to be dialyzed is separated from the dialyzed blood returned through the inflow port and lumen. A triple-lumen catheter for hemodialysis is now available. The third lumen provides a port for drawing venous blood or administering medication and fluid without interruption of the dialysis lumens.

➤ Hemofiltration

Continuous arteriovenous hemofiltration (CAVH) and continuous arteriovenous hemodialysis and filtration (CAVHD) provide additional renal replacement therapies for clients with ARF. These procedures share some similarities with HD, but their use and indications are specific and limited.

CAVH acts to remove large amounts of plasma water and solutes on a continuous basis. CAVH is used to treat massive fluid overload states when hemodynamic stability is not present. When large volumes of plasma water are removed, electrolytes are also removed. Electrolytes are replaced through prescribed amounts of IV electrolyte solution. A double-lumen dialysis catheter inserted into a large vein (subclavian, jugular) provides access for CAVHD. CAVHD uses a dialysate delivery system to remove nitrogenous or other waste products in addition to fluid in clients with limited cardiac output, those with significant hypotension, or those who have been unresponsive to diuretic therapy. The conventional form of HD would not be tolerated, and PD would probably be inadequate for the fluid removal required. These procedures are performed in a critical care unit, and clients require continuous nursing care.

➤ Post-Hospital Care

The post-hospital care for a client with ARF varies widely, depending on the status of the disease when the client is discharged. The course of ARF varies, with recovery lasting up to several months. If the client's renal failure is resolving, follow-up care is often provided by a nephrologist or by the family physician in consultation with the nephrologist. On occasion, however, ARF results in permanent renal damage and the need for chronic dialysis or even transplantation. In these cases, the post-hospital care may be as extensive and multifaceted as it is for any other client with chronic renal failure (CRF) (see Continuing Care for the client with CRF).

If a client's ARF is still in the process of resolving, the follow-up care may involve a variety of services. Frequent

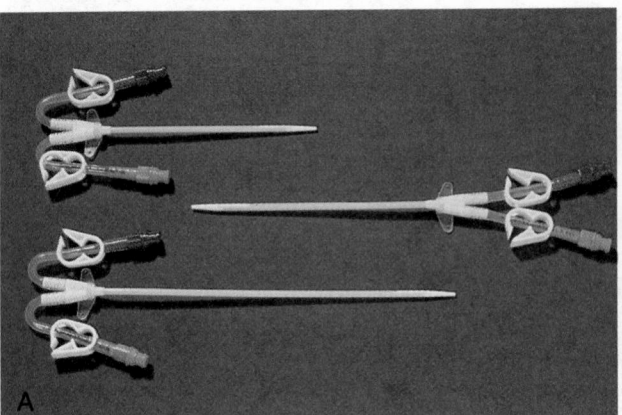
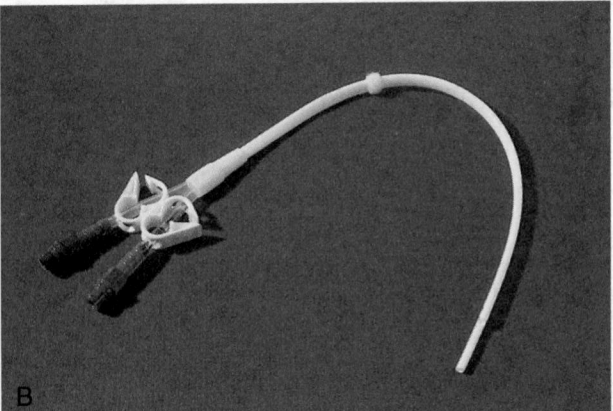

Figure 75–9. Subclavian dialysis catheters. These catheters are radiopaque tubes that can be used for hemodialysis access. The Y-shape tubing allows arterial outflow and venous return through a single catheter. *A,* Mahurkar catheters, made of polyurethane and used for short-term access. *B,* A PermCath catheter, made of silicone and used for long-term access. (Courtesy of Kendall Company, Bothell, WA.)

medical visits are necessary, as are routine laboratory blood and urine tests to monitor renal function. Consultation with a dietitian may be needed to modify the client's diet according to the degree of renal function and the client's ongoing nutritional requirements. Clients continuing dialysis after discharge must be taught to limit foods high in potassium and sodium and to observe protein restrictions. In addition, education concerning the need for limited fluid intake may also be necessary.

Some clients may need some form of temporary dialysis until their kidneys can metabolize fluid and waste products independently. The dialysis begun while the client was hospitalized may be continued at an outpatient dialysis center for as long as necessary. Teaching concerning the type of dialysis, care of vascular access sites, dietary restrictions, fluid restrictions, and prevention of complications are ongoing throughout the recovery phase. Depending on their level of independence and family support, some clients may also need home care nursing or social work assistance.

CASE STUDY of the Client with Acute Renal Failure

■ A 77-year-old female nursing home resident is admitted to the medical-surgical unit with a temperature of 100.8° F, a pulse rate of 96, respirations of 22, and blood pressure of 176/94. The nursing home staff report that she has been lethargic and has had a decline in urine output for the past 2 days. Her medical history includes hypertension and arthritis. Her current medications consist of ibuprofen 400 mg PO tid and captopril 25 mg PO bid. You are about to begin your initial assessment of this client.

QUESTIONS:

1. What risk factors possibly predispose this client to acute renal failure?
2. What measures could be taken to avoid ARF in this client?
3. What circumstances would cause the BUN/creatinine ratio to be elevated in this client?

SELECTED BIBLIOGRAPHY

Albee, B., Beckman, N., & Schell, H. (1996). Patients with end-stage renal disease. In J. Clochesy, C. Breu, S. Cardin, A. Whittaker, & E. Rudy (Eds.), *Critical care nursing* (2nd ed., pp. 949–976). Philadelphia: W. B. Saunders.

Berkoben, M., & Schwab, S. (1995). Maintenance of permanent hemodialysis vascular access patency. *American Nephrology Nurses' Association Journal, 22*(1), 17–24.

Brundage, D., & Linton, A. D. (1997). Age-related changes in the genitourinary system. In M. A. Matteson, E. S. McConnell, & A. D. Linton (Eds.), *Gerontological nursing: Concepts and practice* (2nd ed., pp. 342–343). Philadelphia: W. B. Saunders.

Brunier, G. (1995). Peritonitis in patients on peritoneal dialysis: A review of pathophysiology and treatment. *American Nephrology Nurses' Association Journal, 22*(6), 575–584.

Cotran, R., Kumar, V., & Robbins, S. (1994). *Robbins pathologic basis of disease* (5th ed.). Philadelphia: W. B. Saunders.

Culp, K., Taylor, L., & Hulme, P. (1996). Geriatric hemodialysis pa-

tients: A comparative study of vascular access. *American Nephrology Nurses' Association Journal, 23*(6), 583–591.

Dayer-Berenson, L. (1994). Rhabdomyolysis: A comprehensive guide. *American Nephrology Nurses' Association Journal, 21*(1), 15–20.

Dayton, K., & Lancaster, L. (1995a). The immune system in patients with renal failure part 1: Review of immune function. *American Nephrology Nurses' Association Journal, 22*(6), 523–529.

Dayton, K., & Lancaster, L. (1995b). Part 2: Effects of renal failure and its treatment on the immune system and assessment of immune system function. *American Nephrology Nurses' Association Journal, 22*(6) 530–537.

Dirkes, S. (1994). How to use the new CVVH renal replacement systems. *American Journal of Nursing, 94*(5), 67–73.

Dirkes, S. (1997). A dialysis alternative more nurses can run. *RN, 60*(5), 20–25.

Giuliano, K., & Pysznik, E. (1998). Renal replacement therapy in critical care: Implementation of a unit-based continuous venovenous hemodialysis program. *Critical Care Nurse, 18*(1), 40–51.

Guyton, A., & Hall, J. (1996). *Textbook of medical physiology* (9th ed.). Philadelphia: W. B. Saunders.

Halperin, M., & Goldstein, M. (1994). *Fluid, electrolyte and acid-base physiology: A problem-based approach* (2nd ed.). Philadelphia: W. B. Saunders.

King, B. A. (1994). Detecting acute renal failure. *Nursing94, 24*(3), 34–40.

Levine, D. (1997). *Caring for the renal patient* (3rd ed.). Philadelphia: W. B. Saunders.

McAlpine, L. (1998). CAVH: Principles and practical applications. *Critical Care Nursing Clinics of North America, 10*(2), 179–189.

McCormack, J. (1996). *Drug therapy decision making guide* (pp. 324–326). Philadelphia: W. B. Saunders.

Nelson, J., Moxness, K., Jensen, M., & Gastineau, C., (1994). *Mayo Clinic diet manual: A handbook of nutrition practices* (7th ed.). St. Louis: C. V. Mosby.

Norris, M. K. (1994). Evaluating BUN. *Nursing94, 24*(5), 80.

Port, F., & Young, E. (1996). Fluid and electrolyte disorders in dialysis. In J. Kokko & R. Tannen (Eds.), *Fluids and electrolytes* (3rd ed., pp. 487–532). Philadelphia: W. B. Saunders.

Price, C. (1994). Acute renal failure: A sequelae of sepsis. *Critical Care Nursing Clinics of North America, 6*(2), 359–372.

Radke, K. (1994). The aging kidney: Structure, function and nursing practice implications. *American Nephrology Nurses' Association Journal, 21*(4), 181–189.

Rodriguez, D., & Lewis, S. (1997). Nutritional management of patients with acute renal failure. *American Nephrology Nurses' Association Journal, 24*(2), 232–241.

Sica, D. (1994). Renal disease, electrolyte abnormalities, and acid-base imbalance in the elderly. *Clinics in Geriatric Medicine, 10*(1), 197–211.

Sosa-Guerrero, S., & Gomez, N. (1997). Dealing with end-stage renal disease. *American Journal of Nursing, 97*(10), 44–51.

Stark, J. (1998). Acute renal failure: Focus on advances in acute tubular necrosis. *Critical Care Nursing Clinics of North America, 10*(2), 159–170.

Stark, J. (1994). Acute renal failure in trauma: Current perspectives. *Critical Care Nursing Quarterly, 16*(4), 49–60.

Swartz, R. (1996). Fluid, electrolyte, and acid-base changes during renal failure. In J. Kokko & R. Tannen (Eds.), *Fluids and electrolytes* (3rd ed., pp. 487–532). Philadelphia: W. B. Saunders.

United States Renal Data System (1996). *1996 annual data report.* Washington, DC: U. S. Department of Health and Human Services, Health Care Financing Administration, Bureau of Data Management and Strategy.

White, V. (1997). Hyperkalemia. *American Journal of Nursing, 97*(6), 35.

Whittaker, A. (1996). Patients with acute renal failure. In J. Clochesy, C. Breu, S. Cardin, A. Whittaker, & E. Rudy (Eds.), *Critical care nursing* (2nd ed., pp. 926–948). Philadelphia: W. B. Saunders.

Young, E. (1995). Chronic renal failure. In J. Shayman (Ed.), *Renal pathophysiology* (pp. 155–175). Philadelphia: J. B. Lippincott.

SUGGESTED READINGS

Berkoben, M., & Schwab, S. (1995). Maintenance of permanent hemodialysis vascular access patency. *American Nephrology Nurses' Association Journal, 22*(1), 17–24.

This excellent article focuses attention on a critical element of vascular access patency in hemodialysis. Different types of vascular access grafts are reviewed, along with the potential complications that threaten patency.

Culp, K., Taylor, L., & Hulme, P. (1996). Geriatric hemodialysis patients: A comparative study of vascular access. *American Nephrology Nurses' Association Journal, 23*(6), 583–590.

This research article details the findings of a study comparing vascular access devices used in hemodialysis patients 65 years of age or older with those less than 65 years old. Clinical application and future areas of research are discussed.

Sosa-Guerrero, S., & Gomez, N. (1997). Dealing with end-stage renal disease. *American Journal of Nursing, 97*(10), 44–51.

This article summarizes the pathophysiology and treatment options related to end-stage renal disease. Advantages and disadvantages of major treatment options are presented in a format for nurses to use in guiding clients through decision-making. Self-assessment questions are included.

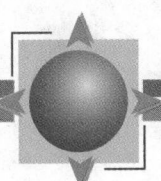

Problems of Reproduction:

Management of Clients

with Problems of the

Reproductive System

ASSESSMENT OF THE REPRODUCTIVE SYSTEM

Assessment of the female and male reproductive systems is an important component of health care. In many instances, the nurse is the first health care professional to assess the client with a reproductive system disorder. The effective nurse is comfortable with his or her own sexuality and is nonjudgmental about variations in sexual practices.

ANATOMY AND PHYSIOLOGY REVIEW
Structure and Function of the Female Reproductive System

Females begin to develop secondary sex characteristics at a wide range of ages. The average age for a girl to begin pubertal development is 11 years. Delayed puberty may be caused by

- A familial history of late growth
- A low percentage of body fat
- Abnormalities of the pituitary gland, the ovaries, or the hypothalamus
- Congenital structural abnormalities
- Chronic illnesses, such as diabetes mellitus and renal disease

External Genitalia

The external female genitalia, or vulva, extends from the mons pubis to the anal opening. The *mons pubis* is a fat pad that covers the symphysis pubis and protects it during coitus (sexual intercourse). The mons becomes prominent and covered with hair during puberty.

The *labia majora* are two vertical folds of adipose tissue that extend posteriorly from the mons pubis to the perineum. Because fatty tissue deposits vary among individuals, the size of the labia majora varies. The skin over the labia majora is usually darker than the surrounding skin and is highly vascular. The labia become prominent during puberty and develop hair on the outer surfaces. The labia majora protect inner vulval structures and enhance sensual arousal.

The labia majora surround two thinner, vertical folds of reddish epithelium, the *labia minora*. The labia minora are highly vascular and have a rich nerve supply. Emotional or physical stimulation produces marked swelling and sensitivity. Numerous sebaceous glands in the labia minora lubricate the entrance to the vagina.

The anterior labia minora form the prepuce (the hood of the clitoris) and the frenulum (a fold connecting the undersurface of the clitoris with the labia minora). The clitoris projects through these branches. The clitoris is a small, cylindric organ that is composed of erectile tissue and has a high concentration of sensory nerve endings. During sexual arousal, the clitoris becomes larger and increases sexual tension. The tissue formed at the merger of the posterior ends of the labia minora folds is called the fourchette.

The *vestibule* is a longitudinal area between the labia minora, the clitoris, and the fourchette. This area contains Bartholin's glands and the openings of the urethra, Skene's glands (paraurethral glands), and the vagina. The two Bartholin's glands, located deeply posterior on both sides of the vaginal opening, secrete lubrication fluid during sexual excitement. Their ductal openings are usually not visible.

The connective tissue that partly or wholly occludes the vaginal opening in the vestibule is called the hymen. The hymen can tear during strenuous exercise, masturbation, coitus, or the insertion of tampons. In some women, hymenal tags remain after the hymen tears; in other women, the tissue disappears.

The area between the fourchette and the anus is the perineum. The skin of the perineum covers the muscles, fascia, and ligaments that support the pelvic structures and provide voluntary control of the vagina and of the urinary and anal sphincters.

Internal Genitalia

The internal female genitalia are shown in Figure 76–1.

Vagina

The vagina is a collapsible hollow tube extending from the vestibule to the uterus. In addition to being the chan-nel for the passage of the menstrual flow, the vagina allows reception of the penis during intercourse and passage of the fetus during childbirth. Squamous epithelium and abundant blood vessels line the thin, muscular vaginal walls of the vagina that lie in transverse folds (rugae) during the female's reproductive years and are highly distensible. Normally, the anterior and posterior vaginal walls lie in contact with each other. There are few sensory nerve endings in the lower vaginal segment near the introitus (opening), which allows the vagina to be relatively insensitive to distention.

The amounts of glycogen and lubricating fluid that are secreted by the vaginal epithelium are influenced by ovarian hormones. Döderlein's bacilli, the normal vaginal flora, interact with the secreted glycogen to produce lactic acid and maintain an acid pH (4–5) in the vagina. The acidity reduces the vagina's susceptibility to infection. Estrogen deprivation occurring during postpartum periods, lactation, and menopause causes the vaginal wall to become dry and thinner and the rugae to become smoother.

Connective tissue forming the vesicovaginal septum separates the anterior wall of the vagina from the urethra and bladder. The posterior wall of the vagina is separated from the rectum by the rectovaginal septum. At the upper end of the vagina, the uterine cervix projects into a cup-shaped vault of thin vaginal tissue. The recessed pockets around the cervix, called fornices, permit palpation of the internal pelvic organs. The posterior area is clinically significant because it provides access into the peritoneal cavity (through Douglas' cul-de-sac) for diagnostic or surgical purposes.

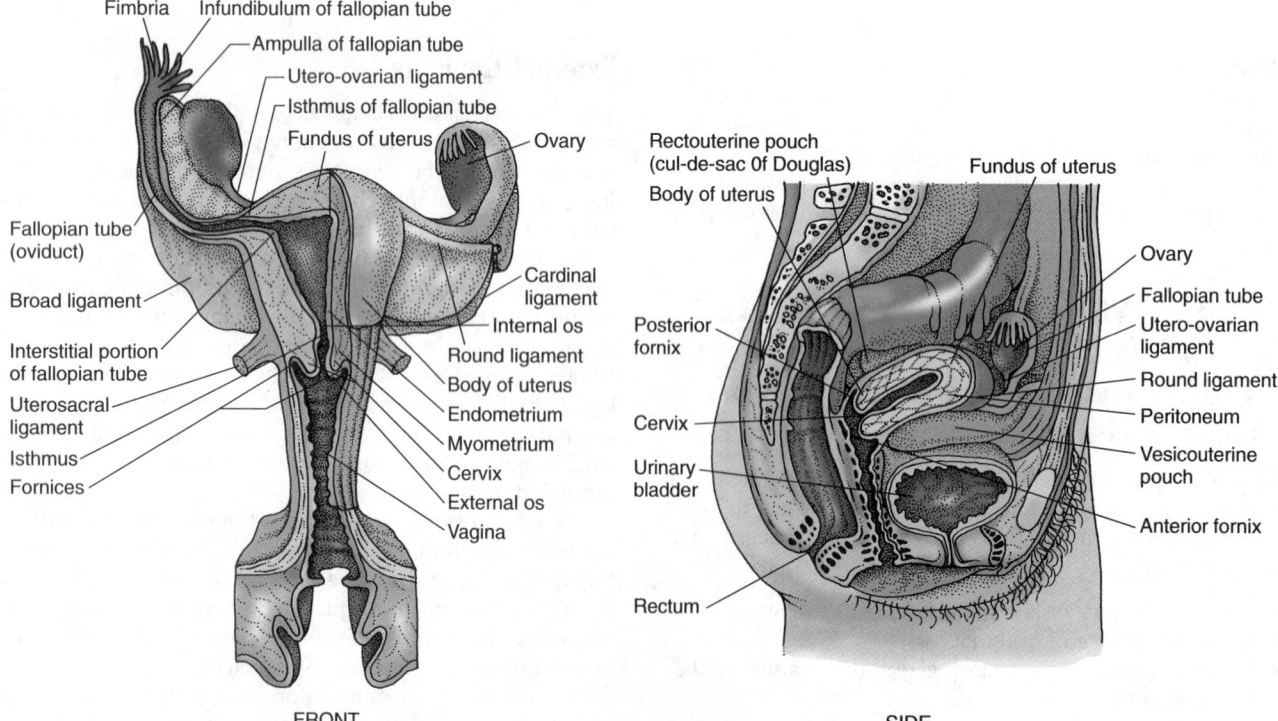

FRONT   SIDE

Figure 76–1. Internal female genitalia.

Uterus

The uterus is a flat, thick-walled, muscular organ attached to the upper end of the vagina. In the nonpregnant woman, the inverted pear-shaped organ is located within the true pelvis, between the bladder and the rectum. Functionally, the uterus responds to hormonal stimulation and prepares to receive, nurture, and finally expel the products of conception.

The size of the uterus depends on the woman's developmental stage and obstetric history. In a woman who has never been pregnant, the average uterine dimensions are $3\frac{1}{2} \times 2 \times 1$ inch ($7.5 \times 5 \times 2.5$ cm).

Gross Anatomic Structure

Anatomically, the uterus is composed of the corpus (body) and the cervix; these areas are separated by a constricted region called the isthmus.

THE CORPUS. The upper segment of the uterine body, between the insertion sites of the fallopian tubes, is referred to as the fundus. Although the uterus is a hollow organ, its walls are in such close proximity in the nonpregnant state that its cavity is merely a slit. The uterine walls are composed of three layers: peritoneum, myometrium, and endometrium.

Peritoneum. This outer layer separates the uterus from the abdominal cavity. The pouch that is formed by the peritoneum, where it lines the anterior uterus and extends to the top of the bladder, is called the vesicouterine pouch. The rectouterine pouch (also referred to as Douglas' cul-de-sac or the posterior cul-de-sac) is the posterior peritoneal pocket, between the rectum and the posterior uterine and vaginal walls.

Myometrium. The thick middle layer of the body of the uterus is made up of three layers of smooth muscle fibers, collectively called the myometrium. These muscle fibers are arranged in opposing directions and are interlaced with blood vessels. Contraction of these muscle fibers can cause the products of conception to be expelled and can then constrict the blood vessels to control postpartum bleeding.

Endometrium. The inner mucosal layer of the uterine body is the endometrium. The cyclic activity of estrogen and progesterone produces great variation in the thickness of this tissue (from 0.5 to 5 mm). The endometrium consists of a single layer of epithelial cells that cover tubular uterine glands, a spongy stroma (connective tissue framework), and a vascular network. The uterine glands secrete an alkaline fluid that keeps the cavity moist. All but the deepest layer of endometrium is shed during menses and after the delivery of a fetus.

CERVICAL PORTION. The cervix is below the isthmus of the uterus and extends into the vagina. The cervix provides a canal for the entry of sperm into the uterus and for the passage of menstrual flow, secretes mucus, and is a barrier to ascending vaginal bacteria. In addition, sphincter-like fibers that comprise the cervix hold the products of conception in the uterine cavity or that stretch to permit vaginal birth.

The cervical portion of the uterus is approximately 1 inch (2.5 cm) long. The upper boundary, the internal os, is approximately at the level where the peritoneal covering of the anterior uterus deflects over the bladder. The lower boundary, the external os, projects into the vaginal fornix. In the nonpregnant woman, the cervix around the external os is usually smooth, firm, and pink. A woman who has borne a child has a small, transverse slit-like external os. The endocervical canal connects the internal os with the external os and provides access from the vagina to the uterine cavity.

CONNECTIVE TISSUE SUPPORT. The uterus is supported by ligaments and muscles of the pelvic floor. The broad ligaments attach to the lateral walls of the uterus, between the insertion of the fallopian tubes and the pelvic floor. Broad ligaments (folds of peritoneum) divide the pelvis into anterior and posterior cavities. The thick portion at the base of each broad ligament is also called the cardinal ligament.

The round ligaments extend outward on each side of the uterus and downward through the inguinal canal. They terminate in the upper portion of the labia majora.

The two uterosacral ligaments are attached to either side of the posterior cervix. They extend posteriorly, around the rectum, to the fascia over the second and third sacral vertebrae. These ligaments exert posterior traction on the cervix and hold the body of the uterus in its anterior position.

Fallopian Tubes

The fallopian tubes (uterine tubes) insert into the upper lateral portion of the body of the uterus and extend laterally to a site near the ovaries. Functionally, the uterine tubes provide a duct between the ovaries and the uterus for the passage of ova and sperm. In most cases, the ovum is fertilized in these tubes.

Each tube, about $3\frac{1}{8}$ to $5\frac{1}{2}$ inches (8 to 14 cm) long, is covered by one of the peritoneal folds of the broad ligament. The tubes are lined with longitudinal folds of ciliated and secretory columnar epithelial cells. Rhythmic contractions of the musculature of the tubes vary in response to the ovarian cycle. The tubal contractions and the current that is produced by the movement of the cilia transport the ovum to the uterus.

The uterine tubes are divided into four anatomic sections (see Fig. 76–1). The interstitial portion is the most proximal to the uterus; the isthmus and the ampulla are the middle segments; and the infundibulum is the most distal portion.

Fimbriated ends of the infundibulum open through the peritoneum into the abdominal cavity. One of the fringe-like fimbriae at the end of each tube is considerably longer than the others. This projection extends nearly to the ovary and facilitates capture of a released ovum.

Ovaries

The ovaries are a pair of almond-shaped organs, approximately $1/8 \times 7/8 \times 3/8$ inch ($0.3 \times 2 \times 1$ cm). They are situated near the lateral walls of the upper pelvic cavity. After menopause, the ovaries are significantly smaller. Functionally, these small organs develop and release ova. This cyclic maturation of a dominant follicle (the graafian follicle) and subsequent release of the ovum is referred to as ovulation. The ovaries also produce the sex steroid hormones (estrogen, progesterone, androgen, and relaxin). Adequate amounts of these steroidal sex hormones are necessary for normal female growth and development and for the maintenance of a pregnancy.

Breasts

The female breasts are a pair of mammary glands that develop in response to secretions from the hypothalamus, the pituitary gland, and the ovaries. Functionally, the breasts are an accessory of the reproductive system meant to nourish the infant after birth.

The breasts are located between the second and sixth ribs, between the edge of the sternum and the midaxillary line. About two thirds of the breast diameter is over the greater pectoral muscle, and one third is superficial to the anterior serratus muscle.

Structure

The structure of a mature female breast is shown in Figure 76–2. The nipple rises from the center of the pigmented areola, which is usually located slightly lateral to the midline of each breast. Montgomery's glands are small, round sebaceous glands that appear as elevations on the areola. These glands are thought to secrete a fatty substance that protects the nipple during breastfeeding.

Breast tissue is composed of a network of glandular and ductal tissue, fibrous tissue, and fat. The proportion of each component of breast tissue depends on genetic factors, nutrition, age, and obstetric history. The breast is supported by Cooper's suspensory ligaments attached to underlying muscles.

The breasts may not develop symmetrically during puberty. By adulthood, both breasts are usually symmetric in size and contour. It is not unusual for the breast on the woman's dominant side (on the basis of right-handedness or left-handedness) to appear larger because of the more developed pectoral muscle base.

In many women, the breasts become slightly larger and tender during the premenstrual period. The tissue may also feel nodular at this time. Increasing levels of estrogen and progesterone 3 to 4 days before menses affect the breasts by increasing vascularity, inducing growth of the ducts and alveoli, and promoting water retention. After menstruation, the cellular growth regresses, the ducts and alveoli decrease in size, and water retention subsides.

Blood Supply

The abundant blood supply to the breasts is from branches of the internal mammary and lateral thoracic arteries. The veins of the breast connect with the superior vena cava. Much of the lymph drains through an extensive network that is radial to the axilla (Fig. 76–3). Lymph may spread cancerous cells directly into the infraclavicular nodes, deeply into the chest or abdomen, or into the opposite breast, depending on the location of a malignant lesion. Lymphatic drainage from the axillary nodes empties into the jugular and subclavian veins. This short route allows cancerous cells to move rapidly into the general circulation and to metastasize to the lungs, pelvis, vertebrae, and brain.

Menstruation and Menopause
Normal Menstrual Cycle

Menstruation is the cyclic shedding of the endometrial lining of the uterus. The term *menarche* refers specifically to the female's first menstruation and is one sign of puberty. Most girls begin to menstruate between the ages of 10 and 16 years.

The occurrence of cyclic menstruation and reproduction depends on maturation of the hypothalamic-pituitary-ovarian-uterine axis. Normally, this cycle is not achieved for the first 1 to 2 years after menarche. The

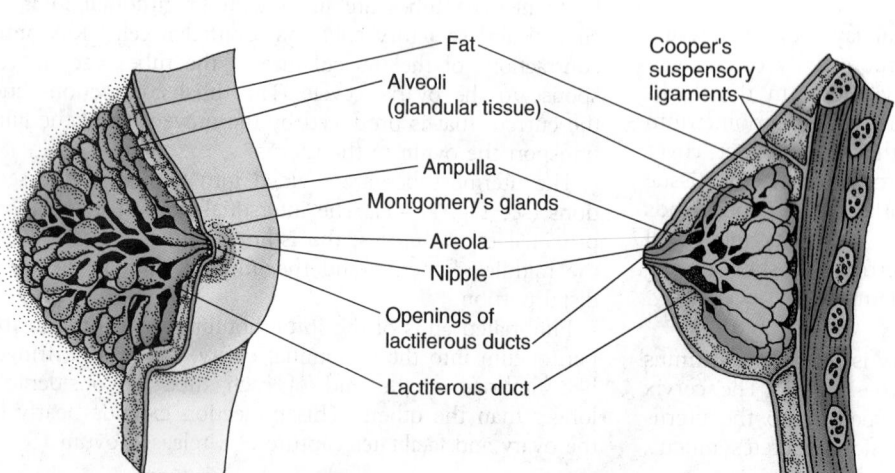

Fat
Alveoli (glandular tissue)
Cooper's suspensory ligaments
Ampulla
Montgomery's glands
Areola
Nipple
Openings of lactiferous ducts
Lactiferous duct

Figure 76–2. Structure of the mature female breast.

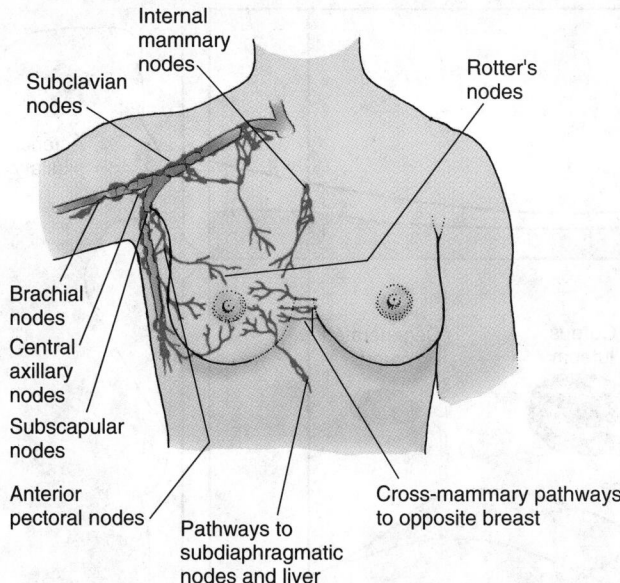

Figure 76–3. Lymphatic drainage of the female breast.

first menstrual cycles are typically anovulatory and irregular.

The menstrual cycle is under a feedback control system of three interrelated cycles:

- The hypothalamic-pituitary cycle
- The ovarian cycle
- The uterine (or endometrial) cycle

The relationship of these cycles is illustrated in Figure 76–4.

The idealized menstrual cycle is 28 days; however, variations are normal. The first day of the menstrual cycle is calculated as the first day of monthly menstrual bleeding. The menstrual flow is referred to as the menses. Ovulation occurs approximately 14 days before the beginning of the next menstrual cycle. Regular menstrual cycles indicate normal sex hormone production and the occurrence of ovulation. Variations in the length of a woman's menstrual cycle occur in response to variations in the length of the preovulatory stage compared with the postovulatory stage.

Menopause and the Climacteric

Natural Menopause

Menopause is the biological end of reproductive ability, but the term applies to only the last menstrual period. The actual date of menopause cannot be determined until at least 1 year has passed without menses. The phase of a woman's life from the initial decline in the amount of estrogen produced by the ovaries to the cessation of symptoms produced by this phenomenon is called the *climacteric*. Lay terminology for this phase is "the change of life." Menopause is only one sign of the climacteric.

During a woman's life span, follicles in the ovary atrophy continuously. The progressive decline in the number of follicles that can produce estrogen in response to pituitary hormones causes the woman (usually between 40 and 50 years of age) to begin to notice physical changes in her body. Levels of estrogen and progesterone diminish gradually until the effect of these hormones on the endometrial lining of the uterus ceases. At the same time, the low levels of the ovarian hormones continue to stimulate the hypothalamic-pituitary axis. The anterior pituitary secretes high levels of follicle-stimulating hormone (FSH) and luteinizing hormone (LH) after menopause has occurred.

For a time, the inner core of the ovary produces androstenedione (a weak male hormone) and testosterone. Eighty percent of the androstenedione is produced by the adrenal glands. When the ovarian core ceases to function, the adrenal cortices are the only source of steroids. The production of androstenedione is significant, especially after menopause, because it is converted to a form of estrogen (estrone) in body fat. Consequently, women with a greater percentage of body fat have higher estrone levels after menopause.

During the climacteric, a woman experiences irregular menstrual and ovarian cycles. Often ovulation fails to occur. The menstrual flow may be lighter or heavier during irregular cycles.

Decreased amounts of estrogen affect multiple sites in the body. The uterus, the cervix, and the ovaries, as well as the labia and the clitoris, shrink in size. The low estrogen levels cause the vagina to narrow and shorten. The vaginal mucosa becomes thin and dry, which makes intercourse uncomfortable.

The muscular support to the pelvis becomes more relaxed. The loss of tone also affects bladder support.

Bone density is a concern after estrogen production decreases. Estrogen is needed by bone tissue for calcium uptake. It also increases the metabolism of vitamin D, which is needed for absorption of calcium from the intestines. In clients with decreased calcium uptake, bone density decreases. The reduction in the amount of bone mass is called *osteoporosis* (see Chap. 53).

One of the most common symptoms occurring during the climacteric are hot flashes, which are caused by vasomotor instability. Their cause is not clear, but it is thought that surges of FSH and LH on the hypothalamus cause vasodilation and increased heat production (Quinn & Lowdermilk, 1995).

Artificial Menopause

Menopause may occur for reasons other than the natural physiologic changes of the climacteric. Artificial menopause is the cessation of menstruation caused by some artificial means, such as an oophorectomy (surgical removal of the ovaries), a hysterectomy (surgical removal of the uterus), or radiation to the ovaries. A premenopausal woman who experiences artificial menopause may need estrogen replacement.

Structure and Function of the Male Reproductive System

External Genitalia

The external male genitalia undergo multiple changes during puberty. The first visible sign of pubescence is

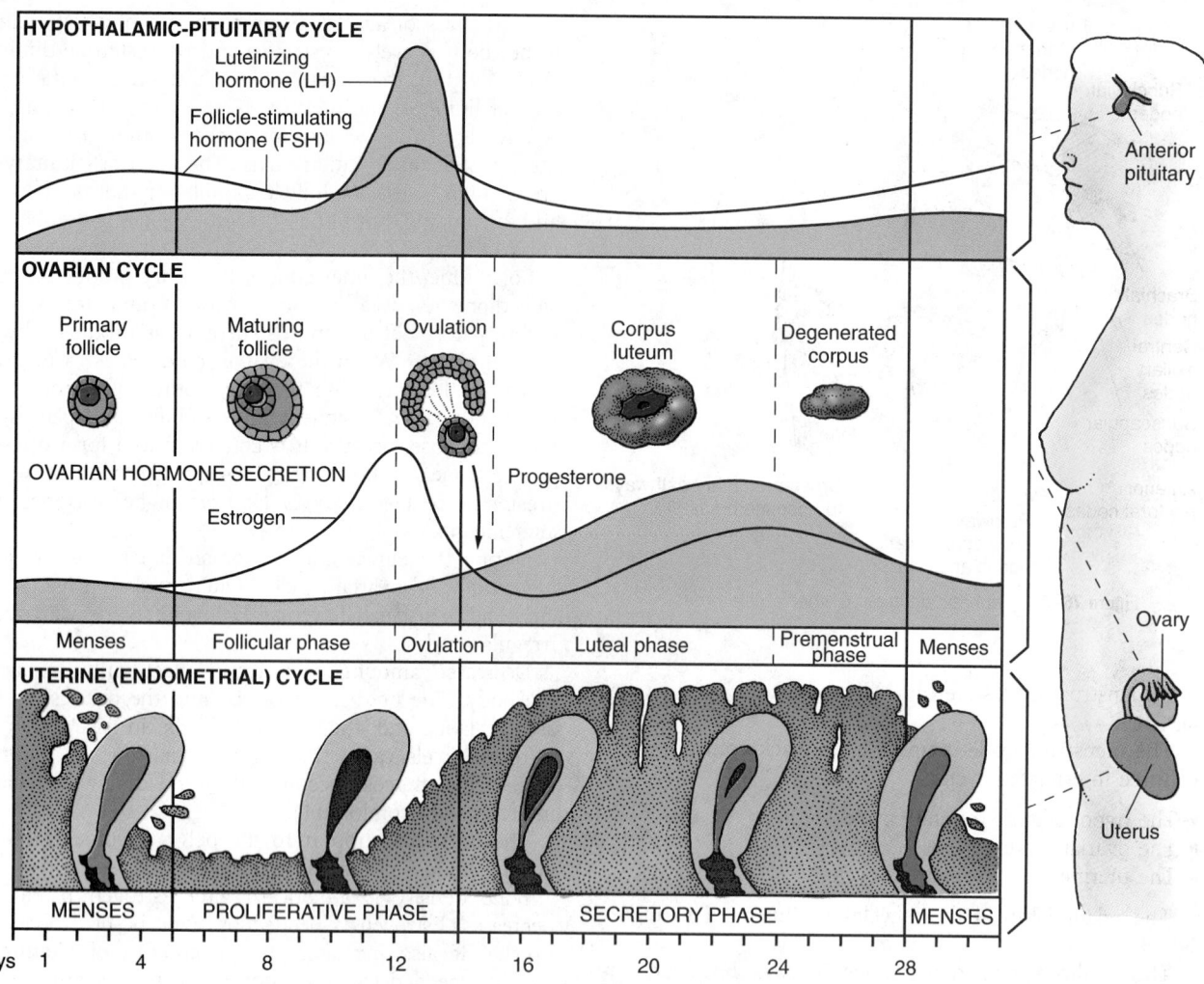

Figure 76–4. Interrelationships of the events of the menstrual cycle.

enlargement of the scrotum and testes, which typically occurs between the ages of 11 and 13½ years.

These changes occur in response to a rise in testosterone production. The release of gonadotropin-releasing hormone (GnRH) from the male's hypothalamus stimulates the anterior pituitary to secrete LH and FSH. As the levels of the gonadotropins increase, the amount of testosterone significantly increases. Other signs of puberty that relate to testosterone production are the growth of axillary hair, lengthening and thickening of the vocal cords, increased sebaceous gland activity, and a general increase in muscle mass and body size.

In the adult male, testosterone production remains relatively constant. Only a slight and gradual reduction of testosterone production occurs in the older adult male. The lower testosterone levels contribute to a decrease in muscle mass, loss of skin elasticity, postural changes, and changes in sexual performance.

Penis

Structure

The penis is the male organ for urination and copulation. The root of the penis is attached to the anterior pubic

arch by a continuation of fascia, a triangular suspensory ligament, and muscle tissue. The root of the penis consists of the posterior ends of the three erectile columns from the body of the penis.

The corpus, or body, is the pendulous, soft-tissue portion that extends from the attached root to the glans penis, the distal end of the penis. Engorgement of the highly vascular, erectile columns with blood during sexual excitement causes the penis to expand and elongate and become firm and erect. A ridge of tissue forms where the glans expands and meets the corpus, called the corona of the glans. The glans tissue surrounds the slit-like opening of the urethral meatus. The male urethra is the pathway for the exit of both urine and semen.

The penis is covered by thin skin that is loosely attached to the underlying fascia. This loose skin allows the penis to enlarge during erections. The skin is darker than that of the rest of the body, and hair is present only at the base of the penis, near its root.

A continuation of penile skin covers the glans and folds back on itself to form the prepuce (foreskin). Adhesions between the foreskin and the glans normally prevent retraction of the foreskin in the newborn. The adhesions gradually disintegrate, and the foreskin can usually be retracted by the time a boy is 3 years old (the range is 4 months to 13 years). Surgical removal of the prepuce (circumcision) is often performed in the newborn period for religious or sociocultural reasons. An adult male may also undergo circumcision.

The penis is richly innervated through branches of the sympathetic and parasympathetic nervous systems and by nerves of cerebral origin. Parasympathetic fibers provide sensory innervation of the penile skin and allow the smooth muscle of the arteries to relax. Parasympathetic stimulation enables blood to flow freely into the cavernous spaces. Sympathetic fibers control the rhythmic muscle contractions that lead to the ejaculation of semen. Sympathetic fibers also constrict the smooth muscle of the arteries to allow blood to flow from the erectile bodies. The cerebral cortex is probably responsible for most of the erogenous stimulation.

Scrotum

The scrotum is a thin-walled, fibromuscular sac that is suspended below the pubic bone. It is posterior to the penis. The pouch protects the testes, the epididymis, and the vas deferens in a space that is relatively cooler than inside the abdominal cavity. Normal spermatogenesis necessitates a controlled temperature. The slightly lower temperature, about 2° C (6° F) less than body temperature, is optimal for sperm production and viability. The left side of the scrotum usually hangs about ⅜ inch (1 cm) lower than the right side.

Scrotal skin is darkly pigmented and contains multiple sweat and sebaceous glands and few hair follicles. The skin is arranged in horizontal folds called *rugae*. The rugae are more apparent when the scrotum is retracted toward the body. The scrotum readily contracts with cold, exercise, tactile stimulation, and sexual excitement.

Internal Genitalia

The internal male genitalia are shown in Figure 76–5.

Testes and Spermatic Cord

The testes are a pair of ovoid organs that produce spermatozoa and testosterone. Each testis is suspended in the scrotum by the spermatic cord, which provides vascular, lymphatic, and nerve supply to the testis. The cord also covers the epididymis and a portion of the vas deferens. The cord and testes are encircled by layers of spermatic fascia and cremaster muscle. Sympathetic nerve fibers are located on the arteries in the cord, and sympathetic and parasympathetic fibers are on the vas deferens. When the testes sustain a trauma, these autonomic nerve fibers transmit excruciating pain and a nauseating sensation.

Epididymis

The epididymis is the first portion of a ductal system that transports sperm from the ductules of the testes to the urethra; it also aids in maturation of the sperm. The epididymis is comma shaped, lies posterolateral to one side of each testis, and is divided into a head, a body, and a tail.

The head of the epididymis attaches to the posterior aspect of the testis. The body descends against the lateral wall of the testis. At the lower border of the testis, the tail folds back over on itself and ascends toward the spermatic cord. The tail merges gradually into the vas deferens and provides storage for sperm.

Vas Deferens

The vas deferens, or ductus deferens, is a firm, muscular tube about 17¾ inches (45 cm) long that continues from the tail of each epididymis. The terminal end of each vas deferens enlarges to form an ampulla, which is a major reservoir for sperm and tubular fluids. The ampulla of each vas deferens merges with a duct from the seminal vesicle to form the ejaculatory ducts at the base of the prostate gland. Sperm from the vas deferens and nutritive secretions from the seminal vesicles are transported

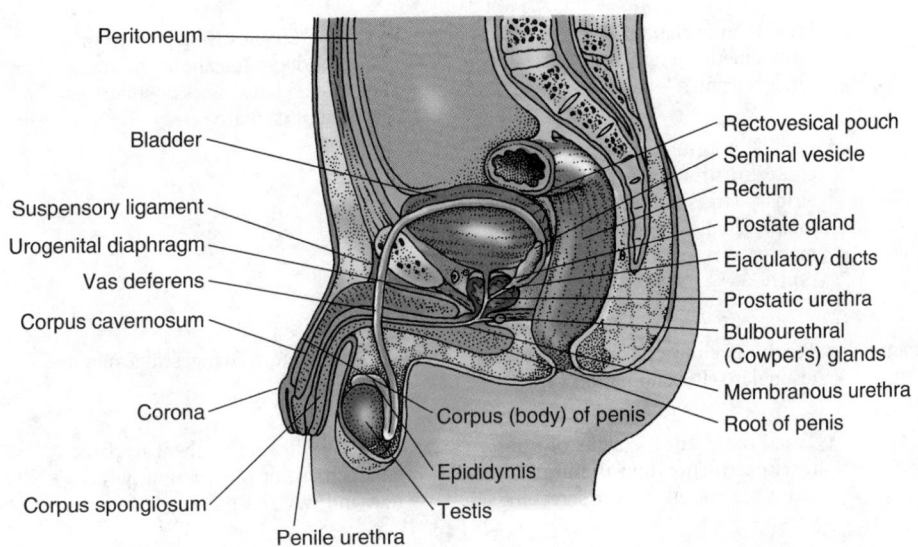

Figure 76–5. Internal male genitalia.

through the ejaculatory duct to mix with prostatic fluids in the prostatic urethra.

The cremaster muscle envelops the vas deferens and the testes within the spermatic cord. The ductus is heavily innervated by autonomic nerve fibers, which cause the expulsive contractions during ejaculation. The hypogastric and pelvic nerves provide the innervation for the contractile movements of the vas deferens.

Although the vas deferens secretes a small amount of fluid to support the sperm, its main function is to transport sperm from the epididymis to the ejaculatory ducts. In contrast to movement of sperm through the epididymis by ciliary action, transport of sperm through the vas deferens occurs by means of peristaltic contractions of the ducts. Thus, a vasectomy, the surgical procedure for male sterilization, prevents only the passage of sperm to the ejaculatory ducts. A vasectomy does not prevent the production of sperm, does not limit the erection of the penis, and does not greatly decrease the total amount of semen. Unexpelled sperm degenerate and are reabsorbed within the epididymis and the distal portion of the vas deferens.

Seminal Vesicles and Ejaculatory Ducts

The seminal vesicles are paired glands that secrete a major portion of the volume of the ejaculate. They are located behind the bladder near the prostate gland and are separated from the rectum by the rectovesical pouch. Each vesicle ends in a small duct, which joins that of the ampulla of the vas deferens to form an ejaculatory duct. The two ejaculatory ducts are slender tubes that descend through the prostate gland; they end in slit-like openings in the prostatic urethra.

Prostate Gland

The prostate gland is the largest accessory gland of the male reproductive system. It is a chestnut-shaped, glandular, and fibromuscular organ. Functionally, it secretes a milky alkaline fluid that adds bulk to the semen, enhances sperm motility, and neutralizes female acidic vaginal secretions.

During emission, the first stage of the male orgasm, the smooth muscle of the prostate gland contracts and secretes its fluid at the same time as the vas deferens. Fluid from the prostate gland contributes 20% to 30% of the total ejaculate. The average pH of the combined secretions of semen is approximately 7.5, whereas secretions from the vagina normally have a pH of 3.5 to 4. Sperm need a surrounding fluid pH of 6 to 6.5 before they become optimally motile.

The prostate gland is approximately 6 inches (15 cm) long. It is situated between the neck of the bladder and the urogenital diaphragm. The prostate gland is separated

---

Chart 76–1

Nursing Focus on the Elderly: Changes in the Reproductive System Related to Aging

Physiologic Change	Nursing Implications	Rationale
Women		
Graying and thinning of the pubic hair.	• Discuss changes with the client (applies to all structures for both women and men).	• Education helps prevent problems with body image (applies to all structures for both women and men).
Decreased size of the labia majora and the clitoris		
Increased flabbiness and fibrosity of the breasts, which hang lower on the chest wall; decreased erection of the nipples	• Teach or reinforce the importance of breast self-examination (BSE).	• BSE may detect lumps or other changes that may indicate the presence of cancer.
Drying, smoothing, and thinning of the vaginal walls	• Provide information about estrogen replacement therapy and water-soluble lubricants.	• Education enables the client to make informed decisions about the treatment of vaginal dryness, which can cause painful intercourse.
Decreased size of the uterus Atrophy of the endometrium Decreased size and marked convolution of the ovaries Loss of tone and elasticity of the pelvic ligaments and connective tissue	• Provide information about Kegel exercises to strengthen pelvic muscles. • Urinary stress incontinence is a major problem. Strengthening exercises may prevent or reduce the condition.	
Men		
Graying and thinning of the pubic hair Increased pedulousness of the scrotum and loss of rugae	• Teach or reinforce the importance of testicular self-examination (TSE).	• TSE may detect changes that may indicate cancer.
Prostate enlargement, with increased likelihood of urethral obstruction	• Teach the client the signs of urethral obstruction and the importance of prostate cancer screening.	• Education helps the client to detect enlargement or obstruction, which may indicate the presence of cancer.

from the anterior wall of the rectum by a thin fascial sheath that is part of the rectovesical septum. The prostate gland can be palpated through the rectum and should not project more than ⅜ inch (1 cm) into the rectal lumen.

As men age, the prostate gland becomes clinically significant. At birth, the gland is small. During puberty, the prostate rapidly enlarges to its normal adult size. By age 50 or 60 years, about 80% of men have an enlarged prostate (benign prostatic hyperplasia), which can cause urinary problems (Seidel et al., 1995).

Prostatic function depends on adequate levels of testosterone. As men age, testicular production of testosterone decreases.

Bulbourethral (Cowper's) Glands

Semen is ejaculated through the prostatic urethra, the membranous urethra, and the penile urethra. The bulbourethral glands are two yellow, pea-sized glands that are located posterior to the membranous urethra within the muscle of the urethral sphincter. They are connected to the penile portion of the urethra by ducts.

The bulbourethral glands secrete an alkaline mucus into the penile urethra during emission. The mucus mixes with the sperm and other glandular secretions to form the semen. The bulbourethral glands contribute about 5% to 6% of the total ejaculate. The alkalinity of the mucus further protects the sperm against the relative acidity within the urethra.

Reproductive Changes Associated with Aging

Age affects the function of the reproductive system in both the male and the female. After puberty, hormones produced by the gonads affect the normal functioning of many body systems. Many changes in the reproductive system are evident in elderly clients (Chart 76–1).

HISTORY
Demographic Data

The nurse uses data about the client's age, sex, and culture to assess the client's risk for certain diseases. The nurse considers the client's age in evaluating the reproductive system. The age at which secondary sex characteristics developed in the client are compared with the established normal ranges for males or females.

TRANSCULTURAL CONSIDERATIONS

Transcultural influences and expectations account for variations in acceptable gender-related and sexual identity. A child's attitude and behavior about the meaning and use of the genitals begin in infancy and are modeled on the behavior of significant adults. Religious dictates often parallel those of a specific culture and strongly affect sexual activity. A person's religious beliefs (Geissler, 1994) often influence specific sexual practices, the acceptable number of partners, contraceptive use, and

specific treatments to terminate a pregnancy, end fertility, or remove barriers to infertility.

Ethnicity often has an epidemiologic influence on particular diseases. For instance, the incidence of cancer of the reproductive system and associated death rates are higher for African-Americans than for Caucasian Americans (American Cancer Society [ACS], 1997). Secondary sex characteristics may differ by ethnicity as well. For example, axillary hair appears at an earlier age in African-Americans than in Caucasians. Asian-Americans have finer, more sparse pubic hair than do people of other races (Seidel et al., 1995).

Personal and Family History
Personal History

The nurse assesses the client's health habits, such as diet, sleep, and exercise patterns. Low levels of body fat may be related to ovarian dysfunction. The nurse also determines the client's alcohol, tobacco, and drug use because libido, spermatogenesis, and potency can be affected by such substances (Quinn & Lowdermilk, 1995).

The client's personal medical history gives data about his or her general health. Certain childhood illnesses are particularly related to the reproductive system. Females need to be screened for sufficient rubella titers and should be treated, if necessary, to prevent possible teratogenic effects on their unborn children. Mumps or smallpox in the postpubertal male may cause orchitis (painful inflammation and swelling of the testes) and occasionally leads to testicular atrophy and sterility.

The nurse also assesses for a history of major adult illnesses or chronic illnesses that may also severely affect reproductive function. For example, endocrine disorders may affect the hypothalamic-pituitary-gonadal axis of the male or female. Almost any disease that disturbs a woman's metabolism or nutrition can depress ovarian function and cause amenorrhea. A history of infertility and failure of ovulation is associated with a greater risk for endometrial cancer. The client with diabetes mellitus may experience physiologic changes, such as vaginal dryness or impotence.

Some pre-existing cancers increase a woman's risk for developing other reproductive system cancers. Chronic disorders of the nervous system, respiratory system, or cardiovascular system can alter the sexual response. Some drugs (antihypertensives, opioids, monoamine oxidase inhibitors, histamine antagonists) may impair fertility (Lowdermilk, 1995a).

Reproductive system dysfunction can also result from radiation, prolonged use of corticosteroids, exogenous estrogen or testosterone use, and chemotherapeutic agents.

In addition, past severe infections can alter a person's reproductive ability. For example, pelvic inflammatory disease or ruptured appendix followed by peritonitis can cause strictures or adhesions in the fallopian tubes and pelvic scarring. Salpingitis (tubal infection) is most frequently caused by *Neisseria gonorrhoeae* infection, commonly resulting in female infertility. In the male, infections or prolonged fever may damage sperm production or cause obstruction of the seminal tract, which leads to infertility. The nurse explores the client's history of surgeries, serious injuries, current medications, and allergies, because each of these can affect reproductive structure or function.

Genitoreproductive History

The nurse completes a genitoreproductive history for both male and female clients. Chart 76–2 lists the key questions that the nurse asks.

Female Client

With a female client, the nurse asks questions about her menses, including age of menarche, cycle frequency and duration, amount of flow, spotting between periods, dysmenorrhea (painful menstrual periods), and premenstrual symptoms.

If the client is of menopausal age, the nurse determines the date of her last menstrual period and the presence of climacteric symptoms. The nurse asks all women about the presence of vaginal discharge, history and treatment of sexually transmitted diseases, the date and the result of her last Papanicolaou (Pap) test, breast self-examination practices, and vulvar self-examination practices.

The nurse also takes an obstetric history. Women who have never had children have higher rates of ovarian, endometrial, and breast cancer than do multiparous women. If the woman has ever been pregnant, the nurse asks about the outcome of the pregnancies. In addition, the nurse collects information about the date and mode of deliveries or termination of the pregnancy; complications during pregnancy, labor, and delivery; birth weight and gestational age of the infants; and the condition of the infants at birth and at present.

The nurse also collects data about sexual activity. Heterosexual activity should not be assumed. Lesbian and gay issues are often not assessed. Early age at first intercourse and multiple sex partners are associated with an increased risk of cervical cancer. The client is asked about satisfaction with sexual response, any pain or bleeding with sexual intercourse, and contraceptive use. Religious beliefs may dictate contraceptive practices for a couple.

Male Client

For male clients, the nurse asks about testicular changes and self-examination practices, problems with urination, discharge from the penis, rectal problems, history and treatment of sexually transmitted diseases, and symptoms related to hernias.

The nurse also inquires about sexual functioning. Reproductive history and contraceptive use, current problems or changes in sexual response, and any occurrence of impotence also direct the physical assessment.

Family History

The family history, including that of the parents, grandparents, siblings, and spouse, helps to determine the client's risk for conditions that affect reproductive system functioning. A seeming delay or precocious development of secondary sex characteristics may be a familial pattern.

Chart 76–2

Nursing Care Highlight: Key Questions in a Genitoreproductive History

For a Female Client

- When did you begin your menstrual period?
- How often do you menstruate (if premenopausal)?
- Do you have premenstrual symptoms?
- How heavy is your menstrual flow?
- Do you experience any spotting between periods?
- Do you experience pain or discomfort during menstruation?
- When was your last menstrual period (if postmenopausal)?
- Do you have or have you had symptoms of menopause, such as hot flashes?
- Have you had any unusual vaginal discharge? If yes, please describe it.
- Have you had any sexually transmitted diseases? If yes, when and what type did you have?
- When was your last Pap test?
- Do you perform monthly breast self-examinations? Have you noticed any abnormality?
- Do you perform monthly vulvar self-examinations? Have you noticed any abnormality?
- How many pregnancies have you had? What was the outcome of each pregnancy?
- How was (were) your baby(ies) delivered?
- What were the weight(s) and health of your baby(ies)?
- How would you describe your "sex life?" Do you have any problems?
- What type of contraception do you use, if any?
- Has any female in your family had cancer of the reproductive organs? Who? What type of cancer?

For a Male Client

- Do you practice monthly testicular self-examination? Have you noticed any abnormality?
- Have you had any discharge from your penis? If yes, describe it.
- Have you had any sexually transmitted disease? If yes, when and what type?
- Have you ever had a hernia?
- Do you use condoms?
- How would you describe your "sex life?" Do you have any problems?
- Has any male in your family had prostate cancer or other type of reproductive cancer? Who? What type of cancer?

The current age and state of health of the living members of the extended family are of interest. Also the cause and age at death of specific family members may be important. Evidence of family members' having serious diseases, such as diabetes, cardiovascular disease, hypertension, renal disease, cancer, and complications of pregnancy, allows the nurse to better interpret the client's presenting symptoms. For example, daughters of women who were given diethylstilbestrol (DES) to control bleeding during pregnancy have an increased risk for infertility and reproductive tract carcinomas.

Diet History

A diet history is often critical for the correct interpretation of presenting symptoms of the reproductive system. For instance, fatigue and lack of sexual interest may be associated with poor diet and anemia. Obesity raises a person's risk for breast and uterine cancer. High-fat diets have been linked with cancer of the breast, the ovary, and the prostate gland (ACS, 1997). The nurse asks the client to recall his or her dietary intake for a recent 24-hour period to estimate the quality of the diet.

The nurse compares the client's height, weight, and body build with the dietary recall. The client may be hesitant to divulge practices such as bingeing, purging, anorexic behaviors, or excessive exercise, although these practices may affect the reproductive system (see Chapter 63 for information on common eating disorders). A certain level of body fat and weight is necessary for the onset of menses and the maintenance of regular menstrual cycles. A decreased amount of body fat is associated with insufficient estrogen levels for the maintenance of normal ovulatory cycles.

In addition, women have special dietary needs. The diet of women who use oral contraceptives should reflect increased sources of folic acid and vitamins B_6, B_{12}, and C. Heavy menstrual bleeding, particularly in women who have intrauterine devices, may necessitate oral iron supplements. All women need to be aware of the female body's need for calcium. Although adequate calcium intake throughout life is optimal, it is especially important during the premenopausal and postmenopausal periods. With the decreased production of estrogen during the climacteric, a woman's bone density decreases, which predisposes her to osteoporosis and fractures (discussed in Chapter 53).

Socioeconomic Status

The social history of the client provides insight into the whole person, including existence of stressors, job history, education, and support systems. All these factors can influence the health of the reproductive system.

Stressors

Stress has long been associated with menstrual and ovulatory irregularities. The nurse asks about leisure time activities that pose a high risk of injury to the reproductive system. For example, men who lounge for long periods in hot tubs or saunas may experience decreased sperm production. Women who are long-distance runners have reduced percentages of body fat and a higher degree of menstrual irregularities.

Occupation

The client's work may directly affect the reproductive system. Routine occupational exposure to potential teratogenic substances (agents capable of producing birth defects in offspring) results in a higher incidence of abnormal sperm morphologic features and low sperm counts in men or of spontaneous abortion (miscarriage) in women. People who work around certain chemicals, radiation, and heavy metals are at risk. Trauma and exposure to extremely high temperatures in the workplace are potential causes of male infertility. In addition, exposure to some industrial agents, such as cadmium, may be related to the development of carcinomas of the reproductive system.

Education

The nurse assesses the educational level of the client to individualize health teaching. Lay language for body parts and functions is commonly used when discussing the reproductive system. The nurse must be familiar with such terms and be comfortable their use. Clients may try to evoke a particular response in the nurse by the use of certain words, or they may have no other terminology to express the problem. The nurse who responds with shock or disdain displays a judgmental attitude that hinders successful data gathering. Health care professionals can use teaching opportunities to provide more appropriate terminology.

Support Systems

The client's general satisfaction with life and the support systems available can directly relate to the current health problem. Questions designed to elicit information about daily routines often give insight into the client's perception of the quality of life and outlook for the future.

Current Health Problem

If a client seeks medical attention for a problem related to the reproductive system, the nurse asks additional questions to explore the chief complaint. Most complaints (Chart 76-3) concern pain, bleeding, discharge, masses, and reproductive functioning.

Pain

Pain related to reproductive system disorders may be confused with that associated with gastrointestinal (GI) or urinary tract problems. The client needs to describe the nature of the pain, including its type; intensity; timing and location; duration; and relationship to menstrual, sexual, urinary, or GI function. Factors that exacerbate or give relief are also assessed.

Reproductive system disorders can be multifaceted; the nurse should not assume that the initial medical diagnosis is conclusive.

Bleeding

Either heavy bleeding or a lack of bleeding may concern the client. The possibility of pregnancy is considered in any sexually active woman presenting with amenorrhea. Any bleeding after the menopause needs to be evaluated. The nurse asks the client to describe the character of abnormal bleeding and amount of blood from the vagina or penis. The nurse asks when the bleeding occurs in relation to certain events, such as the menstrual cycle or menopause, intercourse, trauma, and strenuous exercise. Because many factors can cause bleeding, the nurse considers sources other than the genital tract.

Chart 76–3

Nursing Care Highlight: Assessment of Clients' Complaints Related to the Reproductive System

Complaint	Nursing Assessment
Pain	• Type and intensity of pain • Location and duration of pain • Factors that relieve or worsen pain • Relationship to menstrual, sexual, urinary, or gastrointestinal function
Bleeding	• Presence or absence of bleeding • Character and amount of bleeding • Relationship of bleeding to events or other factors • Onset and duration of bleeding • Presence of associated symptoms, such as pain
Discharge	• Amount and character of discharge • Presence of genital lesions, bleeding, itching, or pain
Masses	• Location and characteristics of mass • Presence of associated symptoms, such as pain • Relationship to menstrual cycle

The nurse also asks about the onset and duration of bleeding, the interval between bleeding episodes, and precipitating factors of the bleeding. The nurse asks the client to describe the character of the bleeding in terms of the amount of blood, its color, its consistency, and changes in the nature of the flow. In addition, the nurse notes the presence of associated symptoms, such as pain, cramping or abdominal fullness, change in bowel habits, urinary difficulties, and weight changes.

Discharge

Discharge from either the male or the female reproductive tract can cause severe irritation of the surrounding tissues, itching, pain, embarrassment, and anxiety.

The nurse asks about the amount, color, consistency, odor, and chronicity of the discharge. Other symptoms may be associated with a discharge and need to be evaluated. Medications (such as antibiotics) and clothing (e.g., tight jeans and noncotton underwear) may also initiate or exacerbate genital discharge. Many types of discharge are caused by sexually transmitted diseases. The localization of these infections in the body depends on the client's sexual practices. The nurse questions the client about lesions, bleeding, itching, pain related to the genitals and orifices used by the client during sexual activity, and presence of symptoms in the sexual partner.

Masses

Any reported masses in the breasts or the testes need to be evaluated. Some masses change in character or size,

and the client can often relate these changes to menstrual cycles or trauma. The nurse inquires about associated symptoms, such as tenderness, heaviness, pain, dimpling, and tender lymph nodes.

PHYSICAL ASSESSMENT
Assessment of the Female Reproductive System

Examination of the breasts, axillae, and lymph nodes often precedes that of the anterior thorax in a complete physical examination. Inspection of the female genitalia and the pelvic examination are usually done at the end of the physical examination. The client is often more apprehensive about these portions of the examination than any other segment. Pain or lack of privacy during previous pelvic or breast examinations may prevent the client from relaxing.

The nurse can show the equipment that is going to be used, along with three-dimensional models to demonstrate the assessment procedures. Relaxation and breathing techniques can be taught to enhance the client's sense of control. The nurse informs the client about what is going to be done and what the client may feel as the examination proceeds. This information allows the client to incorporate learned coping mechanisms more successfully than if she were not expecting any discomfort. If the client displays signs of pain or exceptional concern during the procedures, the nurse should stop and make adjustments in the assessment plan or techniques. The presence of a support person may also be of benefit to the client during the examination.

A pelvic examination is recommended every 1 to 3 years for women older than 19 years as well as for younger sexually active adolescents (Lowdermilk, 1995c). A pelvic examination is indicated to assess

■ Menstrual irregularities
■ Unexplained abdominal pain
■ Vaginal discharge or infection
■ Appropriateness of a desired contraceptive
■ Rape trauma
■ Physical changes in the vagina, cervix, uterus, and adnexa

The woman should not douche for at least 24 hours before the pelvic examination because douching may prevent accurate evaluation of smears, cultures, and cytologic data.

Before the pelvic and breast examinations, the nurse asks the client to empty her bladder and to undress completely. The woman is adequately draped to protect modesty throughout the examination. If the client is not wearing a gown, a small towel, placed over the breasts, can be used under the larger drape. Drapes are removed over only the region that is being examined and are replaced when that area has been examined. Drapes that prevent eye contact between the examiner and the client dehumanize the client and prevent successful assessment of the client's comfort during the examination. Mirrors can be used to facilitate teaching the client if she so desires. The examination is performed in a room that has adequate lighting for body inspection, a comfortable temperature, and the assurance of privacy.

Breast Examination

The physical examination of the reproductive system often includes the breasts (see Chap. 77).

Abdominal Examination

After the breast examination, the examiner generally completes the thorax and cardiovascular examinations and then inspects, auscultates, and palpates the abdomen. The client's arms should be at her sides or over her chest to allow better relaxation of the abdominal muscles. During the gynecologic examination, the health care provider palpates for symptomatic and asymptomatic abdominopelvic masses. A mass can be of reproductive, GI, or urinary tract origin. Careful history taking, combined with the physical examination, can usually determine the origin of a mass. Gynecologic masses, such as ovarian and adnexal masses, can be further differentiated from lesions on the body of the uterus during the bimanual portion of the pelvic examination.

Examination of the External Genitalia

After the abdominal examination, the nurse readies the client for the inspection of the external genitalia and the pelvic examination. The nurse assists the woman into the lithotomy position and asks her to place her arms at her sides or over her chest. The client's buttocks extend slightly beyond the edge of the table, and her thighs are abducted. The nurse prepares all equipment for the vaginal and speculum examination and cytologic studies.

The initial inspection and palpation of the external genitalia provide an assessment of age-appropriate development. Hair color and distribution over the symphysis pubis and vulva suggest the woman's age and hormonal functioning. Pubic hair is inspected for the presence of lice or scabies. The examiner wears gloves to protect against possible disease and potential cross-contamination from other clients. The client is informed that the genitalia will be touched and separated.

The skin and mucosa of the vulva are inspected in a systematic pattern from anterior to posterior for signs of inflammation, infestation, swelling, lesions, and discharge.

The paraurethral glands (Skene's glands) are barely visible on either side of the urethral meatus. If infection is suspected, the urethra should be gently "milked" by inserting the index finger into the vagina and gently pressing its pad against the anterior vaginal wall as the finger is being withdrawn. This procedure usually produces no pain or discharge unless there is inflammation or infection present. The openings of the ducts from the Bartholin's glands cannot be visualized. The examiner carefully palpates the area just outside the lower vaginal orifice to assess for inflammation, tenderness, or swelling. Any discharge elicited from these ducts is cultured because these structures are often involved in gonorrheal infections.

The examination of the external female genitalia is an excellent time for teaching the client about vulvar self-examination (VSE). The incidence of precancerous conditions and infectious diseases of the vulva is increasing, especially in young women (Edge & Miller, 1994). VSE can easily be taught and can lead to early diagnosis of vulvar conditions (Chart 76–4).

Assessment of perineal support and the strength of the vaginal walls is done by asking the woman to squeeze the vaginal opening closed after the examiner has inserted two fingers. The client is then asked to strain downward while the examiner assesses for urinary incontinence or any bulging of the anterior or posterior vaginal walls that, respectively, would indicate a cystocele or rectocele.

Pelvic Examination
Pelvic Examination with a Speculum

Internal examination of the vagina and cervix is first done manually with the index finger to locate the cervix and to determine its size and consistency and dilation of the external cervical os. This procedure also allows the examiner to gauge the size of the speculum that is appropriate for the introitus and to predetermine the placement angle of the speculum for visualization of the cervix. Sterile gloves are used for the internal vaginal examination.

After the correct speculum size is determined, the speculum may be warmed and lubricated with warm water. The examiner's fingers can ease insertion of the speculum by pressing down on the perineal body just inside of the vaginal orifice (Fig. 76–6, step 1). The woman can also be asked to breathe slowly and to bear down. The examiner inserts the closed speculum in an oblique position, with the pressure exerted toward the posterior vaginal wall. The examiner removes his or her fingers. The examiner then rotates the closed blades of the speculum to a horizontal position while inserting the speculum to its full length (see Fig. 76–6, step 2). The blades are opened, and the speculum is maneuvered to enable visualization of the cervix. The examiner locks the blades in

---

Chart 76–4

Health Promotion Guide: Vulvar Self-Examination

- Perform vulvar self-examination monthly between menstrual periods if you are older than 18 years or if you are sexually active.
- Sit in a well-lighted area on a soft surface (on a bed or carpeted floor).
- Use a hand-held mirror to visualize your external genitalia.
- Examine the area around the vaginal opening from the mons pubis to the perianal area.
- Feel as well as visually inspect the area.
- Report to your health care provider new nodes, warts, growths of any kind, ulcers, sores, change in skin color, painful areas, or areas of itching or inflammation.

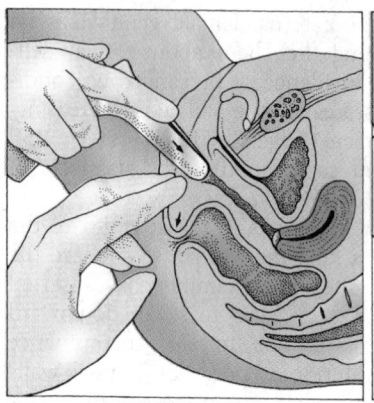
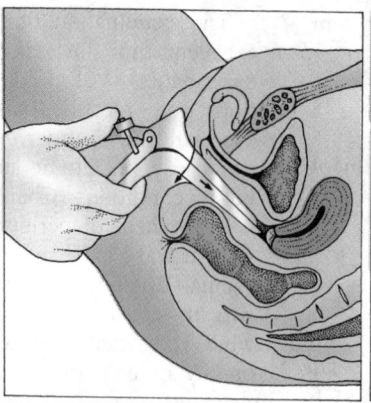
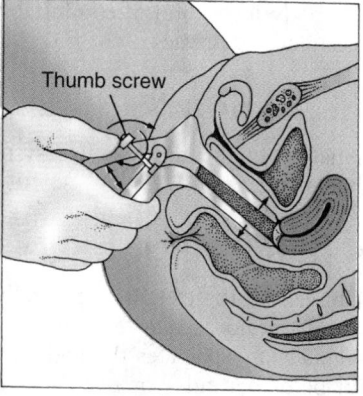
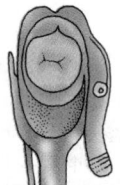

1. With the speculum blades positioned vertically, the nurse presses down on the perineal body just inside the vagina as the speculum is inserted.

2. The nurse removes the fingers from the vagina while continuing to insert the closed blades of the speculum to their full length and rotating them into a horizontal position.

3. The nurse opens the blades and maneuvers the speculum for optimal visualization of the cervix, then tightens the thumb screw to lock the blades in place.

View of the cervix through the speculum

Figure 76–6. Internal examination of the cervix.

place by tightening the thumbscrew of the speculum (see Fig. 76–6, step 3).

The examiner inspects the cervix for color, shape, and dilation of the os; erosions; nodules; masses; discharge; and bleeding.

Herpes simplex, syphilis, and carcinomas can produce characteristic lesions on the cervix. Specimens are obtained from the cervix, endocervix, and vaginal pool for cytologic studies (see discussion of Papanicolaou test). After completion of the cervical examination, the examiner loosens the thumbscrew of the speculum to close the blades and slowly rotates the speculum to a vertical position as it is withdrawn. The examiner inspects the vaginal tissue for lesions or inflammation during withdrawal.

Bimanual Examination

After withdrawing the speculum, the examiner proceeds with a bimanual examination. Using a new glove and lubricant, the examiner stands and inserts one or two fingers of one hand into the client's vagina (Fig. 76–7). The examiner palpates the posterior vaginal wall and checks for masses or tenderness. The cervix and fornix around the cervix are identified. The examiner places the opposite hand on the client's abdomen between her umbilicus and symphysis pubis. The examiner lifts the cervix and uterus with the pelvic hand toward the abdominal hand to trap the uterus between them; this allows examination of the uterus and adnexa. The examiner assesses the size, shape, consistency, and mobility of the uterus as well as any tenderness or masses. To palpate each ovary and tube, the examiner presses the abdominal hand into the right or left lower quadrant. The fingers in the fornix are used to palpate the ovaries and adnexa against the opposite hand.

Obesity or tense abdominal muscles may prevent the examiner from locating the ovaries. If palpable, the ovaries are about 1¾ inches (4 cm), are ovoid, feel firm and smooth, and may feel somewhat tender. Uterine tubes are

not usually palpable. In the premenopausal woman, ovarian cysts may be painful and recurrent. An ovarian cyst smaller than 2 inches (5 cm) in diameter is usually functional and responds to hormonal influence. Cysts larger than 2⅜ inches (6 cm) in diameter are possible neoplasms. Any palpable structure in the adnexa of postmenopausal women suggests cancer; 3 to 5 years after menopause, the ovaries are normally atrophied and not palpable.

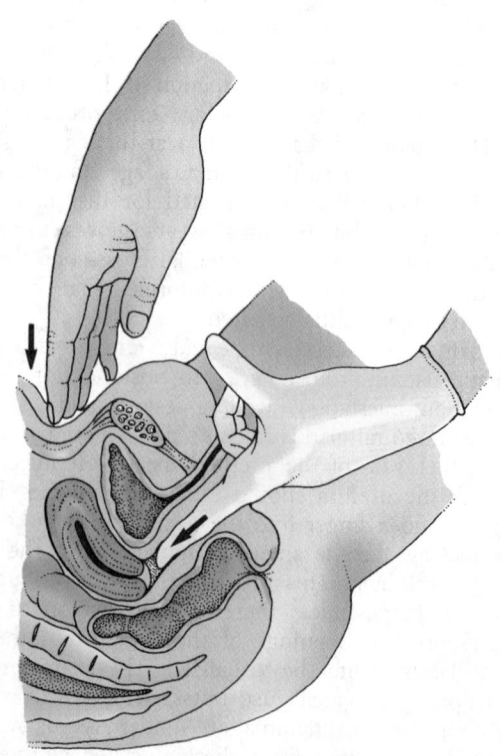

Figure 76–7. Technique of bimanual pelvic examination.

Rectovaginal Examination

A rectovaginal and rectal examination is the last segment of the pelvic examination. The examiner relubricates the glove and places the middle finger in the rectum and the index finger in the vagina. Insertion of the rectal finger is facilitated if the client strains and relaxes the anal sphincter. The procedure for the bimanual examination is repeated. The posterior vaginal and uterine walls are palpated through the rectal mucosa. This examination is especially helpful in assessing a retroflexed or retroverted uterus. The examiner can assess the tissue structure between the vagina and the rectum by palpating between the two fingers. The examiner is careful to avoid cross-contamination between the rectum and the vagina. The examiner's finger is slowly removed from the rectum, and any fecal material that remains on the glove may be tested for occult blood.

After the pelvic examination, the foot of the examining table is raised. The client's feet are lowered from the stirrups at the same time to reduce strain on the perineal muscles and the lumbosacral ligaments. Nurses should be aware that some clients experience orthostatic (postural) hypotension if they sit up too quickly. The nurse evaluates the client for signs of dizziness before letting her get off the examining table. The nurse provides appropriate supplies, such as perineal wipes and perineal napkins or minipads. The nurse allows the client privacy for dressing and is available to answer questions and provide support.

Assessment of the Male Reproductive System

Unless a male client seeks health care for a genital tract problem, inspection and palpation of the male genitalia and rectum may not be performed during routine physical examinations. Male clients are often embarrassed and anxious when the reproductive system is assessed. The concern may be compounded when the examiner is a woman. The client may be concerned about discomfort, the developmental stage of his genitalia, or the likelihood of an erection during the examination. If the client does have an erection, the examiner should assure him that this is a normal response to a tactile stimulus and should continue the examination.

The examination of the male genitalia provides an excellent opportunity to teach the client about contraceptives, testicular self-examination, and the need for regular prostate gland examinations. Testicular cancer is one of the most common cancers in young men and can be treated effectively if it is found early. Prostate cancer is common in older men, and the prognosis is favorable if it is diagnosed early. Annual rectal and prostate gland examinations are recommended for men older than 40 years, although there is debate about the overall effectiveness of this practice for detecting localized disease.

The examiner wears gloves to protect against possible infection. The examination room should offer the client privacy and a comfortable temperature. Proper light sources are mandatory for the inspection. The client undresses completely but should be given a gown to wear because the genitalia and buttocks need to be exposed. As with examinations of other body systems, the examiner explains each step of the assessment procedure before performing it. The client needs to be reassured that if he perceives pain during the examination, the examiner will stop and change the assessment plan or technique. Relaxation techniques and support during the examination can increase the client's tolerance of minimal discomfort.

Examination of the External Genitalia

The client may be in a lying or a standing position for the inspection and palpation of the external genitalia. The examiner is seated on a chair in front of the client. A general observation is made of the secondary sex characteristics. The examiner notes the age appropriateness of the developmental stage, including the distribution pattern of the pubic hair, the descent and size of the testes, and the size of the scrotum and the penis. Pubic hair is inspected for the presence of lice or scabies.

The examiner inspects the skin of the penis for intactness; the dorsal vein should be apparent. Any lesions or ulcers on the penis are noted, and a specimen may be scraped for cytologic study. If the client has not been circumcised, he is asked to retract the foreskin. This should be accomplished easily unless the client has phimosis (a tight prepuce that cannot be retracted). The examiner inspects the glans penis for possible inflammation, fungal infection, syphilitic chancres, and carcinomas. Smegma, a white, cheesy secretion from the sebaceous glands in the glans, may accumulate under the prepuce. This secretion is not present in the circumcised male. The glans is also inspected for the placement of the urinary meatus. Positions other than at the distal end of the glans are abnormal. By compressing the glans between the thumb and index finger, the examiner separates the meatus and can determine whether any discharge is present. Urethral discharge is not normal, and a specimen should be obtained for culture. The foreskin is replaced if it has been retracted. The body of the penis is palpated between the examiner's thumb and first two fingers; the examiner notes tenderness, hard areas under the skin, and signs of inflammation.

Inspection of the scrotum and inguinal areas is best accomplished by having the client hold the penis up and to the side. The examiner documents the shape and contour of the scrotum. Normally, the left side of the scrotum is lower than the right because the left testicle has a longer spermatic cord. Both anterior and posterior surfaces of the scrotum are inspected for lesions, nodules, pain, and edema. Swelling of the scrotum may indicate a hydrocele (an accumulation of serous fluid in the scrotal sac), infection, or torsion (twisting) of the spermatic cord.

Palpation of the scrotum, testes, epididymis, and spermatic cords is best accomplished in a warm environment so that the scrotum hangs low and relaxed. The examiner holds the scrotum gently between the thumb and two fingers. A comparison is made of the contents of each side of the scrotal sac. The examiner locates and examines each testis for size, shape, symmetry, tenderness, nodules, and consistency.

The normal testis has smooth borders, is somewhat sensitive to light palpation, and feels rubbery. The nurse or the examiner should teach self-examination of the testes (see Chap. 79) and encourage men to perform it monthly. The epididymis can be palpated on the posterior surface of the testis. It is examined for size, shape, and tenderness. In clients with infection of the epididymis, its outline is indistinguishable from that of the testis. The examiner palpates the spermatic cord along its length between the epididymis and the superficial inguinal ring; nodules and swelling are noted and further evaluated. Varicose veins of the spermatic cord (varicocele) feel like a "bag of worms" above the testis. If any swelling of the scrotum is observed, the swollen area should be transilluminated. The examining room needs to be darkened for this procedure, and the examiner directs the beam from the penlight through the scrotal swelling from the posterior surface of the scrotum. The light transmits a red glow if the swelling contains a serous fluid. Blood and solid tissue do not transmit the light.

The inner thigh is stroked with a blunt instrument such as the handle of the reflex hammer to elicit the cremasteric reflex. If the reflex is intact, the testicle and scrotum should rise on the stroked side.

Examination for Inguinal Hernia

For palpation for inguinal hernias, the client stands in front of the examiner. The examiner uses the right index finger to examine the client's right side and the left index finger to examine the left side. To provide sufficient mobility of the examining finger, the examiner places his or her fingertip low on the scrotal sac and directs the loose skin of the sac toward the inguinal canal. The slit-like opening of the external inguinal ring is located by following the direction of the spermatic cord. If possible, the examiner gently introduces the finger into the canal, asks the client to cough or bear down, and is alert for a tapping or pushing sensation against the finger.

Examination of the Rectum and Prostate

The final assessment of the male reproductive system includes an examination of the rectum and the prostate gland. Ambulatory clients are best examined by having them stand and lean over the examining table. The man is asked to turn his feet inward to relax his buttocks and to provide better accessibility to the anus during the examination. If a client cannot tolerate this position, he can be directed to lie on his side with his top leg flexed. If a pelvic mass is suspected, a lithotomy position permits a bimanual examination.

Proper lighting is necessary for visualization of the anus and surrounding tissue. The examiner notes any lesions, ulcerations, masses, or fissures.

To assess the prostate gland, the examiner presses the pad of a well-lubricated, gloved index finger against the anus. The finger is slowly inserted, as the sphincter relaxes, in the direction of the umbilicus and is rotated to palpate the anterior rectal wall. The posterior surface of the prostate gland is felt extending less than ⅜ inch (1 cm) into the rectum. The client is informed that he may feel an urge to urinate as the prostate is being examined but that he will not do so. The examiner notes the size of the lateral prostate lobes and their contour, consistency, and mobility. The prostate should feel firm (the consistency has been equated to that of a pencil eraser), smooth, and slightly mobile. It should be nontender across its diameter.

The examiner extends the finger further to attempt to palpate the seminal vesicles, which are palpable only if they are inflamed. If any discharge is secreted from the penis during palpation of the prostate gland and the seminal vesicles, specimens are obtained for culture and microscopic examination. The examining finger is withdrawn, and any fecal material may be tested for occult blood.

PSYCHOSOCIAL ASSESSMENT

The psychosocial assessment may suggest some contributory factors to the client's illness. During the social history, the nurse asks about the client's sources of support, strengths, and likely reactions to illness or dysfunction.

Events in a client's personal history and a client's beliefs may negatively influence the ability to enjoy a satisfactory sexual life. These factors may include

- Sexual trauma or abuse inflicted during childhood or adulthood
- Punishment or reproach for masturbation
- Psychological trauma
- Descriptions of reproductive organs or functions as "dirty"
- Cultural influences, such as the idea of female passivity during intercourse

Fears may affect the client's satisfaction with sexuality or body image. The client may also be concerned about potential or actual reaction of family members to reproductive health problems. (See Chapter 11 on psychosocial assessment and techniques regarding sexuality.)

DIAGNOSTIC ASSESSMENT
Laboratory Tests
Papanicolaou Test

The Papanicolaou test, or Pap smear, is a cytologic study that is effective in detecting precancerous and cancerous cells from the cervix. Health care providers vary in their recommendations for the frequency of routine Pap tests. Many clinicians suggest that the test be performed annually during routine physical examinations. Women in high-risk groups may be advised to have semiannual examinations. The American Cancer Society (ACS) advises all asymptomatic women older than 20 years and younger than 20 years who are sexually active to have a Pap test at least every 3 years after they have had two negative test results 1 year apart (ACS, 1997).

Cytologic examinations can also detect viral, fungal, and parasitic disorders. Examination of cells from the vaginal walls can evaluate the function of steroid hormones.

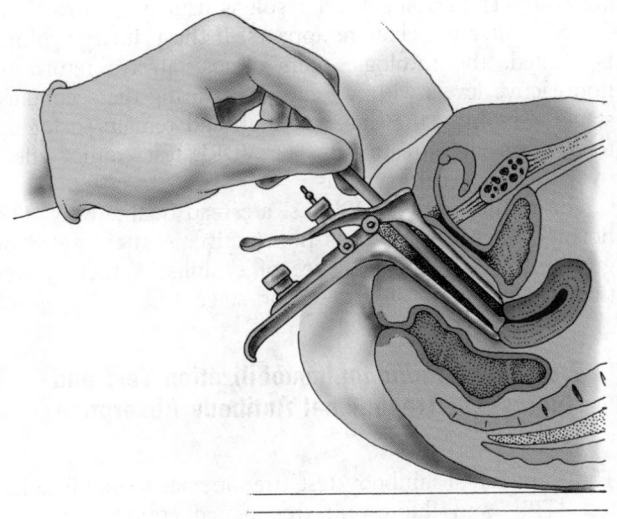
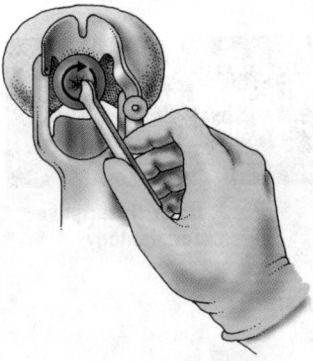
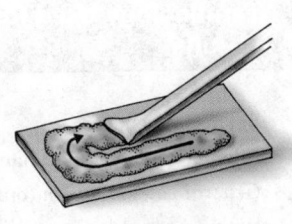

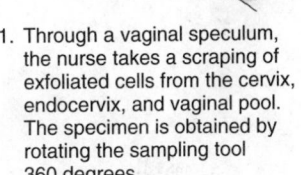

1. Through a vaginal speculum, the nurse takes a scraping of exfoliated cells from the cervix, endocervix, and vaginal pool. The specimen is obtained by rotating the sampling tool 360 degrees.

2. The nurse immediately transfers the specimens to a glass slide and applies a fixative solution.

Figure 76–8. Procedure for obtaining a cervical smear (Pap test).

CLIENT PREPARATION. The Pap test should be scheduled between the client's menstrual periods so that the menstrual flow does not interfere with the test interpretation. The woman should not douche, use vaginal medications or deodorants, or have sexual intercourse for at least 24 hours before the test.

The nurse assists the woman into the lithotomy position. Relaxation techniques, including concentration on breathing patterns or a visual focal point, may be valuable for the apprehensive client. All steps of the examination are explained to the client before they are performed.

PROCEDURE. The examiner first inserts a speculum into the vagina. For the conventional Pap smear, the cervix is visualized and then scraped with one of the various sampling tools available, such as a cytology brush, cotton-tipped applicator, endocervical aspirator, or wooden or plastic spatula.

The examiner takes one sample from the endocervical canal and a second from the ectocervical and squamocolumnar junction (Fig. 76–8). Both specimens are immediately transferred to glass slides and are either sprayed with or immersed in a fixative solution. If the smear is allowed to dry on the slide before the fixative is applied, diagnosis will be inaccurate. The slides are sent to a laboratory, where they are interpreted.

A new method to improve the quality of the sample has been approved by the Food and Drug Administration. Using the new technique, called the ThinPrep Pap Test, the health care provider rinses the cells into a vial filled with a solution that preserves them. The vial is then sent to the laboratory where an automated instrument gently separates the cells from blood and mucus. The thinner layer of cells can then be better visualized under a microscope, which improves the accuracy of the test.

Table 76–1 gives the descriptive terminology currently preferred by clinicians for Pap test results.

FOLLOW-UP CARE. The nurse can provide the client with a perineal pad after the procedure to protect her clothes from any bleeding from the cervix. The results of the test are shared with the client in person, by telephone, or by letter. If a woman's smear has demonstrated atypical cells, she is encouraged to have follow-up testing.

Blood Studies
Pituitary Gonadotropin

Determinations of the quantitative levels of follicle-stimulating hormone (FSH), luteinizing hormone (LH), and prolactin are helpful in the diagnosis of male and female reproductive tract disorders. The serum levels are measured by the radioimmunoassay method. No dietary restrictions are necessary before the test. Chart 76–5 gives the normal values and the significance of abnormal findings.

Steroid Hormones

The radioimmunoassay technique can detect estrogen, progesterone, and testosterone levels at any given time in the menstrual cycle for women and for adult men.

Serologic Tests

Serologic blood studies detect antigen-antibody reactions that occur in response to foreign organisms. This form of diagnostic testing is of benefit only after an infection has become well established. Serologic testing can be used in the evaluation of exposure to organisms causing syphilis and rubella and to herpes simplex virus type 2 (HSV2). Results may be read as nonreactive, weakly reactive, or reactive. A single titer is not as revealing as serial titers, which can detect the rise in antibody reactions as the body continues to fight the intruder.

VDRL Test

The VDRL (Venereal Disease Research Laboratory) test is used to detect, confirm, and monitor cases of syphilis.

TABLE 76-1

Selected Categories from the 1991 Bethesda System Compared with Descriptive Terminology Used for Papanicolaou Test Results	
Bethesda System	**Other Descriptive Terminology**
Adequacy of the specimen	
General categorization (optional)	
Within normal limits	Class I
Benign cellular changes (see Descriptive diagnosis)	
Epithelial cell abnormality (see Descriptive diagnosis)	
Descriptive diagnoses	
Benign cell changes	Class II
Infection (fungal, bacterial viral [CMV, HSV])	
Reactive changes	
Inflammation, radiation effects, intrauterine contraceptive device, atrophic vaginitis	
Epithelial cell abnormalities	
Squamous cell	
Atypical cells	
Squamous intraepithelial lesion (SIL)	
Low grade: HPV, mild dysplasia	Class III, CIN I
High grade: moderate to severe dysplasia	Class III to IV CIS, CIN II, CIN III
Squamous cell carcinoma: invasive	Class V
Glandular cell	
Endometrial: benign in menopausal woman	
Atypical	
Adenocarcinoma	
Hormonal evaluation for vaginal smears	

CMV = cytomegalovirus; HSV = herpes simplex virus; HPV = human papillomavirus.

This nontreponemal antigen test is not absolutely specific or sensitive for syphilis, but it is economical and highly diagnostic. Some acute and chronic conditions that cause false-positive results are

- Tuberculosis
- Infectious mononucleosis
- Recent smallpox vaccination
- Rheumatoid arthritis
- Systemic lupus erythematosus
- Subacute bacterial endocarditis
- Hepatitis

The results of a test vary with the stage of syphilis. During the first week after a chancre appears, the test result is usually negative because the body has not had enough time to produce a sufficiently elevated amount of antibody. The serologic test result is usually positive 1 to 3 weeks after the chancre appears. If the primary syphilis is treated, the serologic titers almost always return to nonreactive levels within 6 months. During the secondary stage of syphilis, the titers are high and remain so for up to 2 years after treatment. The VDRL test cannot effectively detect tertiary syphilis.

The results of the VDRL test are read qualitatively. The normal range is classed as nonreactive. A titer of 1:8 or greater indicates the presence of syphilis. A titer greater than 1:32 can indicate the second stage.

Treponema Pallidum Immobilization Test and Fluorescent Treponemal Antibody Absorption Test

The treponemal antibody test (treponemal immobilization test [TPI]; and fluorescent treponemal antibody absorption test [FTA-ABS]) are specific to *Treponema pallidum*; however, it is more expensive and time consuming than the VDRL test. Samples are usually sent to special laboratories for analysis. This test yields few false-positive results. It is used to confirm or rule out the diagnosis of syphilis after a positive VDRL test result. The test results may remain positive long after treatment.

Urinalysis for Steroid Hormones

The health care provider may order 24-hour urine samples for levels of total estrogens and pregnanediol (a urinary byproduct of progesterone).

Microscopic Studies
Wet Preparation (Wet Smears)

The examiner can obtain secretions from the vaginal pool at the beginning of a speculum examination. Specimens can also be obtained from the vaginal walls, labia, or vulva during the examination. The specimens are placed on glass slides and are treated with a wet preparation such as saline and potassium hydroxide (KOH). The slides are examined under a microscope to confirm or rule out the presence of a pathogen. Table 76-2 presents the common types of wet preparations used to diagnose selected vaginal problems.

Cultures

Cultures identify pathogenic organisms and are used to determine the appropriate antibiotic therapy. The examiner obtains specimens for culture analysis from any discharge or orifice of the male or female reproductive system. When a nonspecific bacterial infection is suspected, the health care provider orders routine bacteriologic cultures and antibiotic sensitivity studies.

The culture to detect *Neisseria gonorrhoeae* is one of the most important in evaluating the reproductive system. The culture is the only means of confirming the diagnosis of gonorrhea in asymptomatic women. Specimens from male clients can be taken directly from any penile discharge. Additional specimens from males or females can

Chart 76–5

Laboratory Profile: Reproductive Assessment

Test	Normal Range for Adults	Significance of Abnormal Findings
Serum Studies		
Follicle-stimulating hormone (FSH) (Follitropin)	• Men: 1.42–15.4 mIU/mL* • Women: follicular phase, 1.37–9.9 mIU/mL; midcycle, 6.17–17.2 mIU/mL; luteal phase, 1.09–9.2 mIU/mL; postmenopause, 19.3–100.6 mIU/mL	• Decreased levels indicate possible infertility, anorexia nervosa, neoplasm • Elevations indicate possible Turner's syndrome
Luteinizing hormone (LH) (Lutropin)	• Men: 1.24–7.8 mIU/mL • Women: follicular phase, 1.68–15 mIU/mL; midcycle, 21.9–56.6 mIU/mL; luteal phase, 0.61–16.3 mIU/mL; postmenopause, 14.2–52.3 mIU/mL	• Decrease levels indicate possible infertility, anovulation • Elevations indicate possible ovarian failure, Turner's syndrome
Prolactin	• Men: 3.0–14.7 ng†/mL • Women: 3.8–23.2 ng/mL	• Elevations indicate possible galactorrhea (breast discharge), pituitary tumor, disease of hypothalamus or pituitary gland, hypothyroidism
Estradiol	• Men: 10–50 pg/mL • Women: follicular phase, 20–350 pg/mL; midcycle, 150–750 pg/mL; luteal phase, 30–450 pg/mL; postmenopause, ≤20 pg/mL	• Elevations of estradiol, total estrogens, and estroil in men indicate possible gynecomastia, decreased body hair, increased fat deposits, feminization
Total estrogens	• Men: 20–80 pg/mL • Women: follicular phase, 60–200 pg/mL; luteal phase, 160–400 pg/mL; postmenopause, <130 pg/mL	• Elevations of estradiol, total estrogens, and estriol in women indicate possible uterine cancer, precocious puberty, cystic breast disease, corpus luteum cysts
Estroil	• Men and nonpregnant women: < 2.0 ng/dL	• Decreased levels of estradiol, total estrogens, and estriol in women indicate possible amenorrhea, climacteric, impending abortion, hypothalamic disorders
Progesterone	• Men: 13–97 ng/mL • Women: follicular phase, 15–70 ng/mL; luteal phase 200–2500 ng/mL	• Decreased levels in women indicate possible inadequate luteal phase, amenorrhea • Elevations in women indicate possible ovarian luteal cysts
Testosterone	• Men: 66–417 ng/dL • Women: 0.6–5.0 ng/dL	• Decreased levels in men indicate possible hypogonadism, Klinefelter's syndrome, hypopituitarism, orchidectomy • Elevations in women indicate possible adrenal neoplasm, polycystic ovaries, ovarian tumors
Urine Studies		
Total estrogens	• Men: 4–23 μg/24 hr • Women: follicular phase, 7–65 μg/24 hr; luteal phase, 8–135 μg/g/24 hr; postmenopause 0–10 μg/24 hr	• Elevations indicate possible testicular tumors, adrenal tumors, ovarian tumors, pregnancy • Decreased levels indicate possible ovarian dysfunction, intrauterine death, menopause
Pregnanediol	• Men: 0.4–2.5 mg/24 hr • Women: follicular phase, 0.1–1.8 mg/24 hr; luteal phase 0.9–2.2 mg/24 hr	• Elevations indicate possible luteal ovarian cysts, ovarian neoplasms, adrenal disorders • Decreased levels indicate possible amenorrhea
17-Ketosteroids	• Men (20–50 yr): 10–25 mg/24 hr • Women (20–50 yr): 6–14 mg/24 hr • Values decrease with age	• Elevations indicate possible Cushing's syndrome, increased androgen or cortisol production, severe stress • Decreased levels indicate possible Addison's disease, hypopituitarism

*mIU/mL = IU/L.
†1 ng = 1 billionth of a gram.

TABLE 76-2

Wet Preparations Used for the Diagnosis of Common Vaginal Problems

Wet Preparation	Problems
Normal saline	• Cervicitis • Trichomoniasis • Bacterial vaginosis
Potassium hydroxide (KOH)	• Candidiasis (*Candidia albicans Monilia*) • Bacterial vaginosis
Gram's stain	• *Haemophilus* vaginitis
Tzanck's test	• Herpes simplex virus (HSV) type 2 infection

also be obtained from the urethra, the rectum, and the oropharynx. The swab is then placed in a culture tube and sent to the laboratory for incubation and analysis.

Cultures to detect *Chlamydia trachomatis* use antigen detection methods. These include a direct immunofluorescent test, a 30-minute test appropriate for screening low-risk populations, and an enzyme-linked immunosorbent assay (ELISA) for high-risk populations (Edge & Miller, 1994).

Radiographic Assessment
General X-Ray Studies

A kidney, ureter, and bladder (KUB) study is an x-ray of the abdomen that shows these structures and is used in the assessment of either male or female reproductive system disorders. Pelvic masses, calcified tumors or fibroids, dermoid cysts, and metastatic bone changes may be evident. Urologic studies may enhance the film by the use of contrast media. No specific client preparation is needed.

Bone scans, intravenous (IV) pyelograms, barium enema studies, and chest films are also included in the work-up of the client with suspected metastatic cancer. They help to determine the extent of the metastasis and obstruction or displacement of the organs. (These tests are discussed elsewhere in this text.)

Computed Tomography

Computed tomography (CT) scans for reproductive system disorders primarily involve the abdomen and the pelvis. They can detect and evaluate masses and lymphatic enlargement from metastasis. This scan can differentiate solid tissue masses from cystic or hemorrhagic structures.

Hysterosalpingography

A hysterosalpingogram is an x-ray of the cervix, uterus, and fallopian tubes that is done after the injection of a contrast medium. This test is used in infertility work-ups to evaluate tubal anatomy and patency and uterine abnormalities, such as fibroids, tumors, and fistulas. The study

can also provide data about the cause of repeated abortions, dysmenorrhea, and postmenopausal bleeding. The study should not be attempted for at least 6 weeks after abortion, delivery, or dilation and curettage. Other contraindications include reproductive tract infection and severe systemic illness. There is a significant incidence of false-positive and false-negative interpretations.

CLIENT PREPARATION. The examination should be scheduled in a radiology department 2 to 5 days after the end of the client's normal menses. The scheduling is important to prevent the accidental flushing of a fertilized ovum from the fallopian tube or the exposure of a fetus to radiation.

The client prepares herself by taking a cathartic the evening before the test, followed by an enema on the morning of the examination, to reduce distortion of the x-rays by gas shadows.

On the day of the examination, the date of the client's last menstrual period is confirmed and recorded in the medical record. The client signs a consent form for the procedure. Because discomfort is anticipated during the examination, she may be premedicated with analgesics or nonsteroidal anti-inflammatory agents. She should be informed that she may experience some nausea and vomiting, abdominal cramping, or faintness. The nurse provides support and assistance with relaxation techniques.

PROCEDURE. The client is placed in the lithotomy position. The health care provider visualizes the cervix through a speculum. The radiologist injects radiopaque oil or water-soluble dye through the cervix to fill and highlight the interior of the cervix, uterus, and fallopian tubes. If the fallopian tubes are patent, the contrast material spills into the peritoneal cavity. Usually, only two or three films are taken to show the path and distribution of the contrast medium.

FOLLOW-UP CARE. The client may experience pelvic pain after the study and should receive medications accordingly. She may also experience referred shoulder pain because of irritation of the phrenic nerve caused by the dye. The nurse provides a perineal pad after the test to prevent the soiling of clothes from dye draining from the cervix. The nurse advises the woman to contact her health care provider if bloody discharge continues for 4 days or longer and to report any signs of infection, such as lower quadrant pain, fever, malodorous discharge, and tachycardia.

Mammography

Mammography is an x-ray of the soft tissue of the breast. Mammograms assess differences in the density of the breast tissue. They are especially helpful in the evaluation of poorly defined masses, multiple masses or nodules, nipple changes or discharge, skin changes, and pain.

Mammography can detect many cancers that are not palpable by physical examination; however, some actual cancers are shown as benign by mammography.

In young women's breasts, there is little difference in

density between normal glandular tissue and malignant tumors, which makes the mammogram less useful for the discovery and diagnosis of breast masses in these women. In older women, the percentage of fatty tissue is higher and the fatty tissue appears lighter than neoplasms. Cancer and cysts may have the same density. However, cysts usually have smooth borders, and neoplasms often have starburst-shaped margins.

CLIENT PREPARATION. No dietary restrictions are necessary before the mammogram. The woman is asked not to use creams, powders, or deodorant on the breasts or underarm areas before the study because aluminum chlorhydrate can mimic calcium clusters. If there is any possibility that the client is pregnant, the test should be rescheduled. The purpose of the examination and its anticipated discomforts should be explained (see Research Applications for Nursing). Adequate privacy for the client to undress above the waist and a cover gown are provided. The client also needs appropriate support and may need time to express her concerns about the mammogram and the presence of any lumps. Because this is a time when the client is anxious about the health of her breasts, it is an excellent opportunity to teach or reinforce the importance of self-examination of the breasts.

PROCEDURE. The technician positions the client next to the x-ray machine with one breast exposed. A film plate and the platform of the machine are placed on opposite sides of the breast to be examined. The technician includes as much breast tissue as possible between the plates. The woman may experience some temporary discomfort when the breast is compressed during the positioning and the test. The test takes approximately 15 minutes; however, the client is usually asked to wait until the films are developed in case a view needs to be repeated. Mammography usually necessitates two low-dose x-ray views of each breast: a view from the side and a view from above each breast.

FOLLOW-UP CARE. The woman should know when to expect the report if results are not communicated at the time of the mammogram. She should be assessed for her knowledge of breast self-examination and given instructions if needed.

Other Diagnostic Tests
Ultrasonography

Ultrasonography is a nonradiographic diagnostic technique that is routinely used for assessing reproductive problems such as uterine fibroids, ovarian cysts, and pelvic masses. It can be used to locate intrauterine devices and to monitor the progress of tumor regression after medical treatment. Ultrasonography is also useful in differentiating solid tumors from cysts in breast examinations (Edge & Miller, 1994).

No specific preparations are necessary for this study. The client should have a full bladder to enable visualization of the uterus and to make the location of other

> ## Research Applications for Nursing
>
> ### Pain Measurement Tools May Need Revision for Mammography Studies
>
> *Baskin-Smith, J., Miaskowski, C., Dibble, S., Weekes, D., & Nielsen, B. (1995). Perceptions of the mammography experience. Cancer Nursing, 18(1), 47–52.*
>
> Early detection of breast cancer is possible with mammography screening, but only 15% to 20% of women older than 50 years have had a screening mammography. Many reasons have been given: fear of pain has been identified.
>
> This descriptive study used an open-ended interview method to sample 272 women about their mammography experiences and whether pain was a deterrent to having the procedure. Most women (37.8%) described the procedure as one without pain or discomfort or as one of pressure (24.1%). About 23% reported some pain or discomfort.
>
> *Critique.* This qualitative research used a fairly large sample size to obtain valid responses from women who actually experienced mammography. Reaction to this diagnostic test has not been studied.
>
> *Possible Nursing Implications.* This study reported that women have very different sensations during a mammography. Nurses should not assume everyone will feel the same thing. Women need to know that the procedure may be painful and should be instructed in ways to cope with the pain, such as relaxation and breathing exercises. The researchers suggest that better pain assessment tools are needed, particularly ones that use a qualitative analytic approach to measurement, because descriptive rating scales may not accurately measure the pain intensity felt by individuals.

structures more distinct with abdominal ultrasonography but not for transvaginal scans.

For an abdominal scan, the technician exposes the client's abdomen and applies oil or gel to the area to be scanned. These substances provide better transmission of the sound waves from the transducer through the client's skin. The transducer is moved in a linear pattern across the abdomen to outline and define soft-tissue masses and to differentiate tumor types, ascites, and encapsulated fluid.

For a transvaginal scan, the transducer is covered with a condom or vinyl glove into which transmission gel has been placed and then inserted in the vagina. The client is often interested in the oscilloscope screen and appreciates a brief explanation of the landmarks and structures visualized. There is no special follow-up care for the client after this procedure except to provide wipes to remove the gel.

Magnetic Resonance Imagery

Magnetic resonance imagery (MRI) uses a magnetic field and radiofrequency energy to scan for pelvic tumors. This scan effectively distinguishes between normal and malignant tissues. MRI is also being investigated for use in the diagnosis of breast cancer (Schneider, 1995).

Endoscopic Studies

Colposcopy

The colposcope allows three-dimensional magnification and intense illumination of epithelium with suspected disease. Colposcopy is suited for inspection of the cervical epithelium, the vagina, and the vulvar epithelium. This procedure can locate the exact site of precancerous and malignant lesions for biopsy. It is an effective tool to screen women at high risk for vaginal changes because of diethylstilbestrol (DES) exposure (Edge & Miller, 1994).

CLIENT PREPARATION. The woman is placed in the lithotomy position and provided the same support as for a pelvic examination. The client should not have douched or used vaginal preparations for 24 to 48 hours before the examination. The relatively painless procedure is usually better tolerated if it is explained in advance and if the instrument is shown to the client (Nugent & Clark, 1996).

Because this procedure provides accurate site selection for tissue biopsy, the client should also be prepared for this test. Materials necessary for cytologic studies and biopsy should be readily available.

PROCEDURE. The physician locates the cervix, or vaginal site, through a speculum examination. Lubricants other than water should not be used. Cells in the area may be stained or left unstained to enhance visualization. The physician cleans the cervix of secretions and moistens the cervix with normal saline. This allows vascular patterns and the junction between the columnar epithelium and the squamous epithelium to be better visualized. Acetic acid, 3%, applied to the cervix acts as a mucolytic agent to draw moisture from the tissue and to accentuate important morphologic features. The physician then uses a colposcope or colpomicroscope to inspect the area in question. A biopsy also may be taken if abnormal cells are seen (see discussion on cervical biopsy).

FOLLOW-UP CARE. The nurse assists the woman after the procedure as for a pelvic examination and provides supplies to clean the perineum. The nurse also gives the client a perineal pad to absorb any dye or discharge. If procedures other than direct visualization were done, follow-up care needs to be revised appropriately.

Laparoscopy

Laparoscopy is a highly accurate diagnostic tool for exploring the pelvic cavity. This procedure can rule out ectopic pregnancy, evaluate ovarian disorders and pelvic masses, and aid in the diagnosis of infertility and unexplained pelvic pain. Laparoscopy is also used during surgical procedures such as

- Tubal sterilization
- Ovarian biopsy
- Cyst or graafian follicle aspiration (to retrieve ova for in vitro fertilization)
- Lysis of adhesions around the fallopian tubes
- Retrieval of "lost" intrauterine devices

The laparoscopy is preferable to laparotomy for minor surgical procedures because it necessitates only a small infraumbilical incision, involves less discomfort, and does not require hospitalization.

CLIENT PREPARATION. The physician explains the procedure, risks (complications associated with the use of general anesthesia, postoperative shoulder pain, and the rare occurrence of infection or electric burns), and anticipated discomforts. The procedure can be performed with regional or general anesthesia. Clients should expect mild discomfort from the incision site and may experience referred shoulder pain from phrenic nerve irritation (Lowdermilk, 1995c).

PROCEDURE. The client is anesthetized and is placed in the lithotomy position. A urinary catheter is inserted to drain the bladder. The operating table is placed in a slight Trendelenburg position to cause the intestines to fall away from the pelvis. The cervix is held with a cannula to allow movement of the uterus during laparoscopy (Fig. 76–9). The surgeon inserts a needle below the umbilicus to infuse carbon dioxide into the pelvic cavity, which distends the abdomen and permits better visualization of the organs. The surgeon inserts a trocar and a cannula into an infraumbilical incision. After the trocar and the cannula are in place in the abdominal cavity, the surgeon removes the trocar and inserts the laparoscope. The surgeon can thus visualize the pelvic cavity and the reproductive organs. Further instrumentation is possible through a second small incision. The laparoscope is removed at the end of the procedure, and the abdomen is deflated. The physician usually closes the incision with absorbable sutures and dresses the area with an adhesive bandage.

FOLLOW-UP CARE. The client requires postoperative care similar to that for other clients after general anesthe-

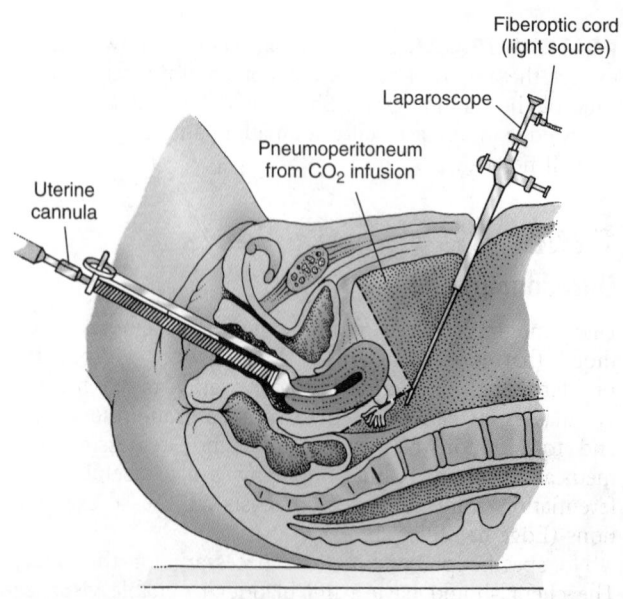

Figure 76–9. Laparoscopy.

sia but is usually discharged on the day of the surgery. The discomfort from the incision is usually alleviated by the administration of oral analgesics. The greatest discomfort is due to referred shoulder pain caused by residual gas in the peritoneal cavity. Most of these sensations disappear within 48 hours. Clients are instructed to change their own dressing and to observe the wound for signs of infection or hematoma. They should be advised to shower, not bathe in a tub, until the umbilical incision has healed. The client should avoid strenuous activity for the first week after the procedure, but ambulation helps to eliminate the gas.

Hysteroscopy

Hysteroscopy is an endoscopic examination that permits visualization of the interior of the uterus and the cervical canal. The hysteroscope includes a lens with fiberoptic lighting; an aqueous solution of carbon dioxide is the medium to distend the uterus. Hysteroscopy can be used for the removal of intrauterine devices and as a complement to other diagnostic tests for infertility and unexplained bleeding.

CLIENT PREPARATION. The surgeon informs the client of all aspects of the procedure. The client receives the same preparation as for a pelvic examination. The procedure is best performed 5 days after menses have ceased to eliminate the possibility of pregnancy. The client is placed in the lithotomy position and is anesthetized with a pericervical or other regional block.

PROCEDURE. After the client is anesthetized, the cervix is dilated. The physician inserts the hysteroscope through the cervix. Because a medium distends the uterus, cells can be pushed through the fallopian tubes and into the pelvic cavity. Hysteroscopy is contraindicated in clients with suspected cervical or endometrial cancer, in clients with infection of the upper reproductive tract, and in pregnant clients.

FOLLOW-UP CARE. Care is the same as that after a pelvic examination. If the client experiences cervical and uterine cramping, the nurse administers analgesics as ordered. Shoulder pain may be present for up to 24 hours if carbon dioxide was used to distend the uterus during the procedure.

Biopsy Studies
Cervical Biopsy

In a cervical biopsy, cervical tissue is removed for additional cytologic study. A biopsy is definitely indicated in a client with an identifiable cervical lesion, regardless of the cytologic findings. The physician usually performs a biopsy in conjunction with colposcopy as a follow-up to a suggestive Pap test finding. The procedure may be done in the physician's office.

The type and extent of the biopsy vary. If a lesion is clearly visible with the use of a colposcope, a punch biopsy may be used to extract a small column of tissue.

Cervical tissue specimens should include a portion of the squamocolumnar epithelial junction because most cervical malignancies occur in this area. Punch biopsy can be done as an office procedure without the use of anesthesia because the cervix has few pain receptors. When no lesions are visible or when the Pap smear results indicate malignancy, an inverted cone biopsy (conization) of the cervix is advised.

CLIENT PREPARATION. The client should be scheduled for the biopsy in the early proliferative phase of the menstrual cycle, when the cervix is least vascular. The procedure that is selected should be explained to the client. Because a biopsy evaluates potentially malignant cells, most women become anxious and need time to discuss their feelings and fears. The use of relaxation techniques may facilitate the woman's comfort. The nurse places the client in the lithotomy position and prepares the client in the same way as for a pelvic examination. Further preparation depends on the type of procedure to be performed.

PROCEDURE. The physician may anesthetize the client according to the needs of the chosen procedure. The physician visualizes the cervix and obtains the tissue sample by needle punch or conization (removal of a cone-shaped tissue specimen with a cold knife scalpel). All specimens are immediately placed into a formalin solution. Cauterization of the biopsy site with a silver nitrate stick usually is sufficient to control light bleeding from the punch biopsy site.

FOLLOW-UP CARE. The type of anesthesia that was used for the procedure determines the type of immediate postoperative care provided by the nurse. Discharge instructions are listed in Chart 76–6.

Endometrial Biopsy and Aspiration

Both endometrial biopsy and aspiration are used to obtain cells directly from the lining of the uterus in women at

---

Chart 76–6

Education Guide: The Client Recovering from Cervical Biopsy

- Do not lift any heavy objects until the site is healed (about 2 weeks).
- Rest for 24 hr after the procedure.
- Leave the postoperative packing in place for 8 to 24 hr or as directed.
- Report any excessive bleeding (more than that of a normal menstrual period) to your health care provider.
- Report signs of infection to your health care provider.
- Do not douche, use tampons, or have vaginal intercourse until the site is healed (about 2 weeks).
- Keep the perineum clean and dry by using antiseptic solution rinses (as directed by your health care provider) and frequently changing pads.

risk for cancer of the endometrium. Endometrial biopsy is also valuable for the assessment of functional menstrual disturbances (especially anovulatory bleeding) and infertility (corpus luteum dysfunction).

When menstrual disturbances are being evaluated, the biopsy is generally done in the immediate premenstrual period to serve as an index of progesterone influence and ovulation. A biopsy done in the second half of the menstrual cycle (approximately days 21 and 22) evaluates corpus luteum function and the presence or absence of a persistent secretory endometrium. Postmenopausal women may have biopsies done at any time.

CLIENT PREPARATION. Menstrual data are obtained from the client and included on the specimen slip for the pathologist. The client is given the same preparation as for a pelvic examination. The nurse advises the client that she may experience some cramping when the cervix is dilated. Analgesia before the procedure and relaxation and breathing techniques during the procedure are often of value.

PROCEDURE. An endometrial biopsy is often done as an office procedure with or without anesthesia. After the uterus is sounded (measured) and the cervix sufficiently dilated, the physician inserts the curette or intrauterine cannula into the uterus. The physician withdraws a portion of the endometrium either with the cup-like end of the curette or with suction aspiration equipment. The client experiences moderate cramping. The specimen is used to evaluate the proliferative or secretory condition of the endometrial cells and to diagnose carcinoma. Women with symptoms suggestive of endometrial cancer need a diagnostic curettage for accurate diagnosis (Edge & Miller, 1994).

FOLLOW-UP CARE. The client is allowed to rest on the examining table until cramping has subsided. A wipe to clean the perineum and a perineal pad are provided. Spotting may be present for 1 to 2 days, but any signs of infection or excessive bleeding should be reported to the physician. The client is informed to refrain from intercourse or douching until all discharge has ceased. Results of the biopsy are usually available within 72 hours.

Breast Biopsy and Aspiration

Figure 76–10 shows three types of breast biopsy:

- Incisional biopsy
- Excisional biopsy
- Aspiration biopsy

An incisional biopsy is the surgical removal of tissue from a breast mass. An excisional biopsy removes the mass itself for histologic evaluation. Aspiration biopsy is the removal of fluid or tissue from the breast mass through a large-bore needle.

Any breast mass needs to be evaluated further for the possibility of cancer. Fibrocystic lesions, as well as fibroadenomas and intraductal papillomas, can be differentiated by biopsy. Any discharge from the breasts is examined histologically.

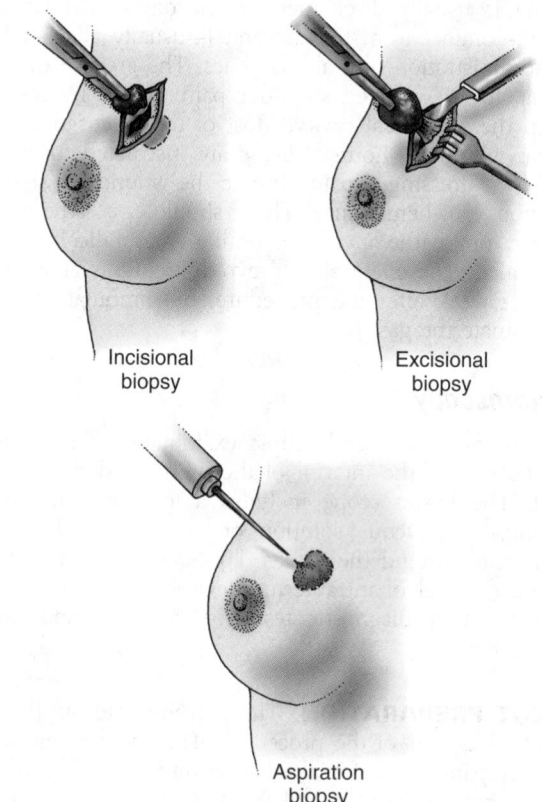

Figure 76–10. Breast biopsy techniques.

Incisional biopsy

Excisional biopsy

Aspiration biopsy

CLIENT PREPARATION. The instructions to the client depend on the type of biopsy and the type of anesthesia. The woman is prepared to expect sensations of pulling or probing during the procedure.

PROCEDURE. Aspiration biopsy is often performed in an outpatient setting without anesthesia. The mass is located by palpation of the breast. The surgeon then directs the needle into the lump and aspirates the contents into the syringe. The contents are placed on a slide for Pap evaluation. Fluid from benign cysts may appear clear to dark green-brown; bloody fluid suggests cancer. If no fluid is aspirated, the tumor should be examined by incisional biopsy.

Incisional or excisional biopsies are typically performed as same-day procedures with local or general anesthesia. The tumor specimen is evaluated by the frozen section technique. If cancer is found, the physician sends the tissue to the laboratory for estrogen receptor analysis.

FOLLOW-UP CARE. Postoperative discomfort is usually mild and is controlled with analgesic administration or use of a heating pad. The client is taught how to assess the incisional site for bleeding and edema. A properly supportive bra should be worn continuously by the woman for 1 week postoperatively. The woman should avoid cold temperatures to prevent nipple contractions that can cause stress on the incision. Numbness around the biopsy site may last 2 to 3 months. The woman should also be assessed about her knowledge of breast self-examination and given instructions if needed. If malignancy is identified, the woman will need emotional support as well as information about follow-up treatment alternatives.

Needle Biopsy of the Prostate

The physician performs a needle aspiration biopsy of the prostate gland to retrieve cells for histologic study when prostate cancer is suspected. The procedure is often done at the same time as cystoscopy, with the client under anesthesia. The physician can perform needle biopsies without anesthesia or with the client under local anesthesia.

CLIENT PREPARATION. Preparation for the procedure depends on the technique to be used to puncture the gland. The nurse provides data on the expected discomforts. The nurse can also teach breathing and relaxation techniques to be used during the examination. Because the purpose of this procedure is to evaluate prostate cells for potential malignancy, the man needs support and time to discuss his fears. Preparation for a transrectal biopsy involves the use of cleansing enemas and the administration of prophylactic antibiotics to reduce the risk of bacterial contamination of the bloodstream or prostate tissue. Local anesthesia is used at the site of transperineal biopsy.

PROCEDURE. The nurse places the client in the same position as for a rectal examination. After the physician injects local anesthetic for the transperineal biopsy, he or she places a finger in the rectum to help guide the needle to the prostate. For the transrectal biopsy, the physician places the needle against the examining finger and then inserts it into the rectum to the prostate. From this site, the needle is advanced through the rectal mucosa and into the prostate gland. The aspiration may be repeated several times to obtain a satisfactory specimen.

FOLLOW-UP CARE. Sepsis is a potentially life-threatening complication of transrectal biopsy. Any signs of infection or septic shock must be reported immediately. The nurse also instructs the man to complete the prophylactic antibiotic regimen.

SELECTED BIBLIOGRAPHY

American Cancer Society. (1997). *Cancer facts and figures 1997.* New York: Author.

*Barkauskas, V., Stoletenberg-Allen, K., Baumann, L., & Darling-Fisher, C. (1994). *Health and physical assessment.* St. Louis: C. V. Mosby.

Baskin-Smith, J., Miaskowski, C., Dibble, S., Weekes, D., & Nielsen, B. (1995). Perceptions of the mammography experience. *Cancer Nursing, 18*(1), 47–52.

*Cook, M. (1994). Nursing assessment for the older woman. RN, 57(9), 40–43.

*Edge, V., & Miller, M. (1994). *Women's health care.* St. Louis: C. V. Mosby.

Fogel, C., & Woods, N. (1995). *Women's health care: A comprehensive handbook.* Thousand Oaks, CA: Sage.

Garrett, C. (1995). Anatomy and physiology of reproduction. In I. Bobak, D. Lowdermilk, & M. Jenson (Eds.), *Maternity nursing* (4th ed., pp. 25–55). St. Louis: C. V. Mosby.

*Geissler, E. (1994). *Pocket guide to cultural assessment.* St. Louis: C. V. Mosby.

*Germain, M., Heaton, R., Erickson, D., Henry, M., Nash, J., & O'Connor, D. (1994). A comparison of the most common Papanicolaou smear collection techniques. *Obstetrics & Gynecology, 84,* 168–173.

Jones, H. (1995). Impact of the Bethesda system. *Cancer, 76,* 1914–1918.

Lowdermilk, D. (1995a). Common reproductive concerns. In I. Bobak, D. Lowdermilk, & M. Jenson (Eds.), *Maternity nursing* (4th ed., pp. 857–895). St. Louis: C. V. Mosby.

Lowdermilk, D. (1995b). Preventive health care for mid-life women, *Capsules and Comments in Perinatal and Women's Health Nursing, 1*(1), 25–34.

Lowdermilk, D. (1995c). Reproductive surgery. In C. Fogel & N. Woods (Eds.), *Women's health care: A comprehensive handbook* (pp. 629–650). Thousand Oaks, CA: Sage.

*Lu, X. (1994). Variables associated with breast self-examination among Chinese women. *Cancer Nursing, 18*(1), 29–34.

*Mettlin, C., & Smart, D. (1994). Breast cancer detection guidelines for women ages 40 to 49 years: Rationale for the American Cancer Society reaffirmation of recommendations. *CA: A Cancer Journal for Clinicians, 44,* 248–255.

Nugent, L., & Clark, R. (1996). Colposcopy: Sensory information for client education. *Journal of Obstetric, Gynecologic, and Neonatal Nursing, 25*(3), 225–231.

Pagana, K., & Pagana, T. (1997). *Diagnostic testing and nursing implications: A case study approach* (3rd ed.). St. Louis: C. V. Mosby.

Quinn, E., & Lowdermilk, D. (1995). Health promotion and screening. In I. Bobak, D. Lowdermilk, & M. Jenson (Eds.), *Maternity nursing* (4th ed., pp. 839–855). St. Louis: C. V. Mosby.

Schneider, D. (1995). Changing the image: Looking to MRI for diagnosing breast cancer. *Scientific American, 272*(4), 42.

Seidel, H. M., Ball, J. W., Dains, J. E., & Benedict, G. W. (1995). *Mosby's guide to physical examination* (3rd ed.). St. Louis: Mosby Year Book.

Shepherd, J., & Fried, R. (1995). Preventing cervical cancer: The role of the Bethesda system. *American Family Physician, 5*(2), 434–437.

Tomaino-Brunner, C., Freda, M. C., & Runowicz, C. D. (1996). "I hope I don't have cancer": Colposcopy and minority women. *Oncology Nursing Forum, 23*(1), 39–44.

*U.S. Department of Health and Human Services, Public Health Service. (1994). *Clinician's handbook of preventive medicine.* Washington, DC: U.S. Government Printing.

*Youngkin, E., & Davis, M. (1994). *Women's health: A primary care clinical guide.* Norwalk, CT: Appleton & Lange.

SUGGESTED READINGS

*Cook, M. (1994). Nursing assessment for the older woman. RN, 57(9), 40–43.

This article provides an overview of interview questions and techniques that a nurse can use to elicit a sexual history in an older woman. Factors that may affect the older woman's interest in sexuality, including physiologic aging and drug effects, are also discussed.

*Lu, X. (1994). Variables associated with breast self-examination among Chinese women. *Cancer Nursing, 18*(1), 29–34.

The largest number of Asians in the United States are Chinese. This article describes self-reported information about the attitudes of a group of Chinese women on breast self-examination. Considerations about the cultural impact on health promotion behaviors such as breast self-examination are addressed.

Tomaino-Brunner, C., Freda, M. C., & Runowicz, C. D. (1996). "I hope I don't have cancer": Colposcopy and minority women. *Oncology Nursing Forum, 23*(1), 39–44.

The results of this research study on determining what women know about colposcopy and their concerns about the test suggest that women need more information before the scheduled test. The article describes nursing implications for educating women about colposcopy and reducing anxiety about the test.

Chapter 77

INTERVENTIONS FOR CLIENTS
WITH BREAST DISORDERS

Breast disorders most frequently affect women. The most common sign and symptom associated with breast disorders is a palpable mass. The discovery of a mass in a woman's breast, whether it is discovered by the woman herself or her health care provider, is a frightening experience. Even if the woman is aware that 90% of all breast lumps are benign, she may fear that the lump is cancerous. This fearful reaction accompanies the woman through the period of diagnosis, decision-making, and treatment. Whether the disease is benign or malignant, the nurse must be aware of the physiologic and emotional factors involved to be effective in nursing care.

SCREENING FOR BREAST MASSES

The American Cancer Society (ACS) and the National Cancer Institute (NCI) have established guidelines for breast cancer screening. Not all cancer agencies support the ACS guidelines, but most, including the Canadian Task Force on the Periodic Health Examination, recom-mend a baseline screening mammogram before the age of 50 years and yearly screening for women over 50. Studies have shown that screening programs can reduce breast cancer deaths by as much as one third in women 50 years and older (Stewart & Carbone, 1994a). However, it is estimated that only 15% to 20% of women 50 years or older have had a screening mammogram (Baskin-Smith et al., 1995).

Nurses have conducted studies to determine what influences mammogram compliance and how compliance rates can be improved (Champion, 1995). Barriers to mammography may include fear of radiation, fear of results, concern about pain, and knowledge deficit. Compliance with mammogram guidelines has been significantly associated with health care provider recommendations for mammography (Champion, 1995).

Other factors influencing whether women have screening mammograms include accessibility and cost. Not all health insurers pay for mammography. A number of state and federal programs that target low-income women are available in many areas of the United States.

In addition to screening mammography, the ACS recommends monthly breast self-examination beginning at age 20 years and clinical breast examination by a health care provider every year for women over 40 years. Nurses need to be familiar with the ACS guidelines as they teach health promotion to their clients in a variety of settings.

Breast Self-Examination

The goal of screening for breast cancer is *early detection*. Detection of breast cancer before the cancer has spread to the axillary nodes increases the chance of survival. Breast self-examination (BSE), used in conjunction with mammography and clinical breast examination (CBE), is extremely effective in detecting early breast cancer and reducing mortality rates. BSE *alone* as a screening technique has not been of value. The ACS recommends that all women older than age 20 years practice BSE monthly. Although most women have heard of BSE, fewer than 33% practice it regularly (Baron & Walsh, 1995). The best methods for teaching BSE and increasing the number of women who perform it on a regular basis are being researched by nurses.

Whether the client seeks health care because she has found a breast lump, because she needs a routine physical examination, or because she has an unrelated health problem, the nurse's encounter with her provides an excellent opportunity to teach BSE. It is erroneous to assume that most women who practice BSE do so competently and regularly. Most women prefer this type of individualized instruction to learning from pamphlets and magazines. Women who are taught by a health care provider on an individual or group basis practice BSE more often, more proficiently, and more confidently.

ELDERLY CONSIDERATIONS

Elderly clients may be more resistant to practicing BSE if they have yearly CBE performed by their health care provider. Health teaching to promote compliance and competence in BSE is extremely important in this high risk group.

TRANSCULTURAL CONSIDERATIONS

One of the national health objectives for the year 2000 is the prevention of cancer in minority ethnic populations. Little research has been done on the variables associated with BSE in minority women. Research results from one study population of Chinese-American women indicated that only 15% of these women practiced BSE monthly, and 48% reported never having done BSE. Although the majority of these women recognized the efficacy of BSE, perceived competency in BSE was the variable that most influenced whether they regularly performed BSE (Lu, 1995). In a similar study of African-American women, findings showed that 63% practiced BSE monthly, and 76% had yearly CBE; however, only 20% had a mammogram according to age-related guidelines (Phillips & Wilbur, 1995). Culturally sensitive strategies need to be utilized to increase breast cancer awareness and screening practices (Brown & Williams, 1994).

Preparation for Teaching Breast Self-Examination

Before teaching breast self-examination (BSE), the nurse assesses the psychological factors influencing the client's motivation to practice BSE. Lack of knowledge about the technique is one reason that women fail to perform BSE regularly. Another reason for failure to do BSE is that many women are not aware of the benefits of early detection. The nurse stresses that treatment for breast cancer is more successful the earlier the disease is found. It is also important that the client develop confidence in her ability to detect breast changes. The nurse emphasizes to the client that a yearly breast examination by a health care provider cannot substitute for BSE. BSE, clinical breast examinations (CBE) by a health care provider, and screening mammography combined can promote early detection of breast cancer.

BSE detects—but does nothing to prevent—breast cancer. Therefore, the asymptomatic woman, when choosing whether to practice BSE, may think, "What's the use? It won't keep me from getting breast cancer." Again, the nurse can emphasize the advantages of early detection in terms of outcome and help the client to review risk factors to determine her risk of developing breast cancer. Women must believe that there are benefits and that the barriers to practicing BSE are minimal. Addressing these issues will increase the client's knowledge and practice of BSE.

The nurse discusses the client's fears, beliefs, and concerns about breast disease and BSE with her. The nurse assesses for the presence of risk factors for breast cancer and a history of previous breast problems (Table 77–1). Proper timing for BSE is also discussed. Premenopausal women should examine their breasts 1 week after the menstrual period. At this time, hormonal influence on breast tissue is minimal so that fluid retention and tenderness are reduced. For these same reasons, the best time of the month to schedule a mammogram is also 1 week after the menstrual period. In addition to being able to state the need for monthly BSE, the client should be able to discuss the need for a yearly CBE and the mammogram recommendations appropriate for her age.

ELDERLY CONSIDERATIONS

Postmenopausal women or women who have had a hysterectomy and no longer menstruate should pick a day each month when they will do BSE, such as the first day of the month.

Teaching Breast Self-Examination

The setting in which BSE is demonstrated should be private and, because little clothing is worn, warm. The nurse asks the woman to undress from the waist up and provides a gown and sheet. Before teaching the technique of breast palpation, the nurse assesses the client's technique by asking her to demonstrate her own method. If the woman is unsure or has not performed BSE before, the nurse can slowly lead her through the examination while explaining the rationale for the techniques and answering

TABLE 77–1

Risk Factors for Breast Cancer

Factor	Degree of Risk	Comments
Female gender	• Increased	• 99% of all breast cancers occur in women and 1% in men.
History of a previous breast cancer	• Increased	• The risk of developing a cancer in the opposite breast is five times greater than for the average population at risk.
Age >40 yr	• Increased	• Incidence increases with age and peaks in the fifth decade.
Menstrual history Early menarche or late menopause or both	• Increased	• The risk of breast cancer rises as the interval between menarche and menopause increases; shortening the interval by castration reduces the risk, especially if performed in women younger than age 35 yrs.
Reproductive history Nulliparity First child born after age 30 yr	• Increased	• Childless women have an increased risk as do women who bear their first child near or after age 30 yr.
Family history Mother or sister or both	• Increased	• Risk increases two to three times if a mother or sister has had breast cancer and is further increased if the relative was diagnosed during the premenopausal state and if the cancer was bilateral.
Diet	• Controversial	• Animal data and descriptive epidemiology of breast cancer incidence strongly suggest an association of dietary factors, specifically a high-fat diet, with an increased risk of breast cancer. The National Academy of Science recommends decreasing total fat intake to 30% of available calories.
Alcohol	• Unknown	• A suggested small increase in risk with moderate alcohol consumption has been reported, although limitations in methodology have been cited, and results require confirmation.
Obesity	• Controversial	• Weight, height, obesity, and increased body mass have been reported to be associated with an increased risk of breast cancer.
Ionizing radiation	• Increased	• Three groups of women who received low-level radiation exposure demonstrated an increased breast cancer risk, which was particularly notable if the exposure occurred in the early years (<30 yr).
Benign breast disease	• None	• Fibrocystic breast disease is not associated with breast cancer. However, biopsy-proven atypical hyperplasia is associated with an increased risk.
Oral contraceptives	• None	• There is no evidence yet to suggest a causal relationship between oral contraceptives and incidence of and survival from breast cancer.
Exogenous hormones	• Controversial	• Several studies report no link with replacement hormones and breast cancer, and those that do appear to identify only subsets of patients at risk: those who have taken replacement estrogens for more than 5 yr and those who have taken large cumulative doses.

Modified from McCorkle, R., Baird, S., and Grant, M. (1996). *Cancer nursing: A comprehensive approach.* Philadelphia: W. B. Saunders.

questions. It is also helpful for the nurse to point out different findings at this time, especially those that the client might perceive as abnormal. For example, nodular breast tissue may normally feel lumpy, which conjures up visions of widespread cancer in the unknowledgeable woman. Placing the client's hand directly on the involved area and showing her precisely what is normal for her can build self-confidence.

The nurse points out the inframammary ridge, the area of the breast where the skin folds under the breast. This thickened area may be perceived as a lump instead of a normal finding. In thin or small-breasted women, the ribs may be mistaken for masses. The nurse shows the client how to follow the rib to the sternum to be sure that it is bone and not breast tissue. The client is taught to stand in front of a mirror to inspect the breast for abnormalities. The client should raise her arms above her head and press her hands on her hips to emphasize any changes in the shape of the breasts. The breasts are examined in a lying position and while bathing or showering.

The nurse also demonstrates two other aspects of the examination: the amount of pressure needed and the correct position of the hands. The finger pads, which are more sensitive than the finger tips, are used when palpating the breasts. The finger pads should press firmly enough to detect the underlying tissue. However, the client should be instructed not to compress the tissue on the ribs, as this may falsely feel like a mass.

Use of teaching models of normal and abnormal breasts is helpful when teaching BSE. The nurse may need more time to teach the older woman about BSE because learning is often slowed by aging. The nurse demonstrates the difference in examining the breasts, especially in large-breasted women, with the arm overhead while lying down instead of having the arm by the side. Showing this difference reveals the advantage of using the correct method, which spreads the tissue over the chest wall for more effective palpation.

Clinical Breast Examination

Advanced practice nurses and physicians typically perform the clinical breast examination. However, if skilled in the technique of CBE, nurses in general practice can perform this examination. The examination can be done before, after, or during the teaching session. The same guidelines of providing a private and warm setting, maintaining dignity, and allowing time for discussion apply.

Taking a breast history is vital. Results may be recorded on a breast evaluation form, which is a part of the client's record (Fig. 77–1). This record helps the nurse establish the relative risk for breast disease and the need for follow-up diagnostic tests, such as mammograms, and teaching.

The physical assessment begins with inspection. The woman undresses from the waist up and first sits or stands with her hands by her sides. The examiner inspects the breasts for symmetry and size, contour, skin

CLIENT'S NAME ____________ Sex ______ Race ______ Age ______

Weight ______ Ideal Weight ______ Marital Status ______

HISTORY	Yes	No	Comments
Family history of breast cancer	____	____	________
Personal history of breast cancer	____	____	________
Previous mammograms	____	____	________
Previous biopsy (findings)	____	____	________
Nipple discharge	____	____	________
Hormone use (specify)	____	____	________
BSE Practice	____	____	________
High-fat diet	____	____	________
ETOH/smoking	____	____	________
Current medications (list)	____	____	________

Age at menses ______ Age at menopause ______

COMMENTS ______

PHYSICAL FINDINGS

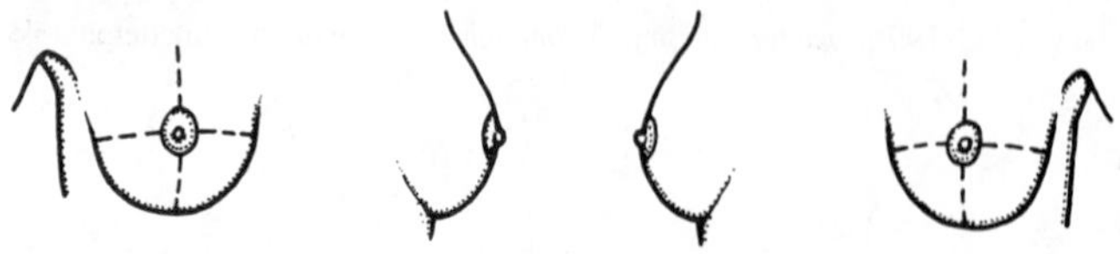

Mammogram Report ______

Biopsy/Cytology Results ______

BSE Return Demonstration ______

Plan ______

CLIENT EDUCATION ______

Figure 77–1. A breast evaluation form.

changes (color, texture, and venous patterns), nipple changes, and lesions.

One breast may be larger than the other, and inverted nipples are not uncommon. The nurse asks the client whether these findings are normal for her. Any change in symmetry may indicate a problem. Contour should be even, and the skin should have a smooth texture. Venous patterns may be visible but should be similar bilaterally. The nipples and areola should be equal or nearly equal in size and be a similar color. The nipples may be wrinkled or smooth, and Montgomery tubercles on the areola are normal. Supernumerary nipples (extra nipples), while rare, are also normal. If a mass is palpated, the examiner notes its position by visualizing the breast as a clock face and noting the "area of the clock" where the mass is located. If it is necessary to move the arms away from the body, the woman should rest her arm on the examiner's to prevent flexion of the underlying muscles. While the arms are by the side and relaxed, the axillae can be palpated. The examiner palpates the axilla and area above and below the clavicle for enlarged lymph nodes. The woman is then asked to raise her hands over her head, which exposes the sides and underneath portions of the breast for inspection. Finally, she is asked to place her hands on her hips and press, thus flexing the pectoral muscles. This action accentuates skin dimpling, retractions, or masses.

The remainder of the examination is done with the client lying supine. The examiner places a pillow or rolled sheet under the client's shoulder, and the arm on that side is raised above the head. Each breast is palpated separately while the other breast remains covered. If the woman has identified a problem in one breast, the other "normal" breast is examined first to establish a baseline for comparison.

To ensure complete coverage of the breast tissue, the examiner palpates in a vertical pattern, in a horizontal pattern, or in concentric circles, which covers every inch of the breast tissue including the tail of Spence, which extends from the upper outer quadrant of the breast into the axilla. Supraclavicular lymph nodes are palpated for the presence of enlarged nodes by hooking the fingers over the clavicle.

Finally, the nipple is gently compressed to detect the presence of a discharge. If a discharge is produced, the examiner notes the "area of the clock" where the breast was compressed when the discharge was released. If there is a history of discharge, the client may be able to express the discharge more successfully than the examiner can and may be asked to do so.

Discovery of a suspicious lesion or discharge during the examination requires consultation or referral to a health care provider who specializes in caring for breast disorders. Follow-up usually involves mammography and possibly ultrasound. If there is a dominant mass or a suspicious clinical picture, the woman should be referred for biopsy even if the mammogram is negative.

ELDERLY CONSIDERATIONS

As women age, the breast tissue becomes flattened and elongated, and it is suspended loosely from the chest wall. On palpation the breast tissue of the elderly woman will have a finer, more granular feel than the lobular feel in a younger woman. The inframammary ridge may be more prominent as a result of atrophy of the breast tissue. Breast examination in the elderly may be easier due to tissue atrophy and relaxation of the suspensory ligaments (Cooper's ligaments).

BENIGN BREAST DISORDERS

Most breast lumps are benign. Because the incidence of breast disease is related to age, breast disorders are described in an age-related order (Table 77–2).

Fibroadenoma

Fibroadenomas are the most common cause of breast masses during adolescence, although they may occur into the 30s. A fibroadenoma is a solid, benign mass of con-

TABLE 77–2

Typical Presentation of Benign Breast Disorders

Breast Disorder	Description	Incidence
Fibroadenoma	• Most common benign lesion; solid mass of connective tissue that is unattached to the surrounding tissue	• During teen-age years into the 30s
Fibrocystic breast disease (FBD)	• *First stage:* Characterized by premenstrual bilateral fullness and tenderness • *Second stage:* Presence of bilateral, multicentric nodules • *Third stage:* Presence of microscopic and macroscopic cysts	• Late teens and 20s
Ductal ectasia	• Hard, irregular mass or masses with nipple discharge, enlarged axillary nodes, redness, and edema; difficult to distinguish from cancer	• Women approaching menopause
Intraductal ectasia	• Mass in duct that results in nipple discharge; mass is usually not palpable	• Women aged 40–55 yr

nective tissue that is unattached to the surrounding breast tissue. It is usually discovered by the client herself. Although the immediate fear is that of breast cancer, fewer than 1% of these masses are malignant. The mass is usually round, firm, easily movable, nontender, and clearly delineated from the surrounding tissue.

Fibroadenomas are usually located in the upper outer quadrant of the breast; multiple masses may be present. The health care provider may order a breast ultrasound examination or may perform a needle aspiration to establish whether the lump is cystic or solid. If the lesion is solid, outpatient excision using local anesthesia is the treatment of choice.

TRANSCULTURAL CONSIDERATIONS

Fibroadenomas are most common in African-American women and tend to occur at an earlier age than in women of other ethnic backgrounds (Tierney et al., 1995).

Fibrocystic Breast Changes

Overview

Fibrocystic changes or physiologic nodularity of the breast, often referred to as *fibrocystic breast disease* (FBD), is the most common breast problem of women in their 20s. Approximately 90% of women will have fibrocystic changes sometime in their lifetime. Fibrocystic changes may proceed through several clinical stages or may present in only one form.

The first stage commonly occurs between the late teens and early 20s. Premenstrual bilateral fullness and tenderness are present, especially in the outer upper quadrant. Symptoms usually resolve after menstruation and then recur before the next menstrual period in a cyclic fashion.

The second stage usually occurs in the late 20s and throughout the 30s. Bilateral multicentric nodular areas that feel like small marbles can be felt and accompany the fullness and soreness.

The third stage generally occurs between the ages of 35 and 55 years. Microscopic or macroscopic cysts generally appear suddenly and are associated with pain, tenderness, or burning. They are usually three dimensional, smooth, mobile, and well delineated. Although the cysts may recede somewhat before menstruation, they do not disappear completely. Mammography is generally indicated, and fine needle aspiration may be performed. Biopsy is indicated if

- The aspirated fluid is bloody
- No fluid is aspirated
- The mammogram shows suspicious findings
- A mass remains palpable after aspiration
- The cytologic study of the aspirated fluid reveals malignant cells

Although the cause of fibrocystic breast changes is unknown, the condition seems to be related to normal fluctuations in estrogen levels during the menstrual cycle. Symptoms usually resolve after menopause in the absence of estrogen supplementation.

ELDERLY CONSIDERATIONS

 Elderly clients on hormone replacement therapy may develop painful, fluid-filled cysts.

Collaborative Management

Medical management of fibrocystic breast changes is generally symptomatic. Hormonal manipulation has been the primary means of pharmacologic intervention. Oral contraceptives can suppress oversecretion of estrogen, and progestins may be used to correct luteal insufficiency. Danazol (Danocrine, Cyclomen♥) suppresses ovarian function and estrogen stimulation of breast tissue. However, because hormonal therapy with danazol will not cure FBD and its side effects are undesirable, it is generally only used in clients with recurrent and unusually severe fibrocystic changes.

Medical management may also include the use of C, E, and B-complex vitamins. The health care provider may prescribe diuretics to decrease premenstrual breast engorgement. Clients are counseled to avoid the use of caffeine; however, the role of caffeine in FBD is controversial.

The nurse encourages the client to continue prescribed medical interventions and monitors the effectiveness of these interventions. The nurse suggests supportive measures, such as the use of mild analgesics or limiting salt intake before menses, to help decrease swelling. The nurse also recommends that the client wear (both day and night) a well-padded, supportive brassiere to decrease tension on ligaments. Local application of ice or heat can be suggested to provide temporary relief of pain. The nurse promotes the practice of BSE and teaches the procedure when necessary.

Ductal Ectasia

Ductal ectasia is a benign breast problem that is usually seen in women approaching menopause. The disease is caused by dilation and thickening of the collecting ducts in the subareolar area. These ducts become distended and filled with cellular debris, which activates an inflammatory response. Two clinical signs result from these changes:

- A mass develops that feels hard, has irregular borders, and may be tender.
- A greenish-brown nipple discharge, enlarged axillary nodes, and redness and edema over the site of the mass are noted.

These masses are often difficult to distinguish from breast cancer. Because the risk for breast cancer is increased in this age group, accurate diagnosis is vital. A microscopic examination of the nipple discharge is performed to detect any atypical or malignant cells, and the affected area is excised. Nursing care is directed at alleviating the anxiety associated with the threat of breast cancer and at supporting the woman through the diagnostic and treatment procedures.

Intraductal Papilloma

Intraductal papilloma, like ductal ectasia and breast cancer, occurs primarily in women aged 40 to 55 years. This benign process in the epithelial lining of the duct forms a papilloma, a pedunculated outgrowth of tissue. As the papilloma grows, it causes trauma and erosion within the duct and results in a serosanguineous or serous nipple discharge. A mass is rarely palpable.

Diagnosis is aimed first at ruling out breast cancer. Microscopic examination of the nipple discharge and surgical excision of the mass and ductal area are usually indicated.

Problems of the Large-Breasted Woman

Although Western society emphasizes the positive attributes of large breasts, women with excessive breast tissue experience difficulties and discomforts. For instance, because fashion is directed at the small-breasted figure, a woman with large breasts may have difficulty finding clothes that fit well and in which she feels attractive. The breast size may be disproportionate to the rest of the body, which adds to the problems of fitting clothes. Brassieres are expensive and may have to be specially ordered, and the straps create large dents in the shoulders. In addition, many large-breasted women experience fungal infections under the breasts because it is difficult to keep this area dry and exposed to air.

Backaches from the added weight are also common. The only alternative for this condition, if well-fitting brassieres do not help and obesity is not part of the problem, may be breast-reduction surgery. The surgeon removes excess breast tissue, repositions the nipple, and repositions the resultant skin flaps to produce the optimal cosmetic effect. This operation is a major surgical procedure and is termed a *reduction mammoplasty.*

The decision to undergo the procedure is usually made after years of living with the discomforts of excessive breast size. The nurse may be involved in the decision-making stage of listening to the client verbalize her feelings and by providing information as appropriate. The postoperative diagnoses and goals are consistent with those for the woman undergoing reconstructive surgery, discussed later in this chapter.

Gynecomastia

Gynecomastia literally means "female breasts" and is a symptom rather than a disease. It is a benign condition of breast enlargement in *men* (Fig. 77–2). However, gynecomastia can be a result of primary cancers such as lung cancer. The enlargement is usually bilateral, but enlargement is asymmetric in about 10% of cases. The condition is caused by proliferation of the glandular tissue, including the mammary ducts and ductal stroma. In many instances, it is difficult to distinguish gynecomastia from breast enlargement related to excess adipose tissue. Etiologic factors of gynecomastia include drugs; aging; obesity; underlying diseases causing estrogen excess, such as malnutrition, liver disease, or hyperthyroidism; and an-

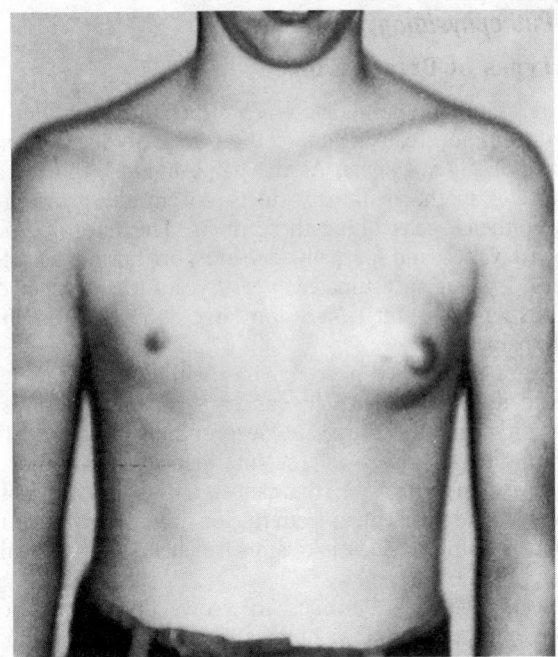

Figure 77–2. Gynecomastia. (From Bland, K. I., & Copeland, E. M. III [1991]. *The breast: Comprehensive management of benign and malignant diseases.* Philadelphia: W. B. Saunders.)

drogen deficiency states, such as age or chronic renal failure.

Although gynecomastia is not common, men with abnormal breast findings, especially a breast mass, are carefully evaluated for breast cancer.

Breast Cancer

Overview

Breast cancer is the second leading cause of breast masses. Because of the high incidence of the disease, almost every woman has had a close personal association with another woman having the disease. Thus, most women have strong reactions to the threat of breast cancer. These reactions greatly influence a woman's health habits, including breast self-examination (BSE) and her readiness to seek care when a suspicious area is discovered.

Until prevention becomes an option, early detection is the key to better treatment and survival. Statistics support the advantages of early detection and treatment. The most reliable indicator of prognosis is related to the stage of the breast cancer at the time of diagnosis. Localized breast cancer with no regional spread is associated with a clinical cure rate of 75% to 90%. If the woman has a small tumor with no evidence of axillary node involvement, the 5-year survival rate is 90%. The 5-year survival rate drops to 40% to 50% when the axillary lymph nodes are involved, with a 10-year survival rate of 25% (Tierney et al., 1995). Breast cancer is the second leading cause of cancer deaths among women in the United States. However, breast cancer is the leading cause of cancer deaths in the 35- to 54-year-old age group.

Pathophysiology

Types of Breast Cancer

There are many pathologic types of breast cancer, but the most common, causing more than 80% of cases, is *infiltrating ductal carcinoma*. As the name implies, the disease originates in the mammary ducts, specifically growing in the epithelial cells lining these ducts. The rate of cancer growth varies and partially depends on hormonal influences. It takes an estimated 5 to 9 years for a cancer cell to divide and result in a lesion large enough to be clinically palpable.

As long as the cancer remains within the duct, it is considered *noninvasive*. The cancer is classified as *invasive* when it penetrates the tissue surrounding the duct. Most breast cancers arise from the intermediate ducts and are invasive. Once invasive, the cancer grows into the tissue around it in an irregular pattern; for this reason, once the lesion is palpable, it is felt as an irregular, poorly defined mass.

As the tumor continues to grow, fibrosis develops around the cancer. This fibrosis may cause shortening of Cooper's ligaments and the resulting characteristic skin dimpling that is seen with more advanced disease.

Complications of Breast Cancer

The tumor also invades the lymphatic channels, blocking skin drainage and causing skin edema and an "orange-peel" appearance of the skin (*peau d'orange*). Invasion of the lymphatic channels carries tumor cells to the lymphatic nodes, including those in the axillary region. For this reason, pathologic examination of the axillary nodes is imperative for staging the disease. The tumor eventually replaces the skin itself, and ulceration of the overlying skin occurs. Metastases result from seeding of the cancer cells into the blood and lymph systems, which permits spread of these cells to distant sites. The most common sites of metastatic disease from breast cancer are bone, lungs, brain, and liver.

The course of metastatic breast cancer is related to the site affected and to the function impaired. (Chapter 26 further describes the pathophysiologic process of cancer.)

Breast Cancer in Men

About 1% of all cases of breast cancer occur in men. The average age of onset is 60 years. Men usually present with a hard, nonpainful, subareolar mass, and gynecomastia may be present. Occasionally the man may present with a nipple discharge, retraction, erosion, or ulceration. Although nipple discharge is not a common presenting symptom, about 75% of the men who present with nipple discharge are diagnosed with breast carcinoma. Breast cancer in men is staged the same as in women. However, the prognosis even for stage I breast cancer is worse for men. Five-year survival rates for stage I breast cancer in men are 58%, decreasing to 38% for stage II disease (Tierney et al., 1995). Breast cancer in men is frequently a disseminated disease, accounting for lower survival rates. Treatment of men with breast cancer parallels that of women at a similar stage of disease.

Etiology

There is no known etiologic agent for breast cancer. Breast cancer probably results from multiple factors.

Women with a familial history of breast cancer, particularly of a first-degree relative (mother, sister, or daughter) with premenopausal breast cancer, have a threefold risk increase. This risk is further increased if the relative had breast cancer bilaterally or before age 50 years. It is important to note that 90% of clients with breast cancer have no familial history. Seventy percent of women over the age of 50 who are diagnosed with breast cancer have no identifiable risk factor for the development of the disease other than age and gender (Shapiro & Clark, 1995). Efforts to utilize genes (*BRCA1, BRCA2, BRCA3*) that predispose women to the development of breast cancer are being investigated (Malone et al., 1998). Breast cancer, however, is not an exclusively inherited, genetic disease. Exposure to high-dose ionizing radiation (especially before the age of 20), early menarche (before age 12 years), and late menopause (after age 50) are associated with increased risk of breast cancer. A history of previous breast cancer, nulliparity, and first birth after age 30 years are also considered to heighten risk.

Questionable risk factors include a diet high in animal fats, a diet low in fiber, alcohol consumption, and long-term estrogen replacement therapy (Leslie, 1995). Studies have shown a small increase in risk of breast cancer in perimenopausal women on hormone replacement therapy (HRT) with 5 or more years of use. The risks must be weighed against the benefits of HRT. The benefits of HRT are decreased risk of heart disease and osteoporosis and the control of menopausal symptoms. Decisions related to use of HRT must be individualized based on the client's risk profile.

Obesity may be a factor associated with the development of breast cancer in postmenopausal women. Other genetic and environmental risk factors are listed in Table 77–1.

ELDERLY CONSIDERATIONS

Ɛ Being an older female is the single most major risk factor, although some women are at higher risk than others. As age increases, so does risk. More than 85% of clients are diagnosed after age 45 years.

Incidence/Prevalence

Each year an estimated 184,000 women and 1,400 men are diagnosed with breast cancer. Of these, approximately 46,000 women and 400 men die from breast cancer (Wingo et al., 1995). While these numbers are staggering, there is a trend toward earlier diagnosis of breast cancer. In 1993, 75% of newly diagnosed breast cancers were stage I or II; additionally, negative nodes were found in one-third of all breast cancers (Moore & Kinne, 1995). Breast cancer accounts for one in four cancers in women.

ELDERLY CONSIDERATIONS

Ɛ Breast cancer occurs most commonly in older adults, and its prevalence increases with age. The risk of developing breast cancer significantly increases as one ages. By age 85 years, each American woman faces a 1-in-9 risk of being diagnosed with breast cancer. One of every eight American women will develop breast cancer in her lifetime (Table 77–3).

TRANSCULTURAL CONSIDERATIONS

 Cancer remains a major public health problem for African-Americans despite decreases in mortality for specific cancers. Although the incidence of breast cancer is lower in African-Americans than in Caucasians, death rates are higher for African-American women at every stage of the disease. The 5-year survival rate for African-Americans is 62% compared with 79% for Caucasians (Allen & Phillips, 1997). Research suggests that poverty, less education, and inadequate access to screening are related to higher cancer morbidity and mortality rates in African-Americans (Wingo et al., 1996).

Like the African-American female population, Latino and Hispanic women have a lower incidence of breast cancer than Caucasians, but have a higher death rate. The differences in survival rates reflect the stage at which the cancer is diagnosed. Breast cancer is the most common cancer among Asian and Pacific Island women; the death rates are higher for Hawaiian women than for all other ethnic groups (Allen & Phillips, 1997).

Collaborative Management

◆ Assessment

➤ History

The initial history may be taken after a mass has been discovered but before definitive diagnosis has been made, or the history may be obtained at the time the woman is seen for treatment of an identified cancer. The history should focus on three major areas: risk factors, history of the breast mass, and health maintenance practices.

TABLE 77–3

Age-Related Risk for Breast Cancer	
Age	**Breast Cancer Risk**
25	1 in 19,608
30	1 in 2,525
35	1 in 622
40	1 in 217
45	1 in 93
50	1 in 50
55	1 in 33
60	1 in 24
65	1 in 17
70	1 in 14
75	1 in 11
80	1 in 10
85	1 in 11
In a lifetime	1 in 8

Source: National Cancer Institute.

Risk Factors. The nurse records age, sex, marital status, weight, and height. Marital status and identification of the client's primary support person provide information about those to be included in the woman's care, teaching, and support. The nurse obtains specific information on personal and family histories of breast cancer. In addition to increasing her own risk, these factors also affect any sister's or daughter's risk and should be incorporated into later counseling.

The hormonal history includes
- Age at menarche
- Age at menopause
- Symptoms of menopause
- Age at first child's birth
- Number of children

It is believed that prolonged hormonal stimulation (e.g., early menses and/or late menopause) increases a woman's risk, as do birth of the first child after age 30 years and nulliparity.

History of the Breast Mass. The second area of assessment focuses on the history of the breast mass. The history reveals not only the course of the disease but also data related to health care–seeking practices and health-promoting behaviors.

Knowledge of how, when, and by whom the mass was discovered and of the interval between discovery and seeking care is crucial. If the woman found the mass, was it discovered through breast self-examination (BSE) or by accident? The answer to this question might alert the nurse to the need for discussion and teaching about BSE regardless of whether the mass proves to be malignant. What was the time interval between discovery and seeing the health care provider? If there was a delay, what caused it? These questions are linked to the psychosocial assessment but also reveal the length of time that the tumor has been present. The nurse notes procedures directed at diagnosing this problem and others in the past. Finally, a review of systems focusing on the most common areas for metastases is made.

Health Maintenance Practices. The third area of assessment includes health maintenance practices. In addition to questioning the client about the knowledge, practice, and regularity of BSE, the nurse takes a mammographic history. The existence of previous mammograms allows the health care provider to compare current with past mammograms and to facilitate diagnosis.

A brief diet history, in which the client is asked to recall a typical day's menu and alcoholic intake per week, reveals the usual intake of fat and alcohol. A high alcohol and fat intake *may* increase the risk of breast cancer.

The nurse asks the client what types of medications she uses, specifically, hormonal supplements. The nurse recalls that estrogen can be administered orally, intravaginally, and via a transdermal patch. The nurse documents the type and form of hormones (birth control pills, supplements) and length of use.

ELDERLY CONSIDERATIONS

Postmenopausal use of estrogen creams intravaginally is not uncommon and should be considered a major source of estrogen.

Chart 77–1

Nursing Care Highlight: Assessment of a Breast Mass

- Identify the location of the mass by the "face of the clock" method.
- Describe the shape, size, and consistency of the mass.
- Assess whether the mass is fixed or movable.
- Note any skin changes around the mass, such as dimpling, *peau d'orange,* increased vascularity, nipple retraction, and ulceration.
- Assess the adjacent lymph nodes, both axillary and supraclavicular nodes.
- Ask the client if she experiences pain or soreness in the area around the mass.

➤ *Physical Assessment/Clinical Manifestations*

The approach to physical assessment has been discussed earlier under Breast Self-Examination and Clinical Breast Examination. The nurse notes specific information about the breast mass (Chart 77–1). The mass is described in the chart in terms of location (using the "face of the clock" method), shape, size, consistency, and fixation to the surrounding tissues.

Any skin change, such as dimpling, *peau d'orange,* increased vascularity, nipple retraction, or ulceration, can indicate advanced disease and needs to be documented. The nurse examines the axillary and supraclavicular areas thoroughly by palpating deeply for enlarged lymph nodes and noting their presence and location in the client's record. The presence of pain or soreness in the affected breast is evaluated. After gathering this information, the nurse draws a diagram on the chart (see Fig. 77–1) that will be helpful for others involved in the client's care.

➤ *Psychosocial Assessment*

The client with potential or diagnosed breast cancer faces three major issues: the fear of cancer; threats to body image, sexuality, intimate relationships, and survival; and decisional conflict related to treatment options.

The woman will need information about how advanced the disease is, likelihood of cure, treatment options and side effects, how treatment will affect her life and self-image, how her family will be affected, and home self-care (Luker et al., 1996). A woman's previous experience with cancer, and especially with other women with breast cancer, influences her reactions to the disease. The nurse asks the client whether she has known anyone with breast cancer and what types of experiences she has had with breast disease and cancer in general. The nurse explores the woman's feelings about the disease because her choices of treatment, her recovery, and her ability to learn are greatly influenced by these emotions. The client's and family's knowledge of breast cancer, stage of disease, and treatment options are assessed. Education level is a significant influencing factor in the client's treatment choices for stage I breast cancer (Graling & Grant, 1995). The client's perception of her situation is often influenced by

outdated information. Perhaps she knew someone who had a Halsted radical mastectomy 30 years ago and associates breast surgery with the chest deformity and lymphedema experienced by that woman. Dispelling misconceptions by providing current information can affect her attitude in a positive way.

The nurse also assesses the client with breast cancer for problems related to sexuality. Three critical areas of distress contribute to the psychosexual morbidity of these clients: psychological, physiologic, and relational. The nurse inquires about frequency of and satisfaction with sexual relations between the client and her partner. The client is asked whether and how the breast cancer has changed the intimate relations, sexual function, or types of touch by the partner. Women who have experienced changes in the areas outlined in Table 77–4 should be referred for counseling.

The need for additional resources is also evaluated at this time. Will extra psychological counseling be needed? Are there financial concerns that need to be discussed with social services? Will her spouse, family, or friends support her throughout this period? How much support

---

TABLE 77–4

Distress Contributing to Psychosexual Morbidity in Breast Cancer

Psychological Distress
- The client may have ineffective strategies for coping with breast cancer.
- Self-esteem may be decreased by the disease.
- The client may suffer changes in body image.
- The client may need to re-evaluate her psychological "investment" in the possibility of conception.

Physiologic Distress
- Physiologic distress varies, depending on the stage of the disease.
- The client may experience pain and other sensations.
- The disease may impose physical limitations on the client.
- Treatment-related complications may cause physiologic distress.

Relational Distress
- Depending on whether the client is single or has a partner, the disease affects relationships differently.
- The stability of the woman's intimate relationships and the degree of support provided by those close to her have a great impact on the effect of the disease on relationships.
- The client's history of sexual satisfaction does much to determine her degree of relational distress after a diagnosis of breast cancer.
- Relational distress also depends in part on the client's flexibility toward different types of sexual expression.

Factors That Indicate a Need for Counseling
- The woman has no committed partner.
- The client is unhappy in her relationships.
- The client wants to bear children after the diagnosis of cancer.
- There is a history of sexual or marital abuse.

and teaching do they need? When does the client expect to hear about her pathology results, and whom would she like to be with her when she hears the results? Answers to these types of questions provide guidelines in establishing expected outcomes and in planning nursing care.

➤ Laboratory Assessment

The diagnosis of breast cancer relies primarily on pathologic examination of tissue from the breast mass. Serum-based laboratory tests are not used routinely to aid in this diagnosis; however, radioimmunoassay (RIA) is being used in research to detect and monitor breast cancer. Studies to identify breast cancer tumor markers are currently being conducted. One possible breast cancer tumor marker is 5-hydroxymethyl-2′-deoxyuridine (Djuric et al., 1996).

After the presence of cancer is established, laboratory tests, including pathologic examination of the lymph nodes, help detect possible metastases. Elevated liver enzyme levels indicate possible liver metastases, and increased serum calcium and alkaline phosphatase levels suggest bone metastases.

➤ Radiographic Assessment

Mammography is the most sensitive tool for screening for breast cancer. However, it must be combined with BSE for optimal early detection and with clinical breast examination (CBE) for full interpretation of the findings. These three methods together are effective in detecting breast cancer as early as possible. The uniqueness of mammography results from its ability to reveal preclinical lesions, masses too small to be palpated manually. (Client preparation and the procedure for mammography are discussed in Chapter 76.)

Other radiographic procedures may be used preoperatively to rule out metastases. A chest x-ray is routine to screen for lung metastases. Bone, liver, and brain scans and computed tomography (CT) scans of the chest and abdomen can reveal distant metastases.

➤ Other Diagnostic Assessment

Ultrasonography of the breast is an additional diagnostic tool used to clarify findings on mammography. If the mammogram reveals a lesion, ultrasonography is helpful in differentiating a fluid-filled cyst from a solid mass.

Postoperative pathologic examination of the breast tissue is the key to diagnosis of breast cancer. It is estimated that as many as 1.8 million breast biopsies are performed each year (Shapiro & Clark, 1995). Breast tissue is obtained by one of several types of *biopsies* (see Chap. 76).

Several other tests are useful for establishing the stage of disease and prognosis after the diagnosis is made. These tests include a pathologic examination of the lymph nodes on the affected side. Other prognostic factors (Donegan & Spratt, 1995) include
- Estrogen and progesterone receptors
- S-phase index, or growth rate (done by flow-cytometric determinations of the S-phase fraction)
- DNA ploidy (the amount of DNA in a tumor cell compared with a normal cell)

- Histologic or nuclear grade

Estrogen and progesterone receptors are cytoplasmic proteins present in and on the surface of breast cancer cells that bind to estrogen and progesterone. When estrogen and progesterone bind to the cell, the cell's activity is thought to change. A tumor that contains receptors capable of binding with circulating hormones, specifically estrogen and progesterone, is estrogen receptor (ER) positive. More postmenopausal women than premenopausal women are ER positive. Women with ER-positive tumors respond better to adjuvant therapy and usually survive longer.

The receptor status also predicts which women will respond to hormonal manipulation as a treatment. Thymidine labeling index, ploidy factor (DNA content), and calculation of the number of cells in S phase by flow cytometry can reveal the growth rate of cells. Tumors with a high growth rate index and altered DNA content are associated with a worse prognosis (Donegan & Spratt, 1995).

Tumor cells are also examined for specialization or differentiation. Because well-differentiated tumors tend to be less aggressive than poorly differentiated ones, a woman with a well-differentiated breast cancer has a better prognosis than the woman with a poorly differentiated tumor.

As mentioned earlier, several procedures related to specific sites of possible metastases also help establish the stage or progression of the breast cancer. Figure 77-3 illustrates the four stages of breast cancer.

 Analysis

➤ Common Nursing Diagnoses and Collaborative Problems

The common nursing diagnosis for the client with breast cancer is Anxiety related to the diagnosis of cancer.

The common collaborative problem is Potential for Metastasis.

➤ Additional Nursing Diagnoses and Collaborative Problems

In clients with advanced breast cancer, the following additional diagnoses may apply:
- Anticipatory Grieving related to loss and possible impending death
- Pain related to tumor compression on nerve endings
- Sleep Pattern Disturbance related to pain and anxiety
- Body Image Disturbance related to loss of body part
- Sexual Dysfunction related to body image or self-esteem disturbance

 Planning and Implementation

➤ Anxiety

Planning: Expected Outcomes. The major expected outcomes are that the client will experience an appropriate level of anxiety and cope effectively throughout the

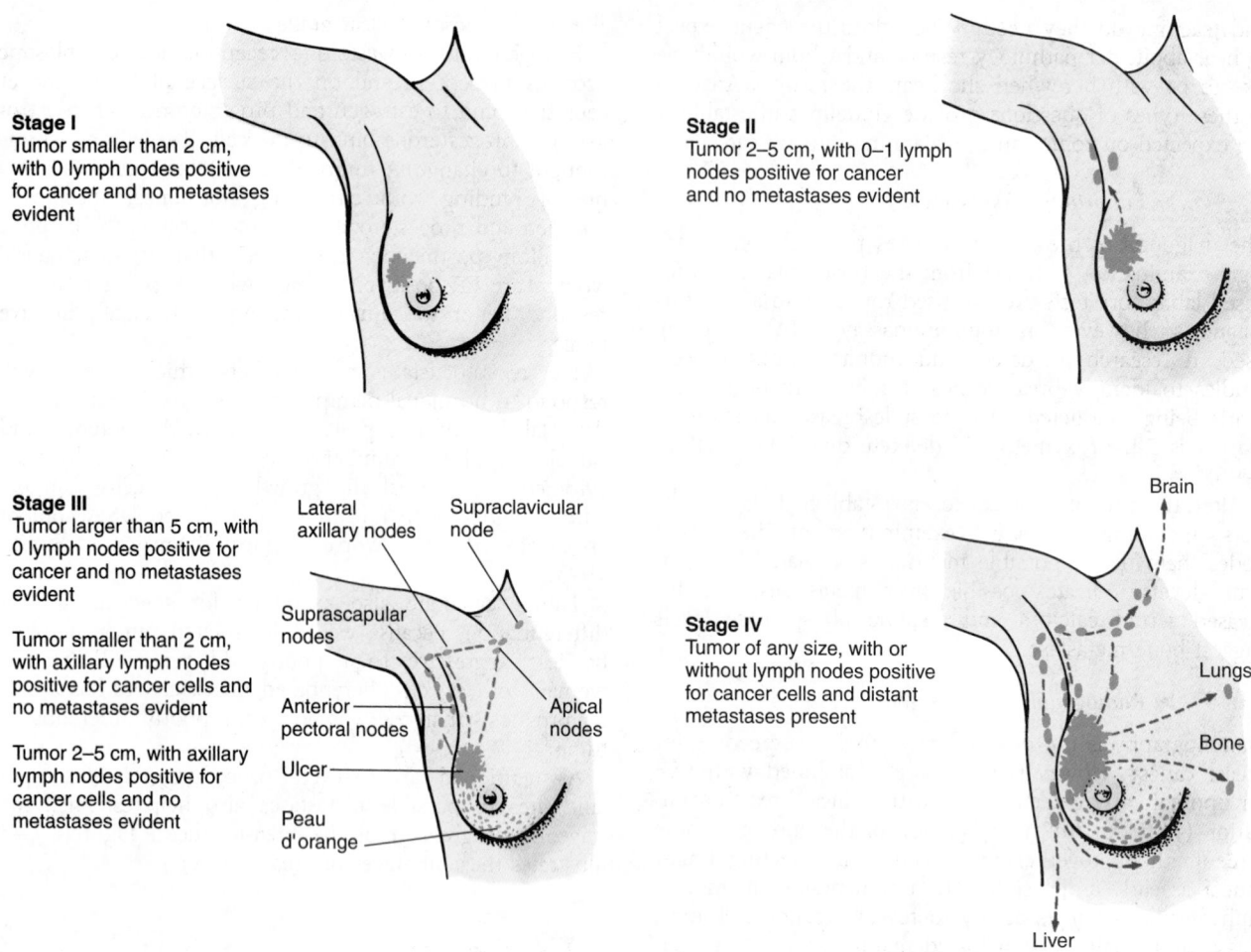

Stage I
Tumor smaller than 2 cm, with 0 lymph nodes positive for cancer and no metastases evident

Stage II
Tumor 2–5 cm, with 0–1 lymph nodes positive for cancer and no metastases evident

Stage III
Tumor larger than 5 cm, with 0 lymph nodes positive for cancer and no metastases evident

Tumor smaller than 2 cm, with axillary lymph nodes positive for cancer cells and no metastases evident

Tumor 2–5 cm, with axillary lymph nodes positive for cancer cells and no metastases evident

Lateral axillary nodes
Supraclavicular node
Suprascapular nodes
Anterior pectoral nodes
Apical nodes
Ulcer
Peau d'orange

Stage IV
Tumor of any size, with or without lymph nodes positive for cancer cells and distant metastases present

Brain
Lungs
Bone
Liver

Figure 77–3. Staging of breast cancer.

treatment period by participating in decision-making, discussing concerns, and learning self-care measures.

Interventions. The woman with breast cancer is usually admitted to the health care facility with a definitive diagnosis established through an outpatient biopsy of the mass. The practice of admitting a woman with a suspicious lesion and using general anesthesia for a biopsy, frozen section, and possible mastectomy has largely been abandoned. Women who have an interval between biopsy and treatment in which they actively participate in the choice of treatment cope more effectively after surgery, no matter which treatment is chosen.

The anxiety for the woman with breast cancer begins the moment the lump is discovered. The level of anxiety may be related to past experiences and personal associations with the disease. Many women also have an intuitive feeling about the diagnosis even before it has been established. The clinical likelihood that the lesion is or is not cancer is irrelevant to the level of fear. The client's perceptions of her own situation and personal level of anxiety are assessed. The nurse allows the client to ventilate these feelings even if a diagnosis has not been established.

If the mass has been diagnosed as cancer, many women feel a partial sense of relief to be dealing with a

known entity. A feeling of shock or disbelief may predominate. It is difficult to accept a diagnosis of cancer when one feels basically well. Clients and their families deal in individual ways with the mix of feelings, which include shock, disbelief, and grief. Some may want to read and discuss any available information. Others may want to know as little as possible and resent attempts at teaching. Although one woman may want to talk at length about her concerns, another may want to be alone. Flexibility is the key to nursing care; the nurse adjusts the approach to care as the client's emotional state changes. An integral part of the plan to meet these emotional needs is the use of outside resources. Most health care providers view such groups as the American Cancer Society's Reach to Recovery as a source of support in the postoperative period, but the nurse can suggest these groups in the preoperative phase.

Health care providers working with breast cancer clients may know other clients willing to make a preoperative visit. These resource people may be chosen on the basis of the client's concerns. The woman who is worried especially about the side effects of radiation therapy may benefit more from talking to someone who has undergone radiation than from talking to the nurse about second-hand experiences.

In addition to Reach to Recovery, formal and informal

community support groups may be available, such as Encouragement, Normalcy, Counseling, Opportunity, Reaching Out, and Energies Revived (ENCORE). These groups can be reached through the health care provider or by word of mouth.

➤ Potential for Metastasis

Planning: Expected Outcomes. The primary expected outcome is that the woman will remain free from metastases or recurrence of disease.

Interventions. There has been significant controversy in the past about the treatment of breast cancer. Until about 1950, the Halsted radical mastectomy was considered the treatment of choice. Gradually, the modified radical mastectomy became popular. More recently, evidence has been presented that supports less traumatic procedures with comparable survival rates. Because of the various options, the woman with breast cancer often faces difficult decisions.

Nonsurgical Management. For clients with late-stage breast cancer, nonsurgical treatment may be the only alternative. If the disease is in a late stage, such as stage IV, with the presence of confirmed metastasis, or if the client cannot withstand a major surgical procedure, the tumor may be removed with a local anesthetic. Follow-up treatment may include chemotherapy and sometimes radiation. If the tumor is attached to the skin or the underlying muscle, resection may be impossible. Follow-up therapy involves radiation, usually in conjunction with chemotherapy. (Chapter 27 describes the nursing care associated with chemotherapy and radiation.)

Surgical Management. The most common types of breast surgery are illustrated in Figure 77–4. Although controversy exists about the best treatment for a malignant mass, many experts agree that the mass itself should be removed to reduce the risk of local recurrence. Removal of the axillary lymph nodes, for staging purposes, may also be recommended. Axillary lymph node dissection (ALND) is usually performed for clients with palpable axillary lymph nodes; it is unclear if clients with nonpalpable nodes should also have ALND.

Preoperative Care. Care of the woman facing surgery for breast cancer focuses on psychological preparation and preoperative teaching. The issues related to anxiety and lack of knowledge are primary. The nurse directs efforts toward the client and the husband or significant other, who may be experiencing similar stress and confusion.

The type of procedure is reviewed. The nurse can initiate the discussion with open-ended questions, such as, What type of surgery are you having? Can you explain what will happen? This questioning helps the nurse assess the client's level of knowledge and allows for additional explanations as needed. The client should be knowledgeable about the type of procedure. The nurse provides specific postoperative information, such as

- The presence of a drainage device
- Location of the incision
- Any mobility restrictions
- Length of hospital stay
- Possibility of additional therapy

- Basic preoperative and postoperative information needed by any surgical client (see Chaps. 20 and 22)

Because of short hospital stays, preoperative teaching should be supplemented with written materials for the client and family to take home as references. The nurse helps the client deal with the threat to body image before surgery to correct misconceptions about postoperative appearance and to begin adjusting to changes after surgery. Clients and their care giver can attend preoperative classes in an outpatient setting such as a surgical clinic to promote successful early discharge from the hospital. Preoperative programs that provide emotional support, information, and opportunities for discussion related to sexuality, body image, preoperative instructions, and postoperative care will enhance the care of the short-stay mastectomy client (Burke et al., 1995).

Operative Procedures. During breast-conserving surgery, the surgeon removes the bulk of the tumor; typically, radiation therapy follows to eradicate residual tumor cells. Types of breast-conserving surgery used as primary treatment for stage I and stage II breast cancer include

- Lumpectomy, also known as tylectomy or local excision
- Partial mastectomy, which includes wide excision, quadrantectomy, or segmental mastectomy

Lumpectomy is gross resection of the tumor; partial mastectomy is removal of the portion of the breast that contains the tumor. Breast-conserving procedures are usually performed in same-day surgical settings.

The breast-conserving approach offers 5- and 10-year survival and local recurrence rates at least equivalent to those of the modified radical mastectomy (Moore & Kinne, 1995). The cosmetic results have been good to excellent, and other long-term problems are comparable with those of more radical procedures. For many women, the psychological benefits of avoiding breast removal are significant and lead them to choose this option.

The modified radical mastectomy does *not* conserve the breast; the affected breast is completely removed. This procedure differs from the older Halsted radical mastectomy in that the surgeon leaves the pectoral muscles and nerves intact. Thus, the breast tissue and skin and the axillary nodes are removed, and the underlying muscles are left in place. The typical incision is a 5- to 6-inch-long elliptical incision from the mid-chest to the axilla (Fig. 77–4). If reconstruction is to follow the procedure, the plastic surgeon may recommend a different location for the incision. When reconstruction is to be performed at the same time as the mastectomy, less invasive techniques have been performed such as incising a 1.5-inch flap of skin around the nipple, excising the same amount of breast tissue as with conventional mastectomy. Skin flaps or implants may be used to create a breast mound at the time of the original procedure.

The use of carbon dioxide laser procedures in place of cutting and cauterizing for mastectomies is an option that is becoming more available. Advantages of laser procedures include less blood loss and faster recuperation.

Postoperative Care. Postoperative and home care of the woman undergoing a modified radical mastectomy or breast-conserving surgery is provided in the Client Care

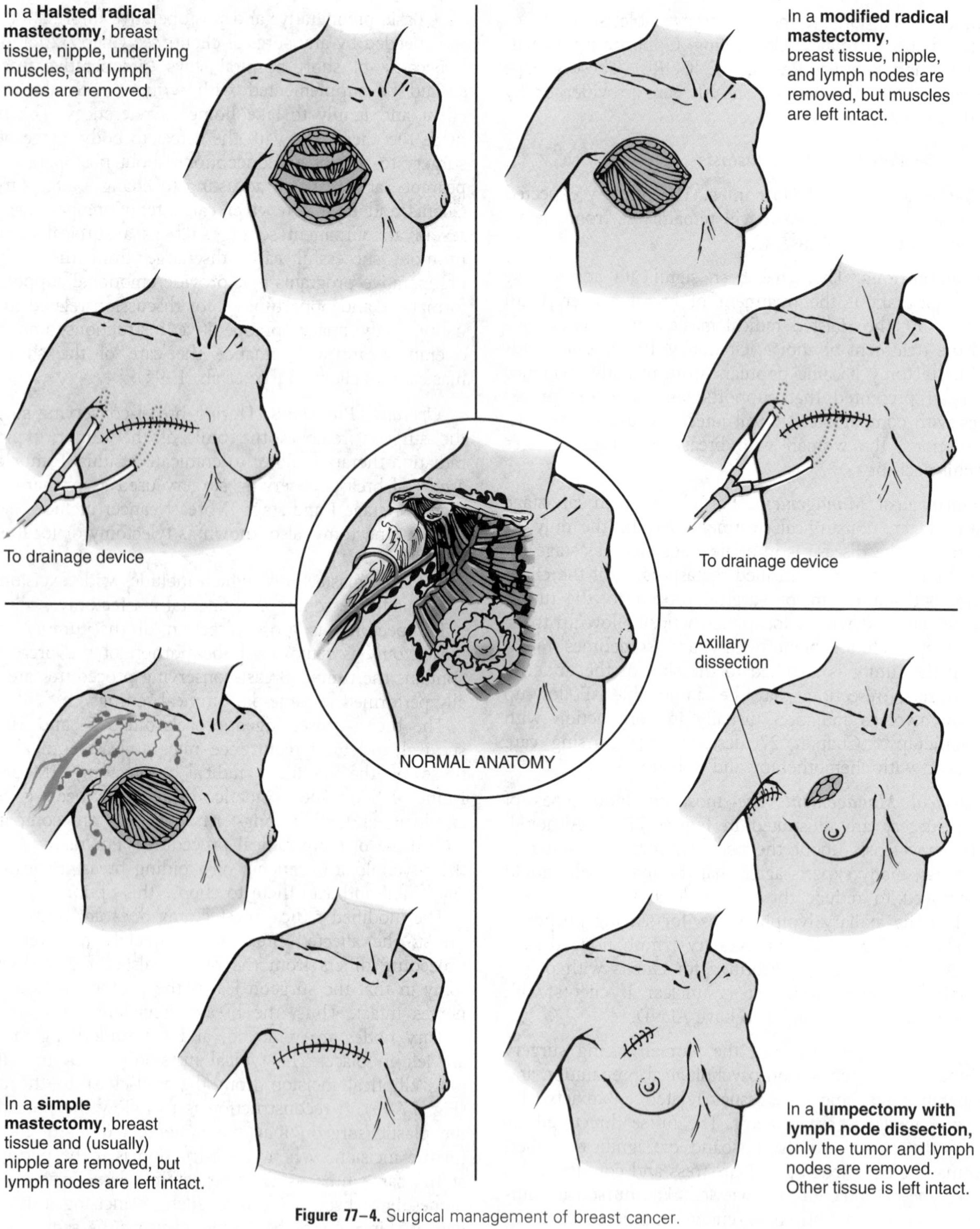

In a **Halsted radical mastectomy**, breast tissue, nipple, underlying muscles, and lymph nodes are removed.

In a **modified radical mastectomy**, breast tissue, nipple, and lymph nodes are removed, but muscles are left intact.

To drainage device

To drainage device

NORMAL ANATOMY

Axillary dissection

In a **simple mastectomy**, breast tissue and (usually) nipple are removed, but lymph nodes are left intact.

In a **lumpectomy with lymph node dissection**, only the tumor and lymph nodes are removed. Other tissue is left intact.

Figure 77–4. Surgical management of breast cancer.

Plan. Before the woman returns from surgery, the nurse places a sign over the client's bed to warn the nurse and assistive personnel to avoid taking blood pressure, giving injections, or drawing blood from the affected arm. The woman returns from the post-anesthesia care unit (PACU) as soon as vital signs return to baseline levels and if no complications have occurred. On the client's return, the nurse focuses on maintaining the client's physiologic sta-

bility and comfort. Vital signs are usually assessed on a schedule of decreasing frequency, such as every 30 minutes for two times, every hour for two times, and then every 4 hours. During these checks, the nurse or assistive personnel assesses the dressing for bleeding.

Care of Drainage Tubes. During a modified radical mastectomy, the surgeon places one or two drainage tubes,

Care of the Client After Mastectomy or Breast-Conserving Surgery

Nursing Diagnosis No. 1: Pain related to tissue trauma from surgery

Expected Outcomes	Nursing Interventions	Rationale
The client will experience no pain or unnecessary discomfort.	■ Assess for pain and identify possible causes. ■ Assess for sensation changes in the arm and the incision. ■ Reduce anxiety by reorienting the client to surroundings and explaining procedures, dressings, drains, and other equipment. ■ Medicate as appropriate with analgesics, as ordered. ■ Position the client on the back or the unaffected side, with the arm on the side of surgery elevated on a pillow. ■ Check drains and dressings for constriction, position, and functioning. ■ Explain the potential for phantom sensations of the missing breast. ■ Explain the potential for numbness in the arm and in the incision.	■ Thorough assessment allows identification of and appropriate intervention for the specific cause of pain. ■ Anxiety and fear of the unknown decrease the pain threshold. ■ Pain medications decrease perception of pain. ■ Elevation of the arm decreases swelling, which might cause discomfort. ■ Impeded circulation or swelling under the skin flap caused by obstruction of the drain causes pain. ■ Previous knowledge of the event decreases anxiety when the event occurs.

Nursing Diagnosis No. 2: Risk for Altered Tissue Perfusion related to edema or bleeding

Expected Outcomes	Nursing Interventions	Rationale
The client will maintain adequate tissue perfusion.	■ Assess the client for signs of shock (decreased blood pressure, increased pulse, decreased urinary output, confusion). ■ Check the dressing and the sheet under the client for bleeding. ■ Empty and record the drainage in the drainage container. Report excessive amounts of and changes in drainage. ■ Assess the operative site for swelling or the presence of fluid collection under the skin flaps.	■ These signs indicate shock. ■ Bleeding may stain the dressing or seep under the dressing and be unnoticed unless the bed is checked. ■ Excessive drainage indicates hemorrhage. ■ Collection of fluid under the skin flaps disrupts healing and may indicate a malfunctioning drainage device or bleeding.

(Continued)

usually Jackson-Pratt drains, under the skin flaps and attached to a small collection chamber. Gentle suction is exerted, and fluid that would accumulate under the flaps and delay healing is collected. Various models are available, but all allow the drainage to be seen and measured. When taking vital signs the nurse or assistive personnel monitors the drain for amount and color of drainage and adds this information to the intake and output record.

Client Care Plan

Nursing Diagnosis No. 3: Impaired Physical Mobility related to pain and tissue trauma

Expected Outcomes	Nursing Interventions	Rationale

The client will experience a return of mobility to her preoperative level.	■ Flexion and extension of the fingers and wrist can begin immediately postoperatively.
	■ Encourage gentle use of the arm for activities of daily living.
	■ Limited exercises include
	  ■ Range of motion for the hand, wrist, and elbow
	  ■ Squeezing a ball
	  ■ Flexing the fingers
	  ■ Touching the hand to the shoulder
	  ■ Circular wrist motion
	■ Teach appropriate exercises and ask the client to begin performing exercises 1 week after surgery or when sutures and drains are removed.
	
	■ Inform the client about Reach to Recovery or a similar organization and contact the organization with the client's permission to arrange a home visit.
	■ Encourage the client to use an upright posture with the shoulders held back and the arm by the side while walking and standing.
		■ Early use of the hand and arm muscles and joints prevents muscle atrophy and contractures and enhances fluid return.
		
		■ Active range-of-motion exercises preserve the range of motion in the client's arm in which axillary dissection was done.
		■ Reach to Recovery provides volunteers and written materials on exercises that are safe to perform at home.
		
		■ The tendency is to hold the arm bent across the waist and to stoop over, which results in elbow and shoulder contractures.

Nursing Diagnosis No. 4: Risk for Infection related to disruption in skin integrity

Expected Outcomes	Nursing Interventions	Rationale
The client will have an incision that remains free from infection.	■ Assess for signs of infection and swelling.	■ Infection and collection of serosanguineous fluid delay wound healing and disrupt adhesion of the skin flaps.

(Continued)

Clients undergoing lumpectomy may also have drainage tubes (usually Jackson-Pratt drains) if the lump is large or if axillary node dissection is performed.

The nurse or assistive personnel continues to measure the amount of wound drainage, although measurements of general fluid intake and output are usually discontinued by the first postoperative day. The nurse observes the wound for signs of swelling and infection throughout the client's recovery. Drainage tubes are removed by the surgeon when drainage is less than 50 mL in 24 hours. With short hospital stays, drainage tubes are usually removed about 1 week after hospital discharge when the client returns for her first postoperative office visit. The nurse informs the client that although these tubes lie just under the skin, removal may be painful.

Comfort Measures. The nurse or assistive personnel assesses the client's position so that the drainage tubes or collection device will not be pulled or kinked. The client should sit with the head of the bed up at least 30 de-

Client Care Plan

Expected Outcomes	Nursing Interventions	Rationale
	■ Teach the client measures to reduce the risk of infection. ■ Avoid taking blood pressure, drawing blood, and giving injections in the operative arm. ■ Avoid injury to the arm, such as burns, scratches, insect bites, and scrapes. ■ Treat injuries immediately to avoid infection.	■ Injury and infection in the operative arm increase the risk of lymphedema related to removal of lymph nodes.
	■ Encourage the client to look at the incision before discharge from the hospital and explain signs of infection, including redness, heat, swelling, and wound discharge.	■ Discharge usually occurs before complete healing. The client or some other responsible person must monitor wound healing.
	■ Instruct the client to notify the physician if swelling, redness, or pain occurs.	■ Early intervention may prevent disruption of the skin flaps.
	■ Instruct the client to avoid the use of creams and ointments on the incision and to avoid the use of deodorant under the affected arm.	■ Chemical irritation may lead to infection and/or inflammation.
	■ Encourage the client to bathe or shower if the wound is healed and the drains have been removed. ■ Instruct the client to avoid restrictive clothing, such as tight jewelry or snug sleeves.	■ Injury and infection in the operative arm increase the risk of lymphedema related to removal of the lymph nodes.

Nursing Diagnosis No. 5: Body Image Disturbance related to loss of all or part of the breast

Expected Outcomes	Nursing Interventions	Rationale
The client will maintain a positive body image.	■ Encourage verbalization of concern about body changes. ■ Discuss the use of a temporary prosthesis and fitting of a permanent prosthesis. ■ Assess brassiere for nonbinding, nonwired structure. ■ Advise the client that the usual time for fitting a permanent prosthesis is 6 to 8 weeks postoperatively.	■ Verbalization decreases anxiety and allows validation of feelings. ■ Maintaining outward appearance promotes positive feelings. ■ Pressure impairs blood supply to healing tissue. ■ Permanent prostheses can be fitted after swelling resolves and wound healing is complete.

(Continued)

grees, with the affected arm (the arm on the same side as the axillary dissection) elevated on a pillow while awake. Keeping the affected arm elevated promotes lymphatic fluid return after removal of axillary lymph nodes and channels.

The nurse provides other basic comfort measures, such

as repositioning and pain medications, as prescribed, on a regular basis until pain ceases.

Mobility and Diet. The hospital stay after the modified radical mastectomy is short, typically 1 to 2 days, and re-

Client Care Plan

Expected Outcomes	Nursing Interventions	Rationale
	■ Provide information about sources of permanent forms (such as department stores and specialty shops) and the need to be fitted by a person with experience.	■ Specific information encourages the client to undergo fitting to obtain the prosthesis.
	■ Inform the client that insurance should cover the cost if the need is validated by the physician.	■ Reducing concerns about cost encourages the client to obtain a prosthesis.
	■ Encourage the client to discuss options for breast reconstruction with the physician if she wishes.	■ Options for breast reconstruction will vary.
	■ Encourage the client to discuss feelings about possible breast reconstruction.	■ The client may feel ambivalent about reconstruction and may need an objective listener.

Nursing Diagnosis No. 6: Impaired Social Interaction related to changes in body image

Expected Outcomes	Nursing Interventions	Rationale
The client will maintain relationships with significant other, family, and friends.	■ Encourage verbalization of concern about possible changes in relationships.	■ Verbalization of concerns decreases anxiety.
	■ Allow the client's significant others to verbalize concerns. Provide information and support.	■ The reaction of the client's significant others to breast cancer and treatment may severely threaten these relationships.
	■ Offer the client and significant others information on breast cancer and what to expect from treatment.	■ Previous knowledge of the treatment may decrease anxiety.

covery is usually not complicated. Because some managed care companies will not authorize an overnight stay in the hospital following a mastectomy, several states have enacted legislation mandating inpatient benefits. The client who chooses an early discharge should have a home health visit within 24 hours of the discharge.

Ambulation and a regular diet are resumed by the day after surgery. While the client is in an upright position, the arm on the affected side may need to be supported at first. Gradually the arm should be allowed to hang straight by the side while the client is walking. The nurse teaches the client to avoid the hunched back position with the arm flexed because of the risk of elbow contractures. Beginning exercises that do not stress the incision can usually be started on the first postoperative day. These exercises include squeezing the affected hand around a soft, round object (a ball or rolled washcloth) and flexion/extension of the elbow. The progression to more strenuous exercises depends on the subsequent pro-

cedures planned (such as reconstruction) and the surgeon's orders.

As soon as the woman is fully ambulatory and eating well and her postoperative pain is under control, she is discharged to continue recuperation at home. Typical instructions for postmastectomy exercises are provided in Chart 77–2.

Breast Reconstruction. The surgeon should offer the option of breast reconstruction before surgery is performed. If the client does not choose immediate reconstructive surgery, a temporary prosthesis is given to the client. Some surgeons allow women to use a temporary prosthesis in the immediate postoperative period as a component of the postoperative dressing. In this instance the client returns from surgery with a surgical brassiere and the temporary sterile prosthesis in place. The nurse or social worker refers the client to the American Cancer Society's Reach to Recovery program. A volunteer who

Chart 77-2

Education Guide: Postmastectomy Exercises

Hand Wall Climbing

1. Face the wall, and put the palms of your hands flat against the wall at shoulder level.
2. Flex your fingers so that your hands slowly "walk" up the wall.
3. Stop when your arms are fully extended.
4. Slowly "walk" your hands back down the wall until they return to shoulder level.

Pulley Exercise

1. Drape a 6-foot-long rope over a shower curtain rod or over the top of a door. If you use a door for this exercise, have someone put a nail or hook at the top of the door so that the rope does not slip off.
2. Grab the ends of the rope, one in each hand, and extend your arms out to your sides until they are straight.
3. Pull down—keeping your arms straight—with your left arm to raise your right arm as high as you can.
4. Pull down with your right arm to raise your left arm as high as you can.

Rope Turning

1. Tie a rope to the knob of a closed door.
2. Hold the other end of the rope and step back from the door until your arm is almost straight out in front of you.
3. Swing the rope in a circle. Start with small circles and gradually increase to larger circles as you become more flexible.

---

has had breast cancer surgery visits the client at home, offering information on breast forms, clothing, and coping with breast cancer. The volunteer should be about the same age as the client and have experienced the same surgical procedure.

The client's level of satisfaction with her prosthesis is evaluated several weeks postoperatively. The nurse assesses the client's attitude by asking about plans for restoring appearance postoperatively. Although reconstruction is not appropriate for some clients and others may not be interested in it, the surgeon should discuss the indications and contraindications, advantages and disadvantages, and typical postoperative recovery. If immediate reconstruction is chosen, the surgeon should be aware of this preoperatively so that the surgeon's plans can be coordinated with those of the plastic surgeon.

Several procedures are available for restoring the appearance of the breast (Table 77-5). Reconstruction may begin during the original operative procedure or later in one to several stages. Some of the more common techniques include

- Use of a flap of skin and muscle from the abdomen, back, or hip to create a breast mound

- Placement of a saline-filled prosthesis
- Use of progressive tissue expanders to slowly create a pocket under the mastectomy site for placement of a permanent implant

If necessary, a new nipple may be created with tissue from the other nipple or from other body tissue, such as the labia or inner thigh. In some cases, the client's natural nipple can be reattached to another part of the body if the reconstruction is planned for a later date.

In June 1992, the U.S. Food and Drug Administration (FDA) restricted use of silicone gel implants to women in FDA-approved safety studies. The studies were open to women seeking implants after breast cancer surgery or traumatic injury (NAACOG, 1992). However, because silicone gel implants have not been manufactured since 1992, this option is essentially unavailable to all women in the United States. The restriction of silicone implants resulted from complaints that silicone leakage caused clients to experience connective tissue diseases, such as lupus, or other vague physical symptoms.

The transverse rectus abdominis myocutaneous (TRAM) flap, a frequently used method of reconstruction, provides women with naturally appearing breasts without the risks associated with the silicone gel implant.

Nursing care of the woman undergoing breast reconstruction is outlined in Chart 77-3.

Adjuvant Therapy. The decision to follow the original surgical procedure with chemotherapy, radiation, or hormonal therapy is based on

- The stage of the disease
- Age and menopausal status of the client
- Client preferences
- Pathologic examination
- Hormone receptor status

The purpose of adjuvant therapy is to decrease the risk of recurrence for the client who has no evidence of but is at risk for metastasis or to prolong survival after metastases occur. Adjuvant therapy for stage I and stage II (early-stage) breast cancer consists of breast-conserving surgery and postoperative radiotherapy or modified radical mastectomy. Women who have estrogen receptor–positive tumors are given tamoxifen (Nolvadex, Tamofen♦). This estrogen antagonist blocks the estrogen receptor sites in the tumor cells, thereby inhibiting growth. When this therapy is appropriate, the response rate is 50% to 60%. The Breast Cancer Prevention Trial, a national study, is currently being conducted to determine the effects of tamoxifen as a chemoprevention agent in women known to be at risk for breast cancer (Gould et al., 1995).

Therapy of stage III, or locally advanced, breast cancer is still controversial. Treatment usually includes surgery, if the tumor is operable, and chemotherapy with or without radiotherapy. Although chemotherapeutic regimens differ among treatment centers, multiple-agent combinations are used. A common example of such a combination is cyclophosphamide (Cytoxan, Neosar, Procytox♦), methotrexate (Folex, Mexate), and fluorouracil (5-FU, Adrucil). The length of treatment may also vary. Autologous and allogeneic bone marrow transplant (stem cell transplantation) and preoperative chemotherapy are being investigated as early treatment for women who have a high risk for

TABLE 77–5

Examples of Breast Reconstruction Procedures

Procedure	Description	Procedure	Description
Implantation	• An implant matching the size of the other breast is placed under the muscle of the operative side to create a breast mound.	Myocutaneous flaps	• A flap of skin, fat, and muscle is transferred from the donor site to the operative area. The flap contains an appropriate amount of fat to match the other breast and is similar in appearance to breast tissue. A blood supply is established by reanastomosis of vessels from the operative area to those with the flap when possible. A new nipple may be created with tissue from the other nipple, labia, or thigh. Nipples can also be created by tattooing.

Latissimus dorsi musculocutaneous flap

Procedure	Description
Tissue expansion	• A tissue expander is placed under the muscle and gradually expanded with saline to stretch the overlying skin and create a pocket. After several weeks, the tissue expander is exchanged for an implant.

Abdominal myocutaneous flap

recurrence or advanced disease (Smith, 1996). Autologous bone marrow transplant (taken from the client's bone marrow), peripheral blood stem cell transplant (taken from the client's circulating blood), or allogeneic bone marrow transplant (taken from a healthy donor's bone marrow or peripheral blood) may be performed as a means of rescue following very high doses of chemotherapy or radiation. These procedures decrease the expected morbidity and mortality related to adjuvant therapy (Jassak & Riley, 1994). Before planning care and teaching for the breast cancer client undergoing chemotherapy, the nurse knows the specific agents to be used and their properties. (A discussion of the care for the client undergoing chemotherapy is given in Chapter 27. A discussion of the care of the client undergoing bone marrow transplantation is given in Chapter 27.)

Chart 77–3

Nursing Care Highlight: Postoperative Breast Reconstruction

- Assess the incision and flap for signs of infection (excessive redness, drainage, odor) during dressing changes.
- Assess the incision and flap for signs of poor tissue perfusion (duskiness, decreased capillary refill) during dressing changes.
- Avoid pressure on the flap and suture lines by positioning the client on her nonoperative side and avoiding tight clothing.
- Monitor and measure drainage in collection devices, such as Jackson-Pratt drains.
- Teach the client to return to her usual activity level gradually and to
  - Avoid heavy lifting.
  - Avoid sleeping in the prone position.
  - Avoid participation in contact sports or other activities that could cause trauma to the chest.
  - Minimize pressure on the breast during sexual activity.
  - Refrain from driving until advised by the physician.
- Remind the client to ask at the 6-week postoperative visit when full activity can be resumed.
- Reassure the client that optimal appearance may not occur for 3 to 6 months postoperatively.
- If implants have been inserted, teach the proper method of breast massage to enhance expansion and prevent capsule formation (consult with the physician).
- Review the breast self-examination procedure and the need to continue this practice monthly.
- Remind the client that mammograms should be scheduled at least yearly for the rest of her life.

 Continuing Care

➤ Home Care Management

Home care preparation should be initiated when the decision to have surgical therapy is made. Referral to a case manager can ensure that the educational needs of the client are met early in the perioperative period. Referrals could be made by the Preadmission Testing Center or the surgeon. Preoperative teaching, home care management, and the need for referrals (Reach to Recovery, social services, home care) can be initiated before hospitalization. Planning ahead for the client's discharge needs facilitates the client's discharge home (Walkenstein, 1995).

The client who has undergone breast surgery can be discharged to the home setting unless other physical disabilities exist. Some clients are discharged 1 to 2 days after surgery, with Jackson-Pratt or other types of drains in place. The current trend, though, is that clients are discharged home on the same day that surgery is performed. These clients need assistance at home with drain care, dressings, and activities of daily living because of impaired range of motion of the affected arm and pain. Summaries of discharge instructions are given in Chart 77–4 and Chart 77–5.

It is not necessary to modify the home for the client

after breast surgery. Activities involving stretching or reaching for heavy objects should be avoided. This restriction can be discussed with a family member who can perform these tasks or place the objects within easy reach of the client.

ELDERLY CONSIDERATIONS

 If fatigue is a major problem and the home has two or more stories, limiting activities to one level may help.

Chart 77–4

Education Guide: Recovery from Breast Cancer Surgery

- There may be a dry gauze dressing over the incision when you leave the hospital. You may change this dressing if it becomes soiled.
- A small, dry dressing will be around the site where a drain is placed. Often there is some leakage of fluid around the drain. Check the gauze dressing for drainage, and change it if it becomes soiled. Some leakage is normal, but if the dressing becomes soaked more than once a day, call your health care provider.
- Your nurse has shown you how to empty the reservoir from your drain and how to measure the volume of drainage. You should empty the drain twice a day and record the measurements.
- Drains are generally removed when drainage is less than 50 mL in 24 hours.
- Drains are often removed at the same time as the stitches or staples, generally 7 to 10 days after surgery.
- You may take sponge baths or tub baths, making certain that the area of the drain and incision stays dry. You may shower after the stitches and drains are removed.
- You can begin using your arm for normal activities, such as eating or combing your hair. Exercises involving the wrist, hand, and elbow, such as flexing your fingers, circular wrist motions, and touching your hand to your shoulder, are very good. You can usually resume more strenuous exercises after the drains have been removed.
- You can expect some discomfort or mild pain after surgery, but within 4 to 5 days most women have no need for pain medication or require medication only at bedtime
- Numbness in the area of the surgery and along the inner side of the arm from the armpit to the elbow occurs in virtually all women. It is the injury to the nerves that causes sensation to the skin in those areas. Women have described sensations of heaviness, pain, tingling, burning, and "pins and needles." These sensations change over the months and usually resolve by 1 year.
- Pamphlets on exercises, hand and arm care, and general facts about breast cancer are available from your nurse or volunteer visitor. The American Cancer Society has volunteers who have had surgery similar to yours and are available to visit you.

Modified from McCorkle, R., Baird, S., & Grant, M. (1996). *Cancer nursing: A comprehensive approach.* Philadelphia: W. B. Saunders.

Chart 77–5

Nursing Care Highlight: Focused Home Care Assessment for Clients Recovering from Breast Cancer Surgery

- Assess cardiovascular, respiratory, and urinary status, including
  - Vital signs
  - Lung sounds
  - Urinary output patterns
- Assess for pain and effectiveness of analgesics
- Assess dressing and incision site for
  - Excess drainage
  - Signs and symptoms of infection
  - Wound healing
  - Intact staples
- Assess drain and site for
  - Drainage around the drain site and in the drain
  - Color and amount of drainage
  - Signs and symptoms of infection
- Review client's recordings of drainage
- Evaluate ability to care for and empty drain
- Assess status of the affected extremity, including
  - Range of motion
  - Ability to perform exercise regimen
  - Lymphedema
- Assess nutritional status, including
  - Food and fluid intake
  - Presence of nausea and vomiting
  - Bowel sounds
- Assess functional ability, including
  - Activities of daily living
  - Mobility and ambulation
- Assess home environment, including
  - Safety
  - Structural barriers
- Assess client's compliance and knowledge of illness and treatment plan, including
  - Follow-up appointment with surgeon
  - Signs and symptoms to report to health care provider
  - Hand and Arm Care Guidelines
  - Referral to Reach to Recovery
- Assess client and caregiver coping skills
  - Determine if client has looked at the incision site
  - Assess client's reaction to incision site

➤ *Health Teaching*

The teaching plan for the client after surgery includes
- Measures to optimize a positive body image
- Information to enhance interpersonal relationships and roles
- Exercises to regain full range of motion
- Measures to prevent infection of the incision
- Measures to avoid injury, infection, and subsequent swelling of the affected arm
- Care of the incision and drainage device

Physical Care. The nurse takes the opportunity to explain incisional care. The client may wear a light dress-

ing to prevent irritation. The nurse explains that no lotions or ointments should be used on the area, and the use of deodorant under the affected arm should be delayed until healing is complete. Although swelling and redness of the scar itself are normal for the first few weeks, swelling, redness, increased heat, and tenderness of the surrounding area indicate infection and should be reported to the surgeon. If a lymph node dissection was performed, the client should elevate the affected arm on a pillow for at least 30 minutes a day for the first 6 months. The nurse asks the client to have a family member bring a loose-fitting, nonwired brassiere or camisole for her to try before discharge with a soft cotton-filled or polyester fiber–filled form supplied by the hospital or by Reach to Recovery. The client wears this form until the incision is completely healed and the health care provider approves the fitting of a more sophisticated prosthesis, usually 6 to 8 weeks after discharge. After going home, the client should be encouraged to dress in loose-fitting street clothes, not pajamas, to further enhance a positive self-image.

Exercises that began in the hospital should continue at home. Active range-of-motion exercises should begin 1 week after surgery or when sutures and drains are removed. The nurse emphasizes that reaching and stretching exercises should continue only to the point of pain or pulling, never higher. ENCORE, a YWCA program, is appropriate for women as early as 3 weeks postoperatively and includes exercise to music, exercise in water, and psychological support. Prior to discharge, the surgeon may prescribe precautions or limitations specific to plans for future procedures, such as reconstruction.

The nurse provides information needed to help the client avoid infection and subsequent lymphedema of the affected arm after mastectomy. The client should avoid having blood pressure taken on, having injections in, and having blood drawn from the arm on the side of the mastectomy. The client can wear a mitt when using the oven, wear gloves when gardening, and treat cuts and scrapes appropriately. If lymphedema occurs, the arm should be elevated when possible and special attention paid to the above-mentioned warnings. Additionally, if lymphedema occurs, it can be managed with the use of an arm sleeve (similar to a Ted or Jobst stocking) or a sequential compression device. Management of lymphedema is directed toward measures that promote drainage of the affected arm; however, prevention is the best cure.

Psychosocial Management. Concerns about appearance after surgery are common and are often a threat to one's self-concept as a woman. Before breast surgery, the woman and her partner can benefit from an explanation of the expected postoperative appearance. After modified radical mastectomy, the chest wall is fairly smooth and has a horizontal incision from the axilla to the mid-chest area. After breast-conserving surgery, scars vary according to the amount of breast tissue removed. Scars may be red and raised at first, but these characteristics diminish in the first few months. After surgery, the nurse encourages

▷ Research Applications for Nursing

Coping Strategies of Breast Cancer Survivors may be Taught to Newly Diagnosed Clients

Fredette, S. L. (1994). Breast cancer survivors: Concerns and coping. Cancer Nursing, 18(1), 35–46.

This descriptive study utilized a convenience sample to determine the long-term characteristics of women who survived breast cancer. Fourteen survivors were interviewed using two instruments. The ages of the participants at interview ranged from 48 to 68 years. The number of years these women had survived breast cancer ranged from 8 to 30 years, with a mean of 13.7 years. All of the women had undergone either modified radical or radical mastectomy. Data were collected on coping strategies, work, spirituality, information-seeking strategies, use of support groups, and the role that family and friends played in the lives of these women. Additionally, data were collected about attitude, impact of cancer, meaning of having cancer, and self-perception about survivorship. Results of the study indicated that these women demonstrated a survival orientation.

Critique. The study used a small convenience sample of self-selected participants who were motivated to share information about their survival. This study validated findings from other studies that particular coping methods appear to be more helpful than others.

Possible Nursing Implications. With further validation, the coping skills that these women used to persevere and survive cancer could be taught to others who are diagnosed with breast cancer. The stories of these women will provide hope for the newly diagnosed client with breast cancer.

the woman to look at her incision before she goes home and offers to be present when she does so.

Much of one's body image is a reflection of how others respond. Therefore, the response of the client's family and partner to the surgery is crucial in determining the effect on self-concept. These people may also need the support of the nurse. They may have concerns about their ability to accept the changes and need to discuss these feelings with an objective listener. They also may need help with communicating their feelings, both negative and positive, with their loved one. Involving them in teaching may also help reinforcement and increase retention.

Sexual concerns should be discussed before discharge. Sexual intercourse can be resumed whenever the client is comfortable. Clients may prefer to lay a pillow over the surgical site or wear a bra or camisole to prevent contact with the surgical site during intercourse. The client may be embarrassed to broach the topic, and the nurse should be sensitive to possible concerns and approach the subject first.

For women of childbearing age (approximately 25% of breast cancer clients), the issues related to childbearing

may be a concern. Some providers believe that the woman who has had breast cancer should wait 2 to 3 years after completing treatment to attempt pregnancy. Others, however, suggest no waiting period as reoccurrences could happen at any time (Shapiro & Clark, 1995). Clients receiving chemotherapy or radiotherapy must use birth control during therapy. The method and length of birth control is discussed with the health care provider.

▷ *Health Care Resources*

Resources available to the client after discharge include personal support and community programs. After discharge, the client's spouse or significant other may need aid in planning support for home responsibilities. For example, a partner who may be assuming additional duties at home and work may feel stressed. Exploring temporary relief resources for child care, cleaning, or cooking may be helpful until the woman regains her previous energy level. Discussing the need for ongoing emotional support is also beneficial to both client and partner. Leaving the hospital and appearing normal do not end the client's anxiety and fear. Identifying a support person with whom the client or couple can explore these feelings and discussing the need to ventilate feelings enhance personal and family recovery (see Research Applications for Nursing).

As mentioned, Reach to Recovery and ENCORE are two community resources for women with breast cancer. Reach to Recovery provides a volunteer who visits the client in the hospital or at home. She brings a personal message of hope, informational materials on breast cancer recovery, and a soft, temporary breast form. Some communities offer additional resources, such as support groups and exercise classes (see Appendix).

 Evaluation

The processes of care planning and implementation are important, but it is only through evaluation that practice can improve. The process of evaluation is based on the identified nursing diagnoses. The expected outcomes may include that the client will

- Demonstrate the correct method of breast self-examination (BSE)
- Practice BSE on a monthly basis
- Comply with guidelines for mammography and professional examination
- Be able to cope with the diagnosis, as shown by her use of social support, use of information to deal with uncertainty, absence of physical signs of anxiety, and verbal confirmation of feeling calm
- State that she feels positive about her self-image
- Regain full range of motion of the affected arm
- Remain free from lymphedema or infection

CASE STUDY for the Client Having Breast Surgery

■ A 67-year-old female presented to her health care provider with a chief complaint of a "lump in my right breast" found when performing BSE. She was worried that the lump is cancer. Several years ago her mother had a mastectomy for breast cancer. Her mammogram revealed a suspicious lesion. A biopsy of the lesion and axillary lymph nodes confirmed a stage I carcinoma of the right breast with negative lymph nodes. The client's health care provider gave her the option of having a total mastectomy with complete axillary node dissection or breast conservation with lumpectomy, complete axillary node dissection, and radiation therapy. Ms. N. chose breast conserving therapy, and her surgery was performed today. She has returned to your unit for postoperative nursing care. The critical pathway indicates that if her status is stable she will be discharged to home tomorrow.

QUESTIONS:

1. What are the preoperative and postoperative informational needs of this client?
2. How can the nurse support this client in the decision-making process regarding her surgical options?
3. What community resources are available to meet the needs of this client?
4. What are the home care needs of this client?
5. During your home visit Ms. N. asks you to do a presentation on breast cancer at the local senior center she attends. What information will you include in your presentation?

SELECTED BIBLIOGRAPHY

Allen, K. M., & Phillips, J. M. (1997). *Women's health across the lifespan.* Philadelphia: J. B. Lippincott.

Baron, R. H., & Walsh, A. (1995). 9 Facts everyone should know about breast cancer. *American Journal of Nursing, 95*(7), 29–33.

Baskin-Smith, J., Miaskowski, C., Dibble, S., Weekes, D., & Nielsen, B. (1995). Perceptions of the mammography experience. *Cancer Nursing, 18*(1), 47–52.

Bostwick, J. (1995). Breast reconstruction following mastectomy. *CA: A Cancer Journal for Clinicians, 45*(5), 289–303.

Brown, L., & Williams, R. (1994). Culturally sensitive breast cancer screening program for older black women. *Nurse Practitioner, 19*(3), 21–35.

Burke, C., Zabka, C., & McCarver, K. (1995). Patients respond positively to nurse-initiated short stay program following breast cancer surgery. *Oncology Nursing Forum, 22*(1), 148–149.

Champion, V. (1995). Development of a benefits and barriers scale for mammography utilization. *Cancer Nursing, 18*(1), 53–59.

Danforth, J., D'Angelo, D., Pierce, S., Lichter, L., & Okunieff, P. (1995). Ten-year results of a comparison of conservation with mastectomy in the treatment of stage I and II breast cancer. *New England Journal of Medicine, 332*(14), 907–911.

Djuric, Z., Heilbrum, L., Simon, M., Smith, D., Luongo, D., LoRusso, P., & Martino, S. (1996). Levels of 5-hydroxymethyl-2'-deoxyuridine in DNA from blood as a marker of breast cancer. *Cancer, 77*(4), 691–696.

Donegan, W., & Spratt, J. (1995). *Cancer of the breast.* Philadelphia: W.B. Saunders.

Fredette, S. L. (1994). Breast cancer survivors: Concerns and coping. *Cancer Nursing, 18*(1), 35–46.

Giomuso, C. B., & Suster, V. (1994). Free flap breast reconstruction. *MEDSURG Nursing, 3,* 9–22.

Gould, K., Gates, M. L., & Miaskowski, C. (1995). Breast cancer prevention: A summary of the chemoprevention trial with tamoxifen. *Oncology Nursing Forum, 21*(5), 835–840.

Graling, P. R., & Grant, J. M. (1995). Demographics and patient treatment choice in stage I breast cancer. *AORN Journal, 62*(3), 376–384.

Ivey, C. L., & Gordon, S. I. (1994). Breast reconstruction: New image, new hope. *RN, 7,* 48–53.

Jacobson, J. A., Danforth, D. N., Cowan, K. H., D'Angelo, T., Steinberg, S. M., Pierce, I., Lippman, M. E., Lichter, A. S., Glastein, E., & Okunieff, P. (1995). Ten-year results of a comparison of conservation with mastectomy in the treatment of stage I and II breast cancer. *New England Journal of Medicine, 332*(14), 907–911.

Jassak, P. F., & Riley, M. B. (1994). Autologous stem cell transplant. *Cancer Practice, 2*(2), 141–145.

Jeffries, E. (1997). Home healthcare for patients receiving one-day mastectomy. *Home Healthcare Nurse, 115*(1), 31–37.

Johnson, J. R. (1994). Caring for the woman who's had a mastectomy. *American Journal of Nursing, 94*(5), 25–31.

Knobf, M. T. (1994). Decision-making for primary breast cancer treatment. *MEDSURG Nursing, 3,* 169–174, 180.

Knobf, M. T. (1994). Treatment options for early stage breast cancer. *MEDSURG Nursing, 3*(4), 249–257, 328.

Leslie, N. S. (1995). Role of the nurse practitioner in breast and cervical cancer prevention. *Cancer Nursing, 18*(4), 251–257.

Lessick, M., Wickham, R., & Rehwaldt, M. (1997). Breast and ovarian cancer: Genetic update and implications for nursing. *MEDSURG Nursing 6*(6), 341–349.

Lu, Z. J. (1995). Variables associated with breast self-examination among Chinese women. *Cancer Nursing, 18*(1), 29–34.

Luker, K. A., Beaver, K., Leinster, S. J., & Owens, R. G. (1996). Information needs and sources of information for women with breast cancer: A follow up study. *Journal of Advanced Nursing, 23,* 487–495.

Malone, K., Daling, J., Thompson, J., et al. (1998). BRCA1 mutations and breast cancer in the general population. *JAMA, 279,* 922–929.

McCorkle, R., Baird, S. B. (1996). *Cancer nursing: A comprehensive textbook.* Philadelphia: W. B. Saunders.

McDaniel, R., Rhodes, V., Nelson, R. A., & Hanson, B. (1995). Sensory perceptions of women receiving tamoxifen for breast cancer. *Cancer Nursing, 18*(3), 215–221.

Melnikow, J. (1995). Hormone replacement therapy and breast cancer risk. *Journal of Family Practice, 41*(5), 501–502.

Mittra, I. (1994). Breastscreening: The case for physical examination without mammography. *Lancet, 343,* 342–344.

Moore, M. P., & Kinne, D. (1995). The surgical management of primary invasive breast cancer. *CA: A Cancer Journal for Clinicians, 45*(5), 278–288.

*NAACOG. (1992). FDA limits access to breast implants. *NAACOG Newsletter, 19*(6), 3.

Newschaffer, C., Penberthy, L., Desch, C., Retchin, S., & Whittemore, M. (1996). The effect of age and comorbidity in the treatment of elderly women with nonmetastatic breast cancer. *Archives of Internal Medicine, 156*(1), 85–90.

Phillips, J. M., & Wilbur, J. (1995). Adherence to breast cancer screening guidelines among African-American women of differing employment status. *Cancer Nursing, 18*(4), 258–269.

*Pierce, P. F. (1993). Deciding on breast cancer treatment: A description of decision behavior. *Nursing Research, 42*(1), 22–28.

Shapiro, T., & Clark, P. (1995). Breast cancer: What the primary care provider needs to know. *Nurse Practitioner, 20*(3), 39–40, 42.

Smith, R. J. (1996). Buying more time in less time: Case management and bone marrow transplantation. *Case Manager, 7*(1), 77–83.

Steele, G. D., Osteem, R. T., Winchester, D. P., Murphy, G. P., & Menck, H. R. (1994). Clinical highlights from the National Cancer Data Base: 1994. *CA: A Cancer Journal for Clinicians, 44*(2), 71–81.

Stewart, J. A., & Carbone, P. P. (1994a). Breast cancer: 1. Screening and early management. *Hospital Practice, 2,* 81–90.

Stewart, J. A., & Carbone, P. P. (1994b). Breast cancer: 2. Recurrent disease. *Hospital Practice, 3,* 59–64.

Tierney, L., McPhee, S. J., & Papadakis, M. A. (Eds.). (1995). *Current medical diagnosis and treatment.* Norwalk, CT: Appleton & Lange.

Walkenstein, M. (1995). Surgical clinical nurse specialist facilitates discharge of patients undergoing breast surgery. *Oncology Nursing Forum, 22*(1), 147–148.

Weber, E. S. (1997). Questions and answers about breast cancer diagnosis. *AJN, 97*(10), 34–38.

Wehrwein, T., & Eddy, M. (1995). A two-part study of the breast health promoting behaviors of mid-life women. *Gynecologic Oncology Nursing, 5*(1), 34–35.

Wingo, P. A., Bolden, S., Tong, T., Parker, S. L., Martin, L. M., & Heath, C. W. Jr. (1996). Cancer statistics for African Americans, 1996. *CA: A Cancer Journal for Clinicians, 46*(2), 113–125.

Wingo, P. A., Tong, T., & Bolden, S. (1995). Cancer statistics, 1995. *CA: A Cancer Journal for Clinicians, 45*(1), 8–30.

SUGGESTED READINGS

Johnson, J. R. (1994). Caring for the woman who's had a mastectomy. *American Journal of Nursing, 94*(5), 25–31.

This article provides a complete overview of the physical, emotional, and informational needs of the client who has had a mastectomy. Surgical options, reconstruction, teaching plans, and potential complications are included.

Sciartelli, C. H. (1995). Using a clinical pathway approach to document client teaching for breast cancer surgical procedures. *Oncology Nursing Forum, 22*(1), 131–137.

This article provides a standardized, comprehensive teaching plan for breast cancer surgical procedures using a clinical pathway approach. Members of the health care community can reproduce the tool for noncommercial use.

Chapter 78

INTERVENTIONS FOR CLIENTS WITH GYNECOLOGIC PROBLEMS

Nurses can play an important role in assessing gynecologic disorders by being sensitive to the client's complaints and by encouraging discussion about menstrual or other reproductive problems. Educating women about their bodies, helping them to recognize when professional help should be sought, and teaching them how to make informed decisions about treatments are major goals for nurses working with female clients in any setting.

MENSTRUAL CYCLE DISORDERS

Primary Dysmenorrhea

Overview

Dysmenorrhea, or painful menstrual flow, is one of the most common gynecologic problems. More than 50% of all women report some degree of dysmenorrhea and 10% are incapacitated. However, one study reported that 75% of women had some degree of discomfort and 15% were incapacitated (Somani, 1995). Dysmenorrhea is usually classified as primary or secondary.

Primary dysmenorrhea is not associated with pelvic pathologic changes, whereas secondary dysmenorrhea usually begins with an underlying disease condition.

Primary dysmenorrhea usually occurs after ovulation is established. Dysmenorrhea is painful uterine cramping. It is characterized by spasmodic lower abdominal pain that begins with the onset of menstrual flow and lasts 12 to 48 hours. The pain often radiates to the lower back and thighs, and nausea and vomiting frequently occur. Less common clinical manifestations include headache, syncope, nervousness, fatigue, diarrhea, bloating, and breast tenderness.

Primary dysmenorrhea occurs more frequently in women in their late teens or early 20s (Ling, 1995). The symptoms may be alleviated after vaginal childbirth.

Most researchers believe that the cause of primary dysmenorrhea is increased production and release of uterine prostaglandins. Prostaglandins are produced by the endometrium during the luteal phase of the menstrual cycle, and the levels peak at the onset of menses. Excessive prostaglandin levels stimulate the myometrium and cause severe spasms, which constrict uterine blood flow, resulting in ischemia and pain.

Collaborative Management

 Assessment

A thorough history of the client includes
- The age at menarche
- Characteristics of menstruation

1981

- Obstetric history
- Contraceptive history
- Type of pain
- Previous therapy

The nurse asks the client whether she has any conditions suggestive of pelvic problems. To plan nursing care, the nurse assesses emotional factors, such as the individual woman's response to dysmenorrhea, her attitudes about menstruation, and the extent to which dysmenorrhea is perceived to disrupt her life.

 Interventions

Interventions for primary dysmenorrhea include prevention, therapeutic measures, education, and support that are tailored to each woman's needs. Prostaglandin synthetase inhibitors (nonsteroidal antiinflammatory drugs) are currently recommended for pain relief. Prescription drugs approved for dysmenorrhea include ibuprofen (Motrin, Apo-Ibuprofen✦), naproxen sodium (Anaprox, Naprosyn), and mefenamic acid (Ponstel, Ponstan✦). Additionally, numerous over-the-counter ibuprofen products, such as Advil and Nuprin, provide pain relief for many clients with primary dysmenorrhea. Aspirin is a mild prostaglandin synthetase inhibitor and may relieve mild dysmenorrhea. All of these drugs can cause gastrointestinal (GI) distress and should, therefore, be taken with meals or milk.

To treat primary dysmenorrhea, the health care provider also uses ovulation inhibitors that decrease prostaglandin activity. Oral contraceptives, especially combination agents, may be prescribed for women who desire contraception as well as pain relief.

Complementary Therapies. Complementary therapies that may alleviate or prevent pain include acupressure, aerobic exercise, swimming, yoga or other meditation, application of heat or cold, massage, biofeedback, and relaxation techniques. Chapter 4 discusses most of these therapies. Nutritional measures for the prevention of pain include increasing the intake of vitamin B₆, calcium, magnesium, and protein and reducing the intake of sodium.

Premenstrual Syndrome

Overview

Millions of women experience emotional problems and physical discomfort associated with the menstrual cycle. These range from a mild awareness to disabling symptoms. The phenomenon, known as premenstrual syndrome (PMS), affects 5% to 95% of all women; about 38% are seriously affected (Klock, 1995).

Premenstrual syndrome is a collection of symptoms that are cyclic in nature, occurring each month during the luteal phase of the menstrual cycle; these symptoms are followed by relief with menses and a symptom-free phase. PMS affects women of all races, socioeconomic levels, and educational levels. It seems to be more prevalent in women 30–40 years old. The severity increases with aging until menopause. Women are at greater risk for PMS after pregnancy, childbirth, and tubal ligation; during the perimenopausal years; and during major life stresses.

The cause of PMS is not well understood. Neuroendocrine mechanisms seem to be involved, but whether there is a single syndrome or several is not known. The symptoms appear only in the luteal phase and disappear with menopause. Etiologic theories (Klock, 1995) include

- Estrogen-progesterone imbalance
- Vitamin and mineral deficiencies (e.g., of vitamin B₆ and magnesium
- Hypoglycemia (from altered carbohydrate intolerance in the luteal phase)
- Fluid retention (from high levels of aldosterone)
- Increased prolactin levels in the luteal phase
- Endogenous hormone allergy
- Prostaglandin imbalance
- Psychogenic and stress-related factors
- Thyroid abnormality
- Serotonin deficiency

Collaborative Management

 Assessment

There is no reported objective means of diagnosing PMS. Some researchers have attempted to differentiate premenstrual patterns (see Research Applications for Nursing). Determining the timing of the symptoms is as critical as noting the type of symptoms. The most effective and readily available assessment tool is a menstrual chart. The nurse instructs the client to keep a chart for at least three consecutive cycles, showing the length of the menstrual cycle, duration of bleeding, and occurrence of symptoms. If the woman has PMS, the symptoms recur during the luteal phase (from ovulation to menstruation), followed by a symptom-free time (at least 7 days). When taking a menstrual history, the nurse also assesses to what extent the woman feels that her activities of daily living (ADLs) are disrupted by the symptoms. Often reassurance that the symptoms are legitimate and that other women share these problems can help the client learn more about PMS.

Clinical manifestations vary greatly among women and affect many body systems (Chart 78–1).

 Interventions

Management of PMS focuses on eliminating the uncomfortable symptoms. Management is highly individualized; however, one of the most important interventions is education. Each woman needs information about her body, especially the menstrual cycle, so that she can begin to understand the physiologic basis of PMS.

Women may need to express their feelings and discuss their experiences with PMS; self-help groups and support groups are helpful resources. These groups also encourage significant others to participate, because PMS usually affects not only the woman but also her family and friends. For example, increased family conflict, communication problems with family and friends, and decreased family cohesion occur. Other coping strategies for the woman with PMS may include spiritual support, especially partic-

Research Applications for Nursing

Various Perimenstrual Symptom Patterns Exist Among Women

Mitchell E. S., Woods, N. F., & Lentz, M. J. (1994). Differentiation of women with three perimenstrual symptom patterns. Nursing Research, 43(1), 25–30.

The prevalence of premenstrual syndrome (PMS) among women of reproductive age ranges from 50% to more than 90%. Of these women with PMS, 2% to 17% experience disabling premenstrual symptoms. This study of 142 women from a community-based sample used retrospective self-reporting to differentiate women into one of three groups based on three perimenstrual symptom severity patterns. The three perimenstrual symptom severity patterns included premenstrual syndrome (PMS), premenstrual magnification (PMM), and low symptom (LS).

The profile for women with PMS compared with LS included more psychological distress, more years of education, and a mother with more premenstrual symptoms than the LS group. The PMM group also showed more psychological distress and mothers with premenstrual symptoms when compared with the LS group. The differentiating characteristics between PMS/LS and PMM/LS groups was that the PMM group had more negative effects from stressful life events, and these women were younger. Five variables were identified that differentiated women with PMS from PMM. PMS women tend to be older, have more education, engage in healthier behaviors, and have more nontraditional attitudes about the roles of women. PMM women have more stress than women with PMS.

Critique. This study, based on a moderate sample size, demonstrates a significant statistical difference between women with PMS and women with PMM. Although this study initially identified a large group of women to study, the final sample size was a limitation. Additionally, the study used retrospective self-reporting, a possible limitation of data collection.

Possible Nursing Implications. The identification of two distinct groups of women, those with PMS and those with PMM, has implications for diagnosis and treatment of women with perimenstrual symptoms. The nurse should assist the woman experiencing PMS and PMM with physical, psychological, and behavioral responses to health and illness. However, the best therapeutic interventions for these two distinct groups needs to be studied by nurse researchers.

ipating in religious services and seeking advice from spiritual leaders.

➤ Diet Therapy

Diet and nutrition are also important in managing PMS. If hypoglycemia occurs, the nurse instructs the woman to eat six small meals a day and to limit her intake of sugar, red meats, alcohol, coffee, tea, and chocolate.

Eliminating caffeine may help reduce irritability. Salt and sodium intake should be limited if edema occurs. Calcium, magnesium, and vitamins A, B_6, and C have been suggested for relief of PMS.

➤ Drug Therapy

Drug therapy remains controversial, but some treatments have been effective. Diuretics taken for 10 days before menstruation can provide relief for some women. Women may need to increase their intake of potassium-containing foods if they are receiving this therapy.

Progesterone may relieve physical and psychological symptoms. Natural progesterone is preferable to synthetic progesterone, even though the drug must be specially made by a pharmacist at the time it is prescribed. The daily dosage is 50 to 100 mg intramuscularly from ovulation to menstruation. Long-term side effects are unknown.

Bromocriptine mesylate (Parlodel), 2.5 mg two or three times a day with meals during the luteal phase, can relieve breast symptoms. The side effects (lightheadedness and hypotension) may not be well tolerated. Other drugs

---

Chart 78–1

Key Features of Premenstrual Syndrome

Dermatologic Manifestations
- Acne
- Urticaria
- Herpes

Respiratory Manifestations
- Sinusitis
- Asthma
- Rhinitis
- Colds

Urologic Manifestations
- Oliguria
- Cystitis
- Enuresis
- Urethritis

Ophthalmologic Manifestations
- Conjunctivitis
- Styes
- Glaucoma

Neurologic Manifestations
- Headaches
- Migraine
- Syncope
- Vertigo
- Numbness of hands and feet
- Epilepsy (if susceptible)

Metabolic Manifestations
- Edema
- Breast tenderness

Emotional or Psychological Manifestations
- Depression
- Irritability
- Tension
- Panic attacks
- Change in libido
- Mood swings
- Anxiety

Behavioral Manifestations
- Lowered work performance
- Food cravings
- Alcohol and drug overindulgence
- Confusion
- Sleeplessnses
- Lack of coordination
- Suicide
- Lethargy
- Child abuse
- Assaultive behavior

Other Manifestations
- Allergies
- Hypoglycemia
- Joint pain
- Backache
- Palpitations
- Water retention

for PMS that have been studied include birth control pills, gonadotropin-releasing hormone (GnRH) agonists, antidepressants, and prostaglandin inhibitors.

Amenorrhea

Overview

Amenorrhea (the absence of menstrual periods) can be either primary (menstruation that has failed to occur by age 16 years) or secondary (menstruation that has started but has since stopped and has not recurred for at least 3 months). Primary amenorrhea is often associated with anomalies of the reproductive tract, and the prognosis for fertility is usually poor. Secondary amenorrhea is probably due to a functional disorder, and the prognosis for fertility is better. Amenorrhea can cause a woman much distress and concern.

Menstruation is a complex series of events that rely on the interplay of the hypothalamic, pituitary, ovarian, and endometrial functions. Dysfunction related to any of these four factors may cause amenorrhea (Table 78–1). Primary amenorrhea is relatively uncommon. Congenital factors are responsible for about two thirds of cases, and the remaining one third of cases are caused by ovarian, pituitary, or hypothalamic disease. Pregnancy, lactation, and menopause are the most common physiologic causes of secondary amenorrhea.

TABLE 78–1

Common Causes of Amenorrhea

Primary
- Congenital anomalies
- Hypothalamic and pituitary disorders, such as delayed puberty
- Systemic disease
  - Thyroid and adrenal dysfunction
  - Diabetes mellitus
  - Extreme malnutrition
- Ovarian disease
- Malformations of the reproductive tract

Secondary
- Pregnancy
- Menopause
- Lactation
- Cervical stenosis
- Polycystic ovary disease
- Pituitary tumor or insufficiency
- Psychogenic stress
- Excessive physical activities
- Medications
  - Antihypertensive agents
  - Birth control pills
  - Phenothiazines
- Nutritional disorders
  - Obesity
  - Anorexia nervosa
  - Sudden weight loss
- Ovarian disease, failure, or destruction

Collaborative Management

 Assessment

The nurse asks about the family history, because girls tend to start menstruation within 2 years of the age when their mothers started. The nurse considers other factors when assessing primary amenorrhea:
- A family history of genetic abnormalities
- Ambiguous genitalia at birth
- Development of secondary sex characteristics
- Nutritional habits
- Past surgery
- Emotional stress

Physical assessment is extremely important in the evaluation of primary amenorrhea. The nurse notes certain factors associated with anomalies of the genital tract or hormonal causes (Laufer & Goldstein, 1995), such as lack of breast development, lack of pubic and axillary hair, and abnormality of the external genitalia.

Diagnosis can also be aided by pelvic examination, chromosomal studies, determination of serum prolactin levels, and hormone withdrawal tests.

The health care provider prescribes progesterone, 10 mg/day orally for 7 days, to stimulate withdrawal bleeding. Withdrawal bleeding usually indicates normal function of the hypothalamus, the pituitary gland, the ovary, and the uterus. Abnormal test results or dysfunction of these organs must be investigated further.

Assessment for secondary amenorrhea is similar to that for primary amenorrhea, but the nurse considers additional factors. Menstrual and obstetric histories are important. The nurse asks about possible sexual activity and symptoms of pregnancy. A medical history may identify a systemic disease as a cause of amenorrhea. The nurse asks about current eating habits and history of dieting because both obesity and starvation (e.g., anorexia nervosa) can contribute toward amenorrhea. Strenuous exercise associated with competitive athletics, such as long-distance running, can cause stress or a reduction in body fat, resulting in amenorrhea. The nurse assesses hormone deficiencies, such as those associated with menopause that can cause hot flashes and vaginal dryness. Women should be questioned about their ingestion of drugs (e.g., oral contraceptives, phenothiazines, and antihypertensives). The nurse is also alert for signs of galactorrhea (watery or milky breast secretions in nonbreastfeeding or nulliparous women) and hirsutism (unusual hair growth in women), both of which are related to polycystic ovary disease.

Interventions

The nurse's primary roles in implementing care are to explain amenorrhea in easily understandable terms and to answer questions about tests and treatments. The nurse also provides counseling and emotional support. Amenorrhea may be a threat to a woman's self-concept; she usually needs to ventilate her feelings about sexuality or fertility.

Interventions for specific causes of amenorrhea must be

based on each woman's needs. Medical and surgical management of amenorrhea is directed at the underlying causes. Treatment includes hormone replacement, ovulation stimulation, and periodic progesterone withdrawal.

Postmenopausal Bleeding

Overview

Postmenopausal bleeding (vaginal bleeding occurring after a 12-month cessation of menses after the onset of menopause) is a symptom rather than a medical diagnosis. Bleeding is considered serious and should be evaluated. Gynecologic cancer occurs in 20% to 40% of women who experience postmenopausal bleeding.

Postmenopausal bleeding can be caused by numerous benign and malignant conditions (Table 78–2). The three most common causes are atrophic vaginitis, cervical polyps, and endometrial abnormalities.

In a client with atrophic vaginitis, the vaginal mucosa is thin and dry and is easily traumatized by intercourse and infection, causing spotting. Cervical polyps are usually soft, red, oval tissue masses that appear within the cervical canal, and they may bleed spontaneously or after intercourse.

The most serious cause of postmenopausal bleeding is endometrial hyperplasia, a precursor of endometrial cancer. Bleeding is caused by declining ovarian function that leads to prolonged estrogen stimulation, producing the hyperplasia that eventually breaks down and bleeds. Estrogen stimulation can also be caused by estrogen replacement therapy (ERT).

Because many women who report postmenopausal bleeding need medical or surgical interventions, assessment is the nurse's major focus. The nurse assesses the menstrual and family history initially, including

- The client's age at menopause
- The frequency and amount of bleeding
- Previous bleeding episodes
- The use of medications (especially estrogen-only [unopposed estrogen] replacement therapy [ERT])
- The presence of gastrointestinal (GI) or genitourinary symptoms

TABLE 78–2

Common Causes of Postmenopausal Bleeding
Benign
• Estrogen therapy
• Endometrial hyperplasia
• Cervical polyps
• Uterine fibroids
• Atrophic vaginitis
• Cervical erosion
Maligant
• Endometrial cancer
• Cervical cancer
• Ovarian cancer
• Vaginal cancer
• Tubal cancer

The nurse also identifies women who are at high risk for endometrial cancer (e.g., women who are obese, hypertensive, or diabetic or who have never had children).

Urine and stool specimens can be collected and tested for blood to differentiate other sources of bleeding. Blood specimens may be drawn for hemoglobin or hematocrit determinations, because clients are often anemic as a result of excessive bleeding. The nurse can prepare the woman for physical and pelvic examinations, including obtaining specimens for a Papanicolaou test (Pap smear), which are usually done to evaluate the cause of bleeding.

Collaborative Management

Nursing interventions focus on providing information and support for diagnostic and treatment procedures directed at the specific causes of bleeding. An endometrial biopsy can evaluate the presence of malignancy. A diagnostic dilation and curettage (D&C) procedure can be used to determine malignancy (see Dysfunctional Uterine Bleeding later). Atypical hyperplasia is frequently treated with a hysterectomy (see Uterine Leiomyomas). Malignancy is usually treated with a combination of surgery, radiation therapy, and chemotherapy (see Endometrial Cancer).

The medical treatment of a woman receiving unopposed estrogen therapy may include the monthly administration of progesterone daily for the last 10 days of the estrogen therapy (days 16 to 25) or a one-time intramuscular (IM) progesterone injection. This treatment can reduce the abnormal endometrial proliferation and is suggested for the prevention of endometrial and breast cancer.

Atrophic vaginitis is managed by the administration of estrogen via vaginal, oral, transdermal, or subdermal route (Chart 78–2). Women who use vaginal estrogen cream need to be aware that it can cause systemic effects. Women who take estrogen may be at risk for gallbladder disease, hypertension, breast cancer, and endometrial cancer.

Endometriosis

Overview

Endometriosis is usually a benign disease characterized by implantation of endometrial tissue outside the uterine cavity. The tissue typically appears on the ovaries and the cul-de-sac and less commonly on other pelvic organs and structures (Fig. 78–1). A "chocolate" cyst is an area of endometriosis inside an ovary.

Endometrial tissue located outside the endometrium responds similarly to the endometrium to hormonal stimulation and goes through the same cyclic changes. Bleeding occurs at the site of implantation, and the blood is trapped in the tissues; scarring and adhesions result as the blood is reabsorbed. Endometriosis progresses slowly; it regresses during pregnancy and at menopause. Rarely does endometriosis become a malignant disease.

Etiology

The cause of endometriosis is unknown. The most accepted theories of causation are transportation and forma-

> **Chart 78–2**
>
> ### Education Guide: Estrogen Replacement Therapy
>
> **For All Types of Estrogen Replacement Therapy**
> - Call your health care provider if you have pain in your calves or groin, if you suddenly become short of breath, if you have abnormal vaginal bleeding, if you feel a lump in your breast, if you have a severe headache, or if you feel weak or numb in your arms or legs.
> - Use sunscreen if you are in the sun for a prolonged period.
> - Keep appointments for checkups.
> - If your health care provider has prescribed progesterone to decrease your risk of endometrial cancer, take it as prescribed.
>
> **For Oral Therapy**
> - Take one pill a day for the first 25 days each month.
> - If you feel nauseated or have intestinal upset, take your medication with food.
>
> **For Transdermal or Subdermal Administration**
> - Rotate the sites for the patches or injections to avoid skin irritation.
> - Change the patches twice a week, according to your prescribed schedule.
>
> **For Vaginal Therapy**
> - Use an applicator to insert the suppository or cream daily as prescribed.
> - You may need to wear a minipad to protect your clothing from soiling or staining by the drug.

tion. There are two transportation theories: (1) implantation and (2) vascular and lymphatic dissemination. The implantation theory holds that endometrial tissue flows back through the fallopian tubes during menstruation and then implants on pelvic structures. Proponents of the vascular and lymphatic dissemination theory say that endometrial glands are transported through the vascular and lymphatic system to foreign locations. This latter theory may explain implantation in areas outside the pelvis, such as the lungs and the kidneys. Formation theories propose that endometrial tissue develops spontaneously outside the uterus.

Incidence/Prevalence

Endometriosis occurs most frequently in women in their 30s and 40s; rarely does it appear before age 20. It is most common in nulliparous women and in those whose mothers had endometriosis. The prevalence of endometriosis in women of reproductive age is about 1% (Hornstein & Barbieri, 1995).

ELDERLY CONSIDERATIONS

 Endometriosis is rare after menopause, although it has been diagnosed in postmenopausal women on hormone replacement therapy (Weiss, 1995).

TRANSCULTURAL CONSIDERATIONS

 Compared with Caucasian women, African-American women have endometriosis less frequently.

Collaborative Management

 Assessment

The nursing assessment should be as detailed as possible and include the client's menstrual history, sexual history, and the characteristics of bleeding. Pain is the most common symptom of endometriosis. The peak of pain usually occurs just before the menstrual flow. Pain is usually located in the lower abdomen, causing many women to feel a sense of rectal pressure. The degree of pain is not related to the extent of the endometriosis, but it is related to the site. Often women with minimal disease have more severe pain than do women with extensive disease. Other clinical manifestations include dyspareunia (painful intercourse), painful defecation, sacral backache, hypermenorrhea (excessive, prolonged, or frequent bleeding), and infertility.

A pelvic examination may reveal pelvic tenderness, nodular uterosacral ligaments, and fixed or limited movement of the uterus. Psychosocial assessment may reveal anxiety because of uncertainty about the diagnosis. The woman may also have concerns about her self-concept if she is infertile and desires to become pregnant.

Diagnostic studies include blood tests (erythrocyte sedimentation rate [ESR] and white blood cell [WBC] count) to rule out pelvic inflammatory disease (PID) and ultrasonography to confirm or delineate pelvic masses that might be mistaken for endometriosis. Laparoscopy is the key diagnostic procedure for pelvic endometriosis. Examination of tissue specimens obtained during laparoscopy can confirm the diagnosis.

Interventions

Medical (hormonal) and surgical management may be used, depending on the symptoms, extent of disease, and

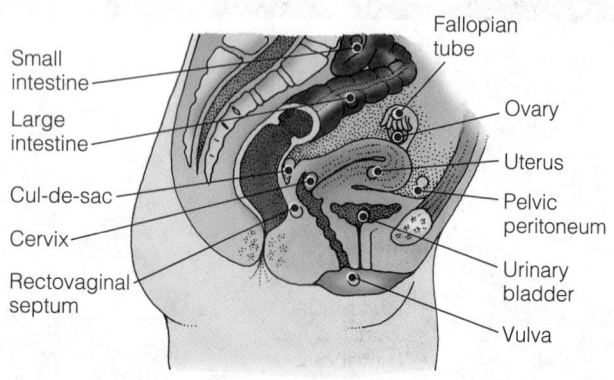

Figure 78–1. Common sites of endometriosis.

client's desire for childbearing. Nursing management is aimed at

- Reducing pain
- Restoring sexual function that was impaired by dyspareunia
- Alleviating anxiety related to the clinical manifestations of the disease and the uncertainty of the diagnosis
- Eliminating the client's knowledge deficit about the disease or its treatment
- Alleviating fear related to the possibility of laparoscopy or surgery
- Preventing self-esteem disturbance related to infertility

Several organizations such as the Endometriosis Society and RESOLVE (an organization for infertile couples) offer additional information on endometriosis that may be helpful in planning care.

Nonsurgical Management. Nonsurgical management involves the use of mild analgesics or prostaglandin synthetase inhibitors for pain relief. The health care provider also uses hormonal therapies to relieve pain by suppressing ovulation. The hormonal therapies produce pseudopregnancy, pseudomenopause, or medical oophorectomy.

Pseudopregnancy is induced with oral contraceptives or progesterone. The health care provider usually prescribes a 6-month course of a low-dose estrogen oral contraceptive, followed by cyclic oral contraceptive use or therapy with progesterone alone.

The second hormonal treatment causes ovarian suppression, or pseudomenopause, by the use of danazol (Danocrine, Cyclomen*), an antigonadotropin testosterone derivative. This therapeutic approach is the current choice of many health care providers, but it is expensive ($120–$180/month) and may cause undesirable side effects. Side effects include acne, hirsutism (abnormal hair growth in unwanted areas), weight gain, decreased breast size, and hot flashes.

The third hormonal treatment is use of gonadotropin-releasing hormone (GnRH) agonists to produce a reversible medical oophorectomy. The drug can be administered by intramuscular or subcutaneous injection or by nasal spray. Side effects include hot flashes, vaginal dryness, and insomnia.

Complementary Therapies. Complementary therapies that can relieve pain include the application of a heating pad to the abdomen or sacrum, relaxation techniques, yoga, and biofeedback.

These approaches may decrease muscle tissue hypoxia and hypertonicity and relieve ischemia by increasing blood flow to the affected areas.

Surgical Management. Surgical management of endometriosis for a woman who wants to remain fertile is conservative and involves removal of endometrial implants and adhesions. The surgeon may use a carbon dioxide laser to treat endometriosis by vaporizing adhesions and endometrial implants. If the client does not wish to have children, the uterus and ovaries may be removed.

Dysfunctional Uterine Bleeding

Overview

Dysfunctional uterine bleeding (DUB), a nonspecific diagnostic term, is bleeding that is excessive or abnormal in amount or frequency without predisposing anatomic or systemic conditions. It is estimated that DUB is responsible for 10% to 15% of the complaints of abnormal bleeding reported by women seeking gynecologic care (Dawood, 1995).

Normally, the menstrual cycle represents a series of complex hormonal events related to balanced hypothalamic, pituitary, ovarian, and uterine functions. Menses, the sloughing of the endometrial lining, is an expected result. DUB occurs when there is a breakdown of these functions, causing hormonal imbalance.

The mechanism of DUB is unknown, but several theories have linked it with endometrial or myometrial dysfunction. Excessive fibrinolytic activity in the endometrium and changes in prostaglandin production in the uterus may also cause DUB.

Generally, DUB occurs in the absence of ovulation that is associated with ovarian dysfunction. Estrogen stimulation of the endometrium is prolonged, and the endometrium grows past its hormonal support, causing bleeding and desquamation.

Anovulatory DUB during the reproductive years is associated with

- Polycystic ovary disease
- Stress
- Extreme weight changes
- Long-term drug use (e.g., of anticholinergics, reserpine, morphine, and oral contraceptives)

Ovulatory causes of DUB are uncommon and are related to a dysfunctional corpus luteum, irregular maturation, and shedding of the endometrium.

Dysfunctional uterine bleeding occurs most often at either end of the span of a woman's reproductive years, when ovulation is becoming established or when it is becoming irregular at menopause. DUB most commonly occurs in adolescents and women older than 50 years (Dawood, 1995).

Collaborative Management

 Assessment

When interviewing a woman with DUB, the nurse takes a complete menstrual history. The nurse also asks about illnesses, variations in weight or diet, exercise, drug ingestion, and presence of pain.

During the physical assessment, the nurse observes for symptoms of anemia or systemic disease, such as

- Renal or hepatic disease
- Obesity
- Undernutrition
- Abnormal hair growth related to hormonal dysfunction
- Evidence of abdominal pain or masses

An examination that includes inspection of the external

TABLE 78-3

Nursing Care of Clients Undergoing Surgery for Dysfunctional Uterine Bleeding		
	Dilation and Curettage (D&C)	**Endometrial Ablation**
Usual site	• Outpatient	• Outpatient
Anesthesia	• Local, regional, general	• Regional, general
Procedure	• The cervical os is dilated; the endometrium is scraped.	• The laser fiber is passed into the uterus through a hysteroscope; the endometrium is destroyed by laser energy, and tissues are removed by irrigating the uterine cavity with saline.
Preoperative care	• Assess the client's knowledge of the procedure.	• Same as for D&C
	• The client is NPO after midnight.	• The client may be given danazol or GnRH agonist for 1 month before surgery to decrease endometrial thickness.
	• Teach postoperative expectations.	• Counsel the client about the likelihood of sterility as a result of uterine scarring.
Postoperative care	• Monitor vital signs every 15 minutes until they are stable.	• Same as for D&C
	• Assess the need for pain relief.	• Same as for D&C
	• Assess for vaginal bleeding.	• Assess for spotting and vaginal drainage.
	• Expect discharge when the client is stable.	• Same as for D&C

genitalia and bimanual pelvic and rectal examination is essential to identify lesions or tenderness. A physician, a nurse practitioner, or a nurse-midwife performs the internal pelvic examination.

Pelvic ultrasonography and hysteroscopy may be performed. In addition, the surgeon usually does an endometrial biopsy by suction aspiration or dilation and curettage (D&C). These are important procedures for women older than 40 years, who are at greater risk for endometrial cancer.

 Interventions

Nonsurgical management is usually the treatment of choice, although surgery may be needed to treat DUB.

Nonsurgical Management. Most women can be treated successfully with hormonal manipulation. For women with anovulatory DUB, the health care provider typically prescribes medroxyprogesterone acetate (Depo-Provera) or combination oral contraceptives. If the client takes oral contraceptives, she should take one pill a day for 21 or 28 days, beginning on the first day of the menstrual cycle. Medroxyprogesterone is taken on days 16 to 25 of each month. Monthly withdrawal bleeding is expected with both therapies.

Women with ovulatory DUB may be treated with progestins during the luteal phase, oral contraceptives, prostaglandin inhibitors, or danazol. The nurse explains the desired and side effects of these drugs and evaluates the woman's knowledge of the effects, dosage and administration schedule.

Surgical Management. Surgical management includes D&C, laser endometrial ablation, and hysterectomy. A D&C procedure is usually used to treat an acute episode

of bleeding. Endometrial ablation is used for women who do not respond to medical management or who do not need a hysterectomy. A hysterectomy is usually performed only after other treatments have failed. Table 78-3 com-

Chart 78-3

Education Guide: Endometrial Ablation and Dilation and Curettage

Endometrial Ablation
• Spotting and vaginal drainage are normal for several days after the procedure.
• If you have abdominal cramping take mild analgesics, such a acetaminophen (Tylenol), or prostaglandin inhibitors, such as ibuprofen (Motrin).
• You can return to your normal activities within 2 or 3 days.
• You will probably be sterile because of uterine scarring.

Dilation and Curettage
• Take your temperature once a day for the next 2 days. If your oral temperature is more than 100° F (38° C), call the clinic or your doctor.
• Avoid sexual intercourse, tub bathing, and the use of tampons for 2 weeks to allow healing and prevent infection.
• Slight bleeding is normal. However, if bleeding is as heavy as during your normal menstrual period or if bleeding lasts longer than 2 weeks, call the clinic or health care provider.
• You can use a heating pad or hot water bottle to relieve abdominal cramping if it occurs.
• You can take mild analgesics, such as acetaminophen (Tylenol, Atasol✦), for pain.

pares the preoperative and postoperative care of clients undergoing D&C or endometrial ablation. Hysterectomy is discussed later under Uterine Leiomyomas.

If the woman has a D&C or laser ablation, the nurse gives the client postoperative instructions (Chart 78–3).

INFLAMMATIONS AND INFECTIONS

Vaginal discharge and itching are two of the most common complaints of female clients. Women may need information from their health care provider about the normal vaginal physiology, causes of symptoms, and methods of treatment. The nurse must be well informed about these topics to provide comprehensive care to clients with vaginal infections.

Vaginal infections are sometimes considered sexually transmitted diseases (STDs) because their causative organisms may be transmitted to sexual partners. However, infections can develop without sexual contact, and sexual partners do not always become infected. (Other true STDs, such as gonorrhea, syphilis, chlamydial infection, and herpes simplex virus infection, are discussed in Chapter 80. Acquired immunodeficiency syndrome [AIDS] is covered in Chapter 25.)

Simple Vaginitis

Overview

Vaginitis can develop whenever there is a disturbance of the balance of hormones and bacterial interaction in the vagina caused by

- Changes in the normal flora
- Alkaline pH
- Insertion of foreign bodies, such as tampons and condoms
- Chemical irritations, such as from douches or sprays
- Medications, especially antibiotics

Vaginitis is an inflammation of the lower genital tract. The nurse completes the assessment of vaginitis by asking questions about the symptoms, assisting with a pelvic examination, and obtaining vaginal smears for laboratory testing (Chart 78–4). The nurse is nonjudgmental and reassuring during the assessment because the client may be embarrassed or afraid to discuss her symptoms.

Collaborative Management

Interventions for vaginitis depend on the causes and the specific vaginal infection (Table 78–4). A woman's proper health habits can be beneficial to treatment. Therefore, she should get enough rest and sleep, observe good nutritional habits, get regular exercise, and use good personal hygiene. Popular, but not scientifically tested, hygiene practices to prevent vaginitis include

- Perineal cleaning (wiping front to back) after urinating or defecating
- Wearing cotton underwear
- Avoiding strong douches and feminine hygiene sprays
- Avoiding tight-fitting pants

Chart 78–4

Nursing Care Highlight: The Client with Simple Vaginitis

- In taking a client history, ask about
  - Onset of symptoms
  - Characteristics of the discharge, especially the color and odor
  - Associated symptoms such as itching and dysuria
  - Types of contraceptives used
  - Recent use of antibiotics
  - Client's sexual activity
  - Any history of vaginal infection
  - Client's hygiene practices: douching and using tampons
- In performing a physical examination,
  - Palpate the abdomen for tenderness or pain.
  - Inspect the external genitalia for erythema, edema, excoriation, odor, and discharge.
  - If you are qualified, perform a speculum examination to visualize the vagina and cervix, and note the source of any discharge or inflammation.
- If you are qualified, perform the following laboratory tests, as ordered: a saline or potassium hydroxide wet smear and a nitrazine paper test of vaginal pH.

If antibiotics are prescribed, eating yogurt or taking *Lactobacillus* culture (Lactinex) tablets may help restore the natural flora (Döderlein's bacilli) of the vagina.

Education of the client focuses on preventive measures and on information about infection transmission (Chart 78–5).

Vulvitis

Overview

Vulvitis is an inflammatory condition of the vulva that is associated with symptoms of pruritus (itching) and a burning sensation. The vulvar skin is sensitive to hormonal, metabolic, and allergic influences. Symptoms can be caused by systemic conditions, direct contact with irritants, and extension of infections from the vagina.

The most common skin disease affecting the vulva is contact dermatitis, which can be caused by an irritant, such as feminine hygiene sprays, fabric dyes, soaps and detergents, and allergens. Primary infections that affect the vulva include herpes genitalis and condyloma acuminatum (venereal wart) (see Chap. 80). Secondary infections of the vulva are caused by organisms responsible for the numerous types of vaginitis, including candidiasis in diabetic women. Pediculosis pubis (crab lice infestation) and scabies (itch mite infestation) are common parasitic infestations of the skin of the vulva. Other causes of vulvitis include

- Atrophic vaginitis (see earlier)
- Vulvar kraurosis (a postmenopausal disorder causing dryness and atrophy)
- Vulvar leukoplakia (postmenopausal atrophy and thickening of vulvar tissues)

TABLE 78–4

Common Vaginal Infections

Etiology	Sexual Transmission	Assessment		Drug Therapy
		Physical Findings	Laboratory Findings	
Candida albicans infection	• Unlikely	• Odorless, white, curd-like discharge • Patches on vaginal walls and cervix • Inflamed vaginal walls and cervix • Itching	• Hyphae and spores visible on potassium hydroxide wet slide • Vaginal pH 4.5 or less	• Miconazole nitrate (Monistat), clotrimazone (Gyne-Lotrimin), or nystatin (Mycostatin) vaginal creams or suppositories for 7 days • Terconazol (Terazol) cream or suppositories for 7 days or double strength for 3 days • Tioconazole (Vagistat) single-dose vaginal application
Trichomonas vaginalis infection	• Yes	• None or fishy • Itching • Strawberry spot on vaginal surface and cervix	• Flagellated, pear-shaped protozoa on saline wet slide • Vaginal pH 6–7	• Oral metronidazole (Flagyl), single 2-g dose for client and sexual partners
Bacterial vaginosis/ *Gardnerella vaginalis* infection	• Yes	• Gray-white or green discharge • Fishy odor • Itching • Normal vaginal mucosa • 10%–40% asymptomatic	• "Clue" cells on examination of saline wet slide • Positive "whiff" test finding • Vaginal pH 5–6	• Oral metronidazole, 500 mg qid for 7 days, or ampicillin or tetracycline • Clindamycin, 450 mg qid for 7 days
Cervicitis	• Yes	• Mucopurulent discharge from endocervix • Pelvic pain, postcoital and intermenstrual bleeding • The cervix may be inflamed and bleed when touched	• Need to rule out herpes, gonorrhea, and chlamydia infection • Vaginal pH 4.5 or less	• Depends on diagnosis
Atrophic vaginitis	• No	• Pale, thin, dry mucosa • Itching • No odor • Scant white, yellow, gray, or green discharge • Dyspareunia, postcoital bleeding	• Parabasal cells • Leukocyte predominance • Vaginal pH 6	• Topical conjugated estrogen cream, $\frac{1}{2}$ to 1 application at night for 7 nights, then twice weekly

■ Cancer
■ Urinary incontinence

Collaborative Management

Assessment of the woman usually identifies symptoms of itching and burning sensation. Erythema, edema, and superficial skin ulcers also may be present. Some women may have an itch-scratch-itch cycle, in which the itching leads to scratching, which causes excoriation that then must heal. As healing takes place, itching occurs again, which leads to further scratching. If the cycle is not interrupted, the condition can become chronic, causing the vulvar skin to become white and thickened (leathery). This skin is dry and scaly and cracks easily, increasing the woman's chances of infection.

Medical treatment of clients with vulvitis depends on the cause. Nursing interventions to relieve itching include applying wet compresses (Burow's solution diluted 1:20) to the affected area for 30 minutes several times a day, followed by cool air–drying with a hair dryer. Other helpful measures include sitz baths for 30 minutes several times a day and the application of prescribed topical medications, such as hydrocortisone and fluorinated corticosteroids (betamethasone valerate [Valisone, Betaderm✦] or fluocinolone acetonide [Synalar, Fluoderm✦]).

The health care provider prescribes oral antibiotics if infection is the underlying cause. Removal of any irritant or allergen should be accomplished, such as by changing detergents. Treatment of pediculosis and scabies can be instituted if appropriate. This entails the application of lindane (1% gamma benzene hexachloride [Kwell, Kwellada✦]) lotion, shampoo, or cream to the affected area as directed; cleaning affected clothes, bedding, and towels; and disinfecting the home environment (lice cannot live more than 24 hours away from the body).

If the vulvitis is chronic or severe, laser therapy (see Cervical Cancer later) or "skinning" vulvectomy (see Vulvar Cancer) may be performed. Preventive measures that may be helpful for vulvitis are listed in Chart 78–6.

Toxic Shock Syndrome

Overview

Toxic shock syndrome (TSS) was infrequently recognized by health care providers until 1980, when it was found to be related to menstruation and tampon use. Other conditions that have been associated with TSS include surgical wound infection, nonsurgical focal infections, postpartum conditions, and nonmenstrual vaginal conditions.

The pathophysiology of TSS is not clearly understood. Certain strains of *Staphylococcus aureus* produce a toxin that has been associated with the symptoms of TSS. Numerous theories have been reported to explain the mechanism of *S. aureus* absorption in TSS. The vagina may be highly susceptible to the toxin released by *S. aureus*.

In menstrually related TSS, the theories about the mechanisms of absorption focus on tampon use. Risk for TSS is related to the degree of absorbency of the tampon. Possible explanations include the following:

- Toxins readily cross the vaginal mucosa.
- Highly absorbent tampons rub the vaginal walls and cause ulceration, which allows transport of the toxins.

Health Promotion: Prevention of Toxic Shock Syndrome

Tampon Use

- Wash your hands before inserting a tampon.
- Do not use a tampon if it is dirty.
- Insert the tampon carefully to avoid injuring the delicate tissue in your vagina.
- Change your tampon every 3 to 6 hours.
- Do not use superabsorbent tampons.
- Use sanitary napkins at night.
- Call your health care provider if you suddenly experience a high temperature, vomiting, or diarrhea.
- Do not use tampons at all if you have had toxic shock syndrome.
- Not using tampons almost guarantees that you will not get toxic shock syndrome.

Vaginal Sponge Use

- Wash your hands before inserting a vaginal sponge.
- Use only clean water to wet the sponge.
- Do not use the sponge if it is dirty.
- Do not use the sponge for more than 30 hours at a time.
- Call your health care provider if you have two or more symptoms of toxic shock syndrome.

Diaphragm Use

- Wash your hands and the diaphragm before insertion.
- Remove the diaphragm within 24 hours after intercourse.
- Do not use the diaphragm during your menstrual period.
- After you take out the diaphragm, wash it with mild soap, rinse it, and dry it. Coating the diaphragm with a small amount of cornstarch will absorb any excess water and prevent damage to the latex rubber. Store it in a clean, dry place.

- Prolonged or continued tampon use can cause chronic vaginal ulcerations through which *S. aureus* is absorbed.
- Plastic tampon inserters can cause ulceration through which toxins are transported.
- Toxin producing *S. aureus* has a growth requirement for magnesium (some tampons contain magnesium) (Tuomala, 1995).

Use of the diaphragm, cervical cap, and vaginal contraceptive sponge has also been linked to TSS.

Collaborative Management

Influenza-like symptoms for the first 24 hours are common. The abrupt onset of a high temperature associated with a headache, sore throat, vomiting, diarrhea, generalized rash, and hypotension are often present. The most common clinical manifestations are skin changes (initially a rash resembling a severe sunburn that changes to a macular erythema similar to a drug-related rash). Because not all women experience all these clinical manifestations, the criteria established by the U.S. Centers for Disease Control and Prevention (CDC) are used in epidemiologic studies to verify cases of TSS (Chart 78-7).

Management in the primary care setting focuses on client education and prevention. The nurse instructs the client on the prevention of TSS related to the use of tampons, vaginal sponges, and diaphragms (Chart 78-8).

Primary treatment in the acute care setting includes fluid replacement, because dehydration and electrolyte imbalance result from vomiting and diarrhea. The health care provider also prescribes antibiotics, such as nafcillin and cephalosporins, if the penicillin-resistant strain of *S. aureus* is the cause of TSS. Other measures may include administering transfusions to reverse low platelet counts, corticosteroids to treat skin changes, and drugs to treat hypotension.

PROBLEMS RELATED TO PELVIC SUPPORT TISSUES

Uterine Displacement

Overview

Normally, the uterus lies in the midline of the pelvis and is freely movable. The cervix is located posteriorly in the vagina, and the body of the uterus has a slight degree of anterior flexion (Fig. 78-2). Variations from this position can result from congenital or acquired weakness of the pelvic support structures. The most common variation is posterior displacement of the uterus (retroversion). The uterus is tilted posteriorly, and the cervix rotates anteriorly. Other variations include retroflexion, anteversion, and anteflexion (Fig. 78-3).

Collaborative Management

The woman with uterine displacement may be asymptomatic, or she may report a history of backaches, secondary amenorrhea, infertility, dyspareunia (painful intercourse), and feelings of pelvic pressure of heaviness.

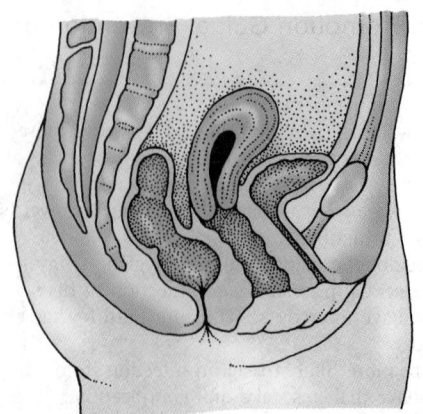

Figure 78-2. The normal position of the uterus.

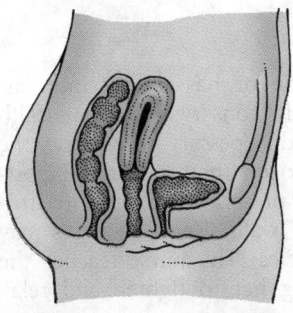
In **retroversion**, the uterus *tilts posteriorly*, and the cervix rotates anteriorly.

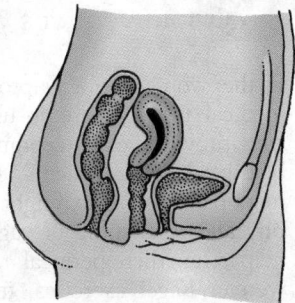
In **retroflexion**, the uterus *bends posteriorly.*

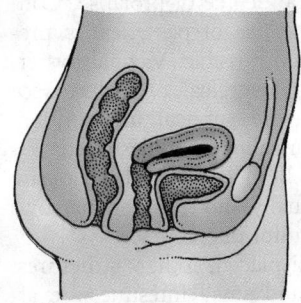
In **anteversion**, the uterus *tilts anteriorly.*

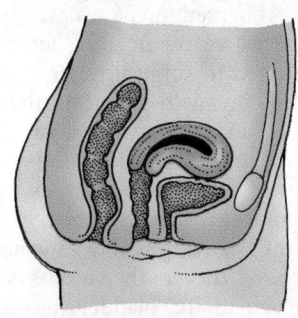
In **anteflexion**, the uterus *bends anteriorly.*

Figure 78–3. Types of uterine displacement.

If symptoms are uncomfortable, several interventions may be implemented. To correct a mildly retroverted uterus, a woman may assume a knee-chest position for a few minutes several times a day. The health care provider may insert a vaginal pessary (a rubber, donut-shaped device) in the vagina to hold the uterus in correct position. A pessary that is inserted correctly should not be felt by the woman. However, the vaginal mucosa may become irritated, and measures to keep the vaginal pH at 4 to 4.5 are implemented. For example, the nurse suggests commercially prepared douches or solutions of 1 tablespoon (15 mL) of vinegar to 1 quart (about 1 L) of water for use twice a week.

Uterine Prolapse

Overview

Three stages of uterine prolapse have been described according to the degree of descent of the uterus (Fig. 78–4). Prolapse of the uterus can be caused by congenital defects, persistent high levels of intra-abdominal pressure related to heavy physical labor or exertion, or any other event that weakens the pelvic supports.

ELDERLY CONSIDERATIONS

Prolapse is often a complication of childbirth injuries, and repetitive stresses occurring many years later, but it also occurs in elderly nulliparas. The pelvic floor that supports the uterus is weakened by aging.

TRANSCULTURAL CONSIDERATIONS

The incidence of prolapsed uterus is high in Caucasian women and low among African-American and Asian-American women.

Collaborative Management

Certain data may alert a nurse that a client may have a prolapsed uterus. These assessment findings include a feeling that the client relates (e.g., "something is in my vagina"), dyspareunia, backache, a feeling of heaviness or pressure in the pelvis, and bowel or bladder problems (if cystocele or rectocele is also present). A pelvic examination may reveal a protrusion of the cervix when the woman is asked to bear down.

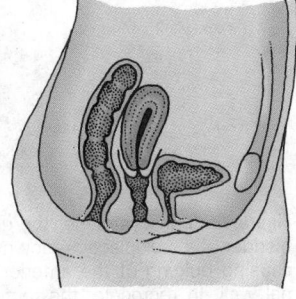
In **grade I uterine prolapse**, the uterus bulges into the vagina, but the cervix does not protrude through the entrance to the vagina.

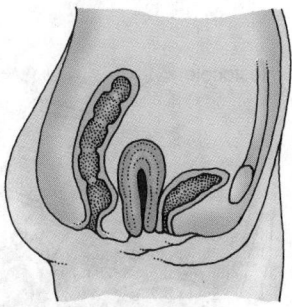
In **grade II uterine prolapse**, the uterus bulges farther into the vagina, and the cervix protrudes through the entrance to the vagina.

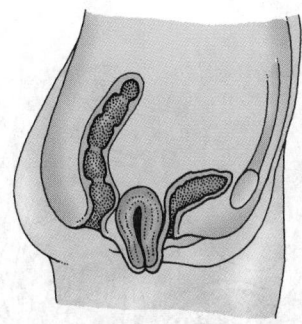
In **grade III uterine prolapse**, the body of the uterus and the cervix protrude through the entrance to the vagina. The vagina is turned inside out.

Figure 78–4. Types of uterine prolapse.

Interventions are based on the degree of prolapse. Conservative treatment, such as the use of pessaries, is preferred to surgical treatment when possible. Vaginal hysterectomy with repair is the usual surgical procedure (see Uterine Leiomyomas later). Before surgical intervention, the nurse questions the woman about her desire for future childbearing (surgery may be delayed) and her desire for coital activities. Surgery usually shortens and narrows the vagina, possibly causing painful intercourse.

Whenever the uterus is displaced, other structures, such as the bladder, rectum, and small intestine, are affected and can protrude through the vaginal walls.

Cystocele

Overview

A cystocele is a protrusion of the bladder through the vaginal wall (Fig. 78–5). It is due to weakened pelvic structures. This protrusion can be caused by obesity, advanced age, childbearing, or genetic predisposition.

The development of a cystocele is more noticeable in the postmenopausal years, when estrogen loss also weakens tissue supports and can cause relaxation of the supports.

Collaborative Management

 Assessment

Assessment findings may include
- Difficulty in emptying the bladder
- Urinary frequency and urgency
- Urinary tract infection
- Stress urinary incontinence (loss of urine during stressful activities such as laughing, coughing, sneezing, and lifting heavy objects)

A pelvic examination reveals a significant bulge of the anterior vaginal wall when the woman is asked to bear down. Diagnostic tests that may be ordered include cystography (to show the presence of bladder herniation), measurement of residual urine by catheterization, and urine culture and sensitivity testing (which may reveal infection caused by urinary retention).

 Interventions

If the woman is asymptomatic or has mild symptoms, medical management is usually conservative. The health care provider may recommend a pessary to support the bladder in some clients. Estrogen therapy for the postmenopausal woman might be prescribed to prevent atrophy and weakening of vaginal walls. Kegel exercises may help strengthen perineal muscles. The nurse teaches the woman Kegel exercises, telling her to tighten and relax the perineal muscles; the woman presses the buttocks together and holds the position for at least 5 seconds. The woman should repeat the exercise frequently throughout the day. An alternative exercise is having the woman try to stop the flow of urine after she has started urinating, holding the position for a few seconds before letting the urine flow again.

The health care provider may recommend surgery for severe symptoms. An anterior colporrhaphy (anterior repair) tightens the pelvic muscles for better bladder support. A vaginal surgical approach is used. Nursing care of a woman having an anterior repair is similar to that for a woman having surgery for vaginal hysterectomy (see Uterine Leiomyomas later).

Postoperatively, the nurse instructs the client to limit her activities, not lift anything heavier than 5 pounds, avoid strenuous exercises, and avoid sexual intercourse for 6 weeks. The woman should notify her health care provider if she has signs of infection: fever, persistent pain, and purulent, foul-smelling discharge. The nurse stresses the importance of keeping the follow-up appointment.

Rectocele

Overview

A rectocele is a protrusion of the rectum through a weakened vaginal wall (see Fig. 78–5). It can result from the pressure of a baby's head during a difficult delivery, a traumatic forceps delivery, or a congenital defect of the supporting tissues. Symptoms do not usually appear until the woman is older than 35 years.

Cystocele

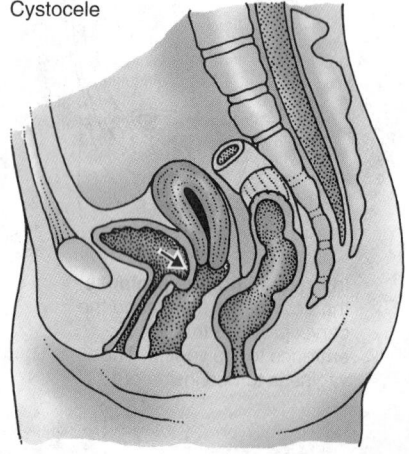

Rectocele

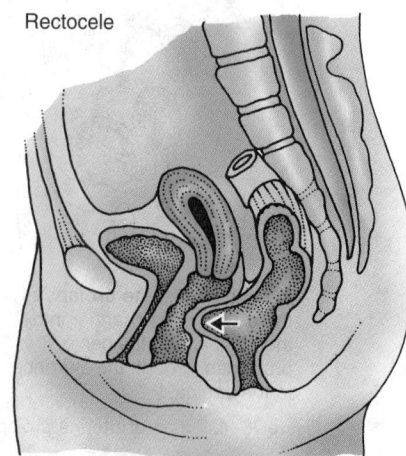

Figure 78–5. In cystocele, the urinary bladder is displaced downward, causing bulging of the anterior vaginal wall. In rectocele, the rectum is displaced, causing bulging of the posterior vaginal wall.

Collaborative Management

The woman's history may reveal symptoms of constipation, hemorrhoids, fecal impaction, and feelings of rectal or vaginal fullness. A pelvic examination may show a bulge of the posterior vaginal wall when the woman is asked to bear down. A rectal examination reveals the presence of a rectocele. A barium enema study also confirms the presence of a rectocele.

Medical management focuses on promoting bowel elimination. The health care provider usually orders a high-fiber diet, stool softeners, and laxatives. The surgical procedure that strengthens pelvic supports and reduces the bulging is posterior colporrhaphy (posterior repair). If both a cystocele and rectocele are present, an anterior and posterior colporrhaphy (anterior and posterior [A&P] repair) is performed.

The nursing care after a posterior repair is similar to that after rectal surgery. Postoperatively, the woman is usually given a low-residue diet to prevent bowel movements and allow time for the incision to heal. The woman is informed not to strain when she does have a bowel movement so that she does not put pressure on the suture line. Bowel movements are often painful, and the client may need pain medication before having a bowel movement. Sitz baths may relieve discomfort. Postoperative instructions for the client having a posterior repair are similar to those for anterior repair.

Fistulas

Overview

Fistulas are abnormal openings between two adjacent organs and are infrequent complications of gynecologic surgery. Vaginal fistulas can occur between the vagina and the urethra (urethrovaginal), the bladder (vesicovaginal), and the rectum (rectovaginal) (Fig. 78–6). Trauma is the primary cause of fistulas, although they can result from complications of surgery, obstetric complications, the spread of malignancy, and radiation therapy for cancer.

Collaborative Management

Symptoms depend on the location of the fistula. A fistula should be considered as a possible cause if a woman's history includes the following complaints:

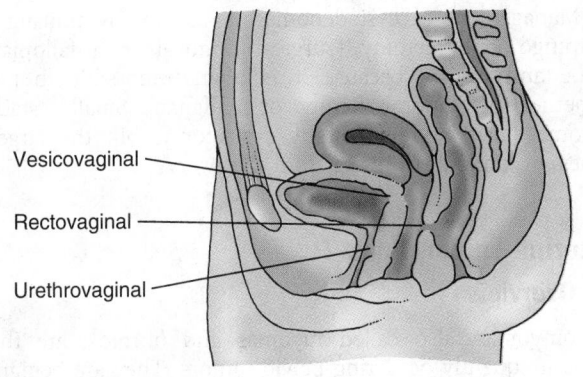

Figure 78–6. Sites of vaginal fistulas.

- Urine, flatus, or feces leaking into the vagina
- Irritation or excoriation of the vulva and vaginal tissues
- Unpleasant odor (fecal or urine) in the vagina
- Feeling wet or dribbling in the vagina

Women who have fistulas may be embarrassed to seek help until symptoms are severe. The client may withdraw from social activities or from relationships with significant others as the symptoms become more difficult to manage.

Management depends on the fistula's location. Surgery is not recommended if infection or inflammation is present. Surgery may not be successful. Nursing care focuses on assisting the woman with the frequent and time-consuming perineal hygiene: sitz baths, perineal cleaning with mild unscented soap and water, and low-pressure douching with commercial deodorizing solutions or homemade solutions (1 teaspoon [5 mL] of nonchlorine household bleach to 1 quart [approximately 1 L] of water). The woman may need to wear sanitary napkins or undergarments (such as Depends) if there is leakage of urine or feces. Other beneficial treatments may include the use of heat lamps for irritated areas and the application of A and D ointment to excoriated tissues.

If the fistula is repaired surgically, the nurse focuses on preventing infection and avoiding stress on the repaired area (low-residue diet and administration of stool softeners for 2 weeks after rectovaginal fistula repair). Nursing care and postoperative teaching are similar to the care and teaching of the client who has a cystocele or rectocele repair (see earlier).

BENIGN NEOPLASMS
Functional Ovarian Cysts

Functional ovarian cysts can occur in a woman of any age but are rare after menopause.

Follicular Cysts

Follicular cysts usually occur in young, menstruating females. These cysts are non-neoplastic and do not grow without hormonal influences. A cyst can develop when a mature follicle fails to rupture or an immature follicle fails to reabsorb follicular fluid during the second half of the menstrual cycle. The cyst is usually small (< 2.4–3.2 inches [6–8 cm]) and may be asymptomatic unless it ruptures. Rupture of a follicular cyst or torsion (twisting) may cause acute, severe pelvic pain. The pain usually resolves after several days of bed rest and administration of mild analgesics. If the cyst does not rupture, it usually disappears within two or three menstrual cycles without medical intervention. If the cyst does not shrink, the health care provider may prescribe oral contraceptive pills for one or two menstrual cycles to depress ovulation. Follow-up care is necessary when the cyst is managed conservatively to confirm that it has disappeared.

If the cyst is larger than 6 to 8 cm, a neoplasm may be suspected, and further evaluation by ultrasonography or laparoscopy is necessary. Larger cysts are often associated with menstrual irregularities.

Surgery is recommended only before puberty, after menopause, or when cysts are larger than 3.2 inches (8 cm). A cystectomy (removal of the cyst) is recommended instead of an oophorectomy (removal of the ovary).

Corpus Luteum Cysts

Corpus luteum cysts occur after ovulation and are often associated with increased secretion of progesterone. The cysts are usually small, averaging 1.5 inches (4 cm). They are purplish-red as a result of hemorrhage within the corpus luteum. Corpus luteum cysts are associated with a delay in the onset of menses and irregular or prolonged flow. They may also be accompanied by unilateral low abdominal or pelvic pain that is usually described as dull or aching. If the cyst ruptures, intraperitoneal hemorrhage can occur.

Corpus luteum cysts may disappear in one or two menstrual cycles or with suppression of ovulation. The treatment is the same as that for follicular cysts.

Theca-Lutein Cysts

Theca-lutein cysts are the least common of the functional cysts. They are associated with hydatidiform mole (molar pregnancy), occurring in 50% of these complicated pregnancies. Theca-lutein cysts develop as a result of prolonged stimulation of the ovaries by excessive amounts of human chorionic gonadotropin (hCG).

Theca-lutein cysts regress spontaneously within 3 months with the removal of the molar pregnancy or the source of excessive hCG. No other treatment is usually necessary.

Polycystic Ovary

Polycystic ovary, or Stein-Leventhal syndrome, results when elevated levels of luteinizing hormone (LH) cause hyperstimulation of the ovaries, which produces multiple cysts on one or both ovaries. High levels of estrogen are produced by these cysts and are unopposed by postovulatory progesterone. Endometrial hyperplasia or even carcinoma may result.

A typical client is obese, is hirsute (hairy), has irregular menses, and may be infertile because of anovulation. Treatment depends on which disorder is of greatest concern to the woman. The best treatment is the administration of oral contraceptives because they inhibit LH production. The health care provider may advise a woman who is older than 35 years and no longer desires childbearing to have a bilateral salpingo-oophorectomy (BSO) (removal of both tubes and ovaries) and hysterectomy (removal of the uterus and cervix). Women who desire fertility can be treated with drugs such as clomiphene citrate (Clomid) to stimulate ovulation.

Other Benign Ovarian Cysts and Tumors

Dermoid Cysts

Dermoid cysts are the most common germ cell tumors and are benign in more than 99% of cases. These cysts are the most common ovarian tumors of childhood, although they can develop in a female of any age.

Dermoid cysts may contain hair, sebaceous material, teeth, and other calcifications. They are usually asymptomatic unless they grow large and put pressure on other organs, such as the bladder and the bowel. The cysts develop bilaterally in 10% to 25% of cases. They are often attached to the ovary by a pedicle (stalk).

Management of dermoid cysts is by surgical removal (cystectomy). If they are not removed, they usually continue to grow and rupture, causing hemorrhage and infection.

Ovarian Fibromas

Fibromas are the most common benign, solid ovarian neoplasms. These pearly-white tumors of connective tissue origin have a low potential for becoming malignant. Fibromas can range in size from a small nodule to a mass weighing more than 50 pounds (22.7 kg). The average size is 2.4 inches (6 cm) in diameter, slightly smaller than a tennis ball. Ninety percent of fibromas are unilateral. On examination, they feel firm, have a slightly irregular contour, and are mobile. Fibromas greater than 6 cm in diameter may be associated with ascites and may cause feelings of pelvic pressure or abdominal enlargement. Unless rupture or torsion occurs, the neoplasm is usually asymptomatic. Fibromas often occur postmenopausally.

Solid ovarian neoplasms are surgically removed. The surgeon may perform an oophorectomy for borderline tumors (when there is a question of possible malignancy). Nursing care of a woman having an oophorectomy is similar to that for a woman having a tubal ligation (see later). When both ovaries are removed, surgery-induced menopause occurs in a premenopausal women. As a result, a woman frequently experiences decreased vaginal lubrication, hot flashes, and atrophy of the vaginal epithelium. These symptoms may be treated with estrogen replacement therapy (see Chart 78–2).

Epithelial Ovarian Tumors

Epithelial ovarian tumors—serous and mucinous cystadenomas—occur in women between the ages of 30 and 50 years. Serous cystadenomas usually occur bilaterally and are more likely to become malignant than mucinous cystadenomas. Both tumors can be irregular and smooth, but mucinous cystadenomas tend to grow large, some to more than 100 pounds (45 kg).

Management of cystadenomas is usually by unilateral salpingo-oophorectomy (surgical removal of a fallopian tube and ovary), because it is often impossible to tell whether the tumor is benign or malignant. Small cystadenomas may be removed by cystectomy, but the larger ones are difficult to resect from the ovary.

Uterine Leiomyomas

Overview

Leiomyomas, also called myomas and fibroids, are the most frequently occurring pelvic tumors. They are benign, slow-growing solid tumors of the uterus.

Pathophysiology

Leiomyomas initially develop from the uterine myometrium. As they grow, fibroids stay attached to the myometrium by means of a pedicle. Leiomyomas are classified according to their position in the layers of the uterus and their anatomic position. The most common types of leiomyomas (Fig. 78–7) are intramural, submucosal, and subserosal.

Intramural leiomyomas are contained in the uterine wall within the myometrium. Submucosal leiomyomas protrude into the cavity of the uterus. Subserosal leiomyomas protrude through the outer surface of the uterine wall. Subserosal leiomyomas may grow laterally and extend to the broad ligament.

Although most fibroids develop within the uterine wall, about 5% may appear in the cervix. Rarely, a fibroid breaks off the pedicle and attaches to other tissues (parasitic fibroid).

Etiology

The cause of leiomyomas is not precisely known. Leiomyomas usually result from a localized proliferation of smooth muscle cells in their initial stages. The stimulus for proliferation may be physical or mechanical and may operate at points of maximal stress within the myometrial layer of the uterine wall. Because there are multiple points of stress caused by the contractions of the uterine muscle, multiple fibroids develop.

The growth of leiomyomas may be related to estrogen stimulation, because fibroids often enlarge during pregnancy and diminish in size after menopause.

Incidence/Prevalence

Leiomyomas occur in approximately 20% to 30% of women older than 30 (Brooks, 1995). It is not clear why leiomyomas develop in some women and not in others.

ELDERLY CONSIDERATIONS

 Fibroids are more common in women in their older reproductive years and postmenopausally if the woman is taking hormone replacement therapy.

TRANSCULTURAL CONSIDERATIONS

The incidence of leiomyomas is two to five times higher in African-American and Asian-American women compared with Caucasian women (McCance & Huether, 1995). The reason for this difference is not known.

Collaborative Management

Assessment

➤ *History*

Although most women with uterine leiomyomas are asymptomatic, abnormal bleeding is the most common complaint. Because African-American women and premenopausal women are at greatest risk for leiomyomas, the nurse questions them about the presence of abnormal bleeding. There may be an increase in menstrual bleeding (menorrhagia), or the bleeding may occur between menstrual periods (metrorrhagia) or be continuous.

➤ *Physical Assessment/Clinical Manifestations*

Women with fibroids do not usually complain of pain, although acute pain may occur with torsion of the fibroid on the pedicle. A woman may report a feeling of pelvic pressure, constipation, or urinary frequency or retention. These symptoms result when an enlarged fibroid presses on other organs. The client may also notice that her abdomen has increased in size with or without noticeable weight gain. Dyspareunia (painful intercourse) and infertility have also been associated with leiomyomas.

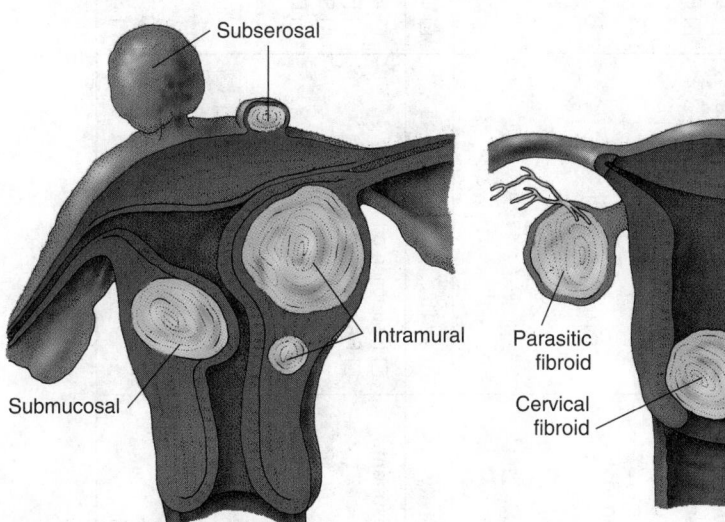

CLASSIFICATION BY POSITION WITHIN UTERINE LAYERS

CLASSIFICATION BY ANATOMIC POSITION

Figure 78–7. Classification of uterine leiomyomas.

CARE PATH NAME: TOTAL ABDOMINAL HYSTERECTOMY
☐ With Burch   ☐ Without Burch

DRG: 353-358   ELOS: 3 Days
Expected Disposition: Home

Collaborative Problem List
1. Discharge Planning
2. Pain/Comfort Management
3. Coping Response to Surgery/Diagnosis
4. _____

Focus	Preadmission	Day of Surgery	Post-Op Day 1	Post-Op Day 2	Post-Op Day 3
Laboratory/ tests/ procedures	☐ Bloodwork ☐ <40 years Hct ☐ >40 years SMA 6, CBC ☐ EKG if > 40 years ☐ CXR if > 60 years ☐ Type and screen		☐ CBC		
Consults/ referrals/	☐ Anesthesia Consult ☐ Nursing Consult		☐ Primary RN		
Physical assessment	☐ H & P obtained	☐ VS per post-op routine ☐ Routine post-op assessment ☐ I/O	☐ VS Q shift ☐ Q shift assessment ☐ I/O ☐ Weight ☐ Fever assessment (if temp > 39° C) ☐ Exam ☐ Cultures of surgical area ☐ CBC with diff ☐ Blood cultures	☐ VS Q shift ☐ Q shift assessment ☐ I/O ☐ Weight ☐ Fever assessment (if temp > 38.5° C) ☐ Exam ☐ Cultures of surgical area ☐ CBC with diff ☐ Blood cultures	☐ VS Q shift ☐ Q shift assessment ☐ I/O ☐ Weight ☐ Fever assessment (if temp > 38.5° C) ☐ Exam ☐ Cultures of surgical area ☐ CBC with diff ☐ Blood cultures
Diagnosis:					
Activity	☐ Ad lib	☐ Dangle at bedside	☐ OOB to chair	☐ Ambulate QID	☐ Ad lib
Treatments	☐ Instruction on IS ☐ Review of procedure	☐ IS/C&DB Q 1 h WA ☐ Foley ☐ SCD's ☐ Drains: BURCH ONLY: ☐ Suprapubic Catheter	☐ IS/C&DB Q 1 h WA ☐ Foley ☐ SCD's ☐ Drains: BURCH ONLY: ☐ Suprapubic Catheter	☐ IS/C&DB Q 1 h ☐ Foley ☐ SCD's ☐ Drains: BURCH ONLY: ☐ Suprapubic Catheter ☐ Monitor postvoid residuals ☐ Begin clamp routine 24 h after surgery if no hematuria	☐ IS/C&DB Q 1 h ☐ D/C Drains: BURCH ONLY: ☐ D/C Suprapubic catheter if PVR < 100 × 2 voids (voids > 250) ☐ Suprapubic catheter

Diet	☐ NPO pre-op	☐ Ice chips ☐ Clear liquids	☐ Advance as tolerated	☐ House diet	☐ House diet
Medications		☐ PCA protocol ☐ Epidural protocol ☐ IV pain meds ☐ IV antibiotics: ☐ IVF:	☐ D/C PCA at 08:00 ☐ D/C Epidural ☐ IV pain meds to PO ☐ IVF: ☐ Heplock when taking PO	☐ PO meds ☐ HL	☐ PO meds ☐ D/C Heplock
Discharge Planning/ Teaching	☐ Discharge Planning Review: ☐ Pre-op checklist ☐ Advanced directives ☐ Patient care path pamphlet ☐ Determine services needed ☐ Patient lives alone ☐ Patient lives with others Support person: Phone number:	☐ Patient lives alone ☐ Patient lives with others Support person: Phone Number:	Provide Homegoing Instructions: ☐ Hysterectomy PI-128 ☐ "Women and AIDS" pamphlet ☐ Breast self exam pamphlet ☐ Hormone replacement therapy ☐ Instruct on pericare **BURCH ONLY:** ☐ Clamp Routine PI Sheets	☐ Review home-going instructions.	☐ Discharge summary completed ☐ Review prescriptions
Individualized Care Focus					
Intermediate Outcomes	☐ Patient able to explain home-going plan ☐ Patient able to describe procedure(s) to be performed ☐ Patient states she has participated in decision making and plan	☐ Afebrile ☐ Patient states pain is adequately controlled ☐ Patient shows no evidence of post-op complications	☐ Able to void without difficulty ☐ Afebrile or temp < 38° with normal WBC ☐ Tolerating PO fluids ☐ Ambulates with assistance ☐ Patient states pain is adequately controlled with PO pain medication	☐ Ambulates independently ☐ Has had a bowel movement and/or passed flatus ☐ Tolerates house diet ☐ Patient able to describe procedure(s) performed ☐ Patient able to describe pericare **BURCH ONLY:** ☐ Able to measure and record postvoid residuals	☐ Patient able to explain home-going plan ☐ Patient able to explain temporary sexual limitations and alternate expressions of sexuality ☐ Patient able to explain use of homegoing medications **BURCH ONLY:** ☐ Patient able to demonstrate clamp routine
Date					
RN Signature Days					
RN Signature Evenings					
RN Signature Nights					

(Continued)

CARE PATH NAME: TOTAL ABDOMINAL HYSTERECTOMY (Continued)
☐ With Burch   ☐ Without Burch

DRG: 353-358   ELOS: 3 Days
Expected Disposition: Home

Collaborative Problem List
1. Discharge Planning
2. Pain/Comfort Management
3. Coping Response to Surgery/Diagnosis
4. _____

Discharge Outcomes:	Met	Not Met	Comments	Date/Initials
1. Abdominal incision approximated and healing				
2. Has minimal, odorless vaginal discharge				
3. Able to describe/perform pericare				
4. Has functional pattern for bladder and bowel				
5. Maintains adequate nutritional intake				
6. Pain controlled by oral medication				
7. States use of homegoing medications				
8. Describes plan for follow-up care				
9. Describes feeling about effects of surgery on health and sexuality				
10. Identifies support systems and resources available to her after discharge				
11. Afebrile or Temp < 38° C with normal WBC				
12. **BURCH ONLY:** Able to demonstrate clamp routine				

University Hospitals' carepaths have been developed to assist clinicians in patient management and clinical decision-making. The carepaths are intended to meet the needs of patients in most circumstances.
They are not intended to replace a clinician's judgement or establish a protocol for all patients with that diagnosis.

SP-12219 (11/19/96)

Abdominal, vaginal, and rectal examinations usually establish the presence of a uterine enlargement that may indicate a leiomyoma. However, other diagnostic procedures may be ordered to differentiate benign from malignant lesions.

> ### ➤ Psychosocial Assessment

A woman who is asymptomatic may fear that she has a malignancy. She may be anxious about abnormal bleeding or her failure to conceive. She may also be concerned if surgical procedures are recommended. The nurse assesses the woman's feelings and concerns about her symptoms and fears of the unknown. If surgery is recommended, the nurse assesses the significance of the loss of the uterus for the woman.

> ### ➤ Laboratory Assessment

A complete blood count identifies iron deficiency anemia (related to bleeding). A pregnancy test may be done to determine whether pregnancy is the cause of the uterine enlargement. An endometrial biopsy may be performed to determine whether the lesion is malignant.

> ### ➤ Radiographic Assessment

Computed tomography (CT) may be of some value. However, CT scans do not differentiate between benign and malignant myomas.

> ### ➤ Other Diagnostic Assessment

Ultrasonography may be useful in differentiating other causes of pelvic masses, including ovarian masses and pregnancy. Culdoscopy or laparoscopy may also be of value in differentiating a uterine fibroid from an ovarian mass.

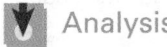 Analysis

> ### ➤ Common Nursing Diagnoses and Collaborative Problems

The most common collaborative problem for women with leiomyomas is potential for hemorrhage.

> ### ➤ Additional Nursing Diagnoses and Collaborative Problems

The woman with leiomyomas may also have one or more of the following nursing diagnoses:
- Fear and Anxiety related to an uncertain diagnosis and potential surgical treatment
- Pain related to pressure from tumors
- Anticipatory Grieving or Dysfunctional Grieving related to perceived or actual loss of the uterus or reproductive function
- Sexual Dysfunction related to dyspareunia
- Ineffective Individual Coping related to depression in response to treatment

 Planning and Implementation

> ### ➤ Potential for Hemorrhage

Planning: Expected Outcomes. The major outcome is that the client is expected to be free of complications, such as hemorrhage and severe anemia from abnormal bleeding.

Interventions. Observation of the leiomyoma over time, myomectomy, and hysterectomy are the methods of management. The choice depends on the size and symptoms of the fibroids and the woman's desire for future childbearing.

Nonsurgical Management. If the client is asymptomatic or desires childbearing, the health care provider typically suggests observation and examination every 4–6 months. If the woman is menopausal, the fibroids usually shrink and surgical intervention may not be necessary. However, a client who is receiving estrogen replacement therapy for menopausal symptoms should know that the fibroids may continue to grow because of the estrogen stimulation.

Surgical Management. The treatment of leiomyomas depends on whether future childbearing is desired, the age of the woman, the size of the fibroids, and the clinical manifestations. If the woman desires childbearing, the surgeon may perform a myomectomy (the removal of leiomyomas with preservation of the uterus) regardless of the size, number, or location of the fibroids. The surgeon may use a laser to remove the tumors. Myomectomy is usually performed in the proliferative phase of the menstrual cycle to minimize blood loss and to avoid the possibility of interrupting an unsuspected pregnancy. Ten percent of the leiomyomas removed recur (Brooks, 1995). Nursing care is similar to that of a woman having a hysterectomy, as described later.

ELDERLY CONSIDERATIONS

A hysterectomy is the usual surgical management in the older woman who has multiple symptomatic leiomyomas. (A sample clinical pathway for a woman having a total abdominal hysterectomy [TAH] is found on pp. 1998 to 2000.)

PREOPERATIVE CARE. Preoperative teaching by the physician begins in his or her office. The physician's office nurse makes sure that the client can describe all the options for surgery, the advantages and risks of having surgery, preoperative and postoperative procedures, and recovery needs. With this information, the woman can make an informed consent to surgery.

The nurse is responsible for psychological as well as physiologic preparation of the woman scheduled for a hysterectomy. Preoperative teaching is usually done on an individual basis. The nurse should explain routine preoperative procedures, including
- Surgical preparation (bowel prep, abdominal mons or perineal shave)

- Laboratory tests for baseline data
- The administration of medications such as prophylactic antibiotics

The client will need preparation for postoperative measures, including turning, coughing, and deep breathing exercises (TCDB) and incentive spirometry; early ambulation; and the need for pain relief. (Chapter 20 describes general preoperative care in detail.)

Psychological assessment is essential. The nurse first explores the significance of the loss of the uterus for the woman. She may feel a great loss if she wishes to retain her childbearing ability, relate her uterus to her self-image and femininity, or feel that her sexual function is related to her uterus. Often a woman has misconceptions about the effects of hysterectomy (e.g., associating it with masculinization and weight gain). The nurse identifies misconceptions so that correct information can be provided, and assesses a woman's support system for adequate support. The client may fear rejection by her husband or sexual partner. The nurse encourages inclusion of the partner in teaching sessions.

OPERATIVE PROCEDURES. A total abdominal hysterectomy (TAH) is usually performed for leiomyomas larger than the gestational size of a 12-week pregnancy. The uterus and cervix are removed through a midline (vertical) or a horizontal incision.

A uterus that has smaller fibroids may be removed via a total vaginal hysterectomy (TVH). The surgeon removes the uterus and cervix through the vagina without an external surgical incision.

In both vaginal and abdominal hysterectomies, the surgeon removes the uterus from the five supporting ligaments, which are then attached to the vaginal cuff so that normal depth of the vagina is maintained (Table 78–5).

In some cases (e.g., treatment of submuous fibroids and menorrhagia), hysterectomy has been replaced by minimally invasive uterine surgery such as transcervical endometrial resection (TCER). A hysteroscope is inserted into the uterus, and the endometrium is destroyed, usually with a diathermy resectoscope (similar to the scope used with prostate surgery) (Baird, 1996). Complications specific to hysteroscopic surgery include

- Fluid overload (fluid used to distend the uterine cavity can be absorbed)
- Embolism
- Hemorrhage
- Perforation of the uterus, bowel, or bladder and ureter injury
- Persistent menorrhagia (10–25%)
- Incomplete suppression of menstruation

These complications occur less frequently when the procedure is performed by an experienced surgeon. Additionally, there is a small risk of subsequent pregnancy and the possibility of cancer developing in the scar. Hysterectomy is still the procedure of choice for women who have coexisting problems, especially those with malignancy or symptomatic uterovaginal prolapse (Baird, 1996).

POSTOPERATIVE CARE. Postoperative care of the woman having a total abdominal hysterectomy is similar to that

TABLE 78–5

Surgical Techniques Used to Remove the Uterus	
Type of Procedure	**Description**
Total hysterectomy	• All of the uterus, including the cervix, is removed. The procedure may be vaginal or abdominal.
Subtotal hysterectomy	• All of the uterus, except the cervix, is removed. This procedure is rarely performed.
Bilateral salpingo-oophorectomy	• Fallopian tubes and ovaries are removed.
Panhysterectomy	• Total abdominal hysterectomy and bilateral salpingo-oophorectomy. The uterus, ovaries, and fallopian tubes are removed abdominally.
Radical hysterectomy	• All of the uterus is removed abdominally. The lymph nodes, the upper third of the vagina, and the surrounding tissues (parametrium) are also removed.

of any client having abdominal surgery (see Chap. 22). For clients who have undergone abdominal hysterectomy, the nurse

- Assesses vaginal bleeding (there should be less than one saturated pad in 4 hours)
- Assesses abdominal bleeding at the incision site (a small amount is normal)
- Checks the incision for intactness
- Maintains the urethral catheter (Foley catheter), usually for 24 hours or less
- Offers pain medications as ordered for the abdominal pain (Chart 78–9)

Specific interventions for a vaginal hysterectomy include

- Assessment of vaginal bleeding (there should be less than one saturated pad in 4 hours)
- Foley catheter care
- Perineal care (sitz baths, heat lamps, or ice packs)

The surgeon usually removes the abdominal sutures or clips at the time of the first postoperative visit, whereas vaginal sutures are usually absorbed. The nurse recognizes and monitors for complications associated with hysterectomies (Table 78–6).

ELDERLY CONSIDERATIONS

Older women are more at risk for all complications, particularly pulmonary embolism. Obese women are more at risk for thromboembolism.

Psychological complications can occur with both abdominal and vaginal procedures. Depression is the most frequent reaction reported. Other reactions are perceived loss of femininity and decreased libido. Loss of femininity

Chart 78–9

Focused Assessment for the Client with a Total Abdominal Hysterectomy

Assess cardiovascular, respiratory, renal and gastrointestinal status, including

- Vital signs
- Auscultate heart, lung, and bowel sounds
- Monitor urinary output
- Assess temperature and color of the skin
- Monitor red blood cell, hemoglobin, and hematocrit levels
- Monitor activity tolerance
- Assess dressing and drains for color and amount of drainage
- Assess peripads for vaginal bleeding and clots
- Monitor fluid intake (IVs until bowel sounds return and client is tolerating oral intake)
- Assess for signs of thrombophlebitis

Use the following interventions to prevent postoperative complications:

- Cough and deep-breathing exercises
- Incentive spirometry
- Sequential compression devices
- Ambulation
- Avoid heavy lifting or strenuous activity

Assess the home care teaching needs of the client related to the illness and surgery, including

- Physiologic effects of the surgery
- Signs and symptoms to report
- Side or toxic effects of medications
- Activity limitations related to driving and use of stairs
- Follow-up care
- Postoperative restrictions related to sexual activity, use of tampons, and bathing
- Care of wound and/or drains

Assess the client's coping skills and reaction to the diagnosis and surgical procedure.

---

may be the problem if a woman before surgery was interested in her appearance but afterward has no interest, even when she is feeling better. Decreased sexual desire is often temporary, if it occurs, and is usually related to discomfort.

 Continuing Care

The client with uterine leiomyomas is managed on an ambulatory basis unless surgical intervention is required. After hospital discharge, the client typically returns to her home.

➤ Home Care Management

Planning for home care management begins at the time of admission. The woman is usually discharged to the home setting 2 days after a traditional TAH. TVH or TCER may be performed as same-day surgery in an ambulatory setting. The client having a hysterectomy should be told to

avoid or limit stair climbing for 1 month. The nurse advises her to avoid tub baths (which may promote infection) and sitting for long periods (which causes pooling of blood in the pelvic vessels). The nurse also teaches the client to avoid engaging in strenuous activity or lifting anything weighing more than 5 pounds (2.3 kg). Some health care providers also restrict driving for 4–6 weeks.

➤ Health Teaching

The nurse teaches the woman who has had a hysterectomy about

- The physical changes to be expected
- Exercise and activities
- Diet
- Sexual activity
- Wound care (if any)
- Complications
- Follow-up care (see Chart 78–9)

The physical changes include cessation of menses, inability to become pregnant, weakness and fatigue during convalescence (may last 2–3 months), and absence of menopausal symptoms unless the ovaries are also removed. Moderate exercise, such as walking, is encouraged, but active sports, such as jogging and aerobic exercise, should be avoided for at least 1 month.

The nurse teaches the client to consume foods that aid in healing tissues, such as foods high in protein, iron, and vitamin C. The nurse also reminds the client to avoid sexual intercourse for 4–6 weeks. The first coital activity may cause some tenderness or pain because the vaginal walls are tight and need to be stretched out. Water-soluble lubricants can decrease discomfort. The client should be taught the signs of complications, particularly infection. An appointment for follow-up medical care is scheduled 1 week postoperatively.

Women who have had a hysterectomy need information about possible emotional reactions. Generally, women adjust well to surgery if they

- Have completed childbearing
- Work
- Have interests outside the home

TABLE 78–6

Common Postoperative Complications of Abdominal and Vaginal Hysterectomies

Abdominal Hysterectomy

- Intestinal obstruction (paralytic ileus)
- Thromboembolism
- Atelectasis
- Pneumonia
- Wound dehiscence (especially in obese clients)
- Urinary retention

Vaginal Hysterectomy

- Hemorrhage
- Urinary tract complications, especially infection or retention
- Wound infection
- Urinary retention

- Have no misconceptions about the effects of hysterectomy
- Have support from the family, especially the husband or sexual partner

Reactions may be different after vaginal and abdominal procedures, because women who have had a vaginal hysterectomy have no external focus (no obvious change in body image) for their feelings.

Psychological reactions can occur 3 months to 3 years after surgery. Women identified as being at high risk for psychological problems may need long-term follow-up care or referral. Women may need to be counseled about signs of depression. Intermittent sadness is normal, but continued feelings of low self-esteem or loss of interest or pleasure in usual activities and pastimes is not normal and should be evaluated. The incidence of psychological reactions often decreases after the nurse provides written materials and discusses the positive forces in her life with the client and her significant others.

➤ Health Care Resources

Usually no special home equipment is needed for a woman who has had a hysterectomy. A home care nurse may be needed to assess and monitor the elderly client's postoperative progress if other conditions, such as uncontrolled diabetes, are present. Financial assistance may be needed, and referral to the hospital's department of social services or case management department may be indicated if the woman has no insurance coverage. The nurse can provide a referral for psychological or sexual counseling if potential problems are identified before discharge.

 Evaluation

On the basis of the identified nursing diagnoses and collaborative problems, the nurse evaluates the care of the woman who has had surgery for leiomyomas. The expected outcomes may include that the client will

- Be free of hemorrhage
- State the role of the reproductive system and the changes that occur after hysterectomy (without misconceptions)
- Recover from surgery without complications
- Demonstrate a positive psychological adjustment to surgery as evidenced by the absence of depression and the presence of a positive self-concept
- Resume sexual activities at her previous level of satisfaction

Bartholin's Cysts

Overview

Bartholin's cysts are one of the most common disorders of the vulva. The cysts result from obstruction of a duct. The secretory function of the gland continues, and the fluid fills up the obstructed duct. The cause of the obstruction may be infection, congenital stenosis or atresia, thickened mucus near the ductal opening, or mechanical trauma, such as lacerations or episiotomy.

Collaborative Management

 Assessment

The woman may be asymptomatic if the cyst is small, but a history may reveal complaints of dyspareunia, inadequate genital lubrication, or a mass in the perineal area. A large cyst usually causes constant localized pain and may cause difficulty walking or sitting. A physical examination of the vulva reveals a swelling immediately beneath the skin in the posterior portion of the vulva (Figure 78–8). The cyst may appear brown or sanguineous, depending on its contents. Usually the cyst is unilateral and ranges from 3/8 to 4 inches (1–10 cm) in size.

If the cyst is draining, the health care provider usually requests that the fluid be sent to the laboratory for culture (for gonorrhea and aerobic and anaerobic organisms) and sensitivity testing. If the woman is older than 40 years, a specimen of the cyst should be sent for pathologic examination to determine whether the lesion is benign or malignant.

 Interventions

If the woman is asymptomatic, no interventions are necessary. If the cysts are symptomatic, simple incision and drainage (I&D) may provide temporary relief; however, cysts tend to recur as the opening of the duct becomes obstructed again. Usually the health care provider establishes a permanent opening for drainage. Marsupialization (formation of a pouch that is a new duct opening) is accomplished under local, regional, or general anesthesia. Any postoperative discomfort may be relieved by the administration of analgesics and sitz baths. The health care provider may prescribe prophylactic antibiotics.

Bartholin's cysts may become infected. Abscesses are formed when bacteria (*Escherichia coli*, *Neisseria gonorrhoeae*, *Staphylococcus aureus*, *Streptococcus*, *Trichomonas vaginalis*, or *Mycoplasma hominis*) enter the duct, resulting in infection that closes the duct. An abscess usually ruptures spontaneously within 72 hours of formation. Inter-

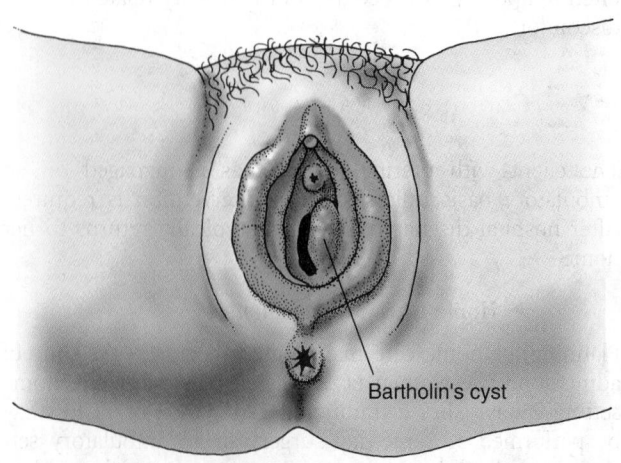

Figure 78–8. Bartholin's cyst.

ventions for the woman with an abscess include bed rest, administration of analgesics, and application of moist heat (sitz baths or hot wet packs) to the vulva. The health care provider usually orders broad-spectrum antibiotics to treat the infection. I&D of the abscess may provide temporary relief.

The health care provider may totally excise the Bartholin's glands in women older than 40 years when cancer is suspected or if repeated infections with abscess formation occur. Postoperative interventions include

- The use of heat lamps, the application of ice packs, or sitz baths several times a day for comfort and promotion of healing
- Administration of analgesics for pain, if needed
- Prophylactic administration of antibiotics
- Assessment of the incision for signs of healing or infection

Cervical Polyps

Cervical polyps are pedunculated (on stalks) tumors arising from the mucosa and extending to the opening of the cervical os. The cause is unknown, although polyps result from a hyperplastic condition of the endocervical epithelium. They may also be due to inflammation. Polyps are the most common benign neoplastic growth of the cervix. Cervical polyps are most common in multiparous women older than 40 years.

A woman may be asymptomatic, or a history may reveal complaints of premenstrual or postmenstrual bleeding or bleeding after coitus. A speculum examination may reveal small (⅜–1½ inches [1–4 cm]), single or multiple polyps. They are bright red; have a soft, fragile consistency; and may bleed when touched.

Polyp removal is easily accomplished as an office procedure. The base of the polyp can be grasped with a clamp, and the polyp can be twisted off and sent to the pathology laboratory for evaluation. Electrocautery or chemical cautery usually stops any bleeding at the site of removal. After the procedure, the nurse may instruct the client to avoid tampon use, douches, and sexual intercourse for a week or until healing has taken place.

MALIGNANT NEOPLASMS
Endometrial Cancer
Overview

Endometrial cancer (cancer of the uterus) is the most frequently occurring reproductive cancer (American Cancer Society, 1996). It is asymptomatic in its early development, and has a good prognosis in 80% to 90% of cases.

ELDERLY CONSIDERATIONS

Endometrial cancer is a slow-growing tumor primarily occurring in postmenopausal women. The average age at onset is 61 years. The incidence declines after the age of 70 years (DeStefano & Bertin-Matson, 1996).

Pathophysiology

Adenocarcinoma of the endometrium accounts for 75% to 80% of all endometrial cancers. It arises from the glandu-

lar component of the endometrial mucosa and may be preceded by endometrial hyperplasia. The initial growth of the cancer is within the uterine cavity, followed by extension into the myometrium and the cervix. Spread outside the uterus (Fig. 78–9) occurs

- Through lymphatic spread to the ovaries and parametrial, pelvic, inguinal, and para-aortic lymph nodes
- By hematogenous metastasis (spread by blood) to the lungs, liver, or bone
- By transtubal or intra-abdominal spread to the peritoneal cavity

Etiology

Risk factors associated with endometrial cancer include obesity, diabetes mellitus, hypertension, history of uterine polyps, history of infertility, nulliparity (no pregnancies), and polycystic ovary disease. Estrogen stimulation, including unopposed menopausal estrogen replacement therapy, late menopause (after age 52 years), postmenopausal bleeding, and a family history of uterine cancer also predispose a woman to endometrial cancer.

Table 78–7 compares the risk factors for endometrial cancer with those for other female reproductive cancers.

Incidence/Prevalence

The National Cancer Institute (NCI) estimates that more than 32,000 new cases of endometrial cancer will occur

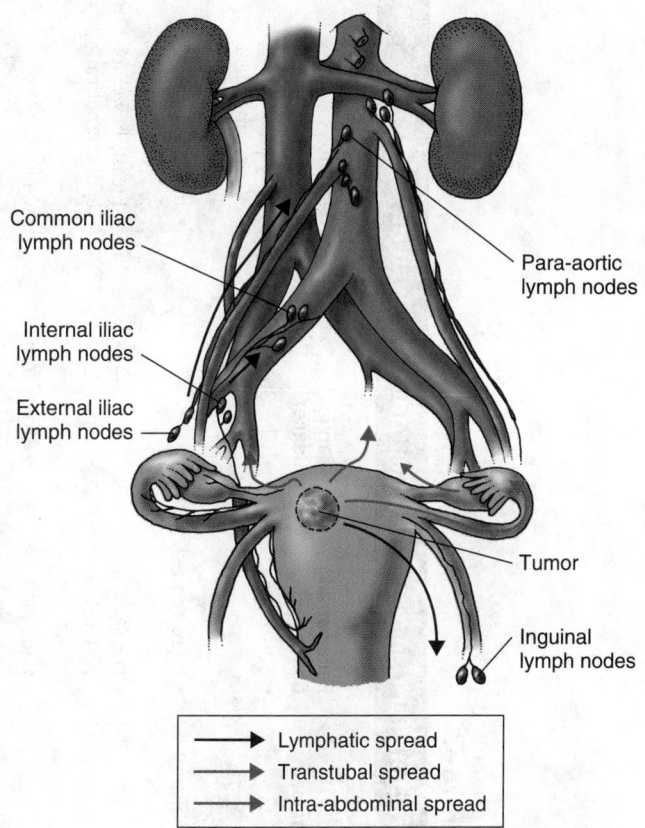

Figure 78–9. Extrauterine spread of endometrial cancer. From Herbst, A. L., Mishell, D. R., Jr., Stenchever, M. A., & Droegemueller, W. (1992). *Comprehensive gynecology* (2nd ed.). St. Louis: C. V. Mosby. Used with permission.

Labels within figure:
Common iliac lymph nodes
Para-aortic lymph nodes
Internal iliac lymph nodes
External iliac lymph nodes
Tumor
Inguinal lymph nodes

Legend:
→ Lymphatic spread
→ Transtubal spread
→ Intra-abdominal spread

TABLE 78–7

Risk Factors for Cancers of the Reproductive System*

Risk Factor	Endometrial Cancer	Cervical Cancer	Ovarian Cancer	Vulvar Cancer	Vaginal Cancer	Fallopian Tube Cancer	Gestational Trophoblastic Disease
Age	50–65 yr	CIS: 30–40 yr; Invasive: 40–60 yr	Infrequent before 35 yr; range usually is 40–65 yr	After 40 yr, peak 60–70 yr	Most after 50 yr; adenocarcinoma 14–30 yr	After 50 yr, range 18–80 yr	After 40 yr, before 20 yr
Family history	Increased risk	—	Increased risk	—	DES exposure in utero	—	—
Personal history	Diabetes, hypertension	—	Breast, bowel, or endometrial cancer	Cervical cancer, diabetes, vulvar disease	Vulvar or cervical cancer	Ovarian or uterine cancer, infertility	Previous molar pregnancy (3%–5%)
Race	Caucasian	African-American, Native American	Caucasian	—	—	—	Asian-American, Mexican-American
Mother's age at birth	—	<18 yr	>30 yr	—	—	—	—
Body size	Obesity	—	—	Possibly obesity	—	—	—
Parity	Nulliparity	Multiparity	Nulliparity	—	Multiparity	Nulliparity	—
Estrogen use	Prolonged use >3 yr menopausally	Possibly long-term birth control pill use	—	—	—	—	—
Smoking	Possible increased risk	Possibly double the risk	—	—	—	—	—
Infection (STD)	—	Possibly STD (herpes simplex virus type 2 or papillomavirus infection)	—	Possibly STD, papillomavirus infection	STD, herpes simplex virus type 2 and papillomavirus infection	PID, chronic salpingitis	Exposure to infectious agents

*CIS = carcinoma in situ; DES = diethylstillbestrol; PID = pelvic inflammatory disease; STD = sexually transmitted disease.

annually in the United States (American Cancer Society, 1996). Thus, about 1 of every 100 women in the United States has endometrial cancer.

TRANSCULTURAL CONSIDERATIONS

 Endometrial cancer occurs more frequently in Caucasian women than in African-American women and typically in postmenopausal women aged 50 to 65 years. Survival rates differ between Caucasian and African-American women with endometrial cancer; Caucasian women have higher survival rates (Barrett et al., 1995). The difference in survival rates appears to be related to higher grade lesions and more aggressive cell types that occur in African-American women (Barrett et al., 1995).

Collaborative Management

Assessment

The primary symptom of endometrial cancer is postmenopausal bleeding. In addition, the woman may complain of a watery, serosanguineous vaginal discharge, low back or abdominal pain, and low pelvic pain (caused by pressure of the enlarged uterus). A pelvic examination may reveal the presence of a palpable uterine mass or uterine polyp. The uterus is enlarged if the cancer is in an advanced stage.

Before a diagnosis is made, the client may deny that the symptoms are related to cancer. During the diagnostic phase, the woman may express fears and concerns about having a malignancy. After the diagnosis is confirmed, she may express disbelief, anger, depression, anxiety, or withdrawal behaviors.

The health care provider orders basic diagnostic tests to determine the client's overall status. The results of the tests may also indicate the presence of metastasis. These tests include

- Chest x-ray to detect metastasis
- Intravenous pyelography (IVP), or excretory urography, to assess renal function and for renal metastasis
- Barium enema study to assess for intestinal metastasis
- Computed tomography (CT) of the pelvis to identify the origin and spread of the tumor
- Lymphangiography to assess for lymph node metastasis
- Liver and bone scans to assess for distant metastasis

Fractional dilation and curettage (D&C [scraping individual sections of the uterus]) and endometrial biopsy are the definitive diagnostic procedures for endometrial cancer. Other tests that may be useful for some clients include proctosigmoidoscopy, ultrasonography, and hysteroscopy (examination of the uterus via an endoscope).

Interventions

Nonsurgical interventions (radiation therapy and chemotherapy) and surgery may be used alone or in combination, depending on the stage of the cancer.

Nonsurgical Management. Radiation therapy and chemotherapy are the two major nonsurgical methods used to treat endometrial cancer.

Radiation Therapy. The health care provider orders radiation therapy (external and internal) if the stage of cancer is hard to determine and if surgery is planned for stage II and III cancers. Clients usually receive radiation therapy for 6 weeks preoperatively to destroy cancer cells in the pericervical lymphatics and to inhibit recurrence.

Intracavitary Radiation. If intracavitary radiation therapy (IRT [brachytherapy]) is selected, the radiologist places an applicator within the woman's uterus through the vagina while she is anesthetized (Fig. 78–10). After the correct position of the applicator is confirmed by x-rays, the woman is taken to the hospital room and a radiologist places a radioactive isotope in the applicator, which remains for 1–3 days. Before the procedure, the nurse instructs the client on postprocedure activities, such as deep breathing and leg exercises. While the radioactive implant is in place, the woman is strictly isolated, usually in a private room. The nurse informs the client that she is restricted to bed rest on her back with the head of the bed flat or slightly elevated (20 degrees or less). Movement in bed is restricted to prevent dislodgment of the radioactive source.

The nurse inserts a Foley catheter into the bladder to prevent dislodgment of the implant, which can be caused by a full bladder or attempts to void. The nurse carefully assesses the skin for breakdown over bony pressure points during the client's activity restriction period. The client is usually placed on a low-residue diet (to prevent bowel movements that might dislodge the implant), and fluid intake is encouraged (to prevent stasis of urine and

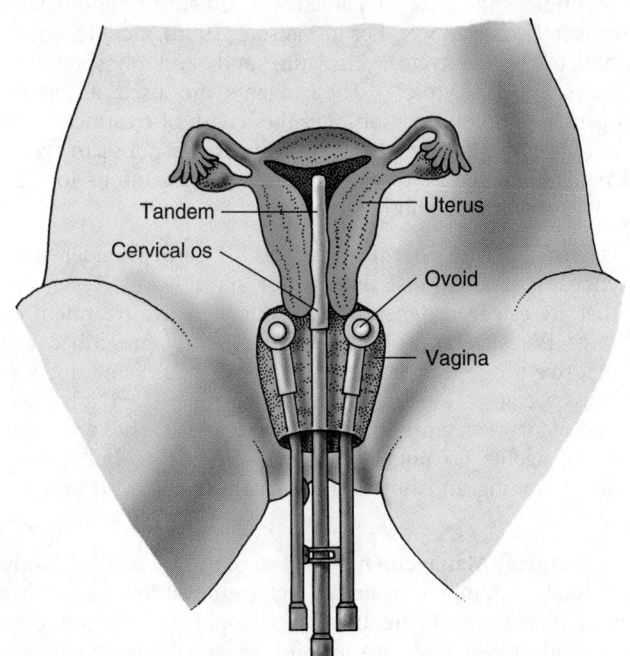

Figure 78–10. Intrauterine placement of an applicator for intracavitary radiation therapy.

possible infection). The health care provider usually prescribes

- Antiemetics
- Broad-spectrum antibiotics (to prevent bladder infections)
- Tranquilizers (to help the client relax)
- Analgesics
- Heparin (to prevent thromboembolism)
- Antidiarrheal medications (to prevent bowel movements)

Radiation precautions are practiced while the implant is in place. The nurse organizes care so that minimal time is spent at the bedside. Care is given as far away from the radioactive source as possible and behind lead shields when possible. Nurses who are pregnant or attempting to become pregnant should not be assigned to these clients. Visitors are restricted to brief visits, and pregnant women and children younger than 18 years should not be allowed to visit.

External Radiation. External radiation therapy may be used to treat all stages of endometrial cancer. It is usually used in combination with surgery, preoperatively or postoperatively. Depending on the extent of the tumor, external radiation is given on an outpatient basis for 4–6 weeks. The lateral extensions of the tumor in the parametrium and pelvic wall nodes are irradiated (see also Chap. 27). Specific instructions for the woman having external radiation for endometrial cancer include watching for signs of skin breakdown, especially in the perineal area, no sunbathing, and no bathing over the markings outlining the treatment site. The nurse informs the woman that cystitis and diarrhea are common complications, as are nutritional problems that result from anorexia.

Chemotherapy. Chemotherapy is used as a palliative treatment in advanced and recurrent disease. Chemotherapeutic agents used for palliative treatment of endometrial cancer (DeStefano & Bertin-Matson, 1996) include doxorubicin (Adriamycin), cisplatin, and cyclophosphamide (Cytoxan, Proxytox♣). These agents are used as single agents or in combination, and the length of treatment and dosage are determined by the woman's response to treatment. (Chapter 27 discusses nursing interventions for clients receiving chemotherapy.)

Other Drug Therapy. The health care provider may choose progestational therapy for stage I and II cancers that are estrogen dependent and for palliative treatment of stage IV cancer. The hormones frequently prescribed are medroxyprogesterone acetate (Depo-Provera) and megestrol acetate (Megace). Tamoxifen citrate (Nolvadex, Tamofen♣), an antiestrogen, is also used. The progestational agents do not cause acute side effects, but nausea and vomiting and hot flashes are associated with tamoxifen.

Surgical Management. The surgeon typically performs a total abdominal hysterectomy (removal of the uterus and cervix) and bilateral salpingo-oophorectomy (removal of both tubes and ovaries) for stage I tumors without cervical involvement. A radical hysterectomy (see Table 78–5) with bilateral pelvic lymph node dissection is performed for stage II cancer. Nursing care is essentially the same as that for hysterectomy (see Uterine Leiomyomas earlier), except that the woman's hospitalization is usually longer and her convalescence may be extended.

Psychosocial Support. Women need to discuss their concerns about the presence of cancer and the potential for recurrence. The nurse provides emotional support and tries to create an atmosphere that encourages the woman to ask questions or express her fears and concerns. Significant others are included in discussions when possible.

Reactions to radiation therapy vary. Some women may feel radioactive or "unclean" after treatments and may exhibit withdrawal behaviors. The nurse needs to correct such misconceptions.

Women who have chemotherapy may be upset if alopecia (hair loss) occurs. The nurse warns the client of this possibility before treatment starts. Wigs, scarves, or turbans can be worn until regrowth occurs.

 Continuing Care

The client with endometrial cancer is managed at home unless surgery is indicated. After surgery, the client is usually discharged to her home.

➤ *Home Care Management*

Home care after surgery for endometrial cancer is the same as that after hysterectomy (see Uterine Leiomyomas). Women who are receiving chemotherapy or external radiation therapy are usually treated on an outpatient basis, which may mean that a woman and her family may have to plan daily activities around trips to the clinic or the health care provider's office. If the tumor recurs and cure is not likely, the client and her family need to think about hospice care and whether the woman can be cared for in the home.

➤ *Health Teaching*

For the woman who has had a hysterectomy for endometrial cancer, the teaching plan is the same as that for the woman who has had a hysterectomy for uterine leiomyomas (see earlier discussion). Side effects to report to the health care provider include vaginal or rectal bleeding, foul-smelling discharge, abdominal pain or distention, and hematuria.

The high dose of radiation causes sterility, and vaginal shrinkage can occur. Vaginal dilators can be used with water-soluble lubricants for 10 minutes/day until sexual activity resumes (in 10 days to 6 weeks). The woman is not radioactive, and her partner will not "catch" cancer from engaging in sexual intercourse. A normal diet may be resumed.

The nurse explains any medications prescribed in terms of dosage, schedule of administration, therapeutic effects, and side effects. The nurse also emphasizes the importance of keeping appointments for follow-up care.

Often women experience emotional crises because of the physical effects of cancer treatments. Radical hysterectomy may be seen as mutilating, and chemotherapy may affect the woman's body image if hair loss occurs. A woman may exhibit a grief reaction to this perceived change in body image. The feelings of loss depend on the visibility of the loss, the function of the loss, and the amount of emotional investment. The nurse may need to help the woman adapt to the body changes. One way to do this is to encourage self-care as soon as the woman's condition is stable. A calm, accepting attitude may also be helpful.

Death can occur with or without treatment. Women and their families have concerns about recurrence. All want to pass the 5-year survival mark without a recurrence. If there is recurrence, the woman may be hostile and may exhibit characteristics of a grief reaction. The nurse encourages clients to ventilate their feelings. (Chapter 12 discusses response to loss and grieving.)

➤ Health Care Resources

In the United States, local American Cancer Society chapters provide written materials about endometrial cancer as well as information about local support groups. If the client is in the terminal stages of cancer, hospice care may be appropriate. If nursing care is needed at home, the hospital nurse or case manager refers the client and her family to a community health or home care agency. A referral to a social services agency may be needed if the woman is unable to meet the financial demands of treatment and long-term follow-up.

Cervical Cancer

Overview

Cervical cancer is the third most common reproductive cancer, after endometrial and ovarian cancers. Cervical cancer is also the third most common cause of death related to reproductive cancers (American Cancer Society, 1996). Death rates for cervical cancer have dropped 50% in the past two decades, primarily because of the availability of Pap tests for screening of premalignant cervical changes. However, the incidence of preinvasive cervical cancer has increased as a result of early diagnosis.

Pathophysiology

Cervical cancer may be described as preinvasive or invasive. Preinvasive cancer is limited to the cervix; invasive cancer is in the cervix as well as other pelvic structures. Preinvasive lesions usually originate in the area called the *transformation zone* (Fig. 78-11). This area includes the squamocolumnar junction, which is located near the external cervical os, where squamous and columnar (glandular) epithelium changes normally occur. Abnormal squamous epithelium can also be found in this zone. These cells can develop into invasive carcinoma.

These premalignant changes can be described on a continuum from dysplasia—the earliest premalignant change—to carcinoma in situ (CIS)—the most advanced premalignant change. Preinvasive cancers can also be described by the term *cervical intraepithelial neoplasia* (CIN) and classified according to severity:

- CIN I, mild
- CIN II, moderate
- CIN III, severe to carcinoma in situ

Squamous cell cancers spread by direct extension to the vaginal mucosa, lower uterine segment, parametrium, pelvic wall, bladder, and bowel. Metastasis is usually confined to the pelvis, but distant metastases can occur through lymphatic spread and, rarely, via the circulatory system to the liver, lungs, or bones. Table 78-8 shows the clinical stages of cancer of the cervix.

Etiology

The exact cause of squamous cell cervical cancer is unknown, but numerous factors may be involved. An association has been identified with early and frequent sexual contact and with viral infections of the cervix, such as herpes simplex virus type 2, cytomegalovirus, and papillomavirus.

Risk factors associated with cervical cancer include low socioeconomic status, early age at first sexual contact or first pregnancy, multiple sexual partners, and intrauterine exposure to diethylstilbestrol (DES). Other possible risk factors include intercourse with men whose previous sexual partners had cervical cancer, use of oral contraceptives, cigarette smoking, and vitamin A and C deficiencies. Nulliparity (no pregnancies) and diabetes mellitus are also associated with adenocarcinoma of the cervix.

TRANSCULTURAL CONSIDERATIONS

The rate of cervical cancer is twice as high for African-American women as for Caucasian women. The mortality rate is more than twice as high for African-American women as for Caucasian women (American Cancer Society, 1996).

Incidence/Prevalence

The National Cancer Institute estimates that there are more than 14,000 new cases of cervical cancer (excluding CIS) and more than 4400 deaths in the United States annually. Although the rate of invasive cervical cancer has decreased over the last several decades, it has increased in recent years in women younger than 50 years (American Cancer Society, 1996).

Cervical intraepithelial neoplasia occurs mainly in young women; the peak incidence of dysplasia occurs in clients in their mid-20s. CIS occurs in women about 30 years old, and invasive cancer occurs most commonly in the late 40s.

ELDERLY CONSIDERATIONS

Cervical adenocarcinoma occurs most often in women in their 50s, and no relationship to sexual transmission or viral infection has been found.

Collaborative Management

 Assessment

The woman who has preinvasive cancer is often asymptomatic. The classic symptom of invasive cancer is painless vaginal bleeding. The bleeding may start as spotting between menstrual periods or after coitus or douching. As

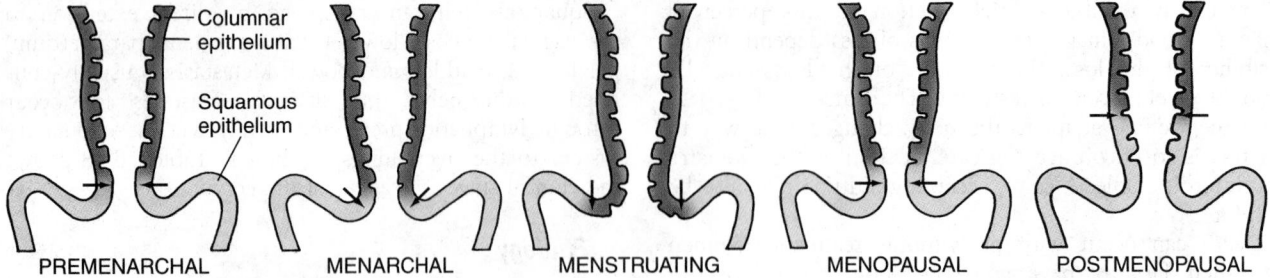

Figure 78–11. The location of the transformation zone at various stages of adult development.

the malignancy grows, the bleeding increases in frequency, duration, and amount. It may become continuous.

The woman may also complain of a watery, blood-tinged vaginal discharge that may become dark and foul smelling as the disease progresses. Leg pain (along the sciatic nerve) or unilateral swelling of a leg may be a late symptom or may indicate recurrent disease. Other signs of recurrence or metastasis (spread) may include unexplained weight loss, pelvic pain (caused by pressure of the tumor on the bladder or the bowel), dysuria (painful urination), hematuria (bloody urine), rectal bleeding, chest pain, and coughing.

A physical examination may not reveal any abnormalities, for early preinvasive cervical cancer, although the internal pelvic examination may identify late-stage disease.

Laboratory assessment of the woman begins with a Pap smear. If the results are abnormal, the smear is repeated before further studies are done. If abnormal tissue is detected on a subsequent Pap test, further testing is done. Figure 78–12 illustrates one common method of evaluating the client with abnormal Pap smear results. If invasive cervical cancer is diagnosed, laboratory tests such as those described earlier for the investigation of endometrial cancer are performed.

The health care provider may perform a colposcopic examination to view the transformation zone, where dysplasia, cervical intraepithelial neoplasia (CIN), and carcinoma in situ (CIS) usually originate. If abnormal tissue is recognized, multiple biopsies of the cervical tissue are performed (see Chap. 76).

The health care provider usually performs an endocervical curettage (scraping of the endocervix from the internal to the external os) as well. Because this procedure is uncomfortable, the nurse may need to encourage the woman to use relaxation or breathing exercises to cope

TABLE 78–8

FIGO Clinical Stages of Cancer of the Cervix (Revised 1985)

Stage	Characteristics
I	• Carcinoma is strictly confined to cervix (extension to corpus should be disregarded)
IA	• Preclinical carcinoma
IA1	• Minimal microscopically evident stromal invasion
IA2	• Microscopic lesions no more than 5-mm depth measured from base of epithelium surface or glandular from which it originates, and horizontal spread not to exceed 7 mm
IB	• All other cases of stage I; occult cancer should be marked "occ"
II	• Carcinoma extends beyond cervix but has not extended to pelvic wall; it involves vagina, but not as far as lower third
IIA	• No obvious parametrial involvement
IIB	• Obvious parametrial involvement
III	• Carcinoma has extended to pelvic wall; on rectal examination, there is no cancer-free space between tumor and pelvic wall; tumor involves lower third of vagina; all cases with hydronephrosis or nonfunctioning kidney should be included, unless they are known to be due to another cause
IIIA	• No extension to pelvic wall, but involvement of lower third of vagina
IIIB	• Extension to pelvic wall, or hydronephrosis or nonfunctioning kidney due to tumor
IV	• Carcinoma has extended beyond true pelvis or has clinically involved mucosa of bladder or rectum
IVA	• Spread of growth to adjacent pelvic organs
IVB	• Spread to distant organs

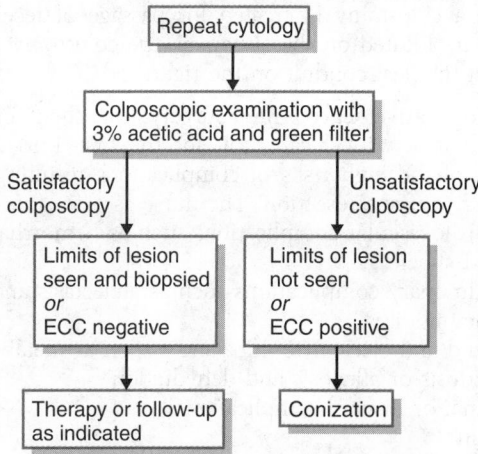

Figure **78–12.** One method of evaluating women who have abnormal Pap smear results. ECC = endocervical curettage. From Herbst, A. L., Mishell, D. R., Jr., Stenchever, M. A., & Droegemueller, W. (1992). *Comprehensive gynecology* (2nd ed.). St. Louis: C. V. Mosby. Used with permission.

with the cramping and pain. A small amount of bleeding is expected and may occur for up to 2 weeks after the biopsies.

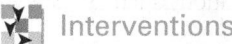 Interventions

Nursing care of the client with cervical cancer is similar to that of the client with endometrial cancer. The only interventions discussed here are those that differ from those for the client with endometrial cancer.

Nonsurgical Management. Nonsurgical interventions for cervical cancer depend on the stage of disease and may include laser therapy, cryosurgery, radiation therapy, chemotherapy, or hysterectomy.

Laser Therapy. Laser therapy is an outpatient procedure that is used whenever all the boundaries of the lesion are visible under colposcopic examination and the endocervical curettage findings are normal. In laser therapy, the invisible beam is directed to the abnormal tissues, where energy from the beam is absorbed by the fluid in the tissues, causing them to vaporize. There is usually a small amount of bleeding associated with the procedure. The woman may have a slight vaginal discharge, and healing occurs in 6 to 12 weeks.

Cryosurgery. Cryosurgery is another common treatment for CIN. A probe is placed against the cervix to cause freezing of the tissues and subsequent necrosis. Although this treatment can also be considered a type of surgery, no anesthesia is required. After the procedure, the client may experience slight cramping. The woman has a heavy watery discharge for several weeks after the procedure; she should avoid intercourse and the use of tampons while discharge is present because the cervix is friable and these precautions will decrease the risk of infection.

Radiation Therapy. Most women with invasive cervical cancer are treated with radiation. For cancer that has extended beyond the cervix but not to the pelvic wall, radiation therapy is as effective as a radical hysterectomy. Intracavitary and external radiation therapies are used in combination, depending on the extent and location of the lesion. Intracavitary implants (brachytherapy) are usually used for lesions that have extended beyond the pelvic wall. External therapy is often given first to shrink the tumor and increase the effectiveness of the implant. (Nursing care related to radiation therapy is presented in the earlier discussion of endometrial cancer and in Chapter 27.)

Chemotherapy. Chemotherapeutic agents have generally performed poorly for cervical cancer. These agents are usually reserved for unresectable recurrent tumors or disseminated metastatic disease (DeStefano & Bertin-Matson, 1996). Two drugs that have shown some response are cisplatin and fluorouracil (5-FU).

Surgical Management. The surgical procedure for cervical cancer depends on the extent of the disease and whether the client wants to have children.

Conization. Conization is the definitive treatment for clients with microinvasive cervical cancer. This procedure is done when the lesion cannot be visualized by colposcopic examination. A cone-shaped area of cervix is removed surgically (Fig. 78–13) and sent to the laboratory to determine the extent of the malignancy. Potential complications associated with conization include hemorrhage, uterine perforation, incompetent cervix, cervical stenosis (hardening), and preterm labor for future pregnancies.

Conization may be used therapeutically for women with CIN who desire further childbearing or less extensive surgical treatment. Long-term follow-up care is needed because new lesions can develop.

Hysterectomy. A hysterectomy may be performed as treatment of microinvasive cancer if the client does not desire childbearing. A vaginal approach is commonly

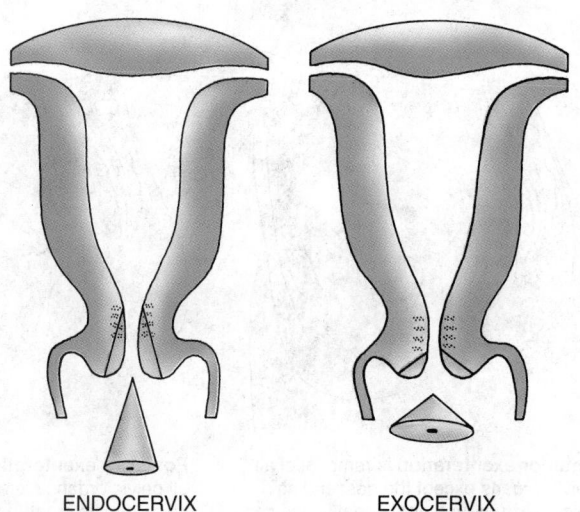

ENDOCERVIX   EXOCERVIX

Figure **78–13.** Conization biopsy for CIN of the endocervix and cervix. From DiSaia, P. J., & Creaseman, W. T. (1989). *Clinical gynecologic oncology* (3rd ed.). St. Louis: C. V. Mosby. Used with permission.

used. A radical hysterectomy and bilateral pelvic lymph node dissection is as effective as radiation for treating clients with cancer that has extended beyond the cervix but not to the pelvic wall. Information about hysterectomy is found under Uterine Leiomyomas.

Pelvic Exenteration. One of the most radical surgical procedures is pelvic exenteration. It is performed for recurrent cancers if there is no evidence of tumor outside the pelvis and no lymph node involvement.

Preoperative Care. Nursing care of the woman scheduled for exenteration includes assessment of preoperative anxiety, concerns about the impact on sexual function, and the ability to adjust to her altered body image. The nurse involves significant others in discussions about postoperative expectations. Physical preparation includes selection of stoma sites, extensive bowel preparation, and extensive radiographic and laboratory tests to assess for spread of cancer outside the pelvis. The nurse teaches the client about

- Postoperative recovery in a critical care unit
- Pain management
- Presence of numerous intravenous (IV) and arterial catheters
- Nasogastric suction
- Colostomy and/or urinary diversion (e.g., ileal conduit, Kock ileal urinary pouch)

Operative Procedures. There are three types of exenteration (Fig. 78–14): anterior, posterior, and total.

Anterior exenteration is the removal of the uterus, cervix, ovaries, fallopian tubes, vagina, bladder, urethra, and pelvic lymph nodes. Posterior exenteration is the removal of the uterus, cervix, ovaries, fallopian tubes, descending colon, rectum, and anal canal. Total exenteration is a combination of anterior and posterior procedures. When the bladder is removed, urine is diverted through a urinary diversion (e.g., ileal conduit or Kock ileal urinary pouch). When the colon, rectum, or anal canal are removed, a colostomy is created for passage of feces. The stomas are located on the abdomen, the colostomy on the left, and the ileal conduit on the right.

Postoperative Care. After surgery, the client often is admitted to a critical care unit for the first 1 to 2 days because of the high risks of complications resulting from the massive tissue resection. The nurse assesses for

- Cardiovascular complications such as hemorrhage and shock
- Pulmonary complications such as atelectasis and pneumonia
- Fluid and electrolyte imbalances such as metabolic acidosis or alkalosis and dehydration
- Renal or urinary complications
- Pain

The nurse or assistive nursing personnel also assists with deep breathing and coughing hourly, monitors urinary output and specific gravity, monitors parenteral nutrition, and provides colostomy and urinary diversion care.

After the client's condition is stable, she returns to the regular postoperative unit. The nurse continues postoperative interventions. During the recovery period, the nurse assesses for

- Late cardiovascular complications such as deep venous thrombosis and pulmonary emboli
- Gastrointestinal (GI) complications such as paralytic ileus
- Wound infections
- Wound dehiscence or evisceration
- Pain

The nurse administers prophylactic heparin and maintains the use of antiembolism stockings or sequential compression devices (SCDs) for the prevention of thrombosis, as ordered. The nurse also auscultates the lungs frequently, assesses for the presence of bowel sounds and wound infection, administers antibiotics as prescribed, and manages pain with a gradual withdrawal of opioid analgesics.

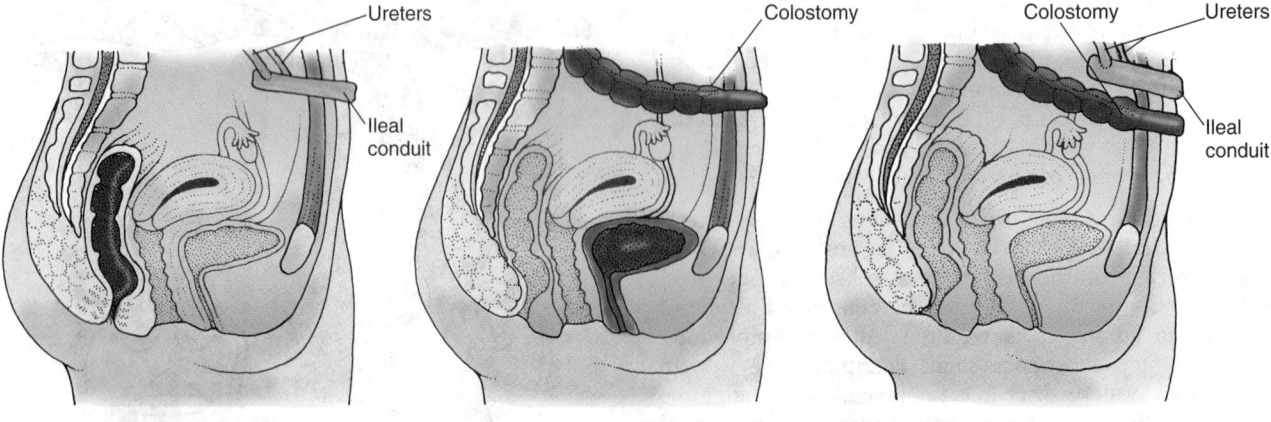

Anterior exenteration is removal of all pelvic organs except the descending colon, rectum, and anal canal. Urine can be diverted into an ileal conduit or urinary Kock pouch.

Posterior exenteration is removal of all pelvic organs except the bladder. A colostomy is created for the passage of feces.

Total exenteration is removal of all pelvic organs with creation of an ileal conduit or urinary Kock pouch and a colostomy.

Figure 78–14. Pelvic exenteration.

After the surgeon removes the operative dressings, perineal irrigations may be implemented. Irrigation is usually done with a normal saline applied with an Asepto syringe. This is followed by drying of the perineum with a heat lamp (25 W at a distance of 18 inches [45 cm]) or a hair dryer (using warm air). Care must be taken to avoid burning the client. Sitz baths may be ordered as tolerated. (Postoperative care of clients with colostomies and urinary diversions is discussed elsewhere in this text).

 Continuing Care

If the client has had a hysterectomy, the discharge planning is similar to that described for endometrial cancer. For the client who has had a pelvic exenteration, the discharge planning is more involved.

➤ Home Care Management

The client with a pelvic exenteration is usually in the hospital for at least 1 week postoperatively. She may be discharged to a nursing home or subacute unit for continued recovery and care or may be discharged directly to home. When the client returns home, she needs assistance. She is not able to engage in strenuous activities associated with most household work for up to 6 months. The family may need to consider outside help if there is no one in the family who can assume household responsibilities.

No special equipment is needed in the home, although an "egg crate" mattress or other special pressure-relieving device may be placed on the bed to prevent skin breakdown and to increase comfort. Colostomy and ureterostomy pouches and equipment for changing the pouches can be purchased in local pharmacies.

➤ Health Teaching

The nurse teaches the woman who has had a pelvic exenteration how to manage new functions with equipment (colostomy and urinary diversion) and to perform activities of daily living (ADLs) and self-care. The perineal opening may drain mucus for several months to a year. The client can wear sanitary napkins (minipads or maxipads) if they are beltless (so as not to interfere with the stomas). The woman may need help in adjusting her diet to maintain high nutritional requirements for healing while selecting foods that are tolerated. The woman should be able to state the effects, dosages, and side effects of all medications prescribed.

Sexual function is different after exenteration (even if an artificial vagina is constructed), and the couple may need counseling about alternatives to intercourse. Even with vaginal reconstruction, the use of vaginal dilators is necessary to achieve desired sexual function.

Physical activities may be limited during convalescence. If walking is not permitted, the nurse encourages range-of-motion exercises. Follow-up care is important. The nurse counsels the client about keeping all follow-up appointments. Information about late complications (e.g., infection and bowel obstruction) is needed so that the woman can seek medical care promptly.

Usually by 3 to 5 days after surgery, the woman begins expressing grief about her body changes. At first she may deny changes by refusing to look at the wound or stoma sites. Later she may become depressed or withdrawn or even angry or hostile. She may then move to reality testing by asking questions about her care, watching the nurses do wound care, and becoming actively involved in self-care.

The woman may have mood swings, and the nurse is alert when the woman becomes depressed so that interventions can be implemented. The woman needs intense emotional support if she is to adapt to her altered body image and functions.

Unless the woman has a vaginal reconstruction after anterior or total pelvic exenteration, she is not able to have vaginal intercourse. The nurse must assess the need for sexual counseling by listening for cues about altered perceptions of body image and anxiety about her sexual partner's response. Further sexual counseling may be needed to provide information on alternative methods of sexual gratification.

➤ Health Care Resources

Resources for the woman who has cervical cancer are similar to those for the woman with endometrial cancer.

Ovarian Cancer

Overview

Ovarian cancer is the leading cause of death from female reproductive malignancies. Death rates have risen during the past four decades, and it is projected that 1 of every 70 women will develop ovarian cancer sometime in her life (American Cancer Society, 1996). Survival rates continue to be low because ovarian cancer is poorly detected in its early stages.

Of all ovarian cancers, 85% are epithelial tumors; the most common type is serous adenocarcinoma. These tumors grow rapidly, spread fast, and are often bilateral. Of all epithelial tumors, ovarian tumors are associated with the worst prognosis.

The cancer spreads by several mechanisms:

- Direct spread to other organs in the pelvis that are in close proximity to the ovary (e.g., uterus, bladder, and colon)
- Distal spread through lymphatic drainage (via para-aortic and iliac lymph nodes to the rest of the pelvis, abdomen or liver, lung, or bones)
- Peritoneal seeding (malignant spread of free-floating cells usually after the development of ascites)

The cause of ovarian cancer is not precisely known. Suggested etiologic theories include a familial association; an environmental association related to products of industry in countries such as the United States and those of western Europe; and a hormonal association, as evidenced by increased incidence with menopause, nulliparity, and breast cancer and decreased incidence with oral contraceptive use.

Risk factors include a family history of ovarian cancer; a history of breast, bowel, or endometrial cancer; nulliparity (no pregnancies); infertility; and a history of dysmenorrhea or heavy bleeding. Diets high in animal fat have been linked to ovarian cancer (DeStefano & Bertin-Matson, 1996).

Ovarian cancer ranks second to endometrial cancer in incidence. The incidence increases in women older than 40 years and peaks at 50 to 55 years.

TRANSCULTURAL CONSIDERATIONS

 Ovarian cancer is seen more frequently in Caucasian women than in African-American women (Herbst et al., 1992).

Collaborative Management

Assessment

Women with ovarian cancer may complain of abdominal pain or swelling or have vague symptoms of abdominal discomfort, such as dyspepsia, indigestion, gas and distention, and other mild gastrointestinal (GI) disturbances. The woman may have a history of ovarian imbalance, such as evidenced by premenstrual tension, heavy menstrual flow, or dysfunctional bleeding.

The only sign may be an abdominal mass, which may

be noticed only after it reaches a size of 6 inches (15 cm). Most pelvic examinations do not identify abnormalities. However, an enlarged ovary found postmenopausally should be evaluated as though it were malignant.

The woman with ovarian cancer has concerns similar to those described for the woman with endometrial cancer. Because the malignancy is usually diagnosed in an advanced stage, fears of death and dying are frequent and may be more of a concern than the proposed treatments.

Cytologic examination has limited application because a Pap smear is abnormal in only 20% to 30% of women, even in advanced cases. Diagnosis depends on surgical exploration. Usually, a complete laboratory work-up is done before exploratory surgery, including a complete blood count, urinalysis, and liver studies if ascites occurs.

The level of ovarian antibody designated as CA-125 may be elevated if ovarian cancer is present. This test may be useful to monitor a woman's progress after treatment but may not be as useful for diagnostic purposes.

Ultrasonography, intravenous pyelography (IVP), computed tomography (CT), and radiography are used in detecting ovarian tumors. In addition, a barium enema study and an upper GI radiographic series can be performed to rule out tumor in the adjacent structures.

Exploratory laparotomy is performed to diagnose and stage ovarian tumors. Ovarian cancer is the only neoplasm that is staged when it is removed (Table 78–9).

TABLE 78–9

FIGO Staging Classification of Ovarian Cancer	
Stage	**Characteristics**
I	• Growth limited to the ovaries
Ia	• Growth limited to one ovary; no ascites. No tumor on the external surface; capsule intact
Ib	• Growth limited to both ovaries; no ascites. No tumor on the external surfaces; capsules intact
Ic	• Tumor either stage Ia or Ib, but with tumor on surface of one or both ovaries, or with capsule ruptured, or with ascites present containing malignant cells, or with positive peritoneal washings
II	• Growth involving one or both ovaries with pelvic extension
IIa	• Extension and/or metastases to the uterus and/or tubes
IIb	• Extension to other pelvic tissues
IIc	• Tumor either stage IIa or IIb, but with tumor on surface of one or both ovaries, or with capsule(s) ruptured, or with ascites present containing malignant cells or with positive peritoneal washings
III	• Tumor involving one or both ovaries with peritoneal implants outside the pelvis and/or positive retroperitoneal or inguinal nodes. Superficial liver metastasis but with histologically proven malignant extension to small bowel or omentum
IIIa	• Tumor grossly limited to the true pelvis with negative nodes but with histologically confirmed microscopic seeding of abdominal peritoneal surfaces
IIIb	• Tumor of one or both ovaries with histologically confirmed implants of abdominal peritoneal surfaces, none exceeding 2 cm in diameter. Nodes are negative.
IIIc	• Abdominal implants greater than 2 cm in diameter and/or positive retroperitoneal inguinal nodes
IV	• Growth involving one or both ovaries with distant metastases. If pleural effusion is present, there must be positive cytologic findings to allot a case to stage IV. Parenchymal liver metastasis equals stage IV.

Interventions

Nursing care of the woman with ovarian cancer is similar to that of the woman with endometrial or cervical cancer. The options for treatment depend on the extent of the cancer and include chemotherapy (systemic or intraperitoneal), immunotherapy, radiation therapy (external or intraperitoneal), and surgery.

Nonsurgical Management. Chemotherapy and radiation therapy are the two most common nonsurgical options for ovarian cancer.

Chemotherapy. The health care provider usually prescribes chemotherapeutic agents postoperatively for all stages of ovarian cancer, although their purpose is usually palliative for stage IV tumors. Cisplatin, carboplatin, paclitaxel (Taxol), isofamide, doxorubicin (Adriamycin), hexamethylmelamine, methotrexate, and 5-fluorouracil (5-FU) have been used as single agents for treating ovarian cancer (DeStefano & Bertin-Matson, 1996). Combinations of agents seem to obtain higher response rates, especially if cisplatin is one of the drugs used.

Chemotherapy is usually administered every 3 to 4 weeks for 1 week and can be administered on an inpatient or an ambulatory basis. Intraperitoneal chemotherapy is the instillation of chemotherapeutic agents into the abdominal cavity. By using this method, it is believed that the cytotoxic effects of the drugs on the tumor are increased. Immunotherapy is also used to treat ovarian cancer. It alters the immunologic response of the ovary and promotes tumor resistance.

Radiation Therapy. External radiation therapy is used postoperatively if tumors have invaded other organs. It may be given with chemotherapy or alone (see Chap. 27). Radioactive colloids have also been injected into the abdomen to increase survival rates. A primary beta-emitter, ^{32}P, is injected through a catheter placed during surgery. After instillation, the woman is asked to turn frequently for 1½ to 2 hours to facilitate the distribution of the radioactive colloids throughout the peritoneal cavity (e.g., turning to the right, to the left, head down, feet down, prone, and supine).

Surgical Management. A total abdominal hysterectomy and bilateral salpingo-oophorectomy is the surgical procedure for all stages of ovarian cancer. In clients with stage III and IV cancer, the goal is to remove as much as possible because it has spread to adjacent organs. Nursing care of the woman is similar to that of the woman having hysterectomy for uterine leiomyomas.

A second-look procedure (laparoscopy or laparotomy) is performed, usually after 1 year of chemotherapy, to confirm the absence or presence of tumor and to remove any new or residual tumor if it was too large to be removed at the first operation. Nursing care is similar to that of the client after any major abdominal surgery.

The woman who is faced with the diagnosis of advanced ovarian cancer may be concerned about dying. She needs to be encouraged to ventilate her feelings about her diagnosis. Realistic assurance, as well as accurate information about treatments, can be provided. Often providing the woman with information about ovarian cancer and its treatment decreases her fears. Providing continuity of care, with at least one regular caregiver, may be helpful. The nurse encourages the client to use her support system, including family members, friends, and a spiritual leader, such as a rabbi or other clergy members. A visit from another woman who has survived a similar disease may decrease fears.

If there is recurrence, the woman may deny symptoms at first or express feelings of anger and grief. The family is often fearful of the outcome. The nurse needs to provide encouragement and support during this difficult time and help the family and the woman work through their grief and prepare for death.

Vulvar Cancer

Overview

Vulvar cancer represents only 4% of all gynecologic malignancies, even though it ranks fourth in occurrence. Vulvar cancer is slow growing, stays localized for a long time, and metastasizes late.

ELDERLY CONSIDERATIONS

Vulvar cancer occurs most frequently in women 50–70 years of age. More than 50% of the cases of vulvar cancer occur in women older than 60 years.

Of all vulvar cancers, 90% are squamous cell carcinomas. The other 10% consist of adenocarcinomas, sarcomas, and Paget's disease. Most vulvar cancers develop in the absence of premalignant changes in the epithelium, but occasionally they develop and spread similarly to cancer of the cervix.

The first change is usually vulvar atypia or mild dysplasia (vulvar intraepithelial neoplasia [VIN] I), followed by moderate dysplasia (VIN II) and severe dysplasia or carcinoma in situ (VIN III) until the lesion becomes invasive. Vulvar cancer can spread directly to the urethra, the vagina, or the anus and through the lymphatic system to the inguinal, femoral, and deep iliac pelvic nodes (Figure 78–15).

The cause of vulvar cancer is unknown. There is no proven relationship to sexually transmitted diseases (STDs), although a history of condylomata acuminatum (venereal warts) may be present. A strong relationship exists between vulvar cancer and herpes simplex type II, human papillomavirus, and capsid antigen (Stefano & Bertin-Matson, 1996). Obesity, hypertension, diabetes, smoking, and granulomatous disease of the vulva have been suggested as possible causes, but no scientific data support these suggestions.

Vulvar cancer seldom occurs before age 40 years, although studies have found premalignant change in women in their 20s and 30s. This increase may be linked to the increase in sexually transmitted infections.

The prognosis for vulvar cancer is related to the stage of the cancer and whether cancer is present in the lymph nodes. Guidelines for the early detection and prevention of vulvar cancer include performing monthly vulvar self-examination, having an annual pelvic examination, and practicing "safe sex."

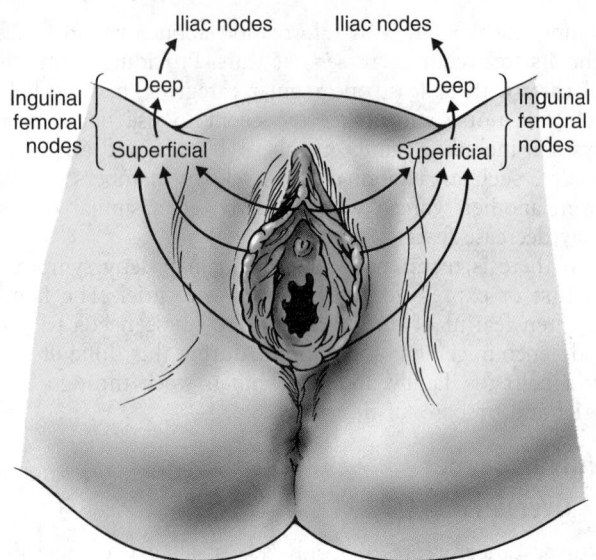

Figure 78–15. The spread of vulvar cancer: a schematic representation of the major lymphatic drainage channels of the vulva. Redrawn from Herbst, A. L., Mishell, D. R., Jr., Stenchever, M. A., & Droegemueller, W. (1992). *Comprehensive gynecology* (2nd ed.). St. Louis: C. V. Mosby. Used with permission.

Collaborative Management

 Assessment

Women with vulvar lesions are likely to report irritation or itching in their perineal area. Sometimes they describe a "sore that will not heal." Bleeding is a late symptom. Women usually try to treat themselves before seeking medical help. Often a lesion has been present for months. Embarrassment has been suggested as the reason why older women delay seeking medical attention.

Pelvic examinations usually reveal multifocal lesions, the majority of which develop on the labia. The lesions may be whitish or reddish, and the vulvar skin may be excoriated owing to irritation.

The woman may be anxious or fearful about the diagnosis of cancer. She may have fears that her partner will reject her because of the diagnosis, or she may worry about disfigurement related to surgery. The nurse needs to assess the woman's past experiences in coping with stressful situations and whether she has the psychological resources to cope with the present crisis.

A Pap smear and colposcopic examination of the vulva (see Cervical Cancer earlier) may aid in diagnosis. A toluidine blue test may be used to identify abnormal cells for biopsy. A 1% aqueous solution of toluidine blue is applied to the vulva and allowed to dry. Then a 1% acetic acid solution is applied. Biopsy of the areas that remain blue is performed. The test chemical stains nuclei in the superficial epithelium, where cells do not normally contain nuclei. An abnormal finding does not necessarily indicate malignancy, because ulcerations also stain.

A biopsy of the lesion is necessary for diagnosis. This is easily accomplished with a Keyes dermal punch (a device that removes a disk of tissue). Depending on the site of the lesion, one or more biopsies may be taken.

 Interventions

Nursing care of the client with vulvar cancer is similar to that of the client who has endometrial cancer; only the interventions that differ are discussed.

Nonsurgical Management. Nonsurgical management of vulvar cancer depends on the extent of the spread and may include laser therapy, chemotherapy, and radiation therapy.

Laser Therapy. If a woman has premalignant vulvar lesions, laser therapy may be used (see Cervical Cancer earlier). The treatment is usually done on an outpatient basis; local, regional, or general anesthesia is used. Healing occurs over several weeks, and usually the lesions are removed without scarring.

Chemotherapy. Chemotherapy in the form of a topical application of 5-FU has been used to treat carcinoma in situ successfully. However, the treatment causes severe vulvar edema and pain and is not often used.

Radiation Therapy. External radiation therapy to the deep pelvic nodes may be used postoperatively (see earlier discussion of endometrial cancer and Chapter 27). Radiation treatments cause ulceration and dermatitis, which can be uncomfortable for the woman.

Surgical Management. The surgeon performs a vulvectomy to remove the cancerous vulvar lesions.

Preoperative Care. The woman needs a complete explanation of the extent of the surgical procedure to be performed and information about preoperative and postoperative procedures (see Chaps. 20 and 22). Specific preoperative procedures for vulvectomy may include abdominal or perineal shave, enema, douche, and insertion of an indwelling catheter into the bladder.

Operative Procedures. Several surgical procedures are effective for the treatment of vulvar cancer. A local wide excision may be used to remove the abnormal area (for CIS). A simple vulvectomy (removal of vulva, the labia majora, the labia minora, and possibly the clitoris) may also be performed for CIS, but this disfiguring surgery is used less frequently today. Instead, a skinning vulvectomy—the removal of superficial vulvar skin (without removal of the clitoris) and replacement of removed skin with split-thickness grafts—is performed (Fig. 78–16). Sexual function is less affected, and the appearance of the vulva is less changed.

For invasive cancer, the surgery most often recommended is the modified radical or radical vulvectomy (removal of the entire vulva—skin, labia, clitoris, subcutaneous tissues, and possibly inguinal and femoral node dissection), depending on node involvement (see Fig. 78–16).

Postoperative Care. Postoperatively, the woman can expect multiple (4–5) suction drains (Hemovac or Jackson-Pratt drains) in the inguinal or vulvar areas for

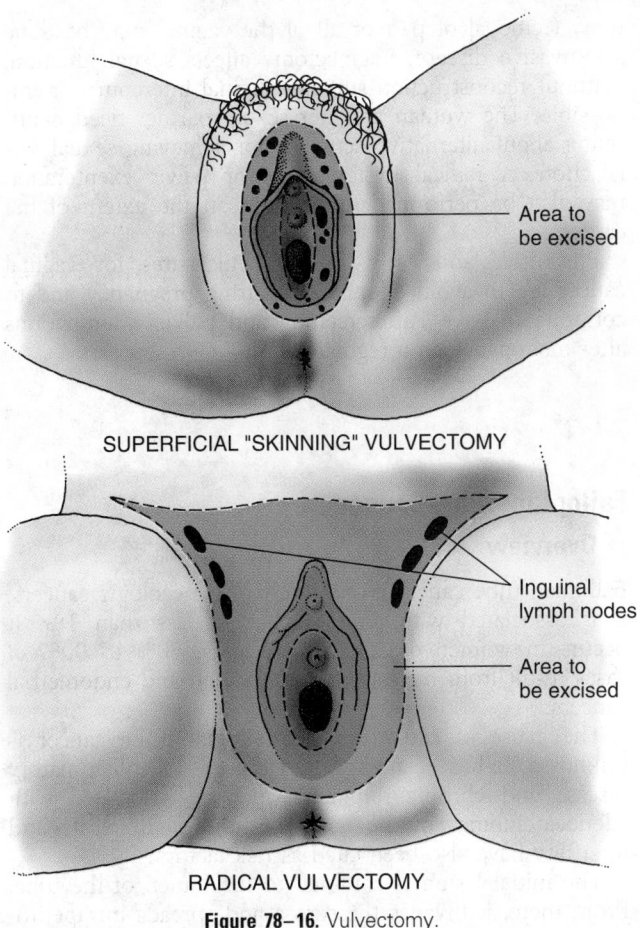

SUPERFICIAL "SKINNING" VULVECTOMY

Area to be excised

Inguinal lymph nodes

Area to be excised

RADICAL VULVECTOMY

Figure 78–16. Vulvectomy.

wound drainage for 7 to 10 days. An air mattress or egg crate mattress may be placed on the bed to prevent pressure sores and increase comfort. A bed cradle can be used to keep linens off the incision site. The client usually wears antiembolism stockings or sequential compression devices to prevent thromboembolism and leg edema.

Providing Wound Care. The major focus of nursing care is wound healing. The nurse changes the dressings over the incision frequently because of the amount of wound drainage and the risk of infection. Wound complications, such as infection and dehiscence, frequently occur after vulvectomies; subsequently, the healing process may take up to 6 months. Meticulous wound care is necessary and usually involves debridement. The nurse typically uses a normal saline solution that may be applied with an Asepto bulb syringe or a water pick (on low speed). The wound is then dried with a heat lamp or air dried with a hair dryer (using warm air). Wound care is usually done three or four times a day.

Diet in the postoperative period should include foods rich in vitamin C, iron, and protein to promote wound healing.

Promoting Urinary and Bowel Elimination. The Foley catheter remains in the bladder for 7 to 10 days to prevent ureteral stenosis and incontinence. After the catheter is removed, the urine stream may be deflected down

the leg due to edema or even may be uncontrolled. Having the woman stand while voiding may decrease the incidence of these annoying problems. Antiperistaltic medications are usually given for 7 to 10 days to prevent defecation and decrease the risk of wound infection. Then, stool softeners can be given to prevent straining and decrease discomfort related to bowel movements. Perineal care or sitz baths after voidings or bowel movements may prevent contamination of the incision site.

Managing Pain. Postoperative discomfort is usually controlled with analgesics during the first couple of days after surgery. Medicating for pain before wound care may help the woman relax and tolerate the procedure with less distress.

Addressing Sexuality. The woman needs complete explanations of the changes that occur as a result of surgery. If a radical vulvectomy is done, the clitoris is removed, and loss of orgasm usually occurs. Dyspareunia may result from any of the surgical procedures. Vaginal dilators may be useful to stretch the remaining vaginal tissues. Discomfort can also be reduced during intercourse by having the couple use water-soluble lubricants or a side-lying position. The couple may need counseling about alternatives to vaginal intercourse. The woman may need to be encouraged to express feelings of grief related to her loss of normal sexual function.

A vulvectomy can be devastating to a woman's self-concept. She frequently has a grief reaction related to the loss of the vulva and subsequent disfigurement. She may fear rejection from her sexual partner and significant others and may be reluctant to make herself vulnerable by getting involved in any relationship. Fears of recurrence or metastasis may be present. The nurse's role is one of support. The woman needs encouragement to vent her feelings and concerns about her perceived or actual losses and body changes. Significant others should be encouraged to share their feelings and concerns with the woman. A visit by a woman who has successfully recovered from similar surgery could be beneficial.

Vaginal Cancer

Overview

Primary invasive vaginal cancer is rare, accounting for less than 2% of all gynecologic cancers. Usually vaginal cancer is an extension of cervical, endometrial, or vulvar cancers. Most vaginal cancers are squamous cell carcinomas that develop in the upper one third of the vagina. They occur most frequently in women older than 50 years; 90% of cases are found postmenopausally. Adenocarcinoma of the vagina is found in females between the ages of 14 and 30 years and is associated with intrauterine exposure to diethylstilbestrol (DES) as a result of maternal ingestion during pregnancy.

The cause of vaginal cancer is unknown. Predisposing factors include repeated pregnancies, vaginal trauma, sexually transmitted disease (especially syphilis and herpes simplex virus type 2 and papillomavirus infections), and prior radiation.

The spread of vaginal cancer depends on the location of the tumor. Upper vaginal lesions spread in the same manner as cervical cancer, whereas lower lesions spread similarly to vulvar cancer. Because of the rich lymphatic drainage in the vaginal area, metastasis can occur early.

Collaborative Management

 Assessment

Premalignant lesions (vaginal intraepithelial neoplasia) are usually asymptomatic. An abnormal Pap smear is the most common presenting problem. Uncommon or late symptoms include pain, foul-smelling vaginal discharge, painless vaginal bleeding, pruritus, and urinary symptoms attributable to the pressure of the lesion on the bladder.

A pelvic examination may reveal a lesion. Premalignant changes are diagnosed through colposcopic examination and biopsy.

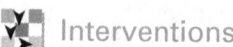 Interventions

Both nonsurgical and surgical interventions may be used to treat women with vaginal cancer.

Nonsurgical Management. Noninvasive malignancy and early-stage vaginal cancers may be treated nonsurgically with a variety of techniques. Laser therapy (see Cervical Cancer earlier) may be used. The health care provider stains the abnormal tissues with an iodine solution to identify the area for treatment. A vaginal discharge may be present for several days after treatment, and healing normally takes a few weeks. Close follow-up is necessary: a Pap smear and colposcopic examination every 4 months for 1 year and then every 6 to 12 months.

Local application of 5-fluorouracil (5-FU) cream to the vagina daily for 1 week is another treatment option. This chemotherapeutic agent is irritating to the skin, and often zinc oxide ointment is recommended for application to the vulvar area. The treatment is repeated in 3–4 weeks, and follow-up is the same as that for laser therapy.

Radiation therapy can be used for all stages of vaginal cancer. Intracavitary radiation therapy (IRT, brachytherapy) is usually used alone for the treatment of cancer limited to the vaginal wall, and external radiation therapy is combined with IRT for the treatment of cancer that extends beyond the vaginal wall. Complications of radiation therapy include vaginal stenosis, adhesions, and discharge. Women need to use vaginal dilators after treatment, and assessment for sexual dysfunction is suggested.

Chemotherapy may be used for recurrent disease, although there is no effective therapy.

Surgical Management. A local wide excision may be performed for localized lesions. A partial or total vaginec-

tomy (removal of part or all of the vagina) may be done for invasive disease. Vaginectomy affects sexual function. Without reconstruction surgery, vaginal intercourse is impossible. The woman and her sexual partner need counseling about alternative activities for achieving sexual satisfaction. A radical hysterectomy or pelvic exenteration may also be performed, depending on the extent of the cancer.

Preventive and early detection measures for vaginal cancer are to avoid taking DES during pregnancy and to continue to have Pap screening and pelvic examinations after menopause on a regular basis.

Fallopian Tube Cancer

Overview

Fallopian tube cancer is the rarest of gynecologic cancers; it is associated with an incidence of less than 1%. It occurs in women older than 50 years; 80% to 90% of cases result from metastasis from ovarian and endometrial cancers.

The cause of squamous cell fallopian tube cancer is unknown. It has been suggested that pelvic inflammatory disease and chronic salpingitis may be associated with adenocarcinomas of the fallopian tubes. Nulliparity and infertility have also been cited as risk factors.

The initial lesion is confined to the lumen of the tube. From there, it invades the serosa and spreads intraperitoneally to the bowel, the omentum, and the peritoneum. Lymphatic spread is to the para-aortic and retroperitoneal lymph nodes.

Collaborative Management

Women are usually asymptomatic until the tumor is in a late stage. In 50% of the cases, bleeding is present. Other symptoms include clear vaginal discharge, lower abdominal pain or distention, and feelings of pressure. A history of abnormal bleeding, adnexal pain, and watery vaginal discharge in a postmenopausal woman may suggest fallopian tube cancer, and further evaluation is needed.

Diagnosis is rare preoperatively. Pap smear has reportedly been abnormal in only 10% of cases. A mass may be felt on examination in late stages. Vaginal ultrasonography, computed tomography (CT), or laparoscopy may be used to confirm a mass.

Chemotherapy may be used postoperatively in later stages or for recurrence. The lesions respond to alkylating agents (see Chap. 27). External radiation therapy has also been used postoperatively for late-stage tumors. The usual treatment of cancer limited to the fallopian tube is a total abdominal hysterectomy and bilateral salpingo-oophorectomy with omentectomy (removal of the connective tissues covering these organs). Care of the woman with fallopian tube cancer is similar to that described earlier for cancer of the ovary.

CASE STUDY for the Client Having an Abdominal Hysterectomy

■ Ms. C. is a 44-year-old Caucasian woman who was diagnosed with squamous cell carcinoma of the cervix. Today she underwent a total abdominal hysterectomy (TAH) and bilateral salpingo-oophorectomy (BSO). She had an estimated blood loss of 300 mL during surgery. Her vital signs and postoperative status are stable. She is to be transferred to your unit for postoperative nursing care.

QUESTIONS:

1. What initial postoperative assessments should the nurse perform?
2. What are the possible nursing diagnoses for the client who has just had a TAH-BSO?
3. What information should be included in this client's discharge teaching plan?

SELECTED BIBLIOGRAPHY

American Cancer Society. (1996). *Cancer facts and figures—1996.* Atlanta: Author.

Baird, G. (1996). Advances in gynaecology. *The Practitioner, 240,* 90–95.

Barrett, R. J., Harlan, L. C., Wesley, M. N., Hill, H. A., Chen, V. W., Clayton, L. A., Kotz, H. L., Eley, J. W., Robboy, S. J., & Edwards, B. K. (1995). Endometrial cancer: Stage at diagnosis and associated factors in black and white patients. *American Journal of Obstetrics and Gynecology, 173*(2), 414–422.

Brooks, S. E. (1995). Uterine leiomyomas. In P. L. Carr, K. M. Freund, & S. Somani (Eds.), *The medical care of women* (pp. 121–125). Philadelphia: W. B. Saunders.

Chuong, C. J., Pearsall-Otey, L. R., & Rosenfeld, B. L. (1995). A practical guide to relieving PMS. *Contemporary Nurse Practitioner, 1*(3), 31–37.

Dawood, M. Y. (1995). Menstrual abnormalities. In D. H. Nichols & P. J. Sweeney (Eds.), *Ambulatory gynecology* (pp. 51–79). Philadelphia: J. B. Lippincott.

DeStefano, M. S., & Bertin-Matson, K. (1996). Gynecologic cancers. In R. McCorkle, M. Grant, M. Frank-Stromborg, & S. B. Baird (Eds.), *Cancer nursing: A comprehensive textbook* (pp. 698–727). Philadelphia: W. B. Saunders.

*Herbst, A. L., Mishell, D. R., Jr., Stenchever, M. A., & Droegemueller, W. (1992). *Comprehensive gynecology* (2nd ed.). St. Louis: C. V. Mosby.

Hornstein, M. D., & Barbieri, R. L. (1995). Endometriosis. In K. Ryan, J. Berkowitz, & R. Barbieri (Eds.), *Kistner's gynecology: Principles and practices* (6th ed., pp. 251–277). St. Louis: C. V. Mosby.

Hutchins, F. L. (1995). Abdominal myomectomy as a treatment for symptomatic uterine fibroids. *Obstetrics & Gynecology Clinics of North America, 22*(4), 781–789.

Ivey, C. L. (1994). When your client has ovarian cancer. *RN, 57*(11), 26–31.

Jarrett, M., Cain, K. C., Heitkemper, M., & Levy, R. L. (1996). Relationship between gastrointestinal and dysmenorrheic symptoms at menses. *Research in Nursing and Health, 19*(1), 45–51.

Jarrett, M., Heitkemper, M., & Shaver, J. F. (1995). Symptoms and self-care strategies in women with and without dysmenorrhea. *Health Care for Women International, 16*(2), 167–178.

Kammerer-Doak, D. N., & Saito, G. E. (1996). What's new in gynecology and obstetrics. *Journal of the American College of Surgeons, 182*(2), 107–114.

Klock, S. C. (1995). Psychosomatic issues in obstetrics and gynecology. In K. Ryan, J. Berkowitz, & R. Barbieri (Eds.), *Kistner's gynecology: Principles and practices* (6th ed., pp. 391–411). St. Louis: C. V. Mosby.

Laufer, M. R., & Goldstein, D. P. (1995). Pediatric and adolescent gynecology. In K. Ryan, J. Berkowitz, & R. Barbieri (Eds.), *Kistner's gynecology: Principles and practices* (6th ed., pp. 571–628). St. Louis: C. V. Mosby.

Lessick, M., Wickham, R., & Rehwaldt, M. (1997). Breast and ovarian cancer: Genetic update and implications for nursing. *MedSurg Nursing, 6*(6), 341–349.

Ling, F. W. (1995). Pelvic pain. In D. H. Nichols & P. J. Sweeney (Eds.), *Ambulatory gynecology* (pp. 200–212). Philadelphia: J. B. Lippincott.

Lowdermilk, D. L. (1995). Reproductive surgery. In C. I. Fogel & N. F. Woods (Eds.), *Women's health care* (pp. 629–650). Springhouse, PA: Springhouse.

McCance, K. L., & Huether, S. E. (1998). *Pathophysiology: The biological basis for disease in adults and children* (3rd ed). St. Louis: Mosby–Year Book.

McGourty, M. K. (1995). Vaginal infections: Keys to treatment. *Contemporary Nurse Practitioner, 1*(3), 18–23.

Mitchell, E. S., Woods, N. F., & Lentz, M. J. (1994). Differentiation of women with three perimenstrual symptom patterns. *Nursing Research, 43*(1), 25–30.

Morrow, C. P., & Curtin, J. P. (1996). *Gynecologic cancer surgery.* New York: Churchill Livingstone.

Rose, P. G. (1996). Endometrial carcinoma. *New England Journal of Medicine, 335*(9), 640–649.

Scura, K. W., & Whipple, B. (1997). How to provide better care for the postmenopausal woman. *American Journal of Nursing, 97*(4), 36–44.

Shurpin, K. (1997). Clinical snapshot: Ovarian cancer. *American Journal of Nursing, 97*(4), 34–35.

Somani, S. (1995). Evaluation and management of pelvic pain. In P. L. Carr, K. M. Freund, & S. Somani (Eds.), *The medical care of women* (pp. 55–66). Philadelphia: W. B. Saunders.

Tuomala, R. (1995). Gynecological infections. In K. Ryan, J. Berkowitz, & R. Barbieri (Eds.), *Kistner's gynecology: Principles and practices* (6th ed., pp. 496–523). St. Louis: C. V. Mosby.

Weiss, R. M. (1995). Endometriosis. In P. L. Carr, K. M. Freund, & S. Somani (Eds.), *The medical care of women* (pp. 67–75). Philadelphia: W. B. Saunders.

SUGGESTED READINGS

Ivey, C. L. (1994). When your client has ovarian cancer. *RN, 57*(11), 26–31.
    This article describes ovarian cancer and the related nursing care. Nonsurgical and surgical options are discussed with associated nursing implications.

McGourty, M. K. (1995). Vaginal infections: Keys to treatment. *Contemporary Nurse Practitioner, 1*(3), 18–23.
    This article describes common vaginal infections, including bacterial vaginosis, vaginal candidiasis, and vaginal trichomoniasis. Classic signs and symptoms and treatment choices are also described.

Scura, K. W., & Whipple, B. (1997). How to provide better care for the postmenopausal woman. *American Journal of Nursing, 97*(4), 36–44.
    This excellent article focuses on health promotion strategies for postmenopausal women, including nutrition, breast self-examination, and osteoporosis prevention. A continuing education quiz is found at the end of the article.

Chapter 79

INTERVENTIONS FOR MALE CLIENTS WITH REPRODUCTIVE PROBLEMS

Nurses need to know about the anatomy and physiology of male reproductive functions so that they can instruct clients about the impact of a disease process or treatment on their reproductive ability. The nurse includes the client and his spouse, sexual partner, or significant other in the decision-making process and works with members of the interdisciplinary team in providing collaborative care.

Benign Prostatic Hyperplasia

Overview

The prostate gland is the major accessory sex gland of the male. It is frequently a site of infection and benign and malignant neoplasms, all of which can affect urinary elimination.

Pathophysiology

In a young adult male, the prostatic capsule is thin and is attached to the underlying tissue. As a male ages, the glandular units in the prostate begin to undergo tissue *hyperplasia* (an abnormal increase in the number of cells),
resulting in prostatic *hypertrophy* (enlargement). Although prostatic hypertrophy is the more common term used to describe this phenomenon, prostatic hyperplasia is the correct term for the pathologic process.

When the prostate gland enlarges, it extends upward, into the bladder, and inward, narrowing the prostatic urethral channel, and obstructs the outflow of urine by encroaching on the bladder opening (Fig. 79–1). In response to this outlet resistance, the bladder is affected in several ways (Fig. 79–2). First, it may become hyperirritable, which produces urgency and frequency. As the bladder tries to compensate for its increased workload, muscles in the bladder wall hypertrophy (trabeculation) and may develop cellules and diverticula. If allowed to continue, this obstruction of urine flow can also cause a gradual dilation of the ureters (hydroureter) and kidneys (hydronephrosis). The enlarged prostate may also obstruct the bladder neck or the prostatic urethra, leading to urinary retention or incomplete bladder emptying. Overflow urinary incontinence is common; the urine "leaks" around the enlarged prostate, causing dribbling. Urinary stasis can result in urinary tract infections.

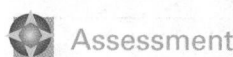

Figure 79–1. Benign prostatic hyperplasia grows inward, causing narrowing of the urethra.

Etiology

The exact cause of benign prostatic hyperplasia (BPH) remains unknown. Because the development of BPH is almost universal in older men, several theories have been examined:

- The effect of chronic inflammation of the prostate gland
- The role of general metabolic and nutritional factors (diet)
- The possible contribution of atherosclerosis

Demographic data (such as race) and social factors (such as socioeconomic status and heredity) have been examined as predictors for the development of BPH. Although these theories continue to be investigated, it is thought that BPH results from a systemic hormonal alteration. Support for this theory is based on the observations that aging is the major contributing factor, and another is the presence of testicular androgen. BPH does not occur in men who have been castrated before puberty (testicular androgen is absent). Men with BPH experience a regression of BPH after bilateral orchiectomies (testicular androgen is removed).

Incidence/Prevalence

ELDERLY CONSIDERATIONS

The incidence of BPH consistently increases with age. Characteristically, BPH is a disease of men older than 40 years of age, with an increase in incidence occurring with each decade of life. By age 50, at least 50% of all men have some degree of BPH, although not all are symptomatic (Matteson et al., 1997).

TRANSCULTURAL CONSIDERATIONS

Worldwide, BPH seems to be most common in Caucasians in Iceland, Europe, and the United States. The reported incidences of BPH in African-American and in Caucasian men in the United States are similar. The incidence of BPH in Asian countries, such as China and Japan, is lower than that in Caucasian or African-American populations (Giger & Davidhizar, 1995).

Collaborative Management

Assessment

➤ History

The nurse pays particular attention to the client's report of his urinary pattern. Commonly, the client complains of frequency, nocturia, and other symptoms of bladder neck obstruction known as *prostatism*. The symptoms of prostatism include hesitancy, intermittency, diminished force and caliber of stream, a sensation of incomplete bladder emptying, and post-void dribbling. If frequency and nocturia are not accompanied by symptoms of restricted flow, the nurse considers the possibility of a nonobstructive etiology, such as infection.

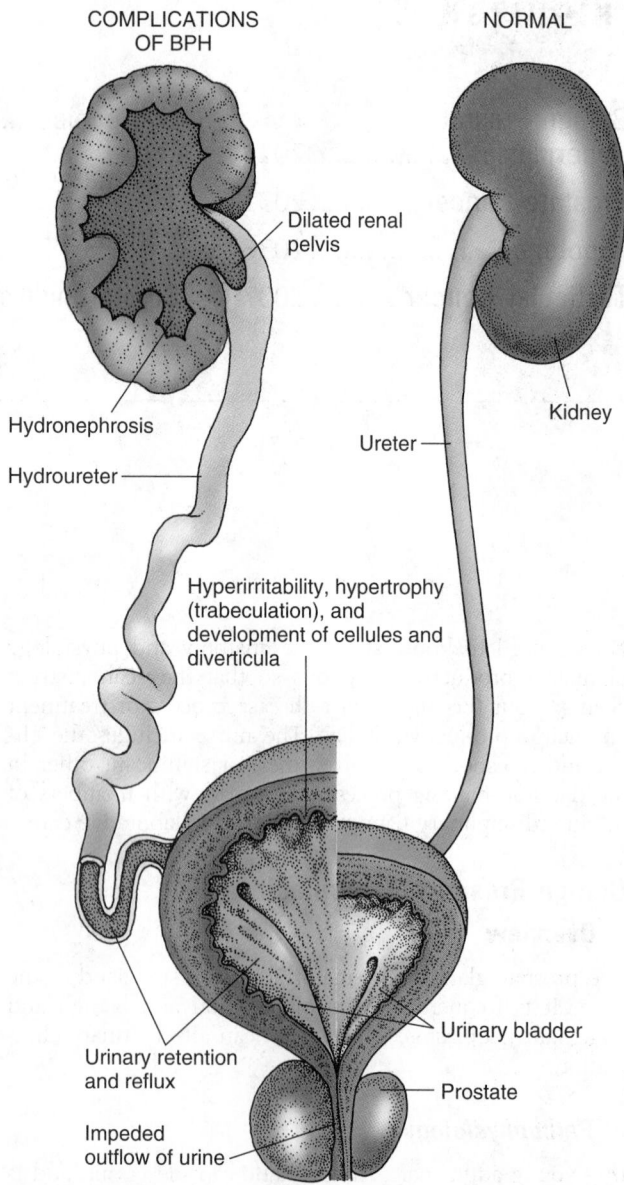

Figure 79–2. Potential complications of benign prostatic hyperplasia. The right side of the illustration shows a normal male urologic system. The left side shows potential complications.

The nurse questions whether the client has experienced any hematuria when initiating or at the end of urination. BPH is a common cause of hematuria in men older than 60 years.

➤ Physical Assessment/Clinical Manifestations

The client is instructed to void before the physical assessment. The nurse inspects, palpates, and percusses the client's abdomen for any evidence of a distended bladder. Normally, the bladder must contain 150 mL of urine to allow its palpation and percussion. A bladder with a larger amount of urine may be visible on inspection. An enlarged bladder may be palpated as a mass in the lower abdomen. If suprapubic pressure on the mass results in a feeling of urgency, the nurse may be able to ascertain that the mass is a distended bladder. The nurse remembers that the bladder of an obese client is best identified through percussion rather than inspection or palpation.

The nurse prepares the client for the examination of the prostate gland. Because the prostate is close to the rectal wall, the nurse explains that the easiest and most satisfactory examination of the prostate is by a digital rectal examination (DRE). The nurse helps the client to bend over the examination table or assume a side-lying fetal position. The nurse explains that the health care provider will examine the prostate for size and consistency. BPH usually presents as a uniform, elastic, nontender enlargement, whereas cancer of the prostate gland usually presents as a stony-hard nodule (Chart 79–1). The nurse advises the client that after the prostate gland is palpated, it may be massaged to obtain a fluid sample for examination to rule out prostatitis.

➤ Laboratory Assessment

The health care provider may order a urinalysis and obtains a urine specimen for culture to detect any urinary abnormality or evidence of urinary tract infection. Urinalysis includes tests for glucose, protein, occult blood, and pH levels. If an infection is present, the specimen may contain white blood cells (WBC) (pus) or red blood cells (RBC).

Blood studies that may be performed at the client's initial evaluation, depending on the client's condition and third-party payer, include

- A complete blood count (CBC) to evaluate any evidence of infection or anemia
- Blood urea nitrogen (BUN) and serum creatinine determinations to evaluate the client's renal function
- A prostate-specific antigen (PSA) and a serum acid phosphatase measurement if a prostatic malignancy is suspected (see Prostate Cancer later)

If the health care provider expresses prostatic fluid during the examination, the fluid is sent to the laboratory for microscopic examination and cultures.

➤ Radiographic Assessment

Radiologic studies that may be conducted in the work-up of the client with suspected benign prostatic hyperplasia (BPH) include x-rays of the kidneys, ureters, and bladder (KUB) and intravenous pyelography (IVP).

The KUB outlines the structure of the urinary tract in the abdomen. The IVP is particularly useful in revealing the structure and function of the urinary tract.

➤ Other Diagnostic Assessment

Urodynamic studies are very important in the diagnosis and evaluation of clients with bladder neck obstruction. Urodynamic flow studies include flow rate analysis (flowmetry) and assessment of residual urine. Flow rate analysis is simply a way of assessing the activity of the bladder and the outlet during the emptying phase of micturition.

During a cystourethroscopic examination, the physician uses a cystoscope to visualize the interior of the bladder, the bladder neck, and the urethra. This examination is necessary to study the presence and effect of bladder neck obstruction. The procedure is usually done in an ambulatory care setting.

Residual urine may be determined by catheterizing the client immediately after he voids. As an alternative, because the client always voids before cystourethroscopy, residual urine may be measured at that time.

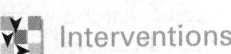 Interventions

Traditionally, the only effective treatment for the relief of the symptoms caused by BPH has been surgical, although attempts are being made to manage clients medically.

➤ Nonsurgical Management

Medical management of BPH includes drug therapy and other measures to minimize obstruction.

Drug Therapy. The health care provider may prescribe finasteride (Proscar) to shrink the prostate gland and improve urine flow. Finasteride lowers the client's level of dihydrotestosterone (DHT), a major cause of prostate growth. In some men, decreasing the DHT levels can shrink the enlarged prostate. The client may need to take the drug for as long as 6 months before any improvement occurs. The major side effects are impotence and decreased libido, although these effects are not common.

The presence of alpha-adrenergic receptors in the prostatic smooth muscle makes it treatable by alpha-blocking

---

Chart 79–1

Key Features of Benign Prostatic Hyperplasia

- Urinary frequency
- Nocturia
- Urinary hesitancy, particularly upon initiation of voiding
- Hematuria
- Diminished force of the urinary stream
- Post-void dribbling (overflow incontinence)
- Bladder distention
- Possible evidence of renal insufficiency, including edema, pallor, and pruritus
- A uniform, elastic, nontender palpable prostate

agents. When alpha-blocking agents are given, the prostate gland constricts, thereby reducing urethral pressure, improving urine flow, and decreasing residual mass. A variety of hormonal agents, including estrogens and androgens, alone or in combination, also have been used in attempts to alter BPH and its effects on voiding. This type of hormonal manipulation has not usually been successful.

Other Measures. Some nonsurgical measures seem to minimize obstructive symptoms, including those that cause the release of prostatic fluid, such as prostatic massage, frequent intercourse, and masturbation. These measures are very helpful for the client whose urinary obstructive symptoms have resulted from an enlarged prostate with a large amount of retained prostatic fluid. The nurse instructs the client to avoid drinking large amounts of fluid in a short time; avoid alcohol, diuretics, and caffeine; and void as soon as the urge is felt. These measures are aimed at preventing overdistention of the bladder, which may result in loss of detrusor muscle tone. Clients should also avoid any medications that can cause urinary retention, especially anticholinergics, antihistamines, and decongestants. The nurse emphasizes the importance of telling the health care provider about the diagnosis of BPH so that these drugs will not be prescribed.

➤ Surgical Management

Because most older men have some evidence of BPH, the mere presence of the condition does not mean that the client requires surgical intervention. In assessment of the client to confirm the need for surgical intervention, some or all of the following criteria are typically present:

- Acute urinary retention
- Chronic urinary tract infections secondary to residual urine in the bladder
- Hematuria
- Hydronephrosis
- Bladder neck obstruction symptoms that are worrisome to the client, such as urinary frequency and nocturia

The goals of surgical intervention are to relieve the symptoms associated with bladder neck obstruction and to improve the quality of the client's life by allowing him to void at normal intervals while retaining adequate urinary control and normal sexual functioning.

Preoperative Care. When planning surgical interventions, the physician considers the client's general physical condition, the size of the prostate gland, and the client's preference.

ELDERLY CONSIDERATIONS

The client is thoroughly evaluated for any other diseases common in the elderly, such as cardiovascular disease, chronic pulmonary disease, diabetes mellitus, and renal disease. If the client has renal disease, the nurse or physician may insert a Foley catheter. The client's intake, output, and serum electrolyte and creatinine levels are closely monitored until renal status has improved. In some cases, a thorough work-up and evalua-

tion of the client's medical condition may indicate that surgery would be too risky. In such cases, bladder neck obstruction may be relieved by permanent Foley drainage. The physician also assesses the client for the presence of urinary tract infection and treats any infection before performing surgery.

Preoperatively, the client may have many fears and misconceptions about prostatic surgery, such as automatic loss of sexual functioning or permanent incontinence. The physician's office nurse assesses the client's anxiety, corrects any misconceptions about the surgery, and provides accurate information to the client and his family. Regardless of the type of surgery to be performed, the nurse informs the client and his family about anesthesia (see Chap. 21). The client may have concurrent medical problems that put him at risk for complications of general anesthesia and may be advised to have epidural anesthesia. An epidural anesthetic may be used for any of the procedures and is the most commonly used type for a transurethral resection of the prostate (TURP). Because the client is awake, it is easier to assess for hyponatremia, fluid overload, and water intoxication.

The nurse also includes the topic of urinary catheters in the preoperative teaching plan for the client and his family. After prostatic surgery, all clients have an indwelling urethral (Foley) catheter for at least a day. The nurse instructs the client that he may also have continuous bladder irrigation (CBI) and traction on the catheter, but this may not be known until the client returns from the postanesthesia care unit (PACU). The nurse also explains before surgery that it is normal postoperatively for the urine to be blood tinged. Small blood clots and tissue debris may pass while the catheter is in place and immediately after it is removed.

Operative Procedures. Several surgical procedures are possible for removing the hypertrophied portion of the prostate gland (Fig. 79–3). In all approaches, the surgeon removes the hyperplastic tissue and leaves the prostatic capsule. The transurethral approach is a "closed" procedure; the others are considered "open" procedures because of the need for a surgical incision. The choice of procedure depends on

- The size of the prostate gland
- The location of the enlargement
- Whether surgery on the bladder is also needed
- The client's age and physical condition

Transurethral Resection of the Prostate. To perform a transurethral resection of the prostate (TURP), the most common type of prostatic surgery, the surgeon inserts a resectoscope (an instrument similar to a cystoscope, but with a cutting and cauterizing loop) through the urethra. The enlarged portion of the prostate gland is then resected in small pieces (prostate chips).

The surgeon chooses the TURP procedure when the major enlargement exists in the medial lobe of the prostate that directly surrounds the urethra and when the amount of tissue to be removed is relatively small. A TURP is safer for the client who is at high risk for surgery because a surgical incision is not necessary. Hos-

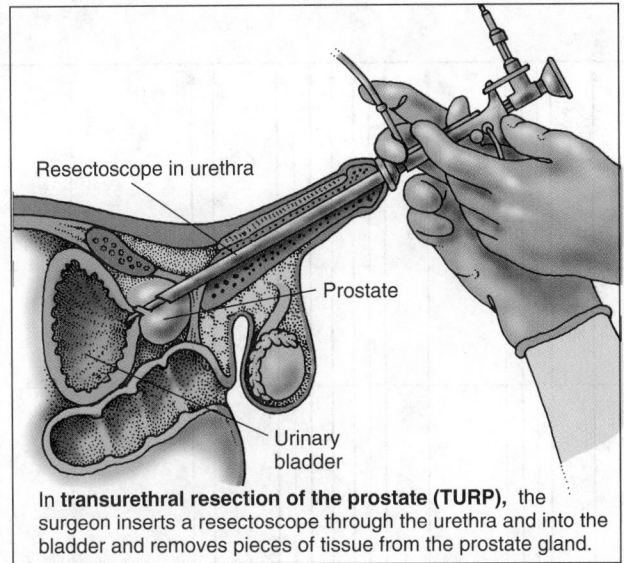

In **transurethral resection of the prostate (TURP),** the surgeon inserts a resectoscope through the urethra and into the bladder and removes pieces of tissue from the prostate gland.

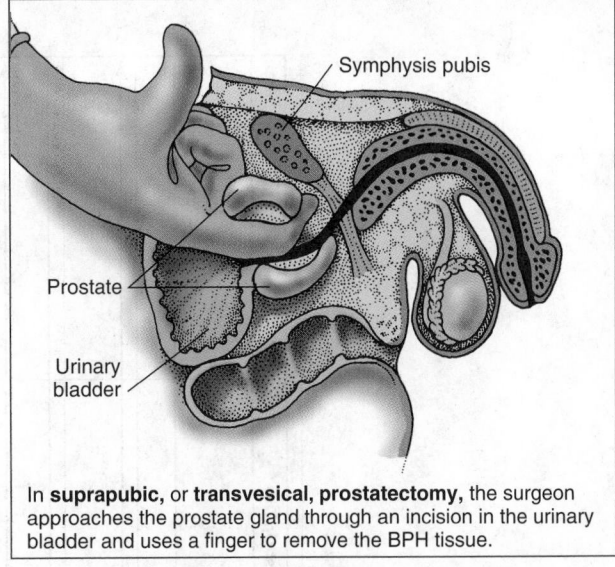

In **suprapubic,** or **transvesical, prostatectomy,** the surgeon approaches the prostate gland through an incision in the urinary bladder and uses a finger to remove the BPH tissue.

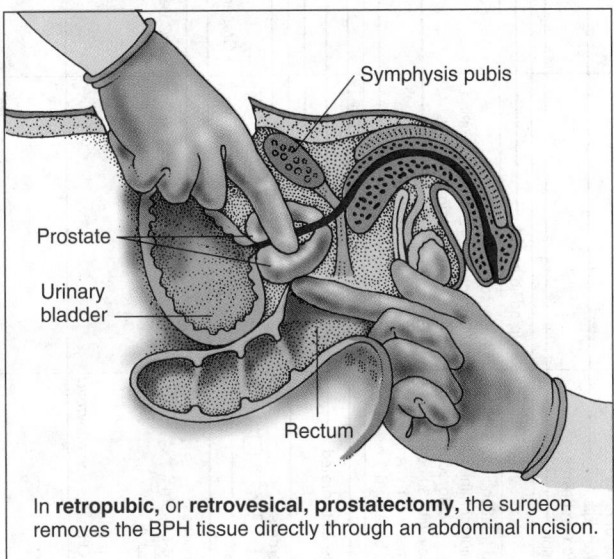

In **retropubic,** or **retrovesical, prostatectomy,** the surgeon removes the BPH tissue directly through an abdominal incision.

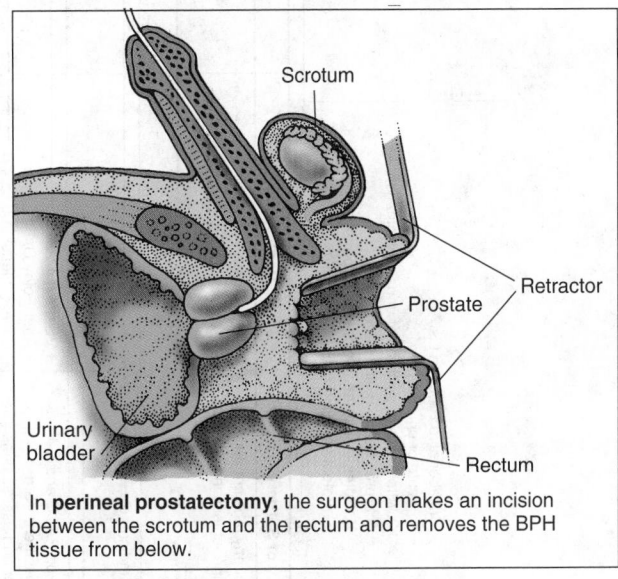

In **perineal prostatectomy,** the surgeon makes an incision between the scrotum and the rectum and removes the BPH tissue from below.

Figure 79–3. Prostatectomy procedures.

pitalization and convalescence are shorter than with any other type of prostatectomy.

The disadvantage of a TURP is that, because only small pieces of the gland are removed, prostatic tissue may grow back, resulting in recurrent urinary obstruction and necessitating additional TURPs. There is also the possibility of urethral trauma from the resectoscope, with resultant urethral strictures.

Suprapubic Prostatectomy. Suprapubic, or transvesical, prostatectomy is performed when the prostate is larger than the surgeon believes can be removed transurethrally and if the client has any coexisting bladder abnormalities that can be treated concurrently.

The surgeon makes a low, horizontal abdominal incision just above the symphysis pubis and exposes the bladder. The bladder is then distended with fluid, and a

small incision is made in the bladder wall. The prostate gland is enucleated through the bladder cavity, and any bladder disease is treated at this time.

The ability to treat bladder problems is the major advantage of suprapubic prostatectomy because an incision is made into the bladder to reach the prostate. Disadvantages are that

- An abdominal incision and an incision into the bladder are necessary.
- The client also has a suprapubic tube in place postoperatively.
- The surgery is more painful.
- Convalescence is longer than with a TURP.

Retropubic Prostatectomy. Retropubic, or extravesical, prostatectomy may be selected when the prostate is too large to be resected via the transurethral approach but no

University Hospitals
of Cleveland

CARE PATH NAME: TURP
DRG: ELOS: 2-3 Days
Expected Disposition: Home

Collaborative Problem List
1. Acute or chronic pain
2. Alterations in patterns of urinary elimination
3. Home health maintenance
4. Potential alteration of sexuality patterns
5. Potential for infection
6.

Focus	Pre-op	Day of Surgery	Post-Op Day 1	Post-Op Day 2	Post-Op Day 3
Laboratory/ Tests/ Procedures	• Chem 7 (Chem 12 if indicated) • CBC • EKG (if not done in last 6 months) • Chest X-Ray (if not done in last 6 months)	• Completion of any labs not done; otherwise, none, unless indicated	• CBC, Chem-7 in AM ☐ Y ☐ N • Only if indicated		
Consults/ Referrals	• Anesthesia	• None unless indicated	• Home RN screen		
Physical Assessment	• H&P	• Routine post-op PACU and Division assessment VS q 4 • I&O, monitor and assess urine output • Monitor patency of Foley • Monitor urine for clots • Assess for bladder spasms, bladder distention	• VS q 8 h if WNL • After Foley D/C monitor urine - at least 200 cc/4 h		
Activity	• Up ad lib	• Up in chair x1	• Up ad lib in AM		
Treatments	• Consent forms signed • Pre-op instruction and incentive spirometer given to patient	• Foley to CD and traction • 3-way NS irrigation continuously; Maintain for ___ colored urine • May irrigate Foley with 30 cc NS prn • Incentive Spirometry q 1 WA or cough and deep breathe q 1 h WA	• Foley to CD • D/C traction. D/C 3-way irrigation and continuous irrigation	• D/C Foley	
Diet	• NPO after MN	• NPO after MN • Clears - advance as tolerated	• Push fluids		
Medications		• IV per post-op orders • PCA order sheet ☐ Y ☐ N or IM/IV analgesics • Stool softeners • IV antibiotics x3 doses • B&O Supp. 1 q 4-6 h prn ☐ Y ☐ N • Antiemetics • Resume pre-op meds • Prn sedatives/PO analgesic/antipyretic	• D/C IV if tolerating fluids/diets • Begin PO antibiotics	• Oral analgesic • D/C B&O	
Psychosocial	• Identify supports • Assess patient/family concerns and coping				

					Discharge →
Discharge Planning/ Teaching	• Begin homegoing instructions - TURP PI sheet Kegel Exercises (PI-1049) • Initiate discussions on social supports, body image, sexual concerns	• Orient to room/unit • Reinforce teaching of post-op routines	• Reinforce home going instructions per PI-507 • Patient maintains urine flow with minimal irrigation • Assess services needed; consult if needed • Evaluate for special needs	• Discharge • Give supplies if patient is dribbling Review discharge instructions and need to push fluids • Provide appointment card; complete discharge form/Gold form if necessary	
Intermediate Outcomes	1. Pre-op testing within normal limits and complete 2. Patient/Family teaching complete 3. Consent signed	1. Pre-op testing within normal limits and complete 2. Patient/Family teaching complete 3. Consent signed 4. D/C'd from PACU per D/C criteria 5. Up in chair x 1 6. Pain/spasm controlled 7. Tolerating diet	1. Pain/spasm controlled 2. Tolerating diet 3. Home going teaching begun 4. Maintains urine flow and unobstructed by clots/minimal bleeding 5. Resuming pre-op ADLs 6. Increasing ambulation	1. Pain/spasm controlled 2. Tolerating diet 3. Home going teaching continues 4. Maintains urine flow and unobstructed by clots/minimal bleeding 5. Resuming pre-op ADLs 6. Increasing ambulation 7. Resumes pre-op diet 8. Using PO analgesia to control pain	1. Pain/spasm controlled 2. Tolerating diet 3. Home going teaching continues 4. Maintains urine flow and unobstructed by clots/minimal bleeding 5. Increasing ambulation 6. Using PO analgesia to control pain
Intermediate Outcomes **RN Signature** **Days**	☐ Met ☐ Not Met (see notes) #s not met ____ Signature ____	☐ Met ☐ Not Met (see notes) #s not met ____ Signature ____	☐ Met ☐ Not Met (see notes) #s not met ____ Signature ____	☐ Met ☐ Not Met (see notes) #s not met ____ Signature ____	
Intermediate Outcomes **RN Signature** **Evenings**	☐ Met ☐ Not Met (see notes) #s not met ____ Signature ____	☐ Met ☐ Not Met (see notes) #s not met ____ Signature ____	☐ Met ☐ Not Met (see notes) #s not met ____ Signature ____	☐ Met ☐ Not Met (see notes) #s not met ____ Signature ____	
Intermediate Outcomes **RN Signature** **Nights**	☐ Met ☐ Not Met (see notes) #s not met ____ Signature ____	☐ Met ☐ Not Met (see notes) #s not met ____ Signature ____	☐ Met ☐ Not Met (see notes) #s not met ____ Signature ____	☐ Met ☐ Not Met (see notes) #s not met ____ Signature ____	

Discharge Outcomes:	Met	Not Met	Comments	Date/Initials
☐ Performing ADLs at pre-op level				
☐ Tolerating regular diet				
☐ Pain control with po analgesia				
☐ Spontaneous urination				
☐ No evidence of infection				
☐ No bright red urine				
☐ Urinating sufficient amount				
☐ Prescriptions/PI Sheets/Follow-up appointments given to patient				

University Hospital's carepaths have been developed to assist clinicians in patient management and clinical decision-making. The carepaths are intended to meet the needs of patients in most circumstances. They are not intended to replace a clinician's judgment or establish a protocol for all patients with this diagnosis.

SP-13283 (09/17/97)

coexisting bladder abnormalities have been identified. The surgeon makes an abdominal incision above the symphysis pubis to expose the prostate gland. A small incision is made in the prostate gland, and the gland is enucleated. The difference between the suprapubic and the retropubic approaches is the bladder incision.

Perineal Prostatectomy. Perineal prostatectomy is performed primarily to

- Remove an enlarged prostate gland that is filled with calculi
- Treat prostatic abscesses that have not responded to conservative treatment
- Repair complications, such as lacerations in the prostatic capsule that may have occurred during a different type of prostatectomy
- Treat clients who are poor surgical risks

The client is placed in an exaggerated lithotomy position, and the knees are positioned on the chest. The surgeon makes a U-shaped incision between the ischial tuberosities, the scrotum, and the rectum. The prostatic capsule is then opened and enucleated. This type of prostatectomy provides a direct anatomic approach to the prostate gland.

The major disadvantage is the loss of sexual potency resulting from damage to the pudendal nerve. Clients with peripheral vascular disease or chronic pulmonary problems cannot tolerate the exaggerated lithotomy position and are not candidates for a perineal prostatectomy. Other disadvantages of this procedure include a greater risk for infection, the possibility of damage to the client's rectum and anal sphincter, and the possibility of urinary incontinence. For these reasons, this surgical approach is not commonly used.

Postoperative Care. The general postoperative care for the client who has had prostatic surgery is the same regardless of the type of procedure done and the type of anesthesia used (see Chap. 22). However, the nurse is aware of several differences as they affect nursing care. The Clinical Pathway on TURP on pages 2026–2027 highlights client care during the hospital stay.

Nursing Care After TURP. After a TURP, the surgeon inserts a three-way Foley catheter with a 30- to 45-mL retention balloon through the urethra into the bladder (Fig. 79–4). The catheter is pulled down into the prostatic fossa to help prevent bleeding. The surgeon often applies traction on the client's catheter by pulling the catheter taut and taping it to the client's abdomen or thigh.

Catheter Care and Continuous Bladder Irrigation. If the catheter is taped to the client's thigh, the nurse instructs him to keep his leg straight. The surgeon determines when the traction should be removed; usually it occurs on the first postoperative day.

The nurse explains that because of the Foley catheter's large diameter and the pressure of the retention balloon on the internal sphincter of the bladder, the client will continually feel the urge to void. The nurse emphasizes that this is a normal event and not a complication. The nurse advises the client not to try to void around the catheter, which causes the bladder muscles to contract and may result in painful bladder spasms. The nurse reassures the client that an antispasmodic medication can be given to keep him comfortable.

ELDERLY CONSIDERATIONS

For elderly clients who may become confused after surgery, the nurse reorients them frequently and reminds them to not pull on the catheter (Chart 79–2). If the client is restless or "picks" at tubes, the nurse may provide a familiar object, such as a family picture or other familiar object, for the client to hold on to for distraction and a feeling of security. If possible, the nurse does not restrain the client.

A continuous bladder irrigation (CBI) with normal saline or other solution, as ordered by the physician, may keep the catheter free of obstruction and facilitates detection of obstruction or other complications. The nurse adjusts the irrigation fluid rate to maintain a colorless or light-pink drainage return. For the nursing care of the client undergoing CBI, see Chart 79–3. The continuous irrigation is usually discontinued 24 hours after a TURP. The Foley catheter is usually removed when the CBI is discontinued.

Post-catheterization Care. When the Foley catheter is removed, the client may experience some burning on urination as well as some urinary frequency, dribbling, and leakage. The nurse reassures the client that these symptoms are normal and will subside. The client may also pass small clots and tissue debris for several days after the TURP. The nurse instructs the client to increase fluid intake to a minimum of 2000–2500 mL/day, which helps to decrease the dysuria and to keep the urine clear. An elderly client who has renal disease or who is susceptible to congestive heart failure may not be able to tolerate this much fluid. By the time of discharge (usually 2–3 days postoperatively), the client should be voiding 150–200 mL of clear yellow urine every 3–4 hours. By discharge, postoperative pain is minimal, and analgesics may not be required.

Complications of TURP. Clients who undergo TURPs or open prostatectomies are at risk for postoperative bleeding or hemorrhage. Bleeding is most common within the first 24 hours postoperatively and may not occur until the client has returned to his room. Bladder spasms or movement may initiate bleeding from previously controlled vessels. This bleeding may be arterial or venous, but venous bleeding is more common.

The nurse or assistive nursing personnel monitors the client's urinary output every 2 hours and vital signs every 4 hours. If the bleeding is arterial, the nurse will notice that the client's urinary drainage is bright red or "ketchup-like" with numerous clots. If arterial bleeding occurs, the nurse notifies the surgeon immediately and increases the CBI rate or intermittently irrigates the catheter with normal saline. The surgeon may order aminocaproic acid (Amicar) to control bleeding. The nurse keeps in mind that if the medication does not work, surgical intervention may be necessary to clear the bladder of clots and to stop the arterial bleeding.

If the bleeding is venous, the client's urinary output

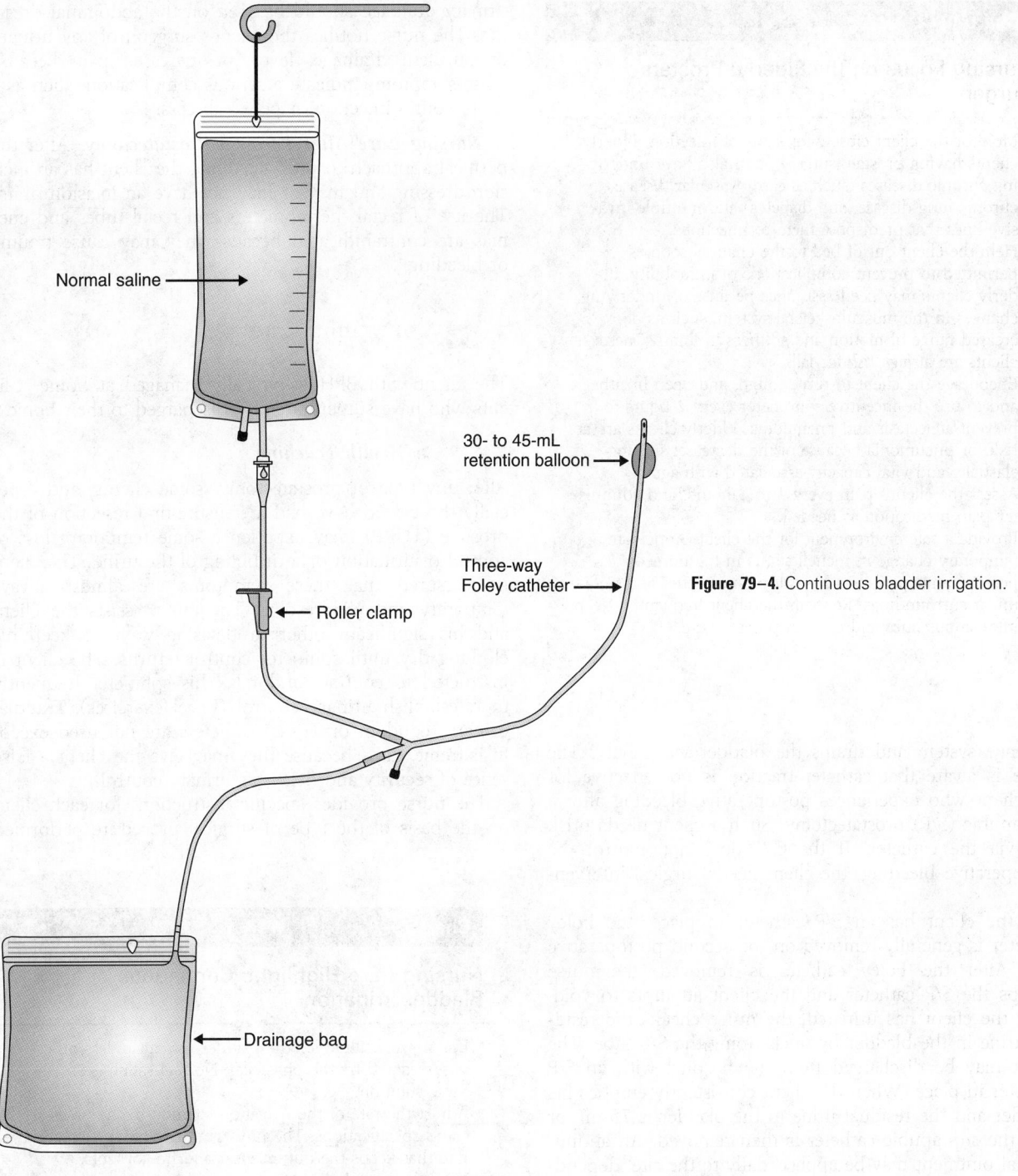

Normal saline

30- to 45-mL
retention balloon

Three-way
Foley catheter

Figure 79–4. Continuous bladder irrigation.

Roller clamp

Drainage bag

will be burgundy, with or without any change in vital signs. The nurse informs the client's surgeon of any of the signs and symptoms of bleeding. The surgeon may apply traction on the client's catheter for a few hours, which may control venous bleeding. The nurse assesses the success of this procedure in stopping the bleeding and is aware that the traction on the client's catheter is quite uncomfortable and increases the risk of bladder spasms. The physician usually orders analgesics or antispasmodics, such as dicyclomine hydrochloride (Bentyl, Antispas, Formulex✦, Lomine✦), oxybutynin (Ditropan), or bella-

donna and opium (B&O) suppositories to decrease painful bladder spasms.

The nurse closely monitors the client's hemoglobin (Hgb) and hematocrit (Hct) levels for anemia as a result of blood loss. Some clients may require blood transfusions to return the Hgb and Hct values to baseline levels.

Nursing Care After Suprapubic Prostatectomy. If the client has had a suprapubic prostatectomy, a suprapubic (S/P) catheter, in addition to a Foley catheter, will be in place. Each catheter is connected to a separate closed

---

Chart 79-2

Nursing Focus on the Elderly: Prostate Surgery

- Monitor the client closely for signs of infection. Elderly clients having prostate surgery often also have underlying chronic diseases (such as cardiovascular disease, chronic lung disease, and diabetes) and multiple invasive lines that predispose them to infections.
- Help the client out of bed to the chair as soon as permitted to prevent complications of immobility. Elderly clients may need assistance because of underlying changes in the musculoskeletal system, such as decreased range of motion and stiffness in joints. These clients are at *high risk* for falls.
- Encourage the client to turn, cough, and deep breathe and to use the incentive spirometer every 2 hours to prevent atelectasis and pneumonia. Elderly clients are at risk for pneumonia because of the decreases in lung elasticity and vital capacity associated with aging.
- Assess the client's pain every 2 to 3 hours, and administer pain medication as needed.
- Provide a safe environment for the client. Anticipate a temporary change in mental status in the immediate postoperative period as a result of anesthetics and unfamiliar surroundings. Reorient the client frequently. Keep intravenous lines and catheter tubes secure.

---

drainage system and drains the bladder via gravity. The nurse is aware that catheter traction is not effective for the client who experiences postoperative bleeding after a suprapubic (S/P) prostatectomy. Such a client needs brisk CBI via the catheter. If the CBI does not control the postoperative bleeding, the client needs surgical intervention.

If the client has an S/P catheter in place, the Foley catheter is generally removed on the second postoperative day. After the Foley catheter is removed, the nurse clamps the S/P catheter and the client attempts to void. After the client has urinated, the nurse checks the residual urine in the bladder by unclamping the S/P tube. The client may be discharged from the hospital with an S/P catheter in place. When the client consistently empties his bladder and the residual urine in the bladder is 75 mL or less, the suprapubic catheter is then removed. An antimicrobial ointment may be applied daily to the site, depending on hospital policy or physician order.

The client with a suprapubic catheter in place is at increased risk for bladder spasms. The incision dressing for these clients should be observed and changed more frequently than for clients who do not have an incision drain because the dressing becomes saturated with urine until the incision heals. If the suprapubic drain is not connected to gravity drainage, the nurse may enclose the drain with an ostomy bag to measure the output accurately and to prevent any skin problems or breakdown.

Nursing Care After Retropubic Prostatectomy. After a retropubic prostatectomy, the urinary sphincter muscles are seldom damaged, the bladder is not entered, and no

urinary drainage should be seen on the abdominal dressing. The nurse notifies the client's surgeon of any urinary or purulent drainage, fever, or increased pain because these symptoms indicate a serious complication, such as a deep wound infection or pelvic abscess.

Nursing Care After Perineal Prostatectomy. After the perineal approach to prostatectomy, the client has an incision dressing and may or may not have an incision drain. The use of rectal thermometers and rectal tubes and enemas are contraindicated because they may cause trauma or bleeding.

➤ Continuing Care

The client with BPH is typically managed at home. Clients who have surgery are also discharged to their home.

➤ *Health Teaching*

After any type of prostatectomy, some clients, and especially those who have had a transurethral resection of the prostate (TURP), may experience some temporary loss of control of urination or a dribbling of the urine. The client is reassured that these symptoms are almost always temporary and will resolve. The nurse assists the client and his significant other in devising ways to keep his clothing dry until sphincter control returns. The client is instructed to contract and relax his sphincter frequently to re-establish urinary control (Kegel exercises). External urinary (condom or Texas) catheters are not used except in extreme cases because they may give the client a false sense of security and delay his urinary control.

The nurse provides specific instructions for each client on the basis of the type of surgical procedure performed

---

Chart 79-3

Nursing Care Highlight: Continuous Bladder Irrigation

- Use normal saline for the bladder irrigant unless otherwise ordered by the physician. Normal saline is an isotonic solution.
- Adjust the rate of the irrigation solution to the physician's specifications. The physician may order a solution rate that keeps the output clear and free of clots.
- Monitor the color, consistency, and amount of urinary output.
- Check the drainage tubing frequently for external obstructions (such as kinks) and internal obstructions (such as blood clots and decreased output).
- Assess the client for complaints of bladder spasms, which may indicate obstruction.
- If the urinary catheter is obstructed, turn off the continuous bladder irrigation (CBI) and irrigate the catheter with 30 to 50 mL of normal saline using a large piston syringe.
- Notify the physician immediately if the obstruction does not resolve by hand irrigation or if the urinary return becomes "ketchupy."

and any further interventions he may need in the future. Discharge instructions for a client undergoing surgery of the prostate gland are listed in Chart 79–4.

The client who undergoes prostatic surgery usually needs emotional support. The client who undergoes a perineal prostatectomy is at risk for permanent sexual dysfunction. The nurse informs the client of the options, such as a penile prosthesis, that are available to treat impotence (see Impotence later).

Other surgical procedures for prostate removal should not cause physiologic impotence. Some clients, though, may have psychological impotence for a short time after surgery during the recovery phase.

➤ Home Care Management

Unless there is a complication of surgery, such as a wound infection or an unusual problem with voiding, the client does not have a dressing or indwelling catheter at the time of discharge. In some cases, the suprapubic tube may remain in place for several weeks after discharge.

➤ Health Care Resources

The nurse may refer clients who have undergone perineal surgery to a support group, such as Impotents Anonymous. These groups do not meet in every community.

Prostate Cancer

Overview

Prostate cancer is the most common cancer among American men, other than skin cancer, and the second leading cause of cancer deaths in this group (Parker et al., 1996; Haas & Sakr, 1997).

Pathophysiology

Of all cancers of the prostate, 95% are adenocarcinomas. These adenocarcinomas arise from the epithelial cells of the prostate and are usually located in the posterior lobe or outer portion of the gland (Fig. 79–5). The remaining types of prostatic neoplasms are classified as *nonepithelial* carcinomas and include ductal carcinomas, transitional cell carcinomas, squamous cell carcinomas, and sarcomas.

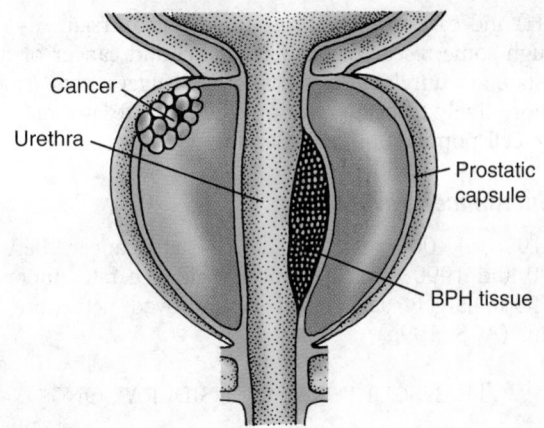

Figure 79–5. The prostate gland with cancer and benign prostatic hyperplasia (BPH). Note that cancer normally arises in the periphery of the gland, while BPH occurs in the center of the gland.

Of all malignancies, prostate cancer is one of the slowest growing and metastasizes in a fairly predictable pattern. The most common sites of metastatic spread are the prostatic and perivesicular lymph nodes; pelvic lymph nodes; bone marrow; and the bones of the pelvis, sacrum, and lumbar spine.

Metastatic involvement of the visceral organs tends to occur late in the natural history of the disease. The most common sites for metastatic prostate cancer are the lungs, liver, adrenals, and kidneys.

Tumor grade is an important variable in the management of prostate cancer. Grading is the pathologist's interpretation of the aggressiveness of the cancer. Usually, the Gleason grading system is used. Normal prostate tissue cells are given a score of 1 (best), and abnormal cells are given a score of 5 (worst). The scores of the two most common cell types found in the specimen are added to give the tumor a grade of between 2 and 10.

Etiology

While the cause of prostate cancer remains unclear, two factors influence its development. First, an intact hypothalamic-pituitary-testicular pathway must be present. Men who have been castrated before puberty are at little risk for prostate cancer. Second, the advancing age of the client increases his risk of prostate cancer.

ELDERLY CONSIDERATIONS

Cancer of the prostate is rare in men younger than 50 years, but the rate of occurrence increases with each decade. The average age at diagnosis is the mid-70s (American Cancer Society, 1996).

Other contributing factors include family history of prostate cancer, heavy metal exposure, and history of vasectomy or sexually transmitted disease. Several viruses, including cytomegalovirus and herpesvirus type 2, are present more frequently in cancerous prostatic tissue than in noncancerous tissue.

The relationship between benign prostatic hyperplasia

Chart 79–4

Education Guide: TURP Care

- Drink 12 to 14 glasses of water each day, preferable before 8 PM, *unless otherwise contraindicated.*
- Use alcohol, caffeinated beverages, and spicy foods in moderation to avoid overstimulation of your bladder.
- If your urine becomes bloody, rest quietly and increase your fluid intake. If the bleeding does not subside shortly, contact your doctor.
- Avoid strenuous activities, such as driving and working, during the first 2 to 3 weeks after surgery.
- Schedule a follow-up appointment with your doctor after you leave the hospital.

(BPH) and cancer of the prostate is controversial. Although some researchers say that BPH and cancer of the prostate are unrelated diseases, others suggest that cancer is more likely to occur within or adjacent to any proliferative cell population (Haas & Sakr, 1997).

Incidence/Prevalence

In 1996, 41,000 men died of prostate cancer. Between 1980 and 1990, prostate cancer incidence rates increased by 50%, largely as a result of improved detection programs (ACS, 1996).

TRANSCULTURAL CONSIDERATIONS

 African-American men have the highest prostate cancer incidence rates in the world. Associated mortality rates are twice those of Caucasian men (von Eschenbach et al., 1997). African-American men tend to be affected at an earlier age and have more advanced disease at the time of diagnosis. Lack of cancer awareness has been identified as a cause of increased mortality rates (Collins, 1997). Prostate cancer also occurs more frequently in Scandinavians than Caucasians.

Hispanic and Asian-American men have lower rates of prostate cancer than Caucasian men and lower mortality rates, implying cultural, genetic, or lifestyle variables (ACS, 1996).

Collaborative Management

Assessment

As with any cancer, accurate staging is necessary for treatment planning and monitoring the clinical course of the disease. As in benign prostatic hyperplasia (BPH), the first symptoms that the client may experience are related to bladder neck obstruction, such as difficulty in initiating urination, recurrent bladder infections, and urinary retention. Gross, painless hematuria is the most common presenting clinical manifestation.

At times, a client may be undergoing intervention for BPH and is discovered to have cancer of the prostate. Bone pain is a symptom of a more advanced stage of prostate cancer. The client who has symptoms of urinary obstruction (urinary hesitancy, back pain) and bone pain is most likely to have metastatic disease at diagnosis.

➤ Prostate Cancer Screening

The most effective procedures for screening for cancer of the prostate are the digital rectal examination (DRE) and the prostate-specific antigen (PSA) test. In 1997, the ACS updated its guidelines for cancer screening (Chart 79–5). Beginning at age 50 years, all men should have an annual DRE and PSA test (Mettlin, 1997). On rectal examination, a prostate that is found to be stony hard and with palpable irregularities or indurations is suspected to be malignant.

Prostate-specific antigen (PSA) is a highly immunogenic glycoprotein produced solely by the prostate. The normal level of PSA established by the American Cancer Society

---

Chart 79–5

Health Promotion Guide: Updated 1997 American Cancer Society Prostate Screening and Detection Guidelines

- An annual digital rectal examination (DRE) and prostate-specific antigen (PSA) test should be offered to
  - Men beginning at age 50 years
  - Men who have a life expectancy of at least 10 years
  - Younger men who are at high risk (at least by age 45 years)
- Men at high risk include those with a strong familial predisposition (e.g., two or more first-degree relatives have prostate cancer) and African-American men.
- DRE should be performed by health care professionals skilled in recognizing subtle prostate abnormalities.
- DRE is less effective than PSA in detecting prostate cancer. An abnormal PSA test result is a value above 4.0 ng/mL.

---

is a value of less than 4 ng/mL. PSA levels are elevated in clients with increased prostatic tissue as a result of various conditions, including carcinoma of the prostate, benign prostatic hyperplasia (BPH), prostatic infarction, and prostatitis.

PSA blood levels should never be used as a screening test without a physical examination of the prostate. The PSA serum level was never meant to replace the DRE, but to be used in conjunction with it (Gelfand et al., 1995). Twenty-five percent of clients with prostate cancer have PSA levels less than 4 ng/mL (Mettlin, 1997).

PSA is not elevated in healthy men or in men with carcinomas other than prostate carcinoma. However, the normal PSA level is slightly higher in the elderly and in African-Americans. An elevated PSA level should decrease a few days after prostatectomy surgery. An increase in the PSA level at postoperative visits usually indicates that the disease has recurred.

TRANSCULTURAL CONSIDERATIONS

The participation rate of African-American men in prostate cancer screening programs remains very low. Lack of knowledge, fear of cancer, and subsequent negative attitudes about DRE may account for low participation (Gelfand et al., 1995). A nursing study by Collins (1997) showed that educational intervention had a positive effect on short-term knowledge and awareness of prostate cancer by African-American men (see Research Applications for Nursing).

After screening by DRE and PSA, some clients undergo a transrectal ultrasound study of the prostate, although its effectiveness is controversial. The urologist inserts a small probe into the client's rectum and obtains an ultrasonogram of the prostate. A specimen for biopsy may also be obtained by the rectal probe.

When the diagnosis of prostatic cancer is suspected, a

Research Applications for Nursing

Educating African American Men About Early Detection of Cancer

Collins, M. (1997). Increasing prostate cancer awareness in African American men. Oncology Nursing Forum, 24, 91–95.

The intent of this study was to assess the effect of an educational program about prostate cancer on the knowledge level of African-American men. A convenience sample of 75 men between the ages of 23 and 83 years completed a pre- and postintervention questionnaire. The findings were positive in that test scores improved after the educational session.

Critique. Although a convenience sample was used, the researcher addressed a major health concern, that is, the lack of knowledge and participation of African-American men in prostate screening programs. Unfortunately, only short-term retention was evaluated. A follow-up test weeks or months later could determine the lasting effects of education. The sample could also be followed to see if they participated in prostate screening as a result of learning more about prostate cancer.

Possible Nursing Implications. Nurses have to continue their efforts to educate the public, especially high-risk groups, about the need for prevention and early detection of all types of cancers. African-American men are at the highest risk for prostate cancer.

biopsy is necessary for confirmation. Prostatic ultrasonography may be performed to isolate the area of the prostate for biopsy. One of several procedures may be used to obtain the biopsy specimen. The most common procedure is the needle-core or aspiration biopsy, described in Chapter 76.

After the diagnosis of prostate cancer is made, the client undergoes radiographic and blood studies to ascertain the extent of the disease. Common tests include computed tomography (CT) of the pelvis and abdomen to assess the status of the pelvic and para-aortic lymph nodes and a bone scan to ascertain any evidence of metastatic disease. Hepatomegaly or abnormal results of liver function studies indicate a need for further evaluation for the presence of liver metastases.

Most clients with advanced prostate cancer also have elevated levels of serum acid phosphatase. Approximately 90% of clients with prostate cancer metastatic to the bone have elevated serum alkaline phosphatase levels.

 Interventions

Management of the client with prostate cancer includes surgery, radiation therapy, and drug therapy. Management is based on the extent of the disease and the client's physical condition. The client may undergo surgery for a tumor biopsy, staging and removal of the tumor, or palliation to control the spread of disease or relieve distressing symptoms.

Surgical Management

Because as many as 30% of localized prostate cancers are resistant to radiation, surgery is the standard treatment. The surgical approaches for prostatectomy in the client with prostate cancer are similar to those for the client with benign prostatic hyperplasia (BPH) (see earlier). In most cases, however, the surgical procedure is much more extensive and includes a pelvic lymphadenectomy (removal of pelvic lymph nodes).

Clients who have stage 0 cancer of the prostate require only close follow-up by their health care provider. If obstruction recurs, repeated needle biopsies or transurethral resections of the prostate (TURPs) should be part of the screening.

Radical Prostatectomy. Clients with more severe disease typically undergo a radical prostatectomy via a retropubic, perineal, or suprapubic approach. In the radical prostatectomy, instead of enucleating only the prostate gland, as in the procedure for BPH, the surgeon removes the entire gland along with the prostatic capsule, the cuff at the bladder neck, the seminal vesicles, and the regional lymph nodes. The remaining urethra is anastomosed to the bladder neck. The removal of tissue at the bladder neck allows the seminal fluid to travel upward into the bladder rather than down the urethral tract, resulting in retrograde ejaculations. The client is sterile, but his ability to have an erection and an orgasm should not be permanently impaired.

Sexual Dysfunction. The surgeon advises clients who undergo radical perineal prostatectomy that they may have an erectile dysfunction (impotence) after the surgery. This consequence is directly related to any damage done to the pudendal nerve (which is necessary for erection and orgasm) during the surgery.

The surgeon may perform a nerve-sparing prostatectomy:

- If there is no evidence of disease in adjacent lymph nodes
- If serum acid phosphatase levels are not elevated
- If there is no clinical evidence of cancer extension beyond the prostate gland

As the name of the procedure implies, the surgeon keeps the nerves responsible for penile erection intact. After surgery, the client may experience temporary impotence, but normal function usually returns in 3–12 months.

Urinary Incontinence. Because the internal and external sphincters of the bladder lie close to the prostate gland, urinary incontinence can be another complication of a radical prostatectomy. The nurse teaches the client perineal exercises to help facilitate the return of urinary continence after surgery or after the removal of the Foley catheter. To perform the exercises, the client contracts and relaxes the perineal and gluteal muscles in several ways. For one of the exercises, the nurse teaches the client to

1. Tighten the perineal muscles for 3–5 seconds as if to prevent voiding, then relax

2. Bear down as if having a bowel movement
3. Relax and repeat the exercise

The nurse shows the client how to inhale through pursed lips while tightening the perineal muscles and how to exhale when he relaxes. To regain urinary control, the client can also practice holding an object, such as a pencil, in the fold between the buttock and the thigh. The client may also sit on the toilet with his knees apart while voiding and start and stop his stream several times. Chart 79–6 summarizes the most important aspects of postoperative nursing care for the client undergoing a radical prostatectomy.

Complementary Therapies. Biofeedback has been successfully used as a noninvasive treatment for incontinence after radical prostatectomy. In a nursing study by Jackson et al. (1996), 27 postoperative radical prostatectomy clients were treated by biofeedback for urinary incontinence. Forty-eight percent of the sample had complete success, 26% had significant improvement but were not completely dry, and 26% experienced failure. The authors concluded that biofeedback training can work as a first-line option for most clients if they are motivated to decrease their incontinence.

If the client cannot recover urinary continence, an artificial urinary sphincter may be surgically implanted (Fig. 79–6). Artificial sphincters have been more successful in males than in females, possibly because of the difference in urethral length.

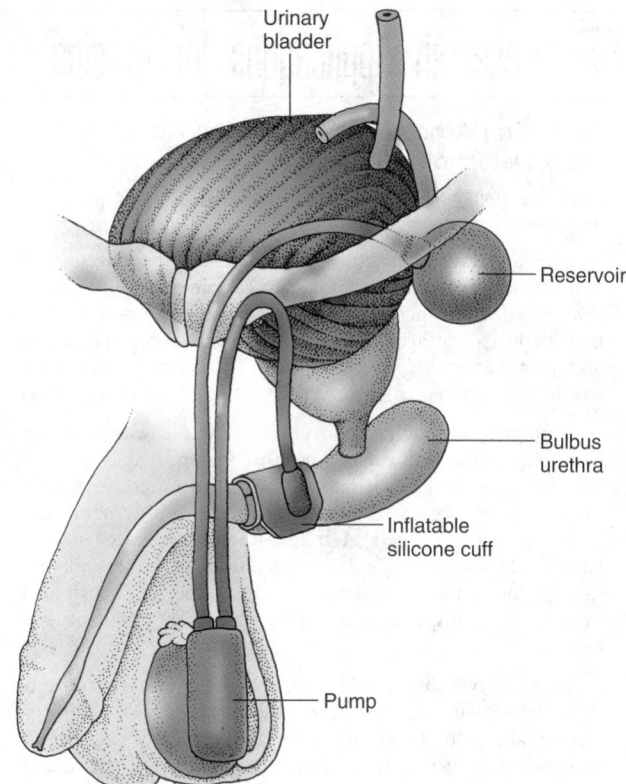

Figure 79–6. An artificial urinary sphincter is a fluid-filled system with a silicone cuff that surrounds the urethra and functions as a urinary sphincter. A pump is placed in the scrotum, and a fluid reservoir is placed in the abdomen. When the pump is squeezed, fluid leaves the urethral cuff and flows into the reservoir, allowing the client to empty his bladder.

Chart 79–6

Nursing Care Highlight: Radical Prostatectomy

• Encourage the client to use patient-controlled analgesia (PCA) as needed. The PCA device may be used through the second postoperative day.
• Keep the client on bed rest on the day of surgery. Help the client to get out of bed and ambulate for a short distance by the first postoperative day.
• Keep the client on NPO status as ordered, usually until the first or second postoperative day.
• Maintain the sequential compression device until the client begins to ambulate. Apply antiembolic stockings until discharge.
• Monitor the client for deep vein thrombosis and pulmonary embolus.
• Keep an accurate record of intake and output, including Jackson-Pratt or other drainage device drainage.
• Keep the urinary meatus clean using soap and water.
• Avoid rectal procedures or treatments.
• Teach the client how to care for the urinary catheter because he will be discharged with the catheter in place.
• Teach the client how to use a leg bag.
• Emphasize the importance of not straining during bowel movement. Advice the client to avoid suppositories or enemas.
• Remind the client about the importance of follow-up appointments with the physician to monitor progress.

After the sphincter has been implanted, the nurse instructs the client to report any complications, such as fever, pain on inflation of the device, edema or cellulitis in the genitalia, or recurrence of incontinence, indicating a possible mechanical malfunction in the system.

Cryosurgical Ablation. A newer, minimally invasive procedure that is becoming more popular as an alternative to radical prostatectomy is cryosurgical ablation of the prostate. During surgery, the client is placed in the lithotomy position to facilitate placement of the transrectal ultrasound probe. The probe helps determine the size of the prostate and the subsequent number of small cryoprobes that are positioned around the prostate gland. Liquid nitrogen freezes the gland, whose dead cells are then absorbed by the body.

The primary advantages of this procedure are minimal blood loss, minimal postoperative pain, decreased risk for postoperative urinary incontinence, and a 1- to 2-day hospital stay versus a 5-day stay for the traditional radical prostatectomy. Most clients are permitted to return to their usual activity level in about 1 week after surgery. The procedure can be repeated if necessary (Brenner & Krenzer, 1995).

Bilateral Orchiectomy. Unlike a radical prostatectomy, a bilateral orchiectomy (removal of both testes) is palliative surgery. The intent of the surgery is not to cure the disease but to arrest its spread by removing testosterone. This procedure is described later in this chapter under Testicular Cancer.

Nonsurgical Management

Nonsurgical management is usually done as an adjunct to surgery, but may be done as an alternative intervention. Modalities include radiation therapy and drug therapy.

Radiation Therapy. External beam radiation therapy is important in the treatment of prostate cancer. It is performed as

- An alternative curative treatment to surgery for locally contained tumors
- An adjunct to radical prostatectomy when surgical margins or regional lymph nodes show malignancy postoperatively
- Palliation of the client's symptoms

Palliative radiation therapy alleviates pain caused by skeletal metastases and relieves ureteral or bladder neck obstruction.

Interstitial radiation therapy, or radioactive seed implantation, with ^{198}Au or ^{125}I may be a treatment option for some clients. Clients who may be candidates for interstitial radiation therapy include those with limited local tumors who have had no previous treatment and those who have had external radiation or surgery but have small areas of tumor remaining (see also Chap. 27).

Drug Therapy. Drug therapy may consist of either hormonal therapy or chemotherapy.

Hormonal Therapy. Because prostate cancer is hormone dependent, clients with extensive tumors or those with metastatic disease are usually managed by androgen deprivation. Manipulating the hormonal environment in the client may be accomplished in two ways:

- The testosterone influence can be removed by a bilateral orchiectomy.

- Estrogens or gonadotropin-releasing hormone (GnRH) agonist analogs can be administered (Chart 79–7).

Estrogens such as diethylstilbestrol (DES) inhibit the release of luteinizing hormone (LH) from the pituitary gland. Clients with significant cardiovascular disease may not be candidates for estrogen therapy because of the side effects of estrogens, such as sodium and water retention and thromboembolic episodes.

Leuprolide acetate (Lupron), a GnRH agonist analog (which suppresses LH release by the pituitary), also reduces serum testosterone levels without any of the estrogenic side effects of DES. Flutamide (Eulexin, Euflex✣), an oral androgen-blocking agent, inhibits tumor progression by blocking the uptake of testicular and adrenal androgens at the prostate tumor site.

The health care provider may prescribe goserelin acetate (Zoladex), a potent GnRH agonist analog, for palliation of advanced prostatic carcinoma. This drug is an alternative treatment when orchiectomy or estrogen administration is neither acceptable nor indicated for the client.

Chemotherapy. Systemic cytotoxic chemotherapy has not proved effective in the treatment of prostate cancer. It is used for the client who fails to respond to hormonal manipulation. Unfortunately, only a small percentage of clients respond to cytotoxic chemotherapy with a partial shrinkage of their tumors, and the response usually lasts only a few months. (See Chapter 27 for a discussion of chemotherapy.)

➤ Continuing Care

Nursing management of the client with prostate cancer always includes the client's spouse or sexual partner. Clients with prostate cancer may require nursing interventions in a wide variety of settings—at the hospital, the

Chart 79–7		
Drug Therapy for Prostate Cancer		
Drug	**Usual Dosage**	**Nursing Interventions**
Leuprolide acetate (Lupron)	7.5 mg IM q month	• Use at least a 22-gauge needle. • Mix the solution well; it is a milky suspension. • Observe for side effects, including "hot flashes" and sweating. Be aware that the client's symptoms may temporarily worsen, caused by a temporary testosterone increase.
Flutamide (Eulexin, Euflex)	750 mg PO in 3 daily divided doses	• Teach the client that side effects include "hot flashes," loss of libido, and impotence. Diarrhea and nausea with vomiting are less common.
Gosereline acetate (Zoladex)	3.6 mg SC every 28 days	• The prefilled syringe cannot be aspirated. If a blood vessel is damaged, blood will enter the syringe. • Teach the client that side effects include "hot flashes," sexual dysfunction, and decreased erections.

radiation therapy department, the oncologist's office, or home—and at any stage of the disease process. Major quality-of-life issues facing the client with prostate cancer include body image, sexuality, and the impact of the cancer diagnosis on his life.

Impotence

Overview

An erection is an involuntary reaction in response to sexual stimulation and excitement. Impotence, the inability to achieve or maintain an erection, is caused by several disorders. It was once believed that 90% of impotence was of psychological origin, but it is now thought that at least 50% of men with impotence have an underlying physical disorder. Health care professionals must correctly identify the underlying cause of impotence so that the proper treatment can be recommended to help the client return to a satisfying sexual life.

Most men, in certain situations or at some time during their sexual life, find themselves unable to achieve or maintain an erection. This is normal and does not indicate a problem. However, a man who cannot achieve or maintain an erection firm enough for sexual intercourse more than 25% of the time is considered to be impotent or to have an erectile dysfunction (see Chap. 11).

Erectile impotence is attributed to psychological factors, physical factors, or a combination of both. The causes of psychological impotence are varied and include anxiety, fatigue, boredom, depression, guilt, and pressure to perform well sexually.

Emotional stress can lead to impotence, just as it can lead to many other forms of illness. Persistent psychological impotence also can be triggered by one incident of sexual failure. A man who is worried about achieving an erection may not be able to relax and thereby may find it difficult to achieve an erection.

Physiologic impotence is caused by a physical disorder, for example, an injury, a disease, a hormonal imbalance, or surgery (Table 79–1). Diabetes mellitus is one of the most common causes of physical impotence. Impotence occurs in over 50% of diabetic men of any age.

Collaborative Management

 Assessment

Assessment begins with a sexual and medical history. The client with *psychological* impotence usually reports

- Acute onset
- Selectivity
- Periodicity
- Nocturnal erections and emissions
- An ability to masturbate
- An ability to have an erection and to function sexually under certain circumstances
- Retention of testicular sensitivity

The client with *physical* impotence usually reports a gradual loss of erectile function, some degree of erectile dysfunction in all sexual circumstances, and absence of nocturnal erections and emissions.

TABLE 79–1

Common Causes of Physiologic Impotence

Pathologic Causes
- Diabetes mellitus
- Thyroid disorders
- Adrenal disorders
- Hypothalamic-pituitary-gonadal disorders
- Decreased testosterone secretion
- Multiple sclerosis
- Amyotrophic lateral sclerosis
- Alzheimer's disease
- Stroke
- Arteriosclerosis
- Pelvic fracture
- Hypertension
- Brain or spinal cord injury

Iatrogenic Causes
- Prostatectomy or other surgery of the prostate or rectum
- Cystectomy
- Abdominoperineal resection
- Pelvic irradiation
- Sympathectomy
- Antihypertensive drugs
- Opioids
- Barbiturates
- Tranquilizers
- Monoamine oxidase inhibitors and other antidepressants
- Estrogens
- Antihistamines

Other Causes
- Alcohol, tobacco, and illicit drugs
- Normal changes of aging
  - Loss of tissue elasticity
  - Decreased levels of circulating testosterone

The client is also asked about the presence of common causes of impotence. The nurse investigates whether there is a family history of impotence or a family history of any physiologic or psychological conditions that may contribute to erectile dysfunction. The nurse gathers information about any symptoms associated with diabetes or hypertension.

Laboratory and other diagnostic studies are done to rule out any genitourinary disease. Cholesterol and triglyceride levels are examined to assess the client for arteriosclerosis. A glucose tolerance test is usually ordered to rule out diabetes mellitus. Serum follicle stimulating hormone (FSH), luteinizing hormone (LH), and testosterone levels are measured to exclude a hypothalamic-pituitary-gonadal cause.

Doppler ultrasound arterial flow studies of the penile arteries can determine whether the client has penile vascular disease, one of the causes of organic impotence. The nocturnal penile tumescence test is used to record and measure nocturnal erections to help distinguish between physiologic and psychological impotence.

A simple variation of the nocturnal penile tumescence test is the stamp test. Stamps are wrapped snugly around the penis with the overlapping stamp moistened to seal the ring. The test is positive if the stamps are broken along the perforations when the client awakens. Depending on his age, a man usually has three or four erections, each lasting about 20–30 minutes, during a night's sleep. If the client experiences normal erections during sleep, erectile dysfunction while he is awake is most likely psychological.

 Interventions

Management of impotence may be nonsurgical or surgical, depending on its cause.

Nonsurgical Management

Nonsurgical management focuses on the underlying cause of the problem. The client may need psychosocial intervention, changes or adjustments in medications that he may be taking, or control of any underlying disease. The client with psychogenic impotence is referred, with his partner, to a sex therapist (see Chap. 11). If a medication is discovered to be the cause of impotence, the health care provider may change the medication. However, depending on the client's illness, this may not be possible, and the client's erectile dysfunction may be managed surgically.

If an underlying disease is causing the impotence, interventions are aimed at controlling the disease. Impotence resulting from hypothalamic-pituitary-gonadal dysfunction may be reversed with proper hormonal therapy, such as testosterone replacement or the administration of gonadotropin-releasing factor or pituitary gonadotropins.

Because impotence often results from inadequate blood flow into the penis and/or the inability of blood vessels to retain the blood flowing into the penis, a vacuum-pump device can be used to treat erectile dysfunction. The client places the penis into a vacuum cylinder. An erection is achieved by a vacuum or suction, which mechanically draws blood into the cavernous bodies. Blood flow from the penis is then reduced with a simple retention device, such as a tension ring, which thus prevents the loss of the erection.

A pharmacologic injection can also be a nonsurgical treatment for impotence. Clients are taught to inject a vasodilator, such as papaverine (Pavabid) or phentolamine (Regitine, Rogitine✦), directly into the corporeal bodies of the penis. This increases arterial blood flow, which creates subsequent venous blood trapping, thus causing an erection.

The newest drug for impotence, Viagra, is taken orally. Although it is a successful treatment for both men and women, men with cardiovascular disease who take nitroglycerin are not candidates for the drug. A number of deaths have been reported in this group either during or after sexual intercourse.

Surgical Management

Surgery may be indicated for clients who are impotent because of physical causes. Clients with insufficient blood flow to the penis may benefit from an arterial bypass or other vascular procedure.

Some clients may be candidates for a penile prosthesis if they meet the following criteria:
- Irreversible physiologic impotence demonstrated by history and diagnostic testing
- Strong desire to sexually satisfy himself or his partner
- The presence of some penile sensation
- The absence of any prostatic or genitourinary problems

Several types of penile prostheses are available (Fig. 79–7), including the semirigid, self-contained, and inflatable prostheses. The semirigid and self-contained prostheses are easier to insert, are less expensive, and necessitate fewer days in the hospital than inflatable prostheses.

The *semirigid* prosthesis has two silicone rods that simulate a normal erection. These rods are implanted into the corpora cavernosa via a perineal or dorsal penile incision. This type of prosthesis has no moving parts that can break or malfunction. Because the penis remains in a constant state of semierection, this intervention may be unacceptable to the client or his sexual partner.

The *self-contained* prosthesis is a newer variation of the semirigid type. Like the semirigid prosthesis, this device is totally contained in the penis but allows the penis to hang in a more natural position. A self-contained prosthesis consists of a cylinder, a pump, and a reservoir filled with fluid. By pumping the prosthesis behind the head of the penis, the client can transfer fluid from the reservoir in the rear portion of the device to the part of the device in the shaft of the penis. The cylinder then becomes enlarged and produces an erection. When an erection is no longer desired, the fluid is returned to the reservoir when the client presses a release valve located behind the pump.

The *inflatable* prosthesis includes two hollow silicone cylinders, a reservoir, and a pump. The cylinders are surgically implanted into the corpora cavernosa. The reservoir containing radiopaque fluid is placed under the abdominal fascia, and the pump is placed in the scrotum. When the pump in the scrotum is compressed, the fluid flows from the reservoir into each cylinder, causing an erection. A one-way valve keeps the fluid in the cylinders until a release valve in the pump is compressed, allowing the fluid to return to the reservoir. This type of prosthesis simulates natural erections and flaccidity, but mechanical problems may occur. Inflatable prostheses cost more than the other types.

Postoperatively, the nurse observes the client with a penile prosthesis for complications, such as shock, atelectasis, pneumonia, fever, deep vein thrombosis, signs of wound infection, and urinary retention. Before discharge, the nurse gives the client instructions for home care. These instructions are similar to postoperative instructions for any client, including observation for bleeding and infection.

Testicular Cancer
Overview

Although malignant tumors of the testis are rare and represent less than 2% of all cancers in men, testicular cancer is the most common malignancy in men aged 15

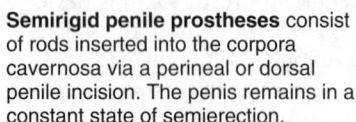

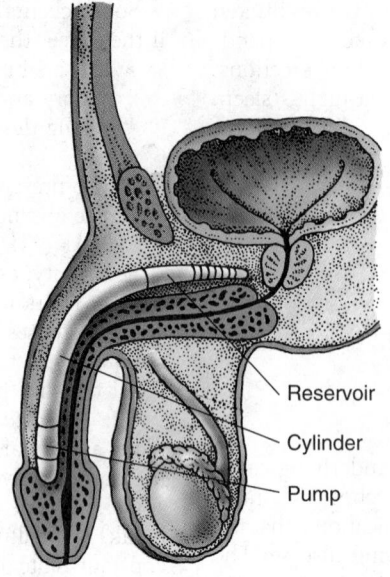

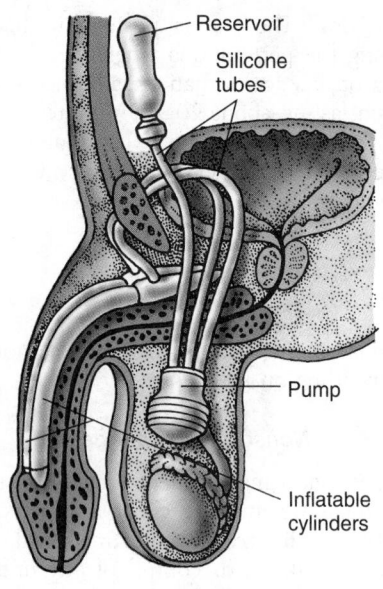

Semirigid penile prostheses consist of rods inserted into the corpora cavernosa via a perineal or dorsal penile incision. The penis remains in a constant state of semierection.

Self-contained penile prostheses consist of a pump, a cylinder, and a reservoir, all in a single unit. The client squeezes the pump just below the head of the penis to fill the cylinder and achieve erection.

Inflatable penile prostheses consist of two hollow silicone cylinders, an abdominal reservoir, and a scrotal pump. The client squeezes the pump to fill the cylinders and achieve erection.

Figure 79–7. Penile prostheses.

to 35 years (American Cancer Society [ACS], 1996). Testicular cancer strikes young men at a productive time of life and thus has significant economic, social, and psychological impact on the client and his family. However, with the advent of combination chemotherapy and earlier detection by testicular self-examination (TSE) (Chart 79–8), this form of cancer can be one of the most curable solid neoplasms.

Pathophysiology

Primary testicular cancers fall into two major groups:

■ Germinal tumors arising from the sperm-producing germ cells

■ Nongerminal tumors arising from the other structures in the testes

Germinal tumors are the most common type of testicular tumors, accounting for more than 95% of the cases.

Germinal Tumors

Germinal tumors of the testis are classified into two broad categories: seminomas and nonseminomas (Table 79–2).

SEMINOMAS. The most common type of testicular tumor is the seminoma. Clients with pure seminomatous tumors have the most favorable prognoses because the tumors generally remain localized and metastasize late. In

---

Chart 79–8

Health Promotion Guide: Testicular Self-Examination

- Examine your testicles monthly immediately after a bath or a shower, when your scrotal skin is relaxed.
- Examine each testicle by gently rolling it between your thumbs and fingers. Testicular tumors tend to appear deep in the center of the testicle.
- Report any lump or swelling to your doctor as soon as possible.

TABLE 79–2

Classification of Testicular Tumors

Germinal (Germ Cell) Tumors
- Seminoma
- Nonseminoma
  - Embryonal carcinoma
  - Teratoma
  - Choriocarcinoma

Nongerminal (Non–Germ Cell) Tumors
- Intestitial cell tumor
- Androblastoma

most clients with seminomatous testicular tumors, seminomas are diagnosed when they are confined to the testicles and retroperitoneal lymph nodes. These tumors also respond extremely well to radiation therapy. Clients with early-stage seminomas have about a 95% 5-year survival rate with surgery (orchiectomy) and radiation therapy (ACS, 1996).

NONSEMINOMAS. Nonseminomatous germ cell tumors include three types: embryonal carcinoma, teratoma, and choriocarcinoma.

These tumors are made up of cells that are not as sensitive to treatment with radiation therapy. They are treated with surgery or chemotherapy, depending on the extent of the disease at presentation.

Pure embryonal carcinomas are common in young men between the ages of 19 and 26 years. Embryonal carcinoma tends to spread earlier than seminoma and usually first affects the retroperitoneal lymph nodes. This type of tumor may also spread via the bloodstream to other sites in the body, such as the lung or the liver. Pure teratomas rarely occur. They are usually found mixed with other types of testicular tumors. Choriocarcinoma is a lethal type of nonseminomatous cancer, which spreads rapidly throughout the body. Clients with choriocarcinoma almost always have metastatic disease at the initial diagnosis because choriocarcinoma spreads via the hematogenous route rather than via the lymphatic system.

MIXED CELL TYPES. Testicular cancers with a mixture of cell types are also common. Almost any combination of germ cell tumors is possible, but the most common combination is embryonal carcinoma and teratoma (*teratocarcinoma*). About 25% of all testicular cancers are teratocarcinomas.

Nongerminal Tumors

The remaining 5% of testicular tumors arise from the nongerminal elements in the testes, such as the interstitial cells or cells that comprise fibrous or vascular networks. Nongerminal testicular neoplasms are classified as either *interstitial cell tumors* or *androblastomas* (testicular adenomas).

Interstitial cell tumors arise from the Leydig cells, which secrete testosterone into the bloodstream. These tumors are rare and usually benign. They may secrete an excessive amount of androgenic hormones, which cause young boys with such tumors to undergo early puberty.

Androblastomas are also rare and usually benign. They sometimes secrete estrogen, which accounts for the feminization and gynecomastia (breast enlargement) occasionally seen in these clients.

Etiology

The cause of testicular cancer is unknown. The risk for testicular tumors is reported to be higher in males who have an undescended testis (cryptorchidism). In cryptorchid males, the testicular cancer usually develops in the undescended testis (80%), and there is a 25% chance of cancer developing in the normally descended testis. Semi-

noma is the most common type of testicular cancer associated with cryptorchidism. The undescended testis undergoes gradual involution and degeneration over time, which may contribute to tumor development. It is not known why the normally descended testis is at risk for cancer. Brothers and close male relatives of clients with testicular cancer have a slightly greater risk of testicular cancer than the general population.

Although a history of trauma or infection is common in clients with testicular cancer, neither has been established as a cause of testicular cancer and may be coincidental findings at the time of the testicular examination. Therefore, the client with a history of trauma or infection should be examined by a health care provider after the acute episode subsides to rule out the existence of a tumor.

Testicular cancer is rarely bilateral. There is only a minute chance that a client with a tumor in one testis will have another primary testicular tumor in the other testis. In rare instances, leukemias, lymphomas, plasmacytomas, and metastatic carcinomas may involve the testes. A client with bilateral testicular tumors is more likely to have metastatic disease to the testes than bilateral primary testicular tumors.

Incidence/Prevalence

In the United States, testicular cancer occurs in 2 to 3 per 100,000 males (American Cancer Society, 1996). This cancer is the most common solid tumor diagnosed in men between the ages of 15 and 40 years. Testicular cancer can occur during infancy and middle age (after age 50); however, the peak incidence is between the ages of 18 and 40 years (American Cancer Society, 1996).

TRANSCULTURAL CONSIDERATIONS

 Testicular cancer occurs most frequently in Caucasians and is rare in African-Americans (American Cancer Society, 1996).

Collaborative Management

◆ Assessment

➤ *History*

When taking a history from a client with a suspected testicular tumor, the nurse keeps the risk factors in mind. Basic but important data to collect are age and race because the disease occurs most frequently in young Caucasian males. The nurse is also alert to other risk factors, including a history or presence of an undescended testis and a family history of testicular cancer.

The nurse then assesses the client's family situation. Is the client married? Does the client have children? Does he want children in the future? Depending on the treatment plan chosen, would he be interested in sperm storage in a sperm bank?

If the client has one healthy testis, he can function sexually and may not have any reproductive dysfunction. If the client undergoes a retroperitoneal lymph node dissection or chemotherapy, he may become sterile because of treatment effects on the sperm-producing cells or surgical trauma to the sympathetic nervous system, resulting in retrograde ejaculations.

► Physical Assessment/Clinical Manifestations

The testes, lymph nodes, and abdomen are thoroughly examined. The health care provider or nurse palpates the testes for lumps or swelling (Chart 79–9). The presence of any palpable lymphadenopathy, abdominal masses, or gynecomastia (enlarged breasts) usually indicates metastatic disease.

► Psychosocial Assessment

Because the diagnosis of testicular cancer usually occurs in the young adult, the nurse pays close attention to the psychosocial ramifications of the disease. Even if the cancer is detected at an early stage and the client is cured after orchiectomy, he may be afraid that he will be sexually handicapped. Even if the client's disease is arrested with surgery, radiation, or chemotherapy, he may think of himself as less than a whole man. These fears can disrupt the psychosocial and sexual development of the young male and can threaten the identity of adult males. The client may be afraid that he will not be able to perform sexually, will no longer be sexually attractive or desirable, and will face rejection. Feelings of sexual inadequacy may be denied, repressed, or displaced, causing increased stress on his personal and work relationships.

The nurse performs a psychosocial assessment of these clients on a routine basis because problems may arise at any time. The nurse also makes referrals to other re-

sources as appropriate. (See Chapter 11 for a further assessment of sexuality.)

► Laboratory Assessment

An important diagnostic indicator for the client with a testicular mass is the presence of any serum or urinary marker proteins (tumor markers) that are often produced by testicular cancers. Benign testicular tumors *never* cause an elevation in the levels of any of these marker proteins.

The primary tumor markers for testicular cancer are alpha-fetoprotein (AFP) and the beta subunit of human chorionic gonadotropin (hCG-β). Approximately 90% of clients with nonseminomatous testicular tumors (embryonal carcinoma, teratoma, or choriocarcinoma) initially have elevated serum levels of AFP, hCG-β, or both. Clients with pure seminoma do not have an elevated AFP level, and only 10% have a slightly elevated hCG-β) level. This level resolves after orchiectomy.

If a client has a diagnosis of seminoma and also has an elevated alpha-fetoprotein level, the tumor specimen must be re-examined for evidence of a component of nonseminomatous cancer. This step is necessary because the treatments differ for seminomatous and nonseminomatous tumors.

Alpha-fetoprotein and hCG-β determinations are also used to evaluate responses to therapy for testicular cancer and to document the presence of residual or recurrent disease. With effective treatment, the levels of abnormal markers fall. The persistence of elevated levels of markers after orchiectomy is substantive evidence that the client has metastatic disease, even if results of clinical staging procedures (x-rays and scans) are normal. The reappearance of the tumor markers heralds a recurrence of the cancer. Therefore, marker levels must be monitored regularly during the follow-up of clients treated for testicular cancer.

► Radiographic Assessment

After the diagnosis of testicular cancer, the client should have a computed tomography (CT) scan of the abdomen and the chest, or chest tomograms, to identify any small lesions not apparent on conventional x-ray films or physical assessment.

Clients with pure seminoma may undergo bipedal lymphangiography as part of the staging work-up to assess for any evidence of retroperitoneal lymph node involvement. Lymphangiograms are also valuable in determining the extent of radiation therapy fields.

 Analysis

► Common Nursing Diagnoses and Collaborative Problems

The nursing diagnosis that is common in men with testicular cancer is Risk for Sexual Dysfunction related to disease or treatment.

The common collaborative problem is Potential for Metastasis.

Chart 79–9

Focused Physical Assessment of a Male Client with a Testicular Lump

1. Obtain a medical history from the client:
   When was the lump discovered?
   Are there any other symptoms?
      sensation of heaviness, dragging in testicle, pain, discharge from penis
   Is there a history of cryptorchidism?
2. Assess the genital system. Always wear gloves during the examination of the male genitalia.
      Inspect and palpate the scrotal contents. Have the client perform a Valsalva maneuver and palpate for varicocele.
      Any lump or enlargement that does not transilluminate should be suspected as malignant.
3. Palpate for any enlarged lymph nodes. Most common lymphadenopathy is in the inguinal or supraclavicular regions.
4. Assess the abdomen for a possible mass or hepatomegaly.

➤ *Additional Nursing Diagnoses and Collaborative Problems*

Depending on the extent of malignancy and the type of treatment selected, the following diagnoses may also be appropriate:

- Dysfunctional Grieving or Anticipatory Grieving related to loss of a body part or changes in body function
- Body Image Disturbance and altered role performance related to the diagnosis of cancer
- Pain related to tumor compression or effects of metastasis
- Anxiety related to diagnosis of cancer

 Planning and Implementation

Risk for Sexual Dysfunction

Planning: Expected Outcomes. The major outcomes are that the client is expected to identify potential or actual alterations in reproductive function and identify alternate methods of meeting reproductive needs if needed.

Interventions. At the time of diagnosis, the incidence of oligospermia (low sperm count) and azoospermia (minimal sperm) is increased in clients with testicular cancer. This finding may be due to the disease process itself and to stress, but the exact reasons are unknown. The client may not discover that he is oligospermic or azoospermic until he has a presurgery sperm count.

Male cancer clients who are not candidates for sperm storage in a sperm bank may select from other options, such as donor insemination, adoption, and not fathering children. The nurse initiates health teaching about reproduction, fertility, and sexuality in the pretreatment phase. The nurse reviews normal reproductive function and explains the possible effects of cancer and its treatment on reproductive function. The nurse explains various reproductive options, for example, sperm banks and artificial insemination (Chart 79–10). The sperm bank facility provides comprehensive information on semen collection, storage of semen, the storage contract, costs, and the insemination process.

Chart 79–10

Education Guide: Sperm Banking

- You may want to investigate sperm storage in a sperm bank as a way to preserve your sperm for future use.
- No one knows how long sperm can be stored successfully, but pregnancies have resulted from sperm that have been stored for longer than 10 years.
- Check with the sperm bank to see how much it charges to process and store your sperm and to see whether you must pay when the service is provided.
- Investigate whether your health insurance company will reimburse you for sperm collection and storage.

When preparing the client for the collection and storage of sperm, the nurse assumes the role of client advocate and keeps in mind the effect of the cancer diagnosis on the client. The psychological benefit of having stored sperm may be important for the client and influence his response to treatment. Knowing that the potential for being a father still exists may help the client cope with other assaults to his masculinity, such as alopecia or erectile dysfunction.

The client should arrange for semen storage as soon as possible after diagnosis. Sperm collection should be completed *before* the client begins radiation therapy or chemotherapy or undergoes a radical retroperitoneal lymph node dissection. After radiation therapy or chemotherapy has been implemented, the client may be at increased risk for producing mutagenic sperm, which may not be viable or may result in fetal abnormalities.

The recommended number of samples to optimize the chances of later fertilization is three to six ejaculates, collected 2–4 days apart. The process of sperm collection can delay treatment for as long as 1 month, especially if the client is still recovering from surgery and multiple procedures or tests. The client's diagnosis (e.g., acute leukemia, sarcoma, advanced lymphoma, or testicular cancer) and his physical condition may not allow treatment to be postponed, thus making sperm storage an unfeasible reproductive option.

Potential for Metastasis

Planning: Expected Outcomes. The desired outcome is that the client will not experience complications of the tumor, including metastasis or recurrence of disease.

Interventions. A combination of nonsurgical and surgical management is often necessary to prevent metastatic disease (or to alleviate symptoms associated with it) and to bring about tumor regression. The nurse explains the interventions for treating testicular cancer.

Nonsurgical Management. Chemotherapy and radiation therapy are indicated for nonsurgical management of clients at high risk for metastatic disease or those with metastatic disease.

Chemotherapy. Combination chemotherapy may be used as adjuvant therapy for *nonseminomatous* testicular tumors or as primary treatment when there is evidence of metastatic disease. Combination chemotherapy is dramatically effective in treating nonseminomatous testicular cancer, particularly if cisplatin (Platinol) is used. This agent is necessary in any successful combination chemotherapy regimen for treating testicular cancer.

Other drugs commonly used in combination with cisplatin are

- Bleomycin sulfate (Blenoxane)
- Vinblastine sulfate (Velban, Velbe✢)
- Etoposide (VP-16, VePesid)
- Dactinomycin (Cosmegan)
- Cyclophosphamide (Cytoxan, Proxytox✢)
- Doxorubicin (Adriamycin)

The specific combination of drugs; the route of administration; and the frequency, cycling, and duration of treatment can vary considerably from client to client, depending on the extent of the disease and the protocol being followed by the health care provider. (Chapter 27 discusses the nursing care of the client receiving chemotherapy.)

Radiation Therapy. After orchiectomy (removal of one or both testes), external beam radiation therapy is the treatment of choice for clients with pure seminomatous testicular cancer because of the marked radiosensitivity of this type of testicular cancer. If radiation therapy is administered, a staging lymphangiogram is used to determine the treatment portals. An advantage of using radiation therapy instead of radical lymph node dissection is that reproductive function is preserved because surgical dissection of the sympathetic ganglia is avoided.

For the client undergoing radiation therapy to the retroperitoneal lymph nodes, the remaining testis is shielded with a lead cup to preserve reproductive function. Yet, even with these precautions, the client may have transient oligospermia (a decreased sperm count) as a result of radiation scatter. Normally, the client's sperm count returns to the pretreatment level 24–30 months after the radiation treatment is completed. If metastases develop outside the lymphatic system, the client may still be cured with radiation therapy if the area of involvement is limited. If lymphatic involvement is extensive, or if the visceral organs are involved, the health care provider uses combination chemotherapy similar to that for nonseminomatous testicular cancer.

Surgical Management. The physician performs a unilateral orchiectomy for diagnosis and uses primary surgical management. Clients with testicular cancer may also undergo a radical retroperitoneal lymph node dissection. Using this procedure, the physician can accurately stage the disease and debulk (reduce) the tumor volume so that chemotherapy or radiation therapy is more effective.

Preoperative Care. Like most clients with cancer, the client with testicular cancer is usually apprehensive. The nurse offers support and reinforces the teaching provided by the surgeon.

The client's postoperative needs should be anticipated and planned for before surgery. The physician's office nurse or case manager informs the client and his family about what to expect after surgery. The surgical incision for a retroperitoneal lymph node dissection is extensive. Depending on the extent of the dissection and the need for surgical exploration, the surgeon might make not only a midline incision but also a transthoracic incision or a combination of the two incisions (thoracoabdominal).

The nurse informs the client that radical retroperitoneal lymph node dissections are relatively long operations, lasting 6–12 hours. These clients need close and frequent observation, which may be done by nurses in a critical care unit.

Operative Procedures. To perform a radical retroperitoneal lymph node dissection, the surgeon removes the retroperitoneal nodes in the iliac and lumbar regions. Because the blood supply and the lymphatic vessels of the testes and kidneys are directly related, an extensive midline incision from the xiphoid process to the pubis is

necessary. After mobilization of the colon, the surgeon removes the perinephric nodes along with the nodes near the aorta and both renal hila. The node dissection also includes the inguinal area on the affected side. During the lymphadenectomy, the sympathetic ganglia around the lower lumbar lymphatics are dissected. The removal of the sympathetic ganglia abolishes peristalsis in the ductus deferens and contractions of the seminal vesicles. This disruption results in sterility because the client's ejaculate no longer contains sperm. The surgery, however, usually does not interfere with the client's ability to have a normal erection and does not affect his ability to experience orgasm.

A gel-filled silicone prosthesis can usually be surgically implanted into the scrotum at the time of the orchiectomy or later, if the client desires. The nurse reassures the client that this procedure does not impair fertility or sexual function; the client cosmetically appears to have two testes.

Postoperative Care. Because of the length of the surgery, the manipulation of the abdominal and retroperitoneal viscera, and the loss of a major part of the lymphatic fluid, nodes, and channels, the nurse observes and assesses the client for any of the complications of major abdominal surgery. The nurse intervenes for any of the following expected problems:

- Pain from surgical incisions
- Immobility related to prolonged maintenance of surgical positioning and postoperative pain
- Injuries related to any invasive catheters or tubes

The client is usually hospitalized for 3 to 4 days after a radical retroperitoneal lymph node dissection. During this time, the nurse explains care after discharge.

 Continuing Care

After an orchiectomy, the client is typically hospitalized for 1–2 days. This period may need to be extended if the client must undergo additional surgery or chemotherapy. Because it may not be known until after the orchiectomy whether the client has cancer, what type of testicular cancer he has, or if he needs additional surgery or treatment with radiation therapy or chemotherapy, specific discharge planning may need to be deferred until the postoperative period.

> *Health Teaching*

For the client who has had testicular surgery, the nurse emphasizes the importance of scheduling a follow-up visit with the physician, who will examine the incision for healing and complications. The nurse instructs the client to notify the physician if any of the following symptoms occurs before the scheduled appointment: chills, fever, increasing tenderness or pain around the incision, drainage, or dehiscence of the incision.

These symptoms may indicate the presence of an infection for which medical attention is needed. The nurse instructs the client that he will be able to resume most of his usual activities within 1 week after discharge, except for lifting heavy objects (weighing 20 pounds [9.1 kg]) or stair climbing. The nurse also reminds the client to ask his physician when strenuous activities may be resumed.

The client who has had an orchiectomy is informed that he may make arrangements with his physician to have a silicone prosthesis inserted into the scrotum if a prosthesis was not inserted during the orchiectomy.

The nurse also explains the importance of performing monthly testicular self-examination (TSE) on the remaining testis and scheduling follow-up examinations with the physician. The client who has had testicular cancer should schedule determinations of urinary and serum levels of tumor markers and computed tomography (CT) or magnetic resonance imaging (MRI) studies as part of his routine follow-up for a minimum of 3 years.

Depending on the pathologic findings and the stage of the cancer, the client may need further treatment. This information may not be available at the time of discharge. If it is known that the client needs further surgery, he and his family need information about the future surgery. If it is known that the client must undergo radiation therapy or chemotherapy, he needs education about a radiation therapy and chemotherapy regimen.

The client who undergoes treatment for testicular cancer may need emotional support. If permanent sterility occurs and sperm storage has not been feasible, the man may need counseling about other reproductive options.

➤ *Home Care Management*

After a unilateral orchiectomy, unless the client has a wound complication, he is discharged without a dressing on the inguinal incision. The client may want to wear a dressing to prevent his clothing from rubbing on the sutures and producing irritation. Because his sutures are intact at the time of discharge, he is told that they will be removed in the physician's office 7–10 days postoperatively.

➤ *Health Care Resources*

The client may be referred to agencies or support groups, such as the American Fertility Society or RESOLVE (an organization for infertile couples).

 Evaluation

On the basis of the identified nursing diagnoses, the nurse evaluates the care of the man who has been treated for testicular cancer. The expected outcomes may include that the client will

- Not experience a recurrence of cancer or metastases
- Accept body image changes and show adaptation to his altered self-concept
- Verbalize feelings of grief
- Recover from surgery, chemotherapy, or radiation therapy without complications
- Verbalize an understanding of the effects of surgery or radiation therapy on sexual function and identify alternative methods of meeting reproductive needs

OTHER COMMON PROBLEMS AFFECTING THE TESTES AND ADJACENT STRUCTURES

Problems that develop inside the scrotum usually occur as a mass or as scrotal edema. Some problems produce pain, but others do not. Figure 79–8 shows some of the most frequent conditions found in the male, including hydrocele, spermatocele, varicocele, and scrotal trauma.

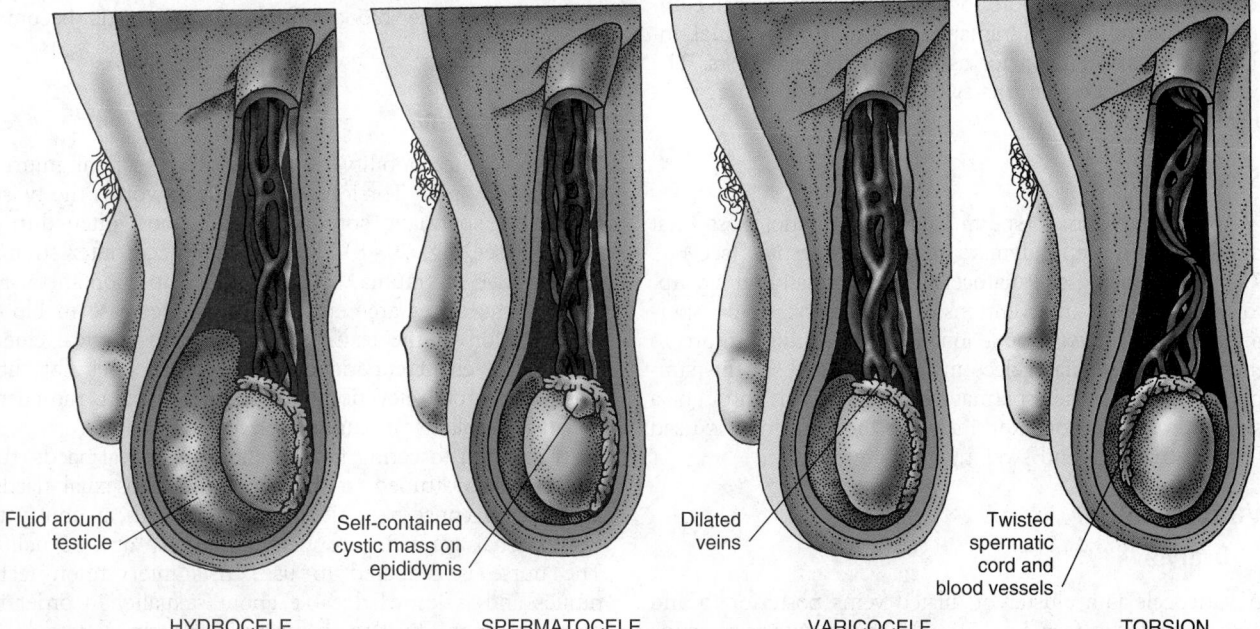

Fluid around testicle

Self-contained cystic mass on epididymis

Dilated veins

Twisted spermatic cord and blood vessels

HYDROCELE   SPERMATOCELE   VARICOCELE   TORSION

Figure 79–8. Common problems affecting the testes and adjacent structures.

Hydrocele

Overview

A hydrocele (see Fig. 79–8) is a cystic mass, usually filled with straw-colored fluid, that forms around the testis. It results from a disorder in the lymphatic drainage of the scrotum, causing a swelling of the tunica vaginalis, which surrounds the testes. Unless the swelling becomes large and uncomfortable or begins to compromise the circulation to the testis, no treatment is necessary.

Collaborative Management

A hydrocele may be aspirated via a needle and syringe, or it may be removed surgically. To correct a hydrocele surgically, the physician makes an incision in the scrotum and removes the hydrocele. The client may or may not return from the operating suite with a drain at the incision site. Typically, hydrocelectomies are performed on an outpatient basis; if the client requires hospitalization, it is for only 1 or 2 days. The nurse instructs the client that if an incision drain is present, there may be some serosanguineous drainage for the first 24–48 hours after surgery. The nurse also explains the importance of wearing a scrotal support. The scrotal support keeps the scrotal dressing in place and keeps the scrotum elevated, which helps to prevent edema.

Clients vary considerably in the degree of pain that they experience with this surgery. The nurse assesses and observes the client for pain every 2–3 hours in the immediate postoperative period. Moderate incision pain is expected for approximately 24 hours after surgery and should markedly decrease within 1 or 2 days. If the client's pain does not resolve within this time, the nurse is alert to the possible development of wound complications.

The nurse instructs the client to schedule a follow-up visit with the surgeon to have the wound evaluated for healing. The nurse stresses the importance of continuing to wear a scrotal support to promote drainage and comfort. The scrotum can remain swollen from residual inflammation and edema for as long as several weeks. The client is reassured that this swelling is normal and eventually subsides.

Spermatocele

A spermatocele is a sperm-containing cystic mass that develops on the epididymis alongside the testicle (see Fig. 79–8). Normally, spermatoceles remain small and asymptomatic, and no interventions are necessary. If the spermatocele becomes large enough to cause discomfort to the client, a spermatocelectomy is performed. In this simple procedure, the spermatocele is excised through a small scrotal incision. Routinely, no incision drain is used because drainage and swelling are minimal.

Varicocele

Overview

A varicocele is a cluster of dilated veins posterior to and above the testis (see Fig. 79–8). The diagnosis is made by scrotal palpation, particularly when the client performs a Valsalva maneuver. The scrotum feels "worm-like" when palpated. Varicoceles can be either unilateral or bilateral, but most are unilateral and on the left side of the scrotum. In many cases, varicoceles are asymptomatic, with no treatment required. In a few men, varicoceles are painful and must be removed surgically.

Varicoceles can also cause infertility. It is thought that the increase in scrotal temperature resulting from the venous stasis near the testis is the cause of the altered spermatogenesis.

Collaborative Management

A varicocelectomy (surgical removal of the varicocele) is usually performed through an inguinal incision, in which the spermatic veins are ligated in the cord, or through an incision adjacent to the superior iliac spine, in which the spermatic veins are ligated in the retroperitoneal space. A varicocelectomy may be done on an outpatient basis, or the client may be hospitalized overnight.

Prior to surgery, the nurse explains to the client that persistent venous congestion of the scrotum is common after this type of surgery because of the changed circulation in the area. To promote drainage of the scrotum, a rolled towel is placed under the scrotum while the client is in bed. The nurse may also apply ice to the scrotum if necessary. Any intervention that facilitates drainage and decreases swelling from the area promotes relief. The nurse instructs the client about the importance of wearing a scrotal support while ambulating.

At the time of discharge, the nurse instructs the client to make a follow-up appointment with the surgeon to have the sutures removed. The nurse also reminds the client to notify the physician of any increasing discomfort at the incision site or in the scrotum, which might indicate an infection. Increasing scrotal discomfort can mean that the circulation to the testis has been impaired. Testicular atrophy, a rare complication of a varicocelectomy, may occur if the blood supply to the testis becomes insufficient.

Scrotal Trauma

Because of the mobility of the scrotum, scrotal injuries are relatively rare. Torsion of the testes involves the twisting of the spermatic cord and occurs most often during puberty (see Fig. 79–8). Torsion may occur after strenuous exercise or trauma, or it may develop spontaneously. Because the testes are sensitive to any decrease in blood flow, torsion of the testis is considered a surgical emergency. The client experiences pain, which does not subside with scrotal elevation. In addition to pain, the client usually complains of nausea and vomiting.

In addition to caring for the client's physical needs, the nurse is also attuned to the client's psychosexual needs. Of primary concern to the male client with an injury to his external genitalia are his masculinity and sexuality. The nurse is prepared to use crisis intervention techniques and is knowledgeable about sexuality in order to help the client adjust to an injury in the genital area.

Cryptorchidism

An undescended testis, or cryptorchidism, is mainly a pediatric problem. Three percent of full-term male infants and 20% of premature infants have an undescended testis. In 80% of cases, the undescended testis descends spontaneously during the infant's first year. If an adult has cryptorchidism, an *orchidopexy* (surgical placement of the testicle into the scrotum) may be performed for cosmetic and psychosexual reasons. The surgery may also prevent the adverse effect of body temperature on spermatogenesis and reduce the risk of testicular cancer. As an alternative, an orchiectomy of the cryptorchid testicle may be recommended.

During an orchidopexy, the client is placed in a supine position. The surgeon makes an inguinal incision, and the spermatic cord is released from the surrounding fascia to obtain maximal length. The surgeon then creates a dartos pouch and places the testis between the skin and the dartos muscle of the scrotum. The tunica albuginea of the testis is sutured to the dartos muscle of the scrotum. The inguinal incision and the scrotal incision (if there is one) are then closed, and a dressing is applied. If there is an incision in the scrotum, it is also covered with a dressing and the client is instructed to wear a scrotal support.

Carcinoma of the Penis

Overview

Carcinoma of the penis represents less than 1% of all malignancies in men in the United States.

TRANSCULTURAL CONSIDERATIONS

 Epidermoid carcinoma is the most common cancer of the penis. In countries where circumcision is not practiced, such as India, China, and Africa, this type of cancer represents 12% of all cancers (American Cancer Society, 1996).

Collaborative Management

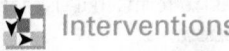 Assessment

Carcinoma of the penis usually occurs as a painless, wart-like growth or ulcer on the glans under the prepuce (foreskin) and may initially be mistaken for a venereal wart. A penile carcinoma may also appear as a reddened lesion with plaque.

Interventions

Small lesions involving only the skin may be controlled by excisional biopsy. When the lesion is not curable by excisional biopsy or radiation therapy, a *penectomy* (partial or total removal of the penis) may be required.

Partial Penectomy

When the lesion is limited to the glans, a partial penectomy is performed. The client is placed in a lithotomy position, and a tourniquet is applied around the penis. The surgeon makes an incision to amputate a portion of the corpus cavernosum and the corpus spongiosum. The urethra is anastomosed to the skin, and a dressing is applied. A Foley catheter is in place for 3–5 days after surgery until the edema surrounding the urethra subsides. The nurse assesses the dressing for drainage, which should be minimal. The catheter is checked for patency every 4 hours for the first postoperative day.

Total Penectomy

A total penectomy is required when the lesion has penetrated the shaft of the penis or when the tumor has recurred after a partial penectomy or radiation therapy. The client is placed in a lithotomy position. The surgeon makes an incision from the pubic bone, which encircles the penis and extends into the perineum. The bases of both corpora cavernosa are exposed and excised, and the penis is amputated. The surgeon places an incision drain in the wound before it is sutured. Clients who undergo a total penectomy also have a perineal urethrotomy (anastomosis of the urethra to the skin in the perineum) for urinary drainage.

After a total penectomy, the nurse observes the incision dressing every 2–4 hours during the first 24–48 hours. There may be a moderate amount of serosanguineous drainage from the incision drains.

The nurse is aware that regardless of how accepting the client may appear preoperatively, he may experience severe emotional problems postoperatively. After a partial penectomy, the client must adjust to considerable changes in body image and sexuality. The nurse encourages the client to verbalize his feelings about the loss of his penis. After a total penectomy, the client can no longer have penile-vaginal or penile-anal intercourse and cannot urinate in a standing position. It is difficult for most clients to accept the possibility that they might die because of a lesion on the penis, especially because they are rarely experiencing any systemic cancer symptoms and are otherwise healthy. The nurse helps the client realize that the removal of his penis may save his life. The nurse is aware of the possibility of suicide attempts, as the client's penis may be more important to him than his life. The nurse may be the one to detect the need for professional psychological assistance for the client or his partner. Early interventions by the nurse can make a tremendous difference in the client's or partner's well-being.

Circumcision (the surgical removal of the prepuce from the penis) in infancy almost eliminates the possibility of penile cancer in that chronic irritation and inflammation of the glans penis predispose uncircumcised men to penile cancer. Because of the ongoing controversy about neonatal circumcision, the nurse teaches both men and new mothers of boys that strict personal hygiene is an important preventive measure against penile cancer.

Phimosis

In a man with phimosis, the prepuce is constricted so that it cannot be retracted over the glans. Because of the recent trend away from routine circumcision of newborns, the nurse instructs new mothers, male children, and adult men about the importance of cleaning the prepuce. Phimosis is corrected by circumcision.

Circumcision

Overview

Circumcision (the surgical removal of the prepuce or foreskin) in the adult male is usually done for medical reasons, such as to correct phimosis and to eliminate the infections that frequently result from this condition.

Collaborative Management

Circumcision in the adult male is usually performed in a same-day surgical setting. If the client has a dressing, the nurse instructs him to soak in a warm bath that evening and allow the dressing to float off the next day. If the dressing falls off before the next day, the client is cautioned not to replace it. The nurse explains that the sutures will be absorbed and need not be removed. No residual or side effects result from this surgery, and the client should be able to resume his normal activities within 1 week; sexual intercourse may be resumed after 1–2 weeks.

The client may be discharged with a prescription for a barbiturate sleeping medication to be taken for several nights postoperatively. The nurse emphasizes that barbiturate sleeping medication suppresses the rapid-eye-movement (REM) phase of sleep so that normal nocturnal erections do not occur. This prevents any tension on the sutures by an erection.

Nonbarbiturate sleeping medications do not inhibit the nocturnal erection pattern. The nurse explains the relationship between barbiturate sleeping medication and nocturnal erections because the client may not comply with the instructions to take the medication, especially if he is not having any difficulty sleeping.

The nurse advises the client to notify his physician if he has any wound complications, such as swelling at the incision area of drainage, and to schedule a postoperative office visit.

Priapism

Overview

Priapism is an uncontrolled and long-maintained erection without sexual desire, which causes the penis to become large, hard, and painful. Priapism affects the two corpora cavernosa; the corpus spongiosum and glans penis are not affected.

Priapism can occur from neural, vascular, or pharmacologic causes and commonly include

- Thrombosis of the veins of the corpora cavernosa (usually resulting from trauma)
- Leukemia
- Sickle cell anemia
- Diabetes
- Malignancies

Sickle cell disease causes priapism by the accumulation of erythrocytes within the corporal bodies. Leukemia may cause priapism because the increased number of white blood cells (WBC) permits persistent engorgement of the corporal bodies. Malignancies may also infiltrate the corporal bodies, causing persistent engorgement. Priapism can also result from an abnormal neurogenic reflex, psychotropic medications, antidepressants, and antihypertensive medications.

Collaborative Management

Priapism is considered a urologic emergency because the circulation to the penis may be compromised and the client may not be able to void with an erect penis. The goal of medical intervention is to improve the venous drainage of the corpora cavernosa. Conservative measures involve prostatic massage, sedation, and bed rest.

Meperidine (Demerol) is usually administered immediately because of its hypotensive effect. Warm enemas may be given to bring about venous dilation and thus increase the outflow of the trapped blood. Urinary catheterization is required if the client cannot void.

If conservative therapy is unsuccessful, treatment may proceed to aspiration of the corpora cavernosa with a large-bore needle or surgical intervention. The priapism should be resolved within the first 24–30 hours to prevent penile ischemia, gangrene, fibrosis, and impotence. If a cause of priapism is identified, treatment is directed toward that underlying cause.

The nurse who is caring for the client with priapism is sensitive to his emotional needs. The client may be uncomfortable and in crisis but at the same time embarrassed by his erection and loss of control. The nurse reassures the client that he or she understands that the client is not in control of his erection and provides him with privacy.

Prostatitis

Overview

A number of inflammatory conditions can affect the prostate gland. The most common is abacterial prostatitis.

ABACTERIAL PROSTATITIS. Abacterial prostatitis can occur after a viral illness or can result from a sudden decrease in sexual activity, especially in young males. In many instances, an exact cause of the perineal discomfort cannot be found. The prostatitis can be related to psychosexual problems. *Prostodynia* is a term that is sometimes used to described this condition.

BACTERIAL PROSTATITIS. Bacterial prostatitis is usually associated with urethritis or an infection of the lower urinary tract. Organisms may reach the prostate via the bloodstream or the urethra. The most common organisms are *Escherichia coli, Enterobacter, Proteus,* and group D streptococci. Acute bacterial prostatitis may be manifested by fever, chills, dysuria (painful urination), urethral discharge, and a boggy, tender prostate.

Gentle palpation of the prostate usually results in a urethral discharge, which is evidenced by white blood cells in the prostatic secretions.

Collaborative Management

The client with chronic prostatitis usually complains of backache, perineal pain, mild dysuria, and urinary frequency; hematuria may be present. The prostate may feel irregularly enlarged, firm, and slightly tender when palpated. Complications of prostatitis are epididymitis (inflammation of the epididymis) and cystitis (inflammation of the bladder). A rare complication is a prostatic abscess. The client with either acute or chronic bacterial prostatitis is likely to experience urinary tract infections. Sexual functioning may be diminished because of discomfort.

Early diagnosis and treatment of prostatitis with antimicrobials such as carbenicillin indanyl sodium (Geocillin, Geopen Oral✦) or the newer fluoroquinolones (ciprofloxacin [Cipro]) can help prevent an abscess. The nurse emphasizes the importance of comfort measures, such as sitz baths, and taking prescribed antibiotics on schedule. The physician orders stool softeners to prevent straining and rectal irritation of the prostate during a bowel movement. Analgesics may be used for symptomatic relief.

The nurse instructs the client with chronic prostatitis about the long-term nature of the problem. Because prostatitis can cause other urinary tract infections, the nurse explains the importance of increasing fluid intake and long-term antibiotic therapy (for 30 days). Because trimethoprim (Protprin) diffuses into the prostatic fluid, it is the antibiotic of choice. The nurse instructs the client about activities that drain the prostate (intercourse, masturbation, and prostatic massage), which may help in the management of chronic prostatitis.

Epididymitis

Overview

Epididymitis, an infection of the epididymis, may result from an infection of the prostate. It used to be a frequent complication of gonorrhea. Although not common, epididymitis can also be a complication of long-term use of an indwelling Foley catheter, prostatic surgery, or a cystoscopic examination.

In men younger than 35 years of age, the major causative organism in epididymitis is *Chlamydia trachomatis,* which is transmitted sexually (see Chap. 80). The infective organism passes upward through the urethra and the ejaculatory duct, then along the vas deferens to the epididymis.

The client with epididymitis usually complains of pain along the inguinal canal and along the vas deferens, followed by pain and swelling in the scrotum and the groin. If epididymitis is untreated, the epididymis becomes swollen and painful, and the client's temperature may become elevated. Pyuria and bacteriuria may develop, with result-

ant chills and fever. An abscess may form, necessitating an orchiectomy (removal of one or both testes).

Collaborative Management

The nurse instructs the client with epididymitis to remain in bed with his scrotum elevated on a towel to prevent traction on the spermatic cord, to facilitate venous drainage, and to relieve pain. The client may be given antibiotics until all acute symptoms of inflammation are gone. If the epididymitis is chlamydial or gonorrheal in origin, the client's sexual partners are also treated with antibiotics.

The client may find other comfort measures effective, such as applying cold compresses or ice to the scrotum intermittently and taking sitz baths. The nurse advises the client to avoid lifting, straining, or sexual activity until the infection is under control (which may take as long as 4 weeks).

In clients with epididymitis, there must always be the suspicion of a testicular tumor, especially if the condition does not resolve in a week or two. Ultrasound study is frequently employed to rule out an abscess or tumor. Clients with recurrent or chronic painful conditions may require an epididymectomy (excision of the epididymis from the testicle).

Orchitis

Orchitis, or acute testicular inflammation, may result from trauma or infection. The infection may be caused by the direct spread of bacteria through the urethra or by an infection elsewhere in the body, such as pneumonia, tuberculosis, gonorrhea, syphilis, or mumps. It is rare that the testes alone are involved; usually, both the testes and the epididymis are involved (epididymo-orchitis).

Orchitis may be unilateral or bilateral. If the orchitis is bilateral, the client is at increased risk for sterility because of the testicular atrophy and fibrosis that occur during healing.

The signs and symptoms of orchitis are the same as those of epididymitis (scrotal pain and edema). In addition, the client may experience nausea and vomiting and pain radiating to the inguinal canal.

The treatment of orchitis is the same as for epididymitis:

■ Bed rest with scrotal elevation
■ Application of ice
■ Administration of analgesics and antibiotics

Mumps orchitis, which occurs in approximately 20% of males who have mumps after puberty, is usually bilateral, and orchitis symptoms develop 4–6 days after the parotitis. Any postpubertal male who has not had mumps and is exposed to or contracts mumps is usually given gammaglobulin. Although gammaglobulin does not prevent mumps, the clinical course of the disease is likely to be less severe, with fewer complications. Childhood vaccination against mumps is an important preventive measure.

CASE STUDY for the Client with Urinary Retention Secondary to Prostate Enlargement

■ A 73-year-old man comes to the Ambulatory Urgent Care center with complaints of burning on urination, urgency, dribbling of urine, and a feeling of bladder fullness. He states that he has noticed a gradual change in his urinary pattern over the past few months but attributes it to "old age." He adds that he would not have come in at all except that he noticed some burning when he urinated today. He also says his back has been hurting, but he attributes that to yard work and gardening.

Q U E S T I O N S :

1. When interviewing this client, what questions should be asked?
2. What areas should be the focus of the nursing assessment?
3. What laboratory tests and/or procedures can be expected for this client?

SELECTED BIBLIOGRAPHY

American Cancer Society (ACS). (1996). *Cancer facts and figures—1996.* Atlanta: American Cancer Society.

*American Joint Committee on Cancer. (1992). *Manual for staging of cancer.* Philadelphia: J. B. Lippincott.

Brenner, Z. R., & Krenzer, M. E. (1995). Update on cryosurgical ablation for prostate cancer. *AJN, 95*(4), 44–49.

Collins, M. (1997). Increasing prostate awareness in African American men. *Oncology Nursing Forum, 24,* 91–95.

Davison, B. J., Degner, L. F., & Morgan, T. R. (1995). Information and decision-making of men with prostate cancer. *Oncology Nursing Forum, 22,* 1401–1408.

Gelfand, D. E., Parzuchowski, J., Cort, M., & Powell, I. (1995). Digital rectal examinations and prostate cancer screening: Attitudes of African American men. *Oncology Nursing Forum, 22,* 1253–1255.

Giger, J. N., Davidhizor, R. E. (1995). *Transcultural nursing: Assessment and intervention* (2nd ed.). St. Louis: C. V. Mosby.

Haas, G. P., & Sakr, W. (1997). Epidemiology of prostate cancer. *CA: A Cancer Journal for Clinicians, 47*(5), 273–285.

Jackson, J., Emerson, L., Johnston, B., et al. (1996). Biofeedback: A noninvasive treatment for incontinence after radical prostatectomy. *Urology Nursing, 16*(2), 50–54.

Johnson, J. E. (1996). Coping with radiation therapy: Optimism and the effect of preparatory interventions. *Research in Nursing & Health, 19,* 3–12.

Karlowitz, K. A. (Ed). (1995). *Urologic nursing principles and practice.* Philadelphia: W. B. Saunders.

Matteson, M. A., McConnell, E. S., & Linton, A. D. (1997). *Gerontological nursing: Concepts and practices* (2nd ed). Philadelphia: W. B. Saunders.

Mettlin, C. (1997). The American Cancer Society National Prostate Cancer Detection Project and national patterns of prostate cancer detection and treatment. *CA: A Cancer Journal for Clinicians, 47*(5), 265–272.

*Murphy, G. (1994) Report on the American Urologic Association/American Cancer Society Scientific Seminar on the Detection and Treatment of Early-Stage Prostate Cancer. *CA: A Cancer Journal for Clinicians 44,* 91–95.

Otto, S. (1995) *Oncologic nursing.* St. Louis: C. V. Mosby.

Parker, S., Tong, T., Bolden, S., & Wingo, P. (1996). Cancer statistics, 1996. *CA: A Cancer Journal for Clinicians, 46,* 5–27.

Sweet, V., Servy, E. J., & Karow A. M. (1996). Reproductive issues for men with cancer: Technology and nursing management. *Oncology Nursing Forum, 23,* 51–58.

von Eschenbach, A., Ho, R., Murphy, G. P., et al. (1997). American Cancer Society guideline for the early detection of prostate cancer: Update 1997. *CA: A Cancer Journal for Clinicians, 47*(5), 261–264.

SUGGESTED READINGS

Brenner, Z. R., & Krenzer, M. E. (1995). Update on cryosurgical ablation for prostate cancer. *AJN, 95*(4), 44–49.
    This article provides a review of a new, minimally invasive surgical intervention for prostate surgery—cryosurgery. The advantages of the procedure are discussed, and a case study is presented. The article has a post-test for receipt of CEUs.

Gelfand, D. E., Parzuchowski, J., Cort, M., & Powell, I. (1995). Digital rectal examinations and prostate cancer screening: Attitudes of African American men. *Oncology Nursing Forum, 22,* 1253–1255.
    This descriptive study explored the relationship between attitudes toward digital rectal examination and participation in prostate cancer screening programs by African-American men. A self-administered questionnaire was completed by 613 African-American men between the ages of 40 and 70 years.

Jackson, J., Emerson, L., Johnston, B., et al. (1996). Biofeedback: A noninvasive treatment for incontinence after radical prostatectomy. *Urology Nursing, 16*(2), 50–54.
    This nursing research article discussed how a noninvasive intervention can help treat urinary incontinence as a postoperative complication of radical prostatectomy. Complementary therapies are being used more frequently in health care as safer and less costly alternatives to conventional management.

Chapter 80

INTERVENTIONS FOR CLIENTS WITH SEXUALLY TRANSMITTED DISEASES

INTRODUCTION TO SEXUALLY TRANSMITTED DISEASES

Sexually transmitted diseases (STDs) are caused by infectious organisms that have been passed from one person to another through anal, oral, or vaginal intercourse. Some organisms that cause these diseases are transmitted only through sexual contact; others are transmitted in other ways, such as parenteral exposure to infected blood, intrauterine transmission to the fetus, and perinatal transmission from mother to neonate.

Historically, five classic diseases were known to be sexually transmitted: syphilis, gonorrhea, chancroid, lymphogranuloma venereum, and granuloma inguinale. The list of STDs continues to grow because of improved diagnostic techniques, an increased number of organisms and systemic diseases that can be sexually transmitted, and changes in sexual attitudes and practices (Table 80–1).

The prevalence of STDs is a major health concern worldwide. Changing patterns of climate, hygiene, culture, population density, and economics affect the prevalence of STDs in any given geographic area (Holmes, 1994). Sexual attitudes and preferences (e.g., frequent sexual contact with casual sexual partners, anal inter-

course) and a lack of preventive health behaviors (e.g., nonuse of condoms, noncompliance with treatments) place clients at greatest risk (Adimora et al., 1994). STDs also cause complications that can contribute to severe physical and emotional suffering, including infertility, ectopic pregnancy, cancer, and death. Complications caused by sexually transmitted organisms are listed in Table 80–2.

Cases of the classic STDs are reportable to local health authorities, but some STDs, such as genital herpes and chlamydial infections, may or may not be reported, depending on local legal requirements. Rigorous reporting and follow-up efforts by federal and local public health departments and health care providers is one key in decreasing the incidence of STDs.

Nurses in advanced practice in a variety of community settings, in collaboration with physicians, are primarily responsible for identifying and caring for clients with STDs. Nurses in secondary and tertiary care settings, such as hospitals, however, also have a responsibility to recognize clients who are at risk or who have symptoms of STDs. In addition, nurses provide care to those clients who may be hospitalized with complications related to STDs.

WOMEN'S HEALTH CONSIDERATIONS

w Women seem to be at greatest risk for morbidity from sexually transmitted diseases. Many adolescents and young women still do not use condoms because of their belief that they cannot become infected, need to fit in with their peer group, and feeling of invulnerability regarding risky behaviors (Braverman & Strasburger, 1994). Many women will use a condom to prevent pregnancy but fail to protect themselves from STDs. One act of intercourse carries more risk of infection for the woman (presumably from infectious semen) than for the man.

Additionally, women tend to have more asymptomatic infections, which may delay diagnosis and treatment. This delay increases the likelihood of more serious problems, including irreversible damage to reproductive organs and systemic illness. Embarrassment or fear about STDs may further delay treatment, increasing the potential for serious sequelae.

Acquired Immunodeficiency Syndrome

Acquired immunodeficiency syndrome (AIDS), a disease thought to be caused primarily by infection with the human immunodeficiency virus (HIV), is a disorder of immunoregulation affecting the body's ability to fight disease. HIV is primarily transmitted through infected body fluids (e.g., semen, vaginal secretions, blood and blood products, breast milk infected with HIV). People at risk include

- Sexually active men who are bisexual or homosexual with multiple sexual partners

TABLE 80–1

Sexually Transmitted Diseases

- Human immunodeficiency virus infections
- Chancroid
- Syphilis
- Lymphogranuloma venereum
- Genital herpes simplex virus infections
- Genital warts
- Gonococcal infections
- Chlamydial infections
- Nongonococcal urethritis
- Mucopurulent cervicitis
- Epididymitis
- Pelvic inflammatory disease
- Sexually transmitted enteritis
- Sexually transmitted proctitis
- Trichomoniasis
- Candidal infections
- Bacterial vaginosis
- Viral hepatitis
- Cytomegalovirus infections
- Ectoparasitic infections
  - Pediculosis pubis
  - Scabies

From Centers for Disease Control and Prevention. (1993). 1993 Sexually transmitted diseases treatment guidelines. *Morbidity and Mortality Weekly Report, 42*(No. RR-14), 1–102.

TABLE 80–2

Complications Caused by Sexually Transmitted Organisms

Complication	Causative Organisms
Salpingitis, infertility, and ectopic pregnancy	• *Neisseria gonorrhoeae* • *Chlamydia trachomatis* • *Mycoplasma hominis*
Reproductive loss (abortion/miscarriage)	• *Neisseria gonorrhoeae* • *Chlamydia trachomatis* • Herpes simplex virus • *Mycoplasma hominis* • *Ureaplasma urealyticum* • *Treponema pallidum*
Puerperal infection	• *Neisseria gonorrhoeae* • *Chlamydia trachomatis*
Perinatal infection	• Hepatitis B virus • Human immunodeficiency virus • Human papillomavirus • *Neisseria gonorrhoeae* • *Chlamydia trachomatis* • Herpes simplex virus • *Treponema pallidum* • Cytomegalovirus • Group B streptococcus
Cancer of genital area	• *Chlamydia trachomatis* • Herpes simplex virus • Human papillomavirus
Male urethritis	• *Mycoplasma hominis* • Herpes simplex virus • *Neisseria gonorrhoeae* • *Chlamydia trachomatis* • *Ureaplasma urealyticum*
Vulvovaginitis	• Herpes simplex virus • *Trichomonas vaginalis* • Bacteria causing vaginosis • *Candida albicans*
Cervicitis	• *Neisseria gonorrhoeae* • *Chlamydia trachomatis* • Herpes simplex virus
Proctitis	• *Neisseria gonorrhoeae* • *Chlamydia trachomatis* • Herpes simplex virus • *Campylobacter jejuni* • *Shigella* species • *Entamoeba histolytica*
Hepatitis	• *Treponema pallidum* • Hepatitis A virus
Dermatitis	• *Sarcoptes scabiei* • *Phthirus pubis*
Genital ulceration or warts	• *Chlamydia trachomatis* • Herpes simplex virus • Human papillomavirus • *Treponema pallidum* • *Haemophilus ducreyi* • *Calymmatobacterium granulomatis*

- Women with persistent and recurrent STDs
- Intravenous drug users
- Infants born to women who are infected with HIV
- People with hemophilia
- People receiving blood transfusions from 1978 to 1985
- Sexual partners (of both sexes) of anyone at risk for HIV

Because HIV affects the immune system and can be transmitted in ways other than by sexual contact, it is discussed in detail in Chapter 25.

Infections Associated with Ulcers

Syphilis

Overview

Syphilis is one of the *classic* sexually transmitted diseases (STDs). It ranks third in incidence behind gonorrhea and chickenpox among reportable communicable diseases in the United States. The use of new techniques for diagnosis and treatment, particularly the discovery of penicillin in the 1940s, has resulted in a decline in the incidence of syphilis. However, in 1990 the number of cases increased to a post–World War II peak of more than 50,000.

The primary population that is infected with syphilis is young adults in their early 20s. The rate of syphilis in males has declined since 1990, but rates for females have not declined as rapidly. This slower decline may be due in part to the practice of exchanging sex for money to support illicit drug habits and subsequent reinfection (Thompson et al., 1996) or delayed diagnosis and treatment.

The causative organism of syphilis is *Treponema pallidum,* a spirochete with a slender, spiral shape that resembles a corkscrew. Nonpathogenic members of *Treponema* are found in the mouth, intestinal tract, and genital areas of people and animals. Although the organism can be seen only with a darkfield microscope, several serologic tests may be used to screen for the presence of syphilis antigen/antibody. *T. pallidum* is susceptible to dry air or to any known disinfectant. The organisms die within hours at temperatures of 41° to 42° C and are not airborne. The infection is usually transmitted by sexual contact, but transmission can occur through close body contact and kissing.

Syphilis progresses through a number of stages: primary, secondary, early and late latent, and late.

Primary Syphilis

The appearance of an ulcer, called a *chancre,* is the first and primary clinical manifestation of syphilis. The chancre develops at the site of inoculation, or entry, of the organism between 10 and 90 days after exposure. Chancres may be found on the genitalia, the lips, the nipples, and the fingers and hands and in the oral cavity, the anus, and the rectum.

During this highly infectious stage, the chancre begins as a small papule. Within 3 to 7 days, it breaks down into its characteristic appearance: a painless, indurated, smooth weeping lesion. Regional lymph nodes enlarge, feel firm, and are not tender. Without treatment, the chancre usually disappears within 6 weeks; however, the organism will have disseminated throughout the body. The client is still considered infectious.

Secondary Syphilis

Secondary syphilis develops 6 weeks to 6 months after the onset of primary syphilis. Secondary syphilis is a systemic disease because the spirochetes circulate throughout the bloodstream. Clinical manifestations include malaise, low-grade fever, headache, muscular aches and pains, and sometimes a sore throat.

These symptoms are frequently mistaken for those of influenza. A generalized rash develops; unlike any other rash, it involves the palms and soles of the feet. Although there is no typical appearance of the rash, it tends to evolve sequentially from papules to squamous papules to pustules. Other skin lesions can include psoriasiform rashes, wart-like lesions, and mucous patches. The lesions are highly contagious and should not be touched with the bare skin. The rash subsides spontaneously in 4 to 12 weeks, but 25% of clients have recurrences within 6 months.

Early and Late Latent Syphilis

After the second stage of syphilis, there is a period of latency. *Early* latent syphilis occurs during the first year after infection and infectious lesions can recur. *Late* latent syphilis is a disease of more than 1 year's duration after infection. This stage is noninfectious except to the fetus of a pregnant woman. Clients with latent syphilis may or may not have reactive serologic test findings.

Late Syphilis

Late syphilis occurs after a highly variable period, from 4 to 20 years. This stage develops in untreated cases and can mimic almost any pathologic condition. Manifestations of late syphilis include

- Benign lesions (gummas) of the skin, mucous membranes, and bones
- Cardiovascular syphilis, usually in the form of aortitis and aneurysms
- Neurosyphilis, which includes central nervous system involvement

Collaborative Management

 Assessment

Assessment of the client presenting with symptoms of syphilis begins with a history, which should include a risk assessment and sexual history (see Chap. 11), information about the lesions noticed, and whether previous testing or treatment for syphilis or other STDs has ever been done (Chart 80–1). The nurse asks about allergic reactions to drugs, especially penicillin. A physical examination, including inspection and palpation, is then given to identify manifestations of syphilis. Women frequently

Focused Assessment for the Client with a Sexually Transmitted Disease

- Assess client's history
  - Chief complaint
  - Symptoms by quality and quantity, precipitating and palliative factors
  - Any treatments taken (self-prescribed or over-the-counter)
- Assess medical history
  - Major health problems
  - Menstrual problems
  - Contraceptive history
  - History of STDs/PID
- Assess sexual history
  - Type and frequency of sexual activity
  - Number of sexual contacts
  - Sexual preferences
- Assess general health
  - Allergies
  - Lifestyle risks
- Assess preventive health care practices
  - Having Pap smears
  - Using contraceptives
- Assess physical findings
  - Vital signs
  - Abdominal examination
  - Genital, pelvic, rectal, and oral examinations
- Assess laboratory data
  - Urinalysis
  - Hematology
  - Samples for microbiology/virology

have the chancre on areas that are invisible to them (e.g., the vagina or cervix). A woman may present with complaints of inguinal lymph node enlargement, the location that drains the area of the vagina and cervix. She may state a history of a sexual contact with a male who had an ulcer that she noticed during the encounter. Men usually discover the chancre on the penis or scrotum.

After the physical examination, the physician, nurse practitioner, or nurse-midwife obtains a specimen of the chancre for examination under a darkfield microscope. Diagnosis of primary or secondary syphilis is confirmed if *Treponema pallidum,* the characteristic spirochete, is present. If the first slide is negative for *T. pallidum,* the procedure should be repeated in 3 days because many conditions can cause a false-negative result.

Blood tests are also used to diagnose syphilis. The usual screening test is the Venereal Disease Research Laboratory (VDRL) serum test. This test is based on an antibody-antigen reaction that determines both the presence and the amount of antibodies produced by the body in response to an infection by *T. pallidum.* The VDRL test becomes reactive 2 to 6 weeks after infection. VDRL titers are also used to monitor the effectiveness of treatment. The antibodies are not specific to *T. pallidum,* and false-positive reactions can occur free from such conditions as

drug addiction, cancer, hepatitis, some viral diseases, and systemic lupus erythematosus (SLE).

If a positive VDRL result is obtained, the health care provider may order a more specific test such as the *fluorescent treponemal antibody absorption* (FTA-ABS) test or the *microhemagglutination assay for T. palladium* (MHA-TP). These tests are more sensitive for all stages of syphilis, although false-positive results may still occur.

 Interventions

The health care provider prescribes antibiotic therapy for the client with syphilis. The drug therapy of choice for syphilis is penicillin. (Note: While other antibiotics may be used to treat syphilis, they should only be offered to clients who will comply with the treatment regimen and be available for follow-up.) Allergic reactions to the antibiotic occur frequently, and the nurse is alert for these signs and symptoms. Penicillin desensitization is recommended for penicillin-allergic clients. The client who has never had penicillin previously should have a skin test before receiving a penicillin injection. All clients who have received injections of antibiotics should remain at the health care agency for at least 30 minutes so that signs of a severe and immediate allergic reaction can be detected. If an allergic reaction does occur, treatment can begin immediately. The most severe reaction is anaphylaxis. All nurses working in clinics or physicians' offices where injections of penicillin are given should be familiar with the symptoms and treatment of anaphylaxis.

The Jarisch-Herxheimer reaction may also follow antibiotic therapy for syphilis. This reaction is due to the rapid release of products from the disruption of the cells of the organism. Onset occurs within 2 hours after therapy, with a peak at 4 to 8 hours. Symptoms include generalized aches and pain at the injection site, vasodilation and hypotension, and a rise in temperature. These symptoms do not always occur and generally are benign. This reaction may be treated symptomatically with analgesics and antipyretics.

Nursing interventions are based on assessments. Common nursing diagnoses for clients with syphilis as well as STDs in general are listed in Table 80-3.

The nurse reinforces the information provided to the client about treatment, including side effects, possible complications of untreated or incompletely treated disease, and the need for follow-up care. All sexual partners must be treated adequately as soon as possible, and the client must be encouraged to provide accurate information for this follow-up. The nurse informs the client that the disease must be reported to the local health authority and that all information will be held in strict confidence. The nurse gathers information and teaches in a setting that offers privacy and encourages open discussion.

The client is encouraged to comply with the treatment regimen, especially if oral antibiotics are included. The nurse stresses the contagiousness of the disease and frankly discusses the client's role in preventing spread to sexual partners (Chart 80-2).

The emotional responses to syphilis vary and may include feelings of shame, fear, depression, and anxiety.

TABLE 80–3

Selected Nursing Diagnoses for Clients with Sexually Transmitted Diseases

- High Risk for Injury related to the disease process
- Ineffective Individual Coping related to guilt, shame, or anger
- Noncompliance related to treatment and/or partner follow-up
- Sexual Dysfunction related to fear of transmission
- Impaired Skin Integrity related to the presence of genital ulcer, warts, or rash
- Altered Health Maintenance related to Knowledge Deficit about the mode of transmission, disease process, or need for treatment
- Impaired Social Interaction related to social stigma
- Pain related to the infection process
- Anxiety related to possible infertility as a result of having an STD
- Self Esteem Disturbance related to the effects of having an STD

Clients may feel guilt if they have infected others or anger if they have been infected by a partner. If further psychosocial interventions are necessary, the nurse encourages the client to discuss these feelings or refers the client to other resources such as psychotherapy groups, self-help support groups, or STD clinics.

Genital Herpes Simplex

Overview

Genital herpes is the most frequent cause of genital ulcer in Western Europe and North America (Mroczkowski & Martin, 1994). Two types of herpes simplex virus (HSV) affect the genitalia: type 1 (HSV-1) and type 2 (HSV-2). Most nongenital lesions, such as cold sores, are caused by HSV-1; HSV-2 causes most of the genital lesions. However, either type can produce oral or genital lesions through oral-genital contact with an infected person.

The incubation period is 2 to 20 days, with the average period being 1 week. Many people are asymptomatic during the primary infection, but symptoms, if they occur, are usually most severe during this first infection.

Itching or a tingling sensation may be felt in the skin 1 to 2 days before an outbreak. These sensations are followed by the appearance of vesicles (blisters) in a characteristic cluster on the penis, scrotum, vulva, perineum, vagina, cervix, or perianal region. The vesicles rupture spontaneously in a couple of days and leave painful erosions. These lesions can become extensive, and other symptoms, such as headaches, fever, general malaise, and inguinal lymphadenopathy, may be present. Urination may be painful, and clients with urinary retention may require catheterization. Lesions resolve within 2 to 6 weeks.

After the lesions heal, the virus remains in a dormant state in the nerve ganglia (specifically, in genital herpes, in the sacral ganglia). Periodically, the virus may activate, and episodes of infection recur. These recurrences may be stimulated by many factors, including stress, fever, sunburn, menses, and sexual activity.

Recurrences are not usually caused by reinfection. These episodes of recurrent infection are usually less severe and shorter than the primary infection; they may not even occur at all. Occasionally, HSV infection may become active without producing apparent clinical manifestations. However, there is viral shedding, and the client is infectious. Clients with frequent symptomatic recurrences may be at high risk for transmitting HSV (Benedetti et al., 1994; Wald et al., 1995).

Long-term complications of genital herpes include the risk of cervical cancer, the risk of neonatal transmission, and an increased risk of acquiring HIV infections.

An association between HSV-2 infections and cervical cancer has been demonstrated, especially in women with recurrent infections. Women with genital herpes should be encouraged to have an annual Papanicolaou (Pap) test. The risk of transmission to the neonate is greater in a pregnant woman who has a primary infection than in one who has recurrent herpes.

Collaborative Management

 Assessment

The diagnosis of genital herpes is usually based on the client's history and physical examination (see Chart 80–1) and is confirmed through viral culture. Cultures are

---

Chart 80–2

Health Promotion Guide: Prevention of Sexually Transmitted Diseases

- Know that the only way to be certain that you will not get a human immunodeficiency virus (HIV) infection or some other sexually transmitted disease is to abstain from all forms of sex.
- Do not have sex with people who have HIV infection or hepatitis B.
- Do not have sex with people who have unusual fluids coming from their genitals. Do not have sex with people who have warts on their genitals, herpes on their genitals, or anything else unusual on their genitals.
- Do not have sexual intercourse with many different people, people you do not know well, prostitutes, or other people who have sex with many different people.
- Avoid oral-anal sex.
- Don't let anyone touch your genitals with a cold sore on his or her mouth.
- Use a latex condom or diaphragm, together with a cream that kills sperm, with each new act of intercourse.
- If your health care provider tells you that you are in danger of getting HIV or some other sexually transmitted disease, get regular checkups for these diseases.

Modified from Centers for Disease Control and Prevention. (1993). 1993 Sexually transmitted diseases treatment guidelines. *Morbidity and Mortality Weekly Report, 42* (No. RR-14), 3–6.

most accurate if specimens are obtained within 48 hours of the first outbreak of the blisters.

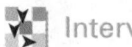 Interventions

Management of HSV infection focuses on
- Decreasing pain and promoting comfort
- Promoting healing without secondary infection
- Decreasing viral excretions
- Preventing transmission of the infection

Treatment is usually symptomatic (Chart 80–3).

➤ Drug Therapy

Acyclovir is an antiviral drug that is used to treat genital herpes. The drug is not a cure, but it partially controls outbreaks and accelerates healing. Topical therapy is not as effective as oral therapy. The recommended dosage of acyclovir is 200 mg orally five times a day for 7 to 10 days, during the first infection. Recommended treatment for recurrent episodes is acyclovir 200 mg orally five times a day for 5 days or 800 mg twice a day for 5 days. Most recurrent episodes do not benefit from treatment, but therapy for severe recurrent disease may be beneficial if it is started within 2 days of the appearance of lesions.

Clients who have frequent recurrences (more than six in a year) may benefit from daily treatment with acyclovir 200 mg two to five times a day. Long-term (more than 3 years) safety of this treatment is unknown. Clients receiving continuous therapy should stop after 1 year for reassessment of recurrences.

Chart 80–3

Nursing Care Highlight: The Client with Genital Herpes

- Administer oral analgesics as prescribed.
- Apply topical steroids to the herpes lesions.
- Apply local anesthetic sprays or ointments as prescribed.
- Apply ice packs or warm compresses to the client's lesions.
- Administer sitz baths three or four times a day.
- Encourage an increase in fluid intake.
- Encourage frequent voidings.
- Pour water over the client's genitalia while the client is voiding, or encourage voiding while the client is sitting in a tub of water or standing in a shower.
- Catheterize the client as necessary.
- Encourage genital hygiene and encourage keeping the skin clean and dry.
- Wash hands thoroughly after contact with lesions.
- Wear gloves when applying ointments.
- Advise the client to avoid sexual activity when lesions are present.
- Advise the client to use latex condoms during all sexual exposures.

Chart 80–4

Education Guide: Use of Condoms

- Use latex condoms rather than natural membrane condoms.
- Keep condoms in a cool, dry place, out of direct sunlight.
- Do not use condoms that are in damaged packages or that are brittle or discolored.
- Always handle a condom with care to avoid damaging it with fingernails, teeth, or other sharp objects.
- Put condoms on before any genital contact. Hold the condom by the tip and unroll it on the penis. Leave a space at the tip to collect semen.
- If you use a lubricant with condoms, make sure that the lubricant is water based—that it washes away with water.
- Use condoms that contain spermicide.
- If a condom breaks, replace it immediately.
- After ejaculation, withdraw the erect penis carefully holding the condom at the base of the penis to prevent the condom from slipping off.
- Never use a condom more than once.

Modified from Centers for Disease Control and Prevention. (1993). 1993 Sexually transmitted diseases treatment guidelines. *Morbidity and Mortality Weekly Report, 42*(No. RR-14), 4.

➤ Nursing Management

Nursing management includes client counseling and education about the infection and the potential for recurrent episodes. Counseling about sexual activity is extremely important. The nurse tells clients to abstain from sexual activity while lesions are present. Condom use during all sexual exposures is encouraged because of the increased risk of HSV transmission (Chart 80–4). Additionally, HSV infections can be transmitted during viral shedding, even when lesions are not present.

The nurse emphasizes the risk of fetal infection to all clients. Women who have genital herpes need to inform their maternity care provider of their history during future pregnancies.

The nurse also assesses the client's psychological responses to the diagnosis of genital herpes. Many clients are initially shocked and need reassurance that they can manage the disease. Feelings of disbelief, uncleanliness, isolation, and loneliness have been reported by infected clients. Clients have also reported anger at their partners for transmitting the infection or fear of rejection by partners because they have the infection. The nurse helps clients cope with the diagnosis by being sensitive and supportive during assessments and interventions. Social supports should be encouraged, and referrals to support groups, such as HELP (see Appendix), may be beneficial.

Lymphogranuloma Venereum
Overview

Lymphogranuloma venereum (LGV) is caused by serotypes of *Chlamydia trachomatis*. The incubation period is 3 to 30 days. The primary lesion is transient and painless and is not usually noticed by the client. The lesion usually appears on the penis in men and on the vaginal wall in women; however, sores may also be located in the mouth and rectum.

Lesions vary in form from herpes-like blisters to ulcers, vesicles, papules, or pustules. Within 1 to 2 weeks after the appearance of the primary lesion, secondary signs of infection appear. Lymphadenopathy (primarily inguinal) is present, and symptoms of headache, malaise, arthralgia, and anorexia may occur. Lymphadenopathy can recede or develop into abscesses. When the abscesses rupture, healing occurs slowly. Sinus tracts formed as a result of the infection drain thick, viscous pus for several weeks, leaving behind deep scars.

Complications of the infection can cause chronic lymphadenopathy, fistulas, rectal strictures, and proctitis. Systemic involvement can also cause carditis, arthritis, and pneumonia.

TRANSCULTURAL CONSIDERATIONS

Lymphogranuloma venereum has a worldwide distribution, but it occurs primarily in South America, the West Indies, Southeast Asia, India, and Africa. Cases in the United States usually occur in clients who have visited these countries, such as military personnel and other travelers.

Collaborative Management

The usual treatment of LGV is doxycycline (Vibramycin, Novodoxylin✦) 100 mg orally twice a day or tetracycline (Tetracyn, Nu-Tetra✦) 500 mg orally four times a day for at least 3 weeks. Incision and drainage of infected lymph nodes are contraindicated, but the nodes may be aspirated by needle. Surgical intervention may be required for late complications, such as strictures and fistulas. Client education is similar to that for the client with syphilis. Sexual partners should be identified and treated.

Chancroid

Overview

Although chancroid has a worldwide distribution, it is most common in developing tropical and subtropical countries (Mroczkowski & Martin, 1994). Recent spread of the causative organism, *Haemophilus ducreyi,* has made chancroid an important sexually transmitted disease in the United States because the open lesions of chancroid have been associated with the spread of HIV. Uncircumcised men may be at greater risk for infection than are circumcised men (Adimora et al., 1994).

The incubation period for chancroid varies from 3 to 10 days. A tender papule appears at the site of inoculation. This lesion rapidly breaks down to form an irregularly shaped, deep ulcer that has a purulent discharge and bleeds easily.

Complications include inguinal adenitis, balanitis, phimosis, and urethral fistulas. Chancroids differ from chancres caused by syphilis in that chancroids are soft and painful. Transmission of the disease is through contact with the ulcer or with the discharge from the infected local lymph glands during sexual activity.

Collaborative Management

Treatment for chancroid consists of azithromycin (Zithromax) 1 g orally in a single dose; erythromycin (E-Mycin, Apo-Erythro✦) 500 mg orally four times a day for 7 days; or ceftriaxone (Rocephin) 250 mg intramuscularly in a single dose. Clients should be observed by a physician or nurse practitioner until ulcers heal. Client education is similar to that for the client with syphilis. Sexual contacts must be located and treated whether or not they are symptomatic.

Granuloma Inguinale

Overview

The causative organism of granuloma inguinale or donovanosis is *Calymmatobacterium granulomatis.* A nodule appears at the site of inoculation after 1 to 12 weeks. This lesion ulcerates, and others are formed; they grow together, becoming a spreading ulcer on the genitalia. Left untreated, these lesions can be mutilating. Although pregnancy may accelerate the disease, there is no evidence of transmission to the fetus.

TRANSCULTURAL CONSIDERATIONS

Granuloma inguinale is endemic in parts of Australia among the central aborigines and common in Africa, Southeast Asia, southern India, and New Guinea. Occurrence in the United States, Japan, and Europe is rare.

Collaborative Management

Granuloma inguinale is treated with an antibiotic, usually tetracycline 500 mg orally four times a day for at least 10 days or until lesions heal. Clients need long-term follow-up on a yearly basis because these lesions may recur (Adimora et al., 1994).

The nurse's responsibility in management of the client with LGV, chancroid, and granuloma inguinale is similar to that for clients with other sexually transmitted diseases (STDs). An adequate history is taken (see Chart 80–1), including physical signs and symptoms and travel abroad. Information about sexual partners is also obtained. Physical examination and laboratory results confirm the diagnosis.

The nurse explains the correct way to take prescribed medications and stresses the importance of taking the entire amount prescribed. Possible side effects and what to do if they occur are described. The nurse also provides information on the disease, including how it is acquired, how it is spread, and the prognosis with and without adequate treatment.

The client should be encouraged to provide sexual contacts for follow-up and treatment. Concerns about coping with the disease may arise; the nurse encourages the client to verbalize concerns and/or refers the client for further counseling.

Infections of Epithelial Surfaces

Condylomata Acuminata

Overview

Condylomata acuminata (also known as venereal or genital *warts*) are caused by certain types of human papillomavirus (HPV). Genital warts are the most commonly sexually transmitted viral disease and are often seen with other infections, such as gonorrhea and trichomoniasis. Sites commonly affected include the urinary meatus, vulva, labia majora, vagina, cervix, penis, scrotum, anus, and perineal area. The infection is exacerbated in pregnant women and the elderly. The incubation period is usually 2 to 3 months. Genital warts are thought to be highly contagious and have been reported in more than 50% of sexual partners of infected persons.

The genital warts are initially single, small papillary growths that may grow into large cauliflower-like masses. Some women also experience a profuse, foul-smelling vaginal discharge. Bleeding may occur. If there are only a few warts, they may regress spontaneously without treatment.

Genital warts are strongly associated with genital dysplasia and cervical carcinoma. A Pap smear is useful in the isolation and diagnosis of HPV from the cervix. HPV can also be detected in genital swab specimens using a more sensitive polymerase chain reaction (PCR) assay. A specimen for biopsy is obtained from any atypical, pigmented, or persistent warts.

Collaborative Management

The diagnosis of condylomata is made by examination of the lesions, which appear wart-like. To rule out the presence of other infections, such as syphilis and gonorrhea, a VDRL test is done and a specimen for gonorrheal culture is obtained. Wet mounts are done if vaginitis is present, and a Pap smear is obtained to assess cervical abnormalities. If lesions bleed easily or appear to be infected, a biopsy may be done to rule out other pathologic conditions. Colposcopy is recommended for assessment of lesions that are not visible to the naked eye.

The goal of management is to remove the warts and to treat the symptoms. No therapy has been shown to eradicate HPV; therefore, recurrences after treatment are likely (Stone, 1995). Treatment of choice for external warts is cryotherapy with liquid nitrogen or a cryoprobe. The nurse explains that anesthesia is not required and scarring does not usually result. Extensive warts have been treated with the carbon dioxide laser or surgery.

As an alternative therapy, podophyllum resin, 10% to 25% in compound tincture of benzoin or trichloroacetic acid (80% to 90%), may be applied to external warts 2 cm or less in diameter located on the external genitalia. Podophyllum resin is teratogenic, and its use is contraindicated in pregnancy. Before podophyllum is applied, the surrounding skin or tissues are covered with petrolatum jelly or a paste of baking soda and water for protection from the caustic effects of the treatments. These treatments are left in place for 1 to 4 hours, after which they are washed off. Treatment may be repeated weekly if necessary. Adverse effects include nausea, diarrhea, lethargy, paralysis, or possibly coma.

Electrocautery or surgical removal may also be used to treat external warts. The type of surgery depends on the site of the warts, such as cone biopsy for cervical lesions and "skinning" vulvectomy for vulvar lesions. (See Chapter 78, under Vulvar Cancer, for a discussion of these procedures.)

For effective management of condylomata, sexual partners must also be treated. Clients should avoid intimate sexual contact until external lesions are healed.

Nursing management focuses on client education about the mode of transmission, incubation period, treatment, and complications.

Condoms are recommended to help reduce transmission (see Chart 80–4). Clients need to know that recurrence is likely and that repeated treatments may be necessary. The nurse encourages women who have had condylomata to have an annual Pap smear. As with other STDs, emotional support for the client is needed, and referral for counseling may help.

Gonorrhea

Overview

Gonorrhea continues to be the most reported communicable disease in the United States. The incidence is highest among sexually active people between the ages of 15 and 34 years. This bacterial infection occurs in men and women, and infants can be infected during childbirth. The causative organism is *Neisseria gonorrhoeae,* a gram-negative diplococcus. *N. gonorrhoeae* cannot survive long outside of the host and is infrequently transmitted by inanimate objects, such as towels and clothing. Transmission is most often by direct sexual contact (vaginal intercourse or orogenital or anogenital contact) and through an infected birth canal to the neonate.

The initial symptoms of gonorrhea may appear 3 to 10 days after sexual contact with an infected person. The infection can be asymptomatic in both males and females, but women have asymptomatic, or silent, infections more often than men do. If symptoms are present, men most likely notice dysuria and a penile discharge that can be either profuse yellowish-green fluid or scant clear fluid. The urethra is the site most commonly affected, but infection can extend to the prostate, the seminal vesicles, and the epididymis. Women may report a change in vaginal discharge, urinary frequency, or dysuria. The cervix and urethra are the most common sites of infection, but ascending spread can cause pelvic infection (pelvic inflammatory disease [PID]), endometritis (endometrial infection), salpingitis (fallopian tube infection), and/or pelvic peritonitis.

Anal manifestations may include anal itching and irritation, rectal bleeding or diarrhea, and painful defecation. Oral manifestations are related to pharyngeal infection. Symptoms are seldom noted but may include a sore throat, ulcerated lips, tender gingivae, and vesicles in the oropharynx. Figure 80–1 shows common sites of gonococcal infections.

Asymptomatic clients may present to the health care

THROAT

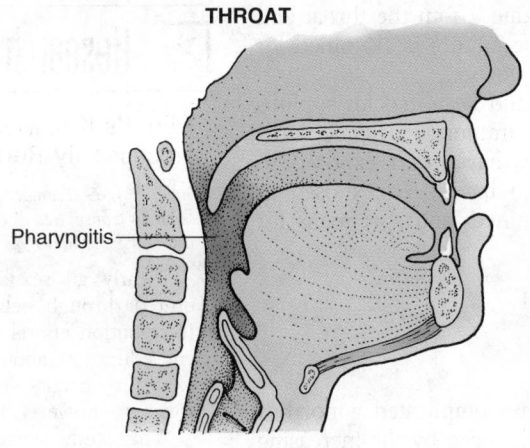

Pharyngitis

PELVIC/GENITAL

MEN

Prostatitis   Urethritis

Proctitis

Epididymitis

Purulent
discharge

WOMEN

Endometritis   Salpingitis

Cervicitis

Proctitis

Urethritis

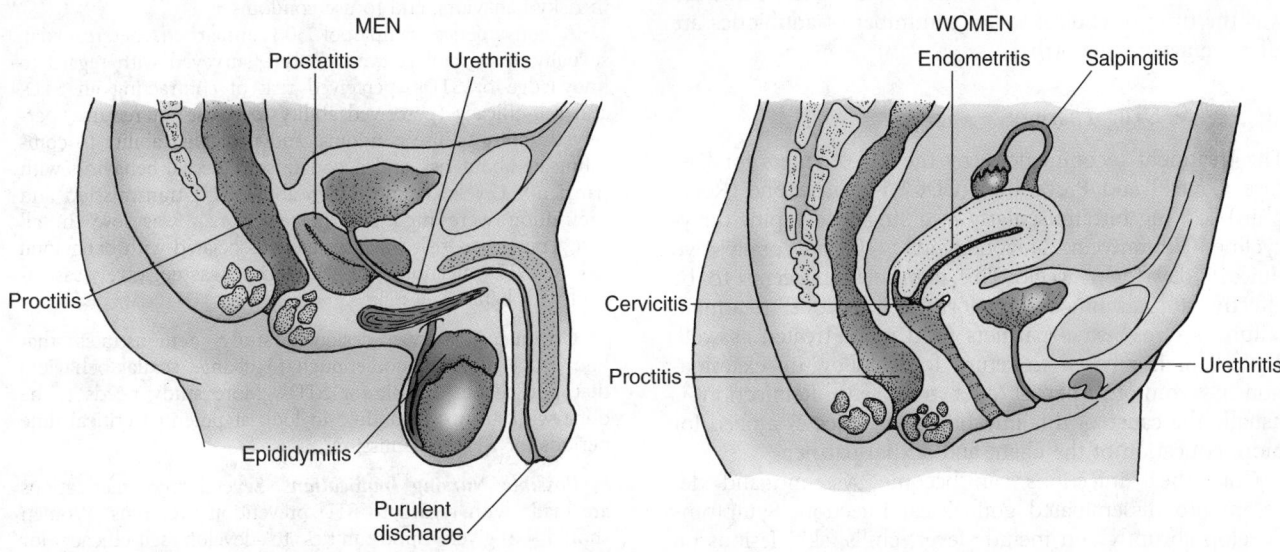

Figure 80–1. Some areas of involvement with gonorrhea in men and women.

facility for routine physical examination or for hospital admission or preoperative examinations, when they may be found to have positive culture results for gonorrhea. Other clients may come to the health care agency because the sexual partner has been diagnosed with the infection and assessment for transmission is needed.

Collaborative Management

 Assessment

A complete history includes allergies to drugs (such as penicillin), signs and symptoms, and a sexual history (see Chart 80–1). The nurse uses a nonjudgmental approach in eliciting information and avoids assumptions about sexual orientation. These techniques may decrease the client's anxiety and embarrassment about having a sexually transmitted disease (STD).

Physical assessment includes inspection for lesions, rashes, and discharges from the urethra, vagina, and rectum. Palpation of affected areas may reveal tenderness. Fever may be present, especially in complicated infections.

Definitive diagnosis involves laboratory tests. Identification of gonorrhea in men can be made with smears of the discharge that has been swabbed on a glass slide, dried, and stained with Gram stain. The presence of gram-negative diplococci is diagnostic for gonococcal urethritis.

Smears do not confirm the diagnosis in women because the female genital tract normally harbors organisms that resemble *Neisseria gonorrhoeae*. Cultures provide a more definitive diagnosis and are the most reliable method of confirming a diagnosis.

A specimen is obtained from the male urethra or the female cervix, and a Thayer-Martin culture medium is inoculated and placed in a carbon dioxide–rich environment. Depending on the history given by the client, culture specimens may also be obtained from the throat and rectum. After 24 to 48 hours, the culture is examined for the presence of gram-negative diplococci.

All clients with gonorrhea should be tested for syphilis and should be offered human immunodeficiency virus (HIV) testing because they may have been exposed to these STDs. Sexual partners who have been exposed in the last 30 days should be examined, and specimens for culture should be obtained.

Interventions

The health care provider treats uncomplicated gonorrhea with antibiotics. Treatment is influenced by the increasing numbers of organisms that have become resistant to antibiotics, especially penicillin and tetracycline; it is also influenced by the high frequency of chlamydial infections found in clients with gonorrhea. In the past, penicillin was the drug of choice; today, a number of antibiotics are effective against gonorrhea.

➤ Drug Therapy

The treatment recommended by the U.S. Centers for Disease Control and Prevention (CDC) is ceftriaxone (Rocephin) 125 mg intramuscularly in a single dose plus doxycycline (Vibramycin, Novodoxylin✻) 100 mg orally two times a day for 1 week. This combination seems to be effective for all mucosal gonorrhea infections; treatment failure is rare. Sexual partners need to be treated as well. The client is advised to return for a follow-up examination if symptoms persist after treatment. Reinfection is usually the cause of this infection and indicates a need for more education of the client and sexual partner.

Gonorrheal infections can become systemic and develop into disseminated gonococcal infection. Symptoms develop abruptly and include fever, chills, skin lesions on distal parts of extremities, and arthritis-like joint involvement with or without swelling, heat, or erythema.

Meningitis and endocarditis occur rarely. Hospitalization for these clients is recommended for the initial treatment, especially if endocarditis or meningitis is suspected.

Treatment is with intravenous antibiotic therapy (ceftriaxone 1 g every 24 hours). If symptoms resolve within 24 to 48 hours, the client may be discharged to home to continue oral antibiotic therapy for at least 1 week. If meningitis or endocarditis is present, therapy may be continued for 2 to 4 weeks.

➤ Health Teaching

Nursing interventions focus on health teaching about transmission and treatment of gonorrhea. However, knowledge alone may not change the client's behavior (see Research Applications for Nursing). Clients must understand why medications should be taken for the prescribed time for maximal effectiveness. The nurse discusses the possibility of reinfection. Clients should avoid sexual activity until the infection is cured. Men are told to wear condoms if abstinence is not possible, and women

▷ Research Applications for Nursing

Client's Knowledge of STDs Does Not Necessarily Reduce the Risk of Infection

Hale, P. J., & Trumbetta, S. L. (1996). Women's self-efficacy and sexually transmitted disease preventive behaviors. Research in Nursing and Health, 19(2), 101–110.

Nearly all sexually transmitted diseases (STDs) are acquired through behavior that can be avoided or modified. Intervention efforts have primarily focused on increasing client education about STDs. Knowledge of STDs is high—exposure occurs in schools and through many media sources—however, infection rates remain high as well.

This study suggests that knowledge of STDs alone does not change behavior. Other factors may be involved in producing behavioral changes, including self-efficacy (a belief in one's own ability to perform a behavior) and belief in one's ability to communicate with a partner, to refuse to participate in risky behaviors, and to use condoms.

A convenience sample of 308 unmarried, heterosexual, sexually active college women were surveyed with regard to knowledge of STDs, perceived risk of contracting an STD, and self-efficacy (perceived ability to refuse intercourse, perceived ability to use condoms, and perceived ability to communicate about risk and negotiate safer sexual behaviors with partners). Levels of knowledge about STD transmission and prevention were high and perceived risk was low. In all cases, perceived risk was positively associated with behavioral risk for STD infection, and self-efficacy was negatively associated with behavioral risk.

Critique. This well-designed study demonstrates that knowledge alone is not enough to change sexual behaviors that put clients at risk for STDs. More study needs to be done with groups over time to look at potential critical time periods for STD transmission.

Possible Nursing Implications. Several recommendations are made with regard to STD prevention programs. Women should be given opportunities to develop self-efficacy for STD prevention behaviors. Modeling, role playing, or video scenarios may help build self-efficacy. Furthermore, women's awareness of what constitutes risky behavior needs to be increased. Women also need to learn to appraise risk more realistically. Education efforts could target messages about STD risk to personal circumstances.

are told to make sure that their partner uses condoms. The nurse explains that gonorrhea is a reportable disease. All sexual contacts need to be examined and treated, according to culture findings.

When a diagnosis of gonorrhea is made, the client may have feelings of shame and guilt. Clients may also see the disease as a punishment for promiscuity or "unnatural" sex acts. Clients may believe that acquiring gonorrhea (or any STD) is a risk that they must take to pursue their desired lifestyle. Such feelings can impair relationships with sexual partners. The nurse encourages expression of feelings during assessments and teaching sessions. Privacy for client teaching and maintenance of confidentiality of medical records are important nursing interventions in meeting the client's psychosocial needs.

Chlamydial Infection

Overview

Chlamydia trachomatis is the most commonly transmitted bacterium in the United States. The disease is not reportable, but more than 5 million acute infections are estimated annually. In men, about half of the cases of nongonococcal urethritis and epididymitis are caused by *C. trachomatis*. In women, about 40% of the cases of pelvic inflammatory disease (PID) are caused by *C. trachomatis*, and 8% to 12% of pregnant women have the infection (Adimora et al., 1994). Transmission to the newborn can occur during vaginal delivery, with resultant neonatal eye infections and pneumonia.

C. trachomatis invades the columnar epithelial tissues in the reproductive tract and causes clinical manifestations similar to those of gonorrheal infections. The incubation period ranges from 1 to 3 weeks, but the pathogen may be present in the genital tract for months or years without producing symptoms.

In men, the primary symptom is nongonococcal urethritis, accompanied by dysuria, frequency of urination, and a mucoid discharge that is more watery and less copious than a gonorrheal discharge. Some men have the discharge only in the morning on arising. Complications include epididymitis, prostatitis, infertility, and Reiter's syndrome, a type of connective tissue disease (see Chap. 24).

In contrast, up to 75% of women may have no symptoms. Some have a mucopurulent cervicitis with symptoms of a change in vaginal discharge, urinary frequency, and soreness in the affected area. Complications include salpingitis, PID, ectopic pregnancy, and infertility.

Collaborative Management

 Assessment

A complete history, including medical, menstrual, and sexual history (see Chart 80–1), is obtained from the client. The nurse asks about
- The presence of symptoms
- A history of sexually transmitted diseases (STDs)
- Whether sexual partners have suspicious symptoms or have a history of STDs

The nurse remembers that many women with chlamydial infections are asymptomatic, and a history may reveal only risk factors associated with *Chlamydia trachomatis*. These factors include pregnancy, sexual activity during adolescence, use of a nonbarrier method of birth control, and a history of multiple sexual partners.

As with all interviews concerning sexual behavior, the nurse uses a nonjudgmental approach and provides privacy and confidentiality.

Diagnosis of chlamydial infections is usually made by excluding gonorrhea on a urethral Gram stain and culture. The presence of polymorphonuclear leukocytes and the absence of gram-negative intracellular diplococci suggest a chlamydial infection. Absolute diagnosis may be made with a tissue culture from the endocervix and urethra of a female client and from the urethra of the male

client. Special media are needed for the culture, and the procedure is expensive. Many laboratories are not equipped to do these tests; therefore, routine cultures may not be available in all health care settings. Screening asymptomatic women who are at high risk for having chlamydial infections is strongly encouraged.

There are two enzyme immunoassay tests that can be performed easily, less expensively, and more quickly than cultures: the Chlamydiazyme, an enzyme-linked immunoassay, and the MicroTrak, a direct fluorescent antibody test. For both tests, urogenital secretions are used for specimens. The Chlamydiazyme test depends on antigen-antibody reactions that are read with a spectrophotometer. A reading of optical density that is equal to or more than 0.1 is considered positive. In the MicroTrak test, stained urogenital secretions are studied under a fluorescent microscope.

The newest, and perhaps most sensitive, laboratory test is the polymerase chain reaction (PCR) assay. This test has higher sensitivity and specificity than the enzyme immunoassay tests (Bowie et al., 1994).

 Interventions

The treatment of choice for chlamydial infections is doxycycline (Vibramycin, Novodoxylin♦) 100 mg two times a day for 7 days or azithromycin (Zithromax) 1 g in a single dose. For clients who are allergic to these drugs, ofloxacin (Floxin) 300 mg two times a day for 7 days is recommended. Sexual partners should be tested for *Chlamydia trachomatis* and treated if infection is present.

Client education is an important nursing intervention. The nurse explains the following:
- Mode of transmission
- Incubation period
- Signs and symptoms
- Treatment
- Possible complications of untreated or inadequately treated infection

Psychosocial support is similar to that discussed in the section on gonorrhea.

Other Gynecologic Conditions

Pelvic Inflammatory Disease

Overview

Pelvic inflammatory disease (PID) is considered the major gynecologic health problem in the United States affecting over 1 million women annually (Kottmann, 1995). PID is an infectious process that may involve one or more pelvic structures, although the most common site is the fallopian tube.

Many practitioners use the terms "PID" and "salpingitis" synonymously for acute infections. PID is one of the leading causes of infertility and seems to relate to the rise in the number of ectopic pregnancies reported in the United States. PID is generally viewed as an acute syndrome resulting in tenderness in the tubes and ovaries (adnexa) and low, dull abdominal pain. However, many women experience only mild discomfort or menstrual irregularity; others experience no symptoms at all. Diagnosis and treatment of PID in these women is a challenge to health care providers. Irreversible scarring or stricture may occur before PID is diagnosed causing sterility.

Pathophysiology

PID is a complex process in which organisms from the lower genital tract migrate from the endocervix upward through the endometrial cavity to the fallopian tubes. The spread of infection to other organs of the upper genital tract occurs by way of direct contact with mucosal surfaces or through the fimbriated ends of the tubes to the ovaries, parametrium, and peritoneal cavity (Fig. 80–2). Resultant infections include

- Endometritis (infection of the endometrial cavity)
- Salpingitis (inflammation of the fallopian tubes)
- Oophoritis (ovarian infection)
- Parametritis (infection of the parametrium)
- Peritonitis (infection of the peritoneal cavity)
- Tubal or tubo-ovarian abscess

Etiology

Many different pathogens are linked to PID (Jossens et al., 1994; Sweet, 1995). Three sexually transmitted organisms are most often responsible for PID: *Neisseria gonorrhoeae, Chlamydia trachomatis,* and *Mycoplasma hominis.*

Chlamydia is the most common causative agent in PID in the United States and Europe (Adimora et al., 1994). In addition to these bacteria, *Staphylococcus, Streptococcus, Escherichia coli,* and other aerobic and anaerobic organisms have been identified in clients with PID. These organisms most likely invade the pelvis from an ascending infection from the vagina or cervix. Infections have

been spread during sexual intercourse, childbirth (including the postpartum period), and after abortion. Rarely do infections result from transperitoneal spread from a ruptured appendix or intra-abdominal abscess.

Incidence/Prevalence

The incidence of pelvic inflammatory disease (PID) is on the rise. Accurate rates are unavailable because PID is not a reportable disease. Many of the same factors that place women at risk for STDs also place them at risk for PID. Sexually active women who have multiple new or casual sexual partners have an increased risk as do women who delay seeking care. Other factors that increase a woman's risk include

- Age less than 20 years
- Contraceptive choice (i.e., intrauterine device [IUD])
- Use of vaginal douches
- Smoking
- History of STDs
- History of PID

TRANSCULTURAL CONSIDERATIONS

 The influence of race as a risk factor for STDs and PID continues to be controversial. Does race alone make a client susceptible, or does the environment that minorities find themselves in make them susceptible? In the early 1990s, the largest increases in STDs were among inner-city, poor, non-Caucasian populations. The highest prevalence of illicit drug use and trafficking is in the same urban areas (Adimora et al., 1994). However, African-Americans have been associated with PID from sexually transmitted microbes (Jossens et al., 1994). Further study is necessary to clarify the role of race in STDs and PID.

Collaborative Management

Assessment

➤ History

The nurse obtains a complete medical, family, menstrual, obstetric, and sexual history, including a history of previous episodes of PID or other infections (see Chart 80–1). The nurse also assesses for contraceptive use (especially the intrauterine device), history of reproductive surgery, and other risk factors previously identified. Symptoms of acute PID most often develop during or after menstruation.

➤ Physical Assessment/Clinical Manifestations

On physical assessment, the nurse may note lower abdominal tenderness with rigidity or rebound pain. One of the most frequent symptoms of PID is lower abdominal pain and tenderness. Other symptoms include menstrual irregularities/abnormal vaginal bleeding, dysuria, increase or change in vaginal discharge, dyspareunia, malaise, fever, and chills.

A pelvic examination may reveal uterine or cervical tenderness with motion and swollen adnexa (tubes and ovaries). If the client is using an IUD for contraception,

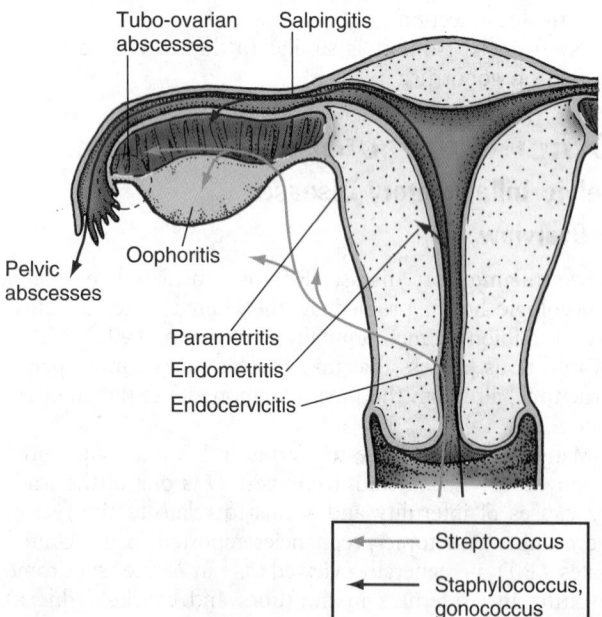

Tubo-ovarian abscesses
Salpingitis
Pelvic abscesses
Oophoritis
Parametritis
Endometritis
Endocervicitis

⟵ Streptococcus
⟵ Staphylococcus, gonococcus

Figure 80–2. The spread of PID.

the device should be removed. Characteristics of vaginal and cervical discharges, if present, are assessed. Ectopic pregnancy and appendicitis must be ruled out as potential etiologies.

➤ *Psychosocial Assessment*

The woman who presents with symptoms of PID is usually anxious and fearful of the examination and unknown diagnosis. She may need much reassurance and support during the physical examination because the abdomen is likely to be quite tender and she may wish to avoid further pain. Explanations of what is taking place often help promote cooperation during the examination.

If the PID is associated with a sexually transmitted disease (STD), the woman may feel embarrassed or guilty. The nurse uses a nonjudgmental approach in making assessments and encourages expression of feelings and concerns.

➤ *Laboratory Assessment*

The health care provider typically orders cultures of the cervix, urethra, and rectum to evaluate the presence of *Neisseria gonorrhoeae* or *Chlamydia*. The white blood cell (WBC) count and erythrocyte sedimentation rate (ESR) may be elevated but are not sensitive enough for sole diagnosis of PID. Gram stains of endocervical secretions may show the presence of *N. gonorrhoeae*. A sensitive test that detects human chorionic gonadotropin in urine or blood should be performed to determine if the client is pregnant.

➤ *Other Diagnostic Assessment*

Abdominal ultrasonography has been more accurate in assessing pelvic abscesses than in assessing enlargements and abscesses related to ovaries and fallopian tubes. Transvaginal ultrasound has been used in some cases to detect tubal enlargement and tubal wall thickening associated with PID. Laparoscopy is most definitive, giving an immediate, accurate diagnosis through direct inspection of the tubes and ovaries.

Culdocentesis is a technique that is performed to aspirate peritoneal fluid or pus from the cul-de-sac. Culture of this fluid may assist the physician in the diagnosis of PID.

 Analysis

➤ *Common Nursing Diagnoses and Collaborative Problems*

The following nursing diagnoses are common for the woman with pelvic inflammatory disease (PID):
1. Pain related to the effects of the infectious process
2. Anxiety related to possible infertility as a result of infection

➤ *Additional Nursing Diagnoses and Collaborative Problems*

In addition to the common nursing diagnoses, some women may have the following problems:

- Self Esteem Disturbance related to guilt of having PID (associated with sexual transmission)
- Chronic Pain after recurrent PID episodes
- Sexual Dysfunction related to the effects of the infectious process
- Altered Health Maintenance related to knowledge deficit about risks, prevention, symptoms, treatment, and effects of PID

 Planning and Implementation

➤ *Pain*

Planning: Expected Outcomes. The client is expected to experience reduced pain and increased comfort.

Interventions. Nonsurgical management (pain management and antibiotic therapy) or surgical management can be used, depending on the symptoms and the extent of the disease.

Nonsurgical Management. Pain management of PID is based on the severity of the symptoms. Relief measures include taking analgesics or sitz baths and applying heat to the lower abdomen or back. Bed rest in a semi-Fowler's position promotes gravity drainage and consolidation of the infection that may relieve pain as well.

Treatment of the infection relieves pain, and a variety of antibiotics are used (Chart 80–5). Two-thirds to three-fourths of women with uncomplicated PID are usually treated on an outpatient basis with oral and intramuscular antibiotics. Therapy consists of one or two antibiotic injections followed by oral antibiotics for 10 to 14 days. These clients should be re-evaluated 48 to 72 hours after antibiotic therapy is started. If the infection has not responded to treatment, the client may need to be hospitalized for intravenous antibiotic therapy and further evaluation.

Inpatient therapy initially involves a combination of several intravenous antibiotics for 4 to 5 days, until the patient is afebrile and improving. Intravenous therapy is discontinued, and oral antibiotic therapy is initiated for 7 to 10 days. Some women may complete intravenous therapy at home with the assistance of a home care agency. When a client is treated at home, she should be encouraged to rest, abstain from sexual intercourse, and check her temperature twice a day. The home care nurse visits every day or every other day, and follow-up with the health care provider is scheduled as needed.

Surgical Management. In a small number of clients, the pain and tenderness may not be relieved by antibiotic therapy. The surgeon may perform a laparotomy to remove an abscess or a pelvic mass. The surgeon usually performs a laparotomy through a subumbilical incision that is several inches long to provide better access to the fallopian tubes.

Preoperatively, the nurse provides information about hospital routines and procedures. (General preoperative care is described in Chapter 20.)

The postoperative care of the woman with PID is similar to that of any client after abdominal surgery. One difference is that the client with PID may have a wound

Chart 80–5

Drug Therapy for Acute Pelvic Inflammatory Disease

Drug*	Visual Dosage	Nursing Interventions	Rationale
Inpatient Treatment			
Regimen A			
Cefoxitin	• 2 g qid IV for 4 days	• Assess the client for rash, itching, and hypotension. • Observe the IV site for signs of redness, heat, and tenderness.	• Assessment detects adverse reactions. • Phlebitis can be detected.
plus Doxycycline	• 100 mg bid IV or PO for 4 days	• Do not give with iron or antacids.	• This precaution avoids inhibition of drug absorption.
followed by Doxycycline	• 100 mg bid PO for 10–14 days	• Assess the client for rashes, nausea, and diarrhea. • Encourage fluid intake.	• Assessment detects drug side effects. • Fluid intake decreases esophageal irritation.
Regimen B			
Clindamycin	• 900 mg tid IV	• Observe the client for rash and urticaria. • Observe the client for hypotension, dyspnea, and restlessness. • Observe the client for diarrhea. • Observe the IV site for redness, heat, and tenderness.	• Adverse reactions are detected. • Anaphylactic reaction is detected. • This precaution avoids pseudomembranous colitis. • Phlebitis can be detected.
plus Gentamicin	• 2 mg/kg IV once followed by 1.5 mg/kg tid for 4 days	• Encourage oral intake of fluids. • Observe the IV site for redness, heat, and tenderness. • Measure fluid intake and output.	• Fluid intake prevents irritation to renal tubules. • Phlebitis can be detected. • Oliguria or anuria can be detected.
then Doxycycline	• 100 mg bid PO for 10–14 days	• See above for doxycycline.	
or Clindamycin	• 450 mg 5 times a day PO for 10–14 days	• Give with 8 oz of water. • See above for clindamycin.	• Water decreases esophageal irritation.
Outpatient Treatment Cefoxitin	• 2 g IM once	• Give deep IM injection in the outer upper quadrant of the gluteus maximus. • Watch for fever, chills, and nausea. • Tell the client that the injection may be painful.	• Local irritation is avoided, and drug absorption is increased. • Allergic reactions can be detected. • The client is prepared for discomfort related to inflammatory reaction.
plus Probenecid	• 1 g PO once	• Give with food. • Encourage fluid intake (10 glasses a day).	• Taking the medication with food avoids gastrointestinal upset. • Fluid intake prevents formation of kidney stones.
or Ceftriaxone	• 250 mg IM once	• Give deep IM injection in the outer upper quadrant of the gluteus maximus. • Watch for fever, chills, and nausea.	• Local irritation is avoided, and drug absorption is increased. • Allergic reactions can be detected.
followed by Doxycycline	• 100 mg bid PO for 10–14 days	• See above for doxycycline.	

Modified from Centers for Disease Control and Prevention (1993). 1993 Sexually transmitted diseases treatment guidelines. *Morbidity and Mortality Weekly Report,* 42(No. RR-14), 78–79.

*These are examples of combinations of drugs recommended by the CDC. No single drug is active against all the pathogens causing PID.

drain in place for drainage of abscess fluid that may not have been completely removed during surgery. The nurse observes, measures, and records wound drainage every 4 to 8 hours as ordered.

➤ Anxiety

Planning: Expected Outcomes. The major outcome is that the client is expected to use effective coping mechanisms to reduce anxiety about infertility.

Interventions. Infertility is the most common complication of PID and affects at least 15% to 25% of women who have had at least one episode of PID. Nursing interventions are aimed at assessing the client for her knowledge of PID and its relation to infertility and for verbal and nonverbal clues to anxiety about this potential problem.

If the client has anxiety, the nurse tries to provide an atmosphere in which the client feels comfortable in expressing her feelings and in asking questions. The nurse encourages emotional support from significant others. Providing information about the advantages of early diagnosis and treatment—possibly limiting damage to one area of the pelvis—and the advances in surgery for infertility may reassure the client.

➤ Continuing Care

The client with PID is typically managed at home and requires health teaching to prevent further episodes of infection.

➤ Health Teaching

Client teaching focuses on providing information about PID, identifying recurrences (persistent pain, dysmenorrhea, low backache, fever) and practicing meticulous perineal hygiene. The nurse also reviews teaching for oral antibiotic therapy (Chart 80–6).

The client needs to be counseled to contact her sexual partner(s) for examination and possible treatment of a sexually transmitted disease (STD). The nurse reminds her about follow-up care and counsels her about the complications that can occur after an episode of PID, including increased risk for recurrence of PID, increased risk for ectopic pregnancy, increased risk for infertility, and chronic pelvic pain.

If the client desires contraceptive measures, the nurse discusses methods that may decrease the risk of future episodes of PID, such as oral contraceptive pills, barrier methods in combination with spermicides containing nonoxynol 9, and tubal ligation.

Counseling is also given to help the client understand lifestyle factors that heighten the risk for recurrent episodes of PID, including sexual intercourse with multiple partners, vaginal douching, and poor genital hygiene.

Psychosocial concerns may require teaching and counseling as well. A client who has PID may exhibit feelings of guilt about having a condition that may have been transmitted to her sexually. These guilt feelings may affect her relationship with significant others. She may also have

---

Chart 80–6

Education Guide: Oral Antibiotic Therapy for Sexually Transmitted Diseases

- Understand the importance of taking your medicine the number of times a day and for the specific number of days prescribed.
- Know that your sexual partner must be tested and may have to be treated.
- Be sure to return for your follow-up appointment after completing your antibiotic treatment.
- Call if you have any questions or concerns.
- Do not have sex until after you complete your antibiotic therapy. If your partner is being treated, you can go back to having sex together 48 hours after he or she starts taking antibiotics if you use a condom.
- Drink at least 8 to 10 glasses of fluid a day while taking your antibiotics.
- Do not take antacids containing calcium, magnesium, or aluminum, such as Tums, Maalox, or Mylanta.
- Take your antibiotics on an empty stomach unless your health care provider instructs you to take them with food.

---

concerns about future fertility if PID has caused major damage or scarring of the fallopian tubes and other reproductive organs. The nurse provides emotional support and allows time for the client to express her feelings.

➤ Home Care Management

No special home care preparation is necessary for women whose treatment for PID is complete. For the client who receives antibiotic therapy at home, see previous section on nonsurgical management of PID pain.

➤ Health Care Resources

If infertility is a result of PID, the client may need referral to a clinic specializing in infertility treatment and counseling. The client can also contact support groups, such as RESOLVE, for infertile couples that exist in many local communities.

Evaluation

On the basis of the identified nursing diagnoses, the expected outcomes may include that the client will

- Report that pain is relieved/reduced and that she feels more comfortable
- Relate that her anxiety about future infertility has decreased
- Describe the risk factors, signs and symptoms, treatments, and effects of PID
- Resume usual sexual activities without discomfort
- Express her feelings about having an infection that was probably caused by a sexually transmitted organism

Vaginal Infections

Vaginal infections are associated with discharge and are frequent and recurring problems for sexually active women. Common causes of vaginal infection are

- *Trichomonas vaginalis*
- *Candida albicans*
- Bacteria that produce bacterial vaginosis, including *Gardnerella vaginalis* and *Mycoplasma hominis*

These infections can be spread by sexual contact. Men can also acquire these infections, but they usually do not present with symptoms and often are not treated. Because these infections are usually seen in women, assessments and interventions are discussed with other causes of vaginitis in Chapter 78.

 CASE STUDY For the Client with a Sexually Transmitted Disease

■ A 22-year-old married woman presents with low abdominal discomfort, dysuria, and menstrual irregularities for 1 month. Her history is noteworthy for past episodes of sexually transmitted diseases (gonorrhea, chlamydia, herpes). She seems nervous and distracted during the visit.

Q U E S T I O N S :

1. What other critical client history questions should you ask?
2. What other physical assessment and laboratory data should you obtain?

■ Your client has been diagnosed with PID and must be admitted to the hospital for intravenous antibiotics. She begins to cry.

3. What assessments/interventions should be completed first?
4. What assessments/interventions should be completed in 24 to 48 hours?

SELECTED BIBLIOGRAPHY

Adimora, A. A., Hamiliton, H., Holmes, K. K., & Sparling, P. F. (1994). *Sexually transmitted diseases* (2nd ed.). New York: McGraw-Hill.

American College of Obstetrics and Gynecology. (1994). Gonorrhea and chlamydial infections. ACOG Technical Bulletin, 190. *International Journal of Obstetrics and Gynaecology, 45*(2), 169.

Anderson, J. E., Brackbill, R., & Mosher, W. D. (1996). Condom use for disease prevention among unmarried U.S. women. *Family Planning Perspectives, 28*(1), 25–28, 39.

Baken, L. A., Koutsky, L. A., Kuypers, J., Kosorok, M. R., Lee, S. K., Kiviat, N. B., & Holmes, K. K. (1995). Genital human papillomavirus infection among male and female sex partners: Prevalence and type-specific concordance. *Journal of Infectious Diseases, 171*(2), 429–432.

Bar-Chama, N., Goluboff, E., & Fisch, H. (1994). Infection and pyospermia in male infertility. Is it really a problem? *Urologic Clinics of North America, 21*(3), 469–475.

Benedetti, J., Corey, L., & Ashley, R. (1994). Recurrence rates in genital herpes after symptomatic first-episode infection. *Annals of Internal Medicine, 121*(11), 847–854.

Braverman, P., & Strasburger, V. (1994). Sexually transmitted diseases. *Clinical Pediatrics, 33*(1), 26–37.

Bowie, W. R., Hammerschlag, M. R., & Martin, D. H. (1994). STDs in '94: The new CDC guidelines. *Patient Care, 28*(7), 29–53.

*Centers for Disease Control and Prevention. (1991). Pelvic inflammatory disease: Guidelines for prevention and management. *Morbidity and Mortality Weekly Report, 40* (No. RR-5), 1–25.

*Centers for Disease Control and Prevention. (1993). 1993 Sexually transmitted diseases treatment guidelines. *Morbidity and Mortality Weekly Report, 42* (No. RR-14), 1–102.

Chin, V. P. (1996). Pelvic inflammatory disease. In C. Havens, N. Sullivan, & P. Tilton (Eds.), *Manual of outpatient gynecology* (3rd ed., pp. 35–42). Boston: Little, Brown.

Corey, L. (1994). The current trend in genital herpes. Progress in prevention. *Sexually Transmitted Diseases, 21*(suppl 2), S38–S44.

Eschenbach, D. A. (1994). Pelvic infections and sexually transmitted diseases. In Scott, J. R., et al. (Eds.), *Danforth's obstetrics and gynecology,* (7th ed.). Philadelphia: J. B. Lippincott.

Ferenczy, A. (1995). Epidemiology and clinical pathophysiology of condylomata acuminata. *American Journal of Obstetrics and Gynecology, 172*(4 pt 2), 1331–1339.

Grodstein, F., & Rothman, K. J. (1994). Epidemiology of pelvic inflammatory disease. *Epidemiology, 5*(2), 234–242.

Hemsell, D. L., Little, B. B., Faro, S., Sweet, R. L., Ledger, W. J., Berkeley, A. S., Eschenbach, D. A., Wolner-Hanssen, P., & Pastorek, J. G., 2nd. (1994). Comparison of three regimens recommended by the Centers for Disease Control and Prevention for the treatment of women hospitalized with acute pelvic inflammatory disease. *Clinical Infectious Diseases, 19*(4), 720–727.

Hoffman, I. F., & Schmitz, J. L. (1995). Genital ulcer disease. Management in the HIV era. *Postgraduate Medicine, 98*(3), 67.

Holmes, K. K. (1994). Human ecology and behavior and sexually transmitted bacterial infections. *Proceedings of the National Academy of Sciences of the United States of America, 91*(7), 2448–2455.

*Holmes, K. K., Per-Anders, M., Sparling, P. F., & Wiesner, P. J. (Eds.). (1990). *Sexually transmitted diseases* (2nd ed.). New York: McGraw-Hill.

Jamison, J. H., Kaplan, D. W., Hamman, R., Eagar, R., Beach, R., & Douglas, J. M., Jr. (1995). Spectrum of human papillomavirus in a female adolescent population. *Sexually Transmitted Diseases, 22*(4), 236–243.

Jossens, M. O., Schachter, J., & Sweet, R. L. (1994). Risk factors associated with pelvic inflammatory disease of differing microbial etiologies. *Obstetrics and Gynecology, 83*(6), 989–997.

Kee, J. L., (1995). *Laboratory and diagnostic tests with nursing implications* (4th ed.). Norwalk, CT: Appleton & Lange.

Kottmann, L. M. (1995). Pelvic inflammatory disease: Clinical overview. *Journal of Obstetric, Gynecologic, and Neonatal Nursing, 24*(8), 759–767.

Kupesic, S., Kurjak, A., Pasalic, L., Benic, S., & Ilijas, M. (1995). The value of transvaginal color Doppler in the assessment of pelvic inflammatory disease. *Ultrasound in Medicine and Biology, 21*(6), 733–738.

Landers, D. V., & Sweet, R. L. (1996). Pelvic inflammatory disease. New York: Springer.

Lynch, P. J. (1994). *Genital dermatology.* New York: Churchill-Livingstone.

Madrid, E., & Swanson, J. (1995). Psychoeducational groups for young adults with genital herpes: Training group facilitators. *Journal of Community Health Nursing, 12*(4), 189–198.

Marion, L. N., & Cox, C. L. (1996). Condom use and fertility among divorced and separated women. *Nursing Research, 45*(2), 110–115.

Martin, D. H., & Mroczkowski, T. F. (1994). Dermatologic manifestations of sexually transmitted diseases other than HIV. *Infectious Disease Clinics of North America, 8*(3), 533–582.

Morse, S. A., Moreland, A. A., & Holmes, K. K. (1996). *Atlas of sexually transmitted diseases and AIDS* (2nd ed.). London: Mosby-Wolfe.

Mroczkowski, T. F., & Martin, D. H. (1994). Genital ulcer disease. *Dermatologic Clinics, 12*(4), 753–764.

Paisarntantiwong, R., Brockmann, S., Clarke, L., Landesman, S., Feldman, J., & Minkoff, H. (1995). The relationship of vaginal trichomoniasis and pelvic inflammatory disease among women colonized with *Chlamydia trachomatis. Sexually Transmitted Diseases, 22*(6), 344–347.

Peipert, J. F., Boardman, L., Hogan, J. W., Sung, J., & Mayer, K. H. (1996). Laboratory evaluation of acute upper genital tract infection. *Obstetrics and Gynecology, 87*(5 pt 1), 730–736.

Prasad, C. J. (1995). Pathobiology of human papillomavirus. *Clinics in Laboratory Medicine, 15*(3), 685–704.

Rice, R., Schwartz, D., Knapp, J., & Paavonen, J. (1996). Pelvic inflammatory disease. In S. A. Morse, A. A. Moreland, & K. K. Holmes (Eds.), *Atlas of sexually transmitted diseases and AIDS* (2nd ed., pp. 134–147). London: Mosby-Wolfe.

Scholes, D., Stergachis, A., Heidrich, F. E., Andrilla, H., Holmes, K. K., & Stamm, W. E. (1996). Prevention of pelvic inflammatory disease by screening for cervical chlamydial infection. *New England Journal of Medicine, 334*(21), 1362–1366.

Soper, D. E. (1994). Pelvic inflammatory disease. *Infectious Disease Clinics of North America, 8*(4), 821–840.

Sparling, P. F., Elkins, C., Wyrick, P. B., & Cohen, M. S. (1994). Vaccines for bacterial sexually transmitted infections: A realistic goal? *Proceedings of the National Academy of Sciences of the United States of America, 91*(7), 2456–2463.

Stastny, J. F., Ben-Ezra, J., Stewart, J. A., Kornstein, M. J., Kay, S., & Frable, W. J. (1995). Condyloma and cervical intraepithelial neoplasia of the endometrium. *Gynecologic and Obstetric Investigation, 39*(4), 277–280.

Stone, K. M. (1995). Human papillomavirus infection and genital warts; update on epidemiology and treatment. *Clinical Infectious Diseases, 20*(suppl 1), S91–S97.

Swanson, J. M., Dibble, S. L., & Trocki, K. (1995). A description of the gender differences in risk behaviors in young adults with genital herpes. *Public Health Nursing, 12*(2), 99–108.

Sweet, R. L. (1995). Role of bacterial vaginosis in pelvic inflammatory disease. *Clinical Infectious Diseases, 20*(suppl 2), S271–S275.

Thompson, S., Larsen, S., & Moreland, A. (1996). Syphilis. In S. A. Morse, A. A. Moreland, & K. K. Holmes (Eds.), *Atlas of sexually transmitted diseases and AIDS* (2nd ed., pp. 21–46). London: Mosby-Wolfe.

Turrentine, M., & Gonik, B. (1994). Herpes simplex virus. *Current Opinion in Obstetrics and Gynecology, 6*(4), 377–382.

Wald, E. R. (1996). Pelvic inflammatory disease in adolescents. *Current Problems in Pediatrics, 26*(3), 86–97.

Wald, A., Zeh, J., Selke, S., Ashley, R. L., & Corey, L. (1995). Virologic characteristics of subclinical and symptomatic genital herpes infections. *New England Journal of Medicine, 333*(12), 770–775.

Whittington, W., Ison, C., & Thompson, S. (1996). Gonorrhea. In S. A. Morse, A. A. Moreland, & K. K. Holmes (Eds.), *Atlas of sexually transmitted diseases and AIDS* (2nd ed., pp. 99–117). London: Mosby-Wolfe.

Youngkin, E. Q. (1995). Sexually transmitted diseases: Current and emerging concerns. *Journal of Obstetric, Gynecologic, and Neonatal Nursing, 24*(8), 743–758.

SUGGESTED READINGS

Adimora, A. A., Sparling, P. F., & Cohen, M. S. (1994). Vaccines for classic sexually transmitted diseases. *Infectious Disease Clinics of North America, 8*(4), 859–876.

Vaccines for infectious diseases are not uncommon; however, vaccines for sexually transmitted diseases (STDs) remain a public health challenge. Many STDs are human-species specific so there are no comparable animal model studies. Furthermore, most STD microbes have complex structures and impart only limited host immunity after infection. This article reviews the status of vaccine research for five STDs: gonorrhea, genital herpes, syphilis, chancroid, and chlamydia.

Briggs, L. P., Patnaude, P., Scavron, J., Whelan, M., & Etkind, P. (1995). The importance of social histories for assessing sexually transmitted disease risk. *Sexually Transmitted Diseases, 22*(6), 348–350.

The identification of STD risk groups is helpful in the development of focused treatment, education, and/or prevention efforts. This article reminds the nurse that assumptions regarding age and other risk factors can lead to missed diagnoses and opportunities for STD treatment, education, and prevention. Although there may be some discomfort when asking the sensitive questions involved in taking a social and/or sexual history, these questions are critical in the recognition of a client's STD infection risk.

Swanson, J. M., Dibble, S. L., & Chenitz, W. C. (1995). Clinical features and psychosocial factors in young adults with genital herpes. *Image—the Journal of Nursing Scholarship, 27*, 16–22.

Reports about genital herpes often describe clinicians' observations of the impact of this disease. This study seeks to describe the impact from the client's point of view. Clients with genital herpes were compared with nonclient controls on physical and psychosocial factors. Stress was reported as the major cause of recurrences and headache as the major stress symptom. Clients with genital herpes had a lower self-concept, more psychological issues, a greater frequency of daily hassles, and less intense uplift in moods. Implications for client instruction and nursing practice and research are discussed.

Appendix 1

Abbreviations

AAA	abdominal aortic aneurysm
AACN	American Association of Critical Care Nurses
AAKP	American Association of Kidney Patients
ABC	airway, breathing, and circulation
ABG	arterial blood gas
ABI	ankle/brachial index
ABPM	ambulatory blood pressure monitoring
ABVD	Adriamycin, bleomycin, vinblastine, dacarbazine
AC	assist-control; alternating current
ACE	angiotensin-converting enzyme
ACh	acetylcholine
AChRAb	acetylcholine receptor antibody
ACL	anterior cruciate ligament
ACLS	advanced cardiac life support
ACS	acute compartment syndrome; American Cancer Society
ACTH	adrenocorticotropic hormone
ADC	AIDS dementia complex
ADH	antidiuretic hormone
ADL	activities of daily living
ADP	adenosine diphosphate
ADPKD	autosomal-dominant polycystic kidney disease
AED	automatic external defibrillation
aFP	alpha-fetoprotein
AGC	absolute granulocyte count
AGN	acute glomerulonephritis
AGR	abdominal/gluteal ratio
AHA	American Heart Association
AHCPR	Agency for Health Care Policy and Research
AIDS	acquired immunodeficiency syndrome
AIVR	accelerated idioventricular rhythm
AJCC	American Joint Committee on Cancer
AKA	above-knee amputation
AL	ascending limb
ALA	American Lung Association
ALG	antilymphocyte globulin
ALL	acute lymphocytic leukemia
ALP	alkaline phosphatase
ALS	amyotrophic lateral sclerosis
AMI	antibody-mediated immunity
AML	acute myelocytic leukemia
AMSN	Academy of Medical-Surgical Nurses
ANA	American Nurses' Association; anti-nuclear antibody
ANC	absolute neutrophil count
ANOVA	analysis of variance
ANP	atrial natriuretic peptide
ANS	autonomic nervous system
AORN	Association of Operating Room Nurses
AP	anteroposterior
APSAC	anisoylated plasminogen streptokinase activator complex
APSGN	acute post-streptococcal glomerulonephritis
APTT	activated partial thromboplastin time
ara-A	adenine arabinoside
ARDS	adult respiratory distress syndrome
ARF	acute renal failure
ASA	acetylsalicylic acid
ASPEN	American Society of Parenteral and Enteral Nutrition
AST	aspartate aminotransferase
ATG	antithymocyte globulin
ATN	acute tubular necrosis
ATP	adenosine triphosphate
ATPase	adenosine triphosphatase
AV	atrioventricular; arteriovenous
AVM	arteriovenous malformation
AVN	avascular necrosis
AZA	azathioprine
AZT	azidothymidine (zidovudine)
BBIAT	Baird Body Image Assessment Tool
BC	Bowman's capsule
BCG	bacille Calmette-Guérin
BCNU	carmustine
BCS	Body Cathexis Scale
BE	barium enema
BGMS	blood glucose monitoring strip
bid	*bis in die* (twice a day)
BKA	below-knee amputation
BMI	body mass index
BMT	bone marrow transplantation
BP	blood pressure
BPEG	British Pacing and Electrophysiology Group
BPH	benign prostatic hyperplasia (hypertrophy)
BPM	breaths per minute; beats per minute
BRM	biologic response modifier
BSE	breast self-examination
BSI	body substance isolation
BSO	bilateral salpingo-oophorectomy
BUN	blood urea nitrogen
c	cup(s)
C & S	culture and sensitivity
CABG	coronary artery bypass graft
CAD	computer-assisted design; coronary artery disease
CAH	chronic active hepatitis
CAL	chronic airflow limitation
CALLA	common acute lymphoblastic leukemia antigen
CAM	computer-assisted manufacturing
cAMP	cyclic adenosine monophosphate
CAPD	continuous ambulatory peritoneal dialysis
CAVH	continuous arteriovenous hemofiltration
CAVHD	continuous arteriovenous hemofiltration and dialysis
CBC	complete blood count
CBD	common bile duct
CBE	charting by exception
CBI	continuous bladder irrigation
CBS	chronic brain syndrome
CCA	circumflex coronary artery
CCP	chronic calcifying pancreatitis
CCPD	continuous-cycle peritoneal dialysis

CD	Cotrel-Dubousset; collecting duct	DJD	degenerative joint disease
CD4	cluster of differentiation 4	dL	deciliter(s)
CDC	Centers for Disease Control and Prevention; cheno-deoxycholic acid	DL	descending limb
		DLCO	diffusion capacity for carbon monoxide
CEA	carcinoembryonic antigen	DLE	discoid lupus erythematosus
CFU	colony-forming unit	DNA	deoxyribonucleic acid
CGN	chronic glomerulonephritis	DNP	dinitrophenol
CHF	congestive heart failure	DNR	do not resuscitate
CIC	Certified in Infection Control	DOE	dyspnea on exertion
CIN	cervical intraepithelial neoplasia	DP	dopamine
CIS	carcinoma in situ	DPOA	durable power of attorney
CK	creatine kinase	DRE	digital rectal examination
CLE	centrilobular emphysema	DRG	diagnosis-related group
CLL	chronic lymphocytic leukemia	DS	double-strength
cm	centimeter(s)	DSA	digital subtraction angiography
CMG	cystometrogram	DTIC	dacarbazine
CMI	cell-mediated immunity	DTR	deep tendon reflex
CML	chronic myelocytic leukemia	DUB	dysfunctional uterine bleeding
CMS	circulation, movement, sensation	DVT	deep venous thrombosis
CMV	cisplatin, methotrexate, vinblastine; cytomegalovirus	EAT	Eating Attitudes Test
		EBL	estimated blood loss
CNS	central nervous system	EBV	Epstein-Barr virus
CO	cardiac output	ECCC	Emergency Cardiac Care Committee
COHb	carboxyhemoglobin	ECCE	extracapsular cataract extraction
COLD	chronic obstructive lung disease	ECF	extracellular fluid
COPD	chronic obstructive pulmonary disease	ECG	electrocardiogram
COPES	Family Crisis–Oriented Personal Evaluation Scale	EDI	Eating Disorder Inventory
		EGD	esophagogastroduodenoscopy
CPAP	continuous positive airway pressure	EHDP	etidronate disodium
CPB	cardiopulmonary bypass	EIA	enzyme immunoassay
CPK	creatine phosphokinase	ELISA	enzyme-linked immunosorbent assay
CPM	continuous passive motion	EMD	electromechanical dissociation
CPN	chronic pyelonephritis	EMG	electromyography
CPO	certified prosthetist-orthotist	EMS	emergency medical services
CPR	cardiopulmonary resuscitation	EMT	Emergency Medical Technician
cps	cycles per second	ENCORE	encouragement, normalcy, counseling, opportunity, reaching out, revived energies
CQI	continuous quality improvement		
CREST	calcinosis, Raynaud's phenomenon, esophageal dys-motility, sclerodactyly, telangiectasia	ENG	electronystagmography
		ENT	ear, nose, and throat
CRF	chronic renal failure	EOM	extraocular movement
CRH	corticotropin-releasing hormone	EPO	erythropoietin
CRI	chronic renal insufficiency	EPS	electrophysiologic study
CRNA	Certified Registered Nurse Anesthetist	ER	estrogen receptor
CS	crush syndrome	ERCP	endoscopic retrograde cholangiopancreatography
CSA	cyclosporine A	ERS	erythrocyte sedimentation rate
CSF	cerebrospinal fluid	ERT	estrogen replacement therapy
CST	Certified Surgical Technologist	ESR	erythrocyte sedimentation rate
CT	computed tomography	ESRD	end-stage renal disease
CTD	connective tissue disease	ET	Enterostomal Therapist; endotracheal tube
CTS	carpal tunnel syndrome		
CVA	cerebrovascular accident (stroke); costovertebral angle	ETDR	early treatment diabetic retinopathy
		ETT	exercise tolerance test
CVC	central venous catheter	EVS	early vitrectomy study
CVP	central venous pressure	FACT	fruits, animals, colors, and towns
D&C	dilation and curettage	FAM	fluorouracil, Adriamycin, and mitomycin C
DARE	Drug Awareness Resistance Education	FANA	fluorescent antinuclear antibody
dB	decibel(s)	FAST	fluoroallergosorbent test
DCCT	Diabetes Control and Complications Trial	FBD	fibrocystic breast disease
DCM	dilated cardiomyopathy	FBSS	failed back surgery syndrome
DCT	distal convoluted tubule	FDA	(US) Food and Drug Administration
DDAVP	desmopressin acetate	FEF	forced expiratory flow
ddI	dideoxyinosine (didanosine)	FES	fat embolism syndrome
DDS	dapsone	FEV	forced expiratory volume
DES	diethylstilbestrol	FEV_1	forced expiratory volume in one second
DHE	dihydroergotamine	FEV_1/FVC	ratio of expiratory volume in one second to forced vital capacity
DHHS	(US) Department of Health and Human Services		
DHT	dihydrotestosterone	FFP	fresh frozen plasma
DI	diabetes insipidus	FIM	Functional Independence Measure
DIC	disseminated intravascular coagulation	FIO_2	fraction of inspired oxygen
DIP	distal interphalangeal joint		

FNB	Food and Nutrition Board	IBS	irritable bowel syndrome
FNCR	Family Nursing Chart Review	IBW	ideal body weight
FOBT	fecal occult blood test	ICD	implantable cardioverter-defibrillator
FR	flutter rate	ICE	Institutional Ethics Committee
Fr	French	ICF	intracellular fluid
FRC	functional residual capacity	ICHD	Intersociety Commission for Heart Disease
FS	full-strength	ICP	intracranial pressure
FSBS	fingerstick blood sugar	ICS	intercostal space
FSH	follicle-stimulating hormone	ICU	intensive care unit
ft	foot (feet)	IF	interstitial fluid
FTA-ABS	fluorescent treponemal antibody absorption test	Ig	immunoglobulin
5-FU	5-fluorouracil	IHSS	idiopathic hypertrophic subaortic stenosis
FUDR	floxuridine	IL	interleukin
FVC	forced vital capacity	IL-3	interleukin-3
FWB	full weight-bearing	IL-4	interleukin-4
g/day	gram(s) per day	IL-5	interleukin-5
g	gram(s)	IL-8	interleukin-8
G6PD	glucose-6-phosphate dehydrogenase	IM	intramedullary rod; intramuscular
GABA	gamma-aminobutyric acid	IMF	intermaxillary fixation
GAS	general adaptation syndrome	IMV	intermittent mandatory ventilation
GB	gallbladder	INF	interferon
GBS	Guillain-Barré syndrome	INR	international normalized ratio
GCS	Glasgow Coma Scale	IOL	intraocular lens
GCSF	granulocyte colony-stimulating factor	IOP	intraocular pressure
GDM	gestational diabetes mellitus	IP	intraperitoneal
GE	gastroenteritis	IPD	intermittent peritoneal dialysis
GF	glomerular filtrate	IPG	impedance plethysmography
GFR	glomerular filtration rate	IRT	intracavitary radiation therapy
GH	growth hormone	IS	incentive spirometer
GH-IH	growth hormone–inhibiting hormone	ITH	idiosyncratic toxic hepatitis
GH-RH	growth hormone–releasing hormone	ITP	idiopathic thrombocytopenic purpura
GI	gastrointestinal	IU	International Unit(s)
GM-CSF	granulocyte-macrophage colony-stimulating factor	IUD	intrauterine device
Gn-RH	gonadotropin-releasing hormone	IU/L	International Unit(s) per liter
GSW	gunshot wound	IV	intravenous
GVHD	graft-versus-host disease	IVC	inferior vena cava
Gy	Gray(s)	IVP	intravenous pyelography
h	hour(s)	JCAHO	Joint Commission on the Accreditation of Health-care Organizations
HAT	hearing assessment test	JGC	juxtaglomerular cell
Hb	hemoglobin	JVP	jugular venous pressure
HBIG	hepatitis B immunoglobulin	KCS	keratoconjunctivitis sicca
HBO	hyperbaric oxygen	kg	kilogram(s)
HBV	hepatitis B virus	kJ	kilojoule(s)
hCG	human chorionic gonadotropin	KS	Kaposi's sarcoma
HCM	hypertrophic cardiomyopathy	KUB	kidneys, ureters, and bladder
Hct	hematocrit	KW	Keith-Wagener classification
HCV	hepatitis C virus	LAC	long arm cast
HD	hemodialysis	LAD	left anterior descending
HDL	high-density lipoprotein	LAK	lymphokine-activated killer (cell)
HDV	hepatitis delta virus	LAP	leukocyte alkaline phosphatase
HEPA	high-efficiency particulate air	LAS	localized adaptation syndrome
HEV	hepatitis E virus	LATS	long-acting thyroid stimulator
Hgb	hemoglobin	LBP	low back pain
HIDA	hepatobiliary iminodiacetic acid analog (radionuclide labeled with technetium-99m)	LCA	left coronary artery
HIP	Help for Incontinent Persons	LDH	lactate dehydrogenase
HITT	heparin-induced thrombocytopenia	LDL	low-density lipoprotein
HLA	human leukocyte antigen	LE	lupus erythematosus; lower extremity
HMO	health maintenance organization	LES	lower esophageal sphincter
HPA	hypothalamic-pituitary-adrenal	LGV	lymphogranuloma venereum
HPV	human papillomavirus	LH	luteinizing hormone
HR	heart rate	LL	left lateral
HSV	herpes simplex virus	LLC	long leg cast
5-HT	5-hydroxytryptamine (serotonin)	LLQ	left lower quadrant
HTLV	human T-cell lymphotropic virus	LMN	lower motor neuron
Hz	Hertz	LOA	leave of absence
I&D	incision and drainage	LOC	level of consciousness
IABP	intra-aortic balloon pumping	LORS	Level of Rehabilitation Scale

LP	lumbar puncture; light perception	MVAC	methotrexate, vinblastine, Adriamycin, cisplatin
LPS	lipopolysaccharide	NANDA	North American Nursing Diagnosis Association
LR	lactated Ringer's (solution)	NAON	National Association of Orthopaedic Nurses
LRD	living related donor	NAPHT	National Association of Patients on Hemodialysis and Transplantation
LTC	long-term care		
LUQ	left upper quadrant	NASPE	North American Society for Pacing and Electrophysiology
LVD	left ventricular dysfunction		
LVEDP	left ventricular end-diastolic pressure	NCI	National Cancer Institute
M-CSF	monocyte-macrophage colony-stimulating factor	NE	norepinephrine
mA	milliampere(s)	ng	nanogram(s)
MAC	*Mycobacterium avium* complex	NG	nasogastric
MAO	monoamine oxidase	NHANES	National Health and Nutrition Examination Survey
MAP	mean arterial pressure		
MAST	military antishock trousers	NHIF	National Head Injury Foundation
MAT	multifocal atrial tachycardia	NIC	Nursing Interventions Classification
MB-CAPD	multiple-bag continuous ambulatory peritoneal dialysis	NK	natural killer (cell)
		NKF	National Kidney Foundation
MCA	middle cerebral artery	NLN	National League for Nursing
MCH	mean corpuscular hemoglobin	NRC/NAS	National Research Council/National Academy of Sciences
MCHC	mean corpuscular hemoglobin concentration		
MCL	modified chest lead	NS	nephrotic syndrome; normal saline
MCP	metacarpophalangeal	NSAID	nonsteroidal anti-inflammatory drug
MCV	mean corpuscular volume	NSNA	National Student Nurse Association
MD	muscular dystrophy	NSR	normal sinus rhythm
MDF	myocardial depressant factor	NTP	noninvasive temporary pacing
MDI	metered-dose inhaler	NWB	non–weight-bearing
MEN	multiple endocrine neoplasia	NYHA	New York Heart Association
mEq	milliequivalent(s)	OA	osteoarthritis
mEq/L	milliequivalent(s) per liter	OBS	organic brain syndrome
MFH	malignant fibrous histiocytoma	OCG	oral cholecystogram
mg	milligram(s)	OD	oculus dexter (right eye)
MG	myasthenia gravis	OFP	Optimal Functioning Plan
mg/dL	milligram(s) per deciliter	OI	osteogenesis imperfecta
MH	malignant hyperthermia	OR	operating room
MHAUS	Malignant Hyperthermia Association of the United States	ORIF	open reduction, internal fixation
		ORT	oral rehydration therapy; operating room technician
MHC	major histocompatibility complex	OS	oculus sinister (left eye)
MI	myocardial infarction	OSHA	(US) Occupational Safety and Health Administration
MICU	medical intensive care unit		
MIH	melanocyte-inhibiting hormone	OT	occupational therapist
min	minute(s)	OTC	over-the-counter
mL	milliliter(s)	oz	ounce(s)
mL/kg	milliliter(s) per kilogram	PA	posteroanterior
mm	millimeter(s)	PAB	prealbumin
mmHg	millimeter(s) of mercury	PAC	premature atrial complex
mmol	millimole(s)	PaCO$_2$	partial pressure of arterial carbon dioxide
mmol/L	millimoles per liter	PACU	postanesthesia care unit
MMPI	Minnesota Multiphasic Personality Inventory	PaO$_2$	partial pressure of arterial oxygen
MMSE	Mini-Mental State Examination	Pap	Papanicolaou (test, smear)
MMV	maximum mandatory ventilation	PAP	pulmonary artery pressure
MODY	maturity-onset diabetes of the young	PASG	pneumatic antishock garment
MOPP	mechlorethamine, Oncovin, procarbazine, prednisone	PAT	paroxysmal atrial tachycardia
		PAWP	pulmonary artery wedge pressure
mOsm	milliosmole(s)	PCA	patient-controlled analgesia
mOsm/L	milliosmole(s) per liter	PCAC	Patient Care Advisory Committee
MRB	manual resuscitation bag	PCM	protein-calorie malnutrition
MRC	Medical Research Council	PCN	penicillin
MRI	magnetic resonance imaging	PCP	*Pneumocystis carinii* pneumonia
MS	multiple sclerosis; morphine sulfate	PCR	polymerase chain reaction
msec	millisecond(s)	PCT	proximal convoluted tubule
MSH	melanocyte-stimulating hormone	PD	peritoneal dialysis
MTP	metatarsophalangeal	PE	pulmonary embolism
MTX	methotrexate	P-E	pharyngoesophageal
mU	milliunit(s)	PEA	pulseless electrical activity
mU/mL	milliunit(s) per milliliter	PEEP	positive end-expiratory pressure
MUGA	multigated angiography	PERRLA	pupils equal, round, and reactive to light and accommodation
mV	millivolt(s)		
MVA	motor vehicle accident	PES	problem, etiology, symptoms

PES-EO-IO	problem, etiology, signs and symptoms; expected outcome, interventions, outcome	qod	every other day
PET	positron emission tomography	QOL	quality of life
PFT	pulmonary function test	QOLY	Quality of Life Year(s)
PGE$_2$	prostaglandin E$_2$	RA	rheumatoid arthritis
PGI$_2$	prostaglandin I$_2$ (prostacyclin)	rad	radiation absorbed dose
pH	the negative logarithm of the hydrogen ion concentration	RAI	radioactive iodine
		RAIU	radioactive iodine uptake
PHP	plasma hydrostatic pressure	RAS	reticular activating system
PHS	Public Health Service	RBC	red blood cell
PICC	peripherally inserted central catheter	RCA	right coronary artery
PID	pelvic inflammatory disease	RDA	recommended daily allowance; recommended dietary allowance
PIE	plan, interventions, evaluation		
PIH	prolactin-inhibiting hormone	REM	rapid eye movement
PIP	proximal interphalangeal; peak inspiratory pressure	RFUT	radiofibrinogen uptake test
PJC	premature junctional complex	RIA	radioimmunoassay
PJT	premature junctional tachycardia	RIND	reversible ischemic neurologic deficit
PKD	polycystic kidney disease	RL	right lateral
PLE	panlobular emphysema	RLQ	right lower quadrant
PLP	phantom limb pain	RNA	ribonucleic acid
PMI	point of maximal impulse	RNI	Recommended Nutrient Intake
PMN	polymorphonuclear cell	ROM	range of motion
PMR	progressive muscle relaxation; polymyalgia rheumatica	RPGN	rapidly progressive glomerulonephritis
		RSD	reflex sympathetic dystrophy
PMS	premenstrual syndrome	RTA	renal tubular acidosis
PMT	premenstrual tension	RUQ	right upper quadrant
PND	paroxysmal nocturnal dyspnea	RV	residual volume
PNS	parasympathetic nervous system	SA	sinoatrial
PO	*per os* (by mouth)	SAC	short arm cast
POAG	primary open-angle glaucoma	SAECG	signal-averaged electrocardiography
POC	point-of-care	SAM	smoking-attributable mortality
POR	problem-oriented record	SaO$_2$	arterial oxygen saturation
PPD	purified protein derivative	SBE	subacute bacterial endocarditis
ppm	parts per million	SBFT	small bowel follow-through
PPM	pulses per minute	SC	subcutaneous
PPN	partial parenteral nutrition	SCD	sequential compression device
PPS	post-polio sequelae (syndrome)	SCI	spinal cord injury
PRL	prolactin	SCID	severe combined immunodeficiency
PRN	*pro re nata* (as needed)	SCS	Self-Cathexis Scale
PSA	prostate-specific antigen	SDA	same-day admission
PSE	portal-systemic encephalopathy	SDAT	senile dementia Alzheimer's type
PSS	progressive systemic sclerosis	SDS	same-day surgery
PSV	pressure support ventilation	SEAPort	side-entry access port
PSVT	paroxysmal supraventricular tachycardia	sec	second(s)
PT	physical therapy; physical therapist; prothrombin time	SEP	somatosensory evoked potential
		SF6	sulfahexafluoride
PTA	percutaneous transluminal angioplasty; peritonsillar abscess	SFA	superficial femoral artery
		SGOT	serum glutamic-oxaloacetic transaminase
PTC	peritubular capillary	SI	Système International d'Unites
PTCA	percutaneous transluminal coronary angioplasty	SIADH	syndrome of inappropriate antidiuretic hormone
PTFE	polytetrafluoroethylene	SIMV	synchronized intermittent mandatory ventilation
PTH	parathyroid hormone (parathormone)	SLC	short leg cast
PTT	partial thromboplastin time	SLE	systemic lupus erythematosus
PTU	propylthiouracil	SLP	speech/language pathologist
PUD	peptic ulcer disease	SLR	straight-leg raise
PULSES	physical condition, upper limb function, lower limb function, sensory components, excretory function, support factors	SMI	sustained minimal inspiration; self-management inventory
		SMR	submucous resection
PUVA	psoralen and ultraviolet A	SMX	sulfamethoxazole
PV	polycythemia vera	SNF	skilled nursing facility
PVC	premature ventricular complex	SNS	sympathetic nervous system
PVD	peripheral vascular disease	SOAP	subjective data, objective data, analysis, plan
PVR	postvoiding residual	SOAPIER	subjective data, objective data, analysis, plan, interventions, evaluation, revision of plan
PVS	persistent vegetative state		
PWB	partial weight-bearing	S/P	suprapubic
q	*quaque* (every)	SPD	supply processing and distribution
qd	*quaque die* (every day)	SPECT	single photon emission computed tomography
qid	*quater in die* (four times a day)	SPEP	serum protein electrophoresis
		SPF	sunburn protection factor

SSKI	saturated solution of potassium iodide		TSE	testicular self-examination
STA	superior temporal artery		TSH	thyroid-stimulating hormone
STD	sexually transmitted disease		TSI	thyroid-stimulating immunoglobulin
STS	serologic test for syphilis		TSM	transparent semipermeable membrane
STSG	split-thickness skin graft		tsp	teaspoon(s)
SV	stroke volume		TSS	toxic shock syndrome
SVC	superior vena cava		TTD	transtelephonic defibrillation/monitoring
T & A	tonsillectomy and adenoidectomy		TTO	transtracheal oxygen
T_3	triiodothyronine		TTP	thrombotic thrombocytopenic purpura
T_3RU	triiodothyronine resin uptake		TURBT	transurethral resection of bladder tumor
T_4	thyroxine		TURP	transurethral resection of the prostate
TAF	tumor angiogenesis factor		TVH	total vaginal hysterectomy
TAH	total abdominal hysterectomy		μg	microgram(s)
TB	tuberculosis		UGI	upper gastrointestinal
TBI	total body irradiation		UMN	upper motor neuron
TBSA	total body surface area		UPJ	ureteropelvic junction
tbsp	tablespoon(s)		UPP	urethral pressure profilometry
TCDB	turn, cough, and deep breathe		US	ultrasonography
TCT	thyrocalcitonin		USDA	United States Department of Agriculture
TDT	terminal deoxynucleotidyl transferase		UTI	urinary tract infection
TED	thromboembolic device		UV	ultraviolet
TEE	transesophageal echocardiography		UVA	ultraviolet A
TEF	tracheoesophageal fistula		UVB	ultraviolet B
TEN	toxic epidermal necrolysis		UVJ	ureterovesical junction
TENS	transcutaneous electrical nerve stimulation		VAD	venous access device
THA	tetrahydroaminoacridine		VADS	Visual Analog Dyspnea Scale
THP	tissue hydrostatic pressure		VAS	visual analog scale
THR	total hip replacement		VC	vital capacity
TIA	transient ischemic attack		VCUG	voiding cystourethrogram
TIBC	total iron-binding capacity		VDRL	Venereal Disease Research Laboratory (test)
tid	*ter in die* (three times a day)		VEP	visual evoked potential
TJR	total joint replacement		VF	ventricular fibrillation
TKR	total knee replacement		VLS	vascular leak syndrome
TLC	total lung capacity; total lymphocyte count		VMA	vanillylmandelic acid
TLS	tumor lysis syndrome		$\dot{V}O_2$	oxygen consumption
TLSO	thoracic lumbar sacral orthosis (thoracolumbosacral orthosis)		VOD	veno-occlusive disease
			VPB	ventricular premature beat
TMJ	temporomandibular joint		$\dot{V}/\dot{Q}$	ventilation-perfusion
TMP	trimethroprim		VR	vasa recta
TNF	tumor necrosis factor		VSE	vulvar self-examination
TNM	tumor, node, metastasis		VT	ventricular tachycardia
TOP	tissue osmotic pressure		V_T	tidal volume
TOPS	Take Off Pounds Sensibly		VZV	varicella-zoster virus
t-PA	tissue plasminogen activator		WAIS	Wechsler Adult Intelligence Scale
TPI	treponemal immobilization (test)		WBC	white blood cell
TPN	total parenteral nutrition		WHO	World Health Organization
TQM	total quality management		WHR	waist-to-hip ratio
TRH	thyrotropin-releasing hormone			

Appendix 2

Screening Guidelines for Secondary Prevention of Selected Cancers in Asymptomatic People

Cancer	Screening Test*
Breast cancer	Breast self-examination (monthly)
	Clinical examination (yearly)
	Mammography (baseline at age 35, every 2 years for ages 40–49, yearly after age 50)
Cervical cancer	Papanicolaou test and pelvic examination (yearly for sexually active women)
Ovarian cancer	Pelvic examination (yearly for women over age 40)
	Pelvic ultrasonography and blood test for CA-125 (yearly for women at high risk)
Prostate cancer	Digital rectal examination and blood test for prostate-specific antigen (yearly starting at age 40)
Testicular cancer	Testicular self-examination (monthly after puberty)
	Clinical examination (yearly)
Colorectal cancer	Digital rectal examination and stool blood test (yearly starting at age 40)
	Colonoscopy (yearly starting at age 50)
Skin cancer	Visual self-examination of skin lesions (monthly for all ages)
	Clinical examination (yearly)

* Recommended frequency of screening tests varies by agency, preference of the health care provider, and individual client risk.

Appendix 3

MINIMUM DATA SET (MDS) — *VERSION 2.0*
FOR NURSING HOME RESIDENT ASSESSMENT AND CARE SCREENING
BASIC ASSESSMENT TRACKING FORM

SECTION AA. IDENTIFICATION INFORMATION

1.	RESIDENT NAME ✱	a. (First) b. (Middle Initial) c. (Last) d. (Jr./Sr.)
2.	GENDER ✱	1. Male 2. Female
3.	BIRTHDATE ✱	☐☐ — ☐☐ — ☐☐ Month Day Year
4.	RACE/ ✱ ETHNICITY	1. American Indian/Alaskan Native 4. Hispanic 2. Asian/Pacific Islander 5. White, not of 3. Black, not of Hispanic origin Hispanic origin
5.	SOCIAL ✱ SECURITY AND ✱ MEDICARE NUMBERS [C in 1st box if non Med. no.]	a. Social Security Number ☐☐☐ — ☐☐ — ☐☐☐☐ b. Medicare number (or comparable railroad insurance number)
6.	FACILITY PROVIDER NO. ✱	a. State No. b. Federal No.
7.	MEDICAID NO. ["+" if pending, "N" if not a Medicaid ✱ recipient]	

8.	REASONS FOR ASSESS- MENT	[Note—Other codes do not apply to this form]
		a. Primary reason for assessment
		  1. Admission assessment (required by day 14)
		  2. Annual assessment
		  3. Significant change in status assessment
		  4. Significant correction of prior assessment
		  5. Quarterly review assessment
		  0. *NONE OF ABOVE*
		b. *Special codes for use with supplemental assessment types in Case Mix demonstration states or other states where required*
		  1. 5 day assessment
		  2. 30 day assessment
		  3. 60 day assessment
		  4. Quarterly assessment using full MDS form
		  5. Readmission/return assessment
		  6. Other state required assessment

9.	SIGNATURES OF PERSONS COMPLETING THESE ITEMS:	

a. Signatures	Title	Date
b.		Date

GENERAL INSTRUCTIONS
Complete this information for submission with all full and quarterly assessments (Admission, Annual, Significant Change, State or Medicare required assessments, or Quarterly Reviews, etc.).

✱ = Key items for computerized resident tracking

▓ = When box blank, must enter number or letter

☐a. = When letter in box, check if condition applies

Code "NA" if information unavailable or unknown.

TRIGGER LEGEND

1 - Delirium	10A - Activities (Revise)
2 - Cognitive Loss/Dementia	10B - Activities (Review)
3 - Visual Function	11 - Falls
4 - Communication	12 - Nutritional Status
5A - ADL-Rehabilitation	13 - Feeding Tubes
5B - ADL-Maintenance	14 - Dehydration/Fluid Maintenance
6 - Urinary Incontinence and Indwelling Catheter	15 - Dental Care
7 - Psychosocial Well-Being	16 - Pressure Ulcers
8 - Mood State	17 - Psychotropic Drug Use
9 - Behavioral Symptoms	17* - For this to trigger, O4a, b, or c must = 1-7
	18 - Physical Restraints

Form 1728HF R196 © 1995 Briggs Corporation, Des Moines, IA 50306 (800) 247-2343 PRINTED IN U.S.A.
Copyright limited to addition of trigger system.

1 of 8   MDS 2.0 10/18/94N

Resident _____   Numeric Identifier _____

MINIMUM DATA SET (MDS) — *VERSION 2.0*
FOR NURSING HOME RESIDENT ASSESSMENT AND CARE SCREENING
BACKGROUND (FACE SHEET) INFORMATION AT ADMISSION

SECTION AB. DEMOGRAPHIC INFORMATION

1.	DATE OF ENTRY	Date the stay began. Note — Does not include readmission if record was closed at time of temporary discharge to hospital, etc. In such cases, use prior admission date.

Month — Day — Year

2. ADMITTED FROM (AT ENTRY)
1. Private home/apt. with no home health services
2. Private home/apt. with home health services
3. Board and care/assisted living/group home
4. Nursing home
5. Acute care hospital
6. Psychiatric hospital, MR/DD facility
7. Rehabilitation hospital
8. Other

3. LIVED ALONE (PRIOR TO ENTRY)
0. No 1. Yes 2. In other facility

4. ZIP CODE OF PRIOR PRIMARY RESIDENCE

5. RESIDENTIAL HISTORY 5 YEARS PRIOR TO ENTRY
(Check all settings resident lived in during 5 years prior to date of entry given in item AB1 above.)
- Prior stay at this nursing home — a.
- Stay in other nursing home — b.
- Other residential facility — board and care home, assisted living, group home — c.
- MH/psychiatric setting — d.
- MR/DD setting — e.
- NONE OF ABOVE — f.

6. LIFETIME OCCUPATION(S) *(Put "/" between two occupations)*

7. EDUCATION *(Highest level completed)*
1. No schooling 5. Technical or trade school
2. 8th grade/less 6. Some college
3. 9-11 grades 7. Bachelor's degree
4. High school 8. Graduate degree

8. LANGUAGE *(Code for correct response)*
a. Primary Language
0. English 1. Spanish 2. French 3. Other
b. If other, specify

9. MENTAL HEALTH HISTORY Does resident's RECORD indicate any history of mental retardation, mental illness, or developmental disability problem?
0. No 1. Yes

10. CONDITIONS RELATED TO MR/DD STATUS *(Check all conditions that are related to MR/DD status that were manifested before age 22, and are likely to continue indefinitely)*
- Not applicable — no MR/DD (Skip to AB11) — a.
- MR/DD with organic condition
  - Down's syndrome — b.
  - Autism — c.
  - Epilepsy — d.
  - Other organic condition related to MR/DD — e.
- MR/DD with no organic condition — f.

11. DATE BACKGROUND INFORMATION COMPLETED
Month — Day — Year

▨ = When box blank, must enter number or letter
a. = When letter in box, check if condition applies
Code "NA" if information unavailable or unknown.

SECTION AC. CUSTOMARY ROUTINE

1. CUSTOMARY ROUTINE *(In year prior to DATE OF ENTRY to this nursing home, or year last in community if now being admitted from another nursing home)*

(Check all that apply. If all information UNKNOWN, check last box only)

CYCLE OF DAILY EVENTS
- Stays up late at night (e.g., after 9 pm) — a.
- Naps regularly during day (at least 1 hour) — b.
- Goes out 1+ days a week — c.
- Stays busy with hobbies, reading, or fixed daily routine — d.
- Spends most of time alone or watching TV — e.
- Moves independently indoors (with appliances, if used) — f.
- Use of tobacco products at least daily — g.
- NONE OF ABOVE — h.

EATING PATTERNS
- Distinct food preferences — i.
- Eats between meals all or most days — j.
- Use of alcoholic beverage(s) at least weekly — k.
- NONE OF ABOVE — l.

ADL PATTERNS
- In bedclothes much of day — m.
- Wakens to toilet all or most nights — n.
- Has irregular bowel movement pattern — o.
- Showers for bathing — p.
- Bathing in PM — q.
- NONE OF ABOVE — r.

INVOLVEMENT PATTERNS
- Daily contact with relatives/close friends — s.
- Usually attends church, temple, synagogue (etc.) — t.
- Finds strength in faith — u.
- Daily animal companion/presence — v.
- Involved in group activities — w.
- NONE OF ABOVE — x.

UNKNOWN — Resident/family unable to provide information — y.

END

SECTION AD. FACE SHEET SIGNATURES
SIGNATURES OF PERSONS COMPLETING FACE SHEET:

a. Signature of RN Assessment Coordinator — Date
b. Signatures — Title — Sections — Date
c. — Date
d. — Date
e. — Date
f. — Date
g. — Date

NOTE: Normally, the MDS Face Sheet is completed once, when an individual first enters the facility. However, the face sheet is also required if the person is reentering this facility after a discharge where return had not previously been expected. It is **not** completed following temporary discharges to hospitals or after therapeutic leaves/home visits.

Resident _____ Numeric Identifier_____

MINIMUM DATA SET (MDS) — *VERSION 2.0*
FOR NURSING HOME RESIDENT ASSESSMENT AND CARE SCREENING
FULL ASSESSMENT FORM
(Status in last 7 days, unless other time frame indicated)

SECTION A. IDENTIFICATION AND BACKGROUND INFORMATION

1. RESIDENT NAME

a. (First)   b. (Middle Initial)   c. (Last)   d. (Jr./Sr.)

2. ROOM NUMBER

3. ASSESSMENT REFERENCE DATE
a. *Last day of MDS observation period*

Month   Day   Year
b. Original (0) or corrected copy of form (enter number of correction)

4a. DATE OF REENTRY
Date of reentry from most recent temporary discharge to a hospital in last 90 days (or since last assessment or admission if less than 90 days)

Month   Day   Year

5. MARITAL STATUS
1. Never married   3. Widowed   5. Divorced
2. Married   4. Separated

6. MEDICAL RECORD NO.

7. CURRENT PAYMENT SOURCES FOR N.H. STAY
(Billing Office to indicate; check all that apply in last 30 days)
Medicaid per diem — a.
Medicare per diem — b.
Medicare ancillary part A — c.
Medicare ancillary part B — d.
CHAMPUS per diem — e.
VA per diem — f.
Self or family pays for full per diem — g.
Medicaid resident liability or Medicare co-payment — h.
Private insurance per diem (including co-payment) — i.
Other per diem — j.

8. REASONS FOR ASSESSMENT
[Note—If this is a discharge or reentry assessment, only a limited subset of MDS items need be completed]

a. Primary reason for assessment
1. Admission assessment (required by day 14)
2. Annual assessment
3. Significant change in status assessment
4. Significant correction of prior assessment
5. Quarterly review assessment
6. Discharged—return not anticipated
7. Discharged—return anticipated
8. Discharged prior to completing initial assessment
9. Reentry
0. NONE OF ABOVE

b. Special codes for use with supplemental assessment types in Case Mix demonstration states or other states where required
1. 5 day assessment
2. 30 day assessment
3. 60 day assessment
4. Quarterly assessment using full MDS form
5. Readmission/return assessment
6. Other state required assessment

9. RESPONSIBILITY/ LEGAL GUARDIAN
(Check all that apply)
Legal guardian — a.
Other legal oversight — b.
Durable power of attorney/health care — c.
Durable power of attorney/ financial — d.
Family member responsible — e.
Patient responsible for self — f.
NONE OF ABOVE — g.

10. ADVANCED DIRECTIVES
(For those items with supporting documentation in the medical record, check all that apply)
Living will — a.
Do not resuscitate — b.
Do not hospitalize — c.
Organ donation — d.
Autopsy request — e.
Feeding restrictions — f.
Medication restrictions — g.
Other treatment restrictions — h.
NONE OF ABOVE — i.

SECTION B. COGNITIVE PATTERNS

1. COMATOSE
(Persistent vegetative state/no discernible consciousness)
0. No   1. Yes (If yes, skip to Section G)

2. MEMORY
(Recall of what was learned or known)
a. Short-term memory OK—seems/appears to recall after 5 minutes
0. Memory OK   1. Memory problem **2**
b. Long-term memory OK—seems/appears to recall long past
0. Memory OK   1. Memory problem **2**

▨ = When box blank, must enter number or letter.

a. = When letter in box, check if condition applies

Code "NA" if information unavailable or unknown.

Form 1728HF   © 1995 Briggs Corporation, Des Moines, IA 50306 (800) 247-2343 PRINTED IN U.S.A.
Copyright limited to addition of trigger system.

3. MEMORY/ RECALL ABILITY
(Check all that resident was normally able to recall during last 7 days)
Current season — a.
Location of own room — b.
Staff names/faces — c.
That he/she is in a nursing home — d.
NONE OF ABOVE are recalled — e.

4. COGNITIVE SKILLS FOR DAILY DECISION-MAKING
(Made decisions regarding tasks of daily life)
0. INDEPENDENT—decisions consistent/reasonable
1. MODIFIED INDEPENDENCE—some difficulty in new situations only **2**
2. MODERATELY IMPAIRED—decisions poor; cues/ supervision required **2**
3. SEVERELY IMPAIRED—never/rarely made decisions **2, 5B**

5. INDICATORS OF DELIRIUM— PERIODIC DISORDERED THINKING/ AWARENESS
(Code for behavior in the last 7 days.) [Note: Accurate assessment requires conversations with staff and family who have direct knowledge of resident's behavior over this time.]
0. Behavior not present
1. Behavior present, not of recent onset
2. Behavior present, over last 7 days appears different from resident's usual functioning (e.g., new onset or worsening)

a. EASILY DISTRACTED—(e.g., difficulty paying attention; gets sidetracked) 2 = **1, 17***
b. PERIODS OF ALTERED PERCEPTION OR AWARENESS OF SURROUNDINGS—(e.g., moves lips or talks to someone not present; believes he/she is somewhere else; confuses night and day) 2 = **1, 17***
c. EPISODES OF DISORGANIZED SPEECH—(e.g., speech is incoherent, nonsensical, irrelevant, or rambling from subject to subject; loses train of thought) 2 = **1, 17***
d. PERIODS OF RESTLESSNESS—(e.g., fidgeting or picking at skin, clothing, napkins, etc.; frequent position changes; repetitive physical movements or calling out) 2 = **1, 17***
e. PERIODS OF LETHARGY—(e.g., sluggishness; staring into space; difficult to arouse; little body movement) 2 = **1, 17***
f. MENTAL FUNCTION VARIES OVER THE COURSE OF THE DAY—(e.g., sometimes better, sometimes worse; behaviors sometimes present, sometimes not) 2 = **1, 17***

6. CHANGE IN COGNITIVE STATUS
Resident's cognitive status, skills, or abilities have changed as compared to status of **90 days ago** (or since assessment if less than 90 days)
0. No change   1. Improved   2. Deteriorated **1, 17***

SECTION C. COMMUNICATION/HEARING PATTERNS

1. HEARING
(With hearing appliance, if used)
0. HEARS ADEQUATELY—normal talk, TV, phone
1. MINIMAL DIFFICULTY when not in quiet setting **4**
2. HEARS IN SPECIAL SITUATIONS ONLY—speaker has to adjust tonal quality and speak distinctly **4**
3. HIGHLY IMPAIRED/absence of useful hearing **4**

2. COMMUNICATION DEVICES/ TECHNIQUES
(Check all that apply during last 7 days)
Hearing aid, present and used — a.
Hearing aid, present and not used regularly — b.
Other receptive comm. techniques used (e.g., lip reading) — c.
NONE OF ABOVE — d.

3. MODES OF EXPRESSION
(Check all used by resident to make needs known)
Speech — a.
Writing messages to express or clarify needs — b.
American sign language or Braille — c.
Signs/gestures/sounds — d.
Communication board — e.
Other — f.
NONE OF ABOVE — g.

4. MAKING SELF UNDERSTOOD
(Expressing information content—however able)
0. UNDERSTOOD
1. USUALLY UNDERSTOOD—difficulty finding words or finishing thoughts **4**
2. SOMETIMES UNDERSTOOD—ability is limited to making concrete requests **4**
3. RARELY/NEVER UNDERSTOOD **4**

5. SPEECH CLARITY
(Code for speech in the last 7 days)
0. CLEAR SPEECH—distinct, intelligible words
1. UNCLEAR SPEECH—slurred, mumbled words
2. NO SPEECH—absence of spoken words

6. ABILITY TO UNDERSTAND OTHERS
(Understanding verbal information content—however able)
0. UNDERSTANDS
1. USUALLY UNDERSTANDS—may miss some part/ intent of message **2, 4**
2. SOMETIMES UNDERSTANDS—responds adequately to simple, direct communication **2, 4**
3. RARELY/NEVER UNDERSTANDS **2, 4**

7. CHANGE IN COMMUNICATION/ HEARING
Resident's ability to express, understand, or hear information has changed as compared to status of **90 days ago** (or since last assessment if less than 90 days)
0. No change   1. Improved   2. Deteriorated **17***

MDS 2.0   10/18/94N

Resident _____   Numeric Identifier _____

SECTION D. VISION PATTERNS

1.	VISION	*(Ability to see in adequate light and with glasses if used)* 0. *ADEQUATE*—sees fine detail, including regular print in newspapers/books 1. *IMPAIRED*—sees large print, but not regular print in newspapers/books 2. *MODERATELY IMPAIRED*—limited vision; not able to see newspaper headlines, but can identify objects 3 3. *HIGHLY IMPAIRED*—object identification in question, but eyes appear to follow objects 4. *SEVERELY IMPAIRED*—no vision or sees only light, colors, or shapes; eyes do not appear to follow objects
2.	VISUAL LIMITATIONS/ DIFFICULTIES	Side vision problems—decreased peripheral vision (e.g., leaves food on one side of tray, difficulty traveling, bumps into people and objects, misjudges placement of chair when seating self) a. Experiences any of following: sees halos or rings around lights; sees flashes of light; sees "curtains" over eyes b. *NONE OF ABOVE* c.
3.	VISUAL APPLIANCES	Glasses; contact lenses; magnifying glass 0. No 1. Yes

SECTION E. MOOD AND BEHAVIOR PATTERNS

1.	INDICATORS OF DEPRESSION, ANXIETY, SAD MOOD	*(Code for indicators observed in last 30 days, irrespective of the assumed cause)* 0. Indicator not exhibited in last 30 days 1. Indicator of this type exhibited up to five days a week 2. Indicator of this type exhibited daily or almost daily (6, 7 days a week)

VERBAL EXPRESSIONS OF DISTRESS
a. Resident made negative statements—e.g., "Nothing matters; Would rather be dead; What's the use; Regrets having lived so long; Let me die" 1
b. Repetitive questions—e.g., "Where do I go; What do I do?" 1 or 2 = 8
c. Repetitive verbalizations—e.g., calling out for help ("God help me") 1 or 2 = 8
d. Persistent anger with self or others—e.g., easily annoyed, anger at placement in nursing home; anger at care received 1 or 2 = 8
e. Self deprecation—e.g., "I am nothing; I am of no use to anyone" 1 or 2 = 8
f. Expressions of what appear to be unrealistic fears—e.g., fear of being abandoned, left alone, being with others 1 or 2 = 8
g. Recurrent statements that something terrible is about to happen—e.g., believes he or she is about to die, have a heart attack 1 or 2 = 8

h. Repetitive health complaints—e.g., persistently seeks medical attention, obsessive concern with body functions 1 or 2 = 8
i. Repetitive anxious complaints/concerns (non-health related) e.g., persistently seeks attention/reassurance regarding schedules, meals, laundry/clothing, relationship issues 1 or 2 = 8

SLEEP-CYCLE ISSUES
j. Unpleasant mood in morning 1 or 2 = 8
k. Insomnia/change in usual sleep pattern 1 or 2 = 8

SAD, APATHETIC, ANXIOUS APPEARANCE
l. Sad, pained, worried facial expressions—e.g., furrowed brows 1 or 2 = 8
m. Crying, tearfulness 1 or 2 = 8
n. Repetitive physical movements—e.g., pacing, hand wringing, restlessness, fidgeting, picking 1 or 2 = 8, 17*

LOSS OF INTEREST
o. Withdrawal from activities of interest—e.g., no interest in longstanding activities or being with family/friends 1 or 2 = 7, 8
p. Reduced social interaction 1 or 2 = 8

2.	MOOD PERSISTENCE	One or more indicators of depressed, sad or anxious mood were not easily altered by attempts to "cheer up", console, or reassure the resident over last 7 days 0. No mood indicators 1. Indicators present, easily altered 8 2. Indicators present, not easily altered 8
3.	CHANGE IN MOOD	Resident's mood status has changed as compared to status of 90 days ago (or since last assessment if less than 90 days) 0. No change 1. Improved 2. Deteriorated 1, 17*
4.	BEHAVIORAL SYMPTOMS	*(A) Behavioral symptom frequency in last 7 days* 0. Behavior not exhibited in last 7 days 1. Behavior of this type occurred 1 to 3 days in last 7 days 2. Behavior of this type occurred 4 to 6 days, but less than daily 3. Behavior of this type occurred daily *(B) Behavioral symptom alterability in last 7 days* 0. Behavior not present OR behavior was easily altered 1. Behavior was not easily altered (A) (B)

a. WANDERING (moved with no rational purpose, seemingly oblivious to needs or safety) A = 1, 2, or 3 = 9, 11
b. VERBALLY ABUSIVE BEHAVIORAL SYMPTOMS (others were threatened, screamed at, cursed at) A = 1, 2, or 3 = 9
c. PHYSICALLY ABUSIVE BEHAVIORAL SYMPTOMS (others were hit, shoved, scratched, sexually abused) A = 1, 2, or 3 = 9
d. SOCIALLY INAPPROPRIATE/DISRUPTIVE BEHAVIORAL SYMPTOMS (made disruptive sounds, noisiness, screaming, self-abusive acts, sexual behavior or disrobing in public, smeared/threw food/feces, hoarding, rummaged through others' belongings) A = 1, 2, or 3 = 9
e. RESISTS CARE (resisted taking medications/injections, ADL assistance, or eating) A = 1, 2, or 3 = 9

5.	CHANGE IN BEHAVIORAL SYMPTOMS	Resident's behavior status has changed as compared to status of 90 days ago (or since last assessment if less than 90 days) 0. No change 1. Improved 2. Deteriorated

SECTION F. PSYCHOSOCIAL WELL-BEING

1.	SENSE OF INITIATIVE/ INVOLVEMENT	At ease interacting with others a. At ease doing planned or structured activities b. At ease doing self-initiated activities c. Establishes own goals 7 d. Pursues involvement in life of facility (e.g., makes/keeps friends; involved in group activities; responds positively to new activities; assists at religious services) e. Accepts invitations into most group activities f. *NONE OF ABOVE* g.
2.	UNSETTLED RELATIONSHIPS	Covert/open conflict with or repeated criticism of staff 7 a. Unhappy with roommate b. Unhappy with residents other than roommate c. Openly expresses conflict/anger with family/friends 7 d. Absence of personal contact with family/friends e. Recent loss of close family member/friend f. Does not adjust easily to change in routines g. *NONE OF ABOVE* h.
3.	PAST ROLES	Strong identification with past roles and life status 7 a. Expresses sadness/anger/empty feeling over lost roles/status 7 b. Resident perceives that daily routine (customary routine, activities) is very different from prior pattern in the community 7 c. *NONE OF ABOVE* d.

SECTION G. PHYSICAL FUNCTIONING AND STRUCTURAL PROBLEMS

1. **(A) ADL SELF-PERFORMANCE**—*(Code for resident's **PERFORMANCE OVER ALL SHIFTS** during last 7 days—Not including setup)*
0. *INDEPENDENT*—No help or oversight—OR—Help/oversight provided only 1 or 2 times during last 7 days
1. *SUPERVISION*—Oversight, encouragement or cueing provided 3 or more times during last 7 days—OR—Supervision (3 or more times) plus physical assistance provided only 1 or 2 times during last 7 days
2. *LIMITED ASSISTANCE*—Resident highly involved in activity; received physical help in guided maneuvering of limbs or other nonweight bearing assistance 3 or more times—OR—More help provided only 1 or 2 times during last 7 days
3. *EXTENSIVE ASSISTANCE*—While resident performed part of activity, over last 7-day period, help of following type(s) provided 3 or more times:
—Weight-bearing support
—Full staff performance during part (but not all) of last 7 days
4. *TOTAL DEPENDENCE*—Full staff performance of activity during entire 7 days
8. *ACTIVITY DID NOT OCCUR* during entire 7 days

(B) ADL SUPPORT PROVIDED—*(Code for MOST SUPPORT PROVIDED OVER ALL SHIFTS during last 7 days; code regardless of resident's self-performance classification)*
0. No setup or physical help from staff
1. Setup help only
2. One person physical assist
3. Two+ persons physical assist
8. ADL activity itself did not occur during entire 7 days

			(A) SELF-PERF	(B) SUPPORT
a.	BED MOBILITY	How resident moves to and from lying position, turns side to side, and positions body while in bed A = 1 = 5A; A = 2, 3, or 4 = 5A, 16; A = 8 = 16		
b.	TRANSFER	How resident moves between surfaces—to/from: bed, chair, wheelchair, standing position (EXCLUDE to/from bath/toilet) A = 1, 2, 3, or 4 = 5A		
c.	WALK IN ROOM	How resident walks between locations in his/her room A = 1, 2, 3, or 4 = 5A		
d.	WALK IN CORRIDOR	How resident walks in corridor on unit A = 1, 2, 3, or 4 = 5A		
e.	LOCOMOTION ON UNIT	How resident moves between locations on same floor. If in wheelchair, self-sufficiency once in chair A = 1, 2, 3, or 4 = 5A		
f.	LOCOMOTION OFF UNIT	How resident moves to and returns from off unit locations (e.g., areas set aside for dining, activities, or treatments). If facility has only one floor, how resident moves to and from distant areas on the floor. If in wheelchair, self-sufficiency once in chair A = 1, 2, 3, or 4 = 5A		
g.	DRESSING	How resident puts on, fastens, and takes off all items of street clothing, including donning/removing prosthesis A = 1, 2, 3, or 4 = 5A		
h.	EATING	How resident eats and drinks (regardless of skill). Includes intake of nourishment by other means (e.g., tube feeding, total parenteral nutrition) A = 1, 2, 3, or 4 = 5A		
i.	TOILET USE	How resident uses the toilet room (or commode, bedpan, urinal); transfers on/off toilet, cleanses, changes pad, manages ostomy or catheter, adjusts clothes A = 1, 2, 3, or 4 = 5A		
j.	PERSONAL HYGIENE	How resident maintains personal hygiene, including combing hair, brushing teeth, shaving, applying makeup, washing/drying face, hands, and perineum (EXCLUDE baths and showers) A = 1, 2, 3, or 4 = 5A		

Resident _____   Numeric Identifier_____

2.	**BATHING**	How resident takes full-body bath/shower, sponge bath, and transfers in/out of tub/shower (EXCLUDE washing of back and hair). *Code for most dependent* in self-performance and support.

A = 1, 2, 3 or 4 =**5A**

(A) BATHING SELF-PERFORMANCE codes appear below.

		(A)	(B)
0. Independent—No help provided			
1. Supervision—Oversight help only			
2. Physical help limited to transfer only			
3. Physical help in part of bathing activity			
4. Total dependence			
8. Activity itself did not occur during entire 7 days			

(Bathing support codes are as defined in Item 1, code B above)

3.	**TEST FOR BALANCE** (See training manual)	*(Code for ability during test in the last 7 days)* 0. Maintained position as required in test 1. Unsteady, but able to rebalance self without physical support 2. Partial physical support during test; or stands (sits) but does not follow directions for test 3. Not able to attempt test without physical help

a. Balance while standing		
b. Balance while sitting—position, trunk control 1, 2, or 3 = **17***		

4.	**FUNCTIONAL LIMITATION IN RANGE OF MOTION** (see training manual)	*(Code for limitations during last 7 days that interfered with daily functions or placed resident at risk of injury)*

(A) RANGE OF MOTION	(B) VOLUNTARY MOVEMENT
0. No limitation	0. No loss
1. Limitation on one side	1. Partial loss
2. Limitation on both sides	2. Full loss

	(A)	(B)
a. Neck		
b. Arm—Including shoulder or elbow		
c. Hand—Including wrist or fingers		
d. Leg—Including hip or knee		
e. Foot—Including ankle or toes		
f. Other limitation or loss		

5.	**MODES OF LOCOMO-TION**	*(Check all that apply during last 7 days)*

Cane/walker/crutch	a.	Wheelchair primary mode of locomotion	d.	
Wheeled self	b.			
Other person wheeled	c.	NONE OF ABOVE	e.	

6.	**MODES OF TRANSFER**	*(Check all that apply during last 7 days)*

Bedfast all or most of time **16**	a.	Lifted mechanically	d.	
Bed rails used for bed mobility or transfer	b.	Transfer aid (e.g., slide board, trapeze, cane, walker, brace)	e.	
Lifted manually	c.	NONE OF ABOVE	f.	

7.	**TASK SEGMEN-TATION**	Some or all of ADL activities were broken into subtasks during last 7 days so that resident could perform them 0. No 1. Yes

8.	**ADL FUNCTIONAL REHABILITA-TION POTENTIAL**		
		Resident believes he/she is capable of increased independence in at least some ADLs **5A**	a.
		Direct care staff believe resident is capable of increased independence in at least some ADLs **5A**	b.
		Resident able to perform tasks/activity but is very slow	c.
		Difference in ADL Self-Performance or ADL Support, comparing mornings to evenings	d.
		NONE OF ABOVE	e.

9.	**CHANGE IN ADL FUNCTION**	Resident's ADL self-performance status has changed as compared to status of 90 days ago (or since last assessment if less than 90 days) 0. No change 1. Improved 2. Deteriorated

SECTION H. CONTINENCE IN LAST 14 DAYS

1.	CONTINENCE SELF-CONTROL CATEGORIES *(Code for resident's PERFORMANCE OVER ALL SHIFTS)*

0. *CONTINENT*—Complete control *(includes use of indwelling urinary catheter or ostomy device that does not leak urine or stool)*
1. *USUALLY CONTINENT*—BLADDER, incontinent episodes once a week or less; BOWEL, less than weekly
2. *OCCASIONALLY INCONTINENT*—BLADDER, 2 or more times a week but not daily; BOWEL, once a week
3. *FREQUENTLY INCONTINENT*—BLADDER, tended to be incontinent daily, but some control present (e.g., on day shift); BOWEL, 2-3 times a week
4. *INCONTINENT*—Had inadequate control. BLADDER, multiple daily episodes; BOWEL, all (or almost all) of the time

a.	**BOWEL CONTI-NENCE**	Control of bowel movement, with appliance or bowel continence programs, if employed 1, 2, 3 or 4 = **16**	
b.	**BLADDER CONTI-NENCE**	Control of urinary bladder function (if dribbles, volume insufficient to soak through underpants), with appliances (e.g., foley) or continence programs, if employed 2, 3 or 4 = **6**	

2.	**BOWEL ELIMIN-ATION PATTERN**	Bowel elimination pattern regular—at least one movement every three days	a.	Diarrhea	c.	
				Fecal impaction **17***	d.	
		Constipation **17***	b.	NONE OF ABOVE	e.	

3.	**APPLIANCES AND PROGRAMS**				
		Any scheduled toileting plan	a.	Did not use toilet room/commode/urinal	f.
		Bladder retraining program	b.	Pads/briefs used **6**	g.
		External (condom) catheter **6**	c.	Enemas/irrigation	h.
		Indwelling catheter **6**	d.	Ostomy present	i.
		Intermittent catheter **6**	e.	NONE OF ABOVE	j.

4.	**CHANGE IN URINARY CONTI-NENCE**	Resident's urinary continence has changed as compared to status of **90 days ago** (or since last assessment if less than 90 days) 0. No change 1. Improved 2. Deteriorated

SECTION I. DISEASE DIAGNOSES

Check only **those diseases that have a relationship** to current ADL status, cognitive status, mood and behavior status, medical treatments, nursing monitoring, or risk of death. (Do not list inactive diagnoses)

1.	DISEASES	*(If none apply, CHECK the NONE OF ABOVE box)*

ENDOCRINE/METABOLIC/NUTRITIONAL				
Diabetes mellitus	a.	Hemiplegia/Hemiparesis	v.
Hyperthyroidism	b.	Multiple sclerosis	w.
Hypothyroidism	c.	Paraplegia	x.
HEART/CIRCULATION		Parkinson's disease	y.
Arteriosclerotic heart disease (ASHD)	d.	Quadriplegia	z.
Cardiac dysrhythmias	e.	Seizure disorder	aa.
Congestive heart failure	f.	Transient ischemic attack (TIA)	bb.
Deep vein thrombosis	g.	Traumatic brain injury	cc.
Hypertension	h.	**PSYCHIATRIC/MOOD**	
Hypotension **17***	i.	Anxiety disorder	dd.
Peripheral vascular disease **16**	j.	Depression **17***	ee.
Other cardiovascular disease	k.	Manic depression (bipolar disease)	ff.
MUSCULOSKELETAL		Schizophrenia	gg.
Arthritis	l.	**PULMONARY**	
Hip fracture	m.	Asthma	hh.
Missing limb (e.g., amputation)	n.	Emphysema/COPD	ii.
Osteoporosis	o.	**SENSORY**	
Pathological bone fracture	p.	Cataracts **3**	jj.
NEUROLOGICAL		Diabetic retinopathy	kk.
Alzheimer's disease	q.	Glaucoma **3**	ll.
Aphasia	r.	Macular degeneration	mm.
Cerebral palsy	s.	**OTHER**	
Cerebrovascular accident (stroke)	t.	Allergies	nn.
Dementia other than Alzheimer's disease	u.	Anemia	oo.
		Cancer	pp.
		Renal failure	qq.
		NONE OF ABOVE	rr.

2.	INFECTIONS	*(If none apply, CHECK the NONE OF ABOVE box)*

Antibiotic resistant infection (e.g., Methicillin resistant staph)	a.	Septicemia	g.
Clostridium difficile (c. diff.)	b.	Sexually transmitted diseases	h.
Conjunctivitis	c.	Tuberculosis	i.
HIV infection	d.	Urinary tract infection in last 30 days **14**	j.
Pneumonia	e.	Viral hepatitis	k.
Respiratory infection	f.	Wound infection	l.
		NONE OF ABOVE	m.

3.	**OTHER CURRENT OR MORE DETAILED DIAGNOSES AND ICD-9 CODES**	Dehydration 276.5 = **14**		
		a. _____		| | | |•| | |
		b. _____		| | | |•| | |
		c. _____		| | | |•| | |
		d. _____		| | | |•| | |
		e. _____		| | | |•| | |

SECTION J. HEALTH CONDITIONS

1.	**PROBLEM CONDITIONS**	*(Check all problems present in last 7 days unless other time frame is indicated)*

INDICATORS OF FLUID STATUS				
Weight gain or loss of 3 or more pounds within a 7 day period **14**	a.	Dizziness/Vertigo **11, 17***	f.
Inability to lie flat due to shortness of breath	b.	Edema	g.
Dehydrated; output exceeds input	c.	Fever **14**	h.
		Hallucinations **17***	i.
Insufficient fluid; did NOT consume all/almost all liquids provided during last 3 days **14**	d.	Internal bleeding **14**	j.
		Recurrent lung aspirations in last 90 days **17***	k.
		Shortness of breath	l.
OTHER		Syncope (fainting) **17***	m.
Delusions	e.	Unsteady gait **17***	n.
		Vomiting	o.
		NONE OF ABOVE	p.

Form 1728HF © 1995 Briggs Corporation, Des Moines, IA 50306 (800) 247-2343 PRINTED IN U.S.A.
Copyright limited to addition of trigger system.

MDS 2.0   10/18/94N

Resident _____ Numeric Identifier_____

2.	PAIN SYMPTOMS	(Code the **highest level of pain** present in the **last 7 days**)		
		a. FREQUENCY with which resident complains or shows evidence of pain	**b. INTENSITY** of pain	
		0. No pain *(skip to J4)* 1. Pain less than daily 2. Pain daily	1. Mild pain 2. Moderate pain 3. Times when pain is horrible or excruciating	

3.	PAIN SITE	(If pain present, **check all sites** that apply in **last 7 days**)		
		Back pain	a.	Incisional pain	f.
		Bone pain	b.	Joint pain (other than hip)	g.
		Chest pain while doing usual activities	c.	Soft tissue pain (e.g., lesion, muscle)	h.
		Headache	d.	Stomach pain	i.
		Hip pain	e.	Other	j.

4.	ACCIDENTS	*(Check all that apply)*			
		Fell in **past 30 days** **11, 17***	a.	Hip fracture in last **180 days 17***	c.
		Fell in **past 31-180 days 11, 17***	b.	Other fracture in last **180 days**	d.
				NONE OF ABOVE	e.

5.	STABILITY OF CONDITIONS	Conditions/diseases make resident's cognitive, ADL, mood or behavior patterns unstable—(fluctuating, precarious, or deteriorating)	a.
		Resident experiencing an acute episode or a flare-up of a recurrent or chronic problem	b.
		End-stage disease, 6 or fewer months to live	c.
		NONE OF ABOVE	d.

SECTION K. ORAL/NUTRITIONAL STATUS

1.	ORAL PROBLEMS	Chewing problem	a.
		Swallowing problem **17***	b.
		Mouth pain **15**	c.
		NONE OF ABOVE	d.

2.	HEIGHT AND WEIGHT	Record **(a.)** height in inches and **(b.)** weight in pounds. Base weight on most recent measure in **last 30 days**; measure weight consistently in accord with standard facility practice— e.g., in a.m. after voiding, before meal, with shoes off, and in nightclothes.		
		a. HT (in.)	**b. WT (lb.)**	

3.	WEIGHT CHANGE	**a. Weight loss**—5% or more in **last 30 days**; or 10% or more in **last 180 days**	
		0. No 1. Yes **12**	
		b. Weight gain—5% or more in **last 30 days**; or 10% or more in **last 180 days**	
		0. No 1. Yes	

4.	NUTRITIONAL PROBLEMS	Complains about the taste of many foods **12**	a.	Leaves 25% or more of food uneaten at most meals **12**	c.
		Regular or repetitive complaints of hunger	b.	*NONE OF ABOVE*	d.

5.	NUTRITIONAL APPROACHES	*(Check all that apply in last 7 days)*			
		Parenteral/IV **12, 14**	a.	Dietary supplement between meals	f.
		Feeding tube **13, 14**	b.	Plate guard, stabilized built-up utensil, etc.	g.
		Mechanically altered diet **12**	c.	On a planned weight change program	h.
		Syringe (oral feeding) **12**	d.	*NONE OF ABOVE*	i.
		Therapeutic diet **12**	e.		

6.	PARENTERAL OR ENTERAL INTAKE	*(Skip to Section L if neither 5a nor 5b is checked)*	
		a. Code the proportion of **total calories** the resident received through parenteral or tube feedings in the **last 7 days**	
		0. None 3. 51% to 75% 1. 1% to 25% 4. 76% to 100% 2. 26% to 50%	
		b. Code the average **fluid intake** per day by IV or tube in last **7 days**	
		0. None 3. 1001 to 1500 cc/day 1. 1 to 500 cc/day 4. 1501 to 2000 cc/day 2. 501 to 1000 cc/day 5. 2001 or more cc/day	

SECTION L. ORAL/DENTAL STATUS

1.	ORAL STATUS AND DISEASE PREVENTION	Debris (soft, easily movable substances) present in mouth prior to going to bed at night **15**	a.
		Has dentures or removable bridge	b.
		Some/all natural teeth lost—does not have or does not use dentures (or partial plates) **15**	c.
		Broken, loose, or carious teeth **15**	d.
		Inflamed gums (gingiva); swollen or bleeding gums; oral abscesses; ulcers or rashes **15**	e.
		Daily cleaning of teeth/dentures or daily mouth care—by resident or staff Not ✓ = **15**	f.
		NONE OF ABOVE	g.

SECTION M. SKIN CONDITION

1.	ULCERS (Due to any cause)	(Record the number of ulcers at each ulcer stage— regardless of cause. If none present at a stage, record "0" (zero). Code all that apply during **last 7 days**. Code 9 = 9 or more.) [Requires full body exam.]	Number at Stage
		a. Stage 1. A persistent area of skin redness (without a break in the skin) that does not disappear when pressure is relieved.	
		b. Stage 2. A partial thickness loss of skin layers that presents clinically as an abrasion, blister, or shallow crater.	
		c. Stage 3. A full thickness of skin is lost, exposing the subcutaneous tissues—presents as a deep crater with or without undermining adjacent tissue.	
		d. Stage 4. A full thickness of skin and subcutaneous tissue is lost, exposing muscle or bone.	

2.	TYPE OF ULCER	(For each type of ulcer, **code for the highest stage** in the last 7 days using scale in item M1—i.e., 0=none; stages 1, 2, 3, 4)	
		a. Pressure ulcer—any lesion caused by pressure resulting in damage of underlying tissue 1 = **16**; 2, 3, or 4 = **12, 16**	
		b. Stasis ulcer—open lesion caused by poor circulation in the lower extremities	

3.	HISTORY OF RESOLVED ULCERS	Resident had an ulcer that was resolved or cured in **LAST 90 DAYS** 0. No 1. Yes **16**	

4.	OTHER SKIN PROBLEMS OR LESIONS PRESENT	*(Check all that apply during last 7 days)*	
		Abrasions, bruises	a.
		Burns (second or third degree)	b.
		Open lesions other than ulcers, rashes, cuts (e.g., cancer lesions)	c.
		Rashes—e.g., intertrigo, eczema, drug rash, heat rash, herpes zoster	d.
		Skin desensitized to pain or pressure **16**	e.
		Skin tears or cuts (other than surgery)	f.
		Surgical wounds	g.
		NONE OF ABOVE	h.

5.	SKIN TREATMENTS	*(Check all that apply during last 7 days)*	
		Pressure relieving device(s) for chair	a.
		Pressure relieving device(s) for bed	b.
		Turning/repositioning program	c.
		Nutrition or hydration intervention to manage skin problems	d.
		Ulcer care	e.
		Surgical wound care	f.
		Application of dressings (with or without topical medications) other than to feet	g.
		Application of ointments/medications (other than to feet)	h.
		Other preventative or protective skin care (other than to feet)	i.
		NONE OF ABOVE	j.

6.	FOOT PROBLEMS AND CARE	*(Check all that apply during last 7 days)*	
		Resident has one or more foot problems—e.g., corns, calluses, bunions, hammer toes, overlapping toes, pain, structural problems	a.
		Infection of the foot—e.g., cellulitis, purulent drainage	b.
		Open lesions on the foot	c.
		Nails/calluses trimmed during **last 90 days**	d.
		Received preventative or protective foot care (e.g., used special shoes, inserts, pads, toe separators)	e.
		Application of dressings (with or without topical medications)	f.
		NONE OF ABOVE	g.

SECTION N. ACTIVITY PURSUIT PATTERNS

1.	TIME AWAKE	*(Check appropriate time periods over last 7 days)* Resident awake all or most of time (i.e., naps no more than one hour per time period) in the:			
	10B only if BOTH N1a = ✓ and N2 = 0	Morning **10B**	a.	Evening	c.
		Afternoon	b.	*NONE OF ABOVE*	d.

(IF RESIDENT IS COMATOSE, SKIP TO SECTION O)

2.	AVERAGE TIME INVOLVED IN ACTIVITIES	*(When awake and not receiving treatments or ADL care)*	
		0. Most—more than 2/3 of time **10B** 1. Some—from 1/3 to 2/3 of time	2. Little—less than 1/3 of time **10A** 3. None **10A**

3.	PREFERRED ACTIVITY SETTINGS	*(Check all settings in which activities are preferred)*			
		Own room	a.		
		Day/activity room	b.	Outside facility	d.
		Inside NH/off unit	c.	*NONE OF ABOVE*	e.

4.	GENERAL ACTIVITY PREFERENCES (Adapted to resident's current abilities)	*(Check all PREFERENCES whether or not activity is currently available to resident)*			
		Cards/other games	a.	Trips/shopping	g.
		Crafts/arts	b.	Walking/wheeling outdoors	h.
		Exercise/sports	c.	Watching TV	i.
		Music	d.	Gardening or plants	j.
		Reading/writing	e.	Talking or conversing	k.
		Spiritual/religious activities	f.	Helping others	l.
				NONE OF ABOVE	m.

Form 1728HF © 1995 Briggs Corporation, Des Moines, IA 50306 (800) 247-2343 PRINTED IN U.S.A.
 Copyright limited to addition of trigger system.

MDS 2.0 10/18/94N

Resident _____ Numeric Identifier _____

| 5. | PREFERS CHANGE IN DAILY ROUTINE | Code for resident preferences in daily routines
0. No change   1. Slight change   2. Major change
a. Type of activities in which resident is currently involved 1 or 2 = **10A**
b. Extent of resident involvement in activity 1 or 2 = **10A** | ☐ |

SECTION O. MEDICATIONS

1.	NUMBER OF MEDICATIONS	*(Record the number of different medications used in the last 7 days; enter "0" if none used)*	☐
2.	NEW MEDICA-TIONS	*(Resident currently receiving medications that were initiated during the last 90 days)* 0. No 1. Yes	☐
3.	INJECTIONS	*(Record the number of DAYS injections of any type received during the last 7 days; enter "0" if none used)*	☐
4.	DAYS RECEIVED THE FOLLOWING MEDICATION	*(Record the number of DAYS during last 7 days; enter "0" if not used. Note—enter "1" for long acting meds used less than weekly)* (NOTE: For **17** to actually be triggered, O4a, b, or c MUST = 1-7 AND at least one additional item marked **17*** must be indicated. See sections B, C, E, G, H, I, J, and K.) **a.** Antipsychotic 1-7 = **17** **d.** Hypnotic **b.** Antianxiety 1-7 = **11, 17** **e.** Diuretic 1-7 = **14** **c.** Antidepressant 1-7 = **11,17**	☐☐

SECTION P. SPECIAL TREATMENTS AND PROCEDURES

1.	SPECIAL TREAT-MENTS, PROCE-DURES, AND PROGRAMS	**a. SPECIAL CARE**—*Check treatments or programs received during the last 14 days*

TREATMENTS		PROGRAMS	
		Ventilator or respirator	l.
Chemotherapy	a.	**PROGRAMS**	
Dialysis	b.	Alcohol/drug treat-ment program	m.
IV medication	c.	Alzheimer's/dementia special care unit	n.
Intake/output	d.	Hospice care	o.
Monitoring acute medical condition	e.	Pediatric unit	p.
Ostomy care	f.	Respite care	q.
Oxygen therapy	g.	Training in skills required to return to the community (e.g., taking medications, house work, shopping, transportation, ADLs)	r.
Radiation	h.		
Suctioning	i.		
Tracheostomy care	j.		
Transfusions	k.	NONE OF ABOVE	s.

b. THERAPIES—*Record the number of days and total minutes each of the following therapies was administered (for at least 15 minutes a day) in the last 7 calendar days (Enter 0 if none or less than 15 min. daily)* [Note—count only post admission therapies]

(A) = # of days administered for 15 minutes or more

(B) = total # of minutes provided in last 7 days

	DAYS (A)	MINUTES (B)
a. Speech-language pathology and audiology services		
b. Occupational therapy		
c. Physical therapy		
d. Respiratory therapy		
e. Psychological therapy (by any licensed mental health professional)		

2.	INTERVEN-TION PROGRAMS FOR MOOD, BEHAVIOR, COGNITIVE LOSS	*(Check all interventions or strategies used in last 7 days—no matter where received)*

Special behavior symptom evaluation program	a.
Evaluation by a licensed mental health specialist in last 90 days	b.
Group therapy	c.
Resident-specific deliberate changes in the environment to address mood/behavior patterns—e.g., providing bureau in which to rummage	d.
Reorientation—e.g., cueing	e.
NONE OF ABOVE	f.

3.	NURSING REHABILI-TATION/ RESTOR-ATIVE CARE	*Record the NUMBER OF DAYS each of the following rehabilitation or restorative techniques or practices was provided to the resident for more than or equal to 15 minutes per day in the last 7 days (Enter 0 if none or less than 15 min. daily.)*

a. Range of motion (passive)		**f.** Walking	
b. Range of motion (active)		**g.** Dressing or grooming	
c. Splint or brace assistance		**h.** Eating or swallowing	
TRAINING AND SKILL PRACTICE IN:		**i.** Amputation/ prosthesis care	
		j. Communication	
d. Bed mobility		**k.** Other	
e. Transfer			

4.	DEVICES AND RESTRAINTS	*(Use the following codes for last 7 days:)* 0. Not used 1. Used less than daily 2. Used daily

Bed rails	
a. —Full bed rails on all open sides of bed	☐
b. —Other types of side rails used (e.g., half rail, one side)	☐
c. Trunk restraint 1 = **11, 18**; 2 = **11, 16, 18**	☐
d. Limb restraint 1 or 2 = **18**	☐
e. Chair prevents rising 1 or 2 = **18**	☐

5.	HOSPITAL STAY(S)	Record number of times resident was admitted to hospital with an overnight stay in **last 90 days** (or since last assessment if less than 90 days). *(Enter 0 if no hospital admissions)*	☐
6.	EMERGENCY ROOM (ER) VISIT(S)	Record number of times resident visited ER without an overnight stay in **last 90 days** (or since last assessment if less than 90 days). *(Enter 0 if no ER visits)*	☐
7.	PHYSICIAN VISITS	In the **LAST 14 DAYS** (or since admission if less than 14 days in facility) how many days has the physician (or authorized assistant or practitioner) examined the resident? *(Enter 0 if none)*	☐
8.	PHYSICIAN ORDERS	In the **LAST 14 DAYS** (or since admission if less than 14 days in facility) how many days has the physician (or authorized assistant or practitioner) changed the resident's orders? *Do not include order renewals without change. (Enter 0 if none)*	☐
9.	ABNORMAL LAB VALUES	Has the resident had any abnormal lab values during the **last 90 days** (or since admission)? 0. No 1. Yes	☐

SECTION Q. DISCHARGE POTENTIAL AND OVERALL STATUS

1.	DISCHARGE POTENTIAL	**a.** Resident expresses/indicates preference to return to the community 0. No 1. Yes	☐
		b. Resident has a support person who is positive toward discharge 0. No 1. Yes	☐
		c. Stay projected to be of a short duration—discharge projected **within 90 days** (do not include expected discharge due to death) 0. No 2. Within 31-90 days 1. Within 30 days 3. Discharge status uncertain	☐
2.	OVERALL CHANGE IN CARE NEEDS	Resident's overall self sufficiency has changed significantly as compared to status of **90 days ago** (or since last assessment if less than 90 days) 0. No change 1. Improved—receives fewer supports, needs less restrictive level of care 2. Deteriorated—receives more support	☐

SECTION R. ASSESSMENT INFORMATION

1.	PARTICI-PATION IN ASSESSMENT	**a.** Resident: 0. No 1. Yes	☐
		b. Family: 0. No 1. Yes 2. No family	☐
		c. Significant other: 0. No 1. Yes 2. None	☐

2. SIGNATURES OF PERSONS COMPLETING THE ASSESSMENT:

a. Signature of RN Assessment Coordinator (sign on above line)

b. Date RN Assessment Coordinator signed as complete

☐☐	—	☐☐	—	☐☐
Month		Day		Year

c. Other Signatures	Title	Sections	Date
d.			Date
e.			Date
f.			Date
g.			Date
h.			Date

TRIGGER LEGEND

1 - Delirium	5B - ADL-Maintenance	10A - Activities (Revise)	14 - Dehydration/Fluid Maintenance
2 - Cognitive Loss/Dementia	6B - Urinary Incontinence and Indwelling Catheter	10B - Activities (Review)	15 - Dental Care
3 - Visual Function	7 - Psychosocial Well-Being	11 - Falls	16 - Pressure Ulcers
4 - Communication	8 - Mood State	12 - Nutritional Status	17 - Psychotropic Drug Use
5A - ADL-Rehabilitation	9 - Behavioral Symptoms	13 - Feeding Tubes	17* - For this to trigger, O4a, b, or c must = 1-7
			18 - Physical Restraints

Form 1728HF © 1995 Briggs Corporation, Des Moines, IA 50306 (800) 247-2343 PRINTED IN U.S.A.
Copyright limited to addition of trigger system.

MDS 2.0   10/18/94N

SECTION V. RESIDENT ASSESSMENT PROTOCOL SUMMARY Numeric Identifier_____

Resident's Name:	Medical Record No.:

1. Check if RAP is triggered.

2. For each triggered RAP, use the RAP guidelines to identify areas needing further assessment. Document relevant assessment information regarding the resident's status.

   • Describe:
   —Nature of the condition (may include presence or lack of objective data and subjective complaints).
   —Complications and risk factors that affect your decision to proceed to care planning.
   —Factors that must be considered in developing individualized care plan interventions.
   —Need for referrals/further evaluation by appropriate health professionals.

   • Documentation should support your decision-making regarding whether to proceed with a care plan for a triggered RAP and the type(s) of care plan interventions that are appropriate for a particular resident.

   • Documentation may appear anywhere in the clinical record (e.g., progress notes, consults, flowsheets, etc.).

3. Indicate under the Location of RAP Assessment Documentation column where information related to the RAP assessment can be found.

4. For each triggered RAP, indicate whether a new care plan, care plan revision, or continuation of current care plan is necessary to address the problem(s) identified in your assessment. The Care Planning Decision column must be completed within 7 days of completing the RAI (MDS and RAPs).

A. RAP Problem Area	(a) Check if Triggered	Location and Date of RAP Assessment Documentation	(b) Care Planning Decision—check if addressed in care plan
1. DELIRIUM	☐		☐
2. COGNITIVE LOSS	☐		☐
3. VISUAL FUNCTION	☐		☐
4. COMMUNICATION	☐		☐
5. ADL FUNCTIONAL/ REHABILITATION POTENTIAL	☐		☐
6. URINARY INCONTINENCE AND INDWELLING CATHETER	☐		☐
7. PSYCHOSOCIAL WELL-BEING	☐		☐
8. MOOD STATE	☐		☐
9. BEHAVIORAL SYMPTOMS	☐		☐
10. ACTIVITIES	☐		☐
11. FALLS	☐		☐
12. NUTRITIONAL STATUS	☐		☐
13. FEEDING TUBES	☐		☐
14. DEHYDRATION/FLUID MAINTENANCE	☐		☐
15. ORAL/DENTAL CARE	☐		☐
16. PRESSURE ULCERS	☐		☐
17. PSYCHOTROPIC DRUG USE	☐		☐
18. PHYSICAL RESTRAINTS	☐		☐

B. _____

1. Signature of RN Coordinator for RAP Assessment Process

2. ☐☐ — ☐☐ — ☐☐☐☐
   Month   Day   Year

_____

3. Signature of Person Completing Care Planning Decision

4. ☐☐ — ☐☐ — ☐☐☐☐
   Month   Day   Year

MDS 2.0 10/18/94N

Appendix 4

Summary of Omaha Classification System

Environmental Domain

Income
Signs/Symptoms

- Low/no income
- Uninsured medical expenses
- Inadequate money management
- Able to buy only necessities
- Difficulty buying necessities
- Other

Sanitation
Signs/Symptoms

- Soiled living area
- Inadequate food storage/disposal
- Insects/rodents
- Foul odor
- Inadequate water supply
- Inadequate sewage disposal
- Inadequate laundry facilities
- Allergens
- Infectious/contaminating agents
- Other

Residence
Signs/Symptoms

- Structurally unsound
- Inadequate heating/cooling
- Steep stairs
- Inadequate/obstructed exits/entries
- Cluttered living space
- Unsafe storage of dangerous objects/substances
- Unsafe mats/throw rugs
- Inadequate safety devices
- Presence of lead-based paint
- Unsafe gas/electrical appliances
- Inadequate/crowded living space
- Homeless
- Other

Neighborhood/Workplace Safety
Signs/Symptoms

- High crime rate
- High pollution level
- Uncontrolled animals
- Physical hazards
- Unsafe play areas
- Other

Psychosocial Domain

Communication with Community Resources
Signs/Symptoms

- Unfamiliar with options/procedures for obtaining services
- Difficulty understanding roles/regulations of service providers
- Unable to communicate concerns to service providers
- Dissatisfaction with services
- Language barrier
- Inadequate/unavailable resources
- Other

Social Contact
Signs/Symptoms

- Limited social contact
- Uses health care provider for social contact
- Minimal outside stimulation/leisure time activities
- Other

Role Change
Signs/Symptoms

- Involuntary reversal of traditional male/female roles
- Involuntary reversal of dependent/independent roles
- Assumes new role
- Loses previous role
- Other

Interpersonal Relationship
Signs/Symptoms

- Difficulty establishing/maintaining relationships
- Minimal shared activities
- Incongruent values/goals
- Inadequate interpersonal communication skills
- Prolonged, unrelieved tension
- Inappropriate suspicion/manipulation/compulsion/aggression
- Other

Spiritual Distress
Signs/Symptoms

- Expresses spiritual concerns
- Disrupted spiritual rituals
- Disrupted spiritual trust
- Conflicting spiritual beliefs and medical regimen
- Other

Grief
Signs/Symptoms

- Fails to recognize normal grief responses
- Difficulty coping with grief responses
- Difficulty expressing grief responses
- Conflicting stages of grief process among family/individuals
- Other

Emotional Stability
Signs/Symptoms

- Sadness/hopelessness/worthlessness
- Apprehension/undefined fear
- Loss of interest/involvement in activities/self-care
- Narrowed perceptual focus
- Scattering of attention
- Flat affect
- Irritable/agitated
- Purposeless activity
- Difficulty managing stress
- Somatic complaints/chronic fatigue
- Expresses wish to die/attempts suicide
- Other

Human Sexuality
Signs/Symptoms

- Difficulty recognizing consequences of sexual behavior
- Difficulty expressing intimacy
- Sexual identity confusion
- Sexual value confusion
- Dissatisfied with sexual relationships
- Other

Caretaking/Parenting
Signs/Symptoms

- Difficulty providing physical care/safety
- Difficulty providing emotional nurturance
- Difficulty providing cognitive learning experiences and activities
- Difficulty providing preventive and therapeutic health care
- Expectations incongruent with stage of growth and development
- Dissatisfaction/difficulty with responsibilities
- Neglectful
- Abusive
- Other

Neglected/Child/Adult
Signs/Symptoms

- Lacks adequate physical care
- Lacks emotional nurturance/support
- Lacks appropriate stimulation/cognitive experiences
- Inappropriately left alone
- Lacks necessary supervision
- Inadequate/delayed medical care
- Other

Abused Child/Adult
Signs/Symptoms

- Harsh/excessive discipline
- Welts/bruises/burns
- Questionable explanation of injury
- Attacked verbally
- Fearful/hypervigilant behavior
- Violent environment
- Consistent negative messages
- Assaulted sexuality
- Other

Growth and Development
Signs/Symptoms

- Abnormal results of development screening tests
- Abnormal weight/height/head circumference in relation to growth curve/age
- Age-inappropriate behavior
- Inadequate achievement/maintenance of developmental tasks
- Other

Physiological Domain
Hearing
Signs/Symptoms

- Difficulty hearing normal speech tones
- Absent/abnormal response to sound
- Abnormal results of hearing screening test
- Other

Vision
Signs/Symptoms

- Difficulty seeing small print/calibrations
- Difficulty seeing distant objects
- Difficulty seeing close objects
- Absent/abnormal response to visual stimuli
- Abnormal results of vision screening test
- Squinting/blinking/tearing/blurring
- Difficulty differentiating colors
- Other

Speech and Language
Signs/Symptoms

- Absent/abnormal ability to speak
- Absent/abnormal ability to understand
- Lacks alternative communication skills
- Inappropriate sentence structure
- Limited enunciation/clarity
- Inappropriate word usage
- Other

Dentition
Signs/Symptoms

- Abnormalities of teeth
- Sore/swollen/bleeding gums
- Ill-fitting dentures
- Malocclusion
- Other

Cognition
Signs/Symptoms

- Diminished judgment
- Disoriented to time/place/person

- Limited recall of recent events
- Limited recall of long-past events
- Limited calculating/sequencing skills
- Limited concentration
- Limited reasoning/abstract thinking ability
- Impulsiveness
- Repetitious language/behavior
- Other

Pain
Signs/Symptoms

- Expresses discomfort/pain
- Elevated pulse/respirations/blood pressure
- Compensated movement/guarding
- Restless behavior
- Facial grimaces
- Pallor/perspiration
- Other

Consciousness
Signs/Symptoms

- Lethargic
- Stuporous
- Unresponsive
- Comatose
- Other

Integument
Signs/Symptoms

- Lesion
- Rash
- Excessively dry
- Excessively oily
- Inflammation
- Pruritus
- Drainage
- Ecchymoses
- Hypertrophy of nails
- Other

Neuro-Muscular-Skeletal Function
Signs/Symptoms

- Limited range-of-motion
- Decreased muscle strength
- Decreased coordination
- Decreased muscle tone
- Increased muscle tone
- Decreased sensation
- Increased sensation
- Decreased balance
- Gait/ambulation disturbance
- Difficulty managing activities of daily living
- Tremors/seizures
- Other

Respiration
Signs/Symptoms

- Abnormal breath patterns
- Unable to breathe independently

- Cough
- Unable to cough/expectorate independently
- Cyanosis
- Abnormal sputum
- Noisy respirations
- Rhinorrhea
- Abnormal breath sounds
- Other

Circulation
Signs/Symptoms

- Edema
- Cramping/pain of extremities
- Decreased pulses
- Discoloration of skin/cyanosis
- Temperature change in affected area
- Varicosities
- Syncopal episodes
- Abnormal blood-pressure reading
- Pulse deficit
- Irregular heart rate
- Excessively rapid heart rate
- Excessively slow heart rate
- Anginal pain
- Abnormal heart sounds/murmurs
- Other

Digestion-Hydration
Signs/Symptoms

- Nausea/vomiting
- Difficulty/inability to chew/swallow/digest
- Indigestion
- Reflux
- Anorexia
- Anemia
- Ascites
- Jaundice/liver enlargement
- Decreased skin turgor
- Cracked lips/dry mouth
- Electrolyte imbalance
- Other

Bowel Function
Signs/Symptoms

- Abnormal frequency/consistency of stool
- Painful defecation
- Decreased bowel sounds
- Blood in stools
- Abnormal color
- Cramping/abdominal discomfort
- Incontinent of stool
- Other

Genitourinary Function
Signs/Symptoms

- Incontinent of urine
- Urgency/frequency
- Burning/painful urination
- Difficulty emptying bladder

- Abnormal urinary frequency/amount
- Hematuria
- Abnormal discharge
- Abnormal menstrual pattern
- Abnormal lumps/swelling/tenderness of male/female reproductive organs
- Dyspareunia
- Other

Antepartum/Postpartum
Signs/Symptoms

- Difficulty coping with pregnancy/body changes
- Inappropriate exercise/rest/diet/behaviors
- Discomforts
- Complications
- Fears delivery procedure
- Difficulty breastfeeding
- Other

Health-Related Behaviors Domain
Nutrition
Signs/Symptoms

- Weighs 10% more than average
- Weighs 10% less than average
- Lacks established standards for daily caloric/fluid intake
- Exceeds established standards for daily caloric/fluid intake
- Unbalanced diet
- Improper feeding schedule for age
- Nonadherence to prescribed diet
- Unexplained/progressive weight loss
- Hypoglycemia
- Hyperglycemia
- Other

Sleep and Rest Patterns
Signs/Symptoms

- Sleep/rest pattern disrupts family
- Frequently awakes during night
- Somnambulism
- Insomnia
- Nightmares
- Insufficient sleep/rest for age/physical condition
- Other

Physical Activity
Signs/Symptoms

- Sedentary lifestyle
- Inadequate/inconsistent exercise routine
- Inappropriate type/amount of exercise for age/physical condition
- Other

Personal Hygiene
Signs/Symptoms

- Inadequate laundering of clothing
- Inadequate bathing

- Body odor
- Inadequate shampooing/combing of hair
- Inadequate brushing/flossing/mouth care
- Other

Substance Use
Signs/Symptoms

- Abuses over-the-counter/street drugs
- Abuses alcohol
- Smokes
- Difficulty performing normal routines
- Reflex disturbances
- Behavior change
- Other

Family Planning
Signs/Symptoms

- Inappropriate/insufficient knowledge of family-planning methods
- Inaccurate/inconsistent use of family-planning methods
- Dissatisfied with present family-planning method
- Other

Health Care Supervision
Signs/Symptoms

- Fails to obtain routine medical/dental evaluation
- Fails to seek care for symptoms requiring medical/dental evaluation
- Fails to return as requested to physician/dentist
- Inability to coordinate multiple appointments/regimens
- Inconsistent source of medical/dental care
- Inadequate prescribed medical/dental regimen
- Other

Prescribed Medication Regimen
Signs/Symptoms

- Deviates from prescribed dosage/schedule
- Demonstrates side effects
- Inadequate system for taking medication
- Improper storage of medication
- Fails to obtain refills appropriately
- Fails to obtain immunizations
- Other

Technical Procedure
Signs/Symptoms

- Unable to demonstrate/relate procedure accurately
- Does not follow/demonstrate principles of safe/aseptic technique
- Procedure requires nursing skill
- Unable/unwilling to perform procedure without assistance
- Unable/unwilling to operate special equipment
- Other person(s) unable/unavailable to assist
- Other

Appendix 5

Health Care Organizations and Internet Resources

Nursing Organizations

Academy of Medical-Surgical Nurses
East Holly Ave.
Box 56
Pitman, NJ 08071
(609) 256-2323
www.amsn.inurse.com

American Academy of Ambulatory Care Nurses
East Holly Ave.
Box 56
Pitman, NJ 08071-0056
(609) 256-2350
aaacn.inurse.com

American Academy of Nurse Practitioners
P.O. Box 12846
Austin, TX 78711
(512) 442-4262
www.aanp.org

American Association of Critical-Care Nurses
101 Columbia
Aliso Viejo, CA 92656
(800) 899-2226
www.aacn.org

American Association of Diabetes Educators
100 West Monroe, 4th Floor
Chicago, IL 60603
(312) 424-2426
www.aadenet.org

American Association of Neuroscience Nurses
224 North Des Plaines
Suite 601
Chicago, IL 60661
(312) 993-0043
www.aann.org

American Association of Nurse Anesthetists
222 South Prospect Ave.
Park Ridge, IL 60068-4001
(847) 692-7050
www.aana.com

American Association of Occupational Health Nurses
2920 Brandywine Rd.
Suite 900
Atlanta, GA 30341
(800) 241-8014
www.aaohn.org

American Association of Spinal Cord Injury Nurses
7520 Astoria Blvd.
Jackson Heights, NY 11370
(718) 803-3782
www.epva.org

American College of Nurse Practitioners
503 Capitol Ct. NE
Suite 300
Washington, DC 20002
(202) 546-4825
www.nurse.org/acnp

American Nephrology Nurses' Association
East Holly Ave.
Box 56
Pitman, NJ 08071
(609) 256-2320
www.anna.inurse.com

American Nurses Association
600 Maryland Ave. SW
Suite 100 West
Washington, DC 20024-2571
(800) 274-4ANA
www.ana.org

American Society of Ophthalmic Registered Nurses
655 Beach St.
P.O. Box 193030
San Francisco, CA 94119
(415) 561-8513

American Society of PeriAnesthesia Nurses
6900 Grove Rd.
Thorofare, NJ 08086
(609) 848-1881
www.aspan.org

American Society of Plastic and Reconstructive Surgical Nurses
East Holly Ave.
Box 56
Pitman, NJ 08071-0056
(609) 256-2340
www.asprsn.inurse.com

American Thoracic Society Nursing Assembly
1740 Broadway
New York, NY 10019
(212) 315-8700
www.thoracic.org/nur

Association of Nurses in AIDS Care
11250 Roger Bacon Dr.
Suite 8
Reston, VA 20190-5202
(800) 260-6780
www.anacnet.org/aids/

Association of Operating Room Nurses
2170 South Parker Rd.
Suite 300
Denver, CO 80231-5711
(303) 755-6300
www.aorn.org

Association of Professionals in Infection Control and Epidemiology, Inc.
1016 Sixteenth St. NW
Sixth Floor
Washington, DC 20036
(202) 296-5645
www.apic.org

Association of Women's Health, Obstetric, and Neonatal Nurses
2000 L St. NW
Washington, DC 20036
(202) 261-2400
www.awhonn.org

Dermatology Nurses Association
East Holly Ave.
Box 56
Pitman, NJ 08071-0056
(609) 256-2330
www.dna.inurse.com

Emergency Nurses Association
216 Higgins Rd.
Park Ridge, IL 60068-5736
(847) 698-9400
www.ena.org

National Association of Orthopaedic Nurses
East Holly Ave.
Box 56
Pitman, NJ 08071-0056
(609) 256-2310
www.naon.inurse.com

National League for Nursing
61 Broadway
New York, NY 10006
(800) 669-1656
www.nln.org

National Student Nurse Association
555 W. 57th St.
New York, NY 10019
(212) 581-2211
www.nsna.org

Oncology Nursing Society
501 Holiday Dr.
Pittsburgh, PA 15220-2749
(412) 921-7373
www.ons.org

Sigma Theta Tau International
550 West North St.
Indianapolis, IN 46202
(317) 634-8171
http://stti-web.iupui.edu

Society of Gastroenterology Nurses and Associates, Inc.
401 North Michigan Ave.
Chicago, IL 60611-4267
www.sgna.org

Society of Urologic Nurses and Associates
East Holly Ave.
Box 56
Pitman, NJ 08071-0056
(609) 256-2335
www.suna.inurse.com

WorldWide Nurse
www.wwnurse.com

Wound, Ostomy, and Continence Nursing Society
1550 South Coast Highway
Suite 201
Laguna Beach, CA 92651
(888) 224-9626
www.wocn.org

Community Organizations and Other Resources

Alternative and Complementary Therapies

Alternative Medicine
http://galaxy.tradewave.com/galaxy/Medicine/therapeutics/Alternative-Medicine.html

Alternative Medicine (Health A-to-Z)
www.healthatoz.com/categories/AM.htm

American Holistic Nurses Association
P.O. Box 2130
Flagstaff, AZ 86003-2130
(800) 278-AHNA
www.ahna.org

American Massage Therapy Association
820 Davis St.
Suite 100
Evanston, IL 60201-444
(847) 864-0123
www.amtamassage.org

Complementary Therapies
www.wholenurse.com

Healing Touch International, Inc.
198 Union Blvd.
Suite 202
Lakewood, CO 80228
(303) 989-7982
www.healingtouch.net

Nurses Certification Program in Interactive Imagery
P.O. Box 8177
Foster City, CA 94404
(650) 570-6157
http://members.aol.com//NCPII/NCPII.html

The Wellness Center
(704) 683-3369
www.newfrontiers.com/wellness

Cancer/Death and Dying

American Brain Tumor Association
2720 River Rd.
Suite 146
Des Plaines, IL 60018
(800) 886-2282
www.abta.org

American Cancer Society
1599 Clifton Rd. NE
Atlanta, GA 30329
(404) 320-3333
www.cancer.org

Breast Cancer Information Clearing House
http://nysernet.org/bcic

Breast Care Helpline
(800) 462-9273

Canadian Cancer Society (National Office)
10 Alcorn Ave.
Suite 200
Toronto, Ontario
Canada M4V 1E4
(416) 961-7223
www.cancer.ca

Cancer Information Hotline
(800) 4-CANCER

CDC's Tobacco Information and Prevention Source Page
www.cdc.gov/nccdphp/osh/tobacco.htm

Choice in Dying
1035 30th St. NW
Washington, DC 20007
(202) 338-9790
www.choices.org

Funeral and Memorial Societies of America
P.O. Box 10
Hinesburg, VT 05461
(802) 482-3437
www.funerals.org

Hospice Association of America
228 7th St. SE
Washington, DC 20003
(202) 546-4759
www.nahc.org

Leukemia Society of America
600 Third Ave.
New York, NY 10016
(212) 573-8484
www.leukemia.org

National Cancer Institute
Building 82
9000 Rockville Pike
Bethesda, MD 20892
(301) 496-8880
www.nih.gov/nci

NCI's CancerNet
www.nci.nih.gov

National Hospice Organization
P.O. Box 903
Falls Church, VA 22040-0903
(703) 243-5900
www.nho.org

National Ovarian Cancer Coalition
www.ovarian.org

The Quitnet
www.quitnet.org

Rory Foundation
12411 Ventura Blvd.
Studio City, CA 91604-2407
(888) RORY123
www.roryfoundation.org

Susan G. Komen Breast Cancer Foundation
www.komen.org

Cardiovascular and Hematologic Problems

American Association of Blood Banks
8101 Glenbrook Rd.
Bethesda, MD 20814-2749
www.aabb.org

American Heart Association
7272 Greenville Ave.
Dallas, TX 75231
(800) AHA USA1
www.americanheart.org

American Heart Association Women's Website
7272 Greenville Ave.
Dallas, TX 75231
(888) MY HEART
www.women.americanheart.org

Heart Information Network
www.heartinfo.org

Mended Hearts, Inc.
www.mendedhearts.org

National Hemophilia Foundation
116 West 32nd St.
11th Floor
New York, NY 10001
(212) 328-3700
www.hemophilia.org

Sickle Cell Disease Association of America, Inc.
3345 Wilshire Blvd.
Suite 1106
Los Angeles, CA 90010-1880
(800) 421-8453

Diabetes Mellitus

American Diabetes Association
1660 Duke St.
Alexandria, VA 22314
www.diabetes.org

American Dietetic Association
216 West Jackson Blvd.
Suite 800
Chicago, IL 60606
(312) 899-0040
www.eatright.org

CDC—Diabetes Home Page
www.cdc.gov/nccdphp/ddt/ddthome.htm

National Institute of Diabetes and Digestive and Kidney Disease
www.niddk.nih.gov

Elderly/Gerontology

Alcohol Rehab for the Elderly
PO Box 267
Hopedale, IL 61747
(800) 354-7089
www.hmc.net

Alzheimer's Association
919 N. Michigan Ave.
Suite 1000
Chicago, IL 60611-1676
www.alz.org

American Association of Retired Persons
601 E St. NW
Washington, DC 20049
(800) 424-3410
www.aarp.org

American Federation for Aging Research
1414 Avenue of the Americas
18th Floor
New York, NY 10019
(212) 752-2327
www.afar.org

National Institute on Aging
www.nih.gov.nia

Eye and Ear Problems

American Foundation for the Blind
11 Penn Plaza
Suite 300
New York, NY 10001
(212) 502-7600
www.afb.org

American Speech–Language–Hearing Association
10801 Rockville Pike
Dept. AP
Rockville, MD 20852
(301) 897-5700
www.asha.org

Deafness Research Foundation
Nine East 38th St.
7th Floor
New York, NY 10016
(800) 535-3323
www.drf.org

Eye Bank Associations of America
1001 Connecticut Ave. NW
Suite 601
Washington, DC 20036
(202) 775-4999
www.restoresight.org

Meniere's Network of the Ear Foundation
2000 Church St.
Box 111
Nashville, TN 37236
(800) 545-4327
www.theearfound.org

Self-Help for Hard of Hearing People
7910 Woodmont Ave.
Suite 1200
Bethesda, MD 20814
(301) 657-2248
www.shhh.org

Gastrointestinal Problems

American Anorexia/Bulimia Association, Inc.
members.aol.com/amanba/index.html

American Liver Foundation—Hepatitis Hotline
1425 Pompton Ave.
Cedar Grove, NJ 07009
(800) 223-0179
www.liverfoundation.org

Crohn's and Colitis Foundation of America
386 Park Ave. South
17th Floor
New York, NY 10016-8804
(800) 932-2423
www.ccfa.org

Healthy Weight
www.healthyweight.com

Immunologic Problems/Infection Control and Prevention

AIDS Treatment Data Network
www.aidsnyc.org

Allergy, Asthma, and Immunology Online
http://allergy.mcg.edu

American Academy of Allergy, Asthma, and Immunology
611 East Wells St.
Milwaukee, WI 53202
www.aaaai.org

Center for Disease Control and Prevention
1600 Clifton Rd. NE
Atlanta, GA 30333
(404) 639-3311
www.cdc.gov

HIV/AIDS Surveillance Report
Center for Disease Control and Prevention
1600 Clifton Rd. NE
Atlanta, GA 30333
(404) 639-3311
www.cdc.gov/nchstp/hiv_aids/stat

Immune Deficiency Foundation
3565 Ellicott Mills Dr.
Unit B-2
Ellicott City, MD 20104
(800) 296-4433
www.primaryimmune.org

Latex Allergy Homepage
http://allergy.mcg.edu/physician/ltxhome.html

National AIDS Treatment Advocacy Project
580 Broadway
Suite 403
New York, NY 10012
(212) 219-0106
www.natap.org

The Safer Sex Page
www.safersex.org

Musculoskeletal Problems

Ankylosing Spondylitis Association
511 North La Cienega
Suite 216
Los Angeles, CA 90048
(800) 777-8189
www.spondylitis.org

Arthritis Foundation
1330 West Peachtree St.
Atlanta, GA 30309
(404) 872-7100
www.arthritis.org

Backpain Hotline
Texas Back Institute
3801 West 15th St.
Plano, TX 75075
(800) 247-2225
www.texasback.com

National Institute of Arthritis and Musculoskeletal and Skin
  Diseases
1 AMS Cir.
Bethesda, MD 20892-3675
(301) 495-4484
www.nih.gov/niams

Osteoporosis and Related Bone Diseases—National Resource
  Center
1150 17th St. NW
Suite 500
Washington, DC 20036-4603
(800) 624-BONE

Neurologic Problems and Rehabilitation

American Paralysis Association
500 Morris Ave.
Springfield, NJ 07081
(800) 225-0292
www.apacure.com

Amyotrophic Lateral Sclerosis Association
21021 Ventura Blvd.
Suite 321
Woodland Hills, CA 91364
(800) 782-4747
www.alsa.org

Epilepsy Foundation of America
4351 Garden City Dr.
Suite 406
Landover, MD 20785
(800) 332-1000
www.efa.org

Epilepsy Ontario
1 Promenade Cir.
Suite 338
Thornhill, Ontario
Canada L4J 4P8
(416) 229-2291
epilepsyontario.org

Huntington's Disease Society of America
140 West 22nd St.
6th Floor
New York, NY 10011-2420
(800) 345-4372
dsa.mgh.harvard.edu

Migraine Resource Center
www.migrainehelp.com

National Headache Foundation
5252 North Western Ave.
Chicago, IL 60625
(800) 843-2256
www.headaches.org

National Multiple Sclerosis Society
733 Third Ave.
6th Floor
New York, NY 10017
(800) 344-4867
www.nmss.org

National Stroke Organization
www.stroke.org

Parkinson's Disease Foundation
Columbia–Presbyterian Medical Center
650 West 168th St.
New York, NY 10032
(800) 457-6676
www.parkinsons-foundation.org

Reproductive Health Problems

All About Menopause
www.menopause.org

Atlanta Reproductive Health Center
www.ivf.com/endohtml.html

Bair PMS Home Page
www.bairpms.com

Center for Human Reproduction
www.centerforhumanreprod.com

Endometriosis Association
8585 North 76th Pl.
Milwaukee, WI 53223
(800) 992-3636
www.endometrios.org

Planned Parenthood Federation of America, Inc.
www.ppfa.org

The Safer Sex Page
www.safersex.org

Respiratory Problems

American Lung Association
1740 Broadway
New York, NY 10019-4374
(800) LUNG-USA
www.lungusa.org

Cystic Fibrosis Foundation
6931 Arlington Rd.
Bethesda, MD 20814
(800) 344-4823
www.cff.org

Urinary and Renal Problems

American Urogynecologic Society
www.augs.org

National Association for Continence
www.nafc.org

National Kidney Foundation
30 East 33rd St.
New York, NY 10016
(800) 622-9010
www.kidney.org

The Simon Foundation for Continence
www.simonfoundation.org

United Network for Organ Sharing
1100 Boulders Parkway
Suite 500
Richmond, VA 23225-8770
www.unos.org

Miscellaneous Resources

Agency for Health Care Policy and Research (AHCPR)
www.ahcpr.gov

American Academy of Dermatology
930 N. Mecham Rd.
Schaumburg, IL 60173
(888) 462-3376
www.aad.org

American Academy of Pain Management
13947 Mono Way # A
Sonora, CA 95370
(209) 533-9744
www.aapainmanage.org

American Council on Alcoholism
5024 Campbell Blvd.
Suite H
Baltimore, MD 21236
(800) 527-5344
www.aca-usa.org

American Hospital Association
www.aha.org

American Red Cross
430 17th St.
Washington, DC 20006
(202) 737-8300
www.crossnet.org

American Thyroid Association
Montefiore Medical Center
111 East 210th St.
Bronx, NY 10467
www.thyroid.org

Case Management Society of America
8201 Cantrell, Suite 230
Little Rock, AR 72227
(501) 225-2229
www.cmsa.org

Commission for Case Manager Certification
1835 Rohlwing Road
Rolling Meadows, IL 60008
(847) 818-1967

Department of Health and Human Services (DHHS)
www.os.dhhs.org

Federal Drug Administration (FDA)
www.fda.gov

Lupus Foundation of America
Four Research Pl.
Suite 180
Rockville, MD 20850
(800) 558-0121
www.lupus.org/lupus

Medicare
www.medicare.gov

Medic Alert Foundation
Turlock, CA 95381
(800) 825-3785
www.medicalert.org

National Graves' Disease Foundation
www.ngdf.org

National Institutes of Health (NIH)
www.nih.gov

National Institute of Nursing Research (NINR)
www.nih.gov/ninr/

National Psoriasis Foundation
6600 SouthWest 92nd Ave.
Suite 300
Portland, OR 97223
(800) 248-0886
www.psoriasis.org

World Health Organization
www.who.org

Women's Health Consideration Resources

A forum for Women's Health
www.womenshealth.org

All About Menopause
www.menopause.org

American Heart Association Women's Website
7272 Greenville Ave.
Dallas, TX 75231
(888) MY HEART
www.women.americanheart.org

Bair PMS Home Page
www.bairpms.com

Breast Cancer Information Clearing House
http://nysernet.org/bcic

Breast Care Helpline
(800) 462-9273

Endometriosis Association
8585 North 76th Pl.
Milwaukee, WI 53223
(800) 992-3636
www.endometrios.org

Healthy Weight
www.healthyweight.com

National Ovarian Cancer Coalition
www.ovarian.org

National Women's Health Hotline
www.womenshealth.com

Osteoporosis and Related Bone Diseases—National Resource
    Center
1150 17th St. NW
Suite 500
Washington, DC 20036-4603
(800) 624-BONE

Planned Parenthood Federation of America, Inc.
www.ppfa.org

The Safer Sex Page
www.safersex.org

The Simon Foundation for Continence
www.simonfoundation.org

Susan G. Komen Breast Cancer Foundation
www.komen.org

Women's Health Interactive
www.womens-health.com

Women to Woman America
www.wtwa.com

WWWomen!
www.wwwomen.com

Search Engines and Online Directories

Alta Vista
www.altavista.digital.com

Big Yellow
www.bigyellow.com

Excite
http://search.excite.com

Galaxy
http://galaxy.tradewave.com

Health A-to-Z
www.healthatoz.com

HotBot
www.search.hotbot.com

National Women's Health Research Center
www.healthywomen.org/links.html

WebCrawler
www.webcrawler.com

WWWomen!
www.wwwomen.com

Yahoo
www.yahoo.com

Index

Anions, 220
definition of, 208t
Anisocoria, 1009, 1158
Anisoylated plasminogen-streptokinase activator complex (APSAC). See also *Thrombolytic therapy*.
for myocardial infarction, 910–912, 912t
Ankle, assessment of, 1236
examination of, 1236
fractures of, 1297
replacement of, 417
Ankle-brachial index (ABI), 731, 854
in amputation, 1302
Ankylosing spondylitis, 436, *437*
Anorectal abscess, 1456–1457
in inflammatory bowel disease, 1442t
Anorectic drugs, 1565
Anorexia, in cancer, 494, 495t
Anorexia nervosa, 1521–1534
assessment in, 1524–1528, 1525c
family, 1526–1527
history in, 1524–1525
family, 1525
sexual, 1524
laboratory, 1527t, 1527–1528
mental status, 1527, 1528
of sexual adjustment, 1527
physical examination in, 1525t, 1525–1526
psychosocial, 1526–1527, 1528, *1528*
binge-eating/purging type, 1521
biological factors in, 1523
biopsychosocial model of, 1523, *1523*
body image in, 151, 1522, 1524, 1526, 1532
body's response to, 1522, 1525t, 1525–1526
bulimia nervosa and, 1535, *1535*
case study of, 1540
clinical manifestations of, 1525t, 1525–1526
complications of, 1526
continuing care in, 1533–1534
contributing factors in, 1522t
cultural influences in, 1522–1523
diagnostic criteria for, 1522, 1522c
etiology of, 1522t, 1522–1523
evaluation in, 1534
health care resources for, 1534
health teaching in, 1533–1534, 1534c
home care in, 1533–1534, 1534c
incidence/prevalence of, 1523–1524
intervention(s) in, dietary, 1529–1530, 1531
fluid management, 1530–1531
for anxiety, 1531–1532
for body image disturbance, 1532
for bowel elimination, 1531
for coping, 1532
for family, 1533
for noncompliance, 1532–1533
for pain, 1529–1530
for refeeding edema, 1531
psychologic counseling/therapy, 1532–1533, 1534
laxative abuse in, 1521, 1526, 1527, 1531
mortality in, 1524
nursing diagnoses for, 1528–1529
pathophysiology of, 1521, 1522

Anorexia nervosa (*Continued*)
personality factors in, 1524–1525, 1526
prevention of, 1523c
restricting type, 1521
with bulimic features, 1521, 1526
Anovulation, dysfunctional uterine bleeding and, 1987
ANP. See *Atrial naturietic peptide (ANP)*.
Ansaid (flurbiprofen), for connective tissue disease, 409t
Anscal. See *Aspirin*.
Antacids, 1380c, 1388–1389
calcium carbonate, for chronic renal failure, 1894, 1895c
for osteoporosis, 1247, 1250c
for acute pancreatitis, 1509
for gastritis, 1381, 1382c–1383c
for gastroesophageal reflux disease, 1358, 1359c–1360c
for peptic ulcer disease, 1380c, 1382c, 1388–1389
Antalgic gait, 1234
Anteflexion, uterine, 1992–1993, *1993*
Anterior chamber, blood in, 1188
Anterior choroidal artery, 998t
Anterior cord syndrome, 1066, *1067*
Anterior cruciate ligament, injuries of, 1307
Anterior inferior cerebellar artery, 997, 998t
Anterior spinal artery, 998, *1000*
Anterior spinocerebellar tract, 997–998, *999*, *1000*
Anterior temporal lobe resection, for epilepsy, 1034
Anterior uveitis, 1183–1184
Anterior vaginal repair, for urinary incontinence, 1835t
Anteversion, uterine, 1992–1993, *1993*
Anthralin (Drithocreme, Lasan), for psoriasis, 1740
Anthropometric measurements, 1549–1552. See also *Height; Weight*.
Antiandrogens, for cancer, 509–510, 511t
Antianxiety agents, 634
for chronic airflow limitation, 634
for pain, 128, 134, 375
Antiarrhythmics. See *Antidysrhythmics*.
Antibacterial baths, 1713t
Antibiotic resistance, 529, 529t
Antibiotic sensitivity, tests for, 532
Antibiotics, allergy to, 536, 536t
antitumor, 502t, 503. See also *Chemotherapy*.
candidiasis and, 1335
Clostridium difficile infection and, 523
compliance with, 536
for brain abscess, 1148, 1148t
for chancroid, 255
for chlamydial infection, 2059
for cystitis, 1824, 1825c
for febrile neutropenia, 972
for fever, 534
for gonorrhea, 2058
for *Helicobacter pylori* infection, 1381
for infective endocarditis, 829
for leukemia, 965, 966c, 971–973, 972
for lymphogranuloma venereum, 255
for meningitis, 1038, 1038t
for osteomyelitis, 1260
for pelvic inflammatory disease, 2061, 2062c

Antibiotics (*Continued*)
for peritonitis, intraperitoneal administration of, 1905
for pharyngitis, 667
for pneumonia, 673, 674t
for prostatitis, 2047
for rheumatic carditis, 832
for septic shock, 896
for sexually transmitted diseases, 2063c
for sprue, 1431
for syphilis, 2052
for urolithiasis, 1842–1843
health teaching for, 536
in chronic renal failure, 1894–1895
in home care, 536, 537
incomplete therapy with, 530
intraperitoneal administration of, 1905
intravenous, in home care, 536, 537
nephrotoxic, 1919, 1919t
noncompliance with, 530
ototoxic, 1199, 1199t
prophylactic, in chronic renal failure, 1893
in infective endocarditis, 830, 830t
in leukemia, 971–972, *972*
in sickle cell disease, 956
in total hip replacement, 411
in valvular heart disease, 824, 826, 827
perioperative, 372
topical, 1734c
for burns, 1778, 1779c–1780c
for ocular disorders, 1169c
Antibody(ies). See also under *Antigen-antibody*.
antigen binding to, 396, 396–397
classification of, 397, 398t
for septic shock, 896–897
production and release of, 396
structure of, 396, *396*
Antibody tests, in AIDS, 448
Antibody-mediated immunity, 387, *387*, 387t. See also *Immunity, antibody-mediated*.
Anticholinergics, for chronic airflow limitation, 625t, 627t, 628
for irritable bowel syndrome, 1407
for Parkinson's disease, 1042
for urinary incontinence, 1833c, 1834
Anticholinesterases, cholinergic crisis and, 1093, 1094, 1095, 1095t
for myasthenia gravis, 1094–1095
Anticipatory grieving, 178, 182
in Guillain-Barré syndrome, 1090
Anticoagulants, after myocardial infarction, 912
antidotes for, 874
bleeding and, health teaching for, 874c, 876
prevention of, 688, 689c, 874c, 876
for acute arterial insufficiency, 862–865
for deep vein thrombosis, 874–875
for pulmonary embolism, 686c–687c, 686–687
for prevention, 685, 685c
for septic shock, 897
for stroke, 1120–1121
for total hip replacement, 414
health teaching for, 689, 689c
in elderly, 876
in hemodialysis, 1899, 1902
in peritoneal dialysis, 1905
in surgical client, 311t

Flovent (fluticasone), for chronic airflow limitation, 626t
Flow-by ventilation, 702
Flowmeter, urinary, 2023
Floxuridine (FUDR), for cancer, 502t
Flu, 668–669, 670
Fluconazole (Diflucan), for opportunistic infections, 451c
Fludarabine (Fludara), for cancer, 502t
Fludrocortisone (Florinef), for adrenal insufficiency, 1604, 1605c
Fluid(s), body, 218–220
    capillary transport of, 210, *211*, 214–217, *215*
    chemistry of, 286–287
    constituents of, 218, 220, *220*
    distribution of, 218, *218*
    electroneutral, 221
    extracellular, 208t, 218
    filtration of, blood pressure and, 210
        edema and, 210
    functions of, 219
    hypertonic, 209t, 213
    hypotonic, 209t, 213
    infection transmission via, 527, 527t
    interstitial, 209t
    intracellular, 209t, 218
    isotonic, 209t, 213
    transcellular, 209t
    viscosity of, 208, 209t
    joint, in degenerative joint disease, 407
    renal reabsorption of, 1794, *1975*
    titration of, 1770
Fluid and electrolyte balance, 207–228, 219t.
        See also *Electrolyte(s); Electrolyte imbalance; Fluid imbalance.*
    active transport in, 209t, 213–214, 214t
    assessment of, 226–228, 227t
        postoperative, 365–366
    capillary dynamics in, 210, *211*, 214–217, *215*
    diffusion in, 208t, 210–212, 214t
    filtration in, 207–210, 209t, *210, 211*, 214t
    hormonal influences on, 217–218, *218*
    hydrostatic pressure in, 208t, 208–210, 209t, *210*, 216
    in blood pressure regulation, 843
    in elderly, 225t, 225–226
    in mechanical ventilation, 707
    membrane processes in, 210–211, *211*
    osmosis in, 209t, *212*, 212–213, 214t
    osmotic pressure in, 208t, 209t, 215–216
    physical and biological influences on, 207–217
    regulation of, 220
    terminology for, 208t–209t
    thirst in, 213, 219
    tissue forces in, 216
Fluid challenge, in acute renal failure, 1921
Fluid deprivation test, in diabetes insipidus, 1598t
Fluid imbalance, acute renal failure and, 1918
    dehydration and, 229–239. See also *Dehydration.*
    diagnosis of, 227t, 227–228
    in acid-base imbalances, 298c, 298–299
    in bulimia, 1537

Fluid imbalance (*Continued*)
    in burns, 1759, 1766
    in chronic renal failure, 1881, 1882t, 1883
    in diabetes, 1637
    in elderly, 225t, 225–226
    in intestinal obstruction, 1420, 1424
    in intravenous therapy, 277t
    in liver disease, *1467*
    in parenteral nutrition, 1560
    in transfusion, 986
    in tube feeding, 1558
    interventions for. See *Fluid management.*
    overhydration and, *239*, 239–241, 240c, 240t. See also *Overhydration.*
    post-craniotomy, 1142–1143, 1146
Fluid intake. See also *Diet.*
    in elderly, 63
    sources of, 219, 219t
Fluid loss. See also *Dehydration.*
    assessment of, 227
    insensible, 209t, 220, 227
    routes of, 219t, 219–220
Fluid management. See also *Intravenous therapy; Transfusion(s).*
    after prostatectomy, 2028
    in acute renal failure, 1921
    in alkalosis, 303–304
    in anorexia nervosa, 1530–1531
    in ARDS, 694
    in ascites, 1470
    in benign prostatic hyperplasia, 2024
    in bladder training, 201
    in burns, 1769–1771, 1770t
    in chronic airflow limitation, 632
    in chronic renal failure, 1892t, 1893
    in constipation, 202
    in coronary artery bypass graft, 919–921
    in cystitis, 1824
    in dehydration, 235–236
    in diabetes, 1677, 1678
    in dying client, 180
    in elderly, 63, 201
    in fever, 535
    in gastroenteritis, 1440
    in heart failure, 816
    in hyperparathyroidism, 1630–1631
    in hyponatremia, 252
    in intestinal obstruction, 1424
    in overhydration, 241
    in peritonitis, 1437
    in pneumonia, 673
    in renal transplant, 1909
    in renal trauma, 1875
    in shock, 891
    in syndrome of inappropriate antidiuretic hormone, 514, 1601
    in tube feeding, 1558
    in tumor lysis syndrome, 516–517
    in urinary incontinence, 1836
    intravenous therapy in, 269–274. See also *Intravenous therapy.*
    postoperative, 366
    titration in, 1770
Fluid overload. See *Overhydration.*
Fluid remobilization, in burns, 1759
Fluid retention. See also *Edema.*
    in heart failure, 808, 810, 811, 816–817

Fluid retention (*Continued*)
    in mechanical ventilation, 705
    in syndrome of inappropriate antidiuretic hormone, 1599
Fluid shift(s), in burns, 1758–1759, *1759*
    in dehydration, 230
    in overhydration, 230
    in peritonitis, 1435
Fluid volume deficit. See *Dehydration.*
Fluid volume excess. See *Overhydration.*
Flunisolide (AeroBid), for chronic airflow limitation, 626t
Fluocinolone acetonide (Fluonid, Synalar), 1735c, 1736c
Fluocinonide (Lidex, Topsyn gel), 1735c
Fluoderm. See *Fluocinolone acetonide (Fluonid, Synalar).*
Fluorescein angiography, in ocular assessment, 1165
Fluorescent treponemal antibody absorption test, 1946
Fluoroplex. See *5-Fluorouracil.*
Fluoroscopy, cardiac, 738
5-Fluorouracil, for cancer, 502t
    of pancreas, 1516
    of skin, 1744
    topical, for vaginal cancer, 2018
    for vulvar cancer, 2016
Fluothane (halothane), 343, 346t
Flurandrenolide (Cordran), 1736c
Flurbiprofen (Ansaid), for connective tissue disease, 409t
Flutamide (Eulexin), for prostate cancer, 2035c, 2305
Fluticasone (Flovent), for chronic airflow limitation, 626t
Fluvastatin (Lescol), for hyperlipidemia, 842, 842c
Foam build-ups, 197t
Foam dressings, 1724t
Focal seizures, 1031, 1031t
Focus charting, 17, *17*
Folex. See *Methotrexate (Folex, Mexate).*
Foley catheter, in prostatectomy, 2028, 2030
Folic acid, 958t
    for chronic renal failure, 1894c
Folic acid deficiency anemia, 952t, 959c, 959–960
    autoimmunity in, 470t, 471
    gastritis in, 1379, 1380
    malabsorption and, 1429–1431
Folk medicine, 10. See also *Complementary therapies.*
Follicle, hair, 1691, *1692*
Follicle-stimulating hormone (FSH), 1577t
    deficiency of, 1590t, 1590–1591
    in reproductive assessment, 1945, 1947c
    tests for, 1591
Follicular cysts, of ovary, 1995–1996
Follicular thyroid cancer, 1628–1629
Folliculitis, 1730, *1730*, 1732c
Follow-up data base, 12
Fomite, 523
Food. See also *Diet; Feeding; Nutrition.*
    allergy to, 465–468, 466t
    calcium-rich, 223t
    carcinogenic, 487, 487c

Mechanical ventilation *(Continued)*
  synchronized intermittent mandatory, 702, 707
  tidal volume in, 702
  T-piece for, in weaning, 707
  tube removal in, 370, 708
    accidental, 698
  ventilator dependence in, 707
  ventilator management in, 705
  ventilator modes for, 701–704
  ventilator settings in, 702–704, *703*
  ventilator types for, *700,* 700–702
  weaning in, 696t–697t, 707, 707t
    in laryngectomy, 598
Mechlorethamine (Mustargen), for cancer, 502t
Meclofenamate (Meclomen), 126t, 133t
Median nerve, injuries of, 1100–1103
  intraoperative, 355t
Median nerve entrapment, in carpal tunnel syndrome, 1268–1270, *1269*
Mediastinitis, after coronary artery bypass graft, 926
Mediastinoscopy, 559, 562t
  in lung cancer, 646
Medicaid, 71
Medical diagnoses, vs. nursing diagnoses, 14t
Medical history, 12
Medical records, 12–14
Medical-surgical nurse. See *Nurse(s), medical-surgical.*
Medicare, 10, 70–71
  for home care, 25
  for nursing home care, 25
  for oxygen therapy, 571–572
  Minimum Data Set for, 12
Medihaler-Iso. See *Isoproterenol (Isuprel).*
Meditation, 106–107
Medrol. See *Methylprednisolone (Solu-Medrol).*
Medroxyprogesterone (Depo-Provera), for dysfunctional uterine bleeding, 1988
MEDSURG Nursing, 6
Medulla, structure and function of, 995, 996t
Medullary thyroid cancer, 1628–1629
Mefenamic acid (Ponstel), 133t
  for connective tissue disease, 409t
Megaloblastic anemia, 952t, 959, 959c
Melanocyte, 1690
Melanocyte-stimulating hormone (MSH), 1577t
Melanoma, *1743,* 1743–1746, 1745t
  metastasis in, 483t
  ocular, 1189–1191
Melena, in cirrhosis, 1468
  in peptic ulcer disease, 1385
Melphalan (Alkeran), for cancer, 502t
Membrane, cell, properties of, 384–385
  impermeable, 209t, 211
  permeable, 209t
Membrane filter, 267
Membrane proteins, 384–385
Memory, assessment of, 1006–1007
  in elderly, 1004, 1005c
Memory cell, 387t, *395,* 395–396, 397
  function of, 938t
Memory loss, in stroke, 1112c, 1122–1123
MEN. See *Multiple endocrine neoplasia (MEN).*
Menarche, 1932
  age at, breast cancer risk and, 1957t, 1962

Mended Hearts, 930
Meniere's disease, 1196t, 1217
Meningeal irritation, 1036, *1037*
Meninges, 994
Meningioma, 1074–1078, 1077t, 1140. See also *Brain tumors.*
Meningitis, 1035t, 1035–1038
  cryptococcal, in AIDS, 446, 451c, 1036
  headache in, 1029t
  postcraniotomy, 1146
Meningococcal meningitis, 1035t, 1035–1038
Meniscus injuries, 1307
Menopause, 51, 1933
  artificial, 1933, 1996
  hormone replacement therapy in, breast cancer and, 1957t, 1962
    client teaching for, 1986c
    for osteoporosis, 1247, 1251c, 1253
    postmenopausal bleeding and, 1985
    progesterone in, 1985
  late-onset, breast cancer risk and, 1957t, 1962
  uterine bleeding after, 1985, 1985t
Menses, 1933
Menstrual cycle, 1932–1933, *1934*
  breast changes in, 1932
Menstrual disorders, 1981–1989
Menstrual history, 1938
  in hematologic assessment, 943
Menstruation, 1932–1933
  absence of, 1984t, 1984–1985
  body weight and, 1525, 1530t
  cessation of, 1933
  in anorexia nervosa, 1525, 1530t
  painful, 1981–1982
  premenstrual syndrome and, 1982–1984, 1983b, 1983c
  toxic shock syndrome and, 1991c, 1991–1992, 1992c
Mental problems, in elderly, 68t, 68–69, 69t
Mental status assessment. See also *Neurologic assessment.*
  attention in, 1007
  brief, 234c
  cognition in, 1007
  in Alzheimer's disease, 1046
  in anorexia nervosa, 1527
  in elderly, 1004, 1005c, 1006
  in multiple sclerosis, 1080
  in shock, 889–890
  in stroke, 1111, 1113b
  language and copying in, 1007
  level of consciousness and orientation in, 1006
  memory in, 1006–1007
  Mini-Mental State Examination in, 1046
  postoperative, 365
  preoperative, 314
Meperidine (Demerol), 125–126
  dosage of, 127t, 135t
  for acute pain, 125–126, 127t
  for acute pancreatitis, 1509
  for chronic pain, 134, 135t
  for chronic pancreatitis, 1512
  in elderly, 126
  in general anesthesia, 345

Meperidine (Demerol) *(Continued)*
  in patient-controlled analgesia, 129
  postoperative, 373, 374c
Mepivacaine (Carbocaine), 349t
6-Mercaptopurine (Purinethol), for cancer, 502
  for ulcerative colitis, 1443–1444
Mercy killing, 182–183
Meridians, acupuncture, 140, *141*
Mesalamine (Asacol, Pentasa), for ulcerative colitis, 1443
Mesangial cells, 1792
Meshed grafts, 1778, *1778*
Mesothelioma, 639
Mestinon (pyridostigmine), for myasthenia gravis, 1094–1095
Metabolic acidosis
  anion gap in, 369
  assessment in, 296–299
  base deficit, 295
  clinical manifestations of, 297, 297c
  compensation in, 284t, 287–290, 289t, 290, *291*
  etiology of, 294t, 294–296
  hyperkalemia in, 298c, 299, *299*
  in burns, 1759
  in chronic renal failure, 1881, 1882t, 1890c
  in diabetes, 1637. See *Diabetic ketoacidosis.*
  in elderly, 290–292, 292c, 296c, 296–297
  in shock, 884, 890t
  incidence/prevalence of, 296
  interventions for, 299
  laboratory findings in, 288c
  lactic, 295
    in diabetes, 1637
    in shock, 884, 890t
  nerve impulse transmission and, 992
  pathophysiology of, 293–294
  pH in, 293
    urinary, 1804, 1805c
  relative, 293, *294*
  with respiratory acidosis, 296
Metabolic alkalosis, 300–303
  actual, 300, *300*
  assessment in, 301–302
  clinical manifestations of, 301–302, 302c
  collaborative management in, 301–303
  compensation in, 284t, 287–290, 289t, 290, *291*
  etiology of, 301, 301t
  in burns, 1759
  interventions in, 302–303
  laboratory findings in, 288c
  nerve impulse transmission and, 992
  pathophysiology of, 300–301
  relative, 300, *300*
  urinary pH in, 1804, 1805c
Metabolic bone disease, 1243–1258
Metabolic status, in burns, 1759, 1760
Metabolism, anaerobic, definition of, 284t
  lactic acidosis and, 295
Metacarpals, fractures of, 1297
Metacarpophalangeal joint, *1236*
Metaproterenol (Alupent, Metaprel), for anaphylaxis, 466, 467c
  for chronic airflow limitation, 624t
Metastasis, *482,* 482–483, 483t
  bloodborne, 483

Renal medulla, *1790*, 1791
Renal osteodystrophy, 1253, 1254t
  in chronic renal failure, 1882, *1882*
Renal parenchyma, *1790*, 1791
Renal pelvis, *1790*, 1791
Renal pyramid, *1790*, 1791
Renal replacement therapy, definition of, 1880.
  See also *Dialysis; Renal transplantation.*
Renal reserve, diminished, 1880, 1880t
Renal system. See *Renal/urinary system.*
Renal transplantation, 1907–1914
  care path for, 1909, 1910t–1913t
  complications of, 1909–1914
  continuing care in, 1914–1916
  donor selection for, 1908–1909
  graft rejection in, 1909–1914
  health teaching for, 1916
  home care in, 1915
  immunosuppression in, 1914
  in elderly, 1908
  operative procedure in, 1909
  patient selection for, 1908
  postoperative care in, 1909, 1910t–1913t
  preoperative care in, 1908–1909
  psychosocial aspects of, 1916
  renal artery stenosis and, 1914
  surgical team for, 1909
  tissue typing for, 1908
Renal trauma, *1874*, 1874–1876
Renal tuberculosis, 1862–1863
Renal ultrasonography, 1810t, 1815
  in urolithiasis, 1840
Renal vein thrombosis, in nephrotic syndrome,
  1867
Renal/urinary assessment, 1799–1817
  blood tests in, 1803c, 1803–1804
  computed tomography in, 1810t, 1813
  creatinine clearance test in, 1808, 1809c
  cystography in, 1810t, 1813
  cystometrography in, 1817
  cystoscopy in, 1810t, 1815–1816
  cystourethrography in, 1810t, 1813
  cystourethroscopy in, 1815–1816
  diagnostic, 1803–1817
  electromyography in, 1817
  excretory urography in, 1810t, 1811–1813,
    1812c
  history in, 1799–1801
    demographic data in, 1799
    diet, 1800
    of current health problem, 1800–1801
    personal and family, 1799–1800
    socioeconomic, 1800
  in burns, 1766
  intravenous urography in, 1810t, 1811–
    1813, 1812c
  kidney, ureter, and bladder x-ray in, 1810t,
    1811
  laboratory tests, 1803c, 1803–1811, 1805c–
    1807c, 1809c
  physical examination in, 1801–1802
  postoperative, 366
  preoperative, 313–314, 315
  psychosocial, 1802–1803
  radiographic, 1810t, 1811–1813, 1812c
  renal arteriography in, 1810t, 1813–1814
  renal biopsy in, 1814–1815

Renal/urinary assessment *(Continued)*
  renography in, 1815
  retrograde procedures in, 1816
  terminology for, 1801t
  ultrasonography in, 1810t, 1815
  urethral pressure profile in, 1817
  urine stream test in, 1817
  urine tests in, 1804–1811, 1805c–1807c
  urodynamic studies in, 1816–1817
Renal/urinary system, age-related changes in,
    55c, 56, 1798c, 1798–1799
  in blood pressure regulation, 723, 843–844,
    844
  in chronic illness/disability, 189, 189t
  in fluid and electrolyte balance, 217–218,
    218, 219, 219t, 220–222
  in sodium regulation, 221
  structure and function of, 1789–1798
Renin, 1578
  functions of, 1578
  renal production of, 1796, 1796t
  secretion of, 1578
Renin-angiotensin-aldosterone system, 1578,
    1796. See also *Aldosterone; Angiotensin.*
  in blood pressure regulation, 843–844, *844*
  in fluid and electrolyte balance, 217, *218*,
    843
  in shock, 885, 885t
Renography, 1815
Renovascular disease, 1868c, 1868–1869
Renovascular hypertension, 845
Repetitive rhythms, 764–765
Reporting, of gastroenteritis, 1440
  of hepatitis, 1483
  of professional misconduct, 89
  of sexually transmitted diseases, 2049
Reproductive assessment, 1937–1953
  blood tests in, 1945–1946
  breast biopsy and aspiration in, *1952*, 1952–
    1953
  cervical biopsy in, 1951, 1951c
  colposcopy in, 1950
  computed tomography in, 1948
  cultures in, 1946–1948
  diagnostic, 1944–1953
  endometrial biopsy and aspiration in, 1951–
    1952
  fluorescent treponemal antibody absorption
    test in, 1946
  history in, 1937–1939, 1938c
    of current health problem(s), 1930b,
    1939–1940
  hysterosalpingography in, 1948
  hysteroscopy in, 1951
  laboratory tests in, 1944–1948, 1947c
  laparoscopy in, *1950*, 1950–1951
  magnetic resonance imaging in, 1949
  mammography in, 1948–1949, 1949b
  microscopic studies in, 1946–1948, 1948c
  Pap test in, 1944–1945, *1945*, 1946c, 1946t
  pelvic examination in, 1940, 1941–1943,
    1942
  physical examination in, 1940–1944
    in female, 1940–1943
    in male, 1943–1944
  psychosocial, 1944
  radiographic, 1948–1949

Reproductive assessment *(Continued)*
  Treponema pallidum immobilization test in,
    1946
  ultrasonography in, 1949
  VDRL test in, 1945–1946
  x-ray studies in, 1948
Reproductive disorders, female, 1981–2018
  bleeding in, 1939–1940, 1940c
  discharge in, 1940, 1940c
  in AIDS, 445, 446
  masses in, 1940, 1940c
  pain in, 1939, 1940c
  male, 2021–2048
Reproductive function, hyperthyroidism and,
    1613–1614
  hypopituitarism and, 1590, 1591
  hypothyroidism and, 1624
  in liver disease, 1468
  in spinal cord injury, 164, 1068–1069,
    1072–1073
  in testicular cancer, 2041
  transcultural considerations in, 1937
Reproductive system, as infection portal of en-
    try, 523, 524t
  female, age-related changes in, 1936c
    structure and function of, 1929–1933,
    1930
  host defenses in, 525
  male, age-related changes in, 1936c
    structure and function of, 1933–1937
Residential facilities, 25. See also *Long-term
    care.*
Residents, nursing home, 25
Residual volume (RV), 560t
  in chronic airflow limitation, 619, 620t
Resol, 236t
Resolution phase, in sexual response cycle,
    158, 159t, *160*
Resonance, pulmonary, 552t
Respiration. See also *Breathing.*
  accessory muscles of, 545
  Cheyne-Stokes, 1130t
  hypoxic drive and, 566, *566*
  Kussmaul's, in acidosis, 297
    in chronic renal failure, 1881, 1885
    in dehydration, 233
    in diabetes, 1637
  paradoxic, 709
Respiratory. See also under *Lung(s); Pulmonary.*
  HEPA, 677, *679*
Respiratory acidosis, 293–300
  assessment in, 296–299
    history in, 296–297
    laboratory, 288c, 298c, 299
    physical examination in, 297
    psychosocial, 297–298
  clinical manifestations of, 297, 297c
  compensation in, 284t, 287–290, 289t, *291*
  complications of, prevention of, 300
  etiology of, 294t, 295–296
  in chronic airflow limitation, 613
  in elderly, 290–292, 292c, 296c, 296–297
  incidence/prevalence of, 296
  interventions for, 299–300
  pathophysiology of, 293
  pH in, 293
  with metabolic acidosis, 296

CONTENTS IN BRIEF